W9-AEI-360

CAMPBELL'S UROLOGY

■

Edited by

Patrick C. Walsh, M.D.

David Hall McConnell Professor and Director
The Johns Hopkins University School of Medicine
Urologist-in-Chief
Brady Urological Institute
The Johns Hopkins Hospital
Baltimore, Maryland

Alan B. Retik, M.D.

Professor of Surgery (Urology)
Harvard Medical School
Chief, Department of Urology
Children's Hospital
Boston, Massachusetts

E. Darracott Vaughan, Jr., M.D.

James J. Colt Professor of Urology
Cornell University Medical College
Urologist-in-Chief
The New York Hospital–Cornell Medical Center
New York, New York

Alan J. Wein, M.D.

Professor and Chair, Division of Urology
University of Pennsylvania School of Medicine
Chief of Urology
University of Pennsylvania Medical Center
Philadelphia, Pennsylvania

■

CAMPBELL'S UROLOGY

Seventh Edition

VOLUME

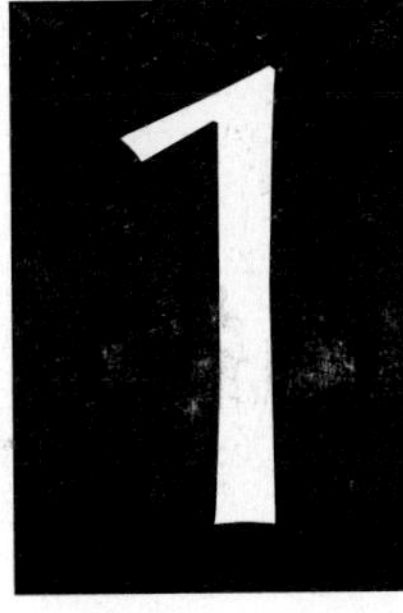

W.B. SAUNDERS COMPANY
A Division of Harcourt Brace & Company
Philadelphia London Toronto Montreal Sydney Tokyo

W.B. SAUNDERS COMPANY
A Division of Harcourt Brace & Company

The Curtis Center
Independence Square West
Philadelphia, Pennsylvania 19106

ESKIND BIOMEDICAL LIBRARY

SEP 0 2 1997

VANDERBILT UNIVERSITY
NASHVILLE, TN 37232-8340

Library of Congress Cataloging-in-Publication Data

Campbell's Urology / [edited by] Patrick C. Walsh [et al.].—7th ed.

p. cm.

Includes bibliographical references and index.

ISBN 0–7216–4461–9

1. Urology. I. Campbell, Meredith F. (Meredith Fairfax). II. Walsh, Patrick C. [DNLM: 1. Urogenital Diseases. 2. Urology—methods. WJ 100 C192 1997]

RC871.C33 1998 616.6—dc21

DNLM/DLC 96–40836

Campbell's Urology

Volume 1 ISBN 0–7216–4462–7
Volume 2 ISBN 0–7216–4463–5
Volume 3 ISBN 0–7216–4464–3
Set ISBN 0–7216–4461–9

Copyright © 1998, 1992, 1986, 1978, 1970, 1963 by W.B. Saunders Company

Copyright © 1954 by W.B. Saunders Company

Copyright renewed 1982 by Evelyn S. Campbell

All rights reserved. No part of this publication may be reproduced or transmitted in any form or by any means, electronic or mechanical, including photocopy, recording, or any information storage and retrieval system, without permission in writing from the publisher.

Printed in the United States of America

Last digit is the print number: 9 8 7 6 5 4 3 2 1

CONTRIBUTORS

Mark C. Adams, M.D.
Associate Professor of Urology and Pediatrics, Vanderbilt University School of Medicine, Vanderbilt University and The Vanderbilt University Children's Hospital, Nashville, Tennessee
AUGMENTATION CYSTOPLASTY

Ahmed Alkhunaizi, M.D.
Renal Fellow, University of Colorado School of Medicine, Denver, Colorado
ETIOLOGY, PATHOGENESIS, AND MANAGEMENT OF RENAL FAILURE

Rodney A. Appell, M.D.
Head, Section of Voiding Dysfunction and Female Urology, Department of Urology, The Cleveland Clinic Foundation, Cleveland, Ohio
PERIURETHRAL INJECTION THERAPY

Anthony Atala, M.D.
Assistant Professor, Harvard Medical School; Assistant in Surgery, Children's Hospital, Boston, Massachusetts
VESICOURETERAL REFLUX AND MEGAURETER

David M. Barrett, M.D.
Professor and Chair, Department of Urology, Mayo Clinic, Rochester, Minnesota
IMPLANTATION OF THE ARTIFICIAL GENITOURINARY SPHINCTER IN MEN AND WOMEN

John M. Barry, M.D.
Professor of Surgery and Chairman, Division of Urology and Renal Transplantation, The Oregon Health Sciences University; Staff Surgeon, University Hospital, Portland, Oregon
RENAL TRANSPLANTATION

Stuart B. Bauer, M.D.
Associate Professor of Urology, Harvard Medical School; Senior Associate in Surgery (Urology), The Children's Hospital, Boston, Massachusetts
ANOMALIES OF THE KIDNEY AND URETEROPELVIC JUNCTION
NEUROGENIC DYSFUNCTION OF THE LOWER URINARY TRACT IN CHILDREN

Arie Belldegrun, M.D.
Professor of Urology, Chief, Division of Urologic Oncology, and Director of Urological Research, Department of Urology, University of California, Los Angeles, School of Medicine, Los Angeles, California
RENAL TUMORS

Mitchell C. Benson, M.D.
Professor of Urology, Columbia University College of Physicians and Surgeons; Director, Urologic Oncology, Columbia-Presbyterian Medical Center, New York, New York
CONTINENT URINARY DIVERSION

Richard E. Berger, M.D.
Professor of Urology, University of Washington, Seattle, Washington
SEXUALLY TRANSMITTED DISEASES: THE CLASSIC DISEASES

Jerry G. Blaivas, M.D., FACS
Clinical Professor of Urology, Cornell University Medical College, The New York Hospital–Cornell Medical Center, New York, New York
URINARY INCONTINENCE: PATHOPHYSIOLOGY, EVALUATION, TREATMENT OVERVIEW, AND NONSURGICAL MANAGEMENT

David A. Bloom, M.D.
Professor of Surgery and Chief of Pediatric Urology, University of Michigan Medical School; Chief of Pediatric Urology, Mott Children's Hospital, Ann Arbor, Michigan
SURGERY OF THE SCROTUM AND TESTIS IN CHILDREN

Jon D. Blumenfeld, M.D.
Associate Professor of Medicine, Cornell University Medical College, New York, New York; Associate Attending in Medicine, Department of Medicine, The New York Hospital–Cornell Medical Center, New York, New York
RENAL PHYSIOLOGY
THE ADRENALS

Michael K. Brawer, M.D.
Professor, University of Washington; Chief, Urology Section, Seattle Veterans Administration Medical Center, Seattle, Washington
ULTRASONOGRAPHY OF THE PROSTATE AND BIOPSY

Charles B. Brendler, M.D.
Professor and Chief, Section of Urology, University of Chicago Hospitals and Pritzker School of Medicine, Chicago, Illinois
EVALUATION OF THE UROLOGIC PATIENT: HISTORY, PHYSICAL EXAMINATION, AND URINALYSIS

Gregory Broderick, M.D., FACS
Associate Professor of Surgery in Urology, University of Pennsylvania School of Medicine; Director of the Center for the Study of Male Sexual Dysfunction, University of Pennsylvania Health Systems, Philadelphia, Pennsylvania
EVALUATION AND NONSURGICAL MANAGEMENT OF ERECTILE DYSFUNCTION AND PRIAPISM

James D. Brooks, M.D.
Instructor of Urology, Department of Urology, Johns Hopkins Medical Institute, Baltimore, Maryland
ANATOMY OF THE LOWER URINARY TRACT AND MALE GENITALIA

H. Ballentine Carter, M.D.
Associate Professor of Urology and Oncology, The Johns Hopkins University School of Medicine; Department of Urology, The Johns Hopkins Hospital and Bayview Medical Center, Baltimore, Maryland
INSTRUMENTATION AND ENDOSCOPY
DIAGNOSIS AND STAGING OF PROSTATE CANCER

William Catalona, M.D.
Professor and Director, Division of Urology, Washington University School of Medicine, St. Louis, Missouri
UROTHELIAL TUMORS OF THE URINARY TRACT

Thomas S.K. Chang, Ph.D.
Associate Professor of Urology, Johns Hopkins School of Medicine, Baltimore, Maryland
PHYSIOLOGY OF MALE REPRODUCTION: THE TESTIS, EPIDIDYMIS, AND DUCTUS DEFERENS

Michael P. Chetner, M.D.
Associate Clinical Professor of Surgery and Oncology, University of Alberta; Director, Division of Urology, University of Alberta Hospital, Edmonton, Alberta, Canada
ULTRASONOGRAPHY OF THE PROSTATE AND BIOPSY

Robert L. Chevalier, M.D.
Genentech Professor of Pediatrics, University of Virginia School of Medicine; Director of Research, Children's Medical Center, University of Virginia, Health Sciences Center, Charlottesville, Virginia
RENAL FUNCTION IN THE FETUS, NEONATE, AND CHILD

Ashok Chopra, M.D.
Fellow of Reconstruction, Neurourology and Female Urology, Center for Health Sciences, University of California School of Medicine, Los Angeles, California
VAGINAL RECONSTRUCTIVE SURGERY FOR INCONTINENCE AND PROLAPSE

Ralph V. Clayman, M.D.
Professor of Urologic Surgery and Radiology, Washington University School of Medicine, St. Louis, Missouri
ENDOUROLOGY OF THE UPPER URINARY TRACT: PERCUTANEOUS RENAL AND URETERAL PROCEDURES

Donald S. Coffey, Ph.D.
Professor of Urology, Oncology, Pharmacology, and Experimental Therapeutics, Department of Urology, The Johns Hopkins Medical Institute, Baltimore, Maryland
THE MOLECULAR BIOLOGY, ENDOCRINOLOGY, AND PHYSIOLOGY OF THE PROSTATE AND SEMINAL VESICLES

Arnold Colodny, M.D.
Clinical Professor of Surgery, Harvard Medical School; Senior Surgeon and Associate Director of Urology, Boston Children's Hospital, Boston, Massachusetts
SURGERY OF THE SCROTUM AND TESTIS IN CHILDREN

Carlos Cordon-Cardo, M.D., Ph.D.
Associate Professor, Cornell University Medical Center; Director, Division of Molecular Pathology, Memorial Sloan-Kettering Cancer Center, New York, New York
AN OVERVIEW OF CANCER BIOLOGY

Jean B. deKernion, M.D.
Professor of Surgery/Urology, University of California, Los Angeles, School of Medicine; The Fran and Ray Stark Professor of Urology and Chairman, Department of Urology, UCLA Medical Center, Los Angeles, California
RENAL TUMORS

Charles J. Devine, M.D.
Professor of Urology, Eastern Virginia Medical School, Norfolk, Virginia
SURGERY OF THE PENIS AND URETHRA

William C. De Wolf, M.D.
Professor of Surgery, Harvard Medical School; Urologist-in-Chief, Division of Urology, Beth Israel Deaconess Medical Center, Boston, Massachusetts
PRINCIPLES OF MOLECULAR GENETICS

David A. Diamond, M.D.
Associate Professor of Surgery (Urology), Harvard Medical School; Associate in Surgery (Urology), Children's Hospital, Boston, Massachusetts
NEONATAL UROLOGIC EMERGENCIES

Giulio J. D'Angio, M.D.
Professor of Radiation Oncology Emeritus, University of Pennsylvania School of Medicine, Philadelphia, Pennsylvania
PEDIATRIC ONCOLOGY

George W. Drach, M.D.
Professor of Urology, University of Texas, Southwestern School of Medicine, Dallas, Texas
URINARY LITHIASIS: ETIOLOGY, DIAGNOSIS, AND MEDICAL MANAGEMENT

John W. Duckett, M.D.
Professor of Urology, University of Pennsylvania; Director of Pediatric Urology, Children's Hospital of Philadelphia, Philadelphia, Pennsylvania
HYPOSPADIAS

James A. Eastham, M.D.
Assistant Professor of Urology and Director of Urologic Oncology, Louisiana State University School of Medicine–Shreveport, Shreveport, Louisiana
RADICAL PROSTATECTOMY

Charles L. Edelstein, M.B., Ch.B., M.Med.
Renal Fellow, University of Colorado School of Medicine, Denver, Colorado; Senior Consultant Physician, Renal Unit, Department of Internal Medicine, University of Stellenbosch and The Tygerberg Hospital, Tygerberg, South Africa
ETIOLOGY, PATHOGENESIS, AND MANAGEMENT OF RENAL FAILURE

Mario A. Eisenberger, M.D.
Associate Professor of Oncology and Urology, Johns Hopkins Medical Institute, Baltimore, Maryland
CHEMOTHERAPY FOR HORMONE-RESISTANT PROSTATE CANCER

Jack S. Elder, M.D.
Professor of Urology and Pediatrics, Case Western Reserve University School of Medicine; Director of Pediatric Urology, Rainbow Babies and Children's Hospital, Cleveland, Ohio
CONGENITAL ANOMALIES OF THE GENITALIA

Jonathan I. Epstein, M.D.
Professor of Pathology, Urology, and Oncology, Johns Hopkins University School of Medicine; Associate Director of Surgical Pathology, The Johns Hopkins Hospital, Baltimore, Maryland
PATHOLOGY OF ADENOCARCINOMA OF THE PROSTATE

Audrey E. Evans, M.D.
Professor of Pediatrics, University of Pennsylvania School of Medicine, Philadelphia, Pennsylvania
PEDIATRIC ONCOLOGY

William R. Fair, M.D.
Professor of Urology, Cornell University Medical College; Chief of Urology and Vice-Chairman, Department of Surgery, Memorial Sloan-Kettering Cancer Center, New York, New York
AN OVERVIEW OF CANCER BIOLOGY

Diane Felsen, Ph.D.
Associate Research Professor of Pharmacology in Urology, Cornell University Medical College, The New York Hospital–Cornell Medical Center, New York, New York
PATHOPHYSIOLOGY OF URINARY TRACT OBSTRUCTION

Jeffrey Forman, M.D.
Professor of Radiation Oncology, Wayne State University School of Medicine, Detroit, Michigan
RADIOTHERAPY AND CRYOTHERAPY FOR PROSTATE CANCER

Jenny J. Franke, M.D.
Assistant Professor, Department of Urologic Surgery, Vanderbilt University, Nashville, Tennessee
SURGERY OF THE URETER

John P. Gearhart, M.D.
Professor of Pediatric Urology and Pediatrics, The Johns Hopkins University School of Medicine; Director of Pediatric Urology, The Johns Hopkins Hospital and Johns Hopkins Children's Center, Baltimore, Maryland
EXSTROPHY-EPISPADIAS COMPLEX AND BLADDER ANOMALIES

Robert P. Gibbons, M.D.
Chief of Staff, Section of Urology and Renal Transplantation, Virginia Mason Medical Center; Clinical Professor of Urology, University of Washington, Seattle, Washington
RADICAL PERINEAL PROSTATECTOMY

Kenneth I. Glassberg, M.D.
Professor of Urology, State University of New York, Health Science Center at Brooklyn; Director, Divisions of Pediatric Urology at University Hospital of Brooklyn, Kings County Hospital Center, Long Island College Hospital, Brooklyn; and Staten Island University Hospital, Staten Island, New York
RENAL DYSPLASIA AND CYSTIC DISEASE OF THE KIDNEY

Marc Goldstein, M.D.
Professor of Urology, Cornell University Medical College; Staff Scientist, Center for Biomedical Research, The Population Council; Attending Urologist and Director, Center for Male Reproductive Medicine and Microsurgery, Department of Urology, The New York Hospital–Cornell Medical Center, New York, New York
SURGICAL MANAGEMENT OF MALE INFERTILITY AND OTHER SCROTAL DISORDERS

Edmond T. Gonzales, Jr., M.D.
Professor of Urology, Scott Department of Urology, Baylor College of Medicine; Head, Department of Surgery, and Chief, Urology Service, Texas Children's Hospital, Houston, Texas
POSTERIOR URETHRAL VALVES AND OTHER URETHRAL ANOMALIES

Rafael Gosalbez, M.D.
Assistant Professor of Urology and Pediatrics and Chief of Pediatric Urology, Jackson Memorial Hospital, University of Miami, Miami, Florida
NEONATAL UROLOGIC EMERGENCIES

James E. Gow, M.D., Ch.M., FRCS
Late Clinical Lecturer, University of Liverpool, Liverpool, United Kingdom
GENITOURINARY TUBERCULOSIS

David Grignon, M.D.
Director of Anatomic Pathology, Harper Hospital; Associate Professor of Pathology, Detroit, Michigan
RADIOTHERAPY AND CRYOTHERAPY FOR PROSTATE CANCER

Frederick A. Gulmi, M.D.
Clinical Assistant Professor of Urology, State University of New York Health Sciences Center at Brooklyn; Associate Attending, Brookdale University Hospital and Medical Center, Brooklyn, New York
PATHOPHYSIOLOGY OF URINARY TRACT OBSTRUCTION

Philip Hanno, M.D.
Professor and Chairman, Department of Urology, Temple University School of Medicine, Philadelphia, Pennsylvania
INTERSTITIAL CYSTITIS AND RELATED DISEASES

W. Hardy Hendren, M.D., FACS, FAAP, FRCS(I)Hon.
Robert E. Gross Professor of Surgery, Harvard Medical School; Chief of Surgery, Massachusetts General Hospital; Visiting Surgeon, Children's Hospital, Boston, Massachusetts
CLOACAL MALFORMATIONS
URINARY UNDIVERSION: REFUNCTIONALIZATION OF THE PREVIOUSLY DIVERTED URINARY TRACT

Terry W. Hensle, M.D.
Professor of Urology, Columbia University, College of Physicians and Surgeons; Director of Pediatric Urology, Babies and Children's Hospital of New York, New York, New York
SURGICAL MANAGEMENT OF INTERSEXUALITY

Dianne M. Heritz, M.D., FRCSC
Lecturer, University of Toronto, Women's College Hospital, Toronto, Ontario, Canada
URINARY INCONTINENCE: PATHOPHYSIOLOGY, EVALUATION, TREATMENT OVERVIEW, AND NONSURGICAL MANAGEMENT

Harry W. Herr, M.D.
Associate Professor, Department of Urology, Cornell University Medical College; Associate Attending Surgeon, Urology Service, Department of Surgery, Memorial Sloan-Kettering Cancer Center, New York, New York
SURGERY OF PENILE AND URETHRAL CARCINOMA

Warren D. W. Heston, Ph.D.
Director, George M. O'Brien Urology Research for Prostate Cancer, Memorial Sloan-Kettering Cancer Center, New York, New York
AN OVERVIEW OF CANCER BIOLOGY

Stuart S. Howards, M.D.
Professor of Urology and Physiology, University of Virginia, Charlottesville, Virginia
MALE INFERTILITY
RENAL FUNCTION IN THE FETUS, NEONATE, AND CHILD

Jeffrey L. Huffman, M.D., M.H.A.
Professor of Urology, School of Medicine, and Associate Vice President for Health Affairs, University of Southern California, Los Angeles, California
URETEROSCOPY

Robert D. Jeffs, M.D.
Professor of Pediatric Urology and Pediatrics, The Johns Hopkins University School of Medicine, The Johns Hopkins Hospital, and Johns Hopkins Children's Center, Baltimore, Maryland
EXSTROPHY-EPISPADIAS COMPLEX AND BLADDER ANOMALIES

Gerald H. Jordan, M.D.
Professor of Urology, Eastern Virginia Medical School, Norfolk, Virginia
SURGERY OF THE PENIS AND URETHRA

John N. Kabalin, M.D.
Assistant Professor of Urology, Stanford University School of Medicine, Stanford, California
SURGICAL ANATOMY OF THE RETROPERITONEUM, KIDNEYS, AND URETERS

Louis R. Kavoussi, M.D.
Associate Professor and Director, Division of Endourology, Brady Urological Institute, The Johns Hopkins School of Medicine; Chief of Urology, Johns Hopkins Bayview Medical Center, Baltimore, Maryland
LAPAROSCOPY IN CHILDREN AND ADULTS

Michael A. Keating, M.D.
Private Practice, Orlando, Florida
VESICOURETERAL REFLUX AND MEGAURETER

William A. Kennedy II, M.D.
Fellow in Pediatric Urology, Children's Hospital of Philadelphia, Philadelphia, Pennsylvania
SURGICAL MANAGEMENT OF INTERSEXUALITY

Joseph M. Khoury, M.D.
Associate Professor of Surgery and Director, Urophysiology Division of Urology, Department of Surgery, University of North Carolina School of Medicine, Chapel Hill, North Carolina
RETROPUBIC SUSPENSION SURGERY FOR FEMALE SPHINCTERIC INCONTINENCE

Stephen A. Koff, M.D.
Professor of Surgery, The Ohio State University Medical Center; Chief, Section of Urology, Children's Hospital, Columbus, Ohio
ENURESIS

Karl J. Kreder, M.D.
Associate Professor of Urology, Department of Urology, University of Iowa Hospital and Clinics, Iowa City, Iowa
THE NEUROUROLOGIC EVALUATION

John N. Krieger, M.D.
Professor, Department of Urology, University of Washington School of Medicine; Attending Surgeon, University of Washington Medical Center, Seattle Veterans Administration Medical Center, Harborview Medical Center, and Children's Orthopedic Hospital, Seattle, Washington
ACQUIRED IMMUNODEFICIENCY SYNDROME AND RELATED CONDITIONS

Elroy D. Kursh, M.D.
Department of Urology, Cleveland Clinic, Cleveland, Ohio
EXTRINSIC OBSTRUCTION OF THE URETER

Gary E. Leach, M.D.
Associate Clinical Professor of Urology, University of California, Los Angeles; Chief of Urology, Kaiser-Permanente Medical Center, Los Angeles, California
SURGERY FOR CERVICOVAGINAL AND URETHROVAGINAL FISTULA AND URETHRAL DIVERTICULUM

Herbert Lepor, M.D.
Professor and Chairman, Department of Urology, and Professor, Department of Pharmacology, New York University School of Medicine; Urologist-in-Chief, New York University Medical Center, New York, New York
NATURAL HISTORY, EVALUATION, AND NONSURGICAL MANAGEMENT OF BENIGN PROSTATIC HYPERPLASIA

Ronald Lewis, M.D.
Professor of Surgery (Urology), Medical College of Georgia; Chief, Section of Urology, Medical College of Georgia Hospital, Augusta, Georgia
SURGERY FOR ERECTILE DYSFUNCTION

John A. Libertino, M.D.
Clinical Assistant Professor, Harvard Medical School, Boston; Chairman of Urology, Lahey Hitchcock Medical Center, Burlington, Massachusetts
RENOVASCULAR SURGERY

Mark R. Licht, M.D.
Head, Section of Sexual Dysfunction, and Staff, Department of Urology, Cleveland Clinic Florida, Ft. Lauderdale, Florida
IMPLANTATION OF THE ARTIFICIAL GENITOURINARY SPHINCTER IN MEN AND WOMEN

Peter Littrup, M.D.
Associate Professor of Radiology, Urology, and Radiation Oncology, Wayne State University School of Medicine, Detroit, Michigan
RADIOTHERAPY AND CRYOTHERAPY FOR PROSTATE CANCER

Tom F. Lue, M.D.
Professor of Urology, University of California School of Medicine, San Francisco, California
PHYSIOLOGY OF PENILE ERECTION AND PATHOPHYSIOLOGY OF ERECTILE DYSFUNCTION AND PRIAPISM
EVALUATION AND NONSURGICAL MANAGEMENT OF ERECTILE DYSFUNCTION AND PRIAPISM

Donald F. Lynch, Jr., M.D.
Associate Professor, Department of Urology, Eastern Virginia Medical School, Norfolk, Virginia
TUMORS OF THE PENIS

Max Maizels, M.D.
Professor of Urology, Northwestern University School of Medicine; Attending Pediatric Urologist, The Children's Memorial Hospital, Chicago, Illinois
NORMAL AND ANOMALOUS DEVELOPMENT OF THE URINARY TRACT

James Mandell, M.D.
Professor of Surgery and Pediatrics and Chief, Division of Urology, Albany Medical College, Albany, New York
PERINATAL UROLOGY
SEXUAL DIFFERENTIATION: NORMAL AND ABNORMAL

David J. Margolis, M.D.
Assistant Professor of Dermatology, University of Pennsylvania School of Medicine, Philadelphia, Pennsylvania
COLOR ATLAS OF GENITAL DERMATOLOGY
CUTANEOUS DISEASES OF THE MALE EXTERNAL GENITALIA

Fray F. Marshall, M.D.
Professor of Urology and Professor of Oncology, The Johns Hopkins University School of Medicine; Director, Division of Adult Urology, James Buchanan Brady Urological Institute, The Johns Hopkins Medical Institute, Baltimore, Maryland
SURGERY OF THE BLADDER

Thomas V. Martin, M.D.
Yale–New Haven Medical Center, New Haven, Connecticut
SHOCK-WAVE LITHOTRIPSY

John D. McConnell, M.D.
Professor and Chairman, Department of Urology, University of Texas Southwestern Medical Center, Dallas, Texas
EPIDEMIOLOGY, ETIOLOGY, PATHOPHYSIOLOGY, AND DIAGNOSIS OF BENIGN PROSTATIC HYPERPLASIA

David L. McCullough, M.D.
William H. Boyce Professor and Chairman of Department of Urology, Bowman Gray School of Medicine of Wake Forest University; Chief of Urology, North Carolina Baptist/Wake Forest University Medical Center, Winston-Salem, North Carolina
MINIMALLY INVASIVE TREATMENT OF BENIGN PROSTATIC HYPERPLASIA

W. Scott McDougal, M.D.
Walter S. Kerr, Jr., Professor of Urology, Harvard Medical School; Chief of Urology, Massachusetts General Hospital, Boston, Massachusetts
USE OF INTESTINAL SEGMENTS AND URINARY DIVERSION

Elspeth M. McDougall, M.D., FRCSC
Associate Professor of Urologic Surgery, Washington University School of Medicine, St. Louis, Missouri
ENDOUROLOGY OF THE UPPER URINARY TRACT: PERCUTANEOUS RENAL AND URETERAL PROCEDURES

Edward J. McGuire, M.D.
Professor and Director, Division of Urology, The University of Texas Health Science Center, Houston, Texas
PUBOVAGINAL SLINGS

Mani Menon, M.D.
Professor and Director, Division of Urology, University of Massachusetts, Worcester, Massachusetts
URINARY LITHIASIS: ETIOLOGY, DIAGNOSIS, AND MEDICAL MANAGEMENT

Edwin M. Meares, Jr., M.D.
Professor of Urology, Emeritus, Tufts University School of Medicine; Chairman, Department of Urology (Retired), New England Medical Center, Boston, Massachusetts
PROSTATITIS AND RELATED DISORDERS

Winston K. Mebust, M.D.
Valk Professor of Surgery/Urology and Chairman, Section of Urologic Surgery, University of Kansas Medical Center, Kansas City, Kansas
TRANSURETHRAL SURGERY

Edward M. Messing, M.D.
Winfield W. Scott Professor of Urology and Chairman, Department of Urology, University of Rochester Medical Center, Rochester, New York
UROTHELIAL TUMORS OF THE URINARY TRACT

James E. Montie, M.D.
Professor of Urology, University of Michigan, Ann Arbor, Michigan
RADIOTHERAPY AND CRYOTHERAPY FOR PROSTATE CANCER

Randall E. Morris, M.D.
Research Professor of Cardiothoracic Surgery and Director of Transplantation Immunology in the Department of Cardiothoracic Surgery, Stanford University School of Medicine, Stanford, California
TRANSPLANTATION IMMUNOBIOLOGY

Stephen Y. Nakada, M.D.
Assistant Professor of Surgery (Urology) and Head, Section of Endourology and Stone Disease, University of Wisconsin Medical School and University of Wisconsin Hospital and Clinics, Madison, Wisconsin

ENDOUROLOGY OF THE UPPER URINARY TRACT: PERCUTANEOUS RENAL AND URETERAL PROCEDURES

H. Norman Noe, M.D.
Professor of Urology and Chief of Pediatric Urology, University of Tennessee, Memphis; Chief of Pediatric Urology, LeBonheur Children's Medical Center, Memphis, Tennessee
RENAL DISEASE IN CHILDHOOD

Andrew C. Novick, M.D.
Professor of Surgery (Urology) Ohio State University School of Medicine; Chairman, Department of Urology, Cleveland Clinic Foundation, Cleveland, Ohio
SURGERY OF THE KIDNEY

Helen E. O'Connell, M.D.
Senior Lecturer, University of Melbourne, Department of Surgery; Attending Urologist, Royal Melbourne Hospital, Melbourne, Australia
PUBOVAGINAL SLINGS

Joseph E. Oesterling, M.D.
Professor and Urologist-in-Chief and Director, The Michigan Prostate Institute, University of Michigan, Ann Arbor, Michigan
RETROPUBIC AND SUPRAPUBIC PROSTATECTOMY

Carl A. Olsson, M.D.
John K. Lattimer Professor and Chairman, Department of Urology, College of Physicians and Surgeons of Columbia University; Director, Squier Urologic Clinic at The Columbia Presbyterian Hospital, New York, New York
CONTINENT URINARY DIVERSION

Nicholas Papanicolaou, M.D.
Professor of Clinical Radiology, Cornell University College of Medicine; Chief, Division of Abdominal Imaging, The New York Hospital–Cornell Medical Center, New York, New York
URINARY TRACT IMAGING AND INTERVENTION: BASIC PRINCIPLES

Alan W. Partin, M.D., Ph.D.
Associate Professor of Urology, Department of Urology, The Johns Hopkins Medical Institute, Baltimore, Maryland
THE MOLECULAR BIOLOGY, ENDOCRINOLOGY, AND PHYSIOLOGY OF THE PROSTATE AND SEMINAL VESICLES
DIAGNOSIS AND STAGING OF PROSTATE CANCER

Bhalchondra G. Parulkar, M.D.
Chief Resident, Division of Urological and Transplant Surgery, University of Massachusetts Medical Center, Worcester, Massachusetts
URINARY LITHIASIS: ETIOLOGY, DIAGNOSIS, AND MEDICAL MANAGEMENT

Craig A. Peters, M.D.
Assistant Professor of Surgery, Harvard Medical School; Assistant in Surgery, Children's Hospital, Boston, Massachusetts
PERINATAL UROLOGY
LAPAROSCOPY IN CHILDREN AND ADULTS

Paul C. Peters, M.D.
Professor Emeritus, University of Texas Southwestern Medical Center, Dallas, Texas
GENITOURINARY TRAUMA

Kenneth J. Pienta, M.D.
Associate Professor, University of Michigan School of Medicine, Ann Arbor, Michigan
ETIOLOGY, EPIDEMIOLOGY, AND PREVENTION OF CARCINOMA OF THE PROSTATE

Arthur T. Porter, M.D., FRCPC
Professor and Chairman, Wayne State University; Director of Clinical Care, Barbara Ann Karmanos Cancer Institute, Detroit, Michigan
RADIOTHERAPY AND CRYOTHERAPY FOR PROSTATE CANCER

Jacob Rajfer, M.D.
Professor of Surgery/Urology, University of California, Los Angeles, School of Medicine, Los Angeles; Chief, Division of Urology, Harbor–UCLA Medical Center, Torrance, California
CONGENITAL ANOMALIES OF THE TESTIS AND SCROTUM

R. Beverly Raney, M.D.
Professor of Pediatrics, University of Texas, M.D. Anderson Cancer Center, Houston, Texas
PEDIATRIC ONCOLOGY

Shlomo Raz, M.D.
Professor of Surgery/Urology, Center for Health Sciences, University of California School of Medicine, Los Angeles, Los Angeles, California
VAGINAL RECONSTRUCTIVE SURGERY FOR INCONTINENCE AND PROLAPSE

Martin I. Resnick, M.D.
Lester Persky Professor and Chairman, Department of Urology, Case Western Reserve University School of Medicine; Director, Department of Urology, University Hospitals of Cleveland, Cleveland, Ohio
EXTRINSIC OBSTRUCTION OF THE URETER

Neil M. Resnick, M.D.
Assistant Professor of Medicine, Harvard Medical School; Chief of Gerontology, Brigham and Women's Hospital, Boston, Massachusetts
GERIATRIC INCONTINENCE AND VOIDING DYSFUNCTION

Alan B. Retik, M.D.
Professor of Surgery/Urology, Harvard Medical School; Chief, Department of Urology, Children's Hospital, Boston, Massachusetts
PERINATAL UROLOGY
ANOMALIES OF THE URETER

Jerome P. Richie, M.D.
Elliott C. Cutler Professor of Surgery, Harvard Medical School; Chief of Urology, Brigham and Women's Hospital, and Chairman, Harvard Program in Urology (Longwood Area), Boston, Massachusetts
NEOPLASMS OF THE TESTIS

Richard C. Rink, M.D.
Associate Professor of Urology and Chief, Pediatric Urology, James Whitcomb Riley Hospital for Children, Indiana University School of Medicine, Indianapolis, Indiana
AUGMENTATION CYSTOPLASTY

Lauri J. Romanzi, M.D., FACOG
Assistant Professor, Cornell University Medical College; Director of Urogynecology, The New York Hospital–Cornell Medical Center, New York, New York
URINARY INCONTINENCE: PATHOPHYSIOLOGY, EVALUATION, TREATMENT OVERVIEW, AND NONSURGICAL MANAGEMENT

Shane Roy III, M.D.
Professor of Pediatrics, Section of Pediatric Nephrology, University of Tennessee, Memphis; Chief, Pediatric Nephrology, LeBonheur Children's Medical Center, Memphis, Tennessee
RENAL DISEASE IN CHILDHOOD

Thomas Rozanski, M.D.
Chief of Urology and Chief of Pediatric Urology, Brooke Army Medical Center, Ft. Sam Houston, Texas
SURGERY OF THE SCROTUM AND TESTIS IN CHILDREN

Daniel B. Rukstalis, M.D.
Chief of Urology, Allegheny University Hospital/Hahnemann, Philadelphia, Pennsylvania
PRINCIPLES OF MOLECULAR GENETICS

Arthur I. Sagalowsky, M.D.
Professor and Chief, Urologic Oncology, Department of Urology, The University of Texas Southwestern Medical Center; Attending, Zale Lipshy University Hospital, Dallas, Texas
GENITOURINARY TRAUMA

Jay I. Sandlow, M.D.
Assistant Professor, Department of Urology, The University of Iowa, Iowa City, Iowa
SURGERY OF THE SEMINAL VESICLES

Peter T. Scardino, M.D.
Russell and Mary Hugh Scott Professor and Chairman, Scott Department of Urology, Baylor College of Medicine; Chief, Urology Service, The Methodist Hospital, Houston, Texas
RADICAL PROSTATECTOMY

Anthony J. Schaeffer, M.D.
Professor and Chairman, Department of Urology, Northwestern University Medical School, Chicago, Illinois
INFECTIONS OF THE URINARY TRACT

Paul F. Schellhammer, M.D.
Professor and Chairman, Eastern Virginia Medical School, Norfolk; Active Staff, Sentara Health System: Norfolk General Hospital, Leigh Memorial Hospital, and Bayside, Norfolk and Virginia Beach, Virginia
TUMORS OF THE PENIS

Peter N. Schlegel, M.D.
Associate Professor of Urology, Cornell University Medical College; Staff Scientist, The Population Council; Associate Attending Urologist, The New York Hospital; Associate Visiting Physician, The Rockefeller University Hospital, New York, New York
PHYSIOLOGY OF MALE REPRODUCTION: THE TESTIS, EPIDIDYMIS, AND DUCTUS DEFERENS

Steven M. Schlossberg, M.D.
Professor of Urology, Eastern Virginia School of Medicine, Norfolk, Virginia
SURGERY OF THE PENIS AND URETHRA

Richard N. Schlussel, M.D.
Assistant Professor of Urology, Mount Sinai School of Medicine; Chief, Pediatric Urology, Mount Sinai Medical Center, New York, New York
ANOMALIES OF THE URETER

Robert W. Schrier, M.D.
Professor and Chairman, Department of Medicine, University of Colorado School of Medicine, Denver, Colorado
ETIOLOGY, PATHOGENESIS, AND MANAGEMENT OF RENAL FAILURE

Fritz H. Schröder, M.D.
Professor and Chairman, Department of Urology, Erasmus University, Rotterdam, The Netherlands
ENDOCRINE TREATMENT OF PROSTATE CANCER

Joseph I. Shapiro, M.D.
Associate Professor of Medicine and Radiology, University of Colorado School of Medicine, Denver, Colorado
ETIOLOGY, PATHOGENESIS, AND MANAGEMENT OF RENAL FAILURE

Linda M. Dairiki Shortliffe, M.D.
Professor and Chair of Urology, Stanford University School of Medicine; Chief of Pediatric Urology, Lucile Salter Packard Children's Hospital, Stanford, California
URINARY TRACT INFECTIONS IN INFANTS AND CHILDREN

Mark Sigman, M.D.
Assistant Professor of Urology, Brown University; Staff, Rhode Island Hospital, Veterans Administration Hospital, Providence, Rhode Island
MALE INFERTILITY

Donald G. Skinner, M.D.
Professor and Chairman, Department of Urology, University of Southern California School of Medicine, Los Angeles, California
SURGERY OF TESTICULAR NEOPLASMS

Eila C. Skinner, M.D.
Associate Professor of Clinical Urology, University of Southern California, Department of Urology, School of Medicine, Los Angeles, California
SURGERY OF TESTICULAR NEOPLASMS

Edwin A. Smith, M.D.
Assistant Clinical Professor of Surgery (Urology), Emory University School of Medicine; Attending, Egleston Children's Hospital and Scottish Rite Children's Medical Center, Atlanta, Georgia
PRUNE-BELLY SYNDROME

Jerome Hazen Smith, M.S.(Anat), M.Sc.Hyg., M.D.
Professor in Pathology, University of Texas Medical Branch; Pathologist, University of Texas Medical Branch Hospitals, Galveston, Texas
PARASITIC DISEASES OF THE GENITOURINARY SYSTEM

Joseph A. Smith, Jr., M.D.
William L. Bray Professor and Chairman, Department of Urologic Surgery, Vanderbilt University, Nashville, Tennessee
SURGERY OF THE URETER

Howard M. Snyder III, M.D.
Professor of Surgery in Urology, University of Pennsylvania School of Medicine, Philadelphia, Pennsylvania
PEDIATRIC ONCOLOGY
PRINCIPLES OF CONTINENT RECONSTRUCTION

R. Ernest Sosa, M.D.
Associate Professor of Urology, Cornell University Medical College; Associate Attending Urologist, The New York Hospital–Cornell Medical Center, New York, New York
RENOVASCULAR HYPERTENSION AND OTHER RENAL VASCULAR DISEASES
SHOCK-WAVE LITHOTRIPSY

William D. Steers, M.D.
Chairman and J.Y. Gillenwater Professor of Urology, University of Virginia School of Medicine, Charlottesville, Virginia
PHYSIOLOGY AND PHARMACOLOGY OF THE BLADDER AND URETHRA

Lynn Stothers, M.D., M.H.Sc.
Fellow of Reconstruction, Neurology, and Female Urology, Center for Health Sciences, University of California, Los Angeles, School of Medicine, Los Angeles, California
VAGINAL RECONSTRUCTIVE SURGERY FOR INCONTINENCE AND PROLAPSE

Stevan B. Streem, M.D.
Head, Section of Stone Disease and Endourology, Department of Urology, Cleveland Clinic Foundation, Cleveland, Ohio
SURGERY OF THE KIDNEY

Terry B. Strom, M.D.
Professor of Medicine, Harvard Medical School; Medical Director, Renal Transplant Service, and Director, Division of Immunology, Beth Israel Hospital; Physician, Brigham and Women's Hospital, Boston, Massachusetts
TRANSPLANTATION IMMUNOBIOLOGY

Manikkam Suthanthiran, M.D.
Professor of Medicine, Biochemistry, and Surgery, Cornell University Medical College; Chief, Division of Transplantation Medicine and Extracorporeal Therapy, and Chief, Division of Nephrology, Department of Medicine, The New York Hospital–Cornell Medical Center; Director, Immunogenetics and Transplantation Center, The Rogosin Institute, New York, New York
TRANSPLANTATION IMMUNOBIOLOGY

Ronald S. Swerdloff, M.D.
Professor of Medicine, University of California, Los Angeles, School of Medicine, Los Angeles; Chief, Division of Endocrinology, Harbor–UCLA Medical Center; Director, World Health Organization Collaborating Center of Reproduction, Torrance, California
PHYSIOLOGY OF HYPOTHALAMIC-PITUITARY FUNCTION

Brett A. Trockman, M.D.
Clinical Instructor, Department of Urology, Loyola University Medical Center, Maywood, Illinois
SURGERY FOR CERVICOVAGINAL AND URETHROVAGINAL FISTULA AND URETHRAL DIVERTICULUM

E. Darracott Vaughan, Jr., M.D.
James J. Colt Professor of Urology, Cornell University Medical College; Chairman, Department of Urology, and Attending Urologist-in-Chief, The New York Hospital–Cornell University Medical Center, New York, New York
RENAL PHYSIOLOGY
PATHOPHYSIOLOGY OF URINARY TRACT OBSTRUCTION
RENOVASCULAR HYPERTENSION AND OTHER RENAL VASCULAR DISEASES
THE ADRENALS

Franz von Lichtenberg, M.D.
Professor Emeritus of Pathology, Harvard Medical School; Senior Pathologist, Brigham and Women's Hospital, Boston, Massachusetts
PARASITIC DISEASES OF THE GENITOURINARY SYSTEM

R. Dixon Walker III, M.D.
Professor of Surgery and Pediatrics, University of Florida College of Medicine; Chief of Pediatric Urology, Shands Children's Hospital, Gainesville, Florida
EVALUATION OF THE PEDIATRIC UROLOGIC PATIENT

Patrick C. Walsh, M.D.
David Hall McConnell Professor and Director, Department of Urology, Johns Hopkins University School of Medicine; Urologist in Chief, James Buchanan Brady Urological Institute, Johns Hopkins Hospital, Baltimore, Maryland
THE NATURAL HISTORY OF LOCALIZED PROSTATE CANCER: A GUIDE TO THERAPY
ANATOMIC RADICAL RETROPUBIC PROSTATECTOMY

Christina Wang, M.D., FRACP, FRCP(Glas.)
Professor of Medicine, University of California, Los Angeles, School of Medicine, Los Angeles; Director, Clinical Study Center, Harbor–UCLA Medical Center, Torrance, California
PHYSIOLOGY OF HYPOTHALAMIC-PITUITARY FUNCTION

George D. Webster, M.B., Ch.B., FRCS
Professor of Surgery, Department of Surgery, Division of Urology, Duke University School of Medicine, Durham, North Carolina
THE NEUROUROLOGIC EVALUATION
RETROPUBIC SUSPENSION SURGERY FOR FEMALE SPHINCTERIC INCONTINENCE

Alan J. Wein, M.D.
Professor and Chair, Division of Urology, University of Pennsylvania School of Medicine; Chief of Urology, University of Pennsylvania Medical Center, Philadelphia, Pennsylvania
COLOR ATLAS OF GENITAL DERMATOLOGY
PATHOPHYSIOLOGY AND CHARACTERIZATION OF VOIDING DYSFUNCTION
NEUROMUSCULAR DYSFUNCTION OF THE LOWER URINARY TRACT AND ITS TREATMENT

Robert M. Weiss, M.D.
Professor and Chief, Section of Urology, Yale University School of Medicine, New Haven, Connecticut
PHYSIOLOGY AND PHARMACOLOGY OF THE RENAL PELVIS AND URETER

Richard D. Williams, M.D.
Professor and Head, Rubin H. Flocks Chair, Department of Urology, The University of Iowa, Iowa City, Iowa
SURGERY OF THE SEMINAL VESICLES

Gilbert J. Wise, M.D.
Professor of Urology, Health Science Center, State University of New York; Director of Urology, Maimonides Medical Center, Brooklyn, New York
FUNGAL INFECTIONS OF THE URINARY TRACT

John R. Woodard, M.D.
Clinical Professor of Surgery (Urology) and Director of Pediatric Urology, Emory University School of Medicine; Chief of Urology, Egleston Hospital for Children at Emory University, Atlanta, Georgia
PRUNE-BELLY SYNDROME

Subbarao V. Yalla, M.D.
Associate Professor of Surgery (Urology), Harvard Medical School, Boston, Massachusetts
GERIATRIC INCONTINENCE AND VOIDING DYSFUNCTION

Muhammad M. Yaqoob, M.D., Ph.D., MRCP
Consultant Nephrologist, The Royal London and St. Bartholomew's Hospitals, London, United Kingdom
ETIOLOGY, PATHOGENESIS, AND MANAGEMENT OF RENAL FAILURE

PREFACE
Seventh Edition of Campbell's Urology

The seventh edition of *Campbell's Urology* perpetuates over 70 years of association between the W.B. Saunders Company and the field of urology. In 1926, the classic textbook by Hugh Hampton Young, *Young's Practice of Urology* was first published. This was followed in 1935 by Frank Hinman Sr.'s *Textbook of Urology.* The first edition of *Campbell's Urology,* which was published in 1954, was edited by Meredith Campbell, Professor and Chairman of Urology at New York University. After his first and second editions he invited J. Hartwell Harrison to join him as a co-editor of the third edition. When Dr. Harrison expanded the editorial board for the fourth edition, the editors believed that Dr. Campbell's contribution to urology should be recognized in perpetuity by officially naming the textbook in his honor. This tradition continues today with the publication of the seventh edition.

With the field of urology undergoing rapid transformation, the editors believed that a major complete revision of *Campbell's Urology* was necessary within 5 years of publishing the last edition. This edition has been greatly expanded with the addition of 22 new chapters and 32 new authors. Dr. Alan Wein, Professor and Chairman of Urology at the University of Pennsylvania, has joined as a new editor and has added immeasurably to the sections on neuromuscular dysfunction of the urinary tract and incontinence.

In this edition we have used an organ systems orientation attempting wherever possible to aggregate physiology, pathophysiology, and medical and surgical management into individual sections, thereby providing a "mini" textbook for each subspecialty. We also believed that multidisciplinary authorship of some areas was very important, especially oncology. For this reason, you will note that prostate cancer is now subdivided into multiple chapters written by basic scientists, surgeons, medical oncologists, and radiation therapists. We have maintained an encyclopedic approach to each topic, but have encouraged the authors to use bold type to emphasize important concepts, thus making it easier to glean the essence from each chapter. Also, to make this edition more user friendly we have expanded the use of algorithms and decision trees wherever possible. Finally, this book will be accompanied by a study guide, which we have created to provide a structured approach to urologic education for residents, program directors, and certified urologists. At present, there is no structured curriculum for this purpose and it is the hope of the editors that this study guide will provide a systematic way to review many of the important areas in each field.

As we enter the 21st century it seemed appropriate to begin the book with the principles of molecular genetics, followed by the more traditional basic sciences such as anatomy. We have grouped renal physiology and pathophysiology together so that the reader can review the entire spectrum from normal physiology to the management of end-stage renal disease and hypertension. By building on a firm base of renal physiology, the reader can better understand the current thinking on acute renal failure, urinary tract obstruction, and renovascular disease.

Section V deals with the transport of urine to the lower urinary tract, normal and abnormal lower urinary tract storage and emptying, and the treatment of voiding dysfunction. Urinary incontinence is such an important topic that it and its treatment are considered in separate chapters in this section even though some overlap with other material is inevitable. Reconstructive and prosthetic surgery for sphincter incontinence are also considered separately here as well as other topics specifically related to female urology. Geriatric voiding dysfunction is likewise important enough to be accorded a separate chapter.

Sexual function and dysfunction, as well as reproductive function and dysfunction, follow in separate sections combining physiology, pathophysiology, and surgery. Benign prostatic hyperplasia represents one of the most common disorders managed by urologists. For this reason, it is now represented as a separate section with six chapters.

The entire section on pediatric urology has been reorganized, with new chapters "Evaluation of the Pediatric Urologic Patient" and "Renal Disease in Childhood." The chapter on "Normal and Anomalous Development of the Urinary Tract" has been expanded to include a section on molecular biology, and the chapter "Neonatal Urologic Emergencies" has been totally reorganized and stresses the most common conditions. In the chapter "Urinary Tract Infections in Infants and Children," there are now new sections discussing the management of girls with recurrent urinary tract infections without anatomic abnormalities and the incidence and detection of pyelonephritis in the absence of vesicoureteral reflux. Congenital disorders of the urinary tract have been subdivided into anomalies of the kidney and ureter, and the chapter "Vesicoureteral Reflux and Megaureter" has been totally rewritten with new authorship. Long-term results are now emphasized in the chapters on prune-belly syndrome, exstrophy of the bladder, cloacal malformations, and urinary undiversion.

The current approach to urinary stone disease as well as the use of emerging techniques in endourology and laparoscopy is now condensed. The chapter on the pathogenesis of urinary stone disease is immediately followed by alternatives for therapy including ESWL, ureteroscopy, and percutaneous approaches. These sections conclude with the chapter on percutaneous approaches for indications other than stone disease and an updated overview of the role of laparoscopy in both adults and children with urological problems. These chapters interface well with the following section, which is a compendium of the current status of urologic surgery, and includes open approaches to stone disease.

The editors are grateful for the support of the W.B. Saunders Company and especially to Richard Zorab, the editorial manager, who has facilitated our interactions. We also wish to express our thanks to Faith Voit, Hazel Hacker, Linda R. Garber, and the staff of the W.B. Saunders Company for their patience and help in bringing this ambitious undertaking to publication.

PATRICK C. WALSH, M.D.
For the Editors

CONTENTS

Volume 1

DRUG NOTICE

Medicine is an ever-changing field. Standard safety precautions must be followed, but as new research and clinical experience broaden our knowledge, changes in treatment and drug therapy become necessary or appropriate. Readers are advised to check the product information currently provided by the manufacturer of each drug to be administered to verify the recommended dose, the method and duration of administration, and contraindications. It is the responsibility of the treating physician, relying on experience and knowledge of the patient, to determine dosages and the best treatment for the patient. Neither the Publisher nor the editor assumes any responsibility for any injury and/or damage to persons or property.

The Publisher

I
MOLECULAR GENETICS AND ANATOMY

1
PRINCIPLES OF MOLECULAR GENETICS

William C. De Wolf, M.D.
Daniel B. Rukstalis, M.D.

Deoxyribonucleic acid (DNA) is the molecule of life. It contains within its elegantly simple structure the coded information that ultimately dictates all structure and function and, with it, the record book of evolution. The past decade has provided the scientific community with the tools and techniques to extract valuable information from this code in such a way that the urologic community may for the first time begin to understand the basis for disease and, in some cases, treatment. In fact, this rapid increase in understanding of the "biochemistry of life" has created an impact on society enough to generate serious ethical issues, ranging from gene ownership to job and insurability discrimination against phenotypically normal individuals with a known genetic predisposition for certain diseases. The ensuing pages provide a historical perspective, an explanation for the basic genetic anatomy, and a description of some of the tools and strategies used for its manipulation and identification; also provided are specific examples of the genetic basis for urologic disease, as well as a look into the future.

HISTORICAL PERSPECTIVE: THE OLD AND THE NEW

More than 100 years ago, two events occurred that would eventually launch biology and medicine into their most productive phase of scientific achievement. One event took place at an Austrian monastery, where a monk named Gregor Mendel recorded the types of offspring that he obtained by crossing different varieties of peas. Out of this work came the "laws of Mendel," first published in an obscure local journal in 1866 but largely ignored until the turn of the century, when the manuscript was rediscovered simultaneously by three botanists; each had independently confirmed Mendel's principles and cited Mendel's work in their own publications (Gardner and Snostad, 1981). From those laws arose the science of *genetics,* a term coined by William Bateson (an Englishman) in 1905 and derived from the Greek verb *gennân* (to beget or to generate). Mendel's discovery, expressed in modern terms, is that discrete hereditary traits, as defined by color, shape, and other features, are transmitted by units (**genes**) that always function in pairs, or **alleles** (Greek *allos,* other) (Table 1–1), one of which is provided by the male parent and the other by the female parent. The **phenotype** (or character) of the offspring depends on which alleles, dominant or recessive, are received from the two parents. Individuals in whom the two alleles are the same are designated **homozygous;** individuals with different alleles are **heterozygous** and express the dominant trait. This is what Mendel (1866) found more than a century ago. Inevitably, however, newer exceptions have been recognized. For example, it is now known that genes may not exist as independent units but are inherited as sets, a phenomenon termed **linkage**, or coupling between genes.

The second major event took place in 1869 in the laboratory of a German chemist of physiology, Felix Hoppe-Seyler, at the University of Tübingen, where Friedrick Miescher isolated a previously unknown substance from nuclei. The new substance contained a large amount of phosphorus. Miescher named his discovery *nuclein,* a word that was later changed to **nucleic acid** after the strongly acidic character of the substance (Sturtevant, 1965).

Table 1–1. GLOSSARY OF TERMS

Allele:	An alternative form of a gene. For example, the sickle-cell mutation is one of the beta-globin gene alleles. Alleles that differ from one another only at the gene sequence level–i.e., they do not produce an altered gene product—can also be recognized.
Blotting:	The process of using a radioactive single-stranded DNA or RNA molecule (a probe) to detect a complementary polynucleotide sequence that is bound (or blotted) to a solid support, usually a sheet of nitrocellulose paper. Usually, blotting is used to identify DNA restriction endonuclease fragments or specific mRNAs from a mixture of molecules that have been separated on the basis of their length by electrophoresis in a semisolid gel (agarose).
cDNA:	Complementary DNA copied from an mRNA molecule.
Denaturation:	A process whereby the two strands of a DNA molecule are separated by interrupting the hydrogen bonds that (weakly) hold the two strands of DNA together. The process, which is reversible (renaturation or annealing), occurs when pH is lowered (from alkaline) or temperature is lowered.
Exon:	A gene sequence that corresponds to part of the mature mRNA (sometimes also called a coding sequence).
Fragment:	The DNA cleavage product of a restriction endonuclease; a specific length (fragment) of DNA between two cleavage sites.
Genomic clone:	A selected host cell with a vector containing a fragment of genomic DNA from a different organism.
Genomic DNA:	All DNA sequences of an organism.
Host cell:	A cell (usually a bacterium) in which a vector can be propagated.
Hybridize:	To anneal two complementary single-stranded polynucleotides, either DNA or RNA, to one another.
Intron:	An intervening sequence that is spliced out of a primary RNA gene transcript to form mature mRNA.
Library:	A complete set of genomic clones from an organism (genomic library) or of cDNA clones from one cell type (cDNA library).
Plasmid:	A small, circular, extrachromosomal DNA molecule capable of reproducing independently in a host cell.
Polymorphisms:	Different forms of the same gene maintained in a population.
Probe:	A piece of DNA of varying length that is homologous to a specific DNA sequence within a genome. Hybridization of the probe to DNA (or RNA) preparations allows for localization of the sequence.
Restriction enzyme:	A restriction endonuclease, one of a class of enzymes that digest DNA at specific sites.
Reverse transcriptase:	The RNA-dependent DNA polymerase enzyme that catalyzes the synthesis of a DNA strand on an RNA template. The resultant single strand of DNA is complementary to its RNA template and is called cDNA.
Vector:	The genetically simple carrier element, usually a plasmid, bacteriophage, or animal virus, into whose genome a foreign segment of DNA has been inserted. There are two major types of vectors used in human genetics (although more are available): (1) A *plasmid* vector is an element consisting only of a double-stranded circular DNA genome that is capable of replicating in the cytoplasm of a bacterial host. It is usually genetically simple (it has few genes) and can be used as an acceptor (vector) for foreign DNA. Because it is replicated independently of its host's chromosome, is usually present as several copies per host cell, and can be introduced into its host as naked DNA (transformation), it is a useful vector system. It is especially useful for secondary cloning operations. (2) A *viral* vector is an animal virus used as a DNA cloning vehicle. The major advantage of viral vectors is that they can be used to infect animal cells and carry cloned genes into a living cell, in which their function can be assayed.

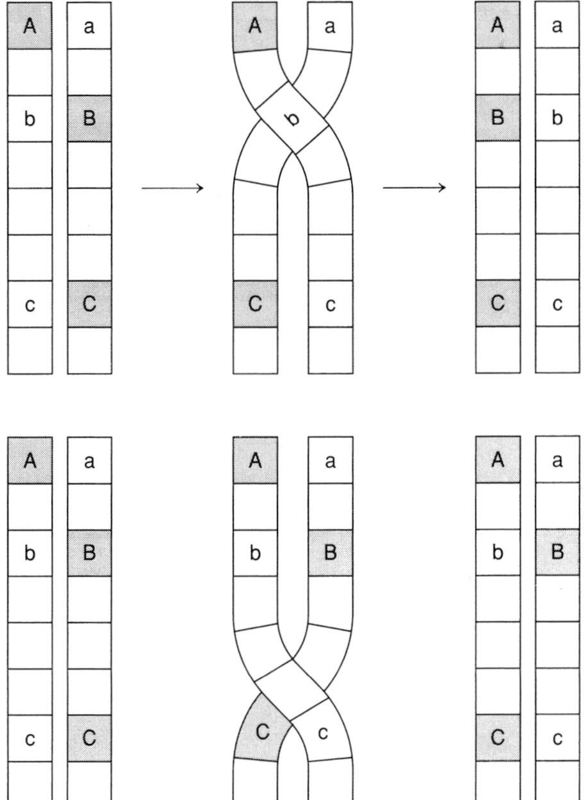

Figure 1–1. Genes situated on homologous chromosomes become recombined by crossing over. In both cases, dominant allele C recombines with A; B, which is situated closer to the A locus, recombines with A only in the first case. Thus the probability that two genes situated on distinct homologous chromosomes will recombine on the same chromosome by crossing over is *proportional* to the distance separating the loci; hence the measurement of recombination frequencies can be used for chromosomal mapping.

What brought the studies of Mendel's units and Miescher's nuclein together was the work of the cytologists who discovered chromosomes and described the behavior of these structures in mitotic division and their numerical halving in meiosis. The size and shape of chromosomes were consistent with the concept of a linear association of many genes, as indicated by the linkage phenomenon. This concept was furthered by a Belgian biologist, Frans Janssens, who observed that during meiosis, paired chromosomes "cross over" each other and exchange large segments before separating again (Fig. 1–1).

This phenomenon provided an explanation for the puzzling fact that linkage is not an all-or-none phenomenon. The first quantitative measurement of the "tightness of linkage" between two genes was provided by Thomas Hunt Morgan, who devised a method for mapping genes (in relative distances) on the four chromosomes of the small fruit fly, *Drosophila melanogaster.* Genes could actually be localized relative to bands on these chromosomes, and Mendel's "units" began to take on a physical reality.

The actual nature of that reality still remained a mystery. Again, the problem was solved with cytology, this time combined with chemistry. Through various investigations, scientists attempted to chemically characterize the structures that were visualized through the microscope. The end result, led by Oswald Avery from Rockefeller Institute in 1944, demonstrated that chromosomes consist mainly of DNA and protein. Most important, it was the DNA—not the protein—that was the actual bearer of genetic information. The search finally ended on April 25, 1953, when an American, James Watson, aged 25, and an Englishman, Francis Crick, aged 37, published a small, unobtrusive paper occupying fewer than two pages of the British scientific journal *Nature* (Watson and Crick, 1953). Interestingly, this paper had only one figure (Fig. 1–2) and six references and, as such, introduced the double helix to the world. The importance of this paper cannot be overstated; it allowed, for the first time, the laws of chemistry and physics to be applied to almost all questions of disease etiology and hence to the recently coined term *molecular medicine*. Francis Crick characterized this best when he later wrote that DNA represents the sole biochemical basis for information storage and information transfer; in a sense, it is the very heart of the biologic communication system.

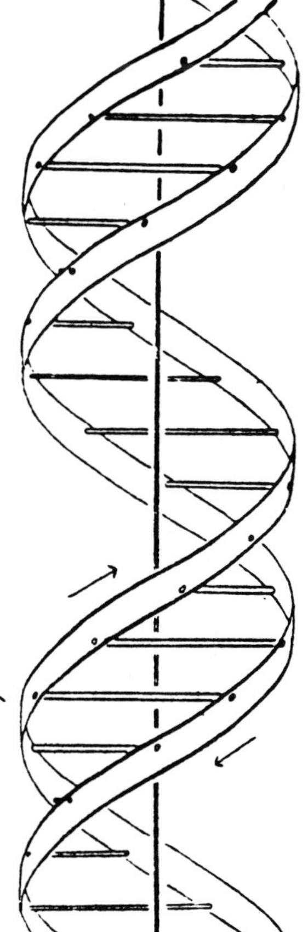

This figure is purely diagrammatic. The two ribbons symbolize the two phosphate—sugar chains, and the horizontal rods the pairs of bases holding the chains together. The vertical line marks the fibre axis

Figure 1–2. The double helix with corresponding legend from the original description (Watson and Crick, 1953). This was the only figure in that article!

GLOSSARY OF TERMS: THE BASICS

DNA Structure

How can DNA successfully hold such a position of power and influence? Surprisingly, one of the reasons lies in its elegantly simple structure. **In a way, DNA resembles proteins in the sense that it is constructed of many building blocks with a repeating fundamental structure, and the blocks are linked end to end. In the case of proteins, the building blocks are amino acids; in the case of DNA, they are nucleotides** (Fig. 1–3*A*). Nucleotides consist of three components: a phosphate group, a sugar group (i.e., ribose), and a base that is either a purine (adenine [A] or guanine [G]) or a pyrimidine (thymine [T] or cytosine [C]). In ribonucleic acid (RNA), thymine is replaced by uracil. Amazingly, the protein "alphabet" consists of 20 amino acids, whereas the DNA "alphabet" consists of only four bases (A, T, G, or C). The triphosphate of the nucleotide is a high-energy compound that can react with polymerases to form a polymer (i.e., RNA or DNA). These acidic polymers of polynucleotides are termed **nucleic acids.** The DNA molecule is then made up of two chains of polynucleotides, with the sugar phosphate backbones on the outside of the DNA molecule and the purine and pyrimidine bases on the inside, as Watson and Crick (1953) originally described (see Fig. 1–3). Of importance is that the bases are oriented in such a way that they hydrogen-bond to bases on the opposing chain; for example, a purine on one chain is always hydrogen-bonded to a pyrimidine on the other chain. The bonding is extremely specific: adenine (A) can pair only with thymine (T), and guanine (G) can pair only with cytosine (C) (see Fig. 1–3*A*). The hydrogen bonding also allows the two chains to temporarily split like a "nature's Velcro." This occurs, for example, in the making of RNA (transcription) when the two chains temporarily separate. **If the sequence of one chain is known, the other can be deduced, and the opposing sequences are referred to as *complementary*** (see Fig. 1–3*D*). Despite the relative weakness of the hydrogen bonds holding the base pairs together, each DNA molecule contains so many base pairs that the complementary chains never spontaneously separate under physiologic conditions. Experimentally, however, if DNA is exposed to near-boiling temperatures or to extremes of pH (<3 or >10), the base pairs quickly fall apart, and the double helix separates into its **complementary** strands—a process called **denaturation** (see Table 1–1). This is referred to in later sections.

Perhaps more important is the fact that denaturation is reversible such that at cooler temperatures at near-neutral pH, complementary single strands recombine to form native double helices. This annealing process is called **renaturation** and forms the basis for Southern and Northern blotting, as described later in this section. Because three hydrogen bonds link guanine to cytosine, whereas only two link adenine to thymine, there is some interchain variability with respect to how "sticky" the two strands really are.

Another simplistic feature of DNA that adds to its "strength" is that **its structure is independent of its sequence.** In other words, the sequence of nucleotides from which DNA is constructed is important, not to determine the general structure of DNA, but rather to code for the sequence of amino acids that constitutes the corresponding polypeptide. The relationship between the sequence of DNA and the sequence of the corresponding protein is the **genetic code** (see Fig. 1–3*D*). A **gene** includes a series of triplets (three nucleotides that encode an amino acid), or **codons**, that are read in a series from a starting point at one end to a termination point at another, always in a 5′-to-3′ direction (direction in the polynucleotide chain as indicated by carbon atoms on the deoxyribose ring; see Fig. 1–3*C*). In any given region, only one of the two strands of DNA codes for a protein. Another feature of the "constant structure" of the backbone of the helix is that general enzymes can copy, cleave, and repair the DNA structure anywhere along its entire length, irrespective of the specific genetic information carried within a particular region of the molecule.

One important consequence of the strict rule that adenine pairs only with thymine and cytosine only with guanine is that the sequence of nucleotides on one strand of the double helix determines the nucleotide sequence on the other strand. The base pairing rule is thus critical for the storage, retrieval, and transfer of genetic information. It guarantees that the instructions encoded by the base sequences of the double helix will be faithfully transmitted whether DNA is being copied (replication) or read (transcription).

This simplicity of structure allows for several other interesting properties besides renaturation. For example, base pairing forms not only between bases on opposing strands but also between bases on single strands that have nearby inverted repetitive sequences that allow the formation of hydrogen-bonded hairpin loops called *palindromes.* These loops are then able to act as "guideposts" to interact with DNA-binding proteins that are important in regulating DNA activity. Regulator protein binding to DNA can be affected by other epigenetic changes in the DNA structure (i.e., changes that do not involve the actual architectural structures of DNA). For example, cytosine residues can exist in a modified form in which a methyl group is attached to the 5′ carbon atom of the pyrimidine ring to make 5-methyl cytosine (Fig. 1–4). Such methyl groups do not affect the way their respective molecules can hydrogen-bond (i.e., the base pairs formed by the 5-methyl cytosine with guanine are equivalent in strength to those formed by cytosine). In eukaryotic DNA, cytosine residues that contain methyl groups are always located next to guanine residues on the same chain—that is, CpG (p is the phosphodiester bond between adjacent nucleotides). The importance of methylation is that it seems to hinder regulatory protein binding to DNA in the sense that highly methylated DNA is usually genetically silent.

As can be imagined, the structure of DNA with its relatively simple construction allows it to be pliable and durable (see Fig. 1–3). Externally there are two outer grooves, a major (larger) one and a minor (smaller) one, that are important because regulatory proteins fit into these grooves. The bases are perpendicular to the axis of symmetry, and there are 10 base pairs per turn; the diameter of the double helix is 20 Å (the diameter of a hydrogen molecule is 1 Å, and the diameter of a human red blood cell is 8×10^4 Å). **This type of construction renders the DNA molecule extremely resistant to all types of denaturing substances as phenol and chloroform, sizable temperature shifts, and pH changes that are not too extensive. Because of**

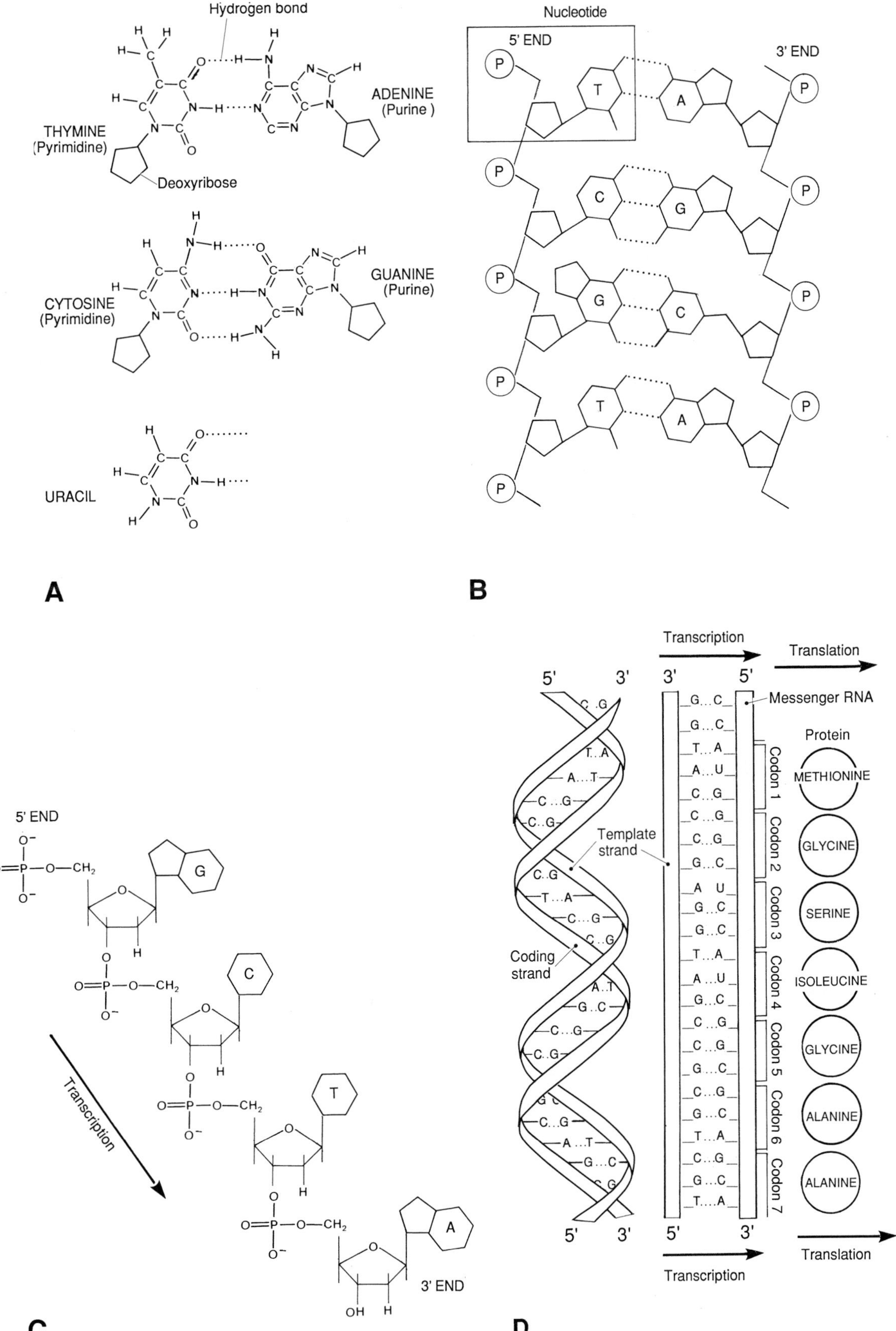

Figure 1–3. The structure of DNA. *A,* The alphabet consists of four bases: the purines adenine (A) and guanine (G) and the pyrimidines thymine (T) and cytosine (C). Uracil (U) is substituted for thymine in the case of RNA. The combination of a base and sugar (deoxyribose) is referred to as a **nucleoside**. *B* and *C,* The combination of a sugar phosphate group and a base constitutes a **nucleotide**. The double helix is made from two polynucleotide chains, each of which consists of a series of 5′- to 3′-sugar phosphate links that form a backbone from which the bases protrude. The double helix maintains a constant width because purines always face pyrimidines in complementary A-T and G-C base pairs, respectively. *D,* During transciption the coding strand conveys its message through the template strand to make mRNA that is eventually translated into polypeptides by ribosomes. The relationship between DNA sequence and corresponding protein is called the **genetic code**, which is read in triplets, or **codons**.

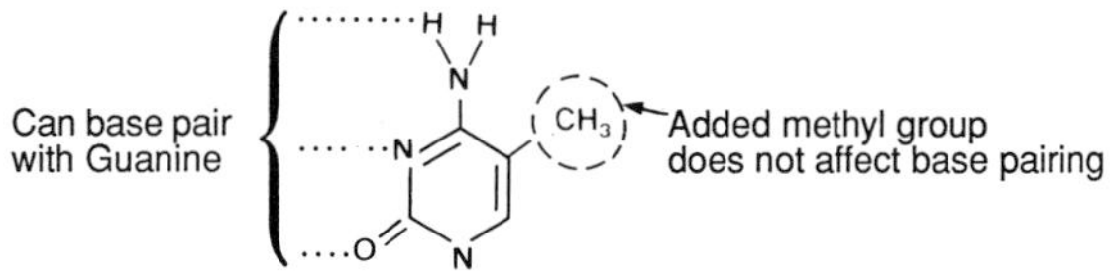

Can base pair with Guanine

Added methyl group does not affect base pairing

Figure 1–4. 5-Methylcytosine.

this, evolutionary biologists have been able to routinely study DNA from properly preserved biologic tissues and organisms that lived several thousands of years ago. So far, three types of super-old DNA have been reported: compression fossils of leaves from Idaho dated at approximately 17 million years; insects encased in amber (which helps prevent oxidative damage with hydrolysis of purines), such as those found in the Dominican Republic that date back 25 to 30 million years and a weevil from Lebanese amber dating back up to 135 million years; and of course dinosaur DNA dated more than 65 million years (Williams, 1995).

As noted, DNA is a long, thin molecule; in fact, each chromosome consists of a single molecule of DNA, and the total length of DNA with a nucleus is about 2 m! All of the DNA within a diploid cell contains 6 billion (6×10^9) base pairs to make the DNA content of each cell, which is called the **genome.** The genome is the same within each cell of an organism; cells from different tissues of the body are genetically distinguished from one another not by their DNA (which is the same) but by which parts of the genome are active—that is, which genes are operational. This notion of tissue-specific differential gene expression is currently challenging the best genetic laboratories in the world with regard to a proper mechanistic explanation. The actual amount of information represented by number of bases per nucleus, however, is almost beyond imagination. If the genome were compared to a book, there would be 6×10^9 letters (A, T, G, C, or bases) in the book; assuming 2000 letters per page, there would be 3 million pages, or 3000 volumes of 1000 pages each!

With this information, the real challenge, then, is how 2 m of DNA gets packaged into a 10-μm (or 10^{-6}-m) nucleus. Also, the mechanism by which this is done must allow replication into 46 daughter chromosomes without tangling. The key to packaging is the **histone** proteins (Fig. 1–5). **The double helix is wound twice around a spool of eight histone molecules to form nucleosomes, which are the fundamental repeating units of chromatin. Six of these nucleosomes form a solenoid to make a 30-μm-diameter fiber that forms the chromatin thread** (Richmond et al, 1984; Arents et al, 1991). These fibers then undergo a series of coordinated loops attached to the nuclear matrix (which is like an internal nuclear skeleton) in such a way that the packaging ratio or the fold condensation of the length of packaged DNA is 10^5.

From this information, it is easy to imagine how this "tight" DNA packaging may have an important regulatory effect on how genetic material is transcribed. Not only must the active genes be exposed for processing, but also transcriptional regulatory proteins and the transcriptional apparatus (see later discussion) must be able to access the DNA for transcription to occur. For example, it is easy to see how DNA in its resting state actually represses transcription: Consider that one side of the double helix is occluded because it faces the core histones (see Fig. 1–5). The solenoid thereby renders large segments of DNA invisible to DNA-binding proteins (which regulate transcription). In a sense, this may be advantageous in reducing the amount of DNA that a eukaryotic transcription factor has to search in order to find its binding site (Lin and Riggs, 1975). Moreover, each transcription complex that does form may, by disrupting the fiber, act as a highly visible signpost to RNA polymerase (the enzyme that binds to DNA to begin transcription) (Wolffe and Brown, 1988). Whatever the answer to these issues, it is apparent that alterations in histone sequence, nucleosome structure, and folding of chromatin fiber influence both activation and repression of genes through alteration of accessibility of DNA to both transcriptional factors and RNA polymerase and influence progression of RNA polymerase along the chromatin fiber (for reviews, see Wolffe, 1992; Lewin, 1994).

Genes and Transcription

The genome of the mammalian cell is quite large, as mentioned, and carries approximately 6 billion base pairs of information within its chromosomal DNA. These sequences contain between 50,000 and 100,000 genes, and each of these is deciphered or transcribed by a complex apparatus (which is still not totally understood) that stands between nucleic acid and protein. This process, called **transcription,** involves the formation of a template in the form of messenger RNA (mRNA), which faithfully duplicates the coding sequence of one of the DNA strands. Once the mRNA is

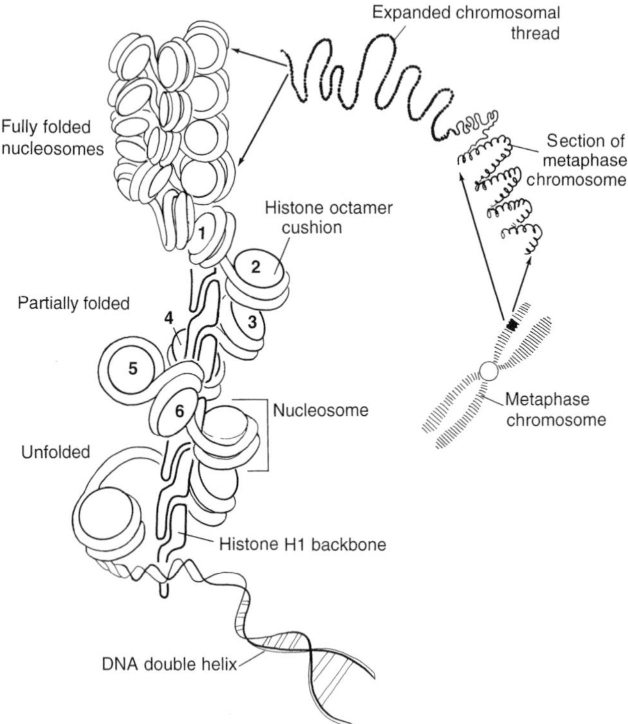

Figure 1–5. The "chromatin thread" is actually a solenoid with a string of nucleosomes coiled helically with a pitch of six nucleosomes per turn in an axial manner. Each nucleosome has an octaneric protein core and is cylindrical in shape. DNA runs continuously from nucleosome to nucleosome.

made, it is shipped to the cytoplasm, where it directs the production of protein (a process called **translation**). Transcription, then, is a process or mechanism whereby DNA information is copied into RNA language. The only difference between DNA and RNA is that uracil (U) replaces thymine (T) in RNA (see Fig. 1–3*D*) (Darnell, 1985; Ross, 1989).

Exons and Introns

Surprisingly, most DNA, estimated at 90%, does not code for proteins but acts as "filler." In fact, it is usually found that genes themselves contain interrupting noncoding sequences that do not code for protein. The reason for this circumstance of nature is not known, although some of the noncoding portion is used for certain regulatory activities (Perlman and Butow, 1989; Augustin et al, 1990). The coding portions of genes are called **exons,** and the noncoding interrupting portions of genes are called **introns.** For proper transcription, the noncoding portion of mRNA (i.e., the message from DNA) must be excised from the coding portion of mRNA (Fig. 1–6). The existence of this anatomic genetic arrangement, with exons and introns, has intrigued evolutionary biologists with regard to the origins of genes and the proteins that they encode. This schema has led to an interesting hypothetical repertoire of mechanisms for the evolution of "new genes." It is generally thought that gene duplication with mutation is the most common mechanism for new gene formation. Because duplicated gene regions are generally unstable (and, if the duplicated sequence were to be functional, it is usually not significantly different from the parent gene), other mechanisms have been popularized. For example, "exon shuffling" refers to a new gene that is formed by addition of new segments (exons) derived from pre-existing exons encoding functional protein domains (Gilbert, 1978). This theory assumes that each exon encodes a protein domain (Go and Nosaka, 1987). Through the combination of different domains into a single protein, the creation of more distinctly unusual proteins is possible, while a high likelihood of functionality is still retained. Both of these mechanisms (duplication and shuffling) are limited in their ability to generate truly unique and unusual gene sequences, which may be necessary for evolution. Another mechanism that circumvents this limitation makes use of intron sequences and is aptly called "intron capture." This mechanism simply involves addition of an intron sequence (or a piece of an intron) to an existing exon to make a new exon and thus a new or improved protein (Golding et al, 1994).

Strangely enough, evolutionary biologists have not yet decided in which evolutionary direction introns are traveling! In other words, some data support the hypothesis that introns are actually ancient and have been subsequently lost in bacteria (bacteria do not have introns) (Cavalier-Smith, 1985), whereas other data show that introns are recent and have been inserted into eukaryotic genes (Sudhof et al, 1985). But whatever their evolutionary course, introns have permitted some genes to be constructed from combinations of exons of other genes (Roger and Doolittle, 1993).

Although the word *intron* implies intervening sequence, presumably without function, it is interesting that linguistic analysis casts a different picture of introns (Mantegna et al, 1994). Zipf analysis calculates a histogram of the number of occurrences of each word in a text and arranges these values in a log:log plot against the rank order of each word. For all human languages, this produces a plot with a slope of −1. When extensive DNA sequences were analyzed in this fashion, with "word" lengths of 3 to 8 bases, linear plots were obtained. The interesting feature was that noncoding regions in human and other DNAs consistently yielded larger negative scores than did coding regions. A second analysis was directed at redundancy. Changing or removing some letters or words did not make the meaning indecipherable. Again, noncoding DNA scored higher than coding DNA. These observations suggest that large stretches of noncoding human DNA may contain information in other "languages"!

Mechanics of Transcription

As previously stated, DNA basically has two jobs: the first is to self-replicate, which is required to make a new

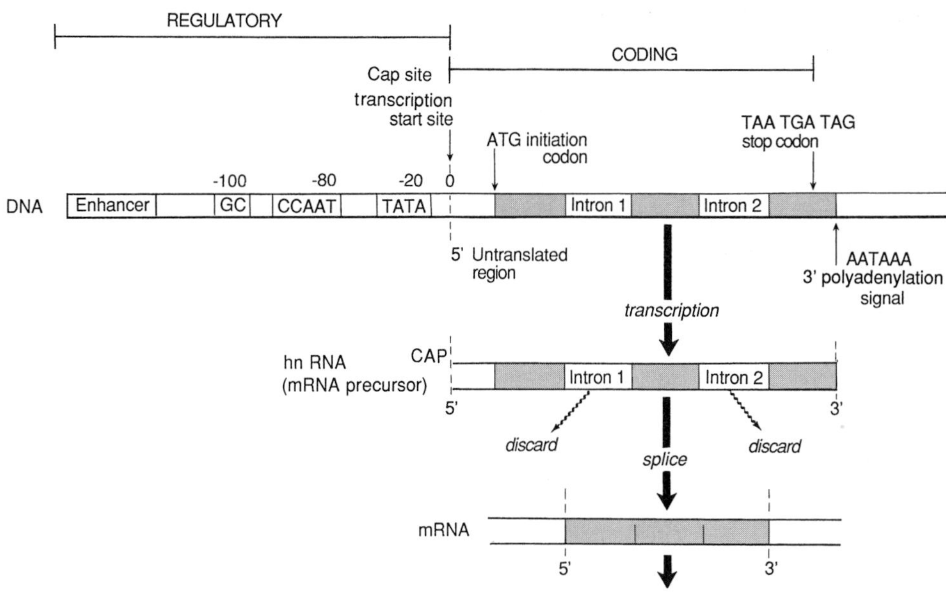

Figure 1–6. Structural landmarks in the transcription of mRNA from DNA.

cell, and the second is to transcribe its code into RNA for delivery to the cytoplasm. The RNA "message" from DNA or mRNA originates in the nucleus, where a polymerase enzyme copies, base by base, a gene sequence in one of the two complementary DNA strands. The nomenclature here is often incorrect or at least confusing in many texts and so must be carefully stated. When DNA transcription is taught, a distinction must be made between the two strands of duplex DNA: One is transcribed and the other is not. Two sets of terms are commonly used: coding/noncoding and sense/antisense. The coding (or "sense") DNA strand is the strand of duplex DNA which is transcribed into a complementary RNA strand. The DNA strand that is not transcribed, having the same sequence as the mRNA, is referred to as the noncoding (or "antisense") strand (see Fig. 1–3*D*).

The enzymes that copy DNA are called **polymerases.** Logically, those that make more DNA from DNA are called DNA polymerases, and those that make RNA from DNA are called RNA polymerases. All eukaryotic cells (cells containing a nucleus; organisms without a nucleus are called prokaryotic) contain three distinct types of RNA polymerase. Each is responsible for making a different kind of RNA. For example, RNA polymerase I (Pol I) synthesizes ribosomal RNA; Pol II transcribes protein-coding genes; and Pol III is responsible for the synthesis of small RNA species such as transfer RNA (tRNA) and ribosomal (5S) RNA. It is not known exactly why the job of RNA synthesis is divided among three enzymes, but the roles of the RNAs clearly differ as to the sites of synthesis. In general, Pol I and Pol III act to produce RNA that will act as the machinery to be used in translating the Pol II product (mRNA) into protein (Fig. 1–7).

The question of how transcription is executed and, in particular, which genes in the cell are transcribed addresses one of the most fundamental questions in molecular genetics and perhaps in all biology: If all cells in the body contain the same genetic content, how does the cell know which gene to turn on? The exact answer is not clear, but enough is known to offer a good perspective. In the nucleus, free Pol II molecules collide randomly with DNA, sticking only weakly to most DNA. However, the polymerase binds very tightly when it collides with a specific DNA sequence, called a **promoter,** that contains the start site for RNA synthesis and signals where RNA synthesis should begin (see Fig. 1–6). Two principal DNA promoter elements located upstream (5′) of the gene are commonly used for transcription. The first is an AT-rich region located approximately 28 base pairs (bp) 5′ from the gene start site. This region contains a consensus sequence (a conserved sequence found in all DNA samples) of TATAAA or ATAAA, which is commonly known as the TATA box (Fig. 1–8; see also Fig. 1–6). This sequence can serve as a recognition site for binding of proteins that control the transcription of DNA. In fact, the first step during formation of a transcription-competent complex on a TATA-containing promoter is the association of a protein called a TATA-binding protein (TBP) with the TATA sequence. **Binding of TBP provides the site to which Pol II and the rest of the general transcription factors can sequentially associate to form a transcriptionally competent complex.** Some promoters, however, do not have TATA sequences to direct transcription initiation. These genes have a second type of sequence called the initiator (Inr) element, which encompasses the transcription start site. The multiprotein complex that directs transcription from this start site is not completely understood but also involves participation from the TBP (for reviews, see Conaway and Conaway, 1993; Zawel and Reinberg, 1995).

Other regulatory sequence elements are located farther upstream and can enhance or repress initiation of transcription. Examples include the CCAAT consensus (CAAT box) and the GGGCC consensus, which were among the first such sequences identified. These have been called **promoter-proximal sequences** because of their "proximal position" to the gene. These elements are conserved in several, but not all, known promoters, where they are often located approximately 80 base pairs 5′ to the gene. However, they can function at distances that vary considerably from the gene start point. It is possible that within the cell there exist hundreds of as-yet-unidentified proteins that interact with these sequences to regulate transcription.

The second major class of gene-activating elements consists of **enhancers** (Fig. 1–9). Like promoters, these sequences bind specific proteins that positively or negatively regulate transcription. The difference, however, is that the enhancer can be positioned in unusual ways relative to the gene: They can be in reverse orientation, they can be located at great distances from the gene (~40 kb) either upstream or downstream from the gene, and they can be located even within the gene, usually within introns. It is thought that enhancer elements form loops in DNA to exert their effect.

The initiation of transcription, then, involves a Pol II recognition of a specific promoter-enhancer region near the start site of a gene followed by the subsequent generation of an mRNA. The process has been arbitrarily divided into five steps:

1. Pre-initiation complex formation.
2. Initiation.
3. Promoter clearance.
4. Elongation.
5. Termination.

The first step, pre-initiation complex formation, is the process whereby the genetics within a cell decides which promoter/gene the Pol II will activate; that is, it is a process that tells the Pol II where to "stick" and initiate transcription. In mammals, there are at least 20 polypeptides that go into making seven transcription factors that act as a "signpost" for Pol II (see Fig. 1–8). The TATA box and the initiator, alluded to earlier, constitute promoter elements that mediate the nucleation (or aggregation) at the pre-initiation complex. Understanding of complex assembly on TATA-containing promoters is more defined than that of promoters that contain only an initiator. In general, TAF II (general transcription factors for polymerase II) and RNA Pol II assemble on the promoter DNA through protein-DNA and protein-protein interactions (see Fig. 1–8) in a highly ordered manner.

The actual initiation of transcription is incompletely understood but apparently is regulated by proteins that bind the promoter region of genes; that is, some of the proteins repress transcription, whereas others activate it. The process of activation involves at least two steps: the removal of factors that maintain a gene in the transcriptionally silent state, and a true activation step, which is a direct

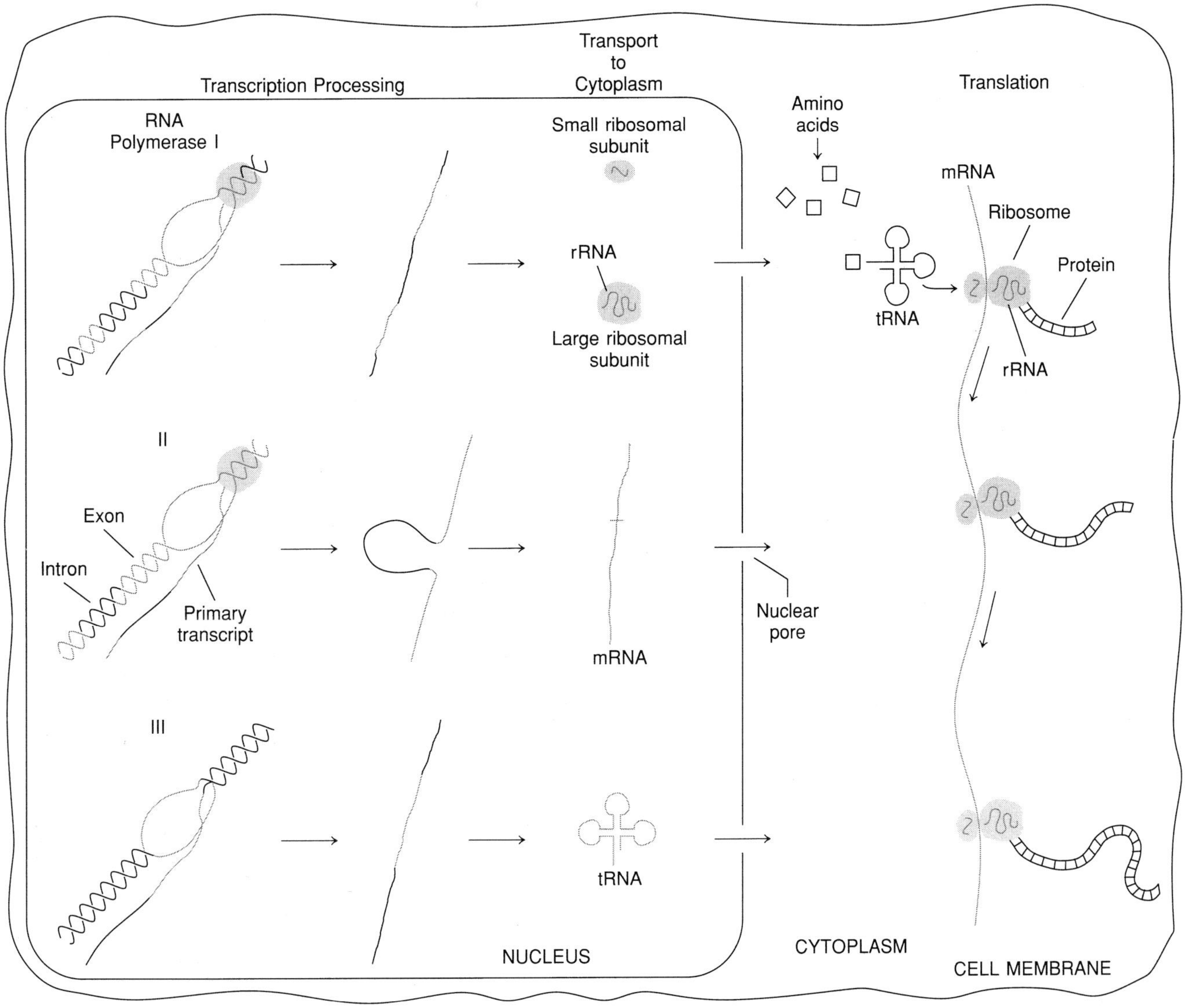

Figure 1–7. Protein synthesis involves three types of RNA. Ribosomal RNA (rRNA), messenger RNA (mRNA), and transfer RNA (tRNA) are made by transcription initiated from one strand of the DNA double helix. The enzymes catalyzing their production are Pol I, Pol II, and Pol III, respectively. The RNA molecules thus formed must be further processed (i.e., cut and spliced) to make an end product. The ends of the tRNA transcript are cut, and the molecule assumes a looped structure. A single rRNA transcript is cut in several places to form two major types of rRNA that are bound to protein molecules to form ribosomal subunits. The mRNA is also "spliced" with removal of introns. After the exons are spliced within the nucleus, the mature mRNA exits the nucleus through pores in the nuclear envelope. In the cytoplasm (endoplasmic reticulum), the mature mRNA, tRNA, and ribosomes are united to begin translation.

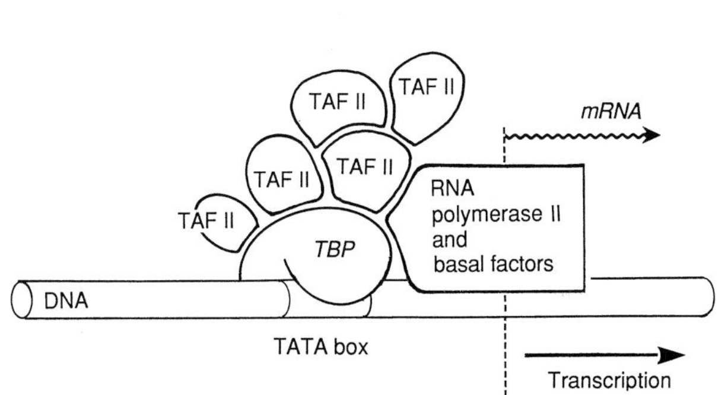

Figure 1–8. Transcriptional apparatus for polymerase II. Distinct multiprotein complexes with a common subunit, the TATA-binding protein (TBP), participate in specific promoter recognition by Pol II. Several other "TBP-associated factors" (TAFs) are required.

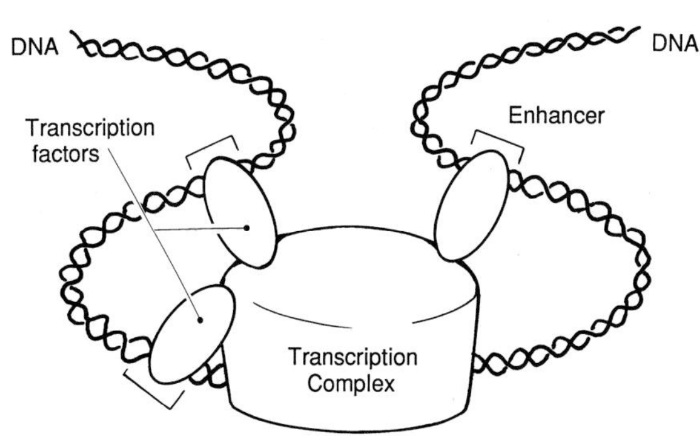

Figure 1–9. A conceptual illustration of how transcriptional factors can bind to DNA recognition sites distant from a gene (enhancer sites) and then, by simultaneously binding to the transcriptional complex, loop out large pieces of DNA. This may help "unwind" DNA in the transcriptional process.

effect on one or more steps of the transcription cycle, presumably through effect of TBP-associated factors (TAFs). These and other proteins act in a yet-to-be-defined way to initiate transcription.

Once RNA polymerase II has "escaped" from the promoter (promoter clearance), it faces the formidable task of elongating the transcript through blocks within genes. In general, the RNA polymerase proceeds by opening up a local region of the DNA double helix with the aid of such enzymes as helicases, gyrases, and topoisomerases to expose nucleotides on a short stretch of DNA on each strand. One of the two exposed DNA strands acts as a template for complementary base pairing with incoming ribonucleoside triphosphate monomers, two of which are joined together by the polymerase to begin an RNA chain. The RNA polymerase molecule then moves stepwise along the DNA, unwinding the DNA helix just ahead to expose a new region of template for complementary base pairing. In this way, the growing RNA chain is extended by one nucleotide at a time in a 5′-to-3′ direction. **The rate of progression is approximately 1 μm/min, which means either that the RNA chain grows at a rate of 50 nucleotides per second or that it takes RNA polymerase no more than two hundredths of a second to try various nucleoside triphosphates for fit, find the right one, substitute one bond for another, move on through the next base pair in the DNA double helix, and get ready for another round of the same kind.** Although this may seem fast, consider the fact that transcription of some large genes, such as the giant dystrophin gene, would take more than 1 hour to complete! Overall, this rate of transcription has strategic implications during embryogenesis, in which cell division is often measured in minutes, thus preventing some genes from ever getting transcribed.

Interestingly, the movement of Pol II involves certain "pause" sites along the genome, perhaps to allow for certain steps of the new mRNA formation to be completed. Although the complete regulatory mechanics that control Pol II "idling" on the genome are not worked out, the principal elements are the elongin proteins, which are separated into three subunits (i.e., elongins A, B, and C). The three-subunit molecule allows the transcriptional apparatus to move ahead without pausing; when the triple complex is not present, the transcriptional apparatus pauses normally, and in this way, regulation of transcriptional "movement" occurs. The importance of this to urologists is that the von Hippel–Lindau (VHL) protein complexes to elongins B and C, preventing the association of the three-unit molecule, and therefore allows normal "pausing" (Aso et al, 1995; Duan et al, 1995; Kibel et al, 1995). Individuals with germ line mutations of the VHL gene are predisposed to multiple forms of cancer, including renal cell carcinoma, hemangioblastoma, and pheochromocytoma (Latif et al, 1993). Many questions still remain unanswered; for example, which genes are targeted by VHL? Patients with a mutated VHL gene have only a few abnormal cell types, and therefore VHL is not a global regulator of transcriptional elongation. However, several genes implicated in the pathogenesis of malignancies (such as *N-myc* and *C-fos)* are regulated at the level of elongation and are thus prime candidates for targets of VHL.

For the most part, mRNA transcripts begin and end in a uniform way. For example, most sequences begin with an AUG that codes for methione; usually this sequence is followed by a purine-rich sequence (e.g., AGGA) that may help to position the starting AUG opposite the ribosomal cavity containing the initiating amino acid tRNA complex (see later discussion). **All mRNA is ordered in such a way that the first codons encode the amino terminal amino acids and finish with the carboxyl terminal amino acid of the polypeptide that is eventually encoded.** One or several amino terminal amino acids that were encoded by the initiating AUG and associated sequences are frequently cleaved away by proteolytic (protein-degrading) enzymes to produce functional polypeptide products whose amino terminal amino acids are different from those of the primary translation products.

Within about 1 second after initiation of transcription, before the RNA is more than 30 nucleotides long, a chemically protective cap is added to the nucleotide at the beginning of the chain (the 5′ end). The cap, which consists of a methylated guanosine (a nucleotide incorporating the base guanine), is linked to the first nucleotide by a triphosphate bridge (see Fig. 1–6). After the cap is attached, the polymerase continues to add nucleotides to the 3′ end of the chain until the enzyme encounters a second special sequence in DNA, the **termination signal,** in the form of the sequence AAUAAA (poly A) located 10 to 30 nucleotides upstream from the actual site of cleavage. Usually the RNA polymerase overshoots the actual end of the gene, and as the poly A sequence is transcribed (in addition to other less well-understood events), cleavage occurs, and a poly A polymerase enzyme adds 100 to 200 residues of adenylic acid (as poly A) to the 3′ end of the RNA chain to complete the primary RNA transcript. Meanwhile, the Pol II fruitlessly continues transcribing for hundreds or thousands of nucleotides until termination occurs at one end of several later sites. The extra mRNA is quickly degraded, presumably because it lacks the methylated guanosine cap that is on the functional mRNA. The function of the poly A tail is not known for certain, but it may play a role in the export of mature mRNA from the nucleus. It also may stabilize mRNA by retarding degradation in the cytoplasm. In general, transcription is usually unidirectional—a one-sided process in which only one side of the two DNA strands is transcribed.

To make a mature mRNA to be exported to the cytoplasm for translation into protein, the primary transcript, called pre-mRNA, must be processed to remove the introns and join the coding sequences into a contiguous mRNA molecule (see Fig. 1–6). **This process is appropriately called *splicing* and is extremely important because if an exon is missed, or if a splice occurs even one nucleotide away from the correct location, the correct protein will not be translated from the resulting mRNA because a base pair will be either added or subtracted from the reading frame (DNA coding sequence). When that happens, a mutation occurs.** For example, when a base pair is added or subtracted, the codon reading frame is "offset" (remember that every third base pair forms a codon that codes for an amino acid). If the start site is moved over by one base pair, a "frame shift" mutation occurs. The splicing process takes place in spliceosomes, which are large ribonucleoprotein particles akin to ribosomes. Although the exact mechanism is not completely clear, it is understood that splicing is a two-step process. First, the 5′ splice site is cut, freeing the upstream exon and generating a lariat molecule containing the intron still joined to the downstream exon. In the second step, the 3′ splice site is cut and the exons are joined, freeing the intron as a lariat (Maniatis and Reed, 1987). Many factors are involved in this process, both small nuclear ribonucleoproteins (sn RNPs) and several protein components.

The process of transcription is not reversible under normal circumstances. Once mRNA molecules are made, they serve as templates that order the amino acids within the peptide chains of proteins during the process of **translation**—so named because the nucleotide language of nucleic acids is translated into amino acid language of proteins. **This schema—that information flows from DNA to RNA to protein—has become known as the central dogma of molecular biology.** In general, the only exception to this rule involves retroviruses, whose genomes consist of single-stranded RNA molecules. During infection, RNA is converted to single-stranded DNA and then to double-stranded DNA by a process called **reverse transcription.** This process is commonly employed in experiments in which DNA probes are made from mRNA transcripts by using the **reverse transcriptase** enzyme.

DNA-Binding Proteins

The initiation of transcription, then, involves a Pol II recognition of a specific promoter-enhancer region near the start site for transcription of a gene, followed by the generation of mRNA. The exact specificity, that is, *which* gene to activate in a cell, is regulated by sequence-specific DNA-binding proteins that "direct traffic" (Levine and Manley, 1989; Ptashne, 1989; Peterson et al, 1990).

DNA-binding proteins, in general, exhibit a limited number of structural designs. These are termed *helix-turn-helix* proteins, *zinc finger* proteins, *leucine zipper* proteins, and *helix-loop-helix* proteins (Fig. 1–10).

1. The **helix-turn-helix** proteins all bind as dimers. They are found principally associated with homeotic genes that regulate spacial development and embryogenesis. Helix 3 (see Fig. 1–10*A*) is the "recognition sequence" that makes the major contacts with DNA. Helices 1 and 2 lie on top of helix 3 and are able to make contact with other proteins.

2. The **zinc finger** protein motif was discovered as part of the first well-characterized eukaryotic positive-acting regulatory protein, transcription factor IIIA (TFIIIA), which is

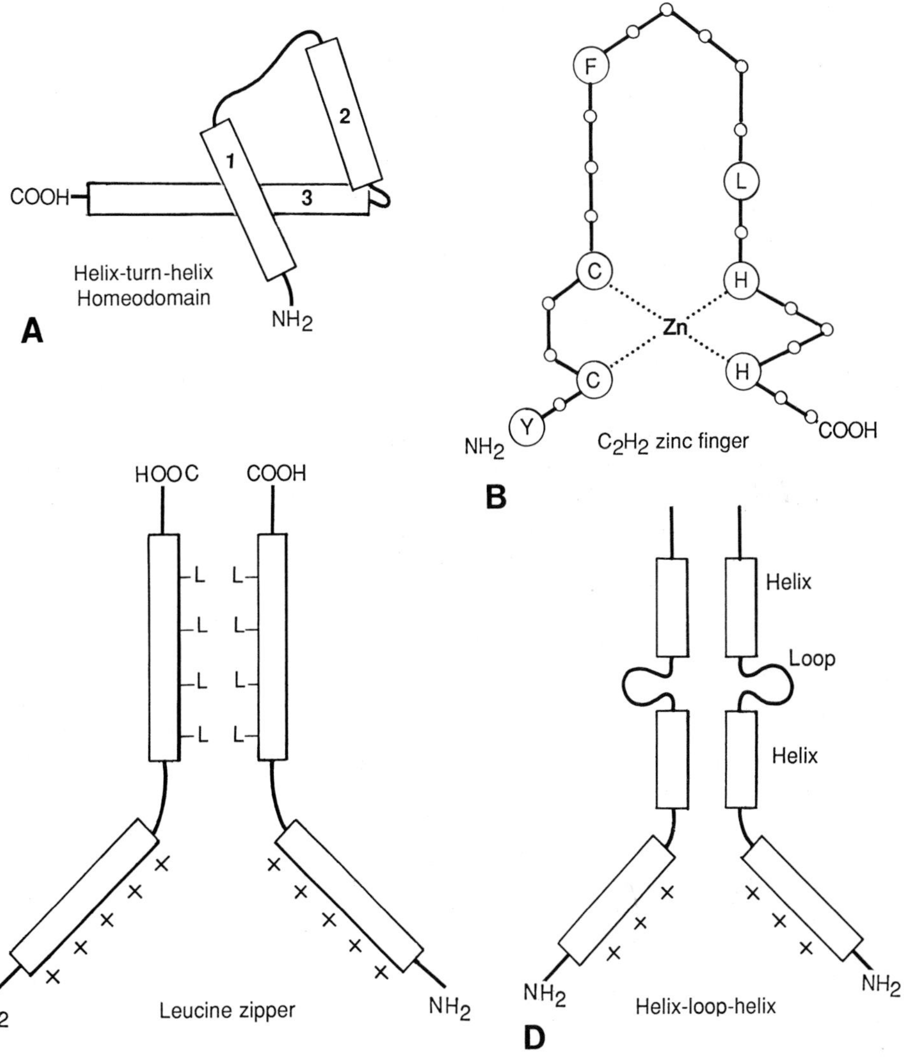

Figure 1–10. DNA binding motifs. *A,* **Helix-turn-helix** motif found in several prokaryotic regulatory proteins and the homeotic proteins of eukaryotes. Helix 3 is the "recognition helix" that contacts the DNA. *B,* **Zinc finger** motif. The helix (*right*) is believed to contact the major groove of the DNA molecule. *C,* The **leucine zipper** motif is formed as a dimer of two subunits. The amino terminal to the interdigitating leucines is a region rich in positively charged amino acids believed to contact DNA. *D,* **Helix-loop-helix** protein motif contains two helices linked by a loop of unknown structure that allows protein dimer formation.

required for RNA polymerase III transcription of the 5S RNA genes. The basic molecule consists of two cysteine residues (C) and two histidine residues (H) coordinated around a zinc molecule. In the structural model of this protein, the helix on the right (see Fig. 1–10*B*) is believed to contact the major groove of molecule (Rhodes and Klug, 1993).

3. The **leucine zipper** protein family act as dimers of two subunits (see Fig. 1–10*C*). At the carboxyl terminus of each subunit, there is a stretch of about 35 amino acids that contains four to five leucine residues, separated from each other by 6 amino acids (Vinson et al, 1989). The leucines are located on one side of the protein helix, and the leucines on two such helices interdigitate, leading to dimerization. The "zipper" is immediately preceded by a region rich in positively charged amino acids, and it is thought that the dimerization arranges the basic regions of the subunits in a configuration that allows specific interaction with a DNA recognition sequence. It is this type of bond that is responsible for joining different proteins as heterodimers that then bind DNA as regulators. An example includes the *fos-jun* proto-oncogene heterodimer, which together acts as a powerful regulatory complex (O'Shea et al, 1989). The finding that leucine zippers are responsible for specific heterodimer formation provides a conceptual framework for understanding combinatorial modes for gene regulation. In this case, dimerization, which is becoming a unifying property of sequence-specific DNA-binding proteins, physically allows DNA-binding proteins to bind to their targets at far more dilute concentrations than monomers. The complexity involved in achieving a highly specific pattern of gene activation required for growth and development of eukaryotic organisms is staggering; this specificity may be achieved, at least in part, by novel protein-protein interactions made possible by dimerization of regulatory proteins.

4. **Helix-loop-helix** proteins constitute the fourth transcription factor family. These proteins are similar to the leucine zipper family in that they bind DNA as dimers—either heterodimers or homodimers—and they have a positively charged domain that recognizes the DNA site. They also contain two helices linked by a loop of unknown structure (see Fig. 1–10*D*). This family includes several proteins with important roles in the control of cell growth and division. Among them is the protein encoded by the *c-myc* proto-oncogene.

A feature common to most of these proteins is that DNA binding and transcription activation reside within discrete domains and thus consist of independently functioning modules. Experimentally, the activation domain of one factor can be joined to the DNA-binding domain of the other, and the resulting hybrid is fully active in cells. However, as previously noted, the exact mechanism of action of transcription factors and how they interact with Pol II (and its associated transcription factors to make the transcription apparatus) is not exactly clear. It is thought that they can do one of three things: help RNA polymerase bind to the promoter, accelerate the rate at which bound RNA polymerase initiates transcription, or block transcription. It is important to remember that chromosomal DNA is tightly packed into higher order nucleoprotein structures; it is possible that transcription factors may act to free DNA from nucleosomes so that the promoter is accessible to the large transcription complex. In this process it is possible that transcription factors bind to enhancers (at distant sites) and to the transcription complex, which then efficiently "loops out" intervening DNA (see Fig. 1–9).

Mutations

If, during the process of DNA replication, a "mistake" is made and results in a change in the coding sequence of a gene, a **mutation** occurs. The occurrence of mutations is important not only because they are responsible for inherited diseases and other diseases such as cancer, but also because they are the source of phenotypic variation on which natural selection acts. The processes by which mutation produces variability and the fact that natural selection favors any resulting advantageous variants are the driving forces in evolution.

There is a wide variety of terminology to describe mutations. For example, **transition** refers to a base substitution by a base of the same class, such as a purine by a purine or a pyrimidine by a pyrimidine. Conversely, **transversion** refers to a base substitution by another class base, such as a purine by a pyrimidine. A **nonsense** mutation refers to a point mutation that converts a codon to a stop codon and therefore results in a premature termination of the polypeptide chain. Similarly, a **missense** mutation occurs when a mutation alters the codon so that an incorrect amino acid is produced. Often this has little effect on the function of the protein unless it is in a critical portion of the protein.

Finally, **deletions** and **insertions** usually have drastic effects on proteins because they alter the triplet groupings in which the bases are read.

RNA Editing

Thus far, regulation of gene expression has been discussed in the context of the transcriptional apparatus. An additional regulatory "compartment" that is post-transcriptional and figuratively termed *RNA editing* has been elucidated. To review, mRNAs are produced in the nucleus from the primary transcripts of protein coding genes, pre-mRNAs or heterogeneous nuclear RNAs (hnRNAs) by a series of processing reactions that typically include capping, pre-mRNA splicing, and polyadenylation.

The mRNAs are then transported to the cytoplasm (see Fig. 1–7), where the protein synthesis machinery is located and the translation and stability of mRNAs are subject to regulation. These processes are mediated by numerous RNA binding proteins and by small RNAs as stable ribonucleoprotein. It now appears that the 3′ untranslated region (UTR) of mRNAs plays a remarkably varied role in the control of gene expression. For example, control of translation of specific mRNAs has been shown to involve regulatory sequences located in their 3′ UTR. These regulatory sequences may also be involved in subcellular localization, its association with polysomes (and thereby its translation), and rate of decay. In general, the 3′ UTR elements can have either a positive or negative effect on the fate of mRNA (Jackson, 1993; St. Johnston, 1995).

Translation

In the process of translation, mRNA molecules serve as templates that order the amino acids within the polypeptide chain. *Translation* is an appropriate name because the nucleotide language of nucleic acids is translated into the amino acid language of proteins. In simplistic terms, the mRNA is read within the **ribosome**, a structure that is composed principally of RNA. Translation begins with a stepwise assembly of a functional ribosome into an mRNA. In brief, the 7-methyl guaninosine cap at the 5′ end of the mRNA is bound by a large complex of proteins, including the cap-binding proteins of eIF-4E and the RNA helicase eIF-4A. After binding the RNA, the small ribosomal subunit-initiation factor complex scans the 5′ UTR until it finds the AUG initiator codon in a favorable sequence context. Once an AUG is selected, the large ribosomal subunit joins the complex, and peptide synthesis begins (Hershey, 1991).

Each amino acid is attached to tRNA, which serves as a reading device through base pairing (see Fig. 1–7). Each tRNA recognizes and binds to a single one of the 20 different amino acids found in proteins (Fig. 1–11). At the opposite end of the tRNA molecule is a loop containing the anticodon, which is a nucleotide triplet that is complementary to a specific mRNA codon. The tRNA molecules carrying an amino acid are brought in contact with an mRNA molecule on the surface of a ribosome. As the ribosome moves along the mRNA one codon at a time, tRNAs with the appropriate anticodons are selectively bound to the mRNA, and the amino acids that they carry are linked to a growing polypeptide chain. The sequence of codons on the mRNA dictates the amino acid sequence. The process of translation is complex, involving perhaps 100 components, and is not yet completely understood. It is known, however, that both the concentration of active initiation factors and the primary sequence of the 5′ UTR can affect the rate of translation. Ribosome binding is most sensitive to secondary structure near the cap, but stable loop structures anywhere in the 5′ UTR can block ribosome scanning. The sequence of the 5′ UTR thus establishes the intrinsic rate of initiation (of translation) of mRNA (Fig. 1–12) (Kozak, 1989; Hess and Duncan, 1994).

Other, less defined mechanisms controlling translational initiation exist. For example, 3′ UTR sequences can repress or activate translation by modulating the length of the poly (A) tail, which in turn regulates the rate of translational initiation of an mRNA.

Factors that bind such sequences may interact with the cap-binding complex or the small ribosomal subunit. Finally, as previously mentioned, sequences in the 3′ UTR can direct mRNAs to specific regions of the cell from which repressor proteins are excluded, thereby activating their translation (Manley, 1995).

The Tools of Molecular Genetics

Southern and Northern Blotting; Restriction Enzymes

Two of the most commonly used methods in a molecular biology laboratory are Southern and Northern blotting, de-

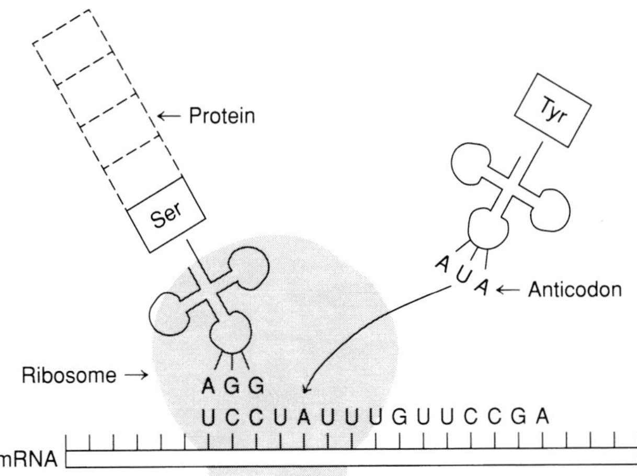

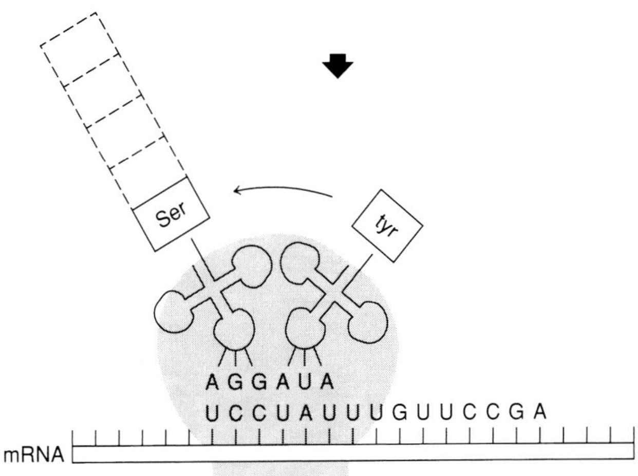

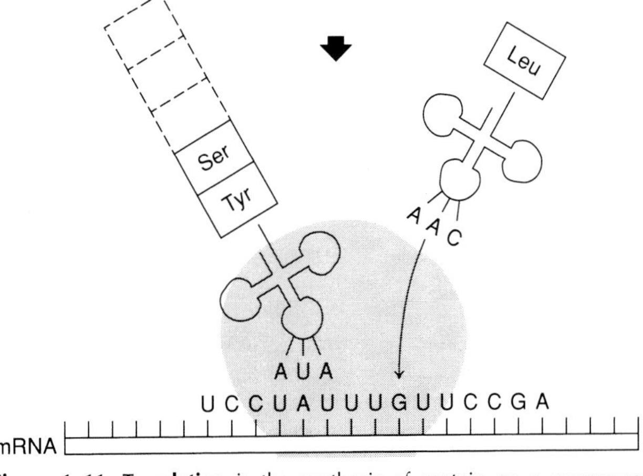

Figure 1–11. Translation is the synthesis of protein on a messenger RNA (mRNA) template. Each nucleotide triplet, or **codon**, on the mRNA chain encodes a specific amino acid. Each molecule of transfer RNA (tRNA), in turn, binds only the amino acid corresponding to a particular codon. A tRNA molecule recognizes a codon by means of a complementary nucleotide sequence called an **anticodon**. The addition of one amino acid to a protein chain is shown here. An incoming tRNA molecule carrying the amino acid tyrosine binds to the codon exposed at a binding site on a ribosome. The tyrosine forms a peptide bond with the serine, the last amino acid on the peptide chain. As the ribosome advances one codon, exposing the binding site to the next incoming tRNA, the serine tRNA is released.

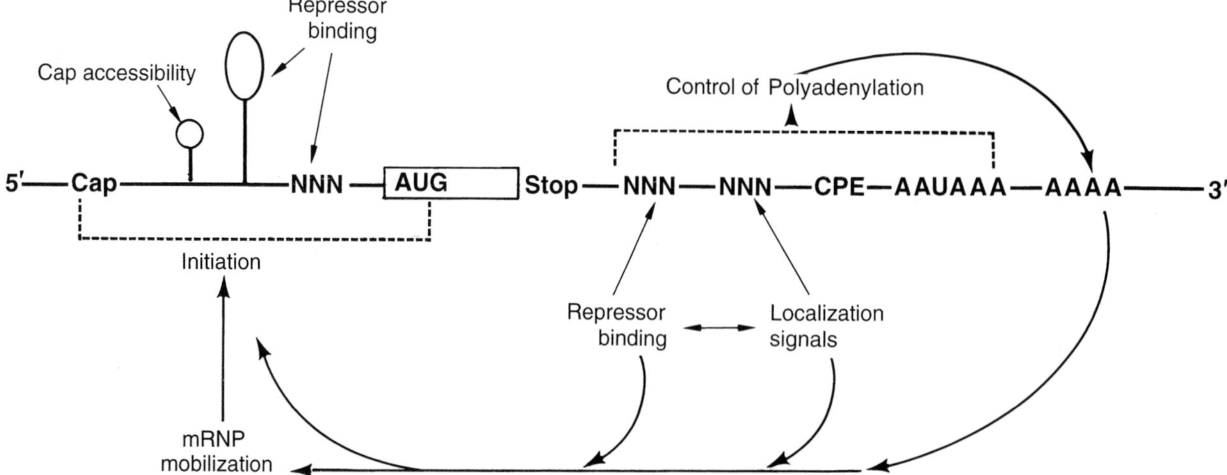

Figure 1–12. The primary factors regulating translational initiation are diagrammed with reference to their sites of action on an mRNA molecule. Brackets indicate that a number of independently acting processes might coordinately regulate a single output, such as cytoplasmic polyadenylation or ribosome binding. (From Curtis D, Lehman K, Zamore P: Cell 1995; 81:171–178.)

veloped by E.M. Southern of the University of Edinburgh (Southern, 1975). The procedures are used to determine the presence of specific base pair sequences in samples of DNA (Southern blotting) or RNA (Northern blotting), as defined by a probe that contains sequences complementary to those that are sought (Fig. 1–13; see Table 1–1 for a review of terms.)

The ability of the DNA double helix to separate and reform during replication, for example, without disrupting covalent bonds (only hydrogen bonds are disrupted; see Fig. 1–3), is an important physical property called **denaturation** (see Table 1–1). In Southern blotting, as described later, DNA strands are separated and then join complementary sequences on the probe. The double strand is broken simply by disrupting the noncovalent forces that stabilize the double helix through the use of heat, exposure to high salt, or high pH. As expected, **renaturation** is the ability of the two separate complementary strands to be reformed into a double helix. It would therefore be expected that the success of an artificially made segment of single-stranded DNA (the probe) to undergo renaturation to a piece of single-stranded genomic DNA (DNA from the native genome) would depend on how well matched the complementary sequences are between the genomic DNA (in Southern blotting) or RNA (in Northern blotting) and the probe.

The renaturation process (probe annealing to genomic DNA strands [Southern] or RNA strands [Northern]) occurs in two stages. First, DNA single strands in solution encounter one another by chance. If the sequences are complementary, the two strands form base pairs to generate a short double-helical region. Then additional base pairing occurs along the molecule by a zipper-like effect through hydrogen bonding (the "Velcro effect") to form a long double-helix molecule. **The renaturation of the DNA helix forms the basis for one of the most important phenomena in DNA technology, known as hybridization. *Hybridization* refers to the tendency of any two complementary single-stranded nucleic acid sequences, whether from DNA or RNA, to anneal with each other to form a duplex structure. In other words, the ability of two nucleic acid preparations to hybridize constitutes a precise test for their complementary sequences.** Molecular biologic investigations are able to exploit this property of DNA in studies designed to locate particular regions of DNA within the human genome.

The strength of interaction between the strands of nucleic acid and the probe is important to understand and is dependent on numerous factors such as temperature, ionic strength of the reaction, molar percentage of G-C base pairs in the probe, probe length, percentage of noncomplementary bases between the probe and the target (percent mismatch), and percentage of formamide (a duplex-destabilizing agent) in the solution. Increasing the ionic strength, probe length, and G-C content increases duplex stability. Increasing temperature, percentage of formamide, and percentage of mismatch decreases duplex stability. The **stringency** of a hybridization reaction refers to the degree to which the reaction conditions favor duplex dissociation; high stringency conditions include high temperature, as well as low salt or high formamide concentrations. Duplexes formed when the two strands have a high degree of base homology withstand a higher stringency wash than do duplexes of a lesser homology. Although seemingly "technical," these factors can play a major role in data analysis, leading to erroneous conclusions to important experiments.

Restriction enzymes are an important tool and are used in almost every experiment of molecular genetics. These are extremely important enzymes, isolated from bacteria, that cut DNA at specific sequences, usually specified by either four- or six-base sequences (Table 1–2). Enzymes that bind to only four bases cut many more times in a given DNA molecule than the ones that have to recognize a specific group of six. A six-base restriction sequence may not exist even once in a given viral DNA molecule. For example, the GAATTC recognition sequence from the *Escherichia coli* *Eco*RI enzyme is not present in phage T7 DNA, which is 40,000 base pairs long! Currently, over 250 restriction endonucleases, with more than 100 different cut sites, are known.

In order to analyze and identify the fragments that result

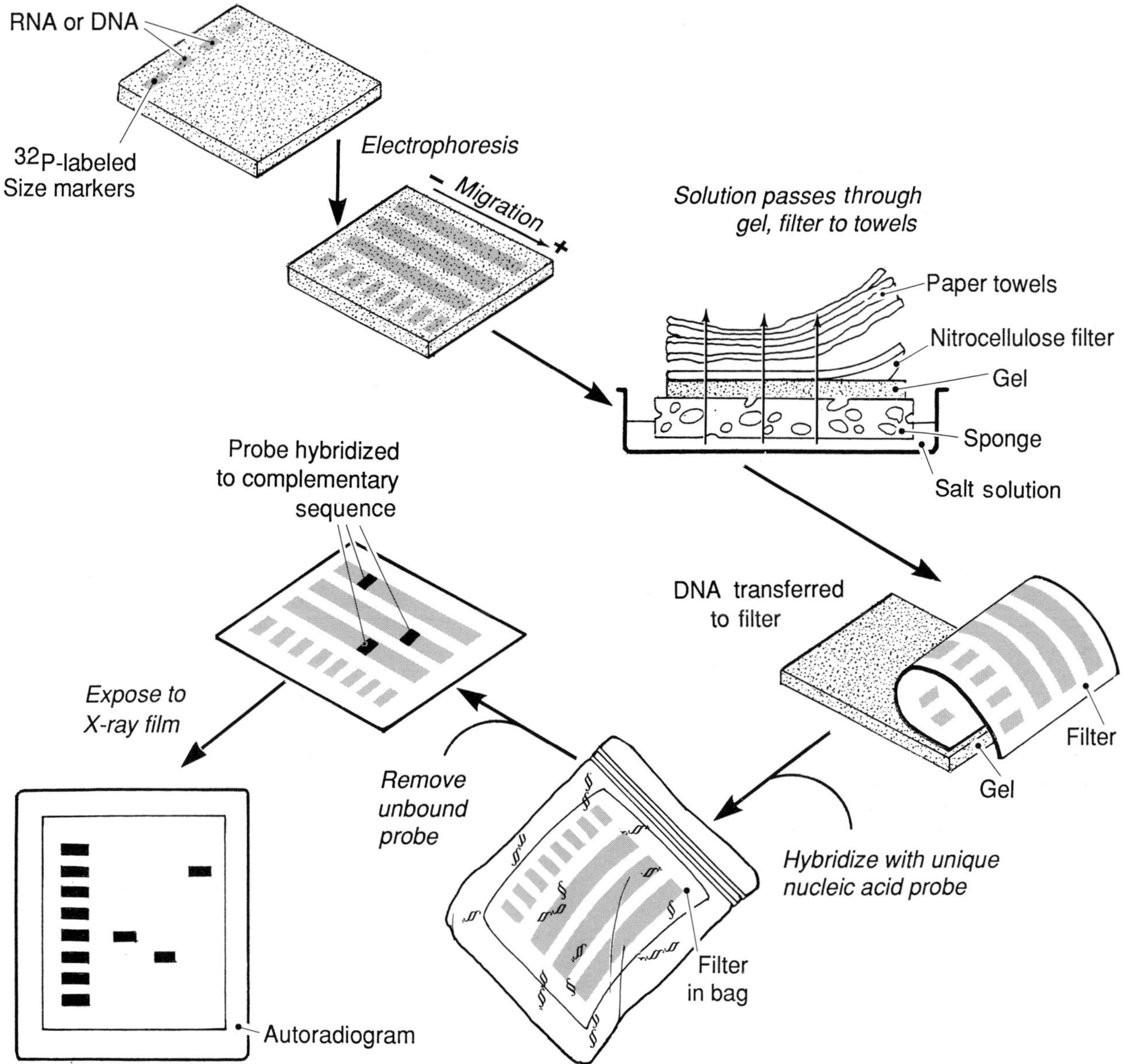

Figure 1–13. Southern and Northern blotting. DNA cleaved with restriction enzymes (or RNA isolated from cells) is applied to an agarose gel and electrophoretically separated by size. The single-stranded nucleic acids in the gel are then transferred to a nitrocellulose filter to make a precise replica of the gel. When transferring DNA, the nitrocellulose acts to "fix" the single strands of DNA in such a way that they will not reanneal, thereby making them accessible to probes. The transfer is usually done by placing the gel atop a sponge sitting in a tray of buffer. The nitrocellulose filter is laid over the gel and covered with a stack of paper towels that act as a wick, pulling buffer up through the sponge, gel, and filter. DNA (or RNA) fragments from the gel are carried up onto the filter, where they are fixed by heating. The filter is then hybridized with a radiolabeled probe. Hybridization thereby specifically tags the sequence of interest, even though it may constitute a very minute fraction of nucleic acid on the filter. Unbound probe is washed off, and the filter exposed to x-rays; the position of the DNA fragment (or RNA fragment) that is complementary to the probe appears as a band on the film. The procedure is termed **Southern blotting** when DNA is transferred to nitrocellulose, **Northern blotting** when RNA is transferred, and Western blotting when protein is transferred from an SDS-polyacrylamide gel. In **Western blotting**, the protein of interest is identified by using an antibody that specifically recognizes it.

from digestion of genomic DNA with restriction enzymes, the resultant fragments must be separated from one another. This is easily accomplished by using agarose gel electrophoresis (see Fig. 1–13), which is the first step in performing a Southern blot. The mixture of DNA fragments after digestion with a designated restriction endonuclease is loaded at one end of a horizontally placed agarose gel that is submerged within an electrophoresis tank; an electric current is then passed through the gel (see Fig. 1–13). The fragments move through the gel at a rate proportional to their length: The smaller fragments move quickly and the larger fragments move slowly. Staining the gels with dyes that bind to DNA generates a series of bands, each corresponding to a restriction fragment (or a cut piece of DNA) whose base pair length can be estimated by calibrating the gel, using DNA molecules with known base pair lengths. It therefore follows that different restriction enzymes display different "restriction patterns" or series of bands for the same digested molecule.

A **Southern blot** is performed to determine the presence

Table 1–2. SOME RESTRICTION ENZYMES AND THEIR CLEAVAGE SEQUENCES

Microorganism	Enzyme	Abbreviation Sequence
Thermus aquaticus	*TaqI*	5′ . . . T | C G A . . . 3′ 3′ . . . A G C | T . . . 5′
Haemophilus haemolyticus	*HbaI*	5′ . . . G C G | C . . . 3′ 3′ . . . C | G C G . . . 5′
*Moraxella bovis**	*MboII*	5′ . . . G A A G A $(N)_8$ | . . . 3′ 3′ . . . C T T C T $(N)_7$ | . . . 5′
Escherichia coli†	*Eco*RV	5′ . . . G A T | A T C . . . 3′ 3′ . . . C T A | T A G . . . 5′
	*Eco*RI	5′ . . . G | A A T T C . . . 3′ 3′ . . . C T T A A | G . . . 5′
Providencia stuarti	*Pst*I	5′ . . . C T G C A | G . . . 3′ 3′ . . . G | A C G T C . . . 5′
Microcoleus‡	*Mst*II	5′ . . . C C | T N A G G . . . 3′ 3′ . . . G G A N T | C C . . . 5′
Nocardia otitidis-caviarum§	*Not*I	5′ . . . G C | G G C C G C . . . 3′ 3′ . . . C G C C G | G C G . . . 5′

*The enzyme cuts, not within the recognition sequence, but at whatever sequence lies eight nucleotides 3′ to the recognition site.
†Enzyme produces blunt ends.
‡The base pair *N* can be any purine or pyrimidine pair.
§*Not*I has an eight-base recognition sequence and cuts mammalian DNA very infrequently.

of a genomic nucleotide sequence or an alteration of a sequence within DNA that has been digested. To actually perform a Southern blot, genomic DNA is cut with one or several restriction enzymes, and the resultant fragments are separated by size on an agarose gel (see Fig. 1–13). Because double-stranded DNA does not undergo hybridization, the DNA, while still in the agarose gel, is denatured by alkaline treatment to yield single-stranded fragments.

The gel is then overlaid with a sheet of nylon or nitrocellulose filter, and a flow of buffer is drawn up through the gel toward the nitrocellulose filter. This causes the DNA fragments to be carried out of the gel onto the filter, where they bind. This is necessary not only to form a replica of the DNA that was on the gel but also to provide a "scaffolding" to permanently hold apart the complementary DNA strands, which, if in a solution (other than alkaline), would tend to renature. It is important that the two strands remain apart so that a labeled probe specific for the gene (or nucleotide sequence) that is being sought can be hybridized to the single-stranded DNA on the nitrocellulose paper (or nylon membrane). The probe can be a purified RNA, a cloned DNA that has been made single-stranded, or a short synthetic oligonucleotide. The labeled probe hybridizes to the specific molecules containing a complementary sequence; thus each complementary sequence gives rise to a labeled band at a position determined by the size of the DNA fragment.

This technique can also be performed with RNA immobilized on the nitrocellulose paper—for example, to determine whether a certain mRNA is being produced by a specific cell type. In this case, the RNA is mixed with formaldehyde or a similar agent to prevent hydrogen bonding between base pairs and to ensure that RNA is in unfolded linear form. In accordance with laboratory jargon, the procedure is then known as **Northern blotting.** (When proteins are fixed to nitrocellulose and probed with antibodies, the procedure is called **Western blotting.**) These procedures form some of the backbone of molecular genetics.

Genetic Polymorphisms

The identification of genetic polymorphisms is another important tool of molecular genetics. Polymorphisms represent normal variance or normally occurring slight changes in DNA structure (base pair change) (Botstein et al, 1980; Gusella, 1986; Housman, 1995). Examination of DNA from any two persons will reveal variations in the DNA sequences involving approximately one nucleotide in every 200 to 500 base pairs. These polymorphic sequences occur more frequently in DNA than in proteins, and most produce no observable effect. Some of these DNA sequence changes are detectable by the digestion of DNA with restriction endonucleases, which, as previously mentioned, cleave DNA whenever a specific sequence (defined by the nuclease used) occurs (Fig. 1–14). For example, a **restriction endonuclease** will cut DNA at a particular site on one chromosome and may not cut the DNA at the same site on another chromosome, if there is a difference between the two chromosomes in the nucleotide sequence. This difference in cleavage is reflected as a difference in size of the DNA fragments on a gel. This is of great importance because the two homologous chromosomes can be marked: One has a restriction site (or a cleavage site) and the other does not.

If a DNA polymorphism is located next to a disease gene, it may serve as a "disease marker" in genetic studies of families with certain diseases. The DNA polymorphism is not a mutation that causes the disorder, but it merely marks the abnormal gene on the two different chromosomes. An example is given in Figure 1–14; in this case, one chromosome has an "extra" recognition site that represents a polymorphism. If the DNA from that individual is digested with the appropriate restriction enzyme and then hybridized with the indicated probe, a heterozygous pattern (I,II) will appear with three bands. However, if the restriction sites on both chromosomes are the same, a homozygous or uniform pattern will appear on the Southern gel: I,I or II,II. Because DNA polymorphisms are abundant, several polymorphisms are usually found either within the gene or very close to it when a gene that is responsible for a disease is cloned and characterized. These polymorphisms can thus be used as markers for the defective gene in the disorder. This method is also important in identifying gene loss in cancer cells. For example, if normal DNA (from an individual with cancer) is heterozygous at a given locus, whereas the DNA from the tumor itself, analyzed with the same probe, is missing the bands from one of the chromosomes, tumor-associated DNA loss can be inferred (which may be associated with loss of a "suppressor gene").

In contrast to single-base-pair polymorphisms, which are somewhat cumbersome to use in genetic studies, another kind of polymorphism takes the form of tandem repeats of short oligonucleotide sequences (i.e., two to four base pairs of repeating sequences). These happen to be scattered throughout the genome, and the reason for their existence is not exactly clear, but it appears as though the length (or number of repetitive units) is highly variable within the population. In fact, these segments are called variable number of tandem repeats (VNTR). When these were first described, they were isolated from centrifuged specimens of DNA, whereby gradient collections would pool these small repetitive elements together into what was called "minisatellite" aggregations, hence the current-day terms *hypervariable* or *minisatellite DNA* (Wyman and White, 1980; Jeffreys et al, 1985; Nakamura et al, 1987). In each case the variable region consists of tandem repeats of short sequence of dinucleotides, and polymorphisms result from allelic differences in the number of repeats, which presumably arise from mitotic or meiotic unequal exchanges or by DNA "slippage" during replication. The resulting minisatellite length variation can be detected by using any restriction endonuclease that does not cleave the repeat unit. Of importance is that the frequency of this kind of replication error is high enough to make alternative lengths at the polymorphic site common, but the rate of change in the length of the site is low enough that the size of the DNA at the polymorphic site serves as a stable trait in family studies (Fig. 1–15).

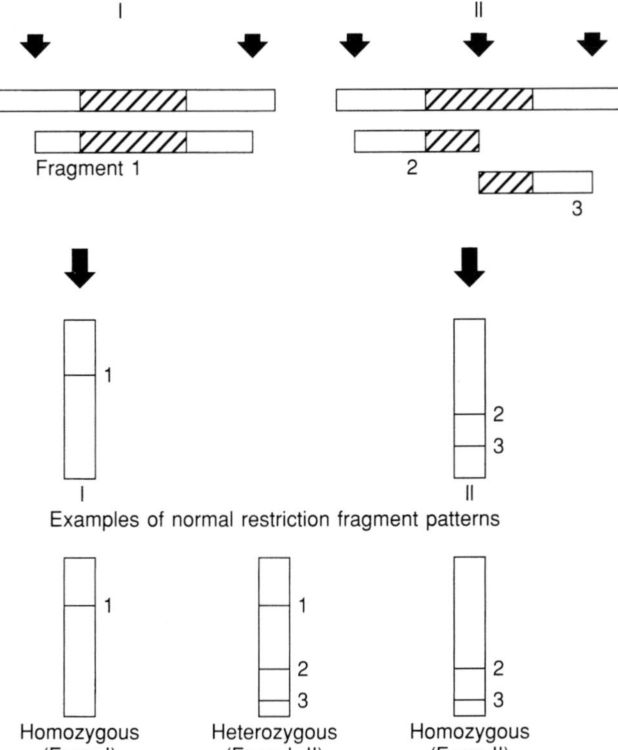

Figure 1–14. Genetic polymorphisms and their recognition by Southern blot analysis; the top row of arrows indicate endonuclease "cut sites"; cross-hatched areas represent the probe recognition sequence. In this case, the polymorphism is represented by the altered cut site (middle arrow) in genotype II that is not present in genotype I, and two genetic forms (I, II) exist normally in the somatic DNA, each producing its own characteristic fragments when cut. After cleavage, three genotypes may exit: I,I; II; and II,II.

Hypervariable regions has come under intense study because it appears as though the genetic machinery that is used to correct natural defects in replication (which understandably tend to occur during replication in these confusing regions of repeats) is the same machinery that, when defective, results in a high incidence of certain cancers. Such replication error–prone individuals are said to have a "mutator phenotype" that is manifested by, among other things, changes in hypervariable regions, noted when their tumors are compared to somatic tissues. The exact mechanisms of malignant transformation are not exactly clear. The term *restriction fragment length polymorphism* has been coined to describe the variation in fragment length generated through either of the aforementioned mechanisms.

DNA Fingerprinting

One of the offshoots of our understanding of polymorphisms is their potential usefulness in forensic analysis. This type of analysis has become increasingly popular in comparison with other protein-based methods designed to detect genetic identity (such as ABO blood groups) because the significance of matches between specimens is greater and the physical stability of DNA (as noted earlier in this chapter) makes it possible to analyze minute amounts of forensic material many years after a criminal incident.

DNA fingerprinting is aimed at identifying polymorphic sites within human DNA, usually VNTR sites. In the forensic laboratory, DNA can be extracted from specimens such as semen from a vaginal swab, blood stains from clothing, or even skin lodged under a victim's fingernails during a struggle with an attacker. The DNA isolated from the forensic specimen is then compared with that derived from the blood of the defendant. The correspondence in position between the VNTR bands from the two samples is the key to identification in DNA fingerprinting. For an apparent match based on conventional analysis of blood type and isotypes of serum enzymes, there is a chance of 1 in 100 to 1 in 1000 that the genetic match between samples may in fact be

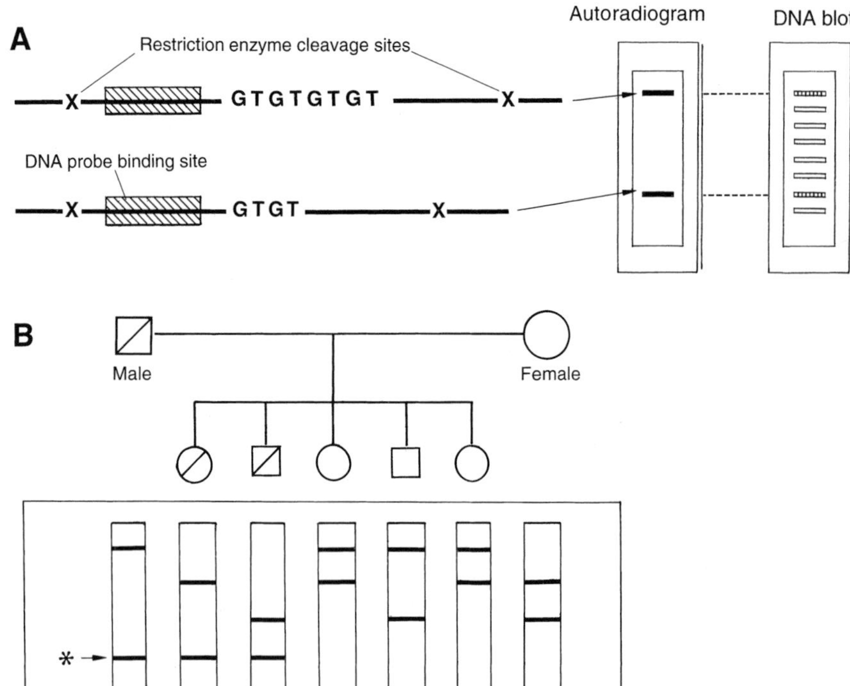

Figure 1–15. *A,* Conceptual drawing of an identical area from each of two homologous chromosomes, showing one of the sections of DNA where variable numbers of tandem repeats (VNTRs) occur: in this, a dinucleotide repeat of GT. A probe that recognizes this "area" is indicated in cross-hatch. In one chromosome, the dinucleotide repeat has two "GTs," and in the other, there are four "GTs"; the difference between the two is easily recognized by Southern blot (*right*), the larger fragment being the upper, slower migrating band and the smaller fragment, the lower, faster migrating band. *B,* This polymorphic marker can be used in family genetic analysis. The origin of each of the two alleles from a given locus in each offspring can be traced back to the father or mother, making the inheritance pattern clear for each parent from this chromosomal site. If the father and the offspring that are marked by cross-hatch have a congenital disease, there is a reasonable likelihood that the disease gene is located somewhere near the polymorphic site marked by the VNTR (*).

due to coincidence. Analogous estimates that an RFLP match is due to coincidence range from 1 in 100,000 to 1 in 1,000,000 (Lander and Budowle, 1994).

Genetic Engineering-Cloning

***DNA cloning* traditionally refers to a process whereby a fragment of DNA is reproduced essentially with unlimited quantities by using the "growth machinery" of either a bacterium or a virus.** Therefore, in theory what is done is fairly simple: A piece of DNA that is to be amplified is obtained either by laboratory synthesis, in which mRNA is reverse-transcribed into a DNA copy (or cDNA), or by digesting nuclear DNA with restriction endonucleases. The selected piece of DNA is then replicated in a foreign cell by putting the DNA into certain genetic carriers (e.g., plasmids or viruses), which nature has endowed with the ability to move from one place within the genome to another or from one to another (see Table 1–1; Fig. 1–16). In a sense, these factors can carry "hitchhiking" genes. A number of techniques are available for introducing the new DNA into recipient cells; collectively, the process is called **transfection.** DNA can be microinjected, helped across the plasma membrane by certain chemical treatments such as calcium chloride, enclosed within small membranous sacs or artificial phospholipid vesicles (liposomes) that fuse to the plasma membrane, or brought into the cell by electrical current. When applicable, the method of choice is to attach the DNA to the DNA of a vector, usually a **plasmid,** which is a self-replicating circular extrachromosomal DNA molecule, or some viral particle that happens to be naturally endowed with the appropriate means for introducing its DNA content into selected cells. This technique has the additional advantage that the vectors used often carry genetic markers, such as resistance to certain antibiotics, that allow recognition and isolation of the transferred cells very easily (see Fig. 1–16) (see the next section, on selectable markers).

The tools for attaching the DNA to its vector are all borrowed from nature. They include restriction enzymes for cutting the DNAs at specific sites; nonspecific terminal deoxynucleotidyltransferases for fitting the vector and its passenger with sticky ends (poly-dG on one and poly-dC on the other); DNA polymerase to fill in the gaps; and DNA ligase to do the final stitching. The passenger DNA may be a simple piece of native DNA, a more complex mixture of such pieces, or the contents of a complete genome fragmented by a restriction enzyme. Bacteria are the obvious recipients for all cloning and manufacturing elements, in view of their rapid generation rate, ease of culture and selection, and large number of possible vectors. Interestingly, some of the initial objections to genetic engineering arose largely from the fear that some bacteria, unwittingly transformed into highly pathogenic species, might escape into the environment. This risk appeared particularly hazardous because the most widely used bacterium is *E. coli,* which is, of course, a natural inhabitant of the human digestive tract. These fears, however, have not been borne out, and no serious accidents have occurred.

Selectable Markers

An important technical requirement for experimental transfection is that a system must be used to identify or isolate cells that have been successfully transfected, because only a small minority of cells undergoing this experimental manipulation actually achieve a stable transfected state. To meet this goal, **selectable markers** have been developed. In bacteria these are commonly drug resistance genes. In other words, a drug resistance gene (e.g., neomycin resistance) is tagged onto the transfected gene of interest, so that after

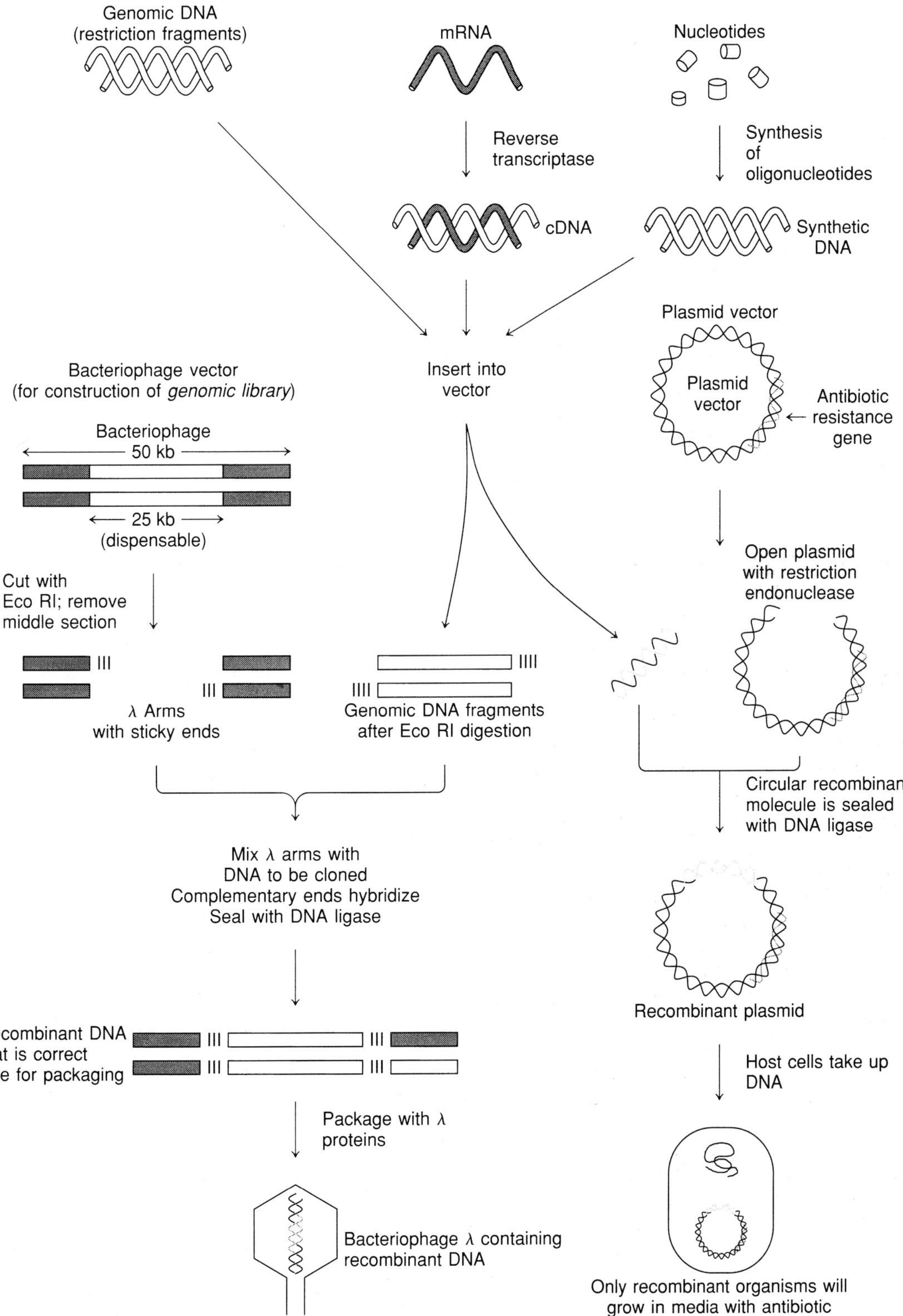

Figure 1–16. DNA recombinant technique: cloning. The passenger DNA to be cloned may consist of fragments cut from the whole genome by means of restriction endonucleases; of complementary DNA (cDNA) transcribed from purified messenger RNA (mRNA) by means of reverse transcriptase; or of completely synthesized DNA. Fragments can be inserted into bacteriophage gamma or into plasmids.

transfection, by whatever technique, the resultant bacterial population that did not take up the transfected gene construct will be killed by the neomycin, leaving only cells that are stably transfected (see Fig. 1–16). Other genes besides neomycin resistance have been used. For example, the thymidine kinase gene allows selective growth of cells transfected with this gene (along with the experimental gene of interest) when the transfected cells are grown in selective hypoxanthine, aminopterine, and thymidine (HAT) medium. Thymidine kinase is an enzyme that catalyzes a step in the synthesis of thymidine triphosphate, one of the four precursor nucleotides for DNA synthesis. Mammalian cells use two distinct routes of synthesizing DNA triphosphates for DNA synthesis: They can make them from scratch, or they can salvage free purine and pyrimidine bases. Aminopterine blocks two steps in the biosynthesis of purines and one in the biosynthesis of thymidine. If cells are provided with hypoxanthine and thymidine, they can survive aminopterine treatment by using the salvage pathways with thymidine kinase. This selection can also be used for the gene that encodes the key salvage enzyme hypoxanthine phosphoribosyltransferase (HPRT) for purines.

Polymerase Chain Reaction

The polymerase chain reaction (PCR) is a rapid procedure for in vitro enzymatic amplification of a specific segment of DNA (Mullis, 1990). Like molecular cloning, PCR has spawned a multitude of experiments that were previously impossible to perform. The importance of the procedure lies in its ability to amplify unpure DNA, either fragmented or intact, by simple chemical, rather than biologic, proliferation of a stretch of DNA. It is possible to amplify DNA sequences from as short as 50 base pairs to over 200 base pairs in length and more than one million–fold in only a few hours. Moreover, the ability to propagate specific DNA (for subsequent analysis) from amounts too minute for standard amplification (i.e., cloning) gives the method such extraordinary power and sensitivity that the DNA from fixed pathologic specimens, from buccal cells in mouthwashes, from human hairs, from a single lymphoid or sperm cell, or from ancient mummies can now be amplified.

The theoretical basis for the PCR is described in three steps and is illustrated in Figure 1–17. The first step of the cycle is the heat denaturation of the native double-stranded DNA, which breaks the hydrogen bonds holding the two strands, thus liberating single strands of DNA (which can hybridize to other DNA with complementary sequences). In the second step, two short DNA primers are annealed to complementary sequences on opposite strands of the target DNA. These primers are chosen to encompass the desired DNA. They define the two ends of the stretch of DNA to be amplified. The final step is the actual synthesis of a complementary second strand of DNA. The primers are designed and annealed in such a way that their 3′ ends are facing each other, so that synthesis by DNA polymerase (which catalyzes growth of new strands in a 5′-to-3′ direction) extends across the segment of DNA between them. A new single strand of DNA is synthesized for each annealed primer. Each new strand consists of the primer and its 5′ end, trailed by a string of linked nucleotides complementary to those of the corresponding template.

An essential feature of PCR is that all previously synthesized products act as template for new primer-extension reactions (i.e., DNA synthesis) in each ensuing cycle. **The result of this aptly named "chain reaction" is the geometric amplification of new DNA products.** Because the primers form the "kernels" of all new DNA strands, each of the two different primers, as well as the four deoxyribonucleoside triphosphates (the building blocks of the DNA molecule), must initially be present in massive amounts, in relation to the quantity of the target (substrate) DNA. The

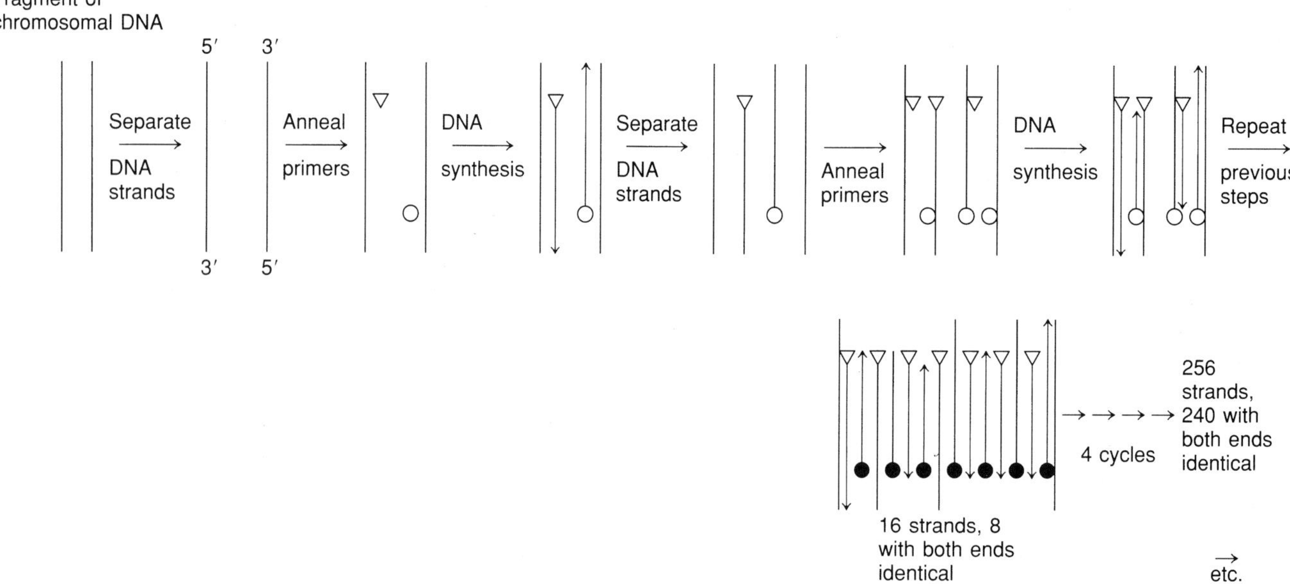

Figure 1–17. The polymerase chain reaction for amplifying specific DNA sequences in vitro. DNA that is isolated from cells is heated to separate its complementary strands. These strands are then annealed with oligonucleotide primers, which "outline" the region to be amplified, generally 50 to 2000 base pairs in length. DNA synthesis is then catalyzed by DNA polymerase, which copies the DNA between the sequences corresponding to the two oligonucleotides. After multiple cycles, a large amount of single-stranded DNA fragments of a specified length is formed.

exquisite **specificity** of the annealing reaction (second step) and the **geometric amplification** of the PCR products (third step) together give the method its extraordinary sensitivity. Each cycle of replication is temperature-controlled; that is, the temperature is raised so that all double-stranded DNAs are converted to single-stranded DNAs (thus aborting any ongoing polymerization); the temperature is then lowered to allow the steps of annealing and extension. Typically, 30 full cycles are completed.

The PCR has the ability to synthesize defined fragments of DNA in unlimited amounts and shares this property with standard gene cloning. The advantage of gene cloning is that it does not require the synthesis of primers that are needed by the PCR, and it therefore remains the method of choice for many experiments, particularly those in which the sequence of the target DNA is unknown. However, PCR surpasses standard cloning in its simplicity, speed, and ability to amplify vanishingly small amounts of impure starting material.

With an understanding of the principles of PCR, it can be seen that this method is potentially useful in any situation that requires examination of DNA. In its most commonly applied form, the PCR is best suited to help answer the often raised question "Does a given sequence of DNA exist in a given clinical specimen?" This approach has numerous clinical applications and in many cases can provide answers that oftentimes can be difficult or impossible to obtain. For example, the PCR is useful in determining the sex of human embryos associated with in vitro fertilization, the prenatal diagnosis of genetic disorders, and the detection of human immunodeficiency virus (HIV) in people whose sera cannot be determined to be HIV-positive by conventional means, such as infants born to HIV-infected mothers and seronegative people at high risk for acquired immunodeficiency syndrome (AIDS).

DNA Sequencing

As described earlier, restriction endonucleases are bacterial enzymes that recognize specific short oligonucleotide sequences four to eight residues long in DNA and then cleave the DNA at each recognition site. The word *restriction* refers to the function of these enzymes in the bacteria of origin: A restriction endonuclease destroys (restricts) incoming foreign DNA by cleaving it at the specific sites (which are not found in the bacteria of origin).

The discovery of restriction endonucleases was an important step that led to general methods for determining the exact nucleotide sequences of long segments of DNA. Two highly successful procedures for DNA sequencing are now in widespread use (Figs. 1–18 and 1–19); both share the same basic principle: A series of DNA molecules (radiolabeled single-stranded or double-stranded but labeled only on one strand) are generated in which each molecule is one base pair longer than the previous one. These molecules, which differ by one base pair, can be separated by careful polyacrylamide gel electrophoresis for molecules up to 500 base pairs long.

To determine the sequence of the DNA molecule, the DNA sample is separated into four tubes, one for each of the four bases that make up DNA. The reaction products undergo electrophoresis in four parallel slots of the same gel, which is then autoradiographed. The radioactive band corresponding to a particular length appears in one of the four slots. The slot position of the band identifies the nucleotide that is present at the corresponding position in the DNA. Thus the DNA sequence is "read" by proceeding from one band to the next, according to the slots in which the bands appear.

One method of DNA sequencing, invented by Maxam and Gilbert (1977), chemically cleaves an end-labeled DNA sample (see Fig. 1–18). The second method, developed by Sanger and colleagues (1977), uses enzymatic synthesis to extend a short sequence of end-labeled DNA (see Fig. 1–19) (for a review, see Rosenthal, 1995).

The DNA Library

A DNA library is a representation of an organism's entire genome. Basically, a total unfractionated set of DNA fragments is converted into a set of stable recombinants that can be stored and used repeatedly.

The DNA is cloned into plasmids or bacteriophages (viruses), which are vectors that are easy to deal with in large numbers and can be stored. Three kinds of libraries are important. One, as mentioned, is constructed from total genomic DNA, and in principle contains all the organism's genes and other DNA sequences. However, this ideal is usually not attained because some of the DNA sequences escape cloning. A second type of library is one representing all the DNA in one particular chromosome. Making such a library requires first fractionating chromosomes by techniques similar to those used in fluorescence activated cell sorting. A third type of library contains sequences representing all the mRNAs found in a particular cell type. In this case, the total mRNA population is converted to cDNAs, which are then cloned. **Genomic libraries** are a source of genes and DNA sequences; **cDNA libraries** represent the expression of those genes in the form of mRNA.

To be useful, a DNA library must be as complete as possible. A library of 300,000 clones in which each clone contained 20,000 base pairs of DNA would contain all the sequences in the human genome. In practice, however, human genomic libraries contain several times that number in order to ensure the representation of all DNA sequences at least once.

To start a library, it is necessary to make recombinant DNA by cleaving the genomic DNA and the vector DNA with the same restriction enzyme and then joining their cut ends with a ligase enzyme. The next step is to introduce the recombinant DNA molecules into a culture of host cells. If the cloning vector contains a gene for resistance to a drug, such as neomycin, the addition of that drug to the culture kills any host cell that has failed to take up the vector (Fig. 1–20).

One of the common uses of a library occurs after the investigator has isolated a small genomic sequence that either is next to the (unknown) gene of interest or is actually part of the gene of interest, and it then becomes necessary to isolate the gene (which has heretofore not been isolated or sequenced). The known isolated genomic sequence previously identified by the investigator must be mixed with all the gene sequences from the library in the hope that it will hybridize to at least one sequence, which will be consider-

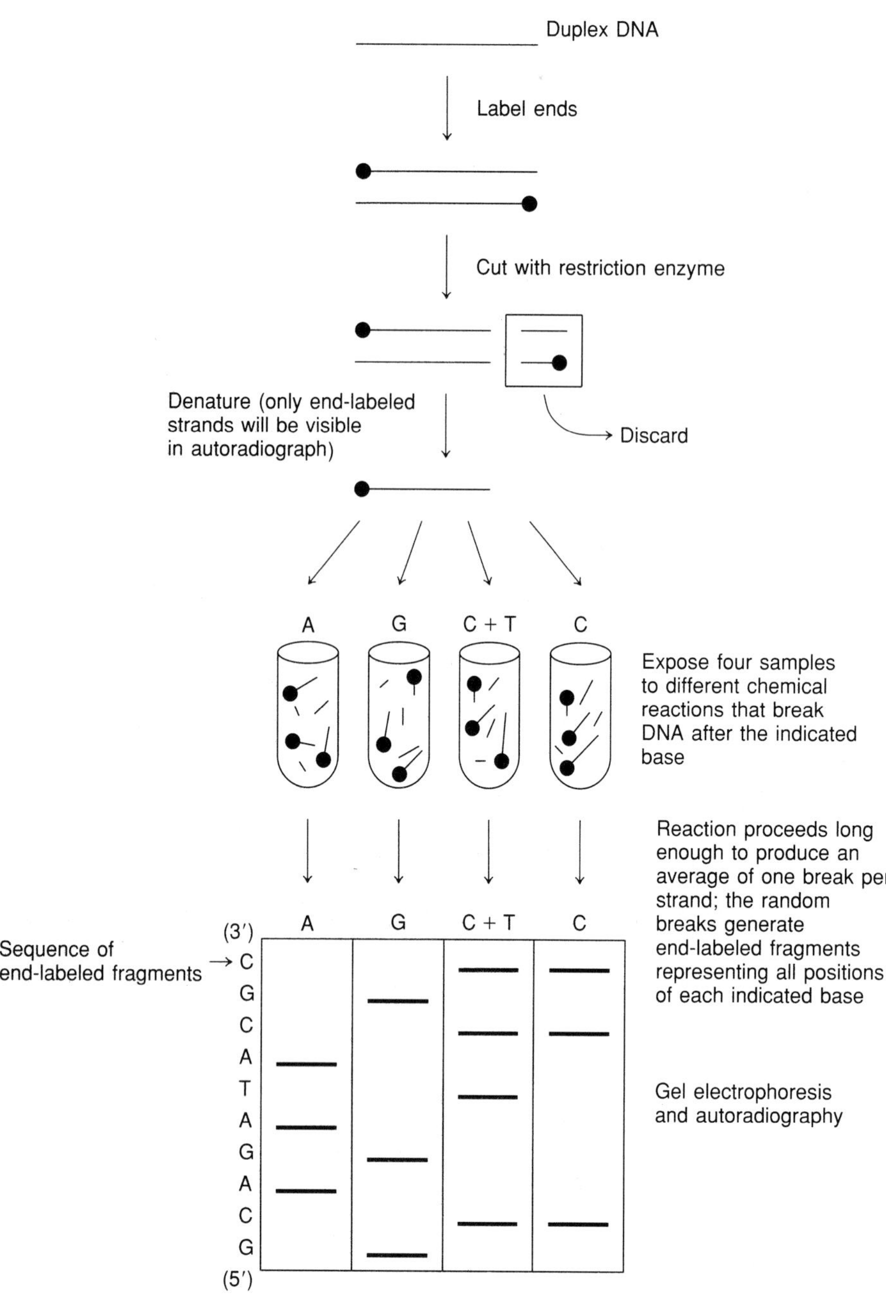

Figure 1–18. DNA sequencing by the Maxam-Gilbert method. The 5′ end–labeled DNA fragment is subjected to controlled digestion at specific base pairs but at random locations on the DNA fragment. After digestion, the resultant fragments are run on a gel that is read by length.

ably larger than the probe, and thus give the investigator either a larger sequence of the unknown gene or at least a better idea of where the sequence of interest lies within the genome. Different microbiologic techniques have been applied to solve this problem. One of them is to use plasmid cloning vectors to introduce a population of recombinant DNA molecules into a bacterial culture en masse under conditions that ensure the uptake of one plasmid per bacterial cell. The transfected bacteria are then spread on a solid growth medium in a Petri dish, and each generates a single colony, resulting in thousands of colonies growing in a single Petri dish. Each colony contains an individual segment of foreign DNA that has been inserted into a cloning vector and is ready for hybridization to the experimental probe. Another, almost identical method is to use a recombinant viral vector to inject the recombinant DNA into a bacterial suspension, which is then spread on growth medium. The viruses lyse their hosts as they replicate, forming clear spots or plaques on the bacterial lawn. With either kind of library (plasmid or viral), thousands of plaques or colonies can grow in a single Petri dish.

The replicate library is then fixed on nitrocellulose or nylon filter and hybridized to the radiolabeled experimental probe. It is hoped that the library will contain a complementary sequence that will contain a sequence or gene of interest in the test colony. The probing process destroys the bacterial or viral hosts on the nylon filter, but the position of the marked clone can be visualized by autoradiography or revealed by an antibody and traced back to the master plate, which harbors live cells (Fig. 1–21). It is then possible to propagate a single colony or plaque simply by picking it off the plate and inoculating it into a new bacterial culture. It

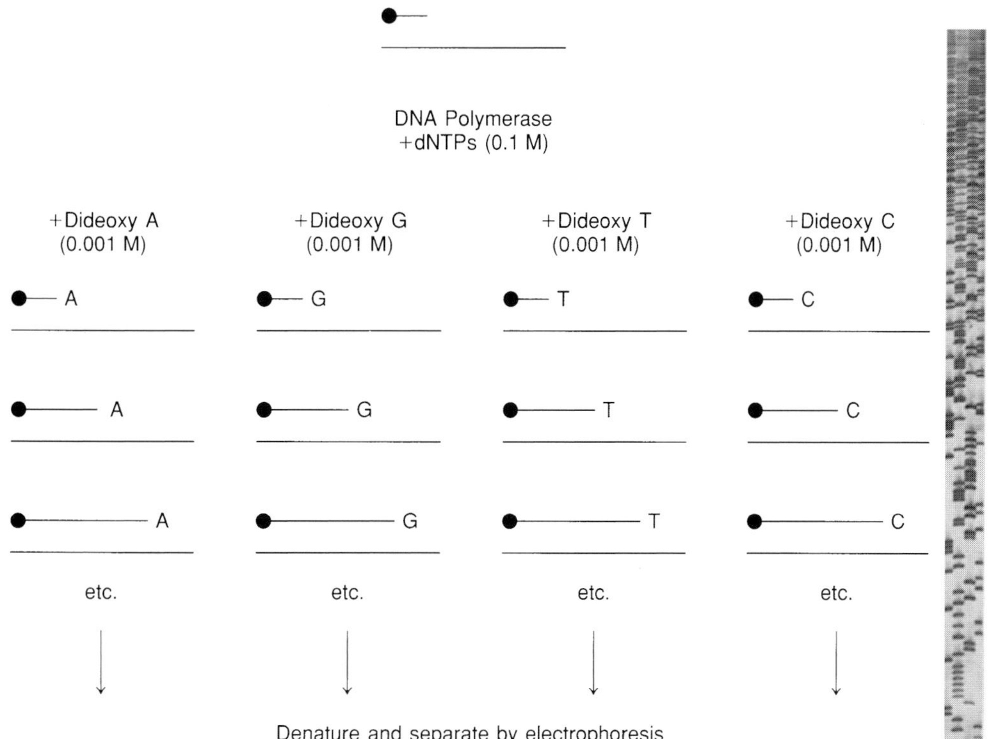

Figure 1–19. DNA sequencing by the Sanger (dideoxy) method. A single strand of DNA to be sequenced is hybridized to a 5′ end–labeled deoxynucleoside primer; four separate reaction mixtures are prepared in which the primer is elongated by a DNA polymerase. Each mixture contains the four normal deoxynucleoside triphosphates plus one of the four dideoxynucleoside triphosphates in a ratio of about 1:100. Because a dideoxynucleoside has no 3′ hydroxyl, no further chain elongation is possible when such a residue is added to the chain. Thus each reaction mixture will produce prematurely terminated chains of varying lengths, ending at every occurrence of the dideoxynucleoside. Each mixture is then separated on a sequencing gel. *Inset,* Actual sequencing gel; lanes represent G, A, T, and C, respectively. (Courtesy of Dr. Glenn Bubley, Boston.)

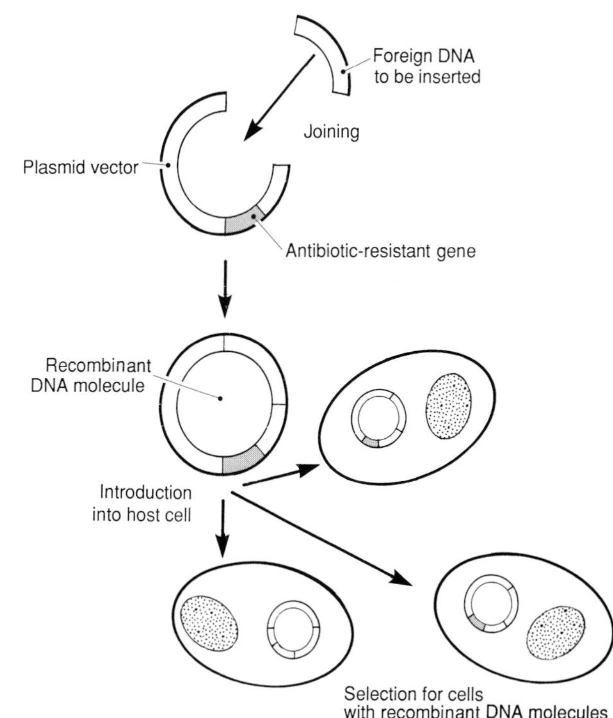

Figure 1–20. Cloning of DNA in a plasmid.

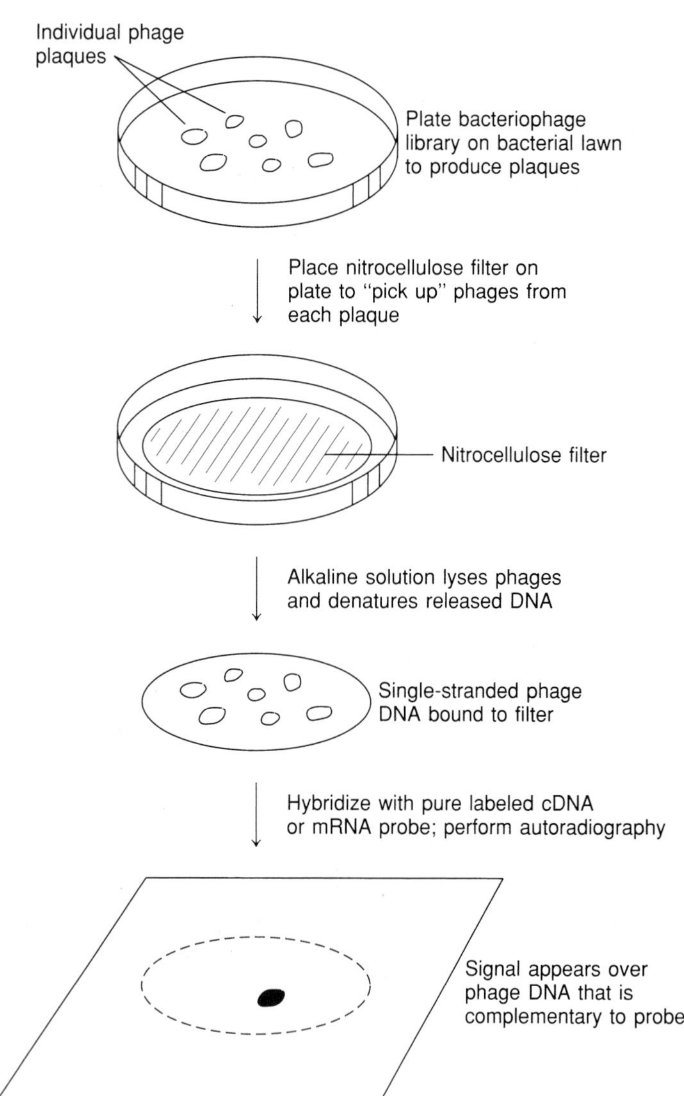
Individual phage plaques
Plate bacteriophage library on bacterial lawn to produce plaques
Place nitrocellulose filter on plate to "pick up" phages from each plaque
Nitrocellulose filter
Alkaline solution lyses phages and denatures released DNA
Single-stranded phage DNA bound to filter
Hybridize with pure labeled cDNA or mRNA probe; perform autoradiography
Signal appears over phage DNA that is complementary to probe

Figure 1–21. Screening a bacteriophage gamma library for a specific DNA sequence. The position of the spot in the autoradiograph identifies the desired plaque on the plate that contains the piece of genomic DNA (or complementary DNA) that is homologous to the probe.

can then be expanded by number and further analyzed, for example, by DNA sequencing.

In Situ Hybridization

A convenient method for detecting the presence (or absence) of specific nucleic acid sequences, of either DNA or RNA origin within cells or on a chromosome, is in situ hybridization (Fig. 1–22). **The principle behind the technique is that labeled nucleic acid probes are hybridized in situ to nucleic acids within cells that have been fixed to glass sides in a manner similar to that of antibody use. This can be done for DNA on chromosomes and mRNA within cells.** The cells are exposed to high pH to disrupt their DNA base pairs. The nucleic acid probes are visualized in one of several ways; the most popular are radiolabeling, fluorescence labeling (hence the name *FISH,* or fluorescence in situ hybridization), and biotin labeling. In the latter case, probes are synthesized with nucleotides that contain a biotin side chain, and the hybridized probes are detected by staining with a network of streptavidin and some type of marker molecule. As mentioned earlier, in situ hybridization methods have also been used to detect specific RNA molecules within cells. In such cases, the tissues are not exposed to high pH, so that the chromosomal-genomic DNA remains double-stranded and cannot bind the labeled nucleic acid probe.

This technique has been so greatly developed that intracellular mRNA signals can first be amplified in situ by PCR and then subjected to probing (Chen and Fuggle, 1993). Such a method has yielded striking results for differential gene expression (Van Ommen et al, 1995).

In general, the advantages of in situ hybridization are localization of the cellular source of mRNA in complex tissues, increased specificity over conventional techniques when the probe is directed at untranslated portions of the gene, and elimination of the need for processing frozen tissue. No freezing that may cause artifact is necessary.

Gel Retardation Assay

The gel retardation assay, also known as the gel-mobility shift assay, is designed to detect the presence of sequence-specific DNA binding proteins. In this assay, a short DNA

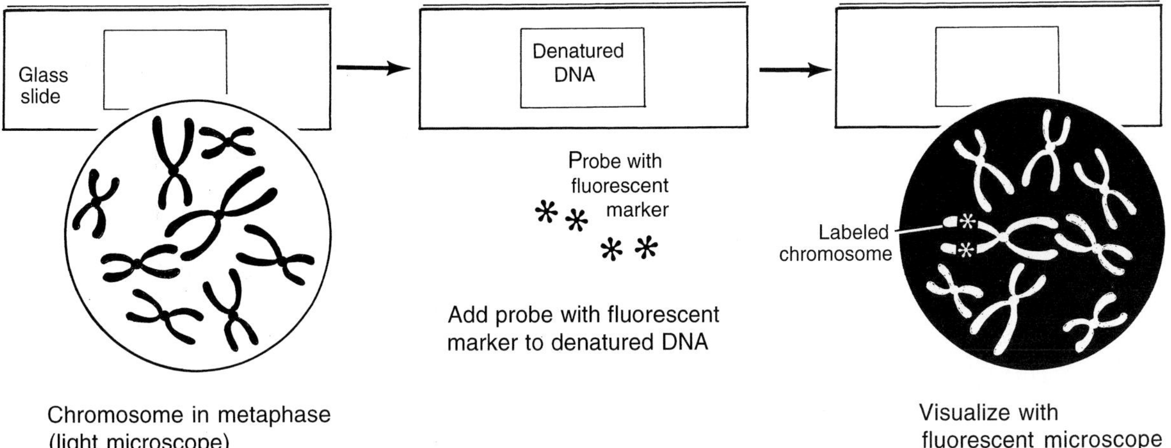

Figure 1–22. Method of fluorescence in situ hybridization. Chromosomes in metaphase are fixed on a microscope slide, and chromosomal DNA is denatured into single strands and hybridized with a cloned piece of DNA labeled with a fluorescent marker. The chromosomal locus of the cloned DNA lights up under ultraviolet light. If there is a deletion, only one copy of the chromosome will show hybridization.

fragment of specific known sequence is labeled and mixed with a cell extract. The mixture is then loaded onto a polyacrylamide gel and is subjected to electrophoresis.

Remember that a DNA molecule is highly negatively charged and will therefore move rapidly toward a positive electrode when it is subjected to an electric field. If the DNA fragment corresponds to the DNA sequence recognized by the protein, the protein, stuck to the DNA, will cause the DNA to move slower than unbound DNA, thus retarding its movement through the gel and producing a characteristic "band" on the gel identified by the labeled DNA fragment (Fig. 1–23). In general, the larger the bound protein, the greater the retardation of the DNA molecule.

DNA binding proteins can be isolated and purified on the basis of this technology. For example, with DNA affinity chromatography, the oligonucleotide is linked to an insoluble porous material such as agarose; this is used to construct a small "column" that, when a cell extract is allowed to run through it, will selectively bind proteins that recognize the particular DNA sequence.

Cytogenetics

The ability to inspect each human chromosome visually in any cell type or disease situation provides an opportunity to step away from the complex nature of individual genes and to delineate a region of interest for further study. In the same sense that visual inspection of a diseased organ allows for subsequent directed microscopic evaluation, the cytogenetic evaluation of cells from diseased organs or patients allows for subsequent directed molecular genetic studies. In addition, karyotypic evaluation of chromosomes allows for prenatal gender determination, provides potential prognostic information about the natural history of several neoplasms, and may be useful in family genetic counseling. Since the field of human cytogenetics is represented by many thorough textbooks, this section provides only a functional overview. The interested reader is referred to the publications by Sandberg (1990, 1994).

Historical Perspectives

More than a century has now elapsed since the term chromosome was first used by Waldeyer (1888) to describe the visible structures that separate during mitosis. Since that time, methodologic developments have led to advances in the understanding of the role of the chromosomes in the normal and disease states. Initial investigations identified both the autosomal chromosomes and the two sex chromosomes. Painter (1921) correctly described the female XX karyotype and the XY karyotype of the male. However, research into human disease was impeded by an inability to demonstrate the normal complement of chromosomes. A crucial breakthrough was provided by Tjio and Levan (1956) with the description of the correct number of normal human chromosomes ($2n = 46$). Subsequent authors quickly described disease syndromes associated with chromosomal numerical anomalies, such as Down's syndrome (Lejeune et al, 1959), Turner's syndrome (Ford et al, 1959), and Klinefelter's syndrome (Jacobs and Strong, 1959).

Despite the importance of these early findings, the study of human chromosomes was limited to evaluations of chromosomal size, number, and any grossly visible structural alterations. The advent of chromosomal banding techniques in the 1970s provided the opportunity to further examine chromosomes for more subtle interstitial changes, such as translocations and deletions. Caspersson and co-workers (1970) demonstrated the procedure for staining chromosomes with fluorochrome quinacrine mustard to produce unique Q-banding patterns. Several other techniques have since been described using agents such as Giemsa (G-banding) to produce individual patterns of visible chromosomal bands. These techniques have allowed the field of modern cytogenetics to associate specific regions of chromosomal alterations with particular disease states.

It is now known, therefore, that each of the 46 human chromosomes can be identified cytogenetically by its distinctive banding pattern (and size). In total, the haploid set of chromosomes comprises 5×10^9 base pairs of DNA. As previously mentioned, less than 5% of this DNA codes for protein, therefore from an organizational standpoint two

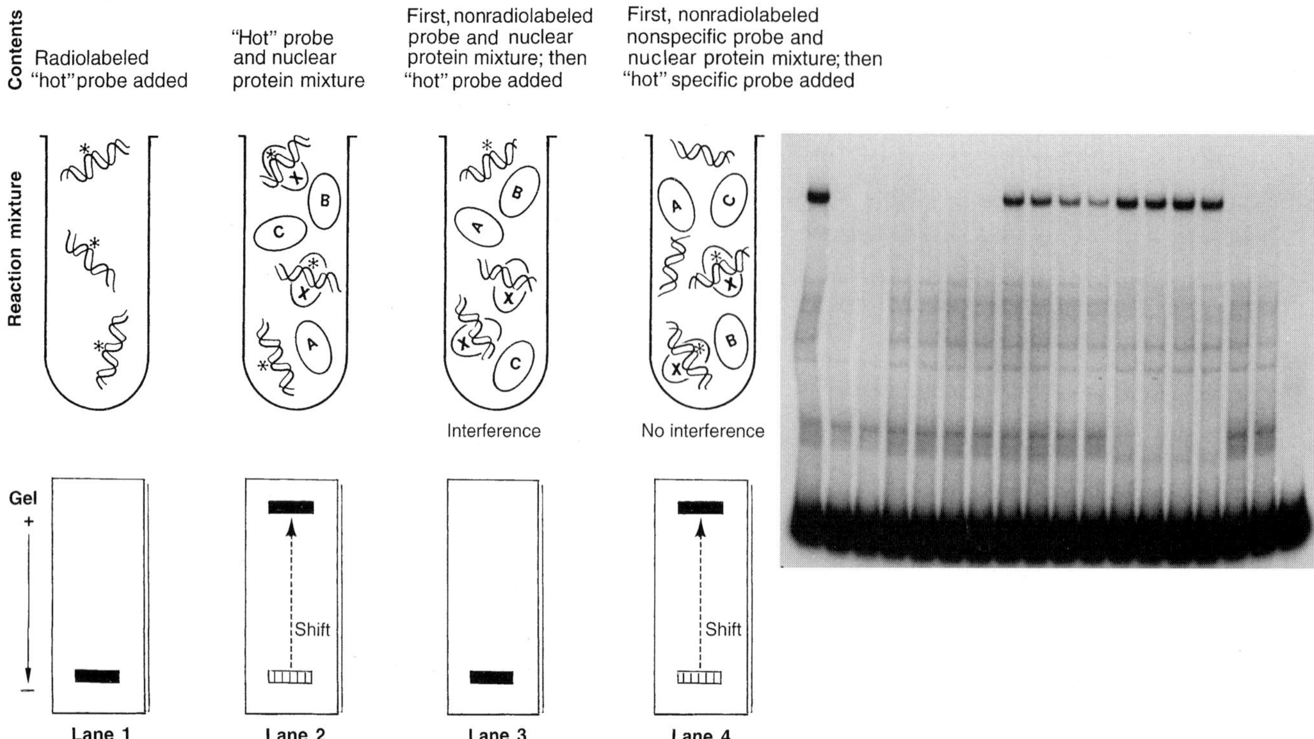

Figure 1–23. Gel retardation assay (also known as electrophoretic mobility shift assay). The principle of the assay is to mix a radioactive DNA probe (carrying the suspected protein-binding sites) with nuclear protein to detect interactions between protein and DNA, which appear as a shifted band in a gel. After a brief incubation, the mixture is loaded onto a gel for electrophoresis to separate molecular complexes of different sizes. Autoradiography of the gel reveals the radiolabeled DNA either by itself (lane 1) or in a protein-DNA complex (lane 2). In the example, protein "X" recognizes a DNA sequence contained within the radiolabeled probe: proteins A, B, and C do not. The additional nonradiolabeled competitor DNA (lane 3) helps to define the specificity of the DNA-protein interaction. If the original interaction between labeled DNA and protein was specific, an unrelated nonspecific competitor should not interfere with the appearance of the shifted band on the gel (lane 4). *Inset,* An actual gel shift assay. The design of the experiment was to look for proteins that bind to the promoter region of the PSA gene in order to help understand how the gene function is regulated. The probe is ^{32}P-labeled, and the nuclear protein extract is from PC-3 (prostatic carcinoma) cells. The dense bands at the bottom are excess labeled probe that "ran through" the gel. Lane 1 (at far left) identified a protein (top dense band) to which the probe "stuck," suggesting specific recognition between the two; other proteins are also identified but appear as weaker bands, suggesting nonspecific reaction (i.e., "background"). Lanes 2 to 7 (counting from left) and 16 to 17 contain increasing concentration of cold specific probe to see whether the reaction (or binding) can be blocked (which it was); lanes 8 to 15 include cold nonspecific probe (irrelevant probe) that did not block reaction, showing specificity of reaction for PSA promoter region in question. Lane 18 contains hot probe only. (Photo courtesy of Dr. Glenn Bubley, Boston.)

questions always come to mind: what is the structural and functional basis for the cytogenetic banding patterns? and how is the <5% protein coding DNA arranged within the chromosomes? Answers to these questions can be obtained from different levels of resolution of cytogenetics or with DNA sequencing and cloning. For a complete understanding of genomic organization, these two levels of resolution must interface.

Cytogenetics and Ploidy

The karyotypic analysis of metaphase chromosomes in cell culture allows for the exact analysis of chromosomal number. Each chromosome, consisting of two identical sister chromatids, can be visualized and counted. Many disease processes have been associated with aberrations of chromosome number. However, the number of chromosomes present in normal tissues had to be established before any conclusions could be reached in particular disease states. Initial cytogenetic studies of normal tissues concentrated on testicular tissue. The germ cells were found to contain 23 chromosomes. This number is considered to be normal for humans and is defined as **haploid (n)**. In mature sperm, the number represents 22 autosomes plus either X or Y; in the ovum, the number represents 22 autosomes plus X. Fertilization of the ovum by a single sperm cell results in a zygote with a **diploid** chromosomal number of 46 (2n).

Numerical alterations are termed variations in **ploidy**—that is, the number of chromosomes as a multiple of the haploid state. **Triploid** and **tetraploid** cells contain 3n and 4n chromosomes; **aneuploid** cells exhibit a chromosomal number that is other than a simple multiple of n. An example of aneuploidy is a prostatic adenocarcinoma cell, which contains 91 chromosomes (Brothman et al, 1990). Numerical alterations also include variations in the number of one particular chromosome; examples include Down's syndrome (three of chromosome 21) and Turner's syndrome (only one sex chromosome, the X). Abnormalities in the number or the structure of sex chromosomes are particularly important in the study of ambiguous genitalia.

In fact, the karyotypic analysis of such patients is a vital facet in the overall management strategy. These situations may also be strictly defined as aneuploid.

Cytogenetics and Banding Techniques

The cytogenetic evaluation of any cell involves the identification of metaphase chromosomes and their arrangement into specific groups. A photographic representation of this arrangement is called the **karyotype** (Fig. 1–24). Early researchers distinguished individual chromosomes only on the basis of size and position of the centromere. In 1970 Caspersson and colleagues employed DNA-binding fluorescent quinacrine to stain individual chromosomes. This produced a unique series of alternating dark and light bands on each chromosome. Specific intrachromosomal regions, unique to each chromosome, could be identified, even if the material was transported elsewhere in the karyotype. This phenomenon allowed Rowley in 1973 to correctly identify the Philadelphia chromosome in chronic myelogenous leukemia as being a translocation between chromosomes 9 and 22. Additional techniques of staining chromosomes that resulted in reproducible banding patterns were developed. These techniques, called G-, R-, T-, and C-banding, were developed independently, yet all have one thing in common: The exact mechanism by which the patterns of bands are created remains a mystery.

Among the most commonly used cytogenetic banding techniques are Giemsa (G-) and reverse (R-) banding. These bands have certain characteristics (Table 1–3), but these characteristics are not necessarily independent. The fact that

Table 1–3. PROPERTIES OF GIEMSA (G) AND REVERSE (R) BANDS

G Bands	R Bands
Stain strongly with Giemsa and quinacrine	Stain weakly with Giemsa and quinacrine
AT rich	GC rich
DNase insensitive	DNase sensitive
Few breakpoints or rearrangements	Many breakpoints and rearrangements
Gene poor	Gene rich
Alu poor	*Alu* rich

R bands are gene rich and therefore of more open chromatin configuration is reflected in their relative sensitivity to DNAases as well as their higher frequency of congenital and radiation-induced rearrangement. In general, chromosomal banding techniques have given indications that the human genome is indeed organized and that functionable characteristics are not randomly distributed.

Cytogenetics and Chromosomal Morphology

Individual chromosomes are subject to many morphologic alterations that may be identified by karyotypic analysis.

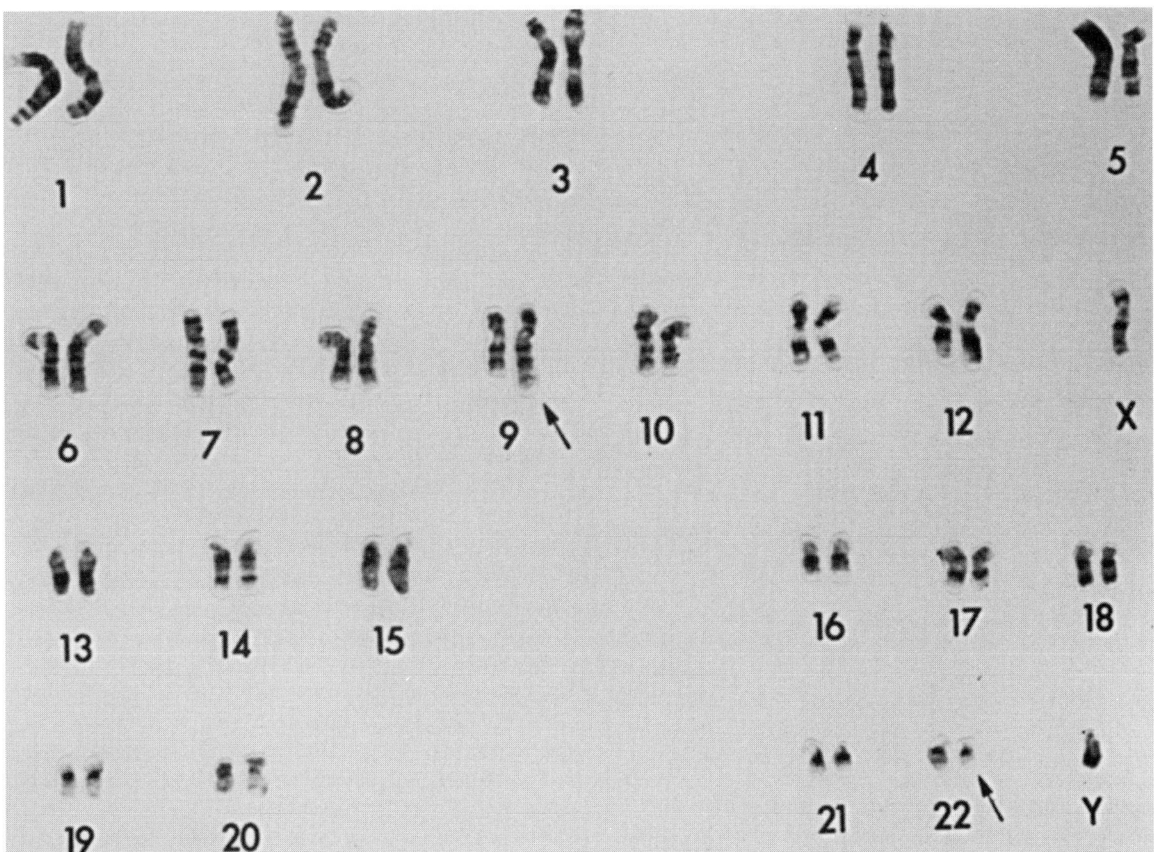

Figure 1–24. Karyotype of the chronic myelogenous leukemia (CML) cell with chromosomes stained to show the Giemsa banding pattern. A morphologic change—translocation—has occurred between chromosomes 9 and 22. The genetic material missing from the Philadelphia (Ph) chromosome has been located to the end of the second chromosome, No. 9; the two abnormal chromosomes are marked by arrows. (Courtesy of Dr. J. D. Rowley, Chicago.)

Although many of these alterations may have little or no pathophysiologic significance, it has become clear that other rearrangements are nonrandom and essential to the disease state. These morphologic changes, in a manner similar to that of numerical abnormalities, may lead to aberrant function of the genes located on a particular chromosome.

During the process of mitosis, loss or deletion of chromosomal material may remove the function of a vital gene. Alternatively, material can be duplicated, potentially increasing the amount of a particularly unwelcome protein. In addition, genetic material may be translocated from one chromosome to another, as with the **Philadelphia chromosome**. In fact, the morphology of a chromosome may become so abnormal, during the evolution of a diseased state, that it can no longer be identified. In this case, it is called a **marker chromosome.**

Each morphologic change has the potential to substantially alter gene function and, therefore, cellular function. It is therefore important to realize that multiple morphologic alterations can be present without affecting the total chromosomal number (i.e., ploidy).

Chromosomal **inversions** and **insertions** are less common. An inversion can be either **pericentric**, resulting from breakage followed by relocation of a segment within a chromosome about the centromere, or **paracentric,** in which case the breaks are on the same arm and the centromere is not involved. Insertion, on the other hand, involves transfer of material from one chromosome to another. Inversions and insertions, like translocations, may lead to an abnormal juxtaposition of genetic materials, which may lead to the formation of chimeric genes, producing abnormal proteins that can initiate neoplasia and contribute to malignant transformation.

Cytogenetics and Malignancy

Chromosomal alterations and the resulting changes in gene function play a fundamental etiologic role in the genesis of a malignancy. A sizable proportion of these alterations is sufficiently large enough to be identified as chromosomal morphologic changes. Mitelman and Heim (1988) subdivided the acquired chromosomal abnormalities in neoplasms into three categories:

1. They may be primary alterations that are pathogenetically essential. By definition, these alterations are present in the earliest disease phase.
2. They may accrue later in the development of a neoplasm. These anomalies are important in generating the genetic variability that gives rise to the clonal evolution of a tumor cell population and to its increasingly malignant phenotype.
3. Alterations may simply represent cytogenetic aberrations without any long-term selection value. It is often difficult to distinguish functionally significant lesions from these background aberrations.

The overall importance of chromosomal alterations in malignancies has been indirectly substantiated by the identification of oncogenes or tumor suppressor genes at the sites of visible chromosomal defects. The cytogenetic analysis of urologic solid tumors, with subsequent molecular genetic investigations, has furthered the understanding of the mechanism of oncogenesis. Wilms' tumor is an example of this process. Franke (1979) identified a consistent cytogenetic deletion of the short arm of chromosome 11 at band 11p13. Other investigators focused on this region and ultimately identified a putative gene responsible for this neoplasm (Call et al, 1990; Gessler et al, 1990; Huang et al, 1990; Rose et al, 1990). This story is being repeated with renal cell carcinoma, which exhibits a primary cytogenetic alteration on the short arm of chromosome 3 (Carroll et al, 1987), as well as with several other urologic neoplasms. The role of cytogenetic analysis in each of these individual malignancies is discussed in greater detail in subsequent chapters (for reviews, see Nowell, 1994; Rabbitts, 1994).

Genetics, Ethics, and Human Values

The first sentence of the chapter states that DNA is the molecule of life. Scientists have long sensed this, which is the basis for the excitement that has been generated; that is, the tools and concepts of molecular genetics have provided new and useful probes toward understanding the answers to several issues about life and disease. Inevitably, however, the same issues are being sensed by society in general, which has raised several moral and ethical issues. The collision between science and society affects us all and therefore at least deserves mention. The issues that are raised deal with moral responsibility and perhaps reflect the enormous power that molecular genetics has in our lives.

One of the major issues at hand concerns gene ownership. In an editorial in the science journal *Nature Medicine*, the severity of the situation was well stated when it was reported that "In the Name of God, a coalition of religious groups that include Christians, Jews, Muslims and Hindus has thrown down the gauntlet against patenting 'life forms' such as human genes and human cell lines" (Culliton, 1995b). This issue suggests that all information arising from human genetic studies should be placed in the public domain. The problem, most simply stated, is that without ownership, the biotechnology industry cannot justify major financial commitment, and such commitment is probably necessary for proper progress to occur. Commercialization is a necessary part of progress, but how it is to fit into gene ownership will take social progress.

Another thorny problem that is developing relates to testing for cancer genes. This issue is not trivial and may involve more people and testing than first apparent. For example, early predictions place the carrier frequencies for predisposing alleles of cancer genes for common cancers such as BRCA 1 and BRCA 2 for breast cancer or MLH 1 and MSH 2 for colorectal cancer at approximately 1 in 500 (Claus et al, 1991; Burt et al, 1992). Eventually, millions of individuals will be eligible for testing for many cancer susceptibility genes. On the surface, such aggressive cancer surveillance seems advantageous; however, such testing poses risks as well as benefits. Individuals at risk must decide whether the increased anxiety of a positive test result, for themselves or their children, would outweigh the relief of a negative outcome. Furthermore, carriers of altered genes must be concerned about the lack of protection adequate to ensure continued access to health, life, and disability insurance. In addition, the issue of job and educational discrimination may also play a role. This issue is so real that there is evidence that people have refused potentially valuable genetic screening for fear of discrimination should they have a gene that predisposes them to cancer or another life-threatening disease. Toward this end, on March 14, 1995, the U.S. Equal Employment Opportunities Commission declared that under the Americans with Disabilities Act (1990), a genetic susceptibility to disease is protected disability within the meaning of the law (Culliton, 1995a). Unfortunately, insurance companies are not controlled by this act, but employers are; it is hoped that through employer negotiations with insurance companies, policies will change with regard to coverage.

At present, it is apparent that before genetic testing, knowledge of inheritance, cancer risk, medical management options, and confidentiality should be established to both protect and benefit all involved.

Genes and Evolution

At the beginning of this chapter, the statement is made that DNA is the "record book of life." Indeed, the concept and basis of genetics and evolution were born almost together. As noted in the introduction, Mendel published his works on genetics in the *Transactions of the Brünn Natural History Society* in 1866, which was 2 years before the publication of Darwin's *Origin of the Species*. Interestingly, neither man knew of the work of the other, yet the roots of what we know of evolution originated from the combination of both. Although the concepts of evolution and genetics are far-reaching and perhaps beyond the scope of this text, a few perspectives and facts are important for a proper understanding of genomic organization and function.

Gene Number and Complexity of Organisms

In general, evolution per se is equated with increasing complexity of living organisms, which is itself a product of increased efficiency. This concept is a bit problematic because there is no theoretical reason to expect evolutionary lineages to increase in complexity with time. The reasons that this happens, however, help us to understand how the genome works.

Although it might be natural to think that accumulation of genes during the evolution of more complex forms has been a gradual process, an estimate of life forms and their genomic organization suggests otherwise (Fig. 1–25). Existing life forms fall into three basic categories: (1) prokaryotes with a few thousand genes, (2) eukaryotes with 7000 to 25,000 genes, and (3) vertebrates with 50,000 to 100,000 genes. Figure 1–25 indicates that the change was not gradual but rather dramatic with two major inflections: one at the prokaryote-eukaryote boundary and the other at the invertebrate-vertebrate boundary. The pattern is not random, and it involved evolutionary forces. The question is, which ones? Although the answers are not entirely clear, there are two likely explanations, one more plausible than the other. The less likely involves mutation rate. It is classically supposed that the rate of mutation imposes strict limitations on genome

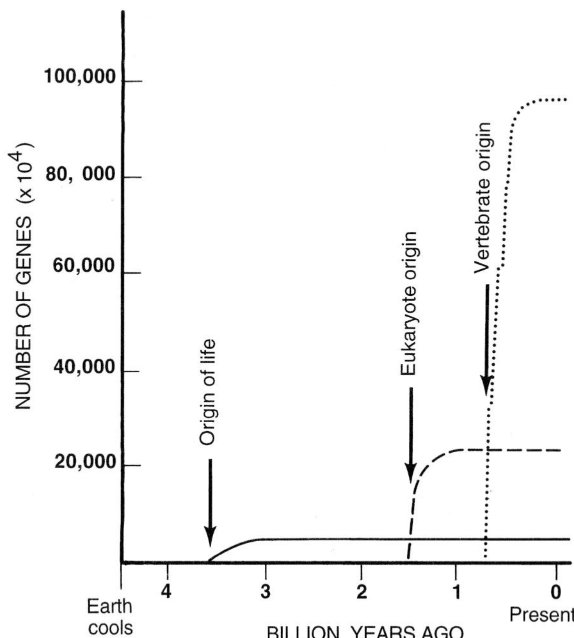

Figure 1–25. An estimate of the evolution of gene number in prokaryotic (*solid lines*), nonvertebrate eukaryotes (*dashed lines*), and vertebrates (*dotted lines*). (Modified from Bird A: Trends Genet 1995; 11:94–99.)

size (Smith and Szathmary, 1995). For a genome to be successful, it must be able to replicate without too many damaged copies. This rate-limiting mechanism, however, does not make complete sense because quantal increases in gene number would require quantal decreases in mutation rates. In fact, there is practically no variation in per-genome mutation rate from phage to fungi despite several variations, in orders of magnitude, in genome size (Drake, 1991). Therefore, it seems unlikely that increases in gene number result solely from reductions in rate of mutation.

The second and perhaps more favorable evolutionary force behind increasing gene complexity involves the hypothesis that maximal gene number is intrinsically limited by the imprecision of the biochemical mechanisms governing gene expression (Bird, 1995).

Most (but not all) genes are tissue specific. The more cell types an organism has, the more tissue-specific genes it requires and, conversely, the greater number of genes that need to be repressed in any one cell type. Thus, biologic complexity can be limited by the efficiency of gene expression/repression mechanisms. In reality, it seems that the level of unscheduled transcription of several silent genes is about one mRNA in 10,000 genes, which if applied to all repressed genes would mean that cells would have about four inappropriate transcripts per cell (assuming a differentiated cell produces 30,000 ubiquitous mRNAs and 10,000 tissue-specific mRNAs; if a total of 80,000 genes are in a cell, then 40,000 genes are repressed per cell). **This argument suggests that the upper limit of genes that an organism can work with is set by the prevailing biochemical machinery to distinguish essential gene expression from background. Essentially, the whole problem is distinguishing signal from noise.**

Two candidate mechanisms for noise reduction at the

prokaryote-eukaryote boundary involve the origin of **histones** and the **nuclear envelope**. Histones and nucleosomes have well described functions in the repression of gene activity. They have regulatory activity particularly with regard to transcriptional activation (Felsenfeld, 1992). Bacteria, in contrast, have no general repression system comparable with that of the nucleosome, and in general, bacterial transcription involves the interaction of RNA polymerase with effectively naked DNA.

Acquisition of a nuclear membrane, on the other hand, would allow transcription to be uncoupled from translation and would certainly introduce a new step in filtering signal from noise. Polyadenylation and capping of RNAs are seen as parts of the filtering process. If this hypothesis is correct, it would be safe to predict that genes inappropriately expressed should be prevented from leaving the nucleus more often than appropriately expressed genes. Interestingly, the evolutionary origin of the nucleus is unknown. Although several theories exist, the most popular is that the nucleus was derived through capture by an engulfing species. In this case, however, the guest (the nucleus), rather than being under the control of the host, actually took control of the host (Lake and Rivera, 1994).

The evolutionary mechanism responsible for the vertebrate-invertebrate transition is thought to be extensive genome-wide methylation, which is well known to repress transcription (see Fig. 1–4). There is no doubt that the vertebrate genome is more heavily methylated than the invertebrate genome. The unique feature of this mechanism is that it is strong enough to prevent spurious interactions between RNA polymerase and DNA but does not interfere with scheduled gene expression. It is still not clear however how the body knows which CpGs to methylate and which to leave open to allow transcription.

Why and how the "new" silencing technology evolved in the first place are unclear. But, once in place, the gene number and complexity increased.

The Origin of DNA

Another problem fundamental to our understanding of molecular genetics concerns the origin of DNA. The answer to this question, according to the first sentence of this chapter, addresses not only a problem of biochemistry but also the most important question of all: namely, what is the origin of life? For a long time it has been clear that the contemporary system could not have been the first but must have replaced an earlier system that had a unitary chemical language to allow catalysis and replication of genetic information to evolve in one molecule. Thus either proteins came first and there was some way for amino acids to be copied or the first molecules were nucleic acids (or nucleic acid–like molecules), RNA in particular, and could have catalytic functions.

Although it is likely that DNA arose from RNA (Fig. 1–26), it is unlikely that RNA represented the beginning step, in view of difficulties with nonenzymatic replication of RNA (Joyce and Orgel, 1993). Most likely, life began with a simpler replicating system that was later replaced by RNA, and the early system was probably capable of self-replication and contained a mechanism for genetic takeover by RNA. Candidates for such molecules are "simpler" nucleotide analogues (Joyce et al, 1989). One example is peptide nucleic acid (PNA), which was first designed and synthesized as an antisense agent (Egholm, 1993). The molecule consists of a polyamide backbone composed of glycine units to which nucleobases are attached by carbonyl methylene linkers. Such molecules have the capability of pairing with DNA and RNA according to Watson-Crick base pairing rules.

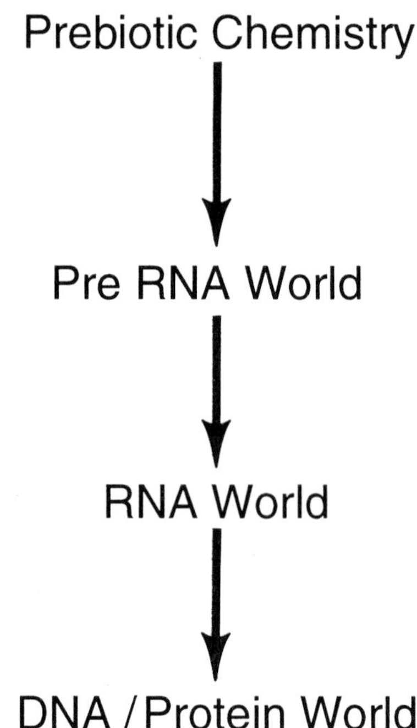

Figure 1–26. Conceptual diagram of the origin of DNA (and life).

DNA and Anthropology

One of the great potentials of DNA analysis is the development of techniques to analyze ancient human DNA. In fact, anthropologists are hoping that genetic analysis of human remains may help in understanding the origin and migration of people around the world over the past 30,000 years. For example, mitochondrial DNA analysis from Native Americans has aroused controversy with regard to old theories concerning the sources and dates of original Asian migrations into the Americas. The most widely held theory is that the first Americans crossed the Bering Strait from Asia within the last 30,000 years in three distinct waves of migration: first the Amerind people 30,000 years ago, followed by the Na-Dene 10,000 years ago, and finally the Eskimo-Aleuts 5000 years ago. Some DNA studies support this plan; for example, Native Americans belong to only four distinct lineages, labeled A to D. In comparison, Asian populations have many more lineages, which suggests that Native Americans were derived from migrants who carried only a small sample of Asian mitochondrial types. Researchers have also found that Native Americans have all four lineages, the Na-Dene have only A, and Eskimos have A and D. This suggests that there were different migrations at different times.

More recent mitochondrial genome analysis, however, suggests more founding lineages in the Americas, and in fact the distribution of the mitochondrial types within the modern Native American populations in both North and South America is better explained by a single wave of migration. Whichever theory is correct is still not known, but it certainly is clear that DNA analysis is adding a new dimension to the study of our heritage.

SPECIAL STRATEGIES IN MOLECULAR GENETICS

Transgenic and Knockout Models

Perhaps the most dramatic example of genetic engineering and its relationship to clinical medicine is the ability to introduce genes into animals (and eventually humans) (Hanahan, 1989; Westphal, 1989). An animal that gains new permanent genetic information from the addition of new foreign DNA is described as **transgenic.** A transgenic animal, or organism for that matter, carries in its genome gene sequences inserted by laboratory techniques.

The design of this approach will eventually be used to cure genetic imperfections and disease; however, at present, technical limitations allow only the construction of transgenic animals as models of disease. There are various ways to do this, but the most common practice is to inject transgene DNA into one of the two pronuclei (the male and female haploid nuclei contributed by the parents) of a fertilized mouse egg before they fuse (Fig. 1–27) (Brinster et al, 1981). The DNA is incorporated into the chromosomes of the diploid zygote. The injected eggs are then transferred to foster mothers, in which normal cell growth and differentiation occur. About 10% to 30% of the progeny contain the foreign DNA in all tissues of the body, including germ cells. Immediate breeding and backcrossing (parent-offspring mating) of the 10% to 20% of these mice that bred normally can produce pure transgenic strains homozygous for the transgene (the newly introduced gene).

The production of transgenic strains of mice provides valuable information, because even if the transgenes are not inserted into the correct chromosomal site, they still function to produce RNA normally during development and differentiation. It is possible for an introduced gene to recombine with the homologous pre-existing gene (as happens with yeast) so that animal genes can be replaced.

Transgenic therapy is still not available clinically because of incomplete understanding of gene targeting (replacing the old gene) as well as regulation of function. For example, in the progeny of injected mice, expression of the donor gene can be quite variable. The level of expression does not always correlate with the number of genes that were integrated.

A natural extension of this approach that has the opposite effect is called the "gene knockout" approach. This procedure allows scientists to switch an abnormal or null gene for a normal one in an embryo with the ultimate goal of watching the development of the new **knockout** animal to determine the effect of the "missing gene." The procedure is outlined in Figure 1–28 (Capecchi, 1989) and is currently used as a popular approach to determine what a certain gene does in the body. The procedure makes use of embryo-derived stem (ES) cells, and it is in these cells that gene "switching" takes place. ES cell lines are derived in culture from blastocyst-stage mouse embryos and can be maintained indefinitely in the undifferentiated state provided that the conditions are carefully controlled. A targeting vector con-

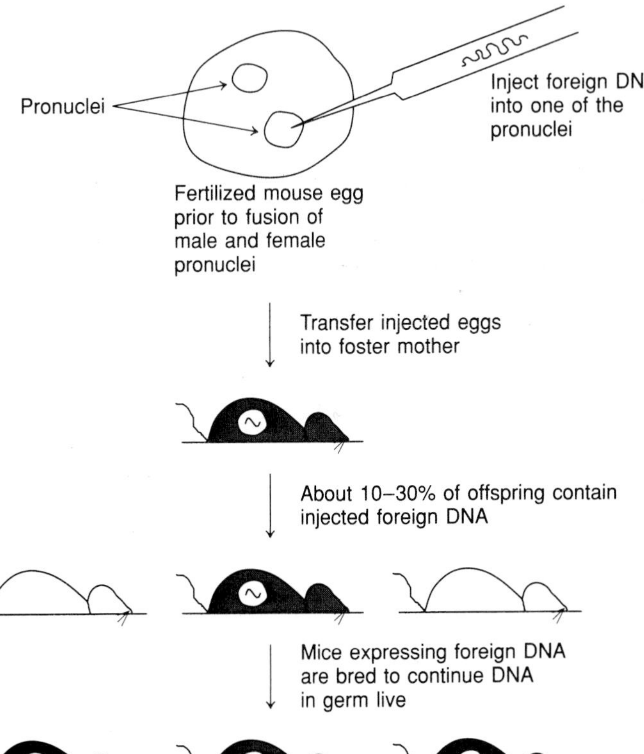

Figure 1–27. Introduction of foreign DNA into a mouse and establishment of a homozygous transgenic mouse strain.

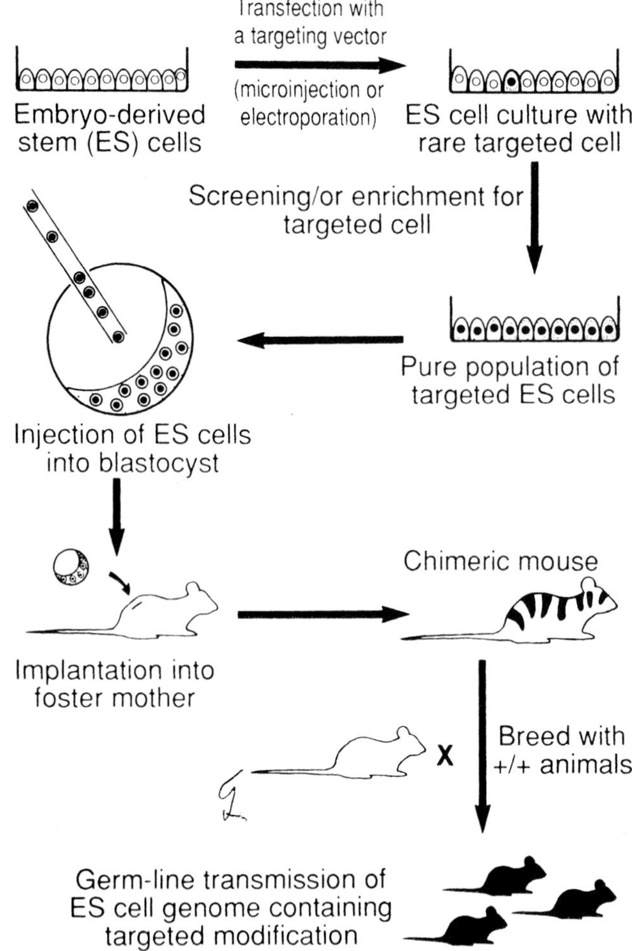

Figure 1–28. Generation of mouse germ line chimeras from embryo-derived stem cells containing a targeted gene disruption. (From Capecchi M: Science 1989; 22:479–488.)

taining the derived gene is introduced into the ES cells. In a small minority of these cells, the "altered experimental" DNA (the altered gene) pairs with the "normal gene" found in the ES cells, and the two genes are switched by natural mechanisms that are not clearly understood (homologous recombination). This of course is the key step and, with our lack of understanding, represents one of the major impediments to progress in human gene therapy. The "altered" ES cell is then reintroduced into an embryo, which is surgically transferred into the uterus of a foster mother. During this time, the ES cell reintegrates into the normal developmental pathway and may differentiate into one or all of several tissues, including the germ line (eggs or sperm), in which case the altered gene will be passed on to future generations. It is not hard to imagine how this technique can be applied to study the function of a cloned gene in the context of the whole organism.

With the knockout gene models, scientists are beginning to understand the relationship among differentiation, development, and cancer. For example, genes that are known to play an important role in malignant transformation are being altered or defunctionalized and introduced back into embryos with the goal of observing the effects on development. A typical example is that of the tumor suppressor gene *wt-1,* the loss of which is believed to cause Wilms' tumor (Haber et al, 1990; Little et al, 1992). Knockout mice were developed for *wt-1* gene mutations (Kreidberg et al, 1993). The mutation resulted in embryonic lethality in homozygotes, and examination of mutant embryos revealed failure of kidney and gonad development. Specifically, at day 11 of gestation, the cells of the metanephric blastema underwent apoptosis. The ureteral bud failed to grow from the wolffian duct, and the inductive events that led to the formation of the metanephric kidney did not occur. Basically, it appears as though initial outgrowth of the ureteric bud is dependent on a signal from the blastema and *wt-1* is required for its expression. These experiments provide a state-of-the-art example of how our understanding of cancer is moving us into other disciplines, including development.

The Two-Hybrid System: An Assay for Protein-Protein Interactions

One of the nice features of molecular genetics is that its biochemistry "nuts and bolts" organization allows for certain laboratory tricks that are applicable to science outside molecular genetics. Perhaps the best example is the two-hybrid system, which is a sophisticated laboratory technique that is designed to determine whether there are proteins in a cell that interact with a given experimental protein. This question is often asked, for example, when a new gene (with unknown function) is found. Its protein sequence is then determined; but to find out what it does, which is one of the toughest assignments given to scientists, one plan of attack is to determine whether it interacts with other proteins in a cell. The two-hybrid system is designed to answer that question and makes use of fundamental molecular genetic principles (Fields and Song, 1989).

The fundamental principle behind this technique is that there exist, as previously noted, DNA-binding proteins that activate transcription of certain genes. Many of these activator proteins are divided into two domains (Fig. 1–29): the DNA-binding domain and the transcription activation domain (Keegan et al, 1986; Hope and Struhl, 1986). It is thought that the activation domain interacts with components of the basal transcription machinery as part of the process of initiation of transcription.

It was later determined that a DNA-binding protein could actually be split, but as long as the two ends were joined by a protein "bridge," the system would still work. Finally, a well-worked-out reporter system was necessary, and several have been described. Usually the study is performed in yeast cells (for technical purposes), and the *Gal 4–lac Z* reporter is used; that is, *Gal 4,* a DNA-binding protein, is split in two. The experimental protein whose function is unknown is fused to the DNA-binding portion of *Gal 4* (by fusing respective genes in such a way that translation results in a fusion protein). The transactivating portion of *Gal 4* is fused to one of several thousand proteins from a cDNA library. If an unknown protein (from the cDNA library) that is fused to the transactivating portion of *Gal 4* associates with protein X, the bridge will be complete and transactivation will occur, which in this case will cause transcription of *lac Z,* which

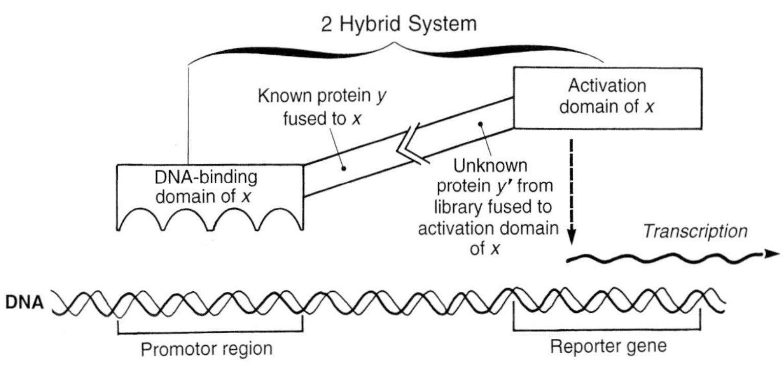

Figure 1–29. The two-hybrid system. *Top,* DNA-binding domain of a DNA-binding protein binds to a promoter-like upstream activating sequence. Usually the DNA binding domain (in this case, of protein "X") is covalently linked to a transcriptional activating domain (of "X") and under experimental conditions can be designed to activate transcription of a "marker" gene, usually lac Z, which turns colonies blue when plated on X-Gal. *Bottom,* The same phenomenon occurs when the DNA-binding domain and the transactivating domain of a DNA-binding protein are linked by two proteins attached by noncovalent means. In this case, the known protein *y* associates with protein *y′*, which was encoded by a pool of plasmids in which total cDNA or genomic DNA was ligated to the activation domain.

produces beta-galactosidase, which produces blue colonies on plates or filters containing X-*Gal.*

From the technical standpoint, the yeast system is usually used because of several advantages: (1) ease of transformation, (2) convenience of retrieving plasmids, (3) availability of several markers and well-characterized reporter genes for direct selection, and (4) the fact that endogenous yeast proteins are less likely to bind mammalian target proteins. Interestingly, the fact that so many pairs of hybrid proteins lead to reporter gene expression argues strongly that activation does not depend on the existence of a defined distance or orientation between the transcription factor domain and the fused X or Y domain. Thus the hybrid proteins might behave as two balls on a short flexible string rather than as two rigidly constrained domains.

Genetic Markers and Linkage Analysis

Genetic Markers

Extraordinary progress has been made in understanding the structure and function of human genes with regard to certain disease states. Most of our understanding has related to disorders associated with a defect in a single gene. **Two basic strategies are used to define a genetic disease with regard to associating an abnormal gene with its abnormal gene product** (Table 1–4). **The most straightforward protocol for genetic analysis assumes that either the abnormal or normal gene product (a protein) is known.** With that prerequisite, amino acid sequence analysis can be performed on part of the protein. From that, an oligonucleotide that is equivalent to a cDNA molecule can be synthetically made. Such a probe can then be used to search a cDNA library from various tissues or chromosomes with resultant identification of the cDNA (or mRNA), the tissue of origin, or the chromosome of origin, according to the experiment done.

This type of approach can also be used when an antibody is available to the protein in question; it can be used to precipitate protein mRNA complexes. After conversion of mRNA to cDNA, an approach identical to that outlined earlier can be used to isolate the gene.

Once the gene is identified, specific abnormalities such as deletions, insertions, rearrangements, or point mutations can be sought in the diseased patient to account for the abnormal protein production (or lack of protein production).

Table 1–4. GENETIC ANALYSIS AND "REVERSE" GENETIC ANALYSIS

From Gene to Protein	From Protein to Gene
Isolate mRNA; make cDNA	Isolate protein
↓	↓
Sequence cDNA	Partial amino acid sequence
↓	↓
Deduce amino acid sequence from cDNA sequence	Make oligonucleotides that correspond to amino acid sequence
↓	↓
Make peptides specified by sequence; inject into animals to produce antibodies	Use labeled oligonucleotides to select cDNA clone from cDNA library
↓	↓
Isolate pure protein by affinity to antibody	Sequence selected gene

Linkage Analysis

For disorders in which the defective protein is unknown, the job of isolating the gene (and then the protein) is a bit more cumbersome. A technique of "reverse genetics" is often used (see Table 1–4). In such circumstances, genes are found through linkage to a marker locus in specific chromosomal regions. Linkage of a disease to a genetic marker locus passed through generations within a family strongly suggests that a nearby gene locus is responsible (at least in part) for the disease in question.

One type of the most commonly used markers, **restriction fragment length polymorphisms (RFLPs),** are nothing more than short DNA sequences that vary from one person to the next. They are sequences that can distinguish one organism from another or even one homologous chromosome from another, they are not associated with any phenotypic change within one individual, and normally they can be mapped to specific chromosomal locations (White and Lalouel, 1988; Marx, 1990). For example, it has been found that examination of DNA from any two persons, or comparing DNA between two homologous chromosomes, will reveal variation in the DNA sequences involving approximately one nucleotide in every 200 to 500 base pairs. Interestingly, these polymorphic sequences occur much more frequently in DNA than in proteins, and most produce no observable effect.

Some of these DNA sequence changes are detectable by digestion of DNA with restriction endonucleases (see Fig. 1–14), producing fragments of discrete length. Single base pair changes may abolish an existing restriction enzyme recognition site (or may create a new one), thereby altering the length of these fragments. Alternatively, change in fragment length can be attributed to variation in "tandem repeat sequences," which are interspaced at various intervals in the human genome; when these repeat sequences occur between enzyme cleavage sites, the lengths of the DNA fragments generated by digestion with the enzyme also vary (Jeffreys et al, 1985; Nakamura et al, 1987). **The idea, then, is to find RFLPs with as much variation as possible and to use them in studies of families who have genetic diseases to see whether all family members who contract the disease carry the same RFLP. If they do, the researchers can conclude that the disease gene and the RFLP are "linked"—that is, that they are inherited together and therefore must be located very near one another on the same chromosome. The RFLP marker is then used as a stepping stone to find the gene itself.** A statistical expression of linkage is the logarithm of the odds (LOD), which statistically measures how close two loci are linked in the genome by comparing the likelihood of an observed association of alleles as a result of varying degrees of linkage versus chance association. Mathematically, LOD scores are defined as the $\log_{10}$ of the ratio of the probability that the data would have arisen from unlinked loci. The conventional threshold for linkage is an LOD score of >3.0, which corresponds to a ratio of 1000:1 in favor of linkage. However, any arbitrary pair of loci is 50 times more likely to be unlinked than linked; thus an LOD score of 3.0 actually provides odds of 20:1 in favor of linkage; with an LOD score of 4.0, the chance of error is only 1 in 200.

The next step in isolating a gene after it has been shown to associate with a certain chromosomal region (by linkage analysis) is to examine ("walk down") the whole genome, beginning with the markers known to be linked to the disease gene; the goal is to eventually find the disease gene (Bender et al, 1983). This is illustrated in Figure 1–30. The examination starts with a clone that was isolated, as mentioned earlier, because it lies near a region of interest. Other clones that overlap the first clone are identified. These other clones are obtained from a genomic library, which as previously mentioned represents a set of cloned fragments (many thousands) together representing the entire genome (see Fig. 1–21). The new second clone, which overlaps the first, extends on one side or the other of the DNA fragment identified by the first clone. The direction of extension (5′ or 3′) can be determined by making a restriction map of each fragment (Fig. 1–31; see also Fig. 1–30). (A restriction

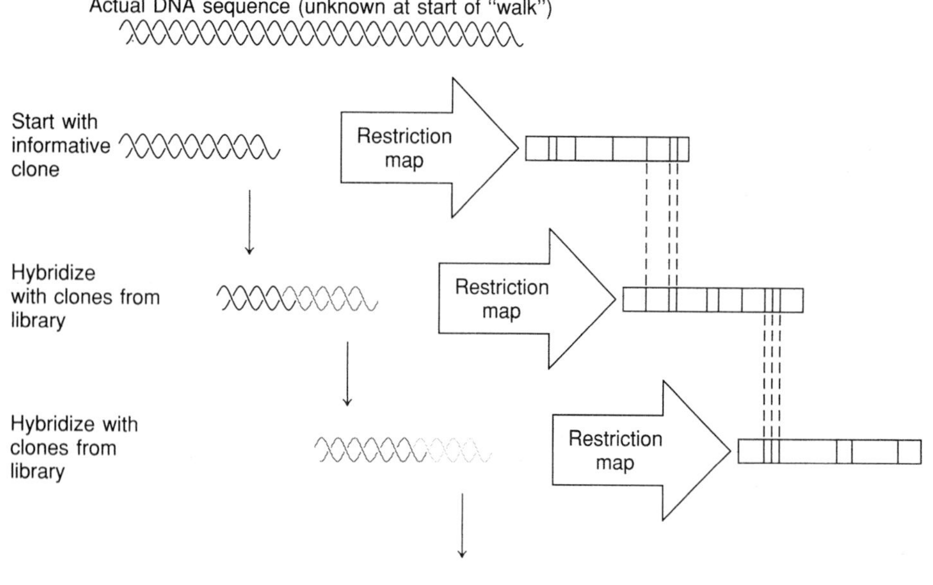

Figure 1–30. Chromosome "walking" is accomplished by successive hybridizations between overlapping genomic clones. The direction of the walk is always checked by restriction mapping of each newly hybridized clone (see Fig. 1–31).

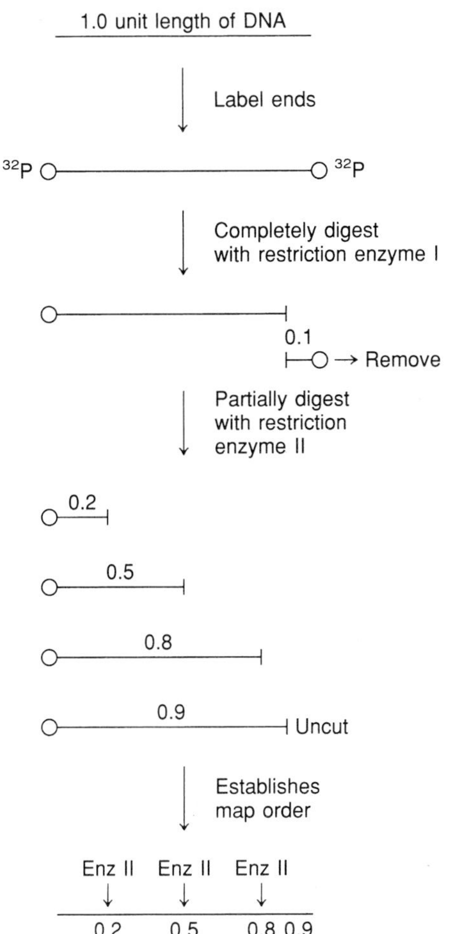

Figure 1–31. Restriction mapping of a specific DNA segment. DNA is labeled at its ends with ^{32}P, and fragments with one labeled terminus can be obtained by cutting off one end with an appropriate enzyme. The mapping procedure is performed with a second enzyme. Complete digestion with the second enzyme would produce only one labeled fragment (0- to 2-unit piece), but brief *partial* digestion in which the enzyme cuts the long piece of DNA in only one of several potential sites produces a labeled fragment for each restriction site. From the lengths of the labeled pieces, the positions of enzyme II restriction sites can be inferred (see Smith HO, Birnsteil M: Nucl Acids Res 1976; 3:2387–2399).

map is a linear array of sites on DNA cleaved by various restriction enzymes.) The map should contain the same fragments as one end of the first clone extended by new material. This process can be repeated indefinitely until the disease gene is found.

Although steady progress in mapping of disease phenotypes is being made, this process is, as expected, labor intensive even for autosomal dominant disorders in which large pedigrees are available. Most common human diseases and traits show complex inheritance in that the phenotype does not display classic mendelian dominant or recessive inheritance attributable to a single locus.

The efficiency of mapping disease phenotypes and hereditary traits (in preparation for chromosomal walking) using conventional linkage strategies is limited by two major steps: acquisition of appropriate study samples and genotyping with the use of genetic markers that span the genome. The first of these steps is often not fully appreciated by those working on the molecular aspects of the project but is a key to any disease-mapping effort. The process includes the identification of individuals and families with the disorder, accurate construction of pedigrees, accurate clinical evaluation to determine the phenotype of each individual, and proper handling of the DNA samples. The second step includes the entire process of genotyping, data entry, and linkage analysis. Because of these drawbacks, more mechanical methods are being developed (see next section), some of which are based on a subtraction-hybridization concept; genetic material from two individuals are mixed with subsequent amplification of unique sequences that differentiate the two individuals. Representational differential analysis and genomic mismatch scanning are still experimental and used largely with animal studies at the present time but may play a role in future genetic analysis (for reviews, see Nelson et al, 1993; Brown, 1995).

RNA Fingerprinting

RNA fingerprinting refers to a composite of several techniques that are designed to detect differences in gene expression between two genetic sources—whether two individuals (with and without a disease) or two tissues within the same individual (e.g., cancerous and noncancerous portions of a diseased organ). The goal is to identify a unique sequence or gene expression that is associated with specific diseases.

The basic idea is to compare pieces of mRNA between two cell populations. Therefore, step one is to obtain template RNA by reverse-transcribing mRNA. In the original description by Liang and Pardee (1992), reverse transcription was performed with an oligo (dT) primer with an AC 2 base anchor at the end (Fig. 1–32). Priming therefore occurs at the 5′ end of the poly (rA) tail and mainly in sequences that end 5′-UpG-poly (rA) $-3'$ with a selectivity approaching 1 of 12 polyadenylated RNAs. After reverse transcription and denaturation, an arbitrary primer of about 10 bases is selected, and PCR is performed on the resulting first strand of cDNA. PCR can now take place to generate a fingerprint of products that best match the primers and that are derived from the 3′ end of mRNAs and polyadenylated heterogeneous RNAs. This protocol has been dubbed *differential display* (Liang and Pardee, 1992).

Alternatively, an arbitrary primer can be used in the first step of reverse transcription to select regions internal to the RNA that have six to eight base matches with the 3′ end of the primer. This is followed by arbitrary priming of the resulting first strand of cDNA with the same or a different arbitrary primer and then PCR (see Fig. 1–32). This particular protocol samples anywhere in the RNA, including open reading frames. In addition, it can be used on RNAs that are not polyadenylated (such as bacterial RNAs).

If arbitrarily primed PCR fingerprinting of RNA is performed on samples derived from isogenic cells that have been subjected to different experimental treatments or have different developmental histories, differences in gene expression between samples can be detected. There are no meaningful relationships between the intensities of bands within a single lane on a gel, which are a function of match and abundance. However, the ratio between lanes is preserved for each sampled RNA, allowing differentially expressed

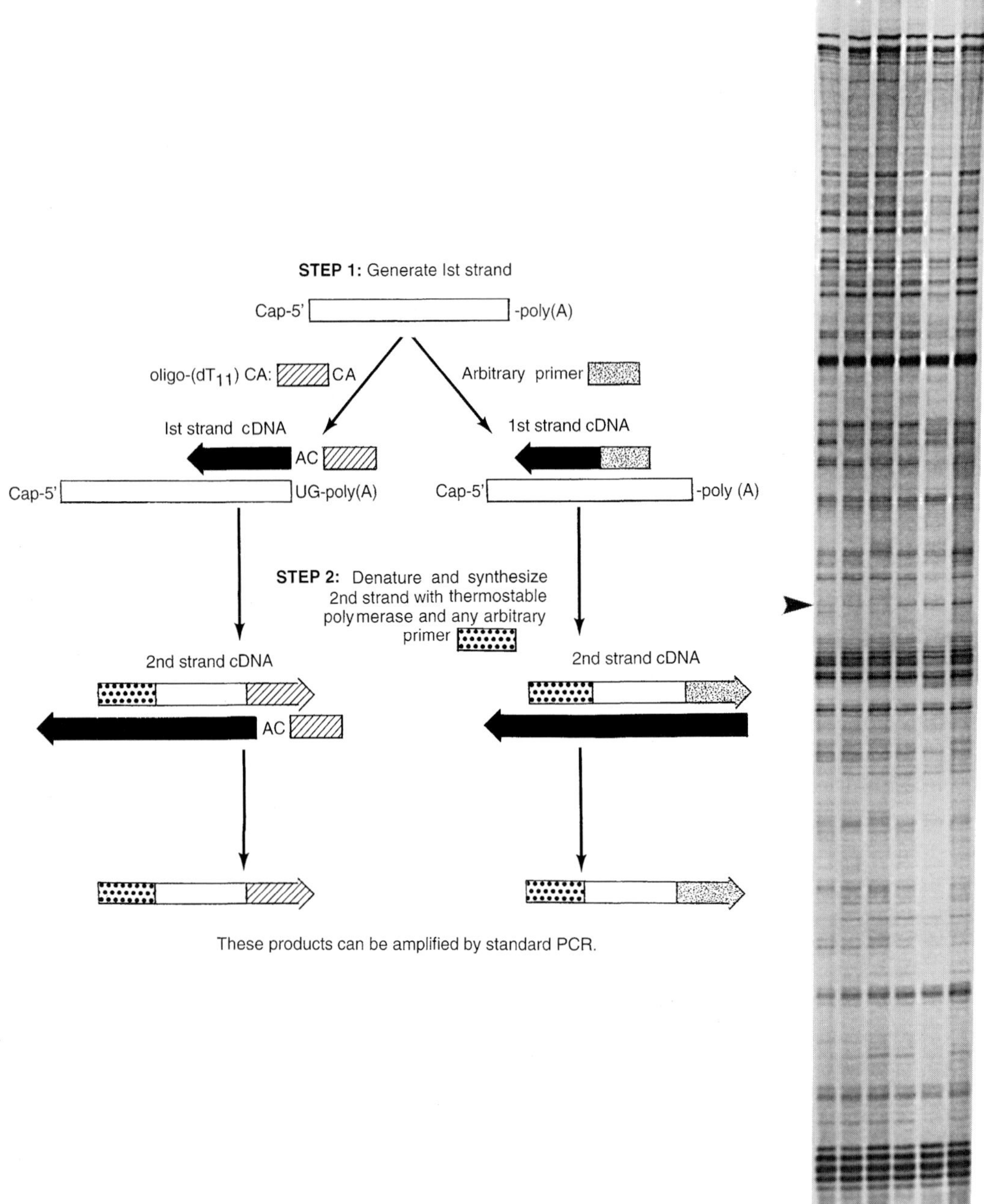

Figure 1–32. Outlines of two RNA fingerprinting strategies. *Left,* An oligo (dt) primer with a CpA-3′ anchor is used to generate the first strand of cDNA. *Right,* An arbitrary primer is used instead. In both cases, an arbitrary primer is then used to synthesize the second strand of cDNA. This second strand of cDNA can be amplified by PCR with the original primers. (Modified from McClelland M, Matthieu-Daude F, Welsh J: Trends Genet 1995; 11:242–246.) *Inset,* Actual differential display comparing RNA samples from the LNCaP-FRG prostate cancer cell line. The six lanes represent samples obtained from cell lines deprived of androgen for 0, 1, 10, 30, 97, and 121 hours. In this case an anchored oligo (dt) primer was used as the first step. The *arrow* marks the appearance of an RNA species according to androgen deprivation. (Photo courtesy of Dr. Lydia Averboukh, Boston.)

RNAs to be detected. One important limitation of RNA fingerprinting is that the probability of observing a product is not only a function of the best primer matches but also a function of the abundance of each RNA. Thus there is good reason to believe that rare RNAs will be under-represented among the visible products on the gel.

Viral Transfection and Gene Therapy

Probably the most logical conclusion for much of genetic research is the hope of gene therapy, a concept based on the assumption that definitive treatment for genetic disease should be possible by directing treatment to the site of the defect itself within the genome (Culliton, 1990).

There are two basic strategies for gene therapy: **gene replacement** and **gene augmentation**. Gene replacement is the more ideal of the two. In what is called *homologous recombination,* the healthy or "therapeutic" gene would replace the damaged copy exactly. The theoretical advantage of this approach is that the introduced gene would function correctly; in addition, there would be a reduced likelihood that random insertion would activate a quiescent oncogene or inactivate a cancer suppressor. This approach, however, is fraught with problems relating to control of fate of the DNA introduced into cells. For every gene spliced into the correct place, more than 1000 fit randomly into the genome.

More established than gene replacement are several techniques of gene augmentation, in which a healthy gene is simply added to the genome without replacement of the defective gene. This approach is helpful especially when a genetic derangement results in little or no production of a protein (each gene encodes a single protein); the approach, however, would not be helpful when a mutated or damaged gene yields overproduction of a protein or synthesis of a destructive substance (e.g., sickle-cell anemia). In that case, therapy would have to include delivery of both a healthy gene and one capable of inactivating the mutated version. At present, gene augmentation strategy requires removal of cells from patients, followed by the introduction of the therapeutic gene into those cells and then reinfusion of the altered cells back into the patient. Nontargeted delivery of genes into cells can be accomplished by chemical or physical means (**transfection**) or by virus (**transduction**). In chemical approaches, many copies of the DNA carrying the healthy gene are mixed with a charged substance, usually calcium phosphate, diethylaminoethyl dextran, or certain lipids. The mixture is then added to the recipient cells. The chemical disturbs the cell membrane and transports the DNA into the interior of the cells. The procedure is simple but with poor efficiency: Usually only 1 cell in 1000 to 100,000 integrates the gene of interest into its genome. Physical methods include microinjection (Capecchi, 1980); this technique can be extremely efficient but tedious. Another technique requires exposure of cells to rapid pulses of high voltage current (electroporation) (Capecchi, 1980). The shock renders cells permeable to DNA in the surrounding medium, but it can also severely damage them.

The final strategy capitalizes on the native ability of viruses to enter cells and to infect virtually every cell in the target population (Gluzman and Hughes, 1988). Viruses can be grouped according to whether their genetic material is RNA or DNA. The first viruses used as gene transfer vectors of mammalian cells were transforming DNA viruses. Because their capacity for foreign sequences was found to be small, other vector systems were developed.

The most useful and popular model vectors for the efficient introduction of foreign genes into target mammalian cells have been derived from murine and avian retroviruses. Retroviruses convert their RNA to DNA in infected cells and then insert the DNA into a chromosome. The integrated DNA (the provirus) then directs the synthesis of viral proteins. Retroviruses can hold more foreign genetic material than can some DNA viruses. They can also infect a broad spectrum of species and cell types. Retroviruses do have drawbacks, however. For example, they can integrate only into cells that are dividing (therefore bypassing cells such as mature neurons).

It is also possible for retroviruses to cause cancer, perhaps through activation of a quiescent oncogene or inactivation of a suppressor gene. The likelihood of this happening seems to be low if the viral vectors are prevented from reproducing. This is accomplished with a clever strategy (Fig. 1–33)**: Retroviral RNA is made by replacing the three major genes (*gag*, *pol*, and *env*, which specify proteins of the viral core, the enzyme reverse transcriptase [allowing the production of viral DNA from RNA], and constituents of the coat of the virus, respectively) with the therapeutic gene. This modified virus is inserted into a packaging cell. The viral DNA directs the synthesis of viral RNA, but lacking viral "housekeeping," genes cannot give rise to proteins needed to package RNA into particles for delivery to other cells. The missing proteins are supplied by a "helper" provirus from which the *psi* region has been deleted. *psi* is critical for the inclusion of RNA in viral particles. Without it, no virus-carrying "helper" RNA can form. The particles that escape the cell then carry therapeutic RNA and no viral genes. They can enter other cells and splice the therapeutic gene into cellular DNA, but they cannot reproduce.**

One type of alternative to retroviruses is adenoviruses, which offer comparative advantages as well as disadvantages. First, they readily infect nondividing cells, unlike retroviruses. Second, they remain extrachromosomal, which reduces the chance of disrupting the cellular genome. However, a disadvantage of the adenovirus vector is that they infect all cells, including the germ line, and thus could affect subsequent generations. Another disadvantage is that they are not as defective as retroviruses and could more readily yield infectious viruses in the body.

The viral vector approach has many therapeutic uses. Probably the most important with urologic relevance involves treatment of cancer. The loss of cancer suppressor genes, as described for kidney cancer (Koufos et al, 1984; Orkin et al, 1984; Zbar et al, 1987; Rukstalis et al, 1989; Aso et al, 1995; Duan et al, 1995; Kibel et al, 1995), bladder cancer (Fearon et al, 1985; Carter et al, 1990), and testis cancer (Rukstalis et al, 1989), provides a perfect setting. These cancers arise in association with inactivation (or alteration) of both alleles of a wild type (normal) gene. Therefore, the cancer phenotype might be suppressed or possibly reversed by restoring functional expression of the wild type gene. This, in fact, has already been done in an animal

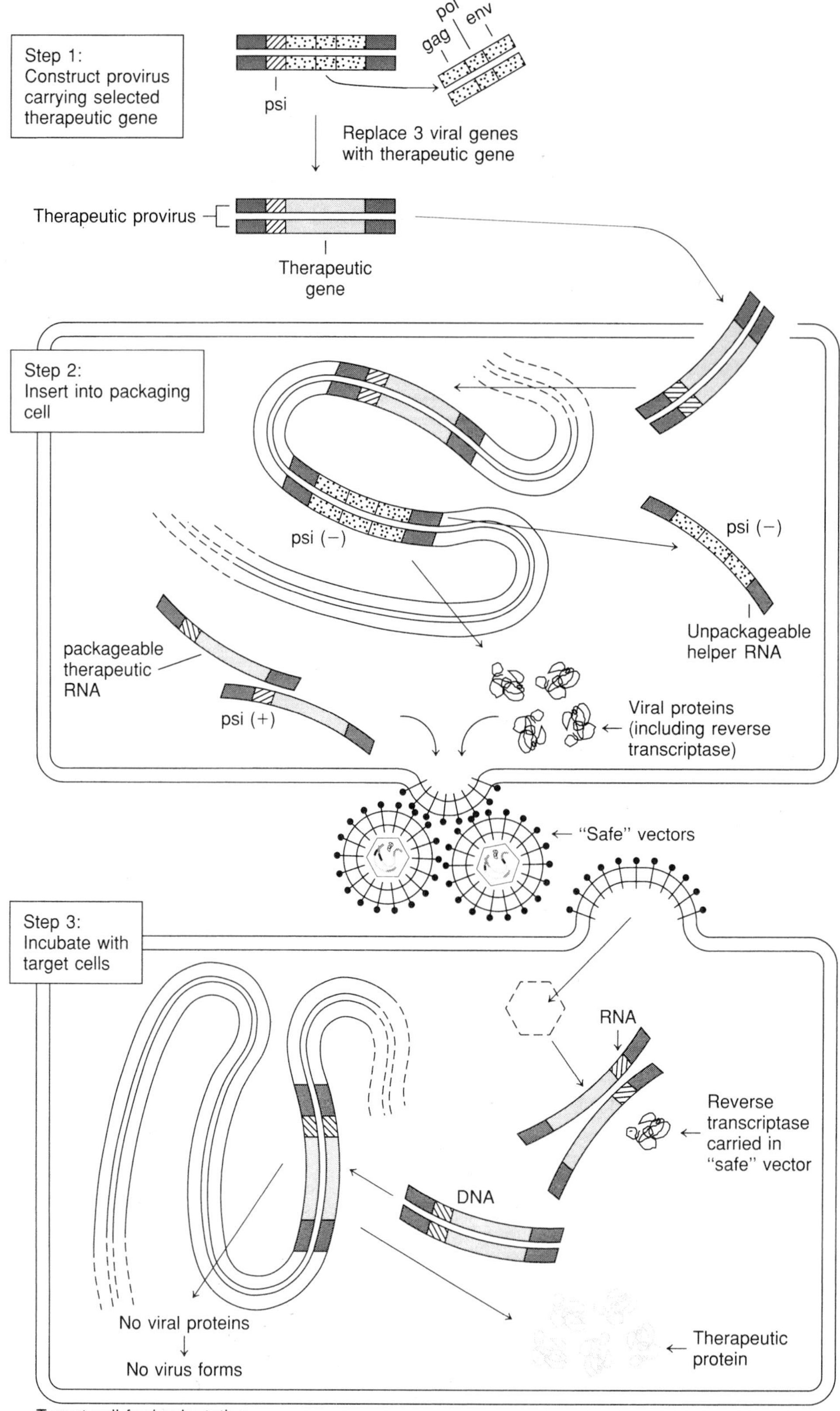

Figure 1–33. Gene therapy may use retroviral vectors to deliver therapeutic genes. In such case, viruses are made in which viral genes (*gag, pol,* and *env,* specifying proteins of the viral core, the enzyme reverse transcriptase, and constituents of the coat, respectively, all of which are necessary for proper packaging of RNA into particles for delivery to other cells) are removed and a therapeutic gene is substituted. The virus is then inserted into a packaging cell. Here, the defective "therapeutic virus" is helped to replicate and repackage with the aid of a "helper" virus, which "lends" the missing viral protein products to the therapeutic virus. The helper virus, however, is also defective because the *psi* region is deleted (necessary for inclusion of RNA into viral particles). It is assumed that the helper virus will not leave the cell. The particles that escape the cell then carry therapeutic RNA and no viral genes. They can enter other cells and splice the therapeutic gene in the cellular DNA, but they cannot reproduce.

model of Wilms' tumor (Weissman et al, 1987) as well as prostate cancer (Bookstein et al, 1990).

Inactivation of dominantly acting oncogenes is conceptually more difficult but may be possible by site-specific target mutagenesis. Several methods have been described for expression of toxin genes in cells (Palmitter et al, 1987; Borrelli et al, 1988). In principle, this would permit the targeted destruction of tumor cells if unerringly specific delivery can be accomplished reproducibly. The potential for modulating the expression of oncogenes and other genes with the use of antisense oligonucleotides suggests another approach to the suppression of the cancer phenotype (Lichenstein, 1988; Weintraub, 1990). The basic concept behind it is quite simple: Antisense RNA or DNA molecules (e.g., oligonucleotides with sequences that are **complementary** to the target) are made and thereby bind specifically with the targeted gene's RNA message, thereby inactivating it. Although the mechanism involved in activation of gene expression by antisense sequences is not thoroughly understood, it is probably necessary in order to deliver large or high concentrations of antisense information to compete either with efficient gene transcription or with the function of transcription factors. Eventually, however, therapy will be directed at correction of abnormal transcriptional elements that are responsible for deregulation. The obvious problems now are identification of those regulatory elements and, once they are identified, tissue-specific targeting. Despite potential technical difficulties and problems, this method has been used to inactivate plant enzymes, with resultant change in color (Vander Krol et al, 1988); in other experiments, antisense *c-raf* transfected Scl-20B squamous cell carcinoma cell lines were found to be less tumorigenic and more radiosensitive in nude mice (Kasid et al, 1989).

PROTEIN KINASES AND PHOSPHATASES

The fundamental information of a cell may be encoded by the DNA and RNA molecules, but the multitude of proteins produced within that cell enact and control the intricate array of metabolic functions chronicled in the genetic code. Each aspect of an individual cell's interaction with its external environment, as well as the routine housekeeping chores, appears to involve a myriad of proteins. Often the function of any individual protein is difficult to discern because of the redundancy of the various mechanisms by which a cell accomplishes its metabolic ends. Multiple proteins may be involved in signaling pathways that overlap in function, or a single protein may serve numerous functions without apparent modification. For example, growth factors such as epidermal growth factor (EGF) and platelet-derived growth factor (PDGF) may stimulate the same cell to replicate in one circumstance but to differentiate in another environment. However, the cellular receptors to which the ligands bind are similar in each case. The method by which the cell recognizes the distinctly different intention of the ligand binding is uncertain but seems to involve a wide array of second-messenger proteins. The challenge of maintaining order in such a potentially chaotic milieu is met with remarkably similar strategies by single-cell organisms as well as by complex multicellular higher vertebrates. This process of organization requires that proteins communicate in some manner so that each protein will be active when its function is required and quiescent when it is no longer necessary.

The communication between individual proteins appears to be based fundamentally on post-translational modifications. The function of one protein may be altered through conformational changes caused by the binding of another regulatory protein. Other mechanisms may include the binding of a cofactor, such as calcium or magnesium, without which the protein would not function. **Perhaps the most common cellular mechanism for the functional control of individual proteins is the addition or removal of phosphate groups on specific amino acids. This process is called *protein phosphorylation* and is the major control mechanism in signal transduction and cell cycle pathways. In fact, exploitation of this mechanism is so widespread in eukaryotic cells that it is often assumed that any protein implicated in a metabolic sequence is modified by phosphorylation.**

When a protein is modified through phosphorylation, the phosphate residues are most often found on three amino acids: serine, threonine, and tyrosine (Ludlow and Nelson, 1995). The phosphorylated state of any protein appears to be a dynamic one wherein phosphate groups are added and removed rapidly. The proteins that add phosphate groups to other proteins (and occasionally to themselves) are called **protein kinases**. Those proteins that then remove the phosphate moiety are named **protein phosphatases**. In addition, proteins such as the EGF receptor possess the ability to phosphorylate themselves during activation (Sunada et al, 1990).

A long-held scientific assumption has been that the 2000 or more protein kinases are activated only when necessary and are therefore tightly regulated. In contrast, protein phosphatases, which are currently fewer in number than the kinases, were thought to be constitutively activated. These proteins were believed to be always turned on so that signals from the protein kinases could be quickly attenuated (Hunter, 1995). Current research information has altered those assumptions by demonstrating that both protein kinases and protein phosphatases are regulated through phosphorylation. For example, a singularly important kinase family, protein kinase C, may be activated by proteolytic cleavage and phosphorylation. The catalytic function of the several members of this family appears to be activated by the addition of phosphate groups to one or all of three threonines (Cazaubon and Parker, 1993). In turn, the activated protein kinase C phosphorylates proteins such as the insulin receptor (Ahn et al, 1993) and cyclic adenosine monophosphate (cAMP)–dependent protein kinase (PKA) (Stabel, 1994). Interestingly, PKA has been shown to phosphorylate the protein phosphatase type 2A (PP2A), which results in an alteration in the substrate specificity of PP2A (Usui et al, 1991). This form of crosstalk provides for exquisite control of function.

For a protein's function to be regulated by phosphorylation, the activities of the protein kinase(s) and protein phosphatase(s) that act on a particular amino acid site in that protein must be in balance. If not, the protein would be either completely phosphorylated or completely dephosphorylated. A cell employs several methods in order to achieve such control of phosphorylation. Kinases

and phosphatases exhibit amino acid specificity in such a way that one group acts on tyrosine, whereas a second group concentrates on serine and threonine. The critical role of protein tyrosine kinases and protein tyrosine phosphatases has been the subject of extensive reviews (Sun and Tonks, 1994). In general, intrinsic protein tyrosine phosphatase activity exceeds that of the protein tyrosine kinases by about two or three orders of magnitude (Hunter, 1995). This differential function can account for the low level of phosphotyrosine (pTyr) in cells and the transient nature of most pTyr responses to stimuli. However, if the protein tyrosine kinase signal pathways are to work effectively the activity of the protein tyrosine phosphatases must be regulated. Additional cellular mechanisms for control of protein tyrosine phosphatase function include subcellular localization and specific phosphorylation on tyrosine or serine and threonine.

Protein serine/threonine kinases and phosphatases are also intimately involved in the cellular control mechanisms. Investigations, begun in the 1950s, into the process of glycogen metabolism illustrate the regulatory role of specific phosphorylation. The requirement for the metabolism of glycogen by a muscle cell stimulates a process of protein phosphorylation. The placement of a phosphate group on glycogen synthase causes inactivation of glycogen synthesis, whereas another enzyme, phosphorylase, is turned on (Brautigan, 1995). Phosphorylase, which catalyzes the key step in the breakdown of muscle glycogen, exists in two forms. The active form of the enzyme is produced by phosphorylation of the inactive protein. The phosphorylase is returned to the inactive state through the subsequent action of a phosphatase. Initially, the phosphatases that remove the phosphate moiety were thought to be constitutively active. However, it has been shown that **phosphorylase phosphatase** may be inhibited by other proteins called inhibitor-1 and inhibitor-2 and is controlled by specific subcellular localization (Hubbard and Cohen, 1993).

SIGNAL TRANSDUCTION

Every individual cell must interact with the external environment. Extracellular messages regarding the availability of food or signals for growth and differentiation must be received at the cell membrane and transduced to the nucleus, where the proper response is encoded in the DNA. The physiologic mechanism by which information from external stimuli is carried to the nucleus is called **signal transduction**. Frequently, the external message arrives in the form of growth factors, such as EGF or PDGF, for which specific transmembrane receptors function as cellular antennae. Binding of the ligand to the receptor on the surface of the cell initiates a complex sequence of intracellular events that culminates ultimately in an increase in transcription and translation. At any given moment, each cell is exposed to an array of external stimuli. Many of these signals bombard the membrane simultaneously. The process by which a cell deciphers this information and arranges an appropriate response is not entirely understood. However, several of the signaling pathways have been identified. In fact, only recently have a sufficient number of proteins been identified so that scientists now have a continuous map from the cell membrane to the nucleus.

Adenylyl Cyclase, cAMP, and G Proteins

The seminal contributions of Rall and Sutherland (1961) established the concept of intracellular second messengers in the late 1950s with the discovery of 3′:5′ cyclic phosphate (cAMP). Stimulation of a cell through an adrenergic receptor results in an amplified production of **cAMP** molecules via the activity of an enzyme called **adenylyl cyclase.** The signal is then attenuated through the activity of another enzyme called phosphodiesterase, which breaks down cAMP. These observations were extended with the observation that binding of an adrenergic agonist was not sufficient to stimulate adenylyl cyclase but required the presence of guanosine triphosphate (GTP) in the reaction mixture (Gilman, 1989). More recent research has demonstrated the existence of guanine nucleotide binding regulatory proteins. These proteins were discovered by Alfred G. Gilman and Martin Rodbell, for which they were awarded the 1994 Nobel Prize in medicine, and are simply called **G proteins** (Hall, 1990).

The G protein family constitutes a group of proteins which bind to guanosine diphosphate (GDP) or GTP and initiate signal transduction from the cell membrane. These proteins are associated with the cell membrane and exist in two interconvertible forms. The inactive G protein is bound to GDP, whereas the active form is tightly attached to GTP. Although these types of proteins are involved in many signaling pathways, they were originally identified as a part of the cAMP system and are further reviewed in this section. The best recognized member of the G protein family is the *Ras* proto-oncogene.

The G proteins exist as a heterotrimer that is composed of three subunits labeled α, β, and γ. The protein complex is intimately associated with the cell membrane, where it communicates with specific receptors (Clapham, 1993). The regulatory pathway of G protein signal transduction is illustrated in Figure 1–34. When GDP is bound to the α subunit, that subunit associates with the βγ subunit to form an inactive G protein, which binds to a receptor. After ligand binding by a receptor such as the adrenocorticotropin hormone (ACTH) receptor or the adrenergic receptors, the receptor becomes activated through either a conformational change or specific phosphorylation. The relationship between the receptor and the receptor-associated G protein is subsequently altered, resulting in a G protein conformational change. The inactive form releases the bound GDP molecule, which is then replaced by a GTP molecule, resulting in activation of a subunit that dissociates from βγ (Neer and Clapham, 1988). The now free αβγ subunits each further activate target effectors such as adenylyl cyclase. The now functional enzyme produces thousands of cAMP molecules, thereby amplifying the original receptor signal.

For every action, there must be an opposite reaction of equal magnitude. This caveat holds true for G protein mediated signaling. The activated α subunit possesses intrinsic GTPase activity, which results in eventual hydrolysis of the GTP to GDP and spontaneous inactivation of the G protein

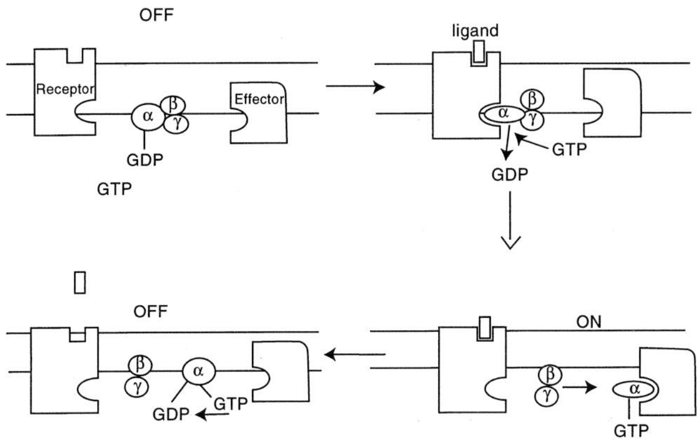

Figure 1–34. The four frames depict the mechanism of activation of the heterotrimeric **G-proteins**. In the nonfunctional state, identified as "off," the alpha subunit is bound to guanosine diphosphate (GDP) and associates with the beta-gamma subunits. The activation of a cell surface receptor by ligand binding causes a conformational change in its juxtaposed G-protein. The alpha subunit releases GDP and binds guanosine triphosphate (GTP). This alteration results in the separation of the alpha subunit from the beta-gamma complex. The alpha polypeptide, as well as the beta-gamma complex, is then capable of activating downstream effector proteins within the cell membrane. The signal is attenuated when the intrinsic GTPase activity of the alpha subunit hydrolyzes GTP to GDP. The G-protein complex then reassociates and is ready for the next signal.

cascade (Neer, 1995). The G protein subunits reassociate and prime the system for the next external signal.

Both the $\alpha\beta\gamma$ subunits appear to modulate the function of adenylyl cyclase in a positive and negative manner. The pattern of regulation appears to be exquisitely specific to the isoform of G protein and adenylyl cyclase involved (Tang and Gilman, 1991). This emphasizes the continuing theme of cellular signal transduction: the multiple layers of control put in place by the cell. Once activated, adenylyl cyclase synthesizes cAMP, which then diffuses as a second messenger to propagate the initial receptor signal. The cAMP molecule conveys its message by impacting on the next protein in the signaling pathway, PKA. The action of cAMP occurs primarily through the activation of the tetrameric (a protein composed of two regulatory R subunits and two catalytic C subunits) PKA holoenzyme. The R subunit binds to cAMP and stimulates the release of the two C subunits that directly mediate the majority of cAMP actions (Beebe, 1994). PKA exists as multiple isoforms, each with potentially different specificity. Because cAMP exhibits various effects on cells such as the stimulation of glycogen metabolism, as well as the positive or negative regulation of growth and differentiation, the list of potential effector proteins altered by PKA phosphorylation is extensive. One particularly important protein, the cAMP regulatory element binding protein (CREB) (Yamamoto et al, 1988), is a transcriptional regulator that binds to the cAMP regulatory element in the promoter of cAMP-responsive genes. The function of CREB is regulated by the now mundane mechanism of phosphorylation by PKA. The stimulation of transcription of specific growth-stimulating or growth-inhibiting genes by CREB completes the signaling pathway that began at the cell membrane when a ligand bound to its cognate receptor.

Inositol Lipids Signaling Pathways

Inositol lipids such as **inositol 1,4,5-triphosphate** (IP_3) and **diacylglycerol (DG)** compete with cAMP for recognition from medical students as biochemical second messengers. In fact, the lipid signaling pathway via the involvement of protein kinase C (PKC) and calcium may well be a system more frequently employed than that of cAMP. What is of particular interest about this pathway is the initial bifurcation into two separate systems. Cell surface binding of growth factors such as PDGF and EGF alter the conformation of their respective receptors (PDGFr and EGFr) and ultimately activate the inositol signaling cascade through one of two potential mechanisms. The first involves the ever-present G proteins, whereas the second is a less understood direct effect. These separate receptor mechanisms activate phospholipase C, which then hydrolyzes the lipid precursor phosphatidylinositol 1,4,5-triphosphate to give both IP_3 and diacylglycerol.

It is at this point that the signaling pathways diverge as the water-soluble IP_3 diffuses into the cytoplasm and binds to an intracellular IP_3 receptor, leading to the release of stored calcium from the endoplasmic reticulum (Berridge, 1993). On the other hand, the neutral diacylglycerol molecule remains in contact with the cell membrane, where it activates protein kinase C (Berridge, 1989). Another important and unique aspect of this signaling pathway is that the two second messengers are released by metabolism of phosphatidylinositol, which is a common component of the lipid layer in the cell membrane. The phosphatidylinositol is phosphorylated by a specific kinase to give rise to phosphatidylinositol 1,4,5-triphosphate, which is the direct parent of IP_3 and diacylglycerol. The casual observer can imagine that with an abundant source of second messengers and a divergent pathway, the inositol lipid signal transduction cascade would be expected to participate in numerous cell processes. The simplified generation of IP_3 and diacylglycerol is illustrated in Figure 1–35. The remainder of this section briefly reviews the role of calcium release and protein kinase C.

The activation of a large family of enzymes collectively known as protein kinase C is accomplished by diacylglycerol often in concert with calcium (Divecha and Irvine, 1995). The exact function of each isoform of protein kinase C is difficult to discern in vitro because the functions overlap. Suffice it to say that the presence of multiple forms of this important kinase provides another layer of substrate specificity to the signal transduction pathway. There is compelling evidence for a role for protein kinase C activity in the release of cellular constituents from endocrine and exocrine cells such as growth hormone, testosterone, and neurotransmitters, as well as modulation of cellular proliferation and differentiation (Nishizuka, 1989). The action of protein kinase C is manifested through phosphorylation of cytoplasmic proteins, as well as nuclear proteins such as *c-fos* and *c-jun* (Boyle et al, 1991). Interestingly, protein kinase C activation appears to increase the activity of both *c-fos* and *c-jun*, which are the two main components of the important

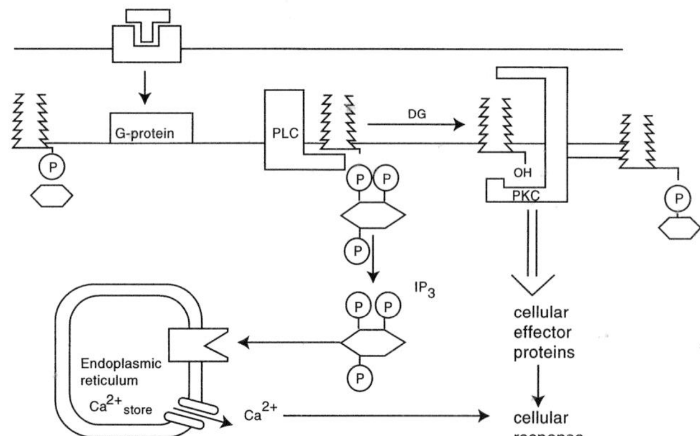

Figure 1–35. The phospholipid signaling system is initiated by the ligand binding of a cell surface receptor communicated through a membrane-bound G-protein. The enzyme **phospholipase C** (PLC) is stimulated to act upon a common membrane constituent called phosphatidylinositol 3,4,5-triphosphate to produce **diacylglycerol** (DG) and **inositol 1,4,5-triphosphate** (IP_3). The DG diffuses within the cellular membrane to activate proteins such as protein kinase C (PKC). Meanwhile, the IP_3 moves into the cytoplasm and binds to a receptor on the surface of the endoplasmic reticulum. The activation of the IP_3 receptor results in the release of sequestered calcium stores.

transcription factor AP-1. Again, the identification of a connection to the nucleus completes the pathway from the cell surface to the DNA molecule.

The divalent calcium molecule is of central importance to cellular metabolism. In fact, its role in metabolism is so far-reaching that the cell expends considerable energy to limit its concentration within the cytoplasm. The cellular requirement to exclude Ca^{2+} from the cytoplasm is likely related to the fact that calcium precipitates phosphate, the energy currency of the cell (Clapham, 1995). Proteins directly bind calcium through interactions with the oxygen atoms on the amino acids. Binding of Ca^{2+} apparently leads to a protein conformational change and activation or inhibition of function. Calcium-specific binding proteins exist in high concentrations in the cell cytoplasm, which serves as a buffer or effector during signal transduction–mediated calcium release. Table 1–5 provides examples of the proteins modulated through calcium binding. One such protein, calmodulin, binds calcium, thereby undergoing a resultant conformational change. The now activated calmodulin modulates the activity of other proteins in the pathway of Ca^{2+} signaling (Clapham, 1995). In view of the significant biologic function of calcium, the cell provides mechanisms to limit the spread of the released Ca^{2+} within the cytoplasm. A high concentration of buffer proteins, such as calsequestrin, maintains calcium as an extremely localized second messenger. In addition, when not required for signaling, the excess calcium is sequestered within the endoplasmic reticulum (Ross et al, 1989).

Table 1–5. CALCIUM-REGULATED PROTEINS

Protein	Protein Function
Troponin C	Modulation of muscle contraction
Caldesmon	Modulation of muscle contraction
Calmodulin	Regulation of protein kinases
Calretinin	Activator of guanylyl cyclase
Phospholipase C	Generates IP_3 and DG
Protein kinase C	Ubiquitous protein kinase
IP_3 receptor	Effector of intracellular Ca^{2+} release
α Actinin	Actin-bundling protein
Gelsolin	Actin-severing protein
Villin	Actin organizer
Calbindin	Ca^{2+} buffer protein
Calsequestrin	Ca^{2+} buffer protein

IP_3, inositol 1,4,5-triphosphate; DG, diacylglycerol.

The excess cytoplasmic calcium that is required for signal transduction is obtained from either intracellular or extracellular sources. The inositol signaling pathway initiates the release of calcium through the process of IP_3 binding to a specific receptor located on the cell membrane and on the endoplasmic reticulum (Berridge, 1989). This receptor opens a Ca^{2+} channel through which Ca^{2+} leaks into the cytoplasm (Merritt and Rink, 1987). Of importance is that whereas previously discussed signaling pathways exerted the majority of impact on effector proteins within the nucleus, this calcium-based system is capable of altering protein function directly within the cytoplasm without initiating transcription. The calcium-dependent kinases and phosphatases are also capable of phosphorylating downstream proteins such as CREB and therefore continuing the signal pathway to the nucleus (Sheng et al, 1991).

Nuclear Hormone Receptors

No discussion of signal transduction would be complete without a mention of the family of nuclear hormone receptors. These proteins are located within the cell cytoplasm, as opposed to being linked to the cell membrane, and bind steroid ligands that are capable of diffusing into the cell. The family includes receptors for glucocorticoids, estrogen, androgen, thyroid hormone, and retinoic acid. The cytoplasmic receptor binds to its respective ligand and translocates to the nucleus, where the receptor-ligand complex acts as a transcriptional regulator. The steroid receptor–mediated induction of gene expression is regulated by the presence and concentration of the ligand (Beato, 1989). Steroid binding results in a wide variety of cellular effects that depend on the cell type and receptor complex involved. These actions range from the stimulation of transcription in prostate epithelium via the androgen receptor to inhibition of gene expression by the glucocorticoid receptor in the pituitary gland (Drouin et al, 1989). In general, this system represents another mechanism for cellular signaling in response to external stimulation. It is important to realize that the pathway of steroid hormone signaling does not function autonomously but rather interacts with the other cell surface–mediated signaling cascades to modulate the cellular activities (Brass et al, 1995).

FUTURE APPLICATIONS OF MOLECULAR BIOLOGY TECHNIQUES

The extraordinary opportunity to isolate and study individual genes and proteins has provided scientists with a much greater understanding of normal cellular physiology. The application of these molecular biologic techniques to disease states such as cancer likewise provides an opportunity for improvements in diagnosis and treatment. This final section briefly identifies several fertile areas for future development.

Molecular Diagnostics

The signature DNA sequence of a neoplastic cell or an infectious bacterial organism may be detected with molecular techniques such as in situ hybridization, Southern blotting, or PCR. The potential for improvement in diagnostic or prognostic information from such an application of sensitive laboratory procedures has opened up the field of molecular pathology (Naber, 1994a).

These techniques have already proved useful in the detection of viral or bacterial organisms in clinical samples. In particular, viral organisms or slow-growing bacterial species such as mycobacteria are identified more rapidly and with improved accuracy in comparison with traditional culture methods. In situ hybridization has been used to identify human papillomavirus subtypes in genital lesions and cytomegalovirus in tissues from immunocompromised hosts. The PCR is even more sensitive and can detect as few as a single organism in samples even if the specimen is poorly preserved. The ability to detect fastidious organisms or to work with suboptimal clinical samples has certain therapeutic advantages. For example, the rapid identification of infectious agents such as mycobacteria can expedite appropriate antibiotic therapy. Similar opportunities in genitourinary infections need to be explored in the future.

Neoplastic cells acquire DNA alterations that are distinct from the normal host cells and may correlate with specific malignant characteristics. The detection of specific genetic abnormalities within a neoplasm may provide a rapid method for diagnosis, as well as a marker for progression (Naber, 1994b). Techniques such as PCR are capable of detecting minute genetic changes in specific genes. The identification of mutations in important genes such as *p53* has been shown to offer diagnostic and prognostic information in neoplasms of the bladder (Sidransky et al, 1991). Interestingly, alterations in *p53* control of apoptosis appear to modulate the cytotoxicity of antineoplastic treatments such as ionizing radiation and chemotherapy (Lowe et al, 1993). Therefore, a potential application of PCR would be to identify cancers that would be unlikely to respond to a particular treatment. This would allow physicians to customize therapy for an individual patient.

Role of Transgenic Models in Treatment Discovery

Transgenic animal technology and the manipulation of germ line DNA for the creation of an experimental animal with a specific gene mutation provide a valuable method for evaluating treatments. The development of murine models with alterations in signal transduction proteins or tumor suppressor genes has already provided useful pathophysiologic information (Viney, 1995). The mice in oncogenic models develop heritable neoplasms in a wide range of tissues; these neoplasms demonstrate predictable patterns of growth and metastasis (Thomas and Balkwill, 1995). The animals represent a model that approximates the ideal investigational system for cancer therapy. The lesions more closely resemble human neoplasms with a natural history that includes local progression and metastases. Of importance is that the lesions develop within an immunocompetent host.

However, investigations into novel therapeutic agents have been limited despite the apparent advantages of a transgenic model for cancer. Certain disadvantages of the murine transgenic model appear to reduce its role in therapeutic research. The primary disadvantage is the wastage of mice. Many neoplasms arise only in one sex and in only a percentage of the animals of that sex. In addition, the genetic background of the animal may affect the tumor type and possibly the response to therapy. Furthermore, the overexpression of the transgene (or the absence of expression in a knockout model) may inhibit the response of the neoplasm to a candidate therapeutic agent. These scientific and economic limitations must be overcome in the future if the oncogenic transgenic murine model is to replace the existing conventional models.

The ability to selectively modulate the expression and function of a gene product in animals is also capable of creating models of benign diseases. For example, targeted germ line alterations in the murine myogenin gene have been found to alter embryologic muscular development. The affected animals survive in utero but die shortly after birth (Hasty et al, 1993). This particular model provides an opportunity to examine embryologic muscular development. However, variations of this model may approximate the human condition of muscular dystrophy and perhaps urologic conditions such as prune-belly syndrome. If such a model could be developed, therapeutic approaches such as fetal intervention or gene therapy could be examined.

Gene Therapy

If future benefit can be predicted by present publicity, the potential of gene therapy approaches to human disease is unparalleled. The development of clinical gene therapy protocols has been exuberant. The first federally approved gene therapy protocol, begun in September 1990, focused on treatment of adenosine deaminase (ADA) deficiency. This rare genetic disorder results in an accumulation of high levels of 2′-deoxyadenosine in the circulation, which is toxic to lymphoid cells and causes a severe immunodeficiency syndrome. Patients have received infusions of their own cells transfected with the gene for ADA with significant success (Miller, 1992). Those initial investigations have been followed with numerous clinical trials of gene marking or gene therapy approaches in diseases ranging from factor IX deficiency to cancer (Anderson, 1992).

The fundamental tenet of any gene therapy protocol is the

transfer of non-native DNA to a patient. As in the case of ADA deficiency, the disease is secondary to a specific alteration in the native DNA molecule. In essence, the altered native function is replaced. Additional creative applications of DNA transfer technology include treatments for cancer and atherosclerosis. In these circumstances, the specific genetic alteration responsible for the disorder may be unknown, and the intention of therapy is to kill the cells. This cytoreductive intention may be accomplished through modification of the host immune system with cytokine gene-induced tumor vaccines or the transfer of drug susceptibility genes (Sanda and Simons, 1994).

The majority of gene therapy protocols remain in the infant stage of preclinical testing. Gene delivery systems must be improved so that the "take" of the transgene is increased while at the same time the potential for collateral injury to normal cells is reduced (Kasahara et al, 1994). In addition, many governmental, regulatory, and economic hurdles must be cleared before a particular vector is available for unrestricted clinical use. Despite this reality, the burgeoning field of gene therapy holds much promise for the future.

REFERENCES

Ahn J, Donner DB, Rosen OM: Interaction of the human insulin receptor tyrosine kinase from the baculovirus expression system with protein kinase C in a cell free system. J Biol Chem 1993; 268:7571–7576.

Anderson WF: Human gene therapy. Science 1992; 256:808–813.

Arents G, Burlingame RW, Wang BW, et al: The nucleosomal core histine octomer at 3.1 Å resolution: A tripartite protein assembly and a left handed superhelix. Proc Natl Acad Sci USA 1991; 88:10148–10152.

Aso T, Lane W, Conaway J, Conaway R: Elongin (SIII): A multisubunit regulator of elongation by RNA polymerase II. Science 1995; 269:1439–1443.

Augustin S, Müller MW, Schweyen RJ: Reverse self splicing group II intron RNAs in vitro. Nature 1990; 343:383–386.

Beato M: Gene regulation by steroid hormones. Cell 1989; 56:335–344.

Beebe SJ: The cAMP-dependent protein kinases and cAMP signal transduction. Semin Can Biol 1994; 5:285–294.

Bender W, Spierer P, Hogness D: Chromosome walking and jumping to isolate DNA from *ace* and *rosy* loci and the bithorax complex in *Drosophila melanogaster.* J Mol Biol 1983; 168:17–33.

Berridge MJ: Inositol triphosphate, calcium, lithium, and cell signaling. JAMA 1989; 262(13):1834–1841.

Berridge MJ: Inositol triphosphate and calcium signaling. Nature 1993; 361:315–325.

Bird A: Gene number, noise reduction and biological complexity. Trends Genet 1995; 11:94–99.

Bookstein R, Shew JY, Chen PL, et al: Suppression of tumorigenicity of human prostate cancer cells by replacing a mutated Rb gene. Science 1990; 247:712–715.

Borrelli E, Heyman R, Hsi M, Evans R: Targeting of an inducible toxic phenotype in animal cells. Proc Natl Acad Sci USA 1988; 85:7572–7576.

Botstein D, White RL, Scolnick M, Davis RW: Construction of a genetic linkage map using restriction fragment length polymorphisms. Am J Human Genet 1980; 32:314–331.

Boyle WJ, Smeal T, Defize LHK, et al: Activation of protein kinase C decreases phosphorylation of *c-Jun* at sites that negatively regulate its DNA binding activity. Cell 1991; 64:573–584.

Brass A, Barnard J, Patai BL, et al: Androgen up-regulates epidermal growth factor receptor expression and binding affinity in PC3 cell lines expressing the human androgen receptor. Cancer Res 1995; 55:3197–3203.

Brautigan DL: Flicking the switches: Phosphorylation of serine/threonine protein phosphatases. Semin Can Biol 1995; 6:211–217.

Brinster PL, Chen H, Trumbauer M: Somatic expression of herpes thymidine kinase in mice following injection of a fusion gene into eggs. Cell 1981; 27:223–231.

Brothman AR, Peehl DM, Patel AM, McNeal J: Frequency and pattern of karyotypic abnormalities in human prostate cancer. Cancer Res 1990; 50:3795–3803.

Brown P: Genome scanning methods. Curr Opin Genet Devel 1995; 4:366–373.

Burt RW, Bishop DT, Cannon-Albright L, et al: Population genetics of colonic cancer. Cancer 1992; 70(6, Suppl):1719–1722.

Call K, Glaser T, Ito C, et al: Isolation and characterization of a zinc finger polypeptide gene at the human chromosome 11 Wilms' tumor locus. Cell 1990; 60:509–520.

Capecchi M: High efficiency transformation by direct microinjection of DNA into mammalian cells. Cell 1980; 22:479–488.

Capecchi M: Altering the genome by homologous recombination. Science 1989; 244:1289–1292.

Carroll PR, Murty VVS, Reuter V, et al: Abnormalities at chromosome region 3p12–14 characterize clear cell renal cell carcinoma. Cancer Genet Cytogenet 1987; 26:253–260.

Carter B, Ewing C, Ward S, et al: Allelic loss of chromosomes 16q and 10q in human prostate cancer. Proc Natl Acad Sci USA 1990; 87:8751–8755.

Caspersson T, Zech L, Modest EJ: Fluorescent labeling of chromosomal DNA: Superiority of quinacrine mustard to quinacrine. Science 1970; 170:762.

Cavalier-Smith T: Selfish DNA and the origin of introns. Nature 1985; 315:283–284.

Cazaubon SM, Parker PJ: Identification of the phosphorylated region responsible for the permissive activation of protein kinase C. J Biol Chem 1993; 268:17559–17563.

Chen RH, Fuggle S: In situ cDNA polymerase chain reaction: A novel technique for detecting mRNA expression. Am J Pathol 1995; 143:1527–1533.

Clapham DE: Mutations in G-protein linked receptors: Novel insights on disease. Cell 1993; 75:1237–1239.

Clapham DE: Calcium signaling. Cell 1995; 80:259–268.

Claus EB, Risch N, Thompson WD: Genetic analysis of breast cancer in the Cancer and Steroid Hormone Study. Am J Hum Genet 1991; 48:232–242.

Conaway RC, Conaway JW: General initiation factors for RNA polymerase II. Annu Rev Biochem 1993; 62:161–190.

Culliton B: Gene therapy. Science 1990; 249:974.

Culliton B: Genes and discrimination. Nature Med 1995a; 1:385.

Culliton B: Biotechnology and God. Nature Med 1995b; 1:489.

Darnell JE Jr: RNA. Sci Am 1985; 253:68.

Divecha N, Irvine RF: Phospholipid signaling. Cell 1995; 80:269–278.

Drake JW: A contrast rate of spontaneous mutation in DNA based microbes. Proc Natl Acad Sci USA 1991; 88:7160–7164.

Drouin J, Trifiro MA, Plante RK, et al: Glucocorticoid receptor binding to a specific DNA sequence is required for hormone dependent repression of proopiomelanocortin gene transcription. Mol Cell Biol 1989; 9:5305–5314.

Duan RD, Pause A, Burgess WH, et al: Inhibition of transcription elongation by the VHL tumor suppressor protein. Science 1995; 269:1402–1406.

Egholm M: DNA hybridizes to complementary oligonucleotides obeying the Watson-Crick hydrogen bonding rules. Nature 1993; 365:566–568.

Fearon E, Feinberg AP, Hamilton SH, Vogelstein B: Loss of genes on the short arm of chromosome 11 in bladder cancer. Nature 1985; 318:377–389.

Felsenfeld G: Chromatin as an essential part of the transcriptional mechanism. Nature 1992; 355:219–224.

Fields S, Song O: A novel genetic system to detect protein-protein interactions. Nature 1989; 340:245–246.

Ford CE, Jones KW, Polani PE, et al: A sex chromosome anomaly in a case of gonadal dysgenesis (Turner's syndrome). Lancet 1959; 1:711–713.

Franke V, Holmes LB, Atkins L, Riccardi VM: Aniridia–Wilms' tumor association evidence for specific deletion of 11p13. Cytogenet Cell Genet 1979; 24:185–192.

Gardner G, Snostad DP: Principles of Genetics, 6th ed. New York, John Wiley and Sons, 1981, p 2.

Gessler M, Poustka A, Cavenee W, et al: Homozygous deletion in Wilms' tumor of a zinc finger gene identified by chromosome jumping. Nature 1990; 343:774–778.

Gilbert W: Why genes in pieces? Nature 1978; 271:501.

Gilman AG: G proteins and regulation of adenylyl cyclase. JAMA 1989; 262(13):1819–1825.

Gluzman Y, Hughes S: Viral Vectors. Cold Spring Harbor, NY, Cold Spring Harbor Laboratory Press, 1988.

Go M, Nosaka M: Protein architecture and the origin of introns. Cold Spring Harb Symp Quant Biol 1987; 52:915–924.

Golding GB, Tsao N, Pearlman R: Evidence for intron capture: An unusual path for the evolution of proteins. Proc Natl Acad Sci USA 1994; 91:7506–7509.

Gusella JF: DNA polymorphism and human disease. Annu Rev Biochem 1986; 55:831–854.

Haber DA, Buckler AJ, Glaser T, et al: The cellular function of small GTP-binding proteins. Science 1990; 249:635–649.

Hall A: The cellular function of small GTP-binding proteins. Science 1990; 249:635–649.

Hanahan D: Transgenic mice as probes into complex systems. Science 1989; 246:1265–1275.

Hasty P, Bradley A, Morris JH, et al: Muscle deficiency and neonatal death in mice with a targeted mutation in the myogenin gene. Nature 1993; 364:501–506.

Hershey JWB: Translational control in mammalian cells. Annu Rev Biochem 1991; 60:717–755.

Hess MA, Duncan RF: RNA/protein interactions in the 5′-untranslated leader of HSP70 mRNA in *Drosophila* lysates. J Biol Chem 1994; 269:10913–10922.

Hope I, Struhl K: Functional dissection of a eukaryotic transcriptional activator protein, GCN4, of yeast. Cell 1986; 46:885–894.

Housman D: Human DNA polymorphism. N Engl J Med 1995; 332:318–320.

Huang A, Campbell C, Bonetta L, et al: Tissue development and tumor-specific expression of divergent transcripts in Wilms' tumor. Science 1990; 250:991–994.

Hubbard MJ, Cohen P: On target with a new mechanism for the regulation of protein phosphorylation. Trends Biochem Sci 1993; 18:172–177.

Hunter T: Protein kinases and phosphatases: The yin and yang of protein phosphorylation and signaling. Cell 1995; 80:225–236.

Jackson RJ: Cytoplasmic regulation of mRNA function: The importance of the 3′ untranslated region. Cell 1993; 74:9–14.

Jacobs PA, Strong JA: A case of human intersexuality having a possible XXY sex determining mechanism. Nature 1959; 183:302–303.

Jeffreys A, Wilson V, Thein S: Hypervariable "minisatellite" regions in human DNA. Nature 1985; 314:67–73.

Joyce GF, Orgel LE. *In* Gesteland R, Atkins JF, eds: The RNA World. Cold Spring Harbor, NY, Cold Spring Harbor Laboratory Press, 1993, pp 1–25.

Joyce GF, Schwartz AW, Miller SL, Orgel LE: The case for an ancestral genetic system involving simple analogues of the nucleotides. Proc Natl Acad Sci USA 1989; 84:4398–4402.

Kasahara N, Dozy AM, Kan YW: Tissue-specific targeting of retroviral vectors through ligand-receptor interactions. Science 1994; 266:1373–1375.

Kasid U, Pfeifer A, Brennan T, et al: Effect of antisense *c-raf-1* on tumorigenicity and radiation sensitivity of a human squamous carcinoma. Science 1989; 243:1354–1356.

Keegan L, Gill G, Ptashne M: Separation of DNA binding from the transcription-activating function of a eukaryotic regulatory protein. Science 1986; 231:699–704.

Kibel A, Iliopoulos O, DeCaprio J, Kaelin W: Binding of the Von Hippel–Lindau tumor suppressor protein to elongin B and C. Science 1995; 269:1444–1446.

Koufos A, Hansen MF, Lamplin BC, et al: Loss of alleles at loci on human chromosome 11 during genesis of Wilms' tumor. Nature 1984; 309:170–172.

Kozak M: Circumstances and mechanisms of inhibition of translation by secondary structure in eukaryotic mRNAs. Mol Cell Biol 1989; 9:5134–5142.

Kreidberg JA, Sariola H, Loring J, et al: WT-1 is required for early kidney development. Cell 1993; 74:679–692.

Lake JA, Rivera MC: Was the nucleus the first endosymbiont? Proc Natl Acad Sci USA 1994; 91:2880–2981.

Lander ES, Budowle B: DNA fingerprinting dispute laid to rest. Nature 1994; 371:735–738.

Latif F, Kalman T, Gnarra J, et al: Identification of the von Hippel–Lindau disease tumor suppressor gene. Science 1993; 260:1317–1320.

Lejeune J, Turpin R, Gautier M: Le mongolism, premier exemple d'aberration autosomique humaine. Ann Genet (Paris) 1959; 1:41.

Levine M, Manley J: Transcriptional repression of eukaryotic promoters. Cell 1989; 59:405–408.

Lewin B: Chromatin and gene expression: Constant questions but changing answers. Cell 1994; 79:397–406.

Liang P, Pardee HB: Differential display of eukaryotic messenger RNA by means of polymerase chain reaction. Science 1992; 267:967–971.

Lichenstein C: Antisense RNA as a tool to study plant gene expression. Nature 1988; 333:801–802.

Lin S-Y, Riggs AD: The general affinity of lac repressor for *E. coli* DNA: Implications for gene regulation in prokaryotes and eukaryotes. Cell 1975; 4:107–111.

Little MH, Prosser J, Cordie A, et al: Zinc finger point mutations within the *wt-1* gene in Wilms' tumor patients. Proc Natl Acad Sci USA 1992; 89:4791–4795.

Lowe SW, Ruley HE, Jacks T, Housman DE: p53-Dependent apoptosis modulates the cytotoxicity of anticancer agents. Cell 1993; 74:957–967.

Ludlow JW, Nelson DA: Control and activity of type-1 serine/threonine protein phosphatase during the cell cycle. Semin Cancer Biol 1995; 6:195–202.

Maniatis T, Reed R: The role of small nuclear ribonucleoprotein particles in pre-mRNA splicing. Nature 1987; 325:673–678.

Manley J: Messenger RNA polyadenylation: A universal modification. Proc Natl Acad Sci USA 1995; 92:1800–1801.

Mantegna RN, Buldyrev SV, Goldberger AR, et al: Linguistic features of noncoding DNA sequences. Phys Rev Lett 1994; 73:3169–3172.

Marx J: Dissecting the complex diseases. Science 1990; 247:1540–1542.

Maxam A, Gilbert W: A new method for sequencing DNA. Proc Natl Acad Sci USA 1977; 74:560–564.

Mendel G: Versuch über pflanzen hybriden. J Hered 1866; 42:1. [English trans: Experiments in plant hybridization. Available from Harvard University Press, Cambridge, MA.]

Merritt JE, Rink TJ: Rapid increases in cytosolic free calcium in response to muscarinic stimulation of rat parotid acinar cells. J Biol Chem 1987; 262:4958.

Miller AD: Human gene therapy comes of age. Nature 1992; 357:455–460.

Mitelman F, Heim S: Consistent involvement of only 71 of the 329 chromosomal bands of the human genome in primary neoplasia-associated rearrangements. Cancer Res 1988; 48:7115–7119.

Mullis K: The unusual origin of the polymerase chain reaction. Sci Am 1990; 262:56–65.

Naber SP: Molecular pathology—Diagnosis of infectious disease. N Engl J Med 1994a; 331(18):1212–1215.

Naber SP: Molecular pathology—Detection of neoplasia. N Engl J Med 1994b; 331(22):1508–1510.

Nakamura Y, Leppert M, O'Connell P, et al: Variable number of tandem repeat (VNTR) markers for human gene mapping. Science 1987; 235:1616–1622.

Neer EJ: Heterotrimeric G proteins: Organizers of transmembrane signals. Cell 1995; 80:249–257.

Neer EJ, Clapham DE: Roles of G protein subunits in transmembrane signaling. Nature 1988; 333:129–134.

Nelson S, McCusker J, Sander M, et al: Genomic mismatch scanning: A new approach to genetic linkage mapping. Nature Genet 1993; 4:11–18.

Nishizuka Y: The family of protein kinase C for signal transduction. JAMA 1989; 262(13):1826–1833.

Nowell P: Cytogenetic approaches to human cancer genes. FASAB J 1994; 8:408–413.

Orkin SH, Goldman DG, Sallan SE: Development of homozygosity for chromosome 11p markers in Wilms' tumor. Nature 1984; 309:172–174.

O'Shea E, Rutkowski R, Stafford W, Kim P: Preferential heterodimer formation by isolated leucine zippers from *fos* and *Jun.* Science 1989; 245:646–648.

Painter TS: The Y chromosome in mammals. Science 1921; 53:503–504.

Palmitter RD, Behringer R, Quaife C, et al: Cell lineage ablation in transgenic mice by cell specific expression of a toxin gene. Cell 1987; 50:435–443.

Perlman PS, Butow RA: Mobile introns and intron-encoded proteins. Science 1989; 246:1106–1109.

Peterson MG, Tanese N, Pugh B, Tijian R: Functional domains and upstream activation properties of cloned human TATA binding proteins. Science 1990; 248:1625–1630.

Ptashne M: How gene activators work. Sci Am 1989; 260:41–47.

Rabbitts TH: Chromosomal translocations in human cancer. Nature 1994; 372:143–149.

Rall TW, Sutherland EW: The regulatory role of adenosine-3′,5′-phosphate. Cold Spring Harb Symp Quant Biol 1961; 26:347–354.

Rhodes D, Klug A: Zinc fingers. Sci Am 1993; 268:56–65.

Richmond TJ, Finch JT, Rushton B, et al: Structure of the nucleosome particle at 7A resolution. Nature 1984; 311:532–537.

Roger A, Doolittle W: Why introns in pieces? Nature 1993; 364:289.
Rose EA, Glaser T, Jones C, et al: Complete physical map of the WAGR region of 11p13 localizes a candidate Wilms' tumor gene. Cell 1990; 60:495–508.
Rosenthal N: Fine structure of a gene—DNA sequencing. N Engl J Med 1995; 332:589–591.
Ross J: The turnover of messenger RNA. Sci Am 1989; 260:48.
Rowley JD: A new consistent chromosomal abnormality in chronic myelogenous leukaemia identified by quinacrine fluorescence and Giemsa staining. Nature 1973; 243:290–293.
Rukstalis D, Bubley G, Donahue J, et al: Regional loss of chromosome 6 in 2 urologic malignancies. Cancer Res 1989; 99:5087–5091.
Sanda MG, Simons JW: Gene therapy for urologic cancer. Urology 1994; 44(4):617–624.
Sandberg AA: The Chromosomes in Human Cancer and Leukemia. New York, Elsevier, 1990.
Sandberg A: Cancer cytogenetics for clinicians. CA Cancer J Clin 1994; 44:136–159.
Sanger R, Nicklen S, Coulsen A: DNA sequencing with chain-terminating 177 inhibitors. Proc Natl Acad Sci USA 1977; 74:5463–5467.
Sheng M, Thompson MA, Greenberg ME.: CREB: A Ca^{2+}-regulated transcription factor phosphorylated by calmodulin-dependent kinases. Science 1991; 252:1427–1430.
Sidransky D, Von Eschenbach A, Tsai YC, et al: Urine samples. Science 1991; 252:706–709.
Smith M, Szathmary E: The Major Transitions in Evolution. Oxford, England, WH Freeman–Spektrum, 1995.
Southern EM: Detection of specific sequences among DNA fragments separated by gel electrophoresis. J Mol Biol 1975; 98:503–517.
St. Johnston D: The intracellular localization of messenger RNA's. Cell 1995; 81:161–170.
Stabel S: Protein kinase C—An enzyme and its relatives. Semin Cancer Biol 1994; 5:277–284.
Sturtevant AH: A History of Genetics. New York, Harper & Row, 1965.
Sudhof TC, Goldstein JL, Brown MS, Russell DW: The LDL receptor gene: A mosaic of exons shared with different proteins. Science 1985; 228:815–822.
Sun H, Tonks NK: The coordinated action of protein tyrosine phosphatases and kinases in cell signaling. Trends Biochem Sci 1994; 19:480–485.
Sunada H, Yu P, Peacock JS, Mendelsohn J: Modulation of tyrosine, serine and threonine phosphorylation and intracellular processing of the epidermal growth factor receptor by antireceptor monoclonal antibody. J Cell Physiology 1990; 142:284–292.
Tang WJ, Gilman AG: Type-specific regulation of adenylyl cyclase by G protein βγ subunits. Science 1991; 254:1500–1503.
Thomas H, Balkwill F: Assessing new anti-tumor agents and strategies in oncogene transgenic mice. Can Metast Reviews 1995; 14:91–95.
Tjio JH, Levan A: The chromosome number of man. Hereditas 1956; 42:1–6.
Usui H, Ariki M, Miyauchi T, Takeda M: Functions and properties of subunits in type-2A protein phosphatase from human erythrocyte. Adv Protein Phosphatases 1991; 6:287–306.
Van Ommen G, Breuning M, Raap A: FISH in V-W genome research and molecular diagnostics. Curr Opin Genet Devel 1995; 5:304–308.
Vander Krol A, Lenting P, Veenstra J, et al: An antisense chalcone synthase gene in transgenic plants inhibits flower pigmentation. Nature 1988; 333:866–869.
Viney JL: Transgenic and gene knockout mice in cancer research. Can Metast Reviews 1995; 14:77–90.
Vinson C, Sigler P, McKnight S: Scissors-grip model for DNA recognition by a family of leucine-zipper proteins. Science 1989; 246:911–916.
Watson JD, Crick FH: Molecular structure of nucleic acid: A structure for deoxyribose nucleic acid. Nature 1953; 171:737–738.
Weintraub H: Antisense RNA and DNA. Sci Am 1990; 262:40–47.
Weissman BE, Saxon PJ, Pasquale SR, et al: Introduction of a normal human chromosome 11 into a Wilms' tumor cell line controls its tumorigenic expression. Science 1987; 236:175–180.
Westphal H: Transgenic mammals and biotechnology. FASEB J 1989; 3:117–120.
White R, Lalouel JM: Chromosome mapping with DNA markers. Sci Am 1988; 258:40–49.
Williams N: The trials and tribulations of cracking the prehistoric code. Science 1995; 269:923–924.
Wolffe AP: New insights into chromatin function in transcriptional control. FASEB J 1992; 6:3354.
Wolffe AP, Brown DD: Developmental regulation of two 5s ribosomal RNA genes. Science 1988; 241:1626–1632.
Wyman H, White R: A highly polymorphic locus in human DNA. Proc Natl Acad Sci USA 1980; 77:6754–6758.
Yamamoto KK, Gonzalez GA, Biggs WH, Montminy MR: Phosphorylation-induced binding and transcriptional efficacy of nuclear factor CREB. Nature 1988; 334:494–498.
Zawel L, Reinberg D: Common themes in assembly of eukaryotic transcription complexes. Annu Rev Biochem 1995; 64:533–561.
Zbar B, Brauch H, Talmadge C, Linehan M: Loss of alleles of loci on the short arm of chromosome 3 in renal cell carcinoma. Nature 1987; 327:721–724.

2

SURGICAL ANATOMY OF THE RETROPERITONEUM, KIDNEYS, AND URETERS

John N. Kabalin, M.D.

As a *surgical* specialty, the practice of urology must begin with a solid foundation and practical knowledge of the anatomy of the urinary tract and its surrounding structures. This chapter reviews in detail the anatomy of the upper urinary tract and adrenal gland as well as the anatomy of the retroperitoneum and abdominal wall, which contain them.

THE RETROPERITONEUM (Fig. 2–1)

Posterior Abdominal Wall

General Description

The retroperitoneum is bounded anteriorly by the peritoneal sac and its contents, is separated from the thorax superiorly by the muscular diaphragm (Fig. 2–2), and is contiguous with the extraperitoneal portions of the pelvis inferiorly. The body wall creates the posterior and lateral limits of the retroperitoneum, and incisions through the posterolateral abdominal wall, or flank, provide the most direct routes to the structures of the retroperitoneum.

Original line drawings appearing in this chapter were created with the assistance and talent of Bayard "Butch" Colyear.

Posterior Musculature and Lumbodorsal Fascia

Beginning in the posterior midline, **the lumbodorsal fascia originates from the lumbar vertebrae** (Figs. 2–3 to 2–5). This is a very strong and thick fascia, which extends anterolaterally from the lumbar spine. **There are three distinct layers of the lumbodorsal fascia.**

The posterior layer extends from the spinous processes of the lumbar vertebrae and lies most superficial to the muscles of the back, forming the posterior covering of the sacrospinalis muscle (see Figs. 2–3 and 2–4). The latissimus dorsi muscle originates medially from this strong aponeurosis to extend obliquely, superiorly, and laterally to the humerus, covering the superomedial muscles of the flank. The middle and anterior layers of the lumbodorsal fascia originate on the transverse processes of the lumbar vertebrae (see Figs. 2–4 and 2–5). The middle layer separates the sacrospinalis from the quadratus lumborum muscle anterior to it, whereas the anterior layer passes anterior to the quadratus lumborum.

All three layers of the lumbodorsal fascia join to form a single thick aponeurosis lateral to the quadratus lumborum muscle before extending further anterolaterally, where they are contiguous with the aponeurosis of the transversus abdominis muscle, the deepest of the three muscle layers of the anterior abdominal wall (see Fig. 2–4). **A vertical incision that parallels the lateral borders of**

Text continued on page 54

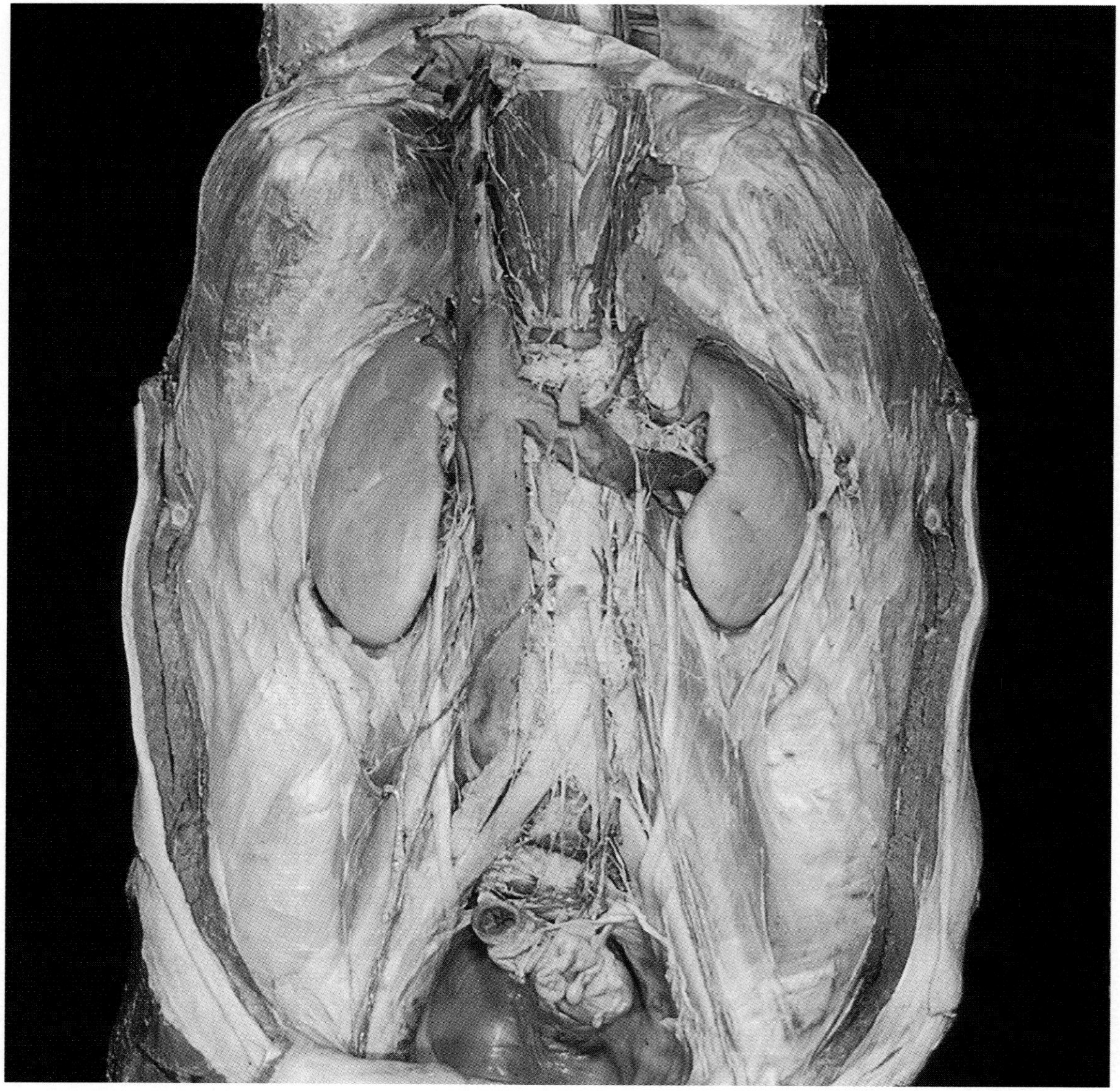

A

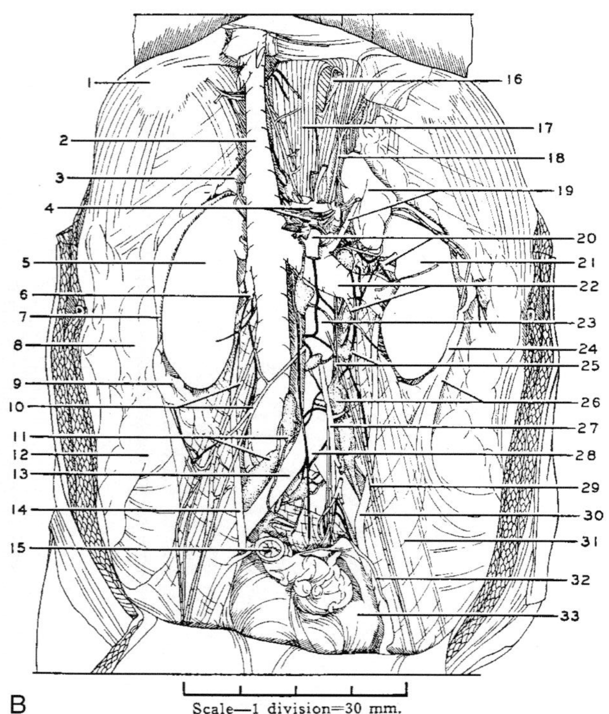

Figure 2–1. *A,* The retroperitoneum dissected. The anterior perirenal (Gerota's) fascia has been removed. *B,* 1, Diaphragm. 2, Inferior vena cava. 3, Right adrenal gland. 4, *Upper pointer,* celiac artery; *lower pointer,* celiac autonomic nervous plexus. 5, Right kidney. 6, Right renal vein. 7, Gerota's fascia. 8, Pararenal retroperitoneal fat. 9, Perinephric fat. 10, *Upper pointer,* right gonadal vein; *lower pointer,* right gonadal artery. 11, Lumbar lymph nodes. 12, Retroperitoneal fat. 13, Right common iliac artery. 14, Right ureter. 15, Sigmoid colon (cut). 16, Esophagus (cut). 17, Right crus of diaphragm. 18, Left inferior phrenic artery. 19, *Upper pointer,* left adrenal gland; *lower pointer,* left adrenal vein. 20, *Upper pointer,* superior mesenteric artery; *lower pointer,* left renal artery. 21, Left kidney. 22, *Upper pointer,* left renal vein; *lower pointer,* left gonadal vein. 23, Aorta. 24, Perinephric fat. 25, Aortic autonomic nervous plexus. 26, *Upper pointer,* Gerota's fascia; *lower pointer,* inferior mesenteric ganglion. 27, Inferior mesenteric artery. 28, Aortic bifurcation into common iliac arteries. 29, Left gonadal artery and vein. 30, Left ureter. 31, Psoas major muscle covered by psoas sheath. 32, Cut edge of peritoneum. 33, Pelvic cavity.

C

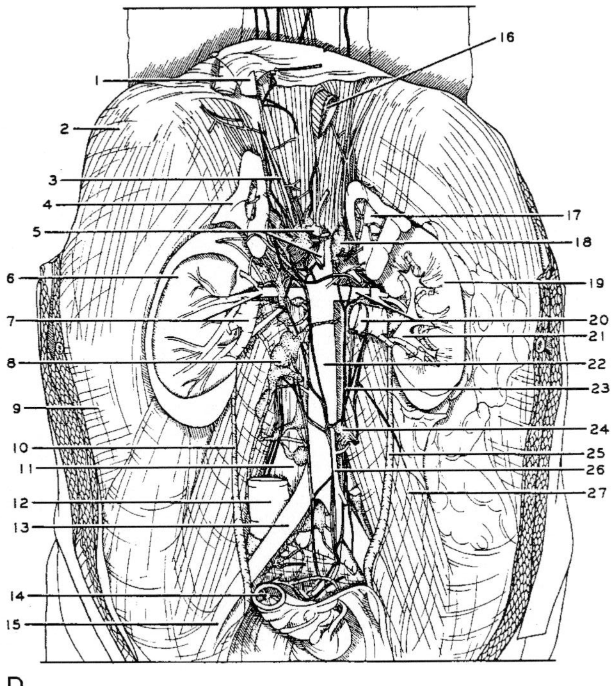

D

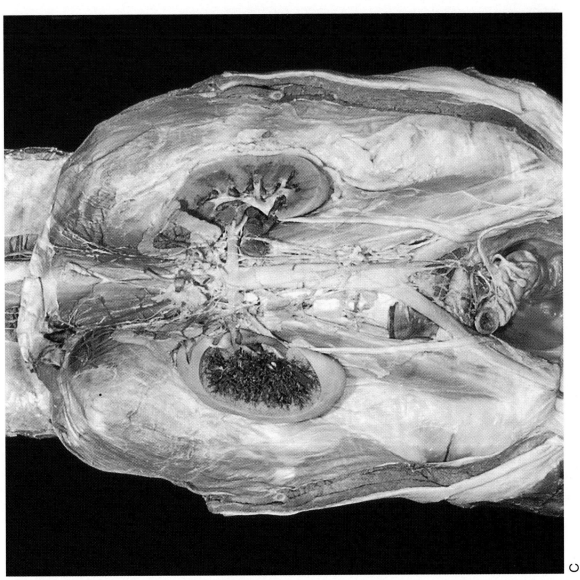

Figure 2–1 *Continued C,* The retroperitoneum dissected. The kidneys and adrenals have been sectioned and the inferior vena cava has been excised over most of its intra-abdominal course. *D,* 1, Inferior vena cava (cut). 2, Diaphragm. 3, Right inferior phrenic artery. 4, Right adrenal gland. 5, *Upper pointer,* celiac artery; *lower pointer,* superior mesenteric artery. 6, Right kidney. 7, *Upper pointer,* right renal artery; *lower pointer,* right renal vein (cut). 8, Lumbar lymph node. 9, Transversus abdominis muscle covered with transversalis fascia. 10, Right ureter. 11, Anterior spinous ligament. 12, Inferior vena cava (cut). 13, Right common iliac artery. 14, Sigmoid colon (cut). 15, Right external iliac artery. 16, Esophagus (cut). 17, Left adrenal gland. 18, Celiac ganglion. 19, Left kidney. 20, *Upper pointer,* left renal artery; *lower pointer,* left renal vein (cut). 21, Left renal pelvis. 22, Aorta. 23, Aortic autonomic nervous plexus. 24, Inferior mesenteric ganglion. 25, Left ureter. 26, Inferior mesenteric artery. 27, Psoas major muscle covered by psoas sheath. (*A* to *D* reproduced from the Bassett anatomic collection, with permission granted by Dr. Robert A. Chase.)

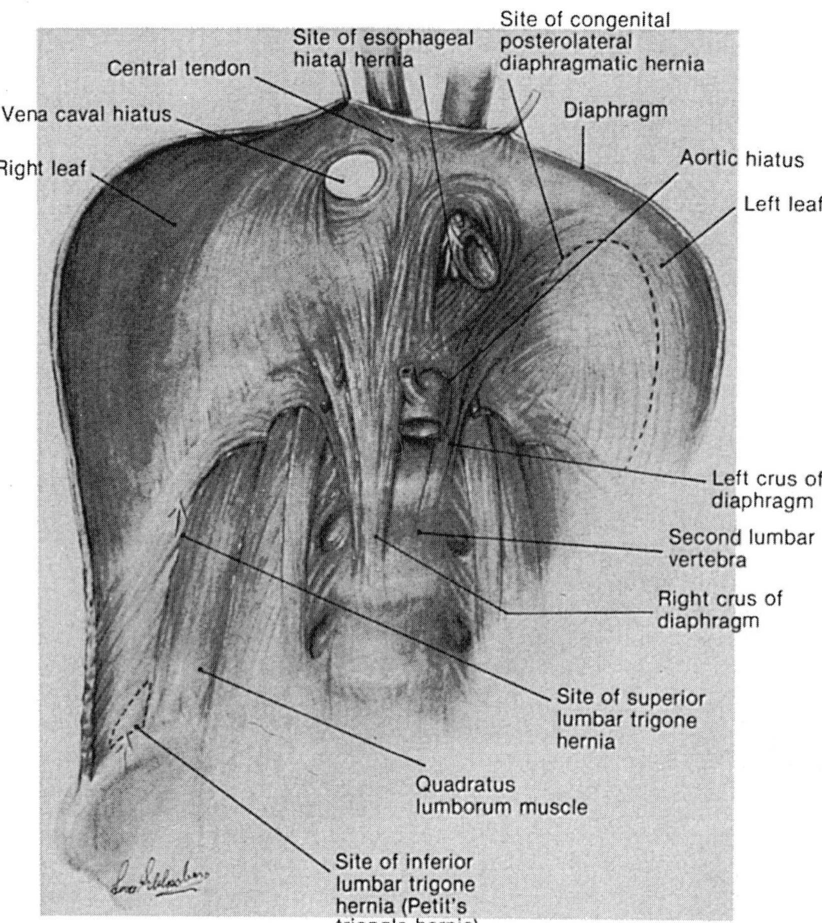

Figure 2–2. The diaphragm, with special attention to the hiatuses of the aorta and vena cava.

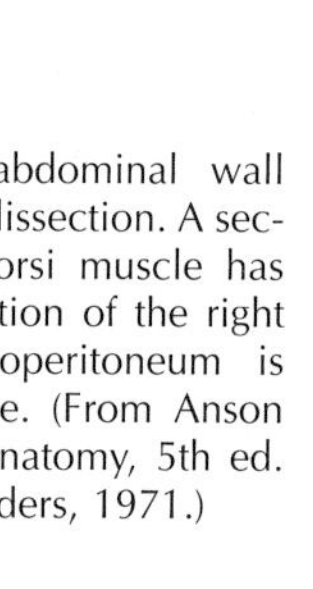

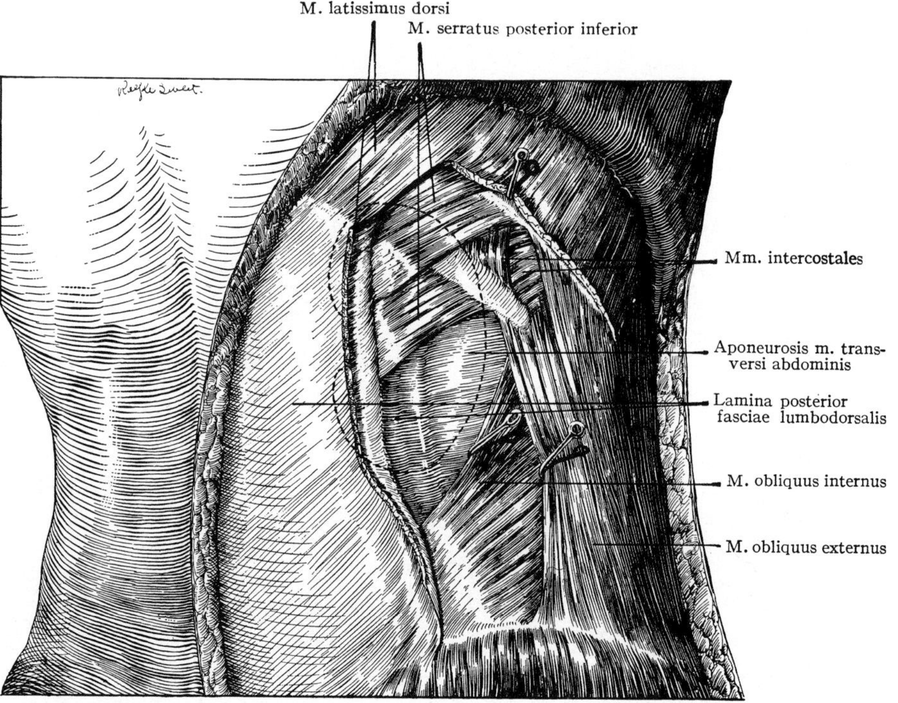

Figure 2–3. Posterior abdominal wall musculature, superficial dissection. A section of the latissimus dorsi muscle has been removed. The location of the right kidney within the retroperitoneum is shown by dashed outline. (From Anson BJ, McVay C: Surgical Anatomy, 5th ed. Philadelphia, W. B. Saunders, 1971.)

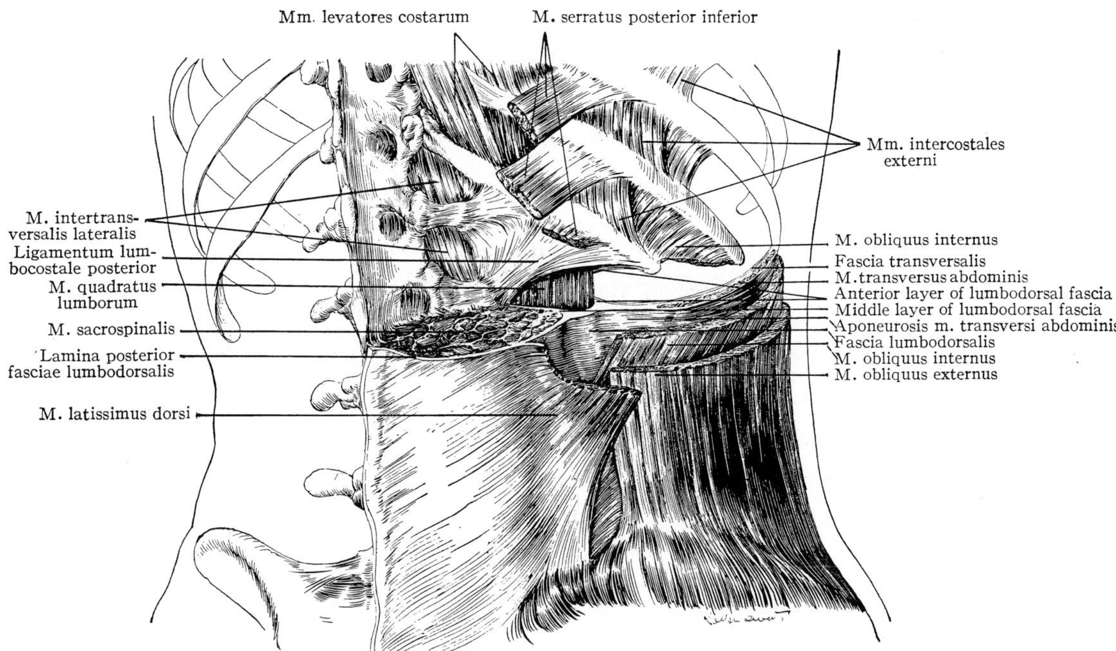

Figure 2–4. Posterior abdominal wall musculature, intermediate dissection. The sacrospinalis muscle and three anterolateral flank muscle layers are seen in cut section, and the three layers of the lumbodorsal fascia posteriorly can be appreciated. (After Kelly, Burnam.) (From McVay C: Anson & McVay Surgical Anatomy, 6th ed. Philadelphia, W. B. Saunders, 1984.)

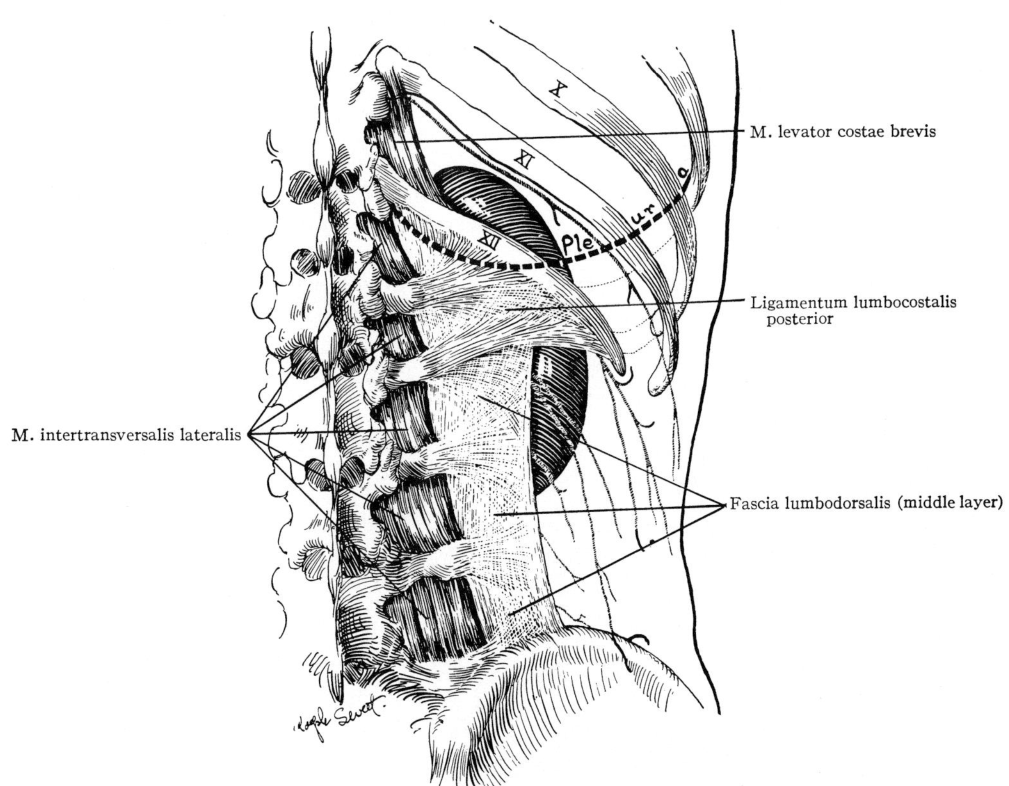

Figure 2–5. Posterior abdominal wall musculature, deep dissection. The lumbodorsal fascia and lumbocostal ligament are visualized, arising from the transverse processes of the lumbar vertebrae. The relation of the kidney and pleura is also shown. (From McVay C: Anson & McVay Surgical Anatomy, 6th ed. Philadelphia, W. B. Saunders, 1984.)

the sacrospinalis and quadratus lumborum can be made through this lumbodorsal fascia, posteromedial to the first transverse muscle fibers of the transversus abdominis, **to gain surgical access to the retroperitoneum and kidney without cutting muscle** (the so-called lumbodorsal approach, or dorsal lumbotomy) (Fig. 2–6). The posterolateral application of the peritoneal reflection also roughly approximates the anterior margin of this lumbodorsal fascia.

Muscles of the Lateral Flank

There are three anterolateral muscle layers of the flank. Most superficial is the external oblique muscle, which arises from the lower ribs to pass obliquely downward and anteriorly to its aponeurotic insertion along the iliac crest laterally; medially, its aponeurosis becomes contiguous with the anterior rectus sheath (see Fig. 2–3). The posterior border of the external oblique muscle is free and can be retracted anteriorly without cutting during some posterior approaches to the retroperitoneum.

The middle layer of the anterolateral flank musculature is formed by the internal oblique muscle, which originates from the iliac crest and lumbodorsal fascia to extend obliquely upward and anteriorly, its fibers roughly perpendicular to those of the external oblique muscle, and which inserts on the lower rib cage (see Fig. 2–3).

The deepest muscle layer in the anterolateral abdominal wall is the transversus abdominis, which runs transversely from the lumbodorsal fascia posteriorly to the lateral margin of the rectus sheath anteriorly (see Fig. 2–4). **The transversalis fascia covers the inner aspect of the transversus abdominis muscle,** lies between the peritoneum and abdominal wall anteriorly, and extends in continuity across the anterior midline behind the rectus muscles. This fascia is thin but strong. The same transversalis fascia extends posteriorly and covers the anterior aspects of the muscles that confine the retroperitoneum.

Psoas and Iliacus Muscles

Lying anteriorly in the groove between the lumbar vertebral bodies and their transverse processes is the psoas major muscle (Fig. 2–7; see also Fig. 2–1). It originates on the 12th thoracic through 5th lumbar vertebrae to run downward and laterally. In about half of the population, a smaller but distinct muscle body, identified as the psoas minor muscle when present, lies on the upper anterior surface of the psoas major. **The psoas major joins the iliacus muscle, which originates broadly over the inner aspect of the iliac wing of the pelvis, to become the iliopsoas and insert on the lesser trochanter of the femur and flex the thigh.**

The posterior surface of the retroperitoneum is thus formed by the lumbar vertebral bodies in the midline, which are covered by the shiny, longitudinal fibers of the anterior spinous ligament (see Fig. 2–7). These are flanked bilaterally by the psoas muscles. The psoas muscles are covered by a glistening white fibrous fascia, the so-called psoas sheath, which is contiguous with transversalis fascia. As one moves laterally, the lateral portion of the quadratus lumborum extends from behind the lateral margin of the psoas. The anterior layer of the lumbodorsal fascia covers this muscle and continues as the aponeurosis of the transversus abdominis muscle. Farther laterally, the transversus abdominis muscle proper is encountered. Superiorly, the posterior wall of the retroperitoneum is formed by the posterior insertion of the diaphragm along the lower ribs (see Figs. 2–2 and 2–3). Inferiorly, below the level of the iliac crest, the iliopsoas muscle forms the posterior confine of the retroperitoneum.

Lower Rib Cage

The 11th and 12th ribs and, in some individuals, the 10th ribs lie behind the diaphragm posterior to the adrenal glands and upper poles of the kidneys bilaterally (see Fig. 2–5). Thus, the rib cage offers protection not only to the organs of the thorax but also to those of the upper abdomen and retroperitoneum. **Any injury that produces fracture of the lower ribs, especially posteriorly, must therefore be evaluated for potential renal injury as well. The costovertebral or lumbodorsal ligament is a strong fascial attachment between the inferior margin of the**

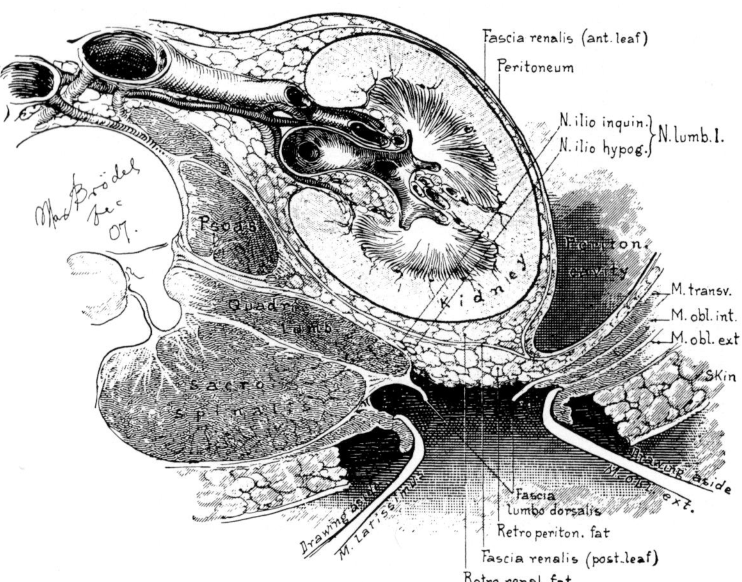

Figure 2–6. Transverse section through the kidney and posterior abdominal wall, showing lumbodorsal fascia incised. Note that through such a lumbodorsal incision the kidney can be reached without incising muscle. (After Kelly, Burnam.) (From McVay C: Anson & McVay Surgical Anatomy, 6th ed. Philadelphia, W. B. Saunders, 1984.)

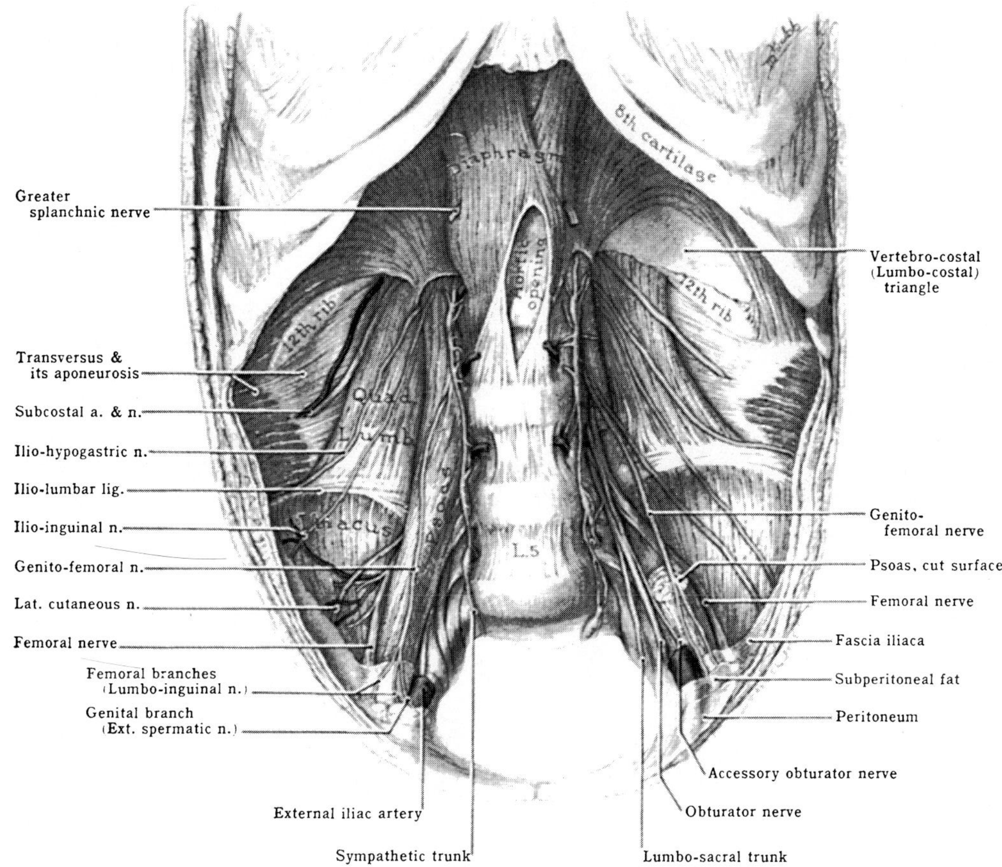

Figure 2–7. Posterior abdominal wall as viewed from anterior with all viscera removed. Muscular anatomy and nervous structures that traverse the retroperitoneum are emphasized. (From Anderson JE: Grant's Atlas of Anatomy, 7th ed. Baltimore, Williams & Wilkins, 1978. Reproduced by permission.)

12th rib and the transverse processes of the first and second lumbar vertebrae (see Fig. 2–5). It is encountered only in posterior approaches to the kidney **and can be incised to produce greater mobility of the 12th rib and provide greater exposure** and access to the structures of the upper retroperitoneum.

Great Vessels

The Abdominal Aorta and Its Branches

The aorta and the inferior vena cava course longitudinally through the central retroperitoneum (Fig. 2–8; see also Fig. 2–1). **The aorta exits the thoracic cavity through the aortic hiatus in the posterior diaphragm, between the muscular slips of the diaphragmatic crura** (see Figs. 2–2 and 2–7). Although anteriorly the aorta enters the retroperitoneum at the level of the thoracolumbar vertebral junction, the crura flank the aorta bilaterally, often to the level of the second or third lumbar vertebral body, at or below the level of the renal vascular pedicles. The aorta lies just to the left of the midline atop the lumbar vertebrae, ending at approximately the lower portion of the fourth lumbar vertebral body, where it bifurcates into the two common iliac arteries.

The first abdominal branches of the aorta are the paired inferior phrenic arteries (Fig. 2–9). These arise anterolaterally from the aorta almost immediately as it exits the aortic hiatus and extend over and supply the inferior surface of the diaphragm. They each also supply multiple superior arterial branches to the ipsilateral adrenal gland. As one proceeds from diaphragm to pelvis, the next branch of the aorta is **the short celiac arterial trunk, which arises in the anterior midline and at once trifurcates into common hepatic, left gastric, and splenic branches.** These three main arteries together **supply the bulk of arterial circulation to the viscera of the upper abdomen, including liver, spleen, stomach, and pancreas.** The next branches from the aorta are paired adrenal vessels, which arise laterally from the aorta and are usually quite small in caliber. At approximately the same level, but in the anterior midline, is **the superior mesenteric artery.** This major vessel **courses inferiorly to supply through multiple branches the entire small intestine and most of the large intestine,** and, via the inferior pancreaticoduodenal artery, it communicates with the celiac system and provides most of the blood supply to the duodenum and a portion of that to the pancreas. All abdominal aortic branches discussed thus far typically occur over the span of the first lumbar vertebra.

Usually overlying the second lumbar vertebral body, but subject to considerable variation, the paired renal arteries next emanate laterally from the aorta. Their take-off may be either slightly anterior or slightly posterior from the great vessel. The renal arteries are discussed further in the section on the kidney.

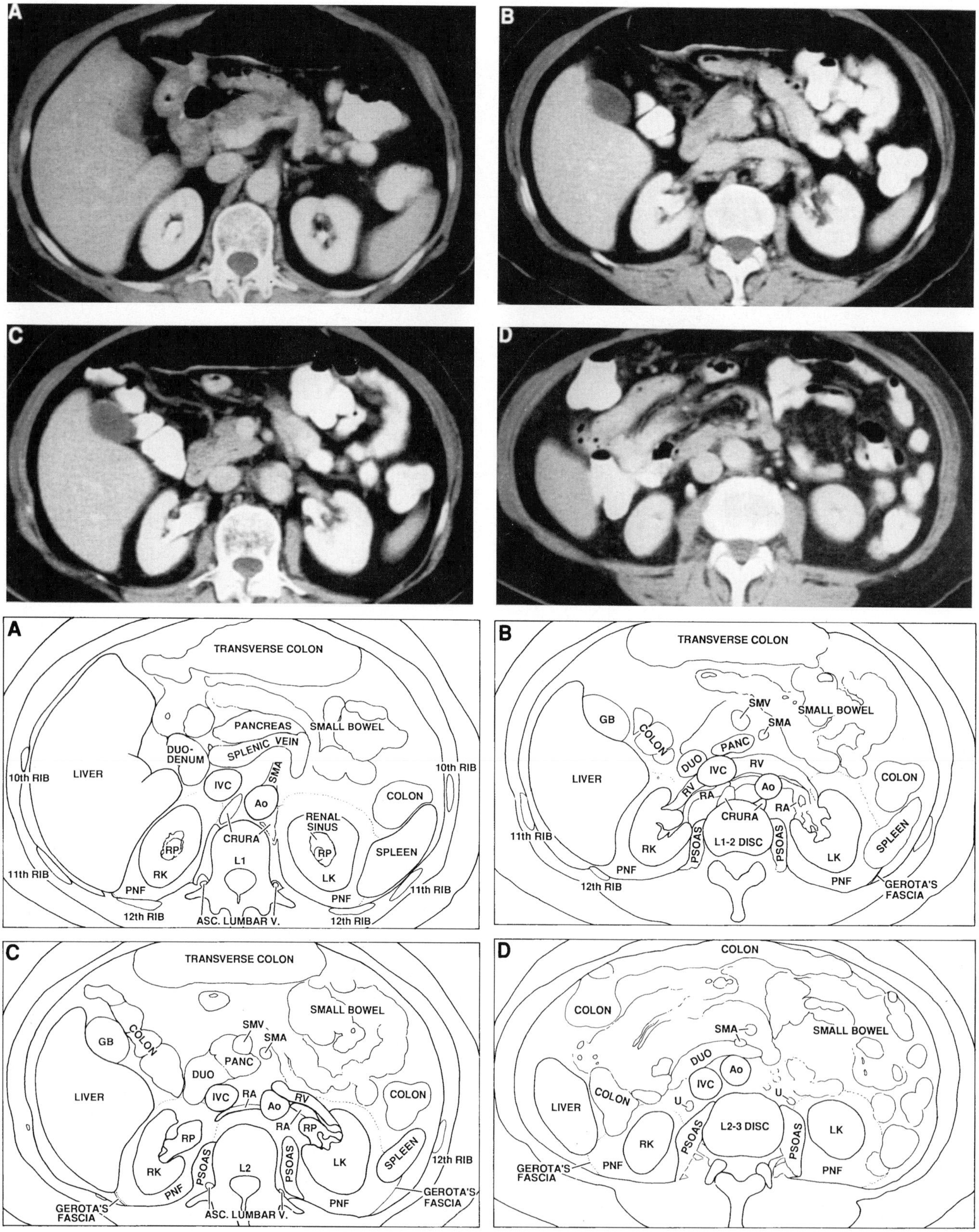

Figure 2–8. Cross-sectional anatomy of the upper abdomen at the level of the kidneys, demonstrated with transverse sections obtained by computed tomography. Sections arranged from most cephalic to caudal. *A*, Section through the upper poles of the kidneys, superior to the renal vascular pedicles. *B*, Section through the level of the renal arteries and veins. *C*, Slightly more inferior section, showing renal pelves and relation of the duodenum to right renal hilum. *D*, Section through the lower poles of the kidneys and showing upper ureters. Ao, aorta; DUO, duodenum; GB, gallbladder; IVC, inferior vena cava; LK, left kidney; PNF, perinephric fat; RA, renal artery; RK, right kidney; RP, renal pelvis; RV, renal vein; SMA, superior mesenteric artery; SMV, superior mesenteric vein; U, ureter.

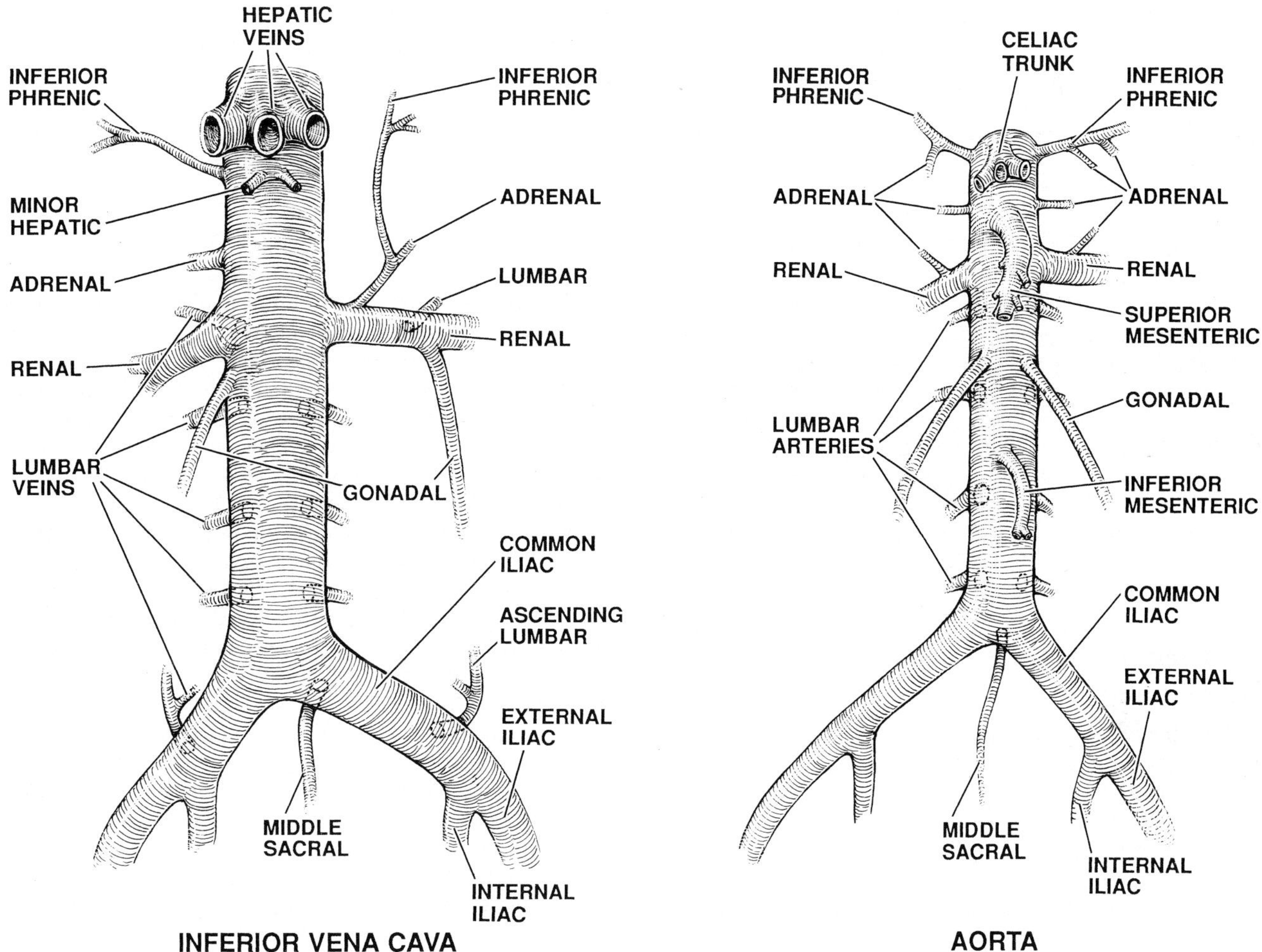

Figure 2–9. Inferior vena cava and abdominal aorta and their branches.

The paired gonadal arteries arise from the anterolateral aorta—in atypical cases, from a single anterior trunk—at a level somewhat below the renal vessels. Occasionally, a gonadal artery may arise from the ipsilateral renal artery or from the aorta above the level of the renal vessels. Duplication of the gonadal arteries on one or both sides may occur. The gonadal arteries are generally of relatively small caliber. **In the male, they are the internal spermatic or testicular arteries; they course inferiorly and laterally to join the structures of the spermatic cord at the internal inguinal ring and thereafter proceed to the ipsilateral testis** (see Fig. 2–1*A* and *B*). In some cases, the artery can be found to initially angle superiorly and arch over either the renal vein or one of its branches before proceeding inferiorly. In their retroperitoneal course, the gonadal arteries pass anteriorly to the ureter on either side and usually provide a small ureteral feeder branch. The right gonadal artery passes anteriorly to the inferior vena cava in most individuals, but in some instances it may pass posteriorly. **In the female, these are the ovarian arteries;** initially, they follow a course in the retroperitoneum similar to that in the male. However, after crossing the ureter anteriorly, rather than exiting the internal ring, these arteries course medially into the pelvis, crossing the external iliac vessels just below their bifurcation from the common iliacs and lateral to the crossing of the ureter. Thereafter, **they enter the suspensory ligament of the ovary and supply the ipsilateral ovary and fallopian tube.** Ligation of the gonadal vessels in their retroperitoneal course in either sex usually produces no ill effect because of rich collateral circulation to the gonads provided by the artery to the vas deferens (deferential) and the external spermatic (cremasteric) artery in the male and by the uterine artery in the female.

Proceeding caudally, **the inferior mesenteric artery next arises from the aorta anteriorly and often to the left of midline, approximately 3 to 5 cm above the aortic bifurcation. It courses inferiorly and to the left to supply the upper rectum, sigmoid colon, descending colon, and variable portions of the left transverse colon.** The inferior mesenteric artery, especially in younger individuals without significant atherosclerotic occlusive arterial disease, can almost always be sacrificed without complication. Adequate collateral circulation is usually provided from below by inferior and middle hemorrhoidal vessels and from above by superior mesenteric arterial branches via the marginal artery ("of Drummond") of the colon.

The terminal branches of the aorta are the common iliac arteries, which themselves then bifurcate into external and internal (hypogastric) branches. The former exit the retroperitoneum via the femoral canal and supply the lower extremities as the femoral arteries; the latter provide multiple branches to the pelvic viscera. These are discussed in the following chapter on pelvic anatomy.

Posteriorly, **the middle sacral artery arises from the terminal aorta just above the bifurcation** of the common iliacs and extends caudally on the anterior surface of the fifth lumbar vertebra and sacrum. This artery can be sacrificed with impunity, but it is often encountered unexpectedly during dissection and may produce troublesome bleeding prior to ligation. **Usually, four pairs of lumbar arteries exit the posterior aspect of the aorta,** any one pair occasionally arising from a single posterior trunk. **These are the lumbar segmental analogs of the intercostal arteries and occur at approximately the levels of the first four lumbar vertebrae and course posteriorly, medial to the psoas muscles, to supply the posterior body wall and spine.** Although the vertebral collateral circulation is generally abundant, in rare instances ligation of all lumbar vessels has produced spinal ischemia and paralysis. A fifth pair of lumbar arteries, often small, may arise from the middle sacral artery or from the posterior aspects of the common iliac arteries.

The Inferior Vena Cava and Its Tributaries

The inferior vena cava (see Figs. 2–1 and 2–9) **arises as the confluence of the common iliac veins,** just below and to the right of the aortic bifurcation. The aorta lies more anteriorly at this point, and the right common iliac artery crosses anteriorly over the junction of the common iliac veins. Both common iliac arteries lie anterolaterally to the associated veins, becoming more lateral as they approach the femoral canal. **Posterior parietal tributaries to the inferior vena cava—the middle sacral and lumbar veins—roughly parallel their arterial counterparts. However, the lumbar veins in particular tend to be more variable in both number and position than do the lumbar arteries.** Ascending lumbar veins run vertically behind the psoas muscles and anteriorly to the transverse processes of the lumbar vertebrae (see Fig. 2–8), variably connecting the lumbar veins and communicating with the hemiazygos (left) and azygos (right) veins in the thorax. The venous drainage of the gastrointestinal tract differs somewhat from that of the arterial circulation, as **inferior mesenteric, superior mesenteric, and splenic veins join to form the portal vein and drain proximally into the liver rather than directly into the inferior vena cava.**

Gonadal veins parallel the gonadal arteries in their inferior course but superiorly tend to lie more lateral and closer to the ipsilateral ureter (see Fig. 2–1*A* and *B*). Also, **gonadal veins are often multiple over their inferior extent (the extension of the "pampiniform plexus" of the spermatic cord in the male) and gradually coalesce to form a single vessel superiorly. The left gonadal vein usually enters the inferior aspect of the left renal vein perpendicularly** (see Fig. 2–9) but rarely may enter the left anterolateral aspect of the inferior vena cava. **The right gonadal vein usually drains obliquely into the right lateral aspect of the inferior vena cava below the level of the right renal vein,** but occasionally it may drain into the right renal vein. The gonadal veins normally contain valves. These may be incompetent or absent and produce the clinical condition of varicocele in the male. The direct perpendicular insertion of the testicular vein into the inferior aspect of the left renal vein is believed to play a role in allowing sufficient back pressure to produce this condition and may explain the preponderance of left-sided varicoceles.

The renal veins are large vessels that drain from the kidneys to enter the inferior vena cava on its lateral aspects at approximately the same level as the renal arteries. These lie anteriorly to the arteries and are of larger caliber, sometimes markedly so. (These, too, are discussed later in greater detail with the kidney.) **The right renal vein is very short and typically receives no branches,** but in some instances a lumbar vein may enter posteriorly or the ipsilateral gonadal vein may enter inferiorly, as noted earlier. **The left renal vein is significantly longer, crossing the aorta anteriorly below the takeoff of the superior mesenteric artery, and commonly receives a lumbar vein (usually the second lumbar) on its posterior aspect. In addition, the left gonadal vein typically drains into its inferior margin and the left adrenal vein into its superior margin.**

The superior extent of the inferior vena cava receives the short right adrenal vein, and usually also a right inferior phrenic vein, on its posterolateral or lateral aspect. On the left, the inferior phrenic vein may enter the inferior vena cava directly but usually joins the left adrenal vein to drain into the left renal vein. The left adrenal vein, although it usually drains to the left renal vein, may in unusual cases also enter the left side of the inferior vena cava directly. **The inferior vena cava is closely applied to the posterior aspect of the liver and here receives multiple very short hepatic veins.** The more inferior of these tend to be of small caliber; however, more superiorly, just below the diaphragm, at least three very large, short hepatic trunks draining into the anterior aspect of the inferior vena cava are typical. After receiving these, the inferior vena cava exits the abdomen through the central tendon of the diaphragm, anterior to the aortic hiatus, and after a very brief thoracic course enters the right atrium directly.

Although the most common anatomy of the great vessels of the retroperitoneum has been described, anomalous development of these blood vessels and their branches is common, and the possible variations are both myriad and far beyond the scope of this text. Brief mention of the most common renal vascular anomalies is made during discussion of the kidney later.

Lymphatics

The lymphatic drainage of the lower extremities, perineum and external genitalia, and pelvic viscera must course through the retroperitoneum. The lymphatics from these large anatomic distributions eventually coalesce into the common iliac lymph vessels and nodes, thereafter forming ascending vertical lumbar lymphatic chains that follow the great vessels superiorly (Fig. 2–10; see also Fig. 2–1). These lumbar nodal chains thus are extraregional or secondary drainage sites for any metastatic process arising from the lower extremity, external genitalia (not including the testes, which are embryologically intra-abdominal organs), or pelvis. **The ascending lumbar lymphatics are closely applied to the great vessels, with**

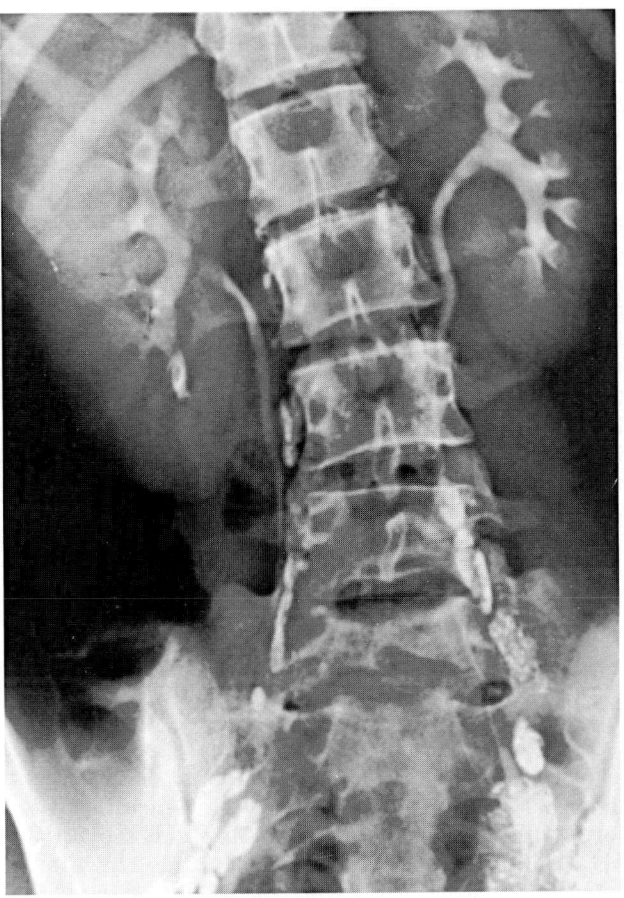

Figure 2–10. Ascending lumbar lymphatic chains following course of the great vessels in the retroperitoneum, as demonstrated by lymphangiography. Simultaneous excretory urogram shows relative position of the kidneys.

multiple transverse communications between ascending lymphatic vessels. It is important that most of the lateral flow between ascending lymphatics moves from right to left ascending lumbar trunks. These ascending trunks are joined by the lymphatic drainage of the gastrointestinal tract, which follows the inferior mesenteric, superior mesenteric, and celiac arteries. **Most, if not all, of these ascending lymphatics finally coalesce posterior to the aorta to form the thoracic duct. In most individuals, the site of this coalescence is marked by a localized dilation of the lymphatic chain, the cisterna chyli.** This latter structure truly lies within the thorax, posterior to the aorta or slightly to the right, in a retrocrural position, usually anterior to the first or second lumbar vertebral body.

The lumbar lymphatics are the primary or regional nodal drainage for two major organs of interest to the urologic surgeon: the kidney and testis. It is easy to visualize the renal lymphatics following the renal blood vessels and draining to paracaval and para-aortic lymph nodes, and this is discussed in detail with the kidney. The testes originally develop in the retroperitoneum in close association with the kidneys, maintaining not only their arterial supply from the abdominal aorta via the testicular arteries but also their lymphatic drainage to the lumbar nodes in the retroperitoneum. They do not normally drain to the iliac chains except indirectly in more advanced disease states. **Although not strictly anatomic, it is of descriptive and practical use for the surgeon to distinguish three major lumbar nodal areas in the retroperitoneum: (1) the left para-aortic nodes, which extend from the midline of this vessel to the left ureter; (2) the right paracaval nodes, which extend from the midline of this vessel to the right ureter; and (3) the interaortocaval nodes, which extend from the midline of the inferior vena cava to the midline of the aorta.** Careful studies of early metastases from testicular tumors have shown that **the left testis drains primarily to the left para-aortic nodal region, including nodes above the left renal hilum, with significant drainage to the interaortocaval region but with essentially no drainage to the right paracaval nodes** (Fig. 2–11). In contrast, **the right testis drains primarily to the interaortocaval region, with significant drainage also to the right paracaval nodes below the right renal hilum and small but real numbers of early metastases from the right testis distributed to the left para-aortic region** (Fig. 2–12). This makes sense in light of the fact that most lateral lumbar lymphatic flow proceeds from right to left. However, in more extensive and advanced testicular malignancies, because of extensive lymphatic communication as well as the possibility of some left-to-right and also retrograde lymphatic flow, metastases may be found in any lumbar lymphatic region and also in common iliac locations.

Nervous Structures

Autonomic

The paired thoracolumbar sympathetic chains initially arise within the thorax as the confluence of preganglionic

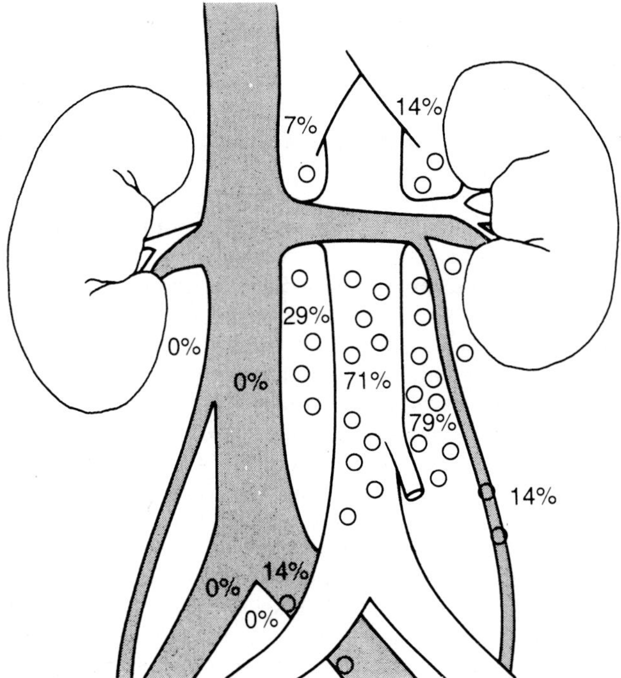

Figure 2–11. Primary sites of lymphatic drainage from the left testis, as defined by early lymph node metastases from left-sided testis tumors. (From Donohue JP: Semin Urol 1984; 2:217.)

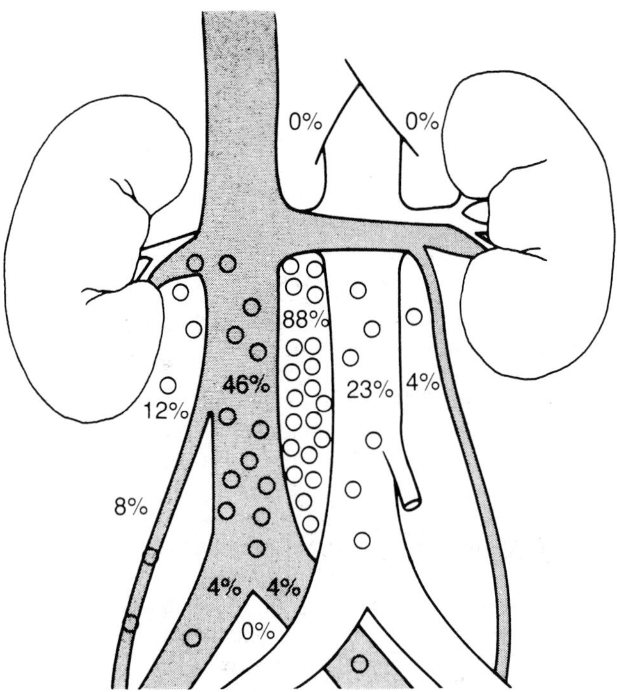

Figure 2–12. Primary sites of lymphatic drainage from the right testis, as defined by early lymph node metastases from right-sided testis tumors. (From Donohue JP: Semin Urol 1984; 2:217.)

fibers extending from the first thoracic through the second or third lumbar spinal nerves. The resulting sympathetic trunks course vertically along the anterolateral aspect of the spinal column, in the retroperitoneum lying within the groove between the medial aspect of the ipsilateral psoas muscle and the spine, in some cases covered by the psoas (see Fig. 2–7). The lumbar arteries and veins, coursing posteriorly, are very closely associated with the sympathetic trunks, crossing them perpendicularly and at times proceeding directly through split portions of the sympathetic chain. **The lumbar sympathetic trunks contain variable numbers of ganglia of variable size and position.** Some of the preganglionic fibers of the sympathetic trunks synapse within these ganglia with postganglionic sympathetic neurons supplying the body wall and lower extremities.

Preganglionic fibers supplying the abdominal viscera exit the lumbar sympathetic trunks via the lumbar splanchnic nerves and course anteriorly over the aorta, forming autonomic nervous plexuses associated with the major branches of the abdominal aorta (see Fig. 2–1). They synapse with postganglionic neurons in ganglia within these plexuses. The exceptions to this are those preganglionic sympathetic fibers to the adrenal, which course without interruption and synapse directly with cells of the adrenal medulla. The abdominal aortic plexuses also receive sympathetic input from the 5th through 12th thoracic spinal nerves via the greater, lesser, and lowest splanchnic nerves, which arise in the thorax and course inferiorly through the diaphragm, as well as parasympathetic input via branches from the vagus nerves.

The first and largest of the autonomic nervous plexuses in the abdomen is the celiac plexus, which lies on the anterior aorta surrounding the celiac arterial trunk. Usually paired celiac ganglia lie on either side of the celiac artery (see Fig. 2–1*C* and *D*). **Through this plexus and these ganglia pass much or all of the autonomic nervous supply to the adrenal, kidney, renal pelvis and ureter,** as well as some sympathetic fibers directed to the testes that travel along the testicular arteries. In addition, a separate aorticorenal ganglion usually exists as an inferior extension of the celiac ganglion, forming part of the renal autonomic plexus. The latter plexus surrounds the renal artery and its branches and is contiguous with the celiac plexus. **At the lower extent of the abdominal aorta, much of the sympathetic input to the pelvic urinary organs and genital tract travels through the superior hypogastric plexus, which lies on the aorta anterior to its bifurcation and extends inferiorly on the anterior surface of the fifth lumbar vertebra. This plexus is contiguous bilaterally with inferior hypogastric plexuses, which extend into the pelvis.** Disruption of the sympathetic nerve fibers that travel through these plexuses during retroperitoneal dissection can cause loss of seminal vesicle emission and/or failure of bladder neck closure that results in retrograde ejaculation.

Somatic

The somatic sensory and motor innervation to the lower abdomen and lower extremities also arises in and courses through the retroperitoneum. **The lumbosacral plexus is formed from branches of all lumbar and sacral spinal nerves, with some contribution from the 12th thoracic spinal nerve** as well (Fig. 2–13). Superiorly, nerves of this plexus form within the body of the psoas muscle and pierce this muscle, with more inferior branches passing medial to the psoas as the pelvis is entered (see Fig. 2–7). **The subcostal nerve is the anterior extension of the 12th thoracic nerve and extends beneath the 12th rib. As one proceeds inferiorly, the iliohypogastric nerve and then the ilioinguinal nerve originate together as a common extension from the first lumbar spinal nerve before splitting. These three somatic nerves cross the anterior or inner surface of the quadratus lumborum muscle before piercing the transversus abdominis muscle and continuing their course between this and the internal oblique muscle. Together they provide multiple motor branches to the muscles of the abdominal wall as well as sensory innervation to the skin of the lower abdomen and genitalia. The lateral femoral cutaneous nerve and the genitofemoral nerve arise from the first through third lumbar nerves and are primarily sensory nerves to the skin of the upper thigh and genitalia; however, the genital branch of the genitofemoral nerve also supplies the cremaster and dartos muscles in the scrotum. The genitofemoral nerve lies directly atop and parallels the psoas muscle throughout most of its retroperitoneal course and is easily identified in this position.**

The femoral nerve is a larger structure arising from the second through fourth lumbar spinal nerves and is largely hidden by the body of the psoas muscle before exiting the abdomen just lateral to the femoral artery. This important nervous structure supplies not only the psoas and iliacus muscles but also the large muscle groups of the anterior thigh as well as sensory innervation of the anteromedi

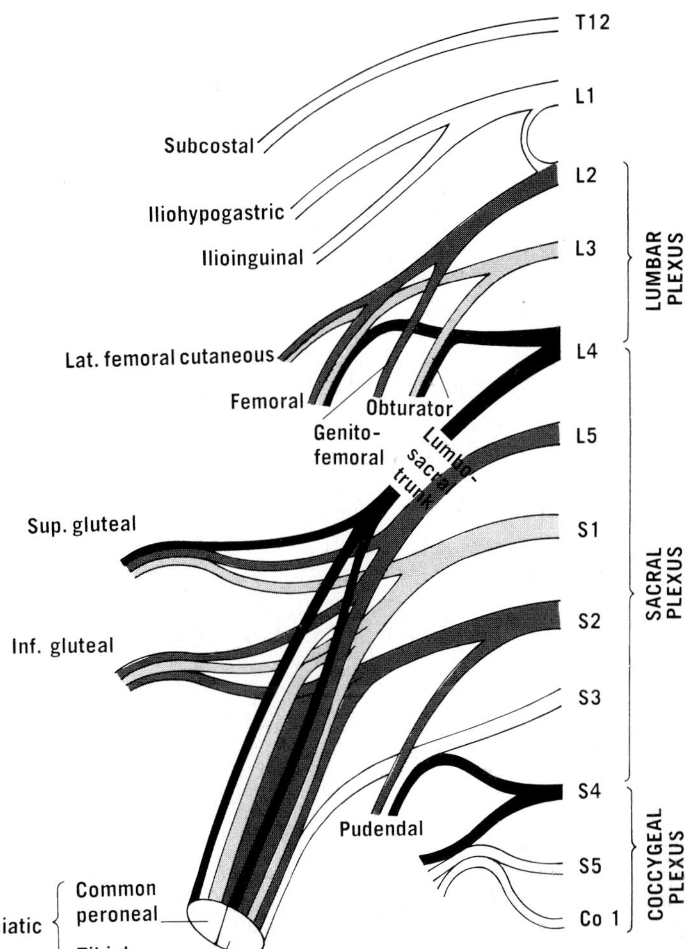

Figure 2–13. Diagrammatic representation of the lumbosacral nervous plexus.

portions of the lower extremity. Intraoperatively, it may be compressed by retractor blades placed inferolaterally against the inguinal ligament in lower abdominal incisions, producing a significant motor palsy that prevents active extension of the knee.

The lumbosacral plexus produces two further nerves that provide key motor and sensory input to the lower extremity. The obturator nerve, an important pelvic landmark, actually arises behind the psoas muscle in the retroperitoneum from the third and fourth lumbar spinal nerves before coursing inferiorly, where its major function is to supply the adductor muscles of the thigh. The sciatic nerve receives input from the fourth lumbar through third sacral spinal nerves, taking final form in the deep posterior pelvis as the body's single largest nerve, supplying the bulk of both sensory and motor innervation to the lower extremity.

Duodenum, Pancreas, and Colon

(Fig. 2–14)

Duodenum

The C-shaped loop formed by the duodenum lies in an almost wholly retroperitoneal position. Only the most proximal portion of the first (ascending) part of the duodenum, just after its takeoff from the gastric pylorus, lies intraperitoneally. **The second (descending) part of the duodenum descends vertically, directly anterior to the right renal hilum, and thus is intimately related on its posterior aspect to the medial margin of the right kidney, right renal vessels, renal pelvis, ureteropelvic junction, and often the upper right ureter.** The common bile duct also lies posterior to and drains into this part of the duodenum. Directly medial and intimately related to the descending duodenum lies the head of the pancreas. Medial and posterior to the descending duodenum is the inferior vena cava. The third (transverse) part of the duodenum crosses from right to left in the retroperitoneum, directly anterior to both the inferior vena cava and aorta, below the takeoff of the superior mesenteric artery from the aorta. The superior mesenteric artery crosses this transverse part of the duodenum vertically as it courses inferiorly into the root of the mesentery of the small bowel. **Surgical reflection of the duodenum (Kocher's maneuver), anteriorly and from right to left, provides anterior operative exposure of the renal vessels and renal pelvis on the right. Reflection of the duodenum is also necessary to expose the upper abdominal portions of the great vessels and the left renal vein in retroperitoneal dissections.**

Pancreas

The pancreas is a solid organ with important endocrine function as the source of insulin as well as important exo-

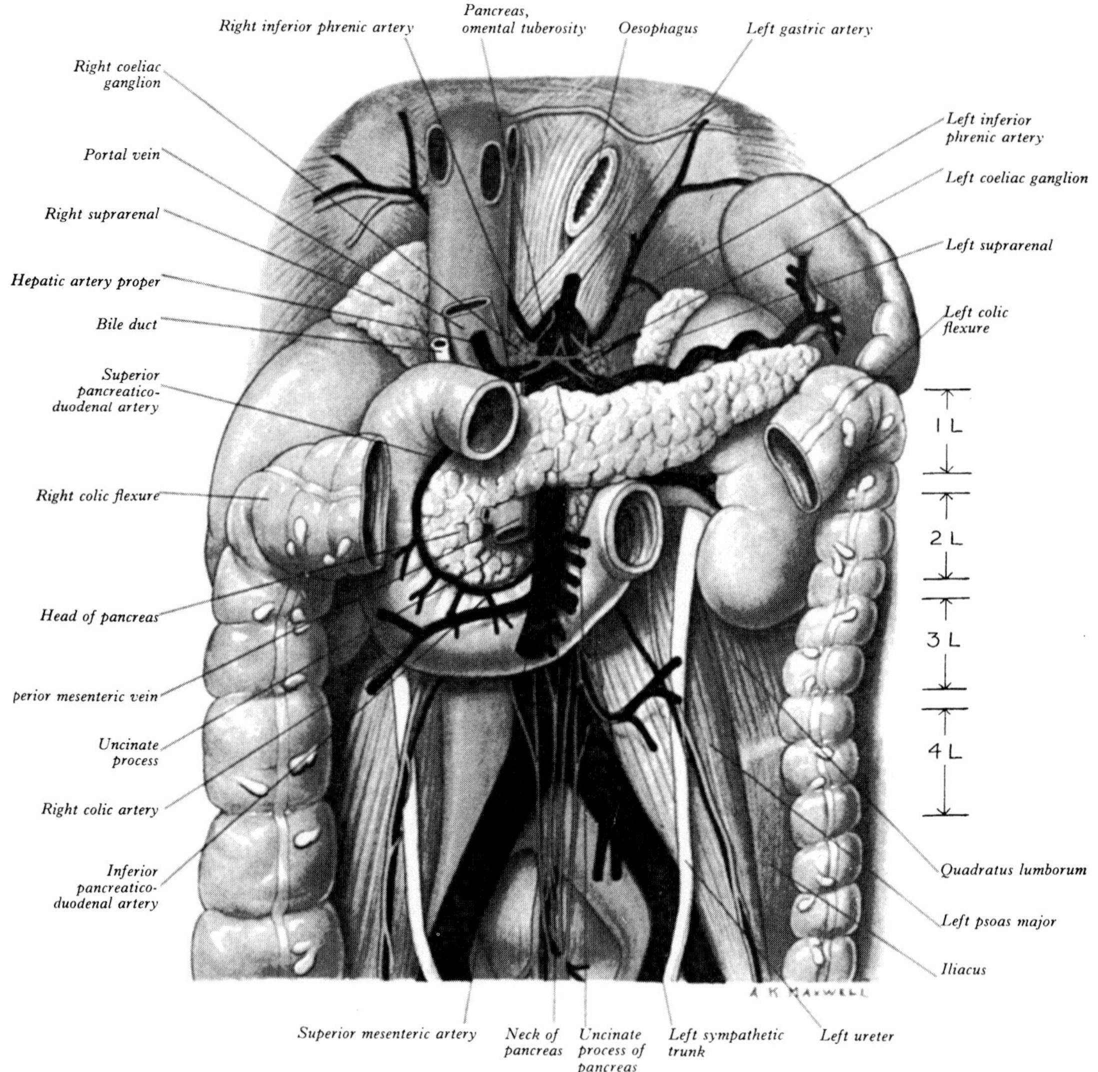

Figure 2–14. Organs of the anterior retroperitoneum, showing relations of the duodenum, pancreas, spleen, and colic flexures to the adrenals, kidneys, and upper ureter. The liver has been removed. Note also the slightly higher position of the right adrenal gland in the retroperitoneum relative to the left adrenal gland. (From Williams PL, Warwick R, eds: Gray's Anatomy, 36th ed. Philadelphia, W. B. Saunders, 1980.)

crine function, secreting numerous digestive enzymes that empty via the pancreatic ductal system into the descending duodenum. With the duodenum, which surrounds the head of the pancreas on the right, it occupies an anterior position in the retroperitoneum. The body of the pancreas crosses the inferior vena cava and aorta below the celiac arterial trunk and above the takeoff of the superior mesenteric artery. **The tail of the pancreas on the left is related posteriorly to the upper portion of the left kidney.** The splenic vein runs directly posterior to the pancreas, and the splenic artery runs just superior to the vein. Thus, both these major vessels are also related to the upper portion of the left kidney. **These relationships are important in that both the pancreas and the splenic vessels are subject to injury during operations on the left kidney.** Injury to the tail of the pancreas, with subsequent release of its powerful digestive enzymes and with the possibility of fistula, is a serious potential complication. Although less common, injury to the duodenum during operations on the right kidney can lead to release of pancreatic enzymes via the duodenum and to similar dire consequences.

Colon

Although the colon is usually considered an intraperitoneal organ, variable portions of this structure may also occupy a retroperitoneal position. In particular, the posterior aspects of the ascending colon and hepatic flexure, and the splenic flexure and descending colon, are generally not covered by the peritoneum. These portions of the colon, for the most part, are fixed to the anterior retroperitoneum and are relatively immobile. **The hepatic flexure of the colon overlies the lower pole of the right kidney. The splenic flexure of the colon overlies the lower pole of the left kidney. The ascending colon is related posteriorly to the right ureter, and the descending and sigmoid colons are related to the left ureter.**

Transabdominal surgical exposure of either kidney or ureter is thus facilitated, in most instances, by medial reflection of the overlying colon. This is accomplished by incision of the reflection of the anterior colonic visceral peritoneum along the line where it joins the posterior parietal peritoneum lateral to the colon on the posterior body wall (the so-called "white line of Toldt"). Either ascending or descending colon may be inadvertently injured during such exposure, resulting in fecal contamination of the operative field. More commonly, **malignant and inflammatory processes of the ascending or descending colon, including retrocecal (i.e., retroperitoneal) appendicitis, may impinge upon the ureter on the involved side.**

Of importance in medial reflection of either ascending or descending colon to expose underlying retroperitoneal structures are their superior fascial attachments. **The hepatic flexure of the colon is variably attached to the right lobe of the liver via the hepatocolic ligament, and the splenic flexure of the colon is more consistently attached to the inferior margin of the spleen via the splenocolic ligament. Excessive traction on these ligaments during manipulation of the colon may result in visceral tears in the liver or spleen and in hemorrhage.** When it is necessary to provide adequate surgical exposure of the ipsilateral kidney, these avascular fascial attachments should be identified early and divided sharply without exerting undue tension during reflection of the colon.

ADRENAL GLANDS (Fig. 2–15)

Anatomic Relations

The adrenal, or suprarenal, glands are paired, yellow-orange, solid endocrine organs that lie within the perirenal (Gerota's) fascia superomedial to either kidney, buried within the perinephric fat. Although closely applied to the upper poles of the kidneys, the adrenals are embryologically and functionally distinct and are physically separated from the kidneys by connective tissue septa in continuity with Gerota's fascia as well as by varying amounts of perinephric adipose tissue. Thus, in cases of renal ectopia, the adrenal usually is found in approximately its normal anatomic position and does not follow the kidney. Similarly, in cases of renal agenesis, the adrenal on the involved side is usually present.

The normal adult adrenal gland weighs approximately 5 g and measures 3 to 5 cm in greatest transverse dimension. In the neonate, the adrenals are relatively much larger in size compared with total body mass and may be one-third the size of the kidney at birth (Fig. 2–16). Both adrenals are somewhat flattened in the anterior-posterior axis, the left more so than the right. The right gland assumes a more pyramidal shape and rests more superior to the upper pole of the right kidney (Figs. 2–17 and 2–18). The left gland has a more crescentic shape and rests more medial to the upper pole of the left kidney; in fact, it may lie directly atop the renal vessels at the left renal hilum (see Fig. 2–15*C* and *D*). **The right adrenal thus tends to lie more superiorly in the retroperitoneum than does the left adrenal** (see Fig. 2–14). This is in contradistinction to the fact that the right kidney lies, in general, slightly more inferiorly than the left, and this fact must be taken into account in the planning of incisions for adrenal surgery.

The diaphragm lies posterior to either adrenal (see Fig. 2–18). The upper aspect of the left adrenal is related anteriorly to the stomach, whereas the tail of the pancreas and the splenic vessels are applied to its inferior aspect (see Fig. 2–17). The right adrenal is related anteriorly on its lateral aspect to the nonperitonealized "bare spot" of the liver. Medially, the right adrenal may be related to the duodenum anteriorly, and there is usually also a retrocaval extension of one wing of the gland, closely applied to the posterior and lateral aspects of the inferior vena cava.

Composition

Each adrenal is a composite of two separate and functionally distinct glandular elements: cortex and medulla (Fig. 2–19). **The medulla, which forms the central core of each adrenal, consists of chromaffin cells derived from the neural crest and intimately related to the sympathetic nervous system. The cells of the medulla produce neuroactive catecholamines, primarily epinephrine and norepinephrine, which are released directly into the blood stream via an extensive venous drainage system. The adrenal cortex is mesodermally derived, completely surrounds and encases the medulla, and forms the bulk of the adrenal gland—80% to 90% by weight. Three cell layers can be identified in the cortex** (see Fig. 2–19). **The outermost layer is the zona glomerulosa, which produces aldosterone in response to stimulation by the renin-angiotensin system. Centripetally located are the zona fasciculata and zona reticularis, which produce glucocorticoids and sex steroids, respectively. Unlike the zona glomerulosa, these latter functions are regulated by pituitary release of adrenocorticotropic hormone (ACTH).** The substance of the adrenal gland is inherently quite friable but is enclosed by a thick, collagenous capsule; yet it still can be readily torn with aggressive handling at time of operation.

Adrenal Vessels and Innervation

The adrenals, concordant with their key role in the body's hormonal milieu, are highly vascularized. The arterial supply is relatively symmetric bilaterally. **Multiple small arteries supply each adrenal gland** (see Fig. 2–15). **These are branch vessels, which can be traced to three major arterial sources for each gland: (1) superior branches from the inferior phrenic artery, (2) middle branches directly from the aorta, and (3) inferior branches from the ipsilateral renal artery** (see Fig. 2–9). **In contrast to the multiple arteries, usually a single large adrenal vein exits each gland from its hilum anteromedially** (see Fig. 2–17). **On the right side, this vein is very short and enters directly into the inferior vena cava on its posterolateral aspect** (see Fig. 2–15*A* and *B*). **The adrenal vein on the left is more elongated and is typically joined by the left inferior phrenic vein before entering the superior aspect of the left renal vein** (see Fig. 2–15*C* and *D* and Fig. 2–9). **The adrenal lymphatics in general exit the glands along the course of the venous drainage and eventually empty into para-aortic lymph nodes.**

The adrenal medulla receives greater autonomic innervation than any other organ in the body. **Multiple preganglionic sympathetic fibers enter each adrenal along the course of the adrenal vein and synapse with chromaffin cells in the medulla.** This rich sympathetic innervation of

Text continued on page 69

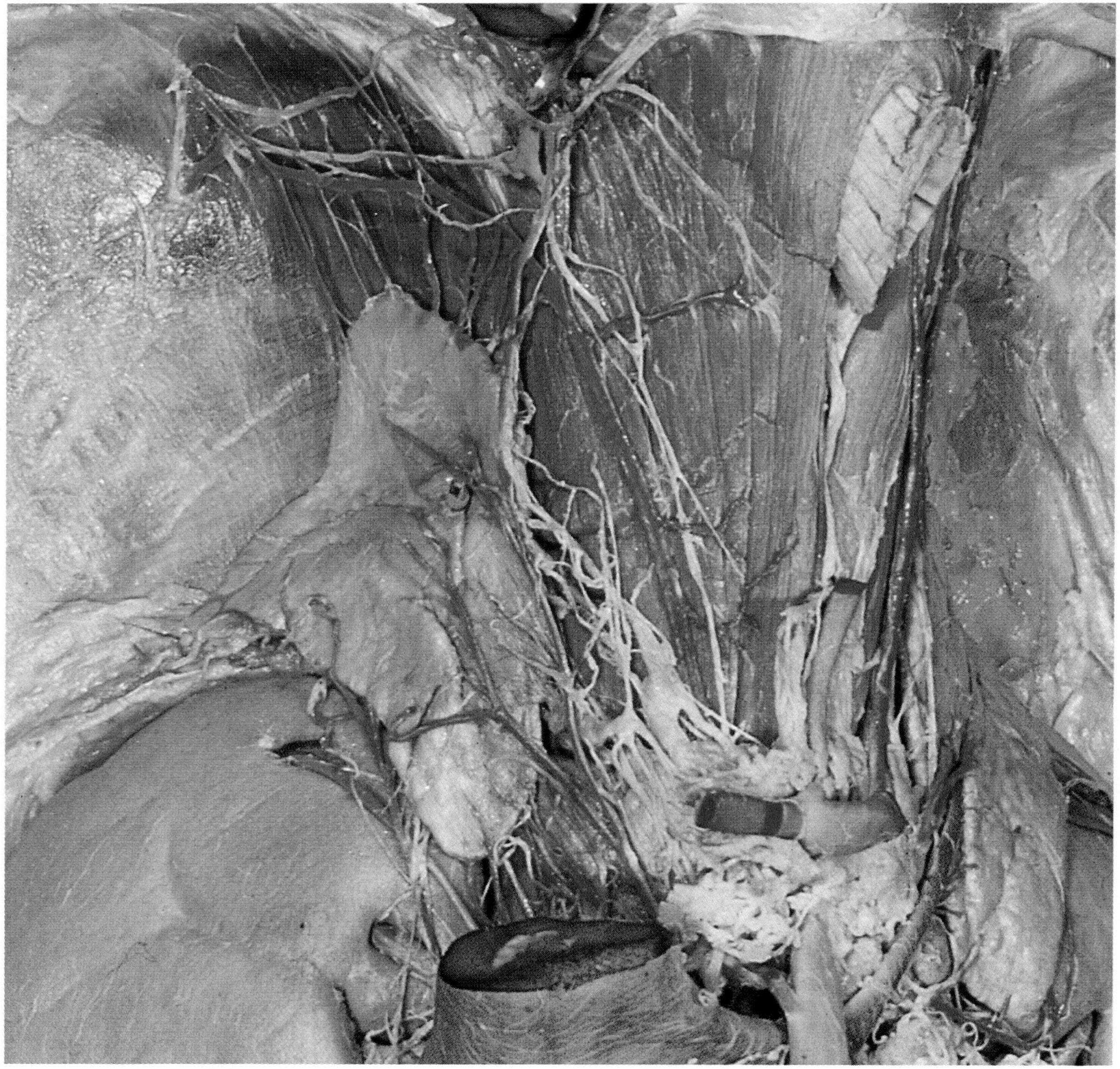

A

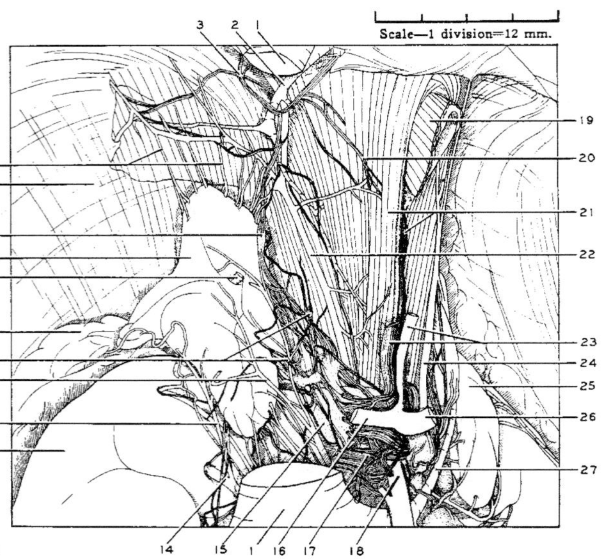

B

Figure 2–15. *A,* Right adrenal gland dissected. The inferior vena cava has been excised to expose the gland. The celiac arterial trunk, its branches, and associated autonomic nervous plexus are also well demonstrated. *B,* 1, Inferior vena cava (cut). 2, Right inferior phrenic vein. 3, Right phrenic nerve. 4, Superior adrenal arteries (branching from right inferior phrenic artery). 5, Diaphragm. 6, Inferior phrenic ganglion. 7, Right adrenal gland. 8, Right adrenal vein (cut). 9, Pararenal retroperitoneal fat. 10, Autonomic nerves to adrenal. 11, Middle adrenal artery (from aorta). 12, Inferior adrenal artery (from renal artery). 13, Right kidney. 14, Branch of right renal artery. 15, Celiac ganglion. 16, Common hepatic artery. 17, Celiac autonomic nervous plexus. 18, Superior mesenteric artery. 19, Esophagus (cut). 20, Branch of phrenic nerve. 21, *Upper pointer,* right crus of diaphragm; *lower pointer,* vagus nerve. 22, Right inferior phrenic artery. 23, *Upper pointer,* left gastric artery; *lower pointer,* superior extension of celiac autonomic nervous plexus. 24, Left inferior phrenic artery. 25, Left adrenal gland. 26, Splenic artery. 27, Left adrenal vein.

C

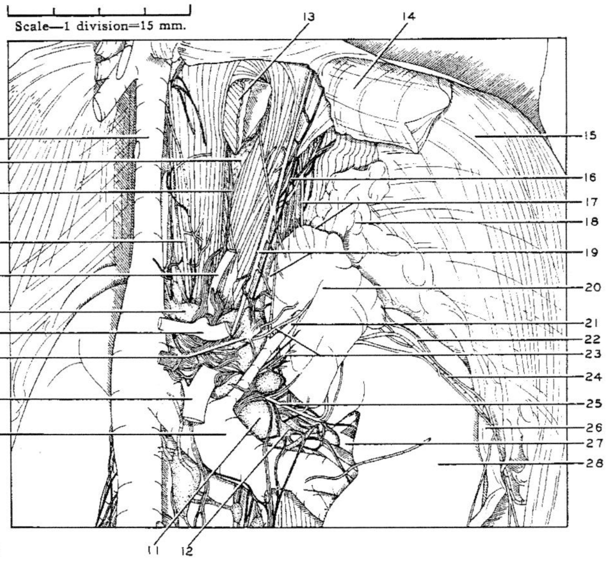

D

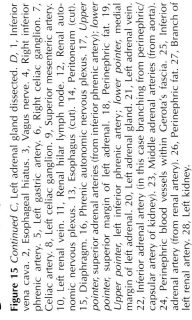

Figure 15 *Continued C,* Left adrenal gland dissected. *D,* 1, Inferior vena cava. 2, Esophageal hiatus. 3, Vagus nerve. 4, Right inferior phrenic artery. 5, Left gastric artery. 6, Right celiac ganglion. 7, Celiac artery. 8, Left celiac ganglion. 9, Superior mesenteric artery. 10, Left renal vein. 11, Renal hilar lymph node. 12, Renal autonomic nervous plexus. 13, Esophagus (cut). 14, Peritoneum (cut). 15, Diaphragm. 16, Phrenic autonomic nervous plexus. 17, *Upper pointer,* superior adrenal arteries (from inferior phrenic artery); *lower pointer,* superior margin of left adrenal. 18, Perinephric fat. 19, *Upper pointer,* left inferior phrenic artery; *lower pointer,* medial margin of left adrenal. 20, Left adrenal gland. 21, Left adrenal vein. 22, Inferior adrenal artery (in this case branching from perinephric/capsular artery of kidney). 23, Middle adrenal arteries (from aorta). 24, Perinephric blood vessels within Gerota's fascia. 25, Inferior adrenal artery (from renal artery). 26, Perinephric fat. 27, Branch of left renal artery. 28, Left kidney.

Illustration continued on following page

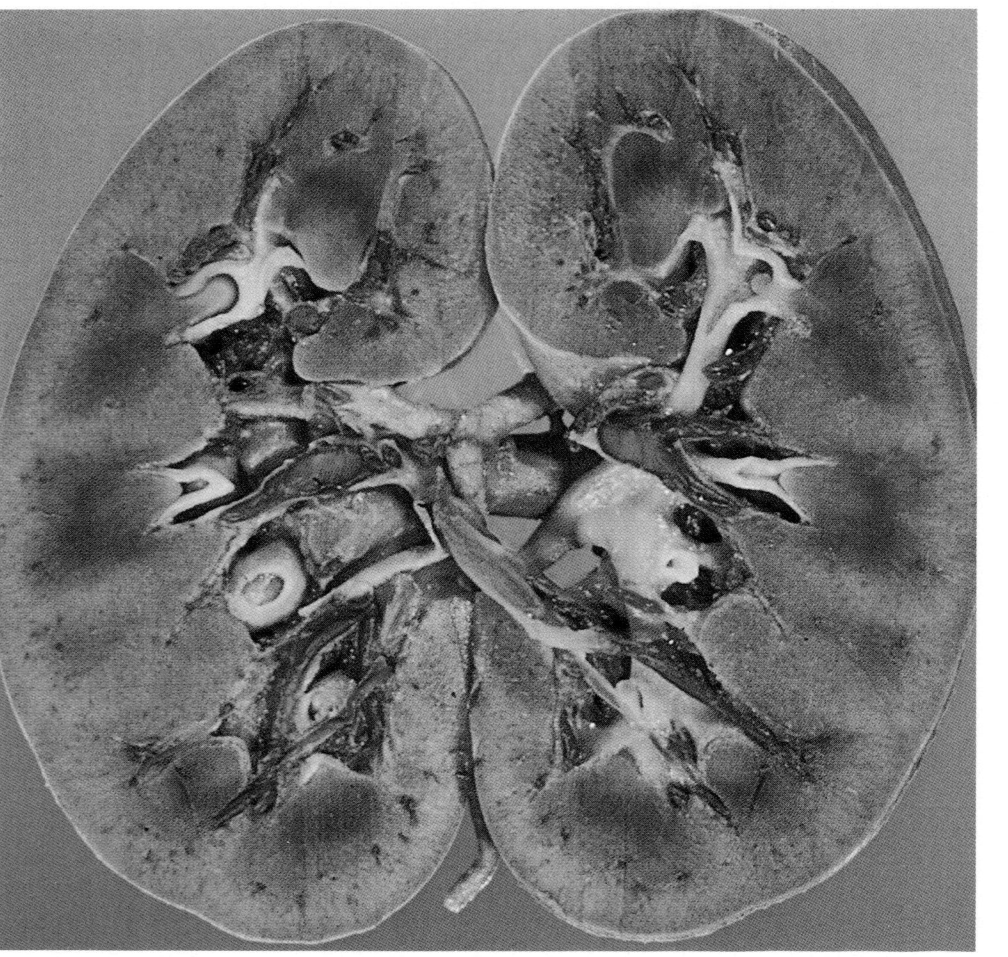

E

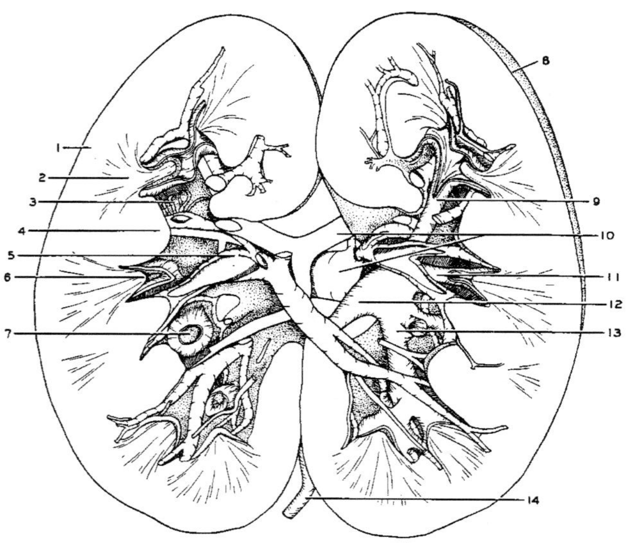

F

Figure 2–15 *Continued E,* Coronal section through the left kidney, with special attention to the renal sinus and contained structures. *F,* 1, Renal cortex. 2, Renal medulla. 3, Renal sinus. 4, Renal column (of Bertin). 5, Branch of renal vein (sectioned). 6, Renal papilla (seen in cut section). 7, Renal papilla (seen end on). 8, Renal capsule. 9, Major calyx to upper pole. 10, *Upper pointer,* main renal artery; *lower pointer,* main renal vein. 11, Minor calyx. 12, Renal pelvis. 13, Major calyx to lower pole. 14, Ureter.

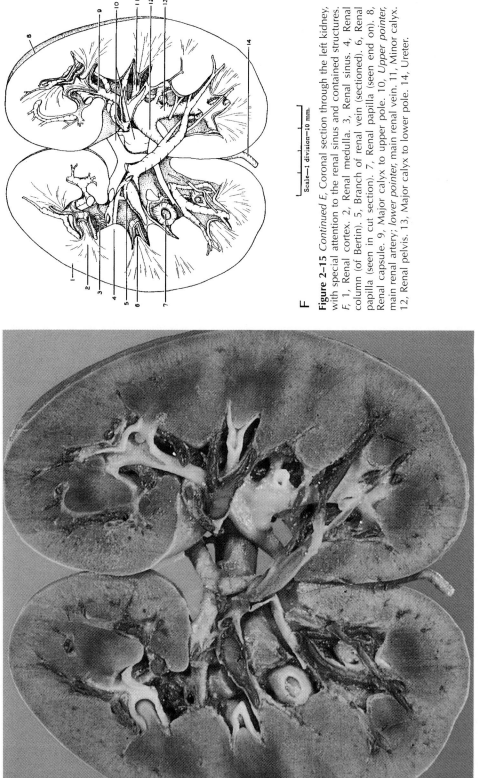

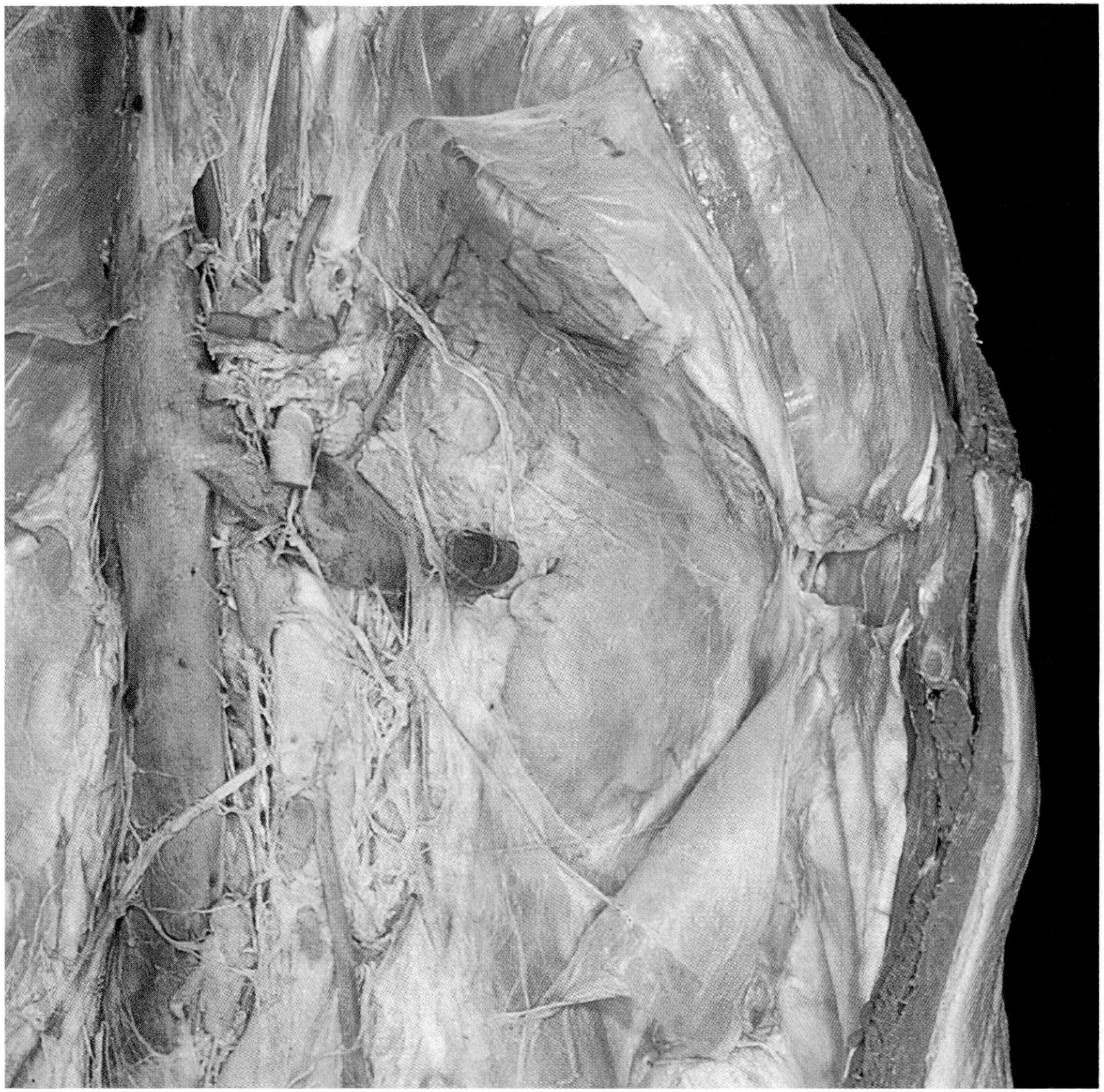

G

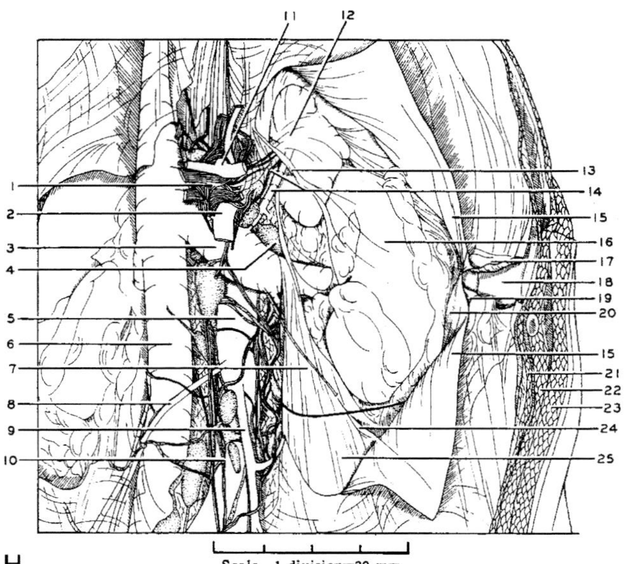

H

Figure 2–15 *Continued G,* Dissection of the left kidney within the retroperitoneum. The anterior perirenal (Gerota's) fascia has been opened and reflected to expose the kidney. *H,* 1, Celiac autonomic nervous plexus. 2, Superior mesenteric artery (cut). 3, Left renal vein. 4, Renal hilar lymph node. 5, Aorta. 6, Inferior vena cava. 7, Fibrous band within Gerota's fascia. 8, Right gonadal artery. 9, Inferior mesenteric artery. 10, Part of aortic autonomic nervous plexus. 11, Celiac artery. 12, Left adrenal gland. 13, Fibrous band within Gerota's fascia. 14, Left adrenal vein. 15, Gerota's fascia. 16, Left kidney. 17, Gerota's fascia. 18, Transversalis fascia. 19, Gerota's fascia. 20, Gerota's fascia. 21, Transversus abdominis muscle (in cut section). 22, Internal oblique muscle (in cut section). 23, External oblique muscle (in cut section). 24, Fibrous band within Gerota's fascia. 25, Psoas major muscle covered by Psoas sheath. (*A* to *H* reproduced from the Bassett anatomic collection with permission granted by Dr. Robert A. Chase.)

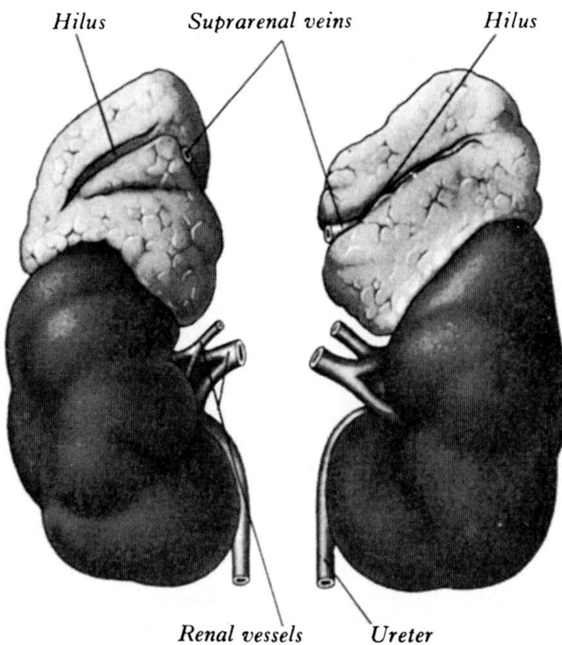

Figure 2–16. Kidneys and adrenals from neonate. Note large size of the adrenal glands relative to the kidneys, and note fetal lobation of the kidneys. (From Williams PL, Warwick R, Dyson M, Bannister LH, eds: Gray's Anatomy, 37th ed. Edinburgh, Churchill Livingstone, 1989.)

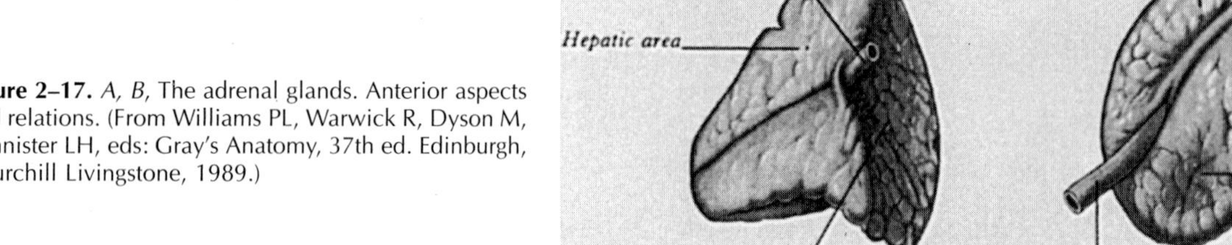

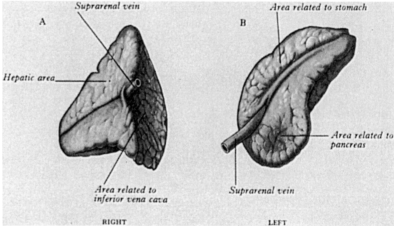

Figure 2–17. *A, B,* The adrenal glands. Anterior aspects and relations. (From Williams PL, Warwick R, Dyson M, Bannister LH, eds: Gray's Anatomy, 37th ed. Edinburgh, Churchill Livingstone, 1989.)

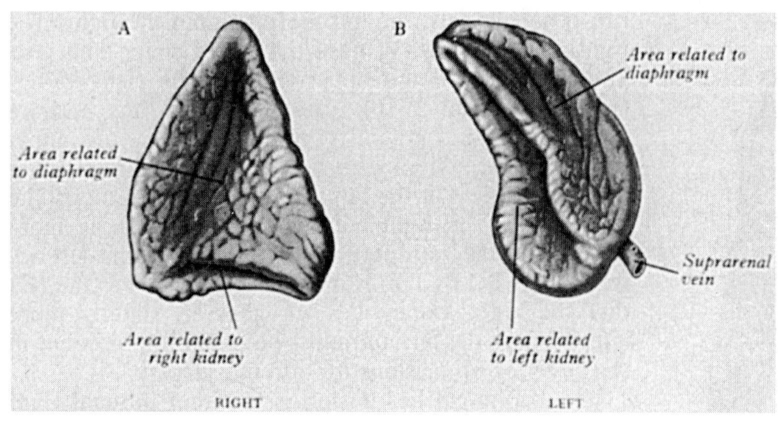

Figure 2–18. *A, B,* The adrenal glands. Posterior aspects and relations. (From Williams PL, Warwick R, Dyson M, Bannister LH, eds: Gray's Anatomy, 37th ed. Edinburgh, Churchill Livingstone, 1989.)

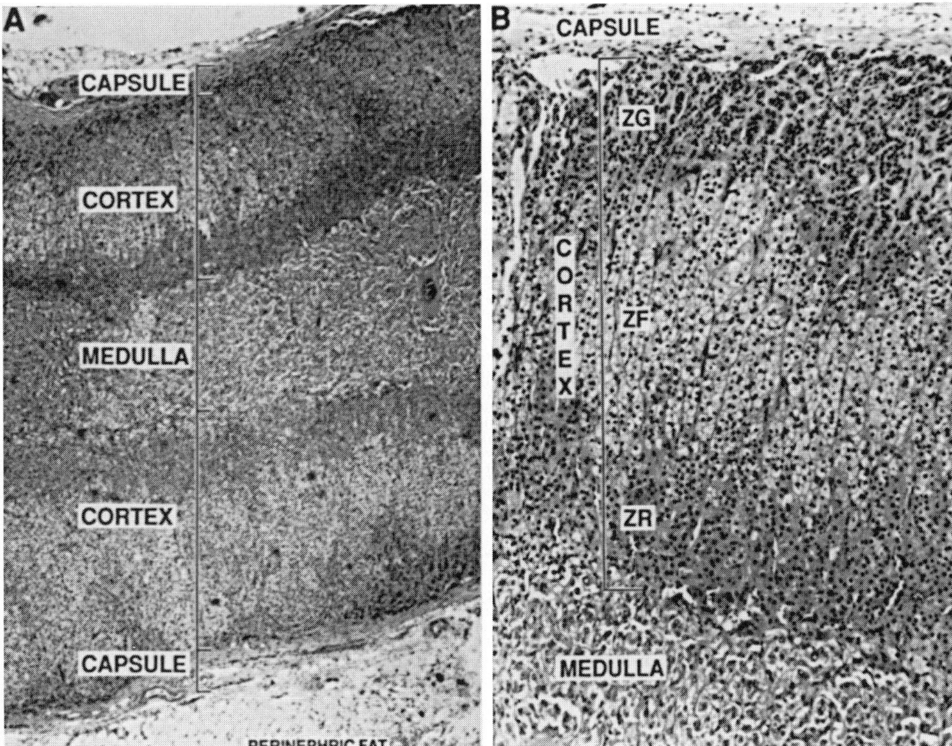

Figure 2–19. Microscopic section through the adrenal gland. *A*, Full-thickness section showing adrenal medulla surrounded by tissue of cortex. Also demonstrated is fibrous capsule of the adrenal, and entire gland is surrounded by perinephric fat. *B*, Section through the adrenal cortex, demonstrating three functionally distinct cellular layers. ZG, zona glomerulosa; ZF, zona fasciculata; ZR, zona reticularis.

the medulla reaches the adrenal via the splanchnic nerves and celiac ganglion. In contrast, the adrenal cortex is believed to receive no innervation.

THE KIDNEYS AND URETERS

Gross and Microscopic Anatomy of the Kidney

Gross Description

The kidneys are paired, reddish-brown, solid organs that lie well protected deep within the retroperitoneum on either side of the spine (see Fig. 2–1). As the organs of urinary excretion, the kidneys play a central role in fluid, electrolyte, and acid-base balance in humans, but they also have important endocrine functions, known to include vitamin D metabolism and the production of both renin and erythropoietin. They are highly vascular organs, receiving one fifth of the total cardiac output under normal conditions, and their parenchyma is friable. A thin but tough fibroelastic capsule encases the parenchyma and, unlike the parenchyma, holds suture. In the normal kidney, the capsule can be readily stripped from the parenchyma by the surgeon or, similarly, can be elevated from the parenchyma by hematoma.

The normal kidney in the adult male weighs approximately 150 g. On the average, it is slightly smaller in the female, weighing approximately 135 g. The normal kidney is typically 10 to 12 cm in vertical dimension, 5 to 7 cm in transverse width, and approximately 3 cm in anterior-posterior thickness. Again, the size in females tends toward the lower ends of these measurement ranges, but these dimensions are related more to overall body size rather than to sex, with smaller individuals having generally smaller kidney mass than larger individuals. The kidneys vary somewhat from right to left, with the right kidney tending to be shorter in vertical dimension and sometimes wider than the longer, more narrow left kidney—a fact attributed to the effect of the hepatic mass on the right.

The kidneys are larger relative to body size in children, as are the adrenal glands, and at birth the kidneys are irregular in contour with multiple "fetal lobations" (see Fig. 2–16). These lobations typically disappear in the first years of life. By adulthood, the lateral surface of the kidney usually forms a smooth convexity with rounded upper and lower poles; however, **it is neither unusual nor abnormal to see persistence of some degree of fetal lobation throughout adult life** (Fig. 2–20). Similarly, **it is not unusual to see a focal bulge in the midlateral contour of the kidney on either side, referred to as a "dromedary hump"** (Fig. 2–21). **This also is a normal variation,** believed to be secondary to downward pressure from spleen or liver on the kidney during development, **and occurs much more commonly on the left than the right side.**

On the medial surface of either kidney is a depression, the renal hilum. The renal hilum opens into the renal sinus, a space that forms the central portion of the kidney and is surrounded by the renal parenchyma (see Fig. 2–15*E* and *F* and Fig. 2–8). The urinary collecting structures and renal vessels occupy the renal sinus and exit the kidney via the hilum medially. Varying amounts of fat surround these structures within the renal sinus.

Microscopic Anatomy

The renal parenchyma is divided into cortex and medulla. The lighter-hued cortex can be readily distinguished

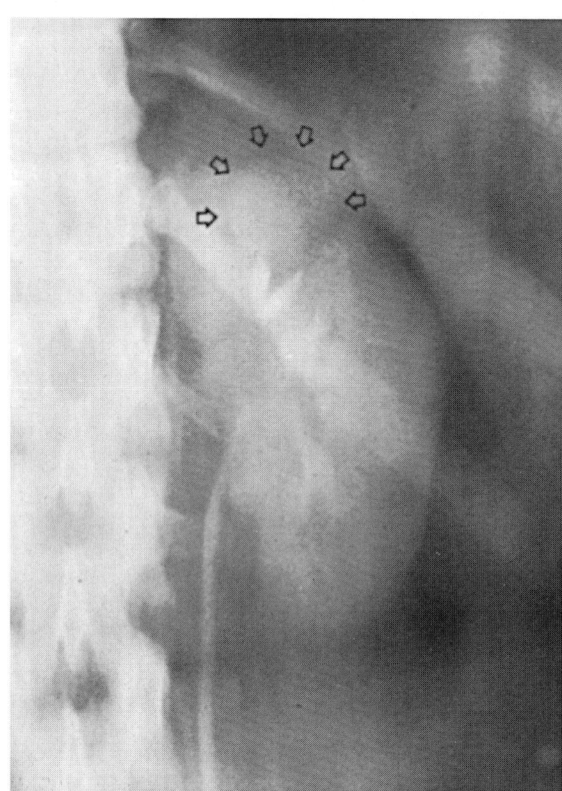

Figure 2–20. Persistent fetal lobation of the upper pole of the left kidney demonstrated on excretory urogram.

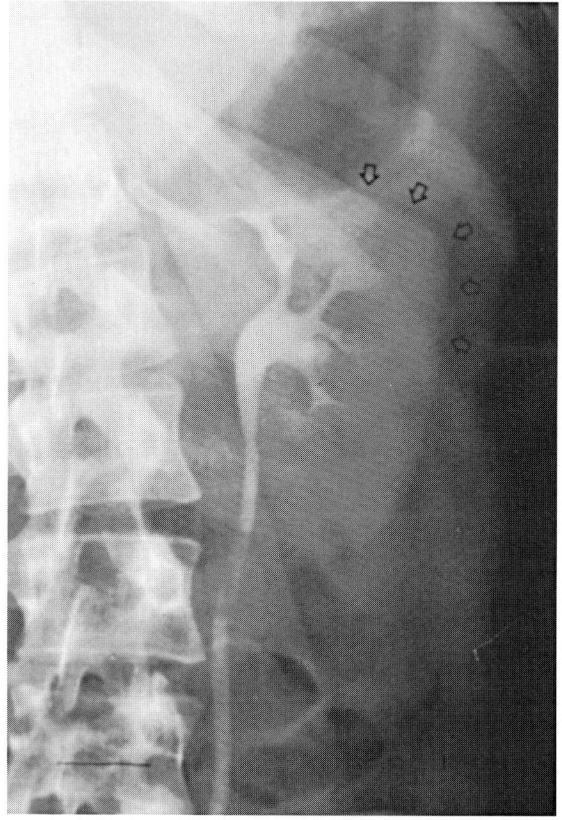

Figure 2–21. Dromedary hump of the left kidney seen on excretory urogram.

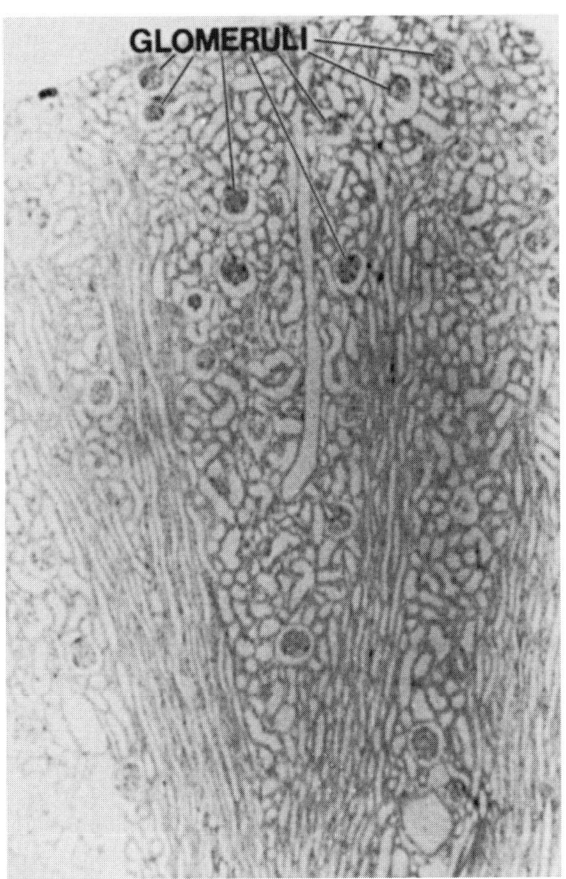

Figure 2–22. Microscopic section through the renal cortex, showing array of vessels and uriniferous tubules, with interspersed glomeruli.

from the darker medulla even on gross inspection of a sectioned kidney (see Fig. 2–15*E* and *F*). **The medulla is not contiguous but consists of multiple distinct conical segments, the renal "pyramids." The rounded apex of each pyramid is the renal papilla, which points centrally into the renal sinus, where it is cupped by an individual minor calyx** of the renal collecting system. Thus, the number of pyramids corresponds to the number of minor calyces. The base of each pyramid roughly parallels the external contour of the kidney. **The renal cortex covers the pyramids, not only peripherally but also extending between the pyramids to the renal sinus. It is through these interpyramidal extensions of cortex—the renal columns ("of Bertin")—that the renal vessels enter and leave the kidney parenchyma.** A renal lobe is defined as a single medullary pyramid and its associated surrounding cortex.

Microscopically, the renal parenchyma consists of multiple tubular structures, in part the kidney's abundant vascular and capillary networks, in part the various tubules that carry the urinary filtrate, with scant intervening interstitial connective tissue in the normal state (Fig. 2–22). In the renal cortex, this tubular array is characteristically peppered by the rounded capillary networks of glomeruli.

Relations and Investing Fascia

Anatomic Relations

As a result of the mass of the liver, in most individuals the right kidney lies 1 to 2 cm lower in the retroperitoneum than does the left; however, this is not invariable, and in some instances the right kidney may be higher than the left. The upper pole of the left kidney typically lies at the level of the 12th thoracic vertebral body, and its lower pole at the level of the 3rd lumbar vertebra. The right kidney usually extends from the top of the first lumbar vertebra to the bottom of the third lumbar vertebra. However, these relationships vary greatly between individuals (Fig. 2–23) and also within the same individual. **The kidneys are remarkably mobile organs, and their positions vary with inspiratory and expiratory movement of the diaphragm as well as with changes in position from upright to supine to head down ("Trendelenburg" position)** (Fig. 2–24).

The posterior relations of the kidneys to the abdominal wall musculature are relatively symmetric (Fig. 2–25). The diaphragm covers roughly the upper third or upper pole of each kidney. With the diaphragm travels the pleural reflection, and thus any direct approach to the upper portion of the kidney, whether percutaneous or open surgical, risks entering the pleural space. The 12th rib on either side crosses the kidney at approximately the lower extent of the diaphragm. The upper border of the left kidney, being higher than the right, usually extends to the upper border of the 11th rib. The medial portion of the lower two thirds of either kidney, with the renal vessels and pelvis, lies against the psoas muscle. Moving from medial to lateral on the posterior surface of the kidney, the quadratus lumborum muscle and then the aponeurosis of the transversus abdominis muscle are encountered. **In part as a result of the contour of the**

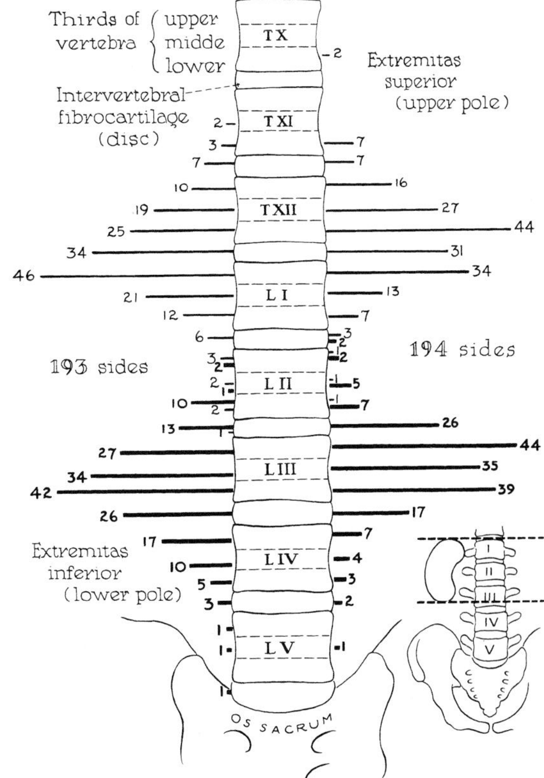

Figure 2–23. Variation between individuals in level of the kidneys relative to the spinal column. Lighter lateral lines represent upper poles of kidneys; darker lateral lines represent lower poles. (From Anson BJ, Daseler EH: Surg Gynecol Obstet 1961; 112:439.)

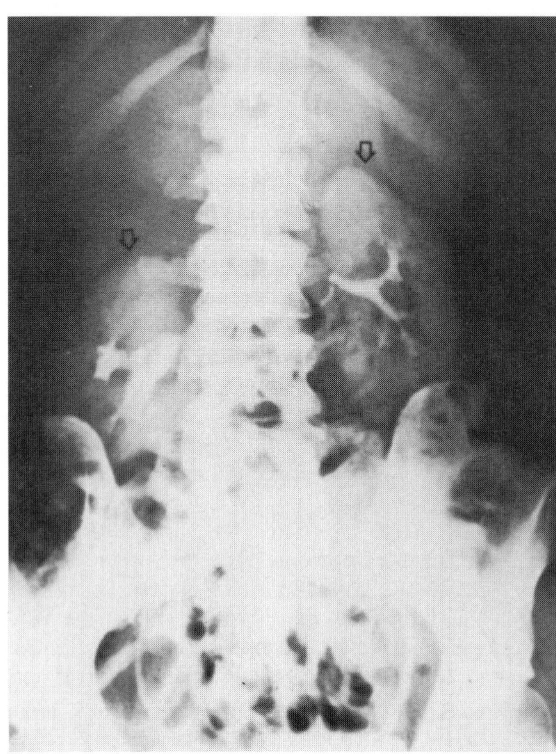

Figure 2–24. Excretory urogram filmed during full inspiration, showing extreme renal mobility with downward displacement (*arrows*) of the kidneys in one individual.

psoas muscle, the lower pole of either kidney lies farther from the midline than does the upper pole, so that the upper poles tilt medially at a slight angle (Fig. 2–26). **Similarly, the kidneys do not lie in a simple coronal plane, but the lower pole of the kidney is pushed slightly more anterior than the upper pole. The medial aspect of each kidney is rotated anteriorly on a longitudinal axis at an angle of about 30 degrees from the true coronal plane, with the renal vessels and pelvis exiting the hilum medially in a relatively anterior direction** (see Figs. 2–8 and 2–26).

Anteriorly, the kidneys differ significantly in their relation-

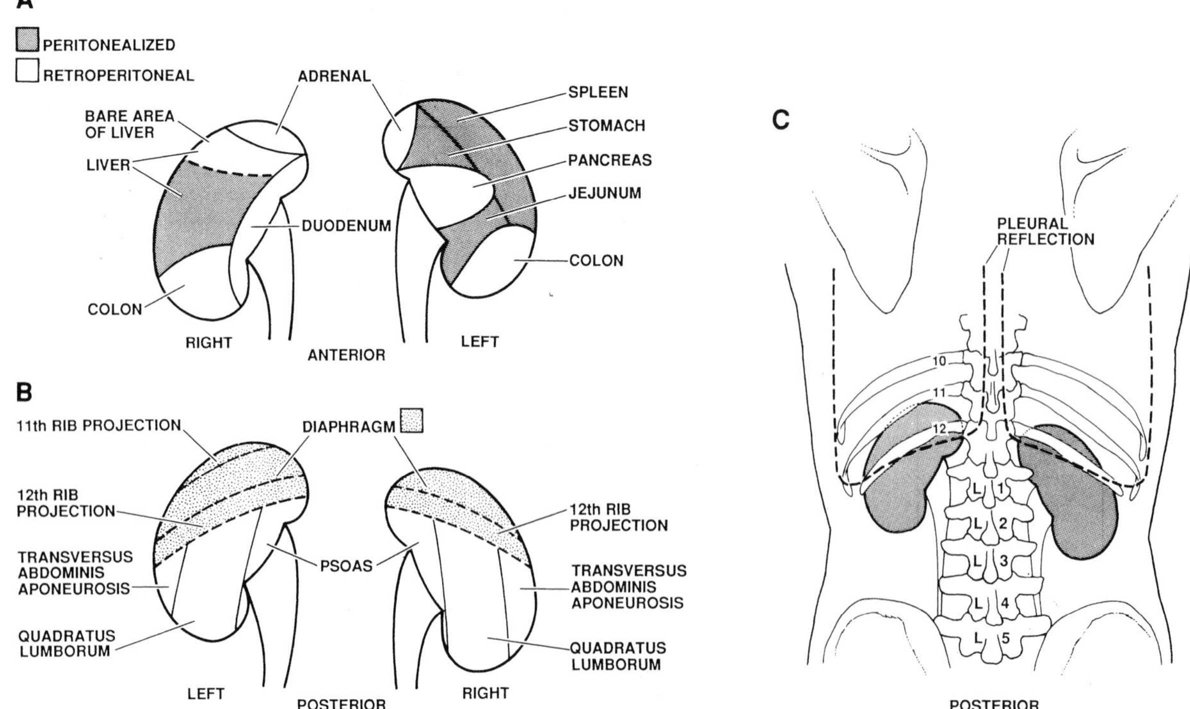

Figure 2–25. Anatomic relations of the kidneys. *A*, Anterior relations to abdominal organs. *B*, Posterior relations to the muscles of posterior body wall and ribs. *C*, Relations to the pleural reflections and skeleton posteriorly.

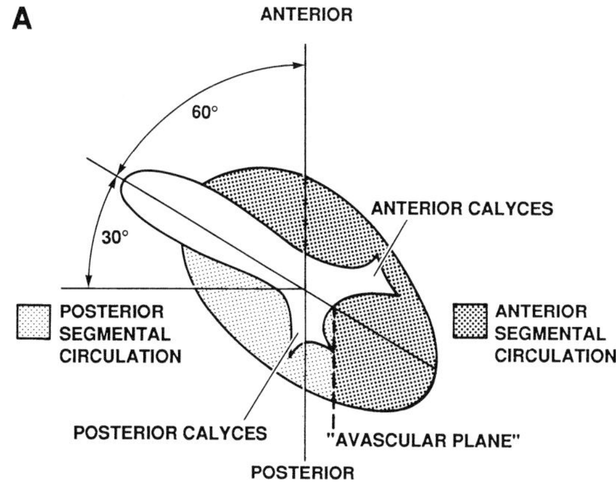

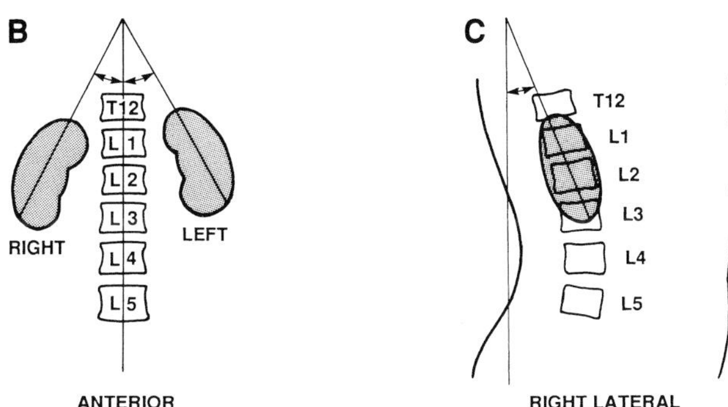

Figure 2–26. Normal rotational axes of the kidney. *A*, Transverse view showing approximate 30-degree anterior rotation of the left kidney from the coronal plane, relative positions of anterior and posterior rows of calyces, and location of the relatively avascular plane separating the anterior and posterior renal circulation. *B*, Coronal section demonstrating slight inward tilt of the upper poles of the kidneys. *C*, Sagittal view showing anterior displacement of the lower pole of the right kidney.

ships to both intraperitoneal and extraperitoneal organs (see Figs. 2–8 and 2–25). The right kidney lies behind the liver; it is separated from the liver by reflection of the peritoneum, except for a small area of its upper pole, which comes into direct contact with the liver's retroperitoneal bare spot. The extent of this peritoneal reflection helps to prevent most, but not all, large right renal cancers from directly invading the liver on the right. **The extension of parietal peritoneum that bridges between the perirenal fascia covering the upper pole of the right kidney and the posterior aspect of the liver is called the hepatorenal ligament. Excessive traction on this attachment or the hepatocolic ligament during right renal surgery may produce hepatic parenchymal tears. The duodenum is applied directly to the medial aspect and hilar structures of the right kidney.** The hepatic flexure of the colon, which also is extraperitoneal, crosses the lower pole of the right kidney. The adrenal gland covers the superomedial aspect of the upper poles of both right and left kidneys, as already discussed.

On the left, the retroperitoneal tail of the pancreas and the related splenic vessels are applied directly to the upper to middle portion and hilum of the kidney. Superior to the pancreatic tail, the left kidney is covered by peritoneum of the lesser sac and here is related to the posterior gastric wall. Below the pancreatic tail, the medial aspect of the kidney is covered by peritoneum of the greater sac and is related to the jejunum. The lower pole of the left kidney is crossed by the splenic flexure of the colon, generally in an extraperitoneal position. The spleen is separated from the upper lateral portion of the left kidney by peritoneal reflection. However, **there is typically a peritoneal extension between the perirenal fascia covering the upper pole of the left kidney and the inferior splenic capsule, called the splenorenal, or lienorenal, ligament. Just as with the adjacent and often contiguous splenocolic ligamentous attachment, care must be taken not to exert undue tension on the splenorenal ligament during operative procedures on the left kidney, in order to avoid inadvertent tearing of the spleen.** Such tearing may necessitate splenectomy during left nephrectomy. Both splenocolic and splenorenal ligaments, and contralateral hepatocolic and hepatorenal ligaments, are avascular and can be divided sharply with safety.

Gerota's Fascia

The kidneys and associated adrenal glands are surrounded by varying degrees of perinephric or perirenal fat, and these together are loosely enclosed by the perirenal fascia, commonly called "Gerota's fascia" (see Figs. 2–15*G* and *H*, 2–6, and 2–8). **The anterior and posterior leaves of Gerota's fascia** (Figs. 2–27 and 2–28), **which extend anterior and posterior to the kidney, become fused on three sides around the kidney laterally, medially, and superiorly.** Superiorly, Gerota's fascia fuses and tapers to disappear over the inferior diaphragmatic surface. Medially, Gerota's fascia extends across the midline and is contiguous

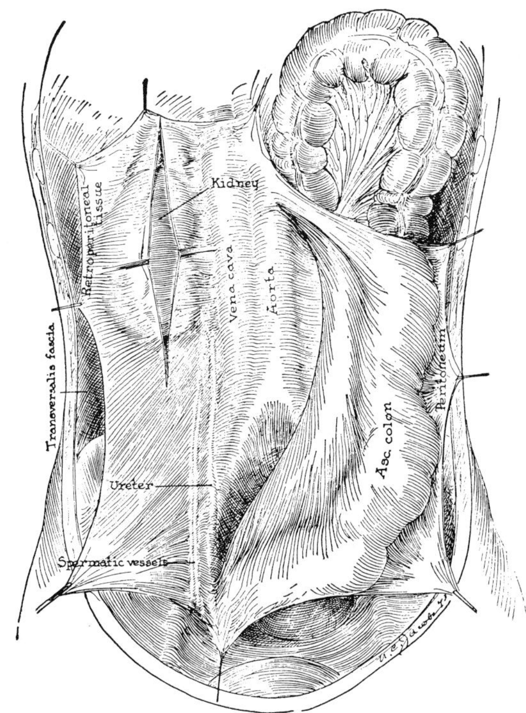

Figure 2–27. Anterior view of Gerota's fascia, split over the right kidney (which it contains), and showing inferior extension enveloping ureter and gonadal vessels. Colon and overlying peritoneum have been reflected medially. (From Tobin CE: Anat Rec 1944; 89:295.)

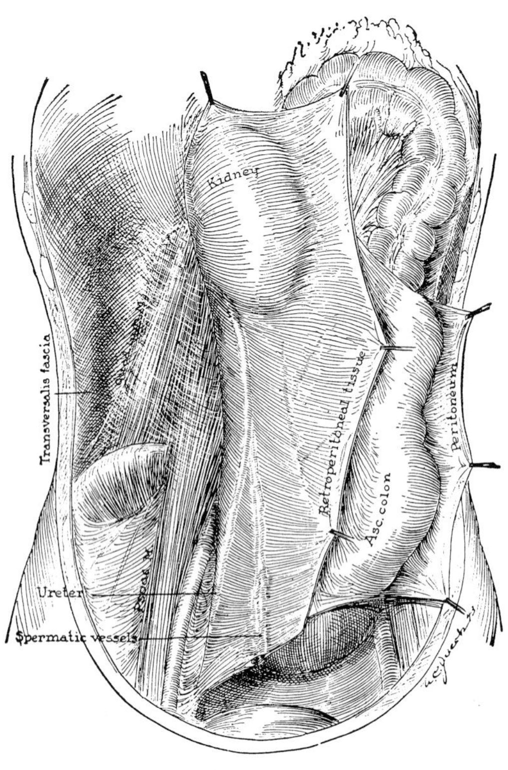

Figure 2–28. Posterior view of Gerota's fascia, rotated medially with contained kidney, ureter, and gonadal vessels, exposing the muscular posterior body wall covered by transversalis fascia. (From Tobin CE: Anat Rec 1944; 89:295.)

with Gerota's fascia on the contralateral side, although the anterior and posterior leaves are generally fused and inseparable as they cross the great vessels. **Inferiorly, Gerota's fascia remains an open potential space, containing the ureter and gonadal vessels on either side.** It thins inferiorly and is contiguous with retroperitoneal fascia, which extends into the pelvis and, in males, also extends with the spermatic vessels and vas deferens into the scrotum. **Around and outside Gerota's fascia are variable amounts of retroperitoneal fat (the *para*renal or *para*nephric fat), distin-**

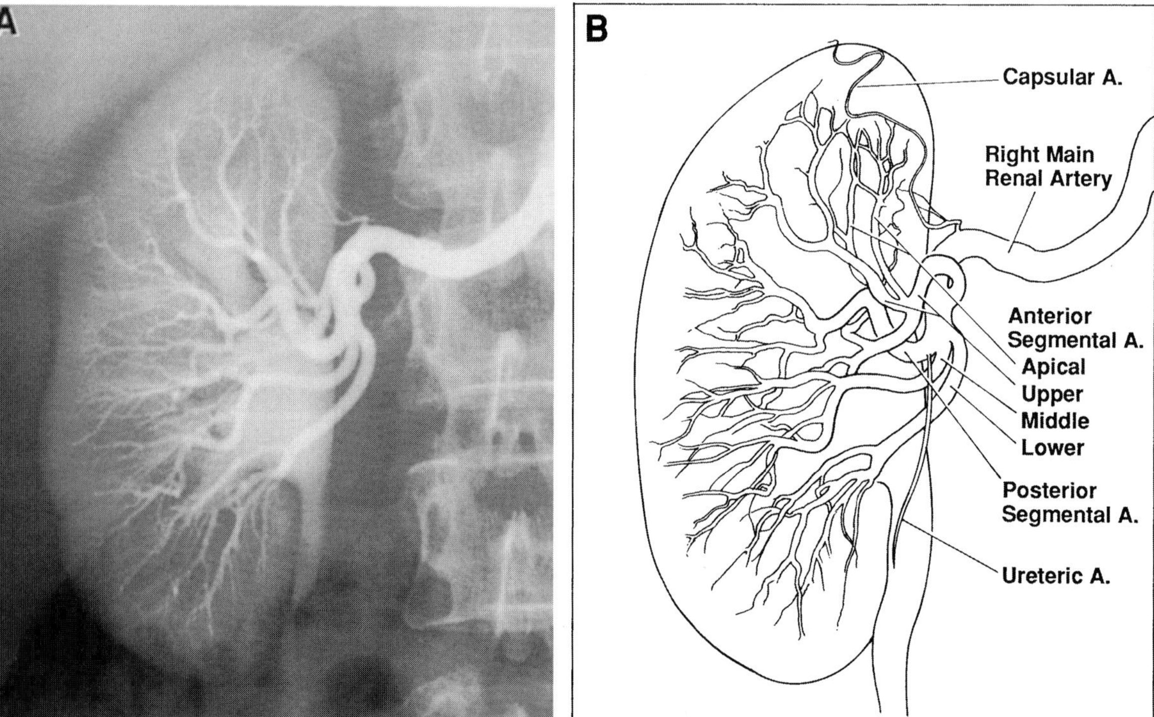

Figure 2–29. Segmental branches of the right renal artery demonstrated by renal angiogram.

guished from the *peri*renal (*peri*nephric) fat that is contained within Gerota's fascia and is immediately adjacent to the kidney.

Gerota's fascia forms an important anatomic barrier around the kidney and tends to contain pathologic processes originating from the kidney. Renal malignancies, early in their course, tend to remain within the fascial capsule formed by Gerota's fascia and can be safely and completely excised by removing the kidney with surrounding Gerota's fascia intact as a single entity. Gerota's fascia usually can be separated from the transversalis fascia overlying the muscles of the retroperitoneum posteriorly (see Fig. 2–28), and from the peritoneum and colon anteriorly (see Fig. 2–27), without great difficulty. Gerota's fascia also serves to contain perinephric fluid collections, whether of pus (abscess), urine (urinoma), or blood (hematoma). These processes rarely cross the midline because of the fusion of Gerota's fascia over the great vessels medially. When very large, such collections can and do, however, extend into the pelvis, following the potential space where Gerota's fascia does not fuse inferiorly. Very extensive and advanced inflammatory or malignant processes may eventually erode through Gerota's fascia and invade adjacent organs or the posterior body wall musculature.

Renal Vasculature

Vascular Pedicle

The renal vascular pedicle, classically described as a single artery and larger vein, enters the kidney via the renal hilum medially (see Fig. 2–1*C* and *D* and Fig. 2–15*E* to *H*). **The renal vein lies most anteriorly, and behind it lies the artery; both normally lie anterior to the urinary collecting system, i.e., the renal pelvis. The renal arteries and veins typically branch from the aorta and inferior vena cava at the level of the second lumbar vertebra below the anterior takeoff of the superior mesenteric artery** (see Fig. 2–9).

Renal Arteries

The right renal artery often leaves the aorta at a slightly higher level than does the left and then must course with a downward slope to reach the usually lower right kidney. **The right renal artery passes behind the inferior vena cava in its course** and is considerably longer than the left renal artery. In rare instances, the right renal artery may arch anteriorly over the inferior vena cava. In contrast, the shorter left renal artery tends to lie in a horizontal plane or to slant slightly upward to reach the left kidney. Because of the normal posterior position and rotation of the kidneys, both renal arteries also course at a slight posterior angle from the aorta (see Fig. 2–8). The renal arteries provide small superior branches to the adrenal gland and small inferior branches that feed the renal pelvis and upper ureter. In addition, tiny arterial branches to the renal capsule and perinephric fat may exit the main renal artery.

The main renal artery typically divides into four or more segmental vessels, with five branches most commonly described (Figs. 2–29 and 2–30). **The first and most constant segmental division is a posterior branch, which usually exits the main renal artery before it enters the renal hilum and proceeds posteriorly to the renal pelvis to supply a large posterior segment of the kidney.** The remaining anterior division of the main renal artery branches as it enters the renal hilum.

Four anterior segmental arterial branches can be described in most kidneys, proceeding from superior to inferior: the apical, upper, middle, and lower anterior segmental arteries. The main renal artery and each segmental artery, as well as their multiple succeeding branch arteries, are all "end arteries," without anastomosis or collateral circulation, and occlusion of any of these vessels produces ischemia and infarction of the corresponding renal parenchyma that it supplies; the entire kidney is lost if the main renal artery is injured prior to its branching.

The segmental arteries course through the renal sinus and branch further into lobar arteries, which divide again and enter the renal parenchyma as interlobar arteries (Fig. 2–31). The latter course radially outward along the junction between the renal pyramid and cortical columns of Bertin. One or more of these large arterial branches often lie in close association with the infundibula of the minor calyces, especially those of the upper and lower poles of the kidney, and may be injured during surgical approaches to the peripheral renal collecting system. Similarly, the lower anterior segmental artery often crosses in close proximity to the anterior aspect of the ureteropelvic junction, and more

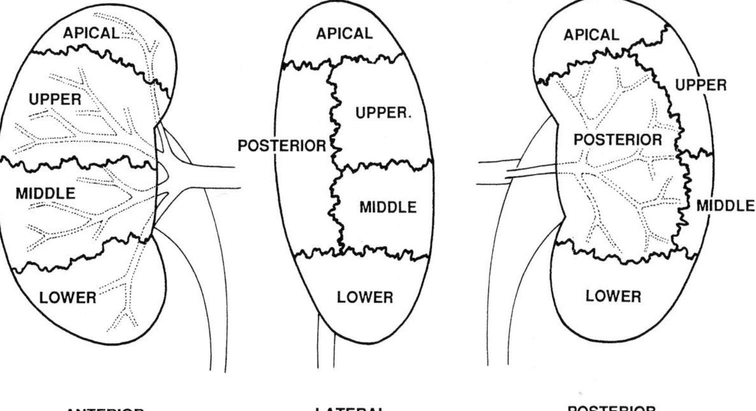

Figure 2–30. Typical segmental circulation of the right kidney, shown diagrammatically. Note that the posterior segmental artery is usually the first branch of the main renal artery and extends behind the renal pelvis.

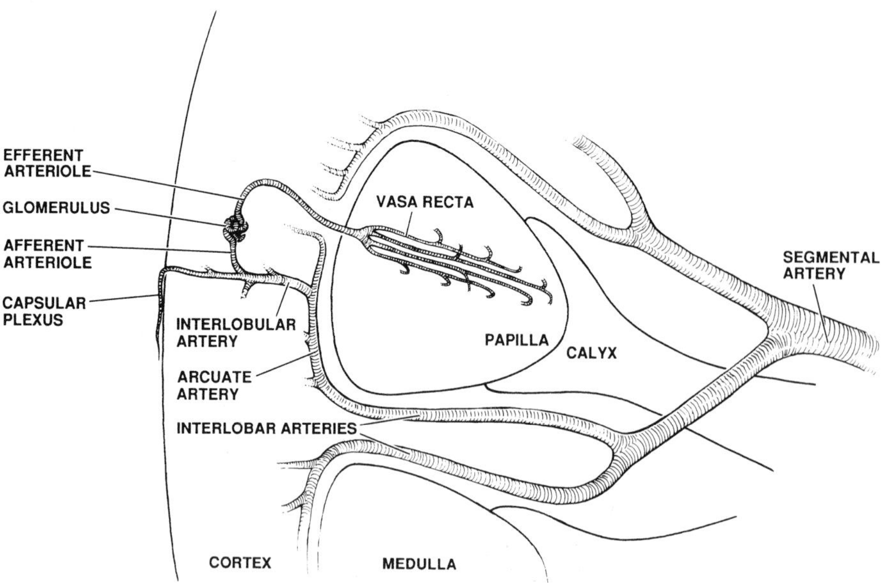

Figure 2–31. Intrarenal arterial anatomy.

rarely the posterior segmental artery may cross the ureteropelvic junction posteriorly, where either artery may be subject to iatrogenic injury. At the base of each pyramid, **the interlobar arteries branch into arcuate arteries, which arc parallel to the renal contour along the corticomedullary junction. The arcuate arteries, in turn, produce multiple radial arterial branches, the interlobular arteries. These have multiple side branches, which are the afferent arterioles to the glomeruli. Each glomerulus, numbering up to 2 million in a single kidney, is a spherical network of fine permeable capillaries through which the urinary filtrate leaves the arterial stream** (Fig. 2–32). **The glomerular capsule ("Bowman's" capsule) surrounds this spherical capillary network and collects the urinary filtrate. Blood leaves the glomerular capillary network via the efferent arteriole, which exits the glomer-**

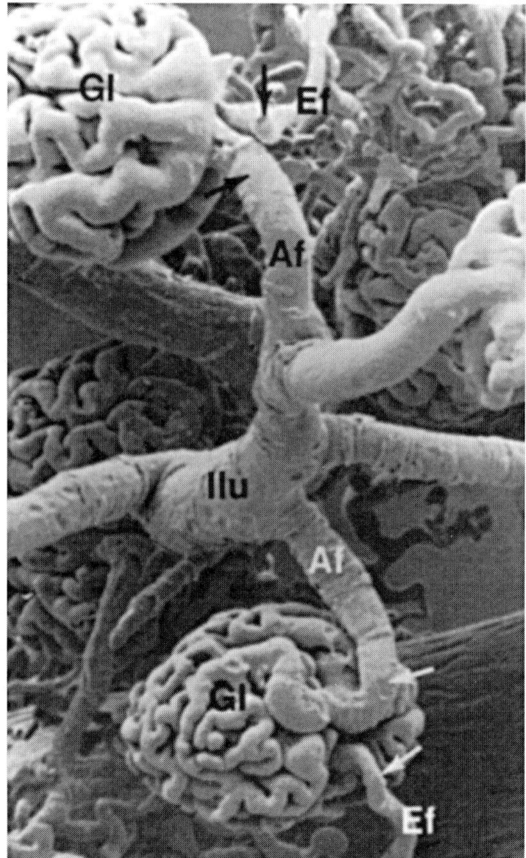

Figure 2–32. Electron micrograph demonstrating the microcirculation of the kidney at the level of the glomerulus. Note that the afferent and efferent arterioles enter and exit the glomerulus together, creating a so-called glomerular hilum. Af, afferent arteriole; Ef, efferent arteriole; Gl, glomerular capillary network; Ilu, interlobular artery. (From Kessel RG, Kardon RH, eds: Tissues and Organs: A Text-Atlas of Scanning Electron Microscopy. Copyright 1979 by W. H. Freeman and Co. Reprinted by permission.)

ulus alongside the afferent arteriole. The efferent arterioles then either form secondary capillary networks around the urinary tubules in the cortex or may descend as long, straight vascular loops into the renal medulla, the "vasa recta."

Renal Veins

The postglomerular capillaries eventually drain into interlobular veins and thus into arcuate, interlobar, lobar, and segmental veins. Usually three large venous trunks, but sometimes as many as five, finally coalesce as the main renal vein, generally within but at times just outside the renal sinus. It is not uncommon for the most inferior of these large segmental venous trunks to lie in close proximity to the ureteropelvic junction. **Unlike the renal arteries, none of which communicate, the renal parenchymal veins anastomose freely,** especially at the level of the arcuate vessels and may form large venous "collars" around the infundibula of many calyces. In addition, the interlobular veins communicate via a subcapsular venous plexus ("stellate" veins) with veins in the perinephric fat.

The right renal vein is short (2 to 4 cm) and enters the right lateral aspect of the inferior vena cava directly, usually without receiving other venous branches. The left renal vein is generally three times the length of the right (6 to 10 cm) and must cross anterior to the aorta to reach the left lateral aspect of the inferior vena cava (see Fig. 2–1). **Lateral to the aorta, the left renal vein typically receives the left adrenal vein superiorly, a lumbar vein posteriorly, and the left gonadal vein inferiorly** (see Fig. 2–9). The left renal vein also tends to enter the inferior vena cava at a slightly higher level than does the right and more anterolaterally, as opposed to a more posterolateral insertion on the right. **Although both renal veins, in general, lie directly anterior to their associated renal arteries, this relation is only approximate, and the more posterior artery may be a centimeter or more superior or inferior to the level of the vein, a disparity that may be exaggerated as one moves medially away from the renal hilum.**

Common Anatomic Variants

Variations of the main renal artery and vein are common, present in 25% to 40% of kidneys. The most common variation is the occurrence of supernumerary renal arteries (two or more arteries to a single kidney, with up to five having been found) (Fig. 2–33). These usually arise from the lateral aorta, occur perhaps slightly more often on the left than the right, and may enter the renal hilum or directly into the parenchyma of one of the poles of the kidney, the upper pole being more common than the lower. Lower pole supernumerary arteries on the right tend to cross anteriorly, rather than posteriorly, to the inferior vena cava. Lower pole arteries on either side must cross anteriorly to the urinary collecting system and may be an extrinsic cause of ureteropelvic junction obstruction. Supernumerary arteries are more common in an ectopic kidney and may, in unusual cases, arise from the celiac, superior mesenteric, or iliac arteries. Multiple renal veins are a less common entity and, when present, usually consist of duplicate renal veins draining the right kidney via the right renal hilum. Polar veins exiting the parenchyma are rare. On the left, it is more common to see the renal vein divide and send one limb anterior and one posterior to the aorta to reach the inferior vena cava (a so-called "renal collar"), representing a persistence of the embryologic state. Only the retroaortic limb of the left renal vein may persist in unusual instances.

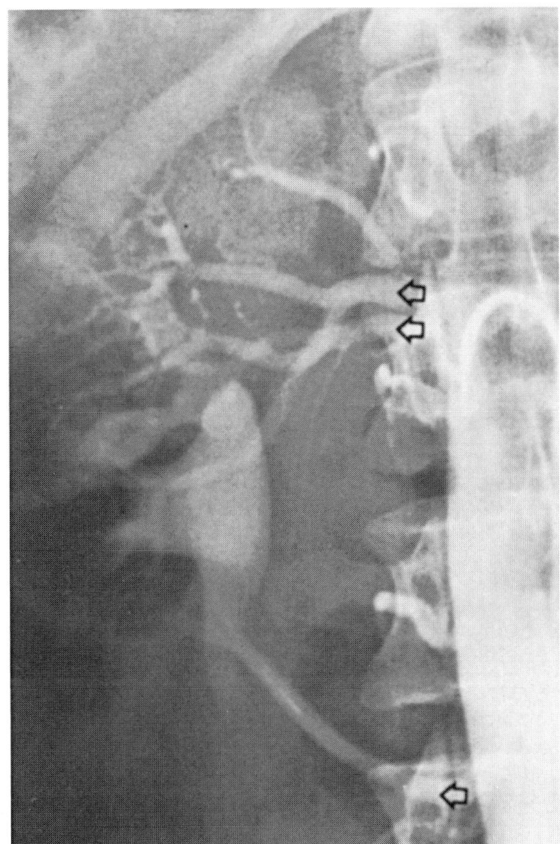

Figure 2–33. Multiple renal arteries (*arrows*) arising from the aorta, demonstrated angiographically.

Surgical Considerations

The presence of extensive renal venous collaterals and absence of arterial collaterals leads to two important surgical considerations. The kidney, because of extensive collateral venous drainage through its subcapsular plexus, which communicates with perinephric vessels, may tolerate amazingly well occlusive processes involving the renal vein, especially if these occur gradually over time, as with slow extension of a tumor or thrombus. On the left side especially, where collateral drainage may occur through adrenal, lumbar, and gonadal veins communicating with the left renal vein (Fig. 2–34), even acute surgical ligation of the vein at the inferior vena cava may be tolerated in some cases. On the other hand, lack of arterial collaterals means that injury or division of any renal arterial vessel at any level will produce some degree of parenchymal loss through infarction. Thus, any incision into the renal parenchyma must take into account the segmental arterial circulation. To this end, a relatively avascular longitudinal plane exists on the posterolateral aspect of the kidney between the posterior segmental circulation and the anterior (see Figs. 2–26 and 2–30). A relatively bloodless vertical incision is feasible here to gain surgical

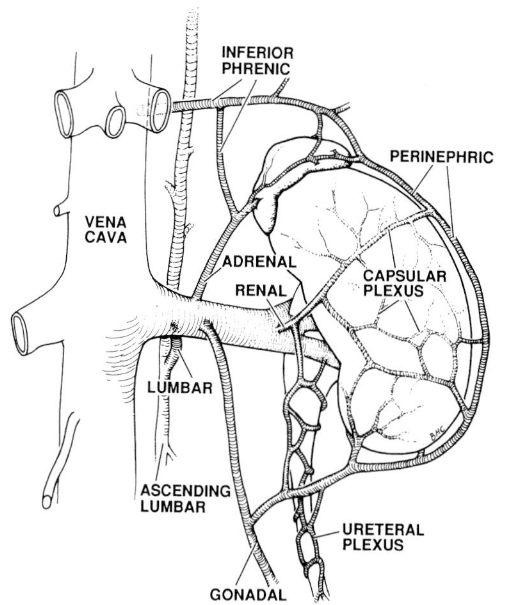

Figure 2–34. Venous drainage of the left kidney, showing potentially extensive venous collateral circulation.

access to the urinary collecting system. Similarly, transverse incisions are usually possible between the posterior segmental circulation and polar segments supplied by the apical or lower segmental arteries of the anterior circulation to gain access to upper or lower pole calyces (see Fig. 2–30). The latter incisions can be extended anteriorly as well to perform a polar partial nephrectomy, as for tumor excision. The segmental circulation varies sufficiently, however, that it must be defined in every individual prior to incision, either with preoperative angiography or with intraoperative segmental injection of a dye, such as methylene blue.

Renal Lymphatics

The renal lymphatic drainage is abundant and follows the blood vessels through the renal columns to exit the renal parenchyma and forms several large lymphatic trunks within the renal sinus. Communicating lymphatics from the renal capsule and perinephric tissues join these trunks as they exit the renal hilum in close association with the renal blood vessels. In addition, lymphatics from the renal pelvis and upper ureter may also join the renal lymphatic trunks. There are often two or more lymph nodes directly at the renal hilum associated with the renal vein, and these, when present, form the very first site of metastatic spread from the kidney (see Fig. 2–15*G* and *H*).

From the left kidney (Fig. 2–35), **the lymphatic trunks then drain primarily into the lateral para-aortic lymph nodes, including nodes anterior and posterior to the aorta, from a level below the inferior mesenteric artery to the diaphragm.** Some lymphatic channels from the left kidney may drain into retrocrural nodes and/or directly into the thoracic duct above the diaphragm. Drainage into the interaortocaval nodes does not generally occur from the left kidney except in advanced disease states.

From the right kidney (Fig. 2–36), **the lymphatic trunks drain primarily into both interaortocaval and right paracaval lymph nodes, including nodes anterior and posterior to the inferior vena cava, extending from a level as inferior as the common iliac vessels on the right to the diaphragm.** Again, some lymphatic channels from the right kidney may drain into retrocrural nodes or

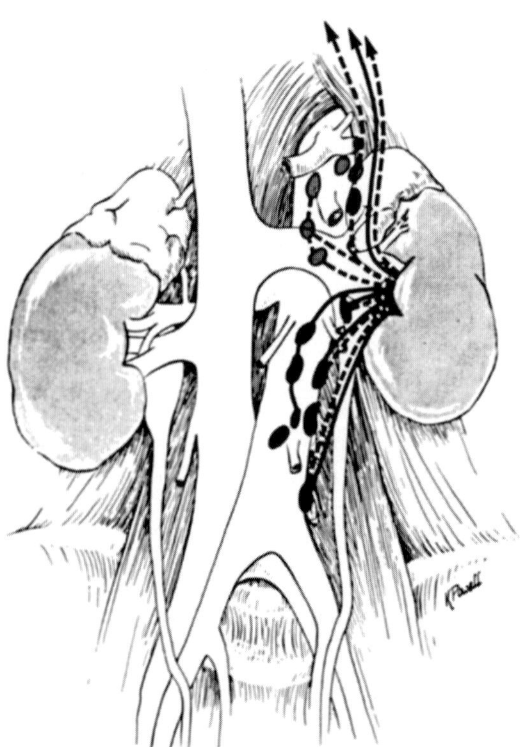

Figure 2–35. Regional lymphatic drainage of the left kidney. *Dark nodes,* anterior; *light nodes,* posterior. *Solid lines,* anterior lymphatic channels; *dashed lines,* posterior lymphatic channels. *Arrows* lead to thoracic duct.

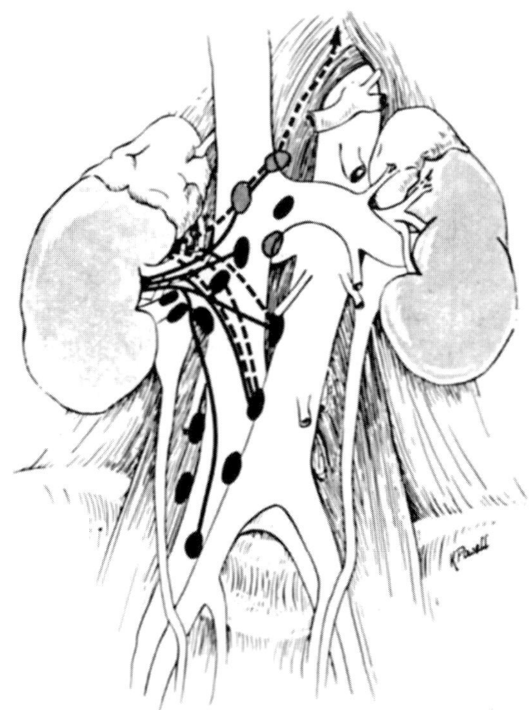

Figure 2–36. Regional lymphatic drainage of the right kidney. *Dark nodes,* anterior; *light nodes,* posterior. *Solid lines,* anterior lymphatic channels; *dashed lines,* posterior lymphatic channels. *Arrow* leads to thoracic duct.

directly into the thoracic duct. In addition, some lymphatics from the right kidney may cross over from right to left and drain primarily into left lateral para-aortic lymph nodes near the left renal hilum, although this is not common.

Renal Collecting System

Microscopic Anatomy from Glomerulus to Collecting Ducts

The renal collecting system has its origins microscopically in the renal cortex at the glomerulus, where the first urinary filtrate enters Bowman's capsule. Together, the glomerular capillary network and associated Bowman's capsule form the renal corpuscle ("Malpighian" corpuscle) (Fig. 2–37). The glomerular capillaries are covered by specialized epithelial cells, the "podocytes," so named because of their characteristic interdigitating foot processes, which enwrap the blood vessels (see Figs. 2–37 and 2–38). With the capillary endothelium, the podocyte foot processes, called "pedicels," help to form the selective filter across which the first urinary filtrate exits the blood. **The fluid flow continues from Bowman's capsule through the proximal convoluted tubule,** composed of a thick, cuboidal epithelium covered with dense microvilli forming a characteristic "brush border" (Fig. 2–39). This brush border creates a vast luminal surface across which most of the urinary filtrate from the glomerulus is reabsorbed. **The proximal convoluted tubule sends a straight, thick descending limb radially inward toward the renal medulla, which is contiguous with the thinner tubule of the loop of Henle. The loop of Henle extends for a variable length, with those originating from juxtamedullary glomeruli reaching the depths of the renal medulla before making a hairpin turn and returning toward the glomerulus. In its outward ascending course, the loop of Henle first thickens, then becomes the distal convoluted tubule, the latter again adjacent to its originating glomerulus and proximal convoluted tubule. The urinary effluent finally enters collecting tubules, which coalesce as collecting ducts as they again extend inward through the renal medulla to empty on the apex of the medullary pyramid, the renal papilla.**

Renal Papillae, Calyces, and Renal Pelvis

The renal papillae may number as few as four or as many as 18, but seven to nine are present in the typical kidney. Each papilla is cupped by a corresponding minor calyx, which receives the urinary output from the collecting ducts. The minor calyces are the first gross structures of the renal collecting system (Fig. 2–40). **There are typically two longitudinal rows of renal pyramids and corresponding minor calyces, roughly perpendicular to one another, extending anteriorly and posteriorly. Because of the natural rotation of the kidney, the anterior calyces typically extend laterally in a coronal plane, whereas the posterior calyces extend posteriorly in a sagittal plane** (see Fig. 2–26). Recognition of this anatomic configuration is important in radiographic interpretation and during percutaneous access to the renal collecting system.

It is common that some renal pyramids fuse during development, thus forming "compound" papillae. This often occurs at the renal poles but can occur throughout the kidney. Such compound papillae result in larger, compound calyces (see Fig. 2–40). **The compound papillae are of physiologic significance in that their configuration permits urinary reflux into the kidney with increased back pressure, also allowing bacterial reflux into the kidney parenchyma in the presence of infected urine** (Fig. 2–41). **Renal parenchymal scarring secondary to infection is typically most severe overlying such compound papillae.**

The minor calyces narrow, creating a neck or infundibulum before joining other minor calyces to form usually two to three major calyces, which in turn coalesce in most individuals to form a single renal pelvis (see Fig. 2–40). **The renal pelvis may be small and completely contained within the renal sinus or may be voluminous and almost entirely extrarenal** (Fig. 2–42). **The renal pelvis is continuous with the ureter and drains into it, the two joined at the anatomically indistinct ureteropelvic junction.** In fact, the entire upper collecting system, from minor calyces to ureter, is a single continuous structure. Any divisions between minor and major calyces, renal pelvis, and ureter are more artificial than real and may be more or less applicable to any one individual's anatomy. Nonetheless, this nomenclature is generally accepted clinically and remains a useful tool for description and communication.

Anatomic Variation

The variations in the gross structure of the renal collecting system are probably as numerous as there are

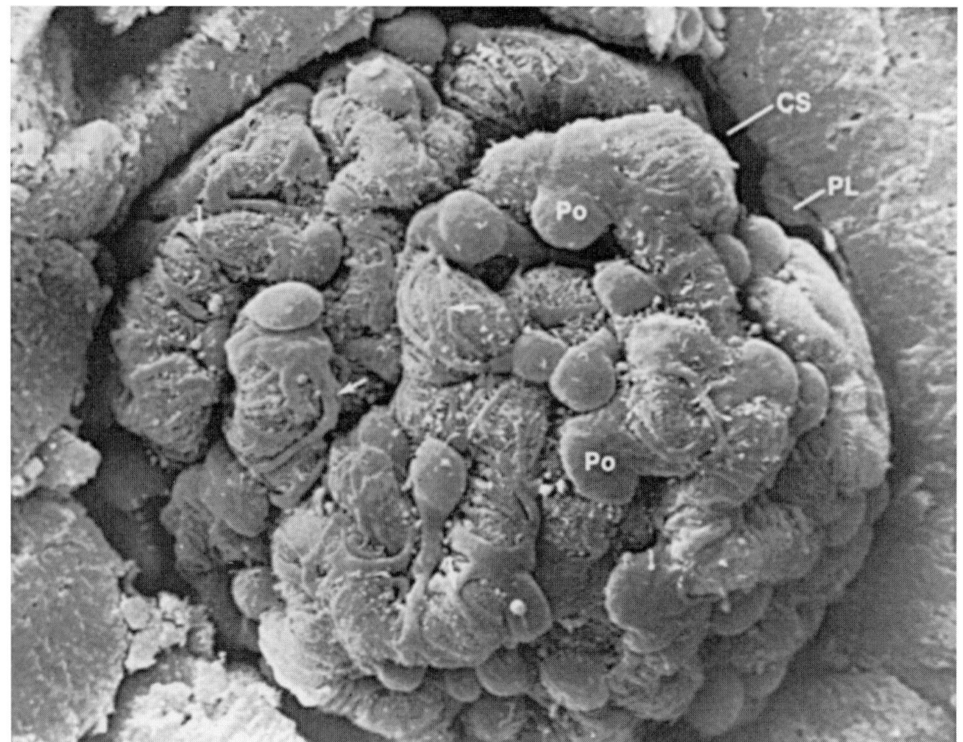

Figure 2–37. Electron micrograph of the renal corpuscle. The glomerular capillary network is enveloped by podocytes and contained within Bowman's capsule. CS, capsular space of Bowman; PL, parietal layer of Bowman's capsule; Po, podocyte. *Arrows* indicate cytoplasmic extensions from podocytes that enwrap the glomerular capillaries. (From Kessel RG, Kardon RH: Tissues and Organs: A Text-Atlas of Scanning Electron Microscopy. Copyright 1979 by W. H. Freeman and Co. Reprinted by permission.)

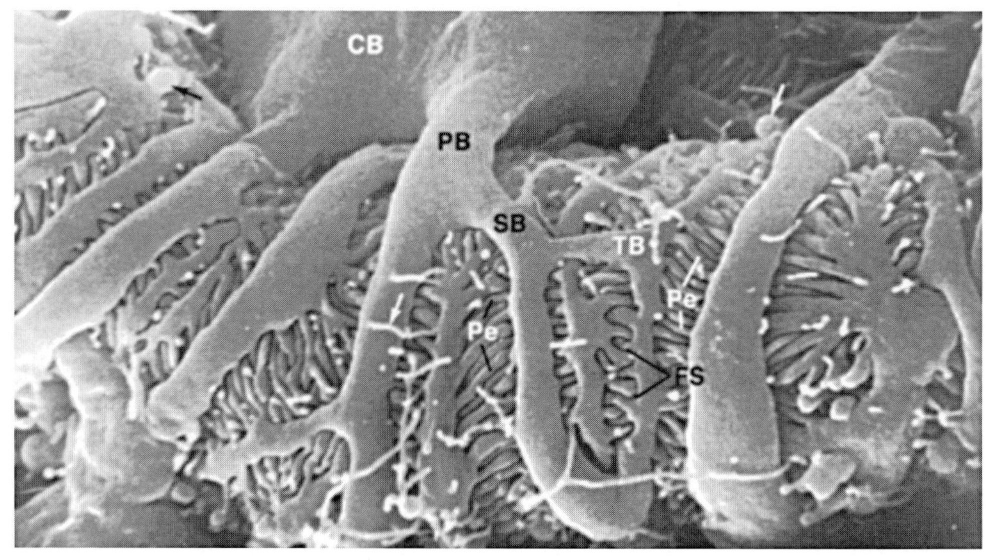

Figure 2–38. Electron micrograph showing close-up view of podocyte foot processes, or "pedicels," covering a glomerular capillary. CB, podocyte cell body; PB, primary branch of podocyte cytoplasm; SB, secondary branch; TB, tertiary branch; Pe, the pedicels, or terminal cytoplasmic extensions; FS, filtration slits between pedicels. (From Kessel RG, Kardon RH: Tissues and Organs: A Text-Atlas of Scanning Electron Microscopy. Copyright 1979 by W. H. Freeman and Co. Reprinted by permission.)

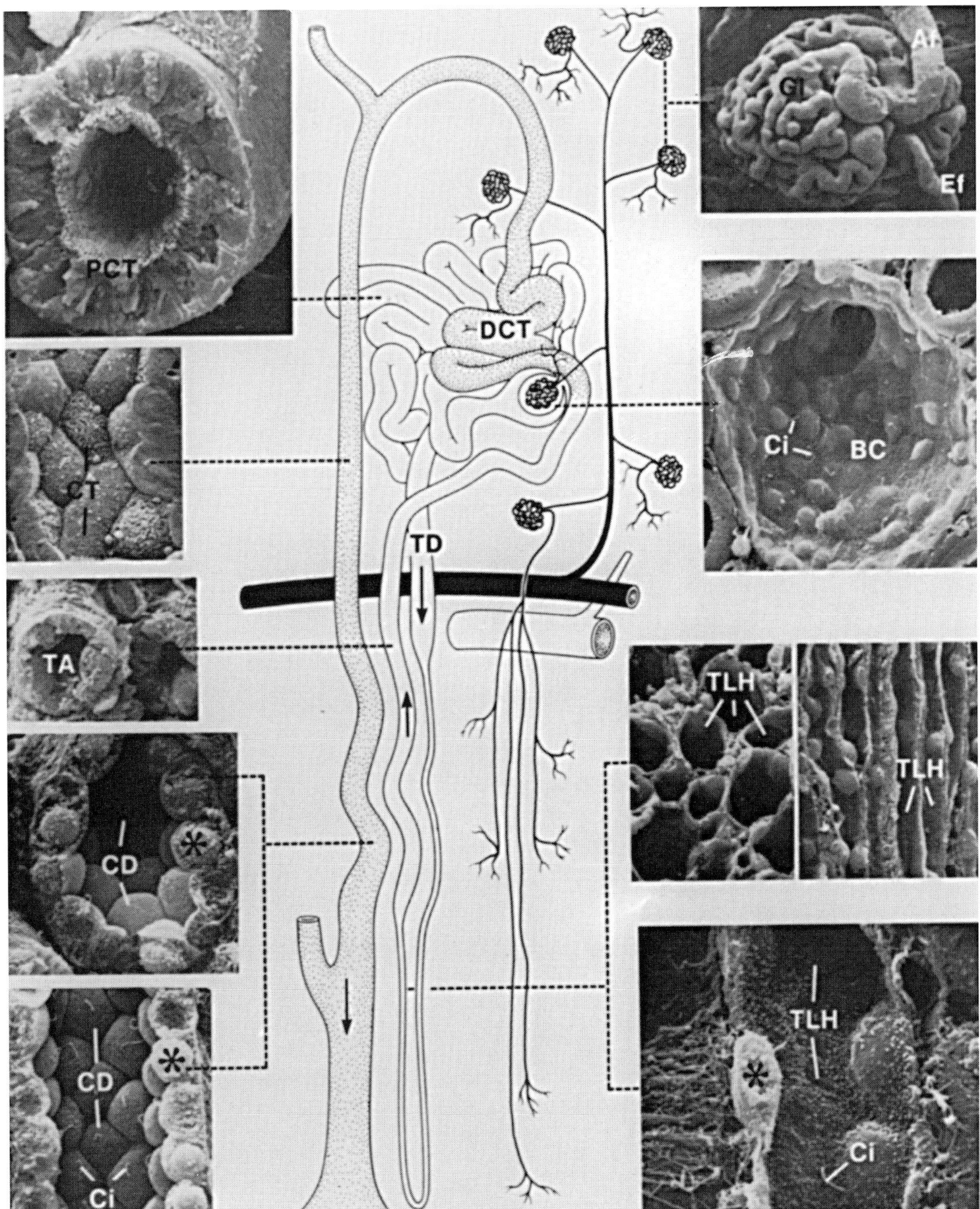

Figure 2–39. The nephron. Serial electron micrographs trace the uriniferous tubules that form the nephron from glomerulus to collecting duct. Af, afferent arteriole; Ef, efferent arteriole; Gl, glomerulus; BC, Bowman's capsule; PCT, proximal convoluted tubule; TD, thick descending segment; TLH, thin limb of loop of Henle; TA, thick ascending limb; DCT, distal convoluted tubule (note proximity to PCT and glomerular hilum); CT, collecting tubule; CD, collecting duct; Ci, cilia. *Asterisks* indicate cell nuclei. (From Kessel RG, Kardon RH: Tissues and Organs: A Text-Atlas of Scanning Electron Microscopy. Copyright 1979 by W. H. Freeman and Co. Reprinted by permission.)

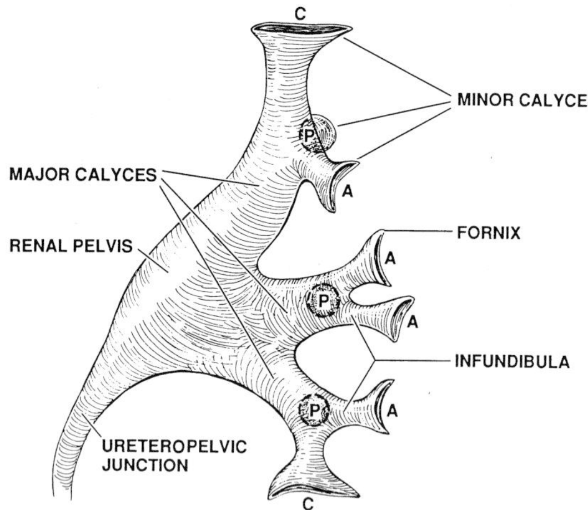

Figure 2–40. The renal collecting system (*left*), showing major divisions into minor calyces, major calyces, and renal pelvis. A, anterior minor calyces; P, posterior minor calyces; C, compound calyces at the renal poles.

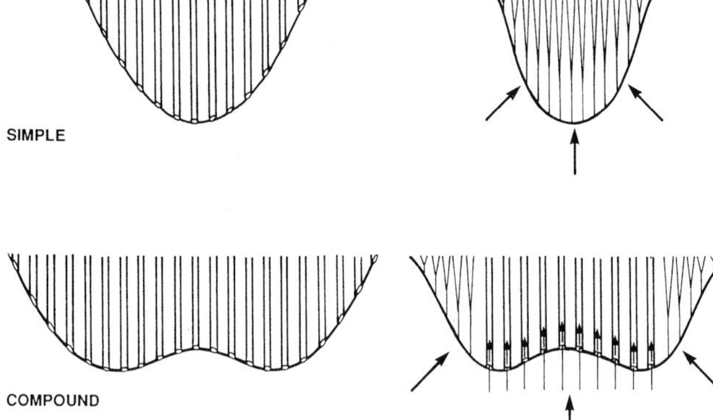

Figure 2–41. Diagram demonstrating structural and functional distinctions between simple and compound renal papillae. Back pressure causes closure of collecting ducts in simple papilla, whereas the structure of the compound papilla allows intrarenal reflux of urine.

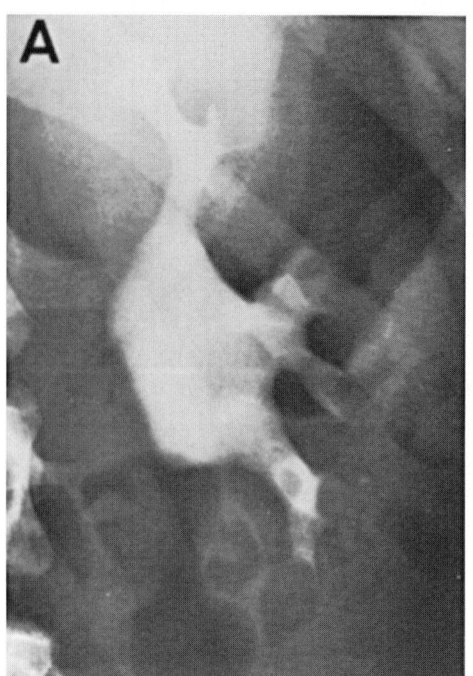

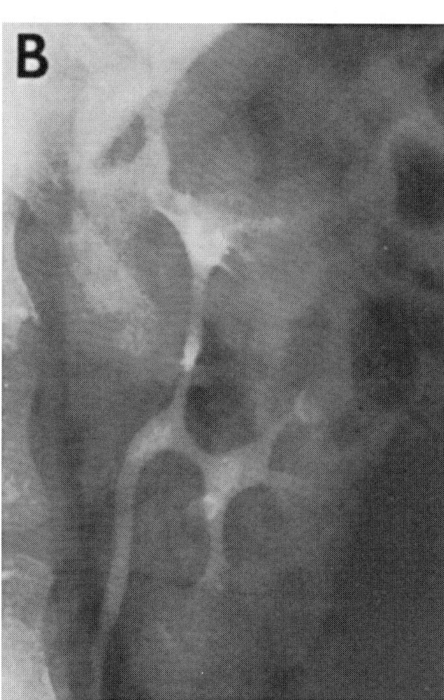

Figure 2–42. Significant variation between two normal renal pelves, demonstrated by excretory urography. *A*, Large, extrarenal pelvis. *B*, Narrow, completely intrarenal pelvis, barely larger in caliber than the ureter.

individuals and thus can be likened to fingerprints. The bilateral collecting systems present in any single individual are often similar (Fig. 2–43) but are rarely identical and not uncommonly may be quite different even from one another. Not only do the numbers and positions of minor calyces vary between individuals; their infundibula may range from absent to extremely elongated (Fig. 2–44). The latter is also true of the major calyces. The renal pelvis may be no wider than the ureter. The entire renal collecting system may be bifid, with two distinct pyelocalyceal systems draining into a single ureter, or the ureter may also be duplicated over varying lengths extending from the kidney. It becomes difficult at times to draw a line between "normal" variants and pathologic formations of the urinary collecting system, and the ultimate criterion must be demonstrated dysfunction, such as obstruction or reflux, resulting from the anatomy.

The Ureters

General Description

Each ureter represents the tubular extension of the renal collecting system, which courses downward and medially to connect the kidney to the urinary bladder (see Fig. 2–1). In the adult, the ureter is generally 22 to 30 cm in total length but varies with body habitus. As noted earlier, its origin at the ureteropelvic junction is often vaguely defined in the normal state. **The ureters and collecting systems extending to the renal papillae are lined by a transitional cell epithelium,** identical to and contiguous with that of the bladder. Beneath this epithelium is a layer of connective tissue, the lamina propria, which together with the epithelium forms the mucosa. When not distended by urine, the ureteral mucosa lies in longitudinal folds. **Smooth muscle covers the renal calyces, pelves, and ureters. In the ureters, this muscle usually can be divided into an inner layer of longitudinally coursing muscle bundles and an outer layer of circular and oblique muscle** (Fig. 2–45). **In the normal state, the urinary effluent does not passively drain but is actively propelled from renal pelvis to bladder by the peristaltic action of the ureteral muscle. A thin layer of adventitia immediately surrounds the ureter and contains an extensive plexus of ureteral blood vessels and lymphatics that course longitudinally with the ureter.**

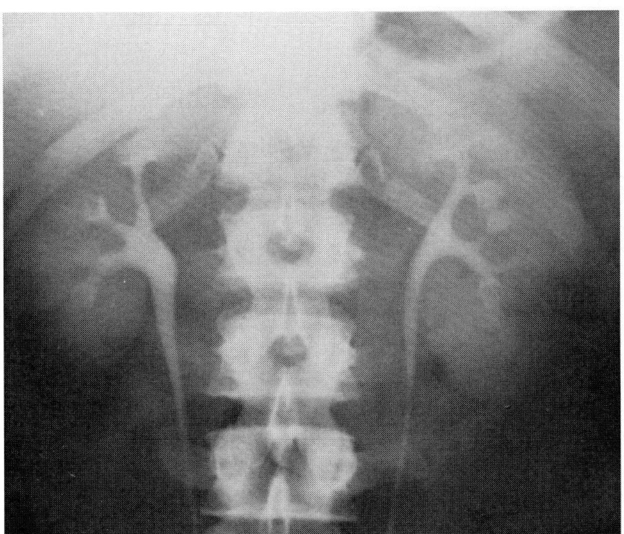

Figure 2–43. Normal bilateral renal collecting systems demonstrated by excretory urography.

Ureteral Blood Supply and Lymphatic Drainage

The ureter receives its blood supply from multiple feeding branches along its course (Fig. 2–46). In the retroperitoneum, the ureter may receive branches from the renal artery, gonadal artery, abdominal aorta, and common iliac artery. After entering the pelvis, additional small arterial branches to the distal ureter may arise from the internal iliac artery or its branches, especially the vesical and uterine arteries, but also from the middle rectal and vaginal arteries. Note that **arterial branches to the upper ureter approach from a medial direction, whereas arterial branches within the pelvis approach the ureter from a lateral direction. After reaching the ureter, the arterial branches course longitudinally within the periureteral adventitia in an extensive anastomosing plexus.** The existence of these longitudinal ureteral arterial communications allows long segments of ureter to be safely mobilized from the surrounding retroperitoneal tissues without compromising the vascular supply, provided that the adventitia is not stripped. The venous and lymphatic drainage of the ureter generally parallels the arterial supply. Thus, **the primary sites of lymphatic drainage from ureteral lesions vary, depending upon the location of the lesion. In the pelvis, the lymphatics drain to internal, external, and common iliac nodes. In the abdomen, the left para-aortic nodes form the primary drainage sites for the left ureter. The abdominal portion of the right ureter is drained primarily to right paracaval and interaortocaval lymph nodes. The lymphatic drainage of the upper ureter and renal pelvis tends to join the renal lymphatics and is identical to the ipsilateral kidney** (described earlier).

Anatomic Relations

The ureter is related posteriorly to the psoas muscle throughout its retroperitoneal course, crossing the iliac vessels to enter the pelvis at approximately the bifurcation of the internal and external iliac arteries (see Fig. 2–1). Rarely, the right ureter crosses behind the inferior vena cava in its course (the "retrocaval" ureter), which may cause ureteral compression and obstruction. Midline retroperitoneal mass lesions, including massive lymphadenopathy or abdominal aortic aneurysm, push the ureter laterally. The gonadal vessels roughly parallel the ureter through much of its retroperitoneal extent, obliquely crossing the ureter from medial to lateral before entering the pelvis. **Anteriorly, the right ureter is related to the terminal ileum, cecum, appendix, and ascending colon and their mesenteries; the left ureter is related to the descending colon and sigmoid and their mesenteries.** Either ureter may be endangered during operations on these structures. The ureter tends to preferentially remain adherent and be reflected with the overlying peritoneum anteriorly rather than remain with the posterior muscu-

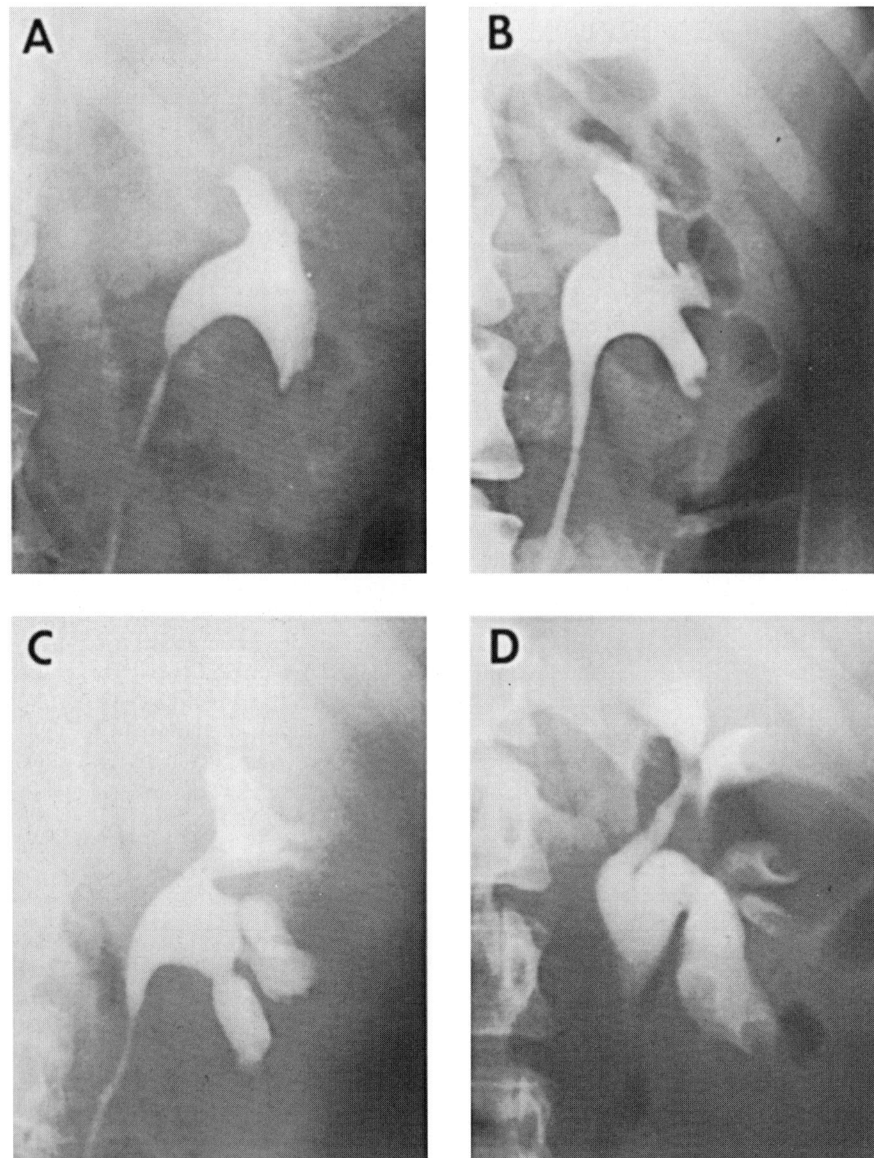

Figure 2–44. Examples of normal variations in the architecture of the renal collecting system demonstrated by excretory urography. *A*, Absence of calyces. *B*, Minor calyces arising directly from the renal pelvis. *C*, Megacalyces. *D*, "Orchid" calyces.

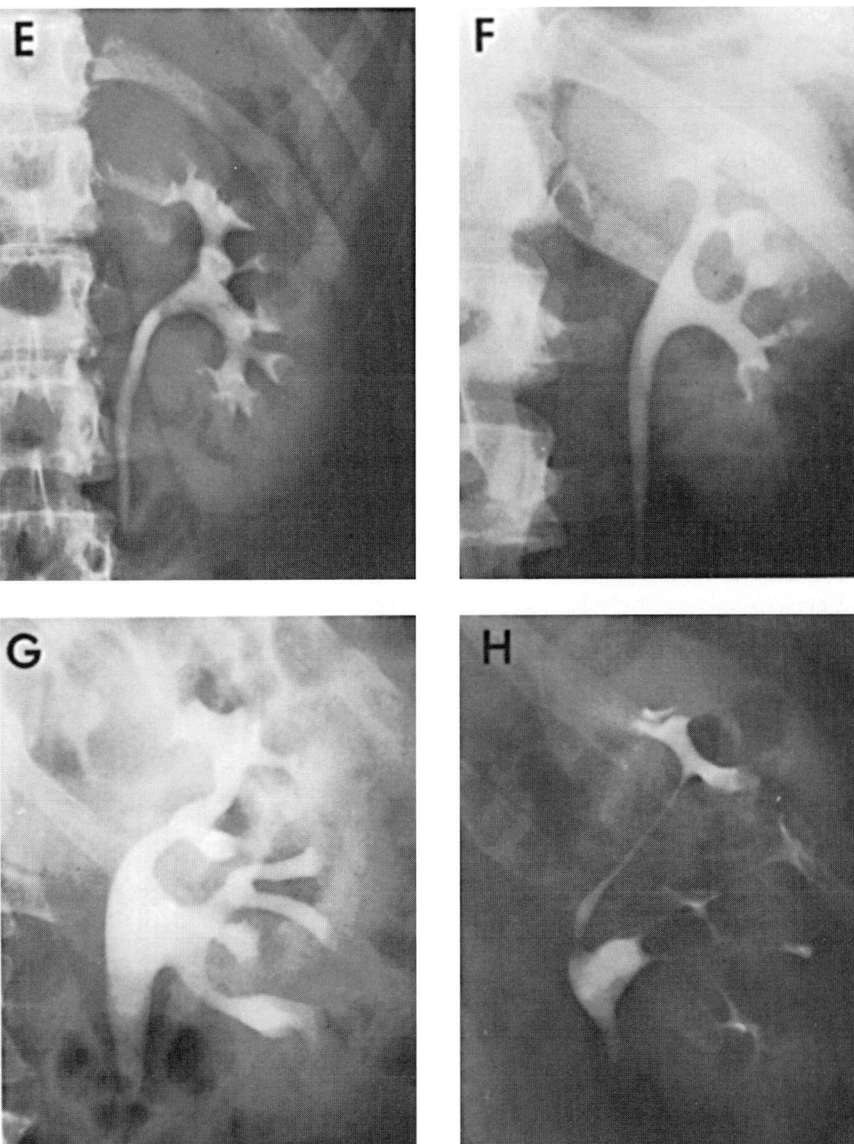

Figure 2–44 *Continued E,* Multiple minor calyces and nearly absent renal pelvis. *F,* "Classic" pyelogram. *G,* Extrarenal extension of infundibula. *H,* Elongated major calyces and infundibula.

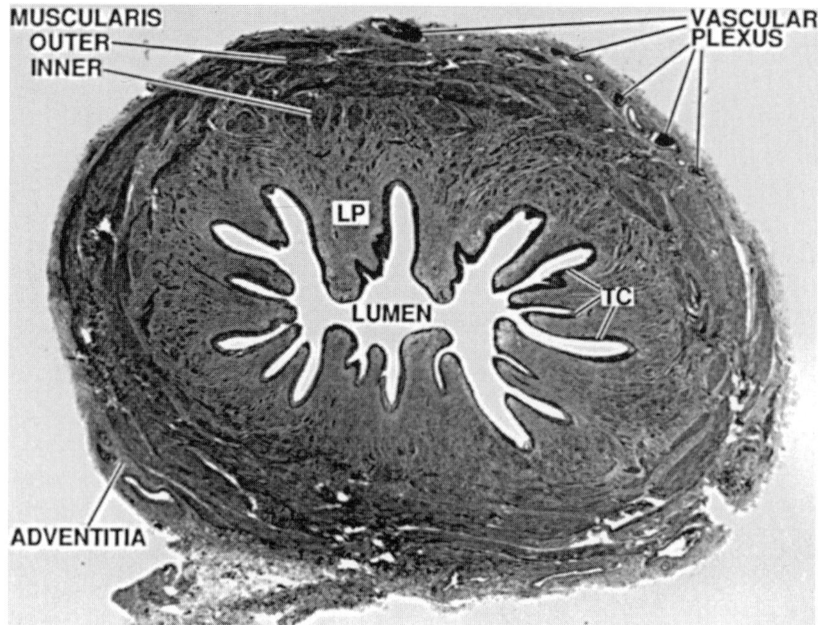

Figure 2–45. Transverse microscopic section through the ureter. Inner longitudinal muscle layer is distinguished from outer circular and oblique muscle fibers. TC, transitional cell epithelium; LP, lamina propria.

lar abdominal wall, thus increasing the likelihood that it may be inadvertently mobilized with the colon. Malignant and inflammatory processes of the terminal ileum, appendix, right or left colon, and sigmoid colon may also directly affect the ipsilateral ureter, with effects ranging from microhematuria to fistula to total obstruction. Within the female pelvis, the ureters are closely related to the uterine cervix and are crossed anteriorly by the uterine arteries and thus are at risk during hysterectomy. Pathologic processes of the fallopian tube and ovary may also encroach upon the ureter at the pelvic brim.

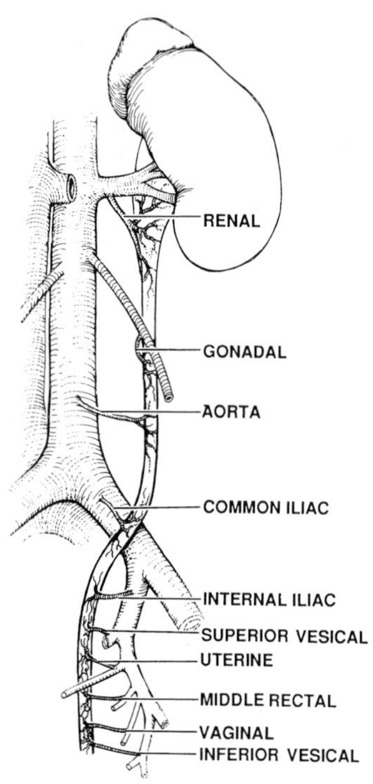

Figure 2–46. Sources of arterial blood supply to the ureter.

Normal Variations in Ureteral Caliber

The ureter is not of uniform caliber, with three distinct narrowings normally present along its course (Fig. 2–47). **The first of these is the ureteropelvic junction, the second**

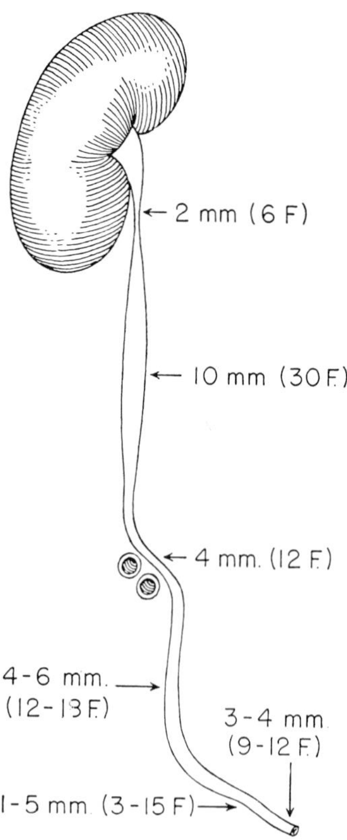

Figure 2–47. The ureter, demonstrating variations in caliber, including three normal anatomic narrowings—at the ureteropelvic junction, the iliac vessels, and the ureterovesical junction. Note also the anterior displacement of the ureter, which occurs over the iliac vessels, shown here diagrammatically.

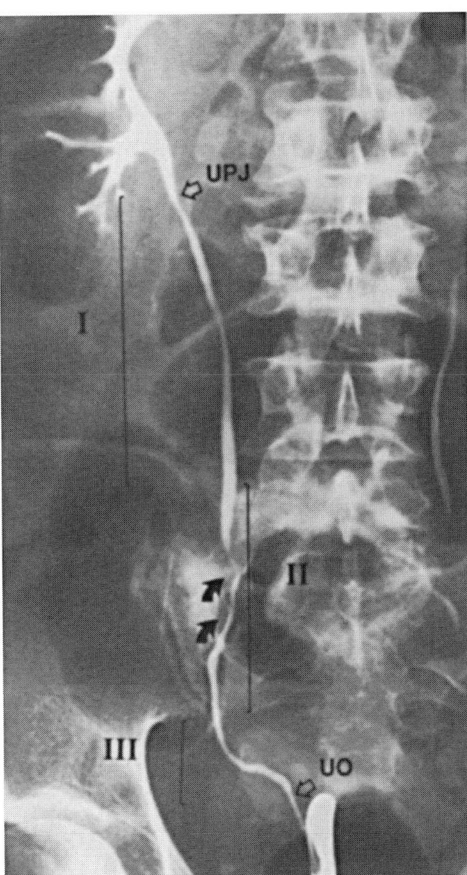

Figure 2–48. The right ureter illustrated by retrograde pyelogram. UPJ, ureteropelvic junction; UO, ureteral orifice in bladder; I, upper ureter, extending to upper border of sacrum; II, middle ureter, extending to lower border of sacrum; III, distal or lower ureter, traversing the pelvis to end in the bladder. Arrows indicate the course of common iliac artery and vein.

is the crossing of the iliac vessels, and the third is the ureterovesical junction in the pelvis. The ureter is narrowest at the ureterovesical junction and as it traverses the intramural tunnel through the bladder wall. These three sites are common locations for urinary calculi to impact during passage, potentially obstructing the flow of urine. **In addition, the ureter angulates anteriorly as it passes over the iliac vessels, then posteromedially again as it enters the pelvis** and courses behind the bladder. Appreciation of this normal angulation, and the three-dimensional course of the ureter in general, has assumed increasing importance with the routine use of ureteroscopy.

Ureteral Segmentation and Nomenclature

The ureter is often arbitrarily divided into segments for purposes of surgical or radiographic description. The "abdominal" ureter extends from renal pelvis to the iliac vessels, and the "pelvic" ureter extends from the iliac vessels to the bladder. The ureter can also be divided into upper, middle, and lower segments, usually for purposes of radiographic description (Fig. 2–48). **The upper ureter extends from the renal pelvis to the upper border of the sacrum; the mid-ureter then extends to the lower border of the sacrum, which roughly corresponds with the iliac vessels; and the lower (or distal or pelvic) ureter extends from the sacrum to the bladder.**

Innervation of Kidneys and Ureters

Renal Innervation

The kidneys receive preganglionic sympathetic input from the eighth thoracic through first lumbar spinal segments. Postganglionic fibers arise primarily from the celiac and aorticorenal ganglia, but they also may reach the kidney through the lesser and lowest splanchnic nerves from the thorax. These, together with parasympathetic input from the vagus nerves, form the renal autonomic plexus, which surrounds the main renal artery and its branches, following these into the substance of the kidney. Small renal ganglia may be present within the renal plexus along the main renal artery in some individuals. Efferent nerve endings within the kidney are primarily vasomotor and end in proximity to renal vessels, glomeruli, and tubules. Sympathetic fibers provide vasoconstrictor activity, whereas parasympathetic fibers produce vasodilation. However, **renal function after**

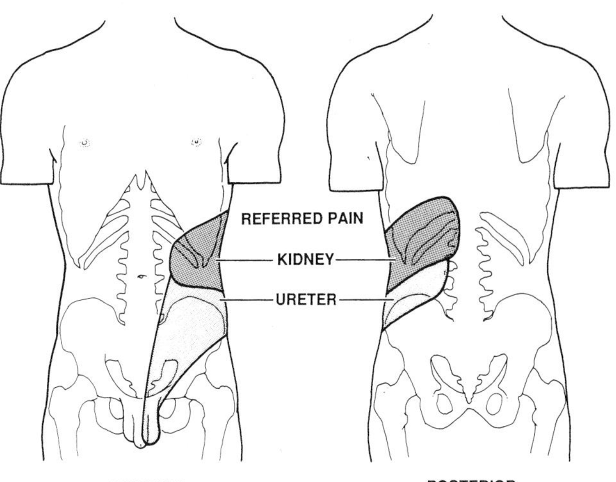

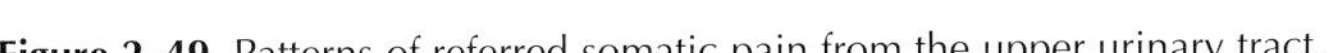
Figure 2–49. Patterns of referred somatic pain from the upper urinary tract.

denervation, as seen after transplantation procedures, is seemingly affected very little.

Ureteral Innervation

The ureters receive preganglionic sympathetic input from the tenth thoracic through second lumbar spinal segments. Postganglionic fibers arise from several ganglia in the aorticorenal, superior, and inferior hypogastric autonomic plexuses. Parasympathetic input is received from the second through fourth sacral spinal segments. However, the exact role of the ureteral autonomic input is unclear. **Normal ureteral peristalsis does not require outside autonomic input but, rather, originates and is propagated from intrinsic smooth muscle pacemaker sites located in the minor calyces of the renal collecting system.** The autonomic nervous system may exert some modulating effect on this process.

Pain Perception and Somatic Referral

Pain fibers leave the kidney, renal pelvis, and ureter, traveling with the sympathetic nerves. They are primarily stimulated by nociceptors sensitive to increased tension (distention) in the renal capsule, renal collecting system, or ureter. Direct mucosal irritation in the upper urinary tract may also stimulate some nociceptors. **The resulting visceral pain is felt directly and is referred to somatic distributions that correspond to the spinal segments providing the sympathetic distribution to ureter and kidney (eighth thoracic through second lumbar).** Pain and reflex muscle spasm are typically produced over the distributions of the subcostal, iliohypogastric, ilioinguinal, and/or genitofemoral nerves, resulting in flank, groin, or scrotal (or labial) pain and hyperalgesia, depending on the location of the noxious visceral stimulus (Fig. 2–49).

BIBLIOGRAPHY

Anson BJ, Daseler EH: Common variations in renal anatomy, affecting blood supply, form, and topography. Surg Gyn Obstet 1961; 112:439–449.

Graves FT: The anatomy of the intrarenal arteries and its application to segmental resection of the kidney. Br J Surg 1954; 42:132–139.

Kaye KW, Reinke DB: Detailed caliceal anatomy for endourology. J Urol 1984; 132:1085–1088.

McVay CB: Anson & McVay: Surgical Anatomy, 6th ed. Philadelphia, W. B. Saunders, 1984.

Parker AE: Studies on the main posterior lymph channels of the abdomen and their connections with the lymphatics of the genitourinary system. Am J Anat 1935; 56:409–443.

Pick JW, Anson BJ: The renal vascular pedicle: an anatomical study of 430 body-halves. J Urol 1940; 44:411–449.

Resnick MI, Parker MD: Surgical Anatomy of the Kidney. Mount Kisco, NY, Futura, 1982.

Sampaio FJB, Aragão AHM: Anatomical relationship between the intrarenal arteries and the kidney collecting system. J Urol 1990; 143:679–681.

Sampaio FJB, Aragão AHM: Anatomical relationship between the renal venous arrangement and the kidney collecting system. J Urol 1990; 144:1089–1093.

Sampaio FJB, Passos MARF: Renal arteries: anatomic study for surgical and radiological practice. Surg Radiol Anat 1992; 14:113–117.

Tobin CE: The renal fascia and its relation to the transversalis fascia. Anat Rec 1944; 89:295–311.

Williams PL, Warwick R, Dyson M, Bannister LH: Gray's Anatomy, 37th ed. New York, Churchill Livingstone, 1989.

3
ANATOMY OF THE LOWER URINARY TRACT AND MALE GENITALIA

James D. Brooks, M.D.

This chapter provides an anatomic framework for apprehending diseases of the pelvis. The bony, ligamentous, and muscular framework of the pelvis is presented first. Next, the pelvic vessels and nerves and the gastrointestinal, urinary, and genital viscera are discussed. Finally, the perineum and external genitalia are reviewed.

BONY PELVIS

The pelvic bones are the sacrum (the termination of the axial skeleton) and the two innominate bones. The latter are formed by the fusion of the ilial, ischial, and pubic ossification centers at the acetabulum (Fig. 3–1). The ischium and pubis also meet below, in the center of the inferior ramus, to form the obturator foramen. The weight of the upper body is transmitted from the axial skeleton to the innominate bones and lower extremities through the strong sacroiliac (SI) joints. As a whole, the pelvis is divided into a bowl-shaped false pelvis, formed by the iliac fossae and largely in contact with intraperitoneal contents, and the circular true pelvis, wherein lie the urogenital organs. **At the pelvic inlet, the true and false pelves are separated by the arcuate line**, which extends from the sacral promontory to the pectineal line of the pubis. The lumbar lordosis that accompanies erect posture tilts the axis of the pelvic inlet so that it parallels the ground; the pelvic inlet faces anteriorly, and the inferior ischiopubic rami lie horizontal (Fig. 3–2). When approaching the pelvis through a low midline incision, the surgeon gazes directly into the true pelvis.

The anterior and posterior iliac spines, the iliac crests, the pubic tubercles, and ischial tuberosities are palpable landmarks that orient the pelvic surgeon (see Fig. 3–1). **Cooper's (pectineal) ligament overlies the pectineal line and offers a sure hold for sutures in hernia repairs and urethral suspension procedures** (see Fig. 3–7). The ischial

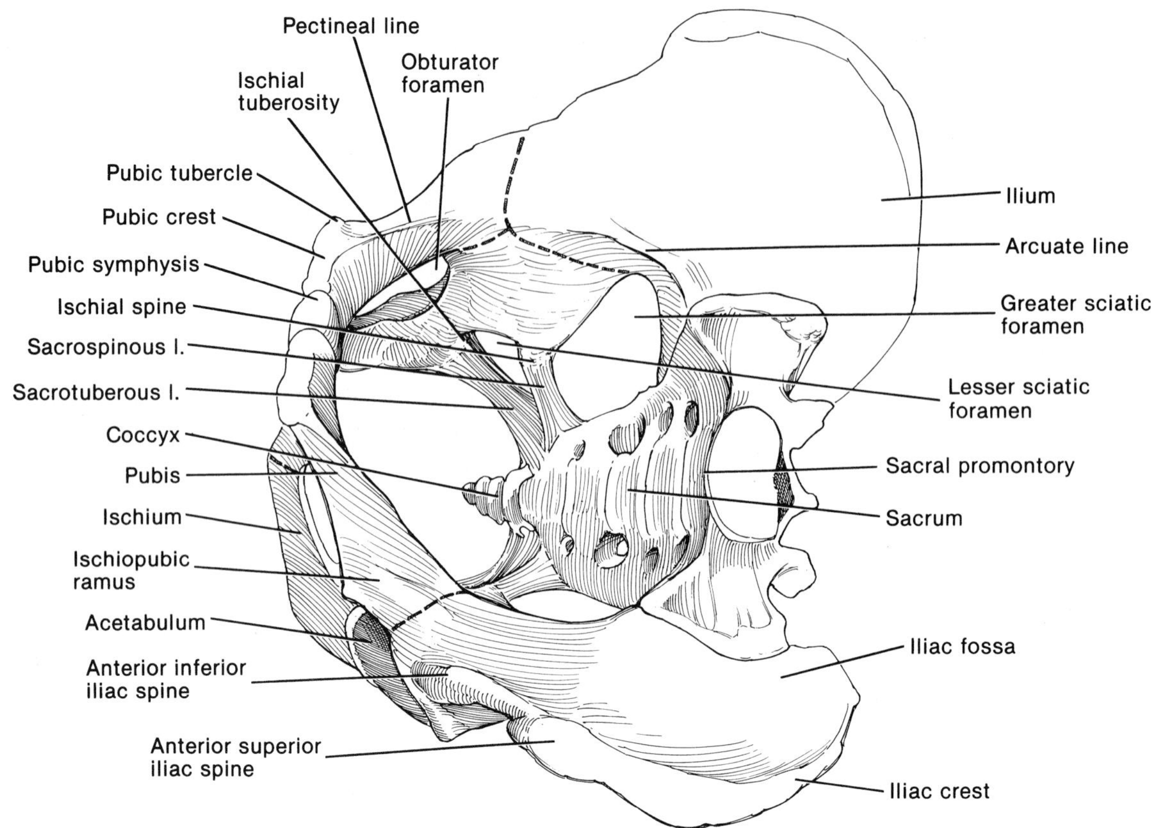

Figure 3–1. The bones and ligaments of the pelvis. (From Hinman F Jr: Atlas of Urosurgical Anatomy. Philadelphia, W.B. Saunders Company, 1993, p 196.)

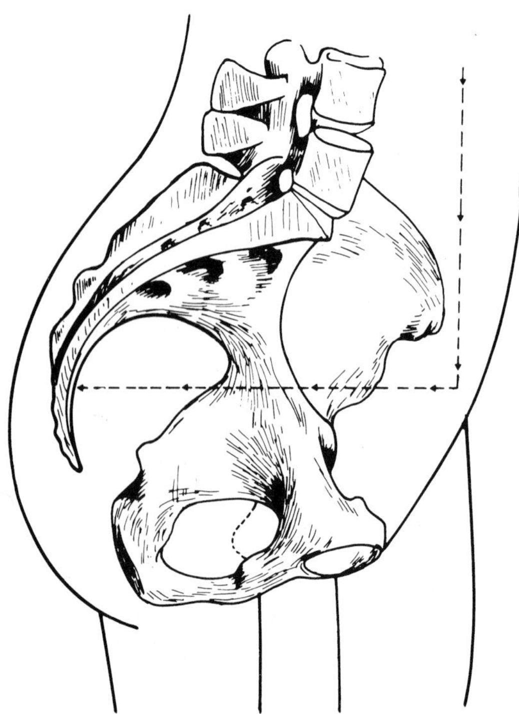

Figure 3–2. The pelvis in standing position. The axis of the pelvic cavity is horizontal because of lumbar lordosis. (From Zacharin RF: Pelvic Floor Anatomy and the Surgery of Pulsion Enterocele. New York, Springer-Verlag, 1985, p 15.)

spine is palpable transvaginally and attaches to the pelvic diaphragm and the sacrospinous ligament. **The sacrospinous ligament separates the greater and lesser sciatic foramina.** Together with the sacrotuberous ligament, it stabilizes the SI joint by preventing downward rotation of the sacral promontory. The SI joint, synovial in type, gains additional strength from anterior and posterior ligaments. In pelvic trauma, fractures virtually never involve this joint, but they occur adjacent to it. The pubes, the thinnest of the pelvic bones, are nearly always fractured, and their fragments may injure the adjacent bladder, urethra, and vagina. Resection or congenital nonunion of the pubes (e.g., bladder exstrophy) does not affect ambulation because of the strength of the SI joint (Golimbu et al, 1990; Waterhouse et al, 1973).

ANTERIOR ABDOMINAL WALL

Skin and Subcutaneous Fasciae

To minimize scarring, incisions of the anterior abdominal wall and flank should follow Langer's lines of cleavage. These lines parallel dermal collagen fibers and are oriented along lines of stress. They correspond to the segmental thoracic and lumbar nerves. **The skin is backed by Camper's fascia, a loose layer of fatty tissue that varies in thickness with the nutritional status of the patient. The superficial circumflex iliac, external pudendal, and superficial inferior epigastric vessels branch from the femoral vessels to run in this layer** (Figs. 3–3 and 3–4). The superficial inferior epigastric vessels are encountered during inguinal incisions and can cause troublesome hemorrhage during placement of pelvic laparoscopic ports.

Scarpa's fascia forms a distinct layer deep to Camper's fascia, although it may be difficult to discern in older patients. Superiorly and laterally, it blends with Camper's fascia. Inferiorly, it fuses with the deep fascia of the thigh 1 cm below the inguinal ligament along a line from the anterior superior iliac spine to the pubic tubercle. **Medially, it is continuous with Colles' fascia of the perineum** (see Fig. 3–3). Colles' fascia attaches to the posterior edge of the urogenital diaphragm and the inferior ischiopubic rami. It is continuous with the dartos fascia of the penis and scrotum. **These fasciae can limit both the spread of infection in necrotizing fasciitis of the scrotum (Fournier's gangrene) and the extent of urinary extravasation in an anterior urethral injury.** These processes do not extend down the leg or into the buttock, but they can freely travel up the anterior abdominal wall to the clavicles and around the flank to the back.

Abdominal Musculature

The abdominal musculature lies immediately below Scarpa's fascia. The origins of these muscles and the orientation of their fibers are presented in the previous chapter. **These muscles terminate on the anterior abdominal wall as broad, tough aponeurotic sheets that fuse in the midline (linea alba) and form the rectus sheath** (see Fig. 3–4). The linea alba is avascular and serves as a convenient point of access to the peritoneal and pelvic cavities. In its upper portion, the anterior rectus sheath is formed by the aponeurosis of the external oblique muscle and a portion of the internal oblique muscle (Fig. 3–5). The posterior sheath is derived from the remaining internal oblique aponeurosis and

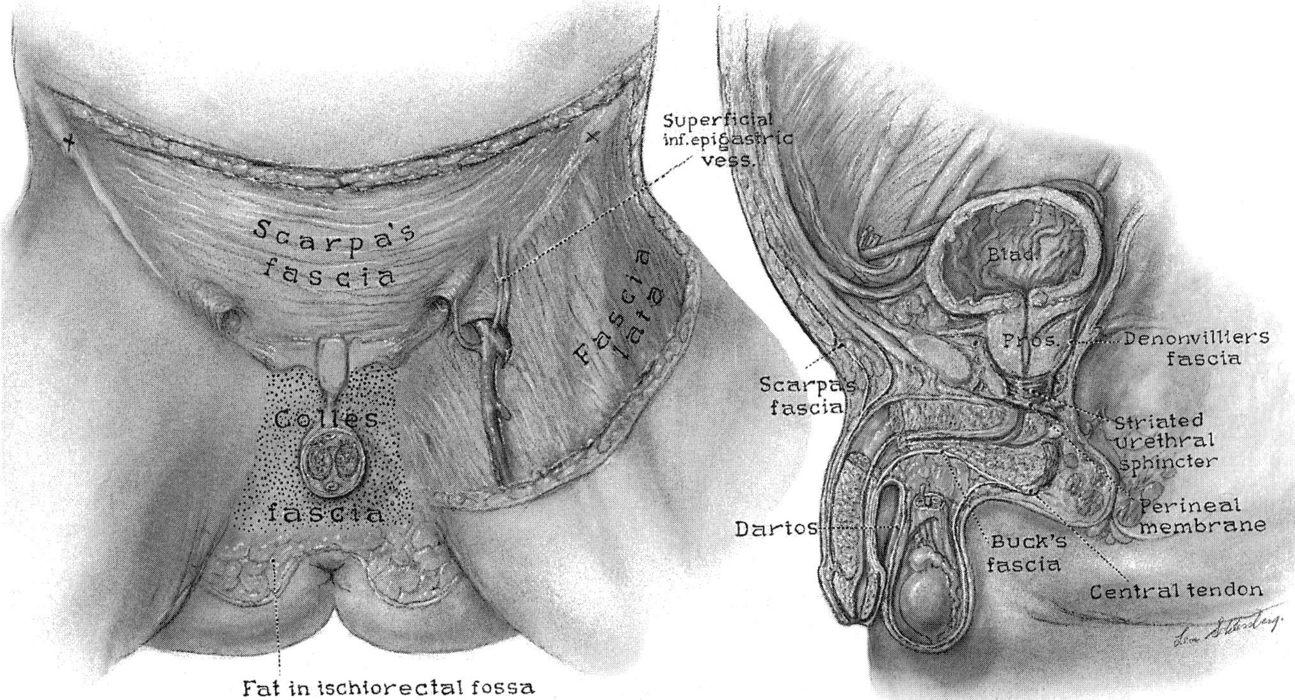

Figure 3–3. *Left,* Anterior view of the deep fasciae of the abdomen, perineum, and thigh. Note the superficial inferior epigastric artery passing superiorly in Camper's fascia. *Right,* Midline sagittal view of the pelvic fasciae and their attachments.

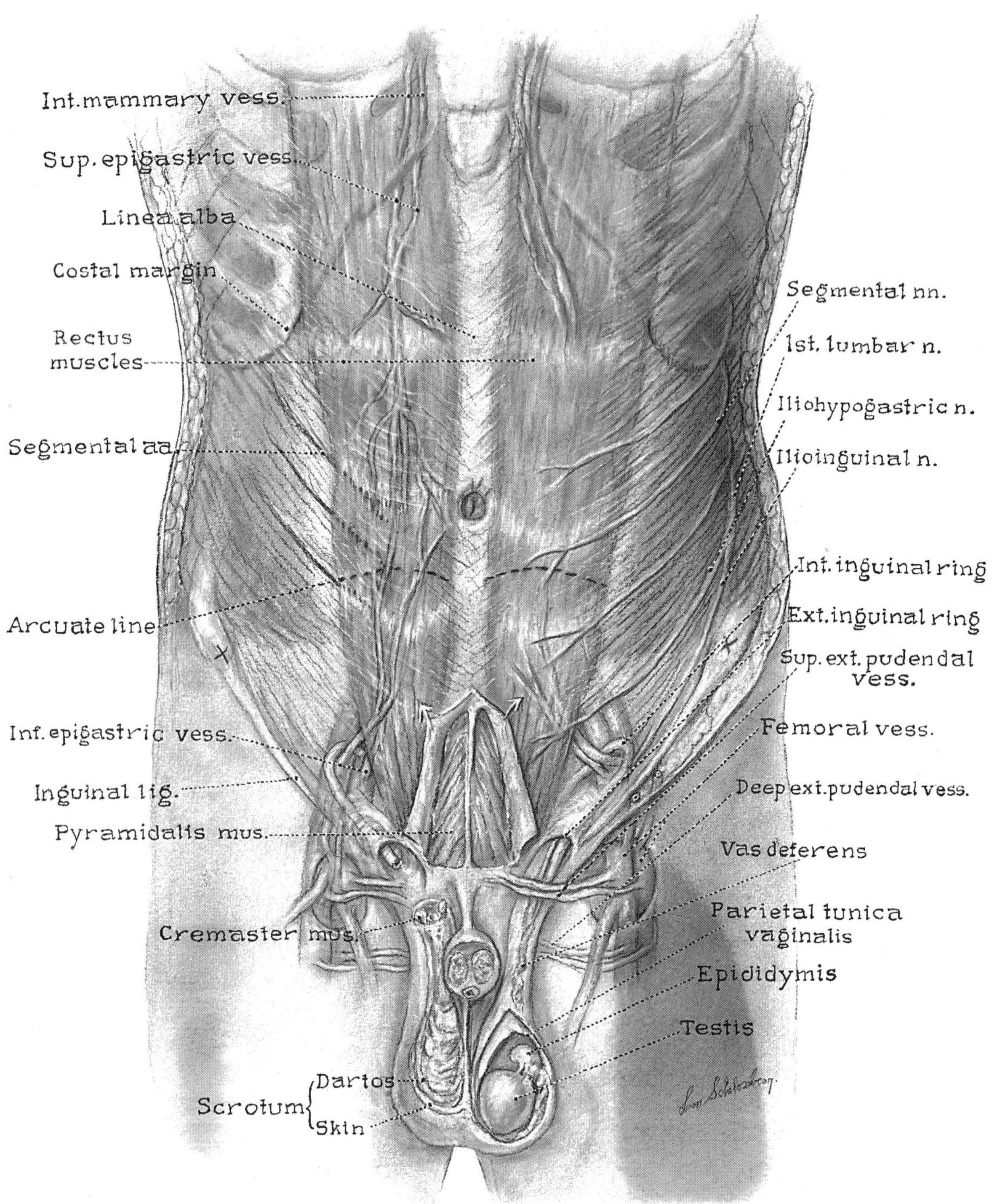

Figure 3–4. Muscles, vessels, and nerves of the anterior abdominal wall.

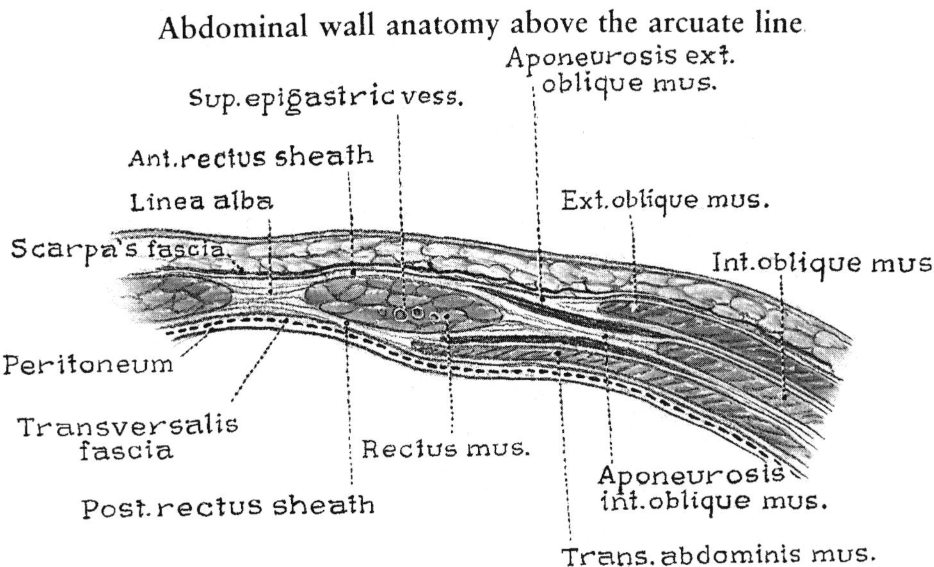

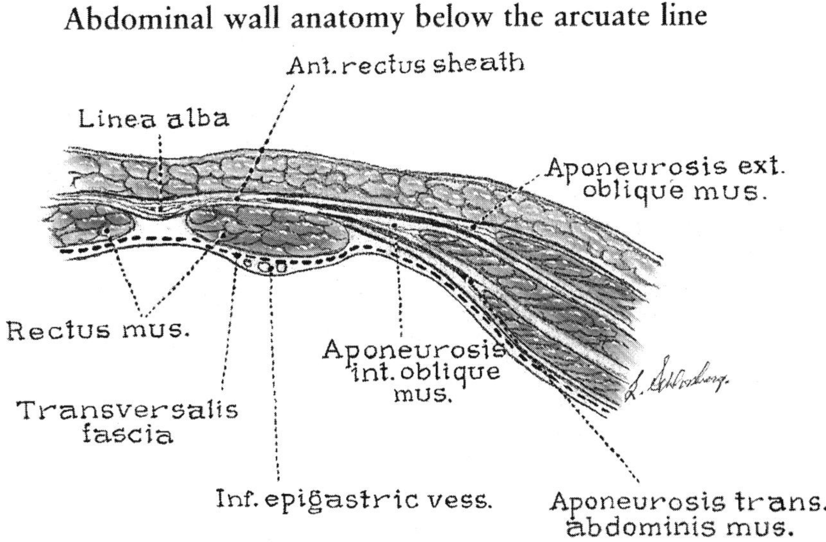

Figure 3–5. Cross section of the rectus sheath. *Top,* Above the arcuate line, the aponeurosis of the external oblique forms the anterior sheath, and the transversus aponeurosis forms the posterior sheath. The internal oblique muscle splits around the rectus to contribute to both the anterior and posterior sheaths. *Bottom,* Below the arcuate line, all aponeuroses pass anterior to the rectus.

that of the transversus abdominis. Two thirds of the distance from the pubis to the umbilicus, the arcuate line is formed as all aponeurotic layers abruptly pass anterior to the rectus abdominis, leaving this muscle clothed only by transversalis fascia and peritoneum posteriorly. **The rectus abdominis arises from the pubis medial to the pubic tubercle and inserts on the xiphoid process and adjacent costal cartilage.** The muscle is crossed by three or four tendinous intersections that are firmly attached to the anterior rectus sheath; thus the muscle can be divided transversely without significant retraction. It is supplied by the last six thoracic segmental nerves that enter it laterally. Paramedian incisions lateral to the rectus belly divide these nerves, cause atrophy of the rectus, and predispose to ventral hernia. Anterior to the rectus and within its sheath, the triangle-shaped pyramidalis muscle arises from the pubic crest and inserts into the linea alba (see Fig. 3–4). It is supplied by the subcostal nerve (T12).

Inguinal Canal

The inguinal canal transmits the spermatic cord in the male, the round ligament in the female, and the ilioinguinal nerve in both sexes (Fig. 3–6; see also Fig. 3–4). **Its anterior wall and floor are formed by the external oblique muscle**, which folds over at its inferior edge as the inguinal ligament. Above the pubic tubercle, the fibers of the external oblique aponeurosis split to form the lateral edges (or crura) of the external inguinal ring. **Transverse (intercrural) fibers bridge the crura to form the superior edge of the external ring.** By dividing the intercrural fibers, the external oblique can be separated along its fibers to gain access to the cord. **The posterior wall of the canal is formed by transversalis fascia, which lines the inner surface of the abdominal wall. The cord structures pierce this fascia lateral to the inferior epigastric vessels at the internal inguinal ring** (see Fig. 3–7). The internal ring lies

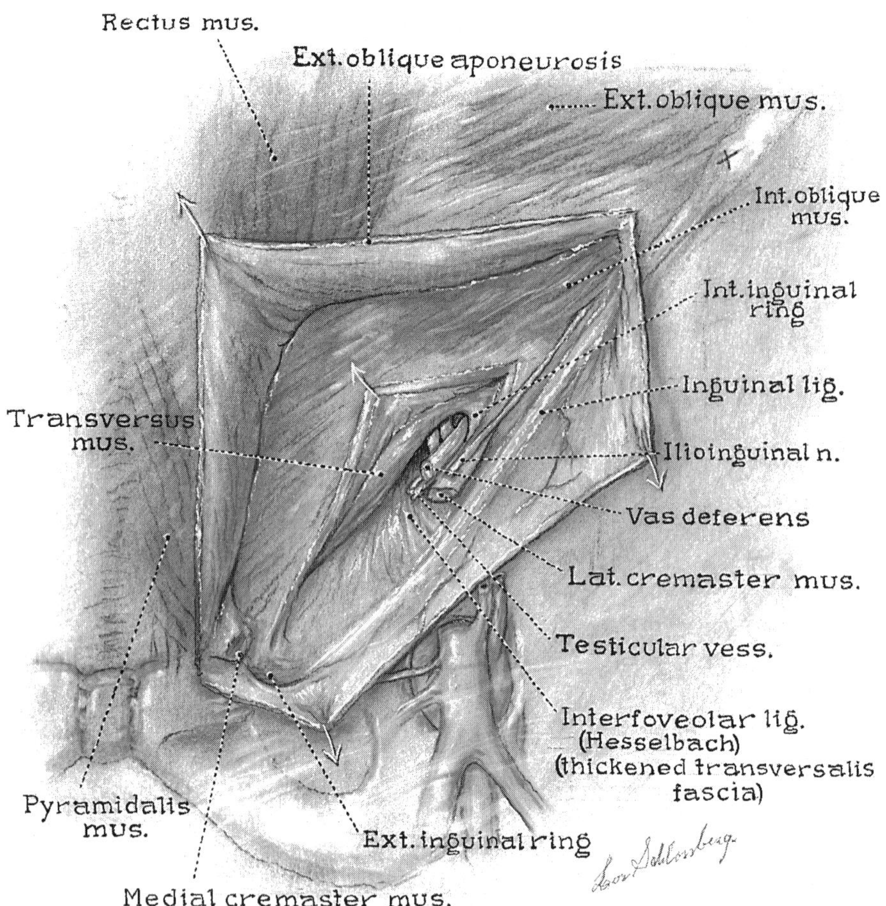

Figure 3–6. Deep structures of left inguinal canal, viewed from the front.

midway between the anterior superior iliac spine and the pubic tubercle, above the inguinal ligament, and 4 cm lateral to the external ring. **Fibers of the internal oblique and transversus abdominis arise from the iliopsoas fascia and inguinal ligament lateral to the internal ring and arch over the canal to form its roof.** They fuse as the conjoint tendon, pass posterior to the cord, and insert into the rectus sheath and pubis. **The conjoint tendon reinforces the posterior wall of the inguinal canal at the external ring.** With contraction of the internal oblique and transversus muscles, the roof of the canal is closed against the floor. Hernias into the canal may occur medial (direct) or lateral (indirect) to the inferior epigastric vessels (see Figs. 3–6 and 3–7).

Internal Surface of the Anterior Abdominal Wall

The peritoneal surface of the abdominal wall has been viewed with increasing frequency since the advent of laparoscopic surgery. **Three elevations of the peritoneum, referred to as the median, medial, and lateral umbilical folds, are visible on the anterior abdominal wall below the umbilicus** (Fig. 3–8). The median fold overlies the median umbilical ligament (urachus), a fibrous remnant of the cloaca that attaches the bladder to the anterior abdominal wall. The obliterated umbilical artery in the medial umbilical fold serves as an important landmark for the surgeon. It may be traced to its origin from the internal iliac artery to locate the ureter, which lies on its medial side. During transperitoneal laparoscopic pelvic lymph node dissection, the obturator packet is accessed by incising the peritoneum lateral to the obliterated umbilical artery. The lateral umbilical fold contains the inferior epigastric vessels as they ascend to supply the rectus abdominis.

SOFT TISSUES OF THE PELVIS

Pelvic Musculature

Muscles and fascia line the true pelvis and form its floor. **The obturator internus arises from the inner surface of the obturator foramen and the obturator membrane and passes through the lesser sciatic foramen to insert on the femur** (see Fig. 3–8). Fascia on the pelvic surface of this muscle is thickened into a tough line extending from the lower half of the pubis to the ischial spine. **This tendinous arc of the levator ani serves as the origin of the muscles of the pelvic diaphragm: the pubococcygeus and iliococcygeus** (Fig. 3–9). These muscles are not truly separable, and they form a diaphragm that closes the pelvic outlet. They pass medial and posterior to meet their counterparts at the perineal body, anococcygeal raphe, and coccyx. Anteriorly, a narrow U-shaped hiatus remains, through which the urethra and rectum exit in the male and the urethra, vagina, and rectum exit in the female. The muscle bordering this

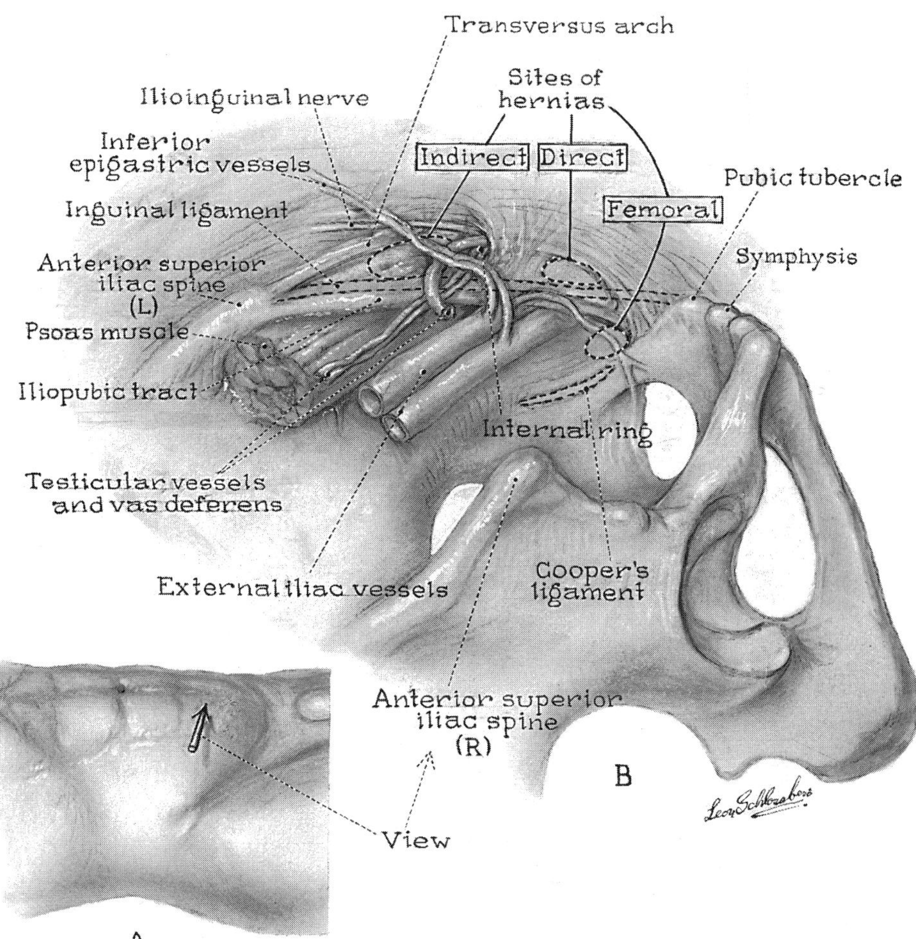

Figure 3–7. Topography *(A)* and posterior wall *(B)* of left inguinal canal, viewed from the preperitoneal space. Location of three types of inguinal hernia is demonstrated. (From Schlegel PN, Walsh PC: J Urol 1987; 137:1181.)

hiatus has been referred to as "pubovisceral" because it provides a sling for (pubourethralis, puborectalis), inserts directly into (pubovaginalis, puboanalis, levator prostatae), or inserts into a structure intimately associated with the pelvic viscera (perineal body) (Lawson, 1974). This pubovisceral group provides strong fixation and support for the pelvic viscera. **The coccygeus muscle extends from the sacrospinous ligament to the lateral border of the sacrum and coccyx to complete the pelvic diaphragm.** Muscles of the pelvic diaphragm contain type I (slow-twitch) fibers, which provide tonic support to pelvic structures, and type II (fast-twitch) fibers, for sudden increases in intra-abdominal pressure (Gosling et al, 1981). The **piriformis muscle** arises from the lateral aspect of the sacrum and passes through and fills the greater sciatic foramen to form the posterolateral wall of the pelvis.

It is important to recognize that the pelvic diaphragm is not flat or bowl-shaped, as it is frequently depicted. At the urogenital and anal hiatus, the muscles lie in a V-shaped configuration and are thickened inferiorly (Fig. 3–10). Behind the anus, they flatten to form a nearly horizontal diaphragm, referred to as the *levator plate*. In the female, the levator plate provides critical support to the pelvic viscera, as discussed later.

Pelvic Fasciae

The pelvic fasciae are not merely collagenous; they are also rich in elastic tissue and smooth muscle. This suggests that they are active in the support, and possibly the function, of the pelvic viscera. **The pelvic fasciae are continuous with the retroperitoneal fasciae** and have been categorized somewhat arbitrarily into outer, intermediate, and inner strata. **The outer stratum, or endopelvic fascia, lines the inner surface of the pelvic muscles** and is continuous with the transversalis layer of the abdomen. It is fixed to the arcuate line of the pelvis, Cooper's ligament, the sacrospinous ligament, the ischial spine, and the tendinous arc of the levator ani. **The intermediate stratum embeds the pelvic viscera in a fatty, compressible layer that accommodates their filling and emptying.** Its tissues are easily swept aside to reveal the retropubic, paravesical, rectogenital, and retrorectal potential spaces. **All pelvic vessels and some pelvic nerves travel in this stratum and are subject to injury when these potential spaces are developed at surgery.** The intermediate stratum coalesces around vessels and nerves supplying the pelvic organs to form named ligaments (e.g., cardinal, uterosacral, lateral, and posterior vesical) that suspend and tether these organs in the pelvis (Fig. 3–11). This fascia also thickens around the pelvic urogenital organs to form their visceral fascia. **The inner stratum lies subjacent to the peritoneum and is associated with the entire gastrointestinal tract. In the pelvis it covers the rectum and the dome of the bladder, and forms the rectogenital septum (Denonvilliers' fascia)** (see Fig. 3–3). This septum is the developmental remains of rectogenital pouch of peritoneum that extended

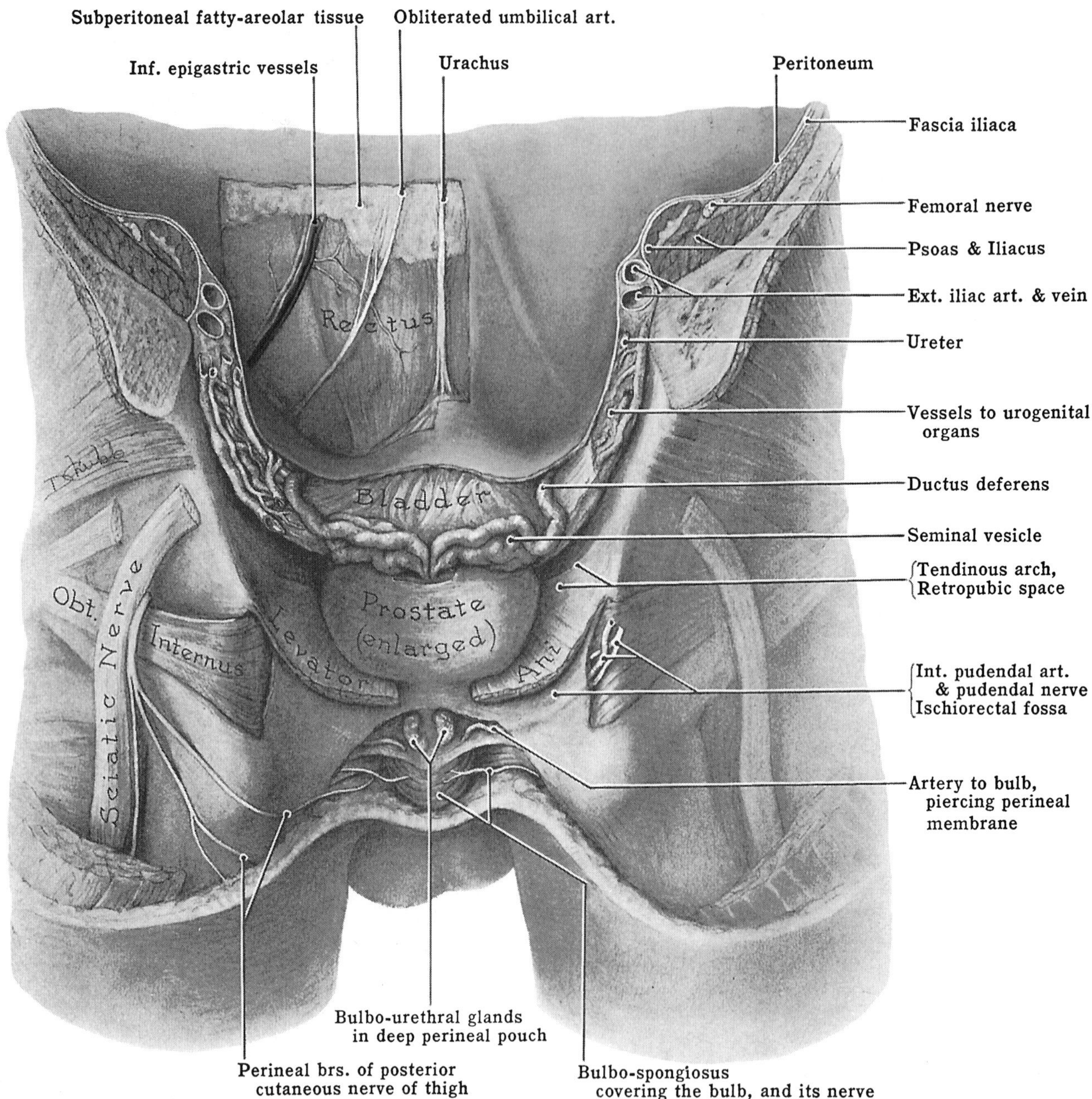

Figure 3–8. The male pelvis and anterior abdominal wall viewed from behind. The sacrum and ilia have been removed. (From Anderson JE: Grant's Atlas of Anatomy, 7th ed. Baltimore, Williams & Wilkins Company, 1978, Fig. 3–41.)

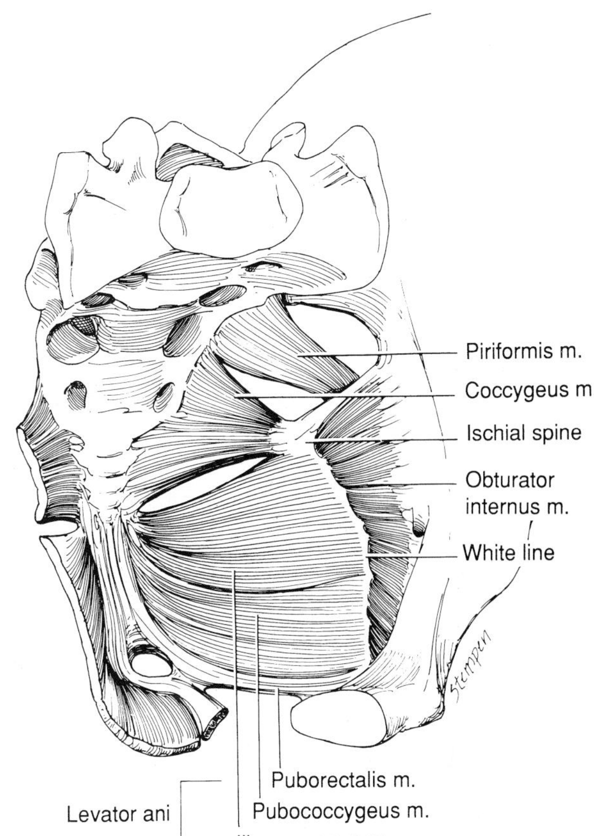

Figure 3–9. Muscles of the true pelvis (three-quarter view).

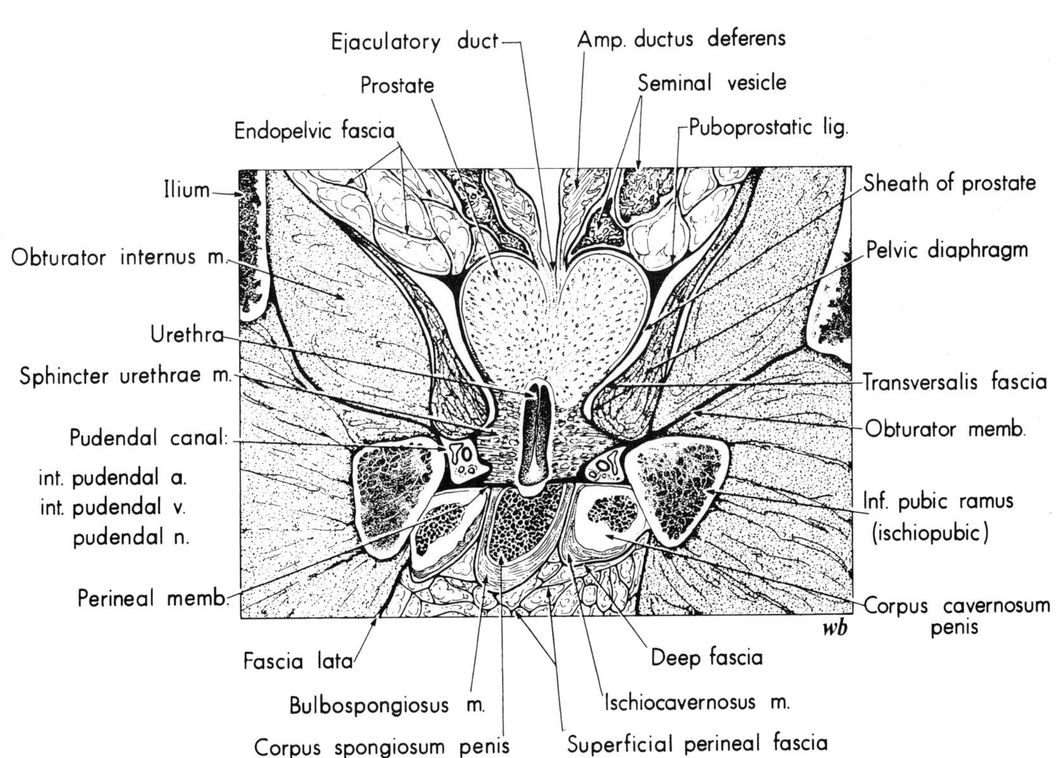

Figure 3–10. Frontal section of the male pelvis through the membranous urethra, perpendicular to the perineal membrane. Note the near-vertical lie of the levator ani, the cone shape of the striated urethral sphincter, and the proximity of Alcock's canal. (From Oelrich TM: Am J Anat 1980; 158:246.)

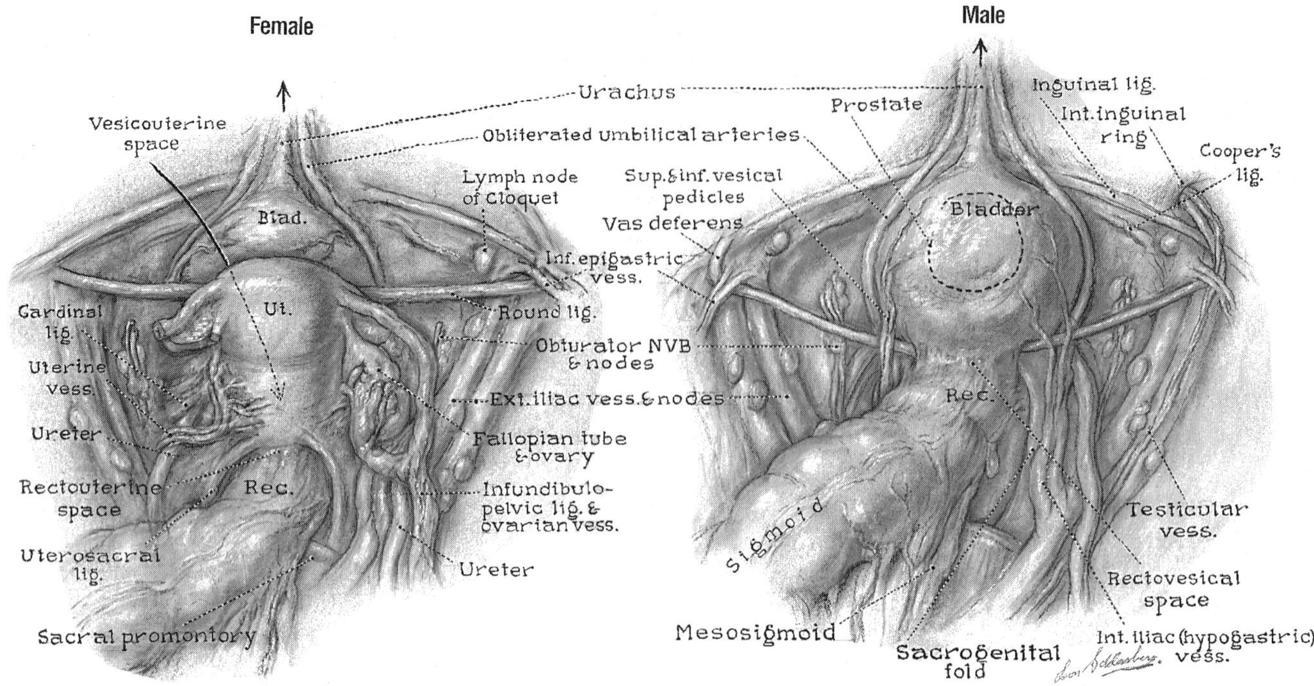

Figure 3–11. The peritoneal surfaces of the female and male pelves. In the female, the ureter passes medial to the ovarian vessels, then deep to the uterine artery within the substance of the cardinal ligament. The sacrogenital and sacrouterine folds represent the posterior portions of pelvic fascial support.

between the rectum and internal genitalia to the pelvic floor.

The pelvic fasciae have been given a confusing array of appellations by anatomists and surgeons interested in female pelvic organ prolapse. To add to the confusion, the strength of these fasciae can differ significantly among individuals and races, and these differences may predispose some individuals to pelvic prolapse (Zacharin, 1985). **There are three important components of the pelvic fasciae: (1) Anteriorly, the puboprostatic ligaments** attach to the lower fifth of the pubis, lateral to the symphysis, and to the junction of the prostate and membranous urethra (see Fig. 3–39). They are called the **pubourethral ligaments in the female** and insert on the proximal third of the urethra (Fig. 3–12). **(2) Laterally, the arcus tendineus fascia pelvis extends from the puboprostatic (pubourethral) ligament to the ischial spine (see Fig. 3–12).** This fascia condensation forms at the junction of the endopelvic and visceral fasciae. It should not be confused with the arcus tendineus levator ani, which lies above its anterior portion (Fig. 3–13). In the male, it is found at the base of a sulcus between the pelvic side wall and the prostate and bladder. In the female, it corresponds to the lateral attachment of the anterior vaginal wall to the pelvic side wall. Paravaginal suspension procedures for stress urinary incontinence entail lateral reapproximation of the vaginal wall to this tendinous arc (Richardson et al, 1981). **The lateral branches of the dorsal venous complex are directly beneath the arcus tendineus fascia pelvis; thus the endopelvic fascia should be opened lateral to this landmark.** In the female, the fascia extending medially from this arch carries a number of names (pubovesical, periurethral, urethropelvic ligament) and provides important support to the urethra and anterior vaginal wall (DeLancey, 1994). Damage to this fascia and its attachments has been implicated in urethrocele, cystocele, and stress urinary incontinence. **(3) Posterior to the ischial spine, the fascia fans out to either side of the rectum and attaches to the pelvic side wall as the lateral and posterior vesical ligaments. In the female, these are the strong cardinal and uterosacral ligaments.** They are not true ligaments; rather, they are condensations of intermediate stratum around visceral neurovascular pedicles. The peritoneum over these ligaments forms discrete folds (rectovesical in the male and rectouterine in the female) that can be appreciated at cystectomy (see Fig. 3–11). Taken as a whole, the pelvic fasciae form a Y-shaped scaffolding for the pelvic urogenital viscera (see Fig. 3–13).

Fasciae of the Perineum and the Perineal Body

The weakest point in the pelvic floor, the urogenital hiatus, is bridged by the urogenital diaphragm, a structure unique to humans. The fibrous perineal membrane lies at the center of, and defines, the urogenital diaphragm (see Fig. 3–3). It is triangular and spans the inferior ischiopubic rami from the pubis to the ischial tuberosities. Posteriorly, it ends abruptly; the superficial and deep transversus perinei muscles run along its free edge (Fig. 3–14). The external genitalia attach to its inferior surface; superiorly, it supports the urethral sphincter (discussed later). The perineal body represents the point of fusion between the free posterior edge of the urogenital diaphragm and the posterior apex of the urogenital hiatus. This pyramid-shaped structure lies at the hub of pelvic support. **Virtually every**

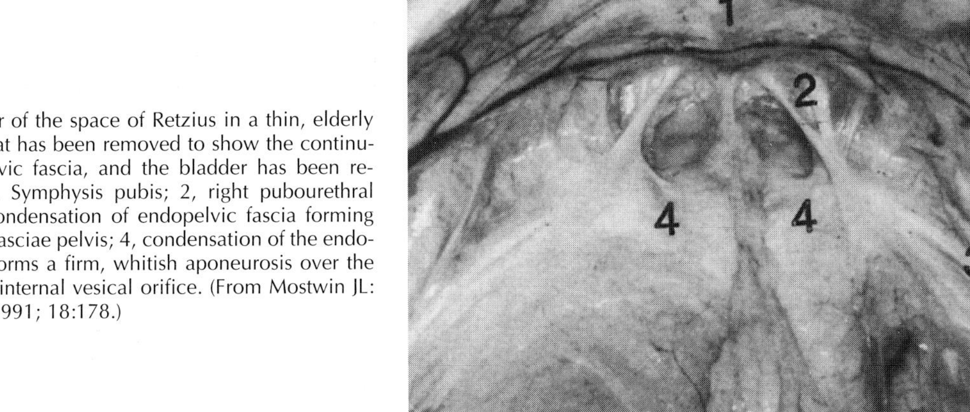

Figure 3–12. The floor of the space of Retzius in a thin, elderly female cadaver. The fat has been removed to show the continuous sheet of endopelvic fascia, and the bladder has been retracted posteriorly. 1, Symphysis pubis; 2, right pubourethral ligament; 3, lateral condensation of endopelvic fascia forming right arcus tendineus fasciae pelvis; 4, condensation of the endopelvic fascia, which forms a firm, whitish aponeurosis over the proximal urethra and internal vesical orifice. (From Mostwin JL: Urol Clin North Am 1991; 18:178.)

pelvic muscle (superficial and deep transversus perinei, bulbospongiosus, levator ani, rectourethralis, external anal sphincter, striated urethral sphincter) and fascia (perineal membrane, Denonvilliers', Colles', and endopelvic) insert into the perineal body. At its core are abundant elastin and richly innervated smooth muscle, which suggests that it may have a dynamic role in pelvic support. Damage to the perineal body during perineal prostatectomy risks postoperative urinary incontinence.

PELVIC CIRCULATION

Arterial Supply

At the bifurcation of the aorta, the **middle sacral artery** arises posteriorly and travels on the pelvic surface of the sacrum to supply branches to the sacral foramina and the rectum. **The common iliac arteries arise at the level of the fourth lumbar vertebra, run anterior and lateral to their accompanying veins, and bifurcate into the external and internal iliac arteries at the SI joint** (Fig. 3–15). The external iliac artery follows the medial border of the iliopsoas muscle along the arcuate line and leaves the pelvis beneath the inguinal ligament as the femoral artery (Fig. 3–16). Its inferior epigastric branch is given off proximal to the inguinal ligament and ascends medial to the internal ring to supply the rectus abdominis muscle and overlying skin. Because the rectus is richly collateralized from above and laterally, the inferior epigastric vessels may be ligated with impunity. A rectus myocutaneous flap based on this artery has been used to correct major pelvic and perineal tissue defects. Near its origin, **the inferior epigastric artery sends a deep circumflex iliac branch laterally and pubic branch medially.** Both vessels travel on the iliopubic tract and may be injured during inguinal hernia repair. **Its cremasteric branch joins the spermatic cord at the internal inguinal ring and forms a distal anastomosis with the testicular**

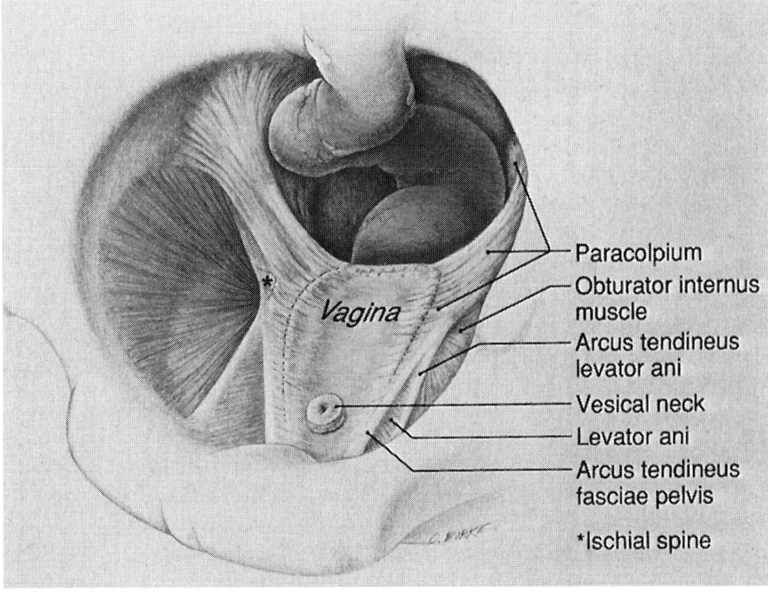

Figure 3–13. The vagina and supportive structures after removal of the bladder and uterus. The arcus tendineus fasciae pelvis and the cardinal and uterosacral ligaments (paracolpium) form a continuous structure that supports the pelvic viscera. (From DeLancey JOL: Am J Obstet Gynecol 1992; 166:1719.)

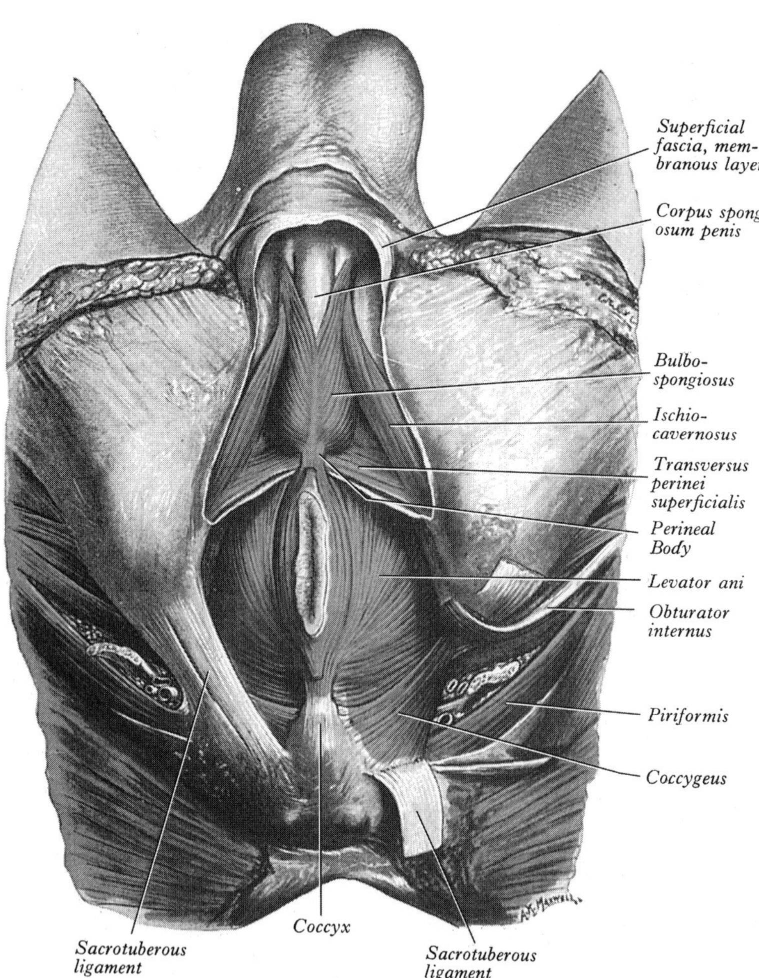

Figure 3–14. Muscles of the male perineum. The transversus perinei and ischiocavernosi frame the urogenital diaphragm. (From Williams PL, Warwick R: Gray's Anatomy, 35th British ed. Philadelphia, W.B. Saunders Company, 1973, p 530.)

artery (see Fig. 3–43). In 25% of people, an **accessory obturator artery** arises from the inferior epigastric artery and runs medial to the femoral vein to reach the obturator canal. This vessel must be avoided during obturator lymph node dissection.

The internal iliac (hypogastric) artery descends in front of the SI joint and divides into an anterior and posterior trunk (see Fig. 3–15). **The posterior trunk gives rise to three parietal branches: (1) the superior gluteal**, which exits the greater sciatic foramen; **(2) the ascending lumbar**, which supplies the posterior abdominal wall; and **(3) the lateral sacral,** which passes medially to join the middle sacral branches at the sciatic foramina. **The anterior trunk gives off seven parietal and visceral branches: (1) The superior vesical artery arises from the proximal portion of the obliterated umbilical artery and gives off a vesiculodeferential branch to the seminal vesicles and vas deferens.** The artery of the vas deferens travels the length of the vas to meet the cremasteric and testicular arteries distally (see Fig. 3–43). Because of these anastomoses, the testicular artery may be sacrificed without compromising viability of the testis. **(2) The middle rectal artery** gives small branches to the seminal vesicles and prostate and anastomoses with the inferior and superior rectal arteries in the rectal wall. **(3) The inferior vesical branches** supply the lower ureter, bladder base, prostate, and seminal vesicles. In the female, they supply the ureter, bladder base, and vagina. **(4) The uterine artery passes above and in front of the ureter** ("water flows under the bridge") to ascend the lateral wall of the uterus and meet the ovarian artery in the lateral portion of the fallopian tube (see Figs. 3–11 and 3–30). The ureter is vulnerable during division of the uterine pedicles. **(5) The internal pudendal artery** leaves the pelvic cavity through the greater sciatic foramen, passes around the sacrospinous ligament, and enters the lesser sciatic foramen to gain access to the perineum. Its perineal course is discussed later. **(6) The obturator artery,** variable in origin, travels through the obturator fossa medial and inferior to the obturator nerve and passes through its canal to supply the adductors of the thigh (Fig. 3–16). **(7) The inferior gluteal artery** travels through the greater sciatic foramen to supply the buttock and thigh.

The internal iliac artery can be ligated to control severe pelvic hemorrhage. Ligation decreases pulse pressure, allowing hemostasis to occur more readily. Internal iliac blood flow does not stop but reverses its direction because of critical anastomoses (lumbar segmentals to iliolumbar, median sacral to lateral sacral, and superior rectal and middle rectal). Bilateral ligation almost invariably produces vasculogenic impotence.

Venous Supply

The dorsal vein of the penis passes between the inferior pubic arch and the striated urethral sphincter to reach

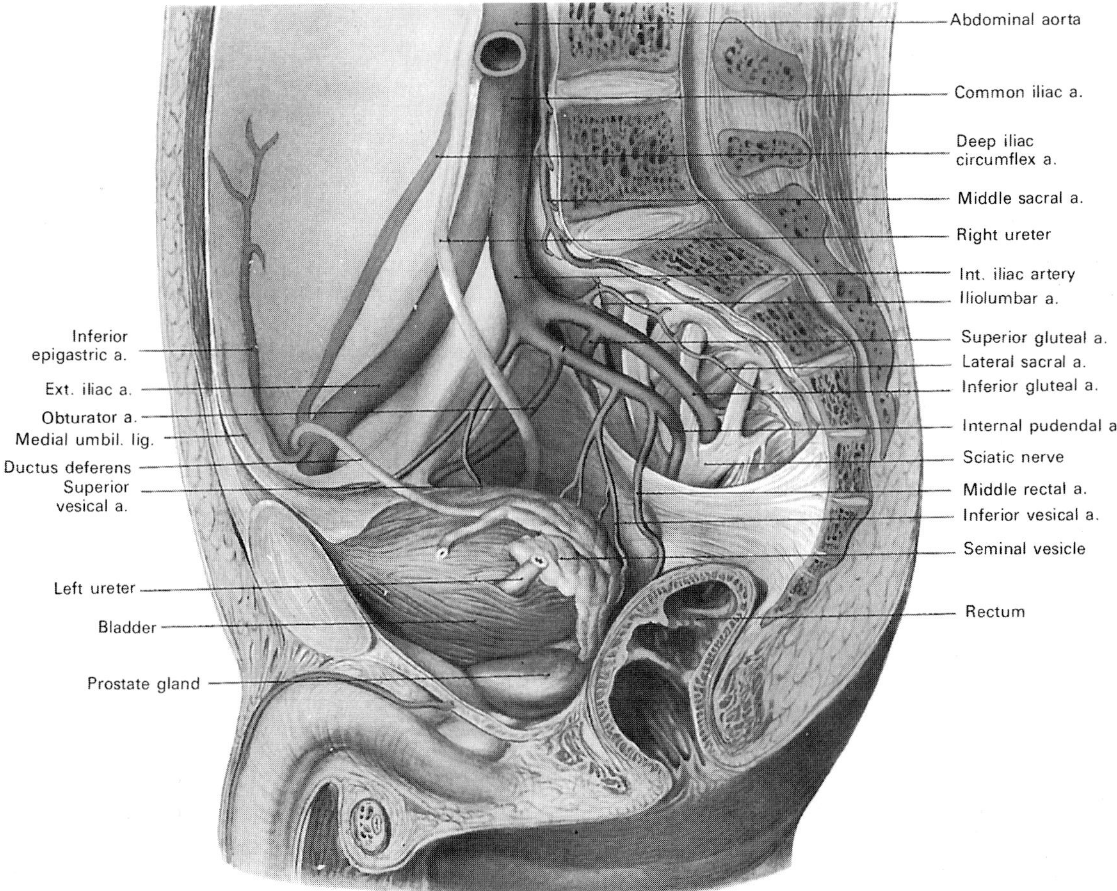

Figure 3–15. The right internal and external iliac arteries. The ureter and vas deferens pass medial to the vessels. (From Clemente CD: Gray's Anatomy, 30th American ed. Philadelphia, Lea & Febiger, 1985, p 750.)

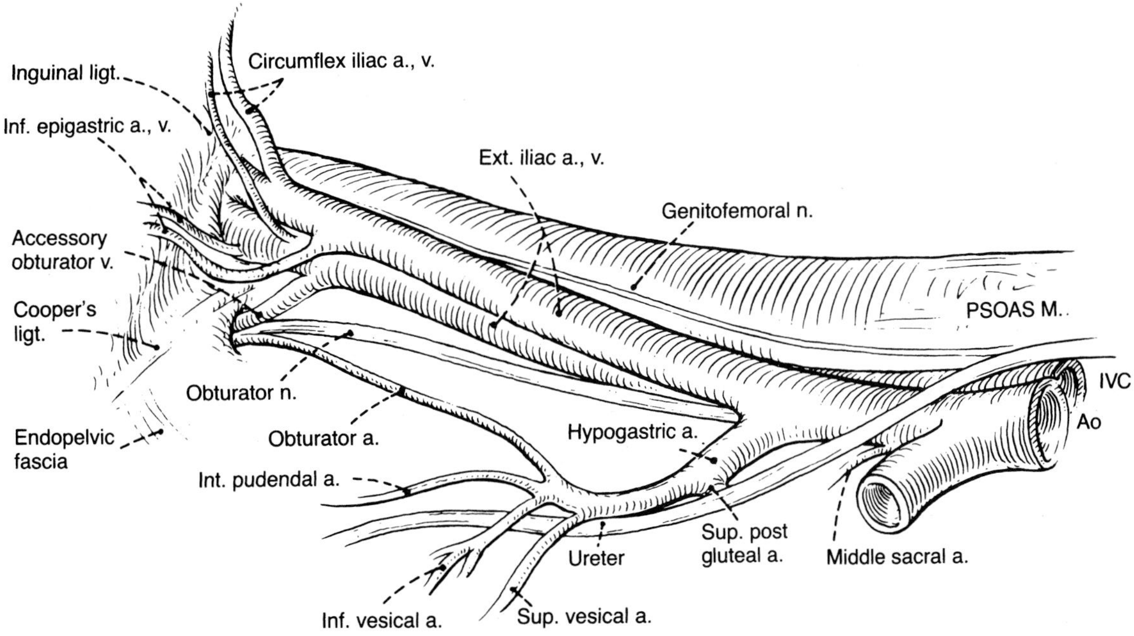

Figure 3–16. The right obturator fossa, showing the iliac vessels and obturator nerve. (From Skinner DG: Pelvic lymphadenectomy. *In* Glenn JF, Ed: Urologic Surgery, 2nd ed. New York, Harper & Row, 1975, p 591.)

the pelvis, where it trifurcates into a central superficial branch and two lateral plexuses (Reiner and Walsh, 1979) (Fig. 3–17). To minimize blood loss at radical retropubic prostatectomy, the dorsal vein complex is best divided distally, before its ramification. It should be recognized that part of this complex runs within the anterior and lateral walls of the striated sphincter; thus care must be taken not to injure the sphincter when securing hemostasis. The superficial branch pierces the visceral endopelvic fascia between the puboprostatic ligaments and drains the retropubic fat, the anterior bladder, and the anterior prostate (see Figs. 3–17 and 3–39).

The lateral plexuses sweep down the sides of the prostate, receiving drainage from it and the rectum, and communicate with the vesical plexuses on the lower part of the bladder. Three to five inferior vesical veins emerge from the vesical plexus laterally and drain into the internal iliac vein. In the female, the dorsal vein of the clitoris bifurcates to empty into the laterally placed vaginal plexuses. These connect with the vesical, uterine, ovarian, and rectal plexuses and drain into the internal iliac veins. **Connections between the pelvic plexuses, emissary veins of the pelvic bones, and the vertebral plexus have been proposed to be routes for dissemination of infection or tumor from the pelvic viscera to the axial and pelvic skeleton** (Batson, 1940).

The internal iliac vein is joined by tributaries corresponding to the branches of the internal iliac artery, and ascends medial and posterior to the artery. This vein is relatively thin-walled and at risk for injury during dissection of the artery or the nearby pelvic ureter. The external iliac vein travels medial and inferior to its artery and joins the internal iliac vein behind the internal iliac artery. In half of patients, one or more **accessory obturator veins drain into the underside of the external iliac vein and can be easily torn during lymphadenectomy** (see Fig. 3–16).

Pelvic Lymphatics

The pelvic lymph nodes can be difficult to appreciate on gross examination because they are embedded in the fatty and fibrous tissue of the intermediate stratum. There are three major pelvic lymph node groups associated with the pelvic vessels (Fig. 3–18). A substantial portion of pelvic visceral lymphatic drainage passes through the **internal iliac nodes and their tributaries: the presacral, obturator, and internal pudendal nodes**. The **external iliac nodes** lie lateral, anterior, and medial to the vessels and drain the anterior abdominal wall, urachus, bladder, and, in part, internal genitalia. The external genitalia and perineum drain into the superficial and deep inguinal nodes (see later discussion). The inguinal nodes communicate directly with the internal and external iliac chains. The **common iliac nodes** receive efferent vessels from the external and internal iliac nodes and the pelvic ureter and drain into the lateral aortic nodes.

PELVIC INNERVATION

Lumbosacral Plexus

The lumbosacral plexus and its rami are well illustrated in the previous chapter; only the pelvic course of its nerves are reviewed here (see Figs. 2–6 and 2–12). The **iliohypogastric nerve** (L1) travels between, and supplies, the internal oblique and transversus muscles and pierces the external oblique 3 cm above the external inguinal ring to supply sensation over the lower abdomen and pubis (see Fig. 3–4). The **ilioinguinal nerve** (L1) passes through the internal oblique muscle to enter the inguinal canal laterally. It travels anterior to the cord and exits the external ring to provide sensation to the mons pubis and anterior scrotum or labia majora (see Figs. 3–4 and 3–6). The **genitofemoral nerve** (L1, L2) pierces the psoas muscle to reach its anterior surface in the retroperitoneum, then travels to the pelvis and **splits into genital and femoral branches**. The latter supplies sensation over the anterior thigh below the inguinal ligament. The genital branch follows the cord through the inguinal canal, supplies the cremaster muscle, and supplies sensation to the anterior scrotum.

For most of its pelvic course, the **femoral nerve** (L2, L3,

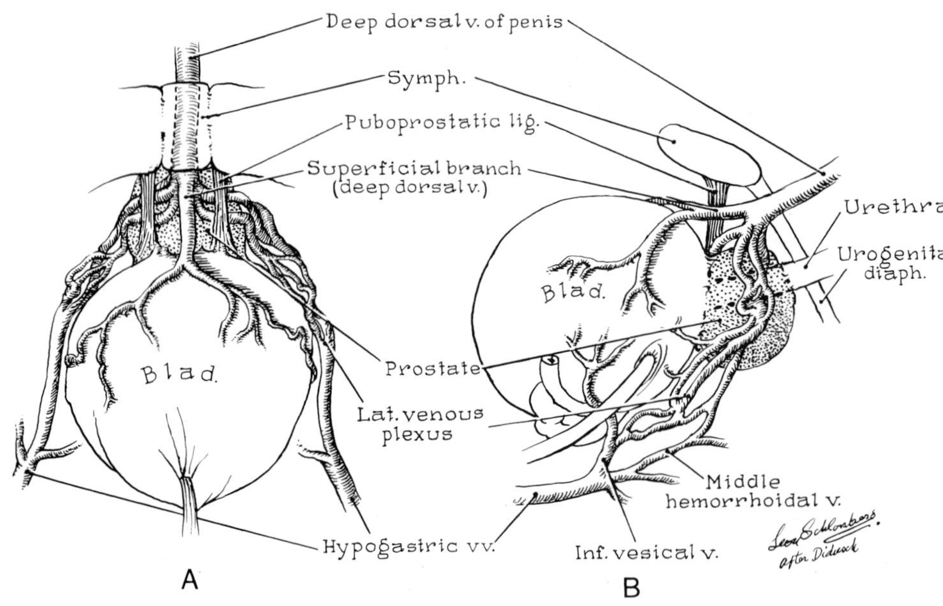

Figure 3–17. The pelvic venous plexus. *A*, Trifurcation of the dorsal vein of the penis, viewed from the retropubic space. Relationship of venous branches to the puboprostatic ligaments is shown. *B*, Lateral view of the pelvic venous plexus after removal of the lateral pelvic fascia. Normally these structures are difficult to see because they are embedded in pelvic fascia. (From Reiner WG, Walsh PC: J Urol 1979; 121:198.)

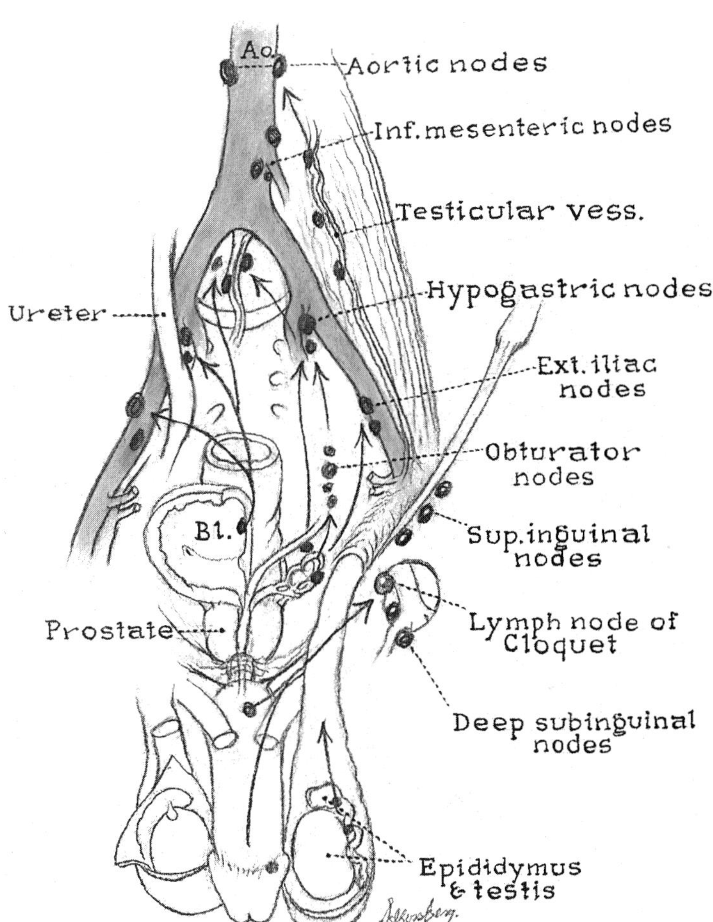

Figure 3–18. Lymphatic drainage of the male pelvis, perineum, and external genitalia.

L4) travels beneath or within the substance of the psoas muscle, then exits its lateral side to pass under the inguinal ligament (Fig. 3–19). It supplies sensation to the anterior thigh and motor innervation to the extensors of the knee. **During a psoas hitch, sutures should be placed in the direction of this nerve (and the psoas muscle fibers) to avoid nerve damage or entrapment. Retractor blades**

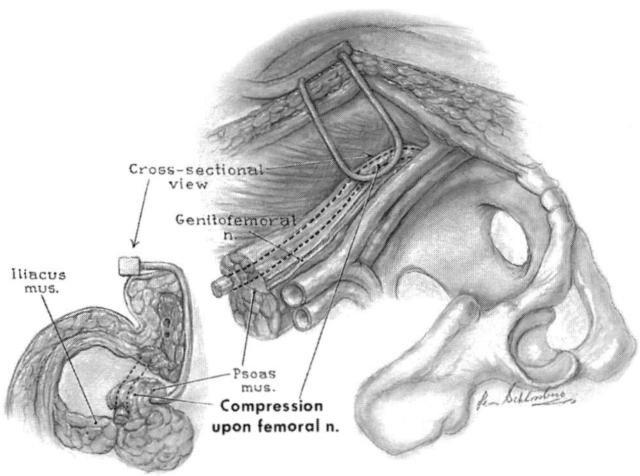

Figure 3–19. The femoral nerve as it relates to the psoas muscle. Retractor blades may compress this nerve to produce a femoral nerve palsy. (From Burnett AL, Brendler CB: J Urol 1994; 151:163.)

must not rest on the psoas muscle because they may produce a femoral nerve palsy, a potentially dangerous setback after pelvic surgery. The lateral femoral cutaneous nerve (L2, L3) may be seen lateral to the psoas in the iliacus fascia.

The **obturator nerve** (L2, L3, L4) emerges in the true pelvis from beneath the psoas muscle, lateral to the internal iliac vessels, and passes through the obturator fossa to the obturator canal (see Fig. 3–16). In the fossa, it is lateral and superior to the obturator vessels and surrounded by the obturator and internal iliac lymph nodes. Damage to this nerve during pelvic lymphadenectomy weakens the adductors of the thigh.

The lumbosacral trunk (L4, L5) passes into the true pelvis behind the psoas and unites with the ventral rami of the sacral segmental nerves to form the sacral plexus. This plexus lies on the pelvic surface of piriformis, deep to the endopelvic fascia and posterior to the internal iliac vessels (see Fig. 3–15). It leaves the pelvis through the greater sciatic foramen immediately posterior to the sacrospinous ligament (where it may be injured during sacrospinous culposuspension) and supplies motor and sensory innervation to the posterior thigh and lower leg. Exaggerated lithotomy position may stretch this nerve or place pressure on its peroneal branch at the fibular head to produce foot drop. **Pelvic and perineal branches of the sacral plexus include (1) the posterior femoral cutaneous branch** (S2, S3), which, after passing through the greater sciatic foramen, gives an anterior sensory branch to the perineum and back of the scrotum (see Fig. 3–8); **(2) the pudendal nerve** (S2, S3, S4), which follows the internal pudendal artery to the perineum (to be discussed); **(3) the nervi erigentes** (S2, S3, S4) to the pelvic autonomic plexus; and **(4) pelvic somatic efferent nerves** from the ventral rami of S2, S3, and S4 (Fig. 3–20). The latter nerves travel on the pelvic surface of the levator ani in close association with the rectum and prostate and are separated from the pelvic autonomic plexus by the endopelvic fascia. They supply the levator ani and extend anteriorly to the striated urethral sphincter (Lawson, 1974; Zvara et al, 1994).

Pelvic Autonomic Plexus

The presynaptic sympathetic cell bodies that project to the pelvic autonomic nervous plexus reside in the lateral column of gray matter of the last three thoracic and first two lumbar segments of the spinal cord. They reach the pelvic plexus by two pathways: (1) The superior hypogastric plexus is formed by sympathetic fibers from the celiac plexus and the first four lumbar splanchnic nerves (see Fig. 2–1). Anterior to the bifurcation of the aorta, it divides into two hypogastric nerves that enter the pelvis medial to the internal iliac vessels, anterior to the sacrum, and deep to the endopelvic fascia. **(2) The pelvic continuation of the sympathetic trunks** pass deep to the common iliac vessels and medial to the sacral foramina and fuse in front of the coccyx at the ganglion impar (see Fig. 2–6). Each chain comprises four to five ganglia that send branches anterolaterally to participate in the formation of the pelvic plexus.

Presynaptic parasympathetic innervation arises from the intermediolateral cell column of the sacral cord. Fibers emerge from the second, third, and fourth sacral spinal nerves as the pelvic splanchnic nerves (nervi erigentes) to join the hypogastric nerves and branches from the sacral sympathetic ganglia to form the inferior hypogastric (pelvic) plexus (Fig. 3–21). Some pelvic parasympathetic efferent fibers travel up the hypogastric nerves to the inferior mesenteric plexus, where they provide parasympathetic innervation to the descending and sigmoid colon.

The pelvic plexus is rectangular, approximately 4 to 5 cm in length, and its midpoint is at the tips of the seminal vesicles (Schlegel and Walsh, 1987). It is oriented in the sagittal plane on either side of the rectum and pierced by the numerous vessels going to and from the rectum, bladder, seminal vesicles, and prostate. **Division of these vessels proximally (the so-called lateral pedicles of the bladder and prostate) risks injury to the pelvic plexus with attendant postoperative impotence** (Walsh and Donker, 1982; Walsh et al, 1983). The right and left components of the pelvic plexus communicate behind the rectum and anterior and posterior to the vesical neck. Branches of the pelvic plexus follow blood vessels to reach the pelvic viscera, although nerves to the ureter may join it directly as it passes nearby. Visceral afferent and efferent nerves travel on the vas deferens to reach the testis and epididymis (see later discussion).

The most caudal portion of the pelvic plexus gives rise to the innervation of the prostate and the important cavernous nerves (Walsh and Donker, 1982). After passing the tips of the seminal vesicles, these nerves lie within leaves of the lateral endopelvic fascia near its juncture with, but outside, Denonvilliers' fascia (Fig. 3–22; Lepor et al, 1985). They travel at the posterolateral border of the prostate on the surface of the rectum and are lateral to the prostatic capsular arteries and veins. Because the nerves are composed of multiple fibers not visible on gross inspection, these vessels serve as a surgical landmark for the course of these nerves (**the neurovascular bundles**). During radical prostatectomy, the nerves are most vulnerable at the apex of the prostate, where they closely approach the prostatic capsule at the 5- and 7-o'clock positions. On reaching the membranous urethra, the nerves divide into superficial branches, which travel on the surface of the striated urethral sphincter at the 3- and 9-o'clock positions, and deep fibers, which penetrate the substance of this muscle and send twigs to the bulbourethral glands. As the nerves reach the hilum of the penis, they join to form one to three discrete bundles, related to the urethra at the 1- and 11-o'clock positions, superficial to the cavernous veins, and dorsomedial to the cavernous arteries (see Fig. 3–40; Lue et al, 1984; Breza et al, 1989). With the arteries, they pierce the corpora cavernosa to supply the erectile tissue (see later discussion). Small fibers also join the dorsal nerves of the penis as they course distally. In the female, the nerves to vestibular bodies and corpora cavernosa of the clitoris travel between the anterior vaginal wall and bladder in association with the lateral venous plexuses.

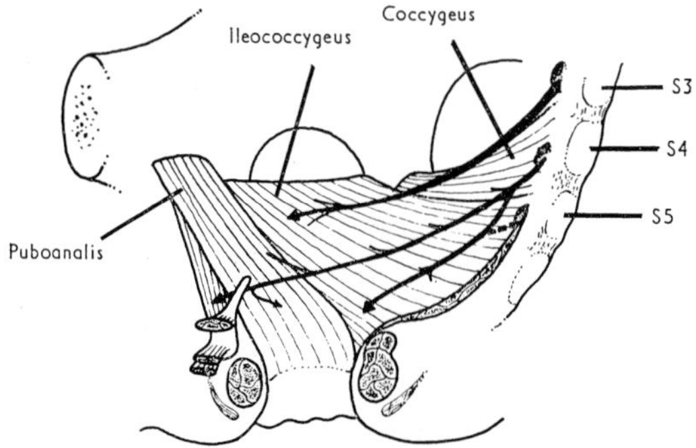

Figure 3–20. Pelvic floor somatic efferent nerves extending anteriorly on the pelvic surface of the levator ani to supply this muscle and the striated urethral sphincter. (From Lawson JON: Ann R Coll Surg Engl 1974; 54:250.)

PELVIC VISCERA

Rectum

The rectum begins with the disappearance of the sigmoid mesentery opposite the third sacral vertebra. **Peritoneum continues anteriorly over the upper two thirds of the rectum as the rectovesical pouch in males and as the rectouterine pouch (of Douglas) in females** (Fig. 3–23; see also Fig. 3–11). This peritoneal pouch extends inferiorly to the tips of the seminal vesicles or to the posterior fornix of the vagina. Inferior to this pouch, the anterior rectum is related to its fascial continuation (the rectogenital, or

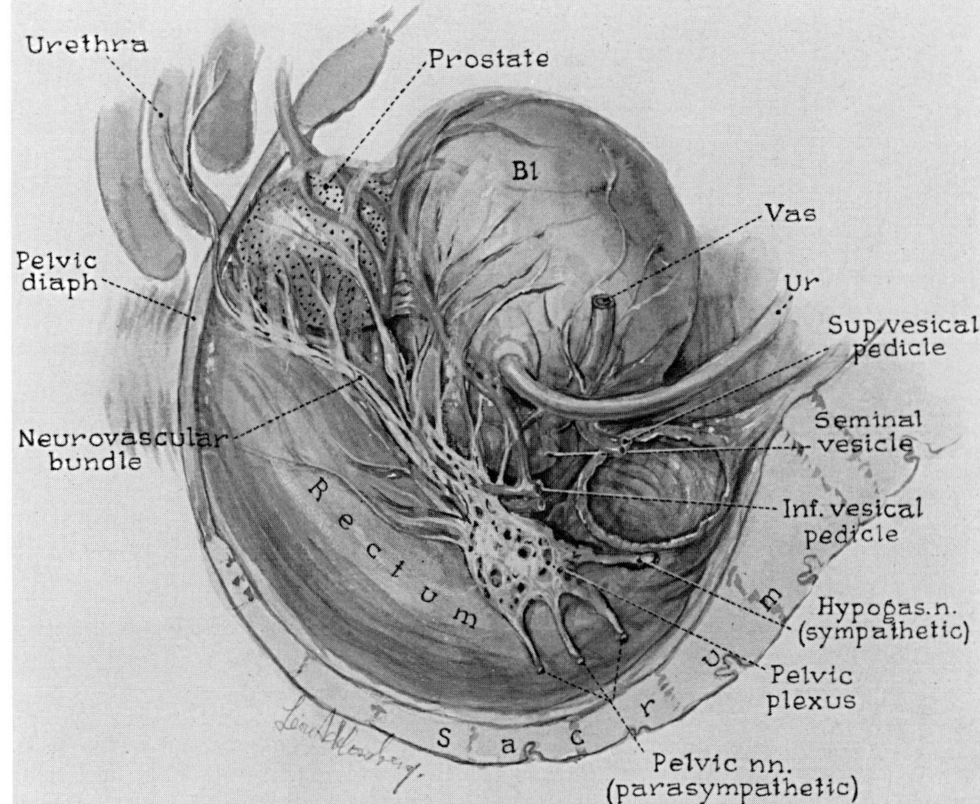

Figure 3–21. Lateral view showing the left pelvic autonomic nervous plexus and its relation to the pelvic viscera. (From Schlegel PN, Walsh PC: J Urol 1987; 138:1403.)

Denonvilliers', fascia) down to the level of the striated urethral sphincter (see Figs. 3–3, 3–23, and 3–32). The rectum describes a gentle curve on the sacrum, coccyx, and levator plate (see Fig. 3–21) and receives innervation from the laterally placed pelvic autonomic plexus and blood supply from the superior (from inferior mesenteric), middle (from internal iliac), and inferior (from internal pudendal) rectal arteries. The rectal walls are composed of an inner layer of circular smooth muscle and a virtually continuous sheet of outer longitudinal smooth muscle derived from the

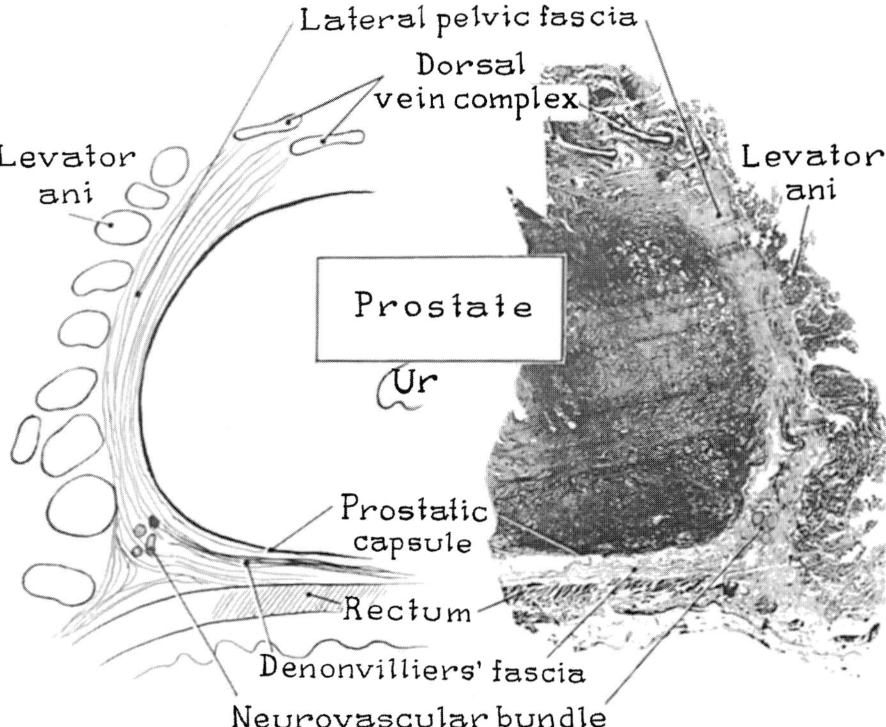

Figure 3–22. Cross section through an adult prostate, showing the relationships between the neurovascular bundle, lateral pelvic fascia, and Denonvilliers' fascia. (From Walsh PC, Lepor H, Eggleston JC: Prostate 1983; 4:477.)

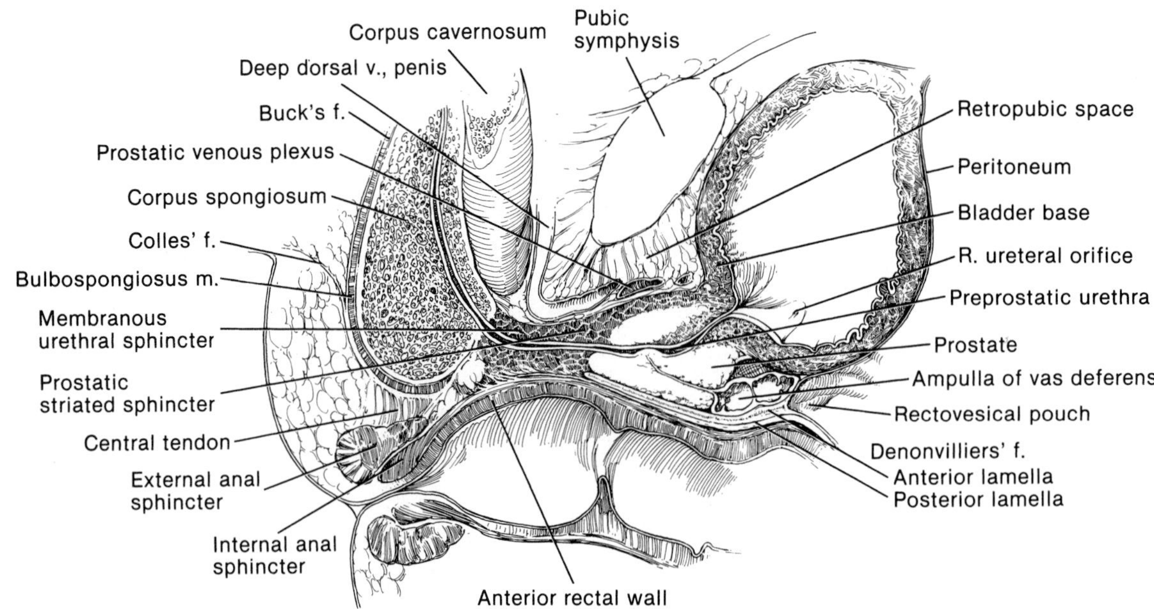

Figure 3–23. Sagittal section through the prostatic and membranous urethra, demonstrating the midline relations of the pelvic structures. (From Hinman F Jr: Atlas of Urosurgical Anatomy. Philadelphia, W.B. Saunders Company, 1993, p 356.)

tenia of the colon. In its lowest part, the rectum dilates to form the rectal ampulla. At the most inferior portion of the ampulla, anterior fibers of the longitudinal muscle leave the rectum to join Denonvilliers' fascia and the posterior striated urethral sphincter in the apex of the perineal body. When approached from below, these fibers, **the rectourethralis muscle, are 2 to 10 mm thick and must be divided to gain access to the prostate** (see Fig. 3–35). **The apices of the prostate and ampulla are in close proximity, and rectal injuries during radical prostatectomy commonly occur at this location.** As the rectourethralis is given off, the rectum makes a right-angle turn posteroinferiorly to exit the pelvis at the anal canal. The anatomy of the anal canal is considered with the perineum.

Pelvic Ureter

The ureter is divided into abdominal and pelvic portions by the common iliac artery. The structure of the ureter and its abdominal course have been reviewed in Chapter 2. Intraoperatively, the ureter is identified by its peristaltic waves and is readily found anterior to the bifurcation of common iliac artery (see Figs. 3–11 and 3–15). At ureteroscopy, pulsations of this artery can be seen in the posterior ureteral wall. **The ovarian vessels (infundibulopelvic ligament) cross the iliac vessels anterior and lateral to the ureter, and dissection of the ovarian vessels at the pelvic brim is a common cause of ureteral injury** (see Fig. 3–11; Daly and Higgins, 1988). **Pyeloureterography discloses a narrowing of the ureter at the iliac vessels**, and ureteral calculi frequently become lodged at this location. Because the ureter and iliac vessels rest on the arcuate line, **the ureter is subject to compression and obstruction by the gravid uterus and by masses within the true pelvis.**

The ureters come within 5 cm of each other as they cross the iliac vessels. On entering the pelvis, they diverge widely along the pelvic side walls toward the ischial spines. The ureter travels on the anterior surface of the internal iliac vessels and is related laterally to the branches of the anterior trunk. Near the ischial spine, the ureter turns anteriorly and medially to reach the bladder. **In men,** the anteromedial surface of the ureter is covered by peritoneum, and the ureter is embedded in retroperitoneal connective tissue, which varies in thickness (see Fig. 3–11). As the ureter courses medially, **it is crossed anteriorly by the vas deferens and runs with the inferior vesical arteries, veins, and nerves in the lateral vesical ligaments.** Viewed from the peritoneal side, the ureter is just lateral and deep to the rectogenital fold. **In women, the ureter first runs posterior to the ovary, then turns medially to run deep to the base of the broad ligament before entering a loose connective tissue tunnel through the substance of the cardinal ligament** (see Fig. 3–11). As in the male, the ureter can be found slightly lateral and deep to the rectouterine folds of peritoneum. It is crossed anteriorly by the uterine artery and is therefore subject to injury during hysterectomy. **As it passes in front of the vagina, it crosses 1.5 cm anterior and lateral to the uterine cervix.** The ureter may be injured at this level during hysterectomy, resulting in a ureterovaginal fistula. The ureter courses 1 to 4 cm on the anterior vaginal wall to reach the bladder. Occasionally, a stone in the distal ureter can be palpated through the anterior vaginal wall. The intramural ureter is discussed with the bladder.

The pelvic ureter receives abundant blood supply from the common iliac artery and most branches of the internal iliac artery. The inferior vesical and uterine arteries usually supply the ureter with its largest pelvic branches. **Blood supply to the pelvic ureter enters laterally; thus, the pelvic peritoneum should be incised only medial to the ureter.** Intramural vessels of the ureter run within the adventitia and generally follow one of two patterns. In approximately 75% of specimens, longitudinal vessels run the length of the ureter and are formed by anastomoses of segmental ureteral vessels. In the remaining ureters, the vessels form a fine interconnecting mesh (plexiform) with less collateral flow (Shafik, 1972). The pelvic ureter appears to have a high preponderance of plexiform vessels, which render it more vulnerable to ischemia and less suitable for ureteroureterostomy (Hinman, 1993). **Lymphatic drainage of the pelvic ureter is to the external, internal, and common iliac nodes.** Pathologic enlargement of the common and internal iliac nodes can encroach on and obstruct the ureter.

The pelvic ureter has rich adrenergic and cholinergic autonomic innervation derived from the pelvic plexus. The functional significance of this innervation is unclear, inasmuch as the ureter continues to contract peristaltically after denervation. Afferent neural fibers travel through the pelvic plexus and account for the visceral quality of referred pain from ureteral irritation or acute obstruction.

Bladder

Relationships

When filled, the bladder has a capacity of approximately 500 ml and assumes an ovoid shape. **The empty bladder is tetrahedral and is described as having a superior surface with an apex at the urachus, two inferolateral surfaces, and a posteroinferior surface or base with the bladder neck at the lowest point** (see Fig. 3–23).

The urachus anchors the apex of the bladder to the anterior abdominal wall (see Fig. 3–8). There is a relative paucity of bladder wall muscle at the point of attachment of the urachus, predisposing to diverticula formation. The urachus is composed of longitudinal smooth muscle bundles derived from the bladder wall. Near the umbilicus, it becomes more fibrous and usually fuses with one of the obliterated umbilical arteries. Urachal vessels run longitudinally, and the ends of the urachus must be ligated when it is divided. An epithelium-lined lumen usually persists throughout life and uncommonly gives rise to aggressive urachal adenocarcinomas (Begg, 1930). In rare instances, luminal continuity with the bladder serves as a bacterial reservoir or results in an umbilical urinary fistula.

The superior surface of the bladder is covered by peritoneum. Anteriorly, the peritoneum sweeps gently onto the anterior abdominal wall (see Fig. 3–11). With distention, the bladder rises out of the true pelvis and separates the peritoneum from the anterior abdominal wall. It is therefore possible to perform a suprapubic cystostomy without risking entry into the peritoneal cavity. Posteriorly, the peritoneum passes to the level of the seminal vesicles and meets the peritoneum on the anterior rectum to form the rectovesical space.

Anteroinferiorly and laterally, **the bladder is cushioned from the pelvic side wall by retropubic and perivesical fat and loose connective tissue. This potential space (of Retzius) may be entered anteriorly by dividing the transversalis fascia and provides access to the pelvic viscera as far posteriorly as the iliac vessels and ureters** (see Fig. 3–12). The bladder base is related to the seminal vesicles, ampullae of the vasa deferentia, and terminal ureter. **The bladder neck**, located at the internal urethral meatus, rests 3 to 4 cm behind the midpoint of the symphysis pubis. **It is firmly fixed by the pelvic fasciae** (see earlier discussion) **and by its continuity with the prostate**; its position changes little with varying conditions of the bladder and rectum.

In the female, the peritoneum on the superior surface of the bladder is reflected over the uterus to form the vesicouterine pouch, then continues posteriorly over the uterus as the rectouterine pouch (see Fig. 3–11). The vagina and uterus intervene between the bladder and rectum, so that the base of the bladder and the urethra rest on the anterior vaginal wall. **Because the anterior vaginal wall is firmly attached laterally to the levator ani, contraction of the pelvic diaphragm (e.g., during increases in intra-abdominal pressure) elevates the bladder neck and draws it anteriorly.** In many women with stress incontinence, the bladder neck drops below the pubic symphysis. **In infants, the true pelvis is shallow, and the bladder neck is level with the upper border of the symphysis.** The bladder is a true intra-abdominal organ that can project above the umbilicus when full. By puberty, the bladder has migrated to the confines of the deepened true pelvis.

Structure

The internal surface of the bladder is lined with transitional epithelium, which appears smooth when the bladder is full but contracts into numerous folds when the bladder empties. This urothelium is usually six cells thick and rests on a thin basement membrane. **Deep to this, the lamina propria forms a relatively thick layer of fibroelastic connective tissue** that allows considerable distention. This layer is traversed by numerous blood vessels and contains smooth muscle fibers collected into a poorly defined muscularis mucosa. **Beneath this layer lies the smooth muscle of the bladder wall. The relatively large muscle fibers form branching, interlacing bundles loosely arranged into inner longitudinal, middle circular, and outer longitudinal layers (Fig. 3–24). However, in the upper aspect of the bladder, these layers are clearly not separable, and any one fiber can travel between each of the layers, change orientation, and branch into longitudinal and circular fibers.** This meshwork of detrusor muscle is ideally suited for emptying the spherical bladder.

Near the bladder neck, the detrusor muscle is clearly separable into the three layers described earlier (Fig. 3–25). Here the smooth muscle is morphologically and functionally distinct from the remainder of the bladder, for the large-diameter muscle fascicles are replaced by much finer fibers. The structure of the bladder neck appears to differ between men and women. In men, radially oriented inner longitudinal fibers pass through the internal meatus to become continuous with the inner longitudinal layer of smooth muscle in the urethra.

The middle layer forms a circular preprostatic sphincter that is responsible for continence at the level of the bladder neck (fundus ring) (see Fig. 3–25). This sphincter has the shape of an inverted cone with its apex projecting down the prostatic urethra nearly to the level of the verumontanum. The fact that perfect continence can be maintained in men in whom the striated urethral sphincter is destroyed attests to the efficacy of this sphincter (Waterhouse et al, 1973). **This muscle is richly innervated by adrenergic fibers,** which, when stimulated, produce closure of the blad-

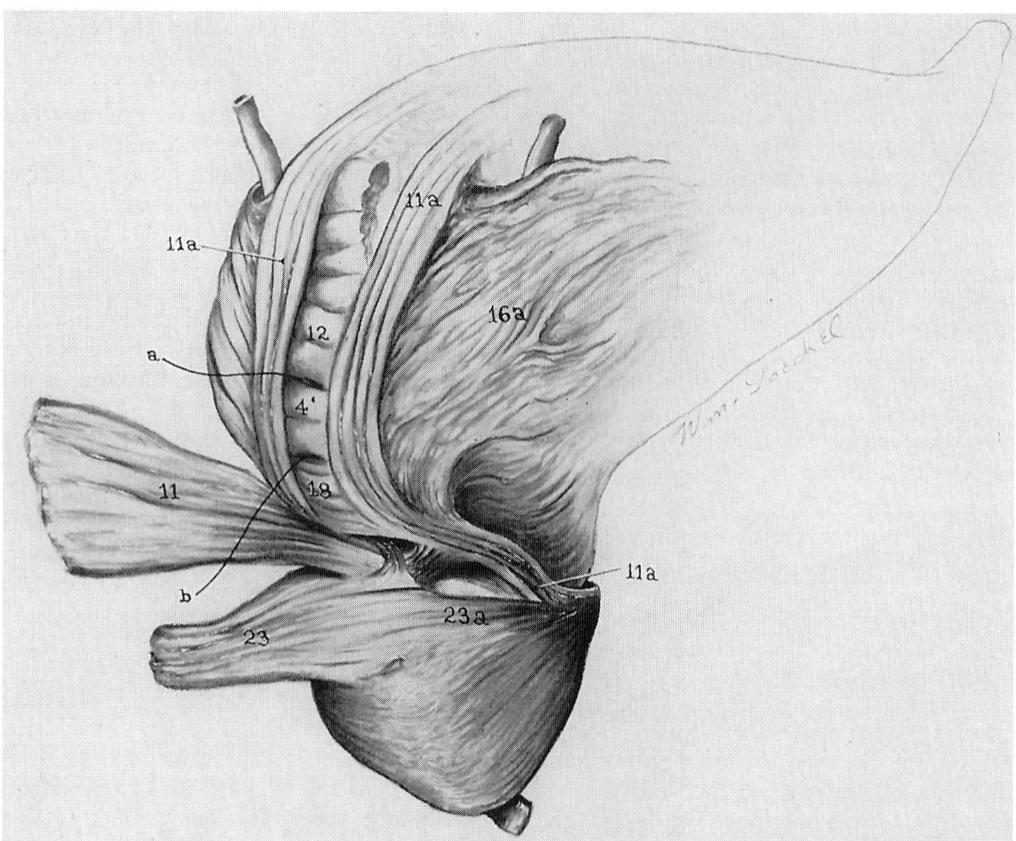

Figure 3–24. Dissection of the male bladder. 11, Posterior outer longitudinal detrusor, which forms backing of the ureters (folded back); 11a, posterolateral portion of outer longitudinal muscle forming loop around anterior bladder neck; 4', 12, and 18, middle circular layer backing the trigone; 23 and 23a, lateral pedicle of the prostate. (From Uhlenhuth E: Problems in the anatomy of the pelvis. Philadelphia, J.B. Lippincott Company, 1953, p 187.)

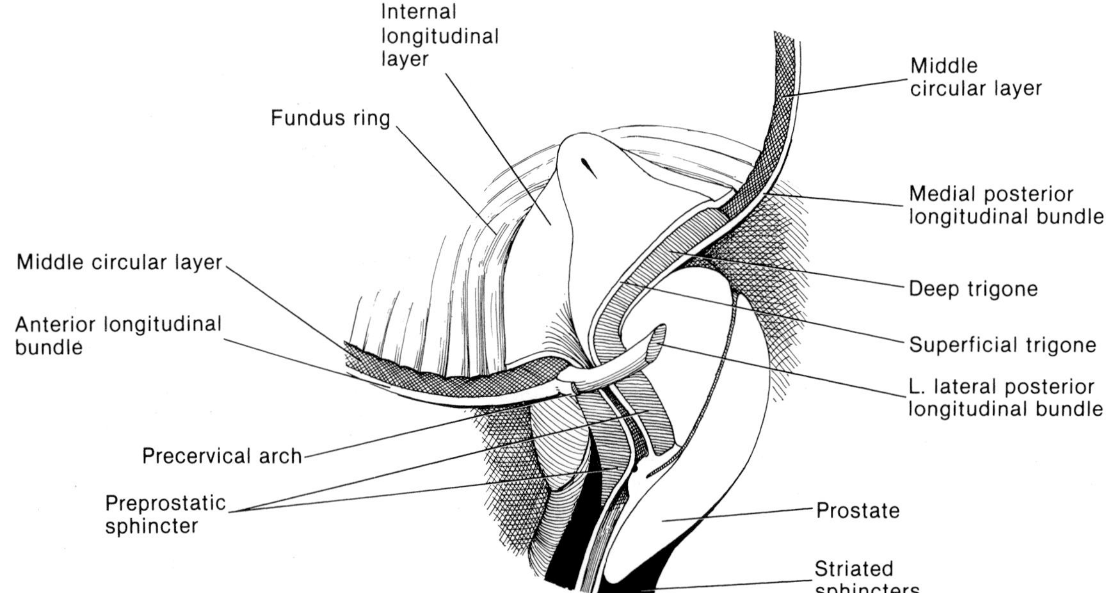

Figure 3–25. The male bladder base and preprostatic sphincter. (From Hinman F Jr: Atlas of Urosurgical Anatomy. Philadelphia, W.B. Saunders Company, 1993, p 336.)

der neck (Uhlenhuth, 1953). Damage to the sympathetic nerves to the bladder, as a result of diabetes mellitus or retroperitoneal lymph node dissection for testis cancer, can cause retrograde ejaculation.

The outer longitudinal fibers are thickest posteriorly at the bladder base. In the midline they insert into the apex of the trigone and intermix with the smooth muscle of the prostate to provide strong trigonal backing. Laterally, **the fibers from this posterior sheet pass anteriorly and fuse to form a loop around the bladder neck** (see Fig. 3–24). This loop is thought to participate in continence at the bladder neck. On the lateral and anterior surfaces of the bladder, the longitudinal fibers are not as well developed. Some anterior fibers course forward to join the puboprostatic ligaments in men and the pubourethral ligaments in women. These fibers contribute smooth muscle to these supports and are speculated to contribute to bladder neck opening during micturition (DeLancey, 1989).

At the female bladder neck, the inner longitudinal fibers converge radially to pass downward as the inner longitudinal layer of the urethra, as described earlier. **The middle circular layer does not appear to be as robust as that of the male**, and several authors have denied its existence altogether (Gosling, 1979, 1985; Williams et al, 1989). Whereas several other investigators have noted an anterior loop of external longitudinal muscle (see Fig. 3–31), the authors just cited have denied the existence of this structure as well. They maintained instead that the external fibers pass obliquely and longitudinally down the urethra to participate in forming the inner longitudinal layer of smooth muscle. Regardless, **the female bladder neck differs strikingly from the male in possessing little adrenergic innervation**. In addition, its sphincteric function is limited; in 50% of continent women, urine enters the proximal urethra during a cough (Versi et al, 1986).

Ureterovesical Junction and Trigone

As the ureter approaches the bladder, its spirally oriented mural smooth muscle fibers become longitudinal. Two to three centimeters from the bladder, a fibromuscular sheath (of Waldeyer) extends longitudinally over the ureter and follows it to the trigone (Tanagho, 1992). The ureter pierces the bladder wall obliquely, near the tip of the seminal vesicle, and travels 1.5 to 2 cm and terminates at the ureteral orifice (Fig. 3–26). **As it passes through a hiatus in the detrusor (intramural ureter), it is compressed and narrows considerably.** This is a common site in which ureteral stones become impacted. **The intravesical portion of the ureter lies immediately beneath the bladder urothelium and therefore is quite pliant; it is backed by a strong plate of detrusor muscle. With bladder filling, this arrangement is thought to result in passive occlusion of the ureter, like a flap valve.** Indeed, reflux does not occur in fresh cadavers when the bladder is filled (Thomson et al, 1994). Vesicoureteral reflux is thought to result from insufficient submucosal ureteral length and poor detrusor backing. Chronic increases in intravesical pressure resulting from bladder outlet obstruction can cause herniation of the bladder mucosa through the weakest point of the hiatus above the ureter and produce a "Hutch diverticulum" and reflux (Hutch, 1961).

The triangle of smooth urothelium between the two ureteral orifices and the internal urethral meatus is referred to as the trigone of the bladder (see Fig. 3–26). The fine longitudinal smooth muscle fibers from the vesical side of the ureters pass to either side of their respective orifices to join the lateral and posterior ureteral wall fibers and fan out over the base of the bladder. **Fibers from each ureter meet to form a triangular sheet of muscle that extends from the two ureteral orifices to the internal urethral meatus.** The edges of this muscular sheet are

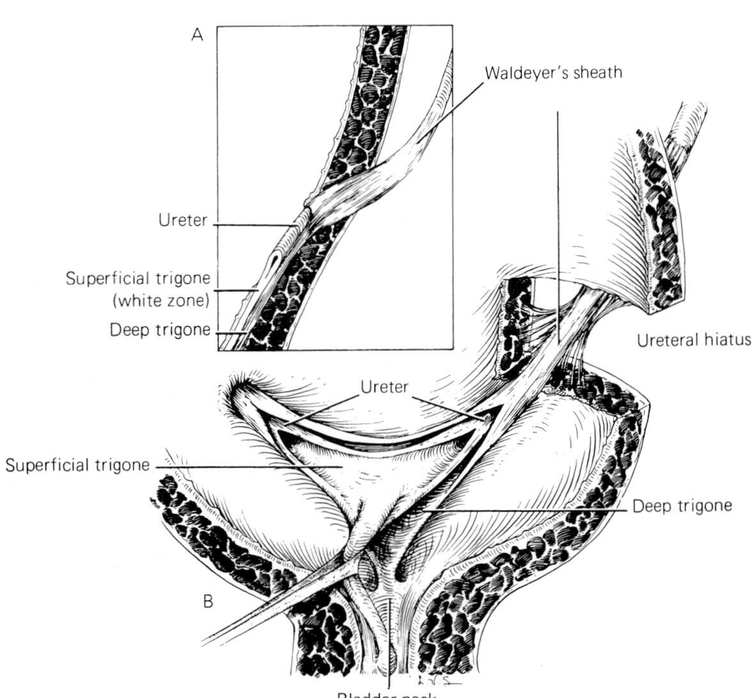

Figure 3–26. The normal ureterovesical junction and trigone. *A,* Section of the bladder wall perpendicular to the ureteral hiatus shows the oblique passage of the ureter through the detrusor and also shows the submucosal ureter with its detrusor backing. Waldeyer's sheath surrounds the prevesical ureter and extends inward to become the deep trigone. *B,* Waldeyer's sheath continues in the bladder as the deep trigone, which is fixed at the bladder neck. Smooth muscle of the ureter forms the superficial trigone and is anchored at the verumontanum. (From Tanagho EA, Pugh RCB: Br J Urol 1963; 35:151.)

thickened between the ureteral orifices (the interureteric crest, or Mercier's bar) and between the ureters and the internal urethral meatus (Bell's muscle).

The muscle of trigone forms three distinct layers: (1) a superficial layer, derived from the longitudinal muscle of the ureter, which extends down the urethra to insert at the verumontanum; **(2) a deep layer, which continues from Waldeyer's sheath** and inserts at the bladder neck; and **(3) a detrusor layer, formed by the outer longitudinal and inner circular smooth muscle layers of the bladder wall.** Through its continuity with the ureter, the superficial trigonal muscle anchors the ureter to the bladder. In a ureteral reimplantation, this muscle is tented up and divided in order to gain access to the space between Waldeyer's sheath and the ureter. In this space, only loose fibrous and muscular connections are found. This anatomic arrangement helps prevent reflux during bladder filling by fixing and applying tension to the ureteral orifice. As the bladder fills, its lateral wall telescopes outward on the ureter, thereby increasing intravesical ureteral length (Hutch, 1961).

The urothelium overlying the muscular trigone is usually only three cells thick and adheres strongly to the underlying muscle by a dense lamina propria. During filling and emptying of the bladder, this mucosal surface remains smooth.

Bladder Circulation

In addition to the vesical branches, the bladder may be supplied by any adjacent artery arising from the internal iliac. For convenience, surgeons refer to the vesical blood supply as the lateral and posterior pedicles, which, when the bladder is approached from the rectovesical space, are lateral and posteromedial to the ureters, respectively. These pedicles are the lateral and posterior vesical ligaments in the male and part of the cardinal and uterosacral ligaments in the female (see Fig. 3–11). The veins of the bladder coalesce into the vesical plexus and drain into the internal iliac veins. Lymphatics from the lamina propria and muscularis drain to channels on the bladder surface, which run with the superficial vessels within the thin visceral fascia. Small paravesical lymph nodes can be found along the superficial channels. **The bulk of the lymphatic drainage passes to the external iliac lymph nodes** (see Fig. 3–18). Some anterior and lateral drainage may go through the obturator and internal iliac nodes, whereas portions of the bladder base and trigone may drain into the internal and common iliac groups.

Bladder Innervation

Autonomic efferent fibers from the anterior portion of the pelvic plexus (the vesical plexus) pass up the lateral and posterior ligaments to innervate the bladder. The bladder wall is richly supplied with parasympathetic cholinergic nerve endings and has abundant postganglionic cell bodies. Sparse sympathetic innervation of the bladder has been proposed to mediate detrusor relaxation but probably lacks functional significance. **A separate nonadrenergic, noncholinergic (NANC) component of the autonomic nervous system participates in activating the detrusor, although the neurotransmitter has not been identified** (Burnett, 1995). As mentioned, the male bladder neck receives abundant sympathetic innervation and expresses alpha$_1$-adrenergic receptors. The female bladder neck has little adrenergic innervation. Nitric oxide synthase (NOS)–containing neurons have been identified in the detrusor, particularly at the bladder neck, where they may facilitate relaxation during micturition. The trigonal muscle is innervated by adrenergic and NOS-containing neurons. Like the bladder neck, it relaxes during micturition. **Afferent innervation from the bladder travels both with sympathetic (via the hypogastric nerves) and parasympathetic nerves to reach cell bodies in the dorsal root ganglia at thoracolumbar and sacral levels.** As a consequence, presacral neurectomy (division of the hypogastric nerves) is ineffective in relieving bladder pain.

Prostate

Relationships

The normal prostate weighs 18 g; measures 3 cm in length, 4 cm in width, and 2 cm in depth; and is traversed by the prostatic urethra (see Fig. 3–23). Although ovoid in shape, **the prostate is referred to as having anterior, posterior, and lateral surfaces, with a narrowed apex inferiorly and a broad base superiorly** that is contiguous with the base of the bladder. **It is enclosed by a capsule composed of collagen, elastin, and abundant smooth muscle.** Posteriorly and laterally, this capsule has an average thickness of 0.5 mm, although it may be partially transgressed by normal glands. **Microscopic bands of smooth muscle extend from the posterior surface of the capsule to fuse with Denonvilliers' fascia.** Loose areolar tissue defines a thin plane between Denonvilliers' fascia and the rectum. **On the anterior and anterolateral surfaces of the prostate, the capsule blends with the visceral continuation of endopelvic fascia** (see Fig. 3–22). Toward the apex, the puboprostatic ligaments extend anteriorly to fix the prostate to the pubic bone (see Fig. 3–39). The superficial branch of the dorsal vein lies outside this fascia in the retropubic fat and pierces it to drain into the dorsal vein complex.

Laterally, the prostate is cradled by the pubococcygeal portion of levator ani and is directly related to its overlying endopelvic fascia (see Figs. 3–8, 3–11, and 3–22). Below the juncture of the parietal and visceral endopelvic fascia (arcus tendineus fasciae pelvis), the pelvic fascia and prostate capsule separate, and the space between them is filled by fatty areolar tissue and the lateral divisions of the dorsal vein complex. During a radical retropubic prostatectomy, the endopelvic fascia should be divided lateral to the arcus tendineus fasciae pelvis to avoid injury to the venous complex. In the process, the endopelvic fascia overlying the levator ani is actually peeled off of the muscle and displaced medially with the prostate. Although this is truly a parietal endopelvic fascia, it is commonly referred to as the lateral prostatic fascia (Myers, 1994). As mentioned earlier, **the cavernosal nerves run posterolateral to the prostate in the substance of the parietal pelvic fascia (lateral prostatic fascia).** Thus, to preserve these nerves, this fascia must be incised lateral to the prostate and anterior to the neurovascular bundle (Walsh et al, 1983).

The apex of the prostate is continuous with the striated

urethral sphincter. Histologically normal prostatic glands can be found to extend into the striated muscle with no intervening fibromuscular stroma or "capsule." At the base of the prostate, outer longitudinal fibers of the detrusor fuse and blend with the fibromuscular tissue of the capsule. As mentioned, the middle circular and inner longitudinal muscles extend down the prostatic urethra as a preprostatic sphincter. **Like the apex, no true capsule separates the prostate from the bladder. In surgically resected prostate carcinomas, this peculiar anatomic arrangement can make interpretation of these margins difficult** and has led some pathologists to propose that the prostate does not possess a true capsule (Epstein, 1989).

Structure

The prostate is composed of approximately 70% glandular elements and 30% fibromuscular stroma. The stroma is continuous with capsule and composed of collagen and abundant smooth muscle. It encircles and invests the glands of the prostate and contracts during ejaculation to express prostatic secretions into the urethra. **The urethra runs the length of the prostate and is usually closest to its anterior surface. It is lined by transitional epithelium,** which may extend into the prostatic ducts. The urothelium is surrounded by an inner longitudinal and an outer circular layer of smooth muscle. **A urethral crest projects inward from the posterior midline, runs the length of the prostatic urethra, and disappears at the striated sphincter** (Fig. 3–27). **To either side of this crest, a groove is formed (prostatic sinuses) into which all glandular elements drain** (McNeal, 1972). At its midpoint, the urethra turns approximately 35 degrees anteriorly, but this angulation can vary from 0 to 90 degrees (see Figs. 3–20, 3–22, and 3–24). **This angle divides the prostatic urethra into proximal (preprostatic) and distal (prostatic) segments that are functionally and anatomically discrete** (McNeal, 1972, 1988). In the proximal segment, the circular smooth muscle is thickened to form the involuntary internal urethral (preprostatic) sphincter described earlier. Small **periurethral glands**, lacking periglandular smooth muscle, **extend between the fibers of the longitudinal smooth muscle to be enclosed by the preprostatic sphincter.** Although these glands constitute less than 1% of the secretory elements of the prostate, they can contribute significantly to prostatic volume in older men as one of the sites of origin of benign prostatic hypertrophy (BPH).

Beyond the urethral angle, all major glandular elements of the prostate open into the prostatic urethra. The urethral crest widens and protrudes from the posterior wall as the verumontanum (see Fig. 3–27). **The small slitlike orifice of the prostatic utricle is found at the apex of the verumontanum** and may be visualized cystoscopically. The utricle is a 6-mm müllerian remnant in the form of a small sac that projects upwards and backwards into the substance of the prostate. In males with ambiguous genitalia, it may

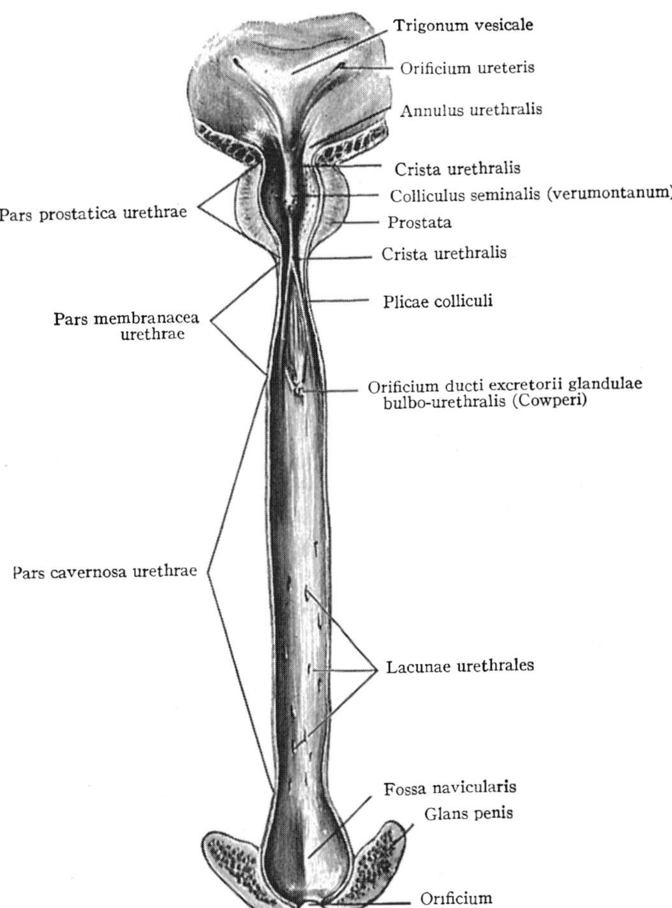

Figure 3–27. Posterior wall of the male urethra. (From Anson BJ, McVay CB: Surgical Anatomy, 6th ed. Philadelphia, W.B. Saunders Company, 1984, p 833.)

form a large diverticulum that protrudes from the posterior side of the prostate. **To either side of the utricular orifice, the two small openings of the ejaculatory ducts may be found.** The ejaculatory ducts form at the juncture of the vas deferens and seminal vesicles and enter the prostatic base where it fuses with the bladder. They course nearly 2 cm through the prostate in line with the distal prostatic urethra and are surrounded by circular smooth muscle (see Figs. 3–23 and 3–28).

In general, **the glands of the prostate are tubuloalveolar with relatively simple branching and are lined with simple cuboidal or columnar epithelium. Scattered neuroendocrine cells, of unknown function, are found between the secretory cells. Beneath the epithelial cells, flattened basal cells line each acinus and are believed to be stem cells for the secretory epithelium.** Each acinus is surrounded by a thin layer of stromal smooth muscle and connective tissue.

The glandular elements of the prostate have been divided into discrete zones, distinguished by the location of their ducts in the urethra, by their differing pathologies, and in some cases by their embryologic origin (see Fig. 3–28). These zones can be demonstrated clearly with transrectal ultrasonography. **At the angle dividing the preprostatic and prostatic urethra, the ducts of the transition zone arise and pass beneath the preprostatic sphincter to travel on its lateral and posterior sides.** Normally, the transition zone accounts for 5% to 10% of the glandular tissue of the prostate. A discrete fibromuscular band of tissue separates the transition zone from the remaining glandular compartments and may be visualized at transrectal ultrasonography of the prostate. **The transition zone commonly gives rise to BPH**, which expands to compress the fibromuscular band into a surgical capsule seen at enucleation of an adenoma. It is estimated that **20% of adenocarcinomas of the prostate originate in this zone.**

The ducts of the central zone arise circumferentially around the openings of the ejaculatory ducts. This zone constitutes 25% of the glandular tissue of the prostate and expands in a cone shape around the ejaculatory ducts to the base of the bladder. The glands are structurally and immunohistochemically distinct from the remaining prostatic glands (which branch directly from the urogenital sinus), which has led to the suggestion that they are of **wolffian origin** (McNeal, 1988). In keeping with this suggestion, **only 1% to 5% of adenocarcinomas arise in the central zone,** although it may be infiltrated by cancers from adjacent zones.

The peripheral zone makes up the bulk of the prostatic glandular tissue (70%) and covers the posterior and lateral aspects of the gland. Its ducts drain into the prostatic sinus along the entire length of the (postsphincteric) prostatic urethra. Seventy percent of prostatic cancers arise in this zone, and it is the zone most commonly affected by chronic prostatitis.

Up to one third of the prostatic mass may be attributed to the nonglandular **anterior fibromuscular stroma.** This region **normally extends from the bladder neck to the striated sphincter**, although considerable portions of it may be replaced by glandular tissue in adenomatous enlargement of the prostate. It is directly continuous with the prostatic capsule, anterior visceral fascia, and anterior portion of the preprostatic sphincter and is composed of elastin, collagen, and smooth and striated muscle. It is rarely invaded by carcinoma.

Clinically, the prostate is often spoken of as having

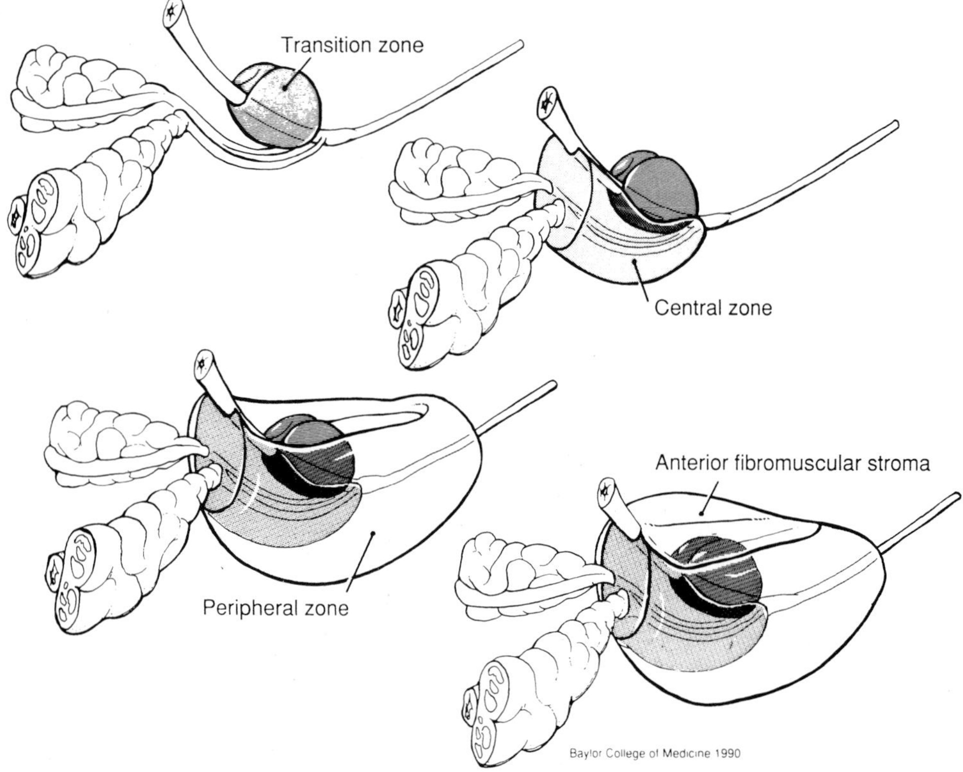

Figure 3–28. Zonal anatomy of the prostate as described by J. E. McNeal (Am J Surg Pathol 1988; 12:619–633). The transition zone surrounds the urethra proximal to the ejaculatory ducts. The central zone surrounds the ejaculatory ducts and projects under the bladder base. The peripheral zone constitutes the bulk of the apical, posterior, and lateral aspects of the prostate. The anterior fibromuscular stroma extends from the bladder neck to the striated urethral sphincter.

two lateral lobes, separated by a central sulcus that is palpable on rectal examination, and a middle lobe, which may project into the bladder in older men. These lobes do not correspond to histologically defined structures in the normal prostate but are usually related to pathologic enlargement of the transition zone laterally and the periurethral glands centrally.

Vascular Supply

Most commonly, **the arterial supply to the prostate arises from the inferior vesical artery.** As it approaches the gland, the artery (often several in number) divides into two main branches (Fig. 3–29). **The urethral arteries penetrate the prostaticovesical junction posterolaterally and travel inward, perpendicular to the urethra.** They approach the bladder neck in the 1- to 5-o'clock and 7- to 11-o'clock positions, with the largest branches located posteriorly. They then turn caudally, parallel to the urethra, to supply it, the periurethral glands, and the transition zone. Thus, **in BPH, these arteries provide the principal blood supply of the adenoma** (Flocks, 1937). **When these glands are resected or enucleated, the most significant bleeding is commonly encountered at the bladder neck, particularly at the 4- and 8-o'clock positions.**

The capsular artery is the second main branch of the prostatic artery. This artery gives off a few small branches that pass anteriorly to ramify on the prostatic capsule. **The bulk of this artery runs posterolateral to the prostate with the cavernous nerves (neurovascular bundles) and ends at the pelvic diaphragm.** The capsular branches pierce the prostate at right angles and follow the reticular bands of stroma to supply the glandular tissues. Venous drainage of the prostate is abundant through the periprostatic plexus (see Fig. 3–17).

Lymphatic drainage is primarily to the obturator and internal iliac nodes (see Fig. 3–18). A small portion of drainage may initially pass through the presacral group or, less commonly, the external iliac nodes.

Nerve Supply

Sympathetic and parasympathetic innervation from the pelvic plexus travels to the prostate through the cavernous nerves. Nerves follow the branches of capsular artery to ramify in the glandular and stromal elements. **Parasympathetic nerves end at the acini and promote secretion; sympathetic fibers cause contraction of the smooth muscle of the capsule and stroma.** Alpha$_1$-adrenergic blockade diminishes prostate stromal, capsular, and preprostatic sphincter tone and improves urinary flow rates in men affected with BPH, which emphasizes that this disease affects both stroma and epithelium. Peptidergic and NOS-containing neurons also have been found in the prostate and may affect smooth muscle relaxation (Burnett, 1995). **Afferent neurons from the prostate travel through the pelvic plexuses to pelvic and thoracolumbar spinal centers.** A prostatic block may be achieved by instilling local anesthetic into the pelvic plexuses.

Membranous Urethra

In its course from the apex of the prostate to the perineal membrane, **the membranous urethra spans on average 2.0 to 2.5 cm** (range, 1.2 to 5.0 cm) (Myers, 1991). It is surrounded by the striated (external) urethral sphincter, which is often incorrectly depicted as a flat sheet of muscle sandwiched between two layers of fascia. **The striated sphincter is actually signet ring–shaped, broad at its base and narrowing as it passes through the urogenital hiatus of the levator ani to meet the apex of the prostate** (see Figs. 3–10 and 3–23). In utero, this muscle forms a vertically oriented tube that extends from the perineal membrane to the bladder neck (Oelrich, 1980). As the prostate grows, posterior and lateral portions of this muscle atrophy, although transverse fibers persist on the entire anterior prostate through adulthood. At the apex of the prostate, circular fibers surround the urethra, and thin posteriorly to insert into a fibrous raphe. Distally, the fibers do not meet posteriorly; rather, they acquire an Ω shape as they fan out laterally over the perineal membrane. Throughout its length, the posterior portion of the striated sphincter inserts into the perineal body. In contrast to the levator ani, **the sphincter consists only of fine, type I (slow-twitch) fibers, rich in acid-stable myosin ATPase, which appear designed for tonic contraction.** The myofibrils are surrounded by abundant connective tissue that blends with adjacent supporting structures.

The striated sphincter is related anteriorly to the dorsal

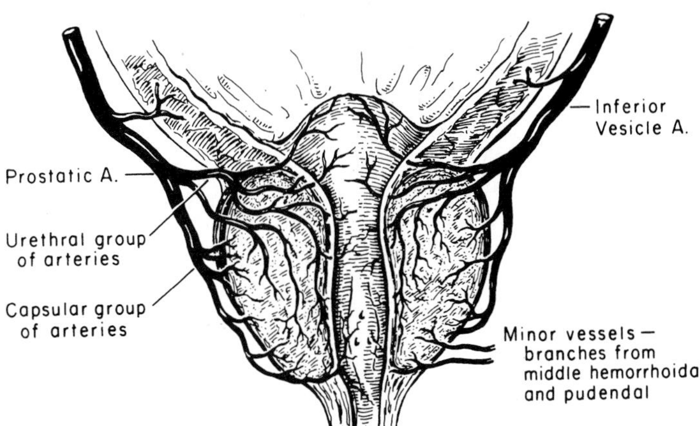

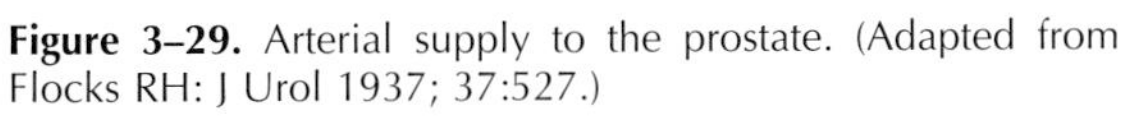
Figure 3–29. Arterial supply to the prostate. (Adapted from Flocks RH: J Urol 1937; 37:527.)

vein complex (which may invade its anterior portion with age) and laterally to levator ani. **Connective tissue from deep within the lateral and anterior walls inserts into the puboprostatic ligaments posteriorly and into the suspensory ligament of the penis anteriorly to form a sling of fibrous tissue that suspends the urethra from the pubis** (see Fig. 3–33; Steiner, 1994). Two **bulbourethral glands lie superior to the perineal membrane and are invested in the broad base of sphincter muscle** (see Fig. 3–8). During sexual excitement, these glands secrete clear mucus into the bulbous urethra.

The striated sphincter corresponds to the location of peak urethral closing pressure and is responsible for continence after prostatectomy. Components involved in generating this closing pressure are (1) the pseudostratified columnar epithelium, which contracts into radial folds as it meets to occlude the lumen; (2) the submucosa, which is rich with blood vessels and soft connective tissue and contributes to urethral sealing (Raz et al, 1972); (3) the longitudinal and circular urethral smooth muscle (intrinsic component of the external sphincter); (4) the striated sphincter; and (5) the pubourethral component of levator ani.

Gross dissection and retrograde axonal tracing techniques have confirmed that **the striated sphincter is supplied by the pudendal nerve** (Tanagho et al, 1982). However, urologists have long been puzzled as to why pudendal nerve block or sectioning does not ablate sphincter activity. Zvara and colleagues (1994) and Lawson (1974) identified **a second source of somatic innervation to the sphincter: a branch of the sacral plexus that runs on the pelvic surface of levator ani** (see Fig. 3–20). They speculated that injury to this nerve at radical prostatectomy may contribute to postoperative urinary incontinence. **Autonomic innervation to the intrinsic smooth muscle of the membranous urethra is likely given by the cavernous nerves** as they pass nearby, although dividing these nerves does not appear to affect urinary continence significantly (Steiner et al, 1991). Afferent fibers from the striated sphincter have not been defined but are sure to have interesting and important functional roles, because this muscle lacks proprioceptive muscle spindles (Gosling et al, 1981).

Vas Deferens and Seminal Vesicle

As it arises from the tail of the epididymis, the vas (ductus) deferens is somewhat tortuous for 2 to 3 cm (see Fig. 3–42). **It runs posterior to the vessels of the cord** and through the inguinal canal and emerges in the pelvis lateral to the inferior epigastric vessels (see Fig. 3–7). At the internal ring, it diverges from the testicular vessels and passes medial to all structures of the pelvic side wall to reach the base of the prostate posteriorly (see Figs. 3–7, 3–11, and 3–15). **The terminal vas is dilated and tortuous (ampulla)** and capable of storing spermatozoa. The vas has a thick wall of outer longitudinal and inner circular smooth muscle and is lined by pseudostratified columnar epithelium with nonmotile stereocilia.

The seminal vesicle is a lateral outpouching of the vas, approximately 5 cm in length, with a capacity of 3 to 4 ml (see Figs. 3–8 and 3–28). Despite its name, it does not store sperm, but it contributes the largest portion of fluid to the ejaculate. The seminal vesicle comprises a single coiled tube with several outpouchings that is lined by columnar epithelium with goblet cells. This tube is encased in a thin layer of smooth muscle and is held in its coiled configuration by a loose adventitia.

The seminal vesicle and ampulla of the vas lie posterior to the bladder. As they join to form the ejaculatory duct, their smooth muscle coats fuse with the prostatic capsule at its base. **Denonvilliers' fascia or, occasionally, the rectovesical pouch of peritoneum separates these structures from the rectum** (see Fig. 3–23). Unless involved by a pathologic process, these structures are not palpable on rectal examination.

Blood supply for both structures comes from the vesiculodeferential artery, a branch of the superior vesical artery. This artery supplies the vas throughout its length, then passes onto the anterior surface of the seminal vesicle near its tip. Additional arterial supply may come from the inferior vesical artery. The pelvic vas and seminal vesicle drain into the pelvic venous plexus. Lymphatic drainage passes to the external and internal iliac nodes (see Fig. 3–18). **Innervation arises from the pelvic plexus, with major excitatory efferents contributed by the (sympathetic) hypogastric nerves** (Kolbeck and Steers, 1993).

Female Pelvic Viscera

The uterus measures 8 × 6 × 4 cm in a normal adult woman and is composed largely of dense smooth muscle (Fig. 3–30). It **has a narrowed neck, the cervix, that opens through the anterior vaginal wall and a broad corpus that is capped by the rounded fundus.** As discussed, it lies in front of the rectum and over the dome of the bladder; its impression may be appreciated cystoscopically (Figs. 3–31 and 3–32). **The fallopian tubes extend laterally from the junction of the corpus and fundus and are draped by leaves of peritoneum called the broad ligaments** (see Figs. 3–11 and 3–30). As they extend to the pelvic side walls, the fallopian tubes angle up and backward to open posteromedially. **The tubes are divided into four segments: uterine, isthmus, ampulla, and infundibulum, which is crowned by the fimbriae. The ovary rests posterior to the elbow of the tube and is supported by its own peritoneal fold, the mesovarium.** The ureter may be found directly posterior to the ovary, covered by pelvic peritoneum. The infundibulopelvic ligament, mentioned earlier, suspends the ovary and lateral fallopian tube from the pelvic side wall and transmits the ovarian vessels to both structures. The round ligament of the ovary passes medially through the broad ligament to fix the ovary to the lateral wall of the uterus. Beneath its point of attachment, **the round ligament of the uterus passes laterally, in the leaves of the broad ligament, to exit through the inguinal canal and attach to the labial fat pad** (see Figs. 3–11 and 3–30).

The uterine artery crosses in front of the ureter and runs in the broad and cardinal ligaments to supply the proximal vagina, uterus, and medial two thirds of the fallopian tube (see Fig. 3–30). It is joined by a rich plexus of uterine veins that freely connect with the ovarian veins. Nerves from the pelvic plexus travel to the female pelvic viscera through the cardinal and uterosacral ligaments

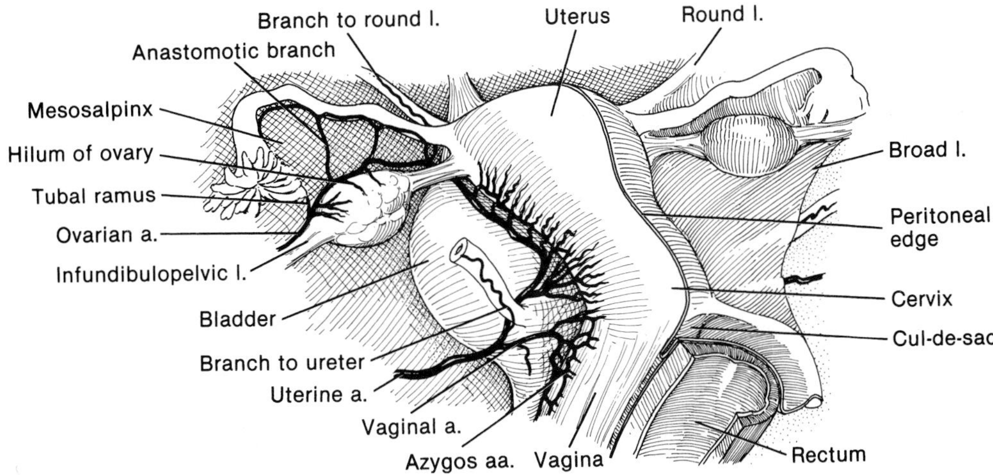

Figure 3–30. Female internal genitalia, from behind. The ureter passes beneath the uterine artery. (From Hinman F Jr: Atlas of Urosurgical Anatomy. Philadelphia, W.B. Saunders Company, 1993, p 402.)

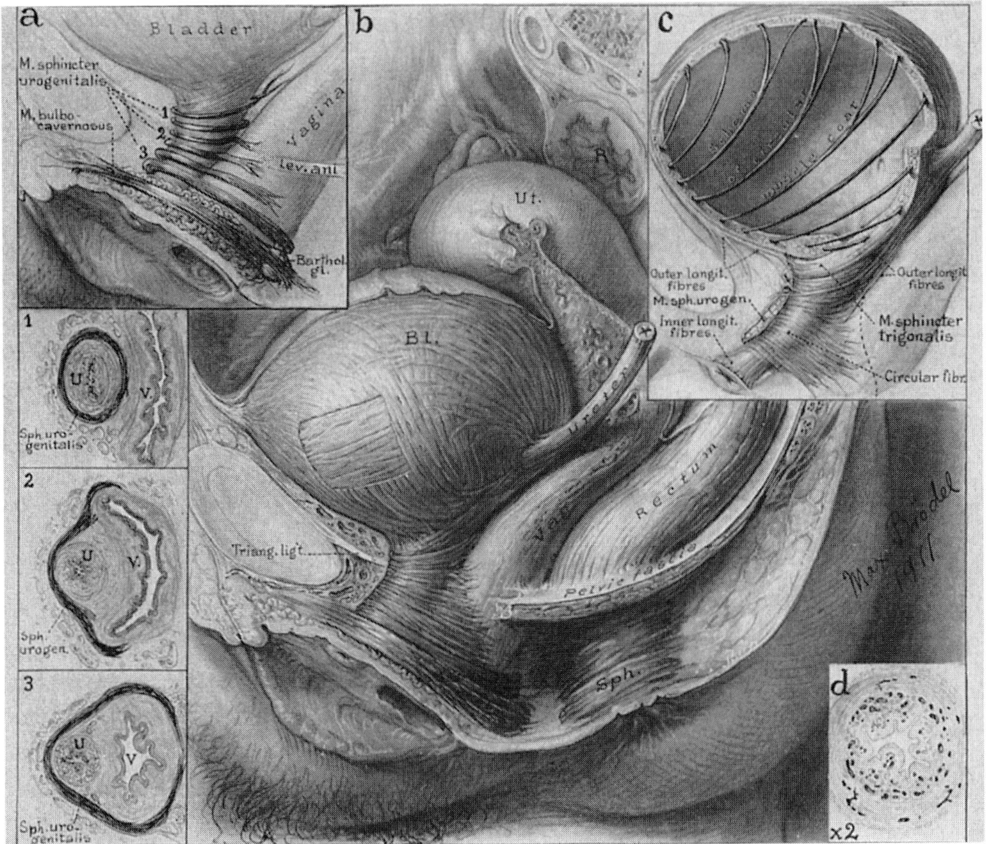

Figure 3–31. The female bladder and striated urethral sphincter. *a,* Diagram of striated urethral sphincter showing disposition of the muscle fibers. *1,* The proximal third of the sphincter encircles the urethra entirely. *2,* The middle bundles surround the urethra in front and pass off the lateral sides to blend with the vaginal wall (compressor urethrae). *3,* The distal portion surrounds the urethra and vagina together and has been called the urethrovaginal sphincter. Bulbocavernosus also acts as a sphincter around the vaginal vestibule. *b,* The urethral sphincter in its entirety. The relationship of pelvic viscera is shown. Interlacing detrusor fibers are also demonstrated. *c,* The posterolateral outer longitudinal detrusor muscle, looping anterior to the bladder neck. Inner longitudinal smooth muscle fibers run the length of the urethra, deep to the striated sphincter. *d,* Cross section of the urethra, showing thick, highly vascularized lamina propria and folded mucosa, which act as a urethral seal. Longitudinal smooth muscle surrounds lamina propria. (From the Brödel Archives, Johns Hopkins School of Medicine, Baltimore.)

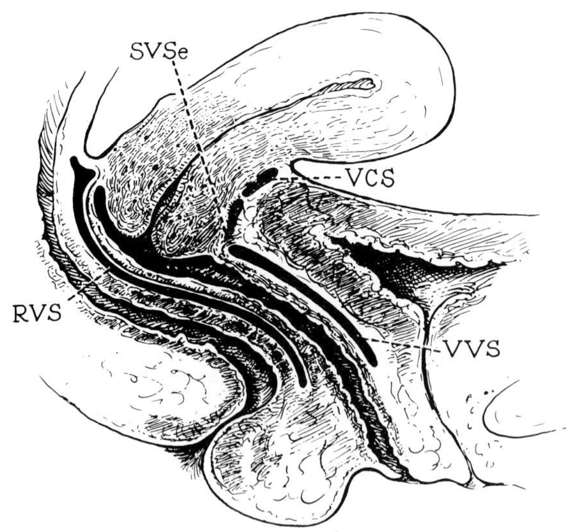

Figure 3–32. Median sagittal section of the female pelvis, showing the potential spaces between the pelvic organs. The posterior two thirds of the vagina lies nearly horizontal and rests with the uterine cervix on the rectum, which is in turn supported by the posterior portion of levator ani (the levator plate, not shown). VCS, vesicocervical space; VVS, vesicovaginal space; SVSe, supravaginal septum, the fusion between the bladder and cervix; RVS, rectovaginal space, the anterior wall is formed by the rectovaginal (Denonvilliers') fascia. (From Nichols DH, Randall CL: Vaginal Surgery, 3rd ed. Baltimore, Williams & Wilkins, 1989, p 34.)

in the company of the vessels; thus after hysterectomy, the bladder may become neurogenic.

The vagina extends inward from the vestibule at a 45° angle, then turns horizontal over the levator plate (see Fig. 3–32). It is lined by rugate nonkeratinized squamous epithelium backed by a thick, well-vascularized lamina propria. It is surrounded by a smooth muscle coat of inner circular and stronger external longitudinal layers. **In cross section, the vagina is H-shaped (Fig. 3–33) as a result of firm attachments of its anterior wall to levator ani at the arcus tendineus fasciae pelvis (see Fig. 3–13) and of its posterior wall to the rectovaginal septum.** The anterior vaginal wall is pierced by the cervix proximally. The shallow fossae around the cervix are referred to as the anterior, lateral, and posterior fornices. Because the apex of the vagina is covered with the peritoneum of the rectouterine pouch, the peritoneal cavity may be accessed through the posterior fornix (see Fig. 3–32).

Immediately in front of the cervix, the base of the bladder rests on the vaginal wall. Smooth muscle fibers tether the posterior bladder wall and base to the uterine cervix and vagina (see Fig. 3–32). Division of these fibers yields posterior access to the **vesicovaginal space**. This space extends distally to the proximal third of the urethra (where the urethra and vagina fuse) and is limited to each side by the lateral ligaments of the bladder. It may be accessed transvaginally through incision of the anterior vaginal wall in front of the cervix. **Incision of the anterior vaginal wall to either side of the urethra leads into the retropubic space** (see Fig. 3–12). The tough leaves of visceral endopelvic fascia are felt medially and should be included in all transvaginal urethral suspension procedures (Mostwin, 1991).

The vagina is separated from the rectum by the rectovaginal septum (see Fig. 3–32), and rectoceles result from a loss of integrity of this septum. Deep to this septum lies a second potential space, the **rectovaginal space**. The bowel may herniate into this space to form an enterocele. On its lateral surfaces, the vagina is related to the levator ani. Near the vestibule, fibers of levator ani blend and fuse with the vaginal muscularis. The vaginal vessels and nerves lie on the anterolateral surface of the vagina deep to the arcus tendineus fasciae pelvis.

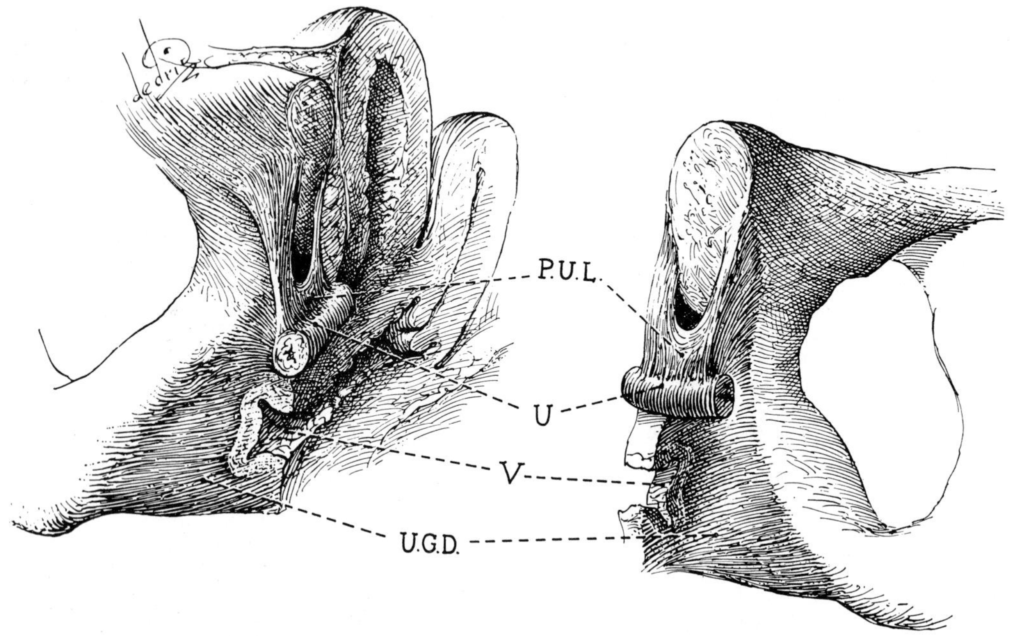

Figure 3–33. The urethral suspensory mechanism. The pubourethral ligament (PUL) is composed of an anterior portion (suspensory ligament of the clitoris), a posterior portion (pubourethral ligament of endopelvic fascia), and an intermediate portion that bridges the other two. (From Milley PS, Nichols DH: Anat Rec 1971; 170:283.)

Female Urethra

On average, the female urethra traverses 4 cm from the bladder neck to the vaginal vestibule. Its lining changes gradually from transitional to nonkeratinized stratified squamous epithelium. Many small mucous glands open into the urethra and can give rise to urethral diverticuli. Distally, these glands group together on either side of the urethra (Skene's glands) and empty through two small ducts to either side of the external urethral meatus. A thick, richly vascular submucosa supports the urethral epithelium and glands (see Fig. 3–31). **Together, the mucosa and submucosa form a cushion that contributes significantly to urethral closure pressure** (Raz et al, 1972). **These layers are estrogen dependent**; at menopause they may atrophy, resulting in stress incontinence. A relatively thick layer of inner longitudinal smooth muscle continues from the bladder to the external meatus to insert into periurethral fatty and fibrous tissue. In contrast to the male proximal urethra, no circular smooth muscle sphincter can be identified. A rather thin layer of circular smooth muscle envelops the longitudinal fibers throughout the length of the urethra.

The striated urethral sphincter invests the distal two thirds of the female urethra (Oelrich, 1983). **It is composed exclusively of delicate type I (slow-twitch) fibers** surrounded by abundant collagen. Proximally, it forms a complete ring around the urethra that corresponds to the zone of highest urethral closure pressure (see Fig. 3–31). Farther down the urethra, the fibers do not meet posteriorly but continue off the lateral sides of the urethra onto the anterior and lateral walls of the vagina. Contraction of these fibers (the compressor urethrae) closes the urethra against the fixed anterior vaginal wall. Near the vestibule, the fibers completely surround the urethra and vagina to form a urethrovaginal sphincter. Contraction of this muscle group, along with bulbospongiosus, tightens the urogenital hiatus.

The suspensory ligament of the clitoris (anterior urethral ligament) and the pubourethral ligaments (posterior urethral ligament) form a sling that suspends the urethra beneath the pubis (see Figs. 3–12 and 3–33; Zacharin, 1963). The striated urethral sphincter likely receives dual somatic innervation, like that in the male, from the pudendal and pelvic somatic nerves. Little sympathetic innervation is found in the female urethra. Parasympathetic cholinergic fibers are found throughout the smooth muscle. **It is thought that the longitudinal smooth muscle of the urethra contracts coordinately with the detrusor during micturition to shorten and widen the urethra** (Gosling, 1979).

Female Pelvic Support

The pelvic muscles and fasciae cooperate to prevent prolapse of the urogenital organs through the hiatus. **Three functional supportive elements are recognized: (1) the pubovisceral and perineal muscles, which form a sphincter around urogenital hiatus** (see Fig. 3–31); **(2) the levator plate,** which acts as a horizontal shelf beneath the bladder, uterine cervix, posterior vagina, and rectum (see Fig. 3–32); and **(3) the cardinal and uterosacral ligaments, which anchor the pelvic viscera over the levator plate** (DeLancey, 1993; Mostwin, 1991; Zacharin, 1985). The pelvic muscles contract tonically to counteract gravitational forces. In response to stress, the levator ani contracts, closing the urogenital hiatus and increasing the anterior-posterior length of the levator plate. Increased intra-abdominal pressure forces the pelvic viscera downward against a fixed levator plate, closing the vagina like a flap valve.

Pelvic and perineal muscles play the greatest role in pelvic support. Damage to the perineal body during parturition destroys the urogenital sphincter, enlarges the urogenital hiatus, and erodes the levator plate. Aging and birth trauma partially denervate and weaken the levator ani (Snooks et al, 1985). With loss of muscular support, intra-abdominal forces impinge directly on the pelvic fasciae; over time, these either tear or stretch. **Procedures to correct pelvic prolapse or urinary incontinence that rely solely on these fasciae may be successful initially but do not fare well over time** (Leach et al, 1995). Repair of a single pelvic defect—a cystocele, for instance—may unmask another (enterocele, rectocele); therefore, **successful repair of pelvic prolapse must address all components of anatomic support** (DeLancey, 1993; Zacharin, 1985).

PERINEUM

The perineum lies between the pubis, thighs, and buttocks and is limited superiorly by levator ani. Viewed from below, the symphysis pubis, ischial tuberosities, and coccyx outline the diamond shape of the perineum; the inferior ischiopubic rami and sacrotuberous ligaments form its bony and ligamentous walls (Figs. 3–34 and 3–35). A line drawn through the ischial tuberosities divides the perineum into an anal and a urogenital triangle.

Anal Triangle

At the apex of the prostate, the rectum turns approximately 90 degrees posteriorly and inferiorly to become

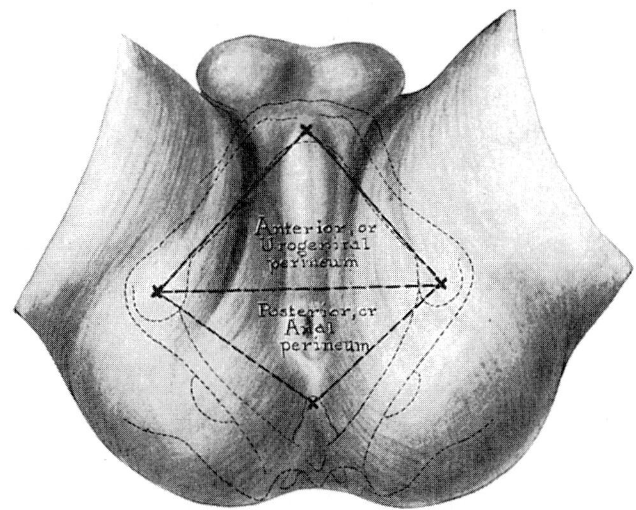

Figure 3–34. The male perineum. (From Anson BJ, McVay CB: Surgical Anatomy, 6th ed. Philadelphia, W.B. Saunders Company, 1984, p 893.)

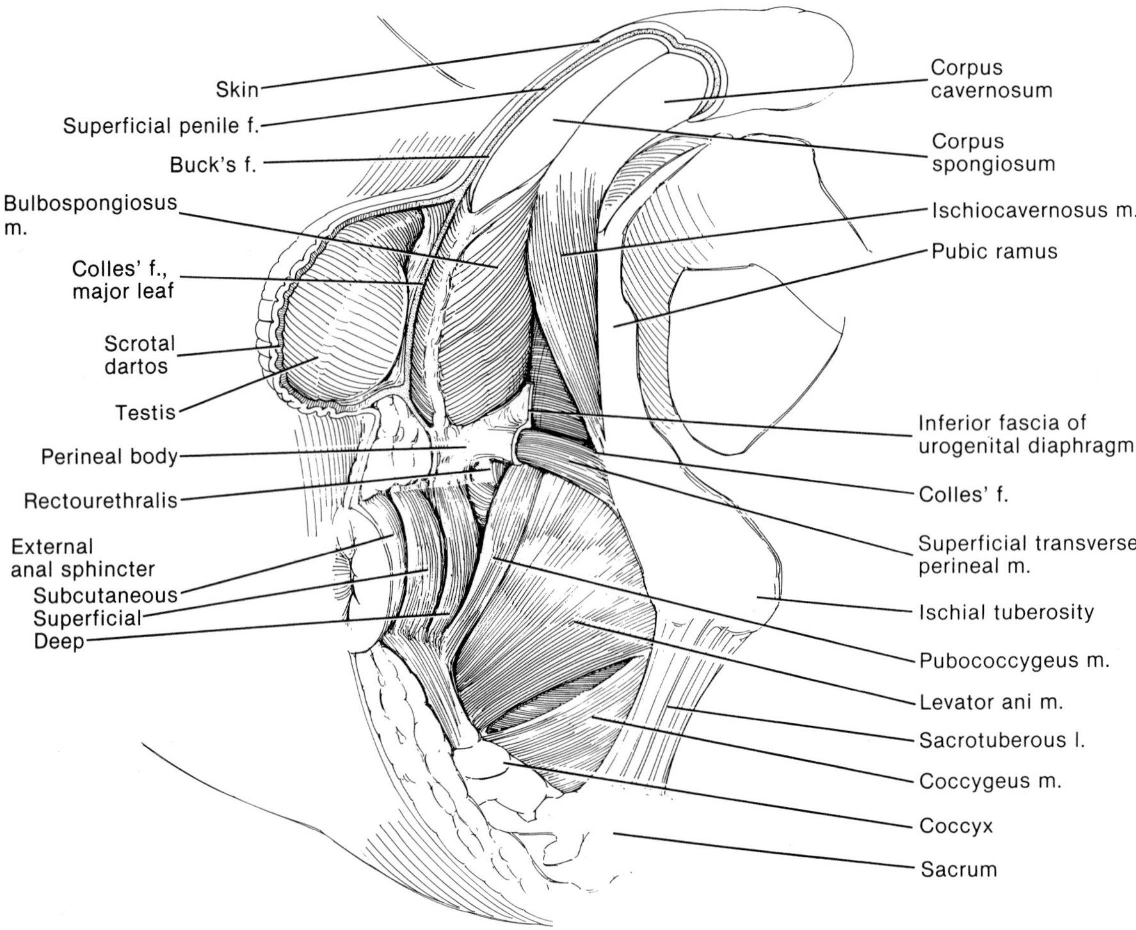

Figure 3–35. Muscles and superficial fasciae of the male perineum. (From Hinman F Jr: Atlas of Urosurgical Anatomy. Philadelphia, W.B. Saunders Company, 1993, p 219.)

the anus (see Figs. 3–23 and 3–35). It traverses 4 cm to reach the skin near the center of the anal triangle. The subcutaneous fat that surrounds the anus is continuous with that of the urogenital triangle, buttocks, and medial thigh. Laterally, the **fat fills the ischiorectal fossa, a space bounded by levator ani medially and by the obturator internus and the sacrotuberous ligament laterally (see Fig. 3–14). Anteriorly, this space extends into a recess above the urogenital diaphragm; posteriorly, it is continuous with the intermediate stratum of the pelvis through the sciatic foramina.** Through this continuity, infections may travel between the perineum and pelvic cavity.

The anal sphincter is divided into internal and external components. **The internal sphincter represents a thickening of the inner circular smooth muscle layer of the rectum.** The outer longitudinal smooth muscle thins beyond rectourethralis and blends with the external sphincter, although a few fibers insert in the skin around the anus (corrugator cutis ani) to give it a puckered appearance. **The external sphincter surrounds the internal and is divided into subcutaneous, superficial, and deep portions.** The subcutaneous part attaches to the perineal body by collagenous and muscular fibers that are thickest superficially and referred to as the central tendon of the perineum. The superficial sphincter attaches to the perineal body and coccyx. At the posterior inflection of the rectum, the deep sphincter blends with the puborectalis sling of levator ani. At this level a firm band may be felt on rectal examination and corresponds to the internal and deep external sphincter. Division of this muscular band results in fecal incontinence. The prostate may be accessed anterior to the sphincter by dividing the central tendon and sphincteric attachments to the perineum (Young's procedure) or by following the anterior rectal wall beneath the external anal sphincter (Belt's procedure).

Male Urogenital Triangle

The entire urogenital triangle is bridged by the urogenital diaphragm. The scrotum is dependent from the anterior aspect of the urogenital triangle; in the posterior aspect, skin and subcutaneous fat overlie Colles' fascia. **The perineal membrane and the posterior and lateral attachments of Colles' fascia limit a potential space known as the superficial pouch (see Figs. 3–3, 3–14, and 3–35). In this space, the three erectile bodies of the penis have their bony and fascial attachments (the root of the penis). The paired corpora cavernosa attach to the inferior ischiopubic rami and perineal membrane and are surrounded by the ischiocavernosus muscles. The corpus spongiosum dilates as the bulb of the penis and is fixed to the center of the**

perineal membrane. It is encompassed by the bulbospongiosus muscles that arise from the perineal body and from a central tendinous raphe and pass around the bulb to attach to the perineal membrane and dorsum of the penis. Contraction of the ischiocavernosus and bulbospongiosus muscles compresses the erectile bodies and potentiates penile erection. The transversus perinei muscles (superficial and deep) run along the posterior edge of the perineal membrane and are thought to stabilize the perineal body. Deep to the perineal membrane rests the striated urethral sphincter (discussed earlier).

Blood supply to the anal and urogenital triangles is derived largely from the internal pudendal vessels (Fig. 3–36). After entering the perineum through the lesser sciatic foramen, the artery runs in a fascial sheath on the medial aspect of obturator internus, the pudendal canal (of Alcock). Early in its course, it gives off three or four **inferior rectal branches** to the anus. **Its perineal branch pierces Colles' fascia to supply the muscles of the superficial pouch and continues anteriorly to supply the back of the scrotum.** The internal pudendal terminates as the common penile artery (to be discussed).

The internal pudendal veins communicate freely with the dorsal vein complex by piercing levator ani. These communicating vessels enter the pelvic venous plexus on the lateral surface of the prostate and are a common, often unexpected source of bleeding during apical dissection of the prostate. **The inferior rectal veins anastomose with the middle and superior rectal veins and produce an important connection between the portal and systemic circulation.** Obstruction of the portal or systemic venous system may cause shunting of collateral venous drainage through the portal system, manifested by hemorrhoids.

The pudendal nerve follows the vessels in their course through the perineum (see Fig. 3–36). Its first branch, the dorsal nerve of the penis, travels ventral to the main pudendal trunk in Alcock's canal. Several **inferior rectal branches** supply the external sphincter muscle and provide sensation to perianal skin. The **perineal branches** follow the perineal artery into the superficial pouch to supply the ischiocavernosus, bulbospongiosus, and transversus perinei muscles. A few branches continue anteriorly to supply sensation to the posterior scrotum. Additional perineal branches pass deep to the perineal membrane to supply the levator ani and striated urethral sphincter.

Penis

As discussed, the root of the penis is fixed to the perineum within the superficial pouch. **The corpora cavernosa join beneath the pubis (penile hilum) to form the major portion of the body of the penis.** They are separated by a septum that becomes pectiniform distally, so that their vascular spaces freely communicate. **They are enclosed by the tough tunica albuginea, which is predominantly collagenous** (Fig. 3–37). Its outer longitudinal and inner circular fibers form an undulating meshwork when the penis is flaccid and appear tightly stretched with erection (Goldstein et al, 1982). **Smooth muscle bundles traverse the erectile**

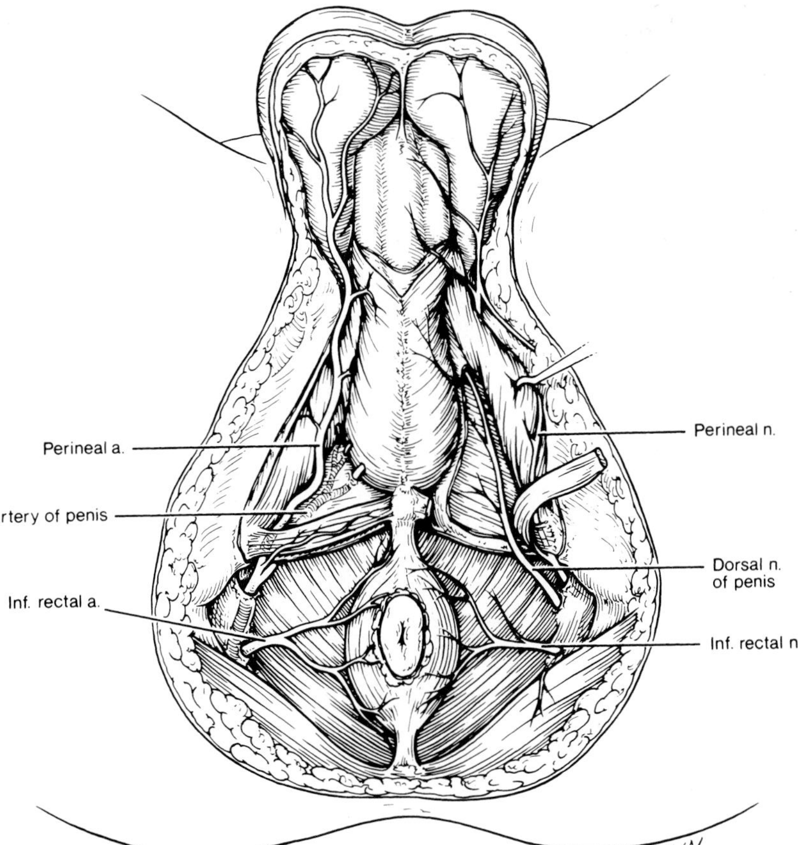

Figure 3–36. The male perineum, illustrating the internal pudendal artery and its branches on the left and the pudendal nerve and its branches on the right.

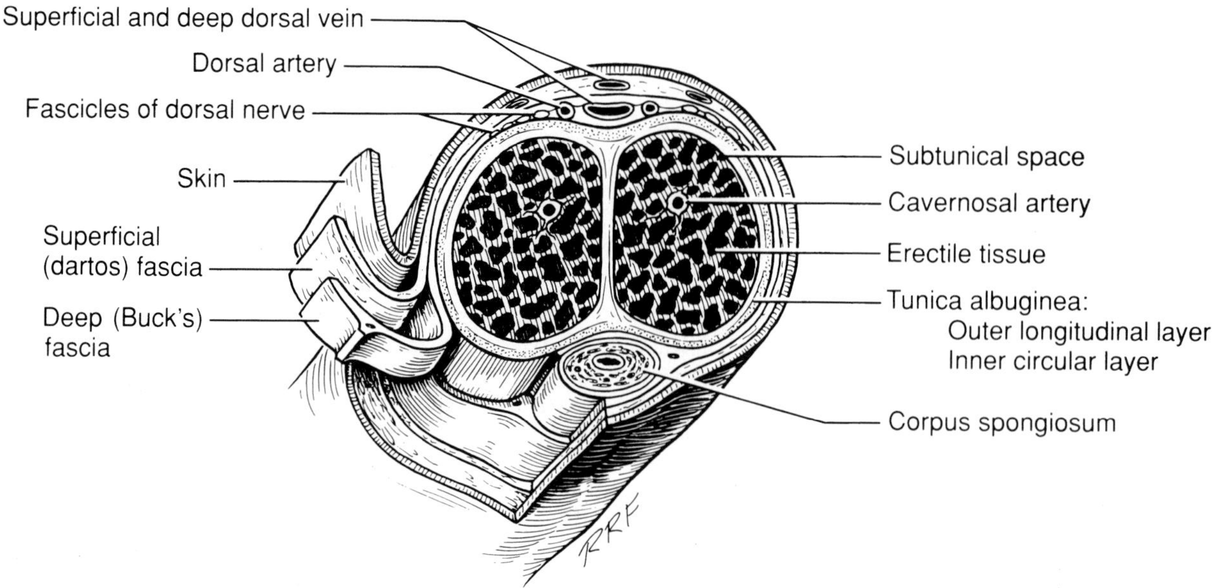

Figure 3–37. Cross section of the penis, demonstrating the relationship between the corporal bodies, penile fascia, vessels, and nerves. (From Devine CJ Jr, Angermeier KW: AUA Update Series, 1994; 13[2]:10.)

bodies to form the endothelium-lined cavernous sinuses. These sinuses give the erectile tissue a spongy appearance on gross examination.

Distal to the bulb, the corpus spongiosum tapers and runs on the underside (ventrum) of the corpora cavernosa, then expands to cap them as the glans penis. The corona separates the base of the glans from the shaft of the penis. The spongiosum is traversed throughout its length by the anterior urethra, which begins at the perineal membrane (see Fig. 3–27). **The anterior urethra is dilated in its bulbar and glanular segments (fossa navicularis) and narrowest at the external meatus.** Proximally, it is lined by stratified and pseudostratified columnar epithelium, distally by stratified squamous. The mucus-secreting glands (of Littre) may be seen as small outpouchings of the mucosa.

Buck's fascia surrounds both cavernosal bodies dorsally and splits to surround the spongiosum ventrally (see Fig. 3–37). Elastic and collagenous fibers from the rectus sheath blend with and surround Buck's fascia as the fundiform ligament of the penis. Deeper fibers from the pubis form the suspensory ligament of the penis. In the perineum, Buck's fascia fuses with the tunica albuginea deep to the muscles of the erectile bodies (Uhlenhuth et al, 1949). Distally, it fuses with the base of the glans at the corona. Bleeding from a tear in the corporal bodies (e.g., penile fracture) is usually contained within Buck's fascia, and ecchymosis is limited to the penile shaft.

The skin of the penile shaft is highly elastic and without appendages (hair or glandular elements), except for the smegma-producing glands at the base of the corona. It is devoid of fat and quite mobile because of the loose attachment of its dartos backing to Buck's fascia. Distally, it folds over the glans as the foreskin and attaches firmly below the corona. **Its blood supply is independent of the erectile bodies and is derived from the external pudendal branches of the femoral vessels** (see Fig. 3–4). These vessels enter the base of the penis to run longitudinally in the dartos fascia as a richly anastomotic network. Thus penile skin may be mobilized on a vascular pedicle as the ideal tissue for urethral reconstruction. The skin of the glans is nonmobile as a result of its direct attachment to the underlying, thin tunica albuginea.

The common penile artery continues in Alcock's canal, above the perineal membrane, and terminates in three branches that supply the erectile bodies (Fig. 3–38). The **bulbourethral artery** penetrates the perineal membrane to enter the spongiosum from above at its posterolateral border. This large, short artery can be difficult to isolate and control during urethrectomy. It supplies the urethra, spongiosum, and glans. The **cavernosal artery** pierces the corporal body in the penile hilum to run near the center of its erectile tissue. It gives off straight and helicine arteries that ramify to supply the cavernous sinuses. The **dorsal artery of the penis** passes between the crus penis and pubis to reach the dorsal surface of the corporal bodies. **It runs between the dorsal vein and dorsal penile nerve and, with them, attaches to the underside of Buck's fascia (see Fig. 3–40).** As it courses to the glans, it gives off cavernous branches and circumferential branches to the spongiosum and urethra. **The rich blood supply to the spongiosum allows safe division of the urethra during stricture repair** (Devine and Angermeier, 1994).

The surgeon contemplating penile revascularization must be aware that **the penile arteries are highly variable in their branching, courses, and anastomoses** (Bare et al, 1994). It is not uncommon for a single cavernosal artery to supply both corporal bodies or to be absent altogether. Alternatively, an **accessory pudendal artery** may supplement or completely replace branches of the common penile artery (Fig. 3–39). This artery usually arises from the obturator or inferior vesical arteries and runs anterolateral to or within the prostate to reach the penis in the company of the dorsal vein. It has been identified in 7 of 10 cadaveric specimens (Breza et al, 1989) and noted at 4% of radical prostatectomies (Polascik and Walsh, 1995); its resection at prostatectomy may adversely affect postoperative potency.

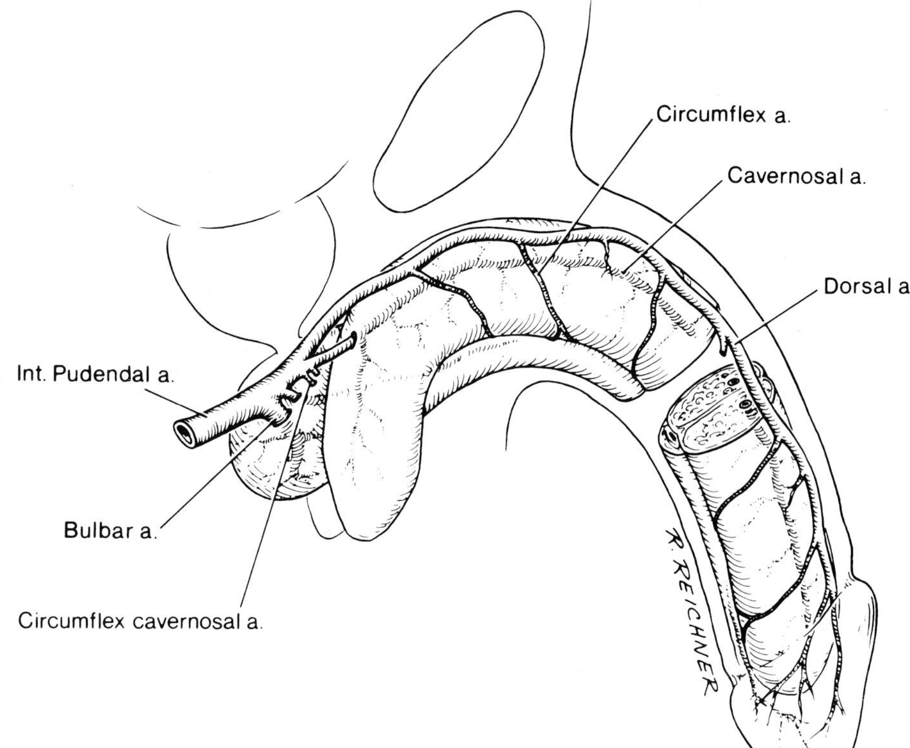

Figure 3–38. Arterial supply of the penis.

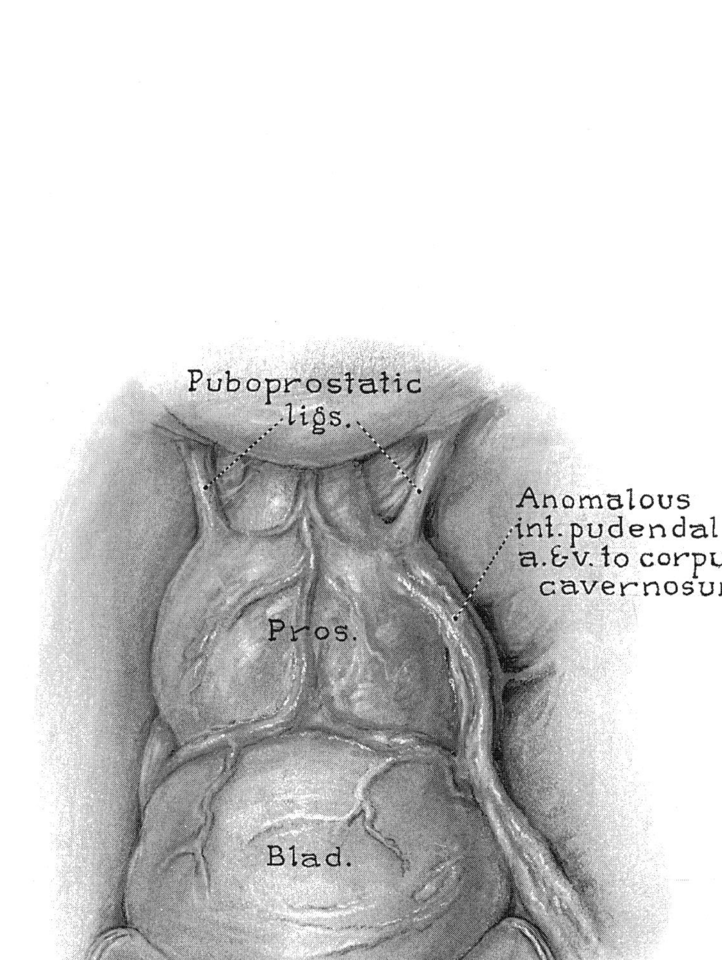

Figure 3–39. Accessory internal pudendal arteries, as seen in the retropubic space. (From Polascik TJ, Walsh PC: J Urol 1995; 153:151.)

At the base of the glans, several venous channels coalesce to form the dorsal vein of the penis, which runs in a groove between the cavernosal bodies and drains into the preprostatic plexus (Fig. 3–40). The **circumflex veins** originate in the spongiosum and pass around the cavernosa to meet the deep dorsal vein perpendicularly. The are present only in the distal two thirds of the penile shaft and are 3 to 10 in number. Intermediary venules form from the cavernous sinuses and drain into subtunical capillary plexuses. These plexuses give rise to **emissary veins**, which commonly follow an oblique path between the layers of the tunica and drain into the circumflex veins dorsolaterally. Emissary veins in the proximal third of the penis join on the dorsomedial surface of the cavernous bodies to form two to five **cavernous veins**. At the hilum of the penis, these vessels pass between the crura and the bulb, receiving branches from each, and join the internal pudendal veins. Valves are found in the emissary, cavernosal, and deep dorsal veins and may thwart attempts to revascularize the penis by arteriovenous anastomosis (Sohn, 1994).

The dorsal nerves provide sensation to the penis. These nerves follow the course of the dorsal arteries and richly supply the glans (see Fig. 3–40). The route of the **cavernous nerves** has been described. After piercing the corporal bodies, they **ramify in the erectile tissue to supply sympathetic and parasympathetic** innervation from the pelvic plexuses. Tonic sympathetic tone inhibits erection. Parasympathetic nerves release acetylcholine, nitric oxide, and vasoactive intestinal polypeptide, which cause the cavernosal smooth muscle and arterial relaxation necessary for erection (Burnett, 1995). It is thought that during erection, the subtunical venules are occluded by being compressed against the nondistensible tunica albuginea. Insufficient venous occlusion, particularly in vessels draining into the deep dorsal and cavernosal veins, is thought to be a cause of vasculogenic impotence.

Scrotum

The scrotal skin is pigmented, hair-bearing, devoid of fat, and rich in sebaceous and sweat glands. It varies from loose and shiny to highly folded with transverse **rugae** depending in the tone of its underlying smooth muscle. A midline raphe runs from the urethral meatus to the anus and represents the line of fusion of the genital tubercles. Deep to this raphe, the scrotum is separated into two compartments by a septum. **The dartos layer of smooth muscle is continuous with Colles', Scarpa's, and the dartos fasciae of the penis** (see Figs. 3–3 and 3–35). The testes are suspended by their cords in the scrotal compartments. **As the testes descend, they acquire coverings from the layers of the abdominal wall, known as the spermatic fasciae**, that form part of the scrotal wall (Fig. 3–41). The **external spermatic fascia** derives from the external oblique fascia and remains firmly attached to the borders of the external ring. The **cremasteric muscle and fascia** arise from the internal oblique muscle and attach laterally to the inguinal ligament and iliopsoas fascia and medially to the pubic tubercle. The **internal spermatic fascia** is a continuation of the transversalis fascia. The **parietal and visceral tunica vaginalis** surround the testis with a mesothelium-lined pouch and are derived from the peritoneum. They are continuous at the posterolateral border of the testis at its mesentery, where it is fixed to the scrotal wall. The testis is also fixed at its lower pole by the gubernaculum. Occasionally, the mesentery and gubernaculum may be deficient, leaving the testis unfixed (bell-clapper deformity) and predisposing to torsion of the cord.

The anterior wall of the scrotum is supplied by the external pudendal vessels and the ilioinguinal and genitofemoral nerves (see Fig. 3–4). The anterior vessels and nerves typically run parallel to the rugae and do not cross the raphe; thus transverse or midline raphe scrotal incisions are most appropriate. The back of the scrotum is supplied by the posterior scrotal branches of the perineal vessels and nerves (see Fig. 3–36). In addition, the posterior femoral cutaneous nerve (S3) gives a perineal branch to supply the scrotum and perineum (see Fig. 3–8). **In accordance with their origin, the spermatic fasciae have a blood supply (cremasteric, vasal, testicular) separate from that of the scrotal wall.** Fournier's gangrene usually does not involve these structures, and they may be spared during débridement.

Perineal Lymphatics

The penis, scrotum, and perineum drain into the inguinal lymph nodes (see Fig. 3–18). These nodes may be

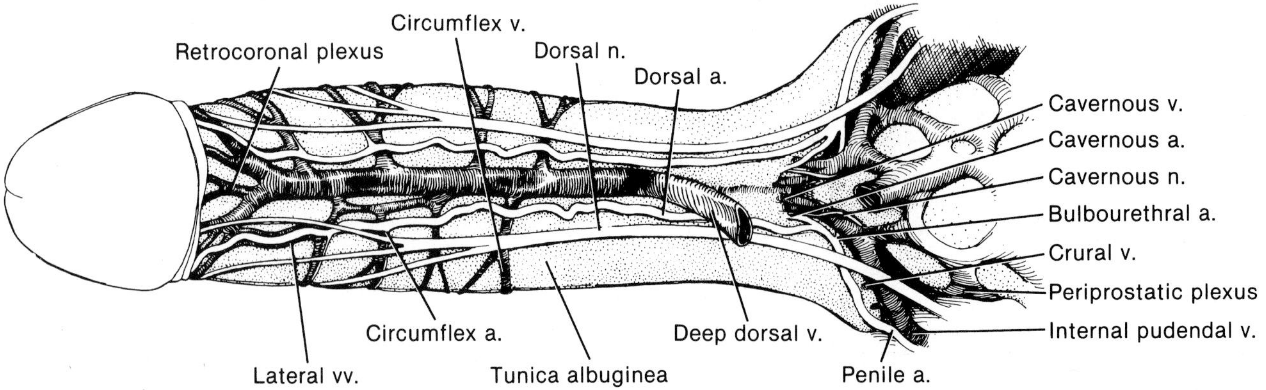

Figure 3–40. Dorsal penile arteries, veins, and nerves. (From Hinman F Jr: Atlas of Urosurgical Anatomy. Philadelphia, W.B. Saunders Company, 1993, p 445.)

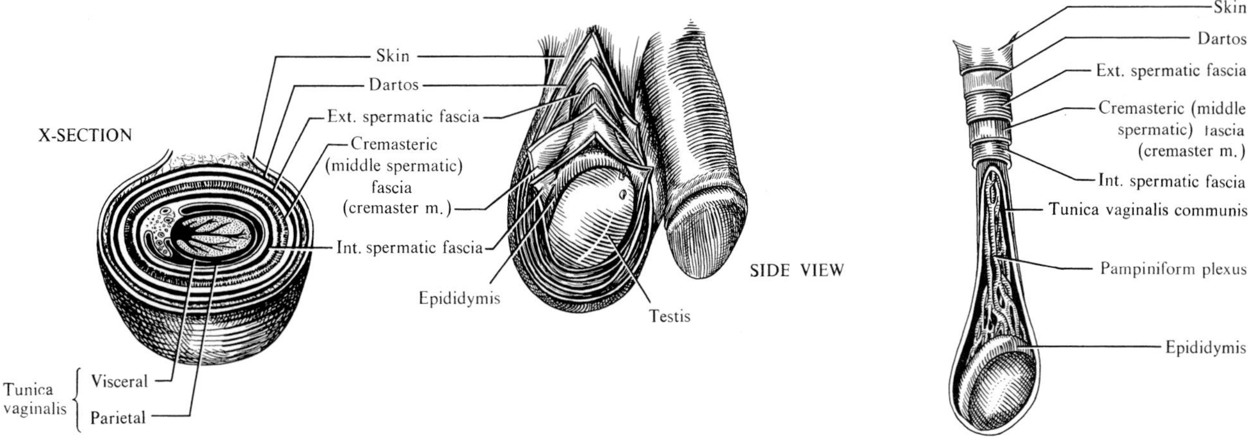

Figure 3–41. The scrotum and its layers. (From Pansky B: Review of Gross Anatomy, 6th ed. New York, McGraw-Hill, 1997, p 483.)

divided into superficial and deep groups, which are separated by the deep fascia of the thigh (fascia lata). The superficial nodes lie in relation with the external pudendal, superficial inferior epigastric, and superficial circumflex iliac vessels at the saphenofemoral junction. At the saphenous opening (fossa ovalis) in the fascia lata, the greater saphenous joins the femoral vein, and the superficial nodes communicate with the deep group. Most of the deep inguinal nodes lie medial to the femoral vein and send their efferents through the femoral ring (beneath the inguinal ligament) to the external iliac and obturator nodes. Just outside the femoral ring, a large node (Cloquet's or Rosenmüller's node) is consistently present.

The scrotal lymphatics do not cross the median raphe and drain into the ipsilateral superficial inguinal lymph nodes. **Lymphatics from the shaft of the penis converge on the dorsum, then ramify to both sides of the groin. Those of the glans pass deep to Buck's fascia dorsally and drain to superficial and deep groups in both sides of the groin.** Direct lymphatic channels from the glans to the pelvic nodes, which bypass the inguinal nodes, have been proposed by anatomists; however, clinical studies have not confirmed their existence. Other studies have suggested that all penile lymphatic drainage passes through "sentinel nodes," which lie medial to the superficial inferior epigastric veins. Clinical studies have also called this speculation into question (Catalona, 1988). The perineal skin and fasciae drain into superficial nodes; the structures of the superficial pouch likely drain into the superficial and deep groups.

Testes

The testes are 4 to 5 cm in length, 3 cm in width, and 2.5 cm in depth and have a volume of 30 ml. **They are enclosed in a tough capsule composed of (1) the visceral tunica vaginalis; (2) tunica albuginea, with collagenous and smooth muscle elements; and (3) the tunica vasculosa.** The epididymis attaches to the posterolateral aspect of the testis. Beneath it, the tunica albuginea projects inward to form the **mediastinum testis**, the point where vessels and ducts traverse the testicular capsule (Fig. 3–42). Septa radiate from the mediastinum and attach to the inner surface of the tunica albuginea to form **200 to 300 cone-shaped lobules, which each contain one or more convoluted seminiferous tubules**. Each tubule is U-shaped and has a stretched length of nearly 1 m. Interstitial (Leydig) cells lie in the loose tissue surrounding the tubules and are responsible for testosterone production. Toward the apices of the lobules, the seminiferous tubules become straight (tubuli recti) and enter the mediastinum testis to form an anastomosing network of tubules lined by flattened epithelium. This network, known as **the rete testis, forms 12 to 20 efferent ductules that pierce the upper pole of the testis and pass into the largest portion of epididymis, the caput.** Here the efferent ductules enlarge, become more convoluted, and form conical lobules. The duct from each lobule drains into a single epididymal duct, which winds approximately 6 m within the fibrous sheath of the epididymis to form its **body** and **tail**. As the duct approaches the tail, it thickens and straightens to become the vas deferens.

The spermatic cord is composed of the vas deferens, testicular vessels, and spermatic fasciae. As discussed in the previous chapter, the testicular arteries arise from the aorta and travel in the intermediate stratum of the retroperitoneum to reach the internal inguinal ring. **Lateral to the internal ring, the attachments of the intermediate stratum form the lateral spermatic fascia**. These attachments may be taken down at orchidopexy to gain cord length. At the internal ring, the vessels are joined by the genital branch of the genitofemoral nerve, the ilioinguinal nerve, the cremasteric artery, and the vas deferens and its artery. **In its course to the testis, the testicular artery branches** into an internal artery and an inferior testicular artery and into a capital artery to the head of the epididymis (Fig. 3–43). **The level of this branching varies and has been noted to occur within the inguinal canal in 31% to 88% of cases** (Jarow et al, 1992; Beck et al, 1992). When performing an inguinal varicocelectomy, the surgeon must remember that there may be two or three arterial branches at this level. **A rich arterial anastomosis occurs at the head of the epididymis, between the testicular and capital arteries, and at the tail, between the testicular, epididymal, cremasteric, and vasal arteries** (see Fig. 3–43). **The testicular arteries enter the mediastinum and ramify in the tunica vasculosa, principally in the anterior, medial, and lateral portions of the**

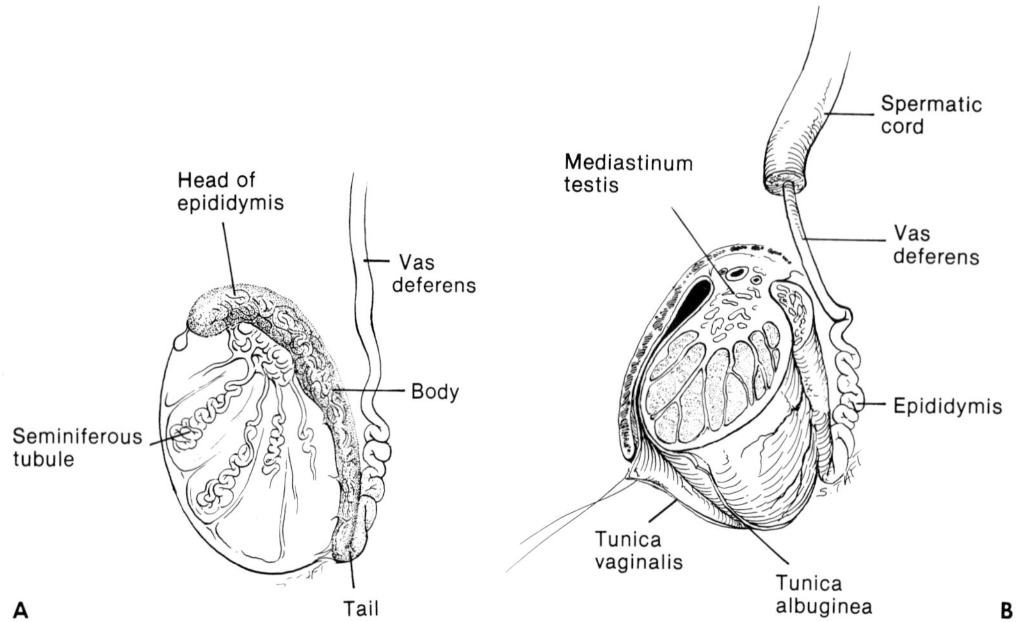

Figure 3–42. The testis and epididymis. *A,* One to three seminiferous tubules fill each compartment and drain into rete testis in the mediastinum. Twelve to 20 efferent ductules become convoluted in the head of the epididymis and drain into a single coiled duct of the epididymis. The vas is convoluted in its first portion. *B,* Cross section of the testis, showing the mediastinum and septations continuous with the tunica albuginea. The parietal and visceral tunica vaginalis are confluent where the vessels and nerves enter the posterior aspect of the testis.

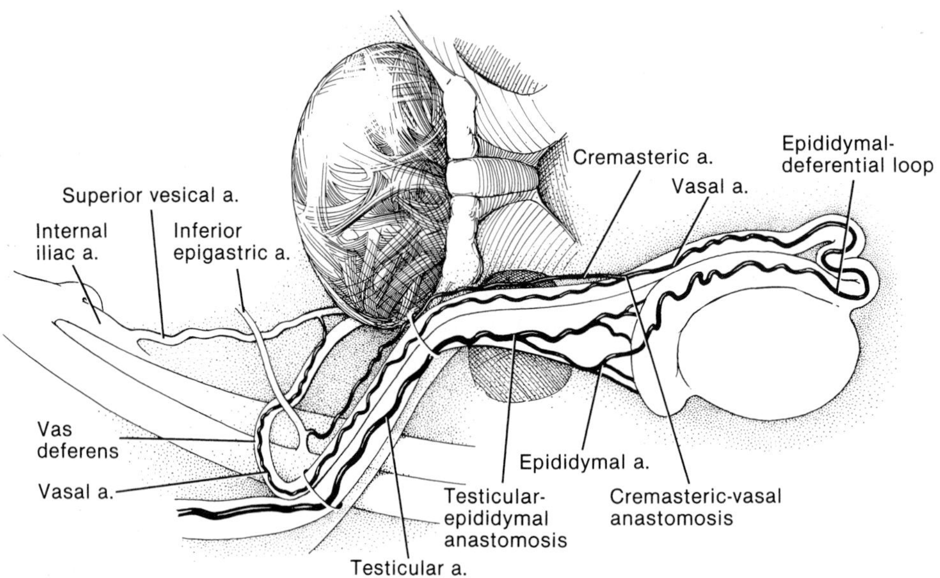

Figure 3–43. Collateral arterial circulation of the testis. (From Hinman F Jr: Atlas of Urosurgical Anatomy. Philadelphia, W.B. Saunders Company, 1993, p 497.)

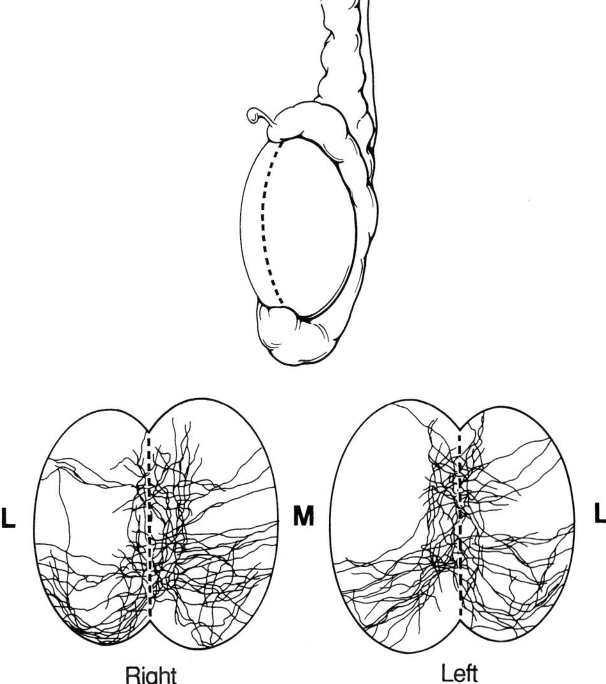

Figure 3–44. Distribution of subtunical testicular arteries compiled from 27 right and 26 left vascular casts. The highest density of subtunical arteries is found at the anterior upper pole and entire lower pole. Lateral and medial sides of the upper pole are relatively free of arterial branches. (From Jarow JP: J Urol 1991; 145:777.)

lower pole and the anterior segment of the upper pole (Fig. 3–44). Thus placement of a traction suture through the lower pole tunica albuginea risks damaging these important superficial vessels and devascularizing the testis (Jarow, 1991). Testicular biopsy should be carried out on the medial or lateral surface of the upper pole, where the risk of vascular injury is minimal.

The testicular veins form several highly anastomotic channels that surround the testicular artery as the pampiniform plexus. This arrangement allows for countercurrent heat exchange, which cools the blood in the testicular artery. At the level of the inguinal canal, the veins join to form two or three channels and then a single vein that drains into the inferior vena cava on the right and the renal vein on the left. **The testicular veins may anastomose with the external pudendal, cremasteric, and vasal veins** (Fig. 3–45). These connections can allow varicoceles to recur after ablative procedures. Testicular lymphatic vessels drain to the para-aortic and interaortocaval nodes as detailed in the previous chapter.

Visceral innervation of the testis and epididymis travels by two routes. A portion arises in the renal and aortic plexuses and travels with the gonadal vessels. Rauchenwald and associates demonstrated that **a major part of gonadal afferent and efferent vessels courses from the pelvic plexus in association with the vas deferens** (Rauchenwald et al, 1995). On the basis of these findings, they successfully treated orchialgia by bupivacaine injection into the pelvic plexus (Zorn et al, 1994). Intriguingly, some afferent and efferent fibers cross over to the contralateral pelvic plexus. This neural cross-communication may explain how pathologic processes in one testis (e.g., tumor or varico-

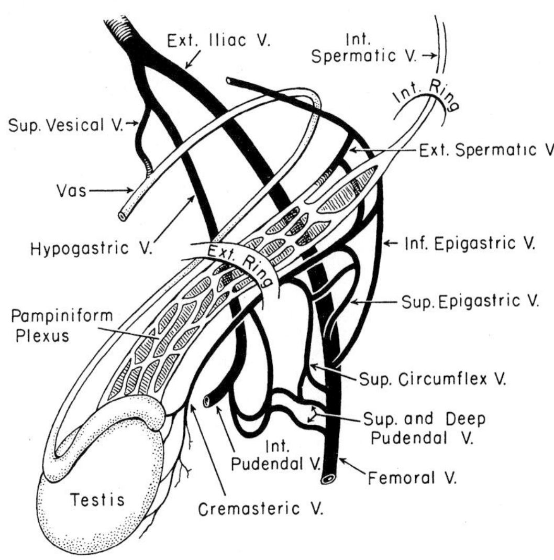

Figure 3–45. Venous drainage of the testis and epididymis. Note connections between the pampiniform plexus and the saphenous, internal iliac, and external iliac veins.

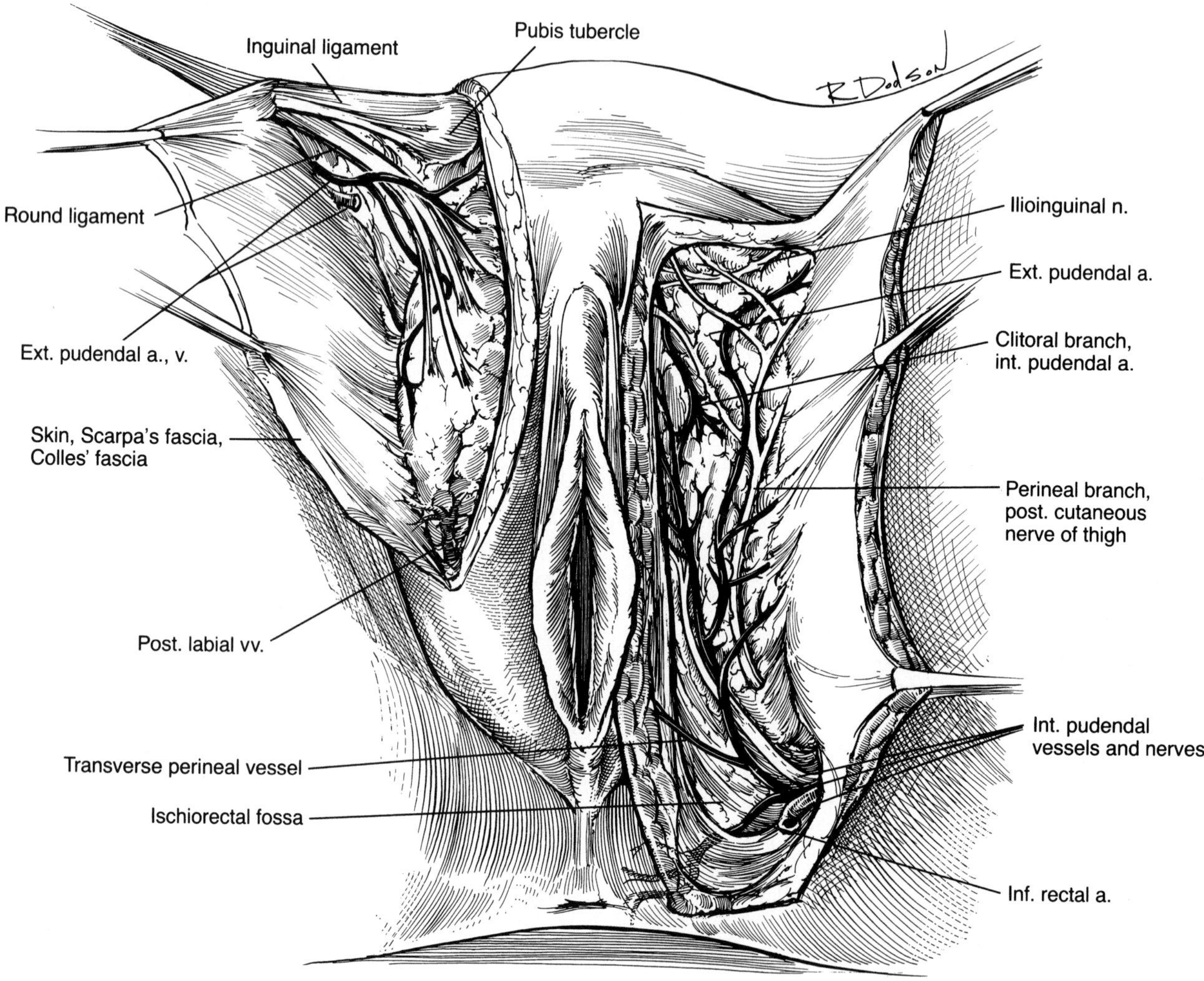

Figure 3–46. Arteries and nerves of the female perineum. (From Doherty MG: Clinical anatomy of the pelvis. *In* Copeland LJ, ed: Textbook of Gynecology. Philadelphia, W.B. Saunders Company, 1993, p 51.)

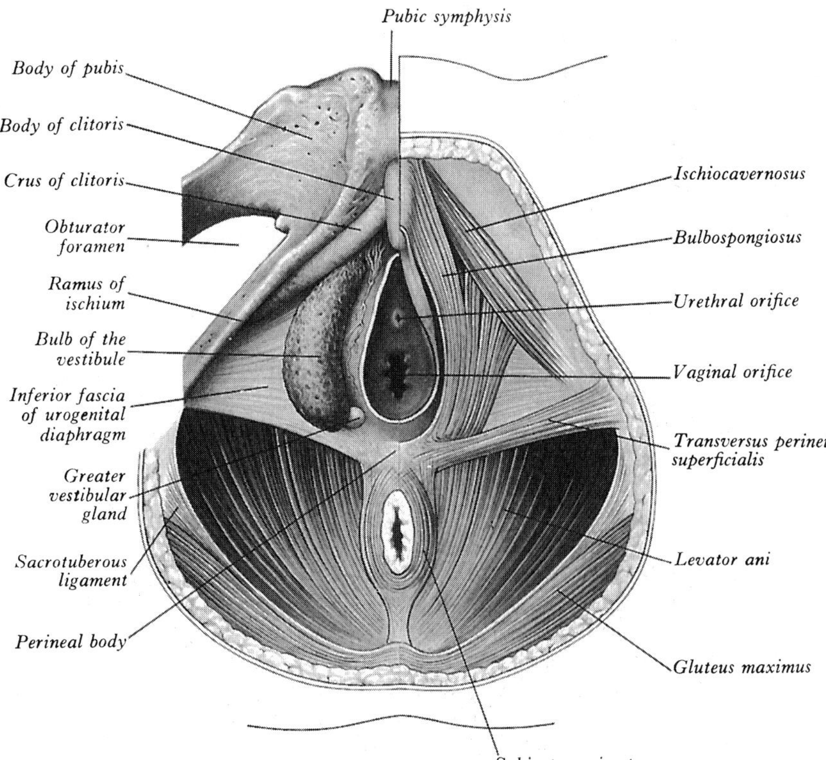

Figure 3–47. The female superficial perineal pouch. On the left side, the muscles have been removed to show the vestibular bulb and Bartholin's gland. (From Williams PL, Warwick R: Gray's Anatomy, 35th British ed. Philadelphia, W.B. Saunders Company, 1973, p 1364.)

cele) may affect the function of the contralateral testis. The genital branch of the genitofemoral nerve supplies sensation to the parietal and visceral tunica vaginalis and the overlying scrotum.

Female Urogenital Triangle

The vestibule of the vagina runs vertically throughout the length of the urogenital triangle. The labia minora form its lateral sides and fuse anteriorly as the hood of the clitoris. The subcutaneous fat pad of the mons pubis continues posteriorly in the labia majora to frame the vestibule. **The labial fat pads receive blood supply from the external pudendal vessels and may be raised on these vessels as a rotational flap for repair of vesicovaginal or urethrovaginal fistulas** (Fig. 3–46). The urethra enters the vestibule between the clitoris and vagina.

The structure of the superficial pouch is similar to that of the male (Fig. 3–47). The crura of the clitoris attach to the inferior ischiopubic rami, surrounded by the ischiocavernosus muscles, and converge to form the body of the clitoris. The vestibular bulbs lie to either side of the vaginal vestibule, covered by the bulbospongiosus muscles. As homologues of the penile bulb, they are composed of erectile tissue and meet anteriorly to form the glans of the clitoris. **The vestibular glands are deep to the vestibular bulbs but, unlike the bulbourethral glands in the male, are superficial to the perineal membrane.** Their ducts travel 2 cm to open in the vaginal vestibule on the posteromedial sides of the labia minora. The perineal membrane, pierced in its center by the vagina, is less developed than that of the male. The innervation, blood supply, and lymphatic drainage of the external genitalia and superficial pouch are similar to those described in the male.

REFERENCES

Bare RL, DeFranzo A, Jarow JP: Intraoperative arteriography facilitates penile revascularization. J Urol 1994; 151:1019–1021.

Batson OV: The function of the vertebral veins and their role in the spread of metastases. Ann Surg 1940; 112:138–149.

Beck EM, Schlegel PN, Goldstein M: Intraoperative varicocele anatomy: A macroscopic and microscopic study. J Urol 1992; 148:1190–1194.

Begg RC: The urachus: Its anatomy, histology and development. J Anat 1930; 64:170–183.

Breza J, Aboseif SR, Orvis BR, et al: Detailed anatomy of penile neurovascular structures: Surgical significance. J Urol 1989; 141:437–443

Burnett AL: Nitric oxide control of lower genitourinary tract functions: A review. Urology 1995; 45:1071–1083.

Catalona WJ: Modified inguinal lymphadenectomy for carcinoma of the penis with preservation of the saphenous veins: Technique and preliminary results. J Urol 1988; 140:306–310.

Daly JW, Higgins KA: Injury to the ureter during gynecologic surgical procedures. Surg Gynecol Obstet 1988; 167:19–22.

DeLancey JOL: The pubovesical ligament: A separate structure from the urethral supports ("pubo-urethral ligaments"). Neurourol Urodyn 1989; 8:53–62.

DeLancey JOL: Anatomy and biomechanics of genital prolapse. Clin Obstet Gynecol 1993; 36(4):897–909.

DeLancey JOL: Structural support of the urethra as it relates to stress urinary incontinence: The hammock hypothesis. Am J Obstet Gynecol 1994; 170:1713–1723.

Devine CJ Jr, Angermeier KW: Anatomy of the penis and male perineum. AUA Update Series 1994; 13(2, 3):10–23.

Epstein JI: The prostate and seminal vesicles. *In* Sternberg SS, ed: Diagnostic Surgical Pathology, 1st ed. New York, Raven Press, 1989, pp 1393–1432.

Flocks RH: The arterial distribution within the prostate gland: Its role in transurethral prostatic resection. J Urol 1937; 37:524–548.

Goldstein AMB, Meehan JP, Zakhary R, et al: New observations on microarchitecture of corpora cavernosa in man and possible relationship to mechanism of erection. Urology 1982; 20:259–266.

Golimbu M, Al-Askari S, Morales P: Transpubic approach for lower urinary tract surgery: A 15 year experience. J Urol 1990; 143:72–76.

Gosling JA: The structure of the bladder and urethra in relation to function. Urol Clin North Am 1979; 6:31–38.

Gosling JA: The structure of the female lower urinary tract and pelvic floor. Urol Clin North Am 1985; 12:207–214.

Gosling JA, Dixon JS, Critchley HOD, Thompson SA: A comparative study of human external sphincter and periurethral levator ani muscles. Br J Urol 1981; 53:35–41.

Hinman F Jr: Atlas of Urosurgical Anatomy. Philadelphia, W.B. Saunders Company, 1993.

Hutch JA, Ayers RD, Loquvam GS: The bladder musculature with special reference to the ureterovesical junction. J Urol 1961; 85:531–539.

Jarow JP: Clinical significance of intratesticular arterial anatomy. J Urol 1991; 145:777–779.

Jarow JP, Ogle A, Kaspar J, Hopkins M: Testicular artery ramification within the inguinal canal. J Urol 1992; 147:1290–1292.

Kolbeck SC, Steers WD: Origin of neurons supplying the vas deferens of the rat. J Urol 1993; 149:918–921.

Lawson JON: Pelvic anatomy: Pelvic floor muscles. Ann R Coll Surg Engl 1974; 54:244–252.

Leach GE, Trockman BA, Sakamoto M, et al: Modified Pereyra bladder neck suspension: Minimum 5 year follow up in 101 patients [Abstract 813]. J Urol 1995; 153(Suppl):432A.

Lepor H, Gregerman M, Crosby R, et al: Precise localization of the autonomic nerves from the pelvic plexus to the corpora cavernosa: A detailed anatomical study of the adult male pelvis. J Urol 1985; 133:207–212.

Lue TF, Zeineh SJ, Schmidt RA, Tanagho EA: Neuroanatomy of penile erection: Its relevance to iatrogenic impotence. J Urol 1984; 131:273–280.

McNeal JE: The prostate and prostatic urethra: A morphologic synthesis. J Urol 1972; 107:1008–1016.

McNeal JE: Normal histology of the prostate. Am J Surg Pathol 1988; 12(8):619–633.

Mostwin JL: Current concepts of female pelvic anatomy and physiology. Urol Clin North Am 1991; 18:175–195.

Myers RP: Male urethral sphincteric anatomy and radical prostatectomy. Urol Clin North Am 1991; 18:211–227.

Myers RP: Radical prostatectomy: Pertinent surgical anatomy. Atlas Urol Clin North Am 1994; 2:1–18.

Oelrich TM: The urethral sphincter in the male. Am J Anat 1980; 158:229–246.

Oelrich TM: The striated urogenital sphincter muscle in the female. Anat Rec 1983; 205:223–232.

Polascik TJ, Walsh PC: Radical retropubic prostatectomy: The influence of accessory pudendal arteries on the recovery of sexual function. J Urol 1995; 153:150–152.

Rauchenwald M, Steers WD, Desjardins C: Efferent innervation of the rat testis. Biol Reprod 1995; 52:1136–1143.

Raz S, Caine M, Zeigler M: The vascular component in the production of intraurethral pressure. J Urol 1972; 108:93–96.

Reiner WG, Walsh PC: An anatomical approach to the surgical management of the dorsal vein and Santorini's plexus during radical retropubic surgery. J Urol 1979; 121:198–200.

Richardson CA, Edmonds PB, Williams NL: Treatment of stress urinary incontinence due to paravaginal fascial defect. Obstet Gynecol 1981; 57:357–362.

Schlegel PN, Walsh PC: Neuroanatomical approach to radical cystoprostatectomy with preservation of sexual function. J Urol 1987; 138:1402–1406.

Shafik A: A study of the arterial pattern of the normal ureter. J Urol 1972; 107:720–722.

Snooks SJ, Badenoch DF, Tiptaft RC, Swash M: Perineal nerve damage in genuine stress urinary incontinence: An electrophysiological study. Br J Urol 1985; 57:422–426.

Sohn MHH: Current status of penile revascularization for the treatment of male erectile dysfunction. J Androl 1994; 15:183–186.

Steiner MS: The puboprostatic ligament and the male urethral suspensory mechanism: An anatomic study. Urology 1994; 44:530–534.

Steiner MS, Morton RA, Walsh PC: Impact of anatomical radical prostatectomy on urinary continence. J Urol 1991; 145:512–514.

Tanagho EA: Anatomy of the lower urinary tract. *In* Walsh PC, Retik AB, Stamey TA, Vaughan ED, eds: Campbell's Urology, 6th ed. Philadelphia, W.B. Saunders Company, 1992, pp 40–69.

Tanagho EA, Schmidt RA, Gomes De Araujo C: Urinary striated sphincter: What is its nerve supply? Urology 1982; 20:415–417.

Thomson AS, Dabhoiwala NF, Verbeek FJ, Lamers WH: The functional anatomy of the ureterovesical junction. Br J Urol 1994; 73:284–291.

Uhlenhuth E: Problems in the Anatomy of the Pelvis. Philadelphia, J.B. Lippincott Company, 1953.

Uhlenhuth E, Smith RD, Day EC, Middleton EB: A re-investigation of Colles' and Buck's fasciae in the male. J Urol 1949; 62:542–563.

Versi E, Cardozo LD, Studd JWW, et al: Internal urinary sphincter in maintenance of female continence. BMJ 1986; 292:166–173.

Walsh PC, Donker PJ: Impotence following radical prostatectomy: Insight into etiology and prevention. J Urol 1982; 128:492–497.

Walsh PC, Lepor H, Eggleston JC: Radical prostatectomy with preservation of sexual function: Anatomical and pathological considerations. Prostate 1983; 4:473–485.

Waterhouse K, Abrahams JI, Gruber H, et al: The transpubic approach to the urinary tract. J Urol 1973; 109:486–490.

Williams PL, Warwick R, Dyson M, Bannister LH: Gray's Anatomy, 37th ed. New York, Churchill Livingstone, 1989.

Zacharin RF: The suspensory mechanism of the female urethra. J Anat Lond 1963; 97(3):423–427.

Zacharin RF: Pelvic Floor Anatomy and the Surgery of Pulsion Enterocele. New York, Springer-Verlag, 1985.

Zorn BH, Watson LR, Steers WD: Nerves from pelvic plexus contribute to chronic orchidalgia. Lancet 1994; 343:1161.

Zvara P, Carrier S, Kour N-W, Tanagho EA: The detailed neuroanatomy of the human striated urethral sphincter. Br J Urol 1994; 74:182–187.

II
RENAL PHYSIOLOGY AND PATHOPHYSIOLOGY

4

EVALUATION OF THE UROLOGIC PATIENT

HISTORY, PHYSICAL EXAMINATION, AND URINALYSIS

Charles B. Brendler, M.D.

Urologists have a unique and interesting position in medicine. Their patients encompass all age groups: prenatal, pediatric, adolescent, adult, and geriatric. Because there is no medical subspecialist with similar interests, **the urologist has the ability to make the initial evaluation and diagnosis and to provide medical and surgical therapy for all diseases of the genitourinary system.** Historically, the diagnostic armamentarium has included urinalysis, endoscopy, and intravenous pyelography. Advances in ultrasonography, computed tomography (CT), magnetic resonance imaging (MRI), and endourology have expanded our diagnostic capabilities. Despite these advances, however, **the basic approach to the patient is still dependent on taking a complete history, executing a thorough physical examination, and performing a urinalysis.** These basics dictate and guide the subsequent diagnostic evaluation.

HISTORY

Overview

The medical history is the cornerstone of the evaluation of the urologic patient, and a well-taken history frequently elucidates the probable diagnosis. However, many pitfalls can prevent the urologist from obtaining an accurate history. The patient may be unable to describe or communicate symptoms because of anxiety, a language barrier, or educational background. Therefore, the urologist must be a detective and lead the patient through detailed and appropriate questioning in order to obtain accurate information. There are practical considerations in the art of history taking that can help to alleviate some of these difficulties. In the initial meeting, an attempt should be made to help the patient feel comfortable. During this time, the physician should project a calm, caring, and competent image that can help foster two-way communication. Impaired hearing, mental capacity, and facility with English can be promptly assessed. These difficulties are frequently overcome by having a family member or, alternatively, an interpreter present during the interview. Patients need to have sufficient time to express their problems and the reasons for seeking urologic care; the physician, however, should focus the discussion to make it as productive and informative as possible. Direct questioning can then proceed logically. The physician needs to listen carefully without distractions in order to obtain and interpret the clinical information provided by the patient. **A complete history can be divided into three major components: the**

chief complaint and history of the present illness, past medical history, and family history. Each segment can provide significant positive and negative findings that contribute to the overall evaluation and treatment of the patient.

Chief Complaint and Present Illness

Most urologic patients identify their symptoms as arising from the urinary tract, and many present to the urologist for the initial evaluation. For this reason, the urologist frequently has the opportunity to act as both primary physician and specialist. The chief complaint must be clearly defined because it provides the initial information and clues to begin formulating the differential diagnosis. Most important, **the chief complaint is a constant reminder to the urologist as to why the patient initially sought care.** This issue must be addressed even if subsequent evaluation reveals a more serious or significant condition that necessitates more urgent attention.

In obtaining the history of the present illness, **the duration, severity, chronicity, periodicity, and degree of disability are important considerations.** The patient's symptoms need to be clarified for details and quantified for severity. Listed next are a variety of typical initial complaints. Specific questions that focus the differential diagnosis are provided.

Pain

Pain arising from the genitourinary tract may be quite severe and is usually associated with either urinary tract obstruction or inflammation. Urinary calculi cause severe pain when they obstruct the upper urinary tract. Conversely, large, nonobstructing stones may be totally asymptomatic. Thus a 2-mm diameter stone lodged at the ureterovesical junction may cause excruciating pain, whereas a large staghorn calculus in the renal pelvis or a bladder stone may be totally asymptomatic. Urinary retention from prostatic obstruction is also quite painful, but the diagnosis is usually obvious to the patient.

Pain caused by inflammation is most severe when the inflammation involves the parenchyma of a genitourinary organ. Pain results from edema and distention of the capsule surrounding the organ. Thus pyelonephritis, prostatitis, and epididymitis are typically quite painful. Inflammation of the mucosa of a hollow viscus such as the bladder or urethra usually produces discomfort, but the pain is not nearly as severe.

Tumors in the genitourinary tract usually do not cause pain unless they produce obstruction or extend beyond the primary organ to involve adjacent nerves. Thus pain associated with genitourinary malignancies is usually a late manifestation and a sign of advanced disease.

Renal Pain

Pain of renal origin is usually located in the ipsilateral costovertebral angle (CVA) just lateral to the sacrospinalis muscle and beneath the 12th rib. **Pain is usually caused by acute distention of the renal capsule, usually from inflammation or obstruction.** The pain may radiate across the flank anteriorly toward the upper abdomen and umbilicus and may be referred to the testis. A corollary to this observation is that renal or retroperitoneal disease should be considered in the differential diagnosis of any man who complains of testicular discomfort but has a normal scrotal examination. **Pain due to inflammation is usually steady, whereas pain due to obstruction fluctuates in intensity.** Thus the pain produced by ureteral obstruction is typically colicky in nature and intensifies with ureteral peristalsis, at which time the pressure in the renal pelvis rises as the ureter contracts in an attempt to force urine past the point of obstruction.

Pain of renal origin may be associated with gastrointestinal symptoms because of reflex stimulation of the celiac ganglion and because of the proximity of adjacent organs (liver, pancreas, duodenum, gallbladder, and colon). Thus renal pain may be confused with pain of intraperitoneal origin; it can usually be distinguished, however, by a careful history and physical examination. Pain that is due to a perforated duodenal ulcer or pancreatitis may radiate into the back, but the site of greatest pain and tenderness is the epigastrium. Pain of intraperitoneal origin is seldom colicky, unlike obstructive renal pain. Furthermore, pain of intraperitoneal origin frequently radiates into the shoulder because of irritation of the diaphragm and phrenic nerve; this does not occur with renal pain. Typically, patients with intraperitoneal pathology prefer to lie motionless to minimize pain, whereas patients with renal pain usually are more comfortable moving around and holding the flank.

Renal pain may also be confused with pain resulting from irritation of the costal nerves, most commonly T10 to T12. Such pain has a similar distribution from the costovertebral angle across the flank toward the umbilicus. The pain, however, is not colicky in nature. Furthermore, the intensity of radicular pain may be altered by changing position; this is not the case with renal pain.

Ureteral Pain

Ureteral pain is usually acute and secondary to obstruction. The pain results from acute distention of the ureter and by hyperperistalsis and spasm of the smooth muscle of the ureter as it attempts to relieve the obstruction, usually produced by a stone or a blood clot. **The site of ureteral obstruction can often be determined by the location of the referred pain.** With obstruction of the midureter, pain on the right side is referred to the right lower quadrant of the abdomen (McBurney's point) and thus may simulate appendicitis; pain on the left side is referred over the left lower quadrant and resembles that of diverticulitis. Also, the pain may be referred to the scrotum in the male or the labium in the female. Lower ureteral obstruction frequently produces symptoms of vesical irritability, including frequency, urgency, and suprapubic discomfort that in men may radiate along the urethra to the tip of the penis. Often, by taking a careful history, the astute clinician can predict the location of the obstruction. **Ureteral pathology that arises slowly or produces only mild obstruction rarely causes pain.** Therefore, ureteral tumors and stones that cause minimal obstruction are seldom painful.

Vesical Pain

Vesical pain is usually produced either by overdistention of the bladder as a result of acute urinary retention or by inflammation. **Constant suprapubic pain that is unrelated to urinary retention is seldom of urologic origin.** Furthermore, patients with slowly progressive urinary obstruction and bladder distention (e.g., diabetics with a flaccid neurogenic bladder) frequently have no pain at all despite residual urine volumes over 1 L.

Inflammatory conditions of the bladder usually produce intermittent suprapubic discomfort. Thus the pain in conditions such as bacterial cystitis and interstitial cystitis is usually most severe when the bladder is full and is relieved at least partially by voiding. Patients with cystitis sometimes experience sharp, stabbing suprapubic pain at the end of micturition, and this is termed *strangury.* Furthermore, patients with cystitis frequently experience pain referred to the distal urethra, which is associated with irritative voiding symptoms such as urinary frequency and dysuria.

Prostatic Pain

Prostatic pain is usually secondary to inflammation with secondary edema and distention of the prostatic capsule. Pain of prostatic origin is localized primarily in the perineum but can be referred to the lower back, inguinal region, or testicles. Prostatic pain is frequently associated with irritative urinary symptoms such as frequency and dysuria, and in severe cases, marked prostatic edema may produce acute urinary retention.

Penile Pain

Pain in the flaccid penis is usually secondary to inflammation in the bladder or urethra, with referred pain that is experienced maximally at the urethral meatus. Alternatively, penile pain may be produced by *paraphimosis*, a condition in which the uncircumcised penile foreskin is trapped behind the glans penis, resulting in venous obstruction and painful engorgement of the glans penis (see later section). Pain in the erect penis is usually due to *Peyronie's disease* or *priapism* (see later section).

Testicular Pain

Scrotal pain may be either primary or referred. **Primary pain arises from within the scrotum and is usually secondary to acute epididymitis, torsion of the testicle, or testicular appendices.** Because of the edema and pain associated with both acute epididymitis and testicular torsion, it is frequently difficult to distinguish these two conditions. Alternatively, scrotal pain may result from inflammation of the scrotal wall itself. This may result from a simple infected hair follicle or a sebaceous cyst, but it may be secondary to Fournier's gangrene, a severe, necrotizing infection arising in the scrotum that can rapidly progress and be fatal unless promptly recognized and treated.

Chronic scrotal pain is usually related to noninflammatory conditions such as a hydrocele or varicocele, and the pain is usually characterized as a dull, heavy sensation that does not radiate. Because the testicles arise embryologically in close proximity to the kidneys, pain arising in the kidneys or retroperitoneum may be referred to the testicles. Similarly, the dull pain associated with an inguinal hernia may be referred to the scrotum.

Hematuria

Hematuria is the presence of blood in the urine; **greater than three red blood cells per high-power microscopic field (HPF) is significant**. Patients with gross hematuria are usually frightened by the sudden onset of blood in the urine and frequently present to the emergency room for evaluation, fearing that they may be bleeding excessively. **Hematuria of any degree should never be ignored and in adults should be regarded as a symptom of urologic malignancy until proven otherwise.** In evaluating hematuria, there are several questions that should always be asked, and the answers will enable the urologist to target the subsequent diagnostic evaluation efficiently: (1) Is the hematuria gross or microscopic? (2) At what time during urination does the hematuria occur? (3) Is the hematuria associated with pain? (4) Is the patient passing clots? (5) If the patient is passing clots, do the clots have a specific shape?

Gross versus Microscopic Hematuria

The significance of gross versus microscopic hematuria is simply that **the chances of identifying significant pathology increase with the degree of hematuria.** Thus it is uncommon for patients with gross hematuria not to have identifiable underlying pathology, whereas it is quite common for patients with minimal degrees of microscopic hematuria to have negative findings in a urologic evaluation.

Timing of Hematuria

The timing of hematuria during urination frequently indicates the site of origin. **Initial hematuria usually arises from the urethra;** it occurs least commonly and usually arises from the prostatic urethra. **Total hematuria is most common and indicates that the bleeding is most likely coming from the bladder or upper urinary tracts. Terminal hematuria occurs at the end of micturition and is usually secondary to pathology in the area of the bladder neck.** It occurs at the end of micturition as the bladder neck contracts, squeezing out the last amount of urine.

Association with Pain

Hematuria, although frightening, is usually not painful unless it is associated with inflammation or obstruction. Thus patients with cystitis and secondary hematuria may experience painful urinary irritative symptoms, but the pain is usually not worsened with passage of clots. More commonly, **pain in association with hematuria usually originates in the upper urinary tracts, resulting from obstruction of the ureters with calculi or blood clots.**

Presence of Clots

The presence of clots usually indicates a more significant degree of hematuria, and the probability of identifying significant urologic pathology increases accordingly.

Shape of Clots

Usually, if the patient is passing clots, they are amorphous and of bladder or prostatic urethral origin. However, **the**

presence of vermiform (wormlike) clots, particularly if associated with flank pain, identifies the hematuria as coming from the upper urinary tract with formation of vermiform clots within the ureter.

It cannot be emphasized more strongly that **hematuria, particularly in the adult, should be regarded as a symptom of malignancy until proven otherwise and mandates immediate urologic examination.** In a patient who presents with gross painless hematuria, cystoscopy should be performed as soon as possible, because frequently the source of bleeding can be readily identified. Cystoscopy determines whether the hematuria is coming from the urethra, bladder, or upper urinary tract. In patients with gross hematuria secondary to an upper tract source, it is very easy to see the jet of reddish urine pulsing from the involved ureteral orifice.

Although inflammatory conditions may result in hematuria, all patients with hematuria, except perhaps young women with acute bacterial hemorrhagic cystitis, should undergo urologic evaluation. Older women and men who present with hematuria and irritative voiding symptoms may have cystitis secondary to infection arising in a necrotic bladder tumor or, more commonly, flat carcinoma in situ (CIS) of the bladder. It should be remembered that **the most common cause of gross hematuria in a patient over 50 years old is bladder cancer.**

Lower Urinary Tract Symptoms

IRRITATIVE SYMPTOMS

Frequency is one of the most common urologic symptoms. The normal adult voids five or six times per day, with a volume of approximately 300 ml with each void. **Urinary frequency is caused either by increased urinary output (polyuria) or by decreased bladder capacity.** If voiding is noted to occur in large amounts frequently, the patient has polyuria and should be evaluated for diabetes mellitus, diabetes insipidus, or excessive fluid ingestion. Causes of decreased bladder capacity include bladder outlet obstruction with decreased compliance, increased residual urine, and/or decreased functional capacity as a result of irritation; neurogenic bladder with increased sensitivity and decreased compliance; pressure from extrinsic sources; or anxiety. **By distinguishing irritative from obstructive symptoms, the astute clinician should be able to arrive at a proper differential diagnosis.**

Nocturia is nocturnal frequency. Normally, adults arise no more than twice at night to void. As with frequency, nocturia may be secondary to increased urine output or decreased bladder capacity. **Frequency during the day without nocturia usually is of psychogenic origin and related to anxiety. Nocturia without frequency may occur in the patient with congestive heart failure and peripheral edema in whom the intravascular volume and urine output increase when the patient is supine. Renal concentrating ability decreases with age; therefore, urine production in the geriatric patient is increased at night, when renal blood flow is increased as a result of recumbency.** Nocturia may also occur in people who drink large amounts of liquid in the evening, particularly caffeinated and alcoholic beverages, which have strong diuretic effects. In the absence of these factors, nocturia signifies a problem with bladder function secondary to either urinary outlet obstruction and/or decreased bladder compliance.

Urgency is the strong, sudden impulse to void. It may be secondary to an inflammatory condition, such as acute bacterial cystitis, which increases bladder sensitivity; a hyperreflexive neurogenic bladder with decreased bladder compliance; or advanced urinary outlet obstruction, which may decrease both functional capacity and compliance. Urinary urgency may also occur because of anxiety without underlying urologic pathology.

Dysuria is painful urination that is usually caused by inflammation. **This pain is usually not felt over the bladder but is commonly referred to the urethral meatus.** Pain occurring at the start of urination may indicate urethral pathology, whereas pain occurring at the end of micturition (strangury) is usually of bladder origin. Dysuria is frequently accompanied by frequency and urgency.

OBSTRUCTIVE SYMPTOMS

Decreased force of urination is usually secondary to bladder outlet obstruction and commonly results from benign prostatic hyperplasia or a urethral stricture. In fact, except for severe degrees of obstruction, **most patients are unaware of a change in the force and caliber of their urinary stream.** These changes usually occur gradually and generally go unrecognized by most patients. The other obstructive symptoms noted as follows are more commonly recognized, and usually are secondary to bladder outlet obstruction in men as a result of either benign prostatic hyperplasia or a urethral stricture.

Urinary hesitancy refers to a delay in the start of micturition. Normally, urination begins within a second after relaxing the urinary sphincter but may be delayed in men with bladder outlet obstruction.

Intermittency refers to involuntary starting-stopping of the urinary stream. It most commonly results from prostatic obstruction with intermittent occlusion of the urinary stream by the lateral prostatic lobes.

Postvoid dribbling refers to the terminal release of drops of urine at the end of micturition. **This is secondary to a small amount of residual urine in either the bulbar or prostatic urethra that normally is "milked back" into the bladder at the end of micturition** (Stephenson and Farrar, 1977). In men with bladder outlet obstruction, this urine escapes into the bulbar urethra and leaks out at the end of micturition. Men frequently attempt to avoid wetting their clothing by shaking the penis at the end of micturition. In fact, this is ineffective, and the problem is more readily solved by manual compression of the bulbar urethra in the perineum and blotting the urethral meatus with a tissue. Postvoid dribbling is often an early symptom of urethral obstruction related to benign prostatic hyperplasia, but by itself it seldom necessitates any further treatment.

Straining refers to the use of abdominal musculature to urinate. Normally, it is unnecessary to perform a Valsalva maneuver except at the end of urination. Increased straining during micturition is a symptom of bladder outlet obstruction.

It is important for the urologist to distinguish irritative from obstructive lower urinary tract symptoms. This most frequently occurs in evaluating men with benign prostatic hyperplasia (BPH). Although BPH is primarily obstructive, it produces changes in bladder compliance that result in increased irritative symptoms. In fact, men with BPH present more commonly with irritative than obstructive symptoms, and the most common presenting symptom is nocturia. **The urologist must be careful not to attribute irritative symptoms to BPH unless there is documented evidence of obstruction.** In this regard, two important examples are mentioned. **Patients with high-grade flat CIS of the bladder frequently present with urinary irritative symptoms.** The urologist should be particularly aware of the diagnosis of CIS in patients who present with irritative symptoms, a history of cigarette smoking, and microscopic hematuria.

The second important example is irritative symptoms resulting from neurologic disease. Most neurologic diseases encountered by the urologist are upper motor neuronal in etiology and result in a loss of cortical inhibition of voiding with resultant decreased bladder compliance and irritative voiding symptoms. The urologist must be extremely careful to rule out underlying neurologic disease before performing surgery to relieve bladder outlet obstruction. Such surgery may not only fail to relieve the patient's irritative symptoms but may also result in permanent urinary incontinence.

A symptom index for BPH has been developed and validated by the American Urological Association (AUA) (Barry et al, 1992). This index includes seven questions regarding frequency, nocturia, weak urinary stream, hesitancy, intermittency, incomplete emptying, and urgency (Table 4–1). The index has been validated and revalidated and found to have excellent test-retest reliability. The index is extremely sensitive to change, with preoperative scores decreasing from a mean of 17.6 to 7.1 by 4 weeks after prostatectomy ($P < .001$). Thus this index is both reliable and valid and is practical for use in patient care and in research protocols.

INCONTINENCE

Urinary incontinence is the involuntary loss of urine. A careful history of the incontinent patient often determines the etiology. Urinary incontinence can be subdivided into four categories:

CONTINUOUS INCONTINENCE. Continuous incontinence refers to the involuntary loss of urine at all times and in all positions. **Continuous incontinence is most commonly caused by a urinary tract fistula that bypasses the urethral sphincter.** The most common type of fistula that results in urinary incontinence is a vesicovaginal fistula, usually secondary to gynecologic surgery, radiation, or obstetric trauma. Less commonly, ureterovaginal fistulas may occur from similar etiologies.

A second major cause of continuous incontinence is an ectopic ureter that enters either the urethra or the female genital tract. An ectopic ureter usually drains a small, dysplastic upper pole segment of kidney, and the amount of urinary leakage may be quite small. Affected patients may void most of their urine normally but have a continuous amount of small urinary leakage that may be misdiagnosed for many years as a chronic vaginal discharge. **Ectopic ureters never produce urinary incontinence in males,** because they always enter the bladder neck or prostatic urethra proximal to the external urethral sphincter.

STRESS INCONTINENCE. Stress urinary incontinence is the sudden leakage of urine with coughing, sneezing, exercise, or other activities that increase intra-abdominal pressure. During these activities, intra-abdominal pressure rises transiently above urethral resistance, resulting in a sudden, usually small amount of urinary leakage. Stress incontinence is most commonly seen in women after childbearing or menopause and is related to a loss of anterior vaginal support. Stress incontinence is also observed in men after prostatic surgery, most commonly radical prostatec-

Table 4–1. THE AUA SYMPTOM INDEX

Question	Not at All	Less Than 1 Times in 5	Less Than Half the Time	About Half the Time	More Than Half the Time	Almost Always
1. During the last month or so, how often have you had a sensation of not emptying your bladder completely after you finished urinating?	0	1	2	3	4	5
2. During the last month or so, how often have you had to urinate again less than 2 hours after you finished urinating?	0	1	2	3	4	5
3. During the last month or so, how often have you found you stopped and started again several times when you urinated?	0	1	2	3	4	5
4. During the last month or so, how often have you found it difficult to postpone urination?	0	1	2	3	4	5
5. During the last month or so, how often have you had a weak urinary system?	0	1	2	3	4	5
6. During the last month or so, how often have you had to push or strain to begin urination?	0	1	2	3	4	5
	None	1 Time	2 Times	3 Times	4 Times	5 or More times
7. During the last month, how many times did you most typically get up to urinate from the time you went to bed at night until the time you got up in the morning?	0	1	2	3	4	5

AUA symptom score = sum of questions 1 to 7. AUA, American Urological Association.
From Barry MJ, Fowler FJ, O'Leary MP, et al: The American Urological Association Symptom Index for benign prostatic hyperplasia. J Urol 1992; 148:1555.

tomy, in which there may be injury to the external urethral sphincter.

URGENCY INCONTINENCE. Urgency incontinence is the precipitous loss of urine preceded by a strong urge to void. This symptom is commonly observed in patients with cystitis, neurogenic bladder, and advanced bladder outlet obstruction with secondary loss of bladder compliance. It is important to distinguish urgency incontinence from stress incontinence for two reasons. First, **urgency incontinence usually is secondary to underlying pathology that should be identified;** treatment of the primary problem, such as infection or bladder outlet obstruction, may result in resolution of urgency incontinence. Second, **patients with urgency incontinence usually are not amenable to surgical correction but, rather, are more appropriately treated with pharmacologic agents** that either increase bladder compliance and/or increase urethral resistance.

OVERFLOW URINARY INCONTINENCE. Overflow urinary incontinence, often called *paradoxical incontinence*, is secondary to advanced urinary retention and high residual urine volumes. In affected patients, the bladder is chronically distended and never empties completely. Urine may dribble out in small amounts as the bladder overflows. This is particularly likely to occur at night, when the patient is less likely to inhibit urinary leakage. **Overflow incontinence has been termed *paradoxical incontinence* because it can often be cured by relief of bladder outlet obstruction.** It is, however, often difficult to make the diagnosis of overflow incontinence by history and physical examination alone, particularly in the obese patient, in whom percussion of the distended bladder may be difficult. Overflow incontinence usually develops over a considerable length of time, and patients may be totally unaware of incomplete bladder emptying. Thus, **any patient with significant incontinence should undergo measurement of postvoid residual urine.**

Enuresis

Enuresis is urinary incontinence that occurs during sleep. It occurs normally in children up to 3 years of age **but persists in about 15% of children at age 5 and about 1% of children at age 15** (Forsythe and Redmond, 1974). Enuresis must be distinguished from continuous incontinence, which occurs during the day as well as at night and which, in a young girl, usually indicates the presence of an ectopic ureter. All children over age 6 with enuresis should undergo a urologic evaluation, although the **vast majority will be found to have no significant urologic abnormality.**

Sexual Dysfunction

The term *male sexual dysfunction* is frequently used synonymously with *impotence*, although *impotence* refers specifically to the inability to achieve and maintain an erection adequate for intercourse. Patients presenting with "impotence" should be questioned carefully to rule out other male sexual disorders, including loss of libido, absence of emission, absence of orgasm, and, most common, premature ejaculation. Obviously, it is important to identify the precise problem before proceeding with further evaluation and treatment.

Loss of Libido

Because androgens have a major influence on sexual desire, a decrease in libido may indicate androgen deficiency, arising from either pituitary or testicular dysfunction. This can be evaluated directly by **measurement of serum testosterone, which, if abnormal, should be further evaluated by measurement of serum gonadotropins and prolactin.** Because the amount of testosterone required to maintain libido is usually less than that required for full stimulation of the prostate and seminal vesicles, patients with hypogonadism may also note decreased or absent ejaculation. Conversely, if semen volume is normal, it is unlikely that endocrine factors are responsible for loss of libido.

Impotence

A careful history often determines whether the etiology is primarily psychogenic or organic. In men with psychogenic impotence, the condition frequently develops rather quickly secondary to a precipitating event such as marital stress or change or loss of a sexual partner. In men with organic impotence, the condition usually develops more insidiously and frequently can be linked to advancing age or other underlying risk factors.

In evaluating men with impotence, it is important to determine whether the problem exists in all situations. Many men who report impotence may not be able to have intercourse with one partner but can with another. Similarly, it is important to determine whether men are able to achieve normal erections with alternative forms of sexual stimulation, such as masturbation, erotic videos, and so forth. Finally, the patient should be asked whether he ever notes nocturnal or early morning erections. In general, **patients who are able to achieve adequate erections in some situations but not in others have primarily psychogenic rather than organic impotence.**

Failure to Ejaculate

There are several causes of anejaculation: (1) androgen deficiency, (2) sympathetic denervation, (3) pharmacologic agents, and (4) bladder neck and prostatic surgery. Androgen deficiency results in decreases in secretions from the prostate and seminal vesicles, causing a reduction or loss of seminal volume. Sympathectomy or extensive retroperitoneal surgery, most notably retroperitoneal lymphadenectomy for testicular cancer, may interfere with autonomic innervation of the prostate and seminal vesicles, resulting in absence of smooth muscle contraction and absence of seminal emission at time of orgasm. Pharmacologic agents, particularly alpha-adrenergic antagonists, may interfere with bladder neck closure at time of orgasm and result in retrograde ejaculation. Similarly, previous bladder neck or prostatic urethral surgery, most commonly transurethral resection of the prostate, may interfere with bladder neck closure, resulting in retrograde ejaculation. Finally, retrograde ejaculation may develop spontaneously in diabetic men.

Patients who complain of absence of ejaculation should be questioned regarding loss of libido or other symptoms of androgen deficiency, present medications, diabetes, and previous surgery. A careful history usually determines the cause of this problem.

Absence of Orgasm

Anorgasmia is usually psychogenic or caused by certain medications used to treat psychiatric diseases. Sometimes, however, anorgasmia may be a result of decreased penile sensation caused by impaired pudendal nerve function. Most commonly, this occurs in diabetics with peripheral neuropathy. Men who experience anorgasmia in association with decreased penile sensation should undergo vibratory testing of the penis and further neurologic evaluation as indicated.

Premature Ejaculation

Men who complain of premature ejaculation should be questioned carefully because this is obviously a very subjective symptom. Many men who complain of premature ejaculation in actuality have normal sexual function with abnormal sexual expectations. There are men, however, with true premature ejaculation who reach orgasm within less than 1 minute after initiation of intercourse. **This problem is almost always psychogenic** and best treated by a clinical psychologist or psychiatrist who specializes in treatment of this problem and other psychologic aspects of male sexual dysfunction. With counseling and appropriate modifications in sexual technique, this problem can usually be overcome.

Hematospermia

Hematospermia refers to the presence of blood in the seminal fluid. The etiology is diverse and poorly understood, but hematospermia most commonly results from nonspecific inflammation of the urethra, prostate, and/or seminal vesicles. Hematospermia also occurs frequently after needle biopsy of the prostate. Most men with hematospermia are young (mean age, 37 years), and hematospermia almost always resolves spontaneously, usually within several weeks. Hematospermia may be associated with infection, particularly tuberculosis, cytomegalovirus, and schistosomiasis, but is rarely secondary to malignancy. Patients with hematospermia that persists beyond several weeks should undergo further urologic evaluation to rule out a specific underlying etiology. The physical examination should include blood pressure measurement, because severe hypertension can be associated with hematospermia. A genital and rectal examination should be done to exclude the presence of tuberculosis; a prostate-specific antigen (PSA) test and rectal examination done to exclude prostatic carcinoma; and a urinary cytologic test done to rule out the possibility of transitional cell carcinoma of the prostate. Transrectal ultrasonography may reveal other significant pathology, including calculi and cysts, involving the prostate, seminal vesicles, or ejaculatory ducts. Finally, cystourethroscopy may be helpful in identifying the source of bleeding, because hematospermia can be secondary to urethral and prostatic pathology. It should be emphasized, however, that **hematospermia almost always resolves spontaneously and rarely is associated with any significant urologic pathology** (Mulhall and Albertsen, 1995).

Pneumaturia

Pneumaturia is the passage of gas in the urine. This almost always **results from a fistula between the intestine and bladder. Common causes include diverticulitis, carcinoma of the sigmoid colon, and regional enteritis (Crohn's disease).** In rare instances, patients with diabetes mellitus may have gas-forming infections, with carbon dioxide formation from the fermentation of high concentrations of sugar in the urine.

Urethral Discharge

Urethral discharge is the most common symptom of venereal infection. A purulent discharge that is thick, profuse, and yellow to gray is typical of gonococcal urethritis; the discharge in patients with nonspecific urethritis is usually scant and watery. A bloody discharge is suggestive of carcinoma of the urethra.

Fever and Chills

Fever and chills may occur with infection anywhere in the genitourinary tract but are most commonly observed in patients with pyelonephritis, prostatitis, or epididymitis. **When associated with urinary obstruction, fever and chills may portend septicemia and necessitate emergency treatment to relieve obstruction.**

Past Medical History

The past medical history is extremely important as it frequently provides clues to the patient's current diagnosis. The past medical history should be obtained in an orderly and sequential manner.

Previous Medical Illnesses with Urologic Sequelae

There obviously are many diseases that may affect the genitourinary system, and it is important to listen and record the patient's previous medical illnesses. **Patients with diabetes mellitus frequently develop autonomic dysfunction, which may result in impaired urinary and sexual function.** A previous history of tuberculosis may be important in a patient presenting with impaired renal function, ureteral obstruction, or chronic, unexplained urinary tract infections. Patients with hypertension have an increased risk of sexual dysfunction because they are more likely to have peripheral vascular disease and because many of the medications that are used to treat hypertension frequently cause impotence. Patients with neurologic diseases such as multiple sclerosis are also more likely to develop urinary and sexual dysfunction. **In fact, 5% of patients with previously undiagnosed multiple sclerosis present with urinary symptoms as the first manifestation of the disease** (Blaivas and Kaplan, 1988). As mentioned earlier, in men with bladder outlet obstruction, it is important to be aware of pre-existing neurologic conditions. **Surgical treatment of bladder outlet obstruction in the presence of detrusor hyperreflexia may result in increased urinary incontinence postoperatively.** Finally, patients with sickle-cell anemia are prone to a number of urologic conditions, including papillary necrosis and erectile dysfunction secondary to recurrent priapism. There are obviously many other diseases with urologic sequelae, and it is important for the urologist to take a careful history in this regard.

Medications

It is similarly important to obtain an accurate and complete list of present medications, because many drugs interfere with urinary and sexual function. For example, **most of the antihypertensive medications interfere with erectile function, and changing antihypertensive medications can sometimes improve sexual function.** Similarly, **many of the psychotropic agents interfere with emission and orgasm.** The list of medications affecting urinary and sexual function is exhaustive, but, once again, each medication should be recorded and its side effects investigated to be sure that the patient's problem is not drug related.

Previous Surgical Procedures

It is important to be aware of previous operations, particularly in a patient for whom surgery is intended. Obviously, previous operations may make subsequent ones more difficult. If the previous surgery was in a similar anatomic region, it is worthwhile to try to obtain the previous operative report. In my own experience, this small additional effort has been rewarded on numerous occasions by providing a clear explanation of the patient's previous surgery, which greatly simplified the subsequent operation. In general, **it is worthwhile obtaining as much information as possible *before* any intended surgery, as most surprises that occur in the operating room are unhappy ones.**

Smoking and Alcohol Use

Cigarette smoking and consumption of alcohol are clearly linked to a number of urologic conditions. **Cigarette smoking is linked to an increased risk of urothelial carcinoma, most notably bladder cancer, and it is also associated with increased peripheral vascular disease and erectile dysfunction. Chronic alcoholism may result in autonomic and peripheral neuropathy with resultant impaired urinary and sexual function. Chronic alcoholism may also impair hepatic metabolism of estrogens, resulting in decreased serum testosterone, testicular atrophy, and decreased libido.**

In addition to the direct urologic effects of cigarette smoking and alcohol consumption, patients who are actively smoking or drinking at the time of surgery are at increased risk for perioperative complications. Smokers are at increased risk for both pulmonary and cardiac complications. If possible, they should **discontinue smoking at least 8 weeks before surgery to optimize their pulmonary function** (Warner et al, 1989). If they are unable to do this, they should quit smoking for at least 48 hours before surgery, because this will result in a significant improvement in cardiovascular function. Similarly, patients with chronic alcoholism are at increased risk for hepatic toxicity and subsequent coagulation problems postoperatively. Furthermore, alcoholics who continue drinking up to the time of surgery may experience **acute alcohol withdrawal during the postoperative period, which can be life-threatening. Prophylactic administration of lorazepam (Ativan) greatly reduces the potential risk of this significant complication.**

Allergies

Finally, medicinal allergies should be questioned because, obviously, they should be avoided in future treatment of the patient. **All medicinal allergies should be marked boldly on the front of the patient's chart** to avoid potential complications from inadvertent exposure to the same medications.

Family History

It is similarly important to obtain a detailed family history because many diseases are genetic and/or familial in etiology. Examples of genetic diseases include adult polycystic kidney disease, tuberous sclerosis, von Hippel–Lindau disease, renal tubular acidosis, and cystinuria; these are but a few common and well-recognized examples.

In addition to these diseases of known genetic predisposition, there are other conditions in which the precise pattern of inheritance has not been elucidated but that clearly have a familial tendency. It is well known that individuals with a family history of urolithiasis are at increased risk for stone formation. More recently, it has been recognized that **about 8% to 10% of men with prostate cancer have a familial form of the disease that tends to develop about a decade earlier in life than the more common type of prostate cancer** (Carter et al, 1993). Other familial conditions are mentioned elsewhere in the text, but suffice it to state again that obtaining a careful history of previous illnesses and a family history of urologic disease can be extremely valuable in establishing the correct diagnosis.

In summary, a careful and thorough medical history that includes the chief complaint and history of present illness, past medical history, and family history should be obtained for every patient. Unfortunately, time constraints often make it difficult for the physician to spend the time necessary to obtain a full history. A reasonable substitute is to have a trained nurse or other health professional see the patient first. With the use of a standard historical form, much of the information discussed earlier in this chapter can be obtained in a preliminary interview. It then remains only for the urologist to fill in the blanks, have the patient elaborate on potentially relevant aspects of the past medical history, and perform a complete physical examination.

PHYSICAL EXAMINATION

A complete and thorough physical examination is an essential component of the evaluation of patients who present with urologic disease. Although it is tempting to become dependent on laboratory and radiologic tests, **the physical examination often simplifies the process and allows the urologist to select the most appropriate diagnostic studies.** Along with the history, the physical examination remains a key component of the diagnostic evaluation and should be performed conscientiously.

General Observations

The visual inspection of the patient provides a general overview. The skin should be inspected for evidence of jaundice or pallor. The nutritional status of the patient should be noted. **Cachexia is a frequent sign of malignancy, and obesity may be a sign of underlying endocrinologic abnormalities.** In this instance, one should search for the presence of truncal obesity, a "buffalo hump," and abdominal skin striae, which are stigmata of hyperadrenocorticism. In contrast, debility and hyperpigmentation may be signs of hypoadrenocorticism. **Gynecomastia may be a sign of endocrinologic disease as well as a possible indicator of alcoholism or previous hormonal therapy for prostate cancer.** Edema of the genitalia and lower extremities may be associated with cardiac decompensation, renal failure, nephrotic syndrome, or pelvic and/or retroperitoneal lymphatic obstruction. Supraclavicular lymphadenopathy may be seen with any genitourinary neoplasm, most commonly prostate and testicle cancer; inguinal lymphadenopathy may occur secondary to carcinoma of the penis or urethra.

Kidneys

The kidneys are fist-sized organs located high in the retroperitoneum bilaterally. In the adult, the kidneys are normally difficult to palpate because of their position under the diaphragm and ribs with abundant musculature both anteriorly and posteriorly. Because of the position of the liver, the right kidney is somewhat lower than the left. **In children and thin women, it may be possible to palpate the lower pole of the right kidney with deep inspiration.** However, it is usually not possible to palpate either kidney in men, and the left kidney is almost always impalpable unless it is abnormally enlarged.

The best way to palpate the kidneys is with the patient in the supine position. **The kidney is lifted from behind with one hand in the costovertebral angle (Fig. 4–1).** On deep inspiration, the examiner's hand is advanced firmly into the anterior abdomen just below the costal margin. At the point of maximal inspiration, the kidney may be felt as it moves downward with the diaphragm. With each inspiration, the examiner's hand may be advanced deeper into the abdomen. Again, it is more difficult to palpate kidneys in men because the kidneys tend to move downward less with inspiration and because they are surrounded with thicker muscular layers. In children, it is easier to palpate the kidneys because of decreased body thickness. **In neonates, the kidneys can be felt quite easily by palpating the flank between the thumb anteriorly and with the fingers over the costovertebral angle posteriorly.**

Transillumination of the kidneys may be helpful in children younger than 1 year of age with a palpable flank mass. Such masses frequently are of renal origin. A flashlight or fiberoptic light source is positioned posteriorly against the costovertebral angle. **Fluid-filled masses such as cysts or hydronephrosis produce a dull reddish glow in the anterior abdomen. Solid masses such as tumors do not transilluminate.** Other diagnostic maneuvers that may be helpful in examining the kidneys are percussion and auscultation. Although renal inflammation may cause pain that is poorly localized, percussion of the costovertebral angle posteriorly more often localizes the pain and tenderness more accurately. Percussion should be done gently, because this may be quite painful in a patient with significant renal inflammation. Auscultation of the upper abdomen or flank during deep inspiration may occasionally reveal a systolic bruit associated with renal artery stenosis or an aneurysm. A bruit may also be detected in association with a large renal arteriovenous fistula.

Every patient with flank pain should also be examined for possible nerve root irritation. The ribs should be palpated carefully to rule out a bone spur or other skeletal abnormality and to determine the point of maximal tenderness. **Unlike renal pain, radiculitis usually causes hyperesthesia of the overlying skin innervated by the irritated peripheral nerve.** This hypersensitivity can be elicited with a pin or by pinching the skin and fat overlying the involved area. Finally, **the pain experienced during the pre-eruptive phase of herpes zoster involving any of the segments between T11 and L2 may also simulate pain of renal origin.**

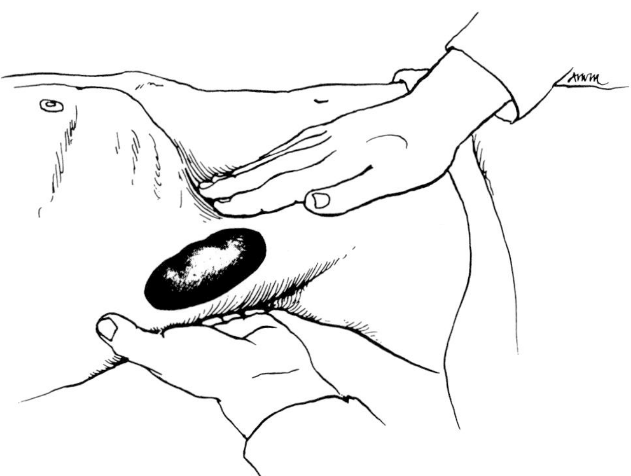

Figure 4–1. Bimanual examination of the kidney. (From Judge RD, Zuidema GD, Fitzgerald FT, eds: Clinical Diagnosis, 5th ed. Boston, Little, Brown & Company, 1989, p 370.)

Bladder

A normal bladder in the adult cannot be palpated or percussed until there is at least 150 ml of urine in it. At a volume of about 500 ml, the distended bladder becomes visible in thin patients as a lower midline abdominal mass.

Percussion is better than palpation for diagnosing a distended bladder. The examiner begins by percussing immediately above the symphysis pubis and continuing cephalad until there is a change in pitch from dull to resonant. Alternatively, it may be possible in thin patients and in children to palpate the bladder by lifting the lumbar spine with one hand and pressing the other hand into the midline of the lower abdomen.

A careful bimanual examination, best done with the patient under anesthesia, is invaluable in assessing the regional extent of a bladder tumor or other pelvic mass. The bladder is palpated between the abdomen and vagina in the female (Fig. 4–2) or between the abdomen and rectum in the male (Fig. 4–3). In addition to defining areas of induration, **the bimanual examination allows the examiner to assess the mobility of the bladder;** such information cannot be obtained by radiologic techniques such as CT and MRI, which convey static images.

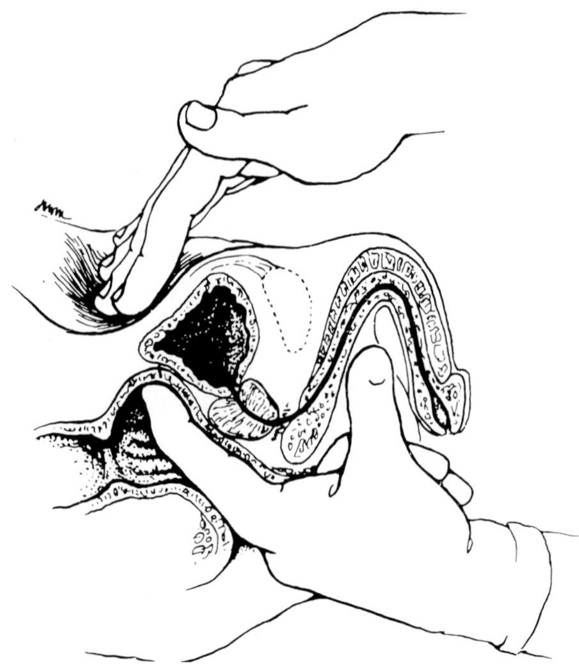

Figure 4–3. Bimanual examination of the bladder in the male. (From Judge RD, Zuidema GD, Fitzgerald FT, eds: Clinical Diagnosis, 5th ed. Boston, Little, Brown & Company, 1989, p 376.)

Penis

If the patient has not been circumcised, the foreskin should be retracted to examine for tumor or balanoposthitis (inflammation of the prepuce and glans penis). **Most penile cancers occur in uncircumcised men and arise on the prepuce or glans penis.** Therefore, in a patient with a bloody penile discharge in whom the foreskin cannot be withdrawn, a dorsal slit or circumcision must be performed to evaluate the glans penis and urethra adequately.

The position of the urethral meatus should be noted. It may be located proximal to the tip of the glans on the ventral surface (hypospadias) or, much less commonly, on the dorsal surface (epispadias). The penile skin should be examined for the presence of superficial vesicles compatible with herpes simplex and for ulcers that may indicate either venereal infection or tumor. The presence of venereal warts (condylomata acuminata), which appear as irregular, papillary, velvety lesions on the male genitalia, should also be noted.

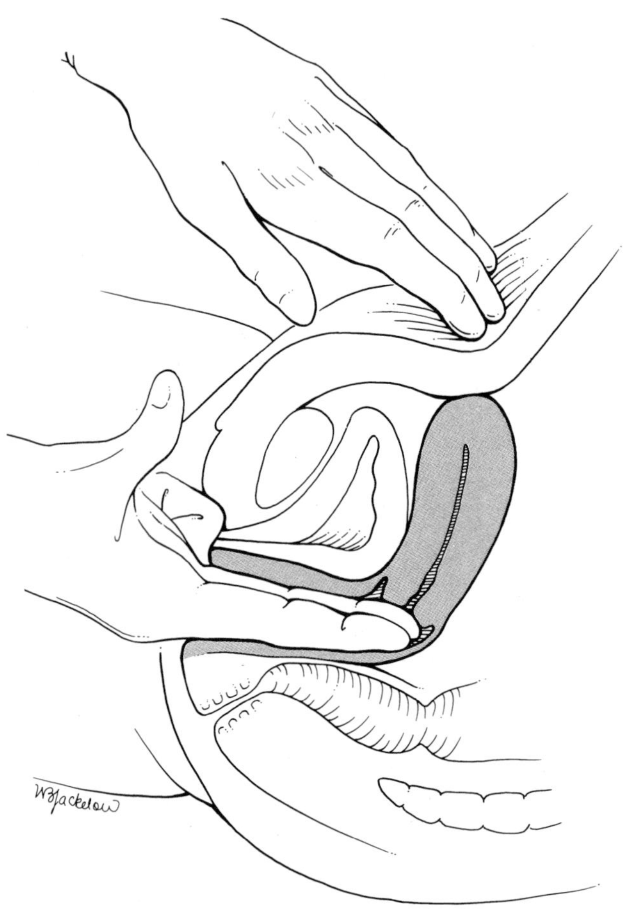

Figure 4–2. Bimanual examination of the bladder in the female. (From Swartz MH: Textbook of Physical Diagnosis. Philadelphia, W.B. Saunders Company, 1989, p 405.)

The urethral meatus should be separated between the thumb and forefinger to inspect for neoplastic or inflammatory lesions within the fossa navicularis. The dorsal shaft of the penis should be palpated for the presence of fibrotic plaques or ridges typical of Peyronie's disease. Tenderness along the ventral aspect of the penis is suggestive of periurethritis, often secondary to a urethral stricture.

Scrotum and Contents

The scrotum is a loose sac containing the testicles and spermatic cord structures. The scrotal wall is made up of skin and an underlying thin muscular layer. The testicles are normally oval, firm, and smooth; in adults they measure about 6 cm in length and 4 cm in width. They are suspended in the scrotum, with the right testicle normally anterior to the left. The epididymis lies posterior to the testicle and is palpable as a distinct ridge of tissue. The vas deferens can be palpated above each testicle and feels like a piece of heavy twine.

The scrotum should be examined for dermatologic abnormalities. **Because the scrotum, unlike the penis, contains both hair and sweat glands, it is a frequent site of local infection and sebaceous cysts.** Hair follicles can become infected and may present as small pustules on the surface of the scrotum. These usually resolve spontaneously but can give rise to more significant infection, particularly in patients with reduced immunity and in diabetics. Patients often become concerned about these lesions, mistaking them for testicular tumors.

The testicles should be palpated gently between the finger tips of both hands. The testicles normally have a firm, rubbery consistency with a smooth surface. Abnormally small testicles suggest hypogonadism or an endocrinopathy such as Klinefelter's disease. **A firm or hard area within the testicle should be considered a malignant tumor until proven otherwise.** The epididymis should be palpable as a ridge posterior to each testicle. **Masses in the epididymis (spermatocele, cyst, epididymitis) are almost always benign.**

To examine for a hernia, the physician's index finger should be inserted gently into the scrotum and invaginated into the external inguinal ring (Fig. 4–4). The scrotum should be invaginated in front of the testicle, and care should be taken not to elevate the testicle itself, which is quite painful. Once the external ring has been located, the physician should place the finger tips of the other hand over the internal inguinal ring and ask the patient to bear down (Valsalva maneuver). A hernia is felt as a distinct bulge that descends against the tip of the index finger in the external inguinal ring as the patient bears down. Although it may be possible to distinguish a direct inguinal hernia, which arises through the floor of the inguinal canal, from an indirect inguinal hernia, which prolapses through the internal inguinal ring, this is seldom possible and of little clinical significance because the surgical approaches are essentially identical for both conditions.

The spermatic cord is also examined with the patient in the standing position. A varicocele is a dilated, tortuous spermatic vein that becomes more obvious as the patient performs a Valsalva maneuver. The epididymis again can be palpated as a ridge of tissue running longitudinally posterior to each testicle. The physician should palpate the testicle again between the fingers of both hands, once again taking care not to exert any pressure on the testicle itself so as to avoid pain.

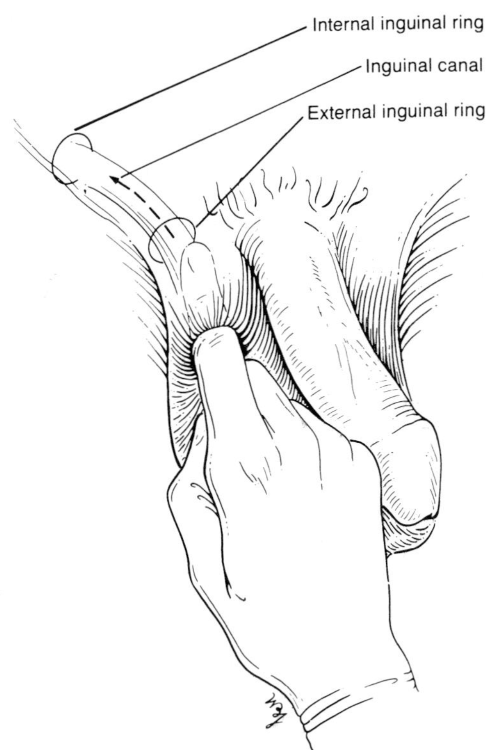

Figure 4–4. Examination of the inguinal canal. (From Swartz MH: Textbook of Physical Diagnosis. Philadelphia, W.B. Saunders Company, 1989, p 376.)

Transillumination is helpful in determining whether scrotal masses are solid (tumor) or cystic (hydrocele, spermatocele). A small flashlight or fiberoptic light cord is placed behind the mass. A cystic mass transilluminates easily, whereas light is not transmitted through a solid tumor.

Rectal and Prostate Examination in the Male

Rectal examination should be performed in every male after age 40 and in men of any age who present for urologic evaluation. Prostate cancer is the second most common cause of cancer deaths in men over age 55 and the most common cause of cancer deaths in men over age 70. Many prostate cancers can be detected in an early curable stage by rectal examination, and about 25% of colorectal cancers can be detected by rectal examination in combination with a stool guaiac test.

Rectal examination should be performed at the end of the physical examination. It is done best with the patient standing and bent over the examining table. The patient should stand with his thighs close to the examining table. His feet should be about 18 inches apart, with the knees flexed slightly. The patient should bend at the waist 90 degrees until his chest is resting on his forearms. The physician should give the patient adequate time to get in the proper position and relax as much as possible. A few reassuring words before the examination are helpful. The physician should place a glove on the examining hand and should lubricate the index finger thoroughly.

Before performing the rectal examination, the physician should place the other hand either on the patient's shoulder or against his lower abdomen. This provides subtle reassurance to the patient by allowing the physician to make gentle contact with the patient before touching the anus. Placing the other hand against the lower abdomen also allows the physician to steady the patient and provide gentle counterpressure if he tries to move away as the rectal examination is being performed.

The rectal examination itself begins by separating the buttocks and inspecting the anus for pathology; hemorrhoids are commonly identified, but occasionally an anal carcinoma or melanoma may be detected. The gloved, lubricated index finger is then inserted gently into the anus. Only one phalanx should be inserted initially to give the anus time to relax and to accommodate the finger easily. Estimation of anal sphincter tone is of great importance; a flaccid or spastic anal sphincter suggests similar changes in the urinary sphincter and may be a clue to the diagnosis of neurogenic disease. If the physician waits only a few seconds, the anal sphincter normally relaxes to the degree that the finger can be advanced to the knuckle without causing pain. The index finger then sweeps over the prostate; the entire posterior surface of the gland can usually be examined if the patient is in the proper position. **Normally, the prostate is about the size of a chestnut and has a consistency similar to that of the contracted thenar eminence of the thumb (with the thumb apposed to the little finger).**

The index finger is extended as far as possible into the

rectum, and the entire circumference is examined to detect an early rectal carcinoma. The index finger is then withdrawn gently, and the stool on the glove is transferred to a guaiac-impregnated (Hemoccult) card for determination of occult blood. Adequate tissues, soap, and towels should be available for the patient to cleanse himself after the examination. The physician should then leave the room and allow the patient adequate time to wash and dress before concluding the consultation.

Pelvic Examination in the Female

Male urologists should always perform the female pelvic examination with a female nurse or other health professional present. The patient should be allowed to undress in privacy and be fully draped for the procedure before the physician enters the room. The examination itself should be performed in standard lithotomy position with the patient's leg abducted. Initially, the external genitalia and introitus should be examined, with particular attention paid to atrophic changes, erosions, ulcers, discharge, and warts, all of which may cause dysuria and pelvic discomfort. The urethral meatus should be inspected for caruncles, mucosal hyperplasia, cysts, and mucosal prolapse. Next, the patient is asked to perform a Valsalva maneuver and is carefully examined for a cystocele (prolapse of the bladder) or rectocele (prolapse of the rectum). The patient is then asked to cough, which may precipitate stress urinary incontinence. Palpation of the urethra is done to detect induration, which may be a sign of chronic inflammation or malignancy. Palpation may also disclose a urethral diverticulum, and palpation of a diverticulum may cause a purulent discharge from the urethra. Bimanual examination of the bladder, uterus, and adnexa should then be performed with two fingers in the vagina and the other hand on the lower abdomen (see Fig. 4–3). Any abnormality of the pelvic organs should be evaluated further with pelvic ultrasonography or a pelvic CT scan.

Common Abnormal Physical Findings

Kidneys

The most common abnormality detected on examination of the kidney is a mass. **In adults, renal masses are difficult to palpate but usually are either benign cysts or malignant renal tumors.** The distinction can seldom be made on physical examination. In children, renal masses may be either cystic and benign (multicystic kidney, polycystic kidney, hydronephrosis) or malignant (Wilms' tumor and neuroblastoma). **In neonates and younger children, the distinction between cystic (benign) and solid (malignant) masses can frequently be made by transillumination.**

Penis

Phimosis

Phimosis is a condition in which the foreskin cannot be retracted behind the glans penis. **In males younger than 4 years of age, it is normal for the foreskin to be unretractable;** in older boys and adults, however, the foreskin can usually be withdrawn easily to the corona (Oster, 1968). Phimosis is usually not painful, but it may produce urinary obstruction with ballooning of the foreskin and may lead to chronic inflammation and carcinoma.

Paraphimosis

Paraphimosis is a condition in which the foreskin has been retracted and left behind the glans penis, constricting the glans and causing painful vascular engorgement and edema. **Paraphimosis is often iatrogenic and frequently occurs after a health professional has examined the penis or inserted a urethral catheter and forgotten to replace the foreskin in its natural position.** Paraphimosis can result in such marked swelling of the glans penis that the foreskin can no longer be drawn forward, which necessitates an emergency dorsal slit or circumcision. If left untreated, paraphimosis can result in necrosis of the glans penis.

Peyronie's Disease

Peyronie's disease is a common condition of unknown etiology that results in **fibrosis of the tunica albuginea,** the tough elastic membrane that surrounds each corpus cavernosum, **producing curvature of the penis during erection.** Peyronie's disease may be difficult to diagnose in the flaccid state; however, the patient's history of curvature with erection establishes the diagnosis. Physical examination reveals fibrous plaques or ridges along the shaft of the penis. Peyronie's disease can be alarming to patients, who may fear that it represents malignancy. They should be reassured that this is always a benign condition that frequently resolves or stabilizes spontaneously without treatment.

Priapism

Priapism is a prolonged painful erection that is not related to sexual activity. **It occurs most commonly in patients with sickle-cell disease but can also occur in those with advanced malignancy, coagulation disorders, or pulmonary disease and without an obvious etiology.** The patient usually presents with a painful, spontaneous erection of several hours' duration. Physical examination reveals the penis to be rigid and mildly tender; the glans penis, however, is usually flaccid.

Hypospadias

Hypospadias is a congenital abnormality in which the urethral meatus is positioned either along the ventral shaft of the penis or on the scrotum or perineum instead of being located at the tip of the penis. **This is a relatively common condition, occurring in about 1 per 300 live male births** (Avellan, 1975). In the more common, less severe forms of hypospadias, the urethra is located at or distal to the corona of the penis; these conditions frequently do not necessitate treatment except for cosmetic purposes. The less common but more severe forms of hypospadias, in which the meatus is located on the penile shaft or in the perineum, may interfere with normal urination in the usual male standing position and may, in adult life, interfere with fertility because the semen is deposited in the distal vagina rather than at the cervix. Such cases are best corrected early in childhood to avoid social embarrassment and psychologic trauma. **Neonates with hypospadias and bilateral cryptorchidism (undescended testicles) should be evaluated for the possibility of intersex, of which the most common cause is adrenogenital syndrome.**

Carcinoma

Carcinoma of the penis usually manifests as a velvety, raised lesion arising on the glans penis or inner surface of the prepuce. Alternatively, it may manifest as an ulcerative lesion. Carcinoma of the penis occurs almost exclusively in uncircumcised men and is more common in underdeveloped nations where hygiene is poor. Penile carcinoma is most commonly a squamous cell tumor and is frequently associated with palpable inguinal lymphadenopathy.

Scrotum and Contents

Testicular Cancer

The most common physical finding in the testicle is a mass. **A useful guideline is that most masses arising from the testicle are malignant, whereas almost all masses arising from the spermatic cord structures are benign.** Thus it is very important to distinguish the testicle and epididymis during the physical examination. Testicular tumors usually manifest as painless, firm, irregular masses on the surface of the testicle. They are usually discovered incidentally by the patient when showering or during self-examination. **Testicular tumors can be readily distinguished from benign masses arising from the spermatic cord by transillumination and scrotal ultrasonography.**

Torsion

Torsion is the twisting of the testicle on the spermatic cord, resulting in strangulation of the blood supply and infarction of the testicle. **Torsion occurs most commonly between the ages of 12 and 20; it also occurs, although less frequently, during the first year of life.** The patient usually presents with the sudden onset of pain and swelling of the involved testicle. The pain may radiate into the groin and lower abdomen; thus it may be confused with appendicitis unless the physician examines the genitalia carefully. On physical examination, it is difficult to distinguish the testicle from the epididymis because of localized swelling. For this reason, the condition is frequently misdiagnosed as epididymitis. **Age is the most useful criterion in distinguishing torsion from epididymitis,** because torsion usually occurs around puberty, whereas epididymitis more often occurs in sexually active males, usually after age 20.

Hydrocele

A hydrocele is a collection of fluid between the tunica vaginalis and the testicle. The patient presents with progressive swelling and local discomfort on the involved side of the scrotum. Physical examination reveals smooth, symmetric enlargement of one side of the scrotum in which it is very difficult to feel the testicle. The diagnosis is made by transillumination of the scrotum. However, **because about 10% of testicular tumors manifest with an associated reactive hydrocele,** it is important to be sure that the hydrocele transilluminates completely and, if there is any doubt, to **confirm the diagnosis with subsequent scrotal ultrasonography.**

Varicocele

A varicocele is an enlarged, tortuous spermatic vein above the testicle that almost always occurs on the left side. The patient presents with a soft mass or swelling above the testicle that is noted when he stands or strains. This mass has been described as a "bag of worms." Varicoceles typically decrease in size and may disappear when the patient is supine. **Patients with the sudden onset of a varicocele, a right-sided varicocele, or a varicocele that does not reduce in size in the supine position should be suspected of having a retroperitoneal neoplasm** with obstruction of the spermatic vein where it enters either the renal vein on the left or the inferior vena cava on the right. Such patients should undergo sonography or CT scanning to rule out malignancy before receiving treatment for the varicocele.

Prostate

Acute Prostatitis

Acute prostatitis most commonly occurs in sexually active men between the ages of 20 and 40. Symptoms include fever, malaise, perineal and rectal discomfort, urinary frequency, urgency, dysuria, and sometimes urinary retention. When acute prostatitis is suspected, rectal examination should be performed extremely gently. Examination reveals the prostate to be warm, tender, and sometimes fluctuant or boggy in consistency. A localized fluctuant, tender region within the prostate may indicate a prostatic abscess, for which surgical drainage is required. **The prostate should never be massaged for secretions in acute prostatitis.** Massage of the acutely infected prostate is not only unnecessary but also extremely uncomfortable for the patient. In addition, massage may disseminate bacteria through the vas deferens, causing secondary epididymitis, or, more significant, may disseminate bacteria into the blood stream, producing gram-negative septicemia.

Benign Prostatic Hyperplasia

The physical findings in BPH are usually limited to the prostate. In BPH the prostate remains rubbery in consistency but may be variably enlarged from normal chestnut size to the size of a lemon or, occasionally, even as large as an orange. There is only a general correlation between prostatic size and degree of symptoms.

Because BPH affects almost all men over age 50, the finding of an enlarged prostate on physical examination is not a reason per se to initiate further urologic evaluation. The severity of the disease and the need for treatment is best determined by the patient's symptoms collaborated with further urologic testing, such as measurement of a urinary flow rate and postvoid residual urine.

CARCINOMA OF THE PROSTATE

Prostate cancer usually arises in the posterior peripheral region of the prostate and, therefore, is frequently palpable in its early stages on rectal examination. On physical examination, **prostatic carcinomas are palpable as firm, indurated nodules or regions within the prostate.** These areas of induration are characterized by having a woodlike consistency. As prostatic carcinomas progress, the entire gland becomes firmer than usual; eventually, these tumors may progress beyond the capsule of the prostate, extending cephalad into the seminal vesicles and laterally toward the pelvic side wall.

It should be emphasized that **men with early, localized carcinoma of the prostate are almost always asymptomatic.** Therefore, a patient should never be allowed to dissuade the urologist from performing a rectal examination simply because the patient is asymptomatic. Urinary obstructive symptoms and skeletal pain are symptoms of advanced, incurable disease.

Detection of early prostatic carcinoma on rectal examination takes practice and has been greatly facilitated by the discovery of PSA. An elevated PSA level should raise the suspicion of prostatic carcinoma, regardless of the findings on rectal examination. Conversely, a normal PSA does not exclude the possibility of early prostate cancer, and, in fact, **30% of men with early prostate cancer have a normal serum PSA level** (Partin et al, 1993).

A prostatic biopsy should be performed for any palpable lesion within the prostate. **About 50% of prostatic nodules detected on rectal examination subsequently prove to be malignant** (Jewett, 1956). Other causes of prostatic induration include calculi (which are typically harder than tumors), inflammation, fibrous BPH, and infarction. Biopsies are now done easily with topical anesthesia under transrectal ultrasound guidance. **There is no excuse for delaying a prostatic biopsy in an otherwise healthy younger man with either an abnormal digital rectal examination or an elevated PSA.** It serves no purpose to have the patient return in 6 months for a repeat examination to see whether the nodule has changed, because prostate cancers usually grow very slowly; the fact that a nodule does not change appreciably with time is of no clinical significance.

URINALYSIS

The urinalysis is a fundamental test that should be performed in all urologic patients. Although in many instances a simple dipstick urinalysis provides the necessary information, **a complete urinalysis includes both chemical and microscopic analyses.**

Collection of Urinary Specimens

Male

In the male patient, a midstream urine sample is obtained. The uncircumcised male should retract the foreskin, cleanse the glans penis with antiseptic solution, and continue to retract the foreskin during voiding. The male patient begins urinating into the toilet and then places a wide-mouth sterile container under his penis to collect a midstream sample. This avoids contamination of the urine specimen with skin and urethral organisms.

In men with chronic urinary tract infections, four aliquots of urine are obtained. **These aliquots have been designated VB1, VB2, EPS, and VB3.** The VB1 is the initial 5 to 10 ml of urine voided; the VB2 is the midstream urine; the EPS is the secretions obtained after gentle prostatic massage; and the VB3 specimen is the initial 2 to 3 ml of urine obtained after prostatic massage. The value of these cultures for localization of urinary tract infections is that **the VB1 sample represents urethral flora; the VB2 sample, bladder flora; and the EPS and VB3 samples, prostatic flora.** The VB3 sample is particularly helpful when little or no prostatic fluid is obtained by massage. To better obtain prostatic secretions, patients should be instructed to attempt to void during prostatic massage and to avoid tightening the anal sphincter and pelvic floor muscles. The four-part urine sample is particularly useful in evaluating men with suspected bacterial prostatitis (Meares and Stamey, 1968).

Female

In the female, it is more difficult to obtain a clean-catch midstream specimen. The female patient should cleanse the vulva, separate the labia, and collect a midstream specimen as described for the male patient. If infection is suspected, however, the midstream specimen is unreliable and should never be sent for culture and sensitivity. **To evaluate for a possible infection in a female, a catheterized urine sample should always be obtained.**

Neonates and Infants

The usual way to obtain a urine sample in a neonate or an infant is to place a sterile plastic bag with an adhesive collar over the infant's genitalia. Obviously, however, these devices may not be able to distinguish contamination from true urinary tract infection. **The best way to obtain an uncontaminated specimen from the bladder is by percutaneous suprapubic aspiration of urine.** With this technique, the suprapubic region immediately above the pubis is cleansed with an antiseptic solution, and urine is obtained from the bladder with a fine-gauge needle.

Whenever possible, **all urine samples should be examined within 1 hour of collection and plated for culture and sensitivity if indicated.** If urine is allowed to stand at room temperature for longer periods of time, bacterial overgrowth may occur, the pH may change, and red and white blood cell casts may disintegrate. If it is not possible to examine the urine promptly, it should be refrigerated at 5°C.

Physical Examination of Urine

The physical examination of the urine includes an evaluation of color, turbidity, specific gravity and osmolality, and pH.

Color

The normal color of urine, pale yellow, results from the presence of the pigment urochrome. **Urine color varies**

most commonly because of concentration, but many foods, medications, metabolic products, and infection may produce abnormal urine color. This is important, because many patients seek consultation primarily because of a change in urine color. Thus it is important for the urologist to be aware of the **common causes of abnormal urine color,** and these **are listed in Table 4–2.**

Turbidity

Freshly voided urine is clear. **Cloudy urine is most commonly a result of phosphaturia,** a benign process in which excess phosphate crystals precipitate in an alkaline urine. Phosphaturia is intermittent and usually occurs after meals or ingestion of a large quantity of milk. Patients are otherwise asymptomatic. The diagnosis of phosphaturia can be accomplished either by acidifying the urine with acetic acid, which will result in immediate clearing, or by performing a microscopic analysis, which will reveal large amounts of amorphous phosphate crystals.

Table 4–2. COMMON CAUSES OF ABNORMAL URINE COLORATION

Colorless	Very dilute urine Overhydration
Cloudy/milky	Phosphaturia Pyuria Chyluria
Red	Hematuria Hemoglobinuria/myoglobinuria Anthrocyanin (in beets and blackberries) Chronic lead and mercury poisoning Phenolphthalein (in bowel evacuants) Phenothiazines (e.g., prochlorperazine [Compazine]) Rifampin
Orange	Dehydration Phenazopyridine (Pyridium) Sulfasalazine (Azulfidine)
Yellow	Normal Phenacetin Riboflavin
Green-blue	Biliverdin Indicanuria (tryptophan indole metabolites) Amitriptyline (Elavil) Indigo carmine Methylene blue Phenois (e.g., IV cimetidine [Tagamet], IV promethazine [Phenergan]) Resorcinol Triamterene (Dyrenium)
Brown	Urobilinogen Porphyria Aloe, fava beans, and rhubarb Chloroquine and primaquine Furazolidone (Furoxone) Metronidazole (Flagyl) Nitrofurantoin (Furadantin)
Brown-black	Alcaptonuria (homogentisic acid) Hemorrhage Melanin Tyrosinosis (hydroxyphenylpyruvic acid) Cascara, senna (laxatives) Methocarbamol (Robaxin) Methyldopa (Aldomet) Sorbitol

From Hanno PM, Wein AJ: A Clinical Manual of Urology. Norwalk, CT: Appleton-Century-Crofts, 1987, p. 67.

Pyuria, usually associated with a urinary tract infection, is another common cause of cloudy urine. The large numbers of white blood cells cause the urine to become turbid. **Pyuria is readily distinguished from phosphaturia by either smelling the urine** (infected urine has a characteristic pungent odor) **or by microscopic examination,** which readily distinguishes amorphous phosphate crystals from leukocytes.

Rare causes of cloudy urine include chyluria (in which there is an abnormal communication between the lymphatic system and the urinary tract, resulting in lymph fluid's being mixed with urine), lipiduria, hyperoxaluria, and hyperuricosuria.

Specific Gravity and Osmolality

Specific gravity of urine is easily determined from a urinary dipstick and usually varies from 1.001 to 1.035. Specific gravity usually reflects the patient's state of hydration but may also be affected by abnormal renal function, the amount of material dissolved in the urine, and a variety of other causes to be mentioned. A specific gravity less than 1.008 is regarded as dilute, whereas a specific gravity greater than 1.020 is considered concentrated. **A fixed specific gravity of 1.010 is a sign of renal insufficiency, either acute or chronic.**

In general, specific gravity reflects the state of hydration but also affords some idea of renal concentrating ability. Conditions that decrease specific gravity include (1) increased fluid intake, (2) diuretics, (3) decreased renal concentrating ability, and (4) diabetes insipidus. Conditions that increase specific gravity include (1) decreased fluid intake; (2) dehydration caused by fever, sweating, vomiting, and diarrhea; (3) diabetes mellitus (glucosuria); and (4) inappropriate secretion of antidiuretic hormone. Specific gravity will also be increased to above 1.035 after intravenous injection of iodinated contrast and in patients taking dextran.

Osmolality is a measure of the amount of material dissolved in the urine and usually varies between 50 and 1200 mOsm/l. Urine osmolality most commonly varies with hydration, and the same factors that affect specific gravity also affect osmolality. Urine osmolality is a better indicator of renal function but cannot be measured from a dipstick and must be determined by use of standard laboratory techniques.

pH

Urinary pH is measured with a dipstick test strip that incorporates two colorimetric indicators, methyl red and bromothymol blue, which yield clearly distinguishable colors over the pH range from 5 to 9. Urinary pH may vary from 4.5 to 8; the average pH varies between 5.5 and 6.5. A urinary pH between 4.5 and 5.5 is considered acidic, whereas a pH between 6.5 and 8 is considered alkaline.

In general, the urinary pH reflects the pH in the serum. In patients with metabolic or respiratory acidosis, the urine is usually acidic; conversely, in patients with metabolic or respiratory alkalosis, the urine is alkaline. **Renal tubular acidosis (RTA) presents an exception to this rule.** In patients with either type I or type II RTA, the serum is acidemic, but the urine is alkalotic because of continued loss of bicarbonate in the urine. **In severe metabolic acidosis in type II RTA, the urine may become acidic, but in type I**

RTA the urine is always alkaline even with severe metabolic acidosis (Morris and Ives, 1991). Urinary pH determination is used to establish the diagnosis of RTA; **inability to acidify the urine below a pH of 5.5 after administration of an acid load is diagnostic of RTA.**

Urine pH determinations are also useful in the diagnosis and treatment of urinary tract infections and urinary calculus disease. **In patients with a presumed urinary tract infection, an alkaline urine sample with a pH greater than 7.5 suggests infection with a urea-splitting organism, most commonly *Proteus*.** Urease-producing bacteria convert ammonia to ammonium ions, markedly elevating the urinary pH and causing precipitation of calcium magnesium ammonium phosphate crystals. The massive amount of crystallization may result in staghorn calculi.

Urinary pH is usually acidic in patients with uric acid and cystine lithiasis. Alkalinization of the urine is an important feature of therapy in both of these conditions, and frequent monitoring of urinary pH is necessary to ascertain adequacy of therapy.

Chemical Examination of Urine

Urine Dipsticks

Urine dipsticks provide a quick and inexpensive method for detecting abnormal substances within the urine. Dipsticks are short plastic strips with small marker pads that are impregnated with different chemical reagents that react with abnormal substances in the urine to produce a colorimetric change. **The abnormal substances commonly tested for with a dipstick are (1) blood, (2) protein, (3) glucose, (4) ketones, (5) urobilinogen and bilirubin, and (6) white blood cells.**

Substances listed in Table 4–2 that produce an abnormal urine color may interfere with appropriate color development on the dipstick. This most commonly occurs in patients taking phenazopyridine (Pyridium) for a urinary tract infection. Pyridium turns the urine bright orange and renders dipstick evaluation of the urine unreliable.

Appropriate technique must be used to obtain an accurate dipstick determination. The reagent areas on the dipstick must be completely immersed in a fresh, uncentrifuged urine specimen and then must be withdrawn immediately to prevent dissolution of the reagents into the urine. As the dipstick is removed from the urine specimen container, the edge of the dipstick is drawn along the rim of the container to remove excess urine. The dipstick should be held horizontally until the appropriate time for reading and then compared with the color chart. **Excess urine on the dipstick or holding the dipstick in a vertical position allows mixing of chemicals from adjacent reagent pads on the dipstick, resulting in a faulty diagnosis.**

Hematuria

Normal urine should contain fewer than three red blood cells per HPF. A positive dipstick reading for blood in the urine indicates hematuria, hemoglobinuria, or myoglobinuria. **The chemical detection of blood in the urine is based on the peroxidase-like activity of hemoglobin.** When in contact with an organic peroxidase substrate, hemoglobin catalyzes the reaction and causes subsequent oxidation of a chromogen indicator, which changes color according to the degree and amount of oxidation. The degree of color change is directly related to the amount of hemoglobin present in the urine specimen. **Dipsticks frequently demonstrate both colored dots and field color change.** If present, free hemoglobin and myoglobin in the urine are absorbed into the reagent pad and catalyze the reaction within the test paper, thereby producing a field change effect in color. Intact erythrocytes in the urine undergo hemolysis when they come in contact with the reagent test pad, and the localized free hemoglobin on the pad produces a corresponding dot of color change. Obviously, the greater the number of intact erythrocytes in the urine specimen, the greater the number of dots that will appear on the test paper, and **a coalescence of the dots occurs when there are more than 250 erythrocytes per milliliter.**

Hematuria can be distinguished from hemoglobinuria and myoglobinuria by microscopic examination of the centrifuged urine; the presence of a large number of erythrocytes establishes the diagnosis of hematuria. If erythrocytes are absent, examination of the serum distinguishes hemoglobinuria and myoglobinuria. A sample of blood is obtained and centrifuged. **In hemoglobinuria, the supernatant will be pink.** This is because free hemoglobin in the serum binds to haptoglobin, which is water insoluble and has a high molecular weight. This complex remains in the serum, causing pink coloration. Free hemoglobin appears in the urine only when all the haptoglobin binding sites have been saturated. In myoglobinuria, the myoglobin released from muscle is of low molecular weight and water soluble. It does not bind to haptoglobin and is therefore excreted immediately into the urine. Therefore, **in myoglobinuria the serum remains clear.**

The sensitivity of urinary dipsticks in identifying hematuria, defined as more than three erythrocytes per HPF of centrifuged sediment examined microscopically, **is over 90%.** On the other hand, **the specificity of the dipstick for hematuria in comparison with microscopy is somewhat lower,** reflecting a higher false-positive rate with the dipstick (Shaw et al, 1985).

False-positive dipstick readings most often result from contamination of the urine specimen with menstrual blood. Dehydration with resultant urine of high specific gravity can also yield false-positive readings as a result of the increased concentration of erythrocytes and hemoglobin. The normal individual excretes about 1000 erythrocytes per milliliter of urine; the upper limits of normal vary from 5000 to 8000 erythrocytes per milliliter (Kincaid-Smith, 1982). Therefore, examining a urine of high specific gravity, such as the first morning-voided specimen, increases the likelihood of a false-positive result. **Other causes of false-positive results include exercise, which can increase the number of erythrocytes in the urine; ingestion of large amounts of ascorbic acid (vitamin C), which inhibits peroxidase reactions; and ingestion of other vitamins and food products with high concentrations of oxidants.**

The efficacy of hematuria screening with the dipstick to identify patients with significant urologic disease is somewhat controversial. Studies in children and young adults have shown a very low rate of significant disease

(Woolhandler et al, 1989). In older adults, one study from the Mayo Clinic of 2000 patients with asymptomatic hematuria showed that only 0.5% had a urologic malignancy and only 1.8% developed other serious urologic diseases within 3 years after identification of the hematuria (Mohr et al, 1986). More recent studies at the University of Wisconsin have found that **26% of asymptomatic men over 50 years old who had a positive dipstick reading for hematuria in a home screening study were subsequently found to have significant urologic pathology, including 5% to 15% who had unsuspected bladder cancer** (Messing et al, 1987). Furthermore, repeat dipstick screening 9 months later in men over 50 whose dipstick urinalysis was initially negative identified an additional 1.8% with significant urologic pathology, including 0.8% with superficial bladder cancer (Messing et al, 1995). Obviously, the age of the population, the completeness of the subsequent urologic evaluation, and the definition of significant disease all influence the benefit of dipstick screening for hematuria in asymptomatic patients. It does appear, however, that dipstick screening for hematuria is cost effective in men over 50 and should be done annually to detect bladder cancer in a superficial stage before invasion occurs.

Differential Diagnosis and Evaluation of Hematuria

Hematuria may reflect either significant renal or urologic disease. **Hematuria of renal origin is frequently associated with casts in the urine and almost always associated with significant proteinuria. Even significant hematuria of urologic origin does not elevate the protein concentration in the urine into the 100- to 300-mg/dl range or the 2+ to 3+ range on dipstick**, and proteinuria of this magnitude almost always indicates glomerular or tubulointerstitial renal disease.

Morphologic evaluation of erythrocytes in the centrifuged urinary sediment also helps localize their site of origin. **Erythrocytes arising from glomerular disease are typically dysmorphic and show a wide range of morphologic alterations. Conversely, erythrocytes arising from tubulointerstitial renal disease and of urologic origin uniformly have a round shape;** these erythrocytes may or may not retain their hemoglobin ("ghost cells"), but the individual cell shape is consistently round. In individuals without significant pathology with minimal amounts of hematuria, the erythrocytes are characteristically dysmorphic, but the number of cells observed is far less than that observed in patients with nephrologic disease. **Erythrocyte morphology is more easily determined through phase contrast microscopy, but with practice, this can be accomplished with a conventional light microscope** (Schramek et al, 1989).

Glomerular Hematuria

Glomerular hematuria is suggested by the presence of dysmorphic erythrocytes, red blood cell casts, and proteinuria. Of patients with glomerulonephritis proved by renal biopsy, however, about **20% have hematuria alone without red blood cell casts or proteinuria** (Fassett et al, 1982).

The glomerular disorders associated with hematuria are listed in Table 4–3. Further evaluation of patients with glomerular hematuria should begin with a thorough history. **Hematuria in children and young adults, usually males, associated with low-grade fever and an erythematous skin rash suggests a diagnosis of immunoglobulin A (IgA) nephropathy (Berger's disease).** A family history of renal disease and deafness suggests familial nephritis or Alport's syndrome. Hemoptysis and abnormal bleeding associated with microcytic anemia are characteristic of Goodpasture's syndrome, whereas the presence of a rash and arthritis suggests systemic lupus erythematosus. Finally, poststreptococcal glomerulonephritis should be suspected in a child with a recent streptococcal infection of the upper respiratory tract or a skin infection.

Further laboratory evaluation should include measurement of serum creatinine, creatinine clearance, and, when proteinuria in the urine is 2+ or greater, a 24-hour urine protein determination. Although these tests quantitate the specific degree of renal dysfunction, further tests are usually required to establish the specific diagnosis and particularly to determine whether the disease has an immune or nonimmune etiology. **Frequently, a renal biopsy is necessary to establish the precise diagnosis, and biopsies are particularly important if the result will influence subsequent treatment of the patient.** Renal biopsies are extremely informative when examined by an experienced pathologist with the use of light, immunofluorescent, and electron microscopy.

An algorithm for the evaluation of glomerular hematuria is provided in Figure 4–5.

IgA NEPHROPATHY (BERGER'S DISEASE). IgA nephropathy, or Berger's disease, is the most common cause of glomerular hematuria, accounting for about 30% of cases (Fassett et al, 1982). IgA nephropathy occurs most commonly in children and young adults, with a male predominance. Patients typically present with hematuria after an upper respiratory tract infection or exercise. Hematuria may be associated with a low-grade fever or a rash, but most patients have no associated systemic symptoms. Gross hematuria occurs intermittently, but microscopic hematuria is a constant finding in some patients. The disease is chronic, but the prognosis in most patients is excellent. Renal function remains normal in the majority, but about **25% subse-**

Table 4–3. GLOMERULAR DISORDERS IN PATIENTS WITH GLOMERULAR HEMATURIA

Disorder	Percentage of Patients
IgA nephropathy (Berger's disease)	30
Mesangioproliferative GN	14
Focal segmental proliferative GN	13
Familial nephritis (e.g., Alport syndrome)	11
Membranous GN	7
Mesangiocapillary GN	6
Focal segmental sclerosis	4
Unclassifiable	4
Systemic lupus erythematosus	3
Postinfectious GN	2
Subacute bacterial endocarditis	2
Others	4
Total	100

IgA, immunoglobulin A; GN, glomerular nephritis.
Adapted from Fassett RG, Horgan BA, Mathew TH: Lancet 1982; 1:1432.

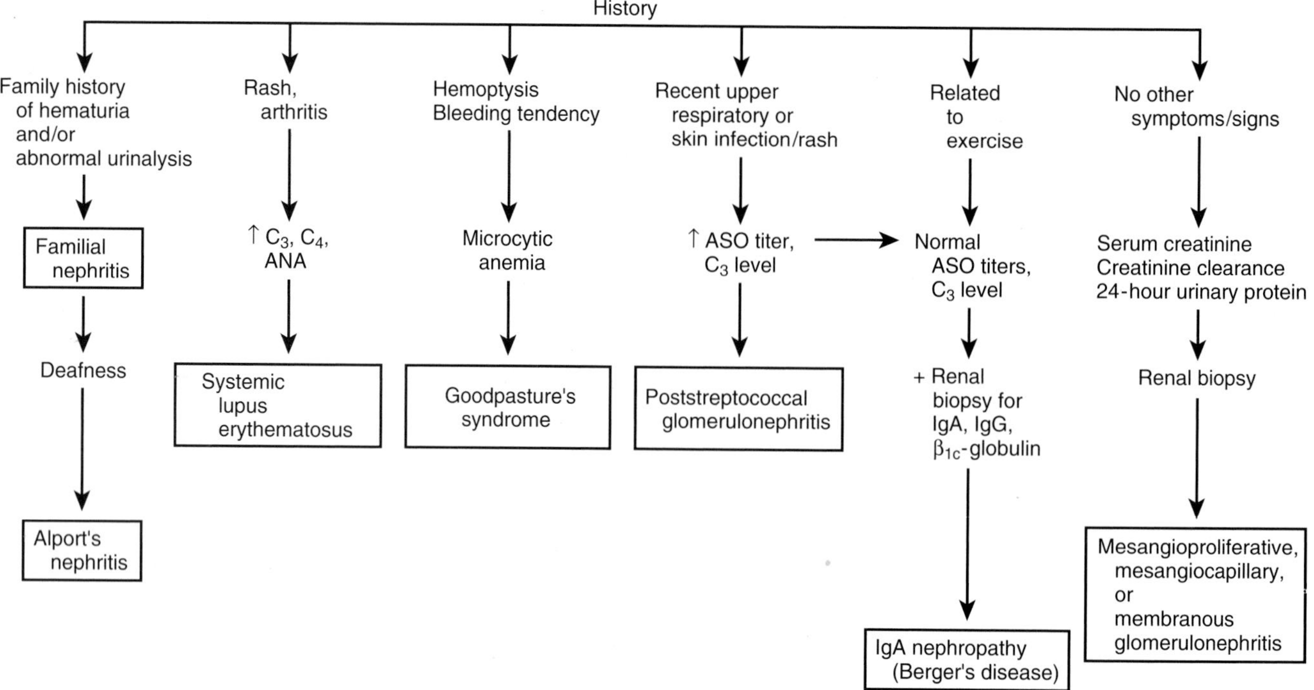

Figure 4–5. Evaluation of glomerular hematuria (dysmorphic erythrocytes, erythocyte casts, and proteinuria).

quently develop renal insufficiency. An older age of onset, initial abnormal renal function, consistent proteinuria, and hypertension are indicators of a poor prognosis (D'Amico, 1988).

The pathologic findings in Berger's disease are limited to either focal glomeruli or lobular segments of a glomerulus. The changes are proliferative and usually confined to mesangial cells (Berger and Hinglais, 1968). Renal biopsy reveals deposits of IgA, immunoglobulin G (IgG), and β_{1c}-globulin, although IgA and IgG mesangial deposits are found in other forms of glomerulonephritis as well. The role of IgA in the disease remains uncertain, although the deposits may trigger an inflammatory reaction within the glomerulus (van den Wall Bake et al, 1989). Because gross hematuria frequently follows an upper respiratory tract infection, a viral etiology has been suspected, but it has not been established. The frequent association between hematuria and exercise in this condition remains unexplained.

The clinical presentation of IgA glomerulonephritis is alarming and similar to certain systemic diseases including Schönlein-Henoch purpura, systemic lupus erythematosus, bacterial endocarditis, and Goodpasture's syndrome. Therefore, a careful clinical and laboratory evaluation is indicated to establish the correct diagnosis. The presence of red blood cell casts establishes the glomerular origin of the hematuria. In the absence of casts, a urologic evaluation is indicated to exclude the urinary tract as a source of bleeding and to confirm that the hematuria is arising from both kidneys. The diagnosis of IgA nephropathy is confirmed by a renal biopsy that demonstrates the classic deposits of immunoglobulins in mesangial cells as described earlier. **Once the diagnosis has been established, repeat evaluations for hematuria are generally not indicated. Although there is no effective treatment of this condition, renal function remains stable in most patients, and there are no other known long-term complications.**

Nonglomerular Hematuria: Medical

Except for renal tumors, nonglomerular hematuria of renal origin is secondary to tubulointerstitial, renovascular, or systemic disorders. **The urinalysis in nonglomerular hematuria is distinguished from that of glomerular hematuria by the presence of circular erythrocytes and the absence of erythrocyte casts.** Like glomerular hematuria, nonglomerular hematuria of renal origin is frequently associated with significant proteinuria, which distinguishes these nephrologic diseases from urologic diseases, in which the degree of proteinuria is usually minimal, even with heavy bleeding.

As with glomerular hematuria, a careful history frequently helps establish the diagnosis. A family history of hematuria or bleeding tendency suggests the diagnosis of a blood dyscrasia, which should be investigated further. A family history of urolithiasis associated with intermittent hematuria may indicate stone disease, which should be investigated with serum and urine measurements of calcium and uric acid. A family history of renal cystic disease should prompt further radiologic evaluation for medullary sponge kidney and adult polycystic kidney disease. **Papillary necrosis as a cause of hematuria should be considered in diabetics, in African-Americans (secondary to sickle-cell disease or trait), and in suspected analgesic abusers.**

Medications, particularly anticoagulants, may induce hematuria. **Anticoagulation at normal therapeutic levels, however, does not predispose patients to hematuria.** In one study, the prevalence of hematuria was 3.2% in anticoagulated patients and 4.8% in a control group. Urologic disease was identified in 81% of patients with more than one episode of microscopic hematuria, and the cause of hematuria did not vary between groups (Culclasure et al, 1994). Thus **anticoagulant therapy per se does not appear to increase the risk of hematuria unless the patient is excessively anticoagulated.**

Exercise-induced hematuria is being observed with increasing frequency. It typically occurs in long-distance (>10 km) runners, usually is noted at the conclusion of the run, and rapidly disappears upon rest. The hematuria may be of renal or bladder origin. An increased number of dysmorphic erythrocytes has been noted in some patients, which suggests a glomerular origin. **Exercise-induced hematuria may be the first sign of underlying glomerular disease such as IgA nephropathy. Also, some patients with calculi in the renal pelvis may first develop hematuria when they run. On the other hand, cystoscopy in patients with exercise-induced hematuria frequently reveals punctate hemorrhagic lesions in the bladder, which suggests that the hematuria is of bladder origin.**

Vascular disease may also result in nonglomerular hematuria. Renal artery embolism and thrombosis, arteriovenous fistulas, and renal vein thrombosis all may result in hematuria. Physical examination may reveal severe hypertension, a flank or abdominal bruit, or atrial fibrillation. In such patients, further evaluation for renal vascular disease should be undertaken.

An algorithm for the evaluation of nonglomerular hematuria is provided in Figure 4–6.

NONGLOMERULAR HEMATURIA: SURGICAL

Nonglomerular hematuria or essential hematuria includes primarily urologic rather than nephrologic diseases. Common causes of essential hematuria include urologic tumors, stones, and urinary tract infections.

The urinalyses in both nonglomerular medical and surgical hematuria are similar in that both are characterized by circular erythrocytes and the absence of erythrocyte casts. Essential hematuria is suggested, however, by the absence of significant proteinuria, which is usually found in nonglomerular hematuria of renal parenchymal origin. It should be remembered, however, that **proteinuria is not always present in glomerular or nonglomerular renal disease.**

An algorithm for the evaluation of nonessential hematuria is provided in Figure 4–7.

Proteinuria

Although healthy adults excrete 80 to 150 mg of protein in the urine daily, the qualitative detection of proteinuria in

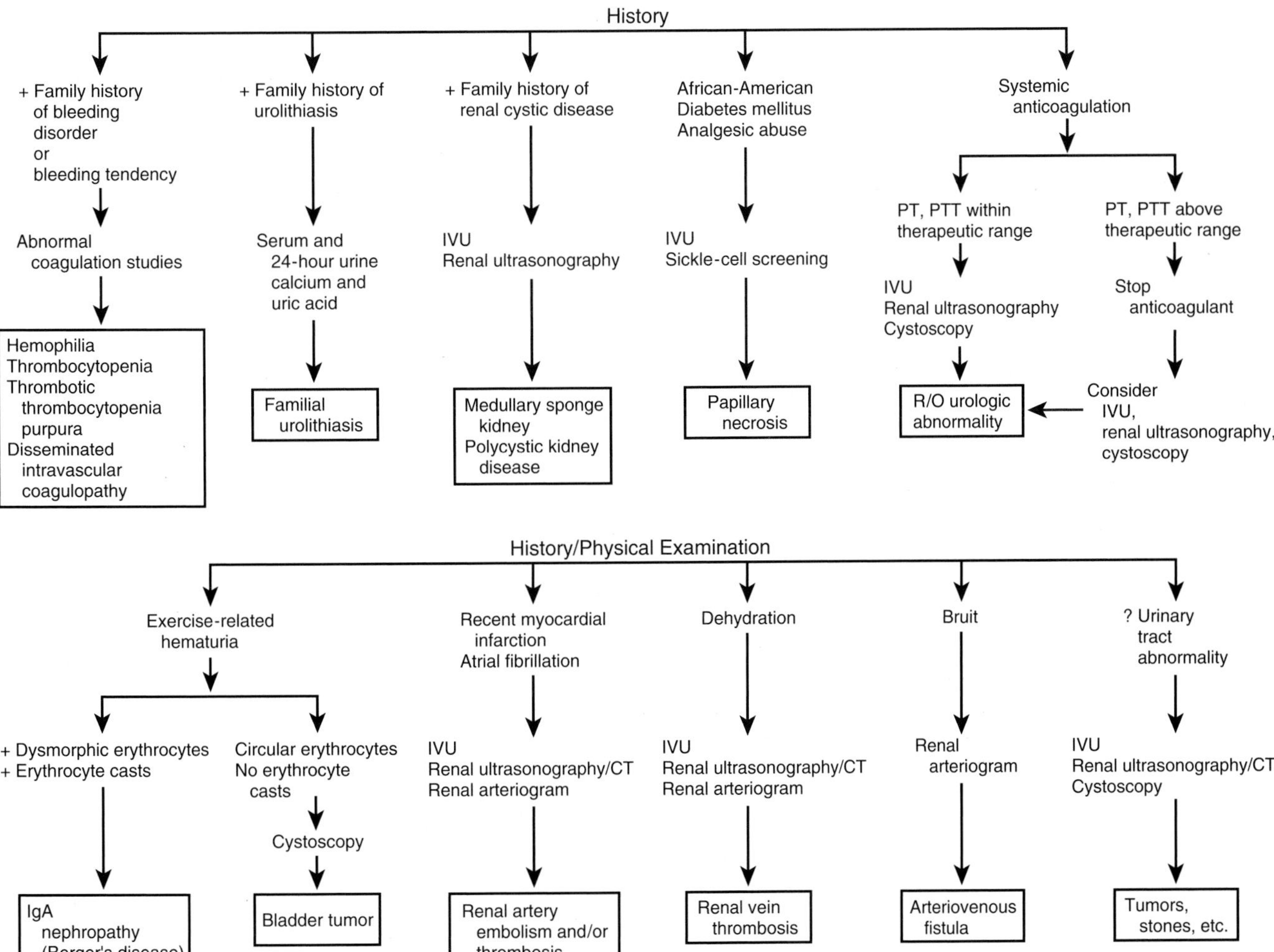

Figure 4–6. Evaluation of nonglomerular renal hematuria (circular erythrocytes, no erythrocyte casts, and proteinuria).

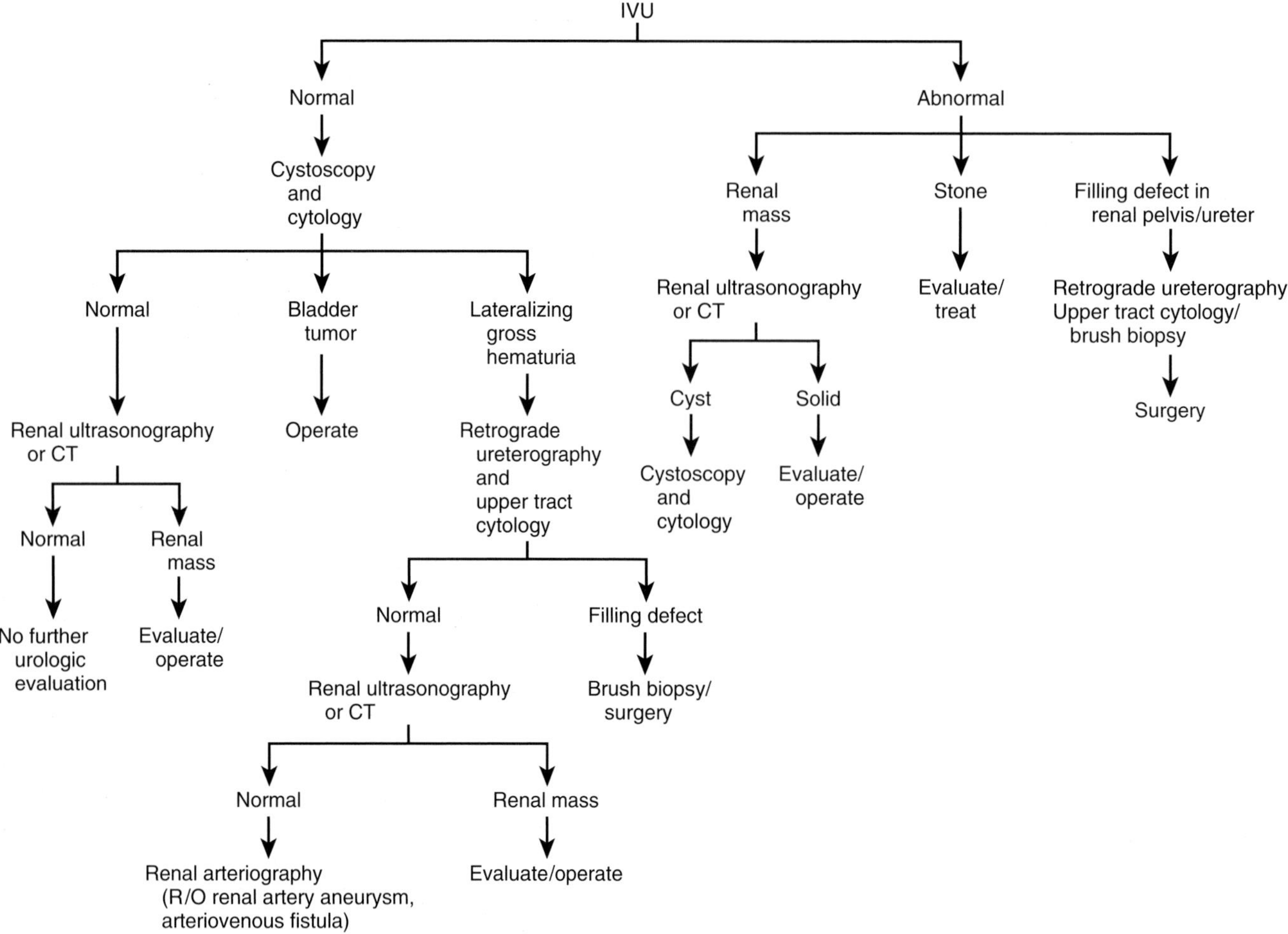

Figure 4–7. Evaluation of essential hematuria (circular erythrocytes, no erythrocyte casts, no significant proteinuria).

the urinalysis should raise suspicion of underlying renal disease. **Proteinuria may be the first indication of renovascular, glomerular, or tubulointerstitial renal disease, or it may represent the overflow of abnormal proteins into the urine in conditions such as multiple myeloma.** Proteinuria also can occur secondary to nonrenal disorders and in response to various physiologic conditions such as strenuous exercise.

The protein concentration in the urine depends on the state of hydration, but it seldom exceeds 20 mg/dl. In patients with dilute urine, however, significant proteinuria may be present at concentrations less than 20 mg/dl. **Normally, urine protein is about 30% albumin, 30% serum globulins, and 40% tissue proteins, of which the major component is Tamm-Horsfall protein.** This profile may be altered by conditions that affect glomerular filtration, tubular reabsorption, or excretion of urine protein, and determination of the urine protein profile by such techniques as protein electrophoresis may help determine the etiology of proteinuria.

Pathophysiology

Most causes of proteinuria can be categorized into one of three categories: glomerular, tubular, or overflow. Glomerular proteinuria is the most common type of proteinuria and results from increased glomerular capillary permeability to protein, especially albumin. Glomerular proteinuria occurs in any of the primary glomerular diseases, such as IgA nephropathy, or in glomerulopathy associated with systemic illness, such as diabetes mellitus. **Glomerular disease should be suspected when the 24-hour urine protein excretion exceeds 1 g and is almost certain to exist when the total protein excretion exceeds 3 g.**

Tubular proteinuria results from failure to reabsorb normally filtered proteins of low molecular weight, such as immunoglobulins. In tubular proteinuria, the 24-hour urine protein loss seldom exceeds 2 to 3 g, and the excreted proteins are of low molecular weight, rather than albumin. Disorders that lead to tubular proteinuria are commonly associated with other defects of proximal tubular function, such as glucosuria, aminoaciduria, phosphaturia, and uricosuria (Fanconi's syndrome).

Overflow proteinuria occurs in the absence of any underlying renal disease and is caused by an increased plasma concentration of abnormal immunoglobulins and other low-molecular-weight proteins. The increased serum levels of abnormal proteins result in excess glomerular filtration that exceeds tubular reabsorptive capacity. **The most common cause of overflow proteinuria is multiple myeloma,** in which large amounts of immunoglobulins are produced and appear in the urine.

DETECTION OF PROTEINURIA

Qualitative detection of abnormal proteinuria is most easily accomplished with a dipstick impregnated with tetrabromphenol blue dye. The color of the dye changes in response to a pH shift related to the protein content of the urine, mainly albumin, leading to the development of a blue color. Because the background of the dipstick is yellow, various shades of green develop, and the darker the green, the greater the concentration of protein in the urine. The minimal detectable protein concentration by this method is 20 to 30 mg/dl. **False-negative results can occur in alkaline urine, in dilute urine, or when the primary protein present is not albumin.** Nephrotic-range proteinuria in excess of 1 g per 24 hours, however, is seldom missed on qualitative screening. Precipitation of urinary proteins with strong acids such as **3% sulfosalicyclic acid** reveals proteinuria at concentrations as low as 15 mg/dl and is more sensitive for revealing other proteins as well as albumin. **Patients whose urine reading is negative on dipstick but strongly positive with sulfosalicylic acid should be suspected of having multiple myeloma, and the urine should be tested further for Bence Jones protein.**

If qualitative testing reveals proteinuria, this should be quantitated with a 24-hour urinary collection. Further qualitative assessment of abnormal urinary proteins can be accomplished by either protein electrophoresis or immunoassay for specific proteins. **Protein electrophoresis is particularly helpful in distinguishing glomerular from tubular proteinuria. In glomerular proteinuria, albumin makes up about 70% of the total protein excreted, whereas in tubular proteinuria, the major proteins excreted are immunoglobulins; albumin constitutes only 10% to 20%. Immunoassay is the method of choice for detecting specific proteins such as Bence Jones protein in multiple myeloma.**

EVALUATION OF PROTEINURIA

Proteinuria should first be classified according to its timing: transient, intermittent, or persistent. Transient proteinuria occurs commonly, especially in the pediatric population, and usually resolves spontaneously within a few days (Wagner et al, 1968). It may result from fever, exercise, or emotional stress. In older patients, transient proteinuria may be caused by congestive heart failure. If a nonrenal cause is identified and a subsequent urinalysis is negative, no further evaluation is necessary. Obviously, if proteinuria persists, it should be evaluated further.

Proteinuria may also occur intermittently, and this is frequently related to postural change (Robinson, 1985). Young males frequently develop mild, intermittent proteinuria as a result of prolonged standing. Total daily protein excretion seldom exceeds 1 g, and urinary protein excretion returns to normal when the patient is recumbent. **Orthostatic proteinuria is thought to be secondary to increased pressure on the renal vein while the patient is standing.** It resolves spontaneously in about 50% of patients and is not associated with any morbidity. Therefore, if renal function is normal in patients with orthostatic proteinuria, no further evaluation is indicated.

Persistent proteinuria necessitates further evaluation, and most cases have a glomerular etiology. A quantitative measurement of urinary protein should be obtained through a 24-hour urine collection, and a qualitative evaluation should be obtained to determine the major proteins excreted. **The findings of greater than 2 g of protein excreted per 24 hours, of which the major components are high-molecular-weight proteins such as albumin, establishes the diagnosis of glomerular proteinuria. Glomerular proteinuria is the most common cause of abnormal proteinuria,** especially in patients presenting with persistent proteinuria. If glomerular proteinuria is associated with hematuria characterized by dysmorphic erythrocytes and erythrocyte casts, the patient should be evaluated as outlined previously for glomerular hematuria (see Fig. 4–5). **Patients with glomerular proteinuria who have no or little associated hematuria** should be evaluated for other conditions, of which the most common is **diabetes mellitus.** Other possibilities include amyloidosis and arteriolar nephrosclerosis.

In patients in whom total protein excretion is 300 to 2000 mg per day, of which the major components are low-molecular-weight globulins, further qualitative evaluation with immunoelectrophoresis is indicated. This determines whether the excess proteins are normal or abnormal. **Identification of normal proteins establishes a diagnosis of tubular proteinuria,** and further evaluation for a specific cause of tubular dysfunction is indicated.

If qualitative evaluation reveals abnormal proteins in the urine, this finding establishes a diagnosis of overflow proteinuria. Further evaluation should be directed toward identifying the specific protein abnormality. The finding of large quantities of light-chain immunoglobulins or Bence Jones protein establishes a diagnosis of multiple myeloma. Similarly, the findings of large amounts of hemoglobin or myoglobin establish the diagnosis of hemoglobinuria or myoglobinuria.

An algorithm for the evaluation of proteinuria is provided in Figure 4–8.

Glucose and Ketones

Urine testing for glucose and ketones is useful in screening patients for diabetes mellitus. Normally, almost all the glucose filtered by the glomeruli is reabsorbed in the proximal tubules. Although very small amounts of glucose may normally be excreted in the urine, these amounts are not clinically significant and are below the level of detectability with the dipstick. If, however, the amount of glucose filtered exceeds the capacity of tubular reabsorption, glucose is excreted in the urine and detected on the dipstick. **This so-called renal threshold corresponds to a serum glucose level of about 180 mg/dl; above this level, glucose is detected in the urine.**

Glucose detection with the urinary dipstick is based on a double sequential enzymatic reaction yielding a colorimetric change. In the first reaction, glucose in the urine reacts with glucose oxidase on the dipstick to form gluconic acid and hydrogen peroxide. In the second reaction, hydrogen peroxide reacts with peroxidase to cause oxidation of the chromogen on the dipstick, producing a color change. **This double oxidative reaction is specific for glucose, and there is no cross reactivity with other sugars.** The dipstick test be-

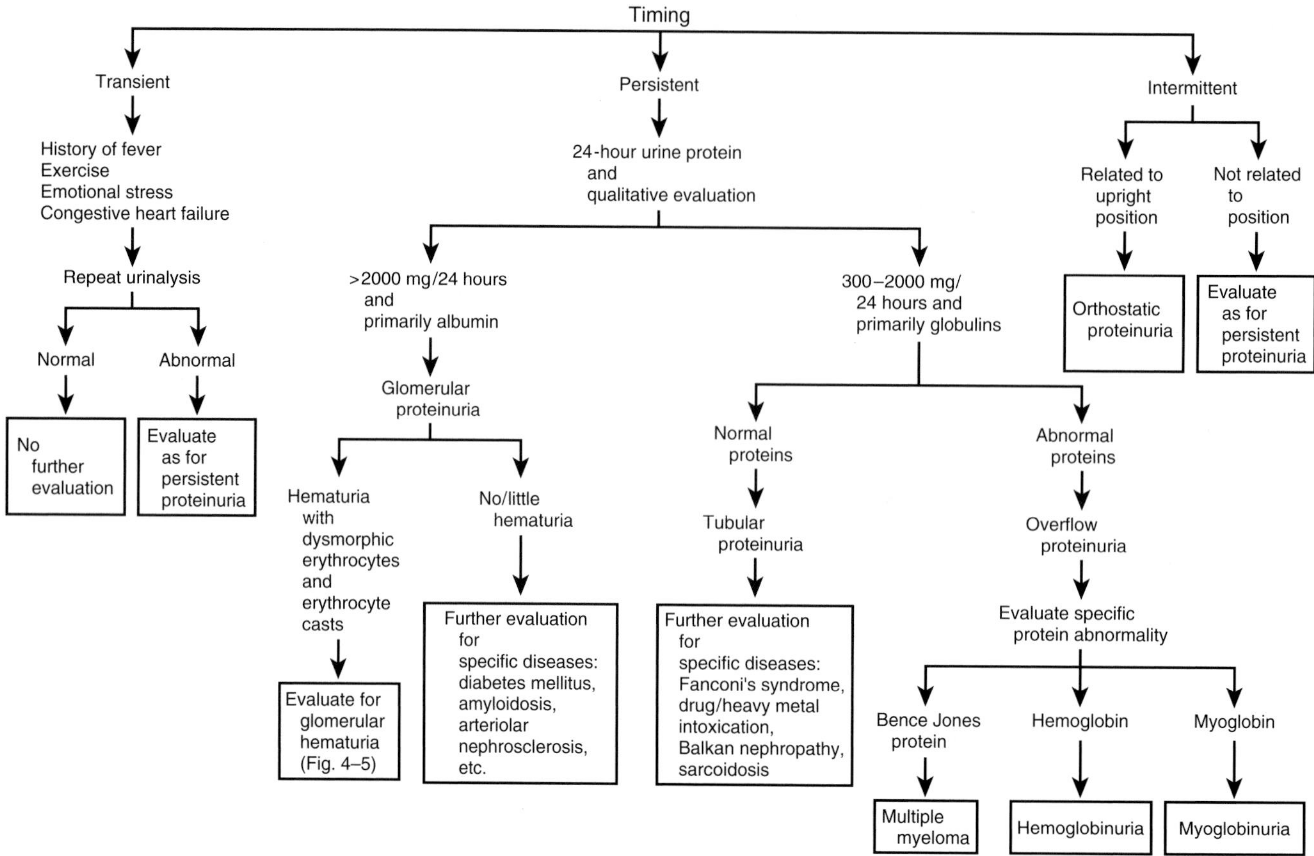

Figure 4–8. Evaluation of proteinuria.

comes less sensitive as the urine increases in specific gravity and temperature.

Ketones are not normally found in the urine, but they do appear when the carbohydrate supplies in the body are depleted and body fat breakdown occurs. This occurs most commonly in diabetic ketoacidosis, but it may also occur during pregnancy and after periods of starvation or rapid weight reduction. **Ketones excreted include acetoacetic acid, acetone, and beta-hydroxybutyric acid. With abnormal fat breakdown, ketones appear in the urine before they appear in the serum.**

Dipstick testing for ketones involves a colorimetric reaction between sodium nitroprusside on the dipstick and acetoacetic acid to produce purple coloration. **Dipstick testing identifies acetoacetic acid at concentrations of 5 to 10 mg/dl but does not detect acetone or beta-hydroxybutyric acid.** Obviously, a dipstick that tests positively for glucose should also be tested for ketones, and the diagnosis of diabetes mellitus should be suspected. False-positive results, however, can occur in very acidic urine of high specific gravity; in abnormal-colored urine; and in urine containing levodopa metabolites, 2-mercaptoethane sulphonate sodium (MESNA), and other sulfhydryl-containing compounds (Csako, 1987).

Bilirubin and Urobilinogen

Normal urine contains no bilirubin and only very small amounts of urobilinogen. There are two types of bilirubin: direct (conjugated) and indirect. Direct bilirubin is made in the hepatocyte, where bilirubin is conjugated with glucuronic acid. **Conjugated bilirubin has a low molecular weight, is water soluble, and normally passes from the liver into the small intestine through the bile ducts, where it is converted to urobilinogen. Therefore, conjugated bilirubin does not appear in the urine except in pathologic conditions in which there is intrinsic hepatic disease or obstruction of the bile ducts.**

Indirect bilirubin is of high molecular weight and bound in the serum to albumin. It is water insoluble and therefore does not appear in the urine even in pathologic conditions.

Urobilinogen is the end product of conjugated bilirubin metabolism. Conjugated bilirubin passes through the bile ducts, where it is metabolized by normal intestinal bacteria to urobilinogen. Normally, about 50% of the urobilinogen is excreted in the stool and 50% is reabsorbed into the enterohepatic circulation. **A small amount of absorbed urobilinogen, about 1 to 4 mg per day, escapes hepatic uptake and is excreted in the urine. Hemolysis and hepatocellular diseases** that result in increased bile pigments can result in **increased urinary urobilinogen.** Conversely, **obstruction of the bile duct or antibiotic usage that alters intestinal flora,** thereby interfering with the conversion of conjugated bilirubin to urobilinogen, **will decrease urobilinogen levels in the urine.** In these conditions, obviously, serum levels of conjugated bilirubin rise.

There are different dipstick reagents and methods to test

for both bilirubin and urobilinogen, but the basic physiologic principle involves the binding of bilirubin or urobilinogen to a diazonium salt to produce a colorimetric reaction. False-negative test results can occur in the presence of ascorbic acid, which decreases the sensitivity for detection of bilirubin. False-positive results can occur in the presence of Pyridium because it causes the urine to turn orange and, as in the colorimetric reaction for bilirubin, to turn red in an acid medium.

Leukocyte Esterase and Nitrite Tests

Leukocyte esterase activity indicates the presence of white blood cells in the urine. The presence of nitrites in the urine is strongly suggestive of bacteriuria. Thus both these tests have been used to screen patients for urinary tract infections. Although these tests may have application in nonurologic medical practice, the most accurate method of diagnosing infection is microscopic examination of the urinary sediment, to identify pyuria, and subsequent urine culture. All urologists should be capable of performing and interpreting the microscopic examination of the urinary sediment. Therefore, leukocyte esterase and nitrite testing are less important in a urologic practice. For purposes of completion, however, both techniques are described briefly as follows.

Leukocyte esterase and nitrite testing are performed with the Chemstrip LN dipstick. Leukocyte esterase is produced by neutrophils and catalyzes the hydrolysis of an indoxyl carbonic acid ester to indoxyl (Gillenwater, 1981). The indoxyl formed oxidizes a diazonium salt chromogen on the dipstick to produce a color change. It is recommended that leukocyte esterase testing be done 5 minutes after the dipstick is immersed in the urine, to allow adequate incubation (Shaw et al, 1985). The sensitivity of this test subsequently decreases with time because of lysis of the leukocytes. Leukocyte esterase testing may also be negative in the presence of infection because not all patients with bacteriuria have significant pyuria. **Therefore, if leukocyte esterase testing is used to screen patients for urinary tract infection, it should always be done in conjunction with nitrite testing for bacteriuria** (Pels et al, 1989).

Other causes of false-negative results with leukocyte esterase testing include increased urinary specific gravity, glycosuria, presence of urobilinogen, medications that alter urine color, and ingestion of large amounts of ascorbic acid. **The major cause of a false-positive leukocyte esterase test is specimen contamination.**

Nitrites are not found normally in the urine, but many species of gram-negative bacteria can convert nitrates to nitrites. Nitrites can readily be detected in the urine because they react with the reagents on the dipstick and undergo diazotization to form a red azo dye. The **specificity of the nitrite dipstick for detecting bacteriuria is over 90%** (Pels et al, 1989). The **sensitivity of the test, however, is considerably less, varying from 35% to 85%.** The nitrite test is less accurate in urine specimens containing fewer than 10^5 organisms per milliliter (Kellog et al, 1987). **As with leukocyte esterase testing, the major cause of a false-positive nitrite test is contamination.**

It remains controversial whether dipstick testing for leukocyte esterase and nitrites can replace microscopy in screening for significant urinary tract infections. **A protocol combining the visual appearance of the urine with leukocyte esterase and nitrite testing has been proposed (Fig. 4–9); it reportedly detects 95% of infected urine specimens and decreases the need for microscopy by as much as 30%** (Flanagan et al, 1989). **Other studies, however, have shown that dipstick testing is not an adequate replacement for microscopy** (Propp et al, 1989). In summary, it has not been demonstrated conclusively that dipstick testing for urinary tract infection can replace microscopic examination of the urinary sediment. In my personal experience, I always examine the urinary sediment whenever I suspect a urinary tract infection, and I subsequently culture the urine when pyuria is identified. Urologists usually have access to a microscope and should be trained and encouraged to examine the urinary sediment.

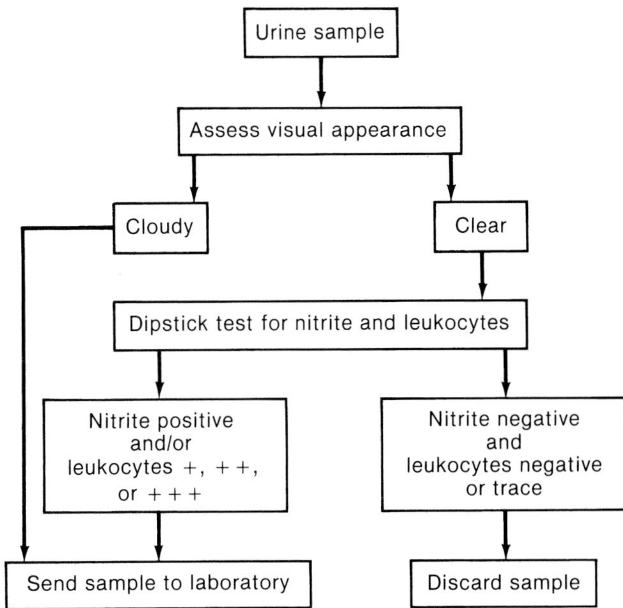

Figure 4–9. Protocol for determining the need for urine sediment microscopy in an asymptomatic population. (From Flanagan PG, et al: Evaluation of four screening tests for bacteriuria in elderly people. Lancet 1989; 1:1117. © by The Lancet Ltd., 1989.)

Urinary Sediment

Obtaining and Preparing the Specimen

A clean-catch midstream urine specimen should be obtained. As described earlier, uncircumcised men should retract the prepuce and cleanse the glans penis before voiding. It is more difficult to obtain a reliable clean-catch specimen in females because of contamination with introital leukocytes and bacteria. If there is any suspicion of a urinary tract infection in a female, a catheterized urine sample should be obtained for culture and sensitivity.

If possible, **the first morning urine specimen is the specimen of choice and should be examined within 1 hour.** A standard procedure for preparation of the urine for microscopic examination has been described (Cushner and Copley, 1989). About 10 to 15 ml of urine should be centrifuged for 5 minutes at 3000 revolutions/minute. The supernatant is then poured off, and the sediment is resuspended in the centrifuge tube by gently tapping the bottom of the tube. Although the remaining small amount of fluid can be poured onto a microscope slide, this usually results in excess fluid on the slide. It is better to **use a small pipette to withdraw the residual fluid from the centrifuge tube and place it directly on the microscope slide.** This usually results in an ideal volume of between 0.01 and 0.02 ml of fluid deposited on the slide. The slide is then covered with a cover slip. **The edge of the cover slip should be placed on the slide first to allow the drop of fluid to ascend onto the cover slip by capillary action.** The cover slip is then gently placed over the drop of fluid; this technique allows for most of the air between the drop of fluid and the cover slip to be expelled. If one simply drops the cover slip over the urine, the urine will disperse over the slide, and there will be a considerable number of air bubbles, which may distort the subsequent microscopic examination.

Microscopy Technique

Microscopic analysis of the urinary sediment should be performed with both low-power (magnification, 100×) and high-power (magnification, 400×) lenses. The use of an oil immersion lens for higher magnification is seldom, if ever, necessary. Under low-power magnification, the entire area under the cover slip should be scanned. **Particular attention should be given to the edges of the cover slip, where casts and other elements tend to be concentrated.** Low-power magnification is sufficient to identify erythrocytes, leukocytes, casts, cystine crystals, oval fat macrophages, and parasites such as *Trichomonas vaginalis* and *Schistosoma haematobium.*

High-power magnification is necessary to distinguish circular from dysmorphic erythrocytes, to identify other types of crystals, and, in particular, to identify bacteria and yeast. In summary, **the urinary sediment should be examined microscopically for (1) cells, (2) casts, (3) crystals, (4) bacteria, (5) yeast, and (6) parasites.**

Cells (Fig. 4–10)

Erythrocyte morphology may be determined under high-power magnification. Although phase-contrast microscopy has been used for this purpose, circular (nonglomerular) erythrocytes can generally be distinguished from dysmorphic (glomerular) erythrocytes under routine bright-field high-power magnification. **This is facilitated by adjusting the microscope condenser to its lowest aperture, thus reducing the intensity of background light. This allows one to see fine detail not evident otherwise and also creates the effect of phase microscopy because cell membranes and other sedimentary components stand out against the darkened background.**

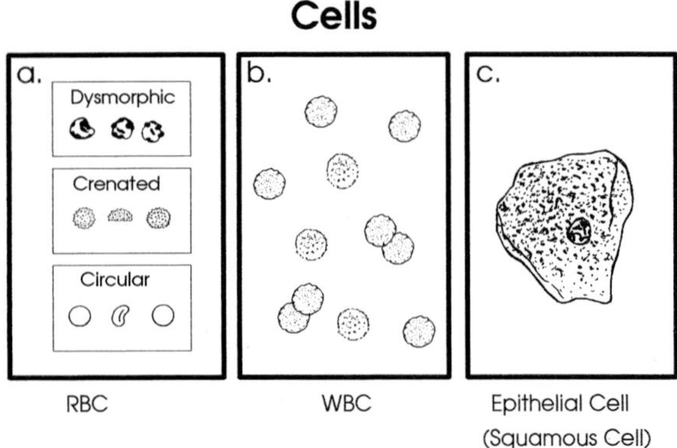

Figure 4–10. High-power magnification (400×) drawing of cells in the urinary sediment. *A,* Red blood cells (RBC): dysmorphic, crenated, and circular. *B,* White blood cells (WBC). *C,* Epithelial cell.

Circular erythrocytes generally have an even distribution of hemoglobin with either a round or crenated contour, whereas dysmorphic erythrocytes are irregularly shaped with minimal hemoglobin and irregular distribution of cytoplasm. Automated techniques for performing microscopic analysis to distinguish the two types of erythrocytes have been investigated but have not yet been accepted into general urologic practice and are probably unnecessary. In one study using a standard Coulter counter, microscopic analysis was found to be 97% accurate in differentiating between the two types of erythrocytes (Sayer et al, 1990). **Erythrocytes may be confused with yeast or fat droplets.** Erythrocytes can be distinguished, however, because yeast shows budding, and oil droplets are highly refractile.

Leukocytes can generally be identified under low-power magnification and definitively diagnosed under high-power magnification. It is normal to find one to two leukocytes per HPF in men and up to five per HPF in woman in whom the urine sample may be contaminated with vaginal secretions. A greater number of leukocytes generally indicates infection or inflammation in the urinary tract. It may be possible to distinguish **old leukocytes, which have a characteristic small and wrinkled appearance** and which are commonly found in the vaginal secretions of normal women, from fresh leukocytes, which are generally indicative of urinary tract pathology. **Fresh leukocytes are generally larger and rounder, and when the specific gravity is less than 1.019, the granules in the cytoplasm demonstrate glitter-like movement, so-called "glitter cells."**

Epithelial cells are commonly observed in the urinary sediment. Squamous cells are frequently detected in female urine specimens and are derived from the lower portion of the urethra, the trigone of postpubertal females, and the vagina. **Squamous epithelial cells are large, have a central small nucleus about the size of an erythrocyte, and have an irregular cytoplasm with fine granularity.**

Transitional epithelial cells may arise from the remainder of the urinary tract. **Transitional cells are smaller than squamous cells, have a larger nucleus, and demonstrate prominent cytoplasmic granules near the nucleus.** Malignant transitional cells have altered nuclear size and morphology, and can be identified either with routine Papanicolaou staining or automated flow cytometry.

Renal tubular cells are the least commonly observed epithelial cells in the urine but are most significant, because their presence in the urine is always indicative of renal pathology. Renal tubular cells may be difficult to distinguish from leukocytes, but they are slightly larger.

Casts (Fig. 4–11)

A cast is a protein coagulum that is formed in the renal tubule and traps any tubular luminal contents within the

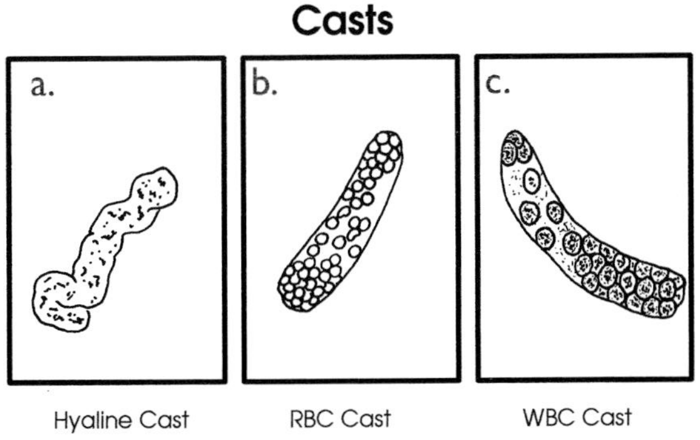

Figure 4–11. High-power magnification (400×) drawing of urinary casts. *A,* Hyaline cast. *B,* RBC cast. *C,* WBC cast.

matrix. **Tamm-Horsfall mucoprotein is the basic matrix of all renal casts; it originates from tubular epithelial cells and is always present in the urine.** When the casts contain only mucoproteins, they are called **hyaline casts** and may not have any pathologic significance. Hyaline casts may be seen in the urine after exercise or heat exposure but may also be observed in pyelonephritis or chronic renal disease.

Red blood cell casts contain entrapped erythrocytes and are diagnostic of glomerular bleeding, most likely secondary to glomerulonephritis. **White blood cell casts are observed in acute glomerulonephritis, acute pyelonephritis, and acute tubulointerstitial nephritis.** Casts with other cellular elements, usually sloughed renal tubular epithelial cells, are indicative of nonspecific renal damage. Granular and waxy casts result from further degeneration of cellular elements. Fatty casts are seen in nephrotic syndrome, lipiduria, and hypothyroidism.

Crystals (Fig. 4–12)

Identification of crystals in the urine is particularly important in patients with stone disease, because it may help determine the etiology. Although other types of crystals may be seen in normal patients, **the identification of cystine crystals, which have a hexagonal benzene ring shape, establishes the diagnosis of cystinuria.** Crystals precipitated in **acidic urine** include **calcium oxalate, uric acid, and cystine.** Crystals precipitated in an **alkaline urine** include **calcium phosphate and triple-phosphate (struvite) crystals.** Cholesterol crystals are rarely seen in the urine and are not related to urinary pH. They occur in lipiduria and remain in droplet form.

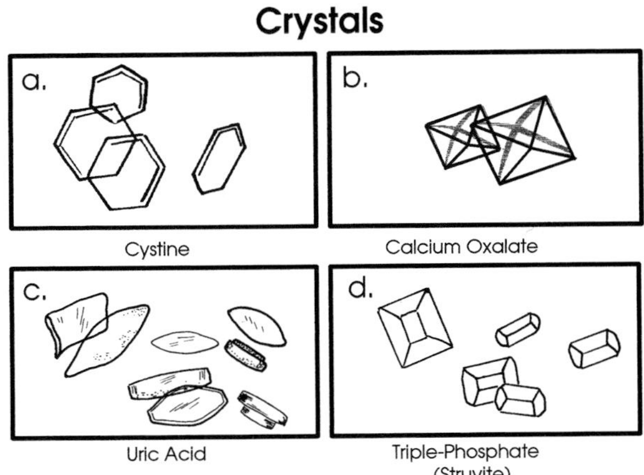

Figure 4–12. Urinary crystals. *A,* Cystine. *B,* Calcium oxalate. *C,* Uric acid. *D,* Triple-phosphate (struvite).

Bacteria (Fig. 4–13)

Normal urine should not contain bacteria, and in a fresh, uncontaminated specimen, the finding of bacteria is indicative of a urinary tract infection. Because each HPF views between 1/20,000 and 1/50,000 ml, each bacterium seen per HPF signifies a bacterial count of more than 20,000/ml. Therefore, **5 bacteria per HPF reflects colony counts of about 100,000/ml.** This is the standard concentration used to establish the diagnosis of a urinary tract infection in a clean-catch specimen. This level should apply only to women, however, in whom a clean-catch specimen is frequently contaminated. **The finding of any bacteria in a properly collected midstream specimen from a male should be further evaluated with a urine culture.**

Under high-power magnification, it is possible to distinguish various bacteria. Gram-negative rods have a characteristic bacillary shape, whereas streptococci can be identified by their characteristic beaded chains, and staphylococci can be identified when the organisms are found in clumps.

Yeast (Fig. 4–14)

The most common yeast cells found in urine are *Candida albicans.* The biconcave oval shape of yeast can be confused with erythrocytes and calcium oxalate crystals, but **yeast can be distinguished by their characteristic budding and hyphae.** Yeast are most commonly seen in the urine of patients with diabetes mellitus or as contaminants in women with vaginal moniliasis.

Parasites (Fig. 4–15)

***Trichomonas vaginalis* is a frequent cause of vaginitis in women and occasionally of urethritis in men.** Trichomonads can be readily identified in a clean-catch specimen under low-power magnification. Trichomonads are large cells with rapidly moving flagella that quickly propel the organism across the microscopic field.

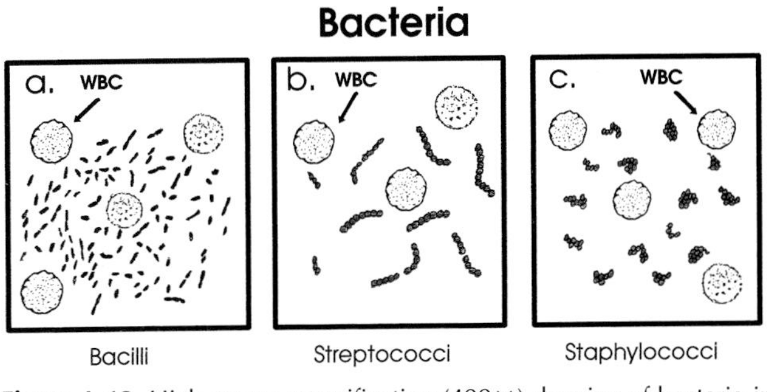

Bacteria

a. WBC | b. WBC | c. WBC

Bacilli | Streptococci | Staphylococci

Figure 4–13. High-power magnification (400×) drawing of bacteria in the urinary sediment. *A,* Bacilli. *B,* Streptococci. *C,* Staphylococci.

Yeast

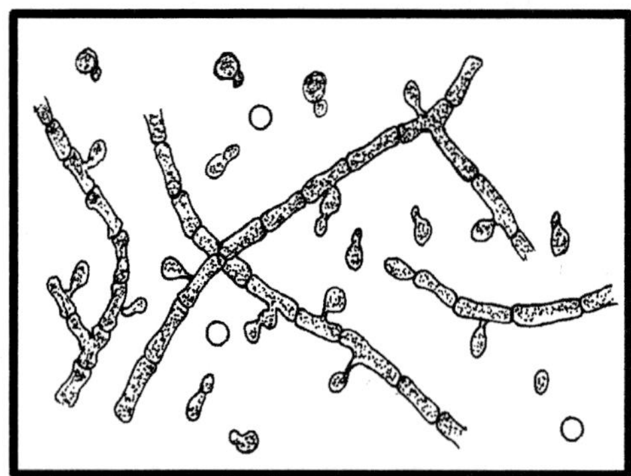

Candida Albicans

(Budding & Hyphae)

Figure 4–14. High-power magnification (400×) drawing of yeast. Note the characteristic budding and hyphae, which distinguish yeast from RBC.

Schistosoma haematobium **is a urinary tract pathogen that is not found in the United States but is extremely common in countries of the Middle East and northern Africa. Examination of the urine shows the characteristic parasitic ova with a terminal spike.**

Expressed Prostatic Secretions

Although not strictly a component of the urinary sediment, the expressed prostatic secretions should be examined in any man suspected of having prostatitis. Normal prostatic fluid should contain few, if any, leukocytes, and the presence of a larger number or clumps of leukocytes is indicative of prostatitis. **Oval fat macrophages are found in postinfection prostatic fluid.** Normal prostatic fluid contains numerous secretory granules that resemble but can be distinguished from leukocytes under high-power magnification because they do not have nuclei.

SUMMARY

This chapter has detailed the basic evaluation of the urologic patient, which should include a careful history, physical examination, and urinalysis. These three basic components form the cornerstone of the urologic evaluation and should precede any subsequent diagnostic procedures. After completion of the history, physical examination, and urinalysis, the urologist should be able to establish at least a differential, if not specific, diagnosis that will allow the subsequent diagnostic evaluation and treatment to be carried out in a direct and efficient manner.

Parasites

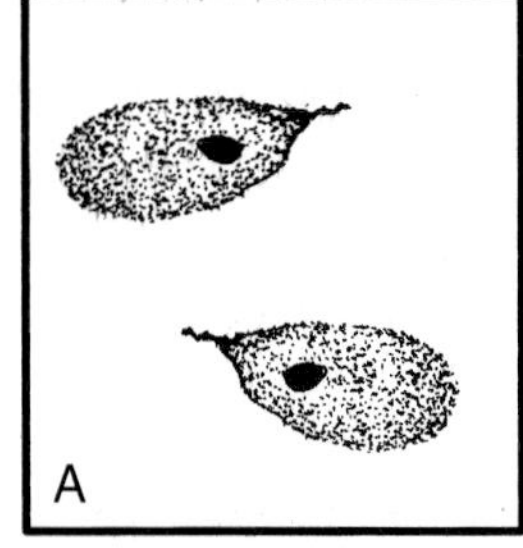

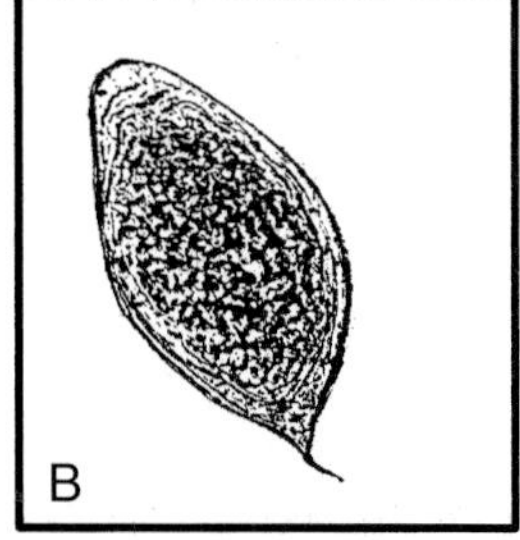

Trichomonas vaginalis — Schistosoma haematobium (ovum)

Figure 4–15. High-power magnification (400×) drawing of urinary parasites. *A, Trichomonas vaginalis. B, Schistosoma haematobium* ovum.

REFERENCES

Avellan L: The incidence of hypospadias in Sweden. Scand J Plast Reconstr Surg 1975; 9:129–138.

Barry MJ, Fowler, FJ, O'Leary MP, et al: The Measurement Committee of the American Urological Association. The American Urological Association symptom index for benign prostatic hyperplasia. Urology 1992; 148:1549–1557.

Berger J, Hinglais N: Les depots intercapillaires d'IgA-IgG. J Urol Nephrol (Paris) 1968; 74:694.

Blaivas JG, Kaplan SA: Urologic dysfunction in patients with multiple sclerosis. Semin Urol 1988; 8:159.

Carter BS, Bova GS, Beaty TH, et al: Hereditary prostate cancer: Epidemiologic and clinical features. J Urol 1993; 150:797–802.

Csako G: False positive results for ketone with the drug MESNA and other free-sulhydryl compounds. Clin Chem 1987; 33:289.

Culclasure TF, Bray VJ, Hasbargen JA: The significance of hematuria in the anticoagulated patient. Arch Intern Med 1994; 154:649–652.

Cushner HM, Copley JB: Back to basics: The urinalysis: A selected national survey and review. Am J Med Sci 1989; 297:193.

D'Amico G: Clinical features and natural history in adults with IgA nephropathy. Am J Kidney Dis 1988; 12:353–357.

Fassett RG, Horgan BA, Mathew TH: Detection of glomerular bleeding by phase-contrast microscopy. Lancet 1982; 1:1432.

Flanagan PG, Davies EA, Rooney PG, Stoot RW: Evaluation of four screening tests for bacteriuria in elderly people. Lancet 1989; 1:1117.

Forsythe WI, Redmond A: Enuresis and spontaneous cure rate: Study of 1129 enurectics. Arch Dis Child 1974; 49:259.

Gillenwater JY: Detection of urinary leukocytes by chemstrip. J Urol 1981; 125:383.

Jewett HJ: Significance of the palpable prostatic nodule. JAMA 1956; 160:838.

Kellog JA, Manzella JP, Shaffer SN, Schwartz BB: Clinical relevance of culture versus screens for the detection of microbial pathogens in urine specimens. Am J Med 1987; 83:739.

Kincaid-Smith P: Hematuria and exercise-related hematuria. BMJ 1982; 285:1595.

Meares EM, Stamey TA: Bacteriologic localization patterns in bacterial prostatitis and urethritis. Invest Urol 1968; 5:492–518.

Messing EM, Young TB, Hunt VB, et al: The significance of asymptomatic microhematuria in men 50 or more years old: Findings of a home screening study using urinary dipsticks. J Urol 1987; 137:919.

Messing EM, Young TB, Hunt VB, et al: Hematuria home screening: Repeat testing results. Urology 1995; 154:57–61.

Mohr DN, Offord KP, Owen RA, Melton LJ: Asymptomatic microhematuria and urologic disease: A population-based study. JAMA 1986; 256:224–229.

Morris RC, Ives HE: Inherited disorders of the renal tubule. *In* Brenner BM, Rector FC Jr, eds: The Kidney, 4th ed, vol 2. Philadelphia, WB Saunders Company, 1991, pp 1596–1656.

Mulhall JP, Albertsen PC: Hemospermia: Diagnosis and management. Urology 1995; 46:463–467.

Oster J: Further fate of the foreskin: Incidence of preputial adhesions, phimosis, and smegma among Danish schoolboys. Arch Dis Child 1968; 43:200.

Partin AW, Pound CR, Clemens JQ, et al: Serum PSA after anatomic radical prostatectomy. Urol Clin North Am 1993; 20:713–725.

Pels RJ, Bor DH, Woolhandler S, et al: Dipstick urinalysis screening of asymptomatic adults for urinary tract disorders: II. Bacteriuria. JAMA, 1989; 262:1221.

Propp DA, Weber D, Ciesta ML: Reliability of a urine dipstick in emerging dipstick patients. Ann Emerg Med 1989; 18:560.

Robinson RR: Clinical significance of isolated proteinuria. *In* Avram MM, ed: Proteinuria. New York, Plenum Medical Book Company, 1985, pp 67–82.

Sayer J, McCarthy JNP, Schmidt JD: Identification and significance of dysmorphic versus isomorphic hematuria. J Urol 1990; 143:545.

Schramek P, Schuster FX, Georgopoulos M, et al: Value of urinary erythrocyte morphology in assessment of symptomless microhematuria. Lancet 1989: 2:1316.

Shaw ST, Pan SY, Wong ET: Routine urinalysis: Is the dipstick enough? JAMA 1985; 253:1956.

Stephenson TP, Farrar DJ: Urodynamic study of 15 patients with post-micturition dribble. Urology 1977; 9:404–406.

van den Wall Bake AW, Daha MR, van Es LA: Immunopathogenetic aspects of IgA nephropathy. Nephrologie 1989; 10:141.

Wagner MG, Smith FG Jr, Tinglof BO, Cornberg E: Epidemiology of proteinuria: A study of 4807 school children. J Pediatr 1968; 73:825.

Warner MA, Offord KP, Warner ME, et al: Role of preoperative cessation of smoking and other factors in postoperative pulmonary complications: A blinded prospective study of coronary artery bypass patients. Mayo Clin Proc 1989; 64:609–616.

Woolhandler S, Pels RJ, Bor DH: Dipstick urinalysis screening of asymptomatic adults for urinary tract disorders: I. Hematuria and proteinuria. JAMA 1989; 262:1215.

5
INSTRUMENTATION AND ENDOSCOPY

H. Ballentine Carter, M.D.

Instrumentation and endoscopy of the lower urinary tract are performed routinely for the diagnosis and treatment of urologic diseases. A basic understanding of lower urinary tract anatomy and available instruments is essential for safe and successful manipulation of the lower urinary tract. This chapter will address basic techniques that are used in the office practice of urology. Ureteroscopy and other endoscopic techniques are addressed elsewhere.

URETHRAL CATHETERIZATION

Indications

Urethral catheterization is performed for both the diagnosis of and therapy for urologic disease. Many types of catheters are available for urethral catheterization, and the choice of a specific type of catheter depends upon the reason for catheterization.

With respect to diagnosis, catheterization is often performed in females for collection of urine for culture to avoid contamination by skin flora. This practice is usually not necessary in males because clean-catch specimens can be obtained without contamination by skin flora. Measurement of the postvoid residual urine can be performed less invasively with ultrasonography; however, catheterization can be performed for this purpose if ultrasound equipment is not available. Instillation of contrast agents into the bladder and urethra for cystourethrography, along with urodynamic studies to assess bladder and urethral function, necessitates urethral catheterization.

Relief of infravesical obstruction is one of the most common therapeutic indications for urethral catheterization. Infravesical obstruction can occur as a result of prostatic enlargement, blood clots within the bladder, postsurgical strictures, and urethral inflammatory processes. In these instances a specialized catheter may be required to relieve the obstruction. Urethral catheters are also used to drain the bladder after surgical procedures involving the lower urinary tract and in both medical and surgical fields to monitor urinary output accurately. Intermittent catheterization performed by the patient or an assistant is a common means of managing neurogenic bladder dysfunction when the bladder functions as a storage organ but no longer empties normally. Although many institutionalized patients are left with indwelling catheters because of urinary incontinence, it is preferable to manage these patients with intermittent catheterization or a condom device for urine collection, if possible, because of the risk of infection with long-term indwelling urethral catheters. Finally, in urologic practice, urethral catheters are often used as stents after surgery to allow healing of an anastomosis or incision involving the bladder neck or urethra.

Types of Catheters (Fig. 5–1)

It should be remembered that catheter size is usually referred to in terms of the French (Fr) scale (circumfer-

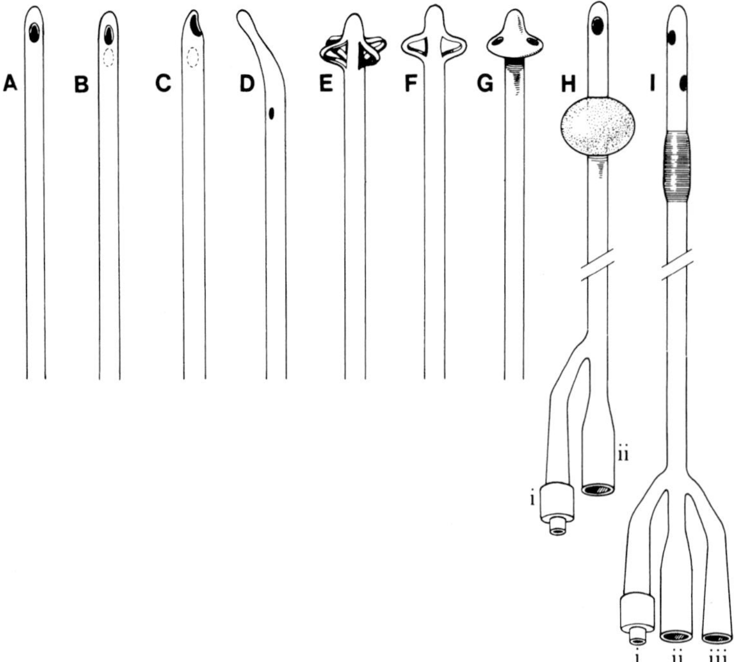

Figure 5–1. Types of large-diameter catheters. *A*, Conical tip urethral catheter, one eye. *B*, Robinson urethral catheter. *C*, Whistle-tip urethral catheter. *D*, Coudé hollow olive-tip catheter. *E*, Malecot self-retaining, four-wing urethral catheter. *F*, Malecot self-retaining, two-wing catheter. *G*, Pezzer self-retaining drain, open-end head, used for cystotomy drainage. *H*, Foley-type balloon catheter. *I*, Foley-type, three-way balloon catheter, with one limb of distal end for balloon inflation (i), one for drainage (ii), and one to infuse irrigating solution to prevent clot retention within the bladder (iii).

ence is in millimeters), whereby No. 1 Fr = 0.33 mm in diameter. For conversion from one scale to the other, it is easier to remember that each millimeter in diameter is approximately No. 3 Fr; thus a No. 18 Fr catheter is about 6 mm in diameter. A No. 20 Fr catheter may have a different luminal size for urinary drainage, depending upon the type of material used for construction and the number of lumens within the catheter (see later discussion).

Straight rubber or latex catheters (see Fig. 5–1*A* to *C*), often referred to as Robinson catheters, are most often used for one-time catheterizations (straight catheterization). These catheters also are available with multiple eyes, making them ideal for irrigating the bladder free of clots. Although these catheters can be left in place for bladder drainage by taping them to the penis, they are not as well tolerated as other catheter materials (e.g., silicone) because they have a tendency to become encrusted with urinary precipitates. Shorter, straight catheters are available for female patients.

Catheters with a curved tip (e.g., coudé catheters; see Fig. 5–1*D*) are specifically designed to help bypass areas of the male urethra that are difficult to negotiate with a straight catheter. The normal S-shaped male bulbar urethra and the prostatic urethra associated with an enlarged prostate can be difficult to bypass with a straight catheter because of the urethral angle associated with the former and bladder neck elevation associated with the latter. Curved tip catheters with balloons on the end (see description of Foley catheters) are available if it is necessary to leave the catheter indwelling after successfully passing a coudé catheter. In addition, coudé catheters can be used to irrigate out bladder clots by cutting additional holes in the end of the catheter if a straight catheter cannot be passed into the bladder.

Self-retaining catheters (see Fig. 5–1*E* to *G*), like the Pezzer and Malecot catheters, are shaped in such a way that after placement at open surgery, the catheter configuration maintains the catheter within a hollow viscus. For insertion, the wings of the catheter (i.e., retention mechanism) are flattened by stretching the catheter with a wire placed inside the catheter or stretching the catheter from outside with a clamp. The advantages of these catheters include the excellent urinary drainage afforded by the single lumen (no balloon mechanism) and the tip design, which make them ideal for use as cystostomy or nephrostomy tubes.

Foley-type catheters (see Fig. 5–1*H* and *I*) are most often used for long-term urethral catheterization. As such, they have a balloon mechanism at the distal end that, when inflated, keeps the catheter from sliding past the bladder neck. Two-way (see Fig. 5–1*H*) and three-way (see Fig. 5–1*I*) Foley catheters are available in multiple sizes. Two-way catheters have a small lumen for inflating the balloon mechanism and a larger lumen for urinary drainage. Three-way catheters have a small lumen for inflating the balloon mechanism, a lumen for instilling irrigant, and a larger lumen for bladder drainage. Two-way catheters are used when an indwelling catheter for urinary drainage is indicated. Three-way catheters are used when bladder irrigation and drainage are necessary, as, for example, in a patient with bladder hemorrhage at risk for forming clots within the bladder that may lead to obstruction of the bladder outlet. It should be remembered that catheters without a lumen for balloon inflation have a larger luminal size for bladder drainage than do Foley catheters of the same outer circumference. Likewise, for a given outer circumference, two-way catheters have a larger luminal size for urinary drainage than do three-way catheters.

Patient Preparation

As with all procedures, the patient should be informed of the reason for catheterization and what to expect in terms of discomfort. Because catheterization is the instrumentation of a potentially sterile tract, it is essential to prepare and drape the urethra and surrounding area as for a surgical procedure.

In the male, retrograde injection of 10 to 15 ml of a water-soluble lubricant anesthetic, such as 2% lidocaine hydrochloride jelly, and placement of a urethral clamp for 5 to 10 minutes to allow the anesthetic to contact the mucosal surfaces are recommended before any urethral instrumentation. In the female, the lubricant anesthetic can be placed directly on the catheter, or a Q-Tip coated with lubricant anesthetic can be placed in the urethra before catheterization.

Technique

In the male, the penis is placed on stretch perpendicular to the body (pointing slightly toward the umbilicus) without compressing the urethra, and the catheter is placed in the urethral meatus by holding the catheter at the tip. Gentle advancement of the catheter causes the least amount of discomfort, and with experience one can feel the natural resistance offered as the catheter traverses the external sphincter. As one approaches the bulbomembranous urethra (i.e., level of external sphincter), one should ask the patient to take slow, deep breaths, which will help relax the patient and often allow easier catheter passage. If resistance is met, one should not attempt forceful catheter insertion but should apply continuous, gentle pressure and ascertain at what level the potential obstruction exists.

In the female, shorter catheters are available for one-time catheterizations. After spreading the labia, one can usually identify the urethral meatus easily, and the catheter is placed gently into the bladder.

If long-term catheterization is anticipated (more than 1 week), it is advisable to use a Foley catheter made of the most biocompatible material. **Catheters made of silicone are in general better tolerated over the long term than those made of materials such as latex and polyurethane.** In addition, one should choose the smallest urethral catheter that will accomplish the purpose of catheterization, because urethral secretions drain more easily around smaller catheters. Allowing egress of urethral secretions lessens the chance of a clinically significant urethral inflammatory response. In the adult, Nos. 16 to 18 Fr catheters are most often chosen for routine bladder drainage; in the pediatric age group, it is often necessary to use Nos. 3 to 5 Fr feeding tubes.

Difficult Catheterizations

Difficulty in catheterizing the male patient can result from a variety of causes. Inability to pass the S-shaped bulbar urethra and resistance to catheter passage at the bulbomembranous urethra with tightening of the external sphincter are common. These problems are easily overcome with a coudé catheter to negotiate the bulb or with slow, gentle pressure to bypass the external sphincter.

Urethral strictures, prostatic enlargement, and postsurgical bladder neck contractures can make urethral catheterization difficult. If one encounters difficulty passing a catheter, it is wise to have a logical stepwise plan to maximize the chances of success in overcoming the difficulty. Often the urologic history will give a clue as to the most likely problem preventing catheterization. For example, the patient with a history of gonococcal urethritis in whom catheterization presents a problem is likely to have a pendulous urethral stricture, whereas the patient who has undergone an open prostatectomy may likely have a bladder neck contracture. The history, together with the clinical observations from the initial unsuccessful urethral manipulation, should give the physician a clue as to the problem.

If difficulty in initial catheterization is encountered, it is advisable to inject retrograde 10 to 15 ml of a water-soluble lubricant anesthetic into the urethra if this has not previously been done. If the catheter is felt to have passed the bulbomembranous urethra and the problem is thought to be a bladder neck contracture, it is helpful to use a latex coudé catheter starting at No. 12 Fr., which will often bypass the obstruction. **The coudé tip may allow negotiation of the lip, which is sometimes present at the 6-o'clock bladder neck position in men with bladder neck contractures.** The curved tip of the catheter must be maintained in the same position during catheter passage with the 12-o'clock position (curved tip pointing up) marked at the connector end of the catheter. If coudé catheterization is not successful, it is sometimes possible to pass a guide wire with a floppy tip into the bladder. Next, an open-ended ureteral catheter is passed over the guide wire, and then a urethral catheter with an end hole (Councill catheter) can be passed over the guide wire and ureteral catheter (Fig. 5–2) (a No. 6 Fr ureteral catheter will pass over 0.038-inch guide wire; a No. 5 Fr catheter will pass over a 0.035-inch guide wire). Any catheter can be used as a Councill catheter if a hole punch is available so that an opening can be made in the catheter tip for insertion of the guide wire–ureteral catheter (see Fig. 5–2). Finally, a filiform catheter may negotiate the bladder neck, which can then be followed gently with a small follower screwed to the filiform (see Fig. 5–5 and see section on urethral dilation). If more than gentle pressure is necessary during an attempt to pass any instrument into the bladder, the procedure should be aborted before urethral trauma occurs.

When it is not possible to gently bypass a bladder neck contracture with a coudé catheter, guide wire, or filiform catheter, percutaneous placement of a cystostomy tube is preferable in order to avoid urethral trauma. Percutaneous cystostomy kits are available with catheter and obturator (Fig. 5–3*A*). Percutaneous puncture of the bladder is accomplished with the obturator and catheter assembled; withdrawal of the obturator leaves the catheter indwelling within the bladder. In preparation for percutaneous cystostomy placement, the suprapubic area is prepped and draped with the patient in the supine position. The percutaneous tract, about 2 inches above the symphysis pubis in the midline, should be anesthetized. Next, a spinal needle with a 10-ml syringe on the end is placed perpendicular to the skin and advanced while withdrawing on the syringe (see Fig. 5–3*B*). Correct placement of the needle is documented by withdrawal of urine into the syringe. The cystostomy catheter and obturator assembly are then placed in the same manner as the spinal needle, and the obturator is withdrawn, leaving the cystostomy catheter in place. The catheter is secured to the abdominal wall with suture material. Before consideration of percutaneous cystostomy placement, one should be certain that a coagulation disorder is not present and that the patient is not taking an anticoagulant. If there has been prior

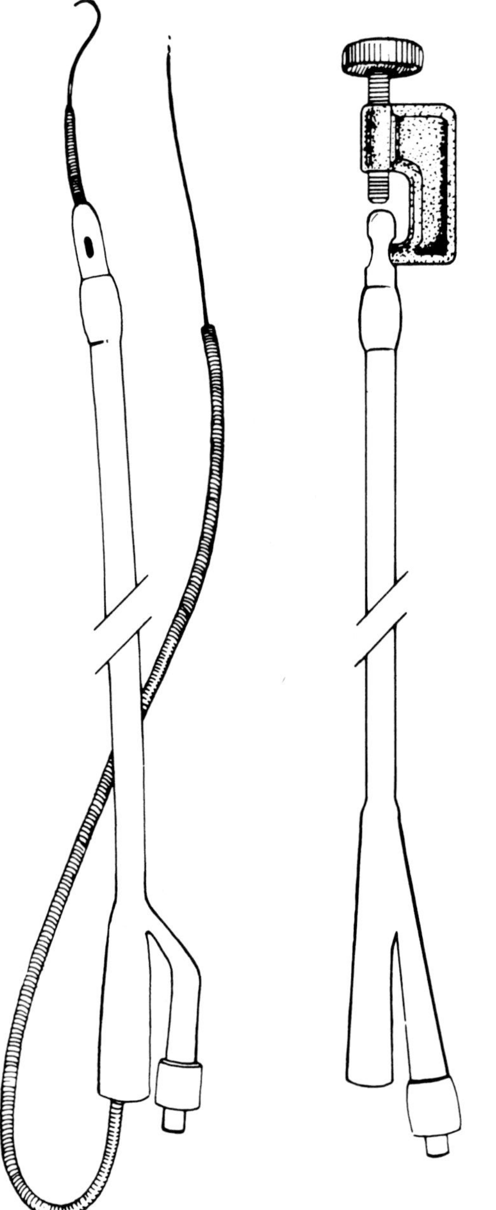

Figure 5–2. Councill catheter—with end hole—passed over a guide wire and ureteral catheter *(left);* creation of end hole in Foley-type catheter with hole punch *(right).*

abdominal or pelvic surgery, or if the bladder is not full, one should consider using ultrasound for bladder localization because the bowel may be in close proximity to the percutaneous tract.

It is not uncommon to encounter difficulty passing a catheter because of tight urethral strictures. Bypassing these areas with a catheter requires patience and gentle technique, because forceful catheterization inevitably results in false passages, bleeding, and the possibility of sepsis. Often there are already false passages from previous attempts at urethral catheterization. If one suspects urethral stricture disease to be the problem that is preventing urethral catheterization, the use of filiform catheters can be most helpful (see section on urethral dilation).

Difficulty in catheterization of the female urethra is uncommon and usually results from extreme obesity and inability to locate the urethral meatus. Placement of a vaginal speculum can aid in localization of the urethra. Also, a catheter can be directed cephalad into the urethra by using the vaginally placed finger as a guide.

URETHRAL DILATION

Indications

Urethral dilation in the male is most commonly performed in preparation for placement of an endoscope or as therapy for a urethral stricture or bladder neck contracture. It is not uncommon for the outer circumference of the instruments used in transurethral surgery (Nos. 24 to 28 Fr) to exceed the diameter of the urethra, especially the urethral meatus and fossa navicularis. In such a case, it is necessary to dilate the urethra gently before passing the endoscope. Dilation for urethral stricture disease and bladder neck contractures is a therapeutic option. However, repeated dilation can result in urethral trauma, which may ultimately increase the inflammatory process and worsen the stricture disease.

True urethral strictures in the female are uncommon without a history of prior urethral or bladder neck surgery. Although dilation of the female urethra as treatment for voiding dysfunction and recurrent infections was once a common practice, there are no objective data to support this form of treatment over other forms (e.g., medication). Occasionally it is necessary to dilate the female urethra gently before the introduction of a larger endoscope.

Patient Preparation

When urethral dilation is required before a transurethral procedure, no specific preparation is necessary because the patient has already been prepared and draped for surgery. Before urethral dilation is begun in an outpatient setting, it is mandatory to ensure sterility and obtain adequate local anesthesia, as described previously for urethral catheterization. If the patient has a urinary tract infection, it must be treated effectively before elective instrumentation.

Technique

Urethral dilation can be accomplished with metal sounds or bougies, urethral catheters of increasing size, filiforms and followers, and balloon expansion. Metal sounds with curved tips (Fig. 5–4) are useful for dilating the male urethra before endoscopy if the endoscope is too large to easily pass transurethrally. The urethra is generally dilated to one French size greater than the endoscopic instrument to be used. In males this is accomplished by holding the penis on stretch and rotating the sound while raising the penis cephalad as the sound approaches the bulbar urethra so that the curve of the sound conforms to the curve of the bulbar urethra. Care should be exercised in passing metal sounds; if resistance is met, it is unwise to exert force because this can result in severe urethral trauma. In the short female urethra, the pas-

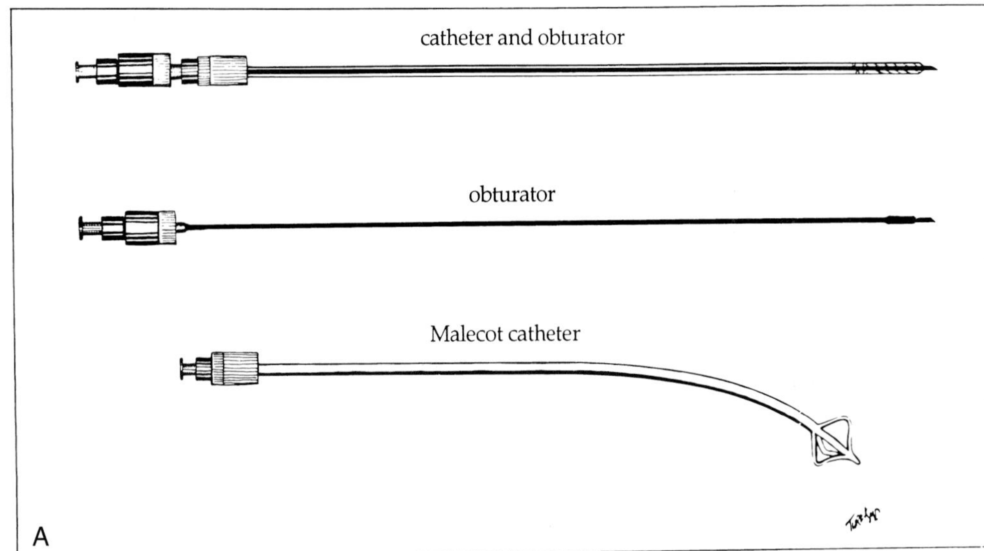

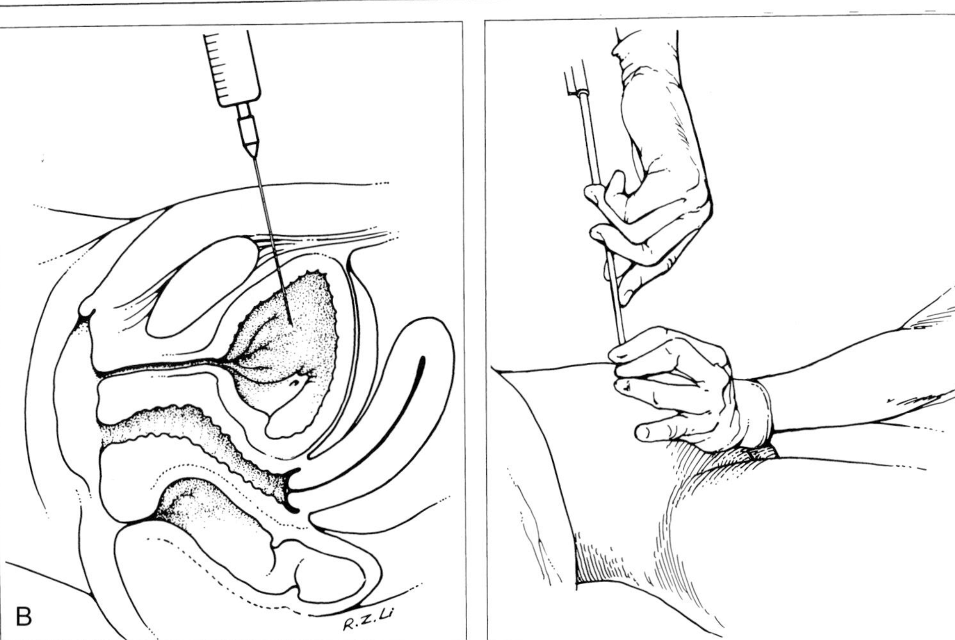

Figure 5–3. *A,* Stamey percutaneous cystostomy set with obturator and catheter. *B,* Localization of bladder with spinal needle placed percutaneously above pubic bone *(left);* placement of percutaneous cystostomy catheter with obturator *(right).* (From Zderic SA, Hanno PM: Suprapubic cystostomy and cutaneous vesicostomy. *In* Fowler JE, ed: Urologic Surgery. Boston, Little, Brown, 1992, pp 235, 236.)

sage of short, straight metal sounds, like that of catheters, is straightforward.

Urethral catheters of increasing size can be used for urethral dilation and are passed as previously described. Patients can be taught self-dilation in order to help prevent strictures from re-forming after treatment. This approach is more appropriate for older patients with strictures that are easily bypassed by urethral catheters after surgical incision of the stricture.

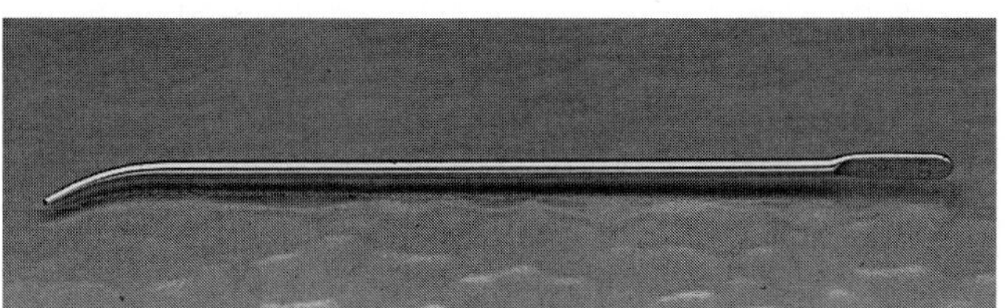

Figure 5–4. Metal sound with curved tip designed for negotiating male urethra and commonly used for urethral dilation. (Courtesy of C.R. Bard, Inc., Covington, GA.)

Filiforms are small-caliber straight- or spiral-tip (No. 5 Fr or smaller) catheters without a lumen, onto which a larger catheter (follower) with a lumen can be attached (Fig. 5–5). The filiform tip is passed without the follower first and maintains access to the bladder once it has been passed by coiling in the bladder. The follower is then screwed onto the filiform and is used to dilate the obstruction by gentle passage behind the filiform. Upon withdrawal of the follower, a larger follower can be placed on the filiform and the catheterization repeated. Filiforms and followers are useful for bypassing and dilating urethral strictures. A single filiform (straight or spiral tip) can occasionally negotiate a tight stricture; however, more commonly the filiform will pass into a false passage associated with the stricture. One can often continue gently passing multiple filiforms into the urethra and eventually occlude the false passage, allowing

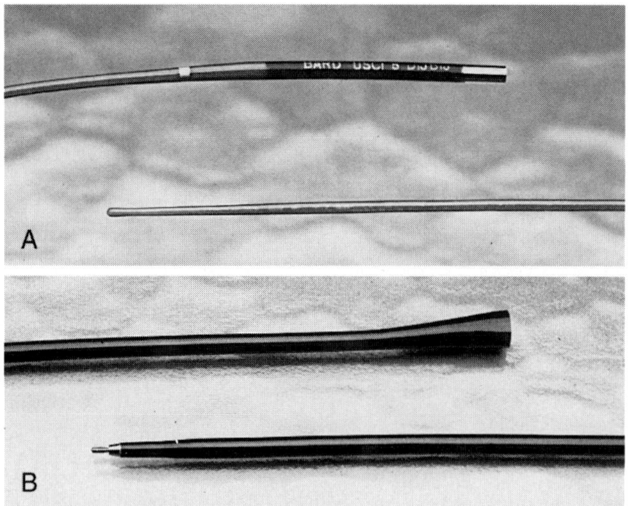

Figure 5–5. *A,* Filiform with grooved metal end to accept follower. *B,* Follower with metal tip designed to screw onto filiform. (Courtesy of C.R. Bard, Inc., Covington, GA.)

one of the filiforms to pass through the strictured area into the bladder. This is most often successful by loading the false passage with straight filiforms and using a spiral-tip filiform to pass into the bladder. Placement of 5 to 10 filiforms may be required to bypass a difficult urethral obstruction. Filiforms and followers can be used for initial dilation of a urethral stricture to allow passage of a catheter, as described previously. However, repeated dilations with filiforms and followers are not recommended for the treatment of urethral strictures. Patients with strictures that require repeated passage of filiforms to bypass the obstruction should undergo some form of definitive treatment.

An angioplasty balloon can be placed over a wire and inflated to accomplish urethral dilation if a wire can be negotiated into the bladder. This method of urethral dilation requires fluoroscopy for proper placement of the balloon and may cause less trauma than other forms of urethral dilation.

CYSTOURETHROSCOPY

Indications

Direct visualization of the anterior and posterior urethra, bladder neck, and bladder is accomplished by cystourethroscopy. The primary indication for cystourethroscopy is the diagnosis of lower urinary tract disease. However, access to the upper urinary tract for diagnosis and treatment can be accomplished cystoscopically.

With regard to the diagnosis of lower urinary tract disorders, signs and symptoms that may be related to the urinary tract are evaluated with cystourethroscopy to directly visualize lower urinary tract anatomy and macroscopic pathology, which may be responsible for the clinical picture under evaluation. In addition, material for both cytologic and histologic examination can be obtained through cystourethroscopic techniques.

One of the most common indications for cystourethroscopy is in the evaluation of microscopic and gross hematuria. By combining radiographic and endoscopic techniques, one can usually determine the source of bleeding in the upper or lower urinary tract (see section on retrograde pyelography). Other indications for cystourethroscopy include evaluation of voiding symptoms (obstructive and irritative), which may be the result of neurologic, inflammatory, neoplastic, or congenital abnormalities.

Access to the upper urinary tract can be obtained cystoscopically. Diagnostic contrast examination of the entire upper urinary tract is accomplished by retrograde injection of contrast agents through small catheters passed cystoscopically (see section on retrograde pyelography). Ureteral stents to bypass or prevent ureteral obstruction as well as ureteral catheters and brushes can be passed cystoscopically to obtain material for cytologic and histologic examination from the upper urinary tract. In most cases, fluoroscopy is used in conjunction with these diagnostic and therapeutic procedures of the upper urinary tract.

Patient Preparation

It is important to ensure that the patient does not have an active urinary tract infection before cystourethroscopy, because of the possibility of exacerbating the infection by instrumentation of the urinary tract. After the patient has been counseled regarding the purpose of the procedure, the preparation is the same in the male as for urethral catheterization. In the female, 5 to 10 ml of lubricant anesthetic jelly should be instilled into the urethra before the procedure. It is important to ensure sterility and obtain adequate urethral anesthesia for diagnostic cystourethroscopy. With local urethral anesthesia, biopsy and cauterization of the urethral and bladder mucosa can be accomplished cystoscopically. In addition, upper urinary tract instrumentation can be performed. More extensive endoscopic procedures should be performed with general or regional anesthesia.

Endoscopic Equipment

Cystourethroscopy can be performed with either rigid or flexible endoscopes (Figs. 5–6 and 5–7). There are many advantages to the use of the rigid endoscope for cystourethroscopy: (1) better optics because of the use of a rod-lens system in rigid instruments, in contrast to the fiberoptic system in flexible instruments; (2) a larger working channel that allows the urologist greater versatility in passage of accessory instruments; (3) a larger lumen for water flow, thus improving visualization; and (4) ease of manipulation and maintaining orientation during inspection within the bladder. The advantages of flexible endoscopes for cystourethroscopy include (1) greater comfort for the patient; (2) the ability to perform the procedure in the supine position; (3) the ease of passing the instrument over an elevated bladder neck; and (4) the ability to inspect at any angle with deflection of the tip of the instrument.

The size of cystourethroscopes is usually given according to the French scale and refers to the outside circumference of the instrument in millimeters. Instruments of different

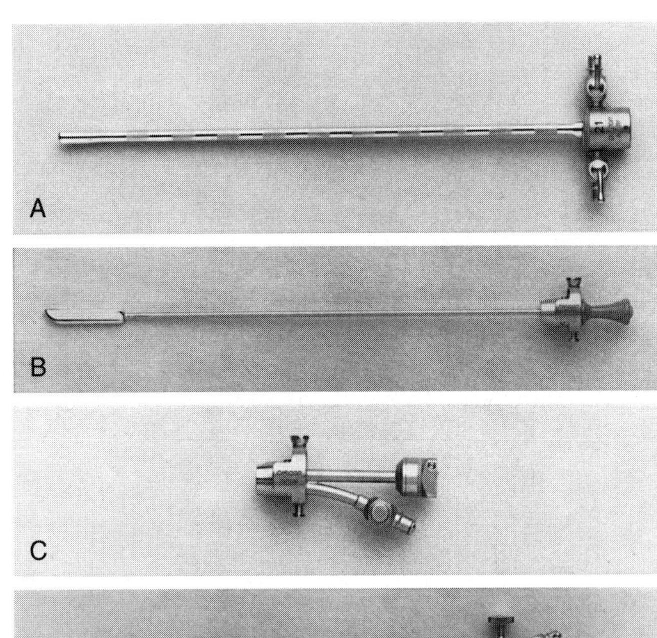

Figure 5–6. Rigid cystoscope consists of metal sheath to which water source is attached *(A);* obturator *(B);* bridge *(C);* deflector system (Albarran lever) *(D);* and lens to which light source is attached *(E).* (Courtesy of Circon Corp., Santa Barbara, CA.)

sizes are available to accommodate pediatric patients (Nos. 8 to 12 Fr) and adults (Nos. 16 to 25 Fr).

Modern rigid cystourethroscopes consist of a sheath, an obturator, a bridge, and telescopes (see Fig. 5–6). The telescopic lens is placed through the sheath by attaching a bridge to the sheath. The bridge allows both passage of the telescope and access to the working channel of the sheath for passage of accessory instruments. A deflector system (Albarran lever) can be placed through the sheath to allow passage and controlled deflection of catheters through the working channel. The irrigant fluid is connected to the sheath, and the fiberoptic light source connects directly to the telescope. Obturators can be placed through the sheath to provide a smooth, blunt tip for easy passage, and obturators through which a telescope can be passed (visual obturators) provide a method of easy direct visual passage of the endoscope.

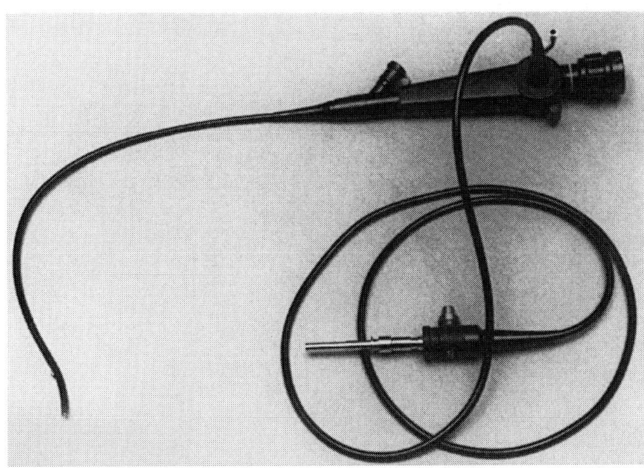

Figure 5–7. Flexible cystoscope with attached light source and deflectable tip. (From Denstedt JD: Cystoscopy: Rigid and flexible. *In* Krane RJ, Siroky MB, Fitzpatrick JM, eds: Clinical Urology. Philadelphia, J.B. Lippincott, 1994, p 529.)

Telescopes consist of illuminating and imaging systems. Modern telescopes use fiberoptic illumination and a rod-lens imaging system. The objective lens at the tip of the instrument collects the light of the image and transmits the image to the eyepiece through the rod-lens system. Telescopes are available with different angles of view for urethroscopy and bladder inspection. A 0-degree lens, which is focused to view straight ahead, is usually used for urethroscopy. A 30-degree lens best affords visualization of the base and anterolateral aspect of the bladder, and a 70- to 90-degree lens is used to view the bladder dome. Retrograde lenses with an angle of view greater than 90 degrees can be used to visualize the anterior bladder neck.

Flexible cystourethroscopes (see Fig. 5–7) contain fiberoptic bundles within a flexible shaft for illumination and visualization. The shaft has an irrigating channel and a working channel for passage of accessory instruments. The tip of a flexible endoscope can be deflected 180 to 220 degrees by a thumb control located near the eyepiece.

The image from a rigid or flexible endoscope can be

transmitted to a TV monitor with the use of a video camera (video-cystourethroscopy) (Fig. 5–8). Modern video cameras may contain an optical device that divides the light into two paths (beam-splitter) to provide simultaneous video-monitor projection and direct viewing through the endoscope. Endoscopic images can be transferred to a video-recording device and taped, allowing documentation and review of a procedure. A video-cystoscopic unit consists of the endoscope, video-camera head and controller, light source, TV monitor, and video-recording device for storage of images on tape (see Fig. 5–8). With a video-cystoscopic unit, the endoscopist can perform the procedure by using the image on the TV monitor to guide movement of the endoscope instead of looking through the eyepiece of the endoscope. The advantages of this approach include (1) avoidance of contact with body fluids; (2) documentation of the procedure by using a video recorder; (3) use of the TV monitor for teaching purposes; and (4) patient education.

Technique

Any urologic irrigant can be used for cystourethroscopy; most often, sterile water or saline is used. **If electrocoagulation is planned, it is necessary to avoid solutions containing electrolytes.**

In general, the choice of an endoscope with respect to size should be the same as for catheter size: the smallest outer circumference that will accomplish the task. If diagnostic cystourethroscopy is being performed, a small instrument (Nos. 16 to 17 Fr) is adequate. If a larger working channel is needed for accessory equipment (e.g., a biopsy device), a larger endoscope is chosen.

Systematic inspection of the entire urethra and bladder should be performed during cystourethroscopy. Before insertion of the instrument, the urethral meatus should be inspected if this has not already been accomplished. If the meatal size appears inadequate to accept the endoscope, it can be dilated with metal sounds (see section on urethral dilation). After the sheath of the cystourethroscope is generously lubricated with a water-soluble anesthetic lubricant, the endoscope can be passed under direct vision with a 0- to 30-degree lens.

In the male, the penis should be grasped and straightened so that it forms almost a right angle to the abdominal wall. The endoscope is passed through the fossa navicularis, and the anterior urethra is inspected as the instrument is gently passed. Any mucosal abnormality should be noted, and the diameter of the urethra should be evaluated. If there is resistance to the passage of the endoscope, a smaller instrument should be used or the urethra should be dilated. As the instrument is advanced and enters the bulbar urethra with its greater diameter, the endoscope and penis are lowered while the instrument is passed until the penis is parallel with the floor. This allows passage of the instrument through the membranous urethra. The external sphincter is easily identifiable at the level of the membranous urethra by the mucosal folds radiating from a narrow lumen ahead of the endoscope. Gentle pressure facilitates passage of the endoscope through this area. When the instrument passes into the prostatic urethra, the verumontanum is noted. The prostatic urethra is inspected, and the size of the prostatic lobes is evaluated together with the length of the prostatic urethra, which can be elongated with prostatic hyperplasia. At the level of the bladder neck, it may be necessary to depress the endoscope gently in order to pass the instrument into the bladder over

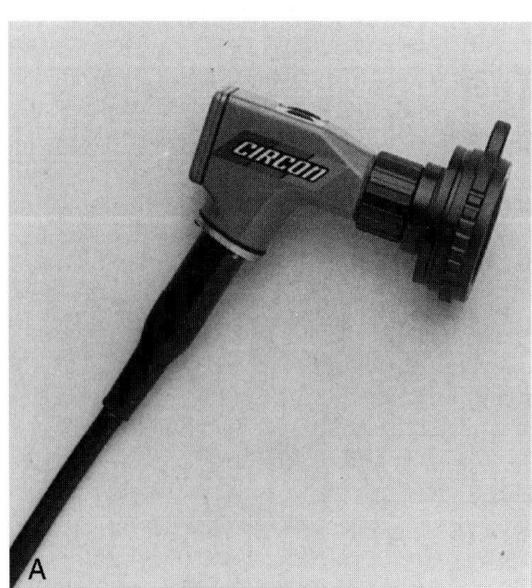

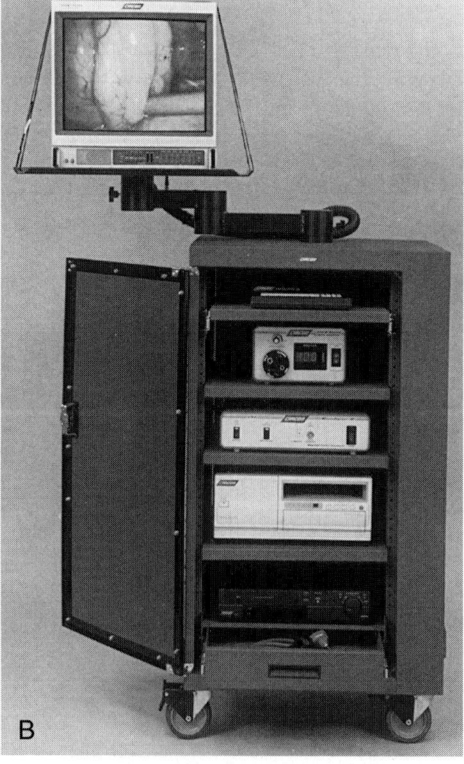

Figure 5–8. Video-cystoscopy unit consists of a camera head, which is placed directly over eyepiece of cystoscopic lens *(A),* and video cart containing TV monitor, light source, video-camera controller, and video-recording device (VCR) *(B).* (Courtesy of Circon Corp., Santa Barbara, CA.)

the bladder neck. An alternative technique is to pass the rigid endoscope "blindly" into the bladder as one would pass a metal dilator, with inspection of the urethra on withdrawal of the endoscope.

Inspection of the female urethra is easily performed by inserting the endoscope under direct vision into the urethral meatus and by directing the instrument cephalad toward the umbilicus.

Once the endoscope is inside the bladder, a systematic evaluation of the entire bladder surface is performed. Using the 30-degree lens with the bladder only slightly filled, one can identify the interureteric ridge just inside the bladder neck along the trigone. Next, the ureteral orifices are visually located several centimeters lateral from the center of the interureteric ridge and should be observed as passage of clear urine occurs bilaterally. The floor of the bladder behind the trigone and posterior bladder wall are inspected. Using the 70- to 90-degree lens, one can systematically inspect the lateral walls of the bladder by moving the endoscope from anterior to posterior and back as the bladder fills slowly. Finally, the dome and anterior bladder wall are evaluated with the 70- to 90-degree lens, with the bladder air bubble instilled at the time of instrumentation as a landmark on the dome of the bladder. The anterior bladder wall just behind the bladder neck is best seen with the bladder only partially filled and with one hand exerting suprapubic pressure to depress the anterior bladder wall. After complete inspection of the urethra and bladder has been accomplished, the bladder is drained and the instrument is gently removed.

It is important to document the procedure in a systematic fashion as it was performed. The urologist should have a systematic method of performing cystourethroscopy that allows careful inspection of the entire lower urinary tract from the urethral meatus to the bladder and that at the same time causes minimal discomfort for the patient.

RETROGRADE PYELOGRAPHY

Retrograde pyelography is a technique of radiographically demonstrating the ureter and renal collecting system (pelves, infundibula, and calyces) by injecting a radiopaque contrast agent under pressure into the ureter. With increasing use of and improvements in other imaging modalities, retrograde pyelography is used less often than in the past. However, specific indications remain for the use of this technique in urologic practice.

Indications

The primary reason for performing retrograde pyelography is to visualize radiographically the ureter or renal collecting system as part of a urologic work-up in which the intravenous urogram has provided inadequate radiographic visualization. Better definition of the upper urinary tract by retrograde pyelography is sometimes required during the evaluation of hematuria, persistent filling defects of the ureter or renal collecting system, an unexplained positive urinary cytologic specimen collected from the upper urinary tract, and fistulas or obstructions involving the ureter. With the advent of nonionic contrast agents, retrograde pyelography is rarely indicated for visualization of the ureter and renal collecting system in a patient who is allergic to intravenous contrast. It should be recognized that retrograde injection of contrast media can result, albeit rarely, in allergic reactions because absorption of contrast agents can occur during retrograde pyelography. In addition, retrograde pyelography can result in urinary sepsis as a result of increased intrapelvic pressures with extravasation of bacteria into the venous or lymphatic system. This occurs when patients with an unrecognized urinary tract infection undergo retrograde studies. Less acute but significant urinary tract infections can be precipitated by introduction of bacteria during retrograde injection above an upper tract obstruction. Consideration should be given to decompression of the urinary tract by retrograde ureteral stent placement or nephrostomy tube placement in the patient with an obstructed upper urinary tract who has undergone retrograde pyelography and in whom poor drainage of contrast is demonstrated on delayed films.

Patient Preparation

Retrograde pyelography is a cystoscopic procedure that can be performed with local intraurethral anesthesia, as previously described. Patient preparation is the same as for cystoscopy. Care should be exercised in ensuring that the urinary tract is sterile before retrograde injection and that patients with poorly draining upper urinary tracts receive preprocedural antibiotics. The patient with sterile urine and a normally draining upper urinary tract does not routinely require preprocedural antibiotics.

Technique

Before retrograde pyelography, cystourethroscopy should be routinely performed. Several types of ureteral catheters (Fig. 5–9) are available for performing retrograde pyelography, and the choice depends upon the preference of the urologist and the purpose of the study. Whistle-, olive-, spiral-, and cone tip catheters can be used for retrograde injection of contrast. The Nos. 4 to 6 Fr whistle-, olive-, or spiral-tip catheters and the Nos. 8 to 12 Fr cone tip catheters are used most often. The cone tip catheter is designed to occlude the ureteral orifice as contrast is injected retrograde, thus filling the ureter and renal collecting system at the same time. The whistle-, olive-, and spiral-tip catheters are placed into the upper tract before injection of contrast, and the renal collecting system and ureter are filled on separate films.

Regardless of the type of catheter chosen, several important points should be kept in mind. A scout film should be routinely performed before injection of contrast material, as with intravenous urography (see discussion on urography). The ureteral catheter should be placed gently without force to prevent submucosal undermining and possible perforation of the ureter. If the study is being performed for evaluation of a possible transitional cell cancer of the upper tract and if collection of urine for cytologic analysis from the upper tract is being considered, it is important to collect the cytologic specimen before retrograde injection of contrast material. Hyperosmolar contrast agents can result in poorly pre-

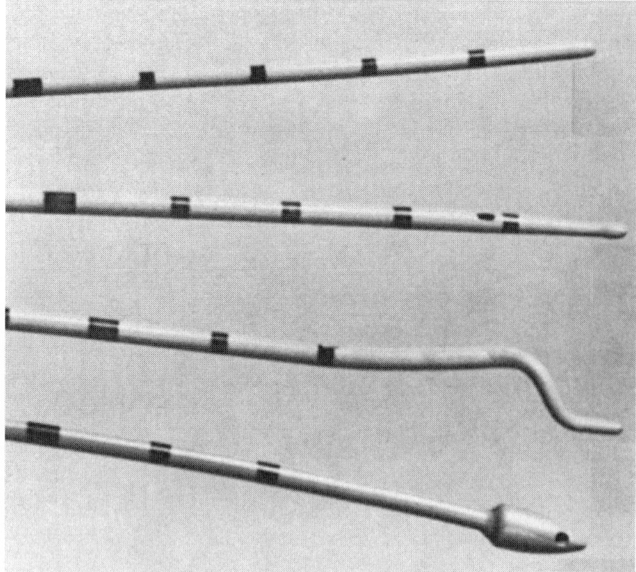

Figure 5–9. Commonly used ureteral catheters, from top to bottom, have round, olive, spiral, and cone or "bulb" tips.

served cytologic specimens, thus making interpretation difficult.

After cystoscopic examination, the ureteral orifice is catheterized with the ureteral catheter after it is certain that any air bubbles have been flushed out of the catheter. An additional film is often obtained at this point to document the location of the ureteral catheter before injection of contrast, especially if the catheter has been passed into the renal pelvis. Ureteral catheters designed for passage into the renal pelvis have markings that can be seen cystoscopically in such a manner that one can ascertain how far the catheter has been passed. The distance from the ureteral orifice to the ureteropelvic junction is between 20 and 25 cm.

A syringe filled with contrast is attached to the ureteral catheter with a needle or an adapter. Approximately 5 to 10 ml of a 50% solution of any routinely used urographic contrast agent is injected slowly and gently into the ureter (cone tip) or renal pelvis (whistle, olive, spiral tip)—unless the upper tract is known to be dilated—and then additional contrast may be needed. After contrast injection, anteroposterior and oblique films are developed as needed to visualize the ureter and collecting system with respect to any abnormality. If fluoroscopy is available, the study can be monitored and the need for additional contrast to fill the collecting system completely will be evident during injection. If a whistle-, olive-, or spiral-tip catheter has been passed into the collecting system for contrast injection, once the renal collecting system has been visualized, a ureterogram is obtained. This is accomplished by injecting several additional milliliters of contrast into the renal pelvis and continuing injection as the catheter is slowly withdrawn (as in a withdrawal ureterogram). A film is developed immediately as the catheter is withdrawn from the ureteral orifice. Alternatively, one can use a cone tip catheter to obstruct the ureteral orifice and fill the ureter with contrast. Once the ureter and renal collecting system have been visualized, a delayed film can be helpful in evaluating upper tract drainage. The patient is instructed to sit or stand for approximately 15 minutes, and an additional film is developed. Retention of contrast material in the upper urinary tract on delayed films is abnormal and suggestive of obstruction.

Ureteral Stents

Indwelling ureteral catheters are commonly used as stents (for urinary drainage) to bypass intrinsic (e.g., stones) or extrinsic (e.g., tumor compression) ureteral obstructions, to prevent obstruction from passage of stone material after shock wave lithotripsy, to promote urinary drainage and healing after ureteroscopic procedures (e.g., stone retrieval), and to bypass urinary fistulas to promote spontaneous closure. Ureteral stents can be placed endoscopically through either rigid or flexible cystoscopy. Because these catheters are often left indwelling for long periods, biocompatibility of stent material is an important aspect of stent choice. Ureteral stents made of hydrophylic-coated synthetic polymers are being used with increasing frequency because of their ease of passage, biocompatibility, and resistance to encrustation with long-term stenting. The most commonly used stent design (Fig. 5–10*A*) has a coil at either end (double-coil stent) that will result in retention of the stent within the ureter when one end is coiled in the renal pelvis and the other end is coiled in the bladder. Indwelling ureteral catheters are available in various French sizes and lengths, but larger sizes (Nos. 6 to 8 Fr) provide better urinary drainage. Stent length in centimeters is determined by measuring the distance from the renal pelvis to the ureterovesical junction from radiographic studies (intravenous pyelogram or retrograde pyelogram).

Before the physician attempts placement of an indwelling ureteral catheter to bypass urinary obstruction, the patient should understand that a percutaneous nephrostomy may be necessary in the event that stent passage is unsuccessful, and the personnel and equipment necessary for percutaneous access should be available. Cystoscopic placement of an indwelling ureteral catheter should begin with carefully performed retrograde pyelography to define the level and nature of the obstruction if this has not been done previously. Next,

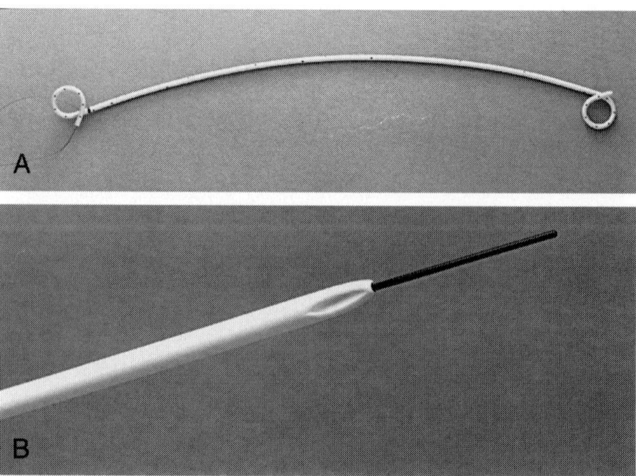

Figure 5–10. *A,* Indwelling ureteral stent with coil at proximal *(right)* and distal *(left)* ends, and suture attached at distal end for easy removal. *B,* Open-ended catheter with guide wire used to bypass ureteral obstruction. (Courtesy of Microvasive, Watertown, MA.)

a flexible-tip guide wire should be placed cystoscopically up the ureter to the renal pelvis—under fluoroscopic guidance—to bypass the obstruction. A hydrophilic guide wire can be utilized if initial attempts with standard guide wires are unsuccessful. Placement of an open-ended catheter up to the obstruction and guide wire placement through the catheter (see Fig. 5–10*B*) can often provide access by increasing the torque and changing the position of the wire relative to the obstruction.

Once guide wire access has been obtained, the ureteral catheter to be left indwelling is placed over the guide wire and advanced to the renal pelvis with a pusher catheter while the guide wire is stabilized by an assistant. Fluoroscopy is used to confirm the correct positioning of the ureteral catheter, and the guide wire is withdrawn while the pusher catheter holds the ureteral catheter in place. Upon withdrawal of the guide wire, the coils on either end of the ureteral catheter form and retain the stent in the correct position. Urinary drainage cannot be ensured unless the stent is properly placed with one coil in the renal pelvis and the other in the bladder. Thus, stent placement with coiling of both ends of the catheter should be radiographically confirmed before completion of the procedure. For short-term stenting (several days), a suture attached to the bladder (distal) end of the stent can be brought out through the urethra for easy removal of the stent without cystoscopy (see Fig. 5–10*A*). The suture can be removed before stent placement if the catheter is to be left indwelling over a long term. Ureteral catheters should be changed approximately every 3 months because of the tendency for encrustation and blockage.

Stent changes in the female can be accomplished by using an endoscopic grasper to withdraw the distal end of the stent outside the urethral meatus. Next, a guide wire is placed through the stent and coiled in the renal pelvis under fluoroscopic guidance. The old stent can then be withdrawn while maintaining access to the kidney by simultaneously advancing the guide wire while withdrawing the old stent. A new stent can be placed over the guide wire as described earlier. In the male, a guide wire must be placed beside the old ureteral stent and advanced into the renal pelvis, because the stent is not long enough to withdraw outside the longer male urethra and still maintain access to the upper urinary tract. Once guide wire access has been obtained, the old stent can be removed with an endoscopic grasper and a new stent can be placed over the guide wire.

6
URINARY TRACT IMAGING AND INTERVENTION: BASIC PRINCIPLES

Nicholas Papanicolaou, M.D.

DIAGNOSTIC URORADIOLOGY

Radiographic investigation of urologic diseases has long been an integral part of patient management. Historically, plain radiography, retrograde pyelography, and intravenous urography (IVU) have been used to screen patients with flank pain, hematuria, or suspected urinary obstruction. New developments in intravascular contrast media, sonography, computed tomography (CT), magnetic resonance imaging (MRI), and percutaneous or endoluminal interventions under imaging guidance have contributed to improved and safe diagnosis and treatment for a variety of urologic disorders. Although physician preference and availability of imaging modalities often dictate the order or choice of procedures, close cooperation between the radiologist and the urologist always benefits the patient and expedites the work-up while keeping the cost under control.

The first part of this chapter analyzes the diagnostic techniques used in clinical practice; the second part presents a number of interventional techniques that, either alone or in conjunction with endourologic (endoscopic) procedures, are used in the treatment of selected urologic problems.

Contrast Media

Contrast media are used in imaging to enhance demonstration of anatomic and/or pathophysiologic changes that cannot be made conspicuous by the mere differences

in tissue attenuation of x-rays, ultrasound waves, or radiofrequency waves.

Intravascular administration of iodinated contrast agents for diagnostic purposes is very common in the practice of uroradiology (Lasser, 1990). IVU, angiography, and CT rely heavily or exclusively on the use of these agents. Furthermore, direct injection of contrast media through needles and catheters into hollow viscera or structures such as the renal pelvis, ureter, and bladder urethra is widespread. MRI often relies on intravenous injection of substances with magnetic susceptibility, called paramagnetic agents, for the purpose of selective enhancement of certain organs and the changes brought upon them by specific disease entities (Watson et al, 1992). The use of contrast agents in sonography is mostly in the investigational stage at this time.

Currently, two classes of iodinated contrast media are available for use in clinical practice: the high-osmolality and the low-osmolality agents. The classification is based on the relative osmolality of these compounds in comparison with that of the serum. The low-osmolality media have been in use longer elsewhere in the world. Both groups of agents are, for practical purposes, cleared through the kidneys by glomerular filtration.

The high-osmolality contrast media (HOCM), also known as conventional contrast media, are meglumine and/or sodium salts of the fully substituted tri-iodobenzoic acid derivatives diatrizoic acid (Renografin or Hypaque) and iothalamic acid (Conray). In solution, all HOCM dissociate or ionize into two osmotically active particles: the radiopaque anion and a cation. Because they all contain three atoms of iodine per molecule, these agents are also referred to as ratio 3:2 or ratio 1.5 media (three iodine atoms with two ions). **The osmolalities of HOCM, therefore, often exceed that of the serum by a factor of 5 to 7.**

The low-osmolality contrast media (LOCM) were developed in an effort to reduce the osmolality of the conventional agents and thus to reduce many of their adverse effects. Iohexol, iopamidol, and ioversol are also tri-iodinated derivatives of benzoic acid; however, they are not salts, as are the conventional media, and therefore **their osmolalities are significantly lower than those of the HOCM, although, depending on the iodine concentration, they can still be two to three times as high as that of serum.** The LOCM agents are known as ratio 3 media, because three atoms of iodine correspond to one particle. Furthermore, **the lack of sodium and meglumine cations eliminates all adverse effects attributed to these ions.**

The LOCM are further divided into dimeric and nonionic media. The representative agent for the former is ioxaglate (hexabrix), an ionic dimer containing two benzoic acid rings (therefore six atoms of iodine) and two particles or ions; thus it is a 6:2, or 3, ratio medium. The other commonly available LOCM are nonionic. They include iohexol (Omnipaque), iopamidol (Isovue), and ioversol (Optiray).

Although iodinated contrast agents are among the most commonly used and safest drugs, **their administration is associated with several well-described reactions, which can be subdivided into minor and major types** (Cohan et al, 1996). **Several of these reactions (e.g., hives, laryngeal and facial edema, and bronchospasm) are idiosyncratic or anaphylactic in nature and may be prevented or lessened by pretreatment with corticosteroids or antihistamines.** Other reactions are clearly not allergic in nature; they include some of the more severe manifestations such as hypotension, pulmonary edema, and dysrhythmia. **Patients with a history of drug allergy, shellfish/seafood allergy, or asthma have an approximately twofold increased risk of contrast reactions. This risk is three to four times as great or about 15% to 20% in patients who have experienced a previous contrast-related reaction.** However, patients who have experienced a prior contrast reaction do not necessarily experience a reaction when reexposed to contrast agents.

There are three strategies for reducing the incidence of contrast-associated reactions: (1) study substitution, (2) use of low-osmolar contrast agents, and (3) pretreatment with corticosteroids and/or antihistamines. If a patient has had a previous moderate or severe reaction, an alternative study without intravascular contrast (e.g., sonography, radionuclide study, CT) could be performed if possible. Pain, nausea, vomiting, and some vascular and cardiac adverse effects are related to the hyperosmolality of conventional contrast agents. The incidence of these reactions can be reduced by using newer low-osmolar contrast agents. However, the cost of these new contrast agents is about 10 to 20 times that of the conventional agents. In patients with a strong allergic diathesis or a history of a reaction after contrast administration, corticosteroid pretreatment can be given. Premedication with corticosteroids (methylprednisolone, 32 mg, given 12 and 2 hours before contrast exposure) has proved effective in reducing the incidence of all reactions that necessitate therapy by 42% and major, life-threatening reactions by 62% (Lasser et al, 1987). However, steroid or antihistamine premedication does not lessen pain or discomfort during intra-arterial administration of contrast or lessen the side effects of contrast agents on the heart.

Contrast agents are potential nephrotoxins, and contrast nephropathy (CN) is the third most common cause of acute renal failure in the hospitalized patient population. CN is defined as an increase in serum creatinine of 0.5 to 1 mg/dl and/or a 25% to 50% decrease in glomerular filtration rate (GFR) after intravascular contrast material administration and appears to be dose-related. In most patients, the acute renal failure is self-limited: creatinine values increase within 24 hours of exposure to iodinated contrast media, peak at 2 to 5 days, and return to normal by 7 to 12 days. Patients usually are not oliguric; however, the presence of oliguria imparts a poorer prognosis for recovery of normal renal function. **Prevention of CN involves identification of patients who are at increased risk. Patients with both kinds of diabetes, particularly the insulin-dependent type, and baseline creatinine level elevated over 3.5 mg/dl are especially prone to contrast-induced renal failure. Patients with severe congestive heart failure and those with markedly elevated uric acid levels are also at a higher risk.** CN is probably not seen with increased frequency in patients with multiple myeloma, dehydration, hypertension, or proteinuria or in those over 65 years of age unless there is preexisting renal insufficiency. **Adequate hydration of high-risk patients before and after the administration of contrast media may have a prophylactic effect on the renal function. Some reports in the literature indicate that the use of LOCM may be less nephrotoxic** than that of HOCM in high-risk patients. Treatment of CN is largely supportive, and only in rare instances is short-term dialysis necessary.

The comparative safety of the two groups of contrast media has been the focus of many clinical studies in the literature, some of them not adequately controlled and randomized. **It is generally agreed that the incidence of mild and moderate adverse reactions is lower with the low-osmolality agents (Katayama et al, 1990).** Reactions do occur, including severe ones and death, with both groups. In view of the high cost of total conversion to LOCM, many hospitals have adopted selective use of the safer agents, mostly in patients with history of significant previous reaction, recent myocardial infarction, and unstable angina and asthma and in children. Also, most neuroradiologic, vascular, diagnostic, and interventional procedures are performed with low-osmolality agents.

Extravasation of contrast media into the soft tissues at or near the site of injection occurs relatively frequently, but it usually resolves without significant consequences. Elderly patients with poor local circulation, such as those with peripheral vascular disease, deep venous thrombosis, Raynaud's phenomenon, or diabetes are more prone to serious complications. Soft tissue necrosis and sloughing of the skin, if extensive, may damage adjacent tendons, nerves, and vessels and cause permanent deformities, scarring, or limb dysfunction. The risk also is higher with the use of high-power injectors for CT imaging or angiography, in which a large amount of contrast material can be rapidly infused into the soft tissues, if the vascular access is compromised. Chemotoxicity, hyperosmolarity, and compression by the large volume of extravasated contrast material are responsible for the local changes. Careful and safe vascular access minimizes the occurrence of extravasation and should be mandatory in every institution where contrast media are given. LOCM produce fewer side effects when extravasated and should be given preference over HOCM in high-risk clinical settings.

Intravenous Urography

Despite occasional although persistent reports in the literature calling for its replacement by sonography or CT, **IVU remains the modality of choice for the visualization of the entire urinary tract and especially the urothelium covering the pyelocalyceal systems, ureters, and bladder** (Dunnick et al, 1991). The examination provides both anatomic and renal physiologic/functional information, although not in a quantitative manner for the latter.

Current indications for the performance of IVU vary with physicians' familiarity and preference, availability of and access to alternative imaging modalities, patients' condition, and the clinical problems under investigation. Most often, **flank pain, hematuria, known symptomatic lithiasis, and abnormal urine cytology are preferably and appropriately evaluated by IVU.** Sonography is the modality of choice in infants and children in whom congenital genitourinary problems are suspected. Renal trauma nowadays is best evaluated by CT. Suspected renal masses may be imaged by IVU; however, sonography and contrast-enhanced CT are superior to IVU in demonstrating masses smaller than 3 cm in diameter, as well as in differentiating solid lesions from cysts. **Screening IVU in patients with prostatism or vague lower urinary tract symptoms should be discouraged.**

There are few contraindications to the performance of IVU. It seems wise that patients with well-documented, previous severe reactions to contrast media undergo an alternative examination, such as sonography, CT, or retrograde pyelography. Premedication with steroids and H_1 and H_2 histamine receptor antagonists or use of LOCM may reduce the risk of a serious reaction, if the examination is truly indicated on sound medical grounds. Patients with **moderate or worse renal failure** probably should not undergo IVU for two reasons: first, the study will likely yield very little information about the urinary tract because excretion is greatly reduced and delayed; second, the intravascular administration of contrast material will almost certainly exacerbate the existing renal insufficiency. Patients with mild renal failure may undergo IVU, if necessary; however, both adequate hydration before and after the injection of the contrast material and a decrease in the amount of contrast material are recommended as prophylactic measures. The use of LOCM may also offer additional protection against nephrotoxicity. Mannitol and/or furosemide often have been given together with hydration to patients receiving intravascular contrast agents. Mannitol is given after, whereas furosemide has been given either before or after the contrast material.

Patients undergoing multiple radiologic examinations requiring intravascular contrast agents on consecutive days are at increased risk for nephrotoxicity. The referring physician and the radiologist should discuss the need, order, and timing of such studies, mindful of the potentially damaging cumulative effect on the kidneys even without pre-existing renal failure. The studies can be prioritized and spread out over a period of a few days while the patient is kept well hydrated.

Pathologic entities such as diabetes and multiple myeloma are not contraindications to IVU unless there is pre-existing renal insufficiency. Adequate hydration is required for patients with multiple myeloma undergoing IVU. Patients with congestive heart failure should be stabilized first and given as low a volume load of contrast as possible.

Preparation of a generally healthy, ambulatory patient before IVU usually includes a mild laxative the night before for cleansing of the colon; regular hydration; and no breakfast for morning appointments and a light breakfast for afternoon appointments. Inpatients and emergency ward patients often are examined without preparation. A recent laboratory evaluation of renal function often is requested of outpatients before the examination.

The choice of contrast material to be given varies greatly from one hospital to another. Low-osmolality agents are safer with regard to mildly and moderately severe adverse reactions. Private offices and small clinics with limited capability for handling emergencies may make use of the safer agents exclusively. Ambulatory patients are asked about risk factors, such as cardiac, pulmonary, or renal disease; allergies; and previous exposure to intravascular contrast media. A decision can be made as to the type of contrast material on the basis of the patient's general present condition and history. If no communication with a patient is possible (language barrier, neurologic problems, etc.), it is advisable to

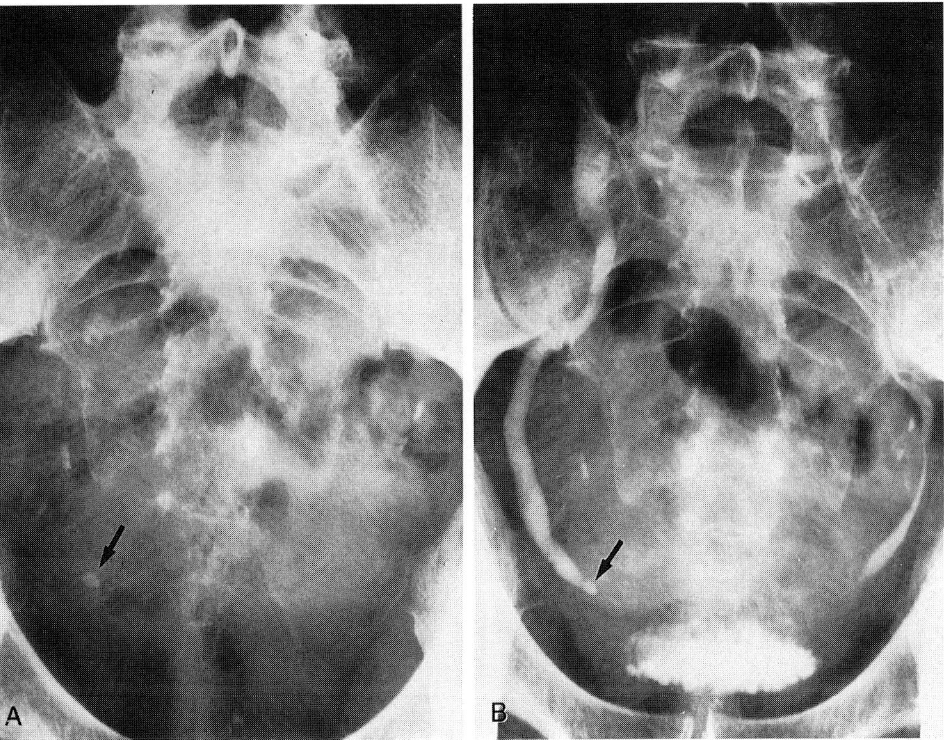

Figure 6–1. Value of plain radiograph in a patient with suspected urolithiasis. *A,* Coned-down view of the pelvis from a plain abdominal radiograph shows a calcification *(arrow)* in the right lower quadrant. *B,* The same calcification is shown to be a partially obstructing right lower ureteral calculus *(arrow)* on subsequent intravenous urogram.

use the LOCM. Requests for specific agents that are made by referring physicians or patients are honored.

The examination begins with a plain radiograph of the abdomen (Pollack and Banner, 1994). This is an essential part of the study because it may be the best or only radiograph to demonstrate urinary calculi (Fig. 6–1). Other calcifications and masses, as well as bony and bowel gas pattern abnormalities, may be present and helpful in establishing the eventual diagnosis (Fig. 6–2).

The intravenous administration of the contrast material is done either rapidly (bolus injection) or, less often, as a slower drip infusion (Hattery et al, 1988). The amount of contrast material given varies, depending on the preference of the radiologist and the size of the patient. Bolus injections usually deliver 50 to 100 ml, and drip infusion delivers 200 to 300 ml.

The filming sequence depends on the technique of injection. With a bolus injection, renal parenchymal opacification occurs fast and lasts a short period of time; therefore, filming begins immediately after the completion of the infusion. With drip infusion, renal parenchymal opacification occurs at a slower pace over several minutes and lasts longer; therefore, imaging usually begins when half of the volume of the contrast material has been infused. **Nephroto-**

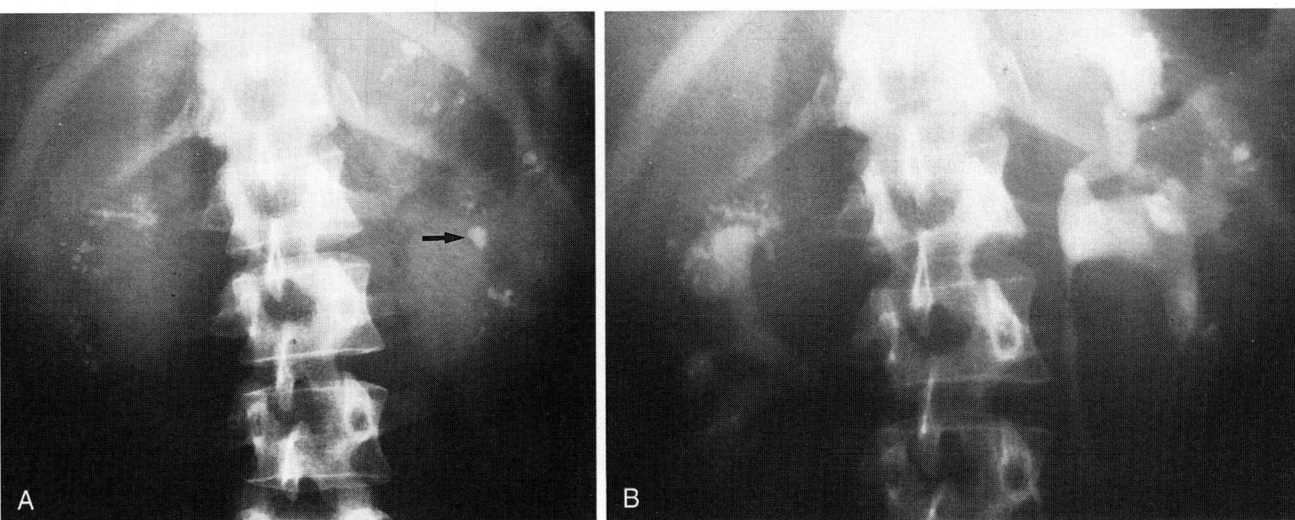

Figure 6–2. Value of plain radiograph in a patient with medullary sponge kidney disease. *A,* Plain radiograph shows multiple small calcifications throughout both kidneys in a distribution that strongly suggests medullary (papillary) nephrocalcinosis. The larger triangular calcification in the left kidney *(arrow)* is a calculus. *B,* The intravenous urogram confirms the papillary location of the calcifications.

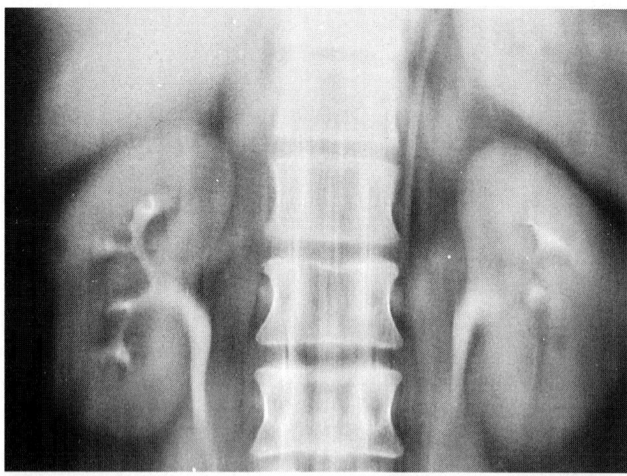

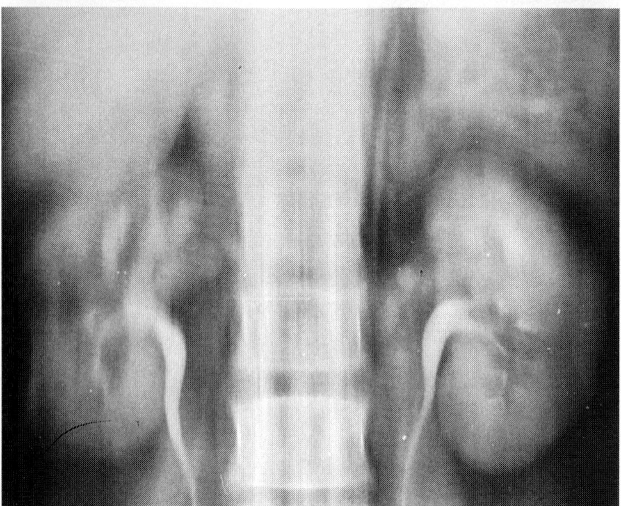

Figure 6–3. Nephrotomography outlines the renal contours and demonstrates the calyceal systems clearly and without interference from overlying bowel loops.

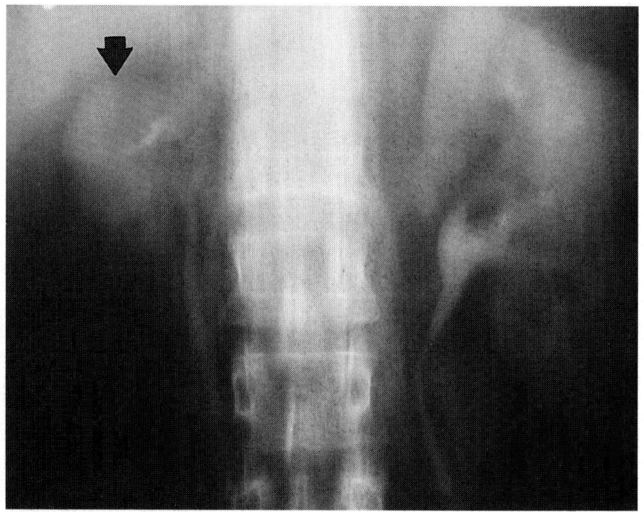

Figure 6–4. Nephrotomography clearly demonstrates a functioning small right kidney *(arrow)* that was difficult to evaluate on overhead radiographs during intravenous urography. There was a long history of recurrent urinary tract infections in childhood secondary to vesicoureteric reflux into the lower pole moiety of the right kidney, leaving the upper pole moiety as the only functioning part of that kidney.

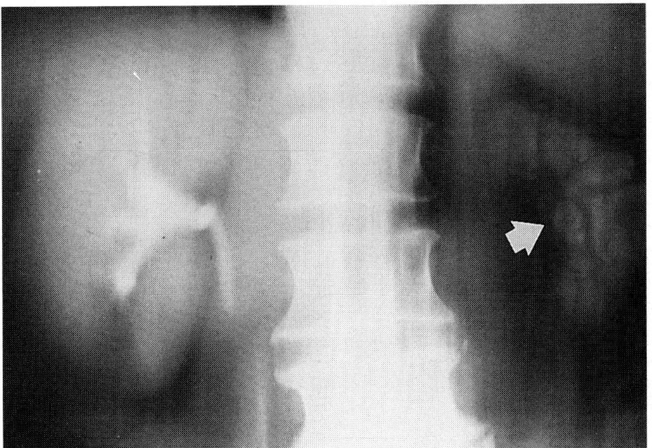

Figure 6–5. Nephrotomography in a patient with a history of renal tuberculosis shows a small, nonfunctioning calcified left kidney *(arrow)* as a result of advanced renal involvement (autonephrectomy).

mograms or a strip film of the kidneys is taken. The former are obtained at different levels to include the more posterior upper and the more anterior lower renal poles and are preferable to plain films because they can outline the kidney, usually without interference from overlying bowel loops or other viscera in the abdomen (Figs. 6–3 to 6–9).

Renal parenchymal opacification alone, referred to as the nephrogram or nephrographic phase of IVU, occurs within the first minute after injection and can be obtained only with the bolus technique (Newhouse and Pfister, 1979) (Fig. 6–10). **The pyelocalyceal system is rapidly opacified within 1 to 2 minutes afterwards, and this is referred to as the pyelogram or pyelographic phase of IVU.** With the drip infusion technique, both the nephrogram and pyelogram are visualized by the time filming begins.

After the opacification of the pyelocalyceal system occurs, full-size abdominal films are obtained within the next several minutes in the supine and both posterior oblique positions to demonstrate the ureters and bladder (Figs. 6–11 to 6–20). **Additional radiographs are taken as dictated by the findings.** Prone films are done to opacify the ureters to a better advantage, when necessary. Erect films may be obtained for evaluation of renal ptosis, ureteral obstruction, bladder hernias, and cystoceles and for detection of air-fluid levels in abscesses or layering milk of calcium in calyceal diverticula. **Delayed views often are necessary in cases of urinary obstruction or unexpected nonvisualization of parts of the urinary tract. A postvoid radiograph is routinely obtained in patients with native and orthotopic bladders** for evaluation of the postvoid residual bladder volume. Also, certain small bladder tumors may be

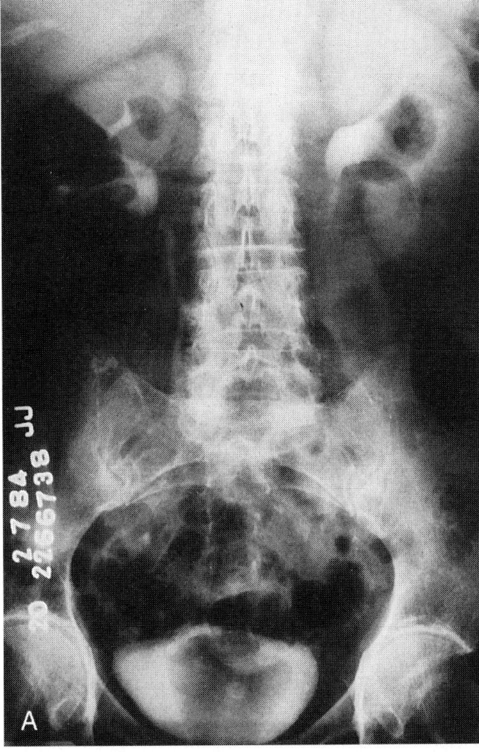

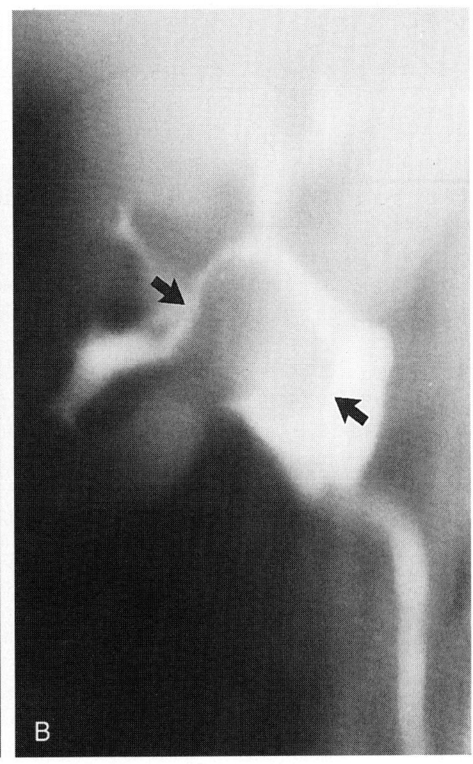

Figure 6–6. Transitional cell carcinoma in the right renal pelvis of an elderly woman. *A,* Overhead radiograph from an intravenous urogram is limited by the presence of bowel loops overlying both kidneys. *B,* Right nephrotomogram clearly shows a large filling defect in the renal pelvis *(arrows).*

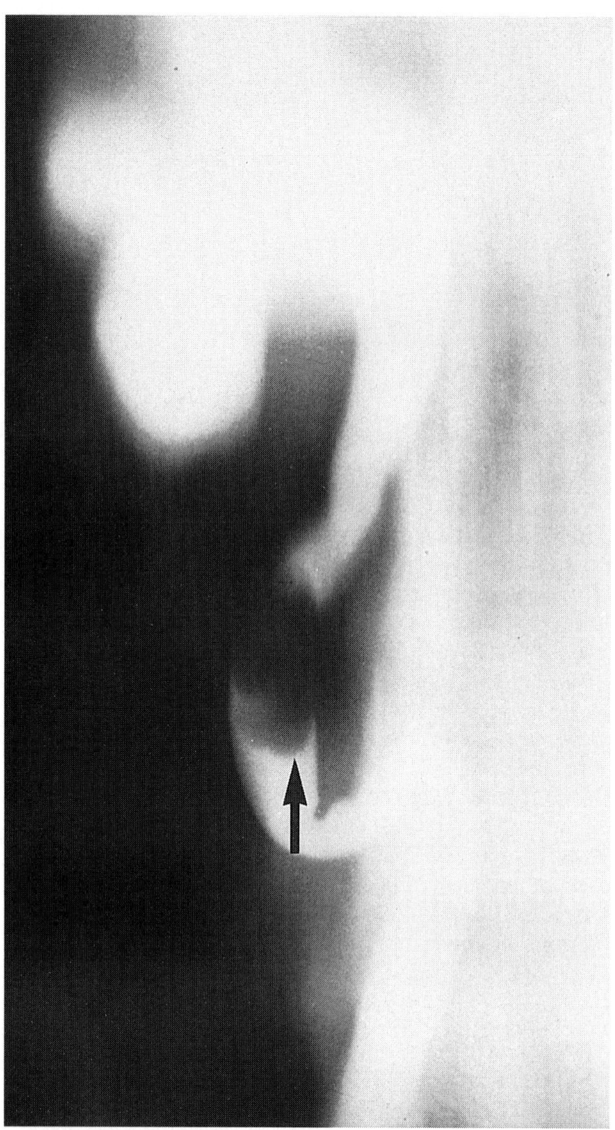

Figure 6–7. Transitional cell carcinoma of the right ureter *(arrow)* is superbly demonstrated on nephrotomography without the interference of overlying bowel loops.

seen to a better advantage on the postvoid film, on which interference from a large amount of radiopaque urine, which may obscure urothelial lesions, is minimized (Fig. 6–21).

Modification in these techniques and filming sequences are appropriate in cases of absent or ectopic kidneys and renal transplants. Patients with one kidney should receive a smaller amount of iodinated contrast material, preferably one half of the full dose. Renal transplants and ectopic kidneys require coned-down imaging of the area in the abdomen where such kidneys are found.

There are two additional modifications of IVU: the diuretic and hypertensive urograms (Pollack and Banner, 1994). Both are currently used on rare occasions, having been replaced by more sensitive radionuclide studies or magnetic resonance angiography in the case of renal artery stenosis.

The **diuretic urogram** may be indicated in cases of suspected borderline ureteral obstruction, often at the ureteropelvic junction, that manifests as intermittent flank pain. As a rule, the standard urogram is normal. The purpose of the study is to demonstrate dilatations of the urinary tract proximal to the narrowing and/or reproduce the symptoms by forced diuresis. Furosemide, usually at an intravenous dose of 40 mg, is given 15 to 20 minutes into the study with the expectation that the increase in urine volume will cause the decompensation of the transport mechanism of the urinary tract at the level of the ureteral narrowing. The diuretic radionuclide renogram is more sensitive, precise, and reproducible than the diuretic urogram and thus is the modality of choice for evaluating patients of all ages with suspected urinary obstruction.

The **hypertensive urogram** may be indicated in cases of suspected unilateral renal artery stenosis as the cause of significant and/or medically difficult to control hypertension (Fig. 6–22). The urographic findings most suggestive of renovascular disease are a slow onset, progressively denser nephrogram of the affected kidney with a corresponding delayed clearance of the nephrographic density, and a pyelogram delayed by 1 minute or more in comparison to the normal contralateral kidney. Eventually, the diseased kidney becomes small and its function decreases. After a bolus injection of the contrast material, strip images of both kidneys are obtained rapidly at 1-minute intervals for 5 minutes or more. This technique has been all but abandoned in

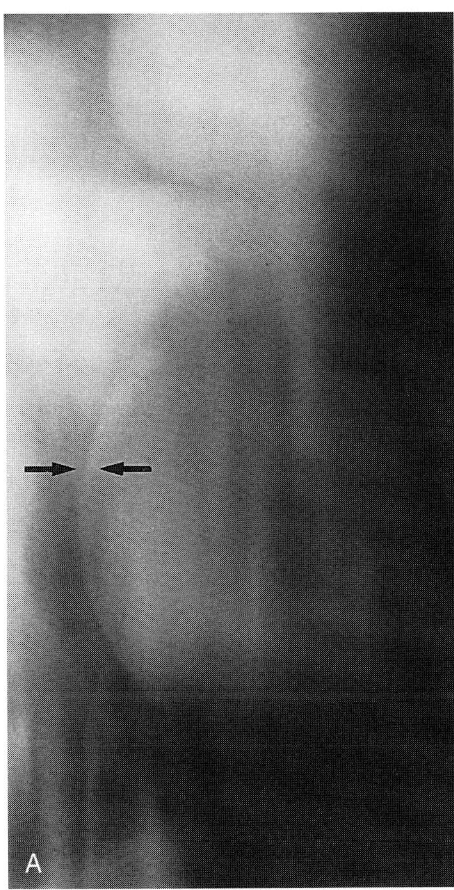

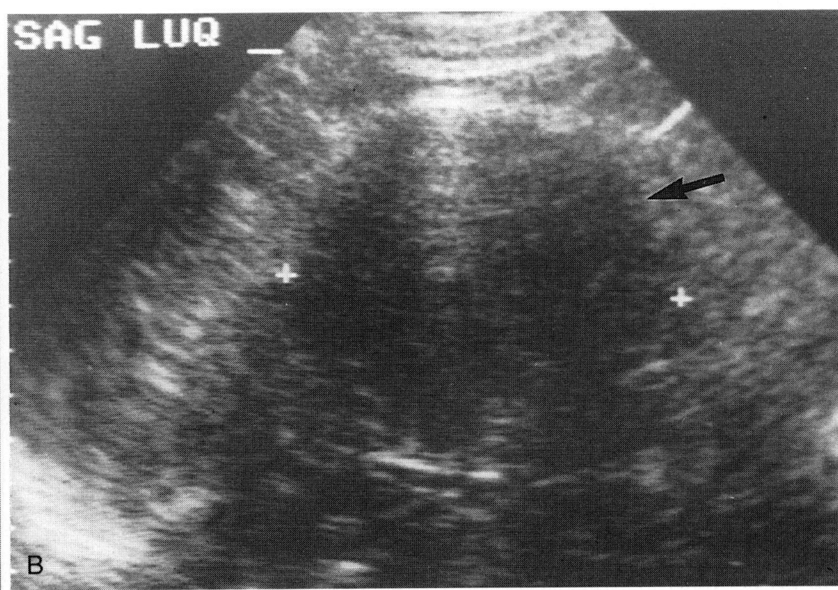

Figure 6–8. Nephrotomography of large left lower renal pole lesion thought to represent a simple cyst. *A,* Nephrotomogram shows a large, low attenuation lesion with a thick wall *(arrows),* which is not consistent with a simple renal cyst. *B,* Renal sonogram shows that the renal lesion contains internal echoes, is not well defined, and does not cause posterior acoustic enhancement *(arrow).* A cystic papillary renal cell carcinoma was found at surgery.

clinical practice because of its low sensitivity. Angiography, radionuclide studies, and magnetic resonance angiography are superior to hypertensive urography and have replaced it.

The nephrogram and pyelogram reveal a wealth of information regarding the structural and functional status of the kidneys (Newhouse and Pfister, 1979). Among the parameters and qualities examined, the most relevant are the absence or time of visualization, homogeneity, and duration of the nephrogram and the absence or time of visualization and density of the pyelogram. In addition, the latter is further evaluated for calyceal dilatation or effacement, ureteral dilatation, and presence of intraluminal filling defects or extravasation of the contrast material anywhere along the urinary tract (see Figs. 6–12, 6–13, and 6–15). With **worsening renal function,** visualization of the nephrogram and the pyelogram is delayed, the latter by several hours to days in severe cases. **Systemic hypotension** causes variable delays in the appearances of both, particularly the pyelogram, which may not be seen until the systolic pressure rises to 70 or 80 mm Hg in normotensive patients and higher in hypertensive patients. **Acute urinary tract obstruction** often appears as a dense, persistent nephrogram caused by reduced effective filtration pressure and glomerular filtration and increased resorption of water and sodium in the proximal convoluted tubules, resulting in increased concentration of the contrast material and increased nephrographic density (Fig. 6–23). In addition, the pyelogram is delayed up to several hours or more, depending on the degree of the obstruction (Fig. 6–24). If the process is at least 1 or 2 days old, some calyceal dilatation may be present. Extravasation of contrast material may be seen, resulting in relief of the symptoms and an impressive radiographic image of the affected kidney (Fig. 6–25). **Acute pyelonephritis** may cause diffuse heterogeneity or decrease in the density of the nephrogram and effacement and/or delayed visualization of the pyelogram. **Renal cysts and masses,** if large enough (3 cm in diameter or more), result in well- and ill-defined nephrographic defects, respectively (Fig. 6–26). The sensitivity of IVU in demonstrating focal renal lesions is inferior to that of sonography and CT. **Nephrotomography is particularly prone to missing anterior or posterior exophytic renal cysts and masses.**

Retrograde Pyelography

The retrograde opacification of the urinary tract after endoscopic cannulation of the ureteral orifice is known as retrograde pyelography or urography (Dunnick et al, 1991). The renal parenchyma is bypassed by the direct instillation of contrast material into the collecting system; therefore, the parenchyma cannot be evaluated. **Urothelial lesions, unusual anatomy of the ureter or pyelocalyceal system, including congenital variations thereof, ureteral obstruction, and the creation of an anatomic map of the urinary tract before a percutaneous or endourologic procedure are the most common indications for the performance of a retrograde pyelogram** (Figs. 6–27, 6–28). **In certain cases, visualization of the urinary tract by means of IVU is limited or suboptimal. The intravenous study**

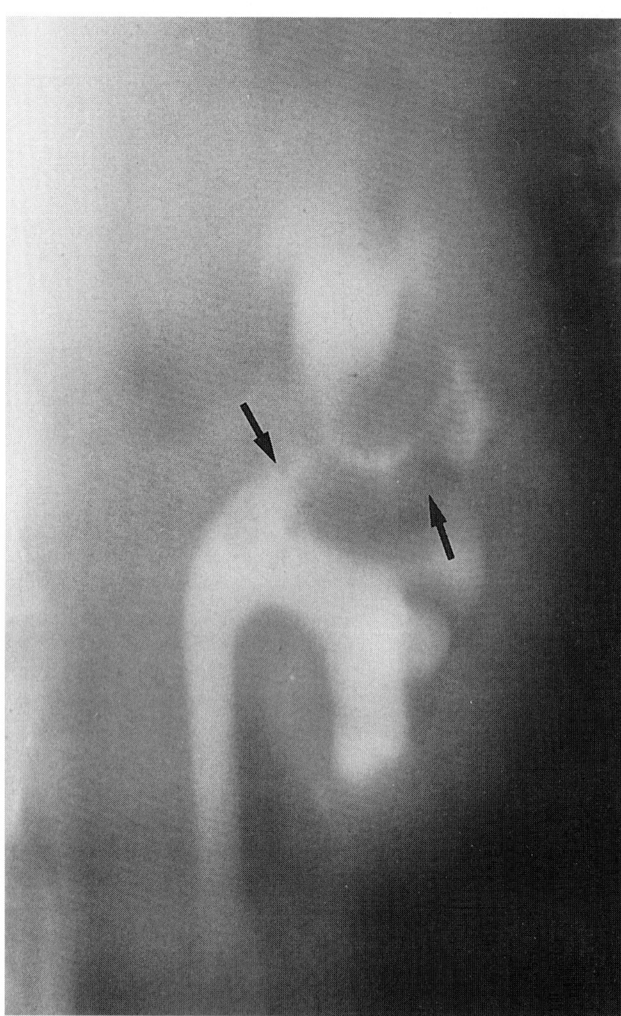

Figure 6–9. Nephrotomogram clearly demonstrates extensive irregularity of the urothelium of the left renal pelvis and upper pole infundibulum and calyces representing transitional cell carcinoma *(arrows)*.

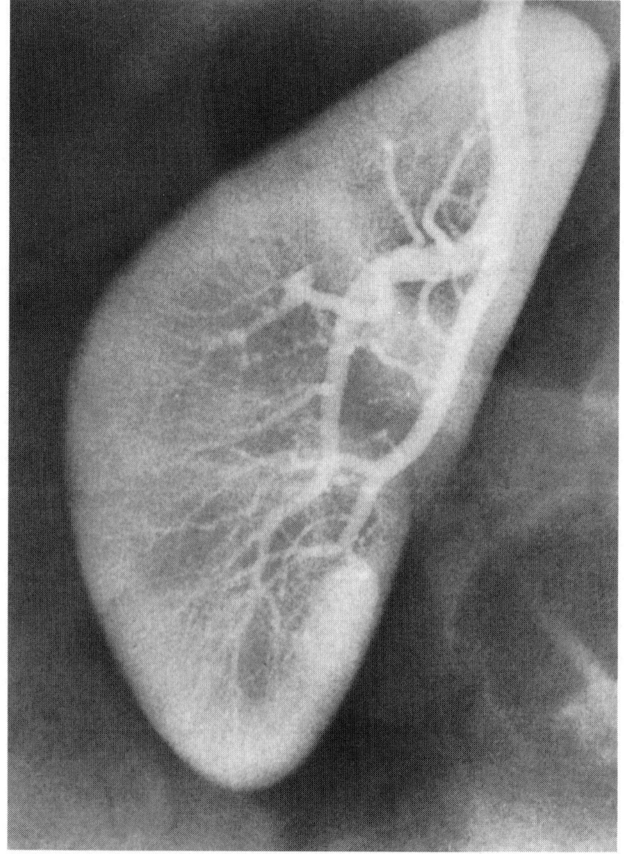

Figure 6–10. Angiographic nephrogram demonstrating differential opacification of the renal cortex and the less enhanced, more centrally located medulla. Although difficult to obtain on intravenous urography even with bolus injection technique, corticomedullary differentiation and the nephrogram effect can be routinely observed on dynamic contrast-enhanced CT scanning.

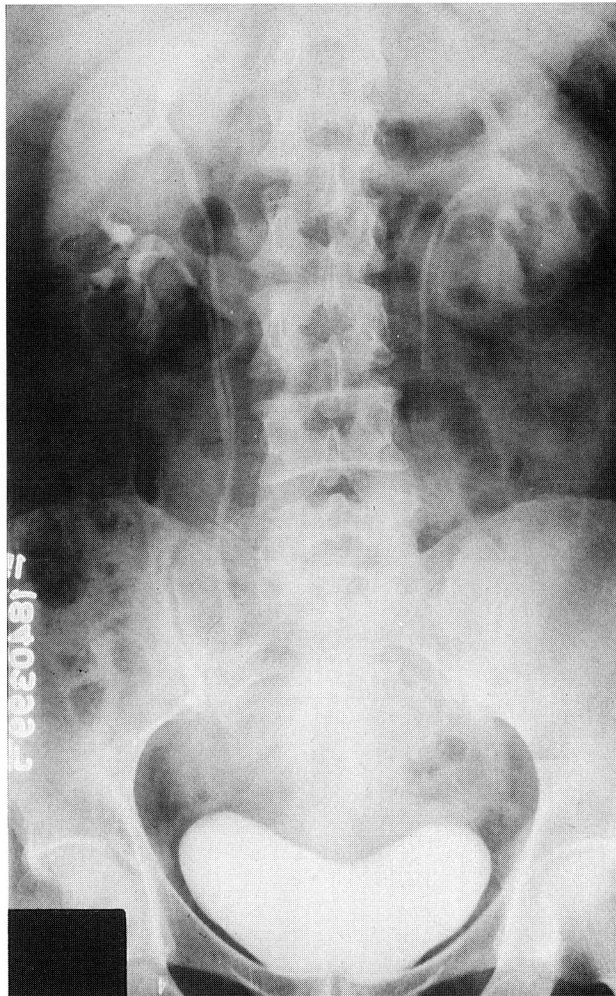

Figure 6–11. Abdominal radiograph 15 minutes into an intravenous urogram shows the kidneys, ureters, and bladder well opacified. Note the right ureteral duplication.

is unsuitable or contraindicated in some patients with significant renal failure or history of severe reaction to contrast media; thus a retrograde pyelogram is appropriate. **Other times, the urologist obtains the retrograde study as a complement to cystoscopy while investigating a patient with hematuria or recurrent or suspected urothelial cancer.** Often, retrograde ureteral stenting and all ureteroscopic procedures may necessitate documentation of the anatomy of the urinary tract and the lesion before an intervention.

The retrograde pyelogram usually is performed after a brief cystoscopy and with general anesthesia. The ureteral orifice is catheterized, and contrast material is injected through a catheter that occludes the orifice at the same time. If the region of concern is in the pyelocalyceal system, the catheter can be advanced up to the renal pelvis before the injection. After a plain abdominal film is taken, the urologist injects the contrast medium, and supine abdominal films are taken without fluoroscopy until the opacification of the urinary tract is satisfactory. Because of the pressure applied and the large volume of contrast material injected, some extravasation may occur. Pyelotubular, pyelosinus, pyelolymphatic, and/or pyelovenous backflow may be seen, and contrast material may be absorbed into the systemic circulation. Because of the latter possibility, the theoretical danger of a reaction to the chemical compound has prompted many clinicians to advocate the use of low-osmolality agents and/or pretreatment of the patient with steroids.

On occasion, the nature and location of a suspected lesion necessitates careful imaging under fluoroscopic control. This can be achieved either in the operating room or by placing a stent and taking the patient to a radiology suite for imaging. Regardless of where the imaging takes place, the operator should be careful not to inject air bubbles into the urinary tract and to subject the films to quality control before the catheter is removed.

In addition to anesthesia- and endoscopy-related complications, such as ureteral injury or ureterovesical junction edema causing transient obstruction, coexisting urinary tract infections may be spread from the bladder or exacerbated by the pressure of the injection and transmitted into the calyces and papillae. Instrument manipulations and pressure must be carefully controlled in infected patients, as must the amount of contrast material injected.

Retrograde pyelography may be contraindicated in the case of very recent lower urinary tract trauma or surgery (urethral or bladder trauma or surgery, ureteral reimplantation). It may not be successful in males with significantly enlarged prostate glands or in patients in whom the anatomy of the trigone is distorted. Infiltrating or fibrotic processes of the bladder wall, such as neoplasms or chronic infections,

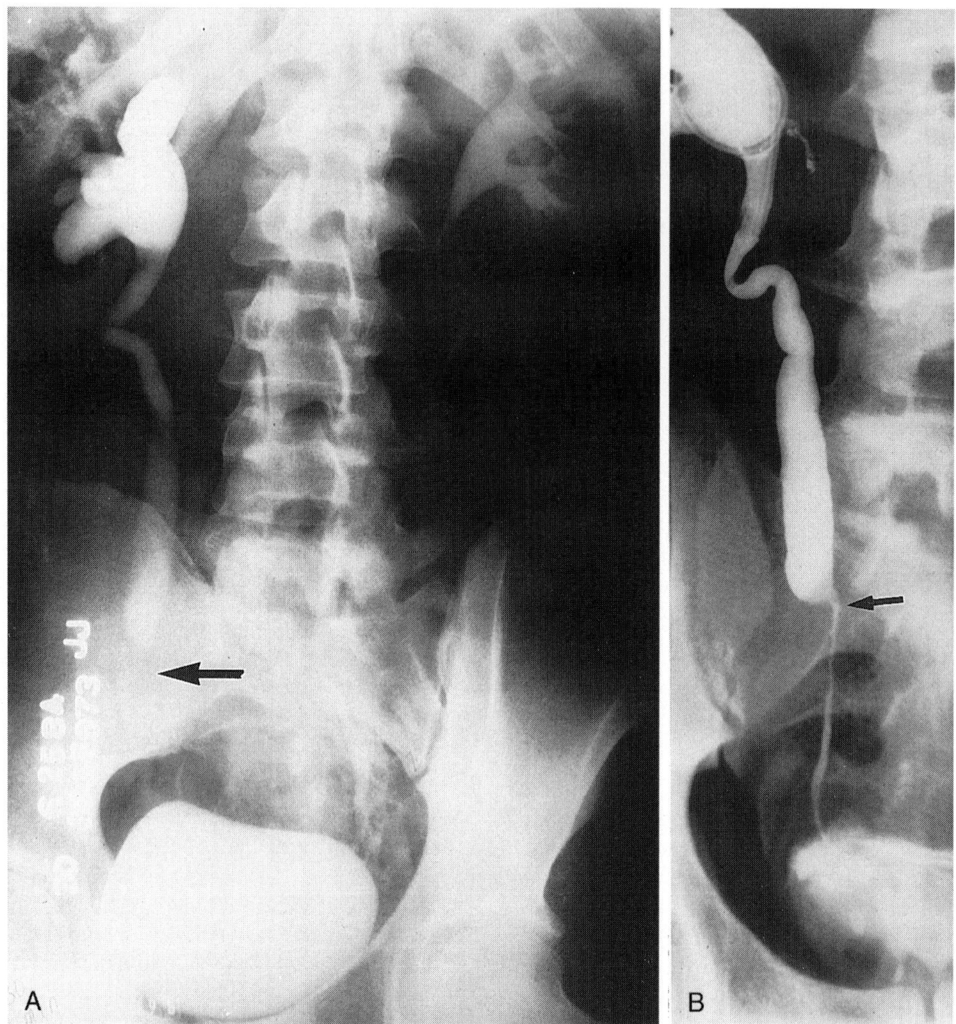

Figure 6–12. Right ureteral obstruction secondary to inflammatory bowel disease in a young man. *A,* There is a transition in the right ureteral caliber at the upper sacral level *(arrow)* on the intravenous urogram. *B,* Nephrostogram shows the exact level of the ureteral stricture *(arrow)* after the obstruction was relieved by the placement of a percutaneous nephrostomy tube.

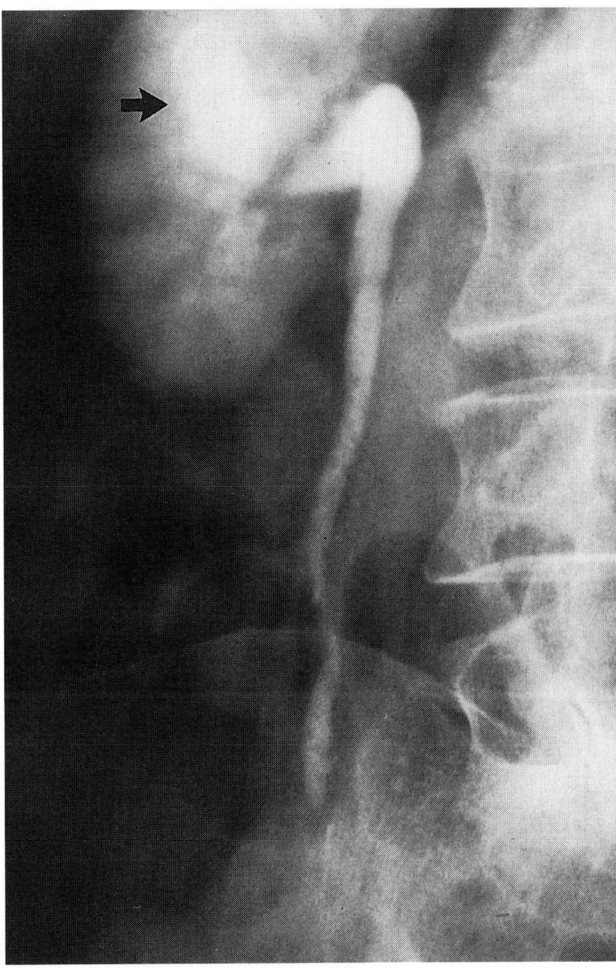

Figure 6–13. Intravenous urogram in a patient with recurrent urinary tract infection and a right renal calculus. The multiple small filling defects seen throughout the proximal right ureter represent ureteritis cystica. The calculus is seen in the midpole renal region *(arrow)*.

sometimes cover or occlude the ureteral orifices so that they cannot be identified at cystoscopy.

Cystography

This examination, imaging of the opacified urinary bladder, is accomplished by the instillation of contrast material into the vesical lumen through a urethral or suprapubic catheter and with fluoroscopically guided filming of the lower pelvis (Pollack and Banner, 1994). Most often, the catheter has already been placed into the bladder after trauma or surgery. Otherwise, a catheter is inserted with the use of sterile technique. A small Foley (Nos. 8 to 12 French) or similar-sized feeding catheter is appropriate.

The main indications for cystography are suspected bladder injury after trauma and anastomotic leak after surgery (Figs. 6–29, 6–30). Adequate distention of the bladder is necessary for optimal evaluation of rupture. Trauma on occasion can be iatrogenic, often after cystoscopic biopsy or resection of a lesion. Postsurgical leakages may result after partial cystectomy, prostatectomy, ureteral reimplantation (ureteroneocystostomy), or renal and/or pancreatic transplantation. **Other indications include investigation for or demonstration of fistulas** between the bladder and adjacent organs, such as the bowel or vagina, **and evaluation of bladder diverticula**—their number, size, and ability to drain well (Fig. 6–31). Stones, neoplasms, fungus balls, and other filling defects within the bladder, as well as cystitis, regardless of etiology, most often are not indications for cystography. On occasion, cystography may be requested to show the exact location of a Foley catheter that does not drain or cannot be irrigated.

Evaluation of the bladder for possible traumatic rupture in the presence of urethral trauma requires that a retrograde urethrogram be performed before the bladder can be catheterized. If the urethra is disrupted, a suprapubic cystostomy catheter is usually placed. If the urethra is intact, a catheter is inserted into the bladder and a cystogram is obtained. An alternative to fluoroscopically performed cystography is CT with intravenous contrast enhancement after direct instillation of contrast material into the bladder.

There are no contraindications to cystography. When a recently operated upon bladder is being evaluated, caution is advised not to overdistend it and not to stretch or disrupt the suture lines.

Iatrogenic complications resulting from the performance of a cystogram are rare. Bladder rupture or urethral injury during the catheterization has on occasion been observed.

After a plain abdominal film is taken, the contrast material is instilled into the bladder, and images of the distended bladder in many different projections are obtained. The bladder then is drained, and a postdrainage film is obtained to evaluate for extravasated contrast material.

Text continued on page 188

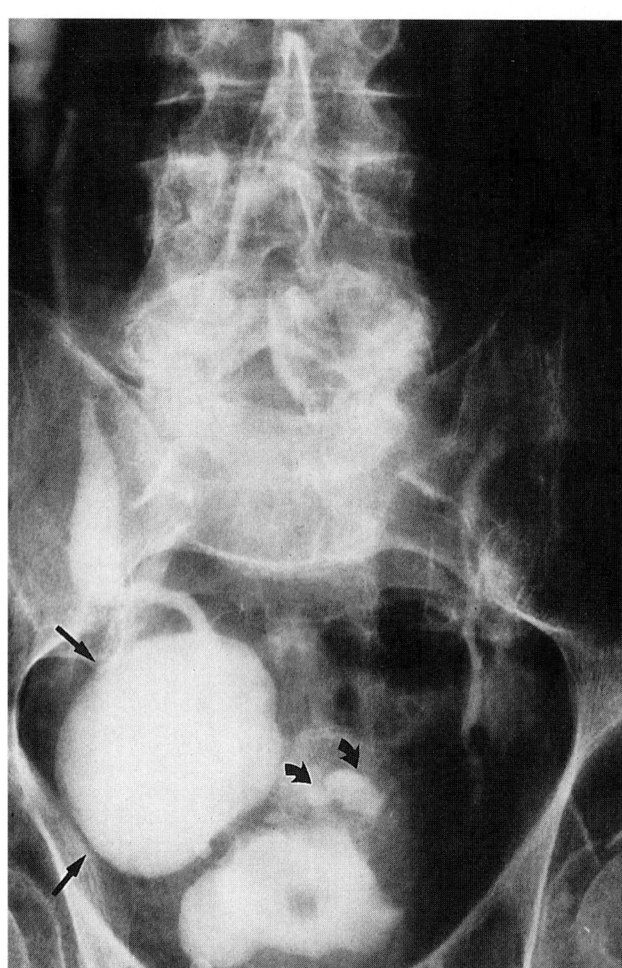

Figure 6–14. Intravenous urogram in an elderly male with urinary frequency shows a large bladder diverticulum causing medial deviation of the right lower ureter *(straight arrows).* Smaller diverticula *(curved arrows)* and thickening of the bladder wall are also present.

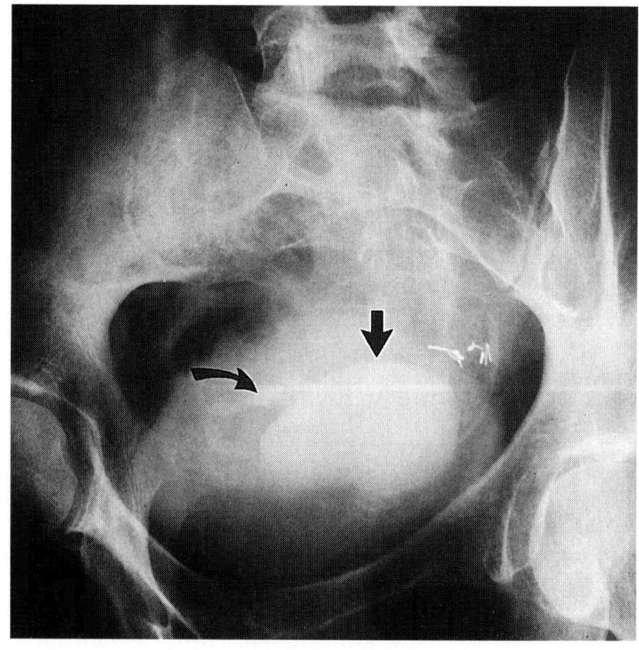

Figure 6–15. Intravenous urogram in a middle-aged woman with vaginal discharge after gynecologic surgery. The fistula between the right lower ureter and the vagina is demonstrated *(curved arrow),* as is the vaginal cavity *(straight arrow).*

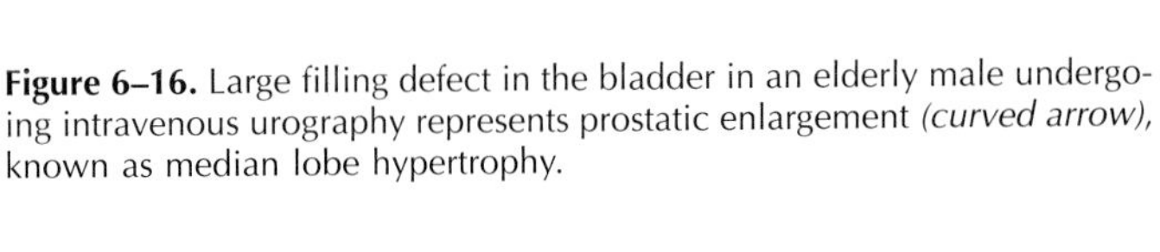

Figure 6–16. Large filling defect in the bladder in an elderly male undergoing intravenous urography represents prostatic enlargement *(curved arrow)*, known as median lobe hypertrophy.

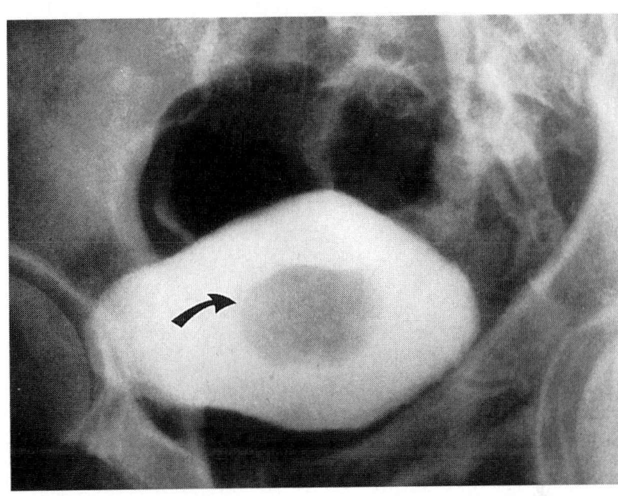

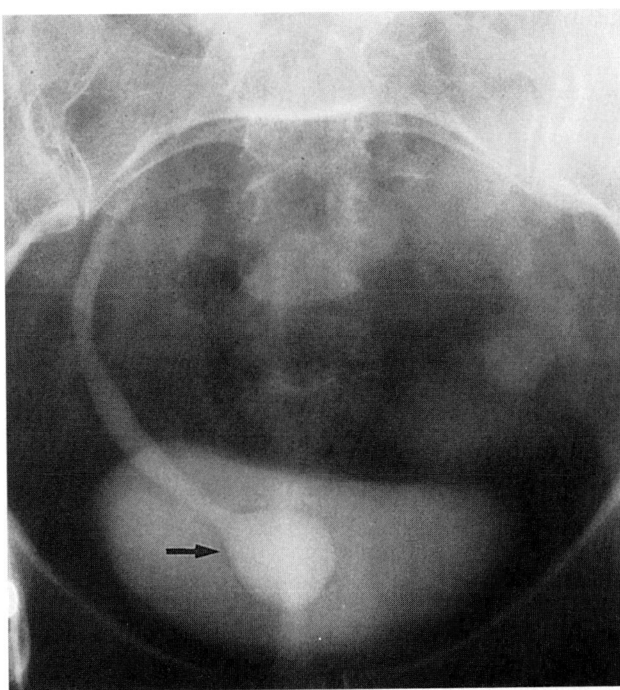

Figure 6–17. Nonobstructing ureterocele in a patient investigated for urinary tract infection *(arrow)*. The well-defined dilatation of the intravesical segment of the right ureter is surrounded by a thin radiolucent halo, which represents the ureteral wall.

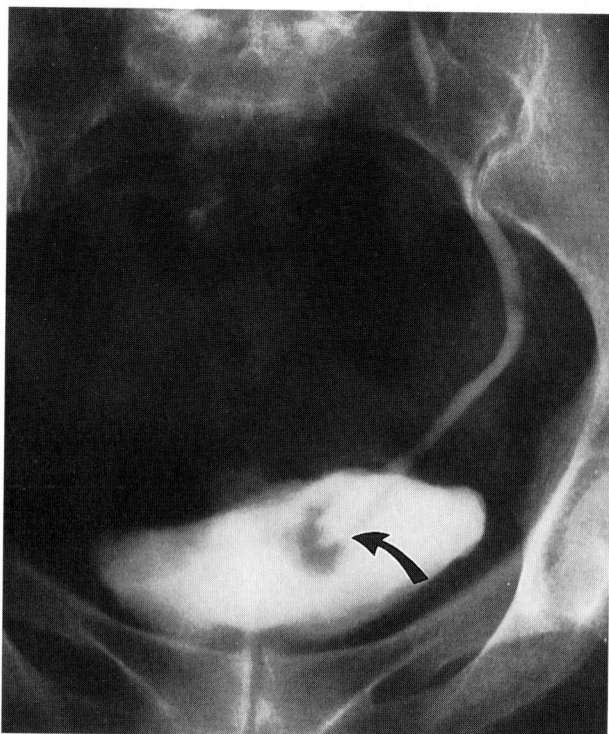

Figure 6–18. Intravenous urogram in an elderly woman with hematuria. An irregular filling defect seen next to the left ureteral orifice *(curved arrow)* represents a urothelial neoplasm.

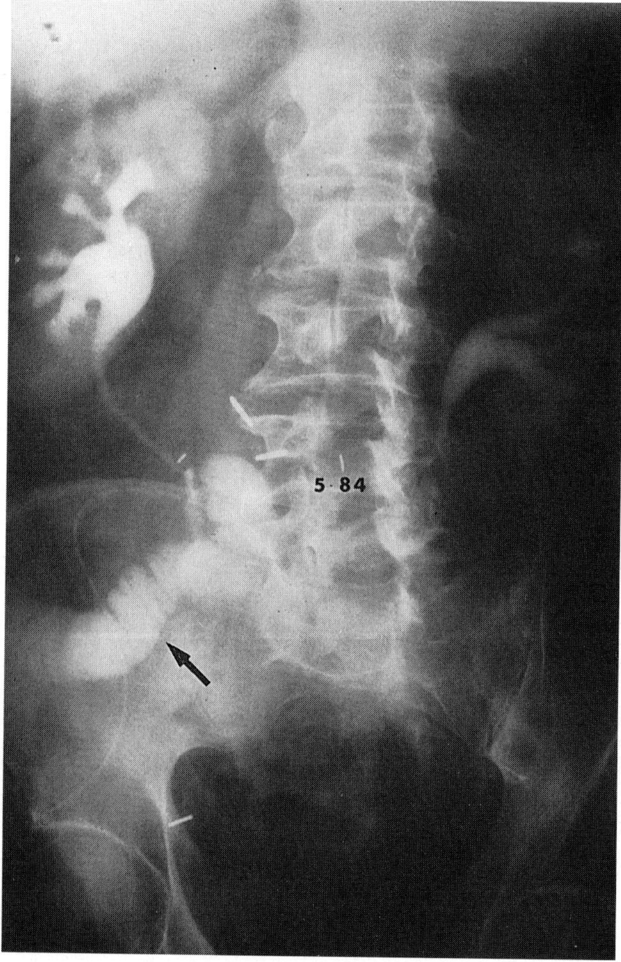

Figure 6–19. Intravenous urogram in a patient with an ileal loop urinary diversion. Both upper urinary tracts appear normal, as does the ileal loop *(arrow)*.

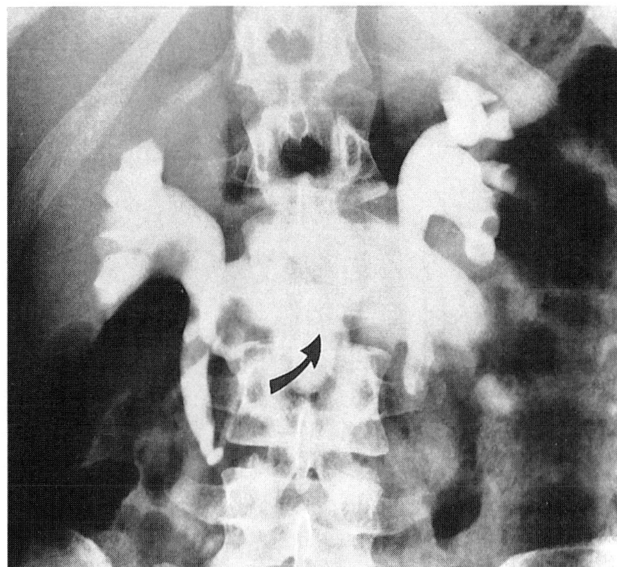

Figure 6–20. Intravenous urogram in a patient with colon loop urinary diversion. The colonic loop is promptly opacified *(curved arrow),* indicating adequate drainage of the upper urinary tract.

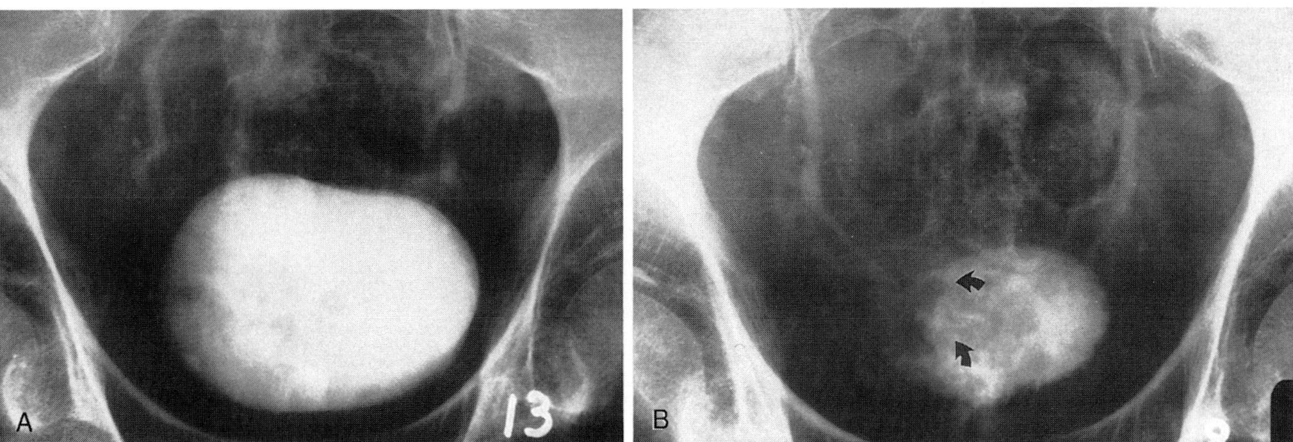

Figure 6–21. Bladder neoplasm demonstrated to a better advantage on postvoid radiography. *A,* The filled bladder radiograph shows a vague mottled density projecting over the right side of the bladder. *B,* The postvoid film clearly demonstrates an irregular mass lesion arising in the right bladder wall, consistent with a malignant neoplasm *(curved arrows).*

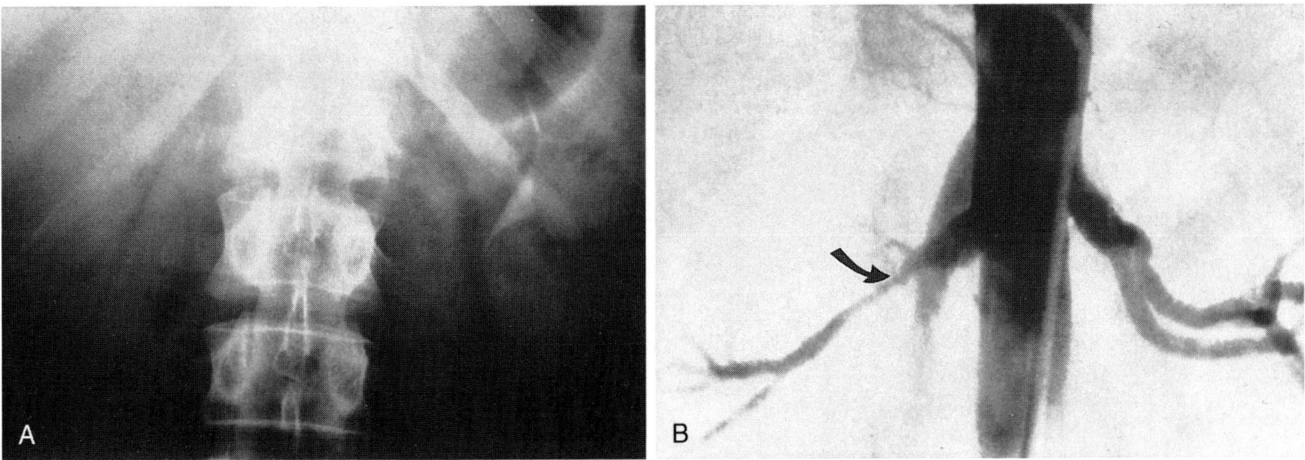

Figure 6–22. Hypertensive intravenous urogram in a hypertensive patient. *A,* There is prompt function of the left kidney and absence of a pyelogram on the right side 3 minutes into the study, suggestive of right renal artery stenosis. *B,* Aortogram confirms right renal artery stenosis secondary to fibromuscular hyperplasia *(curved arrow).*

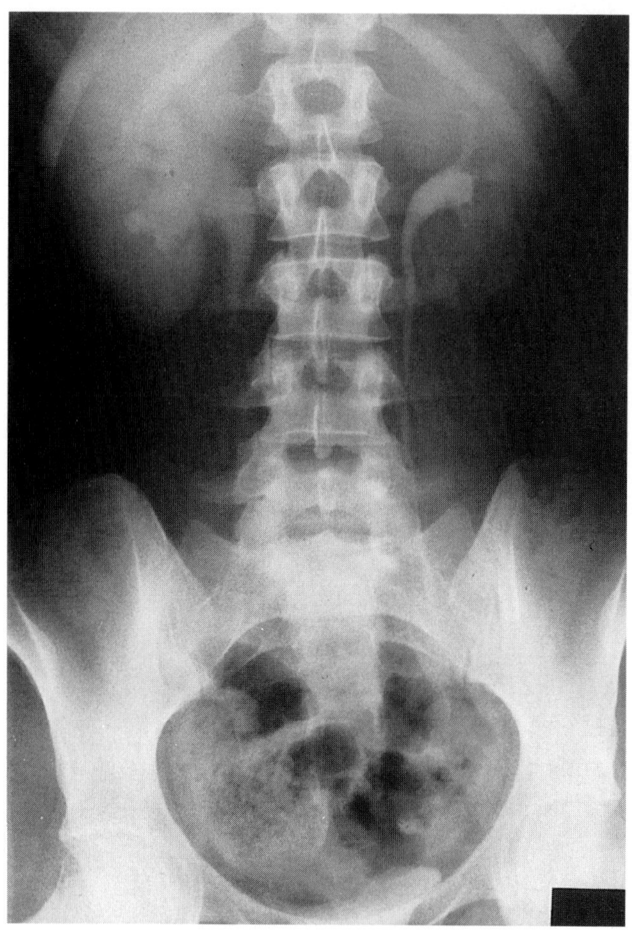

Figure 6–23. Acute urinary obstruction secondary to a ureteral calculus. A dense, persistent right nephrogram is seen together with mild dilatation of the collecting system.

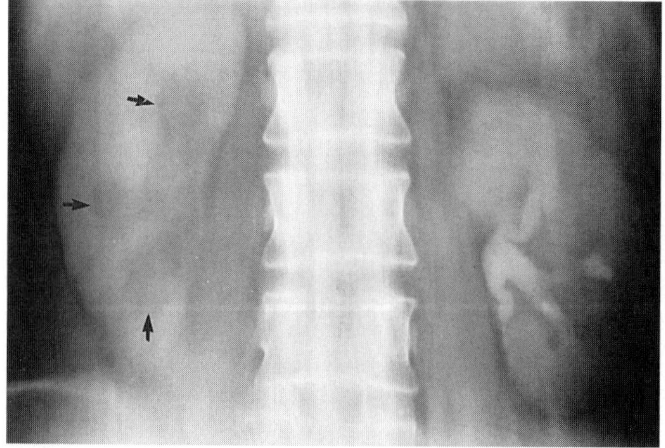

Figure 6–24. Chronic urinary obstruction resulting in absence of excretion of contrast material and moderate dilatation of the right calyceal system *(arrows)* on intravenous pyelogram. The degree of hydronephrosis is such that the obstruction cannot be acute.

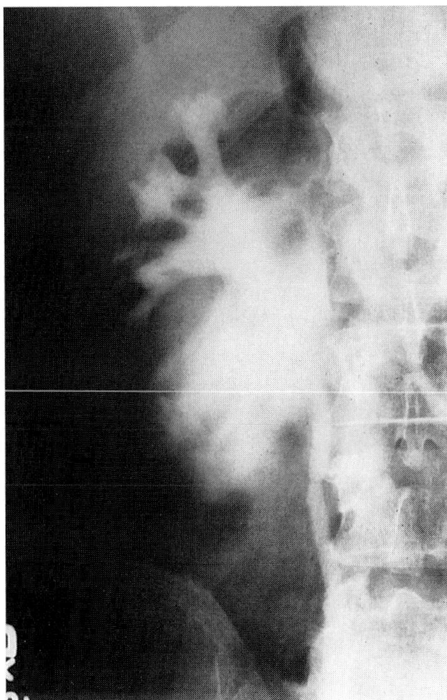

Figure 6–25. Acute urinary obstruction resulting in forniceal rupture and perinephric extravasation of contrast material from the right kidney on intravenous urography.

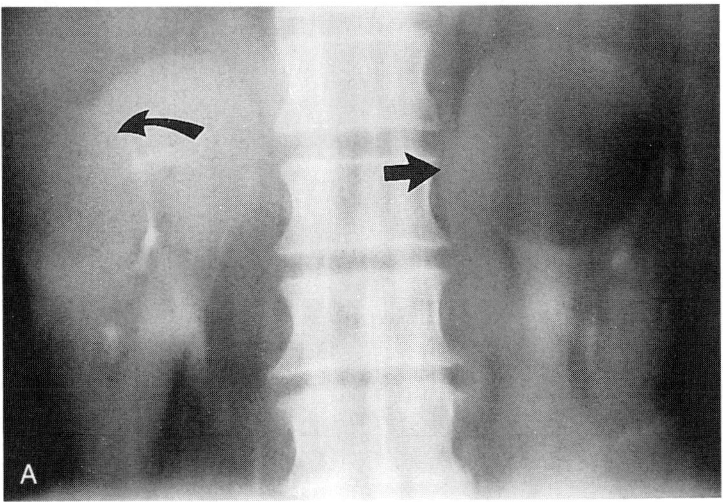

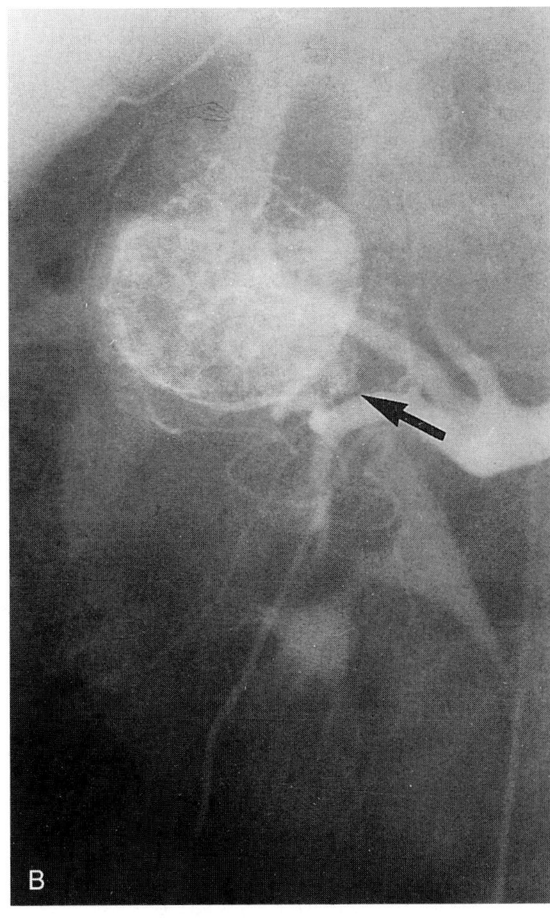

Figure 6–26. Hematuria in a middle-aged patient. *A,* Nephrotomogram shows bilateral renal lesions. The left upper renal pole lesion is of low attenuation with a thin wall *(straight arrow),* consistent with a simple cyst. The right mid- to upper pole lesion is of higher density, consistent with a solid mass *(curved arrow). B,* Angiogram of the right kidney shows a vascular lesion, confirming the presence of a solid mass *(arrow).*

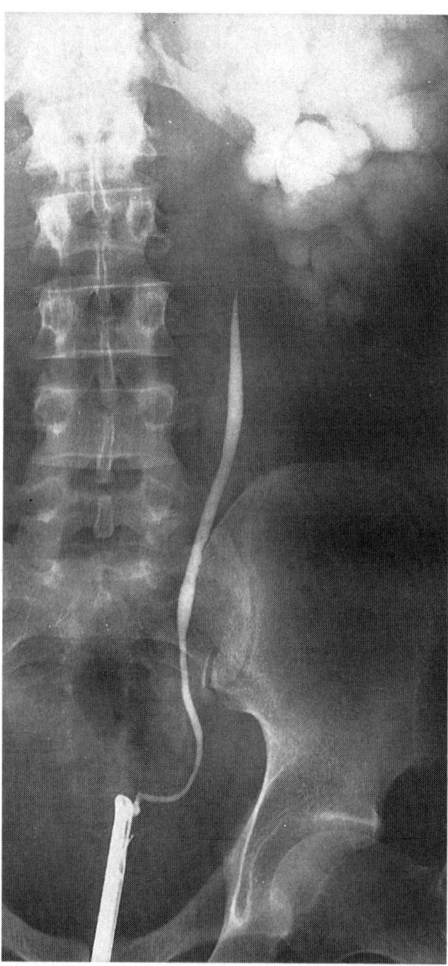

Figure 6–27. Retrograde pyelogram in a patient with left flank pain and a palpable flank mass. Left pyelogram shows a normal ureter with a very tight narrowing at the ureteropelvic junction, diagnostic of ureteropelvic junction obstruction.

Extraperitoneal rupture results in irregular, stellate-shaped, nonmobile, and very slowly absorbed contrast extravasation; the contrast material does not outline specific organs or spaces. Intraperitoneal rupture results in contrast material's surrounding bowel loops and opacifying the subhepatic and perihepatic intraperitoneal spaces. Contrast material is rapidly absorbed and excreted by the kidneys. A fistula is diagnosed when the contrast material from the bladder enters and opacifies adjacent viscera, such as the bowel or the vagina. Because both the bladder and the vagina are midline structures, steep oblique and lateral views of the pelvis are indicated for the clear demonstration of the fistula.

Voiding Cystourethrography

The pathophysiology of micturition and the anatomy of the lower urinary tract are best evaluated both in children and in adults by voiding cystourethrography (VCU). The examination is performed under fluoroscopic control, and images are generated by taking spot films or videotape recording (Fig. 6–32).

Indications often vary with symptoms related to the lower urinary tract dysfunction and suspected anatomic abnormalities (Pollack and Banner, 1994). The female urethra and posterior male urethra are best visualized during VCU; thus a **search for urethral diverticula in women** and **strictures in men or posterior urethral valves in male infants** can be reliably performed (Figs. 6–33, 6–34). Demonstration of the **presence and grade of vesicoureteral reflux** is a common indication, especially in pediatric patients. **Congenital abnormalities** that are well suited for evaluation by VCU include **(1) ureteroceles,** which may on occasion prolapse into the outflow tract and cause obstruction (Fig. 6–35); **(2) paraureteral bladder diverticula,** which often are associated with ureteral reflux; **(3) ectopic drainage of ureters,** which may be associated with ureteral reflux (if the

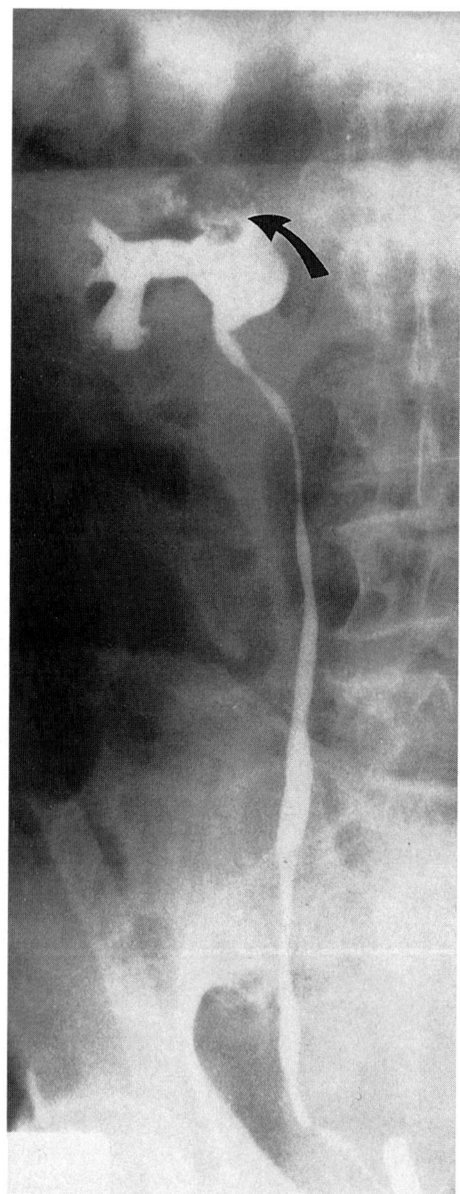

Figure 6–28. Right retrograde pyelogram in a patient with hematuria and positive urine cytology profile shows an irregular mass lesion with faint visualization of the markedly dilated upper pole calyces *(curved arrow).*

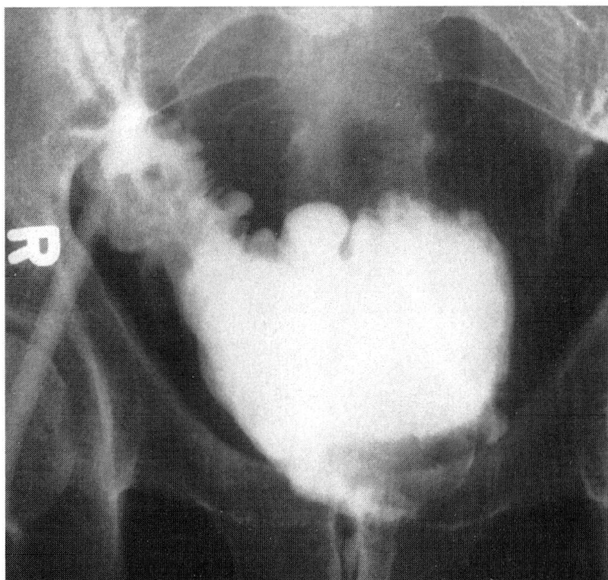

Figure 6–29. Cystogram shows an orthotopic bladder (neobladder) replacing the resected bladder. The study was performed via the suprapubic tube.

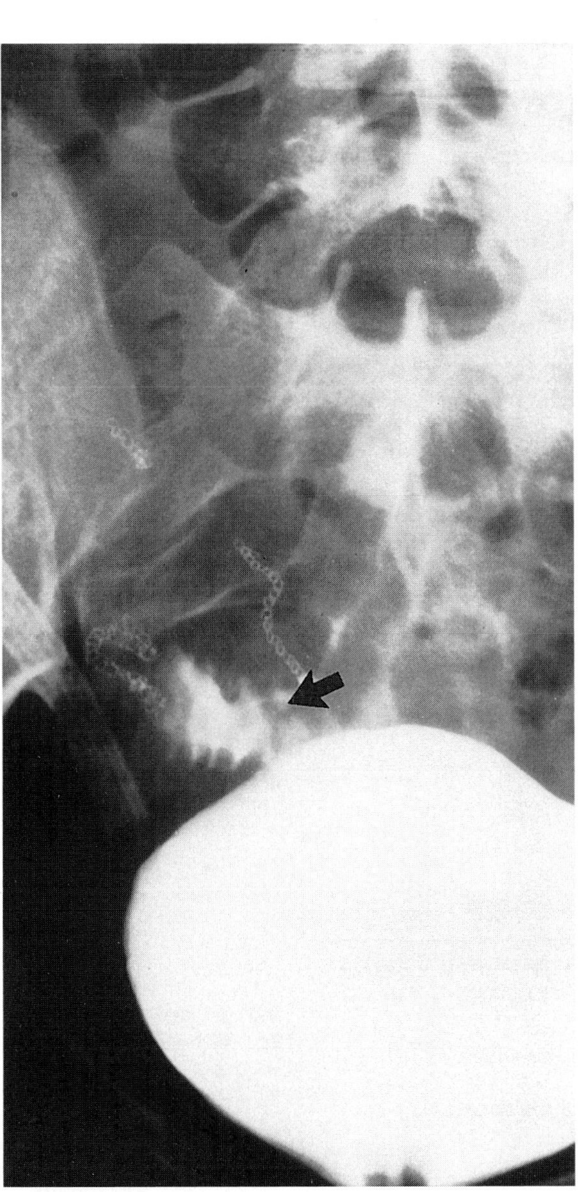

Figure 6–30. Cystogram in a patient who underwent renal and pancreatic transplantation. There is reflux into the short duodenal loop used for the pancreatic transplant *(arrow),* but no extravasation is apparent.

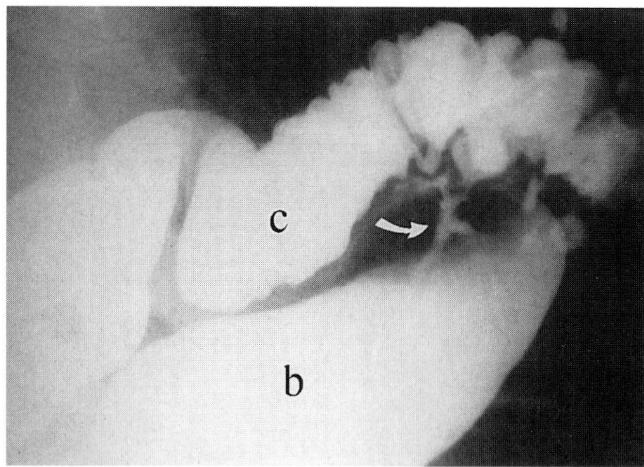

Figure 6–31. Colovesical fistula *(curved arrow)* demonstrated on cystogram. b, bladder; c, colon.

insertion is in the bladder) or with infection, urinary tract obstruction, or enuresis (if the insertion is in the urethra in a female patient) and **(4) the prune-belly syndrome.** The examination often is performed not only to diagnose the abnormalities but also after their repair, for confirmation of a successful outcome.

In older children and adult patients, **voiding difficulties secondary to a neurogenic bladder** may be evaluated by VCU (Fig. 6–36), often in combination with pressure-flow monitoring (videourodynamics; see Chapter 68). **Patients with stress urinary incontinence,** most often women, may benefit from the information obtained from VCU. In these cases, the bladder neck and proximal urethra may descend significantly because of lax muscular and ligamentous support (Fig. 6–37). Measurements of the angle formed between the bladder floor and urethra are made to objectively quantify the degree of incontinence. The normal limits for the posterior urethrovesical angle and the angle formed by the long urethral axis and a vertical plane are 100 and 35 degrees, respectively. Estimation of postvoid residuals is approximate and should not by itself be an indication for performing VCU (sonography or catheterization of the bladder are preferable for postvoid residual measurements). In some instances, acquired or congenital bladder diverticula may enlarge significantly and empty poorly during micturition, leading to incomplete bladder emptying and predisposing to infection. Evaluation with VCU or sonography accurately demonstrates the **presence, number, and size of diverticula, as well as the amount of urine retained within them after voiding** (Fig. 6–38).

The study requires that the bladder be distended with water-soluble contrast material, most often after sterile catheterization or, on occasion, through suprapubic cystostomy catheter. The urethral catheter is removed when the patient begins to urinate. Spot films are taken of the bladder before and of the bladder and urethra during urination. Male patients should be placed in an oblique position for better visualization of the longer urethra. A fluoroscopic search for ureteral reflux is done before and during voiding, and a postvoid film of the bladder is obtained (Fig. 6–39). A number of adult patients may be unable to steadily void on demand at the time of the study, usually because of involuntary inhibition. This results in failure to visualize the urethra and bladder neck during micturition.

Vesicoureteral reflux is of paramount importance to the growth and well-being of the kidneys in pediatric patients.

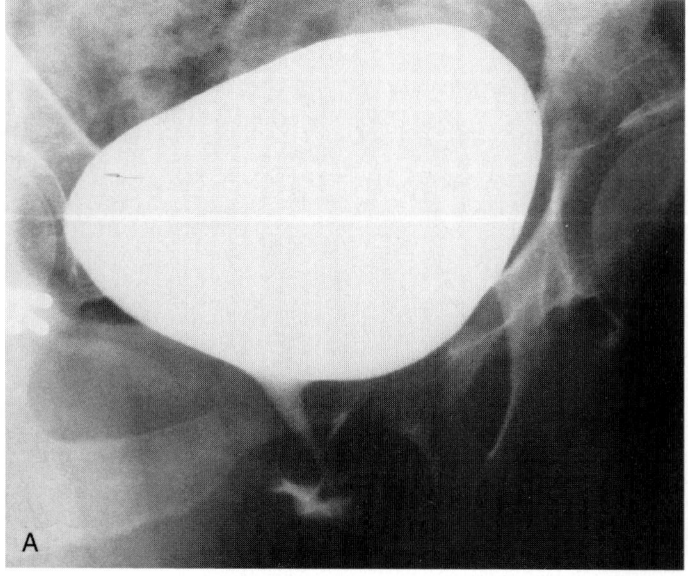

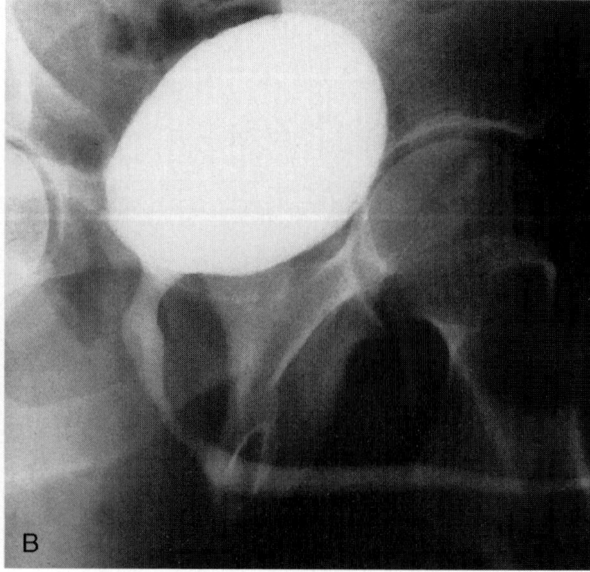

Figure 6–32. Voiding cystourethrograms. *A,* Normal female urethra. *B,* Normal male urethra.

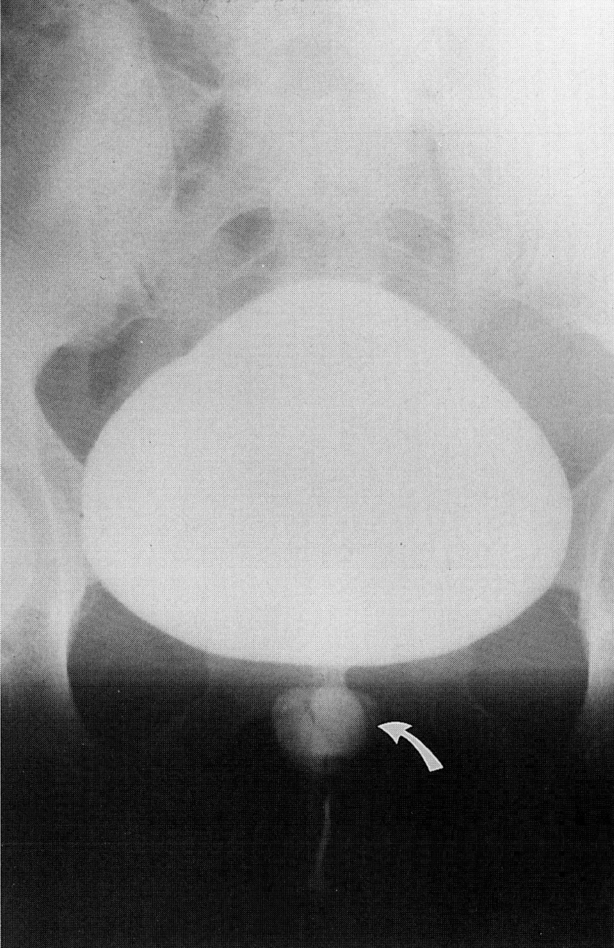

Figure 6–33. Voiding cystourethrogram in a middle-aged woman with recurrent urinary tract infections and urinary dribbling shows a urethral diverticulum *(curved arrow).*

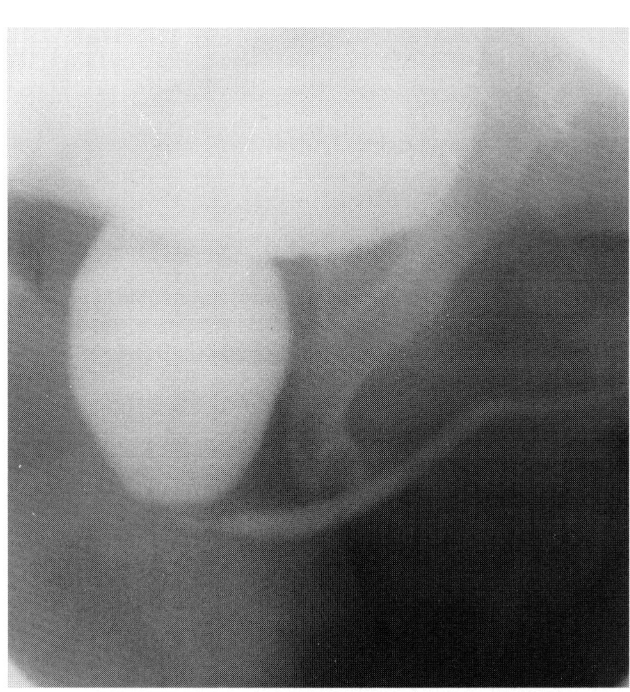

Figure 6–34. Marked enlargement of the posterior urethra in a male infant, suggestive of posterior urethral valves, on voiding cystourethrography.

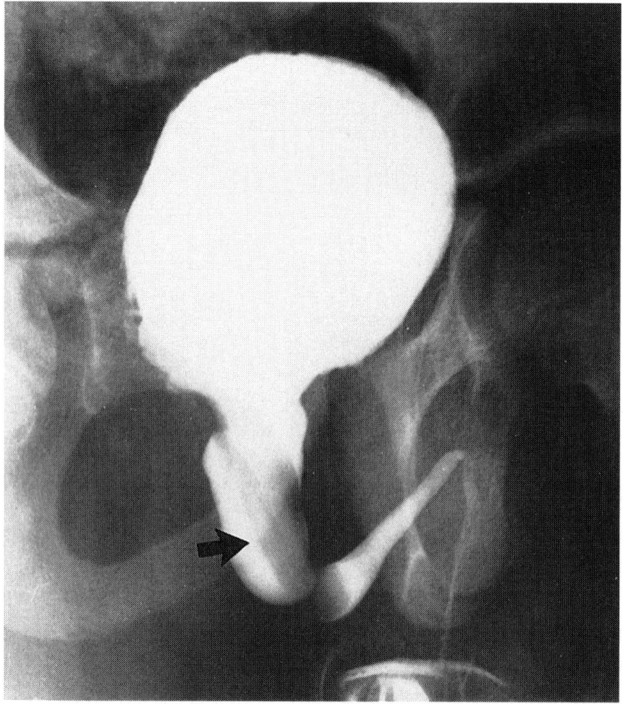

Figure 6–35. Voiding cystourethrogram in a young boy with intermittent decrease in urine stream. A right-sided ureterocele is seen prolapsing into and obstructing the posterior urethra *(arrow)*.

The international grading system has a range of 1 to 5 or I to V. Grade 1 reflux is confined to the normal-appearing ureter without reaching the kidney. Grade 2 reflux extends into the renal calyceal system without dilatation or deformity of the calyces. Grades 3 to 5 are assigned to mild, moderate, and severe dilatation of the urinary tract with blunting of the calyces and intrarenal reflux, especially for grades 4 and 5.

Ureteroceles appear as smooth, round, or oval filling defects within the area of the bladder trigone. Ectopic ureters can be seen only if they exhibit reflux. Urethral strictures often can be diagnosed with precision (Figs. 6–40, 6–41).

The appearance of the bladder in patients after surgery (partial cystectomy, ureteroneocystostomy, etc.) and in patients with neuromuscular disorders varies greatly. Knowledge of the history is very helpful. In cases of neuromuscular disorders, the level of neurologic damage may sometimes result in rather typical appearances of the bladder. Suprapontine lesions may cause mild wall trabeculation and serration of the bladder contour just above the trigone. Spinal lesions more often cause trabeculation, pseudodiverticula, upper tract dilatation, and ureteral reflux. In severe cases, the so-called pine cone or Christmas tree appearance of the bladder may be seen. Sacral cord lesions such as meningomyelocele, spina bifida, tumors, or trauma often result in reduced bladder capacity and compliance, with a thickened wall, pseudodiverticula, and a pine cone appearance. Peripheral neuropathies, such as seen in patients with diabetes, often result in a larger, atonic bladder with large postvoid residual volumes. Many lesions are so complicated and complex that they cause nonspecific or overlapping anatomic changes throughout the urinary tract.

Retrograde Urethrography

This study is an **excellent and, sometimes, the only procedure for visualizing the anterior male urethra.** On occasion, the female urethra may also be imaged in the same manner. Retrograde urethrography may thus complement VCU when the latter fails to visualize the urethra, or it

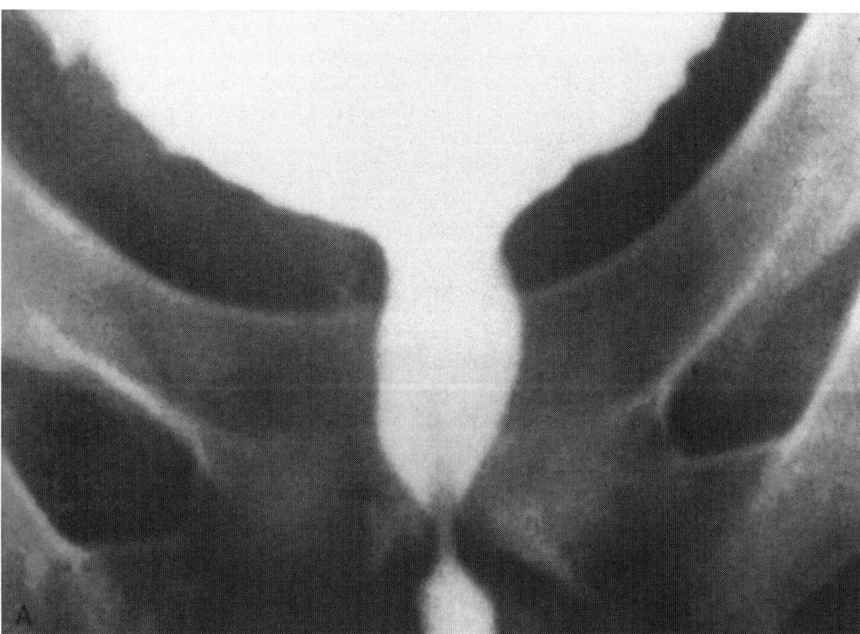

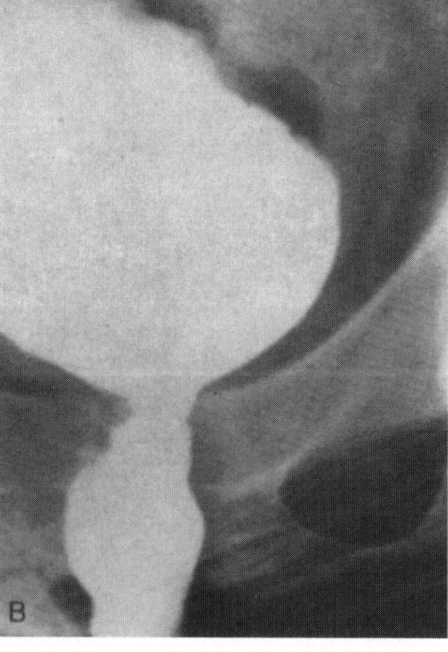

Figure 6–36. Example of a voiding cystourethrogram. *A*, Close-up view of the bladder neck and striated sphincter region in a patient with striated sphincter dyssynergia. The appearance is typical of the narrow sphincter region producing an obstruction. The retained urine, usually under elevated pressure, will eventually cause hydronephrosis. *B*, After sphincterotomy, the area of the striated sphincter has been opened. This was accomplished by resecting the sphincter in the anterior region, in an arc from the 11 o'clock to 1 o'clock positions. The extent of the cut is from the level of the verumontanum to the distal end of the sphincter ring. Doing this seems to disrupt the sphincter fibers adequately.

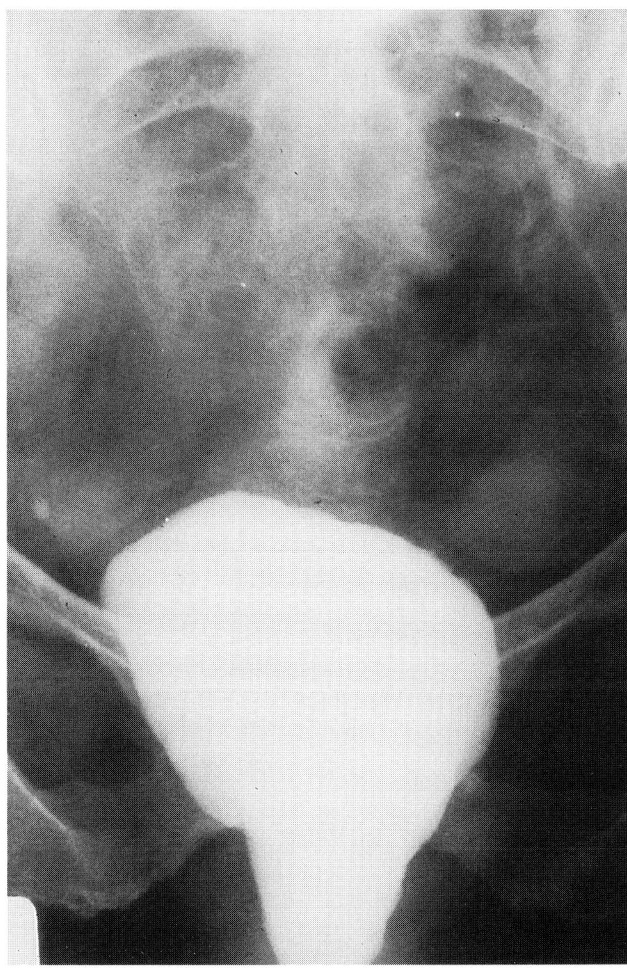

Figure 6–37. Voiding cystourethrogram in an elderly woman with urinary incontinence shows a moderately severe cystocele.

may be performed alone when the pathologic process under investigation is limited to the anterior male urethra or before catheterization of the bladder in cases of trauma.

Primary indications for retrograde urethrography are the **evaluation of strictures in the anterior urethra, before and after treatment** as indicated, and the **diagnosis and staging of urethral injuries after trauma** (Pollack and Banner, 1994) (Fig. 6–42). **In women, a search for suspected urethral diverticula is the main indication when a voiding cystourethrogram is either nonrevealing or cannot be obtained** (patient unable to void on demand). Less often, pseudodiverticula, anterior urethral valves, fistulas, and neoplastic processes can be also evaluated by retrograde urethrography (Fig. 6–43).

The procedure requires the occlusion of the penile urethral orifice, which can be easily accomplished with a Foley balloon catheter. The balloon is inserted into the fossa navicularis and is gently inflated with saline until it effectively tamponades the urethral lumen. The amount of saline required is 1 to 2 ml. Contrast material is then injected under fluoroscopic observation, and images of the distended anterior urethra are taken. The posterior urethra is either incompletely opacified or not visualized at all, depending on the pressure applied and the resistance of the external urethral sphincter. In women, a specially designed double-balloon catheter is necessary in order to occlude both ends of the short urethra. The distal balloon (near the catheter tip) is placed into the bladder, and the proximal balloon is positioned just outside the labia majora. A side hole in the lumen of the catheter between the two balloons allows the contrast material to enter the urethral lumen, and the two inflated balloons provide a temporary, often only partial occlusion of the bladder outlet and the urethral orifice and thus allow for opacification of the urethral lumen.

The amount of water-soluble contrast material necessary to opacify and distend the anterior male urethra usually ranges from 6 to 10 ml. Caution should be exercised not to overdistend the urethra or use undue force during the injection, in order to avoid extravasation of contrast material into the corpus spongiosum and penile veins. Because of the risk of extravasation, the study should not be performed during an episode of acute urethritis.

Sometimes the length and/or number of tight strictures cannot be accurately determined without the combination of a voiding study with a retrograde study. Underfilling of the

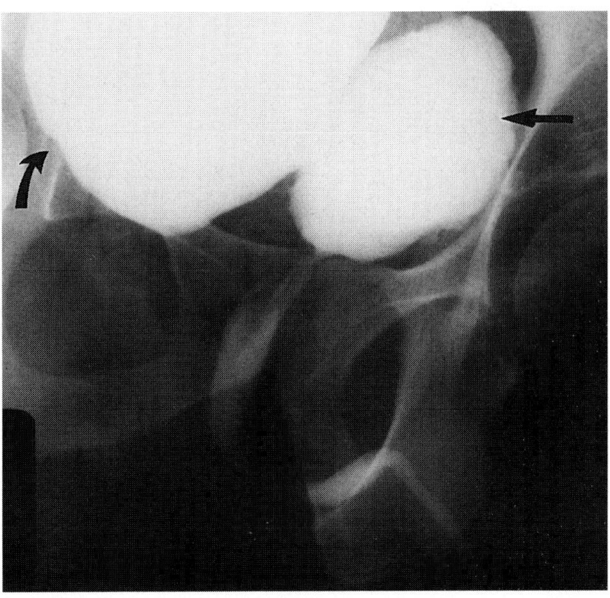

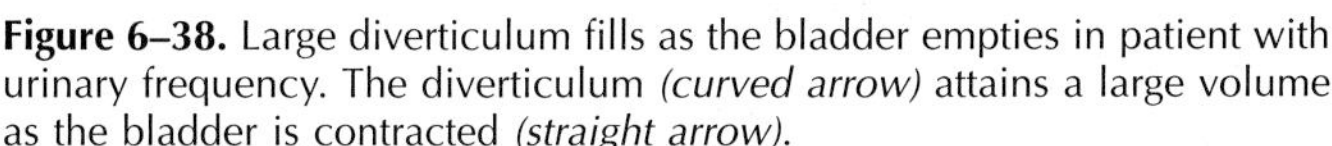

Figure 6–38. Large diverticulum fills as the bladder empties in patient with urinary frequency. The diverticulum *(curved arrow)* attains a large volume as the bladder is contracted *(straight arrow).*

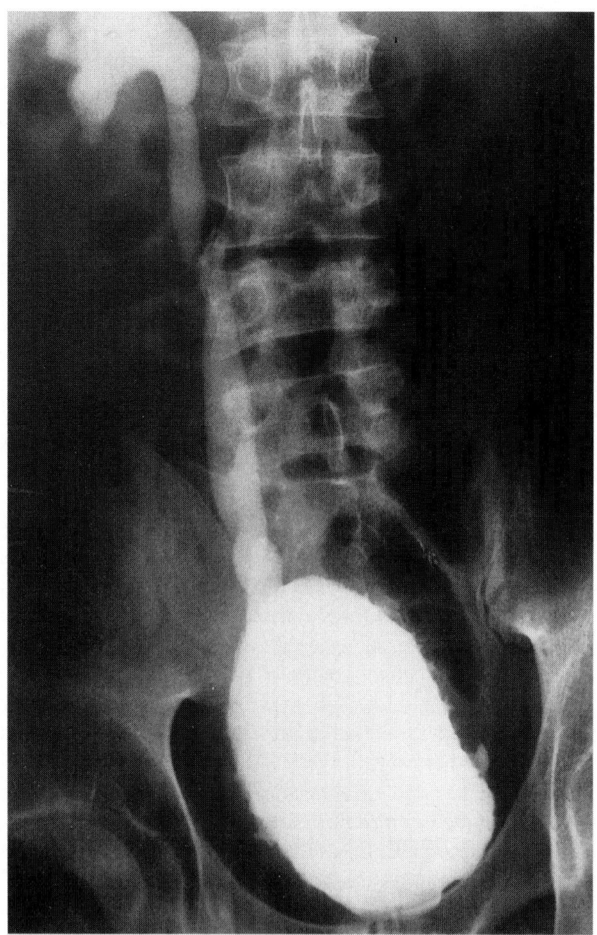

Figure 6–39. Vesicoureteric reflux into a moderately dilated right urinary tract.

urethral lumen distal to the beginning of a stricture may result in overestimation of its length or may obscure the presence of additional strictures. Opacifying the lumen on both sides of the stricture enables the clinician to measure its length reliably. If the urethra cannot be catheterized and a voiding study of the bladder has to be performed, the contrast material can be given intravenously or by direct needlestick into the bladder.

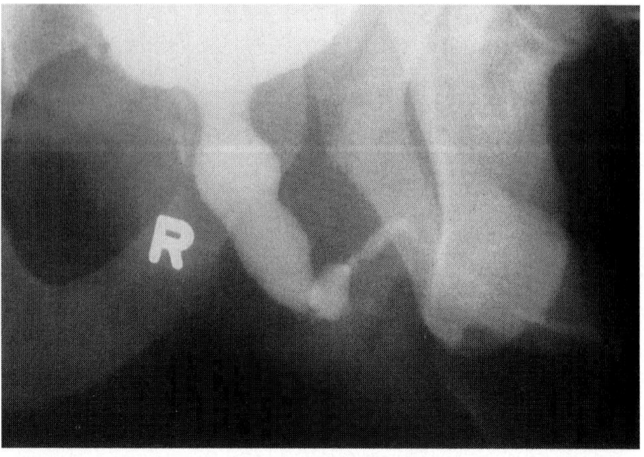

Figure 6–40. Anterior urethral strictures are seen associated with dilatation of the posterior urethra on voiding cystography.

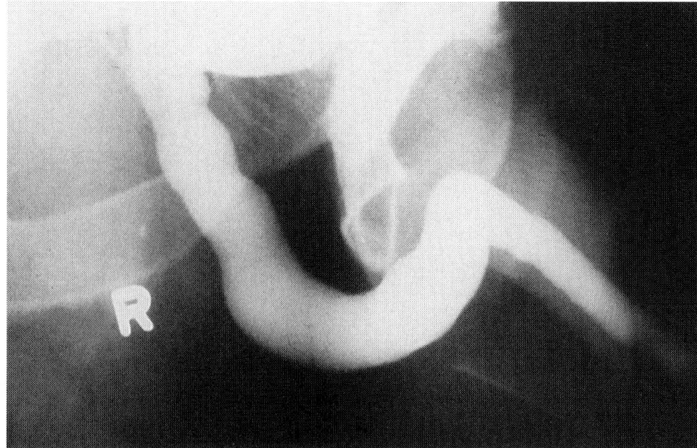

Figure 6–41. Tight urethral meatal stenosis causes dilatation of the entire urethra, as shown on voiding cystourethrography.

Loopography

Urinary diversions and/or reconstruction of, or alterations in, the bladder are common urologic procedures that are performed in patients with congenital or acquired diseases that significantly compromise effective urination. Urinary diversions bypass the bladder, which is usually, but not necessarily, removed. The ureters are anastomosed to a new reservoir, which is made from an isolated segment of bowel and drains through a stoma in the lower anterior abdominal wall. Ileal and colonic loops are incontinent, draining continuously with peristalsis into appliances attached to the stoma. Detubularized bowel segments that can contain urine may be constructed (continent pouches); these are drained by intermittent catheterization. A segment of bowel that replaces a surgically removed bladder and is anastomosed to the urethra, thus preserving urine continence, is called an orthotopic bladder. Sometimes a compromised bladder is augmented by the attachment to it of part of the stomach or a segment of bowel, usually cecum or ascending colon, while the urethra is preserved. Instilling contrast material directly into the diverting loop or pouch or the reconstructed bladder enables imaging of the altered lower urinary tract

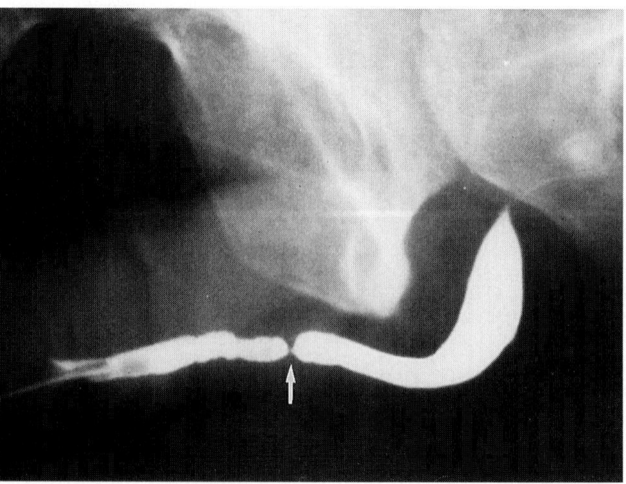

Figure 6–42. Penile urethral stricture is clearly visualized on retrograde urethrography *(arrow)*. The patient had a history of sexually transmitted urethritis, and his bladder could not be catheterized.

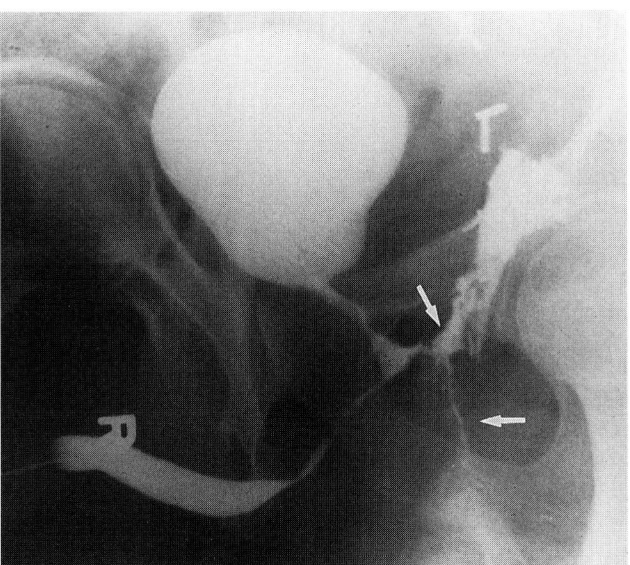

Figure 6–43. Retrograde urethrogram demonstrates fistulous communications between the posterior urethra, bowel, and perineum *(arrows)*.

for evaluation of the surgical results or specific clinical problems.

The indications for loopography or pouchography are related mainly to their function as conduits or reservoirs of urine (Pollack and Banner, 1994). **Capacity, peristaltic activity, presence of strictures, urine leakages, search for filling defects, and emptying capability are parameters that are commonly evaluated. Reflux occurs through ileal loops into the upper urinary tracts; therefore, the question of obstruction after ileal loop diversion can readily be investigated by loopography. Colon loops, continent pouches, or reconstructed bladders as a rule undergo antirefluxing ureteral anastomoses; thus the presence of ureteral reflux, a normal finding in ileal loops, usually indicates failure of the antireflux surgery.** Patients with nonrefluxing ureters and urinary diversion suspect for obstruction should therefore be evaluated by sonography or IVU.

Stenosis of the stoma is easily diagnosed by digital examination and/or attempted catheterization. Strictures of the bowel conduits may be manifested initially by recurrent urinary tract infection or worsening renal function. Longstanding ileal loops often develop strictures that may or may not be causing symptoms. The typical radiographic appearance of the small bowel often is effaced over a period of several years, resulting in a tubular, featureless-appearing ileal loop. Primary carcinomas of the small or large bowel in loops, which are rare, often manifest with hematuria and hydronephrosis. The loopogram usually is diagnostic of a wall lesion, which may then be confirmed by looposcopy and biopsy. Ureterosigmoidostomies, which carry a well-documented risk of bowel cancer at or near the anastomotic site, are rarely performed nowadays.

The procedure requires catheterization of the loop stoma or reconstructed bladder. A Foley balloon catheter is inserted into the loop and the balloon inflated just under the abdominal wall with 3 to 5 ml of saline. Gentle traction on the balloon catheter usually effectively tamponades the stoma and prevents urine from leaking around the stoma. Under intermittent fluoroscopic observation, water-soluble contrast material is infused into the loop until adequate distention of the bowel segment and/or ureteral reflux is seen, the latter in the case of ileal loops only. The amount of contrast material used varies with the capacity of the reservoir. Ileal loops may be filled with 50 to 150 ml, whereas 300 to 400 ml may be required for continent pouches and between 500 and 1000 ml for reconstructed bladders. Instillation is made by gravity or gentle manual injection. After images of the conduit and, possibly, ureters and collecting systems have been taken, the loop or pouch is left for external drainage for 5 to 10 minutes, and a postdrainage image is taken. Patients with a history of recurrent infections should receive prophylactic antibiotics before the study. The risk of urosepsis increases with more fluid infused and higher forces and pressure generated into the loop and the ureters. The hydrostatic pressure within the reservoir should be monitored by means of a simple water manometer, and the pressure should not exceed 30 to 40 cm H_2O during the study.

In addition to the risk of infection, another rare complication of loopography is the creation of tears of the intestinal mucosa by the pressure of the balloon and the pressure within the reservoir. These tears usually occur either at the level of the stoma or at the point where the loop enters the peritoneal cavity just beneath the anterior abdominal wall. The latter can potentially result in peritonitis; therefore, caution is advised during the performance of the study not to overdistend the balloon and not to increase the hydrostatic pressure within the loop to high levels.

Because of the risk of disruption of suture lines after urinary diversion procedures by the high hydrostatic pressure generated during loopography, evaluation of immediate postoperative results is better and safer with IVU. After the healing process is complete, future evaluations of loops can be done safely by loopography.

Nephrostogram and Stentogram

These procedures require that either a percutaneous nephrostomy catheter or a ureteral stent, usually exiting the urethra, are in place in the urinary tract. Water-soluble contrast material can then be injected into catheters, stents, or tubes and the urinary tract imaged.

The indications for the study depend on the indications for the placement of the catheter or stent. Often, a catheter is left in the pyelocalyceal system or ureter because of or after relief of urinary obstruction (see Fig. 6–12). Residual stone fragments or clots, urothelial tumors, fungus balls, ureteral strictures, urine leakages after the perforation of the ureter or renal pelvis, patency of the ureter, and retained foreign bodies (wires, pieces of stents or catheters, etc.) are findings associated with obstruction and efforts to relieve it (Figs. 6–44 to 6–46). The nephrostogram or stentogram may further be used as a map of the urinary tract pending further or additional fluoroscopic or endoscopic procedures and manipulations, such as stone removal, fulguration or biopsy of lesions, and treatment of calyceal diverticula. Sometimes the results of interventions can be evaluated through a nephrostogram or stentogram before the catheter is removed or before the patient is discharged.

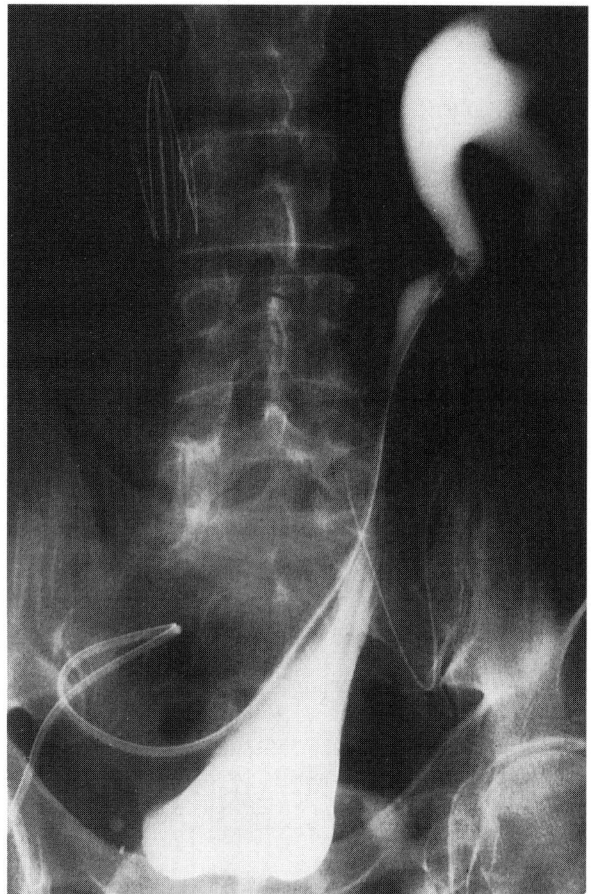

Figure 6–44. Ureteral stentogram after left ureteroneocystostomy with a psoas hitch. The deformed left ureterovesical anastomosis is the result of the procedure. There is no anastomotic leakage.

A plain abdominal film is obtained before opacification of the urinary tract. Water-soluble contrast material is then injected into the catheter or stent, and the collecting system and ureter are imaged under intermittent fluoroscopic control. Oblique, prone, and upright views may be necessary for optimal visualization of the urinary tract. As with the loopogram, caution is advised not to overdistend the system, which usually is infected, so that the risk of pyelonephritis and urosepsis is minimal. Prophylactic antibiotics are advised. Monitoring of the hydrostatic pressure within the renal pelvis is desirable, with the intent not to exceed pressures of 30 to 35 cm H_2O during the study. In most cases of prior reactions to intravascular contrast media, it is still safe to use the less expensive ionic compounds for direct injections into the urinary tract (cystogram, loopogram, nephrostogram).

The findings on the nephrostogram or ureteral stentogram need to be correlated with the plain film findings, history of known or suspected pathology, and the record of recent surgical intervention, if any. Clots often appear as elongated, smooth defects that are radiolucent; fungus balls are radiolucent and round or oval, sometimes with irregular contour; tumors are adherent to the wall and appear as irregular filling defects; stones are usually visible on the plain film. However, the appearances of all these lesions do sometimes overlap with each other; therefore, correlation with the history, and further diagnostic studies, such as sonography or CT, are on occasion indicated.

Sonography

The use of sonography in the investigation of urologic diseases is widespread, and its indications are diverse (Pollack and Banner, 1994). **Its many advantages—such as availability, flexibility, lack of ionizing radiation, and accurate anatomic and, sometimes, physiologic information obtained without the need for intravascular contrast agents—have to be balanced by the great dependency on the operator** to produce consistently high-quality studies and an in-depth knowledge of the yield, indications, and shortcomings of sonography in comparison with other imaging techniques. For example, sonography is **superior to IVU in the evaluation of renal masses but inferior in the detection of most urothelial lesions.** Sonography is **far superior to CT in the evaluation of prostatic and scrotal pathology but inferior in the detection of most retroperitoneal and ureteral lesions.**

Sonography generates images by transducer-emitted short bursts of pulsed sound waves into tissues (Burns, 1991). **Some of the echoes produced as a result of the interaction of the sound beam with the tissues are received**

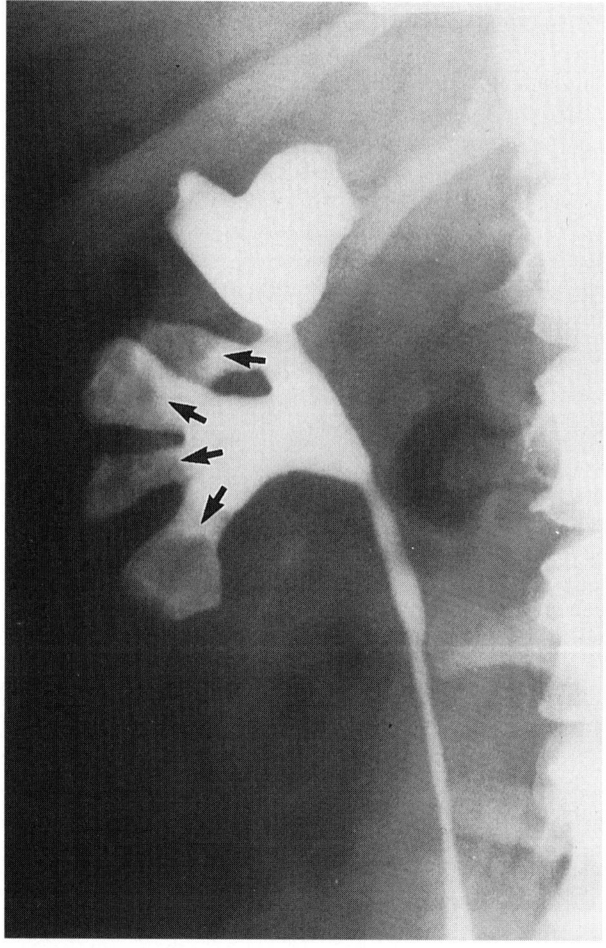

Figure 6–45. Right ureteral stentogram after lithotripsy for stone disease. Several calyces are filled with stone debris *(arrows).*

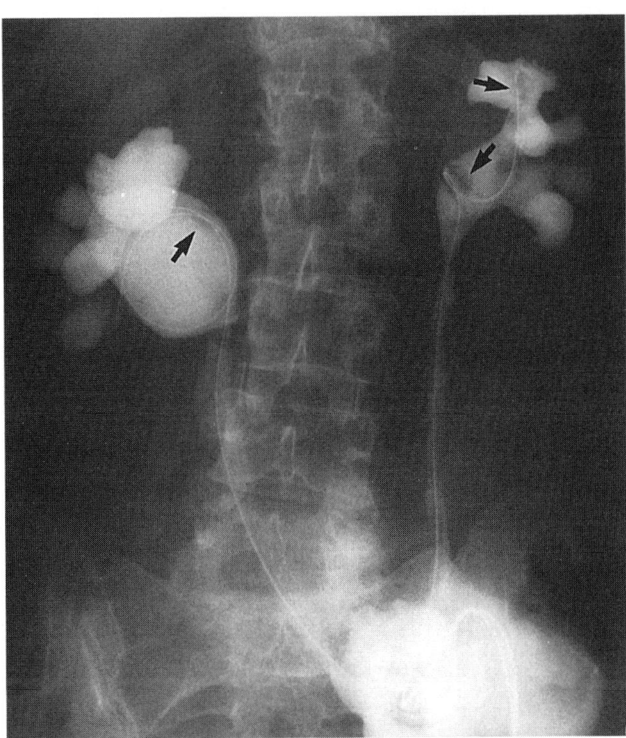

Figure 6–46. Bilateral ureteral stentograms after hysterectomy and pelvic exenteration with urinary diversion. Filling defects in both collecting systems *(arrows)* represent fungus balls.

by the transducer, and this information is digitized and displayed on screen by a built-in computer. Real-time sonography refers to the continuous, very rapid generation of images as the transducer moves over parts of the body, which are then visualized in real time from different projections and depth until optimal imaging is accomplished. Movement of tissues, structures, or contents thereof can be monitored as it happens, allowing the operator to recognize cardiac motion, peristalsis of bowel loops, motion with respiration of organs adjacent to the diaphragm, blood within vessels, and urine expelled into the bladder by the ureters; these are just a few of the physiologic observations made possible by real-time imaging. Individual dynamic images can be frozen on the screen and recorded permanently on film, videotape, or paper for documentation of anatomy or pathology and for future review of pertinent information. A wide choice of transducers makes imaging of most organs possible. **For deep abdominal structures such as the kidneys, adrenal glands, and retroperitoneum, low-frequency transducers provide better tissue penetration. Superficial structures such as the bladder or scrotum are best seen with high-frequency, high-line density-limited field-of-view probes.** Organs or structures such as the **rectum, prostate, and urethra can best be visualized with the use of endoluminal probes especially shaped and constructed to fit into orifices and lumens of hollow viscera.**

Doppler sonography provides information derived from the blood flowing into vessels toward and away from the transducer. The physics principle involved is known as the **Doppler effect or shift** and refers to the changes in frequency of the sound beam that occur when the latter is reflected by a moving target, in this case the blood. This frequency increases when the blood or other moving target moves toward the transducer and decreases when the direction of the motion is away from the transducer. The frequency change is directly proportional to the frequency of the sound, the velocity of the reflector, and the angle between the sound wave and the reflector and is inversely proportional to the velocity of the sound wave in tissues (Burns, 1991). The angle between the sound beam and the moving target should not exceed 90 degrees; optimal angles vary from 45 to 60 degrees. The wave form generated by the combinations of real-time sonography and Doppler techniques is known as duplex Doppler imaging. This technique enables the measurement of the velocity of flow and other parameters from the Doppler shift frequency. The Doppler wave form or spectrum can thus be analyzed for the presence and direction of flow and for identification of arterial and venous flow on the basis of the physical characteristics and direction of flow in the interrogated vessels. Laminar, undisturbed flow can be distinguished from turbulent or disturbed flow on the basis of the spectral tracings.

A numerical index widely used to measure vascular impedance and pulsatility in clinical practice is the **resistive index (RI),** calculated as [peak systolic blood flow velocity minus minimal end-diastolic blood flow velocity] divided by the peak systolic blood flow velocity. Values up to .70 have been considered normal. After much enthusiasm with the early use of the RI in the diagnosis of pathology as diverse as renal transplant rejection, urinary obstruction, and tumor vascularity, the high expectations have been tempered by subsequent reports of lower sensitivity and specificity.

Color Doppler imaging, a newer technique, facilitates the visual recognition of normal and abnormal vascular flow patterns across the spectrum of disease affecting the blood vessels. The color images are obtained by converting the Doppler information from real-time gray-scale imaging to color-encoded images. The assignment of color is usually made on the basis of the direction of flow in relation to the probe. Typically, red indicates flow toward the transducer and blue indicates flow away from the transducer. Increased color shades (lighter colors) indicate higher Doppler frequency shifts. Urologic diseases that can be studied with the use of duplex Doppler and color Doppler imaging are many and are emphasized in the ensuing sections.

Kidney

Sonography can document the presence, location, and size of the kidneys. Furthermore, it may be used to demonstrate the thickness and echogenicity of the renal parenchyma; detect focal parenchymal lesions such as tumors and cysts; assess the appearance of the normally echogenic renal sinus with particular attention to possible dilatation of the pyelocalyceal system and the presence of calculi or, less likely, urothelial neoplasms; evaluate for fluid collections in and around the kidneys; investigate blood flow patterns and certain vascular lesions, such as arteriovenous malformations, aneurysms, occlusions, and bland or tumor thrombosis of the renal vein and inferior vena cava; and guide percutaneous and surgical interventions. Evaluation of the complications and dysfunction of renal transplants often includes sonogra-

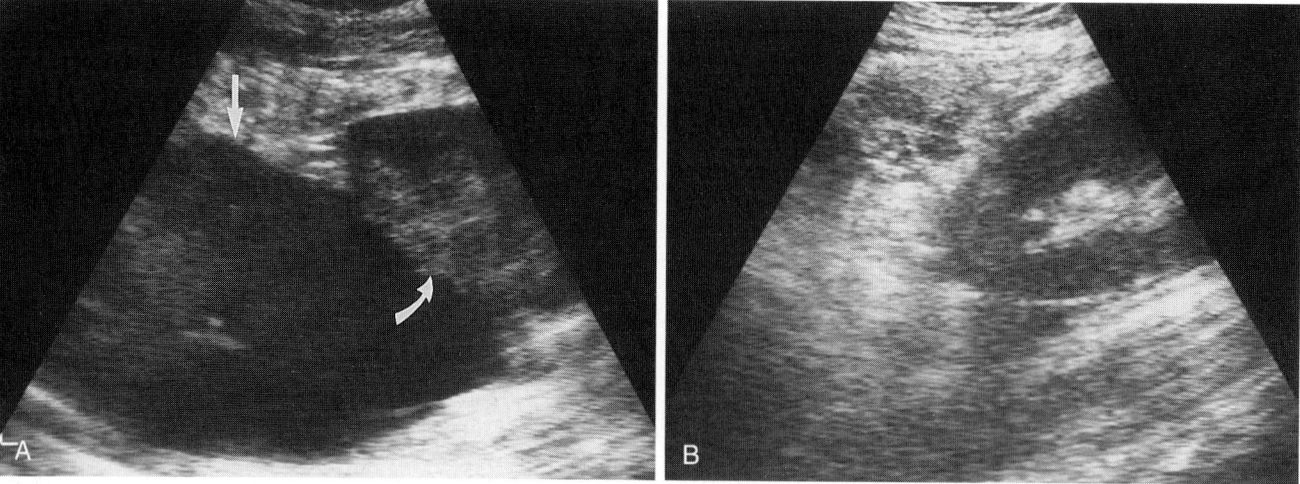

Figure 6–47. Fluid collection after renal transplantation. *A,* A large, mostly anechoic fluid collection *(straight arrow)* is seen on sonography to be adjacent to the upper pole of the renal transplant *(curved arrow). B,* After the collection is drained percutaneously, the perinephric space appears normal.

phy, which is best suited for detecting vascular problems, hydronephrosis, and perinephric fluid collections (Figs. 6–47, 6–48).

The **normal kidney is readily visualized on sonography as a low-echogenic, bean-shaped organ with a bright echogenic center, the renal sinus** (Wolfman et al, 1991) (Fig. 6–49). The echogenicity of the renal parenchyma is typically less than that of the adjacent liver. The kidneys are scanned and imaged in the sagittal, oblique, and transverse planes. Vascular interrogation is often an integral part of the examination. The renal artery and vein may be demonstrated, although not always, on duplex and color Doppler imaging, and blood flow patterns can be recorded. Interrogation of intrarenal vessels is more consistent, reliable, and valuable in clinical practice.

If not found in its usual location, a kidney may be ectopic, absent, or very atrophic and small. A search for an ectopic kidney is mandated if a renal fossa is empty and there is no history of nephrectomy. Ectopic kidneys are most often found in the pelvis and sometimes fused with the contralateral kidney (crossed fused ectopy). Horseshoe kidneys lie more anteriorly and lower in the abdomen than usual. Their lower renal poles converge medially over the spine and great vessels, where they are fused with each other, sometimes mimicking a retroperitoneal mass or lymphadenopathy. They can be recognized by their converging long axes and lower position in the retroperitoneum. Very small kidneys, the result of congenital pathologic processes (as with some multicystic dysplastic kidneys) or acquired pathologic processes (trauma, renovascular insult) may be very difficult to visualize. If the sonogram cannot locate a kidney, CT, angiography, or retrograde pyelography may be further used to elucidate its location. Congenital absence is infrequent. The contralateral kidney is hypertrophied. Surgical nephrectomy should be readily known from the history and flank incision.

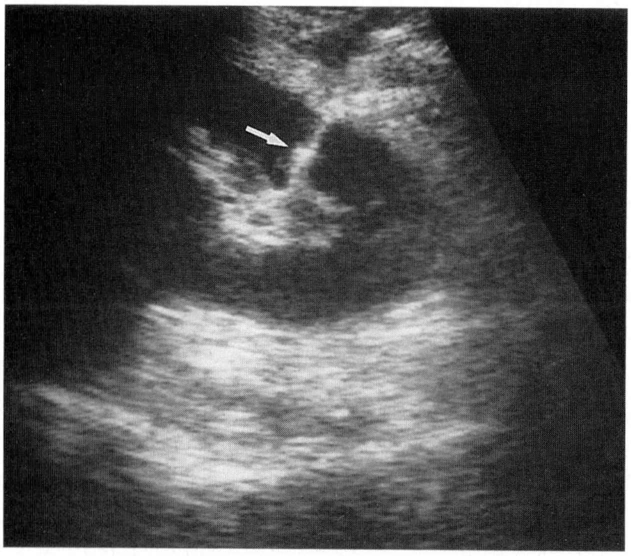

Figure 6–48. Failure of a renal transplant often necessitates biopsy for diagnosis of the specific etiology. Sonography is the imaging guidance procedure of choice for percutaneous needle biopsy. The track of the needle within the cortex can be easily traced *(arrow).*

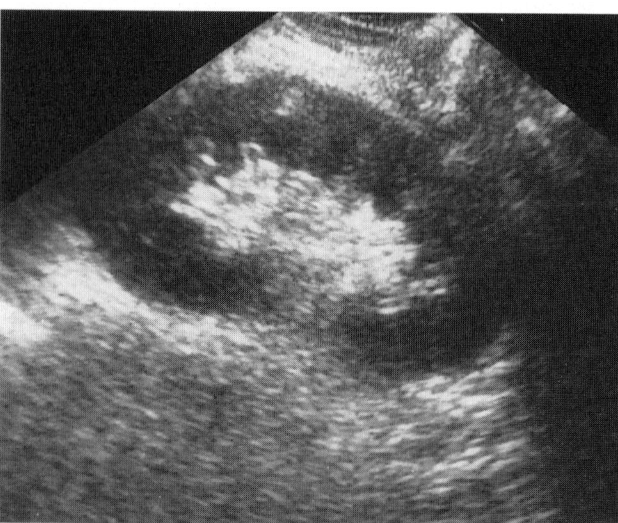

Figure 6–49. Normal longitudinal renal sonogram.

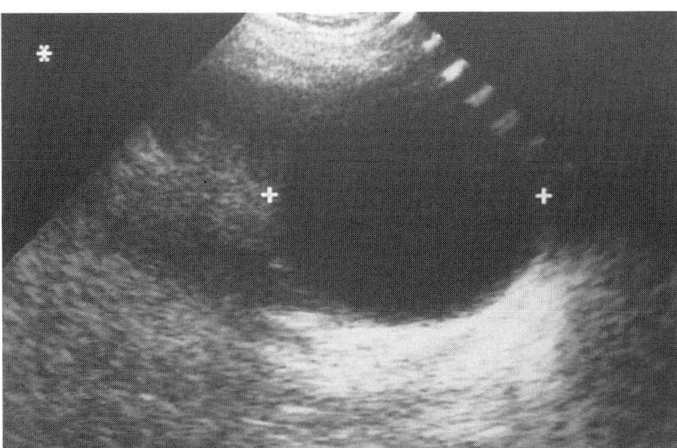

Figure 6–50. Large renal cyst seen on sonography as an anechoic structure with enhanced posterior acoustic transmission.

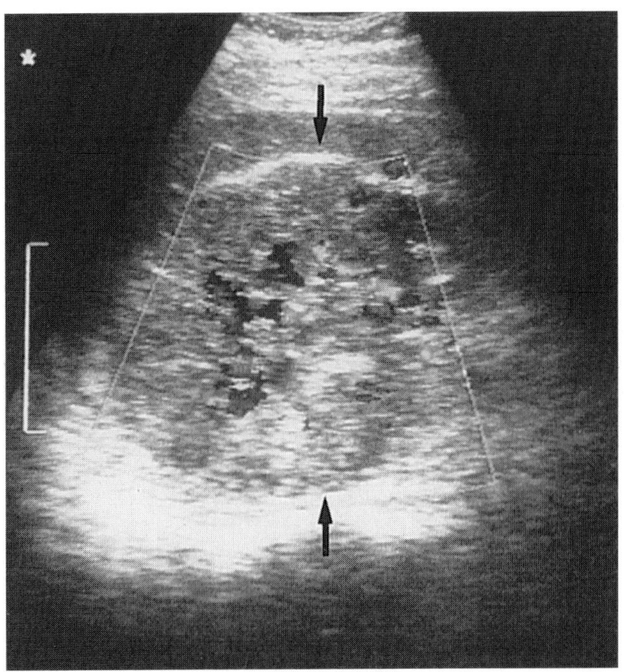

Figure 6–52. Transverse renal sonogram demonstrates a large, heterogeneous solid renal mass, consistent with renal cell carcinoma *(arrows).*

Focal renal masses disrupt the homogeneous appearance of the parenchyma and often distort the renal contours when they are large and/or peripherally located (Drago and Cunningham, 1991). **Renal cysts** are common, especially in elderly patients (Fig. 6–50). The **typical appearance is that of an anechoic, well-defined structure, with very thin walls and clearly enhanced transmission of the sound beam beyond the distal wall of the cyst. On duplex or color Doppler investigation, no vascularity is seen within the cyst.** Simple septa or rim calcification may be seen within the cyst cavity (Fig. 6–51). **Cystic masses** appear as **hypoechoic or mixed anechoic and hypoechoic lesions with thickened walls and irregular or thick septa** (Drago and Cunningham, 1991). **Through transmission of the sound beam is decreased or absent. Solid masses** appear as **well- or ill-defined masses without or with chunky calcifications** (Figs. 6–52, 6–53) and are variably echogenic, from the less echogenic lymphomas to the very echogenic angiomyolipomas. The normal variant of **hypertrophied septa of Bertin** that may simulate a mass on IVU has the **same echotexture on sonography as the adjacent normal parenchyma and can be easily dismissed.**

Several reports in the literature support the use of sonography in the investigation of occult or suspected renal cysts and masses. When the criteria for a simple cyst are carefully adhered to, the accuracy of sonography in detecting cysts is in the 95% range (Fig. 6–54). Obese patients, inexperienced operators, and ectopic kidneys lower that range significantly. The sonogram should be the examination of choice in the initial evaluation of a cystic renal mass, when the presence of a simple cyst is under consideration. Patients who cannot receive intravascular contrast media because of compromised renal function or a history of serious reaction should undergo sonography because of its superior accuracy over nonenhanced CT. Adult polycystic kidney disease can be readily detected on the basis of bilaterally enlarged kidneys that contain innumerable cysts of various sizes (Choyke, 1996). Kidneys with end-stage disease often are investigated with sonography instead of nonenhanced CT for cysts and solid tumors (Levine, 1996). Acquired cystic disease in patients with chronic renal failure is very common, and their kidneys

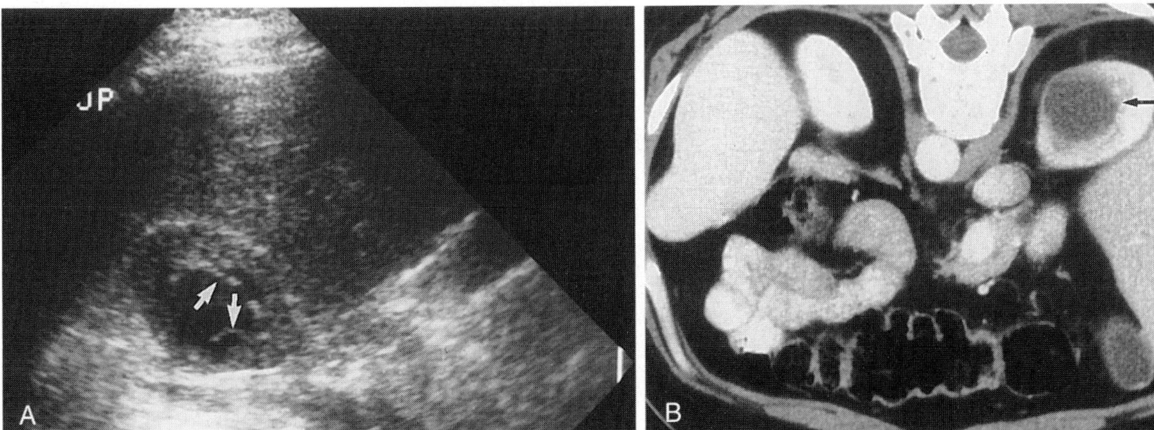

Figure 6–51. Septated renal cyst. *A,* Thin septations are seen within an anechoic lesion in the right upper renal pole on sonography *(arrows). B,* CT correlation shows the lesion to be a simple cyst *(arrow).*

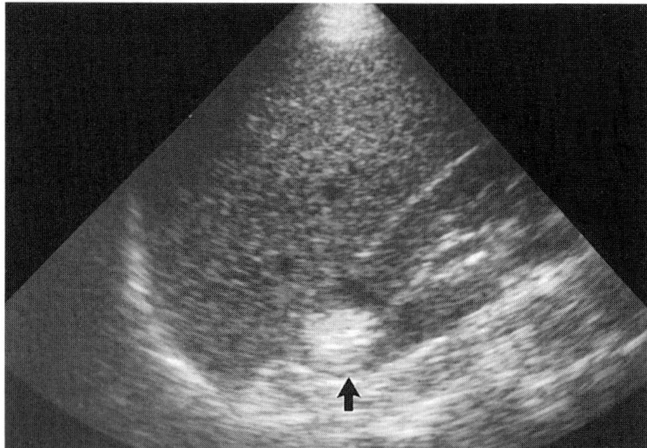

Figure 6–53. Sonogram demonstrates hyperechoic, focal, solid renal mass, consistent with an angiomyolipoma *(arrow)*.

are sometimes difficult to examine because of their small size, irregular contour, and echogenic parenchyma. The major concern is the ability to detect solid tumors amid the cystic and diffuse parenchymal changes.

Sonography is very sensitive in detecting solid masses, particularly those measuring 1.5 to 2 cm or more in largest dimension (Jamis-Dow et al, 1996) (Fig. 6–55). Much like the other cross-sectional imaging techniques, sonography is not very specific in distinguishing benign from malignant tumors. **Accurate staging of renal cell carcinoma and urothelial tumors lags behind that with CT and MRI in regard to lymphadenopathy, capsular invasion, spread into adjacent structures, and distant metastases. The presence or absence of tumor thrombus within the lumen of the inferior vena cava can be reliably investigated by sonography** (Fig. 6–56).

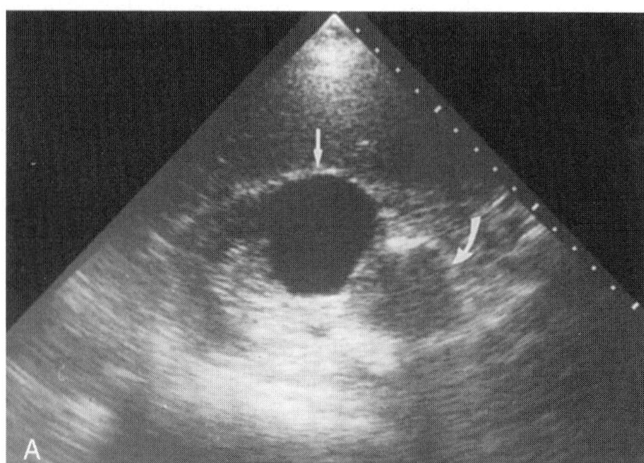

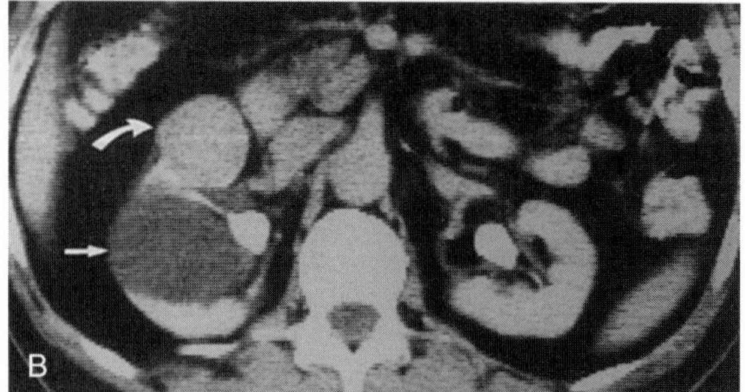

Figure 6–54. Cystic and solid lesions in the right kidney of a middle-aged man. *A,* Longitudinal renal sonogram shows a simple cyst *(straight arrow)* next to a solid mass *(curved arrow)*. *B,* CT scan confirms the cyst *(straight arrow)* and solid mass *(curved arrow)*, which proved to be an oncocytoma.

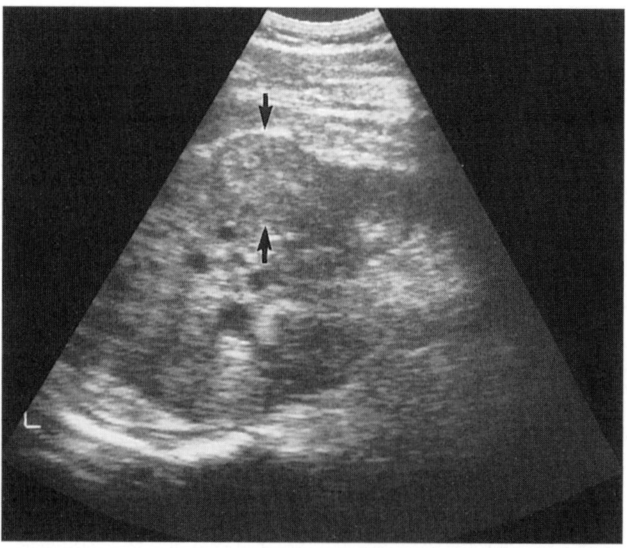

Figure 6–55. Small solid renal mass depicted on sonography in patient with normal nephrotomography *(arrows)*.

Hydronephrosis results in an anechoic (clear urine) or hypoechoic (infected urine, blood clots) fluid collection that splits the bright central echoes of the renal sinus and often assumes the shape of the calyces and renal pelvis (Figs. 6–57, 6–58). Although usually caused by obstruction, hydronephrosis does not invariably indicate that obstruction is present at the time of the examination. Sometimes the dilatation is bilateral and physiologic, usually of mild degree, such as in patients with a distended bladder, pregnant women, or patients with high urine outflow (as in diabetes insipidus or postobstructive diuresis). Furthermore, both dilatation of the

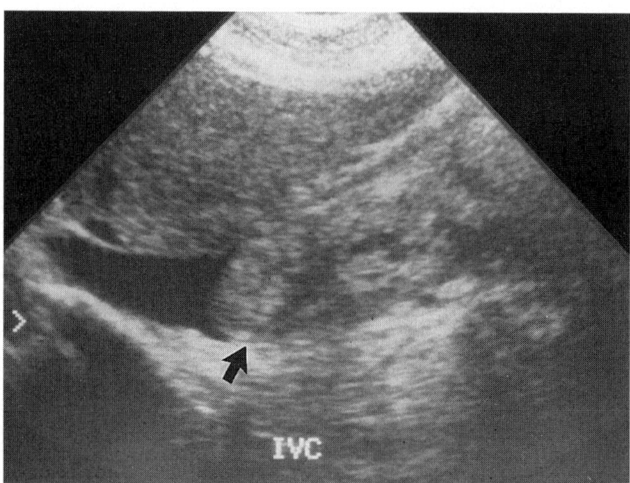

Figure 6–56. Longitudinal sonogram through the inferior vena cava at the level of the liver demonstrates a large tumor thrombus in its lumen from a right renal solid mass *(arrow)*.

urinary tract secondary to ureteral reflux and residual hydronephrosis after relief of obstruction are nonobstructive. **Sonography, however, in the absence of comparison studies or appropriate history cannot by itself distinguish obstructive from nonobstructive hydronephrosis;** therefore, a physiologic or functional study, such as IVU or radionuclide renogram, may be complementary for clarification of the process.

Attempts have been made to combine the gray scale images with Doppler scanning to introduce an element of physiologic investigation to an otherwise anatomic examination. Measurements of the RI have been advocated in clinical practice as a reliable means of separating obstructive from nonobstructive hydronephrosis (Platt et al, 1989). The rationale behind this approach is based on experimental evidence that renal vascular resistance is increased in urinary obstruction. A value above .70 in the presence of hydronephrosis is suggestive of obstruction (Fig. 6–59). After placement of a percutaneous nephrostomy for drainage, the RI value returns to normal levels in patients with acute obstruction. The use of RI in everyday practice is complicated and confounded by medical and technical issues (Cronan, 1991). Tubulointerstitial renal diseases such as interstitial nephritis and acute tubular necrosis have been found to elevate the RI values, whereas glomerular diseases may not. Chronically obstructed kidneys have been reported to yield normal RI levels. Furthermore, the normal aging process has been reported to cause a gradual elevation in the RI values that may become abnormally high over the age of 60 years in the absence of obstruction or a parenchymal renal process. The technique of obtaining reliable RI measurements can be time consuming and tedious in an effort to minimize operator dependence and sampling errors, and the reproducibility of the results has been questioned.

Color Doppler imaging has been used to study the qualitative and quantitative characteristics of ureteral jets in the bladder as a means of detecting ureteral obstruction (Burge et al, 1991). A ureteral jet occurs when denser urine is expelled from the ureteral orifice into the more dilute urine of the bladder and can be detected as a stream of echoes originating in the vicinity of the ureterovesical junction. The different acoustic densities between the urine in the ureter

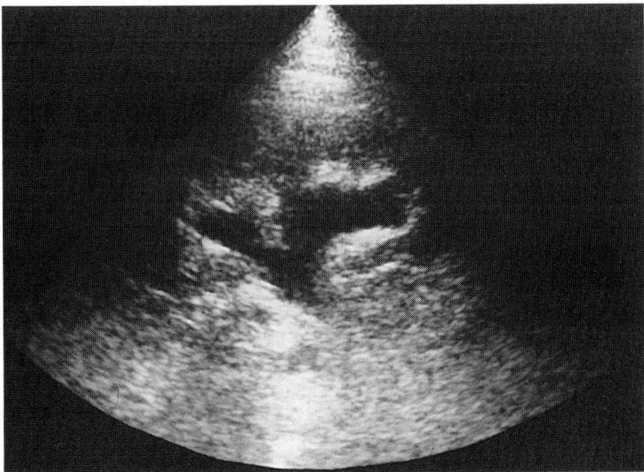

Figure 6–57. Longitudinal renal sonogram shows moderate hydronephrosis.

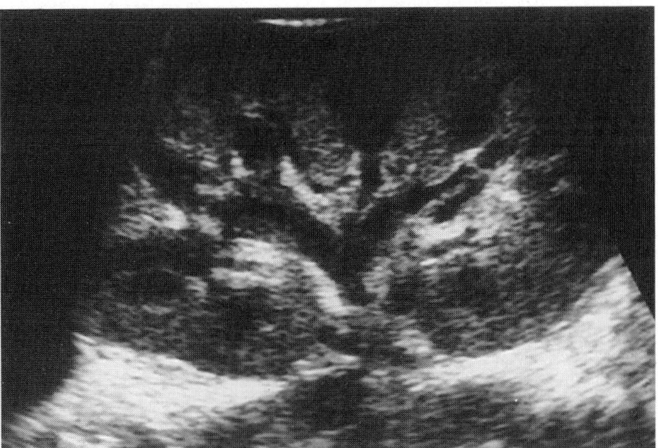

Figure 6–58. Mild degree of hydronephrosis in a renal transplant.

and that of the bladder generate the acoustic reflections detected as ureteral jets. The intensity of these reflections increases with increasing differences in flow rates. A high-grade obstruction is most often associated either with absence of an ipsilateral jet or, less likely, with low-level continuous flow echoes. A low-grade obstruction may have a normal jet pattern. The technique has not gained widespread acceptance in clinical practice because of the overlapping, sometimes nonspecific jet patterns between different grades of obstruction and the significant examination time and patient preparation requirements.

Sonography may not be diagnostic of acute urinary obstruction early after the onset of symptoms. Minimal or no hydronephrosis may be seen for up to 48 hours after the patient becomes symptomatic; therefore, if the clinical suspicion is high and the study normal, an intravenous urogram is indicated for further evaluation. Although evidence is insufficient, the occurrence of a false-negative sonogram in the presence of obstruction is considered uncommon.

False-positive sonographic findings suggestive of hydronephrosis or obstruction are more common (Amis et al, 1982). It has already been mentioned that the demonstration of hydronephrosis on an anatomic study, such as sonography, does not always establish the diagnosis of obstruction. Dilatation of the urinary tract from reflux or previous obstruction that has since been relieved can be seen often enough in everyday practice. Sometimes the false diagnosis of hydronephrosis and/or obstruction is made on sonography. **Peripelvic cysts can mimic pyelocaliectasis,** especially as viewed by inexperienced sonographers (Fig. 6–60). **The difference between the cysts and true hydronephrosis is that the cysts do not communicate with each other, whereas the calyces do.** Careful scanning technique minimizes the risk of incorrect diagnosis, although on occasion the distinction cannot be made with certainty and IVU is required. **A large-capacity extrarenal renal pelvis or anatomic variations in the appearance of the calyceal system may sometimes simulate hydronephrosis.** The anatomic variations occur when the infundibula to the calyces are very short or wide and the renal pelvis appears to be forming most of the collecting system (Fig. 6–61). Scanning peripherally throughout the kidney is likely to show whether the calyces themselves are dilated, which would then make the diagnosis

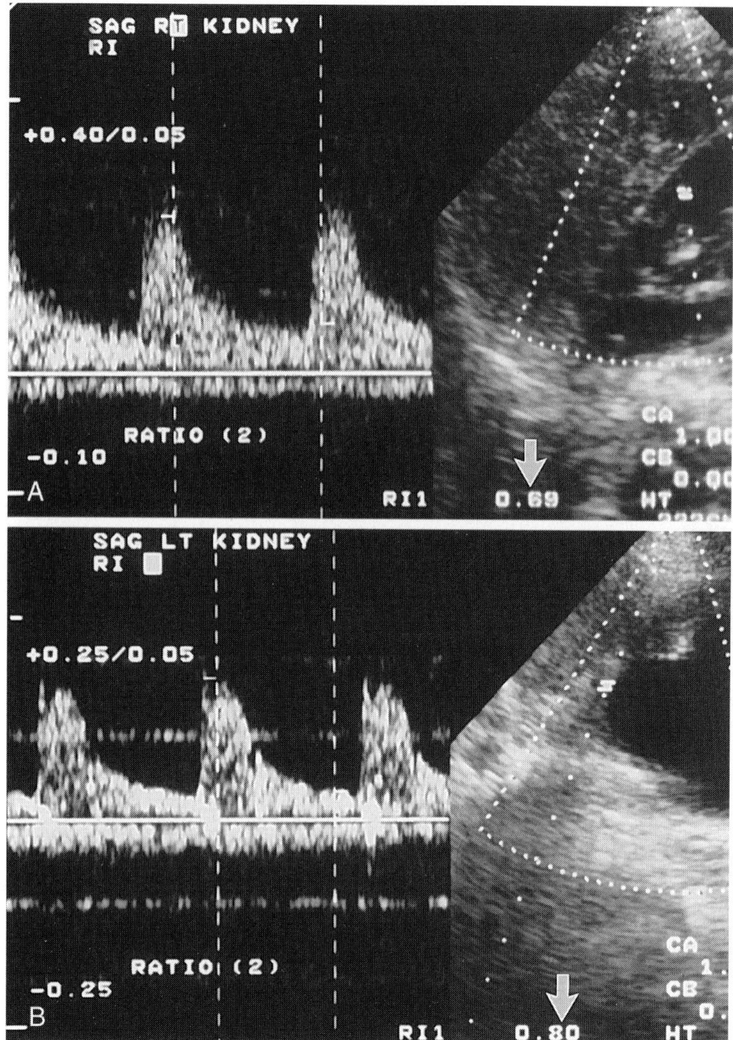

Figure 6–59. Use of the resistive index (RI) measurements in the diagnosis of urinary obstruction. *A,* The normal right kidney has an RI of 0.69 *(arrow)*. *B,* The left kidney, obstructed by a bladder tumor, has an elevated RI *(arrow)*.

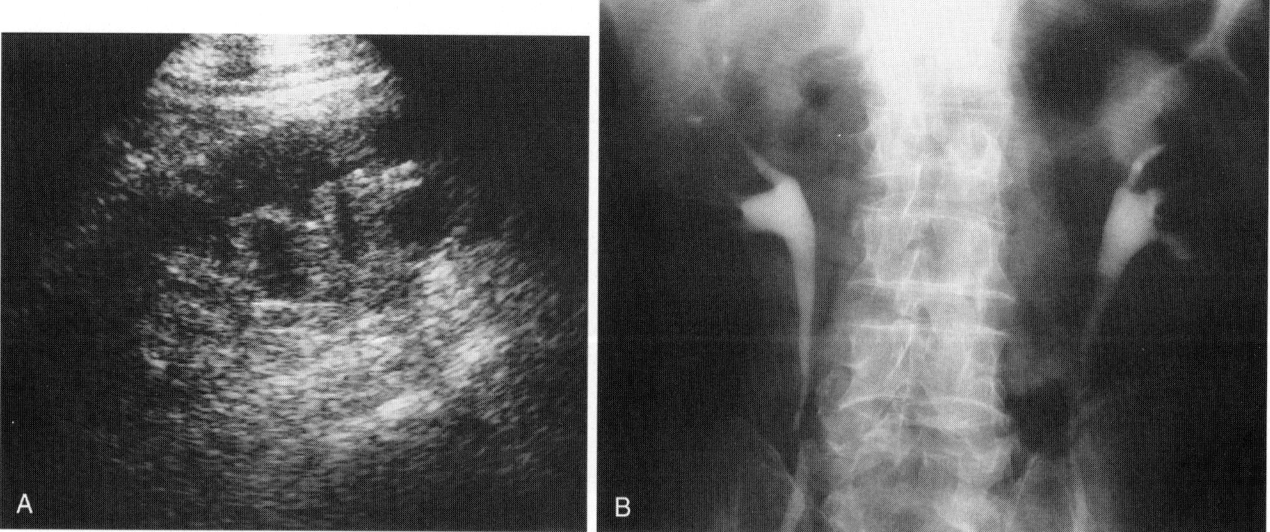

Figure 6–60. Renal false-positive findings for hydronephrosis. *A,* Apparent mild dilatation of the right collecting system was diagnosed on sonography. On re-examination of the patient, the anechoic spaces in the renal sinus did not communicate with each other, which suggested peripelvic cysts. *B,* Intravenous urogram shows no caliectasis.

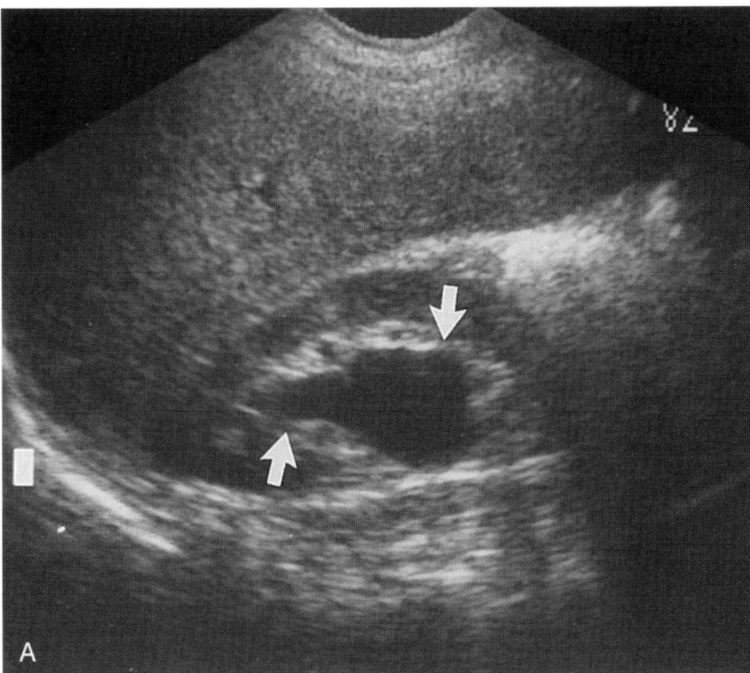

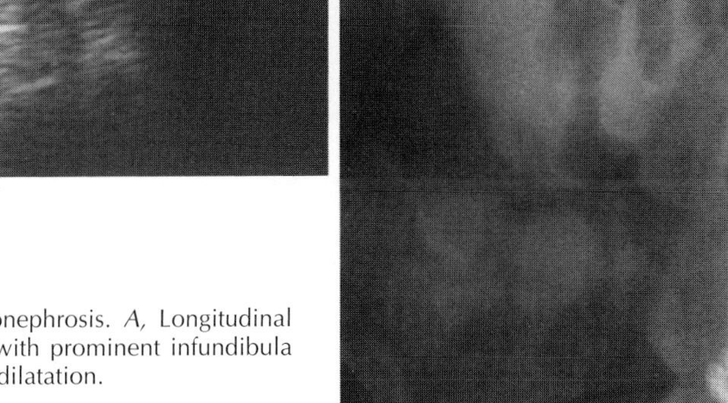

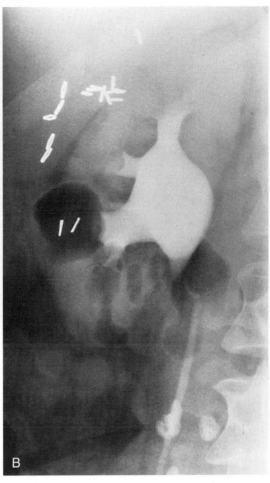

Figure 6–61. Renal false-positive findings for hydronephrosis. *A,* Longitudinal sonogram shows a large-capacity right renal pelvis with prominent infundibula *(arrows). B,* Intravenous urogram shows no calyceal dilatation.

reliable and accurate. On occasions, cystic renal disease, diffuse papillary necrosis changes, and the entity known as congenital megacalyces may simulate the appearance of hydronephrosis on sonography.

Localization of the obstructing process often is limited or impossible. Stones or tumors in the renal pelvis or the ureterovesical junction may be seen in adult patients (Figs. 6–62, 6–63). When bilateral hydronephrosis and hydroureter are associated with a large-capacity trabeculated bladder and an enlarged prostate, the upper tract changes may be attributed to the large size of the prostate. Bladder tumors may be demonstrated on suprapubic sonography. More often than not, however, determining the location and cause of the obstruction requires further investigation by IVU, retrograde pyelography, or CT.

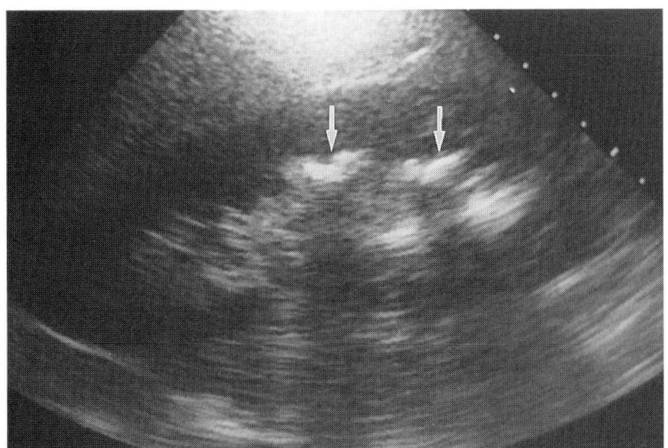

Figure 6–62. Longitudinal renal sonogram shows at least two right-sided renal calculi *(arrows).*

Diffuse parenchymal disease of the kidney, such as glomerulonephritis, interstitial nephritis, certain types of acute tubular necrosis, and vasculitides often result in significant bilateral increased echogenicity of the renal cortex (Wolfman et al, 1991) (Fig. 6–64). The appearance is nonspecific, and the diagnosis is made on clinical grounds or from needle biopsy findings. **Acute and chronic pyelonephritis may also produce changes in the echogenicity of the renal parenchyma. Acute infection usually causes a decrease in echogenicity; chronic infection and scarring cause an increase.** In addition, in chronic pyelonephritis the affected kidney is smaller than the contralateral normal one and has atrophic parenchyma and irregular scarred contour. Small, echogenic kidneys, often with smooth contour, are encountered in cases of renovascular disease or after irradiation of the renal fossa. **Arterial embolic disease** usually results in a normal appearance of the kidney on real-time images, although duplex or color Doppler examination yield strikingly abnormal images. **Renal vein thrombosis** may cause an early decrease in echogenicity, followed by increased parenchymal echoes in the chronic stage. The renal

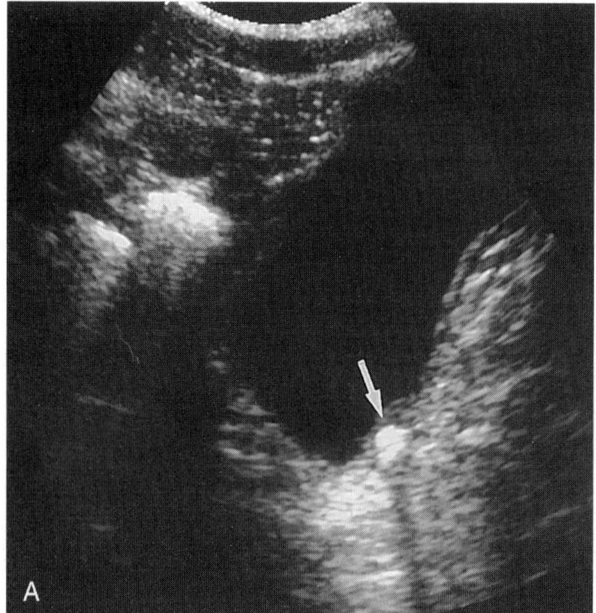

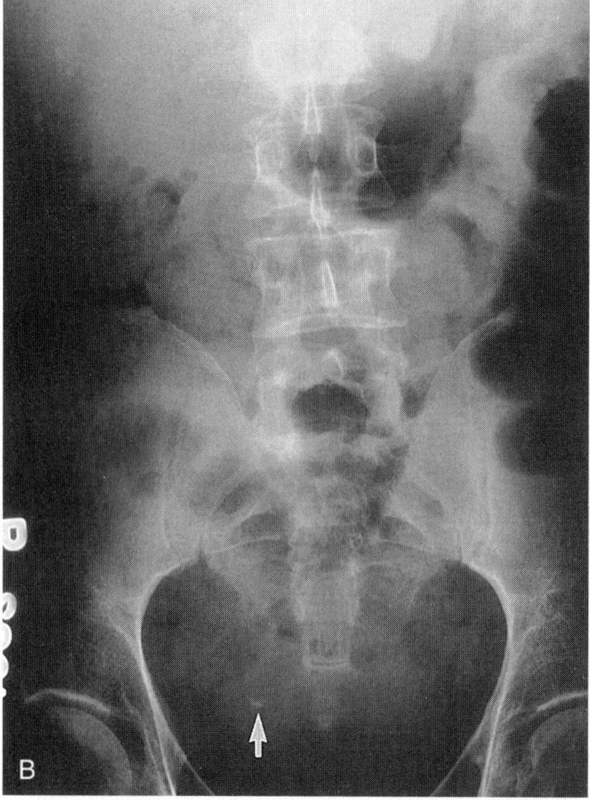

Figure 6–63. Right ureterovesical junction calculus. *A,* Longitudinal sonogram shows an echogenic focus with posterior acoustic shadowing at the ureterovesical junction *(arrow). B,* Plain abdominal radiography also shows the stone in the right lower pelvis *(arrow).*

vein may appear dilated and contains echoes in its lumen, consistent with formation of clot.

The evaluation of **arterial renovascular disease** with sonography is limited (Stavros et al, 1992; Mitty et al, 1996). Localization and interrogation of the entire renal artery, which often is tortuous, is technically difficult or impossible, even by color Doppler techniques. Furthermore, prospective identification of accessory renal arteries is difficult, and the disease sometimes is caused by stenosis of segmental branches, which can be missed, whereas a normal Doppler wave form may be obtained from a nonstenotic artery. Occlusion of the main renal artery or major branches thereof can be successfully diagnosed by the absence of arterial flow on duplex or color Doppler studies. Partial occlusions and their locations, however, remain a problem, despite promising reports of careful and more sophisticated analysis of the Doppler wave form. Patients with renal artery stenosis greater than 75% have been shown to have a significant decrease in systolic acceleration, as measured by the use of the acceleration index, which reflects the rate of velocity increases during the systolic upstroke (Mitty et al, 1996). Results for stenoses ranging from 50% to 75%, still of clinical significance, are very scant. These techniques have not gained widespread acceptance and have not been reproduced successfully by other investigators to resolve the variables and remaining validation questions (Kliewer et al, 1993).

Intrarenal, subcapsular, and perinephric collections can be diagnosed and accurately compartmentalized by sonography. Large perinephric and retroperitoneal collections can be better staged by CT. The nature of the fluid usually cannot be predicted on the basis of sonography alone. Hemorrhage and infection may be more echogenic than a urinoma or lymphocele. Renal abscesses appear as relatively well-defined focal masses, sometimes liquified enough to resemble a complex cystic mass (Drago and Cunningham, 1991). Acute pyelonephritis often appears as a hypoechoic, ill-defined parenchymal process or, less likely, an echogenic mass (Papanicolaou and Pfister, 1996). The increased echogenicity is attributed to hemorrhage. Infected renal cysts and calyceal diverticula are seen as cystic lesions with internal echoes from the inflammatory debris and variable enhancement of the sound beam past the lesion.

Sonography is widely used to guide diagnostic and therapeutic interventions in and around the kidney. Most **renal biopsies,** whether for focal masses or diffuse parenchymal diseases, are performed under ultrasonic guidance (see Figs. 6–47, 6–48). **Fluid collections can be drained** by placing catheters percutaneously under sonographic control. **Renal cysts are safely aspirated,** and **percutaneous nephrostomy** catheters have been placed for drainage of obstructive hydronephrosis in children, pregnant women, and

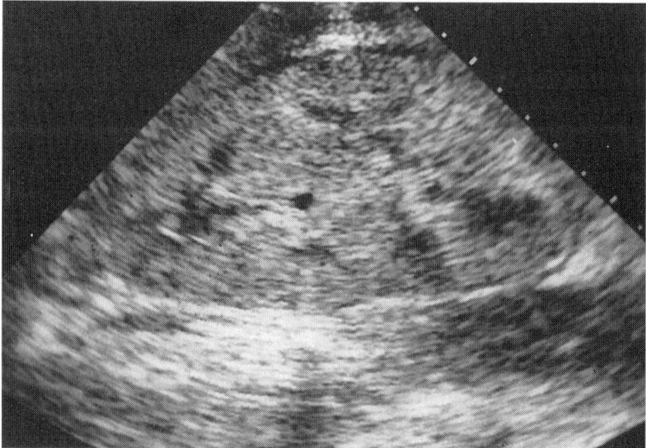

Figure 6–64. Longitudinal renal sonogram in patient with marked renal failure and human immunodeficiency virus (HIV) nephropathy. The renal parenchyma is markedly echogenic.

other patients with the help of ultrasonography. Small, deeply located lesions or collections may be best approached by using CT for guidance.

The superficially located transplanted kidney is very well suited for sonographic investigation (Becker, 1991) (see Figs. 6–47, 6–48, 6–58). Anatomic and physiologic information obtained answers questions about urinary obstruction, perinephric fluid collections, and patency of the vascular pedicle. Despite earlier reports advocating the use of RI values to accurately diagnose acute transplant rejection and distinguish it from acute tubular necrosis and cyclosporine toxicity, subsequent studies have demonstrated limited diagnosis of acute rejection. An abnormal RI often implies allograft pathology but not necessarily rejection.

Anatomic changes that have been described in transplant rejection are renal enlargement, increased cortical echogenicity, poor definition of the echogenic renal sinus, loss of the corticomedullary differentiation, and **swelling of the pyelocalyceal urothelium.** Many of these findings are not pathognomonic of rejection, however, and a renal biopsy remains the ultimate diagnostic study that guides the treatment of the patient.

Renal sonography is the procedure of choice for visualizing the kidneys in patients who cannot receive intravascular contrast material because of the renal dysfunction or history of reaction. Furthermore, it is recommended for the follow-up of renal size, cysts, and survey of the contralateral kidney after unilateral nephrectomy for a neoplasm or of the affected kidney if a partial nephrectomy has been performed. The use of renal sonography for these purposes is particularly well suited for pediatric patients.

Ureter and Retroperitoneum

The ureteropelvic and ureterovesical junctions can be relatively consistently evaluated by sonography (see Fig. 6–63). Ureteroceles, stones, and dilatation of the distal ureteral segment may be demonstrable (Fig. 6–65). The ureteropelvic

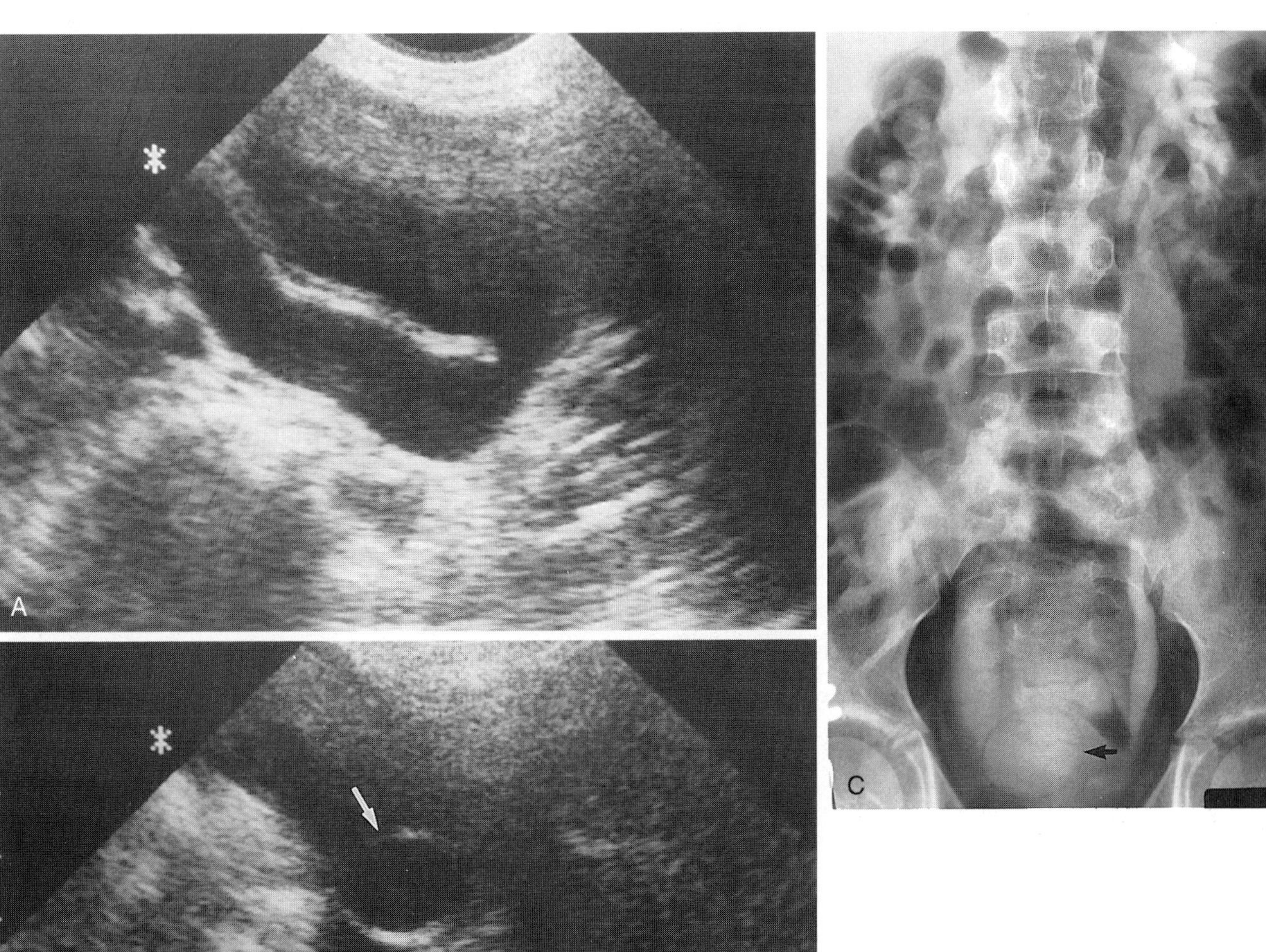

Figure 6–65. Right ureterocele in a young boy. *A,* Longitudinal sonogram reveals ureteral dilatation at the level of the bladder. *B,* The ureterocele is seen at the end of the dilated ureter as a round, anechoic, intravesical structure *(arrow)*. *C,* Intravenous urogram confirms right ureteral dilatation and ureterocele *(arrow)*.

junction usually can be seen; however, the remainder of the ureter cannot unless the patient is thin and the ureter at least moderately dilated. The use of IVU, retrograde pyelography, and/or CT is most appropriate for the complete visualization of the entire ureter.

Likewise, the retroperitoneum usually cannot be adequately investigated by sonography. Large masses and significant adenopathy especially at the level of the kidneys can be seen. Less obvious lesions cannot be detected reliably, and their extent is invariably underestimated or indeterminate on sonography. Patient size and overlying bowel loops filled with gas are commonly to blame for this shortcoming. The use of CT is therefore recommended for demonstration of the extent of lesions, such as adenopathy, retroperitoneal fibrosis, retroperitoneal tumors, and fluid collections and for postoperative complications (Fig. 6–66).

Bladder

Because of its positioning in the pelvis underneath the anterior abdominal wall and its ability to be distended by urine or fluids introduced through the urethra, the bladder can be seen relatively well through a suprapubic abdominal approach. Estimation of postvoid residual urine, search for radiolucent stones, and evaluation of large diverticula with attention to their emptying are the common clinical indications for vesical sonography. Additional applications include detection of neoplasms, confirmation of suspicious filling defects seen on IVU, and guidance for the suprapubic placement of needles or catheters into the bladder (Bodner and Resnick, 1991) (Figs. 6–67 to 6–69).

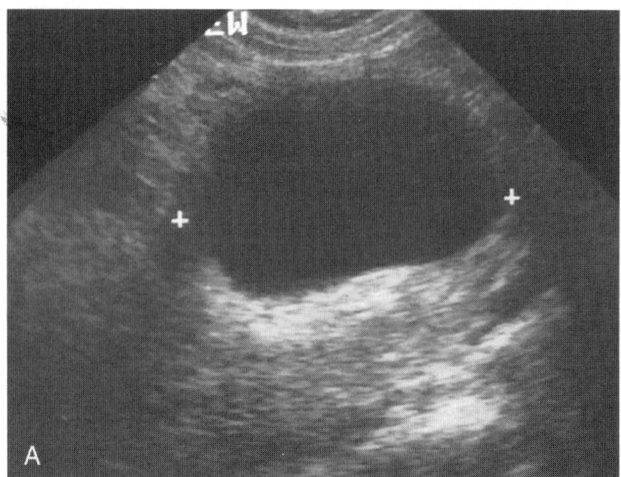

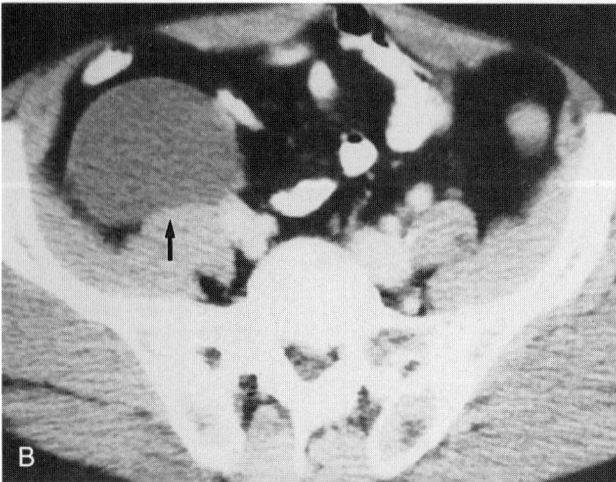

Figure 6–66. Postoperative pelvic lymphocele. *A,* A large fluid collection is seen on sonography. *B,* CT demonstrates the lymphocele in the right lower quadrant after radical prostatectomy *(arrow).*

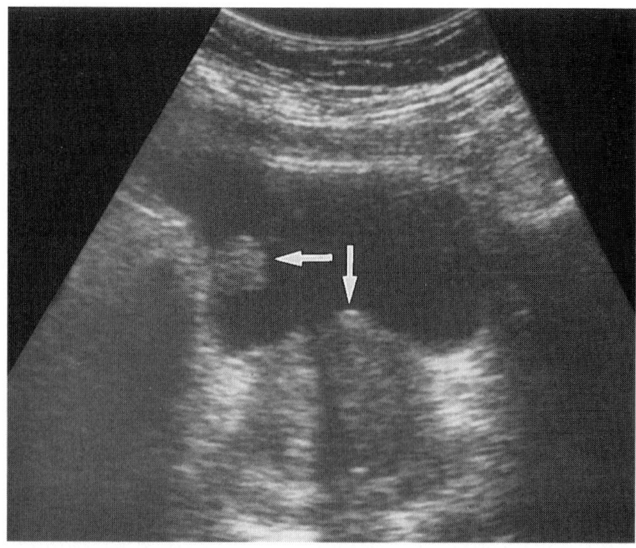

Figure 6–67. Transverse suprapubic sonogram of the bladder reveals two polypoid wall lesions within the lumen consistent with neoplasms *(arrows).*

A few reports in the urologic literature have described the use of (luminal) ultrasonography with appropriate-sized and -shaped probes in the staging of bladder neoplasms. When this is performed by experienced clinicians, the results appear to be satisfactory; however, the technique has not gained widespread acceptance and is practiced in a few specialized centers equipped with the required instruments (Bodner and Resnick, 1991).

Prostate and Seminal Vesicles

Sonography of the prostate gland has become one of the most common urologic applications of the modality and is

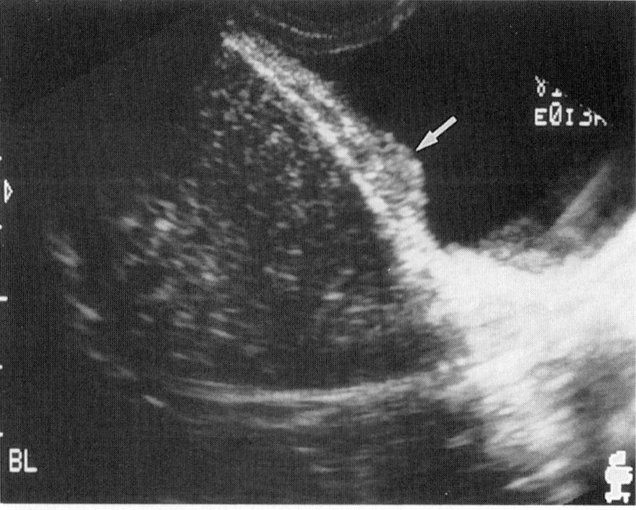

Figure 6–68. Thickening of the bladder wall *(arrow)* represents bladder involvement with schistosomiasis.

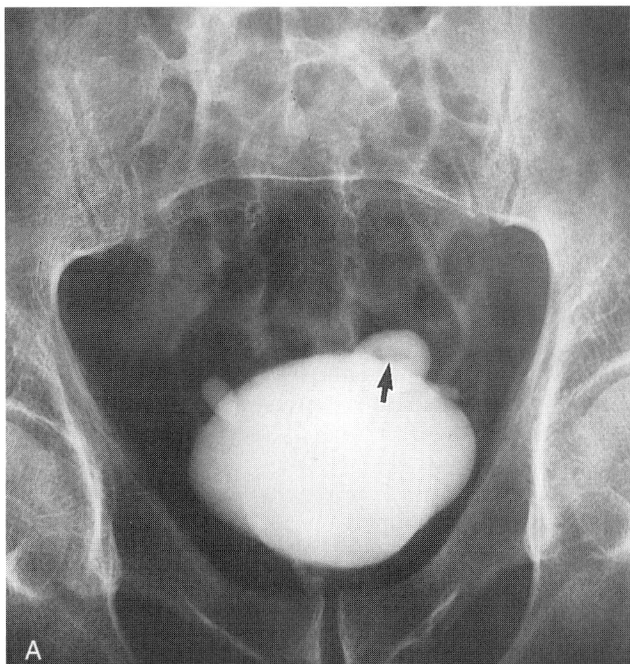

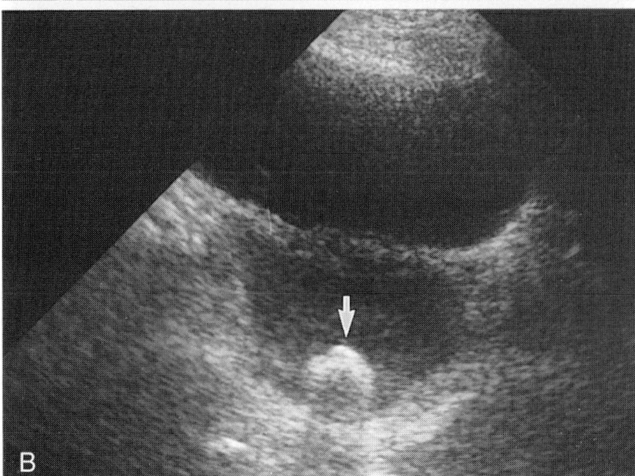

Figure 6–69. Bladder diverticulum with a calculus. *A,* View of the pelvis from an intravenous urogram shows a small filling defect within a bladder diverticulum *(arrow)*. *B,* Transverse suprapubic sonogram demonstrates a calculus within the diverticulum *(arrow)*.

aimed primarily at detecting neoplastic lesions (Rifkin and Resnick, 1991). Currently, after much writing and debate about the sonographic patterns of carcinoma of the prostate, the major indication for transrectal ultrasonography is guiding tissue sampling from the gland for diagnosis and staging of cancer.

The prostate and seminal vesicles are best examined via the endorectal route either with biplane, sagittal, and transverse dual-crystal linear array or with end-firing, single-crystal mechanical or phased-array sector probes. **Most transducers in use today are of high-resolution, sharply focused near-field technology with ultrasonic frequencies in the range of 5 to 7 MHz.** Usually, no patient preparation is necessary for the examination, although a cleansing enema is usually performed before a biopsy.

The normal gland, seen in males up to 45 years of age, is a rather symmetric triangular or ellipsoid structure sur-

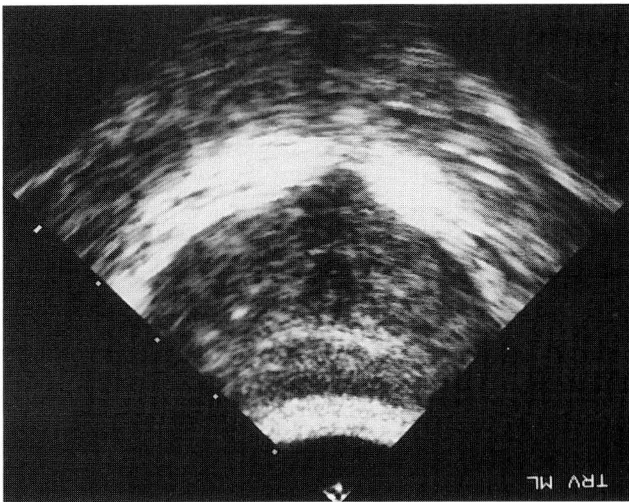

Figure 6–70. Normal transverse endorectal prostatic sonogram.

rounded by the bright, echogenic periprostatic fat (Figs. 6–70 to 6–72). It measures about 4 cm in the transverse dimension by 3 cm in the anteroposterior dimension. The normal volume of the gland is in the range of 10 to 25 cm^3.

Currently, the zonal anatomic model proposed by McNeal (1968) has widespread acceptance in clinical practice, in comparison with the older lobar model. The prostate is divided into three parts: anterior, central, and peripheral. The anterior prostate is composed of a fibromuscular stroma, an extension of which represents the prostatic capsule. The anterior part is free of glandular tissue and contains about one third of the total gland volume in normal young adults. The central gland is made of acinar tissues of the transition zone, situated on both sides of the proximal urethra just above the verumontanum, and of the periurethral zone, or glandular tissue surrounding the urethra. The proximal urethra and internal sphincter are also parts of the central gland, which in the normal young adult encompasses only 5% of the prostatic volume. It is this part of the gland that undergoes striking hypertrophic changes with age and may enlarge many times over its original volume. The peripheral gland contains exclusively glandular tissue and represents about 70% of the prostate volume in the young adult. The periph-

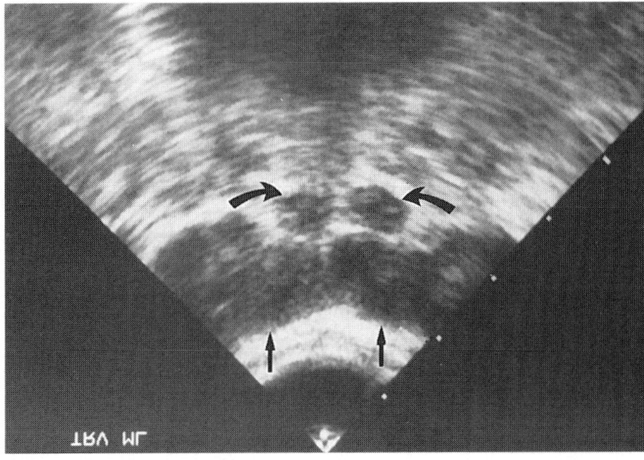

Figure 6–71. Normal ultrasonographic transverse appearance of seminal vesicles *(straight arrows)* and vas deferens *(curved arrows)*.

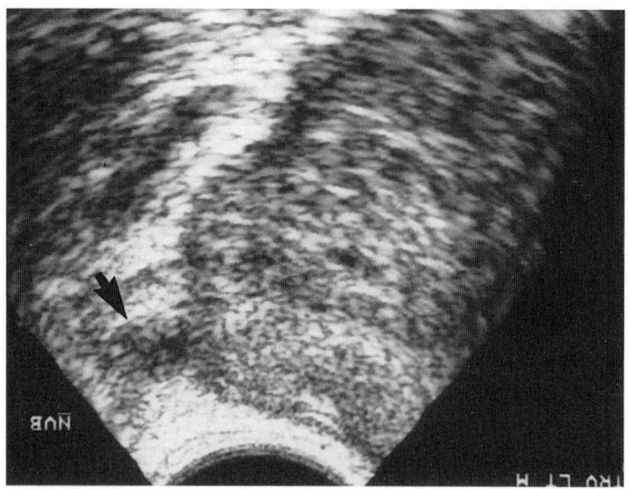

Figure 6–72. Normal ultrasonographic transverse appearance of left neurovascular bundle *(arrow)*.

eral gland makes up the posterior, apical, and lateral aspects of the prostate and is histologically divided into peripheral and central zones, which are sonographically indistinguishable. The central zone surrounds the ejaculatory ducts, extending from the posterior aspect of the base along the midline to the level of the posterior urethra, into which the two ducts drain. The remainder of the peripheral gland posteriorly, inferiorly, and laterally represents the peripheral zone.

The zonal anatomic model of the prostate not only can be, at least in part, demonstrated on sonography and MRI but also makes localization and evaluation of prostatic diseases easier to accomplish (Rifkin and Resnick, 1991). Benign prostatic hypertrophy is a disease of the central gland alone, arising primarily in the transition zone and, to a lesser extent, in the periurethral tissue. Carcinoma obviously originates from glandular tissues of both the peripheral and central gland. Most prostate cancers arise in the peripheral gland (80%); the rest arise in the central gland. Prostatitis can develop in either the peripheral or central gland, predominantly in the former.

The zonal anatomy of the gland is not clearly depicted on sonography in the normal young adult patient, but it becomes much easier to image with age and the gradual development of benign hypertrophy. As the central gland enlarges, it exceeds its original volume by a large margin, and it compresses the tissues of the peripheral gland, which in some advanced cases is reduced to a thickness of a few millimeters. The separation between the peripheral and central glands usually is easy to visualize, and calculi often are seen either randomly within the parenchyma of the central gland or along the surgical capsule. **The sonographic pattern of benign hyperplasia is one of mixed, heterogeneous, mostly hypoechoic parenchyma, often arranged in the form of one or more hyperplastic nodules and sometimes without recognizable internal architecture. This appearance is in contrast to the usually homogeneous, somewhat more echogenic normal peripheral gland,** which undergoes no visible textural changes with age. The enlargement of the parenchyma can be asymmetric and may result in bulging of the contour of the central gland and the prostate itself. Because of the great heterogeneity of the hypertrophic changes, prospective diagnosis of coexisting carcinoma in the central gland by sonography is usually difficult or impossible.

Prostate cancer has a variety of sonographic patterns. The typical appearance is that of a **predominantly hypoechoic lesion in comparison with the normal surrounding peripheral gland tissue** (Rifkin et al, 1990a) (Fig. 6–73). **Lesions as small as 4 to 5 mm may be seen.** A significant percentage of cancers have been found to be isoechoic with the normal parenchyma and are thus indistinguishable from it. The literature suggests that **up to 30% of cancers may be isoechoic.** Finally, **a small percentage of cancers (probably 1% to 3%) may be predominantly hyperechoic.** Mixed patterns and multifocal disease are common. Cancerous lesions often are ill-defined and may infiltrate adjacent tissues and structures. **Capsular bulging and irregularity associated with an adjacent focal hypoechoic lesion often indicate capsular invasion. The neurovascular bundles, seen in most affected patients, should appear symmetric and surrounded by echogenic fat** (see Fig. 6–72). **Asymmetry or extension of a hypoechoic lesion from the peripheral gland into the bundle also raises suspicion of extraprostatic spread of tumor. Invasion of the seminal vesicles by tumors at the base of the gland may appear as unilateral or asymmetric dilatation with loss of the fat plane between the prostate and the involved seminal vesicle.**

Prostatic intraepithelial neoplasia, an often precancerous condition of the prostate, and **a number of benign entities may also appear as hypoechoic lesions.** Examples of the latter include **infarcts, atrophy,** and **infection.** The sensitivity and specificity of prostatic sonography, as well as those of sonography of the hypoechoic lesion, are unacceptably low for screening patients in whom prostate cancer is suspected; therefore, the major indication for prostatic sonography in these patients is the guidance of transrectal biopsies (Fig. 6–74). After radical prostatectomy, patients with rising serum prostate-specific antigen (PSA) levels can be imaged for recurrent disease around the vesicourethral anastomosis and undergo biopsy, if necessary. Irradiation of

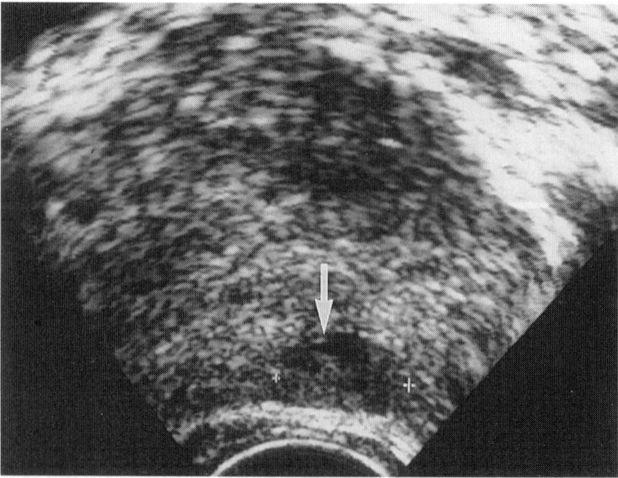

Figure 6–73. Prostatic carcinoma on endorectal transverse sonogram. The lesion has the typical hypoechoic appearance and is located in the peripheral gland *(arrow)*.

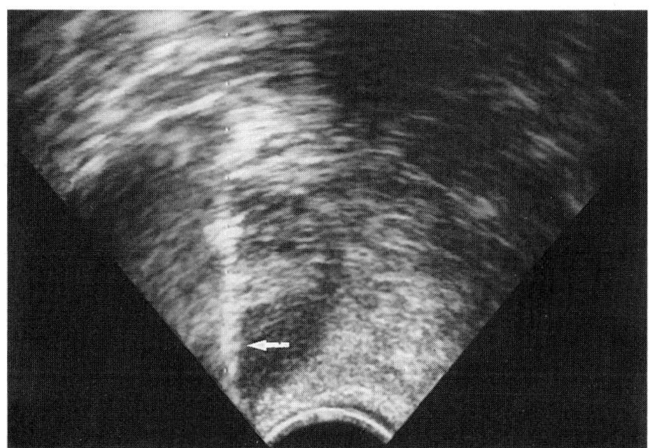

Figure 6–74. Ultrasonographically guided endorectal prostatic biopsy. The needle track is seen traversing a hypoechoic lesion *(arrow)*.

the prostate may cause some decrease in the size and changes in its sonographic appearance, so that ultrasonography cannot be used to evaluate progress of the disease reliably. Often, a hypoechoic lesion may disappear or persist after treatment, or the parenchyma may become diffusely hyperechoic. Reappearance of a hypoechoic lesion or lesions often signifies recurrence. Serial PSA measurements and, when indicated, ultrasonically guided biopsy are the appropriate procedures for monitoring the long-term results of radiation therapy.

Prostatic infection is an infrequent indication for transrectal sonography, often in cases of persistent or recurrent lower urinary tract infection or a painful rectal examination that raises suspicion for prostatic abscess. **Acute prostatitis** usually appears as a hypoechoic, well-defined lesion in either the peripheral or central gland (Rifkin and Resnick, 1991). **Chronic prostatitis** has a variable, nonspecific sonographic appearance, mostly hypoechoic and sometimes in a diffuse manner. An **abscess** can be visualized as a thick-walled, fluid-filled structure that is easily distinguished from the prostatic parenchyma, or it can appear as focal hypoechoic lesions with relatively well-demarcated margins. Transrectal aspiration of the abscess is often an effective treatment, obviating the need for a transurethral resection of the prostate and drainage of the cavity.

Estimation of the prostatic volume by sonography is approximate; the rate of errors is in the range of 10% to 20%. The gland is considered a sphere, an ellipsoid, or a prolate spheroid; the appropriate dimensions are measured, and formulas are used to estimate the volume (Littrup et al, 1991). Most sonographic units currently in use can provide this information after measurement of the dimensions of the gland or tracing of the gland contour. Volumetric measurements of cancerous lesions have been attempted in an effort to stage cancer and monitor the response to treatment of malignant and benign entities, such as benign hypertrophy treated with hyperthermia or oral medications. Ultrasonic guidance has been used in the transperineal implantation of radioactive iodine or palladium seeds for treatment of cancer. More recently, sonography has guided cryotherapy of prostate carcinoma.

The **seminal vesicles** are paired, convoluted tubular structures situated above the base of the prostate and behind the bladder trigone (see Fig. 6–71). They often appear symmetric, although some asymmetry in shape and size may be found in up to a third of normal males. The seminal vesicles appear as hypoechoic or anechoic saccular structures with relatively thick walls (Kuligowska et al, 1992). They measure about 3 cm ± 0.5 cm in length and 1.5 cm ± 0.4 cm in width with an estimated volume of 13.7 ml ± 3.7 ml. Medially and somewhat anteriorly to each seminal vesicle lies the ampullary segment of the **ipsilateral vas deferens.** The two structures merge near the base of the prostate to form the **ejaculatory duct,** which then traverses the prostatic parenchyma surrounded by the central zone to the level of the posterior urethra. The ampullary segment of the vas deferens appears as a tubular structure with a thick wall and anechoic or hypoechoic lumen (see Fig. 6–71). The ejaculatory ducts are often seen in normal males as a pair of tiny hypoechoic or anechoic points on each side of the prostatic midline at the base. Small to medium-sized cystic structures are sometimes encountered along the path of the ejaculatory ducts and often are referred to as ejaculatory duct cysts or müllerian duct cysts. The small ones usually are incidental findings of no clinical significance. Larger cysts may obstruct the outflow of sperm during ejaculation.

Imaging of the seminal vesicles and the sperm transport ductal system has two major clinical indications: the investigation of male infertility and the association of congenital anomalies of the lower genital tract with ipsilateral renal and ureteral anomalies. Evaluation of the seminal vesicles is an integral part of prostatic sonography.

The causes of **male infertility** are numerous and complex. **Sonography may be particularly helpful in ruling out an obstructive lesion** (Carter et al, 1989; Abbitt et al, 1991). Vasography after direct cannulation of the vas deferens and injection of contrast material is the best technique for visualizing the entire sperm transport apparatus; however, it is invasive and carries risks (Fig. 6–75). **Sonography is noninvasive but can evaluate only the distal segment of the transport system from the ampullary segment of the vas deferens to the posterior urethral orifice of the ejaculatory duct.** Lesions of the transport system most often manifest with low-volume ejaculates and oligospermia or neospermia. These lesions may be congenital (such as agenesis of segments or all of the apparatus) or acquired (usually inflammatory strictures or obstruction of the vas deferens, ejaculatory duct, and urethra). Retrograde ejaculation may have a similar clinical picture; however, it can be easily diagnosed by history and discovery of sperm in a urine specimen obtained after ejaculation. Low or undetectable sperm counts with normal-volume ejaculate most often are caused by testicular failure.

Agenesis of the vas deferens commonly is associated with abnormalities of the seminal vesicles. On sonography, a spectrum of anomalies can be detected. Agenesis or hypoplasia of one or both seminal vesicles can be seen, the latter manifesting as a low-volume, usually hypoechoic band of tissue often lacking the typical features of the normal convoluted, cystic seminal vesicle. Congenital cystic dilatation of the seminal vesicle has been described (Fig. 6–76). All these abnormalities, in addition to their adverse effect on fertility, have a significant association with ipsilateral renal anomalies, which range from renal agenesis to dysplasia and ectopia.

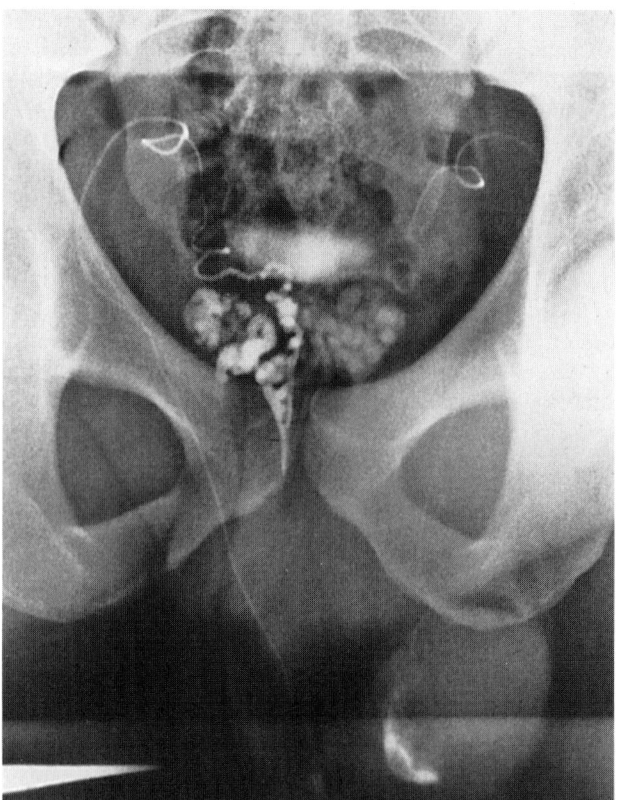

Figure 6–75. Normal bilateral vasogram.

Inflammatory diseases of the lower urinary tract may also produce obstruction to the flow of sperm by causing strictures along the transport apparatus and urethra. The extent of fibrosis, often irreversible, may result in partial or complete obliteration of the lumen with dilatation proximal to the obstruction. Affected seminal vesicles appear smaller and more echogenic than normal. Stones can be formed within and obstruct the seminal vesicles or ducts. They can be diagnosed on sonography as strongly echogenic foci with acoustic shadowing.

The ejaculatory ducts can be readily evaluated for changes in the size of the lumen (dilatation) and presence of echogenic material, such as stones, as already mentioned. **Sonography may accurately determine the presence and level of obstruction,** which is important in the management of certain patients. A blind transurethral resection is often not deep enough to reach and relieve the obstruction within the prostatic parenchyma. Distal obstruction may be amenable to the transurethral resection; however, a high obstructing lesion near the base of the prostate necessitates alternative draining approaches. The results of the sonographic study often guide the choice of treatment. Potential complications of lower genital tract surgery may also be amenable to sonographic detection. Hematomas and abscesses can be demonstrated and drained or aspirated under sonographic guidance.

Testis and Scrotum

A major contribution of sonography to the imaging of the genitourinary tract is the detailed and accurate demonstration of scrotal and testicular pathology (O'Mara and Rifkin, 1991). Because of its superior anatomic visualization of the scrotal contents in comparison with other imaging techniques, MRI being an exception in certain conditions, the indications for sonography cover the whole spectrum of benign and malignant disease, infertility, and trauma.

The **scrotal contents are best examined with a short-focal-zone, high-resolution linear array transducer operating in the frequency range of 5 to 10 MHz.** With the patient in the supine position, the penis is positioned over the suprapubic area, and the scrotum is elevated and supported by a towel placed underneath. After a brief physical examination to confirm and localize the clinical findings, each testis and its appendages are scanned in both the transverse and sagittal planes. The regions of the inguinal canals

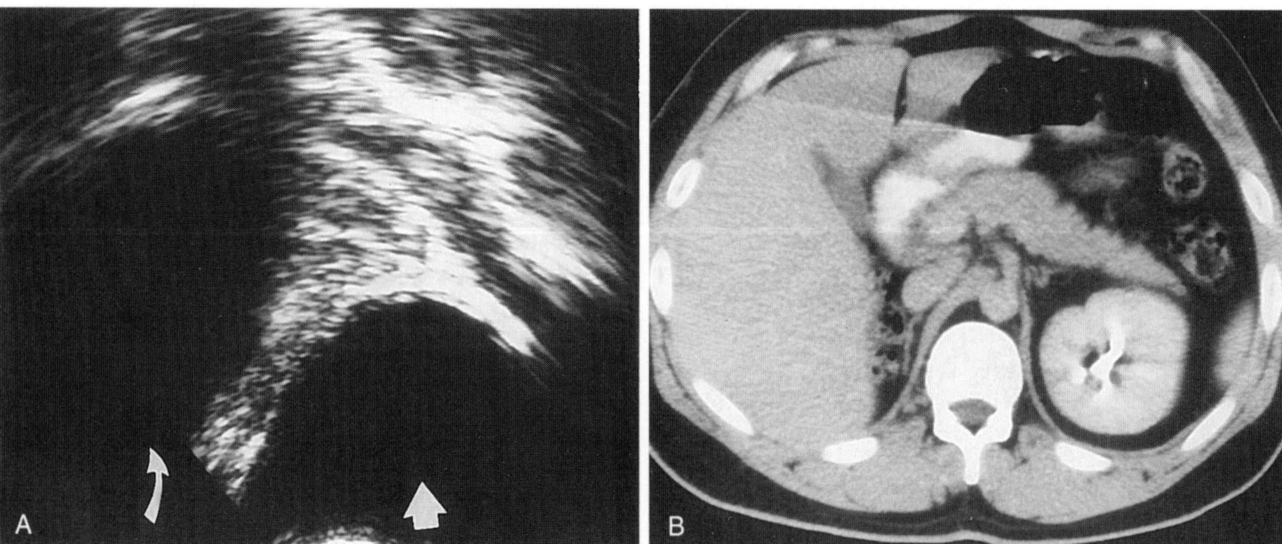

Figure 6–76. Congenital cystic dilatation of the seminal vesicle accompanied by ipsilateral renal agenesis. *A,* Endorectal sonogram shows a large seminal vesicle cyst *(straight arrow)* inferior to the bladder *(curved arrow)*. *B,* CT scan shows absence of the ipsilateral kidney.

are also examined. Both gray-scale and color Doppler examinations are performed.

The **normal testis has a medium-level, homogeneous echotexture with well-defined contour. Often the mediastinum testis appears as an echogenic linear band along the long axis of the testis** (Figs. 6–77, 6–78). The rete testis can be seen only when it is dilated. The **epididymis is easily demonstrable, and its echogenicity is similar to that of the testis.**

The epididymis is divided for anatomic convenience into a head, body, and tail. The head is the widest segment and is triangular or ovoid, located in the superolateral aspect of the testis (see Fig. 6–77). The body is found along the dorsolateral aspect of the testis; the tail is located by the inferior testicular pole. The wider head tapers to a long, tubular body and tail that measure about 3 to 5 mm in diameter, in comparison to a width of 7 to 12 mm for the head.

Both the testis and the epididymis may be accompanied by their own appendixes. The appendix testis is located off the superior testicular pole, whereas the appendix epididymis arises from the epididymal head. Both or either appendage may be sonographically visible. The head of the epididymis represents the confluence of the several efferent ducts from the rete testis into a single duct, which becomes the ductus deferens distal to the epididymal tail.

The testis is covered by a layer of dense connective tissue, the tunica albuginea. An outer cover peripheral to the tunica albuginea is the tunica vaginalis. When large amounts of fluid are accumulated between its two layers (the visceral and the parietal), a hydrocele is formed. A hematocele or herniation of intraperitoneal structures may also be formed between these two layers.

The clinical indications for sonographic evaluation of the scrotal contents vary with the symptoms and age of the patient. Cryptorchidism, testicular torsion, and **trauma** are often encountered among young children and adolescents. **Epididymitis** and **neoplasms** usually affect older males, although torsion and trauma may also be found in this age group.

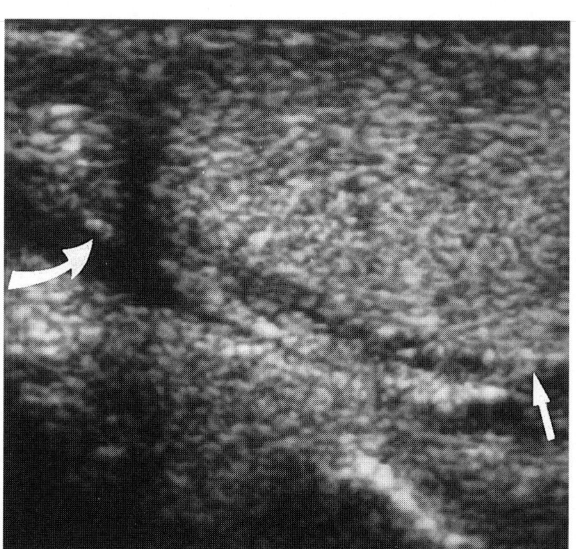

Figure 6–77. Normal sonogram of the testis *(straight arrow)* and epididymal head *(curved arrow).*

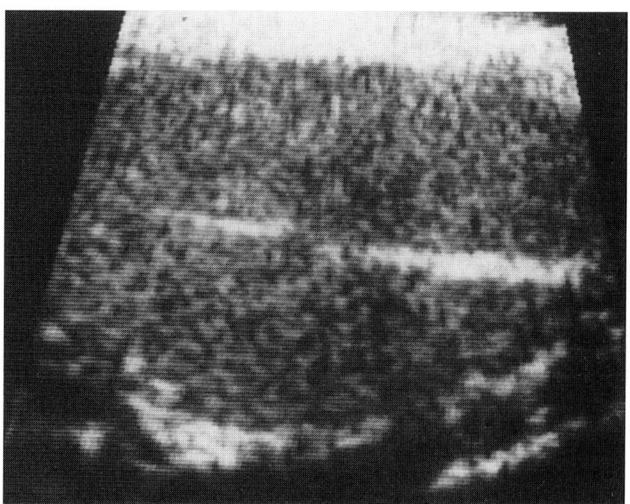

Figure 6–78. Normal testicular sonogram. The bright thin line in the center of the testis represents the mediastinum testis.

Unilateral or bilateral congenital anorchia is rare. Cryptorchidism is seen more often in premature or low-birth-weight neonates. Most undescended testes, however, do migrate into the scrotal sac by the end of the first year of life. The overall incidence of cryptorchidism in the adult male population is in the range of 0.5% to 0.8%. More than 80% of the undescended testes are found high in the scrotal sac or within the inguinal canal. A small number of cryptorchid testes are found close to the internal inguinal ring inside the abdomen. These testes are best identified with CT or MRI after sonographic examination of the inguinal canal fails to visualize the testis. **Sonography is thus best suited for the initial evaluation of the male with an undescended testis.** The inguinal testis is smaller than the contralateral descended testis (Fig. 6–79). An enlarged testis within the inguinal canal raises suspicion of malignant degeneration (Fig. 6–80). It is well established that malignancy occurs up to five times or more frequently in males with undescended testes. The most common type of cancer is seminoma.

Detection of testicular malignancies is a major indication for testicular sonography (Feld and Middleton, 1992). **Often, the clinical dilemma is to decide whether a palpable mass is extratesticular or intratesticular,** the former commonly being benign, the latter likely to be malignant. **The distinction can be made easily with sonography.**

Although not specific enough, the sonographic patterns sometimes accurately predict the histology of the tumor. Seminomas, which account for about half of all germ cell tumors, often manifest as rather well-defined, hypoechoic, homogeneous masses (Fig. 6–81; see also Fig. 6–79). Embryonal cell carcinoma is an aggressive tumor, often invading the tunica albuginea. The sonographic appearance is that of a poorly defined, heterogeneous mass. Teratomas manifest as heterogeneous masses with ill-defined borders and mixed echogenicity. Calcifications may indicate osseous or cartilaginous elements. Necrosis, hemorrhage, and calcification are common features of choriocarcinomas. Sometimes these tumors manifest with metastases, and a small echogenic focus in one of the testes can be the only evidence of the primary site. Clinical evidence usually helps in making the diagnosis in such a case (i.e., of a so-called burned-out neoplasm).

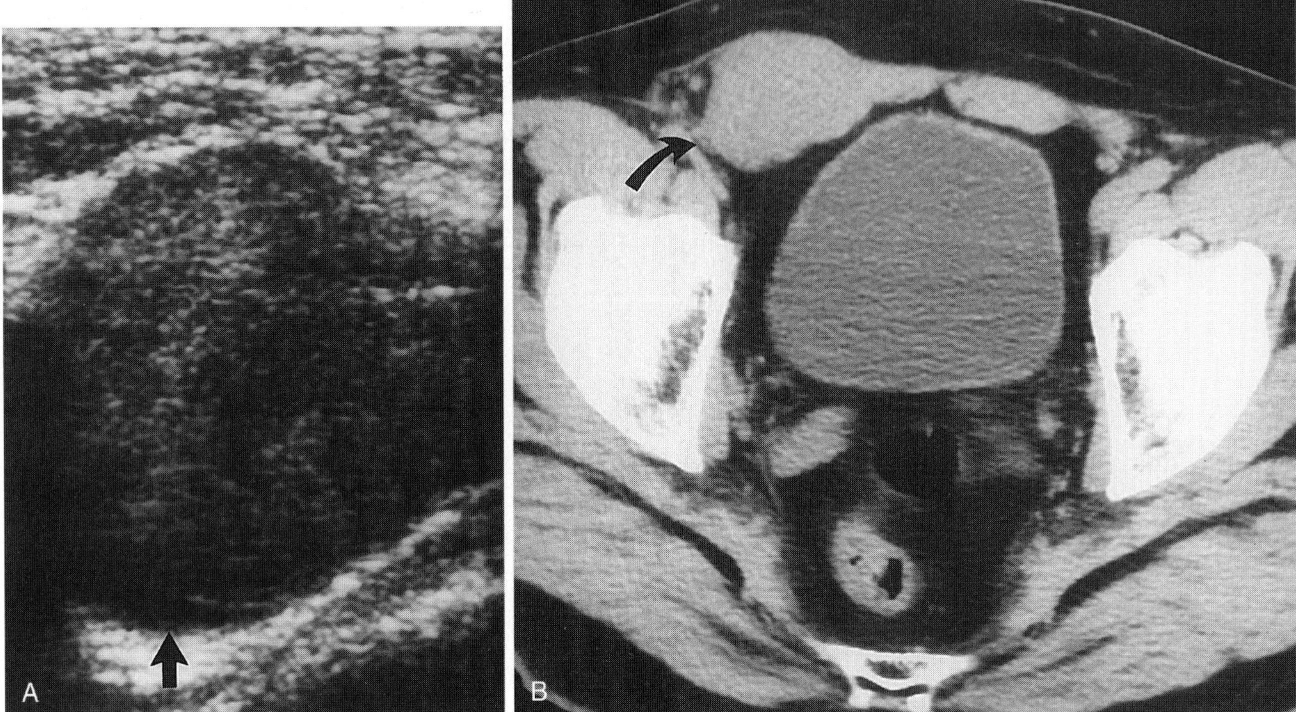

Figure 6–79. Atrophic, nondescended right testis. *A,* Sonogram shows an atrophic testis within the inguinal canal *(arrow),* in contrast to the case seen in Figure 6–80. *B,* CT scan confirms right atrophic undescended testis *(curved arrow).*

Metastases to the testes are relatively common, especially among elderly men. The sonographic appearance is nonspecific. Lymphoma and leukemia can be diagnosed on testicular sonography in children and adults. Leukemia often infiltrates the testicular parenchyma, whereas lymphoma may manifest as multiple, bilateral hypoechoic nodules.

A number of unusual or rare benign testicular lesions may also be discovered on physical examination and/or sonography. **Testicular cysts** are relatively common, found in as many as 8% to 10% of patients, usually as an incidental finding. When they meet the sonographic criteria for a simple cyst, they require no further investigation (Gooding et al, 1987). **Epidermoid testicular cysts** often appear as hypoechoic solid masses with a thick, partially calcified rim. **Dilatation of the rete testis** may mimic a mass lesion on both physical examination and sonography. The lesion, sometimes bilateral, appears as a multicystic area in the expected location of the mediastinum testis, extending to the hilar region of the testis and often accompanied by epididymal cysts (Brown et al, 1992) (Fig. 6–82). Unnecessary orchiectomies have been performed for the treatment of this benign entity. **Testicular abscess or hematoma** is usually associated with infection or trauma, respectively. A hematoma appears as a low-echogenic, ill-defined mass lesion with no discernible blood flow within it. If the trauma is significant enough to cause the lesion, a hematocele may also be present. **Testicular fracture** may coexist with an intratesticular hematoma and appears as a break in the continuity of the smooth contour of the tunica albuginea. If there is concern about a coexisting tumor that may be obscured by the trauma, serial sonograms or an MRI of the testes is indicated. On serial sonography, the hematoma decreases in size over time. A **testicular abscess** may appear as a mixed-echogenic or hypoechoic mass with a greatly vascular hyperemic periphery on color Doppler images. A reactive hydrocele is likely to be seen as well (O'Mara and Rifkin, 1991). A diffusely hypoechoic testis or a focal hypoechoic mass may be the result of **missed torsion** or another ischemic event that leads to testicular infarction. Because the sonographic pattern is similar to that of a malignancy, correlation with history and physical examination is essential.

Patients with the von Hippel–Lindau syndrome are found on occasion to have palpable epididymal cysts or papillary cystadenomas of the epididymis.

Testicular microlithiasis is an uncommon pathologic process with a characteristic diffuse, speckled sonographic pattern. Both testes are involved and contain numerous, small parenchymal echogenic foci without discernible acoustic shadowing. On histologic examination, laminated microcalcifications representing degenerating tubular epithelial cells are scattered either in the lumen of the seminiferous tubules or beneath the epithelium within connective tissues. Testicular microlithiasis is often an incidental finding, although an association with cryptorchidism, precocious puberty, Klinefelter's syndrome, and infertility has been noted (O'Mara and Rifkin, 1991). Case reports of testicular microlithiasis associated with testicular tumors have also appeared in the literature.

Ectopic adrenal rests are relatively common in newborns. Scrotal location is uncommon. The natural evolution of these remnants is regression over time and disappearance; however, in infants with high levels of adrenocortical hormones (congenital adrenal hyperplasia), the rests hypertrophy and may become palpable. On sonography, the adrenal rests appear as multiple hypoechoic mass lesions near or within the testes (Willi et al, 1991; O'Mara and Rifkin, 1991).

Varicoceles—dilatations of the pampiniform venous plexus—are found in 10% to 15% of adult males, mostly on the left side. The incidence of varicoceles in men with impaired fertility varies from 20% to 40%. A clinical grading system divides the varicoceles into three grades: small or grade 1 varicoceles are palpable only during a Valsalva maneuver; moderate or grade 2 varicoceles are palpable without the need for the Valsalva maneuver; and large or grade 3 varicoceles are visible (Dubin and Amelar, 1970).

Sonography has been able to detect palpable and subclinical varicoceles (Fig. 6–83) (McClure et al, 1986). The normal veins of the pampiniform plexus are seen as channels up to 2 mm in diameter (Demas et al, 1991). The sonographic criteria for the diagnosis of a varicocele call for the detection of several venous channels, at least one of which is 3 mm or larger in diameter and is further enlarged with the Valsalva maneuver or with the patient standing. Dilated veins with a diameter of 5 mm or wider are clinically detectable. The use of color Doppler imaging, usually unnecessary, makes the identification of small varicoceles easier.

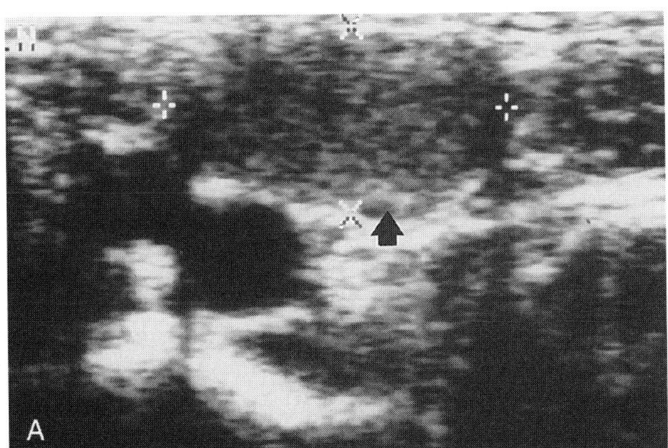

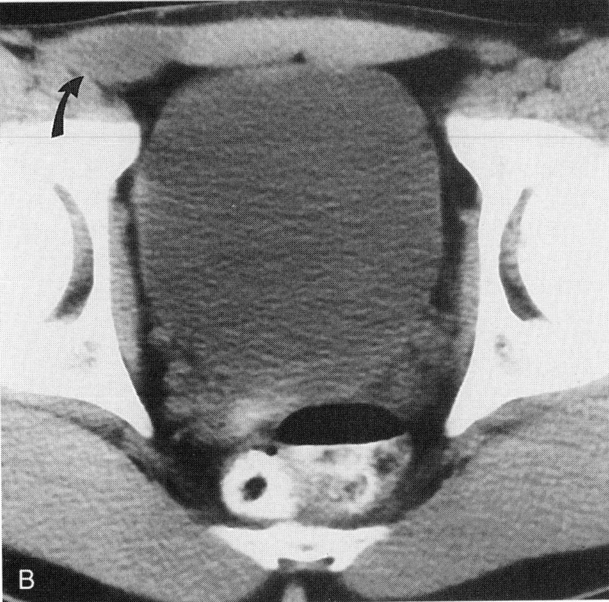

Figure 6–80. Right-sided undescended testis with seminomatous degeneration. *A,* Large, low-echogenic mass in the right inguinal canal *(arrow)* raises suspicion of tumor in undescended testis. *B,* CT scan of the pelvis confirms the presence of a soft tissue density mass in the right inguinal canal *(curved arrow).* A seminoma was found at surgery.

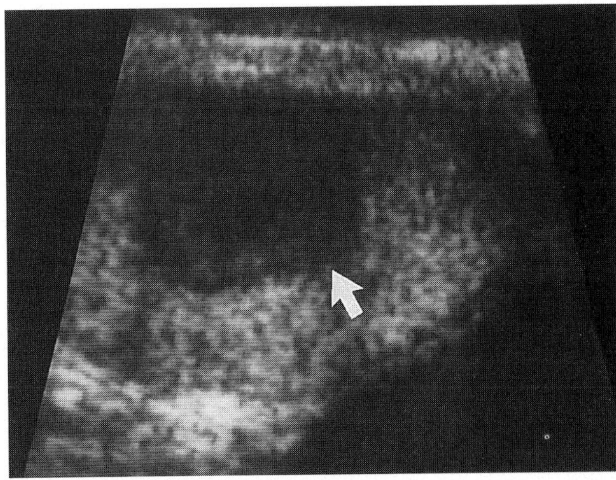

Figure 6–81. Hypoechoic, relatively well-defined testicular mass consistent with seminoma *(arrow).*

The patient most often is scanned supine, and the Valsalva maneuver is routinely used. Sometimes scanning can be performed with the patient standing. Although spermatic venography is the gold standard for the detection of small varicoceles, its invasive nature precludes its use as a screening technique. It is therefore reserved for patients undergoing sclerotherapy. Meanwhile, **sonography remains the most practical and accurate noninvasive modality in the diagnosis of varicocele and follow-up after treatment** (McClure and Hricak, 1986).

The acute scrotum is a clinical problem that very often can be solved with the help of sonography (Feld and Middleton, 1992). The common dilemma of this very painful manifestation is distinguishing between testicular torsion and epididymitis.

The twisting of a testis around the spermatic cord is a

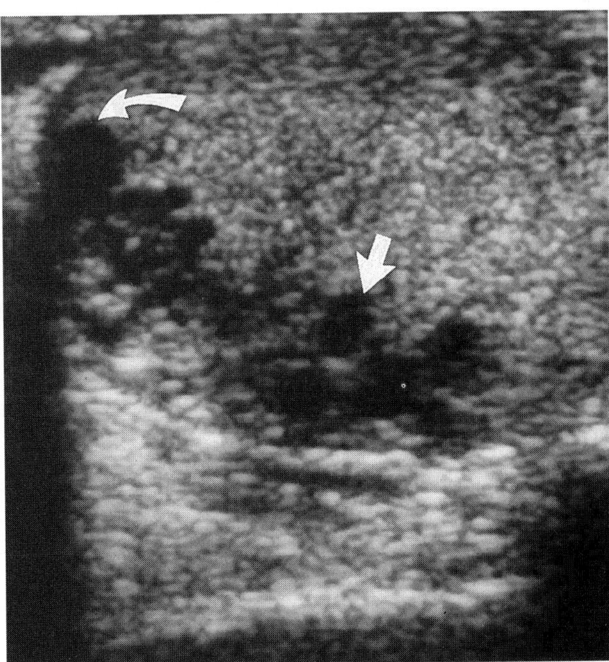

Figure 6–82. Dilatation of the rete testis *(straight arrow)* with small epididymal cyst *(curved arrow).*

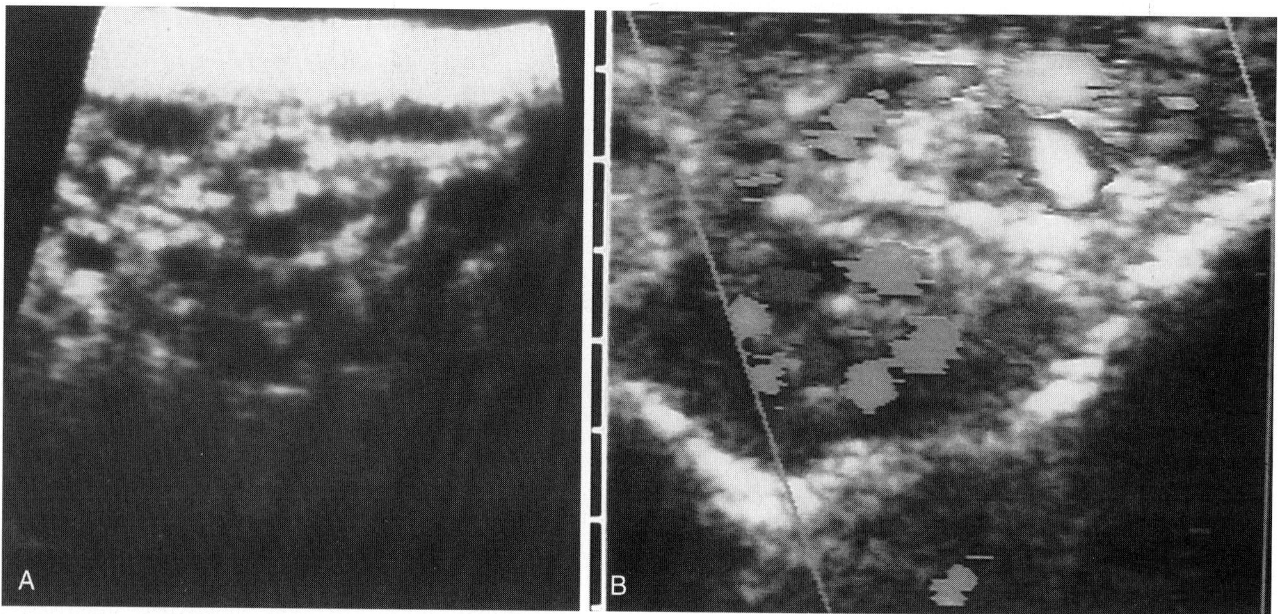

Figure 6–83. Palpable left testicular varicoceles in men evaluated for infertility. *A,* Typical appearance of a varicocele with dilated venous channels. *B,* Doppler sonography shows that most tubular spaces fill with flowing blood (gray in this figure).

surgical emergency. Repair of a complete torsion more than 10 hours after the beginning of the symptoms offers little hope for the salvage of the testis. With intermittent torsion, the chances for recovery may be better. Surgical repair should consist of bilateral orchiopexy because the anatomic abnormality is bilateral. Puberty is the age most often associated with testicular torsion. Neonates are also more prone to testicular torsion, which may be rather asymptomatic.

The adolescent male is at higher risk of torsion when the rapidly growing testes are freely suspended from and twisted around the cord (bell clapper deformity). This is so-called intravaginal torsion, as opposed to extravaginal torsion, which occurs in neonates and is caused by the free rotation of the testis and its layers around the cord at a level above the tunica vaginalis.

The introduction of color Doppler imaging has made sonography a highly accurate and specific technique in diagnosing or ruling out torsion (Middleton et al, 1990). On gray-scale sonography, early on the affected testis may appear normal or slightly enlarged and heterogeneous. Eventually, several days or weeks later, the testis becomes atrophic. Early hyperechoic lesions, when seen, often represent hemorrhage (Bird et al, 1983). A small hydrocele and mild swelling of the epididymis may also be seen. However, the torsed testis more often than not may appear normal for several hours after the vascular strangulation. Therefore, the ability to assess the vascular supply to the testis makes color Doppler imaging an essential element of the sonographic evaluation.

According to all published reports, there is lack of blood flow to the symptomatic testis unless the torsion is intermittent. The examination requires adequate technical skill and is more difficult in neonates and young children because of the small size of the testes.

Torsion of the appendix testis or epididymis may manifest as acute scrotum; however, the event is not a surgical emergency unless the pain does not respond to medication or there is suspicion of testicular torsion.

Epididymitis is the most common cause of acute scrotum. Sometimes epididymal infection may be accompanied by orchitis. Adolescents and middle-aged men are more often afflicted. On sonography the **epididymis appears significantly enlarged, especially in the area of the head, and its echogenicity decreases secondary to edema** (O'Mara and Rifkin, 1991) (Fig. 6–84). A reactive hydrocele of small to moderate size is a common feature. Hypoechoic testicular lesions representing orchitis may be seen in up to 25% of patients with epididymitis. **Color Doppler interrogation and radionuclide flow study invariably demonstrate marked hyperemia** throughout, in contrast to the findings in acute torsion (Fig. 6–85). Neglected or incompletely treated epididymitis may lead to testicular ischemia and scrotal and testicular abscess formation. Focal orchitis may infrequently be diagnosed as a tumor, although the accompanying inflammatory changes usually help distinguish the infection from a neoplasm.

The choice between radionuclide scintigraphy and color Doppler sonography depends on availability of the modalities and personal preference of the imager. Sonography requires less preparation and is radiation free, which is an advantage especially when the patient is young.

Computed Tomography

The diagnostic yield of CT is far superior to that of conventional radiography because the tissue contrast resolution of CT is significantly greater than that of plain radiographs (Pollack and Banner, 1994). Contrast materials are widely used to enhance normal structures and pathologic processes. Oral contrast agents are routinely used, and intravenous enhancement is highly desirable in the investigation of focal renal lesions and pyelonephritis, in staging, in follow-up of neurologic malignancies and other retroperitoneal diseases, and in the evaluation of vascular integrity and patency in the kidneys and the pelvis. Adequate renal function is the prerequisite for the administration of intravascular contrast agents. The patient is screened for serious adverse reactions to past exposure to intravascular contrast material, significant allergies, and recent or active important cardiopulmonary problems; the decision to proceed with the injection, the type of contrast material to be given, and need of pretreatment of the patient is made after the benefits of the procedure are considered. The contrast agent is usually given as a rapid bolus, resulting in a dynamic display of the perfusion patterns of the visualized viscera. Opacification of the calyceal systems often requires repeated imaging through the kidneys several minutes later.

The thickness of the slices obtained can be adjusted, depending on the size and location of the lesion as well as its relationship with important adjacent structures. Helical (spiral) CT technology allows for continuous, rapid, practically breath-hold-time acquisition of scans through large areas of the body such as the abdomen or pelvis. Display of the images is usually in the axial, two-dimensional mode; however, three-dimensional reconstruction is possible and helpful on many occasions. The latter display mode often is used to demonstrate vascular anatomy, such as the renal arteries.

The indications for CT imaging in uroradiologic diagnosis are many. Plain, nonenhanced CT imaging can be used with a high success rate to demonstrate **ureteral calculi** in patients with acute renal colic in the place of the traditional intravenous urogram (Sommer et al, 1995). **Angiomyolipomas** are best detected on plain CT because of their fat content (Bosniak et al, 1988) (Fig. 6–86). **Acute or recent hemorrhage in or around the kidneys and the retroperitoneum** is shown as a high-density collection, in contrast to the lower density urine, ascites, or old blood (Fig. 6–87).

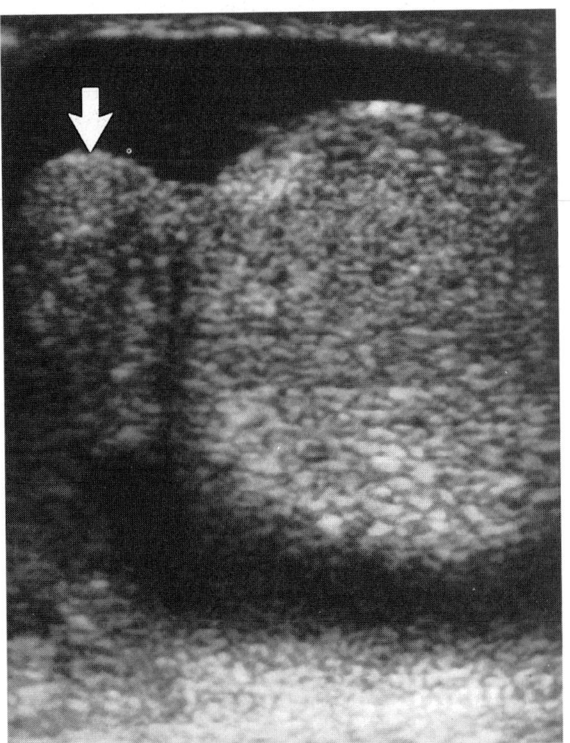

Figure 6–84. Acute epididymitis on sonography. The epididymal head is enlarged *(arrow)*. A reactive hydrocele surrounds the testis.

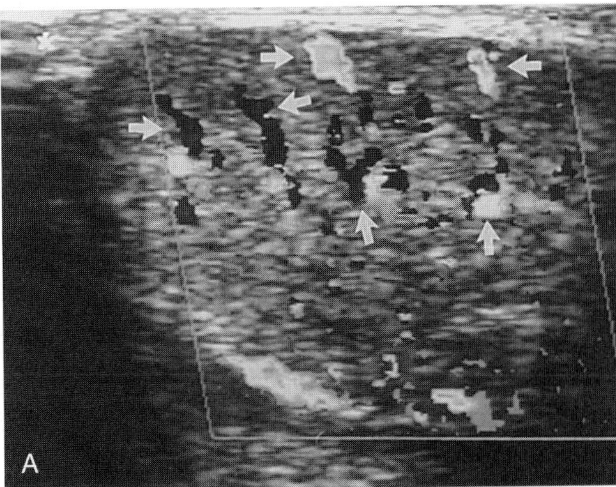

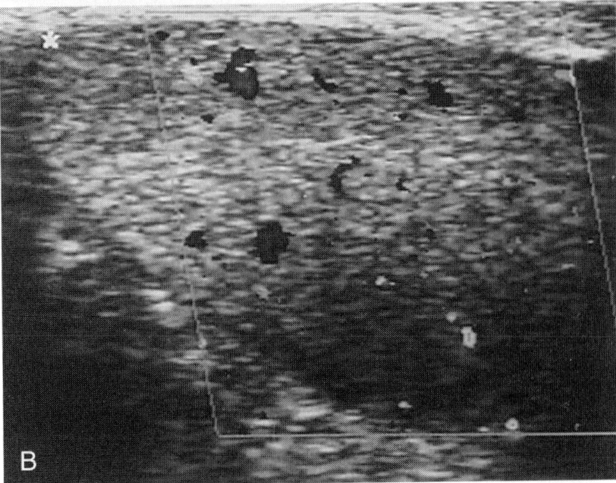

Figure 6–85. Epididymo-orchitis on sonography. *A,* Doppler interrogation shows marked increase in the blood flow (pictured as gray areas in this figure) to the symptomatic side *(arrows)*. *B,* The contralateral normal testis is shown for comparison.

Indeterminate renal masses should be imaged before and after the administration of intravenous contrast material and the enhancement or lack thereof documented (Curry et al, 1986; Bosniak, 1991). **Cysts** are of water density, unless complicated by infection or hemorrhage, and are not enhanced, whereas **solid or mixed cystic and solid masses** are (Bosniak, 1986). **Filling defects in the calyces and renal pelvis** might be viewed on a plain CT scan initially, so that calculi can be safely detected. Calculi that are nonopaque on conventional radiographs appear as high-attenuation foci on nonenhanced CT and are easily demonstrated (Fig. 6–88).

The **evaluation of the indeterminate renal mass** on IVU or sonography, as well as confirmation of a suspected renal cyst, requires the administration of intravenous contrast material after a plain CT of the kidneys has been obtained. The **diagnosis of simple renal cysts can thus be made with a degree of accuracy that exceeds that of sonography and may be as high as 98% of cases** (Bosniak, 1986). **Simple cysts** are not enhanced, appear homogeneous, are well defined, and have a smooth, almost imperceptible wall (Figs. 6–89, 6–90). **Occasional thin septations may be seen** (Fig. 6–91). Calcification occurs in a small percentage of cases

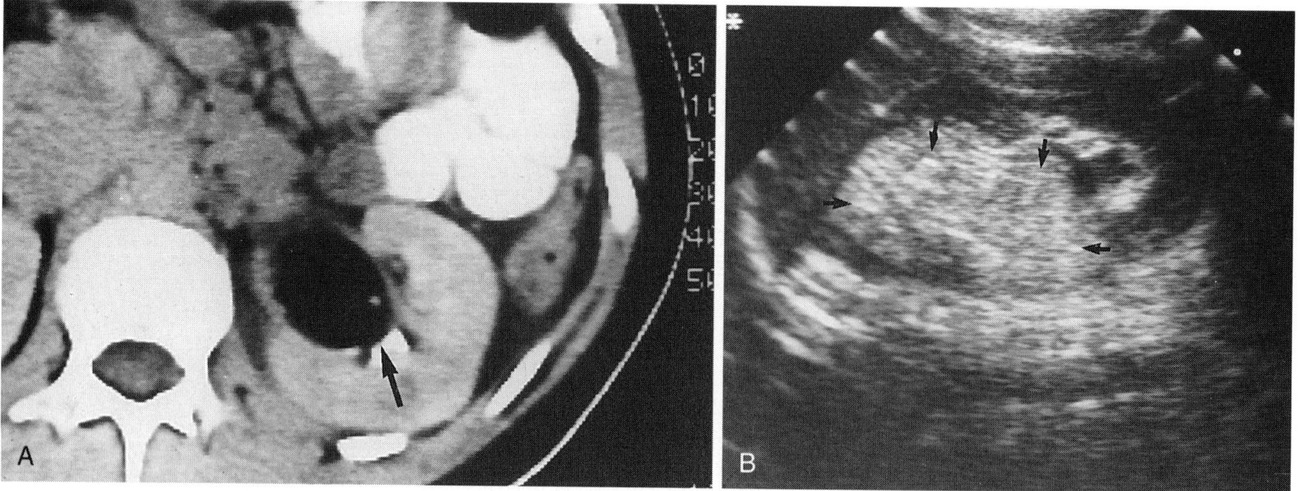

Figure 6–86. Fatty tumor (angiomyolipoma) of the left kidney in a young female. *A,* CT with intravenous contrast enhancement shows a lesion with very low attenuation in the left renal hilar region. The density measurement was diagnostic of fat *(arrow). B,* Longitudinal sonogram shows a large, hyperechoic lesion in the left kidney, corresponding to the angiomyolipoma *(arrows).*

(up to 5%) and most often is thin and conforms to the shape and outline of the cyst wall. **Amorphous calcifications** within a lesion are more likely to suggest a solid mass, whereas **thicker wall calcifications** may be seen in complicated cysts or echinococcal disease. Layering calcified or dense material within an otherwise simple-appearing cyst may represent milk of calcium or small stones within a calyx or calyceal diverticulum. Hemorrhagic cysts also tend to calcify more often and may be of higher overall density than are simple cysts. Further differentiation of complicated cysts from cystic tumors may necessitate follow-up imaging or needle aspiration.

A rather distinct entity known as the **hyperdense cyst** appears infrequently on CT, most often as an incidental finding (Fig. 6–92). The lesion is well defined and homogeneously denser than water, with a smooth wall. Most important, hyperdense simple cysts are not enhanced by contrast material, whereas solid masses, which may have a similar appearance on plain CT, usually display moderate to significant enhancement. Hemorrhage or high protein content is associated with most simple hyperdense cysts. Correlation with sonography often shows these lesions to fulfill the sonographic criteria for simple cysts (Zirinsky et al, 1984).

The **indeterminate renal mass** sometimes generates diagnostic problems with sonographic and CT imaging (Bosniak and Rofsky, 1996). As a rule, the detection of wall nodules, thick septations, and chunky calcification within a lesion strongly suggests that the mass is not a benign cyst, and further work-up or follow-up is advised. Very small (up to 1.5-cm) lesions, which may be difficult to characterize by CT, merit follow-up imaging, especially if they appear to grow faster than expected for a simple cyst. Thin-slice CT imaging with intravenous contrast material enhancement or helical CT is indicated for optimal imaging of these small lesions (Fig. 6–93).

Solid renal lesions are considered to represent renal cell carcinoma until proved otherwise and unless infection, metastatic disease, lymphoma, or hamartoma is suspected. Differentiation between renal cell carcinoma, which is sometimes multifocal and/or bilateral, and mass lesions such as oncocytoma, xanthogranulomatous pyelonephritis, adenoma, and capsular mesenchymal neoplasms is not possi-

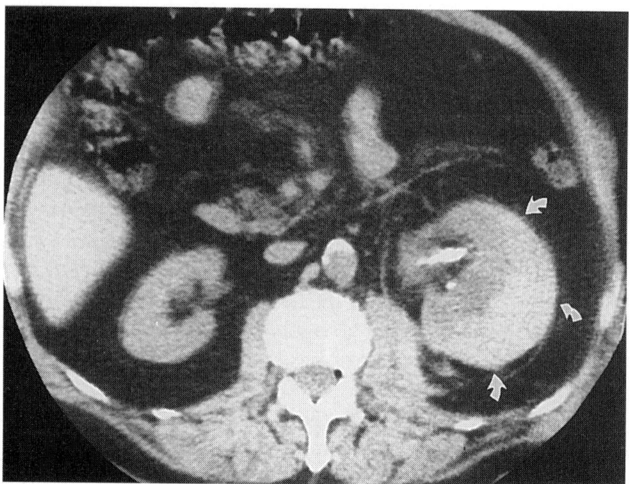

Figure 6–87. Acute hematoma around the left kidney after extracorporeal lithotripsy for renal calculi. The high-density collection surrounding the renal parenchyma on the unenhanced CT is highly suggestive of hematoma *(curved arrows).*

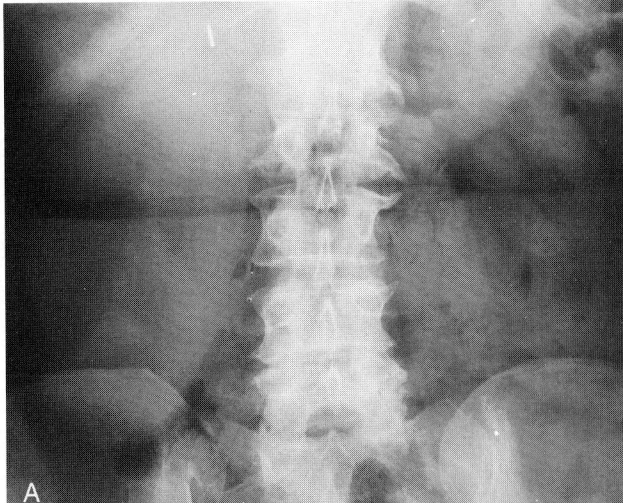

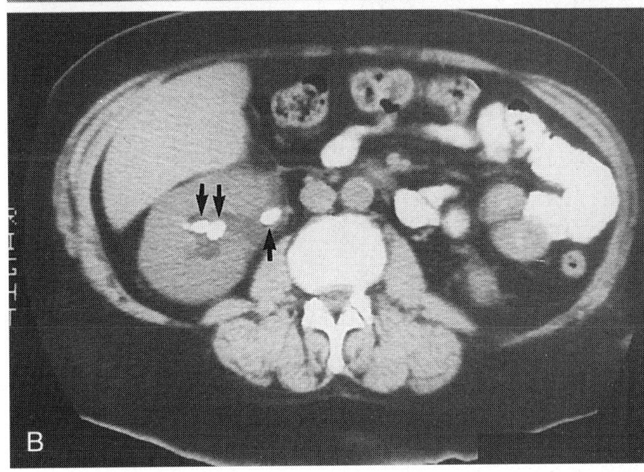

Figure 6–88. Radiolucent renal calculi in solitary right kidney. *A,* Plain radiograph shows no opaque calculi. *B,* Nonenhanced CT demonstrates at least three opaque calculi in right pyelocalyceal system *(arrows).*

ble with any degree of confidence; therefore, surgical exploration may be necessary (Figs. 6–94, 6–95). With improved scanner resolution, many small lesions can be adequately mapped and, therefore, excised locally without a nephrectomy.

Urothelial tumors can be demonstrated with a high degree of accuracy on contrast-enhanced CT. They usually manifest as filling defects within the pyelocalyceal system and, not infrequently, as ill-defined, infiltrating masses around calyces, which are then obstructed and often filled with high-density tumor debris and blood (Fig. 6–96).

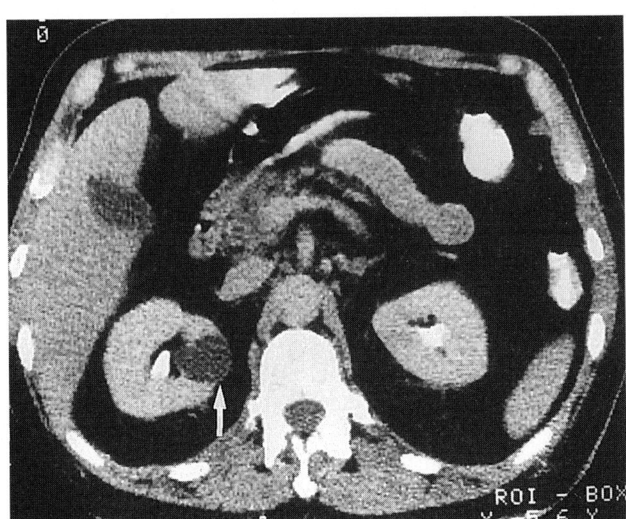

Figure 6–89. Simple renal cyst on contrast-enhanced CT *(arrow).*

Staging of neoplasms of the kidneys can be accurately achieved by CT imaging (Zeman et al, 1988). Infiltration of the renal capsule, regional lymphadenopathy, and tumoral thrombus within the renal vein and inferior vena cava may be detected, as may distant metastases to the lungs, liver, lymph nodes, and other sites in the body (Fig. 6–97; see also Fig. 6–95). Sonography may also detect tumor within the inferior vena cava with a high success rate; however, it may not demonstrate regional or remote lymphadenopathy with the same precision as CT does. MRI appears to be an equal or even slightly better alternative to CT for staging of renal tumors.

Renal infections most often do not necessitate imaging and certainly not CT scanning unless they persist, recur, or progress to abscess formation. **Severe acute pyelonephritis** appears as one or more areas of patchy perfusion defects, often extending from the calyces through the entire thickness of the renal parenchyma as wedge-shaped lesions surrounded by normal tissue (Papanicolaou and Pfister, 1996) (Fig. 6–98). The perinephric fat often is edematous and infiltrated, with or without formation of fluid collections. Delayed CT imaging yields a strikingly striated nephrogram in many cases, as a result of hyperconcentration of contrast material

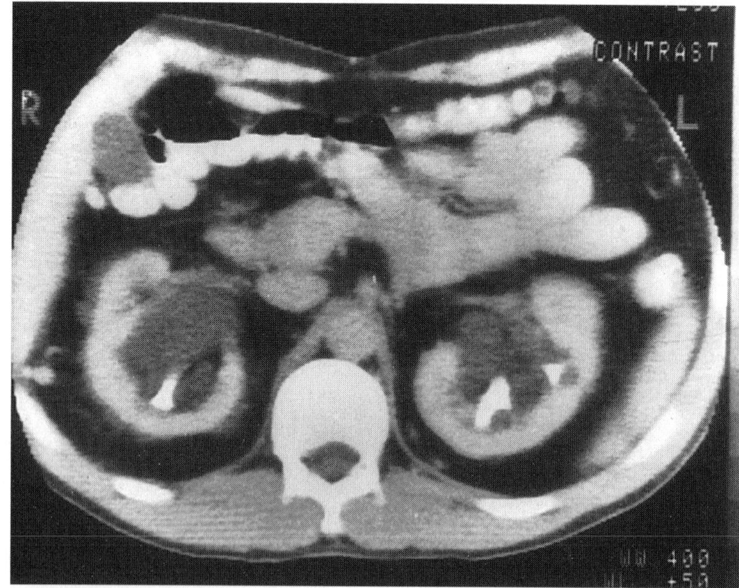

Figure 6–90. Multiple, bilateral peripelvic cysts appear as low-attenuation structures surrounding the opacified calyces. The cysts are not enhanced by contrast material.

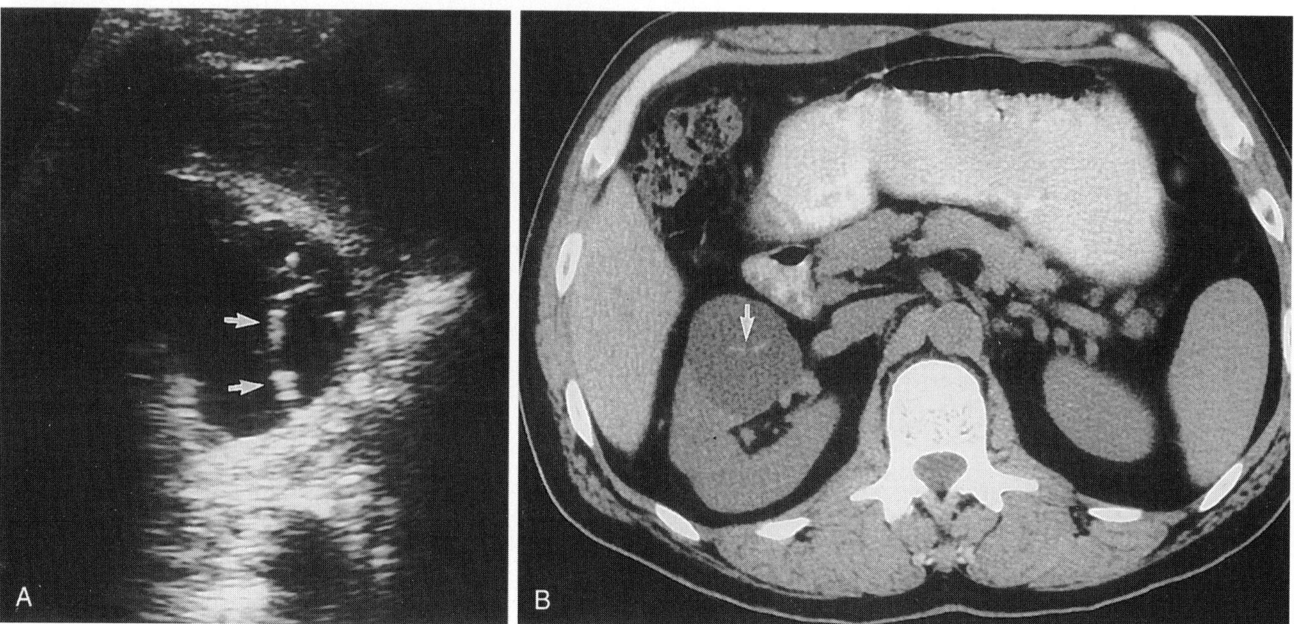

Figure 6–91. Thinly septated simple renal cyst. *A,* Renal sonogram shows the fluid-filled structure with internal septations *(arrows). B,* The septations are barely visible, probably faintly calcified, on the CT scan *(arrow).*

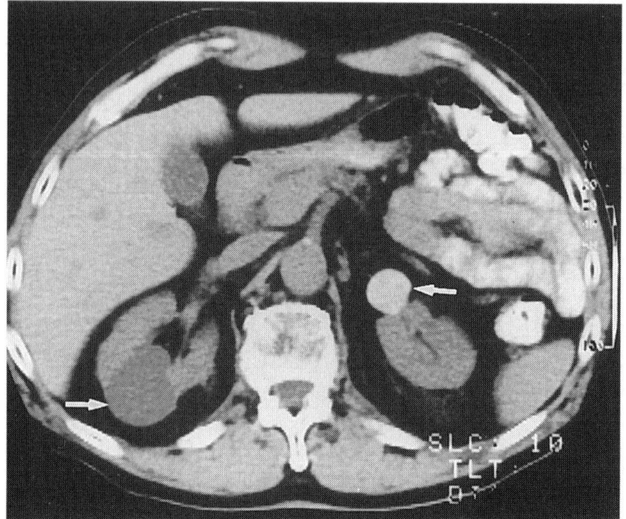

Figure 6–92. Nonenhanced CT of the kidney shows a right midpole simple renal cyst and a hyperdense, left upper pole renal cyst *(arrows).*

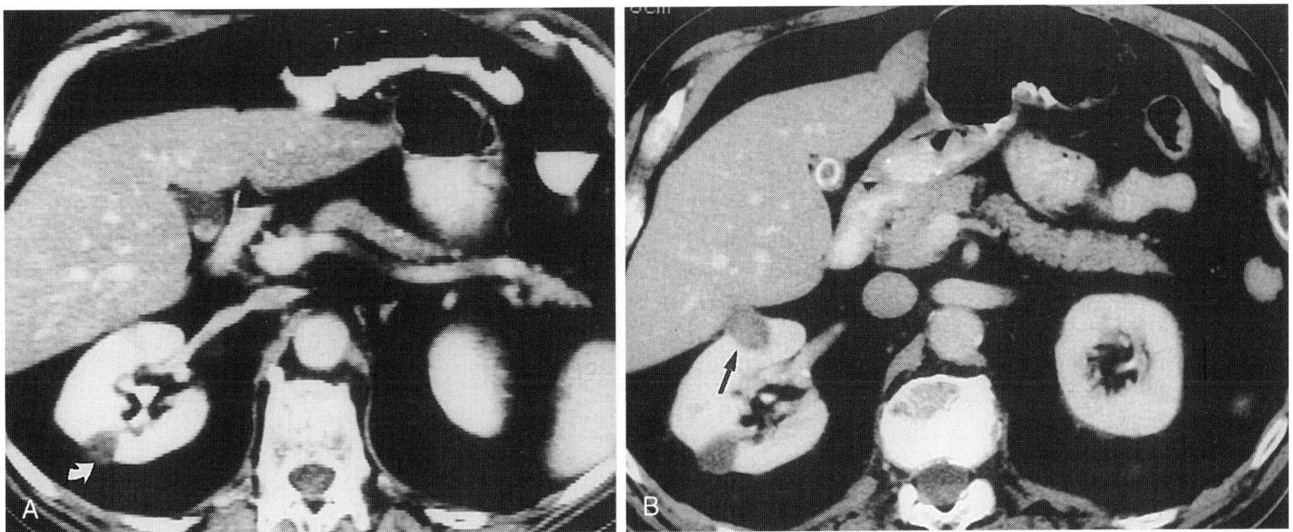

Figure 6–93. Rapid growth of small solid renal mass on follow-up CT. *A,* Small, low-attenuation lesion in posterior aspect of right renal midpole has the appearance of a cyst *(curved arrow)*. A second lesion is not clearly seen. *B,* Six months later, CT shows a 1.5-cm solid renal mass anteriorly in the right kidney *(arrow)*. The previously seen cyst remains unchanged.

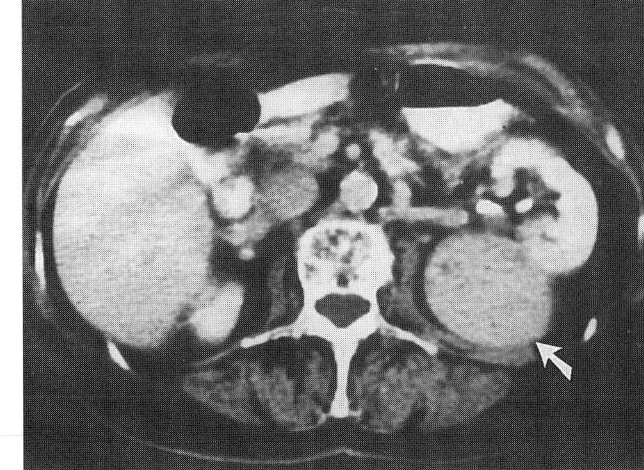

Figure 6–94. Large solid mass arising in the posteromedial aspect of the left kidney *(arrow)*. The postoperative diagnosis was oncocytoma.

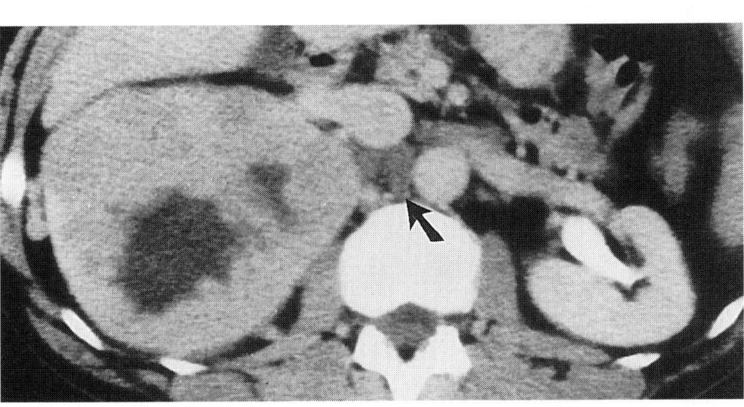

Figure 6–95. Large mass lesion with central necrosis replacing the right kidney. The pathologic diagnosis was renal cell carcinoma. Regional retrocaval adenopathy is also present *(arrow)*.

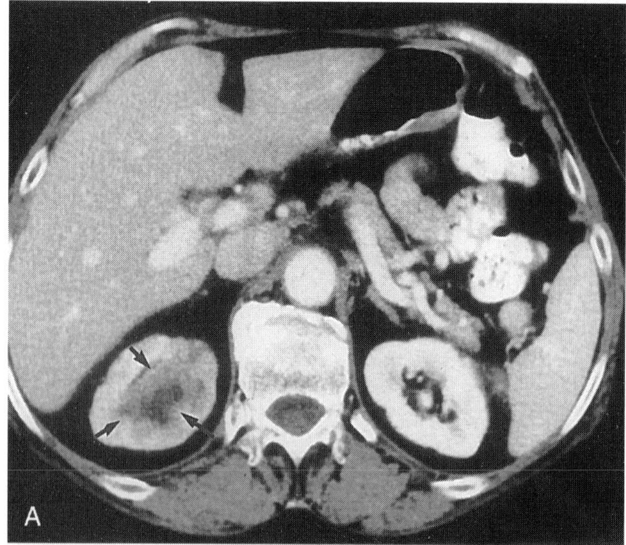

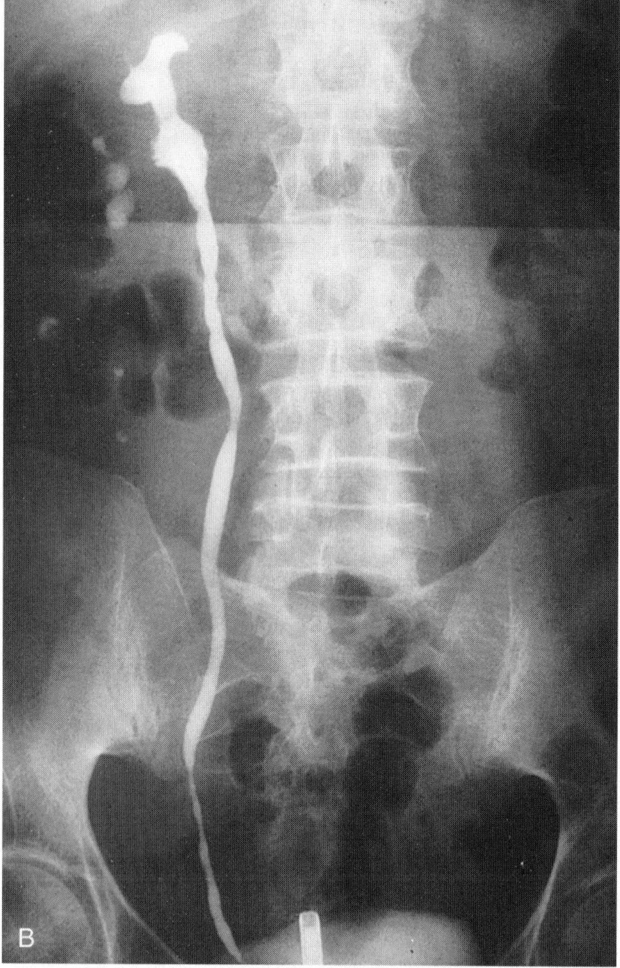

Figure 6–96. Transitional cell carcinoma of the right upper renal pole. *A,* The lesion appears as an infiltrating mass surrounding a dilated calyx *(arrows)*. *B,* Right retrograde pyelogram shows amputation and irregularity of midpole and lower pole calyces.

within collecting tubules and ducts, which are obstructed by surrounding edema and intraluminal infected cellular debris.

Renal abscesses appear as low-density lesions within the parenchyma surrounded by a thick rim of enhanced tissue (pseudocapsule). Infected cysts are not easily differentiated from simple cysts, except when their contents are of higher density. Inflammatory debris (pus) may be more easily demonstrated within an infected cyst or an infected and obstructed pyelocalyceal system on sonography. **Gas-producing infections can be shown very accurately on CT,** and their extent within and around the kidney and/or collecting system may be precisely documented (Figs. 6–99, 6–100). Perinephric abscesses and other fluid collections that may become infected, such as urinomas and hematomas, also are accurately demonstrated on CT scanning. In general, detection of air within or around the kidney is far superior with CT to that with sonography.

Xanthogranulomatous pyelonephritis is an uncommon infectious renal process often associated with indolent symptoms, such as low-grade fevers, vague flank pain, and gradual weight loss. There may be a history of recurrent urinary tract infections. This chronic renal infection may involve the entire kidney or may be focal. When the entire kidney is affected, renal function is often absent, and calculi are seen in many cases. The kidney becomes enlarged, and its contour may be lobulated and deformed, although a reniform shape usually is maintained. Regardless of the imaging modality used, the internal renal architecture and structure are severely altered. The renal parenchyma is replaced by poorly enhanced or nonenhanced masses with lower attenuation centers on CT imaging. The perinephric space is invariably infiltrated, and the perinephric fascia appears thickened. The focal variation of the disease is indistinguishable from a renal cell carcinoma by imaging criteria, whereas the diagnosis can be made with greater certainty when the entire kidney is involved.

Renal trauma is a major indication for CT imaging, although patient selection is strongly advised. Patients with gross hematuria who are symptomatic but stable enough not to require surgery or immediate angiographic intervention are more likely to exhibit findings on CT scanning. **Renal contusions; intrarenal, subcapsular, and perinephric hematomas; lacerations or fractures of the renal parenchyma; and disruption of the pyelocalyceal system are easily demonstrable** (Raptopoulos, 1994; Levine, 1994) (Fig. 6–101). **Adjacent organs, such as the liver and spleen, may also be imaged for trauma. Injury to the renal vascular pedicle can be detected by the lack of perfusion and function of the affected kidney. Additional injuries to bony structures, the ureters, and the bladder can also be assessed** (Levine, 1994). It is strongly recommended that intravenous contrast material be given for optimal enhancement of abdominal, pelvic, and retroperitoneal structures. In the pelvis, the contrast-filled bladder can be evaluated for possible intraperitoneal or extraperitoneal rupture with a great degree of accuracy. Rupture of the posterior urethra may also be seen. The role of IVU in the evaluation of trauma has been debated and questioned vis-à-vis its substitution by CT scanning, analogous to the most recent trend in many medical centers to replace urography with plain CT in patients with acute renal colic who are investigated for a ureteral calculus.

Staging of urologic malignancies and other retroperitoneal tumors is routinely performed with CT, as are follow-up examinations in patients who received treatment for such malignancies. The study ideally should be done after

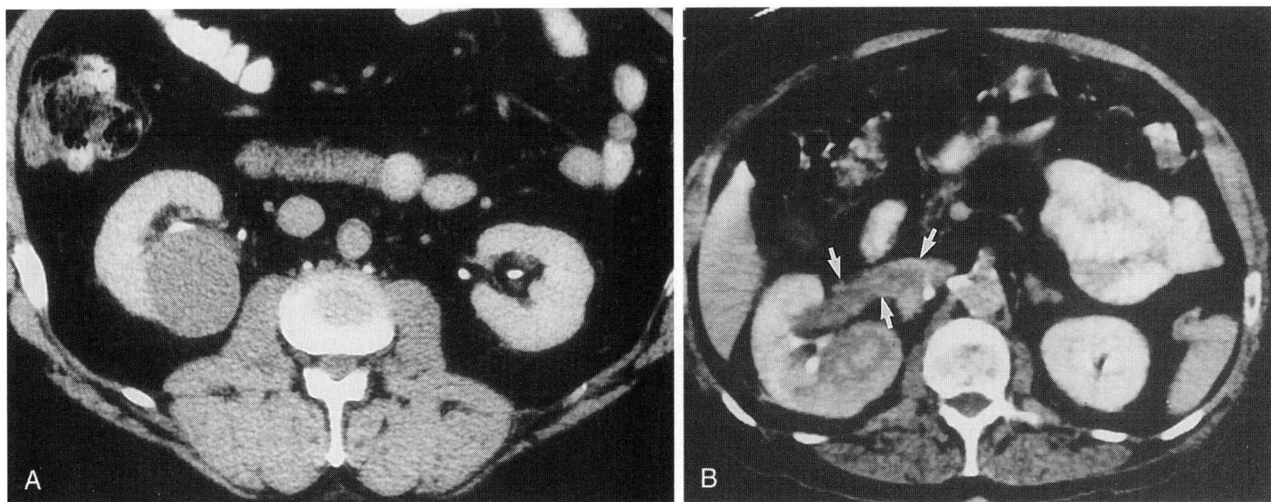

Figure 6–97. Staging of renal cell carcinoma. *A,* Right renal midpole mass is seen without regional adenopathy, caval extension, or perinephric infiltration (stage I Robson). *B,* Right renal cell carcinoma with involvement of the renal vena and inferior vena cava (stage III Robson) *(arrows).*

injection of intravenous contrast material for optimal opacification of the vessels and detection of the surrounding lymph nodes. **Lymphadenopathy sized at over 1 cm in the pelvis and 1.5 cm in the para-aortic region is considered significant,** although scattered reports in the literature suggest nodal sizes as small as 7 mm to be abnormal in the pelvis (Fig. 6–102). A well-known limitation of the technique is its reliance almost exclusively on evaluation of nodal size and hence its inability to detect disease within normal-size nodes. In addition to imaging for diagnostic purposes, CT is widely used to guide needle biopsies and other procedures in the abdomen and pelvis, thus significantly contributing to the staging and demonstration of recurrence in patients with malignancies.

CT is well suited for imaging **retroperitoneal fibrosis.** The fibrous plaques surrounding the retroperitoneal vessels and adjacent structures can be easily shown, because they are often enhanced by contrast material, and their extent can be accurately demonstrated.

Congenital anomalies of the upper urinary tract only occasionally necessitate imaging with CT. Ectopic, fused, dysplastic, or absence of kidneys may be shown on urography, sonography, and retrograde pyelography; thus CT scanning should be reserved for only complicated cases (see Fig. 6–76).

In the pelvis, **benign and malignant diseases of the bladder, prostate, testes, seminal vesicles, and spermatic cords are often evaluated by CT,** although the male genital tract is easily accessible by sonography, which should be the screening imaging modality of choice (Figs. 6–103, 6–104). Staging of bladder and prostate carcinoma often is done with CT, although neither malignancy is well seen within the respective organs on CT scanning, especially prostatic carcinoma. MRI has been found to be superior to CT in the detection and staging of bladder and prostate tumors. **In general, imaging of the lower pelvis with CT for oncologic indications, although still widely performed, has not been very accurate.**

Angiography

The use of angiography as a purely diagnostic radiologic modality has steadily declined since the 1980s. The

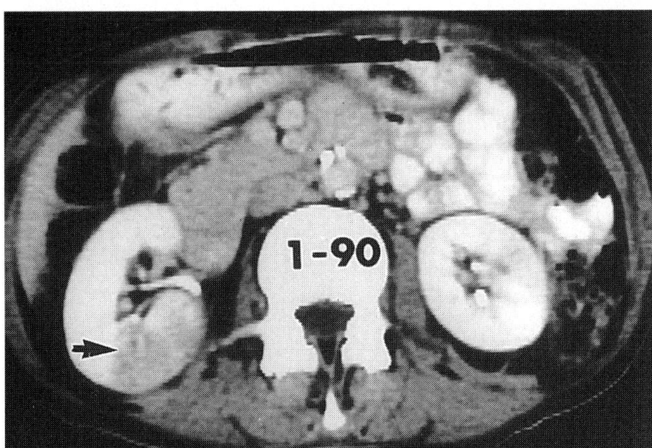

Figure 6–98. Acute pyelonephritis often appears as a perfusion defect extending through the entire thickness of the renal parenchyma *(arrow).*

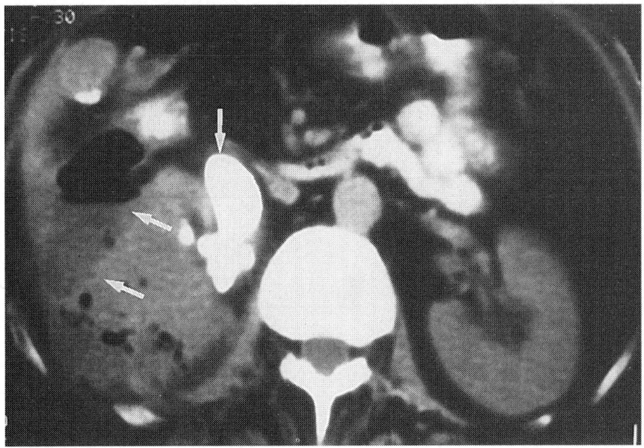

Figure 6–99. Large perinephric abscess with gas formation associated with a staghorn calculus *(arrows).*

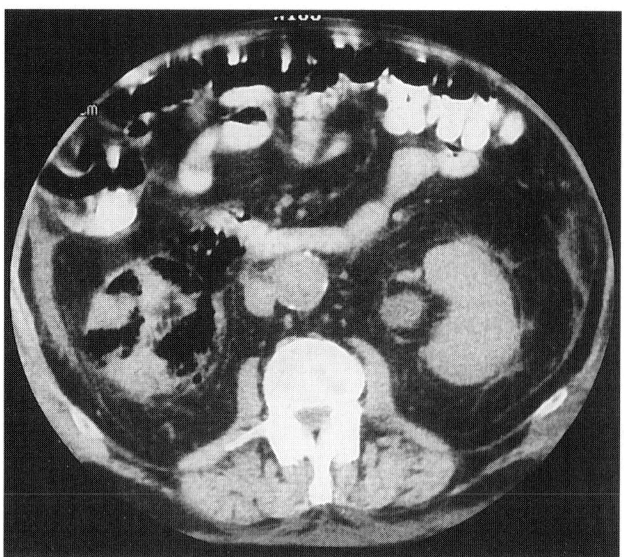

Figure 6–100. Emphysematous pyelonephritis of the right kidney.

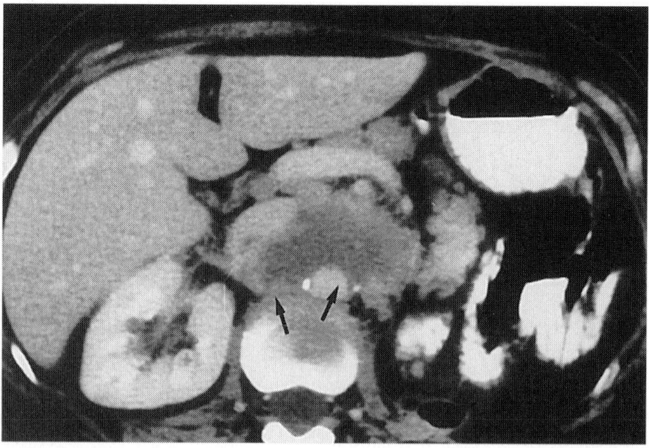

Figure 6–102. Follow-up CT in patient with left nephrectomy for transitional cell carcinoma. Large mass of lymph nodes is seen *(arrows)*.

noninvasive or less invasive cross-sectional imaging techniques (e.g., Doppler sonography, contrast-enhanced CT, and MRI) have in many clinical situations effectively replaced angiography in the diagnostic work-up of urologic disease. However, over the same period of time, **the therapeutic applications of angiography have expanded considerably.** Percutaneous transluminal angioplasty, embolization, thrombolysis, placement of vascular stents, and establishment of venous access are some of the commonly performed vascular procedures. Depending on the location and nature of the clinical problem, the arterial and/or venous aspects of the vascular system can be studied. Access into the major arterial and venous branches in the abdomen and pelvis is gained by means of a percutaneous puncture into the common femoral artery and femoral vein, respectively. Sometimes the brachial or axillary artery may be punctured if the common femoral artery, the iliac artery, or the aorta is occluded (Pollack and Banner, 1994).

Access into the vascular system is obtained in the vast majority of cases through the Seldinger technique. After the vascular structure to be catheterized is identified, antiseptic preparations and local anesthesia are applied to the overlying skin. A needle is then inserted into the lumen of the vessel at a convenient angle (usually approximately 45 degrees), and a guide wire is threaded into the vessel through the needle. The needle is then removed, and a catheter is passed over the wire and positioned within or near the desired anatomic area of the vascular system under fluoroscopic guidance. Accurate and safe placement is guided by the intermittent injection of small amounts of contrast material. Selective catheterization of pelvic, renal, and adrenal vessels is possible for demonstration of the vascular anatomy, for sampling of venous blood for renin or adrenal hormonal levels, and as a guide for percutaneous transluminal interventions. Care is taken to limit the amount of contrast material injected and the total fluoroscopy time. The former can be a major problem in patients with compromised renal function and in need of multiple diagnostic and/or therapeutic studies that require the intravascular administration of iodinated contrast media. Adequate hydration of the patient and prudent use of the contrast material are advised,

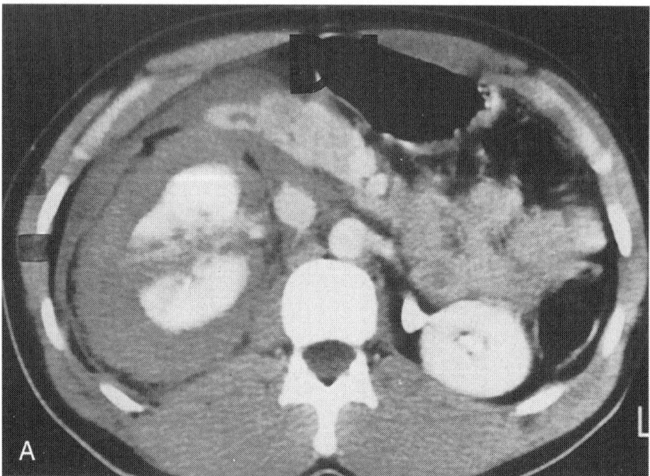

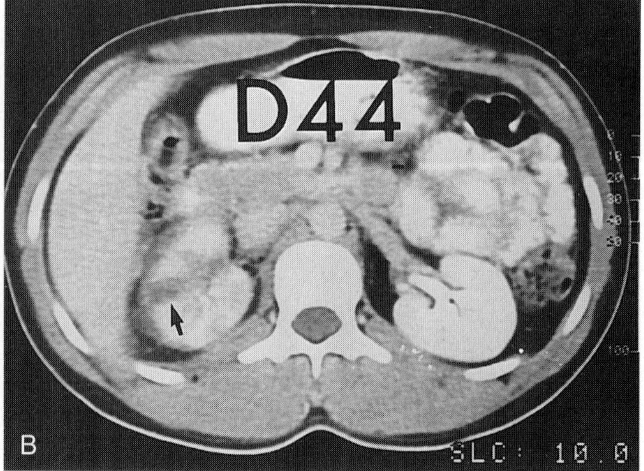

Figure 6–101. Fracture of the right kidney. *A*, Large hematoma surrounds the fractured kidney, which continues to perfuse and excrete. *B*, Follow-up CT 44 days later after conservative treatment shows residual fibrotic and infarcted areas with resolution of perinephric hematoma *(arrow)*.

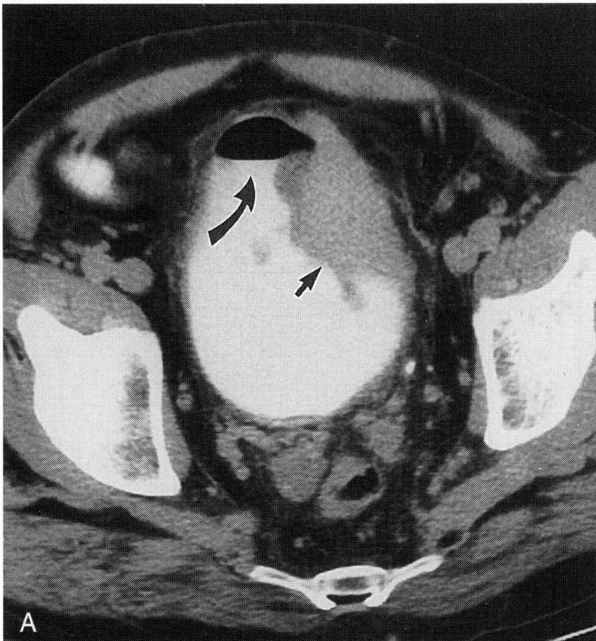

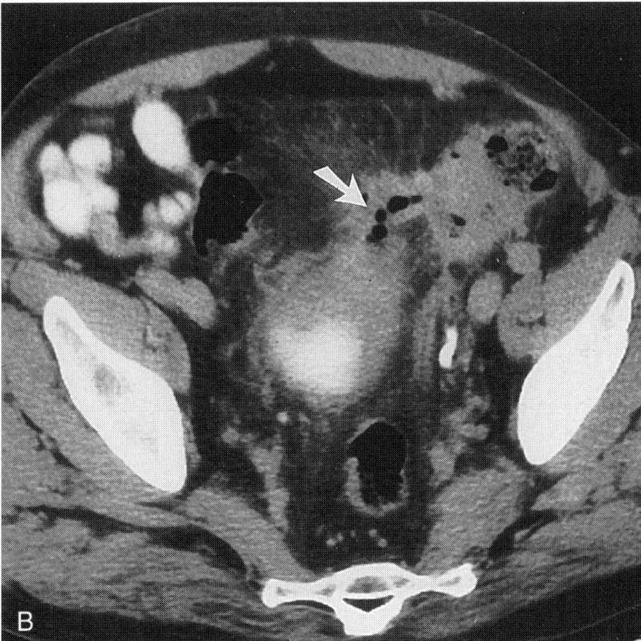

Figure 6–103. Colovesical fistula in patient with diverticulitis and pneumaturia. *A,* The left lateral bladder wall is markedly thickened, simulating the presence of a neoplasm *(straight arrow).* Air-fluid level within the bladder lumen indicates an enterovesical fistula *(curved arrow). B,* Sigmoid colonic inflammation from diverticulitis and fistulous tract are demonstrated *(arrow).*

if it is decided that the benefits from the procedure outweigh its risks.

In most medical centers, routine angiography is nowadays performed in the form of digital subtraction, whereby computerized manipulation of the images makes it possible to obtain good-quality studies with relatively small amounts of intra-arterial contrast material (Dunnick and Sfakianakis, 1991). The same electronically digitized technique may follow opacification of the arterial anatomy after intravenous administration of the contrast material, although the quality of the studies is often inferior to the ones obtained after intra-arterial injections. The direct puncture of the abdominal aorta through a left flank approach, also known as translumbar aortography, is mostly of historical interest but may be useful when no other arterial access is possible.

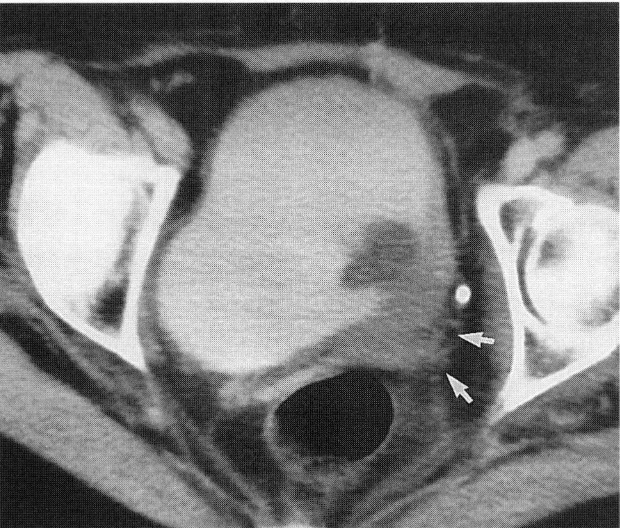

Figure 6–104. Transitional cell carcinoma of the left posterolateral bladder wall with obstruction of the ureter and perivesical fat invasion *(arrows).*

Complications resulting from angiographic procedures are few and mostly minor, such as pain and groin hematomas at the puncture site. **Direct injury to the catheterized vessels is occasionally severe enough to necessitate surgical exploration.** Large hematomas, vascular tears, formation of pseudoaneurysms, dissection, and thrombosis occur infrequently but should be recognized and managed promptly (Pollack and Banner, 1994). It has been suggested that prolonged compression of small pseudoaneurysms with an ultrasonic probe may be curative (Fellmeth et al, 1991). A potentially dangerous but rare complication is massive embolization of small vessels by cholesterol crystals in patients with significant atherosclerotic changes. Foreign bodies—such as pieces of wires, catheters, filters, and other devices—may be lodged within the vascular system; many of them can be retrieved and removed percutaneously. Last but not least important are the complications, idiosyncratic or systemic and nephrotoxic, that result from the use of intravascular contrast materials. The guidelines for use of iodinated media and management of their side effects in angiography are fairly similar to those in IVU or contrast-enhanced CT studies.

The clinical indications for angiography as a diagnostic modality are limited. For instance, characterization of renal masses or staging of renal cell carcinoma, both common indications in the 1980s, have been abandoned in favor of cross-sectional imaging modalities (Figs. 6–105, 6–106). **Some of the clinical problems that may be elucidated by the use of angiography include evaluation for renovascular hypertension** (atherosclerosis, fibromuscular dysplasia, abdominal aortic aneurysm) (Dunnick and Sfakianakis, 1991; Mitty et al, 1996); **certain cases of trauma to the**

kidneys or pelvic organs, often in association with embolization of arterial bleeding or arteriovenous communications; **preoperative evaluation of renal donors; certain postoperative complications of renal transplantation** such as occlusion or stenosis of vascular anastomoses and cases of hyperacute rejection that may be difficult to differentiate from acute arterial thrombosis (Becker, 1991); **suspected renal arterial embolic and venous thrombotic disease** when other modalities are not diagnostic (Fig. 6–107); and the demonstration of **vascular anatomy, arterial or venous, before complicated surgical explorations.** On occasion, angiography may be used to **elucidate the origin of a large suprarenal mass lesion** whether renal or adrenal, **the origin of a retroperitoneal tumor,** and the search for an undescended testis (spermatic venography) that cannot be located by cross-sectional imaging studies, as well as to **confirm the diagnosis of polyarteritis nodosa or other vasculitides or a large, bleeding angiomyolipoma** that may not be clearly seen on CT because of the hemorrhage and a relatively small amount of fat in the tumor.

The opacification of lymph nodes and lymphatic channels after direct cannulation of small lymphatic vessels in the subcutaneous tissues of the toes, known as lymphography, has very limited applications nowadays, being used almost exclusively for the staging of urologic pelvic and testicular malignancies (Pollack and Banner, 1994). This technically difficult procedure may demonstrate metastases within lymph nodes of normal size that are missed on CT imaging. A major pitfall of lymphangiography is its failure to fill certain lymphatic channels and groups of lymph nodes under normal circumstances. Unfortunately, nonfilling of channels and nodes may also be the result of tumor spread; therefore, the nonvisualization of certain segments of the lymphatic system in the abdomen and pelvis may not be helpful in confirming or ruling out metastatic disease. One potential indication for lymphography is testicular seminoma accompanied by a normal CT study in a patient who may nonetheless have metastases to retroperitoneal lymph nodes. Depending on the therapeutic protocols involved, a lymphangiogram may be helpful in the staging and management of such patients.

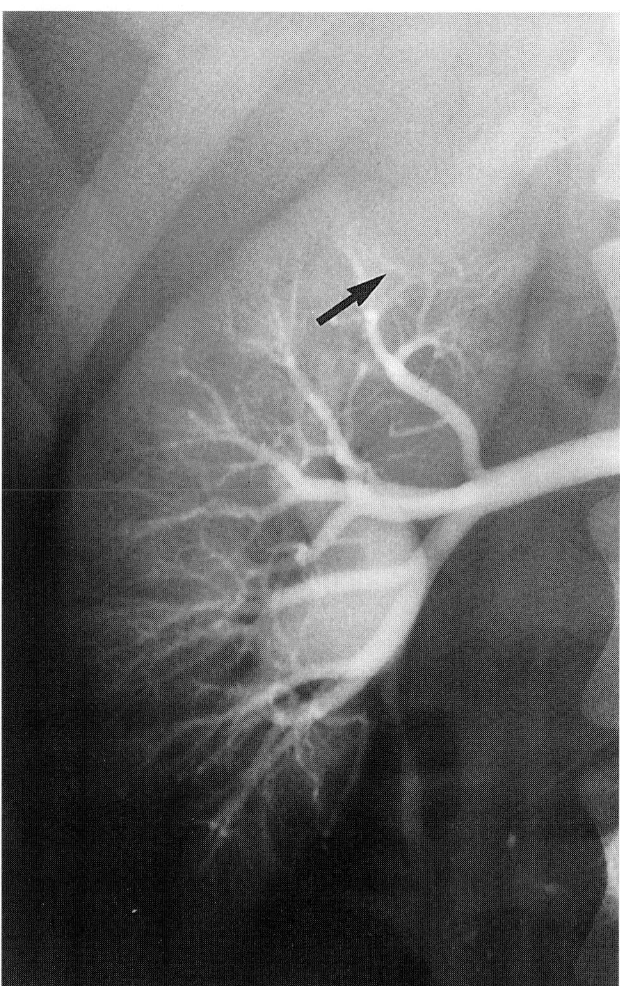

Figure 6–106. Right renal arteriogram demonstrates an avascular mass in the upper pole *(arrow).* The study was performed to support a partial nephrectomy in a young man who was found to have a renal adenoma.

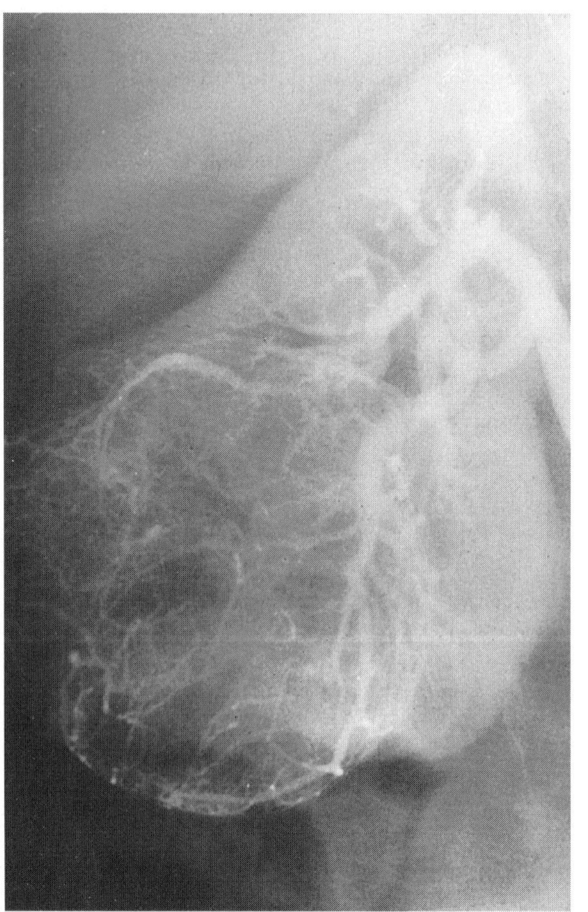

Figure 6–105. Angiographic evaluation of right renal mass demonstrates a hypervascular tumor, most consistent with a renal cell carcinoma. The use of angiography for evaluating renal masses is limited.

Radionuclide Imaging

There are widespread applications for radionuclide imaging in patients with urologic diseases. A large number of radioisotopes have been developed for the investigation of specific anatomic and functional disorders, primarily of the

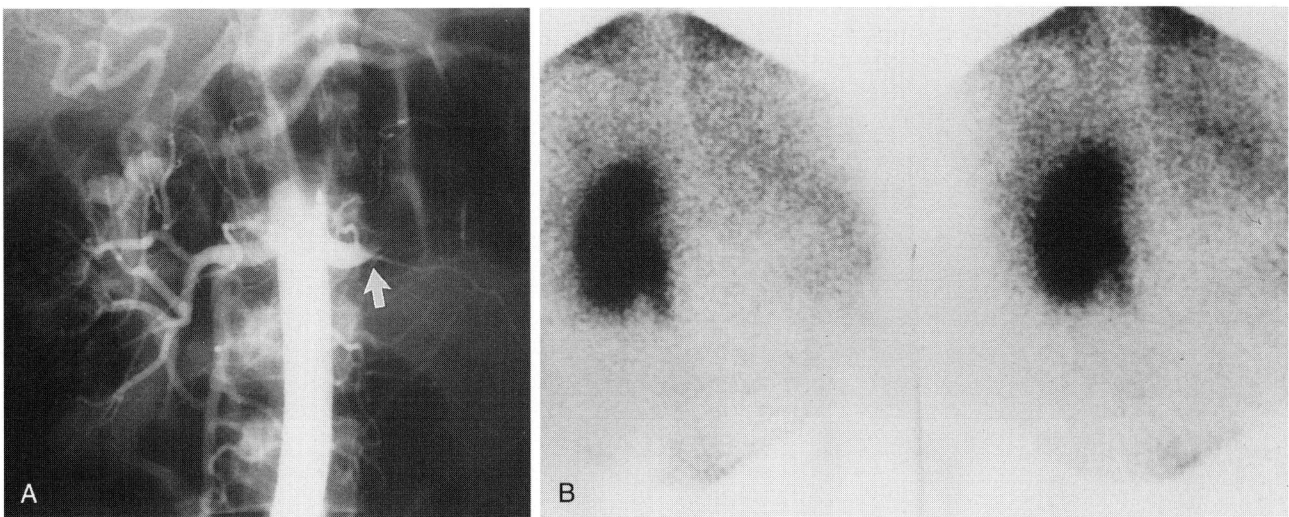

Figure 6–107. Surgical complication after removal of a large left renal cyst. *A,* The left renal artery was abruptly interrupted within 2 cm from its origin by accidental ligation, as shown on aortography *(arrow). B,* Radionuclide renogram shows complete absence of radioactivity over the left kidney (scan inverted). The right kidney functions normally.

kidneys but also of other organs of the genitourinary tract (McBiles and Morita, 1994). Radionuclide studies are best suited for demonstrating pathophysiologic changes that result from abnormalities in the perfusion and function of the organs under scrutiny. Because of the limited spatial resolution of many radioisotopic techniques, detailed delineation of morphologic alterations often is inferior to that of CT, MRI, or sonography. However, the modality often is quite sensitive to certain inflammatory, malignant, and vascular diseases, so that it can detect their presence before other techniques can demonstrate them. A notable example is the use of positron-emitting pharmaceuticals to image a number of genitourinary malignancies and their metastatic spread with specially designed positron-emitting tomography (PET) cameras. The technique requires an on-site cyclotron because the radioisotopes are short-lived, and thus it has limited availability.

With few exceptions, the radionuclides in clinical use are given intravenously. More often than not, a flow study to evaluate perfusion is indicated. Imaging is then obtained at a very rapid sequence such as every one or few seconds over a 30- to 60-second period. Parenchymal transit of the tracer can be imaged at longer intervals over a longer period of time, such as every 1/2 or 1 minute over a 30-minute period. Delayed views are taken as indicated by the kinetics of the radiotracer or the clinical problem or both (McBiles and Morita, 1994). Sometimes the radionuclide accumulates within an organ or disease process slowly, over a period of hours or days; therefore, scanning with the gamma camera is appropriately delayed. Examples here include renal cortical agents (technetium-99m dimercaptosuccinic acid [DMSA]) or infection-seeking isotopes (gallium-67 citrate, indium-111–labeled white blood cells). For the latter agents, imaging often begins at 24 hours and may extend up to 72 hours after injection of the radionuclide. Radionuclide cystography is performed after direct instillation of the radionuclide agent into the bladder after catheterization.

The indications for a radionuclide study vary greatly with the clinical question and the diagnostic algorithm in use. Certain indications are less controversial or more accepted than others. Bone scintigraphy is fairly universally considered as the modality of choice for imaging skeletal metastases from prostate or renal primary tumors (Fig. 6–108). On the other hand, the use of renal cortical agents for the evaluation of certain masses or pseudotumors may be questionable when sonography or CT are available. The choice between contrast-enhanced CT and gallium-67 citrate or indium-111–labeled white blood cells in the search for renal infection can be controversial. The radionuclide studies are very sensitive; however, a 24- or 48-hour delay is required before imaging, and studies may not be able to distinguish pyelonephritis from an abscess. The choice between a radionuclide and a radiologic voiding cystogram may also not be very easy. It appears that because of its superior anatomic resolution, a radiologic study should be the initial examination, especially in males, whereas the radionuclide study with its high sensitivity and somewhat lower radiation exposure to the patient may be suitable for follow-up examinations or studies of siblings of patients with known reflux (Van den Abbeele et al, 1987). Testicular torsion can be evaluated by either radionuclide flow study or color Doppler sonography; both techniques have a high degree of accuracy. The established and potential indications for the use of radioisotopic studies are briefly presented.

Estimation of total and split renal function as well as assessment of the function of a renal transplant are among the commonly requested radionuclide studies (Dubovsky and Russell, 1982). When technetium-99m DTPA (diethylenetriamine-pentaacetic acid), a glomerular filtration excreted agent, is given, an approximate estimation of GFR can be calculated either in vivo, by computer-aided scanning, or in vitro, by collecting one or two blood samples at predetermined time intervals and estimating the clearance of the radiotracer as a function of renal excretion and physical decay. Other agents such as technetium-99m glucoheptonate, iodine-123 iodohippuric acid, and the newest tracer, technetium-99m mercaptoacetyl triglycine (MAG3), are secreted by renal tubular function to a lesser or greater extent and are used to evaluate approximate effective renal plasma flow and other functional parameters with good success

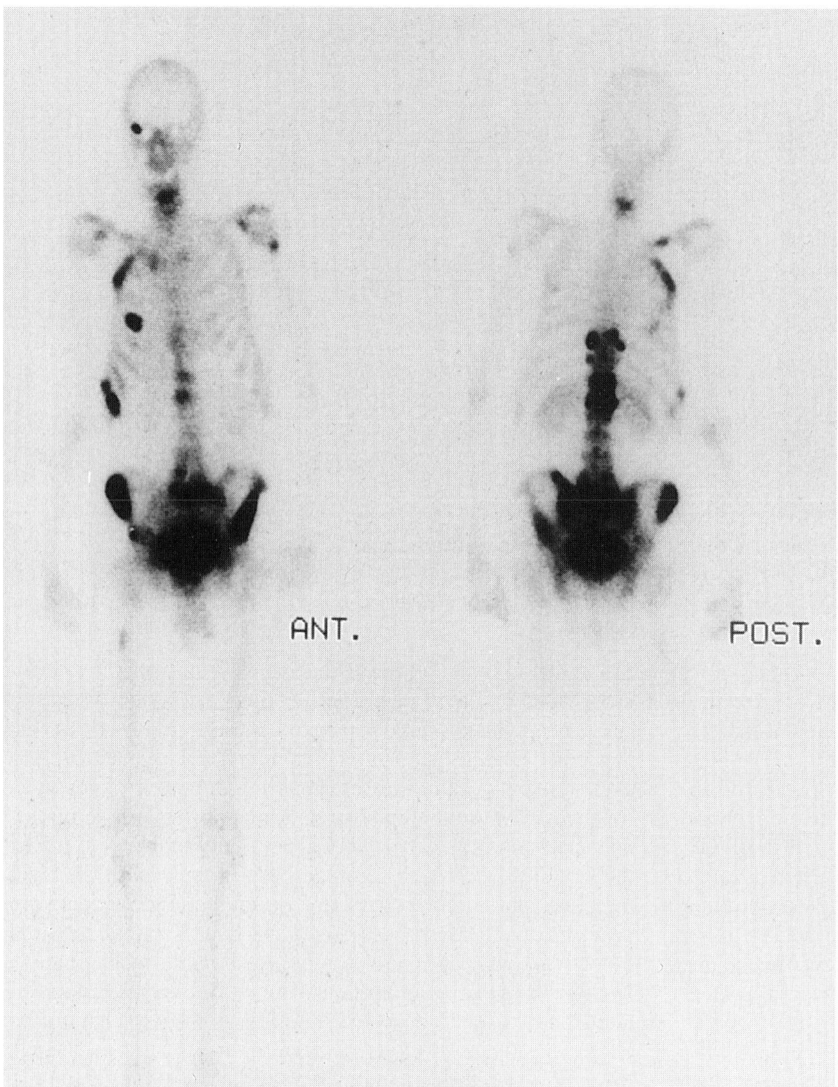

Figure 6–108. Bone scintigraphy with technetium-99m methylene diphosphonate (MDP) demonstrates multiple sites of metastatic disease in a patient with prostate carcinoma.

(Dubovsky and Russell, 1982; Eshima and Taylor, 1992). Estimation of split renal function usually results from the computerized estimation of the relative function (perfusion, excretion, or secretion and clearance) of each kidney. Otherwise, accurate determination of true split renal function requires the presence of a nephrostomy or ureteral stents. In cases of severe hydronephrosis with or without stone disease, the degree of loss of renal function, as well as its partial recovery or lack thereof after decompression through a nephrostomy or stent of the obstructed kidney, can be evaluated by serial radionuclide renograms. This may be particularly crucial in pediatric patients, in whom every effort is made to spare hydronephrotic kidneys if possible.

Renal parenchymal imaging is often not as important as the functional aspect of the study; thus a limited assessment is done with the aforementioned agents. If detailed imaging of the renal cortex is desired, as in pyelonephritis in children, technetium-99m DMSA should be given and the kidneys imaged 3 to 4 hours after the injection. The same agent has limited use in the estimation of split renal function (Taylor, 1982). Use of radionuclide techniques may be made in patients with significant renal dysfunction who are not able to receive intramuscular iodinated contrast material.

The determination of presence or absence of obstruction in a hydronephrotic kidney often necessitates the use of **diuretic renography** (Conway, 1992). Current recommendations indicate that technetium-99m MAG3 is superior to technetium-99m DTPA as the radionuclide agent (Eshima and Taylor, 1992). Furosemide is given 15 to 20 minutes into the study if the washout time–activity curve is still rising or becomes static. The recommended adult dose is 40 mg with a pediatric dose of 1 mg/kg of body weight. Adequate hydration and bladder catheterization for the duration of the study are recommended for all patients, especially children. Visual evaluation of the pyelocalyceal system and computer-generated time-activity curves are used to determine the correct diagnosis (Fig. 6–109). Rising curves 15 minutes or more after the administration of the diuretic indicate obstruction. The **examination is unreliable in patients with poor renal function and/or very dilated urinary tracts.** Combination with the Whitaker test may be helpful in these cases.

Evaluation of renovascular hypertension is another indication for radionuclide studies (Dunnick and Sfakianakis, 1991; Nally and Black, 1992). The time-activity curve over the suspected ischemic kidney often is neither sensitive

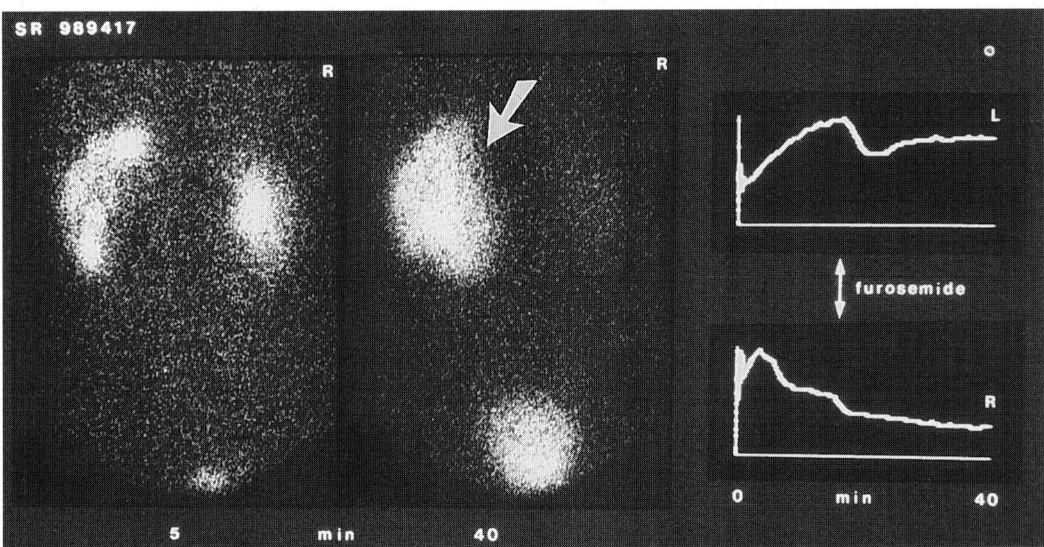

Figure 6–109. Diuretic renogram in a young boy with left ureteropelvic junction obstruction. The time–activity curves indicate lack of washout from the left collecting system after furosemide was given. The scintigraphic images confirm the retention of the radionuclide in the left pyelocalyceal system *(arrow)*.

nor specific enough for renal artery stenosis for plain renography to be used as a screening test in populations in which the prevalence of the disease is very low. **The introduction of captopril-enhanced renography has significantly improved the accuracy of the radionuclide examination.** The aim of the study is to detect, as accurately as possible in a noninvasive manner, potentially reversible renal artery stenosis. Among the clinical findings likely to suggest renal artery stenosis are recent-onset hypertension with a diastolic pressure equal to or higher than 105 mm Hg; long-term well-controlled hypertension that becomes refractory to the treatment without another explanation; hypertension and abdominal bruits; hypertension and unexplained renal dysfunction; hypertension in young, nonobese patients; hypertension refractory to an adequate three-drug antihypertensive regimen; and hypertension accompanied by new or worsened renal failure when treated with an angiotensin converting enzyme (ACE) inhibitor (Nally and Black, 1992).

Although the most impressive results have been reported in cases of unilateral renal artery stenosis, patients with bilateral disease or solitary kidneys with renal artery stenosis may also be studied. Most centers recommend that ACE inhibitors be withheld for a few days before the test but that other antihypertensive medications may be continued. The captopril dose is 25 or 50 mg orally, and the radionuclide of choice is technetium-99m DTPA, although other radioisotopes have also been used. In the presence of renal artery stenosis, the oral ACE inhibitor blocks the angiotensin II–mediated vasoconstriction and high blood pressure, resulting in significant decreases in the filtration pressure and glomerular filtration of the affected kidney. These changes can be shown both visually and by computer-generated curves, the latter indicating a delay in the upslope of the time-activity curve over the affected kidney. A baseline study before the ACE inhibitor is given is not necessary if the captopril study is normal; otherwise, it is recommended that the baseline study be performed if the postcaptopril scan is abnormal. Both the sensitivity and specificity of the test have been reported to be near 90% (Setaro et al, 1991).

Certain complications after renal transplantation can be evaluated with radionuclide studies (Kirchner and Rosenthall, 1982; Becker, 1991) (Fig. 6–110). **Complete renal artery occlusion cannot be distinguished from hyperacute rejection within the first 24 hours after transplantation,** because both pathologic entities result in lack of perfusion of the transplant. A photopenic area corresponding to the kidney surrounded by background activity should be distinguished from a case of uniform activity across the kidney and its background. The former pattern indicates no perfusion, whereas the latter suggests severe depression of renal flow from either rejection and/or acute tubular necrosis, which may improve with treatment. **Urinary obstruction and urine leakage can be diagnosed,** and the latter may appear as a gradually expanding area of increased radioactivity around the transplant, in contradistinction to hematomas or lymphoceles, which appear as photopenic areas. **Acute tubular necrosis** results in decreased perfusion and concentration of the tracer with a very long transit time of the radionuclide through the kidney and into the bladder. **Rejection** often manifests with a similarly decreased perfusion and prolonged parenchymal transit time to the point that differentiation between the two entities may not be possible at first. On serial examinations, however, acute tubular necrosis usually begins to subside, whereas rejection without treatment leads to progressive deterioration of the scintigraphic appearance. The distinction between the two entities may further become more difficult in cases in which both entities coexist.

Imaging of renal infection or occult suppuration in the abdomen or pelvis can be satisfactorily performed by either gallium-67 citrate or indium-111–labeled leukocytes (Papanicolaou and Pfister, 1996). Imaging with gallium-67 citrate is often not complete until 48 to 72 hours after injection, and bilateral symmetric renal activity during the first 24 hours is to be expected (Fig. 6–111). Also, the tracer may be taken up by certain tumors such as lymphomas and hepatomas, which can further confuse the diagnosis in patients with known malignancies who are being evaluated

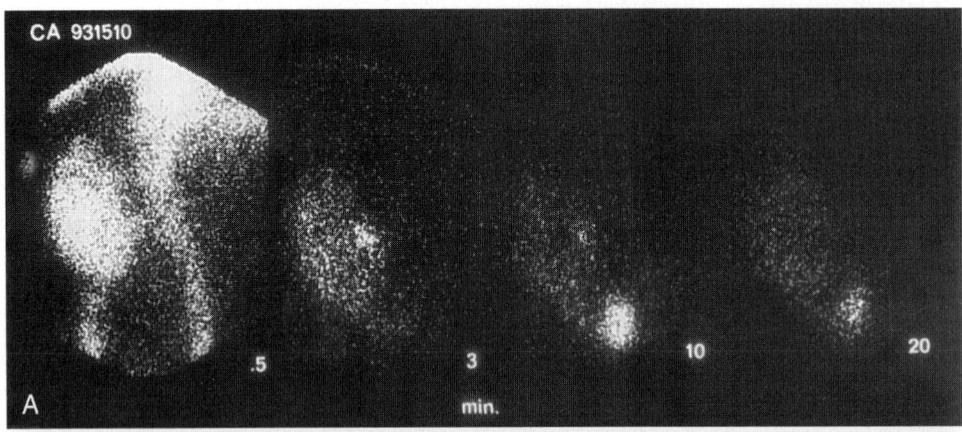

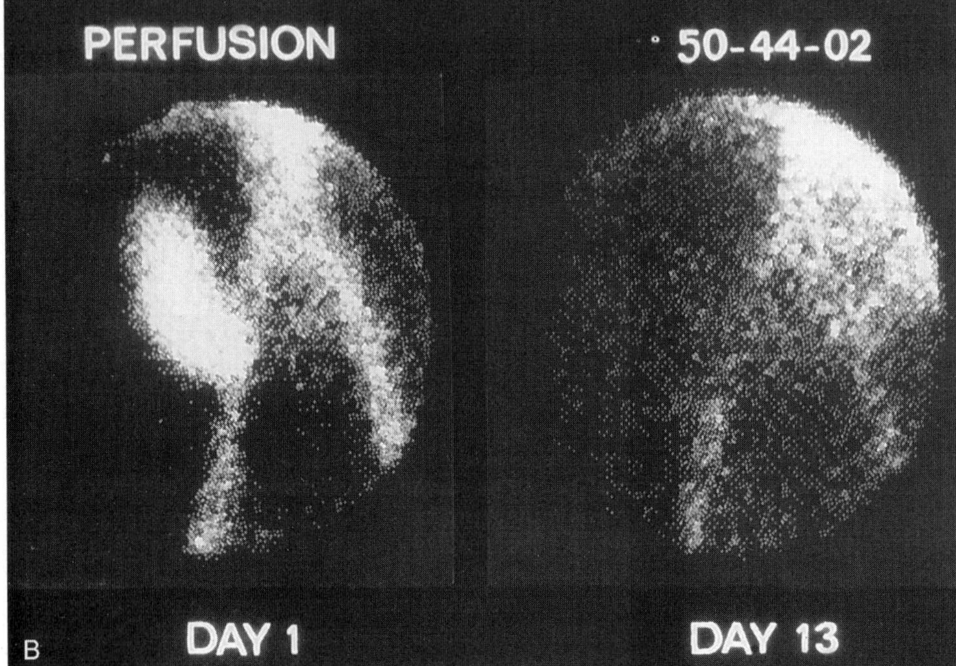

Figure 6–110. Evaluation of renal transplants with iodine-123 iodohippuran. *A,* Normal uptake by and transit time of the radiotracer through the transplanted kidney. *B,* No renal perfusion is seen on day 13 after transplantation, strongly suggesting severe rejection.

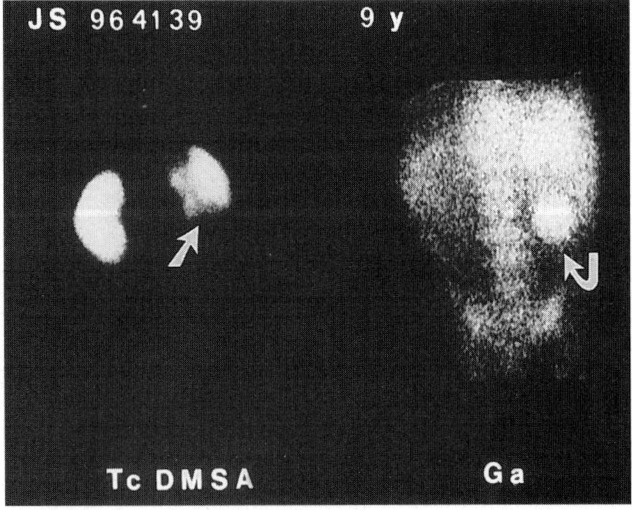

Figure 6–111. Imaging with gallium-67 citrate and technetium-99m dimercaptosuccinic acid (DMSA) of acute pyelonephritis in a young boy. The infection-seeking agent is concentrated in the area of the inflammation *(curved arrow),* whereas the renal cortical agent is absent from the same area within the right kidney *(straight arrow).*

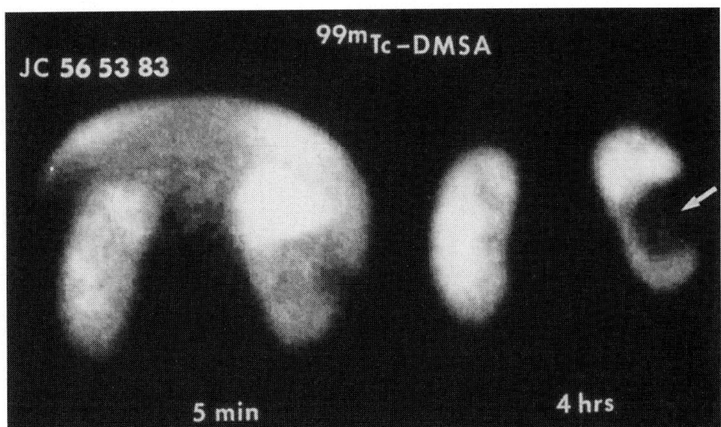

Figure 6–112. Imaging of pyelonephritic scars in children often is done with technetium-99m DMSA. The defect seen in the right renal midpole region is the result of a previous renal abscess *(arrow)*.

for fever and occult sepsis. The choice of indium-111–labeled leukocytes eliminates tumoral uptake and bowel and renal excretion, and they can generate images within 24 hours (McBiles and Morita, 1994). The agent normally is accumulated by the liver, bone marrow, and spleen. Both tracers furthermore generate limited anatomic resolution, which may make accurate localization of the infected focus, as well as the differentiation between pyelonephritis and an abscess or infected cyst, very difficult. Imaging of pyelonephritic renal scars or sequelae of reflux nephropathy in children is best accomplished with technetium-99m DMSA (Majd and Rushton, 1992) (Fig. 6–112).

Vesicoureteric reflux in children can be demonstrated by means of radionuclide cystourethrography (Fig. 6–113). As indicated earlier, the radioisotopic study **most often is used for the follow-up of patients with proven reflux or siblings of children with reflux** and who are at a higher risk for reflux themselves (Van den Abbeele et al, 1987). **Also, girls may undergo imaging by the radionuclide technique from the beginning, whereas it is advisable to obtain a radiologic voiding cystogram as a first study in boys** for adequate documentation of the urethral anatomy.

The **acute scrotum** and, more precisely, differentiating testicular torsion from epididymitis have been clinical problems traditionally evaluated by radionuclide scanning (Lutzker, 1982) (Fig. 6–114). The **radioisotope of choice is technetium-99m pertechnetate given intravenously.** A flow study is performed first with rapid acquisition of images for 1 minute, followed by static scrotal images 5 to 15 minutes later. The tracer is excreted to a large extent by the kidneys into the bladder, which may interfere with the scrotal imaging. Scanning at an early time before the bladder is filled with radioactive urine or after covering of the bladder with a metallic shield minimizes the interference.

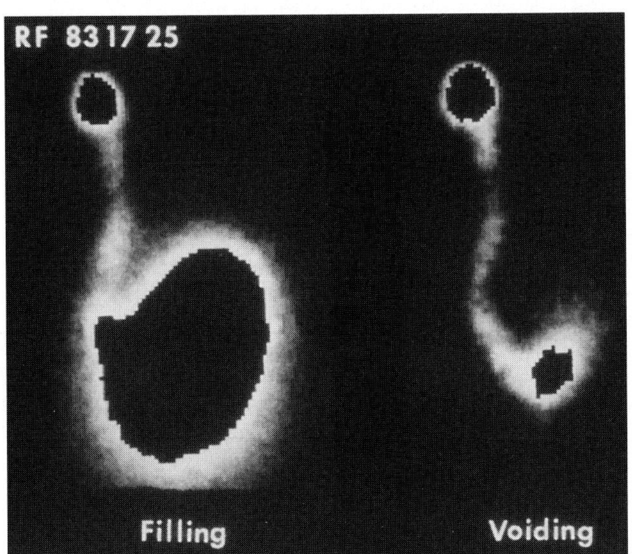

Figure 6–113. Radionuclide demonstration of vesicoureteric reflux.

Flow to a **torsed testis** is virtually absent on the dynamic images. A very faint background activity secondary to scrotal skin circulation may be present. On the static images, likewise, the side of the scrotum with the ischemic testis appears photopenic (see Fig. 6–114*B*). **Missed torsion,** an ischemic event that is several days old, presents typically as a photopenic central area surrounded by a rim of increased radioactivity (doughnut sign) (see Fig. 6–114*C*). A large testicular abscess may also have an appearance similar to that of missed torsion. **Epididymitis,** on the other hand, results in increased blood flow and an area of increased uptake of the tracer by the affected testis and its surrounding appendages and skin (see Fig. 6–114*A*). These findings reflect the intense inflammatory changes present. Testicular sonography likewise shows absence of flow by color Doppler technique in the case of torsion and markedly increased flow in the case of epididymitis. The accuracies of both modalities are comparable, and their use depends on, among other factors, availability, familiarity with the technique, and preference of referring physician and radiologist.

The use of radionuclides in the evaluation of renal trauma has been minimal since the introduction of CT scanning. Radioisotopic imaging may be indicated in selected cases after trauma or surgery to assess the degree of function and amount of functioning renal tissue. The latter is best accomplished by using a renal cortical radionuclide agent.

Magnetic Resonance Imaging

MRI has evolved into a dominant imaging technique for the evaluation of many urologic disorders. Of the many chemical elements in the human body that could be used for imaging, hydrogen is the choice because it is naturally abun-

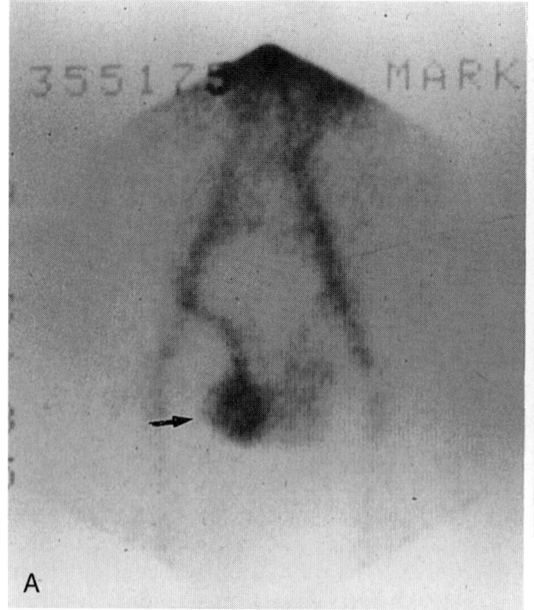

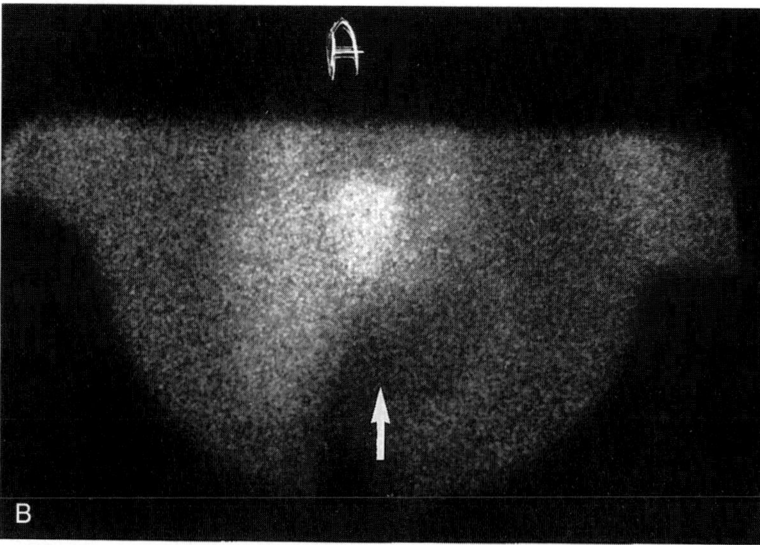

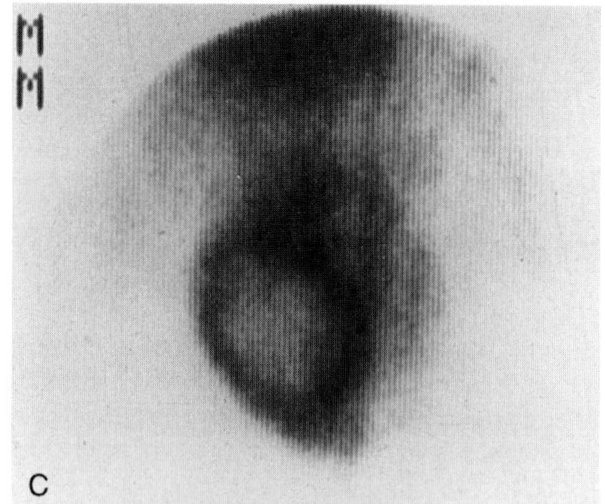

Figure 6–114. Evaluation of the acute scrotum with radionuclides. *A,* Increased flow to the symptomatic right testis is indicative of infection, likely epididymitis *(arrow). B,* Lack of perfusion to the left testis is diagnostic of acute torsion *(arrow). C,* The increased uptake in the periphery of the right hemiscrotum, together with the lack of central perfusion, suggests missed torsion.

dant and its magnetic resonance signal can be easily detected. **In MRI, nonionizing radiofrequency pulses are used to induce brief excitement of the hydrogen protons of the tissues and organs to be imaged, and the signals generated by the protons are converted into digital images.** Typically, the area of clinical interest is placed into the body magnet or a suitable coil, and all its hydrogen protons are aligned by the magnetic field of the magnet. This alignment is then disrupted by the application of appropriately selected radiofrequency pulses, depending on the clinical problem. After the effect of these pulses is over, the protons return to their original alignment, and in the process of relaxing, they emit signals that are proportional to the level of their initial magnetization state. Differences in the signal intensity received by the magnetic resonance computer are translated into different tissue contrast levels and transformed into images of the scanned region of the body.

Although the tissue contrast latitude generated by MRI is wider than that of CT and although blood flow into vascular spaces can often be readily imaged without enhancement, the use of intravascular contrast agents such as gadolinium-DTPA has been increasing steadily in clinical practice. Reactions to the agents used are rare, and the renal function is not as significant a factor as it is for the iodinated contrast materials used for IVU and CT.

Contraindications to an MRI examination are few but may be important (Shellock et al, 1993; Elster et al, 1994). Patients with pacemakers, ferromagnetic intracranial aneurysm clips, cochlear implants, and metallic pieces in vital bodily locations cannot be safely imaged. Certain older heart valves may be a contraindication, as are certain caval filters and shrapnel in or adjacent to vital locations of the body. In general, hip and knee prostheses are safe to image. Clinicians should always check current literature and manufacturer information regarding the safety of uncommon devices worn by patients who may require MRI examinations. Patients on orthopedic or life support devices from the trauma floor or an intensive care unit are often prohibited from entering the magnetic space if they cannot be detached from the equipment. Claustrophobia is a concern for certain patients who are unable to tolerate the scanning experience; if the information gained from the MRI examination is vital and unique, such patients should be sedated.

The ability of MRI to generate multiplanar images is an advantage over conventional CT scanning. This makes MRI particularly helpful in evaluating the pelvis. The indications for magnetic resonance scanning in the urinary tract are outlined as follows.

Characterization of small renal masses can be facilitated by a combination of pulse sequences that may enable distinction between solid lesions and cysts (Fig. 6–115). **Enhancement with gadolinium-DTPA and fat suppression techniques further improve the diagnostic yield** of MRI examinations (Semelka et al, 1991, 1992). Typically, **cysts** appear as lesions of low signal intensity on T1-weighted images and as lesions of high signal intensity on T2-weighted images. The modality is particularly suitable for patients who cannot undergo CT examination with intravenous contrast enhancement (those with renal failure, history of serious reaction to prior contrast material administration) and patients with multiple, small lesions in the kidneys that may be impossible to reliably characterize by any other technique and sometimes small, hyperdense cystic lesions. The classic hyperdense cyst is a high-attenuation lesion on CT secondary to high protein or hemorrhagic contents. Differentiation from solid tumors may be problematic, however, because of the indeterminate nature of the wall and internal structure of some hyperdense lesions. Sonography, when the lesion is at least 1.5 cm in diameter, and MRI for

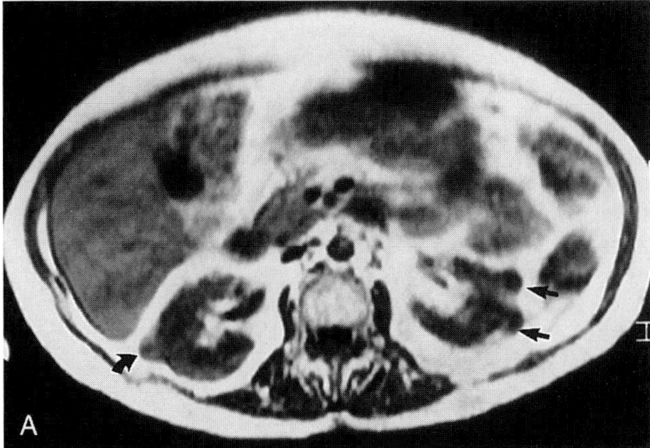

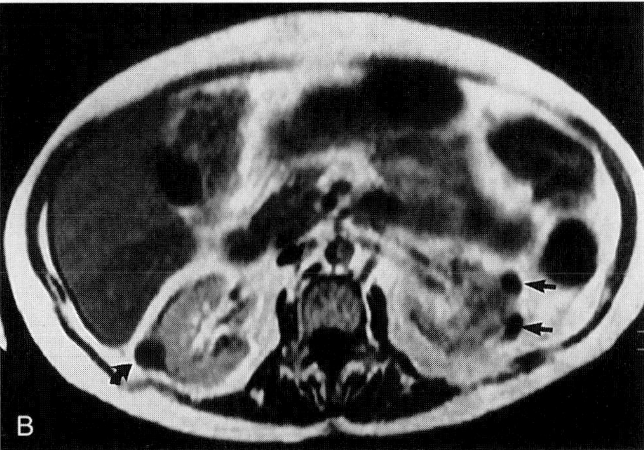

Figure 6–115. Characterization of small renal lesions by MRI. *A,* T1-weighted image shows a small lesion of moderate signal intensity in the right renal midpole *(curved arrow).* Two small lesions of low signal intensity in the contralateral kidney appear to be simple cysts *(straight arrows). B,* Repeated imaging after enhancement with gadolinium-DTPA (diethylenetriamine-pentaacetic acid) shows the lesion to be avascular and therefore a simple cyst *(curved arrow).* The left-sided small lesions are also avascular *(straight arrows).*

smaller lesions can be of help. The simple hyperdense cyst is expected to have a smooth oval or round contour that is sharply marginated and to display no enhancement after intravenous administration of contrast material on CT or MRI examinations.

Staging of renal cell carcinoma can be performed effectively with MRI (Roubidoux et al, 1992) (Fig. 6–116). Anatomic resolution concerning involvement of adjacent organs, regional lymph nodes, and perinephric fat often is superior to that of CT because of multiplanar imaging capability. Furthermore, blood flow pulse sequences with very short acquisition times are well suited for the evaluation of the renal vein and inferior vena cava. The same or similar techniques have been introduced to study renal artery stenosis, renal artery aneurysms, renal vein thrombosis, and arteriovenous shunts. This type of MRI is known as magnetic resonance angiography (MRA) and can be displayed in two- or three-dimensional images (King, 1996) (Fig. 6–117). Although not as well tested by time and experience as captopril scintigraphy, MRA and CT angiography (CTA) are promising new techniques in the evaluation of vascular problems in urologic and nephrologic diseases (Rubin, 1996).

The use of MRI in the retroperitoneum is limited because there is no clear advantage of the modality, with few exceptions, over CT.

In the pelvis, staging of bladder and prostate carcinoma with MRI has received significant attention primarily because of the difficulties with CT accuracy of local staging (Rifkin et al, 1990b; Barentsz et al, 1993; Schiebler et al, 1993). Again, the multiplanar imaging of MRI and superior anatomic display of the pelvis with the use of special transrectal and suprapubic phased array coils make local staging more accurate with MRI (Fig. 6–118). In the case of bladder carcinoma, the study usually requires intravenous administration of gadolinium-DTPA and selection of appropriate planes that display the anatomic relations of the tumor with adjacent perivesical fat and pelvic organs. Differentiation between nodes and vessels often is easier on MRI than on CT. The prostate is imaged in the transverse plane with the addition of coronal or sagittal images when the tumor is near the seminal vesicles or the apex, respectively (Fig. 6–119). No intravenous contrast is required. Macroscopic disease spread beyond the prostatic capsule to the periprostatic fat, neurovascular bundles, nodes, or lateral pelvic wall is often accurately shown, but the modality invariably understages microscopic extension of disease.

The **typical manifestation of prostate carcinoma is one or more lesions of low signal intensity on T2-weighted images that contrast with the usually homogeneous, high–signal intensity peripheral gland** (Schiebler et al, 1993) (Fig. 6–120). Owing to the bright signal of the periprostatic fat, a disruption of the prostatic capsule and invasion of the fat may be seen on the T2-weighted images. A low–signal intensity and asymmetrically enlarged neurovascular bundle raises suspicion for tumor invasion (Fig. 6–121*A*). Involvement of the seminal vesicles, likewise, appears as a low–signal intensity infiltration of these structures, whereas on T2-weighted images they have a bright signal intensity as a result of their fluid content (see Fig. 6–121*B*).

In selected cases, MRI can be used to investigate congenital or acquired benign lesions of the seminal vesicles, vas

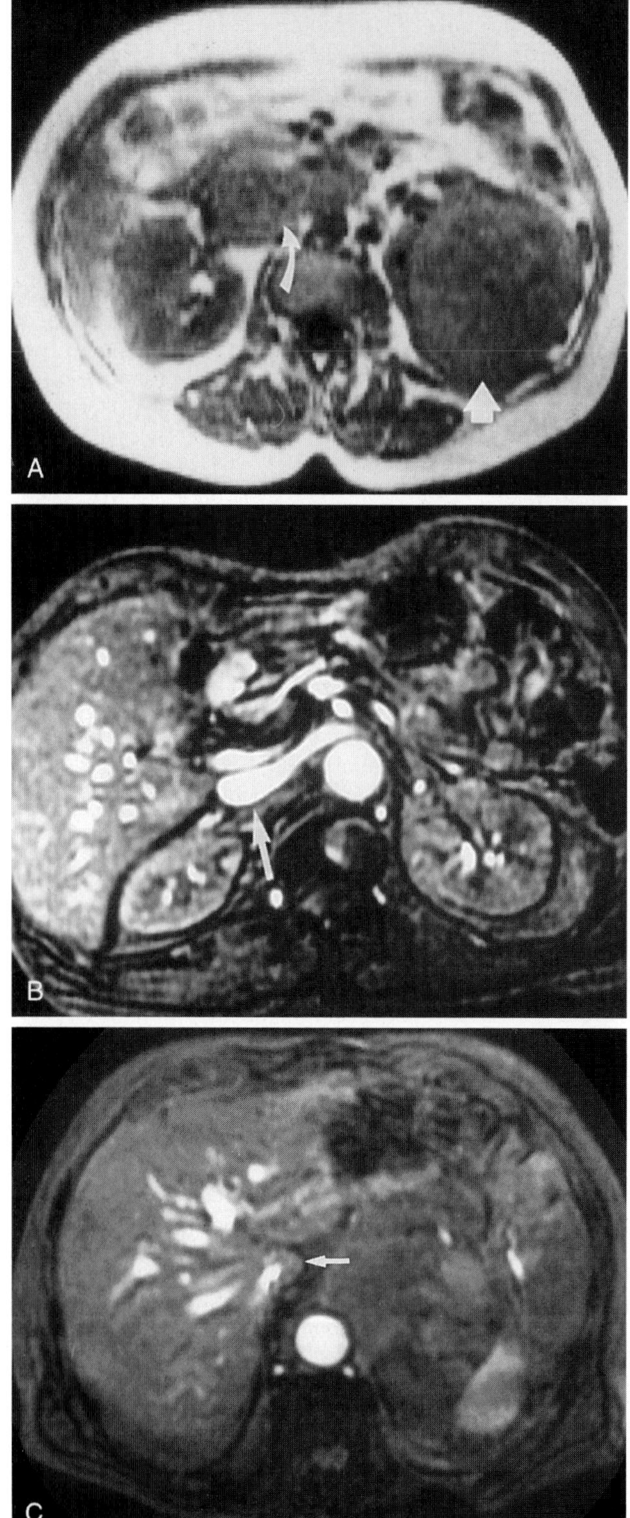

Figure 6–116. Staging of renal cell carcinoma with emphasis on caval involvement. *A,* T1-weighted image shows a large solid renal mass *(arrowhead)* with extension into the inferior vena cava *(curved arrow). B,* Normal appearance of the inferior vena cava and renal vein with use of breath-hold gradient. *C,* Lack of inferior vena caval luminal filling with normal blood flow consistent with caval tumor extension *(arrow).*

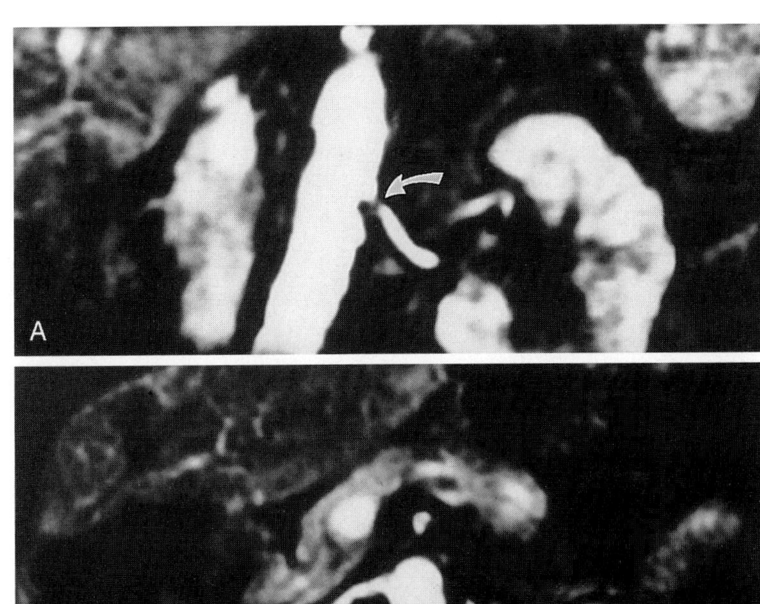

Figure 6–117. Magnetic resonance angiography (MRA) in the evaluation of renal artery stenosis. *A,* Coronal image shows marked narrowing of the take-off of the left renal artery *(curved arrow). B,* Transverse image of the same patient demonstrates a patent right renal artery *(arrow).*

deferens, and prostate when transrectal sonography is noncontributory.

Testicular disorders have traditionally been investigated by sonography, and the role of MRI in the diagnosis of testicular tumors is limited (Mattrey, 1991). Scrotal or testicular hematomas that may simulate testicular tumors can be diagnosed with MRI. The undescended testis is most easily evaluated by sonography or CT; MRI is reserved for specific cases such as abdominal location of the testes in infants and children (nonionizing modality). Varicoceles may also be demonstrated, although sonography is the procedure of choice in the search for the venous disorder implicated in infertility.

Adrenal Imaging

The adrenal glands are well imaged (Fig. 6–122). Abnormalities of the adrenal glands are often classified as function-

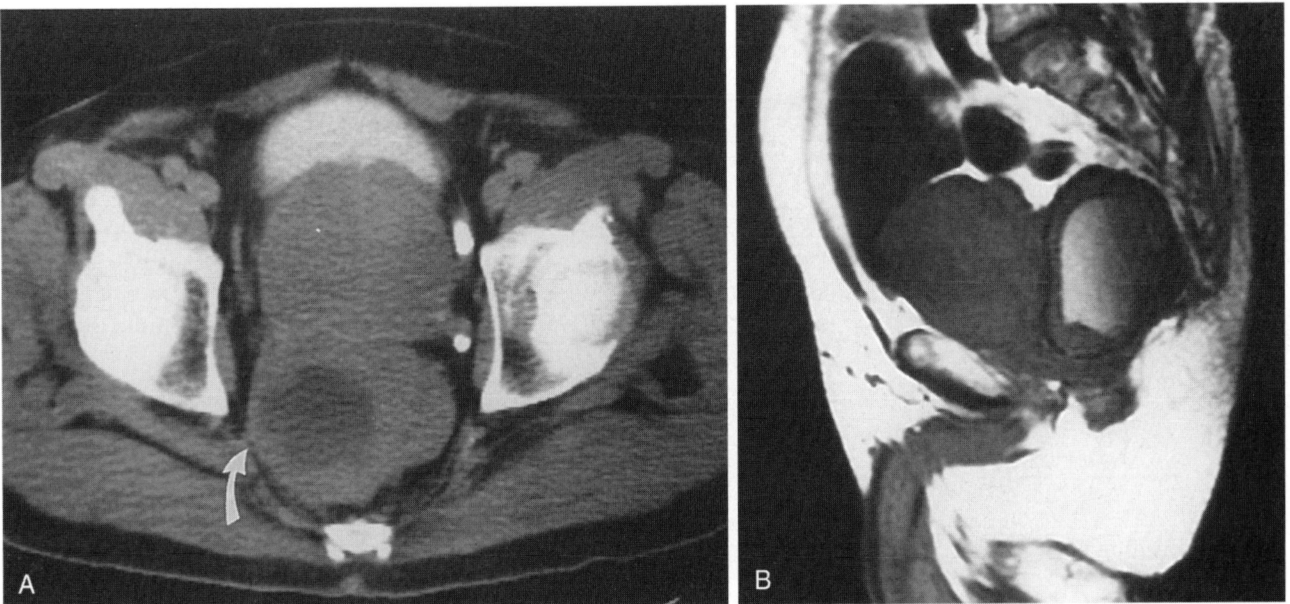

Figure 6–118. Advantage of multiplanar imaging capability of MRI over CT in staging of pelvic tumors. *A,* Large soft tissue tumor posterior to and in contiguity with the prostate gland. No fat plane is seen between the tumor and the gland, and a prostatic origin of the tumor is possible *(curved arrow). B,* Sagittal T1-weighted image of the same patient shows a clear separation of the mass from the prostate. A retroperitoneal sarcoma was found at surgery.

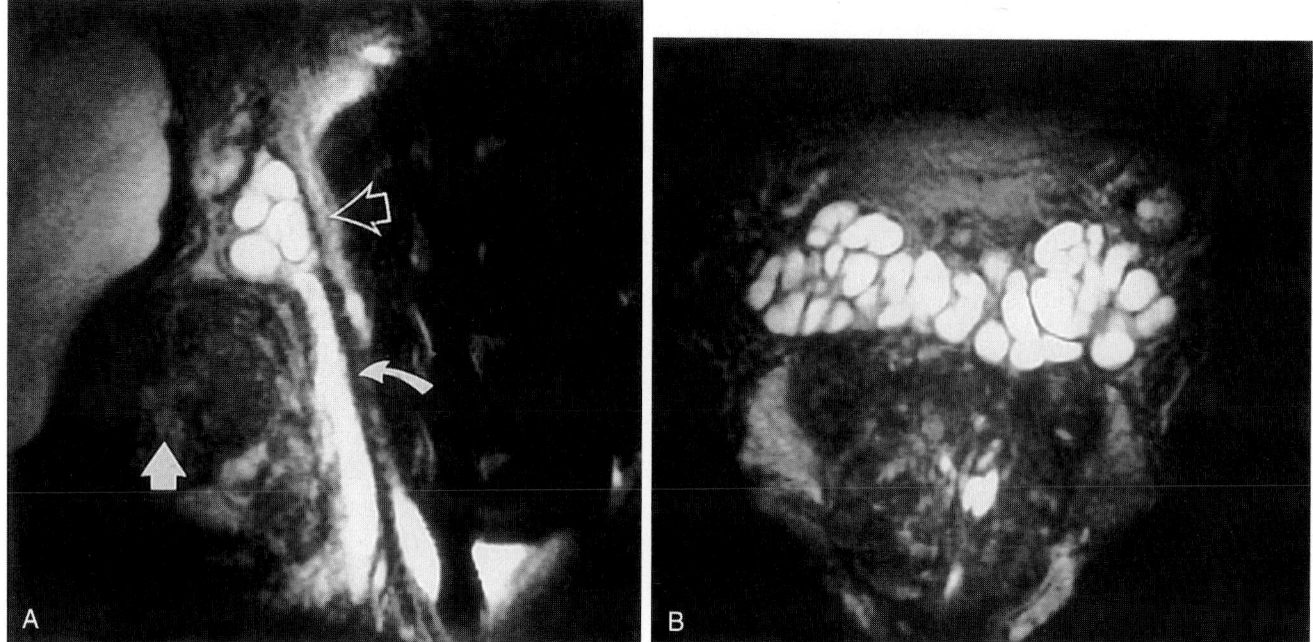

Figure 6–119. Normal prostatic anatomy in an elderly male with slight prostate-specific antigen (PSA) elevation. *A,* Sagittal endorectal fast-spin echo pulse sequence shows the bright sacculations of the seminal vesicles *(open arrow),* the high–signal intensity peripheral gland *(curved arrow),* and the enlarged low–signal intensity central gland *(solid straight arrow). B,* Coronal image of the normal seminal vesicles.

ing and nonfunctioning lesions. Many of the latter masses are incidentally discovered during imaging, usually CT, for other clinical reasons and are referred to as adrenal incidentalomas. Although uncommon, some functioning lesions may be rather silent clinically. Furthermore, both groups of lesions contain benign and malignant masses that may necessitate careful imaging and possible biopsy for accurate diagnosis (Bernardino et al, 1985).

Among the functional adrenal masses, an adenoma is found in about 15% of cases of Cushing's syndrome, and a much smaller percentage of adrenal cortical carcinomas may be responsible for endocrine abnormalities. The adenomas of Cushing's syndrome are masses measuring 2 to 4 cm in diameter, whereas the carcinomas are larger, measuring over 5 cm in diameter. In primary hyperaldosteronism, adenomas are usually the cause of the endocrine disorder (up to 80%), which typically features hypertension, hypokalemia with muscular weakness, and hypernatremia. The size of these lesions varies from a few millimeters to 2 cm. Adrenal hyperplasia is responsible for the remaining cases of Conn's syndrome and may not be easily detected by imaging techniques. The rare cases of feminizing and masculinizing adrenal syndromes in adults are most often caused by large, usually malignant tumors easily detected by imaging studies. Pheochromocytomas arise in the adrenal medulla or other sites of chromaffin cells and are more often than not unilateral and benign. The excessive secretion of catecholamines can manifest with a series of hypertensive crises accompanied by headaches and apprehension. Familial cases of pheochromocytoma often manifest with bilateral tumors, and adrenal pheochromocytomas are part of Sipple's syndrome, together with medullary thyroid cancer and primary hyperparathyroidism. Ectopic pheochromocytomas can be found along sympathetic chromaffin cell chains in the thorax and abdomen in about 10% of cases; the most common extra-adrenal site is an infrarenal organ of Zuckerkandl.

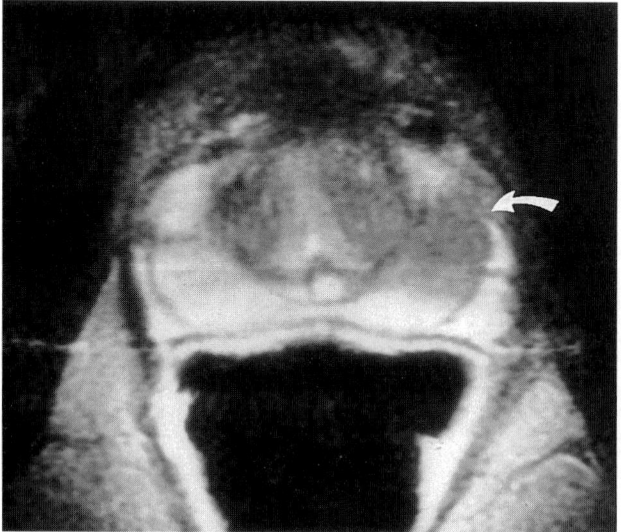

Figure 6–120. Endorectal MRI shows an area of low signal intensity in the left peripheral gland *(curved arrow),* possibly indicative of carcinoma.

Among the non-hyperfunctioning masses, lesions such as cysts, myelolipomas, and hemorrhage are relatively uncommon (Korobkin et al, 1996). Benign, inert adenomas are common, incidentally discovered lesions seen in about 1% to 2% of patients undergoing CT scanning and become diagnostic enigmas in patients in whom metastases are suspected. Metastatic disease to the adrenal glands is relatively common among patients with known primary tumors, especially melanoma, lymphoma, and tumors of the lung, breast, and kidney. Their size varies greatly from one to several centimeters.

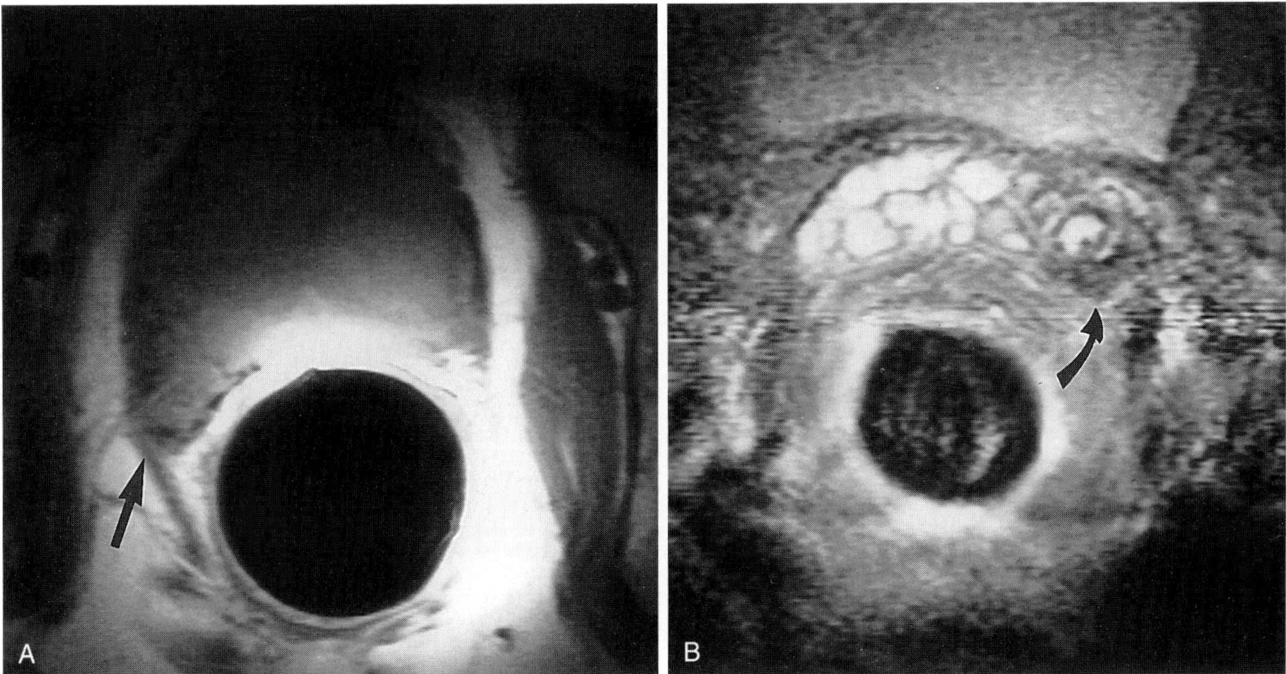

Figure 6–121. Staging of prostate carcinoma. *A,* T1-weighted image shows an asymmetrically enlarged right neurovascular bundle, suggestive of extraprostatic tumor spread *(arrow). B,* T2-weighted image shows abnormally low signal intensity involving the left seminal vesicle in a different patient *(curved arrow).* The finding is very indicative of tumor invasion.

The clinical condition of adrenal insufficiency, or Addison's disease, may be the result of infection, hemorrhage, shock, metastases, and autoimmune diseases. Many causes of adrenal insufficiency may be depicted on imaging studies.

In the pediatric age group, particularly infants and young children, the adrenal glands are larger in relation to the body weight than are the glands of older children and adults; they are therefore easy to detect on sonography. For the other age groups, CT is the modality of choice for the evaluation of most adrenal disorders.

The diagnosis of adrenal cysts and myelolipomas can be very accurate (Figs. 6–123, 6–124). The **cysts** appear on CT as rather large, often lobulated, low-attenuation masses with wall calcification (Tung et al, 1989). The presence of variable amounts of visible fat in the lesion makes the diagnosis of **myelolipoma** likely. Both lesions usually are asymptomatic unless they become very large or are complicated by hemorrhage. **Acute adrenal hemorrhage** appears as high-attenuation collections on CT involving either one or both glands. Care should be exercised not to overlook a bleeding tumor.

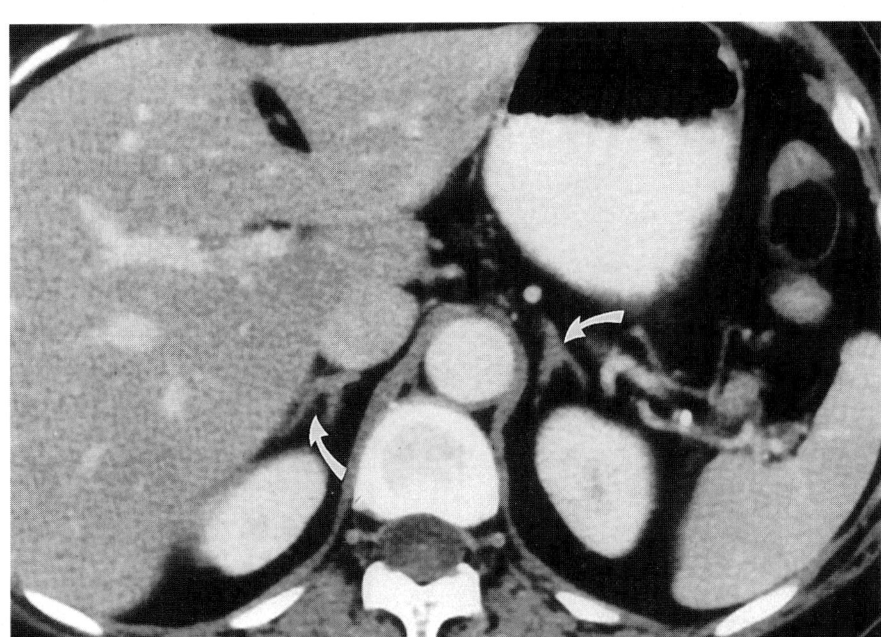

Figure 6–122. CT imaging of normal adrenal glands *(curved arrows).*

Adrenal infection often appears as calcification within the gland and can be bilateral. Tuberculosis and histoplasmosis are common causes. Sometimes the infected glands may become deformed, cystic, or enlarged. Differentiation from solid tumors and hemorrhage may then pose some difficulty.

Adrenal adenomas often manifest on CT as smooth, well defined, homogeneous, smaller than 4 cm in diameter, and low in attenuation (Lee et al, 1991). Several reports in the literature indicate that an adrenal mass with a value of 10 Hounsfield units or fewer on unenhanced CT is very likely to be an adenoma (Lee et al, 1991; McNicholas et al, 1995). The low attenuation of these lesions is attributed to their rich lipid content. On the other hand, **metastases** often are larger, not as well defined, and heterogeneous. Unfortunately, the morphologic overlap between the two lesions is significant, and measurements of their respective attenuation values are strongly recommended as a powerful discriminating feature.

Adrenocortical carcinoma appears as a large, heterogeneous mass with calcification, central necrosis, and ill-defined borders (Fig. 6–125). The differential diagnosis of CT features between an adenoma and an adrenocortical carcinoma should not be based on size alone. Furthermore, it should be kept in mind that adenomas occur much more frequently than carcinomas.

Pheochromocytomas commonly appear as large, low-density masses on CT with central necrosis and infrequent calcifications. They are likely to be enhanced significantly by contrast material. The clinical and biochemical findings distinguish this lesion from a carcinoma or a large metastasis.

Radionuclide scanning has been of limited use in the evaluation of adrenal masses despite its high sensitivity and specificity for certain tumors (Francis et al, 1988). Limited availability of the radioisotopes, high radiation exposure, prolonged patient preparation and imaging, and low anatomic resolution of the modality have curtailed the application of the tracers in clinical practice with few exceptions. **Pheochromocytomas** can be imaged after the administration of metaiodobenzylguanidine (MIBG) containing iodine-131 as the tracer. The specificity of the study for pheochromocytoma or neuroblastoma is high, especially for the former. The examination is particularly indicated for the localization of ectopic or metastatic pheochromocytomas. A second line of chemicals also labeled with iodine-131 are analogues of cholesterol and are used for the imaging of **adrenal adenomas.** The representative of this group is selenomethylnorcholesterol (NP-59). Functioning as well as non-hyperfunctioning adenomas accumulate the radioisotope, whereas primary or metastatic tumors show decreased or no uptake by the adrenal mass. A CT examination usually precedes the radionuclide study for better anatomic localization of the abnormality. Lesions on CT that correspond to areas of increased radionuclide uptake represent adenomas. On the other hand, a discordant lesion—namely, an adrenal mass on CT without radionuclide uptake—is not an adenoma and may well represent metastasis (Francis et al, 1988). Despite the high specificity, these techniques have limited acceptance and are used sparingly for problem cases.

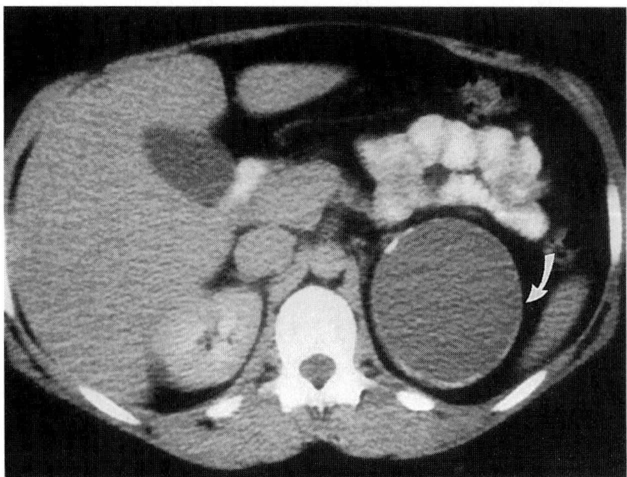

Figure 6–123. Adrenal cysts on CT appear as low-attenuation, well-circumscribed lesions with rim or chunky peripheral calcification *(curved arrow).*

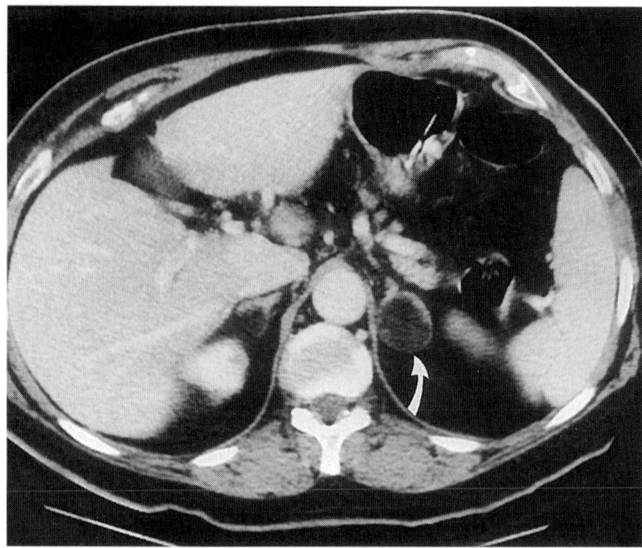

Figure 6–124. Myelolipomas are fatty tumors easily diagnosed by CT scanning *(curved arrow).*

Brief mention is made of the diagnostic contribution of angiographic methods for sampling of venous blood in the evaluation of hyperfunctioning adrenal tumors (Miller, 1993). Adrenal venous sampling can safely distinguish an aldosteronoma, if one exists, from hyperplasia when the CT study suggests bilateral hyperplasia. Sampling of the petrosal sinus can aid in diagnosing a pituitary adenoma in patients with Cushing's syndrome and bilateral adrenal masses or hyperplasia, when adrenocorticotropic hormone (ACTH) levels are found to be elevated.

Last, **the role of MRI in the evaluation of adrenal masses has steadily increased.** A **pheochromocytoma** typically appears as a high-intensity mass on T2-weighted images (Fig. 6–126). Possible pitfalls include significant hemorrhage coexisting with a pheochromocytoma and the use of fast-spin echo-pulse sequences that produce lesions with less intense signal. False-positive results for pheochromocytoma can be obtained with other cystic adrenal masses such as necrotic tumors or benign cysts.

A major contribution of MRI is its ability to differentiate benign adenomas from metastases with high accuracy

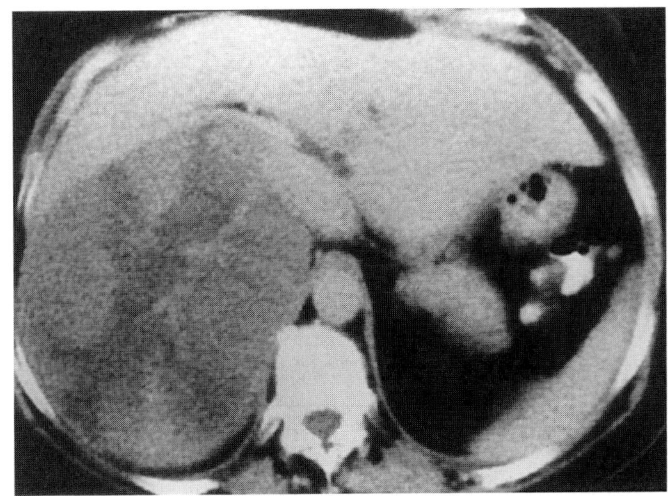

Figure 6–125. Large, partially necrotic mass in the right suprarenal region, consistent with adrenocortical carcinoma.

(Figs. 6–127, 6–128). Out-of-phase or opposed-phase chemical-shift MRI takes advantage of the different resonance frequency peaks for hydrogen protons in water and lipids; lipids are a rich component of most adenomas but are absent from metastases (Mitchell et al, 1992; McNicholas et al, 1995; Korobkin et al, 1996). **A lesion typical of an adenoma displays a loss of signal intensity on opposed-phase imaging, whereas a metastasis does not.** Several reports in the literature have confirmed this observation and established its accuracy. When a nonenhanced CT shows a low-attenuation adrenal mass that meets the criteria for an adenoma (smooth, well defined, rather small, less than 10 Hounsfield units in density, homogeneous), the diagnosis of a benign adenoma seems warranted, and follow-up can be recommended. If an enhanced CT is performed, the study should be repeated without contrast enhancement, or an MRI with in-phase and opposed-phase imaging should be obtained. The latter also should precede a needle biopsy if the nonenhanced CT is equivocal.

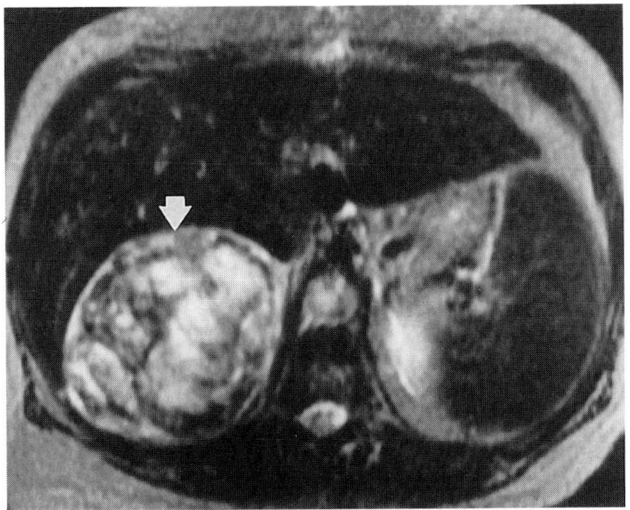

Figure 6–126. Large, mostly high–signal intensity right adrenal mass in a patient with clinical and biochemical evidence of pheochromocytoma *(arrow).*

INTERVENTIONAL URORADIOLOGY

The field of percutaneous, imaging-guided uroradiologic interventions has grown remarkably since the early 1980s. New complex procedures that replaced open surgery were introduced, thus reducing patient morbidity and length of hospital stay. Some of the commonly performed procedures—removal of large renal or upper ureteral calculi, drainage of urinary obstruction and retroperitoneal abscesses, repair of ureteropelvic junction obstruction, dilatation of ureteral strictures, and suprapubic bladder drainage—became feasible and safe without large incisions and prolonged hospitalization, often even without the need for anesthesia.

Furthermore, the almost synchronous development and eventual widespread availability of extracorporeal lithotripsy, as well as a variety of endoscopic techniques, most notably ureteroscopy and flexible endoscopy, has promoted the application of minimally invasive techniques in the management of many urologic diseases.

The most practical and common uroradiologic interventions and their current role in the management of patients are reviewed as follows.

Patient Selection and Preparation

Regardless of the procedure to be performed, certain general principles apply to all patients scheduled to undergo a percutaneous uroradiologic manipulation. The medical indication for the study and overall condition of the patient are the subject of discussion between the referring physician and the interventional radiologist. After the indication and possible contraindications of the study have been thoroughly explored and the decision to proceed with it has been made, the radiologist should explain the rationale of the procedure and its risks, benefits, and alternative methods of treatment to the patient and/or the patient's family or legal custodian (for children and for patients who are unconscious or unable to consent).

The patient's medical records provide information on medications, allergies, medical risks (cardiac, respiratory, etc.), and current coagulation profile. If the bleeding parame-

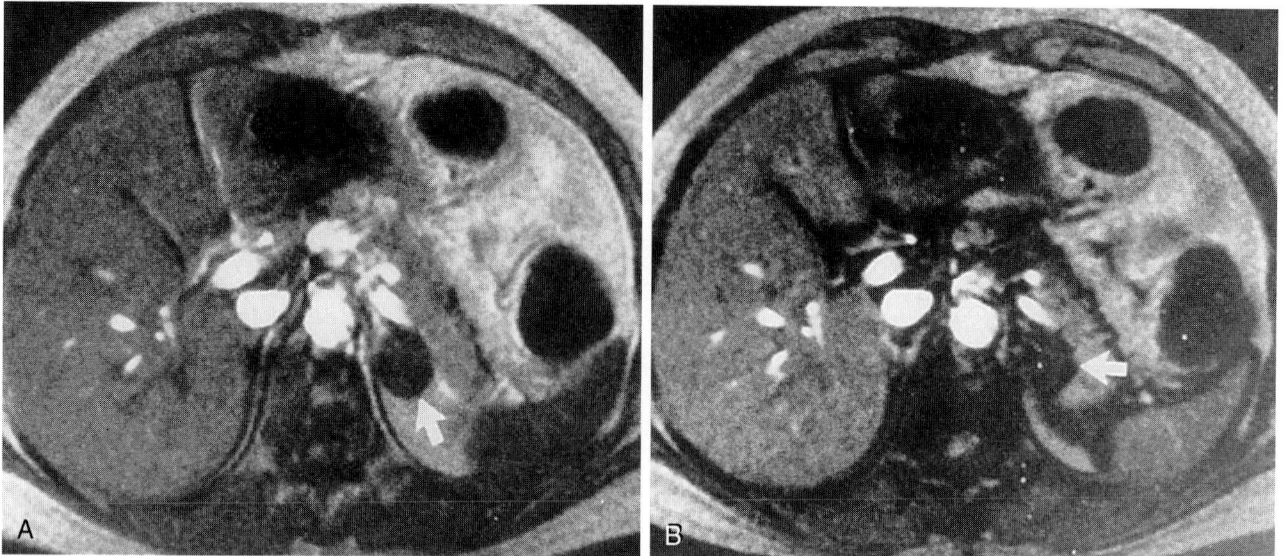

Figure 6–127. Chemical shift imaging can establish the diagnosis of benign non-hyperfunctioning adenoma on the basis of the latter's lipid content. *A,* In-phase T1-weighted image shows a left adrenal lesion that is isointense with the spleen *(arrow)*. *B,* Opposed-phase image shows the same lesion to be hypointense in relation to the spleen after suppression of its fat content *(arrow)*. This is highly suggestive of a benign adenoma.

ters are abnormal, an elective procedure should be postponed until the problem is corrected (Silverman et al, 1990). Emergency procedures necessitate immediate reversal of the coagulation deficit by immediate administration of blood products and/or medications, so that the patient may undergo the study as soon as practicable under the least possible risk of bleeding. Antibiotics are required if infection exists or is suspected. Antibiotics are also advisable in patients with prosthetic heart valves and other implantable devices, which may become seeded with bacteria entering the blood stream during manipulations of wires and catheters. Placement of a peripheral intravenous line is strongly recommended before beginning a procedure, in order to facilitate the administration of antibiotics, contrast material, and analgesics and sedatives. A commonly used antibiotic regimen given in patients suspected of having urinary tract infection is a combination of ampicillin and gentamicin intravenously. Midazolam in 0.5-mg increments and fentanyl in 25- to 50-mg increments are given as needed during interventional procedures. Patients undergoing lengthy procedures should be comfortably sedated from the beginning and given additional analgesics before particularly painful manipulations. Vital signs, including arterial oxygen saturation, are monitored throughout the procedure as well as during the patient's recovery in the radiology unit (outpatients).

With today's strong emphasis on outpatient, minimally invasive care, the interventional radiologist has assumed the responsibility of discharge and postprocedural care of the patient. Patients are advised to bring a companion to the facility, who will then be in charge of returning them home safely. Patients and/or families are told of the main potential side effects or complications and asked to seek care at the nearest health care facility if certain symptoms develop within several hours of the procedure. The daily care of catheters is often left to a visiting nurse and members of the patient's family. The responsibility of caring for catheters in inpatients are shared among the radiologists, the nurses, and the physicians on duty.

Anatomic Considerations Relevant to Interventions

Kidney

Knowledge of the renal anatomy and anatomic relations between the kidney and adjacent organs is essential for the radiologist performing percutaneous renal procedures (Kaye, 1983; Sampaio et al, 1992; Papanicolaou, 1995).

Each kidney is surrounded by retroperitoneal fat and the perinephric fascia and is usually located from the level of the 11th or 12th dorsal to the second or third lumbar vertebrae. Both kidneys are mobile, depending on posture and phase of respiration. Most often, the left kidney lies 1 to 2 cm higher than the right one.

The 12th rib often crosses over the right upper renal pole, whereas the left upper renal pole may be covered by both the 11th and 12th ribs. Both lower renal poles are more anteriorly located than the upper poles. Therefore, **in the prone patient, the lower renal poles are farther from the posterior skin surface.** The pleural reflection and diaphragm project over the upper renal poles superiorly and posteriorly above the 12th rib.

The common patterns or anatomic distribution of the renal vessels and their relationship to the calyceal system are very important to the interventionalist.

In the renal hilum, the renal pelvis lies posterior to the vascular pedicle and is therefore closer than the artery and vein to the posterior skin surface in the prone patient.

The renal artery crosses over from the aorta to the kidney posterior to the renal vein, and as it approaches the hilum, it divides into an anterior and a posterior section. The anterior section is divided into three or four segmental branches, whereas the posterior section usually gives rise to one segmental branch, the posterior one. The corresponding renal segments are the apical segment (medial side of upper renal pole mainly anteriorly); the

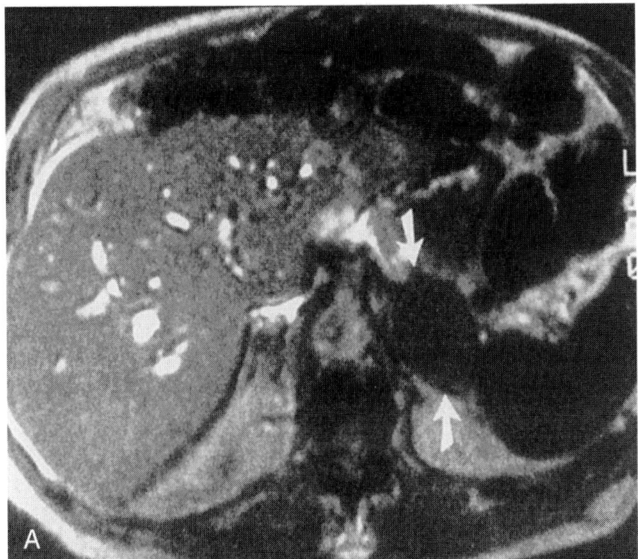

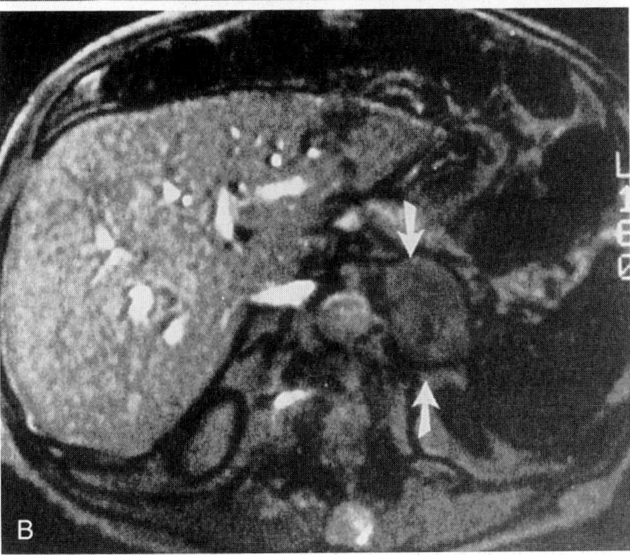

Figure 6–128. Chemical shift imaging of an adrenal metastasis. *A,* In-phase T1-weighted image shows a left adrenal lesion of low signal intensity equal to that of muscle *(arrows). B,* Opposed-phase imaging shows the lesion to remain isointense with muscle without evidence for signal suppression *(arrows).*

anterior segment, covering most of the anterior renal area except for the polar areas; the posterior segment, covering the posterior renal area except for the upper and lower polar areas; and the lower segment, which forms the lower renal pole. Thus each renal pole receives its own arterial supply, whereas the entire anterior aspect of the kidney between the two poles, together with a narrow strip of tissue along the adjacent posterolateral aspect of the kidney, is supplied by one or two anterior segmental arteries. The remainder of the posterior part of the kidney receives its blood supply from the posterior segmental artery, which is found to lie close to the junction of the renal pelvis and the upper pole calyces in about 60% of individuals. In the remaining 40%, the posterior branch courses along the posterior midline of the renal pelvis.

The **segmental renal arteries continue as interlobar arteries in the renal sinus.** The interlobar arteries enter the renal parenchyma through the septa of Bertin and take a course alongside the medullary pyramids, curving around the distal end of the pyramids to divide into the **arcuate arteries.** The latter vessels are distributed around the convex bases of the pyramids, giving off **interlobular arteries,** which supply the peripheral renal cortex toward the surface of the kidney. **The renal artery and its branches are considered end arteries,** with very little, if any, anastomotic connections to each other and without significant collateral circulatory support. This pattern of arterial distribution explains the subsegmental or segmental infarction of the renal parenchyma, after an interruption of the arterial supply to that region, regardless of its etiology.

Brödel's line is an area of the kidney in its posterolateral aspect, along the border between the posterior and inferior interpolar vascular territories. This area is **relatively free of large arterial branches and, therefore, safer for the placement of catheters or performing surgical nephrostomy.**

The renal veins do not follow the pattern of the arterial network, although they form stellate veins in the periphery, followed by the more central arcuate and interlobar veins. Extensive venous plexuses are found around the polar calyces and infundibula. The major tributaries to the renal vein lie anterior to their corresponding arteries in the area of the hilus. A retropelvic renal vein was found in about 70% of cases in a series of cadaveric kidneys. In one half of these kidneys, the retropelvic vein had a close relationship to the junction of the renal pelvis with the upper calyx (Sampaio et al, 1992).

Percutaneous access directly into the renal pelvis is undesirable; the likelihood of causing significant hemorrhage is high, because of its proximity to large arterial and venous branches and the lack of effective tamponading of such bleeding in an area unprotected by renal parenchyma.

As a rule, the periphery of the kidney contains smaller vessels and is close to the line of Brödel; therefore it is safer to direct needle punctures and catheter placement there by targeting calyceal fornices. Anterior segmental arterial injuries are attributed to a through-and-through puncture of both walls of the collecting system by a needle or catheter and may be minimized by the use of biplane fluoroscopic guidance during the intervention. Clinicians should also keep in mind the location of the intercostal or subcostal neurovascular bundles, when performing percutaneous renal procedures. The intercostal (subcostal) vessels course along the inferior margin of the corresponding rib; therefore, intercostal access, as well as angle with the needle or catheter caudad, should remain at least 2 cm below the 12th rib or close to the superior margin of the inferior rib, when possible.

An important first step in planning a percutaneous nephrostomy access route is the study of the calyceal anatomy of the kidney requiring the intervention (Kaye and Reinke, 1984; Sampaio et al, 1992). **With few exceptions, it is technically sound and safe to gain access into the collecting system through a posterior middle or lower pole calyx because the obtuse angle between the inserted needle or wire and the calyceal infundibulum facilitates the manipulations.** A similar entry through an anteriorly located calyx results in manipulations and exchanges of instruments at a sharp angle, which may often be technically difficult and more likely to cause renal injury.

On intravenous or retrograde urography, the anterior calyces are often found to be laterally placed within the kidney, whereas the posterior calyces are more medial and are seen en face. However, calyceal orientation within the renal parenchyma is sometimes difficult to determine accurately on the basis of two-dimensional images. Furthermore, calyceal orientation in relation to the lateral renal contour varies considerably. Two types of calyceal distribution within a kidney have been described: one by Brödel, who proposed that anterior calyces are located medially and posterior calyces laterally, and the second by Hodson, who proposed a mirror-image type of calyceal orientation with the anterior calyces being laterally located (Papanicolaou, 1995).

Kaye and Reinke (1984), using CT imaging, studied calyceal location along the interpolar area of the kidneys. They found that right-sided kidneys often resemble the Brödel type, whereas left-sided kidneys more often correspond to the Hodson type. Their results were confirmed by a study of three-dimensional cadaveric pyelocalyceal casts. All these efforts to document and classify calyceal orientation underline **the importance of understanding the calyceal anatomy with regard to percutaneous procedures and of anticipating or trying to prevent technical problems that may arise during the placement of a nephrostomy catheter.**

Despite these efforts to classify and predict calyceal orientation, there is general agreement that calyceal location varies greatly, particularly at the renal polar areas. Oblique views, biplane fluoroscopy, and/or use of gravity (anterior calyces trap contrast material, whereas posterior calyces retain air or carbon dioxide) are recommended for distinguishing anterior from posterior calyces during difficult and complicated attempts at placing a percutaneous nephrostomy catheter.

In practical terms, **most percutaneous nephrostomy catheters can be placed easily and safely by a posterior or posterolateral subcostal approach between the posterior axillary and posterior midclavicular lines, entering the kidney laterally and aiming at a middle or lower pole calyx.** In certain cases mostly related to endoscopic stone removal, direct access into a specific calyx or calyceal diverticulum may necessitate meticulous localization of these structures. Also, **optimal access to the renal pelvis (endopyelotomy) or ureter (ureteral stenting) necessitates upper or middle pole calyceal entry in order to avoid technical problems sometimes associated with lower pole calyceal entry,** such as buckling of the wire within the renal pelvis during ureteral stenting and inadequate exposure of the posterolateral aspect of the ureteropelvic junction in patients undergoing percutaneous endopyelotomy.

Organs and structures adjacent to the kidneys have to be spared transgression during percutaneous renal and ureteral procedures. Often, the posterior reflection of the pleura may extend below the 12th rib medially during inspiration, but almost always remains above it laterally. In many patients, especially elderly or obese persons, the posterior pleural reflection can be located above the 11th or 10th rib, allowing for safer intercostal percutaneous access to the kidney through the last intercostal space. In some patients, the inferior extension of the pleura can be seen on fluoroscopy with the patient lying prone, and a safe route can thus be planned in order to avoid transgression of the pleural space.

Typically, the liver and spleen are located anteriorly and laterally to the corresponding kidneys and may be safely avoided by selecting a posterolateral lower pole or superomedial upper pole route. The spleen may on occasion be situated behind the upper pole of the left kidney (retrorenal spleen). Because of the relative safety in percutaneous instrumentation of the liver for a number of interventions, transgression is considered less hazardous in the liver than in the spleen, which may require surgical repair if injured by a large catheter. In general, injury to either organ during percutaneous nephrostomy procedures is rare. Unusual positioning of either the liver or spleen cannot be predicted on the basis of plain film findings. If doubt exists, imaging with sonography or CT may be advisable before a percutaneous renal intervention.

The colon may be positioned lateral or even posterior to the kidney in rare instances. Lateral colonic location is frequent enough to warrant avoiding a lateral percutaneous route (Papanicolaou, 1995). Posterolateral or posterior colonic location is rare and may result in colonic transgression. Posterior colonic position is more common in thin patients with very little retroperitoneal fat. The routine use of either CT or barium enema before placement of a percutaneous nephrostomy catheter has not generally gained acceptance by most clinicians, because it is neither cost-effective nor practical.

The horseshoe kidney presents unusual anatomic problems to the interventionist. Access to the preferred lower renal pole entry is not as easy or safe because the lower poles are positioned farther anteriorly and medially in the abdomen. Furthermore, because of its vertical long axis, each renal unit of a horseshoe kidney has to be approached via a route more medial than that used for the usual kidney. Also, the anterior location of the lower pole calyces in the horseshoe kidney makes ureteral access quite difficult, whereas upper or midpole calyceal entrance into the collecting system facilitates such access.

Ectopic, fused, or nonfused kidneys should be approached cautiously and on an individual basis. Obviously, posterior retroperitoneal access, if possible, is preferred. The ectopic pelvic kidney is often off limits to the interventionist, because the bony pelvis posteriorly and loops of bowel anteriorly make a percutaneous approach unsafe and impossible. The transplanted kidney is easily accessible percutaneously via an anterolateral route, because of its superficial location within the iliac fossa.

Ureter

The ureters often are instrumented during percutaneous renal interventions, since ureteral purchase is desirable either as an added safety factor for the performance of renal manipulations or to secure access for treatment of certain ureteral processes (stone removal, stent placement, dilatation of stricture, endopyelotomy, occlusion of fistula, etc.). On occasion, retrograde catheterization of the ureters may be feasible under fluoroscopic guidance alone either through the bladder transurethrally or through a refluxing ureteroileal anastomosis, most often in patients with ileal loop urinary diversion.

Each ureter descends from the abdomen into the pelvis along the anteromedial surface of the ipsilateral psoas muscle, enveloped by the layers of the perinephric fascia. As it enters the pelvis, the ureter assumes a slightly medial course while passing over the common iliac artery at or near the bifurcation of that artery into external and internal iliac arteries. In the pelvis, the ureter initially descends posterolaterally, separated from the iliopsoas muscle by the internal iliac vessels. In the lower pelvis, the ureter turns medially as it approaches the bladder. The **ureteral lumen displays three areas of physiologic narrowing: the ureteropelvic junction, the crossing over the common iliac artery, and the ureterovesical junction.**

Congenital variations or anomalies in the number and course of the ureters may interfere with certain interventions. Duplication of the ureter should be recognized on prior imaging studies or on the antegrade pyelogram performed at the time of the intervention, so that the appropriate calyceal moiety and ureter are accessed. Herniations of the pelvic ureter (primary or the result of herniation of the bladder) are rare, occurring more often through the inguinal and sciatic regions. They may result in significant technical difficulties during intervention that require placement of wires and/or catheters from the kidney to the bladder and vice versa. A retrocaval ureter often causes dilatation of the urinary tract proximal to its medial deviation under the inferior vena cava at the lower lumbar level and may resist instrumentation unless the appropriate wires and catheters are used. Ureters displaced or narrowed by a number of pathologic processes (lymphadenopathy, retroperitoneal fibrosis, vascular aneurysms, prostatic enlargement, intraluminal tumor growth or encasement by adjacent malignancies, inflammatory and infectious collections) are frequently encountered in a busy interventional practice and require experience and the appropriate instruments for successful cannulation.

Bladder

The empty urinary bladder is directly behind the symphysis pubis. In infants, small children, and elderly males with significant prostatic enlargement, the bladder lies higher.

The superior wall (dome) of the bladder is in close contact with loops of ileum and the colon (more often sigmoid, sometimes cecum) in the male and loops of ileum and the uterus in the female. **Only the superior wall of the bladder is covered by peritoneum, together with the superior aspect of the posterior wall in the male, and it should be avoided during percutaneous catheter procedures.** The neck of the bladder is rather stable in position, and filling of the vesical lumen results in distention and elevation of the rest of the bladder well above the symphysis pubis, thus allowing for a safe percutaneous suprapubic access. The **major arterial branches supplying the bladder enter through the posterior and lateral aspects of the wall, thus making the anterior wall relatively safe for placement of catheters.** The inferior epigastric vessels running down the anterior abdominal wall are located farther laterally to the midline and can be avoided by selecting an entry site just off the midline.

After radical prostatectomy or in the case of significant relaxation of the pelvic floor or cystocele in the female, the bladder descends farther behind the bony pelvis, and its percutaneous access may be quite difficult. Likewise, bladder hernias, although uncommon, may cause significant shift or displacement of the bladder from its expected midline position. Most bladder hernias occur into the inguinal canals (more often in men) and femoral canals (more often in women). Preprocedural localization and distention of the bladder are essential for safe access. Retrograde or antegrade cystogram and/or sonography may be necessary. Bladder diverticula, regardless of their size, should not be targeted as entry sites for catheter placement. Their thinner walls are more likely to be perforated during the manipulations than is the true bladder wall.

Imaging Guidance Systems

Personal experience and preference, as well as the type of procedure, usually dictate the choice of the imaging modality for guiding placement of needles and catheters. Drainage of perinephric, retroperitoneal, or pelvic collections can be accomplished easily under sonographic or CT guidance. Sonography may be used as a complement to fluoroscopy for localization of the kidneys and bladder and to search for and avoid adjacent organs (bowel, liver, spleen, etc.) that may be interposed along the catheter path to the calyces or vesical lumen. CT guidance is reserved for cases involving difficult access, such as ectopic kidneys or severe spinal deformities. Often, nephrostomy catheter placement is safely done under sonographic guidance alone. When fluoroscopy is used, precautions should be taken to protect both the patient and the operator from unnecessary radiation exposure.

Radiation Protection

Medical personnel and patients are potentially at risk for significant radiation exposure from fluoroscopy-guided interventional procedures. Among medical personnel, the exposure to direct and scattered radiation varies greatly, depending on the type and duration of the procedure, the equipment used, and the protective measures taken (Marx, 1996). As a rule, the extremities, often the hands, neck, and head of the operator receive much higher doses than the trunk, which is invariably shielded by a lead apron. In the case of the patient, the skin at the x-ray beam entry site is the body part exposed to the highest amount of radiation.

Whereas simple diagnostic procedures, such as VCU or injection of a nephrostomy tube, may require no more than 1 to 5 minutes of fluoroscopy time, complex interventions such as percutaneous ureteral stenting or nephrostomy track preparation for removal of renal calculi may require more than 1 hour. The U.S. Food and Drug Administration has warned against prolonged use of fluoroscopy during complex interventional procedures, after receiving reports of radiation-induced skin injuries to patients. **The onset of the radiation damage to the skin often is delayed, and the severity of the injury may vary** from transient erythema or hair loss (exposures of 200 to 300 rad, or 2 to 3 Gy) to dermal necrosis and ulceration (exposures of 1500 to 2000 rad, or 15 to 20 Gy). The typical absorbed dose in the skin as a result of direct fluoroscopic x-ray beam exposure from a given fluoroscopic unit is in the range of 1 to 5 R/min. Tailoring and shortening the use of fluoroscopy and using equipment that minimizes the amount of transmitted radiation are strongly recommended (Marx, 1996). The patient should be kept far from the x-ray tube and close to the image intensifier, the equipment should be maintained in optimal working order, and fluoroscopy time should be limited to a minimum.

In regard to risks to the operator from radiation exposure, several factors are essential in order to minimize such an exposure. The equipment used should be of high quality and in optimal working condition (Marx, 1996). Units with an over-the-table x-ray tube result in excessive backscatter from the incoming primary beam to the operator and should be avoided in favor of under-the-table x-ray tube units. Interventionists should exercise great caution to distance themselves from the primary beam. Personal shielding is of paramount importance, as is limited use of the fluoroscope. Thyroid shields and leaded glasses offer additional protection necessary to busy interventionists. Yearly doses to the lenses approaching 15 rad, or 0.15 Gy, or more are a strong indication for protective glasses that may prevent development of cataracts (which are caused by a cumulative lifetime dose of 400 rad, or 4 Gy). Exposure to the hands should be limited to around 50 rad (0.5 Gy) per year. Vigorous adherence to and compliance with federal and institutional radiation and occupational protection protocols is mandatory for the safety of the patient and medical personnel.

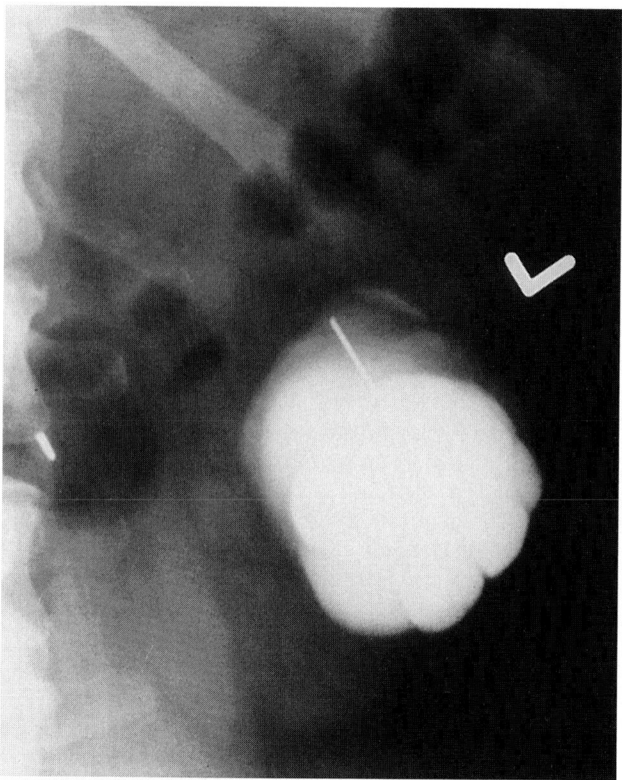

Figure 6–129. Percutaneous renal cyst aspiration. After placement of the needle into the cyst and obtaining samples of the fluid for cytology, contrast material is injected and the inner wall of the cyst is evaluated. Fluoroscopic guidance was used in this case.

Percutaneous Renal Intervention

Renal Cyst Aspiration and Ablation

Before the widespread use of sonography and CT, a large number of renal cysts were subjected to angiography and percutaneous needle aspiration primarily for diagnostic purposes. The high accuracy of cross-sectional imaging techniques in making the diagnosis of simple cysts has eliminated the use of angiography and has greatly reduced the need for percutaneous needle aspiration of such lesions. Currently, the **indications** for the procedure are limited to **(1) diagnostic (cytologic) aspiration of the fluid of cystic renal lesions that cannot be definitively diagnosed as simple cysts by cross-sectional imaging, (2) aspiration, and (3) obliteration of large symptomatic renal cysts** (Amis et al, 1987).

The patient is placed prone, and the cyst is aspirated under fluoroscopic, sonographic, or CT guidance (Fig. 6–129). The usual anatomic precautions are taken with regard to the pleural space, adjacent organs, or the renal vascular pedicle (for lesions situated in the renal hilar region). Thus a posterior subcostal entry site is safer. Local anesthesia to the skin entry site of the needle suffices for patient comfort. Needle sizes used for the aspiration vary from 18 to 22 gauge, depending primarily on the volume of the cyst. Fluid is aspirated and samples are sent to the cytology laboratory. Chemistry and bacteriology consultations are obtained only in the appropriate clinical setting. The fluid retrieved after uncomplicated aspiration of simple cyst should be clear, straw-colored, and free of abnormal cells. Hemorrhagic or infected cysts contain cloudy, dark red or brown fluid. Bright red blood in the cyst fluid usually results from a bloody tap.

An alleged symptomatic cyst should be aspirated dry first, and the **cytology results should be obtained and improvement or relief of the symptoms evaluated before cyst ablation is undertaken. Only if the cytology profile is benign and the pain or discomfort subsides should the ablation proceed when the cyst recurs. For cysts causing pyelocalyceal obstruction, the ablation is indicated as soon as the diagnosis is made if the cytology profile is benign.**

The **cyst ablation is preceded by the removal of a large amount of the cyst fluid** while the inserted needle or sheath is still safely within the cyst cavity. **Injection of the cyst cavity with contrast material is recommended before the instillation of the sclerosing agent,** especially if more than one pass was made before the cyst was entered. **This ensures that no communication with the calyceal system exists** and that the sclerosing agent can be safely instilled. **Absolute ethanol is used in a volume equal to one third to one half the estimated cyst volume.** The ethanol is left inside the cyst for up to 20 minutes, the patient is turned from side to side to denature as much of the lining epithelium of the cyst cavity as possible, and then the ethanol is removed via the needle. The procedure usually is painless.

Follow-up imaging is not necessary unless symptoms recur or monitoring of the hydronephrosis, if the cyst caused obstruction, is indicated. Complications secondary to cyst aspiration are rare. Hematuria, retroperitoneal hemorrhage, or pneumothorax have occasionally been described. Extravasation of the sclerosing agent can result in tissue necrosis or calyceal obliteration, depending on whether the spill is perinephric, intrarenal, or intracalyceal.

Antegrade Pyelography

Percutaneous needle puncture and injection of contrast material into the pyelocalyceal system remain the essential first step for many procedures in the upper urinary tract (Pfister et al, 1986) (Fig. 6–130*A*). When IVU fails to demonstrate the anatomy, whether in the setting of a congenital anomaly or in acquired pathology, antegrade pyelography clearly outlines the appearance of the urinary tract and enables sampling of the urine for cytologic and bacteriologic examination. Antegrade pyelography is an essential part of percutaneous upper urinary tract urodynamics in the evaluation of hydronephrosis (Whitaker test) (see Fig. 6–130*B*,*C*). Furthermore, the procedure precedes all percutaneous intrarenal interventions that require access into specific calyces because of its calyceal mapping capability (Pfister et al, 1986).

The patient is positioned prone, and local anesthesia is administered. The choice of needle gauge (20 versus 22) most often depends on the distance of the calyceal system from the skin. The larger (20-gauge) needles can be directed through muscles and retroperitoneal adipose tissues more easily than the thinner (22-gauge) needles, which are more suitable for use in children and small adults.

Review of previously obtained studies of the urinary tract is advisable before the antegrade needle is inserted into the kidney. An intravenous urogram or retrograde pyelogram, sonogram, or CT scan may help localize the kidney and provide information on the location of adjacent organs. For nonobstructed calyceal systems, intravenous contrast material is given, and one of the opacified calyces is targeted for the needle placement. The antegrade needle should preferably be placed in a calyx or in the lateral aspect of the renal pelvis and kept in the collecting system throughout the procedure, to distend the calyceal system and preserve visual access to it.

For the moderately to severely dilated urinary tract, sonography or fluoroscopy alone is adequate for renal localization. In the case of mild hydronephrosis, sonography is complementary to fluoroscopy for the initial localization of the kidney. Subsequent manipulations within the collecting system require fluoroscopic guidance. Pyelocalyceal radiopaque stones can be used as anatomic landmarks to guide insertion of the antegrade needle next to or on top of them. The needle should preferably be placed laterally to a renal pelvic stone for better opacification of the calyces, because placement medial to the stone often results in the contrast material preferentially flowing down the ureter.

An obstructed collecting system must not be overdistended via the antegrade needle, especially in the presence of cloudy urine. The risk of inducing urosepsis by parenchymal and vascular backflow of infected urine is not trivial. An obstructed collecting system should be decompressed before contrast material is injected into it via the needle.

Ureteral Pressure-Flow Study (Whitaker Test)

Hydronephrosis may be simulated by the calyceal dilatation of congenital megacalycosis or by papillary necrosis. The dilated extrarenal pelvis may be a problem in determining whether there is obstruction in association with

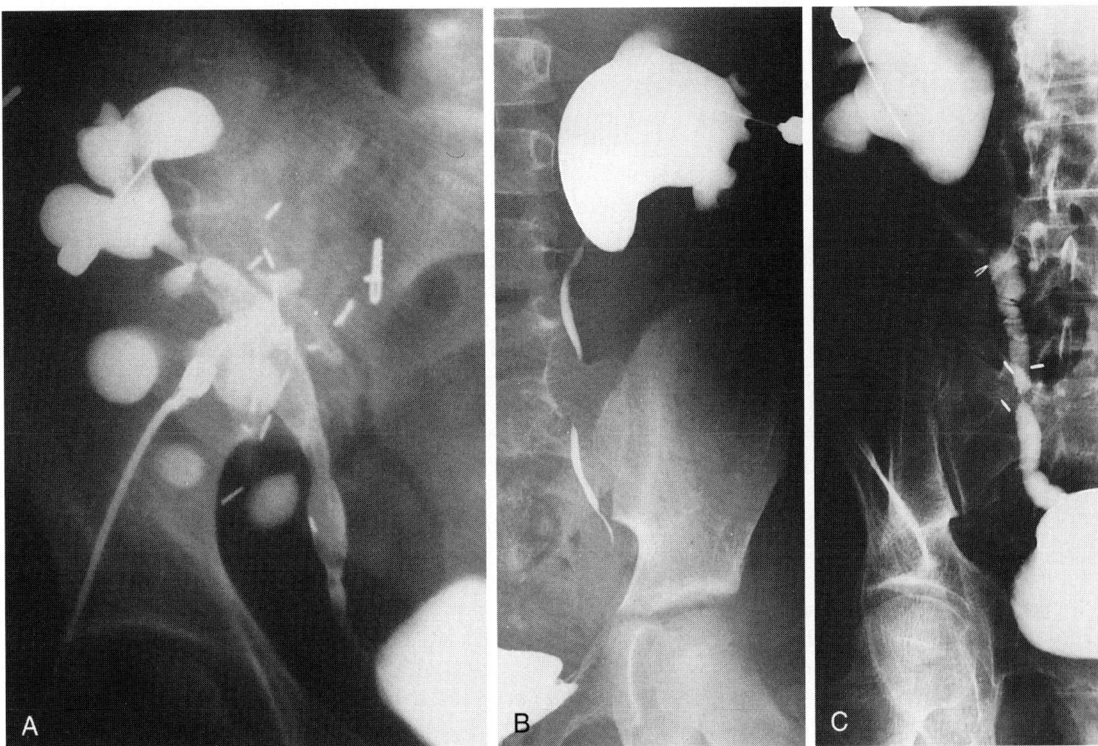

Figure 6–130. Percutaneous antegrade pyelography requires placement of the needle into the pyelocalyceal system and opacification of the upper urinary tract. *A*, Renal transplant obstructed by calculi. The antegrade study demonstrates the calyceal anatomy before a nephrostomy catheter is placed. *B*, Tight left ureteropelvic junction obstruction is evaluated by means of pressure measurements through the antegrade needle. *C*, Demonstration of the anatomy after ileal ureteral interposition on the right side.

it. **Generalized dilatation of the intrarenal collecting system and ureter may reflect only a high fluid output from the kidney; an atonic, inflamed ureter; permanent dilatation from previous obstruction that has since been repaired; ureteral reflux; or recurrent obstruction.** Furthermore, there are several causes of a nonrefluxing megaureter; it may result from intrinsic ureteral disease or may be related to abnormalities of the lower urinary tract, as in posterior urethral valves or the occult neurogenic bladder.

As a result of these and other factors, the evaluation of current or ongoing obstruction by glomerular filtered agents (urography and radionuclide renography with or without diuretic stimulation) or by contrast medium washout rates after retrograde or antegrade pyelography may be unreliable. **Particularly difficult to evaluate by these techniques for the presence or absence of obstruction are cases in which renal function is poor, the ureter is markedly dilated with reduced elasticity, or dilatation of the upper urinary tract persists after surgical or percutaneous correction of an obstructing lesion and in patients with concomitant high-pressure bladders** (Pfister et al, 1986).

Opening or resting pressures of the kidney obtained during antegrade pyelography are helpful only when they are significantly elevated; in acute ureteral obstruction of a previously normal kidney, intrarenal pressures in excess of 50 cm H_2O are common. As obstruction continues toward a chronic state, intrarenal pressure falls toward lower levels as a result of reduced renal function, altered compliance of the dilated ureter, and renal backflow with fluid absorption into venous and lymphatic channels.

The urodynamic antegrade pyelogram, ureteral perfusion test, or pressure-flow Whitaker examination directly measures the ureters' resistance to a known flow rate with simultaneous pressure measurements from the kidney and bladder. The examination is performed with a small catheter in the bladder and a thin antegrade pyelogram needle in the kidney. A simple water manometer is interfaced in each extension tubing to record pressure, and a variable rate pump continuously delivers diluted contrast material through the antegrade needle (Pfister et al, 1986).

The Whitaker test is reproducible and unaffected by the kidney's GFR. It provides good anatomic definition of the dilated ureter and enables direct measurement of the resistance to various known flow rates (10, 15, or 20 ml/minute) with controlled bladder volume and pressure. The lower urinary tract pressure reading is necessary for accurately interpreting the upper tract pressures, particularly in the high-pressure bladder of outlet obstruction or neurogenic disease, and after ureteral reimplantation or any other type of urinary diversion (loop) or undiversion.

The subtraction of absolute bladder pressure from absolute renal pressure provides the relative, differential, or step-off pressure. **At a flow rate of 10 ml/minute, with the bladder empty, a differential pressure below 13 cm H_2O is normal; arbitrary values of 14 to 20 cm H_2O indicate mild obstruction; 21 to 34 cm H_2O, moderate obstruction; and above 35 cm H_2O, severe obstruction.**

When the normal bladder is filled, intravesical pressure rises, so that the absolute renal pelvic pressure increases as well, although the differential pressure drops. The kidney that is subjected to intermittent (reflux) or continuous (bladder obstruction) high absolute pressure above 20 cm H_2O may be at risk even in the absence of true ureteral obstruction. **It is not clear whether percutaneous ureteral perfusion answers all questions about the dilated upper urinary tract. Particularly bothersome is the compliant, atonic, and progressively distensible pyeloureteral unit that can accommodate large fluid volumes and thus dampen pressure response to induced flow rates.** However, this type of upper tract abnormality cannot be definitively evaluated by any single technique. Finally, the Whitaker examination must be carefully performed, without shortcuts or a slipshod approach, if technical errors that alter pressure values are to be avoided.

Nephrostomy

The principal indication for the placement of a percutaneous nephrostomy catheter is the relief of urinary obstruction, which usually is clinically manifested by flank pain, leukocytosis, pyuria, and worsening renal function in the presence of hydronephrosis and/or fever (Barbaric, 1984). In selected cases, the percutaneous nephrostomy tract is used to provide access to the collecting system for a number of fluoroscopic and endoscopic procedures used to treat pathologic processes in a manner less invasive than conventional surgery (stone removal, biopsy or removal of tumors, endopyelotomy, etc.).

The first step toward establishing percutaneous access to the urinary tract is antegrade pyelography. The anatomic information gained from this study allows the safe and appropriate placement of the percutaneous catheter. Fluoroscopy or ultrasonography or, on occasion, CT can be used to guide the procedure. However, catheter placement and all guide wire/catheter/dilator manipulations and tube positioning in nondilated or mildly dilated collecting systems are best done under fluoroscopic control for safety purposes. Sonography enables accurate assessment of renal depth, and such guidance is indicated for pregnant women, for patients at risk from reactions to intravenous contrast media, or at the bedside. Moderate or severe hydronephrosis makes sonographically guided nephrostomy catheter placement easier.

Antegrade pyelography and subsequent percutaneous nephrostomy are performed with the patient in the prone or prone oblique (the side to be punctured elevated 30 degrees) position. In either approach, **the catheter tract should be posterolateral through the renal parenchyma rather than directly into the free wall of the renal pelvis** (Fig. 6–131). **The transparenchymal renal tract ensures entry through the relatively avascular zone (Brödel's line) of the kidney and provides a tight seal around the nephrostomy catheter.** A direct renal pelvic approach reduces intrarenal catheter length and increases the possibility of tearing the renal pelvis or lacerating a major vessel in the renal hilum.

For simple drainage, the calyx through which the nephrostomy catheter enters the kidney is of little concern. Pressure is the same within all areas of the collecting system, and the catheter will drain adequately if it is not wedged into the fornix of a calyx or a tapered obstructed segment of the ureter. If segmental obstruction is present, however, the obstructed calyx must be selectively drained, and this requires careful planning of the percutaneous tract.

The Seldinger technique is used for placement of all nephrostomy catheters. It consists of inserting a guide wire

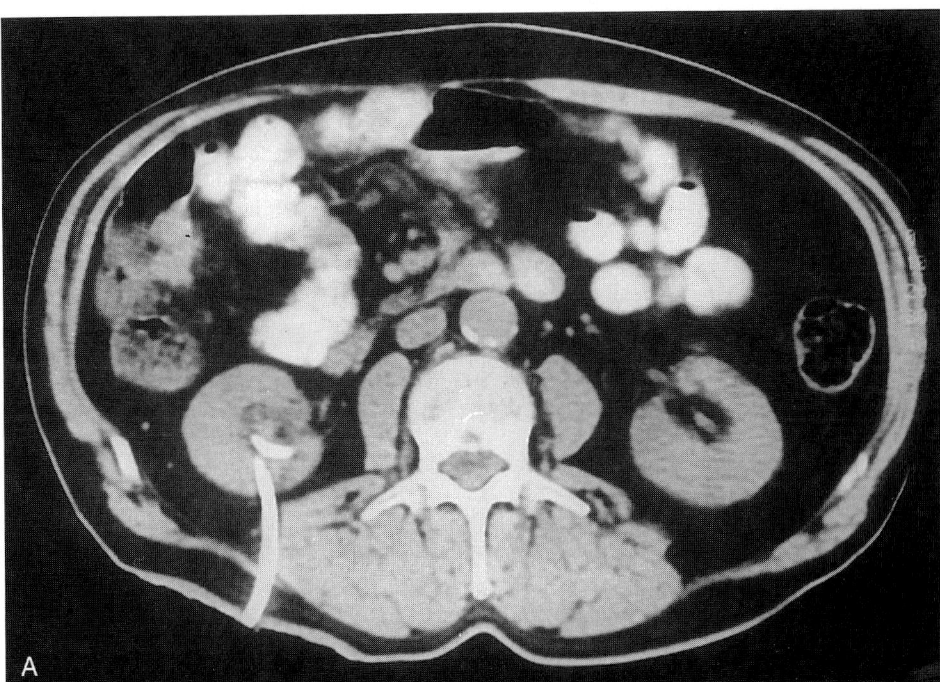

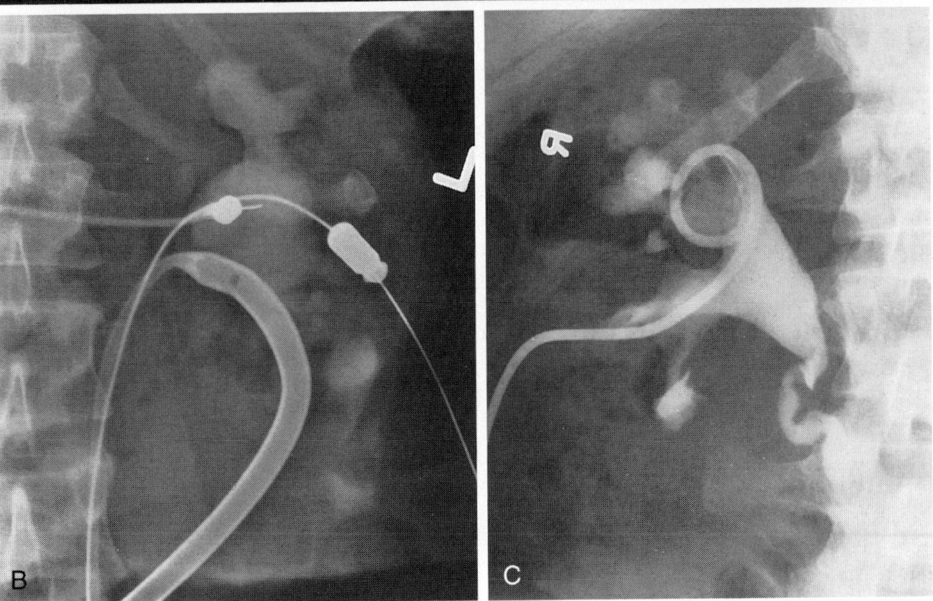

Figure 6–131. Percutaneous nephrostomy tube placement. *A,* CT demonstration of the anatomic relations of the catheter with the retroperitoneum and kidney. *B,* Large-bore nephrostomy tube placement before percutaneous debulking of a staghorn calculus. *C,* Fluoroscopic placement of No. 8 French pigtail nephrostomy catheter for relief of obstruction.

into the collecting system first, followed by dilatation of the newly created percutaneous tract to the desired caliber and placement of the nephrostomy catheter. The usual working guide wire is a torque, 0.038 inch, and the sizes of the nephrostomy catheters vary from No. 8 to 12 French. Larger catheters may be placed, if so indicated, usually for long-term or permanent nephrostomy drainage.

Once the nephrostomy catheter is in the collecting system, adequate urine return and/or a nephrostogram confirm satisfactory tube position. The catheter then is placed for external drainage and is fixed to the skin with a variety of devices, from skin sutures to self-adhesive ostomy discs.

Anterior calyces should be avoided for placement of a nephrostomy catheter. Often after the wire is coiled into an anterior calyx, access into the renal pelvis or ureter is technically difficult or impossible to obtain because of the sharp angle formed between the inserted wire and the calyceal infundibulum leading to the renal pelvis. A curved-tip catheter may be instrumental in getting the wire out of an anterior calyx, if patience and gentle manipulation fail to do so. A posterior calyceal access, however, allows the wire to slide out of the calyx at an obtuse angle with ease and greatly facilitates renal pelvic and ureteral access.

If the guide wire is kinked or offers significant resistance to manipulations, it should be exchanged for a new one if access into the calyces can be preserved, or removed together with the sheath, dilator, or catheter as a unit, even if access is sacrificed. If a sheared-off wire tip is left in the collecting system, endoscopic or open renal surgery may be required for removal. Sometimes if the length of the wire within the urinary tract is sufficient, the kinked segment can be either pushed further into the collecting system or pulled out of the percutaneous tract to a point where it does not interfere with instrument exchanges or manipulations. Such kinks often develop from pushing stiff dilators or catheters over the wire against points where the wire changes direction from a straight course to a curved or angled one as it traverses retroperitoneal structures and enters the kidney or goes around an infundibulum into the renal pelvis or the ureter. Careful, gentle manipulations that transmit the pushing force along the path of the wire often prevent wire kinks.

With some experience, placement of a nephrostomy catheter should be successful in 95% to 98% of adult and pediatric cases. The success rate may be lower (80% to 90%) with nondilated collecting systems or when the targeted calyx or entire pyelocalyceal system is filled with calculi. In such situations, the collecting system can be distended by an antegrade needle or a retrograde ureteral catheter, and a second attempt can be made the next day.

Minor complications such as postnephrostomy transient bleeding and local transient extravasation of contrast material are to be expected. Significant complications from percutaneous nephrostomy catheter placement are infrequent and fewer than those from surgical nephrostomy. Many complications of percutaneous nephrostomy such as pneumothorax, urinoma, and some catheter problems can be prevented, whereas many of those resulting in bleeding cannot. **The most frequent severe complication is hemorrhage; significant vascular trauma may occur in 1% to 2% of patients.** Significant bleeding may be immediate, may be delayed (occurring with the formation of pseudoaneurysms and arteriovenous fistulas), or may occur late when the nephrostomy catheter is removed or exchanged.

Early arterial injury is manifested clinically by continued hematuria for several days and by the formation of new clots. Alternatively, if a significant drop in the hematocrit occurs, a perirenal or subcapsular hematoma should be suspected and investigated by CT or ultrasonography. **If bleeding persists or spontaneously recurs after percutaneous nephrostomy catheter placement, renal angiography is indicated for diagnostic and therapeutic purposes.** Selective embolization of the involved segmental renal artery can be performed while most of the remaining renal parenchyma is preserved.

About 15% of all patients undergoing percutaneous drainage may have pyonephrosis, and many of these patients may suffer an exacerbation of the urosepsis from the manipulations. Shaking chills, worsening fever, and transient hypotension are not infrequent; septic shock can occur in 7% of cases. Overinjecting contrast material into an infected system should be avoided until several days after drainage.

The patient with a percutaneous nephrostomy catheter requires regular monitoring. Most patients tolerate the catheter very well and continue to live a relatively normal life style. Patients or their families can be instructed to take care of the catheter and to recognize a pending or existing malfunction or complication. **When long-term drainage is anticipated, regular change of the catheter is advised every 3 months;** exchange of the initial catheter for a soft rubber balloon tube in this situation may be desirable.

Technical problems may be encountered during a routine or emergency change of a previously inserted nephrostomy catheter. Ordinarily, the catheter is easily replaced over a guide wire after the locking mechanism of the pigtail is released. In drainage units with an intraluminal string responsible for forming and maintaining the pigtail end, the string should be cut about 2 cm above the hub of the catheter. When an exchange is desired, the loose end of the string should be held tight until the guide wire exits the pigtail end of the catheter into the collecting system. Failure to hold onto the string may result in the wire's intussuscepting the string into the lumen of the catheter, which then becomes obstructed and blocks the wire from exiting.

A similar situation may occur when encrustations and other debris block the catheter lumen and prevent an orderly exchange of the catheter over a wire. This often happens when a catheter change is delayed. Three solutions to this technical problem are offered. A short attempt can be made with a slightly curved end wire to exit through a patent side hole of the catheter, in which case the removal and replacement of the old tube can proceed without difficulty. If this fails, a peel-away sheath may be placed coaxially over the catheter into the collecting system, using the catheter itself as a guide wire. Usually, a peel-away sheath one French size larger than the catheter is appropriate. The bulky connecting hub of the catheter is cut off to allow coaxial placement of the sheath over the catheter. Once the sheath is within the calyceal system, the catheter is removed and replaced with a new one of similar size. The third and least recommended intervention may be used with caution and only if the percutaneous tract has been in place for several weeks or months and is mature. The blocked catheter can be pulled out and exchanged for a new one, which is blindly placed into the calyceal system through the tract.

A mature tract may remain patent for several hours after accidental removal of a nephrostomy catheter and may be salvageable, if the patient seeks help immediately. The tract should be probed with a moderately stiff but smooth and round-tipped catheter such as a feeding tube or a small Foley catheter that can be further reinforced with a coaxial wire. Probing the tract with a sharp wire often results in creating false passages into the retroperitoneum. If access is reestablished, a wire is inserted and a new catheter is placed. Otherwise, a nephrostomy catheter is inserted de novo.

Large-Bore Nephrostomy Access for Stone Removal and Other Endoscopic Interventions

Symptomatic and/or large renal stones necessitate treatment because of their associated problems with obstruction, potential infection, and permanent renal damage.

The choice of treatment depends on stone size and location. Today, 80% to 90% of renal and upper ureteral stones necessitating treatment are successfully managed with extracorporeal lithotripsy (EL) alone. **Factors that decrease the likelihood of successful EL include size, location, and composition of the stone or stones.** Cystine, matrix, and some calcium phosphate stones may not respond well to EL. Stones situated proximal to an obstruction in the urinary tract, such as a calyceal diverticulum, calyceal infundibular stenosis, or ureteropelvic junction narrowing, may not pass after fragmentation with EL. For stones within an anatomically normal intrarenal collecting system, stone size greater than 2.5 cm is generally an indication for percutaneous removal, followed by EL of the retained fragments, if any. Stones located in the upper ureter are amenable to EL.

Partial or complete staghorn calculi, as well as smaller renal or upper ureteral calculi unsuitable for EL or ureteroscopic removal are best managed primarily by percutaneous nephrolithotomy (Segura et al, 1985). This results in either complete removal or debulking of large stones. In the latter case, the additional use of EL is recommended for further disintegration and passage of retained stone fragments. The technique used in the percutaneous removal of stones can be applied to a number of other interventions requiring fluoroscopic or endoscopic guidance, including biopsy and/or removal of urothelial tumors from the kidney and upper ureter; removal of retained foreign bodies (Woodhouse et al, 1986); percutaneous endopyelotomy for ureteropelvic junction obstruction (Motola et al, 1993); and treatment of calyceal infundibular stenosis or dilatation of the narrow neck of a symptomatic calyceal diverticulum.

Rapid dilatation of the percutaneous nephrostomy tract is painful, and epidural or general anesthesia is usually required. The procedure can be performed in a single stage or can be staged in two separate sessions. Single-stage procedures, in which the percutaneous establishment and dilatation of the tract is immediately followed by the endoscopic intervention, usually require conscious intravenous sedation for the fluoroscopic part of the intervention and general or epidural anesthesia for the tract dilatation and endoscopy in the operating room. In two-stage procedures, there is usually an interval of one or more days between the establishment and dilatation of the tract and subsequent endoscopic intervention. **The advantage of a two-stage procedure may be less hemorrhaging in the tract,** which makes the endoscopy easier and may reduce operative bleeding. **Disadvantages are the need for two anesthesia sessions,** if the percutaneous tract is dilated during the initial session, **and a longer hospital stay,** by at least one more night.

A nephrostomy catheter for endoscopic stone retrieval is placed through specific calyces, which allows for optimal access to the stone. Available imaging studies are reviewed before the procedure and evaluation for stone size and location, as well as for anatomy of the calyceal system, the posterior pleural space, and adjacent abdominal structures. **Placement of the catheter directly into a stone-bearing calyx ensures the best endoscopic access to the stone.** Because of stone location, an intercostal approach, usually through the 11th to 12th rib intercostal space or even a higher one, is at times necessary. Again, this is performed after review of prior imaging studies and with the help of fluoroscopy to avoid a transpleural puncture, which may result in pneumothorax.

The patient is placed prone on the fluoroscopic table. A posterior or posterolateral approach is preferred; such an approach minimizes the risk of transgressing adjacent organs. Antegrade pyelography is first performed by placing a thin needle into the calyceal system. This is then used as a calyceal map to direct placement of the needle-sheath system, through which further manipulations can be performed. In rare instances when difficulty entering the collecting system (severe spinal deformity, radiolucent stones, nondilated calyceal system, etc.) is encountered or anticipated, ultrasonographic guidance and/or administration of intravenous contrast material for opacification of the calyces is helpful. After the antegrade study, a 19-gauge needle sheath unit is then inserted into the targeted calyx, preferably the stone-bearing calyx. The antegrade needle is left in place, and contrast material is injected during insertion of the needle sheath unit when it becomes necessary to distend the calyx for placement of the wire. Wire and catheter exchanges can then be performed to gain ureteral access, which facilitates further manipulations. A torquable catheter with a curved tip often is used to manipulate an 0.038-inch glidewire into the ureter and bladder. Once ureteral access is safe, the glidewire is replaced by a stiff wire.

Subsequently, the percutaneous tract is dilated. Options include the use of serial fascial dilators or a high-pressure balloon dilation catheter. Waists in the balloon are typically seen during inflation at the renal capsule and at the skin. The skin incision can be extended after the balloon dilatation, if necessary. Persistent, tight waists at the renal level require additional dilatation with vascular or fascial dilators up to size 30 French.

Percutaneous stone removal can be performed at this juncture as a one-step procedure or as a two-step procedure, allowing the tract to mature for 1 to 2 days before the percutaneous lithotripsy. A No. 24 French tapered to No. 8 French nephroureterostomy catheter is left in place to maintain patency of the large-bore tract. For staghorn calculi occupying multiple calyces, two percutaneous tracts are often necessary, each entering the collecting system through a different calyx.

In the operating room, a No. 30 French Amplatz sheath is placed through the nephrostomy tract over a wire with the tip of the sheath positioned into the collecting system and/or against the stone (Fig. 6–132*A*). A second safety wire may be placed in the ureter before the beginning of the endoscopic part of the procedure. The rigid or flexible nephroscope is advanced into the calyceal system through the sheath, until the stone is visualized. Fragmentation of the stone or stones is achieved by ultrasonic, electrohydraulic, or laser lithotripsy, all performed under endoscopic visualization and control. A balloon catheter can be placed near the ureteropelvic junction to occlude the upper ureter and thus prevent distal migration of fragments (see Fig. 6–132*B*). Large stone fragments are retrieved with graspers or baskets. At the end of the procedure, the patient is left with a nephrostomy or nephroureterostomy catheter that preserves access to the collecting system for any further assessment or intervention and allows for drainage should the ureter be temporarily obstructed by edema, stones, or clot.

The technique for other interventions within the calyceal system, such as biopsy of suspicious urothelial lesions or removal of foreign bodies, is similar (Woodhouse et al, 1986) (Figs. 6–133, 6–134). **The percutaneous approach to the treatment of ureteropelvic junction obstruction (endopyelotomy) requires posterior upper or midpole calyceal access for the best endoscopic visualization of the renal pelvis and ureteropelvic junction** (Motola et al, 1993). The technique is successful except when the obstruction is caused by a crossing branch of the renal artery. Ureteral access with a guide wire is usually accomplished

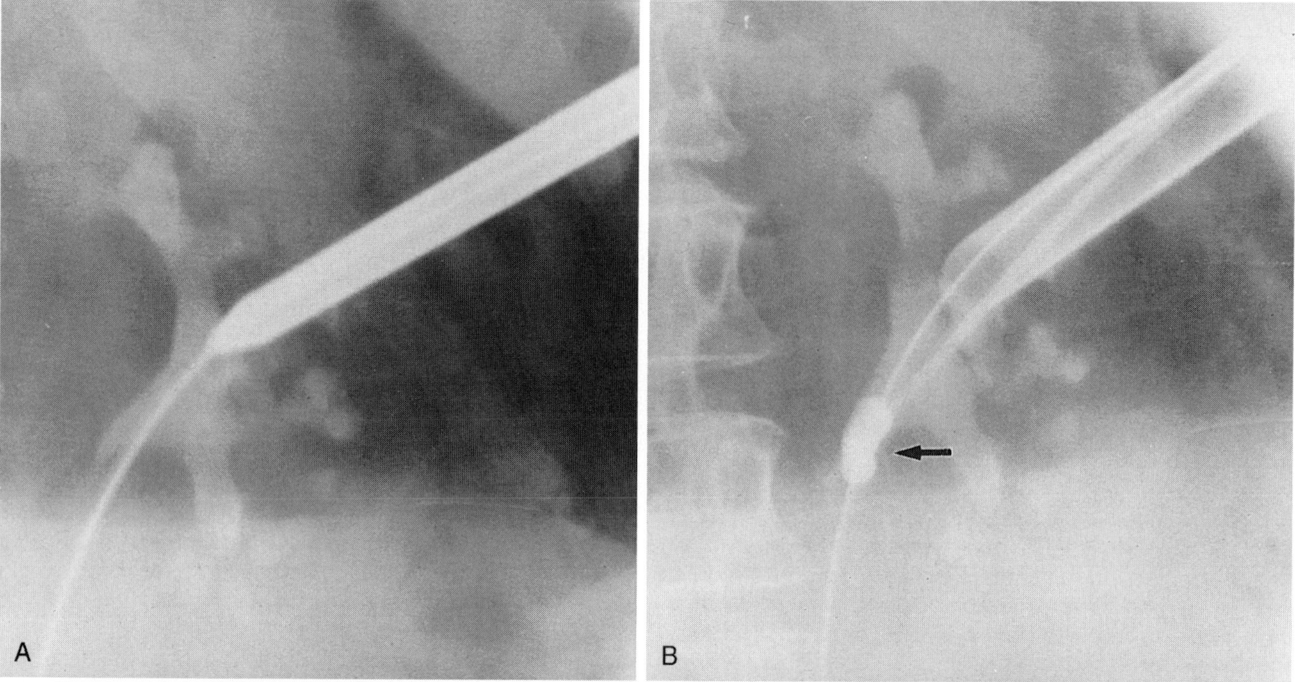

Figure 6–132. Percutaneous stone removal. *A,* After calyceal and ureteral access are achieved, the percutaneous tract is dilated to a size similar to the nephroscope to be used by inserting successively larger dilators through the tract. *B,* Before the lithotripsy begins, a balloon occlusion catheter is placed at the ureteropelvic junction to prevent migration of stone fragments down the ureter *(arrow).*

by retrograde placement of a ureteral stent exiting through the urethra. With the wire under control from both ends (nephrostomy tract and urethra), the posterolateral wall of the ureteropelvic junction is fully incised with a cold knife until retroperitoneal fat is visible. The posterolateral wall is chosen to avoid injury to renal hilar vessels located anterior and medial to the ureteropelvic junction. After incision, a tapered nephroureteral stent (No. 14 or 16 French to 8 French) is placed with the large-bore segment through the incised area and left in place for 4 to 6 weeks.

Percutaneous treatment of symptomatic calyceal diverticula or obstruction due to a stenotic infundibulum usually is performed as a single-stage procedure (Fig. 6–135). Direct access into the diverticular cavity is most helpful,

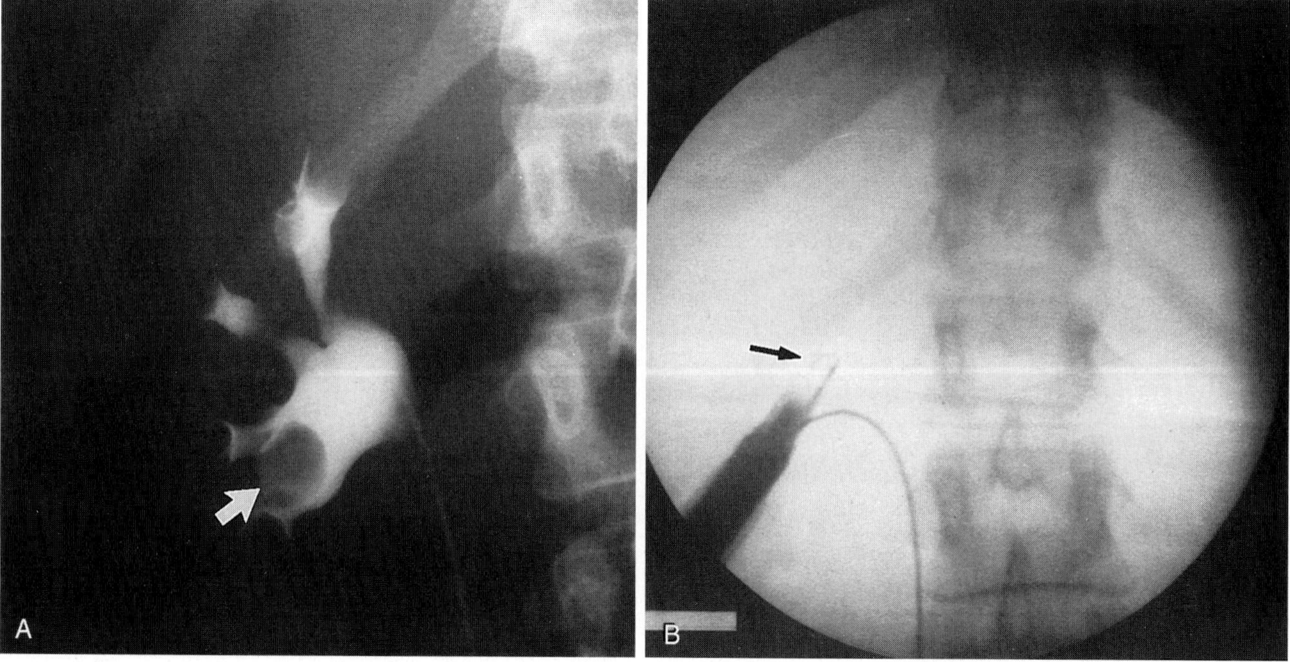

Figure 6–133. Percutaneous biopsy of urothelial lesion. *A,* Retrograde study demonstrates large filling defect in lower pole calyces *(arrow). B,* After percutaneous access into the collecting system, biopsy samples are taken *(arrow)* under endoscopic guidance.

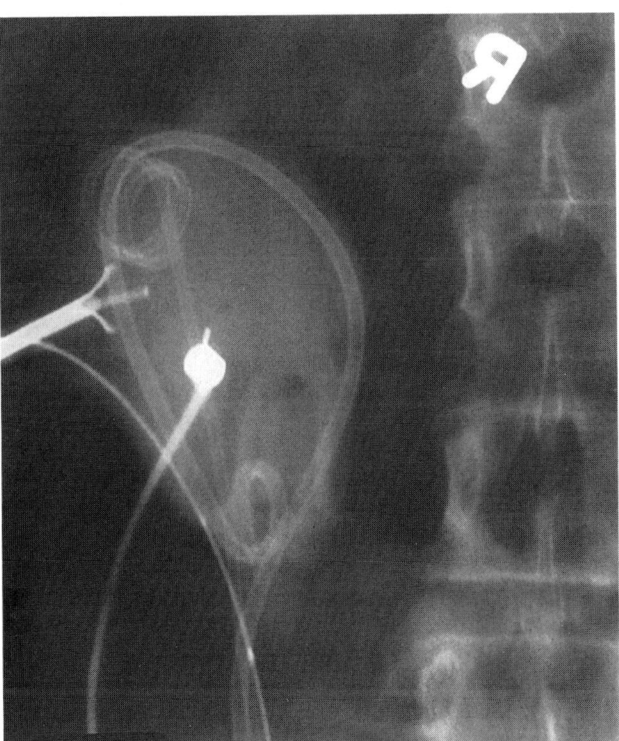

Figure 6–134. Percutaneous removal of foreign body. Three-pronged grasper is placed through the percutaneous tract to extract a malpositioned stent that could not be retrieved by retrograde means.

because the opening into the collecting system may be too small and difficult to find via an adjacent calyx. Once access into the cavity is secure, an attempt is made to cannulate the neck of the diverticulum by passing a wire through it and into the calyceal system. If this is successful, the communication between the diverticulum and its calyx is dilated and stented. Alternatively, a combined percutaneous fluoroscopic and endoscopic approach may be undertaken. A ureteral stent is placed in a retrograde manner and is used to opacify the diverticulum. A direct percutaneous stick into the cavity is then performed, and enough wire length is coiled in it. The tract is dilated to the desirable size of the endoscope to be used, which is then inserted into the diverticulum, preferably through an appropriately sized Amplatz sheath. Methylene blue injected via the ureteral stent enables direct visualization of the orifice of the diverticular neck, and a wire can be placed through the neck under endoscopic control. The communication between the diverticulum and the adjacent calyx is then dilated or incised. Coexisting stones within the cavity are removed at the same time.

Complications resulting from percutaneous nephrostomy catheter placement and associated interventions are infrequent. **Renal hemorrhage is the most common complication** (Clayman et al, 1984; Segura et al, 1985). **The incidence of severe bleeding after percutaneous instrumentation and/or endoscopic manipulations varies from 1% to 11% of patients.** Lee and associates (1986) reported that 12% of their patients required transfusions after percutaneous stone removal. **Arteriovenous fistulas and pseudoaneurysms have been reported to occur in 0.5% to 1% of patients;** Segura and co-workers (1985; Patterson et al, 1985) encountered 6 cases among their first 1000 patients who underwent stone removal via a percutaneous nephrostomy tract. These complications often necessitate angiographic embolization of the injured arterial branch. Parenchymal bleeding often occurs secondary to venous injuries and may be successfully controlled by tamponading the nephrostomy tract with a sheath, a balloon catheter, or a large Foley catheter.

Postprocedural urosepsis occurs in up to 1% to 2% of patients and may either prolong hospitalization or cause delay in further management. Patients with infected urinary obstruction (pyonephrosis) or infected stones (struvite) are more prone to sepsis after a procedure, often despite adequate antibiotic coverage.

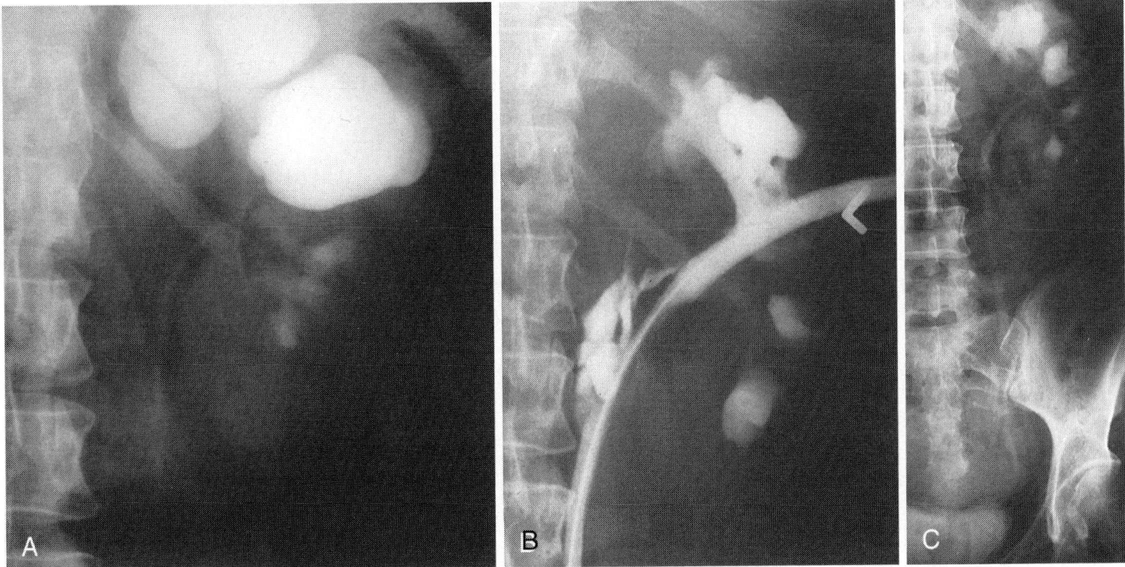

Figure 6–135. Percutaneous infundibulectomy and dilatation. *A,* Solitary left kidney with marked dilatation of upper pole calyces causing recurrent urinary tract infections. *B,* Percutaneous access into the renal pelvis was achieved through the narrow infundibulum, which was cut open, dilated, and stented under endoscopic guidance. *C,* Satisfactory result of the infundibuloplasty.

Pneumothorax is uncommon, and its risk can be minimized by following a subcostal access route. An intercostal approach clearly carries a higher risk. The overall incidence of pneumothorax was 0.1% in a series of 1000 patients evaluated by Segura and co-workers (1985); two other series with mostly intercostal approach to the kidneys reported the incidence of pneumothorax or hydrothorax in the range of 4% to 12% (Young et al, 1985; Picus et al, 1986).

Injuries to the liver and spleen are rare and usually can be avoided if a posterior approach is used. The retrorenal colon is a potential source of serious injury and may be impossible to recognize prospectively. It occurs very infrequently, and performing a barium enema study or CT scan on patients undergoing percutaneous renal interventions is impractical and very expensive. Again, a more posterior approach may be advisable for minimizing risk of injury to a colon that is posterolateral or lateral to the kidney. Posterior colonic position is thought to be more common in thin patients with very little retroperitoneal fat. Fortunately, the retroperitoneal location of the colonic perforation often results in less severe complications than would an intraperitoneal perforation, and some cases in the literature have been successfully managed without exploration.

Injury to organs or structures anterior to the kidneys (duodenum, jejunum, gallbladder, pancreas) is the result of through-and-through puncture of the kidney, which should be avoided.

Occasionally, strictures of the ureteropelvic junction or upper ureter have been described as the result of perforations caused by the endoscopic procedure. Ureteral stenting, when performed in a timely manner, may help prevent strictures. Also rare is the retention of foreign bodies in the calyceal system or ureter during percutaneous and endoscopic interventions. The foreign bodies are usually pieces of wires, baskets, graspers, or ultrasonic, electrohydraulic, or laser lithotrodes or fibers. Endoscopic or surgical intervention is required for their removal. Careful inspection of a postprocedural plain radiograph of the abdomen or nephrostogram may result in the timely discovery and removal of these foreign bodies, before the percutaneous tract is obliterated.

Percutaneous Ureteral Intervention

Ureteral Stenting

Percutaneous (antegrade) internal and/or external ureteral stent placement is a well-established technique for the treatment of malignant ureteral obstruction and a number of benign ureteral diseases. **Internal stenting is better tolerated and preferred by most patients than is external stenting because it improves quality of life by obviating the need for a urine bag and eliminating problems associated with external drainage, such as leakage, skin infection, accidental removal of the stent, and continuous infection of the urinary tract by an infected foreign body** (the stent itself). On rare occasions, ureteral stents cause significant bladder irritation and spasms and have to be replaced by a percutaneous nephrostomy catheter for drainage. Once they are inserted, internal ureteral stents have to be replaced cystoscopically by the urologist.

Percutaneous ureteral stenting usually is requested after a failed attempt at cystoscopic retrograde stenting. Sometimes a percutaneous nephrostomy catheter is in place, and its conversion to internal ureteral stent is requested. The patient with ureteral obstruction and ileal loop urinary diversion usually undergoes percutaneous nephrostomy drainage initially, which may then be converted to ureteral stent placement in an antegrade manner, if the obstructed segment can be negotiated with a wire (Mitty et al, 1988; Lu et al, 1994). On occasion, retrograde transloop ureteral stenting may be accomplished under fluoroscopic guidance. In any case, the **ureteral stent in patients with intestinal diversions should be brought out through the stoma and left within the urine collection bag.** The purpose of this is twofold: first, to prevent clogging of the stent by proteinaceous material secreted by the intestinal loop, and second, to facilitate subsequent stent exchanges.

The main obstacle to be dealt with for successful ureteral stenting is negotiating the tight obstruction with a wire (Fig. 6–136). After steps previously described, a percutaneous nephrostomy tract is established, preferably via an upper- or midpole calyx, to enhance the eventual sliding of the stent over a wire across the point of obstruction. A wire is directed toward the ureteropelvic junction and down the ureter until the obstruction is encountered. A glidewire often is the only wire to slide through a tight narrowing of the ureteral lumen. If the wire passes through, it is followed by a small-bore catheter (No. 5 to 7 French), which serves as a dilator of the stricture and allows the glidewire to be exchanged with an extra stiff wire. The latter is then coiled into the bladder to secure safe ureteral access. The percutaneous tract is then dilated to two French sizes larger than the size of the stent to be placed. The assembled stent-pusher unit is then advanced over the stiff wire until there is enough length of the stent within the bladder for the formation of the distal pigtail. The proximal pigtail is formed in the renal pelvis after the disengagement of the inner stiffener, pusher, and wire from the stent itself.

A temporary percutaneous nephrostomy catheter is left for external urinary diversion after a technically difficult ureteral stent placement. The catheter may be clamped unless internal drainage via the stent is compromised by clots or stent migration. If there is persistent or increasing flank pain possibly in association with fever, the urinary tract should be drained externally via the nephrostomy catheter until the problem with the stent has been satisfactorily addressed. Except in rare instances, the nephrostomy catheter is just an added safety step and is usually removed within 24 hours from the insertion of the stent.

Ureteral stents usually need to be replaced every 3 to 4 months. Periodic evaluation of renal function and renal sonography may provide early evidence of stent malfunction and prompt its replacement.

Complications associated with ureteral stenting are few. Most of them are common to all percutaneous renal interventions, such as hemorrhage, urosepsis, laceration of the renal pelvis, pneumothorax, and retention of foreign bodies. Complications specifically connected with the stent placement are related mostly to malpositioning of either or both pigtails, ureteral injury, and inability to place a stent past the obstruction. The last case is managed by inserting a nephros-

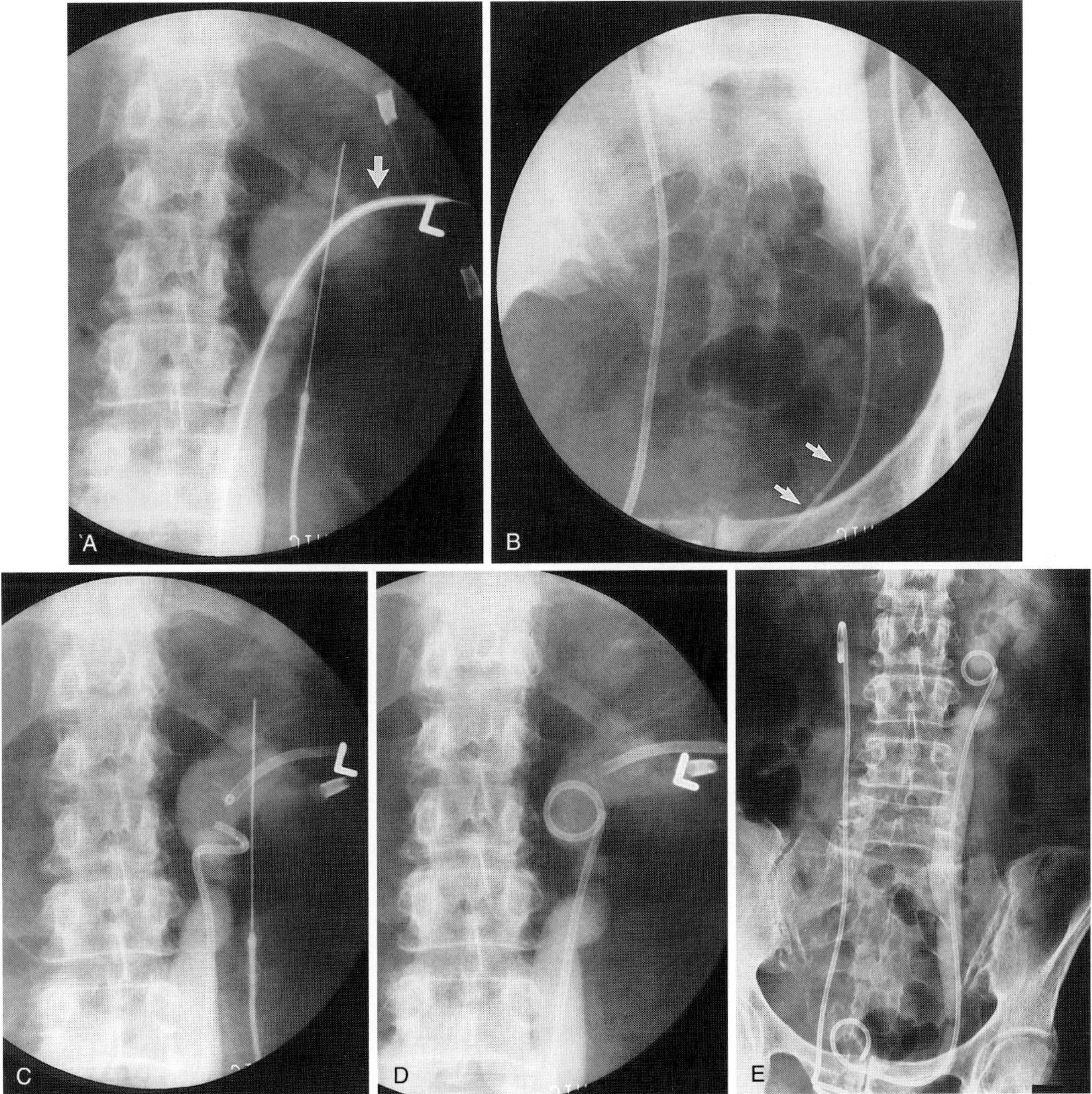

Figure 6–136. Percutaneous ureteral stenting. *A,* Percutaneous access into the collecting system is gained preferably through a midpole calyx *(arrow).* A guide wire is placed down the ureter. *B,* The tight stricture in the lower ureter is crossed, and access into the bladder is gained *(arrows).* *C,* After the stent enters the bladder and the distal pigtail is curled into the vesical lumen, the proximal pigtail is released into the renal pelvis. *D,* The proximal pigtail is formed. *E,* The entire stent is placed, and the percutaneous access is discontinued.

tomy catheter for drainage. A misplaced stent should be removed percutaneously, if possible, or cystoscopically if the distal pigtail is in the bladder. In the latter case, access into the ureter may be salvaged by inserting a wire through the stent before its removal. On rare occasions, renal or retroperitoneal exploration may be necessary for retrieval of an otherwise inaccessible misplaced stent.

Dilatation of Ureteral Strictures

Percutaneous dilatation of benign ureteral strictures has been performed since the early 1980s with variable success rates. Malignant strictures are kept patent by permanent ureteral stenting for the rest of the patient's life. For benign strictures, the goal of the intervention is to sufficiently dilate the narrow ureteral segment so that neither long-term stenting nor surgery is required. For many patients, however, chronic ureteral stenting cannot be avoided even after repeated dilatation sessions.

With regard to percutaneous dilatation of benign ureteral strictures, the general consensus from the literature is the following: **Fresh or recent strictures (up to 3 months) respond well to the dilatation; a great majority of patients recover fully** (Banner and Pollack, 1984; Beckmann et al, 1989). **Older strictures, strictures that develop after gynecologic surgery and radiation for pelvic malignan-**

cies, and strictures involving long, devascularized ureteral segments more often than not do not respond to balloon dilatation. Transplanted kidney ureteric strictures and strictured ureteropelvic junction pyeloplasties, as well as ureteroenteric strictures after ileal or colon urinary diversion, show variable, low long-term success rates after dilatation (Shapiro et al, 1988). **Many strictures, regardless of age and etiology, often necessitate repeat dilatations** and may eventually be treated surgically (Kramolowsky et al, 1988).

It is generally agreed that malignant etiology for a stricture should be ruled out before dilatation is performed. Brush biopsy of the ureteral urothelium and needle aspiration biopsy of periureteral tissues have been suggested. The next step involves the documentation of the appearance, length, and number of the strictures. This is best accomplished by antegrade injection of contrast material, preferably after percutaneous access into the collecting system is achieved, and placement of a small-bore catheter close to the stricture in the ureter. Next, a guide wire is manipulated through the narrowed lumen of the ureter and is coiled in the bladder or the intestinal conduit. A glidewire often is the wire of choice, because it tends to slide through tight strictures more easily than most other wires. Next, a small-bore catheter is passed across the stricture over the glidewire, which is then exchanged with an 0.038-inch extra stiff wire. The balloon dilatation catheter then is positioned across the stricture. The diameter of the balloon varies from 4 to 6 mm (No. 12 to 18 French). The balloon is inflated for 1 to 3 minutes. Initially, a waist in the balloon is evident at the site of the stricture. The waist eventually disappears as the dilatation progresses. More than one dilatation may be necessary until the narrowing is completely resolved.

After the dilatation, an internal/external No. 8 or 10 French ureteral stent is left across the stricture to maintain patency until the healing is completed. The stent further provides internal drainage of the urine, if capped. The stent is left in place for about 2 weeks and then is replaced with a nephrostomy catheter to allow ureteral edema to subside. Antegrade ureteral opacification and urodynamic studies (Whitaker test) are obtained to evaluate the result of the dilatation. If the pressures are high and/or the patient becomes symptomatic with the nephrostomy catheter capped, further dilatation sessions can be performed. Periodic imaging evaluation of the ureter is recommended by means of IVU, Lasix radionuclide renography, or the Whitaker study.

Ureteral stricture dilatation may also be performed with the use of successively larger stents placed across the stricture over a period of several days to a few weeks. The final stenting catheter is left in place for 4 to 8 weeks. The progressively tapered van Andel dilating catheter may also be used. Caution is advised to avoid excessive force when placing the van Andel catheter across the stricture, because it may cause laceration or avulsion of the ureter.

Complications resulting from ureteral dilatation are rare. Ureteral perforation or intimal disruption can be treated adequately by stenting.

Occlusion of Ureteral Fistulas

Benign iatrogenic or traumatic ureteral perforations and fistulas can often be managed by simple antegrade or retrograde ureteral stenting. The result is preservation of ureteral patency, prevention of stricture formation, and continuous drainage of urine into the bladder. If a stricture is formed after removal of the stent, early recognition leads to balloon dilatation with good results. Management of a malignant ureteral fistula, however, can be complicated and technically difficult. Often, the patient has undergone surgery and/or radiation therapy to the fullest extent and presents with local recurrence and a lower ureteral fistula. Because further surgery and radiation cannot be considered, percutaneous palliative occlusion of the fistula is a reasonable and safe alternative to surgical ureteral ligation or ileal loop urinary diversion. The intervention aims at improving the patient's quality of life and preserving ipsilateral renal function.

Occlusion of the ureteral lumen can be accomplished by a number of methods, whereas preservation of the renal function requires a permanent nephrostomy catheter.

Transrenal ureteral occlusion has been attempted with embolizing material (butyl-2-cyanoacrylate), detachable and nondetachable balloons, nylon plugs, silicone cone (Harzmann olive), endoscopic fulguration, and endoscopic ureteral ligation (Reddy et al, 1987; Huebner et al, 1992). All these methods are heavily dependent on operator preference and experience, and the number of patients reported is small. Results are variable and often transient, necessitating repeat or additional procedures. Nondetachable balloons and embolizing material (Gianturco coils, Gelfoam, and butyl-2-cyanoacrylate) have been used with mixed results. After percutaneous access into the ureter is gained, the balloon, embolizing material, or silicone cone are positioned proximal and close to the ureteral leakage and then released into the ureteral lumen under fluoroscopic guidance. Depending on the system used, the percutaneous tract is dilated to the size of a No. 12 to 16 French catheter. Injection of contrast material into the ureter confirms satisfactory sealing of the fistula. A nephrostomy catheter is left on a permanent basis to externally divert the urine.

Failures result from proximal migration of balloons, cones, and plugs, necessitating repositioning or recanalization of the ureteral lumen after long-term exposure of the embolizing material to the urine.

The decision to attempt percutaneous transrenal ureteral occlusion heavily depends on operator experience, the wishes of the patient, and the availability and advisability of surgical alternatives such as ureteral ligation or palliative supravesical urinary diversion; concomitant rates of morbidity and mortality are 7% to 14% for the former and 1% to 3% for the latter.

Percutaneous Bladder Intervention

Suprapubic Cystostomy

Percutaneous suprapubic cystostomy has long been used for the treatment of acute urinary retention regardless of cause, when urethral catheterization is either impossible or contraindicated. Insertion of a small-bore catheter with the trocar technique is fast and safe and necessitates only local anesthesia. Although effective in urgent situations, the small catheter cystostomy system is not suitable for long-term bladder drainage. The latter is best accomplished by placement of a large-bore (No. 16 French or larger) cystostomy catheter. Surgical suprapubic cystostomy is seldom performed as an isolated procedure. **The percutaneous approach under fluoroscopic and sonographic guidance is preferable to surgery (cystostomy or prostatectomy) for the typical patient who benefits from the procedure: namely, an elderly male with cardiovascular risk factors who either has marked enlargement of the prostate gland alone or is convalescing from a cerebrovascular accident** and has a large postvoid residual that necessitates long-term intermittent catheterization. On occasion, young patients who have sustained extensive pelvic injuries and urethral trauma and men and women with neurogenic bladders as the result of a number of diseases may benefit from the procedure as well. The catheters are well tolerated, ease nursing care of the patient considerably, preserve urethral integrity, and can be easily replaced in a medical office without imaging guidance after maturation of the suprapubic tract.

A suprapubic approach is used for either simple or large-bore cystostomy catheter placement. Local anesthesia suffices for trocar, small-bore catheter insertion. Conscious sedation (intravenous) is given to patients undergoing a large-bore cystostomy catheter placement (Papanicolaou et al, 1989).

Bleeding parameters and safe access to the bladder are evaluated before the intervention. The bladder is distended as much as possible to displace the loops of small bowel superiorly. The distention is accomplished either by urethral catheterization, if possible, or by placing a 20-gauge needle directly into the bladder and injecting diluted contrast material. Sonographic imaging confirms the absence of overlying small bowel from the interventional path. A sheath-needle system is placed into the bladder lumen via a paramedian suprapubic approach through the anterior wall at a point between the floor and the dome of the bladder (extraperitoneal surface). A 0.038-inch extra stiff guide wire is inserted through the sheath and coiled into the lumen of the bladder. The percutaneous tract is then dilated to No. 20 to 24 French size with a balloon dilatation catheter (Fig. 6–137). Additional dilatation of the tract may be required with the use of rigid fascial dilators. A peel-away sheath is necessary for delivering the soft Foley catheter into the vesical lumen through the fresh tract. The sheath should be at least 2 French sizes larger than the catheter to be placed. The peel-away sheath is inserted into the bladder coupled with a dilator, which is then removed, allowing for the cystostomy catheter to be advanced into its final position. A 5- or 30-ml balloon Foley catheter, No. 16 to 20 French in diameter, is adequate. If large diverticula are present, the catheter should be placed through the true wall of the bladder and not the thin wall of a diverticulum, which may be perforated or lacerated.

Transient hematuria is common but clears rapidly. Urosepsis is uncommon, inasmuch as many of the patients have been taking antibiotics for lower urinary tract infections. Bladder laceration or perforation can be avoided by use of careful technique. **The risk of injury to adjacent loops of small bowel can be minimized by adequate bladder distention and sonographic guidance.** Malfunction of the catheter may necessitate cystography for evaluation and replacement. The inflated balloon of the Foley catheter has been sufficient to safely keep the catheter in the bladder without the need for skin sutures of adhesive- or ostomy-type discs or devices (Papanicolaou et al, 1989).

Percutaneous Needle and Brush Biopsy

The minimally invasive techniques of obtaining tissue or fluid samples from deeply situated organs or areas under imaging guidance are widely used in clinical practice to diagnose benign and malignant processes, as well as to stage neoplasms before or after treatment (Sandler et al, 1986; Pollack, 1990). Percutaneous biopsy is an effective and safe procedure with few complications and contraindications (Fig. 6–138).

Abnormal or prolonged coagulation is a major contraindication to any biopsy or aspiration. Whether secondary to a systemic deficiency or to medications that may interfere with the clotting mechanism (heparin, warfarin [Coumadin], aspirin, etc.), the bleeding disorder should be documented and reversed before any procedures are performed.

Lack of safe access to a lesion or an area to be sampled may be a relative contraindication to proceeding with the biopsy. On rare occasions, a deeply situated lesion may not be safely approached, although the thin 22- to 25-gauge needles used to obtain cytologic material cause little damage to the tissues they traverse.

As a rule, traversing the colon with a needle is avoided because of the possibility of peritonitis from fecal contamination. Small bowel loops are sometimes needled during retroperitoneal or mesenteric biopsies without significant risk to the patient. Puncturing of large blood vessels with larger needles is not desirable, although accidental entrance into the inferior vena cava or aorta with a needle is usually benign. Before the specimen is obtained, the operator should aspirate first through the needle and withdraw it if blood returns into the syringe.

Small-gauge needles (21- to 25-gauge) are used to obtain material for cytologic examination, and larger gauge needles (14- to 20-gauge) are used to obtain tissue cores for histopathologic evaluation. For certain diseases, larger cores are necessary for detailed pathologic examination. Such examples include prostate carcinoma, for which a Gleason score is desirable information (18-gauge); cases of lymphoma for subtyping (14- or 16-gauge); and complications of renal transplantation such as rejection (16- to 18-gauge). The presence of malignant cells in lymph nodes or focal parenchymal mass lesions is often established by the cytologic examination alone which is performed with thinner needles.

Imaging guidance can be in the form of fluoroscopy, sonography, CT scanning, and, more recently, MRI. Sonography and CT are the most commonly used modalities. Availability of a modality, personal preference by the radiologist, and the size and location of the lesion determine the choice of the imaging modality. Small or deeply situated lesions can be sampled with higher success rates under CT guidance, whereas superficial lesions or structures can easily be approached under sonographic control.

Biopsy may also be performed with the use of special brushlike devices that can obtain cells from the surface of suspicious lesions within the urinary tract (calyces,

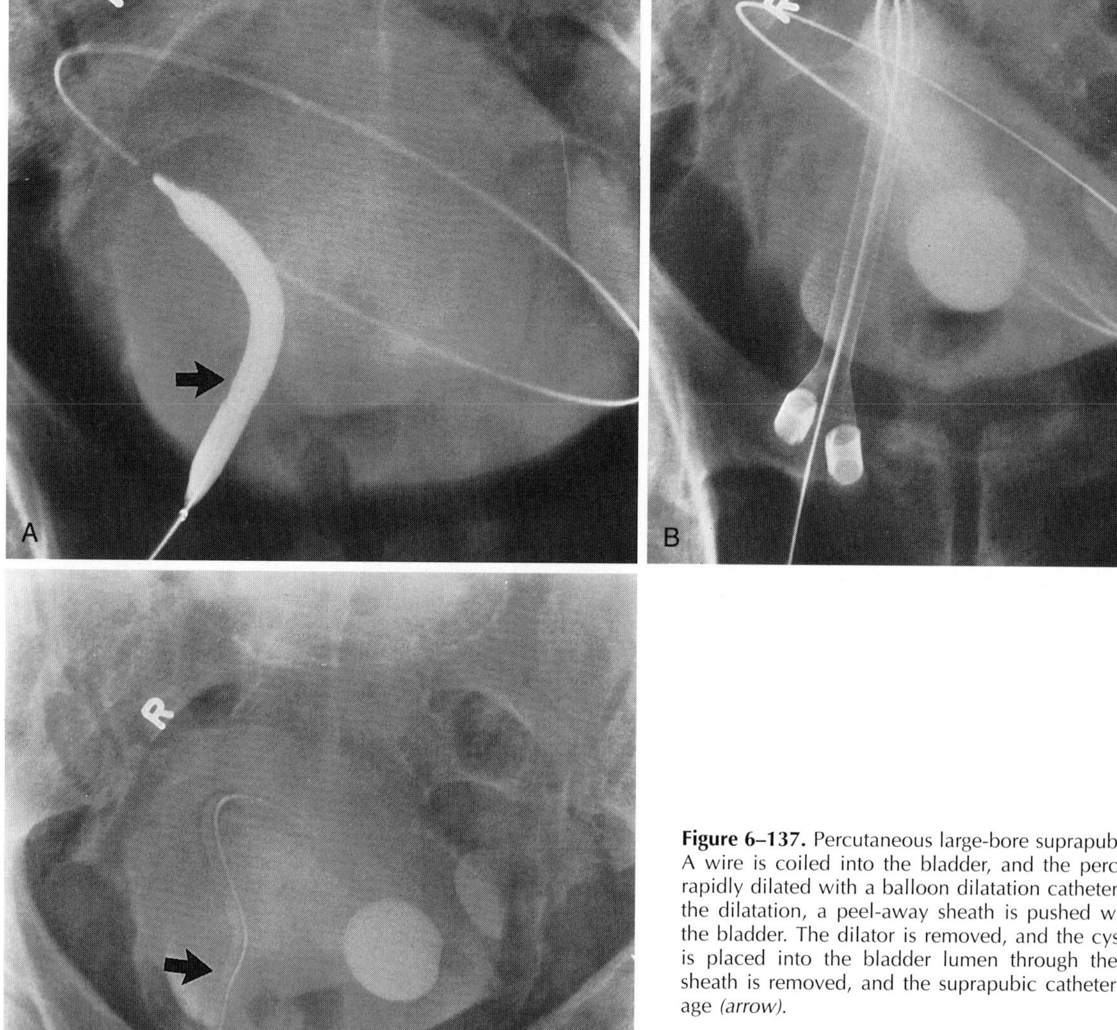

Figure 6–137. Percutaneous large-bore suprapubic cystostomy. *A,* A wire is coiled into the bladder, and the percutaneous tract is rapidly dilated with a balloon dilatation catheter *(arrow). B,* After the dilatation, a peel-away sheath is pushed with a dilator into the bladder. The dilator is removed, and the cystostomy catheter is placed into the bladder lumen through the sheath. *C,* The sheath is removed, and the suprapubic catheter is left for drainage *(arrow).*

renal pelvis, ureter) (Pollack, 1990). The cells retrieved by the brushing device are submitted for cytologic evaluation. The brush is positioned within the vicinity of the lesion either percutaneously through a sheath or catheter or through an endoscope or an endoscopically placed catheter into the upper urinary tract.

Renal biopsies may target either a focal mass lesion or any part of the renal parenchyma, the latter in patients with undiagnosed acute or chronic renal failure or transplantation complications (Nadel et al, 1986). **Renal mass lesions usually do not necessitate biopsy because they are resected. Exceptions to this rule are lesions that may represent metastases or lymphoma in the appropriate clinical settings.** These lesions usually do not undergo surgical excision and may be treated with chemotherapy. Benign renal lesions such as oncocytomas or adenomas should not be subjected to biopsy because the pathologic diagnosis cannot be definitive and accurate on the basis of the small amounts of sampled tissue.

Retroperitoneal and periureteral lymph nodes and tumors can easily be accessed and sampled, usually under CT guidance. Masses or nodes indicative of recurrence of renal cell or transitional cell carcinomas can be sampled for biopsy. Staging of renal cell carcinoma may sometimes necessitate biopsy if metastatic disease is likely and, therefore, if a nephrectomy is unnecessary.

Pelvic masses and lymph nodes can be sampled for biopsy through either a transgluteal or an anterior abdominal

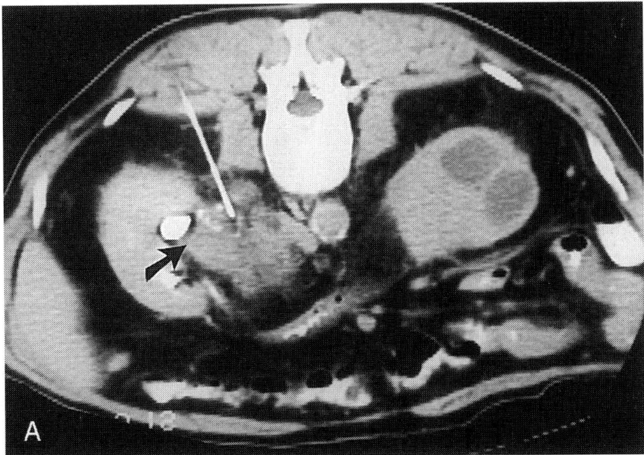

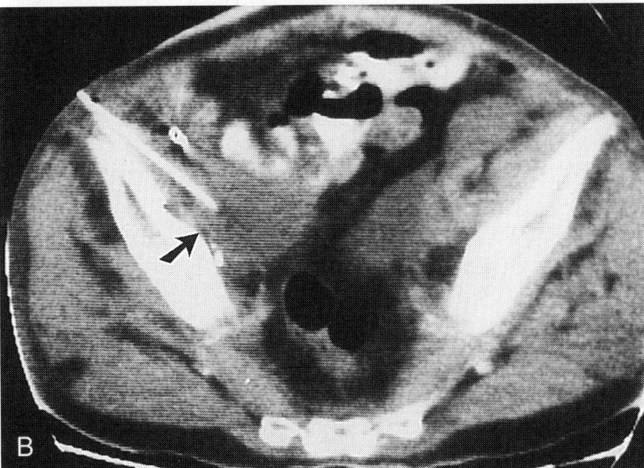

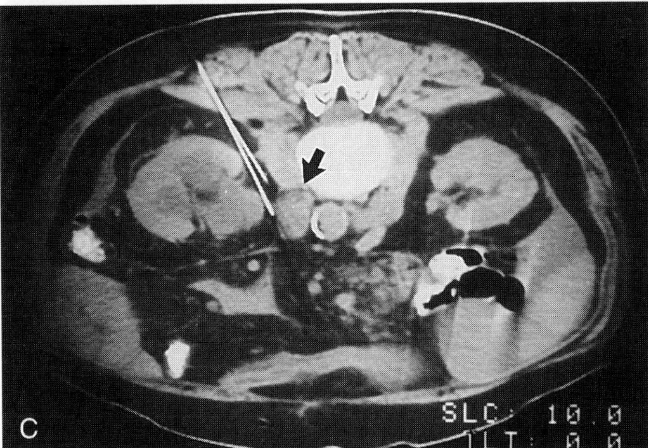

Figure 6–138. Percutaneous needle biopsy. *A,* CT-guided biopsy of retroperitoneal tumor *(arrow). B,* CT-guided biopsy of external iliac nodes *(arrow). C,* CT-guided biopsy of para-aortic nodes *(arrow).* CT scans in *A* and *C* are inverted.

approach in a manner similar to that for sampling retroperitoneal para-aortic nodes. Perivesical nodes or masses may be sampled when no other means of obtaining tissue diagnosis is possible. The bladder can be traversed, if necessary, by a needle aiming at a retrovesical lesion. Prostate and seminal vesicle biopsies are performed under endorectal sonographic guidance except when the rectum has been surgically removed (Resnick, 1988). The transgluteal or transperineal approach may then be used to obtain a biopsy sample of the prostate (Papanicolaou et al, 1996).

Percutaneous access into the upper urinary tract for brush biopsies of suspicious urothelial lesions can be effected transureterally or in a manner similar to that for placement of a nephrostomy tube. In the latter circumstance, care should be taken to target the calyx with the lesion or a calyx with easy access to the lesion for the insertion of the catheter that will direct the brushing device to the abnormal area in the upper urinary tract. The positioning of the nephrostomy catheter and the brush is easily accomplished under fluoroscopic guidance.

Complications resulting from needle or brush biopsy procedures are uncommon. Hemorrhage is the most frequent complication. Peritonitis from colonic injury and pneumothorax from a high abdominal or retroperitoneal biopsy are rare. Arteriovenous fistulas in the kidney have been reported after biopsy or cyst aspiration and can be diagnosed by Doppler sonography, MRI, or angiography. Brush biopsies of the calyceal system or ureter may sometimes result in perforations, which are usually insignificant and can be treated with external or internal drainage via a nephrostomy catheter or ureteral stent, respectively. **Tumor seeding of the percutaneous needle tract is exceedingly rare but may be an issue with transitional cell carcinomas.**

Percutaneous Abscess Drainage

Renal and perinephric abscesses may be the result of untreated or inadequately treated pyelonephritis. Immunocompromised and diabetic patients, as well as those with infected renal calculi, are at higher risk for abscess formation (Roberts, 1986). Gram-negative bacteria in an abscess suggest an ascending route of infection, whereas gram-positive bacteria suggest a hematogenous spread of infection.

Rupture of a renal abscess or infected cyst through the renal capsule spreads the process into the perinephric space. A perinephric abscess often is formed by the decompression of obstructed pyohydronephrosis, by direct extension of peritoneal or retroperitoneal infection, or as the sequela of iatrogenic (surgical, percutaneous, or endoscopic) intervention. When the urinary tract is not obstructed, renal abscesses and infected cysts often drain spontaneously into adjacent calyces or the ureter. Once an abscess is diagnosed, prompt drainage is usually required, by either percutaneous or surgical intervention. Small renal abscesses can be managed conservatively with intravenous antibiotics. Prostatic abscesses may be drained transrectally under sonographic guidance. Pyocystis necessitates drainage via a urethral or suprapubic catheter.

There is general agreement that **percutaneous drainage of a renal or perinephric abscess is preferable to surgery as the initial and potentially definitive procedure, especially for unilocular collections** (Fig. 6–139). Cure rates are high (Deyoe et al, 1990; Lang, 1990); for the remaining patients, the percutaneous route serves as a temporizing measure that stabilizes the condition of the patient and renders subsequent surgery safer and more effective. **Surgery alone may be indicated for the treatment of extensive and multiloculated abscesses with involvement of adjacent organs.**

Percutaneous drainage requires a safe, posterior retroperitoneal approach that spares the pleural and peritoneal spaces

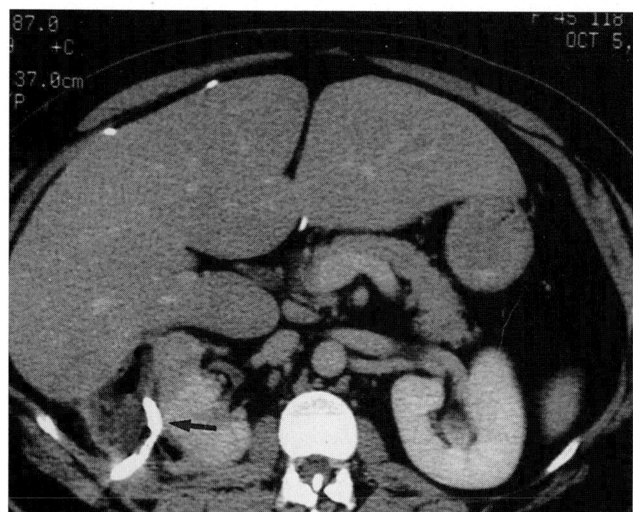

Figure 6–139. Percutaneous catheter drainage of right perinephric abscess *(arrow).*

(Deyoe et al, 1990; Lang, 1990). Sonography and CT are excellent guiding modalities for superficial collections, including renal transplants, and deep collections, respectively. Loculated collections should be drained separately if they do not communicate with each other. If an infected perinephric collection coexists with urinary obstruction, both should be drained.

The Seldinger technique is used for deeper and smaller collections, whereas the trocar technique is safer for superficial and larger collections. The size of the catheter depends on the nature and amount of the fluid to be drained. Clinical improvement is often impressive. Patients who continue to be febrile should undergo reimaging with CT to search for undrained collections or collections that communicate with adjacent organs. Persistent or inaccessible collections should be managed by surgery.

Cure rates with the percutaneous approach range from 60% to 93% (Deyoe et al, 1990; Lang, 1990). Predictably, immunocompromised and diabetic patients fare worse; one series reported only a 20% cure rate (Deyoe et al, 1990). Severe chronic pyelonephritis complicated by acute abscess formation may be appropriately treated by nephrectomy.

Vascular Intervention

Embolization of arteries and/or veins with percutaneous angiographic techniques has applications in the management of certain urologic disorders (McLean and Meranze, 1986). The aim of the procedure is to place a vascular catheter, arterial or venous, depending on the problem, as close to the selected site as possible and deliver the appropriate embolic material safely to the lesion or area to be occluded. Fluoroscopic guidance is essential. A preoperative embolization angiogram maps the vascular anatomy and indicates the best route to be followed by the catheter. The embolic material is chosen according to the desired outcome of the procedure. Biodegradable particles provide short-term vascular occlusion; metallic devices, polymers, and sclerosing agents provide long-term or permanent vascular occlusion.

The **major indications for the procedure include, in brief** (Banner and Pollack, 1994), **significant and difficult-to-control hemorrhage from the kidneys or pelvis secondary to trauma; iatrogenic vascular injuries; large bleeding tumors; and complicated aneurysms and large arteriovenous malformations. Preoperative embolization of large renal, retroperitoneal, or pelvic neoplasms can be performed to decrease operative blood loss and facilitate excision** (Fig. 6–140). **Renal ablation is occasionally indicated** and can be performed angiographically as an alternative to surgical nephrectomy in patients with end-stage renal disease and significant proteinuria or hypertension that is refractory to conservative management and in patients with ureteral fistulas to the skin or pelvic organs secondary to irradiated or unresectable pelvic tumors. Postradiation hemorrhagic cystitis may, likewise, be treated by embolization of the vascular supply to the bladder when cystoscopic or chemical sclerosing control has failed and surgery is not indicated.

Embolization of varicoceles in males with semen abnormalities has been shown to improve sperm count and motility in up to 75% of patients, and reported pregnancy rates after ablation of varicoceles vary from 30% to 60% (Wheatley et al, 1991). The dilatation of the pampiniform plexus is thought to be secondary to incompetent valves within the internal spermatic vein that allow retrograde blood flow. Either the femoral or the internal jugular approach may be used for access into the spermatic veins. The left spermatic vein is catheterized via the left renal vein, whereas the right spermatic vein is entered directly from the inferior vena cava. Selective spermatic venography is then performed to demonstrate the venous anatomy and the presence and location of the collateral veins that may also need to be occluded at the same time as the spermatic vein for a successful outcome. Metallic embolic material (such as coils) or sclerosing agents (such as alcohol, glue, or boiling contrast material) are used (McLean and Meranze, 1986). A postembolization venogram confirms the satisfactory occlusion of the vein and the lack of retrograde flow. Careful technique minimizes the possibility of migration of the embolic material.

Percutaneous transluminal angioplasty (PTA) of the renal arteries is an excellent alternative to surgical grafting in certain patients with proven renovascular hypertension (Sos et al, 1983; Tegtmeyer et al, 1984; Weibull et al, 1993) (Fig. 6–141). The procedure begins with a diagnostic arteriogram of the renal artery in question, followed by placement of a guide wire past the stenosis, after selective catheterization of the renal artery. Dilatation of the stenotic arterial segment is then performed with a balloon catheter centered over the lesion and inflated with contrast material. The waist in the middle of the inflated balloon is obliterated and fully distended after successful dilatation of the lumen. A postangioplasty arteriogram should confirm that the lumen is patent and blood flow across the stenotic lesion has increased. If the flow is delayed, repeated balloon angioplasty is performed. Measurements of the pressure gradient across the lesion before and after PTA are routinely obtained. Antispasmodic and vasodilating agents often are given before the placement of the balloon across the stenosis to prevent or lessen the arterial spasm frequently seen as the result of the manipulation. Pre- or postdilatation thrombi may be

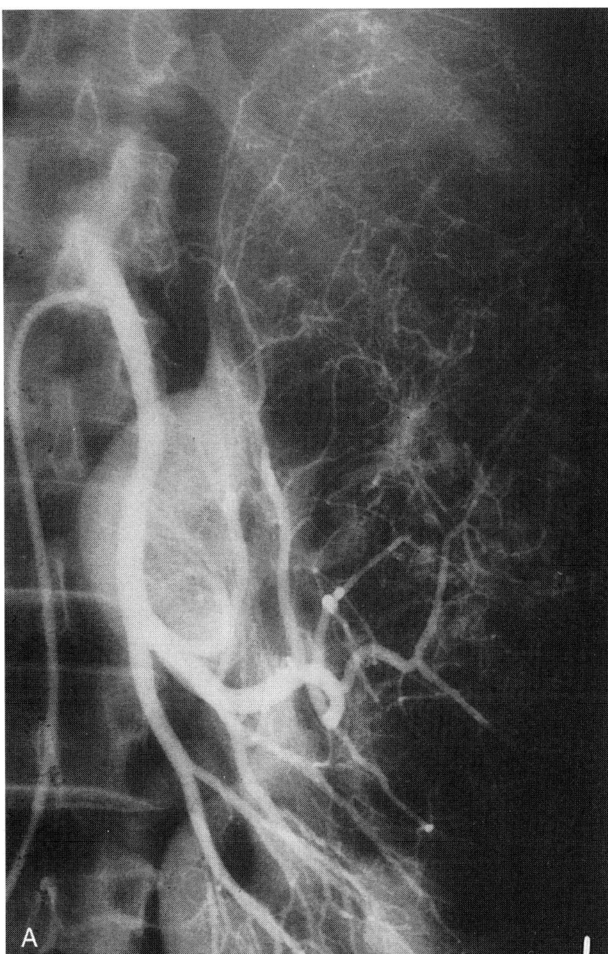

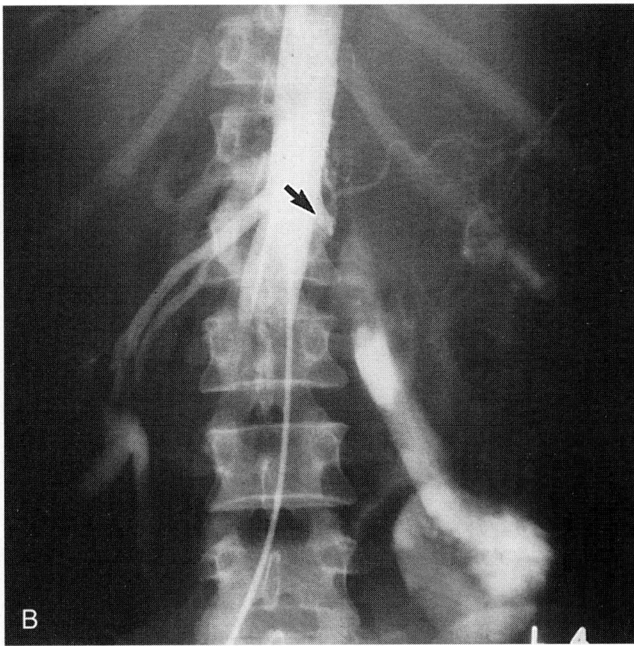

Figure 6–140. Preoperative embolization of large renal cell carcinoma. *A,* Preoperative embolization in selective renal arteriogram shows the large, moderately vascular mass. *B,* After embolization of the artery, blood supply to the tumor is interrupted pending surgery *(arrow).*

treated with thrombolytic agents such as streptokinase. Antihypertensive medications, if given before PTA, are discontinued before the angioplasty to prevent harmful hypotension after dilatation. The patient is given anticoagulants before, during, and after the procedure.

The overall success rate of renal PTA has been reported to be approximately 70% to 90% of cases (Mitty et al, 1996). Repeated dilatations are often successful when there is recurrence of the stenosis. **Long-term patency of the arterial lumen is better in patients with fibromuscular disease than in patients with atherosclerotic lesions. Technical failures occur relatively more often in renal arterial**

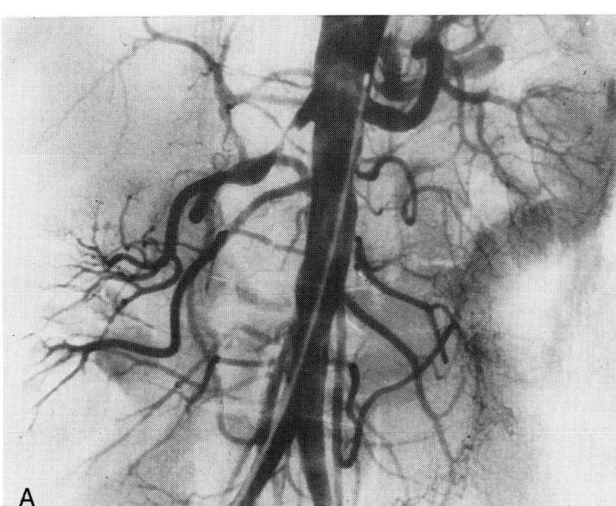

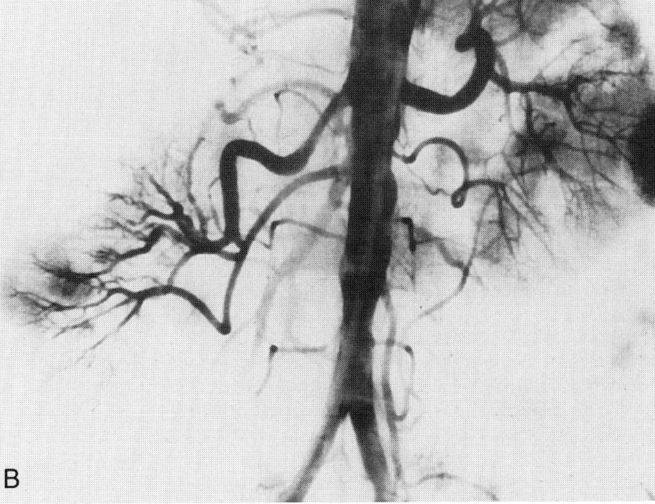

Figure 6–141. Percutaneous transluminal angioplasty of renal artery stenosis. *A,* Preangioplasty arteriogram demonstrates tight narrowing of the proximal right renal artery secondary to atherosclerosis. *B,* Excellent result after the balloon angioplasty.

ostial lesions and stenoses at surgical anastomoses. If the stenosis cannot be crossed with the wire or catheter, the procedure is abandoned and the patient is managed surgically.

Complications occur infrequently. Hematomas or pseudoaneurysms at the femoral or axillary entry puncture site are usually small. Thrombosis of the puncture site or the renal artery may necessitate surgical intervention. Rupture of the renal artery is rare and is a surgical emergency. Dissection of the arterial lumen is most often handled with surgical bypass, on an emergency basis if it results in luminal occlusion. Cholesterol emboli may be the cause of significant morbidity. Last, the nephrotoxic effect of the contrast material often results in transient or, less likely, permanent renal failure. The amount of renal contrast injected should be limited as much as possible, in view of the fact that many patients with atheromatous vascular disease and long-standing hypertension have already sustained a degree of irreversible renal damage.

Renal PTA in general is indicated for patients with proven renovascular hypertension and/or worsening renal failure because it reduces or eliminates the need for antihypertensive regimens and reverses or stabilizes renal dysfunction secondary to renal artery stenosis. The procedure is best suited for fibromuscular arterial disease, short nonostial atherosclerotic lesions, and arterial stenoses after renal transplantation (Roberts et al, 1989). Renal artery disease secondary to aortic aneurysm is not amenable to PTA management. Severe arterial stenoses associated with marked renal dysfunction are not likely to respond to PTA by reversal of the renal failure. Patients with bilateral, atherosclerotic, nonostial renal artery disease or postsurgical stenoses with or without mild to moderate renal failure may improve after PTA, although the improvement may not be long-lasting.

REFERENCES

Abbitt PL, Waston L, Howards S: Abnormalities of the seminal tract causing infertility: Diagnosis with endorectal sonography. AJR 1991; 157:337–339.

Amis ES Jr, Cronan JJ, Pfister RC: Ultrasonic inaccuracies in diagnosing renal obstruction. Urology 1982; 19:101–105.

Amis ES Jr, Cronan JJ, Pfister RC: Needle puncture of cystic renal masses: Survey of the society of uroradiology. AJR 1987; 148:297–299.

Banner MP, Pollack HM: Dilation of ureteral stenoses: Techniques and experience in 44 patients. AJR 1984; 143:789–793.

Banner MP, Pollack HM: Interventional uroradiology. *In* Hanno PM, Wein AJ, eds: Clinical Manual of Urology, 2nd ed. New York, McGraw-Hill, 1994, pp 137–178.

Barbaric ZL: Percutaneous nephrostomy for urinary tract obstruction. AJR 1984; 143:803–809.

Barentsz JO, Ruijs SH, Strijk SP: The role of MR imaging in carcinoma of the urinary bladder. AJR 1993; 160:937–947.

Becker JA: The role of radiology in evaluation of the failing renal transplantation. Radiol Clin North Am 1991; 29:511–526.

Beckmann CF, Roth RA, Bihrle W III: Dilation of benign ureteral strictures. Radiology 1989; 171:437–441.

Bernardino ME, Walther MM, Phillips VM, et al: CT-guided adrenal biopsy: Accuracy, safety and indications. AJR 1985; 144:67–70.

Bird K, Rosenfield AT, Taylor KJW: Ultrasonography in testicular torsion. Radiology 1983; 147:527–534.

Bodner DR, Resnick ML: Ultrasonography of the urinary bladder. *In* Resnick ML, Rifkin MD, eds: Ultrasonography of the Urinary Tract, 3rd ed. Baltimore, Williams & Wilkins, 1991, pp 250–281.

Bosniak MA: The current radiologic approach to renal cysts. Radiology 1986; 158:1–10.

Bosniak MA: The small renal parenchymal tumor: Detection, diagnosis, and controversies. Radiology 1991; 179:307–317.

Bosniak MA, Megibow AJ, Hulnick DH, et al: CT diagnosis of renal angiomyolipoma: The importance of detecting small amounts of fat. AJR 1988; 151:497–501.

Bosniak MA, Rofsky NM: Problems in the detection and characterization of small renal masses. Radiology 1996; 198:638–641.

Brown DL, Benson CB, Doherty FJ, et al: Cystic testicular mass caused by dilated rete testis. AJR 1992; 158:1257–1259.

Burge HJ, Middleton WD, McClennan BL, Hildebott CF: Ureteral jets in healthy subjects and in patients with unilateral ureteral calculi: Comparison with color Doppler US. Radiology 1991; 180:437–442.

Burns PN: Ultrasound imaging and Doppler: Principles and instrumentation. *In* Resnick ML, Rifkin MD, eds: Ultrasonography of the Urinary Tract, 3rd ed. Baltimore, Williams & Wilkins, 1991, pp 1–33.

Carter SSC, Shinohara K, Lipshultz LI: Transrectal ultrasonography in disorders of the seminal vesicles and ejaculatory ducts. Urol Clin North Am 1989; 16:773–788.

Choyke PL: Inherited cystic disease of the kidney. Radiol Clin North Am 1996; 34:925–964.

Clayman RV, Surya V, Hunter D, et al: Renal vascular complications associated with the percutaneous removal of renal stones. J Urol 1984; 132:228–230.

Cohan RH, Leder RA, Ellis JH: Treatment of adverse reactions to radiographic contrast media in adults. Radiol Clin North Am 1996; 34:1055–1076.

Conway JJ: The well-tempered diuresis renography: Its historical development, physiological and technical pitfalls, and standardized technique protocol. Semin Nucl Med 1992; 22:74–84.

Cronan JJ: Contemporary concepts in imaging urinary tract obstruction. Radiol Clin North Am 1991; 29:527–542.

Curry NS, Schabel SI, Betsill WL Jr: Small renal neoplasms: Diagnostic imaging, pathologic features and clinical course. Radiology 1986; 158:113–117.

Demas B, Hricak H, McClure RD: Varicoceles: Radiologic diagnosis and treatment. Radiol Clin North Am 1991; 29:619–627.

Deyoe LA, Cronan JJ, Lambiase RE, Dorfman GS: Percutaneous drainage of renal and perirenal abscesses: Results in 30 patients. AJR 1990; 155:81–83.

Drago JR, Cunningham JJ: Ultrasonography of renal masses. *In* Resnick ML, Rifkin MD, eds: Ultrasonography of the Urinary Tract, 3rd ed. Baltimore, Williams & Wilkins, 1991, pp 152–203.

Dubin L, Amelar RD: Varicocele size and results of varicocelectomy in selected subfertile men with varicocele. Fertil Steril 1970; 21:606–609.

Dubovsky E, Russell C: Quantitation of renal function with glomerular and tubular agents. Semin Nucl Med 1982; 12:308–329.

Dunnick NR, McCallum RW, Sandler CM: Textbook of Uroradiology. Baltimore, Williams & Wilkins, 1991.

Dunnick NR, Sfakianakis GN: Screening for renovascular hypertension. Radiol Clin North Am 1991; 29:497–510.

Elster AD, Liuk KM, Carr JJ: Patient screening prior to MR imaging: A practical approach synthesized from protocols at 15 U.S. medical centers. AJR 1994; 162:195–199.

Eshima D, Taylor A Jr: Technetium-99m mercapto acetyltriglycerine: Update on the new Tc-99m renal tubular function agent. Semin Nucl Med 1992; 22:61–73.

Feld R, Middleton WD: Recent advances in sonography of the testis and scrotum. Radiol Clin North Am 1992; 30:1033–1051.

Fellmeth BD, Roberts AC, Bookstein JJ, et al: Post angiographic femoral artery injuries: Nonsurgical repair with US-guided compression. Radiology 1991; 178:671–675.

Francis IR, Smid A, Gross MD, et al: Adrenal masses in oncologic patients: Functional and morphologic evaluation. Radiology 1988; 166:353–357.

Gooding GAW, Leonhardt W, Stein R: Testicular cysts: US findings. Radiology 1987; 163:537–538.

Hattery RR, Williamson B Jr, Hartman GW, et al: Intravenous urographic technique. Radiology 1988; 167:593–599.

Huebner W, Knoll M, Porpaczy D: Percutaneous transrenal ureteral occlusions: Indication and technique. Urol Radiol 1992; 13:177–180.

Jamis-Dow CA, Choyke PL, Jennings SB, et al: Small renal masses: Detection with CT versus US and pathologic correlation. Radiology 1996; 198:785–788.

Katayama H, Yamaguchi K, Kozuka T, et al: Adverse reactions to ionic and nonionic contrast media: A report from the Japanese Committee on the Safety of Contrast Media. Radiology 1990; 175:621–628.

Kaye W: Renal anatomy for endourologic stone removal. J Urol 1983; 130:647–648.

Kaye W, Reinke DB: Detailed caliceal anatomy for endourology. J Urol 1984; 132:1085–1088.

King BF Jr: MR angiography of the renal arteries. Semin Ultrasound CT MR 1996; 17:398–403.

Kirchner PT, Rosenthall L: Renal transplant evaluation. Semin Nucl Med 1982; 12:370–386.

Kliewer MA, Tupler RH, Carroll BA, et al: Renal artery stenosis: Analysis of Doppler waveform parameters and tardus-parvus pattern. Radiology 1993; 189:779–787.

Korobkin M, Francis IR, Kloos RT, et al: The incidental adrenal mass. Radiol Clin North Am 1996; 34:1037–1054.

Kramolowsky EU, Clayman RV, Weymann PJ: Management of ureterointestinal anastomotic strictures: Comparison of open surgical and endourologic repair. J Urol 1988; 139:1195–1198.

Kuligowska E, Baker C, Oates RD: Male infertility: Role of transrectal US in diagnosis and management. Radiology 1992; 185:353–360.

Lang EK: Renal, perirenal and pararenal abscesses: Percutaneous drainage. Radiology 1990; 174:109–113.

Lasser EC: Contrast media for urography. *In* Pollack HM, ed: Clinical Urography. Philadelphia, W. B. Saunders Company, 1990, pp 23–36.

Lasser EC, Berry CC, Talner LB: Pretreatment with cortical steroids to alleviate reactions to intravenous contrast material. N Engl J Med 1987; 317:845–847.

Lee MJ, Hahn PF, Papanicolaou N, et al: Benign and malignant adrenal masses: CT distinction with attenuation coefficients, size and observer analysis. Radiology 1991; 179:415–418.

Lee WJ, Smith AD, Cubelli V, et al: Percutaneous nephrolithotomy: Analysis of 500 consecutive cases. Urol Radiol 1986; 5:61–66.

Levine E: Acquired cystic kidney disease. Radiol Clin North Am 1996; 34:947–964.

Levine E: Acute renal and urinary tract disease. Radiol Clin North Am 1994; 32:989–1004.

Littrup PJ, Williams CR, Egglin TK, et al: Determination of prostate volume with transrectal US for cancer screening: The accuracy of in vitro and in vivo techniques. Radiology 1991; 179:48–53.

Lu DSK, Papanicolaou N, Girard M, et al: Percutaneous internal ureteral stent placement: Review of technical issues and solutions in 50 consecutive cases. Clin Radiol 1994; 49:256–261.

Lutzker LG: The fine points of scrotal scintigraphy. Semin Nucl Med 1982; 12:387–393.

Majd M, Rushton HG: Renal cortical scintigraphy in the diagnosis of acute pyelonephritis. Semin Nucl Med 1992; 22:98–111.

Marx MV: Interventional procedures: Risks to patients and personnel. *In* Radiation Risk: A Primer. Reston, VA, American College of Radiology, 1996, pp 23–25.

Mattrey RF: Magnetic resonance imaging of the scrotum. Semin Ultrasound CT MR 1991; 12:95–108.

McBiles M, Morita ET: Radionuclide imaging of the kidney, urinary tract and adrenals. *In* Davidson AJ, Hartman DS, eds: Radiology of the Kidney and Urinary Tract, 2nd ed. Philadelphia, W. B. Saunders Company, 1994, pp 33–51.

McClure RD, Hricak H: Scrotal ultrasound in the infertile man: Detection of subclinical unilateral and bilateral varicoceles. J Urol 1986; 135:711–715.

McLean GK, Meranze SG: Embolization techniques in the urinary tract. Radiol Clin North Am 1986; 24:671–682.

McNeal JE: Regional morphology and pathology of the prostate. Am J Clin Pathol 1968; 49:347–357.

McNicholas MMJ, Lee MJ, Mayo-Smith WN, et al: An imaging algorithm for the differential diagnosis of adrenal adenomas and metastases. AJR 1995; 165:1453–1459.

Middleton WD, Siegel BA, Melson GL, et al: Acute scrotal disorders: Prospective comparison of color Doppler US and testicular scintigraphy. Radiology 1990; 177:177–181.

Miller DL: Endocrine angiography and venous sampling. Radiol Clin North Am 1993; 31:1051–1067.

Mitchell DG, Crovello M, Matteucci T, et al: Benign adrenocortical masses: Diagnosis with chemical shift MR imaging. Radiology 1992; 185:345–352.

Mitty HA, Rackson ME, Dan SJ, et al: Experience with a new ureteral stent made of biocompatible polymer. Radiology 1988; 168:557–559.

Mitty HA, Shapiro RS, Parsons RB, et al: Renovascular hypertension. Radiol Clin North Am 1996; 34:1017–1036.

Motola JA, Badlani GH, Smith AD: Results of 212 consecutive endopyelotomies: An 8 year follow-up. J Urol 1993; 149:453–456.

Nadel L, Baumgertner BR, Bernardino ME: Percutaneous renal biopsies: Accuracy, safety, and indications. Urol Radiol 1986; 8:67–71.

Nally JV Jr, Black HR: State-of-the-art review: Captopril renography—Pathophysiological considerations and clinical observations. Semin Nucl Med 1992; 22:85–97.

Newhouse JH, Pfister RC: The nephrogram. Radiol Clin North Am 1979; 17:213–226.

O'Mara EM, Rifkin MD: Scrotum and contents. *In* Resnick ML, Rifkin MD, eds: Ultrasonography of the Urinary Tract, 3rd ed. Baltimore, Williams & Wilkins, 1991, pp 386–435.

Papanicolaou N: Renal anatomy relevant to percutaneous interventions. Semin Intervent Radiol 1995; 12:163–172.

Papanicolaou N, Eisenberg PJ, Silverman SG, et al: Prostatic biopsy after proctocolectomy: A transgluteal, CT-guided approach. AJR 1996; 166:1332–1334.

Papanicolaou N, Pfister RC: Acute renal infections. Radiol Clin North Am 1996; 34:965–995.

Papanicolaou N, Pfister RC, Nocks BN: Percutaneous, large-bore suprapubic cystostomy: Technique and results. AJR 1989; 152:303–306.

Patterson DE, Segura JW, LeRoy AJ, et al: The etiology and treatment of delayed bleeding following percutaneous lithotripsy. J Urol 1985; 133:447–451.

Pfister RC, Papanicolaou N, Yoder IC: Diagnostic morphologic and urodynamic antegrade pyelography. Radiol Clin North Am 1986; 24:561–571.

Platt JF, Rubin JM, Ellis JH: Distinction between obstructive and nonobstructive pyelocaliectasis with duplex Doppler sonography. AJR 1989; 153:997–1000.

Picus D, Weyman PJ, Clayman RV, et al: Intercostal-space nephrostomy for percutaneous stone removal. AJR 1986; 147:393–397.

Pollack HM: Brush biopsy of the upper urinary tract. *In* Pollack HM, ed: Clinical Urography. Philadelphia, W. B. Saunders Company, 1990, pp 2845–2853.

Pollack HM, Banner MP: Diagnostic uroradiology. *In* Hanno PM, Wein AJ, eds: Clinical Manual of Urology, 2nd ed. New York, McGraw-Hill, 1994, pp 89–136.

Raptopoulos V: Abdominal trauma: Emphasis on CT. Radiol Clin North Am 1994; 32:969–987.

Reddy PK, Moore L, Hunter D, Amplatz K: Percutaneous ureteral fulguration: A nonsurgical technique for ureteral occlusion. J Urol 1987; 138:724–726.

Resnick ML: Transrectal ultrasound guided versus digitally directed prostatic biopsy: A comparative study. J Urol 1988; 139:754–757.

Rifkin MD, Daehnert W, Kurtz AB: Progression radiology; state of the art: Endorectal sonography of the prostate. AJR 1990a; 154:691–700.

Rifkin MD, Resnick ML: Ultrasonography of the prostate. *In* Resnick ML, Rifkin MD, eds: Ultrasonography of the Urinary Tract, 3rd ed. Baltimore, Williams & Wilkins, 1991, pp 297–335.

Rifkin MD, Zerhouni EA, Gatsonis CA, et al: Comparison of magnetic resonance imaging and ultrasonography in staging early prostate cancer. N Engl J Med 1990b; 323:621–626.

Roberts JA: Pyelonephritis, cortical abscess, and perinephric abscess. Urol Clin North Am 1986; 13:367–374.

Roberts JP, Ascher NL, Fryd DS, et al: Transplant renal artery stenosis. Transplantation 1989; 48:580–583.

Roubidoux MA, Dunnick NR, Sostman HD, et al: Detection of venous extension of renal cell carcinoma by magnetic resonance imaging with gradient recalled echo sequences. Radiology 1992; 182:269–272.

Rubin GD: Spiral (helical) CT of the renal vasculature. Semin Ultrasound CT MR 1996; 17:374–397.

Sampaio FJB, Zanier JFC, Aragao AHM, et al: Intrarenal access: 3-dimensional anatomical study. J Urol 1992; 148:1769–1773.

Sandler CM, Houston GK, Hall JT, et al: Guided cyst puncture and aspiration. Radiol Clin North Am 1986; 24:527–537.

Schiebler ML, Schnall MD, Pollack HM, et al: Current role of MR imaging in the staging of adenocarcinoma of the prostate. Radiology 1993; 189:339–352.

Segura JW, Patterson DE, LeRoy AJ, et al: Percutaneous removal of kidney stones: Review of 1,000 cases. J Urol 1985; 134:1077–1081.

Semelka RC, Hricak H, Stevens SK, et al: Combined gadolinium-enhanced and fat saturation MR imaging of renal masses. Radiology 1991; 178:803–809.

Semelka RC, Shoenut JP, Kroeber MA, et al: Renal lesions: Controlled comparison between CT and 1.5 T MR imaging with nonenhanced and gadolinium-enhanced, fat-suppressed spin-echo and breath-held FLASH techniques. Radiology 1992; 182:425–430.

Setaro JF, Saddler MC, Chen CC, et al: Simplified captopril renography in diagnosis and treatment of renal artery stenosis. Hypertension 1991; 18:289–298.

Shellock FG, Morisoli S, Kanal E: MR procedures and biomedical implants, materials, and devices: 1993 update. Radiology 1993; 189:587–599.

Shapiro MJ, Banner MP, Amendola MA, et al: Balloon catheter dilatation of ureteroenteric strictures: Long-term results. Radiology 1988; 168:385–387.

Silverman SG, Mueller PR, Pfister RC: Hemostatic evaluation before abdominal interventions: An overview and proposal. AJR 1990; 154:233–238.

Sommer FG, Jeffrey RB Jr, Rubin GD: Detection of ureteral calculi in patients with suspected renal colic: Value of reformatted noncontrast helical CT. AJR 1995; 165:509–513.

Sos TA, Pickering TG, Sniderman K, et al: Percutaneous transluminal renal angioplasty in renovascular hypertension due to atheroma or fibromuscular dysplasia. N Engl J Med 1983; 309:274–279.

Stavros AT, Parker SH, Yakes WF, et al: Segmental stenosis of the renal artery: Pattern recognition of tardus and parvus abnormalities with duplex sonography. Radiology 1992; 184:487–492.

Taylor A Jr: Quantitation of renal function with static imaging agents. Semin Nucl Med 1982; 12:330–344.

Tegtmeyer CJ, Kellum CD, Ayers C: Percutaneous transluminal angioplasty of the renal artery: Results and long-term follow-up. Radiology 1984; 153:77–84.

Tung GA, Pfister RC, Papanicolaou N, et al: Adrenal cysts: Imaging and percutaneous aspiration. Radiology 1989; 173:107–110.

Van den Abbeele AD, Treves ST, Lebowitz RE, et al: Vesicoureteral reflux in asymptomatic siblings of patients with known reflux: Radionuclide cystography. Pediatrics 1987; 79:147–151.

Watson AD, Rocklage SM, Carvlin MJ: Contrast agents. *In* Stark DD, Bradley WG Jr, eds: Magnetic Resonance Imaging, 2nd ed. St. Louis, Mosby–Year Book, 1992, pp 347–372.

Weibull H, Bergquist D, Bergentz SE, et al: Percutaneous transluminal renal angioplasty versus surgical reconstruction of atherosclerotic renal stenosis: A prospective randomized study. J Vasc Surg 1993; 18:841–852.

Wheatley JK, Bergman WA, Green B, et al: Transvenous occlusion of clinical and subclinical varicoceles. Urology 1991; 37:362–365.

Willi UV, Atares M, Prader A, et al: Testicular adrenal-like tissue in congenital adrenal hyperplasia: Detection by sonography. Pediatr Radiol 1991; 21:284–287.

Wolfman NT, Bechtold RE, Watson NE: Ultrasonography of the normal kidney and diffuse renal disease. *In* Resnick ML, Rifkin MD, eds: Ultrasonography of the Urinary Tract, 3rd ed. Baltimore, Williams & Wilkins, 1991, pp 109–151.

Woodhouse CBJ, Kellett MJ, Bloom HJG: Percutaneous renal surgery and local radiotherapy in the management of renal pelvic transitional cell carcinoma. Br J Urol 1986; 58:245–249.

Young AT, Hunter DW, Castaneda-Zuniga WR, et al: Percutaneous extraction of urinary tract calculi: Use of the intercostal approach. Radiology 1985; 154:633–638.

Zeman RK, Cronan JJ, Rosenfield AT, et al: Renal cell carcinoma: Dynamic, thin-section CT assessment of vascular invasion and tumor vascularity. Radiology 1988; 167:393–396.

Zirinsky K, Auh YH, Rubenstein WR, et al: CT of the hyperdense renal cyst: Sonographic correlation. AJR 1984; 143:151–155.

III
RENAL PHYSIOLOGY AND PATHOPHYSIOLOGY

7
RENAL PHYSIOLOGY

Jon D. Blumenfeld, M.D.
E. Darracott Vaughan, Jr., M.D.

Regardless of whether at the bedside, in the operating room, or on the laboratory bench, the urologist is routinely challenged by problems that involve perturbations of kidney function and their metabolic sequelae. The purpose of this chapter is to review advances in renal physiology and thus provide a fundamental basis for the approach to the broader issues that are discussed throughout this textbook.

RENAL HEMODYNAMICS

Under resting conditions, the blood flow to the kidney is approximately 20% of the cardiac output. When expressed as flow per tissue weight, renal blood flow (RBF) is eight times greater than coronary blood flow. This reflects the low resistance of the renal circulation (Dworkin and Brenner, 1991). Blood enters the kidney through serial branches of the renal artery (interlobar, arcuate, and interlobular arteries) and enters the glomeruli through the afferent arterioles. Approximately 20% of the plasma reaching the glomeruli is filtered into renal tubules; the plasma that is not filtered exits the glomerulus through the efferent arteriole into the postglomerular capillaries. In nephrons located in the kidney cortex, these capillaries travel in close proximity to the tubules and modulate solute and water reabsorption by the kidneys. In juxtamedullary nephrons, located deeper in the medulla, the efferent arterioles branch out to form vasa recta, which participate in the countercurrent mechanism through which urine is highly concentrated and body water conserved (see later discussion).

The glomerular circulation promotes ultrafiltration of large volumes of fluid as a result of the excess transcapillary hydraulic pressure relative to oncotic pressure (Maddox and Brenner, 1996). The rate at which glomerular filtration proceeds is result of these opposing forces and can be expressed as

$$\begin{aligned} GFR &= K_f[(P_{gc} - P_B) - (\Pi_{gc} - \Pi_B)] \\ &= K_f(\Delta P - \Delta \Pi), \end{aligned}$$

where

GFR = the glomerular filtration rate
K_f = the glomerular ultrafiltration coefficient; related to the total surface area and water permeability of the capillary membrane
P_{gc} = glomerular capillary pressure
P_B = Bowman's space pressure
Π_{gc} = glomerular colloid osmotic pressure
Π_B = colloid osmotic pressure of the filtrate

Normally, the size and charge characteristics of the glomerular membrane are highly restrictive against the filtration of proteins so that the colloid osmotic pressure of the glomerular filtrate is negligible. P_{gc} and P_B remain relatively constant along the length of the glomerulus, whereas Π_{gc} increases progressively because of the filtration of protein-free fluid into Bowman's space. As Π_{gc} increases without an accompanying change in P_{gc}, the glomerular transcapillary pressure gradient decreases progressively from approximately 15 mm Hg (at the afferent arteriole) toward zero (at the efferent arteriole). The point at which filtration ceases is referred to as filtration pressure equilibrium (Arendhorst and Navar, 1992). During filtration pressure equilibrium, if renal plasma flow (RPF) decreases, there is more time for fluid transfer across the glomerular capillary. As a result, Π_{gc} increases rapidly, net filtration pressure is dissipated more proximally along the glomerular capillary, and GFR is decreased. It occurs at low RPF and is important because, in this setting, GFR is flow dependent and thus changes in proportion to changes in plasma flow.

Because the glomerulus is located between the afferent and efferent arterioles, selective changes in the arteriolar resistances that are caused by vasoactive substances will have a significant impact on glomerular hemodynamics (Figs. 7–1 and 7–2; Maddox et al, 1974a, 1974b; Casellas, 1984; Maddox and Brenner, 1996; Inman et al, 1994). **Afferent arteriolar vasoconstriction decreases both GFR and glomerular plasma flow.** When the afferent arteriole dilates, more arterial perfusion pressure is transmitted to the glomerulus, and both capillary flow and GFR increase. **In contrast, a selective increase in efferent arteriolar reduces glomerular plasma flow but increases glomerular pressure, and thus GFR increases.** This augmentation of GFR by efferent constriction will be limited by the associated decrease in plasma flow and the increase in plasma oncotic pressure (Arendhorst and Navar, 1992).

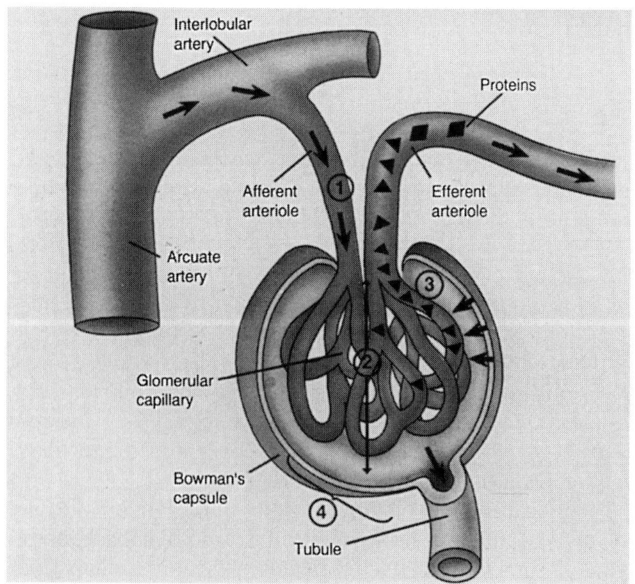

Figure 7–1. The renal microcirculation, highlighting factors that influence glomerular filtration. (From Inman S, Brouhard BH, Stowe NT: Cleve Clin J Med 1994; 61:179–185.)

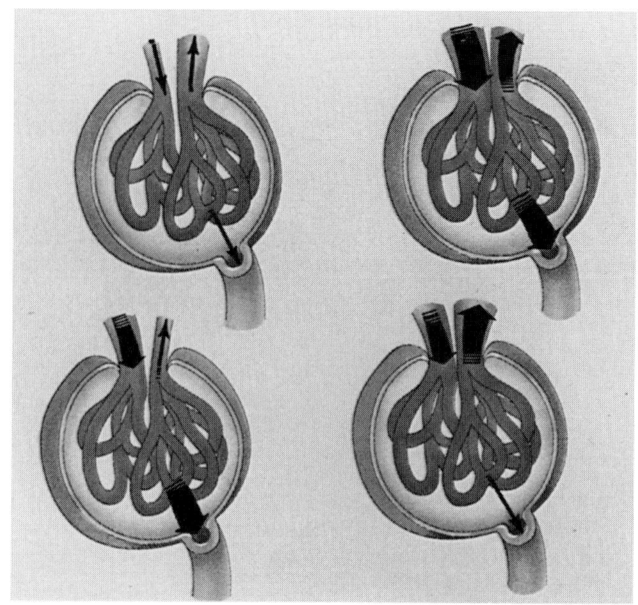

Figure 7–2. Effects of changes in diameter of the afferent and efferent arterioles on glomerular filtration and renal blood flow. *Top left:* constriction of afferent arteriole decreases RBF and GFR; *Top right:* dilatation of the afferent arteriole increases RBF and GFR; *Bottom left:* constriction of the efferent arteriole decreases RBF but increases GFR; *Bottom right:* dilatation of the efferent arteriole increases RBF but decreases GFR. (From Inman S, Brouhard BH, Stowe NT: Cleve Clin J Med 1994; 61:179–185.)

At the level of the whole kidney, arteriolar resistance accounts for approximately 85% of the total renal vascular resistance. The relation between these parameters and RPF can be expressed in the following equation:

$$RPF = \frac{\text{aortic pressure} - \text{renal venous pressure}}{\text{renal vascular resistance}}$$

Accordingly, increases in either afferent or efferent arteriolar tone will increase resistance and decrease RPF (Hall et al, 1995). However, the relation between RPF and GFR depends on whether the predominant change in tone occurs at the afferent or efferent arteriole. GFR and RPF change in parallel during afferent constriction, and so no change occurs in the filtration fraction, defined as the ratio GFR/RPF. In contrast, during efferent constriction, reciprocal changes in GFR and RPF occur. The resulting change in the ratio of GFR/RPF signifies that in general, a change in the filtration fraction accompanies constriction of the efferent but not afferent arteriole (Rose, 1989).

Autoregulation of Glomerular Filtration Rate

GFR and RBF are maintained within a narrow range despite relatively wide variations in blood pressure and, hence, renal perfusion pressure (Fig. 7–3). **As renal perfusion pressure increases, afferent arteriolar resistance increases proportionately so that glomerular hydraulic pressure and GFR do not change** (Maddox and Brenner, 1991). **Conversely, when blood pressure falls, afferent arteriolar resistance decreases, efferent arteriolar resistance increases, and GFR and RBF are preserved.** The mechanisms responsible for renal autoregulation are not completely understood. However, this process can occur in denervated, isolated perfused kidney preparations and in the absence of an intact macula densa–glomerular feedback system, and so it does not appear to be dependent upon these mechanisms (Maddox et al, 1974b).

Neural Control of Glomerular Filtration Rate

The kidney is innervated by adrenergic neurons arising primarily from the celiac plexus. Nerve fibers have been identified in the juxtaglomerular apparatus (afferent arteriole and juxtaglomerular cells, efferent arteriole, mesangium) and proximal and distal tubules and collecting duct (Tisher and Madsen, 1991). At very-low-frequency stimulation, renal sympathetic nerves selectively increase renin secretion (Fig. 7–4; Kopp et al, 1992; Zayas et al, 1993). This process is mediated through beta$_1$-adrenergic receptors on juxtaglomerular cells (Osborne et al, 1981). At slightly higher frequency stimulation, sodium reabsorption is enhanced through alpha-adrenergic receptors on the proximal tubule (see later discussion; Osborne et al, 1982). At higher frequency stimulation, GFR and RBF are reduced as a consequence of the predominant increase in preglomerular resistance (Kopp et al, 1992).

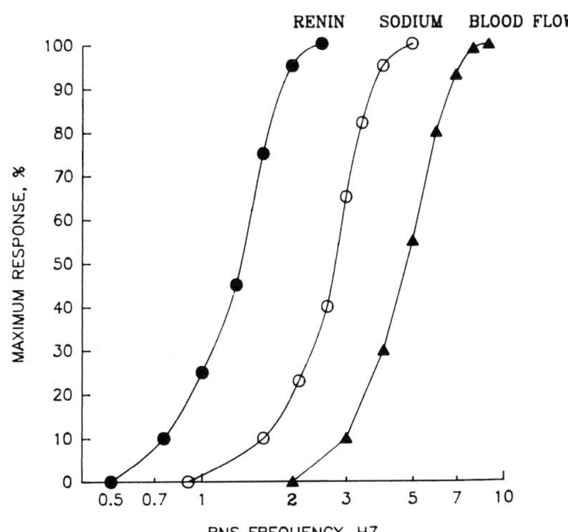

Figure 7–4. Relationship of effects of renal sympathetic nerve stimulation on responses of renin secretion (increase), urinary sodium excretion (decrease), and renal blood flow (decrease). (From DiBona GF, Kopp UC: Neural control of renal function: Role in human hypertension. *In* Laragh JH, Brenner BM, eds: Hypertension: Pathophysiology, Diagnosis, and Management, 2nd ed. New York, Raven Press, 1995, pp 1349–1358.)

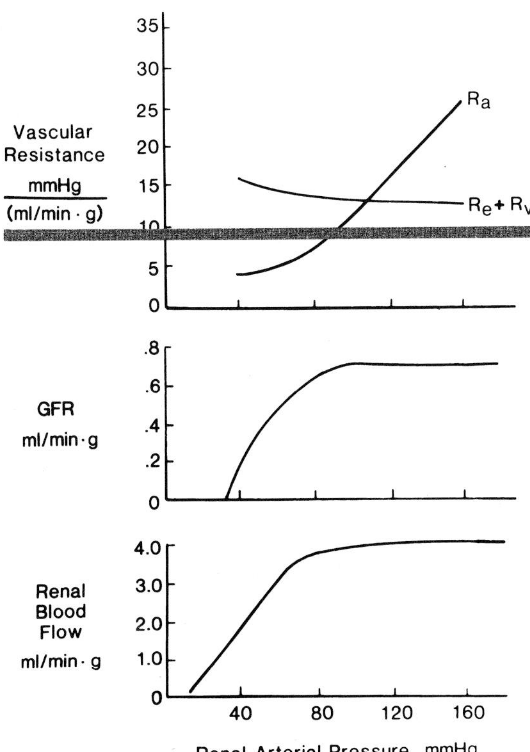

Figure 7–3. Relationships between renal arterial pressure and renal blood flow *(lower panel),* glomerular filtration rate (GFR; *middle panel*) and afferent arteriolar vascular resistance *(upper panel).* R_a = afferent arteriolar resistance; R_e = efferent arteriolar resistance; R_v = capillary and venous resistance. (From Arendhorst WJ, Navar LG: Renal circulation and glomerular hemodynamics. *In* Schrier RW, Gottschalk CW, eds: Diseases of the Kidney, 5th ed. Boston, Little, Brown, 1992, pp 65–117.)

Tubuloglomerular Feedback

The tubuloglomerular feedback response is defined by the increase in afferent arteriolar resistance, an increase that occurs when there is an increase in the delivery of fluid out of the proximal tubule to the loop of Henle. **Accordingly, this is a negative feedback system in which glomerular capillary pressure, a major determinant of GFR, is inversely related to fluid delivery to the distal nephron** (Briggs and Schnermann, 1995). The specialized cells of the juxtaglomerular apparatus (macula densa, juxtaglomerular cells, and extraglomerular mesangium) participate in this response (Barajas et al, 1995). The factors that determine the magnitude of the tubuloglomerular feedback include the chloride content of tubule fluid reabsorbed by the macula densa cells and the osmolality of distal tubular fluid. Afferent arteriolar constriction appears to occur in response to increased intracellular calcium in juxtaglomerular cells. Renin secretion decreases during tubuloglomerular feedback, possibly in response to the increased intracellular calcium (Bell et al, 1987). This reduction in renin-angiotensin, in the setting of ongoing volume expansion, is adaptive in that it allows GFR to increase and reduces reabsorption of tubular fluid. Nitric oxide synthase has been identified in macula densa cells, and local production of nitric oxide generation by these cells has been found to vasodilate the afferent arteriole (Wilcox et al, 1992b). These findings suggest that local production of nitric oxide by an individual nephron can modulate the tubuloglomerular feedback response.

Hormones and Vasoactive Substances

RBF and, in turn, GFR are modified by a variety of hormones and vasoactive substances that have direct actions on arcuate and interlobular arteries and on afferent and efferent arterioles. In addition, important alterations in the ultrafiltration coefficient (K_f), a primary determinant of GFR, occurs in response to the direct actions of some of these substances on glomerular capillaries and mesangial cells (Maddox et al, 1996; Romero et al, 1995).

Vasoconstrictors

The renal vasoconstrictor substances, including angiotensin II, norepinephrine, leukotrienes, endothelin, vasopressin, and epidermal growth factor have similar pathways for their physiologic actions (Maddox et al, 1991). Upon binding to their specific cell surface receptors, membrane-bound phospholipase C is activated by the related guanine nucleotide–binding proteins (G proteins). This catalyzes the formation of phosphoinositides inositol 1,4,5-trisphosphate (IP_3) and 1,2-diacylglycerol (DAG). There is a rapid increase in the concentration of intracellular free calcium in vascular smooth muscle and mesangial cells. In addition to their vasoconstrictor effects, these hormones and vasoactive molecules also share the ability to stimulate the formation of vasodilator prostaglandins, such as prostaglandin E_2 (PGE_2) and prostaglandin I_2 (PGI_2).[52] This provides a mechanism for attenuating the vasoconstrictor effects.

ANGIOTENSIN II. During intravenous infusion at pressor doses, angiotensin II (Ang II) stimulates vasoconstriction of the efferent arteriole and, to a lesser magnitude, the afferent arteriole (Fig. 7–5; Hall and Brands, 1992). In addition, pressor and nonpressor doses of Ang II decrease K_f through its actions on the glomerular mesangium (Scharschmidt et al, 1986). Although RBF and K_f decrease, GFR does not change significantly because the transcapillary hydraulic pressure difference (ΔP) increases. However, in certain experimental settings, such as the model of unilateral hydronephrosis, Ang II can stimulate marked vasoconstriction of both the preglomerular and postglomerular vasculature (Steinhausen et al, 1987). **Elevated levels of Ang II are important for maintaining GFR in physiologic conditions (i.e., dietary Na⁺ restriction) and in disease states** (i.e., congestive heart failure; see the sections on the renin-angiotensin-aldosterone system and volume homeostasis).

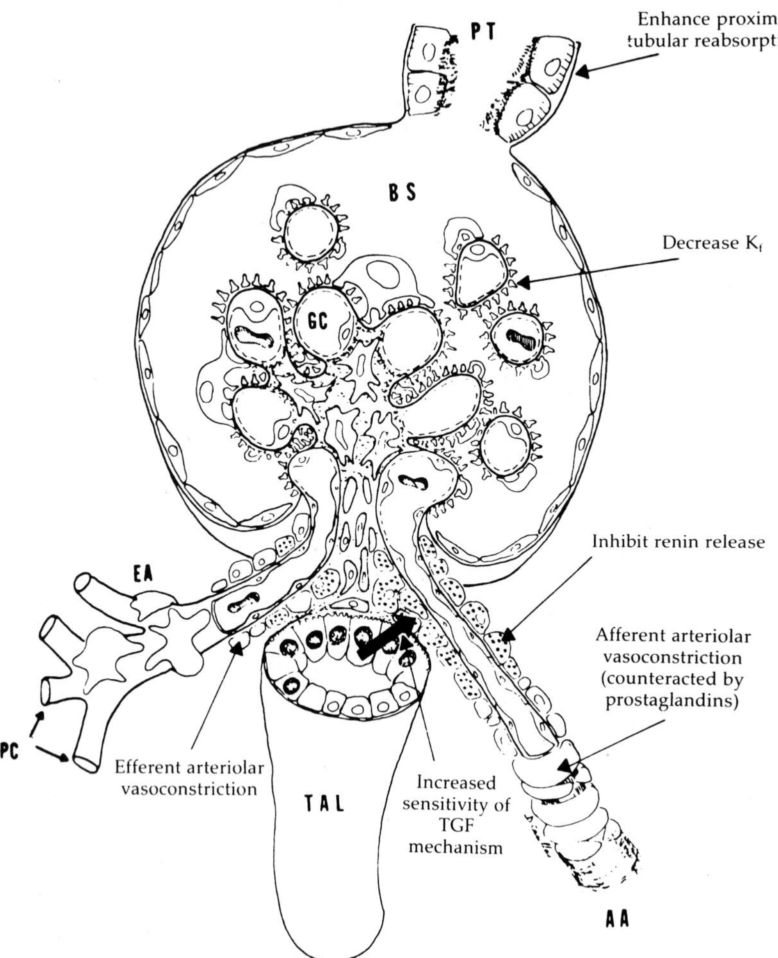

Figure 7–5. Multiple actions of angiotensin II on renal function. PT = proximal tubule; BS = Bowman's space; GC = glomerular capillary; EA = efferent arteriole; PC = peritubular capillaries; TAL = thick ascending limb of Henle; AA = afferent arteriole; TGF = Tubuloglomerular feedback. (From Arendhorst WJ, Navar LG: Renal circulation and glomerular hemodynamics. *In* Schrier RW, Gottschalk CW, eds: Diseases of the Kidney, 5th ed. Boston, Little, Brown, 1992, pp 65–117.)

NOREPINEPHRINE. Norepinephrine vasoconstricts interlobular, afferent, and efferent vessels in vitro (Carmines et al, 1986). The vasoconstrictor effects of norepinephrine are mediated through alpha$_1$-adrenergic receptors. Another alpha-adrenergic receptor–mediated action of norepinephrine is mesangial cell contraction (Maddox et al, 1996). Like Ang II, norepinephrine also stimulates production of vasodilator prostaglandins such as PGE_2 (Mene and Dunn, 1992).

Norepinephrine also has beta$_1$-adrenergic receptor mediated actions at the renal microvasculature. It stimulates renin secretion by juxtaglomerular cells located at the afferent arteriole (Osborne et al, 1981; Zayas et al, 1993) and thus promotes Ang II formation.

ENDOTHELIN. Endothelin (ET) is the most potent renal vasoconstrictor yet identified: it is more than 10 times as potent as Ang II and norepinephrine (Clavell and Burnett, 1994). ET is a 21–amino acid polypeptide with biosynthetic precursors that include proendothelin (big endothelin), which is cleaved by ET converting enzyme to the active peptide (Yanagisawa et al, 1988). There are three isoforms: ET-1, ET-2, and ET-3; ET-1 was the first to be discovered, and its physiologic actions have been characterized more fully than the other isoforms (Luscher, 1994). It is produced de novo primarily in endothelial cells, without apparent sites for intracellular storage. Secretion from these cells occurs predominantly at the basal surface, so that 80% of the total amount is directed toward the underlying vascular smooth muscle rather than toward the lumen of the vessel (Simonson and Dunn, 1993). Accordingly, the plasma levels of ET are normally very low. Furthermore, ET is cleared very rapidly after an infusion. These features suggest that the response to ET is determined by its local concentration rather than the level in the peripheral circulation.

In the kidney, ET has been identified in the vascular endothelium of arcuate arteries, arterioles, veins, glomerular capillaries, peritubular capillaries, and vasa recta (King, 1995). ET synthesis has also been identified in non-endothelial cells, including glomerular mesangial cells. ET has also been localized to renal tubule epithelial cells in cell culture systems derived from microdissected nephron segments; the greatest abundance has been found in medullary collecting duct cells.

ET actions are mediated through highly specific receptors located on the cell surface (Fig. 7–6; Luscher, 1994). There are at least two receptor subtypes, ET_A and ET_B, that belong to the G-coupled receptor family. The ET_A receptor is expressed by renal vascular smooth muscle cells, and ET_B receptors are located on endothelial cells of the glomerulus and vasa recta. ET is produced by the kidney and also has its actions there, supporting the concept that ET can exert its effects by paracrine or autocrine modes. For example, glomerular endothelial cells can synthesize ET and have receptors for it, which suggests an autocrine action. In addition, ET may also diffuse from glomerular endothelial cells

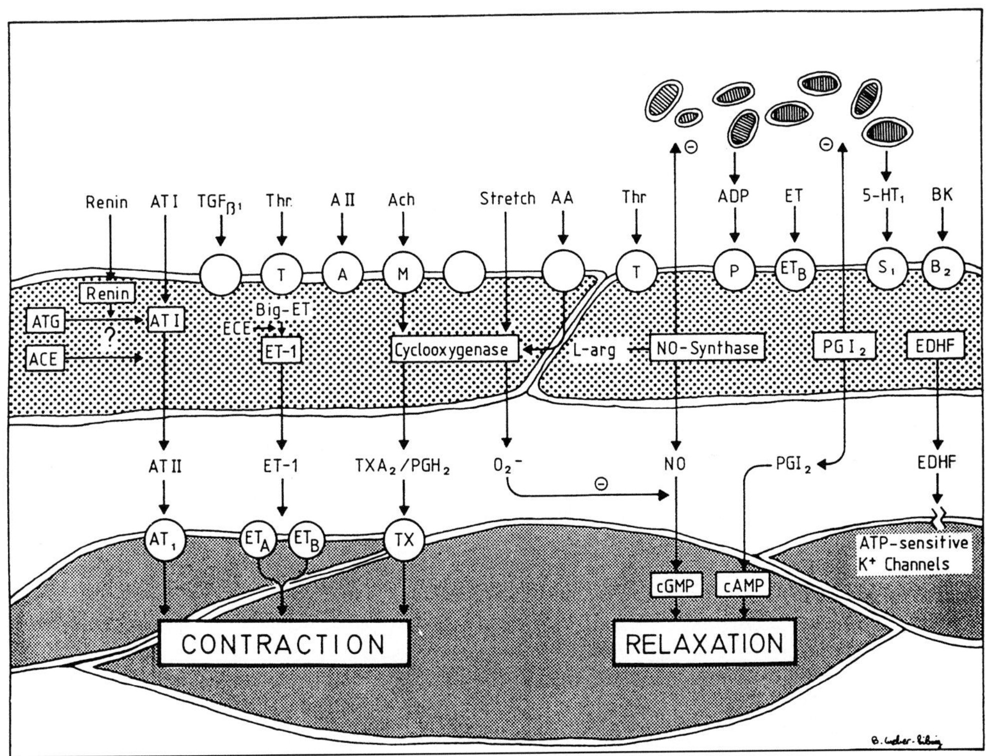

Figure 7–6. Endothelium-derived relaxing factors (right) and contracting factors (left). ATI, angiotensin I; $TGF_{\beta 1}$, transforming growth factor β^1; Thr, thrombin; AII, angiotensin II; Ach, acetylcholine; AA, arachidonic acid; ADP, adenosine diphosphate; ET, endothelin; 5-HT$_1$, 5-hydroxytryptamine; BK, bradykinin; T, thrombin receptor; AT_1, A angiotensin receptor; M, acetylcholine (muscarinic) receptor; P, purinergic receptor; ET_B, endothelin subtype B; S_1, serotonin receptor; B_2, bradykinin receptor; ATG, angiotensinogen; ACE, angiotensin converting enzyme; Big-ET, big endothelin; ECE, endothelin converting enzyme; ET-1, endothelin-1; L-arg, L-arginine; NO, nitric oxide; PGI_2, prostaglandin I_2; EDHF, endothelin derived hyperpolarizing factor; ATII, angiotensin II; TxA_2PGH_2, thromboxane A_2–prostaglandin H_2; ET_A, endothelin subtype A; TX, thromboxane; cGMP, cyclic 3′,5′-guanosine monophosphate; cAMP, cyclic 3′,5′-adenosine monophosphate; ATP, adenosine triphosphate. (From Luscher TF, Duben RK: Endothelium and platelet-derived vasoactive substances: Role in the regulation of vascular tone and growth. *In* Laragh JH, Brenner BM, eds: Hypertension: Pathophysiology, Diagnosis, and Management, 2nd ed. New York, Raven Press, 1992, pp 609–630.)

and bind to mesangial cell receptors, in which case a paracrine mode of action would be operative. However, the factors that regulate ET receptors and determine how the cells are specifically targeted have not been completely defined.

ET has significant effects on renal hemodynamic and excretory function when assessed in a variety of experimental models (Kon and Badr, 1991). Systemic infusion leads to an initial, transient fall in blood pressure and decreased renal vascular resistance that is caused by release of the endothelial vasodilators nitric oxide and prostacyclin. This is followed by intense systemic and renal vasoconstriction, decreased renal blood flow, reduced GFR, and elevated blood pressure that are augmented by inhibitors of prostaglandin synthesis. Endothelin also has been reported to increase cardiac output, possibly through a direct inotropic effect that is not attenuated by blockade of adrenergic receptors.

In addition to these hemodynamic effects, ET also has complex effects on sodium and water balance (Simonson and Dunn, 1993). In vivo systemic infusion of ET decreases sodium excretion. However, this response reflects the aggregate effects of (1) the reduced filtered load of sodium that occurs as the GFR decreases and (2) the stimulation of renin secretion by intrarenal baroreceptor and macula densa mechanisms that augment aldosterone secretion. However, in vitro studies, such as those demonstrating that ET specifically inhibits arginine vasopressin (AVP)–mediated cyclic adenosine monophosphate (cAMP) accumulation in the collecting duct, suggest that ET may promote excretion of sodium and water.

It is apparent from this discussion that the integrated effects of ET on blood pressure homeostasis are not yet established. However, several interesting observations point to a possible role of ET in the pathophysiology of certain hypertensive disorders. For example, cyclosporin-induced hypertension is associated with renal vasoconstriction (Kon and Badr, 1991). Studies in animal models have shown that local infusion of an anti-ET antibody prevents cyclosporine-associated renal hypoperfusion and the accompanying glomerular dysfunction. ET has also been proposed as an important mediator of postischemic acute renal failure and radiocontrast nephropathy (Oldroyd et al, 1994; King, 1995). However, the role of ET in these disorders and in the growing number of pathologic states associated with elevated plasma levels ET has yet to be established.

VASOPRESSIN. Vasopressin contracts mesangial cells in a way similar to that observed with Ang II. However, this vasopressin action is not dependent on Ang II and appears to be mediated by the V_1 receptor subtype. This response contributes to the reduction in K_f described by Ichikawa and Brenner (1977). No change in renal blood flow occurred in those studies. However, single-nephron GFR was maintained because of a decrease in proximal tubule hydraulic pressure and, hence, a net increase in ΔP. The V_1 receptor does not participate directly in the vasopressin-mediated increase in hydraulic permeability of the collecting duct (see later discussion).

LEUKOTRIENES AND LIPOXINS. Leukotrienes are compounds formed from arachidonic acid by the 5-lipoxygenase enzymes (Maddox et al, 1996) from activated inflammatory cells. Leukotriene C_4 (LTC_4) and leukotriene D_4 (LTD_4) are two molecules in this class that have vasoconstrictor actions that are qualitatively and quantitatively similar to those of Ang II (Badr and Jacobson, 1991). Intravenous infusion increases efferent and afferent arteriolar vasoconstriction, decreases renal blood flow and K_f, and reduces GFR. These compounds also appear to participate in the renal hemodynamic responses to endotoxin that result in acute renal failure (Badr et al, 1986). In addition, leukotrienes also appear to promote formation of inflammatory exudate by increasing permeability of the vasculature to macromolecules (Badr, 1992).

Lipoxins are arachidonic acid metabolites formed by 15-lipoxygenase enzymes in polymorphonuclear neutrophils. Lipoxin A specifically vasodilates the afferent arteriole and decreases K_f, without altering postglomerular resistance (Badr et al, 1987). The net result is an increase in single-nephron GFR.

ATRIAL NATRIURETIC PEPTIDE. Atrial natriuretic peptide (ANP) is a vasoactive natriuretic hormone synthesized primarily by the atria in response to stretching, such as that which occurs during physiologic levels of volume expansion (Fig. 7–7). There are two types of ANP receptors (Maack, 1995). The biologic receptor mediates the actions of ANP through activation of membrane-associated guanylate cyclase and the second messenger, cyclic guanosine monophosphate (cGMP). The clearance receptor is far more abundant and is not associated with cGMP. Its main role is in the regulation of circulating levels of ANP.

The natriuretic action of ANP is the consequence of in-

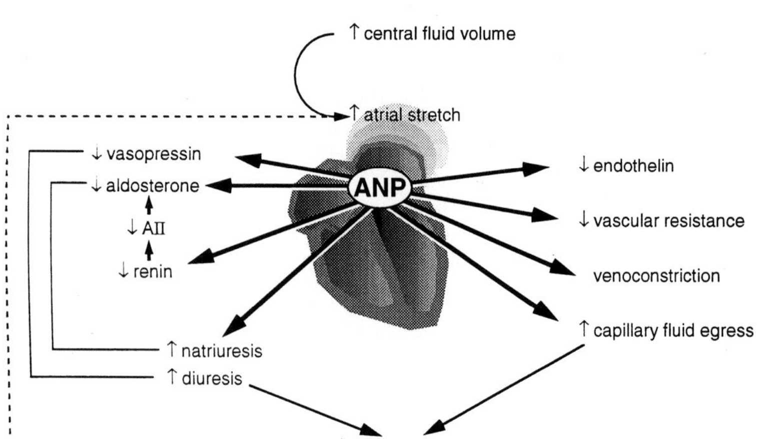

Figure 7–7. A schematic representation of the fundamental biologic processes of atrial natriuretic peptide (ANP). AII, angiotensin II. (From Lewicki JA, Protter AA: Physiologic studies of the natriuretic peptide family. *In* Laragh JH, Brenner BM, eds: Hypertension: Pathophysiology, Diagnosis, and Management, 2nd ed. New York, Raven Press, 1995, pp 1029–1054.)

creases in GFR and a direct effect on the inner medullary collecting duct (Lewicki and Protter, 1995). **ANP can independently increase GFR without a corresponding increase in RBF as a consequence of simultaneous afferent arteriolar vasodilatation, efferent arteriolar constriction, and increases in K_f.** This action accounts for the associated increase in the filtration fraction. In addition, ANP dilates vessels that have been preconstricted by norepinephrine, Ang II, vasopressin, and other agents. Redistribution of intrarenal blood flow to the medulla may also contribute to solute washout, although a direct effect of ANP on inner medullary collecting ducts to decrease sodium reabsorption may also contribute to this response.

ANP also exerts its natriuretic action by suppressing renin secretion (Laragh, 1985). This action is partly the result of the increased filtered load of sodium and chloride reaching the macula densa. Renin secretion is also inhibited in vitro when cGMP levels in juxtaglomerular cells are increased by ANP. Furthermore, ANP selectively reduces basal secretion of aldosterone and blocks aldosterone secretion induced by Ang II, but it has no effect on cortisol production.

Levels of ANP and its second messenger, cGMP, are increased in heart failure (Cody et al, 1986). However, the renal responses to ANP, including urinary sodium excretion, are attenuated in severe heart failure. Nevertheless, results of some studies suggest that despite the kidney's refractoriness to ANP, many extrarenal responses are preserved. Specifically, ANP infusion lowers plasma aldosterone in human heart failure, despite persistently elevated plasma renin activity. Also, short-term infusions have been shown to decrease systemic vascular resistance and cardiac preload, as well as to raise cardiac output in both clinical and experimental heart failure. Thus, the preservation of these extrarenal actions suggests that increased ANP secretion by the failing heart could provide a compensatory mechanism that to some extent mitigates against circulatory overload.

PARATHYROID HORMONE. Administration of parathyroid hormone (PTH) in parathyroidectomized animals caused a significant decrease in single nephron GFR by reducing K_f, and there was no change in renal blood flow in that model (Ichikawa, 1978). Furthermore, the decrement in GFR in hypercalcemia is dependent on the fall in K_f that is related to PTH and can be abolished by parathyroidectomy (Humes et al, 1978). Pretreatment with the Ang II receptor antagonist saralasin abolishes this PTH-related fall in K_f. Therefore, the glomerular effects of PTH appear to be mediated by Ang II, which is stimulated by cAMP production (Brenner et al, 1982).

Vasodilators

Nitric Oxide

In 1980, Furchgott and Zawadski reported that acetylcholine-induced vasorelaxation was not prevented by inhibitors of the vasodilator prostacyclin in vessels with an intact endothelium. It has subsequently become clear that nitric oxide is the endothelium-derived relaxing factor (EDRF) responsible for this response. **Synthesis of nitric oxide by the vascular endothelium is an important determinant of vascular tone that, under normal conditions, contributes to the regulation of systemic blood pressure and blood flow to regional circulations** (Umans and Levi, 1995).

Nitric oxide (NO) production occurs in many cell types in response to a variety of different stimuli (Moncada and Higgs, 1993). NO synthase is the enzyme responsible for NO synthesis from its precursor arginine. Each of the isoforms of this enzyme contain heme and have in common arginine as a substrate, which is oxidized to NO and citrulline coproducts. **The endothelial isoform is stimulated through receptor operator mechanisms by vasoactive compounds, including acetylcholine, bradykinin, serotonin, and other substances derived from platelets and the coagulation system.** In addition, NO production by this isoform is also stimulated by mechanical forces, such as shear stress exerted by circulating blood. Other isozymes of NO synthase include the inducible form (iNOS) and the neuronal form (nNOS). The inducible enzyme is expressed in several cell types, including macrophages and vascular smooth muscle in response to mediators of inflammation (Nathan, 1992).

After its formation in endothelial cells, NO diffuses to adjacent vascular smooth muscle, where it stimulates soluble guanylyl cyclase, increases cGMP, and consequently dilates blood vessels. NO is rapidly inactivated by superoxide anion, by oxygen, and by binding to hemoglobin (Simonson and Dunn, 1993). **Competitive inhibitors of NO synthase (e.g., N^G-monomethyl-L-arginine [L-NMMA]) decrease NO production and are potent vasoconstrictors that can decrease regional blood flow and elevate systemic blood pressure.** These findings indicate that NO-mediated vasodilatation contributes importantly to the basal vascular tone (Umans and Levi, 1995; Cowley et al, 1995).

EFFECTS ON KIDNEY FUNCTION. Several experimental findings indicate that NO has direct effects on renal vascular and tubular function. For example, when competitive antagonists of NO synthase are given to experimental animals acutely by intravenous injection or are administered for several weeks in their drinking water, there are profound effects on the glomerular microcirculation. Characteristic changes that occur during NO synthase inhibition include marked increases in resistances in afferent and, predominantly, in efferent arterioles that result in elevated glomerular capillary pressure and reduced renal blood flow. The K_f also declines significantly during NO synthase inhibition (Simonson and Dunn, 1993; Romero et al, 1995; Cowley et al, 1995). These microvascular changes are accompanied by a significant reduction in sodium reabsorption by the proximal tubule. Furthermore, systemic hypertension occurs in concert with these changes in renal hemodynamic and excretory function.

The acute rise in blood pressure that occurs during systemic NO synthase inhibition promotes an increase in urinary Na^+ excretion. However, when intrarenal perfusion pressure is not permitted to increase, NO synthase inhibition is antinatriuretic and antidiuretic (Umans and Levi, 1995). The renal medulla appears to be an important locus for this NO-mediated pressure natriuresis (Cowley et al, 1995). For example, infusion of an inhibitor of NO synthase directly into the renal medullary interstitium decreased medullary blood flow, medullary interstitial pressure, and excretion of Na^+ and water. However, no changes in GFR, RBF, or arterial blood pressure occurred. Conversely, intrarenal infusion of bradykinin increases medullary blood flow and promotes natriuresis and diuresis (Roman et al, 1988). These bradykinin effects appear to be mediated by NO as they are blocked by NO synthase inhibition (Cowley et al, 1995). A role for NO in maintenance of Na^+ balance is also suggested by the direct relationship between dietary Na^+ intake and urinary excretion of the NO degradation products nitrate and nitrite (Umans and Levi, 1995).

NO synthase has been localized in the macula densa cells of the thick ascending limb of Henle and is activated by tubule fluid reabsorption (Wilcox et al, 1992b). These cells are components of the juxtaglomerular apparatus that regulates renin secretion and contributes to the tubuloglomerular feedback response (Briggs and Schnermann, 1995). This feedback system has been implicated in the regulation of renin release, renal autoregulation, and the long-term body fluid and pressure homeostasis. However, the role of NO as a potential regulator of renin secretion is incompletely defined.

Glucocorticoids

GFR increases during prolonged administration of glucocorticoids (Baylis and Brenner, 1978). This increase is caused primarily by the significant reductions in afferent and efferent arteriolar resistances and the related increase in RBF.

Role of Peritubular Capillaries in Fluid Reabsorption

Approximately 99% of the 180 L of glomerular filtrate that is formed each day is reabsorbed by the renal tubules, where it subsequently enters the postglomerular circulation. Reabsorption of fluid by peritubular capillaries is analogous to the process of filtration described earlier, in as much as it is the net result of an imbalance of hydrostatic and osmotic forces between the interstitial space and capillaries. This relationship can be expressed as follows:

$$PR = K_f [(\Pi_c - \Pi_i) - (P_c - P_i)],$$

where

PR = peritubular capillary reabsorption
K_f = the reabsorptive coefficient
Π_c = capillary osmotic pressure
Π_i = interstitial fluid osmotic pressure
P_c = capillary fluid hydrostatic pressure
P_i = interstitial fluid hydrostatic pressure

The Π_i and P_i are approximately equal (approximately 6–8 mm Hg) and therefore tend to cancel each other out. In contrast, as plasma emerges from the efferent arteriole, it has a higher colloid osmotic pressure (35 mm Hg) and a lower hydrostatic pressure (20 mm Hg) than when it entered the glomerulus. Consequently, there is a net reabsorptive force at the initial portion of the peritubular capillary. Fluid is reabsorbed along the length of these vessels, with a decrease in Π_c accompanied by a small reduction in P_c. Changes in filtration fraction will alter these physical forces and thus influence the rate of peritubular capillary reabsorption (Fig. 7–8). An increase in filtration fraction promotes reabsorption by increasing Π_c and decreasing P_c; a decrease

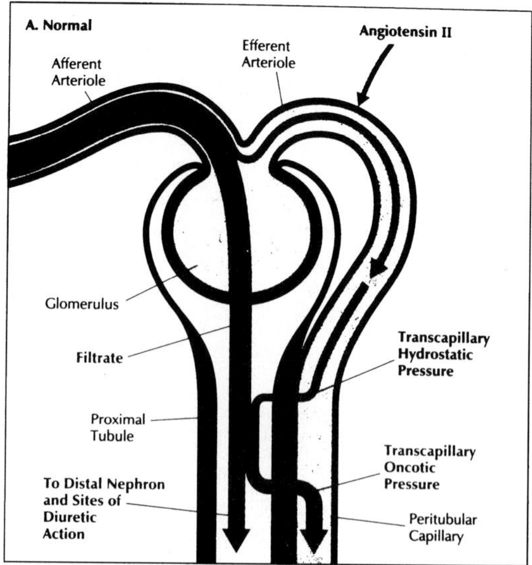

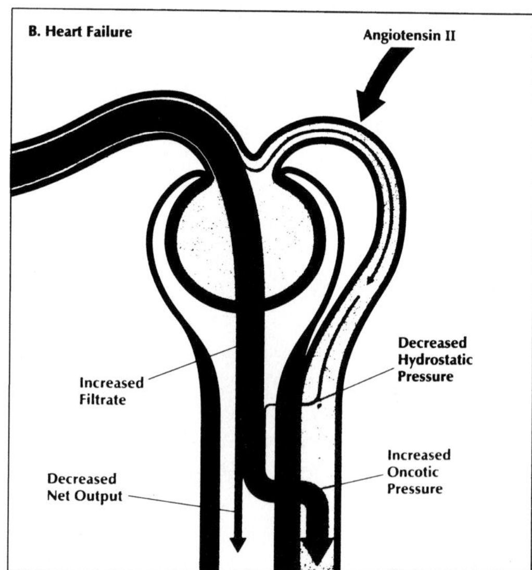

Figure 7–8. Effects of angiotensin II on glomerular and peritubular capillary hemodynamics in kidney from normal subjects *(A)* and subjects with congestive heart failure *(B)*. The renal hemodynamic responses in *B* are similar to those in patients with high plasma angiotensin II associated with a decreased effective extracellular fluid volume level, such as sodium depletion, cirrhosis, and nephrotic syndrome. (From Smith TW, Kelley RA: Hosp Pract 1991; 26[11]:127.)

in filtration fraction attenuates reabsorption (Arendhorst and Navar, 1992). Perturbations in these responses contribute to excessive sodium retention in edematous states such as congestive heart failure, cirrhosis, and nephrotic syndrome (Schrier, 1988; Blumenfeld and Laragh, 1994).

As with the glomerular capillary membrane, the peritubular capillary is relatively impermeable to protein. This is in contrast to the lymphatic capillaries, located primarily in the cortex, which are highly permeable for protein and fluid. **Protein that has leaked out of the capillaries is returned to the circulation by the renal lymphatics.** Under normal circumstances, the rate of renal lymphatic flow is only 1% of that of plasma, although it increases in the settings of increased renal venous pressure, increased ureteral pressure, and other conditions in which interstitial pressure is augmented (Arendhorst and Navar, 1992).

Efferent arterioles from juxtamedullary nephrons branch to form vasa recta, which descend deep into the medulla and are intimately associated with the loops of Henle and collecting ducts. The medullary circulation is characterized by low blood flow and an efficient countercurrent exchange. This system promotes shunting of fluid from descending to ascending limbs while trapping fluid and low-molecular-weight solutes at a hairpin turn in the inner medulla, after they have been reabsorbed from the tubules (Dworkin and Brenner, 1991).

Clinical Assessment of Glomerular Filtration Rate

The renal clearance of a substance, defined as the virtual volume of plasma per unit time from which the substance is completely removed, is expressed by the equation

$$C_i = U_i x V / P_i,$$

where x is the substance; U_i and P_i are the concentrations of the substance in urine and plasma, respectively; V is urine flow; and C_i is the clearance (Schuster and Seldin, 1992).

For a substance that is cleared solely by glomerular filtration and is neither reabsorbed nor secreted by the tubules, renal excretion is determined exclusively by the GFR and concentration of the substance in plasma:

$$U_i x V = GFR x P_i$$
$$GFR = U_i x V / P_i$$
$$GFR = C_i$$

Inulin

Inulin, a 5200-dalton polymer of fructose obtained from plants, is an example of a substance that is cleared solely by glomerular filtration. Inulin clearance, and thus GFR, is determined by measuring the concentration of inulin in urine and plasma samples obtained during intravenous inulin infusion.

Creatinine

Although inulin clearance is the most precise measurement of GFR, it is cumbersome and necessitates specific laboratory expertise (Levey et al, 1991); therefore, it is not used for the routine clinical assessment of GFR. Instead, levels of the endogenous compounds (e.g., creatinine) are measured more commonly to provide estimates of GFR. Creatinine is generated by the nonenzymatic conversion from creatine and phosphocreatine, which are present in muscle. Creatinine is a small molecule (113 daltons) that is freely filtered by the glomerulus and is not metabolized by the kidney. However, creatinine is secreted by the organic cation transporter of the proximal tubule. **Therefore, creatinine clearance (Ccr) is not solely due to glomerular filtration, but also reflect tubular secretion** (Doolan et al, 1962). **In other words, Ccr exceeds GFR at all levels of renal function** (Levey et al, 1991).

The levels of creatinine in serum, plasma, and urine are falsely elevated by about 20% when measured by the traditional colorimetric assay because of cross-reacting materials (e.g., glucose, protein, urate, pyruvate) normally found in those body fluids (Levey et al, 1991). In addition, other non-creatinine chromogens (i.e., cephalosporins) can falsely elevate the serum creatinine level. The autoanalyzer and imidohydrolase methods, now widely used, have been modified to remove most of these interfering substances (Osberg and Hammond, 1978). In addition to these methodologic issues, there is significant variability in the measurement of serum creatinine; the coefficient of variation for repeated measurements in an individual is 11% when the GFR is greater than 30 ml/minute (Levey et al, 1991). Coincidentally, the overestimation of creatinine in serum (but not urine) by Jaffe's reaction compensates for the excess contribution of creatinine to the urine by tubular secretion.

The absolute difference between Ccr and GFR is greatest within the GFR range of 40–80 ml/minute/1.73m², where the Ccr/GFR ratio is 1.5–2.0. At a GFR below this range, the absolute difference between Ccr and GFR is less, but the ratio of Ccr/GFR may increase further (Shemesh et al, 1985).

Ccr is assessed by collecting a 24-hour urine sample and measuring the creatinine concentration from that sample and from a serum sample drawn at the end of the 24-hour urine collection. The major source of error is derived from the timed urine collection. The following formulas, derived from patients without renal or hepatic disease, can be used to estimate whether the amount of creatinine that is collected is appropriate for the individual's age and body weight and thus to determine whether the 24-hour urine sample has been collected correctly:

$$\text{for men:}\quad U_{cr}V = 28.2 - 0.172 \times \text{age}$$
$$\text{for women:}\quad U_{cr}V = 21.9 - 0.115 \times \text{age}$$

where creatinine excretion ($U_{cr}V$) is expressed as milligrams/kilograms/day and age is in years. This estimate is influenced by factors that modify the creatinine pool, including animal protein intake and the presence of muscle-wasting disorders (Levey et al, 1991).

Ccr for an individual can be calculated from the formula described by Cockcroft and Gault (1976), in which the estimation is based on age, sex, and lean body mass:

$$\text{for men:}\quad Ccr = (140 - \text{age}) \times \frac{\text{weight}}{(Pcr \times 72)}$$

$$\text{for women:}\quad Ccr = (140 - \text{age}) \times \frac{\text{weight}}{(Pcr \times 85)}$$

where Ccr is expressed as milliliters/minute, age as years, weight as kilograms, and plasma creatinine as milligrams/deciliter. Several assumptions are made when this formula is employed: (1) lean body mass is used in the calculation, and thus an overestimate can occur in obese or edematous patients, and (2) creatinine production and volume of distribution are in steady state, but this may not be true in certain situations such as rhabdomyolysis (Levey et al, 1991).

Urea

As discussed earlier, urea clearance is normally less than GFR because urea is reabsorbed by the nephron. The ratio of urea clearance to GFR is related to the state of hydration and ranges from 0.65 during diuresis to 0.35 during antidiuresis (Chasis and Smith, 1938). In addition, blood urea nitrogen level is influenced by several other factors, including age and dietary protein intake. Thus, urea clearance is not an accurate measurement of GFR. However, a low ratio of urea to creatinine clearance may be useful in assessing the mechanism of renal insufficiency (see Chapter 8).

Sites of Sodium Reabsorption in the Nephron

Proximal Tubule

The proximal tubule reabsorbs approximately 60%–70% of the glomerular filtrate (Fig. 7–9). Reabsorption by this segment is isosmotic and is driven by primarily the sodium-potassium-adenosine triphosphatase (Na-K-ATPase) pump located at the basolateral membrane (Berry and Rector, 1991). **This pump maintains a low intracellular sodium concentration and thereby establishes an electrochemical driving force for transepithelial transport of sodium together with other filtered solutes.** Sodium entry is passive and occurs eletrogenically through luminal channels or can be associated with other solutes by carrier-mediated mechanisms. One example is the Na-H antiporter, which is the second most important determinant of proximal tubular sodium and water reabsorption, in addition to its role in bicarbonate reabsorption. Furthermore, Ang II directly stimulates Na-H exchange, which accounts for part of this hormone's action in the regulation of body volume. Fluid and solutes reabsorbed by the proximal tubule enter the intercellular

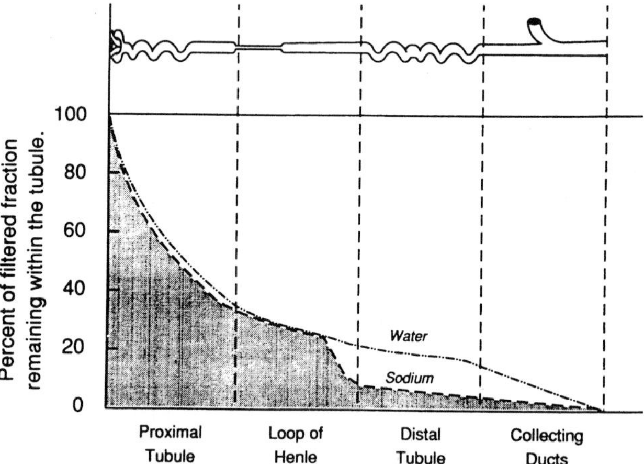

Figure 7–9. Percentage of filtered fractions of sodium and water remaining within the tubule at various nephron segments. Note that in the proximal tubule there is concomitant reabsorption of sodium and water. From the end of the proximal tubule on, sodium and water are reabsorbed independently. (From Gonzalez-Campoy JM, Knox FG: Integrated responses of the kidney to alterations in extracellular fluid volume. *In* Seldin DW, Giebisch G, eds: The Kidney: Physiology and Pathophysiology, 2nd ed. New York, Raven Press, 1992, pp 2041–2097.)

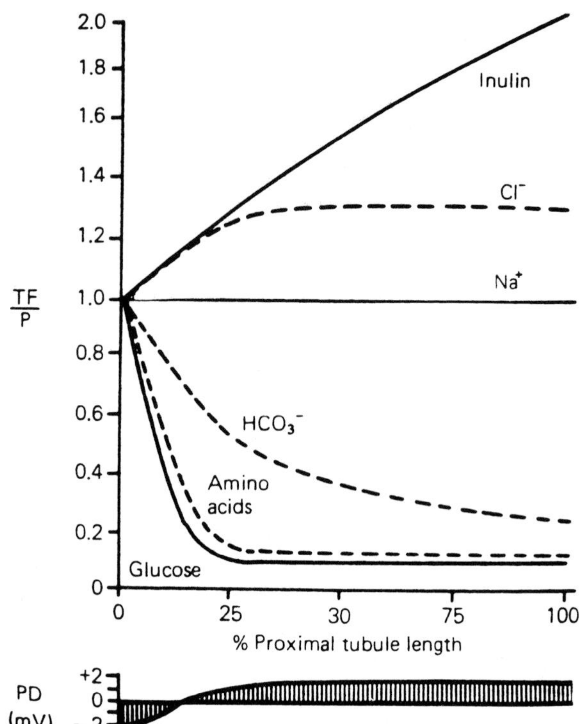

Figure 7–10. Changes in the composition of proximal tubule fluid along the mammalian nephron. TF/P, ratio of tubule fluid to plasma concentration; PV, plasma volume. (From Rector FC: Am J Physiol 1983; 244:F461–F471.)

space (see later discussion). Depending on the peritubular capillary hemodynamics, either reabsorption by these capillaries or leakage back into the tubular lumen may occur (Weinstein, 1992).

Although most of the glomerular filtrate is reabsorbed by the proximal tubule, there are substantial differences in the amounts of individual solutes that are reabsorbed by this segment: almost all of the filtered glucose and amino acids are reabsorbed, but only about 70% of filtered sodium is reclaimed here (Fig. 7–10; Berry and Rector, 1991; Rose, 1989). The amount of filtrate reabsorbed by the proximal tubule is closely linked to the GFR by a process referred to as glomerulotubular balance. Accordingly, alterations in GFR are matched by proportionate changes in proximal reabsorption so that the fractional tubular reabsorption remains constant (Rose, 1989; Wilcox et al, 1992).

Loop of Henle

The loop of Henle is composed of four segments: the descending limb, the thin ascending limb, the medullar thick ascending limb, and the cortical thick ascending limb. These segments combine to reabsorb approximately 25%–40% of the filtered load of sodium (Reeves and Andreoli, 1992).

Fluid entering the loop from the proximal tubule is isotonic to plasma. Unlike the proximal tubule, the thin ascending limb and medullary thick ascending limb are relatively impermeable by water (Hebert et al, 1981, 1987). As sodium is reabsorbed along the medullary thick ascending

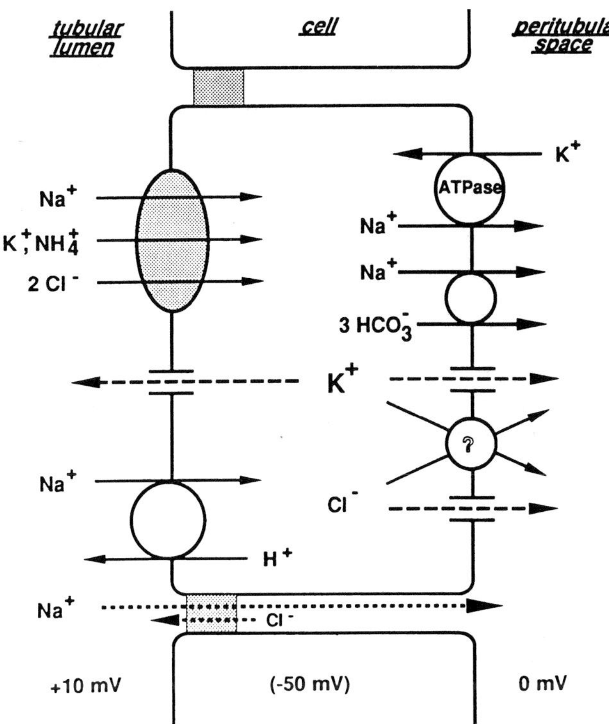

Figure 7–11. A model depicting the major elements of the mechanism of NaCl absorption by the medullary thick ascending limb. Dashed lines indicate passive ion movements down electrochemical gradients. (From Reeves WB, Andreoli TE: Sodium chloride transport in the loop of Henle. *In* Seldin DW, Giebisch G, eds: The Kidney: Physiology and Pathophysiology, 2nd ed. New York, Raven Press, 1992, pp 1975–2002.)

limb by the Na-K-2Cl cotransporter, the osmolality of the tubule fluid decreases to approximately 50 mOs/kg as it exits the loop (Fig. 7–11). **Solute reabsorbed by the loop of Henle of juxtamedullary nephrons accumulates in the medulla, thereby increasing the tonicity of the medullary interstitium. This process permits the excretion of a maximally dilute urine during water loading when AVP levels are low or maximally concentrated urine during dehydration when AVP levels are high** (see later discussion).

Approximately 10%–15% of the filtered load of NaCl exits the loop of Henle and enters this distal nephron. This portion of the nephron includes the distal convoluted tubule, connecting segment, and cortical and medullary collecting tubules. It is at this point that the characteristics of the final urine are established, including magnitude of potassium secretion, urinary acidification, and maximal osmolality (Rose, 1989; see later discussion). These segments have the capacity to generate large transepithelial concentration gradients but have a limited total reabsorptive capacity, in part because of the lower level of Na-K-ATPase present, in comparison with the proximal nephron segments.

Cortical Collecting Duct

This segment is composed of two cell types: principal cells and intercalated cells. Principal cells account for approximately 65% of the cells in this segment. They transport sodium and potassium and are important in determining the final urinary concentration of sodium and potassium. AVP increases the permeability of these cells to water, allowing them to regulate the osmolality of the final urine.

Reabsorption of sodium occurs through channels at the luminal membrane, down an electrochemical gradient established by Na-K-ATPase (Koeppen and Stanton, 1992). Movement of sodium into the cell from the lumen through an Na^+ channel, without an accompanying anion, generates a lumen-negative potential difference and is therefore electrogenic (Fig. 7–12; Palmer et al, 1982, 1993; Pacha et al, 1993). This creates a driving force for secretion of potassium from the cell into the lumen. As sodium enters the cell, it is exchanged for potassium at the basolateral membrane by Na-K-ATPase, and the resulting cell-to-lumen potassium gradient promotes potassium secretion. **When sodium channels are blocked with amiloride, the electrochemical gradient is abolished and potassium secretion ceases** (O'Neil and Boulpaep, 1979). Maneuvers that increase this electrochemical potential, such as high urinary flow (by decreasing luminal potassium concentration) and high serum potassium levels, enhance potassium secretion.

Aldosterone directly stimulates sodium reabsorption by increasing Na^+ conductance by the principal cell (Fig. 7–13; Pacha et al, 1993). This hormone binds to a cytoplasmic receptor and is then translocated to the nucleus, where it interacts with a hormone response element that is present on DNA (Rossier and Palmer, 1992). Through a subsequent series of steps that are not yet well defined but may include the synthesis of aldosterone-induced proteins, the open probability of sodium channels increases. Na-K-ATPase activity increases as a consequence of increased Na^+ entry into the cell rather than a direct effect of aldosterone on the Na-K-ATPase pump (Palmer et al, 1993). Potassium secretion is also stimulated, although this does not appear to be a direct effect of aldosterone on the K^+ channel (Pacha et al, 1993).

In contrast to the principal cells, intercalated cells in the cortical collecting duct contain a K-ATPase pump at the luminal membrane (Wingo and Armitage, 1993; see later section on regulation of potassium excretion). This may contribute to net potassium reabsorption by this segment in the setting of a large total body potassium deficit (see later discussion).

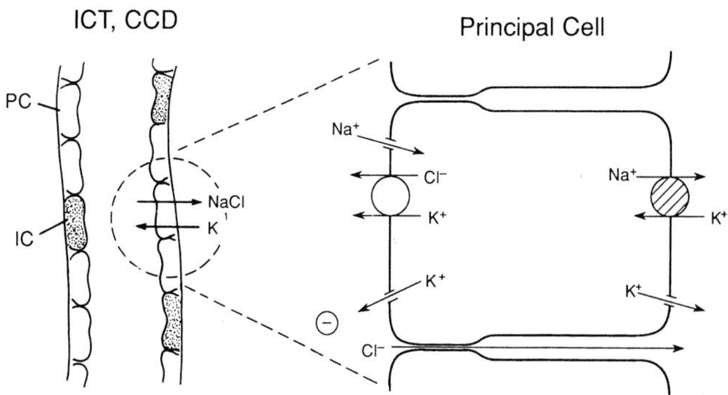

Figure 7–12. Model for principal cell of initial cortical collecting tubule (ICT) and cortical collecting duct (CCD). PC, principal cell; IC, intercalated cell. (From Giebisch G, Malnic G, Berliner RW: Renal transport and control of potassium excretion. *In* Brenner BM, Rector FC, eds: The Kidney, 4th ed. Philadelphia, W.B. Saunders Company, 1991, pp 283–317.)

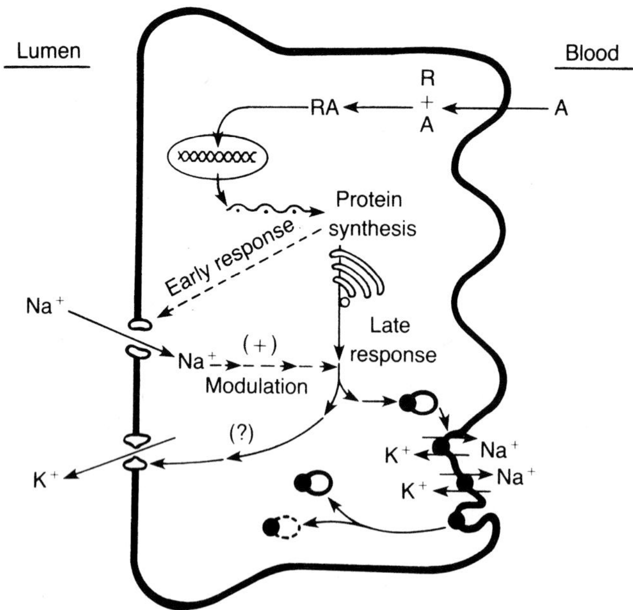

Figure 7–13. Schema of aldosterone effect on potassium secreting cells. A, aldosterone; R, receptor. (From Giebisch G, Malnic G, Berliner RW: Renal transport and control of potassium excretion. *In* Brenner BM, Rector FC, eds: The Kidney, 4th ed. Philadelphia, W.B. Saunders Company, 1991, pp 283–317.)

Medullary Collecting Tubule

This segment of the nephron can be subdivided in outer and inner medullary segments according to their location. The outer medullary collecting duct is composed of cells that function like intercalated cells found in the cortical collecting duct (see later section on potassium excretion).

The inner medullary segment contributes primarily toward concentrating urinary maximally. This segment, like the cortical and outer medullary collecting tubules, is permeable to water only in the presence of AVP. **However, the cortical and outer medullary segments are impermeable to urea in either the presence or absence of AVP.** This differs from the inner medullary collecting duct, in which there is higher basal urea permeability that is increased further by AVP (see later section on regulation of water balance).

Sodium reabsorption occurs in the inner medullary collecting duct through amiloride-sensitive sodium channels similar to those described in the principal cells of the cortical collecting duct (Koeppen and Stanton, 1992). In addition, ANP decreases sodium reabsorption in this segment by decreasing the number of open sodium channels through a mechanism that is cyclic mediated by cGMP (Lewicki and Protter, 1995).

Renin-Angiotensin-Aldosterone System

The renin-angiotensin-aldosterone system is a set of interacting and mutually regulated hormones secreted from the kidney and adrenal cortex and acts as the long-term regulator of (1) sodium balance and extracellular fluid volume, (2) potassium balance, and (3) effective arterial blood pressure (Fig. 7–14). As such, it responds to all influences, external and internal, that affect any of these three parameters, and particularly to dietary salt (Laragh and Sealey, 1992). The kidneys secrete the enzyme renin in response to a variety of normal and abnormal phenomena that reduce arterial blood pressure, renal perfusion, or sodium chloride load in the distal renal tubule. These phenomena include changes in effective blood volume occurring in sodium depletion, shock, hemorrhage, alimentary fluid loss, or heart failure.

Renin is an aspartyl protease belonging to the same family as pepsin and cathepsin (Laragh and Sealey, 1992). It is synthesized by specialized cells, referred to as juxtaglomerular cells, that are located at the afferent arteriole of each nephron (see Fig. 7–5). **The juxtaglomerular cells are in close proximity to the macula densa cells of the ascending limb of Henle and extraglomerular mesangium at the hilum of the glomerulus, where together they form the juxtaglomerular apparatus (JGA;** Barajas et al, 1995). Renin synthesis is not limited to the JGA; renin-producing cells are recruited in the preglomerular circulation close to the junction of the interlobular arteries and also in the postglomerular circulation in efferent arterioles (Taugner et al, 1981). Renin secretion is regulated by intrarenal hemodynamic, hormonal, and biochemical signals that are integrated at the JGA. The mechanisms that regulate renin secretion include the following:

Macula densa mechanism: It is well established that reduced delivery of sodium chloride to the macula densa stimulates renin secretion and increased loads suppress it. This appears to be a chloride-dependent effect, inasmuch as other anions fail to reproduce it. The major determinants of chloride delivery to the macula densa include the filtered load (i.e., GFR) and the extent of reabsorption by the proximal tubule and loop segments (Vander and Miller, 1964; Abboud et al, 1979; Briggs and Schnermann, 1995).

Baroreceptor mechanism: Experimental studies have pro-

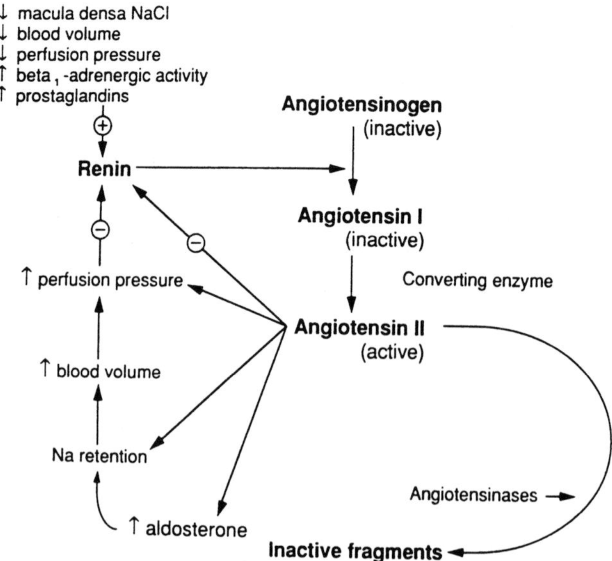

Figure 7–14. The renin-angiotensin-aldosterone system. (Adapted from Arendhorst WJ, Navar LG: Renal circulation and glomerular hemodynamics. *In* Schrier RW, Gottschalk CW, eds: Diseases of the Kidney, 5th ed. Boston, Little, Brown, 1992, pp 65–117.)

vided evidence for a baroreceptor located in the juxtaglomerular cell that controls renin secretion (Fray and Lush, 1984; Laragh and Sealey, 1992). Accordingly, stretch of juxtaglomerular cells causes depolarization, which increases calcium influx through voltage-sensitive calcium channels. Increases in cytosolic calcium suppress renin secretion, decreases in calcium stimulate it.

Neural control: Low levels of renal sympathetic nerve activity, which do not alter renal perfusion pressure, stimulate renin secretion (DiBona and Kopp, 1995; Zayas et al, 1993). A variety of cardiopulmonary and other reflexes stimulate renin secretion through this efferent pathway. This response is mediated through beta$_1$-adrenoceptors and the related activation of adenylate cyclase and cAMP synthesis (Osborne et al, 1981).

When renin enters the blood stream, it splits off the inactive decapeptide, angiotensin I (Ang I), from angiotensinogen (renin substrate; see Fig. 7–14; Laragh and Sealey, 1992). **Ang I is converted to the octapeptide Ang II by angiotensin converting enzyme (ACE), primarily in a single pass through the pulmonary circulation. However, ACE is also located on the endothelial surface through the vasculature and circulating in plasma.** No role for Ang I other than as the precursor to Ang II has been identified.

Ang II is the first effector of the renin system. Its actions include the following:

Arteriolar vasoconstriction: Ang II is bound to a membrane-bound receptor, termed the AT$_1$ receptor, located on arteriolar vascular smooth muscle (Smith and Timmermans, 1994; Harris and Inagami, 1995). Subsequent activation of phospholipase C and the related increases in inositol triphosphate and diacylglycerol lead to increased levels of cytosolic calcium (de Gasparo et al, 1995). Vasoconstriction occurs in response to this increase in cytosolic calcium. Other components of Ang II–mediated vasoconstriction include (1) synthesis of prostaglandins and leukotrienes, (2) inhibition of adenylate cyclase and decreased cAMP formation, and (3) augmentation by adrenergic activity.

Renal hemodynamics: Ang II decreases renal blood flow and increases the filtration fraction, both of which reflect the predominant vasoconstriction of the efferent arteriole (Laragh and Sealey, 1992). However, afferent arteriolar vasoconstriction by Ang II has also been demonstrated (Mitchell and Navar, 1995). This effect has been shown to amplify the autoregulatory tubuloglomerular feedback mechanism, through which increases in tubular flow lead to afferent arteriolar vasoconstriction.

Sodium and water excretion: In keeping with a basic hemodynamic relationship between arterial pressure and renal sodium excretion, low levels of Ang II cause sodium retention, whereas Ang II becomes natriuretic in the presence of arterial hypertension (Laragh et al, 1963; Laragh and Sealey, 1992). Ang II stimulates sodium reabsorption in several ways. First, in response to an increased filtration fraction, peritubular capillary osmotic pressure increases and hydrostatic pressure decreases. Second, binding of low concentrations of Ang II to AT$_1$ receptors at the S$_1$-segment of the proximal tubule stimulates sodium reabsorption via the Na-H antiporter by a process in which adenylate cyclase is inhibited and cAMP levels reduced (Liu and Cogan, 1989). In contrast, higher concentrations of Ang II inhibits sodium reabsorption at this segment. Third, Ang II directly stimulates aldosterone biosynthesis and secretion by the zona glomerulosa of the adrenal cortex (Laragh and Sealey, 1992). Fourth, Ang II promotes thirst and stimulates the nonosmotic release of AVP (Schrier, 1988; Fitzsimons, 1992).

There has been considerable interest in the possible existence and physiologic operation of local tissue renin systems with novel functions. Prorenin, the biosynthetic precursor of renin, has been identified in ovarian, placental, and adrenal tissue, in which its role as an autocoid has been proposed. However, plasma renin activity falls nearly to zero after binephrectomy, which indicates that both conversion to renin and secretion of renin occur only by the kidney (von Lutteroti et al, 1995). Therefore, only renin of renal origin has been shown to participate in the cardiovascular responses described earlier.

Role of the Kidney in Volume Homeostasis

The discussion thus far has outlined the mechanisms through which the long-term regulation of blood pressure and body volume are tightly regulated by the hemodynamic properties of the kidney. In this section, the important role of the renin-angiotensin-aldosterone system as a mechanism for governing these renal hemodynamic responses will be discussed.

Studies by Guyton and coworkers have shown that the ability to maintain normal blood pressure at a wide range of sodium intakes is dependent on circulating levels of Ang II (Guyton et al, 1995; Hall et al, 1995). Figure 7–15 illustrates

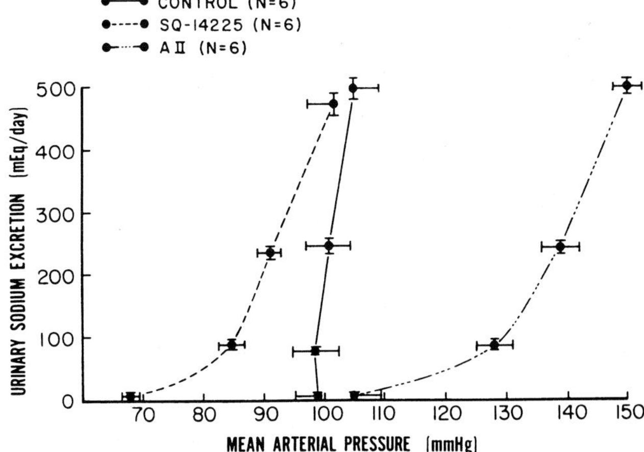

Figure 7–15. The salt-loading renal function curve illustrates the steady-state relationships between arterial pressure and sodium excretion in dogs infused with either angiotensin II or SQ-14225 (captopril). (From Hall JE, Guyton AC, Smith MJ, Coleman TJ: Am. J. Physiol. 1980; 239:F271–F280.)

these effects of Ang II on the salt-loading renal function curve. When salt intake is increased in a normal individual, circulating Ang II levels decrease and blood pressure remains normal. Conversely, when sodium intake is decreased, Ang II levels increase without a significant deviation in blood pressure. **Thus, in the normotensive individual, blood pressure is kept relatively constant even when sodium intake is varied from 10 to 1500 mEq per day because of the reciprocal change in Ang II levels.** In contrast, when the plasma Ang II concentration is fixed at a relatively high level by a constant infusion of exogenous Ang II, increases in sodium intake result in marked increases in blood pressure. Furthermore, when angiotensin levels are suppressed by infusion of the ACE inhibitor captopril, the salt-loading renal function curve is shifted to the left so that blood pressure decreases profoundly at low levels of sodium intake but remains normal when sodium intake is increased.

The relevance of the sodium-volume mechanism and the renin-angiotensin-aldosterone system in the pathogenesis of hypertension can be clearly seen from the results of a series of studies done by Hall and coworkers (Hall et al, 1995; Fig. 7–16). These investigators devised an experimental model in which an electronically controlled hydraulic constrictor was placed around the aorta above the renal arteries in awake animals. With this technique, the renal artery pressure could be maintained at a normal level even though the systemic blood pressure was increased by the simultaneous infusion of vasoactive hormones. When Ang II or aldosterone was infused at a constant rate for 2 weeks, during which the renal perfusion pressure maintained at the normal baseline levels, sodium retention occurred and the systemic pressure rose significantly. By the end of the infusion period, signs of volume overload, including pulmonary edema, were apparent. **The rise in systemic pressure was caused initially by sodium retention resulting from the direct renal effects of aldosterone and, in the latter stages, by the impaired pressure natriuresis caused by the inability to transmit the elevated pressure to the renal circulation.** When the suprarenal constriction was relieved and the renal perfusion pressure allowed to increase to the level of the systemic pressure, a brisk natriuresis and diuresis occurred, and systemic pressure decreased back to the level appropriate for the rate of aldosterone excretion. Similar responses were also observed when other vasoactive hormones causing salt and water retention (Ang II or vasopressin) were infused and a rise in renal perfusion pressure was prevented. Accordingly, Guyton and colleagues postulated that in order for hypertension to occur, vascular resistance must be increased at some point between the aortic valve and the glomerulus, including the glomerular capillary membrane. This locus has been referred to as the "resistance axis of hypertension" (Guyton et al, 1995).

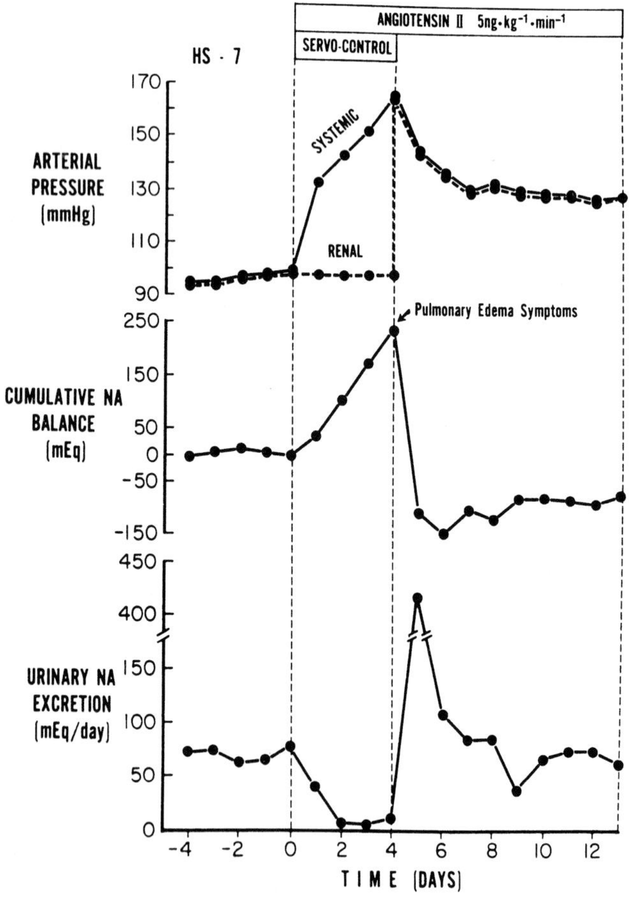

Figure 7–16. Effects of angiotensin II infusion when renal perfusion pressure was servo-controlled at the normal level. After 4 days, retention of sodium and water caused severe hypertension and pulmonary edema. When the renal perfusion pressure was permitted to increase, pressure natriuresis occurred and pulmonary edema resolved. (From Hall JE, Granger JP, Hester RL, et al: Am. J. Physiol. 1984; 246:F627–F634.)

Coordinated Control of Blood Pressure and Volume Homeostasis by the Renin System

A cybernetic control mechanism for the maintenance of blood pressure and volume homeostasis has been described, on the basis of the reciprocal relationship of sodium intake and plasma renin activity (Laragh and Sealey, 1992). Accordingly, at high levels of sodium intake, intravascular volume, renal perfusion pressure, and macula densa NaCl delivery are normal and renin secretion is not required in order to maintain blood pressure. In contrast, during sodium depletion, macula densa delivery and renal perfusion pressure are decreased, and efferent renal sympathetic nerve activity is augmented (Fig. 7–17). These multiple effects, dominated by vasoconstriction, combine to raise blood pressure and restore fluid volume to the point where the initial signal for renin release (lowered blood pressure and perfusion in the kidney) is reversed or dampened. The feedback loop has been completed, and the renin system's role in maintaining blood pressure and electrolyte homeostasis has been served.

REGULATION OF POTASSIUM EXCRETION

Potassium is the most abundant cation in the body, with total body K^+ stores of approximately 3000–4000 mEq. Approximately 98% of the total K^+ content is intracellular;

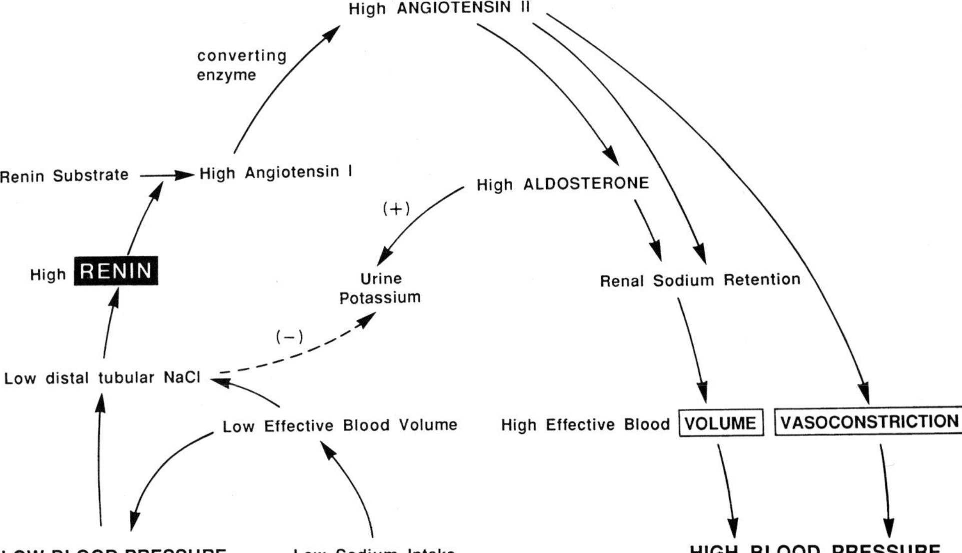

Figure 7–17. The renin-angiotensin-aldosterone system as it works to defend blood pressure and sodium balance during low sodium intake. (From Laragh JH, Sealey JE: Renin-angiotensin-aldosterone system and the renal regulation of sodium, potassium, and blood pressure homeostasis. *In* Windhager EE, ed: Handbook of Physiology, Section 8: Renal Physiology. New York, Oxford University Press, 1992, pp 1409–1541.)

the intracellular K^+ concentration is about 140 mEq/L, and the extracellular K^+ concentration is 4.0 mEq/L (Fig. 7–18). These characteristics differ from those of Na^+, which is predominantly distributed in the extracellular space (Rastegar and DeFronzo, 1992). This high intracellular-to-extracellular ratio (K_i:K_0), which is maintained by Na^+-K^+-ATPase, is essential for normal cell function. **Specifically, this high ratio is the major determinant of the resting cell membrane potential required for normal neuromuscular function, for establishing electrochemical gradients essential for transepithelial transport, and for maintaining the high potassium concentration necessary for cellular metabolism.**

Processes that regulate the internal distribution of K^+ play a major role in maintaining acute K^+ homeostasis. For example, only about half of a K^+ load administered orally or intravenously is excreted by the kidney within the first 4 hours. However, the rise in serum K^+ is blunted because about 80% of the retained K^+ enters the intracellular space (DeFronzo et al, 1978, 1980). The internal distribution of potassium is governed by several factors, including insulin, catecholamines, mineralocorticoids, acid-base balance, and plasma osmolality (see later discussion).

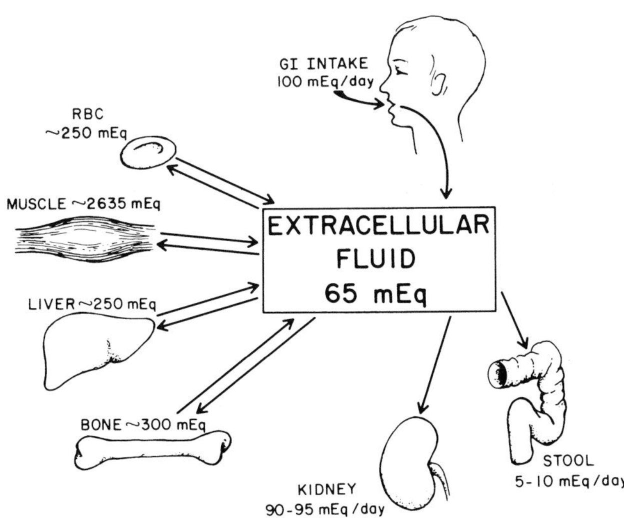

Figure 7–18. Internal and external potassium balance in humans. GI, gastrointestinal; RBC, red blood cells. (From Rastegar A, DeFronzo RA: Disorders of potassium metabolism associated with renal disease. *In* Schrier RW, Gottschalk CW, eds: Diseases of the Kidney, 5th ed. Boston, Little, Brown, 1992, pp 2645–2661.)

Although the acute response to a K^+ load involves redistribution from the extracellular to intracellular compartments, long-term K^+ homeostasis is normally maintained by renal potassium excretion. A normal individual in metabolic balance excretes approximately 90% of the daily dietary K^+ intake by the kidney. The renal processes that govern K^+ excretion include glomerular filtration, tubular reabsorption, and secretion. However, the primary mechanism for renal K^+ excretion is secretion of K^+ by the distal nephron (Wright and Giebisch, 1992).

GLOMERULAR FILTRATION. Potassium is freely filtered by the glomerulus. In an individual with normal renal function, approximately 700 mEq K^+ is filtered daily ([GFR 150 L/day] × [serum K^+: 4 mEq/L]). Only about 10%–15% of this filtered K^+ load is excreted daily in urine (Rastegar and DeFronzo, 1992).

PROXIMAL TUBULE. Approximately 70% of the filtered load of potassium is reabsorbed by the proximal convoluted and proximal straight segments (Giebisch et al, 1991). Potassium reabsorption is dependent on Na^+ and fluid transport, decreasing while proximal fluid reabsorption is reduced or reversed by an osmotic diuretic (Bomsztyk and Wright, 1986; Weinstein, 1988). Diffusion of K^+ through a paracellular pathway contributes to this reabsorptive process (Wright and Giebisch, 1992). Active transport of K^+ has also been proposed in the early portion of the proximal tubule to account for the observation that reabsorption occurs even though the luminal K^+ concentration is below that in plasma and there is a lumen-negative transepithelial potential. A cell model for K^+ reabsorption by the proximal tubule has been proposed (Fig. 7–19). It includes a Na^+-K^+-ATPase "pump" in the basolateral membrane, a potassium conductance ("leak") in the apical membrane, and a pathway for transport between cells.

LOOP OF HENLE. Potassium reabsorption occurs along

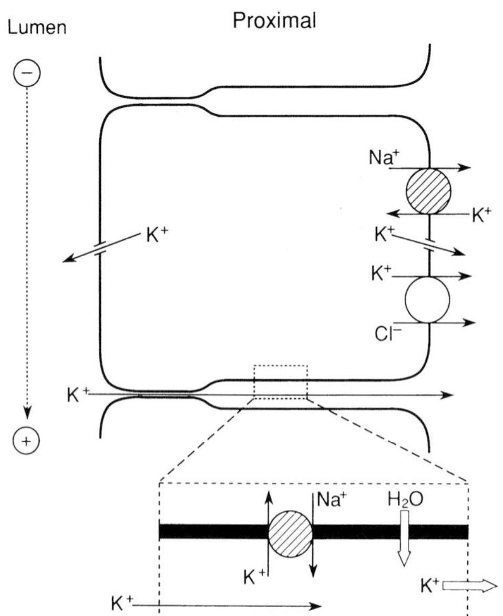

Figure 7–19. Model for proximal tubule cell potassium transport. Enlargement of lateral membrane and intercellular space illustrates postulated mechanism permitting potassium absorption against a concentration gradient. (From Wright FS, Giebisch G: Regulation of potassium excretion. *In* Seldin DW, Giebisch G, eds: The Kidney: Physiology and Pathophysiology, 2nd ed. New York, Raven Press, 1992, pp 2209–2247.)

this segment so that approximately 90% of the filtered load of K^+ is reabsorbed by the time tubular fluid enters the distal nephron (Malnic et al, 1966). However, net K^+ reabsorption at the loop of Henle reflects two opposing processes: passive secretion into the descending limb and active reabsorption from the thick ascending limb. A cell model for K^+ transport is shown in Figure 11. Potassium reabsorption is driven by the Na^+ gradient established across the apical cell membrane. The Na-K-2Cl cotransport mechanism couples K^+ entry with one Na^+ and two Cl^- ions. Back-diffusion of K^+ from the cell to lumen down the concentration gradient provides a continuous luminal supply of K^+ for cotransport with Na^+ and Cl^- (Hebert and Andreoli, 1984; Greger, 1985; Wright and Giebisch, 1992). Basolateral pathways for K^+ reabsorption include a K^+ conductance and K^+-Cl^- cotransporter. Potassium reabsorption also occurs through a paracellular pathway, driven by lumen-positive transepithelial voltage (Greger and Schlatter, 1983; Greger, 1985). Transport of K^+ by the thick ascending limb is abolished when Na-K-2Cl cotransporter activity is inhibited by the presence of a loop diuretic (i.e., furosemide) in the lumen (Burg, 1982).

DISTAL TUBULE AND COLLECTING TUBULE. Distal tubule fluid is dilute, with NaCl concentrations about 20–40 mEq/L. Potassium concentration is also low, and K^+ is secreted down an electrochemical gradient (Schnermann et al, 1987; Velasquez et al, 1987). **The cortical collecting duct is the main site of regulated K^+ secretion.** This segment is composed of principal cells and intercalated cells (see section on acid-base homeostasis); K^+ is secreted by principal cells and reabsorbed by intercalated cells (Wright and Giebisch, 1992).

The cell model for K^+ transport by the principal cell of the cortical collecting duct is illustrated in Figure 7–12. The basolateral Na^+-K^+-ATPase pump maintains high intracellular K^+ concentration and promotes the coupling of Na^+ reabsorption and K^+ secretion. Sodium diffusion from lumen to cell through apical Na^+ channels occurs down a concentration gradient. **The resulting lumen negative transepithelial potential difference promotes K^+ secretion down the electrochemical gradient** (O'Neil and Boulpaep, 1982; O'Neil and Sansom, 1984; Sansom et al, 1987). An electroneutral apical K^+-Cl^- cotransport mechanism that promotes K^+ secretion into the distal tubule when the luminal Cl^- concentration is low has also been identified (Velasquez et al, 1982).

A-type intercalated cells secrete H^+ ions and appear to be able to reabsorb K^+ through active K^+-H^+ exchange (Wingo and Armitage, 1993). This process is attenuated by inhibition of K^+-ATPase (Fig. 7–20; Doucet and Marsy, 1987; Wright and Giebisch, 1992).

MEDULLARY COLLECTING TUBULE. The medullary collecting tubule in the outer stripe of the medulla, like the cortical collecting duct, is composed of principal and intercalated cells. Overall, this segment reabsorbs Na^+ and secretes K^+ (Stokes, 1982). In contrast, the medullary collecting tubules in the inner stripe of the medulla lack an active K^+-secretory mechanism (Stokes et al, 1981; Wingo, 1987). Whether passive K^+ secretion or reabsorption occurs is dependent on the lumen K^+ concentration and electrical potentials. Accordingly, K^+ reabsorption is stimulated by the lumen positive potential generated during H^+ secretion (see section on acid-base homeostasis). Reabsorption and secretion can also occur at the inner medullary collecting duct, through a cation channel. The direction of ion flux depends on the apical electrochemical driving forces (Stanton and Giebisch, 1992).

The K^+ concentration of tubule fluid in Henle's loop at the tip of the papilla is tenfold higher than that of plasma in the systemic circulation (Jamison et al, 1976; Jamison, 1987). Potassium is concentrated in this region by countercurrent multiplication: K^+ is reabsorbed by the medullary thick ascending limb and the medullary collecting tubule. Amplifying the amount of K^+ in the medullary interstitium

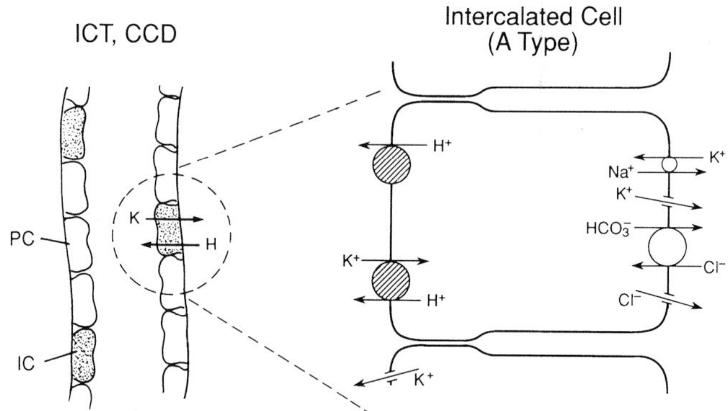

Figure 7–20. Model for acid secreting (A-type) intercalated cells in the initial collecting tubule (ICT) and cortical collecting duct (CCD). These cells are probably the site of potassium reabsorption via an H^+,K^+-ATPase. Proton secretion is also driven by an H^+-ATPase. PC, principal cell; IC, intercalated cell. (From Wright FS, Giebisch G: Regulation of potassium excretion. *In* Seldin DW, Giebisch G, eds: The Kidney: Physiology and Pathophysiology, 2nd ed. New York, Raven Press, 1992, pp 2209–2247.)

promotes K^+ secretion into the descending limb of Henle and the cortical collecting duct and thereby facilitates renal K^+ excretion during K^+ loading (Wright and Giebisch, 1992).

Factors Regulating Renal Potassium Excretion

ALDOSTERONE. **Potassium secretion by the principal cells of the cortical and medullary collecting tubule is directly stimulated by aldosterone** (Field et al, 1984; Field and Giebisch, 1985; O'Neil and Helman, 1977). Accordingly, at any level of serum K^+, urinary K^+ will increase as aldosterone levels rise (Young and Paulsen, 1983; Young, 1988). Aldosterone binds to a cytoplasmic receptor, forming an aldosterone-receptor complex that subsequently activates gene transcription and synthesis of aldosterone-induced proteins (see Fig. 7–13; O'Neil, 1990; Schaefer et al, 1990). **During the early phase of mineralocorticoid action, a greater number of apical Na^+ channels are in the open state, so that sodium entry into principal cells increases** (Sansom and O'Neil, 1986; Rossier and Palmer, 1992; Wright and Giebisch, 1992; Pacha et al, 1993; Palmer, 1993). During this phase, Na^+-K^+-ATPase *activity* increases with Na^+ entry into these cells, although the maximal activity of the enzyme is not increased initially. This electrogenic reabsorption of Na^+ increases the lumen-negative transepithelial potential. **During the late phase of aldosterone action, more Na^+-K^+-ATPase units are added to the basolateral membrane** (Palmer et al, 1993). Together, these aldosterone responses augment the electrochemical gradient for K^+ secretion. The primary importance of the Na^+ reabsorption in this aldosterone effect is illustrated by the effect of amiloride, which blocks the apical Na^+ channel and abolishes aldosterone-stimulated K^+ secretion (Duarte et al, 1971; Pacha et al, 1993; Palmer et al, 1993).

LUMINAL SODIUM SUPPLY AND FLOW RATE. Renal K^+ excretion requires delivery of an adequate amount of Na^+ to the cortical collecting duct and distal nephron. **When the luminal concentration of Na^+ falls below about 15 mEq/L, an amount that is attainable during states of maximal sodium retention, the kaliuretic response to mineralocorticoids is attenuated and urinary K^+ excretion falls** (Good and Wright, 1979; Giebisch et al, 1991; Laragh and Sealey, 1992). Conversely, renal K^+ secretion is enhanced by increasing Na^+ delivery to the distal nephron during volume expansion with saline or high dietary Na^+ intake. However, the kaliuretic stimulus of volume expansion is normally offset by reduced activity of the renin-angiotensin-aldosterone system so that K^+ balance can be maintained across a wide spectrum of Na^+ balance. Under normal conditions, Na^+ reabsorption by the distal nephron is not a rate-limiting factor for K^+ secretion (Wright and Giebisch, 1992).

Potassium secretion increases directly with flow rate at distal nephron segments. Although flow rate usually increases together with Na^+ delivery, and thus enhanced K^+ secretion at high flow may be influenced by increased Na^+ reabsorption, in vitro studies have demonstrated that the effects of these two variables can be separated (Good and Wright, 1979). Because more than 90% of the filtered load of K^+ is reabsorbed from the filtrate by the time it enters the distal tubule, the tubule fluid K^+ concentration is low in the early portion of this nephron segment. **At high flow rates, luminal K^+ concentration is diluted, and the cell-to-lumen electrochemical gradient favors K^+ secretion.**

DIURETICS (Fig. 7–21). Diuretics can be classified according to their effects on potassium excretion (Unwin et al, 1995). **Kaliuretic diuretics include loop diuretics (furosemide, torsemide, bumetanide), thiazide-type diuretics (hydrochlorothiazide, chlorthalidone, metolazone), carbonic anhydrase inhibitors (acetazolamide), and osmotic diuretics (mannitol). Potassium-sparing diuretics include spironolactone, amiloride, and triamterene.**

Kaliuretic diuretics increase renal K^+ excretion in several ways (Fig. 7–22). Loop and thiazide-type diuretics directly inhibit tubular reabsorption of K^+ and Na^+, thereby increasing delivery of potassium to more distal nephron segments (Burg et al, 1973). **These diuretics also decrease extracellular fluid volume and consequently stimulate the renin-angiotensin-aldosterone system** (Laragh and Sealey, 1992). The combined increase in Na^+ delivery to the cortical collecting duct, together with increased aldosterone levels, amplify the amount of K^+ secreted by the distal nephron at any level of serum K^+. Antidiuretic hormone (ADH) secretion is also enhanced by the nonosmotic stimulus of decreased extracellular volume (Schrier, 1988). Both ADH and aldosterone promote K^+ secretion by the distal and cortical collecting ducts (Schaefer et al, 1990). Carbonic anhydrase inhibition stimulates K^+ secretion at the distal nephron by increasing flow rate and also increases electronegativity of the lumen as a result of increased distal HCO_3^+ delivery (Malnic and Giebisch, 1964; Malnic et al, 1971).

Potassium-sparing diuretics (amiloride, triamterene, spironolactone) reduce K^+ secretion by the cortical collecting duct. Furthermore, they can attenuate the kaliuretic effects of loop diuretics without abolishing their natriuretic effects (Hropot et al, 1985). The action by which these K^+-sparing diuretics attenuate K^+ secretion is mediated by the blockade of Na^+ entry into principal cells of the distal tubule and cortical collecting duct and by the subsequent reduction in the electrochemical driving force generated by Na^+ reabsorption (O'Neil and Boulpaep, 1979).

POTASSIUM INTAKE. When K^+ intake is increased acutely or chronically, K^+ secretion by the cortical collecting duct is stimulated and renal K^+ excretion increased. Factors that contribute independently to these responses include plasma levels of potassium, aldosterone, and luminal flow rate (Stanton and Giebisch, 1982; Stanton et al, 1985b, 1987). Glucocorticoids stimulate K^+ secretion indirectly by increasing GFR (reducing free water reabsorption) and thus by augmenting luminal flow rate (Field and Giebisch, 1985). These physiologic responses are accompanied by morphologic and biochemical changes, including amplification of the basolateral membrane surface area, which reflects increased Na^+-K^+-ATPase content. These alterations are evident within 24 hours of the increase in K^+ intake (Wright and Giebisch, 1992; Stanton et al, 1981, 1985a)

ACID-BASE BALANCE. Renal K^+ excretion is modified during derangements in acid-base homeostasis (Toussaint and Vereerstraeten, 1962). Potassium secretion is stimulated by alkalosis and attenuated during acidosis. These direct effects can occur independently of other factors that influence K^+ secretion, such as distal flow rate and serum

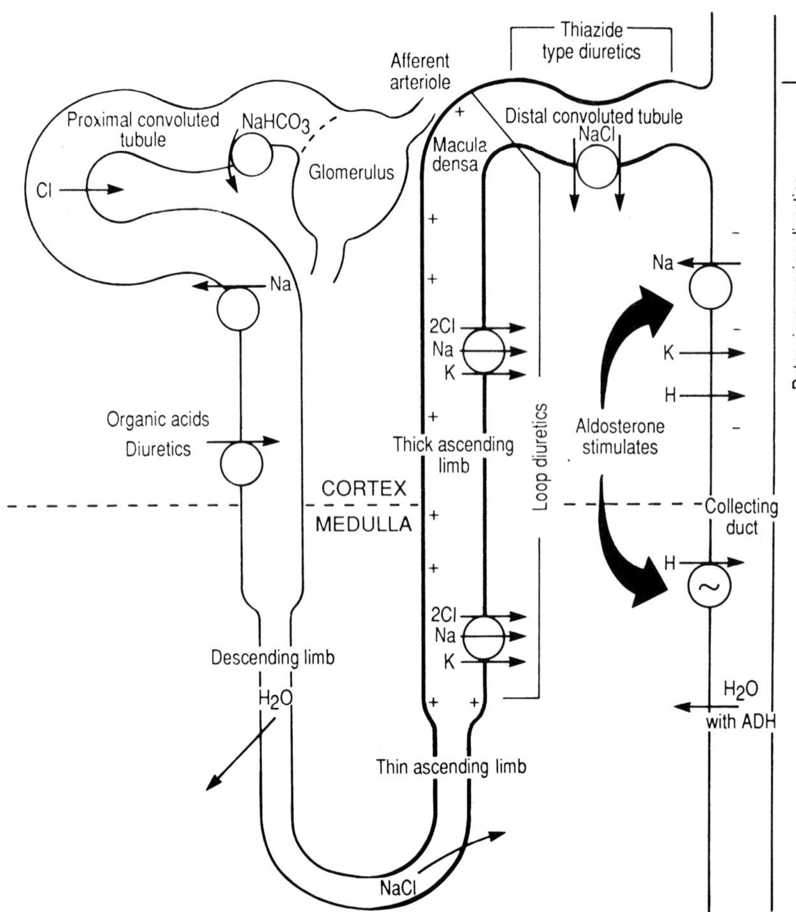

Figure 7–21. Model of major transport processes in the nephron, with sites of diuretic action. (From Pecker MS: Pathophysiologic effects and strategies for long-term diuretic treatment of hypertension. *In* Laragh JH, Brenner BM, eds: Hypertension: Pathophysiology, Diagnosis, and Management, 1st ed. New York, Raven Press, 1990, pp 2143–2167.)

K^+ or aldosterone level (Wright and Giebisch, 1992). However, these effects of pH may be masked by these other determinants of K^+ secretion. For example, in proximal renal tubular acidosis, hypokalemia occurs because K^+ secretion is stimulated by the increased delivery of HCO_3^- at the distal nephron (see earlier section on acid-base homeostasis; Rose, 1989).

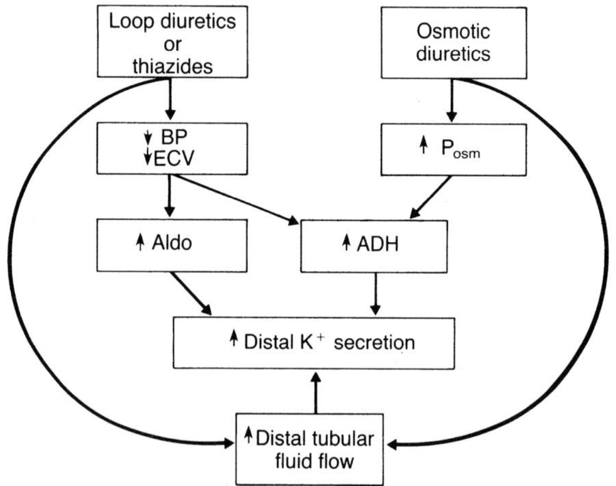

Figure 7–22. Mechanisms that influence renal potassium excretion during diuretic use. BP, blood pressure; ECV, extracellular volume; P_{Osm}, plasma osmolality; Aldo, aldosterone; ADH, antidiuretic hormone. (From Giebisch G, Malnic G, Berliner RW: Renal transport and control of potassium excretion. *In* Brenner BM, Rector FC, eds: The Kidney, 4th ed. Philadelphia, W.B. Saunders Company, 1991, pp 283–317.)

Potassium transport by cell membranes is directly influenced by alterations in acid-base homeostasis. There is a reciprocal relationship between pH and the open probability of apical K^+ channels in principal cells of cortical collecting duct. Accordingly, at a low pH, K^+ secretion is attenuated, and at a high pH, K^+ secretion is enhanced (Wang et al, 1990).

MAGNESIUM BALANCE. Magnesium depletion commonly accompanies clinical states associated with Mg^{2+} deficiency, such as diuretic use, alcoholism, and diabetic ketoacidosis (Whang et al, 1979, 1985). Like K^+, Mg^{2+} is primarily distributed intracellularly; therefore, total body deficits may be underestimated by the serum Mg^{2+} concentration (Ladefoged and Hagen, 1988). **Renal K^+ wasting occurs when body stores of Mg^{2+} are reduced. Furthermore, when hypokalemia is accompanied by Mg^{2+} deficiency, K^+ repletion cannot occur until the associated Mg^{2+} deficiency is corrected** (Shils, 1969).

Disorders of Potassium Homeostasis

(Tables 7–1 and 7–2)

Potassium homeostasis is maintained by the processes that regulate distribution of K^+ between the extracellular fluid and the intracellular space and by the factors that control renal K^+ excretion (Rose, 1989). As discussed, the initial response to an acute K^+ load requires redistribution into cells. This process is facilitated by beta$_2$-adrenergic stimuli (e.g., epinephrine) and insulin (DeFronzo et al, 1981; Brown et al, 1983, Williams et al, 1985; Rosa et al, 1992). When these mechanisms are attenuated by beta-adrenergic receptor antagonists or diabetes mellitus, respectively, increases in the basal serum K^+ concentration may occur (DeFronzo et al, 1980; Lim et al, 1981). However, renal K^+ excretion is the predominant mechanism for controlling K^+ balance and can adapt to a wide range of levels of long-term K^+ intake. Therefore, marked hyperkalemia will occur only if there is a defect in renal or adrenal function (Rastegar and DeFronzo, 1992; Rose, 1989).

The diagnostic approach to the patient with disorders of K^+ homeostasis is outlined in Figures 7–23 and 7–24.

Table 7–1. ETIOLOGIES OF HYPOKALEMIA

Renal Potassium Loss

Diuretics: Thiazide, Loop

Mineralocorticoid Excess

Hypertensive

Primary
  Adrenal adenoma, nonadenomatous adrenal hyperplasia
Secondary
  Glucocorticoid-remediable aldosteronism
  Accelerated and malignant hypertension
  Renin secreting tumor: juxtaglomerular cell, ovarian, renal clear cell, sarcoma
Nonaldosterone mineralocorticoid excess
  Adrenal deoxycorticosterone production
    17-α-hydroxylase deficiency
    11-β-hydroxylase deficiency
Cushing's syndrome: ectopic ACTH
Adrenal carcinoma
  11-β-hydroxysteroid dehydrogenase deficiency
    Acquired: licorice (glycyrrhizic acid) or carbenoxolone
    Congenital: apparent mineralocorticoid excess syndrome (type I)

Normotensive

Bartter's syndrome
Renal tubular acidosis: types I and II

Tubulointerstitial disease

Postobstructive diuresis

Acute tubular necrosis: diuretic phase

Magnesium depletion

Nonreabsorbable anions: penicillins, diabetic ketoacidosis, alkali loading

Liddle's syndrome

Gastrointestinal Potassium Loss

Diarrhea

Laxative or cathartic abuse
Inflammatory bowel disease
Colonic villous adenoma
VIP-producing tumors
Vomiting

Miscellaneous

Lysozymuria of leukemia
Dietary deficiency

ACTH, adrenocorticotropic hormone; VIP, vasoactive intestinal polypeptide.

Adapted from Mujais SK, Katz AI: Potassium deficiency. *In* Seldin DW, Giebisch G, eds: The Kidney: Physiology and Pathophysiology, 2nd ed. New York, Raven Press, 1992, pp 2249–2278.

Table 7–2. ETIOLOGY OF HYPERKALEMIA

Factitious

Laboratory error
Pseudohyperkalemia: in vitro hemolysis, thrombocytosis, leukocytosis

Increased Input

Exogenous: diet, salt substitutes
Endogenous: hemolysis, GI bleeding, catabolic states, crush injury, tumor lysis

Renal Failure

Acute: especially tubulointerstitial disease
Chronic: GFR < 15–20 ml/min

Impaired Renin-Aldosterone Axis

Addison's disease
Congenital adrenal enzyme deficiencies (e.g., corticosterone methyl oxidase deficiency)
Drug induced: heparin, prostaglandin inhibitors, ACE inhibitors, pentamidine, beta blockers
Hyporeninemic hypoaldosteronism
Primary hypoaldosteronism (normal renin)

Primary Renal Tubular Potassium Secretory Defect

Sickle-cell disease
Systemic lupus erythematosis
Postrenal transplantation
Obstructive uropathy
Tubulointerstitial renal disease
Pseudohypoaldosteronism
Hyperkalemic distal renal tubular acidosis

Inhibitors of Tubular Secretion

Diuretics: amiloride, spironolactone, triamterene
Cyclosporine
Lithium
Digitalis

Abnormal Potassium Distribution

Metabolic acidosis
Insulin deficiency
Hypertonicity (e.g., hyperglycemia)
Aldosterone deficiency
Beta-adrenergic receptor blockade
Alpha-adrenergic receptor agonist
Exercise
Periodic paralysis
Digitalis
Succinylcholine

GI, gastrointestinal; GFR, glomerular filtration rate; ACE, angiotensin converting enzyme.

Adapted from Rastegar A, DeFronzo RA: Disorders of potassium metabolism associated with renal disease. *In* Schrier RW, Gottschalk CW, eds: Diseases of the Kidney, 5th ed. Boston, Little, Brown, 1992, pp 2645–2661.

REGULATION OF CALCIUM EXCRETION

Calcium is the most abundant divalent cation in the body, accounting for about 2% of the body weight and is present in extracellular fluid at a concentration of 10 mg/dl (equal to 5 mEq/L and 2.5 mmol/L). This level is tightly regulated despite the wide range of dietary calcium intakes (500–1200 mg/day). **Calcium homeostasis is accomplished through the integration of intestinal absorption, bone remodeling and reabsorption, and renal processes, including glomerular ultrafiltration and tubular reabsorption.** PTH and vitamin D are important participants in these processes, with actions at the target organs that regulate calcium metabolism (Suki and Rouse, 1991).

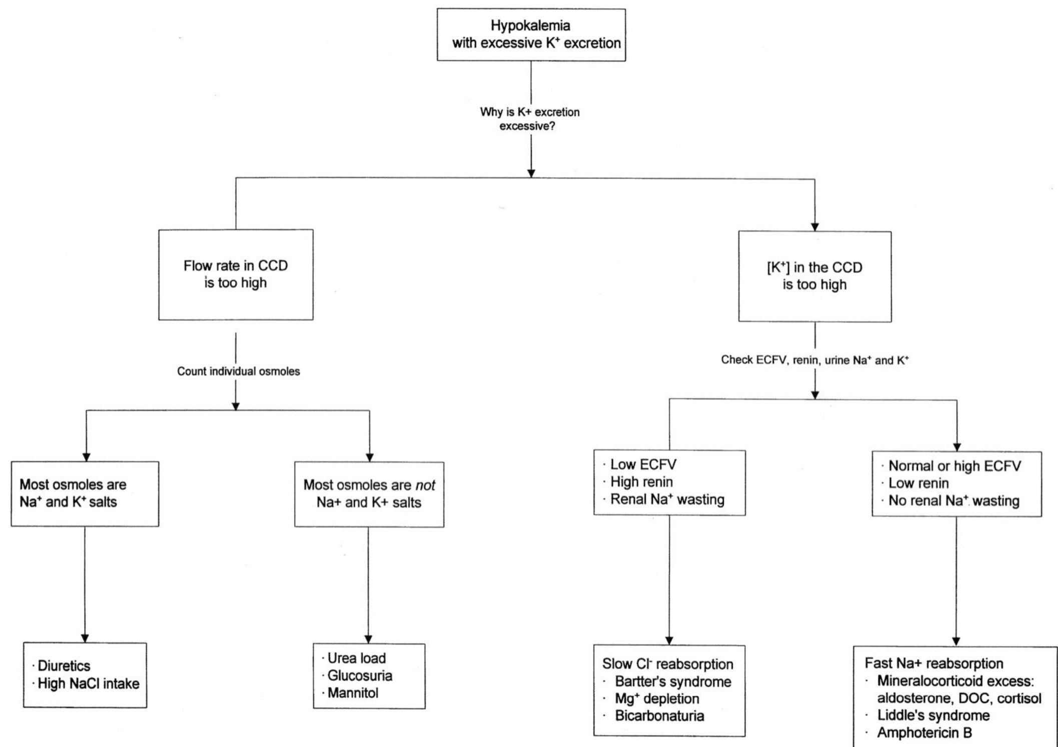

Figure 7–23. Clinical evaluation of the patient with hypokalemia. CCD, cortical collecting duct; ECFV, extracellular fluid volume; DOC, deoxycorticosterone. (From: Halperin ML, Goldstein MB: Fluid, Electrolyte and Acid-Base Physiology: A Problem-Based Approach, 2nd ed. Philadelphia, W.B. Saunders Company, 1994.)

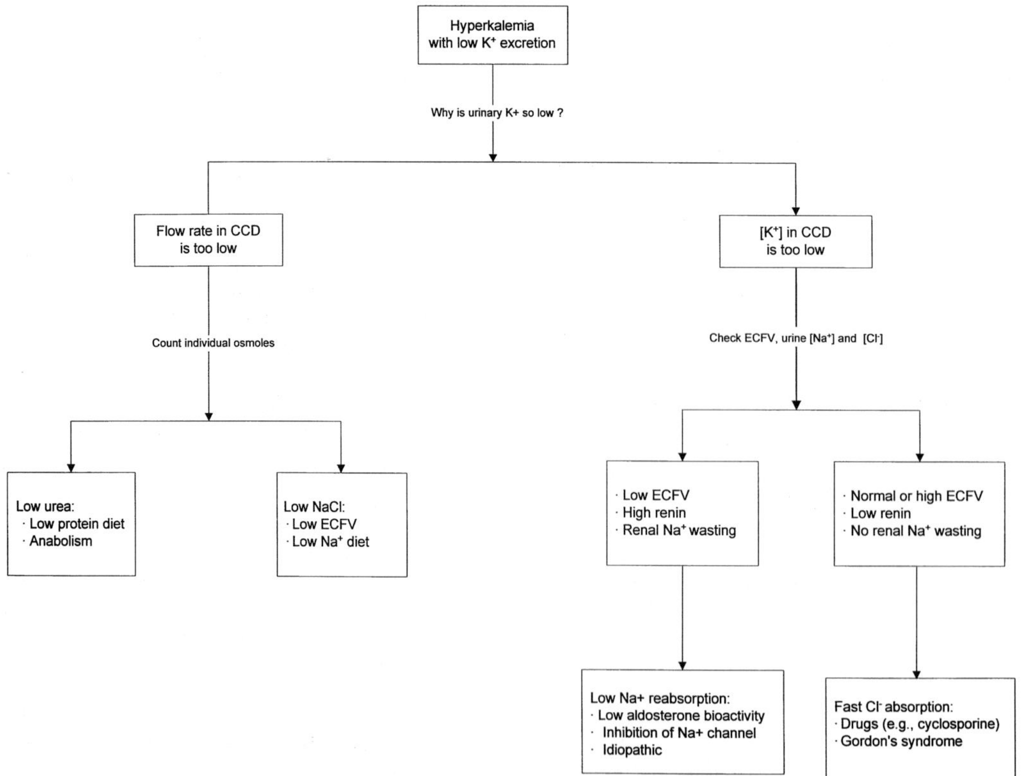

Figure 7–24. Clinical evaluation of the patient with hyperkalemia and low potassium excretion. CCD, cortical collecting duct; ECFV, extracellular fluid volume. (From: Halperin ML, Goldstein MB: Fluid, Electrolyte and Acid-Base Physiology: A Problem-Based Approach, 2nd ed. Philadelphia, W.B. Saunders Company, 1994.)

Approximately 40% of plasma calcium is bound to proteins, predominantly albumin, and the remaining 60% is unbound and can be filtered across the glomerulus (Costanza and Windhager, 1992; Toribara et al, 1957). Of this ultrafilterable Ca^{2+}, 90% is free, nonionized Ca^{2+} (5 mg/dl or 1.25 mmol/L) and the remaining 10% forms complexes with phosphate, HCO_3^-, and other anions. **The relative amount of ultrafilterable calcium is influenced by blood pH: it decreases with severe alkalemia (pH >7.6) and increases with acidemia (pH <7.3;** Peterson et al, 1961). This occurs because calcium binding to albumin and inorganic anions decreases as plasma H^+ increases. Ultrafilterable Ca^{2+} also increases in parallel with the total serum Ca^{2+} concentration until the total serum Ca^{2+} reaches approximately 15 mg/dl, at which point there is a relative decline in ultrafilterable Ca^{2+} (Le Grimellec et al, 1974). Conversely, ultrafilterable Ca^{2+} decreases when the serum Ca^{2+} concentration falls below 6 mg/dl (Terepka et al, 1957; Hopkins et al, 1952).

Sites of Calcium Transport

Less than 2% of the daily filtered load of calcium is excreted in urine; this amount is equivalent to dietary intake when the individual is in calcium balance (Suki and Rouse, 1991). This reflects avid renal tubular reabsorption (Fig. 7–25).

PROXIMAL TUBULE. Approximately 65% of filtered calcium is reabsorbed in the proximal convoluted tubule. Micropuncture studies have demonstrated that calcium reabsorption by this segment, and in the kidney as a whole, parallels that of Na^+ and water (Walser, 1961; Costanza and Weiner, 1974; Costanza and Windhager, 1992). Passive forces for calcium reabsorption include electrical and chemical gradients. In this nephron segment, the transepithelial difference is positive, and the calcium concentration increases to above that of plasma, thus contributing to net calcium reabsorption (Bomsztyk et al, 1984). However, a small amount of calcium reabsorption occurs when the passive driving forces are abolished, which suggests that active transport of calcium also occurs at this segment. Similar mechanisms of calcium reabsorption are in operation at the proximal straight tubule (Bourdeau and Burg, 1986).

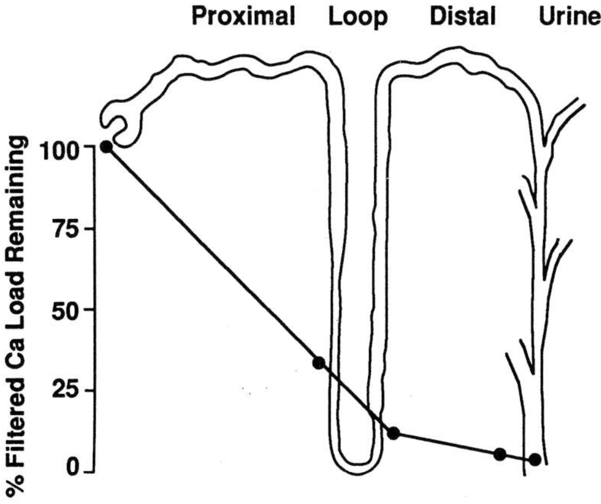

Figure 7–25. Profile of calcium reabsorption along the mammalian nephron. (From Sutton RAL, Dirks JH: Calcium and magnesium: Renal handling and disorders of metabolism. *In* Brenner BM, Rector FC, eds: The Kidney, 3rd ed. Philadelphia, W.B. Saunders Company, 1986, p 592.)

LOOP OF HENLE. Tubule perfusion studies suggest that significant calcium reabsorption does not occur in the thin descending or ascending limbs of Henle (Rocha et al, 1977; Quamme and Dirks, 1980). In contrast, approximately 25% of the filtered load of Ca^{2+} is reabsorbed by the thick ascending limb (Sharegi and Stoner, 1978; Costanza and Windhager, 1992). At the cortical segment, the positive lumen voltage is an important driving force for calcium reabsorption (Bourdeau and Burg, 1979). However, an active component of calcium reabsorption by this segment is likely because calcium efflux continues after passive driving forces have been abolished experimentally (Friedman, 1988). Calcium transport by the medullary thick ascending limb appears to be dependent primarily on passive driving forces similar to those in the cortical segment (Suki et al, 1980).

DISTAL CONVOLUTED TUBULE. Approximately 8% of filtered calcium is reabsorbed by this segment, located between the macula densa and the collecting tubule (Suki and Rouse, 1991). Several features suggest that this involves active transport: (1) the Ca^{2+} concentration in tubule fluid entering this segment from the thick ascending limb is relatively low because relatively more Ca^{2+} than water is reabsorbed from the thick limb (Costanza and Windhager, 1978), and (2) the distal collecting tubule has a lumen-negative transepithelial potential difference (Wright, 1971). As in the proximal tubule and the thick ascending limb, Na^+ and Ca^{2+} reabsorption occur in parallel in this segment. However, these transport processes can be dissociated by modifications in parathyroid hormone levels and during a variety of pathologic conditions to be discussed.

COLLECTING TUBULE. A relatively small amount of calcium is reabsorbed by the collecting tubule under physiologic conditions (Bourdeau and Hellstrom-Stein, 1982).

Mechanisms of Calcium Transport by Tubule Epithelium

Several features of renal epithelial cells indicate that they possess one or more mechanisms for calcium extrusion that are necessary to maintain calcium homeostasis. For example, extracellular Ca^{2+} concentration (10^{-3} mol) greatly exceeds cytosolic (10^{-7} mol), renal cell membranes are permeable to Ca^{2+}, and the intracellular compartment is electrically negative (approximately -70 mV) in relation to the extracellular space (Costanza and Windhager, 1992). Among the mechanisms that participate in efflux of Ca^{2+} from these cells include a Ca^{2+}-ATPase and Na^+-Ca^{2+} exchanger, located on the basolateral membrane. In addition, cytosolic Ca^{2+} is buffered by its binding to calmodulin and other intracellular proteins, and the major fraction of nonionized Ca^{2+} is sequestered within mitochondria and endoplasmic reticulum (Johnson and Kumar, 1994).

Factors Regulating Calcium Transport
(Table 7–3)

PARATHYROID HORMONE. Parathyroid hormone (PTH) directly stimulates calcium reabsorption by the kidney

Table 7–3. FACTORS AFFECTING CALCIUM REABSORPTION

Factor	Nephron Segment		
	Proximal	*Thick Ascending Limb*	*Distal*
Volume expansion	Decreased	?	Decreased
Acidosis	Decreased	?	Decreased
Alkalosis	Increased	?	?
Hypercalcemia	Decreased	Decreased	Decreased
Hypermagnesemia	Decreased	Decreased	?
Phosphate depletion	Decreased	?	Decreased
Parathyroid hormone	Increased	Increased	Increased
Insulin, glucose	Decreased	?	Decreased

?, Unknown.

Adapted from Suki WN, Rouse D: Renal transport of calcium, magnesium, and phosphorus. *In* Brenner BM, Rector FC, eds: The Kidney, 4th ed. Philadelphia, W.B. Saunders Company, 1991, pp 380–423.

(Fig. 7–26). This effect is mediated by PTH-sensitive adenylate cyclase and increased production of cAMP in the proximal tubule, cortical thick ascending limb of Henle, distal tubule, and connecting tubule (Chabardès et al, 1975; Morel, 1981; Costanza and Windhager, 1992). In contrast, there is no PTH effect on Ca^{2+} transport in the medullary thick ascending limb (Friedman, 1988).

The major effect of PTH on Ca^{2+} regulation by the kidney occurs at the distal tubule, where active calcium reabsorption is stimulated independently of Na^+ and water (Costanza and Windhager, 1980). PTH increases adenylate cyclase activity via a stimulatory G-protein that is coupled to the PTH receptor on the basolateral membrane (Bourdeau, 1993). This leads to activation of dihydropyridine-sensitive calcium channels. The related increase in intracellular Ca^{2+} concentration has been attributed predominantly to luminal Ca^{2+} entry rather than to Ca^{2+} release by intracellular stores (Le Grimellec et al, 1974; Backasi and Friedman, 1990; Costanza and Windhager, 1992). This response is mediated by a cAMP-mediated protein kinase (Lau and Bourdeau, 1989).

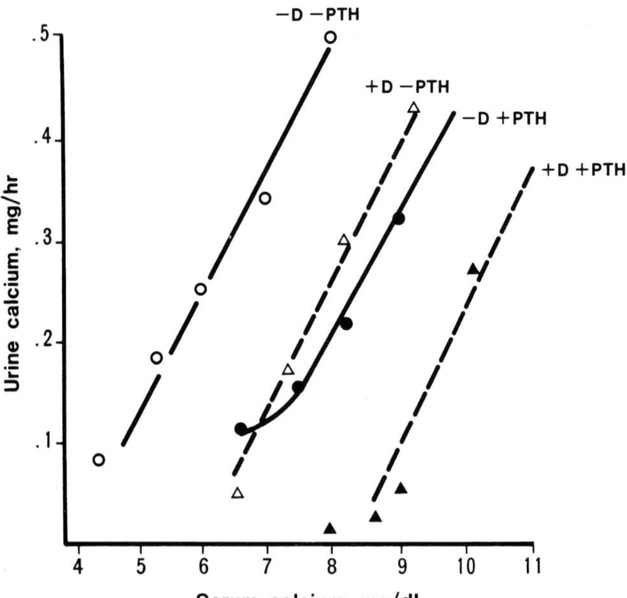

Figure 7–26. Effects of parathyroid hormone (PTH) and vitamin D on renal tubular handling of calcium. (Data from Seldin DW, Giebisch G: The Kidney: Physiology and Pathology, 2nd ed. New York, Raven Press, 1992, p 1358.)

VITAMIN D. The kidney is the major site of production of the most active form of vitamin D: 1,25-dihydroxyvitamin D_3 (calcitriol; 1,25-$[OH]_2D_3$; Fraser and Kodicek, 1970). The enzyme responsible for the production of 1,25-$(OH)_2D_3$ from 25-(OH)D is 25-(OH)D-1α-hydroxylase, a cytochrome P450 monoxygenase. This enzyme is located in the proximal convoluted and straight tubule segments (Ghazarian et al, 1974): 1α-hydroxylase activity is stimulated directly by PTH in the proximal convoluted tubule and by calcitonin in the proximal straight tubule (Akiba et al, 1980).

Vitamin D increases renal calcium reabsorption at distal nephron segments (Costanza et al, 1974). It induces production of calbindin-D_{28}, a vitamin D–dependent calcium binding protein that appears to enhance diffusion of calcium across renal tubule epithelial cells (Taylor et al, 1982; Bronner and Stein, 1988; Costanza and Windhager, 1992; Bourdeau, 1993).

EXTRACELLULAR FLUID VOLUME. Proximal tubular reabsorption of sodium is reduced during volume expansion and is increased when extracellular fluid (ECF) volume is reduced. As discussed, calcium and Na^+ reabsorption occur in parallel in the proximal tubule; hence Ca^{2+} reabsorption is augmented when EFC volume is reduced and attenuated when ECF volume is expanded (Walser, 1961).

DIURETICS (see Fig. 7–21)

- Carbonic anhydrase inhibitors: This class of diuretic inhibits proximal tubular reabsorption of Na^+ and Ca^{2+} (see section on acid-base homeostasis) but does not increase urinary excretion of calcium (Beck and Goldberg, 1973). This dissociation of Na^+ and Ca^{2+} by the kidney most likely reflects augmented Ca^{2+} reabsorption by distal nephron segments (Costanza and Windhager, 1992; Walser, 1961).
- Loop diuretics: These agents promote diuresis by inhibiting the Na-K-2Cl transporter at the thick ascending limb (see section on renal potassium excretion). In addition, they abolish the lumen-positive transepithelial potential that normally serves as a driving force for passive calcium reabsorption (Bourdeau and Burg, 1979). The result is increased excretion of both Na^+ and Ca^{2+}. **However, this effect may be attenuated if ECF volume decreases and filtration fraction increases, because Ca^{2+} reabsorption is increased by the proximal tubule.**
- Thiazide-type diuretics: Unlike loop diuretics, thiazide-type diuretics inhibit NaCl reabsorption at the cortical diluting segment (Costanza, 1985). **Furthermore, these agents do not inhibit calcium reabsorption; instead they have a hypocalciuric effect both acutely and during chronic administration, regardless of the ECF volume.** The mechanism of action involves inhibition of neutral NaCl cotransport by the distal tubule, thereby reducing intracellular Na^+. As a consequence of the decreased intracellular Na^+ concentration, Na^+-Ca^{2+} exchange by the basolateral membrane is stimulated, and Ca^{2+} reabsorption is enhanced (Costanza and Windhager, 1992; Friedman et al, 1981).

- Potassium-sparing diuretics (amiloride, triamterene, spironolactone): These diuretics reduce calcium clearance by the kidney (Costanza, 1984), and this action is additive with thiazide-type diuretics (Alon et al, 1984).

REGULATION OF MAGNESIUM EXCRETION

Magnesium is a predominant intracellular divalent cation, distributed primarily in bone and soft tissues (Alfrey, 1992). Normal plasma Mg^{2+} concentration ranges from 1.7 to 2.3 mg/dl, of which 70% is ultrafilterable and the remainder is bound to albumin and other proteins (Quamme, 1992). Of the 2100 mg of Mg^{2+} filtered daily by the glomerulus, 97% is reabsorbed along the nephron: 20%–30% by proximal convoluted tubule, 15% by the proximal straight tubule, 65% in the thick ascending limb of Henle, and 2%–5% in the distal tubule (Suki and Rouse, 1991). **As with Ca^{2+}, Mg^{2+} reabsorption in the thick ascending limb occurs in parallel with sodium and chloride reabsorption.** A major driving force for Mg^{2+} reabsorption by this segment is the lumen-positive transepithelial potential (Sharegi and Agus, 1982). Hence, Mg^{2+} reabsorption is decreased by loop diuretics and ECF volume expansion (Quamme, 1980, 1981).

The factors affecting Mg^{2+} reabsorption are outlined in Table 7–4.

REGULATION OF PHOSPHATE EXCRETION

The total plasma phosphate level is 14 mg/dl; inorganic phosphate (P_i) accounts for 3.0–4.5 mg/dl, and the remainder is in complexes with lipids and other compounds (Suki and Rouse, 1991). About 90% of the plasma P_i is ultrafiltered by the glomerulus, half of which is in free ionic form (Berndt and Knox, 1992). As discussed later, P_i is present in extracellular fluid as either the divalent or monovalent anion (see section on acid-base homeostasis). At pH 7.4, the ratio HPO_4^{2-}:$H_2PO_4^-$ is 4:1. The relative amount of ultrafilterable P_i decreases when plasma P_i and Ca^{2+} levels increase, such as in primary hyperparathyroidism and hypercalcemia of malignancy, most likely because of the formation of $Ca_3(PO_4^{2-})$ complexes (Cuche et al, 1976; Suki and Rouse, 1991).

Approximately 80%–95% of the filtered phosphate is reabsorbed by the kidney. The plasma concentration at which P_i reabsorption occurs (T_mP) is close to the fasting plasma P_i concentration (Suki and Rouse, 1991). The tubule reabsorptive capacity is most accurately expressed by the ratio GFR/T_mP. When GFR exceeds 40 ml/minute, T_mP varies proportionately with GFR. At a lower GFR, P_i and T_mP/GFR increase, and at a high GFR, they decrease (Anderson and Parsons, 1963; Yanagawa et al, 1983).

Table 7–4. FACTORS AFFECTING MAGNESIUM REABSORPTION

Factor	Nephron Segment		
	Proximal	*Thick Ascending Limb*	*Distal*
Volume expansion	Decreased	Decreased	?
Acidosis	Decreased	Unchanged	Decreased
Alkalosis	Increased	Unchanged	Increased
Hypercalcemia	Decreased	Decreased	Unchanged
Hypermagnesemia	Increased	Decreased	Unchanged
Phosphate depletion	Unchanged	Decreased	Decreased
Parathyroid hormone	Unchanged	Increased	?
Vasopressin	Unchanged	Increased	Unchanged

?, Unknown.

Adapted from Suki WN, Rouse D: Renal transport of calcium, magnesium and phosphorus. *In* Brenner BM, Rector FC, eds: The Kidney, 4th ed. Philadelphia, W.B. Saunders Company, 1991, pp 380–423.

Factors That Influence Phosphorus Excretion

PARATHYROID HORMONE. PTH is the predominant hormonal regulator of urinary phosphate excretion: PTH infusion is phosphaturic; parathyroidectomy decreases phosphate excretion by the kidney (Beck and Goldberg, 1973; Kuntziger et al, 1974). **The major site of PTH-sensitive P_i transport is the proximal tubule, but activity is also present in the distal nephron** (Agus et al, 1971; Greger et al, 1977; Peraino and Suki, 1980). PTH stimulates adenylate cyclase activity in these segments, and the actions of PTH are believed to be mediated by cAMP (Murer and Biber, 1992).

DIETARY PHOSPHATE. The kidney adapts to dietary phosphate intake, with the amount of P_i excretion directly related to P_i intake. Fractional P_i reabsorption increased during low P_i diet independently of PTH, serum Ca^{2+}, or other determinants of P_i excretion (Anderson and Draper, 1972). The site of this adaptation is the proximal convoluted tubule, where V_{max} of Na-dependent P_i transport is affected (Brazy et al, 1980).

REGULATION OF URATE EXCRETION

Uric acid is the byproduct of purine degradation. It is a weak acid (see section on acid-base homeostasis) for which, at physiologic pH in body fluids, 98% is present as monosodium urate (Kippen et al, 1974). Therefore, the term "uric acid" is used as a general term when purine metabolism is discussed, whereas "urate" is specifically referred to in the discussion of renal tubule transport and clinical syndromes. **Saturation of human plasma occurs at a urate concentration of approximately 6.5%–7.0% mg/dl, with lower solubility at lower temperatures and higher sodium concentrations.** Normally, only 5% of urate in plasma is bound to protein (Grantham and Chonko, 1991).

Urate is filtered by the glomerulus, and the fractional excretion of urate in humans ranges from 7% to 12%. Reabsorption of urate by the proximal tubule occurs predominantly in the S_1 segment, where it enters the cytoplasm in exchange for hydroxyl anions, HCO_3^-, Cl^-, hippurate, and lactate (Kahn and Aronson, 1983; Weinman et al, 1976).

Urate secretion also occurs in the proximal tubule, with the secretory rate exceeding reabsorption in the S_2 segment of the proximal tubule (Chonko, 1980; Senekjian et al,

1981). Urinary excretion of urate is markedly reduced, and plasma urate levels are increased by pyrazinamide, an inhibitor of urate secretion. Thus the major component of urate in urine arrives via tubule secretion (Rieselbach et al, 1970; Weiner and Tinker, 1972; Grantham and Chonko, 1991).

Factors Affecting Urate Transport

EXTRACELLULAR FLUID VOLUME. Urate clearance is increased by volume expansion and decreased by ECF volume reduction (Steele and Oppenheimer, 1969; Diamond and Meisel, 1975). The magnitude of proximal reabsorption of urate changes in parallel with ECF volume and thus contributes substantially to its reabsorption. The relative predominance of ECF volume over urinary flow rate as a determinant of urate excretion is illustrated by the comparison of the syndrome of inappropriate antidiuretic hormone secretion (SIADH; see later discussion) with diabetes insipidus. In SIADH, ECF volume is expanded, urate clearance is increased, and serum urate levels are reduced to below normal (Mees et al, 1971; Beck, 1979) despite the low urinary flow rate. In diabetes insipidus, ECF volume is reduced and serum urate levels are high despite the high urine flow rate. These observations also suggest that urate reabsorption by the distal nephron is of relatively minor importance (Grantham and Chonko, 1991). Thus volume expansion can be beneficial in patients at risk for uric acid nephropathy.

URINARY pH. Uric acid is relatively insoluble (15 mg/dl) in its nonionized form in acidified urine (pH 4.5). By contrast, its solubility increases markedly (200 mg/dl) at alkaline pH, when it is dissociated to urate (Grantham and Chonko, 1991).

OTHER SUBSTANCES. Drugs and other compounds that influence urate excretion by the kidney are listed in Table 7–5.

Table 7–5. SUBSTANCES THAT ALTER RENAL URATE EXCRETION

Hyperuricemic Substances
Substances That Inhibit Secretion
Salicylates (low dose, 5–10 mg/dl serum)
Pyrazinamide
Nicotinic acid
Ethambutol
Ethanol (through lactate production)
Certain "secreted" diuretics (furosemide)
Substances That Stimulate Reabsorption
Most diuretics (indirectly when ECF volume is diminished)
Chronic lead intoxication
Chronic beryllium intoxication
Hypouricemic Substances
Substances That Inhibit Reabsorption
Probenecid
Sulfinpyrazone
Salicylates (high dose ≥ 15 mg/dl serum)
Phenylbutazone
Radiocontrast agents
Mannitol
Ascorbic acid (high dose ≥ 4 g)

ECF, extracellular fluid.

Adapted from Grantham JJ, Chonko AM: Renal handling of organic ions and cations; excretion of uric acid. *In* Brenner BM, Rector FC, eds: The Kidney, 4th ed. Philadelphia, W.B. Saunders Company, 1991, pp 483–509.

REGULATION OF WATER BALANCE

The total body solute concentration is maintained within very narrow limits by homeostatic mechanisms that alter the rate of water intake and excretion (Robertson, 1992). Deviations of total body osmolality are usually caused by changes in water balance and are manifested by variations in serum Na^+ concentration, the major determinant of plasma osmolality. When total body osmolality increases or decreases by more than a small percentage from the normal range, serious neurologic complications can occur. The kidney plays a central role in the integrated responses that are essential for maintaining normal water balance and thus defends against these life-threatening consequences.

Composition of Body Fluids

Water constitutes the largest component of the human body, accounting for about 60% of total body weight in men and 50% in women; the gender difference reflects the higher relative body fat content in women. Sixty percent of the total body water is distributed intracellularly, and 40% is in the extracellular compartment. Plasma water accounts for 20% of the ECF volume (Robertson and Berl, 1991).

The total solute concentrations in the intracellular and extracellular compartments are equal, because of the high permeability of cell membranes to water. However, the solute compositions of the extracellular and intracellular fluids are quite different because of the ion transport mechanisms (i.e., Na^+-K^+-ATPase) located on cell membranes (Rose, 1989). Consequently, Na^+, Cl^-, and HCO_3^- are located primarily in extracellular fluid, whereas K^+, Mg^{2+}, and phosphates are predominant in the intracellular space. Glucose is metabolized in cells and thus is present in significant amounts only in extracellular fluid. Each of these solutes is referred to as an effective osmole because they exert an osmotic force that determines the distribution of water throughout the body (Zerbe and Robertson, 1983).

When the solute concentration becomes higher in one compartment, the related increase in osmotic pressure drives water influx from the adjacent compartment across the highly water-permeable cell membranes until a new osmotic equilibrium is established (Kirk and Schaefer, 1992). An increase in effective extracellular fluid osmolality causes cellular dehydration, whereas a decrease causes cellular overhydration. This is clinically relevant because neurologic clinical signs and symptoms occur as a consequence of the associated water fluxes to and from brain cells (Arieff, 1987; Sterns et al, 1986). In contrast, when isosmotic fluid (i.e., normal saline) is added to the ECF, there are no changes in osmolality or shifts in water between body compartments.

The total osmolality of body fluids is defined as

$$P_{Osm} = 2 \times \text{plasma } [Na^+] + \frac{[\text{glucose}]}{18} + \frac{\text{BUN}}{2.8},$$

where plasma sodium is multiplied by 2 to account for the accompanying anion (predominantly Cl^- and HCO_3^-) and glucose and BUN (blood urea nitrogen) are expressed as millimoles per liter.

However, urea is unlike Na^+ and K^+ because it diffuses freely across cell membranes and is present in equal concentrations in the extracellular and intracellular spaces. Urea is referred to as an ineffective osmole because it does not generate an osmotic gradient and therefore does not affect the distribution of water (Rose, 1989). Effective osmolality is thus expressed as

$$P_{Osm} = 2 \times \text{plasma } [Na^+] + \frac{[\text{glucose}]}{18}.$$

This relationship indicates that sodium is the major determinant of normal plasma osmolality ($P_{Osm} = 275 - 290$ mOsm/kg). It follows that serum Na^+ concentration is proportional to total body osmolality because the body compartments are in osmotic equilibrium. Similarly, the concentration of K^+ in cells is also directly proportional to total body osmolality because K^+ is the predominant intracellular effective osmole. Therefore, alterations in total body osmolality, and thus in serum Na^+ concentration, reflect changes in the *ratio* of the body content of K^+, Na^+, and total body water (Edelman et al, 1958). This linear relationship is expressed as

$$\text{Plasma } [Na^+] = \frac{Na^+_e + K^+_e}{TBW},$$

where $Na^+_e + K^+_e$ refer to exchangeable Na^+ and K^+ ions that are not sequestered in body tissues and TBW is total body water.

The central point of the discussion thus far is that the plasma Na^+ concentration does *not* correlate with body volume, and so the plasma Na^+ concentration does not provide information for predicting a patient's volume status: hyponatremia can occur when total body volume is increased (e.g., as in congestive heart failure) or decreased (e.g., as in gastrointestinal losses). As described earlier, the effective circulating blood volume is normally regulated by adjustments in isotonic sodium reabsorption by the kidney in response to signals from volume receptors in the cardiopulmonary circulation and kidneys (Table 7–6). This isosmotic change in body volume has no effect on plasma osmolality.

Total body osmolality and thus the serum sodium concentration are narrowly regulated by factors that influence water balance. Water intake is normally related to consumption and metabolism of food, but it may vary widely among individuals for reasons that are unrelated to diet. **Water intake usually exceeds the volume required for the maintenance of water balance and is not usually dictated solely by thirst when the body osmolality is normal (285–290 mOsm/kg;** Lassiter and Gottschalk, 1992). Within this range, vasopressin is directly correlated with plasma and urine osmolality. Furthermore, a 2% increase in TBW reduces vasopressin to threshold levels and results in maximally dilute urine, whereas a 2% rise in plasma osmolality increases the vasopressin level sufficiently to produce maximally concentrated urine (Robertson and Berl, 1991). These findings, together with the rapid onset of vasopressin action and its short half-life, indicate that **vasopressin plays a more dominant role than thirst in maintaining normal water balance.**

Table 7–6. FACTORS GOVERNING REGULATION OF BODY VOLUME AND OSMOLALITY

	Osmoregulation	Volume Regulation
Signal	Plasma osmolality	Effective circulating volume
Sensors	Hypothalamic osmoreceptor	Carotid sinus Juxtaglomerular cell Atria
Effectors	Vasopressin	Renin-angiotensin-aldosterone system
	Thirst	Sympathetic nervous system Peritubular capillary hemodynamics Atrial natriuretic peptide Vasopressin
What Is Affected	Urine osmolality, water intake	Urine sodium excretion

From Rose BD: Clinical Physiology of Acid-Base and Electrolyte Disorders, 3rd ed. New York, Raven Press, 1992, pp 2837–2872.

However, thirst is a powerful stimulus for water intake when cellular dehydration is produced by water deprivation or during administration of hyperosmotic sodium chloride or other solute that is excluded from the intracellular compartment. This first occurs when the plasma osmolality reaches 295 mOsm/kg, a point at which the vasopressin level is already at a point at which renal compensation is maximal: urine volume is minimized, and it is maximally concentrated. **Total body osmolality can increase significantly when the thirst mechanism is impaired or when access to water is restricted, even though the secretion and renal response to vasopressin are appropriate** (see later discussion). In contrast, urea does not stimulate thirst or vasopressin secretion when it accumulates in acute and chronic renal failure, because it equilibrates across cell membranes and does not cause cellular dehydration (Robertson, 1992; Fig. 7–27).

Thirst may also be increased even though effective osmolality of body fluid is normal or reduced. This phenomenon occurs when the effective circulating volume is reduced. The ECF is a component of blood volume to which regulatory systems respond by modulating sodium and water excretion (Schrier, 1988; Blumenfeld and Laragh, 1994). It is an incompletely defined parameter that reflects the relation between cardiac output and peripheral arterial vascular resistance that is perceived by baroreceptors in capacitance and arterial vessels.

Examples of nonosmotic stimuli of thirst associated with decreased ECF volume are acute blood loss, gastrointestinal losses, congestive heart failure, ascites, and unilateral renovascular hypertension (Schrier, 1988). The renin-angiotensin-aldosterone system is intensely activated in each of these conditions, and Ang II has been demonstrated to be one of the mediators of this potent dipsogenic response through its actions at central nervous system structures located near the third ventricle (Lassiter and Gottschalk, 1992).

There are also several nonosmotic stimuli that influence the rate of vasopressin release. As with thirst, inadequate delivery of blood to the peripheral circulation stimulates

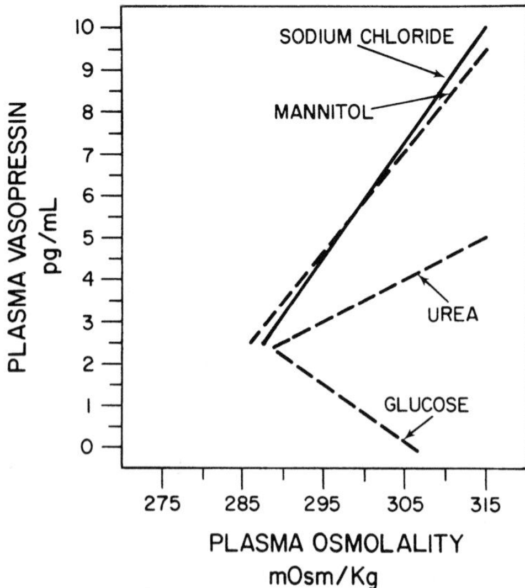

Figure 7–27. Solute specificity of the osmoreceptor. The lines represent the relationship of plasma vasopressin to plasma osmolality in healthy adults during intravenous infusion of hypertonic solutions of different solutes. (From Robertson GL, Berl T: Pathophysiology of water metabolism. *In* Brenner BM, Rector FC, eds: The Kidney, 4th ed. Philadelphia, W.B. Saunders Company, 1991, pp 677–736. Redrawn from Zerbe RL, Robertson GL: Am J Physiol 1983; 224:E607.)

secretion of vasopressin. However, the vasopressin response to changes in ECFV is relatively insensitive. **A decrease in blood volume of 15% is required before this can become the dominant stimulus for vasopressin secretion, in comparison with the 2% change in osmolality** (Fig. 7–28; Dunn et al, 1973). Other nonosmotic stimuli include Ang II (Mouw et al, 1971), nausea (Rowe et al, 1979), pain, and several pharmacologic agents, including general anesthetics (Table 7–7).

In contrast to water intake, water excretion is tightly regulated by the kidney and is normally influenced by the level of vasopressin and the rate of solute excretion. The

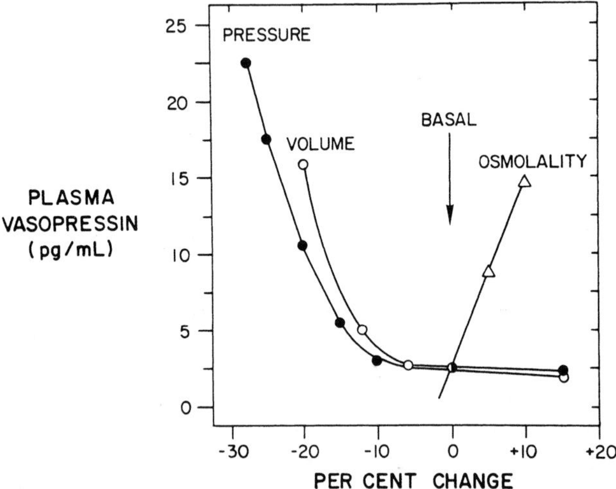

Figure 7–28. Comparative sensitivities of the osmoregulatory and baroregulatory mechanisms. Note that vasopressin secretion is much more sensitive to changes in blood osmolality than volume. (From Gougoux A, Jinay P, et al: Immediate adaption of the dog kidney to acute hypercapnia. Am J Physiol 243:F227–F234, 1982.)

Table 7–7. DRUGS ASSOCIATED WITH WATER RETENTION

Drug	Hyponatremia	ADH Release	Renal Action*
Chlorpropamide	+	−	+
Vincristine	+	+	−
Cytoxan	+	−	+
Carbamazepine	+	+	?
Clofibrate	−	+	−
Narcotics	?	+	−
Haloperidol	+	?	?
Fluphenazine	+	?	?
Amitriptyline	+	?	?
Thioridazine	+	?	?
NSAIDs	−	−	+
Diuretics	+	+	+

?, Unknown.
*Refers to ADH-like action or potentiation of ADH action on the kidney.
ADH, antidiuretic hormone; NSAIDs, nonsteroidal anti-inflammatory drugs.
Adapted from Robertson GL, Berl T: Pathophysiology of water metabolism. *In* Brenner BM, Rector FC, eds: The Kidney, 4th ed. Philadelphia, W.B. Saunders Company, 1991, pp 677–736.

amount of solute that must be excreted daily is related to solute intake; the predominant components include Na^+ and K^+ salts and urea. The volume of urine that is required each day to excrete this obligate solute load depends on the availability of vasopressin and the kidney's responsiveness to it.

Insensible water loss, which is the amount of water lost by evaporation from the skin and respiratory tract, is usually about 14 ml/kg/day but may vary significantly according to factors that include temperature, exercise, and antidiuretic hormone level (Robertson, 1992). Sweat contains significant amounts of Na^+ (30–65 mEq/l; Rose, 1989) and so is referred to as a sensible loss, with volumes exceeding 1 l/day during exercise or in hot weather.

Renal Mechanisms for Concentration and Dilution of Urine

The kidney maintains total body osmolality within a narrow range despite the wide range of fluid intake, variable extrarenal fluid losses, and requirement of urinary excretion of the daily solute load that is generated by metabolism of nutrients. To achieve this goal, the excretion of solutes and water is regulated independently by the kidneys. Consequently, a small volume of hyperosmotic urine is produced when water must be conserved, and a larger volume of hypoosmotic urine is produced when there is excess water (Lassiter and Gottschalk, 1992).

The countercurrent multiplier principle, which provides the basis for urinary concentration and dilution, states that when an exchange of material or energy occurs between two parallel columns of fluid moving in opposite directions, dissipation of energy or material is reduced (Lassiter and Gottschalk, 1992). When this principle is applied to the kidney, the loops of Henle function as the countercurrent multiplier that generates and maintains a longitudinal solute gradient that increases in tonicity from the corticomedullary junction to the tip of the papilla (Fig. 7–29). Urine is initially concentrated in the descending limb of the loop of Henle by the diffusion of water into the medulla. In the medullary

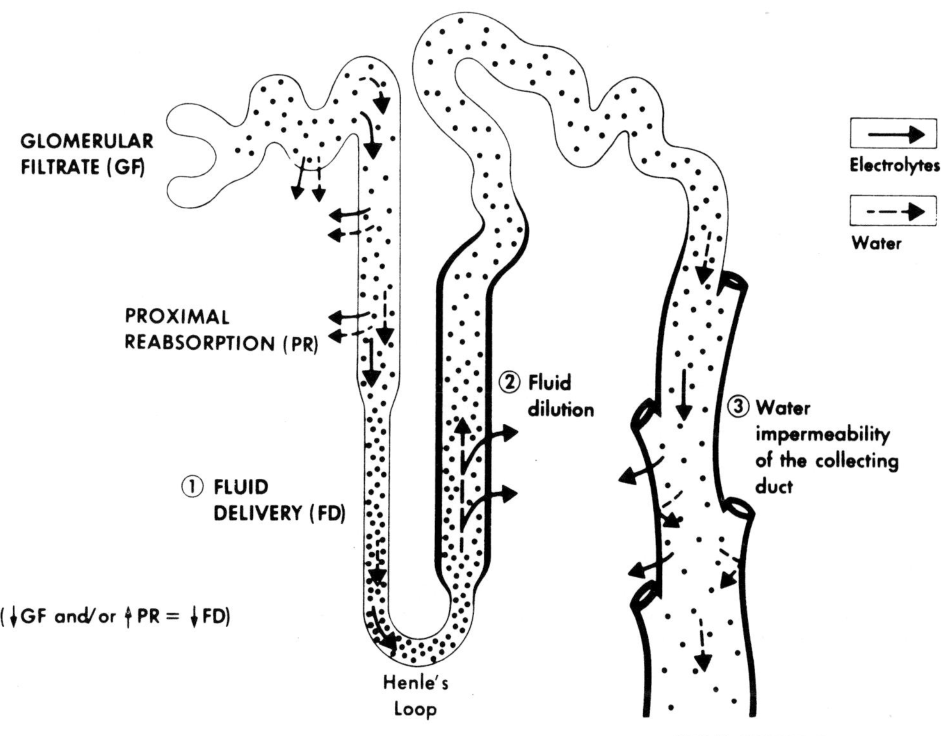

Figure 7–29. The components of the normal urine diluting mechanisms. (From Berl T, Schrier RW: Water metabolism and the hypo-osmolar syndrome. *In* Brenner BM, Stein JH, eds: Sodium and Water Homeostasis. New York, Churchill Livingstone, 1978, pp 1–23.)

thick ascending limb, NaCl is reabsorbed by active transport (Knepper and Rector, 1991). However, this nephron segment is relatively impermeable to water, so that the osmolality of the tubule lumen is reduced to below that of the surrounding medullary tissue and the interstitial solute gradient is not dissipated by water fluxes. During water diuresis, when vasopressin secretion is reduced, tubular fluid hypotonicity is maintained in the distal tubule and collecting ducts because water permeability in these segments is low. During antidiuresis, when vasopressin levels are high, the collecting duct epithelium is highly permeable to water and diffusion of water occurs from the collecting duct lumen into the hyperosmotic medulla. **Thus the major role of vasopressin is related to its effects on water permeability by the collecting ducts** (Roy et al, 1992).

Sites of Urinary Concentration and Dilution

PROXIMAL TUBULE. The osmolality of the glomerular ultrafiltrate is identical to that of plasma (Lassiter and Gottschalk, 1992). In the proximal convoluted tubule, there is isosmotic reabsorption of solutes (e.g., electrolytes, amino acids, and HCO_3^-) and water. Transport of these solutes is coupled to the active transport of Na^+ driven by the Na^+-K^+-ATPase pump. The mechanisms governing passive water transport from the proximal tubule lumen are not completely understood, but it is caused partly by differences in reflection coefficients of the various solutes that affect solute-solvent coupling (Berry and Rector, 1991). This process is not altered by the presence of ADH. Approximately two thirds of the glomerular filtrate is reabsorbed in the proximal tubule.

THIN DESCENDING LIMB OF HENLE. Osmolality of tubule fluid in this section increases as it descends into the medulla. This occurs mainly because water diffuses from the lumen into the hypertonic interstitium. In some species, small quantities of solutes (e.g., Na^+, Cl^-, urea) diffuse into the tubule lumen. This segment is not capable of significant amounts of active transport of solutes because of the low Na^+-K^+-ATPase activity (Knepper and Rector, 1991)

THIN ASCENDING LIMB OF HENLE. Thin ascending limbs are not present in short-loop nephrons that originate in the cortex. In long-loop nephrons that originate at the corticomedullary junction, the thin ascending limb segment originates at the bend of the loop in the inner medulla. The tubular fluid in this segment has a lower osmolality than does that in the adjacent descending limb, which indicates that this segment has a diluting capacity. This is accounted for by low permeability to water. As in the thin descending limb, Na^+-K^+-ATPase activity is low, so that only a small amount of NaCl is reabsorbed in this segment (Knepper and Rector, 1991; Roy et al, 1992). In the passive model proposed by Kokko and Rector (1972), the ascending limb fluid becomes progressively diluted because passive NaCl efflux out of the lumen exceeds urea influx from the medullary interstitium.

THICK ASCENDING LIMB OF HENLE. Tubular fluid becomes progressively more dilute as it flows from the thin ascending limb through the thick ascending limb of Henle and is hypoosmotic to plasma when it enters the distal tubule, regardless of whether vasopressin is present. **This diluting process occurs because active Na^+ reabsorption occurs unaccompanied by water. Two properties of the thick ascending limb make this possible: (1) it has the highest Na^+-K^+-ATPase pump activity of all nephron segments, thus driving high rates of coupled ion transport via Na^+-K^+-$2Cl^-$ cotransporter** (Hebert et al, 1981;

Hebert and Andreoli, 1984), **and (2) it has very low permeability to water** (Blumenfeld, 1989a; Knepper and Rector, 1991). As a consequence of this "single effect," NaCl is the predominant solute in the inner medullary interstitium. Vasopressin stimulates the rate of NaCl reabsorption in this segment, thereby enhancing countercurrent multiplication, the process responsible for generating and maintaining the corticomedullary gradient.

COLLECTING DUCT. The concentration of tubular fluid entering this segment from the distal tubule is approximately 100 mOsm/kg. During water diuresis, the cortical collecting duct is impermeable to water, and thus urine osmolality decreases because of ongoing Na^+ reabsorption. During antidiuresis, vasopressin increases water permeability of this segment and also augments aldosterone-stimulated Na^+ reabsorption, thereby promoting water efflux from the tubule into the interstitium (Roy et al, 1992). By contrast, urea permeability is low and is not increased by vasopressin. **Therefore, the osmolality of tubular fluid is higher when it leaves the cortical collecting duct and enters the medullary collecting duct, because water is reabsorbed and the urea concentration in the tubule is augmented.** The properties of the outer medullary collecting duct are similar to those of the cortical collecting duct.

The initial portion of the inner medullary collecting duct, in the presence of vasopressin, is highly permeable to water but not to urea, so that the urea concentration reaches its maximum (Chou et al, 1993). **However, at the terminal third of this segment, urea permeability increases markedly, and there is a rapid efflux of urea into the medullary interstitium.** The tremendous increase in magnitude of urea transport suggests that facilitated diffusion by a specific urea carrier may occur solely in this segment (Gillin and Sands, 1993). As a consequence of this substantial amount of urea reabsorption, the urea content and osmolality of the inner medulla increase and thereby promote additional reabsorption of water. In addition to urea, Na^+, K^+, and NH_4^+ also accumulate in the medullary interstitium. Studies have also demonstrated that organic, osmotically active compounds, referred to as *osmolytes,* also accumulate in the inner medulla (Gullans et al, 1988, 1989; Blumenfeld et al, 1989a, 1989b; Knepper and Rector, 1991).

VASA RECTA. The vasa recta are hairpin-shaped vessels that arise from efferent arterioles of juxtaglomerular nephrons. They are organized as parallel channels through which blood enters and leaves the medullary interstitium (Roy et al, 1992). This arrangement provides a countercurrent diffusion mechanism in which solutes reabsorbed by the loop of Henle and collecting duct diffuse from the ascending to descending limbs of the vasa recta and are trapped in the medullary interstitium. This mechanisms is made more efficient by the low blood flow through the medulla. When medullary blood flow is abnormally increased (e.g., as in osmotic diuresis), medullary osmolality decreases and urinary concentrating ability is impaired (see later discussion).

WATER CHANNELS. Within minutes after vasopressin binds to basolateral V_2 receptors on the principal cells of the collecting duct, aggregates of intramembranous particles appear in the membrane facing the lumen (Zeidel et al, 1993; Bichet, 1994). These particles contain water channels that are inserted into the apical membrane in response to vasopressin stimulation and that increase water permeability by the collecting duct. When vasopressin is withdrawn, endocytosis of the membrane-containing water channels breaks their contact with the aqueous luminal surface, and water permeability decreases markedly (Zeidel et al, 1993). These particles are structurally similar to, although not identical to, channel-like integral membrane protein with a molecular weight of 28,000 daltons (CHIP28) that are abundant in erythrocytes and other kidney tubules (e.g., proximal tubule, thin descending limb). However, several features distinguish CHIP28, now referred to as aqueporin-1, from aqueporin-2, the vasopressin-dependent water channel, including its absence from the collecting duct, lack of vasopressin-responsiveness, and other biophysical properties (e.g., proton permeability). The link between aqueporin-2 and vasopressin-mediated water transport by the kidney was established with the discovery that the aqueporin-2 gene is mutated in patients with congenital nephrogenic diabetes insipidus (see later; Deen et al, 1994; Knoers and Os, 1995).

In summary, the kidney maintains total body osmolality by the coordinated regulation of solute reabsorption and water excretion. This process requires an adequate GFR, sufficient delivery of filtrate to the loop of Henle and collecting tubules, and appropriate vasopressin secretion and responsiveness by the distal nephron segments.

Measurement of Renal Water Excretion and Reabsorption

The volume of urine excreted each day is normally related to the availability of vasopressin and the amount of solute present in the urine, which under steady-state conditions is related to dietary intake (Rose, 1989). If the normal range of urine osmolality is between approximately 100 and 1200 mOsm/kg and an individual's obligate daily solute load is 600 mOsm, the volume of urine required ranges from 500 ml/day (when the vasopressin effect is maximal) to 6 L/day (when vasopressin is absent). It is apparent from this example that urinary osmolality is related to the daily intake and excretion of solute. Accordingly, if the same individual's solute intake and excretion decrease from 600 to 500 mOsm/day because of dietary protein restriction, the range of urine volume decreases to 420 ml/day (when the vasopressin effect is maximal) to 5 L/day (when vasopressin is absent). Therefore, at any level of vasopressin, the volume of urine output is dependent on the solute load and can vary widely at any given level of urine osmolality (Rose, 1989; Robertson and Berl, 1991). For this reason, urine osmolality does not accurately quantify the amount of water that is excreted or retained.

To calculate the amount of water excreted or retained by the kidney, it is useful to consider that urine has two components: one that contains all of the solute in an isotonic solution (termed C_{Osm}, or osmolar clearance) and another that contains only solute-free water (termed C_{H_2O} or free water clearance). The total urine volume (V) (e.g., liters per day) is the sum of C_{Osm} and C_{H_2O}:

$$V = C_{Osm} + C_{H2O}$$

where

$$P_{Osm} = \text{plasma osmolality}$$

U_{Osm} = urine osmolality

$$C_{Osm} = \frac{U_{Osm} \times V}{P_{Osm}}$$

$$C_{H2O} = V - C_{Osm}$$

$$= V \times \left(1 - \frac{U_{Osm}}{P_{Osm}}\right)$$

When the urine is hypoosmotic to plasma, C_{H2O} is a positive value. **Hyponatremia occurs when one or more of these requirements are not fulfilled, such as when GFR is reduced, when diuretics impair NaCl reabsorption, or when vasopressin is in excess (i.e., SIADH).** If water intake exceeds the kidney's capacity to form solute-free water (greater than 10–20 L/day), hyponatremia also occurs.

Urine that is hyperosmotic to plasma consists of an isoosmotic solution and also a volume of solute-free water that was reabsorbed by the kidney to raise the urine osmolality (Rose, 1989). The expression T^c_{H2O} refers to this volume of water removed from the urine and can be expressed as follows:

$$T^c_{H2O} = -C_{H2O}$$

This relationship includes urea as a major component of urinary osmolality. However, plasma Na^+ concentration is determined mainly by the body contents of extracellular osmoles (Na^+ salts) and intracellular ions (K^+ salts); urea is not an effective osmole because it diffuses freely across cell membranes and does not contribute to plasma Na^+ concentration. Therefore, serum Na^+ is not affected by the amount of urea excreted in urine. A more accurate representation of the effect of urine output on serum Na^+ concentration is determined by the quantity referred to as electrolyte-free water reabsorption (T^e; Rose, 1989). In this relationship, the value for U_{Osm} is substituted for by $U_{Na^+ + K^+}$ (the sum of the urine Na^+ and K^+ concentrations) and P_{Osm} is substituted for by P_{Na} (the plasma Na^+ concentration):

$$T^e_{H2O} = V \times \left(\frac{U_{Na^+ + K^+}}{P_{Na^+}} - 1\right)$$

In summary, several conditions are required for the formation of solute-free water by the kidney, including (1) adequate GFR and delivery of filtrate to the loop of Henle, where (2) tubule fluid is diluted because NaCl is reabsorbed without water, and (3) collecting ducts that are impermeable to water.

Disorders of Osmoregulation

Hyponatremia (Fig. 7–30)

Hyponatremia, defined as a plasma sodium concentration below about 135 mEq/L, is present in 1%–2% of hospitalized patients and is the most common electrolyte disturbance encountered in clinical practice (Anderson, 1986; Bichet et al, 1992). In the setting of a normal GFR (144 L/day), about 15%–20% (25 L/day) of the filtrate

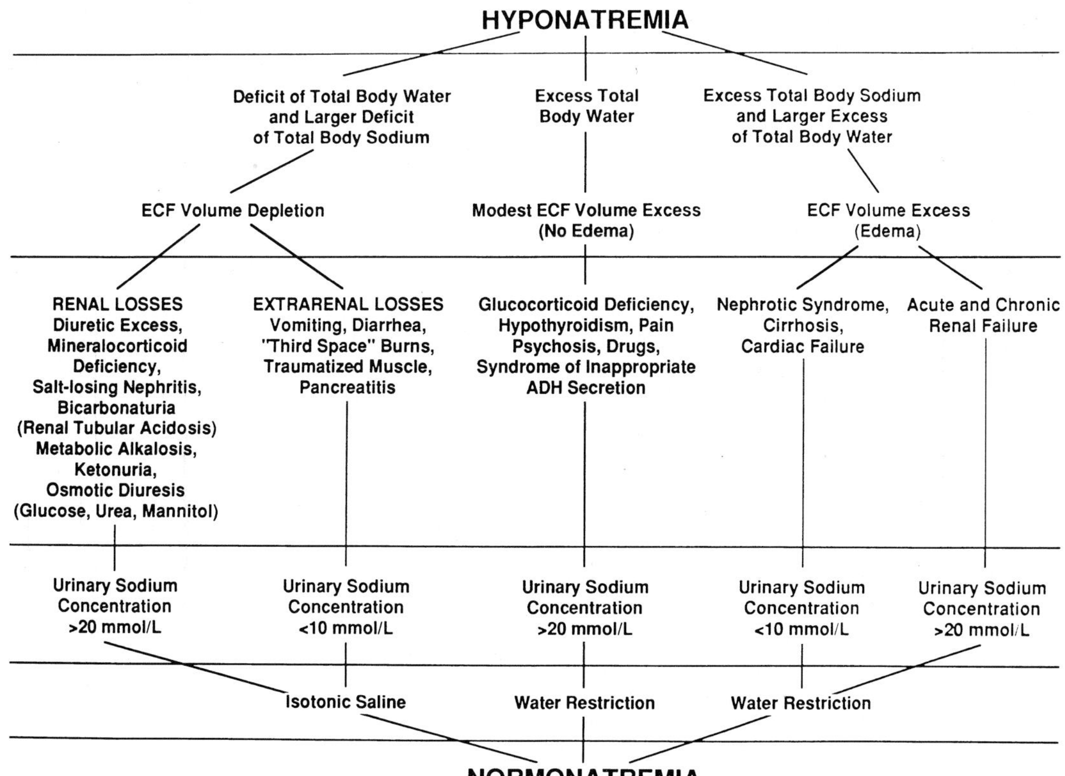

Figure 7–30. Approach to the hyponatremic patient. ECF, extracellular fluid; ADH, antidiuretic hormone. (From Berl T, Anderson RJ, McDonald KM, et al: Kidney Int 1976; 10:117.)

reaches the thick ascending limb of the loop of Henle, where it becomes hypotonic because of reabsorption of NaCl that is unaccompanied by water (Bichet et al, 1992). Under these conditions, up to 25 L of water may be consumed daily without development of hyponatremia. However, hyponatremia occurs with less water intake when the capacity of the kidney to generate solute-free water is impaired. This happens when one or more of the following conditions are present: (1) GFR is reduced, (2) delivery of filtrate to the distal diluting segment is inadequate or its function is impaired by tubulointerstitial disease or diuretics, and (3) the vasopressin level is excessive for the concurrent serum Na^+ concentration (Bichet et al, 1992). This abnormality in solute-free water clearance in hyponatremic patients is reflected by the failure to excrete maximally dilute urine ($U_{Osm} \leq 100$ mOsm/kg).

To adequately diagnosis and treat hyponatremia, the underlying cause and perpetuating factors must be identified. General considerations include whether the hyponatremia truly reflects a hypoosmolar state and whether total ECFV is reduced, normal, or increased.

HYPONATREMIA WITH NORMAL PLASMA OSMOLALITY

Pseudohyponatremia. Ninety-three percent of plasma is water, and the remaining nonaqueous phase is composed primarily of proteins and lipids. **The Na^+ concentration in the aqueous phase is normally about 151 mEq/L; however, the value reported by the clinical laboratory is lower (i.e., 140 mEq/L) because it is expressed as the ratio of Na^+ in total plasma volume** (Bichet et al, 1992). When the proportion of the nonaqueous phase increases, such as in disorders associated with hyperlipidemia or hyperproteinemia, the Na concentration in the *total* plasma volume is decreased, although both the Na^+ concentration in plasma *water* and the total body osmolality are normal (Halperin and Goldstein, 1994). Therefore, hyponatremia associated with normal osmolality is referred to as *pseudohyponatremia.* Examples of pseudohyponatremia include multiple myeloma and other hyperproteinemias, in which the plasma protein is greater than 10 g/dl, and the hyperlipidemias associated with nephrotic syndrome or diabetes mellitus when plasma lipids exceed 4.6 g/dl. This can be detected by comparing the osmolality reported by the laboratory with the value calculated from the plasma levels of Na^+, BUN, and glucose (Rose, 1989; Bichet et al, 1992; see previous discussion).

HYPONATREMIA WITH INCREASED PLASMA OSMOLALITY

When the osmolality of the ECF is increased by the addition of an impermeable solute, an osmotic gradient is established wherein water is drawn from the intracellular compartment, thereby lowering the serum Na^+ concentration. This occurs most commonly in poorly controlled diabetes mellitus, in which the plasma Na^+ concentration is reduced by 1.6 mEq/L for every 100-mg/dl rise in blood glucose above the normal range (Bichet et al, 1992). Other solutes cause a similar reduction in plasma sodium concentration, including mannitol, glycerol, and diatrizoate sodium (Iseri et al, 1965; Kirschenbaum, 1979).

HYPONATREMIA WITH REDUCED PLASMA OSMOLALITY

As discussed, hypoosmolality can occur when there is an excess or a deficit in total body sodium content. Because body sodium content is the major determinant of extracellular volume, physical examination and measurement of urinary sodium concentration are important for the diagnosis and treatment of hyponatremia (Bichet et al, 1992). The release of vasopressin is influenced by osmoreceptors and baroreceptors, which may provide opposing signals for vasopressin secretion. The ability of nonosmotic stimuli (e.g., baroreceptor stimulation in congestive heart failure) to stimulate vasopressin often predominates.

Hyponatremia with Volume Depletion. Volume depletion occurs when there is negative balance of Na^+ and water, usually as the consequence of excess renal or extrarenal losses (e.g., gastrointestinal, skin). In this setting, thirst is normally stimulated, vasopressin release occurs, and water reabsorption continues despite the reduced body osmolality. Physical evidence of volume depletion includes postural changes in blood pressure and pulse, decreased jugular venous pressure, and dry mucous membranes. These findings, together with a relevant clinical history, provide the basis for the diagnosis of hyponatremia.

Measurement of urinary sodium concentration can provide important diagnostic information about whether the fluid losses are renal or extrarenal (Table 7–8). A urinary sodium concentration less than 20 mEq/L reflects a normal renal response to volume depletion and indicates that extrarenal fluid loss has occurred. In contrast, when urine Na^+ concentration is greater than 20 mEq/L in the patient with hypovolemic hyponatremia, volume loss by the kidney has occurred.

Diuretic use is among the most common causes of hyponatremia. The mechanisms that contribute to the development and maintenance include loss of solute (Na^+ and K^+) in excess of water, volume depletion, decreased delivery of filtrate to the diluting segment and impaired function at this nephron site, and K^+ depletion (Bichet et al, 1992). **Hyponatremia occurs primarily with thiazide-type diuretics, which inhibit NaCl reabsorption by the distal tubule but do not interfere with the accumulation of solute into the medullary interstitium or reabsorption of water by vasopressin** (Rose, 1989). Consequently, thiazide-type diuretics impair the excretion of maximally dilute urine, whereas urinary concentrating ability is maintained, thus perpetuating hyponatremia by enabling reabsorption of solute-free water. Hyponatremia associated with thiazide-type diuretics usually occurs within first 2–3 weeks and is most

Table 7–8. URINARY SODIUM VALUES IN HYPOVOLEMIC HYPONATREMIA

Urinary $Na^+ > 20$ mEq/L: Renal Losses	Urinary $Na^+ < 20$ mEq/L: Extrarenal Losses
Diuretic excess	Gastrointestinal (vomiting, diarrhea)
Mineralocorticoid deficiency	"Third space sequestration" (burns, pancreatitis, muscle trauma, peritonitis)
Na^+-losing nephritis	
Osmotic diuresis (glucose, urea, mannitol, ketones)	
Bicarbonaturia (renotubular acidosis, severe metabolic alkalosis)	

Adapted from Robertson GL, Berl T: Pathophysiology of water metabolism. *In* Brenner BM, Rector FC, eds: The Kidney, 4th ed. Philadelphia, W.B. Saunders Company, 1991, pp 677–736.

often relatively mild. However, severe hyponatremia can develop if an intercurrent illness occurs (Ashraf et al, 1981). Loop diuretics, which inhibit NaCl reabsorption by the medullary thick ascending limb, decrease accumulation of solute in the medullary interstitium and thus impair the gradient for water reabsorption from the collecting duct (Suki et al, 1967; Szatalowicz et al, 1982; Rose, 1989).

Hyponatremia with Volume Excess (Edema). In the hyponatremic disorders associated with edema, vasopressin secretion is stimulated by reduced effective circulating volume perceived by baroreceptors in arterial and capacitance vessels (see earlier discussion) despite the excess total body Na^+ and water content. These disorders are associated with avid renal sodium reabsorption, as indicated by a urine Na^+ concentration of less than 20 mEq/L (Table 7–9). However, the urinary sodium concentration is usually above this level when hyponatremia and edema accompany acute and chronic renal failure.

Congestive heart failure, cirrhosis, and nephrotic syndrome are common examples of hypervolemic hyponatremia (Schrier, 1988). Vasopressin contributes importantly to the pathophysiology of hyponatremia in these disorders. In congestive heart failure, the excess vasopressin level is reached without concurrent diuretic use (Szatalowicz et al, 1981). **Nonosmotic stimuli, including increased activities of the adrenergic nervous system and renin-angiotensin-aldosterone system promote vasopressin secretion in these disorders.** The mortality rate for congestive heart failure is directly related to the severity of the hyponatremia, renin-angiotensin-aldosterone and adrenergic activity, and vasopressin (Swedberg et al, 1990; Bichet et al, 1992; Blumenfeld and Laragh, 1994). Improvements in patient survival, cardiac performance, and renal function occurs when these hormone levels are reduced during treatment with ACE inhibitors (Garg and Yusuf, 1995).

Solute-free water excretion in patients with renal failure remains normal until the GFR falls to very low levels (Bichet et al, 1992). At that point, the relative water excretion (i.e., C_{H_2O}/GFR) is reduced because there is an insufficient number of functioning nephrons to excrete the normal daily water load (Rose, 1989).

Hyponatremia with Normal Body Volume. Hyponatremia in hypothyroidism has been related to the associated decreases in GFR and renal blood flow (Robertson and Berl, 1991). In selective glucocorticoid deficiency, in which mineralocorticoid levels are normal, water excretion is also impaired (Boykin et al, 1978). This effect appears to be a result of systemic and renal hemodynamic changes rather than a direct effect by glucocorticoids on vasopressin release or vasopressin-mediated water reabsorption by the collecting duct. Replacement with physiologic amounts of exogenous glucocorticoid restores the capacity to excrete water normally (Rayson et al, 1978).

Postoperative hyponatremia is relatively common, occurring in approximately 4% of patients (Anderson, 1986). In general, these patients are euvolemic and have measurable levels of vasopressin (Chung et al, 1986; Robertson et al, 1991). Neurologic complications, heralded by confusion, nausea, vomiting, and seizures, have been reported to occur postoperatively in a subgroup of women (Arieff, 1986).

Symptomatic hypervolemic hyponatremia has been reported within a few hours after transurethral resection of the prostate (Norris et al, 1973). This syndrome is characterized by marked volume expansion caused by absorption of large amounts of osmotically active irrigant by the prostate. In one prospective study, significant hyponatremia did not occur when a non-irrigating resectoscope was used (Goel et al, 1992).

A variety of medications are associated with water retention and can produce significant hyponatremia (see Table 7–7).

Syndrome of Inappropriate Antidiuretic Hormone Secretion. The characteristic features of this syndrome include (1) hyponatremia with excretion of urine that is not maximally dilute (greater than 100 mOsm/kg), (2) Na^+ balance maintained so that urine sodium reflects intake and is usually high, and (3) hypouricemia with plasma uric acid concentration less than 4 mg/dl, which is indicative of increased urate clearance (Beck, 1979). The pathogenesis of hyponatremia is related to the decreased body solute content caused by the natriuresis and kaliuresis that occurs early in its course (Verbalis and Dutaroski, 1988). However, excess water intake is required for hyponatremia to develop in this syndrome. Therefore, hyponatremia does not develop in SIADH if water intake is restricted despite the high vasopressin level (see later discussion).

The disorders associated with SIADH include malignancies, pulmonary diseases, and central nervous system disorders (Table 7–10). It occurs most commonly with bronchogenic tumors and is found in 8% of patients with small cell carcinoma of the oat cell type (Azzopardi et al, 1970). Robertson and Berl (1991) characterized four osmoregulatory defects in patients with SIADH.

Diagnosis of Hyponatremia: Clinical Features

Hyponatremic patients are usually not symptomatic until the serum Na^+ concentration decreases to significantly be-

Table 7–9. URINARY SODIUM VALUES IN EUVOLEMIC OR HYPERVOLEMIC HYPONATREMIA

Normal ECFV: Urinary $Na^+ > 20$ mEq/L Renal Losses	Increased ECFV	
	Urinary $Na^+ < 20$ mEq/L	*Urinary $Na^+ > 20$ mEq/L*
SIADH	Nephrotic syndrome	Acute renal failure
Primary polydipsia	Cirrhosis	Chronic renal failure
Renal failure	Congestive heart failure	
Reset osmostat		

ECFV, extracellular fluid volume; SIADH, syndrome of inappropriate antidiuretic hormone.

Data from Robertson GL, Berl T: Pathophysiology of water metabolism. *In* Brenner BM, Rector FC, eds: The Kidney, 4th ed. Philadelphia, W.B. Saunders, 1991, pp 677–736.

Table 7–10. DISORDERS ASSOCIATED WITH THE SYNDROME OF INAPPROPRIATE ADH SECRETION

Carcinomas	Pulmonary Disorders	CNS Disorders
Bronchogenic	Pneumonia (viral, bacterial)	Encephalitis (bacterial, viral)
Duodenum	Pulmonary abscess	Meningitis (viral, bacterial, tubercular, fungal)
Pancreas	Tuberculosis	Head trauma
Thymoma	Aspergillosis	Guillain-Barré syndrome
Ureter	Positive pressure breathing	Subarachnoid hemorrhage
Lymphomas	Asthma	Subdural hematoma
Ewing's sarcoma	Pneumothorax	Cerebellar or cerebral atrophy
Mesothelioma	Cystic fibrosis	Cavernous sinus thrombosis
Bladder		Hydrocephalus
Prostatic		Shy-Drager syndrome
		Rocky Mountain spotted fever
		Delirium tremens
		Olfactory neuroblastoma
		Hypothalamic sarcoidosis
		Multiple sclerosis

ADH, antidiuretic hormone; CNS, central nervous system.
Adapted from Levi M, Berl T: Water metabolism. *In* Gonick HC, ed: Current Nephrology (1983–1984), vol 9. Chicago, Year Book, 1986.

low 130 mEq/L. However, symptoms are more likely to occur when the level falls rapidly, especially in the elderly and in young children (Arieff et al, 1976). Signs and symptoms may include lethargy, nausea, vomiting, seizures, coma, and death. These manifestations probably reflect cerebral edema that occurs when ECF osmolality is acutely lowered. Symptoms are less marked when serum Na^+ is reduced more gradually; this perhaps reflects the loss of electrolytes and osmotically active organic solutes from brain cells (Verbalis and Dutaroski, 1988; Heilig et al, 1989).

Treatment of Hyponatremia

There is controversy regarding the relationship between the occurrence of neurologic complications and the rate at which hyponatremia is corrected. **Patients at greatest risk are those in whom serum Na^+ is corrected rapidly, increased to above 140 mEq/L, or are hypoxic before correction.** It has been recommended that the serum Na^+ concentration in symptomatic be increased by 1 mEq/L/hour to a target level of 125 mEq/L. Patients with chronic hyponatremia should be corrected more gradually ($\leq$0.6 mEq/L/hour) (Sterns et al, 1986; Ayus et al, 1987; Robertson and Berl, 1991).

The method of treatment also depends on the volume status. Hypovolemic hyponatremia resulting from renal or extrarenal losses can be corrected with isotonic NaCl. In this setting, serum Na^+ concentration decreases slowly at first because vasopressin secretion persists until ECF volume is restored. When this nonosmotic hypovolemic stimulus for vasopressin is removed, solute-free water can be excreted and serum Na^+ increases more rapidly. In acutely symptomatic patients, hypertonic saline can be administered initially to increase serum Na^+ more rapidly. However, hypotonic fluids should not be used because they will further decrease the serum Na^+ concentration (Rose, 1989).

The amount of Na^+ that is required to raise the serum Na^+ to a target value (i.e., 125 mEq/L) is calculated as follows:

$$Na^+ \text{ deficit} = 0.5 \times \text{body weight (in kg)} \times (125 - \text{actual plasma } [Na^+]),$$

where 0.5 is the volume of distribution of plasma Na^+ in men (0.6 for women).

In edematous patients, the risk of treatment with NaCl addition is exacerbation of volume overload. Therefore, the treatment strategy involves restricting water intake rather than adding sodium. When hyponatremia is asymptomatic, it can be corrected by restricting water intake to less than that excreted in urine (C_{H_2O}) and insensible losses. In addition, treatment of the underlying condition may also improve the hyponatremia (e.g., ACE inhibitors in heart failure). Loop diuretics decrease urinary concentrating ability by inhibiting NaCl reabsorption at the loop of Henle and also reduce ECF volume by promoting natriuresis. Therefore, in symptomatic patients with hypervolemic hyponatremia, treatment with loop diuretics and hypertonic saline increases serum Na^+ concentration rapidly. If the patient is not responsive to the loop diuretic, hypertonic saline should not be administered, because of the risk of exacerbation of volume overload; dialysis may be required. Thiazide-type diuretics are contraindicated because they can worsen the hyponatremia by increasing excretion of Na^+ and K^+ in excess of water (Rose, 1989; see earlier discussion).

The excess water that must be excreted to achieve a safe level (125 mEq/L) in order to correct the hyponatremia can be calculated as follows:

$$\text{Excess water} = \text{TBW} \times \left(1 - \frac{\text{actual plasma } Na^+}{125}\right)$$

where TBW = body weight (in kg) × 0.6 (or 0.5 for women).

Pharmacologic antagonists that can be used to treat patients with SIADH include lithium and demeclocycline. Lithium inhibits vasopressin action both proximal and distal to cAMP formation in the collecting duct (Forrest et al, 1974, 1978). Complications of lithium treatment include interstitial nephropathy. Uptake of lithium by the amiloride-sensitive Na^+ channel appears to contribute to its nephrotoxicity, as evidenced by the beneficial effect of amiloride to reduce lithium-induced polyuria. Demeclocycline, in doses ranging from 600 to 1200 mg/day, induces vasopressin-resistant diabetes insipidus that corrects the serum sodium with 1–2 weeks (Robertson and Berl, 1991).

Urine flow is directly related to daily solute load (see earlier discussion). Supplementing urea in the diet (30–60 g dissolved in 100 ml of water) increases water excretion and can reduce serum Na^+ in patients with SIADH (Decaux et al, 1980).

Hypernatremia (Fig. 7–31, Table 7–11)

Hypernatremia is indicative of hyperosmolality and is the consequence of water loss in excess of sodium or, alternatively, of increased body sodium in relation to water. As discussed, plasma osmolality is maintained at approximately 280–290 mOsm by variations in vasopressin secretion, whereas the threshold for thirst is approximately 5% above this range (Robertson and Berl, 1991). However, thirst defends against the development of hypernatremia. This is evident in patients with impaired thirst or impaired accessibility to water (e.g., as in altered mental status) in whom severe hypernatremia occurs despite maximal vasopressin secretion, whereas plasma sodium concentration is rarely seen in an alert patient when water is available (Rose, 1989). Hypernatremia can also caused by administration of hypertonic solutions, such as $NaHCO_3^-$, or by feeding hypertonic formula to infants (Davies et al, 1979).

NEUROGENIC DIABETES INSIPIDUS (CENTRAL DIABETES INSIPIDUS). Vasopressin deficiency is most commonly caused by destruction of the neurohypophysis. To produce symptomatic polyuria, 80%–90% of the neurosecretory neurons must be destroyed at or above the level of the infundibulum, so that smaller lesions that are limited to the sella turcica usually do not produce symptomatic diabetes insipidus (Randall et al, 1966; Robertson and Berl, 1991).

As a consequence of the reduced vasopressin level, the kidney excretes a high volume of dilute urine. This leads to a reduction in total body water, a rise in total body osmolality, and thus hypernatremia. The related cellular dehydration stimulates thirst. Compensatory water intake decreases plasma osmolality (and Na^+ concentration) towards normal, but they stabilize at the threshold level for thirst, which is slightly above normal (Howard et al, 1992).

As in all forms of diabetes insipidus, the ability of the kidney to maximally concentrate the urine in response to vasopressin is also impaired in neurogenic diabetes insipidus. This abnormality occurs because the medullary osmotic gradient is reduced by the high urine flow (Epstein, et al, 1957; Harrington and Valtin, 1968).

NEPHROGENIC DIABETES INSIPIDUS. In this disorder, of which congenital and acquired forms exist, secretion of vasopressin by the neurohypophysis is normal, but renal responsiveness to the hormone is attenuated or absent, and urinary concentrating ability is impaired. Linkage studies showed that the gene responsible for the congenital form of nephrogenic diabetes insipidus is located on the long arm of X chromosome (Holzman et al, 1993). Several different mutations of the vasopressin V_2 receptor gene have been identified, although the specific mechanisms by which these mutations cause this phenotype are incompletely defined.

OSMOTIC DIURESIS, ELECTROLYTE ABNORMALITIES. When nonreabsorbable solutes (e.g., glucose, mannitol) are present in the tubule lumen, urine flow increases because water reabsorption is impaired. Polyuria is caused by the high urine osmolality, increased urine flow, and diminished amount of water reabsorption along the nephron. In addition, the medullary concentrating gradient may also decrease, which further limits urinary concentration.

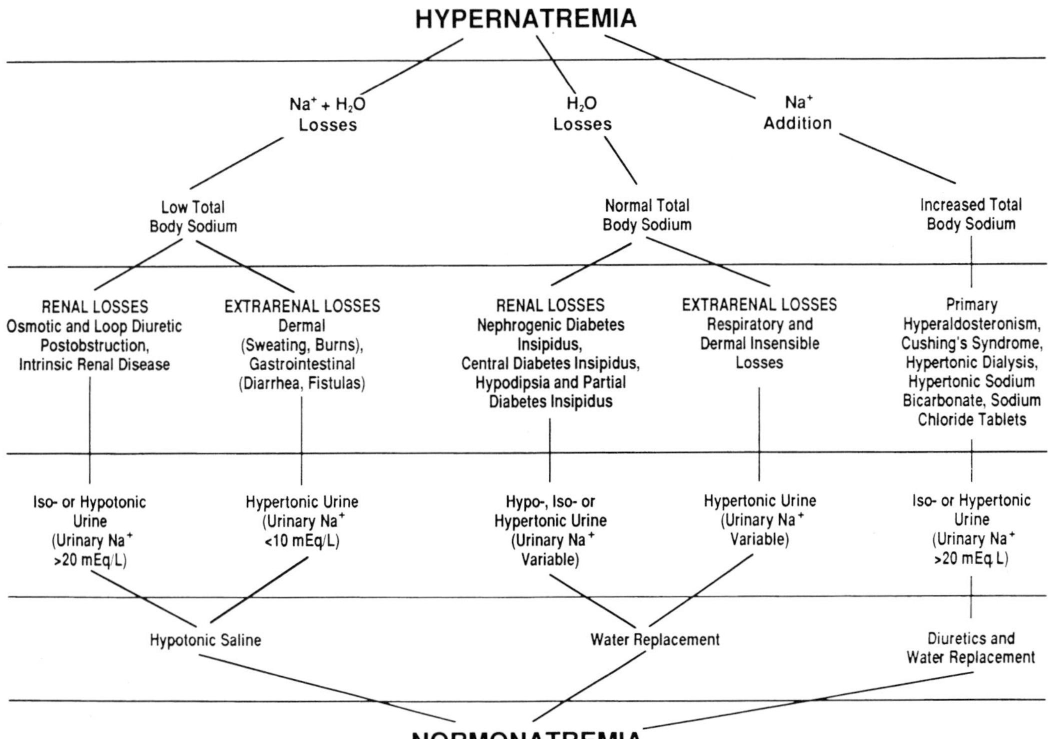

Figure 7–31. Approach to the hypernatremic patient. (From Berl T, Anderson RJ, McDonald KM, et al: Kidney Int 1976; 10:117.)

Table 7–11. ETIOLOGIES OF DIABETES INSIPIDUS

Congenital
Advanced Renal Failure
Electrolyte Disturbances
Hypokalemia
Hypercalcemia
Systemic Disorders
Sickle-cell anemia
Sjögren's syndrome
Amyloidosis
Fanconi's syndrome
Sarcoidosis
Renal tubular acidosis
Light-chain nephropathy
Dietary Abnormalities
Excessive water intake
Decreased solute intake: NaCl, protein
Drugs
Amphotericin B
Colchicine
Demeclocycline
Glyburide, acetohexamide, tolazamide
Lithium
Methicillin
Methoxyflurane
Osmotic diuretics
Propoxyphene
Vinblastine
Miscellaneous
Postobstructive diuresis
Diuretic phase of acute tubular necrosis

Adapted from Levi M, Berl T: Water metabolism. *In* Gonick HC, ed: Current Nephrology (1983–1984), vol 9. Chicago, Year Book, 1986.

Hypercalcemia causes impaired urinary concentrating. The mechanisms that contribute to this include decreased GFR with increased solute load per nephron, reduced medullary solute as a result of impaired NaCl reabsorption, decreased vasopressin sensitivity by the collecting duct caused by increased PGE_2 production, and attenuated vasopressin-sensitive adenylate cyclase activity (Howard et al, 1992). Hypokalemia also leads to a vasopressin-resistant concentrating defect, usually when the serum K^+ concentration is below 3 mEq/L and the total body deficit is in excess of 300 mEq (Fig. 7–32; Berl et al, 1977).

Diagnosis and Evaluation of Hypernatremia

As with hyponatremia, the symptoms of hypernatremia are neurologic, including lethargy, seizures, and coma. The increase in serum Na^+ initially promotes cellular dehydration. However, within 24–48 hours, osmotically active organic solutes, referred to as *osmolytes,* accumulate in the brain and normalize brain water content (Heilig et al, 1989). This increase in solute within the brain has important implications regarding treatment of chronic hypernatremia, because rapid correction can cause cerebral edema and neurologic complications (Trachtman et al, 1988).

Measurement of urine osmolality provides useful information for the differential diagnosis of hypernatremia (Fig. 7–33). When the serum Na^+ concentration exceeds 295 mOsm/kg, the effects of vasopressin on the kidney are maximal (see earlier discussion). Therefore, if the U_{Osm} is less than 800 mOsm/kg, there is a defect in vasopressin release or response by the kidney. Furthermore, exogenous vasopressin will increase U_{Osm} only if vasopressin secretion is reduced. **In the polyuric patient, U_{Osm} below 250 mOsm/kg usually indicates water diuresis, and an evaluation for diabetes insipidus is needed. Conversely, a U_{Osm} greater than 300 mOsm/kg most commonly reflects solute diuresis (e.g., high-protein feedings, glucose).**

The water restriction test is a standard method for evaluating the basis for hypernatremia. While patients are monitored closely, water is withheld; urine volume, U_{Osm}, and body weight are measured hourly and P_{Osm} and serum Na^+ concentration are measured every 4 hours until the P_{Osm} reaches 295 mOsm/kg or the U_{Osm} reaches a plateau (Rose, 1989). Vasopressin is then administered, and measurements continue. However, there may be some ambiguity between the responses in patients with partial central diabetes insipidus and those in patients with primary polydipsia. This is important because an incorrect interpretation could lead to the treatment of primary polydipsia with exogenous vasopressin and thereby result in severe hyponatremia (Rose, 1989).

Treatment of Hypernatremia

When hypernatremia is caused by a water deficit, the volume of water required to correct it can be estimated by the following formula:

$$\text{Water deficit} = 0.4 \times \text{lean body weight} \times \left(\frac{\text{plasma [Na}^+\text{]}}{140} - 1\right)$$

This calculation determines the amount of water required to re-establish abnormal body osmolality, but it does not establish the amount of isoosmotic fluid required to correct the losses of isoosmotic fluid that may also occur. The type of fluid replacement required depends on the hemodynamic status, the source of the water deficit, and whether there are ongoing losses at the time of therapy. **For example, isotonic saline should be used if the patient is hypotensive, because correcting the hemodynamic instability takes precedence over correcting derangements in osmolality. Once blood pressure is stabilized, hypotonic saline infu-**

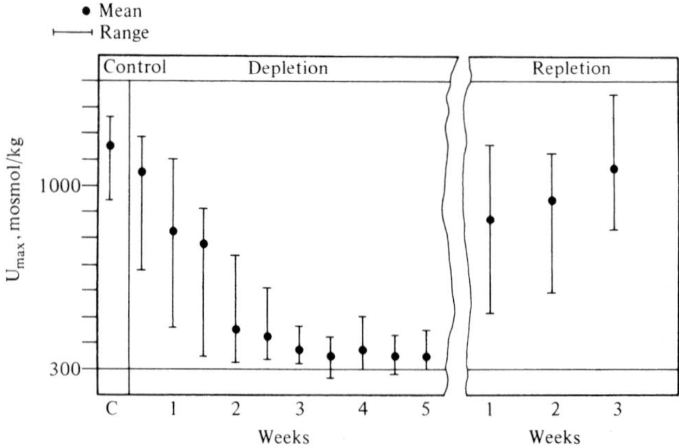

Figure 7–32. Urinary concentrating ability is diminished in patients with progressive potassium depletion. The average potassium deficit was 350 mEq. (From Rubini J: J Clin Invest 1961; 20:2215.)

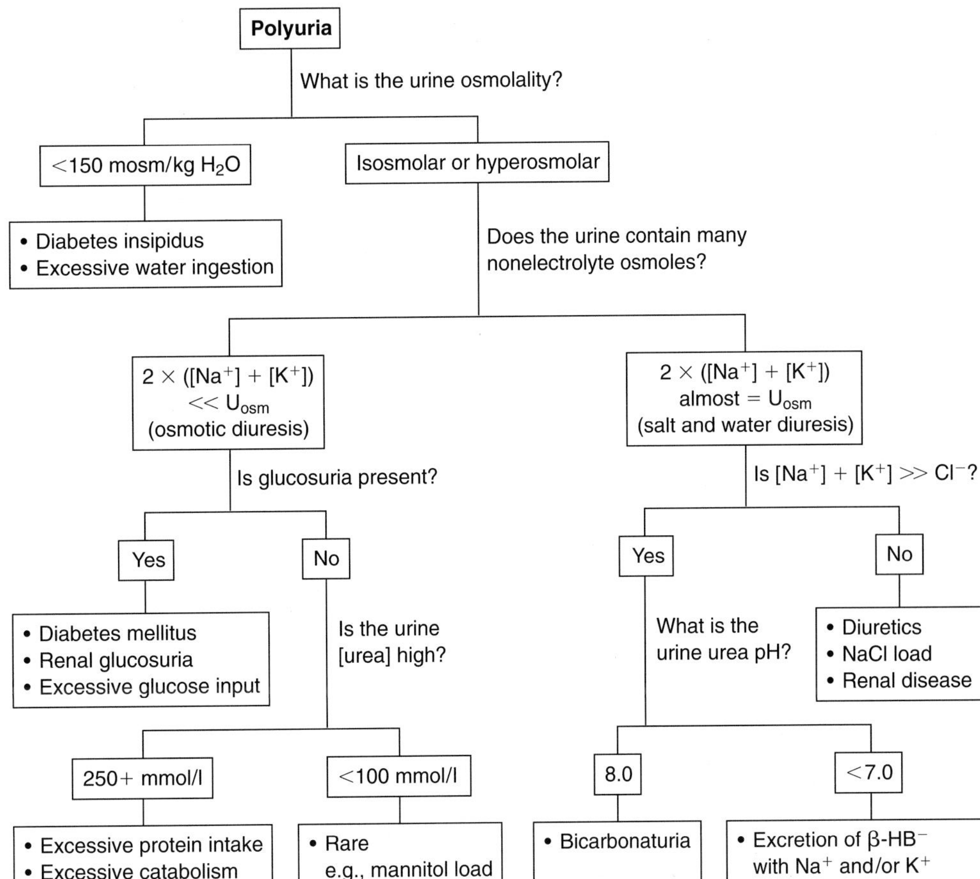

Figure 7–33. Approach to the patient with polyuria. (From Halperin ML, Goldstein MB: Fluid, Electrolyte and Acid-Base Physiology: A Problem-Based Approach, 2nd ed. Philadelphia, W.B. Saunders Company, 1994.)

sion may be appropriate to correct the water deficit and replace ongoing losses.

Rapid replacement of the water deficit is necessary only when symptoms are severe (Howard et al, 1992). In general, half of the calculated water deficit can be replaced within 24 hours. The remainder of the deficit can be replaced over 48 hours with the goal of decreasing osmolality by not more than 2 mOsm/hour.

ACID-BASE HOMEOSTASIS

Blood pH is among the most tightly controlled of all physiologic characteristics, despite the continuous addition of acids and bases to the extracellular fluid from cellular metabolism and exogenous sources. This is evident from the fact that normal blood pH (7.35–7.46) reflects an extracellular hydrogen ion (H^+) concentration of 40 nanOsm/L, which is approximately one-millionth the millimolar concentration of the extracellular ions sodium, potassium, chloride, and bicarbonate ions. Acid-base balance is maintained by extracellular and intracellular chemical buffers, respiratory responses, and renal mechanisms.

Bicarbonate Buffer System

The bicarbonate buffer is predominant in humans and is defined by the following reactions (Henderson-Hasselbalch equation), whereby bicarbonate (HCO_3^-) is the proton acceptor (base) and carbonic acid (H_2CO_3) is the proton donor (acid):

$$H^+ + HCO_3^- \longleftrightarrow H_2CO_3 \xleftrightarrow{\text{carbonic anhydrase}} CO_2 + H_2O$$

$$pH = 6.1 + \log \frac{[HCO_3^-]}{0.03\ P_{CO_2}},$$

where 0.03 is the solubility of CO_2 in plasma.

In general, optimal buffering occurs within 1.0 pH unit of the pK_a. Therefore, the $pK_a = 6.1$ of bicarbonate buffer does not appear to be the most efficient for maintaining pH 7.4 that is required for normal homeostasis. However, one important feature of the bicarbonate system that makes it ideally suited as a body buffer is that the components of this system are regulated independently: HCO_3^- concentration is maintained at 24 mmol/dl by the kidneys, and P_{CO_2} is fixed at 40 mm Hg by the lungs. The ability to regulate alveolar ventilation over a wide range enhances the buffering capacity of the bicarbonate system. The importance of this buffer system is also evident from the fact that approximately 12,000 mmol of CO_2 is produced daily by the metabolism of dietary carbohydrates and fats. This CO_2 load is transported as hemoglobin-generated bicarbonate and hemoglobin-bound carbamino groups to the lungs, where it is excreted by alveolar ventilation (Rose, 1989; Cogan and Rector, 1991).

Homeostatic Response to Volatile Acid

Distribution and Cellular Buffering

The normal American diet results in the production of approximately 1 mEq/kg of acid daily (Harrington and Lemann, 1970). The components of this acid load are not ingested directly but are generated by metabolism of neutral dietary components such as proteins and fats. Examples of these acids are sulfuric, phosphoric, hydrochloric, and organic acids. Carbonic acid ($H_2CO_3^-$), the major product of cellular oxidation, does not normally contribute significantly to the acid content of the body because it is metabolized to CO_2 and H_2O. The proton of carbonic acid is then excreted by the lungs as CO_2.

The time course of the compensatory response to an acid load is illustrated in Figure 7–34. The initial response to an acid load is the distribution of hydrogen ions in the extracellular fluid. In the extracellular fluid, protons are buffered primarily by HCO_3^-. This process can buffer approximately 45% of the acid load and is completed within 30 minutes (Cogan and Rector, 1991).

However, extracellular buffering is insufficient, and additional buffering of approximately 50% of the acid load occurs intracellularly within a few hours. As the duration of the acid loading increases, the amount of intracellular buffering can increase in relation to extracellular buffering, so that more than twice as much buffering occurs intracellularly (Schwartz et al, 1957). Bone is a major site of intracellular buffering, and acidosis appear to lead to increased bone resorption and loss of calcium and potassium (Bushinsky and Lechleider, 1987).

Intracellular buffering requires transcellular ion transport, including sodium/proton, potassium/proton, and chloride/bicarbonate exchanges (Hamm and Alpern, 1992). This response has added significance because the transcellular exchange of potassium for protons can cause significant hyperkalemia. During an acute load with an inorganic acid, plasma potassium increases by approximately 0.6 mEq/L for each 0.1 unit decrease in pH (Sterns et al, 1981; Adrogue and Madias, 1981). By contrast, during organic acidoses (e.g., ketoacidosis), transcellular potassium shifts are minor because the proton is accompanied into the cell by the organic anion rather than in exchange for potassium. **Therefore, hyperkalemia does not usually occur during organic acidoses despite reductions in pH, which are comparable with those in mineral acidoses** (Fulop, 1979; Rose, 1989).

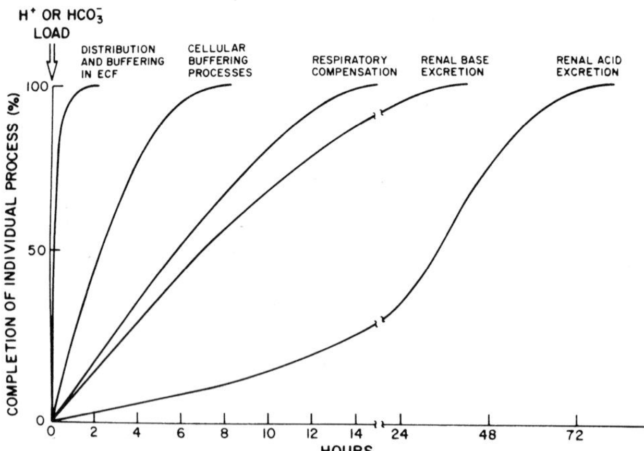

Figure 7–34. Time course of acid-base compensatory mechanisms. (From Cogan MG, Rector FC Jr: Acid-base disorders. *In* Brenner BM, Rector FC, eds: The Kidney, 4th ed. Philadelphia, W.B. Saunders Company, 1991, pp 737–804.)

Respiratory Compensation

When the blood pH decreases (i.e., as in acidemia) during an acid load, chemoreceptors that control respiration are stimulated (Kazemi and Hitzig, 1992). During this compensatory process, which is fully operational within about 14 hours (see Fig. 7–34), alveolar ventilation increases and P_{CO_2} declines. The P_{CO_2} falls approximately 1.25 mm Hg for each mEq/L decrease in HCO_3^-, thus increasing the ratio $[HCO_3^-]$: $[CO_2]$ toward normal (Table 7–12; Bushinsky et al, 1982). Respiratory compensation in response to a pure metabolic acidosis cannot reduce CO_2 to below 10 mm Hg and is therefore unable to maintain pH in the setting of a large acid load. Thus when CO_2 values deviate from those predicted, a combined acid-base disturbance may be present (see later discussion).

Renal Acid Excretion

Renal acid excretion is normally about 50–100 mEq/day, equivalent to the net acid production from metabolism of dietary substrates. To maintain plasma HCO_3^- levels during ongoing acid production, the kidney must accomplish two tasks: (1) reabsorption of the HCO_3^- that is filtered daily by the glomerulus and (2) regeneration of the HCO_3^- that is decomposed by the reaction with metabolic acids (Cogan and Rector, 1991).

HCO_3^- REABSORPTION

A normal individual, with a GFR of 180 L/day and a plasma $[HCO_3^-]$ level of 24 mEq/L, filters 4300 mEq of HCO_3^- daily from the glomerulus into the proximal tubule. Of this filtered load, less than 0.1% normally appears in the urine. **The bulk of the filtered bicarbonate is reclaimed in the proximal nephron, with approximately 80% of the filtered HCO_3^- reabsorbed within the proximal convoluted tubule** (Cogan and Rector, 1991). Hydrogen ion secretion into the tubule lumen by the Na^+-H^+ exchanger is driven by the sodium gradient between the lumen and proximal tubule epithelial cell. This is an energy-dependent process that is powered by the basolateral Na^+-K^+-ATPase. When the secreted H^+ and filtered HCO_3^- combine, carbonic acid is formed and then dehydrated to CO_2 by membrane-bound carbonic anhydrase IV (Wistrand and Knuutila, 1989). CO_2 diffuses into the cell and combines with a hydroxyl ion to form a bicarbonate ion. This process is catalyzed by carbonic anhydrase II. Bicarbonate then exits the cell by a Na^+-$3HCO_3^-$ transport mechanism at the basolateral membrane and enters the blood stream. Carbonic anhydrase minimizes the H^+ concentration in the tubule lumen, thereby providing a favorable gradient for H^+ secretion by

Table 7–12. COMPENSATORY RESPONSES TO ACID-BASE DISORDERS

Disorder	Primary Alteration	Compensatory Response
Respiratory		
Acute acidosis	For each ↑ 1 mm Hg P_{CO_2}	↑ [HCO_3^-] by 0.1 mEq/L ↑ [H^+] by 0.8 nmol/L ↓ pH by 0.008 units
Chronic acidosis	For each ↑ 1 mm Hg P_{CO_2}	↑ [HCO_3^-] by 0.5 mEq/L ↑ [H^+] by 0.25 nmol/L ↓ pH by 0.0025 units
Acute alkalosis	For each ↓ 1 mm Hg P_{CO_2}	↓ [HCO_3^-] by 0.25 mEq/L ↓ [H^+] by 0.7 nmol/L ↑ pH by 0.007 units
Chronic alkalosis	For each ↓ 1 mm Hg P_{CO_2}	↓ [HCO_3^-] by 0.5 mEq/L ↓ [H^+] by 0.3 nmol/L ↑ pH by 0.003 units
Metabolic		
Acidosis	For each ↓ 1 mEq/L [HCO_3]	↓ P_{CO_2} by 1.25 mm Hg ↑ [H^+] by 1.2 nmol/L ↓ pH by 0.012 units
Alkalosis	For each ↑ 1 mEq/L [HCO_3]	↑ P_{CO_2} by 0.2–0.9 mm Hg ↓ [H^+] by 0.3–0.8 nmol/L ↑ pH by 0.003–0.008 units

Adapted from Cogan MG, Rector FC Jr: Acid-base disorders. *In* Brenner BM, Rector FC, eds: The Kidney, 4th ed. Philadelphia, W.B. Saunders Company, 1991, pp 737–804.

the proximal tubule cell. Inhibition of carbonic anhydrase (e.g., by acetazolamide) reduces hydrogen ion secretion rate by approximately 80% (Cogan et al, 1979). A relatively minor proportion of filtered bicarbonate is reabsorbed from the proximal tubule by an H^+-ATPase–dependent process.

The remainder of the filtered bicarbonate that escapes the proximal tubule is reabsorbed in the distal nephron. In the loop of Henle, approximately 10%–20% of the filtered bicarbonate is reabsorbed. As in the proximal tubule, this requires an apical Na^+-H^+ exchanger and, possibly, H^+-ATPase. At the distal convoluted tubule, approximately 3%–5% of filtered bicarbonate is reabsorbed by an H^+-ATPase–dependent process that does not require carbonic anhydrase (Capasso et al, 1987; Gennari and Maddox, 1992).

The cortical collecting duct reabsorbs the remaining filtered bicarbonate and also forms titratable acids (see later discussion). It is composed of distinct segments: cortical, outer medullary, and inner medullary collecting tubules. Each of these segments contains intercalated cells, a cell type that is uniquely responsible for acid secretion. There are two subtypes of intercalated cells in which H^+ secretion is oriented in opposite directions (Hamm and Alpern, 1992; Wingo and Armitage, 1993). In type A cells, the H^+-ATPase is located on the luminal membrane with the chloride/bicarbonate exchanger on the basolateral membrane, secreting H^+ into the lumen and HCO_3^- into the blood. Conversely, type B cells have similar transporters oriented so that protons are secreted into the blood and HCO_3^- into the urine. The relative proportions of these cell types vary according to species; human kidneys apparently have only acid-secreting cells.

NET ACID EXCRETION

In addition to its role in reclaiming filtered HCO_3^-, the kidney is also responsible for excreting the 50–100 mEq of acid produced daily by the body. Both of these processes are accomplished by the secretion of H^+ from the tubule cell into the lumen. Although very steep gradients for H^+ can be maintained in the medullary collecting duct, the urinary pH cannot decrease to below 4.5, which is equivalent to an H^+ less than 0.1 mEq/L. Therefore, urinary buffering by titratable acid and ammonium (NH_4^+) is required (Gennari and Maddox, 1992).

Net acid excretion is defined as follows:

$$\text{Net acid excretion} = \text{titratable acidity} + \text{urinary } NH_4^+ - \text{urinary } HCO_3^-$$

For each H^+ ion excreted with urinary buffers, a new HCO_3^- ion is generated and reabsorbed. This replaces HCO_3^- that was lost when it combined with the daily acid load and was excreted as CO_2 by the lungs.

TITRATABLE ACID EXCRETION. The buffering capacity of a weak acid is optimal within one pH unit of its pK_a. Filtered phosphates are ideal urinary buffers for two reasons: (1) 80% is present in dibasic form (HPO_4^{-2}) with a pK_a of 6.8, and (2) the rate of phosphate excretion is approximately 40–60 mmol/day, leading to the excretion of about 30–40 mEq/L titratable acid daily. **Titratable acid excretion increases two- to three-fold during metabolic acidosis** (see later discussion).

The term *titratable acidity* refers to the quantity of NaOH required to titrate urine back to a pH 7.40, which is similar to that of blood. Other buffers, such as uric acid (pK_a, 5.75) and creatinine (pK_a, 4.97) contribute to the titratable acidity, but only to a minor extent (Rose, 1989).

AMMONIUM (NH_4^+) EXCRETION. In the kidney, two NH_4^+ ions are formed by deamination of glutamine to alpha-ketoglutarate, predominantly in proximal tubular epithelial cells (S_1 segment). Two "new" HCO_3^- ions are formed by the metabolism of alpha-ketoglutarate to CO_2 and H_2O, rather than by the secretion of NH_4^+ into the urine (Halperin et al, 1992). Renal ammonium production is stimulated during acute and chronic metabolic acidosis, but not by respiratory acidosis, which suggests that this is not simply a response to reduced pH. Hypokalemia also can also markedly stimulate renal ammoniagenesis (Tannen and McGill, 1976).

The urinary excretion of NH_4^+ is a complex process. In the proximal tubule, NH_4^+ is secreted into the lumen by replacing H^+ on the Na^+-H^+ exchanger. Upon entering the medullary thick ascending limb of Henle, approximately 50%–80% of the NH_4^+ present in the lumen is then reabsorbed by replacing K^+ on the Na^+-K^+-$2Cl^-$ cotransporter (Buekert et al, 1982; Kikeri et al, 1989). This accounts for the "single effect" of the countercurrent mechanism, whereby very large amounts of NH_3 accumulate in the medulla. NH_3 then diffuses into the cortical collecting duct. The low pH of urine in the cortical collecting duct, together with the high pK_a (9.3) of NH_3, leads to the formation of NH_4^+ and its accumulation in the tubule lumen.

Factors Affectng Acid Excretion

LUMINAL HCO_3^- CONCENTRATION. There is a linear relationship between luminal HCO_3^- concentration and the rate of proton secretion as long as the HCO_3^- concentration is within the physiologic range. This relationship plateaus when the luminal HCO_3^- concentration reaches 45 mmol (Alpern et al, 1982).

EXTRACELLULAR VOLUME AND BODY CONTENTS OF K^+ AND Cl^-. Serum HCO_3^- concentration increases in humans when K^+ stores are massively reduced during dietary restriction (Jones et al, 1982; Hernandez et al, 1987). In this setting, HCO_3^- reabsorption increases in the proximal tubule, loop of Henle, and distal nephron without an associated reduction in GFR (Hernandez et al, 1987).

Dietary chloride intake modulates the effects of K^+ depletion on HCO_3^- reabsorption in humans. When body stores of K^+ are reduced by approximately 400 mEq, the serum HCO_3^- concentration increases by only about 2 mEq/L as long as chloride intake is maintained in the normal range (Jones et al, 1982; Hernandez et al, 1987). In contrast, when chloride intake is restricted in the setting of K^+ depletion, serum $[HCO_3^-]$ increases by about 7.5 mEq/L. This effect is similar to that observed during vomiting or gastrointestinal drainage (see later discussion).

The relative effects of chloride depletion and volume contraction on enhanced bicarbonate reabsorption are incompletely defined. Although GFR and distal tubular delivery of Na^+ and Cl^- also decrease in this setting, it has been demonstrated that chloride repletion without volume expansion can reduce renal bicarbonate reabsorption despite persistent elevations in renin and aldosterone (Kassirer et al, 1967; Rosen et al, 1988). An apical Cl^--HCO_3^- exchanger in the cortical collecting duct may contribute to this effect of Cl^- to stimulate HCO_3^- secretion in this setting (Gennari and Maddox, 1992).

PERITUBULAR HCO_3^-, P_{CO_2}, AND pH. There is an inverse relationship between peritubular HCO_3^- concentration and proton secretion. When the serum HCO_3^- and pH decrease, there is a corresponding decrease in cell pH. The increase in cell H^+ concentration drives the Na^+-H^+ antiporter and H^+-ATPase at a faster rate. In addition, at low cell pH, Na^+-H^+ antiporter activity exceeds that predicted solely by the change in driving force and has been attributed to an allosteric effect associated with low cell pH (Aronson et al, 1983; Alpern, 1992).

ALDOSTERONE. The primary effect of aldosterone is to increase electrogenic transport of Na^+ by the principal cells of the collecting duct. Unlike the intercalated cells in this segment, principal cells do not secrete H^+. However, electrogenic Na^+ transport promotes H^+ secretion by making the electrochemical gradient more favorable (Gennari and Maddox, 1992). This effect can be blocked by restricting sodium intake and thereby decreasing Na^+ delivery to the cortical collecting duct. Aldosterone may also indirectly stimulate H^+ secretion indirectly by stimulating potassium secretion. In this setting, H^+-K^+-ATPase is inserted into apical membranes of the cortical collecting duct, thereby augmenting H^+ secretion. Results of in vivo and in vitro studies in animal models suggest that aldosterone can promote H^+ secretion by the medullary thick ascending limb (Good, 1993). Despite its effects on distal tubule H^+ secretion, aldosterone normally has only a minor effect on acid-base homeostasis in humans (check Kassirer et al, 1970; Sebastian et al, 1980).

ANGIOTENSIN II. Ang II has direct, receptor-mediated effects on sodium reabsorption and H^+ secretion by the proximal nephron. While at relatively low concentrations (10^{-12} to 10^{-10} mol) in the peritubular capillary, Ang II stimulates H^+ secretion by increasing Na^+-H^+ exchange by the proximal convoluted tubule through a process mediated by enhanced production of protein kinase C and reduced cAMP (Harris and Young, 1977; Liu and Cogan, 1989, 1990). At higher Ang II concentrations ($>10^{-7}$ mol), proximal transport of Na^+ was inhibited. The relative contribution of Ang II toward H^+ secretion under physiologic conditions is uncertain.

PARATHYROID HORMONE. When exogenous PTH is administered acutely to humans, renal HCO_3^- reabsorption decreases at the proximal tubule and medullary thick ascending limb of Henle, with compensatory increases in reabsorption at more distal segments (Bichara et al, 1986). PTH inhibits of HCO_3^- reabsorption by decreasing Na^+-H^+ exchange. This effect is mediated by increases in cytosolic calcium via the phosphoinositide signaling system and by increases in cAMP (Hruska et al, 1987). During prolonged administration, serum HCO_3^- increases in humans, which suggests that these effects can be overridden by other factors (Hulter and Peterson, 1985).

NEURAL AND ADRENERGIC EFFECTS. Activation of $alpha_1$- or $alpha_2$-adrenergic receptors directly increase Na^+-H^+ exchange in the proximal tubule, which accounts for the increase bicarbonate reabsorption stimulated directly by renal sympathetic nerves or peritubular administration of agonists. It occurs without associated changes in GFR. This response is mediated via a specific guanine nucleotide–binding peptide, which in turn activates the phosphoinositide signaling pathway (Chiu et al, 1987; Baines et al, 1990). Dopamine, the precursor of norepinephrine, also inhibits Na^+-H^+ exchange by the proximal tubule (Felder et al, 1990). This occurs through a type 1 dopamine (DA_1) receptor–mediated process that also involves activation of phosphoinositide signaling pathway and is associated with increases in intracellular concentrations of [Ca^{2+}] and cAMP.

ATRIAL NATRIURETIC PEPTIDE. Although ANP has no direct action on H^+ secretion that is independent of its effects on renal hemodynamics, some studies have demonstrated that ANP attenuates Ang II–induced stimulation of Na^+-H^+ exchange in the proximal tubule (Harris et al, 1987; Liu and Cogan, 1988).

Excretion of Alkaline Load

When confronted with an alkaline load, the strategies used by the body to eliminate the excess base include distribution and buffering in the extracellular and intracellular compartments and respiratory and renal responses (see Fig. 7–34; Cogan and Rector, 1991).

DISTRIBUTION AND INTRACELLULAR BUFFERING. As with an acid load, a bicarbonate load is distributed throughout the extracellular compartment within 30 minutes. However, a greater proportion of the base load remains in the ECF; only about 30% is buffered in the intracellular compartment.

RESPIRATORY COMPENSATION. When a bicarbonate load is buffered, additional CO_2 is produced and alveolar ventilation increases. This is often followed by hypoventilation, during which carbon dioxide partial pressure (P_{CO_2}) increases, thereby compensating for the persistently elevated bicarbonate concentration. This respiratory response occurs over several hours.

RENAL EXCRETION. Renal excretion of the excess base is necessary for restoring base stores to normal. This process occurs rapidly in comparison with the renal response to an acid load (see Fig. 7–34; Cogan and Rector, 1991), and the kidney has a high capacity for excretion of base. Several intrarenal factors promote bicarbonate excretion by the kidney. As the plasma bicarbonate level increases, the concentration of HCO_3^- in glomerular filtrate increases. However, acidification of the proximal tubular lumen is attenuated because of the associated alkalemia, and so absolute proximal bicarbonate reabsorption does not increase in proportion to the filtered load. As a consequence, bicarbonate delivery to the distal nephron increases. Acidification of the distal nephron is prevented because of the decreased excretion of ammonium and titratable acids, and so urinary excretion of bicarbonate is augmented (Cogan and Rector, 1991). In addition, direct secretion of bicarbonate in the collecting tubule may also contribute to the efficiency of bicarbonate excretion in this setting.

Clinical and Laboratory Diagnosis of Acid-Base Disorders

Appropriate treatment of the patient with an acid-base disorder requires a coordinated response to information obtained from the history, physical examination, and laboratory data (Rose, 1989; Cogan and Rector, 1991). The *clinical history* is important for identifying the etiology of the disturbance in acid-base balance and may be particularly useful in interpreting the results of arterial blood gas measurements in the patient with a mixed acid-base disturbance. For example, a history of vomiting provides the basis for loss of acid in the patient with a metabolic alkalosis, and the physical examination indicates that extracellular volume is present and must be corrected to restore normal acid-base balance. **Essential information provided by the clinical laboratory include blood levels of bicarbonate, potassium, and chloride, in addition to the arterial blood P_{CO_2}, pH, and oxygen partial pressure (P_{O_2}).**

Interpretation of Acid-Base Values

Blood pH is determined by the relationship between the P_{CO_2} and HCO_3^- according to the Henderson-Hasselbalch equation defined earlier. For simplicity, the relationship between the components of the bicarbonate buffer system can be expressed in nonlogarithmic terms:

$$[H^+] = 24 \times \frac{P_{CO_2}}{[HCO_3^-]}$$

When pH = 7.40,

$$\begin{aligned} [H^+] &= 40 \text{ nanOsm/L} \\ P_{CO_2} &= 40 \text{ mm Hg} \\ HCO_3^- &= 24 \text{ mmol} \end{aligned}$$

As discussed in the previous section, plasma HCO_3^- is regulated by renal secretion of H^+. For each H^+ ion secreted by the renal tubules, one HCO_3^- molecule is reabsorbed and returned to the extracellular fluid. As H^+ secretion continues after all the filtered bicarbonate is reabsorbed, additional HCO_3^- is generated. In contrast with HCO_3^- regulation by the kidney, P_{CO_2} levels are regulated by alveolar ventilation so that P_{CO_2} is decreased by hyperventilation and increased by hypoventilation (Rose, 1989; Gennari and Maddox, 1992).

Acidosis is defined as a process that tends to elevate blood H^+ concentration and decrease pH. According to the Henderson-Hasselbalch relationship, this can be the consequence of an elevated P_{CO_2} level or decreased HCO_3^- concentration. In contrast, *alkalosis* is defined as a process that tends to decrease blood H^+ and raise blood pH. This can be caused either by decreased P_{CO_2} or by increased HCO_3^-. The simple acid-base disorders include metabolic acidosis, metabolic alkalosis, respiratory acidosis, and respiratory alkalosis. The primary disorders and their compensatory responses are illustrated in Table 7–12. It is evident that the serum HCO_3^- concentration value alone does not provide sufficient information to determine the primary disturbance: it is elevated in both metabolic alkalosis and respiratory acidosis. Similarly, the P_{CO_2} value alone is insufficient to define the underlying acid-base disorder: it is elevated in both respiratory acidosis and metabolic alkalosis. The blood pH value distinguishes these processes. A further analysis of the Henderson-Hasselbalch equations indicates that to return the pH toward normal, the compensatory response occurs in the same direction as the primary abnormality (e.g., both HCO_3^- and P_{CO_2} are low in metabolic acidosis).

The acid-base map provides the 95% confidence limits for the relationships between P_{CO_2}, H^+, and arterial blood pH for the simple acid-base disorders (Fig. 7–35). Although this map can be quite useful, it does not provide adequate diag-

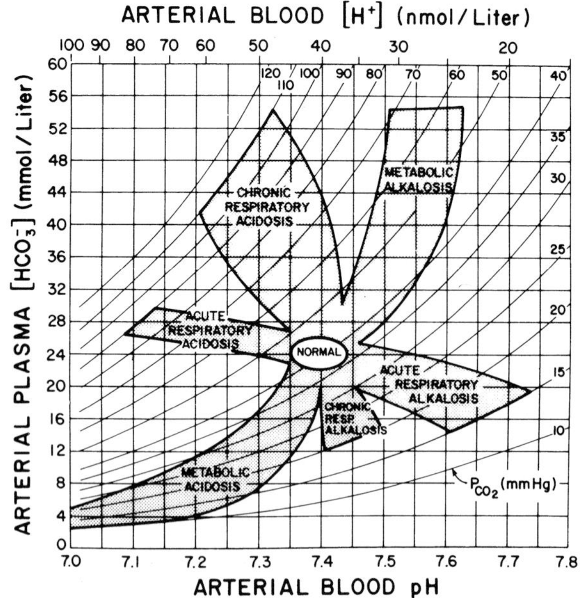

Figure 7–35. Acid-base nomogram. Shown are the 95% confidence intervals of the normal respiratory and metabolic compensations for primary acid-base disturbances. (From Cogan MG, Rector FC Jr: Acid-base disorders. *In* Brenner BM, Rector FC, eds: The Kidney, 4th ed. Philadelphia, W.B. Saunders Company, 1991, pp 737–804.)

nostic information under certain circumstances. **For example, a value may fall outside the bounds of the nomogram if the adequate time has not passed for the compensatory responses to occur. Conversely, a value may be in the shaded region as the consequence of two simultaneous acid-base disorders rather than a simple disorder** (Cogan and Rector, 1991). Other information, discussed as follows, can be useful for distinguishing simple from mixed acid-base disturbances.

The magnitude of the compensatory responses to the acid-base disorders can be estimated from the formulas in Table 7–12.

Metabolic Acidosis

Metabolic acidosis is caused by an inadequate excretion of H^+. This may be the consequence of impaired renal function, whereby a proportion of the daily acid load (50–100 mEq) accumulates. Alternatively, acute generation of large amounts of H^+ (e.g., lactic acidosis) or loss of HCO_3^- (e.g., proximal renal tubular acidosis [RTA]) can exceed the normal mechanisms for acid excretion by the kidney.

ANION GAP ACIDOSIS. The anion gap is defined as the difference between the levels of routinely measured cations (Na^+) and anions ($Cl^- + CO_2$) in blood:

$$\text{Anion gap} = \Delta = Na^+ - (Cl^- + HCO_3^-)$$

$$= 140 - (105 + 24) = 11$$

The normal range is 9–14 mEq/L. It represents the difference between levels of cations and anions that are not measured by the autoanalyzer (Cogan and Rector, 1991; Emmett and Narins, 1977). The predominant unmeasured anions include albumin, each gram of which has a charge equivalence of approximately 2 mEq/L, and phosphate (also 2 mEq/L). The major unmeasured cations include calcium (5 mEq/L), magnesium (1.8 mEq/L), and gamma globulins; potassium (4.5 mEq/L) is not a component, although it is measurable.

In an anion gap acidosis, the anion gap increases when non–chloride-containing acids are added to the blood (e.g., lactic acid; Table 7–13). In this case, bicarbonate is buffered, and the unmeasured anion is retained to maintain electroneutrality. The plasma chloride concentration is unchanged, and so the anion gap is increased. This type of acidosis is often acute and severe, with rapid generation of large amounts of acid. If the unmeasured anion is not excreted, the concentration of the unmeasured anion can be equivalent to the decrease in HCO_3^-. However, this is often not the case, because more than 50% of the acid load is buffered intracellularly rather than extracellularly by HCO_3^-, whereas the charged anion can be relatively impermeable. Thus the [Δ anion gap/Δ plasma HCO_3^-] commonly exceeds unity (Cogan and Rector, 1991). Alternatively, if the anion is filtered and excreted by the kidney, ECF contraction and chloride retention occur, and hyperchloremic acidosis ensues. This process can be exacerbated by volume expansion with saline (Emmett et al, 1992).

The anion gap also provides a clue that a mixed acid-base disturbance is present whereby HCO_3^- is modified by concurrent disorders. For example, in an alcoholic patient with ketoacidosis (beta-hydroxybutyrate is unmeasured anion, lowers HCO_3^-, lowers CO_2) and vomiting (metabolic alkalosis, increases HCO_3^- and $Paco_2$), the anion gap can be elevated despite normal serum levels of bicarbonate and CO_2 and normal pH. Conditions that alter the anion gap are listed in Table 7–14.

HYPERCHLOREMIC (NORMAL ANION GAP) ACIDOSIS. In this form of metabolic acidosis, extracellular HCO_3^- is consumed and replaced by an equivalent amount of chloride; thus the anion gap remains within the normal range. It occurs in the following settings (Table 7–15): (1) when excess HCO_3^- is lost from the gastrointestinal tract (e.g., as in diarrhea) or the kidney (e.g., as in RTA), (2) dilution of HCO_3^- during saline infusion, and (3) during exogenous acid load. In contrast to the non-anion gap acidosis, hyperchloremic acidoses are often less severe and tend to be more chronic processes.

Serum potassium concentration provides important information for the differential diagnosis of the hyperchloremic metabolic acidoses. Hypokalemia occurs during gastrointestinal HCO_3^- loss and in the proximal and distal RTA because

Table 7–13. DISORDERS WITH ALTERATIONS IN THE ANION GAP

Decreased Anion Gap	Increased Anion Gap
Hypoalbuminemia	Increased anions (not Cl^- or HCO_3^-):
	Organic: lactate, ketones, uremic
	Inorganic: phosphate, sulfate
Increased cations (not Na^+):	Toxins: salicylate, methanol, ethylene glycol
K^+, Ca^{2+}, Mg^{2+}, Li^+	
Immunoglobulins	Hyperalbuminemia
IgG	Decreased cations: K^+, Ca^{2+}, Mg^{2+}

Adapted from Cogan MG, Rector FC Jr: Acid-base disorders. *In* Brenner RM, Rector FC, eds: The Kidney, 4th ed. Philadelphia, W.B. Saunders Company, 1991, pp 737–804.

Table 7–14. ETIOLOGIES OF METABOLIC ACIDOSIS WITH AN ELEVATED ANION GAP

Lactic acidosis
Ketoacidosis: β-hydroxybutyrate
Renal failure: sulfate, phosphate, urate, hippurate
Ingestions
Salicylate: ketones, lactate, salicylate
Methanol or formaldehyde: formate
Ethylene glycol: glycolate, oxylate
Paraldehyde: organic anions
Toluene: hippurate
Sulfur
Massive rhabdomyolysis

Adapted from Rose BD: Clinical Physiology of Acid-Base and Electrolyte Disorders, 3rd ed. New York, Raven Press, 1989, pp 2837–2872.

extracellular volume is decreased and, thus, renin and aldosterone secretion are stimulated. Alternatively, in disorders associated with mild to moderate azotemia or generalized tubular dysfunction in which the renin system may be suppressed, the serum potassium level is commonly normal or elevated (Cogan and Rector, 1991).

In contrast to the renal tubular acidoses, segmental nephron function is normal in patients with gastrointestinal bicarbonate wasting. However, distal tubular acidification may appear to be impaired when ECF volume is markedly reduced during gastrointestinal losses, because delivery of sodium to the distal nephron may be reduced. Urinary pH higher than 5.5 can occur during gastrointestinal bicarbonate wasting and thus incorrectly points to a diagnosis of distal RTA. This relatively high urinary pH develops because ammonium production is stimulated by hypokalemia and acidosis associated with gastrointestinal base loss. These disorders can be distinguished by estimating the rate of urinary ammonium excretion—which is decreased in distal RTA (Halperin and Goldstein, 1994).

Table 7–15. HYPERCHLOREMIC METABOLIC ACIDOSIS (NORMAL ANION GAP)

Acid Loads
Ammonium chloride
Hyperalimentation
Ketoacidosis with renal ketone loss
Bicarbonate Losses
Diarrhea
Pancreatic, biliary, or small bowel drainage
Ureterosigmoidostomy
Drugs
Cholestyramine
Calcium chloride
Magnesium sulfate
Posthypocapnia
Defects in Renal Acidification
Proximal: decreased HCO_3^- reclamation
Distal: decreased net acid excretion
Primary mineralocorticoid deficiency
Hypereninemic hypoaldosteronism
Mineralocorticoid-resistant hyperkalemia
Dilutional

Adapted from Cogan MG, Rector FC Jr: Acid-base disorders. *In* Brenner BM, Rector FC, eds: The Kidney, 4th ed. Philadelphia, W.B. Saunders Company, 1991, pp 737–804.

The ammonium excretion rate can be estimated by the urinary anion gap, under the assumptions that the major urinary cations are NH_4^+, sodium, and potassium and that chloride is the predominant anion (Batlle et al, 1988). The anion gap is defined as

$$(Na^+ + K^+ - Cl^-) \cong NH_4^+,$$

so if $[Cl^-] > [Na^+] + [K^+]$, then $[NH_4^+]$ is high, and if $[Cl^-] < [Na^+] + [K^+]$, then $[NH_4^+]$ is low or NH_4^+ excretion is with anion other than Cl^-.

The urinary anion gap value is (1) normally approximately zero because other unmeasured electrolytes are present, (2) markedly negative during gastrointestinal losses of bicarbonate when the NH_4^+ excretion rate can exceed 200 mEq/day, and (3) inappropriately near zero in the RTAs (Batlle et al, 1988).

Proximal (Type II) Renal Tubular Acidosis. Approximately 80% of filtered bicarbonate is reabsorbed in the proximal convoluted tubule (Cogan and Rector, 1991). In proximal renal tubular acidosis, this process is impaired, and the augmented delivery of bicarbonate to more distal nephron segments exceeds their capacity to reabsorb the bicarbonate load. This leads to increased fractional excretion of HCO_3^- (≥10%–30%), bicarbonaturia with a reduction in net acid excretion, and ECF contraction (Fig. 7–36). Stimulation of renin-angiotensin-aldosterone promotes NaCl reabsorption and hyperchloremic metabolic acidosis. Ultimately, a new steady state is reached in which serum HCO_3^- is

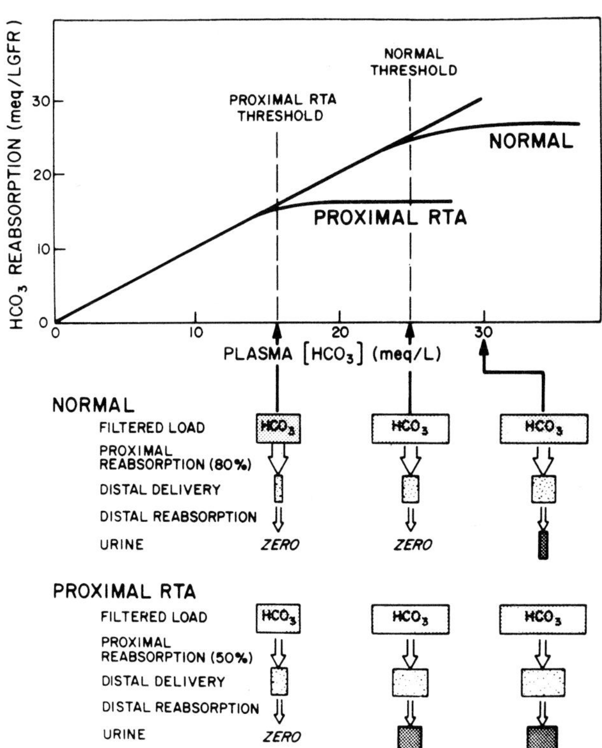

Figure 7–36. Schematic representation of the single-nephron correlates of the whole-kidney bicarbonate titration curves *(top portion)* in normal subjects and in patients with proximal renal tubular acidosis (RTA). (From Cogan MG, Rector FC Jr: Acid-base disorders. *In* Brenner BM, Rector FC, eds: The Kidney, 4th ed. Philadelphia, W.B. Saunders Company, 1991, pp 737–804.)

decreased and hence the filtered load, distal delivery, and urinary excretion of HCO_3^- are all reduced. **The acidosis is self-limited because acid production and excretion are equivalent at this reduced pH; the plasma HCO_3^- remains at 15–20 mEq/L** (Emmett et al, 1992). The diagnosis is confirmed by infusion of a sufficient amount of exogenous bicarbonate to raise the serum HCO_3^- to the normal range, at which point the maximal tubular reabsorptive capacity of the proximal tubule is surpassed. Bicarbonaturia then occurs, and the urinary pH increases to above 7.0. In metabolic acidoses resulting from other causes, the pH will not increase to this level. Glycosuria, aminoaciduria, hypouricemia, and hypophosphatemia may all be present in this disorder.

Another feature of this disorder is hypokalemia, which reflects the high rates of urinary potassium excretion resulting from secondary hyperaldosteronism and increased delivery of an impermeable ion (HCO_3^-) to the collecting duct. Calcium excretion is also elevated, leading to abnormal calcium metabolism, rickets, and osteomalacia in children and to osteopenia in adults. However, nephrocalcinosis and renal calculi do not occur commonly (Cogan and Rector, 1991).

Distal (Type I) Renal Tubular Acidosis. The collecting ducts normally have the capacity to secrete H^+ into the lumen against a concentration gradient to produce minimum urinary pH of 4.5, approximately three pH units lower than that of blood. This feature, together with the titration of weak (titratable) acids and ammonium, enable net acid excretion to occur. In distal RTA, the ability of the collecting duct to secrete H^+ against this gradient is impaired, and urinary pH cannot be reduced to below 5.3 despite the low blood pH. Net acid excretion is reduced because this defect in H^+ secretion impairs excretion of titratable acids and ammonia, even though ammonia production is normal. The buffering capacity of NH_3 is decreased at the higher urinary pH. In addition, the relatively small fraction of filtered bicarbonate that is delivered to the distal nephron is not reabsorbed. **As a consequence, metabolic acidosis develops because the kidney is unable to excrete the entire daily load of acid generated by the diet (50–100 mEq/day) and additional acid is retained daily.** This situation differs from that in proximal RTA, in which the acidosis is self-limited. In distal RTA, the acidosis is progressive and may be severe because the urine cannot be maximally acidified (Halperin et al, 1985; Caruana and Buckalew, 1988). Hypokalemia occurs in distal RTA because of the increased delivery of non-reabsorbable anions (e.g, HCO_3^-) to the distal nephron and the concurrent secondary hyperaldosteronism (Sebastian et al, 1971).

There is controversy regarding the precise mechanism responsible for this abnormal response; however, two hypotheses have been proposed: (1) limitation of H^+ secretion as a result of attenuated cell-lumen H^+ gradient and (2) back-leakage of H^+ from the lumen or increased secretion of HCO_3^- into lumen (Cogan and Rector, 1991; Emmett et al, 1992).

The diagnosis should be suspected in patients with hyperchloremic metabolic acidosis in whom the spontaneous urinary pH exceeds 5.3. In some patients with incomplete distal RTA, the urinary pH remains at a level that is sufficient to maintain normal acid-base balance. In this condition, the defect in distal acidification is expressed when acidosis is induced by infusion of an acid load (i.e., NH_4Cl, arginine HCl, sulfate) and the urinary anion gap is zero or positive (Batlle et al, 1988; Halperin et al, 1988). Other indices of abnormal distal acidification include an inability to generate a normal PCO_2 gradient between blood and urine (Cogan and Rector, 1991).

Other features of distal RTA include abnormal calcium metabolism with hypercalciuria, nephrocalcinosis, and nephrolithiasis. This can be both the cause and the consequence of the distal RTA, in as much as tubulointerstitial disease is associated with primary disorders of calcium metabolism (Brenner et al, 1982; Caruana and Buckalew, 1988; see Chapter 91, on urinary lithiasis).

Impaired Net Acid Secretion and Hyperkalemia. Aldosterone stimulates electrogenic sodium reabsorption by the collecting duct, thereby establishing a favorable electrochemical gradient for secretion of K^+ and H^+ (see earlier section on regulation of potassium excretion). This process can be disrupted when aldosterone secretion is impaired—either as a consequence of decreased renin secretion or through a primary adrenal defect in aldosterone production. Alternatively, it can be disrupted by diminished responsiveness of the collecting duct to aldosterone. For example, selective mineralocorticoid deficiency in humans and in animal models leads to hyperkalemia, hyperchloremic metabolic acidosis with salt wasting, and increased plasma renin levels. The reduced net acid excretion is caused by decreased capacity for distal H^+ secretion at each level of ammonia production and reduced ammoniagenesis related to hyperkalemia (Hutler et al, 1977; Dubose and Calflisch, 1988).

By contrast, most patients with hyporeninemic hypoaldosteronism have mild to moderate renal insufficiency caused by diabetic nephropathy or tubulointerstitial disease, with the hyperkalemia disproportionate to the impairment in GFR (DeFronzo, 1980; Emmett et al, 1992). The mechanism for suppression of renin secretion is not established. About one third of these patients are hypertensive, and the low renin level may reflect the effect of ECF volume expansion. However, most patients are not hypertensive and appear to have normal ECF volume. Net acid excretion can be enhanced by administration of exogenous mineralocorticoids or Ang II, which indicates the potential for aldosterone synthesis by the adrenal glands and H^+ secretion by the distal nephron. Correction of hyperkalemia by furosemide diuresis and ion exchange resin improves the acidosis by enhancing ammonia production and by reducing H^+-K^+ exchange (Cogan and Rector, 1991). The distal nephron may be unresponsive to mineralocorticoids in patients with tubulointerstitial diseases, during treatment with drugs that antagonize the effects of mineralocorticoids (e.g., spironolactone, amiloride), or when the mineralocorticoid receptor is deficient (Emmett et al, 1992; Verrey, 1990).

Acidosis with Reduced Glomerular Filtration Rate. Hyperchloremic metabolic acidosis is commonly observed in patients when the GFR decreases to approximately 20–30 ml/minute. The impaired net acid excretion is caused by reduced NH_4^+ excretion caused either by reduced ammoniagenesis or by a failure to effectively concentrate NH_4^+ in the medulla and secrete it into the collecting duct. Titratable acidity is normal because of the decrease in tubular reabsorption of phosphates that results from secondary hyperparathyroidism (Cogan and Rector, 1991). **Anion gap acidosis**

develops when GFR decreases below 15–20 ml/minute because of the accumulation of anions in blood (i.e., phosphates, sulfates).

Treatment of Metabolic Acidosis

Metabolic acidosis can cause abnormalities in cardiovascular, respiratory, and neuromuscular function and in regulation of the skeletal system and growth. Severe acidosis (i.e., pH less than 7.2) can predispose to life-threatening cardiac arrhythmias and impair cardiac contractility. These changes can occur gradually (e.g., as in chronic renal insufficiency) or more rapidly (e.g., as in diabetic ketoacidosis).

The goals of treatment are to identify and correct the underlying causes of the acidosis and restoring acid-base balance to a safe level. The base deficit can be calculated as follows:

$$HCO_3^- \text{ deficit} = (HCO_3^- \text{ space}) \times (HCO_3^- \text{ deficit per liter})$$

The HCO_3^- space in metabolic acidosis is approximately 50% of the body weight, although the volume of distribution increases with the severity of the acidosis (Emmett et al, 1992) and the normal plasma HCO_3- concentration is 24 mEq/L, so that

$$HCO_3^- \text{ deficit} = 0.5 \text{ (body weight)} \times (24 - \text{plasma } [HCO_3^-]).$$

The goal of therapy in the acute situation is to increase the blood pH to above 7.2 over several hours. In general, only 50% of the calculated amount of bicarbonate should be given before the arterial pH is reassessed. Furthermore, the administered bicarbonate is buffered intracellularly over a few hours, so that the blood pH is higher within the first few minutes after HCO_3^- administration than after a few hours of equilibration. Complications of HCO_3^- therapy include volume overload, hyperosmolality, alkalosis, and exacerbation of lactic acidosis (Cogan and Rector, 1991).

Metabolic Alkalosis

This disorder is characterized by an elevation in blood pH caused by a primary increase in HCO_3^- with compensatory hypoventilation and increase in P_{CO_2}. In order to adequately diagnose and treat the metabolic alkalosis, it is important to determine why the patient became alkalotic and which factors are perpetuating the alkalosis (Table 7–16; Rose, 1989; Alpern et al, 1992).

The common causes of metabolic alkalosis are listed in Table 7–17. In general, an alkali load occurs when acid is lost from the gastrointestinal tract (e.g., as in nasogastric drainage) or kidney (e.g., as in mineralocorticoid excess) or when an exogenous base is added. However, base loads normally are effectively buffered and excreted by the kidney, and so other mechanisms that decrease HCO_3^- excretion and thus retain the excess base must also be operative (see earlier section on excretion of an alkaline load).

HCO_3^- excretion is reduced by factors that increase its reabsorption by the kidney. One mechanism is ECF volume reduction caused by the loss of sodium and chloride. When this occurs, glomerular filtration decreases, fractional reabsorption of HCO_3^- by the proximal tubule increases, renin-angiotensin-aldosterone secretion is stimulated, and H^+ and K^+ secretion by the distal nephron is augmented (see section on regulation of potassium excretion). This situation occurs commonly in patients during treatment with thiazide-type and loop diuretics because they inhibit reabsorption of Na^+, K^+, and Cl^- by the distal tubule and thick ascending limb of Henle, respectively, and promote H^+ and K^+ secretion by the collecting duct (Laragh and Sealey, 1992).

Posthypercapnic alkalosis is another situation in which decreased ECF volume perpetuates the alkalosis. This occurs in patients with chronic respiratory acidosis after rapid reduction in P_{CO_2}. In that setting, plasma HCO_3^- is chronically elevated as the compensatory response to hypoventilation. When P_{CO_2} is rapidly decreased (e.g. as in mechanical ventilation), urinary bicarbonate excretion decreases proportionately with the fall in CO_2. Metabolic alkalosis occurs because K^+ and Na^+ accompany HCO_3^- in the urine, leading to K^+ deficit, reducing ECF volume, and stimulating renin-angiotensin-aldosterone secretion (Turino et al, 1974; Cogan, 1984). When the degree of ECF volume contraction is mild, $NaHCO_3$ excretion may occur, and therefore the urine Na^+ concentration may be relatively high despite the volume deficit. **Metabolic alkalosis with concurrent volume contraction is identified by a low urinary chloride level and,**

Table 7–16. GENERATION OF METABOLIC ALKALOSIS

Excess Acid Loss

Nonrenal Acid Loss

Gastric fluid loss
Intestinal acid loss
Translocation of acid into cells: potassium deficiency

Renal Acid Loss

Persistent mineralocorticoid activity with
  Potassium deficiency
  Distal delivery of sodium, especially with poorly reabsorbable anions

Excess Bicarbonate Gain

Ingestion or infusion of bicarbonate
Metabolism of lactate, ketones, or other organic anions to bicarbonate

Contraction Alkalosis (Minimal)

Adapted from Alpern RJ, Emmett M, Seldin DW: Metabolic alkalosis. *In* Seldin DW, Giebisch G, eds: The Kidney: Physiology and Pathophysiology, 2nd ed. New York, Raven Press, 1992, pp 2733–2758.

Table 7–17. DIFFERENTIAL DIAGNOSIS OF METABOLIC ALKALOSIS

Measurement	Saline Responsive	Normotensive: Saline Unresponsive	Hypertensive: Saline Unresponsive
Urinary [Cl⁻]	<15 mEq/L	>15 mEq/L	>15 mEq/L
Blood pressure	Normal	Normal	Increased
Differential diagnosis	Vomiting	Diuretics	Primary mineralocorticoid excess
	Nasogastric suction	Bartter's magnesium deficiency	

Adapted from Alpern RJ, Emmett M, Seldin DW: Metabolic alkalosis. *In* Seldin DW, Giebisch G, eds: The Kidney: Physiology and Pathophysiology, 2nd ed. New York, Raven Press, 1992, pp 2733–2758.

because it can be corrected by addition of NaCl and fluid, is referred to as "chloride-responsive" metabolic alkalosis (see Table 7–17).

Metabolic alkalosis also occurs when ECF volume expansion is stimulated by mineralocorticoid excess (i.e., primary aldosteronism). The mineralocorticoid effect increases the electrochemical gradient for H^+ and K^+ secretion, promotes K^+ depletion, and thereby stimulates tubule acidification in the collecting duct (see earlier discussion). Sodium reabsorption leads to ECF volume expansion and hypertension with a very low plasma renin activity level (Blumenfeld, 1993; Blumenfeld et al, 1994). The alkalosis tends to be self-limited. **In contrast to the chloride-responsive type, metabolic alkaloses associated with expanded ECF have high urinary Cl^- concentrations and are referred to as "chloride resistant" because they are not corrected by addition of NaCl and water.** Urinary chloride measurements distinguish these mechanisms and can help direct treatment (see Table 7–17).

Evaluation of the respiratory compensation in a patient with metabolic alkalosis may be confounded when a concurrent respiratory disorder (e.g., chronic obstructive pulmonary disease) is present. Hypoxia becomes an important stimulus for ventilation at Po_2 below 60–70 mm Hg (Rose, 1989). Therefore, respiratory compensation for metabolic alkalosis is limited when the Po_2 falls below this level.

Respiratory Acidosis

Under normal circumstances, Pco_2 is the predominant stimulus for ventilation and the level in arterial blood is maintained within a narrow range around 40 mm Hg. Changes in Pco_2 are sensed in the chemosensitive centers in the brain stem, so that when Pco_2 increases, ventilation is stimulated, and when Pco_2 decreases, ventilation is reduced. In contrast, ventilation is stimulated at arterial oxygen tension (Po_2) below 60–70 mm Hg and therefore normally plays a relatively minor role in its regulation. Respiratory acidosis occurs when hypoventilation increases Pco_2 and reduces blood pH (Madias and Cohen, 1992). The metabolic compensation is an increased plasma HCO_3^- level.

When ventilation is impaired, CO_2 retention occurs and H_2CO_3 formation is increased, thereby causing blood pH to fall. Buffering by intracellular proteins (e.g., hemoglobin) is required because extracellular HCO_3^- cannot buffer H_2CO_3. This acute response is inefficient, with a compensatory rise in HCO_3^- of 1 mEq/L for every 10 mm Hg rise in Pco_2 (see Table 7–12; Cogan and Rector, 1991).

When Pco_2 is elevated for more than 3–5 days, renal H^+ secretion and HCO_3^- reabsorption increase. This renal compensatory response adds more HCO_3^- to extracellular fluid, so that during chronic respiratory acidosis, serum HCO_3^- increases approximately 3.5 mEq/L for every 10 mm Hg rise in Pco_2. Therefore, the renal response (increase in H^+ secretion) is the major compensatory mechanism in chronic respiratory acidosis.

Interpretation of an elevated Pco_2 can be difficult when metabolic alkalosis and respiratory acidosis occur simultaneously. **Measuring the alveolar-arterial oxygen (A-a) gradient can sometimes be helpful in distinguishing whether an elevated Pco_2 is related to underlying lung disease and is thus related to a primary respiratory acidosis or whether it is a pulmonary compensation for metabolic alkalosis.** The normal range for the A-a gradient is 5–15 mm Hg (Rose, 1989) and can be calculated from the following:

$$\text{(A-a) } O_2 \text{ gradient} = Pio_2 - 1.25\ Pco_2 - Po_2,$$

where Pio_2 = partial pressure of oxygen (150 mm Hg in room air) and Pco_2 and Po_2 are arterial levels of CO_2 and O_2, respectively, expressed in millimeters of mercury. The gradient is usually increased in patients with intrinsic pulmonary disease. Thus when the A-a gradient is normal in the setting of elevated Pco_2 and HCO_3, hypoventilation represents the *compensatory* respiratory response to metabolic alkalosis rather than the primary disorder.

Respiratory Alkalosis

Respiratory alkalosis is defined as an elevation in blood pH that is caused by a primary decrease in Pco_2 and a compensatory decrease in plasma HCO_3^- (see Table 7–12). Within minutes of the fall in Pco_2, H^+ leaves the intracellular compartment and lowers the plasma HCO_3^- level. This acute response is inefficient. However, after a few days of persistent hypocapnia, HCO_3^- reabsorption by the kidney is reduced and urinary excretion of bicarbonate increases (Madias and Cohen, 1992; Cogan and Rector, 1991). This compensatory response by the kidney further reduces the serum HCO_3^- level and attenuates the rise in pH.

REFERENCES

Renal Hemodynamics

Abboud HE, Luke RG, Galla JH, Kotchen TA: Stimulation of renin by acute selective chloride depletion in the rat. Circ Res 1979; 44:815–821.

Arendhorst WJ, Navar LG: Renal circulation and glomerular hemodynamics. *In* Schrier RW, Gottschalk CW, eds: Diseases of the Kidney, 5th ed. Boston, Little, Brown, 1992, pp 65–117.

Badr KF: 5′-Lipoxygenase products in glomerular immune injury. J Am Soc Nephrol 1992; 3:907–915.

Badr KF, Jacobson HR: Arachidonic acid metabolites and the kidney. *In* Brenner BM, Rector FC, eds: The Kidney, 4th ed. Philadelphia, W.B. Saunders Company, 1991, pp 584–622.

Badr KF, Kelley VE, Rennke HA, Brenner BM: Roles of thromboxane A_2 and leukotrienes in endotoxin-induced acute renal failure. Kidney Int 1986; 30:474.

Badr KF, Serhan CN, Nicolao KC, Samuelsson B: The action of lipoxin A on glomerular microcirculatory dynamics in the rat. Biochem Biophys Res Comm 1987; 145:408.

Barajas L, Salido EC, Liu L, Powers KV: The juxtaglomerular apparatus: A morphologic perspective. *In* Laragh JH, Brenner BM, eds: Hypertension: Pathophysiology, Diagnosis, and Management, 2nd ed. New York, Raven Press, 1995, pp 1335–1348.

Baylis C, Brenner BM: Mechanism of the glucocorticoid-induced increase in glomerular filtration rate. Am J Physiol 1978; 234:F166–F170.

Bell PD, Franco M, Navar LG: Calcium as a mediator of tubuloglomerular feedback. Annu Rev Physiol 1987; 49:275–293.

Berry CA, Rector FC: Renal transport of glucose, amino acids, sodium, chloride, and water. *In* Brenner BM, Rector FC, eds: The Kidney, 4th ed. Philadelphia, W.B. Saunders Company, 1991, pp 245–282.

Blumenfeld, JD, Laragh JH: Congestive Heart Failure: Pathophysiology, Diagnosis and Treatment. New York, Professional Communications, Inc., 1994.

Brenner BM, Schor N, Ichikawa I: Role of angiotensin II in the physiologic regulation of glomerular filtration. Am J Cardiol 1982; 49:1430.

Briggs JP, Schnermann J: Control of renin release and glomerular vascular tone by the juxtaglomerular apparatus. *In* Laragh JH, Brenner BM, eds: Hypertension: Pathophysiology, Diagnosis, and Management, 2nd ed. New York, Raven Press, 1995, pp 1359–1383.

Carmines PK, Morrison TK, Navar LG: Angiotensin II effects on microvascular diameters in in vitro blood perfused juxtamedullary nephrons. Am J Physiol 1986; 251:F610.

Casellas D, Navar LG: In vitro perfusion of juxtamedullary nephrons in rats. Am J Physiol 1984; 246:F349–F358.

Chasis H, Smith WH: The excretion of urea in normal man and in subjects with glomerulonephritis J Clin Invest 1938; 17:347.

Clavell AC, Burnett JC: Physiology and pathophysiologic roles of endothelin in the kidney. Curr Opin Nephrol Hypertens 1994; 3:66–72.

Cockcroft DW, Gault MW: Prediction of creatinine from serum creatinine. Nephron 1976; 16:31.

Cody RJ, Atlas SA, Laragh JH, et al: Atrial natriuretic factor in normal subjects and heart failure patients. J Clin Invest 1986; 78:1362–1374.

Cowley AW Jr, Mattson DL, Lu S, Roman RJ: The renal medulla and hypertension. Hypertension 1995; 25(part 2):663–673.

de Gasparo M, Bottari S, Levens N: Characteristics of angiotensin II receptors and their role in cell and organ physiology. *In* Laragh JH, Brenner BM, eds: Hypertension: Pathophysiology, Diagnosis, and Management, 2nd ed. New York, Raven Press, 1995, pp 1695–1720.

DiBona GF, Kopp UC: Neural control of renal function: Role in human hypertension. *In* Laragh JH, Brenner BM, eds: Hypertension: Pathophysiology, Diagnosis, and Management, 2nd ed. New York, Raven Press, 1995, pp 1349–1358.

Doolan PD, Alpen EL, Theil GB: A clinical appraisal of the plasma concentration and endogenous clearance of creatinine. Am J Med 1962; 32:65.

Duc C, Farman N, Canessa CM, et al: Cell-specific expression of epithelial sodium channel alpha, beta, and gamma subunits in aldosterone-responsive epithelia from the rat: Localization by in situ hybridization and immunocytochemistry. J Cell Biol 1994; 127:1907–1921.

Dworkin LD, Brenner BM: The renal circulations. *In* Brenner BM, Rector FC, eds: The Kidney, 4th ed. Philadelphia, W.B. Saunders Company, 1991, p 164.

Fitzsimons JT: Physiology and pathophysiology of thirst and sodium appetite. *In* Seldin DW, Giebisch G: The Kidney: Physiology and Pathophysiology, 2nd ed. New York, Raven Press, 1992, pp 1615–1648.

Fray JCS, Lush DJ: Stretch receptor hypothesis for renin secretion: The role of calcium. J Hypertension 1984; 2(suppl. 1):19–23.

Furchgott RF, Zawadski JV: The obligatory role of endothelial cells in the relaxation of vascular smooth muscle by acetylcholine. Nature 1980; 288:373–376.

Guyton AC, Hall JE, Coleman TG, et al: The dominant role of the kidneys in long-term arterial pressure regulation in normal and hypertensive states. *In* Laragh JH, Brenner BM, eds: Hypertension: Pathophysiology, Diagnosis, and Management, 2nd ed. New York, Raven Press, 1995, pp 1311–1326.

Hall JE, Brands MW: The renin-angiotensin-aldosterone systems: Renal mechanisms and circulatory homeostasis. *In* Seldin DW, Giebisch G, eds: The Kidney: Physiology and Pathophysiology, 2nd ed. New York, Raven Press, 1992, pp 1455–1504.

Hall JE, Guyton AC, Brands MW: Control of sodium excretion and arterial pressure by intrarenal mechanisms and the renin-angiotensin system. *In* Laragh JH, Brenner BM, eds: Hypertension: Pathophysiology, Diagnosis, and Management, 2nd ed. New York, Raven Press, 1995, pp 1451–1475.

Harris RC, Inagami T: Molecular biology and pharmacology of angiotensin receptor subtypes. *In* Laragh JH, Brenner BM, eds: Hypertension: Pathophysiology, Diagnosis, and Management, 2nd ed. New York, Raven Press, 1995, pp 1721–1738.

Hebert SC, Culpepper RM, Andreoli TE: NaCl transport in mouse medullary thick ascending limbs. I. Functional nephron heterogeneity and ADH-stimulated NaCl cotransport. Am J Physiol 1981; 241:F412–F431.

Hebert SC, Reeves WB, Molony DA, Andreoli TE: Function and modulation of the single-effect multiplier. Kidney Int 1987; 31:580–588.

Humes HD, Ichikawa I, Troy JL, Brenner BM: Evidence for a parathyroid hormone–dependent influence of calcium on the glomerular ultrafiltration coefficient. J Clin Invest 1978; 61:32–40.

Ichikawa I, Brenner BM: Evidence for glomerular action of ADH and dibutryl cyclic AMP in the rat. Am J Physiol 1977; 233:F102.

Ichikawa I, Humes HD, Dousa TJ, Brenner MM: Influence of parathyroid hormone on glomerular ultrafiltration in the rat. Am J Physiol 1978; 234:F393.

Inman S, Brouhard BH, Stowe NT: Preglomerular and postglomerular blood flow: Relationship to kidney disease and treatment. Cleve Clin J Med 1994; 61:179–185.

King AJ: Endothelins: Multifunctional peptides with potent vasoactive properties. *In* Laragh JH, Brenner BM, eds: Hypertension: Pathophysiology, Diagnosis, and Management, 2nd ed. New York, Raven Press, 1995, pp 631–672.

Koeppen BM, Stanton BA: Sodium chloride transport: Distal nephron. *In* Seldin DW, Giebisch G, eds: The Kidney: Physiology and Pathophysiology, 2nd ed. New York, Raven Press, 1992, pp 2003–2039.

Kon V, Badr K: Biological actions and pathophysiologic significance of endothelin in the kidney. Kidney Int 1991; 40:1–12.

Kopp U, DiBona GF: The neural control of renal function. *In* Seldin DW, Giebisch G, eds: The Kidney: Physiology and Pathophysiology, 2nd ed. New York, Raven Press, 1992, pp 1157–1204.

Laragh JH: Atrial natriuretic hormone and the renin-aldosterone axis and blood pressure–electrolyte homeostasis. N Engl J Med 1985; 313:1330–1340.

Laragh JH, Cannon PJ, Bentzel CJ, et al: Angiotensin II, norepinephrine, and the renal transport of electrolytes and water in normal man and in cirrhosis with ascites. J Clin Invest 1963; 42:1179–1192.

Laragh JH, Sealey JE: Renin-angiotensin-aldosterone system and the renal regulation of sodium, potassium, and blood pressure homeostasis. *In* Windhager EE, ed: Handbook of Physiology, Section 8: Renal Physiology. New York, Oxford University Press, 1992, pp 1409–1541.

Levey AS, Madaio MP, Perrone RD: Laboratory assessment of renal disease: Clearance, urinalysis, and renal biopsy. *In* Brenner BM, Rector FC, eds: The Kidney, 4th ed. Philadelphia, W.B. Saunders Company, 1991, pp 919–968.

Lewicki JA, Protter AA: Physiologic studies of the natriuretic peptide family. *In* Laragh JH, Brenner BM, eds: Hypertension: Pathophysiology, Diagnosis, and Management, 2nd ed. New York, Raven Press, 1995, pp 1029–1054.

Liu F-Y, Cogan MG: Angiotensin II stimulates early proximal bicarbonate reabsorption in the rat by decreasing cyclic adenosine monophosphate. J Clin Invest 1989; 84:83–91.

Luscher TF: Endothelin, endothelin receptors, and endothelin antagonists. Curr Opin Nephrol Hypertens 1994; 3:92–98.

Maack T: Receptors of natriuretic peptides. *In* Laragh JH, Brenner BM, eds: Hypertension: Pathophysiology, Diagnosis, and Management, 2nd ed. New York, Raven Press, 1995, pp 1001–1020.

Maddox DA, Brenner BM: Glomerular ultrafiltration. *In* Brenner BM, Rector FC, eds: The Kidney, 4th ed. Philadelphia, W.B. Saunders Company, 1996, pp 236–333.

Maddox DA, Deen WM, Brenner BM: Dynamics of glomerular ultrafiltration: VI. Studies in the primate. Kidney Int 1974a; 5:271.

Maddox DA, Troy JL, Brenner BM: Autoregulation of filtration rate in the absence of macula densa–glomerular feedback. Am J Physiol 1974b; 227:123.

Mene P, Dunn MJ: Vascular, glomerular, and tubular effects of angiotensin II, kinins, and prostaglandins. *In* Seldin DW, Giebisch G, eds: The Kidney: Physiology and Pathophysiology, 2nd ed. New York, Raven Press, 1992, pp 1205–1248.

Mitchell KD, Navar LG: Intrarenal actions of angiotensin II in the pathogenesis of experimental hypertension. *In* Laragh JH, Brenner BM, eds: Hypertension: Pathophysiology, Diagnosis, and Management, 2nd ed. New York, Raven Press, 1995, pp 1437–1450.

Moncada S, Higgs A: The L-arginine–nitric oxide pathway. N Engl J Med 1993; 329:2002–2012.

Nathan C: Nitric oxide as a secretory product of mammalian cells. FASEB J 1992; 6:3051–3064.

Oldroyd S, Slee SJ, Haylor J, et al: Role for endothelin in the renal responses to radiocontrast media in the rat. Clin Sci 1994; 87:427–434.

O'Neil RG, Boulpaep EL: Effects of amiloride on the apical cell membrane cation channels of a sodium-absorbing, potassium-secreting renal epithelium. J Membr Biol 1979; 50:365–387.

Osberg IM, Hammond KB: A solution to the problem of bilirubin interference with the kinetic Jaffe method for serum creatinine. Clin Chem 1978; 24:1196.

Osborne JL, DiBona JF, Thames MD: Beta-1 receptor mediation of renin secretion elicited by low frequency renal nerve stimulation. J Pharmacol Exp Ther 1981; 216:265.

Osborne JL, DiBona JF, Thames MD: Role of renal α-adrenoceptors mediating renin secretion. Am J Physiol 1982; 242:F620.

Pacha J, Frindt G, Antonian L, et al: Regulation of Na channels of the rat cortical collecting tubule by aldosterone. J Gen Physiol 1993; 102:25–42.

Palmer LG, Antonian L, Frindt G: Regulation of the Na-K pump of the rat cortical collecting tubule by aldosterone. J Gen Physiol 1993; 102:43–57.

Palmer LG, Li JHY, Lindemann B, Edelman IS: Aldosterone control of the density of sodium channels in the toad urinary bladder. J Membr Biol 1982; 57:59–71.

Reeves WB, Andreoli TE: Sodium chloride transport in the loop of Henle. *In* Seldin DW, Giebisch G, eds: The Kidney: Physiology and Pathophysiology, 2nd ed. New York, Raven Press, 1992, pp 1975–2002.

Roman RJ, Kaldunski ML, Scicli AJ, Carretero OA: Influence of kinins and angiotensin II on the regulation of papillary blood flow. Am J Physiol 1988; 255:F690–F698.

Romero JC, Lahera V, Ruilope L: Role of nitric oxide on the intrarenal regulation of nephron function and its relevance to hypertension. In Laragh JH, Brenner BM, eds: Hypertension: Pathophysiology, Diagnosis, and Management, 2nd ed. New York, Raven Press, 1995, pp 1385–1404.

Rose, BD: Clinical Physiology of Acid-Base and Electrolyte Disorders, 3rd ed. New York, McGraw-Hill, 1989.

Rossier BC, Palmer LG: Mechanisms of aldosterone action on sodium and potassium transport. *In* Seldin DW, Giebisch G, eds: The Kidney: Physiology and Pathophysiology, 2nd ed. New York, Raven Press, 1992, pp 1373–1410.

Scharschmidt LA, Douglas JG, Dunn MD: Angiotensin II and eicosanoids in the control of glomerular size in the rat and human. Am J Physiol 1986; 250:F348.

Schrier RW: Pathogenesis of sodium and water retention in high-output and low-output cardiac failure, nephrotic syndrome, cirrhosis and pregnancy. N Engl J Med 1988; 319:1065–1127.

Schuster VL, Seldin DW: Renal clearance. *In* Seldin DW, Giebisch G, eds: The Kidney: Physiology and Pathophysiology, 2nd ed. New York, Raven Press, 1992, pp 943–978.

Shemesh O, Golbetz H, Kriss JP, Myers BD: Limitations of creatinine as a filtration marker in glomerulopathic patients. Kidney Int 1985; 28:830.

Simonson MS, Dunn MJ: Endothelin peptides and the kidney. Annu Rev Physiol 1993; 55:249–265.

Smith RD, Timmermans PBMWM: Human angiotensin receptor subtypes. Curr Opin Nephrol Hypertens 1994; 3:112–122.

Steinhausen M, Sterzel RB, Fleming JT, et al.: Acute and chronic effects of angiotensin II on the vessels of the split hydronephrotic kidney. Kidney Int 1987; 31(suppl 20):S64.

Taugner RE, Hackenthal R, Nobiling M, et al: The distribution of renin in the different segments of the renal arterial tree. Histochemistry 1981; 73:75–88.

Tisher CC, Madsen KM: Anatomy of the kidney. *In* Brenner BM, Rector FC, eds: The Kidney, 4th ed. Philadelphia, W.B. Saunders Company, 1991, p 164.

Umans JG, Levi R: The nitric oxide system in circulatory homeostasis and its possible role in hypertensive disorders. *In* Laragh JH, Brenner BM, eds: Hypertension: Pathophysiology, Diagnosis, and Management, 2nd ed. New York, Raven Press, 1995, pp 1083–1095.

Vander AJ, Miller R: Control of renin secretion in the anesthetized dog. Am J Physiol 1964; 207:537–546.

von Lutteroti N, Catanzaro DF, Sealey JE, Laragh JH: Renin is not synthesized by cardiac and extrarenal vascular tissues: A review of experimental evidence. *In* Laragh JH, Brenner BM, eds: Hypertension: Pathophysiology, Diagnosis, and Management, 2nd ed. New York, Raven Press, 1995, pp 1797–1812.

Weinstein AM: Sodium and chloride transport: Proximal nephron. *In* Seldin DW, Giebisch G, eds: The Kidney: Physiology and Pathophysiology, 2nd ed. New York, Raven Press, 1992, pp 1925–1974.

Wilcox CS, Baylis C, Wingo CS: Glomerular-tubular balance and proximal regulation. *In* Seldin DW, Giebisch G, eds: The Kidney: Physiology and Pathophysiology, 2nd ed. New York, Raven Press, 1992a, pp 1807–1842.

Wilcox CS, Welch WJ, Murad F, et al: Nitric oxide synthase in macula densa regulates glomerular capillary pressure. Proc Natl Acad Sci USA 1992b; 7:743–749.

Wingo CS, Armitage FE: Potassium transport in the kidney: Regulation and physiological relevance of H^+, K^+-ATPase. Semin Nephrol 1993; 13:213–224.

Yanagisawa M, Kurihara H, Kimura S, et al: A novel potent vascoconstrictor peptide produced by vascular endothelial cells. Nature 1988; 332:411–415.

Zayas VM, Blumenfeld JD, Bading B, et al: Adrenergic regulation of renin secretion and renal hemodynamics during deliberate hypotension in humans. Am J Physiol 1993; 265(5 Pt 2):F686–F692.

Regulation of Potassium Excretion

Bomsztyk K, Wright FS: Dependence of ion fluxes on fluid transport by rat proximal tubule. Am J Physiol 1986; 250:F680–F689.

Brown MJ, Brown DC, Murphy MB: Hypokalemia from $beta_2$-receptor stimulation by circulating epinephrine. N Engl J Med 1983; 309:1414–1419.

Burg M, Stoner L, Cardinal J, Green N: Furosemide effects on isolated perfused tubules. Am J Physiol 1973; 225:119–124.

Burg MB: Thick ascending limb of Henle's loop. Kidney Int 1982; 22:454–464.

DeFronzo RA, Bia M, Birkhead G: Epinephrine and potassium homeostasis. Kidney Int 1981; 20:83–91.

DeFronzo RA, Lee R, Jones A, Bia M: Effect of insulinopenia and adrenal hormone deficiency on acute potassium tolerance. Kidney Int 1980; 17:586–594.

DeFronzo RA, Sherwin RS, Dillingham M, et al: Influence of basal insulin and glucagon secretion on potassium and sodium metabolism. J Clin Invest 1978; 61:472.

Doucet A, Marsy S: Characterization of K-ATPase activity in distal nephron: Stimulation by potassium depletion. Am J Physiol 1987; 253:F418–F423.

Duarte CG, Chomety F, Giebisch G: Effect of amiloride, ouabain and furosemide on distal tubular function in the rat. Am J Physiol 1971; 221:632–639.

Field MJ, Giebisch G: Hormonal control of potassium excretion. Kidney Int 1985; 27:379–387.

Field MJ, Stanton BA, Giebisch G: Differential acute effects of aldosterone, dexamethasone and hyperkalemia on distal tubular potassium secretion in the rat kidney. J Clin Invest 1984; 74:1792–1802.

Giebisch G, Malnic G, Berliner RW: Renal transport and control of potassium excretion. *In* Brenner BM, Rector FC, eds: The Kidney, 4th ed. Philadelphia, W.B. Saunders Company, 1991, pp 283–317.

Good DW, Wright FS: Luminal influences on potassium secretion: Sodium concentration and luminal flow rate. Am J Physiol 1979; 236:F192–F205.

Greger R: Ion transport mechanisms in thick ascending limb of Henle's loop of mammalian nephrons. Physiol Rev 1985; 65:760–797.

Greger R, Schlatter E: Properties of the lumen membrane of the cortical thick ascending limb of Henle's loop of rabbit kidney. Pflugers Arch 1983; 396:315–324.

Hebert SC, Andreoli TE: Control of NaCl transport in the thick ascending limb. Am J Physiol 1984; 246:F745–756.

Hropot M, Fowler N, Kalmark B, Giebisch G: Tubular actions of diuretics: Distal effects on electrolyte transport and acidification. Kidney Int 1985; 28:477–489.

Jamison RL: Potassium recycling. Kidney Int 1987; 31:695–703.

Jamison RL, Lacy FB, Pennell JP, Sanjana VM: Potassium secretion by the descending limb of pars recta of the juxtamedullary nephron in vivo. Kidney Int 1976; 9:323–332.

Ladefoged K, Hagen K: Correlation between concentrations of magnesium, zinc, and potassium in plasma, erythrocytes and muscles. Clin Chim Acta 1988; 177:157–166.

Laragh JH, Sealey JE: Renin-angiotensin-aldosterone system and the renal regulation of sodium, potassium, and blood pressure homeostasis. *In* Windhager EE, ed: Handbook of Physiology, Section 8: Renal Physiology. New York, Oxford University Press, 1992, pp 1409–1541.

Lim M, Linton RAF, Wolff CB, Band DM: Propranolol, exercise and arterial plasma potassium. Lancet 1981; 2:591.

Malnic G, DeMello-Aires M, Giebisch G: Potassium transport across renal distal tubules during acid-base disturbances. Am J Physiol 1971; 221:1192–1208.

Malnic G, Giebisch G: Some electrical properties of distal tubule epithelium in the rat. Am J Physiol 1964; 206:674–686.

Malnic G, Klose RM, Giebisch G: Micropuncture study of distal tubule potassium and sodium transport in rat nephron. Am J Physiol 1966; 211:529–547.

O'Neil RG: Aldosterone regulation of sodium and potassium transport in the cortical collecting tubule. Semin Nephrol 1990; 10:365–374.

O'Neil RG, Boulpaep EL: Effects of amiloride on the apical cell membrane cation channels of a sodium-absorbing, potassium-secreting renal epithelium. J Membr Biol 1979; 50:365–387.

O'Neil RG, Boulpaep EL: Ionic conductive properties and electrophysiology of the rabbit cortical collecting tubule. Am J Physiol 1982; 243:F81–F95.

O'Neil RG, Helman SI: Transport characteristics of renal collecting tubules: Influence of DOCA and diet. Am J Physiol 1977; 233:544–558.

O'Neil RG, Sansom SC: Characterization of apical cell membrane Na^+ and K^+ conductances of cortical collecting duct using microelectrode techniques. Am J Physiol 1984; 247:F14–F24.

Pacha J, Frindt G, Antonian L, et al: Regulation of Na channels of the rat cortical collecting tubule by aldosterone. J Gen Physiol 1993; 102:25–42.

Palmer LG, Antonian L, Frindt G: Regulation of the Na-K pump of the rat cortical collecting tubule by aldosterone. J Gen Physiol 1993; 102:43–57.

Palmer LG, Antonian L, Frindt G: Regulation of apical K^+ and sodium channels and Na^+/K^+ pumps in rat cortical collecting tubule by dietary K^+. J Gen Physiol 1994; 104:693–710.

Rastegar A, DeFronzo RA: Disorders of potassium metabolism associated with renal disease. *In* Schrier RW, Gottschalk CW, eds: Diseases of the Kidney, 5th ed. Boston, Little, Brown, 1992, pp 2645–2661.

Rosa RM, Williams ME, Epstein FH: Extrarenal potassium metabolism. *In* Seldin DW, Giebisch G, eds: The Kidney: Physiology and Pathophysiology, 2nd ed. New York, Raven Press, 1992, pp 2165–2190.

Rose BD: Clinical Physiology of Acid-Base and Electrolyte Disorders, 3rd ed. New York, McGraw-Hill, 1989.

Rossier BC, Palmer LG: Mechanisms of aldosterone action on sodium and potassium transport. *In* Seldin DW, Giebisch G, eds: The Kidney: Physiology and Pathophysiology, 2nd ed. New York, Raven Press, 1992, pp 1373–1410.

Sansom S, Muto S, Giebisch G: Na-dependent effects of DOCA on cellular transport properties of CCDs from ADX rabbits. Am J Physiol 1987; 253:F753–F759.

Sansom SC, O'Neil RG: Effects of mineralocorticoids on transport properties of cortical collecting duct basolateral membrane. Am J Physiol 1986; 251:F743–F757.

Schaefer JA, Troutman SL, Schlatter E: Vasopressin and mineralocorticoid increase apical membrane driving force for K^+ secretion in rat CCD. Am J Physiol 1990; 258:F199–F210.

Schnermann J, Steipe B, Briggs JP: In situ studies of distal convoluted tubule in rat. II. K secretion. Am J Physiol 1987; 252:F970–F976.

Schrier RW: Pathogenesis of sodium and water retention in high-output and low-output cardiac failure, nephrotic syndrome, cirrhosis and pregnancy. N Engl J Med 1988; 319:1065–1127.

Shils, ME: Experimental human magnesium depletion. Medicine 1969; 48:61–65.

Stanton B, Janzen A, Klein-Robbenhaar G, et al: Ultrastructure of rat initial collecting tubule: Effect of adrenal corticosteroid treatment. J Clin Invest 1985a; 75:1327–1334.

Stanton B, Klein-Robbenhaar G, Giebisch G, et al: Effects of adrenalectomy and chronic adrenal corticosteroid replacement on potassium transport in rat kidney. J Clin Invest 1985b; 75:1317–1326.

Stanton B, Pan L, Deetjen P, et al: Independent effects of aldosterone and potassium on induction of potassium adaptation in rat kidney. J Clin Invest 1987; 79:198–206.

Stanton BA, Biemesderfer D, Wade JB, Giebisch G: Structural and functional study of the rat distal nephron: Effects of potassium adaptation and potassium depletion. Kidney Int 1981; 19:36–48.

Stanton BA, Giebisch G: Potassium transport by the distal renal tubule: Effects of potassium loading. Am J Physiol 1982; 243:F487–F493.

Stanton BA, Giebisch G: Renal potassium transport. *In* Windhager EE, ed: Handbook of Physiology, Section 8: Renal Physiology. New York, Oxford University Press, 1992, pp 813–874.

Stokes JB: Na and K transport across the cortical and outer medullary collecting tubule of the rabbit: Evidence for diffusion across the outer medullary portion. Am J Physiol 1982; 242:F514–F520.

Stokes JB, Ingram MJ, Williams MD, Ingram D: Heterogeneity of the rabbit collecting tubule: Localization of mineralocorticoid hormone action to the cortical portion. Kidney Int. 1981; 20:340–347.

Toussaint C, Vereerstraeten P: Effects of blood pH changes on potassium excretion in the dog. Am J Physiol 1962; 202:768–772.

Unwin RJ, Ligueros M, Shakelton C, Wilcox CS: Diuretics in the management of hypertension. *In* Laragh JH, Brenner BM, eds: Hypertension: Pathophysiology, Diagnosis, and Management, 2nd ed. New York, Raven Press, 1995, pp 2785–2800.

Velasquez H, Ellison DH, Wright FS: Chloride-dependent potassium secretion in early and late renal distal tubules. Am J Physiol 1987; 253:F555–F562.

Velasquez H, Wright FS, Good DW: Luminal influences of potassium secretion: Chloride replacement with sulfate. Am J Physiol 1982; 242:F46–F55.

Wang W, Geibel J, Giebisch G: Regulation of the small conductance K channels in the apical membrane of rat cortical collecting tubule. Am J Physiol 1990; 259:F494–F502.

Weinstein AM: Modeling of the proximal tubule: Complications of the paracellular pathway. Am J Physiol 1988; 254:F297–F305.

Whang R, Flink EB, Dyckner R, et al: Magnesium depletion as a cause of refractory potassium repletion. Arch Intern Med 1985; 145:1686–1689.

Whang R, Oei TO, Hamiter T: Frequency of hypomagnesemia associated with hypokalemia in hospitalized patients. Am J Clin Pathol 1979; 71:610.

Williams ME, Gervino EV, Rosa RM, et al: Catecholamine modulation of rapid potassium shifts during exercise. N Engl J Med 1985; 312:823–827.

Wingo CS: Potassium transport by the medullary collecting tubule of the rabbit: Effects of variation in K intake. Am J Physiol 1987; 253:F1136–F1141.

Wingo CS, Armitage FE: Potassium transport in the kidney: Regulation and physiological relevance of H^+, K^+-ATPase. Semin Nephrol 1993; 13:213–224.

Wright FS, Giebisch G: Regulation of potassium excretion. *In* Seldin DW, Giebisch G, eds: The Kidney: Physiology and Pathophysiology, 2nd ed. New York, Raven Press, 1992, pp 2209–2247.

Young DB: Quantitative analysis of aldosterone role in potassium regulation. Am J Physiol 1988; 255:F1269–F1275.

Young DB, Paulsen AW: Interrelated effects of aldosterone and plasma potassium on potassium excretion. Am J Physiol 1983; 244:F28–F34.

Regulation of Calcium Excretion

Akiba T, Endou H, Koseki C, et al: Localization of 25-hydroxy-vitamin D_3-1α-hydroxylase activity in mammalian kidney. Biochem Biophys Res Commun 1980; 94:313–318.

Alon U, Costanza LS, Chan JCM: Additive hypocalciuric effects of amiloride and hydrochlorothiazide in patients treated with calcitriol. Miner Electrolyte Metab 1984; 10:379–386.

Backasi BJ, Friedman PA: Activation of latent Ca^{++} channels in renal epithelial cells by parathyroid hormone. Nature 1990; 347:388–391.

Beck LH, Goldberg M: Effects of acetazolamide and parathyroidectomy on renal transport of sodium, calcium, and phosphate. Am J Physiol 1973; 224:1136–1142.

Bomsztyk K, George JP, Wright FS: Effects of luminal fluid anions on calcium transport by proximal tubule. Am J Physiol 1984; 246:F600–F608.

Bourdeau JE: Mechanisms and regulation of calcium transport in the nephron. Semin Nephrol 1993; 13:191–201.

Bourdeau JE, Burg MB: Calcium transport across the pars recta of cortical segment 2 proximal tubules. Am J Physiol 1986; 251:F718–F724.

Bourdeau JE, Burg MB: Effect of PTH on calcium transport across the cortical thick ascending limb of Henle's loop. Am J Physiol 1980; 239:121–126.

Bourdeau JE, Burg MB: Voltage dependence of calcium transport in the thick ascending limb of Henle's loop. Am J Physiol 1979; 236:357–364.

Bourdeau JE, Hellstrom-Stein RJ: Voltage-dependent calcium movement across the cortical collecting duct. Am J Physiol 1982; 242:285–292.

Bronner F, Stein WD: CaBP facilitates intracellular diffusion for Ca pumping in distal convoluted tubule. Am J Physiol 1988; 255:F558–F562.

Chabardès D, Imbert M, Clique A, et al: PTH sensitive adenyl cyclase activity in different segments of the rat nephron. Pflugers Arch 1975; 354:229–239.

Costanza LS: Comparison of Ca and Na transport in early and late distal tubules: Effect of amiloride. Am J Physiol 1984; 246:F937–F945.

Costanza LS: Localization of diuretic action in microperfused rat distal convoluted tubules: Ca and Na transport. Am J Physiol 1985; 248:F527–F535.

Costanza LS, Sheehe PR, Weiner IM: Renal actions of vitamin D in D-deficient rats. Am J Physiol 1974; 226:1490–1495.

Costanza LS, Weiner IM: On the hypocalciuric action of chlorothiazide. J Clin Invest 1974; 54:628–637.

Costanza LS, Windhager EE: Calcium and sodium transport by the distal convoluted tubule of the rat. Am J Physiol 1978; 235:F492–F506.

Costanza LS, Windhager EE: Effects of PTH, ADH, cyclic AMP on distal tubular Ca and Na reabsorption. Am J Physiol 1980; 239:F478–F485.

Costanza LS, Windhager EE: Renal regulation of calcium balance. *In* Seldin DW, Giebisch G, eds: The Kidney: Physiology and Pathophysiology, 2nd ed. New York, Raven Press, 1992, pp 2375–2393.

Fraser DR, Kodicek E: Unique biosynthesis by kidney of a biologically active vitamin D metabolite. Nature 1970; 228:764–766.

Friedman PA: Basal and hormone-activated calcium absorption in mouse renal thick ascending limbs. Am J Physiol 1988; 254:F62–F70.

Friedman PA, Figueiredo JF, Maack T, Windhager EE: Sodium-calcium interactions in the renal proximal convoluted tubule of the rabbit. Am J Physiol 1981; 240:F558–568.

Ghazarian JG, Jefcoate CR, Knutson JC, et al: Mitochondrial cytochrome P-450: A component of chick kidney 25-hydroxycholecalciferol-1-α-hydroxylase. J Biol Chem 1974; 249:3026–3033.

Hopkins T, Howard JE, Eisenberg H: Ultrafiltration studies on calcium and phosphorus in human serum. Bull Johns Hopkins Hosp 1952; 91:1–21.

Johnson JA, Kumar R: Renal and intestinal calcium transport: Roles of vitamin D and vitamin D–dependent calcium binding proteins. Semin Nephrol 1994; 14:119–128.

Lau K, Bourdeau JE: Evidence for cAMP-dependent protein kinase in mediating the parathyroid hormone–stimulated rise in cytosolic free calcium in rabbit connecting tubule. J Biol Chem 1989; 264:4028–4032.

Le Grimellec C, Roinel N, Morel F: Simultaneous Mg, Ca, P, K, Na and Ca analysis in rat tubular fluid. III. During acute Ca loading. Pflugers Arch 1974; 346:171–188.

Morel F: Sites of hormone action in the mammalian nephron. Am J Physiol 1981; 240:F159–F164.

Peterson NA, Feigen GA, Crimson JM: Effect of pH on interaction of calcium ions with serum proteins. Am J Physiol 1961; 201:386–392.

Quamme GA, Dirks JH: Intraluminal and contraluminal magnesium on magnesium and calcium transfer in the rat nephron. Am J Physiol 1980; 238:F187.

Rocha AS, Magaldi JB, Kokko JP: Calcium and phosphate transport in isolated segments of rabbit Henle's loop. J Clin Invest 1977; 59:975–983.

Sharegi GR, Stoner LC: Calcium transport across segments of the rabbit distal nephron in vitro. Am J Physiol 1978; 235:367–375.

Suki WN, Rouse D: Renal transport of calcium, magnesium, and phosphorus. *In* Brenner BM, Rector FC, eds: The Kidney, 4th ed. Philadelphia, W.B. Saunders Company, 1991, pp 380–423.

Suki WN, Rouse D, Ng RC, Kokko JP: Calcium transport in the thick ascending limb of Henle. Heterogeneity of function in the medullary and cortical segments. J Clin Invest 1980; 66:1004–1009.

Taylor AN, McIntosh JE, Bourdeau JE: Immunocytochemical localization of vitamin D–dependent calcium binding protein in renal tubules of rabbit, rat, and chick. Kidney Int 1982 21:765–773.

Terepka AR, Toribara TY, Dewey PA: The ultrafilterable calcium of human serum. II. Variation in disease states and under experimental conditions. J Clin Invest 1957; 36:749–759.

Toribara TY, Terepka AR, Dewey PA: The ultrafilterable calcium of human serum. I. Ultrafiltration methods and normal values. J Clin Invest 1957; 36:738–748.

Walser M: Calcium clearance as a function of sodium clearance. Am J Physiol 1961; 200:1099–1104.

Wright FS: Increasing magnitude of electrical potential along the distal renal tubule. Am J Physiol 1971; 220:624–638.

Regulation of Magnesium Excretion

Alfrey AC: Disorders of magnesium metabolism. *In* Seldin DW, Giebisch G, eds: The Kidney: Physiology and Pathophysiology, 2nd ed. New York, Raven Press, 1992, pp 2357–2373.

Quamme GA: Effect of furosemide on calcium and magnesium transport in the rat nephron. Am J Physiol 1981; 241:340–347.

Quamme GA: Influence of volume expansion on Mg influx into the superficial proximal tubule. Kidney Int 1980; 17:721A.

Quamme GA: Magnesium: Cellular and renal exchanges. *In* Seldin DW, Giebisch G, eds: The Kidney: Physiology and Pathophysiology, 2nd ed. New York, Raven Press, 1992, pp 2339–2356.

Sharegi GR, Agus ZS: Magnesium transport in the cortical thick ascending limb of Henle's loop of the rabbit. J Clin Invest 1982; 69:759–769.

Suki WN, Rouse D: Renal transport of calcium, magnesium, and phosphorus. *In* Brenner BM, Rector FC, eds: The Kidney, 4th ed. Philadelphia, W.B. Saunders Company, 1991, pp 380–423.

Regulation of Phosphate Excretion

Agus ZS, Puschett JB, Senesky D, Goldberg M: Mode of action of parathyroid hormone and cyclic adenosine 3′-5′-monophosphate on renal tubular phosphate reabsorption in the dog. J Clin Invest 1971; 50:617–626.

Anderson GH, Draper HH: Effect of dietary phosphorus on calcium metabolism in intact and parathyroidectomized adult rats. J Nutr 1972; 102:1123.

Anderson J, Parsons V: The tubular maximal rebasorption rate of inorganic phosphorus in normal subjects. Clin Sci 1963; 25:431.

Beck LH, Goldberg M: Effects of acetazolamide and parathyroidectomy on renal transport of sodium, calcium, and phosphate. Am J Physiol 1973; 224:1136–1142.

Berndt TJ, Knox FG: Renal regulation of phosphate excretion. *In* Seldin DW, Giebisch G, eds: The Kidney: Physiology and Pathophysiology, 2nd ed. New York, Raven Press, 1992, pp 2511–2532.

Brazy PC, McKeown JW, Harris RH, Dennis VW: Comparative effects of dietary phosphate, unilateral nephrectomy, and parathyroid hormone on phosphate transport by the rabbit proximal tubule. Kidney Int 1980; 17:788–800.

Cuche JL, Ott CE, Marchand GR, et al: Intrarenal calcium in phosphate handling. Am J Physiol 1976; 230:790.

Greger R, Lang F, Marchand G, Knox GG: Site of renal phosphate reabsorption: Micropuncture and microperfusion study. Pflugers Arch 1977; 369:111–118.

Kuntziger H, Amiel C, Roinel N, Morel F: Effetcts of parathyroidectomy and cyclic AMP on renal transport of phosphate, calcium, and magnesium. Am J Physiol 1974; 227:905–911.

Murer H, Biber J: Renal tubular phosphate transport: Cellular mechanisms. *In* Seldin DW, Giebisch G, eds: The Kidney: Physiology and Pathophysiology, 2nd ed. New York, Raven Press, 1992, pp 2481–2509.

Peraino RA, Suki WN: Phosphate transport by isolated rabbit cortical collecting tubule. Am J Physiol 1980; 238:358–362.

Suki WN, Rouse D: Renal transport of calcium, magnesium, and phosphorus. *In* Brenner BM, Rector FC, eds: The Kidney, 4th ed. Philadelphia, W.B. Saunders Company, 1991, pp 380–423.

Yanagawa N, Nossenson RA, Edwards B, et al: Functional profile of the isolated uremic nephron: Intrinsic adaptation of phosphate transport in the rabbit proximal tubule. Kidney Int 1983; 23:674–683.

Regulation of Urate Excretion

Beck LH: Hypouricemia in the syndrome of inappropriate secretion of antidiuretic hormone. N Engl J Med 1979; 301:528.

Chonko AM: Urate secretion in isolated rabbit tubules. Am J Physiol 1980; 239:F545–F551.

Diamond H, Meisel A: Influence of volume expansion, serum sodium, and fractional excretion of sodium on urate excretion. Pflugers Arch 1975; 356:47.

Grantham JJ, Chonko AM: Renal handling of organic ions and cations; excretion of uric acid. *In* Brenner BM, Rector FC, eds: The Kidney, 4th ed. Philadelphia, W.B. Saunders Company, 1991, pp 483–509.

Kahn AM, Aronson PS: Urate transport via anion exchange in dog renal microvillus membrane vesicles. Am J Physiol 1983; 244:F56.

Kippen I, Klinenberg JR, Weinberger A, Wilcox WR: Factors affecting urate solubility in vitro. Ann Rheum Dis 1974; 33:313.

Mees EJD, Blom van Assendelft P, Nieuwenhuis MG: Elevation of uric acid clearance caused by inappropriate antidiuretic hormone secretion. Acta Med Scand 1971; 189:69.

Rieselbach RE, Sorenson LB, Shelp WD, Steele TH: Diminished renal urate secretion per nephron as a basis for primary gout. Ann Intern Med 1970; 73:359.

Senekjian HO, Knight TF, Weinman EJ: Urate transport by the isolated perfused S_2 segment of the rabbit. Am J Physiol 1981; 240:F530.

Steele TH, Oppenheimer S: Factors affecting urate excretion following diuretic administration in man. Am J Med 1969; 47:564.

Weiner IM, Tinker JP: Pharmacology of pyrazinamide: Metabolic and renal function studies related to the mechanism of drug-induced urate retention. J Pharmacol Exp Ther 1972; 180:441.

Weinman EJ, Steplock D, Suki WN, Enkoyan G: Urate reabsorption in proximal convoluted tubule of the rat kidney. Am J Physiol 1976; 231:509.

Regulation of Water Balance

Anderson RJ: Hospital-associated hyponatremia. Kidney Int 1986; 29:1237–1247.

Arieff AI: Hyponatremia associated with permanent brain damage. Adv Intern Med 1987; 32:325–344.

Arieff AI: Permanent neurological disability from hyponatremia in healthy women undergoing elective surgery. N Engl J Med 1986; 314:1529.

Arieff AI, Llach F, Massry SG: Neurological manifestations and morbidity of hyponatremia: Correlation of brain water and electrolytes. Medicine 1976; 55:121.

Ashraf N, Locksley R, Arieff AI: Thiazide-induced hyponatremia associated with death or neurological damage in outpatients. Dig Dis 1981; 21:249–256.

Ayus JC, Krothapolli RK, Arieff AI: Treatment of symptomatic hyponatremia and its relation to brain damage: A prospective study. N Engl J Med 1987; 217:1190.

Azzopardi JG, Freeman E, Poole G: Endocrine and metabolic disorders in bronchial carcinoma. BMJ 1970; 4:528.

Beck LH: Hypouricemia in the syndrome of inappropriate secretion of antidiuretic hormone. N Engl J Med 1979; 301:528.

Berl T, Linas SL, Aisenbrey GA, Anderson RJ: On the mechanism of polyuria in potassium depletion. J Clin Invest 1977; 60:620–625.

Berry CA, Rector FC Jr: Renal transport of glucose, amino acids, sodium, chloride, and water. *In* Brenner BM, Rector FC, eds: The Kidney, 4th ed. Philadelphia, W.B. Saunders Company, 1991, pp 245–282.

Bichet D: Molecular and cellular biology of vasopressin and oxytocin receptors and action in the kidney. Curr Opin Nephrol Hypertens 1994; 3:46–53.

Bichet DG, Kluge R, Howard RL, Schrier RW: Hyponatremic states. *In* Seldin DW, Giebisch G, eds: The Kidney: Physiology and Pathophysiology, 2nd ed. New York, Raven Press, 1992, pp 1727–1751.

Blumenfeld JD, Grossman EB, Sun AM, Hebert SC: Sodium-coupled ion cotransport and the volume regulatory increase response. Kidney Int 1989a; 36:434–440.

Blumenfeld JD, Hebert SC, Heilig CW, et al: Organic osmolytes in inner medulla of the Brattleboro rat: Effects of ADH and dehydration. Am J Physiol 1989b; 256:F916–F922.

Blumenfeld JD, Laragh JH: Congestive Heart Failure: Pathophysiology, Diagnosis and Treatment. New York, Professional Communications, Inc., 1994.

Boykin J, de Torrente A, Erickson A, et al: Role of plasma vasopressin in impaired water excretion of glucorticoid deficiency. J Clin Invest 1978; 62:738.

Chou C-L, Knepper MA, Layton HE: Urinary concentrating mechanism: The role of the inner medulla. Semin Nephrol 1993; 13:168–181.

Chung H-M, Kluge R, Schrier RW, Anderson R: Post-operative hyponatremia. Arch Intern Med 1986; 146:333.

Davies DP, Ansari BM, Mandal BK: The declining incidence of infantile hypernatremic dehydration in Great Britain. Am J Dis Child 1979; 133:148–150.

Decaux G, Brimioulle S, Genette F, Mockel J: Treatment of the syndrome of inappropriate secretion of antidiuretic hormone by urea. Am J Med 1980; 69:99–106.

Deen PMT, Verdijk MAJ, Knoers VAM, et al: Requirement of human renal water channel aquaporin-2 for vasopressin-dependent concentration of urine. Science 1994; 264:92–95.

Dunn FL, Brennan TJ, Nelson AE, Robertson GL: The role of blood osmolality and volume in regulating vasopressin secretion in the rat. J Clin Invest 1973; 52:3212–3219.

Edelman I, Leibman J, O'Meara M, Birkenfeld L: Interrelations between serum sodium concentration, serum osmolarity and total exchangeable sodium sodium, total exchangeable potassium and total body water. J Clin Invest 1958; 37:1236.

Epstein FH, Kleeman CR, Hendrikx A: The influence of bodily hydration on the renal concentrating process. J Clin Invest 1957; 36:629–634.

Forrest JN Jr, Cohen AD, Torretti J, et al: On the mechanism of lithium-induced diabetes insipidus in man and the rat. J Clin Invest 1974; 53:1115–1123.

Forrest JN Jr, Cox M, Hong C, et al: Superiority of demeclocycline over lithium in the treatment of chronic syndrome of inappropriate secretion of antidiuretic hormone. N Engl J Med 1978; 298:173–177.

Garg R, Yusuf S: Overview of randomized trials of angiotensin-converting enzyme inhibitors on mortality and morbidity in patients with heart failure. JAMA 1995; 273:1450–1456.

Gillin AG, Sands JM: Urea transport in the kidney. Semin Nephrol 1993; 13:146–154.

Goel CM, Badenoch DF, Fowler CG, et al: Transurethral resection syndrome: a prospective study. Eur Urol 1992; 21:15–17.

Gullans SR, Blumenfeld JD, Balschi SA, et al: Accumulation of major organic osmolytes in rat renal inner medulla in dehydration. Am J Physiol 1988; 255:F626–F634.

Gullans SR, Stromski MD, Blumenfeld JD, Lee JP: Methylamines and polyols in kidney, urine, liver, brain, and plasma. Renal Physiol 1989; 12:91–101.

Halperin ML, Goldstein MB: Fluid, Electrolyte and Acid-Base Physiology: A Problem-Based Approach, 2nd ed. Philadelphia, W.B. Saunders Company, 1994.

Harrington AH, Valtin H: Impaired urinary concentration after vasopressin and its gradual correction in hypothalamic diabetes insipidus. J Clin Invest 1968; 47:502–510.

Hebert SC, Andreoli TE: Control of NaCl transport in the thick ascending limb. Am J Physiol 1984; 246:F745–756.

Hebert SC, Culpepper RM, Andreoli TE: NaCl transport in mouse medullary thick ascending limbs. I. Functional nephron heterogeneity and ADH-stimulated NaCl cotransport. Am J Physiol 1981; 241:F412–F431.

Heilig CW, Stromski ME, Blumenfeld JD, et al: Characterization of the major brain osmolytes that accumulate in salt-loaded rats. Am J Physiol 1989; 257:F1108–F1116.

Holzman EJ, Harris HW, Kolakowski LF, et al: A molecular defect in the vasopressin V2-receptor gene causing nephrogenic diabetes insipidus. N Engl J Med 1993; 328:1534–1356.

Howard RL, Bichet DG, Schrier RW: Hypernatremic and polyuric states. *In* Seldin DW, Giebisch G, eds: The Kidney: Physiology and Pathophysiology, 2nd ed. New York, Raven Press, 1992, pp 1753–1778.

Iseri LT, Kaplan MA, Evans MJ, Nickel ED: Effects of concentrated contrast media during angiography on plasma volume and plasma osmolality. Am Heart J 1965; 69:154–158.

Kirk KL, Schaefer JA: Water transport and osmoregulation by antidiuretic hormone in terminal nephron segments. *In* Seldin DW, Giebisch G, eds: The Kidney: Physiology and Pathophysiology, 2nd ed. New York, Raven Press, 1992, pp 1693–1726.

Kirschenbaum MA: Severe mannitol-induced hyponatremia complicating transurethral prostate resection. J Urol 1979; 121:687–688.

Knepper MA, Rector FC Jr: Urinary concentration and dilution. *In* Brenner BM, Rector FC, eds: The Kidney, 4th ed. Philadelphia, W.B. Saunders Company, 1991, 445–482.

Knoers NVAM, Os CHV: The clinical importance of the urinary excretion of aquaporin-2. N Engl J Med 1995; 332:1575–1576.

Kokko JP, Rector FC Jr: Countercurrent multiplication system without active transport in inner medulla. Kidney Int 1972; 2:214.

Lassiter WE, Gottschalk CW: Regulation of water balance: Urine concentration and dilution. *In* Schrier RW, Gottschalk CW, eds: Diseases of the Kidney, 5th ed. Boston, Little, Brown, 1992, pp 119–138.

Mouw D, Bonjour JP, Malvin RL, Vander A: Central action of angiotensin in stimulating ADH release. Am J Physiol 1971; 220:239–242.

Norris HT, Aasheim GM, Sherrard DJ, Tremann JA: Symptomatology, pathophysiology and treatment of the transurethral resection of the prostate syndrome. Br J Urol 1973; 45:420–427.

Randall RV, Clark EC, Dodge HW: Polyuria after operation for tumors in the region of the hypophysis and hypothalamus. J Clin Endocrinol 1966; 20:1614–1619.

Rayson BMR, Ray C, Morgan T: The effect of adrenal cortical hormones on water permeability of the collecting duct of the rat. Pflugers Arch 1978; 373:105–112.

Robertson GL: Regulation of vasopressin secretion. *In* Seldin DW, Giebisch G, eds: The Kidney: Physiology and Pathophysiology, 2nd ed. New York, Raven Press, 1992, pp 1595–1613.

Robertson GL, Berl T: Pathophysiology of water metabolism. *In* Brenner BM, Rector FC, eds: The Kidney, 4th ed. Philadelphia, W.B. Saunders Company, 1991, pp 677–736.

Rose BD: Clinical Physiology of Acid-Base and Electrolyte Disorders, 3rd ed. New York, McGraw-Hill, 1989.

Rowe JW, Shelton RL, Helderman JH, et al: Influence of the emetic reflex on vasopressin release in man. Kidney Int 1979; 16:729–735.

Roy D, Layton HE, Jamison RL: Countercurrent mechanism and its regulation. *In* Seldin DW, Giebisch G, eds: The Kidney: Physiology and Pathophysiology, 2nd ed. New York, Raven Press, 1992, pp 1649–1692.

Schrier RW: Pathogenesis of sodium and water retention in high-output and low-output cardiac failure, nephrotic syndrome, cirrhosis and pregnancy. N Engl J Med 1988; 319:1065–1127.

Sterns RH, Riggs JE, Schochet SS Jr: Osmotic demyelination syndrome following correction of hyponatremia. N Engl J Med 1986; 314:1535–1542.

Suki W, Rector FC, Seldin DW: The site of action of furosemide and other sulfonamide diuretics in the dog. J Clin Invest 1967; 24:1458.

Swedberg K, Eneroth P, Kjekshus J, Wilhelmsen L: Hormones regulating cardiovascular function in patients with severe congestive heart failure and their relation to mortality. Circulation 1990; 82:1730–1736.

Szatalowicz VL, Arnold PE, Chaimovitz C, et al: Radioimmunoassay of plasma arginine vasopressin in hyponatremic patients with congestive heart failure. N Engl J Med 1981; 305:263–266.

Szatalowicz VL, Miller PD, Gordon JA, Schrier RW: Comparative effects of diuretics on renal water excretion in hyponatremic oedematous disorders. Clin Sci 1982; 62:236–240.

Trachtman H, Del Pizzo R, Sturman JA, et al: Taurine and osmoregulation. II. Administration of taurine analogs affords cerebral osmoprotection during chronic hypernatremic dehydration. Am J Dis Child 1988; 142:1194–1198.

Verbalis JG, Dutaroski MD: Adaptation to chronic hypoosmolality in rats. Kidney Int 1988; 34:351–360.

Zeidel ML, Strange K, Francesco E, Harris HW Jr: Mechanisms and regulation of water transport in the kidney. Semin Nephrol 1993; 13:155–167.

Zerbe RL, Robertson GL: Osmoregulation of thirst and vasopressin secretion in human subjects: Effect of various solutes. Am J Physiol 1983; 224:E607–E614.

Acid-Base Homeostasis

Adrogue HJ, Madias NE: Changes in plasmapotassium concentration during acid-base disturbances. Am J Med 1981; 71:456.

Alpern RJ, Cogan MG, Rector FC Jr: Effects of luminal bicarbonate concentration on proximal acidification in the rat. Am J Physiol 1982; 243:F53.

Alpern RJ, Emmett M, Seldin DW: Metabolic alkalosis. *In* Seldin DW, Giebisch G, eds: The Kidney: Physiology and Pathophysiology, 2nd ed. New York, Raven Press, 1992, pp 2733–2758.

Aronson PS, Suhm MA, Nee J: Interactions of the external H^+ with the Na^+-H^+ exchanger in renal microvillus membrane vesicles. J Biol Chem 1983; 258:6767.

Baines AD, Drangova R, Ho P: Role of diacylglycerol in adrenergic-stimulated ^{86}Rb uptake by proximal tubules. Am J Physiol 1990; 258:F1133–F1138.

Batlle DC, Hizon M, Cohen E, et al: The use of the urinary anion gap in the diagnosis of hyperchloremic metabolic acidosis. N Engl J Med 1988; 318:594–599.

Bichara M, Mercier O, Paillard M, Leviel F: Effects of parathyroid hormone on urinary acidification. Am J Physiol 1986; 251:F444–453.

Blumenfeld JD: Hypertension and adrenal disorders. Curr Opin Nephrol Hypertens 1993; 2:274–282.

Blumenfeld JD, Sealey JE, Schlussel Y, et al: Diagnosis and treatment of primary hyperaldosteronism. Ann Intern Med 1994; 121:877–885.

Brenner RJ, Spring DB, Sebastian A, et al: Incidence of radiographically evident bone disease nephrocalcinosis and nephrolithiasis in various types of renal tubular acidosis. N Engl J Med 1982; 307:217–221.

Buekert J, Martin D, Trigg D: Ammonium handling by superficial and juxtamedullary nephrons in the rat. J Clin Invest 1982; 70:1–12.

Bushinsky DA, Coe FL, Katzenberg C, et al: Arterial P_{CO_2} in chronic metabolic acidosis. Kidney Int 1982:311–314.

Bushinsky DA, Lechleider RJ: Mechanism of proton-induced bone calcium release: calcium carbonate release. Am J Physiol 1987; 253:F998–F1005.

Capasso G, Jaeger P, Giebisch G, et al: Renal bicarbonate reabsorption in the rat. II. Distal tubule load dependence and effect of hypokalemia. J Clin Invest 1987; 80:409–414.

Caruana RJ, Buckalew VM Jr: The syndrome of distal (Type 1) renal tubular acidosis. Clinical and laboratory findings in 58 cases. Medicine 1988; 67:84.

Chiu AT, Bozarth JM, Timmermans PBMWM: Relationship between phosphatidylinositol turnover and Ca^{++} mobilization induced by alpha-1 adrenoceptor stimulation in the rat aorta. J Pharmacol Exp Ther 1987; 240:123–127.

Cogan MG: Chronic hypercapnia stimulates proximal bicarbonate reabsorption in the rat. J Clin Invest 1984; 74:1942–1947.

Cogan MG, Maddox DA, Warnock DG, et al: Effect of acetazolamide on bicarbonate reabsorption in the proximal tubule of the rat. Am J Physiol 1979; 237:F447–F454.

Cogan MG, Rector FC Jr: Acid-base disorders. *In* Brenner BM, Rector FC, eds: The Kidney, 4th ed. Philadelphia, W.B. Saunders Company, 1991, pp 737–804.

DeFronzo RA: Hyperkalemia and hyporeninemic hypoaldosteronism. Kidney Int 1980; 17:118–134.

Dubose TD Jr, Caflisch CR: Effect of selective aldosterone deficiency on acidification in nephron segements of the rat renal medulla. J Clin Invest 1988; 82:1624–1632.

Emmett M, Alpern RJ, Seldin DW: Metabolic acidosis. *In* Seldin DW, Giebisch G, eds: The Kidney: Physiology and Pathophysiology, 2nd ed. New York, Raven Press, 1992, pp 2759–2836.

Emmett M, Narins RG: Clinical use of the anion gap. Medicine (Baltimore) 1977; 56:38–54.

Felder CC, Campbell T, Albrecht F, Jose PA: Dopamine inhibits Na^+-H^+ exchanger activity in renal BBMV by stimulation of adenylate cyclase. Am J Physiol 1990; 259:F297–F303.

Fulop M: Serum potassium in lactic acidosis and ketoacidosis. N Engl J Med 1979; 300:1087.

Gennari FJ, Maddox DA: Renal regulation of acid-base homeostasis: Integrated response. *In* Seldin DW, Giebisch G, eds: The Kidney: Physiology and Pathophysiology, 2nd ed. New York, Raven Press, 1992, pp 2759–2836.

Good DW: The thick ascending limb as a site of renal bicarbonate reabsorption. Semin Nephrol 1993; 13:225–235.

Halperin ML, Goldstein MB: Fluid, Electrolyte, and Acid-Base Physiology: A Problem-Based Approach, 2nd ed. Philadelphia, W.B. Saunders Company, 1994.

Halperin ML, Goldstein MB, Richardson RMA, Stinebaugh BJ: Distal renal tubular acidosis syndromes: A pathophysiologic approach. Am J Nephrol 1985; 5:1.

Halperin ML, Kamel KS, Ethier JH, et al: Biochemistry and physiology of ammonium excretion. *In* Seldin DW, Giebisch G, eds: The Kidney: Physiology and Pathophysiology, 2nd ed. New York, Raven Press, 1992, pp 2645–2679.

Halperin ML, Richardson RMA, Bera BA, et al. Urine ammonium: The key to the diagnosis of distal renal tubular acidosis. Nephron 1988; 50:1–4.

Hamm LL, Alpern RJ: Cellular mechanisms of renal tubular acidification. *In* Seldin DW, Giebisch G, eds: The Kidney: Physiology and Pathophysiology, 2nd ed. New York, Raven Press, 1992, pp 2581–2626.

Harrington JT, Lemann J: The metabolic production and disposal of acid and alkali. Med Clin North Am 1970; 54:1543–1554.

Harris PJ, Thomas D, Morgan TO: Atrial natriuretic peptide inhibits angiotensin-stimulated proximal tubular sodium and water reabsorption. Nature 1987; 326:697–698.

Harris PJ, Young JA: Dose-dependent stimulation and inhibition of proximal tubule sodium reabsorption by angiotensin II in the rat kidney. Pflugers Arch 1977; 367:295–297.

Hernandez RE, Schambelan M, Cogan MG, et al: Dietary NaCl determines severity of potassium depletion–induced metabolic alkalosis. Kidney Int 1987; 31:1356–1367.

Hruska KA, Moskowitz D, Esbrit P, et al: Stimulation of inositol triphosphate and diacylglycerol production in renal tubular cells by parathyroid hormone. J Clin Invest 1987; 79:230–239.

Hulter HN, Ilnicki LP, Harbottle JA, Sebastian A: Impaired renal H^+ secretion and NH_4^+ production in mineralocorticoid-deficient and glucocorticoid-replete dogs. Am J Physiol 1977; 326:F136–F146.

Hulter HN, Peterson JC: Acid-base homeostasis during chronic PTH excess in humans. Kidney Int 1985; 28:187–192.

Jones JW, Sebastian A, Hulter AN, et al: Systemic and renal acid-base effects of chronic dietary potassium depletion in humans. Kidney Int 1982; 21:402–410.

Kassirer JP, Appleton FM, Chazan JA, Schwartz WB: Aldosterone in metabolic alkalosis. J Clin Invest 1967; 46:1558–1571.

Kassirer JP, London AM, Goldman DM, Schwartz WB: On the pathogenesis of metabolic alkalosis in primary aldosteronism. Am J Med 1970; 49:306–315.

Kazemi H, Hitzig B: Central chemical control of ventilation and acid-base balance. *In* Seldin DW, Giebisch G: The Kidney: Physiology and Pathophysiology, 2nd ed. New York, Raven Press, 1992, pp 2627–2644.

Kikeri D, Sun A, Zeidel ML, Hebert SC: Cell membranes impermeable to NH_3. Nature 1989; 339:478–480.

Laragh JH, Sealey JE: Renin-angiotensin-aldosterone system and the renal regulation of sodium, potassium, and blood pressure homeostasis. *In* Windhager EE, ed: Handbook of Physiology, Section 8: Renal Physiology. New York, Oxford University Press, 1992, pp 1409–1541.

Liu F-Y, Cogan MG: Angiotensin II stimulates early proximal bicarbonate reabsorption in the rat by decreasing cyclic adenosine monophosphate. J Clin Invest 1989; 84:83–91.

Liu F-Y, Cogan MG: Atrial natriuretic factor does not inhibit basal or angiotensin II–stimulated proximal transport. Am J Physiol 1988; 255:F434–437.

Liu F-Y, Cogan MG: Effects of intracellular calcium on proximal bicarbonate reabsorption. Am J Physiol 1990; 259:F451–F457.

Madias NE, Cohen JJ: Respiratory alkalosis and acidosis. *In* Seldin DW, Giebisch G, eds: The Kidney: Physiology and Pathophysiology, 2nd ed. New York, Raven Press, 1992, pp 2837–2872.

Rose BD: Clinical Physiology of Acid-Base and Electrolyte Disorders, 3rd ed. New York, McGraw-Hill, 1989.

Rosen RA, Julian BA, Dubovsky EV, et al: On the mechanism by which chloride corrects metabolic alkalosis in man. Am J Med 1988; 84:449–458.

Schwartz WB, Orning KJ, Porter R: The internal distribution of hydrogen ions with varying degrees of metabolic acidosis. J Clin Invest 1957; 373–382.

Sebastian A, McSherry E, Morris RC Jr: Renal potassium wasting in renal tubular acidosis (RTA). Its occurrence in types 1 and 2 RTA despite sustained correction of systemic acidosis. J Clin Invest 1971; 50:667–678.

Sebastian A, Sutton JM, Hulter AM, et al: Effect of mineralocoticoid replacement therapy on renal acid-base homeostasis in adrenalectomized patients. Kidney Int 1980; 18:762–773.

Sterns RH, Cox M, Feig PU, Singer I: Internal potassium balance and the control of the plasma potassium concentration. Medicine 1981; 60:339.

Tannen RL, McGill J: Influence of potassium on renal ammonium production. Am J Physiol 1976; 231:1178–1184.

Turino GM, Goldring RM, Heinemann HO: Renal response to mechanical ventilation in patients with chronic hypercapnia. Am J Med 1974: 56:151–161.

Verrey F: Regulation of gene expression by aldosterone in tight epithelia. Semin Nephrol 1990; 10:410–420.

Wingo CS, Armitage FE: Potassium transport in the kidney: Regulation and physiological relevance of H^+, K^+-ATPase. Semin Nephrol 1993; 13:213–224.

Wistrand PJ, Knuutila K-G: Renal membrane-bound carbonic anhydrase: Purification and properties. Kidney Int 1989; 35:851.

8
ETIOLOGY, PATHOGENESIS, AND MANAGEMENT OF RENAL FAILURE

Charles L. Edelstein, M.B., Ch.B., M.Med.
Ahmed Alkhunaizi, M.D.
Muhammad M. Yaqoob, M.D., Ph.D., M.R.C.P.
Joseph I. Shapiro, M.D.
Robert W. Schrier, M.D.

INTRODUCTION

Description of Renal Functions

The kidney performs a number of important physiologic and hormonal functions. It plays a central role in maintaining acid-base, water, and electrolyte homeostasis, as well as regulating extracellular volume and blood pressure. It produces hormones such as renin, prostaglandins, kallikrein, vitamin D, and erythropoietin. It is the normal route for excreting nitrogenous and other waste products derived from intermediary metabolism. In short, the kidney does considerably more than eliminate nitrogenous wastes, although this is arguably the most important renal function.

Many renal functions can be quantitated clinically. Urinary concentrating or diluting ability may be assessed by measuring urinary osmolality after water deprivation or water load, respectively. Urinary acidification may be assessed by measuring urinary pH in the presence of spontaneous acidemia or acid loading. Urinary electrolyte concentrations and the fractional excretion of these electrolytes may also be monitored to determine whether renal handling of these electrolytes is normal (Schrier, 1992). However, the most important tests of renal function are those that assess the glomerular filtration rate (GFR).

Laboratory Assessment of Renal Function

Most arterial blood delivered to the kidney passes through glomerular capillaries, where a portion, known as the filtration fraction, is filtered. Under normal circumstances, this filtrate is without blood cells and contains only small amounts of protein. This filtered fluid is modified by tubular reabsorption and secretion in order to regulate the quality and quantity of body fluids, as previously discussed. The rate at which fluid is filtered at the level of the glomerulus is the most important clinical parameter of renal function which can be measured (Brenner et al, 1986).

Measurement of GFR can be accomplished by measur-

ing the renal clearance of a substance that is freely filtered by the glomerulus, not reabsorbed or degraded and not secreted by any tubular segment (Carlson and Harrington, 1992). The renal clearance of such a substance, X (ClX), would be calculated as follows:

$$ClX = (UX \times V)/PX,$$

where UX is the urine concentration of X, V is the urine flow rate, and PX is the plasma concentration of X. No endogenous compound that can be easily measured fits this description perfectly. For experimental work, inulin, a polysaccharide not normally found in humans, is infused to achieve a steady-state plasma concentration, and subsequent determination of its clearance by the kidney is the gold standard for GFR measurement (Brenner et al, 1986). Iodothalamate is a compound that can be easily radiolabeled (iodine-125) and can be used in place of inulin clearance for GFR determinations (Gagnon et al, 1971).

Neither of these measurements is practical on a routine clinical basis. The plasma concentration of urea has been used in the past to assess renal function. Urea is a breakdown product of protein catabolism whose plasma levels have an inverse correlation with GFR. Unfortunately, urea production rate is variable and depends on dietary intake and the rate of catabolism as well as on liver function. Moreover, urea is not only filtered by the glomerulus but is also reabsorbed by the tubules to a significant and variable degree, depending on volume status and urine flow rate. Therefore, neither urea clearance nor plasma urea concentration provides an accurate estimation of GFR (Carlson and Harrington, 1992).

In comparison, creatinine, an important compound in energy metabolism, is another nitrogenous compound that is a breakdown product of creatine. Creatinine is produced at a relatively constant rate, dependent on the amount of total creatine in the body. This, in turn, is dependent primarily on the amount of muscle mass. Therefore, for a given individual, daily creatinine production is relatively constant. Creatinine is freely filtered at the level of the glomerulus and is not reabsorbed but is secreted to some extent. Although creatinine secretion accounts for only 10% of total creatinine excretion in patients with normal renal function, tubular creatinine secretion may represent a greater proportion in some patients with renal disease, particularly those with significant proteinuria. Drugs such as triamterene, spironolactone, amiloride, probenecid, cimetidine, and trimethoprim can blunt the tubular secretion of creatinine, leading to a rise in serum creatinine and a decline in measured creatinine clearance. Erroneous measurements of creatinine clearance can arise from inaccuracies in the process of urine collection by the patient. **Despite these drawbacks, plasma creatinine values and renal creatinine clearance measurements are used to estimate GFR (Carlson and Harrington, 1992).**

GFR is not constant throughout the day and is influenced greatly by dietary protein intake. In patients with normal renal function, a marked increase in GFR occurs rapidly and persists for several hours after ingestion of a protein-laden meal. This increase in GFR after protein ingestion may be blunted or absent in patients with chronic renal failure. This ability to increase GFR with protein ingestion, referred to as the "renal reserve," is another sensitive measurement of renal function (Ter-Wee et al, 1987; Notghi and Anderton, 1988; von-Herrath et al, 1988; Losito et al, 1988).

ACUTE RENAL FAILURE

Definition and Clinical Description

Acute renal failure (ARF) is probably best understood as an acute deterioration in renal functions that results in a buildup of nitrogenous wastes in the plasma and/or a failure of the kidney to regulate extracellular fluid volume or composition. Although this definition offers a reasonable understanding of the concept, it is vague and ill suited for reporting clinical data. For example, in clinical reports, definitions of acute renal failure range from a need for dialysis therapy to 0.5-mg/dl increases in plasma creatinine concentrations. Clearly the criterion used to define patient selection greatly influences estimations of incidence and mortality.

Because the most obvious evidence of renal function is the production of urine, the first descriptions of ARF were limited to patients who developed marked reductions in urine flow rate. **Maximal urine osmolality is about 1000 mOsm/l, and obligate solute excretion requirements are about 500 mOsm/day for a 70-kg man. Reductions of urine flow rate to below 500 ml/day at 1000 mOsm/l are not compatible with the maintenance solute balance, and azotemia invariably occurs. In this setting, reduction of urine flow rate below this amount is referred to as *oliguria*. Virtual cessation of urine flow is called *anuria*. Although oliguria and anuria are certainly serious, their absence does not rule out ARF. The acute accumulation of nitrogenous solutes in the blood as daily urine flow exceeding 500 ml/day is referred to as *nonoliguric ARF* (Anderson and Schrier, 1992).**

ARF is still commonly encountered, especially in hospitalized patients. The most common cause of ARF is prerenal azotemia, but acute tubular necrosis (ATN) and urinary obstruction (postrenal azotemia) also occur frequently (Hou et al, 1983). Because ARF is accompanied by marked increases in morbidity and mortality, avoidance and prompt therapy of ARF are extremely important. An understanding of the different causes of ARF, their differential diagnosis, and the appropriate therapy is therefore required.

Etiologies

ARF may be seen with a variety of insults. Often, more than one insult may be implicated (Rasmussen and Ibels, 1982).

Classification

Clinically, it is extremely useful to separate the causes of ARF into prerenal, intrarenal, and postrenal. Assignment of a patient to one of these groups usually requires a combination of clinical and laboratory evaluation and may occasionally require imaging studies and/or invasive measurements of central hemodynamics. Because the clinical management of ARF may be very different in

patients with prerenal, intrarenal (e.g., ATN), and postrenal ARF, this diagnostic determination is of critical importance (Schrier and Conger, 1986).

Prerenal Acute Renal Failure

Prerenal ARF occurs because of inadequate renal perfusion pressure to maintain GFR. Under normal circumstances, the kidney can maintain normal renal blood flow and GFR down to perfusion pressures of 60 mm Hg. This phenomenon is known as autoregulation and requires a complex interplay of physiologic factors for its maintenance. In many patients, not all of these physiologic factors are intact, and decreases in renal blood flow and GFR occur with modest or even no discernible reductions in blood pressure.

In the setting of decreased renal perfusion pressure, angiotensin II, which has selectively greater vasoconstrictor effects on the efferent arteriole than on the afferent arteriole, and vasodilatory prostaglandins, which cause afferent arteriolar vasodilatation, are important in maintaining glomerular hydrostatic pressure and GFR (Brenner et al, 1986). Drugs that selectively block angiotensin II synthesis or action or that inhibit prostaglandin synthesis may therefore cause ARF in some clinical settings in which GFR is already compromised.

The common causes of prerenal ARF, also called prerenal azotemia, are listed in Table 8–1. Of these, the most common is probably simple dehydration. It must be stressed, however, that gross extracellular volume expansion, as seen with liver failure, nephrotic syndrome, and heart failure, may also be associated with prerenal azotemia because of arterial underfilling. Prerenal azotemia due to dehydration or blood loss can be treated quite simply by volume expansion. However, prerenal ARF related to heart failure may necessitate careful titration of diuretics, cardiac afterload reduction, and infusion of inotropic agents to improve renal perfusion. The prerenal ARF associated with liver failure is particularly difficult to treat, in that affected patients are particularly susceptible to ATN or the hepatorenal syndrome (HRS) with overaggressive diuresis.

The HRS is a particularly severe form of prerenal azotemia in which renal vasoconstriction apparently cannot be reversed by manipulation of cardiac filling pressure secondary to volume expansion. Interestingly, this vasoconstriction can be reversed by transplanting the kidney from the patient with HRS into a patient with a well-functioning liver. HRS can also be reversed by liver transplantation (Arroyo et al, 1988).

Table 8–1. MAJOR CAUSES OF PRERENAL AZOTEMIA

Decreased Cardiac Output

Decreased Intravascular Volume

Dehydration
Hemorrhage
Anaphylactic shock

Decreased Venous Tone

Autonomic neuropathy
Spinal injury

Decreased Contractile Function

Ischemic heart disease
Cardiomyopathy
Valvular heart disease
Pericardial tamponade or constriction

Normal or Increased Cardiac Output

Systemic Disorders

Hepatorenal syndrome
Sepsis

Local Renal Disease

Renal artery stenosis

Table 8–2. MAJOR PARENCHYMAL CAUSES OF ACUTE RENAL FAILURE

Primary Renal Disease

Glomerular

Primary acute glomerulonephritis (e.g., membranoproliferative)

Tubulointerstitial

Acute interstitial nephritis
Acute tubular necrosis
Pyelonephritis
Transplant allograft rejection
Nephrolithiasis
Radiation nephritis

Vascular (of left and right vessels)

Renal artery occlusion
Renal vein thrombosis

Systemic Disease

Glomerular

Vasculitis
Goodpasture's syndrome
Secondary acute glomerulonephritis (e.g., bacterial endocarditis)

Tubulointerstitial

Tumor lysis syndrome
Hypercalcemia
Infections
Infiltration (e.g., sarcoid, lymphoma)

Vascular

Vasculitis
Malignant hypertension
Scleroderma
Thrombotic thrombocytopenic purpura

Parenchymal Causes

ARF may have a variety of parenchymal causes. The most important of these are listed in Table 8–2. Clinically, it is useful to separate these causes into those secondary to systemic diseases, primary glomerular renal diseases, and primary tubulointerstitial renal diseases.

Although a variety of systemic diseases have renal manifestations, relatively few of these commonly cause ARF. Of note is that ARF can occur secondary to systemic vasculitides, in particular polyarteritis nodosa, essential cryoglobulinemia, systemic lupus erythematosus, and multiple myeloma (Ballard et al, 1970; Martinez-Maldonado et al, 1971; Hecht et al, 1976; Schrier, 1992). Diabetes, although not a typical cause for ARF on its own, is a significant predisposing factor for ARF from other causes, particularly ARF caused by radiocontrast media (Schrier and Shapiro, 1985). ARF may complicate the hemolytic uremic syndrome) or the syndrome of thrombotic thrombocytopenic purpura. Distinguishing these syndromes from preeclampsia or renal cortical necrosis in pregnancy-associated ARF may be difficult. ARF in the setting of pregnancy has a very guarded prognosis for renal recovery, perhaps because it may involve cortical necrosis (Kelleher and Berl, 1981).

Primary glomerular diseases most commonly associated with ARF are those caused by antiglomerular basement membrane (anti-GBM) antibody either with pulmonary hemorrhage (Goodpasture's syndrome) or without pulmonary hemorrhage, although other forms of primary glomerular disease, such as membranous glomerulopathy or membranoproliferative glomerulonephritis, may have accelerated courses (Schrier, 1992).

Of the primary tubulointerstitial diseases causing ARF, the most important is ATN. ATN may be caused by a variety of insults. Often, ATN cannot be ascribed to any one insult but develops with multiple potential etiologies (Rasmussen and Ibels, 1982). ATN as it was first described secondary to crush injuries followed a rather predictable course with a 10- to 14-day period of oliguria followed by a 10- to 14-day polyuric recovery phase (Swann and Merrill, 1953). It is now known that nonoliguric ATN is about as frequent as oliguric ATN, and both forms of ATN may follow variable courses. The mortality rate associated with oliguric ATN is 60% to 80%, in comparison with about 20% for nonoliguric ATN (Stott et al, 1972; Anderson and Schrier, 1992).

Renal ischemia is the most common predisposing cause for ATN. It can, in fact, result from any of the causes of prerenal azotemia, although some of these, such as congestive heart failure, rarely cause ATN on their own. Renal ischemia leading to ATN is most often related to prolonged hypotension or surgical interruption of renal blood flow, such as during aortic aneurysm resection or in the course of renal transplantation (Morris, 1986). Some drugs such as nonsteroidal anti-inflammatory agents (NSAIAs), angiotensin converting enzyme inhibitors (ACEIs), or cyclosporine may cause ARF by hemodynamic means, especially in settings of reduced renal perfusion pressure. In most cases, these drugs simply cause prerenal azotemia, but in some cases, they can cause frank ATN (Bennett and Pulliam, 1983; Bakris and Kern, 1989; Paller, 1990).

Nephrotoxic antibiotics, particularly the aminoglycosides, are common and important causes of ATN. Aminoglycoside-associated ATN is typically nonoliguric, usually develops after 5 to 7 days of therapy, and is most often seen in patients who have underlying chronic renal insufficiency, have had recent additional courses of aminoglycosides, and have had other renal insults, in particular ischemia (Appel, 1990).

Radiocontrast-induced ATN is also fairly common and is more likely to affect patients with chronic renal insufficiency, especially that resulting from diabetes or multiple myeloma, but in contrast to aminoglycoside nephrotoxicity, it is usually oliguric in nature (Schrier and Shapiro, 1985). Despite the associated oliguria, radiocontrast-induced nephropathy typically runs a short and benign course. Radiocontrast-induced nephrotoxicity is reversible in most cases, and severe renal failure necessitating dialysis is rare. Low-osmolality radiocontrast media (LOM) is safer than high-osmolality radiocontrast media, but the advantage is small and the costs are much higher. It may be reasonable to use LOM in patients with advanced renal insufficiency, especially diabetics. In these patients, a small additional decrement in GFR is more likely to present problems. The serum creatinine level at which LOM should be used has not been established.

Other drugs that may cause ATN include cisplatin (which typically also results in renal potassium and magnesium wasting and whose effects can persist for extremely long durations), amphotericin, and acyclovir. Drug intoxications, especially with acetaminophen or ethylene glycol, may precipitate ATN (Paller, 1990).

Acute interstitial nephritis (AIN) is a relatively uncommon but important cause of ARF. Classically caused by penicillin antibiotics, AIN can complicate therapy with a myriad of drugs; the most important of these are listed in Table 8–3. The classic form of AIN includes fever, eosinophilia, rash, and eosinophiluria. Reports suggest that in many cases, several if not all of these features may be absent, and in some cases biopsy is the only way to make the diagnosis (Neilson, 1989). In particular, NSAIAs may be associated with AIN in concert with heavy proteinuria but without associated fever, eosinophiluria, eosinophilia, or rash (Bakris and Kern, 1989; Porile et al, 1990).

Finding eosinophils in the urine of patients with AIN may be difficult. Nolan and colleagues demonstrated that the Hansel's stain is far superior to the more traditional Wright's stain in evaluating the urine for eosinophils. These investigators also pointed out that eosinophils in the urine may also be seen with other causes of renal failure, particularly with

Table 8–3. DRUGS COMMONLY ASSOCIATED WITH ACUTE INTERSTITIAL NEPHRITIS

Antibiotics
Penicillins*
Cephalosporins
Trimethoprim
Sulfa derivatives
Rifampicin
Acyclovir
Diuretics
Furosemide
Thiazides
Triamterene
Antihypertensives
Captopril
Alpha-methyldopa
Anticonvulsants
Phenytoin
Carbamazepine
Phenobarbital
Valproic acid
Nonsteroidal Anti-Inflammatory Agents†
Miscellaneous
Cimetidine
Allopurinol
Azathioprine
Penicillamine

*Most often seen with methicillin.

†Virtually all nonsteroidal anti-inflammatory agents have been reported to cause acute interstitial nephritis, but the association is strongest with fenoprofen use.

acute glomerulonephritis (Nolan et al, 1986; Nolan and Kelleher, 1988). Although gross and microscopic hematuria may be seen in AIN and acute glomerulonephritis, the presence of red blood cell casts strongly suggests the latter.

Acute pyelonephritis does not typically cause ARF. This is because most patients with this disease have unilateral involvement and a normally functioning contralateral kidney. However, in patients with a solitary native kidney or a transplanted kidney, acute pyelonephritis is a potential cause of ARF. In renal transplant patients, although the major differential diagnosis of ARF is cyclosporine nephrotoxicity, allograft rejection, and ischemic ARF, acute pyelonephritis occasionally causes ARF, with a presentation very similar to that of allograft rejection (Morris, 1986).

Postrenal Acute Renal Failure

Obstruction to the flow of urine may occur at any site, from microscopic obstruction to obstruction of tubular fluid flow to the urethra. The different causes of urinary obstruction are discussed in detail in other chapters in this textbook. However, it should be stressed that the diagnosis of obstruction should be considered in every patient presenting with ARF, especially patients with bland findings on urine microscopy and negative dipstick readings (Schrier and Conger, 1986).

Pathogenesis of Acute Tubular Necrosis

ATN is a major form of ARF. Awareness of the pathogenetic factors involved in its initiation and in maintenance and recovery are important in approaching its prevention and therapy.

The ischemic form of ATN has been best studied and is discussed primarily. **Reductions in GFR during ATN are due to vascular and tubular factors.** The vascular factors include reductions in glomerular perfusion pressure and decreases in the ultrafiltration coefficient of the glomerulus. Reductions in glomerular perfusion pressure might result either from decreases in renal plasma flow or, in the setting of decreased renal plasma flow, from dilatation of the efferent arteriole, as might be observed when an ACEI removes the efferent constrictive effects of angiotensin II. In most cases of ischemic ATN, reductions in renal perfusion pressure from decreased renal plasma flow is a factor in the initiation but not the maintenance of ARF. In experimental models as well as in patients, renal plasma flow increases toward normal 24 to 48 hours after the ischemic insult without functional recovery, and efforts to increase renal plasma flow with vasodilator in the postischemic period do not ameliorate the course of ARF. Thus maintenance factors in ischemic ATN are primarily tubular in origin (Levinsky, 1977).

Tubular factors may involve two separate processes: namely, backleak and tubular obstruction. Although it is clear that backleak may occur in some experimental models of ARF, tubular obstruction appears to be the most important maintenance factor in ATN. Sloughed brush border membranes, cellular debris, Tamm-Horsfall protein, and decreased filtration pressure may all contribute to tubular obstruction after an ischemic insult (Burke et al, 1980).

The mechanisms by which cytosolic or tissue Ca^{2+} increases in underperfused situations and how this increase may contribute to renal tubular injury are the focuses of much recent research. **Although 60% to 70% of all calcium in renal epithelial cells is located in the mitochondria, cytosolic-free ionized calcium is the most critical with regard to regulation of intracellular events. Cytosolic-free calcium is normally kept at about 100 nmol, which is 1/10,000th of the extracellular level (Weinberg, 1991).**

When exposed to anoxia in vitro, primary cultures of proximal and distal tubule cells exhibit cell death after reoxygenation. However, if Ca^{2+} is removed from the bathing medium during the first 2 hours of reoxygenation and then replaced, cell viability is greatly enhanced (Wilson and Schrier, 1986).

Thus at least a portion of cell damage that occurs during reoxygenation is Ca^{2+} dependent. The increased cellular Ca^{2+} could activate calmodulin or other second messenger–mediated events, thereby leading to cell damage. This seems plausible because drugs that are calmodulin antagonists, even in the presence of Ca^{2+} ions during the first 2 hours of reoxygenation, also delay cell death and preserve cell viability (Schwertslag et al, 1986).

Cytosolic-free Ca^{2+} in freshly isolated proximal tubules, as assessed with the dye fura-2, increases significantly after 2 minutes of hypoxia and continues to increase progressively thereafter. This increase in cytosolic-free Ca^{2+} precedes the release of lactate dehydrogenase or the uptake by nuclei of the membrane impermeable dye propidium iodide (Kribben et al, 1994). The reduction in propidium iodide staining and the reduced rate of lactate dehydrogenase (LDH) release observed when hypoxic rat proximal tubules are incubated either in a Ca^{2+}-free medium (Wetzels et al, 1993b) or with the intracellular Ca^{2+} chelator 1,22-Bis(2-aminophenoxy) ethane-N,N,N′,N′-tetraacetic acid (BAPTA) (Kribben et al, 1994), strongly support the hypothesis that a cause-and-effect relationship exists between elevations in cytosolic-free Ca^{2+} and the development of hypoxia-induced membrane damage. Furthermore, this early rise in cytosolic-free Ca^{2+} after 5 to 10 minutes of hypoxia is reversible, because return to a well-oxygenated medium results in a prompt (1-minute) return of cytosolic-free Ca^{2+} to baseline levels.

There is evidence that this rise in cytosolic-free calcium in proximal tubules activates the Ca^{2+}-dependent enzymes nitric oxide, calpain, and phospholipase A_2 (PLA_2), which mediate the hypoxic tubular injury. Nitric oxide (NO) synthase (NOS) activity is increased during hypoxia in freshly isolated rat proximal tubule. Membrane damage, as assessed by LDH release into the medium, is prevented by both an NOS inhibitor (nitro-L-arginine-methyl ester, L-NAME) and an NO scavenger (hemoglobin) (Yu et al, 1994). In addition, a further increase in hypoxic injury is observed when the NOS substrate L-arginine is added to the hypoxic tubule suspension (Yu et al, 1994). Hypoxia also stimulates prompt and sustained NO release in the proximal tubule suspension, as assessed by an NO-selective electrode (Yaqoob et al, in press). However, neither the specific isoform of NOS nor the mechanism of NO-mediated injury during hypoxia in proximal tubules has been elucidated. Immunoblotting tubular extracts with specific antibodies against the neuronal NOS (nNOS), endothelial NOS (eNOS), and the inducible NOS (iNOS) confirmed the presence of nNOS and eNOS but absence of iNOS. The results of this study suggest that both forms of constitutive NOS, nNOS and eNOS, are present in the proximal tubule (Yaqoob et al, 1995). The early hypoxia-induced NO rise and the demonstration of the Ca^{2+}-dependent constitutive form of NOS on immunoblotting is consistent with activation of constitutive NOS by an early cytosolic calcium rise during hypoxia.

Calpain is a Ca^{2+}-dependent cytosolic protease ubiquitously present in most tissues (Saido et al, 1994). Renal brush border membranes are rich in proteases (Scherberich et al, 1988), and calpain has been demonstrated in the proximal tubule in culture (Wilson and Hartz, 1991) and in both distal and collecting tubules in the rabbit (Hayashi et al, 1987). Calpain activity in isolated proximal tubules significantly increases during hypoxia. This increase in calpain activity occurs before cell membrane damage, which is thus suggestive of a cause-and-effect relationship. The cysteine protease inhibitor N-benzyloxycarbonyl-Val-Phe (N-Cbz-Val-Phe) methyl ester markedly decreases membrane injury and completely prevents the rise in calpain activity during hypoxia. The increase in calpain activity during hypoxia and the inhibitor studies with N-Cbz-Val-Phe methyl ester therefore suggest a role for calpain as a mediator of proximal tubular injury (Edelstein et al, 1995).

PLA_2 hydrolyzes the acyl bond at the sn-2 position of phospholipids to generate free fatty acids and lysophospholipids. Release of free fatty acids, which are believed to contribute to the hypoxic injury, have been shown in rat proximal tubules (Wetzels et al, 1993a). This release is thought to be mediated to a large extent by activation of intracellular PLA_2 during hypoxia (Choi et al, 1995). It has been shown that both the messenger RNA for PLA_2 and the PLA_2 enzyme activity are increased in hypoxic rabbit tubules (Portilla et al, 1992). PLA_2 may contribute to tubular injury as follows (Bonventre, 1993): (1) PLA_2-induced changes in phospholipid integrity and the toxic actions of free fatty acids and lysophospholipids may alter plasma membrane and mitochondrial membrane permeability. These products may themselves serve as intracellular second messengers or can be further metabolized as precursors in the production of specific proinflammatory lipid mediators, such as prostaglandins and leukotrienes. (2) Lipid peroxidation that occurs with ischemia and reperfusion causes an increase in the susceptibility of cellular membranes to PLA_2. (3) Arachidonic acid conversion to eicosanoids generates reactive oxygen species. Studies have shown the disappearance of a high-molecular-weight (~100 kD) Ca^{2+}-dependent form of PLA_2 during hypoxia, which coincides with the appearance of a low-molecular-weight (~15 kD) form with the same Ca^{2+} and substrate specificity (Choi et al, 1995). These data suggest the possibility that the high-molecular-weight form is converted to the low-molecular-weight form by a protease such as calpain that is activated during hypoxia. This provides further support that calcium-mediated cellular events, either alone or in combination, mediate hypoxic cellular injury.

Organ ischemia presents a dilemma in which the restoration of perfusion may add to the organ injury. Results of extensive current investigation clearly indicate that the development of organ dysfunction is ascribable to reperfusion. The importance of these findings is in their contribution to clinical features of ARF, myocardial infarction, and cerebral vascular accident and their implications concerning effects of flow diversion in surgical bypass and for function of transplanted kidneys, hearts, lungs, and other organs.

It is now clear that injury induced by ischemia-reperfusion leads to organ dysfunction, in part by direct injury of parenchymal cells. However, abundant evidence indicates a major role for intravascular neutrophil sequestration early in reperfusion with release of oxidants and other injurious substances. Thus it is not surprising that vascular dysfunction is an early and prominent aspect of ischemia-reperfusion injury with consequent impairment of blood flow and its regulation. Basal vascular tone is essential for perfusion of complex and distinct vascular beds. It is clear that both transmural pressure and shear stress from blood flow contribute to basal arterial vascular tone. The predominant effect of vessel wall pressure is to increase tone and that of flow is to reduce tone. The mechanisms mediating the tonal response to these physical forces are only partially understood. Ca^{2+} entry, at least in part through unique stretch-operated channels, is important in pressure-induced vasoconstriction. Transmembrane Na^+ concentrations are a factor in flow-related vasodilation. In addition, endothelial factors (NO, prostaglandins) are involved in flow-related vasodilation. Apart from its role in mediating shear-induced vasodilation, evidence indicates that endothelial-generated NO independently contributes to normal vascular tone. Other neurohumoral factors that contribute to changes in arterial tone dictated by metabolic demand are adenosine, O_2, and CO_2.

The ischemia-reperfusion process has effects on the arterial microvasculature. The early effects of ischemia on the vasculature involve platelets, endothelial cells, and smooth muscle cells (Lefer, 1987). Platelets undergo aggregation, adhesion, and release of agonists and procoagulant mediators, resulting in vasoconstriction and thrombosis. In endothelial cells and smooth muscle cells, there is progressive depletion of adenosine triphosphate (ATP). There is increased cellular lactate, increased cytosolic Ca^{2+}, and decreased membrane Na-K-ATPase activity. Membrane and cytosolic phospholipase A_2 activity is increased with return of oxygenated blood flow through the vasculature, and the ischemic insult is terminated.

However, a secondary series of noxious events that are the consequence of reperfusion ensues. Oxidizing radicals O_2^- and ^-OH may be generated during the respiratory burst of activated neutrophils (polymorphonuclear leukocytes [PMNs]) and from the endothelial cells subjected to ischemia-reperfusion. In endothelial cells, Ca^{2+}-dependent conversion of xanthene dehydrogenase to xanthine oxidase occurs, which generates O_2^- and H_2O_2 from hypoxanthine and available oxygen. Oxygen radicals attack lipid membranes, nucleic acid, proteins, and carbohydrates.

A host of other proteases, vasoactive agonists, and proinflammatory cytokines are also released after reperfusion, both from neutrophils attached to vessel walls and from endothelial cells. Because of its strategic anatomic position, the vascular endothelium is particularly vulnerable to toxin and ischemia-reperfusion injury. After ischemia-reperfusion, the endothelium itself produces proinflammatory substances, including endothelin 1 (ET-1), platelet activating factor (PAF), leukotriene B_4, and oxygen metabolites (Lefer and Lefer, 1993) while down-regulating production of protective substances, including adenosine, NO, and prostaglandin I_2

(PGI_2) (Engler and Gruber, 1991). There is early increased expression of leukocyte components (CD11/CD18, leukocyte adhesion molecule [LAM]–1, L-selectin) and endothelial components (intracellular adhesion molecule [ICAM]–1, P-selectin) of the adhesion molecule system, resulting in leukocyte (primarily neutrophil) adherence and subsequent release of additional proinflammatory mediators from both endothelial cells and neutrophils, including tumor necrosis factor, proteinases, O_2 metabolites, PAF, and other cytokines (Lefer and Lefer, 1993). These mediators cause endothelial detachment and basal lamina disruption and promote diapedesis of PMNs through the endothelium, where they cause injury to the underlying vessel wall cells. The endothelial cells undergo morphologic changes as a consequence of ischemia and ischemia-reperfusion.

There is also vascular dysfunction as a result of ischemia-reperfusion injury. The vascular element of interest is the small arterial resistance component of the circulation. **The kidney model that exemplifies ischemia-reperfusion injury is ischemically induced ARF. A severe form of this disorder, in which the renal artery is clamped for 40 to 70 minutes followed by immediate reflow, and a less severe form, in which high-dose norepinephrine (NE) is infused into the renal artery for 90 minutes with slow spontaneous return of blood flow, have been studied extensively in rats.** In the former model, there is a brief postocclusion hyperemia, then a sustained small reduction in renal blood flow and attenuated response to endothelium-dependent dilators (Lieberthal et al, 1989). In the first few hours after reflow in the latter model, there is a modest reduction in renal blood flow in comparison to the preischemia level without hyperemia, a decreased response to endothelium-dependent vasodilator, and a small but significant reduction in the constrictor response to the NOS inhibitor L-NAME (Conger et al, 1995).

There is partial endothelial cell detachment without ultrastructural changes in individual cells at 6 hours in both the renal artery clamp (RAC) and NE-ARF models. By 48 hours of reperfusion, the basal renal blood flow remains 20% reduced in the RAC-ARF model, and there is a reduced vasoreactive response to changes in renal perfusion pressure, to constrictor agonists, and to endothelium-dependent and endothelium-independent dilators (Conger et al, 1991). The predominant histologic finding at this time in the small resistance arteries and arterioles is smooth muscle cell necrosis present in 55% to 60% of the vessels (Matthys et al, 1983; Ueda et al, 1991). It is assumed that the lack of response to vasoactive stimuli is a result of the diffuse smooth muscle cell injury related to both the relative severity of ischemia and the rapidity of reperfusion.

In the NE-ARF model at 48 hours, the basal renal blood flow also is approximately 20% less than normal (Conger et al, 1991). However, vascular reactivity is strikingly different from that in the RAC-ARF model. The difference likely is a result of less severe ischemia and a slower rate of reperfusion. There is an exaggerated renal vasoconstrictor response to angiotensin II and ET-1 both in vivo and in arterioles isolated from these kidneys (Conger et al, 1991). Response to endothelium-dependent vasodilator is reduced, but the constrictor response to L-NAME is actually increased. cNOS can be identified as at least as strongly reactive, or more reactive, than normal as determined with cNOS monoclonal antibody in the resistance arterial vessels (Conger et al, 1995). Although there is a dilator response to cyclic adenosine monophosphate (cAMP)–dependent PGI_2 in the 48-hour postischemic renal vasculature, there is no increase in renal blood flow to the NO donor sodium nitroprusside. Taken together, these data indicate that 48 hours after ischemia in NE-ARF in the rat kidney, vascular cNOS activity is not diminished but, rather, is maximal so that it cannot be stimulated further by endothelium-dependent vasodilators. The available NO under basal conditions has fully activated smooth muscle cell soluble cyclic guanosine monophosphate (cGMP) so that there is no additional response to an exogenous NO donor.

It has been suggested, but not demonstrated, that the increase in NOS activity may be a "protective" response to an underlying vasoconstrictor stimulus that is the direct consequence of the ischemia-reperfusion injury. The nature of the constrictor stimulus is unknown but is not likely to be ET-1, thromboxane A_2, or angiotensin II, according to pharmacologic inhibition studies (Kelleher et al, 1984). However, the exaggerated constrictor response to NOS inhibition observed both in vivo and in vitro in 48-hour postischemic renal arterial vessels indicates that the constrictor stimulus is potent.

In examining the mechanism for the constrictor hypersensitivity in the 48-hour postischemic vasculature in NE-ARF, measurements of smooth muscle cell cytosolic calcium $[Ca^{2+}]_i$ have been made in the isolated arterioles from these kidneys perfused at physiologic pressures (Conger et al, 1993). In comparison with similar vessels from sham-ARF kidneys, there is a significantly higher baseline and an earlier and greater increase in smooth muscle cell $[Ca^{2+}]_i$ in response to a normal half-maximal constricting concentration (EC_{50}) of angiotensin II, which correlates with the initially lower and more intense reduction in lumen diameter in the postischemic ARF vessels. One week after ischemic injury, the endothelium appears normal and smooth muscle necrosis is less evident, but perivascular fibrosis is marked in the mid- to small-sized arterial vessels (Conger et al, 1991). Functionally, the response to endothelium-dependent dilators is reduced, L-NAME constrictor response is increased, and immunologically detectable NOS is present (Conger et al, 1995)—observations similar to those at 48 hours. By 30 days after the ischemia-reperfusion insult in NE-ARF, there is minimal residual fibrosis of the tunica adventitia; the remainder of the vascular morphology appears normal. The functional responses to constrictor and dilator agonists and to changes in pressure and flow have returned to near normal (Kelleher et al, 1984).

The course of human ischemically induced ARF is highly variable. An important and relevant observation regarding the variable duration and, in particular, the prolonged course in ARF patients was made by Solez and associates (1979). In individuals with ARF duration longer than 3 weeks, a prominent finding in biopsy or autopsy specimens was fresh tubular renal ischemic lesions that could not be related to the remote initial ischemic insult. A possible explanation for the fresh ischemic lesions was altered reactivity of the renal vasculature. Abnormal vascular reactivity in established ischemic ARF animal models includes loss of renal blood flow autoregulation. Modest arterial pressure reduction during the course of this disease, such as frequently occurs with hemodialysis treatment, could actually result in recurrent ischemic injury and prolongation of ARF (Conger, 1990).

Endogenous vasodilators are involved in the hemodynamic changes that occur during the initiation and maintenance of ARF. Exogenously administered vasodilators, with or without diuretics, are agents that have been used in the pharmacologic therapy of ARF. Not only are vasodilators of historic interest in pathogenesis and treatment, but they also continue to represent a major area of focus in investigative efforts in ARF.

The modulating vasodilator effect of prostaglandins in the setting of impending renal ischemia appears to be greater in afferent than efferent arterioles. When PGI_2 and prostaglandin E_2 (PGE_2) were administered exogenously during reduced renal perfusion, the filtration fraction increased with better preservation of GFR than of renal blood flow (Oliver et al, 1981), which suggests that vasodilator prostaglandins preferentially caused preglomerular vasorelaxation under these conditions. Prostaglandin synthesis was found to be increased in animal models of ischemic ARF (Oliver et al, 1981), aminoglycoside nephrotoxicity (Assael et al, 1985), sepsis, and endotoxic shock (Badr et al, 1986). **The indication that an increase in prostaglandin activity was renoprotective by maintaining glomerular hemodynamics was the observation that cyclooxygenase inhibitors in these disorders augmented the reduction in renal blood flow and GFR.** Other evidence of protection in ARF was the finding that infusion of biologic prostaglandins and their analogues in ischemic (Kaufman et al, 1987), mercuric chloride–induced (Papanicolaou et al, 1989), and glycerol-induced ARF (Werb et al, 1978) improved GFR and attenuated tubular necrosis. In all but one of the studies (Casey et al, 1980), the protective effect was observed only when prostaglandins were given before or during ARF induction. **A predisposing role of reduced intrinsic prostaglandin activity to the development of ARF has been considered by several investigators.** For example, low plasma or urine prostaglandin metabolites have been found in cyclosporine administration (Stahl et al, 1985), thrombotic thrombocytopenic purpura (Hensby et al, 1979), Henoch-Schönlein purpura (Turi et al, 1986b), hemolytic uremic syndrome (Turi et al, 1986a), and the HRS (Zipser et al, 1983). **It has been recognized that treatment with nonsteroidal anti-inflammatory drugs, an induced state of reduced cyclooxygenase activity, can precipitate ARF in settings of prerenal azotemia.**

In 1981, deBold et al reported the natriuretic effects of an extract of mammalian atrial myocytes, later called atrial natriuretic peptide (ANP). The most notable effects of ANP are on the kidney. **The natriuresis induced by ANP is associated with an increase in GFR. In addition, there are direct inhibitory effects of ANP on sodium and water reabsorption that appear to be confined to the distal nephron (Anand-Srivastava et al, 1986). Most, but not all, investigators have found that in vivo infusion of ANPs, both synthetic and naturally occurring from a variety of species, markedly increase GFR while having a proportionately smaller effect on renal blood flow (Huang et al, 1985).**

In the late 1980s, a series of reports that demonstrated a positive effect of ANPs on ischemic and nephrotoxic animal models of ARF began to appear (Nakamoto et al, 1987; Shaw et al, 1987). What was most intriguing about the use of ANP in animal models of ARF was that it was effective when given after the initiating insult. In fact, it attenuated the course of ARF when given as late as 2 days after the initiating ischemic event. These pharmacologic properties made ANP a potential agent to counteract two proposed pathophysiologic mechanisms of GFR reduction in ARF: reduced glomerular perfusion and tubular obstruction. A large (500-patient) clinical phase 3 multicenter study on the use of ANP in ARF showed that ANP did not reduce the need for dialysis in the broad nonoliguric and oliguric patient population or reduce mortality. **The study did, however, demonstrate that ANP significantly reduced the need for dialysis and increased 21-day survival in the oliguric subgroup of patients with ARF (Allgren, 1995).**

Calcium channel blockers, which inhibit voltage-gated calcium entry, have been used in a number of ARF models. Burke and colleagues (1984) found both a protective effect of verapamil (5 μg/kg/minute) or nifedipine (2 μg/kg/minute) when given before or after NE-induced ischemia in dogs. Calcium channel blockers can attenuate radiocontrast-induced ARF (Bakris and Burnett, 1985) and cadaveric kidney transplant dysfunction (Wagner et al, 1987).

In most experimental models of ischemic ATN, the major site of injury is the S3 segment of the proximal tubule—that is, the straight portion of the proximal tubule located primarily in the outer stripe of the outer medulla (Venkatachalam et al, 1978). However, it has been suggested that because renal ischemia is encountered clinically in the thick ascending limb of Henle, which normally lives on the edge of anoxia, that segment may be the segment at greatest risk (Brezis et al, 1984a). In experimental preparations, this segment can be shown to have transport-related injury, which Brezis and co-workers (1984b) believed may be operant in the development of clinical ischemic ATN. Morphologic abnormalities of ATN in humans, however, occur primarily in the proximal tubule rather than the thick ascending limb of Henle.

Approach to the Differential Diagnosis

As discussed, the differentiation among causes of ARF is a key step in the clinical management. This is accomplished primarily with a history and a physical examination, although laboratory evaluation, examination of the urine, and in some cases imaging studies and invasive hemodynamic measurements are necessary.

The history in ARF patients comes from the hospital chart as well as from the interview with the patient. A detailed history must include specific attention to possible hypotensive episodes, blood transfusions (especially with hemolytic reactions), intravenous radiocontrast media administered during radiographic studies, and all other medications received. The meticulous listing of medications is important, not only to detect possible direct renal toxins such as cisplatin or possible causes of AIN such as penicillin antibiotics, but also to determine whether any medications that are normally excreted by the kidney are being administered in a dosage inappropriate for the current level of renal function. In the intensive care unit (ICU) setting, it is quite common for a nephrology consultant to observe continued administration of magnesium-containing antacids, which may cause magnesium intoxication; administration of cimetidine or other H_2 blockers at full dose, which may result in central nervous system depression; or administration of nephrotoxic antibiotics such as aminoglycosides without appropriate dosage reduction.

The history is also useful in establishing how much weight the patient has gained or lost during the hospitalization or during the patient's experience outside the hospital. Rapid reductions in weight are most consistent with dehydration, whereas rapid increases in weight are seen with parenchymal ARF and urinary obstruction, as well as heart failure, liver failure, and cirrhosis.

The physical examination is extremely useful for evaluating the volume status of the patient. Evaluation of the neck veins to noninvasively estimate the central venous pressure, auscultation of the lungs and heart to evaluate for signs of heart failure, and evaluation of the extremities and presacral area for edema are all important in directing the physician to the cause of ARF. Cutaneous evidence for vasculitis or other rashes may also provide important clues. Evaluating the bladder size by suprapubic percussion after voiding may also provide an important clue to the cause of the ARF.

It cannot be overstated how important dipstick evaluation and microscopic examination of the urine are in the differential diagnosis of ARF. Prerenal azotemia is usually associated with concentrated urine, which has a relatively high specific gravity. Although some hyaline casts may be noted, few cellular components should be noted. Urinary obstruction may be associated with dilute or isotonic urine, which on microscopy either appears completely benign or may show white blood cells and/or red blood cells if infection or renal calculi are superimposed.

ATN is usually associated with isotonic urine. Microscopic examination shows tubular epithelial cells with coarsely granular casts (renal failure casts) and possibly tubular epithelial cell casts. AIN is usually accompanied by pyuria and white blood cell casts. White blood cell casts may also suggest acute pyelonephritis or acute glomerulonephritis. Acute glomerulonephritis typically is associated with high urine protein concentrations as well as red blood cell casts. In the setting of oliguria, however, high urine concentrations of protein are rather nonspecific and may be observed with other types of ARF (Schrier and Conger, 1986).

Blood tests may be of some help in the differential diagnosis of ARF. As discussed, marked eosinophilia should suggest the possibility of AIN but may also occur with the cholesterol emboli syndrome. Other types of leukocytosis should suggest infection, possibly pyelonephritis, but are relatively nonspecific. **Increases of blood urea nitrogen (BUN) out of proportion to increases in serum creatinine (SCr) so that the ratio of BUN to SCr > 20 suggests prerenal azotemia, urinary obstruction, or increased rates of catabolism, as seen with sepsis, with burns, and in patients receiving large doses of corticosteroids.** The evaluation of renal sodium handling through urine chemistry studies may be particularly helpful.

In some settings, clinical evaluation of volume status through history, physical examination, and laboratory tests (to be described) is simply not adequate for differentiating among adequate and inadequate left ventricular filling pressures. In these settings, typically encountered with patients with severe hepatic, pulmonary, or cardiac disease, invasive measurements of cardiac output and left ventricular end diastolic pressure are necessary for optimal clinical management.

Imaging modalities may be necessary in the differential diagnosis of ARF. In transplant patients, renal scans that measure renal perfusion may help differentiate between rejection, which is usually associated with early decreases in renal perfusion, and ATN or cyclosporine toxicity, both of which are accompanied by less severe decreases in renal blood flow. The HRS, with marked renal vasoconstriction, should also be associated with marked reductions in renal blood flow. These perfusion studies also may be extremely helpful in identifying acute renal arterial thrombosis or dissection. In nuclear studies that measure tubular secretion and GFR, all causes of ARF should produce delayed excretion of these radioactive compounds. However, urinary obstruction may be associated with a characteristic sustained increase in radioactive counts derived from the kidney, reflecting marked delays in collecting system transit. Gallium scans may detect inflammation present with AIN or allograft rejection; however, these changes are relatively nonspecific.

Renal ultrasonography has become extremely important in the evaluation of ARF. Dilatation of the collecting system is an extremely sensitive test for obstruction to urine flow. A 20% false-positive incidence has been reported secondary to extrarenal pelves. With bilateral small, shrunken kidneys or staghorn calculi, false-negative results may occur. With the use of Doppler techniques, ultrasonography may also measure renal blood flow in different vessels within the kidney. Because this test is noninvasive, it is a very reasonable screening test for ruling out urinary obstruction. Magnetic resonance imaging yields similar information as ultrasonography with better anatomic definition. However, its higher cost negates this potential advantage. Experimental data suggest that magnetic resonance spectroscopy with the P-31 nucleus may someday be useful in the differential diagnosis of ARF (Chan and Shapiro, 1987).

Radiocontrast studies such as intravenous pyelography are rarely useful in the setting of ARF and may further complicate the patient's condition with superimposed radiocontrast toxicity. For anatomic localization within the urinary tract, retrograde pyelography or antegrade pyelography from a percutaneous nephrostomy may be necessary for localizing the obstructing lesion.

Tests of Renal Sodium Handling

Our physiologic understanding of the different causes of ARF has led to the incorporation of tests of renal sodium handling into the clinical approach to ARF. With decreased perfusion pressure, the basic renal response is to reabsorb sodium and water avidly, in order to preserve intravascular volume. The effect of this avid sodium reabsorption is a low urine concentration of sodium. The effect of the avid water reabsorption is an increase in the urine osmolality and the concentration of urine creatinine. In contrast, with ATN, both tubular sodium and water reabsorption should be impaired. **The relative clearance of sodium to the clearance**

of creatinine—that is, the fractional excretion of sodium (FENa)—is calculated as follows:

$$\textbf{FENa} = (\textbf{UNa/PNa}) \times (\textbf{PCr/UCr}) \times 100$$
(expressed in %)

where UNa = urinary sodium, PNa = plasma sodium, PCr = plasma creatinine, and UCr = urinary creatinine.

The renal failure index (RFI), which actually was proposed earlier, is calculated in a similar manner, except that the PNa term is dropped and there is no multiplication by 100. In other words, RFI = UNa × (PCr/UCr) (Handa and Madin, 1967). The FENa and RFI are conceptually and quantitatively quite similar (Shapiro and Anderson, 1984).

Miller and colleagues (1978) observed that in patients with ARF, a low FENa or RFI (<1) predicted prerenal azotemia quite well, especially in patients with oliguria, whereas other causes of ARF, especially ATN, were associated with a higher FENa or RFI (>2). These tests are less useful in the setting of nonoliguria; however, a FENa or RFI of >2 is still suggestive of ATN, even when urine flow rates exceed 500 ml/day (Miller et al, 1978).

ATN secondary to radiocontrast or sepsis is typically associated with a low FENa and RFI, which suggests an important vascular component in its pathogenesis. Moreover, pigment nephropathy—that is, ATN caused by rhabdomyolysis or hemolysis—may also be associated with a low FENa and RFI. Also, patients with early acute urinary obstruction, acute glomerulonephritis, or transplant allograft rejection may have a low FENa and RFI (Shapiro and Anderson, 1984). Conversely, patients with marked elevations in serum bicarbonate and resultant bicarbonaturia may have a relatively high FENa or RFI in the setting of prerenal azotemia, because sodium ions accompany the bicarbonate in the urine as obligate cations. Anderson and co-workers (1984) found that a fractional excretion of chloride of less than 1 suggests prerenal azotemia in this setting.

Conservative Approach

The first approach to ARF is to diagnose its cause. Therapy is of course directed toward the cause of ARF. With regard to the entity of ATN, prevention is of course the best therapy. This may be accomplished by avoiding or minimizing insults that can cause ATN, as discussed earlier. Although more clinical work is needed in this area, there are already some data to support the use of osmotic diuretics and calcium channel blockers prophylactically to avoid ARF in the settings of some high-risk surgery, radiocontrast administration to high-risk individuals, and cadaveric renal transplantation (Old and Lehrener, 1980; Wagner et al, 1988).

In terms of therapy of established ATN, there is no proven therapy for improving renal function and/or shortening the course of ARF except the previously cited ANP study in oliguric ARF. Abel and co-workers (1973) reported that administration of "renal failure fluid," a combination of essential amino acids and dextrose, improved renal recovery and lessened the need for dialysis in patients with ARF. These results, although extremely provocative, have not been confirmed in subsequent trials (Leonard et al, 1975). Therefore, at present we cannot recommend aggressive hyperalimentation in the hope of improving renal recovery by nutritional mechanisms. Thus the therapy of ATN is directed at prophylaxis and treatment of the complications of ARF, which are summarized in Table 8–4.

Management of Fluid Disturbances

Patients with ATN may be oliguric. Such patients, if administered large volumes of intravenous fluids (as is typical for hyperalimentation regimens) or allowed free access to oral fluids, are at risk for developing fluid overload. There are currently data to support the use of high doses of loop diuretics (1 to 3 g/day) in order to convert oliguric to nonoliguric ATN in some patients (Cantarovich et al, 1970, 1971; Bailey et al, 1973). It appears that patients who respond to such therapy have a lower FENa than patients who do not respond, which suggests that responders have less severe tubular injury (Anderson et al, 1977).

Dopamine is widely used in the ICU to increase renal blood flow. At doses of 0.5 to 2 μg/kg/minute, dopamine produces vasodilatation through action on dopamine-1 recep-

Table 8–4. COMPLICATIONS OF ACUTE RENAL FAILURE

Fluid Overload
Hypertension
Edema
Acute pulmonary edema
Electrolyte Disturbances
Hyponatremia
Hyperkalemia
Hypermagnesemia
Hyperphosphatemia
Hypocalcemia
Hypercalcemia (postrhabdomyolysis)
Hyperuricemia
Metabolic Acidosis
Uremic Signs and Symptoms
Gastrointestinal
Nausea
Vomiting
Upper gastrointestinal bleeding
Neurologic
Mental status changes
Encephalopathy
Coma
Seizures
Peripheral neuropathy
Cardiac
Pericarditis
Uremic cardiomyopathy
Pulmonary
Pleuritis
Uremic pneumonitis
Hematologic
Bleeding
Anemia
Immunologic
Impaired granulocyte function
Impaired lymphocyte function

tors (Anderson et al, 1984). At doses of 3 to 5 μg/kg/minute, dopamine increases cardiac output. The diuresis and natriuresis seen after dopamine therapy are also known to result from a direct renal tubular effect on sodium and water excretion (Duke and Bernsten, 1994). Higher doses (>5 μg/kg/minute) induce vasoconstriction. Dopamine, when given to patients with stable renal function, increases GFR and effective renal plasma flow (Vendegna and Anderson, 1994). However, a study in critically ill patients showed that low-dose dopamine increased urine output but had little effect on creatinine clearance. In contrast, dobutamine had little effect on urine output but improved creatinine clearance, possibly because of increased cardiac output and mean arterial pressure (Duke et al, 1994). It is clear that dopamine increases urine output in the ICU setting (Flancbaum et al, 1994). Because patients with a reasonable urine output have fewer problems with hyperkalemia and volume overload and are therefore less likely to require dialysis therapy, early use of dopamine may be beneficial in ICU patients who remain oliguric despite restoration of circulating blood volume and exclusion of obstructive uropathy. It has not been established that conversion of the ARF patient from an oliguric to a nonoliguric state decreases mortality or hastens renal recovery. Duke and Bersten (1994)) questioned the routine use of dopamine in the setting of renal dysfunction in the critically ill patient. Further studies need to be done to determine whether dopamine is beneficial in early oliguric states.

Patients who remain oliguric after such therapy either should have their fluids limited to insensible losses and/or titrated to maintain an appropriate left ventricular filling pressure or must have early institution of nonconservative therapy (see following discussion).

If fluid overload presents an acute emergency, it must be remembered that nonconservative therapy such as dialysis requires some finite time to be initiated. It should be stressed that valuable time may be gained by the administration of oxygen, venodilators such as nitroglycerin, and arterial vasodilators to control hypertension. While such nonconservative therapy is being implemented, loop diuretics may provide transient benefit by dilating veins and thus decreasing cardiac preload and pulmonary congestion.

Fluid intake must be carefully monitored in patients with ARF, either oliguric or nonoliguric. Attempts should be made to maintain a euvolemic state by restricting total fluids to no more than urine output plus insensible losses. If invasive monitoring is being used, the pulmonary capillary wedge pressure is the best guideline for volume status; however, it may be normal in states of noncardiogenic cardiac edema.

Management of Electrolyte Disturbances

Patients with ARF, especially secondary to ATN, are prone to developing electrolyte abnormalities such as acidosis, hyperkalemia, hypermagnesemia, hyperphosphatemia, and hypocalcemia. To some degree, these problems can be minimized by the prophylactic institution of a low-potassium, low-protein diet accompanied by a fluid restriction and oral phosphate binders. Despite these precautions, electrolyte disturbances, especially in patients with oliguric ARF, are quite possible. These abnormalities are discussed in some detail later. However, although refractory electrolyte disturbances, like refractory fluid overload, are indications for nonconservative therapy of ARF, the conservative maneuvers must not be overlooked. Even after it is decided to provide nonconservative therapy, these conservative maneuvers may provide valuable time and, in fact, may be lifesaving while nonconservative therapy for these abnormalities is pending.

Hyperkalemia is probably the most common and most dangerous electrolyte abnormality seen with ARF. A serum potassium value over 6.0 mEq/L is an indication for performing an electrocardiogram (ECG), and subsequent therapy should be based on the ECG changes. With hyperkalemia, the earliest changes on the ECG consist of peaking of the T waves. This is followed by diminishment in the amplitude of the P wave, various conduction disturbances, and finally widening of the QRS complex. In severe hyperkalemia, the ECG tracing may resemble a sign wave.

We believe that any of these ECG alterations with hyperkalemia should provoke some form of intravenous therapy. Calcium, administered as the chloride or gluconate salt, ameliorates the effects of hyperkalemia on the cardiac electrical potential and provides valuable time for methods of potassium removal, such as hemodialysis, to be employed. In general, 1 ampule of calcium chloride or 2 ampules of calcium gluconate (9.6 mEq of calcium) is administered in this setting and has immediate effects. This therapy does not alter the serum potassium concentration and is effective for only 20 to 30 minutes.

Intravenous insulin, administered with glucose to avoid hypoglycemia, causes a shift of potassium from the extracellular to intracellular compartment. Alkalinization with bicarbonate also causes such a shift. These approaches have a rapid onset of action but are effective only for a relatively short time. Repeated doses of bicarbonate, as either boluses or an infusion, are accompanied by volume expansion, which may lead to fluid overload. Also, respiratory compensation for metabolic alkalosis may limit the effectiveness of bicarbonate therapy. Bicarbonate is therefore recommended only as an acute intervention to gain time. In contrast, an insulin infusion will continue to shift potassium into cells and may be useful over a prolonged period of time.

Administration of potassium binding resins such as sodium polystyrene sulfonate (Kayexalate) work by removing potassium from the body. This approach may remove a considerable amount of potassium, but it takes several hours to work. It is therefore not adequate alone for treating acute hyperkalemia accompanied by ECG changes. In this setting, emergent therapy with intravenous calcium and/or insulin and bicarbonate is appropriate. Hyperkalemia is a medical emergency, and although hyperkalemia may eventually mandate nonconservative therapy of ARF, every physician must know how to evaluate and treat this entity while such therapy is being considered.

Hyperphosphatemia almost always accompanies ARF. Although some experimental data suggest that it may worsen the course of ARF, this issue is controversial. Hyperphosphatemia is usually treated with oral phosphate binders, especially because clearance of phosphate with hemodialysis or peritoneal dialysis is limited. Extremely severe hyperphosphatemia may in rare instances be accompanied by symptomatic hypocalcemia and, as such, must be considered an indication for hemodialysis. Less severe hypocalcemia is usually best treated by oral phosphate binders, which control the serum phosphate. Magnesium-containing antacids or cathartics should be avoided in ARF to avoid the risk of dangerous hypermagnesemia.

Acidosis attributable to ARF does not generally constitute an emergency, because in general it is relatively slow to develop and is accompanied by respiratory compensation. However, it is possible that acidosis results from another disturbance, such as lactic acidosis secondary to circulatory insufficiency, and in the setting of ARF may rapidly become very severe. This is a very difficult therapeutic situation. The acute infusion of sodium bicarbonate in the setting of lactic acidosis may, in fact, be deleterious to hemodynamic stability and is currently extremely controversial (Stacpoole, 1986; Narrins and Cohen, 1987). Even if one elects to administer bicarbonate, it is possible that it will be difficult to administer sufficient bicarbonate for correction of the acidosis without causing volume overload. Complicating this issue is that nonconservative therapy such as hemodialysis may be extremely difficult to institute because of circulatory instability. Continuous renal replacement therapy, such as arteriovenous hemofiltration (CAVH) or venovenous hemofiltration (CVVH), may be the best therapeutic intervention in this setting (Maguire and Anderson, 1986). When acidosis develops at a slower pace, it may be treated conservatively with oral or slow intravenous infusions of sodium bicarbonate, or it may be addressed by institution of nonconservative therapy.

Nonconservative Approach

Conservative therapy is often inadequate for the management of ARF caused by ATN. Indications for nonconservative therapy are fluid and electrolyte disturbances refractory to conservative management and the development of uremic signs and symptoms. Nausea and vomiting, mental status changes, a bleeding tendency, and decreased ability to defend against infection are characteristic of ARF. **Less commonly, pleural effusion, uremic pneumonitis, pericarditis (symptoms of pericarditis, development of a pericardial effusion, or an asymptomatic friction rub), and uremic seizures occur as complications of ARF.** Uremia is discussed in greater detail in the section of this chapter devoted to chronic renal failure.

In addition to these clear indications, it has become a standard of care to provide nonconservative therapy to maintain the BUN under 100 mg/dl and/or the SCr under 10 mg/dl. The choice of nonconservative therapy is predicated on the physician's experience and the center's experience as much as by the relative advantages and disadvantages of the treatment modalities available. These aspects must be considered in the implementation of nonconservative treatment of uremia.

Basically, nonconservative therapies for ARF are limited to hemodialysis, peritoneal dialysis, and the relatively new techniques of continuous renal replacement therapy. Continuous renal replacement therapies include slow continuous ultrafiltration, CAVH, CVVH, continuous arteriovenous hemodialysis, continuous venovenous hemodialysis, continuous arteriovenous hemodiafiltration, and continuous venovenous hemodiafiltration. We discuss the relative merits and disadvantages of these techniques in the next section (Table 8–5).

Hemodialysis, Peritoneal Dialysis, and Continuous Arteriovenous Hemofiltration

The most widely employed method for treating ARF is hemodialysis. In this technique, blood is removed from the patient by a blood pump and sent to a dialyzer (i.e., artificial kidney), where it comes into close proximity with dialysate, separated by a semipermeable membrane. It is this contact with the dialysate that allows the removal of solutes by the process of diffusion driven by a concentration gradient from blood to dialysate. Fluid and some solute may also be removed by the process of ultrafiltration driven by a pressure gradient across the dialyzer. The dialyzed blood is then returned to the patient.

To perform this procedure, access to the circulation is essential. Most commonly, a venous catheter is placed percutaneously into the subclavian or internal jugular vein, although occasional femoral venous catheterization and, in rare cases, placement of a Scribner shunt are performed. Hemodialysis allows for more rapid removal of fluid and solutes than does peritoneal dialysis or CAVH.

Hemodialysis treatments are quite stressful hemodynamically and may be complicated by hypotension, hypoxia, bleeding related to the anticoagulant administered (usually heparin), and dialysis disequilibrium with its manifestations ranging from cramps and headache to seizures and coma. Although controversial, it is quite possible that recurrent hypotension suffered during the dialysis treatment for ARF may actually prolong the course of this disease. Clinical studies are under way to test this hypothesis. An additional drawback of hemodialysis is the expense of the procedure, in relation to the special equipment necessary as well as to the trained personnel required to perform the treatment (Schetz et al, 1989).

In general, hemodialysis treatments are instituted for the indications discussed earlier and then continued until evidence of renal recovery is apparent. In a small prospective study, it was not possible to show that intensive daily dialysis treatment is superior to more conservative every other day treatments (Conger, 1975). The dialysis prescription is generally tailored to maintain the BUN under 100 mg/dl, keeping the electrolyte, acid-base, and volume statuses of the patient under control, and preventing uremic symptoms and signs (Schrier and Conger, 1986).

Peritoneal dialysis allows the removal of solutes by using the peritoneal membrane as a dialyzer. It does not require access to the circulation and, in general, is hemodynamically less stressful than hemodialysis. With this approach, dialysate is instilled into the peritoneal space via a catheter that is percutaneously placed, allowed to dwell for a period of time, and then removed, taking with it uremic solutes removed by diffusion across the peritoneal membrane. Ultrafiltration of fluid is performed by using an osmotic pressure gradient induced by the addition of relatively high concentrations of glucose to the dialysate. For noncatabolic patients, peritoneal dialysis allows the physi-

Table 8–5. NONCONSERVATIVE APPROACHES TO ACUTE RENAL FAILURE

Modality	Advantages	Disadvantages
Intermittent		
Hemodialysis	Rapid correction of fluid and electrolyte abnormalities	Expensive and hemodynamically stressful Anticoagulation necessary Vascular access necessary
Continuous		
Peritoneal dialysis	Inexpensive and hemodynamically well tolerated No anticoagulation or vascular access needed	Relatively slow correction of fluid and electrolyte disturbances May have associated leaks and infection
CAVH/CAVHD/CVVH/CVVHD	Intermediate expense Continuous progressive removal of fluid with less hemodynamic stress Allows unlimited nutrition because of excellent fluid removal	Continuous anticoagulation Less rapid correction of electrolyte abnormalities Limits patient mobility Requires intensive care setting
CAVH/CAVHD	No blood pump	Requires arterial vascular access
CVVH/CVVHD	Only venous access needed	Pump-driven circulation

CAVH, continuous arteriovenous hemofiltration; CAVHD, continuous arteriovenous hemofiltration and hemodialysis; CVVH, continuous venovenous hemofiltration; CVVHD, continuous venovenous hemofiltration and dialysis.

cian to maintain fluid and electrolyte homeostasis as well as prevent uremic symptoms and signs.

The peritoneal dialysis method offers relatively slower correction of electrolyte imbalance or fluid overload than does hemodialysis. Therefore, it is best utilized before indications for dialysis are urgent. Although safe and generally well tolerated, the procedure may be complicated by peritonitis, leaking of peritoneal dialysate, and occasionally hydrothorax. In general, it is best avoided after recent abdominal surgery. The major advantages of peritoneal dialysis are its relative inexpensiveness, the absence of need for anticoagulation, and the absence of major hemodynamic stress. Disadvantages of this method are related to the relatively slow correction of fluid and electrolyte disturbances (Nolph, 1978).

Continuous renal replacement therapy was first reported by Kramer and co-workers in 1977. This technique utilizes the patient's own blood pressure (venous or arterial) to send blood to a hemofilter, where fluids and solutes are removed by ultrafiltration. Blood then returns to the patient, accompanied by replacement fluid. Ultrafiltration rates of 10 to 12 ml/minute are achievable with this technique. Perhaps more efficient is the administration of dialysate through the filter to enhance solute clearance, thus allowing dialysis to occur with ultrafiltration. This is called *continuous hemodialysis* and *continuous hemodiafiltration*. If adequate arterial access is not available, the external blood pumps used in standard hemodialysis machines can provide the driving force and permit venovenous access for blood delivery to the filter.

Continuous renal replacement therapies have some potential advantages over hemodialysis in that hemodynamic stability is quite good and expensive equipment and trained hemodialysis technicians are not necessary. It is superior to peritoneal dialysis in the volume-overloaded patient in that fluid may be more rapidly removed. The major disadvantages of this technique are that arterial access is necessary and anticoagulation must be continuous (Maguire and Anderson, 1986).

Patients who are hemodynamically unstable, such as those with sepsis, are particularly susceptible to hypotensive episodes. Hemodialysis is a less desirable modality of renal replacement therapy in this group of patients. Continuous renal replacement therapy is popular among nephrologists as a treatment of ARF in patients with hemodynamic instability, such as those with sepsis and multiorgan failure. The choice of modality of continuous renal replacement therapy depends on a variety of factors, including clinical status, availability, the expertise of the clinician, and the desired rapidity of correction of fluid and electrolyte abnormalities. It is hoped that continuous renal replacement therapy will lead to an improvement in patient outcome. There is indirect evidence of that possibility: For example, the mortality rate of critically ill patients with ARF who require mechanical ventilation is close to 100%, as shown in some studies; in comparison, preliminary findings in similarly ill patients managed with continuous renal replacement therapy have shown a better survival rate (Mehta, 1994). Larger prospective clinical studies are, however, needed to answer the question of whether continuous renal replacement therapy has a positive impact on the outcome of patients with ARF.

Other Complications

Despite continued improvements in nonconservative therapy of ARF, the mortality rate remains extremely high. Because of the availability of dialysis and its alternatives as well as awareness of electrolyte, fluid disturbances, and uremic symptoms, patients generally die with, rather than of, ARF. Renal failure is associated with impairments of immune responses and granulocyte function; these factors may contribute to the increased incidence of infections in ARF patients. Hemorrhage secondary to bleeding disturbances also occurs with ARF and may be related to accumulation of nitrogenous wastes such as phenols and guanidosuccinic acid, but it is best correlated with a deficiency of von Willebrand factor multimers. When dialysis does not adequately correct an abnormal bleeding time, 1-desamino-8-D-arginine vasopressin (DDAVP), which causes the release of these von Willebrand factor multimers from endothelial cells, can be administered; infusion of cryoprecipitate that contains these multimers may be useful to acutely correct the bleeding time. If more prolonged therapy directed at a bleeding tendency is necessary, administration of conjugated estrogens appears to increase the synthesis and release of these multimers. Renal failure is associated with impaired immune responses and granulocyte function; these factors may contribute to the increased incidence of infections in ARF patients. The predominant cause of death in patients with ARF is infection. Thus despite the availability of dialytic therapy, ARF is still an extremely adverse condition, and all possible efforts to avoid ARF should be made (Schrier and Conger, 1986).

CHRONIC RENAL FAILURE

Definition and Clinical Description

In a manner analogous to ARF, chronic renal failure (CRF) can be considered a chronic deterioration in renal functions that results in a buildup of nitrogenous wastes in the plasma and/or a failure of the kidney to regulate extracellular fluid volume or composition. CRF is differentiated from ARF chiefly in the time that it takes to develop but also in its generally irreversible and, in fact, generally progressive nature.

CRF develops insidiously, and the onset of symptoms occurs only when the GFR is 30% of normal. Patients often do not know they have CRF until blood assays of BUN and serum creatinine are obtained, either as part of a routine chemical screen or as indicated by complaints of fatigue, sleep disturbances, nausea and vomiting, or pruritus. Proteinuria or microscopic evidence of blood in the urine, however, usually precedes development of CRF from most causes. The urinalysis remains an important screening test for patients during periodic health evaluations. The presence of urinary abnormalities, anemia, and hypertension, especially with left ventricular hypertrophy, should alert the clinician to a diagnosis of CRF. The military as well as insurance companies certainly appreciate the relevance of proteinuria to subsequent morbidity and mortality.

Etiologies

CRF may result from diseases involving the blood supply to the kidney, the urinary collecting system, and the parenchyma of the kidney. The most important of these diseases are reviewed in the following discussion.

Parenchymal Renal Diseases

Parenchymal causes of CRF can best be understood on the basis of their pathologic features. **Our ability to accurately assign a pathologic diagnosis has, in fact, dramatically improved since the mid-1970s with the widespread availability of electron microscopy and immunofluorescence methods to complement standard light microscopy. Renal diseases are often classified on the basis of the histologic characteristics.** However, it must be stressed that this morphologic approach may, in fact, lump a number of pathogenetic processes together if the appearances of the tissue reactions to these processes are similar.

Glomerular Versus Tubulointerstitial Renal Disease

It is useful to separate parenchymal diseases of the kidney into those that affect primarily the glomeruli and those that involve primarily the tubulointerstitial area of the kidney. The pathologic processes affect both glomeruli and tubules. The amount of tubulointerstitial disease observed histologically correlates better with functional derangements (i.e., decreased GFR) of the kidney than does the extent of pathologic glomerular change.

Besides pathologic examination, the causes of CRF may often be separated into glomerular and tubulointerstitial on the basis of the degree of proteinuria. In general, proteinuria exceeding 3.5 g/day (normalized per 1.73 m^2 body surface area) suggests glomerular disease, whereas more modest degrees of proteinuria (i.e., 1 to 2 g/day) suggests tubulointerstitial diseases. Unfortunately, many milder cases of glomerular disease are accompanied by modest degrees of proteinuria, and some forms of tubulointerstitial disease may be accompanied by considerable degrees of proteinuria, particularly when complicated by glomerulosclerosis. In patients who are not candidates for renal biopsy, however, this approach to classification may be useful.

Primary Renal Diseases

Primary renal diseases that cause CRF may be separated into glomerular and tubulointerstitial, as discussed previously. These diseases are summarized in Table 8–6. These histologic appearances may also be associated with systemic diseases involving the kidney.

Minimal change disease, also called nil disease, is a

Table 8–6. MAJOR PRIMARY RENAL DISEASES THAT CAN CAUSE CHRONIC RENAL FAILURE

Classification	Progression to Chronic Renal Failure
Glomerular	
Nil disease (minimal change disease)	Rare
Focal segmental glomerulosclerosis	Very common
Membranous glomerulopathy	Variable
Berger's disease	Uncommon
Poststreptococcal glomerulonephritis	Rare
Membranoproliferative glomerulonephritis	Common
Rapidly progressive glomerulonephritis	Very common
Chronic glomerulonephritis	Very common
HIV-associated nephropathy	Very common
Tubulointerstitial	
Autosomal dominant polycystic kidney	Very common
Juvenile polycystic kidney	Common
Medullary cystic disease	Rare
Reflux nephropathy	Variable
Analgesic nephropathy	Variable

HIV, human immunodeficiency virus.

common cause of nephrotic syndrome. It most often affects children, although it has been reported in virtually all age groups. It most commonly manifests as the nephrotic syndrome with massive proteinuria and anasarca. Hypertension is usually absent. Microscopic examination of the urine may demonstrate fat but generally not red or white blood cells. Histologic evaluation reveals essentially no changes on light microscopy or immunofluorescence and only epithelial foot process fusion on electron microscopy. The pathogenesis of nil disease is unknown, although alterations in cell-mediated immunity are believed to play a role. Nil disease frequently undergoes spontaneous remission and is also usually responsive to corticosteroid therapy. This disease almost never progresses to CRF (Glassock and Babcock, 1990). When progression to CRF does occur, it is likely that the disease process was actually focal and was segmental glomerulosclerosis rather than nil disease.

Focal and segmental glomerulosclerosis (FSGS) is also a common form of nephrotic syndrome and, in contrast to nil disease, often progresses to CRF. Typically, this disease affects older children and young adults, although it can occur at any age. Affected patients are typically nephrotic and may also be hypertensive. This histologic entity of FSGS has been associated with abuse of intravenous drugs as well as with acquired immunodeficiency syndrome (AIDS). The pathologic evaluation of biopsies from afflicted patients generally demonstrates focal and segmental scarring of glomeruli on light microscopy and electron microscopy. Immunofluorescence may show IgM, IgG, and complement as well as fibrin in these scars. The pathogenesis of this disease is also poorly understood, although it is probably safe to say that it is not caused by immune complexes.

In animal models of CRF, reductions of renal mass may lead to this histologic appearance. On the basis of research with these models, a hemodynamic cause of this entity—specifically, increases in glomerular capillary hydrostatic pressure—has been proposed (Brenner et al, 1982, 1986). There is currently no effective therapy for this disease, although it appears rational to treat any associated hypertension aggressively.

Membranous glomerulonephritis (MGN) also usually manifests with the nephrotic syndrome. MGN affects mainly adults in middle age but can occur at any age. Microscopic examination of the urine may show fat but often also demonstrates microscopic hematuria. In general, this disease either undergoes spontaneous remission or progresses to end-stage renal disease (ESRD). Massive proteinuria, presence of hypertension, impaired renal function on presentation, and male sex are all poor prognostic factors. The pathogenesis of this disease is believed related to in situ formation of immune complexes. MGN may be idiopathic or secondary to an underlying disease process. Secondary causes include malignancies (lung, esophagus, stomach, breast, colon, renal cell carcinoma), infections (hepatitis B, secondary syphilis), drugs (gold, penicillamine), and systemic lupus erythematosus.

Research with animal models has demonstrated the importance of complement and leukocytes in the expression of this disease. On light microscopy, glomeruli are noted to have widened glomerular capillary loops without increased numbers of glomerular cells. On electron microscopy, dense deposits are observed in an epimembranous position—that is, on the epithelial side of the basement membrane. Reaction to these deposits involving synthesis of new basement membrane adjacent to these deposits (spiking) or encircling these deposits may be noted. With special light microscopy stains (e.g., silver or trichrome), these deposits and the basement membrane reaction can be detected. Immunofluorescence demonstrates immunoglobulin G (IgG) and complement staining in capillary loops in a "lumpy bumpy" pattern. Treatment of idiopathic MGN with corticosteroids may be efficacious, although this issue is currently debated (Glassock and Babcock, 1990). If MGN follows an aggressive course, a trial of treatment with corticosteroids is worthwhile (Cameron, 1992a). An approach utilizing alternate months of corticosteroids and chlorambucil has also been advocated (Ponticelli et al, 1984). In secondary MGN, treatment of the underlying disease, such as resection of tumor or stopping the responsible medication, can result in resolution of the MGN.

Focal proliferative glomerulonephritis features microscopic hematuria or recurrent episodes of gross hematuria. Urinalysis may demonstrate the presence of red blood cells and red blood cell casts. Typically, this disease affects older children and adolescents. On light microscopy, focal proliferative glomerulonephritis is characterized by predominantly mesangial proliferation and expansion. On immunofluorescence, there are generally deposits of IgG, IgM, and/or IgA and complement within the mesangium.

If the deposits are primarily IgA, the disease is called Berger's disease or IgA nephropathy. **Berger's disease is thought to be the commonest form of glomerulonephritis in the world, at least in developed countries, where post-infectious glomerulonephritis is uncommon.** Berger's disease is closely related to the systemic vasculitis Henoch-Schönlein purpura, which is discussed later. Electron microscopic analysis generally demonstrates electron-dense deposits within the mesangium. Marked proteinuria, hypertension, and renal insufficiency are ominous signs. If these features are absent, progression to CRF is uncommon. No known therapy definitely affects the natural history of this disease. In extremely progressive cases, immunosuppression with corticosteroids and/or cytotoxic agents may be considered, although their efficacy is unproven. Some authors believe that anticoagulation may be beneficial, but, again, this is also unproven (Glassock and Babcock, 1990).

Acute glomerulonephritis is a clinical diagnosis based on clinical features and urinary sediment findings. Patients present with dark urine, oliguria, hypertension, and other evidence of circulatory overload, including edema in the legs and periorbital regions and sometimes pulmonary edema. Urinalysis by dipstick is positive for hemoglobin and protein and, on microscopy, for red blood cells and red blood cell casts, as well as for white blood cells and occasionally white blood cell casts. Elevations in serum creatinine levels generally are part of the initial presentation.

Diffuse proliferative glomerulonephritis (DPGN) is the typical histologic appearance of renal disease that presents with the acute nephritic syndrome. There is commonly a reduction in the serum level of the complement component 3 (C3). The best characterized cause of acute glomerulonephritis is a reaction to nephritogenic group A streptococci; hence its synonym, poststreptococcal glomerulonephritis. DPGN usually occurs 2 to 4 weeks after skin infection with nephritogenic streptococci. On examination of biopsy material in the acute phase, light microscopy demonstrates swollen, congested glomeruli with proliferation and exudation. Cellular crescents may be present and, if extensive, may confer a more guarded prognosis. On immunofluorescence, a "lumpy bumpy" distribution of IgM, IgG, and C3 is noted. In the acute stages, electron microscopy demonstrates massive subepithelial deposits called "humps" composed of electron-dense material. During recovery, these deposits are eliminated, and any deposits tend to be mesangial in location. DPGN may also be secondary to other infectious agents: bacterial (e.g., *Staphylococcus aureus*), viral, fungal, and protozoal; hence the term *postinfectious glomerulonephritis* is sometimes used.

There is no known therapy for DPGN. However, when DPGN presents as a rapidly progressive glomerulonephritis with epithelial crescents in more than 70% of the glomeruli on renal biopsy, treatment with steroids and immunosuppressive agents is indicated. DPGN was previously thought not to progress to CRF, and this may indeed be the case in subclinical, epidemic cases of DPGN in children. However, in the elderly and in sporadic cases, it may progress to end-stage CRF (Edelstein and Bates, 1992).

Membranoproliferative glomerulonephritis (MPGN) occurs most commonly in children but can occur at any age. Patients present with a mixture of nephritic and nephrotic symptoms. This disease is really two entities: MPGN type I, which is believed to be an immune complex disease, and MPGN type II, also called dense deposit disease, which is not believed to be caused by immune complex deposition. Both type I and type II MPGN are associated with reductions in the serum level of C3 as well as in total complement levels. In type I, there are usually parallel reductions in complement component 4 (C4), but in type II, C4 levels are usually normal. In patients with type II MPGN, evidence for alternate complement pathway activation is present. Both type I and type II gradually but inexorably progress to CRF in most patients.

On light microscopy, both type I and type II MPGN have expansion of the mesangium, endocapillary and mesangial proliferation, and compression of capillary loops. Characteristically, deposition of new basement membrane material occurs around interpolating mesangial cells and mesangium, creating a "tram track" appearance on silver stain. On immunofluorescence with type I, deposits that stain for IgG and complement are noted in a mesangial and subendothelial location and rarely in subepithelial and intramembranous locations. This latter appearance is called type III MPGN by some workers, although it is almost certainly a variant of typical type I MPGN. Immunofluorescence shows negative results for type II disease. With type I MPGN, electron microscopy demonstrates the immune complexes noted on immunofluorescence. With type II, electron-dense deposits in the basement membrane of both glomeruli and tubules are noted. Although immunosuppression is of doubtful efficacy for MPGN, antiplatelet agents may be effective for these diseases.

Rapidly progressive glomerulonephritis is another clinical syndrome characterized by a similar manifestation as acute glomerulonephritis but with progressive worsening of renal function. Physicians should suspect this diagnosis in acute glomerulonephritis patients presenting with either increased BUN or serum creatinine and especially when these parameters of renal function worsen progressively over a period of weeks. Early diagnosis is crucial because early treatment with corticosteroids and cytotoxic agents may prevent the progression to CRF.

The pathophysiology of this syndrome may be secondary to vasculitis (to be discussed) but is also seen with anti-GBM antibody formation and forms of glomerulonephritis, such as DPGN. When associated with pulmonary hemorrhage, anti-GBM antibody disease is called Goodpasture's syndrome. Renal biopsy in affected patients demonstrates a proliferative and exudative picture with numerous epithelial crescents on light microscopy. Electron microscopy confirms these findings. Immunofluorescence demonstrates linear deposition of IgG and C3 along the GBM. The prognosis in patients with anti-GBM antibody disease is related to renal function on presentation as well as the amount of crescents and chronic changes noted on renal biopsy. Plasma exchange along with cytotoxic agents and corticosteroids is thought to be helpful in these patients (Kincaid-Smith, 1978).

Chronic glomerulonephritis is a stage in the progression of renal diseases that involves chronic scarring. Unfortunately, patients who present with significant degrees of CRF most often show on biopsy a chronic scarring process that does not allow a diagnosis of the true underlying disorder. For this reason, renal biopsy is rarely performed in patients with significant degrees of CRF. Although chronic glomerulonephritis is the leading diagnosis of patients who come to need dialysis or transplantation for CRF, it is still unclear as to what primary disease actually results in chronic glomerulonephritis in these patients.

Tubulointerstitial diseases that commonly cause CRF are summarized in Table 8–6. The most important causes are now discussed.

Polycystic kidney disease (PKD) is an extremely important cause of CRF. PKD can occur as an adult-onset disease, which displays autosomal dominant genetics (ADPKD), or as a juvenile-onset disease (JPKD), which is usually autosomal recessive. ADPKD is much more common than JPKD.

ADPKD is genetically heterogeneous, with loci mapped to chromosome 16 (PKD1) and to chromosome 4 (PKD2) and the likelihood of a third, unmapped locus (Hughes et al, 1995). PKD1, which accounts for approximately 85% of ADPKD, is a more severe disease than PKD2. ADPKD typically presents in the fourth or fifth decade of life, but considerable variability may exist. It may be associated with hypertension which is believed, after considerable investigation, to be related to activation of the renin-angiotensin-aldosterone system (Chapman et al, 1990). Although no known therapy has been proven efficacious, some data suggest that aggressive control of blood pressure may slow the progression of this disease. ADPKD is a systemic disease. Cystic involvement is not limited to the kidney and may also involve the spleen, liver, and pancreas. Cardiac malformations and cerebral berry aneurysms are associated with APKD.

JPKD usually manifests in infants and small children. This disease typically is associated with hepatic fibrosis, which is usually fatal. In addition to ADPKD and JPKD, other cystic diseases of the kidney occur. These include medullary cystic disease, which manifests in adults and may progress to CRF, and medullary sponge kidney, which is a nondestructive hereditary cystic disorder of the renal papilla that is often complicated by distal renal tubular acidosis, nephrocalcinosis, and renal calculi but usually does not progress to CRF.

Reflux nephropathy or chronic pyelonephritis is another important tubulointerstitial cause of CRF. As discussed elsewhere in this text, urinary reflux and associated parenchymal infections in childhood may be associated with progressive loss of renal parenchyma and lead to CRF. Unfortunately, once substantial proteinuria is established, repair of the reflux does not appear to ameliorate the progression of CRF. In this setting, the glomerular lesion of focal and segmental glomerulosclerosis may be seen in association with reflux nephropathy and CRF.

Analgesic nephropathy may lead to CRF. The incidence of this disease in the United States is debated. The absence of specific diagnostic criteria for defining this entity make it impossible to accurately estimate its incidence and prevalence. It appears that heavy use of phenacetin and aspirin in combination are most likely to cause this disease, with associated papillary necrosis and CRF. Avoidance of further analgesic use is the only recommended therapy (Paller, 1990).

Metal intoxications with lead or cadmium, as well as Balkan nephropathy, a rare interstitial form of renal diseases of unknown etiology, may lead to CRF. The CRF associated with gout, so-called gouty nephropathy, may in fact be related to chronic lead intoxication rather than to elevations in uric acid. CRF may of course complicate prolonged obstructive uropathy. Causes of urinary obstruction as well as the pathophysiology of this disease are discussed elsewhere in this text.

Chronic hypokalemia and hypercalcemia may be associated with progressive tubulointerstitial nephritis and CRF. Whether lithium therapy is a direct cause of tubulointerstitial nephritis that leads to CRF is still debated.

SYSTEMIC DISEASES

Systemic diseases often affect the kidney. The most important systemic diseases that may cause CRF are listed in Table 8–7. These disease entities are discussed as follows.

Table 8–7. MAJOR SYSTEMIC DISEASES THAT MAY CAUSE CHRONIC RENAL FAILURE (CRF)

Disease	Progression to CRF
Diabetes mellitus	Common
Systemic lupus erythematosus	Common
Vasculitis	
Henoch-Schönlein purpura	Uncommon
Polyarteritis nodosa	Common
Hypersensitivity angiitis	Variable
Wegener's granulomatosis	Common
Lymphomatoid granulomatosis	Variable
Sickle-cell anemia	Common*
Multiple myeloma	Common
Amyloidosis	Common
Essential hypertension	Uncommon†
Malignant hypertension	Common

*Among patients with sickle cell anemia who live into the third decade, CRF is quite common.

†Although CRF is an uncommon complication of essential hypertension, episodes of accelerated hypertension may lead to CRF.

Diabetes mellitus is the most common cause of ESRD in the United States. Patients with type I diabetes mellitus typically present with proteinuria after 10 to 15 years of diabetes, which is followed in 2 to 3 years by progressive renal insufficiency. Only about 50% of patients afflicted with diabetes develop kidney disease. Evidence suggests that patients with type 1 diabetes who develop kidney disease have microalbuminuria: a urinary albumin level of between 30 and 300 mg/day, an amount that is not detected by routine dipsticks and is usually measured by sensitive radioimmunoassay. However, dipsticks that can detect microalbuminuria are now available. The total daily urine protein excretion is still within normal limits, and the GFR is supernormal in the first several years after the onset of diabetes.

Intensive blood glucose control, maintaining the blood glucose concentration close to the normal range, delays the onset and slows the progression of diabetic nephropathy, retinopathy, and neuropathy in insulin-dependent diabetes mellitus (Diabetes Control and Complications Trial Research Group, 1993). Aggressive control of blood pressure, especially with agents that may decrease increases in glomerular capillary pressure, such as ACEIs, may slow the rate of progression of renal failure. Captopril protects against the deterioration in renal function independently of blood pressure control in insulin-dependent diabetic nephropathy patients with proteinuria of more than 500 mg/day and mild renal impairment (Lewis et al, 1993).

Although the progression of kidney disease in type 2 diabetes is not as well understood as in type 1, it is likely that type 2 diabetes may ultimately be a more important cause of CRF than type 1 because of its greater prevalence. Specifically, 90% of all diabetic patients have type II diabetes.

Systemic lupus erythematosus (SLE) is another important systemic disease that affects the kidney. Like diabetes, approximately 50% of patients with SLE develop symptomatic renal disease. Renal manifestations of SLE are varied. In mesangial lupus, renal function is usually normal, urinary abnormalities are minimal, and biopsy findings are limited to mesangial expansion and mesangial immune complex deposits.

In the most severe forms of lupus nephritis in which histologic findings are either diffuse proliferative or membranoproliferative, renal function may be impaired, proteinuria is marked, and the renal sediment is extremely active. In this setting, renal biopsy demonstrates cellular proliferation and exudation with immune complex deposits in subendothelial as well as mesangial locations. Other patients with lupus nephritis demonstrate a histologic pattern of focal proliferative or membranous glomerulopathy. In rare instances, SLE affects the kidney in a predominantly tubulointerstitial pattern. The diagnosis of SLE is based on clinical grounds and laboratory data, although renal biopsy may be useful in assessing prognosis and determining therapy. Corticosteroids and cytotoxic agents, specifically cyclophosphamide and azathioprine, are useful in the management of SLE with renal involvement.

A number of vasculitides affect the kidney. Many of these have pathologic manifestations similar to the primary renal diseases already discussed. **Henoch-Schönlein purpura is a leukocytoclastic vasculitis involving small arteries and venules that manifests clinically with lower intestinal bleeding, palpable purpura, and arthralgias, in addition to renal manifestations of gross or microscopic bleeding, proteinuria, and occasionally renal failure. On biopsy, mesangial IgA deposits are noted, which suggests a common link with Berger's disease (discussed earlier).** Progression to CRF does occur. No known therapy is effective.

Polyarteritis nodosa (PAN) in its classic or macroscopic form typically occurs in males in the sixth decade. Patients present with arthralgias, peripheral neuropathy, fever, and hemolytic anemia. Hypertension may be prominent and life-threatening. This vasculitis involves predominantly middle-sized muscular arteries. The classic form of this disease spares the pulmonary system and is not associated with eosinophilia; however, variants of PAN may have pulmonary manifestations, eosinophilia, or both. Spontaneous rupture of the kidney, manifesting as an acute abdomen, has been described in PAN (Edelstein and Welke, 1991).

The diagnosis is usually based on clinical features and detection of microaneurysms of medium-sized arteries, usually in vessels supplying abdominal viscera. Renal involvement occurs in 80% to 90% of affected patients and ranges from microscopic hematuria to rapid loss of renal function. Renal biopsy may demonstrate focal proliferative and necrotizing glomerulonephritis with crescent formation.

If disease is limited to the medium-sized muscular arteries, glomerular abnormalities may include only some focal collapse of glomeruli, indicating glomerular ischemia. This biopsy picture may, in fact, be very difficult to differentiate from that of focal and segmental glomerulosclerosis. Thus the diagnosis of PAN is best made by arteriographic evidence of microaneurysms. Hepatitis B antigen is present in the serum of about 50% of these patients, which suggests an immune complex etiology of this disease. PAN may cause progressive CRF.

Hypersensitivity angiitis is a leukocytoclastic vasculitis that involves predominantly arterioles and venules. Peripheral eosinophilia, urticaria, arthralgias, and fever are common symptoms. Renal manifestations may include proteinuria, microscopic or macroscopic hematuria, and red blood cell casts. Renal biopsy most often demonstrates focal proliferative glomerulonephritis. Rapid deterioration of renal function and extensive crescent formation is generally treated with cytotoxic agents and corticosteroids. Plasmapheresis is used in some cases, although its use is not supported by controlled prospective studies.

Wegener's granulomatosis is another form of vasculitis that can cause CRF. Wegener's granulomatosis is a granulomatous vasculitis that affects small arteries and venules predominantly in upper and lower airways and in the kidney. The clinical manifestation usually involves pulmonary infiltrates or sinusitis. In rare instances, patients present with an active renal sediment or evidence of deteriorating renal function. Renal biopsy usually demonstrates a focal necrotizing glomerulonephritis. Crescent formation is not unusual and, if extensive, confers a poor prognosis. Treatment with cytotoxic agents and corticosteroids is often efficacious. Lymphomatoid granulomatosis is a rare form of vasculitis that has histologic similarities to Wegener's granulomatosis. Many patients afflicted with lymphomatoid granulomatosis eventually develop lymphoproliferative disease.

Sickle-cell anemia is associated with several types of renal disease. Patients with either the heterozygous or the homozygous form of sickle-cell anemia develop progressive infarction of medullary renal tissue with age and concomitant loss of renal concentrating and diluting abilities. In patients with sickle-cell anemia, progressive renal insufficiency may develop later in life, in association with histologic evidence of either focal and segmental glomerulosclerosis, membranous glomerulopathy, or MPGN on renal biopsy.

Other Causes

Multiple myeloma may cause renal failure by a variety of mechanisms, including tubular precipitation of paraproteins, also called myeloma kidney; urinary obstruction secondary to uric acid or calcium-containing stones; hypercalcemia which typically causes acute and reversible renal failure; and renal amyloidosis. Primary amyloidosis or amyloidosis secondary to inflammatory diseases is another cause of CRF. **Ischemic nephropathy attributable to atherosclerosis or fibromuscular dysplasia of the renal arteries may also cause CRF. Therapy with surgical revascularization or angioplasty may sometimes salvage renal function.** Cholesterol emboli syndrome, which typically causes ARF, may also cause CRF. This syndrome usually occurs in older patients with generalized atherosclerosis after an invasive procedure such as aortic angioplasty. Fabry's disease, which is an inherited abnormality in lipid metabolism, may be complicated by renal disease and CRF. Alport's syndrome, also called hereditary nephritis, is a disorder of type IV collagen synthesis that has complex and different genetic patterns in different affected families and is actually a fairly common form of kidney disease. Affected patients, more often males, may develop deafness as part of the syndrome. Ocular abnormalities may also complicate this syndrome. Essential mixed cryoglobulinemia, secondary to hepatitis C, may also be associated with CRF.

Numerous infections may be complicated by renal involvement. The leading cause of CRF worldwide is still infection with *Schistosoma haematobium,* which causes strictures of the collecting system and obstructive uropathy. Many nonbacterial infections, including hepatitis B as discussed earlier, *Schistosoma mansoni* infection, and malaria, as well as more chronic bacterial infections such as seen with endocarditis, ventriculoperitoneal shunt infections, and deep-seated abscesses, may be complicated by immune complex glomerulonephritis, which may progress to CRF. Treatment of the underlying infection is generally associated with improvement in renal function.

Human immunodeficiency virus (HIV)–associated nephropathy may occur in asymptomatic HIV infection, AIDS-related complex, or AIDS. It manifests with no or mild hypertension, nephrotic-range proteinuria, and large kidneys. Distinctive pathologic features on renal biopsy are "collapsed" glomerular capillaries, reactive visceral epithelium with protein droplets, microcystic

tubules with variegated casts, focal tubular "simplification," and endothelial tubuloreticular inclusions. There is an early and rapidly progressive, irreversible azotemia. There is no specific treatment for HIV nephropathy, and the survival of these patients on dialysis is very poor.

Pathogenetic Factors in the Progression of Chronic Renal Failure

Progression to end-stage renal failure necessitating renal replacement therapy, occurs in a large number of patients with CRF. **Progression often occurs well after the acute renal insult has subsided. For instance, in glomerulonephritis, CRF often develops many years after the initial immune-mediated insult has resolved (Baldwin, 1982).** Although progressive renal failure is common, it is not always the rule; some patients with CRF maintain stable renal function over long periods of time (El Nahas and Coles, 1986). Several factors such as underlying nephropathy, degree of proteinuria, hypertension, tubulointerstitial damage, and degree of renal impairment at presentation determine the likelihood and the rate of progression of renal failure in chronic renal disorders. It is thought that once CRF has advanced to a certain point, it usually progresses relentlessly to end-stage renal failure, but the exact point at which progression becomes inevitable has not been determined and is likely to vary with both the disease and the individual.

Although the mechanisms underlying progression have not been determined, the experimental evidence favors a common pathway to terminal renal failure once such extensive renal impairment has occurred. The most debated hypothesis remains that of Brenner and colleagues, who suggested that progressive renal scarring results from raised intraglomerular pressure in the remnant kidney model of progressive renal failure in the rat (Brenner et al, 1982). Other proposed mechanisms include glomerular hypertrophy, which leads to increased tension in the capillary wall (Yoshida et al, 1989); interstitial fibrosis caused by precipitation of calcium phosphate crystals (Ibels et al, 1978); tubular damage by ammonia-induced complement activation (Nath et al, 1987); and glomerular and tubular damage by lipid deposition (Moorhead et al, 1982). The demonstration that one of these mechanisms is active does not exclude the presence of another, and all may have a role.

The pivotal role of glomerular hypertension in the initiation and progression of glomerular sclerosis combines many of these mechanisms. Renal ablation or primary parenchymal disease leads to systemic hypertension and to glomerular hypertension. Other factors, including normal aging, diabetes, and dietary factors, also lead to glomerular hypertension. Once present, glomerular hypertension exerts deleterious effects on all glomerular cell constituents. In analogy with atherosclerosis, increased glomerular hydraulic pressure enhances endothelial cell release of vasoactive substances, such as thromboxanes, lipid deposition, and intracapillary thrombosis. Injury to the mesangial region consists of increased accumulation of macromolecules, which enhance both mesangial cell proliferation and mesangial matrix production. Epithelial cell injury augments glomerular basement membrane permeability and proteinuria. Together, injury to these cells results in glomerular hypertension, thus perpetuating the cycle (Anderson and Brenner, 1989). However, the role of postglomerular microvessels and tubulointerstitial damage in the progression of renal failure caused by this mechanism is poorly understood.

Few published studies have assessed the frequency of progression as opposed to nonprogressive renal failure in relation to underlying pathology. Williams and associates (1988) found that stability was more likely to be associated with hypertensive nephrosclerosis, analgesic nephropathy, and renal impairment after ARF than with other diagnoses. Bergstrom and colleagues (1989) found that stability was more common in patients with interstitial nephritis and after relief of obstructive uropathy than in chronic glomerulonephritis or polycystic kidney disease. The major criticism of such studies is that the duration of follow-up may be too short to assess progression in human renal failure. However, the demonstration that stability of function, even over a limited period, is more likely to be found in some diagnostic categories than in others argues against the theory that a single mechanism causes progression of renal failure.

There are conflicting reports of the effect of the underlying renal pathology on the rate of progression. Mitch and associates (1976), using reciprocal creatinine/time plots, failed to demonstrate an influence of the underlying renal disease. Rutherford and co-workers (1977) found significantly faster progression in patients with glomerulonephritis and diabetic nephropathy than in those with chronic pyelonephritis and polycystic kidneys. Williams and associates (1988) revealed faster progression in glomerulonephritis and diabetic nephropathy than in chronic pyelonephritis or polycystic kidneys. Stenvinkel and colleagues (1989) also found that glomerulonephritis progressed more rapidly than in patients with chronic interstitial disease but, somewhat surprisingly, found more rapid progression in polycystic kidney disease as well. Other authors have shown an effect of the underlying disease on the rate of progression (Ahlem et al, 1975; Gretz et al, 1983). Thus there is general consensus that patients with chronic glomerular diseases tend to have faster rates of progression than do patients with other forms of renal disorders.

In many forms of glomerular and nonglomerular disease, the magnitude of the proteinuria is a strong predictor of progression provided the proteinuria is persistent. Whether proteinuria is simply a sign of renal damage or is itself pathogenic is not known. Some experimental evidence suggests that traffic of protein macromolecules across the mesangium may damage the glomerulus (Couser and Stilmant, 1975). In experimental glomerulonephritis, a significant positive correlation between the magnitude of proteinuria and the number of glomeruli affected by focal segmental glomerulosclerosis has been described (Glasser et al, 1977). Other authors have suggested that proteinuria may be toxic to renal tubules (Cameron, 1990). Heavy proteinuria may conceivably cause renal damage by secondary effects such as hyperlipidemia or abnormal blood rheology (Moorhead et al, 1982; Gordge et al, 1991). Whether protein in the glomerular filtrate does or does not damage the nephron does not detract from the usefulness of proteinuria to the clinician in the management of most forms of renal disease causing chronic progressive renal failure.

The slow evolution of diabetic nephropathy is well documented and is marked by changes in proteinuria. Microalbuminuria—that is, a urinary albumin of between 30 and 300 mg/day that is not detectable by routine dipstick testing—has been shown to be of importance (Viberti et al, 1982). In the first decade after diagnosis of insulin-dependent diabetes, the albumin excretion is not usually elevated, although poor metabolic control or exercise may raise the level, probably by a hemodynamic mechanism (Parving et al, 1976; Vittinghus and Mogensen, 1982). Once microalbuminuria is established, the albumin excretion rate tends to increase over the years until it reaches detectability on dipstick testing. Certainly, when proteinuria is established, the clinical course is of relentless deterioration in renal function.

The significance of proteinuria in other conditions is not as well documented. As discussed earlier, patients who have significant renal impairment after an acute illness and then develop proteinuria may be at risk of progressive renal failure. In these conditions, the only safe level is less than 200 mg/day: that is, undetectable by routine tests. Any measurement over 1 g/24 hours should be watched carefully; further increases over this level may herald a phase of progression.

The importance of control of hypertension in the prevention of vascular disease is well documented (Medical Research Council, 1985). It is generally accepted that hypertension is an important factor in the progression of renal failure and that effective control slows the rate of deterioration.

The role of hypertension in hastening progression is now an established dogma of nephrology, although it is perhaps based more on experimental than clinical work. Clinical research is now focused on the precise level to which blood pressure should be lowered and at which antihypertensive agents should be used.

Protein restriction and blood pressure control delay the progression of renal disease in laboratory animals (Klahr et al, 1983). A multicenter, randomized study, the Modification of Diet in Renal Disease study, tested the hypotheses that two interventions—(1) a reduction in dietary protein and phosphorus intake and (2) the maintenance of blood pressure at a level below that usually recommended—would retard the progression of renal disease. These interventions were found to be safe and acceptable for long-term management of patients with CRF (Klahr et al, 1994). However, no significant benefit of the two interventions was demonstrated at the end of follow-up in the two study groups (patients with GFR of 45 to 25 ml/minute and those with GFR of <25 ml/minute) when patients with diverse renal diseases were considered together. A benefit of low blood pressure in patients with urinary protein excretion exceeding 1 g/day was found, as was a trend toward a greater benefit of low blood pressure in black patients with moderate renal insufficiency. A more rapid decline in GFR in patients with adult polycystic kidney disease was also found in this study.

The relevance of tubulointerstitial scarring to the development of CRF is often underestimated, in spite of a considerable amount of data from animals and humans, which suggests that such scarring correlates better with renal impairment and outcome than does glomerular scarring (Cameron, 1992b). The first indication that this might be the case was the surprisingly poor correlation between morphologic appearances and GFR on renal biopsy. In contrast, the correlation between GFR and the degree of interstitial disease is much better, as first detailed by Risdon and colleagues (1968) and later by Striker and associates (1970). Different opinions have been entertained about the relationship between glomerular damage and tubulointerstitial lesions especially in primary glomerulonephritis: (1) tubulointerstitial damage in glomerular disorders is secondary to glomerular damage and caused by ischemia (Ravnskov, 1988; Molitoris, 1992); (2) any process that leads to an increased interstitial volume may increase glomerular pressure by obstructing the postglomerular capillaries, and the increased pressure may induce glomerular sclerosis; (3) interstitial cellular infiltrate may release biologically active products such as cytokines and growth factors that may be involved in the tissue degradation, organization and fibrogenesis (Nathan, 1987); and (4) renal tubular cells can synthesize several growth factors that may cause interstitial fibrosis and glomerulosclerosis (El Nahas, 1992). Additional studies investigating the mechanisms by which various cells and their products induce fibrosis and the factors (environmental) that trigger this irreversible process should have rational therapeutic implications.

Clinical Approach

Diagnostic Strategies

In the patient who presents with CRF, efforts should be made to assign a diagnosis of the primary disease. Knowledge of the primary disease, in fact, may have important implications regarding other complications, which must be anticipated as considerations for possible transplantation. Careful review of the history, detailed physical examination, and directed laboratory investigations and imaging methods may yield a diagnosis. Differentiation of the disease entities into primary versus systemic and glomerular versus tubulointerstitial narrows the differential diagnosis. If renal failure has not advanced to end-stage and the kidneys are not small, renal biopsy may be undertaken in an effort to find a treatable form of kidney disease.

In all patients who present with CRF, efforts should be made to search for reversible insults to renal function. Virtually any cause of ARF may be applicable to patients with CRF. Moreover, patients with CRF are more sensitive to many of these insults. Specifically, patients with CRF are more sensitive to all forms of prerenal azotemia; many causes of ATN, such as radiocontrast and aminoglycoside nephrotoxicity; and urinary tract obstruction. Reversal of these acute insults may delay the need for renal replacement therapy, including chronic dialysis and transplantation.

Conservative Management

The conservative management of CRF includes the avoidance of any additional insults to renal function, treatment of complications of CRF, and attempts to slow the progression of CRF. Specifically, in patients with CRF, prerenal azotemia from volume depletion and nephrotoxic drugs must be avoided.

Complications of CRF include the signs and symptoms of the uremic syndrome, as well as acute fluid and electrolyte disorders. Electrolyte disturbances to which CRF patients are more susceptible include hyperkalemia, hyperphosphatemia, hypocalcemia, and hypermagnesemia. Metabolic acidosis may also result from CRF. Although many patients do not develop problems with hyperkalemia until CRF has reached end stage, some patients manifest difficulties in potassium homeostasis with relatively minor impairments in GFR. Most of these patients have what is referred to as type 4 renal tubular acidosis and have difficulties in excreting a potassium load in the urine. This may result from a deficiency in aldosterone, which is common in diabetic patients, or an inherent tubular defect, seen commonly in patients with obstructive uropathy.

Other patients with CRF who are more susceptible to hyperkalemia include patients taking medications that impair potassium excretion or the shift of potassium into the intracellular compartment. Specifically, distal potassium-sparing diuretics (such as amiloride, triamterene, or spironolactone), beta blockers, and ACEIs may cause problems with potassium balance in CRF patients and must be used with caution (Shapiro et al, 1990).

Hyperphosphatemia is the direct result of impaired renal phosphate excretion. Even with relatively mild CRF, phosphate homeostasis is preserved only at the expense of relatively high concentrations of parathyroid hormone (PTH). In more severe CRF, even extremely high concentrations of PTH cannot increase phosphate excretion enough to maintain serum phosphate in the normal range.

Because of increases in serum phosphate as well as impaired production of 1,25-dihydroxycholecalciferol with progressive kidney damage, serum calcium levels may fall. Both of these disturbances may be prevented by administration of calcium-containing phosphate binders, such as calcium carbonate, with meals. Administration of 1,25-dihydroxycholecalciferol is generally avoided in patients with CRF before beginning dialysis because of concerns about accelerating progression of CRF. Hypermagnesemia generally results from ingestion of magnesium-based antacids and/or magnesium-containing cathartics. These agents should be avoided in all patients with significant renal impairment. The progressive metabolic acidosis that occurs with CRF may be exacerbated by hyperkalemia, which impairs ammoniagenesis (Halperin, 1989). Dietary protein restriction and administration of oral sodium bicarbonate may be effective in preventing acidosis and its complications, which include skeletal muscle protein wasting and depletion of bone calcium. Citrate, which is readily metabolized to bicarbonate, should probably be avoided in patients with significant CRF because it may increase aluminum absorption and, especially if administered with aluminum-containing antacids, accelerate the development of aluminum intoxication (Molitoris et al, 1989; Froment et al, 1989).

Complications

In addition to the electrolyte disturbances discussed earlier, a large number of disturbances in normal bodily functions accompany CRF. Together, the symptoms of these dysfunctions are called the *uremic syndrome*. **Major manifestations of uremia are summarized in Table 8–4.** Virtually all organ systems of the body are involved.

Specifically, gastrointestinal function is disturbed, with the development of nausea, vomiting, and occasionally gastrointestinal bleeding. Neurologic abnormalities include peripheral neuropathy, as well as mental status changes ranging from sleepiness and mood disturbances to seizures and coma. Hematopoietic function is impaired, with diminished erythropoietin and decreased production of red blood cells as well as decreased red blood cell survival times, which lead to anemia. In uremia, blood clotting is abnormal, with impairments in platelet function resulting from a deficiency of von Willebrand factor multimers and the presence of small molecules that impair platelet function, as discussed earlier.

Other features of the uremic syndrome include autonomic neuropathy, development of pericardial effusion, and hypertensive and uremic cardiomyopathies. Bone development and mineralization may be impaired by the presence of hyperparathyroidism, development of aluminum-associated osteomalacia, demineralization associated with acidosis, and deposition of β_2-microglobulin in bone cysts. β_2-microglobulin deposition may also lead to compression of nerves, such as seen with median nerve entrapment in carpal tunnel syndrome (Alfrey et al, 1968, 1989). β_2-microglobulin deposition may result in destructive arthropathy, usually involving large and medium-sized joints, including the spine. The radiologic signs of arthropathy include erosion of subchondral bone structure, soft tissue swelling, and bone cysts. These cystic lesions can lead to pathologic fractures. Although the diagnosis is suggested by radiologic features, the definitive diagnosis of β_2-microglobulin amyloidosis requires demonstration of β_2-microglobulin in synovial or other biopsy specimens. Immune function in uremia may also be disturbed, as discussed previously. Pruritus is very common in uremic patients and is attributable to calcium/phosphorus deposits in skin, PTH excess, increases in serum levels of phosphate, hypercalcemia, or dry skin.

The pathogenesis of these complications of uremia is, at present, still poorly understood. Three major theories have been proposed to describe the pathogenesis of uremic symptoms and signs: (1) small solute theory, (2) middle molecule theory, and (3) trade-off hypothesis. The small solute theory suggests that increases in small solutes such as urea and creatinine arise from the breakdown of nitrogenous compounds and produce the uremic syndrome. Although modeling of uremic therapy on the basis of removal of these solutes may have some benefit, as discussed later, no well-characterized small solute accounts for the majority of uremic signs and symptoms. The middle molecule theory suggests that molecules in a "middle range" of molecular weight, about 1000 to 10,000 daltons, account for the uremic syndrome. No single such compound to explain all of the uremic symptoms has been identified. Studies on the adequacy of dialysis suggest that lower molecular weight solutes are more important. The trade-off hypothesis basically assumes that hormones that have supranormal concentrations in CRF to maintain homeostasis of electrolytes and fluid balance are, in these high concentrations, toxic to cellular and organ function. The best, and at present only, identified hormone that fits this description is PTH. The most likely explanation for the uremic syndrome is, in fact, that all of these hypotheses have some merit and that the uremic syndrome is multifactorial in its pathogenesis.

Clues to the pathogenesis of some of the features of uremia may come from the results of different therapies.

Hemodialysis and peritoneal dialysis are both quite successful at improving the gastrointestinal signs and symptoms and central neurologic alterations, as well as controlling hypertension and the development of pericardial effusion. Peritoneal dialysis may be more successful in reversing peripheral neuropathy, and neither modality is successful, on its own, in preventing uremic bone disease from aluminum toxicity or parathyroid hormone excess or in normalizing the hematocrit in patients with CRF. The addition of phosphate binders (preferably not containing aluminum hydroxide), the judicious use of 1,25-OH-D3 (Tzamaloukas, 1990), and the approved employment of erythropoietin supplementation (Eschbach and Adamson, 1988) dramatically improves dialytic management. Despite these quantitative improvements in dialytic therapy, most nephrologists agree that in good candidates, renal transplantation is the preferred mode of renal replacement in appropriate candidates.

Patients with CRF, particularly ESRD patients maintained on renal replacement therapy, are prone to develop bilateral and small cysts in their native kidneys. Acquired cystic disease (ACD) was initially thought to affect only dialysis patients; however, it has been described in patients with CRF before the start of dialysis (Bommer, 1980). The pathogenesis of the disease is still obscure, but the incidence of ACD depends on the duration of renal failure. Ishikawa (1991) found that the incidence of ACD was 44% among patients on dialysis for less than 3 years, 79% among those on dialysis for more than 4 years, and 90% among those on dialysis for more than 10 years. ACD has been described with all forms of renal failure. Diabetic patients, however, for unknown reasons are less likely to develop ACD than are patients with ESRD of other etiologies. No difference in the occurrence of ACD has been found between modes of renal replacement therapy.

Kidneys with ACD are not large, in comparison with those with ADPKD, and the cyst size varies from less than 5 mm to 3 cm in diameter. Most of the acquired cysts are located in the cortex, but some are found in the medulla and may replace most of the parenchyma. They are composed of a single or multilayered epithelia. Epithelial hyperplasia is a universal finding in ACD. There may be a histologic continuum from epithelial proliferation to cyst formation to adenoma and then to renal cell cancer.

ACD is usually asymptomatic. **Complications, however, include asymptomatic enlargement of the kidneys; cyst rupture, which may cause flank, abdominal, or back pain; hematuria; retroperitoneal bleeding; cyst infection, sometimes presenting in the form of long-standing fever; and renal tumors. Renal tumors, potentially the most important complication, are usually asymptomatic but can manifest in the form of a palpable abdominal mass, hematuria, fever, flank or back pain, acute decrease or increase in hematocrit, hypercalcemia, hypoglycemia, and metastatic masses (lung, spine, brain).** Most of the tumors found in the autopsy series are nonmalignant adenomas, which may represent a further step in the evolution of epithelial hyperplasia and renal cell carcinomas.

Comparison of the incidence of renal cell carcinomas in dialysis patients with that in the general population is difficult to extrapolate, because all tumor registries refer to the incidence of cancer per 100,000 people rather than the age group of the dialysis population, which in most of the studies is greater than 50 years. There are two subpopulations of dialysis patients who develop renal cell carcinoma. The first group (80%)is composed of younger patients on long-term dialysis who display extensive cystic changes; the other (20%) is composed of older patients with a short history of dialysis and no or few cysts. The incidence of renal cell carcinoma in patients with ACD has varied in different reports, and there is wide variation between autopsy reports and imaging series. There is general agreement in the literature that screening with renal ultrasonography should be performed in patients who have been on dialysis for 3 years and then yearly thereafter. If cystic changes are identified, a more sensitive imaging technique such as computed tomography should be performed to rule out renal tumors at yearly intervals. If a tumor is detected, nephrectomy should be performed, especially for tumors with a diameter larger than 2 to 3 cm or for tumors increasing in size.

Nephrolithiasis appears to be a more frequent complication in patients on long-term hemodialysis than was previously believed (Daudon et al, 1992). Spontaneously passed renal stones have been reported in 5% to 11% of all dialysis patients (Caralps et al, 1979; Oren et al, 1984). However, radiologic data suggest that 20% to 50% of patients on long-term dialysis have asymptomatic renal stones and/or intrarenal calcifications (Koga et al, 1982). Daudon et al (1992) classified renal stones from chronic hemodialysis patients into three types: (1) protein stones, with less than 30% calcium oxalate, in patients with primary glomerular disease; (2) oxaloprotein stones, with a total stone content of more than 30% calcium oxalate, related to metabolic factors such as high urinary oxalate and vitamin D3 and calcium supplementation; and (3) aluminum magnesium urate stones, induced by aluminum overload. Accurate analysis of these stones may give a clue to their pathogenesis and prophylaxis.

Dialysis and Transplantation

Indications for Dialysis or Transplantation

Development of uremic signs and symptoms should result in rapid institution of renal replacement therapy. Pericardial effusion may rapidly progress to life-threatening tamponade. Also, sensory neuropathy may rapidly progress to combined motor and sensory neuropathy. This motor neuropathy does not usually reverse with dialytic therapy; prevention is therefore paramount (Raskin and Fishman, 1976a, 1976b). Initiation of dialysis therapy or the performance of a renal transplant has been recommended at a stage before the development of uremic signs and symptoms. This is generally done when the creatinine clearance falls below 10 ml/minute, which usually corresponds to a BUN value of >100 mg/dl or a serum creatinine level of >10 mg/dl. However, we stress that in patients on a low-protein diet and/or possessing relatively little muscle mass, renal clearances of urea and creatinine are much lower for a given BUN or serum creatinine value.

Hemodialysis

Hemodialysis is the most widely employed modality of renal replacement. In contrast to the setting of ARF, vascular access in CRF is usually accomplished by an arteriovenous fistula or a Gore-Tex graft placed surgically with the radial or ulnar artery and the cephalic vein. In situations in which this form of access cannot be placed or has recently clotted or been removed, temporary access may be accomplished with a Sheldon catheter placed percutaneously into the subclavian, internal jugular, or femoral vein or with a Scribner shunt generally placed in the radial artery and cephalic vein.

Conventional hemodialysis treatment is usually performed with Cupraphane or cellulose acetate membranes with a surface area of approximately 1 m^2, blood flows of 250 ml/minute, and dialysate flows of 500 ml/minute. Dialysate composition may be acetate or bicarbonate based. With such therapy, dialysis prescription is generally for about 4 hours, three times per week. More efficient hemodialysis with larger surface area (1.5 to 2 m^2) Cupraphane or cellulose acetate dialyzers or with standard-size dialyzers made of very porous material (polysulfone or polyacrylonitrile) with relatively high blood flow rates (350 to 500 ml/minute) and faster dialysate flow rates (600 to 750 ml/minute) have been employed in an effort to shorten the treatment time of hemodialysis.

During hemodialysis, the patient may experience adverse reactions dependent on the contact of blood with tubing, sterilants, dialysate, and the dialysis membrane. Blood-membrane interactions include complement activation, leukopenia, platelet activation, hemolysis of red blood cells, and increased β_2-microglobulin synthesis. The number and severity of these reactions define the biocompatibility of the procedure. Polyacrylonitrile, polymethacrylate, and polysulphone membranes are thought to be more biocompatible than Cupraphane membranes. Adverse events thought to be attributable to bioincompatible membranes include hypersensitivity reactions, infection, β_2-microglobulin amyloidosis, and malnutrition. Biocompatible membranes have been shown to affect patient survival and renal recovery in ARF (Hakim et al, 1994; Schiffl et al, 1994). The effect of biocompatibility on the survival of long-term hemodialysis patients is being investigated.

Currently accepted methods to quantify dialysis therapy and define its adequacy rely on the mathematical description of urea kinetics and the evaluation of an index, Kt/V (Barth, 1993). The traditional method of calculating Kt/V requires three blood samples: before and after dialysis and before the next dialysis. Inputs are the three BUN values, dialyzer urea clearance (Kd), dialysis duration (t), interdialytic interval, and pre- and postdialysis weight (Sargent, 1983). A Kt/V of <1.2 is not regarded as optimal dialysis. Evidence is accumulating that mortality and morbidity among hemodialysis patients may decrease as the Kt/V is increased above 1 (Ahmad and Cole, 1990). Mathematical modeling of urea kinetics is a remarkable conceptual advance, which has unquestionably led to greater understanding of the physiology of dialysis and enables the nephrologist to critically evaluate dialysis therapy (Barth, 1993). Water used to mix with dialysate must be purified with either reverse osmosis or deionization methods to avoid intoxication of the patient with copper, nickel, or aluminum (Simon, 1989). Most dialysis units prescribe phosphate binders to normalize the serum phosphate. Calcium carbonate is the preferred binder; however, some patients become hypercalcemic with this agent and must receive aluminum hydroxide to normalize serum phosphate concentrations. Oral and, more recently, intravenous forms of 1,25-dihydroxycholecalciferol are used by many units to reduce parathyroid hyperactivity and normalize serum calcium.

Anemia is a significant problem for patients with CRF, affecting more than 90% of patients with ESRD. It is thought to be the major factor contributing to the debilitating symptoms experienced by these patients. The anemia caused by CRF is the result of decreased erythropoietin production, decreased red blood cell survival, decreased response to erythropoietin, and bone marrow suppression caused by middle molecules or "uremic toxins." Before 1989, the anemia was treated with blood transfusion, accompanied by all its complications in ESRD patients (e.g., hepatitis C, iron overload, development of anti–human leukocyte antigen antibodies). **The availability of recombinant human erythropoietin has changed the approach to the treatment of this chronic problem** (Eschbach et al, 1987; Eschbach and Adamson, 1988; Adamson and Eschbach, 1989). Erythropoietin may be administered intravenously, subcutaneously, or intraperitoneally, as in patients on continuous ambulatory peritoneal dialysis (CAPD). The response to erythropoietin occurs in a dose-dependent fashion. At doses of 500 U/kg given intravenously three times a week, the hematocrit can rise as much as 10% in 3 weeks (Eschbach et al, 1987). By 18 weeks, more than 95% of patients had reached their target hematocrit of between 30% and 38%. Maintaining adequate iron stores is critical for an optimal response when treating patients with erythropoietin. Quality of life is enhanced for these patients, including improvements in fatigue, physical symptoms, reversal of impotence, and exercise tolerance (Korbet, 1993). Adverse effects associated with the rise in hematocrit include hypertension, seizures, clotting of vascular accesses, and a decrease in dialysis efficiency.

Although hemodialysis is a routine treatment carried out by nurses, dialysis technicians, and even the patients themselves, it is associated with a number of complications, some of which may be life-threatening. Episodes of hypotension are the most frequent complications occurring during hemodialysis. Hypotension may be caused by hemorrhage, volume depletion, extracorporeal blood volume, changes in plasma osmolality, cardiac factors, autonomic neuropathy, and medications. Technical and human errors can result in incorrect proportioning in the preparation of dialysate, the most important consequences of which are acute hyponatremia and hypernatremia. Fever during dialysis most commonly results from endotoxemia caused by a pyrogen reaction. It may also be the result of infection. Air embolism is always a potential hazard resulting from leakage of air into the extracorporeal blood circuit. Painful muscle cramps are common in hemodialysis patients. The dialysis equilibrium syndrome remains a hazard for patients with ARF and for some new patients starting maintenance hemodialysis. Cerebral edema resulting from rapid electrolyte and pH changes is thought to be the main cause and can be prevented by shorter and more frequent dialysis or careful dialysis with equipment with ultrafiltration control.

Hemodialysis methods have been improved, and life expectancies on hemodialysis may exceed 10 to 15 years.

Peritoneal Dialysis

Peritoneal dialysis is less widely used as chronic therapy in the United States than hemodialysis, but because of its reduced cost, it is popular in many other places, particularly developing countries. With this modality, access is generally accomplished with a soft Tenckhoff catheter placed either surgically or percutaneously in the midline of the abdomen into the right or left posterior aspect of the peritoneum. The external end is tunneled subcutaneously to exit in the lateral aspect of the lower abdomen. Sterile dialysate is infused into the abdomen, allowed to dwell, and then drained at prescribed intervals. If these intervals are evenly spaced throughout the day, it is called continuous ambulatory peritoneal dialysis (CAPD). If most exchanges occur at night with a machine performing the procedure, it is called continuous cycling peritoneal dialysis (CCPD) (Nolph, 1978).

Dialysis prescription in peritoneal dialysis is also based on solute clearance. In terms of dialysis effectiveness, peritoneal dialysis clears lower molecular weight molecules slightly more poorly, but larger or mid-sized molecules somewhat better, than does hemodialysis. A peritoneal dialysis clearance of creatinine in excess of 40 L/week is generally considered acceptable therapy. Avoidance of uremic symptoms is generally accomplished with such a clearance. Failure to achieve adequate clearance of creatinine may result from either extremely high or low permeability of the peritoneal membrane to small solutes. If permeability is low, larger exchanges with longer dwelling times may be effective in improving clearances. If permeability is too high, shorter and more rapid exchanges may be efficacious. Failure to remove fluid with hydro-osmotic gradients induced by glucose in the dialysate generally results from high peritoneal permeability or from excessive lymphatic reabsorption of peritoneal fluid. Both of these conditions are best addressed by shorter, more frequent exchanges (Penzotti and Mattocks, 1971). Peritoneal dialysis is generally effective and well tolerated and is less expensive than hemodialysis.

In diabetic patients with vascular disease and in patients with severe cardiac disease, CAPD offers advantages over hemodialysis: Its slow, continuous process has the potential advantage of reduced cardiovascular stress and stable hemodynamic status. A steady biochemical state, easier control of hypertension and extracellular volume, and the possibility of intraperitoneal insulin administration for diabetics are additional advantages. Peritoneal access is easy to establish, and this avoids having to access an atherosclerotic blood vessel. Because the procedure can be carried out without a machine, **CAPD is convenient for free mobility and easy to perform at home or work. It is also convenient for a patient who is soon to get a renal transplant.**

Using the peritoneum as an artificial kidney has unavoidable side effects inherent in the dialysis procedure. Although not life-threatening in the short term, some of these undesirable effects are potentially harmful in the long term and should be closely monitored in the case of prolonged use of CAPD. **Peritonitis is the most significant complication of CAPD. It usually follows a benign course and is readily treatable with intraperitoneal antibiotics.** The main pathways of peritoneal infection are through the catheter lumen and across the abdominal wall through the sinus tract surrounding the catheter. Less commonly, infection can arise from the bowel, via the blood stream, and via the female genital tract. The commonest clinical features are abdominal tenderness and a cloudy dialysate. The commonest organisms causing peritonitis are *Staphylococcus epidermidis* and *Staphylococcus aureus*. Fungal and *Pseudomonas* peritonitis necessitate removal of the dialysis catheter. Recurrent episodes of peritonitis may cause peritoneal adhesions and loss of the peritoneal membrane surface area, resulting in inadequate dialysis.

Increasing duration of CAPD may cause loss of ultrafiltration. This results from a reduced volume of dialysate at the end of an exchange, with the inability to remove adequate amounts of extracellular fluid; thus the patient becomes fluid overloaded.

Nutritional complications of CAPD include a state of protein energy malnutrition resulting from protein and amino acid losses in the dialysate, which average 8 to 18 g/day in a stable CAPD patient. During episodes of peritonitis, this protein loss is much increased. The continuous supply of 100 to 200 g/day of glucose in the dialysate may predispose to hypertriglyceridemia, hyperinsulinemia, carbohydrate intolerance, and obesity in some patients. These potentially adverse metabolic effects have been considered factors limiting the widespread use of CAPD (Lindholm and Bergstrom, 1986).

CAPD also is accompanied by complications from the increased intra-abdominal pressure. These include dialysate leaks (which may predispose to peritonitis), massive hydrothorax caused by transdiaphragmatic dialysate leakage into the pleural cavity, abdominal hernias (e.g., umbilical and inguinal in 10% of patients), and back pain caused by alteration of body posture as a result of the presence of 2 to 3 L of dialysate in the peritoneal cavity.

Renal Transplantation

Renal transplantation is the preferred mode of renal replacement for most patients. **Absolute contraindications to a renal transplant are limited both to documented failure to comply with therapy and to critical coronary or cerebral arterial lesions not amenable to therapy.** Virtually all other patients on hemodialysis or peritoneal dialysis or with CRF about to require such therapy should at least be considered for renal transplantation. The surgical and medical aspects of renal transplantation are discussed in some detail elsewhere in this text.

REFERENCES

Abel RM, Beck CH, Abbott WM, et al: Improved survival from acute renal failure after treatment with intravenous essential L-amino acids and glucose. N Engl J Med 1973; 288:695–699.

Adamson JW, Eschbach JW: Management of the anemia of chronic renal failure with recombinant erythropoietin. Q J Med 1989; 73:1093–1101.

Ahlem J: Incidence of human chronic renal insufficiency. A study of the

incidence and pattern of renal insufficiency in adults during 1966–1971 in Gothenberg. Acta Med Scand 1975; suppl 582:1–50.
Ahmad S, Cole JJ: Lower morbidity associated with higher Kt/V in stable hemodialysis patients. (Abstract.) J Am Soc Nephrol 1990; 1:346.
Alfrey AC, Froment DH, Hammond WS: Beta$_2$-macroglobulin amyloidosis. Am Kidney Found Nephrol Lett 1989; 6:1–20.
Alfrey AC, Jenkins D, Groth CG: Resolution of hyperparathyroidism, renal osteodystrophy and metastatic calcification with transplantation. N Engl J Med 1968; 279:1358–1368.
Allgren RL: Randomized, double blind, placebo-controlled multicenter clinical trial of anaritide atrial natriuretic peptide in the treatment of acute renal failure. Presented at the International Society of Nephrology meeting, 1995, Madrid, Spain.
Anand-Srivastava MB, Vinay P, Genest J, et al: Effect of atrial natriuretic factor on adenylate cyclase in various nephron segments. Am J Physiol 1986; 20:F417.
Anderson RJ, Gabow PA, Gross PA: Urinary chloride concentration in acute renal failure. Miner Electrolyte Metab 1984; 10:92–97.
Anderson RJ, Linas SL, Berns AS, et al: Non-oliguric acute renal failure. N Engl J Med 1977; 296:1134–1137.
Anderson RJ, Schrier RW: Acute tubular necrosis. *In* Schrier RW, Gottschalk CW, eds: Diseases of the Kidney. Boston, Little, Brown and Company, 1992, pp 1287–1318.
Anderson S, Brenner BM: Progressive renal disease: A disorder of adaptation. Q J Med 1989; 70:185–90.
Appel BB: Aminoglycoside nephrotoxicity. Am J Med 1990; 159:427–443.
Arroyo V, Bernadi M, Epstein M, et al: Pathophysiology of ascites and functional renal failure in cirrhosis. J Hepatol 1988; 6:239–257.
Assael BM, Chiabrando C, Gagliardi L, et al: Prostaglandins and aminoglycoside nephrotoxicity. Toxicol Appl Pharmacol 1985; 78:386.
Badr KF, Kelley VE, Rennke HG, et al: Roles for thromboxane A_2 and leukotrienes in endotoxin-induced acute renal failure. Kidney Int 1986; 30:474.
Bailey RR, Natale R, Turnbull I, Linton AL: Protective effect of furosemide in acute tubular necrosis and acute renal failure. Clin Sci Mol Med 1973; 45:1–17.
Bakris GL, Burnett JC Jr: A role for calcium in radiocontrast-induced reductions in renal hemodynamics. Kidney Int 1985; 27:465.
Bakris GL, Kern SR: Renal dysfunction resulting from NSAIDs. Am Fam Physician 1989; 40:199–204.
Baldwin DS: Chronic glomerulonephritis: Non-immunological mechanisms of progressive glomerular damage. Kidney Int 1982; 21:109–120.
Ballard HS, Eisinger RP, Gallo G: Renal manifestations of the Henoch-Schoenlein syndrome in adults. Am J Med 1970; 49:328–335.
Barth RH: Urea modelling and Kt/V: A critical appraisal. Kidney Int 1993; 43(suppl 41):S252–S260.
Bennett WM, Pulliam JP: Cyclosporine nephrotoxicity. Ann Intern Med 1983; 305:267–273.
Bergstrom J, Alvestrand A, Bucht H, et al: Is chronic renal failure always progressive? *In* Berlyne GM, Giovannetti S, eds: The Progressive Nature of Renal Disease: Myths and Facts. Basel, Karger, 1989, pp 60–67.
Bommer J: Acquired renal cystic disease in uremic patients—In vivo demonstration by computed tomography. Clin Nephrol 1980; 14:299.
Bonventre JV: Mechanisms of ischemic acute renal failure: Nephrology Forum. Kidney Int 1993; 43:1160.
Brenner BM, Dworkin LD, Ichikawa I: Glomerular filtration. *In* Brenner BM, Rector FC, eds: The Kidney. Philadelphia, WB Saunders Company, 1986, p 93.
Brenner BM, Meyer TW, Hostetter TH: Dietary protein intake and the progressive nature of renal disease: The role of hemodynamically mediated injury in the pathogenesis of progressive glomerulosclerosis in aging, renal ablation and intrinsic renal disease. N Engl J Med 1982; 303:652–659.
Brezis M, Rosen S, Silva P, Epstein FH: Renal ischemia: A new perspective. Kidney Int 1984a; 26:375–383.
Brezis M, Rosen S, Silva P, Epstein FH: Transport activity modifies thick ascending limb damage in the isolated perfused kidney. Kidney Int 1984b; 25:65–72.
Burke TJ, Arnold PE, Gordon JA, et al: Protective effect of intrarenal calcium membrane blockers before or after renal ischemia. J Clin Invest 1984; 74:1830–1841.
Burke TJ, Cronin RE, Duchin KL, et al: Ischemia and tubule obstruction during acute renal failure in dogs: Mannitol in protection. Am J Physiol 1980; 238:F305-F314.
Cameron JS: Proteinuria and progression in human glomerular disease. Am J Nephrol 1990; 10(suppl 1):81–87.
Cameron JS: Membranous nephropathy and its treatment. Nephrol Dial Transplant 1992a; 7:72–79.
Cameron JS: Tubular and interstitial factors in the progression of glomerulonephritis. Pediatr Nephrol 1992b; 6:292–303.
Cantarovich F, Galli C, Benedetti L, et al: High dose furosemide in established acute renal failure. BMJ 1970; 4:449–450.
Cantarovich F, Locatelli A, Fernandez JC, et al: Furosemide in high doses in the treatment of acute renal failure. Postgrad Med J 1971; 47:13–17.
Caralps A, Lloveras J, Andreu J, et al: Urinary calculi in chronic dialysis patients. Lancet 1979; 2:1024.
Carlson JA, Harrington JT: Laboratory evaluation of renal function. *In* Schrier RW, Gottschalk CW, eds: Diseases of the Kidney. Boston, Little, Brown and Company, 1992, pp 364–371.
Casey KF, Machiedo GW, Lyons MJ, et al: Alteration of postischemic renal pathology by prostaglandin infusion. J Surg Res 1980; 29:1.
Chan L, Shapiro JI: NMR in the investigation and differential diagnosis of acute renal failure. Ann N Y Acad Sci 1987; 508:420–421.
Chapman AB, Johnson A, Gabow PA, Schrier RW: The renin-angiotensin-aldosterone system and autosomal dominant kidney disease. N Engl J Med 1990; 323:1091–1096.
Choi KH, Edelstein CL, Gengaro PE, et al: Hypoxia induced changes in phospholipase A_2 in rat proximal tubules. Evidence for multiple forms. Am J Physiol 1995; 269:F846–F853.
Conger JD: A controlled evaluation of prophylactic dialysis in post-traumatic acute renal failure. J Trauma 1975; 15:1056–1063.
Conger JD: Does hemodialysis delay recovery from acute renal failure? Semin Dialysis 1990; 3:146–148.
Conger JD, Falk SA, Robinette JB: Angiotensin II–induced changes in smooth muscle calcium in rat renal arterioles. J Am Soc Nephrol 1993; 3:1792–1803.
Conger JD, Robinette JB, Hammond WS: Differences in vascular reactivity in models of ischemic acute renal failure. Kidney Int 1991; 39:1087–1097.
Conger JD, Shultz P, Robinette JB: Increased NOS activity despite lack of response to endothelium-dependent vasodilators in post-ischemic acute renal failure in rats. J Clin Invest 1995; 96:631–638.
Couser WG, Stilmant MM: Mesangial lesions and focal glomerular sclerosis. Lab Invest 1975; 33:491–500.
Daudon M, Lacour B, Jungers P, et al: Urolithiasis in patients with end stage renal failure. J Urol 1992; 147:977–980.
deBold AJ, Borenstein HB, Veress AT, et al: A rapid and potent natriuretic response to intravenous injection of atrial myocardial extract in rats. Life Sci 1981; 28:89.
Diabetes Control and Complications Trial Research Group: The effect of intensive treatment of diabetes on the development and progression of long term complications in insulin-dependent diabetes mellitus. N Engl J Med 1993; 329:977–986.
Duke GJ, Bersten AD: Dopamine and renal salvage in the critically ill patient. Anaesth Intens Care 1994; 20:277–302.
Duke GJ, Briedis JH, Weaver RA: Renal support in critically ill patients: Low dose dopamine or low dose dobutamine? Crit Care Med 1994; 22:1919–1925.
Edelstein CL, Bates WD: Subtypes of acute postinfectious glomerulonephritis: A clinicopathological correlation. Clin Nephrol 1992; 38:311–317.
Edelstein CL, Welke H: Spontaneous kidney rupture presenting as an acute abdomen. S Afr Med J 1991; 79:52–53.
Edelstein CL, Wieder ED, Yaqoob MM, et al: The role of cysteine proteases in hypoxia-induced rat renal proximal tubular injury. Proc Natl Acad Sci 1995; 92:7662–7666.
El Nahas AM: Growth factors and glomerular sclerosis. Kidney Int 1992; 41(suppl 36):15–20.
El Nahas AM, Coles GA: Dietary treatment of chronic renal failure: Ten answered questions. Lancet 1986; 1:597–600.
Engler RL, Gruber HE: Adenosine; An autacoid. *In* Fozzard HA, ed: The Heart and Cardiovascular System, 2nd ed. New York, Raven Press, 1991, pp 1745–1764.
Eschbach JW, Adamson JW: Recombinant human erythropoietin: Implications for nephrology. Am J Dis Kidney 1988; 11:203–209.
Eschbach JW, Egrie JC, Downing MR, et al: Correction of anemia of end stage renal failure with recombinant human erythropoietin. Results of a combined phase I and II clinical trial. N Engl J Med 1987; 316:73–78.
Flancbaum L, Choban PS, Dasta JF: Quantitative effects of low-dose dopamine on urine output in oliguric surgical intensive care unit patients. Crit Care Med 1994; 22:61–65.
Froment DPH, Molitoris BA, Buddington B, et al: Site and mechanism of

enhanced gastrointestinal absorption of aluminum by citrate. Kidney Int 1989; 36:978–984.

Gagnon JA, Schrier RW, Weis TP, et al: Clearance of iothalamate-I-125 as a measure of glomerular filtration rate in the dog. J Appl Physiol 1971; 30:774–778.

Glasser RJ, Velosa JA, Michael AF: Experimental model of focal sclerosis. I. Relationship to protein excretion in aminonucleoside nephrosis. Lab Invest 1977; 36:519–562.

Glassock R, Babcock S: Glomerular diseases of the kidney. *In* Schrier RW, ed: Renal and Electrolyte Disorders. Boston, Little, Brown, and Company, 1990.

Gordge MP, Leaker BR, Rylance PB, Neild GH: Hemostatic activation and proteinuria as factors in the progression of chronic renal failure. Nephrol Dial Transplant 1991; 6:21–26.

Gretz N, Korb E, Strauch M: Low protein diet supplemented by ketoacids in chronic renal failure: A prospective study. Kidney Int 1983; 24(suppl 16):263–267.

Hakim RM, Wingard RL, Parker RA: Effect of dialysis membrane in the treatment of patients with acute renal failure. New Engl J Med 1994; 331:1338–1342.

Halperin ML: How much new bicarbonate is formed in the distal nephron in the process of net acid excretion? Kidney Int 1989; 35:1277–1281.

Handa SP, Madin PA: Diagnostic indices in acute renal failure. Can Med Assoc J 1967; 96:78–82.

Hayashi M, Kasau Y, Kawashima S: Preferential localization of calcium activated neutral proteases in epithelial tissues. Biochem Biophys Res Comm 1987; 148:567–574.

Hecht B, Siegel N, Adler M, et al: Prognostic indices in lupus nephritis. Medicine 1976; 55:163–181.

Hensby CN, Lewis PJ, Hilgard PJ, et al: Prostacyclin deficiency in thrombotic thrombocytopenic purpura. Lancet 1979; 2:728.

Hou SH, Bushinsky DA, Wish JB, et al: Hospital acquired renal insufficiency: A prospective study. Am J Med 1983; 74:243–248.

Huang CL, Lewicki J, Johnson LK, et al: Renal mechanism of action of rat atrial natriuretic factor. J Clin Invest 1985; 75:769.

Hughes J, Ward C, Peral B, et al: The polycystic kidney disease 1 (PKD1) gene encodes a novel protein with multiple cell recognition domains. Nat Genet 1995; 10:151–159.

Ibels LS, Alfrey AC, Haut L, Huffer WE: Preservation of function in experimental renal disease by dietary restriction of phosphate. N Engl J Med 1978; 298:122–126.

Ishikawa I: Acquired cystic disease: Mechanism and manifestations. Semin Nephrol 1991; 11:671.

Kaufman RP, Anner H, Kobzik L, et al: Vasodilator prostaglandins prevent renal damage after ischemia. Ann Surg 1987; 205:195–198.

Kelleher SP, Berl T: Acute renal failure in pregnancy. Sem Nephrol 1981; 1:61–68.

Kelleher SP, Robinette JB, Conger JD: Sympathetic nervous system in the loss of autoregulation in acute renal failure. Am J Physiol 1984; 15:F379–F386.

Kelleher SP, Robinette JB, Miller F, et al: Effect of hemorrhagic reduction in blood pressure on recovery from acute renal failure. Kidney Int 1987; 31:725–730.

Kincaid-Smith P: Plasmapheresis in rapidly progressive glomerulonephritis. Am J Med 1978; 65:564–568.

Klahr S, Buerkert J, Purkerson ML: Role of dietary factors in the progression of chronic renal disease. Kidney Int 1983; 24:579–587.

Klahr S, Levey AS, Beck GJ, et al: The Modification of Diet in Renal Disease Study Group. N Engl J Med 1994; 330:877–884.

Koga N, Nomura G, Yamagata Y, Koga T: Ureteric pain in patients with chronic renal failure on hemodialysis. Diagnostic approach with ultrasonography and computed tomography. Nephron 1982; 31:55.

Korbet SM: Anemia and erythropoietin in hemodialysis and continuous ambulatory peritoneal dialysis. Kidney Int 1993; 43(suppl 40):S111–S119.

Kramer P, Wigger W, Reiger J, et al: Arteriovenous hemofiltration: a new and simple method for treatment of overhydrated patients resistant to diuretics. Klin Wochenschr 1977; 55:1121–1122.

Kribben A, Wieder ED, Wetzels JFM, et al: Evidence for role of cytosolic free calcium in hypoxia-induced proximal tubule injury. J Clin Invest 1994; 93:1922.

Lefer AM: Physiologic and pathophysiologic role of cyclo-oxygenase metabolites of arachidonic acid in circulating disease states. *In* Mehta JI, ed: Cardiovascular Clinics: Thrombosis and Platelets in Myocardial Ischemia. Philadelphia, F.A. Davis Company, 1987, pp 85–99.

Lefer AM, Lefer DJ: Pharmacology of the endothelium in ischemia—Reperfusion and circulatory shock. Annu Rev Pharmocol Toxicol 1993; 33:71–90.

Leonard CD, Luke RG, Siegel RR: Parenteral essential amino acids in acute renal failure. Urology 1975; 6:154–157.

Levinsky NG: Pathophysiology of acute renal failure. N Engl J Med 1977; 296:1453–1457.

Lewis EJ, Hunsicker LG, Bain RP, Rohde RD: The effect of angiotensin converting enzyme inhibition on diabetic nephropathy. The collaborative study group. N Engl J Med 1993; 329:1456–1462.

Lieberthal W, Wolf EF, Rennke HG: Renal ischemia and reperfusion impair endothelium-dependent vascular relaxation. Am J Physiol 1989; 256: F894–F900.

Lindholm B, Bergstrom J: Nutritional aspects of CAPD. *In* Gokal R, ed: Continuous Ambulatory Peritoneal Dialysis. London, Churchill Livingstone, 1986, pp 228–264.

Losito A, Fortunati F, Zampi I, Del-Favero A: Impaired renal functional reserve and albuminuria in essential hypertension. BMJ 1988; 296:1562–1544.

Maguire WC, Anderson RJ: Continuous arteriovenous hemofiltration in the intensive care unit. J Crit Care 1986; 1:54–56.

Martinez-Maldonado M, Yium J, Suki WN, Eknoyan G: Renal complications in multiple myeloma: Pathophysiology and some aspects of clinical management. J Chronic Dis 1971; 24:221–237.

Matthys E, Patton M, Osgood R, et al: Alterations in vascular function and morphology in ischemic ARF. Kidney Int 1983; 23:717–724.

Medical Research Council: Trial of treatment of hypertension; principal results. BMJ 1985; 291:97–104.

Mehta RL: Therapeutic alternatives to renal replacement for critically ill patients in acute renal failure. Semin Nephrol 1994; 14:64–82.

Miller TR, Anderson RJ, Linas SL, et al: Urinary diagnostic indices in acute renal failure. Ann Intern Med 1978; 89:47–50.

Mitch WE, Walser M, Buffington GA, Lemann J: A simple method of estimating progression of chronic renal failure. Lancet 1976; 2:1326–1328.

Molitoris BA: The potential role of ischaemia in renal disease progression. Kidney Int 1992; 41(36, suppl):21–25.

Molitoris BA, Froment DH, Mackenzie TA, et al: Citrate: A major factor in the toxicity of orally administered aluminum compounds. Kidney Int 1989; 36:949–953.

Moorhead JF, El Nahas AM, Chan MK, Varghese Z: Lipid nephrotoxicity in chronic progressive glomerular and tubulointerstitial disease. Lancet 1982; 2:1309–1312.

Morris PJ: Renal transplantation: Current status. *In* Robinson RR, ed: 9th International Congress of Nephrology. Springer-Verlag, New York, 1986, p 1627.

Nakamoto M, Shapiro JI, Chan L, Schrier RW: The in vitro and in vivo protective effect of atriopeptin III in ischemic acute renal failure in the rat. J Clin Invest 1987; 80:698–705.

Narrins RG, Cohen JJ: Bicarbonate therapy for organic acidosis. The case for its continued use. Ann Intern Med 1987; 106:615–617.

Nath K, Hostetter M, Hostetter T: Pathophysiology of chronic tubulointerstitial disease in rats: Interaction of dietary acid load, ammonia and complement. J Clin Invest 1987; 79:667–675.

Nathan CF: Secretory products of macrophages. Clin Invest 1987; 79:319–326.

Neilson EG: Pathogenesis and therapy of interstitial nephritis. Kidney Int 1989; 35:1257–1265.

Nolan CR, Anger MS, Kelleher SP: Eosinophiluria—A new method of detection and definition of the clinical spectrum. N Engl J Med 1986; 315:1516–1519.

Nolan CR, Kelleher SP: Eosinophiluria. Clin Lab Med 1988; 8:555–565.

Nolph KD: Peritoneal dialysis. *In* Drukker W, Parsons FM, Maher JF, eds: Replacement of Renal Function by Dialysis. Boston, Martinus Nijhoff (Kluwer), 1978, p 2770.

Notghi A, Anderton JL: Effect of nifedipine and mefruside on renal reserve in hypertensive patients. Postgrad Med J 1988; 64:856–859.

Old CW, Lehrener LM: Prevention of radiocontrast induced acute renal failure with mannitol. Lancet 1980; 1:885.

Oliver JA, Sciacca RR, Pinto J, et al: Participation of the prostaglandins in the control of renal blood flow during acute reduction of cardiac output in the dog. J Clin Invest 1981; 67:229.

Oren A, Husdan H, Cheng PT, et al: Calcium oxalate kidney stones in patients on continuous ambulatory peritoneal dialysis. Kidney Int 1984; 25:534.

Paller MS: Drug-induced nephropathies. Med Clin North Am 1990; 74:909–917.

Papanicolaou N, Darlametsos J, Hatziantoniou C, et al: Partial protection against acute renal failure by Efamol. Prog Clin Biol Res 1989; 301:271.

Parving HH, Noer I, Deckert T, et al: The effect of metabolic regulation on microvascular permeability to small and large molecules in short term juvenile diabetes. Diabetologia 1976; 12:161–166.

Penzotti SC, Mattocks AM: Effects of dwell time, volume of dialysis fluid and added accelerators on peritoneal dialysis of urea. J Pharm Sci 1971; 60:1520–1533.

Ponticelli C, Zucchelli P, Imbarciati E, et al: Controlled trial of methylprednisolone and chlorambucil in idiopathic membranous nephropathy. N Engl J Med 1984; 310:946–950.

Porile JL, Bakris GL, Garella S: Acute interstitial nephritis with glomerulopathy due to nonsteroidal anti-inflammatory agents: A review of its clinical spectrum and effects of steroid therapy. J Clin Pharmacol 1990; 30:468–475.

Portilla D, Mandel LJ, Bar-Sagi D, Millington DS: Anoxia induces phospholipase A_2 activation in rabbit renal proximal tubules. Am J Physiol 1992; 262:F354.

Raskin NH, Fishman RA: Neurological disorders in renal failure (part 1 of 2). N Engl J Med 1976a; 294:143–148.

Raskin NH, Fishman RA: Neurological disorders in renal failure (part 2 of 2). N Engl J Med 1976b; 294:204–210.

Rasmussen HH, Ibels LS: Acute renal failure. Multivariate analysis of causes and risk factors. Am J Med 1982; 73:211–219.

Ravnskov U: Focal glomerular lesions in glomerulonephritis may be secondary to interstitial damage. Am J Kidney Dis 1988; 12:250–251.

Risdon RA, Sloper JC, de Wardener HE: Relationship between renal function and histological changes found in renal biopsy specimens from patients with persistent glomerular nephritis. Lancet 1968; 1:363–366.

Rutherford WE, Blondin J, Miller JP, et al: Chronic progressive renal disease: Rate of change of serum creatinine concentration. Kidney Int 1977; 11:62–70.

Saido TC, Sorimachi H, Suzuki K: Calpain: New perspectives in molecular diversity and physiological-pathological involvement. FASEB J 1994; 8:814–822.

Sargent JA: Control of dialysis by a single-pool urea model. The National Cooperative Dialysis Study. Kidney Int 1983; 23(suppl 13):S19–S25.

Scherberich JE, Wolf G, Stuckhardt C, et al: Characterization and clinical role of glomerular and tubular proteases from human kidney. Adv Exp Med Biol 1988; 240:275–282.

Schetz M, Lauwers PM, Ferdinande P: Extracorporeal treatment of acute renal failure in the intensive care unit: A critical view. Intensive Care Med 1989; 15:349–357.

Schiffl H, Lang SM, Konig A, et al: Biocompatible membranes in acute renal failure: Prospective case-controlled study. Lancet 1994; 344:570–572.

Schrier RW: Renal and Electrolyte Disorders, 4th ed. Boston, Little, Brown, and Company, 1992.

Schrier RW, Conger JD: Acute renal failure: Pathogenesis, diagnosis, and management. *In* Schrier RW, ed: Renal and Electrolyte Disorders. Boston, Little, Brown and Company, 1986; p 423.

Schrier RW, Shapiro JI: Drug induced acute renal failure. *In* Serono Symposium on Acute Renal Failure. New York, Raven Press, 1985, p 242.

Schwertslag U, Schrier RW, Wilson PD: Time dependent protective effect of calcium channel blockers on anoxia and hypoxia-induced proximal tubular injury. J Pharmacol Exp Ther 1986; 238:119–124.

Shapiro JI, Anderson RJ: Urinary diagnostic indices in acute renal failure. Am Kidney Found Nephrol Lett 1984; 1:13–16.

Shapiro JI, Mathew A, Whalen M, et al: Different effects of sodium bicarbonate and an alternate buffer [Carbicarb] in normal volunteers. J Crit Care 1990; 5:157–160.

Shapiro JI, Schrier RW: Clinical aspects of acute renal failure. *In* Anonymous, ed: Proceedings of the 30th Congress of the Japanese Society of Dialysis Therapeutics. Raven Press, New York, 1985, p 45.

Shaw SG, Weidmann P, Holder J, et al: Atrial natriuretic peptide protects against acute ischemic renal failure in the rat. J Clin Invest 1987; 80:1232–1237.

Simon P: Evolution of dialytic therapy. Contrib Nephrol 1989; 71:10–16.

Solez L, Marel-Maroger L, Sraer J: The morphology of acute tubular necrosis in man. Analysis of 57 renal biopsies and comparison with glycerol model. Medicine (Baltimore) 1979; 58:362–376.

Stacpoole DW: Lactic acidosis: The case against bicarbonate therapy. Ann Intern Med 1986; 105:276–279.

Stahl RAK, Kanz L, Kudelka S: Cyclosporine and renal prostaglandin E_2 production. Ann Intern Med 1985; 103:474.

Stenvinkel P, Alvestrand A, Bergstrom J: Factors influencing progression in patients with chronic renal failure. J Intern Med 1989; 22:183–188.

Stott RB, Cameron JS, Ogg CS, Bewick M: Why the persistently high mortality in acute renal failure? Lancet 1972; 2:75–79.

Striker GE, Schainuck LI, Cutler RE, Benditt EP: Structural-functional correlations in renal disease. A method for assaying and classifying histopathologic changes in renal disease. Hum Pathol 1970; 1:615–630.

Swann RC, Merrill JP: The clinical course of acute renal failure. Medicine 1953; 32:215–293.

Ter-Wee PM, van-Ballegooie E, Rosman JB, et al: Renal reserve filtration capacity in patients with type 1 (insulin-dependent) diabetes mellitus. Nephrol Dial Transplant 1987; 2:504–599.

Turi S, Beattie TJ, Belch JJF, et al: Disturbances of prostacyclin metabolism in children with hemolytic uremic syndrome and in first degree relatives. Clin Nephrol 1986a; 25:193.

Turi S, Belch JJF, Beattie TJ, et al: Abnormalities of vascular prostaglandins in Henoch-Schönlein purpura. Arch Dis Child 1986b; 61:773.

Tzamaloukas AH: Diagnosis and management of bone disorders in chronic renal failure and dialyzer patients. Med Clin North Am 1990; 74:961–974.

Ueda M, Becker AE, Tsukada T, et al: Fibrocellular tissue response after percutaneous transluminal coronary angioplasty. An immunocytochemical analysis of the cellular composition. Circulation 1991; 83:1327–1332.

Vendegna TJ, Anderson RJ: Are dopamine and/or dobutamine renoprotective in intensive care unit patients? Crit Care Med 1994; 22:1893–1894.

Venkatachalam MA, Bernard DB, Donohoe JF, Levinsky NG: Ischemic damage and repair in the rat proximal tubule: Differences among the S1, S2 and S3 segments. Kidney Int 1978; 14:31–49.

Viberti GC, Hill RD, Jarrett RD, et al: Microalbuminuria as a predictor of clinical nephropathy in insulin dependent diabetes mellitus. Lancet 1982; 1:1430–1432.

Vittinghus E, Mogensen CE: Graded exercise and protein excretion in diabetic men and the effect of insulin treatment. Kidney Int 1982; 21:725–729.

von-Herrath D, Saupe J, Hirschberg R, et al: Glomerular filtration rate in response to an acute protein load. Blood Purif 1988; 6:264–268.

Wagner K, Albrecht S, Neumayer HH: Prevention of post-transplant acute tubular necrosis by the calcium antagonist diltiazem: A prospective randomized study. Am J Nephrol 1987; 7:287.

Wagner K, Albrecht S, Neumayer HH: Prevention of delayed graft function in cadaveric kidney transplantation by a calcium antagonist. Preliminary results of two prospective randomized trials. Transpl Proc 1988; 18:510–517.

Weinberg JM: The cell biology of ischemic renal injury. Kidney Int 1991; 39:476.

Werb R, Clark WF, Lindsay RM, et al: Protective effect of prostaglandins (PGE_2) in glycerol induced acute renal failure in rats. Clin Sci Mol Med 1978; 55:505.

Wetzels JFM, Wang X, Gengaro PE, et al: Glycine protection against hypoxic but not phospholipase A2 induced injury in rat proximal tubules. Am J Physiol 1993a; 264(33):F94.

Wetzels JFM, Yu L, Wang X, et al: Calcium modulation and cell injury in isolated rat proximal tubules. J Pharmacol Exp Ther 1993b; 267:176.

Williams PS, Fass G, Bone JM: Renal pathology and proteinuria determine progression in untreated mild/moderate chronic renal failure. Q J Med 1988; 67:343–354.

Wilson PD, Hartz PA: Mechanisms of cyclosporin A toxicity in defined cultures of renal tubule epithelia: A role for cysteine proteases. Cell Biol Int Reports 1991; 15:1243–1258.

Wilson PD, Schrier RW: Nephron segment and calcium as determinants of anoxic cell death in primary renal cell cultures. Kidney Int 1986; 29:1172.

Yaqoob MM, Edelstein CL, Alkhunaizi A, et al: Identification and subcellular localization of nitric oxide synthase (NOS) in rat proximal tubules. J Am Soc Nephrol 1995; 6:993.

Yaqoob MM, Edelstein CL, Alkhunaizi A, et al: Nitric oxide kinetics during hypoxia in proximal tubules: Effects of acidosis and glycine. Kidney Int. In press.

Yoshida Y, Fogo A, Ichikawa I: Glomerular hemodynamic changes vs. hypertrophy in experimental glomerular sclerosis. Kidney Int 1989; 35:654–660.

Yu L, Gengaro PE, Niederberger M, et al: Nitric oxide: A mediator in rat tubular hypoxia/reoxygenation injury. Proc Nat Acad Sci 1994; 91:1691.

Zipser RD, Radvan GH, Kronborg IT, et al: Urinary thromboxane B_2 and prostaglandin E_2 in the hepatorenal syndrome: Evidence for increased vasoconstrictor and decreased vasodilator factor. Gastroenterology 1983; 84:697.

9

PATHOPHYSIOLOGY OF URINARY TRACT OBSTRUCTION

Frederick A. Gulmi, M.D.
Diane Felsen, Ph.D.
E. Darracott Vaughan, Jr., M.D.

The basic function of the kidney is the formation of an ultrafiltrate that is free of protein and yet contains appropriate amounts of water, electrolytes, and the end products of metabolic pathways to maintain homeostasis. Once this occurs, the remaining portions of the urinary tract function either to eliminate and/or store urine. When there is a structural impedance to the flow of urine anywhere along that tract, it can be described as *obstructive uropathy.* **The term *obstructive nephropathy* should be reserved for the damage to the renal parenchyma that results from an obstruction to the flow of urine anywhere along the urinary tract.** The term *hydronephrosis* is derived from *hydro* (from the Greek *hydor,* water), *nephros* (Greek for kidney), and *osis* (condition) and is therefore defined as dilatation of the renal pelvis and calyces resulting from obstruction to the flow of urine. Because dilatation of the renal pelvis and calyces can occur without obstruction, this definition is not completely accurate. ***Hydronephrosis* should be used as a descriptive term referring simply to the presence of dilatation of the pelvis and calyces and not to the etiology of that dilatation.** The terms *obstructive uropathy* and *hydronephrosis* should not be used interchangeably.

Ureteral obstruction with subsequent hydronephrosis is a common clinical occurrence. The incidence of hydronephrosis was found in a general autopsy series to be 3.1% among 59,064 patients ranging in age from birth to 80 years (Bell, 1946). In women, obstruction is more likely to occur at a younger age as a result of pregnancy or uterine cancer. In men, prostate disease is a major cause of hydronephrosis. More recently, in a general series of 3172 autopsies of children, 2.5% were found to have urinary tract abnormalities, of which 35% were hydronephrosis or hydroureter (Tan et al, 1994). The extrinsic causes of obstruction are detailed in Chapter 10. In this chapter, we describe the pathophysiologic events that take place within the kidney during obstruction of one or both renal units. Obstruction is reviewed in terms of radiologic, anatomic, physiologic, and molecular changes that occur. Much of this information has been presented in previous editions; however, the present chapter has been reorganized and also contains new information on vasoactive and profibrotic mediators that has not been presented previously.

PATIENT PRESENTATION

Symptoms

Urinary tract obstruction can result in a wide range of symptoms, from asymptomatic (incidentally discovered) to the classic picture of renal colic. **The symptom complex varies according to (1) the time interval over which the obstruction occurs (i.e., acute or chronic), (2) whether the obstruction is unilateral or bilateral, (3) the etiology of the obstruction (i.e., intrinsic versus extrinsic), and (4) whether the obstruction is complete or partial.**

Acute obstruction is usually associated with flank pain that may radiate into the groin and/or the ipsilateral thigh. Patients commonly experience nausea, vomiting, and chills. If the renal unit is infected, high fevers may also be present. It is more common to have acute unilateral occlusion than bilateral ureteral occlusion; however, if acute bilateral obstruction occurs, the patient also may experience a sudden onset of anuria. Unilateral and bilateral obstruction can develop over long periods of time, in which case the patients are usually asymptomatic, making the diagnosis of obstruction more difficult and, in many cases, incidental. When the obstruction is bilateral and chronic, the patients may present with nonspecific complaints of an increase in abdominal girth (pants do not fit), ankle edema, malaise, anorexia, headaches, weight gain, fatigue, and shortness of breath. They may also have symptoms reflective of uremia, such as mental status changes, tremors, and gastrointestinal bleeding. Patients with either a solitary kidney or a nonfunctioning contralateral renal unit can present with unilateral obstruction and symptoms of uremia.

When the obstruction is unilateral and chronic, the patient may complain of intermittent flank pain during periods of forced diuresis, such as after the consumption of alcohol, a known diuretic. If there is hydronephrosis associated with blunt trauma, the presenting symptom can also be gross hematuria. The extrinsic causes of obstruction usually have a more insidious and hence symptom-free presentation, whether they are unilateral or bilateral. These obstructions are usually detected incidentally during the routine clinical work-up of the primary disease process.

A history of the patient's voiding habits is also significant. These can vary from symptoms of a weak and intermittent urine stream, urgency, urgency incontinence, overflow incontinence, and nocturia to barely any urination at all (i.e., complete obstruction). **Finally, the patients may also notice rather profound increases in their urine output out of proportion to their fluid intake, which results from poor renal concentrating ability.**

Clinical Signs and Biochemical Findings

The clinical signs of urinary tract obstruction are somewhat nonspecific. Obstruction is occasionally associated with an abdominal mass palpable during physical examination, which on rare occasions can be visible. The patient may also have signs of volume overload, such as bipedal edema, pulmonary congestion, and hypertension. Laboratory data may include hematuria (microscopic and/or gross), proteinuria, crystalluria, pyuria, and urinary casts. When chronic obstruction is the predominant clinical picture, the urinary diagnostic indices are most often similar to those seen with acute tubular necrosis: an elevated urinary sodium concentration, a decreased urine osmolality, and a decreased urine-to-plasma creatinine ratio. If the obstruction is more acute and not accompanied by renal failure, the urinary indices can resemble those of prerenal azotemia: a low urinary sodium concentration and an increased urine osmolality (Wilson and Klahr, 1993). The serum chemistry studies may demonstrate elevations of serum blood urea nitrogen (BUN) and creatinine, hyperkalemia, and acidosis.

When patients experience acute obstruction in the presence of bacterial urinary tract infection, they may present with signs and symptoms of pyelonephritis or systemic sepsis. **Obstruction coexisting with infection is a true urologic emergency, and appropriate imaging studies (excretory urogram or renal ultrasonography) must be**

performed on an emergency basis. The obstruction must be relieved by either percutaneous nephrostomy or a ureteral stent.

The rationale for immediate relief of obstruction is based on the physiology of fluid reabsorption during obstruction. After the onset of obstruction, there is increased intrapelvic pressure, resulting in pyelolymphatic and pyelovenous urine backflow as well as possible fornix rupture and extravasation (Narath, 1940; Stenberg et al, 1988). Accordingly, there is direct movement of urine and bacteria into the vascular system during obstruction, resulting in a life-threatening situation. In chronic obstruction, despite a marked reduction in glomerular filtration rate (GFR) and renal blood flow (RBF) (Vaughan et al, 1970a), urine continues to move into the vascular system (Naber and Madsen, 1974).

DIAGNOSIS

Excretory Urography

For the urologist, the intravenous urogram (IVU) has been the gold standard for the detection of ureteral obstruction in patients who have normal renal function, have no allergies to contrast material, and are not pregnant. The urogram can provide both functional and anatomic details of the obstruction, as opposed to ultrasonography, which provides more anatomic detail.

Acute urinary obstruction is visualized on the IVU by (1) the obstructive nephrogram, (2) a delay in filling of the collecting system with contrast material, (3) dilatation of the collecting system, possibly with an increase in renal size, and (4) possible fornix rupture with urinary extravasation (Talner, 1990).

Chronic cases of ureteral obstruction are usually visualized by ureteral dilatation, tortuosity, and a standing column of contrast material in the ureter to the point of obstruction. The kidney may demonstrate marked parenchymal thinning (either segmental or complete), calyceal crescents, and the soap-bubble nephrogram (Talner, 1990).

Ultrasonography

The renal sonogram is a good starting point for evaluating the renal units of patients who have azotemia, have contrast material–induced allergy, are pregnant, or are in the pediatric age group. Significant information can be obtained about both the renal parenchyma and the collecting system with no exposure to radiation or contrast material–induced nephrotoxicity or anaphylaxis.

Hydronephrosis will appear as a dilated collecting system separating the normally echogenic renal sinus, creating an anechoic central area surrounded by parenchyma. Echoes within the collecting system may indicate an infection (pyonephrosis), hemorrhage, or a lesion of the transitional mucosa, among other diagnoses. The thickness of the renal parenchyma can be measured as an indicator of the duration of obstruction; the degree of hydronephrosis should not be equated with the duration of obstruction.

There are several pitfalls to the use of ultrasonography for diagnosing obstruction. Both the underdiagnosis of hydronephrosis—that is, missing an obstruction (false negative) **and the overdiagnosis of obstruction due to the presence of hydronephrosis** (false positive) **are possible.** Sonograms can be false negative as a result of an acute onset of obstruction, an intrarenal collecting system, dehydration, and the misinterpretation of caliectasis for renal

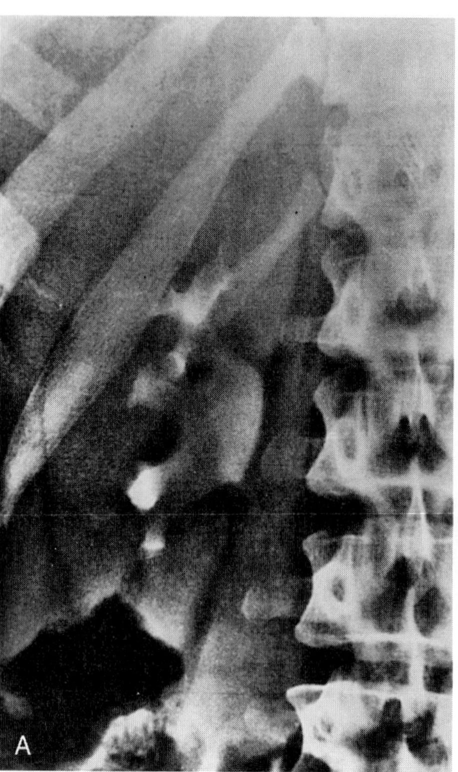

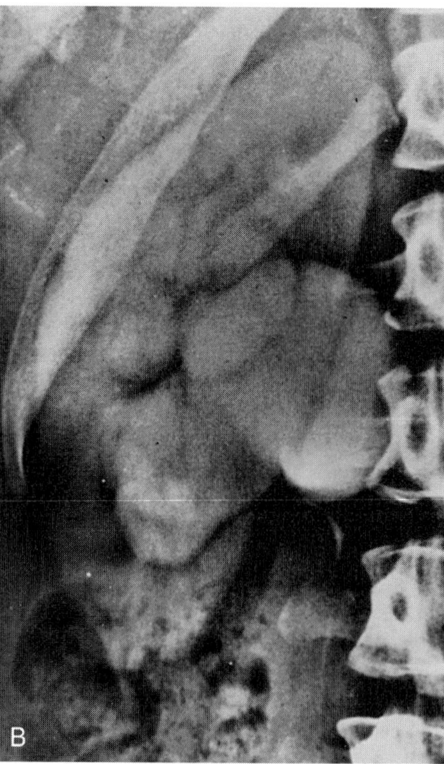

Figure 9–1. Young patient with intermittent flank pain. Intravenous pyelograms show *(A)* normal anatomy before diuresis and *(B)* ureteropelvic junction obstruction after diuretic challenge.

cortical cysts. Sonograms can be false positive for obstruction as a result of a capacious extrarenal pelvis, parapelvic cysts, vesicoureteral reflux, and a high urine flow state (Talner, 1990). Therefore, although an excellent tool for the initial evaluation of selected patients with suspected renal obstruction, the sonogram should be interpreted carefully and must be consistent with the overall clinical picture.

Laing and colleagues (1985) performed a prospective study of 20 patients to evaluate the usefulness of ultrasonography versus excretory urography in patients with acute renal colic. The ultrasonography failed to detect hydronephrosis in 7 of 20 patients (35%) with proven acute obstruction on excretory urography. These investigators concluded that although ultrasonography may be useful for the evaluation of hydronephrosis in the chronically obstructed kidney, it may not be efficacious in the evaluation of patients with acute urinary obstruction. **Accordingly, if a patient initially is evaluated for obstruction with ultrasonography and findings are negative but symptoms persist, excretory urography should follow.**

In order to identify intermittent obstruction as a cause of flank or abdominal pain that is episodic, studies should be obtained while the patient is experiencing symptoms (Fig. 9–1*A* and *B*).

Diuretic Renography

The diuretic renogram is becoming more widely utilized than excretory urography for evaluation of the dilated collecting system. It provides a noninvasive measure of the relative renal function and has the ability to wash out the radiopharmaceutic agent from the dilated collecting system. There is a marked reduction in radiation dose in comparison with excretory urography, and there is no potential for contrast material–induced nephrotoxicity (Taylor and Nally, 1995).

The most widely used radiopharmaceutic agents are (1) tubular tracers—iodine-131-ortho-iodohippurate (OIH) and ^{99m}Tc-mercaptoacetyltriglycine (MAG3)—and (2) glomerular tracers, namely ^{99m}Tc diethylenetriaminepentaacetic acid (DTPA). For evaluating obstruction, the radiopharmaceutic agent of choice today is MAG3, because it is more efficiently extracted by the kidney than is DTPA, delivers a lower dose of radiation to the obstructed kidney than does OIH, and is excreted by the same portion of the tubule that responds to furosemide (Taylor and Eshima, 1988; Taylor and Nally, 1995). MAG3 has been shown to provide better counting statistics and visualization of the anatomy of obstruction than do OIH and other radiopharmaceutic agents (Eshima and Taylor, 1992).

The technique of patient preparation and the timing of the administration of the diuretic when diuretic renography is performed are extremely important. The patients should be well hydrated before the procedure. An intravenous line may be started before the procedure to initiate hydration (Conway, 1992; Taylor and Nally, 1995). Patients who can void spontaneously do not require bladder catheterization. Those who cannot void spontaneously do require bladder catheterization (1) to ensure adequate bladder drainage, (2) to reduce false-positive results, and (3) to decrease the radiation dose to the bladder and gonads. The patient's renal function is extremely important when the results from a diuretic renogram are interpreted. **The ability of the kidneys to generate a sufficient diuretic-induced flow rate to detect renal obstruction depends on the patient's creatinine clearance** (Fig. 9–2). In the presence of a reduced creatinine clearance, it may be necessary to increase the diuretic dose to achieve an adequate flow rate and reduce the possibility of a false-negative result (Upsdell et al, 1988).

The timing of the administration of the diuretic after the administration of the radiopharmaceutic agent has been carefully worked out. Brown and co-workers (1992) determined that the urinary flow rate is 3.5 ml/minute greater at 15 to 18 minutes after intravenous furosemide than at 3 to 6 minutes after a diuretic (Fig. 9–3). **The traditional diuretic renogram is performed by administering the radiopharmaceutic agent and obtaining images, followed 20 minutes later by intravenous administration of the diuretic, and then measuring the $T_{1/2}$ for the clearance of the tracer from the collecting system.** O'Reilly and associates referred to this technique as the F+20 diuretic renogram (O'Reilly et al, 1979; O'Reilly, 1992). Figure 9–4 depicts the various outcomes from the F+20 diuretic renogram. **The diagnostic dilemma arises with the patients who**

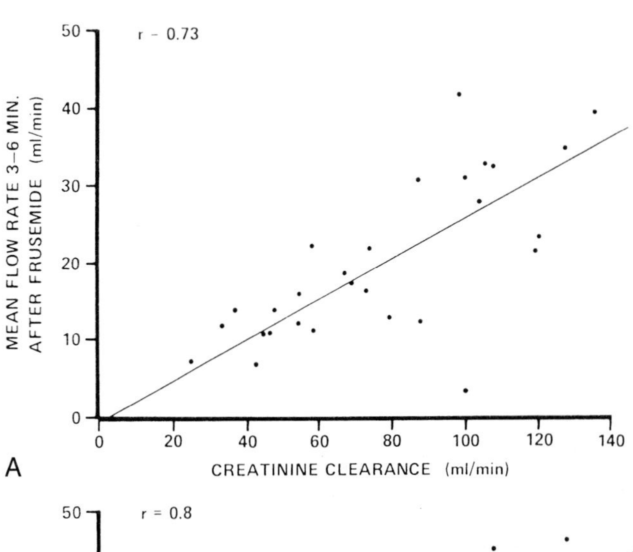

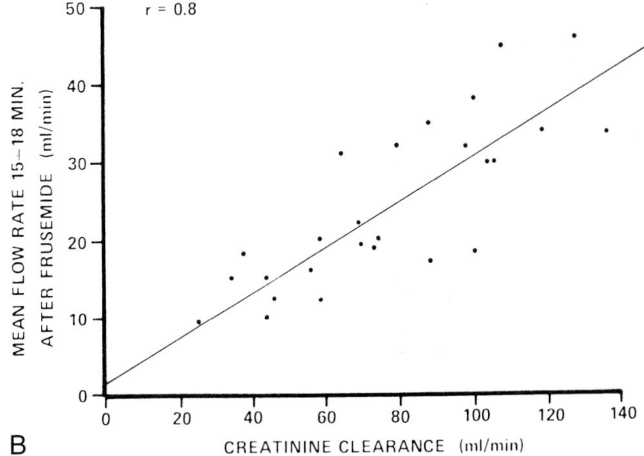

Figure 9–2. *A,* Scattergram of correlation between mean urinary flow rates 3 to 6 minutes after diuretic administration and creatinine clearance in 29 patients. *B,* Scattergram of correlation between mean urinary flow rates 15 to 18 minutes after diuretic administration and creatinine clearance in 29 patients. (From Upsdell SM, Leeson SM, Brooman PJC, O'Reilly PH: Br J Urol 1988; 61:14–18.)

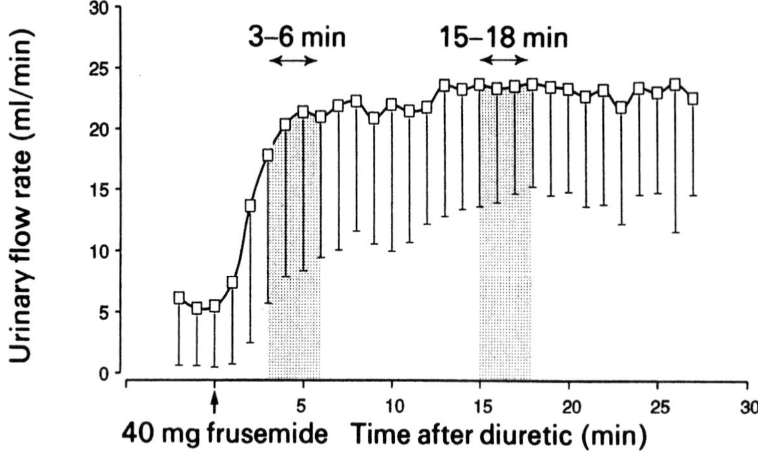

Figure 9–3. Mean urinary flow rates following diuretic injection. Error bars indicate standard deviation. (From Brown SCW, Upsdell SM, O'Reilly PH: Br J Urol 1992; 69:121–125.)

show a partial excretory response; this indicates either an inability to excrete the radioisotope because of poor renal function or a truly partially obstructed system (Group IIIa in Fig. 9–4). Upsdell and associates (1988) were able to convert this equivocal response to the diuretic into a washout response by administering the diuretic 15 minutes before administering the radiopharmaceutic agent (i.e., F − 15) (Fig. 9–5). Some centers now routinely use the F − 15 technique for diuretic renography when renal obstruction is suspected. Others use the F + 20 technique for their routine diuretic renograms, reserving the F − 15 technique for use when the F + 20 method demonstrates partial obstruction.

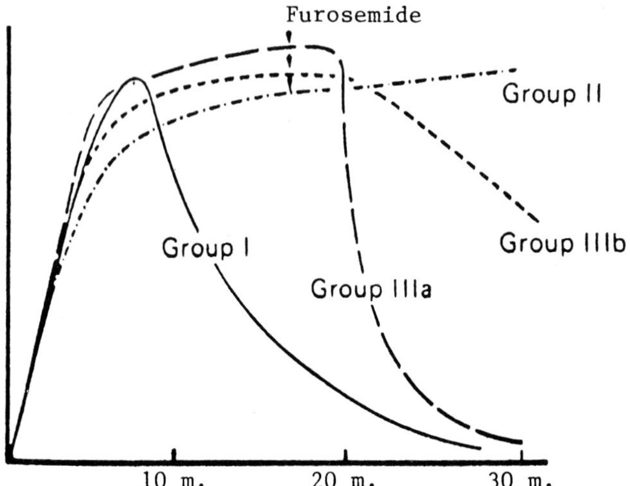

Figure 9–4. Gamma camera renograms obtained from computer-generated regions of interest with ^{123}I-ortho-iodohippurate (OIH) demonstrate four responses. The group I renogram is normal. Because obstruction is sometimes unmasked by diuretic administration, O'Reilly and associates recommended a repeat renogram 15 minutes after diuretic administration. A second normal group I renogram rules out obstruction. Progressive accumulation (group II) despite administration of furosemide at about 20 minutes after tracer injection confirms obstruction. On the other hand, rapid emptying after diuretic administration (group IIIA) despite an initial rise in the renogram curve indicates dilatation without obstruction. Finally, an increasing curve with a partial excretory response may indicate either partial obstruction or renal dysfunction with an inability to respond to the diuretic (group IIIB). (From O'Reilly PH, Shields RA, Testa JH, eds: Nuclear Medicine in Urology and Nephrology, 2nd ed. London, Butterworths, 1986, pp 91–108.)

Data from the diuretic renogram can be interpreted either visually or by quantitative measurements of the $T_{1/2}$ diuretic response (Conway, 1992). There are many factors that influence the $T_{1/2}$, including (1) renal function, which includes the level of renal maturity; (2) compliance of the collecting system; (3) the volume of the collecting system; (4) hydration of the patient; (5) presence or absence of a bladder catheter; (6) the radiopharmaceutic agent; and (7) the dose of the diuretic (Fine, 1991; Taylor and Nally, 1995). It is generally accepted that a clearance of the radiopharmaceutic agent from the renal pelvis with a $T_{1/2}$ of less than 10 minutes is normal; some experts consider a $T_{1/2}$ of less than 15 minutes normal. Clearance of tracer with a $T_{1/2}$ between 15 and 20 minutes is considered equivocal, and a $T_{1/2}$ greater than 20 minutes indicates an obstruction (O'Reilly, 1986; Taylor and Nally, 1995).

Whitaker Test

The Whitaker test was considered the gold standard for the evaluation of upper urinary tract dilatation. It provided urodynamic evidence of a mechanical obstruction of the upper urinary tract at a given flow rate. With the advent of the diuretic renogram and some of the newer radiopharmaceutic agents, the Whitaker test is not often utilized clinically. The Whitaker test is performed with the patient placed on a fluoroscopy table in the prone position. Before the patient is positioned prone, a bladder catheter is placed and connected to a pressure transducer for continuous monitoring of intravesical pressures with changes in renal pressure. A renal cannula (18 gauge) is then inserted and connected to a pressure transducer. A combination of saline and contrast is administered via the renal cannula at a rate of 10 ml/minute. Bladder pressure is monitored throughout the procedure, and its relationship to changes in renal pressure can be significant. Contrast material is given along with the saline, making fluoroscopic monitoring of the anatomic site of the obstruction possible (Whitaker, 1990).

Results are separated into three categories (Whitaker and Buxton-Thomas, 1984):

1. Pressure < 15 cm H_2O = nonobstructed.
2. Pressures of 15 to 22 cm H_2O = equivocal.
3. Pressures > 22 cm H_2O = obstructed.

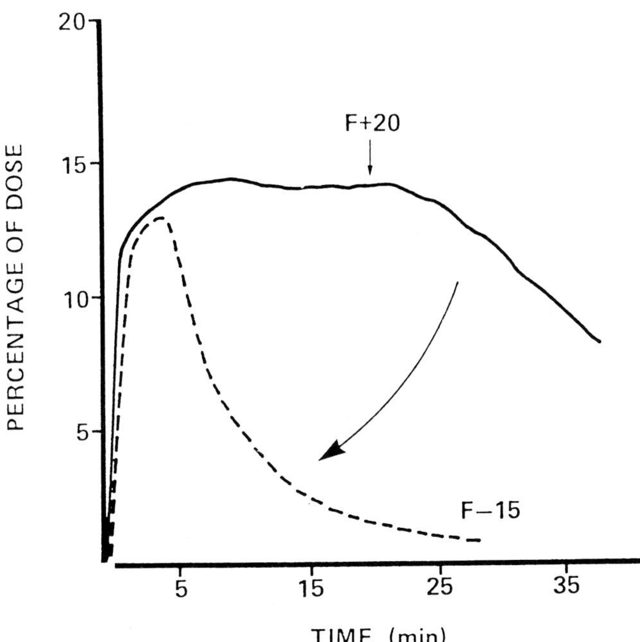

Figure 9–5. Diagram showing conversion of equivocal washout curve on F + 20 diuresis renogram to normal appearance or on F − 15 diuresis renogram; this occurred in 4 of 14 cases. (From Upsdell SM, Leeson SM, Brooman PJC, O'Reilly PH: Br J Urol 1988; 61:14–18.)

Because the diuretic renogram is noninvasive and easily reproducible and provides quantitative evaluation of the split and total renal function with minimal radiation exposure, it is clinically utilized more today than the Whitaker test. However, when there is extreme upper tract dilatation and/or poor renal function precluding an adequate diuretic response, the pressure flow study may still have clinical utility.

Duplex Doppler Ultrasonography and Renal Resistive Index

The use of duplex Doppler imaging during ultrasonographic evaluation of the kidney allows the determination of the renal resistive index (RI), where

$$RI = ([\text{peak systolic velocity}] - [\text{lowest diastolic velocity}]) / [\text{peak systolic velocity}]$$

(Cronan, 1991; Cronan and Tublin, 1995).

A value of 0.70 has been taken as the upper limit of normal (Platt et al, 1991). Resistive indices above 0.70 are used for the diagnosis of obstruction, although this diagnosis is not exclusive for obstruction, inasmuch as medical renal diseases alone can also cause the resistive index to exceed 0.70. A resistive index in the obstructed kidney that is 0.1 greater than the resistive index in the contralateral kidney is considered to be significant enough to indicate obstruction (Palmer and DiSandro, 1995). There is much controversy in the literature regarding the use of the resistive index in obstruction. Platt and co-workers (1993) presented data on 23 patients with acute unilateral ureteral occlusion (UUO) of 36 hours' duration or less, measuring the renal resistive index in the "obstructed" and the contralateral renal units. The mean resistive index in the obstructed kidney was 0.77, as opposed to 0.60 for the normal contralateral kidney. In three obstructed kidneys with a resistive index of less than 0.70, two had pyelosinus extravasation and one had obstruction for less than 4 to 5 hours. Because the vasoconstriction of UUO occurs after 5 to 6 hours, the resistive index may not rise until renal obstruction has been present at least 5 to 6 hours. Platt and co-workers concluded that Doppler determination of renal resistive indices is a valuable addition for improving the accuracy of routine renal ultrasonography in the diagnosis of renal obstruction in patients presenting with acute renal colic and for whom an IVU is not desirable (e.g., pregnant patients and patients with a history of contrast material–induced allergy or renal failure).

Other investigators believe there is no role for the use of duplex Doppler sonography in the detection of acute renal obstruction (Tublin et al, 1994; Cronan and Tublin, 1995). Tublin and co-workers (1994) evaluated 32 patients with acute renal colic. Twelve of the obstructed kidneys had a mean resistive index of less than 0.70, and seven of the nonobstructed kidneys had a mean resistive index of greater than 0.70. Using a resistive index of greater than 0.70 as diagnostic of acute renal obstruction, Tublin and co-workers determined that the sensitivity and specificity of duplex Doppler sonography were 37% and 84%, respectively. When using the difference in the resistive index of greater than 0.10 between the ipsilateral and contralateral renal units to diagnose obstruction, they determined that the sensitivity and specificity were 37% and 100%, respectively. The difference in clinical findings between the two previous studies may result from several factors, including (1) the quality of the examination and the Doppler waveform analysis, (2) the duration of obstruction, (3) the presence of a fornix rupture and extravasation, and (4) the degree of obstruction. Finally, Tublin and co-workers pointed out that the initial management of the acute renal colic with nonsteroidal anti-inflammatory drugs (NSAIDs) could alter the intrarenal vascular tone and hence affect the resistive index.

Chen and co-workers (1993) showed that the degree of renal obstruction affects the renal resistive index. Mildly obstructed kidneys had a mean resistive index of 0.64, as opposed to 0.74 for the severely obstructed kidneys. Three of five kidneys with a prerelease resistive index of greater than 0.70 had a follow-up resistive index of less than 0.70 within 3 days after the relief of obstruction. Prerelease resistive indices of less than 0.70 in two renal units remained less than 0.70 after relief of the obstruction. There may be clinical utility in using the resistive index to decide which patients with hydronephrosis would benefit from surgical intervention to improve RBF and hence preserve renal function. Fung and colleagues (1994) demonstrated a relationship between elevated intrarenal resistive indices and elevated intrapelvic pressures. By increasing intrapelvic pressure with an infusion via a percutaneous puncture, they were able to demonstrate a rise in the intrarenal resistive index. When the pelvic pressure remained low during the percutaneous infusion, the resistive index also remained low. Therefore, an elevated intrarenal resistive index may be able to distinguish obstructive and nonobstructive hydronephrosis. This would indicate which patients will benefit from surgical intervention to preserve and, it is hoped, improve renal function in the future.

Computed Tomography and Magnetic Resonance Imaging

Computed tomography (CT) is an alternative to IVU for patients in whom the immediate use of intravenous contrast material without steroid preparation is contraindicated (e.g., patients with allergy to iodinated contrast or shellfish and patients with asthma) or in patients with elevations in either serum BUN and/or creatinine.

Smith and co-workers (1995) investigated the use of non–contrast-enhanced CT in the diagnosis of acute flank pain. They compared the findings in 20 patients with acute flank pain on both non–contrast-enhanced CT and IVU. The CT and IVU demonstrated ureteric obstruction in 12 patients. In 5 of the 12, a stone was demonstrated on both studies. Six patients had a stone that was seen on the non–contrast-enhanced CT scan and not on the IVU. In one patient, a stone could not be visualized on either study, and no obstruction was demonstrated in eight patients with either investigation. The non–contrast-enhanced CT scan was performed at either 5- or 10-mm cuts, and all studies were completed within 5 minutes. The non–contrast-enhanced CT scan is more sensitive than the IVU in the detection of ureteric stones in acute flank pain ($P < .01$). In addition, the CT scan can provide information about extrinsic causes of ureteral obstruction as well as nonurinary causes for the acute flank pain. Therefore, the patient who is not a candidate for an IVU in the emergency room, and yet for whom a diagnosis for flank pain is warranted, may be a candidate for the non–contrast-enhanced CT scan.

Rothpearl and co-workers (1995) investigated the use of magnetic resonance imaging (MRI) for the simultaneous visualization of the entire urinary tract without the use of intravenous contrast material or ionizing radiation. For all the patients with urinary tract obstruction, a diagnosis of obstruction was made on the magnetic resonance urogram. However, in eight patients in whom ureteral calculi was the source of obstruction, there was no visualization of calculi on the magnetic resonance urogram. This was accomplished by comparing the urogram with a scout radiograph of the kidneys, ureter, and bladder. The point of obstruction was identified in all patients, and other etiologies for obstruction (e.g., intraluminal ureteral neoplasm and ureteral stricture disease) were well visualized. The disadvantages of this technique, in addition to the inability to identify the ureteral calculus, are the acquisition time of 34 minutes for images and the cost of the procedure. Again, for patients with allergies to iodinated contrast material and with renal failure, this technique may have its place.

ANATOMIC CHANGES OF UPPER URINARY TRACT WITH OBSTRUCTION

Gross Changes in the Kidney: Human

The appearance of the kidney after ureteral obstruction varies with the presence of an intrarenal versus extrarenal collecting system, with the length and degree of obstruction, and with the presence or absence of infection. The presence of the renal parenchyma completely around an intrarenal collecting system limits its ability to dilate. Expansion of an extrarenal collecting system, however, is not limited by the renal parenchyma. Therefore, the intrarenal system, although obstructed to the same degree and duration as the extrarenal system, may not exhibit the same degree of hydronephrosis; however, the degree of renal damage may be worse.

Acute complete ureteral occlusion may cause little change in the collecting system, especially if there is an intrarenal collecting system; it may take several days to develop significant dilatation of the collecting system under these conditions. In chronic obstruction, the kidney may be enlarged, normal, or atrophic, again depending on the length and degree of obstruction, as well as on the presence of an intrarenal or extrarenal collecting system (Talner, 1990). Usually the collecting system dilates with time, especially with extrarenal collecting systems, resulting in gradual compression of the renal papilla. Over time, the collecting system enlarges to the point that the tissue between the calyces thins, resulting in calyceal enlargement. Ultimately, the calyces coalesce, with thin septa between them and a "rim" or "shell" of parenchyma remaining peripherally.

Gross Changes in the Kidney: Experimental

There are extensive data on the experimental creation and investigation of hydronephrosis. Hydronephrosis was shown to develop in rabbits as early as 1 day after ureteral ligation in association with an increase in kidney weight and loss of papillary and medullary structures (Sheehan and Davis, 1959). There was a steady and progressive increase in renal weight and pelvic fluid volume in these rabbits up to 4 months after ureteral ligation. This has been confirmed by other investigators utilizing different animal species and models of ureteral occlusion (Scott and Sullivan, 1912; Hinman and Hepler, 1925; Strong, 1940; Huland and Gonnermann, 1983). Strong noted a subsequent decrease in kidney weight and volume of renal pelvic fluid beyond 90 days of complete ureteral obstruction, in contrast with the steady increase in these parameters demonstrated by others. By 231 days of obstruction, the weight and size of the kidney had returned to a baseline value equal to that of the contralateral (nonobstructed) kidney. There was a marked thinning of the renal parenchyma to a shell with little normal architecture at this time, in comparison with the normal kidney. Ladefoged and Djurhuus (1976) also demonstrated a marked decrease in kidney weight in comparison with the contralateral kidney with obstruction of 5 to 6 weeks' duration. On gross examination, the kidney was still enlarged and appeared cystic.

Microscopic Changes in the Kidney: Experimental

Initially, most of the microscopic changes are confined to the tubules with little effect on the glomeruli (Strong, 1940; Sheehan and Davis, 1959). The glomeruli seem relatively resistant to change except for a slight increase in size and a thickening of Bowman's capsule. The development of hyalinization and connective tissue proliferation are not seen until 231 days of ureteral ligation, and only in relatively few glomeruli (Strong, 1940).

The tubules initially undergo dilatation of the lumen with flattening of the epithelium. After approximately 21 days of obstruction, tubules in several areas of the renal parenchyma are barely discernible on microscopic section.

Fibrotic and cellular changes in the rabbit kidney have been examined in kidneys from 1 to 32 days after UUO. Prominent findings included a widening of the cortical interstitial space as early as 1 day after UUO; the interstitial space contained fibroblasts, mononuclear cells, and extravasated red blood cells. The cortical interstitial space widened with time, and fibroblasts and mononuclear cells increased in number (Nagle et al, 1973a; Nagle and Bulger, 1978).

The fibrosis of obstruction has been studied in both rabbits and rats. Nagle and Bulger (1978) used electron microscopy and described the appearance of collagen fibers in the kidney by 7 days after UUO, with an increase up to 32 days. At 32 days, diffuse interstitial collagen was found in the cortex and outer medulla. Sharma and colleagues (1993) studied the immunohistochemical localization of collagen subtypes and used in situ hybridization to localize collagen mRNA in rabbits with UUO for 16 days. In these studies, interstitial volume was increased, as well as interstitial collagen III and IV and fibronectin. Increases in collagen I were only in focal, peritubular accumulations. In situ hybridization for the $alpha_1$ chain of collagen I localized it exclusively to interstitial cells, which formed clusters in association with dilated tubules, arteries, and the periglomerular interstitium. No expression of mRNA for the $alpha_1$ chain of collagen I was seen in tubular epithelium or glomeruli.

Collagen has also been localized immunohistochemically in rats studied from 1 to 28 days after UUO. Increases in the cortical and medullary interstitial space were found; these changes were significant by 7 days after UUO. Collagen III was increased by 3 days in both the cortex and medulla, and medullary collagen was further increased by 7 days after UUO. Prominent changes in collagen I were detected 14 days after UUO. Collagen IV, laminin, and fibronectin also showed prominent changes by 3 days; these components continued to increase through 14 days (Fig. 9–6). Glomerular fibrosis was not prominent; only small changes in glomerular collagen I were found after 14 to 21 days of UUO (Wright et al, 1996).

Collagen synthesis rates have not been measured in rats in UUO. However, collagen degradation has been examined. In rats with 15 days of UUO, collagenolytic activity of renal tissue from obstructed animals was decreased to 10%, in comparison with that of normal and contralateral kidneys (Gonzalez-Avila et al, 1988). The matrix metalloproteinases (MMPs) are a group of enzymes involved in the degradation of both collagen and other extracellular matrix components (Davies et al, 1992). The activity of the MMPs is controlled in part by inhibitors called TIMPs (*t*issue *i*nhibitors of *m*etal*lo*p*roteinases; Denhardt et al, 1993). Beginning 12 hours after UUO, there was a marked increase in the expression of mRNA for TIMP-1 that continues through 4 days; TIMP-2 was unaffected; and TIMP-3 gene expression was actually decreased. Thus, an increase in TIMP-1, which should in-

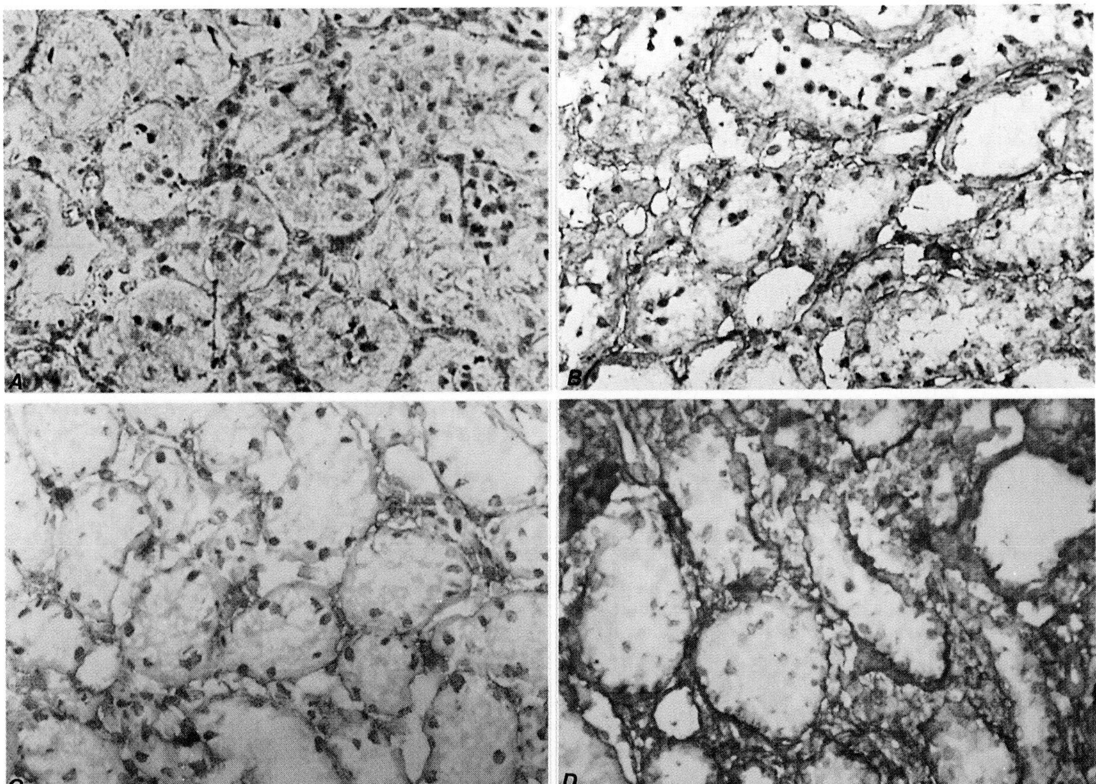

Figure 9–6. Changes in collagen I and IV in UUO in the rat as seen with immunohistochemistry. *A,* Collagen I: sham. *B,* Collagen I: 14 day. *C,* Collagen IV: sham. *D,* Collagen IV: 14 day. Magnification, × 400. Note the increased staining with UUO. (From Wright EJ, McCaffrey TA, Robertson AP, et al: Lab Invest 1996; 74:528–537.)

hibit the MMPs and therefore collagen degradation, could contribute to the fibrotic response (Engelmyer et al, 1995).

Proliferation of interstitial cells has been studied in rabbits with UUO. With the use of [^{3}H]-thymidine, it was found that the majority of labeling occurred in interstitial fibroblasts; in cortex and outer medulla, which had high labeling, cells were separated by a widened interstitial space; and in the inner medulla, where labeling was low, cells maintained their normal spatial relationships (Nagle et al, 1976). The fibroblasts found in the interstitium in obstruction have been shown to be transformed into a myofibroblast type of cell. This has been demonstrated both by morphologic analysis of the cells and by immunohistochemical staining (Nagle et al, 1973b). Studies by Diamond and associates (1995) have confirmed this finding in a rat model. Immunohistochemical localization of smooth muscle actin and desmin (an intermediate filament protein) was detected at 24 hours after UUO and increased through 96 hours; mRNA expression of smooth muscle actin increased by 15.7-fold at 48 hours and had decreased to only 4.1-fold at 96 hours.

The role of interstitial fibrosis in the progression of obstructive nephropathy is unclear. **There is accumulating evidence that this active progressive process may be the cause of renal loss after successful relief of the obstructing event that initiated the process.** The molecular mechanisms of fibrosis are currently under study.

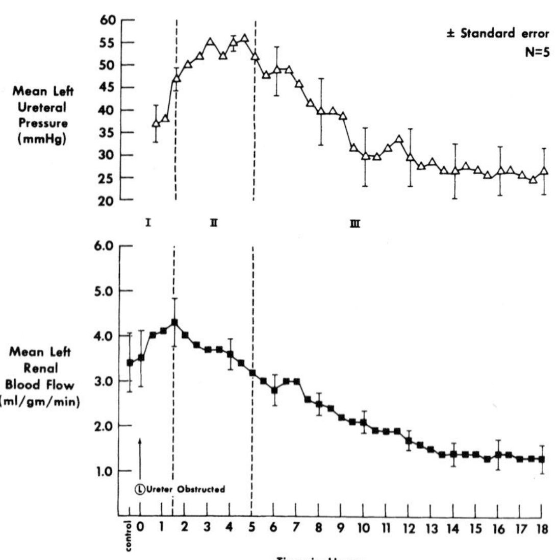

Figure 9–7. The triphasic relationship between ipsilateral renal blood flow and left ureteral pressure during 18 hours of left-sided occlusion. The three phases are designated by Roman numerals and divided by vertical dashed lines. In phase I, renal blood flow and ureteral pressure rise together. In phase II, the left renal blood flow begins to decline, whereas ureteral pressure remains elevated and, in fact, continues to rise. Phase III shows the left-sided renal blood flow and ureteral pressure declining together. (From Moody TE, Vaughan ED Jr, Gillenwater JY: Invest Urol 1975; 13:246–251.)

PHYSIOLOGIC CHANGES IN THE UNILATERAL URETERAL OBSTRUCTION MODEL

Renal Blood Flow, Glomerular Filtration Rate, and Ureteral Pressure

The acute unilateral occlusion of a ureter results in a characteristic triphasic relationship between RBF and ureteral pressure (Moody et al, 1975). **The first phase is characterized by a rise in both ureteral pressure and RBF lasting approximately 1 to 1.5 hours. This is followed in phase 2 by a decline in RBF and a continued increase in ureteral pressure lasting until the fifth hour of occlusion. The final phase ensues with a further decline in RBF accompanied by a progressive decrease in ureteral pressure** (Fig. 9–7). Hemodynamically, phase 1 is characterized by an initial afferent arteriole vasodilatation, followed by an efferent arteriole vasoconstriction in phase 2 and afferent arteriole vasoconstriction in phase 3. The third phase of UUO, the vasoconstrictive phase, is characterized by both pre- and postglomerular vasoconstriction that reduces both RBF and ureteral pressure (Moody et al, 1975).

Harris and Yarger (1974) demonstrated a marked decrease in the perfusion of the superficial cortical tissue and an increase in the perfusion of juxtamedullary glomeruli after 24 hours of UUO. Yarger and Griffith (1974) demonstrated effective renal plasma flow (ERPF) to be 55% of control values in the obstructed kidney after 24 hours of UUO. Utilizing the injection of microspheres during ureteral occlusion, Yarger and Griffith also demonstrated an increase in intrarenal blood flow to the juxtamedullary nephrons with a corresponding decrease in blood flow to the outer cortical nephrons. They believed that an increase in renin in the outer cortex in relation to the inner medulla may explain the shift in intrarenal blood flow. Glomerular cast studies show the poor glomerular perfusion that accompanies UUO (Fig. 9–8). Arendhorst and co-workers (1974) confirmed with micropuncture studies that changes seen in the whole kidney by 24 hours of UUO are found at the single nephron level in association with afferent arteriolar vasoconstriction. More recent studies using a continuous infusion of 51-chromium–ethylenediaminetetraacetic acid (^{51}Cr-EDTA), which allows direct measurement of GFR during obstruction, have shown a 75% decrease in GFR after the onset of UUO (Hvistendahl et al, in press).

Although the physiologic changes characterizing phase I and phase III of UUO have been known for some time, studies are still under way to understand the underlying molecular changes. Early studies invoked local physical interactions to explain changes in afferent and efferent arteriolar tone. As an introduction, the initial studies are described here. However, as it became clear that biochemical mediators were responsible for these changes, there was an explosion of literature, which continues today to determine which mediator (or mediators) is involved in the maintenance of vascular smooth muscle tone during UUO.

The initial hyperemia of acute UUO was originally thought by several investigators to be an autoregulatory phenomenon (Gilmore, 1964; Nash and Selkurt, 1964). They postulated that an acute increase in ureteral pressure is accompanied by an increase in interstitial pressure and compression of the arterioles, causing a reduction in the intravascular pressure. The renal vascular resistance then decreases as the arteriole attempts to increase intravascular flow by relaxation and dilatation (Nash and Selkurt, 1964). This relationship is explained by the Laplace equation:

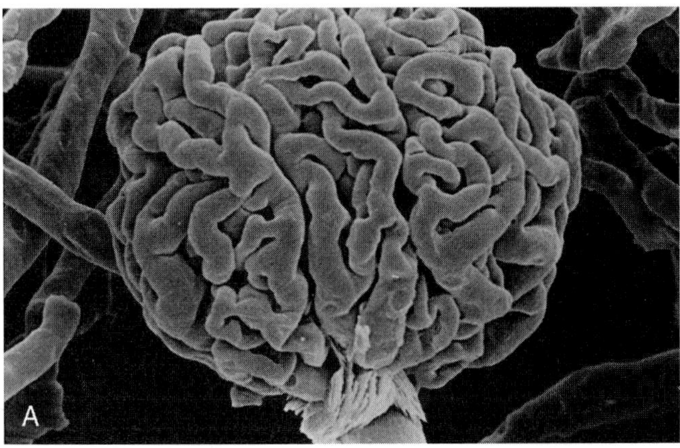

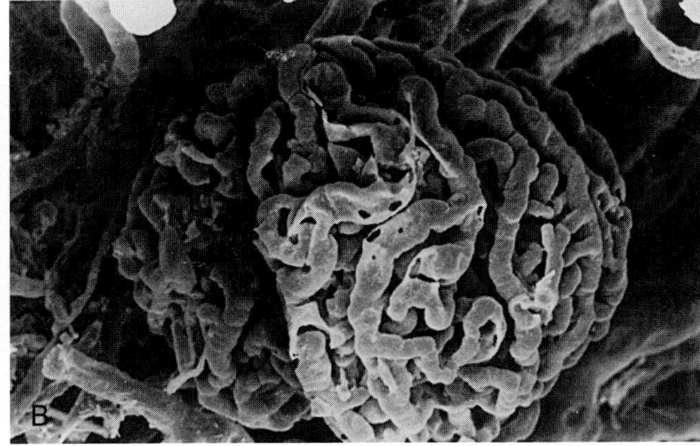

Figure 9–8. *A,* Scanning electron microscopic appearance of normal glomerular cast. Magnification, ×390. *B,* Appearance of glomerular microvascular cast after obstruction, showing capillary collapse and irregularity. Magnification, ×390. (From Leahy AL, Ryan PC, McEntee GM, et al: J Urol 1989; 142:199–203.)

$$T_{wall} = r(P_{in} - P_{out}),$$

where T_{wall} = vascular wall tension, r = inner vessel radius, P_{in} = intravascular pressure, and P_{out} = extravascular pressure (i.e., interstitial pressure). The value for r varies only with the fourth root of resistance changes and can therefore be considered a constant, leaving T_{wall} to vary by $P_{in} - P_{out}$ (Thureau, 1964). Hence increasing interstitial pressures by acute ureteral occlusion decreases wall tension and results in vasodilatation. This logic was used to explain the autoregulatory phenomenon and the initial hyperemia of UUO.

Vaughan and co-investigators (1971) used celiotomy, renal denervation, adrenergic blockade, contralateral nephrectomy, and renin suppression (with deoxycorticosterone acetate and sodium chloride loading) to mitigate the initial hyperemia of UUO. Only celiotomy produced the initial decrease in renal vascular resistance associated with acute ureteral occlusion. They therefore postulated a myogenic response of the arteriolar musculature to the increase in ureteral pressure as the cause for the initial hyperemia of UUO, possibly through an intrarenal action of the renin-angiotensin system (Vaughan et al, 1971). However, Moody and co-workers (1977b) found that the administration of sar^1-ala^8 angiotensin II, a competitive antagonist of angiotensin II (AII), before ureteral occlusion did not alter the initial rise in RBF seen with acute ureteral ligation. They concluded that AII does not seem to play a role in the myogenic response to ureteral occlusion.

Herbaczynska-Cedro and Vane (1973) demonstrated that prostaglandins contribute to the autoregulation of RBF in the isolated perfused canine kidney. Furthermore, they also found that the autoregulation of RBF was not affected by pretreatment with a converting enzyme inhibitor. In 1974, Herbaczynska-Cedro and Vane were able to inhibit the hyperemia that occurred 3 minutes after the release of renal arterial occlusion by the preadministration of indomethacin. The data suggested a role for prostaglandins as mediators of the reactive hyperemia after the release of renal artery occlusion. It thus became apparent that locally or systemically produced mediators could be responsible for autoregulation of RBF and post-UUO renal hemodynamics.

Similarly, the original studies of the vasoconstriction of phase III investigated both physical and humoral mechanism in the obstructed kidney (Kerr, 1956; Vaughan et al, 1968, 1970a). The observed immediate increase in RBF with the release of UUO supported a role for increased interstitial pressure. This increase was not sustained, as would be expected if the increase in interstitial pressure had been the sole factor responsible for the diminished RBF (Shenasky et al, 1971). Hence Shenasky and co-workers investigated the effects of several vasoactive compounds (i.e., both vasodilators and vasoconstrictors) on the RBF in chronic UUO. They demonstrated a marked increase in RBF from 50% to 100% with the intrarenal injection of acetylcholine, dopamine, and isoproterenol. If the decrease in RBF were secondary to compression of the vessels from increased interstitial pressure, administration of vasodilators should not alter the blood flow. Shenasky and co-workers (1971) postulated the existence of a local or circulating humoral agent or a neurogenic stimulus as responsible for the increase in preglomerular vascular tone with chronic UUO. Subsequently, numerous studies, often conflicting, have explored this hypothesis. To understand these studies, a brief review of mediators that are candidates for the observed effects is warranted.

VASOACTIVE AND INFLAMMATORY MEDIATORS AND GROWTH FACTORS INVOLVED IN OBSTRUCTION

Arachidonic Acid Metabolites (Eicosanoids)

The metabolism of the fatty acid arachidonic acid (5,8,11,14-eicosatetraenoic acid) is quite complex, and products include the cyclooxygenase-derived prostaglandins, lipoxygenase-derived leukotrienes, hydroxyeicosatetraenoic acids (HETEs) and lipoxins, and the cytochrome P-450–derived epoxyeicosatrienoic acids (EETs) and dihydroxyeicosatrienoic acids (DHTs). The metabolism of arachidonic acid is depicted in Figure 9–9*A*. **Metabolites of arachidonic acid are known collectively as eicosanoids, and those formed from the cyclooxygenase pathway (see later discussion) are referred to as either *prostaglandins* or *prostanoids*** (Smith et al, 1991; Smith, 1992; Baird and Morrison, 1993; Quilley et al, 1995).

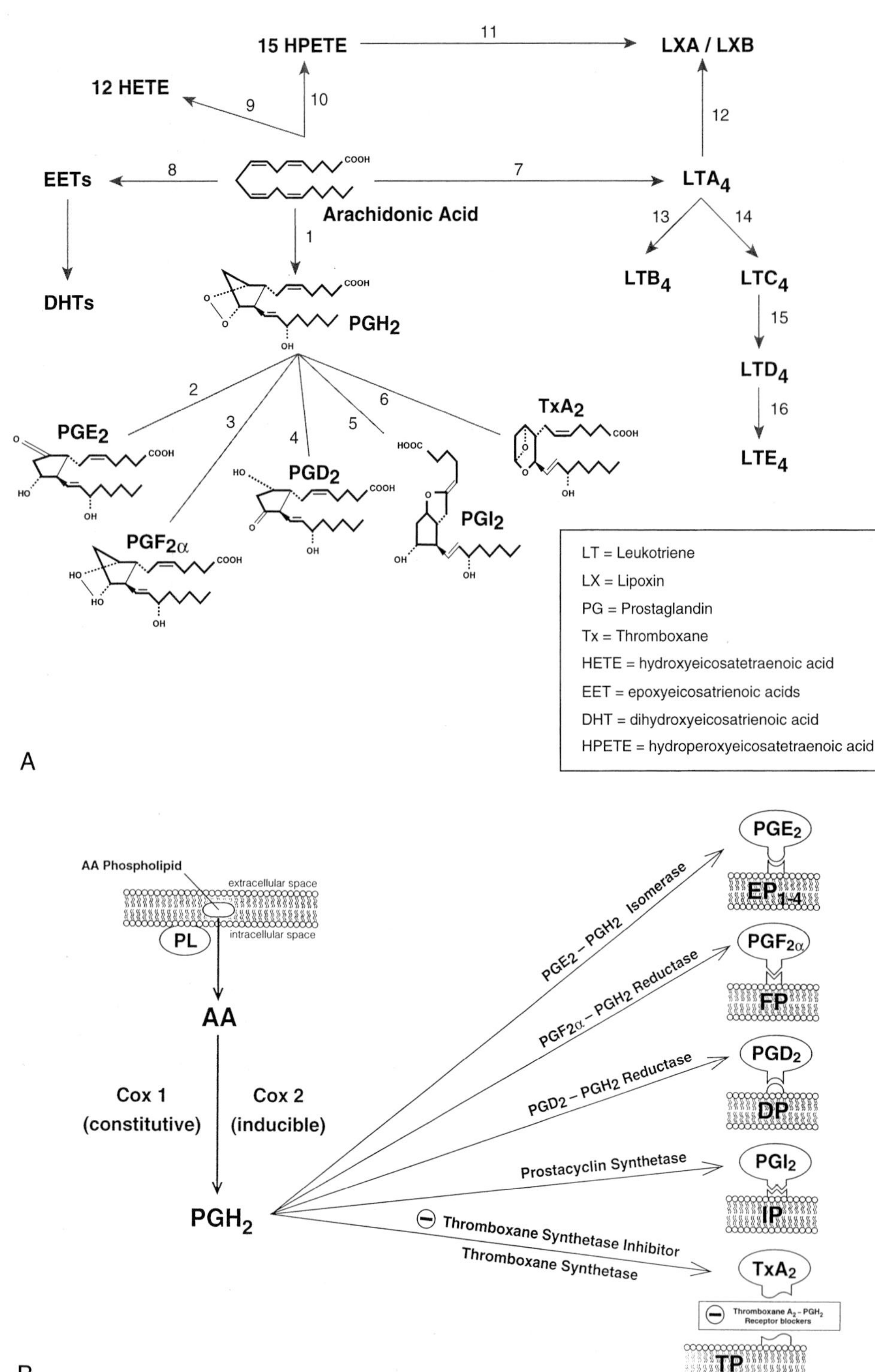

Figure 9–9. *A,* Pathway of arachidonic acid metabolism: metabolism of arachidonic acid to eicosanoids. Enzymes are numbered in the figure: 1, cyclooxygenase; 2, PGE_2 synthase; 3, $PGF_{2\alpha}$ synthase; 4, PGD_2 synthase; 5, prostacyclin synthetase; 6, thromboxane synthetase; 7, 5-lipoxygenase; 8, cytochrome P-450 (pathway); 9, 12-lipoxygenase; 10, 15-lipoxygenase; 11, 5-lipoxygenase; 12, 12- and 15-lipoxygenase; 13, LTB_4 hydrolase; 14, LTC_4 synthetase; 15, γ-glutamyl transferase; 16, dipeptidase. *B,* Terminal pathways of prostaglandin synthesis and prostaglandin receptors: metabolism of arachidonic acid (AA) to prostaglandin H_2 (PGH_2) via cyclooxygenase, which exists in 2 isoforms: COX-1 (constitutive) and COX-2 (inducible). PGH_2 is metabolized via the listed enzymes to the eicosanoid products shown, which interact with specific receptors, as indicated.

Arachidonic acid is found esterified in membrane lipids. It is released from membrane stores by the action of either phospholipase A_2 or phospholipase C. Two types of phospholipase A_2 may be involved: either secretory (found in the pancreas [type I] or in other cells [type II]) or cytosolic (Glaser, 1995). Secretory type II phospholipase A_2 has been found in inflammatory exudates and has also been shown to elicit inflammation after intradermal or intra-articular injection; therefore, it may be the phospholipase involved in inflammatory responses. The more recently characterized cytosolic phospholipase A_2 may be involved in release of arachidonic acid from lipid stores. This enzyme, cloned in 1991 (Clark et al, 1991; Sharp et al, 1991), differs from the well-known secretory phospholipase in several ways: It is much larger, is regulated by phosphorylation, displays a unique preference for arachidonic acid–containing phospholipids, and requires only micromolar (instead of millimolar) levels of calcium to be maximally activated. Thus it is postulated that an agonist-stimulated signal at the cell surface receptor causes changes in intracellular calcium, which result in translocation of the cytosolic phospholipase from the cytosol to the membrane, where it acts to release arachidonic acid intracellularly.

Although there has been interest in inhibitors of phospholipase since the early 1970s, surprisingly few drugs have been added to the clinical armamentarium over the years. A review (Glaser, 1995) suggests that new inhibitors may arise from natural products, molecular modeling of the enzyme, substrate analogues, or anti-sense cDNA. The discovery of the cytosolic phospholipase reveals a new target for phospholipase inhibitors. Further studies on the role of the secretory and cytosolic phospholipase in normal physiology and pathophysiology will result in the design of specific inhibitors. Inhibition of phospholipase, with the concomitant reduction of arachidonic acid release, would reduce the synthesis of all eicosanoids that would be formed by any given stimulus.

Once arachidonic acid is released by the action of phospholipase, it is available for conversion by further enzymes (see Fig. 9–9*B*). The enzyme prostaglandin H (PGH) synthase, also known as cyclooxygenase (COX), converts arachidonic acid to the PGH_2 endoperoxide, which is the immediate precursor of prostaglandins E_2, F_2, and D_2; of prostacyclin (PGI_2); and of thromboxane A_2 (TxA_2). Cyclooxygenase is inhibited by aspirin and other NSAIDs, including meclofenamate and indomethacin. Data demonstrate that cyclooxygenase exists in two forms, designated COX-1 and COX-2. Two forms of cyclooxygenase have been cloned, sequenced, and expressed. Human COX-2 has a 61% sequence homology to human COX-1 (reviewed by Wu, 1995).

A major difference between COX-1 and COX-2 is their regulation. There is cyclooxygenase activity in almost all tissues, due to COX-1, which is constitutively expressed. COX-2, in contrast, is induced by a variety of stimuli in a variety of cells. These stimuli include cytokines, growth factors, hormones, and inflammation. Both COX-1 and COX-2 can be induced; COX-1 may increase two- to fourfold, whereas COX-2 can increase ten- to eightyfold. Although glucocorticoids have very little effect on COX-1, they have been shown to inhibit COX-2. This may be an additional explanation for their anti-inflammatory effects (Masferrer et al, 1994).

Inhibition of prostaglandin synthesis has been studied extensively for some time. Aspirin acetylates the active site of cyclooxygenase and irreversibly inhibits cyclooxygenase. Most other NSAIDs are reversible inhibitors of cyclooxygenase. Studies have suggested that most known NSAIDs either preferentially inhibit COX-1 or are equipotent inhibitors of COX-1 and COX-2. The design of selective inhibitors of COX-2 should lead to the inhibition of the cyclooxygenase associated with inflammation, while leaving the cyclooxygenase associated with constitutive synthesis of eicosanoids undisturbed. Side effects of currently available NSAIDs, such as gastrointestinal or renal, could be avoided (reviewed by Vane and Botting, 1995). Inhibition of cyclooxygenase by NSAIDs reduces the synthesis of prostanoids and could lead to increased appearance of metabolites of arachidonic acid derived from the lipoxygenase and cytochrome P-450 pathways.

The PGH_2 formed by the action of cyclooxygenase is the substrate for a number of enzymes, including prostacyclin synthase, TxA_2 synthase, PGF_2 synthase, PGD_2 synthase, and PGE_2 synthase. The ability to pharmacologically manipulate the various prostanoids varies greatly among the prostanoids. The synthetic enzyme and the receptor for TxA_2 have been the most widely studied of all the prostanoids. The receptor for TxA_2 has been cloned and characterized (Hirata et al, 1991). Other receptors for PGE_2 (EP_2, EP_3) have also been cloned (Thierauch et al, 1993, 1994; Breyer et al, 1996). Extensive studies have been carried out to characterize receptors for TxA_2 (and PGH_2) in many tissues. These receptors have been found in platelets, the vasculature, the brain, and the kidneys (Halushka et al, 1987). Through use of TxA_2 synthase inhibitors and TxA_2 receptor blockers, it has been suggested that TxA_2 is involved in thrombosis, atherosclerosis, and angina (Halushka and Lefer, 1987). There are differences when TxA_2 receptor blockers are used in comparison with TxA_2 synthase inhibitors. TxA_2 receptor blockers are also PGH_2 receptor blockers. PGH_2, the TxA_2 precursor, has intrinsic vasoconstrictor activity, although it is less potent than TxA_2. Thus when TxA_2 synthesis is inhibited, it is possible that vasoconstriction due to TxA_2 inhibition could be offset by vasoconstriction produced by increased PGH_2. The TxA_2 receptor blockers offer advantages over the TxA_2 synthase inhibitors in blocking both PGH_2 and TxA_2 activity and in not changing the profile of products formed.

There are no specific inhibitors of the enzymes that convert PGH_2 to PGE_2, PGD_2, or PGF_2. The involvement of these products is usually surmised by using cyclooxygenase inhibitors and validating that prostaglandin synthesis is decreased. Conversely, addition of exogenous compound and noting its effect have also been done. Receptors for prostanoids have been classified as EP_1-EP_4, FP, or DP to denote interactions characteristic of these prostanoids. Characterization of these receptors is currently under way. The synthesis and availability of inhibitors of individual receptors should help in delineating the role of individual prostanoids in physiology and pathophysiology (see review by Coleman et al, 1994).

The involvement of prostanoids in biologic systems has been studied extensively (Campbell and Halushka, 1996). Relevant to the studies of UUO are prostanoid effects on renal function, pain, cellular proliferation, and fibrosis. Eicosanoids are actively produced by the kidneys and are involved in control of RBF, GFR, free water clearance, tubular transport, and renin release. Under normal conditions, inhibition of prostanoid synthesis has no effect on either RBF or GFR (Sedor et al, 1986). Under conditions in which vasoconstrictor tone is increased, vasodilator eicosanoids are released in an effort to compensate for the vasoconstriction. Prostanoids are known to sensitize pain receptors to stimuli such as bradykinin or histamine, as well as to have central effects that can potentiate peripheral pain mechanisms. In addition, they can either positively or negatively affect cell proliferation, depending on both the prostanoid and the target cell examined.

Other pathways of arachidonic acid metabolism are shown in Figure 9–9*A*. Metabolism of arachidonic acid via the 5-lipoxygenase enzyme (Lewis et al, 1990) results in the formation of the intermediate leukotriene A_4 (LTA_4), which can be converted to the leukotrienes B_4, C_4, D_4, and E_4.

Leukotrienes have been shown to decrease RBF and GFR (Badr et al, 1987; Gulbins et al, 1991).

The LTA_4 intermediate can also be acted on by either a 12-lipoxygenase or 15-lipoxygenase to form lipoxins A and B (see Fig. 9–9*A*) (Serhan, 1994). Alternatively, lipoxins can also be formed by the action of 15-lipoxygenase on arachidonic acid followed by 5-lipoxygenation. Some renal actions of lipoxins have been demonstrated (Badr et al, 1989; Katoh et al, 1992). Specific pharmacologic probes for the lipoxins are not yet available.

A fourth pathway of arachidonic acid metabolism in the kidney is that of the cytochrome P-450 (McGiff et al, 1993), first described by Capdevila and colleagues (1981). This pathway leads to the formation of a number of sets of compounds, including diols, epoxides, and HETEs (see Fig. 9–9*A*). These compounds have numerous biologic activities, including vasoactivity and effects on ion transport and renin release, and they may be important in modulating renal function. The role of the P-450 metabolites has been studied by using typical inducers or inhibitors of the cytochrome P-450–metabolizing enzymes. An additional finding is that the cyclooxygenase enzyme may also be involved in the metabolism of products formed via the P-450 pathway (Escalante et al, 1989; Carroll et al, 1992). Such complex interactions among the pathways of arachidonic acid metabolism make seemingly simple pharmacologic experiments much more complicated.

Angiotensin II

Although pathways of angiotensin II (AII) synthesis, degradation, and receptor interaction have been known for some time, new information in the 1990s led to synthesis of a number of new tools for studying the renin-angiotensin system. Furthermore, the profile of the biologic action of AII has increased from the vascular and metabolic to involvement in fibrosis (Chung et al, 1995). Thus, new probes and new information have pointed to a more global involvement of AII in pathophysiologic processes.

The biologic activation of angiotensin begins with the action of renin on the angiotensinogen substrate. Angiotensinogen is a 14–amino acid $alpha_2$ globulin. Renin cleaves four amino acids, which results in production of the decapeptide angiotensin I (AI). Angiotensin converting enzyme (ACE) converts AI into the active AII, which then acts on AII receptors. AII is then converted to AIII (angiotensin III) by aminopeptidase. The physiology of the renin-angiotensin system is described in Chapters 7 and 11.

Pharmacologic intervention in the renin-angiotensin system includes inhibiting renin, ACE, or the interaction of AII with its receptor. Approaches to inhibiting renin include the following: beta-blockers, angiotensinogen peptide analogues, and antibodies to renin (Cody, 1994). In recent years, analogues utilizing the transition state of angiotensinogen have resulted in smaller, more stable, and less peptidic inhibitors of renin. One of these, enalkiren (Glassman et al, 1990), has been shown to dose-dependently suppress plasma renin activity and to decrease blood pressure in hypertensive patients. Antibodies to renin have been shown to lower blood pressure in experimental animals; this strategy will probably not be clinically useful.

The second step in formation of AII is conversion from AI by ACE. ACE is a carboxypeptidase that not only converts AI to AII but also inactivates bradykinin and other vasodilator peptides (Jackson and Garrison, 1996). Because ACE inactivates bradykinin, experiments using ACE inhibitors result in both a decrease of the constrictor AII and an increase in the vasodilator bradykinin. Therefore, concerns have been raised about the use of ACE inhibitors as specific tools to investigate the renin-angiotensin system.

By inhibiting the action of AII at its receptor, such concerns can be eliminated. Early antagonists of AII, such as saralasin (sar[cosine]^1-ala^8-AII) and sar-ile^8-AII, were used in numerous experimental systems to probe the role of AII. However, saralasin was also a partial agonist (i.e., although it could block AII's actions, it also had intrinsic activity of its own), and no orally active AII antagonists were available. Two developments have once again brought the study of AII physiology and pharmacology to the forefront. One was the development of AII antagonists that are orally active; the second was the cloning of the AII receptor and the discovery of AII receptor subtypes.

It now appears that there are two subtypes of AII receptor: the AT_1 and AT_2 (Griendling et al, 1994; de Gasparo and Levens, 1994). Both receptors have been successfully cloned (AT_1 by Murphy et al, 1992, and Sasaki et al, 1991; AT_2 by Kambayashi et al, 1993, and Mukoyama et al, 1993). Both the AT_1 and AT_2 receptors have high affinity for AII. They differ in several respects. At the AT_1 receptor, AI is more potent than AIII. AT_1 appears to be coupled to phospholipase A_2, C, or D and may be negatively coupled to adenyl cyclase. Dithiothreitol reduces AII's binding capacity and affinity, and Gpp(NH)p (a stable guanosine triphosphate [GTP] analogue) converts the high affinity binding to low affinity. Losartan (DUP 753, MK954), a biphenylimidazole (Chiu et al, 1989), is a prototypical antagonist at this receptor subtype. In contrast, at the AT_2 receptor, AII and AIII have similar affinities, a second messenger has not been well characterized, dithiothreitol increases the binding affinity of AII, and Gpp(NH)p has no effect on AII affinity. PD123177, a tetrahydroimidazopyridine, is the prototypical antagonist (Chiu et al, 1989). Studies have localized AT_1 and AT_2 receptors in many tissues. In the kidney, there are species differences in subtype expression. For example, rat and rabbit kidneys demonstrate only AT_1 binding, whereas human and nonhuman primate kidneys express both AT_1 and AT_2 receptors (de Gasparo and Levens, 1994).

Of interest is the role of the AII receptor subtype in the physiologic effects of AII. It appears that almost all the physiologic effects mediated by AII are done so through the AT_1 receptor. In the kidney, AII vasoconstriction, effects on glomerular hemodynamics, tubular reabsorption, renin secretion, and cell growth are all mediated by the AT_1 receptor. The function of the AT_2 receptor is unknown, but its presence in fetal tissues suggests a role in development.

Atrial Natriuretic Peptide

In 1981, deBold and co-workers demonstrated that intravenous injection of atrial myocardial extracts resulted in a rapid natriuresis. Subsequent studies revealed that the extract contained a substance that has been

variously termed ***atrial natriuretic peptide (ANP), atrial natriuretic factor,* or *atriopeptin.*** ANP is a polypeptide composed of 28 amino acids (ANP_{99-126}). It is synthesized from a pre-pro form of 151 amino acids that is then converted to pro-ANP (ANP_{1-126}). Pro-ANP is stored in secretory granules, where it is the major tissue or cellular form of ANP; ANP_{99-126} is found in the circulation (reviewed by Christensen, 1993; Awazu and Ichikawa, 1993).

Three receptors have been identified for ANP: GC_A, GC_B, and C receptors. GC_A receptors appear to mediate the biologic effects of ANP, whereas the C receptor appears to function as a clearance receptor for ANP. The GC_A receptor is linked to guanylate cyclase to produce cyclic guanosine monophosphate (cGMP), whereas the C receptor acts to decrease basal and hormone-stimulated adenyl cyclase and increases phospholipase C (Maack, 1992).

Glomeruli have the highest concentration of ANP receptors, but there are some in the arterioles, outer medulla, and papilla. More than 95% of ANP receptors in the cortex are C receptors. During examination of ANP-induced cGMP release (as a measure of GC_A-receptor activation), the most prominent response is in the glomerulus and renomedullary interstitial cells; however, some cGMP response or mRNA for GC_A receptors has been detected in almost every nephron segment (Christensen, 1993; Awazu and Ichikawa, 1993).

Administration of ANP results in natriuresis and diuresis. These processes result from numerous actions of ANP, including antagonism of AII actions on renin and aldosterone release and a direct effect to inhibit sodium reabsorption. In addition, ANP decreases inner medullary hypertonicity, leading to renal medullary washout and therefore to natriuresis. ANP's ability to increase GFR also results from multiple effects, including dilatation of the afferent arteriole, constriction of the efferent arteriole, increase in K_f, and enhancement of the glomerular hydrostatic pressure.

Nitric Oxide

Nitric oxide was first described by Stuehr and Marletta (1985) as a product of activated murine macrophages. In addition, the substance known as endothelium-derived relaxing factor (EDRF), described by Furchgott and Zawadzki (1980), has been identified as nitric oxide. Nitric oxide has since been the subject of thousands of research papers in many disciplines in biology. Of particular importance to the discussion of nitric oxide in the kidney is its synthesis by the enzyme nitric oxide synthase (NOS) (see reviews by Billiar, 1995; Kuo and Schroeder, 1995; Clancy and Abramson, 1995). **The combination of molecular oxygen and the amino acid arginine in the presence of reduced nicotinamide–adenine dinucleotide phosphate (NADPH) and NOS yields citrulline and nitric oxide, through a 5-electron oxidation of the guanidine nitrogen of L-arginine** (Fig. 9–10). In biologic systems, nitric oxide has a half-life of 3 to 30 seconds, at which point it is inactivated by superoxide anion and binds to heme-containing proteins. Guanyl cyclase is a heme protein that is a target of nitric oxide. When nitric oxide interacts with guanyl cyclase, cGMP is increased and vascular smooth muscle is relaxed. Other heme protein interactions mediate other actions of nitric oxide (Kuo and Schroeder, 1995). Nitric oxide can be

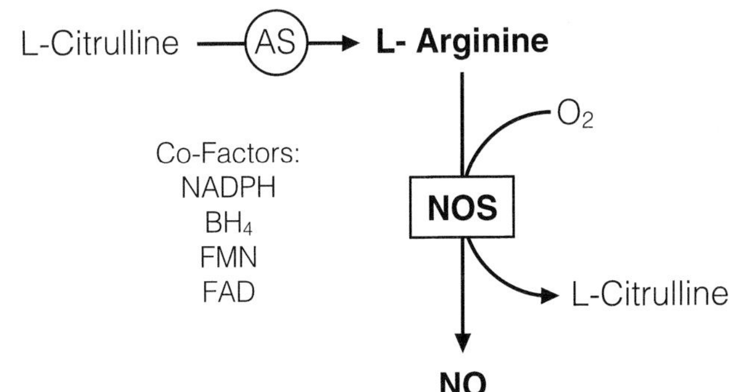

Figure 9–10. Nitric oxide pathway. L-citrulline can be converted by arginine synthetase (AS) to form L-arginine, the precursor for nitric oxide (NO). Nitric oxide synthase (NOS), in the presence of O_2 and the cofactors listed converts arginine to NO, with the formation of citrulline. Cofactors include reduced nicotinamide adenine dinucleotide phosphate (NADPH), tetrahydrobiopterin (BH_4), flavin mononucleotide (FMN), and flavin adenine dinucleotide (FAD). AS, NOS, cofactor, and L-arginine availability are all possible sites of pharmacologic intervention in this pathway.

oxidized by oxygen or superoxide to form other highly reactive products that may be involved in tissue damage. The role of these compounds in the physiologic actions of nitric oxide remains controversial. The short half-life of nitric oxide may be augmented by forming an S-nitroso adduct with albumin or other proteins. Synthetic albumin–nitric oxide adduct has been shown to possess biologic activity similar to that of nitric oxide, but its effect is longer lasting. The role of these adducts in vivo is not yet known.

NOS is found in several forms. A constitutive form of NOS is found in endothelium (cloned by Lamas et al, 1992) and neurons, and is Ca^{2+} dependent. The constitutive NOS found in endothelial cells has been named NOS-3, whereas the constitutive NOS found in neural and epithelial tissue has been named NOS-1. An inducible form of NOS, now designated NOS-2, is calcium independent (cloned by Lyons et al, 1992). It is induced within 4 to 24 hours of the appropriate stimulus and can produce nitric oxide in a 100-fold greater amount than can constitutive NOS.

Nitric oxide is believed to be a major physiologic regulator of basal blood vessel tone. It also appears to play a major role in the pulmonary, gastrointestinal, central nervous, and genitourinary systems (erectile tissue). The role of nitric oxide in renal function is described in Chapter 7. The induction of nitric oxide has been well studied, especially in response to infection and sepsis. Much work has been carried out with endotoxin (lipopolysaccharide [LPS]) used as an inducer in macrophages. However, the stimuli for and target cells of NOS-2 induction are varied. With induction of NOS-2, the capacity to produce nitric oxide can increase up to 100-fold. Many cellular mechanisms can account for this. NOS-1 and NOS-3 are Ca^{2+} dependent, whereas the availability of Ca^{2+} does not affect NOS-2 activity. The cofactor tetrahydrobiopterin is increased when NOS is induced, as is the NADPH generator glucose-6-phosphate dehydrogenase. The availability of the arginine substrate is increased by increased arginine transport and uptake in cells. Each of these enzymes, cofactors, or transport systems could be an eventual target of the pharmacologic intervention in the nitric oxide cascade.

Activation of nitric oxide—for example, during an infection—serves to increase the amount of nitric oxide present to eliminate the pathogen. Furthermore, induction of NOS-2 may increase vasodilatation and maximize tissue perfusion. Unfortunately, excessive NOS induction can lead to vascular collapse and shock. In addition, excessive nitric oxide can lead to chronic inflammatory damage (Billiar, 1995).

Besides the pharmacologic targets just mentioned, the presence of inducible and constitutive forms of NOS should provide specific targets for therapeutic intervention. Currently, inhibitors of NOS are substrate analogues such as N^G-monomethyl-L-arginine (L-NMMA) or N^G-nitro-L-arginine methyl ester (L-NAME). These inhibitors have been indispensable in understanding the role of nitric oxide in various systems. However, use of nonspecific inhibitors is not always beneficial. For example, in both canine and murine models of endotoxemia, survival decreased with NOS inhibition; similarly, in a porcine model of endotoxemia, NOS inhibition potentiated the pulmonary hypertension while ameliorating the arterial pressure and vascular resistance effects (Cobb et al, 1992; Robertson et al, 1994; Minnard et al, 1994). These results suggest that inhibition of both constitutive NOS and NOS-2 amplifies the damage caused by excessive nitric oxide produced by NOS-2, but it also negates the homeostatic mechanisms of nitric oxide produced by constitutive NOS. Specific inhibitors of either the constitutive or inducible nitric oxide synthases will be valuable pharmacologic tools in the future.

Another area of pharmacologic intervention is the availability of substrate for NOS. The nitroprusside and nitroglycerin drugs that have been in use for many years release nitric oxide for vasodilatation (Robertson and Robertson, 1996). Such drugs were discovered well before the description of the nitric oxide pathway. Inhalation therapy with nitric oxide gas may be effective in decreasing pulmonary vascular pressure in children and in adults with mild adult respiratory distress syndrome. As has been shown, physiologic availability of cofactors or substrates that increase with induction may be able to be increased through pharmacologic means.

Endothelin

The production of a coronary vasoconstrictor from cultured endothelial cells (Hickey et al, 1985) was the first demonstration of activity of the peptides that were later identified as endothelins (Yanagisawa et al, 1988). The endothelins are a family of peptides composed of endothelin-1 (ET-1), ET-2, and ET-3, which are coded for by separate genes. ET-1 is produced from a large 203–amino acid precursor called prepro-ET-1, which is then cleaved to a 39–amino acid product referred to as big ET-1. Big ET-1 has 1% of the potency of ET-1 and is cleaved by a metallopeptidase to the 21–amino acid product ET-1 (Rubanyi and Polokoff, 1994; Brown et al, 1996).

The endothelins bind to two types of receptors: ET-A and ET-B (Masaki et al, 1994). The receptors are among the receptors linked with G-proteins and are highly conserved (85% to 90%) across mammalian species. Activation of the ET-A receptor is linked to stimulation of phospholipase C and subsequent inositol triphosphate and diacylglycerol production. The ET-A receptor has a tenfold higher affinity for ET-1 than for ET-3, whereas the ET-B receptor binds both ET-1 and ET-3 with equal affinity. The ET-A receptor appears to mediate most of the vasoconstrictor activities of ET-1; the ET-B receptor appears to be involved in ET-3–supported development of cells derived from neural crest precursors. Transcription of the ET-1 gene to produce prepro-ET-1 is stimulated by many factors, including AII, catecholamines, growth factors, insulin, and hypoxia, among others. Conversely, transcription is inhibited by ANP, ET-3, vasodilator prostaglandins, and nitric oxide (Marsen et al, 1994; Levin, 1995).

Platelet Activating Factor

Platelet activating factor (PAF) was first described by Henson (1970) as a phospholipid mediator released from rabbit leukocytes that induced rabbit platelet aggregation and release of platelet granule contents. Several pathways are involved in the synthesis of PAF: the de novo pathway, the remodeling pathway, and the transacylase pathway (Snyder, 1995). Both the remodeling and transacylase pathways utilize phospholipase A_2, the pivotal enzyme involved in eicosanoid production. The remodeling pathway appears to be active in inflammatory cells, whereas the de novo pathway is active in kidney and central nervous system. The transacylase activity is present in a variety of tissues.

PAF receptors have been studied extensively. The human receptor has been cloned and contains seven transmembrane domains. The guinea pig lung receptor has been cloned and shows 83% homology with the human receptor. The PAF receptor appears to be linked via G-proteins to inositol triphosphate production. Antagonists to the PAF receptor have been synthesized chemically. There are also a number of naturally occurring compounds, many isolated from ginkgolides that have been examined. Well-known PAF antagonists include BN 50739, WEB2086, SRI 63-441, and BN52021. They have been extensively studied and have been shown to be active in a wide variety of systems (Koltai et al, 1994).

PAF has many potent biologic activities, including platelet aggregation, hemoconcentration, bronchoconstriction, hypotension, neutrophil adhesion, and other activities involved in allergic and inflammatory pathways (Bussolino and Camussi, 1995). When given intravenously, PAF decreases RBF, GFR, and urinary volume; other researchers have confirmed this finding, but vasodilatation has also been shown. There are several interactions between PAF and other mediators. An illustrative study of PAF effects on microperfused afferent arterioles showed that PAF's constriction of the vessels was blunted by cyclooxygenase inhibitors and augmented by NOS inhibitors. In preconstricted vessels, low-dose PAF caused a vasodilatation that was unaffected by cyclooxygenase inhibitors but was abolished by NOS inhibitors (Juncos et al, 1993).

Clusterin

Clusterin is a glycoprotein isolated from ram rete testis fluid in 1983. It was named for its ability to cluster Sertoli cells. The rat homologue is called sulfated glycoprotein-2

(SGP-2), and it has been known by diverse names, including glycoprotein III (GPIII), testosterone-repressed message-2 (TRPM-2), complement inhibitor I (CLI), and serum protein-40,40 (sp-40,40). It is an 80-kD heterodimer containing five disulfide bonds. Clusterin is widely distributed in the neuroendocrine system and is also produced in a wide variety of experimental conditions (reviewed by Rosenberg et al, 1993; Dvergsten et al, 1994).

A high concentration of seminal clusterin has been shown to be predictive of successful fertilization, and it may be important in other aspects of sperm development. Clusterin may be involved in lipid transport, is a complement inhibitor, and may also maintain cell-cell and cell-substratum interactions. It has also been found in several renal disease models. However, a definitive role for clusterin still remains ill defined. Clusterin has been found in conjunction with the process of apoptosis (programmed cell death) in prostate (involution after castration), mammary gland (postlactation), and ovarian follicles (luteolysis); however, clusterin is not expressed in all tissues in which apoptosis occurs, and its role, if any, is not clear. In contrast to traditional theory that clusterin was a marker for apoptotic cell death, it has been suggested that clusterin actually is expressed only in cells destined to survive an apoptotic event (French et al, 1994).

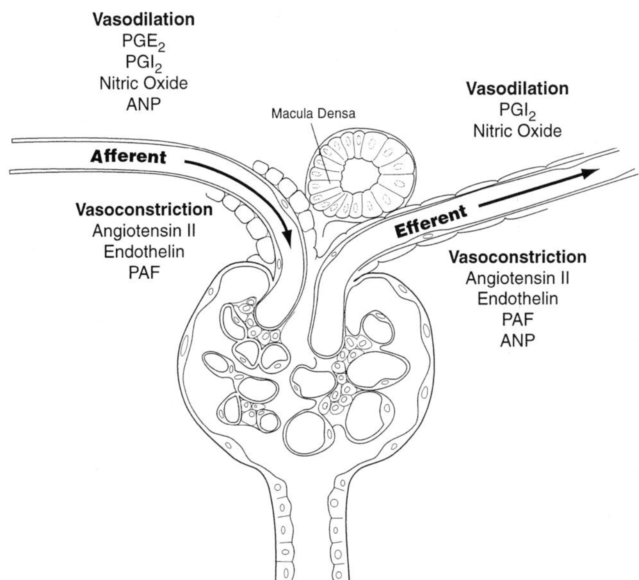

Figure 9–11. Vasoactive mediator effects on the glomerulus. A schematic of a glomerulus is shown, and effects of vasoactive mediators on the afferent and efferent arterioles are indicated. The induction of nitric oxide synthase in the macula densa (Schulsinger et al, unpublished results) may also contribute to the vasoactive effects of nitric oxide. (Adapted from Holley KE: Anatomy of the kidney. *In* Knox FG, ed: Textbook of Renal Pathophysiology. New York, Harper & Row, 1978, pp 25–42. By permission of Mayo Foundation.)

Transforming Growth Factor-β

Transforming growth factor-β (TGF-β) exists in five distinct isoforms and has been shown to increase mRNA levels for matrix proteins and to increase their secretion (Roberts et al, 1992; Border and Noble, 1994). TGF-β also reduces degradation of extracellular matrix. It decreases synthesis of proteases that degrade extracellular matrix or can increase inhibitors of these proteases, the so-called TIMPS (Laiho et al, 1987; Edwards et al, 1987). However, even this simple paradigm is complicated by reports showing that TGF-β may decrease synthesis of some TIMPs (Denhardt et al, 1993). Conversely, extracellular matrix can regulate TGF-β activity by binding it and inactivating it (Andres et al, 1989; Yamaguchi et al, 1990; Paralkar et al, 1991). In vivo, TGF-β has been implicated in the pathophysiology of glomerulonephritis, diabetes, and lung fibrosis. **In glomerulonephritis, administration of either serum-containing antibodies to TGF-β or decorin (a TGF-β antagonist) diminishes extracellular matrix deposition in the kidney** (Border and Noble, 1994; Bruijn et al, 1994). **This suggests a causal relationship between TGF-β and excessive fibrosis.**

To summarize, many different mediators can be synthesized by the kidney and can act locally to affect renal function. These mediators have hemodynamic effects, and may also have effects on fibrosis. A schematic of a glomerulus, listing the major mediators, is shown in Figure 9–11. Their involvement in UUO is detailed in the following section.

MEDIATOR INVOLVEMENT IN THE HEMODYNAMIC CHANGES OF UUO

Eicosanoids

The role of eicosanoids in the response to UUO has been extensively studied. The role of vasodilator eicosanoids in phase I seems to be established and accepted; however, the role of vasoconstrictor eicosanoids in phase III of UUO is still controversial. Eicosanoids, by virtue of their myogenic properties as well as their association with pain pathways, may also play an important role in renal colic.

The first studies to establish a role for eicosanoids in phase I of UUO were carried out by Allen and co-workers (1978). They administered a bolus of indomethacin, followed by a continuous infusion for 50 minutes before and during acute UUO, in conscious dogs. The intravenous administration of indomethacin caused an immediate decline in both ipsilateral and contralateral RBF before obstruction. After ligation of the ipsilateral ureter, there was a further decline in RBF, without the initial vasodilatation seen in the control group after acute ureteral occlusion. The contralateral RBF after obstruction changed minimally from the initial decrease after the infusion of indomethacin. This decrease in RBF was accompanied by a decrease in ureteral pressure. The data suggested that unopposed renovascular constriction follows from the inhibition of prostaglandin synthesis in the acute UUO model. Allen and co-workers further postulated that because there was an associated decrease in ureteral pressure, the afferent arteriole is the site of the increase in vascular resistance. These results have been confirmed by other researchers in dogs and pigs (Blackshear and Wathen, 1978; Frøkiær et al, 1993).

Although eicosanoids were not measured in the experiments by Allen and co-workers (1978), numerous studies since have documented marked changes in eicosanoid synthesis in UUO. Studies by Needleman's group in rabbits demonstrated increased eicosanoid synthesis in the isolated perfused kidney, induction of TxA_2 synthesis in the perfused kidney, and changes in microsomal metabolism of arachidonic acid in obstructed kidneys from rabbits and humans (Morrison et al, 1977, 1981; Currie and Needleman, 1984). Other investigators have noted increased TxB_2 (TxA_2 metabolite) and PGE_2 in tissue slices of kidneys that had undergone obstruction (Whinnery et al, 1982) and in glomeruli from obstructed kidneys incubated in vitro (Yanagisawa et al, 1990). Frøkiær and Sorensen (1995) demonstrated an increase in the urinary excretion of PGE_2 from the contralateral kidney after UUO. Furthermore, the excretion of this eicosanoid was significantly decreased by the intravenous administration of indomethacin before obstruction.

The role of the potent vasoconstrictor eicosanoid TxA_2 has been studied by a number of groups with varying results. In dogs, with the use of either a TxA_2 receptor blocker, SQ 29,548 (Fig. 9–12*A*), or a TxA_2 synthesis inhibitor, OKY-046 (see Fig. 9–12*B*) (Loo et al, 1986; Felsen et al, 1990), no effect was seen on the renal response to UUO. OKY-046, in doses that were documented to inhibit renal TxA_2 synthesis, also had no effect on the renal hemodynamic response in rabbits (see Fig. 9–12*C*) subjected to UUO for 24, 48, or 72 hours (Loo et al, 1987). These studies confirm the results of Balint and Laszlo (1985), who studied both indomethacin and imidazole in dogs after 24 hours of UUO. Using microspheres to measure regional RBF, they showed that outer cortical vasoconstriction predominated. Inner cortical perfusion did not change. Indomethacin led to vasoconstriction in all cortical layers, and imidazole was ineffective. These results suggest that vasodilator prostaglandins modulate a nonprostaglandin vasoconstrictor. Similar results were found by Strand and associates (1981) in the rat and by Frøkiær and associates in the pig (1988).

Other workers, however, have implicated TxA_2 in the decreased RBF associated with UUO. Yarger and colleagues (1980) demonstrated a decrease in the vasoconstriction post-UUO with administration of imidazole, a TxA_2 synthesis inhibitor. In their studies, indomethacin, which decreases synthesis of both vasodilator and vasoconstrictor eicosanoids, had no beneficial effect on RBF in this model. DP-1904, a different TxA_2 synthesis inhibitor, decreased renal TxB_2 production and increased the ratio of prostacyclin to TxA_2 metabolites. Urine volume, GFR, and RPF were all improved when DP-1904 was given 4 days after UUO (Masumura et al, 1991). Rinder and associates (1994), using a TxA_2 receptor blocker, GR32191, 24 hours after UUO in rats, also showed improved renal function (see Fig. 9–12*D*). Histopathologic changes were also attenuated. It is not clear why these discrepancies exist. Possible explanations include differences in species used, time course and doses of the drugs used, and differing pharmacologic profiles of the drugs used.

Leukotriene synthesis in UUO has also been demonstrated. Albrightson and colleagues (1987) found release of leukotrienes B_4, C_4, D_4, and E_4 after stimulation of the isolated perfused obstructed kidney. Release of leukotrienes was associated with vasoconstriction, which was partially blocked by a leukotriene receptor antagonist and completely inhibited by a TxA_2 synthase inhibitor.

Renin-Angiotensin System

The renin-angiotensin system has been studied by many investigators in the pathophysiology of renal vasoconstriction during UUO (Vaughan et al, 1970b; Frøkiær et al, 1992a, 1992b). Elevated levels of plasma renin have been described during UUO (Vaughan et al, 1970b). Frøkiær and colleagues (1992b) described an enhanced intrarenal generation of AII during 15 hours of ureteral occlusion from the obstructed kidney. However, using sar^1-ala^8-AII, an AII antagonist (with partial agonist activity), Moody et al (1977b) failed to demonstrate a beneficial effect of AII blockade on renal hemodynamics in UUO. These results were confirmed by Huland and colleagues (1980), who showed that another AII antagonist, sar^1-ile^8-AII, did not change ipsilateral renal vascular resistance after either 7 hours of UUO or 1, 2, and 3 weeks of ureteral occlusion. Experiments carried out in the ensuing years have suggested a more prominent role for AII in UUO, but there are a number of conflicting reports. Yarger and colleagues (1980) demonstrated that the ACE inhibitor captopril, given 24 hours after UUO, could reverse the decreases in RBF and GFR but would not return them to preobstruction levels; saralasin was ineffective. More recently, Pimentel and associates (1993) pretreated rats with either losartan or the ACE inhibitor lisinopril. Both drugs significantly ameliorated the effects of 24 hours of UUO on GFR and RBF. Franke and McDougal (1991) demonstrated that in animals pretreated with enalapril, there was a trend toward an improvement in RPF and a significant increase in GFR.

Other workers, however, have shown that renin depletion did not alter the increased renal vascular resistance found 24 hours after UUO (Huguenin et al, 1976); furthermore, studies examining the distribution of immunoreactive renin showed no change in chronic obstruction of mouse kidney (Buhrle et al, 1986). Changes in renin gene expression have also been examined in UUO. El-Dahr and co-workers (1990) found no change in the expression of or distribution of renin in the obstructed kidney either 24 hours or 4 weeks after UUO; after 4 weeks of UUO, the contralateral kidney was hypertrophied and showed decreased renin gene expression. Further studies by the same group, however, demonstrated changes in both renin gene expression and AII content of kidneys subjected to UUO for 1 or 5 weeks. The conflict with their previous data was not explained (El-Dahr et al, 1993). Pimentel and associates (1993) demonstrated a marked increase in renin immunoreactivity in the juxtaglomerular apparatus, in the distal third of the afferent arteriole, and in the epithelial cells of the distal tubules, the glomerular tuft, and the mesangial cells of the obstructed kidney. This increase in renin immunoreactivity was not seen in the contralateral unobstructed kidney. The increase in renin immunoreactivity was accompanied by an increase in the expression of mRNA in the corresponding areas of the obstructed kidney, whereas there was essentially an inhibition of mRNA expression in the contralateral kidney.

Pimentel and associates (1994) also reported changes in ACE and angiotensinogen. Studies in pig kidneys, which are polypapillary, have also noted changes in the renin-angiotensin system. Frøkiær and colleagues (1992a, 1992b) demonstrated an enhanced intrarenal generation of AII, as measured both by renal extraction ratios and by sampling renal venous and aortic blood. Thus the demonstration of the effectiveness of some ACE inhibitors or receptor antagonists, together with some data suggesting increases in the

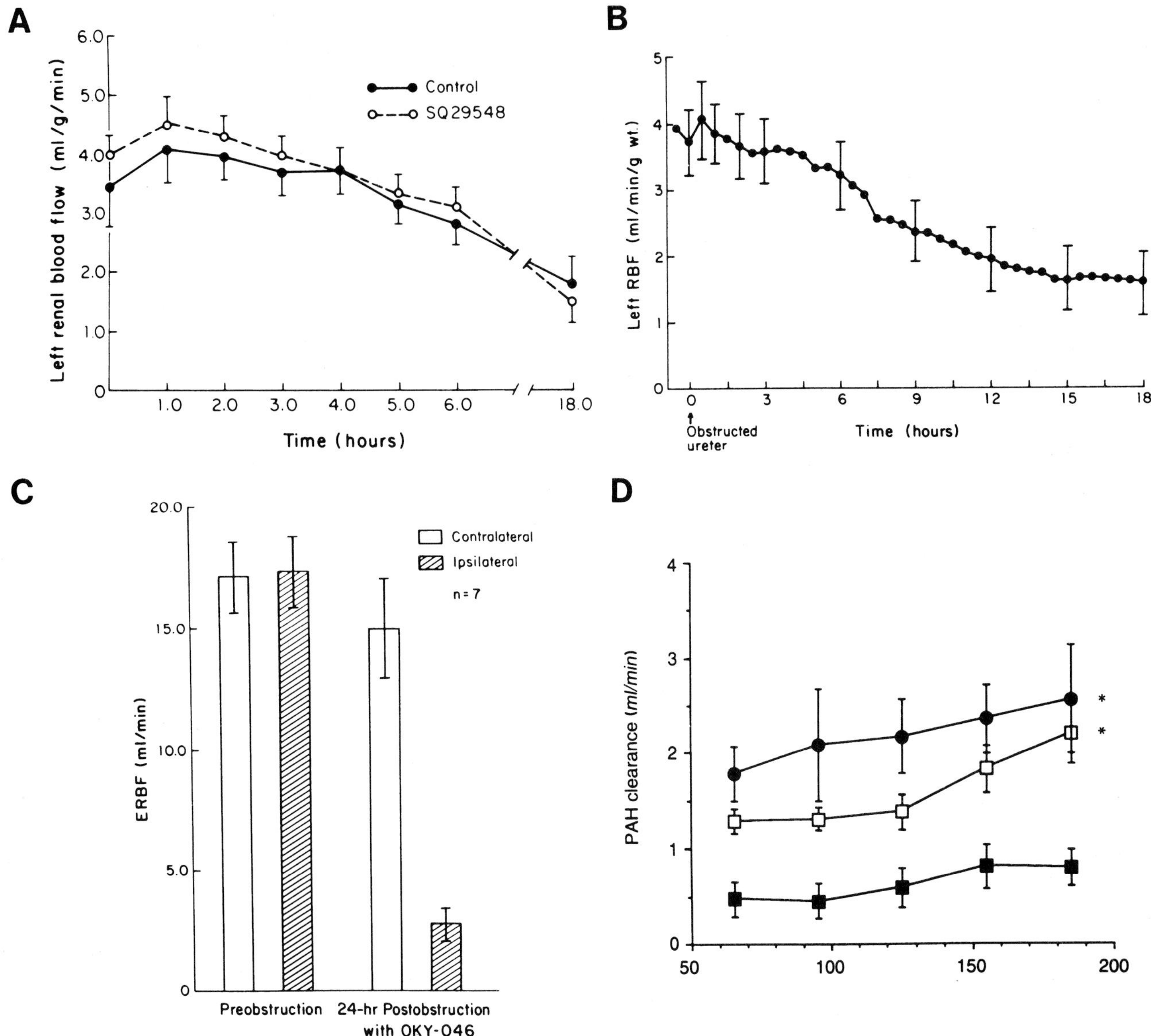

Figure 9–12. Comparison of effects of thromboxane A_2 (TxA_2) receptor blocker and inhibition of renal function in unilateral ureteral occlusion (UUO). *A,* The effect of the TxA_2 receptor blocker SQ29548 on renal blood flow (RBF) in UUO in the dog monitored for 18 hours of UUO. *B,* The effect of the TxA_2 synthetase inhibitor OKY-046 on RBF in UUO in the dog monitored for 18 hours of UUO. (Control obstruction not shown.) *C,* The effect of OKY-046 in UUO in the rabbit. RBF was measured before UUO and at relief of 24 hours of UUO. *A* to *C* demonstrate that either inhibition of TxA_2 synthesis or interaction of TxA_2 with its receptor had no effect on the decreased RBF associated with UUO. *D,* Effect of the TxA_2 receptor blocker GR32191 on RBF in the rat. *Solid squares* represent control UUO; *open squares* represent UUO + GR32191 at 3 mg/kg; *solid circles* represent UUO + GR32191 at 6 mg/kg. Note that GR32191 increases RBF from control obstruction levels. (*A* from Felsen D, Loo MH, Marion D, et al: J Urol 1990; 144:141–145. *B,* from Loo MH, Marion DN, Vaughan ED, et al: J Urol 1986; 136:1343–1347. *C* from Loo MH, Egan D, Vaughan ED Jr, et al: J Urol 1987; 137:571–576. *D* from Rinder CA, Halushka PV, Sens MA, Ploth DW: Kidney Int 1994; 45:185–192.)

intrarenal generation of AII, provide evidence for a role for AII in the hemodynamic response to UUO.

The renin-angiotensin system may play a much more important role in the developing kidney during obstruction. In a series of studies, Chevalier and his group have shown that the renin-angiotensin system is activated in the developing kidney. In addition, the renin-angiotensin system is further activated during UUO and plays a role in renal growth as well as partially mediating the increased renal resistance. Furthermore, the renin-angiotensin system most likely promotes renal interstitial fibrosis and cell death through AT_1 receptors, possibly through stimulation of endogenous TGF-β (Chevalier, 1990; Chung et al, 1995; Peters, 1995).

Nitric Oxide

A number of studies have examined the role of nitric oxide in the hemodynamic response to UUO. In the isolated perfused obstructed rabbit kidney, there was a time-dependent increase in release of NO_2^-, a breakdown product of nitric oxide. Furthermore, bradykinin-stimulated release of prostaglandin E_2 was attenuated by L-NMMA, a NOS inhibitor, which also abolished the NO_2^- release. Aminoguanidine, which in some but not all studies has been shown to be a specific inhibitor of the inducible form of NOS, had effects similar to those of L-NMMA. These studies demonstrate the presence of nitric oxide in the obstructed kidney and also demonstrate that an inducible form of NOS is found in the obstructed kidney (Salvemini et al, 1994).

In rats, infusion of L-NAME, a NOS inhibitor, after 24 hours of UUO results in a decrease in RBF and an increase in the ratio of renal vascular resistance to total vascular resistance (Chevalier et al, 1992). In dogs, administration of L-arginine in the absence of obstruction had no effect on renal hemodynamics; thus, providing additional substrate for NOS either does not provide additional nitric oxide or is unnecessary for maintaining normal hemodynamics (Schulsinger et al, 1993). Nitric oxide may, however, play a role in UUO. **Lanzone and colleagues (1995) demonstrated that administration of L-NMMA before UUO attenuated the initial rise in RBF. When the L-NMMA infusion was discontinued, the rise in RBF was restored within 10 minutes. These findings provide strong evidence for the role of nitric oxide in reducing preglomerular vascular resistance after ureteral occlusion.** Previous micropuncture studies have shown an increase in glomerular capillary hydrostatic pressure after ureteral occlusion (Dal Canton et al, 1977; Ichikawa, 1982). This increase in pressure may provide the stimulus for the release of nitric oxide by physically stretching the endothelium, a known mechanism for the release of nitric oxide in isolated vessels (Marsden and Brenner, 1991).

The interaction between nitric oxide and the prostanoid system has been investigated. **The administration of L-arginine after 140 minutes of ureteral occlusion, in the presence of a cyclooxygenase inhibitor, restored RBF and ureteral pressure to values similar to those of UUO alone** (Schulsinger et al, 1993). Interestingly, the administration of L-arginine in the absence of UUO, with or without prostaglandin synthesis inhibition, did not alter renal hemodynamics. This emphasizes the importance of UUO, and perhaps the associated increase in glomerular hydrostatic pressure, in activating the nitric oxide pathway. Conversely, an activated nitric oxide system appears to contribute to the changes in RBF in UUO, whereas the contribution of nitric oxide to maintenance of normal RBF is limited. This may occur through up-regulation of NOS, the enzyme necessary for the conversion of substrate (i.e., L-arginine) into nitric oxide. Induction of NOS-2 has been found in rat kidneys after UUO. Through use of the polymerase chain reaction, induction of NOS-2 has been found as early as 90 minutes, and immunohistochemical localization of NOS-2 has been demonstrated at 3 days after UUO and continuing through 28 days (Schulsinger et al, 1996).

Endothelin

Administration of endothelin to a normal kidney results in decreases in both RBF and GFR through a locally active preglomerular vasoconstriction (Kon et al, 1989). Kahn and co-investigators (1995) demonstrated an increase in the vasoconstrictor ET-1 in dogs with 19 hours of UUO. Kelleher and colleagues (1992) also demonstrated a significant increase in the urinary excretion of ET-1 from the postobstructive kidney and not from the contralateral kidney in long-standing UUO. However, studies with endothelin antibodies or antagonists have not been carried out to ascertain its specific involvement in the hemodynamic response to UUO.

Endothelin mediates vasoconstriction by increasing the influx of calcium into the smooth muscle cells of the blood vessel. The direct intrarenal infusion of verapamil after relief of UUO significantly increased RBF and GFR associated with a profound ipsilateral diuresis and natriuresis (Kahn et al, 1995). Although the effects of verapamil may result from interactions with endothelin, this remains to be proved.

Platelet Activating Factor

PAF, when given intrarenally, has been shown to decrease RBF, GFR, and urinary volume (Camussi et al, 1990). In the preobstructed kidney, SRI 63-441, a PAF antagonist, had no effect on RBF; in addition, it did not alter the renal hemodynamic response to UUO (Felsen et al, 1990). This suggests that PAF is not involved in maintenance of either baseline RBF or RBF in the presence of UUO.

TUBULAR CHANGES IN UUO

The changes in tubule function after correction of ureteropelvic junction obstruction have been well characterized. Data from a typical patient are shown in Figure 9–13 (J. Gillenwater, unpublished). Gillenwater and associates (1975) presented data on 10 patients with UUO; seven had obstructions secondary to a ureteropelvic junction obstruction, and three had ureteral obstruction. The symptoms lasted from 2 days to 36 months; the average period was about 12 months. The degree of obstruction was graded as moderate to severe in all cases. The patients' ages ranged from 7 to 38 years, with a mean of 23.8 years. Function in the obstructed kidney was evaluated 1 week after relief of obstruction, as shown in Table 9–1. The GFR in the obstructed kidney was significantly less than that in the nonobstructed kidney: 24 versus 60 ml/minute, respectively, $P < .0002$. The GFRs in the obstructed kidneys ranged from 8.0 to 50 ml/minute; the GFRs in only three kidneys were below 20 ml/minute. The mean urine osmolality, absolute osmolar clearance (C_{Osm}), and the absolute and fractional free water clearances were all significantly less in the obstructed kidney. The fractional osmolar clearances (C_{Osm}/GFR) were not different in the two kidneys. Therefore, a true concentrating defect existed between the obstructed and nonobstructed kidneys at 1 week after relief of obstruction. However, no patients experienced a significant postobstructive diuresis. The absolute sodium excretion was lower from the obstructed kidney; however, the fractional sodium excretion was the same. This salt excretion was resistant to pretreatment of the patient with desoxycorticosterone acetate. There was no difference in the fractional titratable acid or ammonia excretion in either kidney in five of the seven patients. Proximal tubular transport, measured by T_{mPAH}, was also impaired after ureteral obstruction. However, when it was adjusted for the decrease in GFR secondary to the obstruction, there was no difference between the two kidneys. **In rare cases in which GFR is**

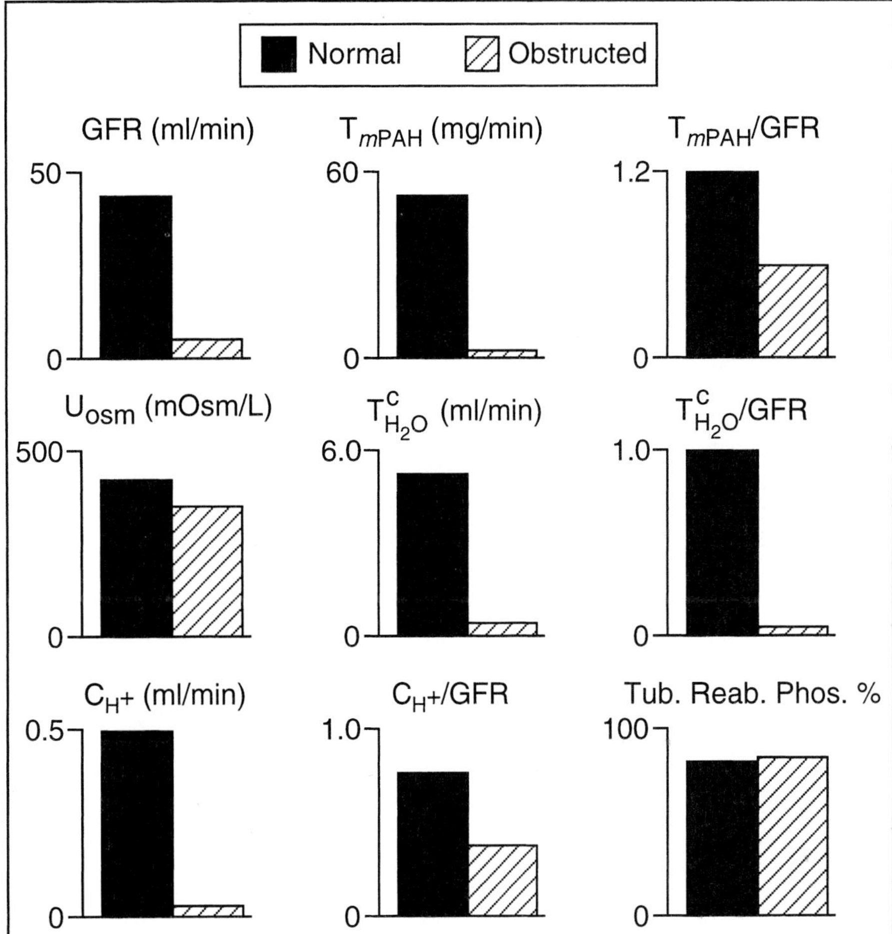

Figure 9–13. Patient tubular function after relief of UUO. (Unpublished data of J. Y. Gillenwater.)

preserved, clinically significant water loss necessitating intravenous replacement can occur (Schlossberg and Vaughan, 1984).

Similar tubular changes have been observed after release of UUO in rats (Harris and Yarger, 1974; Dal Canton et al, 1977). However, during partial UUO, especially early before tubular damage occurs, there actually is a decrease in sodium and water excretion with a resultant increase in urine osmolality, similar to changes found in renal artery stenosis (Suki et al, 1971; Wilson, 1980).

Several studies suggested that the increased excretion of water and salt after UUO occurs in either deep nephrons or the collecting duct of superficial nephrons (Buerkert et al, 1976, 1978). However, Buerkert and co-investigators (1979) were able to show with micropuncture studies that the collecting duct's ability for reabsorption and its permeability to water were not altered by acute ureteral occlusion. Therefore, the more likely location for the increased sodium excretion is the deep juxtamedullary nephron (Table 9–2).

Jaenike and Bray (1960) were able to produce a concentrating defect in the unilaterally obstructed kidney after only 6 minutes of ureteral occlusion. Kessler (1960) was able to demonstrate a concentrating defect in the obstructed kidney within 5 to 8 minutes of ureteral occlusion. The administration of large doses of antidiuretic hormone (ADH) restored the concentrating ability and the papillary chloride concentration in saline-loaded animals. This observation is contrary to that of other investigators, who have found the concentrating defect in the ipsilateral kidney of UUO to be ADH-resistant. Solez and associates (1976) observed a marked decrease in urine osmolality in dehydrated rats after relief of 18 hours of UUO, not in association with a concomitant increase in urine output. They found a significant decrease in inner medullary plasma flow during 18 hours of UUO, and the flow increased after the release of ureteral occlusion. Histologic study revealed necrosis of both the inner and outer medullae. It may be this physical effect of obstruction on the medulla that results in a decreased ability of the post-UUO kidney to concentrate urine.

Wilson (1974) examined the effect of volume expansion on post-UUO renal function and found a significant increase in free water clearance from the obstructed kidney in association with an increase in urine flow rate. Wilson concluded that volume expansion was enhancing an already-present defect in water reabsorption either in distal nephrons and/or deep nephrons or in collecting ducts of the obstructed kidney. Hanley and Davidson (1982) also described an inability of the kidney to concentrate urine after obstruction. This inabil-

Table 9–1. SUMMARY OF MAXIMAL URINE CONCENTRATION STUDIES DURING INFUSION OF INULIN, ADH, MANNITOL, AND 33% NORMAL SALINE (USE OF ONLY SINGLE CLEARANCE DURING MAXIMAL OSMOLALITY)

	GFR (ml/min)		U_{Osm} (mOsm/kg)		C_{Osm} (ml/min)		C_{Osm}/GFR × 100		$T^c_{H_2O}$ (ml/min)		$T^c_{H_2O}$/GFR × 100		$U_{Na}V$ (μEq/min)		$U_{Na}V$/GFR		%Na Rejected	
Patient No.	*N*	*O*	*N*	*O*	*N*	*O*	*N*	*O*	*N*	*O*	*N*	*O*	*N*	*O*	*N*	*O*	*N*	*O*
1	58	23	560	320	4.7	1.8	8.0	7.8	2.1	0.4	6	3	366	152	6.3	6.6	4.6	4.8
2	65	29	548	285	2.6	0.8	4.0	2.7	1.3	0.2	2	0.6	40	41	0.6	1.4	0.5	1.1
3*	58	50	909	385	1.0	0.4	2.0	0.8	0.7	0.1	1.2	0.2	30	8	0.5	0.2	0.4	0.2
4	49	23	460	450	5.7	2.6	12.0	11.0	2.4	1.1	5	4	467	186	9.5	8.0	7.0	6.0
5	60	11	537	441	3.0	1.0	5.0	9.0	1.4	0.4	2	4	210	73	3.6	6.6	2.7	5.0
6†	50	8	419	379	11.0	1.3	22.0	16.0	4.0	0.3	8	3.7	513	54	10.0	6.7	7.5	5.0
7	67	18	484	351	8.2	2.3	12.0	13.0	3.5	0.5	5	3.0	931	219	14.0	12.0	9.6	8.3
8	43	25	509	356	3.3	2.9	7.6	12.0	1.4	0.5	3	2.0	245	240	5.7	9.6	4.0	7.0
9	95	25	544	488	4.6	1.0	4.8	4.0	2.1	0.4	2	1.6	385	88	4.0	3.5	2.8	2.5
10	52	30	484	212	3.4	1.3	6.5	4.3	1.4	−(0.5)	2.7	(1.7)	272	115	5.2	3.8	4.0	2.9
Mean	60	24	545	367	4.8	1.5	8.4	8.1	2.0	0.3	3	2	346	118	5.9	5.8	4.3	4.3
±SEM	±4.5	±3.7	±42.8	±26	±0.9	±0.3	±1.8	±1.6	±0.3	±0.1	±0.8	±0.5	±82.7	±24.9	±1.3	±1.5	±0.9	±0.8
	N = 10		N = 10		N = 10		N = 10		N = 10		N = 10		N = 10		N = 10		N = 10	
P value	P = 0.0002		P = 0.003		P= 0.003		P = 0.36		P = 0.0003		P = 0.02		P = 0.01		P = 0.44		P = 0.48	

ADH, antidiuretic hormone; GFR, glomerular filtration rate; U_{Osm}, urine osmolarity; C_{Osm}, osmolar clearance; $T^c_{H_2O}$, free water clearance; N, normal; O, obstructed; SEM, standard error of the mean.
*GFR = creatinine clearance and before mannitol given.
†GFR = creatinine clearance.

Table 9–2. GFR AND SEGMENTAL REABSORPTION IN SUPERFICIAL (S) AND JUXTAMEDULLARY (J) NEPHRONS AND IN THE COLLECTING DUCTS (CD) IN NORMAL RATS AND AFTER THE RELEASE OF BILATERAL OR UNILATERAL URETERAL OBSTRUCTION

	Values in Individual Nephron			Values in All Functioning Nephrons				
Site	***SNGFR* (nl/min/kg)***	***Fraction of Water Remaining (%)***	***Fraction of Sodium Remaining (%)***	***Number of Nephrons in Group***	***Fraction of Functioning Nephrons (%)***	***GFR of Functioning Nephrons (ml/min/kg)***	***Water in Functioning Nephrons (ml/min/kg)***	***Sodium in Functioning Nephrons (μEq/min/kg)***
				Normal				
S_1	150	100.0	100.0	27,000	100	4.05	4.05	567.0
S_2	150	44.0	44.0	27,000	100	4.05	1.78	249.0
S_3	150	26.0	14.0	27,000	100	4.05	1.05	79.0
S_4	150	9.4	5.0	27,000	100	4.05	0.38	28.0
J_1	330	100.0	100.0	3000	100	1.00	1.00	140.0
J_2	330	12.0	40.0	3000	100	1.00	0.12	56.0
CD_1*	—	3.3	2.0	30,000	100	5.05	0.17	14.0
CD_2	—	0.4	0.6	30,000	100	5.05	0.020	4.2
				$\bar{p}$ Bilateral Obstruction				
S_1	50	100.0	100.0	27,000	80	1.08	1.08	150.0
S_2	50	45.0	45.0	27,000	80	1.08	0.49	68.0
S_3	50	40.0	22.0	27,000	80	1.08	0.43	33.0
S_4	50	25.0	7.0	27,000	80	1.08	0.27	11.0
J_1	100	100.0	100.0	3000	49	0.15	0.15	21.0
J_2	100	42.0	62.0	3000	49	0.15	0.06	13.0
CD_1	—	8.0	6.0	30,000	77	1.23	0.10	10.0
CD_2	—	16.7	12.0	30,000	77	1.23	0.21	21.0
				$\bar{p}$ Unilateral Obstruction				
S_1	50	100.0	100.0	27,000	40	0.54	0.54	75.6
S_2	50	26.0	26.0	27,000	40	0.54	0.14	20.0
S_3	50	21.0	12.0	27,000	40	0.54	0.11	9.1
S_4	50	3.2	1.6	27,000	40	0.54	0.071	1.2
J_1	174	100.0	100.0	3000	20	0.10	0.10	14.0
J_2	174	42.0	52.0	3000	20	0.10	0.04	7.3
CD_1	—	4.2	3.8	30,000	38	0.64	0.027	3.4
CD_2	—	2.9	2.5	30,000	38	0.64	0.018	2.2

SNGFR, single nephron glomerular filtration rate.
*Values for GFR, water, and sodium in the collecting duct result from the combined delivery from both superficial and juxtamedullary nephrons. The values are derived from the many studies referenced in the text.

ity to concentrate the urine was associated with an inability of the cortical collecting tubule to respond to either ADH (vasopressin) or cyclic adenosine monophosphate (cAMP) stimulation with a 76% reduction in the response of the collecting tubule to either stimulus. As previously described, there is an increase in PGE_2 production with UUO. **It is also known that PGE_2 can inhibit the tubular effects of vasopressin, increasing free water losses from the post-UUO kidney** (Grantham and Orloff, 1968).

The kidney after obstruction has an impaired distal hydrogen ion secretion. This is seen as a lack of an increase in carbon dioxide partial pressure (P_{CO_2}) during bicarbonate loading, as well as an impaired urinary acidification with the administration of sodium sulfate. The postobstruction kidney has a higher bicarbonate reabsorption rate than the contralateral kidney (Thirakomen et al, 1976). Walls and co-workers (1975) also demonstrated a low urinary P_{CO_2} during bicarbonate loading in the post-UUO kidney in comparison with the contralateral kidney, as well as an elevation in urinary pH from the postobstruction kidney.

After the release of UUO, the fractional excretion of phosphate is markedly decreased in the obstructed kidney (3.4%), whereas it is increased in the control kidney (35.3%). This was accompanied by a twofold greater fractional excretion of sodium in the obstructed kidney than in the control kidney. However, the decrease in phosphate excretion is believed to be secondary to a decreased filtered load of phosphate. The increased excretion of salt and water is secondary to a decreased reabsorption in the distal nephron without a concomitant decrease in proximal reabsorption (Purkerson et al, 1974).

Harris and Yarger (1975) described a marked decrease in urinary potassium excretion after 24 hours of UUO from the ipsilateral kidney. Yarger and Griffith (1974) found a decrease in both the absolute and fractional excretion of potassium after 24 hours of UUO with micropuncture studies. This suggests that the decrease in potassium excretion does not result from a decrease in the filtered load of potassium. Explanations for the decrease in potassium excretion would be that the distal tubular volume flow rate is low after UUO, the amount of sodium passing through the distal nephron is also decreased during UUO, and the normal potassium secretory mechanism has been interfered with directly as a result of mechanical obstruction. These explanations are supported by the work of Thirakomen and associates (1976), who showed a persistent decrease in absolute potassium excretion despite volume expansion or sodium sulfate administration. These two maneuvers increase distal sodium delivery, but they do not increase the excretion of potassium; this action lends support to the hypothesis of a defect in the distal secretory mechanism of potassium as the cause for the decreased excretion of potassium from the post-UUO kidney.

CELLULAR INFILTRATES AND CYTOKINES IN UUO

Interstitial Cells, Myofibroblasts, and Macrophages

The role of macrophages in the response to obstruction has been studied since the early 1970s. Nagle and co-workers (1973a) showed that macrophages were present in obstructed rabbit kidneys. Much work was done in obstructed rabbit kidneys by Needleman and co-workers (Currie and Needleman, 1984). In their model, the isolated perfused rabbit kidney demonstrated exaggerated eicosanoid synthesis in an ex vivo perfusion system. There is a time-dependent increase in eicosanoid release, as well as an induction in the release of the vasoconstrictor TxA_2. The macrophage stimulant endotoxin causes an exaggerated eicosanoid release. Treatments that decrease the interstitial macrophage population decrease the endotoxin-stimulated release of eicosanoid (Okegawa et al, 1983; Lefkowith et al, 1984).

Macrophages have also been localized in rat kidneys, and their relationship to the fibrotic response of UUO is being actively investigated. Schreiner and associates (1988) described the presence of macrophages in cortical and medullary tissue isolated from rats with UUO of 24 hours' duration; relief of UUO was associated with disappearance of macrophages from tissue isolates. Macrophages have also been localized with monoclonal antibody and have been found in interstitial tissue. Macrophages increased in number by 12 hours later and continued to increase through 96 hours. Macrophages were found in association with TGF-β (Diamond et al, 1994). These results are in contrast to those of Wright and colleagues (1996), who found fewer macrophages in the obstructed rat kidney than did Diamond and associates; these macrophages were not associated with TGF-β staining (Fig. 9–14*A* and *B*).

The influx of macrophages into the kidney may be in response to a specific chemoattractant. A heat-stable lipid with macrophage-attracting ability was found in greater amounts in the obstructed kidney than in the contralateral kidney (Rovin et al, 1990). A peptide known as monocyte chemoattractant peptide-1 (MCP-1) was found in tubules of obstructed, but not contralateral, kidneys (Diamond et al, 1994).

Transforming Growth Factor-β

The involvement of TGF-β in the fibrosis of UUO has been studied by analyzing expression of TGF-β mRNA and by immunohistochemical localization of TGF-β. Increased mRNA expression of TGF-β was found as early as 10 hours after obstruction and was increased through 96 hours (Walton et al, 1992; Diamond et al, 1994). Pretreatment of animals with OKY-046, a TxA_2 synthase inhibitor, had no effect on TGF-β mRNA expression, whereas pretreatment with an ACE inhibitor blunted, but did not completely abolish, the increase in TGF-β mRNA. When tubules and glomeruli from the obstructed kidneys were separated, glomerular TGF-β mRNA was found not to differ from that in the control kidneys, whereas tubular TGF-β mRNA was increased in UUO (Kaneto et al, 1993). TGF-β localization in obstructed kidneys has been studied through immunohistochemistry, and conflicting results have been found. Wright and colleagues (1996) found that tubular TGF-β was increased in the obstructed rat kidney medulla (see Fig. 9–14*C* and *D*); cortical TGF-β was not greatly affected by UUO. This was confirmed in measurement of tissue levels of TGF-β, which were found to be increased in the medulla after UUO. Diamond and associates (1994) found TGF-β in association with interstitial macrophages in early obstruction and not in association with tubules. The reasons for this difference is not clear. However, in studies using the angiotensin receptor antagonist losartan, it was found that losartan treatment decreased the fibrosis of obstruction without decreasing interstitial macrophage number (Ishidoya et al, 1995). Whole-body irradiation lowered cortical macrophage number, TGF-β, and smooth muscle actin mRNA (Diamond et al, 1995). **The involvement of macrophages in the fibrotic response to UUO is unclear at this time.**

The finding by Rinder and associates (1994) of improvement in the histologic appearance of the kidney suggests that TxA_2 (and other eicosanoids) may have a role in the kidney apart from effects on hemodynamics. Comparable results with losartan suggest a similar and expanded role for AII in both the fibrosis and the hemodynamics of UUO. Further studies are needed in this area.

Clusterin

Both cell proliferation and cell death are observed in the obstructed and contralateral kidneys as a result of UUO. Cell death processes may involve necrosis and/or apoptosis, the process of programmed cell death. Apoptosis is also found in embryogenesis and development and may therefore reflect tissue remodeling as well as death. The expression of the gene TRPM-2 and clusterin, the protein product of the SGP-2 gene, have been studied. In the rat kidney, induction of SGP-2 was noted as early as 10 hours after UUO, and the expression continued at least up to 48 hours. No SGP-2 expression was found in normal, sham-operated, or contralateral kidneys at any time (Sawczuk et al, 1989). With in-situ hybridization, SGP-2 expression occurred as early as 30 minutes after UUO. There was labeling in the adventitia of hilar arteries as well as in intrarenal arterioles and interlobular arteries; cortical tubules did not express SGP-2 at 30 minutes. The most intense staining at 24 hours was found over epithelial cells of collecting tubules and distal tubules, coinciding with a slightly dilated, flattened epithelium. At 48 hours, the majority of distal and collecting tubules both were dilated and showed intense SGP-2 staining. Tubules that did not appear to be dilated did not express SGP-2. By 6 days, SGP-2 expression persisted but was decreased in comparison to earlier times. Glomeruli of the obstructed

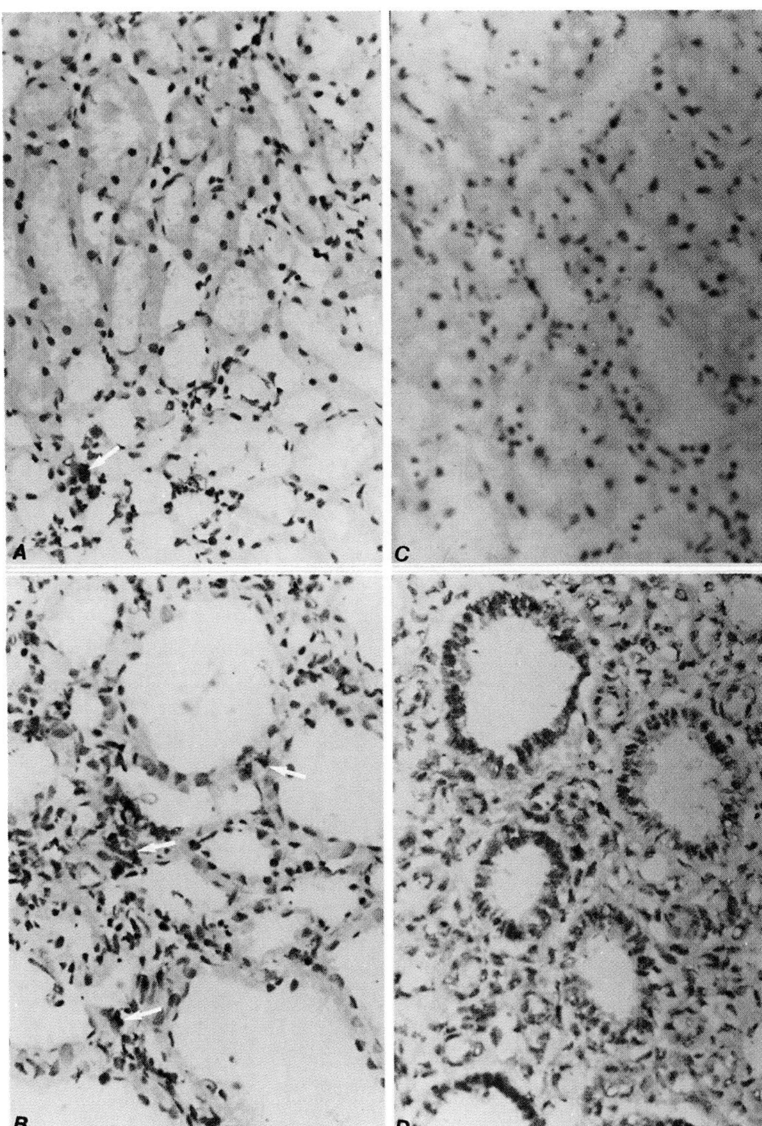

Figure 9–14. Immunohistochemical localization of macrophages and transforming growth factor-β (TGF-β) in an obstructed rat kidney. *A,* Macrophages: sham. *B,* Macrophages: at 7 days. *C,* TGF-β: sham. *D,* TGF-β: 14 days after medullary section. Macrophages increase in the interstitial space with UUO, whereas TGF-β increases are associated with tubular cells. (From Wright EJ, McCaffrey TA, Robertson AP, et al: Lab Invest 1996; 74:528–537.)

kidney did not show SGP-2 expression at any time (Connor et al, 1991).

The expression of clusterin in both renal tissue and urine in relation to renal function after UUO has been studied in rabbits. The studies demonstrated that production of clusterin was associated with decreases in RBF and GFR, as well as in renal concentrating ability, as measured by sodium reabsorption and urine osmolality. As was found in rats, clusterin mRNA was detected in collecting and distal tubules at 12 hours after UUO. After 7 days, increased clusterin expression was detected in proximal tubular epithelium. In rabbits, clusterin gene expression remained elevated in collecting ducts for 60 days after UUO (Schlegel et al, 1992). Whether these cells are destined to survive the obstructive event remains to be studied (French et al, 1994).

PARTIAL OBSTRUCTION MODEL

Although partial ureteral obstruction is commonly found among patients, most studies of experimental models of obstruction have been done in the completely obstructed state. A major problem with studies involving partial obstruction is to be able to reproducibly and accurately determine the degree of obstruction induced. In 1987, Ryan and Fitzpatrick introduced a canine model of partial obstruction in which they created partial obstruction by inserting an obstructing stent into the left ureter. The stent was a semirigid plastic tube, 2 cm long with a 2-mm external diameter; the internal diameter was varied, depending on the degree of obstruction desired. Hydronephrosis was demonstrated in all groups by intravenous urography. Intrapelvic pressure was shown to rise initially after obstruction but was decreased to near normal by 14 days after partial obstruction. Creatinine clearance was decreased in the kidney obstructed by the higher grade obstruction and at 1 month was decreased by about 30% in the highest grade group. At necropsy, both hydroureter and hydronephrosis were confirmed. The ureter showed muscular hypertrophy. Through the use of methacrylate corrosion casts, cortical thinning was noted along with renal segmental arterial constriction.

By 1 week after partial ureteral obstruction, RBF was still

unchanged; at 1 month after obstruction, significant decreases were observed (Ryan et al, 1987). Regional RBF changes measured with labeled microspheres showed that at 5 weeks after partial ureteral obstruction, RBF was decreased on the obstructed (ipsilateral) side but increased by 40% on the unobstructed (contralateral) side. Outer cortical blood was decreased on both sides. In contrast, inner cortical blood flow was increased on both sides. Medullary blood flow was unchanged. Five weeks after reimplantation of the ureters, contralateral RBF was normalized, whereas on the obstructed side, blood flow was not significantly changed from the levels 5 weeks after partial ureteral obstruction. Ipsilateral nephroureterectomy after 5 weeks of partial ureteral obstruction had no effect on contralateral recovery; this suggests that factors that affect the contralateral side are not released from the ipsilateral kidney. Ipsilateral TxB_2 was elevated significantly 5 weeks after partial ureteral obstruction and decreased to normal after reversal of the obstruction. Ipsilateral PGE_2 tended to increase in this model but was significant in only the contralateral kidney; PGE_2 returned to normal after reimplantation.

Reversibility of renal function in this model has been assessed. Animals obstructed for 14 days showed no deficit in function at that time. Animals obstructed for 28 days recovered 31% of function; those obstructed for 60 days recovered only 8% of function (Leahy et al, 1989). In a study on reversibility, Miller and co-workers (1979) created a bilateral partial obstruction in dogs in which one side had severe obstruction and the other side moderate obstruction. There was significantly greater return of function if the more severe obstruction was released first.

In rats, there have been numerous studies of partial ureteral obstruction. Most investigators have used the technique of Ulm and Miller (1962), which involves splitting the psoas muscle longitudinally to form a groove into which the ureter is placed. Whereas most studies in dogs have been in adult animals, in rats studies have been carried out in neonates, weanlings, and older animals. Results of studies of partial obstruction in rats are variable, which may be a result of the severity and duration of the obstruction and also the age at which the obstruction is performed.

In a series of reports, Josephson and colleagues studied partial ureteral obstruction in rats of different ages. Pubescent rats with partial ureteral obstruction studied 1 to 15 weeks after obstruction showed considerable hydronephrosis within 1 week, with a decrease in the number of glomeruli. However, the changes were not progressive, and renal parenchymal weight was not affected (Josephson and Grossman, 1991). When renal function was studied in these animals, decreased urine output and less urinary sodium excretion were noted. Their conclusion was that partial ureteral obstruction in young rats seems to be "relatively harmless." RBF and GFR were not affected (Josephson et al, 1987). In contrast, partial obstruction in weanling rats was associated with substantial increases in mean arterial pressure (Josephson et al, 1992). During normal hydration, the obstructed kidney had lower excretion of urine, which had less osmolality; there was also less excretion of potassium and sodium. Partial ureteral obstruction in 12-week-old rats showed only modest changes at 3 weeks after obstruction, which were more pronounced at 1 year. However, even after 1 year, there was no loss in parenchymal weight in the partially obstructed kidney and no compensatory hypertrophy in the other kidney (Stenberg et al, 1992). Huland and associates (1988) showed in partial ureteral obstruction that atrophy develops only in the first weeks after obstruction and does not progress. If the obstruction is released early, changes can be reversed; later release does not undo damage.

There has been much less information on changes in vasoactive or inflammatory mediators in the partial ureteral obstruction model. In early studies, Ichikawa and Brenner (1979) examined single nephron GFR in rats with partial ureteral obstruction. After 4 weeks, superficial single nephron GFR, total GFR, and glomerular plasma flow rate were unchanged from control values. Administration of either indomethacin or meclofenamate decreased both single nephron GFR and GFR in association with elevations in arteriolar resistance. This suggested that vasodilatory prostaglandins are involved. Other studies have noted changes in eicosanoid excretion (Kekomaki and Vapaatalo, 1989; Sankari et al, 1991), but these have not been correlated with changes in function. Apoptosis and cytokine changes have been studied by Kennedy and colleagues (1994). They found that during the initial 3 weeks after partial ureteral obstruction, there was a progressive increase in the intensity of DNA fragmentation and an increase in apoptotic bodies in the kidney, along with increased SGP-2. TGF-β was increased, and constitutive synthesis of epidermal growth factor was decreased. These changes are comparable with those seen in complete UUO but are delayed 2 to 3 weeks.

PHYSIOLOGIC CHANGES IN BILATERAL URETERAL OBSTRUCTION

Renal Blood Flow, GFR, and Ureteral Pressure

The triphasic pattern of RBF and ureteral pressure changes that characterizes UUO is not seen after bilateral ureteral obstruction (BUO) or unilateral obstruction of a solitary kidney. RBF increases after the first 90 minutes of BUO, as it does with UUO (Moody et al, 1977a). However, between 90 minutes and 7 hours of BUO, the RBF is significantly lower than the RBF during the same time interval of UUO (Fig. 9–15*A*). The decrease in RBF is accompanied by an increase in renal vascular resistance during BUO to a greater level than with UUO (see Fig. 9–15*B*). However, by 24 hours of BUO, the RBF is as low, and renal vascular resistance as high, as with 24 hours of UUO (see Fig. 9–15*A* and *B*). However, ureteral pressure is higher than in UUO (see Fig. 9–15*C*). Gulmi and associates (1995) found effective RBF to be markedly decreased even at 48 hours of BUO. After release of BUO, the RBF remained significantly decreased in comparison with preobstruction values for 11 hours of the study. Jaenike (1972) showed that the distribution of RBF after BUO is much different from that in the UUO model. Using radioactive microspheres, he showed that 55% of RBF remains in the cortical nephrons and only 14% of RBF is shifted to the innermost renal zones. Yarger and co-workers (1972) used micropuncture studies to demonstrate a decrease in both whole kidney as well as single nephron clearance of para-aminohippurate (PAH) (17% and 55%, respectively). Solez and associates (1976), using intravenous [^{125}I]-albumin

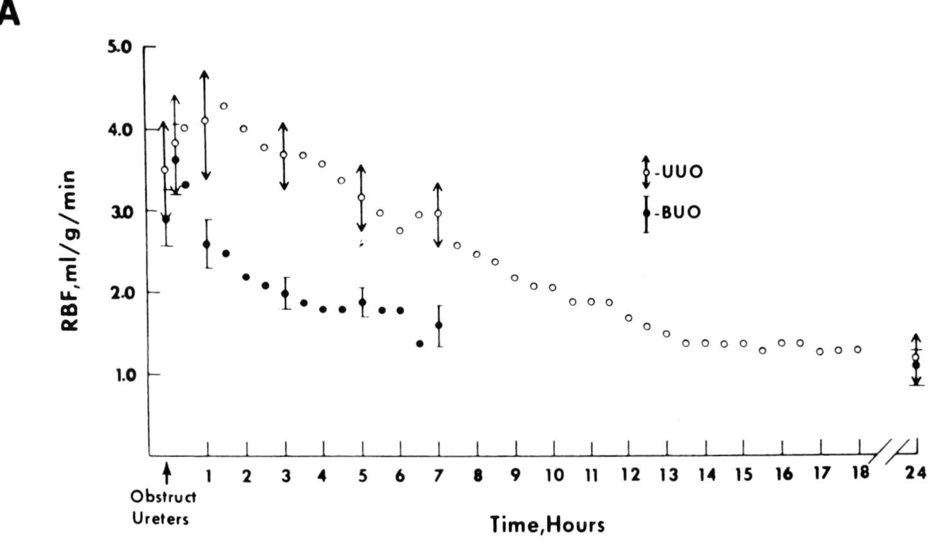

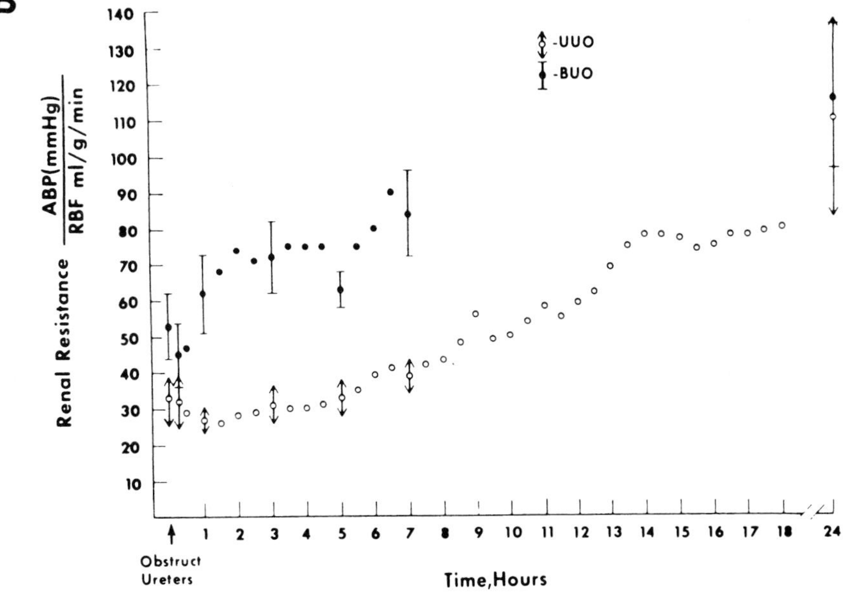

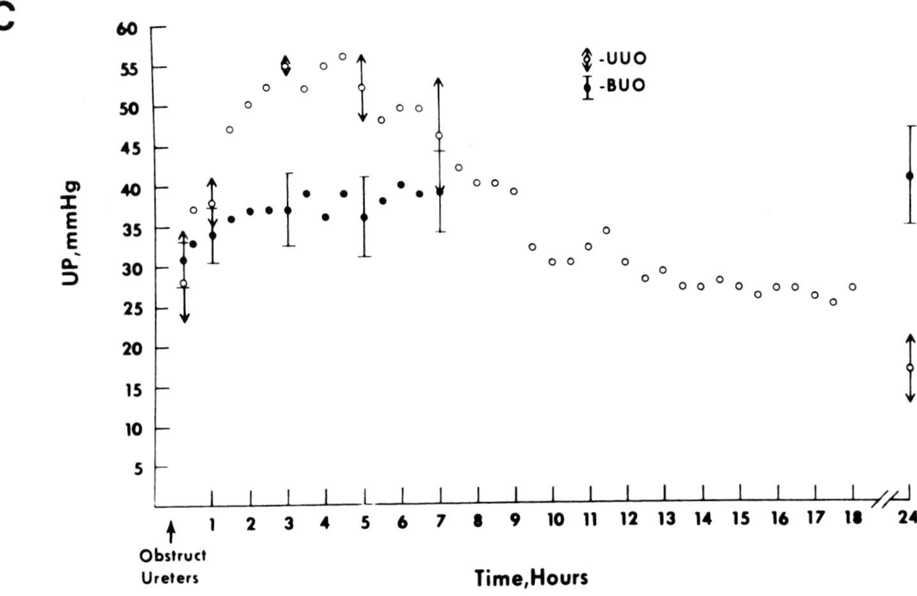

Figure 9–15. *A,* Comparison of renal blood flow (RBF) in unilateral ureteral occlusion (UUO) and bilateral ureteral occlusion (BUO), demonstrating similar patterns of change over the 24-hour period, although the RBF in the bilateral model is below that of the unilateral model from 1½ to 7 hr postobstruction. *B,* Comparison of the renal resistance in UUO and BUO demonstrating similar changes over the 24 hr period. Renal resistance in BUO is higher than in UUO in the early hours, corresponding to the lower renal blood flow at that time in BUO. ABP, arterial blood pressure. *C,* Comparison of ureteral pressure (UP) in UUO and BUO, demonstrating a significant difference in the UP 24 hours after obstruction. (From Moody TE, Vaughan ED Jr, Gillenwater JY: Invest Urol 1977; 14:455–459.)

infusion, showed a marked decrease in inner medullary plasma flow to 8% of normal by 18 hours of BUO.

Ureteral pressure follows a similar pattern for the first 4½ hours of both BUO and UUO: that is, a progressive rise in pressure (see Fig. 9–15*C*). However, after 4½ hours of BUO, the ureteral pressure remains elevated until 24 hours, whereas in UUO, ureteral pressure begins to progressively decline to control levels by 24 hours of ureteral occlusion (see Fig. 9–15*C*). This increase in ureteral pressure has been documented to at least 48 hours of BUO (Gulmi et al, 1995). Dal Canton and associates (1980) demonstrated an increase in intratubular pressure from 14.1 to 28.9 mm Hg, $P < .005$, with micropuncture studies in rats after 24 hours of BUO. This change in intratubular pressure caused a decrease in the hydrostatic pressure gradient from 31.7 to 20.0 mm Hg and in the effective filtration pressure at the afferent end of the glomerulus from 16.6 to 5.4 mm Hg, $P < .001$. Yarger and colleagues (1972) also measured both proximal and distal tubular pressures during micropuncture studies of rats after 24 hours of BUO and found the pressures to be 30 and 27.7 mm Hg, respectively, in comparison with 9.2 and 6.5 mm Hg, respectively, in UUO rats, $P < .001$. The micropuncture studies of both groups have confirmed what other investigators have observed from the monitoring of ureteral pressure: a rise after 24 hours of BUO. Therein lies one of the differences between BUO and UUO: **BUO passes through a phase of preglomerular vasodilatation and then a postglomerular vasoconstriction and remains in this state.** This explains the progressive and persistent rise in ureteral pressure despite a decrease in RBF and an increase in renal vascular resistance. In contrast, during UUO, the kidney passes through three phases: preglomerular vasodilatation, postglomerular vasoconstriction, and, finally, preglomerular vasoconstriction.

The GFR after 48 hours of BUO is significantly decreased (i.e., 22% of control values) in comparison with preobstruction GFR (Gulmi et al, 1995). This decrease was also seen by Jaenike (1972) in rats after 24 hours of BUO; the GFR was reduced to 20% of the control value. With micropuncture studies, Jaenike also found single nephron GFR (SNGFR) to be 34% of normal. However, Yarger and Harris (1985) showed that the number of functioning nephrons, as well as the GFR of those functioning nephrons, is higher for kidneys after BUO than after UUO. Harris and Yarger (1974) also demonstrated that 84% of superficial and 49% of juxtamedullary nephrons filter after 24 hours of BUO, as opposed to 40% of superficial and 12% of juxtamedullary nephrons after 24 hours of UUO.

Dal Canton and colleagues (1980) performed micropuncture studies on rats after 24 hours of BUO. They also observed a decrease in SNGFR after release of BUO to 40% of normal secondary to an increase from 14 to 30 mm Hg in intratubular pressure. There was little change in glomerular capillary pressure (46 and 50 mm Hg pre- and postobstruction, respectively). With relief of obstruction, there was a 52% increase in afferent arteriole resistance, resulting in a low SNGFR in the postrelief period. Therefore, in both BUO and UUO, there is a decline in SNGFR after 24 hours of ureteral occlusion. In UUO this is secondary to an increase in afferent arteriolar resistance, whereas in BUO it is secondary to a rise in intratubular pressure with little change in afferent arteriolar resistance (Table 9–3).

Table 9–3. COMPARISON OF THE EFFECTS OF UNILATERAL URETERAL AND BILATERAL URETERAL OBSTRUCTION ON GLOMERULAR HEMODYNAMICS

	P_T	P_G	AAPF	Ra	SNGFR
24-hr UUL	=	↓	↓↓	↑↑	↓↓
24-hr BUL	↑↑	=	=	=	↓↓

From Dal Canton A, et al: Kidney Int 1980; 17:491. Reprinted from Kidney International with permission.

P_T, intratubular pressure; P_G, hydrostatic pressure gradient across glomerular capillaries; AAPF, afferent arteriole plasma flow; Ra, resistance of single afferent arteriole; SNGFR, single nephron glomerular filtration rate; UUL, unilateral ureteral ligation; BUL, bilateral ureteral ligation.

Involvement of Atrial Natriuretic Peptide in BUO

Several investigators have postulated the accumulation of a "substance" during BUO that would affect the glomerular hemodynamics in such a way that there would be preglomerular vasodilatation and postglomerular vasoconstriction, as seen with late-phase BUO. This substance would not accumulate during UUO, because it could be excreted by the contralateral kidney. Wilson and Honrath (1976) demonstrated such a substance with cross-circulation studies in rats. When the cross-circulation was between a donor rat with 24 hours of BUO and a normal recipient rat, there was an immediate increase in both sodium and water excretion. This did not occur when the donor rat was subject to 24 hours of UUO (Fig. 9–16).

Harris and Yarger (1975) also postulated the existence of a circulating diuretic factor that accumulated only during BUO. They observed an increase in urine flow and sodium excretion after relief of BUO, UUO with contralateral nephrectomy, or UUO with the continuous intravenous reinfusion of urine from the contralateral kidney. In contrast, the UUO-alone animals did not have postobstructive diuresis and natriuresis.

The discovery of ANP paved the way for studies on the role of ANP in BUO. ANP has several physiologic effects, including vascular smooth muscle relaxation (i.e., vasodilatation), natriuresis, and diuresis. **The natriuretic and diuretic actions of ANP have been shown to be caused by (1) an increase in GFR through afferent arteriole vasodilatation and efferent arteriole vasoconstriction, (2) an increase in glomerular capillary ultrafiltration coefficient (K_f), and (3) inhibition of the glomerular-tubular feedback mechanism** (Cogan, 1990). **These glomerular hemodynamic effects point to ANP as the circulating diuretic and natriuretic substance postulated by previous investigators to explain the observed changes in RBF, ureteral pressure, and glomerular filtration during BUO.**

Fried and co-investigators (1987) demonstrated an elevated level of plasma ANP in rats after 24 hours of BUO and not after 24 hours of UUO (393 versus 261 pg/ml, $P < .01$). Purkerson and associates (1989) have shown plasma ANP levels of 400 pg/ml in rats with 24 hours of BUO, in comparison with plasma levels of 71 pg/ml ($P < .01$) in rats with UUO and 81 pg/ml ($P < .01$) in controls. Gulmi and co-workers (1989) demonstrated an augmented release of ANP in a prospective study of nine patients with either BUO

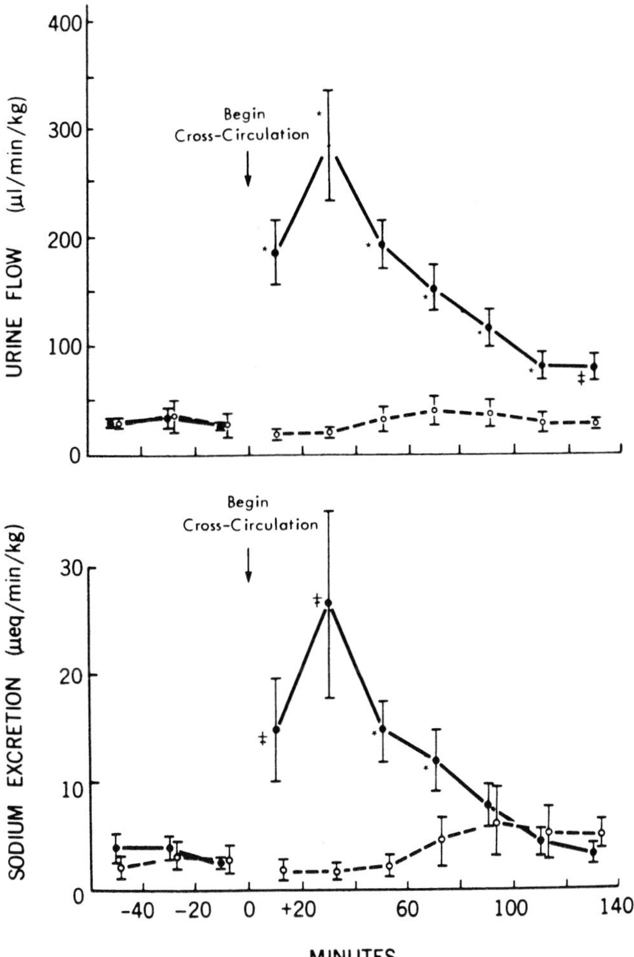

Figure 9–16. Changes in urine flow *(upper panel)* and sodium excretion *(lower panel)* in normal rats undergoing cross-circulation with donor rats that have bilateral (*solid circles,* group A) or unilateral (*open circles,* group B) ureteral ligation of 24 hours' duration. Standard error of mean value is shown; significance of the difference from the mean control value noted as *$P < .01$; $P < .05$. (From Wilson DR, Honrath U: J Clin Invest 1976; 57:380–389.)

or UUO of a solitary kidney. The mean plasma ANP in patients with obstructive uropathy was 130 pg/ml, in comparison with 46 pg/ml in age-matched controls, $P < .01$. Gulmi and associates (1995) also demonstrated markedly elevated levels of ANP in volume-replete dogs after 48 hours of BUO.

With the demonstration of elevated levels of ANP in BUO, it became clear that ANP was likely the factor previously postulated by Wilson and Honrath (1976) and Harris and Yarger (1975). The stimulus for the elevated plasma ANP seems to be an increase in intravascular volume, as determined by an elevation in pulmonary capillary wedge pressure and body weight in volume-replete dogs with BUO (Gulmi et al, 1995). In support, clinical studies on chronic hemodialysis patients show that intravascular volume, and not the degree of renal failure, is the stimulus for an elevation in their plasma ANP levels.

Other Mediators in BUO

Eicosanoid synthesis in BUO has been studied both in vitro and in vivo. Yanagisawa and colleagues (1991) studied glomerular synthesis of several eicosanoids. There was a marked increase in eicosanoid and leukotriene B_4 production in glomeruli of rats with BUO in comparison with that in sham-operated control rats. In addition, there was an increase in the activity of several enzymes involved in arachidonic acid metabolism (Yanagisawa et al, 1993). Hence the entire pathway of arachidonic acid metabolism seems to be increased during BUO, generating both vasodilators and vasoconstrictors.

The involvement of several pathways of eicosanoid synthesis in renal function changes in BUO has been investigated. Cadnapaphornchai and colleagues (1982) improved both inulin and PAH clearances by pretreating dogs with imidazole before 24 hours of BUO. Purkerson and Klahr (1989) demonstrated that the administration of enalapril or OKY-046 for 48 hours before BUO significantly improved both GFR and RPF. Administration of enalapril in BUO abrogated the increase in prostanoids from the isolated glomeruli. When OKY-046 and enalapril were administered together, there was an even greater increase of both GFR and RBF than when either drug was used alone, which suggests that both AII and TxA_2 participate in the diminished RBF and GFR of BUO.

Himmelstein and co-workers (1990) showed increased inulin and PAH clearances in BUO animals in comparison with UUO animals after the release of 24 hours of occlusion. TxB_2 was significantly increased only after UUO. The prostacyclin metabolite 6-keto-$PGF_{1\alpha}$ was markedly elevated in BUO animals in comparison with UUO animals. They demonstrated a dose-dependent increase in 6-keto-$PGF_{1\alpha}$ production with increasing doses of ANP given intrarenally during BUO and UUO, with no effect on sham controls or on renal TxA_2 production. When ANP was infused into UUO and BUO kidneys, there was an accompanying decrease in renal vascular resistance that was mitigated by adding indomethacin to the infusate. Therefore, the vasodilator prostacyclin, stimulated by an elevation in ANP during BUO, may mediate the prolonged preglomerular vasodilatation observed during BUO.

The decrease seen in both GFR and ERPF and the increase in renal vascular resistance after 24 hours of BUO were significantly reversed by pretreatment with MK886, a 5-lipoxygenase inhibitor (Fig. 9–17*A*), and by whole-body irradiation. Both treatments were accompanied by a decrease in LTB_4 (Reyes et al, 1992a). The inhibition and the stimulation of the cytochrome P-450 pathway can be achieved by pretreatment with ketoconazole or 3-methylcholanthrene plus alpha-naphthoflavone, respectively. Inhibition of the pathway caused no change in post-BUO GFR and ERPF, in comparison with BUO alone. However, stimulation of the cytochrome P-450 pathway causes a significant increase in post-BUO GFR and ERPF, as well as a decrease in renal vascular resistance (see Fig. 9–17*B*; Reyes and Klahr, 1992a).

Reyes and co-workers (1992b) examined the role of nitric oxide in BUO. When N-NAME was infused, there was a further decrease in GFR and ERPF in comparison to controls, which suggests that nitric oxide was maintaining GFR and ERPF during BUO. This was confirmed by showing that there was an improvement in GFR and ERPF, as well as a decrease in renal vascular resistance, with the infusion of L-arginine into rats with unilateral release of 24 hours of BUO.

Other endothelial factors may also be involved in BUO. Reyes and Klahr (1992b) demonstrated an elevation in GFR

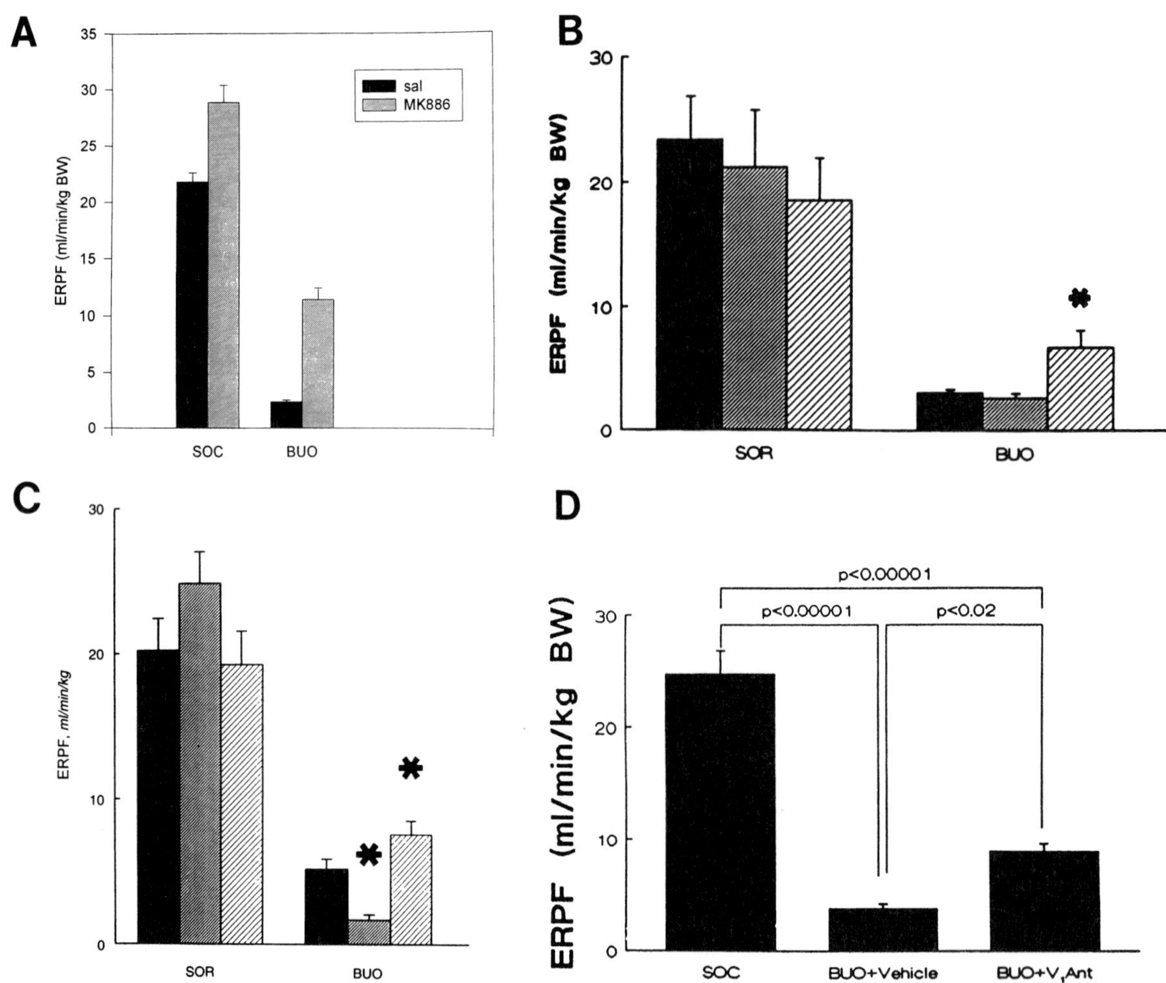

Figure 9–17. Effects of different inhibitors on hemodynamics of bilateral ureteral occlusion (BUO). *A,* Either saline (sal) or the 5-lipoxygenase inhibitor MK886 was administered 4 hours before BUO and in sham-operated controls (SOCs). Effective renal plasma flow (ERPF) was measured at 24 hours. The 5-lipoxygenase inhibitor restores the ERPF in BUO toward control levels. *B,* Rats were treated with vehicle *(solid bar),* an inhibitor (ketoconazole; *gray bar*) or an activator (3-methylcholanthrene; *hatched bar*) of the cytochrome P-450 pathway before BUO. Inhibition of cytochrome P-450 produced no effect, whereas activating cytochrome P-450 restored ERPF in BUO toward control levels. *C,* Rats subject to BUO were either treated with vehicle *(solid bar)* or anti-endothelin antibody *(hatched bar)* or were subject to mechanical denudation of the endothelium of the renal artery *(gray bar).* ERPF was measured at 24 hours. Mechanical denudation of the endothelium significantly decreased ERPF in BUO, whereas anti-endothelin antibody significantly increased ERPF in rats with BUO. *D,* Either vehicle or a vasopressin-V_1 receptor antagonist was administered for 1 week before BUO through an osmotic minipump. The V_1 antagonist restores the ERPF in BUO toward control levels. (*A* adapted from Reyes AA, Lefkowith J, Pippin J, Klahr S: Kidney Int 1992; 41:100–106. *B* from Reyes AA, Klahr S: Proc Soc Exp Biol Med 1992; 201:278–283. *C* from Reyes AA, Klahr S: Kidney Int 1992; 42:632–638. *D* from Reyes AA, Klahr S: Proc Soc Exp Biol Med 1991; 197:49–55.)

and ERPF after release of BUO with the administration of an anti-endothelin antibody before ureteral occlusion, compared to BUO-alone animals. The denudation of the endothelium of the main renal artery before BUO caused significantly lower values for GFR and ERPF in comparison to BUO controls (see Fig. 9–17*C*). These data suggest that endothelin has a vasoconstrictor role in rats with BUO, contributing to the decrease in GFR and ERPF during the release of BUO. The renal artery endothelium seems to have an overall role of vasodilatation.

Additional studies have investigated the role of PAF and vasopressin in the hemodynamics of BUO. Rats given exogenous PAF were found to have a decrease in GFR and ERPF both in sham-operated controls and after relief of 24-hour BUO. Administration of L-659,989, a PAF receptor antagonist, resulted in a dose-dependent decrease in GFR and ERPF after 24-hour BUO (Reyes and Klahr, 1991b). Vasopressin is a known vasoconstrictor of the glomerular efferent arteriole, through binding to V_1 receptors in the postglomerular vascular bed (Edwards et al, 1989). Reyes and Klahr (1991a) demonstrated a fivefold elevation of ADH (vasopressin) in rats with 24-hour BUO, which was not seen in rats with 24-hour UUO or in sham-operated controls. This stimulus for the increase in ADH is most likely a 20% to 25% increase in plasma osmolality in rats with 24-hour BUO, secondary to an elevation in plasma sodium. When animals were pretreated with a V_1 receptor antagonist before BUO, there was an increase in both GFR and ERPF upon release of BUO (see Fig. 9–17*D*).

Tubular Changes in BUO

There are differences between tubular function after release of BUO and UUO, as listed in Table 9–4. Several

Table 9–4. DIFFERENCES IN TUBULAR FUNCTION AFTER RELEASE OF UNILATERAL AND BILATERAL URETERAL OBSTRUCTION (24 HOURS)

	Control	Unilateral	Bilateral
Postobstructive diuresis		Absent	Present
Percent of filtration excreted (V/GFR)	1%	↓ to 0.5%	↑ to 18%
Excreted fraction filtered Na^+	0.6%	↓ to 0.4%	↑ to 13%
Proximal tubular reabsorption		Decrease	Decrease
Distal tubular reabsorption			Decrease
Proximal fraction reabsorption	58%	74%	46%
Distal fraction reabsorption	12%		34%
Fraction K^+ excreted	12.3%	↓ to 7%	↑ to 90%
Concentration U/P	7.6	1.35	1.47

V, volume; GFR, glomerular filtration rate; U, urine; P, plasma.

investigators have described marked diuresis and natriuresis after the relief of either BUO or UUO of a solitary kidney in humans (Wilson et al, 1951; Maher et al, 1963; Vaughan and Gillenwater, 1973; Battle et al, 1981; Gulmi et al, 1989). Maher and colleagues (1963) described a significant increase in urine volume and sodium excretion after relief of obstructive uropathy. The urinary flow more closely followed the osmolar excretion than the sodium excretion in this patient study. The predominant urine solute during this osmotic diuresis was urea, accounting for 37% to 68% of the total urine osmolality (Maher et al, 1963). When serum urea returned to normal, the diuresis ceased. Maher and colleagues therefore postulated that the physiologic diuresis was caused by a high serum urea concentration, which ceased when the BUN returned to normal.

Muldowney and associates (1966) measured total exchangeable sodium to determine whether the postrelease natriuresis of BUO is pathologic or merely a physiologic elimination of excess body sodium. **They found that patients with chronic obstructive uropathy had an increase in total exchangeable body sodium before release of obstruction.** After relief of the obstructive uropathy, total exchangeable body sodium levels returned to normal within 2 to 3 weeks. The loss of sodium in the urine did not result in clinical sodium depletion in any of the patients. Muldowney and associates concluded that the increased loss of sodium in the urine upon release of chronic obstructive uropathy is a physiologic reduction of excess body sodium to normal levels.

Gulmi and co-investigators (1989) also described nine patients with obstructive uropathy and postobstructive diuresis and natriuresis. Patients with obstruction had a significantly elevated plasma ANP, in comparison with the control group of patients (Fig. 9–18). There was an increase in both absolute and fractional excretion of sodium that subsided with improvement in renal function. This natriuresis and diuresis was associated with an elevation of serum ANP in all patients, which decreased as water and salt excretion decreased (see Fig. 9–18). Because ANP is a known diuretic and natriuretic, it may be one of the main factors causing the loss of water and salt in the postobstructive state.

In animals, the release of BUO is accompanied by pro-

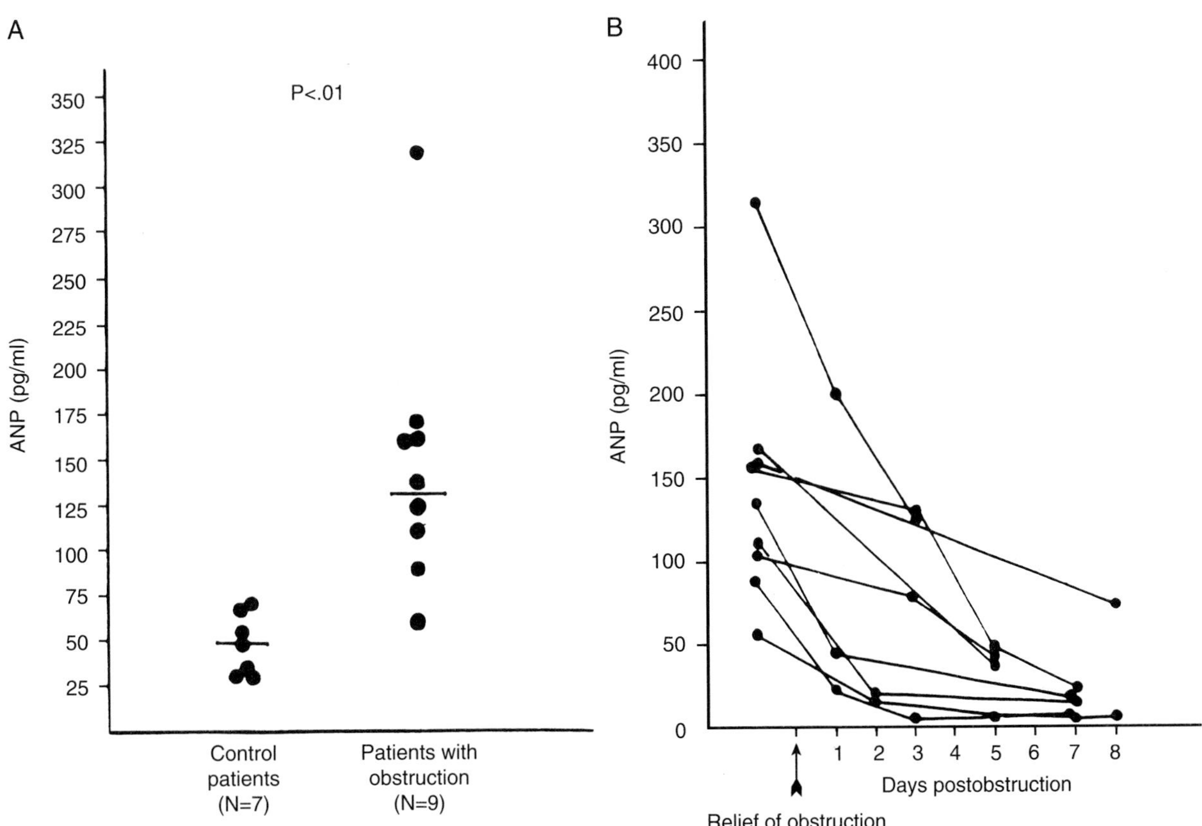

Figure 9–18. Plasma atrial natriuretic peptide levels. *A,* Control group and patients with obstruction. *B,* Before and after relief of obstruction. (From Gulmi FA, Mooppan UMM, Chou S, Kim H: J Urol 1989; 142:268–272.)

found diuresis and natriuresis as well. There seems to be a dual mechanism for the increase in water and sodium loss after release of BUO. Yarger and colleagues (1972) investigated the site of impaired tubular reabsorption of sodium in surface nephrons with micropuncture techniques. They observed impaired fractional sodium reabsorption in the distal tubule, with normal fractional reabsorption of sodium in the proximal tubule. Jaenike (1972) confirmed a postobstructive diuresis and natriuresis in rats after the release of BUO. He also demonstrated that exclusion of sodium intake after obstruction did not decrease the postrelief diuresis and natriuresis of BUO. This contradicts the conclusion of Muldowney and associates (1966) in human studies: that postobstructive diuresis and natriuresis are appropriate responses to increased total body sodium accumulated during obstruction. Jaenike (1972) infused urea into normal rats and into rats after relief of UUO to achieve levels of urea similar to those observed in rats with BUO. This caused no increase in salt and water excretion. Therefore, the postobstructive natriuresis and diuresis do not seem to be secondary to an increased solute load. Jaenike did demonstrate a defect in sodium transport in the distal tubule and suggested that this defect is a direct mechanical effect of obstruction at the distal tubule.

McDougal and Wright (1972) also described an increase in sodium and water excretion that lasted for 24 to 36 hours after relief of 30-hour BUO in rats. However, they observed a reduction in sodium and water reabsorption in both the proximal and distal nephrons. They also observed increased permeability in the tubule wall to both mannitol and inulin. Because there is increased permeability of the tubule after 30 hours of obstruction, it is likely that sodium and other ions have increased permeability, thus elevating their tubular fluid concentration by increasing sodium backflux into the tubule. However, this permeability defect existed only after BUO and not UUO; therefore, it seemed unlikely that a permeability change should occur only when both kidneys are obstructed. McDougal and Wright (1972) suggested the possibility that the accumulation of a substance during BUO is a cause for the permeability defect.

Fried and associates (1987) reported experiments in which animals with UUO were compared with two groups of animals with BUO. One group was given access to water after relief of BUO, and one was not. Fried and associates found elevation of plasma ANP and postobstructive diuresis in both groups of rats with BUO but not in rats with UUO. The two BUO groups lost weight before the relief of BUO, and both groups still demonstrated elevated levels of ANP. Fried and associates postulated decreased renal excretion and/or metabolism or enhanced atrial production of ANP to explain the elevated ANP levels during BUO. However, the acute weight loss seen in these animals should not be associated with volume expansion and consequently atrial stretch. Because atrial stretch is the main stimulus for ANP, this does not seem to be the explanation.

Gulmi and co-workers (1995) performed BUO on dogs, a larger animal model, which allowed the invasive monitoring of pulmonary capillary wedge pressure in addition to monitoring of weight loss or gain during BUO. The BUO animals were subdivided into a volume-replete group, given normal saline during the 48 hours of obstruction, and a second group, not given intravenous saline after ureteral occlusion. **Before release of obstruction, the volume-replete group demonstrated significantly elevated plasma ANP levels in comparison with pre-obstruction values.** This was not seen in the BUO-without-saline group (Fig. 9–19). The elevation of ANP was accompanied by elevations in both pulmonary capillary wedge pressure and weight gain in the volume-replete BUO group. The BUO group not given normal saline did not have an elevation in pulmonary capillary wedge pressure, nor did the animals gain weight. However, both groups of animals did achieve equivalent degrees of renal failure by 48 hours of BUO.

The data strongly suggest that the intravascular volume status during BUO, not the degree of renal failure and consequent inability of the kidney to excrete and/or metabolize ANP, leads to the elevation of ANP via atrial stretch. This has been borne out by clinical studies in chronic renal failure patients on hemodialysis showing that the patient's intravascular volume status, measured by pulmonary capillary wedge pressure and body weight, determined the level of plasma ANP and not the degree of renal failure (Saxenhoffer et al, 1987; Deray et al, 1988). Upon relief of obstruction, both groups of BUO animals exhibited diuresis and natriuresis. However, the group with an elevation of ANP demonstrated prolonged excretion of sodium and water, in comparison with the BUO group, without an increase in plasma ANP. Therefore, an elevated plasma ANP may not be required to achieve the diuresis and natriuresis observed after the release of BUO. A direct effect of obstruction on the tubule itself may contribute to the enhanced excretion of sodium and water of BUO, as suggested in previous studies (McDougal and Wright, 1972; Jaenike, 1972; Sonnenberg and Wilson, 1976).

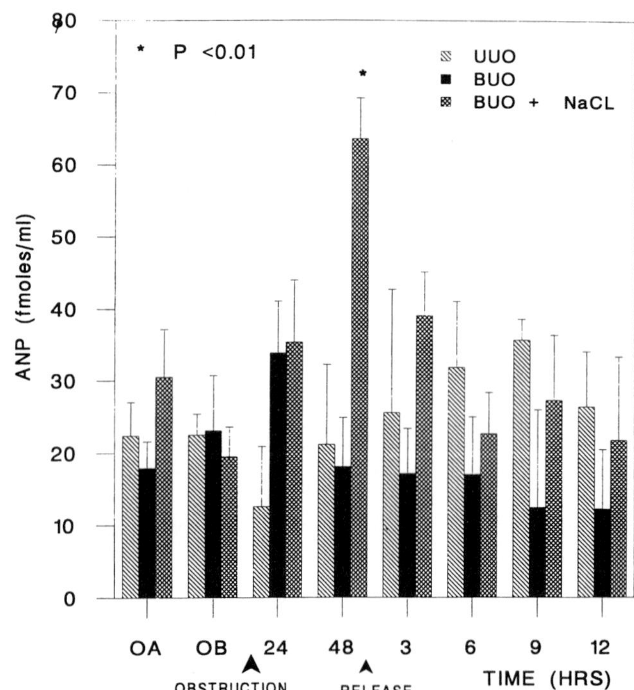

Figure 9–19. Atrial natriuretic peptide (ANP) in all groups both before and after relief of 48-hour obstruction. OA, preclearance time zero; OB, postclearance time zero. (From Gulmi FA, Matthews GJ, Marion D, et al: J Urol 1995; 153:1276–1283.)

There is an enhanced increase in potassium excretion after release of BUO (McDougal and Wright, 1972; Sonnenberg and Wilson, 1976). There is an increase in both the absolute potassium excretion and the fractional excretion of potassium (Buerkert et al, 1977; Yarger and Harris, 1985). The increases in the delivery of sodium, in the tubular fluid flow rate, and in plasma potassium are important stimuli for the enhanced excretion of potassium after the release of BUO (Wilson, 1980; Yarger and Harris, 1985).

There is an impaired ability to acidify the urine and lower the pH in response to acidemia during BUO. This is believed to be secondary to an inability to secrete hydrogen ions against a gradient. The decrease in the tubular reabsorption of sodium distally may contribute to the inability of the kidney to excrete hydrogen ions.

In the postrelief BUO kidney, ability to concentrate urine is impaired. There is an increase in free water clearance (C_{H_2O}) after release of BUO. This is accompanied by an overall increase in total solute excretion (C_{Osm}) (McDougal and Wright, 1972; Gulmi et al, 1989). The major sites affected are the loop of Henle, the distal tubule, and the collecting duct, mostly from the juxtamedullary nephrons (Wilson and Klahr, 1993). The mechanisms most often proposed to explain the decrease in concentrating ability in the kidney after obstruction are an inability of the medullary interstitium to maintain its hypertonicity and an insensitivity of the tubule to vasopressin (Wilson and Klahr, 1993). The inability to establish the medullary tonicity necessary to concentrate urine comes from the inability of the thick ascending limb of the loop of Henle to reabsorb sodium after obstruction (Hanley and Davidson, 1982). This ultimately decreases the tonicity in the medullary interstitium and, consequently, the reabsorption of water. Hanley and Davidson (1982) demonstrated a significant decrease in the response of the cortical collecting tubule to vasopressin. This was also observed by McDougal and Wright in ligated-deligated rats, which showed no changes in either $U_{Na}V$ or $U_{Osm}V$ measured before and after the administration of vasopressin.

Interestingly, the highest density of ANP receptors in the nephron is found in the inner medullary collecting duct (Cogan, 1990). Several investigators have demonstrated that ANP can inhibit both sodium chloride absorption in the inner medullary collecting duct (Nonoguchi et al, 1988; Rocha and Kudo, 1990) and vasopressin-stimulated osmotic water permeability in the same segment of the nephron (Nonoguchi et al, 1988). These factors have previously been invoked to explain the concentrating defect in postobstruction renal function. Therefore, ANP elevated during BUO may be either the primary cause for a concentrating defect in obstructive uropathy or a contributing factor enhancing an already diminished ability of the kidney to concentrate urine in the postobstruction period. This information is summarized in Figure 9–20.

The characterization of the aquaporins, a family of membrane water channels, provides a molecular basis for transmembrane water movement (Knepper, 1994). Aquaporin-2 is the predominant vasopressin-sensitive water channel of the collecting duct. Studies have shown that changes in aquaporins can be documented in BUO. BUO for 24 hours caused a decrease in aquaporin-2 expression in inner medulla to 26% of control; 48 hours after relief of BUO, the reduction in aquaporin expression persisted. Seven days after the release of BUO, renal excretion of water and electrolytes had returned almost to normal. There was only a partial reversal of the decrease in aquaporin-2 at that time, which coincided with a decrease in the urinary concentrating ability (in response to an 18-hour period of thirst). Thus changes in aquaporin-2 may also be involved in the changes in concentrating ability after BUO (Frøkiær et al, 1996).

RENAL FUNCTION AFTER RELEASE OF OBSTRUCTION: UUO AND BUO

Animal Models: UUO and BUO

Early work by Hinman suggested that in order for an obstructed kidney to recover, contralateral nephrectomy would be necessary. The rationale for this concept is the

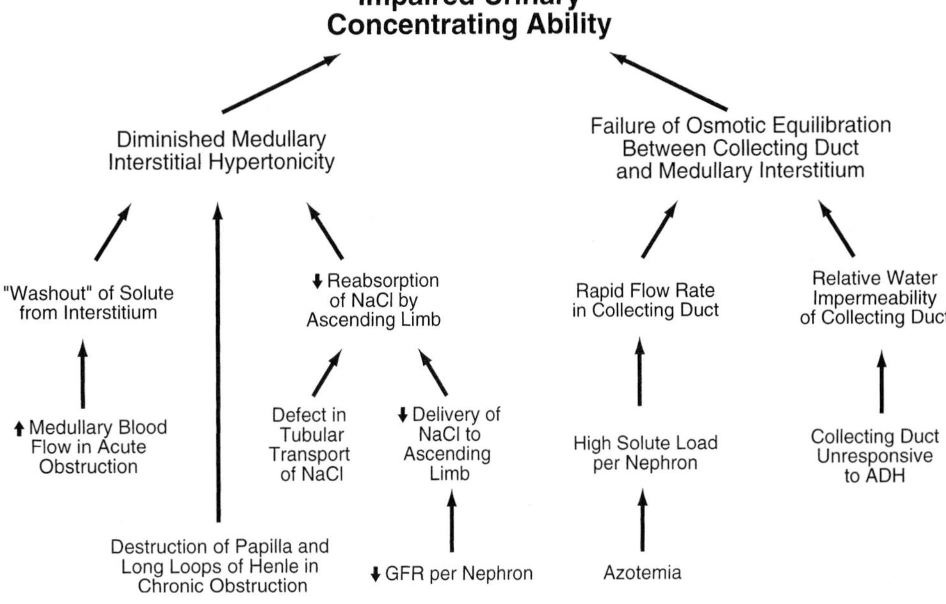

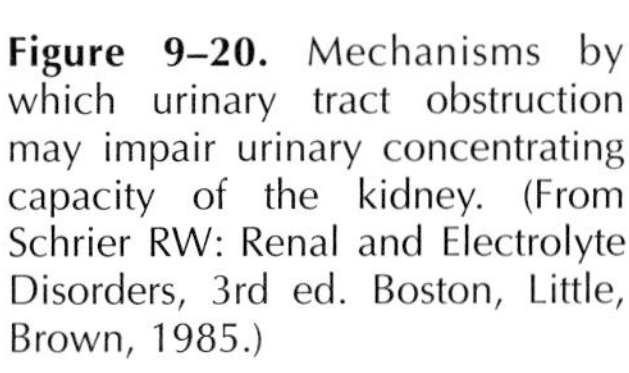
Figure 9–20. Mechanisms by which urinary tract obstruction may impair urinary concentrating capacity of the kidney. (From Schrier RW: Renal and Electrolyte Disorders, 3rd ed. Boston, Little, Brown, 1985.)

observation that the contralateral kidney undergoes compensatory hypertrophy after UUO. Hinman proposed the term *renal counterbalance* to describe the phenomenon (Hinman, 1943). **He postulated that the injured kidney would undergo "disuse atrophy" and would not recover after repair because of the presence of the enlarged healthy mate.** Several studies in the 1950s and 1960s were able to document recovery from obstruction in the presence of contralateral nephrectomy. However, because the contralateral kidney is normally intact in patients, Vaughan and Gillenwater (1971) carried out recovery studies in the presence of the contralateral functioning kidney. Fifteen dogs with kidneys obstructed for various amounts of time were studied. Recovery was monitored for varying lengths of time. Full recovery of renal function after 7 days of UUO was achieved within 2 weeks of the reversal of the obstruction. However, obstruction of 14 days' duration resulted in a permanent decline in renal function to 70% of control levels. Maximal return of function was achieved 3 to 6 months after reversal. Some degree of function was recovered in kidneys obstructed for 4 weeks; obstruction for 6 weeks or more was not followed by any recovery. Prior studies by Kerr (1956) also had demonstrated recovery with the contralateral kidney in situ but had shown greater recovery with contralateral nephrectomy.

Since these early studies, there have been a few other studies on recoverability of function. Fink and co-workers (1980) studied dogs with varying lengths of time of obstruction and recovery and noted similar findings to those just described. There was a progressive loss of renal function (measured by DTPA scans and creatinine clearance) with increasing periods of obstruction. As was noted in the studies of Hinman, contralateral nephrectomy resulted in further improvement.

Several other investigators have examined rats with UUO. One week of UUO followed by 10 days of recovery resulted in a return of function to 71% of control levels (Flam et al, 1984). Yokoyama and colleagues (1984) studied rats with 2 weeks of UUO followed by 2 weeks of recovery. Many tubules showed recovery of structure with normal epithelial lining; however, there was a heterogeneous response of tubules, wherein some actually deteriorated more. Bander and associates (1985) studied the recovery of kidneys obstructed for 24 hours and observed for 3 hours to 60 days after relief. By 14 days, whole kidney GFR had returned to normal. However, as in Yokoyama and colleagues' study, the response of the nephrons was heterogeneous. Thus at 8 days after relief, more than 15% of superficial and juxtamedullary nephrons were not filtering in the kidney after obstruction. At 60 days, a similar percentage of nephrons was still not functional. Remaining nephrons showed hyperfiltration. There have been surprisingly few studies on factors that influence kidney recovery. In one study, the effects of indomethacin and captopril on renal function were studied in rats whose kidneys were obstructed for 1, 2, or 3 weeks, followed by a 3-month recovery. After the 3 months, GFRs were 51.6%, 35.5%, and 16.0% of control levels, respectively. Indomethacin had little effect on GFR, whereas captopril increased function somewhat but to no more than 60.4% in the group obstructed for 1 week. Captopril had less of an effect on ERPF than on GFR. Captopril preserved renal mass somewhat in the obstructed kidneys (McDougal, 1982).

Humans

UUO

One of the challenges facing urologists in treating patients with obstructed kidneys is the decision either to relieve the obstruction to preserve future renal function or to remove the kidney. Diuretic renography, ultrasonography, and possibly even CT are some of the tools necessary for making these decisions. An estimate of renal function with nuclear scans after relief of the obstruction and a view of the architecture of the renal unit through ultrasonography, intravenous pyelography (IVP)/retrograde studies, and CT scans aid urologists in the decision to preserve the kidney or perform a nephrectomy. There is no substitute for the experience of the surgeon and the art of assessing a clinical situation. At times the laboratory data may seem to favor salvage of the renal unit, whereas the experience of the urologist favors nephrectomy, and rightfully so. Duration of obstruction by itself, however, should not influence the urologist to perform a nephrectomy or salvage a renal unit.

Shapiro and Bennett (1976) presented three cases of UUO lasting from 28 to 150 days. They demonstrated return of some renal function on either IVP or hippuran renal scintigraphy. In all three cases, despite demonstration of poor renal function on renal scan or IVP, the cortex was adequate, and hence the decision was to salvage the kidney. Lewis and Pierce (1962) described a case of a 42-year-old woman in whom the right ureter was ligated by several catgut sutures during a hysterectomy for profuse vaginal bleeding. Preoperatively, the kidney was nonvisualized on IVP with delayed films to 195 minutes and nonfunction was shown on an iodine-131 renal scan. The patient underwent a right ureteroneocystostomy, and 6 days after surgery had normal vascular and excretory phases bilaterally on a repeat radioactive renogram. At 19 months postoperatively, a repeat IVP and hippuran scan revealed a normal-functioning right kidney with a decrease in size in comparison with the left kidney. Therefore, the preoperative studies that demonstrated no function were of no value in predicting salvageability of the renal unit.

In animal studies, the duration of obstruction seems important to the return of renal function. Vaughan and Gillenwater (1971) showed little return in renal function in dogs with 40 days of UUO. This discrepancy with the human data just described may exist because the obstruction in the human studies was not as complete or because differences in the lymphatic or venous drainage from the human renal pelvis may provide greater protection than the animal models. Finally, the anatomy of the human kidney and renal pelvis (i.e., intrarenal versus extrarenal) may also afford increased protection from the effects of long-term obstruction in comparison to the animal models. Therefore, the duration of renal obstruction should not dissuade the surgeon from repair of the blockage and possible preservation of some renal function.

BUO

Patients with BUO usually present with a longer duration of the obstruction, because the obstruction is usually secondary to bladder outlet obstruction or a midline retroperitoneal process and is more insidious in nature. There is little or no renal colic associated with BUO, and the uremia is slow and progressive. The patients usually gain weight during this process, which places them in a volume-expanded state, thus differentiating BUO from UUO (Robards and Ross, 1967; Gulmi et al, 1989).

Berlyne (1961) studied seven patients with chronic bilateral hydronephrosis (six of whom were adults after the relief of BUO) to evaluate their distal tubular function. The patients were evaluated for concentrating ability, acidification, ammonia production, total hydrogen excretion, and $T^C_{H_2O}$. Two of the seven patients were able to acidify their urine in response to ammonium chloride 1 and 2 months after the relief of obstruction. Total hydrogen excretion improved in 43% of the patients by 2 months after relief of BUO. As far as the response to vasopressin (Pitressin) and the ability of the kidney to concentrate urine, Berlyne divided the results into three groups: (1) patients who could concentrate urine normally (one patient); (2) those who had an obligatory hyposthenuria and a negative $T^C_{H_2O}$ and had nephrogenic diabetes insipidus (three patients); and (3) those with an impaired urinary concentrating ability and a reduced GFR, in whom the free water clearance may be in the normal range when $T^C_{H_2O}$ is corrected for the GFR (three patients).

Massry and associates (1967) reported on a case of obstructive uropathy secondary to carcinoma of the prostate. Forty-eight hours after the relief of the obstruction, the patient was given increasing doses of vasopressin: 0.1, 1.0, 2.0, and finally 10 milliunits/kg. A decrease in urine volume and an increase in urine osmolality occurred only after the highest dose of vasopressin. However, 2 weeks after relief of obstruction, the urine volume and osmolality responded to the smallest dose of vasopressin, indicating a return to normal urine concentrating ability and distal tubular function with time. The same patient achieved normal ability to acidify the urine by the third day postobstruction.

Gulmi and colleagues (1989) studied nine patients with obstructive uropathy after relief of their obstruction. All patients initially had marked diuresis, natriuresis—both absolute and fractional sodium excretion—and a low urine-to-serum creatinine ratio. Within 7 days after relief of obstruction, the renal function was improved, with a decrease in both absolute and fractional sodium excretion and an increase in the urine-to-serum creatinine ratio.

Human studies do not show any clear relationship between the duration of BUO and expected degree of improvement in renal function after relief of obstruction. There also does not seem to be any prerelease serum chemistry data to predict in which patients renal tubular functions after BUO will return to normal. It is also very difficult to estimate the duration and degree of the obstruction as well as the effect that it has on the overall return of baseline renal function. Therefore, most obstructions warrant relief for attainment of baseline renal function.

Jones and colleagues (1988) studied 21 patients prospectively during and after the relief of obstruction for 3 months. The patients were evaluated for GFR with plasma clearance of ^{99m}Tc-DTPA, iohexol clearance, and/or 24-hour urine collections for creatinine clearance. Two days after the relief of obstruction, there was a rapid increase in creatinine clearance, which then plateaued for 2 weeks. Another increase in function was seen by 3 months after relief of the obstruction. The ^{99m}Tc-DTPA and iohexol clearance values were somewhat different from the creatinine clearance values in that both showed no improvement in GFR until 3 months after relief of the uropathy. There was an immediate increase in absolute and fractional excretion of sodium and urinary volume after the relief of obstruction. There was a gradual decline to baseline fractional excretion of sodium and water with no improvement in their absolute excretion over the next 3 months, which reflects the concomitant improvement in GFR over the same time period. Jones and colleagues therefore describe a two-phase improvement in renal function: the initial or tubular phase, occurring during the first 2 weeks after the relief of obstruction, and the later or glomerular phase, occurring between 2 weeks and 3 months.

IMPLICATIONS OF EXPERIMENTAL MODELS FOR CLINICAL MANAGEMENT OF OBSTRUCTIVE UROPATHY

Postobstructive Diuresis

This phenomenon refers to marked polyuria that occurs after relief of BUO or obstruction of a solitary kidney. The diuresis may be classified as physiologic, caused by retained urea, sodium, and water, or pathologic, caused by impairment of concentrating ability or sodium reabsorption (Earley, 1956; Muldowney et al, 1966; Loo and Vaughan, 1985). In addition, the proximal tubule T_m for glucose can be exceeded, whereby high-volume glucose-containing fluid replacement adds an iatrogenic etiology to continuing diuresis (Fig. 9–21).

The patient most likely to exhibit postobstructive diuresis presents with chronic obstruction, edema, congestive heart failure, hypertension, weight gain, azotemia, and sometimes uremic encephalopathy (Loo and Vaughan, 1985) (see Fig. 9–21). Many patients exhibit a mixed pattern, with both electrolyte and nonelectrolyte solute diuresis as well as a concentrating defect.

The electrolyte portion is accompanied by an increase in sodium, potassium, and possibly magnesium losses in the urine in association with increased water excretion. The nonelectrolyte solute diuresis is caused by osmotically active agents, such as urea, that are accumulated during obstructive uropathy. As the solute diuresis ensues, there is a decrease in urine concentrating ability despite increasing endogenous ADH levels. The mechanisms responsible for this inability to concentrate urine include (1) defective generation of medullary solute gradient secondary to a decreased reabsorption of sodium chloride by the thick ascending limb of Henle's loop and a decreased reabsorption of urea by the collecting tubule; (2) inability to maintain the solute gradient secondary to an increased medullary blood flow (solute washout); and (3) impaired medullary gradient secondary to an increased flow and solute concentration in the distal nephron (Gonzalez and Suki, 1995).

Osmolar clearance (C_{Osm}) is defined as the volume of urine required to excrete urinary solute isoosmotically. If the amount of solute excreted is known, it is possible to calculate the volume of urine necessary to excrete this solute in

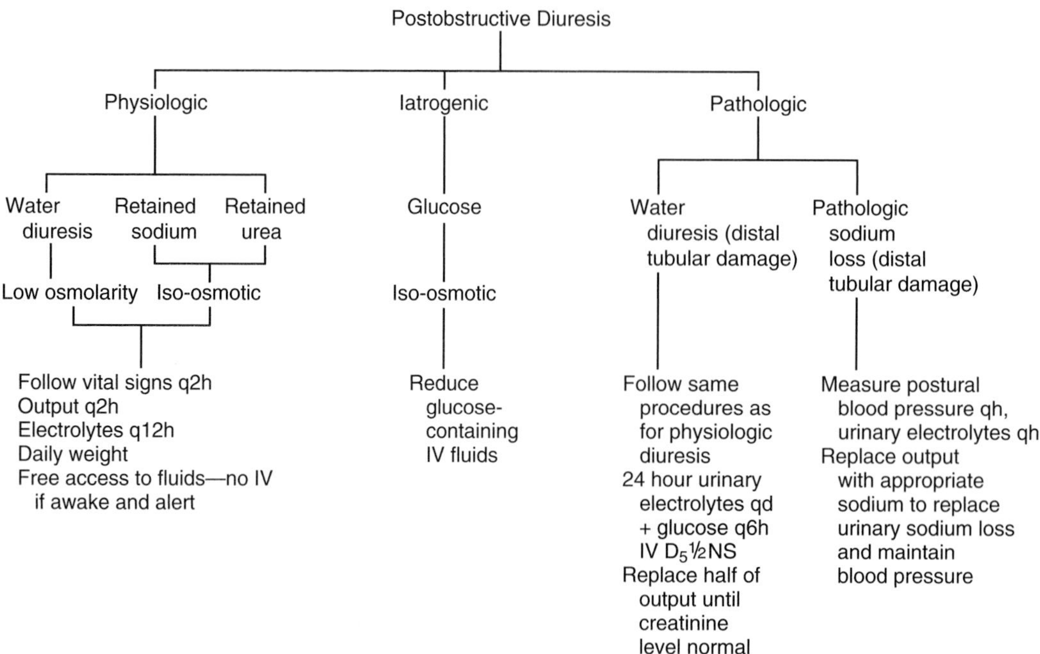

Figure 9–21. Types of postobstructive diuresis (>200 ml/hour for 24 hours).

isoosmotic relation to plasma (i.e., 300 mOsm/L). Therefore, a person would need to make 2 L of urine to excrete the 600 mOsm of solute isoosmotically, and the C_{Osm} would be 2 L/day. To calculate the electrolyte portion of C_{Osm}, $C_{Osm}(e)$, the following formula can be used:

$$C_{Osm}(e) = [2(U_{Na} + U_K)]V/(2P_{Na})$$

or

$$[2(U_{Cl})V]/(2P_{Na}) \text{ if } U_{Cl} > (U_{Na} + UK).$$

By subtracting $C_{Osm}(e)$ from C_{Osm}, the contribution of the nonelectrolyte solute diuresis can be estimated (Gonzalez and Suki, 1995).

Fortunately, most patients do not exhibit postobstructive diuresis after release of obstruction, and those who do have a limited period of physiologic diuresis with rapid return to normal. It is prudent to monitor all patients for an output greater than 200 ml/hour and to notify the physician if this volume occurs for 2 consecutive hours (Fig. 9–22). At this time, urine is collected over a timed period to determine the type of diuresis. Usually, the BUN and creatinine values return to normal within 24 to 48 hours, the patient is alert, and oral replacement suffices, especially if the diuresis is solely physiologic. If the diuresis persists with low urine osmolality, there is most likely a pathologic concentrating defect, and the alert patient can be maintained on oral intake. However, if the BUN and creatinine remain elevated, supplementation with a sodium containing intravenous fluid (5% dextrose in 0.45% saline) may enhance recovery of GFR (Gulmi et al, 1995). The least common but most dangerous form of postobstructive diuresis is pathologic sodium loss, which has been termed *sodium wasting nephropathy* (Howards, 1973). Dramatic fractional sodium loss has been reported; it necessitates copious sodium replacement matching output until the patient stabilizes in order to avoid marked volume depletion and hypotension.

Moreover, maintaining an expanded extracellular fluid volume in dogs with BUO helped them achieve preobstruction baseline serum creatinine levels (Gulmi et al, 1995). In volume-replete dogs, GFR values demonstrated a sequential trend upward toward baseline after relief of BUO, whereas the group of dogs that were not volume replete did not show a trend toward improvement in GFR. Therefore, there may be clinical benefit to maintaining the patient's volume expansion during the postobstructive diuretic phase, ultimately achieving a better return of renal function after relief of the obstruction. This is only a suggestion, and clinical data supporting this experimental observation have thus far not been obtained.

Postobstructive diuresis is only one example of a polyuric state. An acceptable definition of polyuria is a urine output greater than 3 L/day in an individual not drinking large amounts of fluid (Coe, 1994). This amount should be determined through a 24-hour urine collection. The various causes and classifications of polyuria are listed in Table 9–5. Once the diagnosis of polyuria is made, measuring the urine osmolality helps distinguish between solute and water diuresis. The remainder of the work-up can be done according to the flow diagram in Figure 9–23.

Renal Colic

The standard treatment for severe renal colic has been the parenteral administration of narcotic analgesics. This treatment results in the rapid onset of adequate analgesia and avoids oral medication in patients, who frequently are nauseated. However, narcotics can exacerbate gastrointestinal symptoms and can cause excessive sedation. NSAIDs are non-narcotic analgesics that are also available for parenteral

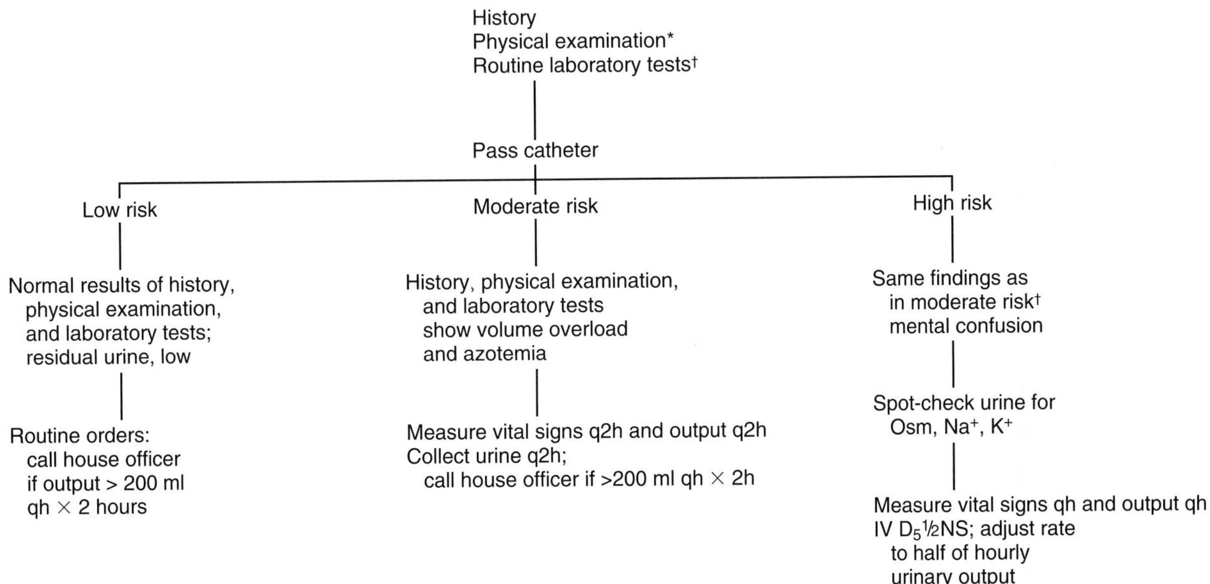

Figure 9–22. Identification of patients at risk for developing a postobstructive diuresis. *At risk: hypertension, congestive heart failure, ankle edema, confusion; †At risk: azotemia, hyperkalemia, high phosphorus, low calcium, low CO_2.

Table 9–5. CAUSES OF POLYURIA

Water Diuresis	Solute Diuresis
Decreased ADH Secretion	***Nonelectrolyte***
Excessive intake of hypotonic fluid	Urea
Psychogenic (compulsive) polydipsia (e.g., schizophrenia)	Metabolic
Thirst Stimulation	Hypercatabolism
Hypercalcemia	High protein diet, nasogastric and gastric tube feeding, TPN
Potassium depletion	Renal disease
Hyperreninemia	Postobstructive diuresis
Organic primary polydipsia (lesion in thirst center)	Diuretic phase of acute tubular necrosis
Central Diabetes Insipidus	Post-transplantation diuresis
Idiopathic (congenital or familial)	Glucose
Secondary to neoplastic, infiltrative, vascular, inflammatory (infectious and noninfectious), traumatic destructive lesions in CNS	Diabetes mellitus
Agents That Inhibit AVP Release	Renal glucosuria
$Alpha_2$-adrenergic agonists, ethanol, opiate antagonist, phenytoin (Dilantin)	Glucose infusions
Cold Diuresis	Mannitol
Impaired Tubular Response to ADH	Glycerol
Hereditary nephrogenic diabetes insipidus	Amino acids
Acquired nephrogenic diabetes insipidus: hypokalemia, hypercalcemia, sickle-cell anemia, chronic tubulointerstitial diseases (obstructive nephropathy, amyloidosis, polycystic disease, medullary cystic disease, Sjögren's syndrome)	***Electrolyte***
Cold diuresis	Saline infusions or excessive dietary salt intake
Drugs: lithium carbonate, methoxyflurane, demethylchlortetracycline (demeclocycline), amphotericin B	Diuretics
	Increased secretion of ANP: paroxysmal tachycardias
	Isolated hypoaldosteronism
	Renal disease: impaired tubular reabsorption
	Salt-losing nephritis
	Postobstructive diuresis
	Diuretic phase of acute tubular necrosis
	Post-transplantation diuresis
	Chronic tubulointerstitial disease (obstructive, cystic, infiltrative, gouty)
	Mixed Water-Solute Diuresis
	Combined uncontrolled diabetes mellitus and chronic renal failure
	Postrelief of obstructive uropathy

ADH, antidiuretic hormone; CNS, central nervous system; AVP, arginine vasopressin; TPN, total parenteral nutrition.

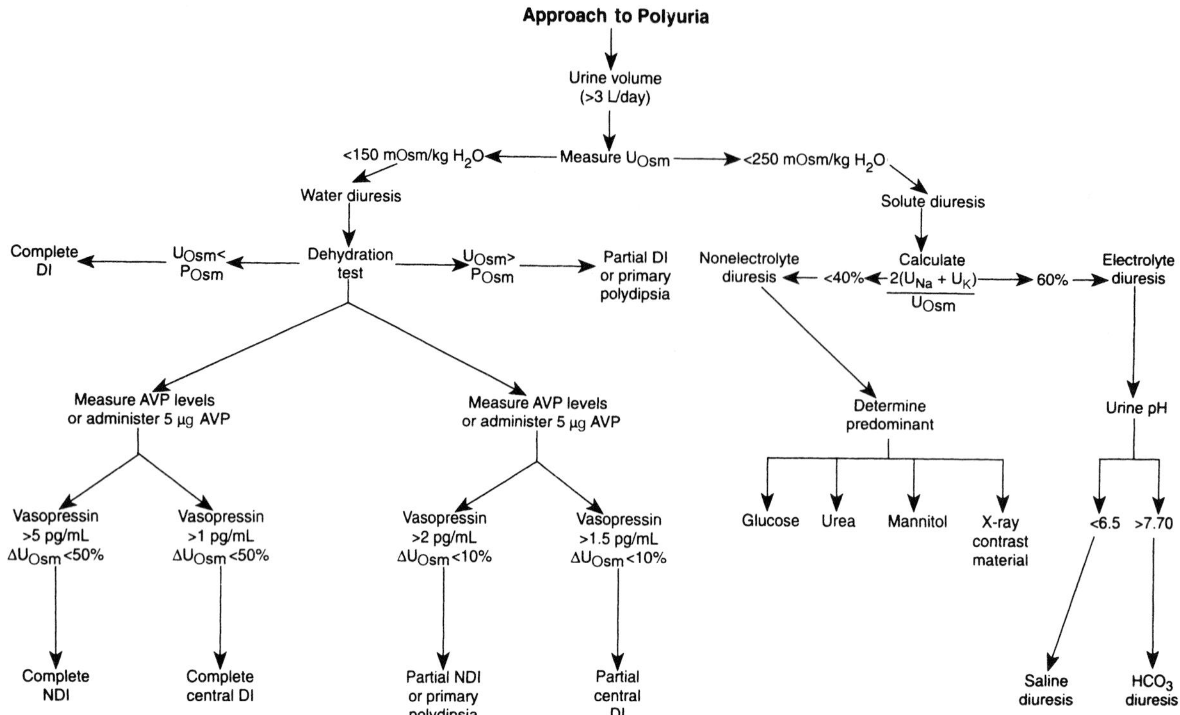

Figure 9–23. A schematic presentation of the approach to the differential diagnosis of polyuria.

administration. NSAIDs are potent inhibitors of cyclooxygenase, and thus their mechanism of pain relief differs from that of the narcotic analgesics. **However, in addition to directly affecting pain pathways, NSAIDs may affect renal function and ureteral pressure. Although beneficial for pain management, such effects may also be detrimental to renal function** (Perlmutter et al, 1993).

Many studies have documented the effectiveness of NSAIDs in the treatment of colic. Holmlund and Sjodin (1978) reported the first results with intravenous indomethacin. Other reports of use of a variety of NSAIDs, including diclofenac (Voltaren) and naproxen, followed. Several subsequent multicenter trials have been reported. A randomized double-blind multicenter trial reported by the Collaborative Group of the Spanish Society of Clinical Pharmacology compared dipyrone (metamizole; an NSAID), diclofenac (an NSAID), and pethidine (a narcotic) in 451 patients. In this study, diclofenac was shown to be as effective as pethidine (Anonymous, 1991). Similar results were found in a multicenter trial in India (Marthak et al, 1991). A meta-analysis of 19 studies assessed results of NSAIDs in colic, using the following criteria: (1) trials were randomized and controlled, (2) NSAIDs were compared with placebo or analgesic agent in the treatment of acute renal colic, and (3) the article was written in English or French. The results demonstrated that parenteral NSAIDs (usually diclofenac or indomethacin) were more effective than placebo and as effective as narcotic analgesics (Labrecque et al, 1994).

The introduction of an intramuscularly administered NSAID, ketorolac (Toradol), has led to numerous studies on its efficacy in colic. Van Laecke and Oosterlinck (1994) presented double-blind studies comparing ketorolac and pethidine. Ketorolac has been shown to be as effective as pethidine, with fewer side effects in both studies.

There are several theories as to the mechanism of action of NSAIDS in the management of colic. Prostaglandins have long been known to sensitize pain receptors to stimuli such as bradykinin and histamine. Furthermore, they have effects on central pain mechanisms (Campbell and Halushka, 1996). Therefore, inhibiting prostaglandin synthesis can interfere with both local and central pain mechanisms. Besides release of local pain mediators, the pain of ureteral colic is likely also from increased pressure and tension in the renal pelvis and ureteral wall secondary to obstruction. Thus mechanisms to reduce pressure would also reduce pain. Allen and coworkers (1978) showed that ureteral pressure in UUO is decreased with indomethacin treatment. Sjodin and associates (1982) studied the effect of indomethacin on glomerular capillary pressure and pelvic pressure during UUO in rats. Their studies showed that indomethacin reduced both renal pelvic pressure and proximal tubule stop-flow pressure by approximately 30%. A study of four NSAIDs in dogs with acute obstruction showed 30% to 50% reductions in renal pelvic pressure after administration of these drugs (Gasparich and Mayo, 1986). Lennon and colleagues (1993) compared the effects of NSAIDs and morphine on contractility of the ureter in vitro. Both pethidine and NSAIDs inhibited spontaneous contractile activity in ureteral segments. Effects on the ureter may relieve colic and also facilitate stone passage.

It is known that in the initial phase of obstruction, prostaglandin synthesis increases in the renal medulla, which increases RBF and has a diuretic effect. Thus NSAIDs could also mediate pain relief by eliminating prostaglandin-mediated increases in RBF and diuresis. Perlmutter and colleagues (1993) measured the effect of ketorolac (Toradol) on RBF and ureteral pressure in a model of acute obstruction. **Toradol given at 4 hours after acute ureteral ob-**

struction in a dog was shown to decrease RBF by 35% in the obstructed kidney; ureteral pressure decreased by 20%.

In summary, NSAIDs have been shown to be as effective as narcotic analgesics in the treatment of colic. NSAID inhibition of prostaglandin synthesis results in decreased prostaglandin-mediated pain pathways, as well as decreases in ureteric contractility, renal pelvic and glomerular capillary pressures, and RBF. The effects on RBF, however, may also be detrimental to renal function in the affected kidney. Therefore, before administering NSAIDs, clinicians should carefully consider the state of renal function in patients experiencing pain.

Calcium Channel Blockers

Kahn and co-workers (1995) showed that the infusion of verapamil into the renal artery of dogs after the relief of 19 hours of UUO increased both the GFR and RBF in a dose-dependent manner. This was associated with profound diuresis and natriuresis. Fleming and co-investigators (1987), using calcium channel blockers, also demonstrated an improvement in RBF in the hydronephrotic rat kidney after 9 to 12 weeks of UUO. Although not clinically proven, calcium channel blockers may be useful in patients with chronic UUO in an attempt to improve postobstructive renal function. This is especially true in patients starting with compromised renal function. This suggestion should be supported by additional clinical data before a definitive practice can be recommended.

HYDRONEPHROSIS AND HYPERTENSION

The incidence of hypertension among patients with ureteral occlusion varies according to whether the renal obstruction is bilateral or unilateral. Vaughan and Gillenwater (1973) reported that of 22 patients with BUO, 17 (77%) had a diastolic pressure greater than 90 mm Hg. The hypertension was reversible in 15 (88%) of the 17 patients. The incidence of hypertension in patients with acute UUO has been reported to be 20% to 30% (Brasch et al, 1940; Schwartz, 1969), whereas the incidence in chronic UUO is significantly lower (Vaughan and Sosa, 1991, 1995). Therefore, a far higher percentage of patients with BUO have hypertension, in comparison with patients with UUO.

In patients with UUO and hypertension, the burden of proof of a cause-and-effect relationship rests on the clinician, who must use criteria developed for identifying patients with renovascular hypertension (see Chapter 11) and must bear in mind that the majority of patients (70% to 80%) will not have clinical proof that hydronephrosis caused the hypertension. **The salient features for a curable patient include (1) increased renin secretion from only the hydronephrotic kidney, (2) decreased renin secretion from the contralateral kidney, and (3) a positive captopril test**

Table 9–6. REPORTED CASES OF CORRECTABLE HYPERTENSION AND HYDRONEPHROSIS

Author	No. Patients	Renin Data	Reference
Belman et al	1	+	N Engl J Med 1968; 278:1133
Garrett et al	2	ND	Am J Med 1970; 49:271
Kluge et al	1	ND; trauma also	Scand J Urol Nephrol 1972; 6:304
Greenhalf and DeVere	1	ND	J Obstet Gynaecol Br Commonw 1973; 80:754
Nemoy et al	1	ND	JAMA 1973; 225:512
Andaloro	1	+	Urology 1975; 5:367
Chapman et al	2	ND	J Pediatr Surg 1975; 10:281
Schift et al	3	2/3+; 1 ND	Urology 1975; 5:178
Wise	1	+	JAMA 1975; 231:491
Carella and Silber	1	+	J Pediatr 1976; 88:987
Ribeiro and Quartey	1	ND	Br J Urol 1976; 48:107
Munoz et al	2	ND	Am J Dis Child 1977; 131:38
Weidman et al	8	5/8+	Ann Intern Med 1977; 87:437
Squitieri et al	3	1/3+; 2 ND	J Urol 1978; 111:284
Uhari et al	1	+ also RAS	J Pediatr 1978; 92:458
Bruckstein et al	1	+	Am J Med 1979; 66:358
Pak et al	1	+	Urology 1980; 16:499
Pranikoff et al	1	+	J Urol 1980; 124:701
Lusher et al	3/6 cured	+	Clin Nephrol 1981; 15:314
Riehle and Vaughan	1	+	J Urol 1981; 126:243
Abramson and Jackson	2	+	J Urol 1984; 132:746
Vrata et al	1	+	Jpn J Med 1985; 24:44
Kawano et al	1	+	Eur Urol 1986; 12:357
Wanner	26 21/26 helped	18/21+	Nephron 1987; 45:236
Kent et al	1	+	J Pediatr Surg 1987; 22:1049
Davis and Schiff	1	ND	J Reprod Med 1988; 33:470
Braren et al	2	1/2+; 1/2 ND	Urology 1988; 32:228
Pezzulli et al	1	+	Urology 1989; 33:70
Hirsch and Jindal	1	+	Can Med Assoc J 1990; 142:1261
Mizuiri et al	1	+	Nephron 1992; 61:217

ND, not done; RAS, renal artery stenosis.

result (Table 9–6). Only patients proved to have lateralized renin secretion and ACE inhibitor–responsive hypertension should undergo correction of the hydronephrosis to achieve a goal of normotension.

The hypertension of BUO is clinically managed very differently. As previously stated, hypertension is reversible in the majority of patients with treatment of the obstruction. When these patients present, they are usually in a state of volume overload (Robards and Ross, 1967; Gulmi et al, 1989; Vaughan and Sosa, 1991). Upon relief of the obstruction, they undergo weight reduction, diuresis, and natriuresis in association with a normalization in their blood pressure. Gulmi and co-workers (1989) described nine patients with significantly depressed plasma renin activity before the relief of BUO, in whom plasma renin activity increased after the release of the obstruction. The decrease in plasma renin activity argues against renin-mediated hypertension during BUO. This decrease in plasma renin is associated with an increase in serum levels of ANP, a hormone known to depress plasma renin activity. With the increase in plasma renin activity and the postobstructive diuresis, there is also a decrease in ANP, which again suggests sodium-/volume-mediated hypertension. These patients do not require the same work-up as the patients with UUO, because relieving the cause of the obstruction most likely results in a cure of the hypertension, if there was no history of hypertension before the onset of BUO. In rare instances after relief of BUO, there is significant hyperkalemia that persists despite return of BUN and creatinine values to normal. The cause is either hyporeninemic hypoaldosteronism or distal tubule refractoriness to aldosterone. The hypokalemia should be treated appropriately, and the entity is self-limiting.

REFERENCES

Albrightson CR, Evers AS, Griffin AC, Needleman P: Effect of endogenously produced leukotrienes and thromboxane on renal vascular resistance in rabbit hydronephrosis. Cir Res 1987; 61:514–522.

Allen JT, Vaughan ED Jr, Gillenwater JY: The effect of indomethacin on renal blood flow and ureteral pressure in unilateral ureteral obstruction in awake dogs. Invest Urol 1978; 15:324–327.

Andres JL, Stanley K, Cheifetz S, Massague J: Membrane-anchored and soluble forms of betaglycan, a polymorphic proteoglycan that binds transforming growth factor-β. J Cell Biol 1989; 109:3137–3145.

Anonymous: Comparative study of the efficacy of dipyrone, diclofenac sodium and pethidine in acute renal colic. Eur J Clin Pharmacol 1991; 40:543–546.

Arendhorst WJ, Finn WF, Gottschalk CW: Nephron stop-flow pressure response to obstruction for 24 hours in the rat kidney. J Clin Invest 1974; 53:1497–1500.

Awazu M, Ichikawa I: Biological significance of atrial natriuretic peptide in the kidney. Nephron 1993; 63:1–14.

Badr KF, Brenner BM, Ichikawa I: Effects of leukotriene D_4 on glomerular dynamics in the rat. Am J Physiol 1987; 253:F239–F243.

Badr KF, DeBoer DK, Schwartzberg M, Serhan CN: Lipoxin A_4 antagonizes cellular and in vivo actions of leukotriene D_4 in rat glomerular mesangial cells: Evidence for competition at a common receptor. Proc Natl Acad Sci USA 1989; 86:3438–3442.

Baird NR, Morrison AR: Amplification of the arachidonic acid cascade: Implications for pharmacologic intervention. Am J Kidney Dis 1993; 21:557–564.

Balint P, Laszlo K: Effect of imidazole and indomethacin on hemodynamics of the obstructed canine kidney. Kidney Int 1985; 27:892–897.

Bander SJ, Buerkert JE, Martin D, Klahr S: Long-term effects of 24-hour unilateral ureteral obstruction on renal function in the rat. Kidney Int 1985; 28:614–620.

Battle DC, Arruda JAL, Kurtzman NA: Hyperkalemic distal renal tubular acidosis associated with obstructive uropathy. N Engl J Med 1981; 304:373–380.

Bell ET: Renal Diseases. Philadelphia, Lea & Febiger, 1946.

Berlyne GM: Distal tubular function in chronic hydronephrosis. Q J Med 1961; 30:339–355.

Billiar TR: Nitric oxide: Novel biology with clinical relevance. Ann Surg 1995; 4:339–349.

Blackshear JL, Wathen RL: Effects of indomethacin on renal blood flow and renin secretory responses to ureteral occlusion in the dog. Miner Electrolyte Metab 1978; 1:271.

Border WA, Noble NA: Transforming growth factor-β in tissue fibrosis. New Engl J Med 1994; 331:1286–1292.

Brasch WF, Walters W, Hammer HJ: Hypertension and the surgical kidney. JAMA 1940; 115:1837.

Breyer MD, Jacobson HR, Breyer RM: Functional and molecular aspects of renal prostaglandin receptors. J Am Soc Nephrol 1996; 7:8–17.

Brown M, Chou S-Y, Poruch JG: Endothelins and kidney diseases. Nephron 1996; 72:375–382.

Brown SCW, Upsdell SM, O'Reilly PH: The importance of renal function in the interpretation of diuresis renography. Br J Urol 1992; 69:121–125.

Bruijn JA, Roos A, de Geus B, de Heer E: Transforming growth factor-β and the glomerular extracellular matrix in renal pathology. J Lab Clin Med 1994; 123:34–47.

Buerkert J, Alexander E, Purkerson ML, Klahr S: On the site of decreased fluid reabsorption after release of ureteral obstruction in the rat. J Lab Clin Med 1976; 87:397–410.

Buerkert J, Head M, Klahr S: Effects of acute bilateral ureteral obstruction on deep nephron and terminal collecting duct function in the young rat. J Clin Invest 1977; 59:1055–1065.

Buerkert J, Martin D, Head M: Effect of acute ureteral obstruction on terminal collecting duct function in the weanling rat. Am J Physiol 1979; 236:F260–F267.

Buerkert J, Martin D, Head M, et al: Deep nephron function after release of acute unilateral ureteral obstruction in the young rat. J Clin Invest 1978; 62:1228–1239.

Buhrle CP, Hackenthal E, Helmchen U, et al: The hydronephrotic kidney of the mouse as a tool for intravital microscopy and in vitro electrophysiological studies of renin-containing cells. Lab Invest 1986; 54:462–472.

Bussolino F, Camussi G: Platelet-activating factor produced by endothelial cells. Eur J Biochem 1995; 229:327–337.

Cadnapaphornchai P, Bondar NP, McDonald FD: Effect of imidazole on the recovery from bilateral ureteral obstruction in dogs. Am J Physiol 1982; 243:F532–F536.

Campbell WB, Halushka PV: Lipid-derived autacoids: Eicosanoids and platelet activating factor. *In* Hardman JG, Limbird LE, eds: Goodman and Gilman's The Pharmacological Basis of Therapeutics, 9th ed. New York, McGraw-Hill, 1996, pp 601–616.

Camussi G, Tetta C, Bussolino F, et al: Involvement of cytokines and platelet-activating factor in renal pathology. J Lipid Mediators 1990; 2(Suppl):S203–S213.

Capdevila J, Chacos N, Werringloer J, et al: Liver microsomal cytochrome P-450 and oxidative metabolism of arachidonic acid. Proc Natl Acad Sci USA 1981; 78:5362–5366.

Carroll MA, Garcia MP, Falck JR, McGiff JC: Cyclooxygenase dependency of the renovascular actions of cytochrome P450–derived arachidonate metabolites. J Pharmacol Exp Ther 1992; 260:104–109.

Chen J, Pu Y, Liu S, Chiu T: Renal hemodynamics in patients with obstructive uropathy evaluated by duplex Doppler sonography. J Urol 1993; 150:18–21.

Chevalier RL: Renal response to ureteral obstruction in early development. Nephron 1990; 56:113–117.

Chevalier RL, Thornhill BA, Gomez RA: EDRF modulates renal hemodynamics during unilateral ureteral obstruction in the rat. Kidney Int 1992; 42:400–406.

Chiu AT, Herblin WF, McCall DE, et al: Identification of angiotensin II receptor subtypes. Biochem Biophys Res Commun 1989; 165:196–203.

Christensen G: Cardiovascular and renal effects of atrial natriuretic factor. Scand J Clin Lab Invest 1993; 53:203–209.

Chung KH, Gomez RA, Chevalier RL: Regulation of renal growth factors and clusterin by AT1 receptors during neonatal ureteral obstruction. Am J Physiol 1995; 268:F1117–F1123.

Clancy RM, Abramson SB: Nitric oxide: A novel mediator of inflammation. Proc Soc Exp Biol Med 1995; 210:93–101.

Clark JD, Ozgur LE, Conway TM, et al: Cloning of a phospholipase A_2-activating protein. Proc Natl Acad Sci USA 1991; 88:5418–5422.

Cobb JP, Natanson C, Hoffman WD, et al: N^{w} amino-L-arginine, an inhibitor of nitric oxide synthase, raises vascular resistance but increases mortality rates in awake canines challenged with endotoxin. J Exp Med 1992; 176:1175–1182.

Cody RJ: The clinical potential of renin inhibitors and angiotensin antagonists. Drugs 1994; 4:586–598.

Coe FL: Alterations in urinary function. *In* Isselbacher KJ, Braunwald E, Wilson JD, et al, eds: Harrison's Principles of Internal Medicine, 13th ed. New York: McGraw-Hill, 1994, pp 235–241.

Cogan MG: Atrial natriuretic peptide. Kidney Int 1990; 37:1148–1160.

Coleman RA, Smith WL, Narumiya S: VIIIth International Union of Pharmacology classification of prostanoid receptors: Properties, distribution, and structure of the receptors and their subtypes. Pharmacol Rev 1994; 46:205–229.

Connor J, Buttyan R, Olsson CA, et al: SGP-2 expression as a genetic marker of progressive cellular pathology in experimental hydronephrosis. Kidney Int 1991; 39:1098–1103.

Conway JJ: "Well-tempered" diuresis renography: Its historical development, physiological and technical pitfalls, and standardized technique protocol. Semin Nucl Med 1992; 22:74–84.

Cronan JJ: Contemporary venous imaging. Cardiovasc Interven Radiol 1991; 14:87–97.

Cronan JJ, Tublin ME: Role of the resistive index in the evaluation of acute renal obstruction. AJR 1995; 164:377–378.

Currie MG, Needleman P: Renal arachidonic acid metabolism. Ann Rev Physiol 1984; 46:327–341.

Dal Canton A, Corradi A, Stanziale R, et al: Glomerular hemodynamics before and after release of 24-hour bilateral ureteral obstruction. Kidney Int 1980; 17:491–496.

Dal Canton A, Stanziale R, Corradi A, et al: Effects of acute ureteral obstruction on glomerular hemodynamics in rat kidney. Kidney Int 1977; 12:403–411.

Davies M, Martin J, Thomas GJ, Lovett DH: Proteinases and glomerular matrix turnover. Kidney Int 1992; 41:671–678.

deBold AJ, Borenstein HB, Veress AT, Sonnenberg H: A rapid and potent natriuretic response to intravenous injection of atrial myocardial extract in rats. Life Sci 1981; 28:89–94.

de Gasparo M, Levens NR: Pharmacology of angiotensin II receptors in the kidney. Kidney Int 1994; 46:1486–1491.

Denhardt DT, Feng B, Edwards DR, et al: Tissue inhibitor of metalloproteinases (TIMP, aka EPA): Structure, control of expression and biological functions. Pharmacol Ther 1993; 59:329–341.

Deray G, Maistre G, Basset JY, et al: Plasma levels of atrial natriuretic peptide in chronically dialyzed patients. Kidney Int 1988; 34:S86.

Diamond JR, Kees-Folts D, Ding G, et al: Macrophages, monocyte chemoattractant peptide-1, and TGF-beta 1 in experimental hydronephrosis. Am J Physiol 1994; 266:F926–F933.

Diamond JR, van Goor H, Ding G, Engelmyer E: Myofibroblasts in experimental hydronephrosis. Am J Pathol 1995; 146:121–129.

Dvergsten J, Manivel JC, Correa-Rotter R, Rosenberg ME: Expression of clusterin in human renal diseases. Kidney Int 1994; 45:828–835.

Earley LE: Extreme polyuria in obstructive uropathy: Report of a case of "water-losing nephritis" in an infant with a discussion of polyuria. N Engl J Med 1956; 255:600.

Edwards DR, Murphy G, Reynolds JJ: Transforming growth factor beta modulates the expression of collagenase and metalloproteinase inhibitor. EMBO J 1987; 6:1899–1904.

Edwards RM, Trizna W, Kinter LB: Renal vascular effects of vasopressin and vasopressin antagonists. Am J Physiol 1989; 256:F274–F278.

El-Dahr SS, Gomez RA, Khare G, et al: Expression of renin and its mRNA in the adult rat kidney with chronic ureteral obstruction. Am J Kidney Dis 1990; 15:575–582.

El-Dahr SS, Gee J, Dipp S, et al: Upregulation of renin-angiotensin system and downregulation of kallikrein in obstructive nephropathy. Am J Physiol 1993; 264:F874–F881.

Engelmyer E, vanGoor H, Edwards DR, Diamond JR: Differential mRNA expression of renal cortical tissue inhibitor of metalloproteinase-1, -2, -3 in experimental hydronephrosis. J Am Soc Nephrol 1995; 5:1675–1683.

Escalante B, Sessa WC, Falck JR, et al: Vasoactivity of 20-hydroxyeicosatetraenoic acid is dependent on metabolism by cyclooxygenase. J Pharmacol Exp Ther 1989; 248:229–232.

Eshima D, Taylor A Jr: Technetium-99m (^{99m}Tc) mercaptoacetyltriglycine: Update on the new ^{99m}Tc renal tubular function agent. Semin Nucl Med 1992; 22:61–73.

Felsen D, Loo MH, Marion D, Vaughan ED Jr: Involvement of platelet activating factor and thromboxane A_2 in the renal response to unilateral ureteral obstruction. J Urol 1990; 144:141–145.

Fine E: Interventions in renal scintirenography. Semin Nucl Med 1991; 21:116–127.

Fink RL, Caridis DT, Chmiel R, Ryan G: Renal impairment and its reversibility following variable periods of complete ureteric obstruction. Aust N Z J Surg 1980; 50:77–83.

Flam T, Venot A, Bariety J: Reversible hydronephrosis in the rat: A new surgical technique assessed by radioisotopic measurements. J Urol 1984; 131:796–798.

Fleming JT, Parekh N, Steinhausen M: Calcium antagonists preferentially dilate preglomerular vessels of hydronephrotic kidney. Am J Physiol 1987; 253:F1157–F1163.

Franke JJ, McDougal WS: The mechanism of the preservation of renal function during obstruction by enalapril. J Urol 1991; 145:466a.

French LE, Wohlwend A, Sappino A-P, et al: Human clusterin gene expression is confined to surviving cells during in vitro programmed cell death. J Clin Invest 1994; 93:877–884.

Fried TA, Ayon MA, McDonald G, et al: Atrial natriuretic peptide, right atrial pressure, and sodium excretion rate in the rat. Am J Physiol 1987; 235:F969–F975.

Frøkiær J, Knudsen L, Nielsen AS, et al: Enhanced intrarenal angiotensin II generation in response to obstruction of the pig ureter. Am J Physiol 1992a; 263:F527–F533.

Frøkiær J, Marples D, Knepper MA, Nielsen S: Bilateral ureteral obstruction downregulates expression of vasopressin-sensitive AQP-2 water channel in rat kidney. Am J Physiol 1996; 270:F657–F668.

Frøkiær J, Nielsen AS, Knudsen L, et al: The effect of indomethacin infusion on renal hemodynamics and on the renin-angiotensin system during unilateral ureteral obstruction of the pig. J Urol 1993; 150:1557–1563.

Frøkiær J, Pedersen EB, Knudsen L, Djurhuus JC: The impact of total unilateral ureteral obstruction on intrarenal angiotensin II production in the polycalyceal pig kidney. Scand J Urol Nephrol 1992b; 26:289–295.

Frøkiær J, Sorensen SS: Eicosanoid excretion from the contralateral kidney in pigs with complete unilateral ureteral obstruction. J Urol 1995; 154:1205–1209.

Frøkiær J, Tagehoj Jensen F, Husted SE, et al: Renal blood flow and pelvic pressure after 4 weeks of total upper urinary tract obstruction in the pig. The effect of a TxA_2 synthetase inhibitor on active preglomerular vasoconstriction. Urol Res 1988; 16:167–171.

Fung LCT, Steckler RE, Khoury AE, et al: Intrarenal resistive index correlates with renal pelvis pressure. J Urol 1994; 152:607–611.

Furchgott RF, Zawadzki JV: The obligatory role of endothelial cells in the relaxation of arterial smooth muscle by acetylcholine. Nature 1980; 228:373–376.

Gasparich JP, Mayo ME: Comparative effects of four prostaglandin synthesis inhibitors on the obstructed kidney in the dog. J Urol 1986; 135:1088–1090.

Gillenwater JY, Westervelt FB Jr, Vaughan ED Jr, Howards SS: Renal function after release of chronic unilateral hydronephrosis in man. Kidney Int 1975; 7:179–186.

Gilmore JP: Influences of tissue pressure on renal blood flow autoregulation. Am J Physiol 1964; 206:707.

Glaser KB: Regulation of phospholipase A_2 enzymes: Selective inhibitors and their pharmacological potential. Adv Pharmacol 1995; 32:31–62.

Glassman HN, Kleinert HD, Boger RS, et al: Clinical pharmacology of enalkiren, a novel dipeptide renin inhibitor. J Cardiovasc Pharmacol 1990; 16:S76–S81.

Gonzalez JM, Suki WN: Polyuria and nocturia. *In* Massry SG, Glassock RJ, eds: Textbook of Nephrology, 3rd ed. Baltimore, Williams & Wilkins, 1995, pp 547–552.

Gonzalez-Avila G, Vadillo-Ortega F, Perez-Tamayo R: Experimental diffuse interstitial renal fibrosis. Lab Invest 1988; 59:245–252.

Grantham JJ, Orloff J: Effect of PGE1 on the permeability response of isolated collecting tubules to vasopressin, adenosine 3′–5′ monophosphate and theophylline. J Clin Invest 1968; 47:1154.

Griendling KK, Lassègue B, Murphy TJ, Alexander RW: Angiotensin II receptor pharmacology. Adv Pharmacol 1994; 28:269–306.

Gulbins E, Parekh N, Rauterberg EW, et al: Cysteinyl leukotriene actions on the microcirculation of the normal and split hydronephrotic rat kidney. Eur J Clin Invest 1991; 21:184–196.

Gulmi FA, Matthews GJ, Marion D, et al: Volume expansion enhances the recovery of renal function and prolongs the diuresis and natriuresis after release of bilateral ureteral obstruction: A possible role for atrial natriuretic peptide. J Urol 1995; 153:1276–1283.

Gulmi FA, Mooppan UMM, Chou S, Kim H: Atrial natriuretic peptide in patients with obstructive uropathy. J Urol 1989; 142:268–272.

Halushka PV, Lefer AM: Thromboxane A_2 in health and disease. Fed Proc 1987; 46:31–32.

Halushka PV, Mais DE, Saussy DL Jr: Platelet and vascular smooth muscle thromboxane A_2/PGH_2 receptors. Fed Proc 1987; 46:149–153.

Hanley MJ, Davidson K: Isolated nephron segments from rabbit models of obstructive nephropathy. J Clin Invest 1982; 69:165–174.

Harris RH, Yarger WE: Renal function after release of unilateral ureteral obstruction in rats. Am J Physiol 1974; 227:806–815.

Harris RH, Yarger WE: The pathogenesis of post-obstructive diuresis. J Clin Invest 1975; 56:880–887.

Henson PM: Release of vasoactive amines from rabbit platelets induced by antiplatelet antibody in the presence and absence of complement. J Immunol 1970; 104:924–934.

Herbaczynska-Cedro K, Vane JR: Contribution of the intrarenal generation of prostaglandin to autoregulation of renal blood flow in the dog. Circ Res 1973; 33:428–436.

Herbaczynska-Cedro K, Vane JR: Prostaglandins as mediators of reactive hyperaemia in kidney. Nature 1974; 247:492.

Hickey KA, Rubanyi G, Paul RJ, Highsmith RF: Characterization of a coronary vasoconstrictor produced by cultured endothelial cells. Am J Physiol 1985; 248:C550–C556.

Himmelstein SI, Coffman TM, Yarger WE, Klotman PE: Atrial natriuretic peptide–induced changes in renal prostacyclin production in ureteral obstruction. Am J Physiol 1990; 258:F281–F286.

Hinman F: The condition of renal counterbalance and the theory of renal atrophy of disuse. J Urol 1943; 49:392–400.

Hinman F, Hepler AB: Experimental hydronephrosis. Arch Surg 1925; 11:917–932.

Hirata M, Hayashi Y, Ushikubi F, et al: Cloning and expression of cDNA for a human thromboxane A_2 receptor. Nature 1991; 349:617–620.

Holmlund D, Sjodin JG: Treatment of ureteral colic with intravenous indomethacin. J Urol 1978; 120:676–677.

Howards S: Postobstructive diuresis: A misunderstood phenomenon. J Urol 1973; 110:537.

Huguenin M, Ott CE, Romero JC, Knox FG: Influence of renin depletion on renal function after release of 24-hour ureteral obstruction. J Lab Clin Med 1976; 87:58–64.

Huland H, Gonnermann D: Pathophysiology of hydronephrotic atrophy: The cause and role of active preglomerular vasoconstriction. Urol Int 1983; 38:193–198.

Huland H, Gonnermann D, Werner B, Possin U: A new test to predict reversibility of hydronephrotic atrophy after stable partial unilateral ureteral obstruction. J Urol 1988; 140:1591–1594.

Huland H, Leichtweib H-P, Augustin HJ: Effect of angiotensin II antagonist, alpha-receptor blockage, and denervation on blood flow reduction in experimental, chronic hydronephrosis. Invest Urol 1980; 18:203–206.

Hvistendahl JJ, Pedersen TS, Jørgensen HH, et al: Renal hemodynamic response to gradated ureter obstruction in the pig. Nephron, in press.

Ichikawa I: Evidence for altered glomerular hemodynamics during acute nephron obstruction. Am J Physiol 1982; 82:F580.

Ichikawa I, Brenner BM: Local intrarenal vasoconstrictor-vasodilator interactions in mild partial ureteral obstruction. Am J Physiol 1979; 236:F131–F140.

Ishidoya S, Morrissey J, McCracken R, et al: Angiotensin II receptor antagonist ameliorates renal tubulointerstitial fibrosis caused by unilateral ureteral obstruction. Kidney Int 1995; 47:1285–1294.

Jackson ED, Garrison JC: Renin and angiotensin. *In* Hardman JG, Limbird LE, eds: Goodman and Gilman's The Pharmacological Basis of Therapeutics, 9th ed. New York, McGraw-Hill, 1996, pp 733–758.

Jaenike JR: The renal functional defect of postobstructive nephropathy. J Clin Invest 1972; 51:2999–3006.

Jaenike JR, Bray GA: Effects of acute transitory urinary obstruction in the dog. Am J Physiol 1960; 199:1219–1222.

Jones DA, George NJR, O'Reilly PH, Barnard RJ: The biphasic nature of renal functional recovery following relief of chronic obstructive uropathy. Br J Urol 1988; 61:192–197.

Josephson S, Aperia A, Lannergren K, Wikstad I: Partial ureteric obstruction in the pubescent rat. J Urol 1987; 138:414–418.

Josephson S, Grossmann G: Partial ureteric obstruction in the pubescent rat: II. Long-term effects on the renal morphology. Urol Int 1991; 47:126–130.

Josephson S, Lannergren K, Eklof AC: Partial ureteric obstruction in weanling rats: II. Long-term effects on renal function and arterial blood pressure. Urol Int 1992; 48:384–390.

Juncos LA, Ren Y, Arima S, Ito S: Vasodilator and constrictor actions of platelet-activating factor in the isolated microperfused afferent arteriole of the rabbit kidney. J Clin Invest 1993; 91:1374–1379.

Kahn SA, Gulmi FA, Chou S-Y, et al: Contribution of endothelin to renal vasoconstriction in unilateral ureteral obstruction: Reversal by verapamil. J Urol 1995; 153:411a.

Kambayashi Y, Bardhan S, Takahashi K, et al: Molecular cloning of a novel angiotensin II receptor isoform involved in phosphotyrosine phosphatase inhibition. J Biol Chem 1993; 268:24543–24546.

Kaneto H, Morrissey J, Klahr S: Increased expression of TGF–beta 1 mRNA in the obstructed kidney of rats with unilateral ureteral ligation. Kidney Int 1993; 44:313–321.

Katoh T, Takahashi K, DeBoer DK, et al: Renal hemodynamic actions of lipoxins in rats: A comparative physiological study. Am J Physiol 1992; 263:F436–F442.

Kekomaki M, Vapaatalo H: Renal excretion of prostanoids and cyclic AMP in chronic partial ureteral obstruction of the rabbit. J Urol 1989; 141:395–397.

Kelleher JP, Shah V, Godley ML, et al: Urinary endothelin (ET1) in complete ureteric obstruction in the miniature pig. Urol Res 1992; 20:63–65.

Kennedy WA, Stenberg A, Lackgren G, et al: Renal tubular apoptosis after partial ureteral obstruction. J Urol 1994; 152:658–664.

Kerr WS Jr: Effect of complete ureteral occlusion in dogs on kidney function. Am J Physiol 1956; 184:521.

Kessler RH: Acute effects of brief ureteral stasis on urinary and renal papillary chloride concentration. Am J Physiol 1960; 199:1215–1218.

Knepper MA: The aquaporin family of molecular water channels. Proc Natl Acad Sci USA 1994; 91:6255–6258.

Koltai M, Guinot P, Hosford D, Braquet PG: Platelet-activating factor antagonists: Scientific background and possible clinical applications. Adv Pharmacol 1994; 28:81–167.

Kon V, Yoshioka T, Fogo A, Ichikawa I: Glomerular actions of endothelin in vivo. J Clin Invest 1989; 83:1762–1767.

Kuo PC, Schroeder RA: The emerging multifaceted roles of nitric oxide. Ann Surg 1995; 221:220–235.

Labrecque M, Dostaler LP, Rousselle R, et al: Efficacy of nonsteroidal anti-inflammatory drugs in the treatment of acute renal colic. A meta-analysis. Arch Intern Med 1994; 154:1381–1387.

Ladefoged O, Djurhuus JC: Morphology of the upper urinary tract in experimental hydronephrosis in pigs. Acta Chir Scand 1976; 472:29–35.

Laiho M, Saksela O, Keski-Oja J: Transforming growth factor-beta induction of type-1 plasminogen activator inhibitor. J Biol Chem 1987; 262:17467–17474.

Laing FC, Jeffrey RB Jr, Wing VW: Ultrasound versus excretory urography in evaluating acute flank pain. Radiology 1985; 154:613–616.

Lamas S, Marsden PA, Li GK, et al: Endothelial nitric oxide synthase: Molecular cloning and characterization of a distinct constitutive enzyme isoform. Proc Natl Acad Sci USA 1992; 89:6348–6352.

Lanzone JA, Gulmi FA, Chou S, et al: Renal hemodynamics in acute unilateral ureteral obstruction: Contribution of endothelium-derived relaxing factor. J Urol 1995; 153:2055–2059.

Leahy AL, Ryan PC, McEntee GM, et al: Renal injury and recovery in partial ureteric obstruction. J Urol 1989; 142:199–203.

Lefkowith JB, Okegawa T, DeSchryver-Decskemeti K, Needleman P: Macrophage-dependent arachidonate metabolism in hydronephrosis. Kidney Int 1984; 26:10–17.

Lennon GM, Bourke J, Ryan PC, Fitzpatrick JM: Pharmacological options for the treatment of acute ureteric colic. Br J Urol 1993; 71:401–407.

Levin ER: Endothelins. New Engl J Med 1995; 333:356–362.

Lewis HY, Pierce JM: Return of function after relief of complete ureteral obstruction of 69 days' duration. J Urol 1962; 88:372–379.

Lewis RA, Austen F, Soberman RJ: Leukotrienes and other products of the 5-lipoxygenase pathway. N Engl J Med 1990; 323:645–655.

Loo MH, Egan D, Vaughan ED Jr, et al: The effect of the thromboxane A_2 synthesis inhibitor OKY-046 on renal function in rabbits following release of unilateral ureteral obstruction. J Urol 1987; 137:571–576.

Loo MH, Marion DN, Vaughan ED Jr, et al: Effect of thromboxane inhibition on renal blood flow in dogs with complete unilateral ureteral obstruction. J Urol 1986; 136:1343–1347.

Loo MH, Vaughan ED Jr: Obstructive nephropathy and postobstructive diuresis: Urology Update Series. 1985:Lesson 9.

Lyons CR, Orloff GJ, Cunningham JM: Molecular cloning and functional expression of an inducible nitric oxide synthase from a murine macrophage cell line. J Biol Chem 1992; 267:6370–6374.

Maack T: Receptors of atrial natriuretic factor. Annu Rev Physiol 1992; 54:11–27.

Maher JF, Schreiner GE, Waters TJ: Osmotic diuresis due to retained urea after release of obstructive uropathy. N Engl J Med 1963; 268:1099–1104.

Marsden PA, Brenner BM: Nitric oxide and endothelins: Novel autocrine/paracrine regulators of the circulation. Semin Nephrol 1991; 11:169–185.

Marsen TA, Schramek H, Dunn MJ: Renal actions of endothelin: Linking cellular signaling pathways to kidney disease. Kidney Int 1994; 45:336–344.

Marthak KV, Gokarn AM, Rao AV, et al: A multi-centre comparative study of diclofenac sodium and a dipyrone/spasmolytic combination, and a single-centre comparative study of diclofenac sodium and pethidine in renal colic patients in India. Curr Med Res Opin 1991; 12:366–373.

Masaki T, Vane JR, Vanhoutte PM: International union of pharmacology nomenclature of endothelin receptors. Pharmacol Rev 1994; 46:137–142.

Masferrer JL, Zweifel BS, Manning PT, et al: Selective inhibition of inducible cyclooxygenase-2 in vivo is anti-inflammatory and noncelcerogenic. Proc Natl Acad Sci USA 1994; 91:3228–3232.

Massry SG, Schainuck LI, Goldsmith C, Schreiner GE: Studies on the mechanism of diuresis after relief of urinary-tract obstruction. Ann Intern Med 1967; 66:149–158.

Masumura H, Kunitada S, Irie K, et al: A thromboxane A_2 synthase inhibitor, DP-1904, prevents rat renal injury. Eur J Pharmacol 1991; 193:321–327.

McDougal WS: Pharmacologic preservation of renal mass and function in obstructive uropathy. J Urol 1982; 128:418–421.

McDougal WS, Wright FS: Defect in proximal and distal sodium transport in post-obstructive diuresis. Kidney Int 1972; 2:304–317.

McGiff JC, Quilley CP, Carroll MA: The contribution of cytochrome P450-dependent arachidonate metabolites to integrated renal function. Steroids 1993; 58:573–579.

Miller JB, Marion DN, Gillenwater JY: Patterns of recovery of renal function after surgical relief of chronic bilateral partial ureteral obstruction. Invest Urol 1979; 17:69–74.

Minnard EA, Shou J, Naama H, et al: Inhibition of nitric oxide synthesis is detrimental during endotoxemia. Arch Surg 1994; 129:142–148.

Moody TE, Vaughan ED Jr, Gillenwater JY: Relationship between renal blood flow and ureteral pressure during 18 hours of total unilateral ureteral occlusion. Invest Urol 1975; 13:246–251.

Moody TE, Vaughan ED Jr, Gillenwater JY: Comparison of the renal hemodynamic response to unilateral and bilateral ureteral occlusion. Invest Urol 1977a; 14:455–459.

Moody TE, Vaughan ED Jr, Wyker AT, Gillenwater JY: The role of intrarenal angiotensin II in the hemodynamic response to unilateral obstructive uropathy. Invest Urol 1977b; 14:390–397.

Morrison AR, Nishikawa K, Needleman P: Unmasking of thromboxane A_2 synthesis by ureteral obstruction in the rabbit kidney. Nature 1977; 267:259–260.

Morrison AR, Thornton F, Blumberg A, Vaughan ED Jr: Thromboxane A_2 is the major arachidonic acid metabolite of human cortical hydronephrotic tissue. Prostaglandins 1981; 21:171–181.

Mukoyama M, Nakajima M, Horiuchi M, et al: Expression cloning of type 2 angiotensin II receptor reveals a unique class of seven-transmembrane receptors. J Biol Chem 1993; 268:24539–24542.

Muldowney FP, Duffy GJ, Kelly DG, et al: Sodium diuresis after relief of obstructive uropathy. N Engl J Med 1966; 1294–1298.

Murphy TJ, Takeuchi K, Alexander RW: Molecular cloning of AT1 angiotensin receptors. Am J Hypertens 1992; 5:236S–242S.

Naber KG, Madsen PO: Renal function in chronic hydronephrosis with and without infection and the role of lymphatics: An experimental study in dogs. Urol Res 1974; 2:1.

Nagle RB, Bulger RE: Unilateral obstructive nephropathy in the rabbit. Lab Invest 1978; 38:270–277.

Nagle RB, Bulger RE, Cutler RE, et al: Unilateral obstructive nephropathy in the rabbit. Lab Invest 1973a; 28:456–467.

Nagle RB, Johnson ME, Jervis HR: Proliferation of renal interstitial cells following injury induced by ureteral obstruction. Lab Invest 1976; 35:18.

Nagle RB, Kneiser MR, Bulger RE, Benditt E: Induction of smooth muscle characteristics on renal interstitial fibroblasts during obstructive nephropathy. Lab Invest 1973b; 29:422–427.

Narath PA: The hydromechanics of the calyx renalis. J Urol 1940; 43:145–176.

Nash FD, Selkurt EE: Effects of elevated ureteral pressure on renal blood flow. Circ Res 1964; 14(15, suppl I):I142–I146.

Nonoguchi H, Sands JM, Knepper MA: Atrial natriuretic factor inhibits vasopressin-stimulated osmotic water permeability in rat inner medullary collecting duct. J Clin Invest 1988; 82:1382–1390.

Okegawa T, Jonas PE, DeSchryer K, et al: Metabolic and cellular alterations underlying the exaggerated renal prostaglandin and thromboxane synthesis in ureter obstruction in rabbits. Inflammatory response involving fibroblasts and mononuclear cells. J Clin Invest 1983; 71:81–90.

O'Reilly PH: Diuresis renography 8 years later: An update. J Urol 1986; 136:993.

O'Reilly PH: Diuresis renography. Recent advances and recommended protocols. Br J Urol 1992; 69:113–120.

O'Reilly PH, Lawson RS, Shields RA, Testa HJ: Idiopathic hydronephrosis—The diuresis renogram: A new non-invasive method of assessing equivocal pelvoureteral junction obstruction. J Urol 1979; 121:153.

Palmer JM, DiSandro M: Diuretic enhanced duplex Doppler sonography in 33 children presenting with hydronephrosis: A study of test sensitivity, specificity and precision. J Urol 1995; 154:1885–1888.

Paralkar VM, Vukicevic S, Reddi AH: Transforming growth factor-β type I binds to collagen IV of basement membrane matrix: Implications for development. Dev Biol 1991; 143:303–308.

Perlmutter A, Miller L, Trimble LA, et al: Toradol, an NSAID used for renal colic, decreases renal perfusion and ureteral pressure in a canine model of unilateral ureteral obstruction. J Urol 1993; 149:926–930.

Peters CA: Urinary tract obstruction in children. J Urol 1995; 154:1874–1884.

Pimentel JL Jr, Martinez-Maldonado M, Wilcox JN, et al: Regulation of renin-angiotensin system in unilateral ureteral obstruction. Kidney Int 1993; 44:390–400.

Pimentel JL Jr, Wang S, Martinez-Maldonado M: Regulation of the renal angiotensin II receptor gene in acute unilateral ureteral obstruction. Kidney Int 1994; 45:1614–1621.

Platt JF, Ellis JH, Rubin JM: Examination of native kidneys with duplex Doppler ultrasound. Semin Ultrasound 1991; 12:308–318.

Platt JF, Rubin JM, Ellis JH: Acute renal obstruction: Evaluation with intrarenal duplex doppler and conventional US. Radiology 1993; 186:685–688.

Purkerson ML, Blaine EH, Stokes TJ, Klahr S: Role of atrial peptide in the natriuresis and diuresis that follows relief of obstruction in rat. Am J Physiol 1989; 256:F583–F589.

Purkerson ML, Klahr S: Prior inhibition of vasoconstrictors normalizes GFR in postobstructed kidneys. Kidney Int 1989; 35:1306–1314.

Purkerson ML, Rolf DB, Chase LR, et al: Tubular reabsorption of phosphate after release of complete ureteral obstruction in the rat. Kidney Int 1974; 5:326–336.

Quilley J, Bell-Quilley CP, McGiff JC: Eicosanoids and hypertension. *In* Laragh JH, Brenner BM, eds: Hypertension: Pathophysiology, Diagnosis, and Management, 2nd ed. New York: Raven Press, 1995, pp 963–982.

Reyes AA, Klahr S: Role of vasopressin in rats with bilateral ureteral obstruction. Proc Soc Exp Biol Med 1991a; 197:49–55.

Reyes AA, Klahr S: Role of platelet-activating factor in renal function in normal rats and rats with bilateral ureteral obstruction. Proc Soc Exp Biol Med 1991b; 198:572–578.

Reyes AA, Klahr S: Cytochrome P-450 pathway in renal function of normal rats and rats with bilateral ureteral obstruction. Proc Soc Exp Biol Med 1992a; 201:278–283.

Reyes AA, Klahr S: Renal function after release of ureteral obstruction: Role of endothelin and the renal artery endothelium. Kidney Int 1992b; 42:632–638.

Reyes AA, Lefkowith J, Pippin J, Klahr S: Role of the 5-lipooxygenase pathway in obstructive nephropathy. Kidney Int 1992a; 41:100–106.

Reyes AA, Martin D, Settle S, Klahr S: EDRF role in renal function and blood pressure of normal rats and rats with obstructive uropathy. Kidney Int 1992b; 41:403–413.

Rinder CA, Halushka PV, Sens MA, Ploth DW: Thromboxane A_2 receptor blockade improves renal function and histopathy in the post-obstructive kidney. Kidney Int 1994; 45:185–192.

Robards VL Jr, Ross G Jr: The pathogenesis of postobstructive diuresis. J Urol 1967; 97:105–109.

Roberts AB, McCune BK, Sporn MB: TGF-β: Regulation of extracellular matrix. Kidney Int 1992; 41:557–559.

Robertson FM, Offner PJ, Ciceri DP, et al: Detrimental hemodynamic effects of nitric oxide synthase inhibition in septic shock. Arch Surg 1994; 129:149–155.

Robertson RM, Robertson D: Drugs used for the treatment of myocardial ischemia. *In* Hardman JG, Limbird LE, eds: Goodman and Gilman's The

Pharmacological Basis of Therapeutics, 9th ed. New York, McGraw-Hill, 1996, pp 759–780.

Rocha AS, Kudo LH: Atrial peptide and cGMP effects on NaCl transport in inner medullary collecting duct. Am J Physiol 1990; 259:F258–F268.

Rosenberg ME, Dvergsten J, Correa-Rotter R: Clusterin: An enigmatic protein recruited by diverse stimuli. J Lab Clin Med 1993; 121:205–214.

Rothpearl A, Frager D, Subramanian A, et al: MR urography: Technique and application. Radiol 1995; 194:125–130.

Rovin BH, Harris KPG, Morrison A, et al: Renal cortical release of a specific macrophage chemoattractant in response to ureteral obstruction. Lab Invest 1990; 63:213–220.

Rubanyi GM, Polokoff MA: Endothelins: Molecular biology, biochemistry, pharmacology, physiology, and pathophysiology. Pharmacol Rev 1994; 46:325–410.

Ryan PC, Fitzpatrick JM: Partial ureteric obstruction: A new variable canine experimental model. J Urol 1987; 137:1034–1038.

Ryan PC, Maher KP, Murphy B, et al: Experimental partial ureteric obstruction: Pathophysiological changes in the upper tract pressures and renal blood flow. J Urol 1987; 138:674–678.

Salvemini D, Seibert K, Masferrer JL, et al: Endogenous nitric oxide enhances prostaglandin production in a model of renal inflammation. J Clin Invest 1994; 93:1940–1947.

Sankari BR, Steinhardt GF, Salinas-Madrigal L, Spry LA: Urinary PGE2 in rats with chronic partial unilateral ureteral obstruction. J Surg Res 1991; 51:253–258.

Sasaki K, Yamano Y, Bardhan S, et al: Cloning and expression of a complementary DNA encoding a bovine adrenal angiotensin II type-1 receptor. Nature 1991; 351:230–233.

Sawczuk IS, Hoke G, Olsson CA, et al: Gene expression in response to acute unilateral ureteral obstruction. Kidney Int 1989; 35:1315–1319.

Saxenhoffer H, Gnadinger MP, Weidmann P, et al: Plasma levels and dialysance of atrial natriuretic peptide in terminal renal failure. Kidney Int 1987; 32:554.

Schlegel PN, Matthews GJ, Cichon Z, et al: Clusterin production in the obstructed rabbit kidney; correlations with loss of renal function. J Am Soc Nephrol 1992; 3:1163–1171.

Schlossberg SM, Vaughan ED Jr: The mechanism of unilateral postobstructive diuresis. J Urol 1984; 131:534–536.

Schreiner GF, Harris KPG, Purkerson ML, Klahr S: Immunological aspects of acute ureteral obstruction: Immune cell infiltrate in the kidney. Kidney Int 1988; 34:487.

Schulsinger DA, Felsen D, Gulmi FA, et al: The expression and localization of inducible nitric oxide synthase (iNOS) following unilateral ureteral obstruction (UUO) in rat kidney. J Urol 1996; 155:561A.

Schulsinger DA, Gulmi FA, Chou S-Y, et al: Endothelium-derived nitric oxide participates in the renal vasodilation induced by acute unilateral ureteral obstruction. J Urol 1993; 149:500A.

Schwartz DT: Unilateral upper urinary tract obstruction and arterial hypertension. N Y J Med 1969; 69:668.

Scott GD, Sullivan I: Experimental hydronephrosis. Surg Gynecol Obstet 1912; 15:296–309.

Sedor JR, Davidson EW, Dunn MJ: Effects of nonsteroidal anti-inflammatory drugs in healthy subjects. Am J Med 1986; 81:58–70.

Serhan CN: Lipoxin biosynthesis and its impact in inflammatory and vascular events. Biochim Biophys Acta 1994; 1212:1–25.

Shapiro SR, Bennett AH: Recovery of renal function after prolonged unilateral ureteral obstruction. J Urol 1976; 115:136–140.

Sharma AT, Mauer SM, Kim Y, Michael AF: Interstitial fibrosis in obstructive nephropathy. Kidney Int 1993; 44:774–788.

Sharp JD, White DL, Chiou XG, et al: Molecular cloning and expression of human Ca^{2+}-sensitive cytosolic phospholipase A_2. J Biol Chem 1991; 266:14850–14853.

Sheehan HL, Davis JC: Experimental hydronephrosis. Arch Pathol 1959; 68:185.

Shenasky JH II, Gillenwater JY, Graham SD Jr, Wooster LD: Effects of vasoactive drugs on renal vascular resistance in obstructive disease. J Urol 1971; 106:355.

Sjodin JG, Wahlberg J, Persson AEG: The effect of indomethacin on glomerular capillary pressure and pelvic pressure during ureteral obstruction. J Urol 1982; 127:1017–1020.

Smith RC, Rosenfield AT, Choe KA, et al: Acute flank pain: Comparison of non–contrast-enhanced CT and intravenous urography. Radiol 1995; 194:789–794.

Smith WL: Prostanoid biosynthesis and mechanisms of action. Am J Physiol 1992; 263:F181–F191.

Smith WL, Marnett LJ, DeWitt DL: Prostaglandin and thromboxane biosynthesis. Pharmacol Ther 1991; 49:153–179.

Snyder F: Platelet-activating factor: The biosynthetic and catabolic enzymes. Biochem J 1995; 305:689–705.

Solez K, Ponchak S, Buono RA, et al: Inner medullary plasma flow in the kidney with ureteral obstruction. Am J Physiol 1976; 231:1315–1321.

Sonnenberg H, Wilson DR: The role of the medullary collecting ducts in postobstructive diuresis. J Clin Invest 1976; 57:1564–1574.

Stenberg A, Bohman SO, Morsing P: Back-leak of pelvic urine to the bloodstream. Acta Physiol Scand 1988; 134:223–234.

Stenberg A, Jacobsson E, Larrson E, Persson AEG: Long-term partial ureteral obstruction and its effects on kidney function. Scand J Urol Nephrol 1992; 26:35–41.

Strand JC, Edwards BS, Anderson ME, et al: Effect of imidazole on renal function in unilateral ureteral-obstructed rat kidneys. Am J Physiol 1981; 240:F508–F514.

Strong KC: Plastic studies in abnormal renal architecture. Arch Pathol 1940; 29:77–119.

Stuehr DJ, Marletta MA: Mammalian nitrate biosynthesis: Mouse macrophages produce nitrite and nitrate in response to *Escherichia coli* lipopolysaccharide. Proc Natl Acad Sci USA 1985; 82:7738–7742.

Suki WN, Guthrie AG, Martinez-Maldonado M, Eknoyan G: Effects of ureteral pressure elevation on renal hemodynamics and urine concentration. Am J Physiol 1971; 220:38–43.

Talner LB: Urinary obstruction. *In* Pollack HM, ed: Clinical Urology: An Atlas and Textbook of Urological Imaging. Philadelphia, W. B. Saunders Company, 1990, pp 1535–1628.

Tan PH, Chiang GS, Tay AH: Pathology of urinary tract malformations in a paediatric autopsy series. Ann Acad Med Singapore 1994; 23:838–843.

Taylor A Jr, Eshima D: Effects of altered physiologic states on clearance and biodistribution of technetium-99m MAG3, iodine-131 OIH, and iodine-125 iothalamate. J Nucl Med 1988; 29:669–675.

Taylor A Jr, Nally JV: Clinical applications of renal scintigraphy. AJR 1995; 164:31–41.

Thierauch K-H, Dinter H, Stock G: Prostaglandins and their receptors: I. Pharmacologic receptor description, metabolism and drug use. J Hypertens 1993; 11:1315–1318.

Thierauch K-H, Dinter H, Stock G: Prostaglandins and their receptors: II. Receptor structure and signal transduction. J Hypertens 1994; 12:1–5.

Thirakomen K, Kozlov N, Arruda JAL, Kurtzman NA: Renal hydrogen ion secretion after release of unilateral ureteral obstruction. Am J Physiol 1976; 231:1233–1239.

Thureau K: Renal hemodynamics. Am J Med 1964; 36:698–719.

Tublin ME, Dodd GD III, Verdile VP: Acute renal colic: Diagnosis with duplex Doppler US. Radiology 1994; 193:697–701.

Ulm AH, Miller F: An operation to produce experimental, reversible hydronephrosis in dogs. J Urol 1962; 88:337–341.

Upsdell SM, Leeson SM, Brooman PJC, O'Reilly PH: Diuretic-induced urinary flow rates at varying clearances and their relevance to the performance and interpretation of diuresis renography. Br J Urol 1988; 61:14–18.

Van Laecke E, Oosterlinck W: Physiopathology of renal colic and the therapeutic consequences. Act Urol Belg 1994; 62:8–15.

Vane JR, Botting RM: A better understanding of anti-inflammatory drugs based on isoforms of cyclooxygenase (COX-1 and COX-2). Ad Prostaglandin Thromboxane Leukot Res 1995; 23:41–48.

Vaughan ED Jr, Gillenwater JY: Recovery following complete chronic unilateral ureteral occlusion: Functional, radiographic and pathologic alterations. J Urol 1971; 106:27–35.

Vaughan ED Jr, Gillenwater JY: Diagnosis, characterization and management of post-obstructive diuresis. J Urol 1973; 109:286–292.

Vaughan ED Jr, Shenasky JH II, Gillenwater JY: Mechanism of acute hemodynamic response to ureteral occlusion. Invest Urol 1971; 9:109–118.

Vaughan ED Jr, Sorenson EJ, Gillenwater JY: Effects of acute and chronic ureteral obstruction on renal hemodynamics and function. Surg Forum 1968; 19:536.

Vaughan ED Jr, Sorenson EJ, Gillenwater JY: The renal hemodynamic response to chronic unilateral complete ureteral occlusion. Invest Urol 1970a; 8:78.

Vaughan ED Jr, Sosa RE: Hypertension and hydronephrosis. AUA Update Series 1991; lesson X:74.

Vaughan ED Jr, Sosa RE: Hypertension and hydronephrosis. *In* Laragh JH, Brenner BM, eds: Hypertension: Pathophysiology, Diagnosis, and Management, 2nd ed. New York, Raven Press, 1995, pp 2103–2110.

Vaughan ED Jr, Sweet RC, Gillenwater JY: Peripheral renin and blood pressure changes following complete unilateral ureteral occlusion. J Urol 1970b; 194:89–92.

Walls J, Buerkert JE, Purkerson ML, Klahr S: Nature of the acidifying defect after relief of ureteral obstruction. Kidney Int 1975; 7:304–316.

Walton G, Buttyan R, Garcia-Montes E, et al: Renal growth factor expression during the early phase of experimental hydronephrosis. J Urol 1992; 148:510–514.

Whinnery MA, Shaw JO, Beck N: Thromboxane B_2 and prostaglandin E_2 in the rat kidney with unilateral ureteral obstruction. Am J Physiol 1982; 242:F220–F225.

Whitaker RH: Perfusion pressure flow studies. *In* O'Reilly PH, George NJR, Weiss RM, eds: Diagnostic Techniques in Urology. Philadelphia, W. E. Saunders Company, 1990, pp 135–141.

Whitaker RH, Buxton-Thomas MS: A comparison of pressure flow studies and renography in equivocal upper urinary tract obstruction. J Urol 1984; 131:446.

Wilson B, Reisman DD, Moyer CA: Fluid balance in the urological patient. Disturbances in the renal regulation of the excretion of water and sodium salts following decompression of the urinary bladder. J Urol 1951; 66:805.

Wilson DR: The influence of volume expansion on renal function after relief of chronic unilateral ureteral obstruction. Kidney Int 1974; 5:402–410.

Wilson DR: Pathophysiology of obstructive nephropathy. Kidney Int 1980; 18:281–292.

Wilson DR, Honrath U: Cross-circulation study of natriuretic factors in postobstructive diuresis. J Clin Invest 1976; 57:380–389.

Wilson DR, Klahr S: Urinary tract obstruction. *In* Schrier RW, Gottschalk CW, eds: Diseases of the Kidney, 5th ed. Boston, Little, Brown, 1993, pp 657–688.

Wright EJ, McCaffrey TA, Robertson AP, et al: Chronic unilateral ureteral obstructions associated with interstitial fibrosis and tubular expression of transforming growth factor-β. Lab Invest 1996; 74:528–537.

Wu KK: Inducible cyclooxygenase and nitric oxide synthase. Ad Pharmacol 1995; 33:179–207.

Yamaguchi Y, Mann DM, Ruoslahti E: Negative regulation of transforming growth factor-β by the proteoglycan decorin. Nature 1990; 346:281–284.

Yanagisawa H, Jin Z, Kurihara N, et al: Increases in glomerular eicosanoid production in rats with bilateral ureteral obstruction are mediated by enhanced obstruction enzyme activities of both the cyclooxygenase and 5-lipoxygenase pathways. Proc Soc Exp Biol Med 1993; 203:291–296.

Yanagisawa M, Kunhara H, Kimura S, et al: A novel potent vasoconstrictor peptide produced by vascular endothelial cells. Nature 1988; 332:411–415.

Yanagisawa H, Morrissey J, Klahr S: Mechanism of enhanced eicosanoid production by isolated glomeruli from rats with bilateral ureteral obstruction. Am J Physiol 1991; 261:F248–F255.

Yanagisawa H, Morrissey J, Morrison AR, Klahr S: Eicosanoid production by isolated glomeruli of rats with unilateral ureteral obstruction. Kidney Int 1990; 37:1528–1535.

Yarger WE, Aynedjian HS, Bank N: A micropuncture study of postobstructive diuresis in the rat. J Clin Invest 1972; 51:625–637.

Yarger WE, Griffith LD: Intrarenal hemodynamics following chronic unilateral ureteral obstruction in the dog. Am J Physiol 1974; 227:816–826.

Yarger WE, Harris RH: Urinary tract obstruction. *In* Seldin DW, Giebisch G, eds: The Kidney: Physiology and Pathophysiology. New York, Raven Press, 1985, pp 1963–1978.

Yarger WE, Schocken DD, Harris RH: Obstructive nephropathy in the rat. J Clin Invest 1980; 65:400–412.

Yokoyama M, Yoshioka S, Iwata H, et al: Paradoxical tubular obstruction after release of ureteral obstruction in rat kidney. J Urol 1984; 132:388–391.

10
EXTRINSIC OBSTRUCTION OF THE URETER

Martin I. Resnick, M.D.
Elroy D. Kursh, M.D.

Extrinsic obstruction of the ureter is a common urologic problem in which the diagnosis may be difficult to establish. It is often associated with significant morbidity, and treatment may present a considerable challenge. On initial presentation, extrinsic or extraluminal obstruction must be differentiated from intrinsic or intraluminal obstruction. The clinician must have a thorough knowledge, not only of different disease processes that often have similar clinical presentations, but also of the available diagnostic procedures that can assist in establishing the appropriate site and cause of the obstruction. The causative process may be acute or chronic and unilateral or bilateral; both symptoms and therapeutic options will vary accordingly. **In most instances, extrinsic ureteral obstruction is a chronic unilateral process that can be managed in a non-emergent manner, but when bilateral obstruction occurs or if the patient is experiencing acute symptoms or has an associated urinary tract infection, rapid intervention is usually mandatory.**

The following section reviews the anatomic basis of obstruction, methods of evaluation, and options for therapy. Specific disorders are discussed in detail, with emphasis on clinical, diagnostic, and therapeutic options.

URETERAL ANATOMY

The ureter is a fibromuscular conduit that traverses the retroperitoneum for a length of approximately 25 cm. During its course from the renal pelvis to the urinary bladder, it is closely approximated to the retroperitoneal musculature posteriorly and multiple abdominal viscera anteriorly. Medial to the ureter are the aorta and inferior vena cava; during its course, it crosses multiple branches of these vessels. **In its retroperitoneal location, the ureter is associated with fat and lymph nodes throughout its course. Disease processes of all of these structures can affect the ureter, and extrinsic obstruction can result from compression and/or inflammation associated with a particular disorder.**

In contrast to anatomic points of narrowing of the ureter

that are important in considering points of intraluminal obstruction, particularly in relation to urolithiasis, areas of extrinsic obstruction are usually associated with the related or contiguous structures. For instance, aortic aneurysm with associated inflammation would result in deviation and obstruction of the midureter, whereas obstruction secondary to gynecologic malignancies usually involves the lower third. Disorders of the ileum typically involve the right ureter and sigmoid colon on the left. Other processes, particularly those originating in the retroperitoneum, such as lymphoma or retroperitoneal fibrosis, can affect various sections of the ureter, and the degree of involvement can be more variable.

PATIENT SYMPTOMS

Presenting symptoms are varied and depend not only on the acuteness or chronicity of the problem but on the cause as well. In most instances, extrinsic obstruction tends to be a unilateral, chronic, slowly developing process, and patient symptoms tend to be nonspecific or nonexistent. Mild flank discomfort, a vague feeling of fullness, or a generally nonspecific lethargy may be the only clinical sign of a problem. If acute obstruction occurs, patients usually experience more intense pain and, like patients with renal colic, may have nausea, vomiting, and other manifestations of acute ureteral obstruction. Symptoms associated with bilateral obstruction can also vary. In cases of chronic obstruction, patients may present with severe hydroureteronephrosis and symptoms secondary to azotemia rather than specifically related to the obstructing disorder.

With acute and bilateral obstruction, marked oliguria or anuria is usually the presenting complaint, but at times, the disorder causing the obstruction may be the predominant reason for which the patients seek medical care. For instance, pain associated with a leaking abdominal aortic aneurysm may cause more symptoms than the associated ureteral obstruction. Pain secondary to a diverticular abscess is another example of this phenomenon. Finally, acute changes, such as the development of infection in an already obstructed system, typically result in sepsis and severe systemic manifestations that necessitate rapid evaluation and intervention.

DIAGNOSTIC STUDIES

Many diagnostic studies, both laboratory and imaging, are available for a thorough assessment of the urinary tract. In many instances, the detection of ureteral obstruction becomes evident when a study is obtained for another reason. For example, the unexpected finding of azotemia resulting from bilateral obstruction necessitates further studies that are likely to result in the identification of the problem. Similarly, an imaging study (e.g., intravenous urogram or computed tomography [CT]) obtained for the assessment of a particular disorder or complaint may lead to the discovery of hydroureteronephrosis. Once the abnormality is identified, other and more appropriate studies are obtained.

Imaging Studies

Intravenous urography is useful not only in identifying the presence of ureteral obstruction but also, if appropriate delayed films are obtained, in determining the location of the obstruction as well. If the location is unclear or if intraluminal obstruction cannot be differentiated from extraluminal disease, retrograde pyeloureterograms are often helpful. Other diagnostic studies, such as ureteral catheterization, ureteral brushing and cytology, and ureteroscopy, are also very helpful, but they usually have more relevance in evaluating intraluminal disorders (e.g., stones and tumors).

Ultrasonography utilizes pulsed ultrasound waves to image various intra-abdominal structures, and it has proved to be a rapid, inexpensive, and accurate means of detecting hydronephrosis. The study usually has little value in precisely pinpointing the site of obstruction, but it may be useful in detecting its cause (e.g., retroperitoneal tumor or abscess). Therefore, ultrasonography's main role is often in screening to identify the presence of urinary obstruction; if it is present, other studies are then utilized. Ultrasonography is also a valuable aid during placement of nephrostomy or drainage tubes percutaneously.

CT with the use of intravenous contrast agents is probably the most common study utilized in the assessment of intra-abdominal disorders. Although not a practical screening procedure, CT often clearly delineates the point of obstruction. In addition, the study has added value in delineating retroperitoneal and intra-abdominal disorders that may be causing ureteral obstruction. As with ultrasonography, CT-guided percutaneous procedures can be used to drain an obstructed kidney and to perform a biopsy so as to establish a correct diagnosis.

Magnetic resonance imaging (MRI) is a relatively new imaging modality that measures changes in molecular energy. Although the study is very useful in assessing the central nervous and musculoskeletal systems, its value in imaging intra-abdominal structures is less dramatic. CT usually provides comparable information, at half the price. MRI does provide detailed imaging of the vascular system, and its value in this area is well recognized. In addition, MRI studies can provide physiologic information regarding renal blood flow and the functional status of the kidney. Despite its limited role in the assessment of extrinsic ureteral obstruction, it does have specific indications, particularly when associated with vascular disease that is believed to be the cause of the difficulty. **MRI also has the potential of differentiating fibrosis from malignant disease when the diagnosis is in doubt.**

Radionuclide imaging also has a limited role in the assessment of patients with extrinsic ureteral obstruction. Anatomic detail is limited with these studies, and much more meaningful information can be obtained with other imaging modalities. Radionuclide studies are of unique value in assessing renal function. Clinical decisions on appropriate treatment are based on useful information regarding renal function and renal reserve that is provided by these studies. Diuretic renograms are standardized studies that often provide critical information regarding not only the presence or absence of obstruction in association with a particular anatomic or imaging finding but also the severity of the problem. Other imaging studies may be used. Angiography and lymphangiography are at times invaluable in determining the presence of specific disorders. In addition, studies may be carried out to assess other organ systems that may be related to the ureteral obstruction (e.g., barium enemas and upper gastrointestinal series).

Some of the studies just described provide unique information, but it is emphasized that redundant details are often obtained from multiple diagnostic studies. The clinician should select those studies that are most appropriate and have the high likelihood of yielding useful information. If these concerns are practiced, cost is reduced and the efficiency of care enhanced.

Laboratory Studies

Certain laboratory studies are invaluable in the assessment of patients with ureteral obstruction. Renal function studies, such as serum creatinine and blood urea nitrogen (BUN), provide a rapid and accurate assessment of the severity of the problem and should be obtained in all patients. A complete blood count (CBC) and serum chemistries also are invaluable in assessing the overall status of the patient. Urinalysis and culture are important, particularly if infection is suspected and may be associated with the obstructed renal unit. Finally, such specific laboratory tests as prostatic specific antigen provide unique information regarding the disease processes either causing or associated with the obstructive process. As with imaging studies, laboratory studies should be obtained for specific reasons and at appropriate time intervals.

THERAPEUTIC OPTIONS

Like various diagnostic studies, many therapeutic procedures are available to manage patients with ureteral obstruction. **Treatment is often dependent on the clinical circumstances and can be nonexistent or limited.** Many would argue that an obstructed kidney in a patient with terminal malignancy requires no treatment provided that the contralateral kidney is functioning satisfactorily. Similarly, all would agree that a unilaterally obstructed but infected kidney in an obviously septic patient requires some drainage procedure. Drainage procedures may be palliative, such as percutaneous nephrostomy or stent placement, and others are therapeutic, such as an open surgical procedure or balloon dilation. Decisions regarding therapy are not only a matter of judgment but also dependent on the desire of the patient and family.

The placement of a ureteral stent is the oldest procedure available to urologists for the relief of upper tract obstruction. With the development of self-retaining stents commonly known as J stents, ureteral obstruction often can be easily and efficiently relieved. Difficulty in stent passage may be encountered when ureteral kinking or significant compression is present. Guide wires of varying composition have been developed primarily by angiographers, but they have proved invaluable to the urologic surgeon in managing some of these problems. **It is also important to remember that well-placed indwelling ureteral stents can be obstructing as well (Docimo and DeWolf, 1989).** This phenomenon is likely to occur in the presence of extrinsic ureteral obstruction; one report noted that 11 of 24 perforated silicone stents placed for extrinsic disease failed and that 9 of 22 perforated polyurethane stents also failed in the presence of extrinsic disease. In the latter group, five of the nine stents failed within 24 hours. The reasons for failure are speculative but are likely related to aperistaltic ureteral segments and ureteral compression against the stent, both interfering with urine drainage. The urologist must remember that the presence of the stent does not ensure proper drainage; if the patient is not responding accordingly, further evaluation must be undertaken and other methods of achieving drainage pursued.

Another method of obtaining renal drainage and relieving obstruction is the placement of a percutaneous nephrostomy. In years past, nephrostomy placement required an open operative procedure, but with new imaging techniques and development of special needles, guide wires, and catheters, direct renal drainage can be effectively obtained with local anesthesia.

The issue of whether to attempt retrograde catheter placement or to insert a percutaneous catheter is much debated. In most instances in which the procedure is being performed electively and the patient has a reasonable life expectancy, an indwelling ureter catheter is preferred. These patients experience minimal discomfort, and stents may remain in place for many months. If a ureteral stent cannot be placed, or in acute situations such as the presence of an infected hydronephrotic kidney, percutaneous drainage may be preferred. Larger drainage catheters can be placed and multiple catheters inserted if needed. In most instances, these procedures can be performed under ultrasound guidance with minimal patient discomfort. Indwelling stents can always be placed at a later date, either antegrade through the nephrostomy tract or in a retrograde manner. If satisfactory internal drainage is achieved, the nephrostomy catheter can then be removed.

Balloon dilation of the ureter is a natural result of endourologic procedures and techniques that have evolved over the past decade. The technique has had the most value in intrinsic obstruction of the ureter, particularly ureteroileal strictures, failed pyeloplasty, and a number of other postoperative conditions (Siegel et al, 1982; Banner et al, 1983; Finnerty et al, 1984). The technique is not as efficacious for dilation of strictures secondary to retroperitoneal fibrosis or strictures associated with gynecologic surgical procedures. Open surgical procedures are not infrequently utilized in definitively correcting extrinsic ureteral obstruction. Obviously, the type of procedure is dependent on the specific disorder, and repair of the ureter is frequently performed in association with a procedure directed at correcting the underlying problem.

There are multiple pathologic conditions that may be responsible for extrinsic obstruction of the ureter. Although extrinsic obstruction of the ureter is a relatively common finding, many of the disease entities that are responsible for this phenomenon obstruct the ureter uncommonly. The following classification was devised to allow patient evaluation to be accomplished in an orderly, methodic fashion. The causes of obstruction are divided into five major categories: (1) vascular lesions, (2) benign conditions of the female reproductive system, (3) diseases of the gastrointestinal tract, and (4) diseases of the retroperitoneum, including retroperitoneal masses. By attempting to place the cause of the ureteral obstruction under one of the five major headings, the urologist can proceed with the work-up in an organized manner and avoid overlooking a major area of consideration.

VASCULAR LESIONS

Arterial Obstruction

Abdominal Aortic Aneurysm

Ureteral obstruction secondary to an abdominal aortic aneurysm may be acute or chronic. In general, when the problem is of a long-standing nature, an aneurysm causes both ureters to deviate, usually pushing the left laterally and drawing the right medially. Because of its size and associated inflammation, a large aneurysm may produce mechanical ureteral obstruction either unilaterally or bilaterally. The scarring and inflammation associated with the aneurysm can also encase and obstruct the ureter.

There are two basic explanations for the development of perianeurysmic fibrosis and retroperitoneal scarring. One is that small leaks develop at the weakest points of the aneurysm. After these seal, a retroperitoneal inflammatory reaction ensues and results in scarring that may extend laterally to encase and subsequently obstruct the ureter. If this theory is true, the fibrous tissue should contain hemosiderin-laden macrophages, which have not been identified. **The second explanation relates to the generalized atherosclerotic process involved in the formation of the aneurysm.** Atherosclerosis often has an associated desmoplastic inflammatory component that extends to involve the adventitia of the scarring in the retroperitoneum (Abbott et al, 1973). The incidence of the association varies from 1% to 10% (Darke et al, 1977; Tracy et al, 1979).

Severe abdominal and low back pain of sudden onset is the symptom most often associated with an acute or dissecting abdominal aortic aneurysm. Patients may also complain of an abdominal mass, vague abdominal pain, and symptoms of peripheral vascular ischemia. **Because an aneurysm may affect the ureter in as many as 10% of cases, the urologist should be aware that these patients may seek care for urologic complaints, such as flank pain, urinary tract infections, and fever.** At times, these symptoms can mimic those secondary to ureteral colic. In rare instances, unexplained azotemia associated with partial or complete obstruction and hydronephrosis may be the presenting problem.

In general, the diagnosis of a suspected aneurysm can be easily made. A pulsatile abdominal mass is almost always palpable. In addition, the examiner may find an abdominal bruit or note the absence of femoral pulses. A plain film of the abdomen usually demonstrates a rim of calcium outlining one wall of the aneurysm. Cross-table and true lateral x-ray films help to delineate the size and position of the aneurysm. Excretory urography with lateral and oblique films establishes the presence of ureteral involvement (Fig. 10–1). Although lateral deviation of the left ureter is more common, medial displacement of the right may occur as well. At times, one ureter may be pushed laterally and the other drawn medially. It is also recognized that ultrasonography, in addition to imaging of the aneurysm, may identify unsuspected retroperitoneal fibrosis associated with aortic aneurysms. A characteristic picture with the fibrous tissue lying anterior and anterolateral has been described (Henry et al, 1978). Although this latter picture may not be demonstrated in all cases, it is clear that ultrasonography is a valuable technique in demonstrating both the aneurysm and the ureteral obstruction with resultant hydronephrosis.

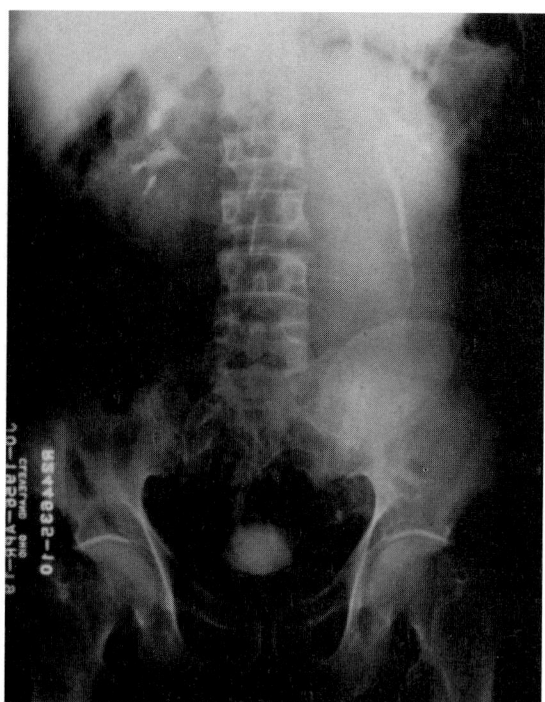

Figure 10–1. Marked deviation of the left ureter caused by a large abdominal aortic aneurysm. The lower pole of the left kidney is also pushed to the left. Note the rim of calcium outlining the left wall of the aneurysm.

If the obstruction is severe enough to compromise kidney function, the surgeon should consider re-establishing adequate drainage of the urinary tract before resecting the aneurysm. Restoration of the best possible renal function is important, because relative renal ischemia with oliguria may be a sequela of aneurysm surgery.

The treatment of choice of an inflammatory aneurysm with ureteral obstruction is aneurysmectomy with ureterolysis. The ureters are generally transplanted intraperitoneally or wrapped with retroperitoneal fat to prevent adherence to the residual inflammatory tissue or aneurysm wall. Care should be taken to preserve ureteral integrity when ureterolysis is performed. If urine from an obstructed, possibly infected kidney is spilled into the retroperitoneum, the hazard of aortic graft infection is increased. Because graft infection is a possible lethal complication of aneurysm surgery, some investigators have suggested that it is preferable to delay the aneurysm resection if a urine leak is suspected (Wagenknecht and Madsen, 1970). Others have advocated continuing with the repair (Spirnak et al, 1989). A possible but controversial alternative to operative ureterolysis in patients who could not tolerate or who refuse surgery is the administration of steroids, which has been shown to relieve ureteral obstruction in a small number of cases. Because spontaneous resolution is not uncommon, the true effect of steroids is difficult to discern (Huben and Schellhammer,

1981). Balloon dilation is another alternative in high-risk patients (Downey et al, 1987).

Iliac Artery Aneurysm

Aneurysms of the internal and common iliac arteries may in rare instances cause lower ureteral obstruction. The mechanism of obstruction is the same as that described for aortic aneurysm. Operative treatment of the aneurysm usually results in relief of the obstruction (Gohji et al, 1988) (Fig. 10–2). Ureteral obstruction has also been reported to occur in a normal iliac artery but with elevated pressure (Yetim and Sener, 1988).

Arterial Anomalies

On rare occasions, a normal vessel taking a normal course and position may cause compression of the ureter (Fig. 10–3).

There are also a number of vascular anomalies that may in rare instances cause ureteral obstruction. Although obstruction may occur at any level, it is more frequent in the lower third of the ureter. The normal vessels may be present but with aberrant courses, or they may be rudimentary embryonic arteries that fail to disappear. The obturator (Bush, 1972), renal (Fletcher and Lecky, 1971), and common iliac arteries (Mehl, 1969) have been reported to cause ureteral obstruction. Development anomalies, such as a persistent umbilical artery, also may cause obstruction of the ureter (Quattlebaum and Anderson, 1985). The use of simultaneous pyelography and angiography is essential in establishing the diagnosis. Occasionally, selective angiography of the branches of the aorta is needed to identify a small persistent embryonic vessel. Angiography done with a retrograde ureteral catheter in place is valuable in helping to demonstrate the point of obstruction. Treatment of a significantly obstructive vascular anomaly requires surgical exploration, at which time the surgeon must decide whether to resect the ureter or the offending vessel. All that is required when dealing with a rudimentary vessel are simple ligation and transection of the artery. The surgeon must ensure that ureteral damage has not occurred, because repair of the ureter may be required as well (e.g., ureteral reimplantation).

Obstruction Phenomena Due to Arterial Repair and Replacement

Reconstructive vascular surgery is being performed with increasing frequency in the aged population for the treatment of peripheral and aortic vascular degenerative disease. **Ureteral obstruction is a recognized complication of these procedures but has a varied incidence. Several reports have shown mild or moderate permanent ureteral ob-**

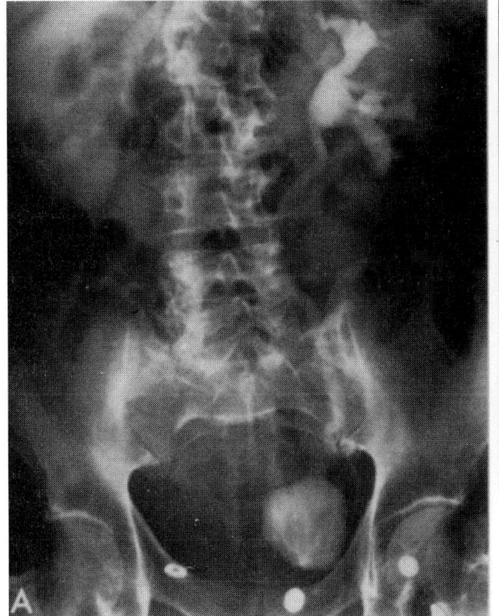

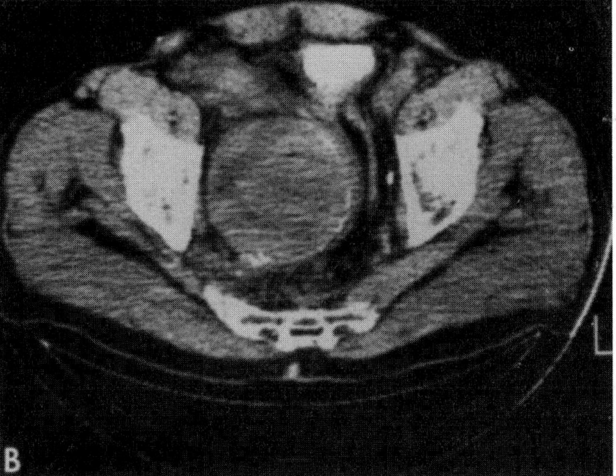

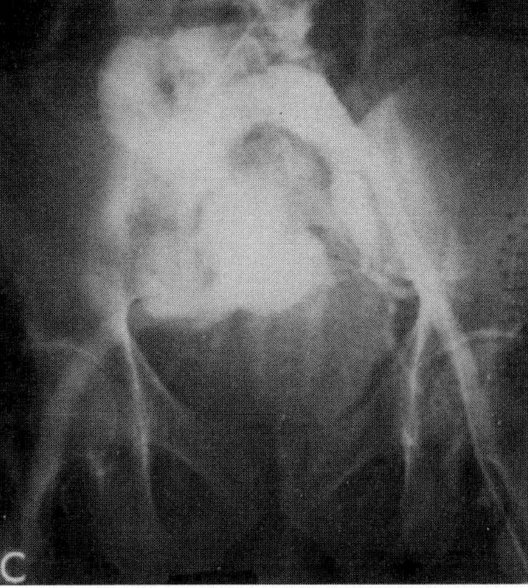

Figure 10–2. Right ureteral obstruction secondary to an aneurysm of the right hypogastric artery. *A,* Intravenous urogram demonstrating delayed visualization of right kidney and marked deviation of urinary bladder. *B,* CT scan demonstrating large aneurysm. Note calcification of wall. *C,* Arteriogram demonstrating extent of aneurysm.

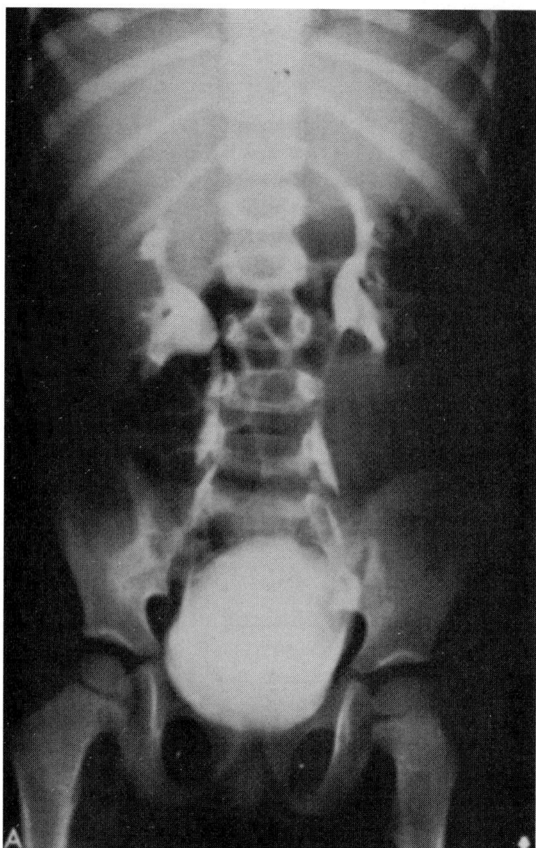

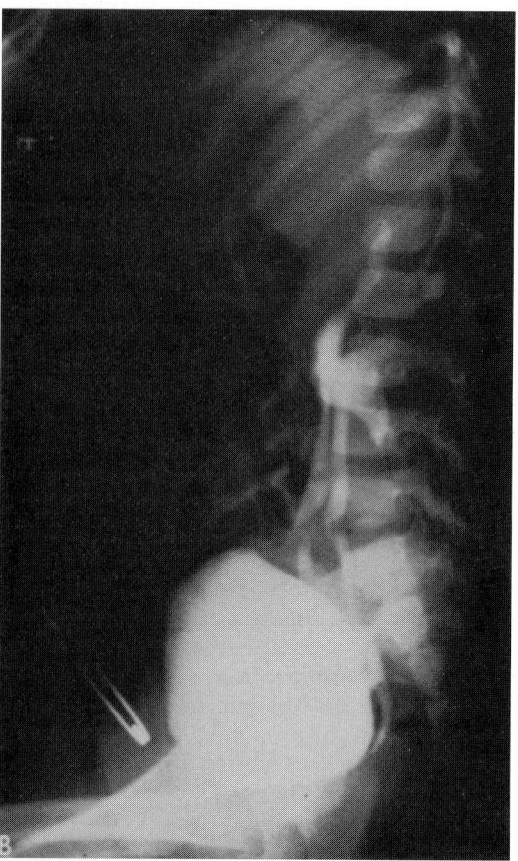

Figure 10–3. *A,* Bilateral compression of the ureters as they course over the bifurcation of the common iliac arteries in a young boy. Although there is mild dilation of the upper ureters, the pelvocalyceal systems are normal. *B,* A lateral x-ray demonstrating the posterior relationship of the offending vessels.

struction in 2% to 14% of patients, and others have noted a 12% to 30% incidence of temporary and asymptomatic hydronephrosis (Goldenberg et al, 1988). Retroperitoneal fibrosis secondary to the surgical procedure is the most common cause of ureteral obstruction. It is likely secondary to bleeding or excessive dissection and resultant fibrosis, but other causes include direct surgical injury (ligation, ischemia), pseudoaneurysm formation, and compression from an anteriorly placed graft (Sant et al, 1983). **Most patients present within 1 year after the vascular procedure, but delays up to 14 years have been reported. It is also of interest that, when evaluated, 13% of the reported patients were free of symptoms, and 30% presented with nonurologic symptoms. Symptoms have included pain, infection, azotemia, and hematuria.**

Treatment of these patients varies on the basis of the patient's symptoms and the surgeon's experience. When repair is contemplated, exact identification of the level of obstruction is essential (Fig. 10–4). Ureterolysis is the most common repair instituted and can be performed with or without intraperitonealization. Ureteral resection and ureteroureterostomy and division and reanastomosis of the vascular graft are less frequently performed reparative procedures.

Venous Obstruction

Ovarian Vein Syndrome

The ovarian veins are formed by multiple, small pelvic venous channels similar to the pampiniform plexus in the male. Joined by uterine branches, the multiple veins fuse to form a single ovarian vein before crossing the pelvic brim. As the ovarian veins course over the iliac vessels, they lie only ½ inch anterior to the ureter in its midportion, crossing it to join the inferior vena cava at the level of the third lumbar vertebra. On the left, the ovarian vein also crosses the ureter to enter the left renal vein. These anatomic relationships make the ovarian veins a potential cause of ureteral obstruction. **The obstruction usually involves only the right ureter, except for conditions that cause stasis in the left renal vein with resultant enlargement of the left ovarian vein, such as encasement by carcinoma or thrombosis.**

Dure-Smith (1979) presented a convincing argument that the ovarian vein syndrome is a myth. It is questionable whether the ovarian veins have ever produced a significant obstruction at any level or whether from theoretical considerations they would ever be expected to do so.

Supposedly, the patient with ovarian vein syndrome usually notes the onset of symptoms during pregnancy and is multiparous, although the entity has been reported in women who have never been pregnant. Patients may also develop symptoms several months to years after pregnancy; not infrequently, the symptoms are worse during menses. The symptoms associated with recurrent urinary tract infections may also represent the presenting complaints. Most patients experience right-sided flank pain, which is generally described as a constant ache but may mimic renal colic. The pain may begin several days before menses and disappear afterward.

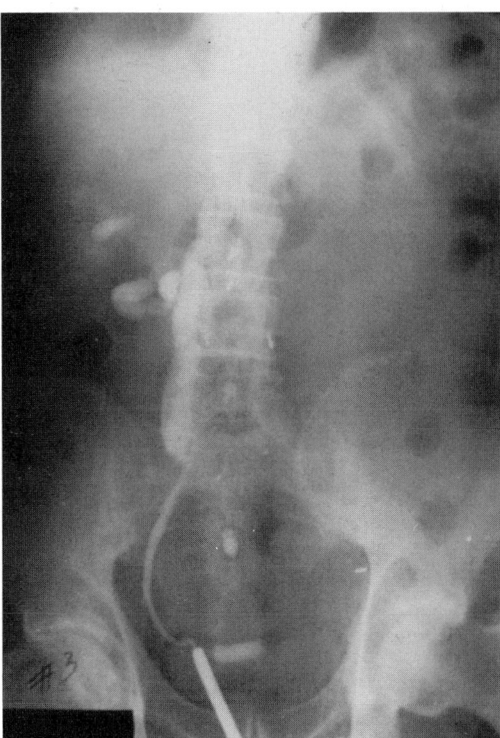
Figure 10–4. Right ureteral obstruction secondary to a vascular graft bypassing the right iliac vessels. Patient presented 2 years after surgery with complaints of dull but persistent right flank pain.

Excretory urography, retrograde pyelography, and simultaneous angiography are utilized to establish the diagnosis. **The obstruction most commonly occurs at the level of the third or fourth lumbar vertebra, where the ovarian vein crosses the ureter (Fig. 10–5).** Operative treatment consists of mobilization of the ureter with ligation of the offending ovarian vein. At the time of surgery, a dilated ovarian vein or network of veins can be seen associated with the ureter at the point of obstruction, and at times both structures are enveloped in a common fibrotic process. It has been emphasized that it is important to lyse the ureter well into its pelvic position to make certain that multiple areas of obstruction caused by a single large ovarian vein or plexus of veins are not overlooked.

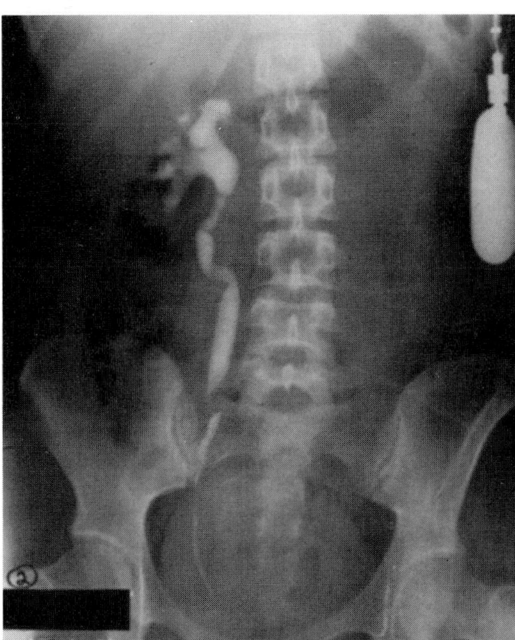
Figure 10–5. A right hydronephrosis extends to the area of the bifurcation of the common iliac artery. In the past, these were thought to be consistent with ovarian vein syndrome.

It is doubtful that the ovarian vein syndrome exists. The ureteral dilation that is supposedly characteristic of the ovarian vein syndrome is identical to the dilation that occurs during pregnancy. These changes may persist as unobstructed dilation postpartum (Dure-Smith, 1979). Experimental and clinical studies have demonstrated that engorged ovarian veins are not associated with ureteral obstruction of pregnancy (Kauppila et al, 1972). Experience has also revealed that many venous anomalies can result in similar clinical and radiographic findings in both men and women (Kretkowski and Shah, 1977).

Postpartum Ovarian Vein Thrombophlebitis

Ovarian vein syndrome should be differentiated from postpartum ovarian vein thrombophlebitis (Dure-Smith, 1979). **Postpartum thrombosis of the ovarian veins had been thought to be an infrequent phenomenon, but more recent evidence indicates that the incidence may be 1 in 600 deliveries.** The entity also has been termed *puerperal septic pelvic vein thrombophlebitis.* It is more common in multiparous women, and a right-sided predominance has been observed. Ten percent of the reported cases are bilateral, and isolated left-sided cases are rare. Patients usually present in the immediate postpartum period with fever, lower abdominal pain, a palpable pelvic mass, and marked leukocytosis.

The etiology of the disease has been ascribed to a variety of coagulation defects that are not uncommonly associated with pregnancy and the immediate postpartum period and that lead to a hypercoagulable state. Ureteral obstruction is not uncommon and results from extension of the inflammatory process to the periureteral tissues.

Postpartum ovarian vein thrombophlebitis is potentially lethal, and pulmonary emboli may originate from the ovarian vein with a thrombus extending into the inferior vena cava (Angell and Knuppel, 1984). Associated thrombosis of the renal vein also has been reported (Bahnson et al, 1985).

The diagnosis can be established with ultrasonography, CT, or MRI (Angell and Knuppel, 1984; Baran and Frisch, 1987). The entity has been misdiagnosed as acute pyelonephritis and acute appendicitis.

The principal differential diagnosis includes thrombosis of an adnexal mass, broad ligament hematoma with abscess formation, appendicitis, and perinephric abscess. Theoretically, treatment by anticoagulation therapy alone may suffice but thus far has been used only as an adjunct to surgery. Operative treatment has consisted of ligation of both ovarian veins and usually extirpation of the veins. Ligation of the inferior vena cava has been undertaken and is considered to be mandatory in suppurative pelvic thrombophlebitis or in the presence of pulmonary embolization.

Retrocaval (Circumcaval) Ureter

The retrocaval ureter is a congenital abnormality in which the right ureter passes behind the inferior vena cava, leading to varying degrees of ureteral compression. It was first reported by Hochstetter in 1893. The etiology of the syndrome relates to the embryologic development of the ureter. The metanephros develops in the pelvis and rises through a ring of embryonic venous channels as it moves to a lumbar position. The major venous channels in the very young embryo are the posterior cardinal veins. The minor venous channels, the subcardinal veins, are connected to the postcardinal veins by numerous prominent anastomotic vessels. The supracardinal veins, which generally develop into the inferior vena cava, become apparent in the 15-mm embryo dorsal to the developing ureters. The posterior cardinal veins and the subcardinal veins lie ventral to the definitive ureteral position. Normally, the posterior cardinal vein undergoes complete regression caudal to the renal vein, allowing the ureter to assume a normal position ventral to the developing infrarenal inferior vena cava (supracardinal vein). The subcardinal vein remains as a tributary of the inferior vena cava, the gonadal vein. **Persistence of the posterior cardinal vein as the major portion of the infrarenal inferior vena cava causes medial displacement and compression of the ureter after the lateral migration of the kidney.** The ureter spirals from a dorsolateral position above to a ventromedial position below around the developing inferior vena cava. Variants of the condition include duplication of the vena cava with the ureter lying beside, behind, or between the vascular limbs. The anomaly develops almost exclusively on the right side except in patients with situs inversus.

The onset of symptoms usually occurs during the fourth decade of life, with men predominating by a ratio of 3:1. Most patients complain of right lumbar pain, which is usually described as a dull intermittent ache but may resemble renal colic. Patients may have associated recurrent urinary tract infections or episodes suggesting recurrent acute right pyelonephritis. Symptoms actually may be attributable to calculi, the incidence of which is increased owing to stasis. Microscopic or gross hematuria is frequently present.

The diagnosis is made by demonstrating the characteristic changes on excretory urography. Typically, the diagnosis is established during imaging studies carried out to investigate the cause of the patient's symptoms. The ureter makes a typical reversed J deformity as it passes from the pelvis under the inferior vena cava at the third or fourth lumbar vertebra. A varying degree of hydronephrosis is noted proximal to the obstruction. A right oblique x-ray film demonstrates the close relationship of the right upper ureter to the inferior vena cava. Retrograde pyelography may show the tortuous ureter to be in the shape of an italic S, beginning just above the pelvic brim and ending below the renal pelvis (Fig. 10–6), but it may not be possible to pass a ureteral catheter beyond the postcaval segment. These findings, coupled with the confirmation of the position of the ureter on an inferior venacavogram, are sufficient to make the diagnosis. It is often helpful to confirm the circumcaval route of the ureter by performing inferior venacavography with a ureteral catheter in place. Ultrasonography and CT scanning are also of value in establishing the diagnosis. Radionuclide imaging is useful to assess the degree of obstruction and functional impairment of the kidney.

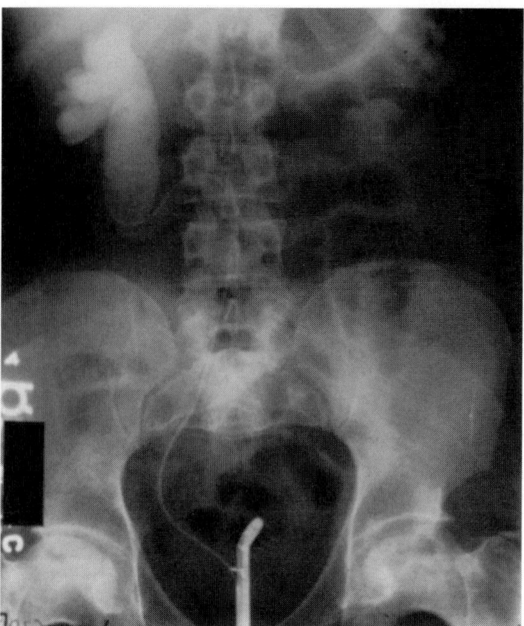

Figure 10–6. Retrograde urography showing the typical reversed-J deformity secondary to a retrocaval ureter. The retrograde catheter takes the shape of an italic S beginning just above the pelvic brim.

Two types of retrocaval ureters have been described (Bateson and Atkinson, 1969) and are to be distinguished from the entity in which only a loop or knuckle of ureter passes behind the inferior vena cava but re-emerges laterally (Talner, 1990). **Type I ("low loop") is the most common, and the dilated proximal ureter assumes a reverse J.** The dilation usually persists 1 to 2 cm past the lateral margin of the inferior vena cava, at which point it turns upward. Possibly a ureteral kink, an adynamic segment, or pressure from the psoas muscle is contributing to the obstruction (Kumar and Bhandari, 1985). The nondilated distal ureter emerges medially, crosses the right iliac vessel anteriorly, and enters the pelvis and bladder in a normal manner.

Type II ("high loop") is rarer and goes behind the ureter at the level of or just above the ureteropelvic junction. The condition can be confused with ureteropelvic junction obstruction. It has been suggested that this latter entity be termed *retrocaval ureter* and that the term *circumcaval ureter* be used to describe the condition in which the ureter crosses behind the inferior vena cava and re-emerges medially.

No therapy other than observation is indicated for patients without symptoms and with minimal or no caliectasis. Occasionally, nephrectomy is the procedure of choice in the presence of marked hydronephrosis and cortical atrophy if the contralateral kidney is normal. Surgery is required for the treatment of the hydronephrosis or related symptomatic problems. Harrill (1940) initially emphasized that the position of the ureter and involved structures makes transection of the pelvis with transposition and reanastomosis the most efficacious surgical treatment. The operation, therefore, is essentially a dismembered pyeloplasty. A transabdominal-transperitoneal operative approach is preferred because of the ease of access to the vital structures, should the need to reach them arise. Considine (1966) suggested that the Harrill procedure should be more appropriately called the caudal division of the dilated segment, because the original ureteropelvic junction is often obliterated by the dilation of the proximal ureter. The performance of the anastomosis as far distal on the dilated segment as possible has the advantage of preserving the blood supply of this segment, which comes from the renal artery. At times, severe adhesions make lysis of the ureter from the inferior vena cava impossible. In this situation, the compressed segment is resected and left in situ. The ureter is then anastomosed to the proximal dilated segment anterior to the inferior vena cava. The retrocaval segment may be scarred and strictured, and a No. 6 to No. 8 French catheter should be routinely passed at the time of repair to test its patency. In all situations, an anastomosis as wide as feasible should be performed. Transection with reanastomosis of the inferior vena cava also has been done, but it is generally not recommended.

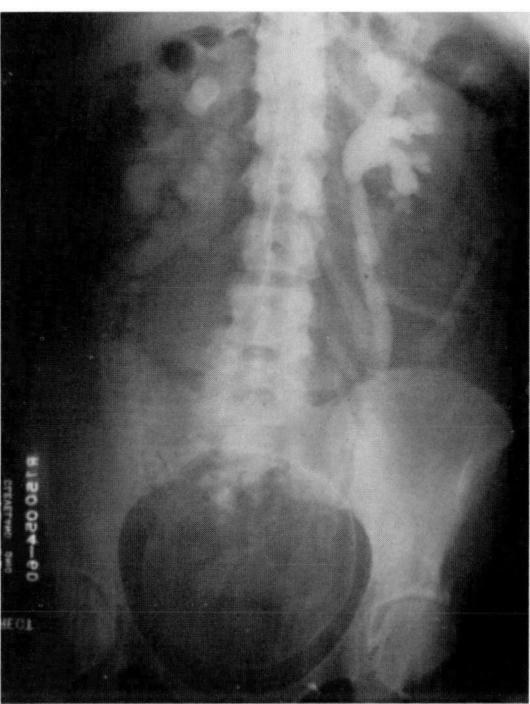

Figure 10–7. Bilateral hydronephrosis resulting from a gravid uterus during the third trimester. After delivery, the hydronephrosis resolved.

BENIGN CONDITIONS OF THE FEMALE REPRODUCTIVE SYSTEM

Benign Pelvic Masses

Pregnancy

Approximately 150 years have passed since Cruveilhier documented that pregnancy can deleteriously obstruct the upper urinary tract. Imaging studies, including intravenous urography and ultrasonography, have documented the dilation of the upper tract in most pregnancies (Cietak and Newton, 1985). **Experience has demonstrated that unilateral or bilateral obstruction occurs by the third trimester in 90% to 95% of asymptomatic pregnant women and that in more than 80% of patients, right-sided hydroureteronephrosis predominates.** Below the pelvic brim the ureters are typically normal, and the dilation usually resolves within weeks after delivery. The degree of obstruction may even be severe enough to cause acute renal failure (Eika and Skajaa, 1988).

The cause of ureteral obstruction during pregnancy is thought to be primarily mechanical compression from the gravid uterus. Right ureteral obstruction is more common than left. One explanation for the increased incidence of right ureteral obstruction in pregnancy is the protection of the left ureter by the interposed sigmoid colon between the ureter and the uterus. Another explanation is related to the asymmetry of the anatomic structures at the pelvic brim, particularly the iliac arteries, making the right ureter more prominent and susceptible to compression. Although rare, bilateral obstruction may also occur (Fig. 10–7) (D'Elia et al, 1982). Other evidence supporting the obstruction theory includes the demonstration of elevated ureteral pressures in the dilated system, the observation of right hydronephrosis being present in association with pelvic masses in nonpregnant females, and the absence of ureteral dilation in pelvic kidneys in which the ureter does not cross the pelvic brim (Erickson et al, 1979).

Several investigators have implicated progesterone and gonadotropins as a cause of ureter stasis and obstruction during pregnancy (Guyer and Delany, 1970). There is laboratory evidence that a large dose of progesterone decreases ureteral peristalsis, but there is no clear-cut evidence that physiologic levels of the hormone have a significant effect on the genitourinary system. In addition, hydroureter has not been observed in the first trimester, before the uterus is large enough to compress the ureter (Dure-Smith, 1979).

The symptoms of ureteral obstruction during pregnancy may be masked by the physiologic changes associated with pregnancy itself. Nausea; pain in the back, flank, and lower abdomen; dysuria; and frequency may be associated with either ureteral obstruction or pregnancy. Progression of symptoms and/or localization to the flank suggests the possibility of significant ureteral obstruction, particularly if there is an associated fever or urinary tract infection. If urine cultures show a persistent urinary tract infection despite appropriate antibiotic therapy, or if the patient has severe flank pain, further evaluation is required. **Because use of ionizing radiation in the pregnant patient is problematic, ultrasonography is the preferred method of determining the presence of ureteral obstruction, and radioisotope renography is a simple, safe means of estimating excretory function.** During the first trimester, renography usually shows normal findings; over the ensuing months, there is a progressive increase in dilation of the urinary tract and a delay in excretion.

If a patient's condition is refractory to medical management, such as antibiotic regimens or analgesics, drainage of the ureter with double-J stents may be necessary. Antimicrobial therapy until the pregnancy is completed is a consideration for patients with significant obstruction and recurrent infections. Post partum, a complete urologic investigation should be undertaken.

Extrauterine Pregnancy

Ureteral obstruction secondary to chronic ectopic pregnancy has been reported but is apparently an extremely rare occurrence. Although ectopic pregnancy is a common problem, occurring in approximately 1 in every 1000 gravid women, chronic ectopic pregnancy is very rare. Ureteral obstruction occurs from the pressure effect of the pelvic mass in association with periureteral fibrosis (Hovatanakul et al, 1971). Bilateral obstruction secondary to a ruptured ectopic pregnancy also has been noted (Cummings, 1988).

Mass Lesions of the Uterus and Ovary

Benign pelvic masses, such as uterine fibroids and ovarian cysts and fibromas, may cause deviation and extrinsic obstruction of the ureter. Uterine fibroids are the most common of these benign tumors to result in extramural ureteral obstruction. Ureteral obstruction secondary to hydrometrocolpos also has been reported. **Years ago, the reported incidence of ureteral involvement due to benign pelvic masses was as high as 50% to 65%. Although the incidence may be less today, it is generally known that ureteral obstruction is a frequent finding with benign masses of the uterus and ovary.** The incidence increases as the size of the mass enlarges, especially if it projects above the pelvic brim.

Because of the frequency of upper urinary tract involvement, excretory urography is an important part of the evaluation of all patients with pelvic masses. Alternatively, ultrasonography and CT not only are valuable in determining the presence of ureteral obstruction and associated hydronephrosis but also provide information regarding the size, shape, and consistency of the mass.

The most common site of obstruction is at the point where the ureter crosses the iliac vessels. Uterine fibroids most commonly affect the right side, but they may cause deviation or obstruction of the left ureter or both ureters (Fig. 10–8). As discussed in the earlier section on pregnancy, **the right ureter is involved more often because of the increased prominence of the right ureter as it crosses the right iliac artery and the protective effect of the interposition of the sigmoid colon between the uterus and the left ureter.** In general, the ureters are deviated laterally. Ovarian cysts, which may push the ureter in a lateral or medial direction, affect the ureters less often. The ureteral obstruction and hydronephrosis are generally relieved after treatment with pelvic laparotomy and excision of the mass.

Ovarian Remnants

Although a rare occurrence, several cases of obstruction of the pelvic ureter secondary to ovarian remnants have been reported. Normally, removal of an entire ovary is a simple procedure. If the ovary and adjacent structures are involved in an extensive disease process that distorts the anatomic relationships and makes the surgical dissection difficult, implantation of a portion of the ovary into the exposed retroperitoneum may occur (Zaitoon, 1987). The functioning ovarian remnant in the retroperitoneum may liberate an ovum. Rupture of an ovarian follicle is thought to be partially dependent on the enzymatic activity of the liquor

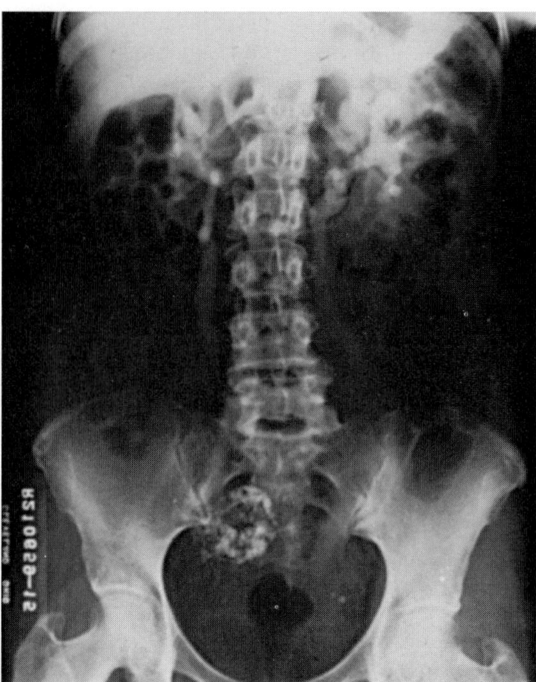

Figure 10–8. Bilateral hydronephrosis secondary to a large calcified fibroid uterus. After a hysterectomy, the upper urinary tracts returned to normal.

folliculi. Possibly, retroperitoneal reaction to the liquor folliculi with associated fibrosis is responsible for the extrinsic ureteral obstruction (Horowitz and Elguezabal, 1966).

Because the establishment of ureteral obstruction may depend on the liberation of an ovum, flank pain of a cyclic nature may be noted. This, in addition to a history of a previous difficult oophorectomy, suggests a possible diagnosis of an ovarian remnant. The diagnosis is confirmed at surgery if a cystic retroperitoneal mass is found. Surgical treatment consists of removal of the mass, along with ureterolysis.

Gartner's Duct Cyst

A Gartner's duct cyst may displace the distal ureter and thus represent a theoretical cause of ureteral obstruction. The wolffian duct drains the original embryonic pronephros and, later, the mesonephros. After the ureters have budded from its distal end, the wolffian duct atrophies in the female. The atrophic wolffian duct is known as Gartner's duct, a vestigial structure extending down the anterolateral margin of the vagina. Incomplete obliteration of the canal with subsequent epithelial secretory activity may lead to the development of retention cysts.

The diagnosis is deduced from the location of the cyst on the anterolateral wall of the vagina, usually near the upper end. No treatment is required for small asymptomatic cysts. Large cysts may protrude through the introitus and may cause local discomfort, dyspareunia, infertility, or dystocia. Transvaginal excision is the treatment for large symptomatic cysts. In rare instances, a large Gartner's duct cyst may displace the distal ureter upward over the cyst wall. If this occurs, an abdominal approach has been recommended to provide improved exposure of the ureter, because the cysts tend to be adherent to the bladder wall.

Pelvic Inflammations

Tubo-Ovarian Abscess and Inflammation

A patient with a tubo-ovarian abscess usually has a history of acute or chronic pelvic inflammatory disease (PID), although occasionally an abscess may develop secondary to the use of an intrauterine device. Inflammation alone can cause ureteral obstruction, and parametritis secondary to an intrauterine device has been reported to cause ureteral obstruction. Hydroureteronephrosis is frequently found in association with tubo-ovarian abscesses. Phillips (1974) reported ureteral dilation and obstruction in 17 of 45 patients with this disorder, and other investigators have described ureteral obstruction with an incidence approaching 40%.

Abdominal pain, fever, nausea, and vomiting are the common presenting symptoms, although tubo-ovarian abscess has been reported in patients who complain of vaginal bleeding alone. The physical examination usually elicits bilateral lower abdominal pain with signs of peritoneal irritation. Pelvic examination reveals a tender adnexal mass or bilateral masses. At times, there may be a purulent exudate from the cervical os.

On roentgenologic examination, the presence of extraluminal pelvic air suggests the diagnosis of an abscess. Because of the high incidence of ureteral obstruction and the risk of iatrogenic ureteral injury at the time of surgery, excretory urography or ultrasonography should be done routinely in a patient with a tubo-ovarian abscess. The ureteral blockage usually occurs at or below the pelvic brim, and in about half of patients, the obstruction is bilateral. The ureter is deviated laterally in most patients, but in approximately one third, medial deviation is found. It is believed that the location of an abscess in the posterior cul-de-sac is responsible for the medial displacement. In this location, the abscess expands in an anterior direction, pushing the ureter medially. The inflammation and fibrosis associated with the abscess also function to pull the ureter medially or laterally.

Treatment of the tubo-ovarian abscess generally consists of total abdominal hysterectomy with bilateral salpingo-oophorectomy. Aggressive surgery is recommended before the abscess perforates intraperitoneally. Although the likelihood of subsequent conception is small, a lesser procedure such as a unilateral salpingo-oophorectomy may be attempted in younger patients who wish to have children. This suboptimal form of surgical therapy mandates careful postoperative follow-up. The deviated ureter increases the risk of ureteral injury, making the preoperative placement of ureteral catheters advisable. Treatment of the abscess generally results in resolution of the ureteral obstruction.

Endometriosis

Endometriosis is a prevalent problem in premenopausal women and occurs in as many as 10% to 20%, with a peak age incidence between 25 and 40 years. The disease is best described as the existence of normal endometrium in an ectopic location. Ureteral obstruction from either an extrinsic or an intrinsic endometrioma is rare, but the urologist and gynecologist must be aware of the possibility of ureteral involvement because of the high rate of unsalvageable kidneys that results from this process (Fig. 10–9). **A variable incidence of urinary tract involvement (ureter and bladder) of up to 24% among women afflicted with endometriosis has been reported** (Williams, 1975).

Involvement of the ureter is much less frequent than that of the bladder; one large series reported only 15 of 151 patients with urinary endometriosis (Abeshouse and Abeshouse, 1960). In another report, only 9 of 77 cases of urinary endometriosis represented ureteral involvement (Williams, 1975). Unilateral involvement is approximately 10 times as common as bilateral involvement (Davis and Schiff, 1988). When the ureter is involved, the process is usually confined to the pelvic ureter. Two types of ureteral involvement have been described: intrinsic and extrinsic. With intrinsic involvement, endometriosis involves the ureteral wall, and the process can extend into the ureteral lumen. Extrinsic involvement results from scarring, fibrosis, and dense adhesions associated with the endometrioma and accounts for 75% to 85% of the reported cases (Al Saleh, 1987).

The symptoms associated with the condition often reflect the organs involved as well as the primary disease process itself. Patients complain of severe dysmenorrhea caused by sloughing of the proliferative endometrium during menstruation. The pain and discomfort abate during pregnancy or when the patients are taking progestational agents that block ovulation and menstruation. When ureteral obstruction is present, symptoms range from mild flank pain to urosepsis and renal failure, but in most instances, urologic signs or symptoms are so subtle that they go unnoticed. Although intrinsic endometriomas of the ureter are rarer than extrinsic lesions, they are more likely to cause cyclic hematuria. Only a minority of patients with ureteral involvement experience hematuria.

The diagnosis of endometriosis is established on the basis of history and pelvic examination. The finding of an adherent ovary or small, indurated, irregular, firm, and tender nodularities in the cul-de-sac or uterosacral ligaments is diagnostic of endometriosis. Because most reported cases have had a paucity of symptoms referable to the urinary tract, the diagnosis of ureteral involvement is difficult to establish unless there is a high index of suspicion. Consequently, when obstruction occurs, a nonvisualizing or severely hydronephrotic kidney is frequently encountered on the excretory urogram (see Fig. 10–9). The routine use of excretory urography and/or ultrasonography in patients with pelvic endometriosis is recommended in an attempt to diagnose ureteral obstruction at an earlier and more salvageable stage. Because the obstruction is often silent, significant renal damage may be present.

The radiographic findings in endometriosis of the ureter are nonspecific, at times resembling stricture or tumor of the pelvic ureter. Retrograde pyelography is helpful in delineating the lower ureter. In general, it is impossible to pass a ureteral catheter beyond the obstruction, located most frequently 3 to 4 cm above the ureteral orifice. In rare instances, a filling defect caused by the endometrioma is identified.

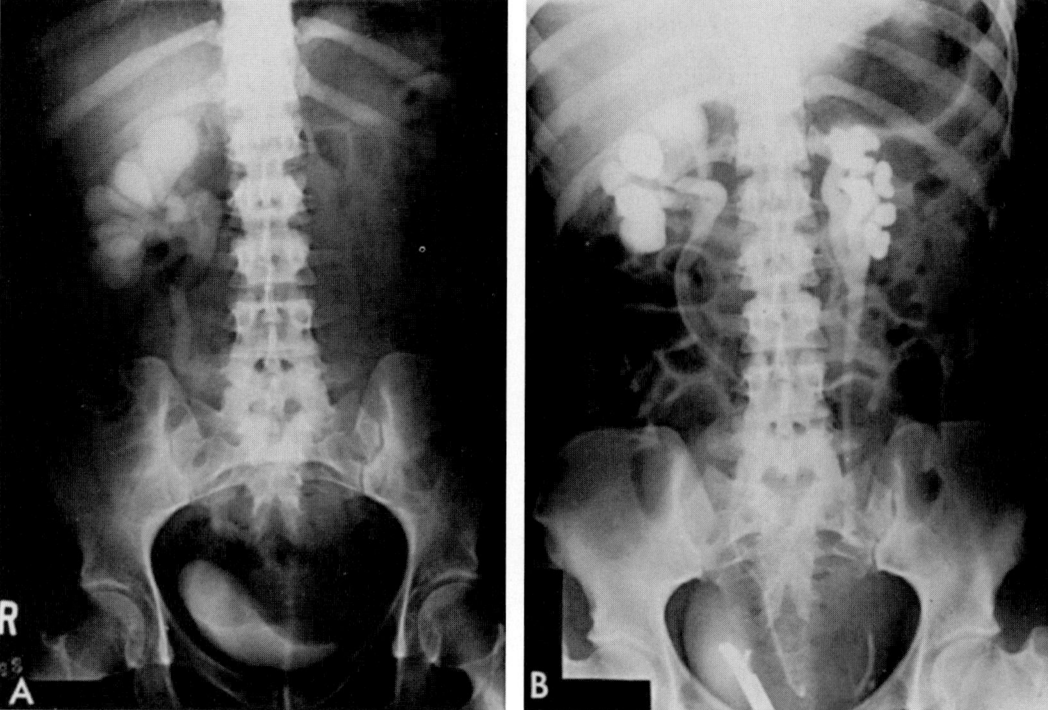

Figure 10–9. *A,* Excretory urogram revealing severe right hydroureteronephrosis and no apparent function of the right kidney in a patient with extensive endometriosis. *B,* Retrograde urography demonstrating obstruction of distal ureters. A right ureteroneocystostomy, total abdominal hysterectomy, and bilateral salpingo-oophorectomy were performed.

Laparoscopy is a diagnostic study that is being used with increasing frequency. At pelvic laparotomy, the presence of the so-called chocolate cyst, which is an ovary filled with old retained blood, alerts the surgeon to the presence of endometriosis.

Hormone therapy with estrogen-progestin combinations or danazol, a testosterone analogue, relieves the primary symptoms associated with endometriosis but only occasionally relieves the ureteral obstruction (Rivlin et al, 1985). Although there have been scattered reports of partial success with nonoperative therapy, this mode of treatment is not recommended, because the ureteral obstruction is secondary to the dense adhesions associated with the endometriosis.

The scarring and inflammatory reaction associated with the disease also make surgical correction of this problem difficult and hazardous. The procedure of choice for patients with severe ureteral obstruction and for women who do not desire further pregnancies is bilateral oophorectomy, total abdominal hysterectomy, and ureterolysis. A lesser procedure may be attempted if the ureteral obstruction is not too severe and the patient wishes to bear more children. The area of involvement dictates the extent of the surgery. Extensive ovarian involvement generally necessitates a unilateral oophorectomy, with meticulous dissection, removal of the endometrioma, and ureterolysis. When a more conservative operative procedure is utilized, careful follow-up is required to ensure relief of the ureteral obstruction and to ensure that the problem does not recur. During ureterolysis, careful inspection of the ureter may demonstrate associated fibrosis and stricture secondary to ureteral involvement by the endometrioma. In these instances, ureterolysis is not sufficient, and partial ureterectomy must be done with ureteroureterostomy (25%). **Nephrectomy is necessary in those patients with severe hydronephrosis, particularly if there is associated sepsis, the rate of which has been reported to vary from 13% to 44%** (Moore et al, 1979).

Ureteral obstruction by extrinsic endometriosis also has been reported in a postmenopausal patient. The administration of conjugated estrogens to the nulliparous patient, who had undergone a previous panhysterectomy, apparently played an etiologic role. The ureteral obstruction was relieved after the hormones were discontinued (Brooks et al, 1969).

Periureteral Inflammation Associated with Contraception

Contraception has become a worldwide concern during the past few decades. Utilization of the intrauterine device (IUD) has led to a number of complications, the most important being infection, perforation, and bleeding. There has been a report of ureteral obstruction secondary to parametritis resulting from long-term use of the IUD. The incidence of PID associated with the IUD is approximately 1.0% to 1.5%. Also, the urologist and gynecologist should consider parametritis associated with the IUD in the differential diagnosis of ureteral obstruction. Treatment with broad-spectrum antibiotics, coupled with removal of the IUD, has led to resolution of both the parametritis and the ureteral obstruction.

A number of cases of ureteral injury associated with laparoscopic tubal ligation have been reported (Grainger et al, 1990). A case of ureteral injury resulting in ureteral obstruction and extravasation of urine secondary to the use of the laparoscope for tubal sterilization is presented in

Figure 10–10. It is thought that during sterilization, ureteral injury is likely a result of the cautery forceps' touching the pelvic side wall while the current is applied. Therefore, it is essential to grasp the tube in the bipolar forceps and move it away from the side wall before applying current. It is erroneous to assume that bipolar coagulation is safe, because five of the reported ureteral injuries occurred during use of this method (Grainger et al, 1990).

Uterine Prolapse

The association of uterine prolapse and ureteral obstruction was first reported in 1923 by Brettauer and Rubin. **The incidence of hydronephrosis associated with uterine prolapse is in the vicinity of 5%; however, hydroureteronephrosis occurs in as many as 30% to 40% of patients with severe uterine prolapse** (Kontogeorgos et al, 1985). In a group of 18 patients with prolapse, 10 had urinary tract infections; 10, severe hydronephrosis; 2, mild hydronephrosis; and 6, normal upper tracts (Jones and Evison, 1977). Older patients are more frequently affected, and bilateral obstruction is more common.

Although the mechanism is not clearly understood, there are several proposed explanations for the ureteral obstruction in these women with procidentia. Obstruction of the urethra secondary to the prolapse has been ruled out as a possible cause, because large residual volumes have not been found. A bowstring effect caused by intramural stretching of the ureter has been considered as a possible cause of obstruction, but radiographic and autopsy studies have failed to demonstrate the occurrence of such a phenomenon. The most reasonable explanation is the compression of the ureters outside the bladder.

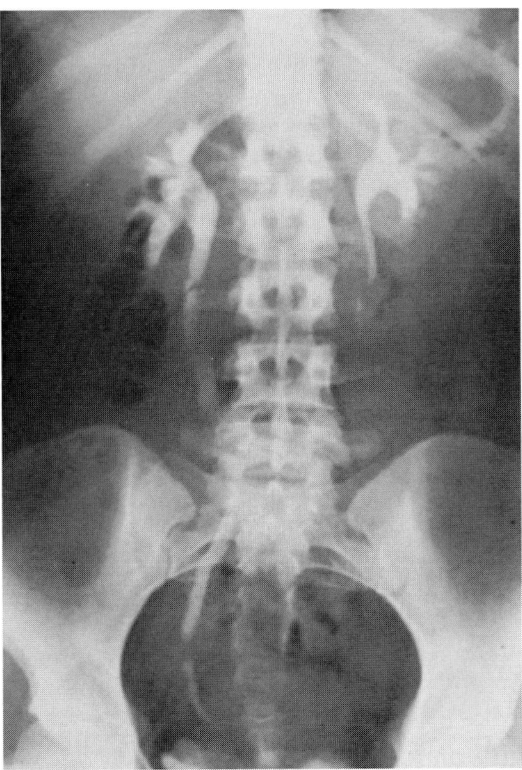

Figure 10–10. Obstruction of short segment of the distal right ureter after laparoscopic sterilization. This obstruction probably resulted from excessive coagulation of the fallopian tube stumps lying against the posterior peritoneum, adjacent to the ureter.

As the bladder, uterus, and ureters are herniated through the weakness in the levator ani muscles, the ureters may be compressed between the fundus of the uterus and the bladder, which is compressed against the levators. Compression by the lateral cervical ligaments of Mackenrodt has also been implicated (Chapman, 1975). The branches of the uterine arteries that cross in front of the distal ureters or the branches of the uterine vessels that form a vascular plexus surrounding the ureters may represent possible points of obstruction by acting as a sling over and around the ureter as the vessels are stretched from the procidentia. Excretory urography and autopsy examination have suggested that the point of obstruction is in the vicinity of the uterine vessels, making the second explanation plausible; however, because it has not been confirmed by pelvic arteriography, this etiology has been discarded. Compression of the ureters against the inferior pubic ramus also has been reported.

Urinary infection, sepsis, pyonephrosis, and renal insufficiency all have been reported to be associated with uterine prolapse. Despite this and the high incidence of hydroureteronephrosis associated with uterine prolapse, urologic investigation is frequently not obtained preoperatively or postoperatively. In one review, excretory urography was done in fewer than 40% of patients with uterine prolapse admitted to a large university medical center (Lattimer, 1974). Both the gynecologist and the urologist must be aware of the need for the routine use of excretory urography or ultrasonography in the evaluation of patients with uterine prolapse. Evaluation is particularly indicated in patients with severe prolapse because of the higher incidence of ureteral obstruction in this group.

Surgical repair of the prolapse by means of a vaginal hysterectomy and vaginoplasty is the preferred therapy. If operative therapy cannot be undertaken, a pessary may be used to reduce the uterine prolapse in an attempt to diminish the ureteral obstruction.

Ureteral Ligation and Intraoperative Injury

Ligation of the ureter is a form of extrinsic obstruction of the ureter that occurs iatrogenically. Because more than 50% of the cases develop during gynecologic procedures, ureteral ligation is included in this section. Ureteral obstruction not only can occur secondary to ligation but also can result from crushing, kinking, laceration, devitalization, and transection. **The incidence of ureteral injury in routine hysterectomy varies from 0.5% to 3%, but, alarmingly, when it occurs it is bilateral in approximately one of every six cases** (Donovan and Ragibson, 1973).

The incidence of injury is much higher after radical hysterectomy and has been reported to vary from 10% to 15% (Whitehouse, 1977). In addition, because of the extensive ureteral dissection often performed during these procedures, ureteral ischemia not infrequently occurs with resultant postoperative hydroureteronephrosis. If tissue necrosis occurs, urinary extravasation, stricture, and fistula formation may result. Ureteral obstruction may result from extrinsic compression by lymphocele that can occur after extensive pelvic dissections; it is most common after radical hysterectomy and cystectomy, renal transplantation, and pelvic lymph node dissection. Extrinsic obstruction and resultant stricture can also form as a result of the urinoma. Ureteral obstruction has been reported to occur after urethropexy for treatment of urinary incontinence (Applegate et al, 1987). In these instances, sutures placed in the region of the bladder neck inadvertently pass through the bladder wall and underlying ureteral orifice. **Although far less often than in gynecologic operations, ureteral ligation may occur during general surgical procedures, such as vascular procedures, orthopedic surgery, neurosurgical (herniated disc) procedures, or colorectal surgery, or during a difficult retrocecal appendectomy.** Ureteral obstruction also has been reported after procedures for correction of scoliosis and placement of a vena caval clip (Wrenn and Assimos, 1988).

After it descends into the true pelvis, the ureter lies in intimate proximity to the female genital organs, making it subject to injury. The ureter is dorsal to the ovary, lateral to the infundibulopelvic ligament, and medial to the ovarian vessels. It enters the broad ligament approximately 9 or 10 cm below the iliac vessels and travels along the lateral aspect of the uterus. It then crosses the vesicovaginal space (¾ inch lateral to the uterine cervix), above the lateral fornix of the vagina. Here it is in intimate proximity to the uterine artery, which crosses above and in front, close to the ureterovesical junction. Most commonly, the ureter is damaged (1) in the ovarian fossa, during excision of large tumors or cysts; (2) in the infundibulopelvic ligament, when this is taken during hysterectomy; (3) where the ureter crosses dorsal to the uterine artery, as the artery is ligated and divided; and (4) in the vesicovaginal space, during the process of reperitonealization (Persky and Hoch, 1972).

Obviously, the best treatment for intraoperative ureteral injury is prophylaxis. In patients with pelvic masses, PID, previous injury adjacent to the ureter, and previous irradiation therapy, preoperative urography is indicated to ascertain the course of the ureter and the presence of ureteral obstruction. It is also advisable to obtain an excretory urogram before surgery if a difficult dissection is anticipated in the vicinity of the ureter. The immediate preoperative placement of ureteral catheters (stents) is helpful if the surgeon expects to encounter difficulty adjacent to the ureter. If catheters are employed, they should be No. 5 or 6 French in size, because smaller catheters are difficult to palpate and larger ones may cause appreciable mucosal edema. The surgeon must not rely on the catheters for more than guidance in determining the presence of the ureter near the field of dissection. They do not prevent ureteral injury; only meticulous dissection in the area of the ureter can avoid such injury.

When the surgeon recognizes that the ureter has been included in a ligature during an operation, the suture should be removed immediately and the injured area inspected. In most instances, nothing further is required. If the ureter appears nonviable, the area is resected and a primary anastomosis performed or, if the injury is sufficiently close to the bladder, a ureteroneocystostomy is done.

In most instances, unfortunately, ureteral ligation is not discovered until the postoperative period. Interestingly, most patients are asymptomatic. If the patient develops flank pain, unexplained fever, leukocytosis, a paralytic ileus, or anuria, excretory urography is indicated. Retrograde pyelography is also helpful in delineating the point of obstruction. The passage of a retrograde catheter may be of therapeutic value if the obstruction is incomplete, as occurs when the ureter is kinked. If a catheter can negotiate the blocked area, further therapy is usually not required. Placement of a percutaneous nephrostomy is an excellent temporizing procedure, but most patients need surgical relief of the obstruction. Formerly, a staged procedure with initial urinary diversion, such as a nephrostomy, was advised before the point of obstruction was repaired. This approach was based on the degree of anatomic distortion, the anticipated inflammatory response, and the threat of hemorrhage in the early postoperative period in the area of the ligated ureter. Reports of the successful early use of the direct approach in such procedures as ureteral deligation or ureteroneocystostomy to relieve the obstruction indicate that the staged procedure is usually no longer required. Preliminary diversion is still advised if a marked inflammatory response or a large hematoma is anticipated in the area of the ligated ureter or if the patient is septic or a poor candidate for surgery. Today, percutaneous techniques are generally used to perform the nephrostomy. A suggested algorithm for patient evaluation and treatment is detailed in Figure 10–11.

Not only do ureteral injuries result from laparoscopic tubal ligation, but injuries are also being reported with the increasing use of the laparoscope for diagnosis and therapeutic modalities. In 1990, Grainger and associates summarized the eight previous reported cases of laparoscopic ureteral injury and presented five additional cases. The indications for laparoscopy were sterilization (four), endometriosis (five), adhesion (two), diagnosis (one), and ureterosacral ligament transection (one). Electrocoagulation was used in each instance of ureteral injury except for a trocar injury in the patient undergoing diagnostic laparoscopy (Grainger et al, 1990).

Grainger and associates emphasize that the ureters cannot be reliably identified in the vicinity of the ureterosacral ligaments, particularly in the presence of diseases such as endometriosis. Thickened nodular ureterosacral ligaments should alert the surgeon to potential distortions of normal anatomy of the ureter. The proximity of the ureter to the cervix is also implicated because this area is difficult to visualize (Grainger et al, 1990).

In the early postoperative period, the common presenting symptoms are abdominal pain with peritonitis, leukocytosis, and fever. As in other forms of ureteral injury, passage of a ureteral stent may lead to resolution of extravasation with ureteral healing, but any of the other options already discussed may be used. Unfortunately, nephrectomy was required in two of the reported cases owing to pyelonephritis and persistent obstruction after treatment (Grainger et al, 1990).

DISEASES OF THE GASTROINTESTINAL TRACT

Granulomatous (Crohn's) Disease of the Bowel

The association of ureteral obstruction and Crohn's disease was first reported in 1943 (Hyams et al, 1943). Other

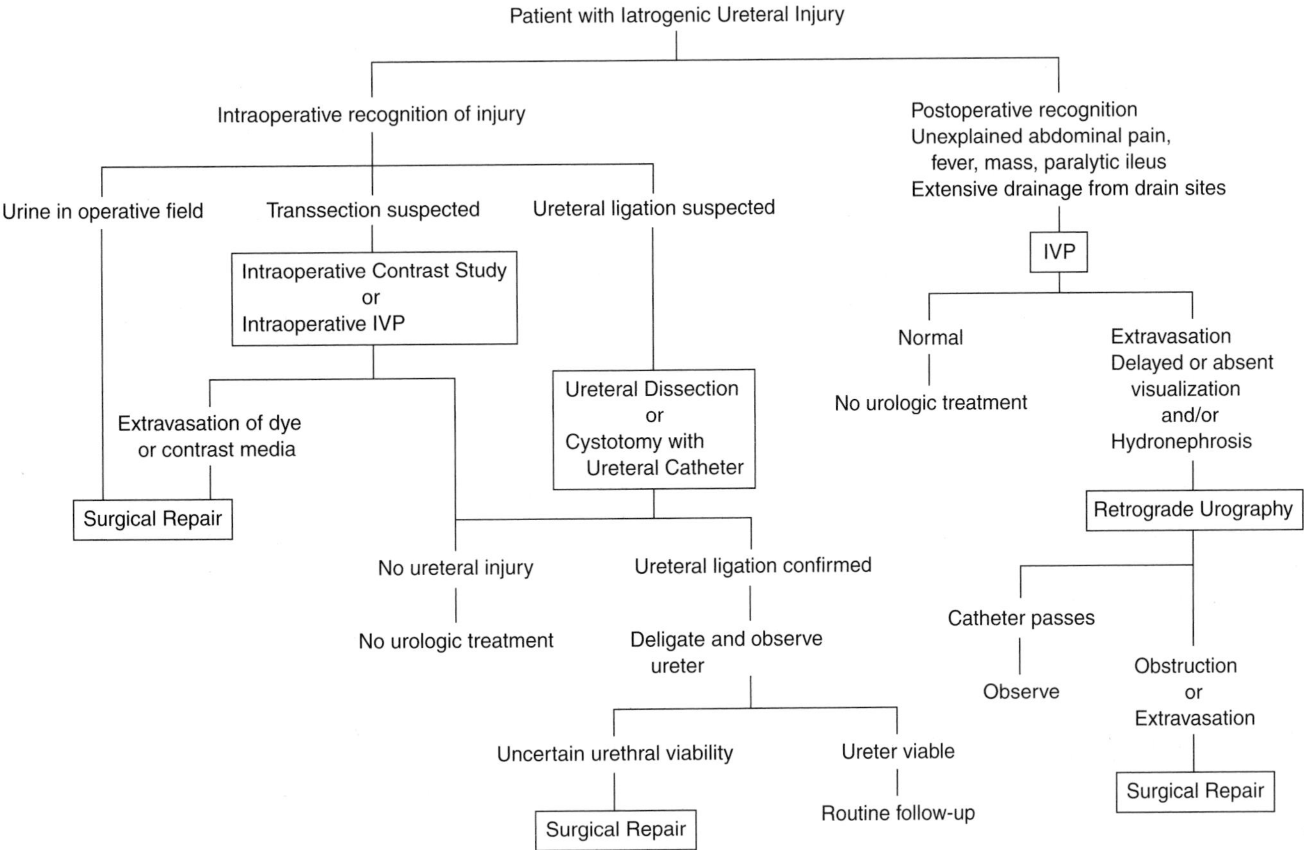

Figure 10–11. Evaluation of patient with iatrogenic ureteral injury. IVP, intravenous urography.

urologic complications of granulomatous disease of the bowel include uric acid calculi, fistulas to the bladder, and the nephrotic syndrome secondary to renal amyloidosis. **Although the reported incidence varies from 0.3% to 50%, the true incidence probably is in the range of 5% to 20%** (Schofield et al, 1968). This discrepancy is likely due to the high incidence of complicated cases of the disease referred to large medical centers. Using radioactive renography as a more sensitive index of ureteral stasis, Schofield and associates (1968) found stasis in 50% of the patients with regional enteritis.

Extrinsic compression of the ureter appears to be caused by the retroperitoneal extension of the severe inflammatory process. The periureteral fibrosis may result from the conveyance of the inflammation from the intestine and mesentery to the retroperitoneum via the lymphatics. Microintestinal perforation with accompanying inflammatory change, with or without retroperitoneal fistula and abscess, is another possible cause of ureteral obstruction. **Because the predominant area of involvement is the terminal ileum, the proximity of the latter to the right retroperitoneum is responsible for the occurrence of extrinsic ureteral compression on the right side in most reported cases.** There have been cases of left ureteral involvement, one of which was related to significant granulomatous disease of the colon (Siminovitch and Fazio, 1980). Bilateral ureteral obstruction also has been noted (Schofield et al, 1968).

Histologic examination of the periureteral fibrotic tissue reveals pseudomyomatous changes with stellate cell formation similar to that seen in liposarcoma. The ureteral mucosa is not involved in the process, and transmural strictures do not occur. Special stains have demonstrated collagen fibers with diffuse edema.

There has been a relatively equal distribution between the sexes, and most patients with ureteral obstruction have been young, with an average age in the mid-20s. The patients almost always have significant gastrointestinal symptoms for a protracted period of time (more than 6 months). It is noteworthy that the majority of patients have no symptoms referable to the urinary tract. Occasionally, a patient may experience frequency or dysuria. Pyuria and laboratory confirmation of a urinary tract infection have been infrequent findings. Present and associates (1963) made special note of the occurrence of pain in the hip, the anterior aspect of the thigh, or the flank, which often resulted in difficulty in walking or bending the hip joint. Many patients have fever, but costovertebral angle tenderness is an uncommon finding. A mass may be palpable, occurring primarily in the right lower quadrant.

Moderate anemia and elevation of both the erythrocyte sedimentation rate and the white cell count are often present. Sigmoidoscopy may reveal evidence of disease, and barium studies show such typical changes as stricture and fistulization, located primarily in the terminal ileum. Because most patients do not experience symptoms referable to the urinary tract, the diagnosis of ureteral obstruction is often an incidental finding when the patient is being evaluated for other reasons. Excretory urography or ultrasonography confirms the presence of ureteral obstruction (Fig. 10–12). **Obstruction occurs almost exclusively in the distal right ureter,**

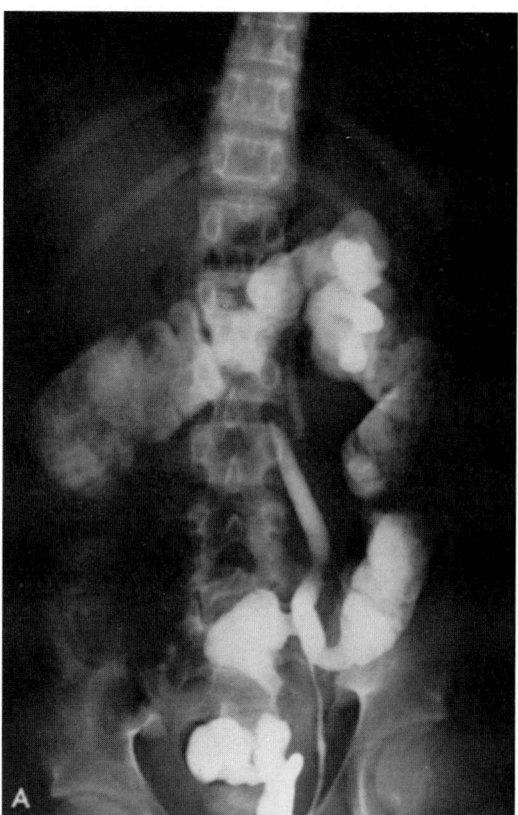

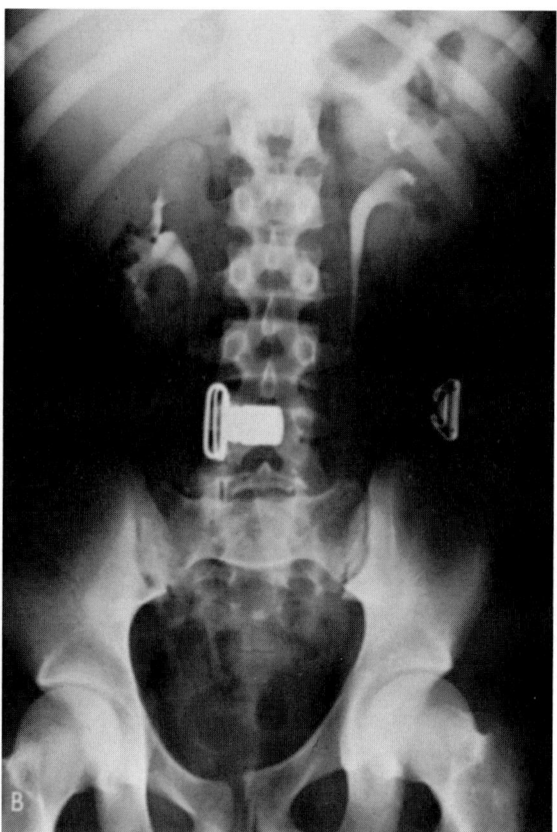

Figure 10–12. *A,* Left ureteral obstruction caused by granulomatous colitis of the sigmoid colon. A long segment of the distal ureter appears to be stenotic on this retrograde pyelogram. Residual barium from a barium enema demonstrates the inflamed sigmoid colon. This case differs from most cases of ureteral obstruction secondary to granulomatous bowel disease, in that the obstruction is on the left side. *B,* Excretory urography 6 months after resection of the diseased bowel and ureterolysis, showing complete resolution of the ureteral obstruction.

usually at the level of the pelvic brim, and results in various degrees of hydroureteronephrosis. In the early stages of obstruction, the ureter takes a normal, relatively straight, downward course, whereas in long-standing obstruction, the ureter becomes tortuous and deviated medially. The extrinsic periureteral process generally causes symmetric tapering of the ureter. **Because ureteral obstruction is generally occult, excretory urography or ultrasonography is essential to the thorough evaluation of all patients with significant involvement of the bowel by Crohn's disease, especially those with ileocecal Crohn's disease or an abdominal mass.**

The primary method of treatment for severe complicated granulomatous bowel disease is surgery. Although diversion of the involved intestinal segment was formerly a frequent procedure, intestinal resection has become the principal form of definitive palliative surgical therapy. Ureteral obstruction is a complication of advanced inflammatory bowel disease that constitutes an indication for surgery. **When ureteral obstruction accompanies granulomatous bowel disease, therapy generally has been directed toward the bowel disease without any attempts made to relieve the ureter.** Experience has indicated that in most instances, ureteral obstruction resolves after bowel resection and/or abscess drainage.

Persistent obstruction is usually secondary to the presence of severe periureteral fibrosis and nearly 30% of patients treated by the above means have failed to improve or have suffered significant renal loss. Siminovitch and Fazio (1980) concluded in a review of 45 patients with ureteral obstruction secondary to Crohn's disease that ureterolysis is rarely indicated. Intestinal resection or staging procedures for complicated Crohn's disease were usually effective in resolving associated obstructive uropathy. It has also been reported that ureteral obstruction resolves with medical therapy alone without any surgical intervention. Accordingly, it appears that ureterolysis is rarely required to relieve hydroureteronephrosis secondary to Crohn's disease but is indicated if there is severe associated retroperitoneal fibrosis with encasement of the ureter. If ureterolysis is contemplated, it is advisable to insert a ureteral catheter (stent) before surgery.

Inflammatory Disease of the Appendix

Appendicitis, appendiceal abscess, and peritonitis can cause hydroureter and hydronephrosis without evidence of mechanical obstruction (Jones and Barie, 1988; Aronson et al, 1994). There is a reported case of a child who developed azotemia and hydronephrosis necessitating bilateral nephrostomy after an appendectomy for an intact inflamed appendix. Izant and associates (1974) described three cases of hydroureteronephrosis in children with peritonitis. Although the mechanism is unclear, the obstruction subsided as the peritonitis resolved.

Appendiceal abscesses may cause both urinary tract symptoms and ureteral obstruction, primarily in the pediatric age group. The incidence of upper urinary tract obstruction secondary to an appendiceal abscess in the adult is not known, but the condition does occur and may be more frequent than is recognized. The diagnosis of appendiceal abscess is often very difficult to establish in the pediatric patient. Dysuria and urinary frequency may occur in children 1 to 2 weeks after the onset of other gastrointestinal symptoms, such as nausea, vomiting, anorexia, diarrhea, and abdominal pain. Urinary retention also has been reported. In addition, patients have experienced ureteral colic and spontaneous urinary extravasation. An abdominal mass is almost always palpable. A scout film of the abdomen often shows a soft tissue shadow obliterating the right psoas margin, with displacement of the bowel gas to the left. Occasionally, a fecalith may be noted in the region of the appendix. Abdominal ultrasonography and CT are usual techniques in determining the extent of the abscess. A barium enema usually shows displacement of the rectum and irregularity of the cecum. The obstruction characteristically occurs on the right side at the level of the pelvic brim but may be left-sided or bilateral. The hydronephrosis resolves after surgical drainage of the abscess.

In rare instances, mucocele of the appendix also has been found to be responsible for extrinsic obstruction of the ureter (Carroll and Laughton, 1973). This entity is usually associated with a postinflammatory appendiceal stricture, carcinoma of the appendix, or carcinoma of the cecum. A case of left ureteral obstruction secondary to a granulomatous mass that developed after appendicitis also has been reported. It was believed that the antibiotic treatment of gonococcal urethritis masked the symptoms of acute appendicitis, leading to the development of a chronic granulomatous mass.

Diverticulitis

Diverticulitis is the most frequent complication of diverticulosis, a condition that affects approximately 5% of the population. The cause of diverticulosis is unclear. A combination of factors, including diet, muscular hypertrophy, and neuromuscular dysfunction of the colon, has been implicated. Diverticulitis results when diverticula are plugged with colonic contents, leading to the establishment of an inflammatory reaction. The disease, which occurs primarily in older patients, is rarely seen in primitive and underdeveloped countries.

Urologic complications are found in approximately 20% of patients with diverticulitis; the most frequent is colovesical fistula. Although rare, there have been reports of ureteral obstruction occurring secondary to diverticulitis (Kubota et al, 1988). The left ureter is involved more often than the right.

The probable mechanism of obstruction is the extension of an inflammatory process from the retroperitoneal perforation of diverticulitis, resulting in a retroperitoneal abscess. The combination of ureteral obstruction and a colon lesion favors the diagnosis of malignancy, especially if there is a palpable mass, but diverticulitis should be considered in the differential diagnosis. It has been suggested that a higher incidence of ureteral obstruction would be noted in association with diverticulitis if more patients were evaluated for this possibility. Accordingly, excretory urography or ultrasonography should be done before surgery to evaluate the upper tracts, to minimize the risk of ureteral injury, and to facilitate planning of the operation. CT is also helpful in assessing the extent of disease. Placement of ureteral catheters is advisable at the time of surgical resection, especially if there is obstructive uropathy. Treatment of the ureteral obstruction associated with diverticulitis consists of treatment of the primary disease. The presence of an inflammatory diverticular mass requires a bowel resection that may be a part of a one-, two-, or three-stage procedure.

Pancreatic Lesions

It is well known that pancreatic lesions occasionally produce changes in the kidney that may be confused with intrinsic renal lesions. Almost all of the lesions have been in the left kidney because of the proximity to the tail of the pancreas. CT studies have shown that 3% of patients with acute pancreatitis have mild right proximal ureteral obstruction (Talner, 1990). Reports have detailed the association of acute inflammatory processes with both unilateral and bilateral obstruction as well (Stone et al, 1989). A pancreatic pseudocyst in rare instances may extend laterally into the perinephric space to displace the kidney or ureter and represent a cause of unilateral or bilateral ureteral obstruction. Also, there have been several reports of ureteral obstruction's being secondary to extension and metastasis from carcinoma of the pancreas.

DISEASES OF THE RETROPERITONEUM

Retroperitoneal Fibrosis

Idiopathic

The noted French urologist Albarran is responsible for the earliest description of retroperitoneal fibrosis (1905), but it was not until Ormond's account, first published in the English literature in 1948, that this disease became an established clinical entity. Ormond reported two patients who presented with anuria, backache, malaise, and anemia associated with retroperitoneal perivascular inflammation. A variety of terms have been used to designate this disease, including periureteritis fibrosa, periureteritis plastica, chronic periureteritis, sclerosing retroperitoneal granuloma, and fibrous retroperitonitis. In the 1960s, the disease became known as retroperitoneal fibrosis, because this term more closely describes the actual nature of the cellular response and the extent of involvement. Accordingly, to avoid confusion, the other terms should no longer be used to refer to this lesion.

Because there is now a greater awareness of this entity, the diagnosis of retroperitoneal fibrosis is being established with increasing frequency. In 1967, Utz and Moghaddam reported 56 cases of retroperitoneal fibrosis in a 6-year period at the Mayo Clinic. More recently, Lepor and Walsh (1979) provided a review of 70 cases. The disease occurs in both sexes and has been reported in an age range extending from 7 to 85 years, with a predominance in the fifth to sixth decades of life. Experience has also indicated that the process is often a generalized one and can involve a variety of anatomic structures and sites, including the mediastinum.

Pathology

On gross examination, retroperitoneal fibrosis appears as an exuberant mass of tan to white, woody, fibrous tissue covering the retroperitoneal structures. The process covers the aorta, inferior vena cava, ureters, and psoas muscles and may extend from the renal pedicle to below the pelvic brim. The center of the plaque is generally located at the level of the fourth or fifth lumbar vertebra, overlying the aortic bifurcation. It is not uncommon for the fibrous tissue to bifurcate and follow the common iliac arteries. In rare instances, the fibrous process may extend into the root of the mesentery or may pass through the crura of the diaphragm to continue as fibrous mediastinitis. An association with sclerosing cholangitis also has been noted in several cases.

The fibrous process envelops the ureter, tending to drag the middle third of the ureter toward the midline in half to two thirds of patients. Fibrous encasement of the ureters eventually leads to hydronephrosis and varying degrees of renal failure. Although there is generally extensive involvement overlying the great vessels, significant arterial obstruction is rare. Venous obstruction is more common, apparently because of the greater compressibility of the thin-walled veins. Obstruction of the inferior vena cava or common iliac veins may cause edema of the lower extremities (Abdel-Dayem et al, 1984; Rhee et al, 1994). Extrahepatic portal vein obstruction has also been reported (Gatanaga et al, 1994). In the past, it was believed that the fibrous tissue enveloped but did not invade the retroperitoneal structures. Reports have emphasized the occasional invasion of the psoas muscles and the ureters by the fibrous process (Heller and Teggatz, 1992). The process may be so hard and extensive that it closely resembles malignant tissue.

On histologic examination, the predominant finding is fibrous tissue consisting of collagen fibrils and fibroblasts. A subacute nonspecific inflammatory reaction is often present, or there may be only complete hyalinized fibrosis. The cellular infiltrate includes polymorphonuclear cells, lymphocytes, eosinophils, or plasma cells. In the more chronic phase of the process, the only finding may be an acellular fibrosis. A necrotizing arteritis has also been observed.

Etiology

In most instances, no etiologic factor is found in patients with retroperitoneal fibrosis (Table 10–1) (Witten, 1990). Hence, the term *idiopathic retroperitoneal fibrosis* is truly applicable. Evidence from the 1980s suggests that this unusual disease is an allergic reaction to insoluble lipid that has leaked through a thinned arterial wall from atheromatous plaques (Bullock, 1988). Some patients with chronic periaortitis have been found to have circulation antibodies to ceroid, and there is a possibility that these antibodies may be used in the future as markers of the activity of the disease (Mitchinson, 1982). **Other reported causes of retroperitoneal fibrosis include hemorrhage, urinary extravasation, trauma, perianeurysmal inflammation, radiation therapy, surgery, inflammatory bowel disease, collagen disease, and fat necrosis.** These are discussed in appropriate sections in this chapter.

Table 10–1. RETROPERITONEAL FIBROSIS: ASSOCIATED FINDINGS IN 491 PATIENTS

Findings	Percent
Idiopathic	67.8
Methysergide	12.4
All malignancies	7.9
Mediastinal fibrosis	3.3
Periaortic inflammation: arteritis	2.4
Mesenteric fibrosis	2.0
Sclerosing cholangitis	1.6
Abdominal aortic aneurysm	1.6
Crohn's disease	1.2
Thrombophlebitis	1.0
Riedel's thyroiditis	0.8
Other	5.3

From Kep L, Zuidema GD: Surgery 1977; 81:250.

There is overwhelming evidence that prolonged use of the drug methysergide (Sansert) for the treatment of migraine headaches is occasionally responsible for retroperitoneal fibrosis. Graham initially noted the occurrence of retroperitoneal fibrosis in patients taking methysergide (Graham, 1964) and later reported a 1% incidence in a large number of patients taking this drug (Graham et al, 1966). Since that time, a number of other authors have noted a causal relationship between methysergide therapy and retroperitoneal fibrosis. Other organ systems are also prone to fibrosis with methysergide treatment, including the heart, lungs, pleura, great vessels, and gastrointestinal tract. Another ergot derivative, lysergic acid diethylamide (LSD), and methyldopa (Aldomet), amphetamines, and phenacetin have been implicated as possible causes of retroperitoneal fibrosis (Iversen et al, 1975). Other medications have been implicated as well (Herzog et al, 1989; Malaquin et al, 1989).

The method by which ergot compounds cause retroperitoneal fibrosis is ill defined. Methysergide and LSD have similar chemical structures and belong to a class of semisynthetic derivatives of ergot alkaloids that are serotonin antagonists, acting by competitive inhibition of receptor sites. Methysergide and LSD therefore cause increased amounts of endogenous serotonin. Elevated serotonin levels have been associated with the fibrosis noted in carcinoid syndrome (Scott et al, 1987). An important relationship between increased serotonin and fibrosis has not been confirmed in the laboratory. The most widely accepted theory about the effect of the ergot alkaloids on the evolution of retroperitoneal fibrosis is that they act as a hapten, setting up a hypersensitivity or an autoimmune reaction. The associated vasculitis occasionally noted in retroperitoneal fibrosis supports this hypothesis.

Clinical Features

Retroperitoneal fibrosis occurs twice as often in males as in females and most commonly affects those from 40 to 60 years of age. The disorder has also been reported in children. Patients with retroperitoneal fibrosis generally present with a group of symptoms that help to classify the disease into one of two stages. In the early stage, the signs and symptoms originate from the disease process itself; in the advanced stage, the clinical features represent the effect of obstructive uropathy and renal failure.

A number of symptoms found in the early stage of the disease are similar to those of any subacute or chronic inflammatory condition: malaise, anorexia, weight loss, moderate pyrexia, nausea, vomiting, and backache. The erythrocyte sedimentation rate (ESR) is usually elevated, and a normocytic normochromic anemia is not uncommon. Hypertension has been reported to be present in 47% of these patients, and 55% have azotemia at time of presentation (Lepor and Walsh, 1979).

A characteristic pain suggesting the diagnosis of retroperitoneal fibrosis occurs as often as 90% of the time, according to Utz and Henry (1966). This distress is insidious in onset, dull, and noncolicky. The pain may have a veritable girdle distribution, because it originates in the lower aspects of the flank or lumbosacral region and extends anteriorly to both lower quadrants, the periumbilical region, or the testes. It is not altered by activity, body position, or increasing intra-abdominal pressure during bowel or bladder function. Later, the pain becomes more severe and unrelenting and suggests a retroperitoneal lesion, such as carcinoma of the pancreas or an abdominal aortic aneurysm. Oddly, the pain is sometimes relieved by aspirin but not by a narcotic. Another observation is that after a simple ureterolysis without any attempts to remove the extensive fibrosis, the perverse pain is relieved. This is most surprising, because the pain is not at all characteristic of that expected with ureteral obstruction. The disease also has been reported to manifest as a large bowel obstruction. Interestingly, most patients have no urinary symptoms.

There may be evidence of compression of the great vessels by the fibrotic process. Many patients exhibit mild edema of the lower extremities. More severe degrees of intrinsic obstruction of the inferior vena cava or iliac veins may lead to the development of thrombophlebitis. Although arterial occlusion and insufficiency are rare, they do occur. The signs and symptoms of reduced circulation, including ischemic pain, may be evident in the lower extremities.

The clinical features of the late stage are attributable to progressive ureteral occlusion. Progressive hydronephrosis may eventuate in complete ureteral obstruction and anuria. Unfortunately, the progression of disease is either very slow or silent, so that the symptoms normally present in the early stage either are not manifested or are so minimal that they are overlooked. In this situation, the patient may present with renal infection or with dull flank pain caused by the increasing hydronephrosis. General deterioration, weakness, weight loss, and gastrointestinal disturbances may constitute the first evidence of disease secondary to progressive uremia.

Diagnosis

The diagnosis of retroperitoneal fibrosis can be made on the basis of the history and the radiologic investigation. At times, the diagnosis is not firmly established until surgical exploration. Several laboratory tests indicative of a subacute or chronic inflammatory process may be helpful, but they are not diagnostic. The ESR is generally increased, and there may be leukocytosis or, occasionally, eosinophilia. Anemia is generally proportionate to the degree of azotemia that is present.

Excretory urography is a beneficial study in helping to establish a diagnosis in the early stage of the disease. **Characteristically, there is medial deviation of the ureter, usually at the middle third, beginning at the level of the third and fourth lumbar vertebrae.** Persky and Huus (1974) emphasized that medial deviation of the ureter is not a constant finding in patients with retroperitoneal fibrosis. Also, it has been demonstrated that almost 20% of patients with normal urograms have medial displacement of the ureters (especially the right) without demonstrable evidence of pathologic change in the urinary tract (Saldino and Palubinskas, 1972). **The medial displacement of the ureter in retroperitoneal fibrosis tends to extend higher than a normally deviated ureter, and the ureter often appears stiff.** Varying degrees of obstruction and hydronephrosis, with tapering of the ureter as it enters the dense plaque, are almost always evident. Most retroperitoneal neoplasms displace the ureters in a lateral direction but, as with normal variation, medial deviation occurs as well. Medial displacement of the pelvic ureters may occur after pelvic surgery, such as an abdominoperineal resection or the removal of a pelvic malignancy. Other causes of medially displaced pelvic ureters include a bladder diverticulum, metastatic tumors, and aneurysms.

More recently, ultrasonography and CT have become valuable techniques for establishing a diagnosis of retroperitoneal fibrosis. The ultrasonic appearance is a smooth-bordered, irregular, relatively echo-free mass centered on the sacral promontory but extending cephalad at least to the level of the aortic bifurcation and caudad into the pelvis. The findings are nonspecific and are less reliable than the image obtained with CT. Sonography can be used to follow response to therapy and detect hydronephrotic changes in the kidneys.

With the superior resolving power of CT, the fibrosis can be shown in more detail (Fig. 10–13). Although lymphoma, metastatic carcinoma, sarcoma, and multiple myeloma may also engulf the aorta and inferior vena cava (Sterzer et al, 1979), the symmetric distribution and geometric shape are highly suggestive of retroperitoneal fibrosis. The attenuation numbers of the mass are similar to those of muscle. **The limits of involvement extend from the renal vessels superiorly to below the level of the bifurcation of the great vessels inferiorly, with the lateral borders reaching or involving the psoas muscles.** The mass is confluent, with encasement of the aorta and inferior vena cava continuously, whereas lymphomas or metastatic disease may demonstrate enlarged lymph nodes separable from the great vessels. Comparable findings have been observed with MRI studies (Arrive et al, 1989). An advantage of MRI is the ability to display the pathologic process in multiple planes (transverse, coronal, sagittal), which provides useful information regarding the relationship of the fibrotic process to adjacent structures. At times, needle biopsy under CT guidance may help to establish a correct diagnosis and avoid an exploratory laparotomy.

As wider segments of the ureter are involved, the hydronephrosis increases. Eventually, complete obstruction and anuria may develop. Typically, hydroureteronephrosis when present extends to the point of ureteral narrowing and ob-

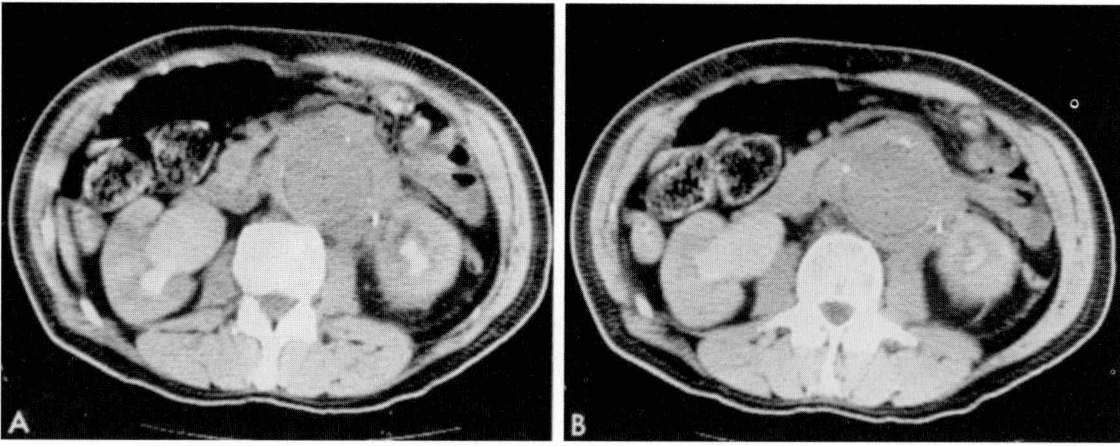

Figure 10–13. *A* and *B*, Computed tomographic scans demonstrating extensive retroperitoneal fibrosis associated with aneurysm of the abdominal aorta.

struction. The obstruction is usually bilateral, but it may be asymmetric and unilateral (Baker et al, 1988). **One third of patients have a nonfunctioning kidney at presentation as a result of long-standing obstruction.** The cause of obstruction has been debated but is believed to be an interference with ureteral peristalsis by the periureteral inflammatory process. Urodynamic evidence of obstruction has been well documented (Whitaker, 1975). Retrograde urography, which is required when there is inadequate demonstration of the pelvocalyceal system and ureter, again demonstrates medial deviation of the ureter and varying degrees of obstruction. Oddly, **in most instances the area of narrowing of the ureter readily permits the passage of a No. 5 or No. 6 French ureteral catheter (Fig. 10–14). This is considered a characteristic feature of retroperitoneal fibrosis,** although it is not a constant finding.

Retrograde studies usually confirm the presence of extrinsic obstruction, and the ureter is often smooth with the obstruction involving several centimeters of urine. If the process extends through the ureteral wall, an irregular or saw-tooth pattern is identified in the ureteral lumen. Percutaneous antegrade pyeloureterography is also a valuable study. Not only is it therapeutic and able to relieve the obstruction in the azotemic patient, but it also provides detailed information regarding the location and extent of the obstruction.

Radioisotope renography may be helpful, particularly for anuric patients or for patients in whom one side does not visualize on routine excretory urography. The curve may confirm the presence of obstructive urography or postrenal failure as opposed to primary renal disease. The height of the curve may also distinguish which kidney is the better functioning of the two when there is no or poor visualization on either side.

Venography is nonspecific but helpful in delineating the area of venous obstruction and the presence of thrombosis if there is significant edema in the lower extremities. Arteriography is employed if there is evidence of arterial insufficiency, but it is usually not needed in patient evaluation. Lymphangiography may be helpful in distinguishing retroperitoneal fibrosis from malignant causes of ureteral obstruction, especially retroperitoneal lymphoma. The presence of enlarged lymph nodes favors the diagnosis of malignant disease.

Treatment

Although surgical treatment is required for most cases of retroperitoneal fibrosis, several medical measures have been found to be worthwhile. Antibiotics and external radiation have virtually no role in the treatment of this disease, in spite of reports to the contrary. If the patient has been taking methysergide, the drug should be stopped immediately. A patient with minimal obstructive changes and renal impairment may show progressive improvement within a few weeks or even days after the drug is discontinued. Close follow-up with careful attention to the upper urinary tract is mandatory. In those patients in whom there has been no resolution of the mild hydronephrotic changes or in whom there is evidence of progression of the disease, surgery is necessary.

Steroids have been found to be helpful in certain instances (Higgins et al, 1988; Harreby et al, 1994). **Resolution of ureteral obstruction has been reported with steroids when used as initial therapy and after ureterolysis of the opposite ureter or in association with perianeurysmal fibrosis** (Feldberg and Hene, 1983). If proper drainage of the upper tracts can be easily accomplished, steroids may be useful in preparing patients for surgery who have renal insufficiency and considerable constitutional disturbance. Operative procedures then can be performed electively on a healthier patient, as opposed to a semiemergent basis. **Patients presenting with much system disturbance, particularly involving the gastrointestinal tract, or with rare extraurinary complications, such as mesenteric ischemia, and laboratory evidence of active inflammation (increased ESR and leukocytosis) are likely to benefit from steroids.**

In elderly patients and patients debilitated from coexistent disease, the need for major surgery may possibly be averted with the aid of steroids. The drugs also have been used concomitantly with the discontinuation of methysergide in patients with mild hydronephrotic changes. Finally, some urologists also advocate the use of steroids after ureterolysis, particularly if the pathologic assessment of the plaque reveals a significant inflammatory component. Determination of the steroid dosage remains empirical. Close observation with interval urography or ultrasonography and determinations of ESR, white blood cell count, serum creatinine level, and creatinine clearance are necessary while the patient is taking the medication. It has been suggested that a good prognostic sign is a decrease in the ESR after steroids are initiated. Persistent hydronephrosis or the lack of improvement as determined from the laboratory studies indicates the need for surgical intervention. In 1993, tamoxifen, an agent that has been effective in treating desmoid tumors, has been reported as a potential agent in treating idiopathic retroperitoneal fibrosis (Loffeld and van Weel, 1993).

Patients with significant renal impairment, evident from the presence of azotemia, oliguria, or anuria, benefit from a course of drainage of the upper urinary tracts. As already emphasized, despite marked hydronephrosis and significant extrinsic ureteral compression, ureteral catheters of sufficient size, or possibly double-J catheters, usually can be passed to the renal pelves. Drainage via percutaneous nephrostomy is also helpful. This affords valuable time to allow for restoration of renal function and to improve fluid, electrolyte, and acid-base balance before surgery.

After the appropriate diagnostic and preoperative therapeutic measures have been instituted, surgical exploration with ureterolysis is required in most cases. Because the disease generally affects both ureters, the best approach is transabdominal through a long midline incision. Incising the posterior peritoneum in the midline between the duodenum and the inferior mesenteric vein has been advocated (Hewitt et al, 1969). Flaps of posterior peritoneum are developed, exposing the entire retroperitoneal area and both ureters. Exposure of the individual ureters also can be achieved by mobilization of the ascending and descending colon, but this is more time consuming. It is generally easiest to locate the ureters by exposing the parts of the dilated proximal ureters that have not been encased in the fibrous plaque. A biopsy of the fibrous tissue is taken for frozen-section analysis.

Ureterolysis is usually accomplished with relative ease if the appropriate plane is found. The ureters are freed with blunt dissection immediately adjacent to the adventitia of the ureter. After the ureters are completely lysed, they are managed in one of several ways: (1) they may be transplanted to an intraperitoneal position; (2) they may be transposed laterally, interposing retroperitoneal fat between the ureters and the fibrosis; or (3) they may be wrapped with omental fat. **The procedure should be performed bilaterally, even in the presence of unilateral disease, because later involvement of the contralateral ureter is almost inevitable.**

On occasion, the fibrotic process may invade the ureter, but this usually occurs over only a short segment of ureter. In this instance, it may be impossible to achieve satisfactory ureterolysis; both resection of the segment of ureter and ureteroureterostomy may be necessary. Some urologic surgeons advocate the use of ureteral catheters during ureterolysis to facilitate dissection of the ureters and to help maintain them in a lateral position after ureterolysis. If the fibrotic process is very extensive and if ureteral invasion has occurred, an ileal ureter may in rare instances be required to provide appropriate drainage. Many innovative approaches

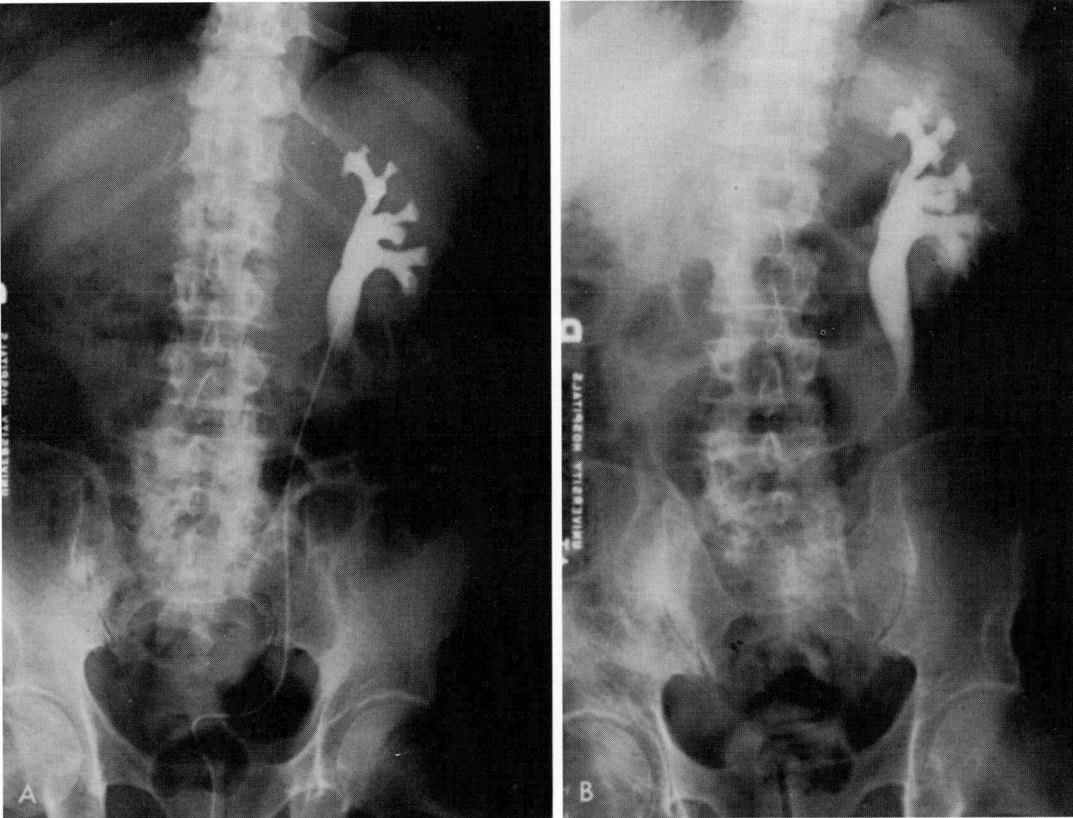

Figure 10–14. *A,* Left retrograde urogram in a patient with retroperitoneal fibrosis. Despite the obstruction, a No. 5 French ureteral catheter passes easily to the kidney. *B,* A pull-out x-ray demonstrates a hydronephrotic kidney with medial deviation of the ureter at the level of the fourth lumbar vertebra. Note the presence of backflow that may be secondary to ureteral obstruction.

have been described in these unusual circumstances (Mikkelsen and Lepor, 1989). A second operative procedure is occasionally required to extend the area of ureterolysis or to free the contralateral ureter.

If significant arterial encroachment is present, aortolysis with lysis of the common iliac arteries also may be required. In most instances, a plane can be established between the fibrotic plaque and the involved vessel with relative ease. On occasion the fibrotic plaque is adherent to the vessel walls, making lysis of the aorta a difficult, time-consuming procedure. Despite this problem, it is possible to free most of the fibrous plaque and to restore blood flow.

Although fatalities do occur, a satisfactory outcome generally can be expected after extensive bilateral ureterolysis if renal impairment is not too severe. In those instances in which ureterolysis is done for only one ureter or over only a short segment of ureter, recurrent disease is not uncommon. Close follow-up is critically important to ensure the absence of progressive or recurrent disease. A suggested algorithm for patient evaluation and treatment is detailed in Figure 10–15.

Secondary to Other Disease Processes

A number of diseases can cause retroperitoneal reaction, inflammation, and fibrosis, and the urologist should be aware of these because of the potential risk of ureteral compression. **Inflammatory processes of the lower extremities with ascending lymphangitis, multiple abdominal surgical procedures, Henoch-Schönlein purpura with hemorrhage, gonorrhea, biliary tract disease, chronic urinary tract infections, urinary extravasation, tuberculosis, and sar-**

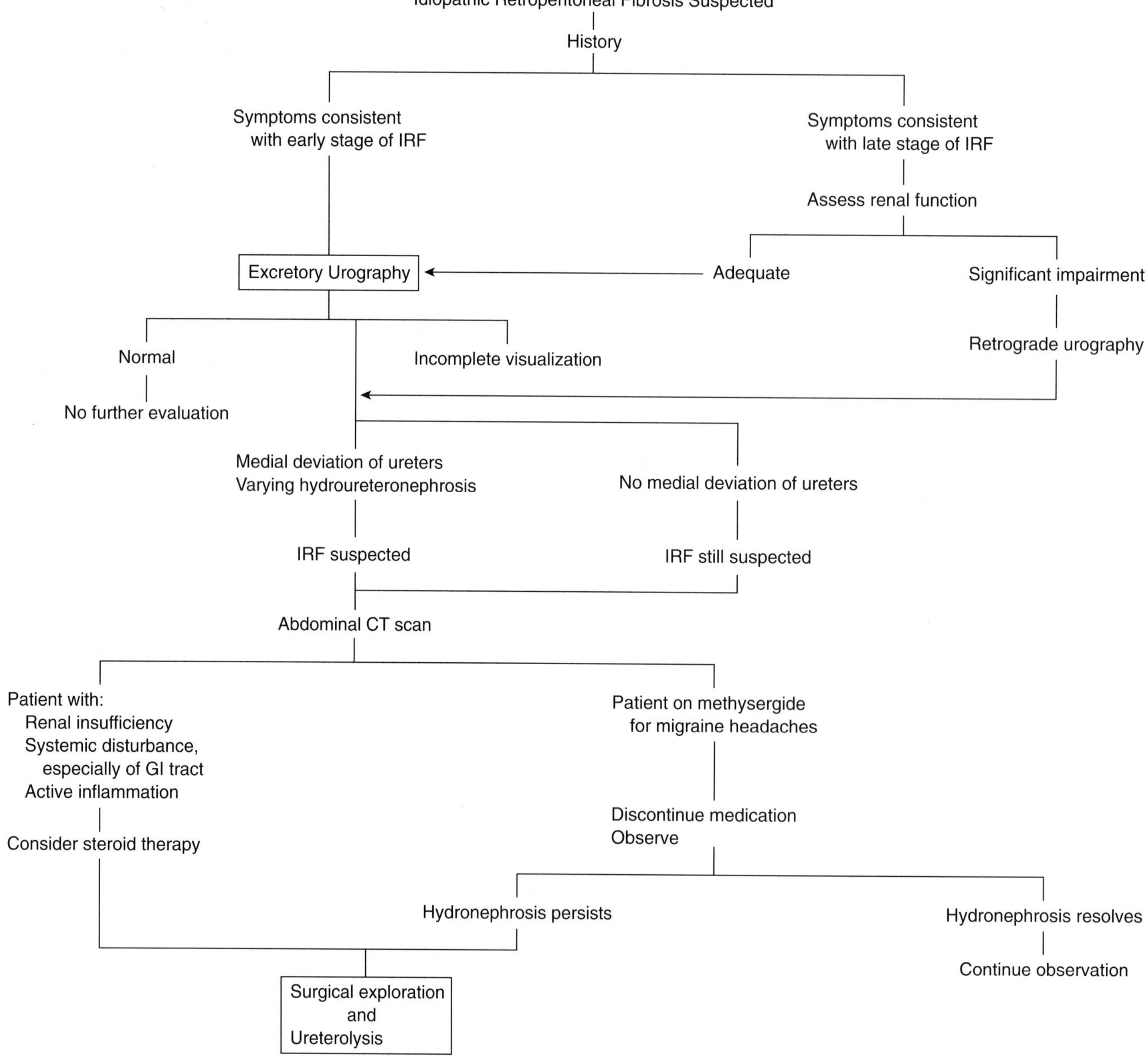

Figure 10–15. Evaluation of patient with suspected retroperitoneal fibrosis. IRF, internal rotation in flexion; CT, computed tomography; GI, gastrointestinal.

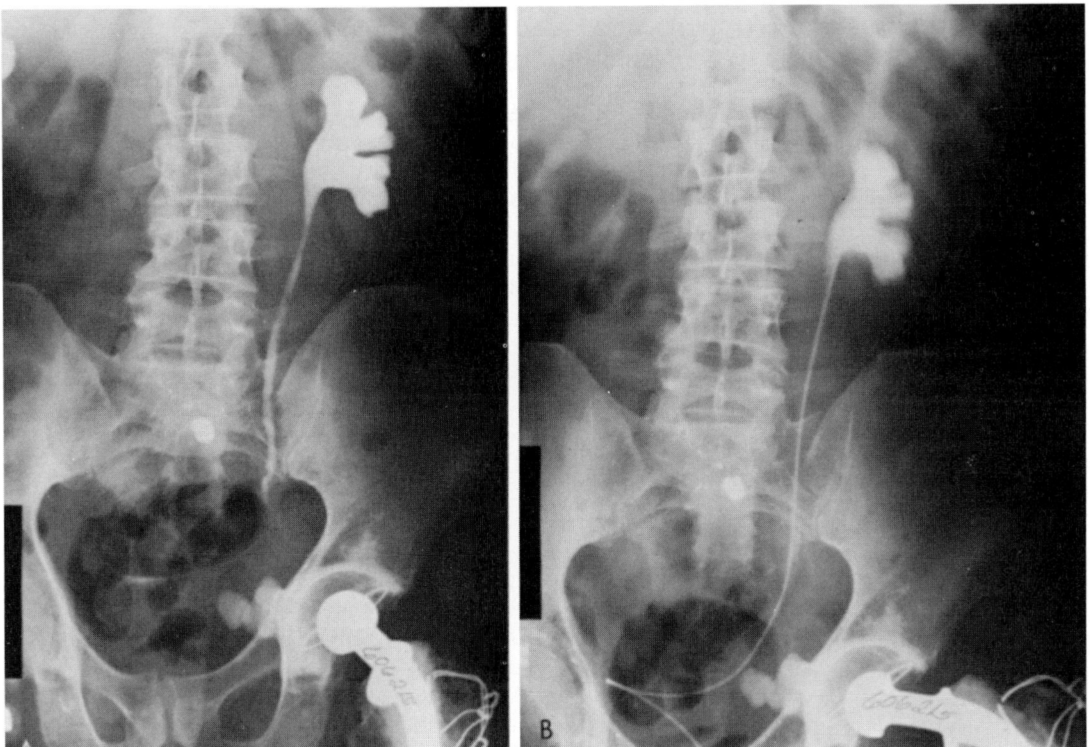

Figure 10–16. *A,* Retrograde urogram demonstrating left hydronephrosis with obstruction where the methyl methacrylate pierced the pelvis. *B,* A catheter placed in the left ureter is immediately adjacent to the methyl methacrylate. Exploration revealed encasement of the ureter in a dense mass of scar tissue, making ureterolysis impossible. A ureteroneocystostomy was performed with a psoas bladder hitch technique.

coidosis all have been associated with retroperitoneal fibrosis on rare occasions. The fibrosis is most commonly found at the level of the sacral promontory and within Gerota's fascia (Scott and Cerny, 1971). Otherwise, the radiologic diagnosis and the treatment are the same as those described earlier for idiopathic retroperitoneal fibrosis.

Methyl methacrylate is a cement commonly used for total joint replacement. A case of arterial occlusion has been reported after the use of methyl methacrylate (Hirsch et al, 1976). We have treated a patient with occlusion of the distal ureter and iliac vein secondary to the use of methyl methacrylate for total hip replacement (Fig. 10–16). Surgical exploration revealed an isolated area of marked fibrosis encasing the distal ureter and iliac vein in the area where the methyl methacrylate pierced the pelvis. It is possible that the heat of polymerization was responsible for this reaction. Because it is not uncommon for a small amount of methyl methacrylate to penetrate through the pelvis during total hip replacement, it is anticipated that additional cases of ureteral obstruction resulting from the use of the cement will be noted in the future.

Other unusual causes of periureteral inflammation and fibrosis include barium granuloma after colon perforation, sclerosing agents for treatment of inguinal hernia and hemorrhoids, mineral oil injection for treatment of vaginal prolapse, and compression by a lumbar subarachnoid peritoneal shunt catheter (Walther et al, 1987).

Radiation-Induced

It has been well documented that under certain conditions, radiation therapy can cause ureteral obstruction. Radiation therapy has been used extensively for the treatment of carcinoma of the cervix. Uremia is the most common cause of death in patients with carcinoma of the cervix, thus indicating that the distal ureters are vulnerable to obstruction. The obstruction is attributable to recurrent cancer in the vast majority of cases, but radiation-induced fibrosis may be the cause (Shingleton et al, 1969). **Upper urinary tract obstruction secondary to the effect of radiation is generally reported to occur in about 5% of patients with ureteral encroachment and in less than 1% of all treated patients.**

The low incidence of ureteral obstruction after radiation therapy, in comparison with the higher incidence of complications affecting the other pelvic organs such as the bladder and rectum, indicates that the ureters are relatively resistant to the effects of radiation. Significant ureteral damage can occur from fibrosis of either the periureteral tissue or the ureter itself. Several mechanisms have been postulated for ureteral obstruction after radiation therapy (Alfert and Gillenwater, 1972):

1. The tumor may incite a pronounced desmoplastic response in the tissue adjacent to the ureter that remains after the neoplasm has been eradicated.
2. It has been shown that infection increases the sensitivity of the ureter and periureteral tissue to radiation; therefore, radiation therapy is hazardous in the presence of PID or urinary tract infection.
3. Necrosis of the tumor invading the ureteral wall may lead to fibrosis and scarring.
4. Direct radiation injury to the ureteral wall may occur.

Ureteral obstruction may become evident near the end of a course of radiation therapy or shortly after its completion. This type of obstruction is caused by ureteral edema and changes in the periureteral tissue, and hydroureteronephrosis has been reported in 50% to 60% of women treated with radiation therapy for carcinoma of the cervix (Sklaroff et al, 1978). In essentially all patients, the obstruction resolves within 3 to 4 months.

Chronic ureteral obstruction can occur 6 to 12 months or even 10 years or more after radiotherapy, but it most often becomes evident in 1 to 3 years after completion (Underwood et al, 1977). The obstruction is related to reduced vascular supply and ischemia secondary to endarteritis obliterans and connective tissue proliferation with contraction of fibrous tissue secondary to the radiation therapy (Alfert and Gillenwater, 1972). Two types of ureteral blockage have been described. One is a localized stricture of the distal ureter caused by fibrosis in the parametrial tissue, and the other is a long, thread-like stenosis of the pelvic portion of the ureter secondary to scarring of the pelvic connective tissue (Altvater and Imholz, 1960).

As noted, the ureter is relatively resistant to radiation, and studies have demonstrated that radiation-induced stricture is unlikely in a normal ureter administered up to 600 rad (Albers et al, 1976). The most common point of ureteral obstruction is where the ureter and uterine arteries cross, which is 3 to 6 cm above the ureterovesical junction and 2 cm from the cervical os (Talner, 1990). **Radiation therapy up to 8000 Gy at this point results in a 40% urologic complication rate, but if the dose is 6000 Gy or less, complications occur in less than 2% of patients** (Underwood et al, 1977). Intracavitary radiation results in a higher incidence of ureteral stricture because, in part, of the ureteral displacement that occurs with vaginal packing. If the ureter is displaced 1 cm, the ureteral dose can be increased by 45%.

The late ureteral obstruction secondary to radiation therapy may be associated with urinary symptoms but more often goes unrecognized until there is severe renal damage. **Because it is slow and insidious in developing, for this reason, it is advisable to follow patients who have received radiotherapy with serial excretory urography, ultrasonography, or radioisotope renography.** Close follow-up is mandatory in patients with pretreatment of renal failure, prior pelvic surgery, infection, or evidence of parametritis.

Prior pelvic surgery increases the potential for development of radiation-induced obstruction, and experience indicates that 5% to 7% of women who receive radiation therapy after surgery develop obstructing symptoms (Goodman and Dalton, 1982). This is likely because of the poor blood supply that may be present in the previously operated patient. Other predisposing factors include urinary infections, PID, and intraoperative ureteral catheterization.

Because infection may be a potent factor predisposing to ureteral damage, several prophylactic measures are advisable. Quiescent salpingitis may be exacerbated with radiotherapy. Accordingly, it is advisable to perform a preliminary bilateral salpingo-oophorectomy before irradiation in patients with a history or physical findings suggestive of PID. In addition, acute infection during radiotherapy should be recognized in the closely followed patient and should be treated with bilateral salpingo-oophorectomy.

As already mentioned, **approximately 90% of late ureteral obstructions after radiation therapy are secondary to recurrent cancer. Only one third to two thirds of obstructions are caused by recurrent cancer when treatment includes both radiation and surgery** (Bahrassa and Ampil, 1987). Recurrent disease is often suspected on physical examination, but imaging studies, especially CT and MRI, are helpful, particularly if a mass is present and the point of ureteral obstruction can be localized. In the absence of positive evidence of recurrent tumor, exploratory laparotomy or laparoscopy and biopsy are mandatory to obtain a tissue diagnosis. Percutaneous biopsy under ultrasound or CT guidance is sometimes helpful, particularly if a diagnosis of malignancy can be established. In a small number of cases, the obstruction is secondary to the radiation therapy, thereby affording an opportunity to salvage renal tissue. If the patient has a normally functioning bladder without significant radiation changes, the pelvic ureter can be lysed from the periureteral fibrotic tissue and reimplanted. A fish-mouth type of ureteroneocystostomy without an antireflux procedure is preferable. When the pelvic ureter or bladder is badly damaged, the use of an ileal ureter or a form of supravesical urinary diversion may be required. Autotransplantation also has been reported (Deane et al, 1983).

Retroperitoneal Abscess, Infections, and Inflammation

The retroperitoneal space is divided into anterior and posterior compartments, with the ureters and kidneys lying in the posterior compartment (Altemeier et al, 1971). Likewise, retroperitoneal abscesses can be divided into anterior and posterior types. The posterior abscess usually results from extravasation behind a ureteral stone or renal caruncle. Anterior abscesses are usually secondary to a gastrointestinal disease, such as appendicitis, diverticulitis, or Crohn's disease. Suppurative iliac adenitis, osteomyelitis, tuberculosis, retroperitoneal brucellosis, suppurative mesenteric adenitis, coccidioidomycosis, disseminated mucormycosis, retroperitoneal malacoplakia, sarcoidosis, actinomycosis, and epidural abscess are other possible etiologic factors (Kuntze et al, 1988; Talner, 1990). A psoas abscess develops if the inflammatory process extends into the psoas muscle. Retroperitoneal inflammatory processes in either compartment may deviate or obstruct the ureter as it courses toward the bladder.

Physical examination usually reveals fever and a tender abdominal mass. As the inflammation spreads, the patient may develop tenderness in the iliac, groin, or upper thigh area. If the musculature is involved, the patient often lies with the hip flexed; extension elicits a positive "psoas sign." On radiologic examination, a lumbar scoliosis with the concavity toward the involved side and air along the fibers of the psoas muscle may be seen on the plain film of the abdomen. Excretory urography can be valuable in helping to establish the diagnosis (Fig. 10–17). **Approximately 2% of all patients with retroperitoneal abscesses and 5% of those with posterior abscesses have displacement or dilation (or both) of the upper urinary tracts** (Stevenson and

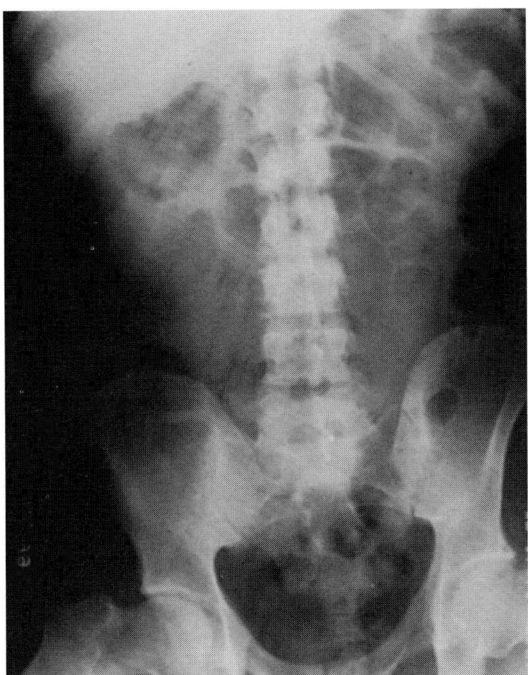

Figure 10–17. There is free retroperitoneal air along the psoas muscle caused by a psoas abscess that resulted from a perirectal infection. This delayed film of an excretory urogram shows considerable dilation and very faint visualization of the right pelvocalyceal system and upper ureter, indicating significant ureteral obstruction.

Ozeran, 1969). Despite this low incidence of secondary involvement of the ureter, excretory urography is essential, because about 70% of the posterior abscesses have a renal origin (Altemeier et al, 1971). Abdominal ultrasonography and CT are excellent radiographic methods of identifying and defining the extent of the abscess.

Surgery consists of prompt extraperitoneal drainage through a large incision. Satisfactory drainage usually results in resolution of the urographic abnormalities. Successful treatment has also been reported with the use of percutaneous drainage techniques (Sacks et al, 1988). Because retroperitoneal scarring can conceivably cause compression of the ureter, adequate follow-up is necessary.

Retroperitoneal Hemorrhage

Primary Retroperitoneal Hematoma

A retroperitoneal hematoma is usually secondary to blunt abdominal trauma, although bleeding in the retroperitoneal space may be attributable to vascular accidents, percutaneous lithotripsy, gynecologic surgery, anticoagulants, blood dyscrasia (e.g., hemophilia anticoagulation), or iatrogenic causes (Farha et al, 1987; Moskovitz et al, 1988; Butt et al, 1994). The physical examination may demonstrate ecchymotic flank discoloration, an adynamic ileus, and hypotension. An accumulation of blood in the retroperitoneum often causes deviation of the ureter and on rare occasions may cause obstruction. Intravenous urography, ultrasonography, CT, and MRI are all useful in delineating the extent of the hematoma and the effect on adjacent structures (Cole-Beuglet et al, 1987). These studies are also useful in monitoring resolution of the process. Iatrogenic hematomas or those secondary to anticoagulants generally resolve spontaneously, but large hematomas caused by abdominal trauma are usually evacuated during exploratory laparotomy. Recurrent retroperitoneal hematoma as occasionally seen in hemophilic patients can calcify and result in fibrosis and chronic ureteral obstruction (Fig. 10–18).

Hematoma of Rectus Abdominis Muscle

A hematoma of the rectus abdominis muscle may cause ureteral obstruction and vesical compression. Most of these hematomas are attributable to muscle exertion, but they also may be caused by degenerative muscle disease, anticoagulants, pregnancy, and direct trauma. The hematoma may extend retroperitoneally; in a few instances, a large amount of bleeding has led to bilateral ureteral obstruction and oliguria. Rupture of the rectus abdominis muscle or of the epigastric vessels, or of both, leads to the acute onset of abdominal pain, tenderness, and rigidity. Immediate evacuation and ligation of the inferior epigastric vessels are essential in the treatment of this entity (Zalar and McDonald, 1969).

Retroperitoneal Masses

Primary Retroperitoneal Tumors

The first description of a retroperitoneal tumor has been credited to Morgagni in 1761, and the term *retroperitoneal*

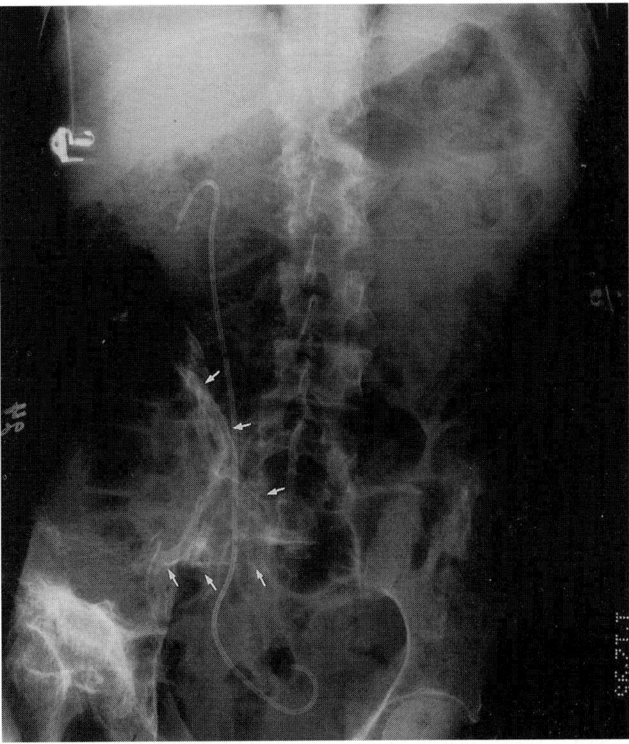

Figure 10–18. Kidney, ureter, and bladder (KUB) view demonstrating retroperitoneal calcification (*arrows*) secondary to recurrent retroperitoneal hematoma in a patient with factor 8 deficiency. Ureteral double-J stents are in place.

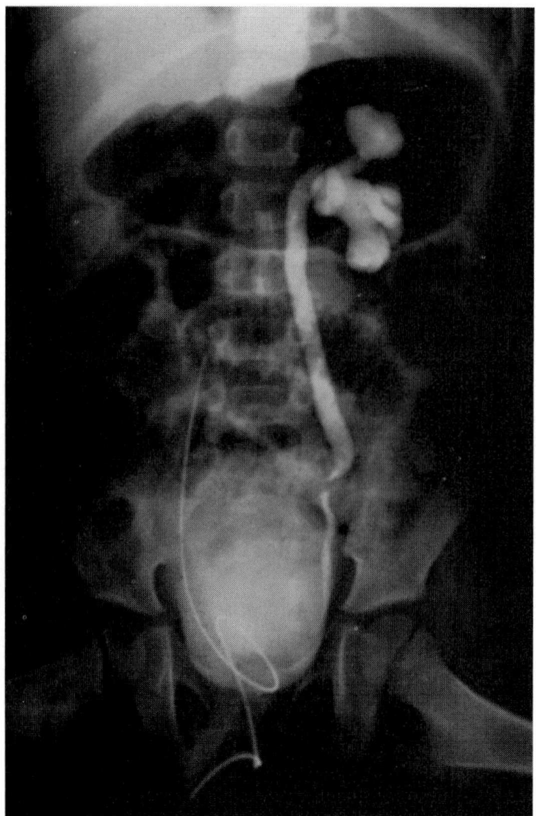

Figure 10–19. Paraganglioma causing obstruction of the midureter in an 8-year-old boy.

tumor was first used by Lobstein in 1834 (Felix et al, 1981). Primary retroperitoneal tumors may arise from the neural, mesodermal, urogenital ridge, or embryonic remnant tissues. They are either benign or malignant, although malignant tumors account for approximately 70% to 80% of the total (Braash and Mon, 1967). **In general, primary retroperitoneal neoplasms are rare, the malignant lesions accounting for only 0.16% of all cancers in a large country hospital during a 15-year period (Braash and Mon, 1967).** The true incidence of these tumors may be higher because, at times, it is difficult to establish the true site of origin.

Because the retroperitoneum contains many structures, including the adrenal glands, kidneys, ureters, bladder, blood vessels, lymphatics, and nerves, tumors in this area can be quite diverse, on the basis of their cell of origin. Most tumors occur in the fourth to fifth decades, and the sex distribution is generally equal (Felix et al, 1981). **Lymphomas predominate (approximately one third), followed in frequency of occurrence by a variety of tumors, including neuroblastomas and liposarcomas. Benign growths include neurofibromas, lipomas, adenomas, and cysts.** The large variety of primary tumors that occur in the retroperitoneal area are listed in Table 10–2. The prognosis is poor for malignant neoplasms, with only 10% to 15% of patients being free of tumor at 5 years (Adams, 1974). Primary retroperitoneal tumors occasionally cause extrinsic obstruction of the ureter. There are rare case reports of ureteral obstruction found in association with such lesions as ectopic pheochromocytoma (Immergut et al, 1970), renal cysts (Evans and Coughlin, 1970), and retroperitoneal xanthogranuloma (Gup, 1972) (Fig. 10–19).

At presentation, patients most often complain of an abdominal mass and pain. Other symptoms may be weight gain, abdominal enlargement, and gastrointestinal and genitourinary complaints or a wide range of symptoms that may include back pain, leg swelling, fever, anorexia, and weight loss (Patel, 1990). The patient's symptoms are often related to the location of the tumor (Fig. 10–20). The abdominal mass is usually most readily palpable in the midline and has variable extensions to the pelvis and flanks. The consistency of the mass may give a clue to the type of tumor; malignancies are hard, whereas benign growths tend to be soft. An abdominal mass in a child most often has a renal or retroperitoneal origin.

Plain abdominal x-rays may demonstrate either calcification or lucency in the region of the tumor, depending on its primary cellular composition. Excretory urography, including lateral and oblique films, is a rewarding diagnostic study. The ureter is usually displaced anteriorly and laterally, and occasionally there may be partial or total obstruction of the ureter. The kidney is often displaced, and the renal pelvis may be distorted, flattened, or rotated (Fig. 10–21). This study is also mandatory for evaluating the contralateral kidney because **25% of patients require nephrectomy for a complete excision of the tumor** (Cody et al, 1981). Retrograde pyelography may be indicated if the upper tracts are inadequately visualized.

Ultrasonography and/or CT scan provide invaluable information regarding the size and shape of the tumor, extent of invasion, and relationship to contiguous structures (Lane et al, 1989). Similar information is often obtained with MRI, and this study can be helpful in delineating the type of tumor present. Gastrointestinal films are often necessary to exclude the intestinal tract as the primary source of the tumor. Arteriography and inferior venacavography are valuable in further delineating the extent of the tumor, particularly in a child (Karp et al, 1980). Venography is occasionally helpful, particularly if marked distortion or infiltration of the inferior vena cava is suspected. Percutaneous biopsy under ultrasound, CT, or fluoroscopic control can be useful in establishing the diagnosis.

In most instances, transperitoneal excision en bloc is the optimal treatment. A bowel preparatory procedure should be carried out preoperatively, because bowel resection may be required to accomplish complete excision. Usually, a transperitoneal approach through a midline incision is used to obtain optimal exposure. Occasionally, removal of adjacent organs (kidney, colon, spleen) is required when they are included within the pseudocapsule of the tumor. **Unfortunately, because of the infiltrative nature of many of these tumors, complete excision can be obtained in only about 50% of cases.**

If the entire tumor cannot be removed, every effort should be made to remove as much as possible. Symptoms may be relieved, and response to adjuvant therapy may be improved. The margins of the remaining tumor should be marked with surgical clips to provide accurate tumor localization. The role of the adjuvant postoperative radiation therapy is unclear, but it may be beneficial. Adjuvant chemotherapy is of value in treating embryonal rhabdomyosarcoma, but its role with other tumors is unknown.

Table 10–2. CLASSIFICATION OF PRIMARY RETROPERITONEAL TUMORS

Origin	Tumors: *Benign*	Tumors: *Malignant*
Tumors of Mesodermal Origin		
Adipose tissue	Lipoma	Liposarcoma
Smooth muscle	Leiomyoma	Leiomyosarcoma
Connective tissue	Fibroma	Fibrosarcoma
Striated muscle	Rhabdomyoma	Rhabdomyosarcoma
Lymph vessels	Lymphangioma	Lymphangiosarcoma
Primitive mesenchyme	Myxoma	Myxosarcoma
Blood vessels	Hemangioma and angiosarcoma Hemangiopericytoma (benign and malignant)	
Uncertain	Xanthogranuloma	
Tumors of Neurogenic Origin		
Nerve sheath	Nonencapsulated neurofibroma Encapsulated neurilemoma Malignant schwannoma	
Sympathetic nervous system	Ganglioneuroma Sympathicoblastoma (ganglioneuroblastoma) Neuroblastoma	
Heterotopic cortical adrenal and chromaffin tissue	Carcinoma arising from cortical adrenal tissue Malignant nonchromaffin paraganglioma Paraganglioma Functioning pheochromocytoma	
Tumors Arising from Embryonic Remnants or Notochord		
Embryonic remnants	Benign and malignant teratomas	
Notochord	Chordomas	

From Ackerman LV: Atlas of Tumor Pathology, Section VI. Fascicles 23 and 24: Tumors of the Retroperitoneum, Mesentery, and Peritoneum. Washington, DC, Armed Forces Institute of Pathology, 1954, pp 12–13.

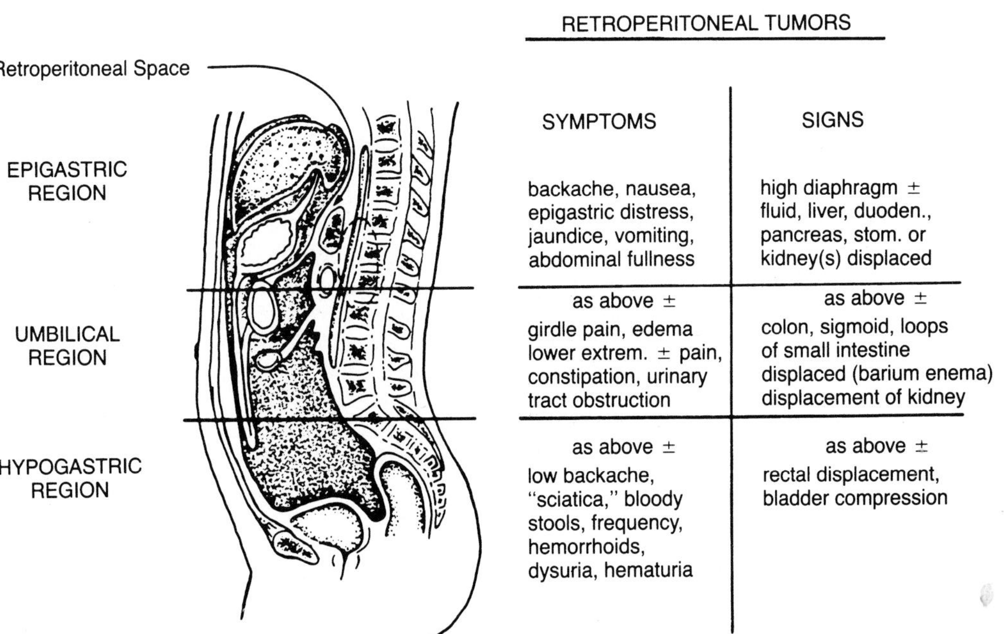

Figure 10–20. Relation of location of retroperitoneal tumors to symptoms and signs (duoden., duodenum; stom., stomach; extrem., extremities). (Modified from Melicow MM: J Int Coll Surg 1953; 19:401, and Patel SK: Retroperitoneal tumors and cysts. *In* Pollack HM, ed: Clinical Urography. Philadelphia, W.B. Saunders, 1990, p 2413.)

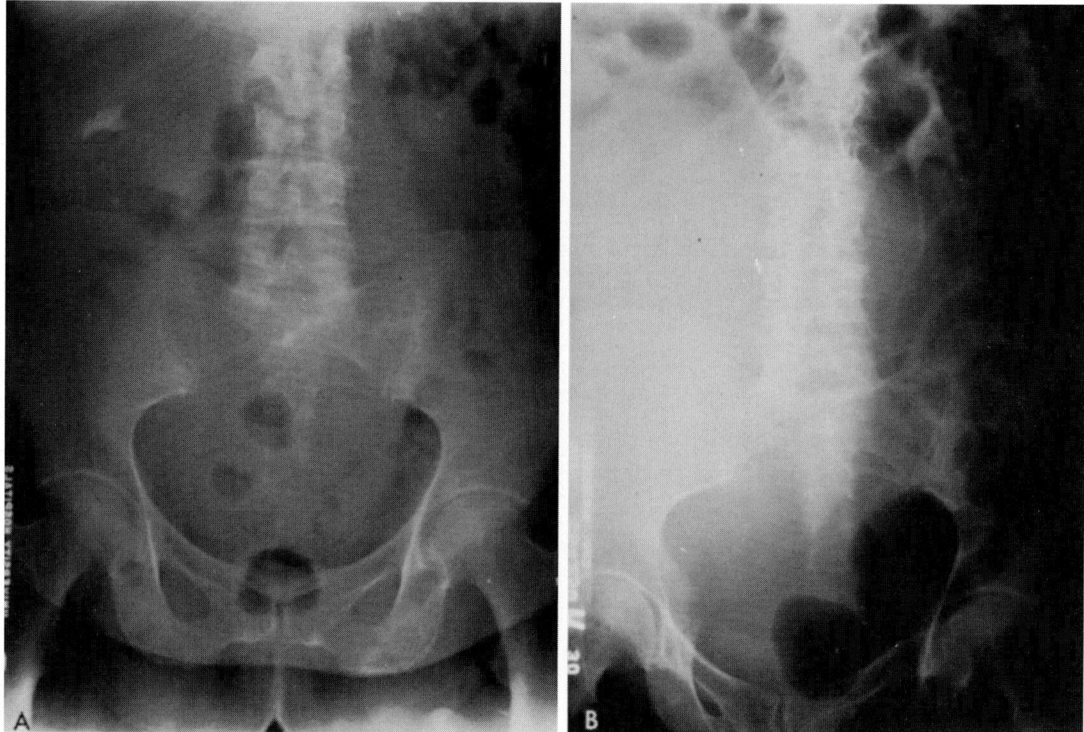

Figure 10–21. *A,* Huge retroperitoneal sarcoma causing lateral deviation of the right ureter and distortion and rotation of the kidney. *B,* Despite surgical excision, recurrent sarcoma resulted in complete obstruction and nonvisualization of the right kidney.

Unfortunately, local recurrence is fairly common, and because these tumors are slow growing, recurrence may be late. Careful follow-up, including appropriate imaging studies, is required. If the tumor recurs, repeat excision should be attempted.

Secondary Retroperitoneal Tumors

Metastases from primary malignancies anywhere in the body can spread to the retroperitoneum and lead to ureteral obstruction. Table 10–3 demonstrates the comparative incidence of various tumors spreading to the retroperitoneum. Secondary involvement of the retroperitoneum by malignant tumors occurs in one of two ways: (1) by direct extension of adjacent malignancy or (2) by metastasis to the retroperitoneal lymph nodes.

Tumors that spread to the retroperitoneum by direct extension usually involve the lower third of the ureter. Typically, these include tumors of the cervix, endometrium, bladder, prostate, sigmoid colon, and rectum. The tumor may simply compress the ureteral wall, but it also can invade the serosa to involve the muscularis and mucosa. Metastatic tumors involving the retroperitoneal and periureteral lymphatics tend to encase the ureter to produce obstruction. Ureteral displacement and angulation often result and can be visualized radiographically. These areas of obstruction may be limited or quite extensive. Tumors of varying origins can progress in this manner and include metastases from carcinomas of the breast, stomach, lung, pancreas, lymphoma, and colon. Tumors arising from pelvic structures can have similar involvement. Theoretically, any secondary tumor spreading to the retroperitoneum can encroach upon the ureter and lead to obstruction (Kaufman and Grabstald, 1969). **Ureteral obstruction occurs within 2 years of the primary diagnosis in 60% to 70% of patients, but it can occur as much as 20 years later** (Brin et al, 1975) (Fig. 10–22). It also can result as a complication after surgery for treatment of these disorders.

Table 10–3. SECONDARY RETROPERITONEAL TUMORS THAT CAUSE EXTRINSIC OBSTRUCTION OF THE URETER*

Cervix†	Lymph nodes
Prostate†	Pancreas
Bladder†	Lung
Colon	Gallbladder
Ovary, uterus	Testis
Stomach	Small bowel
Breast	

*Presented in order of decreasing frequency.
†Account for 70%.

The symptoms associated with metastatic obstruction of the ureter include a wide variety of complaints, but they may be masked by the symptoms associated with the primary tumor and other metastases. Flank pain, sepsis, and fever may herald extrinsic blockage of the ureter. Often, ureteral obstruction is not suspected until the patient develops oliguria or anuria and azotemia as a result of compression of both ureters. In a small number of patients, metastatic obstruction of the ureter is the first evidence of malignancy. The obstruction is usually in the distal or pelvic ureter, although the blockage can occur anywhere along the ureter and may be located at multiple sites (Fig. 10–23) or at a single site (Fig. 10–24).

The diagnosis of secondary retroperitoneal tumors is usually made by imaging studies in association with appropriate

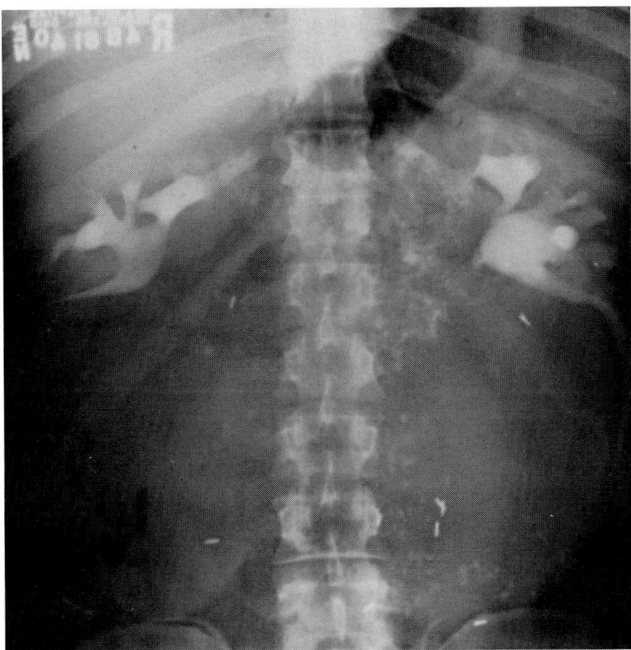

Figure 10–22. Bilateral deviation and obstruction of the ureters as a result of recurrent tumor involving the retroperitoneal nodes in a patient who had undergone an orchiectomy for embryonal cell carcinoma 17 years earlier. The patient had been treated with radiation therapy to the periaortic area after the orchiectomy, but node dissection was not performed.

biopsy. Ureteral obstruction with associated hydronephrosis is usually detected with intravenous urography, and the site and cause of obstruction are delineated with ultrasonography, CT, MRI, or lymphangiography (Jing et al, 1982). Percutaneous transabdominal biopsy under CT guidance has an accuracy of 85% in detecting lymph node invasion by epithelial malignancies.

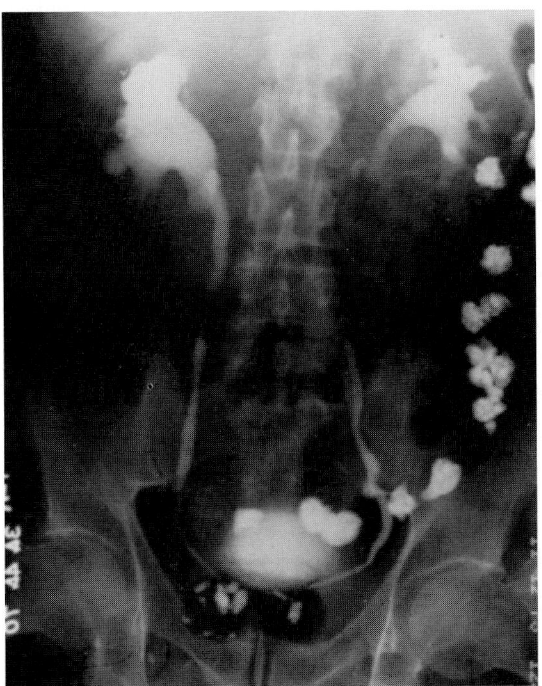

Figure 10–23. Multiple areas of bilateral ureteral obstruction secondary to retroperitoneal metastasis from pancreatic carcinoma.

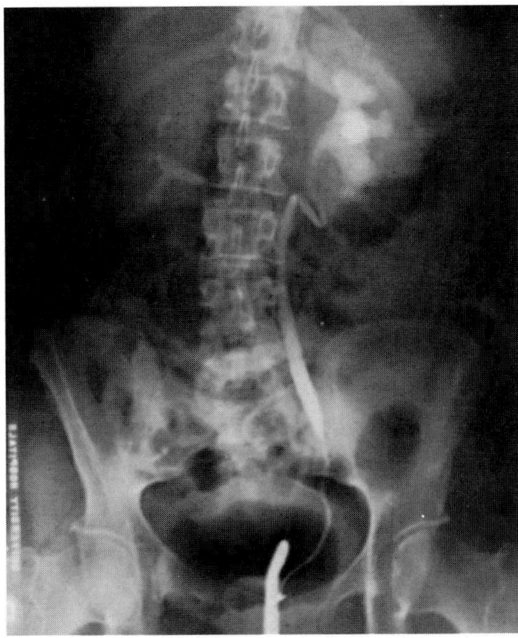

Figure 10–24. Retrograde urogram demonstrating obstruction of a small area of the lower third of the left ureter resulting from a retroperitoneal metastasis from gastric carcinoma.

When the diagnosis is established, the surgeon must decide whether to divert the urinary tract, especially when both ureters are obstructed. The urologist must consider the type of tumor, previous treatment, general condition of the patient, and overall prognosis before proceeding with diversion. **It has been reported that 40% to 50% of patients who undergo diversion for ureteral obstruction never leave the hospital, and the majority of patients live only 3 to 6 months.** As a group, the patients are hospitalized for approximately 60% of the remainder of their lives (Brin et al, 1975). Ulm and Klein (1960) reported on a series of patients with colon cancer, of whom approximately 6% had ureteral obstruction secondary to metastatic disease. None of the patients survived longer than 8 months after diagnosis. On the other hand, later reports indicated that the length of survival was not as dismal after palliative nephrostomy (Bodner et al, 1982).

Several groups of patients tend to fare better than others: patients with carcinoma of the prostate, patients with untreated carcinoma, and patients with bilateral ureteral obstruction from direct extension of pelvic malignancy, as opposed to those with bilateral ureteral obstruction from disseminated disease originating outside the pelvis. Brin and associates (1975) reported that patients with ureteral obstruction caused by prostatic carcinoma were hospitalized for an average of 30% of the remainder of their lives and had a mean survival of 1 year. Khan and Utz (1975) reported comparable figures for patients with prostatic carcinoma and cited two patients who were alive 2 and 4 years after diversion. In those patients who have never been treated for metastatic prostate disease, the response to androgen deprivation treatment is generally more favorable, regardless of the location or type of secondary tumor. Radiation therapy also has proved useful in selected patients.

After deciding to divert the genitourinary system, the urologist must first determine which kidney functions better. This is most effectively done with the radioisotope renogram if it is not apparent on the excretory urogram. Proximal diversion can be accomplished with internal ureteral stents, nephrostomy, or cutaneous ureterostomy. Today, nephrostomy is usually achieved by utilizing percutaneous techniques. Each procedure has drawbacks. Nephrostomies have a significant incidence of associated infection and stone formation. Ureterostomies often result in stomal stenosis unless the ureter is considerably dilated. Zimskind and associates (1967) initially described the use of the long-term indwelling silicone ureteral stent, which was nonreactive and had a low incidence of associated infection. Its use is limited because of the technical difficulties in inserting the stent beyond the obstruction. The double-J ureteral catheter, as described by Finney (1978), has become the preferred long-term ureteral stent because of the relative ease of insertion. At times, placement of the stent does not relieve the obstruction caused by compression of the ureteral wall against the stent, so that drainage around the stent cannot occur.

The lymphoproliferative disorders, such as lymphoma and leukemia, also obstruct the ureter by virtue of lymph node infiltration (Fig. 10–25). In a large autopsy series, 6% of lymphoma patients had evidence of ureteral obstruction secondary to lymph node involvement. The genitourinary tract was involved in approximately 30% of the patients. Ureteral obstruction secondary to lymphoma is therefore a relatively infrequent occurrence and is also a late phenomenon. Death caused by urinary tract involvement accounts for only 0.5% of lymphoma mortalities (Martinez-Maldonado and Romirez DeArellon, 1962).

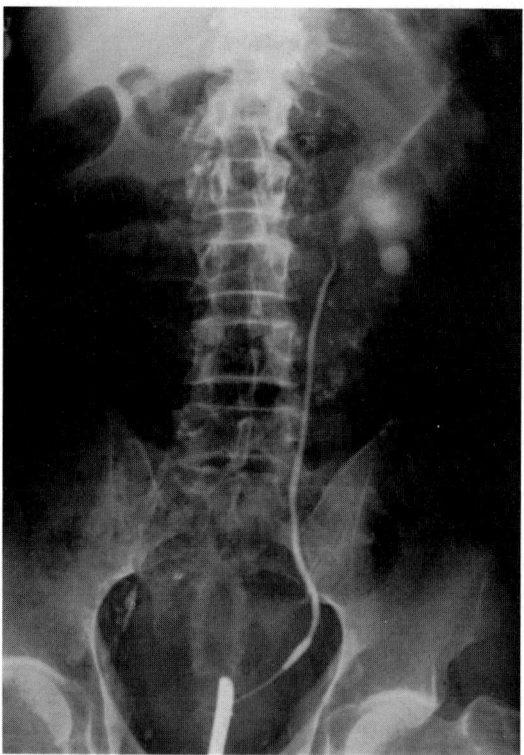

Figure 10–25. Retrograde urogram demonstrating obstruction of the upper third of the left ureter secondary to recurrent lymphoma. Ureterolysis resulted in relief of the hydronephrosis.

Other Mass Lesions of the Retroperitoneum

LYMPHOCELE

A lymphocele, also known as a lymphocyst, is a complication of radical pelvic surgery that may lead to extrinsic obstruction of the ureter. Lymphoceles develop subsequent to pelvic lymphadenectomy and renal transplantation (Brawer et al, 1989). **A variable incidence of 12% to 24% has been reported after pelvic lymphadenectomy, and significant lymphoceles develop in approximately 4% to 5% of renal transplant patients** (Banowsky et al, 1974). Lymphoceles also occur after radical gynecologic surgery (Mann et al, 1989).

Lymphoceles are believed to result from the surgical severance and inadequate closure of afferent lymphatic channels. It has been postulated that the cystic collections develop when the adjacent peritoneum becomes edematous and fibrotic, preventing the resorption of extravasated lymph. **The formation of the cyst is apparently enhanced by extensive dissection, excision of large surgical specimens, the presence of tumor-bearing lymph nodes, and preoperative irradiation.** Surgical preparation of the recipient as well as of the donor kidney may predispose to lymph leakage as a result of the interruption of many lymphatics. In addition, factors related to the transplant state may contribute to the increased and prolonged lymph drainage. Rejection is believed to play an important role, because it causes approximately a 20-fold increase in lymph flow, although it is uncertain whether this is from the donor lymphatics or the recipient lymphatics. Open transplant biopsy may interrupt capsular lymphatics, and ureteral obstruction is also known to increase lymphatic flow. Because the interruption of lymphatics during surgery is believed to be important in the development of lymphoceles, careful attention to the ligation of lymphatics is important in helping to prevent lymph pooling and cyst formation. The role of heparin administration postoperatively in preventing lymphocele formation remains controversial.

Eighty to ninety percent of lymphoceles form within 3 weeks of surgery. Abscesses, urinomas, and hematomas tend to occur earlier in the postoperative period (Letourneau et al, 1988). Small lymphoceles are asymptomatic. The symptoms associated with large lymphatic cysts depend on the size and location of the cysts, which may compress the ureter, bladder, sigmoid colon, and iliac blood vessels. The patients may experience lower abdominal pain, frequency, and constipation. Edema of the genitalia and lower extremities is often present as a result of both venous and lymphatic obstruction. The combination of thigh edema and groin pain may mimic thrombophlebitis. Palpation of the abdomen or bimanual pelvic or rectal examination may reveal a lower abdominal mass. At times, the mass is fluctuant, depending on the size of the cyst and the thickness of the cyst wall. In rare instances, bilateral lymphoceles may be responsible for oliguria and renal failure. Decreased renal function is more often seen in association with lymphoceles in kidney transplant patients.

The excretory urogram often shows anterior and medial displacement of the ureter with varying degrees of obstruction and compression of the bladder. Retrograde urography, particularly with the use of an acorn-tip catheter, is often the best study for demonstrating the displacement of the lower ureter. Indentation of the bladder, if present, also may be displayed on a cystogram. In addition, this study is helpful in excluding extravasation in transplant patients. Ultrasonography or CT is invaluable in demonstrating and following the size of the lymphocele, but it must be recognized that no imaging technique can differentiate a lymphocele from a urinoma. Definitive differentiation can be determined only by measurement of BUN and creatinine in aspirated fluid, although aspiration has the risk of introducing infection. Lymphangiography is a valuable adjunct if the diagnosis remains uncertain, because the puddling of contrast media in the lymphocele is diagnostic.

No surgical treatment is required for most lymphoceles, because spontaneous regression usually occurs. Accordingly, management consists of bed rest, to reduce pain and edema, and antibiotic therapy for pelvic and urinary infections. Elastic stockings help to control edema of the lower extremities and hasten ambulation. If ureteral obstruction is present, careful observation with serial urography or renal ultrasonography is necessary, and ureteral catheterization or stent placement may be required to drain an infected hydronephrotic kidney. Progressive hydronephrosis and pyelonephritis, massive leg edema, or deterioration of renal function indicates the need for surgery.

Aspiration of the cyst alone is not advisable because the fluid rapidly reaccumulates. The necessity for multiple taps also increases the possibility of infection (Burgos et al, 1988). Some clinicians have advocated needle aspiration and percutaneous catheter placement as initial therapy because the risk of this procedure is less than with surgery (Pfister, 1990). Sclerotherapy also has been utilized by irrigating the cavity of the lymphocele percutaneously with tetracycline or povidone-iodine (Cohan et al, 1986; Gilliland et al, 1989).

Internal drainage appears to be the preferred surgical procedure. A transperitoneal window is made by marsupialization of the opened cyst to the peritoneum, and the sigmoid colon or cecum is anchored to the posterior wall of the cyst. Satisfactory drainage has also been accomplished laparoscopically. Incision and drainage by marsupialization of the cyst to the subcutaneous and subcuticular tissue through a small skin incision, with placement of several drains and packing, also have been advocated for renal transplant patients. The latter procedure has the advantages of simplicity, rapidity of performance, lack of injury to the allograft, and prevention of recurrence. In order to reduce the chance of infection, the packing in the cyst cavity is soaked in 1% neomycin solution. The packing is changed daily with a sterile technique, and antibacterial ointment is applied to the skin edges.

Pelvic Lipomatosis

Pelvic lipomatosis is a proliferative process involving the mature fat of the pelvic retroperitoneal space. The proliferating adipose tissue may compress the pelvic viscera, including the pelvic portion of the ureters, in varying degrees. Occasionally, marked bilateral ureteral obstruction may lead to the development of uremia.

Engels, in 1959, first drew attention to this entity. Although the disease is a benign condition, it may have serious consequences and is often mistaken for a pelvic neoplasm. Pelvic lipomatosis is rare—relatively few cases have been reported—but it is probable that many recognized cases have not been included in the medical literature. There have been few reports of pelvic lipomatosis in females (Joshi and Wise, 1983; Honecke and Butz, 1991) and one report in a child (Moss et al, 1972). The latter case was in a child with Cushing's syndrome and did not represent the spontaneous form of the disease. **The disease, therefore, is found almost exclusively in males in the third to sixth decades of life.** An unexplained but definite racial predominance has also been noted, with about two thirds of reported cases occurring in black patients.

The cause of pelvic lipomatosis is unknown (Saxton, 1990). Some authors suggest that it represents a localized form of obesity. Rosenberg and associates (1963) described the process as a manifestation of Dercum's disease (adiposis dolorosa), an entity characterized by the presence of subcutaneous deposits of fat that are irregular and painful. Sclerosing lipogranulomatosis may have a clinical presentation similar to pelvic lipomatosis, but the pathologic findings are those of fat necrosis associated with a granulomatous response (Pallette et al, 1967). Also, involvement often is outside the pelvis and envelops a number of organs that may include the aorta, inferior vena cava, duodenum, colon, small bowel, and common bile duct. Certainly, most reported cases of pelvic lipomatosis have not been associated with the type of involvement described in Dercum's disease and sclerosing lipogranulomatosis. It is interesting to speculate about the possible connection between pelvic lipomatosis and other lipodystrophies, such as mesenteric Weber-Christian disease (relapsing febrile nodular nonsuppurative panniculitis). **Pelvic lipomatosis has been associated with a variety of diverse and often unrelated disorders including: cystitis cystica, cystitis glandularis, adenocarcinoma of the bladder, chronic urinary tract infection, hypertension, superficial thrombophlebitis, constipation, vesicoureteral reflux, retroperitoneal fibrosis, nontropical chyluria, and the *Proteus* syndrome** (Heyns et al, 1991; Gosfield and Siegel, 1992). Until more is known about the cause and natural history of these diseases, pelvic lipomatosis should be considered a separate entity.

On pathologic examination, the lipomatous tissue is found to be composed of mature fatty cells with or without inflammation. The inflammatory response is generally chronic and nonspecific in nature. Varying degrees of fibrosis and adhesions have been reported (Heyns and Allen, 1992). Evidence of a neoplasm is uniformly lacking.

Pelvic lipomatosis is generally found in overweight patients, but most patients have not been grossly obese. Occasionally, the disease is discovered incidentally in an individual who has no presenting symptoms. When symptoms are present, they usually vary and suggest nonspecific disease referable to the pelvis or urinary tract. Symptoms include backache, suprapubic discomfort, perineal pain, low-grade fever, recurrent urinary tract infections, urinary frequency, and dysuria. In a review of the literature, Barry and associates (1973) found that **only half of patients had difficulty with voiding despite gross deformity of the posterior urethra and base of the bladder.** Occasionally, a patient may present with the sequelae of obstructive uropathy and uremia. Although rectal compression frequently occurs, gastrointestinal symptoms are minimal, with the exception of constipation in some patients; only one case of large bowel obstruction has been reported (Jones et al, 1985). Two cases of venous obstruction with complete occlusion of the inferior vena cava and one with left external iliac vein blockage have been reported (Schechter, 1974; Locko and Interrante, 1980).

On physical examination, a suprapubic mass may be palpable. Elevation of the prostate gland may be apparent on rectal examination. Several authors have stressed the frequency of hypertension occurring in patients with pelvic lipomatosis (Moss et al, 1972; Cook et al, 1973), but this finding has been variable. Because of ureteral compression, patients may be azotemic at time of presentation (Crane and Smith, 1977). Cystoscopy is generally difficult or impossible to perform because of elongation and elevation of the trigone and bladder neck. An increased incidence of edema of the bladder and cystitis glandularis has been noted in association with pelvic lipomatosis. Yalla and associates (1975) reported two cases of cystitis glandularis in patients with pelvic lipomatosis and found that six of eight patients in the literature who had undergone endoscopic evaluation were found to have variants of proliferative cystitis, notably cystitis glandularis. They suggested that the majority of patients with pelvic lipomatosis who could not be subjected to cystoscopy for technical reasons may have had proliferative cystitis. The cause of these associated proliferative changes in the bladder remains obscure.

The diagnosis of pelvic lipomatosis is established on radiographic examination. The plain film of the abdomen (kidney, ureter, and bladder [KUB]) may show radiolucent areas of lipomatous tissue in the bony pelvis, but often the degree of lucency is difficult to quantitate. Albert and associates (1972) emphasized that the differentiation of pelvic lipomatosis from malignant neoplasm without laparotomy depends on demonstration of the typical radiolucency surrounding the bladder and rectum.

The intravenous urogram (IVP) usually demonstrates normal upper tracts, but on occasion there may be severe hydroureteronephrosis or, more often, mild distal ureterectasia. Characteristically, the distal ureters are displaced medially, similar to what is observed in retroperitoneal fibrosis. **Elevation of vertical elongation of the bladder is seen best on a cystogram but also may be noted on the IVP (Fig. 10–26).** The bladder is typically pear-shaped as a result of the compression effect on the bladder base. Associated with this change is also marked elevation of the bladder base. Evidence of mucosal thickening secondary to inflammation and edema can be detected, as can other disorders of the bladder (e.g., cystitis glandularis). Classically, there are also straightening and elevation of the rectosigmoid on a barium enema study. The degree of extrinsic compression may vary, but the mucosal pattern is not altered. Typically, the presacral space is widened. Because CT can distinguish between normal fat and other soft tissue densities, it is ideally suited for the diagnosis of pelvic lipomatosis (Jones et al, 1985) (Fig. 10–27). Pelvic and perivesical fat can usually be defined, and other conditions in the differentiated diagnosis can usually be identified.

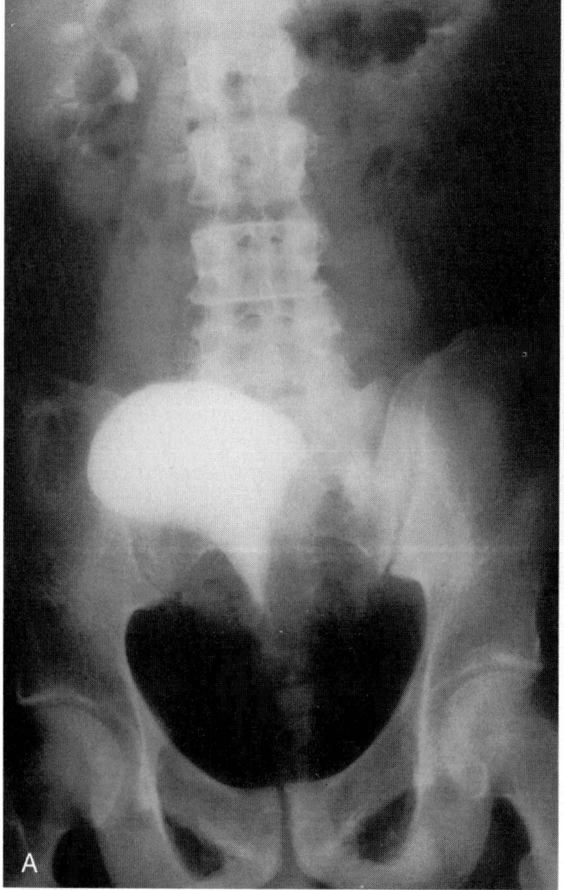

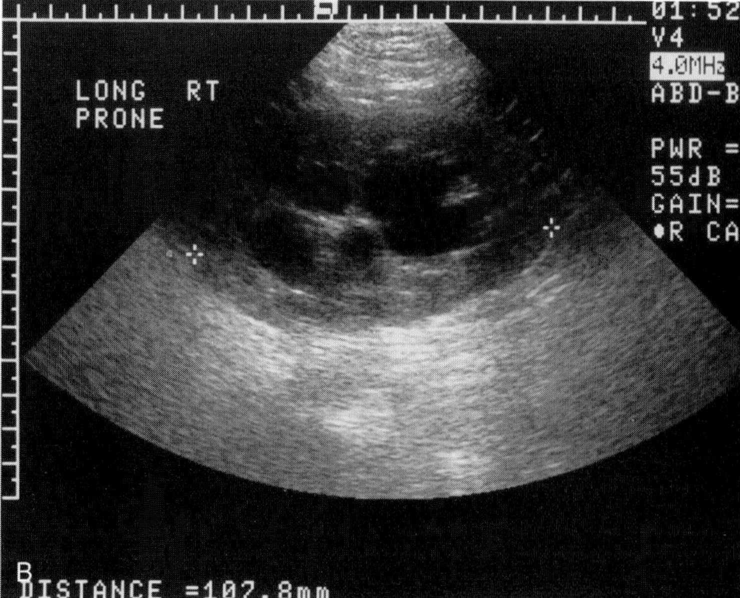

Figure 10–26. *A,* Excretory urogram demonstrating moderately severe right hydronephrosis and the classic vertical elongation of the bladder associated with pelvic lipomatosis. *B,* Abdominal ultrasonogram demonstrating characteristic findings of hydronephrosis. Note hypoechoic areas indicating dilated calyces.

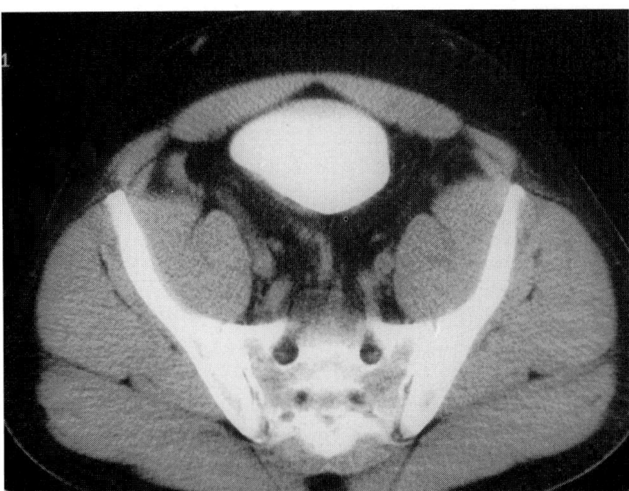

Figure 10–27. Computed tomogram demonstrating typical radiolucent findings associated with pelvic lipomatosis.

MRI is able to detail fatty masses, but it offers little benefit over CT except for definition of fat planes (Demas et al, 1988). Occasionally, ultrasonography is of value, but because of the marked echogenicity associated with fat and bowel gas, a specific diagnosis usually cannot be made (Rizzatto et al, 1982).

Pelvic arteriography is helpful, especially if there is suspicion of pelvic malignancy. Borjsen and Nilsson (1962) stated that arteriography can distinguish inflammatory disease from neoplastic disease. Inflammatory vessels are smaller (less than 0.3 mm in diameter) and the venous phase appears more rapidly in malignancy, whereas in nonmalignant conditions, this phase appears 10 to 15 seconds after injection. Some clinicians also advocate double- or triple-contrast arteriography with the suprapubic perivesical injection of carbon dioxide and intravesical air. This technique clearly demonstrates the pelvic vasculature. An increased vascular supply is always noted in pelvic lipomatosis, but the characteristic larger vessels, rapid venous filling, tumor stain, displacement, and amputation associated with malignancy are not found. Since the advent of CT, arteriographic studies have rarely been indicated.

Table 10–4. CAUSES OF A PEAR-SHAPED BLADDER*

Perivesical hematoma, urinoma, or abscess
Iliopsoas hypertrophy
Pelvic lipomatosis
Lymphoma in pelvic nodes or infiltrating around the bladder
Carcinoma (e.g., prostatic, in pelvic nodes, or infiltrating around the bladder)
Inferior vena cava obstruction
Bilateral lymphocysts or lymphoceles
Bilateral iliac aneurysms
Bilateral hip replacement with extruded cement
Pelvic fibrosis
Pancreatic pseudocysts
Gross prolapse
Scarring or edema
Hypoplastic lymphadenopathy
Ureteral compression balloons

From Saxton HM: Pelvic lipomatosis. *In* Pollack HM, ed: Clinical Urography. Philadelphia, W. B. Saunders, 1990, p 2458. Based on Ambos MA, Bosniac MA, Lefrew RS, Madayag MA: The pear-shaped bladder. Radiology 1977; 122:85. Courtesy of the Radiological Society of North America.

*Other descriptive terms have included *gourd-shaped* and *inverted teardrop* bladder.

A variety of disorders can mimic the bladder deformity typically noted in patients with pelvic lipomatosis (Table 10–4). Oftentimes the clinical history, patient manifestations, and laboratory studies are helpful in establishing the correct diagnosis. Imaging studies, particularly CT, are required to confirm suspicions. In most instances, the disease may be treated conservatively with diet control and massive weight reduction in obese patients. Exploratory laparotomy, which may be necessary if malignancy is suspected, demonstrates adipose tissue surrounding the bladder and rectosigmoid. Most authors have concluded that **the massive amount of fat present, the adherence of the fatty tissue to the pelvic organs, and the inability to find cleavage planes preclude adequate surgical removal.** In several instances, supravesical urinary diversion has been required for the treatment of marked ureteral obstruction (Crane and Smith, 1977). Carpenter (1973) reported the successful removal of fatty deposits in a patient with progressive ureteral dilation secondary to pelvic lipomatosis, in whom the upper tracts returned to normal after surgery. He emphasized that the assumption that the nature of the fatty deposits precludes an adequate operation is no longer warranted. The operation was difficult and time consuming, but with meticulous avoidance of the ureteral blood supply and preservation of a sheath of fat around the ureters, relief of ureteral obstruction was achieved. Others have also reported successful excision of the fatty tissue (Ballesteros, 1977).

Carpenter (1973) also noted that two general clinical groups have emerged from the reported cases. The first consists of young, stocky or obese men with vague pelvic symptoms in whom there is a definite risk of progressive ureteral obstruction developing. The second clinical group is characterized by men more than 60 years old in whom the disease is discovered during evaluation of related problems, often prostatism. There have been no serious sequelae and no significant progression of disease in this second group. Therefore, the patients who belong to the first group must be followed closely for the possibility of development of progressive obstruction of the upper urinary tracts. Patients who demonstrate progressive ureteral obstruction may be considered for surgical extirpation of the lipomatous tissue or, if this is not feasible, for supravesical urinary diversion.

As previously mentioned, **there is a high incidence of cystitis glandularis in patients with pelvic lipomatosis.** The development of adenocarcinoma in a patient with cystitis glandularis has also been noted (Edwards et al, 1972). On the basis of this observation and of the high incidence of adenocarcinoma of the bladder in patients with exstrophy (in whom proliferative cystitis is prevalent), the diagnosis of cystitis glandularis has a definite premalignant connotation. Although no cases of adenocarcinoma have been reported in association with pelvic lipomatosis, patients with this diagnosis should be evaluated and followed for the possibility of cystitis glandularis and the remote possibility of developing adenocarcinoma.

SUMMARY

Extrinsic ureteral obstruction may be discovered during the evaluation of a suspected genitourinary problem or as part of the routine diagnostic work-up for other conditions that are often involved or are associated with the ureter. It is now apparent that there are multiple disorders that may be responsible for extrinsic obstruction of the ureter. When an extrinsic ureteral obstruction is encountered, the urologist must proceed methodically with the diagnostic evaluation to ascertain both the site of occlusion and its cause. The history and physical examination must include a thorough evaluation of the urinary tract, the vascular system, the female reproductive system, and the gastrointestinal tract. As illustrated throughout this chapter, a careful history and physical examination often suggest a specific diagnosis. After the initial physical examination, which helps to subclassify the cause of obstruction, the laboratory and radiographic studies can be done in an intelligent and orderly manner to further confirm or identify the cause of obstruction. The urologist, constantly keeping in mind the classification of the multiple entities responsible for extrinsic ureteral obstruction, must avoid overlooking a possible diagnosis. Although it is not always possible to be entirely certain of the cause of obstruction until an exploratory operation is performed, an orderly evaluation can suggest the best operative approach. A thorough assessment allows a reasonably accurate diagnosis to be made in most instances, thus making appropriate therapy possible.

REFERENCES

Abbott DL, Skinner DG, Yalowitz PA, Mulder D: Abdominal aortic aneurysms: An approach to management. J Urol 1973; 109:987.

Abdel-Dayem HM, Mathew CV, Sahweil A, El-Sayed M: Inferior vena caval obstruction secondary to retroperitoneal fibrosis causing abnormal venous return to left lower limb to portal circulation. Clin Nucl Med 1984; 9:635.

Abeshouse BS, Abeshouse G: Endometriosis of the urinary tract. A review of the literature and a report of 4 cases of vesical endometriosis. J Int Coll Surg 1960; 34:43.

Adams JT: Retroperitoneal tumors. *In* Schwartz S, ed: Principles of Surgery. New York, McGraw-Hill, 1974, p 1339.

Albarran J: Retention renale per periureterite: Liberation externe de l-uretere Assoc Fr Urol 1905; 9:511.

Albers DD, Dee AL, Kalmon EH, et al: Irradiation injury to the ureter and surgical tolerance. Invest Urol 1976; 14:229.

Albert DJ, Herman GP, Persky L: Pelvic lipomatosis: Report of three cases. J Med (Basel) 1972; 3:282.

Alfert HJ, Gillenwater JY: The consequences of ureteral irradiation with special reference to subsequent ureteral injury. J Urol 1972; 107:369.

Al Saleh BMS: Endometriosis: An unusual cause of obstruction in duplex ureters. Br J Urol 1987; 60:469.

Altemeier WA, Culbertson WR, Fuller WD: *In* Welch CE, ed: Advances in Surgery, vol 5. Chicago, Year Book Medical Publishers, 1971.

Altvater G, Imholz G: Ureter Stenosen beim Kollum Karzinom [Ureteral stenosis in carcinoma of the cervix]. Geburtsh Fauenheik 1960; 20:1214.

Angell JL, Knuppel RA: Computed tomography in diagnosis of puerperal ovarian vein thrombosis. Obstet Gynecol 1984; 63:61.

Applegate GB, Bass KM, Kubick CJ: Ureteral obstruction as a complication of the Burch colposuspension procedure: Case report. Am J Obstet Gynecol 1987; 156:445.

Aronson DC, Moorman-Voestermans CGM, Tiel-vanBuul MMC, Vos A: A rare complication of acute appendicitis: Complete bilateral distal ureteral obstruction. Lancet 1994; 344:99.

Arrivé L, Hricak H, Tavares NJ, Miller TR: Malignant versus non-malignant retroperitoneal fibrosis: Differentiation with MR imaging. Radiology 1989; 172:139.

Bahnson RR, Wendel EF, Vogelzang RL: Renal vein thrombosis following puerperal ovarian vein thrombophlebitis. Am J Obstet Gynecol 1985; 152:290.

Bahrassa F, Ampil F: Post-treatment ureteral obstruction in invasive carcinoma of uterine cervix. Int J Radiat Oncol Biol Phys 1987; 13:23.

Baker LRI, Mallinson WJW, Gregory MC, et al: Idiopathic retroperitoneal fibrosis. A retrospective analysis of 60 cases. Br J Urol 1988; 60:497.

Ballesteros JJ: Surgical treatment of perivesical lipomatosis. J Urol 1977; 118:329.

Banner MP, Pollack HN, Ring EJ, Wein AJ: Catheter dilation of benign ureteral strictures. Radiology 1983; 147:427.

Banowsky LH, Francis J, Braun WE, Magnusson MO: Renal transplantation. II. Lymphatic complications. Urology 1974; 4:650.

Baran GW, Frisch KM: Duplex Doppler evaluation of puerperal ovarian vein thrombosis. AJR 1987; 149:321.

Barry JM, Bilbae MK, Hodges CV: Pelvic lipomatosis: A rare cause of a suprapubic mass. J Urol 1973; 109:592.

Bateson EM, Atkinson D: Circumcaval ureter: A new classification. Clin Radiol 1969; 20:173.

Bodner D, Kursh ED, Resnick MI: Palliative nephrostomy for relief of ureteral obstruction secondary to malignancy. Presented at North Central Section of American Urological Association meeting, Marco Island, FL, October 1982.

Borjsen E, Nilsson J: Angiography in the diagnosis of tumors of the urinary bladder. Acta Radiol 1962; 57:241.

Braash JW, Mon AB: Primary retroperitoneal tumors. Surg Clin North Am 1967; 47:663.

Brawer MK, Williams W, Witte CL, et al: Massive lymphocele following pelvic lymphadenectomy for staging of prostate cancer. Lymphology 1989; 22:36.

Brettauer J, Rubin IC: Hydroureter and hydronephrosis: A frequent secondary finding in cases of prolapse of the uterus and bladder. Am J Obstet Gynecol 1923; 6:696.

Brin E, Schiff M, Weiss R: Palliative urinary diversion for pelvic malignancy. J Urol 1975; 113:619.

Brooks RJ Jr, Fraser WE, Lucas WE: Endometriosis involving the urinary tract. J Urol 1969; 102:124.

Bullock N: Idiopathic retroperitoneal fibrosis. BMJ 1988; 23:297.

Burgos FJ, Teruel JL, Mayayo T, et al: Diagnosis and management of lymphoceles after renal transplantation. J Urol 1988; 61:289.

Bush IM: Obstruction of the lower ureter by aberrant vessels in children. J Urol 1972; 110:397.

Butt ZA, Morgan JDT, Osborn DE: Retroperitoneal haematoma causing acute renal failure. Br J Urol 1994; 74:119.

Carpenter AA: Pelvic lipomatosis: Successful surgical treatment. J Urol 1973; 110:397.

Carroll R, Laughton JW: Obstructive uropathy due to unusual pelvic swellings. Proc R Soc Med 1973; 66:1047.

Chapman RH: Ureteric obstruction due to uterine prolapse. Br J Urol 1975; 47:531.

Cietak KA, Newton JR: Serial qualitative maternal nephrosonography in pregnancy. Br J Radiol 1985; 58:399.

Cody HS III, Turnbull AD, Fortner JG, Hajdu SI: The continuing challenge of retroperitoneal sarcomas. Cancer 1981; 47:2147.

Cohan RH, Saeed M, Schwab JJ, et al: Povidone-iodine sclerosis of pelvic lymphoceles. Urol Radiol 1986; 1:203.

Cole-Beuglet C, Aulfrichtig D, Pais MJ, Cohen A: Ultrasound case of the day. Resolving hepatic and duodenal (retroperitoneal) hematoma. Radiographics 1987; 7:600.

Considine J: Retrocaval ureter. A review of the literature with a report on two new cases followed for fifteen years and two years, respectively. Brit J Urol 1966; 38:412.

Cook SA, Hayashi K, Lalli AF: Pelvic lipomatosis. Cleve Clin Q 1973; 40:35.

Crane DB, Smith MJV: Pelvic lipomatosis: 5-year follow-up. J Urol 1977; 118:547.

Cummings JA: Bilateral ureteric obstruction: An unusual late complication of ruptured ectopic pregnancy. Br J Urol 1988; 62:182.

Darke SG, Glass RE, Eadie DG: Abdominal aortic aneurysms, perianeurysmal fibrosis, and ureteric obstruction and deviation. Br J Surg 1977; 64:649.

Davis OK, Schiff I: Endometriosis with unilateral ureteral obstruction and hypertension. A case report. J Reprod Med 1988; 33:470.

Deane AM, Gingell JC, Pentlow BD: Idiopathic retroperitoneal fibrosis—The role of autotransplantation. Br J Urol 1983; 55:254.

D'Elia FL, Brennan RE, Brownstein PK: Acute renal failure secondary to ureteral obstruction by a gravid uterus. J Urol 1982; 128:803.

Demas BE, Avallone A, Hricak H: Pelvic lipomatosis: Diagnosis and

characterization by magnetic resonance imaging. Urol Radiol 1988; 10:198.
Docimo, SG, DeWolf WC: High failure rate of indwelling ureteral stents in patients with extrinsic obstruction: Experience at 2 institutions. J Urol 1989; 142:277.
Donovan AJ, Ragibson R: Identification of ureteral ligation during gynecologic operation. Am J Obstet Gynecol 1973; 116:793.
Downey DB, O'Connell DO, Smith J, Donohoe J: Percutaneous balloon dilatation of a mid-ureteric obstruction caused by retroperitoneal fibrosis. Br J Urol 1987; 60:84.
Dure-Smith P: Ovarian vein syndrome: Is it a myth? Urology 1979; 13:355.
Edwards DD, Hurm RA, Jaeschke WH: Conversion of cystitis glandularis to adenocarcinoma. J Urol 1972; 108:568.
Eika B, Skajaa K: Acute renal failure due to bilateral ureteral obstruction by the pregnant uterus. Urol Int 1988; 43:315.
Engels EP: Sigmoid colon and urinary bladder in high fixation: Roentgen changes simulating pelvic tumor. Radiology 1959; 72:419.
Erickson LM, Nicholson SF, Lewall DB, Frischke L: Ultrasound evaluation of hydronephrosis of pregnancy. J Clin Ultrasound 1979; 7:128.
Evans AT, Coughlin JP: Urinary obstruction due to renal cysts. J Urol 1970; 103:277.
Farha GJ, Hayes KA, Brenneis A: Contralateral retroperitoneal hematoma secondary to percutaneous ultrasonic lithotripsy. Urology 1987; 29:621.
Feldberg MAM, Hene RJ: Perianeurysmal fibrosis and its response to corticosteroid treatment: A computerized tomographic follow-up in 1 case. J Urol 1983; 130:1163.
Felix EL, Wood DK, Das Gupta TK: Tumors of the retroperitoneum. Curr Probl Cancer 1981; 6:1.
Finnerty DP, Trulock TS, Berkman W, Walton KN: Transluminal balloon dilation of ureteral strictures. J Urol 1984; 31:1056.
Finney RP: Experiences with new double J ureteral catheter stent. J Urol 1978; 120:678.
Fletcher EWL, Lecky JW: Retrocaval ureter obstructed by aberrant renal artery. J Urol 1971; 106:184.
Gatanaga H, Ohnishi S, Miura H, et al: Retroperitoneal fibrosis leading to extrahepatic portal vein obstruction. Intern Med 1994; 33:346.
Gilliland JD, Spies JB, Brown SB, et al: Lymphoceles: Percutaneous treatment with povidone-iodine sclerosis. Radiology 1989; 171:227.
Gohji K, Uehara H, Takagi S, et al: Ureteral stenosis secondary to common iliac aneurysm: A case report and review of the literature in Japan. Hinyokika Kiyo 1988; 34:1799.
Goldenberg SL, Gordon PB, Cooperberg PL, McLoughlin MG: Early hydronephrosis following aortic bifurcation graft surgery: A prospective study. J Urol 1988; 140:1367.
Goodman M, Dalton JR: Ureteral strictures following radiotherapy: Incidence, etiology, and treatment guidelines. J Urol 1982; 128:21.
Gosfield E, Siegel A: Renal scintigraphy in a patient with pelvic lipomatosis. Clin Nucl Med 1992; 17:630.
Graham JR: Methysergide for prevention of headache. N Engl J Med 1964; 170:67.
Graham JR, Suby HI, LeCompte PR, Sadowsky NL: Fibrotic disorders associated with methysergide therapy for headache. N Engl J Med 1966; 274:356.
Grainger DA, Soderston RM, Schiff SF, et al: Ureteral injuries at laparoscopy: Insights into diagnosis, management, and prevention. Obstet Gynecol 1990; 75:839.
Gup AJ: Retroperitoneal xanthogranuloma. J Urol 1972; 107:586.
Guyer PB, Delany D: Urinary tract dilatation and oral contraceptives. BMJ 1970; 4:588.
Harreby M, Bilde T, Helin P, et al: Retroperitoneal fibrosis treated with methylprednisolone pulse and disease-modifying antirheumatic drugs. Scand J Urol Nephrol 1994; 28:237.
Harrill HC: Retrocaval ureter. Report of a case with operative correction of the defect. J Urol 1940; 44:450.
Heller JE, Teggatz J: Idiopathic retroperitoneal fibrosis infiltrating ureteral wall. Urology 1992; 40:277.
Henry LG, Doust B, Korns ME, Bernhard VM: Abdominal aortic aneurysm and retroperitoneal fibrosis. Ultrasonographic diagnosis and treatment. Arch Surg 1978; 113:1456.
Herzog A, Minne H, Ziegler R: Retroperitoneal fibrosis in a patient with macroprolactinoma treated with bromocriptine. BMJ 1989; 298:215.
Hewitt CB, Nitz GL, Kiser WS, et al: Surgical treatment of retroperitoneal fibrosis. Ann Surg 1969; 169:610.
Heyns CF, Allen FJ: Pelvic lipomatosis or pericystitis plastica? Br J Urol 1992; 70:327.
Heyns CF, DeKock MLS, Kirsten PH, vanVelden DJJ: Pelvic lipomatosis associated with cystitis glandularis and adenocarcinoma of the bladder. J Urol 1991; 145:364.
Higgins PM, Bennett-Jones DN, Naish PF, Aber GM: Non-operative management of retroperitoneal fibrosis. Br J Surg 1988; 75:573.
Hirsch SA, Robertson H, Gorniowsky M: Arterial occlusion secondary to methyl methacrylate use. Arch Surg 1976; 111:204.
Honecke K, Butz M: Pelvic lipomatosis in a female: Diagnosis and initial therapy. Urol Int 1991; 46:93.
Horowitz M, Elguezabal A: Obstruction of the ureter by recent corpus luteum located in the retroperitoneum. J Urol 1966; 95:706.
Hovatanakul P, Eachempali U, Cavanagh D: Ureteral obstruction in chronic ectopic pregnancy. Am J Obstet Gynecol 1971; 110:311.
Huben RP, Schellhammer PF: Steroid therapy for ureteral obstruction after aortoiliac graft surgery. J Urol 1981; 125:881.
Hyams JA, Weinberg SR, Alley JL: Chronic ileitis with concomitant ureteritis: Case report. Am J Surg 1943; 61:117.
Immergut MA, Boldus R, Kollin CP, Rohif P: Management of ectopic pheochromocytoma producing ureteral obstruction. J Urol 1970; 104:337.
Iversen BM, Norduke E, Thunold SL: Retroperitoneal fibrosis during treatment with methyldopa. Lancet 1975; 2:302.
Izant R, Makker SP, Tucker A, Heymann W: Non-obstructive hydronephrosis. N Engl J Med 1974; 287:535.
Jing B, Wallace S, Zornoza J: Metastases to retroperitoneal and pelvic nodes. Computed tomography and lymphangiography. Radiol Clin North Am 1982; 20:511.
Jones DJ, Dharmeratnam R, Langstaff RJ: Large bowel obstruction due to pelvic lipomatosis. Br J Surg 1985; 72:309.
Jones JB, Evison G: Excretion urography before and after surgical treatment of procidentia. Br J Obstet Gynaecol 1977; 84:304.
Jones WG, Barie PS: Urological manifestations of acute appendicitis. J Urol 1988; 139:1325.
Joshi KK, Wise HA II: Pelvic lipomatosis: 9-year follow-up in a woman. J Urol 1983; 129:1233.
Karp W, Hafstrom LO, Jonsson PE: Retroperitoneal sarcoma: Ultrasonographic and angiographic evaluation. Br J Radiol 1980; 53:525.
Kaufman R, Grabstald H: Hydronephrosis secondary to ureteral obstruction by metastatic breast cancer. J Urol 1969; 102:569.
Kauppila A, Pietila K, Kontturi M: Simultaneous uterine phlebography and retrograde pyelography. A method of investigating ureteric dilatation following pregnancy. Br J Radiol 1972; 45:496.
Khan AU, Utz DL: Clinical management of cancer of prostate associated with bilateral ureteral obstruction. J Urol 1975; 113:816.
Kontogeorgos L, Vassilopoulos P, Tentes A: Bilateral severe hydroureterophrosis due to uterine prolapse. Br J Urol 1985; 57:360.
Kretkowski R, Shah N: Testicular vein syndrome. Unusual cause of hydronephrosis. Urology 1977; 10:253.
Kubota Y, Kawamura S, Ishii N, et al: Ureteral obstruction secondary to sigmoid diverticulitis. Urol Int 1988; 43:359.
Kumar S, Bhandari M: Selection of operative procedure for circumcaval ureter (type I). Br J Urol 1985; 57:399.
Kuntze JR, Park EC, Hardy BE, Herman MH: Acute appendicitis mimicking pelvic neoplasm. Urology 1988; 32:124.
Lane RH, Stephens DH, Reiman HM: Primary retroperitoneal neoplasms: CT findings in 90 cases with clinical and pathologic correlation. AJR 1989; 152:83.
Lattimer JK: Obstructive uropathy associated with uterine prolapse. Urology 1974; 4:73.
Lepor H, Walsh PC: Idiopathic retroperitoneal fibrosis. J Urol 1979; 122:1.
Letourneau JG, Day DL, Asher NL, Castaneda-Zuiniga WR: Imaging of renal transplants. AJR 1988; 150:833.
Locko RC, Interrante AL: Pelvic lipomatosis. Case of inferior vena caval obstruction. JAMA 1980; 244:1473.
Loffeld RJLF, van Weel THF: Tamoxifen for retroperitoneal fibrosis. Lancet 1993; 341:382.
Malaquin F, Urban T, Ostinelli J, et al: Pleural and retroperitoneal fibrosis from dihydroergotamine. N Engl J Med 1989; 321:1760.
Mann WJ, Vogel F, Patsner B, Chalas E: Management of lymphocysts after radical gynecologic surgery. Gynecol Oncol 1989; 33:248.
Martinez-Maldonado M, Romirez DeArellon G: Renal involvement in malignant lymphoma. Am J Med 1962; 32:184.
Mehl RL: Retroiliac artery ureter. J Urol 1969; 102:27.
Mikkelsen D, Lepor H: Innovative surgical management of idiopathic retroperitoneal fibrosis. J Urol 1989; 141:1192.
Mitchinson MJ: Insoluble lipids in human atherosclerotic plaques. Atherosclerosis 1982; 45:11.

Moore JG, Hibbard LT, Growdon WA, Schifrin BS: Urinary tract endometriosis. Am J Obstet Gynecol 1979; 134:162.

Moskovitz B, Braner B, Engel A, et al: Multifocal bleeding due to anticoagulant therapy. Urol Int 1988; 43:53.

Moss AA, Clark RE, Goldberg HI, Pepper HW: Pelvic lipomatosis: A roentgenographic diagnosis. Am J Roentgenol Radium Ther Nucl Med 1972; 115:411.

Ormond JK: Bilateral ureteral obstruction due to envelopment and compression by an inflammatory retroperitoneal process. J Urol 1948; 59:1072.

Pallette EM, Pallette EC, Harrington RW: Sclerosing lipogranulomatosis: Its several abdominal syndromes. Arch Surg 1967; 94:803.

Patel SK: Retroperitoneal tumors and cysts. *In* Pollack HM, ed: Clinical Urography, vol 3. Philadelphia, W. B. Saunders Company, 1990, p 2413.

Persky L, Hoch WH: Genitourinary tract trauma. Curr Probl Surg September 1972, pp 1–64.

Persky L, Huus JC: Atypical manifestations of retroperitoneal fibrosis. J Urol 1974; 111:340.

Pfister RC: Percutaneous sclerotherapy of symptomatic renal cysts and lymphoceles. *In* Pollack HM, ed: Clinical Urography, vol 3. Philadelphia, W. B. Saunders Company, 1990, p 2386.

Phillips JC: Spectrum of radiologic abnormalities due to tubo-ovarian abscess. Radiology 1974; 110:311.

Present DH, Rabinowitz JG, Banks PA, Janowitz HD: Obstructive hydronephrosis in regional ileitis. N Engl J Med 1963; 280:523.

Quattlebaum R, Anderson, A IV: Ureteral obstruction secondary to a patent umbilical artery in a 79-year-old man: A case report. J Urol 1985; 134:347.

Rhee RY, Gloviczki P, Luthra HS, et al: Iliocaval complications of retroperitoneal fibrosis. Am J Surg 1994; 168:179.

Rivlin ME, Krueger RD, Wiser WL: Danazol in the management of ureteral obstruction secondary to endometriosis. Fertil Steril 1985; 44:274.

Rizzatto G, Basadonna P, Delzotto A, et al: Pelvic lipomatosis: Diagnostic role of ultrasound and a case report. Eur J Radiol 1982; 2:313.

Rosenberg B, Hurwitz A, Hermann H: Dercum's disease with unusual retroperitoneal and perivesical fatty infiltration. Surgery 1963; 54:451.

Sacks D, Banner MP, Meranze SG, et al: Renal and related retroperitoneal abscesses: Percutaneous drainage. Radiology 1988; 167:447.

Saldino RM, Palubinskas AJ: Medial placement of the ureter: A normal variant which may simulate retroperitoneal fibrosis. J Urol 1972; 107:582.

Sant GR, Heaney JA, Parkhurst EC, Blaivas JG: Obstructive uropathy—A potentially serious complication of reconstructive vascular surgery. J Urol 1983; 129:16.

Saxton HM: Pelvic lipomatosis. *In* Pollack HM, ed: Clinical Urography, vol 3. Philadelphia, W. B. Saunders Company, 1990, p 2458.

Schechter LS: Venous obstruction in pelvic lipomatosis. J Urol 1974; 111:757.

Schofield PF, Staff WG, Moore T: Ureteral involvement in regional ileitis (Crohn's disease). J Urol 1968; 99:412.

Scott J, Foster R, Moore A: Retroperitoneal fibrosis and nonmalignant ileal carcinoma. J Urol 1987; 138:1435.

Scott T, Cerny JC: Nonidiopathic retroperitoneal fibrosis. J Urol 1971; 105:49.

Shingleton HM, Fowler WC Jr, Pepper FD Jr, Palumbo L: Ureteral strictures following therapy for carcinoma of the cervix. Cancer 1969; 24:77.

Siegel JH, Padula G, Yatto RP, Davis JE: Combined endoscopic and percutaneous approach for the treatment of ureterocolic strictures. Radiology 1982; 146:841.

Siminovitch JMP, Fazio VW: Ureteral obstruction secondary to Crohn's disease. Am J Surg 1980; 139:95.

Sklaroff DM, Gnaneswaran P, Sklaroff RB: Postirradiation ureteric stricture. Gynecol Oncol 1978; 6:538.

Slater JM, Fletcher GH: Ureteral strictures after radiation therapy for carcinoma of the uterine cervix. AJR 1971; 111:269.

Spirnak JP, Hampel N, Resnick MI: Ureteral injuries complicating vascular surgery: Is repair indicated? J Urol 1989; 141:13.

Sterzer SK, Herr HW, Mintz I: Idiopathic retroperitoneal fibrosis misinterpreted as lymphoma by computerized tomography. J Urol 1979; 122:405.

Stevenson E, Ozeran R: Retroperitoneal space abscesses. Surg Gynecol Obstet 1969; 128:1202.

Stone MM, Stone NN, Meller S, Kim U: Bilateral ureteral obstruction: An unusual complication of pancreatitis. Am J Gastroenterol 1989; 84:49.

Talner LB: Specific causes of obstruction. *In* Pollack HM, ed: Clinical Urography, vol 2. Philadelphia, W. B. Saunders Company, 1990, p 1629.

Tracy D, Eisenberg R, Hedgecock M: Urinary obstruction resulting from prosthetic graft surgery. Am J Roentgenol Radium Ther Nucl Med 1979; 132:415.

Ulm AH, Klein E: Management of ureteral obstruction produced by recurrent cancer of rectosigmoid colon. Surg Gynecol Obstet 1960; 110:413.

Underwood PB Jr, Lutz MH, Smoak DL: Ureteral injury following irradiation therapy for carcinoma of the cervix. Obstet Gynecol 1977; 49:663.

Utz DC, Henry JD: Retroperitoneal fibrosis. Med Clin North Am 1966; 50:1091.

Utz DC, Moghaddam A: The clinical guise of retroperitoneal fibrosis. Clin Obstet Gynecol 1967; 10:238.

Wagenknecht LV, Madsen PO: Bilateral ureteral obstruction secondary to aortic aneurysm. J Urol 1970; 103:732.

Walther JM, Romas NA, Lowe FC: Barium granuloma: An unusual cause of unilateral ureteral obstruction. J Urol 1987; 138:614.

Whitaker RH: Urodynamic assessment of ureteral obstruction in retroperitoneal fibrosis. J Urol 1975; 113:26.

Whitehouse GH: The radiology of urinary tract abnormalities associated with hysterectomy. Clin Radiol 1977; 28:201.

Williams TJ: The role of surgery in the management of endometriosis. Mayo Clin Proc 1975; 50:198.

Witten DM: Retroperitoneal fibrosis. *In* Pollack HM, ed: Clinical Urography, vol 3. Philadelphia, W. B. Saunders Company, 1990, p 2469.

Wrenn JJ, Assimos DG: Ureteral obstruction secondary to a vena caval clip. J Urol 1988; 140:1014.

Yalla SV, Duker M, Burkos HM, Dorey F: Cystitis glandularis with perivesical lipomatosis: Frequent association of two unusual proliferative conditions. Urology 1975; 5:383.

Yetim MB, Sener RN: Ureteral obstruction owing to overpressure of a normal right common iliac artery: A case report. J Urol 1988; 140:365.

Zaitoon MM: Ureteral obstruction secondary to retained ovarian remnants: A case report and review of the literature. J Urol 1987; 137:973.

Zalar JA, McDonald JW: Ureteral obstruction and vessel compression secondary to hematoma of rectus abdominis muscle. J Urol 1969; 102:47.

Zimskind PD, Fetter TR, Wilkerson JL: Clinical use of long-term indwelling silicone rubber ureteral splints inserted cystoscopically. J Urol 1967; 97:840.

11 RENOVASCULAR HYPERTENSION AND OTHER RENAL VASCULAR DISEASES

E. Darracott Vaughan, Jr., M.D.
R. Ernest Sosa, M.D.

Renovascular disease is one of the most common causes of secondary hypertension; the rate of detection rises as more definitive diagnostic tests are developed. The need for identification of the entity is apparent. Although this type of hypertension is now more readily controlled with new forms of medical therapy than before (Hunt and Strong, 1973; Textor, 1994), many renal lesions are progressive (Schreiber et al, 1984; Strandness, 1994a), leading to the defined entity ischemic nephropathy (Guzman et al, 1994; Novick et al, 1996; Pickering et al, 1996).

Fortunately, newer diagnostic tests do not require hospitalization to identify these patients (Sosa and Vaughan, 1989; Pohl, 1993; Wilcox, 1993; Nally et al, 1994; Prigent et al, 1994), and the tests have reduced the previous high cost of evaluation, resulting in a more aggressive diagnostic approach. Emphasis has centered on developing accurate tests to identify the **5% of hypertensive patients with this entity**. Criteria for angioplasty or renal revascularization are more clearly defined (Novick, 1995; Pickering and Mann, 1995; Pickering et al, 1996).

HISTORICAL BACKGROUND

Richard Bright, Physician Extraordinary to the Queen of England, was the first to associate proteinuria, fullness and hardness of the pulse, and dropsy with "hardening of the kidneys" (Bright, 1827). In 1856, Traube, from an analysis of pulse tracings, suggested that the abnormality might be high blood pressure, and Mohomed (1874) demonstrated "high tension in the arterial system" in association with renal disease.

The critical experimental work was the discovery of renin by Tigerstedt and Bergmann (1898), who noted an increase in arterial blood pressure in rabbits injected with a saline renal extract. **They reasoned that the renal extract contained a pressor substance and coined the term "renin."** However, the significance of their work was not recognized until the critical experiments by Goldblatt and colleagues (1934), who produced diastolic hypertension in dogs by clamping the main renal arteries and corrected the hypertension by clamp removal.

Soon thereafter, Butler (1937) reported the first reversal of hypertension following nephrectomy in a patient with a small "pyelonephritic kidney"; 1 year later, Leadbetter reported another cure of hypertension in a child with pathologic signs of a renal arterial lesion (Leadbetter and Burkland, 1938).

These clinical observations were paralleled by laboratory investigation, and in 1940 Page and Braun-Menendez independently reported that renin itself was not a pressor substance but acted as an enzyme to release a pressor peptide, now called angiotensin, from a circulating plasma globulin (Braun-Menendez et al, 1940; Page and Helmer, 1940). Goormaghtigh, who had previously described the juxtaglomerular cells, then described increased granularity of these cells in both animals and humans with renal hypertension and postulated that these cells were secreting excessive amounts of renin (Goormaghtigh and Grimson, 1939).

There followed an aggressive but disappointing clinical experience with nephrectomy for cure of hypertension in patients with unilateral renal disease. This experience led to the search for a way of proving that a renal lesion was actually causing the hypertension. Smith (1948), reviewing the literature, reported relief of hypertension in only 19% of 200 patients whose elevated blood pressure was thought to result from unilateral renal disease. Thus it became apparent that even if pressor mechanisms did underlie some forms of renal hypertension, there were no ways to measure them.

This challenge led to studies of the effect of renal artery constriction on renal function. In dogs, renal artery constriction resulted in a marked decrease in sodium and water excretion from the affected kidney (Blake et al, 1950; Pitts and Duggan, 1950). In 1954, Howard used these observations to develop a differential renal function test based on bilateral ureteral catheterization to identify the "ischemic kidney" (Howard and Conner, 1954). Another major advance was the development of translumbar aortography and demonstration of its value in visualizing renal arterial lesions (Smith et al, 1952). By 1957, the first large series of studies of patients with renal arterial lesions was reported (Poutasse and Dustan, 1957).

In addition, interest in what would become known as the renin-angiotensin-aldosterone system was also emerging as new discoveries were made. Accordingly, it was determined that there were two forms of angiotensin (Skeggs et al, 1954), and angiotensin was sequenced (Skeggs et al, 1956) and synthesized (Bumpus et al, 1957). These critical advancements led to accurate radioimmunoassay for angiotensin, the development of angiotensin analogues, and angiotensin converting enzyme inhibitors, all major tools now used to identify the patient with renovascular hypertension. More recently the presence of a family of angiotensin receptors has been clarified (Kang et al, 1994; Goodfriend et al, 1996).

It is now recognized that the renin-angiotensin-aldosterone system is a critical integrated system regulating not only blood pressure, sodium balance, and potassium balance but also regional blood flow and, in particular, glomerular filtration rate (Gunning et al, 1996; Laragh and Blumenfeld, 1996). Moreover, there is an expanding body of literature implicating angiotensin II in cell proliferation and interstitial fibrosis (Mai et al, 1993; Eng et al, 1994; Stoll et al, 1995; Egido, 1996; Gunning et al, 1996).

DEFINITIONS

Hypertension

As strange as it may seem, it has been difficult to establish a precise definition of hypertension. The problem was best stated by Sir George Pickering, who wrote that "there is no dividing line. The relationship between arterial blood pressure and mortality is quantitative; the higher the pressure the worse the prognosis" (Pickering and Pickering, 1995; Pickering et al, 1996). Indeed, cumulative data obtained from insurance companies have validated this point! **Untreated blood pressure in excess of 140/90 is associated with excess mortality, and diastolic pressures below 70 mm Hg are optimal** (Lew, 1973). For operational purposes, the World Health Organization has defined hypertension in adults as a systolic pressure greater than 160 mm Hg and/or a diastolic pressure greater than 95 mm Hg. In addition, consistent elevation of blood pressure should be established

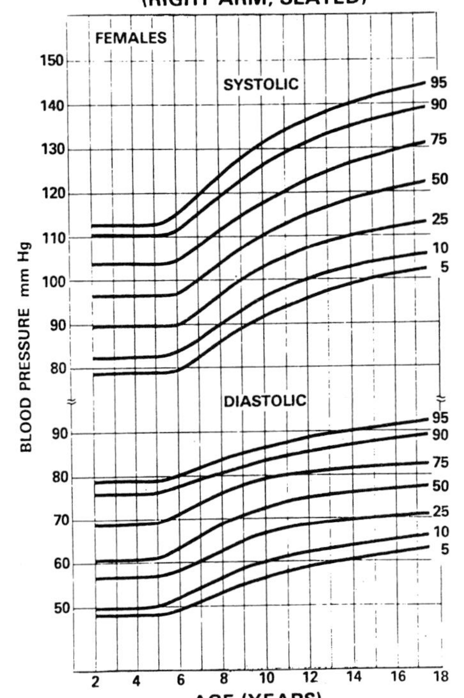

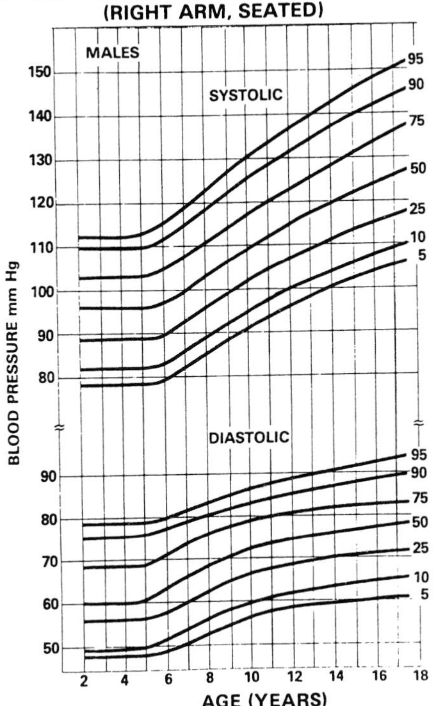

Figure 11–1. Distribution curves for seated blood pressure readings in male and female children from ages 2 to 18 years. (From Loggie JHM: Hypertension in the child and adolescent. *In* Brunner HR, Gavras H, eds: Clinical Hypertension and Hypotension. New York, Marcel Dekker, 1982, pp 351–365.)

with repeated readings before evaluation is instituted. In children, there is a rise in blood pressure with age; an upper normal limit of 130/80 is reached by ages 12 to 15 years. The most accurate evaluation, with the use of an appropriately small cuff, requires comparison of the measured blood pressure with a standard nomogram showing blood pressure related to age (Fig. 11–1) (Sinaiko and Wells, 1990; Sadowski and Falkner, 1996).

Renal Arterial Disease Versus Renovascular Hypertension

The development of arteriography provided an accurate means of identifying renal arterial disease and heralded the advent of renal arterial vascular repair (Freeman et al, 1954), which renewed enthusiasm for surgical management of the disease. However, it soon became apparent that normotensive patients undergoing arteriography for other reasons often had renal arterial disease (Eyler et al, 1962), especially those with arteriosclerotic disease (Wilms et al, 1990), and autopsy figures supported the radiologic findings (Holley et al, 1964). **Accordingly, the finding of renal arterial disease alone is not sufficient justification to warrant correction in a hypertensive patient. The lesion must be functionally significant** (i.e., it must reduce blood flow by an amount sufficient to activate renin release, initiating renovascular hypertension). Hence, a **practical definition of renovascular hypertension is hypertension resulting from a renal arterial lesion that is relieved by correction of the offending lesion or removal of the kidney.**

It is not surprising that not all renal arterial lesions cause renovascular hypertension. Mann and co-workers (1938) showed that the **internal diameter of the carotid artery could be reduced 70% before a significant fall in blood flow occurred** (Fig. 11–2). Similarly, Goldblatt and colleagues (1934) realized that a critical degree of renal arterial stenosis had to be reached before there was sufficient pres-

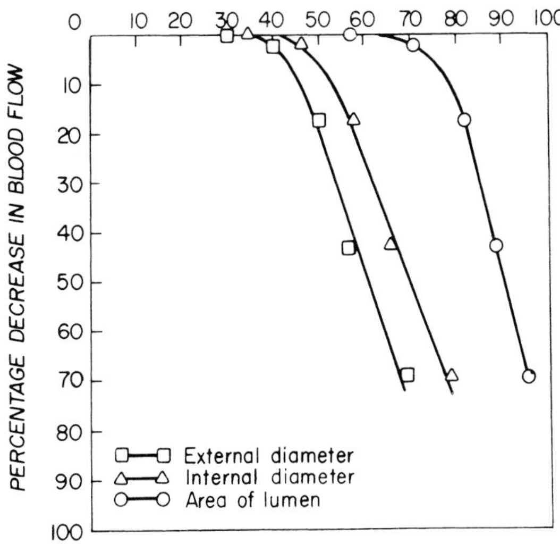

Figure 11–2. The effect of progressive arterial constriction on blood flow distal to the stenotic area. (From Mann FC, Herrick JF, Essex HE, Baldes EJ: Surgery 1938; 4:249.)

Table 11–1. CLASSIFICATION AND NATURAL HISTORY OF RENOVASCULAR DISEASE

Atherosclerosis: Proximal intimal plaques. Seen predominantly in males and usually in older age groups. Progressive in about 40 per cent of patients; may dissect or thrombose. May involve renal arteries only or may involve carotid and coronary arteries, aorta, and other vessels.

Intimal Fibroplasia: Collagenous disease involving intima; seen in children and young male adults. Progressive; may dissect. May involve other vessels.

True Fibromuscular Hyperplasia: Diffusely involves media. Seen in children and young adults. Progressive. Radiographically indistinguishable from intimal fibroplasia. Very rare.

Medial Fibroplasia: Series of collagenous rings involving media of main renal artery, often extending into branches. Usually seen in women in the thirties and forties. Produces typical "string of beads" pattern in angiography. Does not dissect, thrombose, or rupture and seldom progresses after age 40. May involve other vessels.

Perimedial (Subadventitial) Fibroplasia: Dense collagenous collar involving outer media, just beneath adventitia of vessel. Tightly stenotic, with extensive collateral circulation on angiography. Seen mostly in young women ("girlie disease"). Progressive. Involves renal arteries only.

Miscellaneous: Renal artery aneurysms, middle aortic syndrome, periarterial fibrosis, and post-traumatic intimal or medial disease. Variable in location and obstruction; occurs in diverse clinical settings.

From Stewart BH, Dustan HP, Kiser WS, et al: J Urol 1970; 104:231.

sure gradient and flow reduction to initiate hypertension. This observation was carried further by Selkurt (1951), who showed that a 40–mm Hg gradient across a renal artery stenosis was required before there was a change in renal plasma flow, glomerular filtration, sodium excretion, and urinary flow rate. Taken all together, the renal vascular anatomy is important as a guide for choice of transluminal angioplasty or surgical repair, but the demonstration of a renal vascular lesion alone is inadequate for predicting the blood pressure response following correction of the obstructing lesion.

Cure Following Correction of Renal Artery Stenosis

Inherent in the care of patients with renovascular hypertension is close and continuing postoperative blood pressure recording. In fact, sustained blood pressure response at least 1 year after surgical correction or angioplasty is mandatory before the diagnosis of renovascular hypertension is validated. In the past, the definition of "successful" revascularization was often arbitrary, especially in terms of the category "improvement," defined as a 15% decrease in diastolic pressure or "blood pressure easier to control with antihypertensive medications" (Foster et al, 1975).

The definition of a surgical response now should be predicated on reversal of the pathophysiologic abnormalities underlying renovascular hypertension. Hence patients with inadequate blood pressure responses to revascularization or angioplasty intervention require repeat evaluation. **Postintervention renal duplex sonography may prove to be a noninvasive method for monitoring patients** (Hudspeth et al, 1993). We have found that persistence of the criterial characteristics of renovascular hypertension (postoperatively) signifies technical failure of renal revascularization (Vaughan et al, 1979). In contrast, after successful renal angioplasty and normalization of blood pressure, the peripheral plasma renin activity indexed to sodium excretion usually returns to normal, and bilateral symmetric renal renin secretion resumes (Pickering et al, 1984).

PATHOLOGY

The two major pathologic entities that cause renal arterial disease are atherosclerosis and fibromuscular disease. The Cleveland Clinic group has emphasized the importance of the various distinct histologic patterns, identifiable by angiographic techniques, that have predictable natural histories (Schreiber et al, 1984, 1989; Novick et al, 1994). Their classification is shown in Table 11–1.

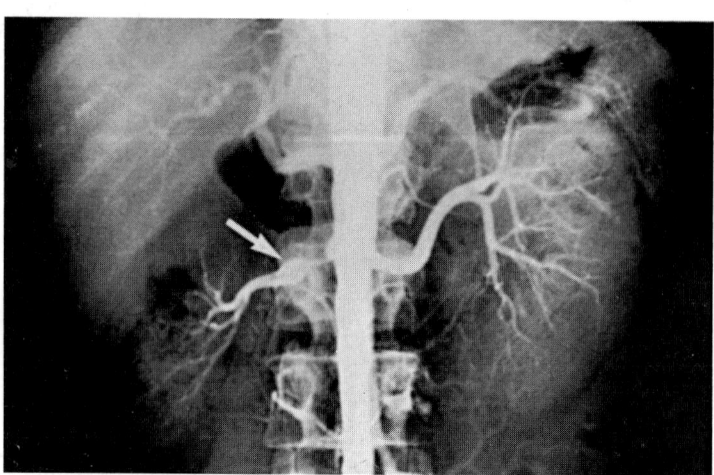

Figure 11–3. Severe atherosclerotic stenosis of the proximal right renal artery in an elderly man. Note the poststenotic arterial dilatation *(arrow).* (From Walter JF, Bookstein JJ: Angiography of renovascular hypertension. *In* Stanley JC, Ernst CB, Fry WJ, eds: Renovascular Hypertension. Philadelphia, W.B. Saunders Company, 1984.)

Atherosclerosis

Atheromatous lesions of the renal artery are common and account for about 60% to 70% of the lesions that cause renovascular hypertension. They usually occur in the proximal 2 cm of the renal artery, including the aorta (ostial lesions), but can involve the distal artery or branches (Fig. 11–3). The natural history of this disease has been described, and the stage of the disease may prove to be a major factor in the response to transluminal renal angioplasty. Atherosclerosis begins as a proliferation of smooth muscle or myointimal cells in the intima. As they proliferate, they form a rounded eccentric mound that protrudes into the lumen. The fully formed initial lesion consists of a mass of smooth muscle cells with a varying amount of connective tissue. Subsequently, lipid deposition occurs, with necrosis, inflammation, and the formation of an atherosclerotic plaque. Local complications of hemorrhage, calcification, or surface erosion with secondary thrombus formation may ensue (Fig. 11–4). Accordingly, the early lesion may be amenable to percutaneous angioplasty, whereas the mature lesion is more difficult to traverse, more rigid, and more likely to shed atheromatous emboli (Ratliff, 1985). Total reversal of hypertension after correction of atherosclerotic lesions is less common than in patients with fibromuscular disease. These patients often have diffuse atherosclerotic disease and underlying essential hypertension. **In the cooperative study of renovascular hypertension, patients with bilateral atherosclerotic disease had the lowest cure rate and the highest morbidity rate of the various groups operated upon** (Foster et al, 1975). However, attention to concurrent carotid and coronary disease before renal revascularization and avoidance of a severely diseased aorta have markedly reduced the morbidity of reconstructive surgery in this group (Novick et al, 1981; Novick, 1981; Novick et al, 1996).

Intimal Fibroplasia

This lesion is characterized by circumferential accumulation of collagen compromising the lumen inside the internal elastic membrane (Fig. 11–5). It occurs in children and young adults and is almost always progressive. It may be complicated by dissection, and it accounts for 10% of the total number of fibrous lesions. Angiography reveals a smooth, fairly focal stenosis that usually involves the midportion of the vessel or its branches (Fig. 11–6). Because of the progression and dissection, the lesion should be corrected when identified.

Fibromuscular Hyperplasia

This rare lesion, composing only 2% to 3% of the total, is the only one in which true hyperplasia of the smooth muscle and fibrous tissue is present. The angiographic picture may be indistinguishable from that of intimal fibroplasia. It also occurs in children and young adults, and because it is progressive, intervention is warranted.

Medial Fibroplasia

This lesion is usually referred to as fibromuscular hyperplasia, a misnomer because it does not consist of true muscle hyperplasia. It has the typical "string of beads" pattern (Fig. 11–7) on angiography, which is caused by the presence of a series of fibrous rings interspersed with aneurysmal dilatations. The aneurysms themselves are larger in diameter than the normal renal artery, and the actual degree of stenosis is difficult to assess. **It is the most common fibrous lesion, constituting 75% to 80% of the total, and characteristically occurs in women between the ages of 20 and 50**

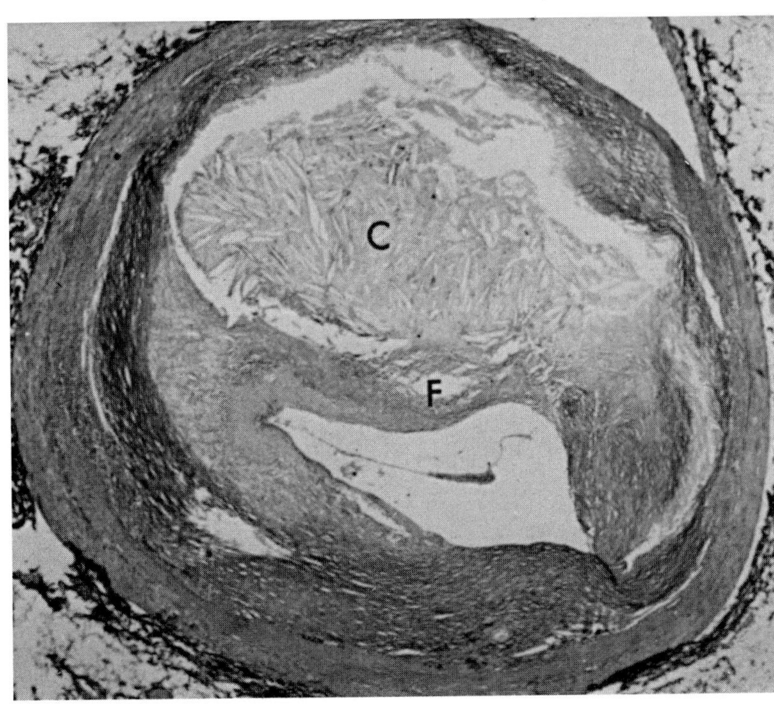

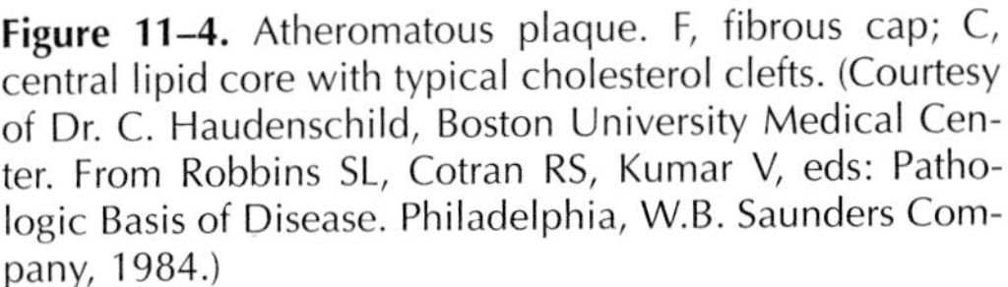
Figure 11–4. Atheromatous plaque. F, fibrous cap; C, central lipid core with typical cholesterol clefts. (Courtesy of Dr. C. Haudenschild, Boston University Medical Center. From Robbins SL, Cotran RS, Kumar V, eds: Pathologic Basis of Disease. Philadelphia, W.B. Saunders Company, 1984.)

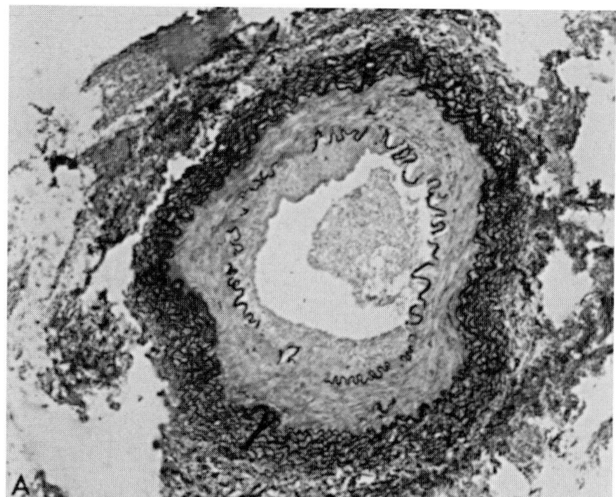

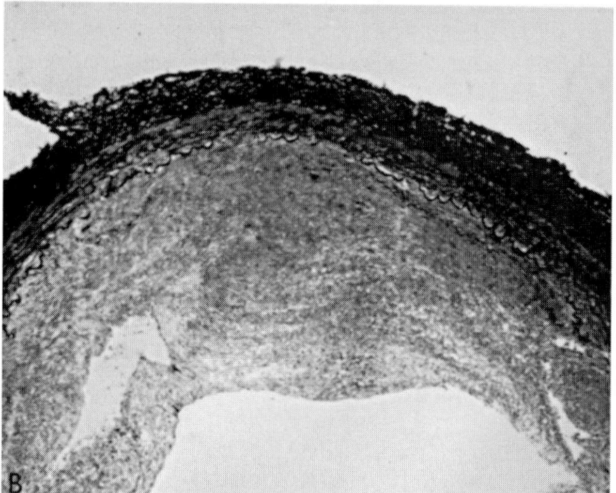

Figure 11–5. *A*, Photomicrograph of cross section demonstrating intimal fibroplasia with focal fragmentation and partial absence of the elastica interna. *B*, Photomicrograph of cross section demonstrating severe renal arterial intimal fibroplasia with a dense cuff of intimal collagen apposed to the luminal surface of a partially disrupted elastica interna. A small recannulized channel is noted in the lower left. (From Novick AC: Renal vascular hypertension in children. *In* Kelalis PP, King LR, Belman AB, eds: Clinical Pediatric Urology. Philadelphia, W.B. Saunders Company, 1984.)

years. The lesion does not hemorrhage or dissect, but it may progress (Schreiber et al, 1984, 1989). Intervention is indicated in younger patients, but older patients probably can be treated with antihypertensive agents if renal function and renal size are carefully monitored.

Perimedial (Subadventitial) Fibroplasia

This is a tightly stenotic lesion with dense collagen within intact adventitia (Fig. 11–8). In this case, the arterial beading is the result of constriction, and the beads are smaller than the diameter of the normal artery (Fig. 11–9). The lesion, accounting for 10% to 15% of the fibrous disorders, is progressive and is seen primarily in young females. It occurs only in the renal artery and predominantly involves the right side. Repair of the lesion is indicated because of progression and the severe hypertension that usually accompanies the disease.

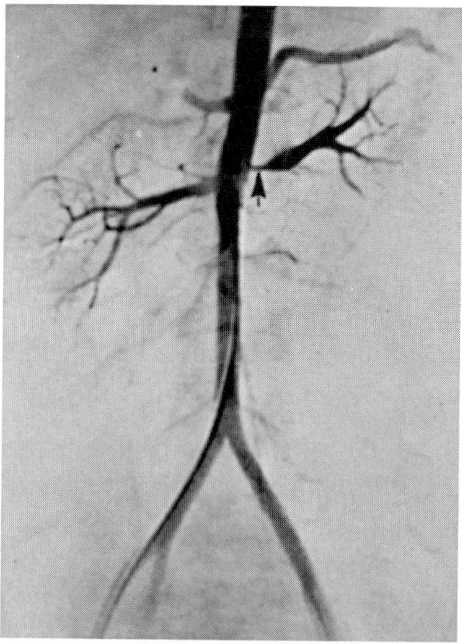

Figure 11–6. Aortogram of a 6-year-old boy demonstrates proximal left renal artery stenosis *(arrow)* from intimal fibroplasia. (From Novick AC: Renal vascular hypertension in children. *In* Kelalis PP, King LR, Belman AB, eds: Clinical Pediatric Urology. Philadelphia, W.B. Saunders Company, 1984.)

Alternative classifications differentiate fibrosis from muscular hyperplasia and suggest different responses to treatment (Alimi et al, 1992). However, the experience is limited. The role of angiotensin II in the fibrotic process is a subject for future study.

Miscellaneous Lesions

Takayasu's aortitis is a chronic sclerosing aortitis of unknown etiology that may involve the renal arteries (Rose

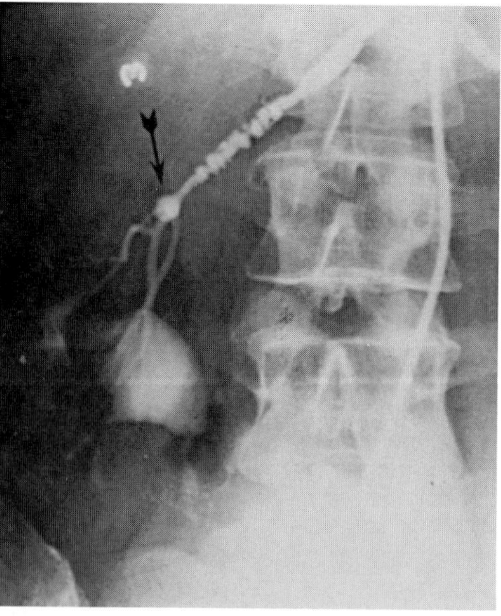

Figure 11–7. Selective right renal arteriogram reveals medial fibroplasia involving the main renal artery with typical "string of beads" appearance. (From Novick AC: Renal vascular hypertension in children. *In* Kelalis PP, King LR, Belman AB, eds: Clinical Pediatric Urology. Philadelphia, W.B. Saunders Company, 1984.)

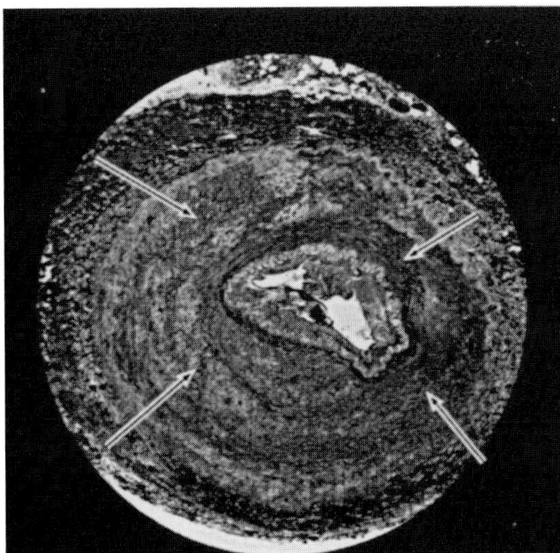

Figure 11–8. Cross section of the main renal artery in a girl with perimedial fibroplasia, demonstrating a dense collagenous collar involving the outer media of the vessel, which causes a severe progressive stenosis. (From Novick AC: Renal vascular hypertension in children. *In* Kelalis PP, King LR, Belman AB, eds: Clinical Pediatric Urology. Philadelphia, W.B. Saunders Company, 1984.)

and Sinclair-Smith, 1980). The disease is progressive and difficult to manage, but it has been treated with angioplasty (Kumar et al, 1990).

Renal vascular lesions can also develop after irradiation (McGill et al, 1979), in association with neurofibromatosis (Halpern and Currarino, 1965) or in association with a variety of other diseases (Gephardt and McCormack, 1982) (Table 11–2). Moreover, hypertension can be caused by a number of unilateral renal parenchymal diseases (Sosa and Vaughan, 1989).

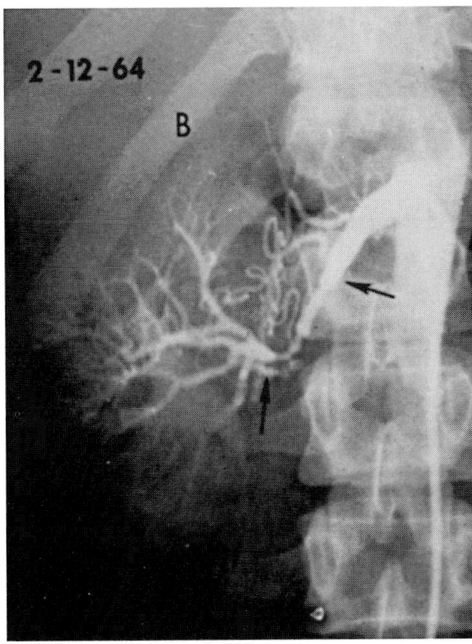

Figure 11–9. Renal arteriogram in patient with perimedial fibroplasia, showing slightly irregular yet severe stenosis of the midrenal artery associated with extensive collateral circulation to the kidney. The small size of the arterial irregularities and the presence of collateral circulation distinguishes this lesion radiographically from medial fibroplasia. (From Novick AC: Renal vascular hypertension in children. *In* Kelalis PP, King LR, Belman AB, eds: Clinical Pediatric Urology. Philadelphia, W.B. Saunders Company, 1984.)

NATURAL HISTORY

Relatively few reports exist on the natural history of renal artery lesions. However, in an important study, Cragg and colleagues (1989) reviewed the results of 1862 renal arteriograms obtained from potential renal donors. Fibromuscular dysplasia was present in 71 patients (3.8%). Of 30 normotensive patients who did not undergo nephrectomy, eight (26.6%) developed hypertension over a mean follow-up period of 7.5 years. This information in normotensive patients complements data from several longitudinal angiographic studies of hypertensive patients showing progression in

Table 11–2. OTHER VASCULAR LESIONS OR DISEASES ASSOCIATED WITH HYPERTENSION

Intrinsic Lesions

Vascular

Aneurysm (Perry: Arch Surg, 102:216, 1971)
Emboli (Arakawa: Arch Intern Med, 129:958, 1972)
Arteritis
  Polyarteritis nodosa (Dornfield, 215:1950, 1971)
  Takayasu's (Kirschbaum: Am Heart J, 80:811, 1970)
Arteriovenous fistula (Bennet: Am J Roentgenol Radium Ther Nucl Med, 95:372, 1965)
Angioma (Farreras-Valenti: Am J Med, 34:735, 1973)
Neurofibromatosis (Halpern: N Engl J Med, 273:248, 1965)
Tumor thrombus (Jennings: Br Med J, 2:1053, 1964)
Renal transplant rejection (Gunnels: N Engl J Med, 274:543, 1966)
Moyamoya disease (Shoskes: J Urol, 153:450, 1995)
AVM in pregnancy (Motta: Urology, 44:911, 1994)

Renal Parenchymal

Vesicoureteral reflux and renal scarring (Savage: Lancet, 1:441, 1978)
Renal tuberculosis (Stockigt: Aust NZ J Med, 6:229, 1976)
Ask-Upmark kidney (Amat: Virchows Arch, 390:193, 1981)
"Page kidney" (Sufrin: J Urol, 113:450, 1975)
Solitary cyst (Kala: J Urol, 116:710, 1976)
Polycystic kidney disease (Nash: Arch Intern Med, 137:1571, 1977)
Radiation nephritis (Shapiro: Arch Intern Med, 137:848, 1977)
Renal cell carcinoma (Hollifield: Arch Intern Med, 135:859, 1975)
Wilms' tumor (Mitchell: Arch Dis Child, 45:376, 1970)
Reninoma (Robertson: Am J Med 43:963, 1967)
Unilateral hydronephrosis (Riehle: J Urol, 126:243, 1981)
Bilateral hydronephrosis (Vaughan: J Urol, 109:286, 1973)
Retroperitoneal paraganglioma (Page kidney) (Nakano: Am J Nephrol, 16:91, 1996)

Extrinsic Lesions

Vascular

Stenosis of celiac axis with "steal of renal blood flow" (Alfidi: Radiology, 102:545, 1972)
Congenital fibrous band (Lampe: Angiology, 16:677, 1965)
Hypoplastic aorta (Kaufman: J Urol, 109:711, 1973)
Postradiation arteritis (McGill: J Pediatr Surg, 14:831, 1979)
Traumatic occlusion (Connell: JAMA, 219:1754, 1972)
Coarctation (Shumaker: N Engl J Med, 295:148, 1976)

Other Lesions

Pheochromocytoma (Rosenheim: Am J Med, 34:735, 1963)
Metastatic tumors (Weidemann: Am J Med, 47:528, 1969)
Ptosis (Derrick: Am J Surg, 106:673, 1963)

about 40%. Thus the limited data available suggest that many patients with both atherosclerotic disease (Wollenweber et al, 1968; Dean et al, 1981) and fibromuscular disease (Meaney et al, 1968) have progressive disease. The important question of progression was addressed by Schreiber and co-workers (1984, 1989), and more precise information is now available.

Serial angiographic studies over a mean interval of 52 months in 85 patients with atherosclerotic disease revealed progressive vascular obstruction in 37 patients (44%). Total arterial occlusion occurred in 14 patients, most commonly in those with greater than 75% stenosis on the initial arteriogram. As would be expected, decline in renal function was more common among patients with progressive disease. Accordingly, the authors suggested that renal revascularization may be indicated for preservation of renal function in individuals whose advanced atherosclerotic disease was a major threat to overall renal function. The disease in these patients is characterized by azotemia and high-grade renal artery stenosis (greater than 75%), bilateral high-grade stenosis, and stenosis involving a solitary kidney (Schreiber et al, 1984, 1989; Novick, 1995).

Sixty patients with medial fibroplasia were also monitored for a mean interval of 45 months. Progressive renal arterial obstruction was observed in 22 (33%) of 66 patients; however, there were no cases of progression to total occlusion. Of particular interest was the similar development of progressive disease in patients older than 40 years of age (15 of 46). Previously it was thought that the disease was stable in this age group (Meaney et al, 1968). Despite

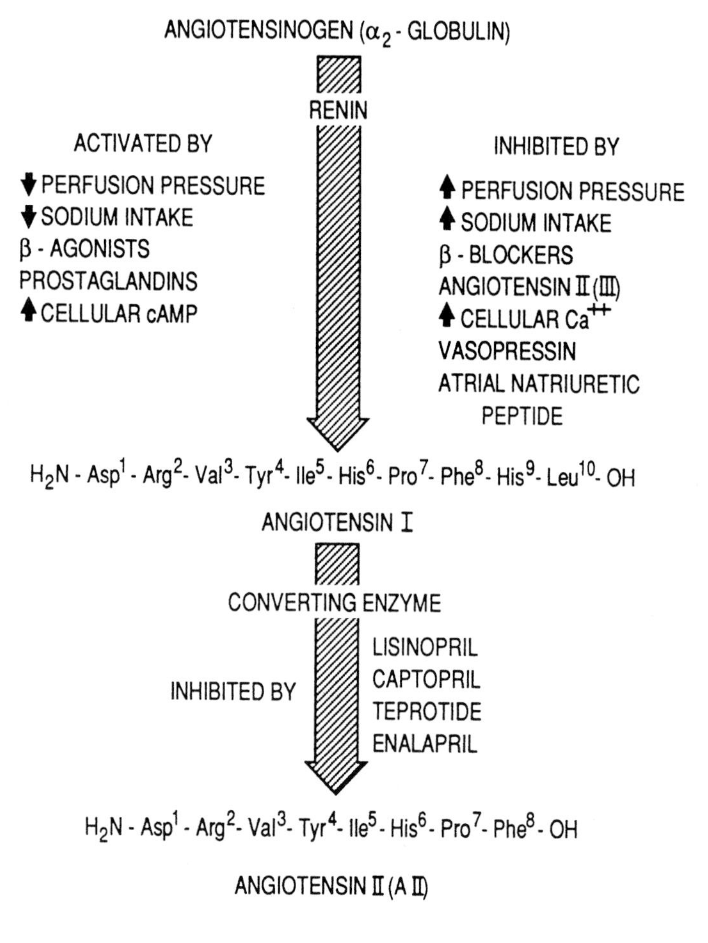

Figure 11–10. The renin-angiotensin system.

the angiographic progression demonstrated, increases in serum creatinine value or reduction in renal size seldom occurred. Accordingly, the authors did not suggest renal revascularization or angioplasty for preservation of renal function alone in this group.

NORMAL PHYSIOLOGY OF THE RENIN-ANGIOTENSIN-ALDOSTERONE SYSTEM

The renin-angiotensin-aldosterone system (RAAS) (Fig. 11–10) is the major renal hormonal system involved in the regulation of systemic blood pressure, sodium and potassium balance, regional blood flow, and perhaps renal growth and development (Gomez and Norwood, 1995; Sealey and Laragh, 1995). Its main components are renin; angiotensin II, an octapeptide that is a pressor agent; and aldosterone, a mineralocorticoid released from the adrenal cortex. The system is thus involved in both the vasoconstriction and the volume and sodium components of blood pressure control (Laragh and Sealey, 1992; Sealey and Laragh, 1995).

Prorenin is the biosynthetic precursor molecule of renin (Inagami and Murakami, 1980). The amino acid sequence of prorenin has been determined from the nucleotide sequence of the human renin gene, and prorenin is thus established as an inactive precursor of renin (Imai et al, 1983; Soubrier et al, 1983). It is believed that prorenin acts through active renin; however, there may be a **second, independent prorenin system functioning at a local level in the kidneys, ovaries, testes, and other organs where it is found, such as a role of prorenin in reproductive function (Sealey et al, 1995)**. Renin is an aspartyl protease with a molecular weight of 37,200 daltons, containing 340 amino acids; a single human renin gene has been determined (Imai et al, 1983; Soubrier et al, 1983). The major source of active renin in humans is the juxtaglomerular apparatus in the kidney, which secretes renin in response to well-defined stimuli (Fig. 11–11) (Barajas et al, 1995). The half-life of plasma renin is usually reported as between 15 and 20 minutes, and its major site of metabolism is in the liver. Release of renin from the juxtaglomerular cells is regulated by several factors to be discussed.

Once in the plasma, renin acts on its substrate angiotensinogen. Angiotensinogen is a glycoprotein (molecular weight 56,800) that is produced by the liver. The cDNA sequence for the rat angiotensinogen has been determined (Ohkubo et al, 1983). Human renin splits a leucyl-valine peptide bond and causes release of the decapeptide angiotensin I. It is generally agreed that angiotensin I itself is basically an inactive species and that its biologic activity results from its conversion to the active species angiotensin II. Angiotensin converting enzyme (ACE), a peptidyl dipeptide hydrolase, also known as kininase II, is a carboxydipeptidase that splits the terminal histidylleucine from angiotensin I, yielding the octapeptide angiotensin II, which is the active peptide in the system (Soffer, 1981). ACE is found in the lungs (Ng and Vane, 1967), plasma, and endothelium of vascular beds, including that of the kidneys. It is the discovery of ACE inhibitors that has contributed much to the understanding of the RAAS. However, with the broad substrate specificity of ACE, it may be unwise to attribute all

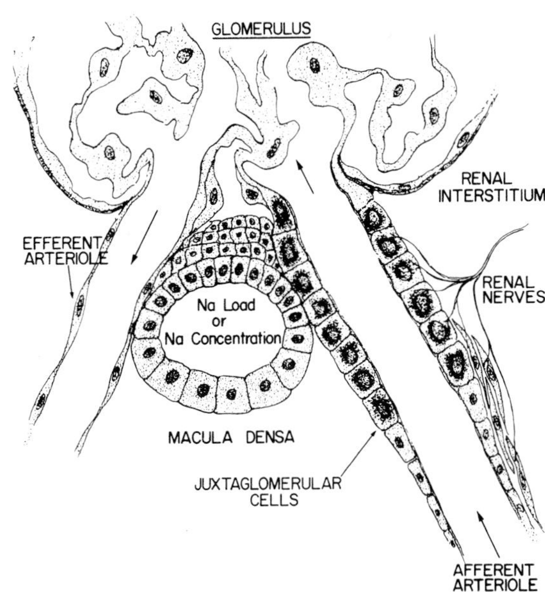

Figure 11–11. Diagram of the juxtaglomerular apparatus. The two intrarenal receptors, the vascular receptor and the macula densa, are depicted in their close physical relationship. According to current theory, the vascular receptor includes the juxtaglomerular cells and adjacent renal afferent arteriole, and this receptor responds to changes in wall tension. A change in renal tubular sodium appears to give the signal for stimulation of the macula densa, with a resulting influence on renin release. The juxtaglomerular cells secrete renin into the lumen of the renal afferent arteriole and into the renal lymph. The renal nerves are shown ending in both the juxtaglomerular cells and the smooth muscle cells of the renal afferent arteriole. Attention is also called to the intimate relationship of the efferent arteriole and the macula densa; granular cells have been observed, but rarely, in the efferent arteriole. (From Davis JO: The control of renin release. *In* Laragh JH, ed: Hypertension Manual. New York, Yorke Medical Books, 1973.)

the effects of ACE inhibitors to ablation of the RAAS. In summary, angiotensinogen is split into angiotensin I by the action of renin. Converting enzyme converts angiotensin I to angiotensin II. Because all the components of the system are present in the kidney, angiotensin II may function as an intrarenal as well as an extrarenal hormone (Gunning et al, 1996).

Angiotensin II is a compound with a wide range of biologic actions. Most of its actions are directed toward maintenance or increase of blood pressure. **This control is accomplished through both its direct effect as a vasoconstrictor and its effect on sodium balance and volume**. The data suggest that the RAAS is activated by sodium depletion to maintain sodium balance and blood pressure by direct vasoconstriction, aldosterone biosynthesis, and renal conservation of salt and water (Laragh and Blumenfeld, 1996) (see Chapters 7 and 96). **In 1960, Laragh and co-workers demonstrated that angiotensin II infusion caused a rise in plasma aldosterone** (Laragh et al, 1960). This is a direct effect of angiotensin II on the adrenals, because angiotensin II increases aldosterone release from isolated adrenal slices and adrenal zona glomerulosa cell suspensions. Aldosterone, an 18-aldehyde steroid, is secreted in nanogram amounts but is a potent regulator of sodium and potassium balance (see Chapter 96). **Aldosterone acts primarily on the renal tubule to promote the reabsorption of sodium and the excretion of potassium**. Fortunately, both plasma and urinary levels of aldosterone can be measured by precise radioimmunoassay (see Chapter 96).

Angiotensin II has also been shown to have a direct sodium-retaining effect, acting at the ascending limb of the loop of Henle (Munday et al, 1971). Mechanisms that serve to dampen the system are feedback-inhibiting loops. The "long" loop involves inhibition of renin release mediated by aldosterone-induced sodium retention and volume expansion and increased blood pressure. A "short" intrarenal loop is also present, in which angiotensin II directly inhibits renin release (Ayers et al, 1977).

Angiotensin II also exerts a number of complex effects within the kidney, which involve endocrine, autocrine, and paracrine mechanisms. Thus the peptide is involved in the autoregulation of glomerular filtration rate (GFR), growth and repair of angiotensin II receptor-containing cells, tubular control of sodium reabsorption, medullary blood flow, and intrarenal hormonal interactions (Gunning et al, 1996). The reader is referred to more comprehensive reviews of this complex topic for more complete information (Laragh and Brenner, 1995; Brenner, 1996).

The identification of a family of angiotensin II receptors and specific receptor antagonists has opened a new avenue to study specific angiotensin II actions and to develop new treatment strategies (Kang et al, 1994; Goodfriend et al, 1996). **At present, the AT_1 receptor appears to be primary for angiotensin II effects on the kidney and vasculature**.

Renin release from the juxtaglomerular cells is controlled indirectly by at least three separate mechanisms—baroreceptor, macula densa, or beta-adrenergic—and directly by various hormones acting at the level of the juxtaglomerular cells. **The baroreceptor mechanism involves changes in renin release in response to changes in pressure at the afferent arteriole** (Tobian et al, 1959). **Increased pressure decreases renin release, and decreased pressure increases renin release** (see Fig. 11–10). The macula densa mechanism involves changes in electrolyte composition detected at the macula densa, a segment of the distal tubule that is in very close proximity to the vascular pole of the glomerulus (Barajas et al, 1995; Briggs and Schnermann, 1995). For many years it was believed that sodium was the ion controlling reactivity of the macula densa. It was known that with decreased salt intake, the filtered fraction of sodium reabsorbed in the proximal tubule increased and less sodium reached the distal tubule. **Decreased salt intake is associated with increased plasma renin activity (PRA). The opposite is true of increased sodium intake**. This observation led to the conclusion that renin secretion is inversely related to sodium load. Data also concerning the role of chloride in regulating the macula densa response have been obtained.

The juxtaglomerular cells of rats, dogs, and humans are innervated by sympathetic fibers. Vander (1965) demonstrated that electrical stimulation of the renal artery and its associated sympathetic nerves causes renin release. Because these studies did not control for other changes in renal function, it was not established that a specific adrenergic receptor was involved. However, later studies established that in dogs with a single nonfiltering kidney, renal nerve stimulation increased renin secretion (Johnson et al, 1971).

Several groups have studied this phenomenon in order to characterize this response pharmacologically. **In general, this receptor appears to have the properties of a beta-adrenergic receptor**. For example, changes in renin release caused by nerve stimulation are blocked by l-propranolol, a beta-blocker, but not by its inactive stereoisomer, D-propranolol. In addition, beta-adrenergic antagonists suppress basal renin release, and these drugs appear to act on the beta-receptors of the juxtaglomerular cells (Buhler et al, 1972).

Changes in renin secretion induced by all these stimuli are mediated by changes in intracellular calcium or cyclic adenosine monophosphate (cAMP) within juxtaglomerular cells (Churchill, 1995). Thus an increase in cytosolic calcium suppresses renin release and an increase in cAMP increases renin release; converse relationships also pertain.

The hierarchy of control of renin release remains under study; however, it appears that the signals are often interdependent (Briggs and Schnermann, 1995).

Mechanisms of Experimental Goldblatt Hypertension

The initial work of Harry Goldblatt stimulated a search for a clearer understanding of the relationship between the renin system and renovascular hypertension. The first advancement was the realization that two models of experimental Goldblatt hypertension can be produced. In one model, a renal artery is clamped and the opposite kidney is left in place; in the other, a renal artery is clamped but the other kidney is removed. Although animals are equally hypertensive in both models, **in the two-kidney, one-clip model, plasma renin activity and renin content are increased in the kidney with the stenosed artery and decreased in the opposite kidney** (Gross, 1971; Mohring et al, 1975). **In the one-kidney, one-clip model, Goldblatt hypertension is characterized by volume expansion and normal or suppressed plasma renin activity and remains a likely subject for dialogue** (Sealey and Laragh, 1991).

A second advance in exposing the role of angiotensin II in these experimental models was the development of compounds that either block the conversion of angiotensin I to angiotensin II or are specific angiotensin II receptor antagonists (Brunner et al, 1971; Miller et al, 1972; Kang et al, 1994). These drugs have been important both in their insights into the role of the RAAS in the normal and abnormal state and, in the case of converting enzyme inhibitors, in their clinical use in renovascular hypertension. Saralasin (sarcosine^1, Val^5, Ala^8) is a prototype of an angiotensin II receptor antagonist with a significant duration of action. Because saralasin is not completely devoid of biologic activity (thus it is a partial agonist), studies in which it is used require careful evaluation (Case et al, 1976a). More recently, an orally active specific angiotensin II receptor antagonist, losartan, has been developed and is available now for clinical use (Brunner et al, 1992; Kang et al, 1994). Clinical use in patients with renovascular hypertension is meager, but it is most effective in high renin animal models (Demeilliers et al, 1995; Siegl et al, 1995).

Captopril (Squibb, 14,225; D-3-mercapto-2-methylpropanoyl-L-proline) **is a clinically used antihypertensive drug that is an ACE inhibitor blocking the formation of angiotensin II** (Rubin et al, 1978). Its synthesis followed by approximately 10 years the discovery of several naturally occurring converting enzyme inhibitors (CEIs) found in snake venom (Bakhle, 1968). The active components of snake venom that were CEIs turned out to be small peptides. Synthesis of large numbers of peptide analogues resulted in synthesis of a nonapeptide CEI (SQ 20881, teprotide), the first CEI used in humans (Cheung and Cushman, 1973). Although useful, SQ 20881 was limited in its effectiveness owing to a lack of oral activity.

In addition, because ACE also participates in the metabolism of bradykinin, the depressor effect of bradykinin is potentiated in the presence of a CEI (Rubin et al, 1978). **The animal model with hypertension that is most analogous to human renovascular hypertension is the one-clip, two-kidney Goldblatt preparation**. The hypertension in this model is initially dependent on increased renin secretion from the kidney with the clipped vessel, leading to angiotensin II formation and arteriolar vasoconstriction. The administration of an angiotensin II analogue (saralasin) (Brunner et al, 1971) or an angiotensin I-converting enzyme inhibitor (captopril) (Weed et al, 1979; Anderson et al, 1990) can prevent or reverse the hypertension. **This early state of one-clip, two-kidney Goldblatt hypertension exhibits four characteristics (Fig. 11–12): increased renin secretion from the damaged kidney; absence of renin secretion from the opposite kidney; decreased renal blood flow to the damaged kidney; and elevated blood pressure resulting from angiotensin II–induced vasoconstriction**. The identification of these characteristics has permitted the development of a rational approach to the use of plasma renin determinations (PRA) and angiotensin blockade in the diagnosis of renovascular hypertension (Vaughan et al, 1973, 1984; Sosa and Vaughan, 1989).

In contrast, the one-kidney, one-clip Goldblatt model rapidly establishes hypertension unresponsive to angiotensin II antagonists (Brunner et al, 1971) or converting enzyme inhibition unless the animal is sodium-depleted (Gavras et al, 1973). On the basis of animal data, the patient most likely to be cured after successful correction of a renal arterial lesion exhibits the characteristics of the early-phase one-clip, two-kidney Goldblatt model. The information gained from the one-kidney model suggests that in any clinical series there are patients who do not meet defined preoperative criteria used to predict curability who will have reversal of the hypertension after successful revascularization because of an increase in GFR and a "pressure" natriuresis after revascularization (Walker et al, 1993). Blood pressure control could result either from restoration of renal blood flow, GFR, and sodium excretion or from reversal of an ill-defined role of angiotensin II in the presence of normal PRA. **It is estimated that 20% of patients with renal artery stenosis whose hypertension is cured by renal angioplasty will have normal peripheral PRA** (Pickering et al, 1984).

IDENTIFYING THE PATIENT WITH RENOVASCULAR HYPERTENSION

Clinical means by which patients with functionally significant renal artery stenosis (RAS) can be identified have proved to be more elusive than might have been predicted. Certainly, there are no pathognomonic clinical characteristics that lead to a reliable diagnosis (Simon et al, 1972; Albers, 1994). However, a number of clinical features should arouse suspicion that renovascular hypertension may be present. These are summarized in Table 11–3. Factors implicated as being of importance in patients with fibromuscular dysplasia

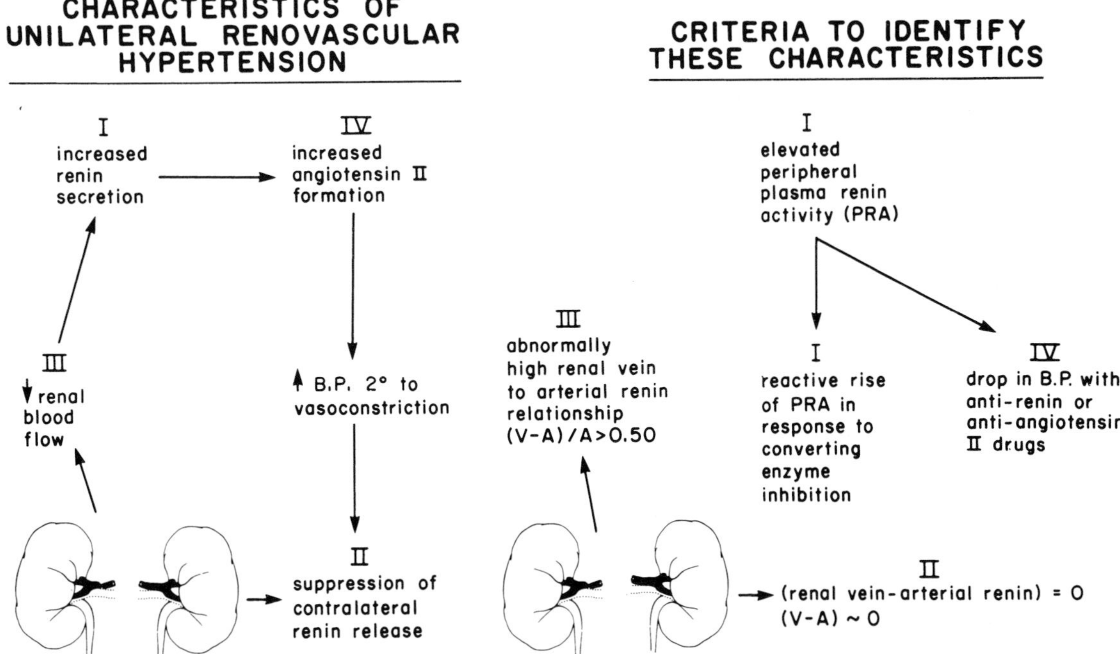

Figure 11–12. Characteristics of the early phase of two-kidney one-clip Goldblatt hypertension in the rat *(left)* and the criteria derived from the animal model that identify the patient with correctable renal hypertension. (From Vaughan ED Jr, Case DB, Pickering TG, et al: Urol Clin North Am 1984; 11:393.)

Table 11–3. CLINICAL CLUES SUGGESTIVE OF RENOVASCULAR HYPERTENSION

History	Comment
Hypertension in the absence of any family history of hypertensive disease	Suspect if family history is negative; however, about one third of patients with renovascular hypertension will have a positive family history.
Age of onset of hypertension: less than 25 years or greater than 45 years	The average age of onset for essential hypertension is 31 ± 10 (SD) years. Children and young adults usually will have fibromuscular disease, whereas adults over 45 years are more likely to have atherosclerotic narrowing of arteries.
Abrupt onset of moderate to severe hypertension	Whereas essential hypertension usually begins with a "labile" phase before mild hypertension becomes established, renovascular hypertension usually has a more telescoped natural history, often first appearing as moderate hypertension of recent onset.
Development of severe or malignant hypertension	Renovascular hypertension often becomes moderately severe and is prone to produce acceleration or malignant phase hypertension; both forms of hypertension involve markedly increased renin release.
Headaches	Essential hypertension is usually asymptomatic. There seem to be more headaches with renovascular hypertension, possibly related to its severity or high levels of angiotensin II, a potent cerebrovascular vasoconstrictor.
Cigarette smoking	In a recent survey, 74 per cent of patients with fibromuscular renal artery stenosis were smokers; 88 per cent of those with atherosclerotic disease smoke (Nicholson et al, 1983).
White race	Renovascular hypertension is uncommon in the black population.
Resistance to or escape from blood pressure control with standard diuretic therapy or antiadrenergic agents	Probably the most typical feature of renovascular hypertension is that it responds poorly to diuretics and often only transiently to antiadrenergic drugs.
Excellent antihypertensive response to converting enzyme inhibitors, e.g., captopril	Converting enzyme inhibitors block the renin-angiotensin system most effectively and are, therefore, highly specified agents.
Flash pulmonary edema	Bilateral renal artery stenosis (Diamond, 1993)
Indeterminate azotemia	Bilateral renal artery stenosis "ischemic nephropathy"
Coronary or carotid disease	Possibility of associated renal arterial disease due to atherosclerosis (Louie et al, 1994; Jean et al, 1994)

Physical Examination and Routine Laboratory Tests	Comment
Retinopathy	Hemorrhages, exudates, or papilledema indicates acceleration or malignant phase.
Abdominal or flank bruit	A helpful clue, but bruits are commonly present in elderly individuals and occasionally present in younger patients who have no apparent vascular stenosis.
Carotid bruits or other evidence of large vessel disease	Commonly, the vascular pathology is not limited to the renal bed.
Hypokalemia—in the untreated state or in response to a thiazide diuretic	Increased aldosterone stimulation by the renin-angiotensin system tends to reduce the serum potassium level. In untreated essential hypertension, this does not occur. Thiazide diuretics accentuate this phenomenon in renovascular hypertension.

Adapted from Vaughan ED Jr, Case DB, Pickering TG, et al: Urol Clin North Am 1984; 11:393.

are cigarette smoking and a genetic predisposition (Sang et al, 1989).

An additional clue to the presence of bilateral RAS is rapid renal deterioration after treatment with ACE inhibitors; this phenomenon, although less dramatic, can occur in patients with unilateral RAS (Hricik et al, 1983). Patients with unexplained azotemia should be evaluated for RAS caused by the presence of ischemic nephropathy. **Recurrent pulmonary edema is more common in patients with bilateral than unilateral disease and may be the first manifestation of renovascular disease** (Pickering et al, 1987).

The only laboratory findings of importance are hypokalemia and azotemia. The low potassium is the result of secondary hyperaldosteronism. However, a low serum K^+ level is found in less than 20% of patients with renovascular hypertension. Renovascular hypertension is less common in blacks (Emovon et al, 1995). **In a review of 819 patients with renal artery stenosis at the Cleveland Clinic, only 40 (4.9%) were black**. However, there were significant differences: more patients with systemic atherosclerotic disease, patients with a smoking history, and male patients were among the black group (Novick et al, 1994).

Eventually the ability to define patients for risk based upon renin-angiotensin gene polymorphisms may lead to early diagnosis or prevention of RAS (Hingorani et al, 1995; Missouris et al, 1996).

In many patients, none of the usual clinical clues are present to prompt a definitive evaluation. Thus the unreliability of clinical information has led to the development of various approaches to screen for the patient with renovascular hypertension.

Differential Renal Function Studies

As previously discussed, the observation in animals that partial occlusion of the renal artery resulted in increased fractional reabsorption of sodium and water (Blake et al, 1950) and increased urinary concentration of non-reabsorbable solute led to the development of differential renal function studies (Howard and Connor, 1954). **The initial criterion for a positive test was a 50% decrease in urine flow and a 15% or greater decrease in sodium concentration from the affected kidney**. The test underwent numerous modifications (Stamey, 1963); the most popular included the infusion of inulin, para-aminohippuric acid (PAH), and antidiuretic hormone during a urea-saline diuresis to accentuate the disparity in salt and water reabsorption between the two kidneys (Stamey et al, 1961).

However, the complexity involved in performing differential split renal function studies coupled with the development of more accurate methods to measure activity of the RAAS has almost eliminated the use of this technique. In general, at this time, differential renal function studies are performed only if the patient has unilateral parenchymal disease. In the setting of unilateral parenchymal disease, differential function studies are now most useful with the use of the isotopic renal scan to obtain renal blood flow (RBF) or GFR values for each kidney. **The treatment choices are nephrectomy and antihypertensive medical management; the latter is preferable if the affected kidney is contributing substantially to the total renal function.**

Intravenous Urogram

The rapid-sequence intravenous urogram is actually a radiographic differential renal function study with the contrast material as the indicator. Reduced renal blood flow is indicated by decreased renal mass or size; decreased GFR by delayed calyceal appearance time of contrast agent; and hyper-reabsorption of water by delayed hyperconcentration of non-reabsorbable solute, the iodinated contrast material. The most reliable abnormality seen in patients with proven unilateral renovascular hypertension is delayed calyceal appearance time on the side of the offending lesion (Bookstein et al, 1972).

However, with the incidence of renovascular hypertension being 5% to 15% and essential hypertension 85% to 95%, a false-positive rate of about 13% and a false-negative rate of 22% make the test unreliable (Maxwell and Lupu, 1968; Thornbury, 1982) (Table 11–4). Thus the intravenous urogram has been abandoned for this purpose.

Similarly, the radionuclide renogram, despite numerous modifications, has been plagued with variability that has led to even less specificity. In fact, review of various techniques disclosed a false-positive rate of 25% (Maxwell et al, 1968), whereas a later study using a refined technique reduced the false-positive rate to 10%, which is still no better than the urogram (Franklin and Maxwell, 1975). **In summary, both the intravenous urogram and the nuclide studies have failed to achieve suitable sensitivity and specificity to be reliable screening tests for renovascular hypertension.** The use of captopril renography is discussed later following definition of the captopril test.

Table 11–4. SENSITIVITY AND SPECIFICITY OF TESTS FOR RENOVASCULAR HYPERTENSION

	% Sensitivity	% Specificity
IVP*	75	86
DIVA*	88	89
PRA†	80	84
Captopril test	100–38‡	100–58
Captopril scan	96–48§	100–41
Doppler flow	93–67	100–98

Assume prevalence of RVH as 5% to calculate predictive value as shown below:

$$\text{Predictive value} = \frac{\text{sensitivity} \times \text{prevalence}}{(\text{sensitivity} \times \text{prevalence}) + \text{false-positive}} \times 100$$

$$\text{Exclusive value} = \frac{\text{sensitivity} \times (100 - \text{prevalence})}{\text{specificity} \times (100 - \text{prevalence}) + (\text{false-negative rate} \times \text{prevalence})} \times 100$$

*Harvey et al, 1985.
†Pickering et al, 1984.
‡Range from 9 studies (Nally, 1994).
§Range from 10 studies (Nally, 1994).

Digital Subtraction Angiography

A major advance was the introduction of computer-assisted digital subtraction angiography (DSA), which allows outpatient definition of renal anatomy at the time of renal venous sampling for renin (Buonocore et al, 1981; Hillman et al, 1982).

However, with further experience there are major disadvantages to DSA. Two studies have compared DSA with conventional angiography, and the sensitivity was 83% to 87% and specificity only 79% to 87% to accurately identify anatomic RAS (Smith et al, 1982; Buonocore et al, 1981). In addition, 5% to 20% of studies are uninterpretable, good patient compliance is necessary, central catheter placement is required, and a large volume of contrast material is given, raising the risk of contrast-induced renal dysfunction. Digital angiography is infrequently used today to identify patients with RAS (Hawkins et al, 1989; Zierler et al, 1994).

Doppler Ultrasound Angiography

Duplex ultrasound scanning combines both B-mode ultrasound imaging with pulsed Doppler ultrasound to provide imaging and velocity of blood flow along vessels. The technique has gained wide acceptance in peripheral vessels and is now being used to detect RAS (Table 11–5). The technique is also used to monitor patients for progression and monitor patients following renal angioplasty or revascularization (Eidt et al, 1988; Soulen et al, 1991; Hudspeth et al, 1993). A number of parameters have been used, including peak systolic velocity, renal aortic ratio, and the renal artery resistive index.

Several studies have shown that a peak systolic velocity higher than 180 to 210 cm/second, coupled with its ratio to the peak velocity of the aorta (RAR) higher than 3.5, correctly identifies high-grade renal artery stenosis (>60%), which is clinically significant (Miralles et al, 1993; Strandness, 1994b; Spies et al, 1995). This truly noninvasive test is conceptually attractive because the patient can be studied in an ambulatory setting and can continue antihypertensive medications, and the test can be utilized safely in azotemic patients (Nally et al, 1994). **However, the technique is technically difficult, requires approximately 1 hour to perform, and is often technically unsuccessful in obese patients, in the presence of excessive bowel gas and in the presence of accessory renal arteries.**

In summary, with increasingly accurate instrumentation, more clinical experience, and perhaps coupled with captopril

Table 11–5. ACCURACY OF DUPLEX ULTRASONOGRAPHIC SCANNING OF THE RENAL ARTERIES

Group	Sensitivity %	Specificity %	Positive Predictive Value %	Negative Predictive Value %
All kidneys (n = 142)	88	99	98	91
Kidneys with single renal arteries (n = 122)	93	98	98	94
Kidneys with multiple renal arteries (n = 21 arteries)	67	100	100	79
All patients (n = 74 patients)	93	100	100	91

From Hansen PB, Tribble RW, Reavis SW, et al: J Vasc Surg 1990; 12:227–236.

administration (Veglio et al, 1992, 1995), duplex sonography may become widely used as a screening test for RAS.

Spiral Computed Tomographic Angiography and Magnetic Resonance Angiography

The development of spiral computed tomography (CT) has permitted data acquisition during a single breath-hold (Kalender et al, 1990). Thus an entire scan can be obtained during the arterial phase of contrast injection, allowing reformation of an arterial segment through any plane. Hence this technique is being used to diagnose RAS (Galanski et al, 1993; Rubin et al, 1994; Brink et al, 1995; Olson and Posniak, 1995). The reconstructions are impressive (Fig. 11–13), especially in patients with proximal stenoses of the main renal artery. The precise role of this technique remains to be determined.

Similarly, magnetic resonance angiography is an evolving technique for noninvasive imaging of the renal vasculature. Moreover, the technique has the potential to measure absolute flow rate, GFR, and tissue diffusion and perfusion rates (Grist, 1994). In contrast to the spiral CT, high-dose iodinated contrast material, which is potentially nephrotoxic, is avoided. The technology is evolving, but faster imaging techniques are being developed, avoiding breath artifacts. The renal arteries appear white because the vascular image is related to the velocity of flow entering the image ("time of flight"). The results from several studies are shown in Table 11–6.

Undoubtedly, one of these new imaging techniques will supplant the arteriogram as we know it and will be used for the evaluation of transplant donors, for anatomic information following angioplasty or revascularization, and for the identification of renal artery stenosis (Kim et al, 1990; Debatin et al, 1991; Kent et al, 1991; Gedroyc, 1994; Hertz et al, 1994; Loubeyre et al, 1994).

Increased Renin Secretion: The Peripheral Plasma Renin

After the initial work of Dr. Harry Goldblatt, it was assumed that excess renin secretion, leading to excess angiotensin II formation, was the underlying derangement in renovascular hypertension. Unfortunately, this possibility was soon challenged when circulating PRA was found to be normal in a large fraction of patients with renovascular hypertension (Marks and Maxwell, 1975). This latter review of the literature revealed the peripheral PRA to be elevated in only 109 of 196 patients (56%) with verified renovascular hypertension. However, upon careful review of the primary papers it is apparent that these samples were often obtained under conditions that are now recognized to invalidate or limit accurate interpretation of the values obtained. For ex-

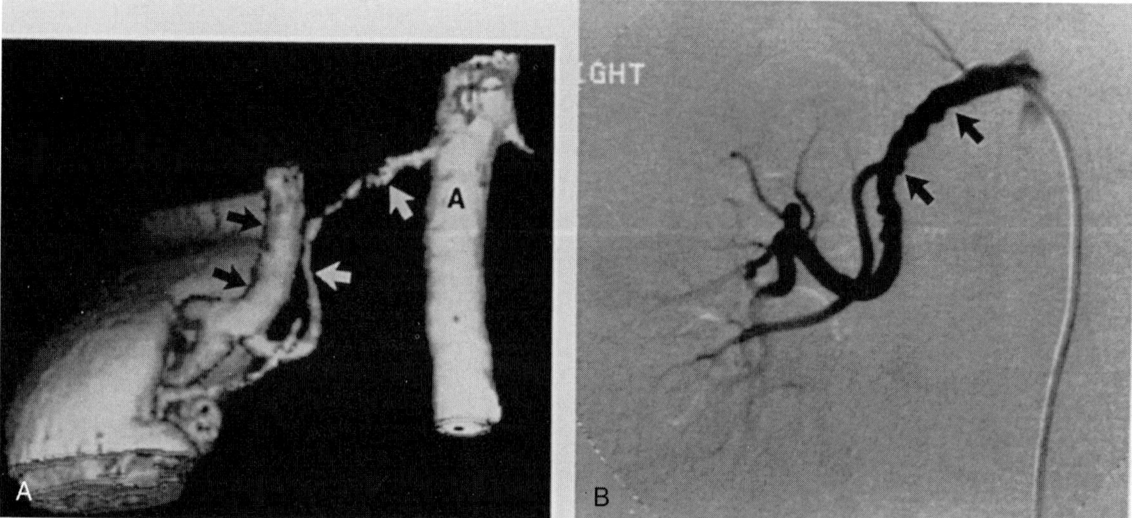

Figure 11–13. Renal artery with fibromuscular hyperplasia. *A*, Shaded surface computed tomographic (CT) display; A, simulated aorta. *B*, Subtraction arteriogram. (From Olson MC, Posniak HV: Techn Urol 1995; 1:141.)

Table 11–6. RESULTS OF RENAL MAGNETIC RESONANCE ANGIOGRAPHY CLINICAL TRIALS

Source	Technique	Sample Size	Sensitivity %	Specificity %
Kim et al, 1990	TOF	25	100	92
Kent et al, 1991	TOF	33	100	94
Debatin et al, 1991	PC, TOF	33	87	97
Grist et al, 1993	PC, TOF	35	89	95
Yucel et al, 1993	TOF	16	100	93
Gedroyc et al, 1992	PC	50*	83	97

*Renal transplant.
TOF, time of flight; PC, phase contrast.
From Grist TM: Am J Kidney Dis 1994; 24:700–712.

ample, it is now recognized that PRA is inversely related to sodium intake and must be indexed in some fashion to the state of sodium balance (Fig. 11–14). Moreover, all antihypertensive drugs influence PRA and must be stopped 2 weeks before blood sampling for PRA.

The peripheral PRA is emphasized because it represents an index of renin secretion (Sealey et al, 1973). A common misconception is that increased renin secretion is determined from differential renal vein renin measurements. Actual renin secretion (renal vein renin concentration minus arterial renin concentration multiplied by renal blood flow) is rarely determined. Accordingly, a high renal venous renin concentration may reflect increased secretion with normal renal blood or, alternatively, a normal amount of renin secreted into reduced renal blood flow (i.e., secretion = concentration × flow).

Increased secretion of renin is characteristic of renovascular hypertension and should therefore be reflected by elevated peripheral PRA, as compared with PRA values obtained from normotensive controls that are collected and analyzed under exactly the same conditions. Peripheral PRA (determined in blood collected at noon after 4 hours of patient ambulation), when indexed against the rate of urinary sodium excretion, is an excellent tool for identifying abnormally high renin secretion. **In a study of patients who subsequently had successful transluminal angioplasty, the**

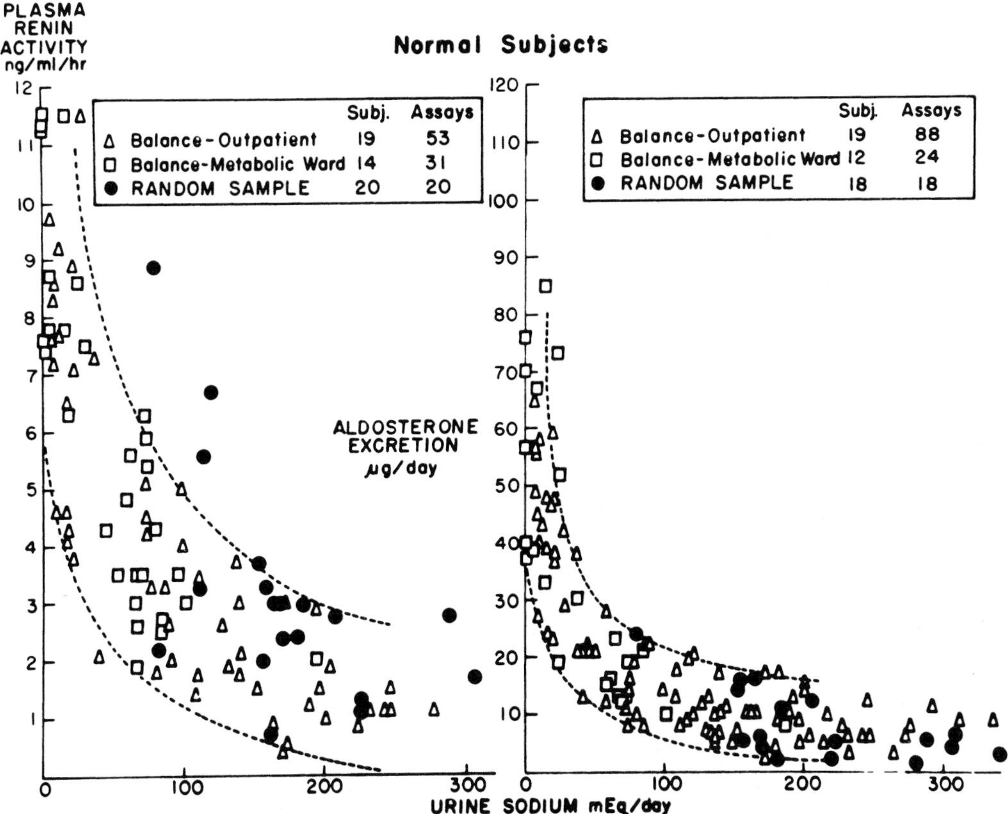

Figure 11–14. Relationship of renin activity in plasma samples obtained at noon and the corresponding 24-hour urinary excretion of aldosterone to the concurrent daily rate of sodium excretion. For these normal subjects, the data describe a similar dynamic hyperbolic relationship between each hormone and sodium excretion. Of note is the fact that subjects on random diets outside the hospital exhibited similar relationships, a finding that validates the use of this nomogram in studying outpatients or subjects not receiving constant diets. (From Laragh JH, et al: The renin-angiotensin-aldosterone system in pathogenesis and management of hypertensive vascular diseases. *In* Laragh JH, ed: Hypertension Manual. New York, Yorke Medical Books, 1973.)

peripheral PRA was elevated in 80% (Fig. 11–15). Moreover, the PRA always decreased and usually returned to normal after successful renal angioplasty, thereby confirming the hypothesis that the peripheral PRA is an indicator of increased renin secretion, which is corrected after relief of the offending stenotic lesion (Pickering et al, 1984).

Measurement of PRA in this manner as a screening test for renovascular hypertension has important limitations (see Table 11–4). In addition to a 20% false-negative rate (i.e., a normal PRA indexed against sodium excretion) in patients with proven renovascular hypertension, there is a technical problem. Many patients with renovascular hypertension have severe life-threatening hypertension or coexistent heart disease that precludes cessation of antihypertensive medication before blood is collected for peripheral PRA determinations. Thus, blood samples taken while patients are taking drugs invalidate the accuracy of peripheral PRA as a practical screening tool. In addition, 16% of the large population of patients with essential hypertension has high PRA (Brunner et al, 1972). Taken all together, these problems have led to the search for additional tests to screen for renovascular hypertension (Wilcox, 1993).

Enhanced Accuracy of Peripheral Plasma Renin Activity by Stimulation with Angiotensin-Blocking Drugs

The first angiotensin-blocking agent used for testing in human hypertension was saralasin. The initial results demonstrated that the compound did, as predicted, lower blood pressure in high-renin forms of hypertension, including renovascular hypertension (Brunner et al, 1973). In a second generation of human studies with saralasin, the partial agonist activity of the drug was exposed (Case et al, 1976b, Carey et al, 1978). Thus, in clinical settings in which PRA was low, the drug actually increased blood pressure.

A second approach to the use of angiotensin blockade to expose renovascular hypertension came from experience following the development of CEIs that block angiotensin II formation. A nonapeptide obtained from the venom of the *Bothrops jararaca* viper, teprotide, or SQ 20881, was shown to block the vasopressor effect of angiotensin I; it was possible to demonstrate a close direct correlation between the pretreatment level of PRA and the magnitude of the depressor response (Case et al, 1976a).

The success of the intravenous CEI was a potent stimulus to the development of an orally active form, the first of which to be used in humans was captopril. Captopril has the potential for use as a diagnostic probe, like teprotide, because it has a rapid onset of action (within 10 to 15 minutes), reaching a peak effect by 90 minutes (Case et al, 1978). Initial studies showed a close relationship between the pretreatment plasma-renin activity and the magnitude of the depressor response induced after the first dose of captopril (Case et al, 1978). During the early studies of the effect of these agents on blood pressure in hypertensive patients, it was noted that angiotensin blockade resulted in a marked rise in PRA in selected patients.

With the availability of the oral converting enzyme inhibitor captopril, we began using single oral test doses instead of intravenous infusions (Case et al, 1978, 1982). An additional advantage was the observation that renovascular hypertensive patients being treated with a beta-adrenergic blocker still responded to oral administration of captopril with a fall in blood pressure and a rise in PRA (Fig. 11–16) (Case et al, 1982).

The protocol for using single oral doses of captopril to screen for renovascular hypertension is shown in Table 11–7. Our current criteria for a positive test result to identify a patient with renovascular hypertension are: a post-captopril PRA of 12 ng/ml or greater per hour and an absolute increase in renin of 10 ng/ml or greater per hour, plus a 400% increase in renin if the baseline PRA was less than 3 ng/ml per hour and greater than 150% if the baseline renin was more than 3 ng/ml per hour (Mueller et al, 1986). In summary, single-dose captopril appears to separate patients with renovascular or renal hypertension from those with essential hypertension. Moreover, a 24-hour urine collection is not necessary and the patient can remain on beta blockade if the baseline PRA is greater than 1 ng/ml per hour. The test is not valid if the PRA is lower than 1 ng/ml per hour. Hence, the test is complementary to the renin-sodium index to identify renin hypersecretion (see Table 11–4).

Numerous other studies now have confirmed the usefulness of converting enzyme inhibition in the identification of renovascular hypertension (Derkx et al, 1987; Wilcox et al, 1988; Gosse et al, 1989) in adults and in children (Willems et al, 1989) (Table 11–8). However, the sensitivity and

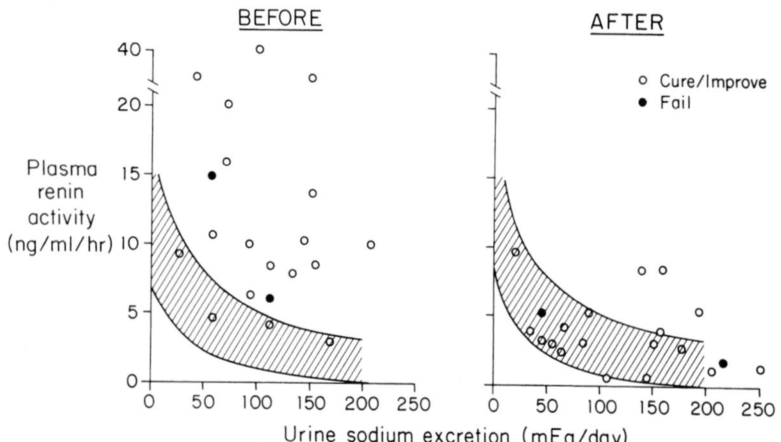

Figure 11–15. Effect of angioplasty on peripheral plasma renin activity indexed against 24-hour sodium excretion. *Left,* Before angioplasty; *right,* 6 months after angioplasty. Hatched area shows normal range. (From Pickering TG, Sos TA, Vaughan ED Jr, et al: Am J Med 1984; 76:398.)

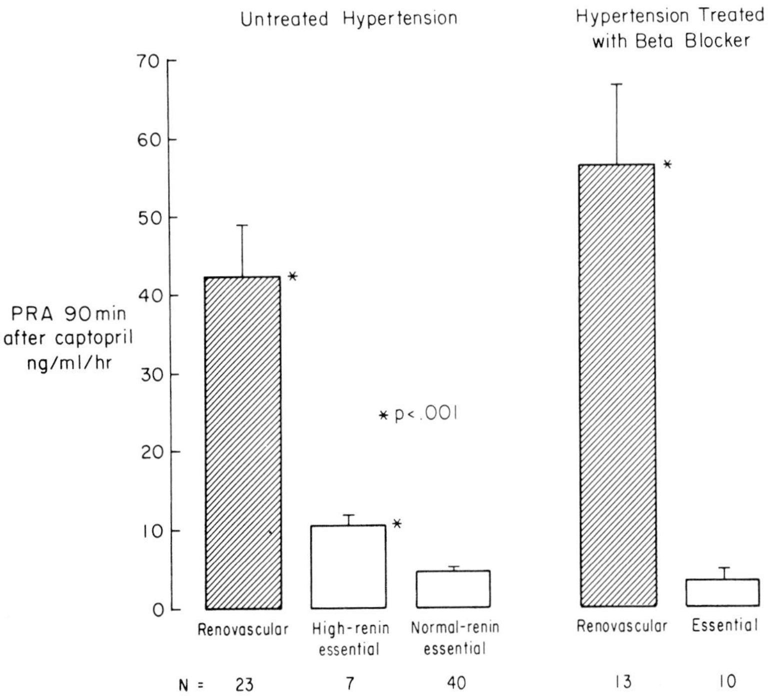

Untreated Hypertension
Hypertension Treated with Beta Blocker

PRA 90 min after captopril ng/ml/hr

*p<.001

	Renovascular	High-renin essential	Normal-renin essential	Renovascular	Essential
N =	23	7	40	13	10

Figure 11–16. Levels of plasma renin activity in renovascular and essential hypertension 90 minutes after a single dose of captopril. A marked reactive hyperreninemia was found in the group with renovascular hypertension whether they were already receiving beta-blocker therapy or not. (From Case DB, Atlas SA, Laragh JH: Physiologic effects and blockade. *In* Laragh JH, Buhler FR, Seldin DW, eds: Frontiers in Hypertension Research. New York, Springer-Verlag, 1982, pp 541–550.)

specificity have varied (Gaul et al, 1989) and the development of the captopril scan has replaced the test in some centers. However, it is a test that can be performed reliably in the physician's office and is safe and inexpensive.

Captopril Renogram

The study of CEI in both the diagnosis and treatment of renovascular hypertension led to the finding of decreased renal function in some patients (Hricik et al, 1983). The response of renal blood flow (RBF) and GFR to CEI in the two-kidney one-clip dog model established in our laboratories (Sosa, 1987) is shown in Figure 11–17. Infusion of enalapril produces a dramatic fall in RBF and GFR in the kidney with the RAS, whereas there is increased RBF in the opposite kidney despite a dramatic fall in blood pressure. These results show that angiotensin II plays a major role in preserving GFR in kidneys with RAS by causing efferent arteriolar constriction, increasing filtration fraction (London and Safar, 1989). Inhibition of angiotensin II by CEI results in a fall in efferent resistance and GFR (Pederson et al, 1989), an effect that is the physiologic basis for the captopril renogram (Meier et al, 1990).

Table 11–7. SINGLE-DOSE CAPTOPRIL TEST

Drugs

The patient should not receive any medications for at least 2 weeks, if possible. Otherwise, the patient may be given a beta-blocker, but omit all diuretics, converting enzyme inhibitors, or nonsteroidal anti-inflammatory drugs for at least 1 week (ideally, 2 weeks).

Diet

A diet with normal or high salt or sodium content is needed. Too low a sodium intake will produce falsely positive results. If there is a question about diet, a 24-hour urine collection for sodium will closely reflect the intake.

Procedure

The patient may be supine, semirecumbent, or seated for the test, but measurements must be made with the patient in the same position. After measurements of blood pressure are stable (this usually takes about 10 to 20 minutes), a blood sample for plasma renin activity is drawn in a lavender-topped Vacutainer kept at room temperature.

Crush a 25-mg tablet of captopril (to ensure that it dissolves) and pour in water to produce a suspension of about 30 ml. Instruct the patient to drink the suspension, wash the contents out twice, and drink those also.

Remeasure blood pressure and plasma renin activity after 1 hour.

From Vaughan ED Jr, Case DB, Pickering TG, et al: Urol Clin North Am 1984; 11:393.

As previously stated, the isotopic renogram has not proved to be an accurate test to identify patients with renovascular hypertension (Maxwell et al, 1968). However, performing the renogram before and after the administration of captopril can induce dramatic falls of GFR and RBF in the involved kidney as well as a fall in blood pressure and reactive rise in renin (Ritter et al, 1990). The test not only screens for renovascular hypertension but also identifies the involved kidney, perhaps obviating the need for renal vein renin determinations (Nally et al, 1986; Geyskes et al, 1987; Nally, 1989; Nally et al, 1994; Meier et al, 1990). However, differential renal vein renin determinations remain the gold standard in identifying the kidney that is the cause of abnormal renin secretion in a patient with renovascular hypertension.

Captopril renography has been shown to have acceptable sensitivity and specificity (Table 11–9) and now plays a major role as a noninvasive diagnostic test. **A number of criteria for a positive test have been used, with a prolonged time to maximal activity being the most common.** This finding is highly specific for renovascular hypertension (Nally et al, 1994; Pickering and Mann, 1995). **The test is less accurate in patients with azotemia or bilateral renal artery stenosis.** At present, patients with a high clinical risk

Table 11–8. SENSITIVITY AND SPECIFICITY OF THE CAPTOPRIL PLASMA RENIN ACTIVITY TEST

Investigator	Number of Patients Studied	Number of Patients with Renal Artery Stenosis	Sensitivity %	Specificity %
Mueller et al, 1986	152	49	100	95
Derkx et al, 1987	179	89	93	84
Frederickson et al, 1990	100	29	100	80
Gosse et al, 1989	114	11	73	84
Hansen et al, 1990a	47	11	91	89
Postma et al, 1990	149	44	38	93
Svetkey et al, 1989	66	11	73	72
Thibonnier et al, 1982	65	14	40	100
Elliott et al, 1993	100	59	76	58

From Nally JV Jr, Olin JW, Lammert GK: Cleve Clin J Med 1994; 61:328–336.

for renovascular hypertension and a positive captopril scan may proceed to arteriography without selective renal vein renins (Fig. 11–18).

Contralateral Suppression of Renin Secretion and an Elevated Renal Vein–to–Arterial Renin Relationship: Use of Differential Renal Vein Renin Determinations

The most common approach for renal vein renin (RVR) analysis has been to calculate the renal vein renin ratio, that is, stenotic divided by normal side PRA values with some arbitrary "positive" ratio (usually 1.5:1) (Judson and Helmer, 1965). The major difficulty with this method is in selecting a ratio that has the accuracy to divide precisely patients with renovascular hypertension from those with essential hypertension (Marks and Maxwell, 1975). In general, a positive renal vein ratio predicts a fall in blood pressure following correction of the vascular lesion in over 90% of cases. However, a negative ratio does not preclude a successful response to revascularization. In the review of Marks and Maxwell (1975), 49% of patients with negative ratio were cured by appropriate surgical intervention. However, these patients were a minority of the total patients studied, and the actual false-negative rate was 15% (62 of 412 patients).

In addition, the collection of renal vein blood alone for PRA is subject to the risk of a sampling error caused either by incorrect catheter placement or sampling from a renal vein that does not subtend the renal area supplied by the stenotic artery. **Sampling from the inferior vena cava below the renal veins is a safeguard against this source of error, and the absence of a 50% renin increment from both kidneys together identifies an inadequate differential renal vein renin study** (Vaughan et al, 1973).

A positive renal vein ratio does not exclude bilateral, albeit asymmetric, renin secretion, which indicates bilateral renal disease. In this setting, correction of a unilateral lesion may not totally correct the underlying pathology, with subsequent failure of total blood pressure control.

In view of these limitations of the traditional renal vein

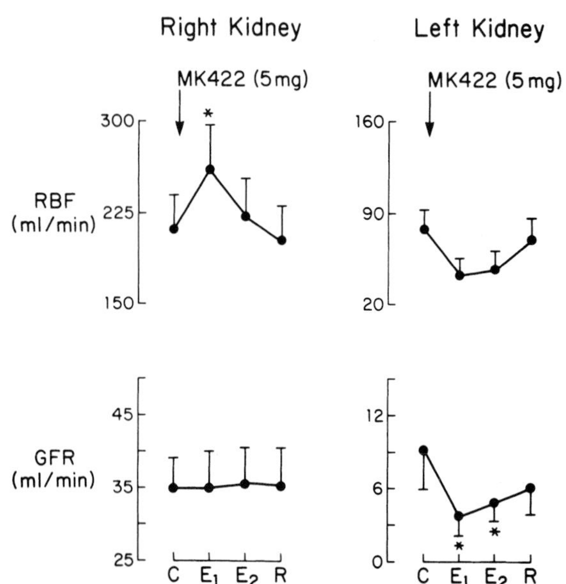

Figure 11–17. Effect of angiotensin converting enzyme inhibition on renal blood flow (RBF) and glomerular filtration rate (GFR), showing a marked fall in GFR in the kidney with renal artery stenosis. C, control; E, experimental periods; R, recovery.

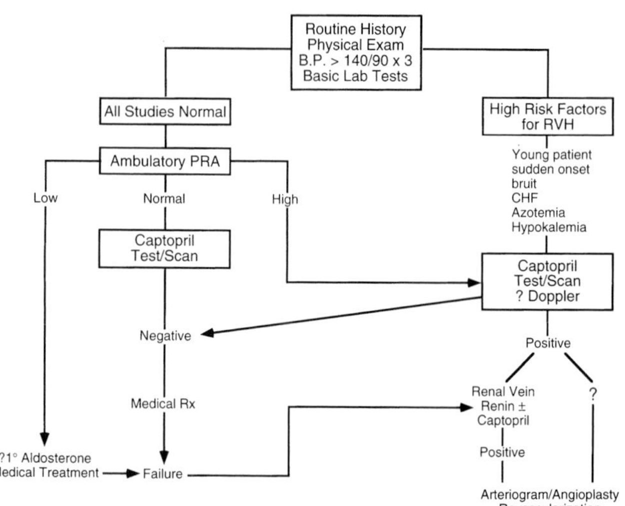

Figure 11–18. Evaluation schema to identify patients with renovascular hypertension.

Table 11–9. SENSITIVITY, SPECIFICITY, AND PREDICTIVE VALUE OF CAPTOPRIL RENOGRAPHY

Investigator	Number of Patients Studied	Number of Patients with Renal Artery Stenosis	Radionuclide Used	Sensitivity %	Specificity %	Predicted Blood Pressure Response
Geyskes et al, 1986	34	15	OIH*	80	100	Yes: 12/15
Sfakianakis et al, 1987	31	16	OIH	67	100	
			Tc-DTPA†	48		
Erbsloh-Moller et al, 1991	40	28	OIH	96	95	Yes: 10/11
Svetkey et al, 1989	61	11	Tc-DTPA	74	44	
			OIH	71	41	
Setaro et al, 1991	90	44	Tc-DTPA	91	94	Yes: 15/18
Mann et al, 1991	55	35	Tc-DTPA	94	95	No: 8/19
			OIH	83	85	
Fommei et al, 1994	472	259	Tc-DTPA (380)	83	91	Yes: 40/43
			Tc-MAG3‡ (74)	83	100	
Dondi et al, 1991	102	54	Tc-MAG3	90	92	Yes
Elliott et al, 1993	100	59	Tc-Pentetate	92	80	Yes: 51/53

*Iodine-131-orthoiodohippurate.
†Technetium-99m-diethylenetriaminepenta-acetic acid.
‡Technetium-99m-mercaptoacetyltriglycine.
From Nally JV Jr, Olin JW, Lammert GK: Cleve Clin J Med 1994; 61:328–336.

ratio analysis, another method for analysis of renin values has been devised. It is based on the characteristics of the experimental one-clip, two-kidney Goldblatt hypertension, as detailed in Table 11–10 and Figure 11–12.

Hypersecretion of renin, as determined by the renin-sodium index or captopril stimulation, serves as the primary criterion for the diagnosis of renovascular hypertension. **A second criterion is the demonstration of the absence of renin secretion from the contralateral (or noninvolved) kidney. Suppression of renin secretion from this kidney can be determined by subtracting the arterial plasma renin activity (A) from the renal venous renin activity (V).** Because the inferior vena caval (IVC) renin and aortic renin are the same, the IVC renin value can be substituted for A in this equation (Sealey et al, 1973). Hence patients with curable renovascular hypertension exhibit an absence of renin secretion from the opposite kidney, that is, $V - A = 0$, also termed *contralateral suppression of renin* (Stockigt et al, 1972; Vaughan et al, 1973; Derkx and Schalekamp, 1994). Contralateral suppression of renin indicates that the noninvolved kidney is responding in an appropriate "normal" fashion to the elevated blood pressure, increased circulating angiotensin II levels, and/or increased sodium chloride at the macula densa by shutting off renin secretion. This phenomenon is at times present not only in patients with unilateral renal arterial lesions but also in patients with bilateral disease (demonstrated by arteriograms) who have a dominant lesion on one side (Gittes and McLaughlin, 1974; Pickering et al, 1986).

A third criterion is based on studies of renal vein and arterial renin relationships in patients with essential hypertension. The mean renal venous renin level has been determined to be about 25% higher than arterial PRA (Sealey et al, 1973). Hence, a total renin increment (both kidneys) of approximately 50% is necessary to maintain a given peripheral renin level $(V - A)/A = 50\%$. However, a reduction

Table 11–10. RENIN VALUES FOR PREDICTING CURABILITY OF RENOVASCULAR HYPERTENSION

Collection of Samples
(moderate sodium intake ± 100 mEq/day)

1. Ambulatory peripheral renin and 24-hour urine sodium excretion under steady-state conditions (i.e., not on day of arteriography)
2. Collection of blood for PRA before and after converting enzyme blockade
3. Collection of supine
   a. Renal vein renin from suspect kidney (V1) and inferior vena cava renin (A1)
   b. Renal vein from contralateral kidney (V2) and inferior vena cava renin (A2)
4. Enhancement of renin secretion by converting enzyme blockade if initial renin sampling is inconclusive

Criteria for Predicting Cure

High PRA in relation to $U_{Na}V$	Measurement of hypersecretion of renin
Contralateral kidney: $(V2 - A2) = 0$	An indicator of absent renin secretion from the contralateral kidney
Suspect kidney: $(V1 - A1)/A1 \geqq 0.50$	As indicator of unilateral renin secretion
$\frac{(V - A)}{A} + \frac{V - A)}{A} < 0.50$	Measurement of reduced renal blood flow
In patients with high PRA	
Means: a. Incorrect sampling b. Segmental disease	Repeat with segmental sampling

From Vaughan ED Jr: In Brenner BM, Stein JM, eds: Hypertension. New York, Churchill Livingstone, 1981.

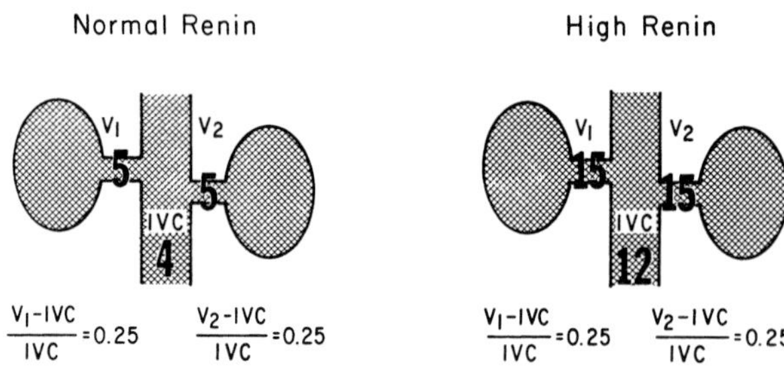

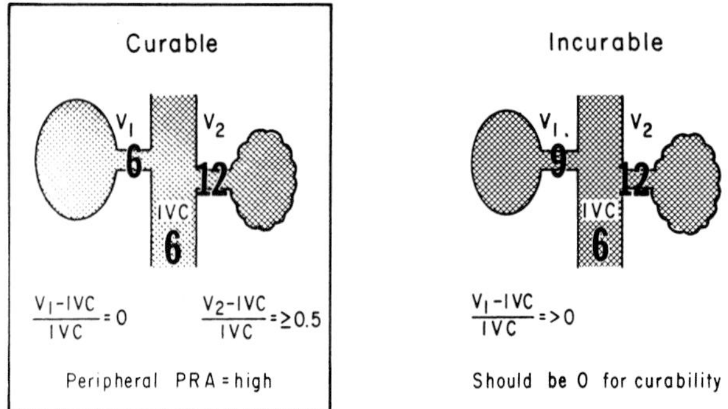

Figure 11–19. Renal vein renin diagnostic patterns. In essential hypertension *(top)* at all levels of renin secretion, the renin level in each renal vein is about 25% greater than either the peripheral arterial or the venous level. In the setting of unilateral renin secretion (curable renovascular hypertension), the active kidney is solely responsible for maintaining the peripheral renin levels. Hence the increment is 50% (0.5) and becomes progressively greater as renal blood flow is reduced. Unequal bilateral renin secretion *(bottom right)* indicates bilateral disease and decreases the chance of cure after corrective unilateral surgery. (From Laragh JH, Sealey JE: Cardiovasc Med 1977; 2:1053. Reprinted with permission from the Physicians World Communications Group.)

in renal blood flow also influences the renal venous renin level. In this setting, the renal venous renin concentration is high, shifting the renal vein–to–arterial renin relationships upward. **Hence, the elevation of the increment above approximately 50% becomes an index of the severity of the reduction in blood flow consequent to the obstructing vascular lesion** (Vaughan et al, 1973; Pickering et al, 1984) (Fig. 11–19).

An additional aid to renal vein sampling is the utilization of segmental renal venous sampling (Schambelan et al, 1974), especially when sampling of blood from the major renal veins fails to demonstrate a combined renin increment of 50% from both kidneys, suggesting either a technical error or segmental disease. This approach may be particularly helpful in children with segmental parenchymal disease (Parrott et al, 1984).

Less emphasis has been placed recently on RVR analysis than on the development of noninvasive tests (Belli, 1994; Prigent and Froissant, 1994; Semple and Dominiczak, 1994). However, the understanding of the physiologic basis of RVR values aids in our knowledge of the physiology of renin release in patients with renovascular hypertension. Moreover, despite limitations, RVR analysis remains the definitive test to demonstrate unilateral renin secretion (Jensen et al, 1995).

Converting Enzyme Inhibition to Enhance the Accuracy of Renal Vein Renin Analysis

Following the initial report of renin stimulation by angiotensin blockade (Re et al, 1978), several groups of investigators have reported increased renin release from the ischemic kidney with converting enzyme inhibition (Lyons et al, 1983; Thibonnier et al, 1984). The magnitude of these induced changes is shown in Figure 11–20. These data were determined from 26 patients with unilateral renovascular hypertension. Not shown in this illustration is the observation that the IVC levels (systemic or peripheral levels) were comparable to those values measured from the normal side, revealing the continued suppression of renin secretion from that kidney even after stimulation. It is clear that renin stimulation by converting enzyme inhibition adds to the analysis in certain specific situations: (1) when patients are already on drug therapy (e.g., beta-blockers) and the renin levels are generally reduced; (2) when there is a question about the reliability of the PRA measurements, particularly if the levels are low; (3) when experience in performing RVR tests is limited and subject to sampling errors; and (4) when equivocal values already exist (Simon and Coleman, 1994).

In summary, RVR sampling after captopril stimulation accentuates renin release from ischemic renal tissue, which is particularly useful when values are equivocal, when branch stenoses are present, or when renovascular disease is superimposed on coexisting hypertension or renal disease.

Validation of the Criteria

In addition to a favorable clinical response to renal angioplasty, we have had the unique opportunity to study the

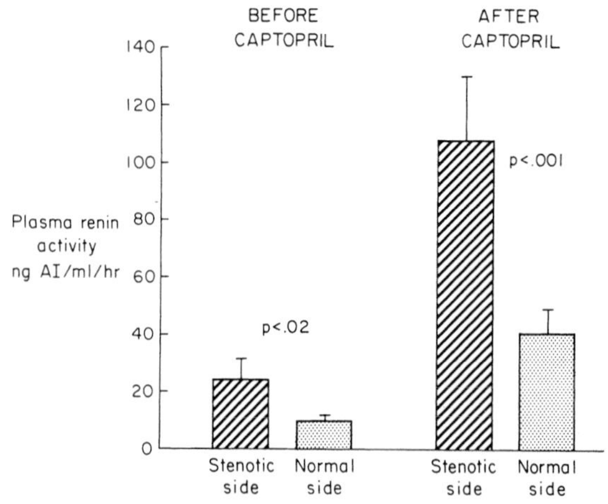

Figure 11–20. Renal vein renin determinations (renal vein levels only) in patients with documented renovascular hypertension before and after captopril stimulation. Captopril accentuates renin secretion from the ischemic kidney. Not shown are the inferior vena cava levels, which are the same as the levels measured from the normal side both before and after captopril stimulation. (From Vaughan ED Jr, Case DB, Pickering TG, et al: Urol Clin North Am 1984; 11:393.)

effect of restoration of blood flow on RVR concentration and renin secretion (Vaughan et al, 1981; Pickering et al, 1984). To accomplish this goal, we have monitored the immediate effect of successful angioplasty on renal renin secretion. Thirty minutes after angioplasty, there was a marked reduction in the renal vein renin from the previously stenotic side (Fig. 11–21). The residual ipsilateral increment of RVR was about 50% above the peripheral level, whereas contralateral renin suppression persisted. This 50% increment had been predicted previously to occur in the setting of unilateral renin secretion and normal RBF (Sealey et al, 1973).

Several months after angioplasty, there was a marked fall in peripheral PRA with a return to normal in most patients, indicating a reduction of renin secretion (see Fig. 11–15). Of equal interest is the restoration of bilateral renin increment of about 25% above the IVC renin level (see Fig. 11–21) (Pickering et al, 1984). Hence contralateral renin suppression was reversed following successful angioplasty. This 25% increment from both kidneys is characteristic of the renin secretory pattern found in patients with essential hypertension (Sealey et al, 1973).

The finding that the renal renin secretory characteristics of renovascular hypertension are reversed after successful angioplasty with correction of the hypertension is strong evidence that they truly reflect the abnormal secretory behavior of renin in curable renovascular hypertension.

Identifying the Potentially Curable Patient: A Cost-Effective Approach

Our current approach is outlined in Figure 11–18. All patients (except those with borderline or mild or moderate hypertension well controlled with mild antihypertensive medications [Pickering, 1995]) with fixed hypertension are candidates for this protocol, because we believe that nearly all patients with renovascular hypertension, when identified, can be best managed by angioplasty or revascularization. With respect to this empirical protocol, it can be argued that patients with highly suspect disease should be screened initially with a captopril scan. If the result is positive, we proceed to arteriography without RVR analysis. However, the functional significance of an anatomic lesion with respect to ischemia-induced renin release confirms the predictive value of the captopril scan, and thus we usually perform RVR analysis.

In general, we begin evaluation with a PRA. In our experience, a low PRA rarely is found in untreated patients with nonazotemic renal arterial disease, and we therefore do not continue this evaluation in those patients unless they demonstrate refractoriness to treatment. Patients with high or normal PRA undergo a peripheral captopril test or captopril renogram. The test cannot be performed if the patient is taking captopril on a long-term basis. If the test is positive, the differential renal vein sampling and digital angiography are performed together. The sampling procedure ideally is done first, and then the catheter is advanced into the superior vena cava for injection of contrast material. This combined study is performed in the radiology suite, following which the patient lies quietly in the hypertension unit for 2 to 4 hours before returning home. After the diagnostic criteria have been established, the patient undergoes selective arteriography and percutaneous transluminal angioplasty or renal revascularization.

We continue to believe that the functional significance of a renal artery lesion must be identified either by captopril renography or RVR analysis before the therapeutic decision is directed toward intervention.

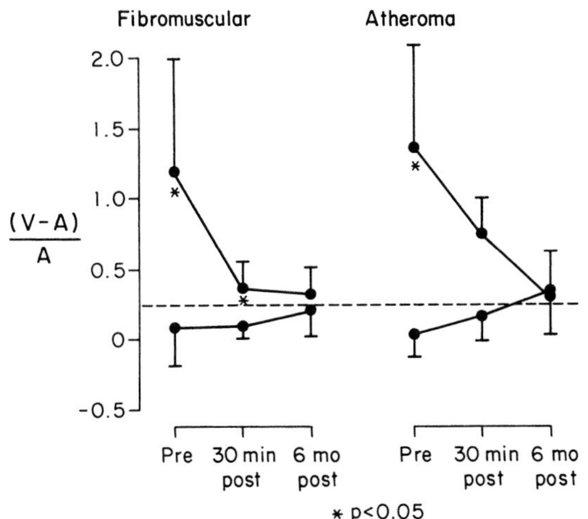

Figure 11–21. Effect of angioplasty on renal vein renin. Samples were taken immediately before angioplasty, 30 minutes after, and 6 months after. The higher values are for the ischemic kidney; the lower values are for the contralateral kidney. *Asterisk* indicates significant difference between the two kidneys, and the *dotted line* is the normal level of (V − A)/A (0.24). (From Pickering TG, Sos TA, Vaughan ED Jr, et al: Am J Med 1984; 76:398.)

Tailored Therapy for Renovascular Hypertension

The rationale for identifying patients with renovascular hypertension is that their management differs from the treatment offered to patients with essential hypertension. Indeed, hypertension of renal origin is difficult to manage with conventional antihypertensive drugs. In a randomized study (Hunt and Strong, 1973), the morbidity and mortality rates were greater in patients with renal hypertension treated in the medical group as contrasted to the surgical group. In addition, as previously discussed, most renovascular lesions are progressive with time, and there is little evidence to suggest that successful control of hypertension influences the natural history of the various pathologic entities (McCormack et al, 1966; Goncharenko et al, 1981; Schreiber et al, 1984). Accordingly, for properly selected cases, surgical management or angioplasty has been the preferable choice.

Medical Management

Effective treatment of renovascular hypertension is possible with specific antihypertensives, such as CEIs, beta-adrenergic blockers, calcium channel blockers, and angiotensin receptor blockers. Medical management is used in patients awaiting angioplasty or revascularization, those who refuse or are too ill for intervention, and those who have failed to respond to intervention (Pickering, 1989; Pickering and Mann, 1995).

The major concern of medical management is the demonstrated progressive deterioration of renal function found in some patients despite adequate blood pressure control (Dean et al, 1981). As previously described during the discussion of the captopril renogram, a major compensatory mechanism to maintain glomerular filtration pressure is efferent arteriolar constriction induced by angiotensin II (London and Safar, 1989; Rosivall et al, 1990). **Accordingly, the administration of CEI to patients with renovascular hypertension can lead to either renal deterioration** (Mason and Hilton, 1983; Chrysant et al, 1983; Ying et al, 1984; Dominiczak et al, 1988, Burnier et al, 1989; Mimran et al, 1991; Toto, 1994) **or total renal artery occlusion** (Postma et al, 1989; Hannedouche, 1991). Moreover, the renal deterioration may not be reversible (Devoy et al, 1992) or may require revascularization (Textor et al, 1983). However, upon review of the world experience of CEI therapy for renovascular hypertension, progressive renal failure sufficient to discontinue treatment occurred in only 5% of patients, whereas there was good blood pressure control in 74% (Hollenberg, 1988).

In summary, CEI is effective in controlling blood pressure in these patients. It is most dangerous in patients with bilateral disease or solitary kidneys. For all patients on medical therapy, careful follow-up must be done and results of serial tests of renal function and size must be monitored. Calcium channel blockers, which induce afferent arteriolar dilatation, can be used alone or with CEIs to maintain GFR in these patients (Fiorentini et al, 1990; Zanchi et al, 1995).

Percutaneous Transluminal Renal Artery Angioplasty

Percutaneous transluminal angioplasty (PTA) was first introduced by Dotter and Judkins in 1964 for the treatment of peripheral vascular stenoses. The difficulties associated with the technique were overcome by the introduction of a flexible, double-lumen balloon catheter by Gruntzig (Gruntzig and Hopff, 1974), permitting the development of percutaneous balloon angioplasty of renal artery stenosis. The fibromuscular dysplasias and unilateral nonosteal nonoccluded atherosclerotic renal artery stenoses are the most suitable lesions for treatment with PTA. In addition, PTA has been used in patients with arteritis (Martin et al, 1980; Kumar et al, 1990), in patients with recurrent stenosis following initially successful PTA, and in patients with anastomotic strictures of the renal artery following surgical correction.

The major groups of patients who do not respond to PTA include those with diffuse atherosclerotic disease primarily involving the aorta, which gives rise to a secondary occlusion of the renal artery ostium. Therefore, in ostial stenosis the success rate of PTA is poor, although an occasional patient has a long-term success (Cicuto et al, 1981; Sos et al, 1983). Patients with total occlusion of the renal artery are also poor candidates for the technique. The management of patients with total renal artery occlusion is discussed in Chapter 12. Patients with multiple branch lesions, particularly at vessel bifurcation, are less likely to respond to angioplasty. This situation is only a relative contraindication to PTA and pertains primarily to patients with atherosclerotic disease.

Taken all together, the ideal patient for PTA is one with unilateral disease, positive renin indices, and fibromuscular dysplasia or nonosteal nonoccluded atherosclerotic renal artery stenosis. A second indication, which will be discussed later, is angioplasty for preservation of renal function.

Advantages of transluminal angioplasty are the ability to avoid a general anesthetic, the relatively low morbidity of the procedure, and short or no interval of hospitalization. It is critical that the procedure be done with a team approach involving not only the radiologist but also medical and surgical teams who are familiar with the management of patients with hypotension and potential surgical complications. Patients often have volume depletion due to their angiotensin II–induced vasoconstriction before angioplasty and often require vigorous hydration to avoid postangioplasty hypotension, electrolyte imbalances, and contrast-induced injury (Katzen et al, 1979; Schwarten, 1987). Some of these complications can be avoided if the patients who are on long-term converting enzyme inhibitors are allowed restoration of vascular volume before angioplasty. In contrast, the patients also may have an increase in blood pressure, requiring medical management after angioplasty, or patients may simply maintain their pre-existing pressure for some period before resolution occurs.

In summary, there is a general consensus at the present time that PTA is the treatment of choice for patients with medial fibroplasia (Tack and Sos, 1989). As shown in Table 11–11, combined results from 10 series reveal a success rate of over 90% (Ramsey and Waller, 1990). Considerably more controversy exists concerning patients with atherosclerotic disease. The technical success rate is lower (70%–80%) and the blood pressure benefit is considerably more variable (see Table 11–11) and less than that found after surgical revascularization (see Chapter 12) (Novick, 1995). Patient selection remains critical and undoubtedly influences whether results are good (Canzanello et al, 1989) or disappointing (Beebe et al, 1988).

The most important new technique that has expanded the use of angioplasty, especially in patients with osteal stenosis, is the renal artery stent (Kuhn et al, 1991; Rees et al, 1991; Wilms et al, 1991; MacLeod et al, 1995). In this technique, a stainless steel balloon-expandable stent is placed across the stenosis to maintain the renal artery lumen (Fig. 11–22). **The primary indications have been osteal stenosis, failure of conventional angioplasty, or intimal tears during the procedure**. The technical success in various series is over 90%. In a cooperative study, follow-up studies at 8 months revealed a 43% restenosis rate (Rees et al, 1991). At 1 year, 47% demonstrated cure or improvement of hypertension, a result dramatically higher than that achieved by angioplasty alone, but also clearly inferior to renal revascularization (Novick, 1995). Whether the success of renal revascularization is limited by stenting is not known. The complications of renal angioplasty and stenting are well defined and occur in about 13%. Fortunately, most do not result in death or renal loss (Trost and Sos, 1994) (Table 11–12).

Angioplasty has also been successfully incorporated in the treatment strategy of children with renovascular hypertension (Guzzetta et al, 1989; Simunic et al, 1990) and the success

Table 11–11. SUMMARY OF OUTCOME AFTER ANGIOPLASTY IN TEN PUBLISHED SERIES OF HYPERTENSIVE PATIENTS ACCORDING TO INDICATION FOR ANGIOPLASTY—ATHEROMATOUS OR FIBROMUSCULAR RENAL ARTERY STENOSIS*

	Atheromatous Renal Artery Stenosis				**Fibromuscular Renal Artery Stenosis**			
	Technically Successful Angioplasty	***Blood Pressure Response***			***Technically Successful Angioplasty***	***Blood Pressure Response***		
Reference		*Cured*	*Improved*	*Failed*†		*Cured*	*Improved*	*Failed*†
Martin et al, 1981	13	2 (15)	4 (31)	7 (54)	8	5 (63)	1 (13)	2 (25)
Colapinto et al, 1982	44	8 (18)	29 (66)	7 (16)	9	4 (44)	5 (56)	0 (0)
Geyskes et al, 1983	44	4 (9)	19 (43)	21 (48)	21	10 (48)	10 (48)	1 (5)
Sos et al, 1983	34	7 (21)	10 (29)	17 (50)	27	16 (59)	9 (33)	2 (7)
Tegtmeyer et al, 1984	61	15 (25)	46 (75)	0 (0)	27	10 (37)	17 (63)	0 (0)
Miller et al, 1985	34	5 (15)	15 (44)	14 (41)	13	11 (85)	2 (15)	0 (0)
Martin et al, 1985	60	9 (15)	30 (50)	21 (35)	20	5 (25)	12 (60)	3 (15)
Kaplan-Pavlobcic et al, 1985	48	11 (23)	21 (44)	16 (33)	21	10 (48)	8 (38)	3 (14)
Kuhlmann et al, 1985	31	9 (29)	15 (48)	7 (23)	22	11 (50)	7 (32)	4 (18)
Bell et al, 1987	22	3 (14)	13 (59)	6 (27)	7	5 (71)	2 (29)	0 (0)
Totals	391	73 (19)	202 (52)	116 (30)	175	87 (50)	73 (42)	15 (9)
Range (%)		9–29	29–75	0–54		25–85	13–63	

*Results are expressed as numbers (percentages) of patients.
†Excludes technical failures.
From Ramsay LE, Waller PC: BMJ 1990; 300:569.

rate utilizing both PTA and revascularization in children is now excellent.

Thus, PTA has assumed a major role in the treatment of renovascular hypertension. In addition, successful surgical correction can be performed without added morbidity in patients who have failed PTA (Martinez et al, 1990). The critical information still lacking is long-term follow-up, which is now available after renal revascularization and

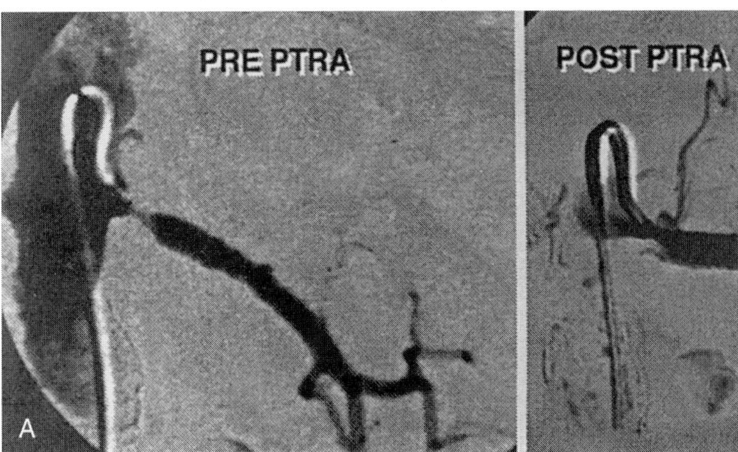

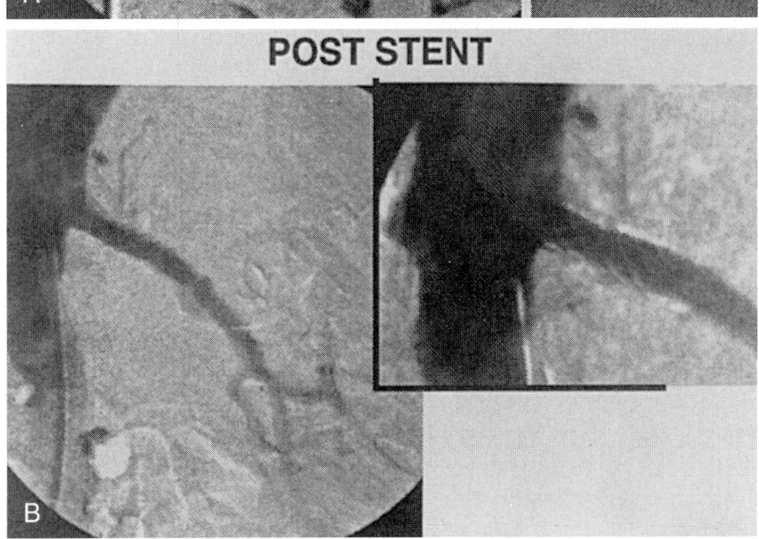

Figure 11–22. *A*, Renal artery stenosis due to atherosclerosis that failed to respond to simple angioplasty. *B*, Treatment with renal arterial stent in the treatment of a proximal renal artery stenosis. (Courtesy of T. Sos.)

Table 11–12. COMPLICATIONS OF RENAL ANGIOPLASTY

		Renal Artery			Distant Problems Puncture Site, Access Route		Renal Failure			
		No. of Operative Repairs								
Study	**No. Patients (Arteries)**	*Dissection*	*Rupture*	*Thrombosis/ Emboli/ Occlusion*	*Major*	*Minor*	*Tran-sient*	*Perma-nent*	**Nephrec-tomy**	**Death**
Katzen et al, 1979	17 (18)	—	—	—	1 (−)	—	1	0	—	—
Martin et al, 1981	31 (36)	—	—	—	2 (−)	—	—	0	0	0
Colopinto et al, 1982	68 (80)	—	—	—	2 (−)	2	1	0	2	0
Sos et al, 1983	89 (104)	5 (−)	0	0	3 (3)	2	6	0	1	0
Tegtmeyer et al, 1984	109 (141)	—	1 (−)	1 (−)	3 (2)	—	6	0	—	—
Martin et al, 1985	100 (137)	5 (4)	0	3 (0)	6 (2)	5	11	0	0	0
Martin et al, 1986	100 (143)	1 (1)	1 (−)	5 (2)	5 (3)	1	5	0	—	—
Gardiner et al, 1986	(77)	5 (−)	2 (−)	4 (−)	—	—	—	0	—	0
Weibull et al, 1987	78 (90)	12	3	6	17	6	11	0	0	1
O'Donovan et al, 1992	17 (19)	1 (1)	—	1 (0)	—	10	—	0	—	1
Lohr et al, 1991	288	7 (6)	5 (4)	2 (2)	2 (2)	—	2	3	—	—

From Trost D, Sos TA: Semin Interven Radiol 1994; 2(2):150–160.

shows effective long-term benefit (Von Knorring et al, 1989; Lawrie et al, 1989; van Bockel et al, 1988, 1989).

Angioinfarction

In rare cases, a patient is too ill for any form of intervention, the kidney has minimal function, and medical management is inadequate. In this unusual setting, percutaneous renal ablation with ethanol can be performed and has been reported to be successful (Iaccarino et al, 1989; Klimberg et al, 1989).

Renal Reconstruction or Angioplasty for Preservation of Renal Function: Ischemic Nephropathy

The work of Schreiber discussed earlier has called attention to the threat of atherosclerotic renal artery disease to overall renal function. This observation is now recognized as an important clinical issue separate from the problem of renovascular hypertension. In addition the Schreiber study suggested that progression occurred primarily within the first 2 years of angiographic follow-up in patients with greater than 50% stenosis on the initial angiogram. Moreover, loss of renal parenchyma could not be attributed to poor blood pressure control. In a separate study, Novick reviewed patients undergoing dialysis over a 10-year period and identified 25 patients with end-stage renal disease as a consequence of atherosclerotic renal artery disease (Novick et al, 1984).

Therefore, a second indication for intervention with angioplasty or revascularization is to preserve renal function, whether or not there is associated renovascular hypertension.

Hypertension is the underlying cause of end-stage renal disease in 29% of patients, second only to diabetes (Klag et al, 1996). Precise studies to define the etiology of the hypertension in these patients are lacking, and the incidence of renal artery disease is unknown although well-recognized (Corradi et al, 1993; Textor, 1994; Appel et al, 1995). However, renal vascular disease was identified in 83 of 687 dialysis patients in one study (Mailloux et al, 1994). Renal Doppler sonography has been suggested in patients with progressive renal insufficiency to identify patients with renal arterial disease or "ischemic nephropathy" (Hansen, 1994). Identification of renal arterial disease in these patients is rational in view of the success of angioplasty or revascularization in preserving renal function (Rimmer and Gennari, 1993; Novick, 1995).

Novick (1984) established the following criteria for angiographic screening of atherosclerotic renal arterial disease: (1) evidence of generalized atherosclerosis; (2) a unilateral small kidney; (3) mild to moderate azotemia (serum creatinine greater than 1.5 mg/dl); and (4) hypertension. If the patient is subsequently found to have a high-grade (greater than 75%) arterial stenosis affecting the entire renal mass, namely where such a stenosis is present bilaterally or involves a solitary kidney, the author recommends intervention.

An additional indicator for intervention is a marked drop in effective renal plasma and glomerular filtration rate when the patient is challenged with the vasodilator sodium nitroprusside (Textor et al, 1985). The mechanism of the fall in blood pressure has previously been discussed.

In a 10-year review of operative patients at the Cleveland Clinic, 161 of 241 patients with atherosclerotic disease underwent surgical revascularization to achieve preservation of renal function. Within this group, renal function was improved in 93 patients (57.7%), stable in 50 patients (31.1%), and deteriorated in 10 patients (6%) (Bedoya et al, 1989).

On the basis of the earlier observations of Novick and Libertino (see Chapter 12), numerous groups have now shown preservation of renal function in these patients after angioplasty (Casarella, 1986; Schwarten, 1987). In the review of six series by Rimmer and Gennari, renal function was improved or stabilized in about 70% of patients after angioplasty, in contrast to 86% of 352 patients undergoing renal revascularization (Rimmer and Gennari, 1993). Thus it is clear that renal arterial disease should be suspected in any azotemic patient without a clearly documented cause of the renal impairment. Renal vascular disease should be excluded before the patient is relegated to medical treatment for renal insufficiency, which actually may be detrimental in this setting. Moreover, it is important to remember that renin determinations and blood response to CEI are inaccurate and often falsely negative in azotemic patients. In this setting, PTA or angioplasty is based on the finding of renal artery disease, not on establishing the kidney as the cause of coexisting hypertension, as described in this chapter.

OTHER RENAL VASCULAR DISEASES

Acute Renal Artery Occlusion

Renal artery embolism is a rare but important cause of hypertension and renal failure. Most emboli are associated with cardiac diseases. **Thirty percent of patients have preexisting coronary artery disease or valvular heart disease; 55% suffer from cardiac arrhythmias** (Gasparini et al, 1992). Atrial fibrillation can induce thrombus formation. Embolic events usually occur in the first year of onset. The prognosis is better for patients with sustained fibrillation than for those with intermittent atrial fibrillation (Morris et al, 1993). Other conditions predisposing to renal artery thrombus formation include blunt trauma, renal artery stenosis, and iatrogenic angiographic manipulation. Rare cases have been noted following cocaine injection, renal transplant, and intra-aortic balloon pump placement. A prior history of cardiac disease, embolic events, hypertension, and peripheral vascular disease is noted in many patients (Gasparini et al, 1992).

Clinical manifestations of renal artery embolism are nonspecific and inconsistent. Because of its rarity and nonspecific presentation the diagnosis of renal artery embolization is often delayed and sometimes missed. The diagnosis of renal infarction was made in 1.4% of autopsies (205 of 14,411) reported by Hoxie and Coggin (1940). However, in only 0.014% of patients was the diagnosis made clinically.

Pain is a frequent finding; it may be acute in onset, sharp, and severe without radiation. Flank pain is found in 61% of cases, abdominal pain in 28%, nausea in 21%. The urinalysis may reveal hematuria (65%), pyuria (50%), and proteinuria (70%). Patients often manifest mild hyperthermia and leukocytosis. Lactate dehydrogenase (LDH) (isoenzymes 1 and 2) is elevated in all patients. Elevations of more than 2000 IU/ml can occur within 24 hours of renal artery occlusion and can persist for up to 14 days. Yet, none of these findings is specific, and a high degree of clinical suspicion is necessary to make the diagnosis in a timely manner.

The differential diagnosis includes nephrolithiasis, pyelonephritis, myocardial infarction, and acute cholecystitis. In a study of 14 patients with renal artery occlusion, Blum and associates (1993) found the admitting diagnosis to be correct in only two patients. The other 12 patients were admitted with diagnoses of nephrolithiasis (eight patients) and mesenteric infarction (four patients). Thirteen of the 14 patients were found to be in atrial fibrillation.

The diagnosis is often suspected on the finding of partial or complete renal ischemia on CT. The presence of renal artery occlusion is confirmed by demonstration of a filling defect or occlusion in the renal artery by angiography. It is recommended that a nonobstructed nonfunctioning kidney be demonstrated before invasive angiography is performed. The angiogram should be carefully evaluated for collateral circulation to the kidney, for the degree of renal artery occlusion, the function of the contralateral kidney, and for evidence of other atherosclerotic or embolic phenomena. Echocardiography is helpful for ruling out intracardiac thrombus as a source of the embolus.

Therapy

Therapeutic intervention for renal artery embolism remains controversial. In the 1960s, surgical embolectomy was commonly attempted (Rohl, 1971). Later, systemic anticoagulation was practiced. In 1973 Moyer and co-workers (1973) compared the results of operative therapy to medical therapy for renal artery emboli. Surgical intervention for unilateral renal artery embolism was found to have greater mortality (18% versus 0%) and greater renal loss (56% versus 23%) than medical management.

More recently, the development of the fibrinolytic agents that can be delivered directly into the thrombosed vessels has introduced new treatment options for renal artery embolism. Sanfelippo and Goldin (1978) demonstrated effective clot lysis with infusion of streptokinase directly into previously embolized canine renal arteries. Fischer first reported the successful lysis of a 7-day-old renal artery thrombus with streptokinase in a 49-year-old woman (Fischer et al, 1981). Selective intra-arterial infusion of thrombolytic agents has proved to be more effective than systemic anticoagulation while decreasing bleeding complications.

Three fibrinolytic agents are in common use at present: streptokinase, urokinase, and recombinant tissue plasminogen activator. Streptokinase is a nonenzymatic protein produced by group C streptococci. It acts by forming a streptokinase-plasminogen activator complex that converts plasminogen to plasmin. Plasmin is a proteolytic enzyme capable of hydrolyzing fibrin into soluble polypeptides, resulting in clot lysis. Streptokinase is the most cost-effective fibrinolytic agent. However, because of its long half-life (27 minutes), a higher incidence of bleeding complications is seen with this agent (Berridge et al, 1989). Moreover, in patients with antistreptococcal antibodies, the initial infusion is neutralized by the formation of antigen-antibody complexes. Clot lysis cannot occur until the dose of streptokinase consumes all the antistreptococcal antibodies. Thus the response to a given dose of streptokinase is variable. Side effects of streptokinase include fever, nausea, hallucinations, and anaphylaxis. Infusion rates of 3000 to 12,000 units/hour are used.

Urokinase is an enzymatic protein produced by human renal parenchymal cells with fibrinolytic function. It does not have antigenicity, as does streptokinase, and it has low pyrogenicity. Infusion rates in the range of 5000 to 75,000 units/hour are used. Urokinase is more expensive than streptokinase.

The third fibrinolytic agent in use today is tissue-type plasminogen activator, a serine protease (Hamilton, 1996). Its DNA structure has been sequenced, and it is now produced by recombinant technology. Tissue plasminogen activator has a high affinity for thrombus-bound plasminogen but low affinity for plasminogen in the absence of fibrin. Therefore, it exerts its clot-lysing effect locally on the intravascular thrombus and not systemically.

At diagnostic angiography, the renal artery catheter can be left in place for fibrinolysis. **The aim of fibrinolytic therapy is to quickly lyse the clot to permit renal reperfusion.** To maximize the interface between the clot and the lytic agent, the percutaneously introduced guide wire and catheter are used to break up the thrombus. Coaxial catheters permit simultaneous delivery of the fibrinolytic agent proximally and distally in the renal artery to further hasten clot lysis. Transcatheter clot aspiration has been attempted to speed up reperfusion of the kidney (Sniderman et al, 1984). However, catheter aspiration is technically difficult to perform and cannot always be achieved. Fibrinolytic therapy is continued until clot lysis is achieved. Prothrombin times are maintained between two and three times normal. At completion of therapy, systemic anticoagulation with heparin and later with warfarin is used to prevent recurrent thrombus formation. Fibrinolytic therapy is contraindicated in patients with bleeding diathesis, in those in the postoperative period, those following significant trauma, or those with an active peptic ulcer.

Technically successful clot lysis is achieved in most cases, but long-term renal function is maintained in only one half the cases. Prompt treatment is stressed because warm ischemia is tolerated by the renal parenchymal for only 60 to 90 minutes. Partial obstruction of the renal artery or occlusion of a segmental branch as well as good collateral renal circulation is associated with a good functional outcome.

Surgical options for treatment of a renal artery thrombus include embolectomy and patch angioplasty, aortorenal bypass graft, renal autotransplant, and excision with end-to-end anastomosis (Spirnak and Resnick, 1987). In their review of cases of complete occlusion of the main renal artery by thrombosis resulting from blunt abdominal trauma, Spirnak and Resnick found only nine successfully performed revascularization procedures. Four of 10 patients with bilateral renal artery occlusion required dialysis support for 3 days to 3 months. Of 35 patients with unilateral occlusion, only five patients had a successful revascularization. All patients were young and had operations within 12 hours of the injury. Postoperatively, three of the five demonstrated either a decrease in size or function of the operated kidney. Of the 35 patients 13 (37%) eventually required a nephrectomy. **The authors concluded that emergency surgery solely for the salvage of renal function in unilateral arterial occlusion in the presence of a normal contralateral kidney is not advocated.** If it is early and surgery is otherwise required and one accepts a 37% chance that delayed nephrectomy will be necessary, it is reasonable to attempt surgery. It should be noted, however, that the patient with a unilateral renal artery thrombus is currently a good candidate for fibrinolysis.

Lacombe (1992) reviewed records of 20 patients having surgery for acute occlusion of the main renal artery 18 hours to 68 days following onset of obstruction. He found a renal salvage rate of 64% and with a mortality rate of 15%. Nephrectomies were performed in three cases and the rest were revascularized. In eight of nine anuric patients, diureses appeared after revascularization. Neither nonfunction of the kidney nor duration of renal artery obstruction was a good predictor of renal function after revascularization. The author surmised that intervention in acute renal artery obstruction is warranted because it is a potentially correctable cause of renal failure.

In a 10-year review of the literature, Gasparini and colleagues found 33 cases of acute renal artery occlusion and reported three additional cases from their own institution. Six patients presented with bilateral renal artery involvement and three with occlusion of a solitary renal unit. Renal artery embolization occurred in a patient with a patent foramen ovale suffering from deep vein thrombosis. In another patient, renal artery embolization followed percutaneous transluminal coronary angioplasty. Treatment included operative embolectomy in 12 patients, intravenous anticoagulation in 12, and intra-arterial streptokinase in nine. Follow-up evaluation was performed by renal scan or intravenous pyelogram (IVP) in unilateral embolism. In bilateral disease or in embolism of a solitary kidney, serum creatinine testing was used. For operative therapy the mortality was 25% with a renal salvage rate of 20%. For systemic anticoagulation the mortality rate was 0% and the renal salvage rate, 30%. With intra-arterial streptokinase, the mortality rate was 0% and the renal salvage rate was 100%. No patient had completely normal renal function on follow-up. Patients with incomplete occlusion or with collateral vessels had better renal salvage.

Several authors have stressed that the considerable delay between the onset of symptoms and the onset of therapy prevents salvage of renal function despite establishment of renal perfusion. (Blum et al, 1993; Gasparini et al, 1992; Spirnak and Resnick, 1987; and Hamilton, 1996). The problem is the delay in formulating the correct diagnosis. In Blum's series it took 12 hours to 8 days to establish the correct diagnosis, far exceeding the warm ischemia time tolerated by the kidney. For treatment, a regional catheter delivery was used for the infusion of the obstructing clot material with streptokinase (30,000 IU/hour), urokinase (30,000–100,000 IU/hour) (Vogelzang et al, 1988), or recombinant tissue type plasminogen activator (2.5–4 mg/hour). Infusion time was 3 to 17 hours (mean 6 hours) accompanied by systemic heparinization (1000 IU/hour). Thrombolysis was successful in 13 of 14 patients. In a mean follow-up period of 27 months, renal function did not improve on the side of complete renal artery occlusion. In incomplete obstruction, or complete obstruction limited to the segmental renal artery branches, renal function did stabilize at pretherapy levels. **In no patient did renal function return to normal. In his review of 82 patients from the literature Blum found that complete occlusion of the main renal artery for more than 3 hours produced irreversible damage of the renal parenchyma.** He hypothesized that in acute embolic renal artery occlusion of greater than 3 hours' duration, thrombolytic therapy does not restore renal function and is therefore not indicated once the ischemic tolerance of the kidney is exceeded. When ischemia lasted less than 3 hours, complete recovery was possible.

Salam and co-workers (1993) performed selective infusion of fibrinolytic agents (streptokinase and urokinase) into the occluded renal artery in 10 patients. In 7 of 10 cases, renal perfusion was restored and in 3 of 10 cases renal function was restored. Morris and associates (1993) reported on a patient who presented with atrial fibrillation and acute anuria resulting from bilateral renal artery embolization from a left atrial thrombus. Embolectomy was performed 30 hours after occlusion. Complete resolution of the renal failure occurred despite the long delay in the onset of therapy. The authors explained that in this patient, the presence of arteriosclerotic occlusion in the proximal portion of both renal arteries induced the formation of a collateral circulation. The metabolic demands of the renal tubular cells were thus satisfied during occlusion by the thrombus. However, the blood flow was inadequate to support glomerular filtration. The authors analyzed Moyer's data (Moyer et al, 1973) and emphasized one patient who survived with a functioning kidney first treated 43 days after the onset of symptoms. Another patient received treatment 12 hours after the onset of symptoms but did not survive. No significant correlation was found between the time to treatment from the onset of symptoms and the outcome, as indicated by functional kidney status and patient survival. The authors recommended that renal revascularization via percutaneous transcatheter thrombolytic therapy or surgical embolectomy be attempted even beyond 24 hours of occlusion.

Conclusion

Renal artery occlusion remains an important cause of acute renal failure and hypertension. **Renal artery embolism should be suspected in any patient with severe acute flank or abdominal pain and a history of cardiac arrhythmia or valvular disease.** In unilateral renal artery occlusion, the presence of urine and the nonspecific presentation may delay diagnosis. The surgeons must keep a high index of suspicion. Treatment goals are renal salvage with minimal morbidity and mortality. Intra-arterial fibrinolytic therapy appears to be the most favorable treatment for unilateral or bilateral renal artery embolism. The potential return of renal function even after 48 hours of anuria emphasizes the importance of renal collateral circulation in preserving glomerular viability. An aggressive interventional approach is indicated, regardless of the time delay. Fibrinolytic therapy appears to be established as a major treatment of thrombotic vascular occlusion. If clot lysis does not occur, surgery may be considered. Aggressive surgical management remains a treatment option.

Cholesterol Embolization

Cholesterol embolization of the kidneys is a rare cause of hypertensive urgency (Van Hoenacker et al, 1994; Simon and Archer, 1995). Renal cholesterol emboli usually affect elderly men with atherosclerotic vascular disease. This rare disease may occur spontaneously or it may be iatrogenic in origin, following angiographic manipulation or cardiovascular surgery. A less frequent cause is use of anticoagulant drugs.

Lye and colleagues (1993) found predisposing factors in 60% of 129 patients with renal cholesterol emboli. Fifty-five (43%) had undergone angiography, 17 (13%) had been started on anticoagulants, and seven (5%) had undergone vascular surgery. The remaining 50 (39%) patients had a severely atherosclerotic abdominal aorta. Clinical findings from Lye and colleagues' review are summarized in Table 11–13. A high incidence of eosinophilia (71%) has been reported (Wilson et al, 1991). Livedo reticularis is present in 32% of patients, digital infarcts in more than 40%. Dialysis for renal insufficiency was necessary in 40% of patients (Koga et al, 1991). Twenty percent recovered sufficiently to discontinue dialysis. Hypertension is a frequent complication of renal cholesterol emboli. It is frequently a consequence of renal ischemia and renal failure. Hypertension is seldom the presenting symptom. It may precede the embolization, being a contributing factor. The mortality rate for patients with renal cholesterol emboli was an alarming 64%.

Table 11–13. DIAGNOSIS OF RENAL CHOLESTEROL EMBOLIZATION IN 129 PATIENTS

Characteristic	Number of Patients	%
Severe hypertension	62	48
Dialysis required	52	40
Digital gangrene	55	43
Livedo reticularis	41	32
Neurologic	15	12
Gastrointestinal	16	12
Retinal emboli	13	10
Eosinophilia (N = 80)	57	71
Recovery of ARF (N = 52)	11	21
Death	82	64

From Lye WC, Cheah JS, Sinniah R: Am J Nephrol 1993; 13:489–493.

Vidt and associates (1989) identified renal cholesterol emboli in 24 renal biopsy specimens. In 19 of these kidneys, renal artery stenosis was present. Clinical manifestations of generalized atherosclerosis were common. Evidence of embolic disease to other organs was also common. These patients were treated with angioplasty or surgical revascularization to improve their renal function.

Extrarenal manifestations of cholesterol embolization are reviewed in Table 11–13. Neurologic manifestations may include cerebrovascular accidents and changes in the level of consciousness. Neurologic manifestations may be a consequence of the effects of embolism, hypertension, or uremia. Gastrointestinal involvement included hemorrhage, infarction, and bowel perforation.

The diagnosis of renal cholesterol emboli is made from the clinical history, physical examination, and laboratory findings. Ultrasound and CT examinations may not yield an explanation for the signs and symptoms. Selective renal angiogram can suggest the diagnosis by showing microemboli in the peripheral renal vessels. The diagnosis is confirmed by biopsy revealing intravascular cholesterol emboli. In Lye and colleagues' (1993) series, the diagnosis was confirmed by renal biopsy as well as muscle and skin biopsies. In the kidneys, intralobular and arcuate arteries are most frequently affected.

The differential diagnosis includes rheumatic heart disease, subacute bacterial endocarditis, diffuse intravascular coagulopathy, Churg-Strauss syndrome, and left atrial myxoma.

The treatment is supportive, providing management of the hypertension and the renal insufficiency and the control of the underlying pathology.

Renal Vein Thrombosis

Renal vein thrombosis (RVT) occurs in 15% to 20% of patients with the nephrotic syndrome, but in up to 50% of those with membranous glomerulonephritis (Rowe et al, 1984). Results of clotting studies contrasting the blood viscosity and fibrinogen content of the renal vein to the elbow vein showed that nephrotic patients are hypercoagulable. Fibrinogen and blood viscosity are both markedly increased (Wu et al, 1994). In 60 nephrotic patients with glomerulonephropathy, 12 were found to have RVT by CT examination. Selective venography confirmed the diagnosis. Treatment with urokinase administration into the renal vein or renal artery in association with dipyridamole (Persantine) and prednisone with warfarin maintenance improved renal function post-treatment.

In children, RVT may have an acute onset presenting with severe flank pain and hematuria. On excretory pyelography there is poor visualization of the kidneys owing to a marked decrease in renal function. The involved kidneys are enlarged with pyelocalyceal abnormalities. Treatment with anticoagulation results in clinical improvement and amelioration of renal function. Rapid and complete resolution of the thrombus through use of thrombolytic agents is possible in acute RVT. Heparin and warfarin maintenance are used in follow-up treatment (Lach et al, 1980). In contrast, chronic RVT in older patients tends to be asymptomatic. Clinical onset is often insidious and barely noticed. The only clinical manifestation may be peripheral edema. Gross hematuria is present, albeit much less often than in acute RVT. Results of pyelography are normal in the majority of patients with chronic RVT. Complications with pulmonary emboli are common. An improvement in renal function is not seen with anticoagulation as in acute RVT, but possibly new thromboembolic episodes are avoided.

Renal Injuries Causing Hypertension

The incidence of hypertension following renal trauma is difficult to establish. In many instances, the kidney has been removed for renal vascular injury. In other cases there may be a delay in presentation and diagnosis, or the diagnosis may be missed altogether. A history of abdominal trauma with flank pain, proteinuria, and hematuria is present in most patients, but findings are variable and nonspecific (Clark et al, 1981). Several reviews report the incidence of hypertension in patients not treated surgically after renal injury to range from 29% to 57% (Cass et al, 1985). Stables and colleagues (1976) noted that five of 10 patients treated conservatively developed hypertension. Clark and associates reported an incidence of hypertension of 18% in patients treated with early revascularization.

Renovascular hypertension associated with renal trauma occurs most often in young males following blunt abdominal trauma. The interval to presentation varies between 2 days and 14 years. However, high blood pressure may present acutely and may be associated with hypertensive encephalopathy (Watts et al, 1987). The mechanisms for hypertension **include renal artery stenosis, renal artery compression, branch artery stenosis, and arteriovenous fistula, which could be intrarenal or extrarenal. External compression of the renal parenchyma may follow trauma and may result in increased renin secretion and hypertension.** Parenchyma compressing hematomas may form in the subcapsular or perirenal spaces. Chronic hematomas may evolve into a fibrous pseudocapsule that compresses the renal parenchyma. (See later discussion of Page kidney.)

No guidelines are available that define when revascularization of the acutely ischemic kidney should be undertaken. Vascular repair is often attempted in patients with limited injuries. Little objective data exist for predicting success. Turner and colleagues (Turner et al, 1983) reviewed the records of 94 patients with 96 renal vessel injuries operated on between 1960 and 1979. The ages ranged from 4 to 67 years with a mean of 30 years. Forty-nine patients had 51 renal artery injuries. There were 78 renal vein injuries. Forty-nine of 51 renal artery injuries were treated operatively. Two patients with renal artery thrombosis were observed. Renal artery repair was successful in one third of cases. Most isolated renal venous injuries were repaired. Thirty-seven percent of the patients died after operative repair of the renal artery injuries, and 28% died after repair of venous injuries. Renal salvage was possible in 10% of patients with renal artery injuries and in 51% of patients with renal vein injuries (see Chapter 99).

The decision to perform revascularization rather than nephrectomy is made with the expectation of renal salvage. Thirty-three percent of arterial repairs and 4% of venous repairs required subsequent nephrectomy. Hypertension developed in 18% of the revascularized patients. Eighty-three percent of these hypertensive patients required nephrectomy. Revascularization of traumatic renal artery occlusions failed in all cases. In these patients, nephrectomy is an option unless the injury is bilateral. In the absence of renal artery occlusion, renal preservation was surgically accomplished in 50% of cases.

The clinical features of 39 patients who developed hypertension after renal trauma are summarized in Tables 11–14 to 11–16. The majority of patients were young males in motor vehicle accidents. The interval between injury and the onset of hypertension varied between 2 days and 13 years. In most instances, hypertension was the first indication of renal artery stenosis. In four cases, stenosis occurred after revascularization had been attempted. Four out of five patients who were hypertensive postoperatively were operated on more than 1 year after the injury. This finding parallels the situation in which late removal of the kidney or clip in the two-kidney one-clip hypertension model fails to cure the hypertension.

Table 11–14. TRAUMA CAUSING RENAL INJURY AND HYPERTENSION

Nature of Trauma	Renal Artery Occlusion	AV Fistula	Page Kidney
MVA	25	0	4
Falls	3	0	7
Blunt	3	2	22
Crush	2	0	0
Penetrating	2	10	1
Others	0	0	3
Unknown	4	0	0

From Massumi RA, Andrade A, Kramer N: Am J Med 1969; 46:635–639.

Table 11–15. INTERVAL BETWEEN ONSET OF INJURY AND DISCOVERY OF HYPERTENSION

Interval	Renal Artery Occlusion	Arteriovenous Fistula	Page Kidney
< 1 year	26	2	18
> 1 year	8	10	11
Unknown	5	0	8

From Massumi RA, Andrade A, Kramer N: Am J Med 1969; 46:635–639.

Arteriovenous Fistula

Renal arteriovenous (AV) fistula formation after trauma is rare. Penetrating injury is the predominant form of trauma associated with AV fistula. Hypertension is a recognized complication of renal AV fistulas and occurs in 50% of cases (McAlhany et al, 1971). In an AV fistula there is ischemia distal to the fistula, increasing renin release from the affected side. Nephrectomy may result in normotension. Experience with vascular reconstruction is limited.

Page Kidney

Perinephric and subcapsular hematomas are common after renal trauma. Renal compression sufficient to cause hypertension is unusual. Most patients are young males who suffer blunt trauma in sports-related injuries. The interval of injury to the presentation of hypertension is variable and in the range of a few days to over 20 years. A review of Page kidney follows in the next section.

Summary

Renal trauma infrequently results in hypertension. Its importance is underlined in that it occurs in young patients. Aggressive evaluation and treatment are justified to reduce the associated morbidity and mortality. Cases presenting within 1 year of injury have a much better prognosis than those presenting later. Although spontaneous resolution may occur, surgery after 1 year following the injury is associated with persistent hypertension. All patients who have suffered renal injury should have their blood pressure monitored closely henceforth.

Page Kidney

In 1934, Page (1939) produced a renin-dependent model of hypertension by wrapping a dog kidney in cellophane.

Table 11–16. BLOOD PRESSURE OUTCOMES OF SURGICAL REVASCULARIZATION

Interval from Injury to Surgery	Postoperative Blood Pressure	Postoperative Blood Pressure
	Normal	Raised
<1 year	25	1
>1 year	6	4
Unknown	2	1

Normal blood pressure is diastolic <90 mm Hg without treatment.
From Massumi RA, Andrade A, Kramer N: Am J Med 1969; 46:635–639.

Hypertension could be reversed by removing the cellophane wrap or the kidney. **The clinical equivalent of this hypertensive model is the kidney compressed by a subcapsular or perirenal process causing renal ischemia, inducing unilateral hypersecretion of renin and contralateral suppression.** Etiologies for the perinephric process include blunt trauma, closed renal biopsy, anticoagulation, or hemorrhage from a tumor (Table 11–17). On surgical exploration renal compression was the result of hematoma in 85% of cases and urinoma in 15% (Suffrin, 1975).

The diagnosis of Page kidney depends on the presence of either a surrounding hematoma or an encasing fibrous pseudocapsule. Imaging with ultrasonography, CTT, or magnetic resonance imaging (MRI) localizes the hematoma or fibrous capsule. Ultrasonography is the least invasive and most cost-effective technique but may lack the resolution for documenting the presence or absence of a smaller hematoma or fibrous capsule. CTT and MRI achieve excellent resolution in the retroperitoneum. When ultrasonography results are equivocal, CTT and MRI should be used.

The treatment of acute Page kidney aims to preserve renal function and cure hypertension. ACE inhibitors plus observation, percutaneous evacuation of the perirenal hematoma, open drainage of the hematoma, and nephrectomy have been performed. A hematoma or fibrous capsule about the kidney can thus be treated in a variety of ways, dictated in large part by the patient's clinical picture. No randomized studies have been done ascertaining the best treatment. Current therapeutic practices are based on case reports and retrospective studies.

Some cases of acute Page kidney with new-onset hypertension have spontaneously resolved. A hematoma may reabsorb, relieving the parenchymal compression without forming an adhesive fibrotic pseudocapsule. Treatment with ACE inhibitors controls the blood pressure until the hematoma resolves. If the hematoma does not resolve, it may be drained percutaneously or surgically.

A chronic hematoma may lead to the formation of a fibrotic pseudocapsule with compression of all or part of the renal parenchyma. Hypertension persists, and there may also be permanent loss of renal function. Conservative surgical therapy such as capsulotomy may preserve renal function and control the hypertension. However, evacuation of the hematoma alone may be frustrated by reaccumulation of fluid or by persistence of the fibrous pseudocapsule, allowing parenchymal compression to persist.

Table 11–17. CAUSES OF PAGE KIDNEY

Cause of Page Kidney	No. of Cases
Contact sports	28
Non-sports trauma	18
Motor vehicle accidents	7
Postoperative complications	5
Renal biopsy	3
Warfarin therapy	2
Renal transplant	2
Lumbar sympathetic block	1
Pancreatitis	1
Tumor	1
Unknown	12

From Sterns RH, Rabinowitz R, Segal AJ, Spitzer RM: Arch Intern Med 1985; 145:169–171.

Nephrectomy has been the most common form of therapy utilized to treat Page kidney. However, nephrectomy may or may not cure the hypertension. Suffrin (1975) found that regardless of the choice of treatment, blood pressure was shown to normalize in approximately 88% of patients treated by observation, evacuation of the hematoma, and nephrectomy. However, these results must be interpreted cautiously because this study represents a small number of patients not stratified as to age, severity of the lesion, or comorbidities. Split renal function studies and renal vein renin levels need to be performed preoperatively. A nonfunctioning or minimally functioning kidney that secretes renin can be considered for removal if the contralateral kidney is capable of supporting renal function on its own.

In some patients, parenchymal compression and renin secretion for too long a period produce contralateral renal injury with chronic hypertension that is no longer renin-dependent. At this point, the hypertension is no longer reversible. In other instances the fibrous pseudocapsule may not be the cause of hypertension but coexists with it. Surgery, in both cases, is not corrective for the hypertension. In the presence of a fibrous capsule, evacuation of the perinephric process has failed to resolve the blood pressure elevation in 6 of 11 patients. However, nephrectomy led to cure of hypertension in 22 patients and improvement in 2 of 26 patients (Sterns, 1985) (Table 11–18). In the management of chronic subcapsular hematoma, simple evacuation of the hematoma often fails to cure the hypertension. It is preferable to attempt percutaneous drainage of the hematoma. If the blood pressure fails to respond to drainage, and RVR lateralizes, surgical drainage with removal of pseudocapsule or nephrectomy can be performed. Alternatively, if the surgical alternative is not appropriate, medical therapy can be used to control the hypertension.

Renal Artery Aneurysm

Renal artery aneurysms are uncommon (Poutasse, 1975). The true prevalence of renal artery aneurysms (RAA) in the general population is unknown. RAA account for 22% of visceral aneurysms. They are diagnosed with an incidence of 0.7% to 1.32% on renal angiograms (Hubert et al, 1980). Because of more widespread use of angiography and CT as well as improved imaging techniques, RAA are diagnosed more frequently. Fibromuscular dysplasia and arteriosclerotic occlusion of the renal artery are believed to be the most frequent causes (Cohen, 1987). Trauma can also be a cause. Children can have saccular RAA at the arterial bifurcations, which is thought to represent a congenital defect. Intrarenal aneurysms are frequently associated with arteritis such as polyarteritis nodosa (PAN) and Wegener's granulomatosis but also can be congenital, traumatic, or associated with atherosclerosis, syphilis, or tuberculosis (Bulbul et al, 1993).

Table 11–18. RESULTS OF THERAPY IN HYPERTENSION DUE TO CHRONIC SUBCAPSULAR HEMATOMA

	Nephrectomy	Evacuation of Hematoma
Total patients	28	11
No. cured (%)	22 (78)	4 (36)
No. improved (%)	2 (11)	1 (9)
No. unimproved (%)	2 (11)	6 (55)

From Sterns RH, Rabinowitz R, Segal AJ, Spitzer RM: Arch Intern Med 1985; 145:169–171.

Dissecting aneurysms are classified etiologically as traumatic, spontaneous, or iatrogenic (resulting from catheterization). Spontaneous dissection has been associated with medial hyperplasia and atherosclerosis.

In general, there are no pathognomonic signs and symptoms of renal artery aneurysms. Nonspecific complaints include flank pain, hematuria, hypertension, and hypotension (suspect rupture of aneurysm). Abnormal findings on IVP suggesting a renal vascular lesion are seen in up to 60% of cases, and more are detected on CT examination. Angiography is needed to confirm the diagnosis.

Rupture, the most lethal complication, is rare. Extrarenal, noncalcified, or incompletely calcified aneurysms are more prone to rupture than those with circumferential calcification. Rupture of RAA during pregnancy has been reported. The results are catastrophic, with a mortality rate of 50% for the mother and 78% for the fetus (Cohen, 1987). In another series (Dayton et al, 1990), 22 cases from the literature revealed a maternal survival in 10 cases and fetal survival in 5. Successful treatment has usually depended on nephrectomy. In situ repair was performed in three cases with satisfactory renal salvage.

Several complications of renal artery aneurysms can occur. Thrombosis of the RAA or distal embolizations are rare complications. Massive hematuria may result from rupture of an aneurysm into the collecting system, by renal infarction, following dissection, thrombosis, or distal embolization. Compression of the collecting system may produce hydronephrosis.

In 56 patients (34 male, 22 female) with 67 renal artery aneurysms, Bulbul (1993) found that 92% were extrarenal. Seventy percent were found to be saccular, 22% fusiform, and 8% dissecting. Most were less than 1 cm in size and noncalcified. Twelve were associated with medial fibroplasia. Associated hypertension was present in 55%, hematuria in 30%, flank pain in 21%, and renal failure in 1.5%. Most were manifestations of medial hyperplasia or atherosclerosis of the renal arteries.

Despite a 70% incidence of hypertension in RAA, a causal relationship has not been well documented. Most aneurysms are found during investigation for renovascular hypertension; therefore, a large number of patients with RAA appear to have hypertension. Cummings (Cummings et al, 1973) recommended an attempt at resection of RAA that is associated with a hemodynamically significant stenosis and elevated PRA (Fig. 11–23). Those without stenosis and PRA are not as likely to be cured despite technically successful surgery.

Patients with fibrodysplasia or arteriosclerotic renal artery occlusions can form a poststenotic fusiform aneurysm. Hypertension associated with the more common saccular aneurysm is less well understood. Saccular aneurysms are present in the main renal branch near the first bifurcation. Ninety percent are extrarenal and 25% to 50% are calcified. Documented renovascular hypertension may be seen with saccular RAA in the absence of renal artery stenosis. The exact mechanism of flow disturbance remains unclear. Throm-

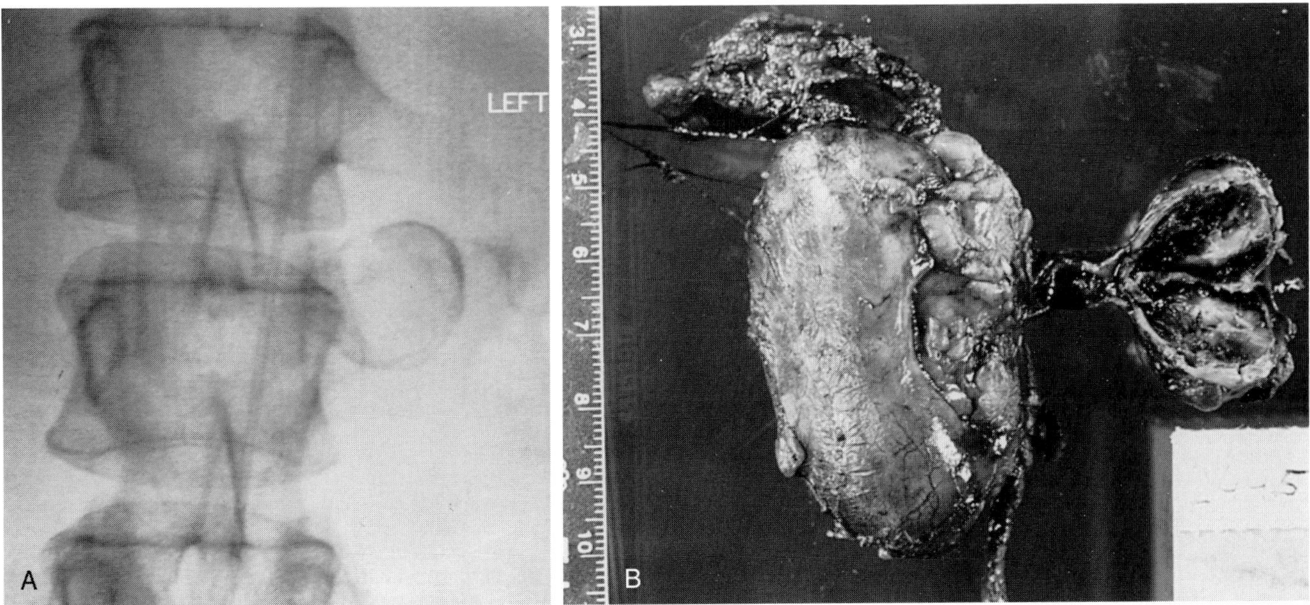

Figure 11–23. Patient with renin-mediated hypertension due to a thrombosed renal artery aneurysm. *A,* Calcified rim of aneurysm shown on an enlarged abdominal plain film. *B,* Specimen showing aneurysm and shrunken kidney.

boembolization distal to the RAA, mechanical compression of adjacent branch arteries, or decreased blood flow due to turbulence within the aneurysm have all been espoused as causing hypertension. (Ruberti et al, 1987).

Treatment of RAA is conservative. **Most reports agree that aneurysms of more than 1.5 cm, calcified or not, should be surgically repaired**. Eighteen hypertensive patients with aneurysms measuring less than 1 cm treated with medication for blood pressure control for more than 10 years did not show complications.

If intervention is indicated, angioinfarction of a segment, surgical reconstruction, or total or partial nephrectomy may be performed. Indications for intervention after RAA include an expanding aneurysm, hypertension, hematuria, renal infarction, and (in women) childbearing age.

Surgical repair options include resection of the aneurysm and direct anastomosis, resection and repair with Dacron patch, aortorenal reconstruction with Dacron or segmental saphenous vein, autotransplantation following resection of the aneurysm, ex vivo reconstruction for multiple anastomoses, partial nephrectomy for intrarenal aneurysm, and nephrectomy (see Chapter 12).

Thirteen hypertensive patients with RAA underwent surgical repair in Bulbul's series (Bulbul, 1993). Nine patients did not require medical treatment postoperatively, three were improved, and one continued unchanged despite good renal blood flow. Surgical repair cured hypertension in 14 of 22 patients (Ruberti, 1987) and improved it in four of 22 for an 82% benefit. In another series (Martin et al, 1989), seven of seven hypertensive patients with RVH improved, and six of 10 with nonrenin-dependent hypertension improved after resection of the aneurysm. The authors recommended that RAA repair in patients with difficult-to-control hypertension should be considered even if renin criteria do not support the diagnosis of RVH.

Patients frequently ask about the risk of rupture of an RAA in pregnancy. It has been suggested that the hormonal changes lead to structural weakness in the arterial wall (Cohen and Shamash, 1987). An increase in renal blood flow and intra-abdominal pressure during pregnancy may further increase the risk of aneurysmal rupture.

Tham and associates (1983) found 83 RAAs in 825 renal angiograms performed over 9 years. Six were bilateral and 11 multiple. Sixty-nine were followed without rupture for a mean of 4.3 years. Fourteen underwent operation, with three of seven hypertensive patients improving blood pressure control. In Sweden in 36,656 autopsies performed over 10 years, no ruptured RAAs were noted. However, aneurysms may thrombose and may be the source of distal emboli, or they may cause obstruction of other renal artery branches. McCarron and colleagues (1975) reported on 19,600 autopsies, without finding a ruptured RAA. He also noted that in 180,000 pregnancies at the New York Hospital, no ruptures of a RAA were observed.

Although the risk for rupture of a RAA is small, the mortality rate for mother and fetus is high. **Most authors recommend repair of a renal artery aneurysm in a woman of childbearing age**.

REFERENCES

Renovascular Hypertension

Albers FJ: Clinical characteristics of atherosclerotic renovascular disease. Am J Kidney Dis 1994; 24:636–641.

Alimi Y, Mercier C, Pellissier J-F, et al: Fibromuscular disease of the renal artery: A new histopathologic classification. Ann Vasc Surg 1992; 6:220–224.

Anderson WP, Ramsey DE, Takata M: Development of hypertension from unilateral renal artery stenosis in conscious dogs. Hypertension 1990; 16:441.

Appel RG, Bleyer AJ, Reavis S, Hansen KJ: Renovascular disease in older patients beginning renal replacement therapy. Kidney Int 1995; 48:171–176.

Ayers CR, Katholi RE, Vaughan ED Jr, et al: Intrarenal renin-angiotensin-sodium interdependent mechanism controlling post clamp renal artery pressure and renin release in the conscious dog with chronic one-kidney Goldblatt hypertension. Circ Res 1977; 40:238.

Bakhle YS: Conversion of angiotensin I to angiotensin II by cell-free extracts of dog lung. Nature 1968; 220:919.

Barajas L, Salido EC, Liu L, Powers KV: The juxtaglomerular apparatus: A morphologic perspective. *In* Laragh JH, Brenner BM, eds: Hypertension Pathophysiology, Diagnosis and Management, 2nd ed. New York, Raven Press, 1995, pp 1335.

Bedoya L, Ziegelbaum M, Vidt DG, et al: The effect of baseline renal function on the outcome following renal revascularization. Cleve Clin J Med 1989; 56:415.

Beebe HG, Chesebro K, Merchant F, Bush W: Results of renal artery balloon angioplasty limit its indications. J Vasc Surg 1988; 8:300.

Belli A-M: New approaches to the diagnosis and management of renal artery stenosis. J Hum Hypertens 1994; 8:593–594.

Blake WD, Wegria R, Ward HP, Frank CW: Effect of renal arterial constriction on excretion of sodium and water. Am J Physiol 1950; 163:422.

Bookstein JJ, Abrams HL, Buenger RE, et al: Radiologic aspects of renovascular hypertension. Part II. The role of urography in unilateral renovascular disease. JAMA 1972; 220:1225.

Braun-Menendez E, Fasciolo JC, Leloir LR, Munoz JM: The substance causing renal hypertension. J Physiol 1940; 98:283.

Brenner BM, ed: The Kidney, 5th ed. Philadelphia, W.B. Saunders Company, 1996.

Briggs JP, Schnermann J: Control of renin release and glomerular vascular tone by the juxtaglomerular apparatus, Chapter 82. *In* Laragh JH, Brenner BM, eds: Hypertension Pathophysiology, Diagnosis and Management, 2nd ed. New York, Raven Press, 1995, p 1359.

Bright R: Reports of medical cases, selected with a view of illustrating symptoms and cure of disease by reference to morbid anatomy. London, Longman Group, 1827.

Brink JA, Lim JT, Wang G, et al: Technical optimization of spiral CT for depiction of renal artery stenosis: In vitro analysis. Radiology 1995; 194:157–163.

Brunner HR, Christen Y, Munafo A, et al: Clinical experience with angiotensin II receptor antagonists. Am J Hypertens 1992; 5:243S–246S.

Brunner HR, Gavras H, Laragh JH, Keenan R: Angiotensin II blockade in man by SAR^1-Ala^8-angiotensin II for understanding and treatment of high blood pressure. Lancet 1973; 2:1045.

Brunner HR, Kirshmann JD, Sealey JE, Laragh JH: Hypertension of renal origin: Evidence for two different mechanisms. Science 1971; 174:1344.

Brunner HR, Laragh JH, Baer L, et al: Essential hypertension: Renin and aldosterone, heart attack, and stroke. N Engl J Med 1972; 286:441.

Buhler FR, Laragh JH, Baer L, et al: Propranolol inhibition of renin secretion. N Engl J Med 1972; 287:1209.

Bumpus FM, Schwarz H, Page IH: Synthesis and pharmacology of the octapeptide angiotensin. Science 1957; 125:886.

Buonocore E, Meaney TF, Borkowski GP, et al: Digital subtraction angiography of the abdominal aorta and renal arteries. Radiology 1981; 139:281.

Burnier M, Waeber B, Nussberger J, Brunner HR: Effect of angiotensin converting enzyme inhibition in renovascular hypertension. J Hypertens 1989; 7(7):S27.

Butler AM: Chronic pyelonephritis and arterial hypertension. J Clin Invest 1937; 16:889.

Canzanello VJ, Millin VG, Spiegel JE, et al: Percutaneous transluminal renal angioplasty in management of atherosclerotic renovascular hypertension: Results in 100 patients. Hypertension 1989; 13:1639.

Carey RM, Vaughan ED Jr, Ackerly JA, et al: The immediate pressor effect of saralasin in man. J Clin Endocrinol Metab 1978; 46:36.

Casarella WJ: Non-coronary angioplasty. Curr Probl Cardiol 1986; 11:3.

Case DB, Atlas SA, Laragh JH: Physiologic effects and blockade. *In* Laragh JH, Buhler FR, Seldin DW, eds: Frontiers in Hypertension Research. New York, Springer-Verlag, 1982, pp 541–550.

Case DB, Atlas SA, Laragh JH, et al: Clinical experience with blockade of the renin-angiotensin-aldosterone system by oral converting enzyme inhibitor (SQ 14225, captopril) in hypertensive patients. Prog Cardiovasc Dis 1978; 21:195.

Case DB, Wallace JM, Keim HJ, et al: Estimating renin participation in hypertension: Superiority of converting enzyme inhibitor over saralasin. Am J Med 1976a; 61:790.

Case DB, Wallace JM, Keim HJ, et al: Usefulness and limitations of saralasin, a weak competitive agonist for angiotensin II, for evaluating the renin and sodium factor in hypertensive patients. Am J Med 1976b; 60:825.

Cheung HS, Cushman DW: Inhibition of homogenous angiotensin-converting enzyme of rabbit lung by synthetic venom peptides of Bothrops jararaca. Biochim Biophys Acta 1973; 293:451.

Chrysant SG, Dunn M, and Marples D: Severe reversible azotemia from captopril therapy. Arch Intern Med 1983; 143:437.

Churchill PC: First and second messengers in renin secretion, *In* Laragh JH, Brenner BM, eds: Hypertension Pathophysiology, Diagnosis and Management, 2nd ed. New York, Raven Press, 1995, pp 1869.

Cicuto KP, McLean GK, Oleaga JA: Renal artery stenosis: Anatomic classification for percutaneous transluminal angioplasty. Am J Roentgenol 1981; 137:599.

Colopinto RF, Stronell RD, Harris-Jones EP, et al: Percutaneous transluminal dilatation of the renal artery: Follow-up studies on renovascular hypertension. AJR Am J Roentgenol 1982; 139:727–732.

Corradi B, Malberti F, Farina M, et al: Chronic renal failure due to atheromatous renovascular disease in the elderly. Contrib Nephrol 1993; 105:167–171.

Cragg AH, Smith TP, Thompson DH, et al: Incidental fibromuscular dysplasia in potential renal donors: Long-term clinical follow-up. Radiology 1989; 172:145.

Dean RH, Kieffer RW, Smith BM, et al: Renovascular hypertension: Anatomic and functional changes during drug therapy. Arch Surg 1981; 116:1408.

Debatin JF, Spritzer CE, Grist TM, et al: Imaging of the renal arteries: Value of MR angiography. AJR Am J Roentgenol 1991; 157:981–990.

Demeilliers B, Jover B, Mimran A: Renal function in one-kidney, one clip sodium-restricted rats: Influence of enalapril and losartan. J Hypertens 1995; 13:1764–1766.

Derkx FHM, Schalekamp MADH: Renal artery stenosis and hypertension. Lancet 1994; 344:237–239.

Derkx FHM, Tan-Tjiong HL, Wentig GJ, et al: Captopril test for diagnosis of renal artery stenosis. *In* Glorioso M, ed: Renovascular Hypertension. New York, Raven Press, 1987, pp 295–305.

Devoy MAB, Tomson CRV, Edmunds ME, et al: Deterioration in renal function associated with angiotensin converting enzyme inhibitor therapy is not always reversible. J Intern Med 1992; 232:493–498.

Diamond JR: Flash pulmonary edema and the diagnostic suspicion of occult renal artery stenosis. Am J Kidney Dis 1993; 21:328–330.

Dominiczak A, Isles C, Gillen G, Brown JJ: Angiotensin converting enzyme inhibition and renal insufficiency in patients with bilateral renovascular disease. J Hum Hypertens 1988; 2:53.

Dondi M: Captopril renal scintigraphy with ^{99m}Tc-Mercaptoacetyltriglycine (^{99m}Tc-MAG$_3$) for detecting renal artery stenosis. Am J Hypertens 1991; 4:737S–740S.

Dotter CT, Judkins MP: Transluminal treatment of arteriosclerotic obstruction. Circulation 1964; 30:654.

Egido J: Vasoactive hormones and renal sclerosis. Kidney Int 1996; 49:578–597.

Eidt JF, Fry RE, Clagett P, et al: Post-operative follow up of renal artery reconstruction with duplex ultrasound. J Vasc Surg 1988; 8:667–673.

Elliott WJ, Martin WB, Murphy MB: Comparison of two non-invasive screening tests for renovascular hypertension. Arch Intern Med 1993; 153:755–764.

Emovon OE, Klotman PE, Dunnick NE, et al: Renovascular hypertension in blacks. Am J Hypertens 1995; 9:18–23.

Eng E, Veniant M, Floege J, et al: Renal proliferative and phenotypic changes in rats with two-kidney, one-clip Goldblatt hypertension. Am J Hypertens 1994; 7:177–185.

Erbsloh-Moller B, Dumas A, Roth D, et al: Furosemide ^{131}I-hippuran renography after angiotensin-converting enzyme inhibition for the diagnosis of renovascular hypertension. Am J Med 1991; 90:23–40.

Eyler WR, Clark MD, Garman JE, et al: Angiography of the renal areas including a comparative study of renal arterial stenosis in patients with and without hypertension. Radiology 1962; 78:879.

Fiorentini C, Galli C, Tamborini G, et al: Hemodynamic and renin responses to nifedipine in renovascular hypertension. Am Heart J 1990; 119:353–356.

Fommei E, Ghione S, Hilson AJW, et al: Captopril radionuclide test in renovascular hypertension. European Multicentre Study. *In* O'Reilly PH, Taylor A, Nally JV, Jr, eds: Radionuclides in Nephro-Urology. Philadelphia, Field & Wood, 1994, pp 33–39.

Foster JH, Maxwell MH, Franklin SS, et al: Renovascular occlusive disease: Results of operative treatment. JAMA 1975; 231:1043.

Franklin SS, Maxwell MH: Clinical workup for renovascular hypertension. Urol Clin North Am 1975; 2:301.

Frederickson ED, Wilcox CS, Bucci CM, et al: A prospective evaluation of a simplified captopril test for the detection of renovascular hypertension. Arch Intern Med 1990; 150:569–572.

Freeman NE, Leeds FM, Elliot W: Thromboendarterectomy for hypertension due to renal artery occlusion. JAMA 1954; 156:1077.

Galanski M, Prokop M, Chavan A, et al: Renal arterial stenoses: Spiral CT angiography. Radiology 1993; 189:185–192.

Gardiner GA, Meyerovitz JF, Stokes KR, et al: Complications of transluminal angioplasty. Radiology 1986; 159:201–208.

Gaul MK, Linn WD, Mulrow CD: Captopril-stimulated renin secretion in the diagnosis of renovascular hypertension. Am J Hypertens 1989; 2:335.

Gavras H, Brunner HR, Vaughan ED Jr, Laragh JH: Angiotensin-sodium interaction in blood pressure maintenance of renal hypertensive and normotensive rats. Science 1973; 180:1369.

Gedroyc WM: Magnetic resonance angiography of renal arteries. Urol Clin North Am 1994; 21:201–214.

Gedroyc WMW, Negus R, Al-Kutoubi A, et al: Magnetic resonance angiography of renal transplants. Lancet 1992; 339:789–791.

Gephardt GN, McCormack LJ: Pathology of the renal artery in hypertension. *In* Breslin DJ, Swinton NW Jr, Libertino JA, Zinman L, eds: Renovascular Hypertension. Baltimore, Williams & Wilkins Company, 1982, pp 63–72.

Geyskes GG, Oei HY, Puylaert CBAJ, et al: Renography with captopril. Changes in a patient with hypertension and unilateral renal artery stenosis. Arch Intern Med 1986; 146:1705–1708.

Geyskes GG, Oei HY, Puylaert CBAJ, Meas EJ: Renovascular hypertension identified by captopril-induced changes in the renogram. Hypertension 1987; 9:451.

Gittes RF, McLaughlin AP: Unilateral operation for bilateral renovascular disease. J Urol 1974; 111:292.

Goldblatt H, Lynch J, Hanzal RF, Summerville WW: Studies on experimental hypertension. I. The production of persistent elevation of systolic blood pressure by means of renal ischemia. J Exp Med 1934; 59:347.

Gomez RA, Norwood VF: Developmental consequences of the renin-angiotensin system. Am J Kidney Dis 1995; 26:409–431.

Goncharenko V, Gerlock AJ, Shaff MI, Hollifield SW: Progression of renal artery fibromuscular dysplasia in 42 patients as seen on angiography. Radiology 1981; 139:45.

Goodfriend T, Elliott ME, Katt KJ: Angiotensin receptors and their antagonists. N Engl J Med 1996; 334:1649–1654.

Goormaghtigh N, Grimson KS: Vascular changes in renal ischemia, cell mitosis in the media of arteries. Proc Soc Exp Biol Med 1939; 42:227.

Gosse P, Dupas JY, Reynaud P, et al: Am J Hypertens 1989; 2:191–193.

Grist TM: Magnetic resonance angiography of renal artery stenosis. Am J Kidney Dis 1994; 24:700–712.

Grist TM, Kennel T, Sproat I, et al: Prospective evaluation of renal MR angiography: Comparison with conventional angiography in 35 patients. Radiology 1993; 189:190.

Gross F: The renin-angiotensin system in hypertension. Ann Intern Med 1971; 75:777.

Gruntzig A, Hopff M: Perkutane rekanalisation chronischer arterieller ver schlusse mit einem neuen dilatations katheter: Modifikation der Dotter technik. Dtsch Med Wochenschr 1974; 99:2505.

Gunning ME, Ingelfinger JR, King AJ, Brenner BM: Vasoactive peptides and the kidney. *In* Brenner BM, ed: The Kidney, 5th ed. Philadelphia, W.B. Saunders Company, 1996, pp 627–712.

Guzman RP, Zierler RE, Isaacson JA, et al: Renal atrophy and arterial stenosis. A prospective study with duplex ultrasound. Hypertension 1994; 23:346–350.

Guzzetta PC, Potter BM, Ruley J, et al: Renovascular hypertension in children: Current concepts and evaluation and treatment. J Ped Surg 1989; 24:1236.

Halpern M, Currarino M: Vascular lesions causing hypertension in neurofibromatosis. N Engl J Med 1965; 73:248.

Hannedouche T, Godin M, Fries D, Fillastre JP: Acute renal thrombosis induced by angiotensin-converting enzyme inhibitors in patients with renovascular hypertension. Nephron 1991; 57:230–231.

Hansen KJ: Prevalence of ischemic nephropathy in the atherosclerotic population. Am J Kidney Dis 1994; 24:615–621.

Hansen PB, Garsdal P, Fruergaard P: The captopril test for identification of renovascular hypertension: Value and immediate adverse effects. J Intern Med 1990a; 228:159–163.

Hansen PB, Tribble RW, Reavis SW, et al: Renal duplex sonography; evaluation of clinical utility. J Vasc Surg 1990b; 12:227–236.

Harvey RJ, Krumlovsky F, DelGroco F, et al: Screening for renovascular hypertension. JAMA 1985; 254:388.

Hawkins PG, McKnoulty LM, Gordon RD, et al: Renal artery duplex ultrasonography: A reliable new screening test for functionally significant renal artery stenosis. Clin Exp Pharm Physiol 1989; 16:293–297.

Hertz SM, Holland GA, Baum RA, et al: Evaluation of renal artery stenosis by magnetic resonance angiography. Am J Surg 1994; 168:140–143.

Hillman BJ, Ovitt PW, Capp MD, et al: The potential impact of digital video subtractions angiography on screening for renovascular hypertension. Radiology 1982; 142:577.

Hingorani AD, Jia H, Stevens PA, et al: Renin-angiotensin system gene polymorphisms influence blood pressure and the response to angiotensin converting enzyme inhibition. J Hypertens 1995; 13:1602–1609.

Hollenberg NK: Medical therapy for renovascular hypertension: A review. Am J Hypertens 1988; 1:338S.

Holley KE, Hunt JC, Brown AL, et al: Renal artery stenosis: A clinical-pathologic study in normotensive patients. Am J Med 1964; 37:14.

Howard JE, Conner TB: Use of differential renal function studies in the diagnosis of renovascular hypertension. Am J Surg 1954; 107:58.

Hricik DE, Browning PJ, Kopelman R, et al: Captopril induced functional renal insufficiency in patients with bilateral renal artery stenosis or renal artery stenosis in a solitary kidney. N Engl J Med 1983; 308:373.

Hudspeth DA, Hansen KJ, Reavis SW, et al: Renal duplex sonography after treatment of renovascular disease. J Vasc Surg 1993; 18:381–390.

Hunt JC, Strong CS: Renovascular hypertension: Mechanism, natural history and treatment. Am J Cardiol 1973; 32:562.

Iaccarino V, Russo D, Niola R, et al: Total or partial percutaneous renal ablation in the treatment of renovascular hypertension: Radiological and clinical aspects. Br J Radiol 1989; 62:593.

Imai T, Miyazaki H, Hirosc S, et al: Cloning and sequence analysis of the cDNA for human renin precursor. Proc Natl Acad Sci USA 1983; 80:7405.

Inagami P, Murakami K: Prorenin. Biomed Res 1980; 1:456.

Jean WJ, Al-Bitar I, Zwicke DL, et al: High incidence of renal artery stenosis in patients with coronary artery disease. Cathet Cardiovasc Diagn 1994; 32:8–10.

Jensen G, Zachrisson B-F, Delin K, et al: Treatment of renovascular hypertension: One year results of renal angioplasty. Kidney Int 1995; 48:1936–1945.

Johnson JA, Davis JO, Witty RT: Effects of catecholamines and renal nerve stimulation on renin release in the non-filtering kidney. Circ Res 1971; 29:646.

Judson WE, Helmer OM: Diagnostic and prognostic values of renin activity in renal venous plasma in renovascular hypertension. Hypertension 1965; 13:79.

Kalender WA, Seissler W, Klotz E, Vock P: Spiral volumetric CT with single-breath-hold technique, continuous transport, and continuous scanner rotation. Radiology 1990; 176:181–183.

Kang PM, Landau AJ, Eberhardt RT, Frishman WH: Angiotensin II receptor antagonists: A new approach to blockade of the renin-angiotensin system. Am Heart J 1994; 127:1388–1401.

Katzen BT, Chang J, Knox WG: Percutaneous transluminal angioplasty with the Gruntzig balloon catheter: A review of 70 cases. Arch Surg 1979; 114:1389–1399.

Kent KC, Edelman RR, Kim D, et al: Magnetic resonance imaging: A reliable test for the evaluation of proximal atherosclerotic renal arterial stenosis. J Vasc Surg 1991; 13:311–318.

Kim D, Edelman RR, Kent KC, et al: Abdominal aorta and renal artery stenosis: Evaluation with MR angiography. Radiology 1990; 174:727–731.

Klag MJ, Whelton PK, Randall BL, et al: Blood pressure and end-stage renal disease in men. N Engl J Med 1996; 334:13–18.

Klimberg IW, Locke DR, Hawkins IF, Drylie TM: Absolute ethanol renal autoinfarction for control of hypertension. Urology 1989; 33:153.

Kuhn F-P, Kutkuhn B, Torsello G, Modder U: Renal artery stenosis: Preliminary results of treatment with the Strecker stent. Radiology 1991; 180:367–372.

Kumar S, Mandalim R, Raovr K, et al: Percutaneous transluminal angioplasty in non-specific aortoarthritis (Takayasu's disease): Experience in 16 cases. Cardiovasc Intervent Radiol 1990; 12:321.

Laragh JH, Angers M, Kelly WG, et al: The effect of epinephrine, norepinephrine, angiotensin II, and others on the secretory rate of aldosterone in man. JAMA 1960; 174:234.

Laragh JH, Brenner BM, eds: Hypertension: Pathophysiology, Diagnosis and Management, 2nd ed, vols. 1 and 2. New York, Raven Press, 1995.

Laragh JH, Blumenfeld JD: Essential Hypertension. *In* Brenner BM, ed: The Kidney, 5th ed. Philadelphia, W.B. Saunders Company, 1996, p 2071.

Laragh JH, Sealey JE: The renin-angiotensin-aldosterone system and the renal regulation of sodium potassium and blood pressure homeostasis. *In* Windhager EE, ed: Handbook of Physiology, New York, Oxford University Press, 1992, p 1409.

Lawrie GM, Morris GC, Gleaser DH, deBakey ME: Renovascular reconstruction: Factors affecting long-term prognosis in 919 patients followed up to 31 years. Am J Cardiol 1989; 63:1085.

Leadbetter WF, Burkland CF: Hypertension in unilateral renal disease. J Urol 1938; 39:611.

Lew EA: High blood pressure, other risk factors and longevity. *In* Laragh JH, ed: The Insurance Viewpoint in Hypertension Manual. New York, Yorke Medical Books, 1973.

Lohr E, Block K-D, Eigler F, et al: Angioplasty of renal arteries: A report of ten years' experience. Angiology 1991; 42:44–47.

London GM, Safar ME: Renal hemodynamics in patients with sustained essential hypertension and in patients with unilateral stenosis of the renal artery. Am J Hypertens 1989; 2:244.

Loubeyre P, Revel D, Garcia P, et al: Screening patients for renal artery stenosis: Value of three-dimensional time-of-flight MR angiography. AJR 1994; 162:847–852.

Louie J, Isaacson JA, Zierler RE, et al: Prevalence of carotid and lower extremity arterial disease in patients with renal artery stenosis. Am J Hypertens 1994; 7:436–439.

Lyons DF, Streck WF, Kem DC, et al: Captopril stimulation of differential renins in renovascular hypertension. Hypertension 1983; 5:65.

MacLeod M, Taylor AD, Baxter G, et al: Renal artery stenosis managed by Palmaz stent insertion: Technical and clinical outcome. J Hypertens 1995; 13:1791–1795.

McCormack LJ, Poutasse EF, Meaney TF, et al: A pathologic arteriographic correlation of renal arterial disease. Am Heart J 1966; 72:188.

McGill CW, Holder TM, and Smith TH: Post-radiation renovascular hypertension. J Pediatr Surg 1979; 14:831.

Mai M, Geiger H, Hilgers KF, et al: Early interstitial changes in hypertension-induced renal injury. Hypertension 1993; 22:754–765.

Mailloux LU, Napolitano B, Bellucci AG, et al: Renal vascular disease causing end-stage renal disease, incidence, clinical correlates, and outcomes: A 20-year clinical experience. Am J Kidney Dis 1994; 24:622–629.

Mann FC, Herrick JF, Essex HE, Baldes EJ: The effect on the blood flow of decreasing lumen of a blood vessel. Surgery 1938; 4:249.

Mann SJ, Pickering TG, Sos TA, et al: Captopril renography in the diagnosis of renal artery stenosis: Accuracy and limitations. Am J Med 1991; 90:30–40.

Marks LS, Maxwell MH: Renal vein renin value and limitations in the prediction of operative results. Urol Clin North Am 1975; 2:311.

Martin EC, Diamond NG, Casarella WJ: Percutaneous transluminal angioplasty in non-atherosclerotic disease. Radiology 1980; 135:27.

Martin EC, Mattern RF, Baer L, et al: Renal angioplasty for hypertension: predictive factors for long-term success. AJR Am J Roentgenol 1981; 137:921–924.

Martin LG, Casarella WJ, Alspaugh JP, Chuang VP: Renal artery angioplasty: Increased technical success and decreased complications in the second 100 patients. Radiology 1986; 159:631–634.

Martin LG, Price RB, Casarella WJ, et al: Percutaneous angioplasty in clinical management of renovascular hypertension: initial and long-term results. Radiology 1985; 155:629–633.

Martinez AG, Novick AC, Hayes JM: Surgical treatment of renal artery stenosis after failed percutaneous transluminal angioplasty. J Urol 1990; 144:1094–1096.

Mason JC, Hilton PJ: Reversible renal failure due to captopril in a patient with transplant artery stenosis. Hypertension 1983; 5:623.

Maxwell MH, Lupu AN: Excretory urogram in renal arterial hypertension. J Urol 1968; 100:395.

Maxwell MH, Lupu AN, Taplin GV: Radioisotope renogram in renal arterial hypertension. J Urol 1968; 100:376.

Meaney TF, Dustan HP, Gilmore JP: Angiotensin I conversion in the kidney and its modulation by sodium balance. Am J Physiol 1973; 224:1104.

Meaney TF, Dustan HP, McCormack LJ: Natural history of renal arterial disease. Radiology 1968; 9:877.

Meier GH, Sumpio B, Black HR, Gusberg RJ: Captopril renal scintigraphy—an advance in the detection and treatment of renovascular hypertension. J Vasc Surg 1990; 11(6):770.

Miller ED Jr, Samuels AI, Haber E: Inhibition of angiotensin conversion in experimental renovascular hypertension. Science 1972; 177:1108.

Mimran A, Ribstein J, DuCailar G: Converting enzyme inhibitors and renal function in essential and renovascular hypertension. Am J Hyperten 1991; 4:7S–14S.

Miralles M, Santiso A, Gimenez A, et al: Renal duplex scanning: Correlation with angiography and isotopic renography. Eur J Vasc Surg 1993; 7:188–194.

Missouris CG, Barley J, Jeffrey S, et al: Genetic risk for renal artery stenosis: Association with deletion polymorphism in angiotensin I-converting enzyme gene. Kidney Int 1996; 49:534–537.

Mohomed FA: The etiology of Bright's disease and the prealbuminuric stage. Med Chir Trans 1874; 57:197.

Mohring J, Mohring B, Naumann JH, et al: Salt and water balance and renin activity in renal hypertension of rats. Am J Physiol 1975; 228:1847.

Motta J, Breslin DS, Vogel F, et al: Congenital renal arteriovenous malformation in pregnancy presenting with hypertension. Urology 1994; 44:911–914.

Mueller FB, Sealey JE, Case DB, et al: The captopril test for identifying renovascular disease in hypertensive patients. Am J Med 1986; 80:633–644.

Munday KA, Parsons BJ, Post JA: The effect of angiotensin on cation transport in rat kidney cortex slices. J Physiol (Lond) 1971; 215:269.

Nakano S, Kogoshi T, Uchida K, et al: Hypertension and unilateral renal ischemia (Page Kidney) due to compression of a retroperitoneal paraganglioma. Am J Nephrol 1996; 16:91–94.

Nally JV: Use of captopril renography for the diagnosis of renovascular hypertension. World J Urol 1989; 7:72.

Nally JV, Clark AHS, Grecos GP, et al: Effective captopril ^{99}Tc-Diethylenetriaminepentaacetic acid renograms in 2-kidney, 1-clip hypertension. Hypertension 1986; 8:685.

Nally JV Jr, Olin JW, Lammert GK: Advances in noninvasive screening for renovascular disease. Cleve Clin J Med 1994; 61:328–336.

Ng KKF, Vane JR: Conversion of angiotensin I to angiotensin II. Nature 1967; 215:762.

Novick AC: Surgical revascularization for renovascular hypertension and preservation of renal function. *In* Laragh JH, Brenner BM, eds: Hypertension: Pathophysiology, Diagnosis, and Management, 2nd ed. New York, Raven Press, 1995, pp 2055–2068.

Novick AC, ed: Renal Vascular Disease. London, W.B. Saunders Company, 1996.

Novick AC, Straffon RA, Stewart BH, et al: Diminished operative morbidity and mortality in renal revascularization. JAMA 1981; 246:749.

Novick AC, Textor SC, Bodie B, Khauli RB: Revascularization to preserve renal function in patients with atherosclerotic renovascular disease. Urol Clin North Am 1984; 11:477.

Novick AC, Zaki S, Goldfarb D, Hodge EE: Epidemiologic and clinical comparison of renal artery stenosis in black patients and white patients. J Vasc Surg 1994; 20:1–5.

O'Donovan RM, Gutierrez OH, Izzo JL: Preservation of renal function by percutaneous renal angioplasty in high-risk elderly patients: Short-term outcome. Nephron 1992; 60:187–192.

Ohkubo H, Kageyama R, Uhihara M, et al: Cloning and sequence analysis of cDNA for rat angiotensinogen. Proc Natl Acad Sci USA 1983; 80:2196.

Olson MC, Posniak HV: Urologic applications of multiplanar and three-dimensional computed tomography. Techniques Urol 1995; 1(3) pp 141–149.

Page IH, Helmer OM: A crystalline pressor substance (angiotonin) resulting from the reaction between renin and renin activator. J Exp Med 1940; 71:29.

Parrott TS, Woodard JR, Trulock TS, Glenn JF: Segmental renal vein renins and partial nephrectomy for hypertension. J Urol 1984; 131:736.

Pederson EB, Sorensen SS, Amdisen A, et al: Abnormal glomerular and tubular function during angiotensin converting enzyme inhibition in renovascular hypertension evaluated by the lithium clearance method. Eur J Clin Invest 1989; 19:135.

Pickering SG, Pickering TG: Part I: Hypertension: Definitions, natural histories and consequences; Part II: Modern definitions and clinical expressions of hypertension. *In* Laragh JH, Brenner BM, eds: Hypertension: Pathophysiology, Diagnosis, and Management, 2nd ed. New York, Raven Press, 1995, pp 3–21.

Pickering TG: Medical management of renovascular hypertension. World J Urol 1989; 7:77.

Pickering TG, Blumenfeld JD, Laragh JH: Renovascular hypertension and ischemic nephropathy. *In* Brenner BM, ed: The Kidney, 5th ed. Philadelphia, W.B. Saunders Company, 1996, pp 2106–2125.

Pickering TG, Herman L, Sotelo JE, et al: Recurrent pulmonary edema as a manifestation of renovascular hypertension and its treatment by renal revascularization. Circulation 1987; 76[Suppl IV]:274.

Pickering TG, Mann SJ: Renovascular hypertension: Medical evaluation and nonsurgical treatment. *In* Laragh JH, Brenner BM, eds: Hypertension: Pathophysiology, Diagnosis, and Management, 2nd ed. New York, Raven Press, 1995, pp 2039–2054.

Pickering TG, Sos TA, Vaughan ED Jr, et al: Predictive value and changes of renin secretion in hypertensive patients with unilateral renovascular disease undergoing successful renal angioplasty. Am J Med 1984; 76:398.

Pickering TG, Sos TA, Vaughan ED Jr, Laragh JH: Differing patterns of renal vein renin secretion in patients with renovascular hypertension, and their role in predicting the response to angioplasty. Nephron 1986; 44([Suppl] 1):8–11.

Pitts RF, Duggan JJ: Studies on diuretics. II. The relationship between glomerular filtration rate, proximal tubular absorption of sodium, and diuretic efficacy of mercurials. J Clin Invest 1950; 29:372.

Pohl MA: The ischemic kidney and hypertension. Am J Kidney Dis 1993; 21:22–28.

Postma CT, Hoefnagels WHL, et al: Occlusion of unilateral stenosed renal arteries—relation to medical treatment. J Hum Hypertens 1989; 3:185.

Postma CT, van der Steen PHM, Hoegnagels HL, et al: The captopril test in the detection of renovascular disease in hypertensive patients. Arch Intern Med 1990; 150:625–628.

Poutasse EF, Dustan HP: Arteriosclerosis and renal hypertension: Indications for aortography in hypertensive patients and results of surgical treatment of obstructive lesions of renal artery. JAMA 1957; 165:1521.

Prigent A, Froissart M: Current recommendations for diagnosis of renovascular hypertension. Kidney: A Current Survey of World Literature 1994; 3:138–144.

Ramsey LE, Waller PC: Blood pressure response to percutaneous transluminal angioplasty for renovascular hypertension: An overview of published series. Br Med J 1990; 300:569.

Ratliff NB: Renal vascular disease: Pathology of large blood vessel disease. *In* Porush JG (ed): Hypertension and the Kidney. New York, Grune & Stratton, 1985.

Re R, Noveline R, Escourrou M-T, et al: Inhibition of angiotensin-converting enzyme for diagnosis of renal-artery stenosis. N Engl J Med 1978; 298:582.

Rees CR, Palmaz JC, Becker GJ, et al: Palmaz stent in atherosclerotic stenoses involving the ostia of the renal arteries: Preliminary report of a multicenter study. Radiology 1991; 181:507–514.

Rimmer JM, Gennari FJ: Atherosclerotic renovascular disease and progressive renal failure. Ann Intern Med 1993; 118:712–719.

Ritter SG, Bentley MD, Fiksen-Olsen MJ, et al: Effect of captopril on renal function in hypertensive dogs with unilateral renal artery stenosis, studied with radionuclide dynamic scintigraphy. Am J Hypertens 1990; 3:591.

Rose AG, Sinclair-Smith CC: Takayasu's arteritis. A study of sixteen autopsy patients. Arch Pathol Lab Med 1980; 104:231.

Rosivall L, Blantz RC, Navar LG, guest eds: Renovascular effects of angiotensin II. Kidney Int 1990[Suppl 30].

Rubin B, Laffan RJ, Kotler DG, et al: SQ 14225 (D-3-mercapto-2-methylpropranoyl-L-proline), a novel orally active inhibitor of angiotensin I-converting enzyme. J Pharm Exp Ther 1978; 204:271.

Rubin GD, Dake MD, Napel S, et al: Spiral CT of renal artery stenosis: Comparison of three-dimensional rendering techniques. Radiology 1994; 190:181–189.

Sadowski RH, Falkner B: Hypertension in pediatric patients. Am J Kidney Dis 1996; 27:305–315.

Sang CN, Whelton PK, Hamper UM, et al: Etiologic factors in renovascular fibromuscular dysplasia. A case control study. Hypertension 1989; 14:472.

Schambelan M, Glickman M, Stockigt JR, Biglieri EG: The selective renal vein renin sampling in hypertensive patients with segmental renal lesions. N Engl J Med 1974; 290:1153.

Schreiber MJ, Pohl MA, Novick AC: The natural history of atherosclerotic and fibrous renal artery disease. Urol Clin North Am 1984; 11:383.

Schreiber MJ Jr, Novick AC, Pohl MA: The natural history of atherosclerotic and fibrous renal artery disease. World J Urol 1989; 7:59.

Schwarten DE: Percutaneous transluminal renal artery angioplasty. *In* Kaplan NM, Brunner BM, Laragh JH, eds: The Kidney and Hypertension. New York, Raven Press, 1987.

Sealey JE, Buhler FR, Laragh JH, Vaughan ED Jr: The physiology of renin secretion in essential hypertension: Estimation of renin secretion rate and renal plasma flow from peripheral and renal vein renin levels. Am J Med 1973; 55:391.

Sealey JE, Laragh JH, co-eds: Symposium: What is the mechanism of one-kidney, one-clip hypertension and its relevance to low renin essential hypertension? Am J Hypertens 1991; 4([Suppl 10, 2]).

Sealey JE, Laragh JH: The renin-angiotensin-aldosterone system for normal regulation of blood pressure and sodium and potassium homeostasis. *In* Laragh JH, Brenner BM, eds: Hypertension: Pathophysiology, Diagnosis, and Management, 2nd ed. New York, Raven Press, 1995, p 1763.

Sealey JE, von Lutteroti N, Rubattu S, et al: The greater renin system: Its prorenin-directed vasodilator limb: Relevance to diabetes mellitus, pregnancy, and hypertension. *In* Laragh JH, Brenner BM, eds: Hypertension: Pathophysiology, Diagnosis, and Management, 2nd ed. New York, Raven Press, 1995, p 1889.

Selkurt EE: The effect of pulse pressure and mean arterial pressure modification of renal hemodynamics and electrolyte and water excretion. Circulation 1951; 4:541.

Semple PF, Dominiczak AF: Detection and treatment of renovascular disease: 40 years on. J Hypertens 1994; 12:729–734.

Setaro JF, Saddler MC, Chen CC, et al: Simplified captopril renography in diagnosis and treatment of renal artery stenosis. Hypertension 1991; 18:289–298.

Sfakianakis GN, Bourgoignie JJ, Daffe D, et al: Single-dose captopril scintigraphy in the diagnosis of renovascular hypertension. J Nucl Med 1987; 28:1383.

Shoskes DA, Novick AC: Surgical treatment of renovascular hypertension in moyamoya disease: Case report and review of the literature. J Urol 1995; 153:450–452.

Siegl PKS, Kivlighn SD, Broten TP: Pharmacology of losartan, an angiotensin II receptor antagonist, in animal models of hypertension. J Hypertens 1995; 13[Suppl 1]:S15–S21.

Simon N, Franklin SS, Bleifer KH, Maxwell MH: Clinical characteristics of renovascular hypertension. JAMA 1972; 220:1209.

Simon G, Coleman CC: Captopril-stimulated renal vein renin measurements in the diagnosis of atherosclerotic renovascular hypertension. Am J Hypertens 1994; 7:1–6.

Simunic S, Winter-Fuduric I, Radanovic B, et al: Percutaneous transluminal renal angioplasty (PTRA) as a method of treatment for renovascular hypertension in children. Eur J Radiol 1990; 10:143.

Sinaiko AR, Wells TG: Childhood hypertension. *In* Laragh JH, Brenner BM, eds: Hypertension: Pathophysiology, Diagnosis, and Management. New York, Raven Press, 1990, p 1853.

Skeggs LT, Marsh WH, Kahn JR, Shumway NP: The existence of two forms of hypertension. J Exp Med 1954; 99:275.

Skeggs LT Jr, Lentz KE, Kahn JR, et al: Amino acid sequence of hypertension II. J Exp Med 1956; 104:193.

Smith CW, Winfield AC, Price RR: Evaluation of digital venous angiography for the diagnosis of renovascular hypertension. Radiology 1982; 144:51.

Smith HW: Hypertension and urologic disease. Am J Med 1948; 4:724.

Smith P, Rush TW, Evans AT: The technique of translumbar arteriography. JAMA 1952; 148:255.

Soffer RL: Angiotensin converting enzyme. *In* Soffer RL, ed: Biochemical Regulation of Blood Pressure. New York, John Wiley & Sons, 1981, p 123.

Sos TA, Pickering TG, Phil D, et al: Percutaneous transluminal angioplasty in renovascular hypertension due to atheroma or fibromuscular dysplasia. N Engl J Med 1983; 309:274–279.

Sosa RE: Effects of converting enzyme inhibition on renal function in chronic 2-kidney, 1-clip hypertensive dogs. J Urol 1987; 137:209A.

Sosa RE, Vaughan ED Jr: Hypertension of renal origin. World J Urol 1989; 7:64.

Soubrier F, Panthier JJ, Corvol P, Rougeon F: Molecular cloning and nucleotide sequence of the human renin cDNA fragment. Nucleic Acid Res 1983; 11:7181.

Soulen MC, Benenati JF, Sheth S, et al: Changes in renal artery Doppler indexes following renal angioplasty. J Vasc Interv Radiol 1991; 2:457–462.

Spies K-P, Fobbe F, El-Bedewi M, et al: Color-coded duplex sonography for noninvasive diagnosis and grading of renal artery stenosis. Am J Hypertens 1995; 8:1222–1231.

Stamey TA: Renovascular Hypertension. Baltimore, Williams & Wilkins Company, 1963.

Stamey TA, Nudelman IJ, Good TH, et al: Functional characteristics of renovascular hypertension. Medicine 1961; 40:347.

Stockigt JR, Noakes CA, Collins RD, et al: Renal-vein renin in various forms of renal hypertension. Lancet 1972; 1:1194.

Stoll M, Meffert S, Stroth U, Unger T: Growth or antigrowth: Angiotensin and the endothelium. J Hypertens 1995; 13:1529–1534.

Strandness DE Jr: Natural history of renal artery stenosis. Am J Kidney Dis 1994a; 24:630–635.

Strandness DE Jr: Duplex imaging for the detection of renal artery stenosis. Am J Kidney Dis 1994b; 24:674–678.

Svetkey LP, Mimmelstein SI, Dunnick NR: Prospective analysis strategies for diagnosing renovascular hypertension. Hypertension 1989; 14:247–257.

Tack C, Sos TA: Percutaneous transluminal renal angioplasty. World J Urol 1989; 7:82.

Tegtmeyer CJ, Kellum CD, Ayers C: Percutaneous transluminal angioplasty of the renal artery: Results and long term follow-up. Radiology 1984; 153:77–84.

Textor SC: Pathophysiology of renal failure in renovascular disease. Am J Kidney Dis 1994; 24:642–651.

Textor SC, Novick AC, Steinmuller DR, Streem SB: Renal failure limiting antihypertensive therapy as an indication for renal revascularization. A case report. Arch Intern Med 1983; 143:2208–2211.

Textor SC, Novick AC, Tarazi RC, et al: Critical perfusion pressure for renal function in patients with bilateral atherosclerotic renovascular disease. Ann Intern Med 1985; 102:308.

Thibonnier M, Joseph A, Sassano P, et al: Improved diagnosis of unilateral renal artery lesions after captopril administration. JAMA 1984; 251:56.

Thibonnier M, Sassano P, Joseph A, et al: Diagnostic value of a single dose of captopril in renin- and aldosterone-dependent, surgically curable hypertension. Cardiovasc Rev Rep 1982; 3:1659–1667.

Thornbury JR, Stanley FC, Freyback DG: Hypertensive urogram: A nondiscriminatory test for renovascular hypertension. AJR, 1982; 138:43.

Tigerstedt R, Bergmann TG: Niere und kreislauf. Scand Arch Physiol 1898; 8:233.

Tobian L, Tomboulian A, Janecek J: Effect of high perfusion pressure on the granulation of juxtaglomerular cells in an isolated kidney. J Clin Invest 1959; 38:605.

Toto RD: Renal insufficiency due to angiotensin-converting enzyme inhibitors. Miner Electrolyte Metab 1994; 20:193–200.

Traube L: Uber den Zusammenhang von Herz- und Nieren-Krankheiten. *In* Gesammelte Beitraege zur Pathologie und Physiologie, vol II, part I, Clinical Investigations. Berlin, A. Hirschwalt, 1856.

Trost D, Sos TA: Complications of renal angioplasty and stenting. Semin Interven Radiol 1994; 2(2):150–160.

van Bockel JH, van Schilfgaar DE, R Felthuis W, et al: Reconstructive surgery for renovascular hypertension secondary to arteriosclerosis and fibrodysplasia. III. The early and late effects of surgery on hypertensive target organ damage. Neth J Med 1988; 32:159.

van Bockel JH, van Schilfgaar DE, van Brummelen P, Terpstra JL: Long-term results of renal artery reconstruction with autogenous artery in patients with renovascular hypertension. Eur J Vasc Surg 1989; 3:515.

Vander AJ: Effect of catecholamines and the renal nerves on renin secretion in anesthetized dogs. Am J Physiol 1965; 209:659.

Vaughan ED Jr, Buhler FR, Laragh JH, et al: Renovascular hypertension; renin measurements to indicate hypersecretion and contralateral suppression, estimate renal plasma flow and score for surgical curability. Am J Med 1973; 55:402.

Vaughan ED Jr, Carey RM, Ayers CR, et al: A physiologic definition of blood pressure response to renal revascularization in patients with renovascular hypertension. Kidney Int 1979; 15:S83.

Vaughan ED Jr, Case DB, Pickering TG, et al: Clinical evaluation for renovascular hypertension and therapeutic decisions. Urol Clin North Am 1984; 11:393.

Vaughan ED Jr, Sos TA, Sniderman KW, et al: Renal venous renin secretory patterns before and after percutaneous transluminal angioplasty: Verification of analytic criteria. *In* Laragh JH, ed: Frontiers in Hypertension Research. New York, Springer-Verlag, 1981.

Veglio F, Frascisco M, Melchio R, et al: Assessment of renal resistance index after captopril test by Doppler in essential and renovascular hypertension. Kidney Int 1995; 48:1611–1616.

Veglio F, Provera E, Pinna G, et al: Renal resistive index after captopril test by echo-Doppler in essential hypertension. Am J Hypertens 1992; 5:431–436.

Von Knorring J, Lepantalo M, Fyhrquist F: Long-term prognosis of surgical treatment of renovascular hypertension. J Intern Med 1989; 225:303.

Walker BR, Jenkins AMcL, Padfield PL: Pressure natriuresis following therapy for "one-clip one-kidney" hypertension in man. Clin Nephrol 1993; 40:321–325.

Weed WC, Vaughan ED Jr, Peach MJ: Prolongation of the saralasin responsive state of two-kidney, one-clip hypertension in the rat by the orally administered converting enzyme inhibitor captopril (SQ 14225). Hypertension 1979; 1:8.

Weibull H, Bergqvist D, Weibull H, et al: Analysis of complications after percutaneous transluminal angioplasty of renal artery stenoses. Eur J Vasc Surg 1987; 1:77–84.

Wilcox CS: Use of angiotensin-converting-enzyme inhibitors for diagnosing renovascular hypertension. Kidney Int 1993; 44:1379–1390.

Wilcox CS, Williams CM, Smith TB, et al: Diagnostic uses of angiotensin-converting enzyme inhibitors in renovascular hypertension. Am J Hypertens 1988; 1:344S.

Willems CED, Shah V, Uchiyama M, Dillon MJ: Arch Dis Child 1989; 64:229.

Wilms G, Marchal G, Peene P, Baert AL: The angiographic incidence of renal artery stenosis in the arteriosclerotic population. Eur J Radiol 1990; 10(3):195.

Wilms GE, Peene PT, Baert AL, et al: Renal artery stent placement with use of the wallstent endoprosthesis. Radiology 1991; 179:457–462.

Wollenweber J, Sheps SG, David DG: Clinical course of atherosclerotic renovascular disease. Am J Cardiol 1968; 21:60.

Ying CY, Tifft CP, Gavras H, et al: Renal revascularization in the azotemic hypertensive patient resistant to therapy. N Engl J Med 1984; 311:1070.

Yucel EK, Kaufman JA, Prince M, et al: Time of flight renal MR angiography: Utility in patients with renal insufficiency. Magn Reson Imaging 1993; 11:925–930.

Zanchi A, Brunner HR, Waeber B, Burnier M: Renal haemodynamic and protective effects of calcium antagonists in hypertension. J Hypertens 1995; 13:1363–1375.

Zierler RE, Bergelin RO, Isaacson JA, Strandness DE Jr: Natural history of atherosclerotic renal artery stenosis: A prospective study with duplex ultrasonography. J Vasc Surg 1994; 19:250–258.

Acute Renal Artery Occlusion and Renal Artery Embolism

Berridge DC, Makin GS, Hopkinson BR: Local low-dose intra-arterial thrombolytic therapy: The risk of stroke and hemorrhage. Br J Surg 1989; 76:1230–1233.

Blum U, Billmann P, Krause T, et al: Effect of local low dose thrombolysis on clinical outcome in acute embolic renal artery occlusion. Radiology 1993; 189:549–554.

Fischer P, Konnack JW, Cho KJ, et al: Renal artery embolism: Therapy with intra-arterial streptokinase infusion. J Urol 1981; 125:402–404.

Gasparini M, Hoffman R, Stoller M: Renal artery embolism: Clinical features and therapeutic options. J Urol 1992; 147:567–572.

Hamilton G: Fibrinolytic therapy in renovascular disease. *In* Novick A, Scoble J, Hamilton G, eds: Renal Vascular Disease. Philadelphia, W.B. Saunders Company, 1996, pp 417–430.

Hoxie HJ, Coggin CB: Renal infarction: Statistical study of two hundred and five cases and detailed report of an unusual case. Arch Intern Med 1940; 65:587–594.

Lacombe M: Acute non-traumatic obstruction of the renal artery. J Cardiovasc Surg 1992; 33:163–168.

Morris D, Kisly A, Stoyka CG, Provenzano R: Spontaneous bilateral renal artery occlusion associated with chronic atrial fibrillation. Clin Nephrol 1993; 39:257–259.

Moyer JD, Rao CN, Wildrich WC, Olsson CA: Conservative management of renal artery embolus. J Urol 1973; 109:138.

Rohl L: First technically successful revascularization procedure in a 25 year old male with traumatic subintimal thrombosis of the left renal artery. Vasc Surg Urol, Proc R Soc Med 1971; 64:589–594.

Salam T, Lumsden AB, Martin LG: Local infusion of fibrinolytic agents for acute renal artery thromboembolism: Report of ten cases. Ann Vasc Surg 1993; 7:21–26.

Sanfelippo CJ, Goldin A: Intra-arterial streptokinase and renal artery embolization. Urology 1978; 11:62–68.

Sniderman KW, Bodner L, Saddekni S, et al: Percutaneous embolectomy by transcatheter aspiration. Radiology 1984; 150:357.

Spirnak JP, Resnick MI: Revascularization of traumatic thrombosis of the renal artery. Surg Gynecol Obstet 1987; 164:22–26.

Vogelzang RL, Moel DI, Cohn RA, et al: Acute renal vein thrombosis: Successful treatment with intraarterial urokinase. Radiology 1988; 169:681–682.

Cholesterol Embolization

Koga T, Okuda S, Takishita S, et al: Renal failure due to cholesterol embolization following percutaneous transluminal renal angioplasty. Jpn J Med 1991; 30:35–38.

Lye WC, Cheah JS, Sinniah R: Renal cholesterol embolic disease. Am J Nephrol 1993; 13:489–493.

Simon G, Archer SL: Hypertensive urgency due to cholesterol embolization of the kidneys. Am J Hypertens 1995; 8:954–956.

Van Hoenacker O, Crolla D, Debakker G, Verbanck J: Renal intravascular cholesterol emboli. J Belge Radiol 1994; 77:225.

Vidt DG, Eisele G, Gephardt GN, et al: Atheroembolic renal disease: Association with renal artery stenosis. Cleve Clin J Med 1989; 56:407–413.

Wilson DM, Salazes TL, Farkouh MF: Eosinophilia in atheroembolic renal disease. Am J Med 1991; 91:186–189.

Renal Vein Thrombosis, Renal Injuries Causing Hypertension, and Page Kidney

Cass AS, Bubrick M, Luxenberg M, et al: Renal pedicle injury in patients with multiple injuries. J Trauma 1985; 25:892.

Clark DE, Gerogitis JW, Ray FS: Renal arterial injuries caused by blunt trauma. Surgery 1981; 90:97–95.

Lach F, Papper S, Massry SG: The clinical spectrum of renal vein thrombosis: Acute and chronic. Am J Med 1980; 69:819–827.

McAlhany JC, Black HC, Hanback LD, Yarbrough DR: Renal arteriovenous fistula as a cause of hypertension. Am J Surg 1971; 122:117–119.

Massumi RA, Andrade A, Kramer N: Arterial hypertension in traumatic subcapsular perirenal hematoma (Page Kidney). Am J Med 1969; 46:635–639.

Page IH: The production of persistent arterial hypertension by cellophane perinephritis. JAMA 1939; 113:2046–2048.

Rowe JM, Rasmussen RL, Mader SL, et al: Successful thrombolytic therapy in two patients with renal vein thrombosis. Am J Med 1984; 77:1111–1114.

Stables DP, Fouche RF, Van Nickkerk JP, et al: Traumatic renal artery occlusions: 21 cases. J Urol 1976; 115:229–233.

Sterns RH, Rabinowitz R, Segal AJ, Spitzer RM: 'Page Kidney': Hypertension caused by chronic subcapsular hematoma. Arch Intern Med 1985; 145:169–171.

Suffrin G: The Page kidney: A correctable form of arterial hypertension. J Urol 1975; 113:450–454.

Turner WW, Snyder WH III, Fry JW: Mortality and renal salvage after renovascular trauma. Am J Surg 1983; 146:848–851.

Vogelzang RL, Moel DI, Cohn RA, et al: Acute renal vein thrombosis: Successful treatment with intraarterial urokinase. Radiology 1988; 169:681–682.

Watts RA, Hoffbrand BI: Hypertension following renal trauma. J Hum Hypertens 1987; 1:65–71.

Wu ZL, Zhou KR, Liao LT: Thrombolytic therapy of renal vein thrombi and follow-up. Clin Nephrol 1994; 42:276–277.

Renal Artery Aneurysm

Bulbul MA, Farrow GA: Aneurysms of the renal artery Urology 1992; 40:124–126.

Cohen JR, Shamash FS: Ruptured renal artery aneurysms during pregnancy. J Vasc Surg 1987; 6:51–59.

Cohen SG, Cashdan A, Burger R: Spontaneous rupture of a renal artery aneurysm during pregnancy. Obstet Gynecol 1972; 39:897–902.

Cummings KB, Lecky JW, Kaufman JJ: Renal artery aneurysms and hypertension. J Urol 1973; 109:144–148.

Dayton B, Helgerson RB, Sollinger HW, Acher CW: Ruptured renal artery aneurysm in a pregnant uninephric patient: Successful ex vivo repair and autotransplantation. Surgery 1990; 107:708.

Hubert JP Jr, Pairolero PC, Kazmier FJ: Solitary renal artery aneurysm. Surgery 1980; 88:557–565.

McCarron JP, Marshall VF, Whitsell JC: Indications for surgery on renal artery aneurysms. J Urol 1975; 114:177–180.

Martin RS, III, Meacham PW, Ditescheim JA, et al: Renal Artery Aneurysm: Selective treatment for hypertension and prevention of rupture. J Vasc Surg 1989; 9:26–34.

Poutasse EF: Renal artery aneurysms. J Urol 1975; 113:443–449.

Ruberti U, Miani S, Scorza R, Mingazzini P, Biasi GM: Aneurysms of the renal artery Int Angio 1987; 6:407–414.

Tham G, Ekelund L, Herrlin K, et al: Renal artery aneurysms. Ann Surg 1983; 197:348–352.

12
RENOVASCULAR SURGERY

John A. Libertino, M.D.

The evaluation and treatment of patients with renovascular lesions has changed dramatically as a result of the availability of new diagnostic studies, such as digital subtraction angiography, the angiotensin converting enzyme inhibitor challenge (Wilcox et al, 1988), and captopril scans, and the advent of new treatment options, such as the newer antihypertensive drugs (Hollenberg, 1988), balloon angioplasty (Sos et al, 1984; Tegtmeyer et al, 1984), stent placement, and alternative surgical bypass procedures (Libertino and Beckmann, 1994).

These technical advances have resulted in the emergence of a new set of contemporary management principles. They include a more aggressive approach to the diagnosis and treatment of renal arterial atherosclerotic disease and, therefore, to the surgical treatment of older patients; the option of revascularization procedures for total renal artery occlusion as well as for renal failure, with preservation of renal function; and bench surgery and autotransplantation for aneurysms, arteriovenous malformations, and segmental branch disease (Libertino et al, 1988).

Many factors must be considered when attempting to determine whether a patient is a candidate for medical therapy, percutaneous transluminal angioplasty, or surgical treatment. The response of blood pressure to medical therapy, the natural history of the offending renal artery lesion, the general medical condition of the patient, the risk of renal parenchymal loss, and the success rates associated with various surgical and radiologic techniques are weighed carefully to arrive at the best treatment option for each individual patient.

Although the true incidence of renovascular hypertension is unknown, it is estimated to be present in 5% to 10% of the 60 million hypertensive individuals in the United States (Sosa and Vaughan, 1987). With the advent of more sensitive and specific diagnostic screening tests for renovascular disease, it may become apparent that the true incidence of renal artery conditions has been underestimated.

The devastating ravages of poorly controlled hypertension, such as myocardial infarction, congestive heart failure, stroke, and renal failure, underscore the importance of identifying and treating all correctable forms of hypertension.

RENAL ARTERY LESIONS

The presence of renal artery stenosis in a hypertensive patient does not establish the diagnosis of renovascular hypertension. Functional tests, such as divided renal vein renin assays and other functional studies, must be performed to determine whether the hypertension is the result of the stenosis. Complications associated with renal angiography and renal vein renin assays occur but are uncommon. These and other studies are essential in determining the functional significance of a renal artery lesion (see Chapter 11, on the natural history and diagnostic evaluation of patients suspected of having renovascular hypertension).

Various lesions can cause stenosis or total occlusion of the main renal artery or its primary branches. The most common lesions are atherosclerosis and the fibrous disorders; however, emboli, traumatic thrombosis, dissection, Takayasu's disease, syphilitic aortitis, thromboangiitis, and periarteritis nodosa have all been described (Kincaid and Davis, 1966).

Atherosclerotic and Fibrous Dysplasias

Atherosclerotic and fibrous dysplasias account for the vast majority of lesions causing renovascular disease. The pathology and natural history of these lesions are discussed comprehensively in Chapter 11. As a result, I present the more unusual causes of renovascular disease: renal artery aneurysms, arteriovenous fistulas, renal artery emboli, renal trauma, arteritis (Takayasu's disease), neurofibromatosis, and renal vein thrombosis.

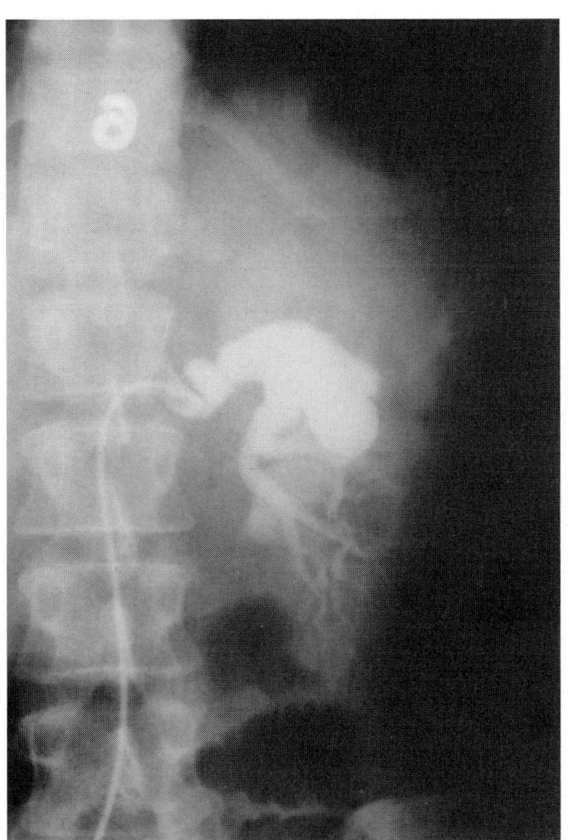

Figure 12–1. Medial fibroplasia with an associated aneurysm.

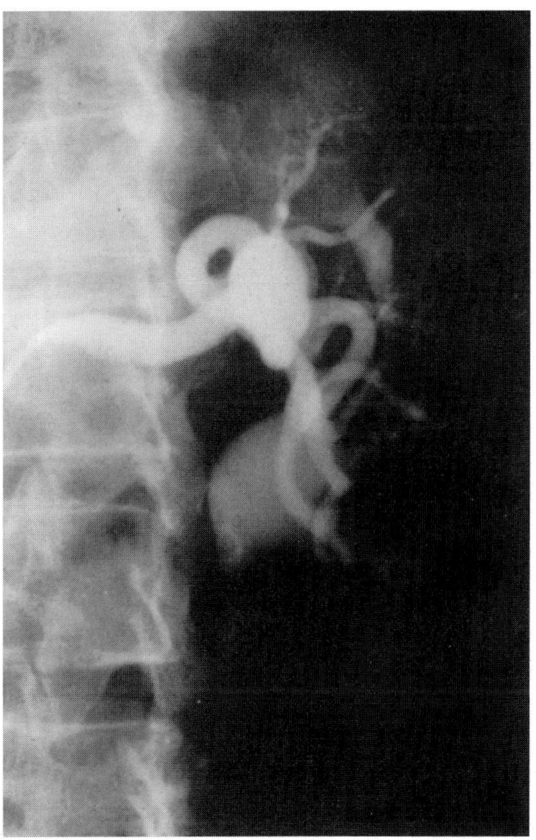

Figure 12–2. Saccular aneurysm in the left renal artery (atherosclerotic).

Renal Artery Aneurysms

Although they are uncommon, renal artery aneurysms are being diagnosed with greater frequency as a result of the advent of standard and digital subtraction angiography. Their true incidence is unknown, but in one study, they were found in 1.5% of potential kidney donors who underwent angiographic evaluation (Harrison et al, 1978). The reported incidence of renal artery aneurysms in patients who are undergoing angiographic evaluation of nonrenal disease has ranged from 0.09% to 0.3% (Stanley et al, 1975; Hageman et al, 1978).

Renal artery aneurysms are clinically significant because they may cause hypertension, be associated with local symptoms, and undergo catastrophic rupture. Four types are known: saccular, fusiform, dissecting, and intrarenal.

Saccular aneurysms usually occur at the bifurcation of the main renal artery or one of its branches (Figs. 12–1 and 12–2) in association with medial fibroplasia and atherosclerosis. In addition to possible spontaneous rupture, these aneurysms may also cause erosion into the renal vein or renal pelvis or thrombosis with peripheral embolization to the renal circulation.

Fusiform aneurysms are usually not calcified and are found in younger hypertensive persons with fibrous mural dysplasia (Fig. 12–3). The major complication of this lesion is thrombosis of the renal artery.

Dissecting aneurysms result from disruption of the internal elastic membrane (Fig. 12–4). This process may be confined to the main renal artery or may extend into the segmental

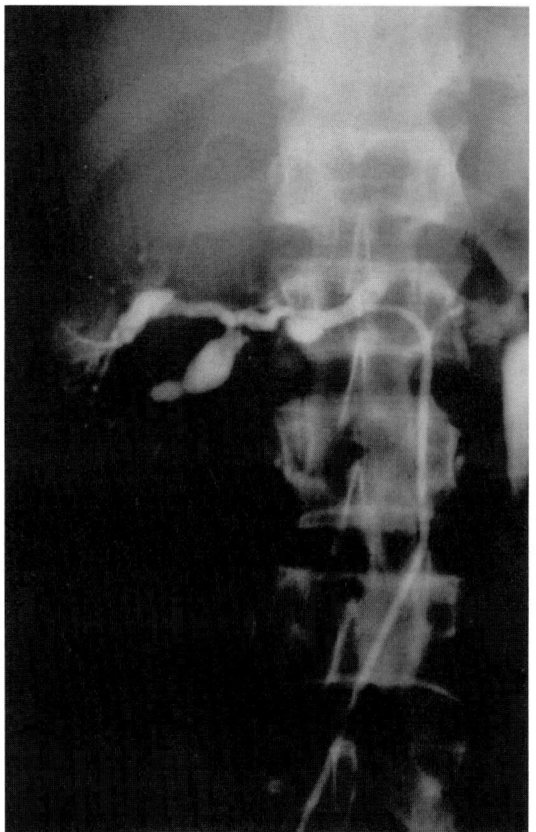

Figure 12–3. Fusiform aneurysms in the right renal artery.

branches. Some dissections re-enter the lumen, and others cause arterial thrombosis with renal infarction or rupture and hemorrhage. Atherosclerosis, intimal fibroplasia, and perimedial fibroplasia are most often associated with dissecting aneurysms of the renal artery. Dissecting aortic aneurysms may also involve the renal vasculature.

Intrarenal aneurysms are caused by atherosclerosis, trauma, congenital vascular malformations, fibrous dysplasia, or needle biopsy of the kidney (Fig. 12–5).

Small (<2 cm), well-calcified aneurysms in a nonhypertensive asymptomatic patient do not require surgical treatment. Surgical intervention is indicated when the aneurysm is causing ischemia or clinical symptoms, is dissecting, or is associated with a functionally significant lesion resulting in decreased renal function or hypertension. Radiologic evidence of expansion or thrombus formation with distal embolization or the clinical presentation of an aneurysm in a woman of childbearing age requires surgical treatment. Various surgical procedures are available, ranging from nephrectomy and partial nephrectomy to resection and in situ or bench revascularization procedures with or without a vein patch graft. Aneurysmectomy with renal preservation is possible in most patients and is described further in this chapter.

Arteriovenous Fistulas

Arteriovenous fistulas are rare and may be congenital, idiopathic, or acquired (Fig. 12–6). Congenital fistulas (cirsoid) have multiple communications, occur equally in both sexes, and usually become manifest in adulthood. Idiopathic fistulas usually have a single communication, are not cirsoid, and have no apparent cause. It has been postulated that they are caused by venous erosion by a large, pre-existing renal artery aneurysm. Acquired fistulas are the most frequently encountered, accounting for 75% of all renal arteriovenous fistulas. The most common cause is iatrogenic injury from a percutaneous needle biopsy or percutaneous nephrolithotomy. Other causes are renal surgery, blunt or penetrating trauma, and renal carcinoma.

The treatment of renal arteriovenous fistulas varies with the cause of the lesion. Nephrectomy is indicated in patients with renal carcinoma. Most fistulas resulting from needle biopsy or other percutaneous procedures and a smaller number resulting from trauma close spontaneously.

Reconstructive surgery or transcatheter occlusion is indicated in patients with hypertension, congestive heart failure, and hematuria. The surgical options range from total nephrectomy for huge arteriovenous fistulas to partial nephrectomy for smaller lesions, as well as extracorporeal or in situ surgery using microvascular techniques to preserve functioning renal parenchyma (Fig. 12–7).

Renal Artery Emboli

Renal artery emboli are a result of an embolic phenomenon from mitral valvular disease, atrial fibrillation, acute myocardial infarction, ventricular aneurysms, subacute bacterial endocarditis, cardiac tumors, and, rarely, a clot originating in the venous system in a patient with an intracardiac septal defect. In addition, atherosclerotic aortic disease, complications of surgical treatment of calcific aortic stenosis or cardiac prosthetic valves, and thrombi originating in renal

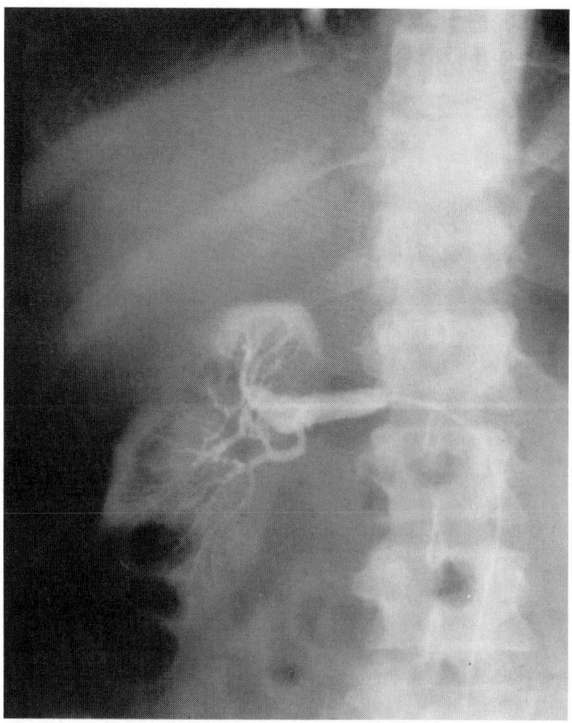

Figure 12–4. Dissecting renal artery lesion.

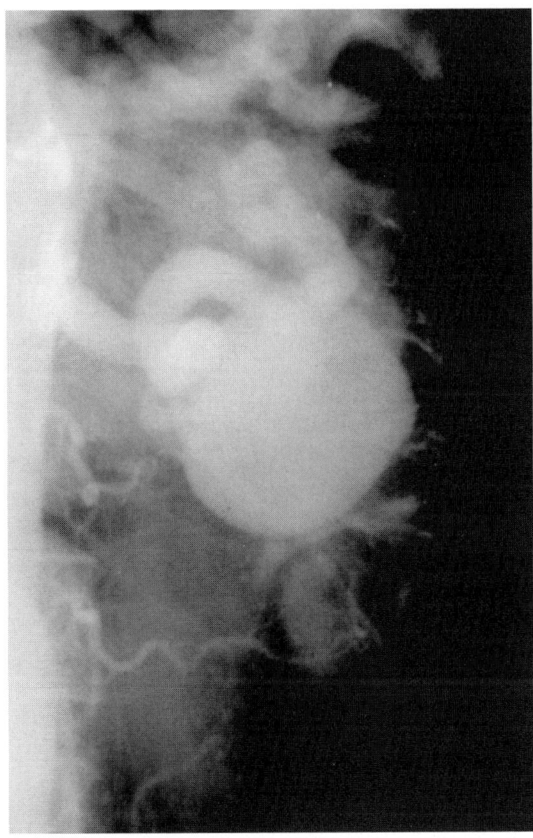

Figure 12–5. Intrarenal aneurysm.

artery aneurysms are known causes of acute emboli and renal artery occlusion (Fig. 12–8).

Renal artery embolization occurs more frequently in the secondary or peripheral vasculature and more commonly affects the left renal artery because of the acute angle that exists between the origin of this artery and the aorta. Iatrogenic emboli to the renal arteries are being seen more frequently with the increasing use of invasive vascular procedures. These emboli may result from angiography or percutaneous transluminal angioplasty.

Operative versus nonoperative treatment for renal artery emboli remains controversial without good therapeutic guidelines because the severity and the extent of renal artery embolization vary greatly (Nicholas and DeMuth, 1984). Patients usually have experienced a recent cardiac event, and their condition is medically unstable. In general, patients who have unilateral complete renal embolic occlusion are best treated by either nonoperative anticoagulant therapy or percutaneous transcatheter thromboembolectomy (Millan et al, 1978). The patient with bilateral renal artery emboli or an embolus to a solitary kidney may be a candidate for anticoagulant therapy, streptokinase catheter embolectomy, supportive hemodialysis, or surgical treatment as determined by the medical status and the response to initial conservative therapy. If the patient is a reasonable surgical risk, preparation for a bypass graft, transection of the renal artery with embolectomy, and reconstruction of the renal circulation by an aortorenal saphenous vein bypass graft gives the surgeon a better chance for salvage.

Renal Trauma

Acute renal artery thrombosis may result from trauma caused by surgical manipulation of a vascular clamp or from external trauma of a blunt or penetrating nature. The left renal artery is more frequently involved in blunt traumatic occlusion, perhaps as a result of deceleration of the mobile kidney with acute angulation of the left renal artery at its aortorenal junction. The more elastic components of the

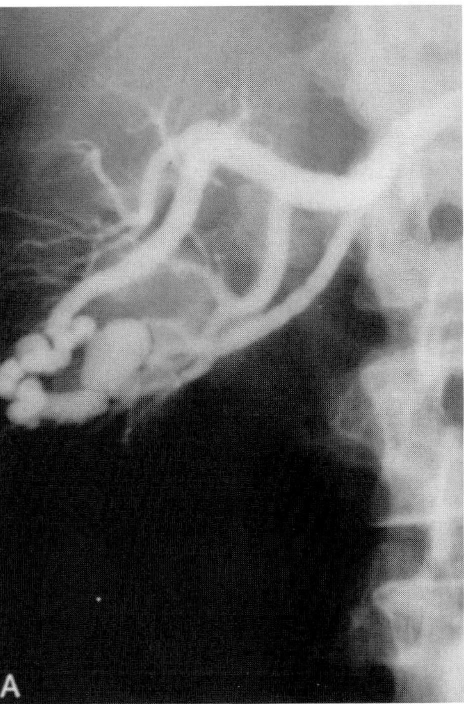

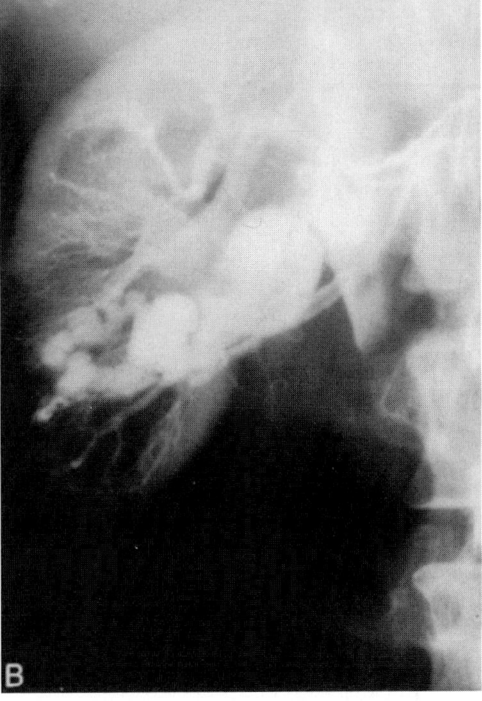

Figure 12–6. *A,* Right renal arteriovenous fistula. *B,* Right arteriovenous malformation with early filling of the renal vein and inferior vena cava.

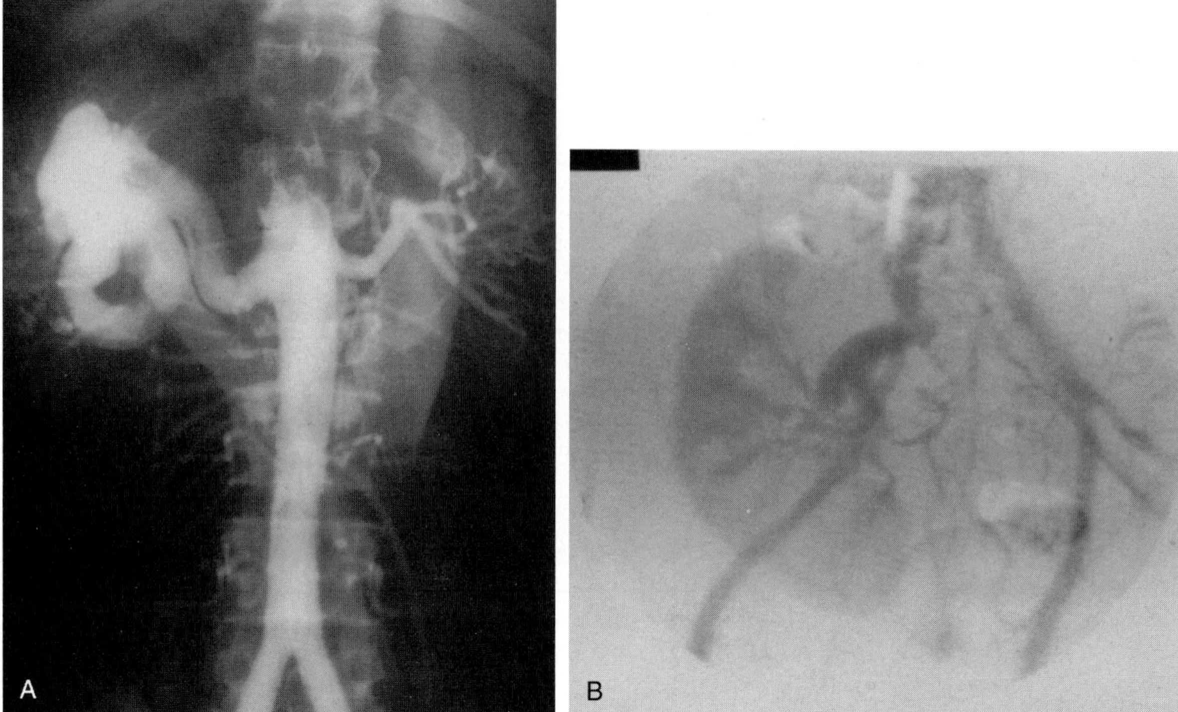

Figure 12–7. *A,* Huge arteriovenous malformation and fistula with early filling of the renal vein and inferior vena cava before bench surgery. *B,* Digital subtraction angiogram of a huge arteriovenous fistula after bench surgery (resection) and autotransplantation.

arterial wall, the adventitia and muscularis, stretch, but the inflexible intima is contused and produces hemorrhage and a propagated thrombus (Fig. 12–9) (Collins and Jacobs, 1961).

The management of traumatic renal artery thrombosis presents the problem of an often irreversible ischemic lesion. In all reported therapeutic successes, the patients have undergone arterial reconstruction within 12 hours of the injury. In one report, only 5 of 35 patients (14%) with a unilateral traumatically obstructed renal artery who underwent revascularization had return of renal function, all with an ischemia time of less than 12 hours (Spirnak and Resnick, 1987). In general, the patient with a traumatic renal artery thrombosis should undergo an attempt at repair only when a solitary kidney is present or when involvement is bilateral. Repair should not be attempted in the patient who has severe associated injuries and a normal contralateral kidney. The historically poor results associated with renal revascularization in this situation should lower the surgeon's expectations in any patient with traumatic renal artery thrombosis.

Arteritis (Takayasu's Disease)

Takayasu's arteritis, an inflammatory disease affecting the aorta and its primary branches, is characterized by stenosis or aneurysmal dilatation of these vessels (Ishikawa, 1978) (Fig. 12–10). The cause of this condition is unclear. It is usually progressive and as a result requires treatment. One study of a series of 32 patients with Takayasu's disease treated with balloon angioplasty reported an 86% beneficial response rate at 6 months (Dong et al, 1987). Until longer follow-up studies are available, surgical intervention appears to be the treatment of choice.

Neurofibromatosis

Neurofibromatosis is characterized by café au lait spots, cutaneous fibromas, and neurofibromas. A hereditary disorder, it is associated with renovascular lesions and pheochromocytomas. The vascular lesions are characterized by intimal endothelial proliferation with or without aneurysmal formation and cellular nodules in the vessel wall. The aorta is frequently involved, and the renal arteries may demonstrate long areas of stenosis (Grad and Rance, 1972) that are probably best treated by revascularization procedures rather than by angioplasty.

Renal Vein Thrombosis

Renal vein thrombosis may occur in a variety of clinical situations. It may arise bilaterally in infants in association with severe dehydration as a result of diarrhea or vomiting or with hyperosmolality related to angiography. In adults, it is more commonly unilateral and is associated with the nephrotic syndrome or invasion of the renal vein by tumor or a primary retroperitoneal process. According to some investigators, renal vein thrombosis occurs in 30% of patients with the nephrotic syndrome because of membranous glomerulonephritis (Llach et al, 1980).

Acute renal vein thrombosis is associated with flank pain, hypertension, and shock. Kidney size is increased, and renal blood flow is decreased to 25% of normal. Macroscopic or microscopic hematuria, proteinuria, and reduced renal function are common. Occasionally, a pulmonary embolus is the presenting sign, and renal failure may occur.

Radiologic studies helpful in making this diagnosis are

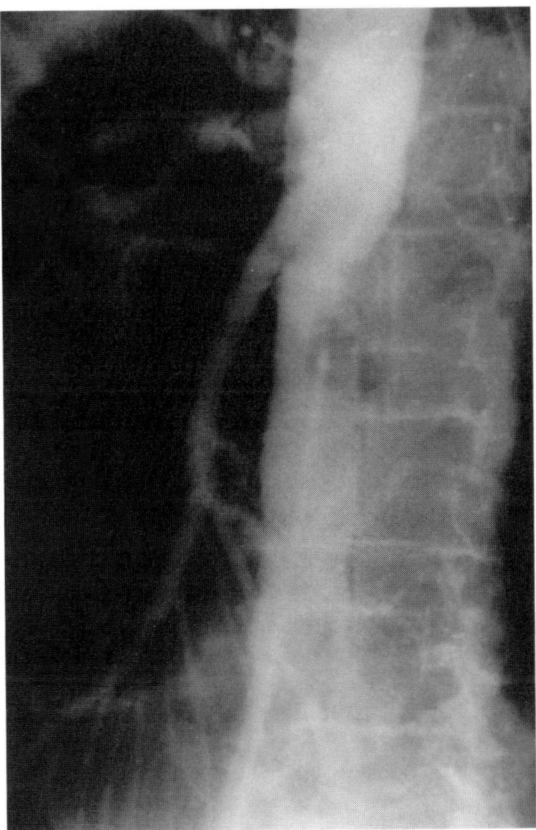

Figure 12–8. Bilateral renal artery emboli with bilateral total renal artery occlusion.

excretory urography (intravenous pyelography [IVP]), which demonstrates an enlarged kidney with poor function. Ultrasonography normally demonstrates a large, hypoechoic kidney with thrombus in the renal vein. Computed tomography (CT) and magnetic resonance imaging (MRI) have been used to confirm the presence of thrombus in the renal vein in association with an enlarged kidney. The definitive diagnostic study, however, is renal venography.

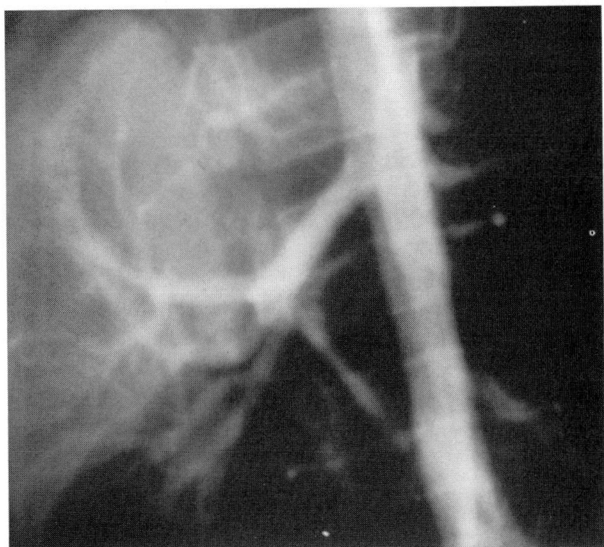

Figure 12–9. Traumatic complete occlusion of dual blood supply to the left kidney.

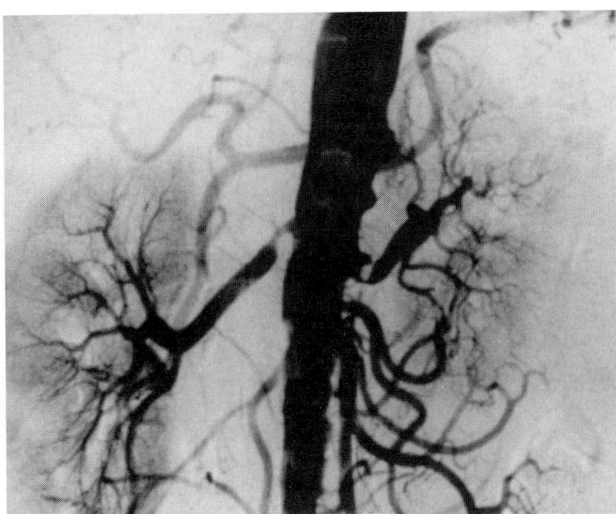

Figure 12–10. Bilateral renal artery stenosis caused by Takayasu's disease.

The management of renal vein thrombosis in infants and children consists of rehydration, fibrinolytic agents, and, occasionally, renal vein thrombectomy (Bromberg and Firlit, 1990).

In adults, anticoagulation therapy should be initiated immediately. Surgical thrombectomy is not indicated because intrarenal venous thrombosis most likely has already occurred.

TREATMENT OF RENOVASCULAR LESIONS: GENERAL PRINCIPLES

Medical therapy, percutaneous transluminal angioplasty, and surgery are the three options currently available for patients with renovascular hypertension. In patients with atherosclerosis, the indications for surgical correction are more limited, owing to the older age of the patients and the presence of extrarenal vascular disease. In these patients, treatment with newer, more potent antihypertensive drugs is warranted initially and may in fact be preferred, especially in patients with generalized atherosclerosis. Our poor results with percutaneous transluminal angioplasty for atherosclerotic lesions prevent us from offering this therapeutic option to our patients unless they have a very short middle main renal artery plaque. Long-term results of angioplasty and stent placement are not yet available; thus, their ultimate role in managing atherosclerotic disease is not known. Surgical treatment is being recommended more frequently in older patients when the hypertension is poorly or inadequately controlled or when renal function is compromised. This circumstance is especially true in the presence of bilateral, high-grade stenotic disease or stenosis in a solitary kidney. Surgical treatment is recommended in these patients not only for control of hypertension but also for preservation of renal function (Libertino et al, 1988).

The choice of treatment in patients with mural dysplasia is determined by the type of the specific dysplastic process present and its natural history. Medial fibroplasia is best treated by antihypertensive medication until the patient "breaks through" on this therapeutic regimen. Excellent results have been achieved with percutaneous transluminal renal angioplasty used for the treatment of mural dysplasias, with 60% cure, 35% improved, and 7% failure rates, as reported by Sos and colleagues (1983 and 1984). A review of our results with this technique revealed an 85% overall success rate. Thus, balloon angioplasty is now our first line of treatment in patients with mural dysplasia. Surgical treatment is reserved for patients in whom percutaneous angioplasty fails and recurrent disease develops or in patients who present with aneurysmal disease or dissection as a component of the mural lesion. If recurrent disease develops after successful dilation, we prefer to proceed with surgical correction rather than redilation. In our experience, complications after percutaneous balloon angioplasty, such as intimal dissection or rupture, have developed only in patients who underwent redilations of mural dysplastic lesions.

SURGICAL TREATMENT

Indications for Operation

Generally, corrective surgery for renovascular hypertension or a renal artery condition should be considered in a patient with significant diastolic hypertension secondary to a functionally significant renal artery lesion who is a reasonable surgical risk. Specifically, a patient with the following manifestations of renovascular disease is clearly a candidate for surgical intervention (Libertino and Zinman, 1987):

- Poor control of hypertension after aggressive, appropriate drug therapy
- Poor compliance
- Total renal artery occlusion or dissection
- Deterioration of renal function as manifested by an elevation of either the blood urea nitrogen or creatinine level
- Pyelographic evidence of renal parenchymal loss
- Angiographic evidence of progressive renal artery disease
- Severely symptomatic or accelerated hypertension
- Anuria from arterial occlusion to a solitary kidney
- Failure of percutaneous transluminal angioplasty
- Any combination of these factors

As previously mentioned, the pathologic entity and its natural history also influence our judgment about who should or should not undergo surgical treatment. Because of the natural history of atherosclerosis, it seems advisable to operate on a patient who is a good surgical risk, with the recent onset of hypertension and a functionally significant unilateral lesion. A patient with long-standing hypertension, evidence of disseminated atherosclerosis, and bilateral disease is a poorer risk. Operation should be advised only when uncontrolled hypertension persists, vascular obstruction progresses, or renal function deteriorates. The mural dysplasias are best treated initially by balloon angioplasty. When this fails, surgical intervention is warranted.

When choosing the proper procedure for a patient with renovascular hypertension, the surgeon should not deal with the complexities of the disease unless nephrectomy, partial nephrectomy, endarterectomy, resection and reanastomosis, bypass grafting, microvascular surgery, and autotransplantation are included in his or her surgical armamentarium. Our large experience with the surgical management of referred complex renovascular problems constitutes the basis for the technical aspects of renovascular surgery described in this chapter.

Preoperative and Intraoperative Adjunctive Aids

Patients with renovascular hypertension may have the complex problems of systemic arteriosclerosis and widespread effects on the vasculature of other organs at the time of presentation. Careful preoperative recording of all distal arterial pulses and bruits in the extremities and the neck should be noted as baseline values. When cerebrovascular or cardiac disease is suspected in a patient with a history of stroke, transient ischemic episode, or angina, cerebral or coronary angiography should be performed. Significant obstructive lesions are repaired before a major procedure on the renal artery is attempted. The reason for this practice is that the perfusion pressure of the heart and brain may be reduced appreciably after successful renal revascularization, and the decreased blood pressure may result in stroke or myocardial injury (Javid et al, 1971). Antihypertensive drugs that deplete catecholamine stores in the nerve end plates are discontinued 2 weeks before operation. Hypokalemia from secondary hyperaldosteronism or long-term use of diuretics should be corrected before operation to avoid the potentiating effects of anesthetic agents.

To protect the already somewhat impaired renal parenchyma from the effects of ischemia, both mannitol and furosemide (Lasix) are given approximately 2 hours before the renal vessels are clamped. In addition, renal dose dopamine may be required to maintain adequate renal perfusion during the surgical procedure. Central venous pressure and Swan-Ganz catheters are required in the elderly atherosclerotic patient to monitor the intraoperative and postoperative hemodynamic status carefully. If cross clamping of the aorta is required and prolonged, sodium bicarbonate and colloid plasma expanders are administered. Systemic anticoagulation is routine: 3000 to 5000 units of heparin are administered intravenously 30 minutes before the renal vessels or aorta is clamped. Without heparinization, thrombi may form proximal to the vascular clamps, with possible embolization to the kidneys or lower extremities. This possibility is even more critical during microvascular surgery on 2- to 3-mm secondary or tertiary branches where anastomotic patency is dependent on adequate heparinization. Generally, I do not reverse the heparinization with protamine but, rather, allow the heparin to be metabolized away within 4 to 6 hours of administration.

Exposure of the Renal Vessels

The patient is placed in a supine position with the arms at the sides. A Foley catheter is introduced into the bladder to monitor urinary output. The skin of the chest, abdomen, and both legs is prepared and draped so that both legs as well as the abdomen and lower part of the chest are exposed.

The feet are wrapped in sterile Lahey intestinal bags so that they can be observed carefully during the procedure. This practice permits access to the lower arterial tree so that the color of the legs and the distal pulses can be assessed during operation should embolization of an atherosclerotic plaque occur. We have also used Doppler monitoring to evaluate the pedal pulses intraoperatively and postoperatively. This method for draping also provides an operative field for saphenous vein procurement.

The type of incision selected to approach the renal circulation is of great importance in safely facilitating dissection and subsequent technical maneuvers. A transverse upper abdominal incision from the lateral border of the contralateral rectus muscle extending across the midline into the ipsilateral flank between the 11th and 12th ribs provides excellent access and greater technical freedom to the high-lying retroperitoneal aortorenal junctions and their covering veins.

The renal vessels are best exposed by reflecting the colon. The right colon is mobilized by entering the retroperitoneal space through an incision in the lateral peritoneal gutter along the white line of Toldt. The peritoneum is incised around the cecum up to the ligament of Treitz. The hepatic flexure and proximal transverse colon are detached from the hepatic peritoneal ligaments.

The avascular space between the colonic mesentery and anterior surface of Gerota's fascia is entered without opening Gerota's fascia. The duodenum is "kocherized," and the right renal vein and inferior vena cava are exposed (Fig. 12–11). The right colon, small bowel, and duodenum are retracted upward and medially, permitting an approach to both renal veins, the aorta, and the infrahepatic portion of the inferior vena cava (Fig. 12–12).

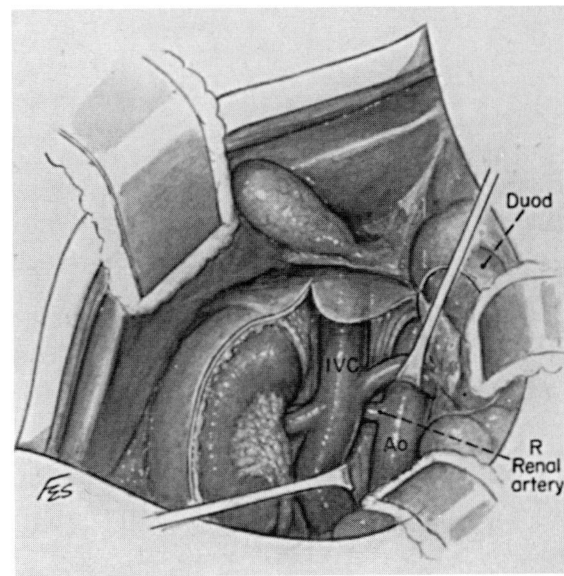

Figure 12–12. Exposure of renal veins and the origin of the right renal artery. IVC, inferior vena cava; Ao, aorta. (From Libertino JA, Zinman L: Surgery for renovascular hypertension. *In* Breslin DJ, Swinton NW Jr, Libertino JA, Zinman L, eds: Renovascular Hypertension. Baltimore, Williams & Wilkins Company, 1982, p 170.)

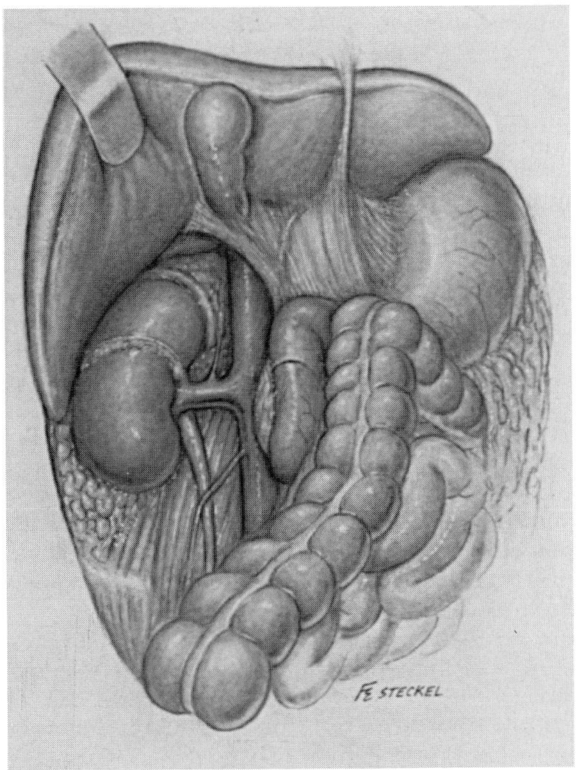

Figure 12–11. Exposure of the right renal vein and inferior vena cava. (Printed by permission of the Lahey Clinic.)

The left descending colon, the splenic flexure, and the distal half of the transverse colon are mobilized by incising the peritoneal reflection along the lateral descending colon to dissect the left renal vasculature. The spleen is protected by dividing the gastrocolic ligament and extending the incision laterally into the avascular space toward the splenocolic attachments, which are then divided. The splenic flexure is retracted downward and medially, exposing the left renal vein, the adrenal gland, and the distal portion of the pancreas (Fig. 12–13). The spleen is retracted with a covering protective abdominal pad. The kidney is not mobilized from its bed so as not to interfere with collateral circulation that may have developed. Great care is taken not to injure the spleen because splenectomy and the attendant rise in the platelet count may occasionally produce hypercoagulability. Nevertheless, splenic lacerations do occur and require either splenorrhaphy or splenectomy.

The extent of the vascular dissection depends largely on the type of reconstructive procedure selected. Bypass techniques require less exposure of the suprarenal portion of the aorta, whereas transaortic endarterectomy requires suprarenal aortic control. The vena cava is retracted laterally and the left renal vein upward to expose the origin of the right renal artery (see Fig. 12–12). Vessel loops are placed around the renal veins so that the veins can be retracted into optimal position for access to the proximal and distal main renal circulation. When renal endarterectomy is planned, the aorta is exposed from just above the superior mesenteric artery to the inferior mesenteric artery. The lumbar arteries are preserved. A space is then developed by careful dissection between the celiac axis and the superior mesenteric arteries. An umbilical tape is placed at this point, marking the site for the proximal aortic clamp. The renal arteries are dissected from their origin to the first major bifurcation of

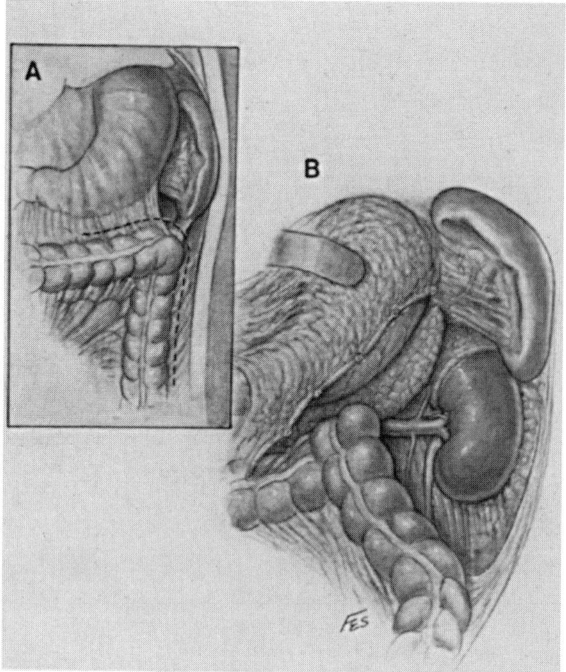

Figure 12–13. *A* and *B*, Exposure of the left renal pedicle. (Printed by permission of the Lahey Clinic.)

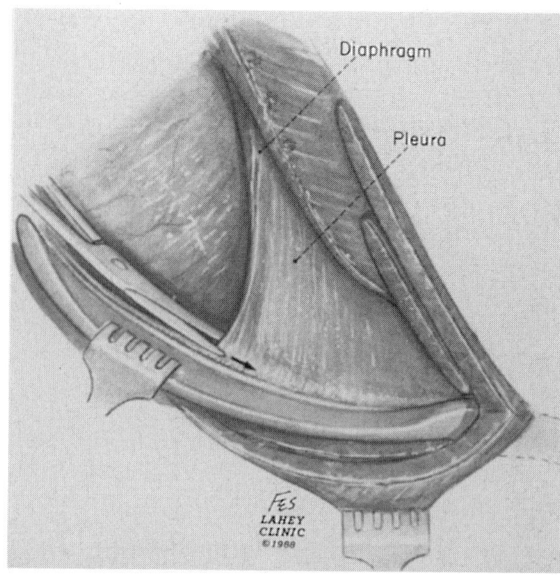

Figure 12–15. Following the intercostal nerve to remain extrapleural back to the intercostal ligament. (Printed by permission of the Lahey Clinic.)

the anterior and posterior divisions. The inferior mesenteric artery should not be divided if occlusive lesions are present in the celiac or superior mesenteric artery because this may be the major blood supply to the entire small and large bowel.

Another surgical approach to left renal artery stenosis is through a supracostal 11th rib incision. The splenic and renal arteries can then be mobilized by a purely retroperitoneal approach (Figs. 12–14 and 12–15) with a direct splenorenal anastomosis. We have performed approximately 100 splenorenal bypass procedures and now prefer this surgical approach.

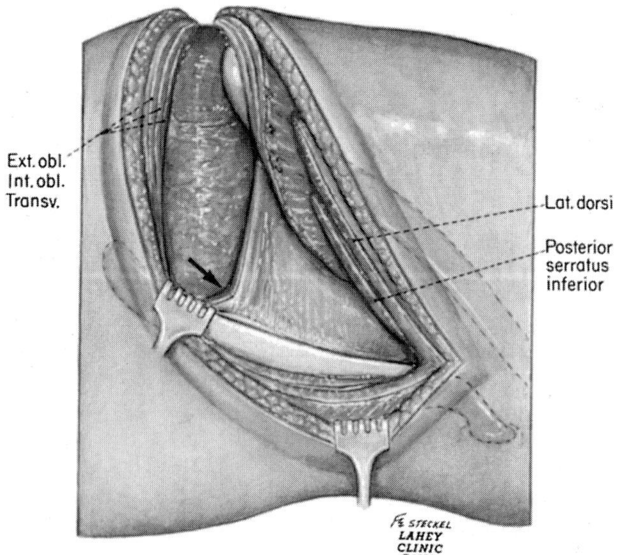

Figure 12–14. Relationship of the flank musculature to the supracostal area. (Printed by permission of the Lahey Clinic.)

ABLATIVE SURGERY

General Considerations

Nephrectomy or partial nephrectomy is indicated in patients who have renovascular disease that is not technically correctable by revascularization and in patients who have technically correctable lesions but who are poor surgical risks. Renal revascularization is advised in all other clinical situations. The indications and type of procedure vary with the nature and extent of the arterial lesion and are described in some detail in the following sections.

Nephrectomy

Reconstructive surgery is clearly preferable to nephrectomy, particularly when the kidney is fundamentally healthy apart from the abnormality in the renal vasculature because both atherosclerosis and mural dysplasia are potentially bilateral entities. However, nephrectomy may be indicated in older patients or patients at high risk. This is especially true when unilateral disease of the segmental vessels is so extensive that reconstruction is not technically feasible (multiple branch lesions). Nephrectomy may also be indicated when arterial reconstruction has failed, resulting in complete graft occlusion; when partial nephrectomy has failed; or when hemorrhage ensues from unilateral renal infarction. Nephrectomy may also be indicated for severe unilateral parenchymal disease and for stenosis or poor flow through a previous vascular repair that has been unresponsive to balloon angioplasty.

The totally occluded renal artery with a nonfunctioning kidney has traditionally been treated by nephrectomy. Since the early 1970s, we have revascularized a large number of patients with both total renal artery occlusion and nonfunctioning kidneys, with restoration or preservation of renal function and cure or improvement of the hypertension (Zinman and Libertino, 1973 and 1977). Therefore, not all pa-

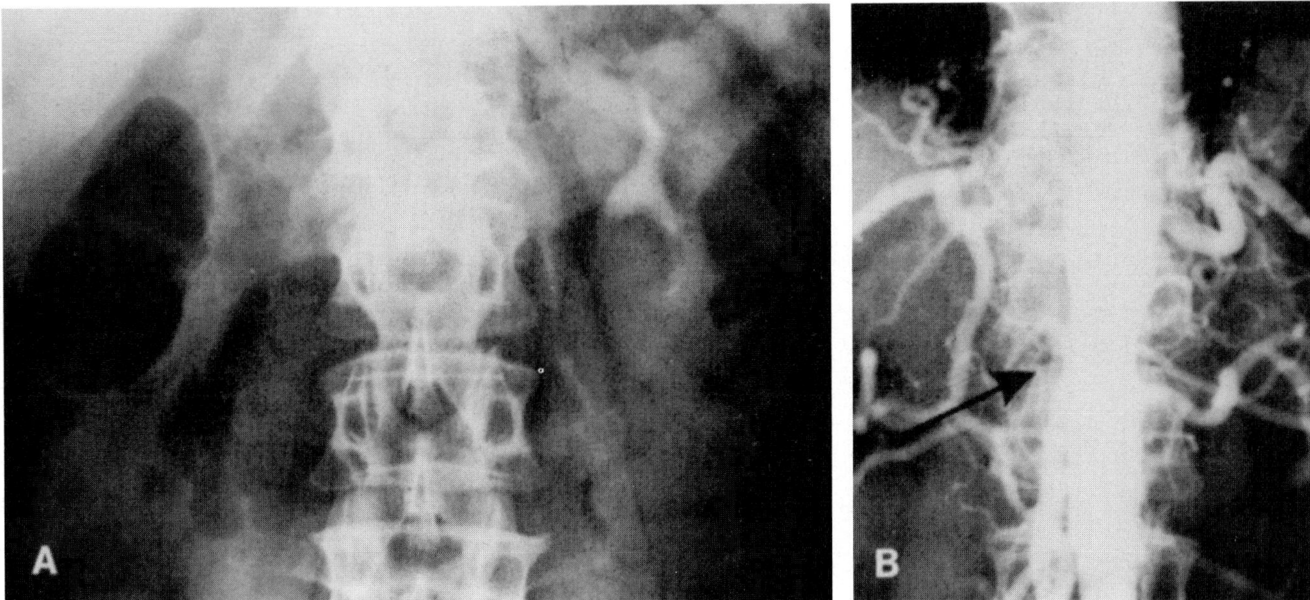

Figure 12–16. *A,* Preoperative intravenous pyelogram showing the right nonfunctioning kidney. *B,* Preoperative arteriogram showing the total right renal artery occlusion with visualization of perihilar collaterals *(arrow).* (From Libertino JA, Zinman L: Surgery for renovascular hypertension. *In* Breslin DJ, Swinton NW Jr, Libertino JA, Zinman L, eds: Renovascular Hypertension. Baltimore, Williams & Wilkins Company, 1982, p 125.)

tients with total renal artery occlusion and a kidney not visible on intravenous pyelography should be treated by nephrectomy. In our experience, certain predictive criteria have emerged that are helpful in deciding whether nephrectomy or a revascularization procedure should be carried out.

The kidney with a totally occluded renal artery may be revascularized if the following criteria are fulfilled: demonstration by arteriography of a nephrogram, visualization of perihilar collaterals, or retrograde filling of the distal renal arterial circulation by collaterals; back bleeding from the renal arteriotomy distal to the total occlusion during operation; and demonstration by intraoperative frozen section biopsy of histologically viable glomeruli (Figs. 12–16 to 12–20) (Libertino et al, 1980).

Nephrectomy is best performed through a supracostal 11th- or 12th-rib incision when operating on a patient at high risk, when multiple branch lesions are not technically reconstructable, when prior arterial reconstruction has failed, or when any of the previously mentioned indications for a nephrectomy exist. In patients with a stenosed graft, poor flow through a previous vascular repair, or a right nonfunctioning or totally occluded renal artery, an anterior approach should be used if revascularization is to be attempted. If nephrectomy is necessary, the renal pedicle that has been isolated is divided and doubly ligated using No. 0 silk ligatures. If microvascular surgery or autotransplantation for peripheral branch lesions is being considered, the ureteral segment is deliberately left long.

Partial Nephrectomy

Removal of a portion of the kidney is based on the premise that the disease process is localized and that preser-

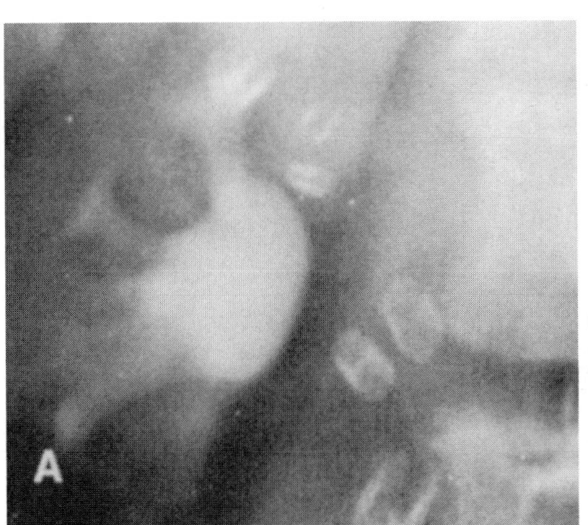

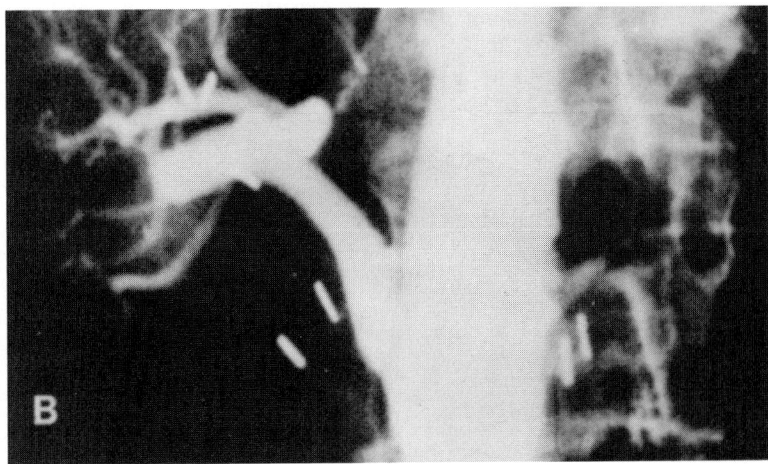

Figure 12–17. *A,* Postoperative intravenous pyelogram showing restoration of right renal function. *B,* Postoperative arteriogram showing patent aortorenal saphenous vein bypass graft. (From Libertino JA, Zinman L: Surgery for renovascular hypertension. *In* Breslin DJ, Swinton NW Jr, Libertino JA, Zinman L, eds: Renovascular Hypertension. Baltimore, Williams & Wilkins Company, 1982, p 125.)

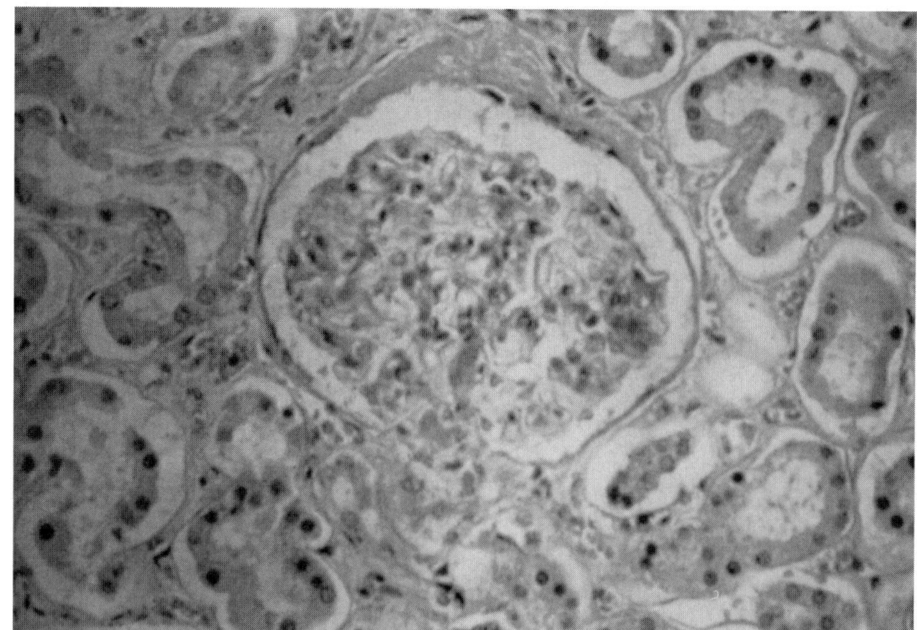

Figure 12–18. Biopsy specimen revealing histologically viable glomeruli. Note the evidence of interstitial fibrosis and tubular atrophy. (From Libertino JA, Zinman L: Surgery for renovascular hypertension. *In* Breslin DJ, Swinton NW Jr, Libertino JA, Zinman L, eds: Renovascular Hypertension. Baltimore, Williams & Wilkins Company, 1982, p 126.)

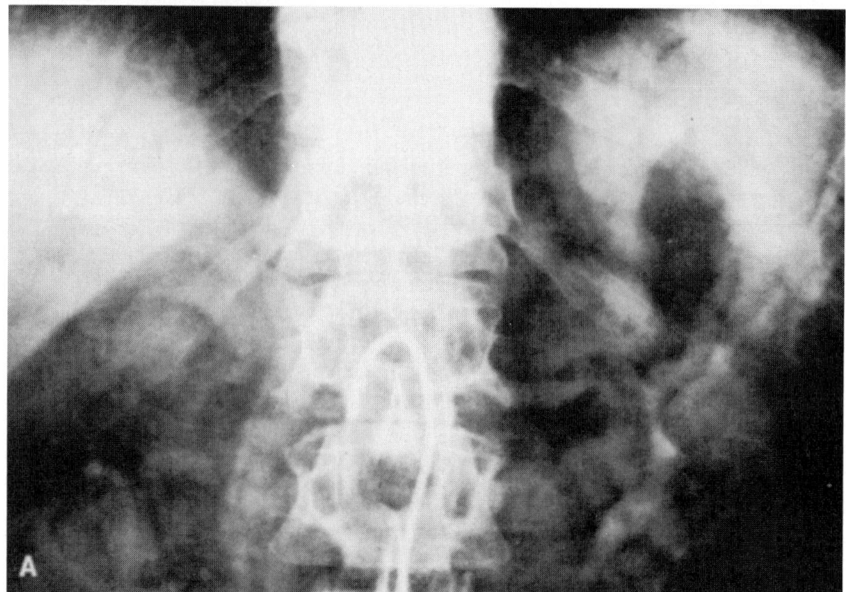

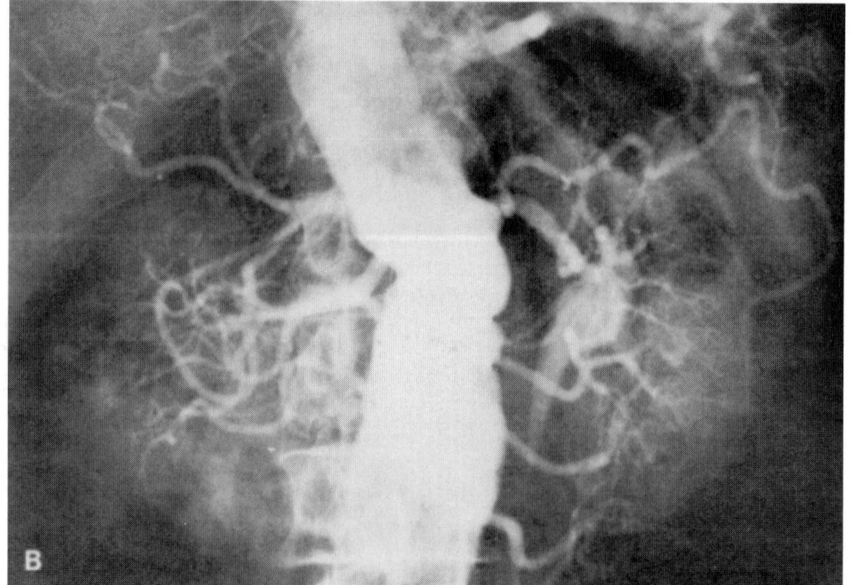

Figure 12–19. *A,* Intravenous pyelogram after angiogram demonstrating the right nonfunctioning kidney with a faint nephrogram. *B,* Arteriogram showing right renal artery occlusion with retrograde filling of the renal circulation via collaterals. Note the aortic aneurysm and right renal nonfunction. (From Libertino JA, Zinman L: Surgery for renovascular hypertension. *In* Breslin DJ, Swinton NW Jr, Libertino JA, Zinman L, eds: Renovascular Hypertension. Baltimore, Williams & Wilkins Company, 1982, p 127.)

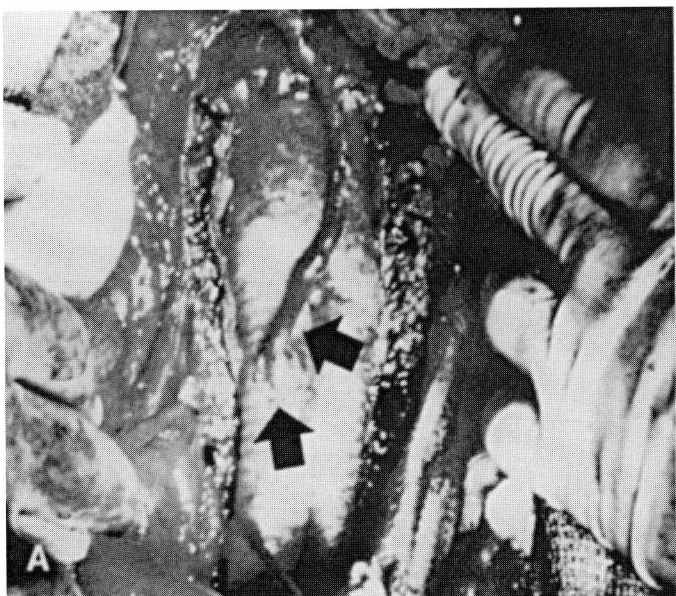

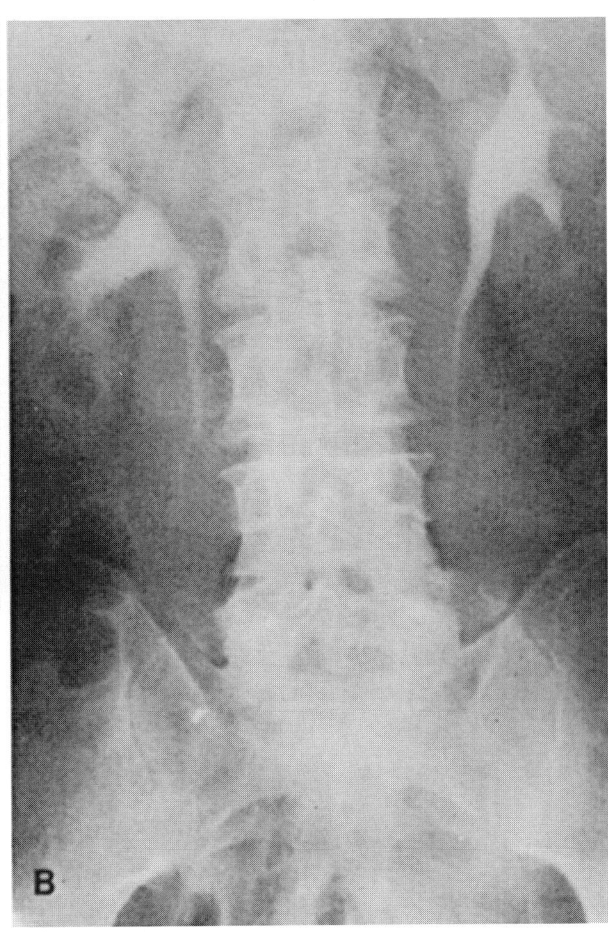

Figure 12–20. *A,* Intraoperative appearance of an aortic replacement graft and saphenous vein bypass graft to the right renal artery *(arrows). B,* Postoperative intravenous pyelogram showing excellent right renal function after revascularization. (From Libertino JA, Zinman L: Surgery for renovascular hypertension. *In* Breslin DJ, Swinton NW Jr, Libertino JA, Zinman L eds: Renovascular Hypertension. Baltimore, Williams & Wilkins Company, 1982, p 128.)

vation of the normal remaining nephrons is worth the increased operative time and surgical risk. Patients with branch lesions producing segmental ischemia and localized overproduction of renin may be treated by arterial bypass if the segmental branch is large enough (Fig. 12–21); by arteriotomy and dilation, especially in pediatric patients; or by partial nephrectomy with an upper, lower, or midsegmental renal resection. Knowledge of the segmental blood supply to the kidney is essential for proper performance of partial nephrectomy (Fig. 12–22).

Polar Nephrectomy

In polar nephrectomy, the kidney is dissected from its perirenal attachments and the renal pedicle exposed. The polar vessel with arterial disease is identified, ligated, and injected distally with a dilute solution of methylene blue dye. This maneuver defines the remaining avascular tissue that might lead to subsequent necrosis, poor healing, or ischemic hypertension. The capsule over the portion of the kidney to be removed is rolled back and preserved for subsequent closure (Fig. 12–23). I prefer not to clamp the main renal artery with instruments or tourniquets to avoid the risk of intimal damage that might result in thrombosis and loss of the viable portion of the kidney.

The collecting system is closed separately with 5–0 chromic catgut sutures. The cut edges of the parenchyma are closed by bringing forward the previously peeled back capsular flaps and suturing their edges over the repaired collecting system. This procedure and the use of double-J stents help prevent the formation of a urinary fistula. The capsular coverings are held in place with separate horizontal mattress sutures. Each suture punctures the capsule eight times before

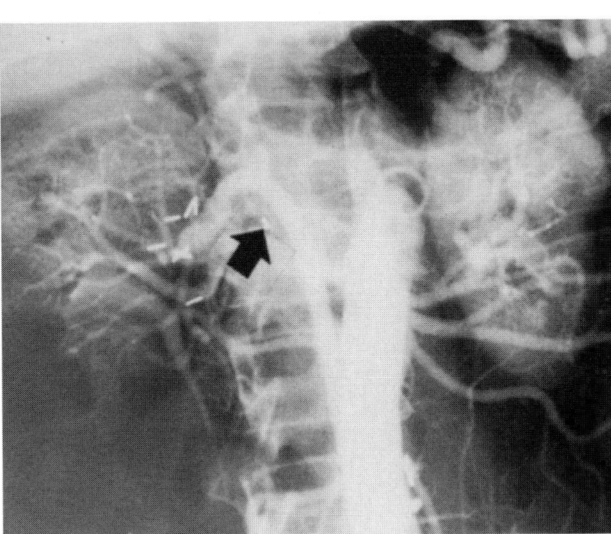

Figure 12–21. Postoperative angiogram; a selective study of an aortorenal saphenous vein bypass graft to the upper polar artery *(arrow).* (From Libertino JA, Zinman L: Surgery for renovascular hypertension. *In* Breslin DJ, Swinton NW Jr, Libertino JA, Zinman L, eds: Renovascular Hypertension. Baltimore, Williams & Wilkins Company, 1982, p 176.)

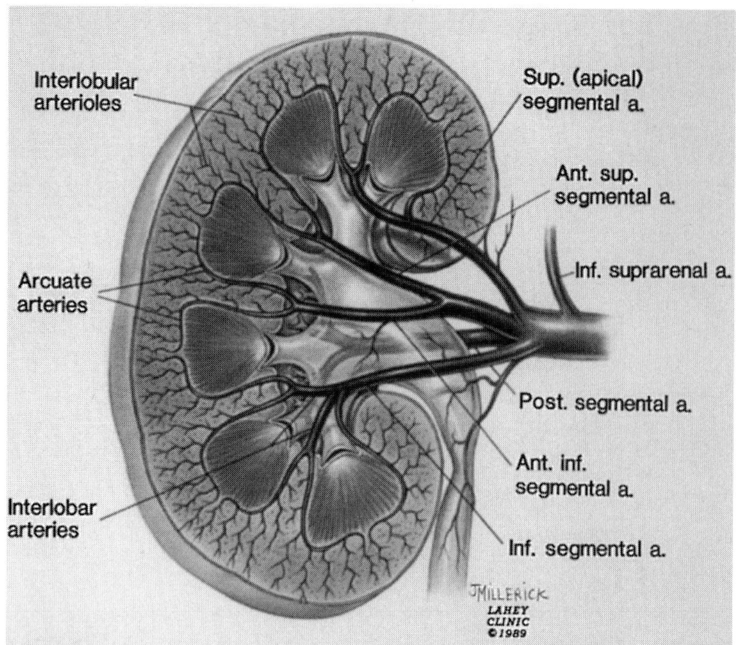

Figure 12–22. Anatomic relationship of cascading intrarenal vessels. (Printed by permission of the Lahey Clinic.)

it is tied (Fig. 12–24). A Penrose drain is left adjacent to the site of the partial nephrectomy, and Gerota's fascia is closed.

Midpolar Partial Nephrectomy

Midpolar partial nephrectomy represents a sophisticated development in tissue-sparing reconstructive surgery. It may be useful in patients with segmental lesions that affect the superior or inferior branches of the anterior segmental renal artery. Painstaking selective arteriography with oblique views is essential to understand the arrangement and distribution of the anterior and posterior arterial branches. Venography and segmental renal venous renin assays are obtained from the venous branches draining the affected tissue. These are helpful when main renal vein renin levels do not lateralize.

The arterial branches are meticulously identified by exposing the renal hilum, isolating the renal pelvis, and gently cleaning the vascular structures of obscuring fat. Silastic loops are placed around the primary and secondary arterial branches to the segment of parenchyma to be removed. The secondary branches with arterial disease are injected with a dilute solution of methylene blue dye or indigo carmine (Fig. 12–25). If the parenchyma demarcated corresponds to that seen on arteriography, vascular tagging is correct and the appropriate segmental arteries are ligated. The secondary veins are doubly tied and divided in like manner, and the caliceal infundibulum draining the targeted tissue is transected and ligated (Fig. 12–26). The capsule is incised in a coronal semicircle and is peeled back on each side to expose the wedge of demarcated central parenchyma. With a scalpel, a full-thickness central wedge is excised,

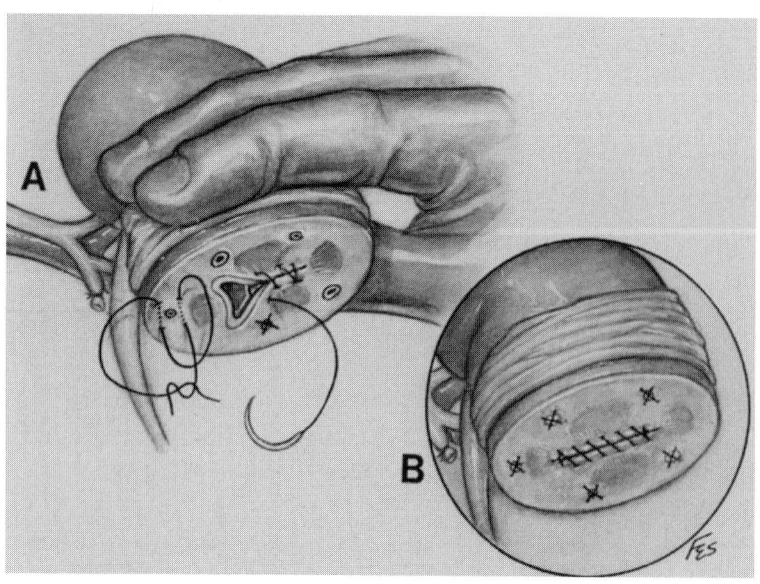

Figure 12–23. *A* and *B*, Hemostasis of the cut surface is achieved with figure-of-eight shallow sutures. Manual pressure by the assistant controls loss of blood. Intermittent release of pressure identifies pulsatile open vessels for ligation by suture. Note the open collecting system and rolled back cuff of the capsular layer. (Printed by permission of the Lahey Clinic.)

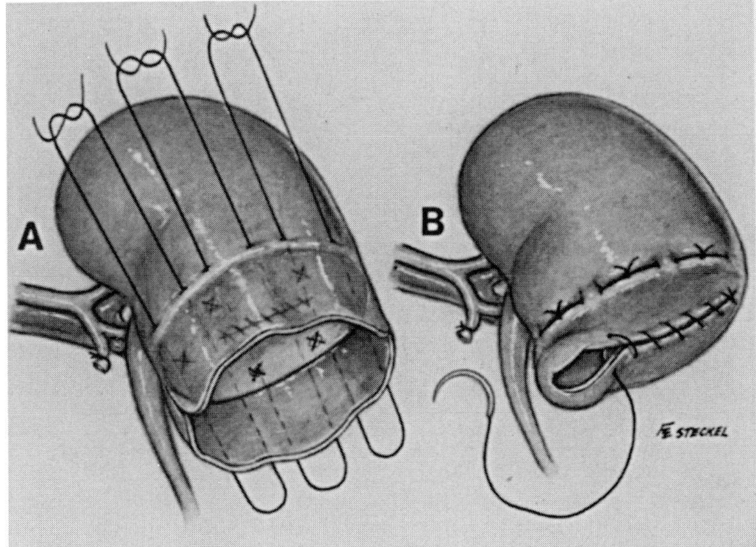

Figure 12–24. *A* and *B*, Closure of the capsular layer over the cut edge of renal parenchyma. Horizontal mattress sutures of 3–0 catgut catch the free edges of the capsule after arterial hemostasis has been completed and after the collecting system has been closed. Gentle compression of these sutures and apposition of the capsular tissue against the cut parenchyma complete hemostasis and prevent postoperative fistula formation. (Printed by permission of the Lahey Clinic.)

enclosing the affected segment. At this point, the surgeon must be assured that no caliceal cavities of the upper or lower pole are left open. The cut surfaces and the hilar branches are checked for significant bleeding.

The collecting system is closed and checked for leaks by injecting dilute methylene blue into the renal pelvis. The capsular apron is draped over the cut edges, and the two poles are approximated with horizontal mattress sutures (Fig. 12–27). Occasionally, partial nephrectomy may be performed judiciously as a component of a bypass procedure. When stenosis of the main renal artery is simply corrected by a bypass procedure, coexisting disease in a branch of the artery may be remedied by simultaneous partial nephrectomy.

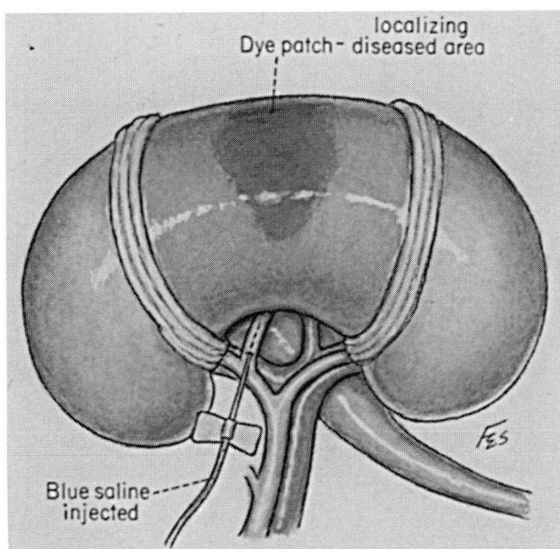

Figure 12–25. Dissection technique in partial nephrectomy of the midsection. Tertiary arterial branches are dissected gently in the renal sinus aided by palpebral retractors of the Gil-Vernet type. Identification of a small blood vessel, such as one that supplies part of the diseased parenchyma, is achieved by injecting a diluted solution of indigo carmine dye into the lumen with a scalp vein needle and correlating the region stained with that seen angiographically. (Printed by permission of the Lahey Clinic.)

RECONSTRUCTIVE SURGICAL PROCEDURES

A great variety of revascularization techniques for the surgical treatment of renovascular lesions have been used during the past two decades. The two procedures that have emerged as applicable and widely used are endarterectomy and aortorenal bypass grafting with synthetic material, autogenous saphenous vein, or splenic or hypogastric artery.

Endarterectomy

Endarterectomy has been advocated as the procedure of choice for renal artery stenosis secondary to atherosclerosis. The pattern of this disease varies from a focal occlusive

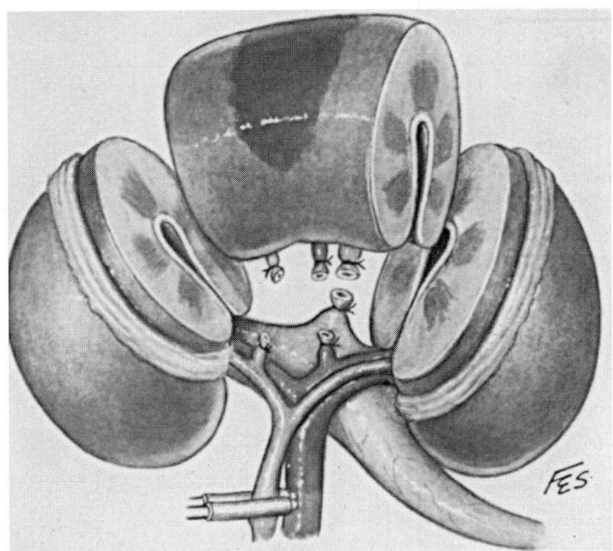

Figure 12–26. Excision is completed by division of tertiary vascular branches and of the infundibulum draining the involved calix. (Printed by permission of the Lahey Clinic.)

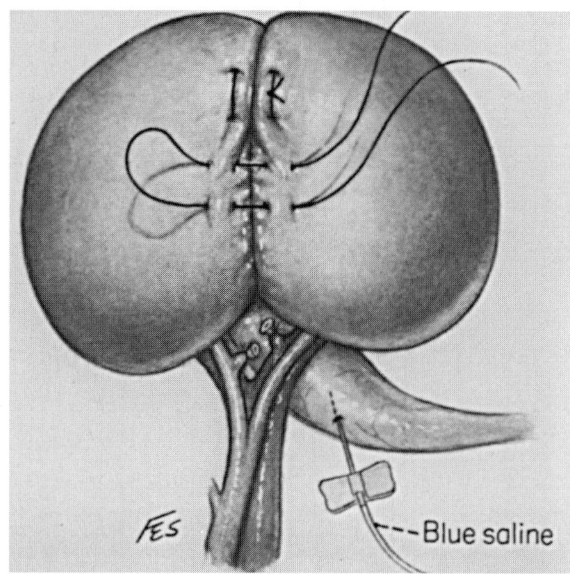

Figure 12–27. Polar remnants are rejoined after releasing the arterial clamp and achieving hemostasis. Closure of the collecting system is tested with blue saline solution. (Printed by permission of the Lahey Clinic.)

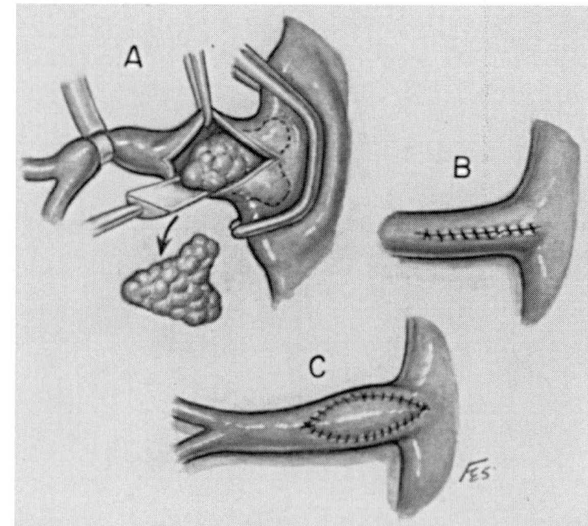

Figure 12–28. *A* to *C*, Technique for renal endarterectomy with or without vein patch closure. (From Libertino JA, Zinman L: Surgery for renovascular hypertension. *In* Breslin DJ, Swinton NW Jr, Libertino JA, Zinman L, eds: Renovascular Hypertension. Baltimore, Williams & Wilkins Company, 1982, p 180.)

plaque at the orifice of the renal artery to extensive involvement of the aorta, renal vasculature, and other visceral branches. Dos Santos, who introduced the technique of endarterectomy in 1949, noted that an occlusive plaque can be removed successfully with its adherent intima and media attached and a patent artery achieved. He destroyed the myth that intimal integrity is necessary for preventing thrombosis and achieving luminal patency.

Renal Endarterectomy

Renal endarterectomy has traditionally been accomplished through a renal arteriotomy with extension into the aorta. The aortic wall is partially occluded with a vascular clamp around the orifice of the renal artery (Fig. 12–28). This approach has distinct disadvantages and should be used only for the management of occlusive atherosclerosis of the renal artery when thrombotic extension involves the distal renal artery and its branches.

The renal artery incision does not afford adequate exposure for the aortic portion of the endarterectomy where the disease originates. It is difficult to continue the point of dissection safely and to obtain a clear demarcation between the renal artery and the aortic lesion. After endarterectomy, the renal artery is often thin-walled and fragile and requires the added complexity of vein patch angioplasty to avoid narrowing. The incidence of thrombosis secondary to a distal intimal flap and recurrent stenosis with this technique is substantial (Kaufman, 1975). For all these reasons, I currently find limited use for this operative technique.

Transaortic Endarterectomy

Transaortic endarterectomy avoids some of the problems inherent in renal endarterectomy. It also permits potential revascularization of a renal artery with multiple lesions, including occluded smaller aberrant vessels, through only one vascular incision.

The surgical technique involves complete mobilization of the aorta from the superior mesenteric artery to the iliac bifurcation (Fig. 12–29). The lumbar vessels are controlled with microvascular bulldog clamps in the proximal portion of the aorta. Vascular clamps are placed proximal to the superior mesenteric artery and distal to the inferior mesenteric artery. Gentle Schwartz microvascular clamps are placed on the distal renal arteries and superior and inferior

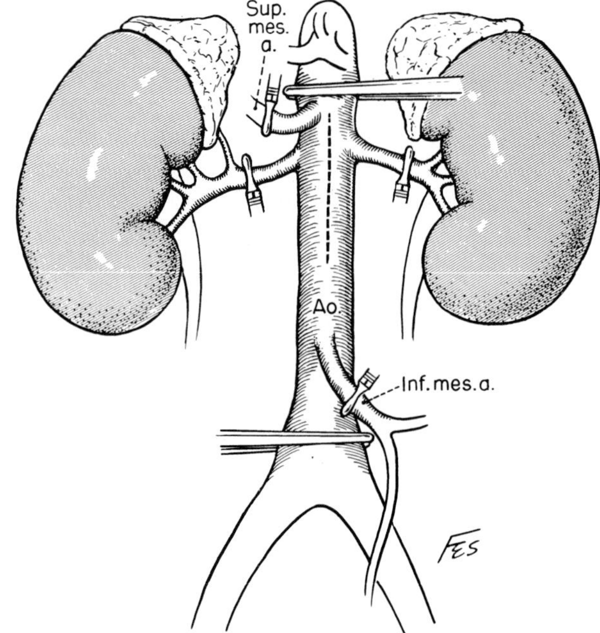

Figure 12–29. The aortotomy for transaortic endarterectomy extends from just above the inferior mesenteric to the level of the superior mesenteric artery. Ao., aorta. (Printed by permission of the Lahey Clinic.)

mesenteric arteries to control backbleeding. Systemic heparin, 3000 to 5000 units, is administered intravenously approximately 30 minutes before the clamps are applied.

The aorta is opened through a vertical anterior aortotomy extending from the level of the inferior mesenteric artery cephalad to a point above and to the left of the superior mesenteric artery (Fig. 12–30). Great care must be taken in establishing the initial plane of the endarterectomy. The proper plane is obtained by starting the dissection with a blunt-tipped, slightly curved instrument, such as a Schnidt clamp or a No. 3 Penfield dural elevator (Fig. 12–30). This procedure should be performed by the gentlest of maneuvers. With a blunt endarterectomy spatula, the plaque is lifted away from the artery, and a plane is developed circumferentially and distal to the lowermost portion of the aortotomy. The plaque is lifted anteriorly and away from the posterior wall with a blunt-tipped right-angle clamp and is transected cleanly with Potts scissors.

To prevent dissection, the distal intima is transfixed with four or five mattress sutures of 6–0 polypropylene (Prolene) tied on the outer aortic wall (Fig. 12–31). The divided plaque is lifted up, and the dissection is continued cephalad to the renal orifices, where the plaque is carefully dissected into the renal artery. With traction on the aortic plaque, the plane is developed within the lumen of the renal artery until the normal intima appears. Usually, the plaque separates easily from the intimal surface of the normal renal artery and can be delivered into the aortic lumen (Fig. 12–32).

A similar procedure is performed on the contralateral renal artery if it is involved, and the dissection is extended cephalad to the superior mesenteric artery, where the plaque is again transected and lifted from the lumen of the aorta. The aortotomy is flushed with a dilute solution of heparin, and the clamps are released momentarily to flush loose plaque or thrombi at their points of coaptation. The intima of the renal artery is inspected through the orifice for residual fragments or any elevated intimal flaps. Gauze pledgets may be used to cleanse the distal renal artery. The renal artery clamps are released momentarily to flush out trapped debris in retrograde fashion. The aortotomy is closed with continuous 4–0 Prolene sutures. If bleeding from the aortotomy persists, it may be buttressed by wrapping a collar of woven Dacron graft around the aorta at the point of the aortotomy. Inspection of the renal artery should reveal a soft wall with no palpable disease and a good pulse. Patency and the absence of an intimal flap can be confirmed by intraoperative angiography or Doppler flow studies. We have just begun to

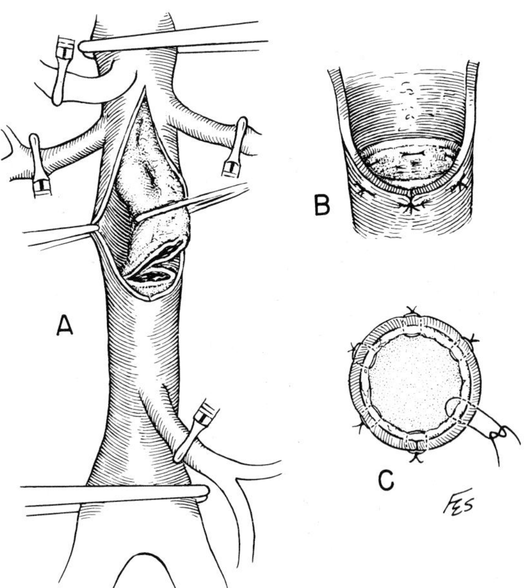

Figure 12–31. Distal intima is transected sharply and tacked to the aortic wall with six mattress sutures to prevent intimal flap dissection. (Printed by permission of the Lahey Clinic.)

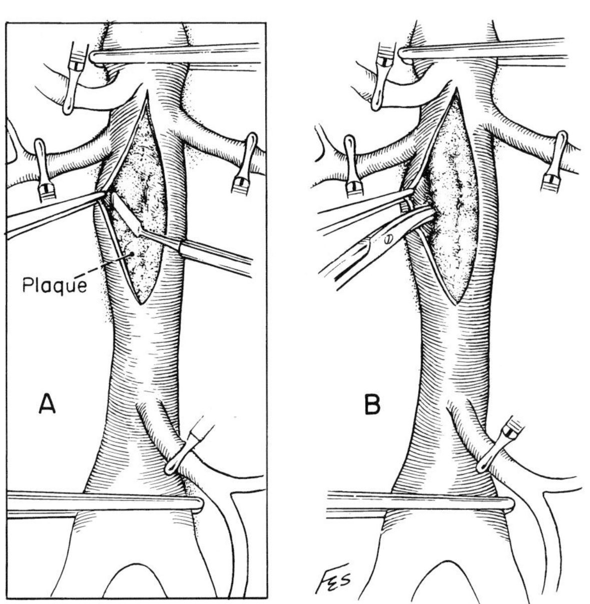

Figure 12–30. *A* and *B,* Transaortic endarterectomy. Initial dissection between the plaque and the aortic wall is done with the tip of the clamp and the dural elevator. (Printed by permission of the Lahey Clinic.)

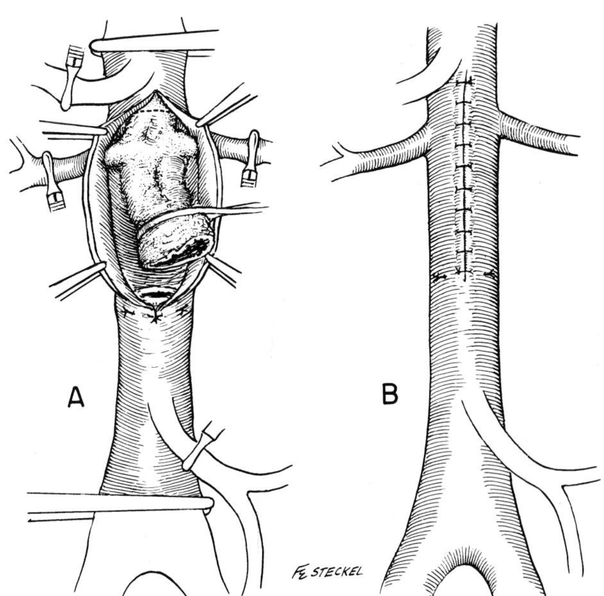

Figure 12–32. *A,* Atherosclerotic plaque is removed from the aorta in continuity with its lateral renal extensions. *B,* Simple closure of aortotomy may occasionally require reinforcing interrupted mattress sutures or prosthetic cuff for hemostasis. (Printed by permission of the Lahey Clinic.)

evaluate intraoperatively Doppler wave form changes before and after revascularization. We note pulsus tardus wave form alterations and increased velocity in the region of the stenosis. Our results are too few and too preliminary to comment on at this time. However, intraoperative Doppler studies may become a useful adjunct in detecting technical difficulties at the time of revascularization.

Endarterectomy should not be undertaken unless the surgeon is experienced and well versed in the nuances of atherosclerotic lesions of the aorta and the renal artery. The procedure has the disadvantage of requiring aortic cross-clamping with bilateral renal ischemia that may be prolonged in a technically difficult situation and may result in renal injury. The denuded medial and intimal surfaces are more prone to early thrombosis, and long-term results in most series reveal a significant incidence of recurrent stenotic disease. The poor results reported in the literature with this procedure as performed by capable surgeons dissuade us from resorting to renal or transaortic endarterectomy as the procedure of choice for atherosclerotic disease of the renal arteries. This procedure should be in the repertoire of a renovascular surgeon but utilized very infrequently.

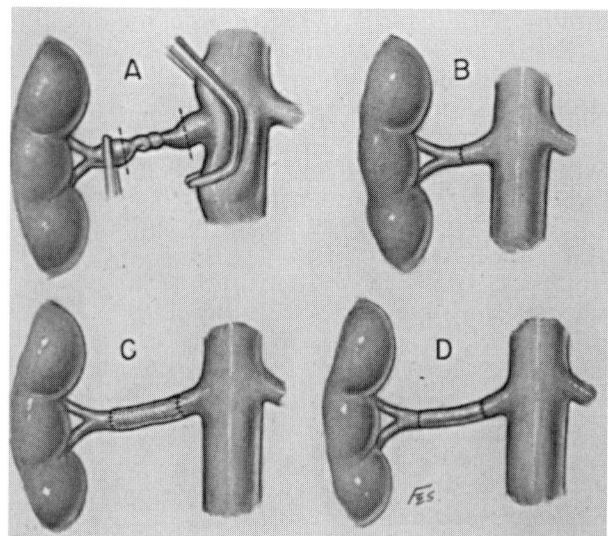

Figure 12–33. *A* to *D*, Resection and reanastomosis with or without interposition grafts of Dacron or saphenous vein. (From Libertino JA, Zinman L: Surgery for renovascular hypertension. *In* Breslin DJ, Swinton NW Jr, Libertino JA, Zinman L, eds: Renovascular Hypertension. Baltimore, Williams & Wilkins Company, 1982, p 184.)

Resection and Reanastomosis

Resection and reanastomosis is occasionally suited for patients with mural dysplasia who have a short, well-defined diseased segment. It may be combined with a Dacron or saphenous vein interposition graft (Fig. 12–33). The true extent of mural disease is not always appreciated or delineated by its angiographic appearance. For this reason and because mural disease left behind after resection and reanastomosis is prone to restenosis, we prefer an aortorenal bypass procedure.

Aortorenal Bypass Graft

The widespread popularity of the bypass graft for renal artery disease was attained by virtue of its technical ease of insertion and the favorable short- and long-term patency rates achieved. Bypass grafts are applicable to almost any disease process involving the main renal artery or its branches. This procedure also eliminates the more hazardous and tedious dissection of the juxtarenal portion of the aorta required in endarterectomy. Bypass grafts are particularly suitable for fibrous lesions that affect long and multiple segments of the renal artery and its branches (Fig. 12–34). Dacron, autogenous artery (hypogastric and splenic), and autogenous saphenous vein may be chosen for aortorenal bypass grafts in properly selected patients.

Dacron has been applied extensively in renal artery reconstruction but has been associated with a relatively high rate of early thrombosis. Excellent long-term patency rates have been reported with a segment of autogenous hypogastric artery. Such a graft matches the size of the renal artery and is sutured more simply than the Dacron prosthesis.

Autogenous hypogastric artery is the most favorable graft material for children with renal artery disease because the saphenous vein is usually too small and is more prone to aneurysmal dilation than in adults. The major disadvantage of the hypogastric artery is that it is often the first to be involved with generalized atherosclerosis and therefore is not suitable graft material in older patients. It is also a short vessel and occasionally technically more difficult to insert between the renal arteries and aorta.

During the past two decades, the autogenous saphenous vein has emerged as our preferred graft material and is the most common source used for restoration of renal blood flow at our medical center (Libertino and Zinman, 1980). Saphenous vein is readily available and closer in size to the lumen of the renal artery than other vascular conduits. Its intima is less thrombogenic than prosthetic material and accommodates the creation of a precise, contoured anastomosis with a delicate, thin-walled distal renal artery. Patent anastomoses can be achieved with the most challenging 2- to 3-mm lumen branches beyond the major bifurcation. Because of its inherent properties and the favorable surgical results obtained, saphenous vein has become the conduit of choice for aortorenal bypass at most major treatment centers. If the saphenous veins are not available, we use cephalic vein and Gore-Tex graft, in that order, as substitutes.

Procurement of Saphenous Vein

The procurement of an adequate segment of the long saphenous vein is critical to the success of the graft procedure. Meticulous technique in exposure and excision of the vein is essential to prevent mural trauma and ischemia. Improper harvesting of the vein may result in the delayed complications of stenosing intimal hyperplasia and aneurysmal dilation. Removal of the saphenous vein should be performed with care as the saphenous vein is critical to the success of the procedure.

The saphenous vein is usually obtained from the thigh opposite the renal lesion so that two surgeons may simultaneously expose the renal vessels and mobilize the graft, shortening the operative time. The vein is mobilized through

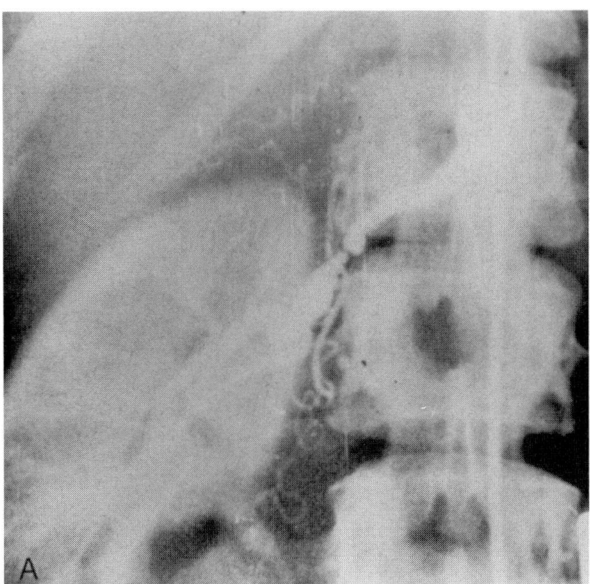

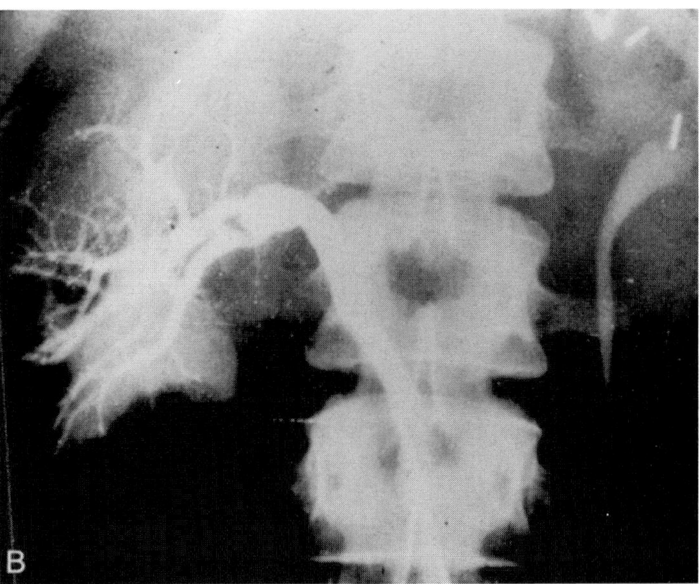

Figure 12–34. *A,* Preoperative arteriogram showing subadventitial disease with involvement of the lower segmental artery and a small aneurysm at the bifurcation of the renal artery. *B,* Postoperative arteriogram showing a saphenous vein graft bypassing the main stem and segmental lesion. This demonstrates the versatility and ease with which saphenous vein can be contoured to the anatomic situation encountered. (From Libertino JA, Zinman L: Surgery for renovascular hypertension. *In* Breslin DJ, Swinton NW Jr, Libertino JA, Zinman L, eds: Renovascular Hypertension. Baltimore, Williams & Wilkins Company, 1982, p 185.)

a single long incision in the upper thigh (Fig. 12–35), which begins parallel to and below the groin crease over the palpable femoral pulses and is extended toward the knee after the junction of the saphenous and femoral veins has been exposed. The incision should be made directly over the vein to avoid producing devascularized skin flaps that can result in necrotic edges and wound sepsis. Finger dissection between the trunk of the vein and the skin is helpful to ensure accurate placement of the incision and thus avoid the development of these flaps (Fig. 12–35). On the day before operation, the course of the saphenous vein is outlined with an indelible pen while the patient is standing.

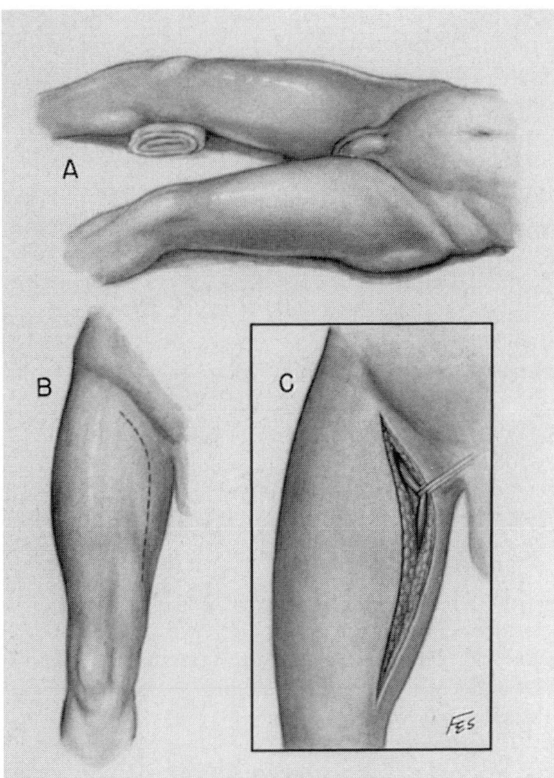

Figure 12–35. *A* to *C,* Procurement of saphenous vein. (Printed by permission of the Lahey Clinic.)

A 20-cm-long vein graft with an outside diameter of 4 to 6 mm is usually adequate for reconstruction of the renal artery. Excess vein should always be available for revision of any procedures because of intraoperative technical problems that may occur during anastomosis. The vein is handled gently without stretching or tearing its branches. The tributaries are tied in continuity with fine silk before they are divided. The areolar tissue is not dissected from the specimen, and the adventitia is left undisturbed.

To decrease transmural ischemia, the vein graft remains in situ until the renal vessels are mobilized and it is ready to be used. If the graft is inadvertently removed prematurely, it is placed in cold Ringer's lactate solution or autologous blood, even when only a short period of time will ensue. The distal end of the vein is transected, cannulated with a Marx needle, and secured with a silk tie (Fig. 12–36). A dilute heparinized solution of autologous blood is used to distend the vein graft before the proximal portion is transected. This step helps to identify any untied tributaries or unrecognized leakage and washes out any residual blood clots. The vein is distended to a minimal diameter of 5 to 6 mm by exerting gentle pressure on the syringe. The proximal end of the vein is transected, and the vein graft is now ready for use. The thigh incision is not closed until the bypass procedure has been completed to ensure that any delayed bleeding caused by the heparinized state is identified and controlled.

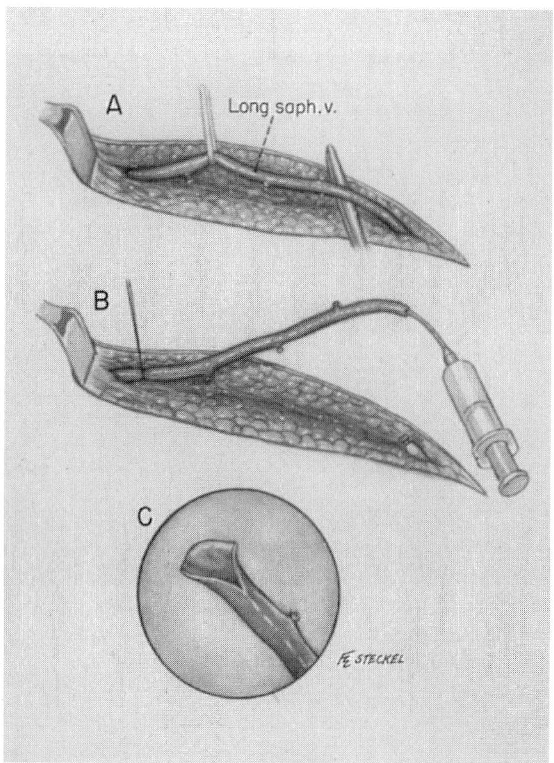

Figure 12–36. *A* to *C*, Harvesting of saphenous vein. (Printed by permission of the Lahey Clinic.)

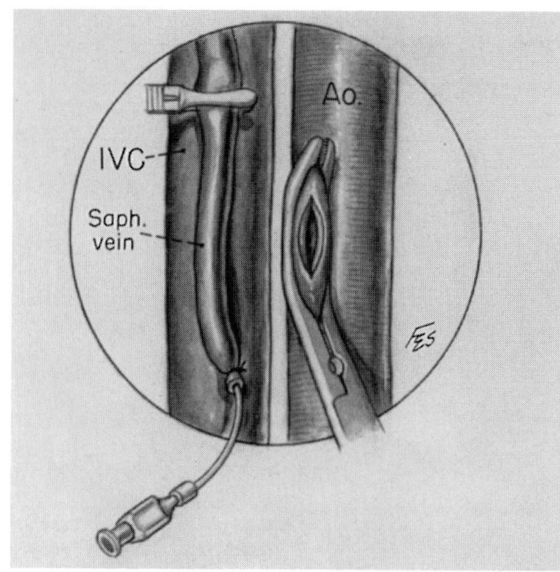

Figure 12–37. An easily accessible segment of the aorta (Ao) is partially occluded with a DeBakey exclusion clamp. A 13- to 16-mm aortotomy incision is made preparatory to constructing the proximal anastomosis. IVC, inferior vena cava; Ao., aorta. (Printed by permission of the Lahey Clinic.)

Technique of Insertion of Saphenous Vein Graft

Heparin is initially given systemically after the surgical dissection has been completed and approximately 30 minutes before the arteries are clamped. The saphenous vein graft should be oriented properly to avoid misalignment during implantation. Either an end-to-end or an end-to-side renal anastomosis can be accomplished, depending on the anatomic situation encountered. An end-to-end anastomosis is preferred under usual circumstances because it permits the best laminar flow.

The aorta, which has already been mobilized and exposed from the renal arteries to the level of the inferior mesenteric artery, is carefully palpated to determine a suitable soft location for the anastomosis that is relatively free of atherosclerotic plaque. A medium-sized DeBakey clamp is placed on the anterolateral portion of the infrarenal aorta in a tangential manner. A vertical 13- to 16-mm aortotomy is made without excising any of the aortic wall or attempting to perform a localized endarterectomy (Fig. 12–37), which may dislodge intimal plaque fragments that can form emboli to the lower extremities when the clamp is released.

Excision of the aortic wall is not necessary because intraluminal aortic pressure spreads the edge of the linear aortotomy to the appropriate dimensions when the clamp is released. The vein graft is anastomosed to the aorta with a continuous 5–0 Prolene suture after it has been spatulated satisfactorily (Fig. 12–38). A microvascular Schwartz clamp is placed on the end of the saphenous vein graft, and the aortic clamp is released. The graft is permitted to lie anterior to the vena cava on the right side or anterior to the renal vein on the left side. Although it is preferable to leave the vein too long than too short, it should not be so long as to bend into an acute angle at any point.

The renal artery is secured distally with a smooth-jawed Schwartz microvascular clamp placed on either the distal main renal artery or its branches. The proper site for the arterial anastomosis is selected. An end-to-end anastomosis is performed using a continuous 6–0 Prolene suture or interrupted sutures of the same material, depending on the diameter of the anastomosis (Fig. 12–39). When the saphenous vein graft is being anastomosed with two branches 3 mm or

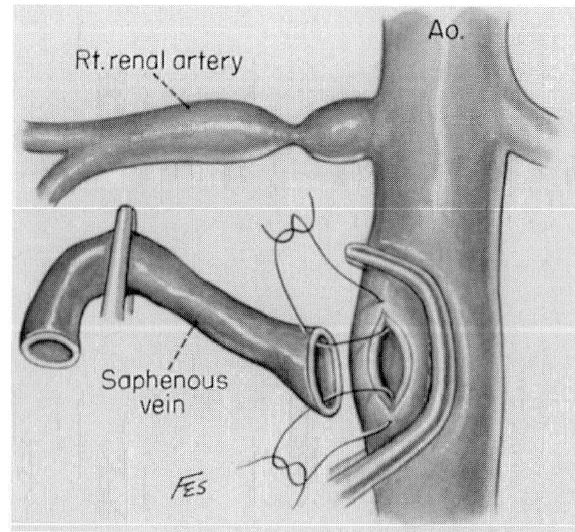

Figure 12–38. Aorta-to-graft anastomosis is carried out before graft-to-kidney anastomosis when an end-to-end anastomosis is desired. Ao., aorta. (From Libertino JA, Zinman L: Surgery for renovascular hypertension. *In* Breslin DJ, Swinton NW Jr, Libertino JA, Zinman L, eds: Renovascular Hypertension. Baltimore, Williams & Wilkins Company, 1982, p 191.)

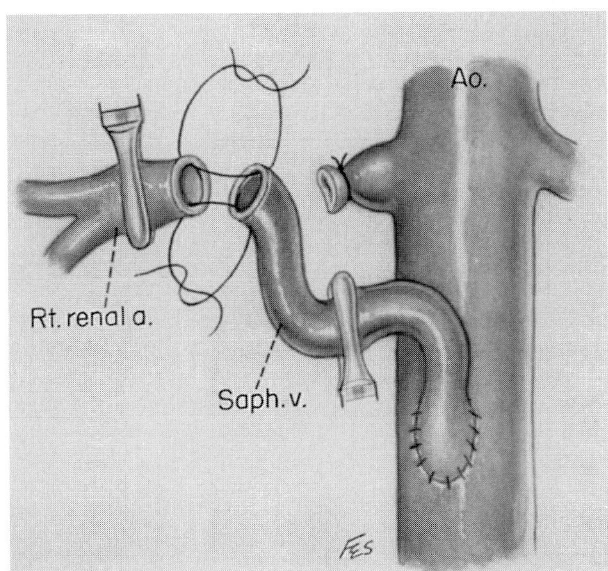

Figure 12–39. Initiation of end-to-end renal anastomosis. Ao., aorta. (From Libertino JA, Zinman L: Surgery for renovascular hypertension. *In* Breslin DJ, Swinton NW Jr, Libertino JA, Zinman L, eds: Renovascular Hypertension. Baltimore, Williams & Wilkins Company, 1982, p 191.)

less, interrupted sutures are used. An interrupted suture line is also selected in children to prevent a purse-string effect with growth of the vessels when the patient becomes older. This effect may also occur with running synthetic monofilament sutures when too much tension is applied during the creation of the anastomosis. The purse-string effect can be avoided by placing sutures at four quadrants in the arterial wall before beginning the anastomosis. Operating loupe magnification and a fiberoptic head lamp are helpful at this point in the operation to permit precise placement of sutures, particularly when exposure in the renal artery is difficult.

The single most important factor responsible for long-term patency is a wide, flawless anastomosis with the renal artery. After completion of the anastomosis, the microvascular bulldog clamps are removed from the distal renal circulation and the saphenous vein graft, permitting reconstitution of the renal circulation (Fig. 12–40).

ALTERNATIVE BYPASS PROCEDURES

When a difficult or troublesome aorta precludes the use of aortorenal revascularization, alternative bypass procedures can be employed for restoration of renal blood flow (Libertino and Selman, 1982).

Splenorenal Bypass

Splenorenal arterial bypass has many desirable features as a substitute for aortorenal bypass in patients with stenosis of the left renal artery. It is particularly suitable for patients with diffuse atherosclerotic disease or thrombosis of the aortic lumen and for patients who have previously undergone difficult aortic reconstructions.

The splenic artery has the advantages of being an autogenous artery that has not been separated from its nutrient vasa vasorum, of being exposed without difficulty by a relatively uncomplicated anatomic dissection, and of requiring only one vascular anastomosis. Carefully monitored oblique and lateral angiography of the celiac axis is required to determine the patency of this artery because atherosclerosis can affect this arterial lumen early in the patient's life. Surgical exploration and intraoperative evaluation by palpation and measurement of splenic blood flow are also helpful in establishing its suitability for renal revascularization. If the blood flow is less than 125 ml/minute, the splenic artery should probably not be used for renal artery bypass.

We now prefer to expose the splenic artery through a supracostal 11th-rib flank incision (see Fig. 12–14). The dissection is continued along the upper border of the rib. The overlying latissimus dorsi, the serratus posterior inferior, and the intercostal muscles are divided. Division of the intercostal ligament permits the rib to move freely. The external, internal oblique, and transversus abdominis muscles are divided in the usual fashion.

The intercostal muscle attachments on the distal 1 inch of the rib are divided carefully until the corresponding intercostal nerve is identified. The investing fascia around the nerve is entered. Dissection in this plane permits an extrapleural approach and generally avoids entry into the pleural cavity. This approach also enables excellent exposure, for the ribs are free to pivot downward in a "bucket-and-handle" fashion (see Fig. 12–15).

The plane between Gerota's fascia and the adrenal gland posteriorly and the pancreas anteriorly is entered. The splenic artery is identified at the upper border of the pancreas. Its enveloping fascia is entered, and the splenic artery is mobilized by a purely retroperitoneal approach. Several small pancreatic branches are identified, isolated, ligated, and divided. The splenic artery can usually be mobilized from the splenic hilum to the celiac axis without difficulty, and it provides sufficient length to reach the left renal artery.

After the splenic artery is mobilized, a sponge soaked

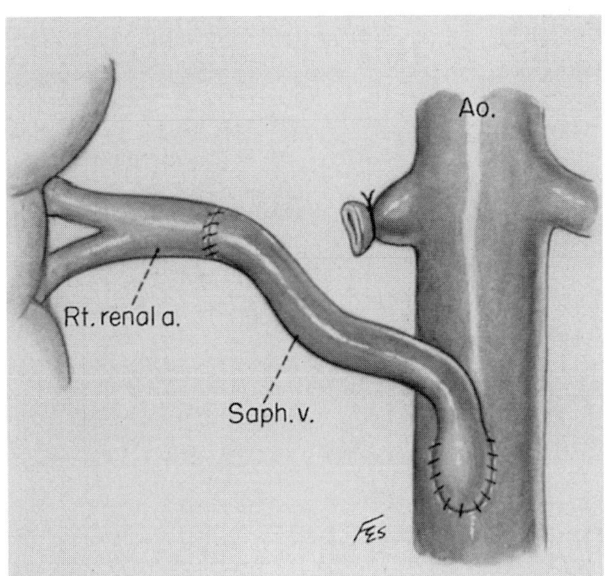

Figure 12–40. Completed end-to-end renal anastomosis. Ao., aorta. (From Libertino JA, Zinman L: Surgery for renovascular hypertension. *In* Breslin DJ, Swinton NW Jr, Libertino JA, Zinman L, eds: Renovascular Hypertension. Baltimore, Williams & Wilkins Company, 1982, p 191.)

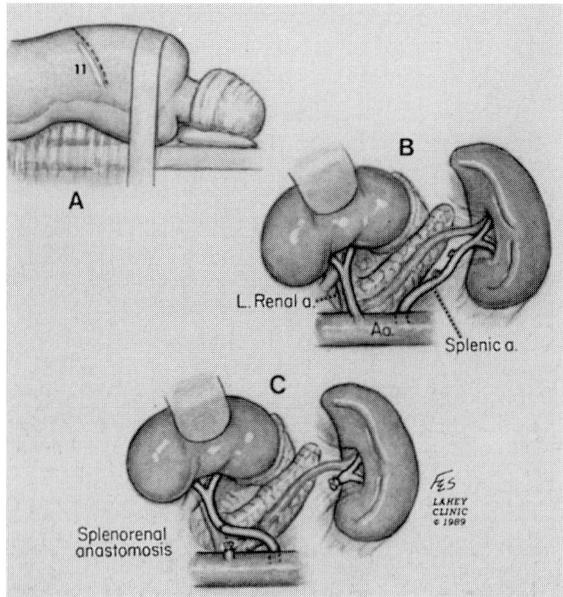

Figure 12–41. *A,* Supracostal 11th-rib flank incision. *B,* Mobilization of splenic and left renal arteries. *C,* Splenorenal bypass procedure. Ao., aorta. (Printed by permission of the Lahey Clinic.)

with papaverine is placed on it to permit it to dilate. The artery is divided just proximal to its primary division in the hilum of the spleen after a suitable vascular clamp has been applied to the origin of the artery. If necessary, the artery may be dilated with a Gruentzig balloon or Fogarty catheter intraoperatively to obtain maximum caliber. Removal of the spleen is not necessary because it continues to receive adequate blood flow from the short gastric arteries. The left kidney is then approached posteriorly, and the left renal artery is identified and mobilized (Fig. 12–41). The renal artery is ligated at the aorta, and an end-to-end anastomosis between the splenic artery and the distal renal artery is carried out using continuous or interrupted 6–0 Prolene sutures (Fig. 12–41). We have employed this approach in nearly 100 patients and now prefer it to our traditional transabdominal technique.

On rare occasions, a sufficient length of splenic artery cannot be achieved. In this instance, an interposition saphenous vein graft from the splenic artery to the renal artery can be used. This maneuver enables the creation of a tension-free anastomosis (Fig. 12–42).

Splenic artery disease, the risk of pancreatitis, and the formation of a pancreatic pseudocyst are some of the limitations that have restricted the use of splenorenal bypass as a routine procedure in the management of disease of the left renal artery.

Hepatic, Gastroduodenal, Superior Mesenteric, and Iliac-to-Renal Artery Bypass Grafts

Extensive atherosclerosis, previous aortic surgery, and complete thrombosis of the aorta may preclude the use of the aortorenal bypass procedure for renal artery reconstruction. When the surgeon is treating a patient with stenosis of the right renal artery in association with these pathologic limitations of the aorta, a hepatic–to–renal artery saphenous vein bypass (Libertino et al, 1976; Chibaro et al, 1984) or a gastroduodenal–to–renal artery bypass procedure (Libertino and Lagneau, 1983) can be selected. The value of these

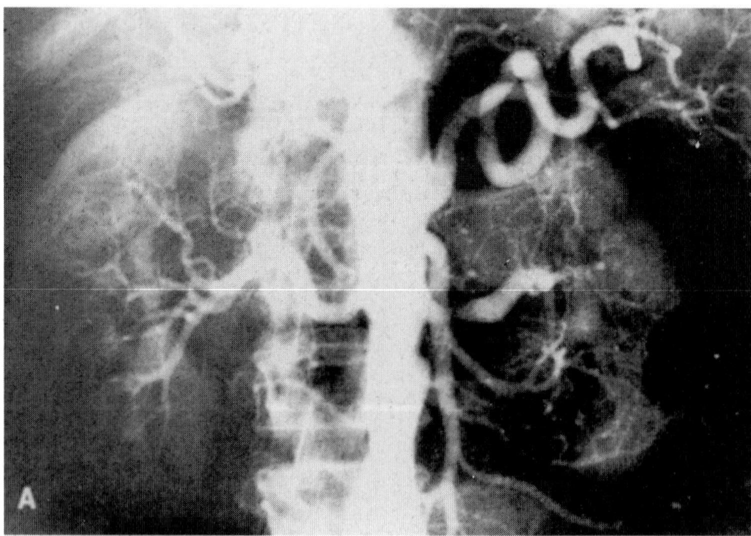

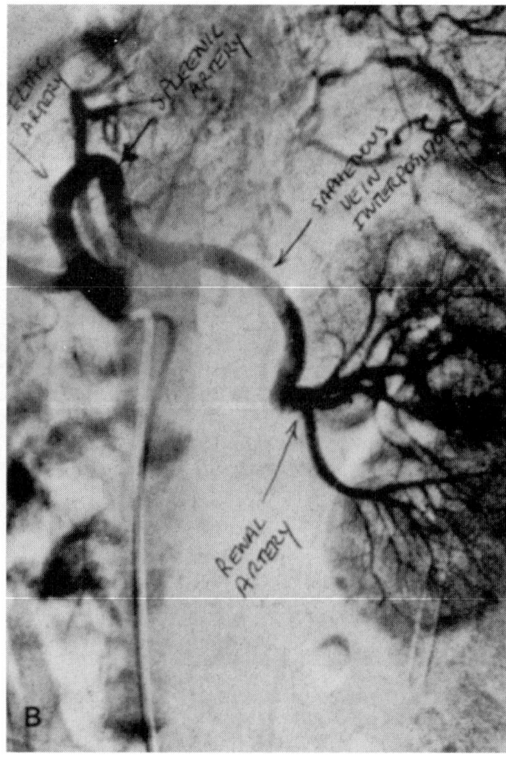

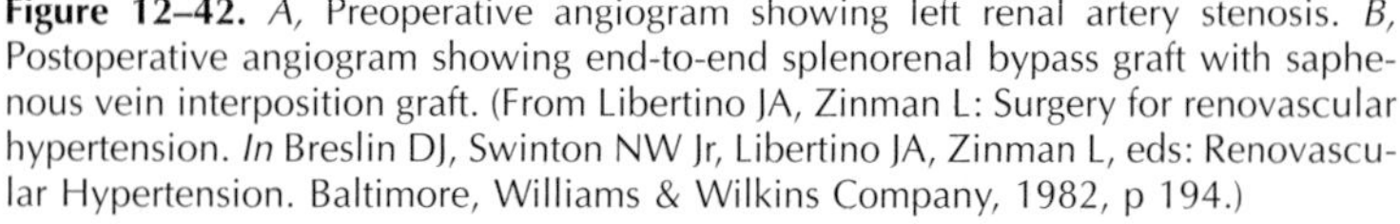

Figure 12–42. *A,* Preoperative angiogram showing left renal artery stenosis. *B,* Postoperative angiogram showing end-to-end splenorenal bypass graft with saphenous vein interposition graft. (From Libertino JA, Zinman L: Surgery for renovascular hypertension. *In* Breslin DJ, Swinton NW Jr, Libertino JA, Zinman L, eds: Renovascular Hypertension. Baltimore, Williams & Wilkins Company, 1982, p 194.)

alternative procedures, initially described by my colleagues and myself, has been confirmed by others (Moncure et al, 1986 and 1988).

Arising from the celiac axis and continuing along the upper border of the pancreas, the hepatic artery reaches the portal vein and divides into an ascending and a descending limb. The ascending limb is a continuation of the main hepatic artery upward within the lesser sac; it lies in front of the portal vein and to the left of the biliary tree. The descending limb forms the gastroduodenal artery. In the porta hepatis, the hepatic artery ends by dividing into the right and left hepatic branches, which supply the corresponding lobes of the liver (Fig. 12–43). The anatomic variations in the hepatic circulation must be appreciated before this procedure can be used. The right hepatic artery is more variable than the left. It may be anterior (24% of patients) or posterior (64% of patients) to the common bile duct, and in 12%, this artery arises from the superior mesenteric artery (Fig. 12–44). The hepatic artery lies anterior (91% of patients) or posterior (9% of patients) to the portal vein. In addition, the left hepatic artery arises from the left gastric artery in 11.5% of patients.

Careful dissection of the porta hepatis is essential. The common hepatic, gastroduodenal, and right and left hepatic arteries should be identified before an anastomotic procedure is attempted. Vascular elastic loops are placed about these vessels, and the common bile duct and portal vein are identified.

After careful dissection and mobilization of the renal artery, clamps are placed on the proximal portion of the common hepatic artery and its distal branches. The gastroduodenal artery is divided (Fig. 12–45). The posterior surface of the hepatic artery is mobilized from the underlying portal vein and the common bile duct (Fig. 12–46). An arteriotomy, 10 to 12 mm in length, is made in the anterior inferior wall of the common hepatic artery beginning at the ostium of the gastroduodenal artery. A reversed autogenous saphenous vein is inserted with an end-to-side anastomosis between the vein graft and the hepatic artery. This maneuver is usually accomplished with a continuous 6–0 Prolene suture. A microvascular clamp is placed on the vein graft after it has been filled with heparin and after the proper alignment and length for the renal artery anastomosis has been determined. The clamps are removed from the hepatic circulation, and a small Schwartz microvascular clamp is placed on the distal renal artery. The vein graft is anastomosed to the right renal artery in an end-to-end fashion (Fig. 12–47). When the

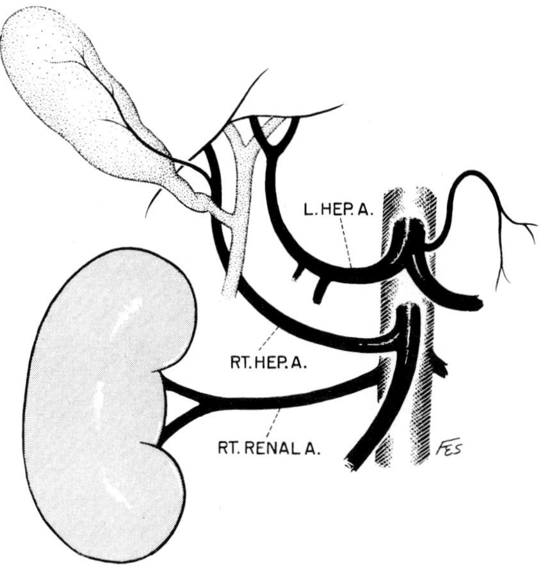

Figure 12–44. The most common variation in the hepatic circulation is to have the right hepatic artery arise from the superior mesenteric artery. (Printed by permission of the Lahey Clinic.)

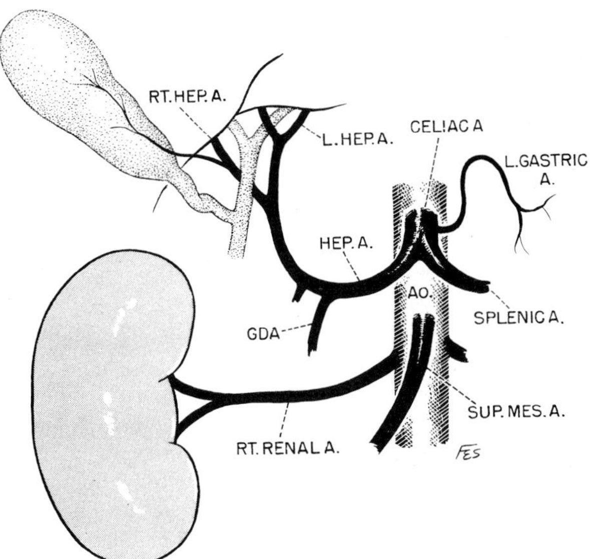

Figure 12–43. Most common pattern of hepatic artery circulation, with the common hepatic artery dividing into the right and left hepatic arteries, which supply the corresponding lobes of the liver. GDA, gastroduodenal artery; Ao., aorta. (Printed by permission of the Lahey Clinic.)

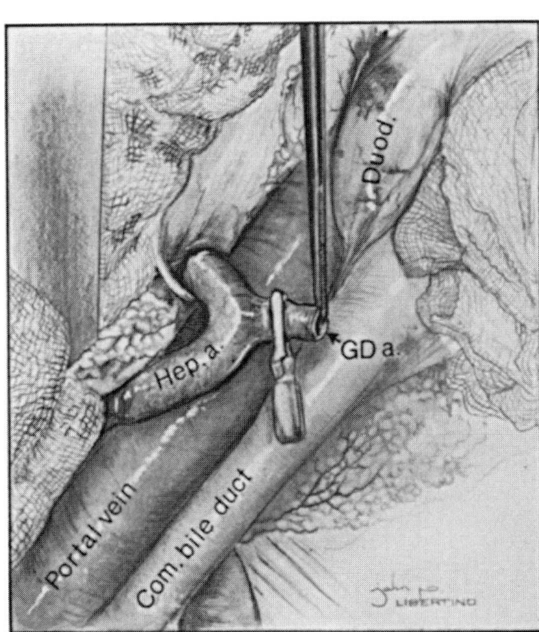

Figure 12–45. Mobilization of the anterior surface of the common hepatic artery. GD a., gastroduodenal artery. (Printed by permission of the Lahey Clinic.)

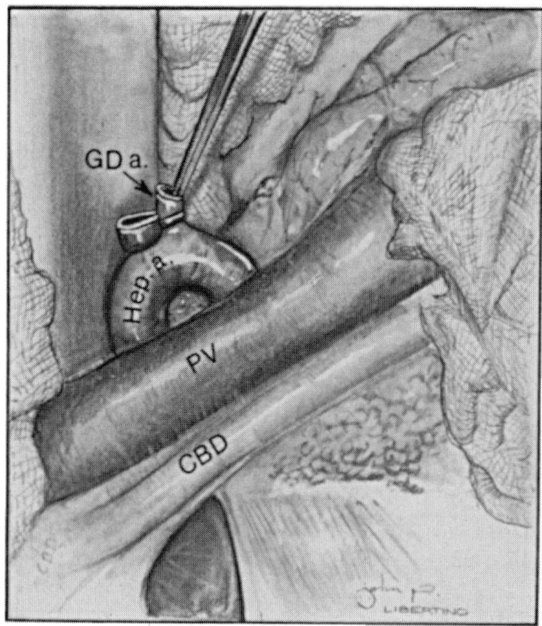

Figure 12-46. Mobilization of the posterior surface of the common hepatic artery. GD a., gastroduodenal artery; PV, portal vein; CBD, common bile duct. (Printed by permission of the Lahey Clinic.)

gastroduodenal artery is used, it is divided, and an end-to-end anastomosis between the gastroduodenal artery and the renal artery is accomplished.

We have employed this procedure in approximately 50 patients with good results. Postoperative angiography has demonstrated the absence of a renal-hepatic steal syndrome. Liver function has not been compromised in any of our patients to date. We no longer advocate the use of the gastroduodenal artery in adult patients, but it is a perfectly acceptable bypass procedure in pediatric patients.

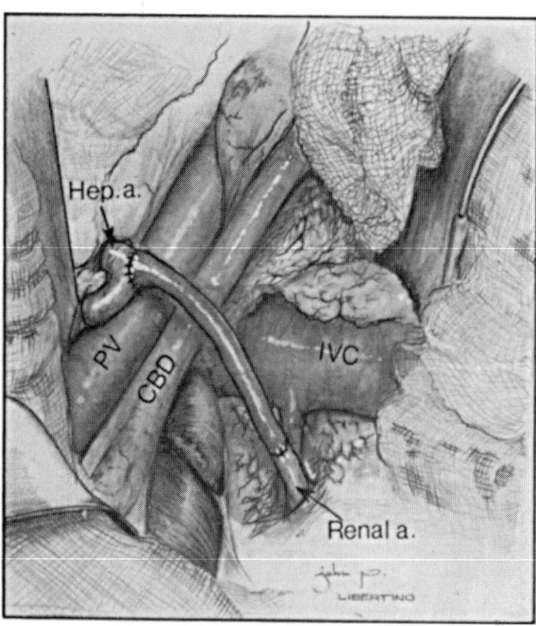

Figure 12-47. Hepatic-to-renal artery saphenous vein bypass graft. PV, portal vein; IVC, inferior vena cava; CBD, common bile duct. (Printed by permission of the Lahey Clinic.)

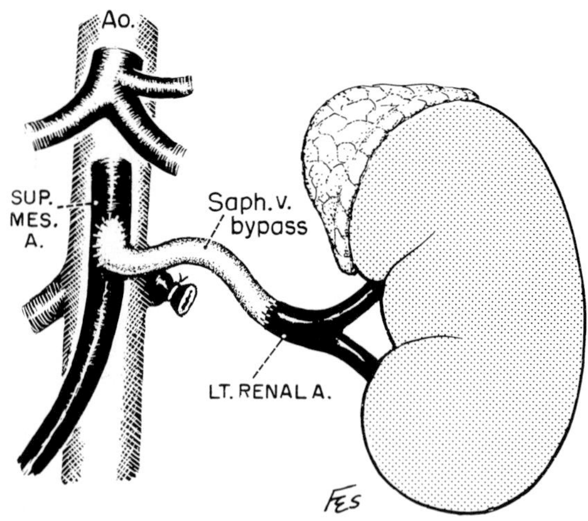

Figure 12-48. Superior mesenteric-to-renal artery end-to-end anastomosis. (From Libertino JA, Zinman L: Surgery for renovascular hypertension. *In* Breslin DJ, Swinton NW Jr, Libertino JA, Zinman L, eds: Renovascular Hypertension. Baltimore, Williams & Wilkins Company, 1982, p 200.)

We have also used the superior mesenteric-to-renal artery saphenous vein bypass as a "bailout procedure" as well, with good results (Fig. 12-48). An iliac-to-renal artery bypass graft has been used as an alternative to the aortorenal bypass procedure in 10 of our patients, with favorable results (Fig. 12-49).

RENAL AUTOTRANSPLANTATION AND EX VIVO BENCH SURGERY

On rare occasions, kidneys with lesions of the renal artery or its branches are not amenable to in situ reconstruction. In these circumstances, temporary removal of the kidney, ex vivo preservation, microvascular repair (workbench surgery), and autotransplantation may permit salvage.

Autotransplantation developed as an outgrowth of the technique used in renal transplantation. Early attempts at this procedure were unsuccessful. In 1963, Hardy successfully autotransplanted a kidney into the ipsilateral iliac fossa in a patient with a severe ureteral injury from previous aortic surgery. The simultaneous development of an apparatus that could preserve kidneys extracorporeally for long periods of time and of preservation solutions led to extracorporeal renal repair (workbench surgery) and subsequent autotransplantation. Ota and colleagues (1967) have been credited with the first successful ex vivo repair and autotransplantation of the kidney. Many other subsequent investigators have reported their experience with these procedures.

Autotransplantation and ex vivo repair should be considered in patients with traumatic arterial injuries, when disease of the major vessels extends beyond the bifurcation of the main renal artery into the segmental branches, and when multiple vessels supplying the affected kidney are involved. Bench surgery may also be required in patients who have large aneurysms, arteriovenous fistulas, or malformations (Fig. 12-50).

Other indications for autotransplantation that usually do not require ex vivo repair include abdominal aortic aneu-

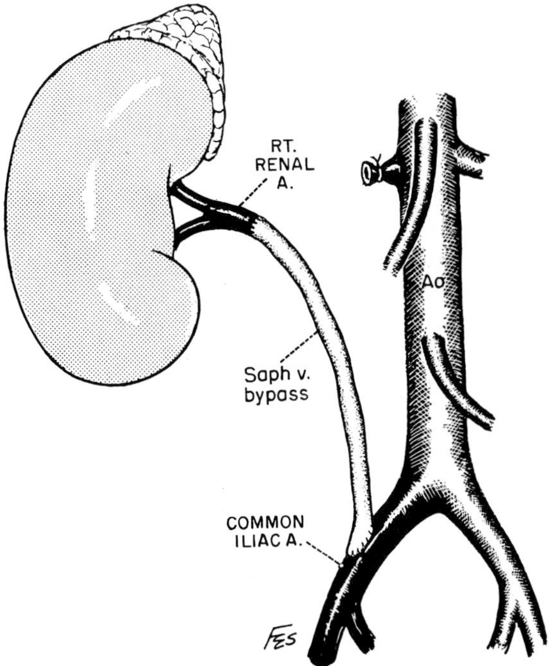

Figure 12–49. Iliac–to–renal artery saphenous vein bypass graft, an alternative to autotransplantation. Ao., aorta. (From Libertino JA, Zinman L: Surgery for renovascular hypertension. *In* Breslin DJ, Swinton NW Jr, Libertino JA, Zinman L, eds: Renovascular Hypertension. Baltimore, Williams & Wilkins Company, 1982, p 201.)

rysms that involve the origin of the renal arteries and extensive atheromatous aortic disease when an operation on the aorta itself may prove hazardous. Patients in the latter group usually have extensive internal iliac artery disease that precludes use of this artery for autotransplantation. However, we have noted that, in these instances, the external iliac artery is spared extensive atherosclerosis and is suitable for autotransplantation with an end-to-side renal artery anastomosis or an iliac–to–renal artery bypass graft (Fig. 12–51).

Techniques for Autotransplantation

Autotransplantation can be accomplished through a large, single midline incision or two separate flank and iliac fossa incisions. Nephrectomy for autotransplantation should be performed with the same degree of care taken in a living-related donor nephrectomy. The longest lengths of artery and vein possible should be preserved, and injury to the renal pelvic and ureteral blood supply avoided (Figs. 12–52 and 12–53). When the transabdominal approach is selected, ureteral continuity can be retained, necessitating only vascular anastomosis after the kidney is flipped over. If ex vivo surgery requires transection of the ureter, ureteroneocystostomy is necessary in addition to vascular anastomosis.

When ureteral continuity is preserved, autotransplantation is performed as illustrated in Figure 12–54. When the kidney has been excised completely, the standard techniques for renal homotransplantation are used.

During dissection of the iliac vessels, meticulous care is taken to ligate the lymphatics in this area to prevent the development of a lymphocele. The external iliac vein is freed to the point where it is crossed by the internal iliac artery (Fig. 12–55*A*). The renal vein is anastomosed end to side to the external iliac vein using 5–0 Prolene sutures (Fig. 12–55*B*). If the internal iliac artery is free of atherosclerotic disease, it is then anastomosed end to end to the renal artery using 6–0 Prolene sutures (Fig. 12–55*C* and *D*). If the internal iliac artery is diseased, the renal artery is anastomosed end to side to the external iliac artery.

When the ureter requires reimplantation, we prefer a modification of the Politano-Leadbetter ureteroneocystostomy. Saline solution, 2 to 3 ml, is injected submucosally, raising a mucosal bleb (Fig. 12–56*A*). A small segment of mucosa

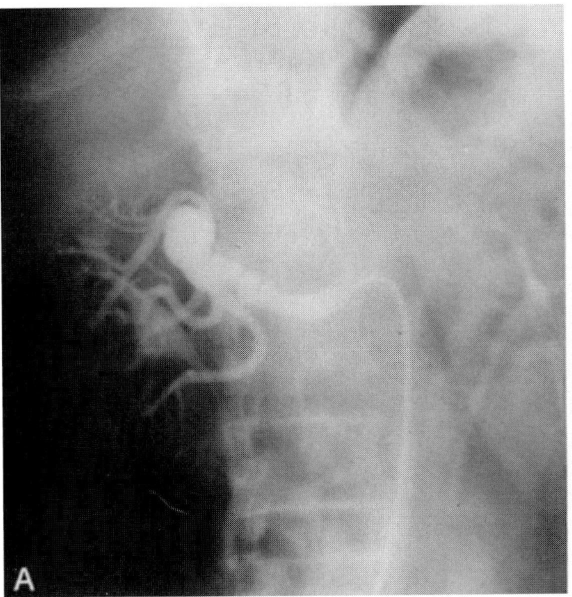

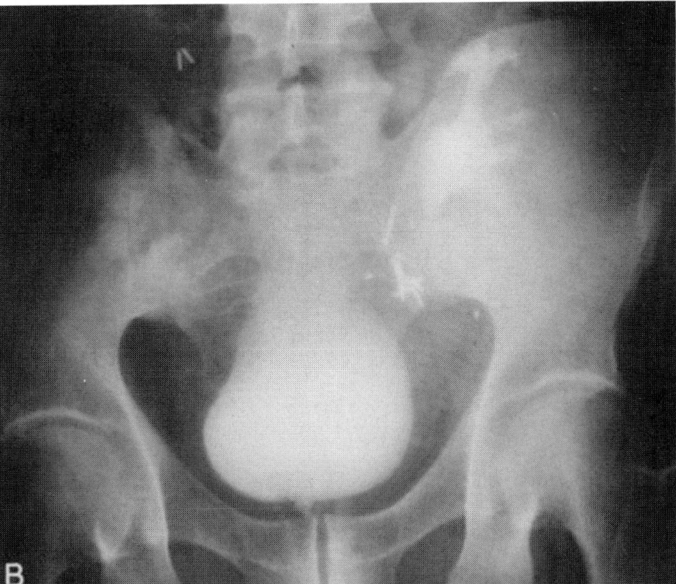

Figure 12–50. *A,* Mural dysplastic aneurysm with segmental branch involvement. *B,* Intravenous pyelogram after bench surgery and autotransplantation.

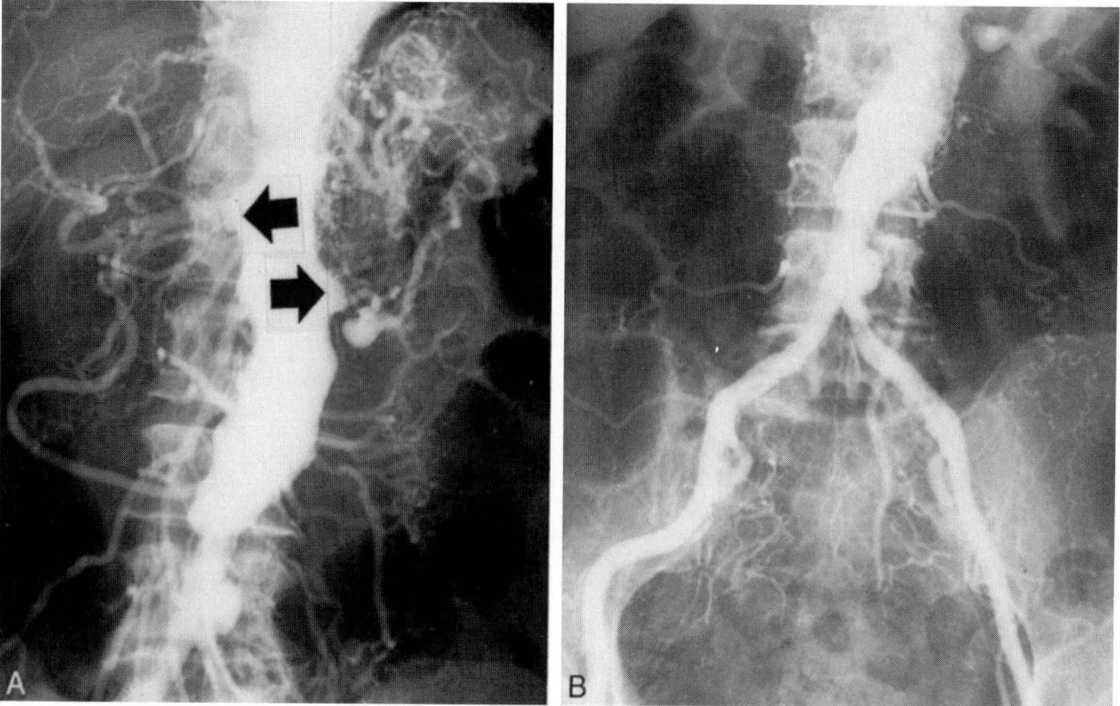

Figure 12–51. *A,* Total right renal artery occlusion *(arrow)*; 95% left renal artery stenosis *(arrow)* with extensive aortic atherosclerosis in an azotemic patient. *B,* External iliac arteries suitable for revascularization. (From Libertino JA, Zinman L: Surgery for renovascular hypertension. *In* Breslin DJ, Swinton NW Jr, Libertino JA, Zinman L, eds: Renovascular Hypertension. Baltimore, Williams & Wilkins Company, 1982, p 202.)

is removed from the inferior portion of the bleb (Fig. 12–56*B*). A right-angle clamp is inserted into this opening, and a 3-cm-long submucosal tunnel is created (Fig. 12–57*A*). At the apex of the tunnel, the right-angle clamp is rotated 180 degrees to pierce the detrusor muscle. The ureter is brought to lie in the submucosal tunnel (Fig. 12–57*B*). The distal ureter is cut at a 45-degree angle, and the ureter is anastomosed to the bladder with interrupted 4–0 or 5–0 chromic catgut or Dexon sutures (Fig. 12–57*C* to *E*).

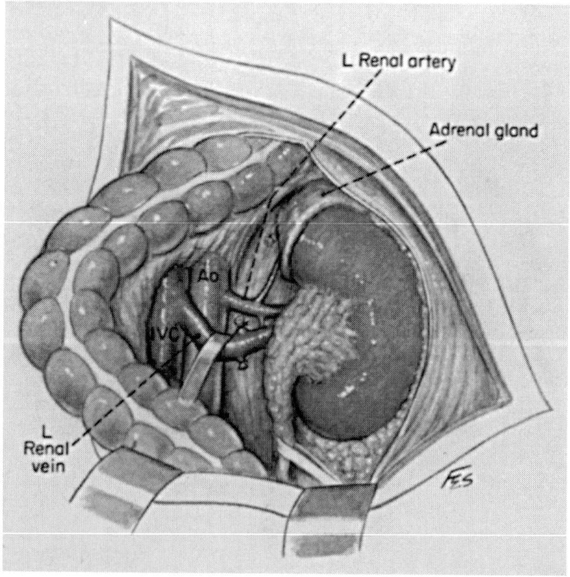

Figure 12–52. Surgical exposure of the left renal artery and left renal vein. Note the mobilization of the left renal vein achieved by ligation of the left adrenal and gonadal veins. (Printed by permission of the Lahey Clinic.)

COMPLICATIONS OF RENAL REVASCULARIZATION

Hemorrhage and thrombosis are the two major problems inherent in any vascular procedure. Serious bleeding from a disrupted anastomosis is fortunately a rare event and is usually associated with approximation of diseased vessels or errors in surgical technique. Prolene sutures, in the renal and aortic anastomosis, have helped to avoid bleeding at the suture line in the presence of systemic heparinization.

Bleeding may occur during the first 24 hours from perihilar collateral vessels, which attain significant size with high-grade renal artery stenosis. Unrecognized venous bleeding can also be encountered from the adrenal vessels during and after a difficult left renal artery dissection because the adrenal gland may be adherent to the anterior portion of the renal vein, renal artery, and perihilar tissue. This has occurred on two occasions in my experience and demands gentle handling of the adrenal gland with compulsive hemostasis during the dissection.

False aneurysms may occur in any vascular anastomosis, including the renal arteries. These occasionally result in intermittent delayed bleeding into the gastrointestinal tract or retroperitoneal space. This complication can be minimized by giving meticulous attention to detail during the anastomosis, by avoiding silk sutures, and by creating a tension-free anastomosis between the graft and a normal undiseased portion of the renal artery.

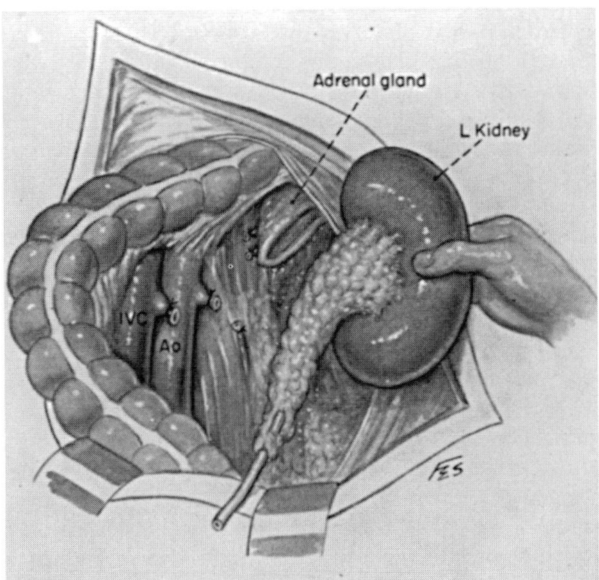

Figure 12–53. Removal of the left kidney when autotransplantation or microvascular workbench surgery is indicated. IVC, inferior vena cava; Ao, aorta. (Printed by permission of the Lahey Clinic.)

Late bleeding has been reported to occur from an aortoduodenal erosion after a prosthetic bypass graft (Cerney et al, 1972). Intestinal hemorrhage is more common with prosthetic replacement when silk has been used for the anastomosis. Delayed bleeding with erosion of the third portion of the duodenum has accounted for most of these instances and could have been prevented with the use of autogenous graft material, synthetic sutures, and interposition of the peritoneum or omentum between the graft and the duodenum.

Renal artery thrombosis is the most prevalent postopera-

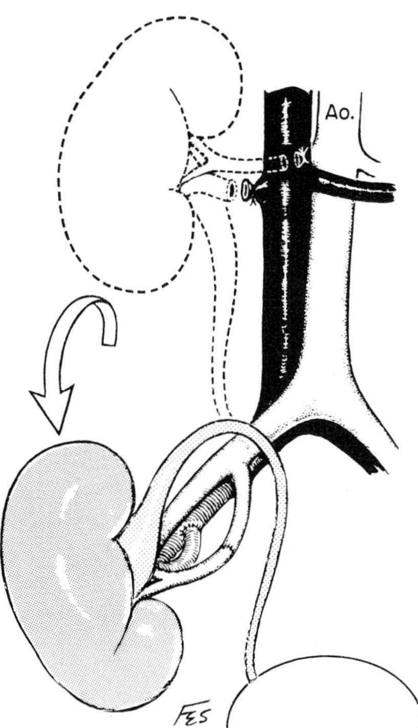

Figure 12–54. Flip-over maneuver for ipsilateral autotransplantation of kidney after workbench surgery with maintenance of ureteral continuity. The renal vessels are turned posteriorly against the recipient vessels, and the pelvis and ureter course unimpeded anteriorly. Ao., aorta. (From Libertino JA, Zinman L: Surgery for renovascular hypertension. *In* Breslin DJ, Swinton NW Jr, Libertino JA, Zinman L, eds: Renovascular Hypertension. Baltimore, Williams & Wilkins Company, 1982, p 203.)

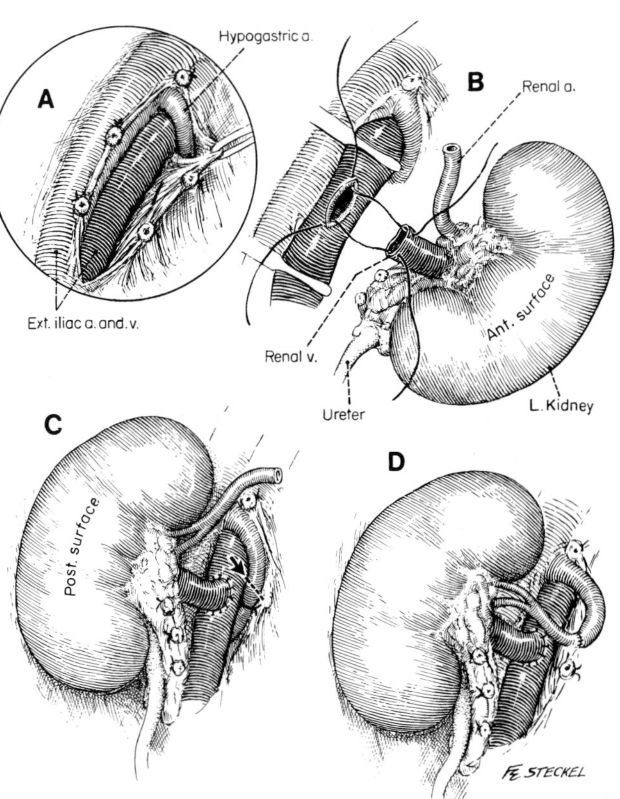

Figure 12–55. *A,* Operative field after exposure of the iliac vessels. *B,* Anastomosis of the renal and external iliac veins. *C,* Preparation of the hypogastric artery for vascular anastomosis. *D,* Appearance of the transplanted kidney after venous and arterial anastomoses are completed. (Printed by permission of the Lahey Clinic.)

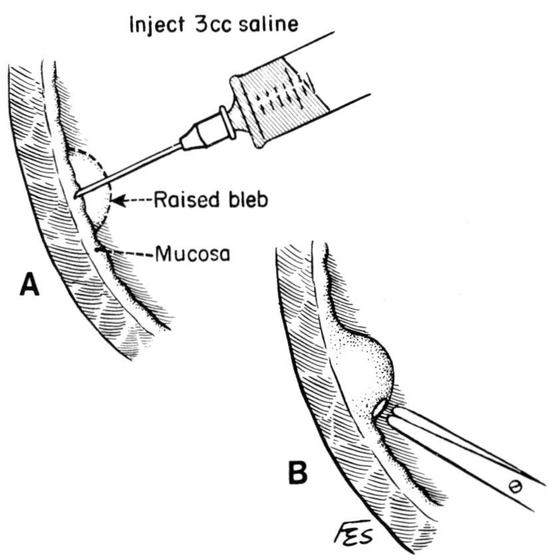

Figure 12–56. *A,* Submucosal injection of saline solution. *B,* Small ellipse of bladder mucosa is excised to permit creation of submucosal tunnel. (Printed by permission of the Lahey Clinic.)

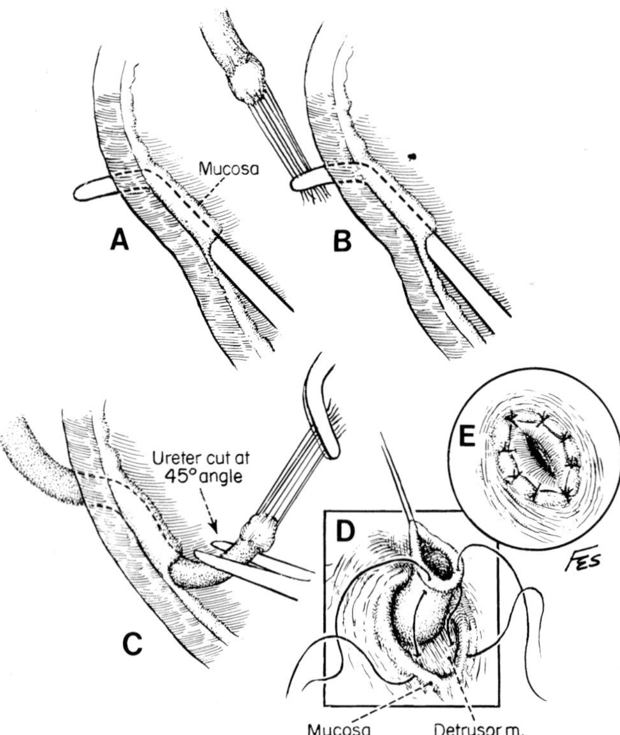

Figure 12–57. *A,* At the apex of the submucosal tunnel the right-angle clamp is turned 180 degrees so as to pierce the detrusor muscle. *B,* The ureter is guided into its new submucosal tunnel. *C,* The distal ureter is cut to a 45-degree angle, creating a new urteral meatus. *D,* The ureter is anastomosed to the bladder detrusor muscle at the 5 and 7 o'clock positions. *E,* Completion of anastomosis of the ureter to the bladder mucosa. (Printed by permission of the Lahey Clinic.)

tive complication. This is more common after renal artery bypass with Dacron prostheses or renal artery endarterectomy. Thrombosis of this type usually occurs early in the postoperative period and may be difficult to detect, especially when an end-to-side anastomosis has been accomplished and when the kidney is being perfused through its native renal artery as well as the bypass graft. Factors that may predispose the patient to the threat of thrombosis are porous Dacron grafts of small caliber, atrophy of the kidneys with a thin-walled diseased main renal artery and high intrarenal resistance, coincidental splenectomy with its associated hypercoagulable sequelae, and any significant hypotension or hypovolemia in the postoperative period. Normal rapid-sequence intravenous pyelography cannot ensure a patent graft. Therefore, when severe unexplained hypertension persists after operation or a serum lactate dehydrogenase level is greater than 1000, digital subtraction angiography is performed to determine graft patency.

Aortic thrombosis and distal extremity embolization from aortic plaque dislodgment and cholesterol microembolization are uncommon but extremely ominous complications that may occur at the time of aortic clamping or unclamping. Systemic heparinization aids in preventing this catastrophe, but the groin and lower extremities should be prepared in the operative field so that the color of the lower legs and distal pulses can be assessed after aortic unclamping.

One should be more acutely aware of the possibility of this complication developing in the patient with a diffusely atherosclerotic aorta and a compromised iliac and femoral circulation. When this event is suspected, iliac thrombectomy and femoral artery embolectomy should be performed, followed by carefully monitored systemic heparinization. When cholesterol microemboli shower, papaverine, systemic heparinization, and fasciotomy may be of help. When vessels, such as digital arteries, are involved, amputation may be required.

Aneurysmal dilation of the autogenous saphenous vein graft and internal iliac artery bypass graft has been shown to occur on late angiographic follow-up studies. Most of these studies demonstrate a uniform increase in the diameter throughout the length of the graft, with a few frank aneurysms noted. We have seen several referred patients with vein graft dilation. When these patients were re-evaluated with posteroanterior and oblique angiography, narrowing at the distal renal artery anastomosis was seen. It is possible that stenosis of the renal artery suture line caused aneursymal dilation of the graft proximal to the stenosis because of the aortic high-pressure inflow. I can find no reports of an instance of rupture of a dilated vein graft, and most patients have remained normotensive with good renal function. Autologous hypogastric artery appears to be superior in this respect, with less dilation seen on long-term follow-up studies.

Despite a patent successful renal artery revascularization, persistent hypertension and hypertensive crisis may occur in the early postoperative period. Hypertension can develop from fluid overload during operation, vasoconstriction from postoperative total body hypothermia, and excessive, poorly controlled incisional pain. When these conditions have been ruled out or when no response to appropriate therapy takes place, control can usually be obtained by intravenous antihypertensive medications or nitroprusside. Patients may remain moderately hypertensive for weeks or even months after successful renal revascularization and should be treated with appropriate antihypertensive medication that can be withdrawn gradually over an appropriate period of time. In fact, 50% of the patients who are ultimately classified as cured, with successful restoration of blood flow to the kidney, have been discharged from the hospital requiring some antihypertensive medication. An early dramatic drop in blood pressure is not always a sequela to successful revascularization, and the blood pressure may take 3 to 4 months to return to normal levels. In contrast, if a patient has unexplained hypertension early in the postoperative period, digital subtraction angiography is performed to rule out graft stenosis or occlusion.

Injury to adjacent organs, such as the spleen and pancreas, can occur even in the hands of the finest surgeon despite meticulous surgical technique, as these organs are friable and delicate. Occasionally splenectomy, splenorrhaphy, and pancreatic repair are required. In these instances intraoperative general surgical consultation may be indicated if the lesions are recognized at the time of surgery.

SURGICAL RESULTS

During the past 25 years, I have treated more than 500 patients with renovascular hypertension using the various surgical techniques described in this chapter. The initial 225 patients had the following clinical characteristics: diastolic hypertension greater than 110 mm Hg while receiving triple-drug therapy (70%), significant preoperative cardiac disease

Table 12–1. CHARACTERISTICS OF PATIENT POPULATIONS I AND II

	Population I (%)*	Population II (%)†
Diastolic hypertension >110 mm Hg while taking multiple drugs	70	55.3
Cardiac disease	20	60.2
Cerebrovascular disease	15	31.7
Azotemia—creatinine level >1.5 mg/dl	20	30.1

*Data from Libertino JA, Zinman L: Surgery for renovascular hypertension. *In* Breslin DJ, Swinton NW Jr, Libertino JA, Zinman L, eds: Renovascular Hypertension. Baltimore, Williams & Wilkins Company, 1982, p 211.

†Data from Libertino JA, Flam TA, Zinman LN, et al: Arch Intern Med 1988; 148:357–359.

(20%), significant preoperative cerebrovascular disease (15%), and azotemia (20%) (Table 12–1). In view of the nature of this high-risk patient population, the mortality rate of 2.1% was acceptable. This result compares favorably with the overall operative mortality rate of 8% reported by the National Cooperative Study Group (Foster et al, 1975). The blood pressure response at 1 year demonstrated either cure or improvement in 97% of the patients; only 3% failed to demonstrate any beneficial response in blood pressure as a result of the operation (Table 12–2). This result also compares favorably with the results reported by the National Cooperative Study Group, with a 66% cure and improvement rate and a 34% failure rate (Foster et al, 1975).

Because we are currently being referred more elderly patients with atherosclerotic disease and fewer young patients with mural disease whose lesions are amenable to balloon angioplasty, our patient profile has changed dramatically. In a later series of 123 patients undergoing 152 surgical procedures (Libertino et al, 1988), the following clinical characteristics were noted: uncontrollable hypertension (55.3%), cardiac disease (60.2%), cerebrovascular disease (31.7%), and azotemia (30.1%) (see Table 12–1). In this second group of higher-risk patients, the cure rate was reduced to 43.5%; the improvement rate increased to 51.5% and the failure rate (no beneficial blood pressure response) to 5% (see Table 12–2). The major reason for the decline in the cure rate with a concomitant increase in the improvement rate is because many of the patients had significant bilateral

Table 12–2. BLOOD PRESSURE RESPONSE TO SURGERY*

	Patient Population I§			Patient Population II		
	Cured† (%)	*Improved† (%)*	*Failure‡ (%)*	*Cured (%)*	*Improved (%)*	*Failure (%)*
Atherosclerosis	66	30	4	43.5	51.5	5
Mural dysplasia	86	14	0	—	—	—
Miscellaneous (arteriovenous malformations and trauma)	77	23	0	—	—	—
Total	72	25	3	43.5	51.5	5

*225 consecutive patients in patient population I and 123 patients (152 procedures) in patient population II.

†Cured and improved: 97%.

‡Failure: 3%.

§Data from Libertino JA, Zinman L: Surgery for renovascular hypertension. *In* Breslin DJ, Swinton NW Jr, Libertino JA, Zinman L, eds: Renovascular Hypertension. Baltimore, Williams & Wilkins Company, 1982, p 211.

Table 12–3. RENAL REVASCULARIZATION FOR PRESERVATION OF RENAL FUNCTION

	Serum Creatinine Level (mg/dl)				
Outcome	*<1.7*	*1.7–2.5*	*2.6–4.0*	*>4.0*	**Total**
Improved	NA	15	19	6	40
Stabilized	16	6	9	0	30
Failed	2	6	2	2	12
Success rate	88% (16/18)	78% (21/27)	93% (27/29)	75% (6/8)	85% (70/82)

NA, not applicable.

disease and underwent only unilateral reconstruction for azotemia and renal preservation.

We have also analyzed another interesting subset of 105 patients who had undergone renal revascularization for preservation of renal function. After a mean follow-up time of 2.2 years, a successful outcome was obtained in 85% of the patients, with stabilization or improvement of renal function (Libertino et al, 1992). The rate of graft occlusion in this group was 6.5%, and the operative mortality rate, 5.7%. Renal revascularization was a successful method for preservation of renal function with acceptable morbidity and mortality in this high-risk patient population, but the preoperative serum creatinine level was not a predictor of surgical outcome (Table 12–3). The results of intraoperative biopsy are more predictive of a successful outcome than serum creatinine levels are. Revascularization with visceral artery bypass procedures was beneficial in reducing the morbidity and mortality in these high-risk patients who had diffuse abdominal aortic atherosclerosis.

The differences in the patient population referred to us have mandated changes in the surgical procedures used and have altered the results that can be expected. Blood pressure response is no longer the sole criterion for the success or failure of renal revascularization. Preservation of renal function must also be taken into account when the surgical results of renal revascularization are analyzed. The concept of ischemic nephropathy and of renal revascularization for preservation of renal function and renal salvage, which we introduced in the early 1970s, has withstood the test of time and has been validated by our surgical experience and that of others (Zinman and Libertino, 1973 and 1977). The predictive criteria to determine whether a kidney is salvageable have also been unaltered by time and subsequent experience (Libertino et al, 1980).

Proper patient selection, performance of an operation individualized to the needs of the patient and the disease, and meticulous surgical technique with adherence to the maneuvers outlined in this chapter are important in achieving a satisfactory result in the treatment of renovascular hypertension.

NEW HORIZONS FOR PERCUTANEOUS RENAL REVASCULARIZATION

Percutaneous transluminal renal angioplasty (PTRA) has emerged as an alternative to surgical renal revascularization and is now in fact the treatment of choice for the initial

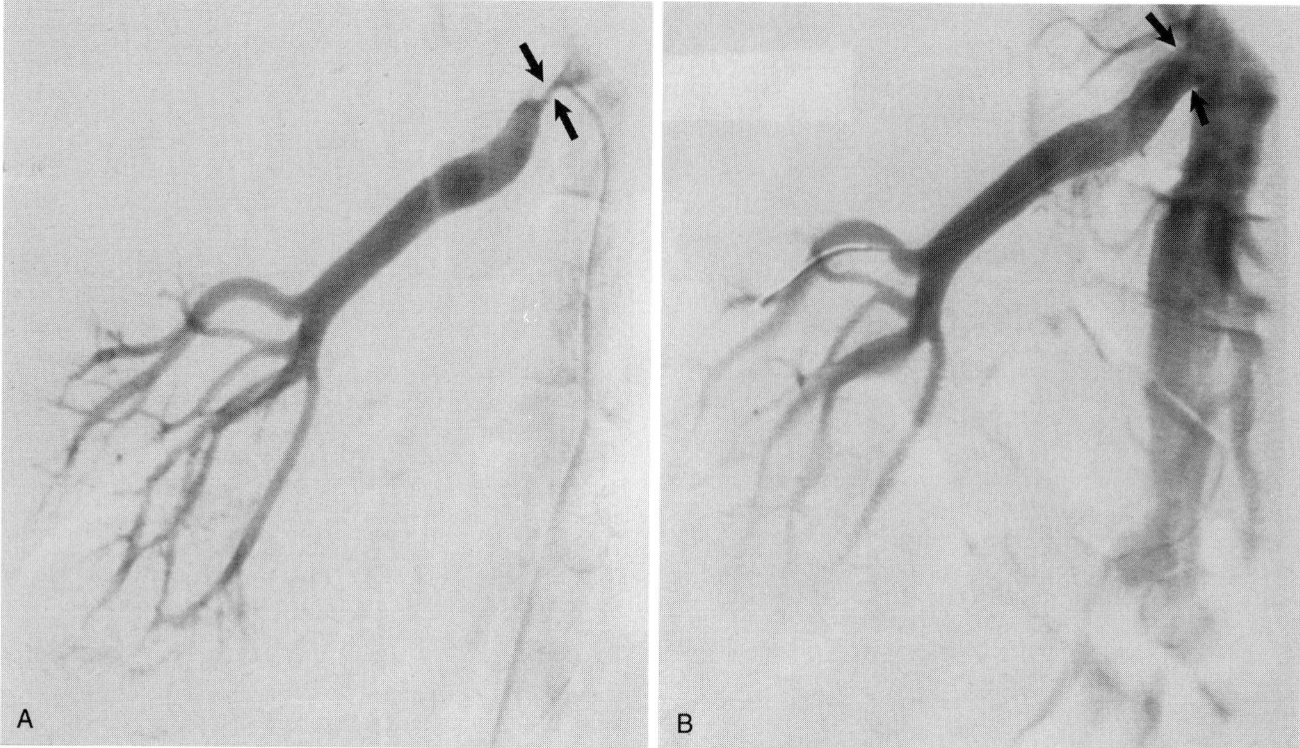

Figure 12–58. *A,* Tight ostial, atherosclerotic right renal artery stenosis before percutaneous transluminal renal angioplasty (PTRA) and stent placement. *B,* After PTRA and stent placement.

management of patients with mural dysplasia. Studies evaluating PTRA for atherosclerotic renovascular disease have reported disparate technical and functional outcomes. For patients with nonostial renal artery stenosis, restenosis occurs in 25% to 60% of patients with variable intervals. In patients with ostial disease, restenosis occurs in 40% to 70% of patients, although few angiographic follow-up data are available. In patients with azotemia, improvement ranges from 30% to 58% (Graor, 1994). The optimal method of renal artery dilation may be debulking of the atheroma and perhaps placing metal stents in the renal artery to prevent elastic recoil and provide the largest lumen possible after PTRA.

Percutaneous Renal Atherectomy

A directional atherectomy device developed by John Simpson has proved to be effective for debulking peripheral and coronary artery stenosis (Simpson et al, 1988). Despite adequate debulking, in our limited experience, restenosis occurred in those patients at 6 months. I believe that the high restenosis rates, approximately 80%, after atherectomy and PTRA for ostial lesions preclude these methods from being considered as viable alternatives to surgical revascularization.

Stenting for Atherosclerosis of the Renal Artery

A great deal of interest has recently emerged in using percutaneously placed metallic expandable stents in the treatment of atherosclerotic ostial renal artery stenosis.

In the largest published series to date using Palmaz stents for ostial and nonostial atheromatous and fibrous lesions in a mixed patient population, 27 of 28 patients were successfully stented. Blood pressure improved in 15 patients and failed to improve in 10 patients. Renal function in 14 azotemic patients improved in 5, stabilized in 5, and deteriorated in 4 patients. Six-month angiography was completed in 18 of 27 patients (39%); 7 of these 18 patients had restenosis (Rees et al, 1991).

Restenosis after stent placement is probably caused by neointimal hyperplasia through the stent struts. Graor (1994) has followed 45 patients with 47 stents in the ostial position. Six-month follow-up renal angiography demonstrated 88% patency. Restenosis occurs, but rates are not reported in this communication (Graor, 1994). Our early results in 20 patients appear to be encouraging in that we too have achieved good patency rates (Fig. 12–58), but our experience is not long enough in duration to know the 6-, 12-, and 18-month restenosis rates.

Angioplasty and stent placement warrant careful investigation and the accumulation of data with special attention to early and late restenosis rates (6 to 48 months). Randomized trials are needed to evaluate the results of this exciting new technique to determine whether this technique is superior to PTRA alone or surgical revascularization.

The future of renal revascularization is in a state of evolution. Developments and the results of randomized trials in the next 5 years will determine the respective roles of percutaneous renal revascularization versus surgical revascularization in the patient with ostial atherosclerotic renal artery stenosis.

REFERENCES

Bromberg WD, Firlit CF: Fibrinolytic therapy for renal vein thrombosis in the child. J Urol 1990; 143:86–88.

Cerney JC, Fry WJ, Gambee J, Koyangyi T: Aortoduodenal fistula. J Urol 1972; 107:12–14.

Chibaro EA, Libertino JA, Novick AC: Use of the hepatic circulation for renal revascularization. Ann Surg 1984; 199:406–411.

Collins HA, Jacobs JK: Acute arterial injuries due to blunt trauma. J Bone Joint Surg 1961; 43(A):193–197.

Dong ZJ, Li SH, Lu XC: Percutaneous transluminal angioplasty for renovascular hypertension in arteritis: Experience in China. Radiology 1987; 162:477–479.

Dos Santos JC: Note sur la désobstruction des anciennes thromboses artérielles. Presse Med 1949; 57:544–545.

Foster JH, Maxwell MH, Franklin SS, et al: Renovascular occlusive disease: Results of operative treatment. JAMA 1975; 231:1043–1048.

Grad E, Rance CP: Bilateral renal artery stenosis in association with neurofibromatosis (Recklinghausen's disease): Report of two cases. J Pediatr 1972; 80:804–808.

Graor RA: New techniques for percutaneous renal revascularization: Atherectomy and stenting. Urol Clin North Am 1994; 21:245–253.

Hageman JH, Smith RF, Szilagyi E, Elliott JP: Aneurysms of the renal artery: Problems of prognosis and surgical management. Surgery 1978; 84:563–572.

Hardy JD: High ureteral injuries: Management by autotransplantation of the kidney. JAMA 1963; 184:97–101.

Harrison LH Jr, Flye MW, Seigler HF: Incidence of anatomic variants in renal vasculature in the presence of normal renal function. Ann Surg 1978; 188:83–89.

Hollenberg NK: Medical therapy for renovascular hypertension: A review. Am J Hypertens 1988; 1(4; pt 2):338S–343S.

Ishikawa K: Natural history and classification of occlusive thromboaortopathy (Takayasu's disease). Circulation 1978; 57:27–35.

Javid H, Ostermiller WE, Hengesh JW, et al: Carotid endarterectomy for asymptomatic patients. Arch Surg 1971; 102:389–391.

Kaufman JJ: Renal vascular disorders. *In* Glenn JF, ed: Urologic Surgery, 2nd ed. Hagerstown, Md, Harper & Row, 1975, pp 874–918.

Kincaid OW, Davis GD, eds: Renal Angiography. Chicago, Year Book Medical, 1966.

Libertino JA, Beckmann CF: Surgery and percutaneous angioplasty in the management of renovascular hypertension. Urol Clin North Am 1994; 21:235–243.

Libertino JA, Bosco PJ, Ying CY, et al: Renal revascularization to preserve and restore renal function. J Urol 1992; 147:1485–1487.

Libertino JA, Flam TA, Zinman LN, et al: Changing concepts in surgical management of renovascular hypertension. Arch Intern Med 1988; 148:357–359.

Libertino JA, Lagneau P: A new method of revascularization of the right renal artery by the gastroduodenal artery. Surg Gynecol Obstet 1983; 156:221–223.

Libertino JA, Selman FJ Jr: Alternatives to aortorenal revascularization. J Cardiovasc Surg (Torino) 1982; 23:318–322.

Libertino JA, Zinman L: Renal revascularization using aortorenal saphenous vein bypass grafting. Surg Clin North Am 1980; 60:487–501.

Libertino JA, Zinman L: Surgery for renovascular hypertension. *In* Libertino JA, ed: Pediatric and Adult Reconstructive Urologic Surgery, 2nd ed. Baltimore, Williams & Wilkins Company, 1987, pp 119–161.

Libertino JA, Zinman L, Breslin DJ, Swinton NW Jr: Hepatorenal artery bypass in the management of renovascular hypertension. J Urol 1976; 115:369–372.

Libertino JA, Zinman L, Breslin DJ, et al: Renal artery revascularization: Restoration of renal function. JAMA 1980; 244:1340–1342.

Llach F, Papper S, Massry SG: The clinical spectrum of renal vein thrombosis: Acute and chronic. Am J Med 1980; 69:819–827.

Millan VG, Sher MH, Deterling RA Jr, et al: Transcatheter thromboembolectomy of acute renal artery occlusion. Arch Surg 1978; 113:1086–1092.

Moncure AC, Brewster DC, Darling RC, et al: Use of the splenic and hepatic arteries for renal revascularization. J Vasc Surg 1986; 3:196–203.

Moncure AC, Brewster DC, Darling RC, et al: Use of the gastroduodenal artery in right renal artery revascularization. J Vasc Surg 1988; 8:154–159.

Nicholas GG, DeMuth WE Jr: Treatment of renal artery embolism. Arch Surg 1984; 119:278–281.

Ota K, Mori S, Awane Y, et al: Ex situ repair of renal artery for renovascular hypertension. Arch Surg 1967; 94:370–373.

Rees CR, Palmaz JC, Becker GJ, et al: Stent in atherosclerotic stenosis involving the ostia of the renal arteries: Preliminary report of a multicenter study. Radiology 1991; 181:505–514.

Simpson JB, Selmon MR, Robertson GC, et al: Transluminal atherectomy for occlusive peripheral vascular diseases. Am J Cardiol 1988; 61:965–1016.

Sos TA, Pickering TG, Saddekni S, et al: The current role of renal angioplasty in the treatment of renovascular hypertension. Urol Clin North Am 1984; 11:503–513.

Sos TA, Pickering TG, Sniderman K, et al: Percutaneous transluminal renal angioplasty in renovascular hypertension due to atheroma or fibromuscular dysplasia. N Engl J Med 1983; 309:274–279.

Sosa RE, Vaughan ED Jr: Renovascular hypertension. *In* Gillenwater J: Adult and Pediatric Urology, vol 1. Chicago, Year Book Medical, 1987, pp 752–776.

Spirnak JP, Resnick MI: Revascularization of traumatic thrombosis of the renal artery. Surg Gynecol Obstet 1987; 164:22–26.

Stanley JC, Rhodes EL, Gewertz BL, et al: Renal artery aneurysms: Significance of macroaneurysms exclusive of dissections and fibrodysplastic mural dilations. Arch Surg 1975; 110:1327–1333.

Tegtmeyer CJ, Kofler TJ, Ayers CA: Renal angioplasty: Current status. Am J Roentgenol 1984; 142:17–21.

Wilcox CS, Williams CM, Smith TB, et al: Diagnostic uses of angiotensin-converting enzyme inhibitors in renovascular hypertension. Am J Hypertens 1988; 1(4; pt 2):344S–349S.

Zinman L, Libertino JA: Revascularization of the totally occluded renal artery. (Abstract.) Circulation 1973; 48(suppl 4):31.

Zinman L, Libertino JA: Revascularization of the chronic totally occluded renal artery with restoration of renal function. J Urol 1977; 118:517–521.

13 TRANSPLANTATION IMMUNOBIOLOGY

Manikkam Suthanthiran, M.D.
Randall E. Morris, M.D.
Terry B. Strom, M.D.

Renal transplantation is the preferred treatment for most patients afflicted with end-stage renal failure. Much has been learned regarding immunobiologic mechanisms responsible for the rejection of organ allografts, including renal allografts. There has also been considerable progress in our understanding of mechanisms responsible for tolerance. A better appreciation of the process involved in allograft rejection and the introduction and judicious use of immunosuppressants such as cyclosporine (CsA) have resulted in excellent patient and graft survival rates after renal transplantation. The principles of tolerance mechanisms are yet to be successfully applied in the clinic. In this chapter, immunobiologic and immunopharmacologic considerations of renal transplantation are reviewed.

IMMUNOBIOLOGY OF THE ANTIALLOGRAFT RESPONSE

Antiallograft response is contingent upon the coordinated activation of alloreactive T cells and antigen-presenting cells (APCs). Through the release of cytokines and cell-to-cell interactions, a diverse assembly of lymphocytes, including CD4+ T cells, CD8+ cytotoxic T cells, antibody-forming B cells, and other proinflammatory leukocytes, are recruited into the antiallograft response (Suthanthiran and Strom, 1994) (Fig. 13–1 and Table 13–1).

T Cell Stimulation

T cell activation, a highly regulated and preprogrammed process, begins when T cells recognize intracellularly processed fragments of foreign proteins (approximately eight amino acids) embedded within the groove of the major histocompatibility complex proteins (MHCs) expressed on the surface of APCs (Unanue and Cerottoni, 1989; Germain, 1994). **Some of the T cells of the recipient directly recognize the allograft—that is, donor antigen(s) presented on**

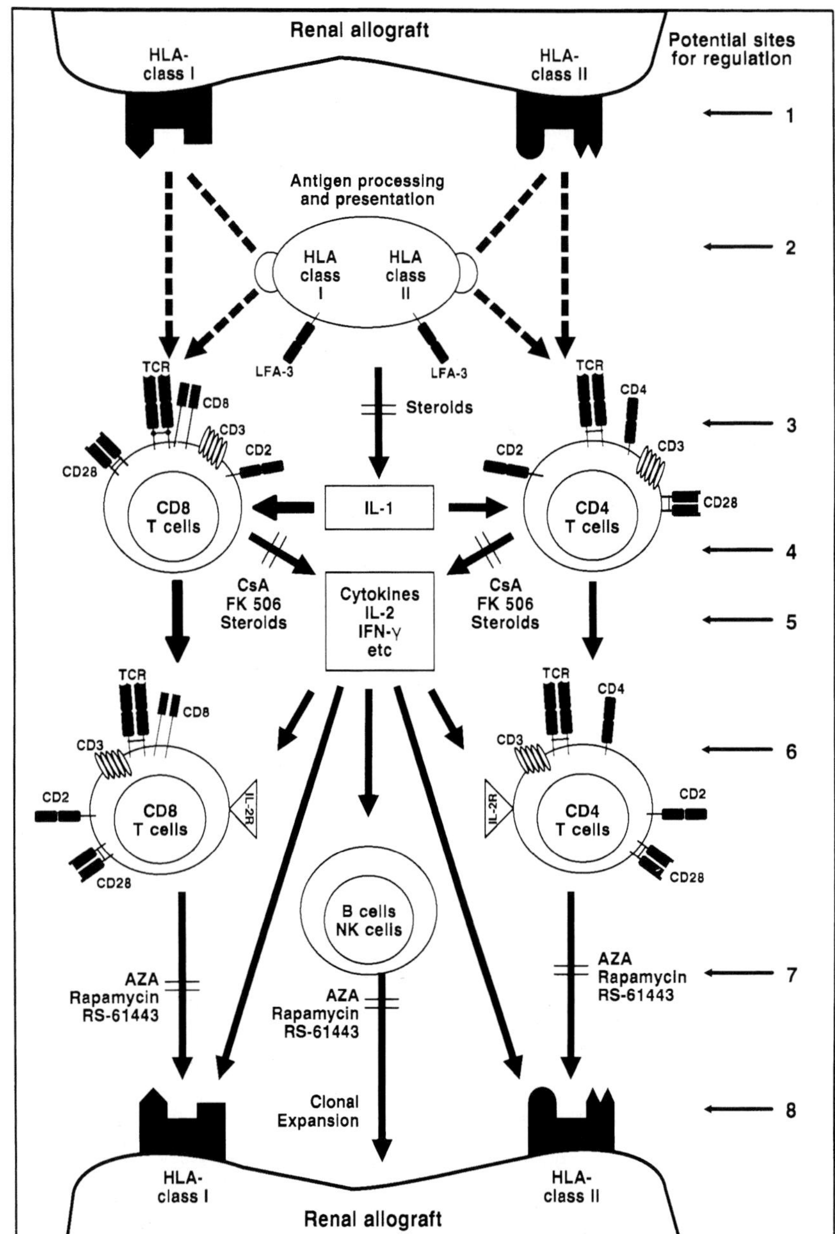

Figure 13–1. The anti-allograft response. Human leukocyte antigen (HLA), the primary stimulus for the initiation of the antiallograft response, cell surface proteins participating in antigenic recognition and signal transduction, and the contribution of the cytokines and multiple cell types to the immune response are all schematically illustrated. The potential sites for the fine regulation of the antiallograft response are also shown. Site 1: minimizing histoincompatibility between the recipients and the donor by HLA matching; site 2: prevention of cytokine production by antigen-presenting cells (APCs) with the corticosteroids; site 3: blockade of antigen recognition (e.g., OKT3 mAbs); site 4: inhibition of T cell cytokine production (CsA, FK506, and steroids); site 5: inhibition of cytokine activity (e.g., anti–interleukin-2 antibody, rapamycin, leflunomide); site 6: inhibition of cell cycle progression (e.g., anti–interleukin-2 receptor antibody); site 7: inhibition of clonal expansion (e.g., azathioprine, mycophenolate mofetil [RS61443], rapamycin, leflunomide); site 8: prevention of allograft damage by masking target antigen molecules (e.g., antibodies directed at adhesion molecules). HLA-class I, HLA-A, -B, and -C antigens; HLA-class II, HLA-DR, -DQ, and -DP antigens; CsA, cyclosporin A; AZA, azathioprine; IL-2, interleukin-2; IFN-γ, interferon-γ; NK cells; natural killer cells; RS61443, mycophenolate mofetil; FK506, tacrolimus; rapamycin: sirolimus. (From Strom TB, Suthanthiran M: Mechanisms of graft rejection. *In* Sayegh MH, Turka LA, eds: ASTP Lectures in Transplantation. Philadelphia, CoMed Communications, Inc, 1996.)

Table 13–1. CELLULAR ELEMENTS CONTRIBUTING TO THE ANTIALLOGRAFT RESPONSE

Cell Type	Functional Attributes
T cells	The CD4+ T cells and the CD8+ T cells participate in the antiallograft response. CD4+ T cells recognize antigens presented by HLA class II proteins, and CD8+ T cells recognize antigens presented by HLA class I proteins. The CD3/TCR complex is responsible for recognition of antigen and generates and transduces the antigenic signal.
CD4+ T cells	CD4+ T cells function mostly as helper T cells and secrete cytokines such as IL-2, a T cell growth factor, and IFN-γ, a proinflammatory polypeptide that can up-regulate the expression of HLA-proteins as well as augment cytotoxic activity of T cells and NK cells. Two main types of CD4+ T cells have been recognized: CD4+ TH1 and CD4+ TH2. IL-2 and IFN-γ are produced by CD4+ TH1 cells, and IL-10 and IL-4 are secreted by CD4+ TH2 cells. Each cell type regulates the secretion of the other, and the regulated secretion is important in the expression of host immunity.
CD8+ T cells	CD8+ T cells function mainly as cytotoxic T cells. A subset of CD8+ T cells expresses suppressor cell function. CD8+ T cells can secrete cytokines such as IL-2 and IFN-γ and can express molecular mediators of cytotoxicity, such as perforin and granzymes.
APC	Monocytes/macrophages and dendritic cells function as potent antigen-presenting cells (APCs). Donor's APCs might process and present donor antigens to recipient's T cells (direct recognition) or recipient's APCs might process and present donor antigens to recipient's T cells (indirect recognition). The relative contribution of direct recognition and indirect recognition to the antiallograft response has not been defined. Direct recognition and indirect recognition might have differential susceptibility to inhibition by immunosuppressive drugs.
B cells	B cells require T cell help for the differentiation and production of antibodies directed at donor antigens. The alloantibodies can damage the graft by binding and activating complement components (complement-dependent cytotoxicity) and/or by binding the Fc receptor of cells capable of mediating cytotoxicty (antibody-dependent cell-mediated cyctoxicity).
NK cells	The precise role of NK cells in the antiallograft response is not known. Increased NK cell activity has been correlated with rejection. NK cell function might also be important in immune surveillance mechanisms pertinent to the prevention of infection and malignancy.

HLA, human leukocyte antigen; TCR, T cell antigen receptor; IFN, interferon; NK, natural killer; Fc, crystallizable fragment.

the surface of donor APCs (direct recognition)—whereas other T cells recognize the donor antigen after it is processed and presented by the self APCs (indirect recognition) (Weiss and Littman, 1994).

TCR/CD3 Complex

The T cell antigen receptor (TCR)/CD3 complex is composed of (1) clonally variant TCR alpha-beta peptide chains that recognize the antigenic peptide in the context of MHC proteins and (2) clonally invariant CD3 chains (gamma, delta, epsilon, and zeta) that initiate intracellular signals originating from antigenic recognition (Clevers et al, 1988; Shoskes and Wood, 1994). The TCR variable, diversity, and junctional and constant region genes (i.e., genes for regions of the clone-specific antigen receptors) are spliced together in a cassette-like manner during T cell maturation. A small population of T cells express TCR gamma-delta chains instead of the TCR alpha-beta chains.

CD4 and CD8 Proteins

CD4 and CD8 proteins, expressed upon reciprocal population of peripheral blood T cell subsets, bind to the monomorphic component of human leukocyte antigen (HLA) class II and class I molecules, respectively (Miceli and Parnes, 1991) (see Fig. 13–1). Antigenic recognition stimulates a redistribution of cell surface proteins and coclustering of the TCR/CD3 complex with the CD4 or CD8 antigens (Miceli and Parnes, 1991). This multimeric complex includes additional signaling molecules, CD2 proteins (Suthanthiran, 1990; Brown et al, 1989), and CD5 proteins (Beyers et al, 1992) and functions as a unit in initiating T cell activation.

Signal Transduction Mechanisms

The TCR/CD3 complex and the CD4 and CD8 proteins, upon stimulation with antigens, physically associate with and activate intracellular protein-tyrosine kinases (Weiss and Littman, 1994; Klausner and Samelson, 1991). **Tyrosine phosphorylation of phospholipase Cγ_1 activates this coenzyme and initiates hydrolysis of phosphatidylinositol 4,5-biphosphate (PIP_2) and generation of inositol 1,4,5-triphosphate (IP_3) and diacylglycerol.** IP_3, in turn, mobilizes ionized calcium from bound intracellular stores, whereas diacylglycerol, in the presence of increased cytosolic free Ca^{2+}, binds to and activates protein kinase C (PKC)—a phospholipid/Ca^{2+}-sensitive protein serine/threonine kinase (Nishizuka, 1992). Sustained activation of PKC is dependent on diacylglycerol generated from hydrolysis of additional lipids such as phosphatidylcholine (Nishizuka, 1992).

The increase in intracellular free Ca^{2+} concentration and the sustained PKC activation function synergistically in promoting the expression of several nuclear regulatory proteins and in the transcriptional activation and expression of genes central to T cell growth.

Calcineurin, a Ca^{2+}- and calmodulin-dependent serine/threonine phosphatase (protein phosphatase 2B) has been shown to participate in signal transduction. Inhibition by CsA and FK506 of the phosphatase activity of calcineurin is considered central to their immunosuppressive activity (O'Keefe et al, 1992; Clipstone and Crabtree, 1992; Liu et al, 1991; Fruman et al, 1992).

Costimulatory Signals

Table 13–2 lists cell surface proteins implicated in T cell signaling. The functional consequences of the physical interactions between the T cell surface proteins and their

Table 13–2. CELL SURFACE PROTEINS IMPORTANT FOR T CELL ACTIVATION

T Cell Surface	APC Surface	Consequence of Blockade
Functional Response: Adhesion		
LFA-1	ICAM-1	Immunosuppression
ICAM-1	LFA-1	Immunosuppression
VLA-4	VCAM-1	Immunosuppression
Functional Response: Antigen Recognition		
CD8, TCR, CD3	MHC-I	Immunosuppression
CD4, TCR, CD3	MHC-II	Immunosuppression
Functional Response: Costimulation		
CD2	LFA-3	Immunosuppression
CD40L	CD40	Immunosuppression
CD5	CD72	Immunosuppression
CD28	B7-1	Anergy
CD28	B7-2	Anergy
Functional Response: Inhibition		
CTLA-4	B7-1	Immunostimulation
CTLA-4	B7-2	Immunostimulation

Pairs of receptors and counter-receptors that mediate interactions between T cells and antigen-presenting cells (APCs) are shown. Inhibition of each protein-to-protein interaction, except the CTLA-4–B7-1, B7-2 interactions, results in an abortive in vitro immune response. Initial contact between T cells and APCs requires an antigen-independent adhesive interaction. Next, the T cell antigen receptor complex engages processed antigen presented within the antigen-presenting groove of major histocompatibility complex (MHC) molecules. Finally, costimulatory signals are required for full T cell activation. An especially important signal is generated by B7-mediated activation of CD28 on T cells. Activation of CD28 by B7-2 may provide a more potent signal than activation by B7-1. CTLA-4, present on activated but not resting T cells, imparts a negative signal.

counter-receptors on APCs, and the consequences of blocking these informative interactions, are also shown in Table 13–2.

Stimulation of T cells via the CD3/TCR complex alone, in the absence of costimulatory signals, induces T cell anergy/paralysis (Schwartz, 1993); T cell activation, as measured by interleukin (IL)–2 production and proliferation in vitro, requires both antigenic and costimulatory signals engendered by cell-to-cell interactions among antigen-specific T cells and APCs (Schwartz, 1993; Suthanthiran, 1993). Interaction of CD2 proteins on the T cell surface with CD58 (LFA-3) proteins on APCs (Suthanthiran, 1993), CD5 proteins with CD72 proteins (Beyers et al, 1992), and CD11a/CD18 (LFA-1) proteins with CD54 (ICAM-1) proteins (Dustin and Springer, 1989) can impart such an activating costimulatory signal.

Delivery of both antigenic and costimulatory signals leads to stable transcription of the IL-2 and other pivotal T cell activation genes (Schwartz, 1993; Suthanthiran, 1993). The foregoing costimulatory signals are PKC-dependent, Ca^{2+}-dependent, and CsA/FK506-sensitive (O'Keefe et al, 1992; Clipstone and Crabtree, 1992; Liu et al, 1991; Fruman et al, 1992).

Potent APCs express CD80 (B7-1) and CD86 (B7-2) surface proteins and many T cells express B7-binding proteins, such as CD28 (June et al, 1990) and CTLA-4 proteins (Linsley et al, 1991). Binding of B7-1/B7-2 by CD28 stimulates a PKC- and Ca^{2+}-independent T cell costimulatory pathway that also leads to stable transcription of the IL-2 and other activation genes, resulting in vigorous T cell proliferation (June et al, 1990). This pathway is relatively resistant to inhibition by CsA/FK506 (Thompson et al, 1989). The interaction of CTLA-4 protein, expressed on activated but not resting cells, with the B7-1/B7-2 proteins, appears to impart a negative signal (Allison and Krummel, 1995).

T cell accessory molecules and their cognate APC surface proteins represent target molecules for antirejection therapy. Indeed, transplantation tolerance has been induced in experimental models by targeting cell surface molecules that transmit costimulatory signals (Isobe et al, 1992; Lenschow et al, 1992).

APC-derived cytokines (e.g., IL-1/IL-6) can also provide costimulatory signals that result in T cell activation in vitro (Williams et al, 1985).

Stimulation of B cells is also dependent on the antigenic signal and the costimulatory signal (Bretcher and Cohen, 1970; Clark and Ledbetter, 1994). The antigenic signal is generated by the interaction between the specific antigen and the cell surface immunoglobulin. T cell–derived cytokines (e.g., IL-2, IL-4) and/or cell-to-cell physical contact between T cells and B cells via specific receptor-coreceptor pairs (e.g., interactions between the CD40 protein and its ligand CD40L) function as costimulatory signals (Clark and Ledbetter, 1994).

IL-2–Stimulated T Cell Proliferation

Autocrine type of T cell proliferation occurs as a consequence of the T cell activation–dependent production of IL-2 and the expression of multimeric high-affinity IL-2 receptors on T cells (Waldmann, 1991; Takeshita et al, 1992). The high-affinity IL-2 receptor complex is formed by the noncovalent association of at least three IL-2 binding peptides (alpha, beta, and gamma chains). The IL-2 receptor alpha chain is expressed only on the surface of activated T cells. Very few T cells constitutively express IL-2 receptor beta chain, and its expression is increased after T cell activation. **The intracytoplasmic domain of the IL-2 beta receptor and gamma chains are required for intracellular signal transduction** (Takeshita et al, 1992; Hatakeyama et al, 1991). **The ligand-activated, but not resting, IL-2 receptors associate with src-like intracellular protein tyrosine kinases** (Fung et al, 1991). Raf-1, a protein serine/threonine kinase, also associates with the IL-2 receptor (Remillard et al, 1991). Activation of phosphatidylinositol-3 kinase and translocation of IL-2 receptor–bound Raf-1 serine/threonine kinase into the cytosol requires IL-2–stimulated protein tyrosine kinase activity (Remillard et al, 1991; Maslinski et al, 1992). The subsequent events leading to IL-2–dependent proliferation are not fully resolved; IL-2-stimulated expression of several DNA-binding proteins, including c-jun, c-fos, and c-myc, contribute to cell cycle progression (Shibuya et al, 1992).

Graft-Destructive Alloreactivity

The net consequence of cytokine production and acquisition of cell surface receptors for these transcellular molecules is the emergence of antigen-specific and graft-destructive T cells (see Fig. 13–1). Cytokines also facilitate the humoral arm of immunity by promoting the production of antibodies that can damage the transplanted organ via one or more complement-dependent and/or antibody-dependent cell-mediated cytotoxicity mechanisms. Moreover, interferon (IFN)–γ and tumor necrosis factor (TNF)–α can amplify the ongoing immune response by up-regulating the expression of HLA molecules as well as costimulatory molecules (e.g., B7) upon graft parenchymal cells and APCs (see Fig. 13–1). **We and others have demonstrated the presence of antigen-specific cytotoxic T lymphocytes (CTL) and anti-HLA antibodies during or before a clinical rejection episode** (Strom et al, 1975; Suthanthiran and Garovoy, 1983). **More recently, we have detected mRNA encoding the CTL-selective serine protease (granzyme B) and IL-2 mRNA and IL-10 mRNA in human renal allografts undergoing acute rejection** (Lipman et al, 1992; Xu et al, 1995).

Granzyme B and perforin are important components of cytolytic machinery of effector T cells and natural killer cells. IL-2 and IL-10 have been demonstrated to increase the cytolytic activity of effector cells. Thus intragraft detection of cytokines capable of promoting cytolytic activity and the presence of molecular mediators of cytotoxicity suggest potential pathways and mechanisms of allograft rejection.

IMMUNOPHARMACOLOGY OF ALLOGRAFT REJECTION

Figure 13–2 illustrates the chemical structure of the new immunosuppressive drugs discussed in this chapter. **On the basis of their primary site of immunoregulatory activity, the immunosuppressants can be classified as inhibitors of transcription (CsA, FK506), inhibitors of growth factor signal transduction (rapamycin, leflunomide), inhibitors of nucleotide synthesis (azathioprine, mycophenolate mofetil, mizoribine, brequinar sodium), and inhibitors of differentiation (15-deoxyspergualin [DSG]).**

Figure 13–3 illustrates, and Table 13–3 describes, the primary site of action of immunosuppressants discussed in this chapter.

CsA and FK506

CsA, a small fungal cyclic peptide, and FK506 (tacrolimus), a macrolide, block T cell activation via similar mechanisms (Schreiber, 1992). **The immunosuppressive effects of CsA and tacrolimus are dependent upon the formation of a heterodimeric complex that consists of the drug (CsA or tacrolimus) and its respective cytoplasmic receptor protein, i.e. cyclophilin and FK-binding protein (FKBP). Both of these complexes bind calcineurin and inhibit its phosphatase activity (O'Keefe, 1992; Clipstone and Crabtree, 1992; Liu et al, 1991; Fruman et al, 1992; Schreiber, 1992), thereby inhibiting, directly or indirectly, de novo expression of nuclear regulatory proteins and T cell activation genes: specifically, those encoding certain cytokines (e.g., IL-2), proto-oncogenes (e.g., H-ras, c-myc), and receptors for cytokines (e.g., IL-2 receptor). The primary mechanism responsible for the immunosup-**

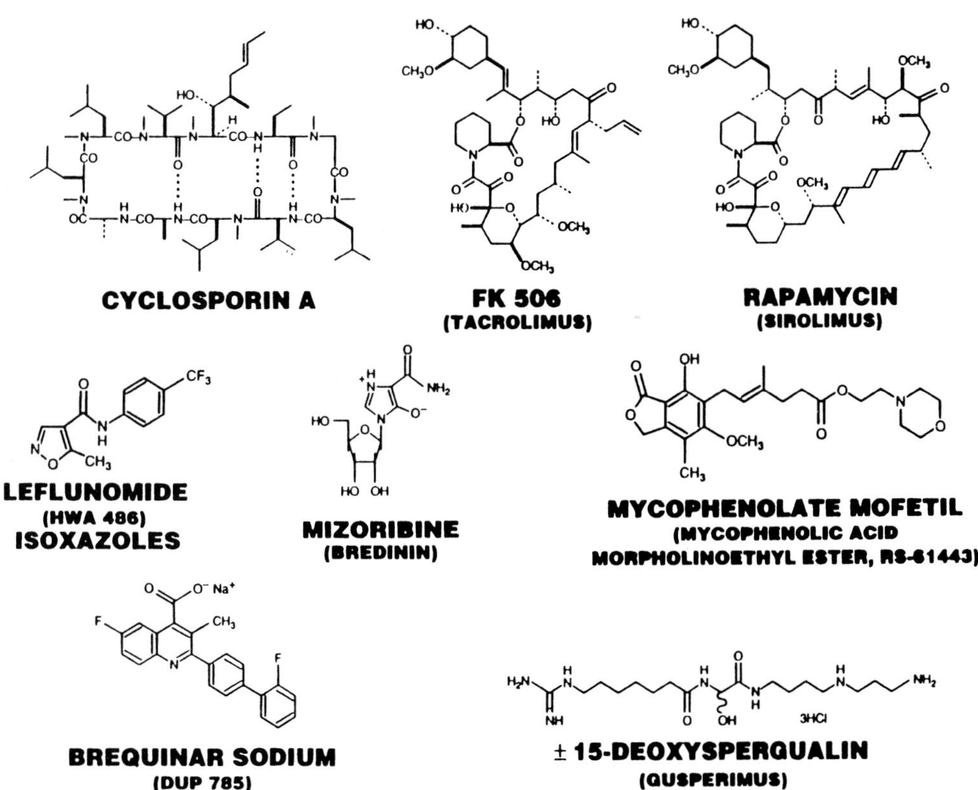

Figure 13–2. The chemical structure of new immunosuppressive drugs.

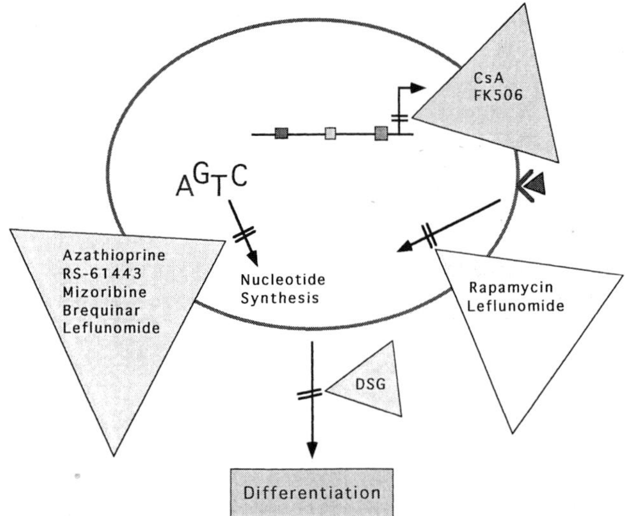

Figure 13–3. Mechanism of action of immunosuppressive drugs. CsA and FK506 inhibit transcription of T cell growth–promoting genes (e.g., interleukin-2); rapamycin and leflunomide block growth factor–initiated signal transduction. Azathioprine, RS61443 (mycophenolate mofetil), and mizoribine inhibit purine biosynthesis, and brequinar and leflunomide inhibit pyrimidine synthesis. DSG (15-deoxyspergualin) is considered an inhibitor of cell differentiation/maturation.

pressive activity of CsA and FK506 is considered to be inhibition of expression of the prototypic T cell growth factor, IL-2.

Corticosteroids

Corticosteroids inhibit T cell proliferation, T cell–dependent immunity, and cytokine gene transcription (including the IL-1, IL-2, IL-6, IFN-γ, and TNF-α genes) (Knudsen et al, 1987; Zanker et al, 1990; Arya et al, 1984). Although no individual cytokine can totally reverse the inhibitory effects of corticosteroids on mitogen-stimulated T cell proliferation, a combination of cytokines is effective in restoring T cell proliferation (Almawi et al, 1991). Inhibition by corticosteroids of cytokine production represents an important rationale for its usage in the control of the antiallograft response.

Some cytokine genes possess a glucocorticosteroid response element in the 5′ regulatory region that serves as a target for the heterodimeric complex formed by the association of corticosteroids with the intracellular glucocorticosteroid receptor protein. Binding of this complex to the glucocorticosteroid response element can, in theory, block gene expression. This mechanism, however, does not fully account for the inhibitory effects of corticosteroids on cytokine gene expression. Blockade of IL-2 gene transcription, for example, involves impairment of the cooperative effect of several DNA-binding proteins (Vacca et al, 1992; Yang-Yee et al, 1990; Palvogianni et al, 1993), although the IL-2 gene does not possess a glucocorticosteroid response element. It has been reported that glucocorticoids can block gene expression through the noncovalent association of the interaction of the activated hormone-receptor complex with the c-jun/c-fos heterodimer (activation protein-1 [AP-1]) (Yang-Yee et al, 1990). The c-jun and c-fos heterodimers bind to an AP-1 site lying within the promoter region of many cytokine genes. In keeping with this observation, glucocorticoids interfere with IL-2 gene expression through prevention of nuclear transcription factors binding to the AP-1 and nuclear factor of activated T cells (NF-AT) sites (Palvogianni et al, 1993).

An additional mechanism for the ability of glucocorticoids to inhibit the transcription of genes that do not contain a glucocorticoid response element has been identified: **Glucocorticoids induce the transcription of IκBα gene; the resultant IκBα protein then binds NF-κB transcription factor and prevents its translocation into the nucleus** (Scheinman et al, 1995; Auphan et al, 1995). Thus genes that are regulated by the DNA-binding protein NF-κB acquire sensitivity to glucocorticoids despite the absence of a cis-acting glucocorticoid response element.

Table 13–3. MECHANISMS OF ACTION OF IMMUNOSUPPRESSANTS

Drug	Subcellular Site(s) of Action
Azathioprine	Inhibits purine synthesis
Brequinar sodium	Inhibits dehydroorotate dehydrogenase and blocks pyrimidine synthesis
Corticosteroids	Block cytokine gene expression
CsA/tacrolimus	Blocks Ca^{2+}-dependent T cell activation pathway via binding to calcineurin
15-Deoxyspergualin (DSG)	Unknown
Leflunomide	Inhibits pyrimidine synthesis; inhibits growth factor receptor-associated tyrosine kinases
Mizoribine	Inhibits purine biosynthesis
Mycophenolate mofetil	Inhibits inosine monophosphate dehydrogenase and prevents de novo guanosine and deoxyguanosine synthesis in lymphocytes
Sirolimus	Blocks interleukin-2 and other growth factor signal transduction; blocks CD28-mediated costimulatory signals

Azathioprine

Azathioprine is the 1-methyl-4-nitro-5-imidzolyl derivative of 6-mercaptopurine (Elion, 1967). **Azathioprine, a purine analogue, functions as a purine antagonist and thereby inhibits cellular proliferation.** Allopurinol blocks the catabolism of azathioprine, causing a dramatic increase in bone marrow suppression. Thus, close monitoring of cell counts and a reduction in the dosage of azathioprine are essential when allopurinol is used in conjunction with azathioprine.

Rapamycin

Rapamycin (sirolimus), a macrocyclic antibiotic produced by *Streptomyces hygroscopicus*, binds to FKBP in a manner similar to that of tacrolimus (Morris, 1992; Sehgal et al, 1995). However, sirolimus and tacrolimus affect different and distinctive sites in the signal transduction pathway. Whereas sirolimus blocks IL-2 and other growth factor–mediated signal transduction (Morris, 1992; Sehgal et al, 1995; Chung et al, 1992), tacrolimus (or CsA) has no such capacity.

Also, the sirolimus-FKBP complex, unlike the tacrolimus-FKBP complex, does not bind calcineurin. **FKBP-12 appears to be a major intracellular receptor for sirolimus.** The cellular receptor or receptors for the sirolimus-FKBP complex are being elucidated. Two proteins, designated as targets of rapamycin (TOR1 and TOR2), each with a relative molecular mass of 282 kD and with 68% homology, were originally identified as receptors for sirolimus (Heitman et al, 1991). Two mammalian proteins, 245 kD and 34 kD, with sequence similarities to yeast TOR1 and TOR2 and homologous to the catalytic domain of p110 subunit of PI-3 kinase, have been identified as putative targets for the drug-immunophilin complex in mammalian cells (Sabatini et al, 1994).

The antiproliferative activity of sirolimus appears to be a consequence partly of the sirolimus-FKBP complex's blocking the activation of the 70-kD S6 protein kinases that are involved in cell proliferation (Morris, 1992; Sehgal et al, 1995; Chung et al, 1992). The kinase activity of additional cell cycle regulatory proteins, cyclin-dependent kinase-2 and -4 (CDK2 and CDK4) is also inhibited by sirolimus. **Sirolimus blocks the Ca^{2+}-independent CD28/B7 costimulatory pathway.** The CD28 pathway participates in the down-regulation of Iκα, a cytosolic protein that prevents nuclear translocation of DNA-binding protein NF-κB, and sirolimus prevents the CD28 costimulatory signal responsible for Iκα down-regulation (Lai and Tan, 1994).

Sirolimus and tacrolimus compete for the occupation of the same cellular receptors; thus they are pharmacologic antagonists in vitro. But in vivo they interact to produce immunosuppression that is additive or synergistic (Morris, 1992). Sirolimus has been shown to prolong the survival of histoincompatible organ allografts in several experimental models of organ transplantation (Morris, 1992; Sehgal et al, 1995). It is also efficacious in disease states characterized by autoimmunity (e.g., insulin-dependent diabetes mellitus, systemic lupus erythematosus) and is capable of constraining not only the proliferation of traditional immune cells (e.g., T cells) but also that of additional cell types such as smooth muscle cells (Gregory et al, 1995). Thus it might be effective in the prevention and/or progression of graft vascular disease (e.g., chronic rejection).

Sirolimus is being evaluated in phase I and phase II clinical trials of organ transplantation (Sehgal et al, 1995). In a preliminary study, supplementation of a CsA-based immunosuppressive regimen with sirolimus was associated with a reduction in the incidence of acute renal allograft rejection. Nephrotoxicity and hypertension have not, thus far, been a serious consideration. Thrombocytopenia and hyperlipidemia appear to respond to a reduction in drug dosage.

Mycophenolate Mofetil

Mycophenolate mofetil (RS-61443), the semisynthetic derivative of the fungal antibiotic, is converted into its active metabolite, mycophenolic acid, which inhibits allograft rejection in rodents, diminishes proliferation of T and B lymphocytes, decreases generation of cytotoxic T cells, and suppresses antibody formation (Morris and Wang, 1991; Allison and Eugui, 1993). **Mycophenolic acid is an effective and reversible inhibitor of inosine monophosphate dehydrogenase.** T cells as well as B cells are dependent on both the de novo and salvage pathways for purine nucleotide synthesis, whereas other cells satisfy their demand for purines via the salvage pathway. Thus **mycophenolic acid is a relatively selective inhibitor of T and B cell proliferation through its ability to prevent guanosine and deoxyguanosine biosynthesis.** The efficacy and safety of mycophenolate mofetil for the prevention of acute rejection during the first 6 months after renal transplantation have been evaluated in a randomized, double-blind multicenter study in Europe and in the United States (European Mycophenolate Mofetil Cooperative Study Group, 1995; Sollinger, 1995). In the European study, mycophenolate mofetil was added to a regimen of CsA and steroids. In the U.S. investigation, mycophenolate mofetil was added to a regimen of CsA, steroid, and antithymocyte globulin induction therapy. The patient and graft survival rates, at 6 months after transplantation, were quite similar with mycophenolate mofetil– or azathioprine-supplemented regimens. The use of mycophenolate mofetil (2 or 3 g/day) resulted in a significant reduction in the incidence and severity of biopsy-proven acute renal allograft rejection. This decrease in acute rejection episodes might be of benefit in long-term outcome of renal allografts, because acute rejection is a risk factor for chronic rejection.

Adverse results after mycophenolate mofetil included a higher incidence of diarrhea, esophagitis, and gastritis (European Mycophenolate Mofetil Cooperative Study Group, 1995; Sollinger, 1995). The incidence of leukopenia and that of opportunistic infections were similar in recipients treated with mycophenolate mofetil or azathioprine. Because leukopenia was not predicted on the basis of the mechanism of action of mycophenolic acid and was not noted in patients with psoriasis or rheumatoid arthritis who were treated with this drug, the reason for leukopenia in transplant patients treated with mycophenolate mofetil remains to be determined. In the U.S. study, 3 of 333 patients enrolled to receive mycophenolate mofetil developed lymphoma or lymphoproliferative disease. Drug toxicity was more frequent with 3 g than with 2 g of mycophenolate mofetil.

Mizoribine

Like azathioprine and mycophenolic acid, this imidazole nucleoside blocks the purine biosynthetic pathway and inhibits mitogen-stimulated T and B cell proliferation (Turka et al, 1991; Kokado et al, 1990). The antiproliferative effect is linked to a decrease in guanine ribonucleotide pools. Mizoribine prolongs graft survival in several preclinical models and is undergoing clinical testing as a substitute for azathioprine in renal transplant recipients in Europe after having been approved in Japan. Mizoribine appears to be safe and, unlike azathioprine, may not be myelotoxic or hepatotoxic.

15-Deoxyspergualin

DSG is a synthetic analog of spergualin that exerts powerful immunosuppressive properties in preclinical transplant models. Although the mechanism by which DSG inhibits immune response is unknown, a member of the heat shock protein 70 family has been identified as an intracellular DSG-binding protein (Takeuchi et al, 1981; Umeda et al, 1985; Nadler et al, 1992). **DSG is unique in that it prevents the differentiation of T and B cells into mature effector cells.** The efficacy of DSG is being tested in the United States in phase III trials, in kidney transplant recipients undergoing rejection, and in highly sensitized recipients. DSG is reported to be effective as a rescue therapy in renal graft recipients who have not responded to high-dose corticosteroid therapy.

Brequinar Sodium

The antimetabolite brequinar sodium is a noncompetitive inhibitor of dihydroorotate dehydrogenase and blocks formation of the nucleotides uridine and cytidine through inhibition of de novo pyrimidine synthesis (Makowka et al, 1993). Lymphocytes are dependent on the pyrimidine pathway for RNA and DNA synthesis; thus brequinar is a potent inhibitor of both T and B cell proliferation. It is quite effective in preclinical transplant models. Clinical trials using combined brequinar and CsA therapy were halted pending review of results that suggested a narrow therapeutic index.

Leflunomide

Leflunomide is an easily synthesized orally bioavailable prodrug immunosuppressant that is being evaluated in phase III trials for rheumatoid arthritis in Europe and the United States. Information from phase II trials has shown it to be an effective disease-modifying antirheumatic drug and to be free from the side effects commonly associated with currently approved immunosuppressive drugs used with transplantation (Fox and Morris, in press; Mladenovic et al, 1995; Cao et al, 1995). In addition to its efficacy in humans and animals with autoimmune diseases, leflunomide has been extensively investigated and found to control acute, ongoing, and chronic allograft rejection of kidney, skin, heart, vessel, and lung tissue in small and large animal models (Cao et al, 1995). In small animal models of xenograft rejection, leflunomide is also an effective agent for prolonging graft survival and suppressing anti–donor antibody production (Yuh et al, 1995; Lin et al, 1995; Xiao et al, 1994).

The active metabolite of leflunomide is A77 1726, and this has been studied in vitro to determine its effects on immune and nonimmune cells. **Study results suggest that A77 1726 mediates at least part of its antiproliferative activity by inhibiting the de novo pathway of pyrimidine biosynthesis** (Cao et al, 1995; Kurtz et al, 1995; Cherwinski et al., 1995a, 1995b; Williamson et al, 1995). **The target of A77 1726 appears to be the enzyme dihydroorotate dehydrogenase** (Greene et al, 1995). Other in vitro data clearly show that the mechanisms of antiproliferative action of A77 1726 are not limited to its effects on pyrimidine biosynthesis; A77 1726 is an inhibitor of tyrosine kinases associated with growth factor receptors (Xu et al, 1995). A component of the efficacy of leflunomide for reduction of intimal thickening in animal models of graft vascular disease may be its direct antiproliferative effects on smooth muscle cells, which also appear to be mediated by inhibition of the pyrimidine biosynthetic pathway in these cells (Nair et al, 1995).

Because of its short patent life and long in vivo half-life, alternatives to leflunomide are being evaluated for use in transplantation (Morris et al, 1995). These molecules, known as malononitriloamides, are structurally similar to A77 1726 but have shorter half-lives in animals. The suitability of these new members of this drug class for clinical use in transplant patients should be better known after more extensive preclinical studies have been completed.

IMMUNOSUPPRESSIVE REGIMENS IN THE CLINIC

Triple Drug Therapy

The basic immunosuppressive protocol involves the use of multiple drugs, each directed at a discrete site in the T cell activation cascade and each with distinct side effects (see Fig. 13–1). CsA, azathioprine, corticosteroids, tacrolimus, and mycophenolate mofetil are already approved by the U.S. Food and Drug Administration for organ transplantation. The clinical efficacy of sirolimus, DSG, mizoribine, and leflunomide are being tested in clinical trials. The best multidrug regimen is not yet established. A representative immunosuppressive protein is described in Chapter 14 (Renal Transplantation). There are several popular embellishments of the basic triple-drug protocol of CsA, azathioprine, and corticosteroids.

Prophylactic Antibody Induction Protocols

Many centers use monoclonal (e.g., OKT3) or polyclonal antilymphocyte antibodies (e.g., antilymphocyte globulin, antithymocyte globulin) as induction therapy for 7 to 14 days immediately after transplantation (Norman, 1992). This strategy establishes an immunosuppressive umbrella that enables early engraftment without CsA usage during the early post-transplantation period. **Antibody induction protocols have reduced the incidence of early rejection** (Norman, 1992; Cecka et al, 1992; Ortho Multicenter Transplant Study Group, 1985) **and are particularly beneficial for patients at high risk for immunologic graft failure, such as broadly presensitized or retransplantation patients** (Cecka et al, 1992).

OKT3 monoclonal antibody binds to the epsilon chain of the T cell CD3 proteins and modulates the T cell antigen receptor/CD3 complex from the cell surface. In a randomized, multicenter trial in the United States, 94% of acute rejections in recipients of primary cadaveric renal transplants were reversed with OKT3, in comparison with 75% reversed with conventional high-dose corticosteroids (Ortho Multicenter Transplant Study Group, 1985).

The first few doses of OKT3 are accompanied by fever, chills, a capillary leak syndrome, hypotension, pulmo-

nary edema, nephropathy, and encephalopathy. A few cases of irreversible graft failure resulting from graft thrombosis have also been observed with OKT3. Cytokines, especially TNF-α, have been implicated as a basis for some of these effects. Rigorous attention to the fluid status of the graft recipient and premedication with high-dose steroids minimize the side effects of OKT3. CsA, pentoxifylline, indomethacin, and anti–TNF-α monoclonal antibodies appear useful (Suthanthiran et al, 1989; First et al, 1993; Chatenoud, 1993). **Monoclonal antibodies that react with the invariant region of the alpha or the beta chains of T cell antigen receptor are also quite effective in reversing rejection** (Waid et al, 1992; Yoshimura et al, 1992). **Anti–IL-2 receptor α (CD25) monoclonal antibodies can also reduce the incidence of early rejection episodes** (Soulillou et al, 1990; Kirkman et al, 1991). **Anti–LFA-1 (CD11a), anti–ICAM-1 (CD54), anti-CD4, and anti-CD45 monoclonal antibodies are currently being tested for clinical efficacy** (Goodman and Hardy, 1993).

Monoclonal antibody usage has been hampered by the recipient's immune response to the monoclonal antibodies. The "humanization" of rodent mAbs (Queen et al, 1989), wherein the antigen-binding sites are genetically engineered onto a human immunoglobulin background, might minimize the problem.

Adjunctive Vasodilation Therapy

CsA toxicity is caused at least in part by intense intrarenal vasospasm (Meyers, 1986; Weir, 1992). Moreover, renal allografts are subject to calcium-dependent ischemic and reperfusion injury (Weir, 1992; Schrier et al, 1987). These considerations have fostered trials of adjunctive calcium antagonists or fish oil during the early post-transplantation period. **Supplementation of a standard immunosuppressive drug protocol with the calcium antagonists diltiazem, verapamil, and nifedipine has resulted in excellent graft outcome after renal transplantation** (Neumayer et al, 1992; Kunzendorf et al, 1991; Dawidson et al, 1991; Suthanthiran et al, 1993; Weir and Suthanthiran, 1994).

Preclinical trials of fish oil have demonstrated immunosuppressive effects—effects that synergize with CsA (Kelley et al, 1989)—and an ability to mitigate CsA-mediated nephrotoxicity (Rogers et al, 1988). A reduction in the incidence of rejection, improved renal blood flow and function, and lower arterial pressure in recipients of renal allografts have been reported with fish oil supplementation of a CsA and prednisolone regimen (Van Der Heide et al, 1993).

HLA AND RENAL TRANSPLANTATION

The genes that code for HLA are located in the short arm of chromosome 6. The class 1 proteins—HLA-A, HLA-B, and HLA-C antigens—are composed of a 41-kD polymorphic chain linked noncovalently to a 12-kD beta-2-microglobulin encoded in chromosome 15. The class 1 molecules are expressed by all nucleated cells and platelets. The class 2 molecules, HLA-DR and DQ, are composed of a 34-kD alpha chain and a 29-kD beta chain. The class 2 molecules are displayed in a much more tissue-restricted manner and are constitutively expressed on the surface of B cells, monocytes/macrophages, and dendritic cells. Additional lymphoid cells, such as T cells, and nonlymphoid cells, such as renal tubular epithelial cells, express class 2 proteins only upon cell activation.

Transplantation from Living Related Donors

The clinical benefits of HLA matching are more easily appreciated in the recipients of renal grafts from living related donors than in the recipients of grafts of cadaveric source. An analysis of the United Network for Organ Sharing (UNOS) scientific renal transplant registry data has revealed that the 1-year graft survival rates are 94% in recipients of two haplotype-matched, HLA-identical kidneys and 89% and 90%, respectively, when a one-haplotype–matched parent or sibling is the donor (Cecka and Terasaki, 1991). The advantage of HLA-matching is maintained beyond the first year of transplantation.

Cadaveric Transplantation

The effect of matching for HLA in recipients of cadaveric grafts has been examined in a prospective study in which kidneys were shared nationally on the basis of matching for HLA-A, HLA-B, and HLA-DR antigens (Takemoto et al, 1992). **In this study, the 1-year graft survival rates were 88% for HLA-matched kidneys and 79% for HLA-mismatched kidneys. Moreover, the benefit of HLA matching persisted beyond the first year of transplantation.**

A stepwise increase in the survival rate of cadaveric renal allografts has also been noted with increasing levels of HLA-A, HLA-B, and HLA-DR antigen matching (Terasaki et al, 1991).

Molecular Typing of HLA-DR

Molecular techniques for the finer resolution of the antigens of the HLA system are being explored. The clinical advantages are suggested by the observation that whereas the 1-year cadaveric renal graft survival rate is 87% in patients who received kidneys that are HLA-DR identical not only by the serologic methods but also by the DNA-RFLP (restricted fragment length polymorphism) method, it is only 69% in patients who received kidneys that are not HLA-DR identical by the molecular methodology (Opelz et al, 1991). **Identification of HLA-DR antigens by molecular techniques has also resulted in the appreciation of a stepwise increase in the survival of cadaveric renal allografts matched for no, one, or two HLA-DR antigens.**

Existing data suggest a very minimal impact of matching for HLA-C locus antigens. Matching for the HLA-DQ antigen, in contrast, appears to be beneficial in early studies (Terasaki et al, 1993).

CROSS-MATCH TESTING

Cross-matches—testing of recipient's serum for antibodies reacting with the donor's HLA-antigens—are always performed before renal transplantation and are beginning to be considered before heart or liver transplantation. The standard cross-match test consists of incubating the serum from the recipient with the donor's lymphocytes in the presence of rabbit serum as a source of complement.

T Cell Cross-Match

The presence in the recipient's serum of cytotoxic antibodies directed at the donor's class 1 antigen (positive T cell cross-match) is an absolute contraindication to renal transplantation, because 80% to 90% of transplantations performed in the presence of a positive cross-match are rejected in a hyperacute manner (Williams et al, 1968). The sensitivity of the standard cross-match test has been increased by the addition of antihuman globulin (AHG) to the test system. **The graft survival rate is about 5% lower in recipients with a positive AHG test result than in recipients with a negative AHG result** (Ogura, 1993).

B Cell Cross-Match

The significance of antibodies reacting with the donor's class 2 antigens (positive B cell cross-match) is not fully resolved. **However, a survival disadvantage—7% of patients with primary transplants and 15% of patients with repeat transplants—has been noted in recipients with a positive B cell cross-match** (Ogura et al, 1993).

Flow Cytometry Cross-Match

Flow cytometry permits detection of complement-fixing as well as noncomplement-fixing antibodies. **A positive flow cytometry cross-match appears to have a negative impact on the survival of transplants, especially retransplants** (Ogura, 1993; Ogura et al, 1993).

TRANSPLANTATION TOLERANCE

Transplantation tolerance can be defined as an inability of the organ graft recipient to express a graft-destructive immune response. True tolerance is antigen-specific, induced as a consequence of prior exposure to the specific antigen, and is not dependent on the continuous administration of exogenous immunosuppressants.

A classification of tolerance on the basis of the mechanisms involved, site of induction, extent of tolerance, and the cell primarily involved, is provided in Table 13–4. Tolerance induction strategies are listed in Table 13–5.

Several hypotheses for the cellular basis of tolerance, not necessarily mutually exclusive and at times even complementary, have been proposed (Suthanthiran, 1993; Nossal, 1989; Roser, 1989; Brent, 1991; Kronenberg, 1991; Miller and Morahan, 1992). **Data from several laboratories support the following mechanistic possibilities for the creation of a tolerant state: (1) clonal deletion, (2) clonal anergy, and (3) suppression.**

Table 13–4. CLASSIFICATION OF TOLERANCE

A. *Based on the Major Mechanism Involved*
   1. Clonal deletion
   2. Clonal anergy
   3. Suppression

B. *Based on the Period of Induction*
   1. Fetal
   2. Neonatal
   3. Adult

C. *Based on the Cell*
   1. T cell
   2. B cell

D. *Based on the Extent of Tolerance*
   1. Complete
   2. Partial, including split

E. *Based on the Main Site of Induction*
   1. Central
   2. Peripheral

From Suthanthiran M, Strom TB: Immunology and genetics of transplantation. *In* Massry SG, Glassock RJ, eds: Textbook of Nephrology, 3rd ed, vol 2. Baltimore, Williams & Wilkins, 1944; pp 1629–1637.

Clonal Deletion

This is a process by which self antigen–reactive cells, especially those with high affinity for the antigens, are eliminated from the organism's immune repertoire. In the case of T cells, this process takes place primarily in the thymus, and the death of the T cells is considered to

Table 13–5. POTENTIAL APPROACHES FOR TOLERANCE INDUCTION

A. *Cell Depletion Protocols*
   1. Whole body irradiation
   2. Total lymphoid irradiation
   3. Panel of monoclonal antibodies

B. *Reconstitution Protocols*
   1. Allogeneic bone marrow cells with or without T cell depletion
   2. Syngeneic bone marrow cells

C. *Combination of Strategies A and B*

D. *Cell Surface Molecule Targeting Therapy*
   1. Anti-CD4 mAb
   2. Anti–ICAM-1 + anti–LFA-1 mAb
   3. Anti-CD3 mAb
   4. Anti-CD2 mAb
   5. Anti–interleukin-2 receptor α (CD25) mAb (also interleukin-2 toxins)

E. *Drugs*
   1. Cyclosporine
   2. Azathioprine
   3. Rapamycin
   4. Mycophenolate mofetil

F. *Additional Approaches*
   1. Donor-specific blood transfusions with concomitant mAb or drug therapy
   2. Intrathymic inoculation of cells/antigens
   3. Oral administration of cells/antigens

From Suthanthiran M, Strom TB: Immunology and genetics of transplantation. *In* Massry SG, Glassock RJ, eds: Textbook of Nephrology, 3rd ed, vol 2. Baltimore, Williams & Wilkins, 1994, pp 1629–1637.

be the ultimate result of high-affinity interactions between a T cell with productively rearranged TCR and the thymic nonlymphoid cells, including dendritic cells that express the self MHC antigen. This purging of the immune repertoire of self-reactive T cells is termed *negative selection* and is distinguished from the positive selection process responsible for the generation of the T cell repertoire involved in the recognition of foreign antigens in the context of self MHC molecules.

Clonal deletion can also occur in the periphery, and tolerance under these circumstances might also involve additional mechanisms, including clonal anergy and suppression mechanisms.

Clonal Anergy

***Clonal anergy* refers to a process in which the antigen-reactive cells are anatomically present but are functionally silent.** The cellular basis for the hyporesponsiveness or nonresponsiveness resides in the anergic cell itself, and the current data suggest that the anergic T cells fail to express the T cell growth factor, IL-2.

T cell clonal anergy appears to result from incomplete signaling of T cells, as mentioned earlier (Schwartz, 1990). The full activation of T cells requires at least two signals: one signal generated via the TCR/CD3 complex, and the second (costimulatory) signal initiated or delivered by the APC. Stimulation of T cells via the TCR/CD3 complex alone or provision of signal 1 without signal 2 can result in T cell anergy or paralysis.

B cell activation, in a manner analogous to T cell activation, requires at least two signals. One signal is initiated via the B cell antigen receptor immunoglobulin, and a costimulatory signal is provided by cytokines of T cell origin. Thus delivery of the antigenic signal alone to the B cells without the instructive cytokines or T cell help can lead to B cell anergy and tolerance (Suthanthiran, 1993; Nossal, 1989).

Suppression Mechanisms

Antigen-specific T or B cells are physically present and are functionally competent in tolerant states resulting from suppressor mechanisms. The immunocompetent and antigen-specific cells are restrained by the suppressor cells or factors.

Each of the major subsets of T cells, the CD4 T cells and the CD8 T cells, has been implicated in mediating suppression. Indeed, a cascade involving MHC antigen–restricted T cells, MHC antigen–unrestricted T cells, and their secretory products have been reported to collaborate to mediate suppression (Dorf and Benacerraf, 1984; Bloom et al, 1992).

At least three distinct mechanisms have been advanced to explain the cellular basis for suppression: (1) **an anti-idiotypic regulatory mechanism,** in which the idiotype of the TCR of the original antigen-responsive T cells functions as an immunogen and elicits an anti-idiotypic response and, in turn, the elicited anti-idiotypic regulatory cells prevent the further responses of the idiotype-bearing cells to the original sensitizing stimulus; (2) **the veto process,** by which recognition by alloreactive T cells of alloantigen-expressing suppressor cells (veto cells) results in the targeted killing (veto process) of the original alloreactive T cells by the veto cells (Miller, 1980); and (3) **the production of suppressor factors** or cytokines, such as transforming growth factor beta (Miller et al, 1992).

Tolerance in the Clinic

It should be emphasized that more than one mechanism might be operative in the induction of tolerance and that a tolerant state is not an all-or-nothing phenomenon but is one that has several gradations (Brent, 1991; Miller et al, 1992; Monaco, 1991). **Of the mechanisms proposed for tolerance, clonal deletion might be of greater importance in the creation of self-tolerance, and clonal anergy and suppression mechanisms might be more applicable to transplantation tolerance.** From a practical viewpoint, a nonimmunogenic allograft (e.g., located in an immunologically privileged site or physically isolated from the immune system) might also be "tolerated" by an immunocompetent organ graft recipient.

Authentic tolerance is difficult to demonstrate in clinical circumstances. Nevertheless, the clinical examples, albeit infrequent, of grafts functioning without any exogenous immunosuppressive drugs (as a result of either noncompliance of the patient or discontinuation of drugs for other medical reasons) do suggest that some long-term recipients of allografts develop tolerance to the transplanted organ and accept the allografts. Also, the in vitro studies conducted with the peripheral blood lymphocytes of the graft recipients in the mixed lymphocyte culture reactions and/or in the cell-mediated lymphocyte assays suggest that some renal allograft recipients do develop antigen-specific hyporesponsiveness. The progress in our understanding of the immunobiology of graft rejection and tolerance and the potential to apply molecular approaches to the bedside hold significant promise for the creation of a clinically relevant tolerant state and transplantation without exogenous immunosuppressants—the cherished goal of the transplant clinician.

ACKNOWLEDGMENT

The authors are grateful to Ms. Linda Stackhouse for meticulous assistance in the preparation of this chapter.

REFERENCES

Immunobiology of the Antiallograft Response

Allison JP, Krummel MF: The yin and yang of T cell costimulation. Science 1995; 270:932–933.

Beyers AD, Spruyt LL, Williams AF: Molecular associations between the T-lymphocyte antigen receptor complex and the surface antigens CD2, CD4, or CD8 and CD5. Proc Natl Acad Sci USA 1992; 89:2945–2949.

Bretcher P, Cohen M: A theory of self-nonself discrimination: Paralysis and induction involve the recognition of one and two determinants on an antigen, respectively. Science 1970; 169:1042–1049.

Brown MH, Cantrell DA, Brattsand G, et al: The CD2 antigen associates with the T-cell antigen receptor/CD3/antigen complex on the surface of human T lymphocytes. Nature 1989; 339:551–553.

Clark EA, Ledbetter JA: How B- and T-cells talk to each other. Nature 1994; 367:425–428.

Clevers H, Alarcon B, Wileman T, Terhorst C: The T-cell receptor/CD3 complex: A dynamic protein ensemble. Annu Rev Immunol 1988; 6:629–662.

Clipstone NA, Crabtree GR: Identification of calcineurin as a key signalling enzyme in T-lymphocyte activation. Nature 1992; 357:695–697.

Dustin ML, Springer TA: T-cell receptor crosslinking transiently stimulates adhesiveness through LFA-1. Nature 1989; 341:619–624.

Fruman DA, Klee CB, Bierer BE, Burakoff SJ: Calcineurin phosphatase activity in T lymphocytes is inhibited by FK 506 and cyclosporin A. Proc Natl Acad Sci USA 1992; 89:3686–3690.

Fung MR, Scearce RM, Hoffman JA, et al: A tyrosine kinase physically associates with the β-subunit of the human IL-2 receptor. J Immunol 1991; 147:1253–1260.

Germain RN: MHC-dependent antigen processing and peptide presentation: Providing ligands for T lymphocyte activation. Cell 1994; 76:287–299.

Hatakeyama M, Kono T, Kobayashi N, et al: Interaction of the IL-2 receptor with the src-family kinase p56lck: Identification of novel intermolecular association. Science 1991; 52:523–528.

Isobe M, Yagita H, Okumura K, Ihara A: Specific acceptance of cardiac allograft after treatment with antibodies to ICAM-1 and LFA-1. Science 1992; 255:1125–1127.

June CH, Ledbetter JA, Linsley PS, Thompson CB: Role of the CD28 receptor in T-cell activation. Immunol Today 1990; 11:211–216.

Klausner RD, Samelson LE: T-cell antigen receptor activation pathways: The tyrosine kinase connection. Cell 1991; 64:875–878.

Lenschow J, Zeng Y, Thistlethwaite R, et al: Long-term survival of xenogeneic pancreatic islet grafts induced by CTLA-4Ig. Science 1992; 257:789–792.

Linsley PS, Brady W, Urnes M, et al: CTLA-4 is a second receptor for the B-cell activation antigen B7. J Exp Med 1991; 174:561–569.

Lipman ML, Stevens AC, Bleackley RC, et al: The strong correlation of cytotoxic T lymphocyte specific serine protease gene transcripts with renal allograft rejection. Transplantation 1992; 53:73–79.

Liu J, Farmer JD Jr, Lane WS, et al: Calcineurin is a common target of cyclophilin-cyclosporin A and FKBP-FK506 complexes. Cell 1991; 66:807–815.

Maslinski W, Remillard B, Tsudo M, Strom TB: Interleukin-2 induces tyrosine kinase dependent translocation of active raf-1 from the IL-2 receptor into the cytosol. J Biol Chem 1992; 267:15281–15284.

Miceli MC, Parnes JR: The role of CD4 and CD8 in T-cell activation. Semin Immunol 1991; 3:133–141.

Nishizuka Y: Intracellular signaling by hydrolysis of phospholipids and activation of protein kinase C. Science 1992; 258:607–614.

O'Keefe SJ, Tamura J, Kincaid RL, et al: FK-506- and CsA-sensitive activation of the interleukin-2 promoter by calcineurin. Nature 1992; 357:692–694.

Remillard B, Petrillo R, Maslinski W, et al: Interleukin-2 receptor regulates activation of phosphatidylinositol 3-kinase. J Bio Chem 1991; 266:14167–14170.

Schwartz RH: T-cell anergy. Sci Am 1993; 269:62–71.

Shibuya H, Yoneyama M, Ninomiya-Tsuji J, et al: IL-2 and EGF receptors stimulate the hematopoietic cell cycle via different signaling pathways: Demonstration of a novel role for c-myc. Cell 1992; 70:57–67.

Shoskes DA, Wood KJ: Indirect presentation of MHC antigens in transplantation. Immunol Today 1994; 15:32–38.

Strom TB, Tilney NL, Carpenter CB, Busch GJ: Identity and cytotoxic capacity of cells infiltrating renal allografts. N Engl J Med 1975; 292:1257–1263.

Suthanthiran M: A novel model for antigen-dependent activation of normal human T-cells. Transmembrane signaling by crosslinkage of the CD3/T cell receptor-αβ complex with the cluster determinant 2 antigen. J Exp Med 1990; 171:1965–1979.

Suthanthiran M: Signaling features of T-cells: Implications for the regulation of the anti-allograft response. Kidney Int 1993; 44:S-3–S-11.

Suthanthiran M, Garovoy MR: Immunologic monitoring of the renal allograft recipient. Urol Clin North Am 1983; 10:315–325.

Suthanthiran M, Strom TB: Renal transplantation. N Engl J Med 1994; 331:365–376.

Takeshita T, Asao H, Ohtani K, et al: Cloning of the chain of the human IL-2 receptor. Science 1992; 257:379–382.

Thompson CB, Lindsten T, Ledbetter JA, et al: CD28 activation pathway regulates the production of multiple T-cell-derived lymphokines/cytokines. Proc Natl Acad Sci USA 1989; 86:1333–1337.

Unanue ER, Cerottoni J-C: Antigen presentation. FASEB J 1989; 3:2496–2502.

Waldmann TA: The interleukin-2 receptor. J Biol Chem 1991; 266:2681–2684.

Weiss A, Littman DR: Signal transduction by lymphocyte antigen receptors. Cell 1994; 76:263–264.

Williams JM, DeLoria D, Hansen JA, et al: The events of primary T-cell activation can be staged by use of sepharose-bound anti-T3 [64.1] monoclonal antibody and purified interleukin-1. J Immunol 1985; 135:2249–2255.

Xu G-P, Sharma VK, Li B, et al: Intragraft expression of IL-10 messenger RNA: A novel correlate of renal allograft rejection. Kidney Int 1995; 48:1504–1507.

Immunopharmacology of Allograft Rejection

Allison AC, Eugui EM: Immunosuppressive and other effects of mycophenolic acid and an ester prodrug, mycophenolate mofetil. Immunol Rev 1993; 136:5–19.

Almawi WY, Lipman ML, Stevens AC, et al: Abrogation of glucocorticosteroid-mediated inhibition of T-cell proliferation by the synergistic action of IL-1, IL-6, and IFN. J Immunol 1991; 146:3523–3527.

Arya SK, Wong-Staal F, Gallo RC: Dexamethasone mediated inhibition of T-cell growth factor and gamma interferon messenger RNA. J Immunol 1984; 133:273–276.

Auphan N, DiDonato JA, Rosette C, et al: Immunosuppression by glucocorticoids: Inhibition of NFB activity through induction of IB synthesis. Science 1995; 270:286–290.

Cao WW, Kao PN, Chao AC, et al: Mechanism of the antiproliferative action of leflunomide: A77 1726, the active metabolite of leflunomide, does not block T cell receptor-mediated signal transduction but its antiproliferative effects are antagonized by pyrimidine nucleosides. J Heart Lung Transplant 1995; 14:1016–1030.

Cherwinski HM, Byars N, Ballaron SJ, et al: Leflunomide interferes with pyrimidine nucleotide biosynthesis. Inflamm Res 1995a; 44:317–322.

Cherwinski HM, Cohn RG, Cheung P, et al: The immunosuppressant leflunomide inhibits lymphocyte proliferation by inhibiting pyrimidine biosynthesis. J Pharmacol Exp Ther 1995b; 275:1043–1049.

Chung J, Kuo CJ, Crabtree GR, Blenis J: Rapamycin-FKBP specifically blocks growth-dependent activation of and signaling by the 70 kd S6 protein kinases. Cell 1992; 69:1227–1236.

Clipstone NA, Crabtree GR: Identification of calcineurin as a key signalling enzyme in T-lymphocyte activation. Nature 1992; 357:695–697.

Elion GB: Biochemistry and pharmacology of purine analogues. Fed Proc 1967; 26:898–904.

European Mycophenolate Mofetil Cooperative Study Group: Placebo-controlled study of mycophenolate mofetil combined with cyclosporin and corticosteroids for prevention of acute rejection. Lancet 1995; 345:1321–1325.

Fox RI, Morris RE: Inhibitors of de novo nucleotide synthesis in the treatment of rheumatoid arthritis. *In* Strand V, ed: Emerging Therapies for Autoimmune Diseases. New York, Marcel Dekker, in press.

Fruman DA, Klee CB, Bierer BE, Burakoff SJ: Calcineurin phosphatase activity in T lymphocytes is inhibited by FK 506 and cyclosporin A. Proc Natl Acad Sci USA 1992; 89:3686–3690.

Greene S, Watanabe K, Braatz-Trulson J, Lou L: Inhibition of dihydroorotate dehydrogenase by the immunosuppressive agent leflunomide. Biochem Pharmacol 1995; 50:861–867.

Gregory CR, Huang X, Pratt RE, et al: Treatment with rapamycin and mycophenolic acid reduces arterial intimal thickening produced by mechanical injury and allows endothelial replacement. Transplantation 1995; 59:655–661.

Heitman J, Movva NR, Hall MN: Targets for cell cycle arrest by the immunosuppressant rapamycin in yeast. Science 1991; 253:905–909.

Knudsen PJ, Dinarello CA, Strom TB: Glucocorticoids inhibit transcription and post-transcriptional expression of interleukin-1. J Immunol 1987; 139:4129–4134.

Kokado Y, Ishibahi M, Jiang H: Low dose cyclosporin, mizoribine and prednisone in renal transplantation: A new triple drug therapy. Clin Transplant 1990; 4:191–197.

Kurtz ES, Bailey SC, Arshad F, et al: Leflunomide: An active antiinflammatory and antiproliferative agent in models of dermatologic disease. Inflamm Res 1995; 44(Suppl 2):S187–S188.

Lai JH, Tan H: CD28 signaling causes a sustained down-regulation of I kappa B alpha which can be prevented by the immunosuppressant rapamycin. J Biol Chem 1994; 269:30077–30080.

Lin Y, Sobis H, Vandeputte M, Waer M: Mechanism of leflunomide-induced prevention of xenoantibody formation and xenograft rejection in the hamster-to-rat heart transplantation model. Transplant Proc 1995; 27:305–306.

Liu J, Farmer JD Jr, Lane WS, et al: Calcineurin is a common target of cyclophilin-cyclosporin A and FKBP-FK506 complexes. Cell 1991; 66:807–815.

Makowka L, Sher LS, Cramer DV: The development of brequinar as an immunosuppressive drug for transplantation. Immunol Rev 1993; 136:51–70.

Mladenovic V, Domljan Z, Rozman B, et al: Safety and effectiveness of leflunomide in the treatment of patients with active rheumatoid arthritis. Results of a randomized, placebo-controlled, phase II study. Arthritis Rheum 1995; 38:1595–1603.

Morris RE: Rapamycins: Antifungal, antitumor, antiproliferative, and immunosuppressive macrolides. Transplant Rev 1992; 6:39–87.

Morris RE, Iluang XF, Shorthouse R, et al: Studies in experimental models of chronic rejection: Use of rapamycin (sirolimus) and isoxazole derivatives (leflunomide and its analogues) for the suppression of graft vascular disease and obliterative bronchiolitis. Transplant Proc 1995; 27:2068–2069.

Morris RE, Wang J: Comparison of the immunosuppressive effects of mycophenolic acid and the morpholinethal ester of mycophenolic acid (RS-61443) in recipients of heart grafts. Transplant Proc 1991; 23:493–506.

Nadler SG, Tepper MA, Schacter B, Mazzucco CE: Interaction of the immunosuppressant deoxyspergualin with a member of the Hsp70 family of heat shock proteins. Science 1992; 258:484–486.

Nair RV, Cao W, Morris RE: Inhibition of smooth muscle cell proliferation in vitro by leflunomide, a new immunosuppressant, is antagonized by uridine. Immunol Lett 1995; 47:171–174.

O'Keefe SJ, Tamura J, Kincaid RL, et al: FK506- and CsA-sensitive activation of the interleukin-2 promoter by calcineurin. Nature 1992; 357:692–694.

Palvogianni F, Raptis A, Ahuja SS, et al: Negative transcriptional regulation of human interleukin-2 (IL-2) gene by glucocorticoids through interference with nuclear transcription factors AP-1 and NF-AT. J Clin Invest 1993; 91:1481–1487.

Sabatini DM, Erdjument Bromage H, Lui M, et al: Raft-1: A mammalian protein that binds to FKBP 12 in a rapamycin dependent fashion and is homologous to yeast TORS. Cell 1994; 78:35–43.

Scheinman RI, Cogswell PG, Lofquist AK, Baldwin AS Jr: Role of transcriptional activation of IB in mediation of immunosuppression by glucocorticoids. Science 1995; 270:283–286.

Schreiber SC: Immunophilin-sensitive protein phosphatase activation in cell signaling pathways. Cell 1992; 70:365–368.

Sehgal SN, Camardo JS, Scarola JA, Maida BT: Rapamycin (sirolimus, rapamune). Curr Opin Nephrol Hypert 1995; 4:482–487.

Sollinger HW for the U.S. Renal Transplant Mycophenolate Mofetil Study Group: Mycophenolate mofetil for the prevention of acute rejection in primary cadaveric renal allograft recipients. Transplantation 1995; 60:225–232.

Takeuchi T, Iinuma H, Kunimoto S, et al: A new antitumor antibiotic, spergualin: Isolation and antitumor activity. J Antibiot (Tokyo) 1981; 34:1619–1621.

Turka LA, Dayton J, Sinclair G, et al: Guanine ribonucleotide depletion inhibits T-cell activation: Mechanism of action of the immunosuppressive drug mizoribine. J Clin Invest 1991; 87:940–948.

Umeda Y, Moriguchi M, Kuroda H et al: Synthesis and antitumor activity of spergualin analogues: I. Chemical modification of 7-guanidine-3-hydroxyacyl moiety. J Antibiot (Tokyo) 1985; 38:886–898.

Vacca A, Felli MP, Farina AR, et al: Glucocorticoid receptor-mediated suppression of the interleukin-2 gene expression through impairment of the cooperativity between nuclear factor of activated T-cells and AP-1 enhancer elements. J Exp Med 1992; 175:637–646.

Williamson RA, Yea CM, Robson PA, et al: Dihydroorotate dehydrogenase is a high affinity binding protein for A77 1726 and mediator of a range of biological effects of the immunomodulatory compound. J Biol Chem 1995; 270:22467–22472.

Xiao F, Chong AS, Foster P, et al: Leflunomide controls rejection in hamster-to-rat cardiac xenografts. Transplantation 1994; 58:828–834.

Xu X, Williams JW, Bremer EG, et al: Inhibition of protein tyrosine phosphorylation in T cells by a novel immunosuppressive agent, leflunomide. J Biol Chem 1995; 270:12398–12403.

Yang-Yee HF, Chambard JC, Sun YL, et al: Transcriptional interference between cp-Jun and the glucocorticoid receptor: Mutual inhibition of DNA binding due to direct protein-protein interaction. Cell 1990; 62:1205–1215.

Yuh D, Gandy KL, Morris RE, et al: Leflunomide prolongs pulmonary allograft and xenograft survival. J Heart Lung Transpl 1995; 14:1136–1144.

Zanker B, Walz G, Wieder KJ, Strom TB: Evidence that glucocorticosteroids block expression of the human interleukin-6 gene by accessory cells. Transplantation 1990; 49:183–185.

Immunosuppressive Regimens in the Clinic

Cecka JM, Cho YW, Terasaki PI: Analysis of the UNOS scientific renal transplant registry at three years—Early events affecting transplant success. Transplantation 1992; 53:59–64.

Chatenoud L: OKT3-induced cytokine-release syndrome: Preventive effect of anti-tumor necrosis factor monoclonal antibody. Transplant Proc 1993; 25:47–51.

Dawidson I, Rooth P, Lu C, et al: Verapamil improves the outcome after cadaver renal transplantation. J Am Soc Nephrol 1991; 2:983–990.

First MR, Schroeder TJ, Hariharan S, Weiskittel P: Reduction of the initial febrile response to OKT3 with indomethacin. Transplant Proc 1993; 25:52–54.

Goodman ER, Hardy MA: Transplantation 1992: The year in review. *In* Terasaki PI, Cecka JM, eds: Clinical Transplants 1992. Los Angeles, UCLA Tissue Typing Laboratory, 1993, pp 285–297.

Kelley VE, Kirkman RL, Bastos M, et al: Enhancement of immunosuppression by substitution of fish oil for olive oil as a vehicle for cyclosporine. Transplantation 1989; 48:98–102.

Kirkman RL, Shapiro ME, Carpenter CB, et al: A randomized prospective trial of anti-Tac monoclonal antibody in human renal transplantation. Transplantation 1991; 51:107–113.

Kunzendorf U, Walz G, Brockmoeller J, et al: Effects of diltiazem upon metabolism and immunosuppressive action of cyclosporine in kidney graft recipients. Transplantation 1991; 52:280–284.

Meyers BD: Cyclosporine nephrotoxicity. Kidney Int 1986; 30:964–974.

Neumayer H-H, Kunzendorf U, Schreiber M: Protective effects of calcium antagonists in human renal transplantation. Kidney Int 1992; 41:S87–S93.

Norman DJ: Antilymphocyte antibodies in the treatment of allograft rejection: Targets, mechanisms of action, monitoring, and efficacy. Semin Nephrol 1992; 12:315–324.

Ortho Multicenter Transplant Study Group: A randomized clinical trial of OKT3 monoclonal antibody for acute rejection of cadaveric renal transplants. N Engl J Med 1985; 313:337–342.

Queen C, Schneider WP, Selick HE, et al: A humanized antibody that binds to the interleukin-2 receptor. Proc Natl Acad Sci USA 1989; 86:10029–10033.

Rogers TS, Elzinga L, Bennett WM, Kelley VE: Selective enhancement of thromboxane in macrophages and kidneys in cyclosporine-induced nephrotoxicity. Dietary protection by fish oil. Transplantation 1988; 45:153–156.

Schrier RW, Arnold PE, Van Putten VJ, Burke TJ: Cellular calcium in ischemic acute renal failure: Role of calcium entry blockers. Kidney Int 1987; 32:313–322.

Soulillou J-P, Cantarovich D, Le Mauff B, et al: Randomized controlled trial of a monoclonal antibody against the interleukin-2 receptor (33B3.1) as compared with rabbit antithymocyte globulin for prophylaxis against rejection of renal allografts. N Engl J Med 1990; 322:1175–1182.

Suthanthiran M, Fotino M, Riggio RR, et al: OKT3-associated adverse reactions: Mechanistic basis and therapeutic options. Am J Kidney Dis 1989; 14:39–44.

Suthanthiran M, Haschemeyer RH, Riggio RR, et al: Excellent outcome with a calcium channel blocker supplemented immunosuppressive regimen in cadaveric renal transplantation: A potential strategy to avoid antibody induction protocols. Transplantation 1993; 55:1008–1013.

Van Der Heide JJH, Bilo HJG, Donker JM, et al: Effect of dietary fish oil on renal function and rejection in cyclosporine-treated recipients of renal transplants. N Engl J Med 1993; 329:769–773.

Waid TH, Lucas BA, Thompson JS, et al: Treatment of acute cellular rejection with T10B9.1A-31 or OKT3 in renal allograft recipients. Transplantation 1992; 53:80–86.

Weir MR: Clinical benefits of calcium antagonists in renal transplant recipients. *In* Epstein M, ed: Calcium Antagonists in Clinical Medicine. Philadelphia, Hanley and Belfus, 1992, pp 391–412.

Weir MR, Suthanthiran M: Supplementation of immunosuppressive regimens with calcium channel blockers. Rationale and clinical efficacy. Clin Immunother 1994; 2:458–467.

Yoshimura N, Takahashi K, Ishibashi M: Treatment of acute cellular rejection with BMA031 in renal transplant recipients—A multicentered trial in Japan [Abstract]. Presented at the Annual Meeting of the American Society of Transplant Surgeons, Chicago, May 1992, p 63.

HLA and Renal Transplantation

Cecka JM, Terasaki PI: The UNOS Scientific Renal Transplant Registry—1991. *In* Terasaki PI, ed: Clinical Transplants 1991. Los Angeles, UCLA Tissue Typing Laboratory, 1992, pp 1–11.

Opelz G, Mytilineos J, Scherer S, et al: Survival of DNA HLA-DR typed and matched cadaver kidney transplants. Lancet 1991; 338:461–463.

Takemoto S, Terasaki PI, Cecka JM, et al: Survival of nationally shared, HLA-matched kidney transplants from cadaveric donors. N Engl J Med 1992; 327:834–839.

Terasaki PI, Cecka JM, Gjertson DW, et al: A ten-year prediction for kidney transplant survival. *In* Terasaki PI, Cecka JM, eds: Clinical Transplants 1992, Los Angeles, UCLA Tissue Typing Laboratory, 1993, pp 501–512.

Terasaki PI, Cecka JM, Lim E, et al: UCLA and UNOS Registries: Overview. *In* Terasaki PI, ed: Clinical Transplants 1990, Los Angeles, UCLA Tissue Typing Laboratory, 1991; pp 409–430.

Cross-Match Testing

Ogura K: Sensitization. *In* Terasaki PI, Cecka JM, eds: Clinical Transplants 1992. Los Angeles, UCLA Tissue Typing Laboratory, 1993, pp 357–369.

Ogura K, Terasaki PI, Johnson C, et al: The significance of a positive flow cytometry crossmatch test in primary kidney transplantation. Transplantation 1993; 56:294–298.

Williams GM, Hume DM, Hudson RP Jr, et al: "Hyperacute" renal homograft rejection in man. N Engl J Med 1968; 279:611–618.

Transplantation Tolerance

Bloom BR, Salgame P, Diamond B: Revisiting and revising suppressor T cells. Immunol Today 1992; 13:131–136.

Brent L: Tolerance: Past, present and future. Transplant Proc 1991; 23:67–72.

Dorf ME, Benacerraf B: Suppressor cells and immunoregulation. Annu Rev Immunol 1984; 2:127–158.

Kronenberg M: Self-tolerance and autoimmunity. Cell 1991; 65:537–542.

Miller A, Lider O, Roberts AB, et al: Suppressor T cells generated by oral tolerization to myelin basic protein suppress both in vitro and in vivo immune responses by the release of transforming growth factor after antigen-specific triggering. Proc Natl Acad Sci (USA) 1992; 89:421–425.

Miller JFAP, Morahan G: Peripheral T cell tolerance. Annu Rev Immunol 1992; 10:51–69.

Miller RG: An immunological suppressor cell inactivating cytotoxic T lymphocyte precursor cells recognizing it. Nature 1980; 287:544.

Monaco AP: Future trends in transplantation in the 1990s: Prospects for the induction of clinical tolerance. Transplant Proc 1991; 23:67–72.

Nossal GJV: Immunological tolerance: Collaboration between antigen and lymphokines. Science 1989; 245:147–153.

Roser BJ: Cellular mechanisms in neonatal and adult tolerance. Immunol Rev 1989; 107:179–202.

Schwartz RH: A cell culture model for T lymphocyte clonal anergy. Science 1990; 248:1349–1356.

Suthanthiran M: Induction of specific transplantation tolerance. *In* Thomson AW, Catto GRD, eds: Immunology of Renal Transplantation. Boston, Edward Arnold, 1993, pp 144–156.

14 RENAL TRANSPLANTATION

John M. Barry, M.D.

Each renal transplantation operation is a study of pelvic anatomy, each cadaver nephrectomy is a study of retroperitoneal anatomy, and each living-donor nephrectomy is an open surgical procedure on a kidney, procedures that are decreasing in frequency because of the development of minimally invasive surgical techniques and of nonoperative methods of treating renal stones and obstruction. Nowhere in urology must the principles of urinary tract reconstruction and infection control be more rigorously applied than in the immunosuppressed kidney transplant recipient. Understanding the molecular mechanisms of antigen-lymphocyte interactions in transplantation should provide insights into other disease processes such as cancer and infection. Renal preservation principles are often applied to parenchyma-sparing renal operations and to complex renovascular reconstruction procedures. As more renal transplantations are performed, more of these patients are apt to present to the practicing urologist for evaluation and preparation of the urinary tract for transplantation, and for the care of urologic problems after transplantation, which may or may not be related to the transplantation surgery or to the consequences of immunosuppression.

END-STAGE RENAL DISEASE

Incidence

In 1995, the estimated number of patients starting renal replacement therapy for end-stage renal disease (ESRD) in the United States was 250 per million population (US Renal Data System [USRDS], 1995). The median age of those new ESRD patients was 63 years. Both the prevalence and the incidence of ESRD are greater in the elderly than in the young, in men than in women, and in black than in white persons. Diabetes is the most frequent cause of ESRD, followed in order by hypertension, glomerulonephritis, and cystic kidney diseases. The incidence rate for hypertension-caused ESRD in blacks is six times that for whites.

Treatment Options

The purposes of renal replacement therapy are to prolong and maintain the quality of life. The treatment or treatments that are chosen for an individual patient are those that allow the longest extension of useful life. Renal replacement therapy is now considered to be a right in the United States and most other developed countries. Permanent renal failure in adults is commonly defined as an irreversible glomerular filtration rate (GFR) of less than 10 ml/minute or a serum creatinine level of greater than 8.0 mg/dl (United Network for Organ Sharing [UNOS], 1994a). Children less than 6 years of age and patients with symptomatic uremia, especially diabetic adults, are considered on an individual basis as meeting criteria for permanent renal failure. A reasonable goal for ESRD treatment programs is the transplantation of all patients in whom the risk is equal to or less than that of remaining on maintenance dialysis. Renal transplantation is the preferred method of therapy for most patients with ESRD because it is more cost-effective (Eggers, 1988) and allows a return to a more normal lifestyle than maintenance dialysis does (Evans et al, 1985; Disney, 1995). When considering comparative costs of renal transplantation and maintenance dialysis, the break-even point is 4½ years when unsuccessful transplants are included in the analysis (UNOS, 1994b). After that, kidney transplantation becomes more cost effective than dialysis. In July 1995, 29,238 patients were still on the UNOS waiting list for cadaver kidney grafts, even though 11,037 kidneys were transplanted in the United States in the preceding calendar year, and 8374 of those were from cadaver donors (UNOS, 1995b, 1995c).

In-center hemodialysis is the predominant form of therapy for ESRD. In the United States it accounts for about 60% of all treated ESRD patients (USRDS, 1995). Transplantation, however, is the predominant mode of care for the young, and it accounts for about 29% of treated patients. About 11% of ESRD patients are treated with chronic peritoneal dialysis. A desire for self-care, a long distance from a hemodialysis unit, difficulties with hemodialysis therapy, serious cardiac disease, diabetes mellitus, and small stature are characteristics of patients especially suited for peritoneal dialysis. Unsuitable characteristics of patients for chronic peritoneal dialysis are considered to be obesity, hernias, poor hygiene, and obliterated peritoneal space (Winearls and Gray, 1994).

The advantages of living related donor renal transplantation over cadaver donor renal transplantation are better graft survivals, less recipient morbidity, specific planning of the operation to allow preemptive transplantation or limitation of the waiting time on dialysis, and partial alleviation of the insufficient supply of cadaver kidneys. The timing of preemptive renal transplantation must be such that the patient does not have months to years of usable function in the failing native kidneys. Objections to transplantation before dialysis are that (1) the procedure removes the experience of dialysis so that the advantages of transplantation are not appreciated and (2) a recipient of preemptive cadaver kidney transplantation may have an unfair advantage over patients already on dialysis, some of whom have been waiting a long time for a kidney graft.

When compared with adults with ESRD, children are more likely to receive chronic peritoneal dialysis, and they are more likely to undergo renal transplantation (USRDS, 1995). Special problems in children with ESRD include growth failure, poor nutrition, and psychiatric problems. They often suffer from a cycle of depression, anxiety, and loss of self-esteem, and these problems can result in family stress and divorce (NIH, 1993). The development of recombinant growth hormone has made possible treatment of short stature in pediatric patients with chronic renal failure and after transplantation (Van Es, 1991), and nutritional supplementation can be done via nasogastric feeding tube or button gastrostomy. There is a relatively greater availability of parental kidney donors, and children receive preferential points when they are listed for cadaver kidney transplantation (USRDS, 1995; UNOS, 1995a).

Results of Treatment

Data from the U.S. Renal Data System (USRDS) indicate that survival after renal transplantation is significantly better than that for patients treated with dialysis (Table 14–1); however, this may simply mean that healthier patients are more likely to be referred for transplantation. A more controlled analysis has indicated a significantly reduced mortality risk for cadaveric renal transplant recipients when compared with acceptable transplant candidates on dialysis (Port et al, 1993). Regardless of whether the treatment modality is dialysis or transplantation, the major causes of death are, in order, heart disease, sepsis, and stroke (USRDS, 1995).

Survival of kidney grafts has improved. The 2-year survival of first grafts from living related donors increased from 79% for transplantations done in 1981 to 89% for those done in 1991 (USRDS, 1995). For first cadaver donor kidney grafts, the 2-year survival increased from 53% to 78% for the same interval. These improvements in kidney graft survivals are due to careful recipient selection and preparation, improvements in donor management and organ procurement, refinement of surgical techniques, improvement and standardization of histocompatibility techniques, improvements in immunosuppression, and careful long-term monitoring of recipients.

Table 14–1. SURVIVAL PROBABILITIES FOR TREATED PATIENTS WITH END-STAGE RENAL DISEASE

	5-Year Survival		10-Year Survival	
Treatment Modality	*No.*	%	*No.*	%
Dialysis	35,135	28	23,205	10
First renal transplant (cadaveric)	5,449	76	3,318	54
First renal transplant (living related)	1,482	88	1,560	76

Data from US Renal Data System: USRDS 1995 Annual Data Report. Bethesda, MD, National Institute of Diabetes and Digestive and Kidney Diseases, April, 1995.

HISTORY OF HUMAN RENAL TRANSPLANTATION

The history of renal transplantation illustrates the successful combination of the fields of surgery, medicine, immunology, and government. Correl established the modern method of vascular suturing at the turn of the 20th century, and he was awarded the Nobel Prize in 1912 for his work on organ grafting (Hamilton, 1994). In 1933, the first human renal allograft was performed by Voronoy in the Ukraine (Hamilton and Reid, 1984). The recipient was a 26-year-old woman who had attempted suicide by ingesting mercuric chloride. The donor was a 66-year-old man whose kidney was removed 6 hours after death. With the recipient under local anesthesia, the renal vessels were anastomosed to the femoral vessels and a cutaneous ureterostomy was performed. A small amount of blood-stained urine appeared, but the patient expired 48 hours after the procedure.

The first long-term success with human renal allografting occurred in Boston in 1954 when a kidney from one twin was transplanted into the other, who had ESRD (Hamilton, 1994). In 1958, the first histocompatibility antigen was described. Radiation was used for immunosuppression in 1959, azathioprine became available for human use in 1951, and glucocorticoids became part of a standard immunosuppression regimen with azathioprine in 1962 (Goodwin et al, 1963). In the same year, the first use of tissue matching to select donor-recipient pairs was done. The direct cross match between donor lymphocytes and recipient serum was introduced in 1966, and heterologous antilymphocyte serum was used as an immunosuppressant in human renal transplantation. In the late 1960s, human renal preservation over 24 hours became possible with either pulsatile machine perfusion (Belzer et al, 1967) or simple cold storage after flushing with an intracellular electrolyte solution (Collins et al, 1969). The beneficial effect of blood transfusions was described by Opelz and colleagues in 1973, and this led to immunologic conditioning with blood products for both cadaveric and living donor renal transplants.

Donor-specific blood transfusions (DST) eventually became part of standardized pretransplantation immunologic conditioning protocols for living donor renal transplantation (Salvatierra et al, 1980). **In the cyclosporine era, the beneficial effects of random blood transfusions and DST protocols have been difficult to establish, and transfusion protocols have been associated with donor-specific sensitization and the transmission of viral illnesses. For these reasons, pretransplantation transfusion protocols are no longer routinely prescribed.** The first clinical trials of cyclosporine were reported by Calne and colleagues in 1978, and this was followed 3 years later by reports of the successful use of monoclonal antibody for the treatment of renal allograft rejection in humans (Cosimi et al, 1981).

Medicare coinsurance for ESRD patients was passed into law in 1972 and instituted in 1973. This removed a significant impediment to renal transplantation in the United States. In the mid-1970s, brain-death laws were passed. This allowed organ retrieval from beating-heart cadaver donors and reduced warm ischemia time. In 1984, Congress passed the National Transplant Act, which authorized a national organ-sharing system and grants for organ procurement. The University of Wisconsin (UW) solution, introduced in the late 1980s, provided one solution for preservation of all transplantable abdominal organs, including kidneys (Belzer and Southard, 1988). Recombinant erythropoietin became available in 1989, and this significantly improved the quality of life for maintenance dialysis patients and reduced the need for blood transfusions (Carpenter, 1990). This has decreased the risk of virally transmitted infections and the risk of the development of anti-HLA (human leukocyte antigen) antibodies in the potential kidney transplant recipient. Thirty-six years after the first long-term success of a human-to-human kidney transplantation, Joseph E. Murray received the Nobel Prize in Medicine in 1990 for his pioneering work in renal transplantation.

SELECTION AND PREPARATION OF KIDNEY TRANSPLANT RECIPIENTS

Nonurologic Evaluation

The pretransplantation evaluation is a multidisciplinary process that is performed well in advance of the renal transplant operation and immunosuppression (Fig. 14–1). Although the criteria for acceptance of candidates for renal transplantation vary among transplant centers (Ramos et al, 1994), the purposes of the evaluation are generally considered to be to diagnose the primary disease; to determine its risk of recurrence in the kidney graft; and to rule out active invasive infection, a high probability of operative mortality, noncompliance, active malignancy, and anatomy unsuitable for technical success (Nohr, 1989; Lemmers and Barry, 1993; Kasiske et al, 1995).

Kidney Disease Recurrence

Patients with focal glomerulosclerosis and hemolytic uremic syndrome need to be counseled about the significant probability of disease recurrence and the risk of secondary graft failure (Cameron, 1991; Artero et al, 1992). Other types of glomerulonephritis have lower probabilities of recurrence and rarely cause loss of the kidney graft. Autosomal dominant **polycystic** kidney disease, renal dysplasia, Alport's syndrome, interstitial nephritis, and chronic pyelonephritis are examples of renal diseases that do not recur in the transplanted kidney. The ESRDs of renal amyloidosis, cystinosis, and Fabry's disease are all potentially treatable with renal transplantation despite significant recurrence. Type I primary hyperoxaluria **rapidly recurs in the kidney graft, and this disease is best treated with combined liver and kidney transplantation** (Watts et al, 1991).

Active Infection

Potential sources of dental sepsis must be treated. Immunizations against pneumococcal pneumonia, hepatitis B, diphtheria, tetanus, and influenza are commonly done before transplantation. Patients who have not had varicella zoster infection can also be immunized before the transplantation. Chest x-ray films and tuberculin skin tests are used to screen for pulmonary infection, and infections or skin test conversions must be satisfactorily treated before the transplantation. Patients with active cholecystitis or diabetics with cholelithiasis should undergo cholecystectomy before transplantation.

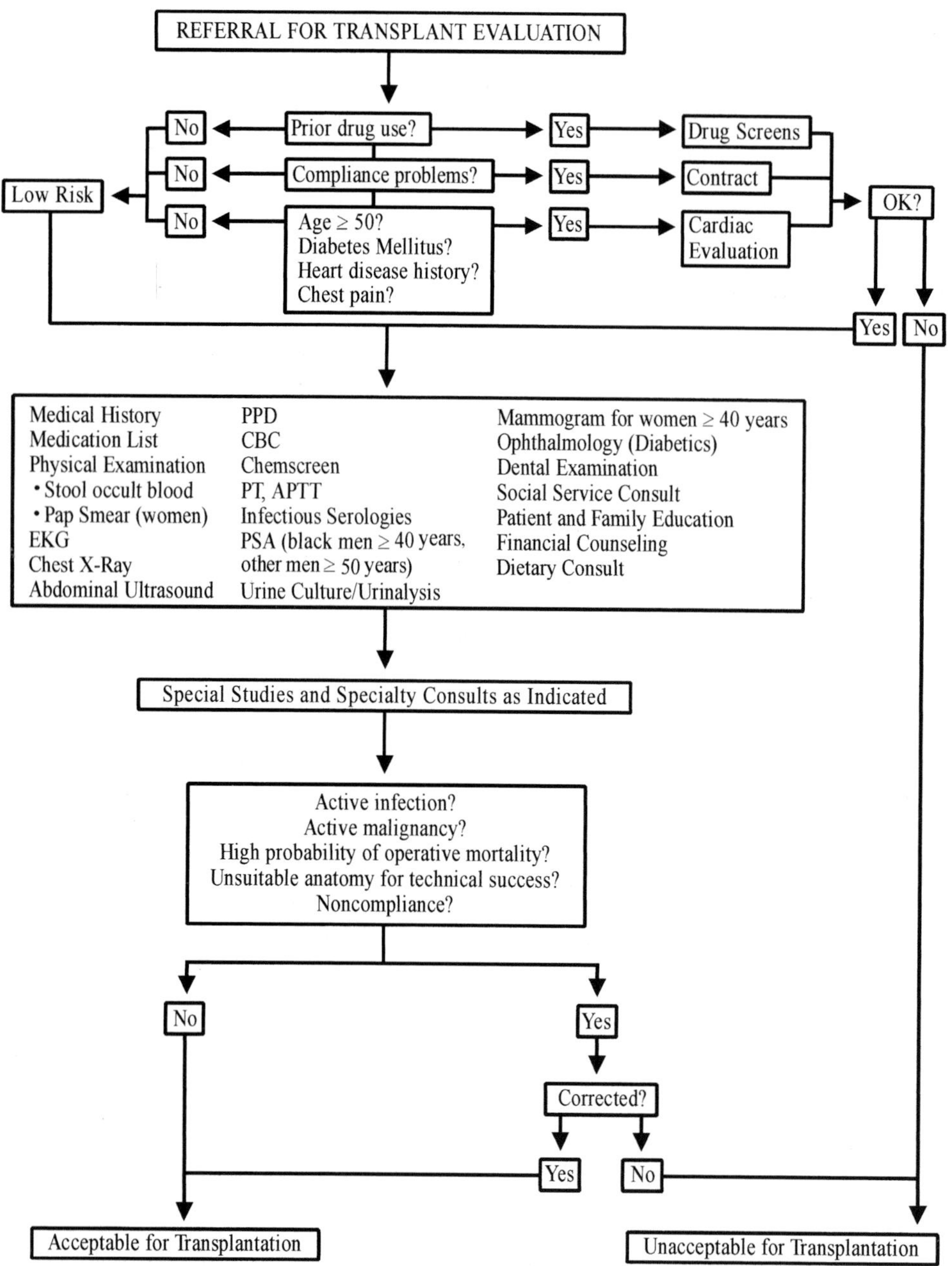

Figure 14–1. Algorithm for the evaluation of renal transplant candidates. Circumstances may change the order in which data are obtained. EKG, electrocardiogram; CBC, complete blood cell count; PPD, tuberculin test; PT, prothrombin time; PSA, prostate-specific antigen; APTT, activated partial thromboplastin time. (Modified from Lemmers MJ, Barry JM: Curr Opin Urol 1993; 3:110.)

Patients who decline cholecystectomy for asymptomatic gallstones should be warned about the possible increased risk of life-threatening cholecystitis with immunosuppression. Prophylactic segmental colectomy is advised for patients with recent diverticulitis (Church et al, 1986). Chronic active hepatitis is a major cause of mortality in the late post-transplantation period. The most common causes of chronic liver disease in renal transplant recipients are hepatitis B and hepatitis C. Patients who are shown on biopsy to have chronic active hepatitis should be advised that they may be at increased risk of dying of hepatic failure after transplantation. Diabetic foot ulcers should be healed to prevent infection through immunosuppression.

Perioperative Morbidity or Mortality

Patients with a history of heart disease or diabetes mellitus or who are over 50 years of age commonly have a cardiac performance evaluation and, if necessary, coronary arteriography (Le et al, 1994). Significant coronary disease is treated before transplantation. Patients with documented cerebrovascular disease within the previous 6 months should be evaluated for medical or surgical therapy, and transplantation should be delayed until they have been symptom-free for at least 6 months. Peptic ulcer disease must be controlled before transplantation.

Compliance Issues

Cigarette smoking increases the risk of surgery, post-transplantation malignancies, and cardiovascular disease. It should be stopped before transplantation. Transplantation candidates with chemical dependency should have a drug- or alcohol-free period of at least 6 months before grafting.

Financial and psychosocial consultations are obtained to

identify and correct problems that could result in noncompliance: for example, the lack of funds to pay for maintenance immunosuppression, or a mental handicap that would prevent the recipient from following a post-transplantation treatment plan.

Malignancy

To reduce the risk of cancer recurrence, a minimal waiting time of 2 cancer-free years from the time of last cancer treatment is recommended for patients who have had malignancies (Kasiske et al, 1995). Shorter intervals from cancer treatment to transplantation are generally accepted for patients who have had low-grade, noninvasive papillary tumors of the bladder; small, incidentally discovered renal cell carcinomas; Clark's level I melanomas; basal cell skin cancers; and in situ carcinomas of the cervix.

Unsuitable Anatomy

Symptoms and signs of lower extremity arterial disease or a history of abdominal or pelvic vascular surgery merit a diagnostic evaluation to be certain that revascularization of a kidney graft is possible and that a steal syndrome will not result from transplantation.

Urologic Evaluation

The purpose of the pretransplantation urologic evaluation is to determine the suitability of the urinary bladder or its substitute for urinary tract reconstruction and to determine the necessity for pretransplantation nephrectomy (Barry and Lemmers, 1989; Reinberg et al, 1990). The urologic evaluation includes a history for urologic disease (tumors, stones, obstruction, reflux, infection, and urinary tract surgeries), physical examination (location of scars and abdominal catheters that may interfere with transplantation), urinalysis, urine or bladder wash culture, and ultrasonography of the abdomen and pelvis to include a postvoid bladder image, the kidneys, and the gallbladder. In the absence of a history suggesting urologic abnormalities, hematuria, bacteriuria, calculi, hydronephrosis, or significant bladder residual urine, further imaging of the urinary tract is unnecessary.

Patients with suspected voiding dysfunction with or without a history of pyelonephritis are commonly screened with a voiding cystourethrogram and then further evaluated with urodynamics and cystoscopy as necessary. If a urinary diversion or continent urinary pouch is present, a retrograde contrast study with antibiotic coverage and drainage films determine its suitability for urinary tract reconstruction during renal transplantation. Many ESRD patients with upper urinary tract diversion have bladders that are acceptable for transplantation, especially if the original reason for diversion was reflux. These defunctionalized bladders usually regain normal volume within weeks of grafting. It is wise to obtain biopsy specimens from the bladders of patients who have small, contracted bladders after multiple lower urinary tract operations. If bladder fibrosis is extensive on histologic examination and the bladder is not compliant, **autoaugmentation or augmentation cystoplasty with the ureter, stomach, ileum, ileocecal segment, or colon may be necessary before renal transplantation (Thomalla et al, 1989; Sheldon et al, 1994). Functionalized augmentation is preferable to dry augmentation because it permits continence and compliance to be documented before transplantation. An advantage of gastrocystoplasty over enterocystoplasty is the absence of metabolic acidosis with the former.** These patients usually require clean intermittent catheterization after grafting. A bladder wash for cytologic examination is recommended for patients with prior cyclophosphamide treatment because of reports of associated transitional cell carcinoma (Pedersen-Bjergaard et al, 1988; Tuttle et al, 1988).

Clean, intermittent catheterization has been used successfully for more than a decade in transplant recipients with diabetes mellitus, meningomyelocele, or transient bladder outlet obstruction (Shneidman et al, 1984). Continent intestinal pouches have been created before transplantation in patients with surgically absent bladders, and renal transplantation has been successful (Hatch, 1994). Before transplantation, these pouches usually require daily irrigations for mucus removal and to maintain volume.

Men with obstructing prostates who require surgical relief of bladder outlet obstruction are managed with pretransplantation prostatectomy or transurethral incision of the bladder neck and prostate. If the patient has oligoanuria, a suprapubic cystostomy placed at the time of bladder outlet surgery allows the patient to instill sterile water and void daily until the operative site has healed, usually within 6 weeks. This prevents scarring or obliteration of the prostatic fossa. An alternative to suprapubic cystostomy and daily bladder instillation is daily intermittent self-catheterization, with bladder filling and then voiding.

Generally accepted indications for pretransplantation nephrectomy are hypertension uncontrolled by dialysis and medications; persistent renal infection; renal calculi; renal obstruction; severe proteinuria; persistent antiglomerular basement membrane antibodies; acquired renal cystic disease with tumors; and polycystic kidney disease with infection, severe bleeding, or significant enlargement that prevents transplantation into the iliac fossa. The incidence of renal cell carcinoma is estimated to be 6 to 30 times higher in patients with acquired renal cystic disease than in the general population, especially when the estimated weight of each involved kidney exceeds 150 g (MacDougall et al, 1990). Severe nephrotic syndrome can be managed by renal infarction and nephrectomy avoided. Pretransplantation nephrectomy is usually performed 6 weeks before transplantation to allow wound healing and the detection and treatment of surgical complications. The use of synthetic erythropoietin has reduced the effects of pretransplantation anemia while the patient awaits transplantation. Although laparoscopic or retroperitoneoscopic nephrectomies have been performed in these patients (Fuchs et al, 1995), bilateral vertical lumbotomies are quickly performed and well tolerated by patients with small kidneys undergoing nephrectomy (Freed, 1976). This procedure is illustrated in Figure 14–2. A flank approach is used when the patient is very obese or very muscular or when a kidney is too large to remove via vertical lumbotomy. The abdominal approach is used when both

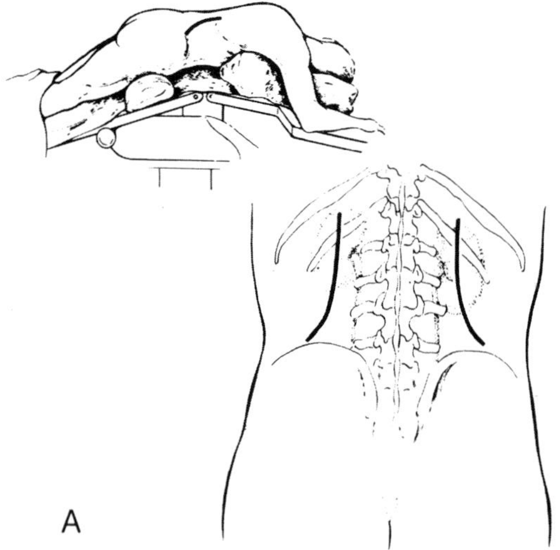

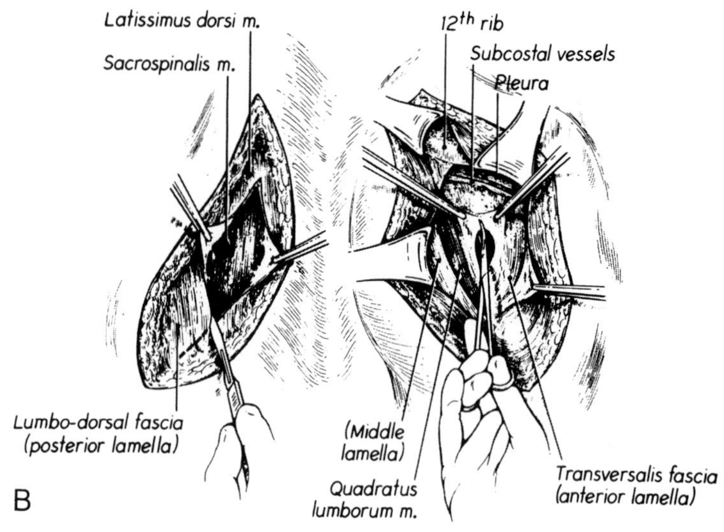

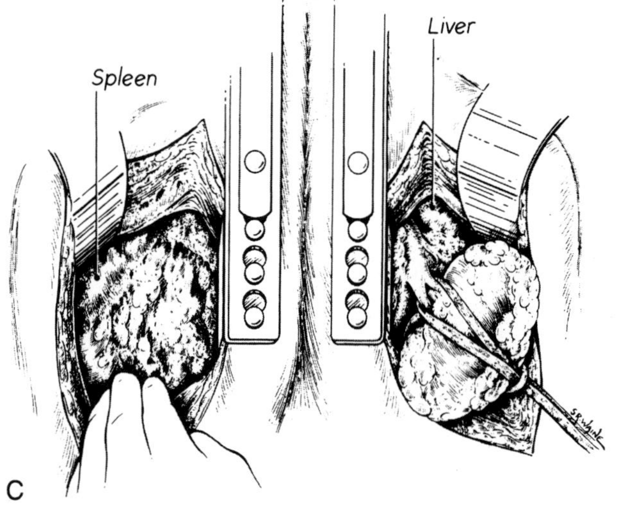

Figure 14–2. *A,* Prone position for bilateral removal of small end-stage kidneys. See text for indications. *B,* Simultaneous bilateral dissection. *C,* Self-retaining retractor with blades reversed facilitates exposure of renal pedicles. The incision can be extended by removing a section of the neck of the 12th rib. (From Freed SZ: J Urol 1976; 115:811.)

kidneys are removed from a large patient, when the kidneys are too large to remove through the back, or when additional procedures, such as total ureterectomy, intestinal conduit removal, augmentation cystoplasty, or the creation of a continent intestinal pouch are planned at the same time.

Impotence is a significant problem in men with ESRD. Contributing factors are the accelerated arteriosclerosis associated with dialysis, hyperprolactinemia with secondary testosterone deficiency, side effects from antihypertensives, and a poor self-image. If penile prosthesis surgery is necessary before renal transplantation, one of the semirigid devices is recommended because the risk of reoperation is less than that with the inflatable devices and because no prevesical reservoir is present to interfere with urinary tract reconstruction. If an inflatable device is selected, one that is self-contained or that has a scrotal reservoir is advisable.

An algorithm for dialysis access is presented in Figure 14–3. The exit site for a chronic ambulatory peritoneal dialysis catheter should be placed well away from any potential kidney transplant incision, and it has been recommended that the external tubing point downward to reduce the risk of tunnel infection.

DONOR SELECTION, PREPARATION, AND SURGERY

Goals

Whether the kidney is removed from a living donor or from a brain-dead cadaver donor, the surgical goals are to minimize warm ischemia time, to preserve renal vessels, and to preserve ureteral blood supply. In the cadaver donor, it is also necessary to obtain histocompatibility specimens. The basic criteria for a renal donor are the absence of renal disease, absence of active infection, and absence of transmissible malignancy.

Living Donor

Evaluation

On the basis of the preoperative evaluation, the physician must be able to assure the donor of nearly normal renal function after unilateral nephrectomy. On evaluation, if one

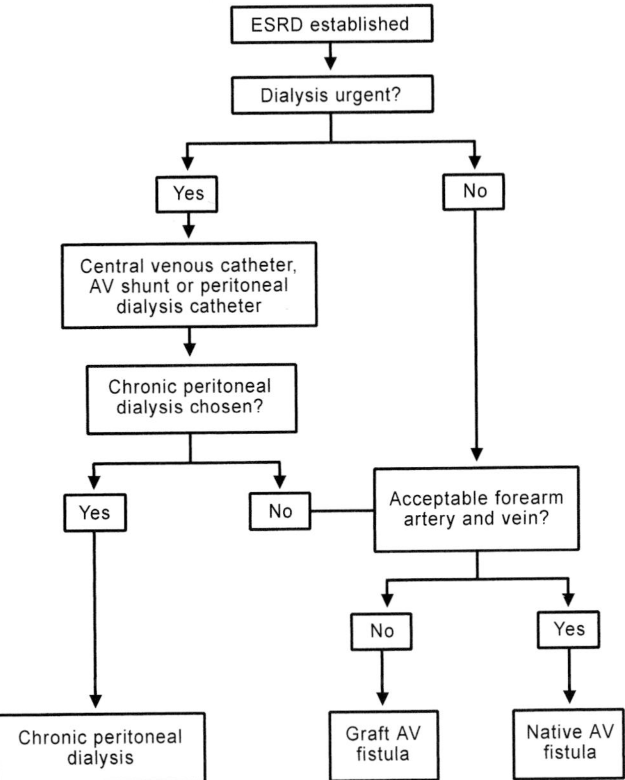

Figure 14–3. Algorithm for decision making in dialysis access surgery. ESRD, end-stage renal disease; AV, arteriovenous.

of the potential donor's kidneys is better than the other, the better kidney is left with the donor. Some surgeons prefer to use the right kidney from women who may become pregnant, because hydronephrosis of pregnancy occurs predominantly in that kidney. An algorithm for the evaluation of a living renal donor is presented in Figure 14–4. Circumstances may change the order in which data are obtained. A living renal donor is considered to be unsuitable when one of the following is present: significant mental dysfunction; significant renal disease; a high risk of perioperative mortality or morbidity; significant transmissible disease; ABO incompatibility; or a positive cross-match between donor lymphocytes and recipient serum. Serologic screening is performed for human immune deficiency virus (HIV), human T-lymphoproliferative virus type I (HTLV-I), hepatitis, cytomegalovirus (CMV), and syphilis. Some programs also screen for Epstein-Barr virus (Bia et al, 1995). When the potential recipient is diabetic, a glucose tolerance test is performed in the prospective donor to exclude, as much as possible, diabetes mellitus. Abdominal ultrasonography can be performed to exclude donors with significant renal abnormalities and to detect incidental intra-abdominal abnormalities. Although excretory urography and abdominal aortography with selected renal arteriography have been the standard studies to determine a living donor's renal anatomy, satisfactory results have been reported with digital subtraction arteriography, magnetic resonance imaging, and, most recently, renal computed tomography (CT) with three-dimensional angiography (Alfrey et al, 1995; Lindgren et al, 1995). In comparison with conventional arteriography, three-dimensional CT angiography offers the advantages of being less invasive, more rapid to perform and less expensive, with less radiation exposure.

Technique

Living donor nephrectomy is usually performed through a flank incision with a rib-resecting or supracostal approach (Fig. 14–5). The donor receives 25 g of mannitol in a 1-hour dose infusion beginning with the skin incision, and intravenous fluids, usually 1 L/hour, are given to maintain diuresis. Overnight hydration of the living donor is unnecessary. Diuresis is confirmed by transecting the ureter and observing urine flow before interrupting renal circulation. After nephrectomy, the kidney is immediately placed in a pan of ice-cold solution and flushed with Ringer's lactate, Collins 2, Euro-Collins, or UW solution at 4°C. It is not necessary to administer heparin to the living renal donor. The kidney is then taken in an ice bath into the recipient's operating room or cold-stored until the time of transplantation if that procedure is delayed. The donor's wound is irrigated and usually closed without drainage, and the donor taken to the recovery room, where a chest x-ray film is obtained to exclude the possibility of pneumothorax. The complications are those of a standard flank nephrectomy. **Hyperfiltration injury has not been a problem for living renal donors.** Endogenous creatinine clearance rapidly approaches 70% to 80% of the preoperative level, and this has been shown to be sustained for more than 10 years (Vincenti et al, 1983; Najarian et al, 1992). The development of late hypertension is nearly the same as for the general population, and the development of proteinuria is negligible (Kasiske et al, 1995; Steckler et al, 1990). The rate of mortality from kidney donation has been estimated to be 0.03% and the risk of a potentially life-threatening or permanently debilitating complication, to be 0.23%; there are isolated reports of ESRD developing in renal donors (Bia et al, 1995). The short-term and long-term risks of living donor nephrectomy are generally considered to be low enough, and the probability of successful graft outcome high enough, to make the risks acceptable for fully informed donors.

Cadaver Donor

Brain Death

The declaration of brain death is the responsibility of the potential cadaver organ donor's physician.

Criteria

The usual criteria for potential cadaver organ donors are ages 18 months to 55 years, no hypertension requiring treatment, no diabetes mellitus, no malignancy other than primary brain tumor or treated superficial skin cancer, no generalized viral or bacterial infection, normal renal function, acceptable urinalysis, and negative assays for syphilis, hepatitis, HIV, and HTLV. Blood cultures are performed if the donor has been hospitalized for more than 72 hours. Eighteen months is the lower age limit for cadaver renal donors because of small anatomic parts and the risk of technical problems, although there are reports of kidneys from

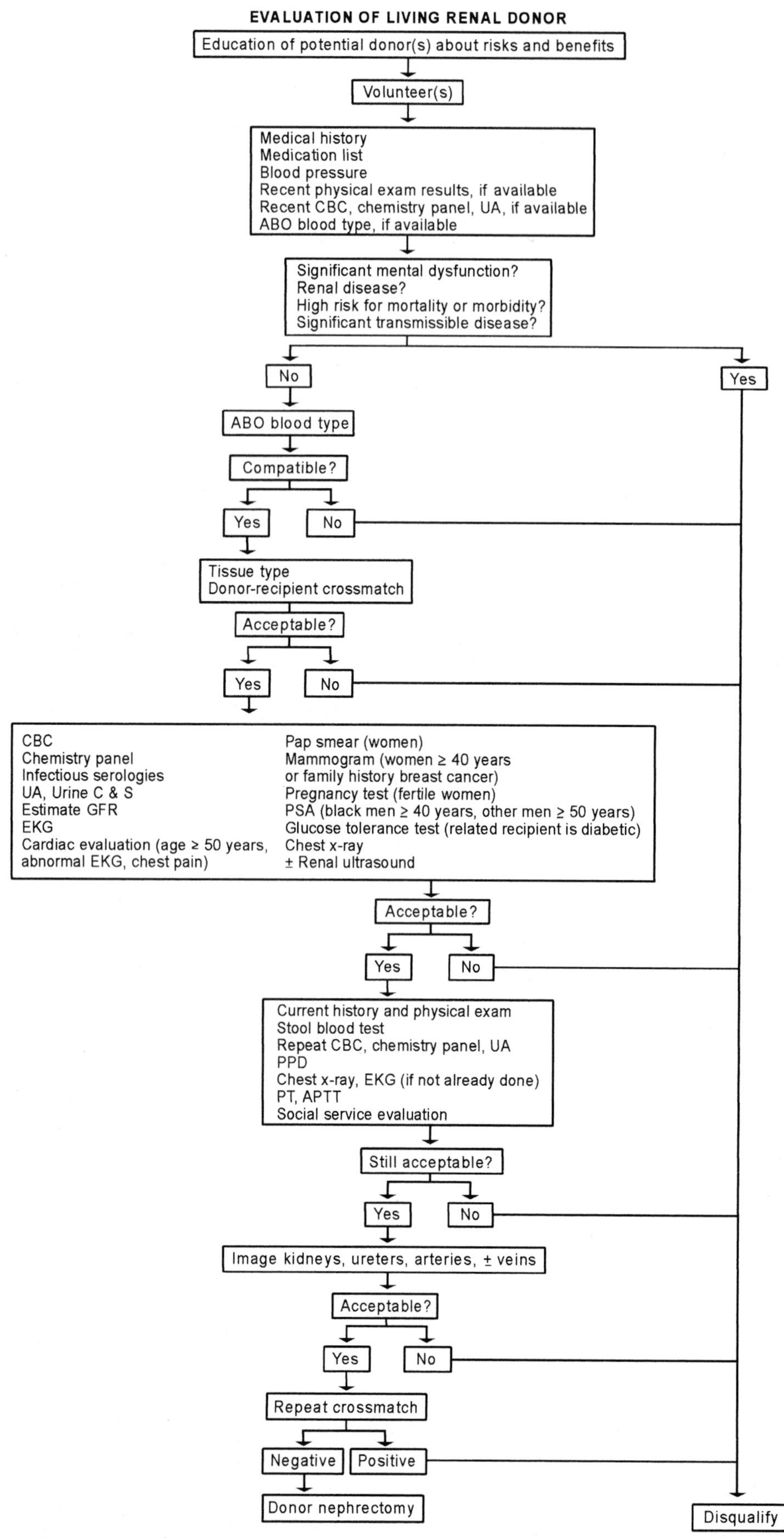

Figure 14–4. Algorithm for the evaluation of living renal donors. CBC, complete blood cell count; EKG, electrocardiogram, PSA, prostate-specific antigen; PT, prothrombin time; PPD, tuberculin test; GFR, glomerular filtration rate; UA, urinalysis; APTT, activated partial thromboplastin time.

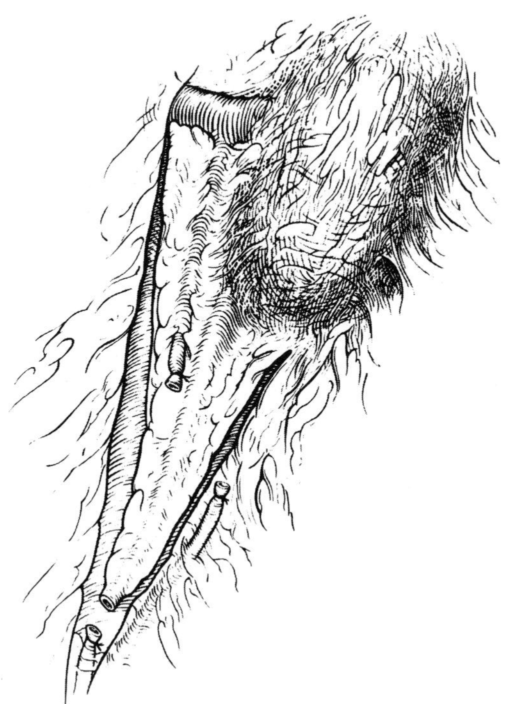

Figure 14–5. Living donor nephrectomy via a flank approach. A generous amount of periureteral tissue remains to preserve ureteral blood supply. Renal circulation is not interrupted until a diuresis is ensured from the proximal end of the divided ureter. (From Streem SB: Live donor nephrectomy. *In* Novick AC, Streem SB, Pontes JE, eds: *Stewart's Operative Urology,* Baltimore, Williams & Wilkins Co., 1989, pp 312–323.)

younger donors functioning satisfactorily (Salvatierra and Belzer, 1975; Hudnall et al, 1989). Fifty-five years is the upper age limit because of nephrosclerosis, although exceptions are made in an effort to expand the donor pool (Alexander et al, 1994). Cadaver kidney grafts from very young ($\leq$5 years) or old (>60 years) donors are not always transplanted because graft survivals are significantly worse than those of cadaver kidney transplants from donors between the ages of 6 and 60 years (Feduska and Cecka, 1995).

Preoperative Care

The initial goals of resuscitation of the brain-dead cadaver donor are systolic blood pressure of 90 mm Hg and urinary output exceeding 0.5 ml/kg/hour. Monitoring of central venous pressure or capillary wedge pressure is helpful for managing fluid administration (Soifer and Gelb, 1989; Boyd, et al, 1991). Serum electrolyte levels are checked every 2 to 4 hours. If the resuscitation goals cannot be met by fluid challenge and the central venous pressure is greater than 15 cm H_2O, dopamine or dobutamine at less than 10 μg/kg/minute can be infused without causing renal vasospasm. If bradycardia does not respond to dopamine or low-dose epinephrine, a temporary pacemaker can be inserted. If intravascular volume expansion and vasopressors are unsuccessful in promoting a diuresis, 1 mg/kg of furosemide with or without 0.5 to 1.0 g/kg of mannitol can be infused. If diabetes insipidus causes unmanageable diuresis, 0.5 to 5 units of aqueous vasopressin per hour can be infused to reduce urinary output. Because hypothermia can cause cardiac irritability and coagulopathy, the head can be wrapped, intravenous fluids can be warmed, and the body can be placed on a warming blanket. Tissue typing and cross-matching can be performed on a peripheral blood sample or groin lymph nodes before organ retrieval. The cadaver donor is maintained in the operating room by the anesthesiology team to ensure ventilation and circulatory support and so that they can administer drugs such as diuretics, heparin, and alpha-blocking agents.

Technique

Most renal donors are now multiple organ donors, and the classic abdominal midline and cruciate incisions have been largely abandoned in favor of the total midline approach with median sternotomy (Fig. 14–6), even when kidneys alone are retrieved (Barry, 1989). The principles of cadaver donor organ retrieval are adequate exposure; control of the great vessels above and below the organs to be removed; initiation of preservation in situ; removal of the organs; separation of the organs; completion of preservation; removal of histocompatibility specimens; removal of iliac vessels for vascular reconstruction of pancreas and liver grafts; and organ packaging. The technical aspects of one en bloc method are illustrated in Figure 14–6 (Nakazato et al, 1992; Barry, 1996). Some retrieval teams prefer to do much more dissection in situ before organ removal. When that occurs, the kidneys are the last transplantable organs to be removed.

KIDNEY PRESERVATION

Cellular Injury

Warm ischemic injury is due to failure of oxidative phosphorylation and cell death due to adenosine triphosphate (ATP) depletion (Belzer and Southard, 1988). ATP is required for the cellular sodium-potassium pump to maintain a high intracellular concentration of potassium and a low internal concentration of sodium. When the sodium-potassium pump is impaired, sodium chloride and water passively diffuse into the cells, resulting in cellular swelling and the "no reflow" phenomenon with renal revascularization. Cellular potassium and magnesium are lost, calcium is gained, anaerobic glycolysis and acidosis occur, and lysosomal enzymes are activated. This results in cellular suicide. During reperfusion, hypoxanthine, a product of ATP degradation, is oxidized to xanthine with the formation of free radicals, which cause further cell damage.

Principles of Simple Cold Storage of Kidneys

Cellular energy requirements are significantly reduced by hypothermia. This is done by surface cooling, hypothermic pulsatile perfusion, or flushing with an ice-cold solution followed by cold storage. Making the flushing solution slightly hyperosmolar with impermeable solutes such as mannitol, lactobionate, raffinose, or hydroxyethyl starch helps prevent endothelial cell swelling and the no-reflow

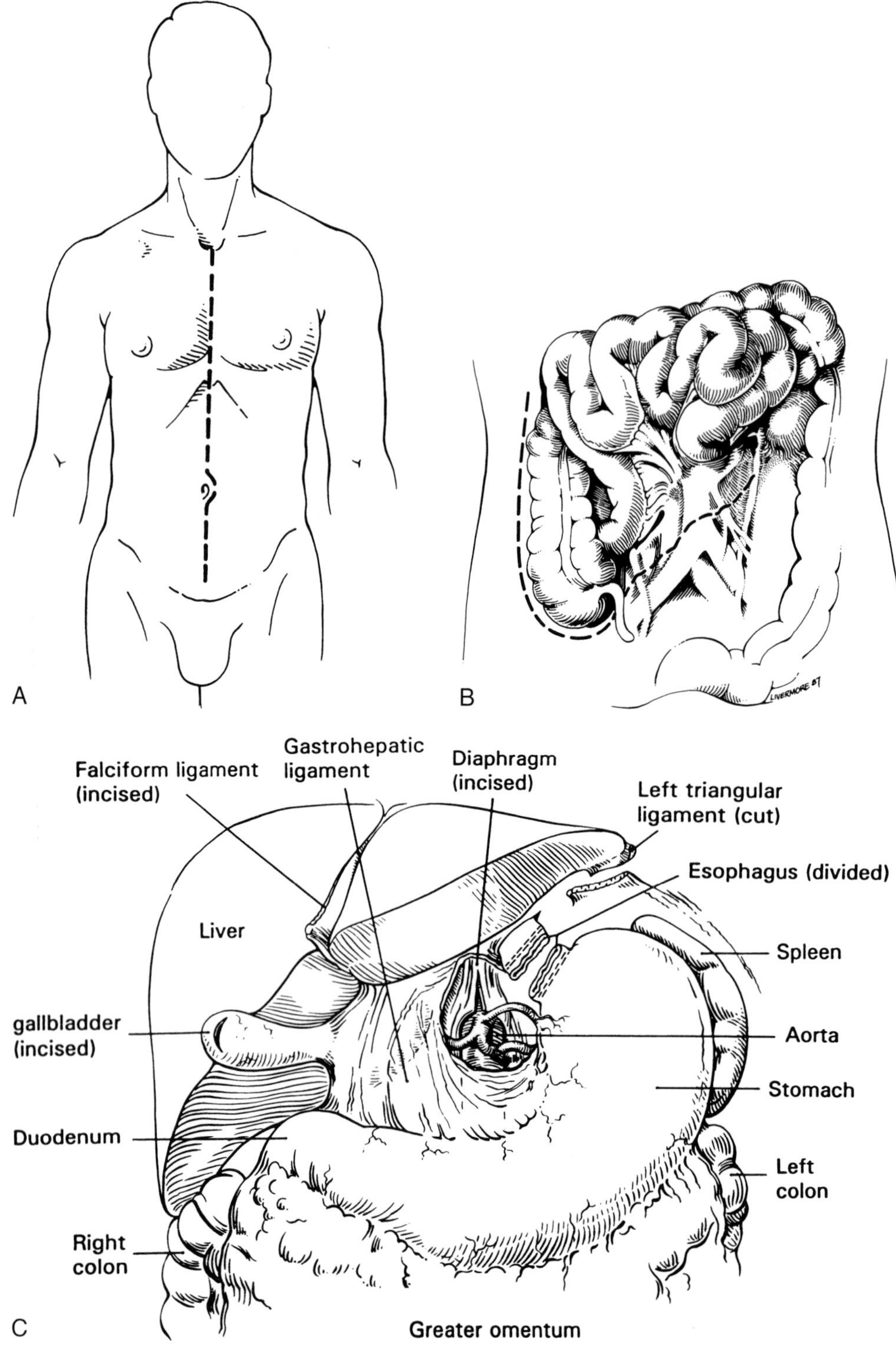

Figure 14–6. *A,* Total midline incision with splitting of the sternum and diaphragm exposes all transplantable organs in the chest and abdomen. It also provides excellent exposure when retrieving only abdominal organs. *B,* The retroperitoneum is exposed as for a retroperitoneal lymphadenectomy. *C,* For multiple abdominal organ retrieval, the aorta is controlled above the celiac axis. The inferior vena cava (IVC) is controlled above the liver (not shown).

phenomenon. When the sodium-potassium pump is impaired, there is passive transfer of ions across the cell membrane, and if the electrolyte composition of the flushing solution is nearly the same as that inside the cell, electrolyte balance is maintained. ATP-$MgCl_2$ infusions have been evaluated as an energy source. Calcium channel blockers, xanthine oxidase inhibitors, free radical scavengers, and lysosome stabilizers such as methylprednisolone have all been used to reduce ischemic injury (Marshall et al, 1994).

Clinical Kidney Transplant Preservation

The basic methods of kidney preservation are pulsatile machine perfusion with a protein-based solution (Belzer et al, 1967) and hypothermic flushing followed by simple cold storage (Collins et al, 1969). After demonstration that the two methods provided equivalent results with ideally harvested dog kidneys after 48 hours of preservation (Halasz and Collins, 1976), simple cold storage became more widely

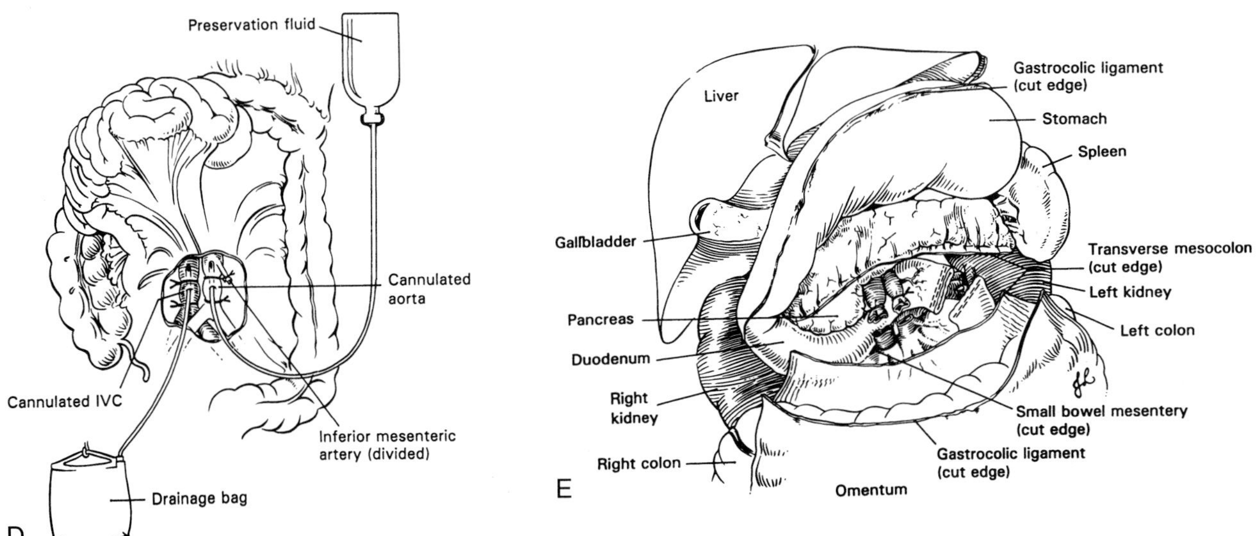

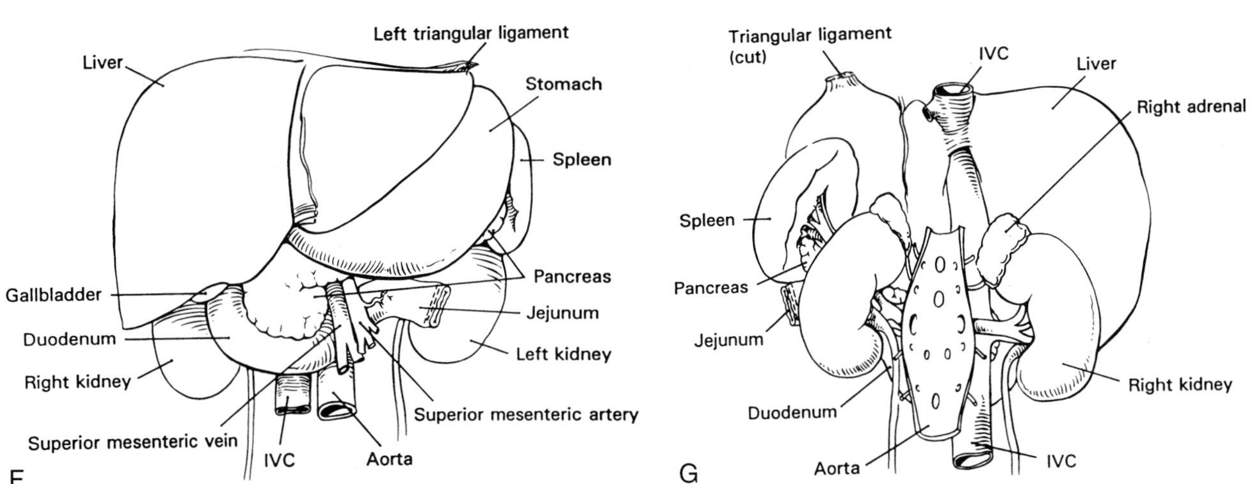

Figure 14–6 *Continued D,* The aorta and IVC are controlled below the renal vessels, heparin is administered to the donor, and the great vessels are cannulated. The proximal aorta is occluded; the IVC is vented into the chest or through the distal IVC cannula; and in situ flushing with an ice cold preservation solution is performed through the aortic cannula. *E,* The gastrocolic ligament is divided, the small bowel mesentery is divided along with the superior mesenteric artery and vein, and the small bowel is divided at the ligament of Treitz. *F,* The esophagus is divided, and, with further dissection, the en bloc specimen consisting of the liver, stomach, spleen, pancreas, both kidneys, aorta, and IVC is removed. *G,* The specimen is placed "face down" in a pan of slush and is separated, first by splitting the aorta posteriorly between the lumbar arteries to identify all renal arteries, second by transecting the aorta between the superior mesenteric artery and the renal arteries, third by splitting the anterior aortic wall between the renal arteries, fourth by transecting the IVC just above the entrance of the renal veins, and fifth by dividing the left renal vein where it enters the IVC. (*A* and *B* from Barry JM: Cadaver donor nephrectomy. *In* Novick AC, Streem SB, Pontes JL, eds: Stewart's Operative Urology. Baltimore, Williams & Wilkins Co., 1989, pp 294–300. *C* to *G* from Barry JM: Donor nephrectomy. *In* Marshall FF, ed: Textbook of Operative Urology. Philadelphia, W. B. Saunders Co., 1996, pp 235–247.)

used for human kidney preservation. Machine perfusion has provided reliable human kidney preservation for 72 hours (Feduska et al, 1978), and there are reports of successfully extending the preservation time for 48 to 95 hours with cold storage alone or in combination with machine perfusion (Haberal et al, 1984). A review of 38,057 cadaver kidney transplants demonstrated no significant differences in graft survivals up to 3 years for kidneys that were preserved by pulsatile machine perfusion or simple cold storage (Gjertson, 1995). The commonly used flushing solutions are compared in Table 14–2. The UW solution (Belzer and Southard, 1988) minimizes cellular swelling with the impermeable solutes lactobionate, raffinose, and hydroxyethyl starch. Phosphate is used for its hydrogen ion buffering qualities; adenosine is for ATP synthesis during reperfusion; glutathione is a free radical scavenger; allopurinol inhibits xanthine oxidase and the generation of free radicals; and magnesium and dexamethasone are membrane-stabilizing agents. A major advantage of this preservation solution has been its utility as a universal preservation solution for all intra-abdominal organs. A prospectively randomized study of 695 cadaver kidney grafts preserved with either UW solution or Euro-Collins solution showed that the UW solution resulted in a significantly more rapid reduction in postoperative serum creatinine levels, a significantly lower postoperative dialysis rate, and a 6% higher 1-year graft survival than did Euro-

Table 14–2. COMMONLY USED HYPOTHERMIC RENAL PRESERVATION SOLUTIONS

UW Solution		Intracellular Electrolyte Flush Solutions		
			Approximate Amount in 1 L	
Substance	***Amount in 1 L***	***Substance***	*Collins 2*	*Euro-Collins*
Potassium lactobionate	100 mmol	KH_2PO_4	15 mmol	15 mmol
KH_2PO_4	25 mmol	$MgSO_4$	30 mmol	0
$MgSO_4$	5 mmol	KCl	15 mmol	15 mmol
Raffinose	30 mmol	K_2HPO_4	42.5 mmol	42.5 mmol
Adenosine	5 mmol	$NaHCO_3$	10 mmol	10 mmol
Glutathione	3 mmol	Glucose	25 g	35 g
Allopurinol	1 mmol			
Hydroxyethyl starch	50 g			
Insulin	100 units			
Dexamethasone	8 mg			
Trimethoprim-sulfamethoxazole solution	5 ml			
or				
Penicillin	200,000 units			

UW, University of Wisconsin.

Collins solution (Ploeg et al, 1992). Animal experiments have shown satisfactory kidney preservation up to 72 hours with UW solution (Ploeg et al, 1988).

The detrimental effects of the events surrounding cadaver kidney retrieval and of preservation injury are shown by the 13% better 1-year graft survival for 256 primary living unrelated donor kidney transplants than for 33,840 primary cadaver kidney transplants (Geffner et al, 1995).

RECIPIENT SELECTION FOR CADAVER KIDNEY TRANSPLANTS

Point System

A point system that has evolved in the United States for the selection of cadaver kidney transplant recipients is presented in Table 14–3 (UNOS, 1995). Initial screening consists of ABO blood group compatibility determination and negative microcytotoxicity lymphocyte cross-matching between donor and recipient. Patients whose serum reacts to a high proportion of lymphocytes on a random or selected panel receive additional points because the probability of obtaining a cross-match–negative kidney for them is decreased in comparison with minimally sensitized transplantation candidates. Time on the waiting list and histocompatibility between donor and recipient result in additional points. For example, assume that there are 20 potential blood group O cadaver kidney recipients for a cross-match–negative blood group O adult kidney graft. Each of the 20 is ranked by the time of waiting on the list. The patient who has been waiting the longest is given 1 point, the one who has been most recently added to the list receives 1/20 point, and the others are assigned fractions of a point depending on their time-of-waiting rank. A patient who has been waiting for 2 years receives an additional 2 × 0.5, or 1, point. If the panel-reactive antibody is ≥80%, 4 more points are added. Histocompatibility points are assigned for HLA mismatches of HLA-B and HLA-DR with the cadaver donor according to the table. Additional points are assigned to potential recipients under the age of 18 years, and each of the potential recipients now has a total point score. The candidates are then placed in rank order by that score, and the patient with the highest score is ranked number 1. The kidney graft is then offered in turn to each of the potential recipients by the final rank. If there is no suitable recipient on the local list, the kidney graft is offered to those on the regional list and, if necessary, the national list. Currently there is mandatory kidney sharing when there are zero HLA-A, HLA-B, and HLA-DR antigens mismatched between a cadaver donor and a recipient on the national waiting list.

Table 14–3. POINT SYSTEM FOR ALLOCATION OF CADAVER KIDNEYS

Parameter	Points	Maximal Points
Time of waiting	—	1
Time of waiting ≥1	—	Additional 0.5/year
year	—	4
Panel reactivity ≥80%	—	7
Histocompatibility		
0 A, B, DR mismatch	Mandatory share	—
0 B, DR mismatch	7	—
1 B, DR mismatch	5	—
2 B, DR mismatch	2	—
Recipient age (years)	—	4
0–10	4	—
11–18	3	—

Adapted from United Network for Organ Sharing (UNOS): Articles of Incorporation, By-Laws and Policies: Policy 3.5, Allocation of Cadaveric Kidneys. Richmond, VA, UNOS, June 28, 1995.

Cytomegalovirus

Some programs do not transplant kidneys from CMV-seropositive donors into CMV-seronegative recipients who have insulin-dependent diabetes or are over the age of 50 years because of the morbidity of new CMV infection in high-risk recipients (Hennel et al, 1989). Prophylaxis is possible with immunoglobulin (Steinmuller et al, 1989), acyclovir (Dunn et al, 1994), or ganciclovir (Markham and Faulds, 1994) when there is significant risk of CMV infection or reactivation of CMV disease.

Admission for Surgery

On urgent admission for cadaver kidney transplantation, a history and physical examination of the recipient focuses on a search for acute invasive infections, interval medical problems such as symptomatic cardiac disease, and the need for additional cross-matching because of recent blood transfusions.

RECIPIENT OPERATION

A prophylactic antibiotic, usually a second-generation cephalosporin, is administered just before surgery and continued postoperatively until the results of intraoperative cultures are known. Immunosuppression is sometimes started 1 week before transplantation in the recipient of a living-donor kidney and just before or during surgery in the recipient of a cadaver kidney.

Technique

After induction of anesthesia and placement of a central venous pressure monitor, the genitalia and skin are prepared, and a Foley catheter is placed in the bladder or bladder substitute. The bladder or bladder substitute is rinsed with a broad-spectrum antibiotic solution, such as neomycin–polymyxin B, and is gravity-filled to capacity, and then the catheter tubing is clamped until the time of the ureteroneocystostomy. It is sometimes helpful to have the catheter attached to a three-way drainage system that allows intraoperative filling and draining of the bladder, especially in a small recipient or in an individual who has a small, defunctionalized bladder. A self-retaining ring retractor bolted to the operating table allows the operation to be performed by a surgeon and one assistant. Antibiotic irrigation is used liberally during the procedure. Central venous pressure is maintained between 5 and 15 cm H_2O with intravenous fluids. If the mean arterial pressure or the systolic blood pressure cannot be maintained at ≥70 mm Hg or ≥90 mm Hg, respectively, with fluid administration, dopamine or dobutamine infusion is started.

In adults and large children, the kidney graft is usually placed extraperitoneally in the contralateral iliac fossa via a rectus muscle–preserving Gibson incision. This allows the renal pelvis and ureter to be the most medial structures in case subsequent urinary tract surgery on the kidney graft is necessary. In men, the spermatic cord is mobilized, preserved, and medially retracted. In women, the round ligament is divided between ligatures. The recipient's blood vessels are dissected, and lymphatics are divided between ligatures to avoid the development of postoperative lymphocele. The surgeon should be careful not to mistake the genitofemoral nerve for a lymphatic. Before the use of donor inferior vena cava to provide extension of the right renal vein in cadaver kidney transplants (Barry and Fuchs, 1978; Corry and Kelley, 1978), the left kidney was preferred because of its longer renal vein. Methods of extending the right renal vein are illustrated in Figure 14–7.

Before temporary vascular occlusion, heparin (30 units/kg) is given intravenously to the recipient. During the vascular anastomosis, an infusion of mannitol (0.5 to 1.0 g/kg) is begun, to act as a free-radical scavenger and to promote diuresis. An electrolyte solution infusion (30 to 50 ml/kg) provides intraoperative volume expansion. The addition of an albumin infusion (1.0 to 1.5 g/kg) has been found to be helpful in promoting early renal function in the cadaver kidney transplant (Dawidson and Ar'Rajab, 1993). The renal artery is usually anastomosed to the end of the internal iliac artery (Fig. 14–8). It is preferable to do the renal artery anastomosis first because it is the more critical of the two vascular anastomoses and iliac venous occlusion can be delayed until after the renal artery anastomosis. This results in decreased iliac venous occlusion time and reduces the risk of iliofemoral venous thrombosis. Techniques for the management of multiple renal arteries are shown in Figure 14–9.

Moderate arteriosclerosis of the internal iliac artery can be managed by endarterectomy. In the event of significant arteriosclerosis of that vessel, the renal artery is anastomosed end to side to the external iliac artery or to the common iliac artery. An aortic punch is useful for creating a round hole in a rigid or arteriosclerotic vessel. When the pelvic vessels are unsuitable for renal revascularization, orthotopic

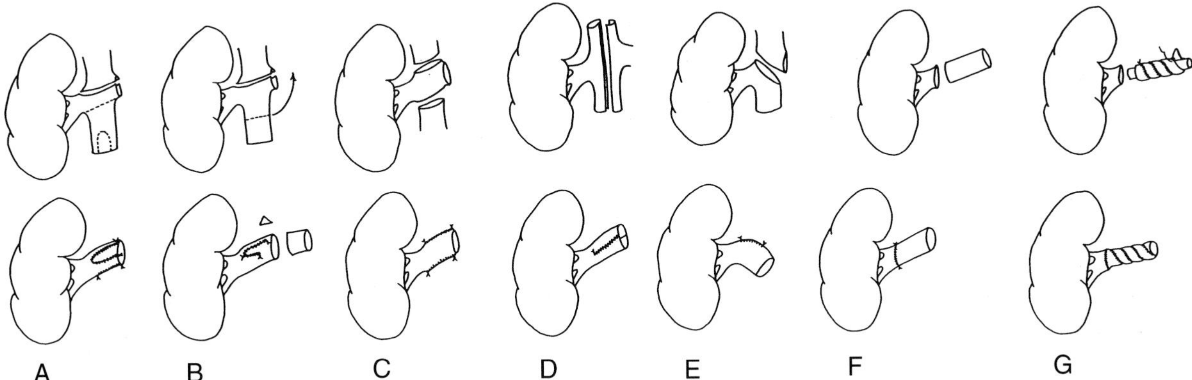

Figure 14–7. Methods of extending the right renal vein include modifications of the inferior vena cava, a free graft of donor external iliac vein, and a spiral graft of recipient gonadal vein. The first two methods are valuable when the cephalad portion of the right renal vein has been compromised by the separation of the liver graft from the kidney grafts. (*A* and *B* from Barry JM, Lemmers MJ: J Urol 1995; 153:1803. *C* from Barry JM, Fuchs EF: Arch Surg 1978; 113:300. *D* and *F* from Barry JM, Hefty TR, Sasaki T: J Urol 1988; 140:1479. *E* from Corry RJ, Kelley SE: Am J Surg 1978; 135:867. *G* from Nghiem DD: J Urol 1989; 142:1525.)

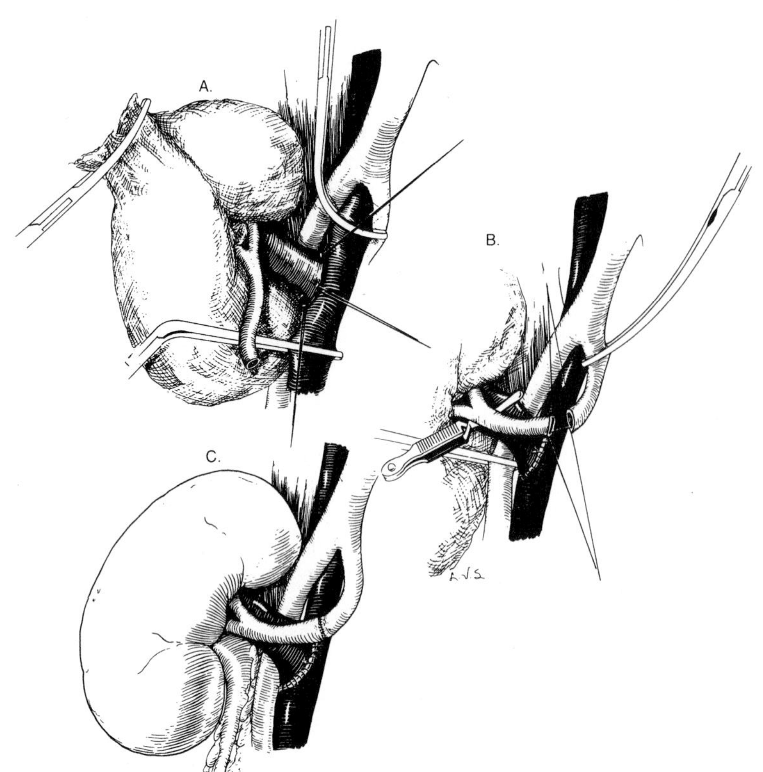

Figure 14–8. *A,* The renal vein is anastomosed to the external iliac vein, usually medial to the external iliac artery. When the recipient has a tortuous external iliac artery, the venous anastomosis is commonly performed lateral to the bowed external iliac artery. *B,* In the absence of significant recipient arteriosclerosis, the renal artery is anastomosed to the internal iliac artery with 5–0 or 6–0 monofilament, nonabsorbable sutures. Many prefer to perform the renal artery anastomosis before the venous anastomosis. *C,* The completed venous and arterial anastomoses. (*A, B,* and *C* from Salvatierra O Jr: Renal transplantation. *In* Glenn JF, ed: Urologic Surgery, 3rd ed. Philadelphia, J. B. Lippincott Co., 1983, pp 362–366.)

renal transplantation with anastomosis of the renal artery to the splenic artery or native renal artery, and venous reconstruction with the renal vein or inferior vena cava, can be done (Gil-Vernet et al, 1989). A male candidate for a second kidney graft whose first transplant was anastomosed to the contralateral internal iliac artery should not have the ipsilateral internal iliac artery used, to ensure a blood supply to the corpora cavernosa and to reduce the risk of arteriogenic impotence (Gittes and Waters, 1979). The renal vein, with or without an extension, is usually anastomosed end to side to the external iliac vein. When the renal vein is short, it is helpful to completely mobilize the external iliac vein by dividing the posterior branches between ligatures. After release of the vascular clamps and control of bleeding, some operators inject up to 10 mg of verapamil, a calcium channel blocker, into the renal arterial circulation of the cadaver kidney graft to protect the kidney from ischemic injury (Dawidson and Ar'Rajab, 1993).

Urinary tract reconstruction is usually by antireflux ureteroneocystostomy. Ureteroureterostomy and pyeloureterostomy are usually reserved for patients with short or ischemic allograft ureters or for patients with very limited bladder capacity. Many surgeons prefer the extravesical rather than the transvesical approach for ureteroneocystostomy because it is faster, a separate cystotomy is not required, and less ureteral length is necessary, thus ensuring distal ureteral blood supply. The transvesical approach is illustrated in Figure 14–10. The two commonly used extravesical techniques are shown in Figure 14–11. Complications requiring reoperation are rare (Gibbons et al, 1992). Regardless of the technique, ureteral stents are used when there is concern about urinary leakage or temporary obstruction due to edema or a thickened bladder, or when ureteroureterostomy or pyeloureterostomy has been performed. A prophylactic ureteral stent for all cases was recommended by Pleass and associates (1995) to reduce the incidence of urologic complications.

Patients with bladder substitutes can undergo transplantation successfully (Hatch et al, 1993; Hatch, 1994). When the transplantation is done in a patient with an intestinal conduit, the kidney graft should be placed in such a way that it does not interfere with the flat surface at the stoma site and contribute to a poor fit of the urinary appliance and subsequent urinary leakage. Standard vascular anastomoses are made, and the ureter is anastomosed to the base of the urinary conduit and protected with a stent that is left in place for 3 to 6 weeks. The technique of ureteral implantation into an intestinal pouch is the same as that for ureteroneocystostomy except that it is usually always protected by a stent. The pouch is irrigated free of mucus with an antibiotic solution, and the best site for the stented ureteral implantation is chosen with the pouch filled. Ureteral implantation into the afferent limb of a Kock pouch has been described (Heritier et al, 1989; Hatch, 1994).

Opinions about wound closure vary. The uncomplicated renal transplant can be closed without drains unless systemic anticoagulation is planned. The iliac wound is well closed by approximating the muscle and fascia as a single layer with interrupted far-far, near-near 0 synthetic absorbable sutures. If the rectus-retracting approach has been used, it is not necessary to place any sutures in the rectus muscle; the anterior rectus sheath is simply closed. A closed suction drain is recommended for the subcutaneous tissues of obese patients. Scarpa's fascia is approximated with a running layer of 3–0 absorbable suture. A running 4–0 or 5–0 absorbable subcuticular suture accurately approximates the skin edges and eliminates the need for subsequent suture or clip re-

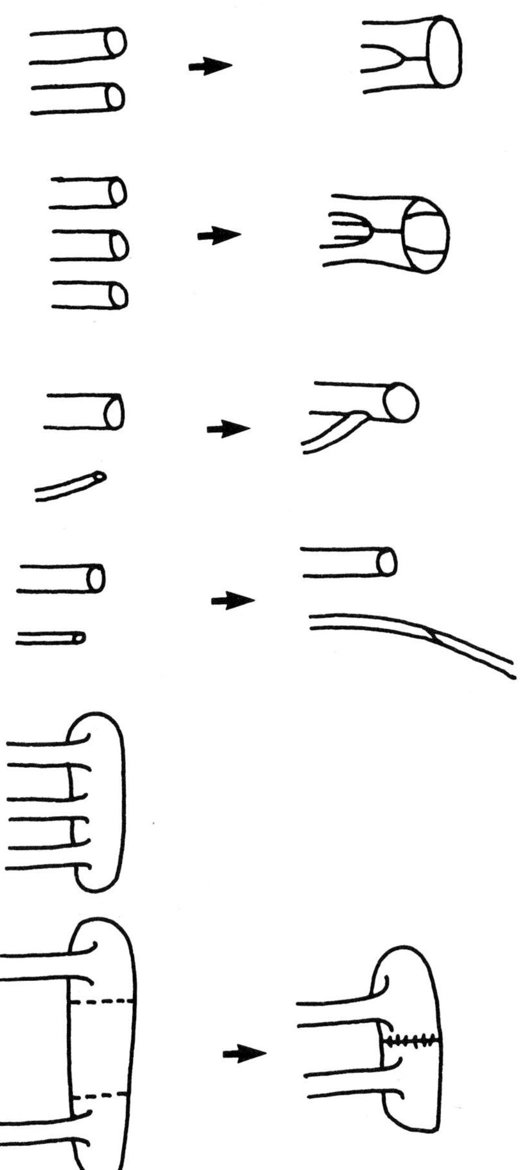

Figure 14–9. Multiple renal arteries are managed by making a "pair of pants" or a three-legged pair of pants; anastomosing a segmental renal artery to the main renal artery; anastomosing a segmental renal artery to the inferior epigastric artery; or, in the case of a cadaveric kidney, using an aortic patch or a modified aortic patch after segmental aortectomy. The main renal artery or aortic patch is then anastomosed to an appropriate-sized iliac artery or the aorta in the recipient. (Modified from Barry JM: Renal transplantation. *In* Krane RJ, Siroky MB, Fitzpatrick JM, eds: Clinical Urology. Philadelphia, J. B. Lippincott Co., 1994, p 329.)

moval. The closed suction drains are removed when the output is less than 50 ml per 24 hours.

Modifications for Pediatric Recipients

When a small child receives an adult kidney, a vertical midline abdominal approach is used; the renal artery and vein are usually anastomosed to the common iliac artery or aorta and inferior vena cava, respectively; and the graft is placed in the retroperitoneal space posterior to the cecum and right colon, as shown in Figure 14–12. Heparin, 30 units/kg, is usually administered just before applying the vascular clamps. When an adult kidney is transplanted into a small child and a hyperkalemic preservation solution has been used, this solution can be rinsed out of the kidney with ice-cold Ringer's lactate solution just before the vascular anastomoses. The renal vein commonly must be shortened before anastomosis to prevent redundancy, kinking, and thrombosis. A mean arterial pressure of ≥70 mm Hg, a systolic blood pressure of ≥90 mm Hg, and a central venous pressure of 10 to 15 cm H_2O are indications of adequate intravascular volume before renal revascularization. In addition to the infusion of mannitol, albumin, and electrolyte solution, it is common to transfuse 100 to 150 ml of packed red blood cells just before releasing the vascular clamps. If the mean arterial pressure does not respond to intravascular volume expansion, a dopamine or dobutamine infusion of ≤5 μg/kg/minute can be administered. Urinary tract reconstruction options are the same as for adult recipients. Long-term results of renal transplantation into the valve bladder have been very satisfactory (Ross et al, 1994).

POSTOPERATIVE CARE

Postoperative fluid and electrolyte management are simple for patients with initial kidney graft function. Intravenous fluid of 0.45% saline in 5% dextrose is given to replace

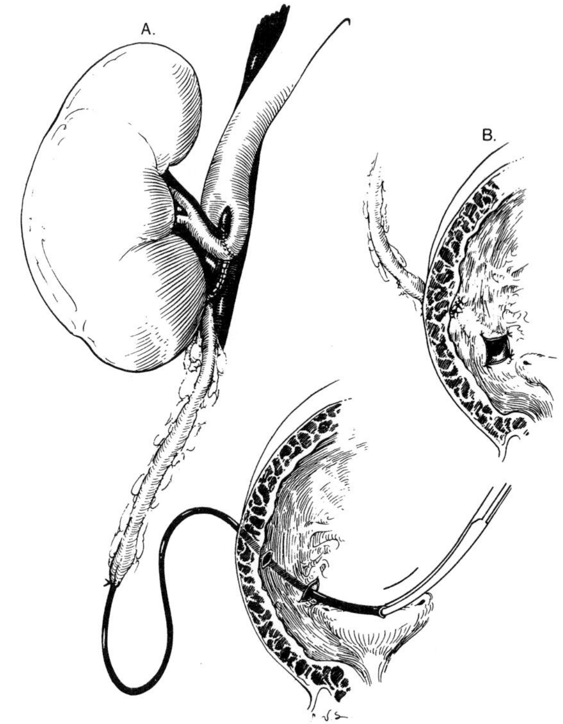

Figure 14–10. Transvesical ureteroneocystostomy. *A,* A No. 8 catheter is passed through the submucosal tunnel and secured to the transplant ureter. *B,* The ureter is drawn into the bladder, transected, spatulated, and secured with interrupted 4–0 or 5–0 absorbable sutures. The distal suture anchors the ureter to the bladder muscularis. The cystotomy is then closed in one or two layers with 3–0 absorbable sutures. (From Salvatierra O Jr: Renal transplantation. *In* Glenn JF, ed: Urologic Surgery, 3rd ed. Philadelphia, J. B. Lippincott Co., 1983, pp 362–366.)

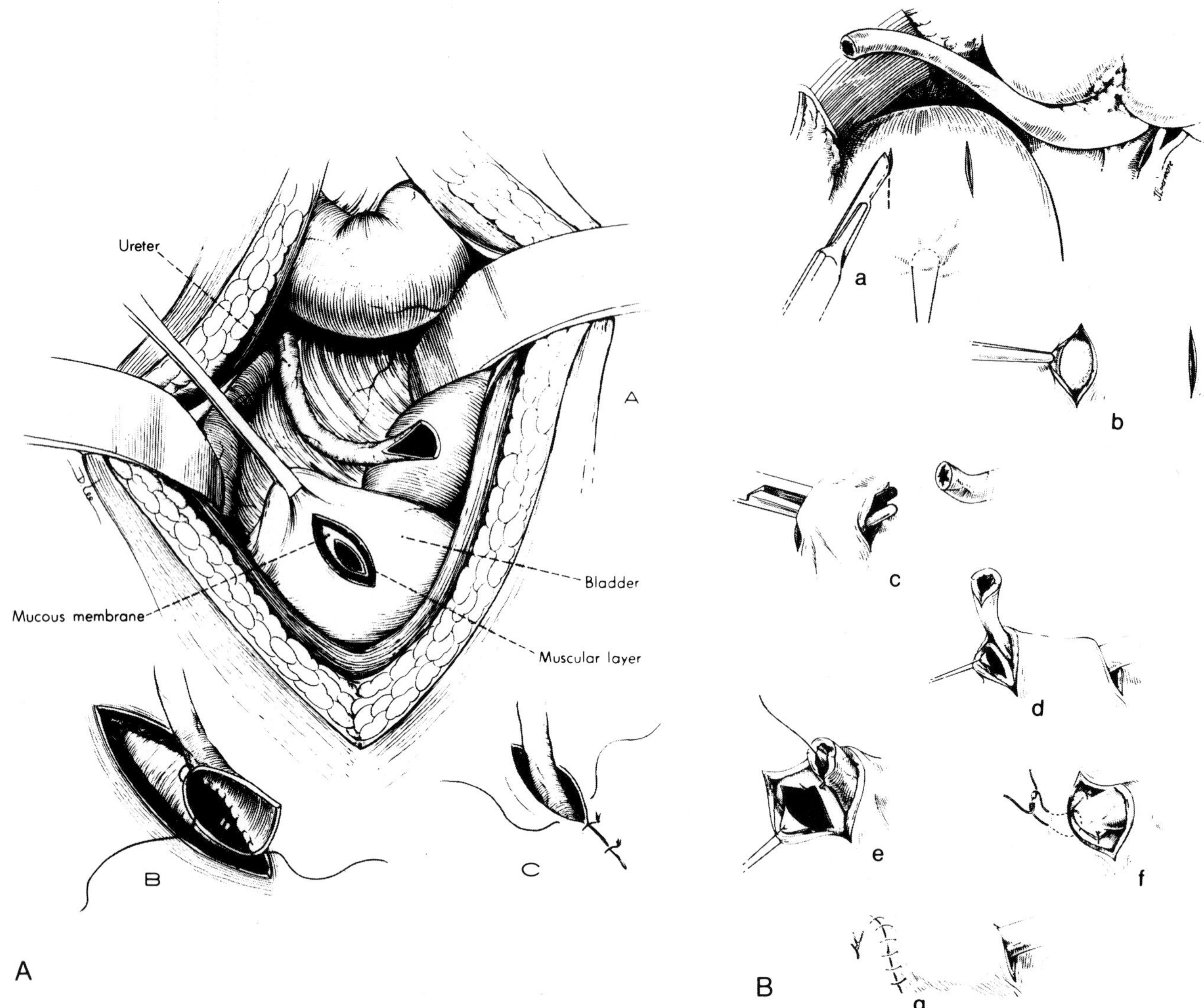

Figure 14–11. Two examples of extravesical ureteroneocystostomy. *A,* An anterolateral seromuscular incision is made down to the bulging bladder mucosa. The bladder is drained, the mucosa incised, and the ureter anastomosed to the bladder (as shown) with fine absorbable sutures. A distal anchoring stitch to hold the ureter to the bladder is sometimes used to prevent proximal migration in the tunnel (not shown). The seromuscular layer is then loosely closed over the ureter. *B,* Steps a through c are completed with the bladder full of an antibiotic solution. The anesthesiologist unclamps the catheter before mucosal incision, and steps d through g are completed with fine absorbable sutures. (*A* from Konnak JW, Herwig KR, Finkbeiner A, et al: J Urol 1975; 113:299–301. *B* from Barry JM: J Urol, 1983; 129:918–919.)

estimated insensible losses, and 0.45% saline in 0% dextrose is given at a rate equal to the previous hour's urinary output. When the urinary output is high, this regimen reduces the probability of a solute diuresis. Serum electrolyte levels are monitored every 4 to 8 hours, and potassium is added to the intravenous solution when the serum potassium level declines to the middle of the normal range. An estimate of the amount of potassium to add is based on a spot check of the urinary potassium concentration. After 24 to 48 hours, the diuresis slows, bowel continuity returns, oral fluids are administered, and the intravenous rate is slowed and then stopped. When delayed graft function occurs, the previously described intravenous fluid is administered at a rate to maintain the central venous pressure at 10 to 15 cm H_2O for 2 to 3 hours, and furosemide, 1 mg/kg, is administered intravenously. After that, the previously described rate is used. The oliguric patient may require urgent treatment of hyperkalemia or fluid overload, which is usually managed by dialysis. High levels of serum potassium can be counteracted by giving intravenous calcium chloride, and the levels are then lowered by using intravenous sodium bicarbonate with or without insulin or glucose. These measures drive potassium into cells for 4 to 6 hours.

If diuresis has ensued and the next day's serum creatinine level is approximately half the baseline level, a baseline radioisotope renogram is probably unnecessary. An ultrasonogram is usually obtained within 48 hours of transplantation to detect urinary extravasation, ureteral obstruction, or fluid collections. When oligoanuria occurs after renal transplantation, radioisotope renograms are commonly performed biweekly until acute tubular necrosis begins to resolve and the serum creatinine level begins to decrease without dialysis. A urine culture is obtained just before catheter removal and the patient given a single dose of a broad-spectrum

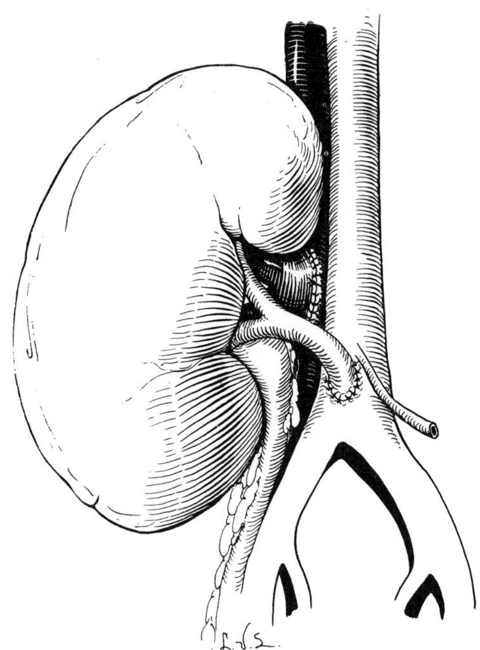

Figure 14–12. Transplantation of an adult kidney into a small child, with anastomosis of the renal vein to the inferior vena cava and of the renal artery to the aorta. The renal vein usually has to be shortened. (From Salvatierra O Jr: Renal transplantation. *In* Glenn JF, ed: Urologic Surgery, 3rd ed. Philadelphia, J. B. Lippincott Co., 1983, pp 362–366.)

antibiotic at that time. If the urine culture is subsequently positive, culture-specific therapy is given for 10 to 14 days.

The timing of catheter removal varies from 12 hours in patients who have had uncomplicated extravesical ureteroneocystostomy (Konnak et al, 1975) to 7 days in diabetic recipients (Barry and Hatch, 1985) to 14 days in recipients of combined cadaver kidney and pancreas transplants with duodenocystostomy. Some physicians prefer to delay catheter removal until a retrograde cystogram documents the absence of extravasation. If a ureteral stent was used to protect the urinary tract reconstruction, it is removed as an outpatient procedure 4 to 6 weeks after the operation. If external skin sutures or staples have been used, they are removed 7 to 14 days postoperatively. Most patients undergoing renal transplantation meet criteria for low-dose anticoagulation to prevent deep venous thrombosis. A simple protocol is the subcutaneous administration of heparin 50 units/kg every 8 hours for 3 to 5 days and then daily low-dose aspirin therapy. Patients with hypercoagulable states receive daily warfarin therapy to maintain the international normalized ratio (INR) between 2 and 3. The heparin dose for children is 5 to 10 units/kg/hour, and this can be given as a constant intravenous infusion.

RENAL ALLOGRAFT REJECTION

Most kidney graft losses are caused by rejection. The antiallograft response, immunopharmacology of allograft rejection, immunosuppressive regimens, histocompatibility, cross-match testing, and transplantation tolerance are discussed in Chapter 13, a companion chapter on renal immunology, and those topics are only briefly reviewed here.

Classification of Rejection

Hyperacute rejection occurs immediately after renal revascularization. It is an irreversible process mediated by preformed circulating cytotoxic antibodies that develop after pregnancy, blood transfusions, or an earlier failed transplant. It is very rare when the cross-match between recipient serum and donor lymphocytes is negative. Accelerated rejection is mediated by humoral and cellular components of the immune response. It occurs within days to weeks and often does not respond to antirejection therapy. Acute rejection occurs within weeks to months after transplantation. The symptoms of acute kidney transplant rejection are those of influenza, accompanied by pain over the kidney graft. Fever; increased blood pressure; decreased urinary output; fluid retention; increased blood urea nitrogen and serum creatinine levels; kidney enlargement; and decreased renal blood flow, glomerular filtration, and tubular function on radioisotope renography are signs associated with acute rejection.

Acute pyelonephritis must be ruled out by urinalysis and subsequently negative urine culture. Fine-needle biopsy of the kidney graft, with or without ultrasonographic guidance, is sometimes necessary to confirm the diagnosis of acute rejection (Belitsky and Gupta, 1990). The typical histologic findings of acute renal allograft rejection are mononuclear cellular infiltration and vasculitis (Fig. 14–13). Chronic rejection is characterized by a gradual decline in renal function associated with interstitial fibrosis, vascular changes, and minimal mononuclear cell infiltration. The incidence and severity of rejection are modified by histocompatibility between donor and recipient, immunosuppression, and pretransplantation immunologic conditioning, most commonly with transfusion of blood products (Suthanthiran and Strom, 1994).

Histocompatibility

The histocompatibility systems of greatest importance in renal transplantation are the ABO blood group and HLA systems. The importance of histocompatibility in kidney graft survival is documented in Table 14–4. There is also a significant beneficial effect of tissue matching in cadaver kidney graft survival, even in the cyclosporine era, when thousands of cases are analyzed (Table 14–5). This effect becomes more significant with time.

Immunosuppression

Immunosuppressive drug regimens include a glucocorticoid in combination with other drugs such as cyclosporine or tacrolimus (formerly known as FK506); azathioprine or mycophenolate mofetil; and antilymphocyte antibody. Triple maintenance immunosuppression with prednisone, cyclosporine or tacrolimus, and azathioprine or mycophenolate mofetil is currently popular to reduce the dosage of each drug and thereby minimize side effects while maintaining immunosuppression. A protocol for immunosuppression and prevention of infection and peptic ulcer disease is presented in Table 14–6. The higher doses of cyclosporine and tacrolimus are usually necessary in children. Maintenance oral

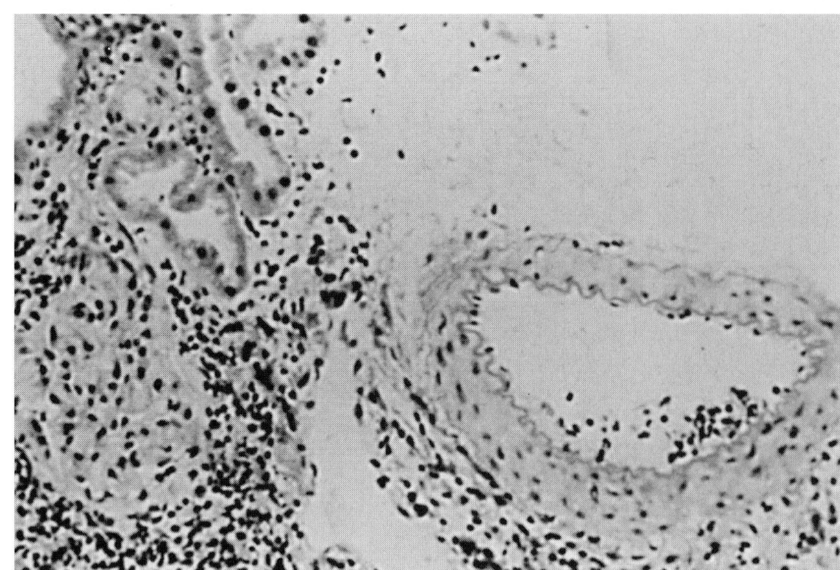

Figure 14–13. Acute renal allograft rejection. Mononuclear cells have infiltrated the interstitium, the tubules, and the small and medium-sized arteries. (From Burdick JF, Strom TB: Immunosuppression and transplantation: The biology and therapeutic modalities. *In* Belzer FO, ed: Transplant Surgical Resource Series. Raritan, NJ, Ortho Pharmaceutical Corporation, 1988, pp 2–28.)

prednisone and azathioprine are administered once per day. Cyclosporine or tacrolimus is administered once or twice a day in adults and two or three times a day in children. Mycophenolate mofetil is given twice a day. Cyclosporine may be unnecessary in recipients of HLA-identical sibling transplants (Stiller and Opelz, 1991). Glucocorticoids are usually started at high doses and then rapidly tapered during the first 6 months after grafting. Cyclosporine and tacrolimus have similar mechanisms of action, and they are not used together. The same reasoning applies to azathioprine and mycophenolate mofetil. Some programs taper patients off one of the maintenance immunosuppressants after many months of stable graft function. Conventional treatment for acute renal allograft rejection includes high-dose pulses of glucocorticoids—for example, prednisone 5 mg/kg/day for 5 days—tapering to maintenance doses. Treatment of steroid-resistant rejection is with antilymphocyte antibody preparations. Side effects from the major immunosuppressants are outlined in Table 14–7.

Both cyclosporine and tacrolimus are metabolized mainly by the cytochrome P-450 enzyme system (Suthanthiran and Strom, 1994; Fulton and Markham, 1996). Substances that inhibit that system usually result in increased whole-blood or plasma levels of those drugs (Table 14–8). Diltiazem and ketoconazole have been used to reduce cyclosporine dosing and cost while maintaining blood levels and immunosuppressive effect (Patton et al, 1994). Drugs known to induce that enzyme system usually result in increased metabolism of cyclosporine and tacrolimus and decreased whole-blood or plasma levels and immunosuppressive effect. Determination of cyclosporine or tacrolimus blood levels is helpful when toxicity is suspected. The characteristics of cyclosporine toxicity and those of acute rejection are contrasted in Table 14–9. Antilymphocyte antibodies such as antithymocyte gamma globulin (ATGAM) or OKT3 are used as part of induction immunosuppressive therapy for up to 2 weeks in some kidney transplant immunosuppressive regimens to allow the graft to recover from preservation injury before the administration of the potentially nephrotoxic drugs cyclosporine or tacrolimus. These antibodies are also valuable for the treatment of steroid-resistant rejection crises.

ATGAM is infused through an inline filter into a central venous line over a 4- to 6-hour period for 5 to 14 days. Potential side effects are fever, chills, thrombocytopenia,

Table 14–4. IMPORTANCE OF HISTOCOMPATIBILITY AND GRAFT SOURCE FOR 1-YEAR KIDNEY TRANSPLANT SURVIVALS

		Survival	
Kidney Source	**Number**	***Patient***	***Graft***
HLA-identical sibling	400	98.3	96.1
Haplo-identical sibling	489	98.2	91.3
Parent	539	97.6	89.3
Offspring	313	94.7	85.3
Cadaver (1st)	6245	94.6	84.0
Cadaver (2nd)	864	95.2	81.8
Cadaver (multiple)	191	92.4	69.4

Adapted from Cecka JM, Terasaki PI: The UNOS Scientific Registry: *In:* Terasaki PI and Cecka JM, eds: Clinical Transplants 1993. Los Angeles, UCLA Tissue Typing Laboratory, 1994, p 3.

Table 14–5. INFLUENCE OF HISTOCOMPATIBILITY ON CADAVER KIDNEY TRANSPLANT SURVIVAL RATES

		Survival		
HLA Antigen Mismatch	**Number**	***1 Year (%)***	***2 Years (%)***	***3 Years (%)***
0	1,774	87.4	84.1	80.2
1	1,216	83.6	79.7	73.9
2	3,821	83.6	78.2	72.9
3	8,191	82.1	76.4	70.5
4	10,339	79.5	73.4	67.8
5	7,438	78.1	72.3	66.1
6	2,932	76.4	69.5	63.8
Not reported	2,918	77.2	71.7	65.6
Overall	38,599	80.3	74.5	68.7

Data from 1994 Annual Report of the US Scientific Registry for Transplant Recipients and the Organ Procurement and Transplantation Network—Transplant Data: 1988–1993. Richmond, VA, UNOS and Bethesda, MD, Division of Organ Transplantation, Bureau of Health Resources Development, Health Resources and Services Administraton, US Department of Health and Human Services, 1994.

Table 14–6. EXAMPLE OF IMMUNOSUPPRESSION PROTOCOL

Postoperative Day	Prednisone* (mg/kg/day)	Cyclosporine‡, §, ** *or* (mg/kg)	Tacrolimus‡, §, ** (mg/kg)	Azathioprine*, † *or* (mg/kg)	Mycophenolate Mofetil†, ¶ (g)
		Prophylactic Immunosuppression			
0	7	5–15 (usually)	0.15–0.30	2–5	0–2
1	1.5	5–10 (usually)	0.15–0.30	2	0–2
2	1.0	5–10	0.15–0.30	2	0–2
3	0.9	5–10	0.15–0.30	2	2
4	0.8	5–10	0.15–0.30	2	2
5	0.7	5–10	0.15–0.30	2	2
6	0.6	5–10	0.15–0.30	2	2
7–30	0.5	5–10	0.15–0.30	2	2
31–181	Taper	Taper	0.15–0.30	2	2
182	0.1	5 (usually)	0.15–0.30	2	2
365	0.1	5 (usually)	0.15–0.30	2	2

Rejection Crisis Treatment

Prednisone: 5 mg/kg/day × 5 days
Steroid-resistant rejection: OKT3: 5 mg/kg/day IV × 10–14 days
Steroid-resistant rejection: ATGAM: 15 mg/kg/day central IV × 10–14 days

Prophylactic Anti-Infective Therapy

Broad-spectrum IV antibiotic perioperatively for skin and urinary tract organisms
Antibiotic into bladder after anesthesia induction
Antibiotic wound irrigation intraoperatively
Trimethoprim-sulfamethoxazole × 3–4 months to prevent UTI and *Pneumocystis* pneumonia
Clotrimazole lozenges × 3 mo to prevent oral *Candida* infection
Clotrimazole vaginal inserts (women) × 1–3 mo to prevent vaginal *Candida* infection
Acyclovir or ganciclovir as necessary to prevent HSV-1, HSV-2, VZV, EBV, and CMV infection††
CMV immune globulin as necessary for risk of primary CMV disease††

Prophylactic Anti–Peptic Ulcer Therapy

Histamine H_2-receptor antagonist††
Antacid as necessary for symptoms††

*IV dose is the same as the oral dose.
†Reduce if leukopenia occurs.
‡Oral dose. Intravenous dose is one-third the oral dose. Reduce if nephrotoxicity or high blood levels occur.
§Higher dose is usually necessary in children.
¶Oral dose. Reduce if leukopenia occurs.
**Delay until postoperative day 5 to 14 if antibody induction with OKT3 or ATGAM is given.
††Reduce dose for decreased renal function.
UTI, urinary tract infection; HSV, herpes simplex virus; VZV, varicella-zoster virus; EBV, Epstein-Barr virus; CMV, cytomegalovirus; ATGAM, antithymocyte gamma globulin.

Table 14–7. POTENTIAL TOXICITY OF IMMUNOSUPPRESSIVE THERAPY

	Prednisone	Cyclosporine	Tacrolimus	Azathioprine	Mycophenolate
Central nervous system	X	X	X	O	O
Gastrointestinal system	X	X	X	X	X
Kidney	O	X	X	O	O
Marrow	O	O	O	X	X
Skin	X	X	X	O	O
Endocrine system	X	X	X	O	O
Cardiovascular system	X	X	X	O	O
Wound healing	X	O	O	O	O

Table 14–8. POTENTIAL DRUG INTERACTIONS WITH CYCLOSPORINE AND TACROLIMUS

Drugs That Affect Plasma or Whole-Blood Concentrations		Drugs with Nephrotoxic Synergy
Decrease	***Increase***	
Rifampin	Diltiazem	Gentamicin
Rifabutin	Verapamil	Tobramycin
Isoniazid	Nicardipine	Vancomycin
Phenobarbital	Erythromycin	Azapropazone
Phenytoin	Clarithromycin	Amphotericin B
Carbamazepine	Ketoconazole	Ketoconazole
	Fluconazole	Melphalan
	Itraconazole	Cimetidine
	Clotrimazole	Ranitidine
	Bromocriptine	Diclofenac
	Danazol	Cisplatin
	Cimetidine	
	Methylprednisolone	
	Metoclopramide	

Modified from Barry JM: Immunosuppressive drugs in renal transplantation: A review of the regimens. Drugs 1992; 44:544–546.

leukopenia, hemolysis, respiratory distress, rash, serum sickness, and in rare instances anaphylaxis. The monoclonal antibody Orthoclone OKT3 (Todd and Brogden, 1989) is administered as a peripheral intravenous bolus daily for 10 to 14 days. The major side effects from this drug are influenza-like symptoms in most of the patients after the first and second doses; increased susceptibility to infection; and hypertension. Severe pulmonary edema has occurred in fluid-overloaded patients. Its principal pharmacologic use is probably the treatment of steroid-resistant rejection; however, a review of more than 60,000 cadaver kidney transplants demonstrated a small but significant advantage for OKT3 prophylaxis in conjunction with delayed cyclosporine therapy for cadaver kidney transplantation (Opelz, 1996).

PROBLEMS

Vascular Complications

Immediate vascular complications include kinking of the kidney graft's artery or vein; suture line stenosis; and thrombosis. These problems are more common with transplantation of the right kidney because of the long right renal artery and the short right renal vein, which limit final positioning of the kidney graft. Blood in the kidney graft may clot because of hyperacute rejection or a recipient hypercoagulable state such as deficiencies of protein C, protein S, or antithrombin III. Hypercoagulable states can be managed with perioperative heparin followed by long-term warfarin administration. Renal artery stenosis is usually diagnosed after renal transplantation because of hypertension, with or without impaired renal function. The causes are atheroma, faulty suture technique, clamp trauma, and immunologic mechanisms (Lacombe, 1988). The finding of a bruit is unreliable because it is a common sign after renal transplantation with or without hypertension. Surgical intervention is difficult, with a significant risk of technical failure, and percutaneous transluminal angioplasty has become the initial treatment of choice (DeMeyer et al, 1989).

Table 14–9. DIFFERENTIATION OF CYCLOSPORINE TOXICITY FROM ACUTE REJECTION

Characteristic	Cyclosporine Toxicity	Acute Rejection
Fever	No	Yes
Urinary output	Maintained	Decreased
Graft tenderness	No	Yes
Graft size	Stable	Increased
Serum creatinine level rise	Slow	Rapid
Cyclosporine blood level	High	Normal or low
Graft biopsy	May be normal	Cellular infiltration, vasculitis, tubulitis

Renal allograft rupture is rare and requires immediate operation. It is usually due to acute rejection or renal vein thrombosis. If it is due to the former, rejection crisis treatment and operative repair with bolstered mattress sutures, administration of topical thrombotic agents, and the use of synthetic glue and polyglactin mesh wrap have resulted in graft salvage (Chopin et al, 1989). If it is due to renal vein thrombosis, graft salvage with thrombectomy and repair of graft rupture are rare, and allograft nephrectomy is usually necessary (Richardson et al, 1990).

Allograft Nephrectomy

The goals of allograft nephrectomy are to remove a symptomatic, irreversibly rejected kidney transplant and, in the case of a chronically rejected, asymptomatic graft, to withdraw immunosuppression and to prevent the development of anti-HLA antibodies that could delay or prevent a subsequent transplant. The usual approach is through the original incision. Within the first month after transplantation, allograft nephrectomy is a straightforward procedure, and it is usually possible to remove all of the transplanted tissue. After 4 to 6 weeks, there is a dense fibrous reaction surrounding the kidney transplant, and the procedure can be a formidable one. It is best accomplished with a subcapsular technique and advanced knowledge of the types of vascular anastomoses and which recipient vessels were used. The surgeon must be prepared to occlude the vascular pedicle with a large vascular clamp, such as a Satinsky clamp; transect the vascular pedicle distal to the clamp; and then either separately ligate the renal veins and arteries or oversew the stumps of the vessels with 4–0 or 5–0 vascular suture. The renal capsule and the intravesical ureteral stump are left behind. The wound is liberally irrigated with an antibiotic solution, a suction drain is placed, and the wound is closed as described in the section on the renal transplantation procedure. Perioperative antibiotics are discontinued, changed, or continued on the basis of intraoperative culture results, and immunosuppression is discontinued within a few weeks. **Cyclosporine is withdrawn immediately; azathioprine is continued for 1 month because of residual allograft tissue, especially in the case of a subcapsular nephrectomy; and prednisone is gradually tapered and withdrawn with the following formula: 1 week of glucocorticoid taper for every month of immunosuppression for a maximum of 6 weeks.**

Hematuria

Immediate post-transplantation hematuria is usually at the ureteroneocystostomy or cystotomy site. If it cannot be controlled with catheter irrigation, endoscopy with fulguration of the bleeding site(s) is necessary. If those treatments fail, transvesical exploration and control of hemorrhage are necessary.

Late hematuria can be due to medical renal disease in the kidney graft, infection, calculus, or malignancy. If hematuria persists after treatment of a documented urinary tract infection, a standard hematuria work-up with phase-contrast microscopy for dysmorphic red blood cells should be done, followed if necessary by imaging of the native kidneys and the kidney transplant, by cystoscopy, by bladder wash for cytologic examination, and by pertinent urothelial biopsies.

Fluid Collections

Most collections after renal transplantation are incidental findings on baseline ultrasonographic examinations and require no treatment (Pollak et al, 1988). An algorithm for the evaluation and management of perigraft fluid collections is shown in Figure 14–14. When fluid collections are large or associated with dilation of the collecting system, pain, fever, or unexplained decline in renal function, ultrasonically guided diagnostic aspiration is necessary. If the fluid is purulent, microscopic examination of the fluid for organisms is done and antibiotic treatment is initiated. Although percutaneously placed tube drainage can be effective, open surgical drainage is usually necessary for fluid collections showing infection. Lymph, urine, and blood can be differentiated from each other by creatinine and hematocrit determinations. Lymph has a creatinine concentration that is the same as that of serum; urine has a creatinine concentration higher than that of serum and approaching that of bladder urine; and blood has a high hematocrit level in comparison with the other two fluids. If urinary tract obstruction is relieved by aspiration and there is no recurrence of the fluid, no further treatment is required. If blood reaccumulates, exploration and control of bleeding are required. If an uninfected lymphocele recurs, it is usually treated by marsupialization into the peritoneal cavity by either open or laparoscopic technique (Schweitzer et al, 1972; Gill et al, 1995), although some authors have reported success with percutaneous sclerosis (Gilliand et al, 1989). If the lymphocele is infected, open drainage is usually necessary.

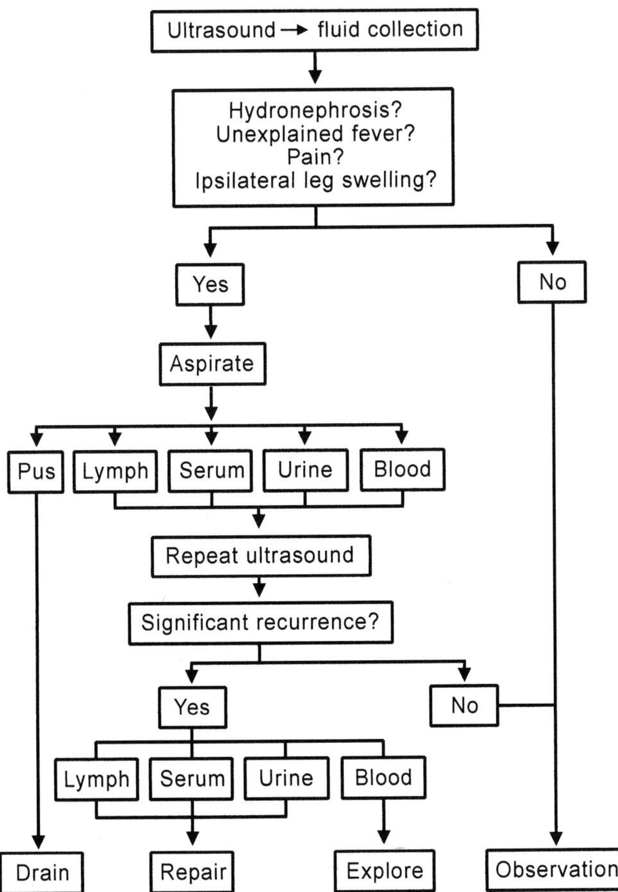

Figure 14–14. Algorithm for evaluation and treatment of perigraft fluid collection. (From Barry JM: Renal transplantation. *In* Krane RJ, Siroky MB, Fitzpatrick JM, eds: Clinical Urology. Philadelphia, J. B. Lippincott Co., 1994; p 325.)

Urinary extravasation often requires open surgical repair. A retrograde cystogram documents leakage at the cystotomy or ureteroneocystostomy site. If a retrograde cystogram does not show extravasation, excretory urography or percutaneous antegrade pyelography documents the site of extravasation from the ureter or renal pelvis. Some urinary leaks at the ureteroneocystotomy site may be managed simply by bladder catheter drainage, with or without percutaneous nephrostomy or with percutaneous or retrograde passage of a double-J ureteral stent, or by performance of another ureteroneocystostomy. If open repair is necessary, retrograde pyelography and passage of a ureteral catheter into the native ureter at the time of repair facilitate identification of that structure if it is needed for ureteroureterostomy or ureteropyelostomy. If the urinary tract repair is extensive, it is often protected with a stent, a small nephrostomy tube, omental wrap, suction drainage, antibiotics based on culture and sensitivity results, and reduction of immunosuppression. Cyclosporine or tacrolimus is usually continued, azathioprine is discontinued, and prednisone is reduced.

Obstruction and Stones

Ureteral obstruction in the immediate postoperative period is due to technical error, edema, blood clot, unsuspected donor calculus, or perigraft fluid collection. Although percutaneous techniques can be successful (Streem, 1994), a technical error is usually repaired with another ureteroneocystostomy. Edema usually resolves within a few days, and ureteral blood clots lyse with naturally produced urokinase. The management of fluid collections is discussed in an earlier section.

Late causes of urinary tract obstruction are periureteral fibrosis, calculi, tumor, fungus ball, lymphocele, and chronic ischemia of the distal ureter with stricture. Figure 14–15 is an algorithm for evaluating ureteral obstruction in the transplanted kidney. Ureteroneocystostomy meatal stenosis can be managed by (1) endoscopic ureteral meatotomy or by

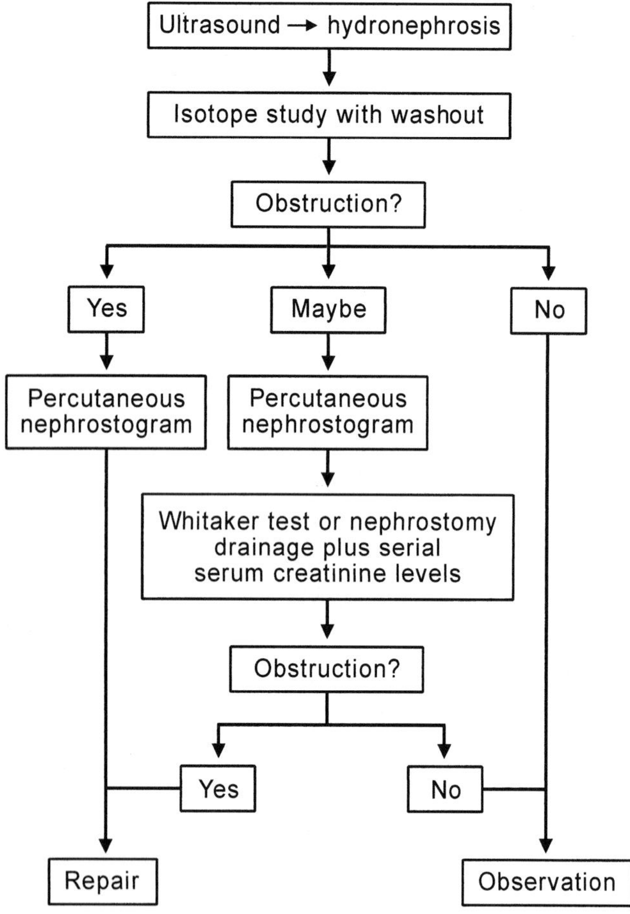

Figure 14–15. Algorithm for evaluation of kidney graft urinary tract obstruction. (From Barry JM: Renal transplantation. *In* Krane RJ, Siroky MB, Fitzpatrick JM, eds: Clinical Urology. Philadelphia, J. B. Lippincott Co., 1994, p 327.)

percutaneous ureteral dilation followed by stent placement (Streem 1994) or (2) open surgical repair. There are reports of long-term success for the endourologic treatment of transplant ureteral stenosis (Streem et al, 1988; Benoit et al, 1993). Failures are usually apparent within 1 year of treatment, and short, anastomotic strictures are the lesions most successfully treated with these techniques. If the stricture is distal and the allograft ureteral length is sufficient, a repeat ureteroneocystostomy is appropriate. For recurrent or long strictures, ureteropyelostomy and ureteroureterostomy as described earlier are reasonable options. Vesicopyelostomy, vesicocalycostomy, and interposition of a small-bowel segment between the renal pelvis and the bladder (Linstedt et al, 1981; Orton and Middleton, 1982; Ehrlich et al, 1983) have all been used as surgical treatments for an obstructed allograft ureter.

Causes of urinary tract calculi after renal transplantation are considered to be persistent hyperparathyroidism; recurrent urinary tract infections; a foreign body such as a suture or staple; obstruction; habitual decreased fluid intake; and distal renal tubular acidosis (Hefty, 1991). Because the renal transplant is denervated, the patient will not experience typical renal colic, and the diagnosis is suspected when renal function suddenly deteriorates or transplant pyelonephritis occurs. Upper tract calculi are managed by the same techniques as calculi in the normal urinary tract; however, negotiation of the transplanted ureter may be difficult or impossible because of tortuosity, and percutaneous techniques are favored (Caldwell and Burns, 1988; Locke et al, 1988; Streem, 1994). Extracorporeal shock-wave lithotripsy has been used successfully with the patient placed prone in the water bath (Wheatley et al, 1991). Bladder calculi are managed by electrohydraulic lithotripsy or, in rare instances, cystotomy.

Infection

Urinary Tract

Urinary tract infections after renal transplantation are common. In addition to immunosuppression and an indwelling bladder catheter, the following risk factors are often present: female sex, diabetes mellitus, and pre-existing urinary tract abnormalities. During the first 3 months after renal transplantation, prophylactic broad-spectrum antibiotics such as trimethoprim-sulfamethoxazole are usually prescribed. Trimethoprim interferes with the tubular secretion of creatinine, and this can cause an increase in serum creatinine levels. Treatment of urinary tract infection is by standard methods with guidance by urine culture and sensitivity. Cases of pyelonephritis should be screened with ultrasonography for obstruction or stone. Graft dysfunction accompanied by fever can be due to either acute pyelonephritis or acute rejection, and it is important to differentiate between the two because increased immunosuppression during an episode of acute pyelonephritis can result in fatal sepsis.

Candida cystitis often responds to bladder irrigations with 5% amphotericin B with or without oral ketoconazole or fluconazole. Cyclosporine and tacrolimus doses usually have to be reduced when ketoconazole or fluconazole is given because they interfere with the metabolism of both of those immunosuppressants. Tissue-invasive infections often require intravenous amphotericin B.

Hemorrhagic cystitis due to adenovirus subtypes 11 and 35 is rare in kidney transplant recipients and more commonly occurs in bone marrow transplant patients (Londergan and Walzak, 1994). The disease is usually self-limited and resolves within a week or two. Treatment is by forced hydration and diuresis. It has been suggested that intravenous ribavirin, an antiviral agent, will suppress the infection.

The urinary tract infections that occur months after transplantation are usually benign and respond readily to conventional antimicrobial therapy.

Lungs

Pneumonia in the immunosuppressed kidney transplant recipient is usually due to common bacterial pathogens; however, *Legionella, Nocardia*, mycobacteria, viruses, parasites *(Pneumocystis)*, and fungi can all be etiologic agents.

Vesicoureteral Reflux

Although there is some controversy about the need for antireflux ureteroneocystostomy in kidney transplantation,

Table 14–10. POTENTIAL CAUSES OF ERECTILE DYSFUNCTION AFTER TRANSPLANTATION

Anatomic Location	Examples	Mechanisms
Central		
Antihypertensives	Clonidine	$Alpha_2$ agonist
	Methyldopa	$Alpha_2$ agonist, ↑ prolactin
	Propranolol	Beta antagonist
Peptides or amino acids	Prednisone	↓ ACTH
↓ Testosterone	Cimetidine	↑ Prolactin
	Cyclosporine	↑ Prolactin
Anxiety		↑ Norepinephrine
Autonomic nerves	Diabetes mellitus	Axon injury
	Uremia	Axon injury
Peripheral nerves	Uremia	Axon injury
	Diabetes mellitus	Axon injury
Cavernosal blood supply		
Internal iliac arterial tree	Renal artery anastomosis	↓ Penile blood flow
Accelerated arteriosclerosis	Prednisone, cyclosporine, propranolol, diabetes mellitus	↑ Cholesterol
Antihypertensives	Any	↓ Penile blood pressure and blood flow
Diuretics	Any	↓ Blood volume and penile blood flow
Cavernosal smooth muscle	Diabetes mellitus, ↑ cholesterol	Impairs nitric oxide–mediated relaxation
	Cyclosporine	↑ Thromboxane A_2
Tunica albuginea of penis	Propranolol	Peyronie's disease

Modified from Barry JM: The evaluation and treatment of erectile dysfunction following organ transplantation. Semin Urol 1994; 12:147.

common urologic thinking is that reflux of infected bladder urine or high-pressure reflux is damaging to a kidney. The indications for antireflux surgery of the ureter in kidney transplant patients are the same as those for nontransplant patients (Reinberg et al, 1990). If the reflux is due to high-pressure voiding, relief of the bladder outlet obstruction (Dorsan et al, 1995) or augmentation cystoplasty with intermittent catheterization must be considered. Ureteral advancement techniques, ureteroureterostomy to the nonrefluxing native ureter, and submucosal injection techniques are all possible therapies.

Erectile Dysfunction

Erectile impotence can be due to the multiple factors outlined in Table 14–10. Treatment options for transplant recipients with this problem are presented in Table 14–11. Intracorporeal injections of vasoactive drugs (Rodriguez et al, 1992) and implantation of penile prostheses have successfully treated this problem (Rome et al, 1993); however, the transplant recipient must be warned of the increased risk of infection with either of these treatment modalities. If a penile prosthesis is chosen as the most appropriate therapy, application of the following criteria is helpful: stable graft function without a rejection crisis for at least 6 months; low doses of maintenance immunosuppressants; a low probability of device malfunction; no intra-abdominal components; minimal tissue dissection; no skin or urinary tract infections; prophylactic antibiotics (parenteral, intraurethral, and wound irrigation); and postoperative oral antibiotics for 1 to 2 weeks (Barry, 1994b). When a stress steroid protocol is used, 25 mg of prednisone (or its equivalent) is given with the preoperative medications and 12 and 24 hours later. Maintenance glucocorticoids are resumed on the second postoperative day. The oral doses of cyclosporine or tacrolimus, and azathioprine or mycophenolate mofetil, are not altered. The intravenous doses of cyclosporine and tacrolimus are one-third the oral doses and are infused over 24 hours. The intravenous dose of azathioprine is the same as the oral dose. Mycophenolate mofetil is an oral preparation.

Pregnancy and Childbearing

Successful renal transplantation usually restores female fertility. In a report of 2309 pregnancies in 1594 women (Davison, 1991), therapeutic abortion was done in 27%, spontaneous abortion occurred in 13%, and 92% of the

Table 14–11. TREATMENT OPTIONS FOR TRANSPLANT RECIPIENTS WITH ERECTILE DYSFUNCTION

Treatment	Examples
Psychotherapy and/or counseling	Suggest alternative sexual techniques
	Urge patient to stop alcohol use
	Urge patient to stop smoking
Medication changes	Treat hypertension with calcium antagonists or $alpha_1$ blockers
	Change cimetidine to ranitidine, famotidine, or nizatidine
	Withdraw glucocorticoids, if possible
Medication additions, if indicated by work-up	Testosterone
	Thyroid replacement
	Bromocriptine
Vacuum erection devices	
Intracavernous injections	Prostaglandin E_1
Vascular procedures	Angiodilation
	Revascularization
Penile prostheses	Semirigid
	Malleable
	Mechanically jointed
	Self-contained inflatable
	Inflatable with scrotal pump-reservoir

Adapted from Barry JM: The evaluation and treatment of erectile dysfunction following organ transplantation. Semin Urol 1994; 12:147.

conceptions that continued beyond the first trimester ended successfully. Permanent renal impairment occurred in 15% of pregnancies, hypertension developed in 30%, preterm delivery occurred in 50%, and there were no frequent or predominant abnormalities in the children. The transplanted kidneys rarely caused dystocia, and they were not injured during vaginal delivery.

Cancer

Immunosuppressed patients are more likely to develop cancer than age-matched control subjects in the general population (Sheil et al, 1993). The acquisition or liberation of oncogenic viruses is facilitated by impaired cellular immunity, and immunosuppressants may have a mutagenic role in tumorigenesis. Among 7119 tumors that occurred in 6635 renal transplant recipients, the common cancers were skin cancers (39%), lymphomas (12%), Kaposi's sarcoma (4%), carcinomas of the cervix (4%), renal tumors (4%), and carcinomas of the vulva and perineum (3%) (Penn, 1995). Lymphoproliferative disorders are associated with Epstein-Barr virus infection. In rare instances, renal malignancy is transplanted with the kidney graft. When this happens, treatment is by removal of the transplanted kidney and discontinuation of immunosuppressive therapy. Calmette-Guérin bacillus vaccine should be avoided for the treatment of superficial transitional cell carcinoma of the bladder in immunosuppressed kidney transplant recipients because of the risk of systemic infection and the likelihood of diminished therapeutic response. Absorbed thiotepa may have an additive myelosuppressive effect if the patient is also taking azathioprine or mycophenolate mofetil.

Medical Vascular Complications

Hypertension after renal transplantation is common. Causes of this include medications (glucocorticoids, cyclosporine, and tacrolimus), intrinsic renal disease, and rejection.

In spite of aggressive preoperative assessment and treatment, myocardial infarction and stroke continue to be leading causes of death in these patients. Prednisone and cyclosporine increase cardiovascular risk because of associated hyperlipidemia, and post-transplantation hyperlipidemia should be treated with dietary changes and, if necessary, antilipid medications.

Diabetes Mellitus

New diabetes occurs in a small percentage of kidney transplant recipients. This is due to the diabetogenic effects of glucocorticoids and cyclosporine.

CONCLUSIONS

Renal transplantation is the best therapy for most patients with ESRD. Morbidity and mortality have been significantly reduced by attention to pretransplantation evaluations, donor surgery, kidney preservation, recipient selection, recipient surgery, histocompatibility, immunosuppression, and successful management of complications. Organ shortage continues to be a significant problem.

REFERENCES

End-Stage Renal Disease

Disney APS, ed: ANZDTA Report 1994. Adelaide, South Australia, Australia and New Zealand Dialysis and Transplant Registry, 1995.

Eggers PW: Effect of transplantation on the Medicare End-Stage Renal Disease Program. N Engl J Med 1988; 318:223.

Evans RW, Manninea DL, Garrison LP, et al: The quality of life of patients with end-stage renal disease. N Engl J Med 1985; 312:553.

NIH Consensus Development Conference: Morbidity and mortality of dialysis. NIH Consens Statement 1993; 11(2):1.

Port FK, Wolfe RA, Mauger EA, et al: Comparison of survival probabilities for dialysis versus cadaveric renal transplant recipients. JAMA 1993; 270:1339.

United Network for Organ Sharing: 1994 Annual Report of the US Scientific Registry for Transplant Recipients and the Organ Procurement and Transplantation Network—Transplant Data: 1988–1993. Richmond, VA, UNOS; and Bethesda, MD, Division of Organ Transplantation, Bureau of Health Resources Development, Health Resources and Services Administration, US Department of Health and Human Services, 1994a.

United Network for Organ Sharing: The UNOS Statement of Principles and Objectives of Equitable Organ Allocation. UNOS Update 1994b; 10(8):20.

United Network for Organ Sharing: Articles of Incorporation, Bylaws, and Policies: Policy 3.5, Allocation of Cadaveric Kidneys. UNOS, June 28, 1995a.

United Network for Organ Sharing: Comparison of 1993 and 1994 US Transplant Statistics. UNOS Update 1995b; 11(2):39.

United Network for Organ Sharing: Patients Waiting for Transplants. UNOS Update 1995c; 11(8):41.

US Renal Data System, USRDS: 1995 Annual Data Report. Bethesda, MD, National Institutes of Health, National Institute of Diabetes and Digestive and Kidney Diseases, April, 1995.

Van Es A: Growth hormone treatment in short children with chronic renal failure and after renal transplantation: Combined data from European clinical trials. Acta Paediatr Scand 1991; 379(suppl)42:42.

Winearls G, Gray D: Chronic renal failure—Renal replacement therapy. *In* Morris PJ, ed: Kidney Transplantation: Principles and Practice, 4th ed. Philadelphia, W. B. Saunders Company, 1994, pp 26–42.

History of Human Renal Transplantation

Belzer FO, Ashby BS, Dunphy JE: 24- and 72-hour preservation of canine kidneys. Lancet 1967; 2:536.

Belzer FO, Southard JH: Principles of solid-organ preservation by cold storage. Transplantation 1988; 45:673.

Calne RY, Wite DJG, Thiru S, et al: Cyclosporine A in patients receiving renal allografts from cadaver donors. Lancet 1978; 2:1323.

Carpenter CB: Blood transfusion effects in kidney transplantation. Yale J Biol Med 1990; 63:435.

Collins GM, Bravo-Sugarman MB, Terasaki PI: Kidney preservation for transportation: Initial perfusion and 30 hours of ice storage. Lancet 1969; 2:1219.

Cosimi AB, Colvin RB, Goldstein G, et al: Treatment of acute renal allograft rejection with OKT3 monoclonal antibody. Transplantation 1981; 32:535.

Goodwin WE, Kaufman JJ, Mims MM, et al: Human renal transplantation. I: Clinical experience with 6 cases of renal homotransplantation. J Urol 1963; 89:13.

Hamilton D: Kidney transplantation: A history. *In* Morris PJ, ed: Kidney Transplantation: Principles and Practice, 4th ed. Philadelphia, W. B. Saunders Company, 1994, pp 1–7.

Hamilton DNH, Reid WA: Yu Yu Voronoy and the first human kidney allograft. Surg Gynecol Obstet 1984; 159:289.

Opelz G, Sengar DF, Mickey MR, et al: Effect of blood transfusions on subsequent kidney transplants. Transplant Proc 1973; 5:253.

Salvatierra O Jr, Vincenti F, Amend WJC, et al: Deliberate donor-specific blood transfusions prior to living related transplantation. Ann Surg 1980; 192:543.

Selection and Preparation of Kidney Transplant Recipients

Ramos EL, Kasiske BL, Alexander SR, et al: The evaluation of candidates for renal transplantation. Transplantation 1994; 57:490.

Reinberg Y, Bumgaardner GL, Aliabadi H: Urological aspects of renal transplantation. J Urol 1990; 143:1087.

Sheldon CA, Gonzalez R, Burns MW, et al: Renal transplantation into the dysfunctional bladder: The role of adjunctive bladder reconstruction. J Urol 1994; 152:972.

Shneidman RS, Pulliam JP, Barry JM: Clean, intermittent self-catheterization in renal transplant recipients. Transplantation 1984; 38:312.

Thomalla JV, Mitchell ME, Leapman SB, et al: Renal transplantation into the reconstructed bladder. J Urol 1989; 141:265.

Tuttle TM, Williams GM, Marshall FF: Evidence for cyclophosphamide-induced transitional cell carcinoma in a renal transplant patient. J Urol 1988; 140:1009.

Watts RWE, Morgan SH, Danpure CJ, et al: Combined hepatic and renal transplantation in primary hyperoxaluria type I: Clinical report of nine cases. Am J Med 1991; 90:179.

Donor Selection, Preparation, and Surgery

Alexander JW, Bennett LE, Green PJ: Effect of donor age on outcome of kidney transplantation: A two-year analysis of transplants reported to the United Network for Organ Sharing registry. Transplantation 1994; 57:871.

Alfrey EJ, Rubin GD, Kuo PC, et al: The use of spiral computed tomography in the evaluation of living donors for kidney transplantation. Transplantation 1995; 59:643.

Barry JM: Cadaver donor nephrectomy. *In* Novick AC, Streem SB, Pontes JE, eds: Stewart's Operative Urology. Baltimore, Williams & Wilkins Company, 1989, pp 294–300.

Barry JM: Donor nephrectomy. *In* Marshall FF, ed: Textbook of Operative Urology. Philadelphia, W. B. Saunders Company, 1996, pp 235–247.

Bia MJ, Ramos EL, Danovitch GM, et al: Evaluation of living renal donors: The current practice of US transplant centers. Transplant 1995; 60:322.

Boyd GL, Phillips MG, Diethelm AG: Donor management. *In* Phillips MG, ed: Organ Procurement, Preservation and Distribution in Transplantation. Richmond, Va, UNOS, 1991, pp 39–51.

Feduska NJ Jr, Cecka JM: Donor factors. *In* Terasaki PI, Cecka JM, eds: Clinical Transplants 1994. Los Angeles, UCLA Tissue Typing Laboratory, 1995, pp 381–394.

Hudnall CH, Hodge EE, Centeno AS, et al: Evaluation of pediatric cadaver kidneys transplanted into adult recipients receiving cyclosporine. J Urol 1989; 142:1181.

Kasiske BL, Ma JZ, Louis TA, et al: Long-term effects of reduced renal function in humans. Kidney Int 1995; 48:814.

Lindgren BW, Posniak HV, Marsan R, et al: Renal computed tomography with three-dimensional angiography and simultaneous measurement of plasma contrast clearance reduce invasiveness and cost of evaluating living renal donor candidates. J Urol 1995; 153:529A.

Najarian JS, Chavers BM, McHugh LE, et al: Twenty years or more of follow-up of living kidney donors. Lancet 1992; 340:807.

Nakazato PZ, Concepcion W, Bry W, et al: Total abdominal evisceration: An en-bloc technique for abdominal organ harvesting. Surgery 1992; 111:37.

Salvatierra O Jr, Belzer FO: Pediatric cadaver kidneys: Their use in renal transplantation. Arch Surg 1975; 110:181.

Soifer BE, Gelb AW: The multiple organ donor: Identification and management, Ann Intern Med 1989; 110:814.

Steckler RE, Riehle RA Jr, Vaughan BD Jr: Hyperfiltration-induced renal injury in normal man: Myth or Reality. J Urol 1990; 144:1323.

Vincenti F, Amend WJC Jr, Kaysen G: Long-term renal function in kidney donors: Sustained compensatory hyperfiltration with no adverse effects. Transplantation 1983; 36:626.

Kidney Preservation

Belzer FO, Ashby BS, Dunphy JE: 24- and 72-hour preservation of canine kidneys. Lancet 1967; 2:536.

Belzer FO, Southard JH: Principles of solid-organ preservation by cold storage. Transplantation 1988; 45:673.

Collins GM, Bravo-Sugarman MB, Terasaki PI: Kidney preservation for transportation: Initial perfusion and 30 hours of ice storage. Lancet 1969; 2:1219.

Feduska NJ Jr, Belzer FO, Stieper KW, et al: A ten-year experience with cadaver kidney preservation using cryoprecipitated plasma. Am J Surg 1978; 135:356.

Geffner SR, D'Alessandro AM, Kalayoglu M, et al: Living-unrelated renal donor transplantation: The UNOS experience, 1987–1991. *In* Terasaki PI, Cecka JM, eds: Clinical Transplants 1994. Los Angeles, UCLA Tissue Typing Laboratory, 1995, p 197.

Gjertson DW: Multifactorial analysis of renal transplants reported to the United Network for Organ Sharing Registry: The 1994 Update. *In* Clinical Transplants, 1994. Los Angeles, UCLA Tissue Typing Laboratory, 1995, p 532.

Haberal M, Oner Z, Karamehmetoglu M, et al: Cadaver kidney transplantation with cold ischemia time for 48 to 95 hours. Transplant Proc 1984; 16:1330.

Halasz NA, Collins GM: Forty-eight hour kidney perfusion: A comparison of flushing and ice storage with perfusion. Arch Surg 1976; 1:175.

Marshall VC, Jablonski P, Scott DF: Renal preservation. *In* Morris PJ, ed: Kidney Transplantation: Principles and Practice, 4th ed. Philadelphia, W. B. Saunders Company, 1994, pp 86–108.

Ploeg RJ, Goossens D, McAnulty JR, et al: Successful 72-hour cold storage kidney preservation with UW solution. Transplantation 1988; 46:191.

Ploeg RJ, Van Bockel JH, Langendijk PTH, et al: Effect of preservation solution on results of cadaveric kidney transplantation. Lancet 1992; 340:129.

Recipient Selection for Cadaver Kidney Transplants

Dunn DL, Gillingham KJ, Kramer MA, et al: A prospective randomized study of acyclovir versus ganciclovir plus human immune globulin prophylaxis of cytomegalovirus infection after solid organ transplantation. Transplantation 1994; 57:876.

Henell KR, Chou S, Norman DJ: Use of cytomegalovirus seropositive donor kidneys in seronegative patients: Results of prospective serotesting and matching in one center. Transplant Proc 1989; 21:2082.

Markham A, Faulds D: Gancyclovir: An update of its therapeutic use in cytomegalovirus infection. Drugs 1994; 48:455.

Steinmuller DR, Graneto D, Swift C, et al: Use of intravenous immunoglobulin prophylaxis for primary cytomegalovirus infection post living related donor renal transplantation. Transplant Proc 1989; 21:2069.

United Network for Organ Sharing: Articles of Incorporation, Bylaws, and Policies: Policy 3.5, Allocation of Cadaveric Kidneys. UNOS, June 28, 1995.

Recipient Operation

Barry JM, Fuchs EF: Right renal vein extension in cadaver kidney transplantation. Arch Surg 1978; 113:300.

Corry RJ, Kelley SE: Technic for lengthening the right renal vein of cadaver donor kidneys. Am J Surg 1978; 135:867.

Dawidson IJA, Ar'Rajab A: Perioperative fluid and drug therapy during cadaver kidney transplantation. *In* Terasaki PI, Cecka JM, eds: Clinical Transplants 1992. Los Angeles, UCLA Tissue Typing Laboratory, 1993, pp 267–284.

Gibbons WS, Barry JM, Hefty TR: Complications following unstented parallel incision extravesical ureteroneocystostomy in 1,000 kidney transplants. J Urol 1992; 148:38.

Gil-Vernet JM, Gil-Vernet A, Caralps A, et al: Orthotopic renal transplant and results in 193 consecutive cases. J Urol 1989; 142:248.

Gittes RF, Waters WB: Sexual impotence: The overlooked complication of a second renal transplant. J Urol 1979; 121:719.

Hatch DA: A review of renal transplantation into bowel segments for conduit and continent urinary diversions: Techniques and complications. Semin Urol 1994; 12:108.

Hatch DA, Belitsky P, Barry JM, et al: Fate of renal allografts transplanted in patients with urinary diversion. Transplantation 1993; 56:838.

Heritier P, Perraud Y, Relave MH, et al: Renal transplantation and Kock pouch: A case report. J Urol 1989; 141:595.

Pleass HCC, Clark KM, Rigg KS, et al: Urologic complications after renal transplantation: A prospective randomized trial comparing different techniques for ureteric anastomosis and the use of prophylactic ureteric stents. Transplant Proc 1995; 27:1091.

Ross JH, Kay R, Novick AC, et al: Long-term results of renal transplantation into the valve bladder. J Urol 1994; 151:1500.

Postoperative Care

Barry JM, Hatch DA: Parallel incision unstented extravesical ureteroneocystostomy: Follow-up of 203 kidney transplants. J Urol 1985; 134:249.

Konnak JW, Herwig KR, Finkbeiner A, et al: Extravesical ureteroneocystostomy in 170 renal transplant patients. J Urol 1975; 113:299.

Renal Allograft Rejection

Belitsky P, Gupta R: Mini-core needle biopsy of kidney transplants: A safer sampling method. J Urol 1990; 144:310.

Fulton B, Markham A: Mycophenolate mofetil: A review of its clinical pharmacology and therapeutic efficacy in renal transplantation. Drugs 1996; 51:278.

Opelz G: Efficacy of rejection prophylaxis with OKT3 in renal transplantation. Transplantation 1996; 60:1220.

Patton PR, Brunson ME, Pfaff WW, et al: A preliminary report of diltiazem and ketoconazole: Their cyclosporine-sparing effect and impact on transplant outcome. Transplantation 1994; 57:889.

Stiller CR, Opelz G: Should cyclosporine be continued indefinitely? Transplant Proc 1991; 23:36.

Suthanthiran M, Strom TB: Renal transplantation. N Engl J Med 1994; 331:365.

Todd PA, Brogden RN: Muromonab CD3: A review of its pharmacology and therapeutic potential. Drug 1989; 37:871.

Problems

Barry J: The evaluation and treatment of erectile dysfunction following organ transplantation. Semin Urol 1994; 12:147.

Benoit G, Alexander L, Moukarzel M, et al: Percutaneous antegrade dilation of ureteral strictures in kidney transplants. J Urol 1993; 150:37.

Caldwell TC, Burns JR: Current operative management of urinary calculi after renal transplantation. J Urol 1988; 140:1360.

Chopin DK, Abbou CC, Lottmann HB, et al: Conservative treatment of renal allograft rupture with polyglactin 910 mesh and gelatin resorcin formaldehyde glue. J Urol 1989; 142:363.

Davison JM: Dialysis, transplantation, and pregnancy. Am J Kidney Dis 1991; 17:127.

DeMeyer M, Pirson Y, Dautrebande J, et al: Treatment of renal graft artery stenosis: Comparison between surgical bypass and percutaneous transluminal angioplasty. Transplantation 1989; 46:784.

Dorsan J, Wiesel M, Mohring K, et al: Transurethral incision of the prostate following renal transplantation. J Urol 1995; 153:1499.

Ehrlich RM, Whitmore K, Fine RN: Calycovesicostomy for total ureteral obstruction after renal transplantation. J Urol 1983; 129:818.

Gill IS, Hodge EE, Munch LC, et al: Transperitoneal marsupialization of lymphoceles: A comparison of laparoscopic and open techniques. J Urol 1995; 153:706.

Gilliland JD, Spies JB, Brown SB, et al: Lymphoceles: Percutaneous treatment with povidone-iodine sclerosis. Radiology 1989; 171:227.

Hefty TR: Complications of renal transplantation: The practicing urologist's role. AUA Update Series 1991; 10(8):58.

Lacombe M: Renal artery stenosis after renal transplantation. Ann Vasc Surg 1988; 2:155.

Lindstedt E, Bergentz SE, Lindholm T: Long-term clinical follow-up after pyelocystostomy. J Urol 1981; 126:253.

Locke DR, Steinbock G, Salomon DR, et al: Combination extracorporeal shock wave lithotripsy and percutaneous extraction of calculi in a renal allograft. J Urol 1988; 139:575.

Londergan TA, Walzak MP: Hemorrhagic cystitis due to adenovirus infection following bone marrow transplantation. J Urol 1994; 151:1013.

Orton KR, Middleton RG: Ileal substitution of the ureter in renal transplantation. J Urol 1982; 128:374.

Penn I: Occurrence of cancers in immunosuppressed organ transplant recipients. *In* Terasaki PI, Cecka JM, eds: Clinical Transplants 1994. Los Angeles, UCLA Tissue Typing Laboratory, 1995, pp 99–109.

Pollak R, Beremis SA, Maddux MS, et al: The natural history of and therapy for peri-renal fluid collections following renal transplantation. J Urol 1988; 140:716.

Reinberg Y, Bumgaardner GL, Aliabadi H: Urological aspects of renal transplantation. J Urol 1990; 143:1087.

Richardson AJ, Higgins RN, Jaskowski AJ, et al: Spontaneous rupture of renal allografts: The importance of renal vein thrombosis in the cyclosporine era. Br J Surg 1990; 77:558.

Rodriguez AA, Morales AM, Andres A, et al: Treatment of erectile impotence in renal transplant patients with intracavernosal vasoactive drugs. Transplant Proc 1992; 24:105.

Rome SJ, Montague DK, Steinmuller DR, et al: Treatment of organic impotence with penile prostheses in renal transplant patients. Urology 1993; 41:16.

Schweitzer RT, Cho S, Kountz SL, et al: Lymphoceles following renal transplantation. Arch Surg 1972; 104:43.

Shiel AGR, Disney APS, Mathew TH, et al: De novo malignancy emerges as a major cause of morbidity and late failure in renal transplantation. Transplant Proc 1993; 25:1383.

Streem SB: Endourological management of urological complications following renal transplantation. Semin Urol 1994; 12:123.

Streem SB, Novick AC, Steinmuller DR, et al: Long-term efficacy of ureteral dilation for transplant ureteral stenosis. J Urol 1988; 140:32.

Wheatley M, Ohl DA, Sonda LP III, et al: Treatment of renal transplant stones by extracorporeal shock-wave lithotripsy in the prone position. Urology 1991; 37:57.

IV
INFECTIONS AND INFLAMMATIONS OF THE GENITOURINARY TRACT

15
INFECTIONS OF THE URINARY TRACT

Anthony J. Schaeffer, M.D.

Urinary tract infections are a common cause of morbidity and can lead to significant mortality. Careful diagnosis and treatment result in successful resolution of infections in most instances. A better understanding of the pathogenesis of urinary tract infection and the role of host and bacterial factors has improved the ability to identify patients at risk and prevent or minimize sequelae. New antimicrobial agents that achieve high urinary levels, that can be administered orally, and that are not nephrotoxic have significantly reduced the need for hospitalization for severe infection. Shorter-course therapy and prophylactic antimicrobials have reduced the morbidity and cost associated with recurrent cystitis in women. Although the vast majority of patients respond promptly and are cured by therapy, early identification and treatment of patients with complicated infections that place them at significant risk remain a clinical challenge to urologists.

DEFINITIONS

Urinary tract infection is an inflammatory response of the urothelium to bacterial invasion that is usually associated with bacteriuria and pyuria.

***Bacteriuria* is the presence of bacteria in the urine, which is normally free of bacteria, and implies that these bacteria are from the urinary tract and are not contaminants from the skin, vagina, or prepuce. The possibility of contamination increases as the reliability of the collection technique decreases from suprapubic aspiration to catheterization to voided specimens.** Significant bacteriuria has a clinical connotation and is used to describe the number of bacteria in a suprapubically aspirated, catheterized, or voided specimen that exceeds the number usually caused by bacterial contamination of the skin, urethra, or the prepuce or introitus, respectively, and hence represents a urinary tract infection. Rarely, bacteria may colonize the urinary tract without causing bacteriuria (Hultgren et al, 1985; Elliott et al, 1985). Bacteriuria can be symptomatic or asymptomatic. When it is detected by population studies (screening surveys), *screening* bacteriuria (scBU) is a more precise and descriptive term than *asymptomatic* bacteriuria, especially since the latter term is clinically useful for describing the presence or absence of symptoms in an individual patient.

***Pyuria* is the presence of white blood cells in the urine and is generally indicative of an inflammatory response of the urothelium to bacterial invasion.** Bacteriuria without pyuria indicates bacterial colonization rather than infection. **Pyuria without bacteriuria warrants evaluation for tuberculosis, stones, or cancer.**

Infections are generally defined clinically by their presumed site of origin.

***Acute pyelonephritis* is a clinical syndrome of chills, fever, and flank pain that is accompanied by bacteriuria and pyuria, a combination that is reasonably specific for an acute bacterial infection of the kidney.** The term should not be used if flank pain is absent; there may be serious difficulties in diagnosing spinal cord–injured and elderly patients who may be unable to localize the site of their discomfort.

Chronic pyelonephritis describes a shrunken, scarred kidney, diagnosed by morphologic, radiologic, or functional evidence of renal disease that may be postinfectious but is frequently not associated with urinary tract infection. Bacterial infection of the kidney may cause a *focal, coarse scar* in the renal cortex overlying a calyx, almost always accompanied by some calyceal distortion (Fig. 15–1), which can be detected radiographically or by gross examination of the kidney. Less commonly, renal scarring from infection can

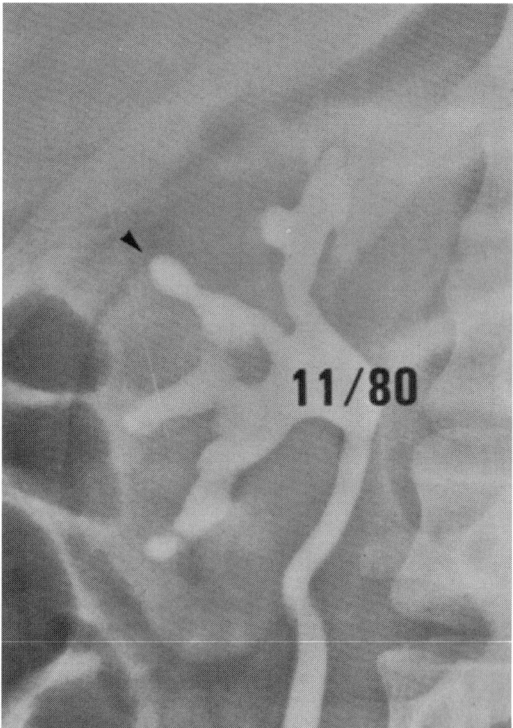

Figure 15–1. Intravenous urogram demonstrating focal, coarse scarring in the right kidney of an 18-year-old girl with a history of many recurrent fevers between 2 months and 2 years of age. A cystogram when the patient was 2 years old established an atrophic left kidney with marked reflux up to the left kidney and slight reflux up to the right kidney. An intravenous urogram at the age of 6 years established severe atrophy of the left kidney. She had no infections between the ages of 6 and 15 years. Several reinfections occurred at the age of 15 years, and they ceased with prophylactic therapy. Her blood pressure has remained normal, and her serum creatinine level was 0.9 mg/dl at the age of 18 years. She is now 21 years old and has stopped antimicrobial prophylaxis for 18 months without infections or introital colonization with Enterobacteriaceae. Note that all calyces are blunted and that one extends to the capsule *(arrow)* because of atrophy of the overlying cortex.

result in atrophic pyelonephritis, or generalized thinning of the renal cortex with a small kidney appearing radiographically similar to one with postobstructive atrophy (Fig. 15–2). When accompanied by vesicoureteral reflux (VUR), these characteristic radiologic changes have been referred to as "reflux nephropathy," emphasizing the role of reflux in the resultant scarring. But because focal, coarse scarring secondary to clinical pyelonephritis is also demonstrable in the absence of reflux, the term "reflux nephropathy" should not be used.

Cystitis is inflammation of the bladder, whether used as a histologic, bacteriologic, or cystoscopic description, or a clinical syndrome that is usually accompanied by an abrupt onset of dysuria, increased frequency, urgency, and suprapubic pain. *Bacterial cystitis*, as opposed to nonbacterial cystitis (e.g., radiation or interstitial), is a useful term.

Urethritis, like cystitis, also refers to inflammation, but of the urethra rather than the bladder. It requires an adjective for modification, for example, nongonococcal urethritis. Symptoms arising from urethritis and cystitis are difficult, if not impossible, to distinguish in the female, but pure urethritis in the female—unlike that in the male—is very rare.

Uncomplicated **is used to describe an infection in a patient with a structurally and functionally normal urinary tract.** The majority of these patients are women with isolated or recurrent bacterial cystitis or acute pyelonephritis, and the infecting pathogens are usually susceptible to and eradicated by a short course of inexpensive oral antimicrobial therapy.

Complicated **describes an infection in a patient with pyelonephritis and/or a urinary tract with a structural or functional abnormality that would reduce the efficacy of antimicrobial therapy.** The infections are frequently caused by bacteria that are resistant to many antimicrobials.

Chronic is a poor term that should be avoided in the context of urinary tract infections, except for chronic bacterial prostatitis, since the duration of the infection is not defined.

Reinfection **is recurrent infection with different bacteria from outside the urinary tract.** Each infection is a new event; the urine must show no growth after the preceding infection.

Bacterial persistence **refers to a recurrent urinary tract infection caused by the same bacteria from a focus within the urinary tract, such as an infection stone or the prostate.** *Relapse* is frequently used interchangeably. Relapse is a useful term when used in the European sense of consecutive infections regardless of the time lapse between them. Unfortunately, investigators in the United States often use the term with a 2-week (or less) limitation between recurrences and thereby imply that the kidney is the site of bacterial persistence. Reinfections of the urinary tract can readily recur within 2 weeks with the same bacterial species that has remained on the vagina and urethra; the relapse then is from the reinfection route of the rectum to vagina to bladder and not from the kidney (Stamey, 1980).

Prophylactic antimicrobial therapy **is the prevention of reinfections of the urinary tract by the administration of antimicrobial drugs.** If the term is used correctly in reference to the urinary tract, it can be assumed that bacteria have been eliminated before prophylaxis is begun.

Suppressive antimicrobial therapy **is the suppression of a focus of bacterial persistence that cannot be eradicated.** A low, nightly dosage of an antimicrobial agent usually results in the urine's showing no growth, as in the case of a small infection stone or in an *Escherichia coli* bacterial prostatitis. *Suppressive* is also a useful term when recurrent acute symptoms are prevented in a poor-risk patient such as one with a large staghorn infection calculus in whom the antimicrobial agent reduces but does not eliminate the bacteria in the urine. In all instances, resorting to suppressive antimicrobial therapy is an admission of defeat (sometimes

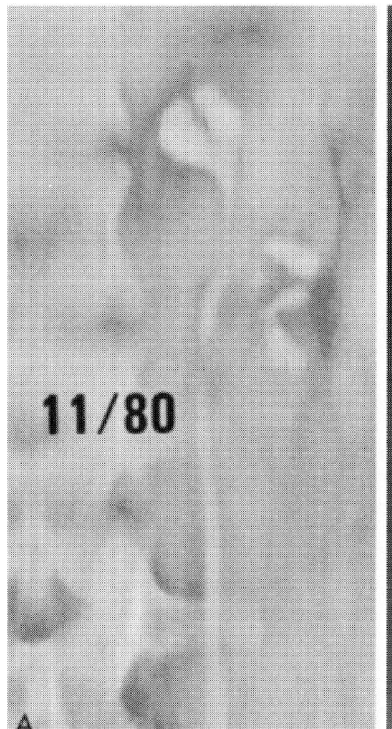

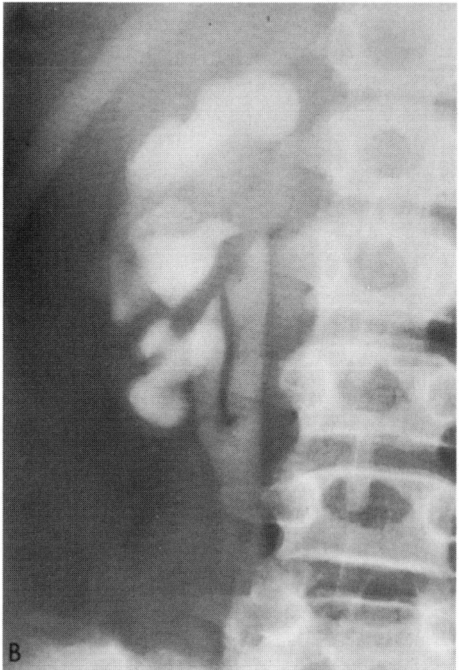

Figure 15–2. *A,* Intravenous urogram of the contralateral left kidney from the same patient as in Figure 15–1. The severe pyelonephritic atrophy, undoubtedly caused by febrile urinary infections during early infancy with reflux into different segments of the kidney, produced irregular cortical scarring. Note how all the calyces extend to the capsule with irregular, intervening areas of cortex. *B,* Pyelonephritic atrophy, suggestive of postobstructive atrophy, in a 20-year-old woman with spina bifida, neurogenic bladder, and many episodes of fever and bacteriuria in early childhood. Observe the uniform, regular atrophy of the renal cortex that suggests reflux of bacteria simultaneously into virtually all nephrons. This type of pyelonephritic atrophy is uncommon compared with that shown in *A* and is characteristic of obstruction with superimposed infection.

in the best interest of the patient) in the challenge of managing difficult urinary tract infections.

Domiciliary urinary tract infections occur in patients who are not hospitalized or institutionalized at the time they become infected. **The infections are generally caused by common fecal bacteria (e.g., Enterobacteriaceae, *Enterococcus faecalis*, or *Staphylococcus epidermidis*) that are susceptible to most antimicrobials.**

***Nosocomial urinary tract infections* occur in patients who are hospitalized or institutionalized and are caused by *Pseudomonas* and other more antimicrobial-resistant strains.**

Table 15–1. CAUSES OF UNRESOLVED BACTERIURIA IN DESCENDING ORDER OF IMPORTANCE

Bacterial resistance to the drug selected for treatment
Development of resistance from initially susceptible bacteria
Bacteriuria caused by two different bacterial species with mutually exclusive susceptibilities
Rapid reinfection with a new, resistant species during initial therapy for the original susceptible organism
Azotemia
Papillary necrosis from analgesic abuse
Giant staghorn calculi in which the "critical mass" of susceptible bacteria is too great for antimicrobial inhibition
Self-inflicted infections or deception in taking antimicrobial drugs (a variant of Munchausen's syndrome)

CLASSIFICATION

Infections in the urinary tract can be divided into four categories: (1) isolated infections, (2) unresolved infections, (3) recurrent urinary tract infections that are reinfections, and (4) recurrent infections resulting from bacterial persistence.

Isolated Infections

First infections or those isolated from previous infections by at least 6 months occur in 25% to 30% of women between the ages of 30 and 40, but occur infrequently in men with a normal urinary tract. About one fourth of such women experience a recurrence in the next few years. Isolated infections in domiciliary patients are usually susceptible to all antimicrobial agents.

Unresolved Bacteriuria During Therapy

The term *unresolved* indicates that the initial therapy has been inadequate. The absence of bacterial growth in the urine during therapy is a prerequisite for successful treatment and for characterization of the type of recurrence. The clinician often fails to recognize this problem because (1) cultures of the urine are not obtained during treatment or (2) if they are obtained, bacterial counts of less than 10^5/ml are misinterpreted as contaminants. Clearly, if *any* of the bacteria that caused the infection are present in the urine during therapy, regardless of how low the number, the bacteria have not been eradicated.

The causes of unresolved bacteriuria, in descending order of importance, are shown in Table 15–1.

The most common cause is that the infecting organisms are resistant to the antimicrobial agent selected to treat the infection. The patient almost invariably has received recent antimicrobial therapy, with the treatment producing resistant organisms among the fecal flora that subsequently infected the urinary tract. Tetracyclines, sulfonamides, and penicillins are notorious for producing resistance in the fecal bacteria. Moreover, through plasmid-mediated resistance transfer factors (R factors), a single course of treatment with one of these drugs may produce bacteria that are simultaneously resistant to such other agents as ampicillin, cephalosporins, streptomycin, and chloramphenicol. Thus, a recent history (3 months or less) of antimicrobial therapy increases the likelihood that resistant fecal flora have colonized the vaginal introitus and produced a urinary tract infection that requires susceptibility testing to select a drug capable of sterilizing the urine. Nitrofurantoin and the quinolones do not cause plasmid-mediated (R factor) resistance and are excellent choices for empirical therapy in patients who have been recently treated with the aforementioned drugs.

The second but less common cause is the development of resistance in a previously susceptible population of bacteria infecting the urinary tract during the course of treatment for the infection. This form of resistance occurs in about 5% of patients treated for urinary tract infections and is easy to recognize clinically. Within 48 to 72 hours of starting therapy a previously susceptible population of 10^5 or more bacteria per milliliter of urine is replaced by an equal population of completely resistant bacteria of the same species through selection of a resistant clone undetected in the original susceptibility testing. When the antimicrobial concentration in the urine is insufficient to kill all the bacteria present, the more resistant strains emerge. This is characteristically seen in patients who are underdosed or noncompliant.

A third cause is the presence of a second unsuspected species that is resistant to the antimicrobial agent chosen to treat the predominant infecting organism. In these mixed infections one of the two organisms acquires dominance over the other and often appears on culture plates as a pure culture of the dominant species. Treatment of the dominant organism unmasks the presence of the second strain.

The fourth cause is rapid reinfection with a new, resistant species before the completion of therapy for the original infecting organism. Fortunately, most reinfections, even in highly susceptible females, do not recur quickly. However, a new resistant strain can reinfect the bladder from introital carriage or an enterovesical fistula on therapy, thus making it appear as if the original bacteriuria were unresolved.

The fifth cause of unresolved bacteriuria is azotemia, in which the bacteriuria continues with susceptible bacteria because the diseased kidney cannot achieve bactericidal concentrations of the antimicrobial agent. Bioassay of the urinary antimicrobial concentration in these cases usually shows the level of the drug to be below the minimal inhibitory concentration of the infecting organism.

The sixth cause is azotemia and papillary necrosis (*analgesic* nephritis). These patients have serum creatinine concentrations greater than 2 mg/dl accompanied by severe defects in medullary concentrating capacity; they can be bacteriuric while taking an antimicrobial agent to which the organism is susceptible. Sometimes the antimicrobial agent can be switched to one with even higher urinary concentrations, while the patient is encouraged not to force fluids, and the bacteriuria can be resolved.

The seventh cause relates to those rare patients with giant staghorn calculi who have an inordinate mass of bacteria that exceeds the antimicrobial activity of the urine. The phenomenon of a *critical density* is well known in susceptibility testing, in which it is recognized that even susceptible bacteria cannot be inhibited once they reach a certain critical density on the agar plate. Although these giant staghorn calculi are rare and smaller calculi do not interfere with eradication of bacteriuria, this is the only circumstance (other than renal failure and the occasional patient with analgesic nephritis) in which susceptible bacteria can continue to cause an unresolved bacteriuria in the presence of proper antimicrobial therapy.

The last cause of unresolved bacteriuria occurs in those patients who have variants of Munchausen's syndrome. These patients secretly inoculate their bladders with uropathogens or omit their oral antimicrobials while steadfastly asserting that they never miss a dose. The patient with Munchausen's syndrome presents with a horrendous clinical history and invariably a normal collecting system on intravenous urography. Careful bacteriologic observations usually indicate the implausibility of the clinical picture.

Recurrent Urinary Tract Infections

The term *recurrent urinary tract infection* applies either to reinfection from *outside* the urinary tract or to bacterial persistence in a focus *within* the urinary tract. It is also clear that until a urinary tract infection is resolved with proper antimicrobial therapy, the type of recurrence—bacterial reinfection or persistence—cannot be classified.

Reinfections

More than 95% of all recurrent infections in females are reinfections of the urinary tract. Reinfections in men are uncommon unless associated with an underlying abnormality of the urinary tract. Vesicointestinal and vesicovaginal fistulas are an unusual, but surgically correctable, cause of reinfections.

Bacterial Persistence

Once the bacteriuria has resolved (i.e., the urine shows no growth for several days after the antimicrobial agent has been stopped), recurrence with the same organism can arise from a site *within* the urinary tract that was excluded from the high urine concentrations of the antimicrobial agent. The 12 correctable urologic abnormalities that cause bacteria to persist within the urinary tract between episodes of recurrent bacteriuria are listed in Table 15–2. The relationship of these abnormalities to bacterial persistence, as well as the documentation that surgical excision removes the infection as a source of recurrent bacteriuria, is presented elsewhere in detail (Stamey, 1980). Once the urologist recognizes that the cause of the patient's recurrent bacteriuria is bacterial persistence, Table 15–2 should serve as a checklist for known, correctable causes. Some of the causes are subtle, and many require cystoscopic localization of the infection with ureteral catheters to accurately define the focus of bacterial persistence.

Table 15–2. CORRECTABLE UROLOGIC ABNORMALITIES THAT CAUSE BACTERIAL PERSISTENCE

Infection stones
Chronic bacterial prostatitis
Unilateral infected atrophic kidneys
Ureteral duplication and ectopic ureters
Foreign bodies
Urethral diverticula and infected paraurethral glands
Unilateral medullary sponge kidneys
Nonrefluxing, normal-appearing, infected ureteral stumps after nephrectomy
Infected urachal cysts
Infected communicating cysts of the renal calyces
Papillary necrosis
Paravesical abscess with fistula to bladder

INCIDENCE AND EPIDEMIOLOGY

Urinary tract infections account for more than 7 million visits to physicians' offices, and necessitate or complicate over 1 million hospital admissions in the United States annually (Patton et al, 1991; Haley et al, 1985). **Urinary tract infections are more common in women than in men except in the neonatal period.**

Surveys screening for bacteriuria have shown that about 1% of schoolgirls (aged 5 to 14 years) (Kunin et al, 1962) **have bacteriuria and that this figure increases to about 4% by young adulthood and then by an additional 1% to 2% per decade of age** (Fig. 15–3). The prevalence in young women is 30 times more than in men. However, **with increasing age the ratio of women to men with bacteriuria progressively decreases.** At least 20% of women and 10% of men over 65 years of age have bacteriuria (Boscia and Kaye, 1987). **The prevalence of bacteriuria also increases with institutionalization or hospitalization and concurrent disease** (Sourander, 1966). In a study of women and men over 68 years of age, Boscia and colleagues (1987) found that 24% of functionally impaired nursing home residents had bacteriuria compared with 12% of healthy domiciliary subjects (Boscia et al, 1986).

Whether bacteriuria is symptomatic or asymptomatic is not always an important distinction for prognosis. Investigators who have traced patients through symptomatic and asymptomatic infections have found that many individuals who have asymptomatic infections become symptomatic at some time and many who experience symptomatic infections then become asymptomatic with time alone. When Mabeck (1972) followed 23 untreated nonpregnant women with acute symptomatic cystitis, 21 lost their symptoms after 4 weeks but before the infection had disappeared. Conversely, when 12 pregnant women with asymptomatic untreated bacteriuria were followed, 7 of the 12 became symptomatic at some time after diagnosis (McFadyen et al, 1973).

A patient who has once had an infection is likely to develop subsequent infections. Many adults had urinary tract infection as children (Gillenwater et al, 1979). Little is known about the natural history of untreated bacteriuria in

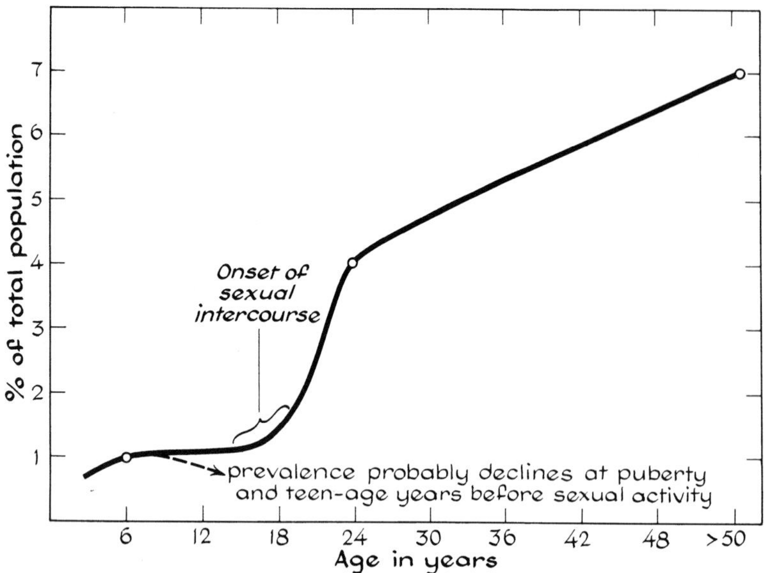

Figure 15–3. Prevalence of bacteriuria in females as a function of age. (From Stamey TA: The Prevention of Recurrent Urinary Infections. New York, Science and Medicine Publishing Company, 1973.)

women because most are treated when they are diagnosed, but a few studies in which treatment with antimicrobials is compared with placebo have been done. These show that 57% to 80% of bacteriuric women who are untreated or treated with placebo clear their infections spontaneously (Mabeck, 1972; Guttman, 1973). Mabeck (1972) found that 8 of 53 bacteriuric women placed on placebo needed treatment with an antimicrobial because of symptoms, but 32 of the remaining 45 women cleared without treatment within a month, and 43 of the 45 had spontaneously cleared of bacteriuria within 5 months; only 2 women remained persistently bacteriuric. Of those who cleared, 10 women became reinfected and another 10 had recurrences with the same organism after a year; that is, 46% of the untreated women had become bacteriuric by a year later.

When women with recurrent bacteriuria were followed after treatment, about one sixth (37 of 219) had a very high recurrence rate (2.6 infections per year), whereas the remaining women had a recurrence rate of only 0.32 per year (Mabeck, 1972). Similar separation was seen in a prospective study, in which only 28.6% of 60 women who experienced their first symptomatic urinary tract infection had recurrent infections over the first 18 months of observation, as opposed to recurrences in 82.5% of 106 women who had had previous urinary tract infections (Harrison et al, 1974). **Other investigators also have found that the probability of recurrent urinary tract infections increases with the number of previous infections and decreases in inverse proportion to the elapsed time between the first and second infections** (Mabeck, 1972). **Of these recurrent infections, 71% to 73% are caused by reinfection with different organisms, rather than recurrence with the same organism** (Mabeck, 1972; Guttmann, 1973).

Women with frequent reinfections have a rate of 0.13 to 0.22 urinary tract infections per month (1.6 to 2.6 infections per year) when the infections are treated with antimicrobials (Mabeck, 1972; Guttmann, 1973; Kraft and Stamey, 1977). **Most reinfections occurred after 2 weeks** (Harrison et al, 1974) **and within 5 months** (Mabeck, 1972), **and most occurred early in this interval** (Kraft and Stamey, 1977) (Fig. 15–4). **Rates of reinfections were independent of bladder dysfunction, radiologic changes of chronic pyelonephritis, and vesicoureteral reflux** (Guttman, 1973). The reinfections did not occur evenly over time. In the Stanford series 23 women with frequent recurrent infections were studied with monthly urine cultures when asymptomatic and with immediate cultures when symptomatic for cystitis, for a mean of 3 years. Thirty-four percent of infections were followed by infection-free intervals of at least 6 months (average 12.8 months), and 22 of the 23 women had such intervals (Fig. 15–5). However, even these long intervals were followed by further infections (Kraft and Stamey, 1977). Similarly, Mabeck (1972) noted that some women who had frequent reinfections showed unpredictable pauses in their recurrences, further evidence to suggest that reinfections may occur in clusters.

When the Stanford data (Kraft and Stamey, 1977) on recurrent urinary tract infections in highly susceptible females are analyzed by examining sets of infections separated by remissions of at least 6 months, 69% of the sets contain only one infection (Fig. 15–6). After this first set the remaining sets show a 33% remission rate in infections, which means a patient who has two or more infections within 6

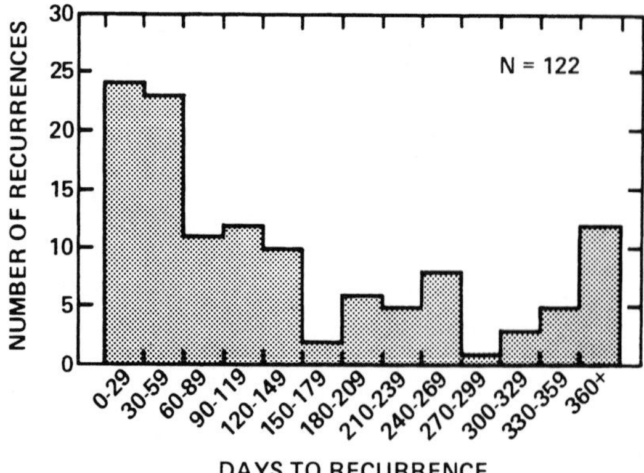

Figure 15–4. Days between recurrent urinary tract infections grouped by 30-day intervals. (From Kraft JK, Stamey TA: Medicine 1977; 56:55.)

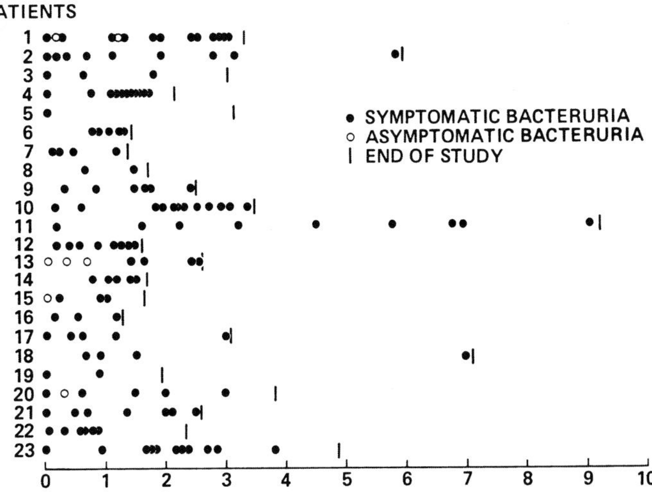

Figure 15–5. Occurrence of urinary tract infections in 23 women with frequent recurrent bacteriuria. (From Kraft JK, Stamey TA: Medicine 1977; 56:55.)

months has only a 33% probability of remaining free of infection for the next 6 months. Therefore, **if antimicrobial prophylaxis is started after the second or any succeeding infection within a set, about one third of the women will be treated unnecessarily. The remaining two thirds of the women still risk more infections.**

Whether a patient receives no treatment at all, or short-term, long-term, or prophylactic antimicrobial treatment, the risk of recurrent bacteriuria remains the same; treatment appears to alter only the time until recurrence. Asscher and associates (1973) found that reinfections occurred in 17 patients (34%) treated with a 7-day course of nitrofurantoin, and 13 patients (29%) receiving placebo during a 3- to 5-year follow-up. Mabeck (1972) found that 46% (20 of 43) of untreated patients had recurrent infections by 12 months compared with about 40% of treated patients who had recurrences. Both studies suggest that it makes little difference whether a urinary tract infection is cured with an antimicrobial or is allowed to clear spontaneously—the susceptibility to recurrent urinary tract infection remains the same. Moreover, patients with frequent urinary tract infection who take prophylactic antimicrobial agents for extended periods (6 months or more) may decrease their infections during the time of prophylaxis, but the rate of infection returns to the pretreatment rate after prophylaxis is stopped (Stamm et al, 1980a; Vosti, 1975). Even long interruptions in the pattern of recurrence, therefore, do not appear to alter the patient's basic susceptibility to infections.

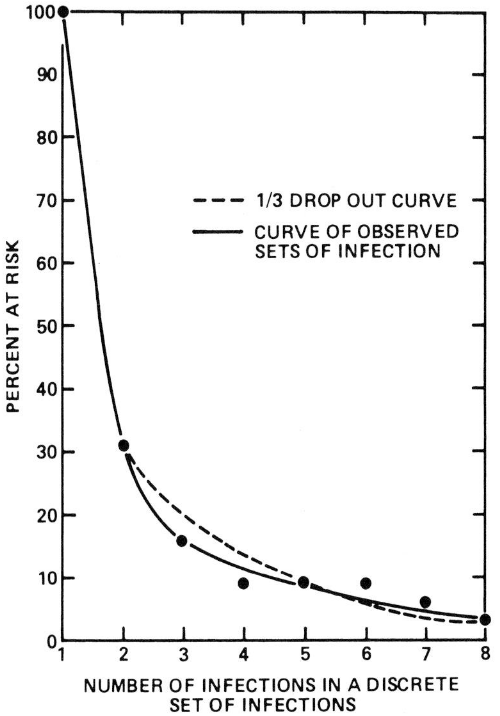

Figure 15–6. Sets of urinary tract infections as a function of the fraction of women who remain at risk of recurrent infection. After two or more infections within a set, there is a two-thirds probability of another infection during the next 6 months. A set is defined as any infection or group of infections preceded and followed by 6 months of remission. (From Kraft JK, Stamey TA: Medicine 1977; 56:55.)

The long-term effects of uncomplicated recurrent urinary tract infections are not completely known, but so far no association between recurrent infections and renal scarring, hypertension, or progressive renal azotemia has been established (Asscher et al, 1973; Freedman, 1975). Indeed, one investigator was unable to find a single case of unequivocal nonobstructive chronic pyelonephritis in 22 patients in whom chronic pyelonephritis was the cause of end-stage renal failure (Schechter et al, 1971). Similar data were reported by Huland and Busch (1982).

Although short-term antimicrobial treatment and prophylaxis do not seem to affect the course of recurrent urinary tract infections, pregnancy does affect this course. **In pregnant women, the prevalence and rate of recurrent infection are the same, but their bacteriuria progresses to acute clinical pyelonephritis more frequently than in nonpregnant women.** This variation in the natural history of recurrent infections in females is discussed in a later section on urinary tract infections in pregnancy.

PATHOGENESIS

Urinary tract infections are a result of interactions between a uropathogen and the host. Increased bacterial

virulence appears to be necessary to overcome strong host resistance, and conversely, bacteria with minimal virulence characteristics are able to infect patients who are significantly compromised.

Routes of Infection

Ascending Route

Most bacteria enter the urinary tract from the fecal reservoir via ascent through the urethra into the bladder. This route is enhanced in individuals with significant soilage of the perineum with feces, women using spermicidal agents (Hooton et al, 1989b), and patients with intermittent or indwelling catheters.

Although cystitis is frequently restricted to the bladder, in approximately 50% of instances there is further extension of the infection into the upper urinary tract (Stamey, 1980). **The weight of clinical and experimental evidence strongly suggests that most episodes of pyelonephritis are caused by retrograde ascent of bacteria from the bladder through the ureter to the renal pelvis and parenchyma. Reflux of urine is not required for ascending infections, but edema associated with cystitis may cause sufficient changes in the ureterovesical junction to permit reflux.** Once the bacteria are introduced into the ureter they may ascend to the kidney unaided. **This ascent, however, is greatly increased if bacteria have special adhesions (i.e., P pili; see below) or by any process that interferes with the normal ureteral peristaltic function.** Gram-negative bacteria and their endotoxins as well as pregnancy and ureteral obstruction have a marked antiperistaltic effect.

Once the bacteria reach the renal pelvis they can enter the renal parenchyma by means of the collecting ducts at the papillary tips and then ascend upward within the collecting tubules. This process is hastened and exacerbated by increased renal pelvic pressure due to ureteral obstruction or vesicoureteral reflux, particularly when it is associated with intrarenal reflux.

Hematogenous Route

Infection of the kidney by the hematogenous route is uncommon in normal individuals. However, **the kidney is occasionally secondarily infected in patients with *Staphylococcus aureus* bacteremia from oral sites or with *Candida*** fungemia. Experimental data indicate that infection is enhanced when the kidney is obstructed (Smellie et al, 1975).

Lymphatic Route

Direct extension of bacteria from the adjacent organs via lymphatics may occur in unusual circumstances such as a severe bowel infection or retroperitoneal abscesses. There is little evidence that lymphatic routes play a significant role in the vast majority of urinary tract infections.

Urinary Pathogens

Most urinary tract infections are caused by facultative anaerobes that are able to grow under either anaerobic or aerobic conditions and usually originate in the bowel flora. Uropathogens such as *S. epidermidis* and *Candida albicans* originate in the flora of the vaginal or perineal skin.

Escherichia coli* is by far the most common cause of urinary tract infection, accounting for 85% of community-acquired and 50% of hospital-acquired infections. Other gram-negative Enterobacteriaceae including** *Proteus* and *Klebsiella*, and gram-positive *E. faecalis* and *Staphylococcus saprophyticus* are responsible for the remainder of most community-acquired infections. **Nosocomial infections are frequently caused by *E. faecalis (Hall et al, 1992) **as well as caused by *Klebsiella, Enterobacter, Citrobacter, Serratia, Pseudomonas aeruginosa, Providencia*, and *S. epidermidis*** (Kennedy et al, 1965).

Less common organisms such as *Gardnerella vaginalis, Mycoplasma* species, and *Ureaplasma urealyticum* may infect patients with intermittent or indwelling catheters (Josephson et al, 1988).

The prevalence of infecting organisms is influenced by the age of the patient. For example, ***S. saprophyticus* is now recognized as causing approximately 10% of symptomatic lower urinary tract infections in young, sexually active females** (Latham et al, 1983), **whereas it rarely causes infection in males and elderly individuals.** A seasonal variation with a late summer to fall peak has been reported (Hovelius and Mardh, 1984; Hedman and Ringertz, 1991).

Fastidious Organisms

Anaerobes in the Urinary Tract

Although symptomatic anaerobic infections of the urinary tract are documented, they are uncommon. The distal urethra, perineum, and vagina are normally colonized by anaerobes. Whereas 1% to 10% of voided urine specimens are positive for anaerobic organisms (Finegold, 1977), anaerobic organisms found in suprapubic aspirates are much more unusual (Gorbach and Bartlett, 1974). Clinically symptomatic urinary tract infections in which only anaerobic organisms are cultured are rare, but these must be suspected when a patient with bladder irritative symptoms has cocci or gram-negative rods seen on microscopic examination of the centrifuged urine (catheterized, suprapubic aspirated, or voided midstream urine), and routine quantitative aerobic cultures fail to grow organisms (Ribot et al, 1981).

Anaerobic organisms are frequently found in suppurative infections of the genitourinary tract. In one study of suppurative genitourinary infections in males, 88% of scrotal, prostatic, and perinephric abscesses included anaerobes among the infecting organisms (Bartlett and Gorbach, 1981). The organisms found are usually *Bacteroides* species including *Bacteroides fragilis, Fusobacterium* species, anaerobic cocci, and *Clostridium perfringens* (Finegold, 1977). The growth of clostridia may be associated with cystitis emphysematosa (Bromberg et al, 1982).

Mycobacterium tuberculosis *and Other Atypical Mycobacteria*

Mycobacterium tuberculosis and other atypical mycobacteria may be found when cultures for acid-fast bacteria are requested; they do not grow under routine aerobic conditions and may be found during evaluation for sterile pyuria. It has been emphasized that the mere presence of mycobacteria may not indicate tissue infection. Therefore, factors such as symptoms; endoscopic or radiologic evidence of infection; abnormal urine sediment; the absence of other pathogens; repeated demonstration of the organism; and the presence of granulomas should be considered before therapy is instituted (Brooker and Aufderheide, 1980; Thomas et al, 1980). (*M. tuberculosis* is discussed in Chapter 24.)

Chlamydia

Chlamydiae are not routinely grown in aerobic culture but have been implicated in genitourinary infections. (Their role in the urinary tract is discussed in Chapter 18.)

Bacterial Virulence Factors

Since the intestine is the ultimate reservoir of *E. coli* for urinary tract infections, as well as for other extraintestinal infection sites, microbiologists have long been interested in the question of whether certain strains have a pathogenic advantage (uropathogenicity or nephropathogenicity) over others in causing disease. Do the *E. coli* that cause urinary tract infections colonize the vagina and urethra in a random fashion, or do only a few strains from the intestinal reservoir have virulence factors that impart a biologic advantage? For example, hemolysis of red blood cells is assumed to be a cytotoxic factor and occurs in a substantial percentage of *E. coli* strains that cause urinary tract infections. McGeachie (1966) found hemolysis in 29% of 534 strains isolated from voided urine and noted also that five common serologic O groups (01, 04, 06, 018, and 075) accounted for 72% of all the hemolytic strains he isolated. Cooke and Ewins (1975) found that hemolytic strains of *E. coli* in the periurethral flora were more likely to occur in subsequent urinary tract infections than were nonhemolytic strains in the same flora. Minshew and her associates (1978) reported that 49% of their urinary tract strains caused hemolysis, in contrast to only 1 of 20 strains (5%) isolated from normal enteric flora. Although the potential virulence that hemolysis imparts to some *E. coli* strains is unknown, Fried and colleagues (1971) demonstrated that a hemolytic *E. coli* (06:H31) commonly caused pyelonephritis in the kidneys of mice and rats, whereas a nonhemolytic mutant of the same *E. coli* did not.

In addition to hemolysin production Minshew and coworkers (1978) showed that the characteristics of colicin V production, the ability to kill allantoically inoculated 13-day-old chick embryos, and hemagglutination of human erythrocytes in the presence of D-mannose, were all more common in extraintestinal *E. coli* infections than in *E. coli* from the normal enteric flora. The ability of *E. coli* to agglutinate human erythrocytes in the presence of D-mannose was demonstrated in 59% of *E. coli* from extraintestinal infections but in only 15% of *E. coli* from the normal enteric flora.

Strains of *E. coli* elaborate envelope or capsular acidic polysaccharide antigens called K antigens. Specific K antigens are associated with *E. coli* strains implicated in infections of many different tissues, including those of the urinary tract, particularly pyelonephritis. In several experimental studies of urinary tract infection in mice, it is quite clear that *E. coli* strains elaborating specific K antigens have a striking propensity to cause pyelonephritis, in contrast to other strains elaborating either no K antigens or K antigens of other serotypes. These observations collectively suggest that specific K antigens endow strains of *E. coli* with enhanced pathogenic potential. Studies indicate that it is not merely the presence of K antigen but the quantity of K antigen synthesized by a given strain of *E. coli* that determines the degree of virulence of that strain (Kaijser et al, 1977).

Achtman and associates (1983) have identified six widespread bacterial clones among several common serotypes of *E. coli* K_1 isolates from a number of centers in Europe and the United States—implying linear descent of each clone from an ancestral cell. Using electrophoretic migration of major outer membrane proteins as their clonal markers, they proposed that O serogroups; hemolysin and colicin production; plasmid content; and metabolic (biochemical) properties are all independent, conserved characteristics of a limited number of clonal groups of *E. coli* K_1. It is interesting that within the K_1 isolates none of these other properties correlated with bacterial virulence.

Bacterial Adherence and Colonization

Because of an accumulating literature in the early 1970s on bacterial adherence to mucosal surfaces in diseases of the intestinal, respiratory, and pharyngeal tracts, investigators began to study the role of bacterial adherence in urinary tract infections. The following passages are modified, with permission, from Schaeffer (1989).

Bacterial Adhesins

Numerous studies have demonstrated that bacteria selectively adhere to mucosal surfaces and that the extent to which they adhere is a critical event in colonization and infection (Savage, 1972; H. Smith, 1977; Ofek and Beachey, 1980). **The bacterial cell structures that seem to be most important in binding of bacteria to epithelium cells are long, filamentous protein appendages called *pili* or *fimbriae*** (Fig. 15–7) (Brinton, 1959). A typical piliated cell may contain 100 to 400 pili (Brinton, 1965; Duguid et

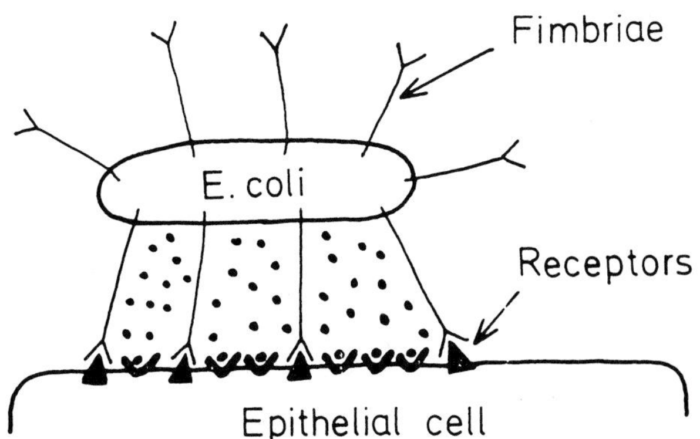

Figure 15–7. Bacterial adherence. Adhesins on pili (fimbriae) mediate attachment to specific epithelial cell receptors.

al, 1966). These supramolecular structures are usually 5 to 10 nm in diameter and up to 2 μm long and appear to be composed primarily of subunits known as pilin, which have molecular masses of 17 to 27 kD, depending on the type of pili (Klemm, 1985). *E. coli* produces a number of antigenically and functionally different types of pili on the same cell; other strains may produce only a single type, and in some isolates, no pili are seen.

Pili are defined functionally by their ability to mediate hemagglutination of specific types of erythrocytes.

Mannose-Sensitive (Type 1) Pili

Type 1 pili of *E. coli* mediate hemagglutination (HA) of guinea pig erythrocytes (Duguid et al, 1979). The reaction is mediated by the addition of mannose and thus termed mannose-sensitive hemagglutination (MSHA) (Duguid et al, 1966; Old, 1972). **Type 1 pili are found in most uropathogenic strains of *E. coli*, and in many nonpathogens.** Type 1C pili are closely related structurally to type 1 pili but do not mediate HA or mannoside binding (Klemm et al, 1982). The genes encoding the common type 1 and type 1C pili have been cloned and sequenced, revealing a 68% amino acid identity between the major pilin subunits of the two types (Hull et al, 1981).

Mannose-Resistant (P) Pili

P pili bind to α-D-Gal-(1–4)-β-D-Gal belonging to the globoseries of glycolipids (Kallenius et al, 1980; Leffler and Svanborg-Eden, 1980), **which are found on P–blood group antigens and on uroepithelium** (Svenson et al, 1983). **P pili, which are found in most pyelonephritogenic strains of *E. coli*, mediate HA of human erythrocytes that is not altered by mannose, and is thus termed mannose-resistant hemogglutination (MRHA)** (Kallenius and Molby, 1979). Polyclonal antisera raised against P pili show considerable cross reactivity with type 1 pili, suggesting that these structures are morphologically and antigenically related (de Ree et al, 1985). The relationship is also reflected at the genetic level, where the nucleotide sequences between the P pilin and type 1 pilin genes share significant homology (Baga et al, 1984). The MRHA adhesins of uropathogenic *E. coli* that do not show the digalactoside-binding specificity have been provisionally named X adhesins (Vaisanen et al, 1981). In some strains of *E. coli*, hemagglutination is mediated by nonpiliated adhesins or hemagglutinins (Duguid et al, 1979).

Svanborg-Eden and associates (1976) were the first to report a correlation between bacterial adherence and severity of urinary tract infections. They showed that *E. coli* strains from girls with acute pyelonephritis had high adhesive ability, whereas strains from girls with asymptomatic bacteriuria or normal feces had low bacterial adherence. Between 70% and 80% of the pyelonephritic strains had adhesive capacity, but only 10% of the fecal isolates adhered. **When 97 children with urinary tract infections and 82 healthy controls were examined for the occurrence of *E. coli* possessing P pili, the pili were present in 91% of urinary strains causing pyelonephritis, 19% of strains causing cystitis, and 14% of strains causing asymptomatic bacteriuria but were in only 7% of fecal isolates from healthy children** (Kallenius et al, 1981).

Although the association of MRHA and digalactoside P specificity with *E. coli* causing pyelonephritis in children is greater than the association of any other laboratory-defined bacterial characteristic, the renal abnormalities in terms of scarring and degree of reflux are not impressive (Vaisanen et al, 1981). **This observation is confirmed by the more recent findings of Lomberg and associates (1983) that in girls, recurrent pyelonephritis with gross reflux (in which most of the scarring historically occurs) is minimally associated with P-piliated *E. coli* strains. Thus, it would appear that P pili in acute pyelonephritis are important mainly in nonrefluxing or minimally refluxing children.**

The role of type 1 pili in urinary tract infections has not been as thoroughly studied probably because (1) type 1 pili are found frequently on nonpathogenic, as well as pathogenic, *E. coli;* (2) urinary isolates frequently do not express type 1 pili in urine in vivo (Harber et al, 1982; Ljungh and Wadstrom, 1983); and (3) previous animal models have indicated that type 1 pili are less important than P pili in the pathogenesis of renal parenchymal infection (pyelonephritis) (Guze et al, 1983; Hagberg et al, 1983a, 1983b; O'Hanley et al, 1985).

Some studies, however, clearly suggest a role for type 1 pili in urinary tract infections. This evidence has been obtained **(1) from the fact that bacteria isolated from the urine of patients with urinary tract infections expressed MS adhesins** (Ljungh and Wadstrom, 1983); **(2) from studies with animal models** (Fader and Davis, 1982; Hagberg et al, 1983a, 1983b; Iwahi et al, 1983; Hultgren et al, 1985) **in which inoculation of type 1 piliated organisms into the bladder resulted in significantly more colonization of the urinary tract than inoculation of nonpiliated organisms; and (3) from the observation that anti–type 1 pili antibodies and methyl-α-D-mannopyranoside protected mice from experimental urinary tract infections** (Aronson et al, 1979; Hultgren et al, 1985).

Bacterial Pili in Vivo

Direct evidence for the role of type 1 and P pili in adherence in urinary tract infections in vivo in humans is limited and partially contradictory. Ljungh and Wadstrom (1983) demonstrated by electron microscopy that pili were present on *E. coli* in the urine of 31 of 37 patients, but the specific pilus type was not determined. Conversely, Ofek and associates (1981) showed no MS adhesins in 22 of 24 urine isolates from patients with indwelling catheters, and Harber and associates (1982) found that 19 of 20 samples from patients with acute urinary tract infections were devoid of pili and nonadherent until subcultured in broth. **Assessment of pili production by clinical *E. coli* isolates is further complicated by the fact that environmental growth conditions can produce rapid changes in pilus expression** (Duguid et al, 1966; Goransson and Uhlin, 1984; Hultgren et al, 1986), **wherein cells switch back and forth between piliated and nonpiliated phases** (Eisenstein, 1981). **This process is called phase variation and has obvious biologic and clinical implications.** For example, the presence of type 1 pili may be advantageous to the bacteria for adhering to and colonizing the bladder mucosa, but disadvantageous because the pili enhance phagocytosis and killing by neutrophils (Silverblatt et al, 1979).

Preliminary evidence in an animal model of ascending urinary tract infections and studies of isolates from different sites in patients with urinary tract infections provide preliminary evidence that phase variation can occur during *E. coli* urinary tract infections in vivo. Type 1–piliated *E. coli* that were capable of phase variation were introduced into the mouse bladder in the piliated phase. Then the bacteria recovered from the bladder and urine 24 or more hours after inoculation were tested for piliation. All the animals had bladder colonization, and 78% of the recovered bacteria showed type 1 piliation. The bacteriologic state of the urine often differed from that of the bladder. The urine was sterile in 59% of the animals with bladder colonization, and the bacteria recovered from the urine were frequently nonpiliated. Phase variation also occurred over time. When bladder and kidney cultures were examined 1, 3, and 5 days after intravesical inoculation of piliated bacteria, organisms recovered from the bladder remained piliated whereas organisms recovered from the kidney and urine showed significantly less piliation (Fig. 15–8).

Recent studies in humans using indirect immunofluorescence of fresh urine bacteria have confirmed in vivo expression and phase variation of pili. Pere and colleagues studied the urine of 20 children with pyelonephritis or cystitis and identified P pili in 17 specimens and type 1 pili in 9 (Pere et al, 1987). More recently, Kisielius and associates (1989) analyzed the urine of adults with lower urinary tract infections and detected type 1 pili in 31 of 41 specimens and P pili in 6 of 18 specimens. The piliation status of the bacterial population in the urine was heterogeneous, varying from predominantly piliated to a mixture of piliated and nonpiliated cells (Fig. 15–9). Strains isolated from different sites in the urogenital tract showed variation in the state of piliation. Thus, results demonstrate that *E. coli* type 1 and P pili are expressed and subject to phase variation in vivo during acute urinary tract infections in children and adults.

Model Adherence Systems

A number of models have been used to study the nature of adherence between bacteria and mammalian cells and their relevance to virulence and the pathogenesis of urinary tract infections. These studies can be difficult to interpret and to compare, because many factors can influence the results. For example, the source of the bacteria in nature; artifacts resulting from conditions of in vitro growth of the bacteria (e.g., phenotypic changes); the phase of growth selected for study or effects of laboratory passage; the nature of the mammalian cells or tissue investigated; the species of the donor; the age of the host; or the integrity of the tissue of in vitro systems each may affect the findings.

To date most adherence assays have been performed in vitro. Suspensions of cells (e.g., epithelial cells) are exposed to a standardized concentration of bacteria for a given period of time (usually 30 to 60 minutes). The unattached bacteria are then separated by centrifugation or filtration and are counted in approximately 40 to 50 epithelial cells with adhering bacteria during visual examination by light microscopy. In addition to being tedious, this type of assay cannot readily distinguish adherent test bacteria from the indigenous bacteria already present on the cell surface before assay. Vigorous washing of the epithelial cells, which is required to remove the indigenous bacteria before incubation, can modify the cell surface and alter its receptivity. Because of these disadvantages, assays were developed using radioisotopically labeled bacteria. Such assays eliminate the problem of distinguishing experimental bacteria from indigenous organisms on epithelial cells. Also, many epithelial cells can be studied in each assay. A disadvantage of this technique, however, is that individual variations in the binding capacities of cells cannot be determined. In vitro systems can assess the effects of various conditions of incubation or of various defined substances on the adherence process. However, the natural physiologic barriers of the intact tissue are bypassed. Therefore, the in vivo significance of in vitro experiments must be interpreted with caution.

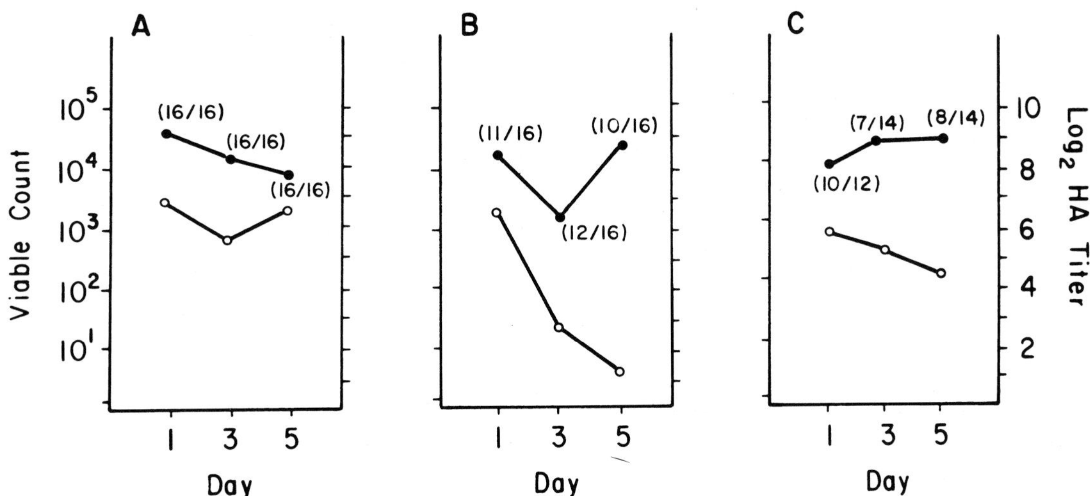

Figure 15–8. Time study after intravesical inoculation with *E. coli* strain I-149 that compared the mean viable bacteria count (○) and hemagglutination (HA) titer (●) for bladders *(A)*, kidneys *(B)*, and urine specimens *(C)* from the same animals. Each point is the mean of all the animals tested. The numbers in parentheses show the proportion of animals inoculated that gave positive cultures. The HA titers were tested after 18 hours of growth on agar. The HA titer of bacteria recovered from the kidney decreased significantly by day 5 ($P < .001$). (From Schaeffer AJ, Schwan WR, Hultgren SJ, Duncan JL: Infect Immun 1987; 55:373–380.)

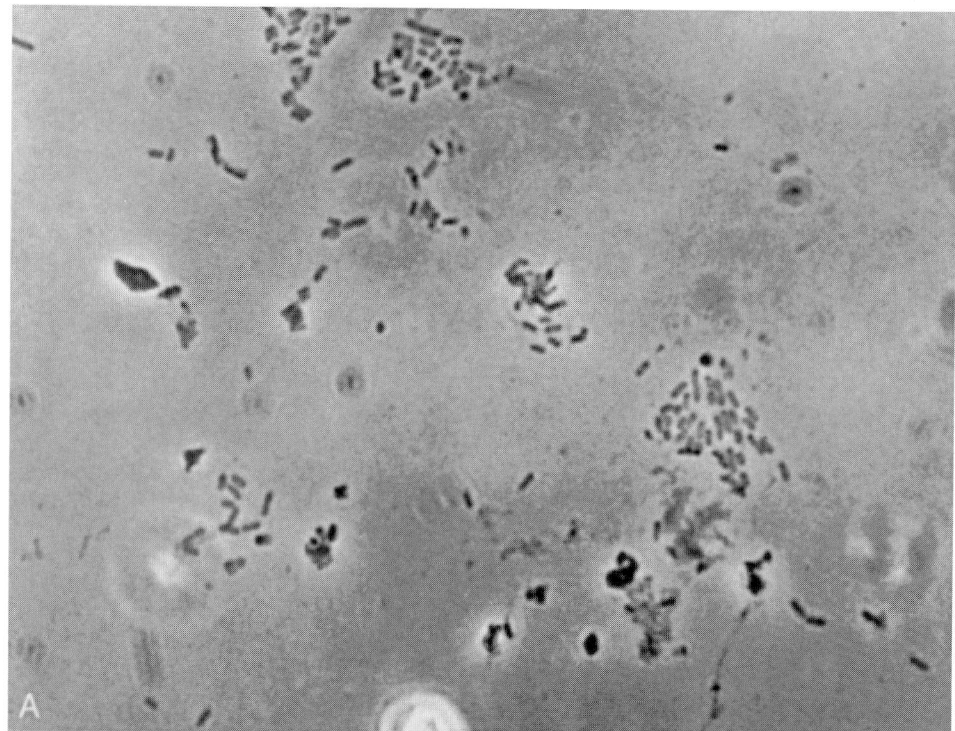

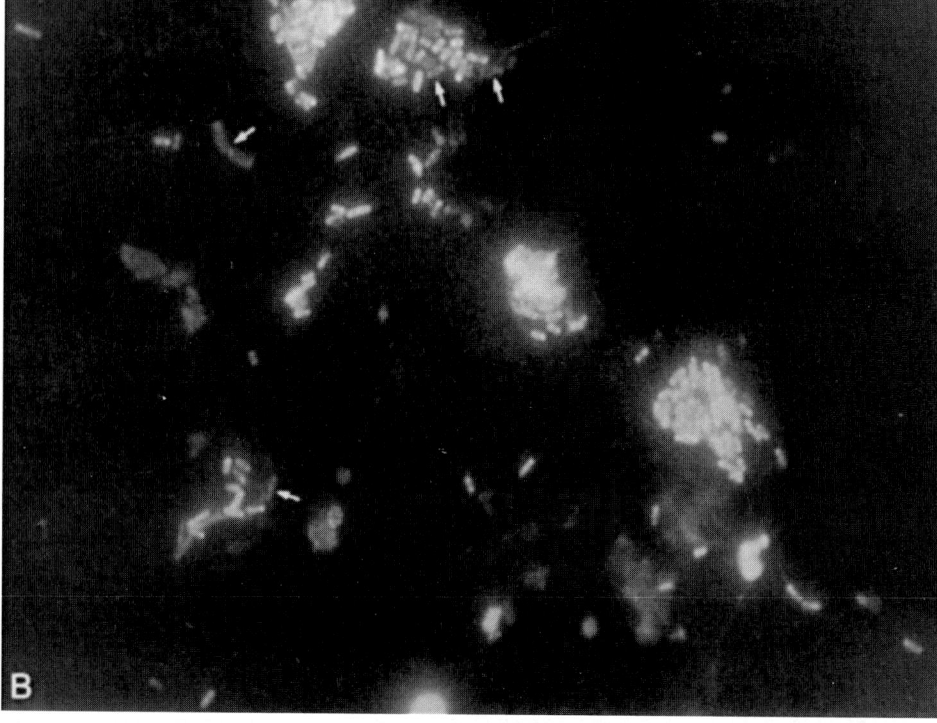

Figure 15–9. Phase-contrast micrograph *(A)* and immunofluorescence micrograph *(B)* of a sample stained with antiserum to type 1 pili of strain I49 and with FITC-conjugated second antibody against nonadherent *E. coli* in the urine of a patient with acute urinary tract infection, showing a mixture of piliated and nonpiliated *(arrows)* cells. (From Kisielius PV, Schwan WR, Amundsen SK, et al: Infect Immun 1989; 57:1656.)

In vivo adherence assays have been developed in which adherence to mucosal surfaces is determined directly by light or electron microscopy, or indirectly by quantification of radiolabeled bacteria. More commonly, the sequela of adherence (i.e., infections) is assessed and judged to be the result of an initial adhesive process.

Epithelial Cell Receptivity

The significance of bacterial adherence in the pathogenesis of ascending urinary tract infection has been studied initially by examining adherence of *E. coli* to vaginal epithelial cells and uroepithelial cells collected from voided urine specimens. **When vaginal epithelial cells were collected from patients susceptible to reinfection and compared with such cells obtained from controls resistant to urinary tract infections, the *E. coli* strains that cause cystitis adhered much more avidly to the epithelial cells from the susceptible women** (Fowler and Stamey, 1977). **These studies established increased adherence of pathogenic bacteria to vaginal epithelial cells as the first demonstra-**

ble biologic difference that could be shown in women susceptible to urinary tract infections.

These findings were confirmed in children by Kallenius and Winberg (1978) and Svanborg-Eden and Jodal (1979). Subsequently, the author and associates (Schaeffer et al, 1981) also confirmed these vaginal differences in women but, in addition, observed that the increased adherence is also characteristic of buccal epithelial cells. As can be seen in Figure 15–10, there is a striking similarity in the ability of both cell types to bind the same *E. coli* strain. **The authors also determined that there is a significant relationship between vaginal cell and buccal cell receptivity.** Seventy-seven different *E. coli* strains were tested for their ability to bind to vaginal and buccal epithelial cells. A direct nonlinear relationship between buccal and vaginal adherence in both controls and patients was confirmed for urinary, vaginal, and anal isolates (Schaeffer et al, 1982). Thus, **high vaginal cell receptivity is associated with high buccal cell receptivity.**

These observations emphasize that the increase in receptor sites for *E. coli* on epithelial cells from women with recurrent urinary tract infections is not limited to the vagina and thus suggest that a genotypic trait for epithelial cell receptivity may be a major susceptibility factor in urinary tract infections. This concept was extended by examining the human leukocyte antigens (HLAs), which are the major histocompatibility complex in humans and have been associated statistically with many diseases (Schaeffer et al, 1983). The HLA types in 35 women with documented recurrent urinary tract infections were compared with those from women having no history of infection. The A3 antigen was identified in 12 (34%) of the patients, a frequency significantly higher than the 8% frequency observed in healthy controls. Thus, HLA-A3 may be associated with an increased risk of recurrent urinary tract infections.

Blood group antigens, carbohydrate structures bound to membrane lipids or proteins, constitute an important part of the uroepithelial cell membrane. The presence or absence of blood group determinants on the surface of uroepithelial cells may influence an individual's susceptibility to urinary tract infections. The author and associates determined the blood group phenotypes in women with recurrent urinary tract infections and compared them with age-matched female controls; **women with Lewis blood group Le(a − b −) and Le(a + b −) (nonsecretor) phenotypes had a significantly higher incidence of recurrent urinary tract infections than women with an Le(a − b +) phenotype.** There was no significant difference in the distribution of ABO or P blood group phenotypes. The Lewis antigen controls fucosylation. The protective effect in women with the Le(a − b +) phenotype presumably is due to fucosylated structures at the cell surface that decrease the availability of putative receptors for *E. coli*. Alternatively, susceptibility among women who do not secrete blood group antigens may be due to specific *E. coli*–binding glycolipids that are absent in women who secrete blood group antigens (Stapleton et al, 1992). **These studies individually and collectively support the concept that there is an increased epithelial receptivity for *E. coli* on the introital, urethral, and buccal mucosae that is characteristic of women and girls susceptible to recurrent urinary tract infections, and this may be a genotypic trait.**

Variation in Cell Receptivity

A small variation in both vaginal cell and buccal cell receptivity may be observed from day to day in healthy

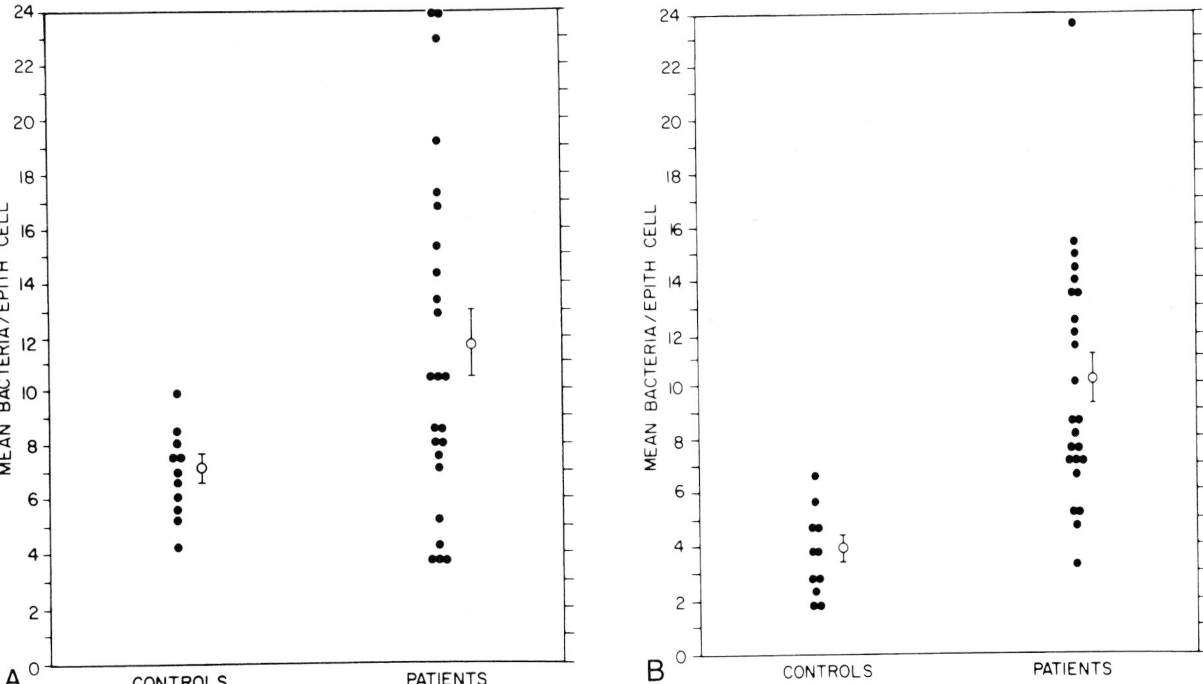

Figure 15–10. In vitro adherence of *Escherichia coli* to vaginal *(A)* and buccal *(B)* cells from healthy controls and patients with recurrent urinary tract infections. Values represent an average of 14 *(A)* and 11 *(B)* determination in each individual. The open circles and bars represent the means + S.E. (From Schaeffer AJ, Jones JM, Dunn JK: N Engl J Med 1981; 304:1062–1066.)

controls. Adherence ranges from 1 to 17 bacteria per cell and appears to be both cyclic and repetitive. When adherence was correlated with the days of a woman's menstrual cycle, higher values were noted in the early phase, but these diminished shortly after the time of expected ovulation (day 14) (Fig. 15–11) (Schaeffer et al, 1979). The number of bacteria per epithelial cell frequently correlated with the value obtained on the same day of the menstrual cycle 1 or 2 months previously. Premenopausal women are particularly susceptible to attachment of uropathogenic *E. coli* and nonpathogenic lactobacilli at certain times during the menstrual cycle and to *E. coli* during the early stages of pregnancy (Reid et al, 1983; Chan et al, 1984). The importance of such hormones as estrogens in the pathogenesis of urinary tract infections is therefore a matter of great interest, especially as the clinical urologist may see women who have recurrent cystitis at regular intervals, possibly in response to these hormonal changes.

Elderly women have low levels of estrogens, yet urinary tract infections are common, especially in hospitalized patients (Brocklehurst et al, 1977). **Reid and associates (1984) found that uropathogens attached in larger numbers to uroepithelial cells from women older than 65 years of age than to cells from premenopausal women aged 18 to 40 years. This enhanced adherence has been associated with increased colonization by *E. coli*** (Raz and Stamm, 1993).

The role of mucopolysaccharides that coat the surface of the uroepithelial cells and of uromucoid in modulating receptivity and preventing bacterial attachment is still a matter for debate. Parsons and associates (1980) described a surface mucin on the bladder mucosa of rabbits that they identified as a glycosaminoglycan that prevents bacterial attachment. **Orskov and colleagues (1980) observed that *E. coli* strains expressing mannose-sensitive (MS) type 1 pili were trapped in vitro by uromucoid (Tamm-Horsfall protein) and thus blocked from attaching to uroepithelial cells; this suggests that type 1 pili may facilitate clearance of bacteria from the urinary tract. However, it is possible that association with surface mucus rather than with the tissue surface itself may be a first stage in bacterial colonization of the urinary tract.** After binding to the mucus, bacteria that also possess the ability to attach to the epithelial cells lining the bladder and the kidney may proceed to induce infection. In asymptomatic patients bacteria could remain associated with the mucus or in residual urine and thus not attach to the tissue surface.

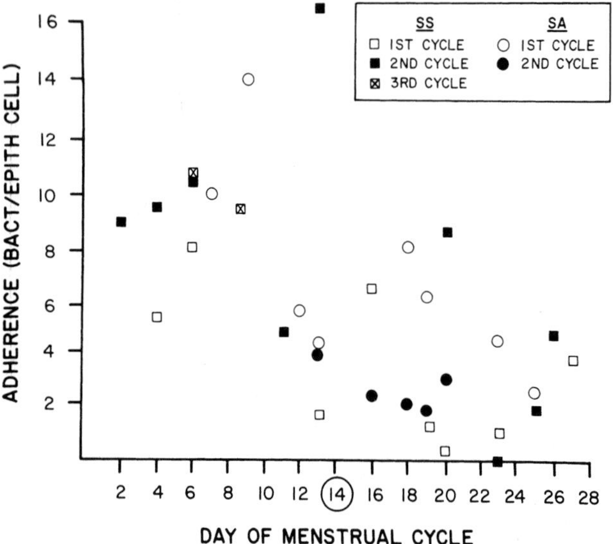

Figure 15–11. Relationship between the adherence of *E. coli* and the day of the menstrual cycle on which uroepithelial cells were obtained from two women with no history of urinary tract infections. Adherence was measured on the same day that the cells were collected. (From Schaeffer AJ, Amundsen SK, Schmidt LN: Infect Immun 1979; 24:753–759.)

DIAGNOSIS

Urine Collection

Diagnostic accuracy can be improved by reducing bacterial contamination when the urine is collected. In order of decreasing complexity: (1) the bladder urine can be aspirated suprapubically in order to provide the highest degree of reliability (Stamey et al, 1965); (2) the female patient can be catheterized; and (3) segmented voided urine specimens can be collected.

Suprapubic Aspiration

Bladder aspiration, although neither painful nor dangerous, is unpleasant for the patient. It is highly useful in newborn infants (Newman et al, 1967) and in patients with paraplegia. A single aspirated specimen reveals the bacteriologic status of the bladder urine without introducing urethral bacteria, which can start a new infection.

Before a suprapubic aspiration (SPA) is performed, the patient should force fluids until the bladder is full. The site of the needle puncture is in the midline, between the symphysis pubis and the umbilicus and directly over the palpable bladder. The full bladder in the male is usually palpable because of its greater muscle tone; unfortunately, the full bladder in the female is frequently not palpable. In such patients, the physician performing the aspiration must rely on the observation that suprapubic pressure directly over the bladder produces an unmistakable desire to urinate. After determining the approximate site for needle puncture, the local area is shaved and the skin is cleansed with an alcohol sponge; a cutaneous wheal is raised with a 25-gauge needle and any local anesthetic (Fig. 15–12). A 3.5 inch spinal, 22-gauge needle is introduced through the anesthetized skin. The progress of the needle is arrested just below the skin within the anesthetized area, and with a quick plunging action, similar to that of any intramuscular injection, the needle is advanced into the bladder. Most patients experience more discomfort from the initial anesthetization of the skin than they feel during the second stage when the needle is advanced into the bladder. After the needle has been introduced, a 20-ml syringe is used to aspirate 5 ml of urine for culture and 15 ml of urine for centrifugation and urinalysis. The obturator is reintroduced into the needle, and both needle and obturator are withdrawn. A small dressing is placed over the needle site in the skin. If urine is not obtained with complete introduction of the needle, the patient's bladder is not full and is usually deep within the

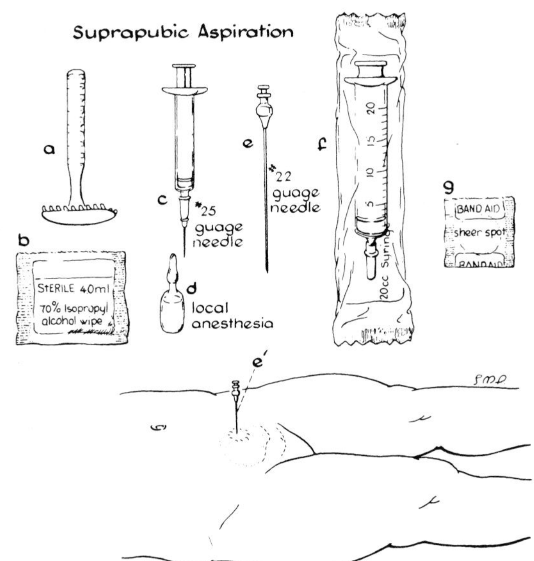

Figure 15–12. Technique of suprapubic aspiration of the bladder. (From Stamey TA: The Prevention of Recurrent Urinary Infections. New York, Science and Medicine Publishing Company, 1973.)

retropubic area. When no urine is obtained on the first attempt, it is probably wise to wait until the bladder is full.

Urethral Catheterization in the Female Patient

Urethral catheterization is useful for many female patients. In a remarkable study that was well ahead of its time, Philpot (1956) obtained catheterized urine samples from 50 volunteer normal women after washing the introitus with green soap and rinsing with potassium mercuric iodide: 66% were sterile, 28% had a count of 1 to 30 bacteria per milliliter, and 6% demonstrated 30 to 400 bacteria per milliliter; none of the contaminating bacteria were gram-negative bacteria or even enterococci. **Regardless of the technique of catheterization, however, some nonbacteriuric bladder urine specimens will be contaminated by urethral bacteria.** A small No. 10 to 14 French, soft plastic catheter should be used for catheterization after the labia and urethral meatus are cleaned with soap and water; the labia minora should be separated during the meatal washing and the catheterization. Of course, it is impossible to remove the bacteria on the distal third of the urethral mucosa, but collecting a midstream catheterized specimen minimizes urethral contaminants. With careful technique, the presence of 100 or more colony-forming units of a uropathogen per milliliter usually indicates infection.

The objection to the catheter, of course, is that it produces a bladder bacteriuria in some patients who were not bacteriuric. **This incidence of infection varies with the type of patient catheterized, from 1% in healthy schoolgirls in the series by Turck and co-workers (1962) to 20% in women hospitalized on a medical ward** (Thiel and Spuhler, 1965). **The incidence of catheter-induced urinary tract infection is determined primarily by the population at risk, with the lowest incidence occurring in nonhospitalized, healthy women. It is inexcusable to catheterize a male patient for a urine culture.**

The easiest way to prevent catheter-induced infections is to give one or two tablets of an oral antimicrobial agent, such as trimethoprim-sulfamethoxazole (TMP-SMX). Ireland and associates (1982) catheterized 100 women immediately before abdominal hysterectomy; 50 of the women each received a single dose of TMP-SMX (160 mg of trimethoprim and 800 mg of sulfamethoxazole). A postoperative urinary tract infection developed in only 2 patients. In contrast, infections developed in 35% of the 50 control patients. The 4% infection rate in the single-dose prophylactic group indicates impressive protection, not only from catheter-induced bacteria but also from the exigencies of postoperative abdominal surgery.

Alternatively, antibacterial solutions can be left in the bladder after catheterization. For example, Pearman (1971) catheterized patients with acute traumatic spinal cord injury every 6 hours until bladder function returned. At each catheterization the urine was cultured; 150 mg of kanamycin with 30 mg of colistin sulfate in 25 ml of sterile water was left in the bladder. Of 1547 catheterizations performed in nine female patients, 9 instances of bacteriuria occurred (an incidence of 1 in 172 catheterizations, or 0.6%); almost all the infections were caused by either enterococci or *S. epidermidis*.

Segmented Voided Urine Specimens

Women are asked to provide a self-caught, midstream voided urine specimen. These women are carefully instructed in the collection technique to spread the labia, wipe the periurethral area from front to back with a moistened, clean gauze sponge, and collect a specimen while holding the labia apart with one hand. No antiseptic is used to prepare the patient because it could contaminate the specimen and cause a false-negative culture. The male patient can produce two-glass (i.e., urethral and bladder) urine specimens that are about as reliable as SPA.

Urinalysis

Indirect dipstick tests for bacteriuria (nitrite) or pyuria (leukocyte esterase) are informative but are less sensitive than microscopic examination of the urine. For example, the leukocyte esterase dipstick has a reported sensitivity of 75% to 96% in detecting pyuria associated with infection (Pappas, 1991; Blum and Wright, 1992). **Indirect tests are most useful for screening urine of asymptomatic patients** (Carroll et al, 1994).

For patients with urinary symptoms, microscopic urinalysis for bacteriuria, pyuria, and hematuria should be performed. The most important error (i.e., a false-negative result) occurs because of the limitation imposed by the microscope on the volume of urine that can be observed. If the volume of urine that can easily rest beneath a standard 22-mm coverglass is carefully measured (0.01 ml) and the number of high dry fields (× 570 magnification) present beneath the coverglass is estimated, it is disturbing to find that one high dry field represents a volume of approximately 1/30,000 ml. There are excellent studies showing that the bacterial count must be approximately 30,000/ml before bacteria can be found in the sediment, stained or unstained, spun or unspun (Sanford et al, 1956; Kunin, 1961). For these reasons, **a negative urinalysis for bacteria never excludes the presence of bacteria in numbers of 30,000/ml and less.** As already pointed out, many circumstances can reduce the bacterial colony count in bladder urine to numbers less than 30,000/ml.

The second error of urinalysis (i.e., a false-positive result) is the reverse of the first error: **Bacteria are seen in the microscopic sediment but the urine culture shows no growth. The voided urine from a female patient can contain many thousands of lactobacilli and corynebacteria. These bacteria are readily seen under the microscope, and although they are gram-positive they often appear gram-negative (gram-variable) if stained.** Strict anaerobes, usually gram-negative bacilli, also make up a significant mass of the normal vaginal flora (Marrie et al, 1978).

In practice these problems can be minimized by using other information provided by urinalysis that can help the clinician to decide whether or not a patient has a urinary tract infection (Stamm et al, 1982). **The validation of the midstream urine specimen can be questioned if numerous squamous epithelial cells (indicative of preputial, vaginal, or urethral contaminants) are present. Pyuria and hematuria are good indicators of an inflammatory response.** Although the number of white blood cells (WBCs) per high-power field (hpf) in a centrifuged urine sample is useful, it is important to remember that other factors can influence the number of cells seen. These include the state of hydration; the intensity of tissue reaction; the method of urine collection; the volume, speed, and time of centrifugation; and the volume in which the sediment is resuspended.

Pyuria, however, can be quantitated in the uncentrifuged urine by measuring either the WBC excretion rate (in a timed urine collection) as WBCs per hour or the WBC concentration as WBCs per milliliter in a random, nontimed urine sample. Both methods require that a fresh, unspun sample of urine be placed in a counting chanber of exact volume, such as the Neubauer hemacytometer, or the Fuchs-Rosenthal chamber, which has twice the depth (0.2 mm) and volume of the Neubauer chamber. Mabeck (1969b) found that women without evidence of urinary tract disease excrete fewer than 400,000 leukocytes per hour. In a nontimed voided urine sample, pyuria has been defined as >10 WBCs/mm^3 of urine (Stamm et al, 1982). Because these methods are more time-consuming than direct urinalysis, they have not achieved widespread clinical acceptance.

The absence of pyuria should cause the diagnosis of urinary tract infection to be questioned until urine culture data are available. Conversely, many diseases of the urinary tract produce significant pyuria in the absence of bacteriuria. Whereas tuberculosis is the well-recognized example of abacterial pyuria, staghorn calculi and stones of smaller size can produce intense pyuria with clumps of WBCs in the absence of urinary tract infection. **Almost any injury to the urinary tract, from chlamydial urethritis to glomerulonephritis and interstitial cystitis, can elicit large numbers of fresh polymorphonuclear leukocytes (glitter cells).** Depending on the stage of hydration, the intensity of the tissue reaction producing the cells, and the method of urine collection, any number of WBCs can be seen in the microscopic sediment in the presence of an uninfected urinary tract. **Microscopic hematuria is found in 40% to 60% of cases of cystitis and is uncommon in other dysuric syndromes** (Stamm et al, 1980b; Wigton et al, 1985).

Urine Culture

Two techniques for urine culture in the office setting are available. The better of the two, although slightly more expensive and troublesome to acquire, is direct surface plating on split-agar, disposable plates. One half is blood agar, which grows both gram-positive and gram-negative bacteria, and the other is desoxycholate or eosin–methylene blue (EMB), which grows gram-negative bacteria (some of them, such as *E. coli*, in a very characteristic manner). Simple curved-tip eye droppers are sufficient to deliver about 0.1 ml of urine onto each half of the plate. After overnight incubation in an inexpensive incubator, the number of colonies is estimated, often identified (after some experience), and multiplied by 10 to report the number of colony-forming units (cfu) per milliliter of urine. The technique has been presented elsewhere in detail (Stamey, 1980).

A simpler but somewhat less accurate technique is the use of dip-slides (Fig. 15–13). These inexpensive plastic slides are attached to screw-top caps; they have soy agar (a general nutrient agar to grow all bacteria) on one side and EMB or MacConkey's agar for gram-negative bacteria on the opposite side. A slide is dipped into urine, the excess is allowed to drain off, and the slide is replaced in its plastic bottle and incubated. The volume of urine that attaches to the slide is between 1/100 and 1/200 ml. Hence, the colony count is 100 to 200 times the number of colonies that become visible with incubation. In actual practice, the growth is compared with a visual standard and reported as such. The species of bacteria is more difficult to recognize when this technique is used, but the technique is completely adequate.

It is emphasized that the urine must be refrigerated immediately upon collection and should be cultured within 24 hours of refrigeration. One advantage to the dip-slide is the ease with which the urine can be immediately cultured without the necessity of refrigeration. Patients can culture their own urine at home, keep the slide at room temperature, and bring it to the office within 48 hours.

Although most bacteria allowed to incubate for several hours in bladder urine reach colony counts of 10^5/ml, this statistical number is fraught with two limitations. The first is that 20% to 40% of women with symptomatic urinary tract infections present with bacteria counts of 10^2 to 10^4/ml of urine (Stamey et al, 1965; Mabeck, 1969a; Kunzet al, 1975; Kraft and Stamey, 1977), **probably because of the slow doubling time of bacteria in urine (every 30 to 45 minutes) combined with frequent bladder emptying (every 15 to 30 minutes) from irritation. Thus, in dysuric patients, an appropriate threshold value for defining significant bacteriuria is $\geq 10^2$cfu/ml of a known pathogen** (Stamm and Hooton, 1993). Fortunately, most of these patients have symptoms of urinary tract infection and most have pyuria on urinalysis.

The second limitation of the 10^5 cutoff is overdiagnosis. **Women susceptible to infection often carry large numbers of pathogenic bacteria on the perineum that contam-**

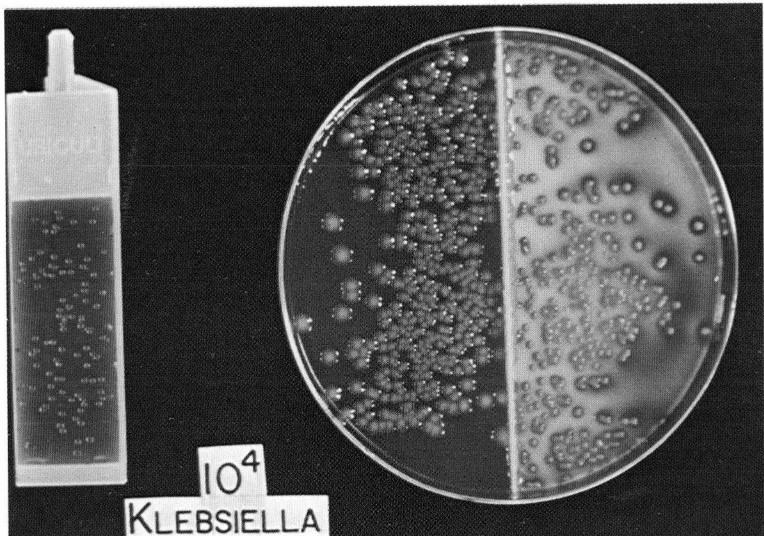

Figure 15–13. The dip-slide on the left is compared with a split-agar surface plate on the right. The urine contained 10,000 colonies of *Klebsiella* per milliliter (about 200 times the number of colonies on the dip-slide and 10 times the number on either side of the split-agar plate).

inate otherwise sterile bladder urine. Uncircumcised men may harbor uropathogenic bacteria on their foreskins. In the original studies by Kass (1960), a single culture of 10^5 cfu's/ml or more had a 20% chance of representing contamination. There is no statistical way to avoid these two major limitations on the interpretation of the midstream voided culture in women and in uncircumcised men without careful preparation.

Localization

Kidney

Fever and Flank Pain

Fever and flank pain are thought to indicate pyelonephritis, but few studies have tested the hypothesis. Aggressive localization studies in children and adults (Huland et al, 1982; Busch and Huland, 1984), as well as in patients with end-stage renal disease (Huland et al, 1983) have shown substantial incidences of fever and even flank pain in bacteriuric patients in whom infection was localized to the bladder (see the later section on acute pyelonephritis).

Ureteral Catheterization

Ureteral catheterization allows not only separation of bacterial persistence into upper and lower urinary tracts but also separation of the infection between one kidney and the other, and even localization of infection to ectopic ureters or to nonrefluxing ureteral stumps (by using saline irrigation) (Stamey, 1980).

Stamey began in 1959 to localize the site of bacteriuria by ureteral catheterization studies; the technique was published in 1963 (Stamey and Pfau, 1963) and the results in 1965 (Stamey et al, 1965). The technique is simple but exacting; the urologist should consult a more detailed description (Stamey, 1980) before actually performing this localization technique. The validity depends on controlling the number of bacteria from the bladder that contaminate the ureteral catheters as they pass through the bladder into the ureteral orifices. The bladder must be thoroughly irrigated before both ureteral catheters are passed into a small volume of residual irrigating fluid. A sample is obtained through both ureteral catheters simultaneously, and then each catheter is passed into the ureter or renal pelvis. Four serial cultures are obtained from each kidney. It is mandatory that the patient be started on the appropriate antimicrobial agent before leaving the cystoscopy room. In addition to quantitative bacterial counts on each specimen, determination of either specific gravity or urine creatinine levels on the renal samples can be very helpful in interpreting a change in diuresis in relation to bacterial counts. Examples of infections localized to the bladder, to one kidney, and to both kidneys have been published (Stamey, 1980). Classic examples of results from each site are shown in Table 15–3.

When this technique was applied to large numbers of bacteriuric patients, 45% were found to have bladder infection only; 27%, unilateral renal bacteriuria; and 28%, bilateral renal bacteriuria (Table 15–4) (Stamey et al, 1965). These figures have been confirmed by at least five investigators in three countries (the United States, England, and Australia) and can be taken as a good approximation for any general bacteriuric adult population. **Although renal stones and other kidney abnormalities in the presence of bacteriuria can increase the proportion of renal infections, the urologist should never assume the kidney is involved if an important decision is to be made.**

Fairley Bladder Washout Test

In 1967 Fairley and associates proposed a method for differentiating kidney from bladder infections by washing the bladder free of bacteria and then collecting serial cultures that would essentially represent upper tract urine. He modified his original 1967 procedure in 1971 (Fairley et al, 1971):

After collecting the initial specimen, the bladder is emptied through a urethral catheter and 40 ml of 0.2% neomycin, together with one ampoule of "Elase," is introduced into the bladder. After 10 minutes the bladder is distended with 0.2% neomycin to reduce the folds in the mucosa and the catheter is clipped off for 20 minutes. The bladder is then emptied and

Table 15–3. CLINICAL EXAMPLES OF URETERAL CATHETERIZATION STUDIES IN LOCALIZING THE SITE OF BACTERIURIA

Source	Bladder Infection (Bacteria/ml)	Left Renal Infection (Bacteria/ml)	Right Renal Infection (Bacteria/ml)	Bilateral Renal Infection (Bacteria/ml)
CB	$>10^5$	5000	$>10^5$	4000
WB	900	300	1000	20
LK_1	20	2000	20	400
LK_2	0	2200	0	350
LK_3	0	2500	0	500
LK_4	0	2200	0	400
RK_1	10	0	10,000	260
RK_2	0	0	10,000	220
RK_3	0	0	8000	300
RK_4	0	0	12,000	250

CB, catheterized patient, cystoscopic specimen; WB, controlled, "wash bladder" specimen collected after copious irrigation of the bladder; LK_1, LK_2, etc., serial cultures of urine from the left kidney; RK_1, RK_2, etc., serial cultures of urine from the right kidney.

washed out with 2 liters of sterile saline solution. Some of the saline of the final washout is collected for culture and, after emptying the bladder, a further three, timed specimens are collected at 10-minute intervals. Bacterial counts are done on all specimens.

Elase is a combination of two lytic enzymes, fibrinolysin and deoxyribonuclease. There are no studies that have demonstrated a beneficial effect of these enzymes. The neomycin, on the other hand, is probably important. In their 1971 paper Fairley and associates gave specific criteria for separating bladder from renal infection:

Renal infection was assumed to be present when the timed specimen collected 20 to 30 minutes after bladder washout contained more than 3,000 bacteria/ml, and in addition this 20- to 30-minute specimen contained more than five times as many bacteria as were present in the final bladder washout specimen. Bladder infection was assumed to be present when the final timed specimen (20 to 30 minutes after the bladder washout) was sterile.

According to these criteria, 21 of 48 patients in this general practice study showed evidence of renal infection, 22 showed the infection was limited to the bladder, and only 5 studies were equivocal. This method may not be valid in spinal cord injury patients with reflux. However, the Fairley washout test is a useful technique in studies of recurrent urinary tract infections in patients without significant underlying abnormalities of the urinary tract.

Immunologic Responses

Although both cellular and humoral immune responses are observed in genitourinary infections, this section focuses primarily on the humoral immune response, which is better understood. The cellular response is mentioned briefly in the later section on pyelonephritis. Humoral immunity is characterized by the formation of antibodies (immunoglobulins) in response to invasive bacterial antigens. These antibodies may be produced and found systemically in the blood or locally within the genitourinary tract. New, more sensitive methods of measuring these antibodies have improved physicians' knowledge of humoral immunity. Knowledge of the response of these antibodies to infecting bacteria (antigen-specific antibodies) is clinically useful because investigators have studied these antibodies as markers to distinguish between acute and chronic pyelonephritis and kidney and bladder infections.

DIRECT AGGLUTINATION TESTS. Bacterial agglutination is performed by mixing dilutions of serum with bacterial suspensions. The presence of serum antibodies to the bacteria (antigen-specific antibodies) is detected by agglutination of particles. Primarily multivalent antibodies, such as immunoglobulin M (IgM) combine with surface bacterial antigens to cause the clumping. Since IgM is seen most commonly during the early phases of an acute infection, this method has limited use in detecting chronic infections, in which IgG is more important.

PASSIVE AGGLUTINATION TESTS. Many bacterial polysaccharide and protein antigens may stick nonspecifically to the surface of red blood cells. When these red blood cells with their attached antigens are mixed with dilutions of serum, antigen-specific antibodies can be detected by measuring agglutination of the red blood cells.

ANTIBODY-COATED BACTERIA. In 1974, Thomas and associates reported a significant advance in the diagnosis of urinary tract infection. They observed that if the bacteria in the urine of a patient with urinary tract infection were centrifuged, washed, and mixed with fluorescein-conjugated anti–human globulin, antibody coating of the bacteria could be seen under a fluorescence microscope as a typical apple-green fluorescence. **Thomas and associates reported that 34 of 35 patients with pyelonephritis had bacteria that were fluorescent antibody–positive (FA$^+$, whereas bacteria from 19 of 20 patients with cystitis were not antibody-coated (FA$^-$).**

Other studies in adults have confirmed the usefulness of this immunofluorescent technique in separating renal from bladder infection (Kohnle et al, 1975; Harding et al, 1978). To be sure, there are some false-negative results in renal

Table 15–4. LOCALIZATION OF URINARY TRACT INFECTIONS IN 95 FEMALES AND 26 MALES WITH BACTERIURIA

Number and Sex	Bladder Only	Unilateral Renal Bacteriuria	Bilateral Renal Bacteriuria
95 females	38 (40%)	27 (28%)	30 (32%)
26 males	16 (62%)	6 (26%)	4 (15%)

From Stamey TA, Govan DE, Palmer JM: Medicine 1965; 44:1.

bacteriuria when there has not been time (if the bacteria are studied very early in the course of an acute infection) to generate local antibody. It is also true that a few asymptomatic ascending infections do not stimulate local antibody formation, but these exceptions are not a great disadvantage to the test.

On the other hand, false-positive findings caused by local production of bladder antibody have virtually invalidated the test in children (Forsum et al, 1976; Hellerstein et al, 1978; Scherf et al, 1978). False positives also may occur with prostatitis, hemorrhagic cystitis, and cystitis associated with many submucosal, lymphoid follicles at cystoscopy (Stamey, 1980).

Despite these few problems in adults, discussed elsewhere in substantial detail (Stamey, 1980), Thomas's antibody-coating test is useful, although it will not replace either ureteral catheterization or the Fairley test. By indicating that the urinary tract infection is severe enough to cause local antibody production (whether in the kidney or in the bladder), it adds a dimension to research on urinary tract infections that is not provided by direct localization techniques.

ENZYME-LINKED IMMUNOSORBENT ASSAYS AND RADIOIMMUNOASSAYS FOR IMMUNOGLOBULINS. The enzyme-linked immunosorbent assay (ELISA) and radioimmunoassay (RIA) are sensitive laboratory procedures that can detect and quantitate many chemicals and proteins. In the urinary tract, they have been used to detect and measure serum, urine, and prostatic fluid, total immunoglobulins, and antigen-specific antibodies. The tests are similar and use specially labeled antisera to the immunoglobulin heavy-chain fractions of IgM, IgG, and IgA to detect antibody to bacteria (antigen-specific antibody). These tests can measure antigen-specific antibodies belonging to any of the immunoglobulin classes (IgM, IgG, and IgA) and are more sensitive and quantitative than agglutination or hemagglutination tests.

IMMUNOGLOBULIN RESPONSE IN PYELONEPHRITIS. In adults with acute pyelonephritis, antibodies to the infecting bacteria can be measured in the serum. **Measurement by bacterial agglutination has revealed that serum levels of antibodies (primarily IgM) against the infecting bacteria are elevated in human acute clinical pyelonephritis; these elevated titers decreased after the pyelonephritis was treated but were persistently elevated when the patient remained infected** (Percival et al, 1964). Similar studies in adults with bacteriuria, proteinuria, pyuria, and radiographic findings of chronic pyelonephritis have shown that serum antigen-specific antibody titers measured by indirect immunofluorescence are persistently elevated; however, it was not proved by using the techniques discussed earlier that these patients had upper tract infections (Nimmich et al, 1976). Some investigators found that passive hemagglutination titers, which favor the measurement of IgM antibodies, are not reliably elevated in patients they have defined to have chronic pyelonephritis (Nimmich et al, 1976; Scarpelli et al, 1979). Other workers, using animal models of pyelonephritis caused by direct renal injection of bacteria, have confirmed elevation of serum antigen-specific antibody levels (measured by agglutination) by the third day, a peak of the antibody level 6 days after infection, and then a decline in antibody production after this time (Miller and North, 1971). Other studies confirm that serum levels of antigen-specific antibodies measured by any technique are elevated more frequently, and to a greater extent, in pyelonephritis than in cystitis (Percival et al, 1964; Hanson et al, 1975; Neter, 1975; Akerlund et al, 1978), but it must be emphasized that levels of serum antibodies are not always elevated in pyelonephritis.

Antigen-specific antibodies stimulated by urinary tract infection have also been identified in human and animal urine both directly and indirectly. Smith and associates (1974), using a sensitive ELISA, detected urinary antibodies in pyelonephritic rabbits (made pyelonephritic by the intravenous injection of *E. coli* while the right ureter was transiently obstructed). They detected urinary antigen-specific IgG and IgA antibodies 11 days after infection and urinary IgM antibodies later. Both antigen-specific IgG and IgM antibodies were present in serum by day 6. These investigators concluded that serum antibody and local urinary antibody are produced independently and that serum antibody is not the result of antibody synthesized in the kidney (Smith et al, 1974). Later it was shown, again in experimental pyelonephritis produced in rabbits as just described, that antibody-coated bacteria appeared by the 11th day after infection, 3 days after serum antibody was detected (Smith et al, 1977). These investigators concluded that a positive test for antibody-coated bacteria indicates that a local immune response to bacterial O antigen has occurred.

In a study of humans, investigators found urinary IgA antibodies to *Mycoplasma* in nine patients 1 to 4 days after acute *Mycoplasma hominis* pyelonephritis; this was followed by urinary IgG antigen-specific antibodies (Erno and Thomsen, 1980). Furthermore, Akerlund's studies (1978) in humans with urinary tract infections show differences in the activities of urinary and serum antibodies to infecting bacteria and no correlation between urinary and serum IgA antibody levels—more evidence that production of antibodies occurs locally in the urinary tract.

DIAGNOSTIC USE OF ANTIBODY TITERS. Serum or urinary antibody titers may be useful in acute urinary tract infection, but they are far from diagnostic. Individual patients cannot be diagnosed as having pyelonephritis or cystitis by using antibody titers or fluorescent antibody–coated bacteria tests. Although patients with acute pyelonephritis usually have positive antibody coating of bacteria and elevated serum or urinary antigen–specific antibody titers, the results of the tests overlap with those of cystitis patients (Hawthorne et al, 1978; Bilges et al, 1979; Budde et al, 1981; Ratner et al, 1981). Since the results of these antibody tests are dependent on the natural history of the immune response, the tests may be negative very early in the infection or when the humoral immune system is incompletely developed, as in infancy (Pylkkanen, 1978; Wientzen et al, 1979). Furthermore, high antibody titers or positive antibody coating of bacteria may reflect the severity of disease (tissue invasion by bacteria) rather than the site of disease. For these reasons, **measurements of antigen-specific antibody in serum or urine may be more useful in chronic bacterial infections than in acute infections.**

Prostate and Urethra Localization Studies

The technique for localizing infections to the urethra or prostate is covered in detail in Chapter 16.

Tissue and Stone Cultures

It is clinically useful to culture stones removed from the urinary tract to document that bacteria reside within their interstices. Tissue cultures are primarily useful for research information.

Using sterile technique at the operating table, the surgeon places the stone or fragment of tissue into a sterile culture tube containing 5 ml of saline; the culture is packed in ice and sent to the bacteriologic laboratory, where, after agitation of the stone or tissue in the 5 ml of saline, 0.1 ml is surface-streaked on both blood agar and EMB agar. The saline is then poured off the specimen; and with sterile forceps the stone or tissue is transferred to a second 5 ml of sterile saline. After agitation to ensure a reasonable washing action, the saline is again decanted and the specimen is transferred to a third 5 ml of saline and finally to a fourth 5 ml of saline. This last saline wash is cultured quantitatively in the same manner as the first. The remainder of this fourth 5 ml of saline is poured with the stone into a sterile mortar and pestle dish. After the stone is crushed (or the tissue is ground in a tissue blender) in the fourth saline wash, 0.1 ml is again cultured on both blood agar and EMB agar. The difference in colony counts between the first and fourth saline washes represents the washing effect of the saline transfers on the surface bacteria of the stone or tissue. The difference between the fourth saline wash before and after crushing (or grinding, for tissue) represents the difference between surface bacteria and bacteria within the specimen. An example of this method of stone culture is shown in Figure 15–14; this middle-age woman had suffered from recurrent *Proteus mirabilis* urinary tract infection secondary to a struvite stone in her right lower pole calyx. The figure shows the culture results of this stone after it was surgically removed.

IMAGING TECHNIQUES

Indications

Radiologic studies are unnecessary for evaluation of most patients with genitourinary infections, but in certain patients they may be useful (Table 15-5). In these patients radiologic imaging studies may determine acute infectious processes that require further intervention or may find the cause of complicated infections.

Table 15–5. INDICATIONS FOR RADIOLOGIC INVESTIGATION IN ACUTE CLINICAL PYELONEPHRITIS

History of calculi, especially infection (struvite) stones
Potential ureteral obstruction (e.g., due to stone, ureteral stricture, tumor)
Papillary necrosis (e.g., patients with sickle cell anemia, severe diabetes mellitus, analgesic abuse)
Poor response to appropriate antimicrobial agents after 5–6 days of treatment
Neuropathic bladder
History of genitourinary surgery that predisposes to obstruction, such as ureteral reimplantation or ureteral diversion
Polycystic kidneys in patients on dialysis or with severe renal insufficiency
Unusual infecting organisms, such as tuberculosis, fungus, or urea-splitting organisms (e.g., *Proteus*)
Diabetes mellitus

First, radiologic procedures are needed in patients with risk factors that may require intervention in addition to antimicrobial treatment. **A urinary tract infection associated with possible urinary tract obstruction must be evaluated.** These are patients with calculi, especially infection (struvite) stones; ureteral tumors; ureteral strictures; congenital obstructions; or previous genitourinary surgery, such as ureteral reimplantation or urinary diversion procedures, that may have caused obstruction. **Patients with papillary necrosis risk impacting necrotic papillae that cause acute ureteral obstruction. Urologic intervention is indicated in patients whose symptoms of acute clinical pyelonephritis persist after 5 to 6 days of appropriate antimicrobial therapy; they often have perinephric or renal abscesses.** Patients with polycystic kidney disease who are on dialysis are particularly prone to developing perinephric abscesses. **Patients with diabetes mellitus can develop special complications from urinary tract infections; they may acquire emphysematous pyelonephritis or papillary necrosis. In addition, patients with unusual organisms, including tuberculosis and fungal and urea-splitting organisms (e.g., *Proteus* species), should be examined for abnormalities within the urinary tract, such as strictures, fungus balls, or obstructing stones.**

The second reason for radiologic evaluation is to diagnose a focus of bacterial persistence. **In patients whose bacteriuria fails to resolve after appropriate antimicrobial therapy or who have rapid recurrence of infection, abnormal-**

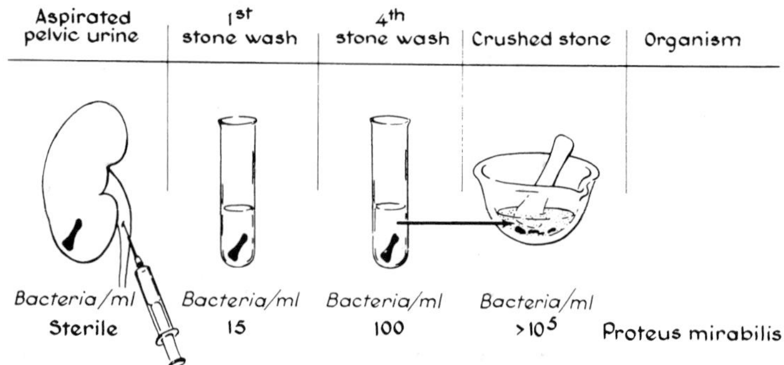

Figure 15–14. Method of culturing stones at surgery. Urine is aspirated to ensure sterility, and a stone (or portion of it) is placed in 5 ml of cold saline. See text for bacteriologic techniques of washing and crushing the stone. In this example, note that the number of *Proteus mirabilis* organisms in the fourth wash was increased 1000 times when the stone was crushed, clearly demonstrating that large numbers of bacteria were inside the stone. (From Nemoy NJ, Stamey TA: JAMA 1971; 215:1470.)

ities that cause bacterial persistence should be sought (see Table 15–2). Several reports of women patients with recurrent urinary tract infections show, however, that excretory urograms are unnecessary for routine evaluation if women who have special risk factors are excluded (Fair et al, 1979; Engel et al, 1980; Fowler and Pulaski, 1981; Fairchild et al, 1982). In none of these studies was information that was useful in the management of these patients obtained from excretory urograms. Furthermore, excluding excretory urograms in the routine evaluation of such patients represents a substantial financial saving.

Imaging techniques that are useful in genitourinary infections are discussed below.

Plain Film of the Abdomen

The plain film of the abdomen (kidney, ureter, and bladder) is useful for the rapid detection of radiopaque calculi and unusual gas patterns in emphysematous pyelonephritis. It may show abnormalities, such as an absent psoas or abnormal renal contour, that suggest perirenal or renal abscess, but these findings are nonspecific.

Plain Film Renal Tomograms

Plain film renal tomograms show small or poorly calcified stones despite overlying gas and fecal shadows. Struvite and uric acid stones that contain small amounts of calcium may be seen on these films but not on routine plain films of the abdomen. Tomograms also localize findings (calcifications or gas) to the kidney.

Excretory Urogram

The excretory urogram has been a routine examination to evaluate patients with complicated infection problems but is not required in uncomplicated infections. The radiologic features of acute clinical pyelonephritis are discussed in a later section on that subject. The excretory urogram study is useful to determine the exact site and extent of urinary tract obstruction; however, it is not the best screening test for hydronephrosis, pyonephrosis, or renal abscess.

Voiding Cystourethrogram

The voiding cystourethrogram is an important examination in assessing VUR. It may be used to evaluate patients with neuropathic bladders and the rare female patient who has a urethral diverticulum causing her persistent infections.

Renal Ultrasonography

The renal ultrasound study is an important renal imaging technique because it is noninvasive, is easy to perform, and offers no radiation or contrast risk to the patient. It is particularly useful in eliminating the concern of hydronephrosis associated with urinary tract infection, pyonephrosis, and perirenal abscesses. A disadvantage is that the study is dependent on the interpretative and performance skills of the examiner. Furthermore, the study may be technically poor in patients who are obese or who have dressings, drainage tubes, or open wounds overlying the area of interest.

Computed Tomography

Computed tomography (CT) is the radiologic modality that offers the best anatomic detail, but its cost prevents it from being a screening procedure. It is more sensitive than excretory urography or ultrasonography in the diagnosis of acute focal bacterial nephritis and renal and perirenal abscesses (Kuhn and Berger, 1981; Mauro et al, 1982; Wadsworth et al, 1982; Soulen et al, 1989). When used to localize renal and perirenal abscesses, CT improves the approach to surgical drainage and permits percutaneous approaches.

Radionuclide Studies

Hippuran I-131 and technetium Tc-99m glucoheptonate scans are used to detect focal parenchymal damage, renal function impairment, and decreased renal perfusion in acute renal infections (McAfee, 1979). Two radionuclides that have been used to detect renal or perirenal infections are gallium 67 and indium 111.

Gallium has been used to distinguish some upper-tract from lower-tract infections (Kessler et al, 1974; Hurwitz et al, 1976; Mendez et al, 1978, 1980; Patel et al, 1980). The exact mode of gallium localization in tissues is not clear. Suggested possible mechanisms include concentration within labeled polymorphonuclear leukocytes, leakage of protein-bound gallium through capillaries, and increased vascularity of the lesion. False-negative and false-positive results limit its usefulness (Hurwitz et al, 1976). This technique has also been useful in the detection of focal bacterial nephritis and infected renal cysts (Hoffer, 1980). Gallium has the disadvantage of being unable to differentiate simple inflammatory processes from pyelonephritis, pyonephrosis, perirenal abscess, or renal tumors (Hampel et al, 1980). False-positive findings may be caused by the accumulation of the radionuclide in the colon and sterile healing tissues, whereas false-negative findings may be caused by the normal accumulation of the substance in liver or spleen, which may obscure small pathologic accumulations.

Indium 111–labeled leukocytes accumulate only in sites of inflammation and not in normal kidneys or in tumors. Thus their presence appears highly specific for inflammation. The indium scan, however, has limitations. From 30 to 40 ml of the patient's blood must be obtained and the white blood cells labeled. Hyperalimentation and hyperglycemia can prevent the accumulation at the site of inflammation, and the distribution of leukocytes is altered in patients who have had splenectomy or bone marrow radiation. Some investigations recommend that this study be combined with abdominal ultrasonography, especially when focal signs are absent (Carroll et al, 1981).

In general, **the radionuclide studies are helpful in cases**

in which an intra-abdominal abscess is suspected but localizing signs are absent, or in cases in which clinical suspicion of abscess remains high but ultrasound and CT studies are equivocal or negative (Biello et al, 1979; Hampel et al, 1980). Furthermore, because the gallium scan is performed 48 hours after injection and the indium scan at 24 hours, there is considerable delay before the studies can be interpreted; therefore, these studies may not be useful in patients who are acutely ill.

PRINCIPLES OF ANTIMICROBIAL THERAPY

Initial Elimination of Bacteriuria

Treatment of each urinary tract infection must result in urine's showing no bacterial growth, an event that occurs within hours if the proper antimicrobial agent is used (Stamey, 1980). If the bacteriuria is only suppressed to low counts, even a few hundred per milliliter or less, higher counts are almost certain to occur; in terms of the classification presented earlier in this chapter, the bacteriuria remains unresolved. **The principle of no bacterial growth in urine during treatment is the basis for successful antimicrobial therapy; without initial elimination of the bacteriuria there can be no successful therapy, and, moreover, there can be no assurance that post-therapy bacteriuria indicates a recurrent urinary tract infection.**

With the duration of therapy now much shorter in symptomatic lower-tract infections and with some regimens requiring only a single dosage, it is often difficult, if not impossible, to confirm no growth in urine during therapy. In these instances, a positive culture within several days of discontinuing therapy probably indicates an unresolved rather than a recurrent infection.

Serum Versus Urinary Levels of Antimicrobial Agents

The cure of urinary tract infection is dependent on the antimicrobial levels achieved in the urine, not in the serum. The concentration of useful antimicrobial agents in the serum and urine of healthy adults is shown in Table 15–6, which demonstrates that the urinary levels are often several hundred times greater than the serum levels.

Clinical studies (McCabe and Jackson, 1965; Stamey et al, 1965; Klastersky et al, 1974; Stamey et al, 1974) have confirmed that urinary levels and not serum concentrations are important in the cure of urinary tract infection. The question of serum levels versus urinary levels is a practical one because the policy of testing antibacterial susceptibility agents at concentrations obtainable only in the serum discourages the physician from using drugs that are effective at the urinary level, for example, oral penicillin G for *E. coli* and *P. mirabilis* and tetracycline for *P. aeruginosa.*

Bacterial Resistance

Table 15–1 shows that the two most common causes of unresolved bacteriuria are two different forms of bacterial resistance. Since the urine must show no growth if the infection is to be cured or if differentiation between bacterial persistence and reinfection is to be made, it is important to understand the mechanisms and implications of bacterial resistance. These have been reviewed in detail elsewhere (Stamey, 1980) but are briefly commented on here.

From the therapeutic view, bacterial resistance can be divided into three categories: (1) "natural" resistance; (2) selection of resistant mutants within the urinary tract during therapy; and (3) transferable, extrachromosomal, plasmid-mediated, (R factor) resistance.

Natural Resistance

Natural resistance simply refers to the absence of drug-susceptible substrate in some species of bacteria. For example, all *Proteus* species are resistant to nitrofurantoin, and *Enterococcus fecalis* is always resistant to cephalexin.

Resistant Mutants

Selection of resistant mutants within the urinary tract during therapy has a simple clinical setting. Susceptibility testing shows that the bacteriuric population is highly susceptible to a specific antimicrobial drug, but within 48 hours of therapy the susceptible population is replaced in the urine by an equal population of bacteria (10^5 or greater) of the original strain, which is now resistant to the antimicrobial agent; susceptibility testing, however, shows that the organism remains susceptible to all antimicrobial drugs except the one used for therapy. It can be shown by elegant bacteriologic studies that the resistant organism (clone) was present before contact with the antimicrobial drug but only in numbers of one resistant clone per 10^5 to 10^{10} organisms, making it impossible to detect its presence clinically before therapy.

How often does the urologist experience this selection of resistant clones in the course of therapy for a previously sensitive bacteriuric population? **It occurs somewhere between 5% and 10% of the time, clearly not an insignificant factor, and one that must be considered in resolving bacteriuria.** The classic way to prevent selection of these resistant clones is to treat a susceptible infection with two or even three antimicrobial agents simultaneously. Although this is necessary in the therapy of tuberculosis, in which a chronic tissue infection imposes great difficulties in exceeding the minimal inhibitory concentration (MIC) of the infecting strain, it is almost never required in urinary tract infection, in which the opportunity to exceed the MIC by a hundred times or more occurs with many antimicrobial agents. **Ideal treatment for urinary tract infection would include acute hydration and diuresis to reduce the total bacterial population before commencing therapy (to reduce the chance of resistant clones), and then doubling or tripling the drug dosage in the first 48 hours to exceed the MIC of the infecting organism by as much as possible despite the hydration. In theory, the clinician should select an antimicrobial agent with a urinary concentration that exceeds the MIC by the widest margin possible, avoid underdosing, and emphasize patient compliance.**

Transferable Resistance

Transferable, extrachromosomal plasmid-mediated (R factor) drug resistance is more important to the urologist

Table 15–6. SERUM AND URINARY ANTIMICROBIAL LEVELS IN ADULTS

Antibiotic	Dose (mg)	Peak Serum Level (μg/ml)	Percentage Bound to Protein	$T_{1/2}$ Serum Peak (h)	Mean (Active) Urine Levels* (μg/ml)	Percentage of Dose Excreted in Urine	Percentage of Dose Active in Urine (if Different)
Ampicillin	250 p.o. q 6 h	3 at 2 h	15	1	350	42	—
Carbenicillin	764 p.o. q 6 h	11–17 at 1.5 h	60	1.2	1000	40	—
Cephalexin	250 p.o. q 6 h	9 at 2 h	12	0.9	800	98	—
Ciprofloxacin	500 p.o. q 12 h	2.3 at 1.2 h	35	3.9	200	30	—
Colistin	75 IM q 12 h	1.8 at 4 h	≃ 10	2	34	75	50
Gentamicin	1 mg/kg IM q 8 h (200 mg/day)	4 at 1 h	Negligible	2	125	80	—
Kanamycin	500 IM q 12 h	18 at 1 h	Negligible	2	750	94	—
Nalidixic acid	1000 p.o. q 6 h	34 at 2–23 h	85	1.5	75	79	5
Nitroflurantoin	100 p.o. q 6 h	< 2		0.3	150	42	—
Norfloxacin	400 p.o. q 12 h	1.5 at 1.5 h	15	3.3	170	27	—
Penicillin G	500 p.o. q 6 h	1 at 1 h	60	0.5	300	20	—
Sulfamethizole	250 p.o. q 6 h		98	10	700	95	85
Tetracycline hydrochloride	250 p.o. q 6 h	2–3 at 4 h	31	6	500	60	—
Trimethoprim-sulfamethoxazole	160/800 p.o. q 12 h	1.7/32 at 2 h	45/66	10/9	150/400	55/50	—/37
Trimethoprim	100 μ p.o. q 12 h	1.0 at 2–4 h	45	10	92	55	—

*These average urinary concentrations are based on the amount of biologically active drug excreted by normal kidneys at a urine flow rate of 1200 ml/24 hours.
IM, intramuscularly; p.o., by mouth; q, every.
From Stamey TA: The Pathogenesis and Treatment of Urinary Infections. Baltimore, Williams & Wilkins Company, 1980, p. 59, with modifications.

than is selection of resistant clones within the urinary tract because (1) it is much more common; (2) the transferable or "infectious" nature of R factors produces multiply resistant strains, making therapy more difficult; and (3) R-factor resistance occurs only in the fecal flora, never within the urinary tract, which makes the latter amenable to the intelligent use of antimicrobial drugs with regard to their influence on the fecal flora. For example, transfer of R-factor resistance to nitrofurantoin is so rare that it is almost never seen; in the case of quinolones (e.g., norfloxacin and ciprofloxacin), R-factor transfer has never been demonstrated. Thus, multiply resistant *E. coli* in the fecal flora that have infected the urinary tract almost always show susceptibility to nitrofurantoin or to the quinolones. Several adverse and favorable effects of specific antimicrobial agents on the fecal flora, especially in relation to transferable extrachromosomal resistance, are covered in detail in the section on prophylaxis.

Antimicrobial Formulary

The mechanism of action; reliable coverage; and common adverse reactions, precautions, and contraindications for antimicrobials used in the treatment of urinary tract infections are indicated in Tables 15–7, 15–8, and 15–9, respectively.

Trimethoprim-Sulfamethoxazole

The combination of trimethoprim (IMP) and sulfamethoxazole (SMX), TMP-SMX, has been the most widely used

Table 15–7. MECHANISM OF ACTION OF COMMON ANTIMICROBIALS USED IN THE TREATMENT OF URINARY TRACT INFECTIONS

Drug or Drug Class	Mechanism of Action	Mechanisms of Drug Resistance
Beta-lactams (penicillins, cephalosporins, aztreonam)	Inhibition of bacterial cell wall synthesis	Production of beta-lactamase Alteration in binding site of penicillin-binding protein Changes in cell wall porin size (decreased penetration)
Aminoglycosides	Inhibition of ribosomal protein synthesis	Downregulation of drug uptake into bacteria Bacterial production of aminoglycoside-modifying enzymes
Quinolones	Inhibition of bacterial DNA gyrase	Mutation in DNA gyrase–binding site Changes in cell wall porin size (decreased penetration)
Nitrofurantoin	Inhibition of several bacterial enzyme systems	Not fully elucidated—develops slowly with prolonged exposure
Trimethoprim-sulfamethoxazole	Antagonism of bacterial folate metabolism	Draws folate from environment (enterococcus)
Vancomycin	Inhibition of bacterial cell wall synthesis (at different point than beta-lactams)	Not fully elucidated—two or three levels of resistance associated with different phenotypes of protein encoded by *van* gene

Table 15–8. RELIABLE COVERAGE OF ANTIMICROBIALS USED IN THE TREATMENT OF URINARY TRACT INFECTIONS OF COMMONLY ENCOUNTERED PATHOGENS

Antimicrobial or Antimicrobial Class	Gram-Positive Pathogens	Gram-Negative Pathogens
Amoxicillin with ampicillin	*Streptococcus* Enterococci	*Escherichia coli* *Proteus mirabilis*
Amoxicillin with clavulanate Ampicillin with sulbactam	*Streptococcus* *Staphylococcus* (not MRSA) Enterococci	*E. coli* *P. mirabilis* *Haemophilus influenzae, Klebsiella* spp.
Antistaphylococcal penicillins	*Streptococcus* *Staphylococcus* (not MRSA)	None
Antipseudomonal penicillins	*Streptococcus* Enterococci	Most including *Pseudomonas aeruginosa*
First-generation cephalosporins	*Streptococcus* *Staphylococcus* (not MRSA)	*E. coli* *P. mirabilis* *Klebsiella* spp.
Second-generation cephalosporins (cefamandole, cefuroxime, cefaclor)	*Streptococcus* *Staphylococcus* (not MRSA)	*E. coli, P. mirabilis* *H. influenzae, Klebsiella* spp.
Second-generation cephalosporins (cefoxitin, cefotetan)	*Streptococcus*	*E. coli, Proteus* spp. (incl. indole +) *H. influenzae, Klebsiella* spp.
Third-generation cephalosporins (ceftazidime, cefoperazone)	*Streptococcus*	Most, including *P. aeruginosa*
Aztreonam	None	Most, including *P. aeruginosa*
Aminoglycosides	*Staphylococcus* (urine)	Most, including *P. aeruginosa*
Fluoroquinolones	None	Most, including *P. aeruginosa*
Nitrofurantoin	*Staphylococcus* (not MRSA) Enterococci	Many Enterobacteriaceae (not *Providencia, Serratia, Acinetobacter*) *Klebsiella* spp.
Trimethoprim-sulfamethoxazole	*Streptococcus* *Staphylococcus*	Most Enterobacteriaceae (Not *P. aeruginosa*)
Vancomycin	All including MRSA	None

MRSA = methicillin-resistant *Staphylococcus aureus*.

antimicrobial for the treatment of acute urinary tract infections. TMP alone is as effective as the combination for most uncomplicated infections and may be associated with fewer side effects (Johnson and Stamm, 1989). The addition of SMX, however, contributes to efficacy in the treatment of upper-tract infection via a synergistic bactericidal effect and may diminish the emergence of resistance (Burman, 1986). **TMP alone or in combination with SMX is effective against most common uropathogens with the notable exception of enterococcus and *Pseudomonas* species. The TMP-SMX–based drugs are inexpensive and have minimal adverse effects on the fecal flora. Disadvantages are relatively frequent adverse effects, consisting primarily of skin rashes and gastrointestinal complaints** (Cockerill and Edson, 1991).

Nitrofurantoin

Nitrofurantoin is effective against most uropathogens including Enterobacteriaceae but it is not effective against *Pseudomonas* and *Proteus* species (Iravani, 1991). **It is rapidly excreted from the urine but does not obtain therapeutic levels in most body tissues including those of the urinary and gastrointestinal tracts. It is therefore, not useful for upper-tract and complicated infections** (Wilhelm and Edson, 1987). It has minimal effects on the resident fecal and vaginal flora and has been used effectively in prophylactic regimens for over 30 years. **Acquired bacterial resistance to this drug is exceedingly low.**

Cephalosporins

All three generations of cephalosporins have oral preparations that have been used for the treatment of acute urinary tract infections (Wilhelm and Edson, 1987). In general, as a group, activity is high against Enterobacteriaceae and poor against enterococci. **First-generation cephalosporins have greater activity against gram-positive organisms, and second-generation cephalosporins have activity against anaerobes. Third-generation cephalosporins are more reliably active against community-acquired and nosocomial gram-negative organisms than other beta-lactam antibiotics.** Their cost should limit their use to situations in which parenteral therapy is required and resistance to standard antibiotics is likely. Cephalosporins produce less resistance among fecal bacteria than the aminopenicillins, but the incidence of *Candida* vaginitis is nearly the same (Iravani, 1991).

Aminopenicillins

Ampicillin and amoxicillin have been used frequently in the past for the treatment of urinary tract infection, but the emergence of resistance in up to 30% of common urinary isolates has lessened the utility of these drugs (Hooton and Stamm, 1991). The effects of these agents on the normal fecal and vaginal flora can predispose to reinfection with resistant strains and frequently lead to *Candida* vaginitis (Iravani, 1991). The addition of the beta-lactamase inhibitor clavulanate to amoxicillin greatly improves activity against beta-lactamase–producing bacteria that are resistant

Table 15–9. COMMON ADVERSE REACTIONS, PRECAUTIONS, AND CONTRAINDICATIONS FOR ANTIMICROBIALS USED IN TREATMENT OF URINARY TRACT INFECTIONS

Drug or Drug Class	Common Adverse Reactions	Precautions and Contraindications
Amoxicillin with ampicillin	Hypersensitivity (immediate or delayed) Diarrhea (esp. with ampicillin), gastrointestinal (GI) upset Antibiotic-associated pseudomembranous colitis (AAPMC) Maculopapular rash (not hypersensitivity) Decreased platelet aggregation	Increased risk of rash with concomitant viral disease, allopurinol therapy.
Amoxicillin with clavulanic acid	Same as amoxicillin with ampicillin	
Ampicillin with sulbactam	Increased diarrhea, GI upset with amoxicillin/clavulanic acid	
Antistaphylococcal penicillins	Same as with amoxicillin/ampicillin GI upset (with oral agents) Acute interstitial nephritis (esp. with methicillin)	
Antipseudomonal penicillins	Same as with amoxicillin/ampicillin Hypernatremia (these drugs are given as sodium salt; esp. carbenicillin, ticarcillin) Local injection site reactions	Use with caution in patients very sensitive to sodium loading.
Cephalosporins	Hypersensitivity (less than with penicillins) GI upset (with oral agents) Local injection site reactions AAPMC Positive Coombs' test Decreased platelet aggregation (esp. with cefotetan, cefamandole, cefoperazone)	**Should not be used in patients with immediate hypersensitivity to penicillins;** may use with caution in patients with delayed hypersensitivity reactions.
Aztreonam	Hypersensitivity (less than with penicillins)	Less than 1% incidence of cross reactivity in penicillin- or cephalosporin-allergic patients; may be used with caution in these patients.
Aminoglycosides	Ototoxicity—vestibular and auditory components Nephrotoxicity—nonoliguric azotemia Neuromuscular blockade with high levels	**Avoid in pregnant patients.** Avoid if possible in patients with severely impaired renal function, diabetes, or hepatic failure. Use with caution in myasthenia gravis patients (due to potential for neuromuscular blockade). Use with caution with other potentially ototoxic and nephrotoxic drugs.
Fluoroquinolones	Mild GI effects Dizziness, lightheadedness	**Avoid in children or pregnant patients due to arthropathic effects.** Concomitant antacid or iron or zinc or sucralfate use dramatically decreases oral absorption—**use another antimicrobial or discontinue sucralfate use while on quinolones;** space administration of quinolones from antacids or iron or zinc products by at least 2 h to ensure adequate absorption. Ensure adequate patient hydration. Can significantly increase theophylline plasma levels (ciprofloxacin and enoxacin seem to have a greater effect than norfloxacin or ofloxacin)—avoid quinolones or monitor theophylline levels closely.

Table continued on following page

Table 15–9. COMMON ADVERSE REACTIONS, PRECAUTIONS, AND CONTRAINDICATIONS FOR ANTIMICROBIALS USED IN TREATMENT OF URINARY TRACT INFECTIONS *Continued*

Drug or Drug Class	Common Adverse Reactions	Precautions and Contraindications
Nitrofurantoin	GI upset Peripheral polyneuropathy—esp. in patients with impaired renal function, anemia, diabetes, electrolyte imbalance, or vitamin B deficiency, and debilitated Hemolysis in patients with glucose-6-phosphate dehydrogenase (G6PD) deficiency Pulmonary hypersensitivity reactions—can range from acute to chronic and include cough, dyspnea, fever, and interstitial changes	**Do not use in patients with low creatinine clearance (<40 ml/min) as adequate urine concentrations will not be achieved.** Use with caution in patients predisposed to peripheral polyneuropathy or with G6PD deficiency. Monitor long-term patients closely. Avoid concomitant probenicid use, which blocks renal excretion of nitrofurantoin. Avoid concomitant magnesium or quinolones, which are antagonistic to nitrofurantoin.
Trimethoprim-sulfamethoxazole	Hypersensitivity, rash GI upset Photosensitivity Hematologic toxicity (acquired immunodeficiency syndrome [AIDS] patients)	Higher incidence of all adverse reaction in AIDS patients, elderly. Avoid in pregnant patients. Avoid in patients receiving warfarin; concomitant use can significantly elevate prothrombin time. Increased risk of hematologic effects in folate- or G6PD-deficient patients. Ensure adequate hydration to avoid crystallization of drug in urinary tract.
Vancomycin	"Red-man's syndrome"—flushing, fever, chills, rash, hypotension (histaminic effect) Nephrotoxicity and/or ototoxicity when combined with other nephrotoxic and/or ototoxic drugs Local injection site reactions	Use with caution with other potentially ototoxic and nephrotoxic drugs.

From McEvoy GK, ed: American Hospital Formulary Service Drug Information. Bethesda, MD, American Society of Health-System Pharmacists, 1995.

to amoxicillin alone (Med Lett, 1984). However, its high cost and frequent gastrointestinal side effects argue against its use for first-line therapy of uncomplicated urinary tract infections. The extended-spectrum penicillin derivatives (e.g., piperacillin, mezlocillin, azlocillin) retain ampicillin's activity against enterococci and offer activity against many ampicillin-resistant gram-negative bacilli. This makes them attractive agents for use in patients with nosocomially acquired urinary tract infections and as the initial parenteral treatment of acute uncomplicated pyelonephritis acquired outside of the hospital, although less expensive agents are equally effective.

Aminoglycosides

Aminoglycosides, when combined with TMP-SMX, or ampicillin, are the first drugs of choice for febrile urinary tract infections. Their nephrotoxicity is well recognized, and hence careful monitoring of patients with renal impairment associated with infection is indicated.

Aztreonam

Aztreonam has a similar spectrum of activity as the aminoglycosides, and, like all beta lactams, it is not nephrotoxic. Its spectrum of activity, however, is less broad than that of the third-generation cephalosporins. **Hence it should be used primarily in patients who have penicillin allergies.**

Fluoroquinolones

The fluoroquinolones share a common predecessor in nalidixic acid and inhibit DNA gyrase, a bacterial enzyme integral to replication. The fluoroquinolones have a broad spectrum of activity that makes them ideal for the empirical treatment of urinary tract infection (Naber, 1989). They are highly effective against Enterobacteriaceae as well as *P. aeruginosa*. Activity is also high against *S. aureus* and *S. saprophyticus*, but in general antistreptococcal coverage is marginal. Most anaerobic bacteria are resistant to these drugs, and therefore the normal vaginal and fecal flora are not altered (Wright et al, 1993). **For most uncomplicated urinary tract infections, the fluoroquinolones are not significantly more effective than less expensive drugs. The fluoroquinolones have distinct advantages in the treatment of complicated urinary tract infections due to host factors, resistant organisms, or difficult-to-treat pathogens such as *P. aeruginosa*** (Dalkin and Schaeffer, 1988). **Bacterial resistance initially appeared to be uncommon, but it is being reported at an increasing rate, due to indiscriminate use of these agents** (Acar and Francoual, 1990; Wright et al, 1993).

These drugs are not nephrotoxic, but renal insufficiency

prolongs the serum half-life, requiring adjusted dosing in patients with creatinine clearances of <30 ml/min. Adverse reactions are uncommon; gastrointestinal disturbances are more frequent. Hypersensitivity, skin reactions, mild central and peripheral nervous system reactions, and even acute renal failure have been reported (Hootkins et al, 1989). **Administration of the fluoroquinolones to immature animals has caused damage to the developing cartilage, and therefore they are currently contraindicated in children, adolescents, and pregnant or nursing women** (Christ et al, 1988). **There are important drug interactions associated with the fluoroquinolones. Antacids containing magnesium or aluminum interfere with absorption of fluoroquinolones** (Davies and Maesen, 1989). **Certain fluoroquinolones (enoxacin and ciprofloxacin) elevate plasma levels of theophylline and prolong its half-life** (Wright et al, 1993). All quinolones can be administered orally, and ciprofloxacin and ofloxacin can also be administered parenterally (Lode, 1989; Madari, 1989).

Choice of Antimicrobial Agents

Many antimicrobial agents have been shown to be effective in the treatment of urinary tract infections. **Factors important in aiding selection of empirical therapy include whether the infection is complicated or uncomplicated; the spectrum of activity of the drug against the probable pathogen; a history of hypersensitivity; potential side effects, including renal and hepatic toxicity; and cost.** In addition, favorable or unfavorable effects of the antimicrobial on the vaginal and fecal flora are important in women with recurrent urinary tract infections. The bacterial susceptibility and antimicrobial cost vary dramatically among inpatient and outpatient settings throughout the country. **It is imperative, therefore, that each clinician keep abreast of changes in bacterial susceptibility and cost and use current information when choosing antimicrobial agents.**

Duration of Therapy

The duration of therapy needed to cure a urinary tract infection appears to be related to a number of variables, including the extent and duration of tissue invasion; the bacterial concentration in urine; the achievable urine concentration of the antimicrobial; and risk factors (see below) that impair the host and natural defense mechanisms. As a guideline, an uncomplicated urinary tract infection occurring in a urinary tract with structural and functional integrity should be treated with 3-day therapy. Acute uncomplicated pyelonephritis in women or complicated urinary tract infections, that is, those occurring in a urinary tract with a structural or functional abnormality or in a host who is significantly compromised by other diseases, require long-term (10 days or more) therapy.

Symptomatic Acute Cystitis

In women, information on 3 days of full-dose therapy is especially well documented by Charlton and associates (1976), Fair and associates (1980), Norrby (1990), Osterberg and associates (1990), and Hooton and colleagues (1991c, 1991d) (Table 15–10). **In general compared with 7 or 10 days of therapy, 3 days appear to be optimal because there is no difference in cure rates, side effects are reduced, and the cost is decreased.** In most incidences the mean time for dysuria and frequency to disappear in bacteriuric patients is 4 to 5 days (Cartwright et al, 1982). The 3-day treatment obviates the need to persuade patients that

Table 15–10. TREATMENT REGIMENS FOR ACUTE CYSTITIS

Circumstances	Route	Drug	Dosage (mg)	Frequency per Dose	Duration (Days)
Women					
Healthy	Oral	TMP-SMX;	160–800	Every 12 h	3
		TMP;	100	Every 12 h	
		Microcrystalline nitrofurantoin;	100	Four times a day	
		Ciprofloxacin;	250	Every 12 h	
		Enoxacin;	400	Every 12 h	
		Lomefloxacin;	400	Every day	
		or			
		Norfloxacin	400	Every 12 h	
		Ofloxacin	400	Every 12 h	
Symptoms for >7 days, recent urinary tract infection, age >65 yr, diabetes, diaphragm use		TMP-SMX	160–800	Every 12 h	7
		or			
		Fluoroquinolone	As above	As above	
Pregnancy	Oral	Amoxicillin;	250	Every 8 h	7
		Cephalexin;	500	Four times a day	
		Microcrystalline nitrofurantoin;	100	Four times a day	
		or			
		TMP-SMX	160–800	Every 12 h	
Men					
Healthy and less than 50 years old	Oral	TMP-SMX	160–800	Every 12 h	7
		or	As above	As above	
		Fluoroquinolone			

TMP, trimethoprim; TMP-SMX, trimethoprim-sulfamethoxazole.
Modified from Stamm WE, Hooton TM: N Engl J Med 1993; 329:1328–1334.

they require further therapy. **It seems reasonable, therefore, to treat most ambulatory women who present with uncomplicated urinary tract infections with 3 days of full-dose therapy and to verify that the original infecting organism is not present in the urine on follow-up urinalysis or culture 7 to 10 days after therapy. A 7-day regimen should be considered in the presence of mitigating circumstances such as symptoms for over 7 days, recent urinary tract infection, age over 65 years, diabetes, or pregnancy.**

The efficacy of single-dose therapy has been studied extensively and reviewed (Kunin, 1981; Souncy and Polk, 1982; Hooton et al, 1985; Philbrick and Bracikowski, 1985; Gleckman, 1987; Zhanel and Ronald, 1988). Single-dose therapy is based on the premise that lower urinary tract infection is a superficial mucosal infection that can be cured with very high antimicrobial concentrations in the urine. **Single-dose therapy is convenient and inexpensive, but the failure** (Saginur and Nicolle, 1992) **and recurrence rates are greater than with longer therapy** (Fihn et al, 1988). Agents that have been used effectively as single-dose therapy include amoxicillin (3-g oral dose), TMP-SMX (TMP, 320 mg, and SMX, 1600 mg; or two double-strength tablets) or enoxacin (600 mg). Good results also have been reported with ampicillin and sulfisoxazole (Rubin et al, 1980; Greenberg et al, 1981; Buckwold et al, 1982; Pontzer et al, 1983; Backhouse and Matthews, 1989). Reports on single-dose cephalosporin therapy have been less promising (Brumfitt et al, 1970; Greenberg et al, 1981). Only 44% and 33%, respectively, of ambulatory symptomatic women were cured.

In men less than 50 years old, urinary tract infections are uncommon. Although an underlying urologic abnormality may be present and thus cause a complicated infection, recent studies suggest that the uropathogenic strains of *E. coli* that cause pyelonephritis in women can also cause uncomplicated infections (usually cystitis) in men (Spach et al, 1992). Young healthy men who have no discernible complicating factors can be treated with a 7-day course of TMP-SMX, trimethoprim, or a fluoroquinolone (Stamm and Hooton, 1993). In older men, all urinary tract infections should be treated as if they are complicated.

Acute Uncomplicated Pyelonephritis in Women

Until the results of the culture and sensitivities are available, broad-spectrum antimicrobial therapy should be instituted (Table 15–11). A Gram stain of the urine sediment is helpful to guide the selection of the initial empirical antimicrobial therapy. **For women without sepsis, nausea, or vomiting, 10 to 14 days of single-drug oral therapy with a fluoroquinolone or TMP-SMX is recommended, except for pregnant women. Parenteral TMP-SMX, a fluoroquinolone, or a third-generation cephalosporin is usually effective for most patients with domiciliary infections. An aminoglycoside plus ampicillin has traditionally been used for compromised hosts with nosocomial infections.** A major advantage of this regimen has been its effectiveness against both *E. faecalis* and against *Pseudomonas* or other nosocomial gram-negative bacilli. However, recently as many as one third of patients have had ampicillin-resistant organisms, whereas TMP-SMX has provided more predictable antibacterial activity (Johnson et al, 1991). Therefore, TMP-SMX plus gentamicin should be considered for treatment of hospitalized patients with acute pyelonephritis.

Table 15–11. TREATMENT REGIMENS FOR ACUTE UNCOMPLICATED PYELONEPHRITIS IN WOMEN

Circumstances	Route	Drug	Dosage	Frequency per Dose	Duration (Days)
Outpatient—moderately ill, no nausea or vomiting	Oral	TMP-SMX	160–800 mg	Every 12 h	10–14
		Ciprofloxacin	500 mg	Every 12 h	
		Enoxacin	400 mg	Every 12 h	
		Lomefloxacin	400 mg	Every day	
		Norfloxacin	400 mg	Every 12 h	
		or			
		Ofloxacin	400 mg	Every 12 h	
Inpatient—severely ill, possible sepsis	Parenteral	TMP-SMX	160–800 mg	Every 12 h	14
		Ampicillin and	1 g	Every 6 h	
		gentamicin	1.5 mg/kg body weight	Every 8 h	
		Ciprofloxacin	200–400 mg	Every 12 h	
		Ofloxacin	200–400 mg	Every 12 h	
		or			
		Ceftriaxone	1–2 g	Every day	
		Take until afebrile, then take oral TMP-SMX or fluoroquinolone			
Pregnant	Parenteral	Ceftriaxone	1–2 g	Every day	14
		Ampicillin and	1 g	Every 6 h	
		gentamicin	1 mg/kg body weight	Every 8 h	
		Aztreonam	1 g	Every 8–12 h	
		or			
		TMP-SMX	160–800 mg	Every 12 h	
		Take until afebrile, then take:			
	Oral	Cephalexin	500 mg	Every 12 h	

TMP-SMX, trimethoprim-sulfamethoxazole.
Modified from Stamm WE, Hooton TM: N Engl J Med 1993; 329:1328–1334.

Patients with Unresolved or Complicated Infections

A 10- to 21-day regimen of antimicrobial therapy should be used in patients who remain bacteriuric on antimicrobial therapy or have structural or functional abnormalities of the urinary tract or abnormal host defenses (Lerner 1987; Ronald 1987) (Table 15–12). If the patient is moderately ill and can be treated as an outpatient, a fluoroquinolone is the drug of choice on the basis of in vitro susceptibility data. If the patient has a more severe infection, broad-spectrum parenteral therapy should be given initially, followed by oral therapy. More extended therapy of up to 6 weeks does not appear to be superior to 14-day therapy. **There is no evidence that parenteral therapy is more effective than oral therapy, but patients who are septic or intolerant of oral therapy should receive parenteral therapy initially. When the patient is stable, parenteral therapy may be converted to oral therapy to complete the 14 to 21 days.**

Antimicrobial Prophylaxis for Transurethral Procedures

Patients who are known preoperatively to have urinary tract infections should have the infections eradicated before the procedure is started; hence, in these patients preoperative antimicrobials are therapeutic and not prophylactic. Failure to eradicate bacteriuria results in bacteremia in 50% of patients (Morris et al, 1976).

Patients with Risk of Endocarditis

There is no question that antimicrobial prophylaxis against infective endocarditis should be given to patients with prosthetic valves or valvular heart disease who are to have genitourinary manipulation. These guidelines are published in many places (Abrabomwicz, 1984; Durack, 1990). For transurethral genitourinary procedures, including catheterization, catheter manipulation, cystoscopy, and urethral dilation, the regimens are as follows:

1. *Adults.* Ampicillin 2 g plus gentamicin 1.5 mg/kg body weight (not to exceed 80 mg) intramuscularly one-half hour before the procedure or intravenously immediately before the procedure, followed by amoxicillin 1.5 g orally, 6 hours after the initial dose. Alternatively, the parenteral regimen may be repeated once, 8 hours after the initial dose.
2. *Adults allergic to penicillin.* Vancomycin 1 g given intravenously slowly over 1 hour plus gentamicin 1.5 mg/kg body weight (not to exceed 80 mg) intramuscularly or intravenously 1 hour before the procedure. This regimen may be repeated once, 8 hours after the initial dose.

Patients Without Risk of Endocarditis

The issue of systemic antimicrobial prophylaxis in patients who are undergoing endoscopic procedures and who do not have cardiac valvular disorders is controversial.

If no preoperative or postoperative antimicrobial agents are used in transurethral resection of the prostate (TURP), postoperative bacteriuria is found in 11% to 45% of patients up to 1 month postoperatively (Morris et al, 1976; Gibbons et al, 1978; Matthew et al, 1978; Hargreave et al, 1982). Thus far, most prophylaxis studies have used various antimicrobials preoperatively and continued them until the catheter was removed (Lacy et al, 1971; Gibbons et al, 1978; Nielsen et al, 1981), or started the antimicrobials preoperatively and continued them for 5 days to 3 weeks postoperatively (Gonzalez et al, 1976; Morris et al, 1976; Matthew et al, 1978; Falkiner et al, 1983). All but one of these studies (Gibbons et al, 1978) suggest that postoperative urinary tract infections decrease from a range of 26% to 42% to a range of 0% to 12% when various antimicrobial agents are used prophylactically (Morris et al, 1976; Lacy et al, 1971; Matthew et al, 1978; Nielsen et al, 1981; Hargreave et al, 1982). In the single study that shows no decrease (Gibbons et al, 1978), the post-TURP incidence of urinary tract infections in patients who received no prophylactic antimicrobials was 11%, which is a very low rate when compared with other

Table 15–12. TREATMENT REGIMENS FOR COMPLICATED URINARY TRACT INFECTIONS

Circumstances	Route	Drug	Dosage	Frequency per Dose	Duration (Days)
Outpatient, moderately ill, no nausea or vomiting	Oral	Ciprofloxacin	500 mg	Every 12 h	10–14
		Enoxacin	400 mg	Every 12 h	
		Lomefloxacin	400 mg	Every day	
		Norfloxacin	400 mg	Every 12 h	
		or			
		Ofloxacin	400 mg	Every 12 h	
Inpatient, severely ill, possible sepsis	Parenteral	Ampicillin	2 g	Every 6 h	14–21
		Gentamicin	1 mg/kg body weight	Every 8 h	
		Ciprofloxacin	200–400 mg	Every 12 h	
		Ofloxacin	200–400 mg	Every 12 h	
		Ceftriaxone	1–2 g	Every day	
		Ticarcillin-clavulanate	3.1 g	Every 8 h	
		Imipenem-cilastatin	500 mg	Every 6 to 8 h	
		or			
		Aztreonam	1 g	Every 8 to 12 h	
		Take until afebrile, then oral fluoroquinolone			

Modified from Stamm WE, Hooton TM: N Engl J Med 1993; 329:1328–1334.

studies. Furthermore, in this study catheters were routinely removed on the second postoperative day; this may account for the low incidence of infections in control subjects. Most of the other studies did not designate the duration of catheter drainage, but it can be inferred that it was usually longer than that cited in the Gibbons study.

From a review of these studies, several observations relating to the prevention of postoperative urinary tract infections may be made. First, in studies in which patients were randomized into groups that received and did not receive antimicrobial prophylaxis, between 6% and 12% of patients who were thought to have no growth in the urine were ultimately excluded because their preoperative urine was unexpectedly infected (Gonzalez et al, 1976; Morris et al, 1976; Gibbons et al, 1978; Hargreave et al, 1982). This 6% to 12% incidence of infections was found in TURP patients after the exclusion of patients with catheters and those with other causes for a high probability of infection. Second, in control patients who had no growth in urine 24 hours after the catheter was removed, 7% to 15% were infected 1 month later (Gonzalez et al, 1976; Gibbons et al, 1978; Matthew et al, 1978). It is inferred that no growth meant that fewer than 10^4 organisms (Gibbons et al, 1978) or 10^5 organisms (Gonzalez et al, 1976; Matthew et al, 1978) were cultured from urine in these studies. These data suggest either that the urine was not actually free of bacteria or that men undergoing TURP have an increased susceptibility to urinary tract infections in the period immediately following removal of the catheter. The latter is suggested by other studies that show indwelling catheters to be associated with increased urethral and meatal colonization (Bultitude and Eykyn, 1973; Garibaldi et al, 1980). Third, no study to date has involved prophylaxis that was started only the evening before or the morning of catheter removal.

Although investigations to date do not give a definitive answer as to whether antimicrobial prophylaxis should be used in the routine healthy patient undergoing TURP, a rational approach to prophylaxis may be made. In order to approach this question, prophylaxis should be broken into two parts: (1) prophylaxis to prevent operative and perioperative bacteremia, and (2) prophylaxis to prevent postoperative urinary tract infections.

For the patient who has no growth in preoperative urine and carries no gram-negative organisms in the urethra, probably no prophylaxis to prevent bacteremia is needed ("no growth" must mean <100 bacteria per milliliter, not <10^4/ml or 10^5/ml). Unfortunately, if this is not known, or if culture results are unavailable preoperatively, 6% to 12% of patients may be considered to have unsuspected bacteriuria and a probability as high as 67% of becoming bacteremic if not treated prophylactically. A first-generation cephalosporin, gentamicin, or a fluoroquinolone may be given several hours before surgery and for 24 hours postoperatively.

It should be assumed that any patient with an indwelling catheter is infected and must achieve no growth in the urine preoperatively through administration of at least two doses of a drug that has broad coverage against gram-negative organisms. (An aminoglycoside will probably result in no growth in most cases, unless multiple previous antimicrobial courses have been given or the patient has had a long hospitalization, in which case antimicrobial susceptibilities need to be obtained.)

To prevent a postoperative urinary tract infection, which is usually catheter-associated, management similar to that for removal of catheters may be followed. A broad-spectrum antimicrobial agent (a fluoroquinolone or TMP-SMX) should be started the evening before the catheter is to be removed and continued for 3 to 5 days after its removal. A urine culture should be obtained at the time the catheter is removed and on the postoperative office visit. This shorter antimicrobial therapy should minimize the creation of in-hospital resistant organisms and decrease patient cost.

Antimicrobial Prophylaxis for Transrectal Prostatic Needle Biopsy

Infectious complications of transrectal biopsy include cystitis, prostatitis, epididymitis, pyelonephritis, local abscess, osteomyelitis, and sepsis. It has been reported that 5 minutes after transrectal biopsy 76% of patients (16 of 21) had bacteremia proved by blood culture (Asbhy et al, 1978). Over half the organisms isolated in this study were anaerobic (mainly *Bacteroides* species and anaerobic streptococci). Simple cleansing enemas with povidone-iodine do not alter the infectious complications associated with the procedure, but several studies have demonstrated that appropriate antimicrobial prophylaxis may (Ashby et al, 1978; Crawford et al, 1982).

Although it is suggested that metronidazole plus either ampicillin or TMP-SMX given postoperatively are satisfactory prophylaxis for transrectal biopsy, organisms resistant to both drugs were noted (Ashby et al, 1978). The author has found that a fluoroquinolone given several hours before the procedure and continued for 24 hours after the procedure is effective.

Asymptomatic Bacteriuria

The distinction between symptomatic infections and those detected on screening surveys for asymptomatic bacteriuria is considered in this chapter and in Chapter 57 (relating to infants and children). There is evidence in adults (Asscher et al, 1969a) and children (Savage et al, 1975; Lindberg et al, 1978) that although 80% of patients with asymptomatic bacteriuria can be cured with a 7-day course of oral antimicrobial therapy, long-term cure rates are no better than placebo therapy because of reinfections in treated patients and spontaneous cures in untreated subjects.

Moreover, treatment of asymptomatic infections, which are often associated with self-agglutinating *E. coli* that have lost their O polysaccharide surface antigens (Lindberg et al, 1975), is frequently followed by a new *E. coli* infection with intact O surface antigens that are apparently responsible for acute symptoms. For this reason, unless a patient is willing to undertake long-term prophylactic regimens to prevent reinfections, a sound argument can be made against treating an asymptomatic infection just to achieve no growth in the urine for a short period of time. This may be especially true for the geriatric patient with asymptomatic bacteriuria, in whom the potential side effects from unnecessary antimicrobial therapy may represent a substantial hazard.

Some patients with asymptomatic bacteriuria may feel better generally when their bacteriuria is treated even though they have no specific urinary tract symptoms. About one third of patients with asymptomatic bacteriuria develop acute symptoms within 12 months of detection if it is left untreated (Asscher et al, 1969a; Gaymans et al, 1976). **Infection from *Proteus* species causes struvite stones if left untreated for long periods of time and therefore should be eradicated. Moreover, patients at risk for increased morbidity from bacteriuria, such as patients with severe diabetes, pregnant women, and others, should not be left with asymptomatic bacteriuria caused by *Proteus* species.** (See the later section on patients at risk of serious morbidity and/or renal scarring for discussion of these subjects.)

FACTORS INCREASING MORBIDITY AND/OR MORTALITY

Table 15–13 indicates those patients who are at risk of either serious morbidity or renal function impairment and/or scarring from urinary tract infections. The urologist should be particularly aggressive in resolving urinary tract infections in patients within these categories. Each is considered briefly in this section.

Obstruction

Obstructions are frequently metabolic or iatrogenic and largely preventable. Included in this category are those calcium oxalate stones that cause acute obstruction but become secondarily colonized during the course of unsuccessful efforts to remove the calculus. Patients who are susceptible to reinfections of the urinary tract and who also form calcium oxalate stones can develop acute obstruction and urinary tract infection in the absence of urologic intervention.

Serious loss of renal function has been noted in men with megaloureters who had adequate to good renal function and no infections before they were operated on to "improve" renal drainage; postoperatively they became obstructed and infected and eventually required dialysis and transplantation. It should not be forgotten that 15 of the 22 patients who presented to Scribner's dialysis unit with end-stage renal failure (Schechter et al, 1971), in whom the primary cause was chronic pyelonephritis, had "significant obstructive or calculous disease, which preceded the initial episode of urinary tract infection in each."

Table 15–13. SPECIAL PROBLEMS THAT PLACE PATIENTS AT RISK OF SERIOUS MORBIDITY OR RENAL SCARRING*

Obstruction
Urea-splitting bacteria that cause struvite renal stones
Congenital urinary tract anomalies that become secondarily infected
Catheter drainage
Renal papillary necrosis
Diabetes, especially with emphysematous pyelonephritis
Spinal cord injury with high-pressure bladders
Pregnancy
Acute bacterial prostatitis

*Acute pyelonephritis, perirenal abscess, and gram-negative septicemia add significant morbidity and risk to any of the conditions.

Urea-Splitting Bacteria that Cause Struvite Renal Stones

If a recurrent urinary tract infection in an adult **is caused by *E. coli*, the consequences other than symptomatic morbidity are usually not serious. However, the physician should be wary of the patient with bacteriuria due to *P. mirabilis* that recurs soon after stopping antimicrobial therapy** (Fig. 15–15). It is true that *P. mirabilis* is a not uncommon cause of bacteriuria (about 25% of people carry this organism in their normal fecal flora), and most patients with *P. mirabilis* cystitis do not form struvite stones. But struvite stones form in those patients who have a protracted infection with *P. mirabilis*, an infection that is often asymptomatic or minimally symptomatic. ***P. mirabilis* causes intense alkalinization of the urine with precipitation of calcium, magnesium, ammonium, and phosphate salts and the subsequent formation of branched struvite renal stones. The bacteriologic consequences are substantial because the bacteria persist inside these struvite stones even when the urine shows no growth** (see Fig. 15–14). **Indeed, struvite infection stones, together with the occasional oxalate or apatite stone that becomes secondarily colonized, constitute the major cause of bacterial persistence in women in the absence of azotemia.** The bacteriuria in most of these patients with struvite stones recurs almost immediately on stopping antimicrobial therapy, usually within 5 to 7 days (see Fig. 15–15).

These stones can cause serious renal damage. Figure 15–16 shows the plain film radiograph from a 52-year-old white woman whose urinary tract disease was uncovered by her family doctor when he found pyuria during an examination for a febrile, flulike illness accompanied by minimal backache. She had never experienced localized flank pain; her urine culture grew only 10^4 *P. mirabilis* organisms per milliliter. Figure 15–17 represents a 20-minute intravenous urogram and Figure 15–18 a biopsy of the left kidney at the time the staghorn calculus was removed. In Figure 15–18, note the hyalinized glomeruli, the destroyed renal tubules, the inflammatory infiltrate, and the early periglomerular sclerosis. At surgery, both the left and the right renal calculi cultured large numbers of *P. mirabilis* when the stones were crushed (see Fig. 15–14). Antimicrobial agents were stopped 4 weeks after the stones were removed, and the urine has shown no growth for 3 years since surgery. The patient's creatinine level has not changed from its preoperative value of 1.2 mg/dl.

When electrohydraulic shock wave lithotripsy (ESWL) is used to fragment infection stones, the patient should be maintained on appropriate antimicrobial therapy until the fragments pass. Occasionally, long-term antimicrobial therapy can result in eradication of bacteriuria even if some fragments persist after ESWL, presumably because the shock waves have rendered the entrapped bacteria more susceptible to antimicrobial therapy (Michaels et al, 1988). **If percutaneous or open surgery is used, all the residual particles**

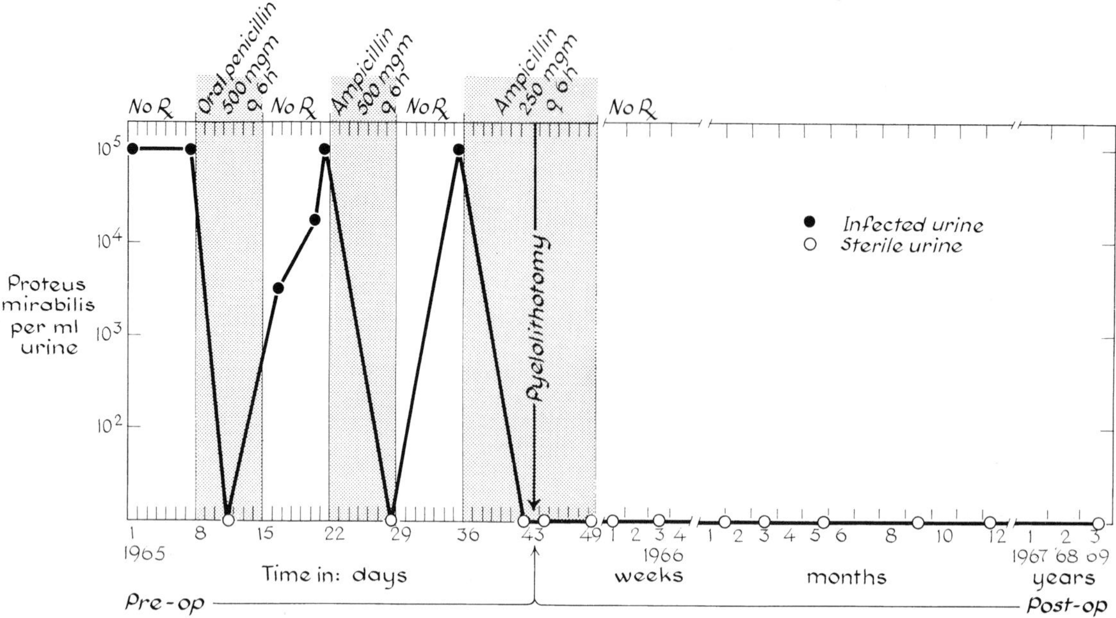

Figure 15–15. Preoperative and postoperative bacteriologic course of a 39-year-old woman with an infection stone caused by *Proteus mirabilis*. Note that eradication of the infection was achieved only after removal of the stone (80% struvite and 20% apatite), and that in the absence of reinfection with urea-splitting bacteria, no further stones have appeared. (From Nemoy NJ, Stamey TA: JAMA 1971; 215:1470.)

of struvite stones must be removed at surgery in order to prevent recurrent bacteriuria from bacterial persistence in the calculus. Rocha and Santos (1969) have shown that soaking these stones in iodine and alcohol for 6 hours will not kill the bacteria within the interior of the stone. The importance of recognizing this fact is twofold: (1) The bacteria cannot be killed by antimicrobial therapy, even though the urine may show no growth for months or even years (Shortliffe et al, 1984), and (2) any fragments left behind at the time of surgical removal leave residual bacteria within the interstices of the stone; these bacteria ensure recurrence of the staghorn calculus with its attendant morbidity.

If fragments remain after surgery, a small multiholed polyethylene catheter should be left for postoperative irrigation with Renacidin or Suby's-G solution. Using this technique and postoperative plain film tomograms to detect residual fragments missed on the intraoperative radiographs, Silverman and Stamey (1983) published results in 44 consecutive kidneys in 40 patients with proven struvite infection stones. With a mean follow-up of 7 years, there was one 4-mm stone recurrence in the left kidney (see Figs. 15–16 to 15–18) in a patient whose urine had consistently shown no growth for 14 months after cessation of therapy and whose calcification was thought to be around a radiolucent papilla. None of the patients had bacterial persistence postoperatively; antimicrobial agents were stopped in all within a few weeks of discharge. Among seven infections in the postoperative years, only one was *P. mirabilis*, an infection that never recurred after 10 days of treatment.

Finally, **it should be emphasized that struvite stones,**

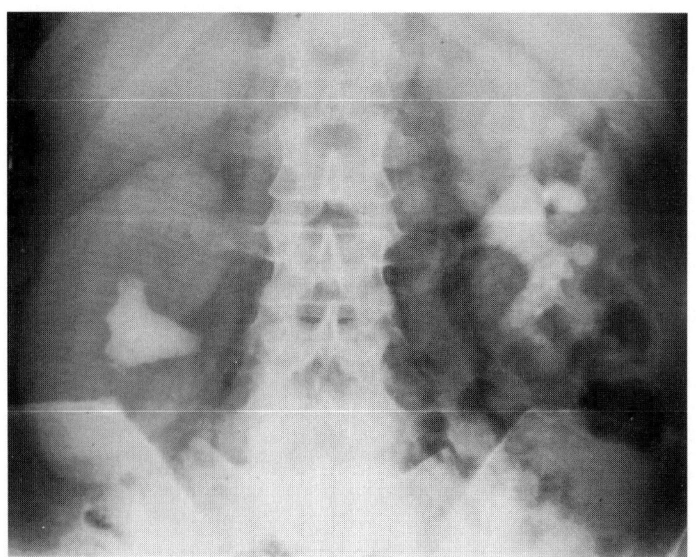

Figure 15–16. Plain film radiograph from a 52-year-old woman with bilateral struvite infection stones caused by *Proteus mirabilis*.

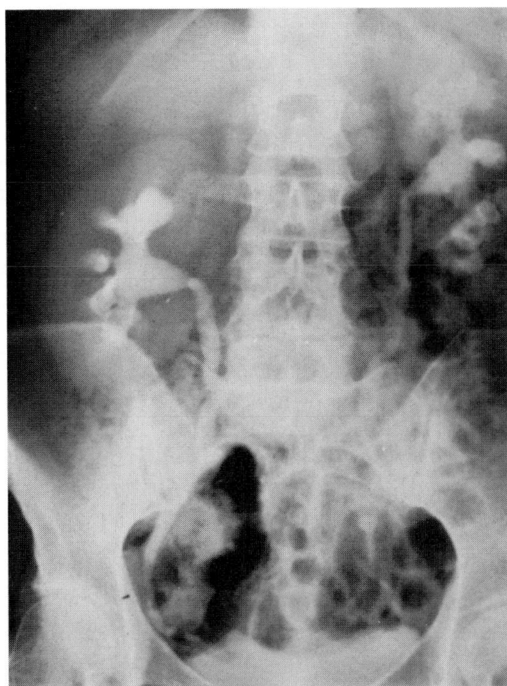

Figure 15–17. A 20-minute film from the preoperative intravenous urogram of the patient shown in Figure 15–11. The left kidney with the staghorn calculus appears to excrete the contrast medium more poorly than the right kidney does. Neither ureter is obstructed below the renal pelves.

usually about 80% struvite and 20% apatite, often contain minimal calcium and are easily obscured on plain film radiographs of the abdomen unless the kidneys are absolutely free of overlying gas and feces. Therefore, most patients with recurrent *P. mirabilis* infection warrant plain film tomography or ultrasonography of the kidneys. In addition, once all fragments have been surgically removed or dissolved and the patient is shown to have no growth in urine after cessation of antimicrobial therapy (the final test of successful surgery), the patient should be followed bacteriologically in case reinfection occurs with a new strain of urea-splitting bacteria.

Congenital Urinary Tract Anomalies

Any woman with a biologic susceptibility to recurrent bacteriuria (see below) or a man with a urinary tract infection who also has a congenital anomaly can develop secondary infection of the anomaly (see Table 15–2). When this occurs, recurrent bacteriuria is characterized by the same organism until the anomalous colonized structure is surgically removed. Almost invariably after surgical resection, however, if a woman is followed long enough, reinfections appear once again. Such anomalies include nonfunctioning duplications of the renal collecting system, which accompany ectopic ureters. Friedland and Stamey (1974) reported one case in which bacteriuria due to *P. aeruginosa* had been constantly present for several years. Complete resection of the ureteral duplication with its ectopic ureteral orifice in the urethra cured the recurrent *P. aeruginosa* urinary infection, but the patient had reinfections with *E. coli* over the next 10 years.

Other anomalies include pericalyceal diverticula that lose their free communication with pelvic urine (but excrete bacteria into the urine), urachal cysts of the dome of the bladder, unilateral medullary sponge kidneys, and occasional congenital obstructions that have produced nonfunctioning kidneys into which effective urinary concentrations of antimicrobial agents cannot be delivered. Clinical examples with bacteriologic documentation of each of these congenital anomalies that can cause bacteria to persist within the urinary tract have been published (Stamey, 1980).

Catheter Drainage

The most common site of hospital-acquired infections is the urinary tract, where approximately 40% of all hospital-acquired infections occur (Stamm, 1975). **The most common predisposing factor for these infections is urethral instrumentation, including catheterization. In fact, between 10% and 15% of all hospitalized patients have indwelling catheters** (Stamm, 1975; Fincke and Friedland, 1976), and there are more than 1 million catheter-associated urinary tract infections per year in the United States (Stamm, 1991).

Catheter-associated bacteriuria is the most common source of gram-negative bacteremia in hospitalized patients (Kreger et al, 1980). Sullivan and associates (1973) reported that 8% (6 in 75) of urethral catheterizations caused bacteremia as documented by a positive blood culture. More-

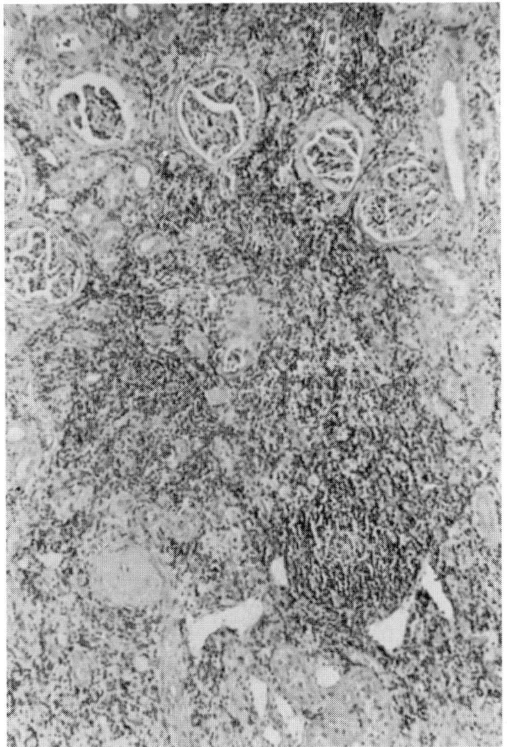

Figure 15–18. Random biopsy from the left kidney at the time of the anatrophic nephrolithotomy. The intense interstitial infiltrate with inflammatory cells, the periglomerular sclerosis, and the hyalinized glomeruli are easily seen.

over, in one study, 46% of adult cases of gram-negative bacteremia resulted from urinary tract infections or prior genitourinary manipulation (DuPont and Spink, 1969). **Other infectious complications associated with urethral catheterization and concomitant urinary tract infections are acute epididymitis-orchitis; bacterial prostatitis; pyelonephritis; periurethral abscesses; and struvite, bladder, and especially renal calculi** (Warren et al, 1988).

To collect a culture specimen one should needle-aspirate the catheter urine from the catheter tubing with an aseptic technique. **A count of 100 or more colony-forming units per milliliter (cfu/ml) indicates significant bacteriuria in a catheterized patient since these counts usually persist or increase within 48 hours** (Stark and Maki, 1984). Cultures taken from Foley tips are useless and show less than 3% correlation with subsequent and simultaneous urine cultures (Gross et al, 1974). **Pyuria does not indicate bacteriuria but may help to differentiate bacterial colonization from bacterial infection of the urinary tract.**

When a urethral catheter is placed in a patient, the patient risks bacteremia from the manipulation and introduction of a urinary tract infection. Any patient who risks endocarditis or who has a prosthesis that might become infected should receive antimicrobial prophylaxis before catheter manipulation.

The incidence of urinary tract infections in patients with indwelling catheters is directly related to the duration of catheterization. When open drainage systems are used, 95% of patients (sex unspecified) became bacteriuric by 4 days (Kass and Finland, 1956). With the advent of closed drainage systems, the average daily rate of acquired bacteriuria is decreased to 4% in males and 10.4% in females (about half the patients received antibiotics with the insertion of the catheter) (Garibaldi et al, 1974). **Also with a closed system, Warren and associates (1978) found the incidence of acquired bacteriuria to be about 5% per day of catheterization.** Other authors have calculated that a patient has only a 50% cumulative probability of remaining free of infection (fewer than 10 bacteria per milliliter) for 4½ days after catheterization even when a closed collecting system is used (Maizels and Schaeffer, 1980).

Etiology

Catheter-associated bacteriuria may originate from three sources: (1) periurethral and perineal organism; (2) organisms colonizing the collecting bag or collecting device; and (3) breaks in the drainage system caused by opening the closed system for irrigation, changes in tubing, or emptying the collecting bag. Kass and Schneiderman (1957) showed that 24 to 72 hours after *Serratia marcescens* was applied to the glans penis or vulva in three semicomatose patients with indwelling catheters, thousands of the organisms could be cultured from the bladder. In another study, investigators found that organisms causing catheter-associated bacteriuria could be isolated from the urethra and perineum before they could be isolated from the bladder most of the time (Brehmer and Madsen, 1972; Bultitude and Eykyn, 1973). **Maizels and Schaeffer (1980) found that bacteriuria could be attributed to the collecting bag in 45% of patients who became infected and to the urethra in 27%.**

Methods to Decrease Catheter-Associated Urinary Tract Infections

In patients on intermittent catheterization, it has been shown by several investigators that the instillation of antimicrobial solutions into the bladder just after catheterization, with or without the administration of prophylactic oral antimicrobials agents, may decrease the rate of infection induced by catheterization to 0.5% to 0.6% or lower (Pearman, 1971; Anderson, 1980). **Routine use of a closed-catheter drainage system has reduced catheter-associated infections from about 90% at 4 days to 30% to 40%.** Other means of decreasing infections have focused on the collecting bag and urethra as sources of infection. Periodic instillations of a chemical such as hydrogen peroxide or glutaraldehyde into the collecting bag may delay the onset of bacteriuria during catheterization (Bloom and Gonick, 1969; Maizels and Schaeffer, 1980), but no devices have been completely effective in eliminating infections in the patient with a long-term indwelling catheter.

Prophylactic antimicrobial irrigations of closed-catheter systems have not decreased the incidence of infections and have only led to infection by more resistant organisms (Warren et al, 1978; Dudley and Barriere, 1981). Moreover, a randomized, controlled trial of repetitive courses of cephalexin for the treatment of bacteriuria sensitive to cephalexin in long-term catheterized patients showed no difference in the prevalence of bacteriuria, incidence of infections, number of bacterial strains present on weekly culture, febrile days, or catheter obstructions (Warren et al, 1982). Not unexpectedly, during the study the proportion of organisms that were cephalexin-resistant increased in the cephalexin-treated group, and these organisms were resistant to many antimicrobial agents.

Antimicrobial Therapy

Whether antimicrobial prophylaxis can or should be used to prevent catheter-associated urinary tract infections depends on the circumstances of the catheterization. If one-time catheterizations are followed by a single dose of an antimicrobial agent, such as nitrofurantoin 100 mg, and/or the instillation of 30 ml of neomycin-polymyxin B solution (160 mg of neomycin and 300,000 units of polymyxin B per liter of sterile water) as Anderson (1980) used during intermittent catheterization, the incidence caused by catheterization is very low.

Patients with indwelling catheters that will be removed after only a few days require the same treatment as patients undergoing transurethral resection of the prostate. In these patients it is reasonable to prevent the onset of infection as long as possible. Such measures as putting hydrogen peroxide into the collecting bags may be helpful. An antimicrobial agent should be given just before catheter removal, and the urine should be cultured after removal of the catheter to verify no growth. Any patient who risks endocarditis must be treated with systemic antimicrobial agents when the catheter is inserted or removed.

In patients with chronic indwelling urethral catheters, no methods totally eliminate catheter-associated infections. Periods of bacteriuria may alternate with periods of urine showing no growth, or bacteriuria may become chronic. The infecting stains frequently change, and bacteriuria is often polymicrobial (Warren, 1987). **Asymptomatic bladder bacteriuria, funguria, or pyuria should not be treated as long as the catheter remains and the patient is asymptomatic. However, if a urea-splitting bacteriuria is identified, it should be eradicated by a 3- to 5-day course of antimicrobial therapy.** If the urea-splitting bacteria return immediately, infection stones should be suspected and appropriate steps instituted to identify and remove them. For catheters that need occasional irrigation, distilled water, acetic acid, or 10% hemiacidrin may be used; antimicrobial irrigation fluids should not be used. **A patient with an elevated temperature or flank pain who has a catheter-associated infection must be treated for clinical acute pyelonephritis with the appropriate antimicrobial agent until asymptomatic. Furthermore, it is important to determine that neither the urinary tract nor the catheter drainage system is obstructed.** Bacteria can become trapped in an indwelling catheter over a period of time. If the catheter has been in place for more than 3 weeks, it is prudent to replace it with a new catheter. **When the catheter is going to be removed, the antimicrobial susceptibility of the colonizing bacteria should be determined and the patient started on specific antimicrobial therapy 8 hours before catheter removal and the drug continued for 24 hours.**

Renal Papillary Necrosis

The role of infection in the development and progression of renal papillary necrosis (RPN) is controversial. Mutiple predisposing conditions have been associated with the development of RPN, particularly diabetes, analgesic abuse, sickle cell hemoglobinopathy, and obstruction (Table 15–14). In the excellent review of RPN by Eknoyan and associates (1982), 67% of the patients (18 of 27) with RPN had an acute or chronic urinary tract infection. In only 4 patients (22%) was pyelonephritis alone associated with RPN. In the remaining 14 patients, several of the conditions that can be associated with RPN were present in addition to the urinary tract infection. All 4 patients with urinary tract obstruction had concomitant urinary tract infection. In 9 of the RPN patients (one third), there was no evidence of infection at all. These figures emphasize that although any of the recognized factors in Table 15–14 alone may cause RPN, the coexistence of multiple factors, such as diabetes or obstruction and infection, increases the risk of developing RPN.

Table 15–14. CONDITIONS ASSOCIATED WITH RENAL PAPILLARY NECROSIS

- Diabetes mellitus
- Pyelonephritis
- Urinary tract obstruction
- Analgesic abuse
- Sickle cell hemoglobinopathies
- Renal transplant rejection
- Cirrhosis of the liver
- Dehydration, hypoxia, and jaundice of infants
- Miscellaneous: renal vein thrombosis, cryoglobulinemia, renal candidiasis, contrast media injection, amyloidosis, calyceal arteritis, necrotizing angiitis, rapidly progressive glomerulonephritis, hypotensive shock, acute pancreatitis

From Eknovan G, Qunibi WY, Grisson RT, et al: Medicine 1982; 61:55.

Clinically, RPN is a spectrum of disease. Patients may have an acute fulminating illness with rapid progression or may have a chronic disease that is incidentally discovered on excretory urography. Some patients may chronically pass necrotic tissue in their urine (Hernandez et al, 1975), and some may never pass papillae (Lindvall, 1978). Although the diagnosis may be made from the passage of necrotic papillae in the urine, most often it is made from the excretory urogram. The radiographs show various degrees of renal involvement with either medullary or papillary changes causing irregular sinuses or medullary cavities or classic ring shadows (Lindvall, 1978; Eknoyan et al, 1982). Retained necrotic papillae may calcify, especially in association with infection. Furthermore, this necrotic tissue may form the nidus for chronic infection. Opportunistic fungal infections have been reported (Madge and Lomvardias, 1973; Juhasz et al, 1980; Vordermark et al, 1980; Tomashefski and Abramowsky, 1981). Renal sonography may be useful to diagnose papillary necrosis (Buonocore et al, 1980; Hoffman et al, 1982).

The early diagnosis of RPN is important to improve prognosis and reduce morbidity. In addition to chronic infection, patients with analgesic abuse–associated papillary necrosis may have an increased incidence of urothelial tumors; routine urinary cytologic examinations may be helpful to diagnose these tumors early (Jackson et al, 1978). In patients who have analgesic abuse–induced RPN, the disease stabilizes if the analgesic intake is stopped (Gower, 1976). Furthermore, adequate antimicrobial therapy to control infection and early recognition and treatment of ureteral obstruction caused by sloughed necrotic tissue can minimize a decline in renal function. **A patient who suffers from an acute ureteral obstruction due to a sloughed papilla and who has a concomitant urinary tract infection is a urologic emergency. In this case, immediate removal of the obstructing papilla by stone basket** (Jameson and Heal, 1973) **or acute drainage of the kidney by ureteral catheter or percutaneous nephrostomy is necessary.**

Diabetes Mellitus

Although some studies have shown that the incidence of urinary tract infections in diabetic girls aged 6 to 15 years (1.6% to 2.0%) (Pometta et al, 1967) and in hospitalized diabetic patients (Huvos and Rocha, 1959) may be no different than in nondiabetic persons, several more recent studies documented that diabetic women have a higher incidence of infections than do nondiabetic women (Vejlsgaard, 1975; Ooi and Chen, 1974; Forland et al, 1977). **Two of these studies found that the incidence of infections in diabetic women ranged from 11.4% to 15.8%, whereas that in matched nondiabetic women ranged from 4.5% to 4.6%** (Vejlsgaard, 1973; Ooi and Chen, 1974), **only 2% of diabetic men were found to have infections** (Forland et al, 1977). **These patients often have a glomerulopathy, with difficulty concentrating antimicrobial agents. In addition, they seem to be predisposed to special complications of**

urinary tract infections—papillary necrosis and emphysematous pyelonephritis.

Papillary Necrosis

Although in diabetic patients urinary tract infection may be a primary or secondary factor in the etiology of papillary necrosis, **diabetics with acute clinical pyelonephritis seem to be particularly predisposed to RPN** (Eknoyan et al, 1982). In the study cited by Eknoyan and associates (1982), 29 of 107 diabetic patients (27.1%) who died of acute renal infection exhibited RPN on gross or microscopic examination. RPN is discussed in a previous section.

Emphysematous Pyelonephritis

Emphysematous pyelonephritis is an uncommon complication of acute pyelonephritis that occurs **in diabetic patients (although 15% of patients have diabetes discovered only when they are found to have emphysematous pyelonephritis), with an overall mortality of 43%** (Freiha et al, 1979). Emphysematous pyelonephritis is discussed below.

Spinal Cord Injury with High-Pressure Bladders

Of all patients with bacteriuria, no group compares in severity and morbidity with those who have spinal cord injury. Nearly all these patients require catheterization early after their injuries becasuse of bladder spasticity of flaccidity, and significant numbers develop ureterectasis, hydronephrosis, reflux, and renal calculi. Bacteriologic and urodynamic advances in the management of these patients have vastly reduced their morbidity and mortality.

Pregnancy

The special problems that relate to bacteriuria of pregnancy, including the effects on the fetus as well as the occurrence of acute pyelonephritis, are presented in a later section on urinary tract infections in pregnancy.

Acute Bacterial Prostatitis

Except in the very elderly or in immunocompromised hosts who are highly susceptible to gram-negative bacteremia, most men with acute bacterial prostatitis suffer mainly from the serious morbidity of chills, and, often, acute urinary retention. These patients at serious risk are discussed in Chapter 16.

Conclusion

The bacteriuric patients described in Table 15–3 represent those who are at substantial risk of either serious morbidity or loss of renal function, or both. They deserve special attention and care by the urologist; they often represent true emergencies. When acute pyelonephritis and especially perirenal abscess or gram-negative septicemia supervene, the potential for mortality is real.

UPPER-TRACT INFECTIONS

Acute Pyelonephritis

Although pyelonephritis is defined as inflammation of the kidney and renal pelvis, the diagnosis is clinical. True infection of the "upper urinary tract" can be proved by catheterization tests (ureteral catheterization or bladder washout) as described in this chapter, but these are impractical and unnecessary in most patients with acute pyelonephritis; none of the noninvasive tests that have been developed to determine infection in the kidney or bladder are totally reliable.

Clinical Presentation

The clinical spectrum ranges from gram-negative sepsis to cystitis with mild flank pain (Stamm and Hooton, 1993). The classic presentation is an abrupt onset of chills, fever, and unilateral or bilateral costovertebral angle tenderness. These so-called upper-tract signs are often accompanied by dysuria, increased urinary frequency, and urgency.

In a large study of 201 women and 12 men with recurrent urinary tract infections, Busch and Huland (1984) showed that fever and flank pain are no more diagnostic of pyelonephritis than they are of cystitis. Of patients with flank pain and/or fever, over 50% had lower-tract bacteriuria. Conversely, patients with bladder symptoms or no symptoms frequently had upper-tract bacteriuria. Approximately 75% of patients give a history of previous lower urinary tract infections.

On physical examination there is frequently tenderness to deep palpation in the costovertebral angle. Variations of this clinical presentation have been recognized. Acute pyelonephritis may also simulate gastrointestinal tract abnormalities with abdominal pain, nausea, vomiting, and diarrhea. Asymptomatic progression of acute pyelonephritis to chronic pyelonephritis, particularly in compromised hosts, may occur in the absence of overt symptoms. Acute renal failure may be present in the rare case (Richet and Mayaud, 1978; Olsson et al, 1980).

Laboratory Findings

Urine cultures are positive, but about 20% of patients have urine cultures with $<10^5$ cfu/ml and therefore negative results on Gram's staining of the urine (Rubin et al, 1992). **Urinary sediment usually shows increased white blood cells, white blood cell casts, and red blood cells.** Bacterial rods or chains of cocci are often seen. Blood tests may show a polymorphonuclear leukocytosis, increased erythrocyte sedimentation rate, elevated C-reactive protein levels, and elevated creatinine levels if renal failure is present. In addition, creatinine clearance may be decreased. Blood cultures may be positive.

Bacteriology

***E. coli*, which constitutes a unique subgroup that possesses special virulence factors, accounts for 80% of**

cases. If VUR is absent, a patient bearing the P blood group phenotype may have special susceptibility to recurrent pyelonephritis caused by *E. coli* that have P pili and bind to the P blood group antigen receptors (Lomberg et al, 1983). Bacterial K antigens and endotoxins also may contribute to pathogenicity (Kaijser et al, 1977). Other members of the Enterobacteriaceae family, including species of *Klebsiella, Proteus, Enterobacter, Pseudomonas, Serratia,* and *Citrobacter*, are also cultured from the urine. Of the gram-positive organisms, only *E. faecalis* and, less commonly, *S. aureus* are important causes of pyelonephritis.

Radiographic Findings

Intravenous Urogram

Radiologic findings characteristic of acute pyelonephritis have been emphasized only recently, because previously it was thought that intravenous urograms in these patients were normal. In 24% (Little et al, 1965) to 28% (Silver et al, 1976) of patients with acute pyelonephritis, abnormal urograms have been attributed to the acute disease. Others have confirmed the radiographic abnormalities that may be found in acute pyelonephritis (Cameron and Azimi, 1974; Barth et al, 1976; Richie et al, 1978; Teplick et al, 1978; Harrison and Shaffer, 1979). Since an intravenous urogram is often obtained in acute pyelonephritis, the urologist should be aware of the radiologic changes that may be seen in this disease.

Generalized or focal renal enlargement during the acute infection was seen in about 20% of the urograms examined by Silver and associates (1976). This renal enlargement is probably caused by inflammation and congestion from the infection. The clinically involved kidney is usually enlarged, but the contralateral kidney may be enlarged as well (Silver et al, 1976). An overall length of 15 cm or a length 1.5 cm greater than that of the unaffected side has been established as consistent with a diagnosis of acute pyelonephritis.

Focal renal enlargement, less common than generalized enlargement, may appear as a renal mass. Indeed, this finding, *focal bacterial nephritis* or *acute lobar nephronia*, has been emphasized as causing a renal mass only since 1978 (Rosenfield et al, 1978). **This mass must be differentiated from a neoplasm or intrarenal abscess** (Little et al, 1965; Barth et al, 1976; Teplick et al, 1978; McDonough et al, 1981; Funston et al, 1982; Konetschnik et al, 1982; Sotolongo et al, 1982). Although other radiologic modalities may be needed to differentiate the lesion from a neoplasm or intrarenal abscess, time and treatment cause the mass to disappear; however, scarring may occur.

Obstruction of the renal tubules from parenchymal edema and vasoconstriction may impair contrast excretion. This is manifested by delayed appearance of contrast material in the calyces and a diminished nephrogram and pyelogram (Silver et al, 1976). In the extreme case, the collecting system may not be visualized (Richie et al, 1978; Teplick et al, 1978). In the nephrogram phase of the urogram (or arteriogram) in acute pyelonephritis, cortical striations may be seen (Davidson and Talner, 1973; Silver et al, 1976; Teplick et al, 1978).

Dilation of the ureter and renal pelvis without any obstructive cause may be seen during acute pyelonephritis (Kass et al, 1976; Silver et al, 1976; Teplick et al, 1978). This may be caused by the bacterial endotoxins that impair ureteral peristalsis. Parallel lucent renal pelvic and ureteral streaks have been seen in acute pyelonephritis (Harrison and Shaffer, 1979). These are probably caused by mucosal edema.

Renal Ultrasonography

Although renal ultrasonography is useful to show renal size and collecting system obstruction and to delineate focal bacterial nephritis, in most infected kidneys no findings are seen on ultrasonography that are not seen on the urogram.

Computed Tomography

CT is not indicated unless the diagnosis cannot be established by an intravenous urogram or if the patient does not respond after 72 hours of therapy. When parenchymal destruction becomes pronounced, a more disorganized parenchyma and abscess formation may be demonstrated.

Renal Angiogram

Angiograms are unnecessary in acute bacterial pyelonephritis, except for the diagnosis of unusual patients. Most angiograms are normal, but they occasionally show attenuated and stretched interlobar arterial branches as well as the cortical striations seen on the urogram (Barth et al, 1976; Teplick et al, 1978).

Pathology

In acute pyelonephritis the kidney may be grossly enlarged (Freedman, 1979). The capsule strips easily, and suppuration may soften areas of parenchyma. There are usually small yellow-white cortical abscesses mixed with parenchymal hyperemia. Histologically, the parenchyma shows a focal, patchy infiltrate of neutrophils. Bacteria are often in the infiltrate. Early in the inflammatory process, this infiltrate is limited to the interstitium, but later linear bands of inflammation extend from the papillae to the cortex in a wedge-shaped manner. Abscesses may cause tubular destruction; the glomeruli are usually spared.

Treatment

Infection in patients with acute pyelonephritis can be subdivided into (1) uncomplicated infection that does not warrant hospitalization, (2) uncomplicated infection in patients with normal urinary tracts who are ill enough to warrant hospitalization for parenteral therapy, and (3) complicated infection associated with hospitalization, catheterization, urologic surgery, or urinary tract abnormalities (Fig. 15–19). In all cases, antimicrobial therapy should be initiated that will be active against potential uropathogens and achieve antimicrobial levels in renal tissue as well as urine. **Oral fluoroquinolones are particularly attractive for individuals who receive outpatient therapy (see Table 15–11).** TMP-SMX is another alternative. For patients requiring parenteral therapy for uncomplicated pyelonephritis, ampicillin and an aminoglycoside have proven efficacy and offer effectiveness against both Enterobacteriaceae, *Pseudomonas*, and

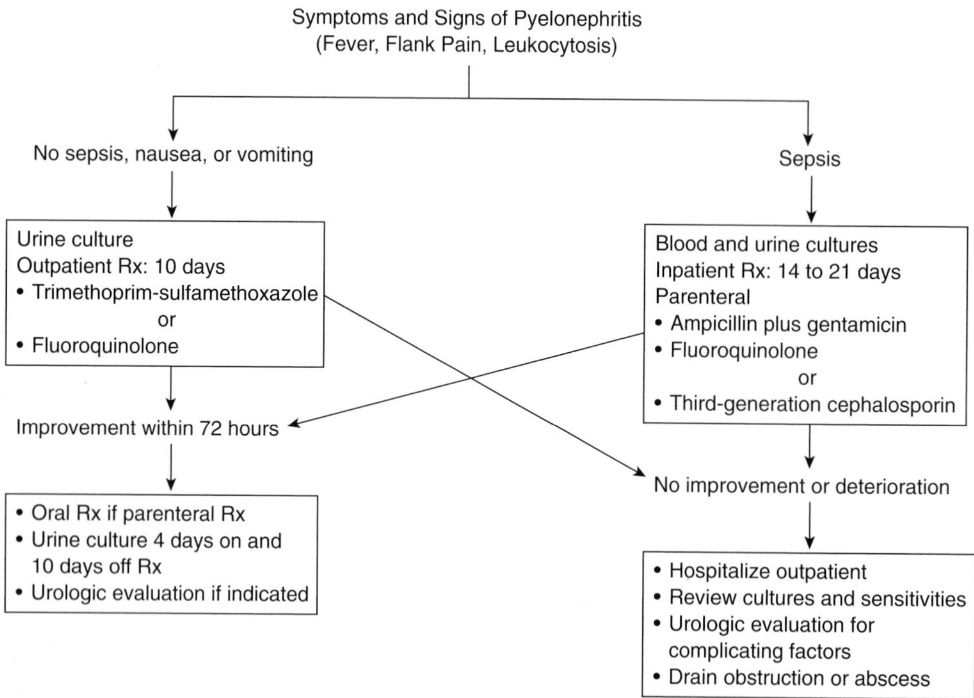

Figure 15–19. Management of acute pyelonephritis.

other gram-negative bacilli. If ampicillin-resistant organisms are suspected, TMP-SMX has more predictable antibacterial activity (Johnson et al, 1991). Fluoroquinolones, TMP-SMX, or third-generation cephalosporins are also effective. Complicated pyelonephritis due to nosocomial pathogens requires aggressive broad-spectrum parental therapy (see Table 15–12). The patient then can be treated with selective parenteral or oral antimicrobial therapy once susceptibility testing is available.

Most patients have persistent fever and flank pain for several days after initiation of successful antimicrobial therapy. If symptoms persist beyond 72 hours, however, the possibility of perinephric or intrarenal abscesses, urinary tract abnormalities, or obstruction should be considered and radiologic investigation with ultrasonography or CT performed (Soulen et al, 1989). **Urine and blood cultures should be repeated at appropriate intervals, and antimicrobial therapy should be adjusted, if necessary, on the basis of susceptibility testing. The duration of therapy for acute uncomplicated pyelonephritis generally should be 14 days** (Ronald, 1987). **Patients with complicated pyelonephritis should be treated for 21 days. Repeat urine cultures should be performed 5 to 7 days after initiation of therapy and 4 to 6 weeks after discontinuation of antimicrobial therapy to ensure that the urinary tract remains free of infection.**

Between 10% and 30% of individuals with acute pyelonephritis relapse after a 14-day course of therapy. Patients who relapse usually are cured by a second 14-day course of therapy, but occasionally a 6-week course is necessary (Tolkoff-Rubin et al, 1984; Johnson and Stamm, 1987).

Chronic Pyelonephritis

The definition of chronic pyelonephritis is controversial. As previously noted in the section on definitions, the term *chronic pyelonephritis* has been used to refer to a variety of chronic renal lesions and has been used synonymously with interstitial nephritis, reflux nephropathy, chronic atrophic pyelonephritis, and focal coarse renal scarring. In contrast to the patient with clinical acute pyelonephritis, the patient with chronic pyelonephritis is diagnosed by radiologic and pathologic means. Even when a patient has a radiographically scarred, shrunken kidney with microscopic evidence of inflammation, there is often no recent or remote history of urinary tract infection and no sign of viable bacteria. This has caused speculation that nonviable bacterial antigens and autoimmune reactions may account for scarring (Aoki et al, 1969; Cotran and Piessens, 1976). So far, however, there is little support for an autoimmune antibody-mediated injury (Cotran and Piessens, 1976). For the purposes of this discussion, **the term *chronic pyelonephritis* refers to the small, contracted, atrophic kidney or to the coarsely scarred kidney that has been produced by bacterial infection, whether recent or remote.**

Since many patients with radiologic or pathologic evidence of pyelonephritic scarring do not have a history of urinary tract infections and bacteria cannot be cultured from their renal tissue or urine, the terms *abacterial pyelonephritis* and *interstitial nephritis* have been used. Work by Aoki and associates (1969) showed that bacterial antigens could be detected in the renal tissue by immunofluorescent localization in six of seven patients with abacterial pyelonephritis.

Pathogenesis

Immunologic Response to Infection

Much knowledge about the immune response to bacterial infection of the kidney has been derived from experimental animal models (Fierer et al, 1971; Brooks et al, 1977; Glauser et al, 1978; Kaijser et al, 1978; Miller and Phillips, 1981; Roberts et al, 1981, 1982; Shimamura, 1981; Bille and Glauser, 1982; Slotki and Asscher, 1982). These studies have tried to relate bacterial infection and subsequent renal scarring.

Bacterial infection of the kidneys in both humans and animals stimulates humoral and cellular immune responses (Miller et al, 1979). **In pyelonephritis the systemic humoral response is characterized by a rise in both total and anti–*E. coli* IgM, IgA, and IgG (Miller et al, 1979); this response, however, does not appear to be associated with the scarring seen in chronic pyelonephritis.** The cause of the renal scarring that unpredictably follows infection is unclear. With a rat model of pyelonephritis that was induced by retrograde injection of *E. coli* in a partially obstructed ureter, Glauser and associates (1978) showed that maximal renal exudation and suppuration occurred 3 days after infection and lasted until the fifth day. During the period of maximal suppuration, the kidneys were enlarged (renal mass increased) and had numerous cortical abscesses, but this period was followed by extensive parenchymal scarring with a 50% loss of renal mass at 21 days and a 70% loss at 75 to 90 days. Similarly, Slotki and Asscher (1982) examined rat kidneys at fixed intervals of time after direct bacterial infection and showed that polymorphonuclear leukocytes infiltrated the tissue as early as 6 hours after infection; mononuclear cells were visible at 16 hours, when macroscopic pustules began to appear on the renal cortex. Maximal suppuration was seen at 3 to 5 days with microabscesses scattered throughout the cortex and medulla, while collagen appeared on the fifth day and cortical depressions on the sixth. Roberts and associates (1981) caused experimental pyelonephritis in monkeys by injecting *E. coli* retrograde into their kidneys until pyelotubular backflow occurred. With this model, they showed that mononuclear cells infiltrated the renal pelvic interstitium in a wedge toward the medulla and cortex. They also showed that similar injection with heat-killed bacteria caused a humoral immune response but no cellular response or subsequent renal scarring.

These animal studies support the theory that the leukocyte response is at least partially responsible for renal scarring. Reducing the acute suppurative response to renal bacterial infection by using antimicrobial and other agents has been shown to decrease and ablate scarring (Glauser et al, 1978; Miller and Phillips, 1981; Shimamura, 1981; Slotki and Asscher, 1982). Glauser and associates (1978), using 10 days of antimicrobial treatment with ampicillin and gentamicin, showed that rat kidneys were sterile at 75 to 90 days and that minimal scarring and loss of renal mass (8%) were observed if antimicrobial treatment was started 28 to 30 hours after the onset of infection. If treatment was started 5 days after infection, the pyelonephritic kidneys, although sterilized, were shrunk to 30% of their original mass and were indistinguishable from untreated kidneys. Similarly, Slotki and Asscher (1982) demonstrated that treatment within 24 hours of infection (amoxicillin and gentamicin for 10 days) prevented or reduced scarring. Miller and Phillips (1981), using an experimental model of pyelonephritis caused by direct bacterial injection in the kidney, showed reduced scarring if treatment was begun within 4 days of infection (ampicillin, carbenicillin, nitrofurantoin, and cephalothin).

Other research suggests that the bactericidal activity of the neutrophils causes the initial damage to the renal tubular cells (Roberts et al, 1982). During bacterial phagocytosis, enzymes, superoxide, and oxygen radicals are released; these investigators have shown that the addition of superoxide dismutase, which inhibits superoxide production, decreases renal inflammation and tubular damage caused by bacteria. From this, they have concluded that superoxide contributes to the renal tubular cell damage seen in acute bacterial infection.

Although most of this work has been done on rats, a species possessing a unicalyceal system, the results support observations in humans. Children under 4 years of age with intrarenal reflux commonly have renal scarring present before they have their first documented urinary tract infection. If histories of undiagnosed febrile illnesses in early childhood do, indeed, represent pyelonephritis, untreated infections may be the cause of scarring in the "chronic pyelonephritic" kidney.

Association with Reflux Nephropathy

The association of the small, scarred, clubbed kidney with VUR is called *reflux nephropathy*. The role that bacterial infection of the urinary tract plays in reflux nephropathy is controversial. Whether the small, scarred kidney is secondary to urinary tract infections is difficult to establish because the occurrence of a bacterial pyelonephritic scar in a previously documented unscarred kidney is a rare event. Moreover, it is often difficult to distinguish a pyelonephritic kidney from a congenially abnormal one. The question why all persons with VUR reflux do not develop reflux nephropathy is complicated, but it was partially addressed by Ransley and Risdon (1979) in experimental studies involving piglets. In their work, they reported intrarenal reflux only in papillae of a particular morphology; they described a *nonrefluxing* papilla, which is conical and has papillary ducts that close when calyceal pressure is increased, and a *refluxing* papilla, which is larger and has papillary ducts that are wide open. Furthermore, they found that renal scarring occurred only in piglet kidneys exposed to reflux with infected urine and only in those areas drained by refluxing papillae. Scars did not occur when the urine was sterile.

The natural history and prevalence of reflux nephropathy found incidentally in adults is unknown. **If adult bacteriuric women are screened, reflux nephropathy is present in 0.6%** (Alwall, 1975) **to 1%** (Kincaid-Smith and Bullen, 1965). In a nephrology clinic, Kincaid-Smith and Becker (1979) studied 55 patients with reflux nephropathy and found that most were under 30 years of age. A urinary tract infection was the diagnostic event in 80%; 20% had had enuresis that had never been investigated. In 27%, reflux nephropathy was diagnosed during pregnancy because of urinary tract infection, hypertension, albuminuria, and postpartum edema. Approximately 50% of the patients had elevated serum creatinine values, 38% had hypertension (diastolic pressure greater than 90), and 35% had proteinuria (greater than 0.2 g in 24 hours). In one half of the patients with proteinuria, renal function declined further during follow-up (a mean of 15.5 months) (Kincaid-Smith and Becker, 1979). The importance of reflux nephropathy in children is discussed in Chapter 57.

Clinical Presentation

Many patients diagnosed as having chronic pyelonephritis have no urologic symptoms, and the condition is discovered incidentally. Pregnant women with chronic pyelonephritis may present with urinary tract infection, but many are diagnosed because of symptoms related to the complications of chronic azotemia, such as hypertension, visual impairment, headaches, increased fatigue, polyuria, and polydipsia; these patients may have VUR or recurrent urinary tract infections.

Laboratory Findings

Urinary sediment may show leukocytes, proteinuria, and, rarely, leukocyte casts. Studies comparing a pyelonephritic kidney with a normal contralateral one have shown that a medullary defect in the pyelonephritic kidney causes the loss of filtered water and sodium (Stamey, 1980); thus, urinary concentrating capacity is impaired. Serum creatinine levels may be increased and creatinine clearance may be decreased.

Radiologic Findings

Intravenous Urogram

The intravenous urogram is the best technique for diagnosing chronic pyelonephritis. The involved kidneys are usually small and atrophic. Focal coarse renal scarring with clubbing of the underlying calyx is characteristic (Witten et al, 1977) (see Figs. 15–1 and 15–2); since the scarring and atrophy commonly affect the renal poles, the renal parenchyma is especially thin in these areas. These findings are unilateral or bilateral. When they are unilateral, the contralateral kidney is often hypertrophied. Even localized areas of normal renal tissue within a scarred kidney may undergo compensatory hypertrophy, suggesting a renal mass (Witten et al, 1977). These pseudotumors sometimes need to be differentiated from neoplasms by other radiologic imaging techniques.

Voiding Cystourethrogram

The voiding cystourethrogram is useful, particularly in children, to show VUR, which may be associated with focal renal scarring.

Pathology

In chronic pyelonephritis, the gross kidney is often diffusely contracted, scarred, and pitted. The scars are U-shaped, flat, broad-based depressions with red-brown granular bases. The scarring is often polar with underlying calyceal blunting. The parenchyma is thin, and the corticomedullary demarcation is lost.

Histologic changes are patchy. There is usually an interstitial infiltrate of lymphocytes, plasma cells, and occasional polymorphonuclear cells. Portions of the parenchyma may be replaced by fibrosis, and, although glomeruli may be preserved, periglomerular fibrosis is often seen. In some affected areas, glomeruli may be completely fibrosed and tubules atrophied. Leukocyte and hyalin casts are sometimes present in the tubules; the latter may cause resemblance to the thyroid colloid—hence, the description *renal thyroidization* (Braude, 1973). In general, the changes are nonspecific; they also may be seen in toxic exposures, postobstructive atrophy, hematologic disorders, postirradiation nephritis, ischemic renal disease, and nephrosclerosis.

Sequelae of Pyelonephritis

Although it is known that certain adults have increased risk of renal damage from bacteriuria (this subject is discussed in detail in a previous section on patients at risk of serious morbidity and/or renal scarring from recurrent bacteriuria), acute clinical pyelonephritis does not cause scarring in most adults with normal urinary tracts. **Most of the changes of chronic pyelonephritis seem to occur in infancy, probably because the growing kidney is most susceptible to scarring. In a review that examined the long-term effect of urinary tract infections in adults, it was concluded that renal damage is rare in nonobstructive urinary tract infections** (Stamey, 1980) **but that it does occur** (Bailey et al, 1969; Davies et al, 1972; Davidson and Talner, 1973; Feldberg, 1982). In most reports of renal change after acute nonobstructive bacterial pyelonephritis, calyceal and papillary distortion similar to that occurring in papillary necrosis is seen, but focal cortical scars characteristic of chronic pyelonephritic changes are absent. Instead, the urograms show generalized shrinkage of the kidneys after the acute infection. Two of the four patients reported by Davidson and Talner (1973) had diabetes in addition to pyelonephritis.

The natural history of patients with chronic pyelonephritis is discussed in Chapter 57, relating to urinary tract infections in infants and children (see the sections on course and prognosis), since these changes are usually discovered in childhood. A few studies have examined the prognosis in cases that were discovered in adults. In a longitudinal study of patients with the radiologic changes of bilateral chronic pyelonephritis defined by focal parenchymal scarring and calyceal clubbing, the calculated 5-year survival rate was 95% and the 10-year survival rate was 86% (Gower, 1976). The survival rate for patients with changes of unilateral chronic pyelonephritis was 100% at both 5 and 10 years. This investigator also observed during the study period of 5 to 135 months that bacteriuria found in patients more than 20% of the time could not be correlated with deteriorating renal function; however, infection was often associated with the appearance or growth of renal calculi.

The relationships of the pyelonephritic kidney with end-stage renal disease and hypertension have been examined. In one report of 161 patients with end-stage renal disease requiring dialysis, 42 patients (26%) had "chronic pyelonephritis" with bacteriuria in the past or at the time they were studied (Huland and Busch, 1982). However, a complicating factor was involved in all of the 42 patients with chronic pyelonephritis and end-stage renal disease: 66.7% had VUR; 14.3%, analgesic abuse; 11.9%, nephrolithiasis; 4.8%, pyelonephritis during pregnancy; and 2.4%, hydronephrosis. The association between hypertension and the pyelonephritic kidney has been addressed by Pfau and Rosenmann (1978), who concluded that the association of chronic pyelonephritis and hypertension is usually coincidental. Their conclusion agrees with a study in 1973 that examined 74 women who had been admitted to the hospital some 10 to 20 years previously for pyelonephritis; only 14.5% of these women had hypertension, a rate similar to that found in a random female population of the same age (Parker and Kunin, 1973).

Emphysematous Pyelonephritis

Emphysematous pyelonephritis is an acute necrotizing parenchymal and perirenal infection caused by gas-forming uropathogens. The pathogenesis is poorly understood. Because the condition usually occurs in diabetic patients, it has been postulated that the high tissue glucose levels provide the substrate for microorganisms such as *E. coli*, which are able to produce carbon dioxide by the fermentation of sugar (Schainuck et al, 1968). Although glucose fermentation may be a factor, the explanation does not account for the rarity of emphysematous pyelonephritis despite the high frequency of gram-negative urinary tract infections in diabetic patients, nor does it explain the rare occurrence of the condition in nondiabetic patients. **In addition to diabetes, many patients have urinary tract obstruction associated with urinary calculi or papillary necrosis and significant renal functional impairment.**

It seems more reasonable to postulate that impaired host response caused by local factors such as obstruction or a systemic condition such as diabetes allows organisms with the capability of producing carbon dioxide to use necrotic tissue as a substrate to generate gas in vivo. **Thus emphysematous pyelonephritis should be considered a complication of severe pyelonephritis rather than a distinct entity. The overall mortality is 43%** (Freiha et al, 1979).

Clinical Presentation

All the documented cases of emphysematous pyelonephritis have been in adults (Hawes et al, 1983). Juvenile diabetic patients do not appear to be at risk. **Women are affected more often than men.**

The usual clinical presentation is severe, acute pyelonephritis that fails to resolve during the first 3 days of treatment. In some instances a chronic infection precedes the acute attack. **Almost all patients display the classic triad of fever, vomiting, and flank pain** (Schainuck et al, 1968). Pneumaturia is absent unless the infection involves the collecting system. Results of urine cultures are invariably positive. ***E. coli* is most frequently identified; *Klebsiella* and *Proteus* are less common.**

Radiologic Findings

The diagnosis is established radiographically. The hallmark is intraparenchymal gas. Tissue gas that is distributed in the parenchyma may appear on abdominal x-ray films as mottled gas shadows over the involved kidney. **This finding is often mistaken for bowel gas.** A crescentic collection of gas over the upper pole of the kidney is more distinctive (Fig. 15–20). **As the infection progresses, gas extends to the perinephric space and retroperitoneum.**

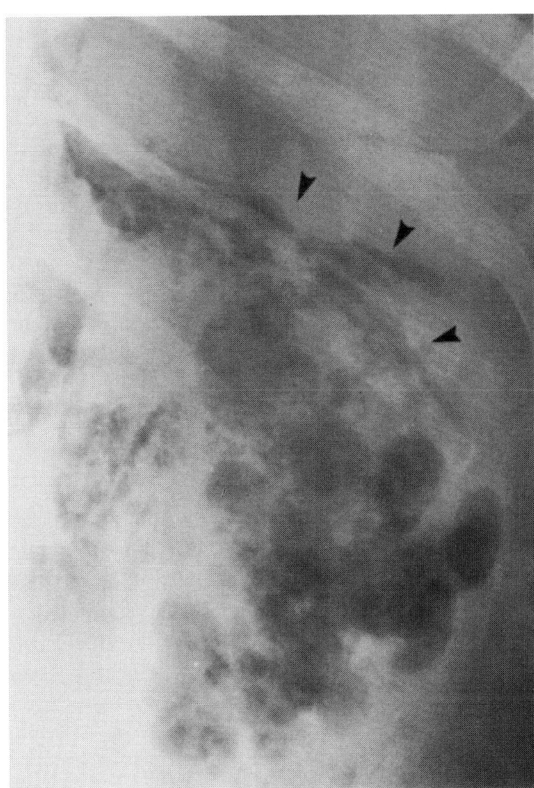

Figure 15–20. Part of an abdominal plain film taken in a woman with diabetes and emphysematous pyelonephritis. The arrows mark the thin crescents of gas found around the kidney. Other areas of the kidney show small gas bubbles extending radially in the parenchyma.

This distribution of gas should not be confused with cases of pyelonephritis in which air is in the collecting system of the kidney. This condition is secondary to a gas-forming bacterial urinary tract infection, frequently occurs in nondiabetic patients, is less serious, and usually responds to antimicrobial therapy.

Excretory urography is rarely of value, since the affected kidney usually is nonfunctioning or poorly functioning. Because of the significant risk of contrast nephropathy in critically ill, dehydrated diabetic patients with abnormal renal function, retrograde pyelography or ultrasonography rather than excretory urography is advisable to demonstrate obstruction. Obstruction is demonstrated in approximately 25% of the cases. **Ultrasonography usually demonstrates strong focal echoes suggesting the presence of intraparenchymal gas** (Brenbridge et al, 1979; Conrad et al, 1979). **CT has also been used to localize the gas and extent of infection** (Paivansalo et al, 1989). **A renal scan should be performed to assess the degree of renal function impairment in the involved kidney and the status of the contralateral kidney.**

Management

Patients with this infectious complication are usually acutely ill, and rapid supportive measures are required. **Patients should be started on appropriate antimicrobial agents, and treatment of diabetes must be initiated. Obstruction of the affected kidney, if present, must be elimi-**

nated, and function of the contralateral kidney must be established, since 10% of the reported cases have been bilateral (Freiha et al, 1979). Since carbon dioxide diffuses rapidly through body tissues, the observation of persistent intraparenchymal renal gas documents ineffective treatment; then surgical drainage or nephrectomy is needed (Schainuck et al, 1968). **Freiha and associates (1979) have emphasized that surgical treatment must be complete extirpation because most attempts at renal sparing have been unsuccessful in retaining renal function or decreasing patient morbidity. In selected cases percutaneous drainage combined with medical therapy can produce complete recovery and preserve renal function** (Hall et al, 1988).

Renal Abscess

Renal abscess or carbuncle is a collection of purulent material confined to the renal parenchyma. Before the antimicrobial era, 80% of renal abscesses were attributed to hematogenous seeding by staphylococci (Campbell, 1930). Although experimental and clinical data document the facility for abscess formation in normal kidneys after hematogenous inoculation with staphylococci, widespread use of antimicrobials in the past 25 years appears to have diminished the propensity for gram-positive abscess formation (DeNavasquez, 1950; Cotran, 1969).

During the past two decades, gram-negative organisms have been implicated in the majority of adults with renal abscesses. Hematogenous renal seeding by gram-negative organisms may occur, but this is not likely to be the primary pathway for gram-negative abscess formation. Clinically there is no evidence that gram-negative septicemia antedates most lesions. Further, gram-negative hematogenous pyelonephritis is virtually impossible to produce in animals unless the kidney is traumatized or completely obstructed (Cotran, 1969; Timmons and Perlmutter, 1976). The partially obstructed kidney rejects blood-borne gram-negative inocula as well as a normal kidney. Thus ascending infection associated with tubular obstruction from prior infections or calculi appears to be the primary pathway for the establishment of gram-negative abscesses. Two-thirds of gram-negative abscesses in adults are associated with renal calculi or damaged kidneys (Salvatierra et al, 1967). Although the association of pyelonephritis with VUR is well established, the association of renal abscess with VUR has been infrequently noted (Segura and Kelalis, 1973). Recent observations, however, indicate that reflux is frequently associated with renal abscesses and persists long after sterilization of the urinary tract (Timmons and Perlmutter, 1976).

Clinical Presentation

The patient may present with fever, chills, abdominal or flank pain, and occasionally weight loss and malaise. Symptoms of cystitis may occur. Occasionally these symptoms may be vague and delay diagnosis until surgical exploration or, in more severe cases, autopsy (Anderson and McAninch, 1980). A thorough history may reveal a gram-positive source of infection 1 to 8 weeks before the onset of urinary tract symptoms. The infection may have occurred in any area of the body. Multiple skin carbuncles and intravenous drug abuse introduce gram-positive organisms into the blood stream. Other common sites are the mouth, lungs, and bladder (Lyons et al, 1972). Complicated urinary tract infections associated with stasis, calculi, pregnancy, neurogenic bladder, and diabetes mellitus also appear to predispose the patient to abscess formation (Anderson and McAninch, 1980).

Laboratory Findings

The patient typically has marked leukocytosis. The blood cultures are usually positive. Pyuria and bacteriuria may not be evident unless the abscess communicates with the collecting system. Because gram-positive organisms are most commonly blood-borne, urine cultures in these cases typically show no growth or a microorganism different from that isolated from the abscess. When the abscess contains gram-negative organisms, the urine culture usually demonstrates the same organism isolated from the abscess.

Radiologic Findings

The urographic findings depend on both the nature and the duration of the infection. Differentiation between early renal abscesses and acute pyelonephritis can be difficult because most of the former are small. **In patients in whom abscess formation has progressed from an episode of acute bacterial nephritis or those in whom the kidney has been seeded by an outside infection, radiologic examination may demonstrate generalized renal enlargement with distortion of the renal contour on the affected side.** Renal fixation on aspiratory and expiratory films and obliteration of the corresponding psoas shadow may also be evident. Scoliosis is often present, with a concavity of the curve facing the affected kidney. If renal involvement is diffuse, the nephrogram is delayed or even absent. When an abscess is more localized, the findings may be similar to those of acute focal bacterial nephritis.

In a more chronic abscess the predominant urographic abnormalities are those of a renal mass lesion. The calyceal system may be poorly defined or show distortion or even amputation (Resnick and Older, 1982). Nephrotomography usually reveals a relative radiolucency in the involved area. Occasionally the excretory urogram appears normal despite the presence of a renal abscess, particularly if the abscess involves the anterior or posterior portion of the kidney without impinging on the parenchyma or collecting system.

Ultrasonography and CT are helpful to distinguish abscess from other inflammatory renal diseases. **Ultrasonography is the quickest and least expensive method to demonstrate a renal abscess. An echo-free or low-echo-density space-occupying lesion with increased transmission is found on the sonogram (Fig. 15–21).** The margins of an abscess are indistinguishable in the acute phase, but the structure contains a few echoes, and the surrounding renal parenchyma is edematous (Fiegler, 1983). Subsequently, the appearance tends to be that of a well-defined mass. The internal appearance, however, may vary from a virtually solid lucent mass to one with large numbers of low-level internal echoes (Schneider et al, 1976). The number of echoes depends on the amount of cellular debris within the abscess. The pres-

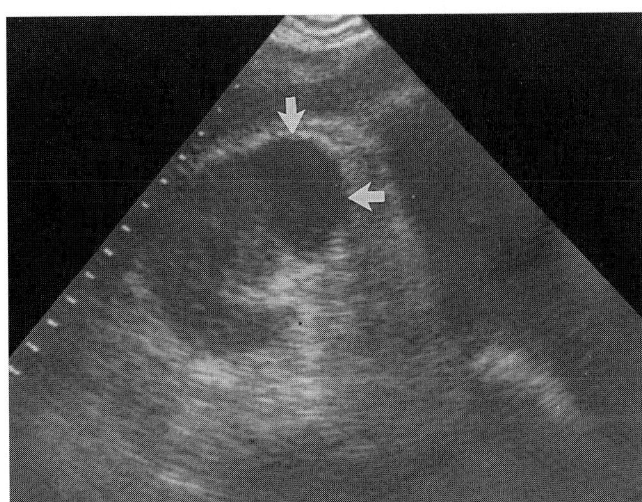

Figure 15–21. Acute renal abscess. Transverse ultrasonographic scan of the right kidney demonstrates a poorly marginated rounded focal hypoechoic mass *(arrows)* in the anterior portion of the kidney.

ence of air results in a strong echo with a shadow. Differentiation between an abscess and a tumor is impossible in many cases. Arteriography is used infrequently to demonstrate abscesses. The center of the mass tends to be hypervascular or avascular, with increased vascularity at the cortical margins and lack of vascular displacement and neovascularity.

CT appears to be the diagnostic procedure of choice for renal abscesses, since it provides excellent delineation of the tissue. On CT, abscesses are characteristically well defined both before and after contrast enhancement. Initially CT shows renal enlargement and focal, rounded areas of decreased attenuation (Fig. 15–22). After several days of the onset of the infection, a thick fibrotic wall begins to form around the abscess. An echo-free or slightly echogenic mass due to the presence of necrotic debris is seen. CT of a chronic abscess shows obliteration of adjacent tissue planes, thickening of Gerota's fascia, a round or oval parenchymal mass of low attenuation, and a surrounding inflammatory wall of slightly higher attenuation that forms a ring when the scan is enhanced with contrast material (Fig. 15–23). The ring sign is caused by the increased vascularity of the abscess wall (Callen, 1979; Gerzof and Gale, 1982).

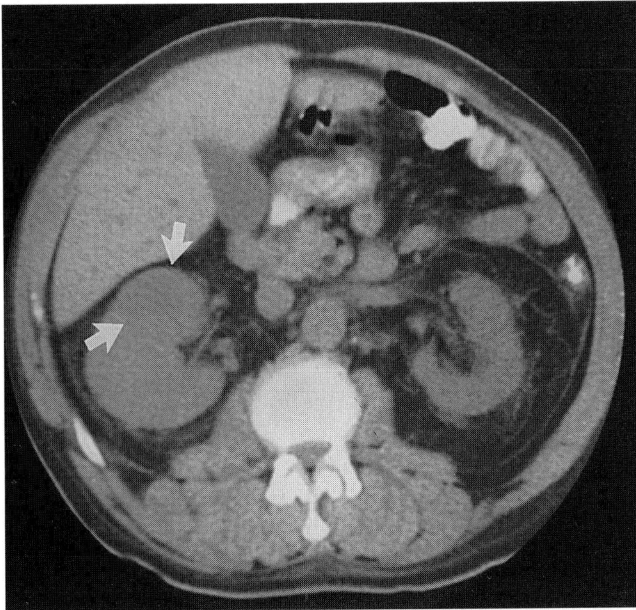

Figure 15–22. Acute renal abscess. Nonenhanced CT scan through the midpole of the right kidney demonstrates right renal enlargement and an area of decreased attenuation *(arrows)*. After antimicrobial therapy, a follow-up scan showed complete regression of these findings.

Radionuclide imaging with gallium or indium is sometimes useful in evaluating patients with renal abscesses (see Chapter 6).

Management

Although the classic treatment for an abscess has been percutaneous or open incision and drainage, in the past few years there has been good evidence that the use of intravenous antimicrobials and careful observations, if begun early enough in the course of the process, may obviate surgical procedures (Hoverman et al, 1980; Levin et al, 1984).

The selection of empirical antimicrobial therapy is depen-

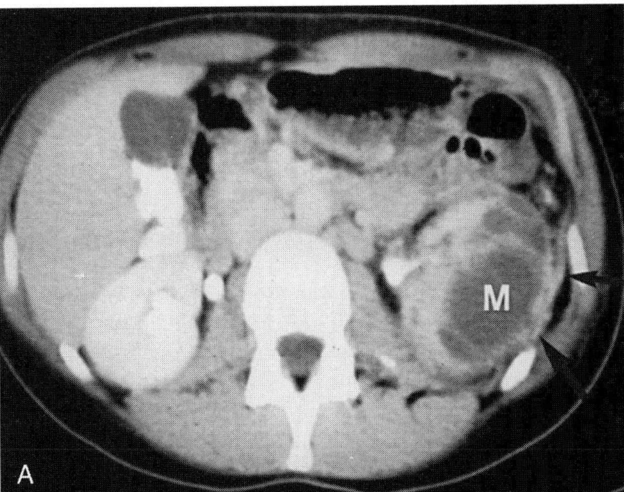

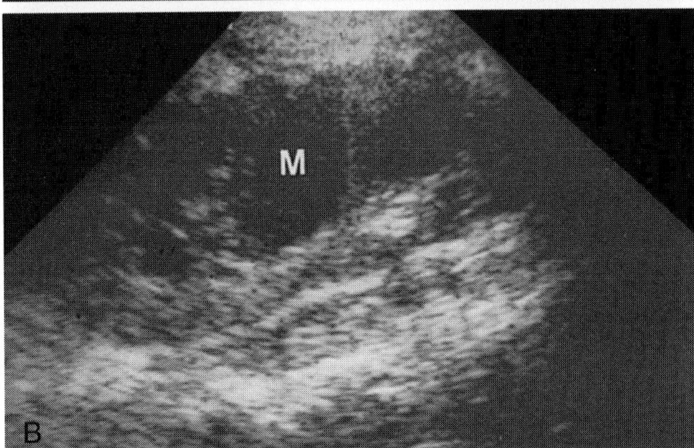

Figure 15–23. *A,* Chronic renal abscess computed tomography. Enhanced scan shows an irregular septated low-density mass (M) extensively involving the left kidney. Note thickening of perinephric fascia *(arrows)* and extensive compression of the renal collecting system. Findings are typical of renal abscess. *B,* Ultrasound longitudinal scan demonstrating septated hypoechoic mass (M) occupying much of the renal parenchymal volume.

dent on the presumed source of the infection. When hematogenous dissemination is suspected, the pathogenic organism most frequently is penicillin-resistant *Staphylococcus*, and the antibiotic of choice therefore is a penicillinase-resistant penicillin (Schiff et al, 1977). If a history of penicillin hypersensitivity is present, the recommended drugs are either cephalosporin or vancomycin. Cortical abscesses that occur in the abnormal urinary tract are associated with more typical gram-negative pathogens and should be treated empirically with intravenous third-generation cephalosporins, antipseudomonal penicillins, or aminoglycosides until specific therapy can be instituted.

CT- or ultrasound-guided needle aspiration may be necessary to differentiate an abscess from a hypervascular tumor. Aspirated material can be cultured and appropriate antimicrobial therapy instituted on the basis of the findings. Patients should have serial examinations with ultrasonography or CT until the abscess resolves. A clinical course contrary to this should lead to the suspicion of misdiagnosis or an uncontrolled infection with the development of perinephric abscess or infection with an organism resistant to the antimicrobial agents used in therapy.

Some renal abscesses may be treated successfully by percutaneous drainage (Finn et al, 1982; Fernandez et al, 1985). These preliminary reports are encouraging and support the use of percutaneous drainage of renal abscess in selected patients. Surgical drainage, however, currently remains the procedure of choice for most renal abscesses.

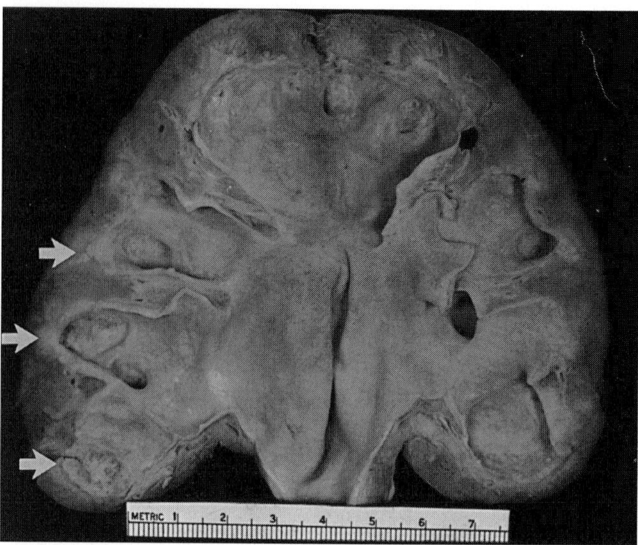

Figure 15–24. Pyonephrosis; gross specimen. The kidney shows marked thinning of renal cortex and medulla, suppurative destruction of the parenchyma *(arrows)*, and distention of the pelvis and calyces. Previous incision released a large quantity of purulent material. The ureter showed obstruction distal to the point of section.

Infected Hydronephrosis and Pyonephrosis

***Infected hydronephrosis* is bacterial infection in a hydronephrotic kidney. The term *pyonephrosis* refers to infected hydronephrosis associated with suppurative destruction of the parenchyma of the kidney, in which there is total or nearly total loss of renal function (Fig. 15–24).** Where infected hydronephrosis ends and pyonephrosis begins is difficult to determine clinically. Rapid diagnosis and treatment of pyonephrosis are essential to avoid permanent loss of renal function and to prevent sepsis.

Clinical Presentation

The patient is usually very ill, with high fever, chills, flank pain, and tenderness. Occasionally, however, a patient may have only an elevated temperature and a complaint of vague gastrointestinal discomfort. A previous history of urinary tract calculi, infection, or surgery is common. Bacteriuria may not be present if the ureter is completely obstructed.

Radiologic Findings

The urographic findings are those of urinary tract obstruction and depend on the degree and duration of obstruction. Excretory urography shows a poorly functioning or nonfunctioning hydronephrotic kidney in 50% of cases (Coleman et al, 1981). **Renal ultrasonography is the most useful procedure to diagnose pyonephrosis. The renal sonogram may show one of four patterns: (1) persistent echoes from the inferior portion of the collecting system, (2) a fluid-debris level with dependent echoes that shift when the patient changes position, (3) strong echoes with acoustic shadowing from air in the collecting system, or (4) weak echoes throughout a dilated collecting system** (Coleman et al, 1981). In contrast, the renal pelvis always shows good ultrasonic transmission in infected hydronephrosis. If ultrasonography is not diagnostic, a retrograde pyelogram should be obtained; it usually shows ureteral obstruction with an irregular filling defect in the renal pelvis caused by purulent sediment.

Management

Once the diagnosis of pyonephrosis is made, the treatment is initiation of appropriate antimicrobial drugs and drainage of the infected pelvis. A ureteral catheter can be passed to drain the kidney, but if the obstruction prevents this, a percutaneous nephrostomy tube should be placed (Camunez et al, 1989). When the patient becomes hemodynamically stable, other procedures are usually needed to identify and treat the source of the obstruction.

Perinephric Abscess

The mortality rate from perinephric abscesses, as high as 56% (Salvatierra et al, 1967), is caused in part by the long delay in making the diagnosis. The diagnosis is difficult to make from a patient's history and physical examination alone because the findings are nonspecific. During the past 20 years, new radiologic techniques and antimicrobial agents have improved the diagnosis and treatment of this condition.

Perinephric abscesses are thought to arise from hematogenous seeding from sites of infection or from renal extension of an ascending urinary tract infection. They are located within Gerota's fascia. When a perinephric infection ruptures through Gerota's fascia into the pararenal space, the abscess becomes paranephric. Paranephric abscesses may also result from infectious disorders of the bowel, pancreas, or pleural cavity. Thorley and associates (1974), in their review of perinephric abscesses, found that the literature about perinephric abscesses had changed since the introduction of antimicrobial agents in the 1940s. They reported that the percentage of cases caused by staphylococci decreased from 45% before 1940 to 6% after 1940, and those cases attributable to *E. coli* and *Proteus* organisms rose from 8% to 30% and from 4% to 44%, respectively. They thought this change reflected the expeditious use of antimicrobial agents to treat skin and wound infections since the 1940s; the use of antimicrobial therapy decreases the chance of hematogenous seeding from the infection. More recent studies support these observations (Merimsky and Feldman, 1981; Saiki et al, 1982).

Clinical Presentation

As emphasized by Thorley and associates (1974), the classic patient who has a cutaneous infection or urinary tract infection that is followed in 1 to 2 weeks by fever and unilateral flank pain is uncommon. In their group of 52 patients, 58% had symptoms longer than 14 days. The most common complaints were fever, flank or abdominal pain, chills, and dysuria; physical findings showed flank or abdominal tenderness and fever (Thorley et al, 1974; Saiki et al, 1982). However, one third of the patients may be afebrile. In the review by Saiki and associates (1982), a flank mass was present in 47% of the patients. In several series, 36% (Thorley et al, 1974) to 42% (Merimsky and Feldman, 1981) of patients had diabetes, and 19% to 50% had calculi (Thorley et al, 1974; Sheinfeld et al, 1989).

Bacteriology and Laboratory Findings

Edelstein and McCabe (1988) have shown that urine cultures identified the infecting pathogen in only one third of cases; blood culture, particularly with multiple organisms, was more frequently indicative of perinephric abscess but identified the pathogen in less than one half of the cases. Therefore, therapy based on urine and blood cultures may be inadequate. Most patients had a white blood count of $\geq 10^4$ (Thorley et al, 1974; Truesdale et al, 1977; Saiki et al, 1982). Surprisingly, admission urinalyses were normal in 25% of the 52 patients with perinephric abscesses evaluated by Thorley and associates (1974).

Radiologic Findings

Recent radiologic imaging techniques have improved the likelihood of diagnosing a perinephric abscess preoperatively. Renal sonography and CT provide new means of diagnosis and treatment. Although the abdominal plain film has been reported normal in 40% of patients with perinephric abscesses (Thorley et al, 1974), abnormalities that may be seen on the affected side are missing psoas shadows; apparent renal masses; absent renal outlines; calculi; and retroperitoneal gas. These same investigators reported that approximately 20% of their patients had normal intravenous urograms. When abnormalities occurred, they were on the side of the abscess and showed a kidney with little or no function in 64% of patients, calicectasis or calyceal stretching in 39%, calculi in 14%, and renal displacement in 4%. Others have stated that intravenous urography may show a displaced renal fascia (anteriorly the fascia of Zuckerkandl and posteriorly Gerota's fascia) and renal arteriography may show displacement of the renal capsular artery away from the kidney (Meyers et al, 1974) (Fig. 15–25).

Although abdominal plain films or intravenous urograms may show abnormalities associated with perinephric abscess, none of these abnormalities are pathognomonic. One radiologic examination that is more specific for a perinephric abscess is assessment of renal mobility by fluoroscopy or inspiration-expiration films. Normal kidneys that have not been operated on should move 2 to 6 cm with respiration, but a kidney with a perinephric abscess is fixed to surrounding tissues and does not move with respiration. In a series of 71 patients with perinephric abscesses, Salvatierra and associates (1967) reported that only 12 patients were assessed for renal mobility and that in 10 of the 12 it was absent.

Currently, renal sonography and CT are the most specific means of evaluating and localizing perinephric abscesses. Ultrasonography can demonstrate a diverse sonographic appearance ranging from a nearly anechoic mass displacing the kidney to an echogenic collection that tends to blend with normally echogenic fat within Gerota's fascia (Corriere and Sandler, 1982). Diagnostic aspiration under ultrasound guidance carries minimal morbidity (Conrad et al, 1977). **CT defines renal distortion and perirenal fluid or gas associated with perinephric abscesses in excellent anatomic detail** (Mendez et al, 1979; Wolverson et al, 1979; Haaga and Weinstein, 1980; Hoddick et al, 1983) (Fig. 15–26). Hoddick and associates (1983), in a series of mixed renal and perirenal abscesses, concluded that CT is more sensitive than sonography for evaluation of severe renal and perirenal infections.

Management

Although antimicrobial agents are useful to control sepsis and to prevent spread of infection, the primary treatment for perinephric abscess is drainage; reports of successful treatment by antimicrobial agents alone are unusual (Herlitz et al, 1981). A detailed analysis of 52 perinephric abscess patients by Thorley and associates (1974) supports this tenet. In this study half the patients were admitted to medical services and the other half to surgical services; 65% of those admitted to medical services died, whereas 23% of those admitted to surgical services died. These mortality rates reflect differences in the population of patients. Those admitted to the medical services were usually sicker and had higher temperatures, more underlying diseases, and vaguer symptoms. More importantly, none of those admitted to medical wards had an admission diagnosis of perinephric abscess, whereas 73% of those admitted to surgical wards did. Although 71% of all the patients had eventual surgical treatment of their perinephric abscesses, the diagnostic delay of those patients admitted to medical services delayed definitive treatment and consequently caused higher mortality.

Although surgical drainage, or nephrectomy if the kid-

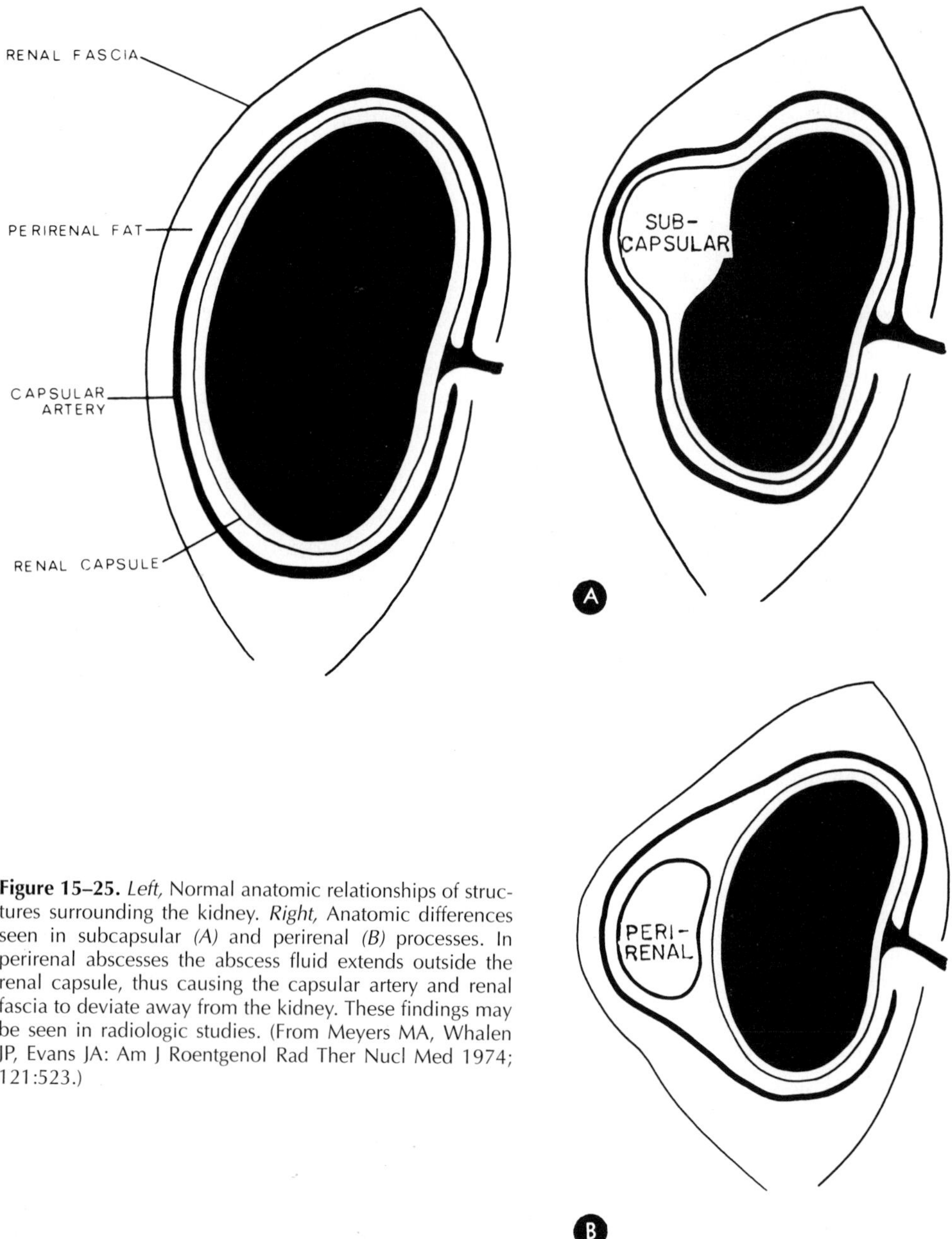

Figure 15–25. *Left,* Normal anatomic relationships of structures surrounding the kidney. *Right,* Anatomic differences seen in subcapsular *(A)* and perirenal *(B)* processes. In perirenal abscesses the abscess fluid extends outside the renal capsule, thus causing the capsular artery and renal fascia to deviate away from the kidney. These findings may be seen in radiologic studies. (From Meyers MA, Whalen JP, Evans JA: Am J Roentgenol Rad Ther Nucl Med 1974; 121:523.)

ney is nonfunctioning or severely infected, is the classic treatment for perinephric abscesses, renal sonography and CT make percutaneous aspiration and drainage of perirenal collections possible (Haaga and Weinstein, 1980; Elyaderani et al, 1981; Edelstein and McCabe, 1988). Haaga and Weinstein (1980), however, consider percutaneous drainage to be contraindicated in large abscess cavities filled with thick purulent fluid.

Once the perinephric abscess has been incised and drained through a retroperitoneal incision, the underlying problem must be dealt with. Some conditions such as renal cortical abscess or enteric communication require prompt attention. Nephrectomy for pyonephrosis may be performed concurrent with drainage of the perinephric abscess if the patient's condition is good. In other instances it is best to drain the perinephric abscess first and correct the underlying problem or perform a nephrectomy when the patient's condition has improved.

Perinephric Abscess Versus Acute Pyelonephritis

It has already been emphasized that the greatest obstacle to the treatment of perinephric abscess is the delay in diagnosis. **In the series of Thorley and associates (1974), a common misdiagnosis was acute pyelonephritis. In their review, they found that two factors differentiated perinephric abscess and acute pyelonephritis: (1) Most patients with uncomplicated pyelonephritis were symptomatic for less than 5 days before hospitalization, whereas**

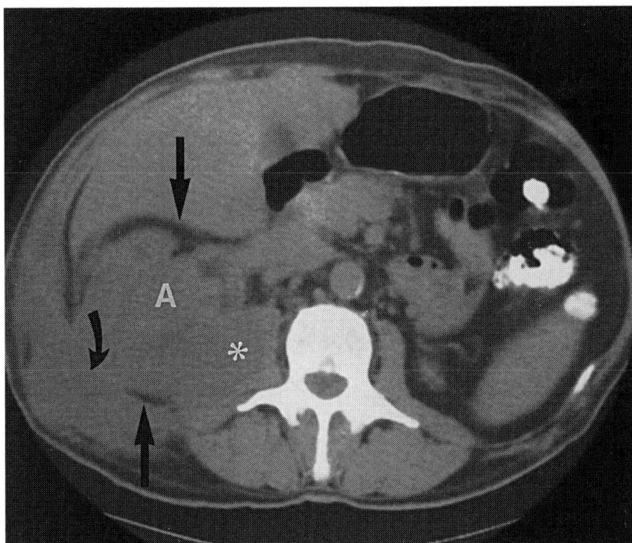

Figure 15–26. Nonenhanced CT scan through the lower pole of the right kidney (previous left nephrectomy), showing extensive perinephric abscess. Extensive abscess (A) distorts and enlarges the renal contour, infiltrates perinephric fat *(arrows),* and also extends into the psoas muscle *(asterisk)* and the soft tissues of the flank *(curved arrow).* Also note that normal renal collecting system fat has been obliterated by the process.

most with perinephric abscesses were symptomatic for longer than 5 days; and (2) no patient with an acute pyelonephritis remained febrile for longer than 4 days once appropriate antimicrobial agents were started. All patients with perinephric abscesses had a fever for at least 5 days, with a median of 7 days.

Patients with polycystic renal disease who undergo hemodialysis may be particularly susceptible to the progression from acute urinary tract infections to perinephric abscess. Of 445 patients undergoing chronic hemodialysis at the Regional Kidney Disease Program in Minneapolis, Minnesota, 5.4% had polycystic kidney disease and 33.3% of these patients developed symptomatic urinary tract infections (Sweet and Keane, 1979). Eight (62.5%) developed perinephric abscesses, and three of these patients died. According to the investigators, all urinary tract infections, even those that progressed to perinephric abscesses, were promptly treated with appropriate antimicrobial agents, and all patients in this group became afebrile and asymptomatic when antibiotics were stopped; yet later, after various times, symptoms attributable to perinephric abscess developed in eight of the patients.

Xanthogranulomatous Pyelonephritis

Xanthogranulomatous pyelonephritis is a rare, severe, chronic renal infection typically resulting in diffuse renal destruction. Most cases are unilateral and result in a nonfunctioning, enlarged kidney associated with obstructive uropathy secondary to nephrolithiasis. In this condition, gross renal examination reveals yellow nodules and pericalyceal granulation. The entity is uncommon and is found in only about 0.6% (Malek et al, 1972) to 1.4% (Ghosh, 1955) of patients with renal inflammation who are evaluated pathologically; it is important, however, because it is "a great imitator" (Malek and Elder, 1978; Tolia et al, 1980). It is often misdiagnosed as a renal tumor (Anhalt et al, 1971; Malek and Elder, 1978; Flynn et al, 1979; Lorentzen and Overgaard, 1980; Tolia et al, 1980).

Although the disease can affect any age group, the peak incidence is in the fifth to seventh decades. Women are affected nearly 3:1 compared with men. Approximately 15% of patients are diabetic.

Pathogenesis

The primary factors necessary for the development of xanthogranulomatous pyelonephritis are obstruction and urinary tract infection. Although the pathogenesis is unknown, it has been proposed that the obstruction is primary and followed by infection with *E. coli*, which leads to tissue destruction and collections of lipid material by histocytes. These lipid-laden macrophages (xanthoma cells) are distributed in sheets around parenchymal abscesses and calyces and are intermixed with lymphocytes, giant cells, and plasma cells. A fibrous tissue reaction ensues to form a granulomatous process initially in the renal pelvis and calyces that infiltrates, destroys, and replaces the renal parenchyma.

Pathology

The pathologic process is usually unilateral, although cases of bilateral disease have been reported. Xanthogranulomatous pyelonephritis may be divided into three extents of retroperitoneal involvement: (1) kidney alone, (2) kidney and perinephric fat, and (3) kidney, perinephric fat, and extensive retroperitoneum (Malek and Elder, 1978). In addition, the disease may involve the kidney diffusely or the pericalyceal tissue alone (Moller and Kristensen, 1980; Tolia et al, 1980).

Grossly, the involved kidney usually shows yellow-white nodules, pyonephrosis, and hemorrhage (Moller and Kristensen, 1980). In addition to xanthoma cells, necrosis and inflammation are often associated, and hemosiderin is commonly in the histiocytes (Moller and Kristensen, 1980). As emphasized by Moller and Kristensen (1980), the xanthoma cells are not specific to xanthogranulomatous pyelonephritis but also appear in other conditions, such as obstructive pneumonia, in which inflammation and obstruction are associated. Transitional cell carcinoma of the renal pelvis has been reported with this disease (McDonald, 1981; Tolia et al, 1981).

In the majority of cases, the diagnosis is made postoperatively by the pathologist. For this reason, a test that offered the promise of preoperative diagnosis would be valuable. In a preliminary report, some investigators have shown that preoperative cytologic studies of the urinary sediment in four of five patients with pathologically proven xanthogranulomatous pyelonephritis showed renal xanthoma cells (Ballesteros et al, 1980). Four other kidneys that had hydronephrosis or chronic inflammation alone had cytologic findings negative for xanthoma cells.

Clinical Presentation

Most patients present with flank pain (69%), fever and chills (69%), and persistent bacteriuria (46%) (Malek

and Elder, 1978). Additional vague symptoms, such as malaise, may be present. On physical examination, 62% of the patients had a flank mass, and 35% had previous calculi (Malek and Elder, 1978).

Bacteriology and Laboratory Findings

Although review of the literature shows *Proteus* to be the most common organism involved with xanthogranulomatous pyelonephritis (Anhalt et al, 1971; Tolia et al, 1981), ***E. coli* is also common.** The prevalence of *Proteus* organisms may reflect their association with stone formation and subsequent chronic obstruction and irritation. Malek and Elder (1978), in their analysis of 26 cases, found that renal tissue cultures grew bacteria in 22 of 23 cases. Anaerobes also have been cultured (Malek and Elder, 1978).

Approximately 10% of patients have mixed cultures. About one third of patients have no growth in their urine, probably because many patients have recently taken or are taking antimicrobial agents when cultures are obtained. The infecting organism may be revealed only by tissue cultures obtained during surgery. Urinalysis usually shows pus and protein. In addition, blood tests often reveal anemia and may show hepatic dysfunction in up to 50% of the patients (Malek and Elder, 1978).

Xanthogranulomatous pyelonephritis is almost always unilateral; therefore, azotemia or frank renal failure is uncommon (Goodman et al, 1979). Recently, Ballesteros and associates (1980) reported accurate preoperative diagnosis of xanthogranulomatous pyelonephritis by serial urine cytologic examination in 80% of their patients.

Radiologic Findings

The intravenous urogram shows renal calculi in 38% (Malek, 1978) **to 70%** (Anhalt et al, 1971) **of patients, lack of excretion in 27%** (Malek and Elder, 1978) **to 80%** (Anhalt et al, 1971), **a renal mass in 62%** (Malek and Elder, 1978), **and calyceal deformity in 46%** (Malek and Elder, 1978) (Fig. 15–27). Renal ultrasonography usually reveals an enlarged kidney with a large central echogenic area and increased parenchymal anechoic pattern (VanKirk et al, 1980).

CT is probably the most useful radiologic technique in evaluating patients with xanthogranulomatous pyelonephritis. **CT usually demonstrates a large, reniform mass with the renal pelvis tightly surrounding a central calcification but without pelvic dilation** (Solomon et al, 1983; Goldman et al, 1984; Hartman, 1985b). Renal parenchyma is replaced by multiple water-density masses representing dilated calyces and abscess cavities filled with varied amounts of pus and debris. On enhanced scans, the walls of these cavities demonstrate a prominent blush owing to the abundant vascularity within the granulation tissue. The cavities themselves, however, fail to enhance, whereas tumors and other inflammatory lesions usually do. The CT scan is particularly helpful in demonstrating the extent of renal involvement and may indicate whether adjacent organs or the abdominal wall are involved by xanthogranulomatous pyelonephritis.

Arteriography shows hypervascular areas, but there may be some hypovascular areas (Malek and Elder, 1978; VanKirk et al, 1980; Tolia et al, 1981). Therefore, radiologic studies, although distinctive, often cannot differentiate between xanthogranulomatous pyelonephritis and renal cell carcinoma.

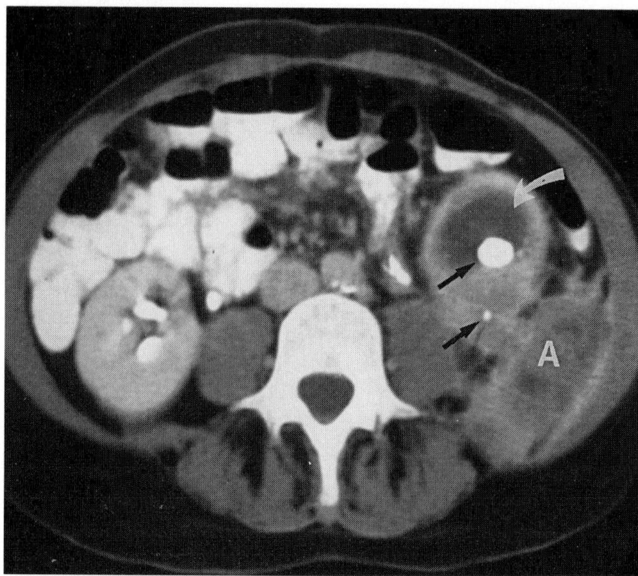

Figure 15–27. Excretory urogram, showing xanthogranulomatous pyelonephritis. Enhanced CT scan shows collecting system and parenchymal calculi *(arrows)* with lower pole pyonephrosis *(curved arrow)* and an irregular, predominantly low-density perinephric abscess (A) extending into the soft tissues of the flank.

Management

The primary obstacle to the correct treatment of xanthogranulomatous pyelonephritis is incorrect diagnosis. In most patients, the diagnosis is made postoperatively. In fact, in Malek's series of 26 patients (Malek, 1978), only 1 of 26 patients was correctly diagnosed preoperatively. Furthermore, because the renal abnormality is often diagnosed preoperatively as a renal tumor, nephrectomy is usually performed. If localized xanthogranulomatous pyelonephritis is diagnosed preoperatively or at exploration, it is amenable to partial nephrectomy (Malek and Elder, 1978; Tolia et al, 1980).

The lipid-laden macrophages associated with xanthogranulomatous pyelonephritis, however, closely resemble clear cell adenocarcinoma and may be difficult to distinguish solely on the basis of frozen section. Further, xanthogranulomatous pyelonephritis has been associated with renal cell carcinoma, papillary transitional cell carcinoma of the pelvis or bladder, and infiltrating squamous cell carcinoma of the pelvis (Schoborg et al, 1980; Pitts et al, 1981; Tolia et al, 1981). Therefore, **if malignant renal tumor cannot be excluded, nephrectomy should be performed.** When diffuse and extensive disease into the retroperitoneum exists, removal of the kidney and perinephric fat may be needed. Under these circumstances, the surgery may be difficult and may involve dissection of granulomatous tissue from the diaphragm, great vessels, and bowel (Malek and Elder, 1978; Flynn et al, 1979). It is important to remove the entire inflammatory mass because in nearly three fourths of patients, xanthogranulomatous tissue is infected. **If incision and drainage alone are per-**

formed rather than nephrectomy, the patient may continue to suffer from protracted debilitating illness and may develop a renal cutaneous fistula; an even more difficult nephrectomy then will be necessary.

Malacoplakia

Malacoplakia, from the Greek word meaning "soft plaque," is an unusual inflammatory disease that was originally described to affect the bladder but has been found to affect the genitourinary and gastrointestinal tracts, skin, lungs, bones, and mesenteric lymph nodes. In a review of 153 cases, the urinary tract was involved in 58% (bladder, 40%; ureter, 11%; renal parenchyma, 16%) and the retroperitoneum was involved in 16% (Stanton and Maxted, 1981). Patients with genitourinary malacoplakia have chronic coliform bacteriuria.

Pathogenesis

The pathogenesis is unknown, but several theories are popular. In 93 patients who had cultures of urine, diseased tissue, or blood, 89.4% had coliform infections (Stanton and Maxted, 1981). Moreover, 40% of the patients in this review had an immune deficiency syndrome, autoimmune disease, carcinoma, or another systemic disorder. This association of coliform infections and compromised health status in patients with malacoplakia is well recognized.

It is hypothesized that bacteria or bacterial fragments form the nidus for the calcium phosphate crystals that laminate the Michaelis-Gutmann bodies. Most investigations into the pathogenesis of this disease support theories that a defect in intraphagosomal bacterial digestion accounts for the unusual immunologic response that causes malacoplakia.

Pathology

The diagnosis is made by biopsy. The lesion is characterized by large histiocytes, known as von Hansemann cells, and small basophilic, extracytoplasmic, or intracytoplasmic calculospherules called Michaelis-Gutmann bodies, which are pathognomonic. Electron microscopy has revealed intact coliform bacteria and bacterial fragments within phagolysosomes of the foamy-appearing malacoplakic histiocytes (Lewin et al, 1976; Stanton and Maxted, 1981). In their review of the subject, Stanton and Maxted (1981) and Esparza and associates (1989) emphasized that although pathognomonic for the disease, Michaelis-Gutmann bodies may be absent in early malacoplakia and are not necessary for the diagnosis.

It has been shown that macrophages in malacoplakia involving the kidney and bladder contain large amounts of immunoreactive alpha$_1$-antitrypsin (Callea et al, 1982). The amount of alpha$_1$-antitrypsin remains unchanged during the morphogenetic stages of the pathologic process. Macrophages from other pathologic processes, closely resembling malacoplakia but without Michaelis-Gutmann bodies, do not contain alpha$_1$-antitrypsin except for a few macrophages in tuberculosis and xanthogranulomatous pyelonephritis. Therefore, immunohistochemical staining for alpha$_1$-antitrypsin may be a useful test for an early and accurate differential diagnosis of malacoplakia.

Clinical Presentation

Most patients are older than 50 years of age. The ratio of females to males with malacoplakia within the urinary tract is 4:1, but this disparity does not occur in other body tissues (Stanton and Maxted, 1981). The patients often are debilitated, are immunosuppressed, and have other chronic diseases. **The symptoms of bladder malacoplakia are bladder irritability and hematuria. Cystoscopy reveals mucosal plaques or nodules.** As these lesions progress they may become fungating, firm, sessile masses that cause filling defects of the bladder, ureter, or pelvis on intravenous urograms. The distal ureter may become strictured or stenotic and cause subsequent renal obstruction or nonfunction (Sexton et al, 1982). A typical patient with renal parenchymal disease may have one or more radiographic masses and chronic *E. coli* infections. Extension of renal parenchymal malacoplakia into the perirenal space is uncommon. Renal parenchymal malacoplakia may be complicated by renal vein thrombosis and inferior vena cava thrombosis (McClure, 1983). When malacoplakia involves the testis, epididymo-orchitis is present. Malacoplakia of the prostate is rare, but when it occurs it may be confused with carcinoma clinically (Shimizu et al, 1981). **Mortality can exceed 50%, and the morbidity can be substantial** (Stanton and Maxted, 1981).

Radiologic Findings

Multifocal malacoplakia on excretory urography typically presents as enlarged kidneys with multiple filling defects (Fig. 15–28*A*). Renal calcification, lithiasis, and hydronephrosis are absent. The multifocal nature is best appreciated by using ultrasonography, CT, or arteriography. Sonographic examination may demonstrate renal enlargement and distortion of the central echo complex. The masses are often confluent, resulting in an overall increase in the echogenicity of the renal parenchyma (Hartman et al, 1980). On CT, the foci of malacoplakia are less dense than the surrounding enhanced parenchyma (Hartman, 1985a). Arteriography typically reveals a hypovascular mass without peripheral neovascularity (Fig. 15–28*B* and *C*) (Cavins and Goldstein, 1977; Trillo et al, 1977).

Unifocal malacoplakia on excretory urography appears as a noncalcified mass that is indistinguishable from other inflammatory or neoplastic lesions. Ultrasonography and CT may demonstrate a solid or cystic structure, depending on the degree of internal necrosis. Angiography may demonstrate neovascularity (Trillo et al, 1977). Extension beyond the kidney, which can occur with either multifocal or uniform malacoplakia, is best demonstrated by CT.

Management

Management of malacoplakia should be directed at control of the urinary tract infections, which should stabilize the disease process. This subject is well reviewed by Stanton and Maxted (1981). Although multiple long-term antimicrobial agents, including many antituberculosis agents, have been used, the sulfonamides, rifampin, doxycycline,

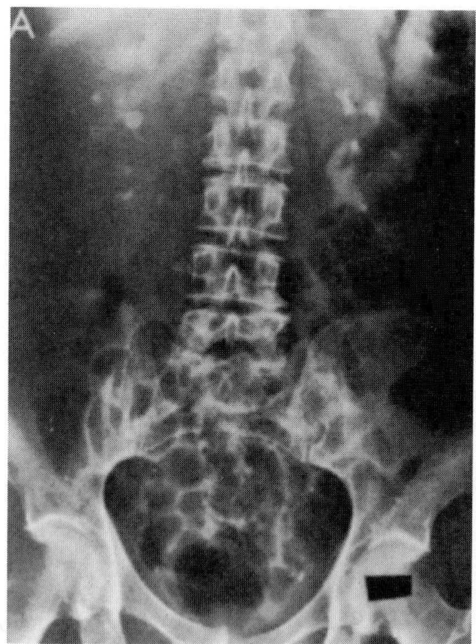

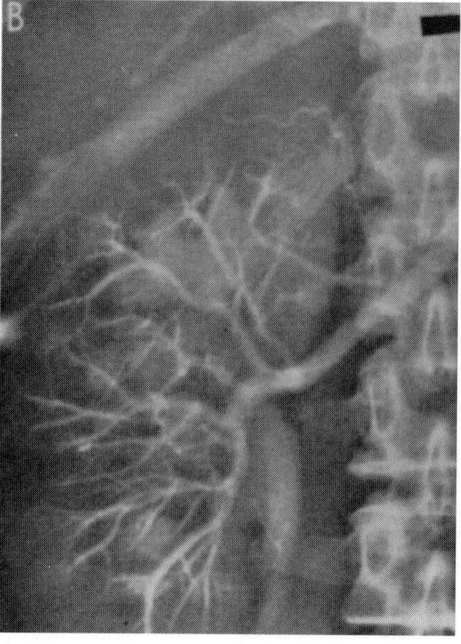

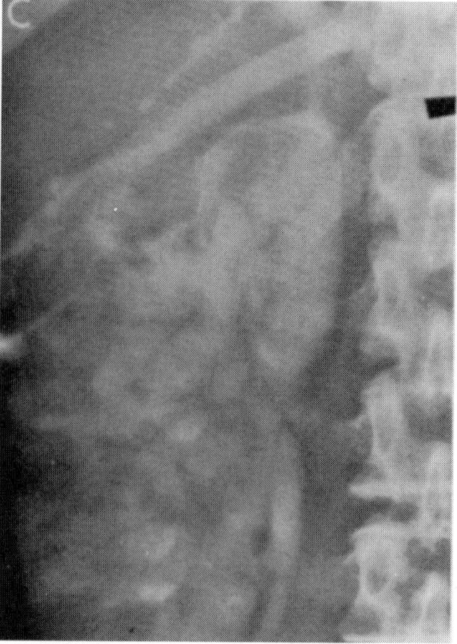

Figure 15–28. Multifocal renal parenchymal malakoplakia. *A,* Excretory urogram, showing that the right kidney is enlarged (16.5 cm) with dilatation of the upper pole calcyes and poor filling of the renal pelvis. *B,* Early angiogram, showing separation of the intrarenal vessels without neovascularity. *C,* angiographic nephrogram, showing multiple irregular filling defects located primarily within the cortex. (Courtesy of Charles E. Bickham Jr, MD, Bethesda, MD. From Hartman DS, Davis CJ, Lichtenstein JE, et al: Radiology 1980; 136:33–42.)

and trimethoprim are thought to be especially useful because of their intracellular bactericidal activity (Maderazo et al, 1979). Other investigators have used ascorbic acid and cholinergic agents, such as bethanechol in conjunction with antimicrobial therapy, and have reported good results. Both agents are thought to increase intracellular cyclic guanine monophosphate levels, which have been postulated as the biologic defect causing macrophage dysfunction. Surgical intervention, however, may be necessary if the disease progresses in spite of antimicrobial treatment. Nephrectomy is usually performed for the treatment of symptomatic unilateral renal lesions.

The long-term prognosis appears to be related to the extent of the disease. When parenchymal renal malacoplakia is bilateral or occurs in the transplanted kidney, death usually occurs within 6 months (Bowers and Cathey, 1971; Deridder et al, 1977). Patients with unilateral disease usually have a long-term survival after nephrectomy.

Renal Echinococcosis

Echinococcosis is a parasitic infection caused by the larval stage of the tapeworm *Echinococcus granulosus.* The disease is prevalent in dogs, sheep, cattle, and humans in South Africa, Australia, New Zealand, Mediterranean countries (especially Greece), and some parts of the Soviet Union. **In the United States the disease is rare, but it is found in immigrants from Eastern Europe or other foreign endemic areas or as an indigenous infection among Native Americans in the Southwest and in Eskimos** (Plorde, 1977).

Pathogenesis and Pathology

Echinococcosis is produced by the larval form of the tapeworm, which in its adult form resides in the intestine of the dog, the definitive host. The adult worm is 3 to 9 mm long. The ova in the feces of the dog contaminate grass and farmlands and are ingested by sheep, pigs, or humans, the intermediate hosts. Larvae hatch, penetrate venules in the wall of the duodenum, and are carried by the blood stream to the liver. Those larvae that escape the liver are next filtered by the lungs. Approximately 3% of the organisms that escape entrapment in the liver and lungs may then enter the systemic circulation and infect the kidneys. The larvae undergo vesiculation, and the resultant hydatid cyst gradually develops at a rate of about 1 cm/year. Thus the cyst may take 5 to 10 years to reach pathologic size.

Echinococosis cysts of the kidney are usually single and located in the cortex (Nabizadeh et al, 1983). The wall of the hydatid cyst has three zones: a peripheral zone of fibroblasts derived from tissues of the host becomes the adventitia and may calcify; an intermediate laminated layer becomes hyalinized; and a single inner layer is composed of nucleated epithelium and is called the germinal layer. The germinal layer gives rise to brood capsules that increase in number, become vacuolated, and remain attached to the germinal membrane by a pedicle. New larvae (scoleces) develop in large numbers from the germinal layer within the brood capsule. The hydatid cyst is also filled with fluid. When brood capsules detach, they enlarge and move freely in the fluid and are then called daughter cysts. Hydatid sand is composed of free larvae and daughter cysts.

Clinical Findings

The symptoms of echinococcosis are those of a slowly growing tumor. Most patients are asymptomatic or have a flank mass, dull pain, or hematuria (Gilsanz et al, 1980; Nabizadeh et al, 1983). Because the cyst is focal, it rarely affects renal function. Rarely the cyst ruptures into the collecting system, and the patient may experience severe colic and passage of debris resembling grape skins in the urine (hydatiduria). **The cyst may also rupture into an adjacent viscus or the peritoneal cavity. The fluid is extremely antigenic** (Hartman, 1985b).

Laboratory Findings

If cyst rupture occurs, the definitive diagnosis can be established by identifying daughter cysts in the urine or by identfying the laminated wall of the cyst (Sparks et al, 1976). Fewer than half of the patients have eosinophilia. **The most reliable diagnostic test uses partially purified hydatid arc 5 antigens in a double-diffusion test** (Coltorti and Varela-Diaz, 1978). Complement fixation, hemagglutination, and the Casoni intradermal skin tests are less reliable but when combined are positive in about 90% of patients (Sparks et al, 1976).

Radiologic Findings

Excretory urography typically shows a thick-walled cystic mass, occasionally calcified (Buckley et al, 1985). If the cyst ruptures into the collecting system, daughter cysts may be outlined in the pelvis as an irregular mass or as multiple solitary lesions (Gilsanz et al, 1980). Occasionally direct filling of the cyst with contrast medium occurs.

Ultrasonography and CT are useful in characterizing the mass. Ultrasonography usually demonstrates a multicystic or multiloculated mass. A sudden change in position may demonstrate bright falling echoes corresponding to hydatid sand, which can be observed during real-time evaluation of hydatid cysts (Saint Martin and Chiesa, 1984).

On CT, several patterns of renal echinococcosis may be recognized. The most specific is a cystic mass with discrete round daughter cysts and a well-defined enhancing membrane (Martorana et al, 1981). The less specific pattern is that of a thick-walled multiloculated cystic mass (Gilsanz et al, 1980). **The presence of daughter cysts within the mother cyst differentiates the lesion from a simple renal cyst and from renal abscesses, infected cysts, and necrotic neoplasm.**

Both CT and ultrasonography are useful in evaluating the liver. Angiography is seldom required. **Diagnostic aspiration should not be performed because of the danger of rupture and spillage of the highly antigenic cyst contents and risk of fatal anaphylaxis** (Roylance et al, 1973).

Management

The prognosis of echinococcosis is good but depends on the site and size of the cysts. Medical treatment with benzimidazole compounds such mebendazole has shown limited success with significant side effects (Nabizadeh et al, 1983).

Surgery remains the mainstay of treatment of renal echinococcosis (Poulios, 1991). **The cyst should be removed without rupture to reduce the chance of seeding and recurrence.** If the cyst wall is calcified, the larvae are probably dead and the risk of seeding is low, although a daughter cyst may be viable. If the cyst ruptures or cannot be removed and marsupialization is required, the contents of the cyst initially should be aspirated and filled with a scolecidal agent such as 30% sodium chloride, 2% formalin, or 1% iodine for approximately 5 minutes to kill the germinal portion (Sparks et al, 1976; Nabizadeh et al, 1983).

Bacteremia, Sepsis, and Septic Shock

Bacteremia and its sequelae (sepsis syndrome and septic shock) are increasingly common and are still potentially lethal diagnoses that have become increasingly important in the last 40 years. Bacteremia is most common among hospitalized patients, particularly those with underlying diseases. The sepsis–septic shock syndromes have recently been defined (Table 15–15).

Recent data from the Centers for Disease Control and Prevention suggest that the incidence of septicemia (which they define as systemic disease associated with the presence and persistence of pathogenic microorganisms or their toxins in the blood) increased 139% between 1970 and 1987 (Hospital Discharge Survey Rates, 1979–1987; Annual Summary of Births, Marriages, Divorces, and Deaths: United States, 1989). Septicemia is now ranked as the 13th leading cause of death in the United States and is estimated to cost $5 to $10 billion per year to treat (Hospital Discharge Survey Rates, 1979–1987; Annual Summary of Births, Marriages, Divorces, and Deaths: United States, 1989). **Septic shock has been traditionally recognized as a consequence of gram-negative bacterial infection, but it may also be caused by gram-positive organisms and fungi and probably by viruses and parasites as well. Although bacteremia can be transient, self-limited, and therefore of little clinical significance (as sometimes occurs with instrumentation of the urinary tract), severe bacteremia constitutes a major emergency.** It calls for an organized diagnostic approach and an aggressive implementation of a therapeutic program directed at eliminating blood stream invasion by the infecting microbe and correction of the pathophysiologic

Table 15–15. DEFINITIONS OF SEPSIS SYNDROME AND SEPTIC SHOCK

Sepsis Syndrome	Septic Shock
Clinical evidence of infection	Sepsis syndrome with hypotension**
Tachypnea*	
Tachycardia†	
Hyperthermia or hypothermia‡	
Evidence of inadequate organ perfusion, including one or more of the following:	
Hypoxemia§	
Elevated plasma lactate concentration‖	
Oliguria¶	

*Respirations > 20/minute; if mechanically ventilated, > 10 L/min.
†Pulse > 90/minute.
‡Core or rectal temperature > 38.3°C or < 35.6°C.
§$PaO_2/FIO_2 \leq 280$ (without other pulmonary or cardiovascular disease as the cause).
‖Exceeding upper limits of normal for the laboratory.
¶Documented urine output < 0.5 ml/kg of body weight for at least 1 hour (in patients with catheters).
**Sustained decrease in systolic blood pressure to <90 mm Hg or drop by >40 mm Hg for at least 1 hour when volume replacement is adequate, the patient is taking no antihypertensive medication, and other causes of shock (such as hypovolemia, myocardial infarction, and pulmonary embolism) are absent.
From Glauser MP, Heumann D, Baumgartner JD, Cohen J: Clin Infect Dis 1994; 18(suppl 2):S205–S216.

sequelae to that event. **Recent studies indicate that the septic syndrome without shock has a mortality of 13%, the sepsis syndrome presenting with shock has a mortality of 28%, and shock developing after the sepsis syndrome has a mortality of 43%** (Bone et al, 1989).

Pathophysiology

Initial studies of pathophysiologic features of septic shock concentrated on the interactions of lipopolysaccharide (LPS) from the gram-negative bacterial cell wall with various humoral pathways. However, attention is now focused on the central role of macrophages, endothelium, and cytokines that are released on stimulation by most, if not all, of the recognized agents of septic shock (Fig. 15–29).

Bacterial Cell-Wall Components in Septic Shock

The exotoxins produced by some bacteria (e.g., exotoxin A produced by *P. aeruginosa*) can initiate septic shock. **However, the bacteria themselves and in particular their cell wall components are primarily responsible for the development of septic shock. These components activate numerous humoral pathways and macrophages and other cells involved in the inflammatory process. The prime initiator of gram-negative bacterial septic shock is endotoxin, an LPS component of the bacterial outer membrane.** Endotoxin circulating in the blood appears to be a predictor of poor outcome in some clinical settings, but the levels of endotoxin required to trigger the cascade of events in septic shock may vary greatly.

As discussed by Glauser and colleagues (1994), the outermost part of the endotoxin molecule consists of a series of structurally and antigenically diverse oligosaccharides that are responsible for the O serotype of gram-negative bacteria. Internal to the O side chains are the core oligosaccharides, which have similar structures in common gram-negative bacteria. **Lipid A, which is bound to the core oligosaccharide, has a highly conserved structure and is responsible for most of the toxicity of endotoxin.** However, some types of natural lipid A and synthetic lipid A analogues that have different sugars and acyl residues are less or not at all toxic. This observation has lead to the development of lipid A analogues that can block the toxic effects of endotoxin or act as endotoxin antagonists (Lynn and Golenbock, 1992; Stutz and Liehl, 1991).

Antibodies to Endotoxin

The O-specific oligosaccharide side chains of endotoxin are highly immunogenic, and antibodies to these side chains inhibit the effects of endotoxin. By virtue of their opsonophagocytic properties, these antibodies can eradicate endotoxin-producing organisms. Because these antibodies are specific, their clinical application is limited. However, an alternative approach has been to develop antibodies to the structurally conserved core glycolipid of endotoxin or to lipid A in the hope that these antibodies will offer cross reactivity or protection against the toxic component of gram-negative bacteria. Recently, clinical trials of two monoclonal antibodies to the core glycolipid of endotoxin have received considerable attention (Greenman et al, 1991; Ziegler et al, 1991). Although the first study showed favorable results, in the second study, treatment did not affect survival among patients with documented gram-negative sepsis. These discrepancies stress the need for extensive characterization of antibodies to core glycolipid before the initiation of further clinical trials.

Cytokine Network

Monocytic cells appear to have a pivotal role in mediation of the biologic effects of LPS (Fig. 15–30). Monocytes can remove and detoxify LPS and be beneficial to the host. However, LPS-stimulated monocytes produce cytokines such as tumor necrosis factor (TNF) and interleukin-1 (IL-1). The intravascular activation of inflammatory systems involved in septic shock is mainly the consequence of an overproduction of these and other cytokines. Several cytokines are produced not only by macrophages, but also by lymphocytes, endothelial cells, and other

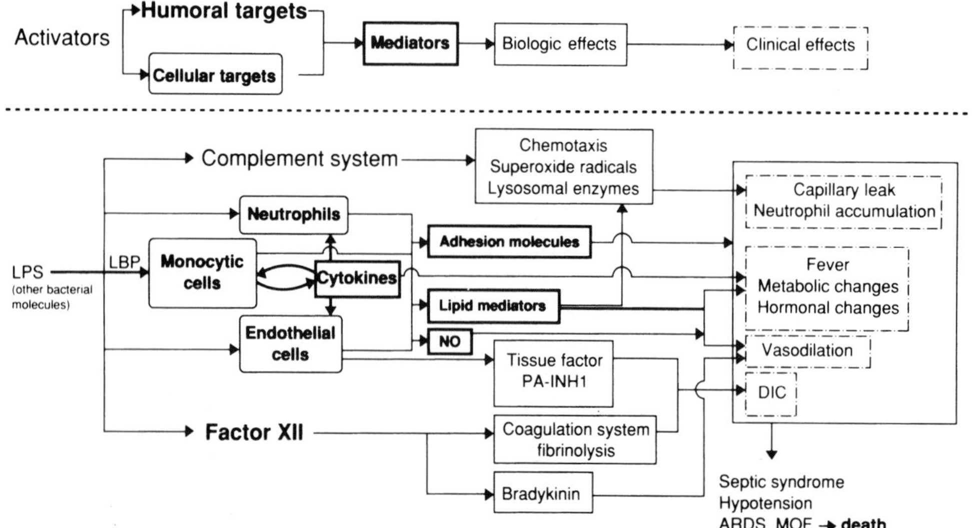

Figure 15–29. Interaction of humoral factors and cytokines in the pathogenesis of septic shock. LPS, lipopolysaccharide; LBP, LPS-binding protein; NO, nitric oxide; PA-INH1, plasmin activator-inhibitor 1; DIC, disseminated intravascular coagulation; ARDS, adult respiratory distress syndrome; MOF, multiple organ failure. (From Glauser MP, Heumann D, Baumgartner JD, Cohen J: Clin Infect Dis 1994; 18[suppl 2]:S205–S216.)

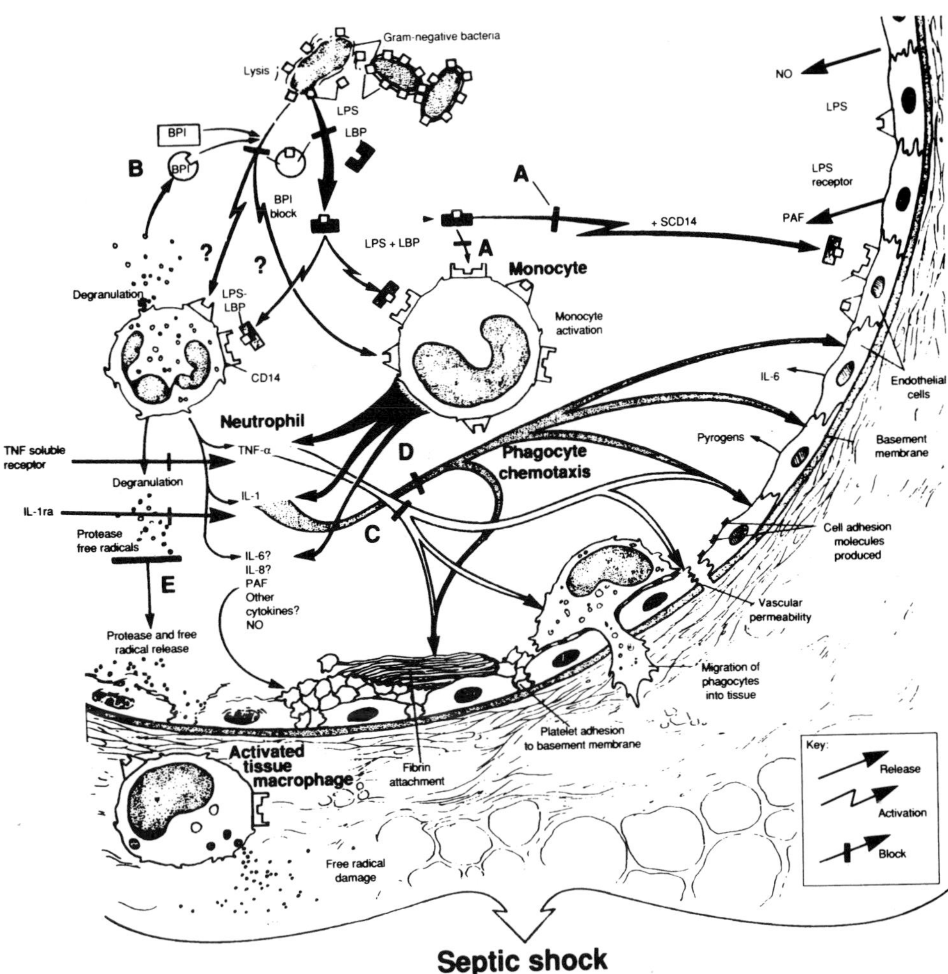

Figure 15–30. Experimental approaches to blocking septic shock. *A,* Monoclonal antibodies to lipopolysaccharide (LPS) prevent LPS from activating inflammatory reactions. *B,* Bactericidal–permeability-increasing protein (BPI), a protein from neutrophil granules, binds LPS. Neither BPI nor antibodies to LPS function when gram-positive organisms invade the blood stream. *C,* Tumor necrosis factor–α receptors. *D,* Interleukin-1 (IL-1) is blocked by soluble IL-1 receptors or IL-1-receptor antagonist (IL-1ra), a naturally occurring human protein. *E,* Tissue damage later in the septic shock cascade is minimized by protease inhibitors and free-radical scavengers or agents blocking other cytokines, including IL-6 and IL-8. LBP, LPS-binding protein; PAF, platelet-activating factor; NO, nitric oxide; SCD14, soluble CD14. (From Glauser MP, Heumann D, Baumgartner JD, Cohen J: Clin Infect Dis 1994; 18[suppl 2]:S205–S216.)

cells stimulated by microbial products. **The systemic release of large amounts of cytokines is associated with death from septic shock in humans** (Waage et al, 1987; Girarin et al, 1988; Calandra et al, 1990).

TNF is regarded as a central mediator of pathophysiologic changes associated with the release of LPS and possibly with septic shock by microorganisms that do not contain LPS. In animal models, antibodies to TNF have effectively increased the rate of survival. Cytokines other than TNF are involved in the induction of a shocklike state. Circulating levels of IL-1 are elevated in shock, and their increased levels correlate with the severity of the disease. Direct proof of the central role of IL-1 in septic shock comes from experiments with animals in which specific blocking of the binding of IL-1 to its cell receptor by IL-1-receptor antagonist (IL-1ra) prevented the detrimental effects of inoculation of LPS or *E. coli* (Alexander et al, 1991; McIntyre et al, 1991; Wakabayashi et al, 1991). Elucidation of these pathophysiologic events has prompted the development of strategies to counteract the production or release of TNF and IL-1 to prevent or treat septic shock. However, TNF, IL-1, and other cytokines are released during the first hour after the injection of LPS or live bacteria. This suggests that the levels of TNF may be elevated before shock develops, and if so, perhaps antibodies to TNF could not be administered soon enough to effectively treat patients with shock. Preliminary trials of studies aimed at inhibiting cytokines are under way and should identify the usefulness of this approach.

Two other cytokines, IL-8 and IL-10, are being evaluated as possible important mediators in shock. IL-8 has been characterized primarily as a polymorphonuclear chemoattractant and a proinflammatory mediator. It has been detected in healthy volunteers after intravenous injection of endotoxin (Martich et al, 1991) and in patients with gram-negative shock (Halstensen et al, 1993). Its precise role in vivo has not been fully elucidated. Recently the anti-inflammatory IL-10 has been suggested as a candidate for treatment of bacterial sepsis.

Clinical Presentation

The classic clinical presentation of fevers and chills followed by hypotension is only manifest in about 30% of patients with gram-negative bacteremia (McCabe and Trendwell, 1983). **Even before temperature elevation and the onset of chills, bacteremic patients often begin to hyperventilate. Thus the earliest metabolic change in septicemia is a resultant respiratory alkalosis.** In critically ill patients the sudden onset of hyperventilation should lead to blood drawing for culture and careful evaluation of the patient. Changes in mental status can also be important clinical clues. Although the most common pattern is lethargy or obtundation, an occasional patient may become excited, agitated, or combative. Cutaneous manifestations such as the bull's eye lesion associated with *P. aeruginosa* may be identified.

Metastatic infections secondary to genitourinary tract bacteremia have been described (Siroky et al, 1976). In this review of 137 patients who developed metastatic infections from bacteremia with a genitourinary source, 79% had undergone prior urologic instrumentation, 59% developed skeletal infections, mainly of the spine; and 29% developed endocarditis, most commonly caused by *E. faecalis.*

Bacteriology

In three recent studies of sepsis syndrome and septic shock, gram-negative bacteria were isolated in 30% to 80% of cases and gram-positive bacteria in 5% to 24% (Ispahani et al, 1987; Calandra et al, 1988; Bone et al, 1992). In one prospective study of sepsis syndrome (Bone et al, 1992), no etiologic agent was identified in more than half of all cases. The severity of septic shock, as reflected by mortality, did not depend on the type of organism responsible.

Although *E. coli* is the most common organism causing gram-negative bacteremia, many nosocomial catheter-associated infections are caused by highly resistant gram-negative organisms—*P. aeruginosa, Proteus, Providencia,* and *Serratia* (Table 15–16). In a large series, *E. coli* caused about one third of the cases; the *Klebsiella-Enterobacter-Serratia* family, approximately 20%; and *Pseudomonas, Proteus-Providencia,* and anaerobic species, approximately 10% each (Kreger et al, 1980). Anaerobic organisms may cause bacteremia when the source is a postsurgical intra-abdominal abscess or transrectal prostatic biopsy.

Diagnosis and Management

The overall mortality associated with septic shock ranges from 10% (Cunnion and Parrillo, 1989) **to 90%** (Bone 1991b). In the evaluation of 612 patients with gram-negative bacteremia, Kreger and associates (1980) reported that approximately 40% of deaths occurred **within 24 hours** and 60% within 48 hours of onset. **Appropriate initial antimicrobial treatment decreases the frequency of shock and improves survival rates.** The use of inappropriate antimicrobial agents to which the organisms were resistant did not improve patients' morbidity or mortality. Therefore early diagnosis and treatment with an agent to which the organism is sensitive is critical (see Table 15–16). **Five factors have been associated with a high probability of bacteremia: (1) temperature, (2) leukocyte count, (3) creatinine level, (4) diabetes mellitus, and (5) low serum albumin level. Septicemia and death were more prevalent in these populations compared with those without these factors** (Leibovico et al, 1992).

Once a presumptive diagnosis of bacteremia is made, multiple blood cultures for aerobic and anaerobic organisms should be obtained (Table 15–17). In addition, all potential sources of bacteremia must be cultured (i.e., urine, sputum, and wounds). **Careful attempts to identify the source of infection should be made, because the**

Table 15–16. FACTORS INFLUENCING ETIOLOGIC AGENTS IN BACTEREMIA

Site of Origin	Precipitating Events	Most Frequent Etiologic Agent	Antibiotic(s) of Choice	Alternative
Genitourinary tract	Indwelling catheters, instrumentation	*Escherichia coli, Klebsiella-Enterobacter-Serratia, Proteus* sp., *Pseudomonas aeruginosa*	Aminoglycoside Amikacin (15 mg/kg/day) Tobramycin (5 mg/kg/day) Gentamicin (5 mg/kg/day)	Cephalosporin
Gastrointestinal tract Bowel	Obstruction, perforation, abscesses, neoplasia, diverticuli	*Bacteroides* sp., *E. coli, Klebsiella-Enterobacter-Serratia, Salmonella*	Aminoglycoside plus clindamycin (600–900 mg every 8 h)	Cefoxitin (2.0 g every 4–6 h) Third-generation cephalosporin
Biliary tract	Cholangitis, obstruction (stones), surgical procedures	*E. coli, Klebsiella-Enterobacter-Serratia*	Aminoglycoside	Cephalosporin
Reproductive system	Abortion, instrumentation, postpartum	*Bacteroides* sp., *E. coli*	Aminoglycoside plus clindamycin	Cefoxitin, third-generation cephalosporin, or chloramphenicol (50 mg/kg/day)
Vascular system	Venous cutdowns, intravenous catheters, intracardiac pacemakers, surgical procedures	*P. aeruginosa, Acinetobacter, Serratia, Enterobacter* sp.	Aminoglycoside plus ticarcillin (200–300 mg/kg/day) or piperacillin (3 g every 4 h)	Third-generation cephalosporin
Decubiti		*E. coli, Bacteroides* sp., *Klebsiella pneumoniae, Proteus* sp.	Aminoglycoside and clindamycin	Second- or third-generation cephalosporin
Respiratory tract	Tracheostomy, mechanical ventilatory assistance	*P. aeruginosa, Klebsiella-Enterobacter-Serratia, Acinetobacter, E. coli*	Aminoglycoside and piperacillin (3 g every 4 h)	Third-generation cephalosporin
	Aspiration	*E. coli, Bacteroides* sp., *Klebsiella-Enterobacter-Serratia*	Aminoglycoside and piperacillin/tozobactam (3.375 g every 4 h) or ticarcillin/clavulanate (3.1 g every 4 h)	Second- or third-generation cephalosporin

From McCabe WR, Treadwell TL: Monogr Urol 1983; 4:November/December.

Table 15–17. MANAGEMENT OF SEPTIC SHOCK

1. Establishment of diagnosis
   a. Diagnosis of bacteremia
      (1) Epidemiologic, clinical, and physical findings
      (2) Collection of blood, urine, and other appropriate specimens for Gram's stain or culture
   b. Diagnosis of cause of shock when preceding bacteremia not recognized
      (1) Hypovolemia
      (2) Hemorrhage
      (3) Cardiac cause
      (4) Hypersensitivity, anaphylaxis
      (5) Endocrine cause (adrenal insufficiency)
      (6) Other cause (pulmonary emobolism)
      (7) Bacteremia
2. Appropriate antibiotic therapy
   a. Check available culture and sensitivity data
   b. Consider diagnosis, possible site of origin, nosocomiality, and possibility of anaerobes
   c. Ensure collection of appropriate cultures before administration of antibiotics
3. Volume expansion: 1000 ml of crystalloid solution over 15–20 min if congestive failure absent
4. Monitoring of volume expansion: insertion of Swan-Ganz or central venous pressure (CVP) catheter
   a. Increase in wedged pulmonary artery pressure of >8 mm Hg or to levels ≥18 mm Hg suggests possible cardiac decompensation
   b. Increase in CVP of >50 mm H_2O or to level >120–140 mm H_2O with volume expansion suggests potential hazard of fluid overload
5. Continuation of volume expansion (15–20 ml/min) until recovery or wedged pulmonary artery pressure ≥ 18 mm Hg or CVP ≥ 120 mm H_2O
6. Vasoactive agents
7. Continued evaluation of mental status and urinary output (indwelling urethral catheter, "closed" sterile drainage system essential)
8. Ventilation: supplemental O_2 with or without intubation and assisted ventilation
9. Digitalis if congestive heart failure develops
10. Drainage of purulent accumulations; removal of foreign bodies
11. Modification of antibiotics as indicated by cultures, susceptibility tests, and renal function

From McCabe WR, Treadwell TL: Monogr Urol 1983; 4:November/December.

choice of appropriate antimicrobial coverage depends on the organisms that are thought most likely to cause the infection. The severity of the underlying disease and the possibility of synergistic interactions are also important considerations. If the urinary tract is the most likely portal of entry, an aminoglycoside (gentamicin, tobramycin, or amikacin) is usually the drug of choice, unless *E. faecalis* is suspected. **Three clinical factors have been predictive of the subsequent isolation of a resistant pathogen: (1) the use of an antibiotic drug in the last month, (2) advanced age, and (3) male sex** (Leibovico et al, 1992). If the infection is hospital-acquired, or if the patient has had multiple infections or is immunocompromised or severely ill, an aminoglycoside and anti-*Pseudomonas* penicillin (carbenicillin, ticarcillin, or piperacillin) or a third-generation cephalosporin should be used. When identification and drug sensitivities of the offending organism are known, antimicrobial therapy should be changed to use the cheapest, least toxic antibiotic with the narrowest antimicrobial coverage. **Antimicrobial treatment should be continued until the patient has been afebrile for 3 to 4 days. Local infections that may have provided the focus for the bacteremia should be treated individually as appropriate.**

Complications, such as hypotension and renal failure, should be monitored and managed with supportive measures, as well outlined by McCabe and Olans (1981). Careful volume expansion monitored by central venous pressure or a Swan-Ganz catheter may be given as needed. If hypotension continues, vasoactive agents may be necessary to maintain adequate cardiac perfusion. Dopamine in doses of 2 to 25 μg/kg/min is commonly used. Other useful agents are listed in Table 15–18. It is still unclear whether corticosteroids are useful in the treatment of gram-negative shock (Bone et al, 1987).

Finally, when the patient is stable, the source of bacteremia must be sought and adequately treated. On occasion, **bacteremia continues until the focus of infection is treated; in fact, surgical treatment may be needed even though the patient is hemodynamically unstable.** For instance, if the infection focus is an abscess or pyonephrosis, it must be drained. Infected venous catheters need to be removed and replaced. On many occasions, however, successful treatment of the bacteremia alone also eliminates the original source of infections.

LOWER-TRACT INFECTIONS

Uncomplicated Cystitis

Uncomplicated urinary cystitis occurs in patients without physiologic or anatomic abnormalities of the urinary tract and in the absence of recent urologic surgery or instrumentation. Uncomplicated cystitis occasionally occurs in prepubertal girls, but it increases greatly in incidence in late adolescence and during the second and fourth decades alike. In the United States an estimated 4 to 6 million cases of acute bacterial cystitis involve young women and 25% to 30% of women between the ages of 20 and 40 years old have had urinary tract infections (Kunin, 1987). Although it is much less common, young men may also experience acute cystitis without underlying structural or functional abnormalities of the urinary tract. These infections are often in association with not being circumcised, with sexual activity, or with human immunodeficiency virus (HIV) infection.

A remarkably narrow spectrum of etiologic agents with highly predictable profiles of antimicrobial susceptibility cause infections in young women with acute uncomplicated cystitis: *E. coli* in 80%, and *S. saprophyticus* in 5% to 15% (Jordan et al, 1980; Stamm and Hooton, 1993). Other organisms less commonly involved include *Klebsiella* species, *P. mirabilis*, or enterococci. In men, *E. coli* and other Enterobacteriaceae are the most commonly identified organisms.

Clinical Presentation

Acute uncomplicated cystitis produces inflammation in the bladder and urethra. **Clinical symptoms include dysuria, frequency, urgency, voiding of small urine volumes, and suprapubic or lower abdominal pain (Fig. 15–31).** Hematuria or foul-smelling urine may develop. Upon examination, suprapubic tenderness may be present. Males with acute

Table 15–18. DRUGS USED IN MANAGEMENT OF SEPTIC SHOCK

Agent	Dose	Effects	Response
Dopamine	2–25 μg/kg/min*	Alpha, beta$_1$, and "dopaminergic" effects; positive inotropic > chronotropic effects; renal and splanchnic vasodilation with doses <8 μg/kg/min without increase in blood pressure or heart rate; vasoconstriction, reversal of renal vasodilation and ↑ in blood pressure with doses per minute of ≥10 μg/kg	↑ in blood pressure; ↑ in urine flow; improved sensorium
Isoproterenol	5 μg/ml/min†	Beta$_1$ and beta$_2$, positive inotropic > chronotropic effects; vasodilation, ↑ strength and rate of cardiac contractions with ↑ cardiac output and venous return	↓ central venous pressure, ↑ cardiac output, ↑ urine output, improved sensorium; risk of tachycardia and arrhythmias
Dobutamine	2–25 μg/kg/min‡	Alpha and beta$_1$; positive inotropic effects > chronotropic effects	↑ cardiac output, ↑ urine output, improved sensorium
Norepinephrine	0.05 μg/kg/min§	Alpha and beta$_1$; positive inotropic effects > chronotropic effects	↑ blood pressure, ↑ cardiac output, ↑ coronary perfusion, marked peripheral vasoconstriction
Corticosteroids as single dose:			
Dexamethasone	6 mg/kg/min	?	Value debatable
Methylprednisolone	30 mg/kg/min	?	Value debatable

*Increase the rate of infusion (5% dextrose in water; or saline) every 15–20 min until the systolic blood pressure exceeds 90 mm Hg and the urine output exceeds 30 ml/h

†Observe the effect within 15–25 min and double the rate of infusion if necessary.

‡Titrate as with dopamine.

§Give a test dose of 0.1–0.2 μg/kg and observe the response (usually in minutes). The normal maintenance dose is delivered via a plastic catheter into a large peripheral or central vein.

Modified from McCabe WR, Olans RN: Shock in gram-negative bacteremia predisposing factors, pathophysiology and treatment. *In* Remington JS, Swartz MN (eds): Current Clinical Topics in Infectious Disease. New York, McGraw-Hill Book Company, 1981, pp 121–150.

cystitis may have a syndrome resembling nongonococcal urethritis (urethral discharge and dysuria).

Laboratory Diagnosis

The presumptive laboratory diagnosis of acute cystitis is based on microscopic urinalysis that indicates bacteriuria, pyuria, and hematuria. Indirect dip-stick tests for bacteriuria (nitrite) or pyuria (leukocyte esterase) may also be informative but are less sensitive than microscopic examination of the urine. **Urine culture remains the definitive test, and in symptomatic patients the presence of 10^2 or more cfu/ml of urine usually indicates infection** (Stamm et al, 1982).

Although many investigators recommend that urine culture and antimicrobial susceptibility testing be done in all patients with suspected uncomplicated cystitis, in practice this is often neither done nor necessary. Indeed, with many patients who have symptoms and urinalysis findings characteristic of uncomplicated cystitis, it may be more cost-effective to manage them without an initial urine culture because treatment decisions are usually made and therapy is often completed before culture results are known (Komaroff, 1986). This position was supported by a cost-effectiveness study (Carlson and Mulley, 1985) in which it was estimated that routine use of pretherapy urine cultures for lower urinary tract infection increased the cost by 40% but decreased the overall duration of symptoms by only 10%.

Thus in women with symptoms and signs suggesting acute cystitis, and in whom no complicating factors are judged to be present, a urinalysis that is positive for pyuria, hematuria, or bacteriuria or a combination should provide sufficient documentation of urinary tract infections, and a urine culture may be omitted. **A urine culture should be obtained, however, for women in whom symptoms and urine examination findings leave the diagnosis of cystitis in doubt. Pretherapy cultures and susceptibility tests are also essential in the management of women with recent antimicrobial therapy or urinary tract infection symptoms for greater than 7 days, age over 65 years, diabetes, or pregnancy.** In these situations various pathogens may be present and antimicrobial therapy is less predictable and needs to be tailored to the individual organisms (Stamm, 1986). **Pretreatment urine culture is recommended in all men.**

Differential Diagnosis

Cystitis must be differentiated from other inflammatory infectious conditions in which dysuria may be the most prominent symptom including vaginitis, urethral infections caused by sexually transmitted pathogens, and miscellaneous noninflammatory causes of urethral discomfort (Komaroff, 1984). Characteristic features of the history, physical examination, and voided urine or other specimens allow patients with dysuria to be assigned to one of these diagnostic categories. Vaginitis is characterized by irritative voiding associated with vaginal irritation and is subacute in onset. A history of vaginal discharge or odor and multiple or new sexual partners is common. Frequency, urgency, hematuria, and suprapubic pain are not present. Physical examination reveals a vaginal discharge, and examination of vaginal fluid demonstrates inflammatory cells. The differential diagnosis includes herpes simplex virus, gonorrhea, *Chlamydia*, trichomoniasis, yeast, and bacterial vaginosis. Urethritis causes dysuria that is usually subacute in

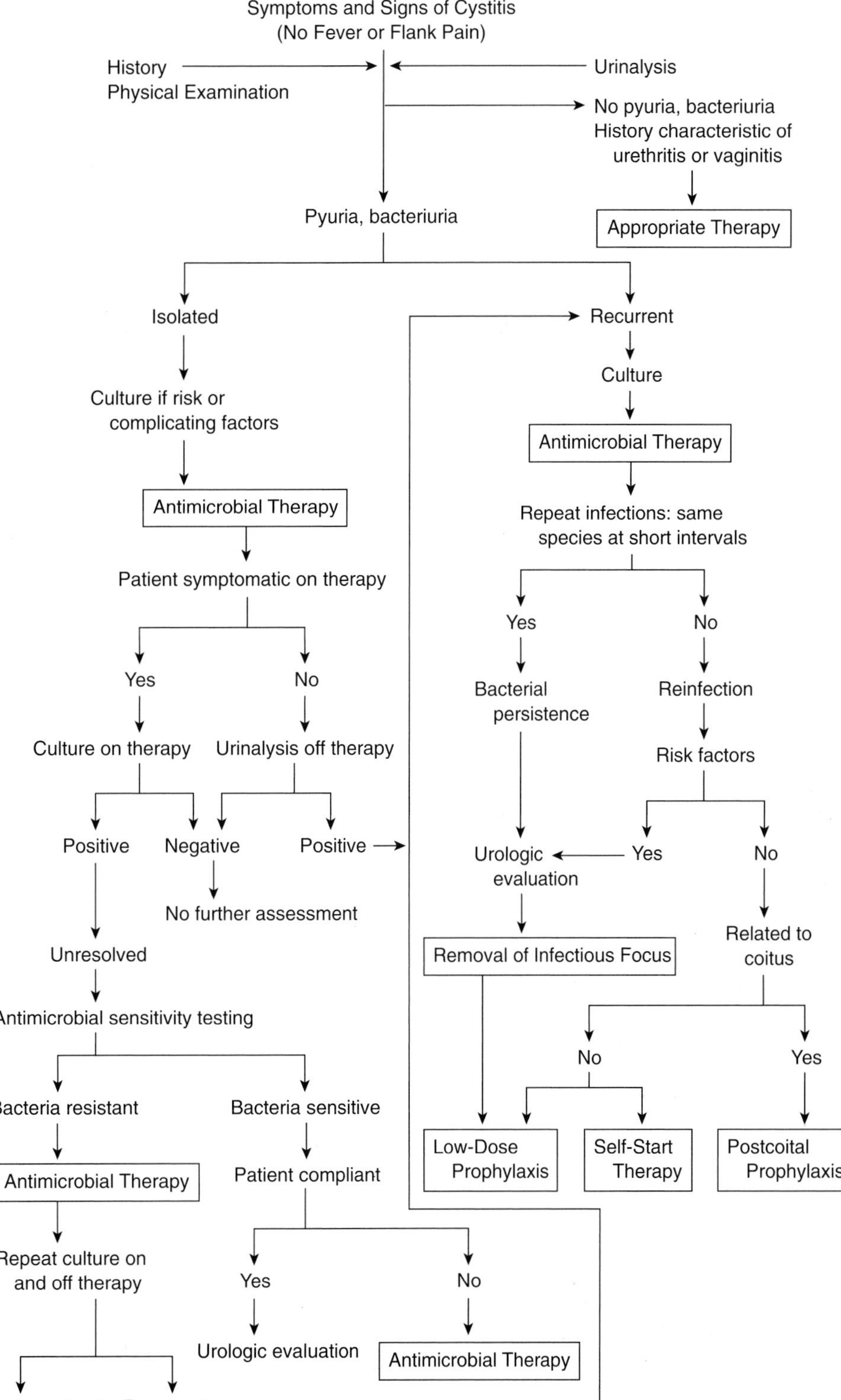

Figure 15–31. Management of acute cystitis.

onset and is associated with a history of discharge and new or multiple sexual partners. Frequency and urgency of urination may be present but is less pronounced than in patients with cystitis, and fever and chills are absent. Urethral discharge with inflammatory cells or initial pyuria in the male are characteristic. The common causes of urethritis include gonorrhea, *Chlamydia* infection, herpes simplex, and trichomoniasis. Appropriate cultures and immunologic tests are indicated. Urethral injury associated with sexual intercourse, chemical irritants, or allergy may also cause dysuria. A history of trauma or exposure to irritants, and a lack of discharge or pyuria is characteristic.

Management

Antimicrobial Selection

Oral antimicrobial agents for the treatment of acute uncomplicated cystitis are listed in Table 15–10. Resistance to TMP and TMP-SMX is 5% to 15%, varies geographically, and appears to be increasing nationwide. TMP, when used alone, is as efficacious as TMP-SMX and is associated with fewer side effects, presumably because of the absence of the sulfa component (Harbord and Gruneberg, 1981).

About one third of bacterial strains causing uncomplicated cystitis in the United States now demonstrate in vitro resistance to amoxicillin and sulfonamides, and 15% to 20% are resistant to nitrofurantoin (Fihn et al, 1988; Inter-Nordic Urinary Tract Infection Study Group, 1988; Johnson and Stamm, 1989; Norrby, 1990; Ronald et al, 1992). The high cost of amoxicillin-balbulanate and the cephalosporins limit their usefulness. These agents, however, are the drugs of choice for treatment of cystitis during pregnancy. The fluoroquinolones offer excellent activity and they are well tolerated. Resistance to the fluoroquinolones remains below 5% in most places (Fihn et al, 1988). Their use for uncomplicated cystitis should be limited to patients with allergy to less costly drugs or with previous exposure to antibiotics causing bacterial resistance.

The effects of an antimicrobial agent on the vaginal flora are also important in achieving eradication of bacteriuria (Fihn et al, 1988). The concentrations of TMP and the fluoroquinolones that have been studied in vaginal secretions are high, eradicating *E. coli,* but minimally altering normal anaerobic and microaerophilic vaginal flora (Hooton, Stamm, 1991). Single-dose regimens using these drugs are less effective than multiple-day regimens in this regard (Fihn et al, 1988), which probably explains why there are more early recurrent infections after single-dose therapy with these drugs. Nitrofurantoin and beta-lactam drugs are generally not effective in eliminating *E. coli* from the vagina.

Duration of Therapy

A number of studies have been conducted in recent years to define the optimal treatment for uncomplicated cystitis in women (Bailey, 1983; Fihn et al, 1988; Inter-Nordic Urinary Tract Infection Study Group, 1988; Johnson, Stamm, 1989; Wolfson, Hooper, 1989; Norrby, 1990; Hooton et al, 1991d; Hooton and Stamm, 1991; Ronald, Nicolle, Harding, 1992). **With most antimicrobial agents, 3-day regimens appear optimal, with efficacy comparable to that of 7-day regimens, but with fewer side effects and lower cost** (Sheen et al, 1984). **Single-dose therapy can be used, but it generally results in lower rates of cure and more frequent recurrences, especially with drugs such as amoxicillin and oral cephalosporins, which are very rapidly excreted and are often ineffective in patients with occult renal infection** (Fihn et al, 1988; Johnson and Stamm, 1989; Norrby, 1990). Even with TMP-SMX and fluoroquinolones, therapy for 3 days or longer has been more effective than single-dose therapy in most trials and in a meta-analysis (Fihn et al, 1988; Johnson and Stamm, 1989; Norrby, 1990; Hooton et al, 1991c).

Considering all the above factors, TMP-SMX and TMP are the optimal choices for empirical 3-day therapy for uncomplicated cystitis in young women. The fluoroquinolones are highly effective and well tolerated in 3-day regimens but are more expensive. In women with uncomplicated cystitis, fluoroquinolones should be used primarily for recurrent infections, treatment failures (unresolved urinary tract infections), infections in patients with allergies to other drugs, and infections caused by strains known to be resistant to other antimicrobials. Additionally, fluoroquinolones should be used where TMP resistance is common among the pathogens causing uncomplicated cystitis. Less satisfactory results have been observed with 3-day courses of amoxicillin, cefadroxil, or nitrofurantoin in the management of acute cystitis (Norrby, 1990; Hooton et al, 1991d) even with susceptible microorganisms, but these regimens may be useful in selected patients or clinical settings. **Young healthy men should be treated with a 7-day regimen of TMP-SMX, TMP, or a fluoroquinolone.** Shorter regimens should be avoided.

No follow-up visit or culture is recommended in young women after therapy unless symptoms persist or recur, in which case a urinalysis and a urine culture should be obtained and the patient treated for 7 days with a fluoroquinolone. A follow-up visit, urinalysis, and urine culture are recommended in older women or those with potential risk factors and in men. Urologic evaluation is unnecessary in women and is usually unnecessary in young men who respond to therapy (Lipsky 1989).

Recurrent Urinary Tract Infections

Recurrent urinary tract infections are most commonly new infections from bacteria outside the urinary tract (reinfection). Recurrent infections due to the re-emergence of bacteria from a site within the urinary tract (bacterial persistence) are uncommon. Reinfections usually occur at differing and sometimes long intervals and frequently are caused by different species. Conversely, bacterial persistence must be due to the same organism, and infections generally occur at close intervals. **The distinction between reinfection and bacterial persistence is important in management because women with reinfection usually do not have an underlying alterable urologic abnormality and usually require long-term medical management.** Reinfections in men are uncommon but may be associated with underlying abnormalities such as urethral stricture. Therefore, at a minimum, endoscopic evaluation is indicated in men. **Conversely, patients with bacterial persistence can usually be cured of recurrent infections by identification and surgical removal or correction of the focus of infection.**

Reinfections

Reinfections in women are associated with increased vaginal mucosal receptivity for uropathogens and ascending colonization from the fecal flora. Reinfections in men may be associated with a urinary tract abnormality. The possibility of a vesicoenteric or vesicovaginal fistula should be considered when there is any history of pneumaturia, fecaluria, diverticulitis, obstipation, previous pelvic surgery, or radiation therapy. Evaluation of the patient with presumed reinfections must be individualized.

Failure to recognize and correct abnormalities that reduce the formation, transmission, and elimination of urine by the urinary tract increases the incidence of reinfections in susceptible patients and reduces the effectiveness of antimicrobial therapy. Abnormalities should be corrected and urinary tract function restored by medical, pharmacologic, or surgical management. **In women diaphragm-spermicide use has been associated with an increased risk of urinary tract infection and vaginal colonization with *E. coli*** (Hooton et al, 1991b). Spermicides containing the active ingredient nonoxynol-9 may provide a selective advantage in colonizing the vagina, perhaps by a reduction in colonization population of vaginal lactobacilli and through enhancement of adherence of *E. coli* to epithelial cells (Hooton et al, 1991a). Thus **spermicidal agents should be discontinued in women with recurrent urinary tract infections, and other forms of contraception should be used.**

Postmenopausal women have frequent reinfections (Hooton et al, 1991d; Raz, Stamm, 1993). These infections are sometimes attributable to residual urine after voiding, which is often associated with bladder or uterine prolapse. In addition the lack of estrogen causes marked changes in the vaginal microflora including a loss of lactobacilli and increased colonization by *E. coli* (Raz and Stamm, 1993). **Estrogen replacement frequently restores the normal vaginal environment, allows recolonization with lactobacilli, and thus eliminates bacterial uropathogenic colonization. A reduced incidence of urinary tract infections has been documented with this approach** (Raz and Stamm, 1993).

In healthy women upper-tract abnormalities associated with reinfections are very rare, and therefore routine excretory urography is not indicated. Excretory urography is useful in patients with risk factors such as a history of unexplained hematuria, obstructive symptoms, neurogenic bladder dysfunction, renal calculi, fistula, analgesic abuse, and/or severe diseases such as diabetes mellitus. Cystoscopy should be performed in men or women who have frequent reinfections and symptoms suggestive of obstruction, bladder dysfunction, and fistula. Dilation of a stenotic urethra to a normal caliber would appear appropriate. There is little evidence, however, that repeated urethral dilation is indicated in the routine management of most women.

Low-Dose Prophylaxis

Prophylactic therapy is given to prevent reinfection. The successful management of virtually all recurrent urinary tract infections is easy if the physician understands the biology of prophylaxis, recognizes the prophylactic effectiveness of the five successful, highly useful antimicrobial agents, and remembers the causes of bacterial persistence in the urinary tract (see Table 15–2).

Biologic Basis of Successful Prophylaxis: Antimicrobial Effect on Bowel and Vaginal Bacterial Flora

The success of prophylaxis depends in large part on the effect an antimicrobial agent has on the introital and fecal reservoirs of pathogenic bacteria. Antimicrobial agents that eliminate pathogenic bacteria from these sites and/or do not cause bacterial resistance at the sites can be effective for antimicrobial prophylaxis of urinary tract infections. Winberg and his colleagues were the first to emphasize that oral antimicrobial therapy causes resistant strains in the fecal flora and subsequent resistant urinary tract infections (Lincoln et al, 1970; Winberg et al, 1973).

With 7- to 10-day therapy, the disadvantage of a resistant fecal flora is not as great because rapid reinfections are relatively uncommon (Kraft and Stamey, 1977). Nevertheless, the increase in resistant strains of *E. coli,* as well as the proliferation of other Enterobacteriaceae species, *C. albicans,* enterococci, and other pathogenic bacteria in the fecal and vaginal flora that accompanies even short-term, full-dose oral administration of tetracyclines, ampicillin, sulfonamides, amoxicillin, and cephalexin, is well documented (Sharp, 1954; Daikos et al, 1968; Hinton, 1970; Lincoln et al, 1970; Datta et al, 1971; Gruneberg et al, 1973; Winberg et al, 1975; Toivanen et al, 1976; Ronald et al, 1977; Preiksaitis et al, 1981). These ecologic changes may interfere with antimicrobial prophylaxis in the urinary tract and must be considered in the choice of prophylactic agents.

Effective Drugs

The oral antimicrobial agents with minimal adverse effects on the fecal and vaginal flora are TMP-SMX or TMP alone, nitrofurantoin, cephalexin (in minimal dosage), and the fluoroquinolones.

TRIMETHOPRIM-SULFAMETHOXAZOLE. TMP-SMX eradicates gram-negative aerobic flora from the gut and vaginal fluid. Because the gut is a reservoir for organisms that may colonize the periurethral area and subsequently cause episodes of acute cystitis in young women, infection is prevented by eliminating the pathogens from this reservoir. In addition vaginal fluid measurements of TMP and SMX in patients showed that TMP infused across the noninflamed vaginal wall and produced concentrations that exceeded serum levels (Stamey and Condy, 1975); SMX was undetectable in vaginal fluid. These observations on diffusion and concentration of TMP and vaginal fluid and on the effects of TMP-SMX in clearing Enterobacteriaceae from the rectal and vaginal flora clearly indicate why TMP-SMX is such a powerful prophylactic agent for the prevention of reinfections in the female. These important biologic effects occur in addition to the bactericidal levels of TMP-SMX that are present in the urine during nightly prophylaxis.

TRIMETHOPRIM. Kasanen and his associates in Finland (1978) studied the fecal flora in volunteers and patients who took 100 mg of TMP per day for periods of 3 weeks to 36 months; 4 of 20 patients treated for long periods developed coliforms resistant to TMP (>8 μg/ml). Svensson and his colleagues (1982) gave 100 mg of TMP once daily for 6 months to 26 patients with recurrent urinary tract infections. The infection recurrence rate before prophylaxis was 26 per 100 months compared with 3.3 recurrences per 100 months during prophylaxis (P <.001). The postprophylactic infection rate returned to 23 recurrences per 100 months. It is important to note that all *E. coli* urinary tract infections after prophylaxis were sensitive to TMP, that the number of rectal enterobacteria was markedly reduced during prophylaxis, and that although a 10% incidence of TMP-resistant organisms from rectal swabs was observed less than 1 month into prophylaxis, there was no significant further accumulation of resistant bacteria. This 10% incidence of TMP-resistant enterobacteria is virtually the same as was found in patients receiving 40 mg of TMP and 200 mg of SMX nightly in combination (Stamey and Condy, 1975).

These studies on TMP alone suggest that it should be as effective as TMP-SMX for prophylactic prevention of recurrent urinary tract infections. Stamm and associates (1980a) noted only one resistant strain of *E. coli* in 316 rectal, urethral, and vaginal isolates from 15 patients receiving 100 mg of TMP and 15 others receiving 40 mg of TMP with 200 mg of SMX nightly for 6 months; their unbelievably low recovery of TMP-resistant *E. coli* was due to their method of sampling, which did not include streaking cultures from these colonization sites directly onto media containing TMP.

These studies on TMP-SMX and TMP prophylactic therapy usually have been limited to 6 months to test continuing susceptibility in patients with reinfections. Two studies (Pearson et al, 1979; Harding et al, 1982), however, continued TMP-SMX prophylaxis from 2 to 5 years without showing any increase in "breakthrough" infections or any increase in TMP-resistant recurrent infections. Indeed, in the 15 patients treated for 2 years with one-half tablet of TMP-SMX thrice weekly (Harding et al, 1982), 100 of 116 cultures from the periurethral area (91%) and 60 of 97 cultures from the anal canal (68%) showed no aerobic gram-negative bacilli at these colonization sites.

In view of all these studies that indicate minimal fecal resistance in patients who take oral TMP-SMX or TMP alone, it is remarkable that Murray and associates (1982) reported TMP-resistant fecal gram-negative bacteria in 42 of 46 students who took TMP-SMX for 2 weeks in a diarrhea-preventive study in Mexico. This study would suggest that TMP-resistant strains are endemic in Mexico and should serve as a precaution to those who want to preserve the prophylactic efficacy of TMP-SMX in the United States.

NITROFURANTOIN. Nitrofurantoin, which does not alter the gut flora, is present for brief periods at high concentrations in the urine and leads to repeated elimination of bacteria from the urine, presumably interfering with bacterial initiation of infection. Either because of its complete absorption in the upper intestinal tract or its degradation and inactivation in the intestinal tract, it produces minimal fecal resistance—about 2% of fecal cultures (Stamey et al, 1977). Unlike the situation in prophylaxis with TMP-SMX, which eliminates colonization, in prophylaxis with nitrofurantoin, colonization of the vaginal introitus with Enterobacteriacae continues throughout therapy. The bacteria colonizing the vagina nearly always remain susceptible because of the lack of bacterial resistance in the fecal flora.

The urologist should know the adverse reactions to nitrofurantoin; according to Holmberg and associates (1980), nitrofurantoin accounted for 10% to 12% of all adverse drug reactions reported in Sweden. The two largest groups consisted of acute pulmonary reactions (43%) and allergic reactions (42%). Neuropathy, blood dysurias, liver damage, and chronic pulmonary reactions constituted the remainder. These appeared to be acute hypersensitivity reactions, with 65% to 83% of the patients showing eosinophilia in the blood smears. **The risk of an adverse reaction increases with age, with the greatest number occurring in patients over 50 years of age. Patients on long-term therapy should be monitored.**

CEPHALEXIN. Fairley and his associates (1974) first reported on the prophylactic efficacy of 500 mg of cephalexin per day in preventing recurrent infections during a 6-month period of observation. Of the 22 patients, 17 remained free of infection, an impressive record because several patients had papillary necrosis, chronic pyelonephritis, and even renal calculi. Gower (1975) treated 25 women with 125 mg of cephalexin nightly for 6 to 12 months and found only one infection, whereas 13 of 25 women receiving a placebo had infection. In a study of hospitalized patients with a mean age of 78 years, 125 mg of cephalexin per day was as effective as 250 mg per day in the 50% of patients whose urine remained sterile (Sourander and Saarimaa, 1975).

Martinez and associates (1985) studied the effect on the vaginal and rectal flora of 250 mg of cephalexin nightly for 6 months in 23 patients with reinfections of the urinary tract. Throughout prophylaxis, 22 of the 23 patients maintained a sterile urine; a single patient developed two enterococcal urinary tract infections, both of which responded to nitrofurantoin. No change was detected in the rectal or vaginal carriage of Enterobacteriaceae. More importantly, not a single resistant strain of *E. coli* was detected in 154 cultures obtained at monthly intervals during cephalexin therapy. All rectal and vaginal cultures were streaked on Mueller-Hinton agar containing 32 of cephalexin per milliliter. These results are in contrast with those of Preiksaitis and associates (1981), who found rectal Enterobacteriaceae resistance in 38% of patients when cephalexin was administered at a dose of 500 mg four times daily for 14 days. **Cephalexin at 250 mg or less nightly is an excellent prophylactic agent because fecal resistance does not develop at this low dosage.**

FLUOROQUINOLONES. With short-course fluoroquinolone therapy (Hooton et al, 1989b), eradication of Enterobacteriaceae from the fecal and vaginal (Nord, 1988; Tartaglione et al, 1988) flora has been documented, observations that have been exploited in the use of these agents for prophylaxis. More recently, Nicolle and colleagues (1989) documented the prophylactic efficacy of norfloxacin for the prevention of recurrent urinary tract infections in women. Of 11 women who completed 1 year of prophylaxis (200 mg orally), all remained free of infection. By comparison, the majority of individuals receiving placebos developed urinary tract infections; the infection rate in the placebo group was similar to that previously reported in populations of women with recurrent urinary tract infections. The drug was well tolerated. In addition to preventing symptomatic urinary tract infections, norfloxacin virtually eradicated periurethral and fecal colonization with aerobic gram-negative organisms. A larger study by Raz and Boger (1991) confirmed these results.

Because the fluoroquinolones are expensive and can be used only in nonpregnant women, the author favors their use only when antimicrobial resistance or patient intolerance to TMP-SMX, TMP, nitrofurantoin, or cephalexin occurs. Further studies are required to determine the minimal effective regimen and efficacy of the fluoroquinolones for prophylaxis of recurrent urinary tract infections in women.

Efficacy of Prophylaxis

Prophylactic therapy has been repeatedly documented as being effective in the management of women with recurrent urinary tract infections, with recurrences decreased by 95% when compared with placebo or with the patients' prior experiences as controls. These reported results of prophylaxis, together with agents and doses, have been summarized by Ronald (1987) (Table 15–19). These studies consistently show a remarkable reduction in the reinfection rate from 2.0 to 3.0 per patient year to 0.1 to 0.4 per patient year with the use of prophylaxis. Urinary antiseptics, such as methenamine mandelate or hippurate, have resulted in some decrease in recurrences, but they are not as effective as antimicrobial agents.

Prophylactic therapy requires only a small dose of an antimicrobial agent, which is generally given at bedtime for 6 to 12 months. If a woman experiences symptomatic reinfection during prophylactic therapy, full therapeutic dosing may be used with the prophylactic agent or another antimicrobial used to treat the infection. Then, antimicrobial prophylaxis may be reinstituted. If a patient experiences symptomatic reinfection immediately after cessation of prophylactic therapy, reinstitution of nightly prophylaxis is an effective alternative and results in no increase in adverse effects (Harding et al, 1982).

Postintercourse Prophylaxis

Sexual intercourse has been established as an important risk factor for acute cystitis in women (Nicolle et al, 1983). Diaphragm users have a significantly greater risk of urinary tract infection than women who use other contraceptive methods (Fihn et al, 1985). **Postintercourse therapy with antimicrobials such as nitrofurantoin, cephalexin, or TMP-SMX taken as a single dose effectively reduces the incidence of reinfection** (Pfau et al, 1983; Stapleton et al, 1990).

Intermittent Self-Start Therapy

Some patients are reluctant to continue long-term antimicrobial prophylaxis. In such cases women may be managed with repeated courses of self-administered, single-dose therapy (Wong et al, 1985). **In this regimen women identify episodes of infection on the basis of their symptoms and treat themselves at the onset of symptoms.** Thirty-five of 38 symptomatic episodes diagnosed by patients as infection were confirmed microbiologically, and 30 of 35 infections responded clinically and microbiologically to patient-administered therapy with single-dose TMP-SMX. In selected patients, self-administered single-dose therapy is efficacious and economical compared with conventional nightly prophylaxis.

With this approach the patient is given a dip-slide device to culture the urine and instructed to perform a urine culture when symptoms of urinary tract infection occur (Schaeffer, 1987). The patient is also provided a 3-day course of empirical full-dose antimicrobial therapy to be started immediately after performing the culture. It is important that the antimicrobial agent selected for self-start therapy has a broad spectrum of activity and achieves high urine levels to minimize development of resistant mutants. In addition there should be minimal or no side effects on the fecal flora. **Fluoroquinolones are ideal for self-start therapy because they have a spectrum of activity broader than that of any of the other oral agents and are superior to many parental antimicrobials, including aminoglycosides. Nitrofurantoin and TMP-SMX are acceptable alternatives although somewhat less effective**. Antimicrobial agents such as tetracycline, ampicillin, sulfamethoxazole, and cephalexin in full doses should be avoided because they can give rise to resistant bacteria (Wong et al, 1985).

The culture is brought to the office as soon as possible. If the culture is positive and the patient is asymptomatic, a culture is performed 7 to 10 days after therapy to determine efficacy. In most cases the therapy is limited to two inexpensive dip-slide cultures and a short course of antimicrobial therapy. If the patient has symptoms that do not respond to initial antimicrobial therapy, a repeat culture and sensitivity testing of the initial culture specimen are performed and therapy is adjusted accordingly. If symptoms of infection are not associated with positive cultures, urologic evaluation should be performed to rule out other causes of irritative bladder symptoms. These include carcinoma in situ, interstitial cystitis, and neurogenic bladder dysfunction. Our experience with this technique has been very favorable, and we find that it is particularly attractive to patients who have less frequent infections and are willing to play an active role in their diagnosis and management.

Bacterial Persistence

Although patients with bacterial persistence are uncommon, their identification is important because they represent the only surgically curable cause of recurrent urinary tract infections (see Table 15–2). Bacterial persistence within the urinary tract is usually caused by a correctable abnormality, the most common being bacterial persistence within infection stones. Systematic radiologic and endoscopic evaluation of the urinary tract is mandatory. **Excretory urography and cystoscopy provide initial screening, but in selected patients CT and bacterial localization cultures are indicated.** For example urea-splitting organisms such as *P. mirabilis* cause infection stones that are relatively radiolucent. If such a stone is suspected, plain film tomograms or CT should be obtained.

Identification of an upper tract abnormality suggests, but does not confirm, that it is the source of bacterial persistence. Therefore, in selected cases ureteral catheterization studies should be performed in order to verify that the abnormality harbors the bacteria. In men, if chronic bacterial prostatitis is suspected, lower urinary tract localization studies should be performed (see Chapter 16). Chronic bacterial prostatitis is treated initially with long-term antimicrobial therapy and in selected cases by radical transurethral resection. Most of the other congenital or acquired abnormalities listed in Table 15–2 require surgical removal for eradication of the source of bacterial persistence.

Table 15–19. LOW-DOSE PROPHYLAXIS FOR RECURRENT URINARY TRACT INFECTIONS IN WOMEN

Investigators	Regimen	Infections per Patient Year
Bailey et al (1971)*	a. Nitrofurantoin, 50 or 100 mg daily	0.09
	b. Nitrofurantoin, 50 mg daily	0.19
	c. Placebo	2.1
Harding and Ronald (1974)†	a. Sulfamethoxazole, 500 mg daily	2.5
	b. TMP-SMX, 40 and 200 mg daily	0.1
	c. Methenamine mandelate, 2 g daily, plus ascorbic acid, 2 g	1.6
	d. No drug	3.6
Kasanin et al (1974)‡	a. Nitrofurantoin, 50 mg daily	0.32
	b. Methenamine hippurate, 1 g daily	0.39
	c. Trimethoprim, 100 mg daily	0.13
	d. TMP-SMX, 80 and 400 mg daily	0.19
Gower (1975)§	a. Cephalexin, 125 mg daily	0.10
Stamey et al (1977)‖	a. TMP-SMX, 40 and 200 daily	0
	b. Nitrofurantoin macrocrystals, 100 mg daily	0.74
Harding et al (1979)¶	a. TMP-SMX, 40 and 200 mg daily thrice weekly	0.1
Stamm et al (1980)**	a. TMP-SMX, 40 and 200 mg daily	0.15
	b. Trimethoprim, 100 mg daily	0
	c. Nitrofurantoin macrocrystals, 100 mg daily	0.14
	d. Placebo	2.8
Brumfitt et al (1981)††	a. Nitrofurantoin, 50 mg twice daily	0.19
	b. Methenamine hippurate, 1 g twice daily	0.57
Harding et al (1982)‡‡	a. TMP-SMX, 40 and 200 mg thrice weekly	0.14
Brumfitt et al (1983)§§	a. Trimethoprim, 100 mg daily	1.53
	b. Methenamine hippurate, 1 g daily	1.38
	c. Povidone-iodine wash, twice daily	1.79
Wong et al (1985)‖‖	a. TMP-SMX, 40 and 200 mg daily	0.2
	b. Self-administered co-trimoxazole, 4 × 80 and 400 mg	2.2
Martinez et al (1985)¶¶	a. Cephalexin, 250 mg daily	0.18
Brumfitt et al (1985)***	a. Trimethoprim, 100 mg daily	1.00
	b. Nitrofurantoin macrocrystals, 100 mg daily	0.16

TMP-SMX, trimethoprim-sulfamethoxazole.

*Bailey RR, Roberts AP, Gower PE, de Wardener HE: Prevention of urinary tract infection with low dose nitrofurantoin. Lancet 1971; 2:1112–1114.

†Harding GKM, Ronald AR: A control study of antimicrobial prophylaxis of recurrent urinary infection in women. N Engl J Med 1974; 291:597–601.

‡Kasanin A, Kaarsolo E, Hiltunen R, Sorni V: Comparison of long-term, low dose nitrofurantoin, methenamine hippurate, trimethoprim-sulfamethoxazole on the control of recurrent urinary tract infection. Ann Clin Res 1974; 6:285–289.

§Gower PE: The use of small doses of cephalexin (125 mg) in the management of recurrent urinary tract infection in women. J Antimicrob Chemother 1975; 1(suppl. 3):93.

‖Stamey RA, Condy M, Mehara G: Prophylactic efficacy of nitrofurantoin macrocrystals and trimethoprim-sulfamethoxazole in urinary infections: Biologic effects on the vaginal and rectal flora. N Engl J Med 1977; 296:780–783.

¶Harding GKM, Ruckwold FJ, Marrie TJ, Thompson L, et al: Prophylaxis of recurrent urinary tract infection in female patients. Efficacy of low-dose, thrice weekly therapy with trimethoprim-sulfamethoxazole. JAMA 1979; 242:1975–1977.

**Stamm WE, Counts GW, Wagner KF, et al: Antimicrobial prophylaxis of recurrent urinary tract infections. A double-blind, placebo-controlled trial. Ann Intern Med 1980; 92:770–775.

††Brumfitt W, Cooper J, Hamilton-Miller JMT: Prevention of recurrent urinary infections in women: A comparative trial between nitrofurantoin and methenamine hippurate. J Urol 1981; 126:71–74.

‡‡Harding GK, Ronald AR, Nicolle LE, et al: Long-term antimicrobial prophylaxis for recurrent urinary tract infection in women. Rev Infect Dis 1982; 4:438.

§§Brumfitt W, Hamilton-Miller JMT, Gargon RA, et al: Long-term prophylaxis of urinary infections in women: Comparative trial of trimethoprim, methenamine hippurate, and topical povidone-iodine. J Urol 1983; 130:1110–1114.

‖‖Wong ES, McKevitt M, Running K, et al: Management of recurrent urinary tract infections with patient-administered single-dose therapy. Ann Intern Med 1985; 102:302.

¶¶Martinez FC, Kindrachuk RW, Stamey TA, et al: Effect of prophylactic, low dose cephalexin on fecal and vaginal bacteria. J Urol 1985; 133:994.

***Brumfitt W, Smith GW, Hamilton-Miller JMT, Gargon RA: A clinical comparison between Macrodantin and trimethoprim for prophylaxis in women with recurrent urinary infection. J Antimicrob Agents Chemother 1985; 16:111–120.

From Nicolle LE, Ronald AR: Infect Dis Clin North Am 1987; 1(4):793–806.

In patients in whom the focus of infection cannot be eradicated, long-term, low-dose antimicrobial suppression is necessary to prevent symptoms of infections. The antimicrobial drugs used for low-dose prophylaxis are also effective for bacterial suppression if the persistent strain is susceptible. These include nitrofurantoin, TMP-SMX, cephalexin, and fluoroquinolones.

Symptomatic Infections Versus Infections Detected on Screening Surveys for Bacteriuria

About 3% to 6% of sexually active women of childbearing age are bacteriuric on screening surveys; when bacteriuria is detected by screening surveys, it is conveniently called screening bacteriuria (ScBU). Three questions need to be answered. What do we know about the urinary tracts of women with ScBU? Do these women represent a separate population from those who have symptomatic infections? Is detection of their ScBU worthwhile?

Are Adult Women with Screening Bacteriuria at Risk of Serious Renal Damage?

In the late 1950s and early 1960s, several excellent epidemiologic studies (see Stamey, 1980, for review) were published on the 3% to 6% of adult women with ScBU; these studies examined such demographic parameters as age, blood pressure, concentrating ability, serologic titers, and proteinuria. Unfortunately, they never answered two critical questions: What do the kidneys look like? and What is the past history of these ScBU patients that can be related to their bacteriuria?

Asscher and his group at Cardiff, Wales (Asscher et al, 1969a; Asscher et al, 1973; Sussman et al, 1969), answered these questions by screening 3578 asymptomatic, nonpregnant women between the ages of 20 and 65 years. Of the 107 bacteriuric subjects 69% (3% of those screened) had had bladder irritative symptoms within a year before their bacteriuria was detected, whereas only 18% of matched controls without bacteriuria had similar symptoms. These observations established that women with ScBU are not asymptomatic.

Of more importance, these investigators obtained intravenous urograms on 87% of the 107 bacteriuric women and 57% of 88 matched nonbacteriuric controls. Every patient had a normal volume of renal cortex. Thirty-four percent of the urograms in bacteriuric women were abnormal, but these abnormalities were minor scars, rarely involving more than a single calyx; small calculi in eight patients (four of them in the scarred kidneys); nonsurgical hydroureter and hydronephrosis; and even less important findings, such as rotation of the kidney or simple cyst. None of these patients had progressive renal cortical destruction, even though one half were over 45 years of age. Moreover, when 90% of the 107 bacteriuric subjects were restudied with intravenous urograms 3 to 5 years later (Asscher et al, 1973), there was no evidence that the bacteriuria had caused hypertension, azotemia, or further renal scarring. These classic studies clearly established that although women with ScBU have three times the number of abnormalities in their kidneys as matched control subjects (of the same age and parity) without bacteriuria, these abnormalities do not represent serious renal disease.

Do Women with Screening Bacteriuria Differ from Those with Symptomatic Bacteriuria?

Gaymans and his colleagues asked this question in their general practice office (Gaymans et al, 1976). They screened 95% of their female patient population over the age of 14 years (1758 women); the prevalence of ScBU was 4.7%, with 2.7% in the age group 15 to 24 years and 9.3% in women 65 years and older. Ninety percent of the infections were caused by *E. coli.* All 1758 women were followed closely for 1 year, during which time 105 women (6%) had symptomatic infections; 29% of those with symptomatic infections had pre-existing ScBU. From these data they calculated that the probability of acquiring a symptomatic infection is seven times greater in women with known ScBU than in those without ($P < .0001$).

In addition to the 29% of patients with ScBU who developed symptomatic infections, one third had only transient bacteriuria. This left only one third of the patients of Gaymans and colleagues who had continuous ScBU; they were older (51.2 years), had fewer upper-tract symptoms, and had fewer abnormalities on intravenous urograms than those patients with ScBU who developed acute symptoms (average age of 41 years).

Is Detection of Screening Bacteriuria in Adult Women a Worthwhile Public Health Effort?

Asscher and his colleagues (1969b) emphasized that the two requirements for a useful screening procedure are that it "detects disease before irreversible damage has occurred and that the disease so detected may be effectively treated." It should be added to the first requirement, of course, that the disease under study be serious enough that detection would be worthwhile. As to the second requirement, the Cardiff study showed that 80% of the subjects with ScBU were cured with 7 days of oral nitrofurantoin therapy; this 80% cure rate is the same as that for treating symptomatic acute infections. At follow-up a year later, however, only 55% of the treated women with ScBU remained without infection, which differed little from the number of women who had spontaneous remission of their infection with placebo. Asscher and his group (1969b) concluded that successful therapy in ScBU was little different in the long run from the natural history of spontaneous remissions. Similar epidemiologic data in children is considered in Chapter 57. However, as seen in a later section on urinary tract infections in pregnancy, screening for bacteriuria in the first trimester of pregnancy probably represents the only time that screening for bacteriuria is worthwhile.

Urethral Syndrome

The urethral syndrome is considered in detail in Chapter 18. However, a brief overview of the approach at Stanford

University, which has been published elsewhere in detail (Stamey, 1980), is presented here. The urethral syndrome, whether acute or chronic, usually refers to any symptoms or combination of symptoms suggestive of urinary tract infection occurring in patients considered to be uninfected. The urethral syndrome for the urologist can be divided for practical purposes into three subgroups: (1) the syndrome with an infectious (microbial) cause, nearly always accompanied by an inflammatory response; (2) interstitial cystitis, rarely accompanied by inflammatory cells; and (3) the "pure" urethral syndrome, which includes patients who have neither a microbial cause nor interstitial cystitis.

Urethral and vaginal infections can be ruled out as discussed above. With this exclusion, the urologist can then concentrate on excluding interstitial cystitis (see Chapter 24). Once interstitial cystitis is excluded, the patient has the "pure" urethral syndrome. Many of these patients have an emotional basis for their discomfort, and the solutions are not easy. Dysfunctional voiding may contribute to the symptoms. It is in this group that urodynamic studies may be useful, but this remains to be seen.

It is hoped that the labels "trigonitis" and "urethrotrigonitis" will soon disappear from our vocabulary of ignorance. The cobblestone or granular appearance of the trigone and floor of the vesical neck represents normal squamous epithelium in the postpubertal female. It should not be scraped off, resected, or coagulated in the false belief that trigonitis is present. The pathologist has encouraged the delusion by reporting biopsy material from these areas as "squamous metaplasia" rather than the normal squamous epithelium that it actually represents. Failure to recognize that vaginal inclusion epithelium covering the trigone and urethra is a normal embryologic development, plus lack of experience in cystoscopic study of normal women without bladder symptoms, is undoubtedly responsible for the cystoscopic terms "trigonitis" and "granular urethrotrigonitis." The distal third of the vagina, the urethra, and the trigone are all derived from the urogenital sinus; thus, the same squamous epithelium of the vagina usually covers the trigone and floor of the urethra (Cifuentes, 1947).

URINARY TRACT INFECTIONS DURING PREGNANCY

Although the prevalence of bacteriuria does not change with the occurrence of pregnancy, certain anatomic and physiologic alterations associated with this state probably do change the course of bacteriuria during pregnancy. These changes may cause pregnant women to be more susceptible to pyelonephritis and may require alteration of therapy. These changes have been well summarized in several reviews (Davison and Lindheimer, 1978; Waltzer, 1981).

Anatomic and Physiologic Changes During Pregnancy

Increase in Renal Size

Renal length increases approximately 1 cm during normal pregnancy. It is thought that this does not represent true hypertrophy but is the result of increased renal vascular

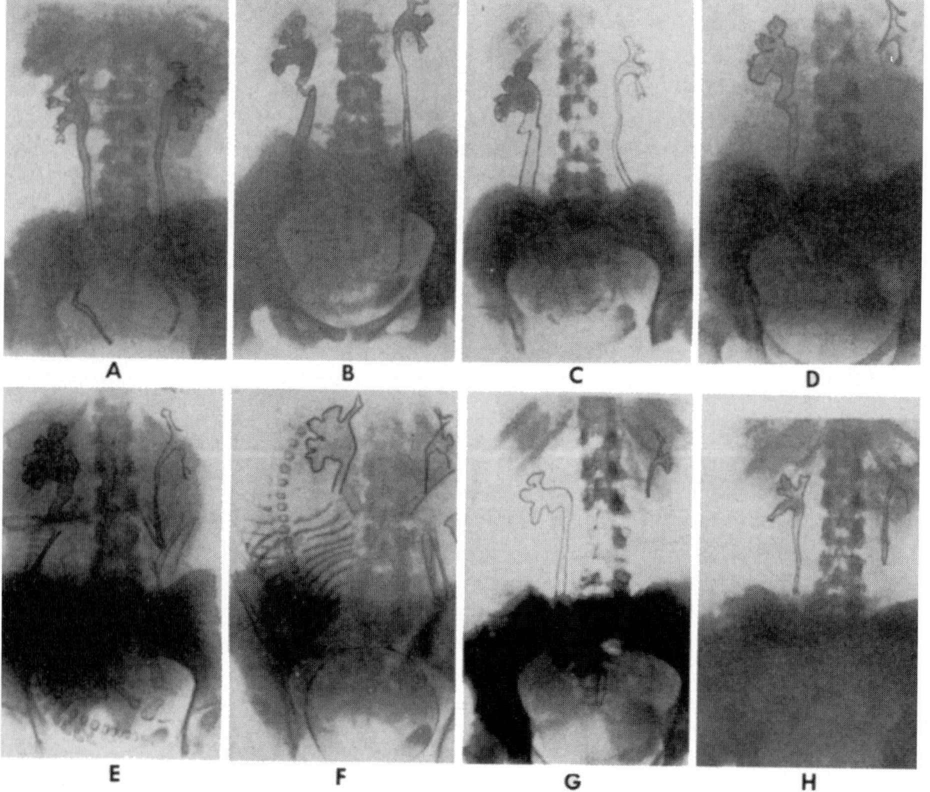

Figure 15–32. Progressive hydroureter and hydronephrosis observed on intravenous urograms during a normal pregnancy. *A,* At 15 weeks; *B,* 18 weeks; *C,* 22 weeks; *D,* 26 weeks; *E,* 34 weeks; *F,* 39 weeks; *G,* 1 week postpartum; *H,* 6 weeks postpartum. Bilateral hydroureter and hydronephrosis are shown as early as 15 weeks *(A).* Successive urograms *B* to *H* are from one patient during a normal pregnancy. Dilation occurs mainly on the right side, and both urinary tracts are normal by 6 weeks after delivery. (From Hundley JM, Walton HJ, Hibbits JT, et al: Am J Obstet Gynecol 1935; 30:625.)

and interstitial volume. No histologic changes have been identified in renal biopsies (Waltzer, 1981).

Smooth Muscle Atony of the Collecting System and Bladder

The collecting system, especially the ureters, undergoes decreased peristalsis during pregnancy, and most women in their third trimester show significant ureteral dilatation (Davison and Lindheimer, 1978; Kincaid-Smith, 1979; Waltzer, 1981) (Fig. 15–32). This hydroureter has been attributed both to the muscle-relaxing effects of increased progesterone during pregnancy and to mechanical obstruction of the ureters by the enlarging uterus at the pelvic brim. Progesterone-induced smooth muscle relaxation also may cause an increased bladder capacity (Waltzer, 1981).

Bladder Changes

The enlarging uterus displaces the bladder superiorly and anteriorly. The bladder becomes hyperemic and may appear congested endoscopically (Waltzer, 1981). Estrogen stimulation probably causes bladder hypertrophy as well as squamous changes of the urethra (Waltzer, 1981).

Augmented Renal Function

The transient increases in glomerular filtration rate and renal plasma flow during pregnancy have been well summarized by several authors and are probably secondary to the increase in cardiac output (Zacur and Mitch, 1977; Davison and Lindheimer, 1978; Kincaid-Smith, 1979; Waltzer, 1981) (Fig. 15–33). Glomerular filtration increases by 30% to 50%, and urinary protein excretion increases. The significance of these physiologic changes is apparent when the normal serum creatinine and urea nitrogen values for pregnant women are surveyed (Table 15–20). Values considered normal in nonpregnant women may represent renal insufficiency during pregnancy.

Davison and Lindheimer (1978) recommend that pregnant patients with serum creatinine levels greater than 0.8 mg/dl or urea nitrogen levels greater than 13 mg/dl undergo further evaluation of renal function. Similarly, urinary protein in pregnancy is not considered abnormal until greater than 300 mg of protein in 24 hours is excreted.

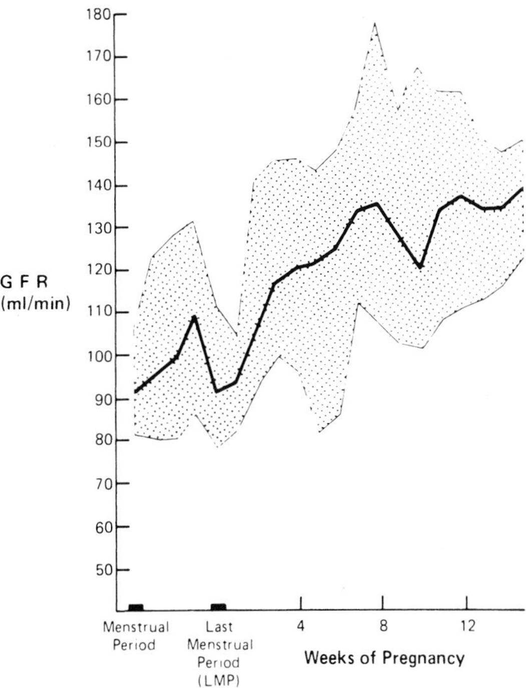

Figure 15–33. Weekly 24-hour creatinine clearance in eight women starting before conception and measured through the 12th gestational week. The solid line represents the mean glomerular filtration rate (GFR) and the stippled area the range. (From Davison JM, Lindheimer MD: Clin Obstet Gynecol 1978; 21:411.)

Screening for Bacteriuria During Pregnancy

The prevalence of bacteriuria found in screening pregnant females (ScBUP) is the same as that in nonpregnant females; this has been well reviewed by Stamey (1980). Beginning with a prevalence of 1.1% in young schoolgirls (Kunin et al, 1962), bacteriuria appears to increase approximately 1% to 2% per decade of age to attain a rate of 10% by 55 to 64 years. From these data, approximately 4% to 6% of females of childbearing age are bacteriuric. In Sweet's extensive review of 26 studies on the prevalence of bacteriuria in pregnant patients, all of which used differing criteria to determine bacteriuria, a rate of 2.5% to 8.7% is cited (Sweet, 1977). Most of the rates ranged between 4% and 7%, rates no different from those found in nonpregnant females. Furthermore, of those female patients who had uninfected urine when first seen, less than 1% (1 of 186 female patients) developed bacteriuria during the pregnancy in one study (McFadyen et al, 1973), and approximately 2% (6 of 279) developed it in another study (Elder et al, 1971). These are the low rates expected if the prevalence of bacteriuria in females is unaffected by pregnancy.

Increased rates of bacteriuria have been associated with duration of pregnancy, lower socioeconomic class, multiparity, and sickle cell traits (Patterson and Andriole, 1987; Stenqvist et al, 1989).

The site of bacteriuria in the pregnant female patients probably also reflects the situation before conception. In two studies that localized the origin of the bacteriuria, one using the Stamey ureteral catheterization technique and the other the Fairley bladder washout, upper-tract infections were found in 44% and 24.5% of pregnant female patients, respectively (Fairley et al, 1966; Heineman and Lee, 1973). In nonpregnant females with recurrent bacteriuria, Stamey has

Table 15–20. AVERAGE VALUES FOR SERUM CREATININE AND UREA NITROGEN

	Nonpregnant Females (mg/dl)	Pregnant Females (mg/dl)
Serum creatinine	0.7	0.5
Urea nitrogen	13.0	9.0

Data from Davison JM, Lindheimer MD: Clin Obstet Gynecol 1978; 21:411.

reported about a 50% probability that the origin is in the upper tracts (Stamey, 1980). With other techniques, which may reflect the severity of tissue infection rather than the location of infection, the results are similar; approximately 50% of women with ScBUP are fluorescent antibody–positive (Fa^+) (Harris et al, 1976). Fairley and associates found that the site of infection is unrelated to the likelihood that pyelonephritis will develop during pregnancy, but localization to the upper tracts may identify those women who are likely to have persistent postpartum bacteriuria (Fairley et al, 1973).

Natural History of Bacteriuria During Pregnancy

Whether treated or not, pregnant females with bacteriuria are at high risk of suffering recurrent bacteriuria. In one study that examined 148 pregnant women placed on placebo for bacteriuria, 18% (27 of 148) developed acute pyelonephritis, 13.5% (20 of 148) spontaneously cleared their infection, and 66% (98 of 148) remained bacteriuric (Elder et al, 1971). When infections were cured by antimicrobial agents, 16% and 27% of the women in two studies developed a recurrent infection later in the pregnancy (Elder et al, 1971; Harris, 1979). Kincaid-Smith (1979) has shown that 6 months after delivery the rate of recurrent bacteriuria in treated women was no different from that in untreated women. Indeed, in a long-term follow-up of women who had ScBUP, 38% were bacteriuric 14 years later regardless of the initial treatment (Zinner and Kass, 1971); others have reported bacteriuria to recur or persist in 20% to 30% of women postpartum (Sweet, 1977). Leveno and associates (1981) have shown that this risk of recurrent infection in pregnant women is independent of the duration of antimicrobial therapy and the site of infection in the urinary tract (Leveno et al, 1981). All this evidence suggests that recurrent bacteriuria in the pregnant female merely reflects a segment of the natural history of recurrent infections in females and is not a peculiarity of pregnancy.

The incidence of acute clinical pyelonephritis in pregnant women with bacteriuria is significantly increased over that in nonpregnant women. Nonpregnant women with uncomplicated urinary infections rarely develop pyelonephritis. Acute bacterial pyelonephritis is frequent in pregnant women, on the other hand, and occurs in 1% to 4% of all pregnant women (Kass, 1973). In his review of 18 papers, Sweet (1977) reported that 13.5% to 65% of women with ScBUP developed acute pyelonephritis during pregnancy; the average was 28%. In women without ScBUP, only about 1.4% developed acute pyelonephritis during pregnancy. Clearly, ScBUP increases a woman's risk of developing pyelonephritis during pregnancy.

Of the women who develop pyelonephritis during pregnancy, 60% to 75% acquire it during the third trimester (Cunningham et al, 1973), **when hydronephrosis and stasis in the urinary tract are most pronounced.** From 10% to 20% of pregnant women who get pyelonephritis develop it again before or just after the delivery (Cunningham et al, 1973; Gilstrap et al, 1981). Moreover, a third of pregnant women who develop pyelonephritis have a documented prior history of pyelonephritis (Gilstrap et al, 1981). Treatment of ScBUP decreases the incidence of acute pyelonephritis during pregnancy from a range of 13.5% to 65% to a range of 0% to 5.3% (Sweet, 1977).

In Sweet's excellent review of bacteriuria and pyelonephritis during pregnancy (1977), he suggests that patients with a renal source of bacteriuria are more likely to have persistent postpartum bacteriuria than those with cystitis alone. In addition, those women with persistent bacteriuria may have an increased incidence of impaired creatinine clearance and urinary concentrating ability, and an increased incidence of radiographic changes compatible with chronic pyelonephritis. His review of 12 studies revealed that follow-up intravenous urograms in pregnant women with bacteriuria showed an 8% to 33% incidence of radiologic changes compatible with chronic pyelonephritis; the incidence of all urinary tract abnormalities in this group was 18% to 80%. Zinner and Kass (1971) estimated that approximately 10% of bacteriuric pregnant females have pyelographic evidence of pyelonephritis, and in their study these abnormalities were most common in women who had bacteriuria 10 to 14 years after pregnancy. The highest incidence of radiographic changes of pyelonephritis was found in women who had their infections localized to their upper urinary tracts (Fairley et al, 1966). In this study, abbreviated intravenous urograms were performed within a few days of localization of the infection by ureteral catheterization. Thirty percent of women (six) with upper urinary tract infections revealed radiographic renal abnormalities compatible with chronic pyelonephritis on the side to which the infection was localized, and 10% (two) had nonexcretion of one kidney with infection in the contralateral one. No patient with an infection localized to the bladder showed radiographic evidence of pyelonephritis.

In their evaluation of renal function, Zinner and Kass (1971) found that women who had had bacteriuria during pregnancy and had it again 10 to 14 years later on follow-up showed significantly lower mean maximal urine osmolalities than those who were not bacteriuric on follow-up; others have found evidence of decreased creatinine clearance and concentrating ability in bacteriuric women postpartum (Sweet, 1977). It is unlikely, however, that uncomplicated bacteriuria in pregnant women produces changes in kidney appearance or function different from those found in nonpregnant bacteriuric women. After following 40 bacteriuric women during pregnancy, Kincaid-Smith (1979) stated that there was no difference in renal size or function between 6 months and 4 years after delivery. Pregnancy, therefore, may provide the opportunity for bacteriuria to be discovered, but this bacteriuria probably reflects only a susceptibility to urinary infection that was present at conception. The increased likelihood that bacteriuria may progress to acute pyelonephritis during pregnancy alters the morbidity of bacteriuria for this group.

Complications Associated with Bacteriuria During Pregnancy

Prematurity and Perinatal Mortality

In the preantibiotic era, pregnant women with bacterial pyelonephritis had a high rate of infant prematurity and associated perinatal mortality (Gilstrap et al, 1981), but now acute pyelonephritis is aggressively treated with antimicrobial agents. **Whether women who have been treated for pyelonephritis or screening bacteriuria during pregnancy still deliver infants with increased prematurity and perinatal mortality is controversial**. Studies designed to answer this question have not done so (Zinner, 1979). Evaluation of these studies is difficult because they define prematurity by different criteria (weight versus gestational age), define bacteriuria in different ways, fail to report statistically significant differences, and fail to mention which patients were treated. Sweet (1977) has critically reviewed these studies and concludes that the conflicting data can suggest only that pregnant women with bacteriuria have an increased incidence of prematurity.

In a recent study of 487 women with acute pyelonephritis and 248 women with asymptomatic bacteriuria, Gilstrap and associates (1981) showed that antepartum renal infections that were treated, whether symptomatic or not, did not affect pregnancy outcome. Intrapartum pyelonephritis was associated with an increased incidence of low-birth-weight babies, but the number of patients studied was too small for significance. In a retrospective analysis of data collected for the Collaborative Perinatal Project of the National Institute of Neurological and Communicative Disorders and Stroke, which analyzed over 50,000 births between 1959 and 1966, only placental growth retardation (defined as placental weight less than 40% of normal) of eight prenatal disorders studied (amniotic fluid infection, congenital malformation, umbilical cord compression, large placental infarcts, abruptio placentae, growth-retarded placenta, Rh disease, and placenta previa) was significantly increased in frequency in pregnant women with pyuria and bacteriuria over that observed in normal pregnant women (Naeye, 1979). When analyzed, the higher combined perinatal mortality rate for these eight common disorders in the infected (42 of 1000 women) compared with the uninfected (21 of 1000) could be attributed to greater mortality from the noninfectious disorders that were accompanied by urinary tract infection within 15 days of delivery. McGrady and co-workers (1985) found that pregnancies complicated by urinary tract infections were associated with 2.4 times the fetal mortality when compared with the overall fetal mortality rates in the same geographic area. They also reported increased risks of prematurity, intrauterine growth retardation, and low birth weight in patients with bacteriuria when compared with controls.

Whether clinical pyelonephritis during pregnancy causes increased risk of prematurity is still unclear, but bacteriuria in the symptomatic or asymptomatic pregnant female should be treated to avoid pyelonephritis and its possible sequelae in the mother.

Maternal Anemia

Although several studies suggest that bacteriuria untreated during pregnancy is associated with maternal anemia, not all studies support this. Some difficulties in interpreting the results of these surveys have been caused by inadequate documentation of bacteriuria. In one survey in which urine cultures were obtained by suprapubic aspiration, the data suggest that pregnant patients requiring three or more treatments for bacteriuria have lower levels of serum hemoglobin and folate than controls (McFadyen et al, 1973). In another study from England, investigators showed a statistically significant difference in the incidence of anemia between 410 bacteriuric pregnant women and 409 control pregnant women (Williams et al, 1973). In this survey, 14.6% of bacteriuric women and 10% of control women were anemic at the first prenatal visit. This separation increased during the third trimester (32 weeks), when 25% of women treated with placebo alone had anemia, but only 16.8% of those women treated with antibiotics had anemia. Furthermore, in the 31 untreated (placebo-treated) bacteriuric women who subsequently developed pyelonephritis, the incidence of anemia was 45.2%. These investigators concluded that "untreated bacteriuria increases the likelihood of developing anemia during pregnancy and that this risk is enhanced by the development of acute pyelonephritis, even if it is treated promptly" (Williams et al, 1973).

Maternal Hypertension and Eclampsia

The data relating bacteriuria during pregnancy to hypertension and toxemia are inconclusive.

Management of Bacteriuria During Pregnancy

Diagnosis of Bacteriuria

Since pregnant women with bacteriuria suffer such an increased risk of developing acute pyelonephritis and other complications, bacteriuria should be sought at the initial prenatal visit (Stenquist et al, 1989; Gratacos et al, 1994). **The risk of bacteriuria increases with the duration of pregnancy. If the culture shows no growth, a repeat culture should be performed at week 16 of gestation because this is the optimal time to screen for bacteriuria** (Stenquist et al, 1989). **A midstream voided urine sample should be obtained. Urethral catheterization, which may introduce bacteria into the bladder, should be avoided in the pregnant female, if possible.** Attempts to localize the infection to the upper or lower urinary tract are not thought to be helpful in the management of the bacteriuria, since recurrence rates are independent of the site of infection (Leveno et al, 1981).

Treatment of Urinary Tract Infections During Pregnancy

When symptomatic or asymptomatic bacteriuria of pregnancy is diagnosed, the bacteriuria should be treated to avoid the complications already discussed. **Selection of an antimicrobial agent to treat the bacteriuria must be made, however, with special considerations given to maternal and fetal toxicity.** The physiologic changes of pregnancy may decrease tissue and serum drug concentrations. Maternal expanded fluid volume, the distribution of the drug in the fetus, increased renal blood flow, and increased glomerular filtration decrease the serum drug concentration.

Although the adverse effects of most antimicrobials are the same whether or not the patient is pregnant, certain antimicrobial agents should be avoided in pregnancy (Ries and Kaye, 1974; Sweet, 1977; Harris, 1980; McGeown, 1981; Schwarz, 1981). Tetracyclines are contraindicated throughout pregnancy because they may cause acute maternal liver decompensation and fetal malformations. The chelating action of tetracycline causes hypoplasia and staining of the child's deciduous teeth. The estolate salt of erythromycin is contraindicated because it can cause cholestatic jaundice in pregnant females. Chloramphenicol, in addition to its adverse affects in adults, may accumulate to toxic concentrations in the neonate because infants may lack the ability to metabolize or excrete the drug; this toxic neonatal effect, "the gray syndrome," may cause cardiovascular collapse and high neonatal mortality. The fluoroquinolones are contraindicated during pregnancy because of potential adverse effects on cartilage formation.

Sulfa preparations, especially long-acting forms, should be avoided during the third trimester of pregnancy because they compete for fetal bilirubin-binding sites on albumin and can cause neonatal hyperbilirubinemia and kernicterus. Although it is undocumented as a teratogen (Brumfitt and Pursell, 1973), most investigators feel that trimethoprim, a folic acid antagonist, should be avoided during the first trimester of pregnancy because of its potential teratogenic activity. The nitrofurantoins, a group of oxidizing drugs, can cause a hemolytic anemia in patients and fetuses with a glucose-6-phosphate dehydrogenase deficiency, a defect found in about 10% of blacks in the United States and in Sardinians, non-Ashkenazi Jews, Greeks, Eti-Turks, and Thais (Thompson, 1969). In these people, regeneration of glutathione, which is partially responsible for maintaining red blood cell integrity, is impaired by the enzyme deficiency, and nitrofurantoin oxidizes the hemoglobin to methemoglobin, which is further degraded. Aminoglycosides have no specific complications associated with pregnancy, but they may cause ototoxicity and nephrotoxicity in both fetus and mother.

Although few data on human fetal toxicity of antimicrobial agents are available, several antimicrobial drugs that appear to be relatively safe during pregnancy have been identified (Sweet, 1977; Weinstein, 1979; Harris, 1980; Schwarz, 1981). Ideally, these drugs should achieve high urinary and low serum concentrations and affect only the bacteria. Since the penicillins and cephalosporins inhibit growth of the bacterial cell wall, and human cells have a cytoplasmic membrane without a cell wall, these drugs act specifically on the bacteria.

Only the penicillins (penicillin, ampicillin, and synthetic penicillins) and cephalosporins, given orally or parenterally, are thought to be safe and effective during any phase of pregnancy (Gerstner et al, 1989). In this situation oral penicillin, with its extremely high urinary concentrations, may be a particularly effective and inexpensive agent. Of course, like any drugs, these drugs may still cause difficulties in women who suffer sensitivities to them. Methenamine mandelate, when excreted in an acid urine, forms formaldehyde, which is nonspecifically bactericidal. Since the activity of this agent is dependent on a urine pH below 5.5, this drug, although safe, has limited use. In fact, in one study in which pregnant women with bacteriuria were either placed in a control group or treated with methenamine mandelate or methenamine hippurate for the remainder of the pregnancy, only a small reduction in the incidence of pyelonephritis was noted in the treated groups. These results are poor when compared with the results of other antimicrobial agents and probably reflect the somewhat low efficacy of the methenamine. **The short-acting sulfonamides can be safely used during the first two trimesters of pregnancy, since the fetus in utero handles excess unconjugated bilirubin through the placenta. Similarly, nitrofurantoin has been commonly used in pregnancy during the first two trimesters but may be contraindicated at term because it can cause a hemolytic anemia in neonates with an immature enzyme system. Although TMP-SMX has been used during all phases of pregnancy without a documented increase in fetal abnormalities related to it** (Brumfitt and Pursell, 1973), **it probably should not be considered the drug of choice for simple infections, particularly during the first and third trimesters.**

Although single-dose beta-lactam therapy in nonpregnant women is usually effective (Gerstner et al, 1989), **it is probably prudent to prescribe a 3-day course of therapy in pregnant women.** Longer-term treatment does not appear to reduce the risk of recurrent bacteriuria (Leveno et al, 1981). **It is important to reculture the urine 1 to 2 days after treatment is completed to ensure that the urine shows no growth.** If it does, the cause of bacteriuria must be determined to be lack of resolution, bacterial persistence, or reinfection. If the infection is unresolved, proper selection and administration of another drug probably will solve the problem. If the problem is bacterial persistence or rapid reinfection, antimicrobial suppression of infection or prophylaxis (Pfau and Sacks, 1992) throughout the remainder of the pregnancy should be considered. Women with severe pyelonephritis requiring hospitalization should be treated parenterally until they become afebrile and then switched to an oral regimen for a total of 14 days. TMP-SMX, ciprofloxacin, ofloxacin, or ceftriaxone is usually effective in most patients with domiciliary infections. The antimicrobial agents and their dosage for this long-term treatment are discussed in a previous section. When a prophylactic or suppressive agent is selected, however, the contraindications imposed by pregnancy still should be considered.

Pregnant women with acute clinical pyelonephritis should be admitted to the hospital for treatment with parenteral agents (Angel et al, 1990). Drugs with adequate serum and urine levels and the least potential maternal and fetal toxicity should be selected. Patients who fail to improve after 2 to 3 days of appropriate antimicrobial therapy should be evaluated for complications, such as obstruction or perinephric abscess.

Since these patients suffer an increased risk of repeated pyelonephritis during the pregnancy (Cunningham et al, 1973; Gilstrap et al, 1981), they should either be monitored closely for recurrent bacteriuria or be given prophylaxis for the remainder of the pregnancy.

Pregnancy in Women with Renal Insufficiency

With current management of recurrent urinary tract infections, infections alone are no contraindication to pregnancy. In patients who have renal insufficiency with or without urinary tract infections, Davison and Lindheimer (1978) emphasize that renal function should be carefully evaluated by both serum creatinine levels and creatinine clearance before a woman is counseled about conceiving or continuing a pregnancy. Although little is known about the outcome of pregnancies with differing degrees of renal insufficiency, it is known that normal pregnancy is rare if the preconception serum creatinine level exceeds 3 mg/dl (about 30 ml/minute clearance) (Davison and Lindheimer, 1978).

One retrospective analysis of 44 pregnancies in women with pre-existing renal disease provides some helpful guidelines about the degree of renal impairment beyond which pregnancy is inadvisable (Bear, 1976). In this study, patients were divided into those with mild renal disease and serum creatinine levels less than 1.5 mg/dl and those with renal disease and serum creatinine levels greater than 1.6 mg/dl. In those with mild renal disease, 34 of 35 pregnancies resulted in normal live births, and although the serum creatinine level remained fixed during the pregnancy (it did not decrease as expected during a normal pregnancy), the pregnancy appeared to have no remote effect on renal function. On the other hand, pregnancy in eight patients with serum creatinine levels greater than 1.6 mg/dl was complicated in all cases, and the incidences of prematurity, delivery by cesarean section, hypertension, and worsening proteinuria and renal insufficiency during pregnancy were increased; four of the eight patients progressed to severe renal failure or death within 18 months. These data have caused Bear to recommend that conception is ill-advised in patients with less than 50% of normal renal function (serum creatinine levels greater than 1.7 mg/dl or less than about 50 ml/minute clearance).

URINARY TRACT INFECTIONS IN THE ELDERLY

Urinary tract infections in the elderly are a major, expanding health problem. Today there are over 28 million Americans older than 65 years (Kaye, 1980; Current Population Reports, 1988). As the life expectancy increases, the diagnosis, treatment, morbidity, and mortality of urinary tract infections in the elderly will assume increasing importance.

The causes of the increased susceptibility to urinary tract infections in the elderly are multiple and include physiologic changes of aging, acquired abnormalities of the urinary tract, and increased exposure to environmental and therapeutic risk factors. The symptoms range from asymptomatic bacteriuria to life-threatening sepsis. A higher mortality in the bacteriuric elderly has been reported in some populations (Sourander and Kasanen, 1972; Dontas et al, 1981), but the explanation for this observation is not clear, nor is there clear evidence that therapy is effective or significantly alters the natural history. Furthermore, therapy is complicated because unusual pathogens are frequently encountered, special considerations are required for antimicrobial administration, and adverse effects are frequent.

Epidemiology

The prevalence of urinary tract infections in the elderly is much higher than in younger populations. **At least 20% of women and 10% of men older than 65 years of age have bacteriuria** (Boscia and Kaye, 1987). **In contrast to young adults, in whom bacteriuria is 30 times more prevalent in women than in men, the ratio in women to men with bacteriuria progressively decreases to 2:1. The prevalence of bacteriuria in the elderly increases with age** (Table 15–21) (Sourander, 1966; Brocklehurst et al, 1968), **and concurrent disease** (Fig. 15–34). **Risk factors can be compounded.** In a study of 373 women and 150 men over the age of 68 years, 24% of functionally impaired nursing home residents had bacteriuria compared with 12% of healthy domiciliary subjects (Boscia et al, 1986).

Longitudinal studies have helped to clarify the dynamic aspects of bacteriuria in the elderly and have established that the cumulative percentage of subjects with at least one positive culture increases with each survey, thus indicating that bacteriuria in the elderly is much more common than is apparent from a single survey (Fig. 15–35). There is only a small pool of elderly patients with persistent bacteriuria (Kaye, 1980). Most patients have transient bacteria, and this fact influences the management of asymptomatic bacteriuria in the elderly (Boscia et al, 1986; Sourander and Kasanen, 1972).

Clinical Presentation

The majority of elderly subjects have asymptomatic bacteriuria (Wolfson et al, 1965; Walkey et al, 1967). Such symptoms as lethargy, confusion, anorexia, and incontinence frequently cause missed or delayed diagnosis and may lead to increased morbidity and mortality. Even severe urinary tract infections may not be associated with fever (Stark and Maki, 1984) or leukocytosis. **Therefore, a high index of suspicion is warranted, particularly when risk factors (e.g., an indwelling urethral catheter) are present.**

Urinalysis and cultures are valid only if the urine has been collected without contamination. If urinalysis of a midstream voided specimen shows epithelial cells, vaginal or preputial contamination should be suspected and another specimen obtained by catheterization in women or after retracting the foreskin and cleansing the glans penis in men.

Pyuria alone is not a good predictor of bacteriuria in this population. More than 60% of women with pyuria ≥ 10 WBC/ml^3 noted in midstream specimens do not have concurrent bacteriuria. **The absence of pyuria, however, was a good predictor of the absence of bacteriuria.** The diagnosis of urinary tract infections is confirmed by quantitative urine culture. Although 10^5 or more bacteria per milliliter constitute the traditional level of significance, counts of 10^3 or more bacteria are clinically significant in carefully collected specimens (Kunin, 1987).

Table 15–21. BACTERIURIA IN TWO POPULATION SURVEYS

Age	Men (%)	Women (%)
65–70 years	2–3	20–21
Older than 80 years	21–22	23–50

Data from Brocklehurst JC, Dillane JB, Griffiths L, et al: Gerontol Clin 1968; 10:242–253; and Sourander LB: Ann Med Intern Fenn 1966; 55(suppl 45):7–55.

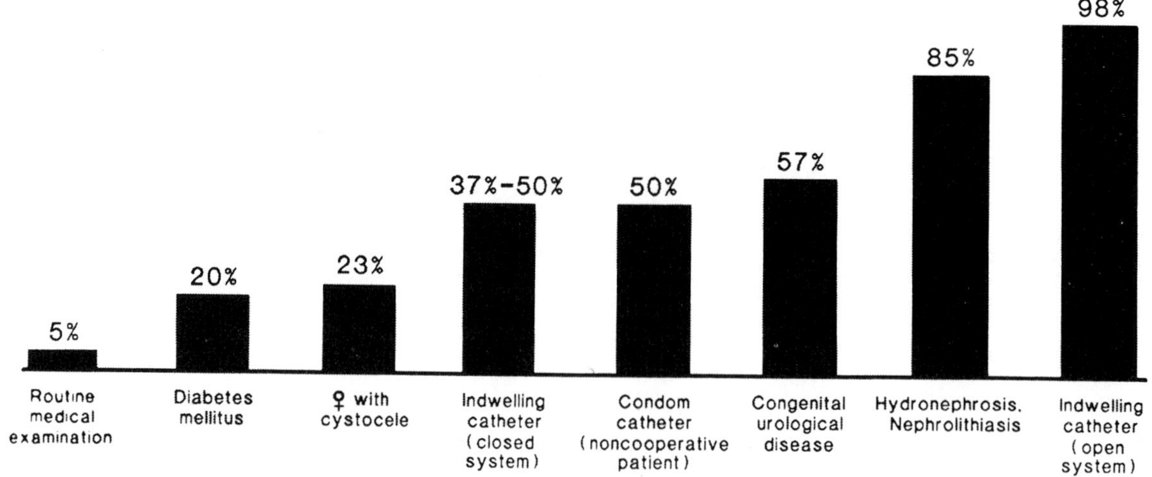

Figure 15–34. Frequency of significant bacteriuria related to underlying disease. (Adapted from Jackson GG, Arana-Sialer JA, Andersen BR: Arch Intern Med 1962; 110:663–675.)

Because urinary tract abnormalities frequently predispose to or complicate urinary tract infections in the elderly, a thorough evaluation should be performed. Renal dysfunction, calculi, hydronephrosis, urinary retention, neurogenic bladder dysfunction, and other abnormalities should be identified by serum creatinine measurement, excretory urography, ultrasonography, urodynamics and/or cystoscopy. The timing and sequence of these tests should be dictated by the clinical setting.

Bacteriology

The bacteriologic features of urinary tract infections in the elderly differ from those in the young. *E. coli* causes only 75% of these infections; *Proteus, Klebsiella, Enterobacter, Serratia*, and *Pseudomonas* species and enterococci (Walkey et al, 1967; Nicolle et al, 1983; Sant, 1987) are also frequently encountered. Bacteriuria due to gram-positive bacteria is much more common in elderly men than in elderly women (Jackson et al, 1962). **The shift in the pattern of uropathogens, the high frequency of polymicrobial infections, and antimicrobial resistance in urinary tract infections in the elderly are due in large part to the high frequency of institutionalization and hospitalization, catheterization, and antimicrobial usage in this population** (Fig. 15–36).

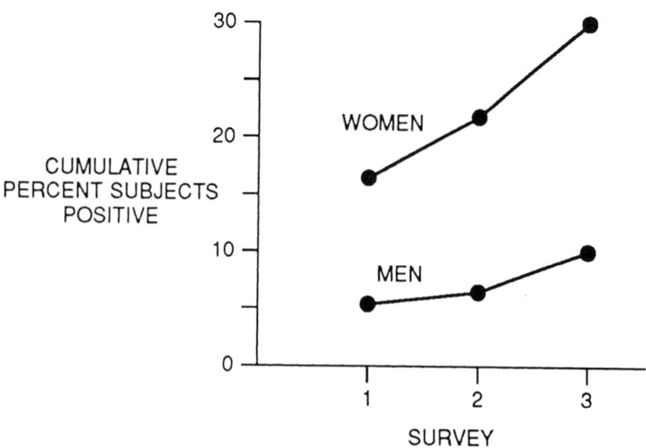

Figure 15–35. Cumulative percentage of subjects with at least one positive urine culture survey result over three surveys performed at 6-month intervals. (From Boscia JA, Kobasa WD, Knight RA, et al: Am J Med 1986; 80:208.)

Pathophysiology

Factors contributing to urinary tract infections in the elderly are complex and poorly understood. Multiple age-related changes include a decline in cell-mediated immunity; altered bladder defenses due to obstructive uropathy; neurogenic dysfunction; increased receptivity of uroepithelial cells (Reid et al, 1984); an increased risk of contamination due to fecal and urinary incontinence and urethral instrumentation and catheterization; and a decrease in prostatic and vaginal antibacterial factors associated with changes in pH and levels of zinc and hormones (Boscia et al, 1986).

Significance

Urinary tract infections in elderly subjects in the presence of underlying structural urinary tract abnormalities or systemic conditions (e.g., diabetes mellitus) are clinically significant, can lead to renal failure, and require prompt therapy. In addition urinary tract infections caused by urea-splitting bacteria, such as *Proteus* or *Klebsiella* species that cause formation of infection stones, may also lead to severe renal damage.

The significance of asymptomatic bacteriuria that is not caused by urea-splitting bacteria is controversial. Some authors have reported decreased renal function in association with bacteriuria (Krieger et al, 1983). Other studies (Wolfson et al, 1965; Klarskov, 1976), however, do not support this concept, and it is now reasonably clear that bacteriuria in the absence of obstruction rarely, if ever, progresses to renal failure. Bacteriuria has also been associated with increased mortality (Sourander and Kasanen, 1972; Dontas et al, 1981; Gleckman et al, 1982; Latham et al,

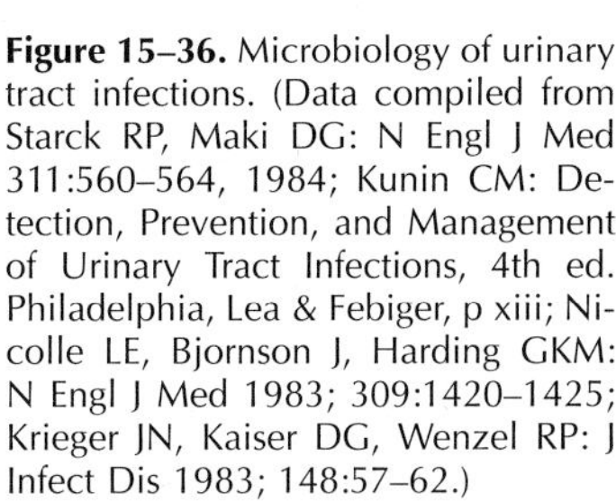

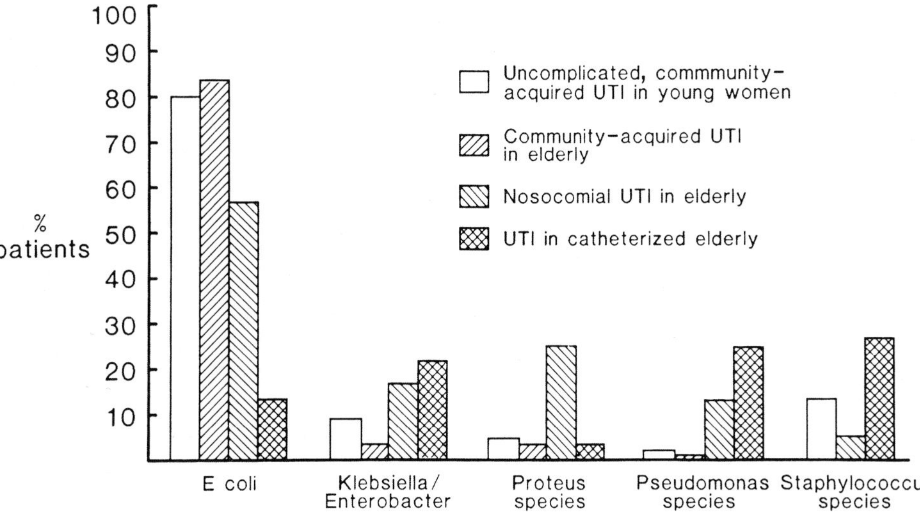

Figure 15–36. Microbiology of urinary tract infections. (Data compiled from Starck RP, Maki DG: N Engl J Med 311:560–564, 1984; Kunin CM: Detection, Prevention, and Management of Urinary Tract Infections, 4th ed. Philadelphia, Lea & Febiger, p xiii; Nicolle LE, Bjornson J, Harding GKM: N Engl J Med 1983; 309:1420–1425; Krieger JN, Kaiser DG, Wenzel RP: J Infect Dis 1983; 148:57–62.)

1985). This association may result either from a direct effect on mortality of the bacteriuria itself or from such factors as aging or underlying disease that increase both bacteriuria and mortality. The distinction is important because treatment can be expected to reduce mortality only if bacteriuria is the direct cause (Dontas et al, 1968).

Studies that have found a significantly increased mortality among persons with bacteriuria have looked at populations that were heterogeneous in terms of age and underlying disease (Dontas et al, 1981; Latham et al, 1985). An age difference of only 2 years increases mortality by 20% (Dontas et al, 1968). Therefore, in the studies mentioned above (Dontas et al, 1968), it is not clear how much of the observed association between bacteriuria and mortality was due to differences in age between the bacteriuric and abacteriuric groups. In a study of bacteriuria and mortality in a homogeneous 70-year-old population, the association between bacteriuria and mortality was weaker and linked to fatal diseases not attributable to bacteriuria (Dontas et al, 1968). Furthermore, when Nicolle and associates (1983) attempted to estimate the contribution of bacteriuria to mortality by treating elderly men, the treatment did not result in prolonged intervals without bacteriuria, and it had no effect on mortality.

It is possible that bacteriuria may lead to bacteremia or accelerate pre-existing renal disease or that pre-existing renal disease may facilitate upper urinary tract infection, but further studies are required to test such hypotheses. Treatment of asymptomatic bacteriuria to improve incontinence has not been justified (Baldassarre and Kaye, 1991). Sepsis and its sequelae (sepsis syndrome and septic shock) are increasingly common in the elderly. This is in part due to the aggressive use of catheters (Kunin et al, 1992) and other invasive equipment; implantation of prosthetic devices; and the administration of chemotherapy to cancer patients or corticosteroids in other immunosuppressed patients with organ transplants or inflammatory diseases. In addition modern medical care has given longer life spans to the elderly and patients with metabolic, neoplastic, or immunodeficiency disorders, who remain at increased risk for infection.

Management

The elderly population is more susceptible than young patients to the toxic and adverse effects of antimicrobial agents (Grieco, 1980; Carty et al, 1981; Boscia et al, 1986) because the metabolism and excretion of antimicrobial agents may be impaired, and resulting increased serum levels can further damage renal function. Interactions with other medications can occur, and the safety margin between therapeutic and toxic doses is significantly narrowed. Therefore, antimicrobials must be used judiciously, and dosing and drug levels should be carefully monitored.

There is no question that symptomatic urinary tract infections should be treated. However, the majority of elderly patients have asymptomatic bacteriuria, and the merit of antimicrobial therapy in this population is debatable. Boscia and associates (1987) demonstrated that in elderly, *nonhospitalized* women, a short course of antimicrobial therapy is effective and can eliminate bacteriuria for 6 months in two thirds of the patients. Conversely, Nicolle and associates (1987) randomized *institutionalized* elderly women to therapy or no therapy and showed no differences in the genitourinary tract related to morbidity or mortality. Despite a lowered prevalence of bacteriuria, no short-term benefits were identified and some harmful effects were observed with treatment. Abrutyn et al (1994) studied asymptomatic bacteriuria in elderly ambulatory women and found that it was not an independent risk factor for mortality and its treatment did not lower the mortality rate. **Until it is determined that elimination of asymptomatic bacteriuria is cost-effective and risk-beneficial and decreases morbidity or lengthens survival, treatment of asymptomatic bacteriuria in the absence of obstruction does not appear warranted.**

OTHER INFECTIONS

Fournier's Gangrene

Fournier's gangrene is a form of necrotizing fasciitis occurring about the male genitalia. It is also known as idiopathic gangrene of the scrotum, streptococcal scrotal gangrene, perineal phlegmon, and spontaneous fulminant gangrene of the scrotum (Fournier 1883, 1884). As originally reported by Baurienne in 1764, and by Fournier in 1883, it was characterized by an abrupt onset of a rapidly fulminating genital gangrene of idiopathic origin in previously healthy young patients, which resulted in gangrenous destruction of the genitalia. The disease now differs from these descriptions in that it involves a broader age range, including older patients (Bejanga, 1979; Wolach et al, 1989), follows a more indolent course, and has a less abrupt onset, and in approximately 95% of the cases, a source can now be identified (Macrea, 1945; Burpee and Edwards, 1972; Kearney and Carling, 1983; Jamieson et al, 1984; Spirnak et al, 1984). Infection most commonly arises from the skin, urethra, or rectal regions. An association between urethral obstruction associated with strictures and extravasation and instrumentation has been well documented. **Predisposing factors include diabetes mellitus, local trauma, paraphimosis, periurethral extravasation or urine, perirectal or perianal infections, and surgery such as circumcision or herniorrhaphy.** In cases originating in the genitalia, the infecting bacteria probably pass through Buck's fascia of the penis and spread along the dartos fascia of the scrotum and penis, Colles' fascia of the perineum, and Scarpa's fascia of the anterior abdominal wall. In view of the typical foul odor associated with this condition, a major role for anaerobic bacteria is likely. **Wound cultures generally yield multiple organisms, implicating anaerobic-aerobic synergy** (Meleney, 1933; Miller, 1983; Cohen, 1986). Mixed cultures containing facultative organisms (*E. coli, Klebsiella*, enterococci) along with anaerobes (*Bacteroides, Fusobacterium, Clostridium*, microaerophilic streptococci) have been obtained from the lesions.

Clinical Presentation

Patients frequently have a history of recent perineal trauma, instrumentation, urethral stricture associated with sexually transmitted disease or urethral cutaneous fistula. Pain, rectal bleeding, and a history of anal fissures suggest a rectal source of infection. Dermal sources are suggested by history of acute and chronic infections of the scrotum, and spreading recurrent hidradenitis suppurativa or balanitis.

The infection commonly starts as cellulitis adjacent to the portal of entry. Early on, the involved area is swollen, erythematous, and tender as the infection begins to involve the deep fascia. Pain is prominent, and fever and systemic toxicity are marked (Paty and Smith, 1992). The swelling and crepitus of the scrotum quickly increase and dark purple areas develop and progress to extensive gangrene. If the abdominal wall becomes involved in an obese patient with diabetes, the process can spread very rapidly. Specific genitourinary symptoms associated with the condition include dysuria, urethral discharge, and obstructed voiding. Alterations in mental status, tachypnea, tachycardia, and temperature greater than 101°F or less than 96°F, suggest gram-negative sepsis.

Laboratory Studies

Anemia occurs secondary to a decreased functioning erythrocyte mass caused by thrombosis and ecchymosis coupled with decreased production secondary to sepsis (Miller, 1983). Elevated serum creatinine levels, hyponatremia, and hypocalcemia are common. The latter is believed to be secondary to bacterial lipases that destroy triglycerides and release free fatty acids that chelate calcium in its ionized form.

Diagnostic Tests

Because crepitus is often an early finding, a plain film of the abdomen may be helpful in identifying air. Scrotal ultrasonography is also useful in this regard. Biopsy of the base of an ulcer is characterized by superficially intact epidermis, dermal necrosis, and vascular thrombosis and polymorphonuclear leukocyte invasion with subcutaneous tissue necrosis. Stamenkovic and Lew (1984) noted that the use of frozen sections within 21 hours after the onset of symptoms could confirm a diagnosis earlier and lead to early institution of appropriate treatment.

Management

Prompt diagnosis is critical because of the rapidity with which the process can progress. The clinical differentiation of necrotizing fasciitis from cellulitis may be difficult since the initial signs including pain, edema, and erythema are not distinctive. **However, the presence of marked systemic toxicity out of proportion to the local finding should alert the clinician. Intravenous hydration and antibiotic therapy are indicated in preparation for surgical debridement.** Antibiotic regimens include combinations of ampicillin plus sulbactam or a parenteral third-generation cephalosporin such as ceftriaxone, gentamicin, and clindamycin. If there is no response to clindamycin, chloramphenicol may be used. Immediate debridement is essential. In the patient in whom diagnosis is clearly suspected on clinical grounds (deep pain with patchy areas of surface hypoesthesia or crepitation, or bullae and skin necrosis), direct operative intervention is indicated. Extensive incision should be made through the skin and subcutaneous tissues going beyond the areas of involvement until normal fascia is found. Necrotic fat and fascia should be excised, and the wound should be left open. A second procedure 24 to 48 hours later is indicated if there is any question about the adequacy of initial debridement. Orchiectomy is almost never required since the testes have their own blood supply independent of the compromised fascial and cutaneous circulation to the scrotum. Suprapubic diversion should be performed in cases where urethral trauma or extravasation is suspected. Colostomy should be performed if there is colonic or rectal perforation. Hyperbaric oxygen therapy has shown some promise in shortening hospital stays, increasing wound healing, and decreasing the gangrenous spread when used in conjunction with debridement and antibiotics (Paty and Smith, 1992). Once wound healing is complete, reconstruction, for example, using myocutaneous flaps, improves cosmetic results.

Outcome

The mortality rate averages approximately 20% (Cohen, 1986; Baskin et al, 1990; Clayton et al, 1990), but ranges from 7% to 75%. **Higher mortality rates are found in diabetics, alcoholics, and those with colorectal sources of infection who often have a less typical presentation, greater delay in diagnosis, and more widespread exten-**

sion. Regardless of the presentation, Fournier's gangrene is a true urologic emergency that demands early recognition, aggressive treatment with antibiotics, and surgical debridement in order to reduce morbidity and mortality.

Periurethral Abscess

Periurethral abscess is a life-threatening infection of the male urethra and periurethral tissues. Initially the area of involvement can be small and localized by Buck's fascia. However, when Buck's fascia is penetrated, there can be extensive necrosis of the subcutaneous tissue and fascia. Fasciitis can spread as far as the buttocks posteriorly and the clavicle superiorly. Rapid diagnosis and treatment are essential to reduce the morbidity and high mortality historically associated with this disease.

Pathophysiology

Periurethral abscess is frequently a sequela of gonorrhea, urethral stricture disease, or urethral catheterization. Frequent instrumentation is also associated with periurethral abscess formation. The source of the infecting organism is the urine. Gram-negative rods, enterococci, and anaerobes are most frequently identified. The presence of multiple organisms is common. Anaerobes, normal residents of the male urethra, are also frequently found in wound cultures.

Clinical Presentation

Presenting signs and symptoms includes scrotal swelling in 94% of patients, fever (70%), acute urinary retention (19%), spontaneously drained abscess (11%), and dysuria or urethral discharge (5% to 8%) (Walther et al, 1987). The average interval between initial symptoms and presentation is 21 days. Urinalysis of the first glass specimen reveals pyuria and bacteriuria.

Management

Treatment consists of immediate suprapubic urinary drainage and wide debridement. Antimicrobial therapy with an aminoglycoside and a cephalosporin is usually adequate for empirical coverage. More selective antimicrobial therapy can be instituted when the antimicrobial susceptibility of the organisms is available. Perineal urethrostomy or chronic suprapubic diversion occasionally has been helpful to prevent recurrences, and it should be considered in patients with diffuse stricture disease. **The presence of a malignancy is unusual, but biopsy is important.**

REFERENCES

Abrabomwicz M: Prevention of bacterial endocarditis. Med Lett 1984; 26:3.

Abrutyn E, Mossey J, Berlin JA, et al: Does asymptomatic bacteriuria predict mortality and does antimicrobial treatment reduce mortality in elderly ambulatory women? Ann Intern Med 1994; 120:827.

Acar JF, Francoual S: The clinical problems of bacterial resistance to the new quinolones. J Antimicrob Chemother 1990; 26(suppl B):207.

Achtman M, Mercer A, Kusecek B, et al: Six widespread bacterial clones among *Escherichia coli* K1 isolates. Infect Immun 1983; 39:315.

Akerlund AS: Urinary antibodies to *Escherichia coli* bacteria in childhood urinary tract infections. Technical Report. University of Goteborg, Sweden, 1978.

Alexander HR, Doherty GM, Buresh CM, et al: A recombinant human receptor antagonist to interleukin 1 improved survival after lethal endotoxemia in mice. J Exp Med 1991; 173:1029.

Alwall N: Screening for urinary tract infection in non-pregnant women. Kidney Int 1975; Suppl 4:S107.

Anderson KA, McAninch JW: Renal abscesses: Classification and review of 40 cases. Urol 1980; 16:333.

Anderson RU: Prophylaxis of bacteriuria during intermittent catheterization of the acute neurogenic bladder. J Urol 1980; 123:364.

Angel JL, O'Brien WF, Finan MA, et al: Acute pyelonephritis in pregnancy: A prospective study of oral versus intravenous antibiotic therapy. Obstet Gynecol 1990; 76:28.

Anhalt MA, Cawood CD, Scott R Jr: Xanthogranulomatous pyelonephritis: A comprehensive review with report of 4 additional cases. J Urol 1971: 105:10.

Annual Summary of Births, Marriages, Divorces, and Deaths; United States. 1988. Hyattsville, Md, US Department of Health and Human Services, Public Health Service, CDC, 1989, p 7. Monthly vital statistics report 1989; 37(13).

Aoki S, Imamura S, Aoki M, et al: "Abacterial" and bacterial pyelonephritis. Immunofluorescent localization of bacterial antigen. N Engl J Med 1969; 281:1375.

Aronson M, Medalia O, Schori L, et al: Prevention of colonization of the urinary tract of mice with *Escherichia coli* by blocking of bacterial adherence with methyl-α-b-mannuside. J Infect Dis 1979; 139:329.

Ashby EC, Rees M, Dowding CH: Prophylaxis against systemic infection after transrectal biopsy for suspected prostatic carcinoma. Br Med J 1978; 2:1263.

Asscher AW, Chick S, Radford N, et al: Natural history of asymptomatic bacteriuria (ASB) in non-pregnant women. *In* Brumfitt W, Asscher AW, eds: Urinary Tract Infection. London, Oxford University Press, 1973, p 51.

Asscher AW, Sussman M, Waters WE, et al: Asymptomatic significant bacteriuria in the non-pregnant woman. II: Response to treatment and follow-up. Br Med J 1969; 1:804.

Asscher AW, Sussman M, Waters WE, et al: The clinical significance of asymptomatic bacteriuria in the nonpregnant woman. J Infect Dis 1969b; 120:17.

Backhouse CI, Matthews JA: Single-dose enoxacin compared with 3-day treatment for urinary tract infections. Antimicrob Agents Chemother 1989; 33:877.

Baga M, Normark S, Hardy J, et al: Nucleotide sequence of the *PapA* gene encoding the PapA pilus subunit of human uropathogenic *Escherichia coli*. J Bacteriol 1984; 157:330.

Bailey RR: Single Dose Therapy of Urinary Tract Infections. Sydney, Australia, AIDS Health Science Press, 1983, pp 1–125.

Bailey RR, Little PJ, Rolleston GL: Renal damage after acute pyelonephritis. Br Med J 1969; 1:550.

Bailey et al, 1971 (T 15–19).

Baldassarre JS, Kaye D: Special problems of urinary tract infections in the elderly. Med Clin North Am 1991; 75:375.

Ballesteros JJ, Faus R, Gironella J: Preoperative diagnosis of renal xanthogranulomatosis by serial urine cytology: Preliminary report. J Urol 1980; 124:9.

Barth KH, Lightman NI, Ridolfi RL, et al: Acute pyelonephritis simulating poorly vascularized renal neoplasm, non-specificity of angiographic criteria. J Urol 1976; 116:650.

Bartlett JG, Gorbach SL: Anaerobic bacteria in suppurative infections of the male genitourinary system. J Urol 1981; 125:376.

Baskin LS, Carroll PR, Cattolica EV, et al: Necrotizing soft tissue infections of the perineum and genitalia: Bacteriology, treatment, and risk assessment. Br J Urol 1990; 65:524.

Baurienne H: Sur une plaie contuse qui s'est terminée par la sphacale de le scrotum. J Med Chir Pharm 1764; 20:251.

Bear RA: Pregnancy in patients with renal disease: A study of 44 cases. Obstet Gynecol 1976; 48:13.

Bejanga BE: Fournier's gangrene. Br J Urol 1979; 51:312.

Biello DR, Levitt RG, Melson GL: The roles of Gallium-67 scintigraphy, ultrasonography, and computed tomography in the detection of abdominal abscesses. Semin Nucl Med 1979; 9:58.

Bilges H, Brod J, Christ M, et al: Diagnosis of renal and urinary tract infection by recent techniques. Contrib Nephrol 1979; 16:27.
Bille J, Glauser MP: Protection against chronic pyelonephritis in rats by suppression of acute suppuration: Effect of colchicine and neutropenia. J Infect Dis 1982; 146:220.
Bloom S, Gonick P: Urine sterilization in catheter drainage bottles. Invest Urol 1969; 6:527.
Blum RN, Wright RA: Detection of pyuria and bacteriuria in symptomatic ambulatory women. J Gen Intern Med 1992; 7:140.
Bone RC: Sepsis, the sepsis syndrome, multi-organ failure: A plea for comparable definitions. (Editorial.) Ann Intern Med 1991a; 114:332.
Bone RC: The pathogenesis of sepsis. Ann Intern Med 1991b; 115:457.
Bone RC, Fisher CJ, Clemmer TP, et al: A controlled clinical trial of high-dose methylprednisolone in the treatment of severe sepsis and septic shock. N Engl J Med 1987; 317:653.
Bone RC, Fisher CJ Jr, Clemmer TP, et al: Sepsis syndrome: A valid clinical entity. Crit Care Med 1989; 17:389.
Boscia JA, Kaye D: Asymptomatic bacteriuria in the elderly. Infect Dis Clin North Am 1987; 1:893.
Boscia JA, Kobasa WD, Knight RA, et al: Epidemiology of bacteriuria in an elderly ambulatory population. Am J Med 1986; 80:208.
Boscia JA, Kobasa WD, Knight RA, et al: Therapy vs no therapy for bacteriuria in elderly ambulatory nonhospitalized women. JAMA 1987; 257:1067.
Bowers JH, Cathey WJ: Malakoplakia of the kidney with renal failure. Am J Clin Pathol 1971; 55:765.
Braude AI: Current concepts of pyelonephritis. Medicine 1973; 52:257.
Brehmer B, Madsen PO: Route and prophylaxis of ascending bladder infection in male patients with indwelling catheters. J Urol 1972; 108:719.
Brenbridge AN, Buschi AJ, Cochrane JA, et al: Renal emphysema of the transplanted kidney: Sonographic appearance. AJR 1979; 132:656.
Brinton CC Jr: Non-flagellar appendages of bacteria. Nature 1959; 183:782.
Brinton CC Jr: The structure, function, synthesis, and genetic control of bacterial pili and a molecular model for DNA and RNA transport in gram-negative bacteria. Trans NY Acad Sci 1965; 27:1003.
Brocklehurst JC, Bee P, Jones D, et al: Bacteriuria in geriatric hospital patients, its correlates and management. Age Ageing 1977; 62:240.
Brocklehurst JL, Dillane JB, Griffiths LL, et al: Prevalence and symptomatology of urinary infection in an aged population. Gerontol Clin 1968; 10:242–253.
Bromberg K, Gleich S, Ginsberg MB: Clostridia in urinary tract infections. South Med J 1982; 75:1298.
Brooker WJ, Aufderheide AC: Genitourinary tract infections due to atypical mycobacteria. J Urol 1980; 124:242.
Brooks SJD, Lyons JM, Braude AI: Immunization against retrograde pyelonephritis. III: Vaccination against chronic pyelonephritis due to *Escherichia coli.* J Infect Dis 1977; 136:633.
Brumfitt W, Pursell R: Trimethoprim-sulfamethoxazole in the treatment of bacteriuria in women. J Infect Dis 1973; 128:S657.
Brumfitt W, Faiers MC, Franklin IN: The treatment of urinary infection by means of a single dose of cephaloridine. Postgrad Med J 1970; 46:65.
Buckley RJ, Smith S, Herschorn S, et al: Echinococcal disease of the kidney presenting as a renal filling defect. J Urol 1985; 133:660.
Buckwold FJ, Ludwig P, Harding GK, et al: Therapy for acute cystitis in adult women: Randomized comparison of single-dose sulfisoxazole vs. trimethoprim-sulfamethoxazole. JAMA 1982; 247:1839.
Budde E, Naumann G, Nimmich W, et al: Antibody-coating of bacteria in the urine in relation to various immunologic indexes. Kidney Int 1981; 19:65.
Bultitude MI, Eykyn S: The relationship between the urethral flora and urinary infection in the catheterised male. Br J Urol 1973; 45:678.
Buonocore E, Vidt DG, Montie JE: Ultrasonography in the diagnosis of obstructive uropathy caused by papillary necrosis. Cleve Clin Q 1980; 47:109.
Burman LG: Significance of the sulfonamide component for the clinical efficacy of trimethoprim-sulfonamide combinations. Scand J Infect Dis 1986; 18:89.
Burpee JF, Edwards P: Fournier's gangrene. Br J Urol 1972; 107:812.
Busch R, Huland H: Correlation of symptoms and results of direct bacterial localization in patients with urinary tract infections. J Urol 1984; 132:282.
Calandra T, Baumgartner JD, Grau GE, et al: Prognostic values of tumor necrosis factor/cachectin, interleukin-1, interferon-alpha and interferon-gamma in the serum of patients with septic shock. Swiss-Dutch J5 Immunoglobulin Study Group. J Infect Dis 1990; 161:982.
Calandra T, Glauser MP, Schellekens J, Verhoef J, the Swiss-Dutch J5 Immunoglobulin Study Group: Treatment of gram-negative septic shock with human IgG antibody to *Escherichia coli* J5: A prospective, double-blind, randomized trial. J Infect Dis 1988; 158:312.
Callea F, Van Damme B, Desmet VJ: Alpha-1-antitrypsin in malakoplakia. Virchows Arch A 1982; 395:1.
Callen PW: Computed tomographic evaluation of abdominal and pelvic abscesses. Radiology 1979; 131:171.
Cameron DD, Azimi F: The value of excretory urography in the diagnosis of acute pyelonephritis. J Urol 1974; 112:546.
Campbell MF: Perinephric abscess. Surg Gynecol Obstet 1930; 51:654.
Camunez F, Echenagusia A, Prieto ML, et al: Percutaneous nephrostomy in pyonephrosis. Urol Radiol 1989; 11:77.
Carlson KJ, Mulley AG: Management of acute dysuria: A decision-analysis model of alternative strategies. Ann Intern Med 1985; 102:244.
Carroll B, Silverman PM, Goodwin DA, et al: Ultrasonography and indium 111 white blood cell scanning for the detection of intraabdominal abscesses. Radiology 1981; 140:155.
Carroll KC, Hale DC, vonBoerum DH, et al: Laboratory evaluation of urinary tract infections in an ambulatory clinic. Am J Clin Pathol 1994; 101:100.
Cartwright KA, Stanbridge TN, Cooper J: Comparison of once daily trimethoprim and standard co-trimoxazole in urinary infections: A clinical trial in general practice. Practitioner 1982; 226:152.
Carty M, Brocklehurst JC, Carty J: Bacteriuria and its correlates in old age. Gerontology 1981; 27:72.
Cavins JA, Goldstein AMB: Renal malakoplakia. Urology 1977; 10:155.
Chan RCY, Bruce AW, Reid G: Adherence of cervical, vaginal, and distal urethral normal microbial flora to human uroepithelial cells and the inhibition of adherence of gram-negative uropathogens by competitive exclusion. J Urol 1984; 131:596.
Charlton CAC, Crowther A, Davies JG, et al: Three-day and ten-day chemotherapy for urinary tract infections in general practice. Br Med J 1976; 1:124.
Christ W, Lehnert T, Ulbrich B: Specific toxicologic aspects to the quinolones. Rev Infect Dis 1988; 10:141.
Cifuentes L: Epithelium of vaginal type in the female trigone: The clinical problem of trigonitis. J Urol 1947; 57:1028.
Clayton MD, Fowler JE Jr, Sharifi R: Causes, presentation, and survival of 57 patients with necrotizing fasciitis of the male genitalia. Surg Gynecol Obstet 1990; 170:49.
Cockerill FR, Edson RS: Trimethoprim-sulfamethoxazole. Mayo Clin Proc 66:1249, 1991.
Cohen MS: Fournier's gangrene. AUA Update Series 1986; 5(6).
Coleman BG, Arger PH, Mulhern CB Jr, et al: Pyonephrosis: Sonography in the diagnosis and management. Am J Roentgenol 1981; 137:939.
Coltorti EA, Varela-Diaz VM: Detection of antibodies against *Echinococcus granulosus* arc 5 antigens by double diffusion test. Trans R Soc Trop Med Hyg 1978; 72:226.
Conrad MR, Bregman R, Kilman WJ: Ultrasonic recognition of parenchymal gas. AJR 1979; 132:395.
Conrad MR, Sanders RC, Mascardo AD: Perinephric abscess aspiration using ultrasound guidance. Am J Roentgenol 1977; 128:459.
Cooke EM, Ewins SP: Properties of strains of *Escherichia coli* isolated from a variety of sources. J Med Microbiol 1975; 8:107.
Corriere JN, Sandler CM: The diagnosis and immediate therapy of acute renal and perirenal infections. Urol Clin North Am 1982; 9:219.
Cotran RS: Experimental pyelonephritis. *In* Rouiller C, Muller AF, eds: The Kidney, Vol 2. New York, Academic Press, 1969, pp 269–361.
Cotran RS, Piessens WF: Pathogenesis of chronic pyelonephritis. *In* Proceedings of the 6th International Congress of Nephrology. Basel, 1976, p 509.
Crawford ED, Haynes AL, Story MW, et al: Prevention of urinary tract infection and sepsis following transrectal prostatic biopsy. J Urol 1982; 127:449.
Cunningham FG, Morris GB, Mickal A: Acute pyelonephritis of pregnancy: A clinical review. Obstet Gynecol 1973; 42:112.
Cunnion RE, Parrillo JE: Myocardial dysfunction in sepsis. Recent insights. Chest 1989; 95:941.
Daikos GK, Kontomichalou P, Bilalis D, et al: Intestinal flora ecology after oral use of antibiotics (terramycin, chloramphenicol, ampicillin, neomycin, paromomycin, aminodidin). Chemotherapy, 1968; 13:146.
Dalkin BL, Schaeffer AJ: Fluoroquinolone antimicrobial agents: Use in the treatment of urinary tract infections and clinical urologic practice. Probl Urol 1988; 2:476.

Datta N, Faiers MC, Reeves DS, et al: R-factors in *Escherichia coli* in feces after oral chemotherapy in general practice. Lancet 1971; 1:312.

Davidson AJ, Talner LB: Urographic and angiographic abnormalities in adult-onset acute bacterial nephritis. Radiology 1973; 106:249.

Davies AG, McLachlan MS, Asscher AW: Progressive kidney damage after non-obstructive urinary tract infection. Br Med J 1972; 4:406.

Davies BI, Maesen FPV: Drug interactions with quinolones. Rev Infect Dis 1989; 11(5):1083.

Davison JM, Lindheimer MD: Renal disease in pregnant women. Clin Obstet Gynecol 1978; 21:411.

DeNavasquez S: Experimental pyelonephritis in the rabbit produced by staphylococcal infection. J Pathol 1950; 62:429.

De Ree JM, Schwillens P, van den Bosch JF: Monoclonal antibodies that recognize the P-fimbriae $F7_1$, $F7_2$, F9 and F11 from uropathogenic *Escherichia coli*. Infect Immun 1985; 50:900.

Deridder PA, Koff SA, Gikas PW, et al: Renal malakoplakia. J Urol 1977; 117:428.

Dontas AS, Kasviki-Charvati P, Papanayiotou PC, et al: Bacteriuria and survival in old age. N Engl J Med 1981; 304:939.

Dontas S, Papanayiotou P, Marketos SG, et al: The effect of bacteriuria on renal functional patterns in old age. Clin Sci 1968; 34:73.

Dudley MN, Barriere SL: Antimicrobial irrigations in the prevention and treatment of catheter-related urinary tract infections. Am J Hosp Pharm 1981; 38:59.

Duguid JP, Anderson ES, Campbell I: Fimbriae and adhesive properties in salmonellae. J Pathol Bacteriol 1966; 92:107.

Duguid JP, Clegg S, Wilson MI: The fimbrial and nonfimbrial haemagglutinins of *Escherichia coli*. J Med Microbiol 1979; 12:213.

DuPont HL, Spink WW: Infections due to gram-negative organisms: An analysis of 860 patients with bacteremia at the University of Minnesota Medical Center, 1958–1966. Medicine 1969; 48:307.

Durack DT: Prophylaxis of infective endocarditis. *In* Mandell GL, Douglas RG, Bennett JE, eds: Principles and Practice of Infectious Diseases, ed 3. New York, Churchill Livingstone, 1990, 716–721.

Edelstein H, McCabe RE: Perinephric abscess. Medicine 1988; 67:118.

Eisentein BI: Phase variation of type-1 fimbriae in *Escherichia coli* is under transcriptional control. Science 1981; 214:337.

Eknoyan G, Quinibi WY, Grissom RT, et al: Renal papillary necrosis: An update. Medicine 1982; 61:55.

Elder HA, Santamarina BA, Smith S, et al: The natural history of asymptomatic bacteriuria during pregnancy: The effect of tetracycline on the clinical course and the outcome of pregnancy. Am J Obstet Gynecol 1971; 111:441.

Elliott TSJ, et al: Bacteriology and ultrastructure of the bladder in patients with urinary tract infections. J Infect 1985; 11:191.

Elyaderani MK, Subramanian VP, Burgess JE: Diagnosis and percutaneous drainage of a perinephric abscess by ultrasound and fluoroscopy. J Urol 1981; 125:405.

Engel G, Schaeffer AJ, Grayhack JT, et al: The role of excretory urography and cystoscopy in the evaluation and management of women with recurrent urinary tract infection. J Urol 1980; 123:190.

Erno H, Thomsen AC: Immunoglobulin classes of urinary and serum antibodies in mycoplasmal pyelonephritis. Acta Pathol Microbiol Scand 1980; 88:237.

Esparza AR, McKay DB, Cronan JJ, et al: Renal parenchymal malakoplakia. Histologic spectrum and its relationship to megalocytic interstitial nephritis and xanthogranulomatous pyelonephritis. Am J Surg Pathol 1989; 13:225.

Fader RC, Davis CP: *Klebsiella pneumoniae*–induced experimental pyelitis: The effect of piliation on infectivity. J Urol 1982; 128:197.

Fair WR, Crane DB, Peterson LJ, et al: Three-day treatment of urinary tract infections. J Urol 1980; 123:717.

Fair WR, McClennan BL, Jost RG: Are excretory urograms necessary in evaluating women with urinary tract infection? J Urol 1979; 121:313.

Fairchild TN, Shuman W, Berger RE: Radiographic studies for women with recurrent urinary tract infections. J Urol 1982; 128:344.

Fairley KF, Bond AG, Adey FD: The site of infection in pregnancy bacteriuria. Lancet 1966; 1:939.

Fairly KF, Bond AG, Brown RB, Habersberge EB: Simple test to determine one site of urinary tract infection. Lancet 1967; 2(513):427–428.

Fairley KF, Grounds AD, Carson NE, et al: Site of infection in acute urinary-tract infection in general practice. Lancet 1971; 2:615.

Fairley KF, Hubbard M, Whitworth JA: Prophylactic long-term cephalexin in recurrent urinary infection. Med J Aust 1974; 1:318.

Fairley KF, Whitworth JA, Radford NJ, et al: Pregnancy bacteriuria: The significance of site of infection. Med J Aust 1973; 2:424.

Falkiner FR, Ma PT, Murphy DM, et al: Antimicrobial agents for the prevention of urinary tract infection in transurethral surgery. J Urol 1983; 129:766.

Feldberg MA: Bilateral adult-onset acute bacterial pyelonephritis and its late unusual sequelae: A case report. Diagn Imaging 1982; 51:296.

Fernandez JA, Miles BJ, Buck AS, et al: Renal carbuncle: Comparison between surgical open drainage and closed percutaneous drainage. Urology 1985; 25:142.

Fiegler W: Ultrasound in acute renal inflammatory lesions. Eur J Radiol 1983; 3:354.

Fierer J, Talner L, Braude AI: Bacteremia in the pathogenesis of retrograde *E. coli* pyelonephritis in the rat. Am J Pathol 1971; 64:443.

Fihn SD, Johnson C, Roberts PL, et al: Trimethoprim-sulfamethoxazole for acute dysuria in women: A single-dose or 10-day course: A double-blind, randomized trial. Ann Intern Med 1988; 108:350.

Fihn SD, Latham RH, Roberts P, et al: Association between diaphragm use and urinary tract infection. JAMA 1985; 254:240.

Fincke BG, Friedland G: Prevention and management of infection in the catheterized patient. Urol Clin North Am 1976; 3:313.

Finegold SM: Urinary tract infections. *In* Finegold SM, ed: Anaerobic Bacteria in Human Disease. New York, Academic Press, 1977, pp 311–349.

Finn DJ, Palestrant AM, DeWolf WC: Successful percutaneous management of renal abscess. J Urol 1982; 127:425.

Flynn JT, Molland EA, Paris AMI, et al: The underestimated hazards of xanthogranulomatous pyelonephritis. Br J Urol 1979; 51:433.

Forland M, Thomas V, Shelokov A: Urinary tract infections in patients with diabetes mellitus: Studies on antibody coating of bacteria. JAMA 1977; 238:1924.

Fournier JA: Étude clinicque de la gangrène-foudroyante de la verge. Semin Med 1884; 4:69.

Fournier JA: Gangrène-foudroyante de la verge. Semin Med 1883; 3:345.

Forsum U, Hjelm E, Jonsell G: Antibody-coated bacteria in the urine of children with urinary tract infections. Acta Paediatr Scand 1976; 65:639.

Fowler JE, Pulaski ET: Excretory urography, cystography, and cystocopy in the evaluation of women with urinary-tract infection: A prospective study. N Engl J Med 1981; 304:462.

Fowler JE Jr, Stamey TA: Studies of introital colonization in women with recurrent urinary infections. VII: The role of bacterial adherence. J Urol 1977; 117:472.

Freedman LR: Natural history of urinary infection in adults. Kidney Int 1975; 8(5):96.

Freedman LR: Interstitial renal inflammation, including pyelonephritis and urinary tract infections. *In* Early LE, Gottschalk CW, eds: Strauss and Welt's Diseases of the Kidney, 3rd ed, Vol 2. Boston, Little, Brown and Company, 1979, pp 817.

Freiha FS, Messing EM, Gross DM: Emphysematous pyelonephritis. J Contin Ed Urol 1979; 18:9.

Fried FA, Vermeulen CW, Ginsburg MJ, et al: Etiology of pyelonephritis; further evidence associating the production of experimental pyelonephritis with hemolysis in *Escherichia coli*. J Urol 1971; 106:351.

Friedland GW, Stamey TA: Recurrent urinary tract infection: With persistent Wolffian duct masquerading as duplicated urethra. Urology 1974; 4:315.

Funston AR, Fisher KS, vanBlerk JP, et al: Acute focal bacterial nephritis or renal abscess? A sonographic diagnosis. Br J Urol 1982; 54:461.

Garibaldi RA, Burke JP, Britt MR, et al: Meatal colonization and catheter-associated bacteriuria. N Engl J Med 1980; 303:316.

Garibaldi RA, Burke JP, Dickman ML, et al: Factors predisposing to bacteriuria during indwelling urethral catheterization. N Engl J Med 1974; 291:215.

Gaymans R, Haverkorn MJ, Valkenburg HA, et al: A prospective study of urinary-tract infections in a Dutch general practice. Lancet 1976; 2:674.

Gerstner GJ, Muller G, Nahler G: Amoxicillin in the treatment of asymptomatic bacteriuria in pregnancy: A single dose of 3 g amoxicillin versus a 4-day course of 3 doses 750 mg amoxicillin. Gynecol Obstet Invest 1989; 27:84.

Gerzof SG, Gale ME: Computed tomography and ultrasonography for diagnosis and treatment of renal and retroperitoneal abscesses. Urol Clin North Am 1982; 9:185.

Ghosh H: Chronic pyelonephritis with xanthogranulomatous change: A report of three cases. Am J Clin Pathol 1955; 25:1043.

Gibbons RP, Stark RA, Correa RJ Jr, et al: The prophylactic use or misuse of antibiotics in transurethral prostatectomy. J Urol 1978; 119:381.

Gillenwater JY, Harrison RB, Kunin CM: Natural history of bacteriuria in school girls: A long-term case-control study. N Engl J Med 1979; 301:396.

Gilsanz V, Lozano G, Jimenez J: Renal hydatid cysts: Communicating with collecting system. AJR 1980; 135:357.

Gilstrap LC, Leveno KJ, Cunningham FG, et al: Renal infection and pregnancy outcome. Am J Ostet Gynecol 1981; 141:709.

Girardin E, Grau GE, Dayer JM, et al: Tumor necrosis factor and interleukin-1 in the serum of children with severe infectious purpura. N Engl J Med 1988; 319:397.

Glauser MP, Heumann D, Baumgartner JD, Cohen J: Pathogenesis and potential strategies for prevention and treatment of septic shock: An update. Clin Infect Dis 1994; 18(Suppl 2):S205–S216.

Glauser MP, Lyons JM, Braude AI: Prevention of chronic experimental pyelonephritis by suppression of acute suppuration. J Clin Invest 1978; 61:403.

Gleckman RA: Treatment duration for urinary tract infection in adults. Antimicrob Agents Chemother 1987; 31:1.

Gleckman R, Blagg N, Hibert D, et al: Community-acquired bacteremic urosepsis in the elderly patients: A prospective study of 34 consecutive episodes. J Urol 1982; 128:79.

Goldman SM, Hartman DS, Fishman EK, et al: CT of xanthogranulomatous pyelonephritis: Radiologic-pathologic correlation. AJR 1984; 141:963.

Gonzalez R, Wright R, Blackard CE: Prophylactic antibiotics in transurethral prostatectomy. J Urol 1976; 116:203.

Goodman M, Curry T, Russell T: Xanthogranulomatous pyelonephritis (XGP): A local disease with systemic manifestations: Report of 23 patients and review of the literature. Medicine 1979; 58:171.

Goransson M, Uhlin BE: Environmental temperature regulates transcription of a virulence pili operon in *E. coli.* EMBO J 1984; 12:2885.

Gorbach SL, Bartlett JG: Anaerobic infections (second of three parts). N Engl J Med 1974; 209:1237.

Gower PE: A prospective study of patients with radiological pyelonephritis, papillary necrosis, and obstructive atrophy. Q J Med 1976; 45:315.

Gower PE: The use of small doses of cephalexin (125 mg) in the management of recurrent urinary tract infection in women. J Antimicrob Chemother 1975; 1(suppl. 3):93.

Gratacos E, Torres PJ, Vila J, et al: Screening and treatment of asymptomatic bacteriuria in pregnancy prevent pyelonephritis. J Infect Dis 1994; 169:1390.

Greenberg RN, Sanders CV, Lewis AC, et al: Single-dose cefaclor therapy of urinary tract infection. Evaluation of antibody-coated bacteria test and C-reactive protein assay as predictors of cure. Am J Med 1981; 71:841.

Greenman RL, Schein RM, Martin MA, et al: A controlled clinical trial of E5 murine monoclonal IgM antibody to endotoxin in the treatment of gram-negative sepsis. The XOMA Sepsis Study Group. JAMA 1991; 266:1097.

Grieco MH: Use of antibiotics in the elderly. Bull NY Acad Med 1980; 56:197.

Gross PA, Harkavy LM, Barden GE, et al: The fallacy of cultures of the tips of Foley catheters. Surg Gynecol Obstet 1974; 139:597.

Gruneberg RN, Smellie JM, Leaky A: Changes in the antibiotic sensitivities of faecal organisms in response to treatment in children with urinary tract infection. *In* Brumfitt W, Asscher AW, eds: Urinary Tract Infection. London, Oxford University Press, 1973, p 131.

Guttmann D: Follow-up of urinary tract infection in domiciliary patients. *In* Brumfitt W, Asscher AW, eds: Urinary Tract Infection. London, Oxford University Press, 1973, p 62.

Guze LB, Silverblatt F, Montgomerie JZ, et al: Lack of significance of pili in experimental ascending *Escherichia coli* pyelonephritis. Scand J Infect Dis 1983; 15:57.

Haaga JR, Weinstein AJ: CT guided percutaneous aspiration and drainage of abscesses. Am J Roentgenol 1980; 135:1187.

Hagberg L, Engberg I, Freter R, et al: Ascending unobstructed urinary tract infection in mice caused by pyelonephritogenic *Escherichia coli* of human origin. Infect Immun 1983a; 40:273.

Hagberg L, Hull R, Hull S, et al: Contribution of adhesion to bacterial persistence in the mouse urinary tract. Infect Immun 1983b; 40:265.

Haley RW, Culver DH, White JW, Morgan WM, Emori TG: The nationwide nosocomial infection rate: A new need for vital statistics. Am J Epidemiol 1985; 121:159.

Hall JR, Choa RG, Wells IP: Percutaneous drainage in emphysematous pyelonephritis—An alternative to major surgery. Clin Radiol 1988; 39:622.

Hall LM, Duke B, Urwin G, et al: Epidemiology of *Enterococcus faecalis* urinary tract infection in a teaching hospital in London, United Kingdom. J Clin Microbiol 1992; 30:1953.

Halstensen A, Ceska M, Brandtzaeg P, et al: Interleukin-8 in serum and cerebrospinal fluid from patients with meningococcal disease. J Infect Dis 1993; 67:471.

Hampel N, Class RN, Persky L: Value of ^{67}gallium scintigraphy in the diagnosis of localized and renal and perirenal inflammation. J Urol 1980; 124:311.

Hanson LA, Ahlstedt S, Jodal U, et al: The host-parasite relationship in urinary tract infections. Kidney Int 1975; suppl. 4:S28.

Harber MJ, Mackenzie R, Chick S, et al: Lack of adherence to epithelial cells by freshly isolated urinary pathogens. Lancet 1982; 1:586.

Harbord RB, Grüneberg RN: Treatment of urinary tract infections with a single dose of amoxycillin, co-trimoxazole, or trimethoprim. Br Med J 1981; 283:1301.

Harding GKM, Marrie TJ, Ronald AR, et al: Urinary tract infection localization in women. JAMA 1978; 240:1147.

Harding GK, Ronald AR, Nicolle LE, et al: Long-term antimicrobial prophylaxis for recurrent urinary tract infection in women. Rev Infect Dis 1982; 4:438.

Hargreave TB, Hindmarsh JR, Elton R, et al: Short-term prophylaxis with cefotaxime for prostatic surgery. Br Med J 1982; 284:1008.

Harris RE: Antibiotic therapy of antepartum urinary tract infections. J Int Med Res 1980; 8:40.

Harris RE: The significance of eradication of bacteriuria during pregnancy. Obstet Gynecol 1979; 53:71.

Harris RE, Thomas VL, Shelokov A: Asymptomatic bacteriuria in pregnancy. Antibody-coated bacteria, renal function, and intrauterine growth retardation. Am J Obstet Gynecol 1976; 126:20.

Harrison RB, Shaffer HA Jr: The roentgenographic findings in acute pyelonephritis. JAMA 1979; 241:1718.

Harrison WO, Holmes KK, Belding ME, et al: A prospective evaluation of recurrent urinary tract infection in women. Clin Res 1974; 22:125A.

Hartman DS: Radiologic pathologic correlation of the infectious granulomatous diseases of the kidney: Parts I and II. Monogr Urol 1985a; 6:3.

Hartman DS: Radiologic pathologic correlation of the infectious granulomatous diseases of the kidney. Parts III and IV. Monogr Urol 1985b; 6:26.

Hartman DS, Davis CJ, Lichtenstein JE, et al: Renal parenchymal malakoplakia. Radiology 1980; 136:33.

Hawes S, Whigham T, Ehrmann S, et al: Emphysematous pyelonephritis. Infect Surg 1983; 2:191.

Hawthorne NJ, Kurtz SB, Anhalt JP, et al: Accuracy of antibody-coated-bacteria test in recurrent urinary tract infections. Mayo Clin Proc 1978; 53:651.

Hedman P, Ringertz O: Urinary tract infections caused by *Staphylococcus saprophyticus:* A matched case control study, J Infect 1991; 23:144–153.

Heineman HS, Lee JH: Bacteriuria in pregnancy: A heterogeneous entity. Obstet Gynecol 1973; 41:22.

Hellerstein S, Kennedy E, Nussbaum L, et al: Localization of the site of urinary tract infections by means of antibody-coated bacteria in the urinary sediments. J Pediatr 1978; 92:188.

Herlitz H, Westberg G, Nilson AE: A perinephric abscess in a diabetic woman: Successful conservative treatment. A case report. Scand J Urol Nephrol 1981; 15:337.

Hernandez GV, King AS, Needle MA: Nephrosis and papillary necrosis after pyelonephritis. N Engl J Med 1975; 293:1347.

Hinton NA: The effect of oral tetracycline HCl and doxycycline on the intestinal flora. Curr Ther Res 1970; 12:341.

Hoddick W, Jeffrey RB, Goldberg HI, et al: CT and sonography of severe renal and perirenal infections. Am J Roentgenol 1983; 140:517.

Hoffer P: Gallium and infection. J Nucl Med 1980; 21:484.

Hoffman JC, Schnur MJ, Koenigsberg M: Demonstration of renal papillary necrosis by sonography. Radiology 1982; 145:785.

Holmberg L, Boman G, Bottiger LE, et al: Adverse reactions to nitrofurantoin: Analysis of 921 reports. Am J Med 1980; 69:733.

Hootkins R, Fenzer AZ, Stephens MK: Acute renal failure secondary to oral ciprofloxacin therapy: A presentation of three cases and a review of the literature. Clin Nephrol 32:75, 1989.

Hooton TM, Fennell CL, Clark AM, Stamm WE: Nonoxynol-9: Differential antibacterial activity and enhancement of bacterial adherence to vaginal epithelial cells. J Infect Dis 1991a; 164:1216.

Hooton TM, Fihn SD, Johnson C, et al: Association between bacterial vaginosis and acute cystitis in women using diaphragms. Arch Intern Med 1989a; 149(9):1932–6.

Hooton TM, Hillier S, Johnson C, et al: *Escherichia coli* bacteriuria and contraceptive method. JAMA 1991b; 265:64.

Hooton TM, Johnson C, Winter C, et al: Single-dose and three-day regimens of ofloxacin versus trimethoprim-sulfamethoxazole for acute cystitis in women. Antimicrob Agents Chemother 1991c; 35:1479.

Hooton TM, Latham RH, Wong ES, et al: Ofloxacin versus trimethoprim-sulfamethoxazole for treatment of acute cystitis. Antimicrob Agents Chemother 1989b; 33:1308.

Hooton TM, Running K, Stamm WE: Single-dose therapy for cystitis in women. A comparison of trimethoprim-sulfamethoxazole, amoxicillin, and cyclacillin. JAMA 1985; 253:387.

Hooton TM, Stamm WE: Management of acute uncomplicated urinary tract infections in adults. Med Clin North Am 1991; 75:339.

Hooton TM, Winter C, Kuwamura L, et al: A comparison of amoxicillin (a), cefadroxil (C), nitrofurantoin (N), and trimethoprim/sulfamethoxazole (T/S) in 3-day regimens for the treatment of uncomplicated UTI in women. (Abstract.) *In* Program and Abstracts of the 31st Interscience Conference on Antimicrobial Agents and Chemotherapy. Chicago, September 29–October 2, 1991. Washington, DC, American Society for Microbiology, 1991d, p 260.

Hospital Discharge Survey Rates: Increase in national Hospital Discharge Survey rates for septicemia–United States 1979–1987. MMWR 1989; 39:31.

Hovelius B, Mardh PA: *Staphylococcus saprophyticus* as a common cause of urinary tract infections. Rev Infect Dis 1984; 6(3):328.

Hoverman IV, Gentry LO, Jones DW, et al: Intrarenal abscess: Report of 14 cases. Arch Intern Med 1980; 140:914.

Huland H, Busch R: Chronic pyelonephritis as a cause of end stage renal disease. J Urol 1982; 127:642.

Huland H, Busch R, Riebel T: Renal scarring after symptomatic and asymptomatic upper urinary tract infection: A prospective study. J Urol 1982; 128:682.

Huland H, Gonnermann D, Clausen C: Bacterial localization in patients with end stage renal disease to avoid bilateral nephrectomy before renal transplantation. J Urol 1983; 129:915.

Hull RA, Gill RE, Hsu P, et al: Construction and expression of recombinant plasmids encoding type 1 or D-mannose-resistant pili from a urinary tract infection *Escherichia coli* isolate. Infect Immun 1981; 33:933.

Hultgren SJ, Porter TN, Schaeffer AJ, et al: Role of type 1 pili and effects of phase variation on lower urinary tract infections produced by *Escherichia coli.* Infect Immun 1985; 50:370.

Hultgren SJ, Schwan WR, Schaeffer AJ, et al: Regulation of production of type 1 pili among urinary tract isolates of *Escherichia coli.* Infect Immun 1986; 54:613.

Hurwitz SR, Kessler WO, Alazraki NP, et al: Gallium-67 imaging to localize urinary-tract infections. Br J Radiol 1976; 49:156.

Huvos A, Rocha H: Frequency of bacteriuria in patients with diabetes mellitus: A controlled study. N Engl J Med 1959; 261:1213.

Inter-Nordic Urinary Tract Infection Study Group. Double-blind comparison of 3-day versus 7-day treatment with norfloxacin in symptomatic urinary tract infections. Scand J Infect Dis 1988; 20:619.

Iravani A: Advances in the understanding and treatment of urinary tract infections in young women. Urology 1991; 37:503.

Ireland D, Tacchi D, Bint AJ: Effect of single-dose prophylactic co-trimoxazole on the incidence of gynaecological postoperative urinary tract infection. Br J Obstet Gynaecol 1982; 89:578.

Ispahani P, Pearson NJ, Greenwood D: An analysis of community and hospital-acquired bacteremia in a large teaching hospital in the United Kingdom. Q J Med 1987; 241:427.

Iwahi T, Abe Y, Nakao M, et al: Role of type 1 fimbriae in the pathogenesis of ascending urinary tract infection induced by *Escherichia coli* in mice. Infect Immun 1983; 39:1307.

Jackson GG, Arana-Sialer JA, Andersen BR, et al: Profiles of pyelonephritis. Arch Intern Med 1962; 110:63.

Jameson RM, Heal MR: The surgical management of acute renal papillary necrosis. Br J Surg 1973; 60:428.

Jamieson NV, Everett WG, Bullock KN: Delayed recognition of intersphincteric abscess as underlying case of Fournier's scrotal gangrene. Ann R Coll Surg Engl 1984; 66:434.

Johnson JR, Lyons MF, Pearce W, et al: Therapy for women hospitalized with acute pyelonephritis: A randomized trial of ampicillin versus trimethoprim-sulfamethoxazole for 14 days. J Infect Dis 1991; 163:325.

Johnson JR, Stamm WE: Diagnosis and treatment of acute urinary tract infections. Infect Dis Clin North Am 1987; 1(4):773.

Johnson JR, Stamm WE: Urinary tract infections in women: Diagnosis and treatment. Ann Intern Med 1989; 111:906.

Jordan PA, Iravani A, Richard GA, et al: Urinary tract infections caused by *Staphylococcus saprophyticus.* J Infect Dis 1980; 142:510.

Josephson S, Thomason J, Sturino IS, et al: *Gardnerella vaginalis* in the urinary tract: Incidence and significance in a hospital population. Obstet Gynecol 1988; 71:245.

Juhasz J, Galambos J, Surjan L Jr: Renal actinomycosis associated with bilateral necrosing renal papillitis. Int Urol Nephrol 1980; 12:199.

Kaijser B, Hanson LA, Jodal U, et al: Frequency of *E. coli* K antigens in urinary tract infections in children. Lancet 1977; 1:663.

Kaijser B, Larsson P, Olling S: Protection against ascending *Escherichia coli* pyelonephritis in rats and significance of local immunity. Infect Immun 1978; 20:78.

Kallenius G, Mollby R: Adhesion of *Escherichia coli* to human periurethral cells correlated to mannose-resistant agglutination of human erythrocytes. FEMS Microbiol Lett 1979; 5:295.

Kallenius G, Mollby R, Svenson SB, et al: Occurrence of P-fimbriated *Escherichia coli* in urinary tract infections. Lancet 1981; 2:1369.

Kallenius G, Mollby R, Svenson SB, et al: The Pk antigen as receptor for hemagglutinin of pyelonephritic *Escherichia coli.* FEMS Microbiol Lett 1980; 7:297.

Kallenius G, Winberg J: Bacterial adherence to periurethral epithelial cells in girls prone to urinary-tract infections. Lancet 2:540, 1978.

Kasanen A, Anttila M, Elfving R, et al: Trimethoprim: Pharmacology, antimicrobial activity, and clinical use in urinary tract infections. Ann Clin Res 1978; 10:1.

Kass EH: The role of asymptomatic bacteriuria in the pathogenesis of pyelonephritis. *In* Quinn EL, Kass EH, eds: Biology of Pyelonephritis. Boston, Little, Brown and Company, 1960, p 399.

Kass EH: The role of unsuspected infection in the etiology of prematurity. Clin Obstet Gynecol 1973; 16:134.

Kass EH, Finland M: Asymptomatic infections of the urinary tract. Trans Assoc Am Physicians 1956; 69:56.

Kass EH, Schneiderman LJ: Entry of bacteria into the urinary tracts of patients with inlying catheters. N Engl J Med 1957; 256:556.

Kass EH, Silver TM, Konnak JW, et al: The urographic findings in acute pyelonephritis: Non-obstructive hydronephrosis. J Urol 1976; 116:544.

Kaye D: Urinary tract infections in the elderly. Bull N Y Acad Med 1980; 56:209.

Kearney GP, Carling PC: Fournier's gangrene: An approach in its management. J Urol 1983; 130:695.

Kennedy RP, Plorde JJ, Petersdorf RG: Studies on the epidemiology of *Escherichia coli* infections. IV: Evidence for a nosocomial flora. J Clin Invest 1965; 44:193.

Kessler WO, Gittes RF, Hurwitz SR, et al: Gallium-67 scans in the diagnosis of pyelonephritis. West J Med 1974; 121:91.

Kincaid-Smith P: Management of renal and urinary tract disorders during pregnancy. *In* Harrison JH, Gittes RF, Perlmutter AD, et al, eds: Campbell's Urology. Philadelphia, W. B. Saunders Company, 1979, p 2518.

Kincaid-Smith P, Becker GJ: Reflux nephropathy in the adult. *In* Hodson J, Kincaid-Smith P, eds: Reflux Nephropathy. New York, Masson Publishing USA, 1979, pp 21–28.

Kincaid-Smith P, Bullen M: Bacteriuria in pregnancy. Lancet 1965; 1:395.

Kisielius PV, Schwan WR, Amundsen SK, et al: In vivo expression and variation of *Escherichia coli* type 1 and P pili in the urine of adults with acute urinary tract infections. Infect Immunol 1989; 57:1656.

Klarskov P: Bacteriuria in elderly women. Dan Med Bull 1976; 23:200.

Klastersky J, Daneau D, Swings G, et al: Antibacterial activity in serum and urine as a therapeutic guide in bacterial infections. J Infect Dis 1974; 129:187.

Klemm, P: Fimbrial adhesins of *Escherichia coli.* Rev Infect Dis 1985; 7:321.

Klemm P, Orskov I, Orskov F: F7 and type 1-like fimbriae from three *Escherichia coli* strains isolated from urinary tract infections: Protein chemical and immunological aspects. Infect Immun 1982; 36:462.

Kohnle W, Vanek E, Federlin K, Franz HE: Localization of urinary-tract infection by demonstrating antibody-coated bacteria in urine. Dtsch Med Wochenschr 1975; 100:2598.

Komaroff AL: Acute dysuria in women. N Engl J Med 1984; 310:368.

Komaroff AL: Urinalysis and urine culture in women with dysuria. Ann Intern Med 1986; 104:212.

Konetschnik F, Goldin AR, Marshall VR: Management of "acute renal carbuncle." Br J Urol 1982; 54:467.

Kraft JK, Stamey TA: The natural history of symptomatic recurrent bacteriuria in women. Medicine 1977; 56:55.

Kreger BE, Craven DE, Carling PC, McCabe WR: Gram-negative bacteremia. III: Reassessment of etiology, epidemiology, and ecology in 612 patients. Am J Med 1980; 68:332–343.

Kreiger JN, Kaiser DL, Wenzel RP: Urinary tract etiology of bloodstream infections in hospitalized patients. J Infect Dis 1983; 148:57.

Kuhn JP, Berger PE: Computed tomography of the kidney in infancy and childhood. Radiol Clin North Am, 1981; 19:445.

Kunin CM: Detection, Prevention, and Management of Urinary Tract Infections, 4th ed. Philadelphia, Lea & Febiger, 1987, Chapter 2.

Kunin CM: Duration of treatment of urinary tract infections. Am J Med 1981; 71:849.

Kunin CM: The quantitative significance of bacteriuria visualized in the unstained urinary sediment. N Engl J Med 1961; 265:589.

Kunin CM, Douthitt S, Dancing J, et al: The association between the use of urinary catheters and morbidity and mortality among elderly patients in nursing homes. Am J Epidemiol 1992; 135:291.

Kunin CM, Zacha E, Paquin AJ Jr: Urinary-tract infections in schoolchildren. I: Prevalence of bacteriuria and associated urologic findings. N Engl J Med 1962; 266:1287.

Kunz HH, Sieberth HG, Freiberg J, et al: Zur Bedeutung der Blasenpunktion für den sicheren Nachweis einer Bacteriurie. Dtsch Med Wochenschr 1975; 100:2252.

Lacy SS, Drach GW, Cox CE: Incidence of infection after prostatectomy and efficacy of cephaloridine prophylaxis. J Urol 1971; 105:836.

Latham RH, Running K, Stamm WE: Urinary tract infections in young adult women caused by *Staphylococcus saprophyticus*. JAMA 1983; 250:3036.

Latham RH, Wong ES, Larson A, et al: Laboratory diagnosis of urinary tract infection in ambulatory women. JAMA 1985; 254:3333.

Leffler H, Svanborg-Eden C: Chemical identification of a glycosphingolipid receptor for *Escherichia coli* attaching to human urinary tract epithelial cells and agglutinating erythrocytes. FEMS Microbiol Lett 1980; 8:127.

Leibovico L, Greenshtain S, Cohen O, et al: Toward improved empiric management of moderate to severe urinary tract infections. Arch Intern Med 1992; 152:2481.

Lerner SA: Optimal duration of treatment of urinary tract infections. Eur Urol 1987; 13(suppl 1):26.

Leveno KJ, Harris RE, Gilstrap LC, et al: Bladder versus renal bacteriuria during pregnancy: Recurrence after treatment. Am J Obstet Gynecol 1981; 139:403.

Levin R, Burbige KA, Abramson S, et al: The diagnosis and management of renal inflammatory processes in children. J Urol 1984; 132:718.

Lewin KJ, Fair WR, Steigbigel RT, et al: Clinical and laboratory studies into the pathogenesis of malacoplakia. J Clin Pathol 1976; 29:354.

Lincoln K, Lidin-Janson G, Winberg J: Resistant urinary infections resulting from changes in the resistance pattern of faecal flora induced by sulfonamide and hospital environment. Br Med J 1970; 3:305.

Lindberg U, Claesson I, Hanson LA, et al: Asymptomatic bacteriuria in schoolgirls. VIII: Clinical course during a 3-year follow-up. J Pediatr 1978; 92:194.

Lindberg U, Hanson LA, Jodal U, et al: Asymptomatic bacteriuria in schoolgirls. II: Differences in *Escherichia coli* causing asymptomatic bacteriuria. Acta Paediatr Scand 1975; 64:432.

Lindvall N: Radiological changes of renal papillary necrosis. Kidney Int 1978; 13:93.

Lipsky BA: Urinary tract infections in men: Epidemiology, pathophysiology, diagnosis, and treatment. Ann Intern Med 1989; 110:138.

Little PJ, McPherson DR, Wardener HE: The appearance of the intravenous pyelogram during and after acute pyelonephritis. Lancet 1965; 1:1186.

Ljungh A, Wadstrom T: Fimbriation of *Escherichia coli* in urinary tract infections: Comparisons between bacteria in the urine and subcultured bacterial isolates. Curr Microbiol 1983; 8:263.

Lode H: Pharmacokinetics and clinical results of parenterally administered new quinolones in humans. Rev Infect Dis 1989; 2(suppl 5):S996.

Lomberg H, Hanson LA, Jacobsson B, et al: Correlation of P blood group, vesicoureteral reflux, and bacterial attachment in patients with recurrent pyelonephritis. N Engl J Med 1983; 308:1189.

Lorentzen M, Overgaard NH: Xanthogranulomatous pyelonephritis. Scand J Urol Nephrol 1980; 14:193.

Lynn WA, Golenbock DT: Lipopolysaccharide antagonists. Immunol Today 1992; 13:271–276.

Lyons RW, Long JM, Litton B, et al: Arteriography and antibiotic therapy of a renal carbuncle. J Urol 1972; 107:524.

Mabeck CE: Studies in urinary tract infections. I: The diagnosis of bacteriuria in women. Acta Med Scand 1969a; 186:35.

Mabeck CE: Studies in urinary tract infections. IV: Urinary leukocyte excretion in bacteriuria. Acta Med Scand 1969b; 186:193.

Mabeck CE: Treatment of uncomplicated urinary tract infection in nonpregnant women. Postgrad Med J 1972; 48:69.

Macrea LE: Fulminant gangrene of the penis. Clinic 1945; 4:796.

Maderazo EG, Berlin BB, Morhardt C: Treatment of malakoplakia with trimethoprim-sulfamethoxazole. Urology 1979; 13:70.

Madge CE, Lomvardias S: Chronic liver disease and renal papillary necrosis with *Aspergillus*. South Med J 1973; 66:486.

Maizels M, Schaeffer AJ: Decreased incidence of bacteriuria associated with periodic instillations of hydrogen peroxide into the urethral catheter drainage bag. J Urol 1980; 123:841.

Malek RS: Xanthogranulomatous pyelonephritis: A great imitator. *In* Stamey TA, ed: Journal of Continuing Education in Urology. Northfield, Ill, Medical Digest, 1978, pp 17–28.

Malek RS, Elder JS: Xanthogranulomatous pyelonephritis: A critical analysis of 26 cases and of the literature. J Urol 1978; 119:589.

Malek RS, Greene LF, DeWeerd JH, et al: Xanthogranulomatous pyelonephritis. Br J Urol 1972; 44:296.

Marrie TJ, Harding GK, Ronald AR: Anaerobic and aerobic urethral flora in healthy females. J Clin Microbiol 1978; 8:67.

Martich GD, Danner RL, Ceska M, Suffredini AF: Detection of interleukin 8 and tumor necrosis factor in normal humans after intravenous endotoxin: The effect of antiinflammatory agents. J Exp Med 1991; 173:1021.

Martinez FC, Kindrachuk RW, Stamey TA, et al: Effect of prophylactic, low dose cephalexin on fecal and vaginal bacteria. J Urol 1985; 133:994.

Martorana G, Gilberti C, Pescatore D: Giant echinococcal cyst of the kidney associated with hypertension evaluated by computerized tomography. J Urol 1981; 126:99.

Matthew AD, Gonzalez R, Jeffords D, et al: Prevention of bacteriuria after transurethral prostatectomy with nitrofurantoin macrocrystals. J Urol 1978; 120:442.

Mauro MA, Balfe DM, Stanley RJ, et al: Computed tomography in the diagnosis and management of the renal mass. JAMA 1982; 248:2894.

McAfee JG: Radionuclide imaging in the assessment of primary chronic pyelonephritis. Radiology 1979; 133:203.

McCabe WR, Jackson GG: Treatment of pyelonephritis: Bacterial, drug, and host factors in success or failure among 252 patients. N Engl J Med 1965; 272:1037.

McCabe WR, Olans RN: Shock in gram-negative bacteremia. Predisposing factors, pathophysiology, and treatment. *In* Remington JS, Swartz MN, eds: Current Clinical Topics in Infectious Diseases. New York, McGraw-Hill Book Company, 1981, pp 121–150.

McCabe WR, Treadwell TL: Gram-negative bacteremia. Monogr Urol 1983; 4(November/December).

McClure J: Malakoplakia. J Pathol 1983; 140:275.

McDonald GS: Xanthogranulomatous pyelonephritis. J Pathol 1981; 133:203.

McDonough WD, Sandler CM, Benson GS: Acute focal bacterial nephritis: Focal pyelonephritis that may simulate renal abscess. J Urol 1981; 126:670.

McFadyen IR, Eykyn SJ, Gardner NHN, et al: Bacteriuria in pregnancy. J Obstet Gynaecol Br Commonw 1973; 80:385.

McGeachie J: Hemolysis by urinary *Escherichia coli*. Am J Clin Pathol 1966; 45:22.

McGeown MG: Treatment of urinary tract infection during pregnancy. Contrib Nephrol 1981; 25:30.

McGrady GA, Daling JR, Peterson DR: Maternal urinary tract infection and adverse fetal outcomes. Am J Epidemiol 1985; 121:377.

McIntyre KW, Stepan GJ, Kolinshy KD, et al: Inhibition of interleukin 1 (IL-1) binding and bioactivity in vitro and modulation of acute inflammation in vivo by IL-1 receptor antagonist and anti-IL-1 receptor antagonist and anti-IL-1 receptor monoclonal antibody. J Exp Med 1991; 173:931–9.

Amoxicillin-clavulanic acid. Med Lett 1984; 26:99.

Meleney FL: A differential diagnosis between certain types of infectious gangrene of the skin, with particular reference to hemolytic streptococcal gangrene and bacterial synergistic gangrene. Surg Gynecol Obstet 1933; 56:842.

Mendez G Jr, Isikoff MB, Morillo G: The role of computed tomography in the diagnosis of renal and perirenal abscesses. J Urol 1979; 122:582.

Mendez G Jr, Morillo G, Alonso M, et al: Gallium-67 radionuclide imaging in acute pyelonephritis. Am J Radiol 1980; 134:17.

Mendez G Jr, Quencer RM, Miale A: Gallium-67 tomographic radionuclide imaging in pyelonephritis: A report of two cases. J Urol 1978; 120:613.

Merinsky E, Feldman C: Perinephric abscess: Report of 19 cases. Int Surg 1981; 66:79.

Meyers MA, Whalen JP, Evans JA: Diagnosis of perirenal and subcapsular masses: Anatomic-radiologic correlation. Am J Roentgenol Rad Ther Nucl Med 1974; 121:523.

Michaels EK, Fowler JE, Jr, Mariano M: Bacteriuria following extracorporeal shock wave lithotripsy of infection stones. J Urol 1988; 140:254.

Miller JD: The importance of early diagnosis and surgical treatment of necrotizing fasciitis. Surg Gynecol Obstet 1983; 157:197.

Miller TE, North D: The cellular kinetics of the immune response in pyelonephritis. J Lab Clin Med 1971; 78:891.
Miller T, Phillips S: Pyelonephritis: The relationship between infection, renal scarring, and antimicrobial therapy. Kidney Int 1981; 19:654.
Miller TE, Stewart E, North JDK: Immunobacteriological aspects of pyelonephritis. Contrib Nephrol 1979; 16:11.
Modai J, The French Multicenter Study Group: Treatment of serious infections with intravenous ciprofloxacin. Am J Med 1989; 87(suppl 5A):243S.
Moller JC, Kristensen IB: Xanthogranulomatous pyelonephritis. A clinicopathological study with special reference to pathogenesis. Acta Pathol Microbiol Scand 1980; 88:89.
Morris MJ, Golovsky D, Guinness MD, et al: The value of prophylactic antibiotics in transurethral prostatic resection: A controlled trial, with observations on the origin of postoperative infection. Br J Urol 1976; 48:479.
Murray BE, Rensimer ER, DuPont HL: Emergence of high-level trimethoprim resistance in fecal *Escherichia coli* during oral administration of trimethoprim or trimethoprim-sulfamethoxazole. N Engl J Med 1982; 306:130.
Naber KG: Use of quinolones in urinary tract infections and prostatitis. Rev Infect Dis 1989; 2(suppl 5):S1321.
Nabizadeh I, Morehouse HT, Freed SZ: Hydatid disease of the kidney. Urology 1983; 22:176.
Naeye RL: Causes of the excessive rates of perinatal mortality and prematurity in pregnancies complicated by maternal urinary-tract infections. N Engl J Med 1979; 300:819.
Neter E: Estimation of *Escherichia coli* antibodies in urinary tract infection: A review and perspective. Kidney Int 1975; suppl 4:S23.
Newman CGH, O'Neill P, Parker A: Pyuria in infancy, and the role of suprapubic aspiration of urine in diagnosis of infection of urinary tract. Br Med J 1967; 2:277.
Nicolle LE, Bjornson J, Harding GKM, et al: Bacteriuria in elderly institutionalized men. N Engl J Med 1983; 309:1420.
Nicolle LE, Harding GKM, Thompson M, et al: Prospective, randomized, placebo-controlled trial of norfloxacin for the prophylaxis of recurrent urinary tract infection in women. Antimicrob Agents Chemother 1989; 33:1032.
Nicole LE, Mayhew WH, Bryan L: Prospective randomized comparison of therapy and no therapy for asymptomatic bacteriuria in institutionalized elderly women. Am J Med 1987; 83:27.
Nielsen OS, Maigaard S, Frimodt-Moller N, et al: Prophylactic antibiotics in transurethral prostatectomy. J Urol 1981; 126:60.
Nimmich W, Budde E, Naumann G, et al: Long-term study of humoral immune response in patients with chronic pyelonephritis. Clin Nephrol 1976; 6:428.
Norrby SR: Short-term treatment of uncomplicated lower urinary tract infections in women. Rev Infect Dis 1990; 12:458.
Nord CE: Effect of new quinolones on the human gastrointestinal microflora. Rev Infect Dis 1988; 10(suppl):193.
Ofek I, Beachey EH: General concepts and principles of bacterial adherence in animals and man, receptors and recognition. *In* Beachey EH, ed: Bacterial Adherence. London, Chapman and Hall, 1980, pp 3–29.
Ofek I, Mosek A, Sharon N: Mannose-specific adherence of *Escherichia coli* freshly excreted in the urine of patients with urinary tract infections, and of isolates subcultured from the infected urine. Infect Immun 1981; 34:708.
O'Hanley P, Lark D, Falkows S, et al: Molecular basis of *Escherichia coli* colonization of the upper urinary tract in BALB/c mice (Gal-Gal pili immunization prevents *E. coli* pyelonephritis in the BALB/c mouse model of human pyelonephritis). J Clin Invest 1985; 75:347.
Old DC: Inhibition of the interaction between fimbrial hemagglutinins and erythrocytes by D-mannose and other carbohydrates. J Gen Microbiol 1972; 71:149.
Olsson PJ, Black JR, Gaffney E, et al: Reversible acute renal failure secondary to acute pyelonephritis. South Med J 1980; 73:374.
Ooi BS, Chen BTM: Prevalence and site of bacteriuria in diabetes mellitus. Postgrad Med J 1974; 50:497.
Orskov I, Ferencz A, Orskov F: Tamm-Horsfall protein or uromucoid is the normal urinary slime that traps type 1 fimbriated *Escherichia coli*. (Letter.) Lancet, 1980; 1:887.
Osterberg E, Aberg H, Hallander HO, et al. Efficacy of single-dose versus seven-day trimethoprim treatment of cystitis in women: A randomized double-blind study. J Infect Dis 1990; 161:942.
Paivansalo M, Hellstrom P, Siniluoto T, et al: Emphysematous pyelonephritis: Radiologic and clinical findings in six cases. Acta Radiologica 1989; 30:311–315.
Pappas PG: Laboratory in the diagnosis and management of urinary tract infections. Med Clin North Am 1991; 75:313.
Parker J, Kunin C: Pyelonephritis in young women: A 10- to 20-year follow-up. JAMA 1973; 224:585.
Parsons CL, Pollen JJ, Answar H, et al: Antibacterial activity of bladder surface mucin duplicated in the rabbit bladder by exogenous glycosaminoglycan (sodium pentosanpolysulfate). Infect Immun 1980; 27:876.
Patel R, Tanaka T, Mishkin F, et al: Gallium-67 scan: Aid to diagnosis and treatment of renal and perirenal infections. Urology 1980; 16:225.
Patterson TF, Andriole VT: Bacteriuria in pregnancy. Infect Dis Clin North Am 1987; 1(4):807.
Patton JP, Nash DB, Abrutyn E: Urinary tract infections: Economic considerations. Med Clin North Am 1991; 75:495.
Paty R, Smith AD: Gangrene and Fournier's gangrene. Urol Clin North Am 1992; (19)1:149.
Pearman JW: Prevention of urinary tract infection following spinal cord injury. Paraplegia 1971; 9:95.
Pearson NJ, McSherry AM, Towner KJ, et al: Emergence of trimethoprim-resistant enterobacteria in patients receiving long-term co-trimoxazole for the control of intractable urinary-tract infection. Lancet 1979; 2:1205.
Percival A, Birumfitt W, De Louvois J: Serum-antibody levels as an indication of clinically inapparent pyelonephritis. Lancet 1964; 2:1027.
Pere A, Nowicki B, Saxen H, et al: Expression of P, type-1 and type 1C fimbriae of *Escherichia coli* in the urine of patients with acute urinary tract infection. J Infect Dis 1987; 156:567.
Pfau A, Rosenmann E: Unilateral chronic pyelonephritis and hypertension: Coincidental or casual relationship? Am J Med 1978; 65:499.
Pfau A, Sacks TG: Effective prophylaxis for recurrent urinary tract infections during pregnancy. Clin Infect Dis 1992; 14:810.
Pfau A, Sacks T, Engelstein D: Recurrent urinary tract infections in premenopausal women: Prophylaxis based on an understanding of the pathogenesis. J Urol 1983; 129:1153.
Philbrick JT, Bracikowski JP: Single-dose antibiotic treatment for uncomplicated urinary tract infections. Less for less? Arch Intern Med 1985; 145:1672.
Philpot VB Jr: The bacterial flora of urine specimens from normal adults. J Urol 1956; 75:562.
Pitts JC, Peterson NE, Conley MC: Calcified functionless kidney in a 51-year-old man. J Urol 1981; 125:398.
Plorde LL: Echinococciasis. *In* Harrison's Principles of Internal Medicine, 8th ed. New York, McGraw-Hill, 1977, pp 1117–1118.
Pometta D, Rees SB, Younger D, et al: Asymptomatic bacteriuria in diabetes mellitus. N Engl J Med 1967; 276:1118.
Pontzer RE, Krieger RE, Boscia JA, et al: Single-dose cefonicid therapy for urinary tract infections. Antimicrob Agents Chemother 1983; 23:814.
Poulios C: Echinococcal disease of the urinary tract: Review of the management of seven cases. J Urol 1991; 145(May):924.
Preiksaitis JK, Thompson L, Harding GK, et al: A comparison of the efficacy of nalidixic acid and cephalexin in bacteriuric women and their effect on fecal and periurethral carriage of Enterobacteriaceae. J Infect Dis 1981; 143:603.
Pylkkanen J: Antibody-coated bacteria in the urine of infants and children with their first two urinary tract infections. Acta Paediatr Scand 1978; 67:275.
Ransley PG, Risdon RA: The pathogenesis of reflux nephropathy. Contrib Nephrol 1979; 16:90.
Ratner JJ, Thomas VL, Sanford BA, et al: Bacteria-specific antibody in the urine of patients with acute pyelonephritis and cystitis. J Infect Dis 1981; 143:404.
Raz R, Boger S: Long-term prophylaxis with norfloxacin versus nitrofurantoin in women with recurrent urinary tract infection. Antimicrob Agents Chemother 1991; 35:1241.
Raz R, Stamm WE: A controlled trial in intravaginal estriol in postmenopausal women with recurrent urinary tract infection. N Engl J Med 1993; 329:753.
Reid G, Brooks HJ, Bacon DF: In vitro attachment of *Escherichia coli* to human uroepithelial cells: Variation in receptivity during the menstrual cycle and pregnancy. J Infect Dis 1983; 148:412.
Reid G, Zorzitto ML, Bruce AW, et al: Pathogenesis of urinary tract infection in the elderly: The role of bacterial adherence to uroepithelial cells. Curr Microbiol 1984; 11:67.
Resnick MI, Older RA: Diagnosis of Genitourinary Disease. New York, Thieme-Stratton, 1982.

Ribot S, Gal K, Goldblat MV, et al: The role of anaerobic bacteria in the pathogenesis of urinary tract infections. J Urol 1981; 126:852.

Richet G, Mayaud C: The course of acute renal failure in pyelonephritis and other types of interstitial nephritis. Nephron 1978; 22:124.

Richie JP, Nicholson TC, Hunting D, et al: Radiographic abnormalities in acute pyelonephritis. J Urol 1978; 119:832.

Ries K, Kaye D: The current status of therapy in urinary tract infection in pregnancy. Clin Perinatol 1974; 1:423.

Roberts JA, Domingue GJ, Martin LN, et al: Immunology of pyelonephritis in the primate model: Live versus heat-killed bacteria. Kidney Int 1981; 19:297.

Roberts JA, Roth JK, Domingue GJ, et al: Immunology of pyelonephritis in the primate model. V: Effect of superoxide dismutase. J Urol 1982; 128:1394.

Rocha H, Santos LCS: Relapse of urinary tract infection in the presence of urinary tract calculi: The role of bacteria within the calculi. J Med Microbiol 1969; 2:372.

Ronald AR: Optimal duration of treatment for kidney infection. Ann Intern Med 1987; 106:467.

Ronald AR, Jagdis FA, Harding GK, et al: Amoxicillin therapy of acute urinary infections in adults. Antimicrob Agents Chemother 1977; 11:780.

Ronald AR, Nicolle LE, Harding GK. Standards of therapy for urinary tract infections in adults. Infection 1992; 20(Suppl 3):S164.

Rosenfield A, Glickman M, Taylor KJ, et al: Acute focal bacterial nephritis (acute lobar nephronia). Radiology 1978; 132:553.

Roylance J, Davies ER, Alexander WD: Translumbar puncture of a renal hydatid cyst. Br J Radiol 1973; 46:960.

Rubin RH, Beam TR, Stamm WE: An approach to evaluating antibacterial agents in the treatment of urinary tract infections [review]. Clin Infect Dis 1992; 14(Suppl 2):S246–S251.

Rubin RH, Fang LST, Jones SR, et al: Single-dose amoxicillin therapy for urinary tract infection. JAMA 1980; 244:561.

Saginur R, Nicolle LE, Canadian Infectious Diseases Society Clinical Trials Study Group: Single-dose compared with 3-day norfloxacin treatment of uncomplicated urinary tract infection in women. Arch Intern Med 1992; 152:1233.

Saiki J, Vaziri ND, Barton C: Perinephric and intranephric abscesses: A review of the literature. West J Med 1982; 136:95.

Saint Martin G, Chiesa JC: "Falling snowflakes": An ultrasound sign of hydatid sand. J Ultrasound Med 1984; 3:257.

Salvatierra O Jr, Bucklew WB, Morrow JW: Perinephric abscess: A report of 71 cases. J Urol 1967; 98:296.

Sanford JP, Favour CB, Mao FH, et al: Evaluation of the "positive" urine culture: An approach to the differentiation of significant bacteria from contaminants. Am J Med 1956; 20:88.

Sant GR: Urinary tract infection in the elderly. Semin Urol 1987; 5:126.

Savage DC: Survival on mucosal epithelia, epithelium penetration and growth in tissues of pathogenic bacteria. *In* Smith H, Pearce JH, eds: Microbial Pathogenicity in Man and Animals. Twenty-Second Symposium of the Society of General Microbiology. London, Cambridge Press, 1972, pp 25–57.

Savage DCL, Howie G, Adler K, et al: Controlled trial of therapy in covert bacteriuria of childhood. Lancet 1975; 1:358.

Scarpelli PT, Lamanna S, Bigioli F, et al: The antibody response in chronic pyelonephritis. Clin Nephrol 1979; 12:7.

Schaeffer AJ: Urinary tract infections in urology: A urologist's view of chronic bacteriuria. Infect Dis Clin North Am 1987; 1(4):875–892.

Schaeffer AJ: The role of bacterial adherence in urinary tract infections. Am Urol Assoc Update Series 1989; 8:18.

Schaeffer AJ, Amundsen SK, Schmidt LN: Adherence of *Escherichia coli* to human urinary tract epithelial cells. Infect Immun 1979; 24:753.

Schaeffer AJ, Jones JM, Duncan JL, et al: Adhesion of uropathogenic *Escherichia coli* to epithelial cells from women with recurrent urinary tract infection. Infection 1982; 10:186.

Schaeffer AJ, Radvany RM, Chmiel JS: Human leukocyte antigens in women with recurrent urinary tract infections. J Infect Dis 1983; 148:604.

Schaeffer JK, Jones JM, Dunn JK: Association of in vitro *E. coli* adherence to vaginal and buccal epithelial cells with susceptibility of women to recurrent urinary tract infections. N Engl J Med 1981; 304:1062–1066.

Schainuck LI, Fouty R, Cutler RE: Emphysematous pyelonephritis, a new case and review of previous observations. Am J Med 1968; 44:134.

Schechter H, Leonard CD, Scribner BH: Chronic pyelonephritis as a cause of renal failure in dialysis candidates: Analysis of 173 patients. JAMA 1971; 216:514.

Scherf H, Kollermann MW, Busch R: Nachweis antikorperbeladener Bakterien im Urinsediment bei kindlichen Harnwegsinfektionen. Monatsschr Kinderheilkd 1978; 126:23.

Schiff M Jr, Glickman M, Weiss RM: Antibiotic treatment of renal carbuncle. Ann Intern Med 1977; 87:305.

Schneider M, Becker JA, Staiano S, et al: Sonographic-radiographic correlation of renal and perirenal infections. AJR 1976; 127:1007.

Schoborg TW, Saffos RO, Urdaneta L, et al: Xanthogranulomatous pyelonephritis associated with renal carcinoma. J Urol 1980; 124:125.

Schwarz RH: Consideration of antibiotic therapy during pregnancy. Obstet Gynecol 1981; 58:95S.

Segura JW, Kelalis PP: Localized renal parenchymal infections in children. J Urol 1973; 109:1029.

Sexton CC, Lowman RM, Nyongo AO, et al: Malacoplakia presenting as complete unilateral urethral obstruction. J Urol 1982; 128:139.

Sharp JL: The growth of *Candida albicans* during antibiotic therapy. Lancet 1954; 1:390.

Sheehan G, Harding GKM, Ronald AR: Advances in the treatment of urinary tract infection. Am J Med 1984; 76:141.

Sheinfeld J, Schaeffer AJ, Cordon-Cardo C, et al: Association of the Lewis blood-group phenotype with recurrent urinary tract infections in women. N Engl J Med 1989; 320:773.

Shimamura T: Mechanisms of renal tissue destruction in an experimental acute pyelonephritis. Exp Mol Pathol 1981; 34:34.

Shimizu S, Takimoto Y, Niimura T, et al: A case of prostatic malacoplakia. J Urol 1981; 126:277.

Shortliffe LM, McNeal JE, Wehner N, et al: Persistent urinary infections in young women with bilateral renal stones. J Urol 1984; 131:1147.

Silver TM, Kass EJ, Thornbury JR, et al: The radiological spectrum of acute pyelonephritis in adults and adolescence. Radiology 1976; 118:65.

Silverblatt FJ, Dreyer JS, Schauer S: Effect of pili on susceptibility of *Escherichia coli* to phagocytes. Infect Immun 1979; 24:218.

Silverman DE, Stamey TA: Management of infection stones: The Stanford experience. Medicine 1983; 62:44.

Siroky MB, Moylan RA, Austen G Jr, et al: Metastatic infection secondary to genitourinary tract sepsis. Am J Med 1976; 61:351.

Slotki IN, Asscher AW: Prevention of scarring in experimental pyelonephritis in the rat by early antibiotic therapy. Nephron 1982; 30:262.

Smith H: Microbial surfaces in relation to pathogenicity. Bacteriol Rev 1977; 41:475.

Smith J, Holmgren J, Ahlstedt S, et al: Local antibody production in experimental pyelonephritis: Amount, avidity, and immunoglobulin class. Infect Immun 1974; 10:411.

Smith JW, Jones SR, Kaijser B: Significance of antibody-coated bacteria in urinary sediment in experimental pyelonephritis. J Infect Dis 1977; 135:577.

Solomon A, Braf Z, Papo J, et al: Computerized tomography in xanthogranulomatous pyelonephritis. J Urol 1983; 130:323.

Sotolongo JR, Schiff H, Wulfsohn MA: Radiographic findings in acute segmental pyelonephritis. Urology 1982; 19:335.

Soulen MC, Fishman EK, Goldman SM, et al: Bacterial renal infection: Role of CT. Radiology 1989; 171:703.

Souney P, Polk BF: Single-dose antimicrobial therapy for urinary tract infections in women. Rev Infect Dis 1982; 4:29.

Sourander LB: Urinary tract infections in the aged: An epidemiological study. Ann Med Intern Fenn 1966; 55(Suppl 45):7.

Sourander LB, Kasanen AA: 5-year follow-up of bacteriuria in the aged. Gerontol Clin 1972; 14:274.

Sourander L, Saarimaa H: Effect of long-term treatment of urinary tract infection with a single dose in the evening. Chemotherapy 1975; 21:52.

Spach DH, Stapleton AE, Stamm WE: Lack of circumcision increases the risk of urinary tract infection in young men. JAMA 1992; 267:679–681.

Sparks AK, Connor DH, Neafie RC: Echinococcosis. *In* Binford CH, Connor DH, eds: Pathology of Tropical and Extraordinary Diseases. Washington, DC, The Armed Forces Institute of Pathology, 1976, pp 530–533.

Spirnak JP, Resnick MI, Hampel N: Fournier's gangrene: A report of 20 patients. J Urol 1984; 131:289.

Stamenkovic I, Lew PD: Early recognition of potentially fatal necrotizing fasciitis: The role of frozen section biopsy. N Engl J Med 1984; 310:1689.

Stamey TA: Pathogenesis and Treatment of Urinary Tract Infections. Baltimore, Williams & Wilkins Company, 1980.

Stamey TA, Condy M: The diffusion and concentration of trimethoprim in human vaginal fluid. J Infect Dis 1975; 131:261.

Stamey TA, Condy M, Mihara G: Prophylactic efficacy of nitrofurantoin macrocrystals and trimethoprim-sulfamethoxazole in urinary infections:

Biologic effects on the vaginal and rectal flora. N Engl J Med 1977; 296:780.
Stamey TA, Fair WR, Timothy MM, et al: Serum versus urinary antimicrobial concentrations in cure of urinary-tract infections. N Engl J Med 1974; 291:1159.
Stamey TA, Govan DE, Palmer JM: The localization and treatment of urinary tract infections: The role of bactericidal urine levels as opposed to serum level. Medicine 1965; 44:1.
Stamey TA, Pfau A: Some functional, pathological, bacteriologic, and chemotherapeutic characteristics of unilateral pyelonephritis in man. II: Bacteriologic and chemotherapeutic characteristics. Invest Urol 1963; 1:162.
Stamm WE: When should we use urine cultures? Infect Control 1986; 7:431–433.
Stamm WE: Catheter-associated urinary tract infections: Epidemiology, pathogenesis, and prevention. Am J Med 1991; 91(suppl 3B):3B–65S.
Stamm WE: Guidelines for prevention of catheter-associated urinary tract infections. Ann Intern Med 1975; 82:386.
Stamm WE, Counts GW, Running KR, et al: Diagnosis of coliform infection in acutely dysuric women. N Engl J Med 1982; 307:463.
Stamm WE, Counts GW, Wagner KF, et al: Antimicrobial prophylaxis of recurrent urinary tract infections: A double-blind, placebo-contracted trial. Ann Intern Med 1980a; 92:770.
Stamm WE, Hooton TM: Management of urinary tract infections in adults. N Engl J Med 1993; 329:1328–1334.
Stamm WE, Wagner KF, Amsel R, et al: Causes of the acute urethral syndrome in women. N Engl J Med 1980b; 303:409.
Stanton MJ, Maxted W: Malakoplakia: A study of the literature and current concepts of pathogenesis. J Urol 1981; 125:139.
Stapleton A, Latham RH, Johnson C, et al: Postcoital antimicrobial prophylaxis for recurrent urinary tract infection. A randomized, double-blind, placebo-controlled trial. JAMA 1990; 264:703.
Stapleton A, Nudelman E, Clausen H, et al: Binding of uropathogenic *Escherichia coli* R45 to glycolipids extracted from vaginal epithelial cells is dependent on histoblood group secretor status. J Clin Invest 1992; 90:965.
Stark RP, Maki DG: Bacteriuria in the catheterized patient: What quantitative level of bacteriuria is relevant? N Engl J Med 1984; 311:560.
Stenqvist K, Dahlen-Nilsson I, Lidin-Janson G, et al: Bacteriuria in pregnancy: Frequency and risk of acquisition. Am J Epidemiol 1989; 129:372.
Stenqvist K, Lidin-Janson G, Sandberg T, et al: Bacterial adhesion as an indicator of renal involvement in bacteriuria of pregnancy. Scand J Infect Dis 1989; 21:193.
Sullivan MN, Sutter VL, Mins MM, et al: Clinical aspects of bacteremia after manipulation of the genitourinary tract. J Infect Dis 1973; 127:49.
Sussman M, Asscher AW, Waters WE, et al: Asymptomatic significant bacteriuria in the nonpregnant woman. I: Description of a population. Br Med J 1969; 1:799.
Svanborg-Eden C, Hanson LA, Jodal U, et al: Variable adherence to normal human urinary tract epithelial cells of *Escherichia coli* strains associated with various forms of urinary tract infections. Lancet 1976; 2:490.
Svanborg-Eden C, Jodal U: Attachment to *Escherichia coli* to sediment epithelial cells from urinary infection-prone and healthy children. Infect Immun 1979; 26:837.
Svenson SB, Hultberg H, Kallenius G, et al: P-fimbriae of pyelonephritis *Escherichia coli*: Identification and chemical characterization of receptors. Infection 1983; 11:61.
Svensson R, Larsson P, Lincoln K: Low dose trimethoprim prophylaxis in long term control of chronic recurrent urinary infection. Scand J Infect Dis 1982; 14:139.
Sweet RL: Bacteriuria and pyelonephritis during pregnancy. Semin Perinatol 1977; 1:25.
Sweet R, Keane WF: Perinephric abscess in patients with polycystic kidney disease and undergoing chronic hemodialysis. Nephron 1979; 23:237.
Tartaglione TA, Johnson CR, Brust P, et al: Pharmacodynamic evaluation of ofloxacin and trimethoprim-sulfamethoxazole in vaginal fluid of women treated for acute cystitis. Antimicrob Agents Chemother 1988; 32:1640.
Teplick JG, Teplick SK, Berinson H, et al: Urographic and angiographic changes in acute unilateral pyelonephritis. Clin Radiol 1978; 30:59.
Thiel G, Spuhler O: Urinary tract infection by catheter and the so-called infectious (episomal) resistance. Schweiz Med Wochenschr 1965; 95:1155.
Thomas E, Hillman BJ, Stanisic T: Urinary tract infection with atypical mycobacteria. J Urol 1980; 124:748.
Thomas V, Shelokov A, Forland M: Antibody-coated bacteria in the urine and the site of urinary tract infection. N Engl J Med 1974; 290:588.
Thompson RB: A Short Textbook of Haematology. Philadelphia, J. B. Lippincott Company, 1969.
Thorley JD, Jones SR, Sanford JP: Perinephric abscess. Medicine 1974; 53:441.
Timmons JW, Perlmutter AD: Renal abscess: A changing concept. J Urol 1976; 115:299.
Toivanen A, Kasanen A, Sundquist H, et al: Effect of trimethoprim on the occurrence of drug-resistant coliform bacteria in the faecal flora. Chemotherapy 1976; 22:97.
Tolia BM, Iloreta A, Freed SZ, et al: Xanthogramulomatous pyelonephritis: Detailed analysis of 29 cases and a brief discussion of atypical presentations. J Urol 1981; 126:437.
Tolia BM, Newman HR, Fruchtman B, et al: Xanthogranulomatous pyelonephritis: Segmental or generalized disease? J Urol 1980; 124:122.
Tolkoff-Rubin NE, Wilson ME, Zuromskis BP, et al: Single dose amoxicillin therapy of acute uncomplicated urinary tract infections in women. Antimicrob Agents Chemother 1984; 25:626.
Tomashefski JF, Abramowsky CR: Candida-associated renal papillary necrosis. Am J Clin Pathol 1981; 75:190.
Trillo A, Lorentz WB, Whitley NO: Malakoplakia of kidneys simulating renal neoplasm. Urology 1977; 10:472.
Truesdale BH, Rous SN, Nelson RP: Perinephric abscess: A review of 26 cases. J Urol 1977; 118:910.
Turck M, Goffe B, Petersdorf RG: The urethral catheter and urinary tract infection. J Urol, 1962; 88:834.
Vaisanen V, Elo J, Tallgren LG, et al: Mannose-resistant haemagglutination and P antigen recognition are characteristic of *Escherichia coli* causing primary pyelonephritis. Lancet 1981; 2:1366.
VanKirk OC, Go RT, Wedel VJ: Sonographic features of xanthogranulomatous pyelonephritis. Am J Roentgenol 1980; 134:1035.
Vejlsgaard R: Studies on urinary infections in diabetes. IV: Significant bacteriuria in pregnancy in relation to age of onset, duration of diabetes, angiopathy and urological symptoms. Acta Med Scand 1973; 193:337.
Vordermark JS, Modarelli RO, Buck AS: Torulopsis pyelonephritis associated with papillary necrosis: A case report. J Urol 1980; 123:96.
Vosti KL: Recurrent urinary tract infections: Prevention by prophylactic antibiotics after sexual intercourse. JAMA 1975; 231:934.
Waage A, Halstensen A, Espevik T: Association between tumor necrosis factor in serum and fatal outcome in patients with meningococcal disease. Lancet 1987; 1:355.
Wadsworth DE, McClennan BL, Stanley RJ: CT of the renal mass. Urol Radiol 1982; 48:85.
Wakabayashi G, Gelfand JA, Burke JF, et al: A specific receptor antagonist for interleukin 1 prevents *Escherichia coli*–induced shock in rabbits. FASEB J 1991; 5:338.
Walkey FA, Judge TG, Thompson J, et al: Incidence of urinary infection in the elderly. Scott Med J 1967; 12:411.
Walther PJ, Adriani RT, Maggio MI: Fournier's gangrene: A complication of penile prosthetic implantation in a renal transplant patient. J Urol 1987; 137:299–300.
Waltzer WC: The urinary tract in pregnancy. J Urol 1981; 125:271.
Warren JW: Catheter-associated urinary tract infections. Infect Dis Clin North Am 1987; 1:823.
Warren JW, Anthony WC, Hoopes JM, et al: Cephalexin for susceptible bacteriuria in afebrile, long-term catheterized patients. JAMA 1982; 248:454.
Warren JW, Muncie HL Jr, Hall-Craggs M: Acute pyelonephritis associated with bacteriuria during long-term catheterization: A prospective clinicopathological study. J Infect Dis 1988; 158:1341.
Warren JW, Platt R, Thomas RJ, et al: Antibiotic irrigation and catheter-associated urinary-tract infections. N Engl J Med 1978; 299:570.
Weinstein AJ: Treatment of bacterial infections in pregnancy. Drugs 1979; 17:56.
Wientzen RL, McCracken GH Jr, Petruska ML, et al: Localization and therapy of urinary tract infections of childhood. Pediatrics 1979; 63:467.
Wigton RS, Hoellerich VL, Ornato JP, et al: Use of clinical findings in the diagnosis of urinary tract infection in women. Arch Intern Med 1985; 145(12):2222.
Wilhelm MP, Edson RS: Antimicrobial agents in urinary tract infections. May Clin Proc 1987; 62:1025.
Williams JD, Reeves DS, Brumfitt W, et al: The effects of bacteriuria in pregnancy on maternal health. *In* Brumfitt W, Asscher AW, eds: Urinary Tract Infections. London, Oxford University Press, 1973, p 103.
Winberg J, Bergstrom T, Lincoln K, et al: Treatment trials in urinary tract infection (UTI) with special reference to the effect of antimicrobials on the fecal and periurethral flora. Clin Nephrol 1973; 1:142.

Witten EM, Myers GH, Utz DG: Emmett's Clinical Urography. Philadelphia, W. B. Saunders Company, 1977.

Wolach MD, MacDermott JP, DeVere White RW: Treatment and complications of Fournier's gangrene. Br J Urol 1989; 64:310.

Wolfson JS, Hooper DC: Treatment of genitourinary tract infections with fluoroquinolones: Activity in vitro, pharacokinetics, and clinical efficacy in urinary tract infections and prostatitis. Antimicrob Agents Chemother 1989; 33:1655.

Wolfson SA, Kalmanson GM, Rubini ME, et al: Epidemiology of bacteriuria in a predominantly geriatric male population. Am J Med Sci 1965; 250:168.

Wolverson MK, Jagannadharao B, Sundaram M, et al: CT as a primary diagnostic method in evaluating intraabdominal abscess. Am J Roentgenol 1979; 133:1089.

Wong ES, McKevitt M, Running K, et al: Management of recurrent urinary tract infections with patient-administered single-dose therapy. Ann Intern Med 1985; 102:302.

Wright AJ, Walker RC, Barrett DM: The fluoroquinolones and their appropriate use in treatment of genitourinary tract infections. *In* Ball TP, Novicki DE, eds: AUA Update Series. Houston, American Urologic Association, 1993, pp 50–55.

Zacur HA, Mitch WE: Renal disease in pregnancy. Med Clin North Am 1977; 61:89.

Zhanel GG, Ronald AR: Single dose versus traditional therapy for uncomplicated urinary tract infections. Drug Intell Clin Pharm 1988; 22:21.

Ziegler EJ, Fisher CJ, Sprung CL, et al: Treatment of gram-negative bacteremia and septic shock with HA-1A human monoclonal antibody against endotoxin. A randomized, double-blind, placebo-controlled trial. N Engl J Med 1991; 324:429.

Zinner SH: Bacteriuria and babies revisited. N Engl J Med 1979; 300: 853.

Zinner SH, Kass EH: Long-term (10 to 14 years) follow-up of bacteriuria of pregnancy. N Engl J Med 1971; 285:820.

16
PROSTATITIS AND RELATED DISORDERS

Edwin M. Meares, Jr., M.D.

Prostatitis remains a common but often confusing ailment that rarely affects prepubertal boys but frequently affects adult men. Whereas little information concerning the true incidence of prostatitis is available, a National Health Center for Health Statistics study indicates that during 1977 and 1978, there were 76 annual office visits per 1000 men for genitourinary tract problems. About 25% of these visits were for prostatitis (Lipsky, 1989). Most patients with chronic prostatitis have a poor understanding of their condition, and many are generally unhappy with the results of treatment. Moreover, many clinicians are frustrated in their attempts to treat patients with prostatitis. Unless the patient responds quickly to therapy, which seldom is the case, the tendency is for the clinician to refer the patient elsewhere or to tell the patient that he must simply learn to live with his condition.

It is now recognized that prostatitis occurs in several distinct forms or syndromes. These syndromes have separate causes, clinical features, and sequelae. Proper clinical management is therefore possible only if the clinician is specific in diagnosis and therapeutic strategy.

TYPES OF PROSTATITIS

A new classification of the most common forms of prostatitis was introduced in 1978: (1) acute and chronic bacterial prostatitis, (2) nonbacterial prostatitis, and (3) prostatodynia (Drach et al, 1978).

Bacterial prostatitis is associated with urinary tract infection (UTI) and excessive numbers of inflammatory cells (leukocytes and macrophages containing fat) in the prostatic secretions; positive cultures localize the bacterial pathogen to the prostatic secretions. Acute bacterial prostatitis (ABP) is a febrile illness with abrupt onset and marked genitourinary tract and constitutional signs and symptoms; chronic bacterial prostatitis (CBP) is a more subtle illness, typified by relapsing recurrent UTI caused by persistence of the pathogen in the prostatic secretory system despite courses of antibacterial therapy. In contrast, patients with *nonbacterial prostatitis* (NBP) have excessive numbers of inflammatory cells in the prostatic secretions despite no history of documented UTI and negative cultures. In patients with *prostatodynia*, there is no history of UTI, cultures are negative, and prostatic secretions typically appear normal.

Even though the relative incidence of these common forms of prostatitis has not been studied thoroughly, an evaluation of approximately 600 men attending a special prostatitis clinic in Germany indicates that 5% had bacterial prostatitis, 64% had NBP, and 31% had prostatodynia (Brunner et al, 1983). Some similarities and differences in clinical features of these common prostatitis syndromes are shown in Table 16–1.

Since the 1980s, **my own experience and that of others (Neal and Moon, 1994) have suggested that there is no reason to distinguish prostatodynia from NBP. Indeed, patients with prostatodynia do at times have excessive leukocytes in the prostatic expressates; moreover, treatment of these two conditions is essentially the same.**

It has been observed that many NBP/prostatodynia patients who fail standard therapy are found to actually have prostatitis associated with interstitial cystitis (Meares and Sant, 1995).

ETIOLOGY AND PATHOGENESIS

The causative organisms in bacterial prostatitis are similar in type and incidence to those responsible for UTI; common strains of *Escherichia coli* clearly predominate. Infections caused by species of *Proteus, Klebsiella, Enterobacter, Pseudomonas, Serratia,* and other less common gram-negative organisms are less common (Meares, 1987). **Obligate anaerobic bacteria seldom cause prostatic infection.** Most prostatic infections are caused by a single pathogen; however, infections involving two or more strains or types of bacteria occur occasionally.

The role played by gram-positive bacteria in the etiology of prostatitis is controversial. Most investigators agree that strains of *Enterococcus fecalis* cause CBP and related recurrent enterococcal bacteriuria. However, the pathogenic role in prostatitis of other gram-positive organisms, such as coagulase-negative staphylococci, streptococci, micrococci, and diphtheroids, is uncertain. Drach (1974, 1975) reported that gram-positive bacteria are frequently localized by culture to the prostatic secretions of men with prostatitis. More recently, Bergman and colleagues (1989) analyzed the bacteriologic findings in patients with chronic prostatitis and reported an apparent causative role for gram-positive bacteria in several patients. These normal "skin inhabitants," however, typically colonize the anterior urethra of normal men and are generally considered commensals, not pathogens (Meares, 1980). Moreover, extended studies of men who have only gram-positive bacteria (other than enterococci) on localization cultures seldom show reproducible patterns that prove CBP or a tendency for these organisms to cause UTI—a hallmark of chronic prostatitis caused by gram-negative bacteria (Meares, 1987). Indeed, most researchers believe that gram-positive bacteria other than enterococci rarely cause bacterial prostatitis (Meares, 1973; Måardh and Colleen, 1975; Pfau and Sacks, 1976; Stamey, 1981; Thin and Simmons, 1983; Pfau, 1986).

Bacterial prostatitis probably evolves from ascending urethral infection or reflux of infected urine into prostatic ducts that empty into the posterior urethra. Other possibilities include invasion by rectal bacteria (by direct extension or lymphogenous spread) and hematogenous infection.

Blacklock (1974) and Stamey (1980) independently observed that for some men with CBP and their female sexual partners, the same pathogen is often found in prostatic fluid and vaginal cultures. This suggests that bacterial prostatitis may develop in some men as a consequence of ascending urethral infection resulting from meatal inoculation during sexual relations. Unprotected anorectal insertive intercourse is a documented cause of urethritis, UTI, and acute epididymitis resulting from coliform bacteria (Berger et al, 1987). Undoubtedly, this sexual practice can also lead to bacterial prostatitis.

The intraprostatic reflux of urine apparently occurs commonly and may play the most important role in the pathogenesis of bacterial prostatitis. Sutor and Wooley (1974) and Rameriz and co-workers (1980), studying prostatic calculi by crystallographic analysis, noted that many calculi contained constituents found only in urine, not in prostatic secretions. This implicates intraprostatic reflux of urine in the formation of these stones. Kirby and colleagues (1982) provided more direct proof of intraprostatic urinary reflux. A carbon-particle solution was instilled into the bladders of ten men immediately before transurethral prostatectomy and into the bladders of five men in whom NBP was diagnosed. The surgical specimens clearly showed carbon particles within the prostatic ductile system in seven (70%) of the ten men who underwent surgery. In each of the five men with NBP, there

Table 16–1. CLINICAL FEATURES OF COMMON PROSTATITIS SYNDROMES

Syndrome	History of Confirmed UTI	Prostate Abnormal on Rectal Examination	Excessive WBCs in EPS	Positive Culture of EPS	Common Causative Agents	Response to Antimicrobial Treatment	Impaired Urinary Flow Rate
Acute bacterial prostatitis	Yes	Yes	Yes	Yes	Coliform bacteria	Yes	Yes
Chronic bacterial prostatitis	Yes	±	Yes	Yes	Coliform bacteria	Yes	±
Nonbacterial prostatitis	No	±	Yes	No	None ? *Chlamydia* ? *Ureaplasma*	Usually no	Yes
Prostatodynia	No	No	No	No	None	No	Yes

UTI, Urinary tract infection; WBCs, white blood cells; EPS, expressed prostatic secretions.

were numerous macrophages studded with intracellular carbon particles in prostatic expressates 3 days after bladder instillation of the carbon-particle solution. It therefore appears that **intraprostatic urinary reflux occurs commonly and probably plays an important role in the pathogenesis of bacterial prostatitis,** that is, the direct inoculation of infected urine into the prostate.

The cause and pathogenesis of NBP remain uncertain; however, this syndrome appears either to be caused by yet-unidentified pathogenic organisms or to represent a noninfectious disease. **It is thought that intraprostatic urinary reflux, causing a "chemical" prostatitis, may play an etiologic role in the pathogenesis of prostatodynia and NBP** (Meares, 1986a).

Because they are frequently associated with urethral colonization with pathogenic bacteria and ascending UTI, drainage systems involving both indwelling urethral catheters and condom catheters can lead to bacterial infection of the prostate. It is commonly known that bacterial prostatitis can develop in men who have untreated infected urine immediately after transurethral prostatic resection.

METHODS OF DIAGNOSIS

The diagnosis of prostatitis is made most often with little substantiation by the clinician. The medical history and physical findings may suggest the diagnosis of a prostatitis syndrome but are not confirmatory. Acute bacterial prostatitis generally is recognized easily because its clinical manifestations are dramatic and characteristic; in contrast, the clinical features of chronic prostatitis syndromes are highly variable and inexact. Indeed, many of the signs, symptoms, and physical findings in cases of CBP, NBP, and prostatodynia are often indistinguishable. Likewise, radiographic studies and cystourethroscopy may assist in differential diagnosis and identifying complicating factors, but they do not confirm the diagnosis of prostatitis.

Histologic examination of prostatic tissue generally is required for diagnosing unusual forms of prostatitis, such as granulomatous prostatitis. However, the histologic changes seen in CBP are not sufficiently specific to confirm a bacterial etiology of the inflammation. Kohnen and Drach (1979) reviewed 162 consecutive cases of surgically resected hyperplastic prostates and found an incidence of inflammation of about 98%. Six distinct morphologic patterns of inflammation were observed, but no significant differences were identified among groups of cases with positive and negative evidence by culture of bacterial prostatic infection. Furthermore, in most instances the inflammatory reaction was quite focal and involved only small portions of the total gland. Prostatic biopsy is therefore seldom indicated in the management of prostatitis. Moreover, tissue culture of specimens obtained by prostatic biopsy is seldom indicated in the diagnosis of CBP. The focal nature of the infection makes sampling errors significant, and tissue specimens are difficult to culture quantitatively and are easily contaminated during procurement.

Examination of the Prostatic Expressate

Microscopic examination of the expressed prostatic secretions is important in the diagnosis and classification of prostatitis but can be misleading. For example, excessive numbers of leukocytes in the prostatic expressate may create false impressions in urethral disease (e.g., urethritis, strictures, condylomata, and diverticula); likewise, noninfectious conditions of the prostate (e.g., uninfected prostatic calculi) may lead to false impressions. The white blood cell (WBC) count in prostatic fluid also rises significantly in healthy men for several hours after sexual intercourse and ejaculation (Jameson, 1967).

To localize the site of an inflammation to the urethra or prostate, the clinician must always compare the microscopic appearance of the prostatic expressate to smears of the spun sediment of the first voided 10 ml of urine (urethral specimen) and the midstream urine (bladder specimen) that are obtained immediately before prostatic massage. What constitutes an excessive number of WBCs in prostatic secretions remains controversial. **Most clinicians agree that more than 20 WBCs per high-power field (hpf) is excessive; some prefer the criterion of more than 15 WBCs per hpf; others believe that more than 10 WBCs per hpf represents leukocytosis** (Drach et al, 1978; Meares, 1980). Studies by Blacklock (1969), Anderson and Weller (1979), and Schaeffer and co-workers (1981) indicate that prostatic fluid normally contains 10 WBCs per hpf or fewer.

The finding of both excessive numbers of leukocytes and macrophages containing fat (oval bodies) is the most convincing sign of prostatic inflammation. The macrophages containing fat seldom are noticed in the prostatic secretions of healthy men, are increased about eightfold in men with NBP, and often are exceedingly prominent in the secretions of men who have bacterial prostatitis (Anderson and Weller, 1979; Meares, 1980; Stamey, 1981). Moreover, macrophages containing fat are not found in exudates arising from anterior urethritis.

Examination of the Semen

Results of isolated analysis or culture of the ejaculate without concomitant study of urethral and bladder specimens may be more misleading than results of isolated examination of the prostatic expressate. The semen not only passes through the urethra but also contains fluids from several accessory glands. Cytologic examination of the semen is also complicated by the difficulty of distinguishing immature sperm from leukocytes. Mobley (1974, 1975, 1981) advocated using semen cultures to diagnose bacterial prostatitis and based some of his clinical studies, at least in part, on this method. Specimens from the urethra (VB1) and bladder (VB2) must be obtained immediately before collection of the semen specimen, and all specimens must be cultured quantitatively. Comparison of the bacterial counts of the three cultures must clearly show excessive counts of bacteria in the semen; otherwise, proper interpretation of the semen culture is impossible and the diagnosis of prostatitis remains speculative. Obviously, urethral organisms of nonprostatic origin can easily contaminate the semen as it passes through the urethra during specimen procurement.

Measurement of the Immune Response

Chodirker and Tomasi (1963) were the first to identify and quantitatively measure immunoglobulins G and A (IgG and IgA) in normal human prostatic fluid. Subsequently, several investigators, using various techniques, demonstrated both a systemic and a local prostatic immune response to bacterial infection of the prostate. These studies were reviewed and summarized by Meares (1986b).

The most important contribution in this area has been the work of Shortliffe and associates (1981a, 1981b), who developed a solid-phase radioimmunoassay to study the immune response in cases of human acute and chronic bacterial prostatitis. **These investigators observed in prostatic fluid a distinct local antibody response, mainly secretory IgA, that is independent of a serum response and is antigen-specific for the infecting pathogen.** In acute bacterial prostatitis that is cured by medical therapy, antigen-specific IgG levels in both serum and prostatic fluid are elevated at the onset of infection but decline slowly during the ensuing 6 to 12 months. In contrast, antigen-specific IgA levels in prostatic fluid become elevated immediately after infection and begin to decline only after about 12 months; after only 1 month, the initial elevation in serum IgA disappears. In CBP, although both antigen-specific IgA and IgG levels in prostatic fluid are elevated, neither immunoglobulin is substantially elevated in serum. In CBP that is cured by medical therapy, the IgA level in prostatic fluid remains elevated for almost 2 years and the IgG level, for 6 months, before levels of each immunoglobulin begin to decline to normal. In men with bacterial prostatitis that is not cured by medical therapy, prostatic fluid antigen-specific IgA and IgG levels remain persistently elevated.

It appears that measurement of antigen-specific IgA and IgG levels in prostatic fluid not only is helpful in diagnostic confirmation but also is useful in determining the response to treatment in patients with bacterial prostatitis.

In 1986, Shortliffe and Wehner reported a study of the antigen-specific antibody response in prostatic fluid of three groups of men: 23 patients with confirmed bacterial prostatitis, 23 men with NBP, and 21 normal men without history of prostatitis or UTI. Two mixes of bacterial antigen were used: mix 1 consisted of eight serogroups of *E. coli*, which is commonly responsible for UTI, and mix 2 consisted of other enteric gram-negative bacteria that commonly cause UTI *(Klebsiella pneumoniae, Proteus mirabilis, Pseudomonas aeruginosa, Enterobacter aerogenes, Serratia marcescens,* and *Citrobacter freundii).* The mean values of the IgA present in the prostatic fluid in patients with bacterial prostatitis, patients with NBP, and normal controls were 60.7, 14.1, and 4.2 mg/dl, respectively. In the same groups, the mean values of the IgG present in the prostatic fluid were 54.3, 26.3, and 14.9 mg/dl, respectively. These differences were statistically significant. Only patients with bacterial prostatitis showed a significant antibody response to mix 1 and mix 2 bacterial antigens. None of the control specimens showed elevated IgA or IgG titers in response to mix 1 or mix 2 antigens. The patients with NBP, however, were unique in that they demonstrated a weak but definite mean antibody response to mix 1 and mix 2 bacterial antigens. The cause of this feeble but measurable elevation, in comparison with normal controls, remains unclear and requires additional study.

Shortliffe and colleagues (1985) also reported insignificant antigen-specific antibody elevations against *Ureaplasma* and *Chlamydia* in the prostatic fluid of male patients with NBP. This raises serious doubt concerning an etiologic role of these organisms in prostatitis.

Diagnostic Bacteriologic Localization Cultures

The diagnosis of bacterial prostatitis is confirmed when quantitative bacteriologic cultures clearly localize pathogenic bacteria to the prostate. It is important to realize that the growth of small numbers of bacteria on culture of prostatic fluid is often found in CBP. Because CBP usually is a focal, not diffuse, tissue infection, no absolute count of bacteria—that is, colony-forming units (cfu) per millimeter—is diagnostic. Rather, the counts of bacteria in concomitantly obtained specimens from the urethra, midstream bladder urine, and prostatic expressate must be compared. Details concerning the collection of specimens, methods of culture, and interpretation of results have been reported previously (Meares and Stamey, 1968). Both the careful collection of segmented specimens plus immediate culturing after collection (Fig. 16–1, Table 16–2) and the application of bacteriologic techniques capable of quantifying small numbers of bacteria are mandatory for the proper diagnosis of CBP.

If the bladder urine is sterile, or nearly so, urethral colonization or infection is indicated by a much higher count in the first-voided 10 ml of urine that is passed (VB1) than is obtained from either the expressed prostatic secretions (EPS) or the first 10 ml of urine that is voided after prostatic massage (VB3). With bacterial prostatitis, the converse occurs. If heavy bacteriuria is observed in the bladder urine (VB2), treatment for 2 or 3 days with an antimicrobial agent that is active in the urine but not in tissues—for example, 500 mg of penicillin G by mouth every 6 hours or 100 mg of nitrofurantoin by mouth every 8 hours—should precede the collection of segmented specimens. Clinical examples of this method in the diagnosis of patients with CBP are shown in Table 16–3. For the accurate diagnosis of CBP, the counts of pathogenic bacteria in the prostatic specimens should exceed by tenfold or more the counts in the VB1 and VB2 specimens.

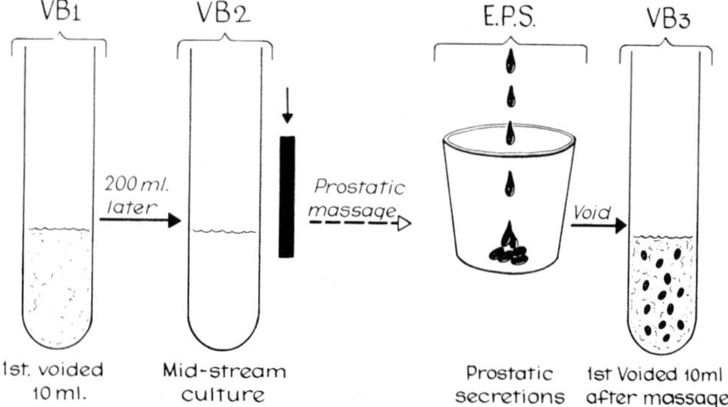

Figure 16–1. Segmented cultures of the lower urinary tract in the male. (Reproduced by permission from Meares EM, Stamey TA: Invest Urol 1968; 5:492. Copyright 1968 by the Williams & Wilkins Company, Baltimore.)

Table 16–2. TECHNIQUE OF SPECIMEN COLLECTION IN PERFORMING DIAGNOSTIC LOCALIZATION CULTURES FOR PROSTATITIS

1. Ensure that the patient has a full bladder and desires to void
2. Prepare the skin of the glans in uncircumcised men (generally unnecessary in circumcised men)
3. Maintain full retraction of foreskin throughout all collections
4. Collect the first 10 ml voided directly into sterile tube (urethral sample)
5. Collect midstream specimen after patient voids about 200 ml (bladder sample)
6. Have the patient stop voiding and bend forward
7. Collect drops of prostatic secretions directly into sterile container during prostatic massage (prostatic sample)
8. Have the patient then void immediatley; collect the first 10 ml (prostatic sample)
9. Refrigerate all samples immediately until cultures are performed

Table 16–3. SEGMENTED CULTURES OF 15 MEN IWTH CHRONIC BACTERIAL PROSTATITIS

		Colonies per ml				
Patient	**Antibiotic**	***VB1***	***VB2***	***EPS***	***VB3***	**Organism**
1	Yes	90	0	800	20	*Escherichia coli*
	No	10	0	1000	20	*E. coli*
2	Yes	0	0	1000	0	*Enterococcus*
	Yes	20	0	4000	10	*Enterococcus*
3	Yes	50	0	165	150	*E. coli*
		0	0	50	20	*Enterobacter aerogenes*
		0	0	560	50	*Proteus mirabilis*
		0	0	140	0	*P. morganii*
	Yes	0	0	660	190	*E. coli*
		10	0	400	40	*E. aerogenes*
		0	0	500	20	*P. mirabilis*
		0	0	200	0	*P. morganii*
4	Yes	20	0	5000	50	*Klebsiella*
	Yes	50	0	100,000	1000	*Klebsiella*
5	No	60	0	1000	20	*E. coli*
	No	640	40	100,000	220	*E. coli*
6	Yes	0	0	5000	100	*E. coli*
	Yes	50	10	10,000	1500	*E. coli*
7	Yes	120	0	3600	370	*E. coli*
	No	2000	200	100,000	4000	*E. coli*
8	Yes	250	20	5000	330	*Klebsiella*
	No	0	0	50	0	*Klebsiella*
	No	20	0	10,000	2000	*Klebsiella*
9	Yes	10,000	150	100,000	10,000	*E. coli*
	Yes	110	0	1500	810	*E. coli*
10	No	2000	60	4000	250	*Enterococcus*
	No	600	60	4000	2000	*Enterococcus*
	No	260	20	7200	90	*Enterococcus*
	Yes	20	20	500	30	*Enterococcus*
11	Yes	30	0	10,000	—	*E. coli*
	Yes	0	0	3600	—	*E. coli*
12	Yes	800	20	—	5000	*E. coli*
	Yes	10,000	800	100,000	10,000	*E. coli*
13	No	0	0	10,000	600	*E. coli*
	Yes	0	0	7000	10	*E. coli*
	Yes	0	0	4000	120	*E. coli*
14	Yes	0	0	700	200	*P. mirabilis*
	Yes	30	0	1000	10	*P. mirabilis*
15	Yes	2500	300	20,000	10,000	*Pseudomonas*
	Yes	110	70	30,000	750	*Pseudomonas*

VB1, the first 10 ml of urine voided (urethral culture); VB2, midstream aliquot (bladder culture); EPS, expressed prostatic secretions from prostatic massage (prostatic culture); VB3, the first 10 ml of urine voided immediately after prostatic massage (prostatic culture).

SECRETORY DYSFUNCTION IN PROSTATITIS

Significant alterations in the secretory products of the prostate occur in patients with prostatitis. The most profound changes are found in patients with documented CBP and are sufficiently inclusive to suggest generalized secretory dysfunction of the prostate (Table 16–4). **Because the relative pH values of prostatic fluid and plasma are thought to be critically important in the nonionic diffusion of drugs across prostatic epithelium, this secretory dysfunction—especially the associated increased alkalinity of the secretions—undoubtedly affects the passage of antimicrobial agents from plasma into prostatic fluid.**

The possibility that dogs and normal men secrete prostatic fluid that is slightly acidic (pH about 6.4) was suggested by Huggins and colleagues (1942) and remained unquestioned for more than three decades. Indeed, Blacklock and Beavis (1974) reported that in normal men, the mean prostatic fluid pH value is 6.6. In contrast, Anderson and Fair (1976) observed that human prostatic fluid is normally alkaline (mean pH: 7.6). In 1978 Pfau and associates noted that the prostatic fluid of normal men is slightly acidic (mean pH: 6.7). Subsequently, Fair and co-workers (1979) observed a mean pH value of 7.28 among 136 specimens of prostatic fluid obtained from 93 normal men and further noted a natural tendency for prostatic fluid to become increasingly alkaline with advancing age. Although these investigators disagreed about the absolute pH value of normal human prostatic fluid, they uniformly agreed that the prostatic fluid of men with CBP is distinctly alkaline. Indeed, the mean pH value of prostatic fluid among their patients generally exceeded that of their controls by about tenfold.

What are the implications concerning pharmacokinetics of increased alkalinity of the prostatic secretions in patients with CBP? Theoretically, a reversal of pH relationships between plasma and prostatic fluid as seen in the experiments performed in dogs must adversely alter the diffusion of antimicrobial bases and favor the diffusion of antimicrobial acids from plasma into prostatic fluid. Because the prostatic secretory dysfunction found in patients with CBP involves multiple factors and not merely

Table 16–4. ALTERATIONS IN PROSTATIC FLUID OF MEN WITH CHRONIC BACTERIAL PROSTATITIS

Increased

pH value
Ratio of LDH isoenzyme 5 to LDH isoenzyme 1*
Immunoglobulins (IgA, IgG, IgM)

Decreased

Specific gravity
Prostatic antibacterial factor (PAF)
Cation concentrations (zinc, magnesium, calcium)
Citric acid concentration
Spermine concentration
Cholesterol concentration
Enzyme concentrations (acid phosphatase, lysozyme)

LDH, lactate dehydrogenase; Ig, immunoglobulin.
*Normal values > 2.
From Meares EM Jr: J Urol 1980; 123:141. Copyright 1980, the Williams & Wilkins Company, Baltimore.

pH changes, however, investigators cannot currently predict with certainty the possible alteration in pharmacokinetics in human patients that may result from this single factor.

PROSTATIC ANTIBACTERIAL FACTOR

The prostatic fluid of dogs, rats, and normal men contains a potent antibacterial factor (PAF) that is bactericidal to most pathogens that commonly cause genitourinary tract infections. Fair and co-workers (1976) initially identified PAF as a zinc compound, but later it was concluded that **PAF is free zinc** (Parrish et al, 1983). **Because zinc concentrations are low and PAF activity is depressed or absent in the prostatic fluid of men who have CBP, some clinicians believe that zinc (PAF) may serve as a natural defense against ascending genitourinary tract infection in normal men.** Whether men become infected because their prostatic secretions contain inadequate levels of zinc (PAF), however, or whether zinc (PAF) is depressed as a consequence of prostatic infection remain unanswered questions. Because the prostatic fluid content of all cations, not merely zinc cations, is depressed in patients with CBP, the low level of zinc observed may represent merely an effect, not an etiologic factor. Additional study is needed in order to resolve this important question. Depressed levels of zinc in prostatic secretions remain unaltered during therapy with oral zinc preparations (Fair et al, 1976).

PHARMACOKINETICS IN PROSTATITIS

Results in Dogs

The results of various antimicrobic diffusion studies in dogs indicate that most agents useful against gram-negative uropathogens diffuse poorly into prostatic secretions (Table 16–5). In contrast, trimethoprim achieves levels in prostatic fluid that exceed plasma levels by severalfold. Dorflinger and associates (1986) investigated the diffusion of various quinolone derivatives into the prostates of dogs. Only enoxacin achieved levels in prostatic fluid (PF) that slightly exceeded the levels in plasma (P): the PF/P ratio was 1.35. The PF/P ratios of ciprofloxacin, amifloxacin, norfloxacin, rosoxacin, and cinoxacin were 0.67, 0.47, 0.34, 0.09, and 0.02, respectively. Although the quinolone levels observed in canine prostatic fluid were generally lower than those in plasma, therapeutic levels against some pathogenic organisms may be achieved in human patients with CBP, especially inasmuch as the prostatic fluid in these patients is usually quite alkaline, not acidic. The new fluoroquinolones are highly active against most pathogens that cause bacterial prostatitis, and their activity is enhanced in alkaline environments (Wolfson and Hooper, 1989).

Factors Determining Diffusion

It is thought that drugs pass from plasma across the prostatic epithelial lipid membrane to enter prostatic fluid by means of nonionic diffusion (Fig. 16–2). Under normal conditions, a drug must be lipid-soluble and not bound to plasma proteins in order to permeate this lipid membrane. Only the nonionized portion of a drug is lipid-soluble; therefore, the dissociation constant of the drug in plasma (pKa) is important in membrane diffusion. This is especially true when the pH values of plasma and prostatic fluid differ significantly, because the acidity or alkalinity of the drug affects nonionic diffusion.

Table 16–5. DIFFUSION AND PROPERTIES THAT AFFECT DIFFUSION OF CERTAIN ANTIMICROBIAL AGENTS FROM PLASMA INTO PROSTATIC FLUID IN DOGS

	Concentration (μg/ml)				
Antimicrobial Agent	***Plasma***	***Prostatic Fluid***	**Dissociation Characteristic**	**Lipid Solubility**	**pKa**
Penicillin G	62	<0.2	Acid	No	2.7
Ampicillin	54	<0.2	Acid	No	2.5
Cephalothin	63	<0.4	Acid	No	2.5
Cephalexin	53	0.7	Amphoteric	Low	5.2, 7.3
Nitrofurantoin	15	3.2	Acid	Low	6.3
Nalidixic acid	53	<5.0	Acid	Yes	6.0
Rifampicin	17	2.0	Acid	Yes	7.9
Chloramphenicol	23	14.0	Nondissociable	Yes	—
Sulfamethoxazole	13	1.3	Acid	Low	6.05
Sulfisoxazole	15	0.3	Acid	Low	5.0
Polymyxin B	14	<0.5	Base	No	8–9
Kanamycin	41	2.0	Base	No	7.2
Erythromycin	16	38.0	Base	Yes	8.8
Oleandomycin	12	39.0	Base	Yes	7.6
Clindamycin	10	76.0	Base	Yes	7.6
Lincomycin	41	10.0	Base	Yes	7.6
Tetracycline	19	4.0	Amphoteric	Yes	3.3, 7.7, 9.7
Oxytetracycline	10	<2.0	Amphoteric	Low	3.3, 7.3, 9.1
Doxycycline	48	7.0	Amphoteric	Low	3.4, 7.7, 9.7
Minocycline	3.6	0.54	Amphoteric	Yes	3.4, 7.8, 9.3
Rosamicin	1.0	8.9	Base	Yes	9.1
Trimethoprim	1.2	10.0	Base	Yes	7.3

From Meares EM Jr: Rev Infect Dis 1982; 4:475.

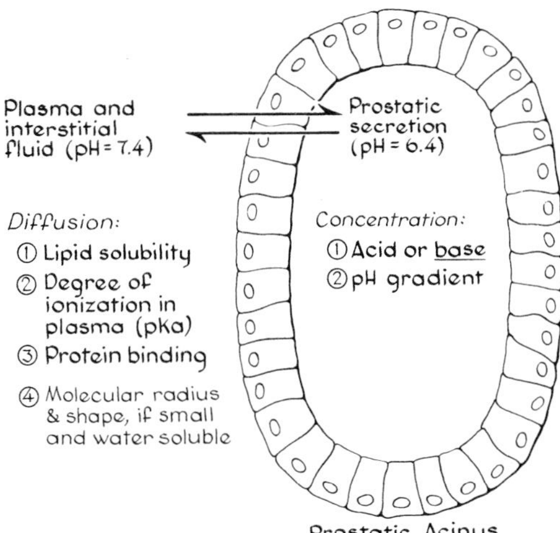

Figure 16–2. Factors determining diffusion and concentration across biologic membranes. (From Stamey TA: Pathogenesis and Treatment of Urinary Tract Infections. Baltimore, Williams & Wilkins, 1980. Copyright 1980 by the Williams & Wilkins Company, Baltimore.)

Drug Diffusion in Chronic Bacterial Prostatitis

The pharmacokinetic studies in dogs (prostatic fluid pH: 6.4 or less; plasma pH: approximately 7.4) have demonstrated, as expected on theoretical grounds, poor accumulation of antimicrobial acids and excellent accumulation of antimicrobial bases in prostatic fluid. The situation concerning pH relationships in human patients with CBP, however, is reversed: prostatic fluid (pH: approximately 8.4) is distinctly more alkaline than plasma (pH: approximately 7.4). In this regard, Stamey and associates (1973) studied the diffusion of trimethoprim into prostatic fluid (pH: approximately 6.4) and salivary fluid (pH: approximately 8.4) of dogs. In each instance, the level of trimethoprim (TMP), a base, found in acidic prostatic fluid was considerably greater than that found in alkaline saliva (Fig. 16–3). One may therefore speculate that levels of antimicrobics found in dog salivary fluid probably correlate better with levels achievable in prostatic fluid of human patients with CBP than do levels found in canine prostatic fluid.

Levels of Antimicrobial Drugs in Prostatic Tissue

Several groups of investigators have studied the prostatic tissue/serum ratios of various antimicrobial agents both in dogs and in human prostatic tissue surgically excised in the treatment of benign prostatic hyperplasia (BPH). In experiments with dogs, Nielsen and co-authors (1980) noted that levels of various penicillanic acid derivatives (including ampicillin, amoxicillin, carbenicillin, and carbenicillin indanyl sodium) in prostatic tissue significantly exceeded levels in prostatic fluid and yet were only 20% to 30% as high as levels in serum. More surprisingly, these investigators found a prostatic interstitial fluid/serum ratio of 0.69 for carbenicillin indanyl sodium, although this drug was not detectable in assays of prostatic tissue or prostatic fluid. Other experiments in dogs have shown that levels of minocycline and rosaramicin in prostatic tissue significantly exceed their levels in serum. More recently, Larsen and colleagues (1986) studied tissue levels of the new fluoroquinolone antimicrobial agents in human prostatic tissue of patients undergoing transurethral prostatectomy; the levels that they observed were sufficiently higher than plasma levels that efficacy against most common prostatic pathogens is suggested.

Human prostatic tissue procured by means of surgical excision or by biopsy of "normal" prostates typically shows prostatic tissue/serum ratios of TMP of 2:1 to 3:1 (Meares, 1982). The concentration of TMP in prostatic tissue therefore exceeds that reached in serum. As with the finding in experiments with dogs, Hensle and associates (1977) found that tissue levels of minocycline exceeded serum levels in men undergoing prostatectomy for BPH. Therapeutic levels of tobramycin and cephalosporins during standard dosing also have been observed in human prostatic tissue obtained by surgical excision. The significance of these observations remains uncertain.

Bacterial infections of the prostate probably involve the interstitium and stroma, not merely the ducts and acini. Whether infection of the interstitium and stroma occurs without simultaneous infection of prostatic ducts and acini cannot, unfortunately, be resolved by current diagnostic methods. Available data imply that many antimicrobial agents attain therapeutic levels in human prostatic interstitium and stroma and may effectively clear infection from those sites. However, **because the pathogens in CBP are readily recovered in EPS cultures, therapeutic levels of antimicrobic agents obviously must be achieved in the secretions, not merely in the stroma and the interstitium.** Indeed, animal and human studies uniformly show TMP levels in prostatic tissue that greatly exceed levels in serum. Treatment failures in bacterial prostatitis therefore cannot logically be attributed to inadequate levels of TMP in prostatic tissue. The most reasonable explanation is the inade-

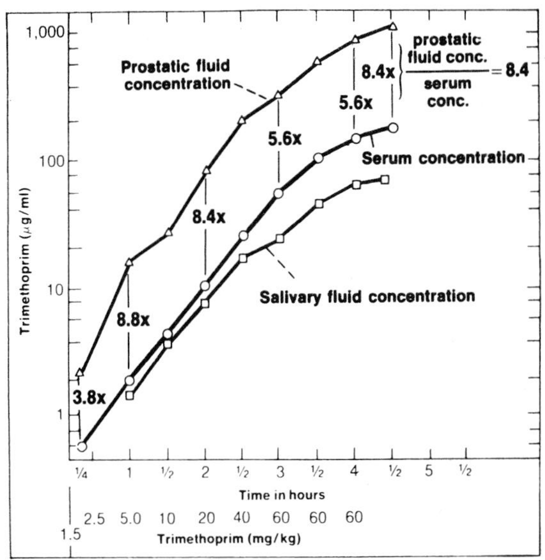

Figure 16–3. Diffusion of trimethoprim from serum into prostatic and salivary fluid in dogs. (From Stamey TA, Bushby SRM, Bragonje J: J Infect Dis 1973; 128[Suppl]:686.)

quate penetration of drugs into the prostatic ducts, acini, and secretions. In addition, infected prostatic calculi cannot be cured by medical therapy alone (Meares, 1986c).

BACTERIAL PROSTATITIS

Acute Bacterial Prostatitis

Clinical Features

Acute bacterial prostatitis is characterized by the sudden onset of moderate to high fever, chills, low back and perineal pain, urinary frequency and urgency, nocturia, dysuria, generalized malaise with accompanying arthralgia and myalgia, and varying degrees of bladder outlet obstruction. Rectal palpation usually discloses an exquisitely tender, swollen prostate gland that is partially or totally firm, irregular, and warm to the touch. The prostatic expressate is packed with leukocytes and fat-laden macrophages, and large numbers of the bacterial pathogen grow on culture. At the onset of illness, however, prostatic massage is not recommended; it is painful for the patient and may lead to bacteremia. **Because bacteriuria usually accompanies ABP, the pathogen generally is identified by culture of the voided urine.**

Pathology

ABP results in marked inflammation of part or all of the prostate gland. Sheets of polymorphonuclear leukocytes are characteristically noted within and around the acini, along with intraductal desquamation and cellular debris. Variable tissue invasion by lymphocytes, plasma cells, and macrophages also is typical. Diffuse edema and hyperemia of the stroma are typical. Microabscesses may occur early in the course of the disease; large abscesses are late complications.

Therapy

Patients who have ABP usually respond readily to therapy with antibacterial agents that normally diffuse poorly from plasma into prostatic fluid. Perhaps, as in acute meningitis, the intense, diffuse inflammatory reaction enhances the passage of these drugs from plasma into the prostatic secretory system. Most patients in whom acute urinary retention develops or who need parenterally administered antimicrobial therapy must be hospitalized. Preferred initial therapy in the nonallergic patient is trimethoprim-sulfamethoxazole (TMP-SMX), 160 mg of TMP and 800 mg of SMX, orally twice daily, or 8 to 10 mg/kg (based on the TMP component) in two to four divided doses every 6, 8, or 12 hours intravenously, until the culture and sensitivity test results are known. If the pathogen is susceptible and the clinical response satisfactory, treatment is continued orally for 30 days to prevent CBP.

There is evidence that the new fluoroquinolone agents ciprofloxacin, norfloxacin, ofloxacin, and enoxacin have excellent efficacy in the treatment of bacterial prostatitis (Naber, 1989; Wolfson and Hooper, 1989). The recommended dosage is ciprofloxacin, 500 mg orally bid; norfloxacin, 400 mg orally bid; ofloxacin, 400 mg orally bid; or enoxacin, 400 mg orally bid. As with TMP-SMX, therapy is continued for 30 days when the clinical response is favorable. If, for some reason, these oral agents cannot be used, initial therapy with intravenous gentamicin plus ampicillin (3 to 5 mg/kg/day gentamicin divided into three intravenous doses; 2 g ampicillin given intravenously every 6 hours) is recommended until the culture and sensitivity test results are available. After the patient is afebrile for 48 hours, a suitable oral agent is administered instead for an additional 30 days. General supportive measures, such as adequate hydration, analgesics, antipyretics, bed rest, and stool softeners, are also employed. Urethral instrumentation should be avoided. Acute urinary retention is best managed by temporary placement of a punch suprapubic tube under local anesthesia. Transurethral catheters are tolerated poorly and may lead to complications.

Chronic Bacterial Prostatitis

Clinical Features

The clinical manifestations of CBP are quite variable. Although chronic prostatitis may evolve from ABP, many men with CBP have no history of prior ABP. Some men are found to have CBP only because asymptomatic bacteriuria is found incidentally. **Most men with CBP, however, complain of variable irritative voiding symptoms, including dysuria, urinary urgency and frequency, nocturia, and pain perceived in various sites within the the pelvis and genitalia.** Chills or fever is unusual, although postejaculatory pain and hemospermia occur occasionally. **No findings on physical examination, rectal palpation of the prostate, cystoscopy, or urography are specifically diagnostic of CBP.**

The hallmark of CBP is recurrent UTI caused by the same pathogen. The organism persists unaltered in prostatic fluid during therapy with most antimicrobial agents because it accumulates poorly in prostatic secretions. The urine may be sterilized and symptoms controlled during medical therapy; however, discontinuation of medication often leads to reinfection of the urine by the prostatic pathogen and recurrence of symptoms.

Patients with CBP typically have prostatic expressates that at microscopy show excessive numbers of leukocytes and fat-laden macrophages. Because "inflamed" prostatic secretions are also typical in cases of NBP, however, this finding is not diagnostic of CBP. Despite the development of certain biochemical and immunologic markers of prostatic bacterial infections, the diagnosis is still best confirmed clinically by performance of bacteriologic cultures that localize the pathogen to the prostatic secretions. Clinical examples of the usefulness of these culture techniques in diagnosis are shown in Table 16–3.

As mentioned previously, both the careful collection of segmented specimens and the application of bacteriologic techniques capable of quantifying small numbers of bacteria are mandatory for the proper diagnosis of CBP. Unless the clinician has made arrangements with the clinical laboratory to carry out these special techniques, it is impractical to attempt to use these cultures in diagnosis. **Because only 5% of cases of prostatitis are caused by an infectious organ-**

ism and because men with no history of documented UTI seldom, if ever, have CBP, prostatitis patients without histories of UTI can be assumed to actually have NBP/ prostatodynia.

Pathology

The histologic findings in cases of CBP are nonspecific. In general, the inflammatory reaction is less marked and much more focal than that seen in cases of ABP. Variable infiltration by plasma cells and macrophages are prominent within and around the acini, along with focal invasion by lymphocytes. Because these changes are frequently found in the prostates of patients who have no clinical or bacteriologic evidence of bacteriuria or bacterial infections, they are not diagnostic of CBP (Kohnen and Drach, 1979).

Infected Prostatic Calculi

Prostatic calculi, most of which cannot be appreciated by means of rectal examination of the prostate or simple plain-film radiographic studies, develop in adult men with amazing incidences. Transrectal prostatic ultrasonography detects calculi of variable size and number in adult prostates with an incidence of about 75% in middle-aged men and about 100% in elderly men (Peeling and Griffiths, 1984). Moreover, transrectal ultrasonography is said to demonstrate prostatic stones in as many as 70% of men who have no other radiologic signs of prostatic calculi. These stones typically are small but tend to occur in clusters. Multiple large calculi are seen most often in men who have chronic bacterial infections of the prostate. Uninfected prostatic calculi usually cause no symptoms or apparent harm; however, in men who have bacterial prostatitis, prostatic stones can become infected and serve as a source of bacterial persistence and relapsing UTI (Eykyn et al, 1974; Meares, 1974, 1986c).

Ductal obstruction associated with adenomatous hyperplasia has traditionally been implicated as the main predisposing factor in the origin of prostatic calculi. The examination of prostatic calculi by crystallographic analysis, however, indicates that some prostatic calculi are composed of constituents commonly found in urine but foreign to prostatic secretions; this observation suggests that intraprostatic reflux of urine is important in the formation of certain prostatic stones. Indeed, it has been suggested that "primary" or "endogenous" stones are composed mainly of constituents of prostatic secretions and that "secondary" or "exogenous" stones are composed mainly of constituents of urine (Sutor and Wooley, 1974; Rameriz et al, 1980).

The clinical histories of men who have CBP with or without infected prostatic calculi are indistinguishable, except that infected prostatic stones have never been cured by medical therapy alone. Proof that prostatic calculi are infected requires bacteriologic culture of the washed and crushed stones; however, the calculi should be presumed infected in men who have stones and documented CBP (Eykyn et al, 1974; Meares, 1974, 1986c). Although appropriate antimicrobial therapy usually controls symptoms and prevents bacteriuria, infected prostatic calculi cannot be sterilized by medical therapy. Permanent cure of infection is achieved only when all infected calculi and prostatic tissue are removed successfully by surgical means, especially by "radical" transurethral prostatectomy (Meares, 1986c).

Medical Treatment

Regardless of concerns and theoretical controversies about the levels of antimicrobial agents that accumulate in human prostatic fluid, carefully documented clinical studies have shown that few drugs actually cure CBP. Fairly good cure rates with TMP-SMX have been documented in reported prospective studies. Among patients who received TMP-SMX continuously for a long term (4 to 16 weeks), the rate of cure in various studies has been about 30% to 40%, which significantly exceeds the rates of cure after short-term therapy (Meares, 1980). The usual dosage is one double-strength tablet (160 mg TMP, 800 mg SMX) orally twice daily. The optimal duration of therapy remains uncertain.

Other agents with reported usefulness in the management of CBP include carbenicillin indanyl sodium, erythromycin, minocycline, doxycycline, and cephalexin. My own experience with these agents has been disappointing. Studies reported from Belgium indicated remarkable success in curing CBP by means of direct injection of antimicrobial agents into the caudal prostate (Baert and Leonard, 1988). Pfau (1986) reported about a 44% cure rate with the injection of kanamycin, 1000 mg intramuscularly twice daily for 3 days, followed by 500 mg twice daily for 11 days, among patients with CBP who had susceptible pathogens. **The fluoroquinolones ciprofloxacin, enoxacin, norfloxacin, and ofloxacin have excellent efficacy in treatment of CBP and now are the drugs of choice.** Ofloxacin has been approved for treatment of prostatitis caused by strains of *E. coli* (Naber, 1989; Wolfson and Hooper, 1989). **Recommended dosing is ciprofloxacin, 500 mg orally twice daily for 30 days; norfloxacin, 400 mg orally twice daily for 30 days; enoxacin, 400 mg orally twice daily for 30 days; or ofloxacin, 300 mg orally twice daily for 6 weeks.**

Infections that are not cured are generally managed satisfactorily by continuous, suppressive, low-dose medication. When the organism is susceptible, TMP-SMX or nitrofurantoin is well suited for long-term use; neither tends to produce bacterial resistance. The usual dosage is TMP-SMX, one single-strength tablet daily, or nitrofurantoin, 100 mg orally once or twice daily. Discontinuation of therapy, however, eventually results in a return of symptoms and relapsing, recurrent UTI.

Surgical Treatment

Patients with CBP, especially those with prostatic calculi that are not cured or adequately controlled by medical therapy, are candidates for surgical therapy. Total prostatovesiculectomy can cure these patients but is seldom indicated. If the resectionist successfully removes all infected tissue and calculi, transurethral prostatectomy can result in cure. It is often difficult to achieve this goal, especially because the peripheral zones of the prostate contain the greatest foci of infection and stones (Blacklock, 1974). My experience with "radical" transurethral prostatectomy in selected patients with CBP, however, has been encouraging (Meares, 1986c).

NONBACTERIAL PROSTATITIS AND PROSTATODYNIA

Clinical Features

NBP is an inflammation of the prostate of indeterminate cause. Prostatodynia has been described as a special type of NBP in which patients have symptoms of NBP, especially those of a "pelvic pain syndrome," but no history of UTI and normal EPS on microscopy and culture (Drach et al, 1978). As mentioned previously, Brunner and associates (1983) studied men attending a special prostatitis clinic and found that 64% had NBP and 31% had prostatodynia. **During the 1980s and 1990s, my own experience and that of others** (Neal and Moon, 1994) **suggest that there is no reason to distinguish prostatodynia from NBP. Patients with prostatodynia at times do have excessive numbers of leukocytes in the EPS** (Meares, 1986a); **furthermore, video-urodynamic studies reveal similar findings in patients with prostatodynia and NBP, and treatment of the two conditions is essentially the same.**

The typical patient with NBP/prostatodynia is a man aged 20 to 45 years who has symptoms of irritative or obstructive voiding dysfunction or both, no history of documented UTI, negative bacteriologic localization cultures, and variable numbers of inflammatory cells in the EPS. A predominant complaint is pain: perineal, suprapubic, scrotal, low back, or urethral, especially pain referred to the tip of the penile urethra. Other common complaints include urinary urgency, frequency, and nocturia, along with a diminished urinary stream, hesitancy, and even interrupted flow (voiding in "pulses"). Examination of the genitourinary tract and neurologic physical examination disclose no specific abnormality, except that **some patients have "tight" anal sphincters, tender prostates, and tender paraprostatic tissues on digital rectal examination.** Cystoscopic examination often suggests mild to moderate bladder neck obstruction and variable degrees of bladder trabeculation. Studies by Kirby and co-workers (1982) indicated that **NBP/prostatodynia probably is a chemical prostatitis caused by the intraprostatic reflux of urine.**

Possible Causative Agents

As discussed earlier in this chapter, gram-positive bacteria, other than enterococci, seem insignificant causative agents in prostatitis. It is thought that gram-positive bacteria occasionally colonize the prostatic fluid without producing infection. This possibility was suggested by the work of Fowler and Mariano (1982), wherein prostatic expressates from 10 uninfected controls, two bacteriuric patients, and two bacterial prostatitis patients were assayed for IgA binding to *Staphylococcus epidermidis.* Despite positive cultures for *S. epidermidis* in 9 of these 14 samples, no binding of IgA to *S. epidermidis* was found in any sample. In contrast, patients with documented chronic gram-negative prostatitis showed uniform binding of IgA to the infectious pathogen.

Studies on the etiology of NBP have generally excluded fungi, obligate anaerobic bacteria, trichomonads, and viruses as causative agents (Meares, 1987).

Most investigators have found that *Mycoplasma* and *Ureaplasma* species are not causative agents in cases of NBP (Meares, 1973; Måardh and Colleen, 1975; Shortliffe et al, 1985; Berger et al, 1989). In 1983, however, Brunner and colleagues found a tenfold or greater increase in quantitative counts of *Ureaplasma urealyticum* in prostatic fluid cultures in comparison with urethral cultures in 82 (13.7%) of 597 patients who appeared to have NBP. Most of these patients were said to respond to therapy with tetracycline. Unfortunately, these investigators failed to measure the immune response in these patients. Because Shortliffe and associates (1985) found insignificant antigen-specific antibody elevations against *Ureaplasma* in their patients with NBP, the etiologic role of these organisms in prostatitis seems doubtful.

The most controversial putative agent in prostatitis is *Chlamydia trachomatis.* Because this organism is the causative agent in about 40% of cases of male nongonococcal urethritis and in most cases of acute epididymitis in men younger than 35, an etiologic role of this organism in prostatitis seems plausible (Berger et al, 1979). Unfortunately, reported studies leave considerable doubt that *C. trachomatis* is an important pathogen in prostatitis.

In 1981, Bruce and associates studied early morning urine specimens of 70 men with histories suggestive of chronic prostatitis and reported isolating *C. trachomatis* in 35 (50%), in comparison with only 1 (2%) of 50 normal controls. Unfortunately, the study design did not allow for localization of this organism to the prostate or for definite conclusions concerning an etiologic role of *Chlamydia* in prostatitis. In contrast, Måardh and co-workers (1978) studied 53 men with nonacute prostatitis by cultural and serologic methods and concluded that *C. trachomatis* appears to play a minor role, if any, in etiology. Indeed, *C. trachomatis* was isolated from the urethra of only 1 of 53 men and from none of 28 specimens of prostatic fluid obtained from these patients. Moreover, an immunofluorescent test showed little or no antibody activity against *Chlamydia* in the serum of most patients and in the prostatic fluid of even fewer patients. More recently, Berger and associates (1989) studied 35 men with apparent NBP in comparison with 50 normal controls and found no evidence that *C. trachomatis* was an etiologic agent in NBP.

Poletti and associates (1985) performed aspiration biopsies of the prostate in 30 men with NBP, all of whom had positive urethral cultures for *C. trachomatis,* and reported isolating *C. trachomatis* in prostatic tissue cultures from 10 men (33%). In an accompanying editorial, however, Schachter (1985) expressed concern about the methods that these researchers used to identify chlamydial organisms and the possibility of specimen contamination. Subsequently, Doble and co-authors (1989) reported a study of 50 men with NBP; in only one of these men was *Chlamydia* detected in the urethra by an immunofluorescence technique. Each patient underwent transperineal prostatic aspiration biopsy under transrectal ultrasonic control. *Chlamydia* was detected in none of these patients despite application of McCoy tissue culture and immunofluorescence techniques. As mentioned previously, Shortliffe and colleagues (1985) detected insignificant elevations in antigen-specific antibody against *Chlamydia* in the prostatic secretions of their patient with NBP.

It must therefore be concluded that *Chlamydia* appears to play an insignificant role in the etiology of prostatitis.

Video-Urodynamic Findings

Clinical and video-urodynamic studies of NBP/prostatodynia patients demonstrate that most have "spastic" dysfunction of the bladder neck and prostatic urethra—that is, the internal urinary sphincter (Barbalias et al, 1983; Meares, 1986a). **The principal findings are depressed urinary flow rates, incomplete relaxation of the bladder neck and prostatic urethra to a point just proximal to the external urinary sphincter, and abnormally high maximal urethral closure pressures at rest.** Electrical silence (normal relaxation) of the external urinary sphincter during voiding is typical in these patients, and uninhibited bladder contractions are unusual (Table 16–6). Because NBP/prostatodynia patients are otherwise normal neurologically, an acquired functional disorder is suggested. This condition is a type of bladder-internal sphincter dyssynergia that has been called a *bladder neck/urethral spasm syndrome* (Meares, 1986a). **The postulated basis of symptoms in these NBP/prostatodynia patients is as follows: Smooth muscle spasm of the bladder neck and prostatic urethra causes elevated pressures in the prostatic urethra, resulting in intraprostatic and ejaculatory duct urinary reflux, which leads to a chemical prostatitis, seminal vesiculitis, and even epididymitis.** In this regard, Hellstrom and co-authors (1987) reported three patients with NBP (probably prostatodynia) whose intraprostatic and ejaculatory duct urinary reflux was severe enough that it was demonstrated easily by voiding cystourethrography.

Some patients with NBP/prostatodynia appear to suffer mainly from tension myalgia of the pelvic floor (Sinaki et al, 1977; Segura et al, 1979). Symptoms in these patients are thought to arise from habitual contraction and spasms of the pelvic floor skeletal muscles. Pelvic pain and discomfort are associated with sitting, running, or other physical activities that lead to fatigue of the perineal muscles. Rectal examination typically demonstrates discomfort from palpation of the anus and paraprostatic tendons and muscles, but a nontender prostate.

Table 16–6. CLINICAL AND VIDEO-URODYNAMIC FINDINGS IN PROSTATODYNIA

Clinical presentation: variable
Neurologic examination: normal
Pudendal neuropathy: absent } by EMG confirmation
Urethral reflexes: intact } by EMG confirmation
Type of voiding: synergistic (no dyssynergia)
Bladder capacity: often increased
Bladder contractions: voluntary (rarely involuntary) and of normal magnitude
VCUG: bladder neck obstructed or incompletely funneled
VCUG: prostatic urethra narrowed in area of EUS despite EMG silence of the EUS
Urethral pressure profile: increased maximal urethral closure pressure (at rest)
Urinary flow rate: decreased peak and average flow

EMG, electromyogaphy; VCUG, voiding cystourethrography; EUS, external urethral sphincter.

From Meares EM Jr, Barbalias GA: Semin Urol. 1983; 1:146. Used by permission.

Most patients with NBP/prostatodynia experience emotional strife and psychosocial or psychosexual abnormalities of variable degree. Many clinicians therefore believe that psychologic factors play a primary role in the etiology of prostatodynia. Blacklock (1986) summarized various psychometric observations in patients with prostatodynia and concluded, "These various studies support a contention that prostatodynia patients have increased levels of self-reported anxiety-related somatic discomfort and pain in comparison with normal subjects and that there is a general behavior pattern of excessive tension." Miller (1988) reported that in many of his patients with apparent NBP and prostatodynia, stress seemed to be a basis for their prostatitis. Indeed, he preferred to call this condition "stress prostatitis."

Regardless of what actually initiates NBP/prostatodynia, the symptoms probably are the result of nonrelaxation (or spasm) of the internal urinary sphincter and nonrelaxation (or spasm) of the pelvic floor striated muscles, alone or in combination, leading to elevated prostatic urethral pressures and intraprostatic (and possibly ejaculatory duct) urinary reflux.

Treatment

Because most men with NBP/prostatodynia show functional obstruction of the bladder neck and prostate on video-urodynamic testing, it is believed by many investigators that this leads to intraprostatic and ejaculatory duct urinary reflux and a chemically induced inflammation within the prostate and ejaculatory system (Blacklock, 1986; Meares, 1986a). **The bladder neck and prostate are rich in alpha-adrenergic receptors; therefore, alpha-adrenergic blocking agents can relax the bladder neck and prostate, improve the voiding dysfunction, eliminate the intraprostatic and ejaculatory duct system urinary reflux, and improve or eliminate the symptoms of NBP/prostatodynia. Indeed, alpha blockers are the most important agents in the management of NBP/prostatodynia.** Because of once-a-day dosing and fewer adverse side effects, newer alpha blockers, such as terazosin and doxazosin, are preferred over older agents, such as prazosin and phenoxybenzamine. **To prevent or minimize adverse side effects, especially postural hypotension, these agents must be given initially at low dosage. The dosage is then increased slowly until the desired relief of symptoms is achieved.**

The manufacturers of terazosin (Abbott Laboratories) and doxazosin (Roerig Division of Pfizer Laboratories) supply free patient starter cards that begin with 1-mg pills and gradually increase the dose to 5 mg (terazosin) or 4 mg (doxazosin). **Attaining an effective dosage that minimizes or eliminates symptoms without causing troublesome adverse side effects is the therapeutic goal. In my experience, most patients need 10 to 15 mg of terazosin or 4 to 8 mg of doxazosin, each taken once daily at bedtime.** Treatment should be continued for at least 6 months. Because most patients experience a return of symptoms when the medication is discontinued, treatment usually must be prescribed indefinitely.

It is important to reassure the patient that his condition is noninfectious and noncontagious and does not lead to serious complications or cancer. Dietary restrictions are unnecessary, unless spicy foods or alcoholic beverages seem to cause or aggravate the symptoms. Hot sitz baths can sooth painful symptomatic episodes, but prostatic massage is probably therapeutic only in men in whom the prostate is "congested" as a result of infrequent sexual activity. Pain and discomfort often respond to short courses of anti-inflammatory agents, such as ibuprofen, 600 mg orally four times daily; irritative voiding dysfunction usually responds to the use of anticholinergics, such as oxybutynin, 5 mg orally three times daily. The efficacy of oral zinc preparations and megavitamins remains unproven.

Patients with tension myalgia of the pelvic floor respond best to treatment with diazepam, 5 mg orally three times daily, alone or in combination with an alpha-adrenergic blocking agent.

Patients who respond poorly to medical management or who have significant emotional problems should be referred to a psychologist or psychiatrist for stress management.

INTERSTITIAL CYSTITIS AND PROSTATITIS

In 1987, Messing suggested that some men with prostatodynia may represent a subset of patients with interstitial cystitis. Later, in 1992, he described five male patients in whom prostatodynia was refractory to treatment and who had the typical cystoscopic features of interstitial cystitis. In 1995, Miller and associates studied 20 men with prostatodynia/nonbacterial prostatitis and observed petechial hemorrhages in the bladder ("glomerulations") in 12 after the patients underwent hydrodistention under general anesthesia. Miller and associates recommended that the **diagnosis of interstitial cystitis should be considered in patients with a clinical diagnosis of prostatodynia or nonbacterial prostatitis that is refractory to treatment.**

Since the 1980s at the New England Medical Center, my colleagues and I have made the diagnosis of interstitial cystitis in more than 30 men who were initially thought to have nonbacterial prostatitis or prostatodynia but whose conditions were refractory to treatment (Meares and Sant, 1995). In all patients, cystoscopy showed some degree of bladder neck obstruction and the typical appearance of mucosal petechial hemorrhages ("glomerulations") after two hydrodistentions. All patients were under general or high spinal anesthesia. Cold-cup bladder biopsies revealed increased numbers of mast cells in the mucosa in all patients and in the detrusor in most patients. All patients who could tolerate the medication responded favorably or extremely well to monotherapy with amitriptyline, 50 to 100 mg once daily at bedtime. One of my patients, a 48-year-old man from Greece, was hospitalized with a 2-year history of marked irritative and obstructive voiding dysfunction and intermittent gross hematuria. Cystoscopy revealed marked bladder outlet obstruction, marked trabeculation, a bladder capacity of only 300 ml, and frank mucosal hemorrhage after hydrodistention (Theoharides et al, 1990). Cold-cup bladder biopsies revealed increased numbers of mast cells (about 150 cells/mm^2) in the submucosal and detrusor layers. Transurethral prostatectomy was performed, and a similar excessive number of mast cells was observed in the prostatic tissue. Our experience with this patient proves that at least some men with refractory NBP/prostatodynia have interstitial cystitis and possibly interstitial prostatitis as well.

OTHER TYPES OF PROSTATITIS

Gonococcal Prostatitis

The incidence of venereal disease caused by *Neisseria gonorrhoeae* remains high throughout the world. Although the rate of isolation of *N. gonorrhoeae* from the urethras of men is usually low, the incidence of urethral infection among contacts of women with gonorrhea is frequent and often symptomatic. Indeed, in one study, *N. gonorrhoeae* was isolated from urethral specimens of 78% of male contacts of women with gonorrhea; about half of these men were asymptomatic (Thelin et al, 1980).

That the gonococcus can infect the prostate was demonstrated in 1931 by Sargent and Irwin, who reviewed 42 cases of prostatic abscess and found that 75% were caused by gonococcal infection. However, whether prostatic infection with *N. gonorrhoeae* remains a significant clinical problem is uncertain. Most studies have suggested that gonococcal prostatitis rarely occurs. Two studies, however, demonstrated positive antibody against *N. gonorrhoeae* in the prostatic fluid of patients whose cultures were negative. Danielsson and Molin (1971) used fluorescent antibody tests and detected apparent persistence of gonococci in the prostatic fluid of 40% of men who were deemed cured, on the basis of ordinary diagnostic techniques, after usual short-term therapy. In another study, six men had repeatedly negative cultures but positive findings of fluorescent antibody tests against *N. gonorrhoeae* in the seminal fluid. After therapy with metacycline, antibody studies were no longer positive in five men (Colleen and Måardh, 1975).

It must be concluded that gonococci may invade the male accessory sex glands during acute urethral infection and that conventional therapy for gonococcal urethritis may occasionally fail to clear the gonococcus from these accessory glands. Symptomatic prostatitis may develop in these patients despite negative cultures for *N. gonorrhoeae.* Therefore, patients with histories of prior gonococcal urethritis in whom apparent NBP develops probably should receive tetracycline therapy, preferably minocycline or doxycycline, 100 mg orally twice daily or ofloxacin, 400 mg orally twice daily for 3 to 4 weeks.

Tuberculous Prostatitis

Granulomatous prostatitis caused by *Mycobacterium tuberculosis* may develop as a sequela of miliary tuberculosis. The diagnosis is confirmed by recovery of the organism from prostatic fluid cultures. The reader is referred to Chapter 24 for a more detailed discussion.

Parasitic Prostatitis

Prostatitic infection caused by parasites is common in certain parts of the world but uncommon in the United States. (See Chapter 22.)

Mycotic Prostatitis

Granulomatous prostatitis caused by fungi associated with systemic mycosis (blastomycosis, coccidioidomycosis, cryptococcosis, histoplasmosis, paracoccidioidomycosis, and candidiasis) are seen occasionally in clinical practice (Schwarz, 1982). Diagnosis is usually confirmed by means of prostatic histology and culture of prostatic fluid and tissue. Therapy is directed toward treatment of the generalized disease. (See Chapter 23.)

Nonspecific Granulomatous Prostatitis

Nonspecific granulomatous prostatitis occurs in two forms: a noneosinophilic variety and an eosinophilic variety. Although neither variety is seen frequently in clinical practice (the eosinophilic variety is especially rare), both types are important clinically because they may be confused with prostatic carcinoma.

NONEOSINOPHILIC VARIETY. Noneosinophilic granulomatous prostatitis apparently represents a tissue response of the foreign body type to extravasated prostatic fluid (O'Dea et al, 1977). Acute signs and symptoms of bladder outlet obstruction associated with an enlarged, firm prostate that feels malignant characterize the clinical presentation. Fever and significant symptoms of irritative voiding dysfunction may or may not be found. Urine cultures often are sterile, but coliforms (mainly *E. coli*) may grow. Histologic examination of prostatic tissue obtained by biopsy or surgical excision and the exclusion of specific forms of infectious granulomatous prostatitis by culture or other means confirm the diagnosis. Some patients respond favorably to antimicrobial agents, corticosteroids, and temporary bladder drainage via a catheter; others require transurethral resection of the prostate.

EOSINOPHILIC VARIETY. Particularly when associated with fibrinoid necrosis and generalized vasculitis, eosinophilic granulomatous prostatitis is a serious illness (Towfighi et al, 1972). Because it occurs almost exclusively in patients with allergies, especially in asthmatic patients, this entity also is known as allergic granuloma of the prostate. In general, affected patients become severely ill, and high fevers develop. Hemograms of the peripheral blood typically show significant eosinophilia. As the prostate gland typically becomes markedly enlarged and indurated, complete urinary retention often develops. Diagnostic confirmation requires histologic examination of prostatic tissue. Because the response to therapy using corticosteroids is usually dramatic, the need for surgical intervention to relieve bladder outlet obstruction is often avoided. The severity of the associated generalized vasculitis and the response to therapy primarily determine the prognosis.

PROSTATIC ABSCESS

Since the 1940s, the incidence of prostatic abscess appears to have declined and the type of infecting organism has changed. In 1931 (the preantibiotic era), Sargent and Irwin noted that *N. gonorrhoeae* caused 75% of 42 cases of prostatic abscess. In 1988, Weinberger and associates reviewed the clinical and bacteriologic features of 269 cases of prostatic abscess that had been reported by various authors during the preceding 40 years (the antibiotic era). During this period, coliforms (chiefly *E. coli*) caused about 70% of the cases. Other significant pathogens included *Pseudomonas* species, staphylococci, and occasionally obligate anaerobic bacteria.

Ascending urethral infection and the intraprostatic reflux of infected urine are thought to initially cause ABP, which then leads to prostatic abscess (Weinberger et al, 1988). A few cases of prostatic abscess have been caused by staphylococci, especially *Staphylococcus aureus,* which suggests a hematogenous pathogenesis (Meares, 1986d). Men especially prone to prostatic abscess include those who are diabetic, those who are on maintenance dialysis for chronic renal failure, those who are immunocompromised for various reasons, and those who undergo urethral instrumentation or require indwelling urethral catheters (Meares, 1986d; Weinberger et al, 1988).

Because of highly variable clinical manifestations, the diagnosis of prostatic abscess has become increasingly elusive. The signs and symptoms of prostatic abscess in 213 adult cases are shown in Table 16–7. On rectal examination, the prostate has been enlarged in about 75% of patients, but prostatic tenderness (in 35% of patients) and fluctuation (in 16% of patients) have been unreliable indicators of prostatic abscess (Weinberger et al, 1988). Most cases of prostatic abscess occur in men who are in the fifth and sixth decades of life; however, nine cases have been reported in infants (ages 14 to 35 days), all of whom were infected with staphylococci alone or in combination with a coliform (Weinberger et al, 1988).

Prostatic imaging (computed tomography or transrectal ultrasonography) is important in the diagnosis of prostatic abscess and also serves as a guide for percutaneous aspiration (for culture), for drainage, and for evaluation after the response to treatment (Fig. 16–4) (Meares, 1986d; Weinberger et al, 1988).

Once the diagnosis of prostatic abscess is confirmed, therapy consists of pathogen-specific antimicrobial agents plus adequate drainage of the abscess. Occasionally, percutaneous drainage suffices, but more often transurethral incision or resection is required. Perineal drainage by means of incision, once the preferred method of drainage, is now seldom used. When properly identified and treated, most prostatic abscesses resolve without recurrence or serious sequelae. Indeed, modern methods of diagnosis and treatment have resulted in a decline in mortality from about 30% (in the

Table 16–7. SIGNS AND SYMPTOMS OF PROSTATIC ABSCESS IN 213 ADULTS

Sign or Symptom	No. of Patients	Percentage
Acute urinary retention	72	34
Fever	70	33
Dysuria	58	27
Urinary frequency	49	23
Perineal pain	49	23
Hematuria	15	7
Urethral discharge	15	7
Pain in low back	2	1

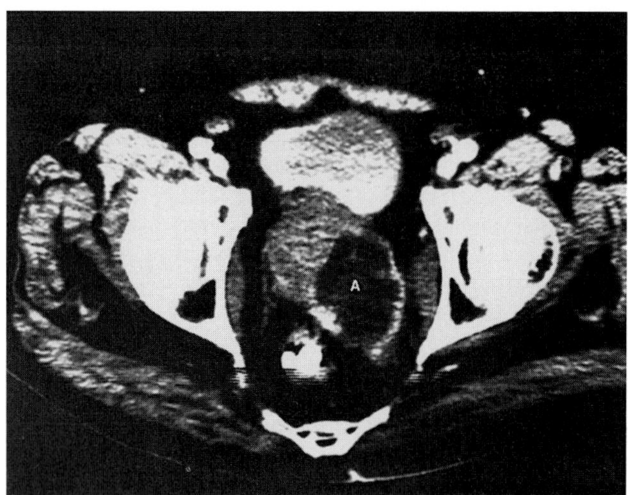

Figure 16–4. Pelvic computed tomographic scan showing prostatic abscess (A).

preantibiotic era) to about 5% (in the antibiotic era) (Weinberger et al, 1988).

PROSTATITIS AND INFERTILITY

Interest in the possible relation of infections of the prostate and seminal vesicles to male subfertility and barren marriages has grown. Despite extensive investigative study, however, controversy prevails.

A review of most studies shows that the addition of live microorganisms to normal fresh ejaculates decreases sperm viability (impairing motility and agglutination) but only when the inocula are massive ($>10^6$ cfu/ml) (Meares, 1980; Fowler, 1981). Because spermatozoa are not likely exposed to such massive concentrations of pathogens as a result of CBP, subfertility in such cases probably does not occur on the basis of a direct effect of the pathogen on spermatozoa. Many clinicians, however, believe that the secretory dysfunction of the prostate that accompanies CBP leads to adverse effects on spermatozoa and resultant subfertility (Homonnai et al, 1978; Caldamone et al, 1980). Additional study of the possible interrelations of infections of the prostate and seminal vesicles, secretory dysfunction of these glands, and subfertility seems warranted.

SEMINAL VESICULITIS

Bacterial infections of the seminal vesicles undoubtedly occur but generally cannot be proved clinically. Whether bacterial seminal vesiculitis occurs without concomitant prostatic infection is unknown. Histopathologic studies of unselected autopsies and of autopsies performed upon men with known terminal UTIs suggest a low incidence of seminal vesiculitis, even when the incidence of prostatitis is high (Hyams et al, 1932; Calams, 1955). However, the incidence of seminal vesiculitis among men with clinical signs and symptoms of prostatitis apparently has not been documented well by histopathologic study.

Because "pure" vesicular fluid is virtually unobtainable for culture and analysis, the challenge of clinically proving a case of seminal vesiculitis is formidable. Semen analyses that show a low volume and subnormal levels of fructose suggest secretory dysfunction of the seminal vesicles but do not confirm an infectious cause of this dysfunction. Likewise, a positive culture or abnormal cytologic findings of the ejaculate cannot be used to confirm a diagnosis of seminal vesiculitis with certainty. Seminal vesiculograms have been reported to correlate poorly with the results of surgery and histologic findings in patients with suspected seminal vesiculitis (Dunnick et al, 1982).

When a bacterial infection of the seminal vesicles is suspected, recommended therapy is the same as that for bacterial prostatitis. That bacterial infections of the seminal vesicles occur was demonstrated by Kennelly and Oesterling (1989), who reported a case of seminal vesicle abscess and cited six other reported cases. Like prostatic abscesses, abscesses of the seminal vesicles are generally managed by appropriate antimicrobics plus adequate abscess drainage.

REFERENCES

Anderson RU, Fair WR: Physical and chemical determinations of prostatic secretion in benign hyperplasia, prostatitis, and adenocarcinoma. Invest Urol 1976; 14:137.

Anderson RU, Weller C: Prostatic secretion leukocyte studies in nonbacterial prostatitis (prostatosis). J Urol 1979; 121:292.

Baert L, Leonard A: Chronic bacterial prostatitis: 10 years of experience with local antibiotics. J Urol 1988; 140:755.

Barbalias GA, Meares EM Jr, Sant GR: Prostatodynia: Clinical and urodynamic characteristics. J Urol 1983; 130:514.

Berger RE, Alexander ER, Harnisch JP, et al: Etiology, manifestations and therapy of acute epididymitis: Prospective study of 50 cases. J Urol 1979; 121:750.

Berger RE, Kessler D, Holmes KK: Etiology and manifestations of epididymitis in young men: Correlations with sexual orientation. J Infect Dis 1987; 155:1341.

Berger RE, Krieger JN, Kessler D, et al: Case-control study of men with suspected chronic idiopathic prostatitis. J Urol 1989; 141:328.

Bergman B, Wedren H, Holm SE: Long-term antibiotic treatment of chronic bacterial prostatitis. Effect on bacterial flora. Br J Urol 1989; 63:503.

Blacklock NJ: Some observations on prostatitis. *In* Williams DC, Briggs MH, Stanford M, eds: Advances in the Study of the Prostate. London, Heinemann, 1969, pp 37–61.

Blacklock NJ: Anatomical factors in prostatitis. Br J Urol 1974; 46:47.

Blacklock NJ: Urodynamic and psychometric observations and their implications in the management of prostatodynia. *In* Weidner W, Brunner H, Krause W, Rothauge CF, eds: Therapy of Prostatitis. Munich, W. Zuckschwerdt Verlag, 1986, pp 201–206.

Blacklock NJ, Beavis JP: The response of prostatic fluid pH in inflammation. Br J Urol 1974; 46:537.

Bruce AW, Willett WS, Chadwick P, et al: The role of chlamydiae in genitourinary disease. J Urol 1981; 126:625.

Brunner H, Weidner W, Schiefer H-G: Studies of the role of *Ureaplasma urealyticum* and *Mycoplasma hominis* in prostatitis. J Infect Dis 1983; 147:807.

Calams JA: A histopathologic search for chronic seminal vesiculitis. J Urol 1955; 74:638.

Caldamone AA, Emilson LBU, Al-Juburi A, et al: Prostatitis: Prostatic secretory dysfunction affecting fertility. Fertil Steril 1980; 34:602.

Chodirker WB, Tomasi TB: Gamma-globulins: Quantitative relationships in human serum and nonvascular fluids. Science 1963; 142:1080.

Colleen S, Mårdh P-A: Effect of metacycline treatment of non-acute prostatitis. Scand J Urol Nephrol 1975; 9:198.

Danielsson D, Molin L: Demonstration of *N. gonorrhoeae* in prostatic fluid after treatment of uncomplicated gonorrheal urethritis. Acta Derm Venereol 1971; 51:73.

Doble A, Thomas BJ, Walker MM, et al: The role of *Chlamydia trachomatis* in chronic abacterial prostatitis: A study using ultrasound guided biopsy. J Urol 1989; 141:332.

Dorflinger T, Larsen EH, Grasser TC, et al: The concentration of various quinolone derivates in the dog prostate. *In* Weidner W, Brunner H, Krause W, Rothauge CF, eds: Therapy of Prostatitis. Munich, W. Zuckschwerdt Verlag, 1986, pp 35–39.

Drach GW: Problems in diagnosis of bacterial prostatitis: Gram-negative, gram-positive and mixed infections. J Urol 1974; 111:630.

Drach GW: Prostatitis: Man's hidden infection. Urol Clin North Am 1975; 2:499.

Drach GW, Fair WR, Meares EM Jr, Stamey TA: Classification of benign diseases associated with prostatic pain: Prostatitis or prostatodynia? J Urol 1978; 120:266.

Dunnick NR, Ford K, Osborne D, et al: Seminal vesiculography: Limited value in vesiculitis. Urology 1982; 20:454.

Eykyn S, Bultitude MI, Mayo ME, et al: Prostatic calculi as a source of recurrent bacteriuria in the male. Br J Urol 1974; 46:527.

Fair WR, Couch J, Wehner N: Prostatic antibacterial factor. Identity and significance. Urology 1976; 7:169.

Fair WR, Crane DB, Schiller N, Heston WDW: A re-appraisal of treatment in chronic bacterial prostatitis. J Urol 1979; 121:437.

Fowler JE Jr: Infections of the male reproductive tract and infertility: A selected review. J Androl 1981; 3:121.

Fowler JE Jr, Mariano M: Immunologic response of the prostate to bacteriuria and bacterial prostatitis: II. Antigen specific immunoglobulin in prostatic fluid. J Urol 1982; 128:165.

Hellstrom WKG, Schmidt RA, Lue TF, et al: Neuromuscular dysfunction in nonbacterial prostatitis. Urology 1987; 30:183.

Hensle TW, Prout GR Jr, Griffin P: Minocycline diffusion into benign prostatic hyperplasia. J Urol 1977; 118:609.

Homonnai ZT, Matzkin H, Fainman N, et al: The cation composition of the seminal plasma and prostatic fluid and its correlation to semen quality. Fertil Steril 1978; 29:539.

Huggins C, Scott WW, Heinen JH: Chemical composition of human semen and of secretions of prostate and seminal vesicles. Am J Physiol 1942; 136:467.

Hyams JA, Kramer SE, McCarthy JF: The seminal vesicles and the ejaculatory ducts: Histopathologic study. JAMA 1932; 98:691.

Jameson RM: Sexual activity and the variations of the white cell content of the prostatic secretion. Invest Urol 1967; 5:297.

Kennelly MJ, Oesterling JE: Conservative management of a seminal vesicle abscess. J Urol 1989; 141:1432.

Kirby RS, Lowe D, Bultitude MI, Shuttleworth KED: Intra-prostatic urinary reflux: An aetiological factor in abacterial prostatitis. Br J Urol 1982; 54:729.

Kohnen PW, Drach GW: Patterns of inflammation in prostatic hyperplasia: A histologic and bacteriologic study. J Urol 1979; 121:755.

Larsen EH, Grasser TC, Dorflinger T, et al: The concentration of various quinolone derivatives in the human prostate. *In* Weidner W, Brunner H, Krause W, Rothauge CF, eds: Therapy of Prostatitis. Munich, W. Zuckschwerdt Verlag, 1986, pp 40–44.

Lipsky BA: Urinary tract infections in men. Ann Intern Med 1989; 110:138.

Mårdh P-A, Colleen S: Search for uro-genital tract infections in patients with symptoms of prostatitis. Studies on aerobic and strictly anaerobic bacteria, mycoplasmas, fungi, trichomonads and viruses. Scand J Urol Nephrol 1975; 9:8.

Mårdh P-A, Ripa KT, Colleen S, et al: Role of *Chlamydia trachomatis* in non-acute prostatitis. Br J Vener Dis 1978; 54:330.

Meares EM Jr: Bacterial prostatitis versus "prostatosis": A clinical and bacteriological study. JAMA 1973; 224:1372.

Meares EM Jr: Infection stones of the prostate gland. Laboratory diagnosis and clinical management. Urology 1974; 4:560.

Meares EM Jr: Prostatitis syndromes: New perspectives about old woes. J Urol 1980; 123:141.

Meares EM Jr: Prostatitis: Review of pharmacokinetics and therapy. Rev Infect Dis 1982; 4:475.

Meares EM Jr: Prostatodynia: Clinical findings and rationale for treatment. *In* Weidner W, Brunner H, Krause W, Rothauge CF, eds: Therapy of Prostatitis. Munich, W. Zuckschwerdt Verlag, 1986a, pp 207–212.

Meares EM Jr: Prostatitis and related disorders. *In* Walsh PC, Gittes RF, Perlmutter AD, Stamey TA, eds: Campbell's Urology, 5th ed. Philadelphia, W. B. Saunders Company, 1986b, pp 868–887.

Meares EM Jr: Chronic bacterial prostatitis: Role of transurethral prostatectomy (TURP) in therapy. *In* Weidner W, Brunner H, Krause W, Rothauge CF, eds: Therapy of Prostatitis. Munich, W. Zuckschwerdt Verlag, 1986c, pp 193–197.

Meares EM Jr: Prostatic abscess. (Editorial.) J Urol 1986d; 136:1281.

Meares EM Jr: Acute and chronic prostatitis: Diagnosis and treatment. Infect Dis Clin North Am 1987; 1:855.

Meares EM Jr, Stamey TA: Bacteriologic localization patterns in bacterial prostatitis and urethritis. Invest Urol 1968; 5:492.

Meares EM Jr, Sant GS: Unpublished observation, 1995.

Messing EM: The diagnosis of interstitial cystitis. Urology 1987; 29(Suppl 4):4.

Messing EM: Interstitial cystitis and related syndromes. *In* Walsh PC, Retik AB, Stamey TA, Vaughan ED Jr, eds: Campbell's Urology, 6th ed. Philadelphia, W. B. Saunders Company, 1992, pp 982–1005.

Miller HC: Stress prostatitis. Urology 1988; 32:507.

Miller JL, Rothman I, Bavendam TG, et al: Prostatodynia and interstitial cystitis: One and the same? Urology 1995; 45:587.

Mobley DF: Erythromycin plus sodium bicarbonate in chronic bacterial prostatitis. Urology 1974; 3:60.

Mobley DF: Semen cultures in the diagnosis of bacterial prostatitis. J Urol 1975; 114:83.

Mobley DF: Bacterial prostatitis: Treatment with carbenicillin indanyl sodium. Invest Urol 1981; 19:31.

Naber KG: Use of quinolones in urinary tract infections and prostatitis. Rev Infect Dis 1989; 11(Suppl 5):S1321.

Neal DE Jr, Moon TD: Use of terazosin in prostatodynia and validation of a symptom score questionnaire. Urology 1994; 43:460.

Nielsen OS, Frimodt-Moeller N, Maigaard S, et al: Penicillanic acid derivatives in the canine prostate. Prostate 1980; 1:79.

O'Dea MJ, Hunting DB, Greene LF: Non-specific granulomatous prostatitis. J Urol 1977; 118:58.

Parrish RF, Perinetti EP, Fair WR: Evidence against a zinc binding peptide in pilocarpine-stimulated canine prostatic secretions. Prostate 1983; 4:189.

Peeling WB, Griffiths GJ: Imaging of the prostate by ultrasound. J Urol 1984; 132:217.

Pfau A: Prostatitis: A continuing enigma. Urol Clin North Am 1986; 13:695.

Pfau A, Perlberg S, Shapira A: The pH of the prostatic fluid in health and disease: Implications of treatment in chronic bacterial prostatitis. J Urol 1978; 119:384.

Pfau A, Sacks T: Chronic bacterial prostatitis: New therapeutic aspects. Br J Urol 1976; 48:245.

Poletti F, Medicin MC, Alinovi A, et al: Isolation of *Chlamydia trachomatis* from the prostatic cells in patients affected by nonacute abacterial prostatitis. J Urol 1985; 134:691.

Rameriz CT, Ruiz JA, Gomez AZ, et al: A crystallographic study of prostatic calculi. J Urol 1980; 124:840.

Sargent JC, Irwin R: Prostatic abscess: Clinical study of 42 cases. Am J Surg 1931; 11:334.

Schachter J: Is *Chlamydia trachomatis* a cause of prostatitis? (Editorial.) J Urol 1985; 134:711.

Schaeffer AJ, Wendel EF, Dunn JK, Graynack JT: Prevalence and significance of prostatic inflammation. J Urol 1981; 125:215.

Schwarz J: Mycotic prostatitis. Urology 1982; 19:1.

Segura JW, Opitz JL, Greene LF: Prostatosis, prostatitis or pelvic floor tension myalgia? J Urol 1979; 122:168.

Shortliffe LMD, Elliott KM, Sellers RG, et al: Measurement of chlamydial and ureaplasmal antibodies in serum and prostatic fluid of men with nonbacterial prostatitis. (Abstract.) J Urol 1985; 133(4, pt 2):276A.

Shortliffe LMD, Wehner N: The characterization of bacterial and nonbacterial prostatitis by prostatic immunoglobulins. Medicine 1986; 65:399.

Shortliffe LMD, Wehner N, Stamey TA: Use of a solid-phase radioimmunoassay and formalin-fixed whole bacterial antigen in the detection of antigen-specific immunoglobulin in prostatic fluid. J Clin Invest 1981a; 67:790.

Shortliffe LMD, Wehner N, Stamey TA: The detection of a local prostatic immunologic response to bacterial prostatitis. J Urol 1981b; 125:509.

Sinaki M, Merritt JL, Stillwell GK: Tension myalgia of the pelvic floor. Mayo Clin Proc 1977; 52:717.

Stamey TA: Pathogenesis and Treatment of Urinary Tract Infections. Baltimore, Williams & Wilkins, 1980.

Stamey TA: Prostatitis. J R Soc Med 1981; 74:22.

Stamey TA, Bushby SRM, Bragonje J: The concentration of trimethoprim in prostatic fluid: Nonionic diffusion or active transport? J Infect Dis 1973; 128(Suppl):S686.

Sutor DJ, Wooley SE: The crystalline composition of prostatic calculi. Br J Urol 1974; 46:533.

Thelin I, Wennstrom A-M, Måardh P-A: Contact tracing in patients with genital chlamydial infection. Br J Vener Dis 1980; 56:259.

Theoharides TC, Flaris N, Cronin CT, et al: Mast cell activation in sterile bladder and prostate inflammation. Int Arch Allergy Appl Immunol 1990; 92:281.

Thin RN, Simmons PD: Chronic bacterial and nonbacterial prostatitis. Br J Urol 1983; 55:513.

Towfighi J, Sadeghee S, Wheller JE, et al: Granulomatous prostatitis with emphasis on the eosinophilic variety. Am J Clin Pathol 1972; 58: 630.

Weinberger M, Cytron S, Servadio C, et al: Prostatic abscess in the antibiotic era. Rev Infect Dis 1988; 10:239.

Wolfson JS, Hooper DC: Fluoroquinolone antimicrobial agents. Clin Microbiol Rev 1989; 2:378.

17
INTERSTITIAL CYSTITIS AND RELATED DISEASES

Philip Hanno, M.D.

GENERAL CONSIDERATIONS

Possibly one of the most challenging diseases in the urologic spectrum, interstitial cystitis (IC) has only recently been recognized as the major health problem that it is (Held et al, 1990). **It encompasses a major portion of the "painful bladder" disease complex, which includes a large group of urologic patients with bladder and/or pelvic pain, irritative voiding symptoms (urgency, frequency, nocturia, dysuria), and negative urine cultures.** Painful bladder diseases with a well-known cause include radiation cystitis, cyclophosphamide cystitis, cystitis caused by microorganisms that are not detected by routine culture methodology, and systemic diseases affecting the bladder.

There appear to be three groups of patients who show symptoms of bladder pain and urinary frequency without an obvious cause. One group develops lower-tract symptoms that resolve before any formal evaluation can be instituted. These appear to be patients who would be diagnosed as suffering from urethral syndrome. A second group of patients has shown the symptom complex long enough to be referred to a urologist, who elects to perform an evaluation including cystoscopy under anesthesia with hydrodistention of the bladder and biopsy. Patients with petechial hemorrhages after distention and a biopsy not suggestive of other abnormalities are considered to have IC. Such patients without the typical findings of IC are in a twilight zone but are generally treated in a similar manner.

One problem with defining IC is that the symptoms are in reality an exaggeration of normal sensations. Urinary frequency patterns can be related to fluid intake and age, and the signal or urge to void is considered an unpleasant or painful sensation by most persons (Burgio et al, 1991). **With no pathognomonic findings on pathologic examination, IC is truly a diagnosis of exclusion.** It may have multiple causes and represent a final common reaction of the bladder to different types of insult. Thus, issues of definition are critical. To understand the current way IC is defined and how this came to be, a look back in time is helpful.

HISTORICAL PERSPECTIVE

Interstitial cystitis was recognized as a pathologic entity in the last century. Skene (1887) used the term to describe an inflammation that has "destroyed the mucous membrane partly or wholly and extended to the muscular parietes."

Early in this century at a New England section meeting of the American Urological Association, Guy Hunner (1915) reported on eight women with a history of suprapubic pain, frequency, nocturia, and urgency lasting an average of 17 years. Hunner drew attention to the disease, and the red, bleeding areas he described on the bladder wall came to have the pseudonym "Hunner's ulcer." As Walsh (1990) points out, this has proved to be unfortunate. In the early part of this century the very best cystoscopes available gave a poorly defined and ill-lit view of the fundus of the bladder. It is not surprising that when Hunner saw red and bleeding areas high on the bladder wall he thought they were ulcers. For the next 60 years, urologists would look for ulcers and fail to make the diagnosis in their absence. The disease was felt to be focal rather than a pancystitis.

Hand (1949) wrote the first comprehensive paper about the disease, reviewing 223 cases. In looking back, his paper was truly a seminal one and ahead of its time. Many of his epidemiologic findings have held up over the years. His description of the clinical findings is eerily familiar to the way we now define it. He writes, "I have frequently observed that what appeared to be a normal mucosa before and during the first bladder distention showed typical interstitial cystitis on subsequent distention." He notes "small, discrete, submucosal hemorrhages, showing variations in form. . . . dotlike bleeding points. . . . little or no restriction to bladder capacity." He portrays three grades of disease, with grade 3 the small-capacity, scarred bladder described by Hunner. Sixty-nine percent of patients were grade 1 and only 13% were grade 3.

Walsh (1978) later coined the term "glomerulations" to describe the petechial hemorrhages that Hand described. But it wasn't until Messing and Stamey (1978) discussed the "early diagnosis" of IC that attention turned from looking for an ulcer to make the diagnosis to the concept that symptoms and glomerulations under anesthesia were the disease hallmarks and that the diagnosis was primarily one of exclusion.

The best historical description of IC comes from Bourque (1951) and is worth recalling. "We have all met, at one time or another, patients who suffer chronically from their bladder; and we mean the ones who are distressed, not only periodically but constantly, having to urinate often, at all moments of the day and of the night, and suffering pains every time they void. We all know how these miserable patients are unhappy, and how those distressing bladder symptoms get finally to influence their general state of health, physically at first, and mentally after a while."

Although dramatic and right on the mark, this description and others like it were not suitable for defining this disease in such a manner as to help physicians make the diagnosis and design research studies to learn more about the problem. Physician interest and government participation in research were sparked through the efforts of a group of frustrated patients led by Dr. Vicki Ratner, then an orthopedic surgery resident in New York City, who founded the patient advocacy group, the Interstitial Cystitis Association (Wein et al, 1990; Ratner et al, 1992). The first step was to develop a working definition of the disease.

DEFINITION

In an effort to define IC so that patients in different geographic areas, under the care of different physicians, could be compared, the National Institute of Arthritis, Diabetes, Digestive and Kidney Diseases (NIADDK) held a workshop in August 1987 (Gillenwater and Wein, 1988) at which consensus criteria were established for the diagnosis of IC. These criteria were not meant to define the disease, but rather to ensure that groups of patients studied would be relatively comparable. After pilot studies testing the criteria were carried out, the criteria were revised at another NIADDK workshop a year later (Wein et al, 1990). These criteria are depicted in Table 17–1.

Although meant initially to serve only as a research tool, the NIADDK "research definition" has become a de facto definition of this disease, diagnosed by exclusion and colorfully termed a "hole in the air" by Hald (George, 1986). Certain of the exclusion criteria serve mainly to make one wary of a diagnosis of IC but should by no means be used for categoric exclusion of such a diagnosis. However, because of the ambiguity involved, these excluded patients should probably be eliminated from

Table 17–1. NIADDK RESEARCH DEFINITION OF INTERSTITIAL CYSTITIS

Required Criteria:

Glomerulations *or* Hunner's ulcer on cystoscopic examination

and

Pain associated with the bladder *or* urinary urgency

Examination for glomerulations should occur after distension of bladder under anesthesia to 80–100 cm H_2O for 1–2 min. Bladder may be distended up to two times before evaluation. Glomerulations must be diffuse—present in at least three quadrants of the bladder—and there must be at least 10 glomerulations per quadrant. Glomerulations must not be along path of cystoscope (to eliminate artifact from contact instrumentation). Presence of any one of the following criteria *excludes* diagnosis of interstitial cystitis:

1. Bladder capacity of greater than 350 ml on awake cystometry using either gas or liquid as filling medium
2. Absence of intense urge to void with bladder filled to 100 ml of gas or 150 ml of water during cystometry, using a fill rate of 30–100 ml/min
3. Demonstration of phasic involuntary bladder contractions on cystometry using fill rate described above
4. Duration of symptoms less than 9 months
5. Absence of nocturia
6. Symptoms relieved by antimicrobials, urinary antiseptics, anticholinergics, or antispasmodics (musculotropic relaxants)
7. Frequency of urination, while awake, of fewer than eight times per day
8. Diagnosis of bacterial cystitis or prostatitis within 3-month period
9. Bladder or lower ureteral calculi
10. Active genital herpes
11. Uterine, cervical, vaginal, or urethral cancer
12. Urethral diverticulum
13. Cyclophosphamide or any type of chemical cystitis
14. Tuberculous cystitis
15. Radiation cystitis
16. Benign or malignant bladder tumors
17. Vaginitis
18. Age less than 18 years

NIADDK, National Institute of Arthritis, Diabetes, Digestive and Kidney Diseases.

research studies or separately categorized. In particular, exclusion criteria 4, 5, 6, 8, 9, 11, 12, 17, and 18 are only relative. What percentage of patients with idiopathic sensory urgency have IC is unclear (Frazer et al, 1990). The specificity of the finding of bladder glomerulations and the percentage of the normal population that would be found to have glomerulations if the bladder were distended under anesthesia to 80 cm H_2O is unknown. Likewise, the number of patients with urethral syndrome who would have findings of IC if they were evaluated with bladder distention under anesthesia is also unknown. **Bladder ulceration is extremely rare and accounts for less than 5% of patients in this author's experience and in the group treated by Sant (1991). Koziol (1994) found 20% of his series in California to have ulceration.** Specific pathologic findings represent a glaring omission from the criteria, as there is a lack of consensus as to which pathologic findings, if any, are required for a tissue diagnosis (Hanno et al., 1990).

EPIDEMIOLOGY

Most epidemiologic information about IC has historically come from anecdotal reports and reviews of series of patients from physicians or programs that see a lot of patients with the disease. Farkas and colleagues (1977) discussed IC in adolescent girls, Hanash and Pool (1969) reviewed their experience with IC in men, and Geist and Antolak (1970) reviewed and added to reports of the disease occurring in childhood. **A childhood presentation is extremely rare and must be differentiated from the much more common and benign-behaving *extraordinary urinary frequency syndrome of childhood,* a self-limited condition of unknown etiology** (Koff and Byard, 1988; Robson and Leung, 1993). Perhaps the largest single clinic survey aimed at determining the natural history of IC was conducted at the Scripps Research Institute and included 374 of their patients as well as some members of the Interstitial Cystitis Association, the large patient support organization (Koziol et al, 1993). Although such reviews provide some information, they would seem to be necessarily biased by virtue of their design.

Population-Based Studies

Two population-based studies have been reported in the literature, and it is these studies that tend to give credibility to reviews of self-selected patients or from individual clinics like the comprehensive follow-up review by Koziol (1994). The first population-based study was conducted by Oravisto (1975), who included "almost all the patients with interstitial cystitis in the city of Helsinki. . . ." This superb, brief report from Finland looked at all diagnosed cases in a population approaching 1 million. The prevalence of the disease in women was 18.1 per 100,000. The joint prevalence of both sexes was 10.6 cases per 100,000. The annual incidence of new female cases was 1.2 per 100,000. **Severe cases accounted for about 10% of the total. Ten percent of the cases were in men. An interesting finding was that the disease onset is commonly subacute rather than insidious, and full development of the classic symptom complex takes place over a relatively short time.** Many patients can remember the day the symptoms began, an unusual situation for a chronic illness. IC does not progress continuously but reaches its final stage rapidly and then continues without significant change in symptomatology. Subsequent major deterioration was found by Oravisto to be unusual.

The duration of symptoms before diagnosis was 3 to 5 years in the Finnish study. Analogous figures in the United States in Hand's classic 1949 paper were 7 to 12 years. Oravisto commented on an increasing incidence of the disease from 1965 to 1975. The apparent increasing incidence may well be secondary to referral patterns, earlier recognition, and increasing awareness of the disease among patients and physicians.

Much of the current interest in IC in the American public health arena and among physicians dates from the only other population-based study of IC. This widely reported comprehensive study of IC in the United States was carried out on a shoestring budget by researchers at the Urban Institute and the University of Pennsylvania and published only as a chapter in a text on the disease (Held et al, 1990). It confirmed many of the findings in the Oravisto study and revealed a wealth of interesting findings. It was based on data from four sources:

1. A random survey of 127 board-certified urologists who supplied material on prevalence and incidence of IC and criteria they used in diagnosis
2. A survey of 64 IC patients selected by the random sample of urologists, divided into those they had last treated and those they had last diagnosed (the newest cohort)
3. A survey of 902 female patients who were members of the Interstitial Cystitis Association
4. A random sample of 119 persons (73 females) from the U.S. population

The data were confirmed by surveying nonresponders to rule out nonresponse bias.

The following findings highlighted the study:

1. In 1987 there were 43,500 (perhaps up to 90,000) diagnosed cases of IC in the United States, approximately twice the prevalence in Finland found by Oravisto 12 years earlier. More interesting, women who were diagnosed by sampled urologists as actually having IC represented only 20% of the cases presenting with symptoms (chronic painful bladder, sterile urine) that were suggestive of this disease. On the basis of these data, **from 250,000 to almost 500,000 patients in the United States might have had IC in 1987, depending on the assumptions used.**
2. The median age of onset is 40 years.
3. Late deterioration in symptoms is unusual (as per Oravisto).
4. **Up to 50% of patients experience spontaneous remissions probably unrelated to treatment with a duration ranging from 1 to 80 months (mean 8 months).**
5. Patients with IC are 10 to 12 times more likely than controls to report childhood bladder problems.
6. Patients with IC are twice as likely as controls to report a history of urinary tract infection; however, over half of all IC patients report fewer than one such infection per year before the onset of IC.

7. The time from symptom onset to diagnosis varied from 24 months for the patients most recently diagnosed to 51 months for members of the Interstitial Cystitis Association.

8. Household size, marital status, number of male sexual partners, and educational status did not seem to significantly differ between those patients diagnosed as having IC and the general adult female population. Fourteen percent of patients were of Jewish origin compared with 3% in the general population sample. This compares with 15% of the Koziol sample (1994) and may demonstrate some genetic predisposition.

9. **Using well-developed quality-of-life indicators that employed responses to subjective statements, female IC patients scored lower on nine such tests, compared with an identical set of tests given to a sample of U.S. women with chronic renal failure undergoing dialysis.**

10. Taking the prevalence figure of 44,000, the IC-related incremental medical care cost in the United States was $116.6 million in 1987 and IC-related lost economic production was $311.7 million.

Put in practical terms, the Held figures suggest that if all IC patients were seen by urologists (a doubtful assumption), on average, board-certified urologists would have 10 diagnosed IC patients in their practice and 78% would have made at least one new diagnosis of IC in the previous year.

Associated Diseases

No discussion of epidemiology is complete without looking at the subject of associated diseases. This is especially relevant for a disorder like IC, in which the diagnosis is one of exclusion and the etiology is unclear. It is possible that clues to etiology and ideas for treatment could be suggested.

Newly diagnosed patients are most concerned with the possibility that IC could be a forerunner of bladder carcinoma. **No reports have ever documented a relationship to suggest that IC is a premalignant lesion.** Utz and Zincke (1973) discovered bladder cancer in 12 of 53 men treated for IC at the Mayo Clinic. Three of 224 women were eventually diagnosed with bladder cancer. From this experience has come the dictum that all patients with presumed IC should undergo cystoscopy, urine cytologic examination, and bladder biopsy to be sure that a bladder carcinoma is not masquerading as IC. Four years later additional cases were reported by Lamm and Gittes (1977). In a follow-up from the Mayo Clinic (Murphy et al, 1982), no additional patients had been diagnosed with carcinoma in situ, strongly suggesting no transition to carcinoma had occurred, but rather that the relationship is indeed one of incorrect diagnosis.

Prostatodynia may masquerade as IC, or vice versa (Miller et al, 1995), but any true association of the two disorders would be almost impossible to prove, given the similarity and nonspecificity of the symptoms and the fact that both are diagnoses of exclusion.

A recent large-scale survey of 6783 individuals diagnosed by their physicians as having IC studied the incidence of associated disease in this population (Alagiri et al, 1995). Data from the 2405 responders were validated with information gleaned from 277 nonresponders (Fig. 17–1). **Allergies were the most common disorder, with 41% diagnosed with allergies and 44% with allergic symptoms.** Allergy was also the primary association in Hand's study (1949). Thirty percent of patients had symptoms of irritable bowel syndrome, a finding confirmed in Koziol's study (1994). Altered visceral sensation has been implicated in **irritable bowel syndrome** in that these patients experience intestinal pain at intestinal-gas volumes that are lower than those that cause pain in healthy persons (Lynn and Friedman, 1993), strikingly similar to the pain on bladder distention in IC.

Fibromyalgia, another disorder frequently considered functional because no specific structural or biochemical cause has been found, is also overrepresented in the IC population. This is a painful, nonarticular condition predominantly involving muscles; it is the commonest cause of chronic, widespread musculoskeletal pain. It is typically associated with persistent fatigue, nonrefreshing sleep, and generalized stiffness. As in IC, women are affected at least 10 times more often than men (Consensus Document, 1993). The association is intriguing as both conditions have nearly identical demographic features, modulating factors, associated symptoms, and response to tricyclic compounds (Clauw et al, 1995).

Vulvodynia, migraine headaches, endometriosis, chronic fatigue syndrome, incontinence, and asthma had a similar prevalence as in the general population. **Several publications have noted an association between IC and systemic lupus erythematosus (SLE)** (Fister, 1938; Boye et al, 1979; Rodriguez de la Serna, 1981; Weisman et al, 1981; Meulders et al, 1992). The question has always been whether the bladder symptoms in this relatively rare group of patients represent an association of these two disease processes or rather are a manifestation of lupus involvement of the bladder. The beneficial response of the cystitis of SLE to steroids (Meulders et al, 1992) tends to support the latter view. No association with discoid lupus has been demonstrated (Jokinen, 1972). Although the actual numbers are small, the Alagiri study demonstrated a 30 to 50 times greater incidence of SLE in the IC group compared with the general population. Overall, the incidence of collagen-vascular disease in the IC population is low. Parsons found only 2 of 225 consecutive IC patients to have a history of autoimmune disorder (1990).

Inflammatory bowel disease was found in over 7% of the IC population Alagiri studied, a figure 100 times higher than in the general population. Although unexplained at this time, abnormal leukocyte activity has been implicated in both conditions (Bohne et al, 1962; Kontras et al, 1971).

Another mysterious disorder that has been associated with IC is focal vulvitis. **Vulvar vestibulitis syndrome** is a constellation of symptoms and findings involving and limited to the vulvar vestibule consisting of (1) severe pain on vestibular touch to attempted vaginal entry, (2) tenderness to pressure localized within the vulvar vestibule, and (3) physical findings confined to vulvar erythema of various degrees (Marinoff and Turner, 1991). McCormack (1990) reported on 36 patients with focal vulvitis 11 of whom also had IC. Fitzpatrick and colleagues (1993) have added three more cases. The concordance of these noninfectious inflammatory syndromes involving the tissues derived from the embryonic urogenital sinus and the similarity of the demographics argue for a common cause.

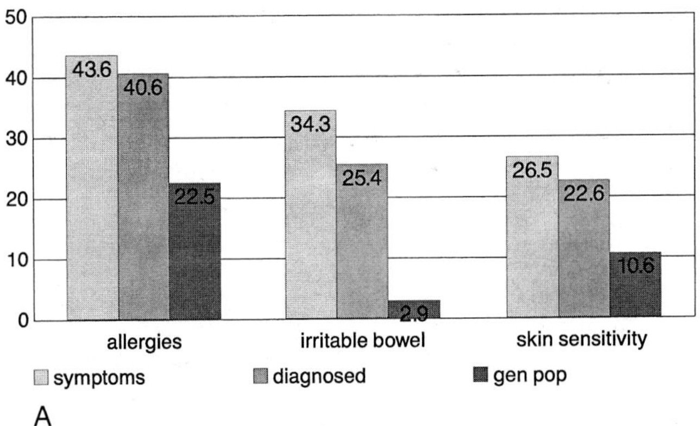

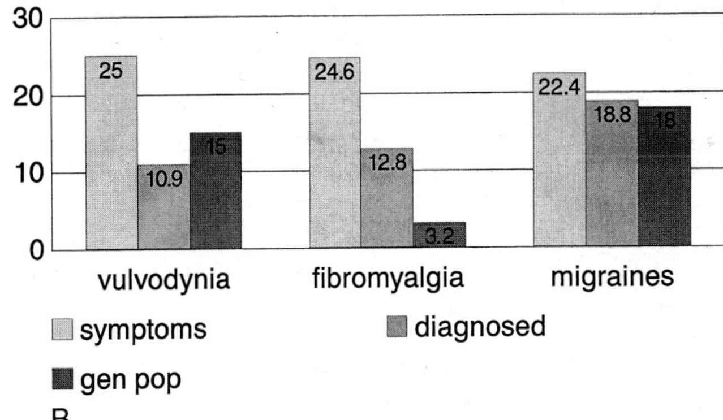

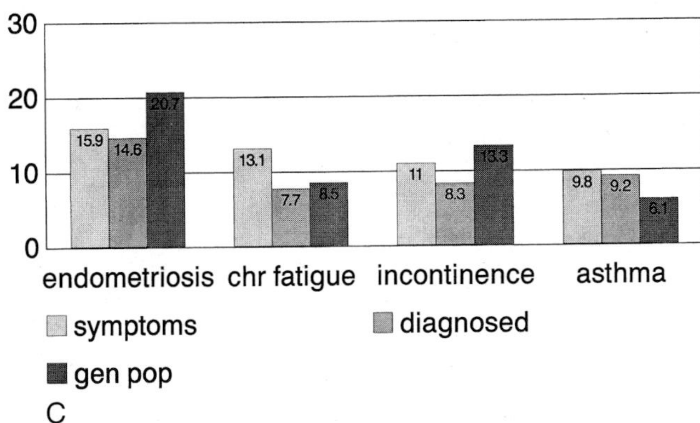

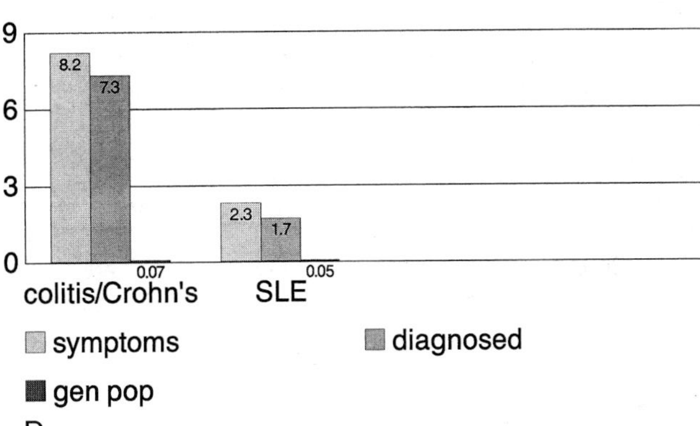

Figure 17–1. Comparison of disease prevalence rates between the Interstitial Cystitis Association (ICA) study group patients who report symptoms of a disorder, who have been diagnosed with a disorder, and the general population. SLE, systemic lupus erythematosus. (From Alagiri M, Chottiner S, Ratner V, et al: J Urol 1995; 153:287A.)

An unexpected association has been reported between IC and **Sjögren's syndrome** (SS), an autoimmune exocrinopathy with a female preponderance manifested by dry eyes, dry mouth, and arthritis, which can also include fever, dry skin, and gastrointestinal and lung problems. Van De Merwe and colleagues (1993) investigated 10 IC patients for the presence of SS. Two patients had both the keratoconjunctivitis sicca and focal lymphocytic sialoadenitis, allowing a primary diagnosis of SS. Only two patients had neither finding.

Finally, a negative correlation with diabetes has been noted. Parsons (1990) had no diabetics in his series of 225 patients. Koziol (1994) reported a 4% incidence of diabetes compared with a prevalence of 8.9% in women aged 45 to 54 years.

The epidemiology of IC may ultimately yield as many clues as the laboratory in trying to understand this condition.

ETIOLOGIC THEORIES

Although there is no lack of theories, the etiology of IC remains obscure. This is not necessarily surprising in a disease as difficult to categorize objectively as this one. As Mulholland and Shupp (1994) and others (Holm-Bentzen et al, 1990) have emphasized, there is no doubt that **multiple factors are capable of causing these symptoms. Therefore, we cannot look at this syndrome as a single disease.** Different initiating insults could result in activation of specific pathogenic pathways that result in the classic symptom complex. We must be careful, at least at this juncture, in trying to explain this disease with one simple theory. A theory may be valid and still only account for a given percentage of patients with the symptom complex. The difference between cause and pathogenesis must be kept in mind. Any marker that seems to be common to most individuals with this condition may reflect a common pathogenesis that can be derived from multiple etiologic mechanisms. Perhaps the bladder has a limited way it can react to injury.

Animal Models

Although it would be nice to have a naturally occurring animal model of IC, up to now researchers have had to devise animal models to study isolated symptoms of IC. The hope is that this compartmentalized approach will yield clues as to the root causes of the symptomatology (Ruggieri et al, 1990).

Abelli and colleagues (1989) have developed a method for studying pain arising from the urinary bladder in conscious, freely moving rats. Potentially helpful in evaluating the action of analgesic drugs, it does not serve as a model for IC etiology.

Two animal models inducible in the laboratory have been developed. Bullock and colleagues (1992) reported a mouse model in which bladder inflammation could be induced by the injection of syngeneic bladder antigen. This demonstrates that a component in the bladder in the Balb/cAN mouse is capable of inducing an adoptively transferrable cell-mediated autoimmune response specific for the bladder that exhibits many characteristics of clinical IC. These include mononuclear infiltration; decreased bladder capacity that is accompanied by fibrosis; edema; increased bladder permeability; hemorrhage on distention; and detrusor mast cell infiltration. The potential exists to study an immune component of the syndrome.

Christensen and colleagues (1990) developed a guinea pig model in which bladder inflammation was induced by the instillation of a solution containing a protein to which the animal had previously been immunized. Further work with this model (Kim et al, 1992) supports the hypothesis that a protein or proteins contained in the urine can gain entry into the bladder wall and induce bladder inflammation consistent with that observed in IC. The type of immune response has not been defined.

The most exciting development in animal model research is the hypothesis put forward by Buffington and associates at Ohio State (1995) that the feline urologic syndrome represents the animal equivalent of IC. Approximately two thirds of cats with lower urinary tract disease have sterile urine and no evidence of other urinary tract disorders (Kruger et al, 1991). A portion of these cats experience frequency and urgency of urination, pain, and bladder inflammation (Houpt, 1991). Glomerulations have been found in the bladder of some cats with this symptom complex. Press and colleagues (1995) recently reported that GP-51, a glycosaminoglycan (GAG) commonly found in the surface mucin covering the mucosa of the normal human bladder and decreased in patients with IC, shows a decreased expression in cats with the feline urologic syndrome. Thus, there now appears to be a common animal malady manifested by urinary urgency, frequency, and pain, with findings of sterile urine, bladder mastocytosis, increased histamine excretion, increased bladder permeability, and decreased urinary GAG excretion (Buffington et al, 1996).

It remains to be seen if the feline urologic syndrome will ultimately yield information useful in prevention or treatment of IC. The many etiologic theories stem primarily from human clinical data.

Infection

Interstitial cystitis usually presents like an infectious disease, and, without a doubt, infection is the diagnosis that physicians and patients assume to be the cause of the bladder symptoms early in the course of IC. By the time the diagnosis has been established, the patient has generally been seen by a number of physicians and treated for a presumed urinary tract infection with a variety of antibiotics, to no avail (Held et al, 1990). IC has facets that make infection appear to be a reasonable cause. The epidemiology of urinary tract infection and its predominance in women mirror the IC data (Warren, 1994). The acute to subacute onset is remarkable for what proves to be a chronic disease. Many patients can remember the morning their symptoms began!

The fact that most patients had been on antibiotics at some point before diagnosis of the disorder led some to speculate that antibiotics might be the cause (Holm-Bentzen et al, 1990). Although it is well known that numerous antibiotics, primarily the penicillins, can induce a cystitis (Bracis et al, 1977; Chudwin et al, 1979; Moller, 1978; Cook et al, 1979), no evidence that these antibiotics or the supposedly "surface active" nitrofurantoins or tetracyclines have any involvement has ever been documented (Levin et al, 1988; Ruggieri et al, 1987).

To determine whether there is an infectious cause of IC, one must use certain procedures (Warren, 1994). Bladder epithelium and not just urine must be cultured for appropriate microorganisms, including bacteria, viruses, and fungi. Because some organisms might be culturable yet fastidious, special culture techniques should be used. Because some organisms in urine or tissue might be viable but nonculturable, specific nonculture techniques for discovery and identification should be employed. Most important, the same procedures must be carried out in a control population.

Up to now, the case for infection has not been a strong one. Hunner (1915) originally proposed that IC results from chronic bacterial infection of the bladder wall secondary to hematogenous dissemination. Harn and colleagues (1973) proposed a relationship between IC and streptococcal and poststreptococcal inflammation. He produced a progressive chronic inflammation in rabbit bladders by injecting small numbers of *Streptococcus pyogenes* in the bladder wall. The discovery that *Helicobacter pylori* is related to the pathogenesis of chronic atrophic gastritis and peptic ulcer disease and that antibiotic treatment can heal ulceration (Parsonnet et al, 1991; NIH Consensus Development Panel, 1994; Sung et al, 1995) has continued to focus attention by researchers in IC on the possibility that an infectious cause is not only reasonable but will ultimately be found. Wilkins and colleagues (1989) found bacteria in catheterized urine specimens and/or bladder biopsies in 12 of 20 patients with IC. However, eight of the isolates were fastidious bacteria, *Gardnerella vaginalis* and *Lactobacillus* sp, and no controls were included in the study. Maskell (1995) continues to believe that infection is a major etiologic component in patients with IC and urethral syndrome. She blames inadequate culture techniques for the failure to document infection. The intriguing suggestion that treatment with up to five sequential antibiotics covering the anaerobic spectrum cured 27 out of 27 IC patients (Durier, 1992) merits further investigation.

The dearth of enthusiasm for an infectious cause is not for lack of trying. Hanash and Pool (1970) performed viral, bacterial, and fungal studies on 30 IC patients and failed to substantiate an infectious cause. Hedelin and colleagues (1980) found only 3 of 19 IC patients to have urine cultures positive for *Ureaplasma urealyticum*, and indirect hemagglutination antibodies to *Mycoplasma hominis* to be no greater than in controls. Fall and associates (1985) could not document a viral cause in 41 consecutive IC patients. Keay and colleagues (1995a) studied urine and bladder tissue from 11 IC patients and 7 controls, finding no evidence that IC is associated with infection or colonization by a single microorganism. Six of the IC patient urine samples did show growth by the sensitive methods employed, but there was no pattern in terms of organisms, and the counts were low, possibly suggesting contamination. The need for controls is obvious, as bladder biopsies from 3 of 6 control subjects grew small numbers of *Pseudomonas* sp or *Staphylococcus epidermidis*.

The development of highly sensitive, rapid, and specific molecular methods of identifying infectious agents by the direct detection of DNA or RNA sequences unique to a particular organism (Naber, 1994) has breathed new life into the search for a responsible microorganism. Hampson and colleagues (1993), using DNA probes, could find no evidence of mycobacterial involvement in eight cases of IC. Alanen and associates (1995) confirmed an absence of bacterial DNA in the bladder of 15 untreated patients with IC. Kiilholma and colleagues (1995) reported an absence of adenovirus and BK virus genomes in urinary bladder biopsies of IC patients. However, Domingue and associates (1995) demonstrated the presence of bacterial 16-S ribosomal RNA genes in bladder biopsies from 29% of IC patients but not from control patients with other urologic diseases. In an unrelated finding, they reported discovering 0.22-μm filterable forms in culture from the biopsy tissue of 14 of 14 IC patients and only 1 of 15 controls. The forms contain nucleic acids, but their significance, if any, is unknown.

The role of infection in the pathogenesis of IC remains a mystery. At this time there are few data to support an infectious cause, but investigators keep coming back to an infectious theory. **Infection could work in concert with other mechanisms, leading to bladder injury and an autoimmune reaction, or leading directly to an autoimmune response and subsequent bladder injury** (Warren, 1994). Either way, urothelial injury could result that persists in the absence of identifiable infection (Elgavish et al, 1995).

Mast Cell Involvement

Although mast cells are thought of primarily in the context of allergic disorders and certain acute inflammatory responses, these cells have also been implicated in biologic responses as diverse as angiogenesis and wound healing; bone remodeling; peptic ulcer disease; atherosclerosis; reactions to neoplasms; and many clinically important chronic inflammatory conditions including scleroderma, rheumatoid arthritis, forms of pulmonary fibrosis, chronic graft-versus-host disease, and inflammatory bowel disease (Galli, 1993).

Mast cells have frequently been reported to be associated with IC both as a pathogenetic mechanism and as a pathognomonic marker (Simmons, 1961; Bohne et al, 1962; Smith and Dehner, 1972; Larsen et al, 1982). Although their role in the disease process is still largely unknown, evidence of their importance is mounting, perhaps serving as the final common pathway through which the symptomatic condition is expressed. Mast cells produce, among other compounds, histamine. Histamine release in tissue causes pain, hyperemia, and fibrosis, all notable features of IC.

Simmons (1961) was the first to suggest mast cells as a cause of IC. **The contribution of mast cells to the cellular infiltrate in IC (Fig. 17–2) has been shown to vary from about 20% in nonulcer IC patients to 65% in patients with ulceration** (Sant et al., 1988; Enerback et al, 1989). Mast cells participate in allergic reactions (hypersensitivity type I) during which immunoglobulin E (IgE) antibody is synthesized in response to specific antigens. IgE binds to mast cell receptors, and antigen binds to the IgE, leading to degranulation (Lagunoff et al, 1983). Other triggers of mast cell activation include acetylcholine, anaphylatoxins, cationic peptides like substance P, chemicals, contrast material, cytokines, opioids, antihistamines, exercise, hormones, viruses, and bacterial toxins (Sant and Theoharides, 1994). Mast cells promote infiltration of neutrophils, T and B lymphocytes, monocytes, and eosinophils. T lymphocytes secrete substances capable of activating mast cells, thus perpetuating the cycle of inflammation (Kaplan et al, 1985).

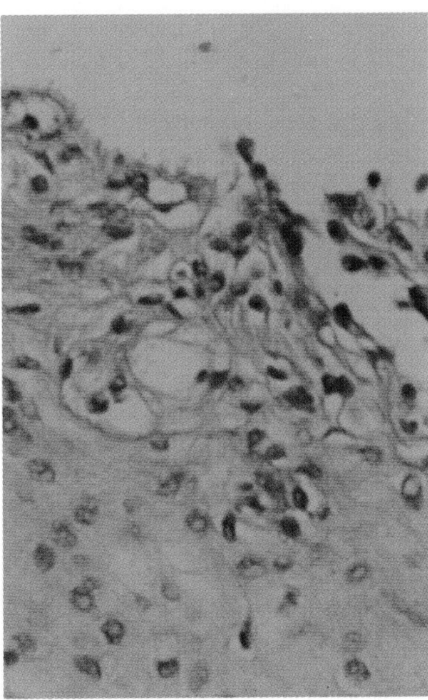

Figure 17–2. Mast cells in the submucosa in a bladder biopsy from a patient with interstitial cystitis (IC). Stain is toluidine blue. Magnification × 40.

Since the presence of mast cells within the bladder wall was first recognized by Simmons and Bunce (1958), numerous investigators have tried to determine whether there is an increase in the number of mast cells in the bladders of patients with IC, or differences in their location or functional state (Larsen et al, 1982; Kastrup et al, 1983; Fall et al, 1987; Feltis et al, 1987; Lynes et al, 1987; Christmas and Rode, 1991). **An increase in urothelial mast cells appears to be part of the generalized inflammatory cell reaction regardless of cause and not a specific feature of IC, whereas the presence of increased numbers of mast cells in the detrusor is more specific for IC.** However, one study did report detrusor mastocytosis in 64% of IC patients and 80% of a control group with other urologic disease, with no statistically significant difference between the mean number of detrusor mast cells in the two groups (Hanno et al, 1990).

Aldenborg and colleagues (1986) reported that mast cells are found predominantly in the detrusor muscle in patients with classic IC, but there is also a secondary population of mast cells in the lamina propria and the bladder epithelium, with staining characteristics distinct from those in the detrusor. None of these epithelial mast cells were found in controls. These findings were interpreted to indicate a transepithelial migration of mast cells in patients with IC. This second population of mast cells does not appear to be involved in the nonulcer type of IC (Aldenborg et al, 1989). This mucosal population of mast cells can also differ from the mast cells found in deeper tissues in physiologic responses and release of secretory products (Sant, 1991). The "mucosal mast cells" are susceptible to aldehyde fixation and require special fixation and staining techniques for proper demonstration. Detrusor mast cells are not susceptible to fixation techniques. Combined with the fact that activated mast cells lose their histologically identifiable granules once degranulation occurs, estimates of mast cell density using standard histologic techniques may underestimate mast cell numbers (Sant and Theoharides, 1994).

Electron microscopy has confirmed that mast cells in IC are more likely to be degranulated or activated than those found in other conditions (Larsen et al, 1982; Theoharides and Sant, 1991; Theoharides et al, 1995). A chronic exposure of detrusor muscle to histamine in IC patients is suggested by the finding of Palea and colleagues (1993) that there is an impairment of the direct contractile response to histamine in detrusor muscle affected by IC in comparison with control detrusor, suggesting a receptor desensitization. **The clinical relationship between an increased number of mast cells and symptoms of IC has not been definitively established.** Some studies have found no correlation (Holm-Bentzen et al, 1987; Lynes et al, 1987). Although mast cell infiltration in intestinal segments used for augmentation has been associated with pain and failure of the procedure (Kisman et al, 1991), other studies have shown that mast cell infiltration in intestine used in the urinary tract is the norm and not pathologic (MacDermott et al, 1990).

Many of the substances that have been shown to induce mast cell secretion are released from neurons that innervate the organ containing the mast cells (Christmas et al, 1990). The capsaicin-sensitive sensory neurons that innervate the bladder are thought to play a dual "sensory-efferent" function, in which a reflex-induced axon release of neuropeptides results in local inflammation (Foreman, 1987; Barbanti et al, 1993). Hand (1949) reported an increase in the submucosal nerve density in IC, a phenomenon confirmed by Christmas and colleagues (1990), who showed an increase in nerve fiber proliferation in IC but not in patients with bacterial or lupus cystitis. Increased innervation by nerves releasing substances affecting mast cells could lead to increased mast cell secretion. Among these substances is acetylcholine. Mast cells can be stimulated by cholinergic agonists to secrete serotonin (Theoharides and Sant, 1991). Substance P–containing fibers have been found to be increased in bladders from IC patients and are found adjacent to mast cells (Pang et al, 1995a). An increase in adrenergic but not cholinergic nerves in IC patients compared with controls was reported by Hohenfellner and colleagues (1992). They also found increased numbers of neurons staining for vasoactive intestinal polypeptide and neuropeptide Y (NPY), both of which are associated with sympathetic nerves. Others have not confirmed the NPY finding and, in fact, have reported a decrease in such staining relative to controls (Schickley et al, 1993).

Could mast cell products be useful in diagnosing IC and/or further indicate a role in pathogenesis? Elevated histamine levels have been found in bladder biopsies of IC patients (Kastrup et al, 1983; Lynes et al, 1987; Enerback et al, 1989) as well as from bladder washings (Lundberg et al, 1993). Holm-Bentzen and colleagues (1987) reported a significantly elevated urinary excretion of 1,4-methylimidazole acetic acid, the major metabolite of histamine. Yun and associates (1992) found no differences between IC patients and controls in random spot tests of urinary histamine. Levels were elevated after hydrodistention in IC patients but not in controls, a possible consequence of hydrodistention and resultant mast cell degranulation. **El-Mansoury and colleagues (1994) found increased levels of methylhistamine, a histamine metabolite, in spot and 24-hour urine samples from IC patients compared with controls. Although such an increase could still be interpreted as indicating a systemic rather than a bladder syndrome, elevated levels of mast cell tryptase in the urine of IC patients, which could only come from the bladder, were subsequently found** (Boucher et al, 1995).

The realization that mast cells are associated with the syndrome of IC by no means diminishes the other multiple etiologic theories. The very presence of mast cells could be related to injury from any of the proposed causes, and degranulation could likewise reflect a final common pathway resulting in pain and frequency from multiple causes. Rickard and Lagunoff (1995) proposed, based on results with mast cell granules and epithelial cells in tissue culture, that mast cells could contribute to failure of epithelialization of the bladder surface after injury by two potential mechanisms: (1) inhibition of epithelial cell replication and (2) interference with epithelial cell spreading, thus resulting in the "leaky epithelium" found in some patients. Mast cells may actually be the mediator through which female hormones play a role, accounting for the 10:1 female-to-male preponderance of the disease (Vliagoftis et al, 1992; Pang et al, 1995b; Patra et al, 1995).

To summarize, the bladder mast cell is a fascinating piece of the IC puzzle. It contains many granules, each of which can secrete many vasoactive and nociceptive molecules. A number of conditions such as extreme cold, drugs, neuropeptides, stress, trauma, and toxins, can trigger the mast cell to secrete some of its contents; they, in turn, can sensitize sensory neurons, which can further activate mast cells by releasing neurotransmitters or neuropeptides. Additionally, the mast cell can directly cause vasodilatation and bladder mucosal damage while also attracting inflammatory cells, thus causing many of the problems seen in IC. There is obviously more to IC than the mast cell, or treatment would be relatively straightforward. There is much individual variation among patients with regard to their presence and their products, and antihistamine treatment has overall proved very disappointing. The words of the group most identified with mast cell research at this time (Sant and Theoharides, 1994) sum it up well: "The mast cell appears to be involved in the pathogenesis of interstitial cystitis. Although it is not pathognomonic of the disease, mastocytosis does occur in a significant subset of interstitial cystitis patients. Because interstitial cystitis is now regarded as a syndrome caused by multiple factors, it is conceivable that one cause of interstitial cystitis is associated with bladder mastocytosis and mast cell activation."

Epithelial Permeability

Until the early 1970s, most investigators thought that the major barrier to free flow of urinary constituents into the bladder interstitium was at the level of the epithelial cells. Tight junctions between urothelial cells, specialized "umbrella cells" lining the surface, and direct bactericidal activity of the vesical mucosa were thought capable of defense of the internal milieu from bacteria, molecules, and ions in the urine (Ratliff et al, 1994). Staehelin and colleagues (1972) proposed that lipid and other hydrophobically bonded materials were important in any barrier to permeability in the luminal membrane because permeants leaked through the interplaque regions if the cell constituents alone limited transport.

It was Parsons who hypothesized and popularized the concept that in a subset of patients, IC is the result of some defect in the epithelial permeability barrier of the bladder surface GAGs (Parsons and Hurst, 1990). The major classes of GAGs include hyaluronic acid, heparan sulfate, heparin, chondroitin 4-sulfate and chondroitin 6-sulfate, dermatan sulfate, and keratan sulfate. These carbohydrate chains, coupled to protein cores, produce a diverse class of macromolecules, the proteoglycans (Trelstad, 1985). GAGs exist as a continuous layer on the bladder urothelium (Dixon et al, 1986; Cornish et al, 1990). Except heparin, all other types of GAGs have been found on the bladder surface (Ruoslahti 1988). The GAG layer functions as a permeability and antiadherence barrier. When impaired, its functions can be duplicated by exogenous GAG (Hanno et al, 1978).

Parsons and Hurst (1990) reported a lower excretion of urinary uronic acid and GAGs in IC patients than in normal volunteers and hypothesized that a leaky transitional epithelium might be absorbing these substances to its surface. The data are interesting in that one might expect urinary GAG levels to increase with injury to the bladder and decrease with resolution (Uehling et al, 1988). The San Diego group (Lilly and Parsons, 1990; Parsons et al, 1990) went on to show experimentally that one can damage the GAG layer with protamine sulfate with resultant backdiffusion of urea through the bladder lumen, and that this urea loss can be prevented with a bladder instillation of exogenous GAG (heparin). By placing a solution of concentrated urea into the bladder of IC patients and measuring absorption versus controls, Parsons and colleagues (1991) presented confirmatory evidence of his theory in patients with IC. Parsons' views are nicely summarized in two recent publications (1993, 1994) and provide a comprehensive, if somewhat imperfect, theory of the disorder. Support for an epithelial abnormality from a different perspective has come from Bushman and colleagues (1994), who found aneuploid DNA profiles on barbotage specimens from IC patients that may signal an underlying abnormality of the epithelial cell population in some patients with IC. Newer methods of culturing bladder epithelium from 4-mm cystoscopic biopsies of IC patients can be expected to yield interesting data in the future (Trifillis et al, 1995).

At this point, however, all is not as simple as it seems. The 1988 paper of Fowler and colleagues provided perhaps the most graphic data to date that the urothelium might be leaky in IC. With immunohistochemical techniques, they assayed the bladder biopsies of 14 IC patients and 10 normal controls for intraurothelial Tamm-Horsfall protein (THP) to indirectly assess the in vivo permeability of the urothelium. Eight pathologic controls were also assessed. Ten of 14 IC patients versus 1 of 18 controls demonstrated intraurothelial THP. In a follow-up study Neal and associates (1991) measured serum THP autoantibody and found high levels versus controls. It is known that excretion rates of THP vary widely, even in repeat samples taken from the same individual (Reinhart et al, 1990). Subsequent studies in IC have failed to show differences in the presence of intraurothelial THP in the IC population versus controls, or in antibody reactivity to THP (Stone et al, 1992; Stein et al, 1993). Thus, one piece of potentially confirmatory evidence that a leaky epithelium is present failed to materialize.

Further data for an abnormal surface mucin came from Moskowitz and colleagues (1994), who studied biopsies from 23 IC patients with regard to the presence of a glycoprotein component of the surface mucin referred to as GP1 and compared the results to those from 11 normal controls. Qualitative GP1 changes in a majority of IC patients were identified. GP1 reactivity was noted in all controls but was absent in 35% of IC patients and diminished in 61%. This study may provide evidence of an abnormal bladder urothelium, but the effects of bladder distention in the IC group is unknown and may have contributed to the results. There were no pathologic controls used, and no attempt was made to correlate GP1 reactivity with IC symptoms (Messing, 1994).

Potentially strong evidence for a population with mucosal leak has recently been reported by Parsons and colleagues (1994). Water or 0.4 mol/L potassium chloride was placed intravesically into normal volunteers and IC patients. Water did not provoke symptoms in either group, but KCl provoked symptoms in 4.5% of normal subjects and 70% of IC patients. Symptomatic responses were reduced in patients on heparinoid therapy. However, even the authors postulate that the same findings might occur in patients with urinary infection, detrusor instability, and carcinogenesis. They may not be specific to IC and do not provide unequivocal evidence of a permeability dysfunction. Could heightened sensitivity to KCl rather than increased permeability of the GAG be responsible for the results?

Finally, we must look at a body of literature that has failed to find GAG abnormality. **Ultrastructural, biochemical, and functional studies of bladder GAG have not supported the increased mucosal permeability theory** (Collan et al, 1976; Dixon et al, 1986; Johansson, 1990; Ruggieri et al, 1991). Nickel and colleagues (1993) did sophisticated electron micrography using a specific antimucus, antisera stabilization technique to study the ultrastructural morphologic appearance of the GAG. No significant difference in the morphologic appearance of the mucus or GAG layer was noted in IC versus controls. That leaves one to postulate an unknown functional abnormality to account for any increase in permeability. Chelsky and associates

(1994) measured bladder permeability in IC using direct measurement by transvesical absorption of technetium Tc-99m diethylenetriamine pentaacetic acid (DTPA). Although some IC patients had a more permeable bladder than others, the same was true for normal volunteers. Increased permeability in the IC group could not be demonstrated. However, three IC patients had marked absorption of DTPA and may represent a subpopulation of patients with increased epithelial permeability.

Overall, it does seem that there is a population of IC patients with increased epithelial permeability, but the issue is far from closed. Increased mucosal permeability is nonspecific and a consequence of bladder inflammation and also occurs with cyclophosphamide-induced bladder injury, bacterial infection, and cystitis after intravesical challenge with antigen after sensitization (Engelmann et al, 1982; Kim et al, 1992). It may also be a consequence of aging itself (Jacob et al, 1978). Whether this represents a primary cause of IC, is a secondary result of IC, or merely reflects the result of an unidentified source of inflammation is unclear. Treatments that tend to *damage* GAG, including transurethral resection and laser of ulcerated areas, bladder distention, silver nitrate administration, oxychlorosene (Clorpactin) administration, and the organic solvent dimethylsulfoxide, have all been used with differing results to *treat* IC. **Increased permeability must be only a part of the story.**

Neurogenic Mechanisms

New etiologic research is focusing on the knowledge that the sensory nervous system can generate some of the manifestations of inflammation (Foreman, 1987; Dimitriadou et al, 1991, 1992). Polymodal nociceptor activation generates axon reflexes in the terminal arborizations of primary afferent neurons. These reflexes cause the C fibers to release neuropeptides that initiate inflammatory changes. Neuropeptides can exert direct effects on vascular smooth muscle and endothelium to increase flow and permeability. Histamines released from mast cells may also participate in neurogenic inflammation. An increase in nerve fibers within the suburothelium and detrusor muscle in ulcerative IC has been noted (Lundberg et al, 1993). A correlation was found between the number of nerve fibers and the number of mast cells as well as between the number of nerve fibers and the amount of histamine. **In a disease manifested primarily by sensory abnormalities, the possibility that the sensory nervous system itself might be the underlying culprit is worth exploring.**

Harrison and colleagues (1990) proposed that small-diameter sensory nerves in the bladder wall may have a role in the transmission of the sensation of pain and in the triggering of inflammatory reactions rather than forming the afferent limb of the micturition reflex. Abelli and colleagues (1991) demonstrated in the rat urethra that mechanical irritation alone can cause neuropeptide release from peripheral capsaicin-sensitive primary afferent neurons resulting in neurogenic inflammation. Hohenfellner and associates (1992) suggest that IC is associated with increased sympathetic outflow into the bladder and altered metabolism of vasoactive intestinal polypeptide and NPY inhibits bladder afferents and therefore may be involved in autonomic disturbances affecting the bladder. Schickly and colleagues (1993) found that hydrodistention in IC patients decreased NPY levels and that predistention levels were lower than in control human bladder tissue. This contrasts with the Hohenfellner findings.

Neurogenic inflammation may be the cause of some cases of IC or may be the result of other initiating etiologic events. It is not incompatible with the central role of the mast cell, nor with the leaky epithelium theory. It conceivably could result in the appearance of autoimmune phenomena or result from an episode of infection. Ongoing immunohistochemical studies on the neuropeptides and muscarinic receptors of the bladder in IC and non-IC populations promise to reveal important data regarding the pathogenesis of IC.

Hypoxia: Reflex Sympathetic Dystrophy

Galloway and colleagues (1991) have proposed that the changes in IC may be explained by an increase in sympathetic discharge, analogous to that seen in reflex sympathetic dystrophy (RSD) of limbs. The abnormality in RSD is the development of abnormal synaptic activity between sensory afferent and sympathetic efferent neurons. Nerve cells in the spinal cord become hypersensitive to sensory input, and this sustains abnormal sympathetic outflow and corresponding vasomotor dysregulation. The excess sympathetic outflow leads to constriction of blood vessels and tissue ischemia, setting up further sensory changes and perpetuating the cycle. In RSD, there is usually a trigger event leading to these changes. Perhaps a urinary infection could trigger such a pathologic cycle in some IC patients.

Herbst and associates (1937) produced bladder lesions resembling the ulceration of IC in a dog by ligating the blood vessels to the posterior bladder wall and infecting the area with α-hemolytic streptococcus. Irwin and Galloway (1993), using laser Doppler flowmetry, showed that when the bladder is distended under anesthesia, blood flow increases in control patients to a statistically significant degree compared with IC patients. However, no difference in flow was noted when the bladder was distended to 100 ml, and any ischemia was a relative phenomenon at unphysiologic filling levels.

No studies performed to date can say any case of IC is related to the syndrome of RSD (Ratliff et al, 1994). Nevertheless, the hypoxia theory of disease is fascinating. We know that hyperbaric oxygen has been effective in the treatment of radiation-induced cystitis (Weiss and Neville, 1989), another disorder manifested by sensory urgency.

Urine Abnormalities

The idea that the urine of IC patients itself is carrying a pathologic substance accounting for the disorder has not escaped the attention of researchers. Indeed, most current theories of pathogenesis involve access of a component of urine to the interstices of the bladder wall, resulting in an inflammatory response induced by toxic, allergic, or immunologic means. **The substance in the urine may be a naturally occurring one—a substance that acts as an**

initiator only in particularly susceptible individuals—or may act like a true toxin, gaining access to the urine by a variety of mechanisms or metabolic pathways (Wein and Broderick, 1994). Clemmensen and colleagues (1988) noted that 8 of 11 IC patients had positive skin reactions to patch tests with their own urine. Immediate reactions were not observed, and the histologic appearance suggested a toxic rather than an allergic reaction. Lynes and colleagues (1990) were unable to find a urinary myotropic substance unique to IC patients. Parsons and Stein (1990) found IC urine to result in higher cell death of cultured transitional cells than normal urine, suggesting a toxic compound in the urine of some IC patients. Balagani and colleagues (1991) were able to induce glomerulations in rabbit bladder after repeated intravesical exposure to the urine of IC patients. However, a follow-up study (Perzin et al, 1991) did not demonstrate increased rabbit urothelial permeability after exposure to either the high- or low-molecular-weight fraction of IC urine. Beier-Holgersen and colleagues (1994) could not demonstrate cytotoxicity of IC urine. Keay and associates (1995b) also found no evidence that a cytotoxin for bladder epithelial cells is present in the urine of symptomatic IC patients compared with controls.

Perhaps the best circumstantial evidence for the toxicity of IC urine relates to the failure of substitution cystoplasty and continent diversions in some of these patients because of the development of pain or contraction of the bowel segment over time (Nielsen et al, 1990; Baskin and Tanagho, 1992; Trinka et al, 1993; Lotenfoe et al, 1994) and to some histologic findings similar to those of IC found to develop in bowel used to augment the small-capacity IC bladder (McGuire et al, 1973). The significance of the latter finding has been questioned by MacDermott and colleagues (1990), who feel those changes are normal for bowel exposed to urine on a long-term basis.

Anecdotal association of IC with certain foodstuffs has spawned the recommendation of various "IC diets" with little in the way of objective, scientific basis. The only placebo-controlled dietary study, although small, failed to demonstrate a relationship between diet and symptoms (Fisher et al, 1993).

Autoimmunity

For many years the possibility that IC may represent some type of autoimmune disorder has been considered. To establish a disease as autoimmune, three types of evidence can be marshaled (Rose and Bona, 1993): (1) direct evidence from the transfer of pathogenic antibody or pathogenic T cells, (2) indirect evidence based on reproduction of the autoimmune disease in experimental animals, and (3) circumstantial evidence from clinical clues. Circumstantial evidence would include (1) association with other autoimmune diseases in the same individual or same family, (2) lymphocytic infiltration of target organ, (3) statistical association with a particular major histocompatibility complex haplotype, and (4) a favorable response to immunosuppression. Circumstantial evidence by itself cannot define an autoimmune disease, and at this point the case for autoimmunity in IC is far from clear.

Silk (1970) found bladder antibodies in 9 of 20 IC patients and none in 35 pathologic or normal control patients. Gordon and associates (1973) found antibladder antibodies present in biopsies from 6 of 8 IC patients and in 3 of 5 control patients. No control patient demonstrated antibodies in the muscle, whereas 3 of 5 IC patients with muscle in the biopsy did so. Jokinen and colleagues (1972) looked at sera from 33 IC patients and found 28 with an antinuclear antibody (ANA) titer of 1:10 or greater, but no bladder-specific antibodies were detected with immunofluorescence. There was poor correlation between ANA titers and symptom severity. The next year (Jokinen et al, 1973) they noted that elevated antibody titers against cell nuclei and crude kidney homogenate decreased within 12 months after cystectomy in three IC patients. All of this provided hints that IC could fall into the autoimmune group of diseases.

Oravisto summarized the world literature on this idea in 1980, concluding that the chronic course of the disease, the absence of detectable infection, the pathologic findings, the occurrence of ANAs, and the reported responses to steroids at that time provided strong circumstantial evidence of autoimmunity. He discounted the paucity of activated lymphocytes, which speaks against an autoimmune process. Mattila (1982) presented evidence of immune deposits in the bladder vascular walls in 33 of 47 IC patients. Studying sera from 41 patients with IC, Mattila and colleagues (1983) concluded that the classic pathway of activation of the complement system was involved, supporting the possibility that a chronic local immunologic process was indeed occurring. Mattila and Linder (1984) determined that the autoantibodies they tested were directed against cytoskeletal intermediate filaments. As the autoantibodies have to gain access to intracellular structures in order to cause in vivo deposits, primary tissue injury of unknown cause has to be postulated.

Anderson and colleagues (1989) studied 26 patients with IC and compared them with a control group, of similar age and sex, with other urologic complaints. They performed a standard autoimmune profile and looked for specific antibodies to normal human bladder in the serum: 65% of IC patients and 36% of controls demonstrated non–organ-specific antibodies; 40% of IC patients and 22% of controls had ANAs; and 75% of IC patients and 40% of controls had antibladder antibodies present in the serum. There was no increase in immunoglobulin deposition in the bladder epithelium in IC patients versus controls. Although IC patients demonstrated a nonspecific increase in antibody formation, this was not significantly different from a similar group of other urologic patients. The lack of specificity indicates that the immunologic findings are likely secondary to inflammation rather than having a primary cause.

In a study looking for active immune cellular deposition in IC patients (Harrington et al, 1990), no statistically significant difference between control and nonulcerative IC patients was identified. In contrast, the ulcerative IC group had focal sheets of plasma cells, aggregates of T cells, B-cell nodules, a decreased or normal helper-to-suppressor cell ratio and suppressor cytotoxic cells in germinal centers. Flow cytometric analysis of peripheral blood lymphocyte subsets showed increased numbers of secretory Ig-positive B cells and activated lymphocytes in the nonulcerative group, and increased numbers of secretory Ig-positive cells and activated lymphocytes in the ulcerative group. These results may suggest a partial role for an immune mechanism in IC.

Hanno and associates (1990) found a CD4 cell predominance in all layers of the bladder in IC patients. MacDermott and colleagues (1991) found a normal distribution of peripheral blood lymphocytes in IC patients, a finding not supportive of an autoimmune mechanism in the disease. The lamina propria showed a predominance of CD4 (helper T cells) lymphocytes over CD8 cells in both IC and other cystitis patients. The same pattern was seen in the epithelium of patients with bacterial or mechanical cystitis, but patients with IC had a predominance of CD8 lymphocytes in the urothelium—identical to controls. The findings suggest that the urothelium is not involved in the inflammatory reaction, as is the lamina propria, making the urothelium an unlikely source for the initiating factor.

Miller and colleagues (1992) investigated the function of peripheral blood lymphocytes from nonulcerative IC patients. They tested the proliferative response and cytokine production of T cells to nonspecific mitogenic stimulation and the proliferative response of T cells to urine components. Proliferation and cytokine production after mitogen stimulation were the same for controls and IC patients. Moreover, no immunologic response to IC urine by autologous peripheral blood lymphocytes in in vitro assays was observed. Their findings cast doubt on theories suggesting that IC is an autoimmune disease. More recently, Christmas (1994) reported increased numbers of CD4+ and CD8+ T cells in bladder biopsies from patients with IC and bacterial cystitis compared with controls. These T cells were present in the urothelium and submucosa but not in the detrusor. Control bladder tissue demonstrated only CD8 cells in the urothelium and both CD4+ and CD8+ cells in the submucosa. The number of plasma cells was significantly greater in IC patients than in normal controls and controls with bacterial cystitis. **Thus the issue of autoimmunity is still controversial.**

Numerous inflammatory mediators have been studied with regard to their relation to interstitial cystitis (Elgebaly et al, 1992; Felsen et al, 1994; Lotz et al, 1994; Steinert et al, 1994; Zuraw et al, 1994), but no consistent data or conclusions have resulted. Urothelial cell activation in IC may result in aberrant immune responses and immune activation within the bladder wall (Liebert et al, 1993) that could relate to pathogenesis of the disease but might not reflect the initiating cause (Ochs et al, 1994). Martins and associates' (1994) report of the absence of urinary interleukin-1b in IC argues against an immunologic or autoimmune cause of the disorder.

Other Suggested Causes

Various other etiologic theories have been proposed (Ratliff et al, 1994), but none have received much scientific support. **There is no question but that voiding almost hourly, always having to be aware of how far the nearest rest room facilities are, and suffering constant pain would lead to psychological stress. However, there are no data to suggest that stress leads to the chronic syndrome of IC.** Speculation that abnormalities in or obstruction of lymphatics or vascular structures is causative has never been borne out. The fact that some of these patients have had hysterectomies probably relates more to the attempts of the physicians to treat chronic pelvic pain than postsurgical changes causing the IC syndrome.

The knowledge that there is a 10:1 female-to-male preponderance immediately makes the role of the hormonal milieu potentially important. Paradoxically, it is known that estrogens can control hematuria in hemorrhagic cystitis, perhaps by decreasing the fragility of the mucosal microvasculature of the bladder (Liu et al, 1990). Estradiol augments, while the estrogen receptor blocker tamoxifen inhibits, mast cell secretion (Vliagoftis et al, 1992). Pang and colleagues (1995b) have shown that bladder mast cells express high-affinity estrogen receptors and that there is a higher number of such cells present in patients with IC compared with controls. Although this may help explain why IC is so common in women, the hormonal role can only account for the propensity of IC to occur in females, not the ultimate cause.

PATHOLOGY

It is interesting that not a word about pathology is mentioned in the definition of IC. Immediately, the observer notices that this sets this disorder apart from the vast majority of other disease entities, most of which are far better understood than IC.

The role of histopathology in the diagnosis of IC is primarily one of excluding other possible diagnoses. One must rule out carcinoma, eosinophilic cystitis (Hellstrom et al, 1979), and tuberculous cystitis as well as any other entities with a specific tissue diagnosis (Johansson and Fall, 1990).

Although earlier reports described a chronic, edematous pancystitis with mast cell infiltration; submucosal ulcerations and involvement of the bladder wall; and chronic lymphocytic infiltrate (Smith and Dehner, 1972; Jacobo et al, 1974), these were cases culled from patients with severe disease and not representative of the majority of cases currently diagnosed. The pathologic findings in IC are not consistent. There has been a great variation in the reported histologic appearance of biopsies from IC patients, and even variation among biopsies taken from the same patients over time (Gillenwater and Wein, 1988).

Lepinard and colleagues (1984) reported a pancystitis affecting the three layers of bladder wall. In nonulcerative disease the vesical wall was never normal, epithelium being thinned and muscle being affected. Johansson and Fall (1990) looked at 64 patients with ulcerative disease and 44 with nonulcerative IC. The former group had mucosal ulceration and hemorrhage, granulation tissue, intense inflammatory infiltrate, elevated mast cell counts, and perineural infiltrates. The nonulcer group, despite the same severe symptoms, had a relatively unaltered mucosa with a sparse inflammatory response, the main feature being multiple, small, mucosal ruptures and suburothelial hemorrhages that were noted in a high proportion of patients. As these specimens were almost all taken immediately after hydrodistention, how much of the admittedly minimal findings in the nonulcer group were purely iatrogenic is a matter of speculation. One can see completely normal biopsies in the nonulcerative IC group (Johansson and Fall, 1994). **Transition from nonulcerative to ulcerative IC is a rare event** (Fall et al, 1987), and pathologically the two types of IC may be completely separate entities. Although mast cells are more commonly seen in the detrusor in ulcerative IC (Holm-Bentzen et al, 1987), they are also common in patients with idiopathic bladder instability (Moore et al, 1992). **Mast cell counts have no place in the differential diagnosis of IC.**

Lynes and colleagues (1990) concluded that biopsy specimens are often not helpful in confirming the diagnosis. Although IC patients in their study had a higher incidence and degree of denuded epithelium, ulceration, and submucosal inflammation, none of these findings were pathognomonic. In addition, these "typical" findings occurred only in IC patients with pyuria or small bladder capacity. Epithelial and basement membrane thickness, submucosal edema, vascular ectasia, fibrosis, and detrusor muscle inflammation and fibrosis were not significantly different in the IC and control patients.

Attempts to differentiate IC from other disorders by electron microscopy have also been very unsuccessful. Collan and associates (1976), in the first such study, wrote that the similarity of the ultrastructure of epithelial cells in controls and IC patients makes it improbable that the disease process originates in the epithelium. Dixon and associates (1986) also found no differences in the morphologic appearances of the glycocalyx and urothelial cells in patients with IC compared with controls. Anderstrom and colleagues (1989) found no surface characteristics specific for IC but believed that the mucin layer covering the urothelial cells seemed reduced in IC patients compared with controls, a fact disputed by Nickel and colleagues (1993) in a very elegant paper.

So what is the place of pathologic examination of tissue in IC? Attempts to classify the painful bladder by the pathoanatomic criteria described by Holm-Bentzen (1989) are of questionable value. There is a group of patients with what she describes as "nonobstructive detrusor myopathy" (Holm-Bentzen et al, 1985), but these patients with degenerative changes in the detrusor muscle often have residual urine, a history of urinary retention, and an absence of sensory urgency on cystometry with bladder capacities over 400 ml. Most would not be clinically confused with IC. **IC is a diagnosis of exclusion, and excluding other diseases that are pathologically identifiable is now the primary use of bladder biopsy in this group of patients.**

DIAGNOSIS

As IC is primarily a diagnosis of exclusion, it is incumbent upon the physician to try to make an accurate diagnosis. This is especially important with a chronic disease like IC that will likely impact on the patient's life for decades. **A diagnosis is the initial step in educating the patient about the disorder and in attempting to give the patient realistic expectations in terms of what can and cannot be done.** To impart the feeling that "the disease will not kill you, there is no cure; therefore we need not worry about a vigorous attempt at diagnosis" shortchanges both the patient and the physician for years to come.

The diagnosis of IC is by its very nature based upon the techniques necessary to elicit the criteria established at the conferences of the NIDDK (Table 17–1). One must rule out infection and less common conditions including but not limited to carcinoma (Utz and Zincke, 1974), eosinophilic cystitis (Sidh et al, 1980; Littleton et al, 1982), malakoplakia, schistosomiasis, and detrusor endometriosis (Sircus et al, 1988).

What is required is a thorough history, a urodynamic evaluation, appropriate urine cultures and cytologic examination, and cystoscopy under anesthesia with hydrodistention of the bladder and bladder biopsy (Hanno et al, 1990; Hanno, 1994). **Many dispute the need for a urodynamic study, but we agree with Siroky (1994) that not only can it help to assess bladder compliance and sensation and reproduce the patient's symptoms during bladder filling, but it can help to rule out bladder instability.** We do not diagnose patients with discrete, involuntary bladder contractions as having IC. These patients often respond to anticholinergic medication and tend not to respond to standard therapy for IC (Perez-Marrero et al, 1987). Cystometry in conscious IC patients generally demonstrates normal function, except for decreased bladder capacity and hypersensitivity, perhaps exaggerated by the use of gas as a filling medium. Siroky (1994) did not find diminished bladder compliance, as hypersensitivity would prevent the bladder from filling to the point of noncompliance.

Cystoscopy is performed with the patient under anesthesia to allow sufficient distention of the bladder to afford visualization of either glomerulations or Hunner's ulcers (Figs. 17–3 and 17–4). After filling to 80 cm H_2O for 1 to 2 minutes, one drains and refills the bladder. The terminal portion of the effluent is often blood-tinged. Reinspection reveals the pinpoint petechial hemorrhages that develop throughout the bladder after distention and are not usually seen after examination without anesthesia. **Glomerulations are not specific for IC, and only when seen in conjunction with the clinical criteria of frequency and pain and/or urgency can the finding of glomerulations be viewed as significant.** Glomerulations can be seen in patients who have had radiation therapy, in patients with carcinoma, in patients exposed to toxic chemicals or chemotherapeutic agents, and often in patients on dialysis or after urinary diversion when the bladder has not filled for prolonged periods. We have speculated that they may simply reflect the response of the bladder to distention after a prolonged period of chronic underfilling because of sensory urgency, rather than result from a primary pathologic process.

Further confusion arises when the patient demonstrates all the symptoms of IC but the cystoscopic findings under anesthesia are completely normal. Is this a disease, a different disease, or IC? Do we need to see glomerulations to diagnose IC? By the NIDDK research definition (or with a Hunner's ulcer) we do, but is this reasonable? The answers are not in, but an intriguing paper by Awad and colleagues (1992) describes an entity almost identical to IC in terms of symptomatology, urodynamic evaluation, histologic appearance, and response to therapy, but with normal findings on cystoscopy. It was termed "idiopathic reduced bladder storage." **Ultimately, disease definitions are helpful only relative to the utility they provide in terms of treatment and prognosis, and it is likely that the definition of IC**

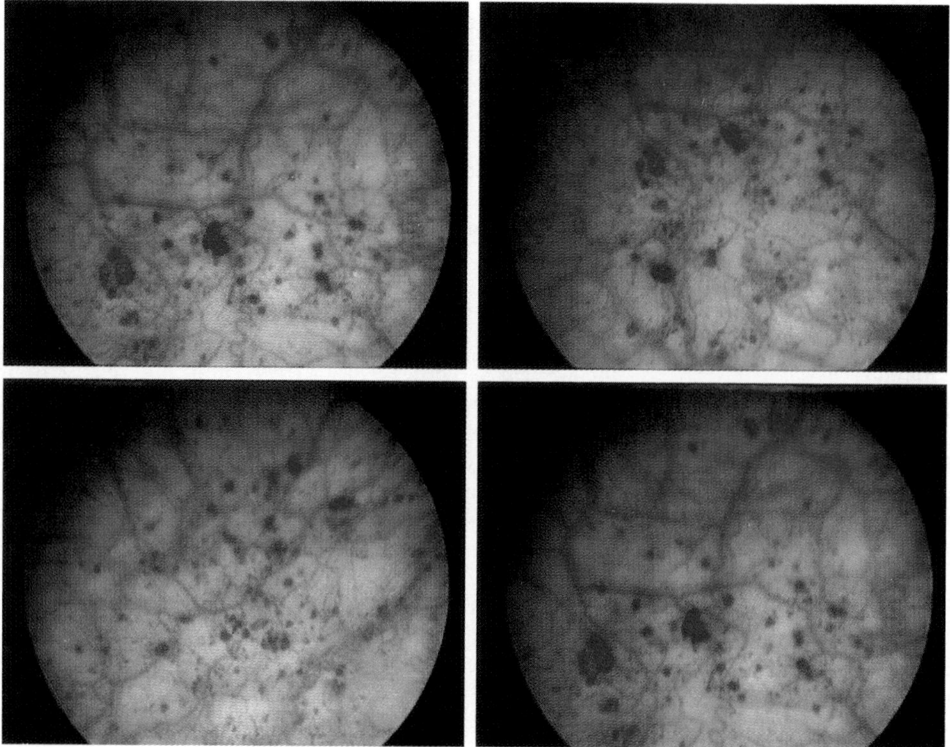

Figure 17–3. Typical appearance of glomerulations after bladder distention in a patient with nonulcerative IC.

and therefore proper methods of diagnosis will continue to evolve.

In just such an effort, numerous investigators have looked at the mast cell as a possible diagnostic marker for IC. The results have been very contradictory, and at this time, in terms of the use of mast cell criteria in diagnosis, the issue remains moot (Kastrup et al, 1983; Feltis et al, 1987; Holm-Bentzen et al, 1987; Lynes et al, 1987; Hanno et al, 1990; Christmas and Rode, 1991; Moore et al, 1992).

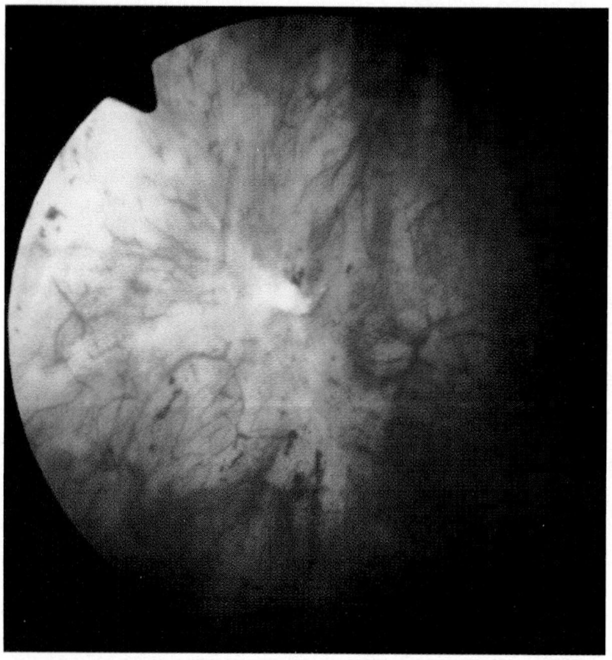

Figure 17–4. Typical appearance of a "Hunner's ulcer" in an IC patient before bladder distention.

Attempts have been made to look at other markers including eosinophil cationic protein (Lose et al, 1987), GAG excretion (Hurst et al, 1993), and urinary histamine and methylhistamine (El-Mansoury et al, 1994). Although such studies may prove to be confirmatory in some patients, their value in a disease diagnosed on the basis of symptoms and exclusion of other pathologic processes remains illusory. Markers may prove more useful in the search for cause and cure than in diagnosis.

One hopes that Benson's somewhat facetious comment on the diagnosis of IC will ring less true as time goes on. He wrote, "We may be doing our patients a disservice by diagnosing 'interstitial cystitis.' I would much prefer to say, 'I believe you have symptoms, I don't know what's wrong with you, but I'll do my best to make you symptomatically better" (Benson, 1990).

TREATMENT

The ultimate goal of therapy of any disease process is to neutralize the factor or factors responsible for the disorder. **As long as causative factors are unknown, treatments will be based on empiricism. Although the symptoms of IC can be controlled with one of a variety of treatments in the overwhelming majority of patients, there is little evidence that treatment accomplishes anything more than influencing the symptomatic expression of the disease rather than curing the condition. In order that the best therapeutic results for an individual patient are achieved, both patient and physician must understand that there is no sure cure for IC, nor is there a single**

treatment that is effective in reducing symptoms for every patient. Most patients, however, can in fact benefit from one treatment or another, or a combination of treatments, and most can be maintained in a satisfied, although definitely not asymptomatic, state, punctuated by exacerbations and remissions (Wein and Broderick, 1994).

Assessing Treatment Results

Although somewhat unconventional, a brief section on critical appraisal of treatment results is in order before getting into the substance of treating IC. IC is not only a difficult condition to diagnose but a difficult condition in which to assess therapeutic impact. **The study by Held and colleagues (1990) documents a 50% incidence of temporary remission unrelated to therapy with a mean duration of 8 months.** In a chronic, devastating condition with primarily subjective symptomatology, no known cause, and no cure, patients are desperate and often seem to respond to any new therapy. They are often victims of unorthodox health care providers with untested forms of therapy, some medical, some homeopathic, and some even surgical.

Placebo effects influence patient outcomes after any treatment, including surgery, that the clinician and patients believe is effective. Placebo effects plus disease natural history and regression to the mean can result in high rates of good outcomes, which may be misattributed to specific treatment effects (Fig. 17–5) (Turner et al, 1994). Unfortunately, few IC treatments have been subjected to a placebo-controlled trial. This is not to say that what seems effective is not, but rather that a high index of skepticism is healthy, even in treatments tested by controlled trials (Schulz et al, 1995). Although in many diseases an argument can be made against using a true placebo control as opposed to an orthodox treatment of approved or accepted value (Rothman and Michels, 1994), a good case for true placebo can readily be made for IC. The vagaries of the natural history, the general lack of progression of symptom severity over time, and the fact that it is not life-threatening mean that there is little to lose and much to gain by subjecting new treatments to the vigorous scrutiny of placebo control. Many patients who volunteer for such trials have already run the gamut of accepted (though generally unproven) therapies. It has long been recognized in protocols that use subjective criteria for assessment that "improvement" may be expected in up to 35% of placebo-treated patients (Benson and Epstein, 1976). The spontaneous remission rate (though temporary) for IC is 11% (Oravisto and Alfthan, 1976) to 50% (Held et al, 1990); combined with the placebo improvement, this makes it difficult to prove true efficacy.

Finally, **when objective changes are considered, the concept of statistical versus clinical significance is paramount.** As Wein and Broderick point out (1994), investigators should, but rarely do, point out differences between statistical improvement and what they consider to be clinically significant improvement. To paraphrase Gertrude Stein, **"A difference, to be a difference, must make a difference."** An increase in bladder capacity of 30 ml may be statistically significant but clinically irrelevant. Various methods for measuring pain (Melzack, 1975) and other

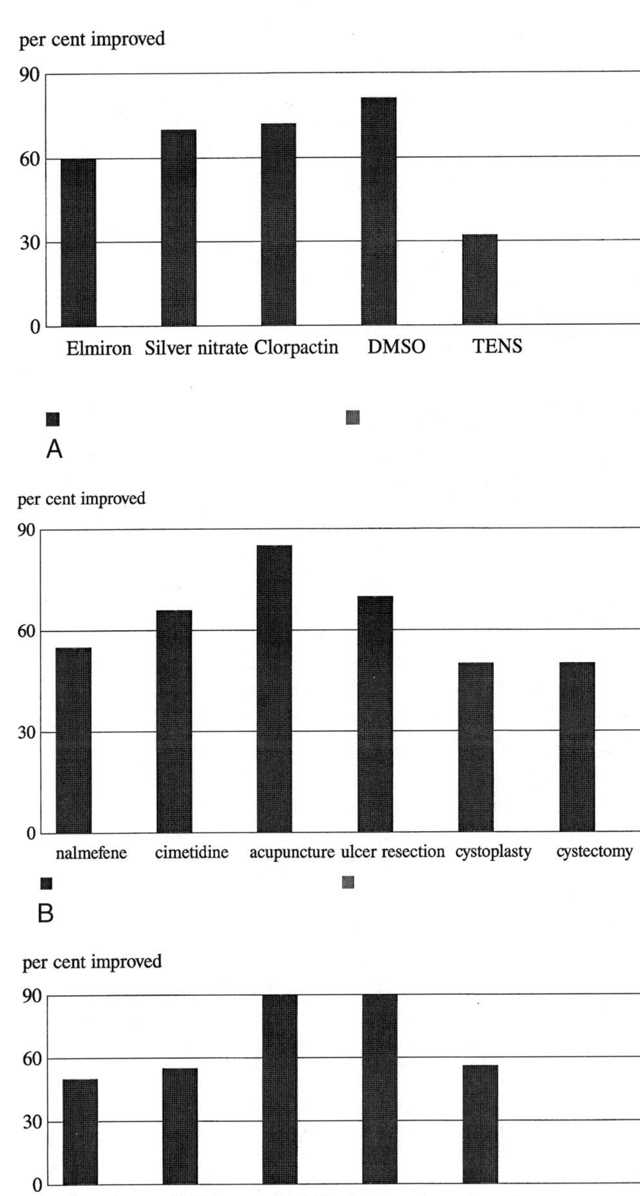

Figure 17–5. Selected reported treatment outcomes in uncontrolled studies in IC literature: Percentage of patients initially improved (see text for details). DMSO, dimethyl sulfoxide; TENS, transcutaneous electric nerve stimulation.

symptoms in IC (Keller et al, 1994) have been developed and will be valuable in future trials. The Interstitial Cystitis Data Base project sponsored by the National Institutes of Health will, it is hoped, provide a longitudinal view of this condition and a more realistic idea of what the effects of therapy might be.

Initial Therapeutic Approach

Hydrodistention of the bladder under anesthesia, although technically a surgical treatment, is usually the first therapeutic modality employed, often as a part of

the diagnostic evaluation. Because there have been no standard methods of distention, results vary markedly. Simple bladder filling at cystoscopy gives relief to some patients (Hald et al, 1986), whereas Dunn and colleagues (1977) reported on 25 patients distended under anesthesia to the level of the systolic blood pressure for up to 3 hours. Sixteen of the patients were symptom-free, with a mean follow-up of 14 months; two patients suffered bladder rupture. The bladder in IC patients can be very thin, and the possibility of perforation or rupture must always be kept in mind and discussed with the patient (Badenoch, 1971; Hamer et al, 1992; Taub and Stein, 1994).

Our method is to perform an initial cystoscopic examination (which is generally unremarkable), obtain urine for cytologic examination, and distend the bladder for 1 to 2 minutes at a pressure of 80 cm H_2O. The bladder is emptied and then refilled to establish the diagnosis. A therapeutic hydraulic distention then follows for another 8 minutes. Biopsy follows the second distention. Therapeutic responses in patients with a bladder capacity of less than 600 ml under anesthesia showed 26% with an excellent and 29% with a fair result compared with 12% excellent and 43% fair in patients with larger bladder capacities (Hanno and Wein, 1991). Most favorable responses were extremely brief, however, with the exceptional patient noting improvement for 6 months, and thus being a candidate for repeat therapeutic distention.

Acute hydrodistention does not seem to result in any long-term bladder dysfunction (Kang et al, 1992; Lasanen et al, 1992), and any efficacy is probably related to damage to mucosal afferent nerve endings (Dunn et al, 1977). It has no benefits in patients with detrusor hyperreflexia (Taub and Stein, 1994). Although many patients with IC have sensory urgency at awake capacities of less than 100 ml, hydrodistention under anesthesia seems to allow "staging" of the disease, giving the clinician some idea of the capacity he or she has to work with when using conservative therapies. **A capacity under anesthesia of under 200 ml would not bode well for the likelihood of success of medical therapy.** Fortunately, these cases are very rare.

Once the diagnosis has been made, one must decide whether to institute therapy or employ a policy of conservative "watchful waiting." **If the patient's symptoms are livable, the withholding of immediate treatment is reasonable.** Although the concept of *livable* is certainly patient-dependent, someone who gets up once or twice a night and voids every 2 to 3 hours during the day with minimal pain would certainly fall into this category. **Educated patients are likely to realize that no treatment will make them perfect, and any therapy is a tradeoff between the inconvenience, chronicity of treatment, side effects, and benefits. One must never forget that "perfect is the enemy of good."**

Patient education and empowerment are an important initial step in therapy. The Interstitial Cystitis Association (Ratner et al, 1992) is an important resource for information and support for patients as well as a clearinghouse for ideas and funding for researchers and clinicians. Patients can keep a voiding diary. There are data that timed voiding and behavioral therapy can be helpful in the short term, especially in patients in whom frequency rather than pain predominates (Parsons and Koprowski, 1991; Chaiken et al, 1993).

Although there are no data to prove it, many clinicians believe that stress reduction, exercise, warm tub baths, and efforts by the patient to maintain a normal lifestyle all contribute to the overall quality of life (Whitmore, 1994). Elaborate dietary restrictions are unsupported by any literature, but many patients do find their symptoms are adversely affected by specific foods and would do well to avoid them. Often this includes caffeine, alcohol, and acidic beverages. However, this is very patient-dependent. Urinary alkalinization may be worth trying, but supporting studies are lacking.

Unfortunately education and self-help are often not sufficient, and most patients require one or more of a variety of therapies.

Medical Therapy

Several oral therapies for IC have been tried and essentially been discarded. Dees (1953) reported temporary improvement with systemic steroids, but these drugs have not been found to be useful (Pool, 1967), and the risks of chronic administration are considerable. Hormones have been used without success (Burford and Burford, 1958; Badenoch, 1971). Vitamin E, anticholinergics, and antispasmodics are not generally efficacious (Burford and Burford, 1958; Pool, 1967). Oravisto and Alfthan (1976) tried immunosuppression and chloroquine derivatives. About 50% of patients responded to some extent, but potential complications are significant and neither therapy has found general usage. Benzydamine, a potent anti-inflammatory drug with strong analgesic effects, was initially reported to have a superb response rate in IC (Walsh, 1977a), but a controlled follow-up trial demonstrated no responses in the first 12 patients, and the trial was discontinued (Walsh, 1977b).

Amitriptyline, one of the tricyclic antidepressants, has become a staple of oral treatment for IC. The tricyclics possess differing degrees of at least three major pharmacologic actions: (1) they have central and peripheral anticholinergic actions at some but not all sites, (2) they block the active transport system in the presynaptic nerve ending that is responsible for the re-uptake of the released amine neurotransmitters serotonin and noradrenaline, and (3) they are sedatives; sedation occurs presumably on a central basis but perhaps is related to their antihistaminic properties. Amitriptyline, in fact, is one of the most potent tricyclic antidepressants in terms of blocking H_1-histaminergic receptors (Baldessarini, 1985). There is also evidence that the tricyclics desensitize alpha-2 receptors on central noradrenergic neurons. Paradoxically, they also have been shown to block alpha-adrenergic receptors and serotonin receptors. Theoretically, tricyclic agents have actions that might tend to stimulate predominantly beta-adrenergic receptors in bladder body smooth musculature, an action that would further facilitate urine storage by decreasing the excitability of smooth muscle in that area (Barrett and Wein, 1987).

Hanno and Wein (1987) first reported a therapeutic response in IC after noting a "serendipitous" response to amitriptyline in one of their patients concurrently being treated for depression. The following year a similar report appeared relating a response to desipramine hydrochloride

(Renshaw, 1988). Reasoning that a drug used successfully at relatively low dosages for many types of chronic pain syndromes, one that would also have anticholinergic properties, beta-adrenergic bladder effects, sedative characteristics, and strong H_1-antihistaminic activity, would seem to be ideal for IC, Hanno and colleagues (1989) carried out the first clinical trial, with promising results. A subsequent follow-up study (Hanno, 1994a) reported that in 28 of 43 patients who could tolerate therapy for at least a 3-week trial at a dosage of 25 mg at bedtime gradually increasing to 75 mg at bedtime over 2 weeks, 18 had total remission of symptoms with a mean follow-up of 14.4 months, 5 dropped out because of side effects, and 5 derived no clinical benefit. Benefits were apparent within 4 weeks. All patients had failed hydrodistention and intravesical dimethyl sulfoxide (DMSO) therapy. Sedation was the main side effect. Kirkemo and associates (1990) treated 30 patients and had a 90% subjective improvement rate at 8 weeks. Both studies noted that patients with bladder capacities over 450 to 600 ml under anesthesia seemed to have the best results. Another uncontrolled study of 11 patients with urinary frequency and pelvic pain (Pranikoff and Constantino, 1995) related success in 9 of the patients, with 5 reporting complete resolution of symptoms and 4 significant relief. Two patients could not tolerate the medication.

The use of antihistamines goes back to the late 1950s and stems from work by Simmons (1961), who postulated that the local release of histamine may be responsible for or accompany the development of IC. He reported on six patients treated with pyribenzamine. The results were far from dramatic, with only half of the patients showing some response. The therapy is notable for this disease in that it was very logically conceived. It has been Theoharides (1994) who has spearheaded mast cell research in this field and been a major modern proponent of antihistamine therapy. He used the unique piperazine H_1-receptor antagonist **hydroxyzine**, which can block neuronal activation of mast cells. In 40 patients treated with 25 mg before bed increasing over 2 weeks (if sedation was not a problem) to 50 mg at night and 25 mg in the morning, virtually every symptom evaluated improved by 30%. Only 3 patients had absolutely no response. As with many IC drug reports, these responses were evaluated subjectively and without being blinded or placebo-controlled. Why an H_2-antagonist would be effective is unclear, but Seshadri and colleagues (1994) reported a 66% response rate in 9 patients treated with cimetidine at a dose of 300 mg twice daily for 1 month.

The calcium channel antagonist **nifedipine** has been tried in an uncontrolled study for IC (Fleischmann et al, 1991). Nifedipine has been reported to inhibit detrusor contractions and depress cell-mediated immune functions. Of nine patients treated for at least 4 months, five showed a 50% decrease in symptom scores and 33% were asymptomatic. Although changes in symptom scores did not correlate with changes in interleukin-2 (IL-2) inhibitor activity, arguing against an immune-mediated effect, Fleischmann (1994) did speculate about a possible increase in bladder blood flow. Similar results were noted in patients treated for urethral syndrome (Fleischmann, 1994).

Parsons' suggestion that a defect in the epithelial permeability barrier, the GAG layer, contributes to the pathogenesis of IC has led to an attempt to correct such a defect with the synthetic sulfated polysaccharide **sodium pentosan polysulfate** (PPS), available in an oral formulation and excreted to some extent in the urine. It is sold under the trade name Elmiron and as of 1996 is available in the United States only from the manufacturer on a compassionate-use basis. Studies have been contradictory.

Fritjofsson and colleagues (1987) treated 87 patients in an open multicenter trial in Sweden and Finland. Bladder volume with and without anesthesia was unchanged. Relief of pain was complete in 35% and partial in 23% of patients. Daytime frequency decreased from 16.5 to 13 and nocturia decreased from 4.5 to 3.5, both figures statistically significant but clinically marginal. Mean voided volumes increased by almost a tablespoon in the nonulcer group. Holm-Bentzen and associates (1987) studied 115 patients in a double-blind, placebo-controlled trial. Symptoms, urodynamic parameters, cystoscopic appearance, and mast cell counts were unchanged after 4 months. Bladder capacity under anesthesia increased significantly in the group with mastocytosis, but this had no bearing on symptoms or awake capacity.

Parsons and colleagues (1983) had a more encouraging initial experience, and subsequently the results of two placebo-controlled multicenter trials in the United States were published (Mulholland et al, 1990; Parsons et al, 1993). In the initial study, overall improvement of greater than 25% was reported by 28% of the PPS-treated group versus 13% in the placebo group. In the latter study the respective figures were 32% on drug versus 16% on placebo. The average voided volume on PPS increased by 20 ml. No other objective improvements were documented. **Side effects with PPS are minimal at the dose of 100 mg three times daily, and it is certainly easily administered. It seems to be effective in some patients.** Positive results in a small trial using the drug for radiation cystitis may make it more applicable for that condition, in which damage to the bladder lining is more readily apparent (Parsons, 1986).

The opiate antagonist **nalmefene** was tried in an uncontrolled trial with promising results (Stone, 1994). It is known that mast cells degranulate and release histamines and other mediators when their endogenous opioid receptors are stimulated. In IC this theoretically could occur because of chronic endorphin release stimulated by the pain. By blocking the patient's own endogenous stimulation of mast cell degranulation, a "vicious cycle" could possibly be broken. Unfortunately, an unpublished, placebo-controlled trial failed to demonstrate the hoped-for efficacy.

The long-term, appropriate use of pain medications forms an integral part of the treatment of a chronic pain condition like IC. Many **nonopioid analgesics**, including acetaminophen and nonsteroidal anti-inflammatory drugs and even **antispasmodic agents** (Rummans, 1994), have a place in therapy along with agents designed to specifically treat the disorder itself.

With the results of major surgery anything but certain, the use of **long-term opioid therapy** in the rare patient in whom all forms of conservative therapy have failed over many years may also be considered. This is a difficult decision that requires much thought and discussion between patient and urologist, and involvement of a pain specialist is often indicated. Opioids are effective for most forms of moderate and severe pain and have no ceiling effect other than that imposed by adverse effects. The common side effects include sedation, nausea, mild confusion, and pruritus. These are generally transient and easily managed. Respiratory depression is extremely rare if the drugs are used as prescribed. Constipation is common, and a mild laxative is generally necessary. The major impediment to the proper use of these drugs when they are prescribed for long-term nonmalignant pain is the fear of addiction. Studies suggest the risk is low (Gourlay, 1994). The long-acting narcotic formulations that result in steady levels of drug over many hours are preferable.

Chronic pain patients often receive inadequate doses of short-acting pain medications, which puts them on cycles of short-term relief, anxiety, and pain. It leads to doctor-shopping and drug-seeking behavior that physicians may confuse with drug addiction. Although physical dependence to opioids is unavoidable, physical addiction, a chronic disorder characterized by the compulsive use of a substance resulting in physical, psychological, or social harm to the user and the continued use despite that harm, is rare. **Chronic opioid therapy can be considered as a last resort in selected patients. It is best administered in a pain clinic setting, requiring frequent reassessment by both patient and physician** (Portenoy and Foley, 1986).

Intravesical Therapy

Intravesical lavage with one of a variety of preparations remains the standard treatment against which other treatments must be measured.

Perhaps the oldest of the intravesical therapies is **silver nitrate.** Pool and Rives (1944) note that the use of silver nitrate can be attributed to Mercier, who reported in 1855 that excellent results with bladder instillations had been obtained in patients suffering from symptoms compatible with IC. Dodson in 1926 advocated the use of solutions of silver nitrate in increasing strengths as the treatment of choice for this condition. In 1944 Pool and Rives reported on 74 patients with IC treated with intravesical silver nitrate. The treatment was carried out as follows:

A urethral catheter is inserted and the contents of the bladder are evacuated. The bladder is then irrigated with a saturated solution of boric acid. Then 30 to 60 cc of a 1:5000 solution of silver nitrate is instilled into the bladder and permitted to remain there for 3 or 4 minutes if it does not cause intolerable irritation. At the end of this period the solution is permitted to run out through the catheter, which is then withdrawn. The patient usually experiences some dysuria and vesical irritability for 2 or 3 hours. Treatments are repeated every other day. At subsequent treatments, the concentration of silver nitrate in the solution is increased to 1:2500, 1:1000, 1:750, 1:500, 1:400, 1:200, and finally 1:100. If at any time the reaction is too severe, the concentration is increased more slowly.

Although the initial treatments are performed under general anesthesia, later treatments are given on an outpatient basis. Ureteral reflux would be a contraindication, and it goes without saying that bladder biopsy would be contraindicated just before instillation for fear of extravasation. Twenty-three years later, Pool (1967) wrote that he still considered this treatment regimen the most efficacious form of treatment.

Pool reported excellent results in 70% of patients with a mean response of 7.6 months. Burford and Burford (1958) reported a 14% cure rate and 79% improved figure. DeJuana and Everett (1977) had a 50% response rate in 102 patients.

O'Conor (1955) reported the use of intravesical **Clorpactin WCS-90.** Clorpactin is a trade name for closely related, highly reactive solutions having a modified derivative of hypochlorous acid (oxychlorosene) in a buffered base. Its activity is dependent on the liberation of hypochlorous acid and its resulting oxidizing effects; wetting and penetrating properties; and detergency. Wishard and colleagues (1957) reported on 20 patients treated with 0.2% Clorpactin gently lavaged in the bladder for 3 to 5 minutes without anesthesia; 14 of them reported subjective improvement. Murnaghan and colleagues (1970) noted improvement in 14 of 17 patients, though 10 required further treatment during the average 2-year follow-up. Most commonly, the treatments are given as described by Messing and Stamey (1978), using 0.4% solution administered at 10 cm H_2O under anesthesia. Multiple instillations can be given, with a 1-month pause after the first two instillations to await a therapeutic response. Their success rate was 72% with an average 6-month duration of response. A case of ureteral fibrosis complicating the treatment prompted the recommendation that vesicoureteral reflux be considered a contraindication to the procedure (Messing and Freiha, 1979).

A mainstay of the treatment of IC is the intravesical instillation of DMSO (Sant, 1987). DMSO is a product of the wood pulp industry and a derivative of lignin. It has exceptional solvent properties and is freely miscible with water, lipids, and organic agents. Pharmacologic properties include membrane penetration, enhanced drug absorption, anti-inflammatory properties, analgesic properties, collagen dissolution, muscle relaxation, and mast cell histamine release. In vitro effects on bladder function belie its positive effects in vivo (Freedman et al, 1989). Tests for DMSO for treatment of human illness began in the 1960s in the areas of musculoskeletal inflammation and the cutaneous manifestations of scleroderma.

Stewart and colleagues (Stewart et al, 1968) are responsible for popularizing the use of intravesical DMSO for IC. In the mid 1960s they applied it to the skin over the suprapubic area in a group of patients refractory to conventional forms of therapy. Results were poor, but intravesical delivery of 50 ml of a 50% solution instilled for 15 minutes by catheter and repeated at intervals of 2 to 4 weeks showed positive effects in 6 of 8 patients, the effects lasting 2 to 12 months. The lack of side effects, other than a garlic-like odor on the breath, and of need for inpatient administration were significant breakthroughs over previous treatments. Further reports by this group confirmed safety and efficacy (Stewart et al, 1971, 1972; Stewart and Shirley, 1976; Shirley et al, 1978) with symptom-free intervals of 1 to 3 months in 73% of patients. Ek and colleagues (1978) reported a 70% success rate but found that most patients ultimately required retreatment or further therapy with other modalities. Prospective series of Fowler (1981) and Barker and colleagues (1987) revealed symptomatic success rates of greater than 80%, although relapse was not uncommon. Fowler noted only minimal improvements in functional bladder capacity and attributed the beneficial effects of DMSO to a direct effect on the sensory nerves of the bladder. Perez-Marrero and associates (1988) compared DMSO to saline and showed a 93% objective improvement and 53% subjective improvement compared with 35% and 18%, respectively, for saline. Patients with bladder instability do not respond (Emerson and Feltis, 1986), making the diagnosis suspect in patients with this finding on urodynamics. **With its ease of administration (Biggers, 1986), lack of side effects, and dependable symptomatic results, DMSO certainly merits its place as one of the first-line treatments for this difficult and often frustrating condition.**

Heparin, which can mimic the activity of the bladder's own mucopolysaccharide lining (Hanno et al, 1978), has anti-inflammatory effects as well as actions that inhibit fibroblast proliferation, angiogenesis, and smooth muscle cell proliferation. Because of its numerous effects, the possibility that heparin could be used for therapeutic reasons other than the control of coagulation has been the subject of much inquiry and speculation (Lane and Adams, 1993). Weaver and colleagues (1963) first reported intravesical heparin for IC treatment. Given intravesically, there is virtually no systemic absorption, even in an inflamed bladder (Caulfield et al, 1995). Although uncontrolled studies suggested some beneficial effect for subcutaneous administration (Lose et al, 1983; Lose et al, 1985), the obvious risks of anticoagulation and osteoporosis have prevented this form of administration from undergoing further trials and general usage. Ten thousand units can be administered intravesically in sterile water either alone or with DMSO at various intervals, with good results reported (Perez-Marrero et al, 1993; Parsons et al, 1994).

In an attempt to bring therapy directly to the bladder, numerous other drugs have been introduced intravesically, but reports to date are sketchy, and no efficacy has been convincingly demonstrated. *Capsaicin* has been administered (Jancso and Lynn, 1987; Barbanti et al, 1993), but local irritation and pain related to the treatment can be intense. Whether it causes true desensitization of primary sensory afferents as intended, or merely a counterirritation is not known. Intravesical *lidocaine* has short-term anesthetic effects (Glanakopoulos and Champilomatos, 1992). Doxorubicin (Khanna and Loose, 1990), the GAG *hyaluronic acid* (Morales and Emerson, 1995), bacillus Calmette-Guérin (Zeidman et al, 1994); and the mast cell stabilizer *cromolyn sodium* (Kennelly and Konnak, 1995) have all been tried in pilot trials with the promising results we have come to expect in such studies. Iontophoretic intravesical delivery potentially could improve results (Gurpinar and Griffith, 1995).

Nerve Stimulation

Pain diversion by transcutaneous electric nerve stimulation (TENS) is routine in a variety of painful conditions (Fall, 1987). Fall and colleagues (1980) were the first to use electric stimulation in IC, reporting on 14 women treated successfully with long-term intravaginal stimulation or TENS. Subsequently McGuire and colleagues (1983) noted improvement in 5 of 6 patients treated with electric stimulation.

The primary intention in applying peripheral electric nerve stimulation in IC is to relieve pain by stimulating myelinated afferents in order to activate segmental inhibitory circuits. As a secondary effect, urinary frequency may also be reduced. In the most complete review of the subject to date, Fall and Lindstrom (1994) report on 33 patients with ulcerative IC and 27 patients with nonulcerative IC treated by means of suprapubic TENS. Electrodes were positioned 10 to 15 cm apart immediately above the pubic symphysis. High- or low-frequency (2 to 50 Hz) TENS was employed. If there was no effect with high-frequency TENS after 1 month, low-frequency TENS was used. Thirty to 120 minutes of TENS was prescribed daily. Pain improved more than frequency. Good results or remission were described in 26% of nonulcer patients and a surprising 54% of patients with ulcerative disease. The authors caution that the experience is based on open studies, relatively few patients, and the knowledge of a significant placebo effect with peripheral pain stimulation.

Acupuncture has been used to treat frequency, urgency, and dysuria (Chang, 1988). Twenty-two of 26 patients treated at the Sp. 6 point had clinically symptomatic improvement. A recent study looking at both acupuncture and TENS in IC showed limited effects of both modalities (Geirsson et al, 1993).

Lumbar epidural blockade (Irwin et al, 1993) has yielded short-term (mean 15 days) pain relief in IC.

Surgical Therapy

The surgical therapy of IC is an absolute last resort after all trials of conservative treatment have failed; this point cannot be overemphasized. Although a cause of significant morbidity, IC is a nonmalignant process with a temporary spontaneous remission rate of 50% (Held et al, 1990) and does not result in death. **Nowhere does the caveat *"primum non nocere"* bear more relevance;** the treatment must be no worse than the disease process (Siegel et al, 1990). **Surgery should be reserved for the motivated and well-informed patient who falls into the category of extremely severe, unresponsive disease, a group that comprises far fewer than 10% of patients** (Irwin and Galloway, 1994).

Many surgical approaches have been employed for IC, and it is worth mentioning a few for historical perspective alone. Sympathectomy and intraspinal alcohol injections have been used to treat pelvic pain (Greenhill, 1947). Differential sacral neurotomy was reported in three patients with good results (Meirowsky, 1969), but like most denervation procedures never gained popularity because of subsequent poor results. Transvesical infiltration of the pelvic plexuses with phenol failed in 5 of 5 patients with IC (Blackford et al, 1984). With a significant complication rate of 17% (McInerney et al, 1991) it is rarely if ever currently used for sensory urgency disorders or detrusor hyperreflexia. There are several reports on cystolysis going back to Richer in 1929 (Bourque, 1951). Worth and Turner-Warwick (1973) reported some short-term benefit but unpredictable long-term results (Worth, 1982). Freiha and Stamey (1979) used it in 6 IC patients with good results in 4. Albers and Geyer (1988) reported long-term followup in 11 IC patients and had only 1 success. Denervation procedures have a notoriously high late-failure rate, and the procedure is not justified for IC (Walsh, 1985; Stone, 1991).

Transurethral resection of a Hunner's ulcer, as initially reported by Kerr (1971), can provide symptomatic relief. Fall (1985) resected ulcerated lesions in 30 patients resulting in initial disappearance of pain in all and a decrease in urinary frequency in 21. Similar results have been attained with the **neodymium-yag laser** (Shanberg et al, 1985; Shanberg, 1989). Extreme caution is critical if using a laser in an IC bladder, as forward scatter through these thin bladders with resulting bowel injury is an ever-present danger. **There would seem to be no justification in the literature for using the laser to treat areas of glomerulation or in the nonulcerative form of the disease** (Malloy and Shanberg, 1994).

Supratrigonal cystectomy and the formation of an enterovesical anastomosis with bowel segments has been a popular surgical procedure for intractable IC. The diseased bladder is resected in its entirety, sparing only a 1-cm cuff around the trigone to which the bowel segment is anastomosed (Worth and Turner-Warwick, 1972; Irwin and Galloway, 1994). Although it is not always clear in the literature how much bladder has been resected, the results reported using this procedure for IC have been mixed at best. Badenoch (1971) operated on 9 patients, with 4 becoming much worse and 3 ultimately undergoing urinary diversion. Flood and colleagues (1995) reviewed 122 augmentation procedures, 21 of which were done for IC. Patients with IC had the poorest results of any group, with only 10 having an "excellent" outcome. Wallack and colleagues (1975) reported 2 successes, Seddon and associates (1977) had success in 7 of 9 patients, and Freiha and colleagues (1980) ended up performing formal urinary diversion in 2 of 6 patients treated with augmentation cecocystoplasty. Weiss and colleagues (1984) had success in 3 of 7 patients treated with sigmoidocystoplasty, and Lunghi and associates (1984) had no excellent results in 2 patients with IC. Webster and Maggio reviewed their data in 1989 in 19 patients and concluded that only patients with bladder capacities less than 350 ml under anesthesia should undergo substitution cystoplasty. (Webster has subsequently become disillusioned with surgical treatment for IC altogether.) Huges and colleagues (1995) have cut the threshold to less than 250 ml.

Not all patients empty the bladder spontaneously after substitution cystoplasty. Although the need for clean intermittent catheterization would not obviate a successful outcome in the patient treated for bladder contraction from tuberculous cystitis, it can be a painful disaster in the IC patient. Nurse and associates (1991) have gone one step further, recommending trigonal biopsy before substitution cystoplasty. Diversion and/or total cystourethrectomy is recommended if the trigone is "affected" by IC. It is not clear how this is determined histologically, as IC has no pathognomonic histologic findings and generally is not a localized process. Nielsen and associates (1990) described eight women treated with substitution cystoplasty. In six of the patients the therapy failed, and the results of postoperative biopsies from the trigone showed no difference in the amount of fibrosis, degree of degenerative changes in the muscle, and mast cell density between the two cured patients and the others.

There has been a controversy over whether the IC process can occur in a transposed bowel patch (McGuire et al, 1973; Kisman et al, 1991). If so, not only would this be a relative contraindication to the procedure, but it would also provide evidence that a substance in the urine might be involved in pathogenesis. In an elegant paper, **MacDermott and colleagues (1990) presented evidence that inflammation and fibrosis are the usual reactions of bowel to exposure to urine and do not represent a specific spread of IC in those patients.**

Augmentation cystoplasty has many potential complications from the rare incidence of bladder neoplasm (Golomb et al, 1989) to the more common complication of upper-tract obstruction (Cheng and Whitfield, 1990). In the best of hands (Khoury et al, 1992) complications can involve almost 50% of patients, requiring surgical intervention in 25%. Although problems are more common in patients operated on for disorders other than IC, **the risk/benefit ratio of substitution cystoplasty seems to have discouraged its use in the last several years.**

Urinary diversion with or without cystourethrectomy is the ultimate surgical answer to the dilemma of IC. If diversion alone is chosen, one must keep in mind potential problems that can befall the remaining bladder including pyocystis, hemorrhage, severe pain, and unremitting feelings of incomplete emptying and spasm (Eigner and Freiha, 1990). Bladder carcinoma has also been reported after urinary diversion but is not specifically associated with IC (Hanno and Tomaszewski, 1982). **Cystourethrectomy is certainly indicated in patients who are miserable and have not only failed all other therapies but have demonstrated chronicity such that remission is considered extremely unlikely.** Fortunately, few patients fall into this category. **Theoretically, conduit diversion seems to be reasonable if one is concerned about disease occurring in any continent storage type of reconstruction.**

Bejany and Politano (1995) reported excellent results in 5 patients treated with total bladder replacement and recommend neobladder reconstruction. Keselman and associates (1995) had 2 failures in 11 patients treated with continent diversion and attributed this to surgical complications. Lilius and colleagues (1973) noted failure in 2 of 4 patients treated with cystectomy and conduit diversion because of persistent pain. Baskin and Tanagho (1992) also cautioned about persistence of pelvic pain after cystectomy and continent diversion, discussing 3 such patients. In a subsequent letter to the editor, Irwin and Galloway (1992) added 4 of their own. Webster and associates (1992) had 10 failures in 14 patients treated with urinary diversion and cystourethrectomy. Ten patients had persistent pelvic pain, and four of them also complained of pouch pain. Only two patients had symptom resolution. Attempts have been made to improve results by limiting the operation to those without detrusor mastocystosis (Trinka et al, 1993) and those without "neuropathic pelvic pain" (Lotenfoe et al, 1994). Based on the experience of the past decades, it is unclear if these efforts will prove any more successful.

Almost 30 years ago Pool (1967) recognized that "surgical treatment has not been the boon many had hoped it would be. Diversion of the urine is not the entire answer to the situation. Removal of the lesion in the bladder has been of no benefit. Likewise, removal of almost all of the mobile portion of the bladder proved to be a failure." When one of the deans of major urologic reconstruction writes, "I find it very difficult to justify

such extensive surgery [continent diversion, cystourethrectomy] with such limited results and for these reasons have not been involved in surgery for IC over the past 3 years" (Webster, 1993), it is obvious that one should think carefully and proceed with surgery only after a complete discussion with a very motivated and well-informed patient.

Principles of Management

There are many different ways to manage IC, some of which have been described (Wein and Hanno, 1992; Hanno, 1994b; Wein and Broderick, 1994). A reasonable approach to diagnosis and treatment is detailed in the algorithms shown in Figures 17–6 and 17–7. **Perhaps the most critical step in management is patient education.** This is an incurable, chronic condition. It is subject to periods when the symptoms wax and wane and also go into remission for varying lengths of time. As such, it lends itself to practitioner abuse, and the uninformed, desperate patient is easy prey. As a general rule, except for the transurethral fulguration or resection of the rare Hunner's ulcer, surgery should be considered a last resort. **Because of the natural history of the disorder, it is best to cautiously progress through a variety of treatments, trying to employ just one at a time, at least initially. One should encourage the patients to maximize their activity and live as normal a life as possible, not becoming a prisoner of the condition. Although some activities or foods may aggravate symptoms, nothing has been shown to negatively affect the disease process itself. Therefore, patients should feel free to experiment and judge for themselves how to modify their lifestyle without the guilt that comes from feeling they have harmed themselves if symptoms flare. Dogmatic restrictions and diet are to be avoided unless they are shown to improve symptoms in a particular patient.**

As a rule, in the patient who does not respond to the initial diagnostic distention, oral therapy with amitriptyline or hydroxyzine is a noninvasive way to begin treatment. Understanding that perfect is the enemy of good, patients need to have realistic expectations, and invasive therapies should be avoided unless symptoms are significant. Other oral medications detailed earlier can also be tried. Intravesical therapies are an important second-line strategy. We mix 50 ml of DMSO with 10,000 units of heparin, 10 mg of triamcinolone, and 44 mEq of bicarbonate and administer it weekly for 6 weeks. In the refractory patients, TENS and/or intravesical Clorpactin administered under anesthesia can be considered. The vast majority of patients respond to these measures. If not, nontraditional medications like PPS or nifedipine can be tried and will certainly "buy time" until the symptoms improve of their own accord. A consultation with a pain center and consideration of analgesic treatment should be considered before a major surgical procedure is entertained.

The knowledge that one is not alone helps both physician and patient deal with the problems of this disorder, and it is in this regard that the Interstitial Cystitis Association is so important. Most patients with IC can be helped to live

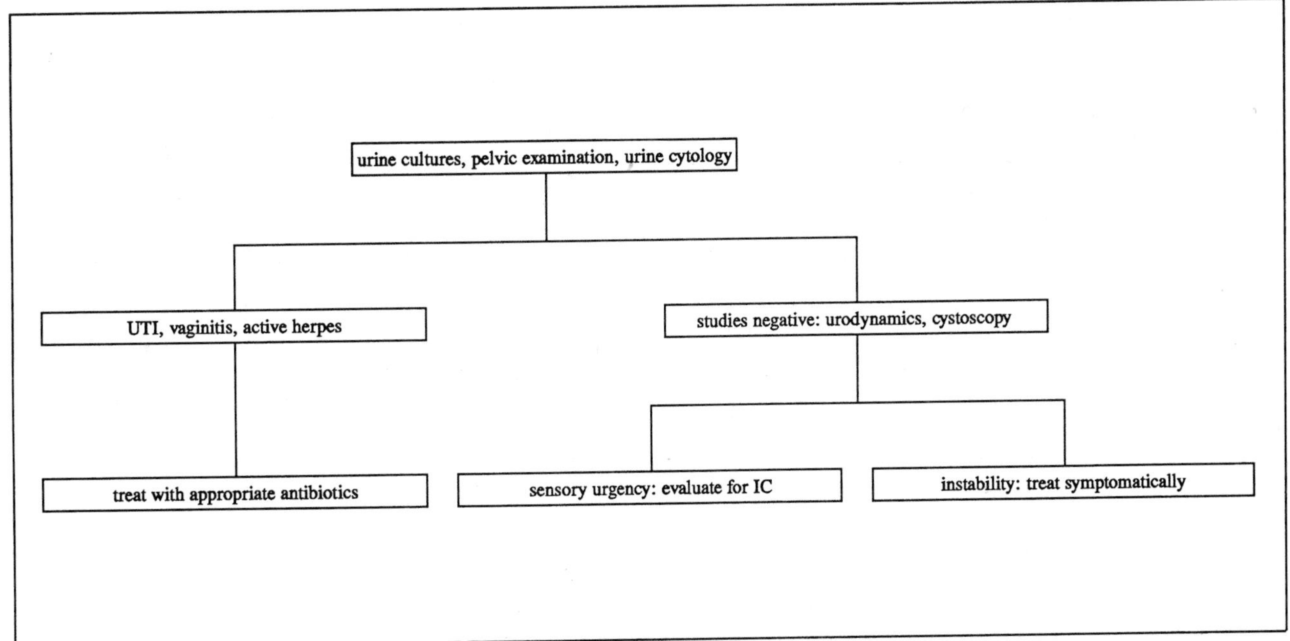

Figure 17–6. Diagnostic schema for interstitial cystitis (IC) and urethral syndrome.

Diagnosed IC/ Chronic urethral syndrome

symptoms tolerable: self-help protocols, mild analgesics

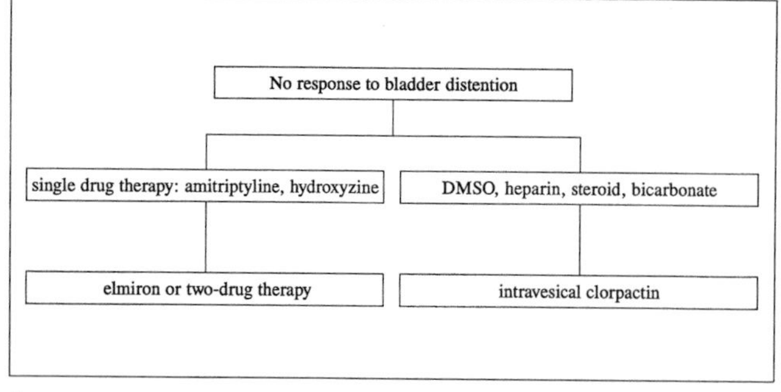

A

Failure of first line therapy

Cross over to intravesical or oral Rx

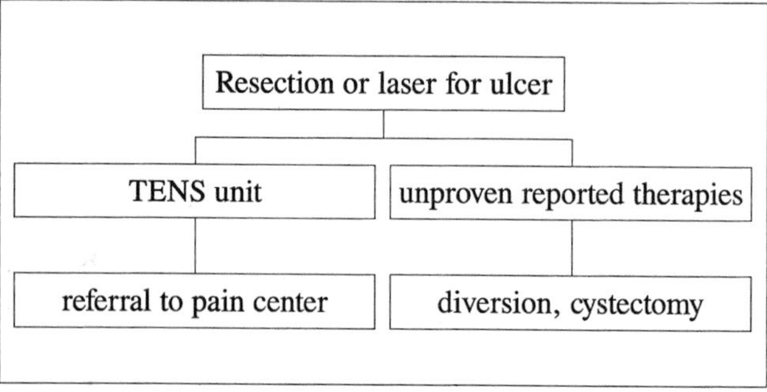

B

Figure 17–7. Treatment algorithms for interstitial cystitis (IC) and urethral syndrome. DMSO, dimethyl sulfoxide; TENS, transcutaneous electric nerve stimulation.

relatively normal lives and, with the aid of various forms of treatment modalities, including self-help, to tolerate their disability.

URETHRAL SYNDROME

Issues of Definition

In 1945 the distinguished American physician Richard Cabot was quoted as having stated that "any pain within two feet of the female urethra for which one cannot find an adequate explanation should be suspected of coming from the female urethra" (Charlton, 1986). The term *urethral syndrome* was first mentioned in a clinicopathologic study of the female urethra in 1949 (Powell and Powell). It appeared in the British literature in 1965 (Gallagher et al, 1965) when a group of New Zealand physicians used it to describe the 50% of their female patients with urinary symptoms without demonstrable infection. **The urethral syndrome comprises a very nonspecific constellation of symptoms including urinary frequency, urgency, dysuria, and suprapubic discomfort without any objective findings of urologic abnormality to account for the symptoms.** Although the symptoms are typically thought to occur in women, there is no reason to assume that a similar entity does not occur in men (Bodner, 1988; Hanno, 1995). The frequency; urgency; and suprapubic, perineal, and low back pain of prostatodynia are certainly reminiscent of the urethral syndrome (Fowler, 1989).

The urethral syndrome can be subdivided into an acute and a chronic condition. In the past, dysuric women with midstream urine cultures containing 10^5 bacteria/ml or greater were usually considered to have cystitis, and those with fewer bacteria were said to have the urethral syndrome. In the last 15 years it has become apparent that infections of the urethra, urinary bladder, and vagina account for a large proportion of patients who develop the symptom complex acutely. **Therefore the term *acute urethral syndrome*, implying as it does a mysterious cause and a urethral origin of the malady, has largely been abandoned in favor of specific etiologic diagnoses** (Latham and Stamm, 1984; Hooton, 1988), many of which will be found in the chapters on urinary tract infection and sexually transmitted disease. The acute urethral syndrome can thus be considered a circle that is invaded by two other circles, one of which is urinary tract infection and the other of which is genital infection (Stamm, 1987). Only a relatively small percentage of patients with acute urethral syndrome are found on investigation to have no cause for the symptoms. It would be more accurate to categorize this group of patients by their symptoms than to give them a diagnosis of "acute urethral syndrome," which ultimately communicates little about what is going on.

Those patients with chronic symptoms and with no discerned cause constitute the *chronic urethral syndrome* category. This phantom diagnosis is one of exclusion and rarely used in modern urology. Because it is rather undefined, it is almost impossible to interpret the literature. It is rather like looking at IC before the National Institutes of Health conferences in 1987 and 1988 defined the disorder (Gillenwater and Wein, 1988). In fact, **the symptomatic manifestations of IC and chronic urethral syndrome are by and large indistinguishable** (Fowler, 1989; Hanno, 1995).

Etiology

Acute dysuria and frequent urination in women whose voided urine is sterile or contains fewer than 10^5 microorganisms/ml is a common problem. Fifty percent of adult women have had an attack of urinary symptoms at some time during their lives, and 25% experience at least one episode each year. About half of the episodes of dysuria or frequency are due to urinary tract infections that can be documented by the growth of 10^5 bacteria/ml or greater (Hamilton-Miller, 1994). This "magic" number dates from classic studies by Kass (1955, 1956, 1957) designed to distinguish contaminated specimens from true bacteriuria in asymptomatic women and in women with acute pyelonephritis. Kass did not report on women with lower urinary tract symptoms. The large number of patients for whom 10^5 bacteria do not grow out with routine culture methods belong in the acute urethral syndrome category.

As reviewed by Latham and Stamm (1984), several epidemiologic and clinical features were observed to be shared by women with acute urethral syndrome and bacterial cystitis. This culminated in an oft-quoted seminal paper by Stamm and colleagues (1980) that compared 59 women with acute urethral syndrome with 35 patients with classically defined cystitis and 66 asymptomatic women. Forty-two of 59 women with urethral syndrome had pyuria, and 37 of these 42 were shown to be infected on urine obtained by catheterization or suprapubic aspiration with coliforms (24), *Staphylococcus saprophyticus* (3), or *Chlamydia trachomatis* (10). Few women without pyuria had demonstrable infection. *U. urealyticum* and *M. hominis* were found in both symptomatic and control groups and were not felt to be associated with the urethral syndrome. Thus 63% of women with acute urethral syndrome in this study had bacterial infection and should not have been given this purely descriptive diagnosis. Wilkins and colleagues (1989) proposed an infectious theory of urethral syndrome and IC, but their finding of fastidious organisms (*G. vaginalis* and *Lactobacillus* sp) in urine specimens or bladder biopsies in a group of 20 patients was not compared with findings in a control group.

An infectious cause in the vast majority of patients is not without its critics. Gillespie and colleagues (1989) were unable to find any difference in the incidence of positive cultures with fastidious organisms in disease and control groups, nor did the number of leukocytes differ. They concluded that the urethral syndrome is not caused by bacterial or chlamydial infection. Stamm's report, although a turning point in the treatment and evaluation of this symptom complex, still leaves a large number of patients with unexplained symptoms (Brumfitt et al, 1991a, 1991b). Some would apply his conclusions only to the group of young, sexually active women that made up his population (Hamilton-Miller, 1994). Maskell's (1991) suggestion that the urethral syndrome is caused by excessive multiplication of lactobacilli in the urethra runs counter to a report by Cooper and associates (1990) showing that antibiotics effective against lactobacilli are no more efficacious than those without such activity.

Sexually transmitted organisms like *Neisseria gonorrhoeae* and *C. trachomatis* can cause dysuria and frequency in 20% of women with these infections (Latham and Stamm, 1984), especially when the infection involves the urethra (Paavonen, 1979). Primary genital herpes (Corey et al, 1983) and vaginitis can also cause frequency and/or dysuria. Although candidiasis and trichomoniasis are other common causes of acute dysuria and frequency, the presence of sexually transmitted pathogens cannot explain the majority of such symptoms (Hamilton-Miller, 1994).

The varied causes of diagnosable and treatable problems that can result in the acute urethral syndrome make an office visit advisable. These patients should not be diagnosed and treated over the telephone.

The causes of chronic symptoms of the urethral syndrome are much more varied and murky. The overlap with the IC syndrome (disease) is almost total, and the reader is referred to the earlier sections of this chapter for a more complete discussion of etiology. As Cardozo (1984) points out, frequency and urgency are only symptoms for which there are many causes. The diagnosis changes from urethral syndrome when the cause is discerned, leaving a rather small group of patients with the diagnosis of chronic urethral syndrome. Aside from IC, some causes of urgency and frequency are detailed in Table 17–2.

Table 17–2. CAUSES OF FREQUENCY AND URGENCY

Urinary tract infection
Upper motor neuron lesion habit
Large fluid intake
Pregnancy
Bladder calculus
Urethral caruncle
Radiation cystitis
Large postvoid residual
Genital condyloma
Diabetes mellitus
Cervicitis
Periurethral gland infection
Chemical irritants:
contraceptive foams, douches, diaphragm, obsesssive washing
Detrusor instability
Vulvar carcinoma
Diuretic therapy
Bladder cancer
Urethral diverticulum
Pelvic mass
Chemotherapy
Bacterial urethritis
Renal impairment
Diabetes insipidus
Atrophic urethral changes

Theories of the cause of the chronic urethral syndrome are varied. Hormonal imbalances, reactions to ingested or environmental chemicals, and allergic conditions have been proposed with little supporting evidence and are not widely accepted (Messing, 1992). Many authors have supported the idea of urethral stenosis and reported good results with urethral dilatation (Davis, 1955; Roberts and Smith, 1968; Richardson, 1969; Splatt and Weedon, 1977; McCannel and Haile, 1982; Testa, 1992). However, diagnostic criteria are inconsistent, histologic studies claiming to document periurethral fibrosis are not reproducible, and a truly stenotic urethra in these patients is probably very rare (Zufall, 1978; Mabry et al, 1981; Splatt and Weedon, 1981; Rutherford et al, 1988).

Latham and Stamm (1984) have extensively evaluated women with chronic urethral symptoms for infectious causes, with results uniformly uninformative. Most urine specimens have lacked evidence of inflammatory cells. Carson and associates (1980) propose that the disorder represents a conversion reaction or psychophysiologic abnormality. Others have found no increase in psychiatric morbidity in these unfortunate patients (Sumners et al, 1992), nor have they found psychological factors to be a predominant cause of the symptoms (Maskell, 1988; Nazareth and King, 1993).

Not surprisingly, with the lack of a meaningful definition, the term *chronic urethral syndrome* conveys very little and has virtually fallen out of use in the American urologic literature in the last decade. One must remember that in few if any papers written about the urethral syndrome were patients clinically evaluated to exclude IC as it is now defined.

Diagnosis

The acute urethral syndrome must be distinguished from infectious processes. Vaginitis and active genital herpes can often be excluded by pelvic examination. If gonorrhea is a possibility, cultures for it should be obtained. As Kunin (1987) warns, it is unwise to treat this syndrome by telephone, at least initially until one has an idea of the cause of the symptoms and a familiarity with the patient. **The presence of pyuria in a midstream urine sample indicates a probable infectious cause. Urine microscopy may miss a low-count infection, and quantitative culture of a midstream sample is necessary to evaluate patients for urinary infection. The presence of even low colony counts of a pure culture of coliforms or *S. saprophyticus* from acutely symptomatic patients should be suspected as indicating a true urethritis or cystitis rather than idiopathic urethral syndrome, leading to appropriate antibiotic treatment.**

Chlamydial cultures are worth obtaining, but if they are not available, the presence of sterile pyuria associated with acute dysuria and frequency in a sexually active woman is certainly suggestive of infection with *C. trachomatis* (Latham and Stamm, 1984). Most physicians empirically treat these patients with antibiotics, and the reader is referred to the chapter on urinary infections for further discussion of empirical therapy. **By definition, the acute urethral syndrome is a self-limited illness, and in the absence of treatable infection in the patient without microhematuria, no further diagnostic studies are routinely indicated.**

In patients with chronic symptoms, the same diagnostic techniques used in the evaluation of IC and detailed in those sections are useful in diagnosing the urethral syndrome. One is hard put to differentiate the two entities. Chronic urethral syndrome may be the term used for patients who have symptoms of IC but do not meet the currently used criteria for diagnosis as outlined in the preceding sections. Indeed, as both are essentially diagnoses of exclusion, one must be sure that specific disease entities (detailed in the National Institutes of Health "research definition" of IC) are not responsible for the symptom complex (Nyberg, 1991). **Although urine and urethral cultures are critical, urodynamic and cystoscopic examination under anesthesia with bladder distention can be postponed until symptoms have persisted for 6 to 9 months, as many patients experience spontaneous and long-lived remission of their symptoms.** Urine cytologic and imaging studies to rule out other conditions can also be withheld assuming the symptoms resolve in a matter of weeks.

If the patient has not already been evaluated gynecologically, **a gynecologic consultation is generally worthwhile in the patient with chronic, unexplained symptoms.** Bogaert (1992) has reported on six patients with female hypospadius whose symptoms were initially triggered by intercourse and who improved after surgical transposition of the urethral meatus. This condition could be easily overlooked on physical examination. Imaging studies in the patient without microhematuria have a low yield and are not routinely indicated (Carson et al, 1980; Mabry et al, 1981). A voiding cystourethrogram is helpful if one suspects a urethral diverticulum as a result of symptoms or physical examination.

A urinary diary is an often overlooked part of the evaluation that is not only helpful diagnostically to confirm the symptoms and differentiate true frequency from polyuria but also tends to "empower" the patient and give her some feeling of taking part in the treatment process (Cardozo, 1984). The value of urodynamics is somewhat controversial (Maskell, 1988; Rutherford et al, 1988). Nevertheless, it will identify a small group of patients with unsuspected detrusor instability, can virtually rule out IC if completely normal, and can suggest a group of patients with smooth and/or striated muscle spasm of the outlet that may be masquerading as chronic urethral syndrome (Raz and Smith, 1976; Kaplan et al, 1980; Barbalias and Meares, 1984). If IC is not suspected, a cystoscopic examination in the office will reassure both the patient and the physician that no obvious, easily treated abnormality exists to account for the chronic, debilitating symptoms. Because of the nature of the symptoms, however, many of these patients require, at least on one occasion, cystoscopy under anesthesia with hydrodistention to rule out IC.

Management

In patients with a culture-documented urinary tract infection, the term *urethral syndrome* does not really apply. These patients should be treated with a short course of appropriate antibiotics. The reader is referred to Chapter 15 for a full discussion of urinary tract infection and to Chapter 18 for a discussion of sexually transmitted diseases. A course of empirical antibiotics would seem to be the mainstay of treatment for acute symptoms of dysuria and frequency even in the absence of positive cultures. Doxycycline, erythromycin, and metronidazole (Flagyl) have been recommended to treat the fastidious organisms and anaerobes potentially missed on routine culture (Messing, 1992). Stamm and colleagues (1981) undertook a randomized, double-blind prospective trial comparing doxycycline with placebo for treatment of the acute urethral syndrome. He found that doxycycline was significantly more effective than placebo in eradicating urinary symptoms, pyuria, and the infecting microorganism in women with the "urethral syndrome" due to coliforms, staphylococci, or *C. trachomatis*. In women without pyuria, no benefit could be ascribed to antibiotic therapy. However, it is the rare physician who will not start a short course of antibiotics pending culture in this clinical situation. Trimethoprim-sulfamethoxazole along with the tetracyclines are reasonable choices (Kunin, 1987). Although women with urethral syndrome due to chlamydial infection more frequently have a history of a new sex partner in the month before the onset of symptoms, less frequently have a history of symptoms of urinary tract infection in the preceding 2 years, and more often use oral contraceptives than those with low-count bladder bacteriuria (Stamm et al, 1980; Andriole, 1983), these features are by no means diagnostic and should not direct therapy. **Overuse of antibiotics and potential proliferation of bacteria resistant to antibiotics is certainly a concern (Brumfitt et al, 1991a, 1991b), but this applies far more to treatment of the chronic urethral syndrome than to treatment of the acute variety.**

Aside from infection, there are other, perhaps less defined but still specific causes of urethral syndrome that lend themselves to directed treatment. Estrogen deficiency may be characterized by recurrent episodes of urinary frequency and urgency with dysuria (Belchetz, 1994). Although estrogen supplementation may be therapeutically effective in this situation, the routine use of local estrogen therapy is not indicated (Parziani et al, 1994). *Female hypospadius* associated with symptoms of urethral syndrome has been successfully treated surgically with meatal transposition (Bogaert, 1992) but likely accounts for only an infinitesimal portion of patients with the syndrome. Patients with urodynamically demonstrated sphincter spasticity and pelvic floor hyperactivity may respond to alpha-blocking agents or diazepam (Raz and Smith, 1976; Kaplan et al, 1980; Barbalias and Meares, 1984).

The treatment of chronic symptoms is much more difficult, and the overlap with IC becomes more pertinent. Virtually the entire gamut of treatments appropriate to IC would apply, and the reader is referred to the relevant sections of this chapter. There is probably no difference between this group and the IC group, and the term *chronic urethral syndrome* is going the way of the dinosaur. As with IC, a group of these patients have fibromyalgia, and some of them respond to the nonspecific therapies, including antihistamines, diazepam, and nonsteroidal anti-inflammatory drugs, used for both illnesses (Paira, 1994).

Urethral dilatation was long a mainstay of urologic therapy because of the belief that distal urethral constriction was the cause of symptoms. This culminated in the "external urethroplasty" described by Richardson (1969) with glowing results in this patient population. The operation was designed to weaken the distal urethral segment by excision of posterior periurethral connective tissue, exposed through an incision of the anterior vaginal mucosa. Splatt and Weedon (1977) felt the procedure helpful in patients with a poor flow rate and trabeculation on endoscopy. However, this procedure as well as routine urethral dilatation have fallen out of favor and are of mainly historical interest (Testa, 1992). **Objective evidence of improvement and strict definitions of the patient population and symptoms studied are missing from most publications.** This author has treated hundreds of patients with this symptom complex and seen only three or four with a truly strictured urethra. Rutherford and colleagues (1988) showed an 80% symptomatic improvement with urethral dilatation to No. 36–42 Fr, a result identical to that of a control group who underwent cystoscopy alone.

Sand and colleagues (1989) utilized a specially designed cryoprobe and reported a 91% success rate compared with 33% for urethral dilatation alone. Urinary retention, incontinence, pain, bleeding, and recurrence of symptoms have prevented cryotherapy from becoming popular. Carson and colleagues (1980) concluded that patient reassurance and psychiatric consultation when necessary should form the mainstay of treatment. Certainly, the former continues to be extremely important, and as with IC, the relationship between the health care provider and patient is all-important.

Perhaps Zufall (1978) summed up the frustration of all physicians who treat this syndrome. Looking at the results of a variety of treatments in 150 patients, he concluded that none of the treatments were clearly superior. Sixty percent of patients were able to go for over 3 months without sufficient symptoms to warrant a repeat office visit. **Treatment should be supportive and harmless.**

REFERENCES

General Considerations

Burgio KL, Engel BT, Locher JL: Normative patterns of diurnal urination across 6 age decades. J Urol 1991; 145:728–731.

Held PJ, Hanno PM, Wein AJ, et al: Epidemiology of interstitial cystitis: 2. *In* Hanno PM, Staskin DR, Krane RJ, Wein AJ, eds: Interstitial Cystitis. London, Springer-Verlag, 1990; pp 29–48.

Historical Perspective

Bourque JP: Surgical management of the painful bladder. J Urol 1951; 65:25–34.

Hand JR: Interstitial cystitis: Report of 223 cases (204 women and 19 men). J Urol 1949; 61:291–310.

Hunner GL: A rare type of bladder ulcer in women; report of cases. Boston Med Surg J 1915; 172:660–664.

Messing EM, Stamey TA: Interstitial cystitis, early diagnosis, pathology and treatment. Urology 1978; 12:381–392.

Ratner V, Slade D, Whitmore KE: Interstitial cystitis: A bladder disease finds legitimacy. J Women's Health 1992; 1:63–68.

Skene AJC: Diseases of the Bladder and Urethra in Women. New York, William Wood, 1887.

Walsh A: Interstitial cystitis. *In* Harrison JH, Gittes RF, Perlmutter AD, et al, eds: Campbell's Urology, 4th ed. Philadelphia, W. B. Saunders Company, 1978; pp 693–707.

Walsh A: Historical perspectives. *In* Hanno PM, Staskin DR, Krane RJ, Wein AJ, eds: Interstitial Cystitis. London, Springer-Verlag, 1990; pp 17–21.

Wein AJ, Hanno, PM, Gillenwater JY: Interstitial cystitis: An introduction to the problem. *In* Hanno PM, Staskin DR, Krane RJ, Wein AJ, eds: Interstitial Cystitis. London, Springer-Verlag, 1990; pp 3–15.

Definition

Frazer MI, Haylen BT, Sissons M: Do women with idiopathic sensory urgency have early interstitial cystitis? Br J Urol 1990; 66:274–278.

George NJR: Preface. *In* George NJR, Gosling JA, eds: Sensory Disorders of the Bladder and Urethra. Berlin, Springer-Verlag, 1986; p vii.

Gillenwater JY, Wein AJ: Summary of the national institute of arthritis, diabetes, digestive and kidney diseases workshop on interstitial cystitis, NIH, Bethesda, Maryland August 28–29, 1987. J Urol 1988; 140:203–206.

Hanno PM, Levin RM, Monson FC, et al: Diagnosis of interstitial cystitis. J Urol 1990; 143:278–281.

Koziol JA: Epidemiology of interstitial cystitis. Urol Clin North Am 1994; 21:7–20.

Sant GR: Interstitial cystitis. Monogr Urol 1991; 12:37–63.

Wein AJ, Hanno PM, Gillenwater JY: Interstitial cystitis: An introduction to the problem. *In* Hanno PM, Staskin DR, Krane RJ, Wein AJ, eds: Interstitial Cystitis. London, Springer-Verlag, 1990; pp 3–15.

Epidemiology

Alagiri M, Chottiner S, Ratner V, et al: Interstitial cystitis: Unexplained associations with other chronic disease and pain syndromes. (Abstract.) J Urol 1995; 153:287A.

Bohne AW, Hodson JM, Rebuck JW, et al: An abnormal leukocyte response in interstitial cystitis. J Urol 1962; 88:387–391.

Boye E, Morse M, Huttner I, et al: Immune complex–mediated interstitial cystitis as a major manifestation of systemic lupus erythematosus. Clin Immunol Immunopathol 1979; 13:67–76.

Clauw J, Schmidt M, Radulovic D, et al: The relationship between fibromyalgia and interstitial cystitis. (Abstract.) Research Symposium on Interstitial Cystitis, 1995; NIDDK, Bethesda, MD, p 103.

Consensus document: Consensus document on fibromyalgia: The Copenhagen declaration. J Musculoskeletal Pain 1993; 1:295–312.

Farkas A, Waisman J, Goodwin WE: Interstitial cystitis in adolescent girls. J Urol 1977; 118:837–839.

Fister GM: Similarity of interstitial cystitis (Hunner ulcer) to lupus erythematosus. J Urol 1938; 40:37–51.

Fitzpatrick CC, DeLancey JO, Elkins TE, et al: Vulvar vestibulitis and interstitial cystitis: A disorder of urogenital sinus-derived epithelium? Obstet Gynecol 1993; 81:860–862.

Geist RW, Antolak SJ: Interstitial cystitis in children. J Urol 1970; 104:922–925.

Hanash KA, Pool TL: Interstitial cystitis in men. J Urol 1969; 102:427–428.

Hand JR: Interstitial cystitis: Report of 223 cases (204 women and 19 men). J Urol 1949; 61:291–310.

Held PJ, Hanno PM, Wein AJ, et al: Epidemiology of interstitial cystitis:

2. *In* Hanno PM, Staskin DR, Krane RJ, Wein AJ, eds: Interstitial Cystitis. London, Springer-Verlag, 1990; pp 29–48.

Jokinen EJ, Lassus A, Salo OP, et al: Discoid lupus erythematosus and interstitial cystitis. Ann Clin Res 1972; 4:23–25.

Koff SA, Byard MA: The daytime urinary frequency syndrome of childhood. J Urol 1988; 140:1280–1281.

Kontras SB, Bodenbender JG, McClave CR, et al: Interstitial cystitis in chronic granulomatous disease. J Urol 1971; 105:575–578.

Koziol JA: Epidemiology of interstitial cystitis. Urol Clin North Am 1994; 21:7–20.

Koziol JA, Clark DC, Gittes RF, et al: The natural history of interstitial cystitis: A survey of 374 patients. J Urol 1993; 149:465–469.

Lamm DL, Gittes RF: Inflammatory carcinoma of the bladder and interstitial cystitis. J Urol 1977; 117:49–51.

Lynn RB, Friedman LS: Irritable bowel syndrome. N Engl J Med 1993; 329:1940–1945.

Marinoff SC, Turner MLC: Vulvar vestibulitis syndrome: An overview. Am J Obstet Gynecol 1991; 165:1228–1234.

McCormack WM: Two urogenital sinus syndromes, interstitial cystitis and focal vulvitis. J Reprod Med 1990; 35:873–876.

Meulders Q, Michel C, Marteau P, et al: Association of chronic interstitial cystitis, protein-losing enteropathy and paralytic ileus with seronegative systemic lupus erythematosus. Clin Nephrol 1992; 37:239–244.

Miller JL, Rothman I, Bavendam TG, et al: Prostatodynia and interstitial cystitis: One and the same? Urology 1995; 45:587–590.

Murphy DM, Zincke H, Utz DC: Interstitial cystitis. (Letter.) J Urol 1982; 128:606.

Oravisto KJ: Epidemiology of interstitial cystitis. Ann Chir Gynaecol Fenniae 1975; 64:75–77.

Parsons CL: Interstitial cystitis: Clinical manifestations and diagnostic criteria in over 200 cases. Neurourol Urodyn 1990; 9:241–250.

Robson WLM, Leung AKC: Extraordinary urinary frequency syndrome. Urology 1993; 42:321–324.

Rodriguez de la Serna A, Alarcon-Segovia D: Chronic interstitial cystitis as an initial major manifestation of systemic lupus erythematosus. J Rheumatol 1981; 8:808–810.

Utz DC, Zincke H: The masquerade of bladder cancer in situ as interstitial cystitis. Trans Am Assoc Genito-urinary Surg 1973; 65:64–65.

Van De Merwe J, Kamerling R, Arendsen E, et al: Sjögren's syndrome in patients with interstitial cystitis. J Rheumatol 1993; 20:962–965.

Weisman MH, McDanald EC, Wilson CB: Studies of the pathogenesis of interstitial cystitis, obstructive uropathy, and intestinal malabsorption in a patient with systemic lupus erythematosus. Am J Med 1981; 70:875–881.

Etiologic Theories

Abelli L, Conte B, Somma V, et al: A method for studying pain arising from the urinary bladder in conscious, freely-moving rats. J Urol 1989; 141:148–151.

Abelli L, Conte B, Somma V, et al: Mechanical irritation induces neurogenic inflammation in the rat urethra. J Urol 1991; 146:1624–1626.

Alanen A, Jalava J, Laato M, et al: Absence of bacterial DNA in the bladder of patients with interstitial cystitis. (Abstract.) J Urol 1995; 153:329A.

Aldenborg F, Fall M, Enerback L: Proliferation and transepithelial migration of mucosal mast cells in interstitial cystitis. Immunology 1986; 58:411–416.

Aldenborg F, Fall M, Enerback L: Mast cells in interstitial cystitis. Ann Urol 1989; 23:165–166.

Anderson JB, Parivar F, Lee G, et al: The enigma of interstitial cystitis—an autoimmune disease? Br J Urol 1989; 63:58–63.

Balagani RK, Hanno PM, Ma M, et al: Induction of glomerulations in rabbit bladder after exposure to IC urine. (Abstract.) J Urol 1991; 145:258A.

Barbanti G, Maggi CA, Beneforti P, et al: Relief of pain following intravesical capsaicin in patients with hypersensitive disorders of the lower urinary tract. Br J Urol 1993; 71:686–691.

Baskin LS, Tanagho EA: Pelvic pain without pelvic organs. J Urol 1992; 147:683–686.

Beier-Holgersen R, Hermann GG, Mortensen SO, et al: The in vitro cytotoxicity of urine from patients with interstitial cystitis. J Urol 1994; 151:206–207.

Bohne AW, Hodson JM, Rebuck JW, et al: An abnormal leukocyte response in interstitial cystitis. J Urol 1962; 88:387–391.

Boucher W, El-Mansoury M, Pang X: Elevated mast cell tryptase in the urine of patients with interstitial cystitis. Br J Urol 1995; 76:94–100.

Bracis R, Sanders CV, Gilbert DN: Methicillin hemorrhagic cystitis. Antimicrob Agents Chemother 1977; 12:438–439.

Buffington CAT, Blaisdell JL, Binns SP, et al: Decreased urine glycosaminoglycan excretion in cats with idiopathic cystitis. J Urol 1996; 155:1801–1804.

Buffington CAT, Sokolov AG, Wolfe SA: Effects of interstitial cystitis on bladder tachykinin receptor concentrations in cats. NIDDK Interstitial Cystitis Symposium 1995; Bethesda, Md, abstract book, p 88.

Bullock A, Becich MJ, Klutke CG, et al: Experimental autoimmune cystitis: A potential murine model for ulcerative interstitial cystitis. J Urol 1992; 148:1951–1956.

Bushman W, Goolsby C, Grayhack JT, et al: Abnormal flow cytometry profiles in patients with interstitial cystitis. J Urol 1994; 152:2262–2266.

Chelsky MJ, Rosen SI, Knight LC, et al: Bladder permeability in interstitial cystitis is similar to that of normal volunteers: Direct measurement by transvesical absorption of technetium DTPA. J Urol 1994; 151:346–349.

Christensen MM, Keith I, Rhodes PR, et al: A guinea pig model for study of bladder mast cell function: Histamine release and smooth muscle contraction. J Urol 1990; 144:1293–1300.

Christmas TJ: Lymphocyte sub-populations in the bladder wall in normal bladder, bacterial cystitis and interstitial cystitis. Br J Urol 1994; 73:508–515.

Christmas TJ, Rode J: Characteristics of mast cells in normal bladder, bacterial cystitis and interstitial cystitis. Br J Urol 1991; 68:473–478.

Christmas TJ, Rode J, Chapple CR, et al: Nerve fiber proliferation in interstitial cystitis. Virchows Arch Pathol Anat 1990; 416:447–449.

Chudwin DS, Chesney PJ, Mischler EH, et al: Hematuria associated with carbenicillin and other semisynthetic penicillins. (Letter.) Am J Dis Child 1979; 133:98–99.

Clemmensen OJ, Lose G, Holm-Bentzen M, et al: Skin reactions to urine in patients with interstitial cystitis. Urology 1988; 32:17–20.

Collan Y, Alfthan O, Kivilaakso E, et al: Electron microscopic histological findings on urinary bladder epithelium in interstitial cystitis. Eur Urol 1976; 2:242–247.

Cook FV, Farrar WE, Kreutner A: Hemorrhagic cystitis and ureteritis, and interstitial nephritis associated with administration of penicillin G. J Urol 1979; 122:110–111.

Cornish J, Nickel JC, Vanderwee M, et al: Ultrastructural visualization of human bladder mucus. Urol Res 1990; 18:263–264.

Dimitriadou V, Buzzi MG, Moskowitz MA, et al: Trigeminal sensory fiber stimulation induces morphological changes reflecting secretion in rat dura mater mast cells. Neuroscience 1991; 44:97–112.

Dimitriadou V, Buzzi MG, Theoharides TC, et al: Ultrastructural evidence for neurogenically mediated changes in blood vessels of the rat dura mater and tongue following antidromic trigeminal stimulation. Neuroscience 1992; 48:187–203.

Dixon JS, Holm-Bentzen M, Gilpin CJ, et al: Electron microscopic investigation of the bladder urothelium and glycocalyx in patients with interstitial cystitis. J Urol 1986; 135:621–625.

Domingue GJ, Ghoniem GM, Bost KL, et al: Dormant microbes in interstitial cystitis. J Urol 1995; 153:1321–1326.

Durier JL: The application of anti-anaerobic antibiotics to the treatment of female bladder dysfunctions. Neurourol Urodyn 1992; 11:418.

El-Mansoury M, Boucher W, Sant GR, et al: Increased urine histamine and methylhistamine in interstitial cystitis. J Urol 1994; 152:350–353.

Elgavish A, Robert B, Lloyd K, et al: Evidence for a mechanism of bacterial toxin action that may lead to the onset of urothelial injury in the interstitial cystitis bladder. (Abstract.) J Urol 1995; 153:329A.

Elgebaly SA, Allam ME, Walzak MP, et al: Urinary neutrophil chemotactic factors in interstitial cystitis patients and a rabbit model of bladder inflammation. J Urol 1992; 147:1382–1387.

Enerback L, Fall M, Aldenborg F: Histamine and mucosal mast cells in interstitial cystitis. Agents Actions 1989; 27:113–116.

Engelmann U, Burger R, Jacobi G: Experimental investigations on the absorption of intravesically instilled mitomycin-C in the urinary bladder of the rat. Eur Urol 1982; 8:176–181.

Fall M, Johansson SL, Aldenborg F: Chronic interstitial cystitis: A heterogeneous syndrome. J Urol 1987; 137:35–38.

Fall M, Johansson SL, Vahlne A: A clinicopathological and virological study of interstitial cystitis. J Urol 1985; 133:771–773.

Felsen D, Frye S, Trimble LA, et al: Inflammatory mediator profile in urine and bladder wash fluid of patients with interstitial cystitis. J Urol 1994; 152:355–361.

Feltis JT, Perez-Marrero R, Emerson LE: Increased mast cells of the bladder in suspected cases of interstitial cystitis: A possible disease marker. J Urol 1987; 138:42–43.

Fisher BP, Bavendam TG, Roberts BW, et al: Blinded placebo controlled evaluation on the ingestion of acidic foods and their effect on urinary pH and the symptomatology of interstitial cystitis. Research Symposium on Interstitial Cystitis, 1993; NIDDK, Orlando, FL, p 53.

Foreman JC: Peptides and neurogenic inflammation. Br Med Bull 1987; 43:386–400.

Fowler JE, Lynes WL, Lau JLT, et al: Interstitial cystitis is associated with intraurothelial Tamm-Horsfall protein. J Urol 1988; 140:1385–1389.

Galli SJ: New concepts about the mast cell. N Engl J Med 1993; 328:257–265.

Galloway NTM, Gabale DR, Irwin PP: Interstitial cystitis or reflex sympathetic dystrophy of the bladder? Semin Urol 1991; 4:148–153.

Gordon HL, Rossen RD, Hersh EM, et al: Immunologic aspects of interstitial cystitis. J Urol 1973; 109:228–233.

Hampson SJ, Christmas TJ, Moss MT: Search for mycobacteria in interstitial cystitis using mycobacteria-specific DNA probes with signal amplification by polymerase chain reaction. Br J Urol 1993; 72:303–306.

Hanash KA, Pool TL: Interstitial and hemorrhagic cystitis: Viral, bacterial and fungal studies. J Urol 1970; 104:705–706.

Hand JR: Interstitial cystitis: Report of 223 cases (204 women and 19 men). J Urol 1949; 61:291–310.

Hanno PM, Fritz R, Wein AJ, et al: Heparin as an antibacterial agent in rabbit bladder. Urology 1978; 12:411–415.

Hanno PM, Levin RM, Monson FC, et al: Diagnosis of interstitial cystitis. J Urol 1990; 143:278–281.

Harn SD, Keutel HJ, Weaver RG: Immunologic and histologic evaluation of the urinary bladder wall after group A streptococcal infection. Invest Urol 1973; 11:55–64.

Harrington DS, Fall M, Johansson SL: Interstitial cystitis: Bladder mucosa lymphocyte immunophenotyping and peripheral blood flow cytometry analysis. J Urol 1990; 144:868–871.

Harrison SCW, Ferguson DR, Hanley MR: Effect of capsaicin on the rabbit urinary bladder. What is the function of sensory nerves that contain substance P? Br J Urol 1990; 66:155–161.

Hedelin HH, Mardh PA, Brorson JE, et al: *Mycoplasma hominis* and interstitial cystitis. Sex Transm Dis 1980; 10S:327–330.

Held PJ, Hanno PM, Wein AJ, et al: Epidemiology of interstitial cystitis: 2. *In* Hanno PM, Staskin DR, Krane RJ, Wein AJ, eds: Interstitial Cystitis. London, Springer-Verlag, 1990; pp 29–48.

Herbst RH, Baumrucker GO, German KL: Elusive ulcer (Hunner) of the bladder with an experimental study of the etiology. Am J Surg 1937; 38:152–167.

Hohenfellner M, Nunes L, Schmidt RA, et al: Interstitial cystitis: Increased sympathetic innervation and related neuropeptide synthesis. J Urol 1992; 147:587–591.

Holm-Bentzen M, Nordling J, Hald T: Etiology: Etiologic and pathogenetic theories in interstitial cystitis. *In* Hanno PM, Staskin DR, Krane RJ, Wein AJ, eds: Interstitial Cystitis. London, Springer-Verlag, 1990; pp 63–77.

Holm-Bentzen M, Sondergaard I, Hald T: Urinary excretion of a metabolite of histamine (1,4-methyl-imidazole-acetic acid) in painful bladder disease. Br J Urol 1987; 59:230–233.

Houpt KA: Housesoiling: Treatment of a common feline problem. Vet Med 1991; 86:1000–1006.

Hunner GL: A rare type of bladder ulcer in women; report of cases. Boston Med Surg J 1915; 172:660–664.

Irwin P, Galloway NTM: Impaired bladder perfusion in interstitial cystitis: A study of blood supply using laser Doppler flowmetry. J Urol 1993; 149:890–892.

Jacob J, Ludgate CM, Forde J, et al: Recent observations on the ultrastructure of human urothelium. Cell Tiss Res 1978; 193:543–560.

Johansson SL: Light microscopic findings in bladders of patients with IC. *In* Hanno PM, Staskin DR, Krane RJ, Wein AJ, eds: Interstitial Cystitis. London, Springer-Verlag, 1990; pp 83–90.

Jokinen E, Alfthan S, Oravisto K: Antitissue antibodies in interstitial cystitis. Clin Exp Immunol 1972; 11:333–339.

Jokinen EJ, Oravisto KJ, Alfthan OS: The effect of cystectomy on antitissue antibodies in interstitial cystitis. Clin Exp Immunol 1973; 15:457–460.

Kaplan AP, Haak-Frendscho M, Fuci A, et al: A histamine-releasing factor from activated human mononuclear cells. J Immunol 1985; 135:2027–2032.

Kastrup J, Hald T, Larsen S, et al: Histamine content and mast cell count of detrusor muscle in patients with interstitial cystitis and other types of chronic cystitis. Br J Urol 1983; 55:495–500.

Keay S, Schwalbe RS, Warren JW, et al: A prospective study of microorganisms in urine and bladder biopsies from interstitial cystitis patients and controls. Urology 1995a; 45:223–229.

Keay S, Trifillis A, Jacobs S, et al: Lack of urine cytotoxicity in interstitial cystitis. NIH Interstitial Cystitis Symposium, Bethesda, MD, 1995b, abstract book p 66.

Kiilholma PJ, Hukkanen V, Haarala M, et al: Viruses and interstitial cystitis: Absence of adenovirus and BK virus genomes in urinary bladder biopsies. (Abstract.) J Urol 1995; 153:289A.

Kim YS, Levin RM, Wein AJ, Longhurst PA: Effects of sensitization on the permeability of urothelium in guinea pig urinary bladder. J Urol 1992; 147:270–273.

Kisman OK, Lycklama AB, Nijeholt A, et al: Mast cell infiltration in intestine used for bladder augmentation in interstitial cystitis. J Urol 1991; 146:1113–1114.

Kruger JM, Osborne CA, Goyal SM, et al: Clinical evaluation of cats with lower urinary tract disease. J Am Vet Med Assoc 1991; 199:211–216.

Lagunoff FD, Martin TW, Read G: Agents that release histamine from mast cells. Ann Rev Pharmacol Toxicol 1983; 23:331–351.

Larsen S, Thompson SA, Hald T, et al: Mast cells in interstitial cystitis. Br J Urol 1982; 54:283–286.

Levin RM, Lavkar RM, Monson FC, et al: Effect of chronic nitrofurantoin on the rabbit urinary bladder. J Urol 1988; 139:400–404.

Liebert M, Wedemeyer G, Stein J, et al: Evidence for urothelial cell activation in interstitial cystitis. J Urol 1993; 149:470–475.

Lilly JD, Parsons CL: Bladder surface glycosaminoglycans is a human epithelial permeability barrier. Surg Gynecol Obstet 1990; 171:493–496.

Liu YK, Harty JI, Steinbock GS, et al: Treatment of radiation or cyclophosphamide induced hemorrhagic cystitis using conjugated estrogen. J Urol 1990; 144:41–43.

Lotenfoe R, Christie J, Parsons A, et al: Absence of neuropathic pelvic pain and favorable psychological profile in the surgical selection of patients with disabling interstitial cystitis. (Abstract.) J Urol 1994; 151:285A.

Lotz M, Villiger P, Hugli T, et al: Interleukin-6 and interstitial cystitis. J Urol 1994; 152:869–873.

Lundberg T, Liedberg H, Nordling L, et al: Interstitial cystitis: Correlation with nerve fibres, mast cells and histamine. Br J Urol 1993; 71:427–429.

Lynes WL, Flynn SD, Shortliffe LD, et al: Mast cell involvement in interstitial cystitis. J Urol 1987; 138:746–752.

Lynes WL, Shortliffe LD, Stamey TA: Urinary myotropic substances in interstitial cystitis. (Abstract.) J Urol 1990; 143:373A.

MacDermott JP, Charpied GL, Tesluk H: Recurrent interstitial cystitis following cystoplasty: Fact or fiction? J Urol 1990; 144:37–40.

MacDermott JP, Miller CH, Levy N, et al: Cellular immunity in interstitial cystitis. J Urol 1991; 145:274–278.

Martins SM, Darlin DJ, Lad PM, et al: Interleukin-1B: A clinically relevant urinary marker. J Urol 1994; 151:1198–1201.

Marx CM, Alpert SE: Ticarcillin-induced cystitis. A J Dis Child 1984; 138:670–672.

Maskell R: Broadening the concept of urinary tract infection. Br J Urol 1995; 76:2–8.

Mattila J: Vascular immunopathology in interstitial cystitis. Clin Immunol Immunopathol 1982; 23:648–655.

Mattila J, Harmoinen A, Hallstrom O: Serum immunoglobulin and complement alterations in interstitial cystitis. Eur Urol 1983; 9:350–352.

Mattila J, Linder E: Immunoglobulin deposits in bladder epithelium and vessels in interstitial cystitis: Possible relationship to circulating anti-intermediate filament autoantibodies. Clin Immunol Immunopathol 1984; 32:81–89.

McGuire EJ, Lytton B, Cornog JL: Interstitial cystitis following colocystoplasty. Urology 1973; 2:28–29.

Messing EM: Interstitial cystitis. (Editorial.) J Urol 1994; 151:355–356.

Miller CH, MacDermott JP, Quattrocchi GA, et al: Lymphocyte function in patients with interstitial cystitis. J Urol 1992; 147:592–595.

Moller NE: Carbenicillin-induced hemorrhagic cystitis. Lancet 1978; 2:946.

Moskowitz MO, Byrne DS, Callahan HJ, et al: Decreased expression of a glycoprotein component of bladder surface mucin (GP1) in interstitial cystitis. J Urol 1994; 151:343–345.

Mulholland SG, Shupp Byrne D: Interstitial cystitis. (Editorial.) J Urol 1994; 152:879–880.

Naber SP: Molecular pathology—diagnosis of infectious disease. N Engl J Med 1994; 331:1212–1215.

Neal DE, Dilworth JP, Kaack MB: Tamm-Horsfall autoantibodies in interstitial cystitis. J Urol 1991; 145:37–39.

Nickel JC, Emerson L, Cornish J: The bladder mucus (glycosaminoglycan) layer in interstitial cystitis. J Urol 1993; 149:716–718.

Nielsen KK, Kromann-Andersen B, Steven K, et al: Failure of combined supratrigonal cystectomy and Mainz ileocystoplasty in intractable interstitial cystitis: Is histology and mast cell count a reliable predictor for the outcome of surgery? J Urol 1990; 144:255–259.

NIH Consensus Development Panel: *Helicobacter pylori* in peptic ulcer disease. JAMA 1994; 272:65–69.

Ochs RL, Stein TW, Peebles CL, et al: Autoantibodies in interstitial cystitis. J Urol 1994; 151:587–592.

Oravisto KJ: Interstitial cystitis as an autoimmune disease. Eur Urol 1980; 6:10–13.

Palea S, Artibani W, Ostardo E, et al: Evidence for purinergic neurotransmission in human urinary bladder affected by interstitial cystitis. J Urol 1993; 150:2007–2012.

Pang X, Cotreau-Bibbo MM, Sant GR, et al: Bladder mast cell expression of high affinity oestrogen receptors in patients with interstitial cystitis. Br J Urol 1995b; 75:154–161.

Pang X, Marchand J, Sant GR, et al: Increased number of substance P positive nerve fibres in interstitial cystitis. Br J Urol 1995a; 75:744–750.

Parsonnet J, Friedman GD, Vandersteen DP, et al: *Helicobacter pylori* infection and the risk of gastric carcinoma. N Engl J Med 1991; 325:1127–1136.

Parsons CL: The role of the glycosaminoglycan layer in bladder defense mechanisms and interstitial cystitis. Int Urogynecol J 1993; 4:373–379.

Parsons CL: A model for the function of glycosaminoglycans in the urinary tract. World J Urol 1994; 12:38–42.

Parsons CL, Boychuk D, Hurst R, Callahan H: Bladder surface glycosaminoglycans: An epithelial permeability barrier. J Urol 1990; 143:139–142.

Parsons CL, Hurst RE: Decreased urinary uronic acid levels in individuals with interstitial cystitis. J Urol 1990; 143:690–693.

Parsons CL, Lilly JD, Stein P: Epithelial dysfunction in nonbacterial cystitis (interstitial cystitis). J Urol 1991; 145:732–735.

Parsons CL, Stein P: Role of toxic urine in interstitial cystitis. (Abstract.) J Urol 1990; 143:373A.

Parsons CL, Stein PC, Bidair M, et al: Abnormal sensitivity to intravesical potassium in interstitial cystitis and radiation cystitis. Neurourol Urodyn 1994; 13:515–520.

Patra PB, Tibbitts FD, Westfall DP: Endocrine status and urinary mast cells: Possible relationship to interstitial cystitis. Proceedings of the Interstitial Cystitis Symposium 1995; NIH, Bethesda, MD, p 70.

Perzin AD, Hanno PM, Ruggieri MR: Effect of protamine and IC urine on dye penetration across urothelium. (Abstract.) J Urol 1991; 145:259A.

Press SM, Moldwin R, Kushner L, et al: Decreased expression of GP-51 glycosaminoglycan in cats afflicted with feline interstitial cystitis. (Abstract.) J Urol 1995; 153:288A.

Ratliff TL, Klutke CG, McDougall EM: The etiology of interstitial cystitis. Urol Clin North Am 1994; 21:21–30.

Reinhart H, Obedeanu N, Hooton T, et al: Urinary excretion of Tamm-Horsfall protein in women with recurrent urinary tract infections. J Urol 1990; 144:1185–1187.

Rickard A, Lagunoff D: A novel model for the role of mast cells in interstitial cystitis. Proceedings of the Interstitial Cystitis Symposium 1995; NIH, Bethesda, MD, p 69.

Rose NR, Bona C: Defining criteria for autoimmune diseases (Witebsky's postulates revisited). Immunol Today 1993; 14:426–430.

Ruggieri MR, Hanno PM, Levin RM: Nitrofurantoin not a surface active agent in rabbit urinary bladder. Urology 1987; 29:534–537.

Ruggieri MR, Monson FC, Levin RM, et al: Interstitial cystitis: Animal models. *In* Hanno PM, Staskin DR, Krane RJ, Wein AJ, eds: Interstitial Cystitis. London, Springer-Verlag, 1990; pp 49–62.

Ruggieri MR, Steinhardt GF, Hanno PM: Antiadherence of IC bladder extracts. Semin Urol 1991; 9:136–142.

Ruoslahti E: Structure and biology of proteoglycans. Ann Rev Cell Biol 1988; 4:229–232.

Sant GR: Interstitial cystitis. Monogr Urol 1991; 12:37–63.

Sant GR, Kilaru P, Ucci AA: Mucosal mast cell contribution to bladder mastocytosis in interstitial cystitis. (Abstract.) J Urol 1988; 139:276A.

Sant GR, Theoharides TC: The role of the mast cell in interstitial cystitis. Urol Clin North Am 1994; 21:41–53.

Shickley TJ, Hanno PM, Whitmore KE, et al: Effect of hydrodistension on human bladder neuropeptide-Y content in interstitial cystitis. (Abstract.) J Urol 1993; 149:507A.

Silk MR: Bladder antibodies in interstitial cystitis. J Urol 1970; 103:307–309.

Simmons JL: Interstitial cystitis: An explanation for the beneficial effect of an antihistamine. J Urol 1961; 85:149–155.

Simmons JL, Bunce PL: On the use of an antihistamine in the treatment of interstitial cystitis. Am Surg 1958; 24:664–667.

Smith BH, Dehner LP: Chronic ulcerating interstitial cystitis. Arch Pathol 1972; 93:76–81.

Staehelin L, Chalpowski F, Bonneville M: Luminal plasma membrane of the urinary bladder: I. Three-dimensional reconstruction of freeze-etch images. J Cell Biol 1972; 53:73.

Stein PC, Santamaria PJ, Kurtz SB, et al: Evaluation of urothelial Tamm-Horsfall protein and serum antibody as a potential diagnostic marker for interstitial cystitis. J Urol 1993; 150:1405–1408.

Steinert BW, Diokno AC, Robinson JE, et al: Complement C3, eosinophil cationic protein and symptom evaluation in interstitial cystitis. J Urol 1994; 151:350–354.

Stone AR, Vogelsang P, Miller CH, et al: Tamm-Horsfall protein as a marker in interstitial cystitis. J Urol 1992; 148:1406–1408.

Sung JJY, Chung SCS, Ling TKW, et al: Antibacterial treatment of gastric ulcers associated with *Helicobacter pylori.* N Engl J Med 1995; 332:139–142.

Theoharides TC, Sant GR: Bladder mast cell activation in interstitial cystitis. Semin Urol 1991; 9:74–87.

Theoharides TC, Sant GR, El-Mansoury M, et al: Activation of bladder mast cells in interstitial cystitis: A light and electron microscopic study. J Urol 1995; 153:629–636.

Trelstad RL: Glycosaminoglycans: Mortar, matrix, mentor. Lab Invest 1985; 53:1–4.

Trifillis AL, Cui X, Jacobs S, et al: Culture of bladder epithelium from cystoscopic biopsies of patients with interstitial cystitis. J Urol 1995; 153:243–248.

Trinka PJ, Stanley BK, Noble MJ, et al: Mast-cell syndrome: A relative contraindication for continent urinary diversion. (Abstract.) J Urol 1993; 149:506A.

Uehling DT, Kelley E, Hopkins J, et al: Urinary glycosaminoglycan levels following induced cystitis in monkeys. J Urol 1988; 139:1103–1105.

Vliagoftis H, Dimitriadou V, Boucher W, et al: Estradiol augments while tamoxifen inhibits rat mast cell secretion. Int Arch Allergy Immunol 1992; 98:398–409.

Warren JW: Interstitial cystitis as an infectious disease. Urol Clin North Am 1994; 21:31–39.

Wein AJ, Broderick GA: Interstitial cystitis: Current and future approaches to diagnosis and treatment. Urol Clin North Am 1994; 21:153–161.

Weiss JP, Neville EC: Hyperbaric oxygen: Primary treatment of radiation-induced hemorrhagic cystitis. J Urol 1989; 142:43–45.

Wilkins EGL, Payne SR, Pead PJ, et al: Interstitial cystitis and the urethral syndrome: A possible answer. Br J Urol 1989; 64:39–44.

Yun SK, Laub DJ, Weese DL, et al: Stimulated release of urine histamine in interstitial cystitis. J Urol 1992; 148:1145–1148.

Zuraw BL, Sugimoto S, Parsons CL, et al: Activation of urinary kalikrein in patients with interstitial cystitis. J Urol 1994; 152:874–878.

Pathology

Anderstrom CRK, Fall M, Johansson SL: Scanning electron microscopic findings in interstitial cystitis. Br J Urol 1989; 63:270–275.

Collan Y, Alfthan O, Kivilaakso E, et al: Electron microscopic histological findings on urinary bladder epithelium in interstitial cystitis. Eur Urol 1976; 2:242–247.

Dixon JS, Holm-Bentzen M, Gilpin CJ, et al: Electron microscopic investigation of the bladder urothelium and glycocalyx in patients with interstitial cystitis. J Urol 1986; 135:621–625.

Fall M, Johansson SL, Aldenborg F: Chronic interstitial cystitis: A heterogeneous syndrome. J Urol 1987; 137:35–38.

Gillenwater JY, Wein AJ: Summary of the National Institute of Arthritis, Diabetes, Digestive and Kidney Diseases workshop on interstitial cystitis, NIH, Bethesda, Maryland August 28–29, 1987. J Urol 1988; 140:203–206.

Hellstrom HR, Davis BK, Shonnard JW: Eosinophilic cystitis: A study of 16 cases. Am J Clin Pathol 1979; 72:777–784.

Holm-Bentzen M: Pathology, pathophysiology, and pathogenesis of painful bladder diseases. Urol Res 1989; 17:203–209.

Holm-Bentzen M, Jacobsen F, Nerstrom B, et al: Painful bladder disease: Clinical and pathoanatomical differences in 115 patients. J Urol 1987; 138:500–502.

Holm-Bentzen M, Larsen S, Hainau B, et al: Nonobstructive detrusor myopathy in a group of patients with chronic abacterial cystitis. Scand J Urol Nephrol 1985; 19:21–26.

Jacobo E, Stamler FW, Culp DA: Interstitial cystitis followed by total cystectomy. Urology 1974; 3:481–485.

Johansson SL, Fall M: Clinical features and spectrum of light microscopic changes in interstitial cystitis. J Urol 1990; 143:1118–1124.

Johansson SL, Fall M: Pathology of interstitial cystitis. Urol Clin North Am 1994; 21:55–62.

Lepinard V, Saint-Andre JP, Rognon LM: La cystite interstitielle aspects actuels. J Urol (Paris) 1984; 7:455–465.

Lynes WL, Flynn SD, Shortliffe LD, et al: The histology of interstitial cystitis. Am J Surg Pathol 1990; 14:969–976.

Moore KH, Nickson P, Richmond DH, et al: Detrusor mast cells in refractory idiopathic instability. Br J Urol 1992; 70:17–21.

Nickel JC, Emerson L, Cornish J: The bladder mucus (glycosaminoglycan) layer in interstitial cystitis. J Urol 1993; 149:716–718.

Smith BH, Dehner LP: Chronic ulcerating interstitial cystitis. Arch Pathol 1972; 93:76–81.

Diagnosis

Awad SA, MacDiarmid S, Gajewski JB, et al: Idiopathic reduced bladder storage versus interstitial cystitis. J Urol 1992; 148:1409–1412.

Benson G: Interstitial cystitis. *In* Hanno PM, Staskin DR, Krane RJ, Wein AJ, eds: Interstitial Cystitis. London, Springer-Verlag, 1990; p 131.

Christmas TJ, Rode J: Characteristics of mast cells in normal bladder, bacterial cystitis and interstitial cystitis. Br J Urol 1991; 68:473–478.

El-Mansoury M, Boucher W, Sant GR, et al: Increased urine histamine and methylhistamine in interstitial cystitis. J Urol 1994; 152:350–353.

Feltis JT, Perez-Marrero R, Emerson LE: Increased mast cells of the bladder in suspected cases of interstitial cystitis: A possible disease marker. J Urol 1987; 138:42–43.

Hanno PM: Diagnosis of interstitial cystitis. Urol Clin North Am 1994; 21:63–66.

Hanno PM, Levin RM, Monson FC, et al: Diagnosis of interstitial cystitis. J Urol 1990; 143:278–281.

Holm-Bentzen M, Jacobsen F, Nerstrom B, et al: Painful bladder disease: clinical and pathoanatomical differences in 115 patients. J Urol 1987; 138:500–502.

Hurst RE, Parsons CL, Roy JB, et al: Urinary glycosaminoglycan excretion as a laboratory marker in the diagnosis of interstitial cystitis. J Urol 1993; 149:31–35.

Kastrup J, Hald T, Larsen S, et al: Histamine content and mast cell count of detrusor muscle in patients with interstitial cystitis and other types of chronic cystitis. Br J Urol 1983; 55:495–500.

Littleton RH, Farah RN, Cerny JC: Eosinophilic cystitis: An uncommon form of cystitis. J Urol 1982; 127:132–133.

Lose G, Frandsen B, Holm-Bentzen M, et al: Urine eosinophil cationic protein in painful bladder disease. Br J Urol 1987; 60:39–42.

Lynes WL, Flynn SD, Shortliffe LD, et al: Mast cell involvement in interstitial cystitis. J Urol 1987; 138:746–752.

Moore KH, Nickson P, Richmond DH, et al: Detrusor mast cells in refractory idiopathic instability. Br J Urol 1992; 70:17–21.

Perez-Marrero R, Emerson L, Juma S: Urodynamic studies in interstitial cystitis. Urology 1987; 29(suppl):27–30.

Sidh SM, Smith SP, Silber SB, et al: Eosinophilic cystitis: Advanced disease requiring surgical intervention. Urology 1980; 15:23–26.

Sircus SI, Sant GR, Ucci AA: Bladder detrusor endometriosis mimicking interstitial cystitis. Urology 1988; 32:339–342.

Siroky MB: Is it interstitial cystitis? Diagnostic distinctions in reduced bladder capacity. Contemp Urol 1994; July:13–22.

Utz DC, Zincke H: The masquerade of bladder cancer in situ as interstitial cystitis. J Urol 1974; 111:160–161.

Treatment

Albers DD, Geyer JR: Long-term results of cystolysis (supratrigonal denervation) of the bladder for intractable interstitial cystitis. J Urol 1988; 139:1205–1206.

Badenoch AW: Chronic interstitial cystitis. Br J Urol 1971; 43:718–721.

Baldessarini RJ: Drugs and the treatment of psychiatric disorders. *In* Gilman AG, Goodman LS, Rall TW, et al, eds: The Pharmacological Basis of Therapeutics, 7th ed. New York, Macmillan Publishing Company, 1985; pp 387–445.

Barbanti G, Maggi CA, Beneforti P, et al: Relief of pain following intravesical capsaicin in patients with hypersensitive disorders of the lower urinary tract. Br J Urol 1993; 71:686–691.

Barker SB, Matthews PN, Philip PF, et al: Prospective study of intravesical dimethyl sulfoxide in the treatment of chronic inflammatory bladder disease. Br J Urol 1987; 59:142–144.

Barrett DM, Wein AJ: Voiding dysfunction: Diagnosis, classification, and management. *In* Gillenwater JY, Grayhack JT, Howards SS, et al, eds: Adult and Pediatric Urology. Chicago, Year Book Medical Publishers, 1987; pp 863–892.

Baskin LS, Tanagho EA: Pelvic pain without pelvic organs. J Urol 1992; 147:683–686.

Bejany DE, Politano VA: Ileocolic neobladder in the woman with interstitial cystitis and a small contracted bladder. J Urol 1995; 153:42–43.

Benson H, Epstein MD: The placebo effect. JAMA 1976; 232:1225–1226.

Biggers RD: Self-administration of dimethyl sulfoxide (DMSO) for interstitial cystitis. Urology 1986; 28:10–11.

Blackford HN, Murray K, Stephenson TP, et al: Results of transvesical infiltration of the pelvic plexuses with phenol in 116 patients. Br J Urol 1984; 56:647–649.

Bourque JP: Surgical management of the painful bladder. J Urol 1951; 65:25–34.

Burford EH, Burford CE: Hunner ulcer of the bladder: A report of 187 cases. J Urol 1958; 79:952–955.

Caulfield J, Phillips R, Steinhardt G: Intravesical heparin instillation: Is there systemic absorption? (Abstract.) J Urol 1995; 153:289A.

Chaiken DC, Blaivas JG, Blaivas ST: Behavioral therapy for the treatment of refractory interstitial cystitis. J Urol 1993; 149:1445–1448.

Chang PL: Urodynamic studies in acupuncture for women with frequency, urgency and dysuria. J Urol 1988; 140:563–566.

Cheng C, Whitfield HN: Cystoplasty: Tubularization or detubularization? Br J Urol 1990; 66:30–34.

Dees JE: The use of cortisone in interstitial cystitis: A preliminary report. J Urol 1953; 69:496–502.

DeJuana CP, Everett JC: Interstitial cystitis; experience and review of recent literature. Urology 1977; 10:325–329.

Dodson AI: Hunner's ulcer of the bladder; a report of ten cases. Va Med Mon 1926; 53:305–310.

Dunn M, Ramsden PD, Roberts JBM, et al: Interstitial cystitis, treated by prolonged bladder distention. Br J Urol 1977; 49:641–645.

Eigner EB, Freiha FS: The fate of the remaining bladder following supravesical diversion. J Urol 1990; 144:31–33.

Ek A, Engberg A, Frodin L, et al: The use of dimethyl-sulfoxide (DMSO) in the treatment of interstitial cystitis. Scand J Urol Nephrol 1978; 12:129–131.

Emerson LE, Feltis JT: Urodynamic factors affecting response to DMSO in the treatment of interstitial cystitis. (Abstract.) J Urol 1986; 135:188A.

Fall M: Conservative management of chronic interstitial cystitis: Transcutaneous electrical nerve stimulation and transurethral resection. J Urol 1985; 133:774–778.

Fall M: Transcutaneous electrical nerve stimulation in interstitial cystitis. Urology 1987; 29:40–42.

Fall M, Carlsson CA, Erlandson BE: Electrical stimulation in interstitial cystitis. J Urol 1980; 123:192–195.

Fall M, Lindstrom S: Transcutaneous electrical nerve stimulation in classic and nonulcer interstitial cystitis. Urol Clin North Am 1994; 21:131–139.

Fleischmann J: Calcium channel antagonists in the treatment of interstitial cystitis. Urol Clin North Am 1994; 21:107–111.

Fleischmann JD, Huntley HN, Shingleton WB, et al: Clinical and immunological response to nifedipine for the treatment of interstitial cystitis. J Urol 1991; 146:1235–1239.

Flood HD, Malhotra SJ, O'Connell HE, et al: Long-term results and complications using augmentation cystoplasty in reconstructive urology. Neurourol Urodyn 1995; 14:297–309.

Fowler JE: Prospective study of intravesical dimethyl sulfoxide in treatment of suspected early interstitial cystitis. Urology 1981; 18:21–26.

Freedman AI, Wein AJ, Whitmore K, et al: In vitro effects of intravesical dimethysulfoxide. Neurourol Urodyn 1989; 8:277–283.

Freiha FS, Faysal MH, Stamey TA: The surgical treatment of intractable interstitial cystitis. J Urol 1980; 123:632–634.

Freiha FS, Stamey TA: Cystolysis: A procedure for the selective denervation of the bladder. Trans Am Assoc Genito-Urinary Surg 1979; 71:50–53.

Fritjofsson A, Fall M, Juhlin R, et al: Treatment of ulcer and nonulcer interstitial cystitis with sodium pentosanpolysulfate: A multicenter trial. J Urol 1987; 138:508–512.

Geirsson G, Wang YH, Lindstrom S, et al: Traditional acupuncture and electrical stimulation of the posterior tibial nerve. A trial in chronic interstitial cystitis. Scand J Urol Nephrol 1993; 27:67–70.

Glanakopoulos X, Champilomatos P: Chronic interstitial cystitis: Successful treatment with intravesical lidocaine. Arch Ital Urol Nefrol Androl 1992; 64:337–339.

Golomb J, Klutke CG, Lewin KJ, et al: Bladder neoplasms associated with augmentation cystoplasty: Report of 2 cases and literature review. J Urol 1989; 142:377–380.

Gourlay GK: Long-term use of opioids in chronic pain patients with nonterminal disease states. Pain Rev 1994; 1:62–76.

Greenhill JP: Sympathectomy and intraspinal alcohol injections for relief of pelvic pain. BMJ 1947; Nov 29:859–862.

Gurpinar T, Griffith DP: Iontophoretic intravesical intraprostatic drug delivery: An animal model and preliminary results. (Abstract.) J Urol 1995; 153:289A.

Hald T, Barnard RJ, Holm-Bentzen M: Treatment of interstitial cystitis. *In* George NJR, Gosling JA, eds: Sensory Disorders of the Bladder and Urethra. Berlin, Springer-Verlag, 1986; pp 73–78.

Hamer AJ, Nicholson S, Padfield CJ: Spontaneous rupture of the bladder in interstitial cystitis. Br J Urol 1992; 69:102.

Hanno PM: Amitriptyline in the treatment of interstitial cystitis. Urol Clin North Am 1994a; 21:89–92.

Hanno PM: Interstitial cystitis. *In* Seidmon EJ, Hanno PM, eds: Current Urologic Therapy, 3rd ed. Philadelphia, W. B. Saunders Company, 1994b; pp 263–266.

Hanno PM, Buehler J, Wein AJ: Use of amitriptyline in the treatment of interstitial cystitis. J Urol 1989; 141:846–848.

Hanno PM, Fritz R, Wein AJ, et al: Heparin as an antibacterial agent in rabbit bladder. Urology 1978; 12:411–415.

Hanno PM, Tomaszewski JE: Bladder carcinoma after urinary diversion. JAMA 1982; 248:2885.

Hanno PM, Wein AJ: Medical treatment of interstitial cystitis (other than Rimso-50/Elmiron). Urology 1987; 29S:22–26.

Hanno PM, Wein AJ: Conservative therapy of interstitial cystitis. Semin Urol 1991; 9:143–147.

Held PJ, Hanno PM, Wein AJ, et al: Epidemiology of interstitial cystitis: 2. *In* Hanno PM, Staskin DR, Krane RJ, Wein AJ, eds: Interstitial Cystitis. London, Springer-Verlag, 1990; pp 29–48.

Holm-Bentzen M, Jacobsen F, Nerstrom B, et al: A prospective double-blind clinically controlled multicenter trial of sodium pentosanpolysulfate in the treatment of interstitial cystitis. J Urol 1987; 138:503–507.

Hughes ODM, Kynaston HG, Jenkins BJ, et al: Substitution cystoplasty for intractable interstitial cystitis. Br J Urol 1995; 76:172–174.

Irwin P, Galloway NTM: Re: Pelvic pain without pelvic organs. (Letter.) J Urol 1992; 148:1265–1266.

Irwin PP, Galloway NTM: Surgical management of interstitial cystitis. Urol Clin North Am 1994; 21:145–151.

Irwin PP, Hammonds WD, Galloway NTM: Lumbar epidural blockade for management of pain in interstitial cystitis. Br J Urol 1993; 71:413–416.

Jancso G, Lynn B: Possible use of capsaicin in pain therapy. Clin J Pain 1987; 3:123–126.

Kang J, Wein AJ, Levin RM: Bladder functional recovery following acute overdistention. Neurourol Urodyn 1992; 11:253–260.

Keller ML, McCarthy DO, Neider RS: Measurement of symptoms of interstitial cystitis: A pilot study. Urol Clin North Am 1994; 21:67–72.

Kennelly MJ, Konnak JW: Intravesical cromolyn sodium for treatment of interstitial cystitis—a double-blind placebo controlled pilot study. (Abstract.) Interstitial Cystitis Symposium 1995; NIDDK, Bethesda, MD, p 64.

Kerr WS: Interstitial cystitis: Treatment by transurethral resection. J Urol 1971; 105:664–666.

Keselman I, Austin P, Anderson J, et al: Cystectomy and urethrectomy for disabling interstitial cystitis: A long term followup. (Abstract.) J Urol 1995; 153:290A.

Khanna OP, Loose JH: Interstitial cystitis treated with intravesical doxorubicin. Urology 1990; 36:139–142.

Khoury JM, Timmons SL, Corbel L, et al: Complications of enterocystoplasty. Urology 1992; 40:9–13.

Kirkemo AK, Miles BJ, Peters JM: Use of amitriptyline in the treatment of interstitial cystitis. (Abstract.) J Urol 1990; 143:279A.

Kisman OK, Lycklama AB, Nijeholt A, et al: Mast cell infiltration in intestine used for bladder augmentation in interstitial cystitis. J Urol 1991; 146:1113–1114.

Lane DA, Adams L: Non-anticoagulant uses of heparin. N Engl J Med 1993; 329:129–130.

Lasanen LT, Tammela TL, Kallioinen M, et al: Effect of acute distension on cholinergic innervation of the rat urinary bladder. Urol Res 1992; 20:59–62.

Lilius HG, Oravisto KJ, Valtonen EJ: Origin of pain in interstitial cystitis. Scand J Urol Nephrol 1973; 7:150–152.

Lose G, Frandsen B, Hojensgard JC, et al: Chronic interstitial cystitis: Increased levels of eosinophil cationic protein in serum and urine and an ameliorating effect of subcutaneous heparin. Scand J Urol Nephrol 1983; 17:159–161.

Lose G, Jesperson J, Frandsen B, et al: Subcutaneous heparin in the treatment of interstitial cystitis. Scand J Urol 1985; 19:27–29.

Lotenfoe R, Christie J, Parsons A, et al: Absence of neuropathic pelvic pain and favorable psychological profile in the surgical selection of patients with disabling interstitial cystitis. (Abstract.) J Urol 1994; 151:285A.

Lunghi F, Nicita G, Selli C, et al: Clinical aspects of augmentation enterocystoplasties. Eur Urol 1984; 10:159–163.

MacDermott JP, Charpied GL, Tesluk H: Recurrent interstitial cystitis following cystoplasty: Fact or fiction? J Urol 1990; 144:37–40.

Malloy TR, Shanberg AM: Laser therapy for interstitial cystitis. Urol Clin North Am 1994; 21:141–144.

McGuire EJ, Lytton B, Cornog JL: Interstitial cystitis following colocystoplasty. Urology 1973; 2:28–29.

McGuire EJ, Shi-chun Z, Horwinski ER, et al: Treatment of motor and sensory detrusor instability by electrical stimulation. J Urol 1983; 129:78–79.

McInerney PD, Vanner TF, Matenhelia S, et al: Assessment of the long-term results of subtrigonal phenolisation. Br J Urol 1991; 67:586–587.

Meirowsky AM: The management of chronic interstitial cystitis by differential sacral neurotomy. J Neurosurg 1969; 30:604–607.

Melzack R: The McGill pain questionnaire: Major properties and scoring methods. Pain 1975; 1:277–299.

Messing EM, Freiha FS: Complication of clorpactin WCS90 therapy for interstitial cystitis. Urology 1979; 13:389–392.

Messing EM, Stamey TA: Interstitial cystitis, early diagnosis, pathology and treatment. Urology 1978; 12:381–392.

Morales A, Emerson L: Treatment of refractory interstitial cystitis with intravesical hyaluronic acid. (Abstract.) J Urol 1995; 153:288A.

Mulholland SG, Hanno PM, Parsons CL, et al: Pentosan polysulfate sodium for therapy of interstitial cystitis. Urology 1990; 35:552–558.

Murnaghan GF, Saalfeld J, Farnsworth RH: Interstitial cystitis—treatment with chlorpactin WCS 90. Br J Urol 1970; 42:744.

Nielsen KK, Kromann-Andersen B, Steven K, et al: Failure of combined supratrigonal cystectomy and Mainz ileocystoplasty in intractable interstitial cystitis: Is histology and mast cell count a reliable predictor for the outcome of surgery? J Urol 1990; 144:255–259.

Nurse DE, Parry JRW, Mundy AR: Problems in the surgical treatment of interstitial cystitis. Br J Urol 1991; 68:153–154.

O'Conor VJ: Clorpactin WCS 90 in the treatment of interstitial cystitis. Q Bull NWU Med Sch 1955; 29:392.

Oravisto KJ, Alfthan OS: Treatment of interstitial cystitis with immunosuppression and chloroquine derivatives. Eur Urol 1976; 2:82–84.

Parsons CL: Successful management of radiation cystitis with sodium pentosanpolysulfate. J Urol 1986; 136:813–814.

Parsons CL, Benson G, Childs SJ, et al: A quantitatively controlled method to study prospectively interstitial cystitis and demonstrate the efficacy of pentosanpolysulfate. J Urol 1993; 150:845–848.

Parsons CL, Housley T, Schmidt JD, et al: Treatment of interstitial cystitis with intravesical heparin. Br J Urol 1994; 73:504–507.

Parsons CL, Koprowski PF: Interstitial cystitis: Successful management by increasing urinary voiding intervals. Urology 1991; 37:207–212.

Parsons CL, Schmidt JD, Pollen JJ: Successful treatment of interstitial cystitis with sodium pentosanpolysulfate. J Urol 1983; 130:51–53.

Perez-Marrero R, Emerson LE, Feltis JT: A controlled study of dimethyl sulfoxide in interstitial cystitis. J Urol 1988; 140:36–39.

Perez-Marrero R, Emerson LE, Maharajh DO, et al: Prolongation of response to DMSO by heparin maintenance. Urology 1993; 41(Suppl):64–66.

Pool TL: Interstitial cystitis: Clinical considerations and treatment. Clin Obstet Gynecol 1967; 10:185–191.

Pool TL, Rives HF: Interstitial cystitis: Treatment with silver nitrate. J Urol 1944; 51:520–525.

Portenoy RK, Foley KM: Chronic use of opioid analgesics in nonmalignant pain: Report of 38 cases. Pain 1986; pp 171–186.

Pranikoff K, Constantino GL: Amitriptyline therapy for patients with urinary frequency and pelvic pain. (Abstract.) Interstitial Cystitis Symposium 1995, National Institutes of Health, Bethesda, MD, p 67.

Ratner V, Slade D, Whitmore KE: Interstitial cystitis: A bladder disease finds legitimacy. J Women's Health 1992; 1:63–68.

Renshaw DC: Desipramine for interstitial cystitis. JAMA 1988; 260:341.

Rothman KJ, Michels KB: The continuing unethical use of placebo controls. N Engl J Med 1994; 394–398.
Rummans TA: Nonopioid agents for treatment of acute and subacute pain. Mayo Clin Proc 1994; 69:481–490.
Sant GR: Intravesical 50% dimethyl sulfoxide (RIMSO-50) in treatment of interstitial cystitis. Urology 1987; 29:17–26.
Schulz KF, Chalmers I, Hayes RJ, et al: Empirical evidence of bias; dimensions of methodological quality associated with estimates of treatment effects in controlled trials. JAMA 1995; 273:408–412.
Seddon JM, Best L, Bruce AW: Intestinocystoplasty in treatment of interstitial cystitis. Urology 1977; 10:431–435.
Seshadri P, Emerson L, Morales A: Cimetidine in the treatment of interstitial cystitis. Urology 1994; 44:614–616.
Shanberg AM: Benign diseases of the bladder. *In* Smith JA, Stein BS, Benson RC, eds: Lasers in Urologic Surgery, 2nd ed. Chicago, Year Book Medical Publishers, 1989; pp 50–56.
Shanberg AM, Baghdassarian R, Tansey LA: Treatment of interstitial cystitis with the neodymium-YAG laser. J Urol 1985; 134:885–888.
Shirley SW, Stewart BH, Mirelman S: Dimethyl sulfoxide in treatment of inflammatory genitourinary disorders. Urology 1978; 11:215–220.
Siegel A, Snyder J, Raz S: Surgical therapy of interstitial cystitis. *In* Hanno PM, Staskin DR, Krane RJ, Wein AJ, eds: Interstitial Cystitis. London, Springer-Verlag, 1990; pp 193–205.
Simmons JL: Interstitial cystitis: An explanation for the beneficial effect of an antihistamine. J Urol 1961; 85:149–155.
Stewart BH, Branson AC, Hewitt CB, et al: The treatment of patients with interstitial cystitis, with special reference to intravesical DMSO. Trans Am Assoc Genito-urinary Surg 1971; 63:69–72.
Stewart BH, Branson AC, Hewitt CB, et al: The treatment of patients with interstitial cystitis, with special reference to intravesical DMSO. J Urol 1972; 107:377–380.
Stewart BH, Persky L, Kiser WS: The use of dimethyl sulfoxide (DMSO) in the treatment of interstitial cystitis. J Urol 1968; 98:671–672.
Stewart BH, Shirley SW: Further experience with intravesical dimethyl sulfoxide in the treatment of interstitial cystitis. J Urol 1976; 116:36–38.
Stone AR: Treatment of voiding complaints and incontinence in painful bladder syndrome. Urol Clin North Am 1991; 18:317–325.
Stone NN: Nalmefene in the treatment of interstitial cystitis. Urol Clin North Am 1994; 21:101–106.
Taub HC, Stein M: Bladder distention therapy for symptomatic relief of frequency and urgency: A ten-year review. Urology 1994; 43:36–39.
Theoharides TC: Hydroxyzine in the treatment of interstitial cystitis. Urol Clin North Am 1994; 21:113–119.
Trinka PJ, Stanley BK, Noble MJ, et al: Mast-cell syndrome: A relative contraindication for continent urinary diversion. (Abstract.) J Urol 1993; 149:506A.
Turner JA, Deyo RA, Loeser JD, et al: The importance of placebo effects in pain treatment and research. JAMA 1994; 271:1609–1614.
Wallack HI, Lome LG, Presman D: Management of interstitial cystitis with ileocecocystoplasty. Urology 1975; 5:51–55.
Walsh A: Benzydamine: A new weapon in the treatment of interstitial cystitis. J Urol 1977a; 68:43–44.
Walsh A: Interstitial cystitis; observations on diagnosis and on treatment with anti-inflammatory drugs, particularly benzydamine. Eur Urol 1977b; 3:216–217.
Walsh A: Cystolysis (supra-trigonal denervation) for intractable interstitial cystitis. Urologists' Correspondence Club 1985; p 142.
Weaver RG, Dougherty TF, Natoli CA: Recent concepts of interstitial cystitis. J Urol 1963; 89:377–383.
Webster GD: Doctor's forum. ICA Update 1993; summer.
Webster GD, MacDiarmid SA, Timmons SL, et al: Impact of urinary diversion procedures in the treatment of interstitial cystitis and chronic bladder pain. Neurourol Urodyn 1992; 11:417.
Webster GD, Maggio MI: The management of chronic interstitial cystitis by substitution cystoplasty. J Urol 1989; 141:287–291.
Wein AJ, Broderick GA: Interstitial cystitis: Current and future approaches to diagnosis and treatment. Urol Clin North Am 1994; 21:153–161.
Wein AJ, Hanno PM: Interstitial cystitis. *In* Resnick MI, Kursh ED, eds: Current Therapy in Genitourinary Surgery, 2nd ed. St. Louis, Mosby-Year Book, 1992; pp 379–382.
Weiss JP, Wein AJ, Hanno PM: Sigmoidocystoplasty to augment bladder capacity. Surg Gynecol Obstet 1984; 159:377–380.
Whitmore KE: Self-care regimens for patients with interstitial cystitis. Urol Clin North Am 1994; 21:121–130.
Wishard WN, Nourse MH, Mertz JHO: Use of Clorpactin WCS90 for relief of symptoms due to interstitial cystitis. J Urol 1957; 77:420–423.
Worth PHL: The treatment of interstitial cystitis by cystolysis with observations on cystoplasty. A review after 7 years. Br J Urol 1982; 52:232.
Worth P, Turner-Warwick R: Interstitial cystitis. (Letter.) BMJ 1972; April 8:111–112.
Worth PHL, Turner-Warwick R: The treatment of interstitial cystitis by cystolysis with observations on cystoplasty. Br J Urol 1973; 45:65–71.
Zeidman EJ, Helfrick B, Pollard C, et al: Bacillus Calmette-Guérin immunotherapy for refractory interstitial cystitis. Urology 1994; 43:121–124.

Urethral Syndrome

Andriole VT: Modern trends in the treatment of sporadic, uncomplicated, lower urinary tract infection in women. *In* Francois B, Perrin P, eds: Urinary Infection. London, Butterworths, 1983; pp 177–178.
Barbalias GA, Meares EM: Female urethral syndrome: Clinical and urodynamic perspectives. Urology 1984; 23:208–212.
Belchetz PE: Hormonal treatment of postmenopausal women. N Engl J Med 1994; 330:1062–1071.
Bodner DR: The urethral syndrome. Urol Clin North Am 1988; 15:699–704.
Bogaert LJV: Surgical repair of hypospadias in women with symptoms of urethral syndrome. J Urol 1992; 147:1263–1264.
Brumfitt W, Hamilton-Miller JMT, Gillespie WA: The mysterious urethral syndrome. BMJ 1991a; 303:1–2.
Brumfitt W, Hamilton-Miller JMT, Gillespie WA: The mysterious urethral syndrome. BMJ 1991b; 303:719–720.
Cardozo L: Urinary urgency and frequency. *In* Stanton SL, ed: Clinical Gynecologic Urology. St Louis, CV Mosby Company, 1984; pp 300–304.
Carson CC, Segura JW, Osborne DM: Evaluation and treatment of the female urethral syndrome. J Urol 1980; 124:609–610.
Charlton CAC: Historical review: Confusions in definition. *In* George NJR, Gosling JA, eds: Sensory Disorders of the Bladder and Urethra. Berlin, Springer-Verlag, 1986; pp 81–83.
Cooper J, Raeburn A, Brumfitt W, Hamilton-Miller JMT: Single dose and conventional treatment for acute bacterial and non-bacterial dysuria and frequency in general practice. Infection 1990; 18:65–69.
Corey L, Benedetti J, Critchlow C, et al: Treatment of primary first-episode genital herpes simplex virus infections with acyclovir: Results of topical, intravenous and oral therapy. J Antimicrob Chemother 1983; 12(suppl B):79.
Davis DM: Vesical orifice obstruction in women and its treatment by resection. J Urol 1955; 73:112–116.
Fowler JE: Nonmicrobial inflammation and noninflammatory disorders. *In* Fowler JE, ed: Urinary Tract Infection and Inflammation. Chicago, Year Book Medical Publishers, 1989; pp 292–293.
Gallagher DJA, Montgomerie JZ, North JDK: Acute infections of the urinary tract and the urethral syndrome in general practice. Br Med J 1965; 1:622–626.
Gillenwater JY, Wein AJ: Summary of National Institute of Arthritis, Diabetes, Digestive and Kidney Diseases workshop on interstitial cystitis. National Institutes of Health, Bethesda, August 1987. J Urol 1988; 140:203–206.
Gillespie WA, Henderson EP, Linton KB, Smith JB: Microbiology of the urethral (frequency and dysuria) syndrome. Br J Urol 1989; 64:270–274.
Hamilton-Miller JM: The urethral syndrome and its management. J Antimicrob Chemother 1994; 33(suppl A):6–73.
Hanno PM: Interstitial cystitis and female urethral syndrome. *In* Stein BS, ed: Clinical Urologic Practice. New York, W. W. Norton and Company, 1995; pp 611–622.
Hooton TM: Epidemiology, definitions, and terminology in urinary tract infections. *In* Neu HC, Williams JD, eds: New Trends in Urinary Tract Infections. Basel, Karger, 1988; pp 5–8.
Kaplan WE, Firlit CF, Schoenberg HW: The female urethral syndrome: External sphincter spasm as etiology. J Urol 1980; 124:48–49.
Kass EH: Chemotherapeutic and antibiotic drugs in the management of infections of the urinary tract. Am J Med 1955; 18:764–781.
Kass EH: Asymptomatic infections of the urinary tract. Trans Assoc Am Physicians 1956; 69:56–63.
Kass EH: Bacteriuria and the diagnosis of infections of the urinary tract: With observations on the use of methionine as a urinary antiseptic. Arch Intern Med 1957; 100:707–714.
Kunin CM: Management of urinary tract infections. *In* Kunin CM: Detection, Prevention and Management of Urinary Tract Infections. Philadelphia, Lea & Febiger, 1987; pp 341–342.
Latham RH, Stamm WE: Urethral syndrome in women. Urol Clin North Am 1984; 11:95–101.

Mabry EW, Carson CC, Older RA: Evaluation of women with chronic voiding discomfort. Urology 1981; 18:244–246.

Maskell R: Urinary Tract Infection in Clinical and Laboratory Practice. London, Edward Arnold, 1988.

Maskell R: The mysterious urethral syndrome. BMJ 1991; 303:361–362.

McCannel DA, Haile RW: Urethral narrowing and its treatment. Intl Urol Nephrol 1982; 14:407–414.

Messing EM: Interstitial cystitis and related syndromes. *In* Walsh PC, Retik AB, Stamey TA, Vaughn ED, eds: Campbell's Urology, 6th ed. Philadelphia, W. B. Saunders Company, 1992; pp 997–1005.

Nazareth I, King MB: The urethral syndrome: A controlled evaluation. J Psychosom Res 1993; 37:737–743.

Nyberg LM: Advances in the diagnosis and management of interstitial cystitis. *In* Rous S, ed: Urology Annual. Norwalk, Conn, Appleton & Lange, 1991; pp 181–191.

Paavonen J: *Chlamydia trachomatis*–induced urethritis in female partners of men with nongonococcal urethritis. Sex Transm Dis 1979; 6:69–71.

Paira SA: Fibromyalgia associated with female urethral syndrome. Clin Rheumatol 1994; 13:88–89.

Parziani S, Costantini E, Petroni PA, et al: Urethral syndrome: Clinical results with antibiotics alone or combined with estrogen. Eur Urol 1994; 26:115–119.

Powell NB, Powell EB: The female urethra: A clinico-pathological study. J Urol 1949; 61:557–570.

Raz S, Smith RB: External sphincter spasticity syndrome in female patients. J Urol 1976; 115:443–446.

Richardson FH: External urethroplasty in women: Technique and clinical evaluation. J Urol 1969; 101:719–723.

Roberts M, Smith P: Non-malignant obstruction of the female urethra. Br J Urol 1968; 40:694.

Rutherford AJ, Hinshaw K, Essenhigh DM, Neal DE: Urethral dilatation compared with cystoscopy alone in the treatment of women with recurrent frequency and dysuria. Br J Urol 1988; 61:500–504.

Sand PK, Bowen LW, Ostergard DR, et al: Cryosurgery versus dilatation and massage for the treatment of recurrent urethral syndrome. J Reprod Med 1989; 34:499–504.

Splatt AJ, Weedon D: The urethral syndrome: Experience with the Richardson urethroplasty. Br J Urol 1977; 49:173–176.

Splatt AJ, Weedon D: The urethral syndrome: Morphological studies. Br J Urol 1981; 52:263–265.

Stamm WE: Relationship of interstitial cystitis to the urethral syndrome. Proceedings of the NIDDK Workshop on Interstitial Cystitis 1987, section 4, pp 21–22.

Stamm WE, Running K, McKevitt M, et al: Treatment of the acute urethral syndrome. N Engl J Med 1981; 304:956–958.

Stamm WE, Wagner KF, Amsel R, et al: Causes of the acute urethral syndrome in women. N Engl J Med 1980; 303:409–415.

Sumners D, Kelsey M, Chait I: Psychological aspects of lower urinary tract infections in women. BMJ 1992; 304:17–19.

Testa GM: The urethral syndrome—Why what we do works or doesn't. Med J Aust 1992; 157:549–553.

Wilkins EGL, Payne SR, Pead PJ, et al: Interstitial cystitis and urethral syndrome: A possible answer. Br J Urol 1989; 64:39–44.

Zufall R: Ineffectiveness of treatment of urethral syndrome in women. Urology 1978; 12:337–339.

18 SEXUALLY TRANSMITTED DISEASES: THE CLASSIC DISEASES

Richard E. Berger, M.D.

The incidence and variety of the known sexually transmitted diseases (STDs) have greatly increased since the 1970s. In addition to the five classic venereal diseases (syphilis, gonorrhea, chancroid, granuloma inguinale, and lymphogranuloma venereum), illness such as "idiopathic epididymitis," Reiter's syndrome, infant pneumonia, the female urethral syndrome, and acquired immunodeficiency syndrome (AIDS) have been shown to be sexually transmitted (Table 18–1). Genital herpesvirus infection, genital warts, and AIDS are increasing at such a rapid rate as to cause panic in sexually active populations.

The explosive increase in STDs has been accompanied by an explosion of information concerning them. The turnover in knowledge has been exceedingly rapid: What is considered accurate today may be incorrect tomorrow. The rapid changes have been due to advances in diagnostic techniques, in treatment methods, and sometimes even in mutations in STD organisms themselves. Changes in sexual behavior also mean that STDs affect more people from a wide variety of social, economic, and ethnic backgrounds.

Thus, it is imperative that the physician treating STDs make special efforts to be sure that his or her methods of diagnosis and treatment reflect the latest knowledge. Recommendations for STD treatment are periodically updated by the Centers for Disease Control and Prevention (CDC). Changes that occur in the interim must come from a review of the current literature. The accurate diagnosis and treatment of an STD patient allows the physician to treat not only the patient but also the sexual partner and even the couple's unborn children.

A major obstacle to the optimal treatment of STDs is, paradoxically, the inappropriate behavior of some health care providers. *All* medical care personnel need to express a nonjudgmental and caring attitude toward patients with STDs. Many patients feel guilt or shame about the disease. Seeking care is often extremely difficult for them. They believe they will be singled out with a lecture on sexual ethics or that the behavior of the physician or nurse will make them feel unclean, undesirable, or unwanted as a patient. It is essential that health care providers approach patients with understanding and sensitivity; otherwise, patients may very likely not return for necessary treatment and their sexual partners may never be treated. Taking a sexual history is one of the most difficult tasks in STD care. Sometimes a proper beginning statement may put both the physician and the patient more at ease. An example might be (1) "To give you the best care I can, I need to ask some specific questions about your lifestyle and sexual behaviors; or (2) "I realize that a person's sexual behavior is very personal, but I need to ask you some questions so we can

Table 18–1. PATHOGENS FOR WHICH SEXUAL TRANSMISSION IS IMPORTANT

Agent	Disease or Syndrome
Bacteria	
Neisseria gonorrhoeae	Urethritis, epididymitis, proctitis, cervicitis, endometritis, salpingitis, perihepatitis, bartholinitis, pharyngitis, conjunctivitis, prepubertal vaginitis, ?prostatitis, accessory gland infection, amniotic infection syndrome, disseminated gonococcal infection, chorioamnionitis, premature rupture of membranes, premature delivery
Chlamydia trachomatis	Urethritis, epididymitis, proctitis, cervicitis, endometritis, salpingitis, perihepatitis, bartholinitis, prepubertal vaginitis, otitis media in infants, ?chorioamnionitis, ?premature rupture of membranes, ?premature delivery, inclusion conjunctivitis, nasopharyngitis, infant pneumonia, trachoma, lymphogranuloma venereum
Mycoplasma hominis	Postpartum fever, ?salpingitis
Ureaplasma urealyticum	Nongonococcal urethritis, ?chorioamnionitis, ?premature delivery, infant pneumonia
Treponema pallidum	Syphilis
Gardnerella vaginalis	*Gardnerella*-associated ("nonspecific") vaginosis, neonatal sepsis
Haemophilus ducreyi	Chancroid
Calymmatobacterium granulomatis	Donovanosis (granuloma inguinale)
Shigella spp	Enterocolitis
Campylobacter spp	Enterocolitis
Streptococcus agalactiae	Neonatal sepsis and meningitis
Viruses	
Herpes simplex virus	Initial and recurrent genital herpes, aseptic meningitis, neonatal herpes, cervical dysplasia and carcinoma, ?carcinoma in situ of the vulva
Hepatitis B virus	Acute hepatitis B, chronic active hepatitis, persistent (unresolved) hepatitis, polyarteritis nodosa, chronic membranous glomerulonephritis, ?mixed cryoglobulinemia, ?polymyalgia rheumatica, hepatocellular carcinoma
Hepatitis A virus	Acute hepatitis A
Cytomegalovirus	Heterophil-negative infectious mononucleosis, congenital infection, gross birth defects and infant mortality, neonatal brain damage, ?cervical dysplasia and carcinoma
Genital papillomavirus	Condyloma acuminatum, laryngeal papilloma, ?cervical dysplasia and carcinoma
Molluscum contagiosum	Genital molluscum contagiosum
Human immunodeficiency virus	Acquired immunodeficiency syndrome
Protozoa	
Trichomonas vaginalis	Vaginitis
Entamoeba histolytica	Enteritis, liver abscess
Giardia lamblia	Enteritis
Fungi	
Candida albicans	Vulvovaginitis, balanitis
Metazoa	
Phthirus pubis	Pubic lice infestation
Sarcoptes scabiei	Scabies
Enterobius vermicularis	Proctitis

From Holmes KK, Handsfield HH: Sexually transmitted diseases. *In* Petersdorf RG, Adams RD, Braunwald E, et al (eds): Harrison's Principles of Internal Medicine. New York, McGraw-Hill, 1983.

explore whether you are at risk for certain medical conditions, such as HIV infection, or other sexually transmitted diseases." The physician needs to pose specific questions in a nonjudgmental manner in words that the patient will understand. Instead of asking, "Are you a homosexual?" ask, "Do you have sex with men, women, or both?" History taking must be looked upon as an opportunity for education. The ultimate goal is to help patients learn to assess their own level of risk so they can make informed choices about future behaviors (Kassler and Cates, 1992).

TRENDS

STDs are, of course, most common in young, sexually active people. The incidence of STDs declines with age (Bell and Hein, 1984). As a result of the "baby boom" at the end of World War II, the sexually active group has been increasing in numbers. Since some of the most serious consequences of STDs, such as ectopic pregnancies and cervical carcinoma, may occur years after exposure to STDs, the sometimes tragic consequences of STD are also beginning to increase (Beral, 1974). Although the threat of human immunodeficiency virus (HIV) infection is becoming greater, high-risk behavior is still very prevalent.

Rates continue to be higher in men than in women (Bell and Hein, 1984). In part, the apparently high STD rate in men may be because symptoms and signs in men may be more obvious, with men more often seeking medical care. Also, men may have more sexual partners than women (Sorensen, 1972; Hunt, 1974). Certain STDs (syphilis, hepatitis, gonorrhea, and HIV infection) occur much more frequently in homosexual men than in heterosexual men (Crawford et al, 1937; William, 1981; Bell and Hein, 1984).

STDs are becoming more frequent in women. Women's sexual behavior may be becoming like men's: More women are having intercourse at an earlier age, and the number of sexual partners a woman is likely to have is increasing. This change in behavior has led to a proportional increase in STDs in women, along with an increase in the serious consequences often associated with STDs: pelvic inflammatory disease (PID), infertility, ectopic pregnancy, and so forth (Bell and Hein, 1984).

Socioeconomic factors affect the prevalence and types of STDs. Persons of lowest socioeconomic status have the highest morbidity rates; in the United States, Asians have the lowest reported incidence of STDs; blacks have the highest, and whites occupy the middle category (Pedersen and Bonin, 1971). Although the rates of STDs may actually be decreasing, the rates of some STDs may actually be increasing. There has been a dramatic increase in STDs among low-income, inner-city, heterosexual racial and ethnic minority populations (Kassler and Cates, 1992). Studies have suggested that illegal drug use, which is often associated with high-risk sexual behaviors, may be contributing to the increase in STDs in some populations (Rolfs et al, 1990).

Certain types of STDs apparently affect some groups more than others (Crawford et al, 1937). Strains of gonorrhea that cause systemic disease are more common in blacks than in whites (Knapp et al, 1978). Genital herpes infection is more common in whites than in blacks. The rate of STDs is higher in urban populations than in rural residents.

Adolescents experience the highest risk for exposure to STDs. Teenagers tend to deny that their partners could have STDs and have more spontaneous rather then premeditated sex. Biologic factors also play a part. In early puberty the columnar epithelium in the uterus extends from the endocervical canal into the vagina and is not protected by cervical mucus. The columnar epithelium is the primary site of invasion for both *Chlamydia trachomatis* and *Neisseria gonorrhoeae* (Ostergard, 1977).

CONTACT TRACING

Examination and treatment of the sexual partners of the patients with STDs are essential to prevent reinfection, to prevent complications in sexual partners, and to limit spread of the disease in the community. Because most microbiologic tests have a less than 100% sensitivity and regular partners run a high risk of being infected, they should always be treated regardless of the culture result. This practice is especially important for infection with *C. trachomatis*, which has a high infectious asymptomatic carrier rate. **Sexual partners (especially those infected with syphilis, *N. gonorrhoeae* or *C. trachomatis*) should be treated on the basis of contact. If partners are treated only if they become symptomatic, as many as 50% of patients would remain untreated** (Johnson, 1979). **Furthermore, if cultures of partners are obtained and if the partner is treated only if the culture is positive, patients will be lost to follow-up, may possibly reinfect their partners, and may have increased risk of possible serious consequences of their infections** (Ramstedt et al, 1991).

Since approximately 60% of patients who have one STD have at least one other, examination of the patients and their partners for other STDs and treatment of that disease are highly recommended (Wentworth et al, 1973). The control of STD is based on the following concepts:

1. Education of the persons at risk on the modes of disease transmission and the means of reducing the risk of transmission
2. Detection of infection in asymptomatic persons and in persons who are symptomatic but unlikely to seek diagnostic and treatment services
3. Effective diagnosis and treatment of persons who are infected
4. Evaluation, treatment, and counseling of sex partners with an STD

The diagnosis of an STD should be considered a "sentinel event" that reflects unsafe sexual activity. Patients with one STD are at a higher risk for having others and should be evaluated for others, including syphilis and HIV infection. Patients with multiple episodes of STD should be targeted for intensive counseling on the methods of reducing risk. Breaking the chain of transmission is crucial to STD control. Urologists must ensure that sexual partners, including those without symptoms, are referred for evaluation. Some studies suggest that treating any regular sexual partner even without examination greatly decreases the rates of reinfection (Ramstedt et al, 1991).

URETHRITIS

Gonococcal Urethritis in Men

Gonococcal urethritis (GU) is associated with the gram-negative diplococcus *N. gonorrhoeae.* The incubation period for GU varies from 3 to 10 days, but exceptions are very common. For example, some strains of gonococci produce symptoms in a period as short as 12 hours; other strains may take as long as 3 months to manifest themselves (Harrison et al, 1984).

Epidemiology

Although the overall rates of gonorrhea have decreased since 1986, gonorrhea remains the most commonly reported communicable disease in the United States. It remains very common in teenagers and racial and ethnic minorities. Most cases of GU are acquired during intercourse. For a man, the risk of acquiring gonorrhea during a single episode of intercourse with an infected partner is approximately 17% (Greenberg, 1979). This risk increases as the number of sexual contacts with an infected partner increases. Not only can the gonococcus be transmitted by direct vaginal exposure, but there is increasing evidence that infection may be transmitted through oral sex with a partner whose pharynx is infected. There have been cases of gonorrhea that have been acquired from secretions without vaginal penetration.

Symptoms and Signs

Classically, GU produces urethral discharge and burning on urination. The discharge is usually profuse and purulent, but it may be scant or even absent. **GU may be asymptomatic in 40% to 60% of the contacts of partners with known gonorrhea** (Crawford et al, 1937; Portnoy et al, 1974; John and Donald, 1978). **Without treatment, even**

symptomatic gonorrhea will improve. However, the host may remain a carrier and may be potentially infective (McCutchan, 1981).

Prevention

Gonorrhea may be prevented by the regular use of condoms, postcontact antibiotics, and intravaginal application of antiseptics and antibiotics. Although condoms can prevent urethrally acquired gonorrhea as well as HIV and other infections, most men still do not use this protection (Hooper et al, 1978).

Unfortunately, the indiscriminate use of prophylactic antibiotics can result in the development of resistant strains of gonococci (Harrison, 1979). The impact of intravaginal bacteriostatic agents is currently unknown (Cates et al, 1982). Researchers are working to develop immunization against *N. gonorrhoeae* (Marx, 1980), but immune vaccines are not yet available.

Diagnosis

Laboratory procedures are essential for the accurate diagnosis of gonorrhea. Because gonococcal infections occur in areas such as the urethra, that have extensive normal bacterial flora, it is extremely important to collect uncontaminated specimens. Urethral specimens must be obtained from within the urethra and not simply from a drop of discharge. One should collect specimens with a calcium alginate (Calgiswab, Inolex) urethrogenital swab, waiting at least 1 hour (preferably 4 hours) after the patient has urinated before swabbing. Swabs need to be inserted 2 to 4 cm into the urethra and rotated gently. Cotton swabs should be avoided because of a bactericidal effect (Kellogg et al, 1976). If there is a history of oral genital contact, pharyngeal specimens should also be collected. In homosexual men (and all women), rectal swabs should be obtained. The swabs are inoculated directly onto the culture medium. The same swab may be used for Gram's staining. If this is not possible, two specimens are collected. The swab should be rolled onto the slide, as white blood cells may be disrupted if roughly rubbed. The slide then can be heat-fixed, air-dried, and examined immediately. Trained laboratory personnel who regularly read Gram's stains can make the diagnosis of gonorrhea with approximately a 99% specificity and 95% sensitivity (Granato et al, 1981).

Because the gonococcus is an extremely friable organism, the preferred method of diagnosis is to plate the urethral swab directly onto modified Thayer-Martin and New York City media (Thayer and Martin, 1964; Riccardi and Felman, 1979; Granato et al, 1981). Transport media should be used to take specimens to the laboratory when direct plating of specimens cannot be done (James-Holmquest et al, 1973). Although there are a number of serologic and fluorescent antibody tests available for diagnosis, the high sensitivity and specificity of Gram's stain make these tests unnecessary in most instances (Harrison et al, 1984). Antigen detection for gonorrhea would be of value (1) in the diagnosis of gonococcal cervical infections in women, (2) in the diagnosis of gonococcal proctitis in homosexual men, and (3) in situations requiring lengthy specimen transport (Stamm, 1986).

Treatment

Gonococcal urethritis was initially treated by instillation of antiseptic agents into the urethra (Kampmeier, 1983). In the mid-1930s, sulfa drugs were used successfully. However, resistance quickly developed (Dees and Colston, 1937; Campbell, 1944). During the 1940s, GU was treated successfully with penicillin. Since then, the amount of penicillin needed to treat gonorrhea has steadily increased (Harrison et al, 1978). In 1976, the gonococcus acquired a plasmid for penicillinase production, making some strains totally resistant to penicillin (John and Donald, 1978). Since 1972, the CDC has issued recommendations for the treatment of gonorrhea.

The current CDC recommendations for treatment of GU with their advantages and disadvantages are summarized in Table 18–2. **Ceftriaxone** (125 mg intramuscularly) is currently the recommended drug of choice for the treatment of all uncomplicated gonococcal infections of the pharynx, anorectum, cervix, and urethra (Judson, 1986). Penicillin and tetracycline are not recommended for primary treatment because of the high resistance of the gonococcus to these agents in the United States. However, the current recommended treatment for GU includes a tetracycline or a tetracycline derivative, because about 30% of men with GU are also infected with *C. trachomatis,* which is not sensitive to ceftriaxone (Martin, 1990).

Nongonococcal Urethritis in Men

The incidence of nongonococcal urethritis (NGU) has increased faster than that of any other STD except, perhaps, herpes simplex II and genital warts (Aral and Holmes, 1984). In 1972, NGU surpassed gonorrhea as the more common diagnosis for patient visits to private physician offices, with the incidence now 2.5 times that of GU (Thompson and Washington, 1983). The morbidity of clinical infections and complications of NGU may be equal to and perhaps greater than that of gonococcal disease (Table 18–3). However, since NGU infections are not often reported to health authorities,

Table 18–2. TREATMENT OF GONOCOCCAL URETHRITIS IN MEN*

Treatment	Treatment Regimens
Ceftriaxone, 125 mg IM	Effective against PPNG
Cefixime, 400 mg orally	—
Spectinomycin, 2 g IM once	Effective against PPNG
Ciprofloxacin, 500 mg orally, or ofloxacin, 400 mg orally	Both effective against PPNG
Norfloxacin, 800 mg orally once	Effective against PPNG
Cefuroxime axetil, 1 g orally once with probenecid, 1 g	Effective against PPNG
Ceftizoxime, 500 mg IM once	Effective against PPNG
Amoxicillin, 3 g orally with 1 g probenecid	—

*All patients must be treated with doxycycline, 100 mg twice a day for 2 days, to treat coexisting chlamydial infection. Erythromycin, 500 mg, four times a day for 7 days or erythromycin ethylsuccinate may be subsituted in patients who cannot take tetracycline (e.g., pregnant women).

PPNG, penicillinase-producing *Neisseria gonorrhoeae*.

Modified from Centers for Disease Control: MMWR Morb Mortal Wkly Rep, 1989; 381:1–43.

Table 18–3. DISEASES ASSOCIATED WITH THE SEXUAL TRANSMISSION OF *NEISSERIA GONORRHOEAE* AND *CHLAMYDIA TRACHOMATIS*

N. gonorrhoeae	*C. trachomatis*
Urethritis	Urethritis
Cervicitis	Cervicitis
Salpingitis	Salpingitis
Bartholinitis	Bartholinitis
Perihepatitis	Perihepatitis
Arthritis	Reiter's syndrome
Urethral syndrome	Urethral syndrome
Proctitis	Proctitis
Conjunctivitis	Conjunctivitis
Asymptomatic urethritis	Pneumonia
	Otitis media
	Asymptomatic urethritis

From Berger RE: Nongonococcal urethritis and related syndromes. Monogr Urol 1982; 3(4):99–122.

the sexual partners of infected patients often are not examined or treated. Therefore, the incidence of NGU and its associated infections will probably continue to increase. Young men are prime candidates for contracting NGU. NGU more often affects men of higher socioeconomic status than does GU (Wiesner, 1977). Urethritis in homosexual men is less likely to be nongonococcal and more likely to be gonococcal.

Etiology

Nongonococcal urethritis is a syndrome with several causes and not an etiologic diagnosis (Table 18–4). The most important and potentially dangerous pathogen involved in NGU is *C. trachomatis*, which can be blamed for 30% to 50% of NGU cases (Alani et al, 1977; Bowie et al, 1977b; Segura et al, 1977; Wong et al, 1977; Bowie, 1978; Csango, 1978; Perroud and Miedzybrodzka, 1978; Ripa et al, 1978; Swartz et al, 1978; Terho, 1978b; Coufalik et al, 1979; Lassus et al, 1979; Taylor-Robinson and McCormack, 1980).

Table 18–4. MANAGEMENT OF NONGONOCOCCAL URETHRITIS (NGU)

Investigation

1. Do a careful physical examination.
2. Demonstrate a polymorphonuclear leukocyte response—Gram's stain or first voided urine sediment.
3. Exclude *Neisseria gonorrhoeae* infection—Gram's stain ± culture.
4. Reassess in the morning before the patient voids if necessary.

Initial Management of NGU if Diagnosed

1. Treat for 7 days with tetracycline, 500 mg q.i.d.; or minocycline or doxycycline, 100 mg twice daily; or erythromycin, 500 mg q.i.d. for 7 days.
2. Treat partner(s) appropriately.

Management of Persistent or Recurrent NGU

1. Question about compliance and re-exposure.
2. Examine carefully for less usual causes of urethritis.
3. Demonstrate urethritis.
4. Treat any specific cause that can be elucidated.
5. If a specific cause is not found or if *Ureaplasma urealyticum* is present, treat with erythromycin base, 500 mg q.i.d. for 14 days.

Modified from Bowie WR: Urol Clin North Am 1984; 11:55.

Bowie and colleagues (1977b) have summarized evidence in favor of *C. trachomatis* in the etiology of NGU:

1. Chlamydia can be isolated from the urethra in 25% to 60% of men who have NGU (Alani et al, 1977; Bowie et al, 1977b; Segura et al, 1977; Wong et al, 1977; Bowie, 1978; Csango, 1978; Paavonen et al, 1978; Perroud and Miedzybrodzka, 1978; Ripa et al, 1978; Swartz et al, 1978; Terho, 1978a; Coufalik et al, 1979; Lassus et al, 1979; Taylor-Robinson and McCormack, 1980). Conversion and the formation of immunoglobulin M (IgM) antibodies against *C. trachomatis* can be demonstrated in men with NGU with positive urethral cultures for *C. trachomatis*.
2. Up to 80% of sexual contacts of men with *C. trachomatis* also have *C. trachomatis* infection (Linder, 1911; Holmes et al, 1975; Richmond and Sparling, 1976).
3. Differential responses to therapy can be demonstrated in chlamydial-positive and chlamydial-negative cases (Handsfield et al, 1975; Bowie et al, 1976; Coufalik et al, 1979).
4. PGU develops in men who contract gonococcal and chlamydial infection simultaneously (Richmond et al, 1972; Oriel et al, 1975; Alani et al, 1977; Segura et al, 1977; Vaughn-Jackson, 1977; Bowie, 1978; Terho, 1978a) and who are treated with penicillin to which *Chlamydia* is not sensitive.

C. trachomatis can be recovered from the urethra in 25% to 60% of heterosexual men with NGU, in 4% to 35% of men with gonorrhea, and in 0% to 7% of men seen in STD clinics without symptoms of urethritis (Schachter, 1978). Although asymptomatic infection seems to be infrequent in men seen in STD clinics, asymptomatic infection occurs in 50% of the contacts of women with chlamydial cervical infections (Thelin et al, 1980). Forty percent of pelvic inflammatory disease in the United States is caused by *C. trachomatis* (Brunham, 1984).

From 20% to 50% of men with NGU may have infections with *Ureaplasma urealyticum*. Information on the pathogenic role of *U. urealyticum* in the etiology of NGU has been difficult to interpret because genital colonization with this organism is directly proportional to the patient's number of previous sexual partners. With three to five partners, specimens from 40% of men and 70% of women contain *Ureaplasma* (Taylor-Robinson and McCormack, 1980).

Evidence for the role of *U. urealyticum* in NGU has come from several sources. When men with relatively few sexual partners and no history of urethritis are examined, the rate of isolation of *U. urealyticum* is significantly higher in those men with negative chlamydial cultures than in those with positive chlamydial cultures (Bowie et al, 1977a). Treatment studies have also shown a pathogenic role for *Ureaplasma.* Bowie and colleagues (1976) found that men with *C. trachomatis*–negative, *U. urealyticum*–positive urethritis responded poorly to sulfonamides but well to aminocyclatal, to which *U. urealyticum* but not *C. trachomatis* is sensitive. It has also been shown that NGU persists in a group of *Chlamydia*-negative patients with NGU who have persistence of *Ureaplasma* (Swartz et al, 1978; Root et al, 1980; Stimson et al, 1981). Furthermore, endourethral inoculation of *Ureaplasma* in nonhuman primates has produced colonization of urethritis (Taylor-Robinson and McCormack, 1980). Some serotypes of *U. urealyticum* may be more pathogenic than others.

In 20% to 30% of cases of men with acute urethritis, the cause cannot be determined. Although these men may show improvement or may even be cured with antibiotics, the cause of their urethral inflammation cannot be definitely determined (Bowie et al, 1981). Herpes simplex virus (Holmes et al, 1975), cytomegalovirus, *Trichomonas vaginalis*, and other organisms have not been convincingly shown to be associated with the majority of these cases (Bowie et al, 1977a; Swartz et al, 1978).

There is no evidence that drinking caffeinated beverages or alcohol causes urethritis, nor has it been shown that stripping the urethra causes urethritis. There is evidence to suggest that smoking may be an independent risk factor for the development of NGU (Pessione et al, 1988). Smith and colleagues (1987) showed that circumcised soldiers were 1.6 times as likely to have NGU as uncircumcised active duty soldiers. Hernandez and colleagues (1988) found insertive genital-oral intercourse to significantly increase the risk of chlamydial-negative, ureaplasmal-negative NGU. Insertive anal intercourse did not increase the risk of chlamydial-negative, ureaplasmal-negative NGU.

Diagnosis

The usual incubation period for NGU is 1 to 5 weeks. Longer incubation periods often occur. The usual symptoms include dysuria and urethral discharge. Diagnosis of NGU requires demonstration of urethritis and exclusion of infection with *N. gonorrhoeae*. Urethral discharge is often scant; however, it may be thick and purulent. Discharge may not be present, and the patient may complain only of urethral itch (Jacobs and Kraus, 1975). Asymptomatic infection is common, especially among contacts of women with known cervical chlamydial infection.

Ideally, a man suspected of having urethritis should be examined after 4 hours of urinary incontinence so that discharge may be reliably demonstrated. On a Gram stain urethral swab, more than four polymorphonuclear leukocytes per field in five 1000-power oil-immersion fields correlate with urethritis. Alternatively, the presence of 15 or more polymorphonuclear leukocytes in five random 400-power fields of the spun sediment of the first-void urine correlates with urethritis (Bowie, 1978; Swartz et al, 1978). The leukocyte esterase urine dipstick test may be useful for screening purposes. A positive test, in the absence of bladder infections, should suggest urethritis, and more specific tests for *N. gonorrhoeae* and *C. trachomatis* should then be obtained (Bell, 1990; Ferris et al, 1991). **When urethritis is suspected but urethral inflammation cannot be detected, the patient should be examined in the early morning before voiding.** Simmons (1978) found that of 200 men with genitourinary symptoms without urethritis on initial examination, 108 had urethritis diagnosed when examined in the early morning.

Cultures for the detection of *C. trachomatis* should be employed when available. Because *C. trachomatis* is an intracellular parasite of columnar epithelium, the appropriate specimen for culture is an endourethral swab rather than urethral exudate or urine. The specimen must be taken carefully from 2 to 4 mm inside the urethra and placed in special transport medium. It then may be frozen to −70°C and stored, or kept at 4°C and delivered to the laboratory, where it should be inoculated promptly. Preliminary culture results are available 2 to 3 days after inoculation. Although many physicians believe that cultures are unnecessary, *C. trachomatis* is a dangerous pathogen, and culture results may serve both as a guide to therapy and as a proof of cure.

Because obtaining rapid, inexpensive, and accurate cell culture results may be difficult or unavailable, other diagnostic tests have been developed. Direct fluorescent antibody (DFA) rapidly identifies *C. trachomatis* elementary bodies using chlamydia-specific monoclonal antibodies conjugated to a fluorescent stain. Urethral material is swabbed onto a glass and kept at room temperature until staining. Enzyme immunoassay (EIA) can also be used to rapidly detect chlamydial infections. A urethral swab is placed in transport medium and can be kept at room temperature several days for evaluation. A positive test is indicated by color change when the specimen is viewed with a spectrophotometer. Results can be available in 24 hours. DFA testing may be slightly more specific than EIA testing, but results seem generally comparable (Stamm, 1988; Grossman et al, 1991). When the diagnostic tests for a specific population are interpreted, consideration of the predictive value of positive tests and the predictive value of the negative test is important. Caution is needed when interpreting test results in low-prevalence (less than 7%) populations. Unexpected positive results should be confirmed by additional testing in general with more specific methods, such as cell culture. For example, with a DFA or EIA test with a sensitivity of 81% and a specificity of 98%, the predictive value of a positive test is 81% when the disease prevalence is 16.8%. However, the predictive value is only 50% when the disease prevalence is 2.5% (in many private practice settings). Nonculture chlamydial testing therefore yields more false-positives in low-risk groups than in high-risk groups (Ridgway and Taylor-Robinson, 1991).

A chemoluminesence-enhanced nucleic acid probe system has been developed. This test detects the presence of chlamydia-specific ribosomal RNA. The polymerase chain reaction (PCR) is a new and highly specific test for the fluorescence of chlamydial nucleic acids. Contamination by foreign DNA is a potential problem (Ridgway and Taylor-Robinson, 1991). A rising antibody titer or IgM response to chlamydial trachomatis can be measured serologically. A low titer of chlamydial antibody, however, only indicates infection sometime in the past (Potts, 1992). Krieger and co-workers (1988) documented that 25% of men with persistent nonchlamydial NGU had structural abnormalities of the urinary tract. Uroflow studies identified all these patients.

Treatment

Since NGU is a syndrome that can be caused by many different organisms that respond differently to treatment, results of therapy are inconsistent. The current recommendations from the CDC are based on chlamydial infection and are given in Table 18–4. Although the quinolone antibiotics adequately treat gonococcal infections, their use is less efficacious for nonspecific urethritis than is doxycycline. Quinolones do have some activity against *C. trachomatis* (Bowie et al, 1986). In a large multi-institutional study (Stamm et al, 1995) it has been shown that azithromycin 1 g orally in a single dose is equivalent in efficacy to doxycycline 100 mg orally two times a day for 7 days in the treatment of chlamydial, nonchlamydial, ureaplasma-related and nonchlamydial- and nonureaplasma-related NGU. Alternative regimens include ofloxacin 300 mg orally 2 times a day for 7 days, erythromycin base 500 mg orally 4 times a day for 7 days, erythromycin ethylsuccinate 800 mg 4 times a day for 7 days, or sulfisoxazol 500 mg orally 4 times a day for 10 days. The safety of azithromycin for persons less than 15 years of age has not been established.

The cause of the urethritis appears to be the best indicator of response to therapy. Men with *C. trachomatis* infection respond the best to therapy, and men with neither *C. trachomatis* nor *U. urealyticum* infection respond the worst (Bowie et al, 1981).

In the absence of culture, NGU should be assumed to be caused by *C. trachomatis. C. trachomatis* can be isolated from 30% to 60% of female partners of men with NGU (Oriel et al, 1975; Alani et al, 1977). Therefore, as part of the management of urethritis, every attempt should be made to treat the patient's sexual partner promptly. In general, the same regimen used to treat men should be used to treat women.

Recurrence

Symptoms may persist in some men, and in other men, polymorphonuclear leukocytes may persist in the absence of infection. A clear or mucoid urethral discharge after therapy is not necessarily abnormal. Sometimes it takes days or weeks after treatment before discharge associated with *N. gonorrhoeae* or *C. trachomatis* disappears. Likewise, symptoms of dysuria or urethral itch in the absence of a polymorphonuclear leukocyte response in the urethra does not constitute failure.

Recurrent or persistent NGU may be due to

1. Reinfection with the initial organism (usually from reexposure to the same sexual partner who has not been treated)
2. Persistence of the original organism because of antibiotic resistance
3. Idiopathic failure, usually in cases in which *Chlamydia* or *Ureaplasma* is not found

Recurrence that is due to reinfection often can be prevented if the sexual partner is treated concurrently. When both male and female partners are treated concurrently with a tetracycline regimen, *C. trachomatis* is almost never isolated at the time of recurrence. Since *C. trachomatis* causes major morbidity whereas the other organisms involved in NGU cause minimal morbidity, every effort should be made to eradicate and confirm the eradication of *C. trachomatis*. Cultures are most helpful in this respect.

Recurrence caused by resistance to tetracycline therapy is almost never due to *C. trachomatis*. However, *U. urealyticum* can be isolated in 20% to 30% of men at the time of recurrence (Bowie et al, 1981). *C. trachomatis* usually is not resistant to tetracycline; however, tetracycline-resistant *U. urealyticum* may be one cause of persistent urethritis (Root et al, 1980; Stimson et al, 1981). To eradicate the infection, patients are treated with erythromycin for 1 to 2 weeks. Treatment of sexual partners with erythromycin also may be indicated (see Table 18–4).

Not surprisingly, the urologist often sees patients with urethral discharge or symptoms who have had multiple courses of antibiotics effective against both *C. trachomatis* and *U. urealyticum*. It is imperative that urethritis and urethral inflammation be properly diagnosed in these patients. Sometimes patients can express a small amount of mucoid material from the urethra; however, this does not contain inflammatory cells, and therefore the patient cannot be considered to have true urethritis. If the patient does continue to have a discharge, cultures for *T. vaginalis* should be performed and smears examined for fungi with 10% potassium hydroxide (KOH). Examination of the sexual partner may be of help in determining the cause, especially with *T. vaginalis* infection. If no pathogens are detected, uroflowmetry and urethroscopy should be performed to detect possible intraurethral lesions (Krieger et al, 1988). A genital examination should be performed to detect unusual causes of urethritis. Urethral genital warts may be suggested by external warts. Tender inguinal adenopathy and localized urethral tenderness could suggest urethral herpes or intraurethral foreign bodies (Bowie, 1990).

When a man has recurrence of persistence of urethritis with polymorphonuclear leukocytes, an evaluation needs to be performed. Urethral swabs for *N. gonorrhoeae* and *C. trachomatis* cultures should be obtained. However, if these are performed too soon (less than 48 hours for *N. gonorrhoeae* and up to three weeks for *C. trachomatis*) false-negatives can be obtained. In the presence of negative cultures, the patient should be retreated with erythromycin base 500 mg orally four times a day, for 2 weeks. This covers the proportion of strains of *U. urealyticum* that are resistant to tetracyclines. If the treatment fails a second time, reevaluation by cultures probably is not indicated. These men need to be reassured that if their cultures are negative they are not a danger to their sexual partners. If their partners have been treated, this persistence of urethritis is probably not due to reinfection and does not indicate "unfaithfulness." They should also be reassured that this is not a manifestation of HIV infection (Bowie, 1990).

Complications in Men

In most cases, *Chlamydia*-negative urethritis does not cause severe complications in men. Some cases of salpingitis and resulting infertility in women are related to neither gonococcal nor chlamydial infection; however, it is not known whether nonchlamydial urethritis in man can lead to transmission and complications in their female partners.

It is essential that male patients with *Chlamydia*-negative urethritis be given correct information and emotional reassurance. Many men are ridden with guilt at the thought of spreading an STD. In general, the physician can tell the patient that *Chlamydia*-negative recurrent urethritis is a nuisance but probably is of no serious consequence to the patient's health or that of his female partner or his children.

Consequences of Transmission to Women of Infections Causing Urethritis in Men

PELVIC INFLAMMATORY DISEASE. Pelvic inflammatory disease (PID) is one of the most severe consequences of STDs in women. The cost of caring for acute infection and its sequelae is over $1 billion per year (Curran, 1980). It has been linked to infection with *N. gonorrhoeae, C. trachomatis*, anaerobic bacteria, and possibly *Mycoplasma*. Since at least three of these four groups of organisms are sexually transmitted, it is essential that the urologist be aware of the serious sequelae of the transmission of the organisms. Untreated male contacts with urethral gonorrhea and/or chlamydial infection are a major source of infection for both initial and recurrent episodes of PID.

More than 80% of the male sexual partners of women with gonococcal PID have gonococcal urethritis. These men are often asymptomatic. Identification and treatment of infected male contacts should decrease the rate of recurrent PID in their partners.

INFERTILITY. Pelvic inflammatory disease can lead to serious and permanent consequences, including infertility. After a single episode of PID, 12% of patients are sterile; after two episodes, 35% are sterile; and after three attacks, 75% are sterile (Westrom, 1975). Of women who have had one episode of salpingitis, 25% incur another (Falk, 1965). The damage caused by the first occurrence may make the patient more susceptible to further problems. In virtually all cases, PID-caused infertility is due to tubal occlusion.

Infertility increases in direct proportion to the severity of the pelvic infection. Infertility is more likely to occur in patients with nongonococcal rather than gonococcal PID (Westrom, 1975). Westrom estimated that of every 29 girls born in 1950, one was sterile because of tubal occlusion by the age of 30.

ECTOPIC PREGNANCY. The most common cause of ectopic pregnancy is fallopian tube damage caused by PID. Approximately half of all women with ectopic pregnancy have had previous PID (Westrom, 1980). Indeed, the risk of ectopic pregnancy in women who have PID is 7 to 10 times greater than in women who never have had this infection (Westrom, 1975; Westrom, 1980). The increasing rate of PID is one factor in the doubling of the number of ectopic pregnancies in the United States in the past decade.

PAIN. Chronic abdominal pain is a sequela of PID in approximately 15% of women who have salpingitis. This pain is probably related to pelvic adhesions around the fallopian tubes and ovaries.

TREATMENT OF SEXUALLY TRANSMITTED DISEASES IN WOMEN. Nonpregnant women should generally be treated with the same antibiotic regimens as men. In pregnant women, quinolones and tetracyclines should be avoided in all trimesters. Aminoglycosides should be avoided in the first and second trimesters. Chloramphenicol should be avoided in the third trimester. Metronidazole should not be used in the first trimester. Sulfonamides should not be used in the second trimester. In general, erythromycin and penicillins can be used in all trimesters. Cephalosporins can be used in all trimesters with the exception of those with the methyltetrazolethiol side chain (moxalactam, cefotetan, and cefoperazone), which should be avoided (Lynch et al, 1991).

PERINATAL INFECTIONS. Of newborns exposed to *Chlamydia* during vaginal delivery, up to 15% contract chlamydial pneumonia and 50% develop chlamydial conjunctivitis (Potts, 1992).

EPIDIDYMITIS

Acute epididymitis is a clinical syndrome resulting from inflammation, pain, and swelling of the epididymis of less than 6 weeks. It should not be confused with chronic epididymitis, which involves long-standing pain in the epididymis and testicle, usually without swelling.

Acute epididymitis has been a major cause of loss of work. In the military, it is a major cause of hospital admissions to urology wards (Hanley, 1966; Shapiro and Breschi, 1973; Sufrin, 1980). Complications from acute epididymitis include abscess formation, testicular infarction, and development of chronic pain and infertility (Pelouze, 1941; Bietz, 1959; Gartman, 1961).

Etiology (Table 18–5)

Until relatively recently, most of the cases of epididymitis in young men were considered to be "idiopathic." Physicians thought that inflammation resulted from sterile urine's being forced down the vas deferens while the patient strained against a closed external urethral sphincter. Graves and Engle (1950) developed a dog model that tended to confirm this theory. However, in military studies, less than 10% of patients with epididymitis had a history of straining (Mittemeyer et al, 1966). In a series of civilian patients, only 2 of 50 patients had a history of straining, and both these patients were concurrently infected with *C. trachomatis* (Berger et al, 1979). Although the reflux of sterile urine down the vas deferens may occur when men with normal urinary tracts strain, such reflux probably would not cause the pyuria and urethritis seen in the vast majority of these young men.

Epididymitis caused by sexually transmitted organisms occurs mainly in sexually active males under the age of 35 years (Berger et al, 1979; Olier, 1981). The majority of cases of epididymitis in children and older men, on the other hand, are due to the common urinary pathogens.

Epididymitis is usually caused by spread of infection from the urethra or bladder. The most common cause of epididymitis in any particular group appears to be the most common cause of genitourinary infection in that group. Although epididymitis is uncommon in children, the most common cause of epididymitis is the coliform organisms that cause bacteriuria. In heterosexual men under the age of 35, bacteriuria is uncommon, whereas urethritis from *N. gonorrhoeae* and *C. trachomatis* is common. The most common cause of epididymitis in young men, therefore, is the organisms that cause urethritis (Berger et al, 1978, 1979; Berger, 1981; Scheibel et al, 1983; Gasparich et al, 1985; Vieras, 1986; Berger et al, 1987; Brehmer et al, 1987; De Jong, 1988; Kaneti et al, 1988; Kojima et al, 1988; Pearson et al, 1988). In approximately two thirds of heterosexual men aged under 35 years with noncoliform, nongonococcal epididymitis, *C. trachomatis* is the cause. On the other hand, in homosexual men who practice anal intercourse, coliform infection may be the most common cause of epididymitis; Berger and associates (1987) found six of nine homosexual men under the age of 35 years to have infection with coliforms or *Haemophilus influenzae*. On the other hand, none of 42 heterosexual men under the age of 35 years had coliform infection. In men aged over 35 years, sexually transmitted urethritis is uncommon. Bacteriuria secondary to

Table 18–5. ETIOLOGY OF ACUTE EPIDIDYMITIS

Study	Total No. of Men	Age <35 (No./Total [%])			Age >35 (No./Total [%])		
		GC	*Ct*	E. coli	*GC*	*Ct*	E. coli
Berger et al (1978)	23		11/13 [85]			8/10 [80]	
Scheibel et al (1983)	52	1/31 [3]	13/31 [42]			6/13 [46]	
Kristensen et al (1984)	16	4/16 [25]	14/16 [88]				
Hawkins et al (1986)	40		13/27 [48]		2/13 [15]	3/13 [23]	
Berger et al (1987)	51	9/51 [28]	19/51 [37]	6/51 [12]*			
Grant et al (1987)	54	2/42 [5]	29/40 [73]	3/42 [7]		3/12 [25]	8/12 [67]
Melekos et al (1987)	31		10/17 [59]	4/17 [24]		3/14 [21]	7/14
Mulcahy et al (1987)	40	4/40 [10]	13/40 [33]	0			6/11 [55]
De Jong et al (1988)	25	1/13 [8]	11/13 [85]	1/13 [8]		1/12 [8]	10/12 [83]
Kojima et al (1988)	45	3/30 [10]	21/30 [70]			10/15 [67]	
Pearson et al (1988)	27	1/27 [4]	7/29 [24]	0			
Doble (1989)	24†	1/24 [4]	10/24 [42]				
Hoosen et al (1993)‡	144	76/134 [57]	46/134 [34]	4/134 [3]	1/10 [10]	2/10 [20]	3/10 [30]

*Six of nine homosexual men had coliform infection; one other had infection with *Haemophilus influenzae*. None of 42 heterosexual men had coliform infections.
†All less than 45 years old.
‡Cut-off between younger and older men was 40 years of age.
GC, gonococcus; Ct, *Chlamydia trachomatis; E. coli, Escherichia coli.* Blank spaces indicate not evaluated.
References not listed in this chapter:
Kristensen JK, Scheibel JH: Etiology of acute epididymitis presenting in a venereal disease clinic. Sex Transm Dis 1984; 11:32–33.
Hawkins DA, Taylor RD, Thomas BJ, Harris JR: Microbiological survey of acute epididymitis. Genitourin Med 1986; 62:342–344.
Grant JB, Costello CB, Sequeira PJ, Blacklock NJ: The role of *Chlamydia trachomatis* in epididymitis. Br J Urol 1987; 60:355–359.
Melekos MD, Asbach HW: Epididymitis: aspects concerning etiology and treatment. J Urol 1987; 138:83–86
Mulcahy FM, Bignell CJ, Rajakumar R, et al: Prevalence of chlamydial infection in acute epididymo-orchitis. Genitourin Med 1987; 63:16–18
Doble A, Taylor RD, Thomas BJ, et al: Acute epididymitis: a microbiological and ultrasonographic study. Br J Urol 1989; 63:90–94.
Hoosen AA, O'Farrell N, van-den-Ende J: Microbiology of acute epididymitis in a developing community. Genitourin Med 1993; 69(5):361–363.

acquired obstructive urinary disease, however, is relatively common. The most common cause of epididymitis in older men is the organisms that cause bacteriuria (Berger et al, 1978, 1979).

A small group of men in all age groups may have epididymitis that is due to systemic disease such as tuberculosis, *Cryptococcus, Brucella*, and other organisms that cause systemic infections (Gottesman, 1974; Kazzaz and Salmo, 1974; Mitchell and Huins, 1974; Thomas et al, 1981).

A truly noninfectious cause of epididymitis has been described secondary to treatment with the antiarrhythmic drug amiodarone (Gasparich et al, 1985). This disorder does not respond to antibiotic therapy, is not associated with ureteral or urinary inflammation, involves only the head of the epididymis, and responds favorably to a decrease in the dosage of amiodarone. It appears to be due to the selective concentration of amiodarone in the epididymis.

Diagnosis

In acute epididymitis, the inflammation and swelling usually begin in the tail of the epididymis and may spread to involve the rest of the epididymis and testicular substance. The spermatic cord is usually tender and swollen. Although men with epididymitis that results from sexually transmitted organisms always have a history of sexual exposure, exposure can be months before the onset. Watson (1979) found that half of the men with gonococcal epididymitis did not have a urethral discharge. If the patient is examined immediately after he produces a urine specimen, urethritis and urethral discharge may be missed because white blood cells and bacteria have been washed out of the urethra during urination.

The microbial cause of epididymitis can usually be determined easily by examination of a Gram-stained urethral smear for urethritis and Gram's stain of a midstream urine specimen for gram-negative bacteriuria. The presence of intracellular gram-negative diplococci on the smear correlates with the presence of *N. gonorrhoeae*. The presence of only white blood cells on urethral smear indicates the presence of NGU. *C. trachomatis* is isolated in approximately two thirds of these patients (Berger et al, 1979).

Differential Diagnosis from Torsion

It is imperative for the physician to make the differential diagnosis between epididymitis and torsion promptly. Delay in accurate diagnosis of torsion can result in the patient's losing a testicle. Mistakes are often made in men younger than 35 years of age, in whom both epididymitis and torsion are common.

The presence of urethritis probably indicates that the patient has epididymitis and not a torsion.

Physical examination in early epididymitis shows swelling limited to the tail of the epididymis. However, in 15% of patients with early torsion, there is also swelling only in the epididymis (Delvillar et al, 1972).

Radionuclide scanning of the scrotum is probably the most accurate method of diagnosis; however, it may not be readily available (Abu-Sleiman et al, 1979; Arrosagaray et al, 1987; Brehmer et al, 1987). Doppler ultrasonography of the scrotum may be of use if the operator is experienced. In order to press the Doppler probe firmly against the testicle, one performs a spermatic cord block with 1% lidocaine (Xylocaine). In men with epididymitis, the arterial pulse of the ipsilateral testicle should be louder than the pulse in the contralateral testicle. If a pulse is heard in the ipsilateral testicle, the testicular artery should be compressed at the external ring. If the pulse disappears, it is truly coming from the testicle and probably a torsion has not occurred. If the

Table 18–6. TREATMENT OF ACUTE EPIDIDYMO-ORCHITIS

Epididymo-orchitis Secondary to Bacteriuria

1. Do urine culture and sensitivity studies.
2. Promptly administer broad-spectrum antimicrobial (e.g., tobramycin, trimethoprim-sulfamethoxazole, quinolone antibiotic).
3. Prescribe bed rest and perform scrotal evaluation.
4. Strongly consider hospitalization.
5. Evaluate for underlying urinary tract disease.

Epididymo-orchitis Secondary to Sexually Transmitted Urethritis

1. Do Gram's stain of urethral smear.
2. Administer ceftriaxone, 250 mg IM once; then tetracycline, 500 mg orally q.i.d. for at least 10 days, or doxycycline, 100 mg orally b.i.d. for at least 10 days.
3. Prescribe bed rest and perform scrotal evaluation.
4. Examine and treat sexual partners.

Adapted from Berger RE: Semin Urol 1983; 1:143.

pulse remains, the impulse may be coming from inflamed scrotal vessels and torsion may still be present (Pederson, 1975). In case of any doubt, it is always safer to perform scrotal exploration promptly.

Color-coded duplex Doppler ultrasonography has recently proved to be a valuable tool in the differential diagnosis of epididymitis and torsion. This method uses visual color coding of flow velocities in blood vessels superimposed on the gray-scale ultrasonography. Increases or decreases in blood flow can be determined. (Middleton et al, 1990; Fitzgerald et al, 1992) Wilbert and colleagues (1993) found that color-coded Doppler ultrasonography had a sensitivity of 82% and a specificity of 100% for torsion. For epididymitis the sensitivity was 70% and specificity was 88%. Falsely negative scans in torsion were generally due to partial torsion with some residual blood flow in the testicle and epididymis. Magnetic resonance imaging has also been found to be accurate in the differential diagnosis of epididymitis and torsion in a small series (Trambert et al, 1990).

Treatment

Treatment for acute epididymitis (Table 18–6) is directed at the specific etiologic organism. One tells the patient to rest in bed, provides pain medication, and makes sure that the patient relaxes with his scrotum elevated on a towel. Elevation improves lymphatic drainage. All patients should be treated with antibiotics. Since GU is associated with

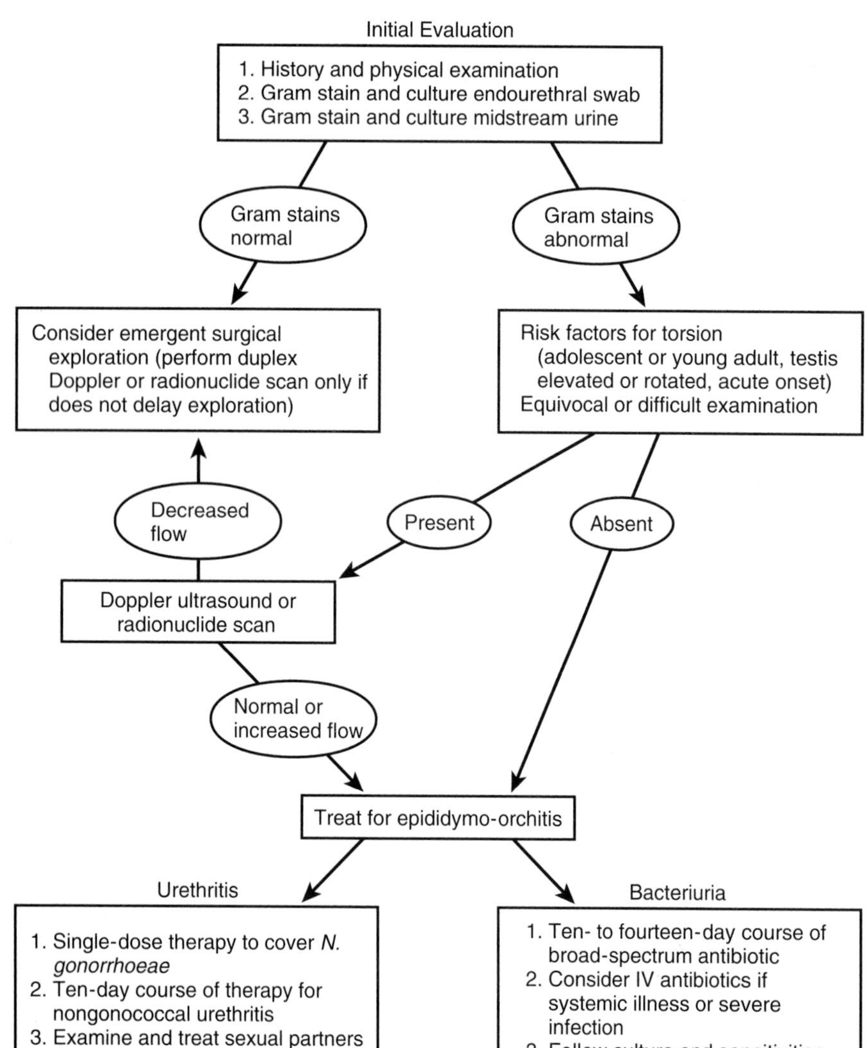

Figure 18–1. Algorithm for management of the acute scrotum. (From Shapiro R, Berger RE: Curr Ther Infect Dis, in press.)

concomitant *C. trachomatis* infection in approximately 30% to 50% of cases, tetracycline or a derivative is the drug of choice in men with *N. gonorrhoeae* or *C. trachomatis* infection (Fig. 18–1). Injection of the spermatic cord with a local anesthetic and oral nonsteroidal anti-inflammatory drugs may be of symptomatic benefit (Lapides et al, 1964; Moore et al, 1971; Smith, 1971; Costas and Van Blerk, 1973). In a controlled trial, Moore and co-workers (1971) found prednisone to be of no value as an adjunct to antibiotic therapy in the treatment of epididymitis.

Men with epididymitis caused by urethritis-causing organisms seldom have structural urinary tract abnormality. Younger boys and older men who have epididymitis secondary to bacteriuria often have structural urologic abnormalities. Men and boys with bacteriuria should undergo radiographic and cystoscopic evaluation for structural urinary tract abnormalities.

GENITAL ULCERS

The diagnosis of acute genital ulcers presents a perplexing problem. The initial clinical impressions of even the most experienced specialist in STDs may be wrong 40% of the time (Chapel et al, 1977). In only three instances is the presentation of the ulcer pathognomonic:

1. A fixed drug eruption is always triggered by the ingestion of one particular medication.
2. A group of vesicles on an erythematous base that does not follow a neural distribution is pathognomonic for herpes simplex infection.
3. A genital ulcer that develops acutely during sexual activity is diagnostic of trauma (Krauss, 1984).

If the clinical picture does not fit any of these pathognomonic presentations, the physician must include premalignant processes, such as erythroplasia of Queyrat; malignant processes, such as squamous cell carcinoma; and nonmalignant processes, such as syphilis, chancroid, genital herpes, lymphogranuloma venereum, granuloma inguinale, fixed drug eruptions, and traumatic ulcers in the differential diagnosis (Table 18–7). Although the symptoms of each of these diseases do differ, the natural variability, influence of secondary infection, and possible coexistence of more than one disease entity make the differential diagnosis extremely difficult. The quest for the proper diagnosis and treatment, therefore, needs to be based largely on laboratory examination. The test most valuable for malignant lesions is biopsy; for genital herpes, it is viral culture; for syphilis, it is darkfield examination and serologic tests; for chancroid, it is selective medium culture for *Haemophilus ducreyi*; for granuloma inguinale, a crush preparation for the cytologic or histologic identification of *Calymmatobacterium granulomatis* is necessary; and for lymphogranuloma venereum, a serologic test and chlamydial culture are required.

Since the treatment for each of these diseases differs significantly (Table 18–8), a correct differential diagnosis is essential (Table 18–9).

Genital Herpes Infections

Genital herpes simplex virus (HSV) is a disease of great concern to physicians and patients. The increasing incidence of the infection in men and women, the risk of transmission to sexual partners, the high morbidity and even mortality of infant infections, the association with cervical cancer, and the absence of curative therapy have made it imperative that all physicians be able to diagnose, counsel, and treat the patient with genital herpes (Nahmias et al, 1973; Nahmias and Roizman, 1973).

HSV is a double-stranded DNA virus that may cause persistent or latent infections. Two antigenic types may be distinguished (Nahmias and Roizman, 1973). Types I and II may be distinguished by DNA restriction enzyme analysis or monoclonal antibodies directed against glycoproteins (Balachandran et al, 1982; Richman et al, 1982; Goldstein et al, 1983; Peterson et al, 1983).

The majority of patients with genital herpes infection have type II virus. However, type I herpes, which is commonly associated with oral infections, has been reported in 10% to 25% of cases (Reeves et al, 1981; Corey et al, 1983a). HSV is seen in 5% of STD clinic visits. In college students, HSV infections are 10 times more common than gonorrhea or

Table 18–7. CLINICAL FEATURES OF GENITAL ULCERS

	Syphilis	Herpes	Chancroid	Lymphogranuloma Venereum	Donovanosis
Incubation period	2–4 wk (1–12 wk)	2–7 days	1–14 days	3 days–6 wk	1–4 wk (up to 6 mo)
Primary lesion	Papule	Vesicle	Papule or pustule	Papule, pustule, or vesicle	Papule
Number of lesions	Usually one	Multiple, may coalesce	Usually multiple, may coalesce	Usually one	Variable
Diameters (mm)	5–15	1–2	2–20	2–10	Variable
Depth	Superficial or deep	Superficial	Excavated	Superficial or deep	Elevated
Edges	Sharply demarcated, elevated, round, or oval	Erythematous	Undermined, ragged, irregular	Elevated, round, or oval	Elevated, irregular
Base	Smooth, nonpurulent	Serous, erythematous	Purulent	Variable	Red and rough ("beefy")
Induration	Firm	None	Soft	Occasionally firm	Firm
Pain	Unusual	Common	Usually very tender	Variable	Uncommon
Lymphadenopathy	Firm, nontender, bilateral	Firm, tender, often bilateral	Tender, may suppurate, usually unilateral	Tender, may suppurate, loculated, usually unilateral	Pseudopathy

Table 18–8. TREATMENT OF SEXUALLY ACQUIRED GENITAL ULCERS

Infection Process	Drug of Choice	Alternative Drug
Chancroid	Erythromycin, 500 mg orally 4 times a day for 7 days or Ceftriaxone, 250 mg IM in a single dose or Azithromycin, 1 g orally in a single dose	Amoxicillin, 500 mg plus clavulanic acid, 125 mg orally 3 times a day for 7 days or Ciprofloxacin, 500 mg orally 2 times a day for 3 days
Genital herpes		
First episode	Acyclovir, 200 mg orally 5 times a day for 10 days	
Suppression therapy	Acyclovir, 400 mg orally 2 times a day	
Granuloma inguinale	Trimethoprim-sulfamethoxazole, 160 and 800 mg orally 2 times a day for 20 days or Tetracycline, 500 mg orally 4 times a day for 20 days	
Lymphogranuloma venereum	Doxycycline, 100 mg orally 2 times a day for 21 days	Erythromycin, 500 mg 4 times a day for 21 days or Sulfisoxazole, 500 mg orally 4 times a day for 21 days
Syphilis (primary)	Benzathine penicillin, 2.4 million units IM	Doxycycline, 100 mg orally 2 times a day for 2 weeks or Tetracycline, 500 mg orally 4 times a day for 2 weeks or Erythromycin, 500 mg orally 4 times a day for 2 weeks

syphilis (Scriba, 1978). Although the risk of transmission from a single exposure is unknown, genital herpes infection may be transmitted by either genital or oral-genital contact.

Although it is not inevitable if one infected partner has genital herpes for the other to acquire it, partners are at risk even when the infection is asymptomatic. The risk of transmission, however, is lower when couples avoid sexual contact during clinical recurrences (Mertz et al, 1981, 1983).

Clinical Course

The signs and symptoms from first-episode genital herpes are much more severe than those from recurrent disease (Table 18–10). HSV types I and II produce primary genital infections of equal severity. First-episode disease is also much more severe in persons without prior HSV oral infection (primary first-episode disease) than is first-episode genital herpes in persons with prior HSV oral infection (nonprimary first-episode disease). Dysuria is present in 44% of men and 83% of women. HSV can be isolated from the urethras of most of these patients, suggesting a true urethritis. The virus may cause NGU in men and urethral syndrome in women in the absence of external lesions (Corey and Holmes, 1983). The clinical illness of primary genital herpes tends to be more severe in women. Recurrent genital herpes is usually milder in either sex. HSV type II causes 99% of recurrent genital herpes. The cases of recurrence with HSV type I primary infections are fewer than those with primary HSV type II infections (Reeves et al, 1981; Corey et al, 1983a). In contrast to primary herpes, which is often bilateral, recurrent disease is often unilateral. Local symptoms are milder, and systemic symptoms are unusual. Urethral isolation can be obtained in less than 2% of men (Corey et al, 1983a). Extragenital skin lesions, usually from autoinoculation, are found in 10% of men and 26% of women with primary genital herpes (Corey et al, 1983a).

Neurologic complications are also common in patients with primary infections. In 13% to 36% of patients, mild meningitis with spinal fluid leukocytosis develops (Brenton, 1980). Of patients with primary genital herpes, severe sacral or autonomic nervous system dysfunction develops in 1% (Goldmeier et al, 1975; Caplan et al, 1977; Oates and Greenhouse, 1978; Goldmeier, 1979; Riehle and Williams, 1979; Jacobs et al, 1980; Corey et al, 1983a), resulting in urinary

Table 18–9. LABORATORY AIDS IN THE DIAGNOSIS OF ACUTE GENITAL ULCERS

Diagnosis	Preferred Test*	Ancillary Tests
Genital herpes	Viral culture, antigen activation	Tzanck smear Fluorescent antibody smear
Syphilis	Dark-field examination	Serologic tests (RPR, VDRL, FTA-ABS, MHA-TP)
Chancroid	Selective medium culture	
Granuloma inguinale	Crush preparation	Histologic examination
Lymphogranuloma venereum	Serologic test (LGV complement fixation or *Chlamydia trachomatis* microimmunofluorescence)	*C. trachomatis* culture
Traumatic ulcer	None	
Fixed drug reaction	None	

*Based on sensitivity, specificity, and availability.

RPR, rapid plasma reagin test; VDRL, Venereal Disease Research Laboratory test; FTA-ABS, fluorescent treponemal antibody absorption test; LGV, lymphogranuloma venereum test; MHA-TP, microhemagglutination test.

From Kraus SJ: Urol Clin North Am 1984; 11:155.

Table 18–10. VIRAL TYPE, SIGNS, AND SYMPTOMS IN PATIENTS WITH GENITAL HERPES SEEN AT THE UNIVERSITY OF WASHINGTON

	First Episode of Genital Herpes		
	Primary	*Nonprimary*	Recurrent Genital Herpes
Number of patients	209	77	362
Percentage female	68	57	40
Percentage with HSV-2	90	99	99
Mean duration of viral shedding (days)	11.3	6.8	4.1
Percentage shedding virus from cervix	87	65	12
Mean number of lesions at onset	16.3	9.5	6.4
Mean lesions area (mm^2) at onset	525	158	59
Percentage with bilateral lesions	84	45	11
Percentage forming new lesions	75	45	37
Mean duration of lesions (days)	19.0	15.5	10.0
Percentage with tender lymphadenopathy	80	—	26
Mean duration of local pain (days)	11.9	8.7	4.7
Percentage with systemic symptoms	62	16	8

Data from Corey L, Adams HG, Brown AZ, et al: Ann Intern Med 1983; 98:958.
Adapted from Mertz GJ, Corey L: Urol Clin North Am 1984; 11:103.

retention. Patients may complain of constipation, weakness, impotence, and sensory loss. Cystometric examination may reveal a hypotonic curve with decreased sensation. Catheterization for a period of weeks may be necessary before bladder function returns. On the other hand, some patients may be unable to urinate because of local pain. These latter patients may be managed by having them void into a tub of warm water (Mertz and Corey, 1984). HSV encephalitis is associated with a mortality rate of 70% and is usually associated with HSV type I (Craig and Nahmias, 1973).

In homosexual men, HSV is the second most common cause of proctitis after gonorrhea (Goldmeier et al, 1975; Goldmeier, 1979; Goodell et al, 1983).

Diagnosis

Vesicles grouped on an erythematous base that do not follow a neural distribution are essentially pathognomonic for genital herpes. Confirmation of the diagnosis and the diagnoses of outpatient cases are based on laboratory methods. Papanicolaou (Pap) smears of lesions demonstrate intranuclear inclusions in 50% to 60% of culture-positive cases (Brown et al, 1979; Corey and Holmes, 1983; Goldstein et al, 1983). Immunofluorescent techniques reveal 70% of culture-positive cases (Moseley et al, 1981).

Virus isolation by culture is the most sensitive technique for diagnosing herpesvirus infections. Results can be available in 5 days (Goldstein et al, 1983). Serum antibody to HSV infections can be measured by a number of methods (Cappel et al, 1980; Ashley and Corey, 1981; Balachandran et al, 1982) and is reliable in differentiating type I from type II infection but may be unreliable when both types of infection are present (Ashley et al, 1991).

Treatment

Acyclovir is a drug of choice for treatment of genital herpes. Other drugs are under investigation. Topical, intravenous, and oral forms of acyclovir are effective for first-episode genital herpes. Oral acyclovir has been shown to be effective therapeutically and prophylactically in recurrent genital herpes infections. Although other forms of therapy may be harmless, patients should be discouraged from using potentially harmful, as well as ineffective, forms of therapy.

Acyclovir acts on viral thymidine kinase as a guanine analogue. It is selectively phosphorylated in the virus, acts as an inhibitor of viral DNA polymerase, and also acts as a chain terminator (Ashley and Corey, 1981).

Oral acyclovir (200 mg five times per day for 5 to 10 days) and intravenous acyclovir (5 to 10 mg/kg every 8 hours for 5 to 7 days) appear more effective than topical therapy (5% acyclovir in polyethylene glycol) in the treatment of primary herpes. Oral acyclovir offers considerable economic advantage over intravenous therapy (Nilson et al, 1981; Wallin et al, 1981; Mertz et al, 1982; Mindel et al, 1982; Corey et al, 1983b). In any form, acyclovir decreases the duration of viral shedding, time to crusting of lesions, time to healing of lesions, and duration of pain and itching in primary genital herpes. Only the oral and intravenous forms decrease dysuria, vaginal discharge, systemic symptoms, and the development of new lesions. Initial systemic delivery of acyclovir does not influence subsequent development of recurrent disease (de Ruiters and Thin, 1994).

In the treatment of recurrent herpes, topical acyclovir has shown little effect (Corey et al, 1982; Spruance et al, 1982; Reichman et al, 1983). However, oral acyclovir has been shown to significantly decrease the duration of viral shedding and time to crusting of recurrent lesions. Oral acyclovir did not significantly decrease the duration of local pain or itching (Reichman et al, 1983). Treatment initiated by patients rather than physicians, and therefore started earlier, appears to enhance significantly both the clinical and the virologic response (Reichman et al, 1983; Goldberg et al, 1986). In some patients, if acyclovir is taken during the prodromal period, the episode will be aborted (Goldberg et al, 1986).

Prophylactic oral acyclovir (400 mg orally twice a day) decreases recurrence (Douglas et al, 1984). Oral acyclovir has been shown to be effective and safe therapy for up to 5 years (Goldberg et al, 1993). Men on prophylactic acyclovir appear to have fewer recurrences than men treated with intermittent therapy. Even on prophylactic therapy asymptomatic viral shedding may occur, causing infection in partners (Strauss et al, 1989). Suppressive therapy should be considered for patients with six to eight or more recurrences per year.

As with treatment for other STDs, resistance to acyclovir has already occurred (Caplan et al, 1977; Burns et al, 1982; Crumpacker et al, 1982). Use of acyclovir outside its prescribed indications should be discouraged.

Primary Syphilis

Etiology

The incidence of syphilis is higher than it has been in more than 30 years. In 1990 more than 55,000 cases of syphilis were reported, reflecting the highest number of cases since 1949 (Rolfs and Nakishima, 1990). Many of these increases are also occurring in populations that have a high prevalence of HIV infection (Felman, 1993). Syphilis is caused by the spirochete *Treponema pallidum* and gains access through skin or mucous membranes. Two to 4 weeks after sexual exposure, a male patient usually presents with a painless penile sore called a "chancre." This chancre usually begins as a small red spot or a papule and then breaks down to form an indurated, punched-out lesion. It may occur on the glans of the penis, foreskin, suprapubic area, or scrotum; it may also occur on other areas of sexual contact such as the lips or the tongue.

Diagnosis

For diagnosis, scrapings should be taken from the base of the chancre and examined by darkfield or fluorescent antibody techniques. For darkfield examination, serous fluid from the base of the lesion is best. The exudate should be examined fresh so that the corkscrew motility of the spirochete can be observed. False-positive results can occur as a result of nonpathogenic spirochetes in oral and anal specimens (Johnson and Farnie, 1994). A monoclonal antibody test to *T. pallidum* can differentiate pathogenic from nonpathogenic spirochetes (Lukehart et al, 1985). Presumptive diagnosis may be made on the basis of serologic tests for *Treponema* with the fluorescent treponemal antibody absorption test (FTA-ABS) and the microhemagglutination assay for antibody to *T. pallidum* (MHATP) or the nontreponemal tests, such as Venereal Disease Research Laboratory (VDRL) and rapid plasma reagin (RPR) tests. None of these tests are sufficient for diagnosis. Treponemal antibody tests, once positive, remain positive for life and do not correlate with disease activity. Nontreponemal antibody titers, such as the quantitative RPR and VDRL, correlate with disease activity. These tests should become negative after 1 year. A fourfold increase in titer is indicative of ineffective therapy or reinfection (Johnson and Farnie, 1994).

Polymerase chain reaction for diagnosis of HSV is an excellent noninvasive method. It is far more sensitive than viral cultures or HSV antibody determination but requires a high degree of laboratory technical expertise (Ehrlick, 1991).

Therapy

Benzathine penicillin G (2.4 million units IM in one dose) is the preferred treatment for early or primary syphilis. For patients with penicillin allergies, skin testing with subsequent desensitization is the best option. Alternative treatments include doxycycline (100 mg orally two times per day for 2 weeks) or tetracycline (500 mg orally four times per day for 2 weeks). Also, erythromycin (500 mg orally four times a day for 2 weeks). With this last regimen, careful follow-up is mandatory because of the preliminary nature of the data on cure. Treatment failures occur with all regimens, and patients need to be re-examined serologically at 3 and 6 months. If the primary antibodies have not declined by fourfold within 6 months of treating early syphilis, patients should undergo cerebrospinal fluid (CSF) examination for CNS syphilis and be re-treated appropriately. The CDC recommends that all syphilis patients receive counseling concerning the risks of HIV infection and be encouraged to be tested for HIV.

Lymphogranuloma Venereum

Etiology

Lymphogranuloma venereum is caused by *C. trachomatis* serotypes L1, L2, and L3. The primary lesion is firm and painless and has low elevated borders. It may be quite transient and not noticed by the patient. It may also be easily confused with the lesions of chancroid. The papule usually appears 5 to 21 days after sexual exposure. As the lesion evolves, painful inguinal lymph nodes become the most prominent sign. Unilateral lymphadenopathy is the most commonly found sign. At the stage of bubo formation, systemic symptoms are often present, including vomiting, nausea, joint pains, headache, fever, and chills. Skin rashes may occur.

Diagnosis

The most specific and best test for the diagnosis of lymphogranuloma venereum is culture of *C. trachomatis*. Culture is best obtained from aspiration of a fluctuant inguinal node. Other serologic tests for *C. trachomatis*, such as the microimmunofluorescent antibody test, are commonly used. The Frei skin test is no longer used. In the course of the disease, the white blood cell count may be quite elevated. Anemia may even be present and gamma globulin levels elevated. Biopsy of the node shows heavy infiltration by neutrophils and plasma cells (Van Dyck and Piot, 1992; Joseph and Rosen, 1994).

Treatment

The preferred treatment is doxycycline, 100 mg orally, two times per day for 21 days. Alternative regimens include erythromycin, 500 mg orally, four times per day for 21 days; or sulfisoxazole, four times per day for 21 days. Complications may occur such as rectal strictures from rectal involvement and may need to be treated by surgical means.

Chancroid

Etiology

Because of recent increases in transmission, chancroid caused by *H. ducreyi* has become an important STD in the

United States. It must be considered in differential diagnosis in any man with a painful genital ulcer. Painful lymphadenopathy is present in about half the cases. Typically, the ulcer has a deep undermined border. It may be soft or indurated and may be purulent. The base of the lesion is often friable and bleeds easily. Chronic inflammation may be seen with enlarged inguinal nodes. Genital lymphedema may occur. In Africa, chancroid infection has emerged as a major risk factor in acquisition of HIV-1 after heterosexual intercourse (Ronald and Plummer, 1989).

Diagnosis

Definitive diagnosis can be made from a Gram stain smear at the base of the lesion. The Gram stain may show gram-negative coccobacilli in chains of clusters with a "school of fish" appearance (Joseph and Rosen, 1994). Definitive diagnosis can also be made using selective cultures for *H. ducreyi*. The optimal culture for *H. ducreyi* may require both supplemented gonococcal base and Mueller-Hinton agar.

Treatment

Treatment for chancroid may be difficult because of regional differences in antibiotic sensitivities. Antibiotic resistance in *H. ducreyi* has been a special concern because this organism acquires both gram-negative and gram-positive resistance determinants. It has been found that some of these determinants can be transferred to other *Haemophilus* species or to *N. gonorrhoeae* (Morse, 1989). The current recommended regimens are erythromycin base (500 mg orally, four times per day for 7 days) or ceftriaxone (250 mg intramuscularly, in a single dose); or azithromycin 1 g orally in a single dose. Sex partners should be treated with the same regimen. If the treatment is successful, ulcers should improve symptomatically within 3 days and objectively within 7 days. Lymphadenopathy resolves more slowly. Patients with coexisting HIV infections seem not to respond as well to antibiotic therapy (CDC Recommendations, 1989).

Granuloma Inguinale

Etiology

Granuloma inguinale is a sexually transmitted chronic infection of the skin and subcutaneous tissue of the inguinal area, perineum, and genitalia. Its usual incubation is 2 to 3 months. The infective agent is *Calymmatobacterium granulomatis* and is related to *Klebsiella pneumoniae*. A small papule is the first sign. It usually forms as a small ulcer protruding above the level of the skin. The base of the ulcer is erythematous and may have hemorrhagic secretions. It is nontender, indurated, and firm (Billstein and Mattaliano, 1990).

Diagnosis

Identification of Donovan bodies in monocytes on a stained smear makes the diagnosis of granuloma inguinale. These organisms appear as bipolar staining rods within the monocytes. A crush specimen for histologic study is prepared by obtaining a small fragment of tissue from the ulcer base and crushing it between two slides. Leishman's stain, Giemsa's stain, or Wright's stain may be used. Multiple sections need to be studied. In case of doubt, biopsy may be performed. A reliable culture for *C. granulomatis* is not available. Chancroid may easily be mistaken for granuloma inguinale, and therefore chancroid must always be ruled out before the diagnosis is made (Van Dyck and Piot, 1992; Joseph and Rosen, 1994).

Treatment

Treatment has been successful with tetracycline (500 mg orally four times per day) or trimethoprim-sulfamethoxazole (one double-strength tablet orally twice daily). There have been no good control trials of treatment with this disease.

GENITAL WARTS

All wart viruses belong to the papilloma species, which are DNA-containing viruses (Dunn and Ogilvie, 1968; Oriel and Almeida, 1970; Oriel, 1971). Papilloma virus infection stimulates rapid cell division and duplication of virus particles. Patients transmit the disease when released viral particles from lesions come in contact with another person (Coggin and zur Hausen, 1979). A relationship between genital warts and cervical carcinoma is now receiving significant research attention (Syrjanen et al, 1981). It is possible that this "minor" veneral disease may cause significant health problems. Visible external genital warts are most often caused by types 6 and 11 of human papillomavirus (HPV). Some other types present in the anogenital region, notably types 16, 18, 31, 33, and 35, have been strongly associated with cervical dysplasia in women and the development of carcinoma. It is recommended that a biopsy be undertaken in all instances of atypical pigmented or persistent warts.

Because of the sexual transmission of HPV in its probable role in the development of carcinoma, investigators have looked for more sensitive ways of detecting wart virus in partners. It has been found that a towel soaked in 5% acetic acid that is then wrapped around the genitals of the male may show subclinical, flat condylomas appearing as whitish areas. With this method, it has been found that most steady sexual male partners of women with HPV infection and/or cervical neoplasia have subclinical HPV infection (Barrasso et al, 1987). Likewise, it has been found that female partners of men with condyloma have a high incidence of HPV infection (Campion et al, 1985). Men and women experience a high prevalence of asymptomatic genital HPV infection. Using polymerase chain reaction studies, Bauer and colleagues (1991) showed that 46% of college women undergoing routine pelvic examination were infected with HPV.

The goal of treatment is removal of exophytic warts and the amelioration of signs and symptoms, and not the eradication of HPV. No therapy has been shown to eradicate HPV, which has been found in tissue after laser treatment as well as other treatment. Acetowhitened areas from the application of 5% acetic acid have been shown to be falsely interpreted as virally infected, and normal areas, not acetowhitened, have been shown to have virus. "The urologist is, however, often asked to examine and eradicate genital wart virus in partners of women with warts and/or cervical dysplasia. At the present time there is no evidence that this is possible. Aggressive treatment of acetowhite areas will not eradicate virus as it is often present in non-acetowhite areas. It is best to reply to the request that you will certainly examine and treat the patient for any exophytic warts, but that extensive diagnostic and treatment regimens have not been shown to be beneficial and will cause unnecessary morbidity. Likewise it has not been shown that any treatment of the woman will eradicate the wart virus and that reoccurrence may more likely be due to autoinfection than infection from her partner" (Cowsert, 1994; Maymon et al, 1994). Therefore, the benefit of treating patients with subclinical HPV infection has not been demonstrated, and recurrence is usual. The goal with treatment in HPV infection, especially in men, is only to remove exophytic warts and to decrease any signs or symptoms the patient may have from the wart infection. Since local cure is probably not possible, expensive therapies or toxic therapies that may result in considerable scarring should be avoided when possible. Patients, however, should be made aware that they are infective to uninfected partners, and the use of condoms must be recommended. Numerous treatments have been used for warts, and the current CDC recommendations are presented in Table 18–11.

Table 18–11. SITE-SPECIFIC TREATMENT OF GENITAL WARTS

Site	Treatment
External genital and perianal	*Primary*
	Cryotherapy with liquid nitrogen or cryoprobe
	Secondary
	10%–25% podophyllin* in compound tincture of benzoin weekly for 4 wks, electrosurgery
	Trichloroacetic acid (80%–90%)† weekly
Vaginal	*Primary*
	Cryotherapy with liquid nitrogen
	Secondary
	10%–25% podophyllin‡ in compound tincture of benzoin weekly
	Trichloroacetic acid (80%–90%)†
Cervical	Rule out dysplasia; consult expert
Meatal	*Primary*
	Cryotherapy
	Secondary
	10%–25% podophyllin in compound tincture of benzoin weekly for 4 wks§
Urethral	Laser therapy
	5% 5-fluorouracil or thiotepa (do not use podophyllin)
Anorectal	*Primary*
	Cryotherapy
	Secondary
	Surgical removal, trichloroacetic acid (80%–90%)
Oral	Cryotherapy, electrosurgery, and surgical removal

*Use <0.5 ml per session. Wash off in 1 to 4 hours. Contraindicated in pregnancy. Treat <10 cm^2 per session.

†Powder with talc or sodium bicarbonate to remove unreacted acid.

‡Treatment area must be dry before speculum is removed.

§Treatment area must be dry before contact with normal mucosa. Wash off in 1 to 2 hours.

From Sexually Transmitted Disease Treatment Guidelines: MMWR Morbid Mortal Wkly Rep 1989; 38(S8):16–19.

SCABIES

Etiology

Scabies is a highly contagious parasitic infection caused by the mite *Sarcoptes scabiei*. The mite is usually contracted from contact with infested clothes, bedding, or other people. Adults or children who have close personal contact may directly transmit it. Sometimes, the infection is transmitted among hospital personnel between infected patients and staff. Some have questioned the concept that scabies is an STD, since 30-year cycles of scabies epidemics exist, correlating, perhaps, with changes in the immune status of the host population. Full mite transmission is rare, and African Americans appear to be resistant to the mite (Burkhart, 1983). Scabies may be an unrecognized cause of recurrent streptococcal or staphylococcal skin infections (Billstein and Mattaliano, 1990).

Symptoms and Diagnosis

Scabies is characterized by profound itching, especially when the patient becomes warm, often under the bedclothes at night. Itching may be so intense that people severely excoriate themselves from the scratching. Reports have linked scabies with immunosuppression, such as in AIDS, and in transplant patients (Lang et al, 1989). The mite can usually be demonstrated if a thin sliver of skin from a papule is removed, placed on a glass slide, and digested with heat and 10% KOH. Oftentimes, the mite can be seen, and, if not, its eggs can usually be identified.

Treatment

The current recommendation for treatment is lindane, 1% (1 oz of lotion or 30 g of cream) applied thinly to all areas of the body from the neck on down and then washed off thoroughly after 8 hours. Pregnant and lactating women and children under 2 years of age should not use lindane. Alternatively permethrin cream (5%), applied to all areas of the body from the neck down and washed off after 8 to 14 hours, can be used. Also alternatively, crotamiton (10%) can be applied to the entire body from the neck down nightly for two consecutive nights and washed off 24 hours after the second application. Sex partners and close contacts should also be treated. Clothing or bed linen that may have been contaminated should be washed and dried by machine on a hot cycle or dry cleaned to kill the mites. It should be noted that itching may persist for several weeks after adequate therapy. Sometimes, a re-treatment after 1 week, if no improvement has occurred, is necessary. If itching continues, a search for live mites should be made before additional treatment is prescribed (Orkin and Maibach, 1993).

PEDICULOSIS PUBIS

Etiology

Pediculosis pubis (phthiriasis) is infection with the crab louse. This disorder should be suspected whenever there is itching of the haired portions of the pubis, thighs, or scrotum.

Diagnosis

The presence of nits attached to the hair shaft near the skin surface or the actual presence of an imbedded louse in the hair follicle is diagnostic. These lice can often be seen with the naked eye or with low-power magnification. Oftentimes, the nits are seen in the axilla, eyelashes, or scalp hair.

Treatment

Treatment should be with permethrin (1% cream rinse), applied to affected areas and washed off after 10 minutes; or with lindane (1% shampoo), applied for 4 minutes and then thoroughly washed off. Patients should be re-evaluated after 1 week if symptoms persist. Re-treatment may be necessary if further lice or eggs are found. Sexual partners and close contacts should also be treated. Clothing and bedclothes that may have been contaminated should be washed and dried in the hot cycle. Although topical insecticidal preparations are the preferred treatment, trimethoprim-sulfamethoxazole can eliminate infections (Hutchinson and Farquhar, 1982).

MOLLUSCUM CONTAGIOSUM

Etiology

Molluscum contagiosum is caused by a virus belonging to the DNA pox family. The worldwide incidence of this disease is 2% to 8%. It most commonly involves the genitalia, although other parts of the body can be involved as well. Intimate skin-to-skin contact is required for transmission. The incubation period is 2 to 3 months.

Diagnosis

Molluscum contagiosum presents as small firm umbilicated papules on the skin. They are smooth and pearly-colored or flesh-colored. They contain a milky white material that contains the virus and epidermal cells. The natural history is to enlarge for a few months, persist, and then in many cases spontaneously resolve. On biopsy eosinophilic hyalin spherical masses, called *molluscum bodies*, are noted.

Treatment

The molluscum may be removed by curettage, liquid nitrogen, or chemical eradication with cantharidin, phenol, tincture of iodine, silver nitrate, or trichloroacetic acid. Close sexual contacts should also be examined (Billstein and Mattaliano, 1990; Epstein, 1992).

HEPATITIS AND ENTERIC INFECTIONS

In the past, viral hepatitis and enteric infections were not viewed as STDs. Now, however, many of these infections are known to be sexually transmitted in some cases (Table 18–12). Hepatitis A and B may be transmitted by sexual contact and through other close physical contact. Enteric infections (amebiasis, giardiasis, shigellosis, and campylobacteriosis) and enteric viruses may be transmitted directly by the oral-fecal route.

Most sexually transmitted enteric infections occur in homosexual men. Fecal contact is made in two ways: through anal-receptive intercourse, and by anilingus. Both these sexual practices are common among homosexuals but are much less frequent among heterosexuals. Approximately 10% of the population may be homosexual or bisexual (Kinsey et al, 1948). In at least one study, 31% of the men who were homosexual also had sexual contact with women (Judson et al, 1980). Enteric diseases contracted by homosexual contact may also be transmitted to female partners.

Approximately one third of hepatitis B cases may be attributable to homosexual contacts; 25% are acquired by heterosexual contact. From 30% to 80% of homosexual men test seropositive for hepatitis B (Judson et al, 1981). Female partners of men with hepatitis B are also at risk; in one study, hepatitis developed 3 to 12 months after exposure in 20% to 27% (Judson et al, 1981).

Hepatitis A is also spread by sexual contact (Corey and Holmes, 1980; Christenson, 1982). Hepatitis A is more prevalent in homosexual men than in heterosexual men. In heterosexuals, the incidence of seropositivity is directly proportional to the number of sexual partners (Corey and Holmes, 1980; McFarlane et al, 1981; Christenson, 1982).

At this time, there is little evidence that non-A, non-B hepatitis, which accounts for 70% of post-transfusion hepatitis, has a sexual mode of transmission (Robinson, 1982; Gilson, 1992).

PROCTITIS

Proctitis is another syndrome found in homosexual men. This syndrome may be caused by *N. gonorrhoeae*, *C. trachomatis*, or HSV. Culture is the best method of diagnosis (Deheragoda, 1977; Klein et al, 1977; Quinn et al, 1981a, 1981b; Klotz et al, 1983).

Acute proctitis of recent onset in an individual who has

Table 18–12. SEXUALLY TRANSMITTED AGENTS THAT CAUSE INFECTIONS OF THE LIVER, INTESTINES, AND ANORECTUM

Target Organ	Infectious Agents
Liver	Hepatitis B virus
	Hepatitis A virus
	Hepatitis non-A, non-B agent(s)
Intestines	*Giardia lamblia*
	Entamoeba histolytica
	Cryptosporidium species
	Shigella species
	Campylobacter fetus
	Strongyloides species
Anorectum	*Neisseria gonorrhoeae*
	Chlamydia trachomatis
	Treponema pallidum
	Herpes simplex virus
	Human papillomavirus

recently practiced unprotected receptive anal intercourse may most often be sexually transmitted. These men should be examined by anoscopy and evaluated for infection with *N. gonorrhoeae, C. trachomatis*, HSV, and syphilis. Enteric treatment should be instituted with ceftriaxone, 125 mg intramuscularly, plus doxycycline, 100 mg orally, two times per day for 7 days (Centers for Disease Control and Prevention, 1993).

REFERENCES

Abu-Sleiman R, Ho JE, Gregory JG: Scrotal scanning: Present value and limits of interpretation. Urology 1979; 13:326.

Alani MD, Darougar S, Burns DC, et al: Isolation of *Chlamydia trachomatis* from the male urethra. Br J Vener Dis 1977; 58:88.

Aral SO, Holmes KK: Epidemiology of sexually transmitted diseases. *In* Holmes KK, Maardh PA, Sparling PF, et al, eds: Sexually Transmitted Diseases. New York, McGraw-Hill Book Company, 1984, pp 126–141.

Arrosagaray PM, Salas C, Morales M: Bilateral abscessed orchiepididymitis associated with sepsis caused by *Veillonella parvula* and *Clostridium perfringens*: Case report and review of the literature. J Clin Microbiol 1987; 25:1579.

Ashley R, et al: Inability of enzyme immunoassays to discriminate between infections with herpes simplex viruses types 1 or 2. Ann Intern Med 1991; 115:520–526.

Ashley RL, Corey L: Analysis of the humoral immune response to HSV in primary genital herpes patients. (Abstract.) Anaheim, Calif, 1981.

Balachandran N, Frame B, Chernesky M, et al: Identification and typing of herpes simplex viruses with monoclonal antibodies. J Clin Microbiol 1982; 16:205.

Barrasso R, Coupez F, Ionescu M, deBrux J: Human papilloma viruses and cervical intraepithelial neoplasia: The role of colposcopy. Gynecol Oncol 1987; 27:197–207.

Bauer HM, et al: Genital human papillomavirus infection in female university students as determined by a PCR-based method. JAMA 1991; 265:472–477.

Bell TA: *Chlamydia trachomatis* infection in adolescents. Med Clin North Am 1990; 74:1225–1233.

Bell TA, Hein K: Adolescents and sexually transmitted diseases. *In* Holmes KK, Maardh PA, Sparling PF, et al, eds: Sexually Transmitted Diseases. New York, McGraw-Hill Book Company, 1984, pp 73–84.

Beral V: Cancer of the cervix: A sexually transmitted infection? Lancet 1974; 1:1037.

Berger RE: Acute epididymitis. Sex Transm Dis 1981; 8:286.

Berger RE, Alexander ER, Harnish JP, et al: Etiology, manifestations and therapy of acute epididymitis: Prospective study of 50 cases. J Urol 1979; 121:750–754.

Berger RE, Alexander ER, Monda GD, et al: *Chlamydia trachomatis* as a cause of acute "idiopathic" epididymitis. N Engl J Med 1978; 298:301.

Berger RE, Kessler D, Holmes KK: The etiology and manifestations of epididymitis in young men: Correlations with sexual orientation. J Infect Dis 1987; 155:1341.

Bietz O: Fertilitatsuntersuchungen bei der unspezifichen epididymitis. Hautarzt 1959; 10:134.

Billstein SA, Mattaliano VJ Jr: The "nuisance" sexually transmitted diseases: Molluscum contagiosum, scabies, and crab lice. Med Clin North Am 1990; 74:1487–1505.

Bowie WR: Comparison of Gram stain and first voided urine sediment in the diagnosis of urethritis. Sex Transm Dis 1978; 5:39.

Bowie WR: Approach to men with urethritis and urologic complications of sexually transmitted diseases. Med Clin North Am 1990; 74:1543–1557.

Bowie WR, Alexander ER, Floyd JF, et al: Differential response of chlamydial and ureaplasma-associated urethritis to sulfafurazole (sulfisoxazole) and aminocyclitols. Lancet 1976; 2:1276.

Bowie WR, Alexander ER, Stimson JB, et al: Therapy for nongonoccal urethritis: Double-blind randomized comparison of two doses and two durations of minocycline. Ann Intern Med 1981; 95:306.

Bowie WR, Pollock HM, Forsyth PS, et al: Bacteriology of the urethra in normal men and men with nongonococcal urethritis. J Clin Microbiol 1977a; 6:482.

Bowie WR, Wang SP, Alexander ER: Etiology of nongonococcal urethritis: Evidence for *C. trachomatis* and *U. urealyticum*. J Clin Invest 1977b; 59:735.

Bowie WR, Yu JS, Jones HD: Partial efficacy of clindamycin against *Chlamydia trachomatis* in men with nongonococcal urethritis. Sex Transm Dis 1986; 13:76–80.

Brehmer B, Grunig F, von Berger L, et al: Radionuclide scrotal imaging: A useful diagnostic tool in patients with acute scrotal swelling? Scand J Urol Nephrol 1987; 104(suppl):119.

Brenton DW: Hypoglycorrhachia in herpes simplex type 2 meningitis. Arch Neurol 1980; 37:317.

Brown ST, Jafee HW, Zaidi A, et al: Sensitivity and specificity of diagnostic tests for genital infection and herpesvirus hominis. Sex Transm Dis 1979; 6:10.

Brunham RC: Mucopurulent cervicitis: The ignored counterpart in women of urethritis in men. N Engl J Med 1984; 311:1–6.

Burkhart CG: Scabies: An epidemiologic reassessment. Ann Intern Med 1983; 98:498–503.

Burns WH, Saral R, Santos GW, et al: Isolation and characterization of resistant herpes simplex virus after acyclovir therapy. Lancet 1982; 1:421.

Campbell DJ: Gonorrhea in North Africa and the central Mediterranean. Br Med J 1944; 2:44.

Campion MJ, Singer A, Clarkson PK, McCance DJ: Increased risk of cervical neoplasia in consorts of men with penile condylomata acuminata. Lancet 1985; 1:943–946.

Caplan LR, Kleman FJ, Berg S: Urinary retention probably secondary to herpes genitalis. N Engl J Med 1977; 297:920.

Cappel R, De Cuyper F, Berg S, et al: Efficacy of a nucleic acid free herpetic subunit vaccine. Arch Virol 1980; 65:15.

Cates W Jr, Weisner PJ, Curran JW: Sex and spermicides: Preventing unintended pregnancy and infection. JAMA 1982; 148:1636.

Centers for Disease Control: Premarital Sexual Experiences Among Adolescent Women—United States 1970–1988. Atlanta, Centers for Disease Control, 1991.

Centers for Disease Control and Prevention: 1993 sexually transmitted diseases treatment guidelines. MMWR 1993; 42(RR-14):1–102.

Chapel TA, Brown WJ, Jeffries C, et al: How reliable is the morphological diagnosis of penile ulcerations? Sex Transm Dis 1977; 4:150.

Christenson B, Brostrom CH, Bottiger M, et al: An epidemic outbreak of hepatitis A among homosexual men in Stockholm. Am J Epidemiol 1982; 116:599.

Coggin J, zur Hausen H: Papillomaviruses and cancer. Cancer 1979; 39:545.

Corey L, Benedetti J, Critchlow C, et al: Treatment of primary first-episode genital herpes simplex virus infections with acyclovir: Results of topical, intravenous and oral therapy. J Antimicrob Chemother 1983a; 12(suppl. B):79–88.

Corey L, Fife KH, Benedetti JK, et al: Intravenous acyclovir for the treatment of primary genital herpes. Ann Intern Med 1983b; 98:914.

Corey L, Holmes KK: Sexual transmission of hepatitis A in homosexual men: Incidence and mechanism. N Engl J Med 1980; 302:435.

Corey L, Holmes KK: Genital herpes simplex virus infections: Current concepts in diagnosis, therapy, and prevention. Ann Intern Med 1983; 98:973.

Corey L, Nahmias ME, Guinan ME, et al: A trial of topical acyclovir in genital herpes simplex virus infections. N Engl J Med 1982; 306:1313.

Costas S, Van Blerk PJP: Incision of the external inguinal ring in acute epididymitis. Br J Urol 1973; 45:555.

Coufalik ED, Taylor-Robinson D, Csonka GW: Treatment of nongonococcal urethritis with rifampicin as a means of defining the role of *Ureaplasma urealyticum*. Br J Vener Dis 1979; 55:36.

Cowsert LM: Treatment of papillomavirus infections: Recent practice and future approaches. Intervirology 1994; 37:226–230.

Craig CP, Nahmias A: Different patterns of neurologic involvement with herpes simplex virus types 1 and 2: Isolation of herpes simplex virus from the buffy coat of two adults with meningitis. J Infect Dis 1973; 127:365.

Crawford G, Knapp JS, Hale J, et al: Asymptomatic gonorrhea in men. Science 1937; 196:1352.

Crumpacker CS, Schnipper LE, Zaia JA, et al: Growth inhibition by acycloguanosine of herpesvirus isolated from human infections. Antimicrob Agents Chemother 1982; 15:642.

Csango PA: *Chlamydia trachomatis* from men with nongonococcal urethritis: Simplified procedure for cultivation and isolation in replicating McCoy cell cultures. Acta Pathol Microbiol Scand B 1978; 86:257.

Curran JW: Economic consequences of pelvic inflammatory disease in the United States. Am J Obstet Gynecol 1980; 138:848.

Dees JE, Colston JAC: The use of sulfonilamide in gonococcis infections: A preliminary report. JAMA 1937; 108:1855.

De Jong Z, Pontonnier F, Plante P, et al: The frequency of *Chlamydia trachomatis* in acute epididymitis. Br J Urol 1988; 62:76.

Deheragoda P: Diagnosis of rectal gonorrhea by blind anorectal swabs compared with direct vision swabs taken via a proctoscope. Br J Vener Dis 1977; 53:311.

Delvillar RG, Ireland GW, Cass AS: Early exploration in acute testicular conditions. J Urol 1972; 108:887.

De Ruiters A, Thin RN: Genital herpes: A guide to pharmacological therapy. Drugs 1994; 47:297–304.

Douglas JM, Critchlow C, Benedetti J, et al: A double-blind study of oral acyclovir for suppression of recurrences of genital herpes simplex virus infection. N Engl J Med 1984; 310:1551.

Dunn AE, Ogilvie MM: Intranuclear virus particles in human genital wart tissue: Observations on the ultrastructure of the epidermal layer. J Ultrastruct Res 1968; 22:282.

Ehrlick GD: Caveats of PCR. Clin Microbiol Newslett 1991; 13:149–151.

Epstein WL: Molluscum contagiosum. Semin Dermatol 1992; 11.3:184–189.

Falk V: Treatment of acute non-tuberculous salpingitis with antibiotics alone and in combination with glucocorticoids. Acta Obstet Gynecol Scand 1965; 44(suppl 6):3.

Felman YM: Sexually transmitted diseases: Selections from the literature since 1990 syphilis: Epidemiology. Cutis 1993; 52:72–74.

Ferris DG, Martin WH, Mathis DM, et al: Non-invasive detection of *Chlamydia trachomatis* urethritis in men by a rapid enzyme immunoassay test. J Fam Pract 1991; 33:73–78.

Fitzgerald SW, Erikson S, DeWire DM, et al: Color Doppler sonography in the evaluation of the adult acute scrotum. [See comments.] J Ultrasound Med 1992; 11:543–548.

Gartman E: Epididymitis: A reappraisal. Am J Surg 1961; 101:756.

Gasparich JP, Mason JT, Greene HL: Amiodarone-associated epididymitis: Drug-related epididymitis in the absence of infection. J Urol 1985; 133:971.

Gilson RJ: Sexually transmitted hepatitis: A review. Genitourin Med 1992; 68:123–129.

Goldberg LH, Kaufman R, Conant MA: Oral acyclovir for episodic treatment of recurrent genital herpes: Efficacy and safety. J Am Acad Dermatol 1986; 15:256–264.

Goldberg LH, Kaufman R, Kurtz TO: Long term suppression of recurrent genital herpes with acyclovir: A five-year benchmark. Arch Dermatol 1993; 129:582–587.

Goldmeier D: Herpetic proctitis and sacral radiculomyelopathy in homosexual men. Br Med J 1979; 2:549.

Goldmeier D, Bateman JRM, Rodin P: Urinary retention and intestinal obstruction associated with anorectal herpes simplex virus infection. Br Med J 1975; 1:425.

Goldstein LC, Corey L, McDougall J, et al: Monoclonal antibodies to herpes simplex viruses: Use in antigenic typing and rapid diagnosis. J Infect Dis 1983; 147:829.

Goodell SE, Quin TC, Mkrtichian EE, et al: Herpes simplex proctitis in homosexual men: Clinical sigmoidoscopic, and histopathological findings. N Engl J Med 1983; 147:829.

Gottesman JE: Coccidioidomycosis of prostate and epididymis. With urethrocutaneous fistula. Urology 1974; 4:311.

Granato PA, Schneible-Smith C, Weiner LB: Use of New York City medium for improved recovery on *N. gonorrhoeae* from clinical specimens. J Clin Microbiol 1981; 13:963.

Graves RS, Engel WJ: Experimental production of epididymitis with sterile urine: Clinical implications. J Urol 1950; 64:601.

Greenberg SH: Nongonococcal urethritis. Arch Androl 1979; 3:321–327.

Grossman JH III, Rivlin ME, Morrison JC: Diagnosis of chlamydial infection in pregnant women using the test pack chlamydial diagnostic kit. Obstet Gynecol 1991; 77:801–803.

Handsfield HH, Alexander ER, Wang SP, et al: Differences in the therapeutic response of chlamydia-positive and chlamydia-negative forms of nongonococal urethritis. J Am Vener Dis Assoc 1975; 2:5.

Hanley HG: Non-specific epididymitis. Br J Surg 1966; 53:873.

Harrison WO: Cefaclor in the treatment of uncomplicated gonococcal urethritis. Postgrad Med J 1979; 55:85.

Harrison WO, Hooper RR, Kilpatrick ME, et al: Penicillin-resistant gonorrhea: Alternative therapy. *In* Seigenthaler W, Luthy R, eds: Current Chemotherapy. Washington DC, American Society for Microbiology, 1978, pp 194–195.

Harrison WO, Sanchez PL, Lancaster DJ: Gonococcal urethritis. Urol Clin North Am 1984; 11:45–53.

Hernandez AI, et al: Oral sex as a risk factor for *Chlamydia*-negative ureaplasma-negative nongonococcal urethritis. Sex Transm Dis 1988; 15:100–102.

Holmes KK, Handsfield HH, Wang SP, et al: Etiology of nongonococcal urethritis. N Engl J Med 1975; 292:1199.

Hooper RR, Wiesner PJ, Harrison WO, et al: Cohort study of venereal diseases. 1: Risk of transmission from infected women to men. Am J Epidemiol 1978; 107:235.

Hunt M: Sexual Behavior in the Seventies. Playboy Press 1974, pp 150–152.

Hutchinson DB, Farquhar JA: Trimethoprim-sulfamethoxazole in the treatment of malaria, toxoplasmosis, and pediculosis. Rev Infect Dis 1982; 4.2:419–425.

Jacobs NF, Kraus SJ: Gonococcal and nongonococcal urethritis in men. Clinical and laboratory differentiation. Ann Intern Med 1975; 82:7.

Jacobs SC, Hebert LA, Piering WF, et al: Acute motor paralytic bladder in renal transplant patients with anogenital herpes infection. J Urol 1980; 123:426.

James-Holmquest AN, Wende RD, Mudd RL, et al: Comparison of atmospheric conditions for culture of clinical specimens of *Neisseria gonorrhoeae*. Appl Microbiol 1973; 26:466.

John J, Donald WH: Asymptomatic urethral gonorrhea in men. Br J Vener Dis 1978;54:322.

Johnson PC, Farnie MA: Testing for syphilis. Dermatol Clin 1994; 12:9–17.

Johnson RE: Epidemiologic and prophylactic treatment of gonorrhea: A decision analysis review. Sex Transm Dis 1979; 6:159.

Joseph AK, Rosen T: Laboratory techniques used in the diagnosis of chancroid, granuloma inguinale, and lymphogranuloma venereum. Dermatol Clin 1994; 12:1–8.

Judson FN: Epidemiology and control of nongonococcal urethritis and genital chlamydial infections: A review. Sex Transm Dis 1981; 8(suppl):117.

Judson FN: Treatment of uncomplicated gonorrhea with ceftriaxone: A review. Sex Transm Dis 1986; 13(suppl):199.

Judson FN, Penley KA, Robinson ME, et al: Comparative prevalence rates of sexually transmitted diseases in heterosexual and homosexual men. Epidemiology 1980; 112:836.

Kampmeier RH: Introduction of sulfonamide therapy for gonorrhea. Sex Transm Dis 1983; 10:81.

Kaneti J, Sarov B, Sarov I: IgG and IgA antibodies specific for *Chlamydia trachomatis* epididymitis diagnosed by fluorescent monoclonal antibody. Urology 1988; 30:395.

Kassler WJ, Cates W Jr: The epidemiology and prevention of sexually transmitted diseases. Urol Clin North Am 1992; 19:1–12.

Kazzaz BA, Salmo NA: Epididymitis due to *Schistosoma haematobium* infection. Trop Geogr Med 1974; 26:333.

Kellogg DS, Holmes KK, Hill GA: Presented at Cumitech 4: Laboratory Diagnosis of Gonorrhea. Washington, DC, 1976.

Kinsey AL, Pomeroy WB, Martin CE: Sexual Behavior in the Human Male. Philadelphia, W. B. Saunders Company, 1948.

Klein EJ, Fisher LS, Chow AW, et al: Anorectal gonococcal infection. Ann Intern Med 1977; 86:340.

Klotz SA, Drutz DJ, Tam MR, et al: Hemorrhagic proctitis due to lymphogranuloma venereum serogroup L. N Engl J Med 1983; 308:1563.

Knapp JS, Thornsberry C, Schoolnik GK, et al: Phenotypic and epidemiologic correlates of auxotype in *Neisseria gonorrhoeae*. J Infect Dis 1978; 138:160.

Kojima H, Wang S-P, Kuo C-C, Grayston T: Local antibody in semen for rapid diagnosis of *Chlamydia trachomatis* epididymitis. J Urol 1988; 140:528.

Krauss SJ: Evaluation and management of acute genital ulcers on sexually active patients. Urol Clin North Am 1984; 11:155.

Krieger JN, Hooton TM, Brust PJ: Evaluation of chronic urethritis. Defining the role for endoscopic procedures. Arch Intern Med 1988; 148:703–707.

Lang E, Humphreys DW, Jaqua SM: Crusted scabies: A case report and review of the literature. S D J Med 1989; 42(4):15–17.

Lapides J, Harwig KR, Anderson EC, et al: Oxphenbutazone therapy for mumps orchitis and acute epididymitis and osteitis pubis. J Urol 1964; 98:526.

Lassus A, Paavonen J, Kousa M, et al: Erythromycin and lymecycline treatment in *Chlamydia*-positive and *Chlamydia*-negative nongonococcal urethritis: A partner-controlled study. Acta Derm Venereol 1979; 59:278.

Linder K: Gonoblennurrhoe, Finehlussblennorrhoe, und Trachoma. Graefes Arch Clin Exp Ophthalmol 1911; 78:345.

Lukehart SA, Tam MR, Horn J, et al: Characterization of monoclonal antibodies to *Treponema pallidum*. J Immunol 1985; 134:585–592.

Lynch CM, Sinnott JT 4th, Holt DA, Herold AH: Use of antibiotics during pregnancy. Clin Pharmacol 1991; 43(4):1365–1368.

Martin DH: Chlamydial infections. Med Clin North Am 1990; 74(6):1367–1387.

Marx JL: Vaccinating with bacterial pili. Science 1980; 209:1103.

Maymon R, Shulman A, Maymon B: Penile condylomata: A gynecological epidemic disease: A review of the current approach and management aspects. Obstet Gynecol Surv Surg 1994; 49:790–800.

McCutchan JA: Gonorrhea and nongonococcal urethritis. *In* Braude AI, ed: Medical Microbiology and Infectious Disease. Philadelphia, W. B. Saunders Company, 1981, pp 1201–1210.

McFarlane ES, Embil JA, Manuel FR, et al: Antibodies to hepatitis A antigen in relation to number of lifetime sexual partners in patients attending an STD clinic. Br J Vener Dis 1981; 57:58.

Mertz GJ, Jourden P, Peterman G, et al: Herpes simplex virus type-2 glycoprotein subunit vaccine: Tolerance and immunogenicity. Presented at American Federation of Clinical Research, Western Section, Carmel, Calif, 1983.

Mertz GJ, Jourden J, Winter C, et al: Sexual transmission of initial genital herpes (HSV): Implications for prevention. (Abstract 622.) Presented at 21st Interscience Conference on Antimicrobial Agents and Chemotherapy, Chicago, 1981.

Mertz GJ, Reichman R, Dolin R, et al: Double-blind placebo controlled trial of oral acyclovir for first-episode genital herpes. Presented at 22nd Interscience Conference on Antimicrobial Agents and Chemotherapy, Miami Beach, 1982.

Middleton WD, et al: Acute scrotal disorders: Prospective comparison of color Doppler US and testicular scintigraphy. Radiology 1990; 177:177–181.

Mindel A, Adler MW, Sutherland S, et al: Intravenous acyclovir treatment for primary genital herpes. Lancet 1982; 1:697.

Mitchell CJ, Huins TJ: Acute brucellosis presenting as epididymo-orchitis. (Letter.) Br Med J 1974; 2:557.

Mittemeyer JT, Lennox KW, Borski AA: Epididymitis: A review of 610 cases. J Urol 1966; 95:390.

Moore CA, Lockett BL, Lennox KW, et al: Prednisone in the treatment of acute epididymitis: A cooperative study. J Urol 1971; 106:578.

Morse SA: Chancroid and *Haemophilus ducreyi*. Clin Microbiol Rev 1989; 2:137–157.

Moseley R, Corey L, Winter C, et al: Comparison of the indirect immunoperoxidase and direct immunofluorescence technique with viral isolation for the diagnosis of genital herpes simplex virus infection. J Clin Microbiol 1981; 13:913.

Nahmias AJ, Naib ZM, Josey WE: Prospective studies of the association of genital herpes simplex virus infection and cervical anaplasia. Cancer Res 1973; 33:1491.

Nahmias AJ, Roizman D: Infection with herpes simplex virus 1 and 2. N Engl J Med 1973; 29:667.

Nilson AE, Aasen T, Halsos AM, et al: Efficacy of oral acyclovir in the treatment of initial and recurrent genital herpes. Lancet 1981; 2:571.

Oates JK, Greenhouse PR: Retention of urine in anogenital herpetic infection. Lancet 1978; 1:691.

Olier C: Diagnosis of acute chlamydial epididymitis. Prog Reprod Biol 1981; 8:161.

Oriel JD: Natural history of genital warts. Br J Vener Dis 1971; 47:1.

Oriel JD, Almeida JD: Demonstration of virus particles in human genital warts. Br J Vener Dis 1970; 37:37.

Oriel JD, Reeve P, Thomas BJ, et al: Infection with *Chlamydia* group A in men with urethritis due to *Neisseria gonorrhoeae*. J Infect Dis 1975; 131:376.

Orkin M, Maibach HI: Scabies therapy—1993. Semin Dermatol 1993; 12:22–25.

Ostergard DR: The effect of age, gravidity, and parity on the location of the cervical squamo-columnar junction as determined by colposcopy. Am J Obstet Gynecol 1977; 129:59–63.

Paavonen J, Kousa M, Saikku P, et al: Examination of men with nongonococcal urethritis and their sexual partners for *Chlamydia trachomatis* and *Ureaplasma urealyticum*. Sex Transm Dis 1978; 5:93.

Pearson RC, Baumber CD, McGhie D, Thambar IV: The relevance of *Chlamydia trachomatis* in acute epididymitis in young men. Br J Urol 1988; 62:72.

Pedersen AHB, Bonin P: Screening females for asymptomatic gonorrhea infection. Northwest Med 1971; 70:255.

Pederson JF, Holm HH, Hald T: Torsion of the testes diagnosed by ultrasound. J Urol 1975; 113:66.

Pelouze PS: Epididymitis. *In* Gonorrhea in the Male and Female. Philadelphia, W. B. Saunders Company, 1941.

Perroud HM, Miedzybrodzka K: Chlamydial infection of the urethra in men. Br J Vener Dis 1978; 54:45.

Pessione F, Dolivo M, Casin I: Sexual behavior and smoking: Risk factor for urethritis in men. Sex Transm Dis 1988; 15:119–122.

Peterson EP, Schmidt OW, Goldstein LG, et al: Typing of clinical HSV isolates using mouse monoclonal antibodies to HSV-1 and HSV-2: Comparison with type-specific rabbit antisera and restriction endonuclease analysis of viral DNA. J Clin Microbiol 1983; 17:92.

Portnoy J, Mendelson J, Clecner B, et al: Asymptomatic gonorrhea in the male. Can Med Assoc J 1974; 110:169.

Potts JF: Chlamydial infection. Screening and management update, 1992. Postgrad Med 1992; 91:120–126.

Quinn TC, Corey L, Chaffee RG: The etiology of anorectal infections in homosexual men. Am J Med 1981a; 71:395–406.

Quinn TC, Goodell SE, Mkrtichian E, et al: *Chlamydia trachomatis* proctitis. N Engl J Med 1981b; 305:195.

Ramstedt K, Forssman L, Johannisson G: Contact tracing in the control of genital *Chlamydia trachomatis*. Int J Study AIDS 1991; 2:116–118.

Reeves WC, Corey L, Adams HG, et al: Risk of recurrence after first episodes of genital herpes: Relation to HSV type and antibody response. N Engl J Med 1981; 305:315.

Reichman RC, Badger GJ, Guinan ME, et al: Topically administered acyclovir in the treatment of recurrent genital herpes simplex genitalis: A controlled trial. J Infect Dis 1983; 147:336.

Riccardi NB, Felman YM: Laboratory diagnosis in the problem of suspected gonococcal infection. JAMA 1979; 242:2703.

Richman DD, Cleveland PH, Oxman MN: A rapid enzyme immunofiltration technique using monoclonal antibodies to serotype herpes simplex virus. J Med Virol 1982; 9:299.

Richmond SJ, Hilton AL, Clark SKR: Chlamydial infection: Role of *Chlamydia* subgroup A in nongonococcal and postgonococcal urethritis. Br J Vener Dis 1972; 48:437.

Richmond SJ, Sparling PF: Genital chlamydial infections. Am J Epidemiol 1976; 103:428.

Ridgway GL, Taylor-Robinson D: Current problems in microbiology: 1. Chlamydial infections: Which laboratory test? Gen Clin Pathol 1991; 44:1–5.

Riehle RA, Williams JJ: Transient neuropathic bladder following herpes simplex genitalis. J Urol 1979; 122:283.

Ripa KT, Mardh PA, Thelin I: *Chlamydia trachomatis* urethritis in men attending a venereal disease clinic: A culture and therapeutic study. Acta Derm Venereol 1978; 58:175.

Robinson WS: The enigma of non-A, non-B hepatitis. J Infect Dis 1982; 145:387.

Rolfs RT, Goldberg M, Sharrar RG: Risk factors for syphilis: Cocaine use and prostitution. Am J Public Health 1990; 80:853–857.

Rolfs RT, Nakishima AK: Epidemiology of primary and secondary syphilis in the United States, 1981–1989. JAMA 1990; 264:1432–1437.

Ronald AR, Plummer FA: Chancroid and granuloma inguinale. Clin Lab Med 1989; 9:535–543.

Root TE, Edwards LD, Spengler PJ: Nongonococcal urethritis: A survey of clinical and laboratory features. Sex Transms Dis 1980; 7:59.

Schachter J: Chlamydial infections. N Engl J Med 1978; 298:423.

Scheibel JH, Anderson JT, Brandenhoff P, et al: *Chlamydia trachomatis* in acute epididymitis. Scand J Urol Nephrol 1983; 17:47.

Scriba M: Protection of guinea pigs against primary and recurrent genital herpes infections by immunization with live heterologous or homologous herpes simplex virus: Implications for herpes virus vaccine. Med Microbiol Immunol 1978; 166:63.

Segura JW, Smith TF, Weed LA, et al: *Chlamydia* and nonspecific urethritis. J Urol 1977; 117:720.

Shapiro SR, Breschi CC: Acute epididymitis in Vietnam: Review of 52 cases. Mil Med 1973; 138:643.

Simmons PD: Evaluation of the early morning smear investigation. Br J Vener Dis 1978; 54:128.

Smith DR: Treatment of epididymitis by infiltration of the spermatic cord with procaine HCl. J Urol 1971; 46:74.

Smith GL, Greenup R, Takafuji ET: Circumcision as a risk factor for urethritis in racial groups. Am J Public Health 1987; 77:452–454.

Sorensen RC: Adolescent Sexuality in Contemporary America. New York, World Publishing Company, 1972, p 122.

Spruance SL, Crumpacker CS, Schnipper LE, et al: Topical 10% acyclovir (ACV) in polyethylene glycol (PEG) for herpes simplex labialis: Results of treatment begun in the prodrome and erythema stages. Presented at the 22nd Interscience Conference on Antimicrobial Agents and Chemotherapy, Miami Beach, October 1982.

Stamm WE: Diagnosis of *Neisseria gonorrhoeae* and *Chlamydia trachomatis* infections using antigen detection methods. Diagn Microbiol Infect Dis 1986; 4(suppl 3):936.

Stamm WE: Diagnosis of *Chlamydia trachomatis* genitourinary infections. Ann Intern Med 1988; 108:710–717.

Stamm WE, Hick CB, Martin DH, et al: Azithromycin for empirical treatment of the nongonococcal urethritis syndrome in men: A randomized double-blind study. JAMA 1995; 274(7):577–579.

Stimson JB, Hale J, Bowie WR, Holmes KK: Tetracycline resistant *Ureaplasma urealyticum*: A cause of persistent urethritis. Ann Intern Med 1981; 94:192.

Strauss SE, Seidland NM, Tikiff HE: Effect of oral acyclovir treatment on symptomatic and asymptomatic virus shedding in recurrent herpes. Sex Transm Dis 1989; 16:107–113.

Sufrin G: Acute epididymitis. Sex Transm Dis 1980; 8:132.

Swartz SL, Kraus SJ, Herrmann KL, et al: Diagnosis and etiology of nongonococcal urethritis. J Infect Dis 1978; 138:445.

Syrjanen KJ, Heinonen UM, Kauraniemi T: Cytologic evidence of the association of condylomatous lesions with dysplastic and neoplastic changes in the uterine cervix. Acta Cytol 1981; 25:17.

Taylor-Robinson D, McCormack WM: The genital mycoplasmas. N Engl J Med 1980; 302:1003.

Terho P: *Chlamydia trachomatis* in gonococcal and post-gonococcal urethritis. Br J Vener Dis 1978a; 54:326.

Terho P: *Chlamydia trachomatis* in nonspecific urethritis. Br J Vener Dis 1978b; 5:93.

Thayer JD, Martin JE: A selective medium for the cultivation of *N. gonorrhoeae* and *N. meningitidis*. Public Health Rep 1964; 79:49.

Thelin I, Wennstrom Am, Mardh PA: Contact tracing in patients with genital chlamydial infection. Br J Vener Dis 1980; 56:93.

Thomas D, Simpson K, Ostojic H, et al: Bacteremic epididymo-orchitis due to *Hemophilus influenzae* type B. J Urol 1981; 126:832.

Thompson SE, Washington AE: Epidemiology of sexually transmitted *Chlamydia trachomatis* infections. Epidemiol Rev 1983; 5:96–123.

Trambert MA, Mattrey RF, Levine D, Berthoty DP: Subacute scrotal pain: Evaluation of torsion versus epididymitis with MR imaging. Radiology 1990; 175:53–56.

Van Dyck E, Piot P: Laboratory techniques in the investigation of chancroid, lymphogranuloma venereum and donovanosis. Genitourin Med 1992; 68:130–133.

Vaughn-Jackson JD, Dunlop EMC, Daroughar S, et al: Urethritis due to *Chlamydia trachomatis*. Br J Vener Dis 1977; 53:180.

Vieras F: Evolution of acute epididymitis to testicular infarction. Scintigraphic demonstration. *Clin Nucl Med* 1986; 11:158.

Wallin JE, Thompson SE, Zaidi A, et al: Urethritis in women attending an STD clinic. Br J Vener Dis 1981; 57:50.

Watson RA: Gonorrhea and acute epididymitis. Mil Med 1979; 144:785.

Wentworth BB, Bonin P, Holmes KK, et al: Isolation of viruses, bacteria and other organisms from venereal disease clinic patients: Methodology and problems associated with multiple isolations. Health Lab Sci 1973; 10:75.

Westrom L: Effect of acute pelvic inflammatory disease on fertility. Am J Obstet Gynecol 1975; 121:707.

Westrom L: Incidence, prevalence, and trends of acute pelvic inflammatory disease and its consequences in industrialized countries. Am J Obstet Gynecol 1980; 1138:880.

Wiesner PJ: Selected aspects of the epidemiology of nongonococcal urethritis. *In* Hobson D, Holmes KK, ed: Nongonococcal Urethritis and Related Oculogenital Infections. Washington, DC, The American Society for Microbiology, 1977, pp 9–14.

Wilbert DM, Schaerfe CW, Stern WD: Evaluation of the acute scrotum by color-coded Doppler ultrasonography. J Urol 1993; 149:1475–1477.

William DC: Hepatitis and other sexually transmitted diseases in gay men and lesbians. Sex Transm Dis 1981; 8(suppl.):330.

Wong JL, Hines PA, Brasher MD, et al: The etiology of nongonococcal urethritis in men attending a venereal disease clinic. Sex Transm Dis 1977; 4:4.

19

ACQUIRED IMMUNODEFICIENCY SYNDROME AND RELATED CONDITIONS

John N. Krieger, M.D.

Acquired immunodeficiency syndrome (AIDS) is the most severe clinical manifestation of infection with human immunodeficiency virus (HIV). The syndrome is defined by development of serious opportunistic infections, neoplasms, or other life-threatening conditions resulting from progressive immunosuppression caused by HIV infection.

The first cases of AIDS were described in 1981, and the number of reported cases has increased rapidly. The first 100,000 AIDS cases were reported during an 8-year period, whereas the second 100,000 cases were reported in a 2-year period. Over 440,000 cases of AIDS were reported in the United States by 1994 (Centers for Disease Control and Prevention, 1994; Chamberland et al, 1995). Dramatic progress has led to specific antiviral chemotherapy and improved management of opportunistic infections. It is now necessary to understand certain basic concepts to provide optimal treatment for increasing numbers of patients with HIV infections encountered in the everyday practice of urology.

The exponential growth of knowledge about AIDS and related conditions means that much of the most current information will be dated within a very short period. This chapter emphasizes basic concepts on which continued progress will be based, rather than the newest forms of chemotherapy or details of clinical management. Thus, I begin with the biology of this infection. Much is now known about this basic subject. Furthermore, understanding basic ideas should help urologists deal with major changes in medical care and social and economic issues. I consider the clinical manifestations and epidemiology briefly. Little emphasis is given to specific issues in treatment since general medical management of patients with AIDS and HIV infections is outside the practice of most urologists. In contrast, I emphasize specific issues of urologic interest.

BIOLOGY OF HIV AND RELATED RETROVIRUSES

The acquired immunodeficiency syndrome was first described in 1981. Early identification of major routes of transmission by sexual contact among homosexual men, and transmission to hemophiliacs and others receiving transfusions, suggested the role of an infectious agent. The use of information and methods based on earlier work with retroviruses led to the development of diagnostic tests and rapid advances in understanding the etiology of the disease and routes of transmission. In addition, effective and specific antiretroviral treatment has substantially improved clinical management. This section defines the unique properties of retroviruses and considers HIV, the causative agent of AIDS in the context of other retroviruses.

Retroviruses

The "usual" flow of genetic information is from DNA to RNA, a process termed *transcription,* and then from the RNA to protein, a process termed *translation.* In retroviruses this flow of genetic information is different. Retroviruses contain their genetic information in RNA. During replication a copy of the viral RNA is transcribed by the viral DNA polymerase (called *reverse transcriptase,* because the flow of information is from RNA to DNA). This process of reverse transcription is the distinctive characteristic of the retroviruses. The viral DNA is integrated into the host cell genome to establish infection (Fig. 19–1) (Watkins et al, 1995). Infection with retroviruses seldom results in lysis of host cells. Thus retroviral infection tends to be permanent. Viral propagation within the infected cell can proceed either through production of new virus particles followed by infection of new cells (horizontal transmission) or by replication of infected cells (vertical transmission).

Retroviruses and Cancers

Retroviruses were first described in leukemias and lymphomas in chickens. In the early 1950s murine leukemia virus, a retrovirus, was shown to cause leukemia in inbred strains of laboratory mice. Many other retroviruses have

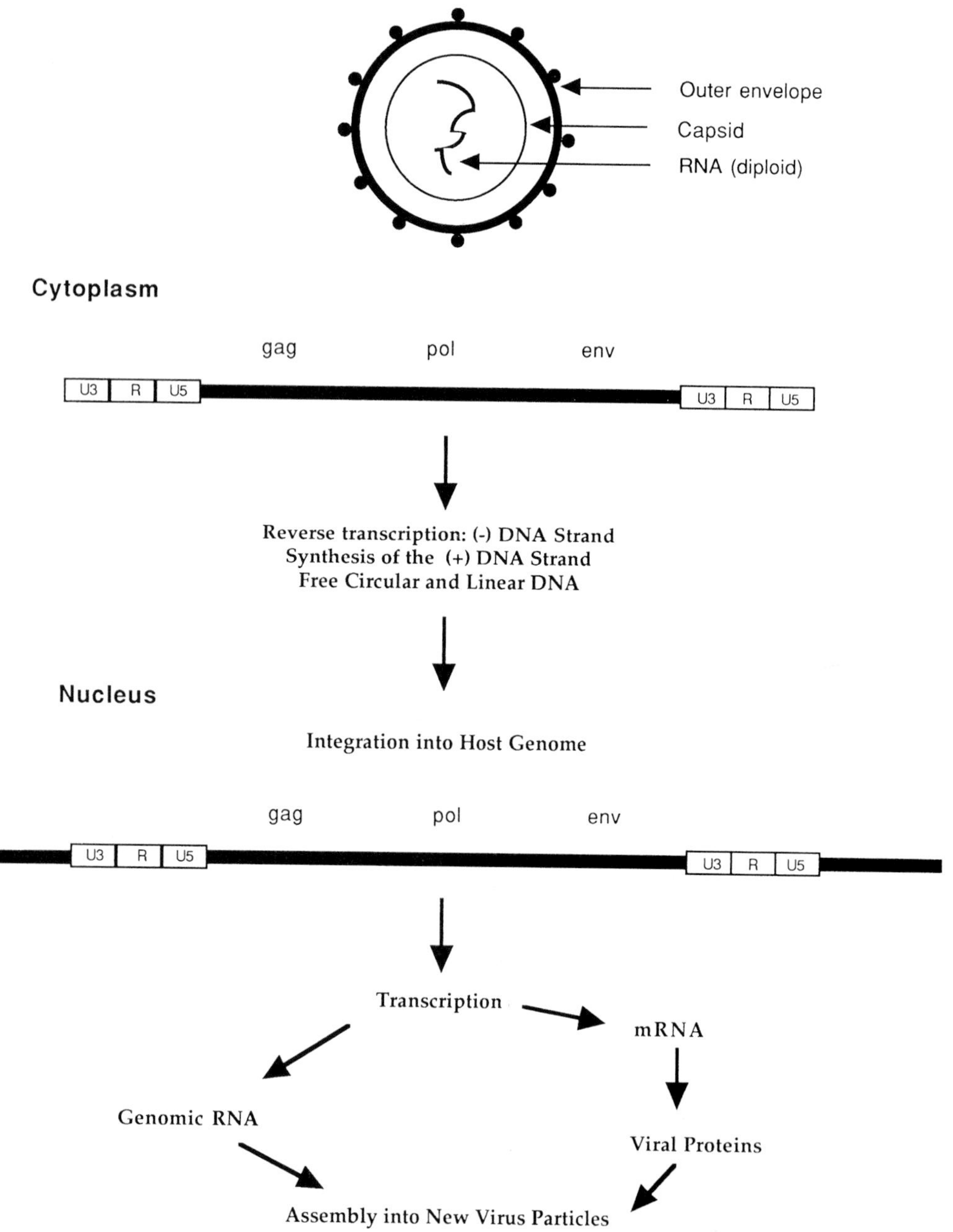

Figure 19–1. The human immunodeficiency virus (HIV) life cycle. The retrovirus attaches to and penetrates the host cell surface. The RNA of the virus is uncoated in the host cell cytoplasm, followed by reverse transcription into linear double-stranded DNA. This viral DNA is transported into the host cell nucleus, where it is first circularized and then integrated into the host genome as proviral DNA. The provirus is transcribed into viral RNA, which can either become viral genomic RNA or serve as a template for messenger RNAs (mRNAs), which are translated into viral proteins. (After Watkins BA, Klotman ME, Gallo RC: Human immunodeficiency viruses. *In* Mandell GL, ed: Principles and Practice of Infectious Diseases, 4th ed. New York, Churchill Livingstone, 1995, pp 1590–1606).

been identified as the causes of malignancies in animals, such as feline leukemia virus, which causes lymphosarcoma in cats after a long latent phase (Watkins et al, 1995). By the early 1970s leukemias in the gibbon apes had proved to have a retroviral cause. To date, however, efforts at identifying human retroviruses associated with leukemias have been disappointing (Watkins et al, 1995).

There was no convincing isolation of a biologically active human retrovirus until 1982. The critical technical advance was the development of a tissue culture system that supported long-term growth of human T cells to establish cultures from a variety of human T-cell neoplasms. Using these methods plus sensitive assays for reverse transcriptase, Poiez and others isolated the first human retroviruses from patients with cutaneous T-cell neoplasms. This virus was termed human T-lymphotrophic virus type I (HTLV-I) (Watkins et al, 1995). These neoplasms were actually a disease that is now termed adult T-cell leukemia. A related virus was isolated from a patient with a T-cell variant of hairy cell leukemia. This virus was termed human T-lymphotrophic virus II (HTLV-II) and was the second human retrovirus.

Identification of HIV

AIDS was first described based on clinical findings, and several features suggested an infectious cause. These features included clustering of cases and transmission by sexual contact and blood products. In addition, a number of findings suggested that a retrovirus might be the causative agent. First, AIDS was a T-cell disease, and the known human retroviruses were T-cell-trophic. Second, a number of animal retroviruses, such as feline leukemia virus, are associated with immunosuppression (Watkins et al, 1995). Third, there was a long delay between transmission and illness, consistent with other retroviral diseases. Finally, because the agent could be transmitted by filtered blood products, it could not be a bacterium or other large microorganism.

In 1983, Barre-Sinoussi and associates (1983) identified a retrovirus that ultimately proved to be the causative agent. Because this virus was highly cytotoxic for T cells, it was difficult to grow in quantity. Characterization of the virus became possible after identification of a T-cell line that permitted replication of the virus. The causative agent is now termed human immunodeficiency virus type 1 (HIV-1). Other names for this virus include lymphadenopathy-associated virus and human T-lymphotrophic virus type III. The fact that the causative agent of AIDS is a retrovirus made it possible to predict many of the unusual virus-host relationships and the formidable difficulties that must be overcome to control a slow virus infection (Hasse, 1995).

Characteristics of HIV

HIV is a retrovirus in the subfamily termed lentiviruses. In Latin, *lentus* means "slow." This is because infections caused by lentiviruses characteristically take months or years between infection of the host and the appearance of symptoms (Hasse, 1995). In contrast, other subfamilies of retroviruses transform cells in culture and induce tumors in a variety of species (oncogenic retroviruses) or establish persistent and inapparent infections. It is now clear that HIV-1 is not closely related to the human T-lymphotrophic viruses, HTLV-I and HTLV-II, as was initially thought (Hasse, 1995).

The lentiviruses are genetically heterogeneous, with great diversity in the region of the genomic areas coding for the viral envelope protein. This diversity is important because the viral envelope is the area that comes in direct contact with the host immune system. Using techniques and probes for HIV-1, researchers identified in humans from western Africa a distantly related virus that also causes AIDS. This virus has been termed human immunodeficiency virus type 2 (HIV-2). HIV-1 and HIV-2 are distinct antigenically and differ in pathogenicity. HIV-2 appears to be transmitted less readily than HIV-1, and the virus appears less virulent. HIV-2 is otherwise similar to HIV-1 in many respects. Both viruses have similar modes of transmission, and HIV-2 also causes an immunodeficiency syndrome. Because very few cases of HIV-2 infection have been identified in the United States, this chapter focuses on infection caused by HIV-1.

Like other lentiviruses, HIV-1 has a spherical shape and an outer envelope, variable surface projections, and an icosahedral capsid containing ribonucleoprotein complexed with a core shell (Fig. 19–2) (Hasse, 1995). Seventy-two knoblike

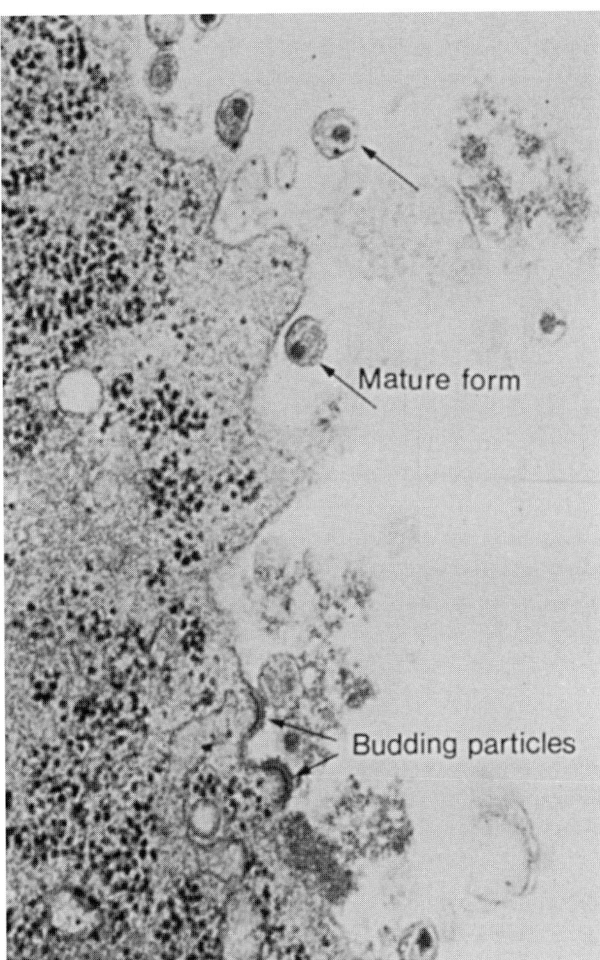

Figure 19–2. Like other lentiviruses, HIV has a spherical shape, an outer envelope, variable surface projections, and an icosohedral capsid containing ribonucleoprotein complexed with a core shell. (Electron micrograph courtesy of Centers for Disease Control and Prevention.)

projections protrude from the virion surface (Watkins et al, 1995). These envelope structures are composed of glycoproteins, termed gp 120 and gp41. The conical core of HIV also appears to be typical of other lentiviruses, with a major structural polypeptide (p24) and other polypeptides derived from a common precursor to form a shell around the core or complex with the virion RNA (Hasse, 1995).

Current evidence suggests that HIV-1 and HIV-2 both originated in other primates with subsequent infection of humans (Hasse, 1995). These data were obtained by comparing HIV-1 and HIV-2 with related retroviruses that infect monkeys and great apes, termed simian immunodeficiency viruses. Genetically, HIV-1 is related most closely to a simian immunodeficiency virus isolated from chimpanzees. HIV-2 is closest to a simian immunodeficiency virus isolated from sooty mangabey monkeys. The close similarity in genetic sequences, documented infection of humans with simian immunodeficiency virus, and benign nature or natural infection in simian hosts suggest that HIV originated in a primate, likely in Africa, with subsequent infection of humans. Such trans-species infections are often associated with increased virulence.

Pathogenesis of HIV-1 (Fig. 19–1)

Establishment of Infection

After gaining entry to the host, the first step in HIV-1 infection is binding of the virus particle to the surface of a target cell. This process is mediated by the gp120 molecule on the envelope of the virion to the CD4 protein found on the surface of most helper T lymphocytes (CD4+ T cells). After binding to the host cell surface, the virus is internalized and its genetic material is released into the host cell cytoplasm. The viral RNA is then transcribed by the reverse transcriptase into a linear double-stranded viral DNA in the host cell cytoplasm. This viral DNA is transported to the nucleus, where it is integrated into the host cell genetic material. After integration of the viral genetic material, the host cell is persistently infected. This means that the only way to "cure" the infection is to eliminate all infected cells in the host.

Production of Virus from Infected Cells

The integrated viral DNA, termed *provirus,* is transcribed into messenger RNA (mRNA) by the host cell's RNA polymerase. The rate of transcription is regulated by viral sequences termed *promoter, enhancer,* and *negative regulatory elements.* The full-length RNA transcript can serve a variety of different functions: (1) it may be packaged within virus particles serving as a genome for progeny virus; (2) it may serve as the mRNA template for synthesis of viral structural gene products; or (3) it may serve a regulatory function (Watkins et al, 1995).

Viral mRNAs are translated into structural polypeptide precursors. HIV-1 contains three genes, termed *gag, pol,* and *env,* that are similar to genes in other retroviruses (see Fig. 19–1) (Stanley and Fauci, 1995). The *gag* translational products are viral core proteins. The *env* gene products form the viral envelope proteins. The *pol* gene products include the reverse transcriptase, a protease, and integrase. Structural components of the virus are assembled at the cell surface. Mature virions then bud from the cell surface and attach to other susceptible cells (see Fig. 19–2). HIV-1 can also induce fusion of host cells with other cells, forming large syncytia. In this fashion, infected and uninfected cells can fuse. Thus, HIV-1 may also be transmitted from one host cell to another without being exposed to the humoral immune system of the host.

Expression of the *gag, pol,* and *env* genes occurs through binding of regulatory proteins to promoter and enhancer sequences in the long terminal repeat (LTR) regions that flank both the 5′ and 3′ ends of the genome (Stanley and Fauci, 1995). The HIV genome also encodes for several regulatory proteins. The best studied regulatory elements include *tat,* the transactivator leading to increased viral transcription; *rev,* which enhances unspliced mRNA levels; and *nef,* which can either increase or decrease viral transcription under different circumstances. Other regulatory genes include *vif,* or virion infectivity factor; *vpu,* or viral protein U, which facilitates envelope processing and viral budding; and *vpr,* or viral protein R, whose function remains unknown. The complexity of the HIV genome endows this virus with a versatility lacking in other viruses. The HIV viral regulatory genes are of great interest to researchers because they represent potential sites for antiretroviral therapy that may be substantially more effective than available agents.

Since the CD4 molecule is the primary receptor for HIV, any cell that expresses this protein is a target for infection with HIV (Stanley and Fauci, 1995). The CD4+ T lymphocyte is extraordinarily susceptible and is the predominant cell type targeted by HIV. However, cells of the monocyte-macrophage lineage also express CD4 and can be infected. Although the hallmark of infection with HIV is progressive depletion of CD4+ T cells, a broad array of defects also occurs in the function of a variety of immune cell types. In some instances, for example, with CD4+ T lymphocytes, these defects are due to direct infection of the cells, whereas other effects on immunologic function are indirect.

Pathogenesis

Depletion of a particular type of T cells (CD4+) is a primary manifestation of HIV-1 infection. HIV-1 can lyse cultured CD4+ T cells, but the basis for this is incompletely understood (Watkins et al, 1995). One aspect appears to be formation of large, multicellular syncytia in which one infected cell can account for the death of many other noninfected cells. This process appears to depend on expression of the CD4 antigen on the surface of susceptible cells. In addition, infected cells can be killed without syncytia formation. Depletion of CD4+ T cells accounts for much of the profound depression in cell-mediated immune function that is characteristic of AIDS. In general, the secondary complications of opportunistic infections and neoplasms develop at levels below 200 cells/mm^3. Monitoring of the total CD4+ T cell count is the standard method for following disease progression because these levels correlate with the severity of immune suppression. The case definition of AIDS was modified recently to include patients with a total CD4+ T cell count below 200/mm^3 without symptoms or any other AIDS-defining illness.

Infected persons develop serum antibodies that neutralize viral infectivity in vitro, but the presence of such antibodies does not lead to protection of the host (Walker et al, 1987). Besides a serologic response, HIV-1 also elicits a cell-mediated immune response, including the production of cytotoxic T cells, but these cells also fail to provide protection against the virus (Walker et al, 1987). Some workers believe that hypervariable regions in the virus envelope mutate quickly, leading to selection of variants of the virus that evade the host immune response. Experimental data supporting this view include the demonstration that growth of cloned virus in the presence of neutralizing antiserum from a healthy infected individual can lead to emergence of a neutralization-resistant variant (Watkins et al, 1995).

An acute illness resembling mononucleosis may occur at the time of seroconversion, but HIV-1 infection is characterized by prolonged clinical latency (Moss and Bachetti, 1989) with the median period of latency estimated to be approximately 10 years (Fig. 19–3) (Stanley and Fauci, 1995). Viral replication continues, associated with a gradual erosion of immune competence, during this clinically quiescent period. Opportunistic infections and malignancies develop as the person becomes progressively immunosuppressed.

Lymphoid Organ Involvement

Data suggest that lymphoid tissues are critical in the pathogenesis and progression of HIV-1 infection (Branson, 1995; Stanley and Fauci, 1995). After HIV-1 enters the body through the blood stream or mucosa, the virus localizes in regional lymph nodes. The viremia during primary infection results in extensive dissemination of HIV-1 to other lymphoid organs. The HIV-1–specific immune response then leads to follicular hyperplasia and sequestration of infected CD4+ cells in the lymphoid organs, with lower levels of viral replication in peripheral blood. During this phase the infection appears to be latent clinically, but active viral replication continues in the lymphoid organs. Up to 25% of CD4+ lymphocytes and fixed-tissue macrophages are infected with HIV-1 at this point, and follicular dendritic cells may transmit infection to additional cells as they migrate through lymphoid follicles. The immune depletion characteristic of AIDS results from slow elimination of latently infected cells as they are recognized and killed by the immune system. With evolution of HIV-1 infection, lymph node architecture is disrupted and follicular dendritic cells die in enormous numbers. The immune response against HIV-1 is lost, and the viral burden in peripheral blood increases, reflecting the spillover of virus from lymphoid organs.

Antiretroviral Strategies

HIV-1 has developed mechanisms that allow it to persist, spread, and cause disease in the presence of natural immunity. As summarized above, these mechanisms include covert infection of cells and tissues, blood, and secretions, as well as refuge in the central nervous system outside the blood-brain barrier. The second major problem is that, like other lentiviruses, HIV-1 can produce antigenic variants that may be freed temporarily from immune restraints. Because of these problems, many workers believe that the only way to

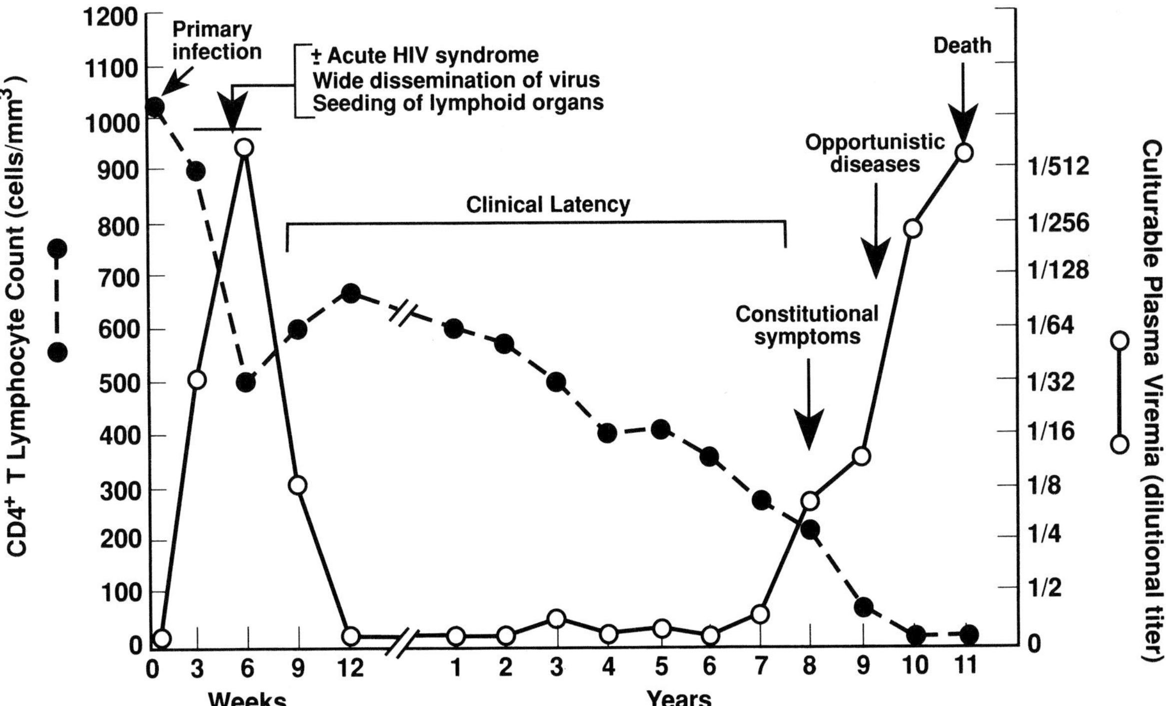

Figure 19–3. Hypothetical course of HIV infection. Wide dissemination of virus occurs during the primary infection associated with a sharp decline in the CD4+ T-cell count. The subsequent immune response is accompanied by lower levels of culturable HIV levels in peripheral blood and a lengthy period of clinical latency. However, the CD4+ T-cell count continues to decline during this period. After a critical reduction in systemic immune function the risk of opportunistic infections or malignancies increases dramatically. (From Stanley SK, Fauci AS: Immunology of AIDS and HIV infection. *In* Mandell GL, ed: Principles and Practice of Infectious Diseases, 4th ed. New York, Churchill Livingstone, 1995, 1203–1217.)

control HIV-1 is to view it as an intracellular pathogen and seek methods to maintain dormancy of the virus and prevent progression to disease.

Another strategy is to develop means to prevent infection in the first place. For example, it may be possible to block entry of the virus into susceptible cells or to block subsequent steps in the viral life cycle. The goals are to limit the number of infected cells, to limit the adverse effects of viral infection in persons who already harbor the virus by preventing replication within infected cells, and to limit the spread of virus within and between individuals.

Avoiding Infection

At present the only means to control HIV-1 infection is to avoid exposure to the virus. For this reason education is critical to persuade people to avoid high-risk behaviors, in particular intravenous drug use and promiscuity. Current programs for screening blood for antibodies to HIV-1 have almost totally eliminated transfusion-associated infections in the United States. The problem remains that many people are already infected and that others will continue to practice high-risk behaviors. Thus, additional strategies are needed for dealing with this infection.

Vaccines

Development of a vaccine to prevent infection by HIV-1 is an attractive strategy. There are many difficult obstacles to be overcome (Dolin and Keefer, 1995). First, the high degree of variability among HIV-1 strains may make development of a vaccine difficult. The most variable region appears to be the viral envelope or surface. Since this is the site of initial interaction with the host immune system, these envelope proteins are major targets for the development of neutralizing antibodies. An effective vaccine must exhibit activity against a broad range of types of this virus. Unfortunately, very small changes in the *env* gene may produce large changes in the viral surface, limiting the ability to develop neutralizing antibodies (Watkins et al, 1995).

A second problem is that there is no good animal model system in which to test vaccines. Use of chimpanzees has been the standard to date, but these large apes are scarce and expensive to maintain, and infected animals do not develop disease. Carrying out studies in humans presents additional problems. Immunized people will test positive for the virus, and those who have received candidate vaccines cannot ethically be challenged with a lethal virus.

A third problem with vaccine development is that persons with natural infections are known to develop antibodies against HIV-1. Such persons develop AIDS despite the presence of these antibodies, suggesting that it may be difficult for many humans to mount a long-lasting, protective response against HIV-1 (Watkins et al, 1995). Humans infected with HIV-1 exhibit humoral and cell-mediated immune responses against a variety of viral antigens. However, correlation of specific immune responses with protection from infection and/or disease has not been accomplished. Many investigators hope that if we could develop higher levels of antibodies before the first exposure to the virus, then protection against infection might occur.

Because of the uncertainty regarding the optimal immune responses, a wide variety of candidate vaccines have been proposed. At least 20 candidate HIV-1 vaccines have reached trials in humans. Most of these trials are phase 1 studies in seronegative volunteers, but in some cases studies have enrolled asymptomatic HIV-1–seropositive individuals.

Antiviral Chemotherapy

Treatment is necessary for persons who are already infected to eliminate or limit the spread of the virus. During the past decade, a number of agents have been developed that have proved useful (Corey, 1995). Established agents are all dideoxynucleoside compounds, including zidovudine (ZDV, AZT), didanosine (ddI), and zalcitabine (ddC). Optimal use of these drugs remains highly controversial (Corey, 1995). The major problem is that these drugs have relatively low potency. This low therapeutic potency is related to the complexity of the HIV-1 life cycle that provides the virus with a unique opportunity for continued persistence within the host (see Fig. 19–1). In addition, the rapid mutational variety of HIV-1 represents a formidable challenge for development of long-standing antiviral therapy. However, the complex life cycle of HIV-1 also provides many potential targets for therapeutic agents.

The enzyme reverse transcriptase is a unique feature of retroviruses such as HIV-1. Thus, inhibition of reverse transcriptase activity represents an attractive target for antiretroviral drugs. This is the target for the dideoxynucleosides. These compounds are essentially prodrugs that are activated metabolically to their respective 5′-triphosphates by cellular enzymes. These compounds are incorporated into the growing HIV-1 DNA chain. Since they lack a 3′ hydroxyl group, this terminates elongation of the DNA chain. Unfortunately, all current dideoxynucleosides inhibit HIV-1 replication only partially. All have significant side effects that complicate long-term use. In addition, resistance has been described for all available dideoxynucleosides that appears to limit their long-term utility.

The problem with antiretroviral drug development is that the life cycle of the virus is intimately connected with cellular processes, making development of selective activity against the virus very difficult. The initial step of viral binding to the host cellular receptor is one unique step in viral replication that may be amenable to therapy. Interference at this point may limit infection. In vitro truncated forms of soluble CD4 can inhibit viral infection without inhibiting T cell function. Dextran sulfate can also selectively inhibit infection by binding to the CD4 site. This approach might prove useful very early after infection. After this stage this approach would not limit the spread of the virus by the formation of cellular syncytia in which there is no cell-free virus. Another site where an antiretroviral drug might act is during integration of the viral DNA into the cellular genome. Many other steps in the viral life cycle, such as transcription of viral DNA to RNA, translation of viral mRNA into proteins, or processing of these proteins, are carried out by cellular components. Such steps are expected to afford few targets for antiviral chemotherapy. In contrast, the regulatory genes appear to be unique to the virus. Some products of these genes may be absolutely necessary for virus replication. Thus, it may be possible to inhibit the gene products of these regulatory genes selec-

Table 19–1. ACQUIRED IMMUNODEFICIENCY SYNDROME CASE DEFINITION

Bacterial infections, multiple or recurrent in children under 13 years old
Candidiasis of bronchi, trachea, lungs, or esophagus
Cervical cancer, invasive*
Coccidioidomycosis, disseminated or extrapulmonary
Cryptococcosis, extrapulmonary
Cryptosporidiosis, chronic intestinal (>1 month's duration)
Cytomegalovirus
Disease other than liver, spleen, or nodes
Retinitis (with loss of vision)
Encephalopathy (HIV-related)
Herpes simplex, chronic ulcers (>1 month's duration)
Bronchitis, pneumonitis, or esophagitis
Histoplasmosis, disseminated or extrapulmonary
Isosporiasis, chronic intestinal (>1 month's duration)
Kaposi's sarcoma
Lymphoid interstitial pneumonia and/or pulmonary lymphoid hyperplasia in children under 13 years old
Lymphoma, Burkitt's (or equivalent term)
Lymphoma, immunoblastic (or equivalent term)
Lymphoma, primary of brain
Mycobacterium avium–intracellulare complex or *M. kansasii*, disseminated or extrapulmonary
Mycobacterium tuberculosis, any site (pulmonary* or extrapulmonary)
Mycobacterium, other species or unidentified species, disseminated or extrapulmonary
Pneumocystis carinii pneumonia
Pneumonia, recurrent*
Progressive multifocal leukoencephalopathy
Salmonella septicemia, recurrent
Toxoplasmosis of brain
Wasting syndrome due to HIV

*Conditions added to the 1993 AIDS surveillance case definition.

From Centers for Disease Control and Prevention: 1993 Revised classification system for HIV infection and expanded surveillance case definition for AIDS among adolescents and adults. MMWR 1992; 41(RR-17):1–19.

HIV, human immunodeficiency virus; AIDS, acquired immunodeficiency syndrome.

tively to limit the infection. Finally, viral proteins are assembled at the host cell surface into mature virions. Interference with this assembly process is another potential site for antiviral intervention.

The feeling of most researchers is that there are many potential ways to interfere with viral infection, expression, and spread within a susceptible host, but that it is unlikely that any one method will be sufficient. Effective antiviral chemotherapy will likely require a combination of approaches.

Opportunistic Infections

Survival has improved dramatically for patients with HIV-1 infection since AIDS was first recognized in the early 1980s. Although much of this improvement reflects effective antiretroviral therapy, a major contribution reflects more effective management of the opportunistic processes complicating HIV-1–related immunodeficiency (Masur, 1995). Patients with HIV-1 infection are highly susceptible to a unique constellation of pathogens (Table 19–1). Most of these opportunistic infections are believed to reflect reactivation of latent infection. Improvements in diagnosis and treatment are responsible for better outcomes for many HIV-1–associated infections. However, familiar pathogens, such as cytomegalovirus, *Candida,* and *Mycobacterium tuberculosis,* are increasingly resistant to the most widely used agents.

DIAGNOSIS, NATURAL HISTORY, AND CLASSIFICATION OF HIV-1 INFECTION

Diagnosis of HIV-1 Infection

Serologic tests that recognize antibodies against HIV-1 antigens are critical for diagnosis. Detecting anti–HIV-1 antibodies by enzyme-linked immunosorbent assay (ELISA) is highly sensitive (greater than 99%) and specific (95% to 99%) (Schleupner, 1995). Current technology is in the second or third generation, with recently developed ELISAs using polypeptide antigens of the HIV-1 core and envelope produced by recombinant DNA technology.

As with any test, the predictive value of a positive result depends on the prevalence of infected persons in the population being tested. Serum samples that are reactive should be retested, and repeatedly positive specimens confirmed with a second highly specific test. The most commonly used test is the Western blot. Immunofluorescence assays are also used for this purpose. When confirmed by one of these tests, specimens are considered as true positives, and individuals should be informed that they are infected and should be counseled about the implications of this infection. The risk of a false-positive result after completing the testing sequence is estimated to be 1 to 5 per 100,000 persons screened. Perhaps more important from a clinical perspective, estimates of the false-negative rate for HIV-1 antibody testing range from 1 in 40,000 to 1 in 1 million.

Other methods for diagnosis of HIV-1 infection include direct detection of viral antigens and cocultivation of the virus in cell culture. The sensitivity of antigen detection systems appears to be less than that of detection of antibodies against HIV-1 in most situations (Chaisson and Volberding, 1995). However, antigen detection schemes might be useful in selected patients shortly after infection (Fig. 19–4).

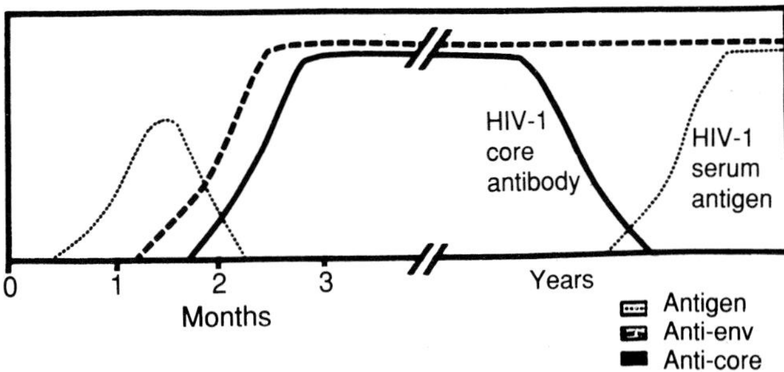

Figure 19–4. Hypothetical time course of immune response to infection with HIV. The chronology of HIV-1 infection is defined by the presence of core antigen (p24) and antibodies to core protein and envelope glycoprotein (gp41). After the initial "window period" there is a humoral immune response. Cell-free virus decreases in blood plasma after establishment of the host immune response. Late in infection cell-free virus may again be isolated from essentially all patients. (From Schleupner C: Detection of HIV-1 infection. *In* Mandell GL, ed: Principles and Practice of Infectious Diseases, 4th ed. New York, Churchill Livingstone, 1995, pp 1253–1267).

Whether this is a practical system for routine use (such as screening donated blood specimens) has yet to be determined. The use of culture systems for the detection of HIV-1 infection requires considerable time and expense as well as technical expertise. Therefore, it is doubtful that such systems will ever be widely used in clinical practice. It is certain that current tests will continue to be improved.

Natural History of HIV-1 Infection

Deficient Cell-Mediated Immunity

Infection with HIV-1 leads to a sequential decline and finally ablation of cell-mediated immunity eventually leading to manifestations of opportunistic diseases. Therefore, HIV-1 infection results in a wide range of clinical presentations ranging from totally asymptomatic carriage of the virus to life-threatening opportunistic infections and malignancies (Chaisson and Volberding, 1995). AIDS is the final stage when the infected host can no longer control opportunistic infections and malignancies that rarely cause illness in immunologic normal individuals (see Fig. 19–3).

At present, AIDS, or the end stage of HIV-1 infection, affects a limited proportion of persons with HIV-1 infections. Although this condition has received tremendous attention in the media, it is important to recognize that we are likely to have seen only the beginning of the clinical manifestations of this epidemic. Most patients who are infected and asymptomatic may not be ill, but they have a chronic progressive disease that may ultimately lead to significant immunologic impairment or death. The Centers for Disease Control and Prevention (CDC) surveillance case definition for AIDS is summarized in Table 19–1. Without other causes of immunosuppression, diagnosis of one of the conditions listed in Table 19–1 is now defined as AIDS for purposes of surveillance of epidemiologic trends. From a clinical standpoint, a useful functional definition of AIDS is the occurrence of certain systemic infections or malignancies in a patient with no other cause of defective cell-mediated immunity.

Clinical Spectrum and Progression

The spectrum of HIV-1 infection ranges from asymptomatic infection to severe immunodeficiency with serious secondary infections, neoplasms, and other conditions (see Fig. 19–3) (Chamberland et al, 1995). Initial or primary infection with HIV-1 is associated with an acute mononucleosis-like illness in 50% to 70% of persons. The acute illness associated with seroconversion is characterized by fever, lymphadenopathy, night sweats, myalgia, arthralgia, rash, malaise, lethargy, and sore throat. The interval between exposure and development of the acute retroviral syndrome illness is usually 2 to 4 weeks, with the duration of illness lasting from 1 to 2 weeks.

Laboratory evaluation of some persons with primary HIV-1 infections found transient high levels of p24 antigen in plasma (see Fig. 19–4) (Chamberland et al, 1995). It has been suggested that the intensity and/or resolution of symptomatic primary HIV-1 infection may be related to the level of viremia, which declines precipitously soon after infection, coincident with increasing levels of antiviral antibodies and a high level of antiviral activity mediated by CD8+ T lymphocytes. Development of detectable HIV-1 antibodies usually occurs within 3 to 12 weeks after infection. Seroconversion beyond 6 months is very uncommon.

The rate of progression from asymptomatic disease to AIDS is high and increases with the length of follow-up (Moss, 1988). The rate at which symptomatic disease develops in seropositive men appears to be approximately 4% to 10% per year of infection. Thus the progression is uncommon during the first several years after infection, but the likelihood of progression increases thereafter (Chamberland et al, 1995). Most cohort studies suggest that without therapy, less than 5% of HIV-1–infected adults develop AIDS after 2 years, approximately 20% to 25% develop AIDS within 6 years after infection, and 50% of HIV-1–infected persons develop AIDS within 10 years. Unusual HIV-1–infected individuals have remained clinically asymptomatic with normal CD4+ T lymphocyte counts for 5 to 10 years after infection.

Laboratory findings may help predict the risk of progression in seropositive persons (Moss, 1988). Among the tests that have been evaluated include CD4+ lymphocyte counts, the ratio of CD4+ to CD8+ lymphocytes, β_2-microglobulin levels, the presence of HIV-1 core antigen in serum (Moss, 1988), and HIV-1 plasma viremia (Coombs et al, 1989). The precise clinical utility of these tests remains to be defined, but it is likely that in the future it may be possible to predict patients at high risk for disease progression and institute therapy based on such prognostic parameters.

Effective antiretroviral therapy and widespread prophylaxis against *Pneumocystis carinii* pneumonia have substantially altered the natural history of AIDS (Chaisson and Volberding, 1995). The median survival in treated AIDS patients ranges from 2 to 3 years. Antiretroviral therapy and prophylaxis against opportunistic infections also extend the clinical incubation from infection with HIV to AIDS. Prophylaxis against opportunistic infections, such as *P. carinii,* means that diseases that occur later during HIV-induced immunodeficiency, such as *Mycobacterium avium–intracellulare* complex bacteremia or cytomegalovirus organ disease, may be the first clinical manifestation of HIV disease.

Classification of HIV-1 Infection

Several systems for classifying HIV-1–associated diseases have been proposed. The CDC system most widely used by clinicians reflects both the evolving knowledge about the spectrum and progression of HIV-1 infection and current standards of medical care for infected persons (Table 19–2). The system is based on a combination of three ranges of CD4+ T lymphocyte counts (>500, 200 to 499, or <200/μl) and three clinical categories (asymptomatic, or category A; mild symptoms, or category B; and AIDS-indicator conditions, or category C). Three clinical conditions accounted for more than 75% of all initial AIDS-indicator conditions reported in 1992: *P. carinii* pneumonia (42%); HIV-1 wasting syndrome (20%); and candidiasis of the esophagus (15%) (Chamberland et al, 1995). Thus the CDC scheme results in a total of nine combinations of CD4+ T cell categories and clinical categories.

Generalized lymphadenopathy is common among HIV-

Table 19–2. CLASSIFICATION SYSTEM FOR HUMAN IMMUNODEFICIENCY VIRUS

CD4+ T-Cell Categories (No./μl)	Clinical Categories		
	A *Asymptomatic, Acute (Primary) HIV, or PGL*	*B* *Symptomatic, But Not A or C Conditions*	*C* *AIDS-Indicator Conditions*
1. ≥500	A1	B1	C1†
2. 200–499	A2	B2	C2†
3. 200*	A3†	B3†	C3†

*AIDS-indicator T-cell count.
†Included in the 1993 AIDS surveillance case definition for adolescents and adults.
HIV, human immunodeficiency virus; AIDS, acquired immunodeficiency syndrome; PGL, persistent generalized lymphadenopathy.
From Centers for Disease Control and Prevention: 1993 Revised classification system for HIV infection and expanded surveillance case definition for AIDS among adolescents and adults. MMWR 1992; 41(RR-17):1–19.

infected persons, often beginning with the acute retroviral syndrome (Chaisson and Volberding, 1995). In the early 1980s, the syndrome of persistent generalized lymphadenopathy (defined as the presence of two or more extrainguinal sites for at least 3 months for which no other explanation could be found) was believed to have prognostic importance. It is now recognized that 50% to 70% of infected persons develop persistent generalized lymphadenopathy and that the natural history of HIV infection associated with persistent generalized lymphadenopathy does not differ from that of HIV infection without generalized adenopathy (Chaisson and Volberding, 1995). Involution of enlarged lymph nodes, reflecting degeneration of follicular germinal centers and loss of hyperplasia, often accompanies progression of HIV infection.

EPIDEMIOLOGY

The AIDS Epidemic

Occasional cases of AIDS occurred in the United States and Europe as early as 1952. In addition, aggressive cases of Kaposi's sarcoma were noted in Africans who had emigrated to Europe during the late 1970s. However, the AIDS epidemic is usually dated from the 1981 description of both *P. carinii* pneumonia (hitherto reported only in immunocompromised patients) and Kaposi's sarcoma (hitherto a rare tumor occurring in elderly men of Mediterranean origin) in previously healthy homosexual men.

The best data on the potential for spread of HIV-1 within a population at risk come from the San Francisco cohort study. From 1978 to 1980, almost 6700 homosexual men participated in a study of the sexual transmission of hepatitis B virus and evaluation of a vaccine (Centers for Disease Control and Prevention, 1987a). In subsequent studies, 1600 men were re-examined. The prevalence of HIV-1 antibody increased from 4.5 per 100 in 1978 to over 70 per 100 in 1986. Since AIDS was recognized as a sexually transmitted disease before the actual agent was identified, and because many of these men changed their behavior, the actual rate of seroconversion peaked in 1982.

By 1992, AIDS/HIV-1 infection was the leading cause of death for men and the fourth leading cause of death for women 25 to 44 years old (Branson, 1995). Because the surveillance system for AIDS cases relies on availability and willingness of physicians to diagnose and report AIDS cases through local regional and national agencies, there is concern that AIDS cases may be considerably under-reported. It is difficult to extrapolate reports of AIDS in limited populations to estimates of HIV-1 infection in the overall population in the United States. For example, in San Francisco, the estimated ratio of HIV-1 seropositive men to men with AIDS was 825 to 1 in 1980 and 28 to 1 in 1984, a substantial decline (Curran et al, 1988). The relative proportions of seropositivity and AIDS in most areas of the United States are probably between these ratios.

By December 31, 1994, 435,319 adolescents and adults and 6209 children with AIDS were reported in the United States (Centers for Disease Control and Prevention, 1994; Chamberland et al, 1995). The number of persons with AIDS increased rapidly. The first 100,000 cases were reported during the first 8 years of the epidemic (1981 to 1989), whereas the second 100,000 cases were reported in the next 2 years (1989 to 1992). In the early 1990s the number of persons reported with AIDS in the United States was expected to increase further, although at a slower rate. An aberration in the temporal trends resulted from expanding the surveillance definition for AIDS to include markers of severe HIV-1–related immunosuppression (Centers for Disease Control and Prevention, 1994; Chamberland et al, 1995). In 1994, 231,031 persons were reported to be living with AIDS in the United States (Centers for Disease Control and Prevention, 1994). Because of the long period between infection with HIV-1 and the development of AIDS, surveillance systems for HIV-1 infection are used to supplement the information on AIDS case surveillance. The U.S. Public Health Service has estimated that approximately 1 million U.S. residents are infected with HIV-1, with at least 40,000 new infections occurring annually (Centers for Disease Control and Prevention, 1990).

Worldwide predictions indicate that the epidemic will continue to grow, with an increasing proportion of infected persons living in developing countries. In 1995, an estimated 17.4 million persons were infected with HIV-1, including 6.4 million persons with AIDS, with the developing world having approximately 84% of all infected persons (Chamberland et al, 1995).

Modes of Transmission and Major Risk Groups

Three modes of transmission have been described for HIV-1: direct sexual contact, exposure to contaminated blood and blood products, and perinatal transmission. These modes of transmission can occur under a variety of circumstances, and many factors influence the spread of HIV-1.

Sexual Transmission

Sexual transmission of HIV-1 infections may occur between homosexual and heterosexual persons.

Homosexual Men

The majority of AIDS patients in the United States have occurred in homosexual and bisexual men, including homosexual and bisexual men who use intravenous drugs. HIV-1 seroprevalence rates in homosexual and bisexual men range from 10% to 70%, with most rates in the range of 20% to 50% (Centers for Disease Control and Prevention, 1987a). However, the HIV-1 infection rates in selected cohorts of homosexual men in major cities have clearly declined, reflecting the efficacy of education efforts in this population (Holmberg and Curran, 1990). This has been attributed to changes in sexual practices, particularly limiting sexual partners, the use of condoms, and other practices to avoid exchange of semen. Supporting data for such changes include the declining incidence of other sexually transmitted diseases, such as gonorrhea, in homosexual men since 1982. The increasing use of effective therapy, such as zidovudine and prophylaxis against *Pneumocystis,* has also delayed the occurrence of AIDS-defining conditions in many HIV-1–infected men.

There are problems with these data. First, in cities such as San Francisco, 50% or more of homosexual men are already infected. Thus, relatively few sexual contacts may lead to exposure to an infected partner. Second, the number of cases in homosexual men will increase as persons who were infected many years ago become ill. Thus, it is expected that the incidence of AIDS cases in homosexual men will continue to be substantial despite major changes in risk factors in this population.

Heterosexual Transmission

Early in the AIDS epidemic it was recognized that some women with AIDS who denied drug use said they had had sexual contact with men who used intravenous drugs, who were bisexual, or who were hemophiliac. Thus it became apparent that heterosexual transmission from infected men to women could occur. It is now recognized that heterosexual transmission is the major route for spread of HIV-1 in Africa (Quinn, 1990). In developed countries, heterosexual transmission appears to be an increasingly common mode of infection. Since 1986 the rate of increase in this group has been higher than the rate of increase of any other exposure category. The increase has been most striking for women infected through heterosexual contact. The number of cases among women infected through heterosexual contact exceeded those infected through injecting drug use for the first time in 1992 (Centers for Disease Control and Prevention, 1992b).

The average risk of HIV-1 infection from a single heterosexual contact may be less than 0.1% (Peterman et al, 1988). However, such statistics obscure well-documented reports of persons who were infected after only one or few sexual contacts with an HIV-1–infected person (Peterman et al, 1988). To date, penetrance of HIV-1 infection into the overall U.S. population has been relatively low (Holmberg and Curran, 1990; Chamberland et al, 1995). In U.S. military recruits, the seroprevalence of HIV-1 antibody has been about 1.3 per 1000 and the seroprevalence among blood donors has been 1.4 per 10,000. Most infected military recruits and blood donors have had identifiable risk factors, such as high-risk sexual practices or intravenous drug use.

Although HIV-1 has had relatively little penetrance into the overall U.S. population, rates of HIV-1 infection among certain populations appear to be high. This is especially true among inner-city minority populations. For example, among patients attending a sexually transmitted disease clinic in Baltimore, the seroprevalence was 6.3% for men and 3.0% for women. Many of the women had been infected by heterosexual contacts with intravenous drug-using men and/or bisexual men. In this population, the seroprevalence appears to be especially high among patients having emergency surgery, in whom the seroprevalence may be 15%.

HIV-1 prevalence for childbearing women was estimated in blinded surveys of residual blood samples on filter paper used to screen neonates for diseases such as phenylketonuria. These studies suggest approximately 7000 annual births to HIV-1–infected women during 1991 to 1992, for an estimated national HIV-1 infection prevalence of 1.7 per 1000 childbearing women (Chamberland et al, 1995). Female commercial sex workers (the politically correct term for what were formerly termed "prostitutes") are at high risk for HIV-1 infection because of exposure to multiple sex partners and frequent use of intravenous drugs. A multicenter study of sex workers found that 10% of 650 women were HIV-1–seropositive, with rates ranging from 0% among prescreened women in Nevada to 69% among sex workers being treated for drug addiction in New Jersey (Chamberland et al, 1995).

Blood-Borne Transmission

Intravenous Drug Users

Intravenous drug users are the second largest category of AIDS patients in developed countries. Risk factors include the extent of drug use since 1978, needle sharing, use of "shooting galleries," and use of crack (Holmberg and Curran, 1990). In some shooting galleries, for example, needles may be shared 50 times or more. In contrast, the use of sterile needles and participation in methadone treatment programs have been associated with lower rates of infection. Geography also appears to be important in HIV-1 transmission among intravenous drug users. Most cases have occurred in the New York City metropolitan area (Holmberg and Curran, 1990). In this region it is estimated that there may be up to half a million intravenous drug users. The total number in the United States is unknown but may be over 1 million. The current seropositivity rate in this population has been estimated to be 60%.

Intravenous drug users also appear to be a potentially important link between the reservoir of HIV-1–infected people and the uninfected heterosexual population. For example, women who acquire HIV-1 infection by sexual contact often have partners in high-risk groups for AIDS, especially intravenous drug users. Female-to-male spread of HIV-1 has been commonly associated with commercial sex workers. Many of these women are either intravenous drug users or the sex partners of intravenous drug users. Finally, approximately 80% of pediatric cases of AIDS have occurred in children born to HIV-1–infected women, who are often injection drug users or their sex partners.

BLOOD AND ORGAN RECIPIENTS

The probability of infection after receiving a single-donor blood product documented to be HIV-1–positive approaches 100% (Chamberland et al, 1995). Before serologic testing was begun, an estimated 29,000 blood or blood-product recipients were exposed to HIV-1 in the United States. Because many died of underlying conditions, 12,000 of these persons were estimated to survive long enough to develop AIDS. Since the spring of 1985, essentially all units of blood collected in the United States and all organ donors have been screened for HIV-1 antibodies. The result has been virtual elimination of new HIV-1 infections from blood transfusions.

Because screening cannot detect every infectious unit, all blood centers have established policies for self-deferral of donors who think they may be at risk for HIV-1 infection. It is still possible for an infected unit to be transfused, and this does occur. It is estimated that the number of such infected units being transfused ranges from 70 to 460 per year in the United States, a risk of 1 in 40,000 to 1 in 250,000 transfused units (Peterman et al, 1988). These infections result from donations from recently infected donors who do not have detectable antibody (Chamberland et al, 1995). This "window period" is estimated to last an average of 6 to 10 weeks, with 95% of infected persons developing detectable antibody within 6 months (see Fig. 19–4). Since approximately 60% of blood and blood components are used for people who do not survive the condition for which they are hospitalized, a worst-case scenario is that the risk of acquiring HIV-1 by receiving a single unit of blood is less than 1 per 100,000. This risk should not deter anyone who needs a unit of blood from receiving it.

HEMOPHILIACS

The typical hemophiliac person receives approximately 70,000 units of clotting factor concentrates per year (Holmberg and Curran, 1990). Thus, hemophiliacs are exposed to many blood-borne infections, particularly viruses. Current studies of hemophiliac men in the United States indicate that the seroprevalence increased from approximately 10% in 1980 to 70% to 80% in 1984. As with homosexual men, the greatest incidence of infection occurred between 1982 and 1983. Frequent users of factor VIII concentrates from those years are virtually all infected. In 1984, heat treatment was found to be effective in eliminating HIV-1 from factor concentrates. This method has been widely adopted, and very few infections currently occur in persons receiving factor concentrates (Holmberg and Curran, 1990).

HEALTH CARE WORKERS

There have been at least 42 well-documented seroconversions among health care workers as a result of occupational exposures to HIV-1 (Chamberland et al, 1989; Centers for Disease Control and Prevention, 1994). "Possible occupational transmission," that is, cases in which transmission is likely but the CDC's strict criteria were not met, was reported in 91 other health care workers (Centers for Disease Control and Prevention, 1994). These cases of occupational transmission included 18 physicians, three of whom were surgeons.

A number of studies evaluated the risk for occupational transmission to health care workers after exposure to HIV-seropositive patients (Holmberg and Curran, 1990). The risk of seroconversion after a needle stick injury appears to be less than 0.5%. The upper limit of the 95% confidence interval for the risk for seroconversion from an accidental needle stick is less than 1% per stick. This rate can be compared with the risk for hepatitis B infection from an accidental needle stick, which is estimated at 12% per stick.

There have been a few documented seroconversions after cutaneous exposures to HIV-infected blood. In 1987, the CDC reported three incidents involving young female health professionals who acquired HIV infection through contact with infected blood. These cases indicated that blood-to-mucosa or blood-to-skin transmission of HIV can occur, but that these cases are very rare.

Perinatal Transmission

Children can acquire HIV infection through breast milk or through any of the mechanisms discussed so far, including transfusion of blood or blood factors, or sexual exposures. However, the great majority of HIV disease in children occurs by transmission from a parent who is at risk for AIDS. Approximately 80% of cases occur from intravenous drug–using mothers. Thus, the characteristics of pediatric AIDS patients resemble those of their parents: 80% are black or Hispanic, and 75% reside in New York, New Jersey, Florida, and California (Holmberg and Curran, 1990). As many as 30,000 births to infected drug-abusing women may have occurred in New York City alone, and the New York State Health Department estimates that approximately 1 in 60 births in New York City is to an HIV-infected woman. Pooled data from a variety of large studies suggest that infants born to infected mothers have an approximately 25% risk of acquiring HIV. Assessment of infection in newborns is complicated by the presence of passively acquired maternal antibody. Thus, HIV antibody tests do not reflect the infection status of the infant before clearance of maternal antibodies.

Other At-Risk Populations

Studies of commercial sex workers in the United States reflect rates of HIV infection ranging from 0% in Las Vegas, where commercial sex workers are screened for HIV, to 50% in cities in northern New Jersey. Overall, it appears that about 20% to 30% of commercial sex workers in most U.S. cities may be infected, but the rates vary considerably depending on the use of intravenous drugs and the types of sexual partners. Another at-risk group is the prison population. Most HIV infections in this population appear to be related to intravenous drug use. The prevalence of infection in one study was 7%.

Unproved Modes of Transmission

There has been considerable investigation of other potential modes of HIV spread, including casual contact, human or insect bites, fomites, food, and water. To date there is no proof that HIV infection can be contracted from such sources (Chamberland et al, 1995). Combining data from several studies (Holmberg and Curran, 1990): approximately 450 family members and household (nonsexual) contacts of AIDS patients have been investigated. None were seropositive although they shared eating utensils, toothbrushes, razors, and toilet articles and kissed AIDS patients on the lips. In addition, more than 30 patients have been reported who have been bitten by AIDS patients, but none seroconverted (Holmberg and Curran, 1990). There has been some concern over the potential for mosquitoes as possible vectors of HIV, but this also appears unlikely. Finally, there are no reports of HIV transmission by food, water, or other articles.

Risk Factors for HIV Transmission

The best studies have been in homosexual men and indicate that large numbers of sexual partners and sexual acts involving receptive anal intercourse unprotected by condoms increase the likelihood of infection with HIV (Polk et al, 1987). The data regarding the risk of HIV infection from insertive anal intercourse and/or oral intercourse are less clear, because it is extremely difficult to find sufficient numbers of persons who engage in just one of these activities. However, since these types of sexual relations involve exchange of semen or mucosal contact, they should not be regarded as safe sex practices.

Genital ulcer disease also appears to be a major risk factor for infection with HIV (Stamm et al, 1988; Holmberg and Curran, 1990). It is possible that much of the difference in transmission patterns between developed countries and Africa may be explained by the high incidence of genital ulcer disease in Africans. In particular, diseases such as chancroid, syphilis, and herpes simplex virus type 2 appear to be associated with a high risk of HIV infection. Genital ulcers appear to be more common in HIV-infected than in non-infected African female commercial sex workers (Kreiss et al, 1986). In addition, a study of homosexual men in Seattle found that antibody-positive men were more likely to have antibodies to herpes simplex virus type 2 than uninfected men (77% versus 39%) (Stamm et al, 1988). Genital ulcer disease may cause breaks in the integrity of the skin that facilitate infection and/or recruit infected and susceptible white cells to the sites of exposure to HIV. Nonulcerative sexually transmitted diseases, such as gonorrhea and chlamydial infection, may also enhance sexual transmission of HIV (Chamberland et al, 1995). The higher frequency of balanitis and epithelial disruptions among uncircumcised men are proposed explanations for the increased risk of HIV infection observed among uncircumcised men in developing countries (Cameron et al, 1989; Jessamine et al, 1990; Piot and Merson, 1995).

AIDS AND HIV INFECTIONS IN UROLOGIC PRACTICE

Genitourinary Tract Involvement

The genitourinary tract may be involved in HIV infections as the site of infections or malignancies, such as Kaposi's sarcoma or non-Hodgkin's lymphoma, or in patients with AIDS-associated renal disease (Table 19–3). Involvement of the reproductive organs may be critical for sexual transmission of infection. The remaining issue concerns the indications for HIV antibody testing.

Opportunistic Infections

Given the systemic nature of AIDS, it is not surprising that the genital tract may be involved. This is especially true in patients who die of opportunistic infections. For example, one study (Shevchuk et al, 1989) of 80 autopsies in AIDS patients demonstrated that 2 of 11 cases with systemic toxoplasmosis involved the testes; 4 of 48 cases of systemic cytomegalovirus infection involved the prostate and one involved the testes; and 1 of 27 cases of systemic candidiasis involved the prostate. The testes in most patients exhibited marked spermatogenic arrest, germ cell degeneration, peritubular fibrosis, and Leydig cell depletion, nonspecific findings that most likely reflect the severe systemic disease in these patients. Other immunocompromised patients develop symptomatic genitourinary tract infections with both common and unusual organisms, for example epididymitis caused by *Candida* (Swartz et al, 1994) or cytomegalovirus (Randazzo et al, 1986). Bacteriuria and scrotal infections are common (see Table 19–3). Clinically, scrotal infection usually presents as nonspecific swelling or epididymo-orchitis. Patients with evidence of systemic infection usually receive systemic therapy (Leibovitch and Goldwasser, 1994). Clinical relapse is common and may result in persistent symptoms or fulminant infection with abscess formation.

Resurgence of tuberculosis is a new problem that is closely related to the HIV epidemic. The number of new cases of tuberculosis in the United States has increased each year since 1986 (Chamberland et al, 1995). This increase is closely associated with the HIV epidemic. More than 100,000 persons in the United States are coinfected with HIV and *Mycobacterium tuberculosis*. Recently, there has been a notable rise in drug-resistant tuberculosis in the United States. Persons with or at risk for HIV infection appear to be at increased risk for active infection with drug-resistant strains of *M. tuberculosis*. Persons coinfected with HIV and *M. tuberculosis* have a much greater likelihood of developing clinical tuberculosis, including extrapulmonary disease, and may be more difficult to diagnose and to treat than non–HIV-infected persons (Selwyn et al, 1989; Chamberland et al, 1995). The importance of these trends is that genitourinary and genital tuberculosis are again considerations in the evaluation and management of urologic patients.

Both men and women with HIV infection are at increased risk for genital tract infections (Chaisson and Volberding, 1995). Genital herpes virus infections may be chronic or recurrent and are associated with increased likelihood of transmission of HIV to sexual partners. Genital warts may also be severe and chronic (Fig. 19–5). Other sexually transmitted diseases, such as syphilis, may have more atypical and prolonged manifestations in people with HIV infection. Pelvic inflammatory disease appears to be more common, be more severe, and require more frequent hospitalization and surgical intervention in HIV-seropositive women.

Table 19–3. UROLOGIC MANIFESTATIONS OF ACQUIRED IMMUNODEFICIENCY SYNDROME AND HUMAN IMMUNODEFICIENCY VIRUS

Clinical and/or Pathologic Finding	Definite or Probable Increase	Case Reports
Kidney		
Nephropathy	✓	
AIDS-associated	✓	
Immune complex	✓	
Treatment-related	✓	
Obstruction	✓	
Tumors		
Renal cell		✓
Lymphoma	✓	
Kaposi's sarcoma		✓
Infections		
Pyelonephritis	✓	
Abscess		✓
Bladder		
Neurogenic	✓	
Neoplasms		
Transitional cell		✓
Kaposi's sarcoma		✓
Cystitis		
Bacteriuria	✓	
Opportunistic*	✓	
Fistulas		✓
Penis and/or Scrotum		
Impotence or Decreased Libido		
Hormonal	✓	
Neurologic	✓	
Psychogenic	✓	
Testicular Problems		
Atrophy	✓	
Orchitis	✓	
Nonspecific	✓	
Opportunistic*	✓	
Neoplasms		
Seminoma	✓	
Nonseminomatous germ cell	✓	
Lymphoma	✓	
Epididymitis		
Nonspecific	✓	
Sexually transmitted	✓	
Opportunistic*	✓	
Kaposi's Sarcoma	✓	
Fournier's Gangrene		✓
Prostate		
Prostatitis		
Nonspecific bacterial	✓	
Opportunistic organisms*	✓	
Abscess		
Nonspecific bacterial	✓	
Opportunistic organisms*	✓	
Benign Hypertrophy		✓
Cancer		✓
Urethra		
Reiter's syndrome		✓
Dysuria, urgency (culture-negative)		✓
Tumors		
Kaposi's sarcoma	✓	
Lymphoma	✓	
Gynecologic		
Cervical carcinoma	✓	
Vulva		
Squamous cell carcinoma		✓
Kaposi's sarcoma	✓	
Sexually Transmitted Diseases†	✓	
Urethritis	✓	
Ulcerative	✓	
Vaginitis	✓	
Cervicitis	✓	
Pelvic inflammatory disease	✓	
Urinalysis		
Hematuria	✓	
Pyuria	✓	
Proteinuria	✓	
Bacteriuria	✓	

*Caused by the opportunistic organisms listed in Table 19–1.
†Ulcerative and nonulcerative sexually transmitted diseases are associated with a twofold to fivefold increase in transmission of human immunodeficiency virus.
AIDS, acquired immunodeficiency syndrome.
Based on data from Pardo et al, 1984; Rao et al, 1984; Kaplan et al, 1987; Stamm et al, 1988; Leport et al, 1989; Miles et al, 1989; Shevchuk et al, 1989; Hirsch, 1990; Volberding, 1990; Wilkinson and Carroll, 1990; Pudney and Anderson, 1991; Wilson et al, 1992; Buzelin et al, 1994; Kreiss et al, 1994; Leibovitch and Goldwasser, 1994; Swartz et al, 1988; Trauzzi et al, 1994; Cespedes et al, 1995; Chaisson and Volberding, 1995; Kwan and Lowe, 1995; Timmerman et al, 1995.

Malignancies

Given the large numbers of HIV-infected persons, it is to be expected that a broad range of malignancies has been described in patients with AIDS and other HIV infections (Volberding, 1990). These malignancies include squamous cell carcinomas in various sites, malignant melanoma, testicular cancers of all histologic types (Wilkinson and Carroll, 1990; Wilson et al, 1992; Buzelin et al, 1994; Leibovitch and Goldwasser, 1994), Hodgkin's disease, and cervical carcinoma (Volberding, 1990; Chaisson and Volberding, 1995).

Selection of the therapy for neoplasms in HIV-seropositive patients may be influenced by several major considerations. The clinical stage of HIV infection is the first consideration. In general, asymptomatic or minimally symptomatic patients should receive standard therapy. For patients with AIDS, decisions about optimal treatment are influenced by the patient's overall medical status and other therapy. Characteristics associated with an increased risk of toxicity after cancer therapy include prior bone marrow suppression due to antiretroviral therapy, leukopenia, and significant immunodeficiency. AIDS-related life expectancy may influence the therapeutic decisions. These considerations are illustrated by management of testicular tumors in men with AIDS (Wilkinson and Carroll, 1990; Wilson et al, 1992; Buzelin et al, 1994; Leibovitch and Goldwasser, 1994; Kwan and Lowe, 1995). Some evidence suggests that there may be an increased incidence of testicular tumors associated

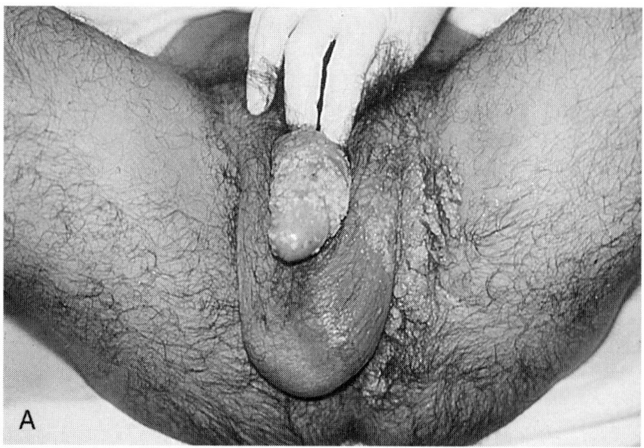

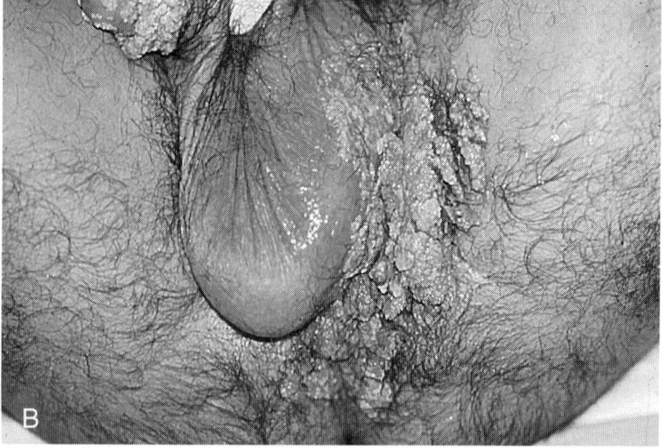

Figure 19–5. Extensive condylomata acuminata associated with areas of dysplasia and carcinoma in a patient with acquired immunodeficiency syndrome and human papillomavirus infection.

with HIV infection. The therapeutic dilemma in patients with AIDS is that the accepted treatments for testicular neoplasms, except surveillance, may result in additional immune suppression. Furthermore, patients with AIDS often do not tolerate radiation or chemotherapy. This may require major modifications of standard treatment protocols, resulting in decreased effectiveness. Despite these limitations, most experts recommend that AIDS patients with testicular neoplasms receive standard treatment as indicated by the tumor histologic appearance and stage (Wilkinson and Carroll, 1990; Wilson et al, 1992; Buzelin et al, 1994; Leibovitch and Goldwasser, 1994).

With the possible exception of Hodgkin's disease, there is minimal evidence that any of these cancers are caused by the HIV-induced immunologic deficits. However, there is a direct relationship between AIDS and Kaposi's sarcoma; primary central nervous system, non-Hodgkin's lymphoma; and high-grade peripheral B-cell lymphomas. Women with HIV infection are also at substantially increased risk for invasive cervical carcinoma. These malignancies are now diagnostic of AIDS in patients with HIV infections (Centers for Disease Control and Prevention, 1985). Although the cause of these AIDS-associated malignancies has not been clearly defined, most authorities believe that deficient immune surveillance is the key factor, perhaps combined with viral activation (Volberding, 1990).

Kaposi's Sarcoma

Kaposi's sarcoma may involve the genitalia in patients with HIV infections, occasionally as the initial manifestation of AIDS. Before 1981, this was an extremely rare tumor in the United States. It occurred only in elderly men and usually affected the feet and lower extremities, occasionally with involvement of the genitalia by lymphedema. This disease, now referred to as "classic Kaposi's sarcoma," ran an indolent course that was not associated with HIV. In the 1960s, it was found that Kaposi's sarcoma was common in central Africa, where it was an aggressive and infiltrating disease that was not associated with underlying immune deficiency. Beginning in the early 1970s cases of Kaposi's sarcoma were described in patients with organ transplants, particularly kidneys. Kaposi's sarcoma was the first tumor linked with AIDS and was seen in some of the initial cases. Kaposi's sarcoma is the most common malignancy in patients with AIDS (Moore and Chang, 1995). The predominant group affected appears to be homosexual men, and in some cohorts the lifetime risk of Kaposi's sarcoma approaches 50%.

Epidemiologic and molecular biologic evidence suggests that the development of Kaposi's sarcoma may be related to coinfection with a second infectious agent, likely a new herpes termed Kaposi's sarcoma–associated herpesvirus (Cesarman et al, 1995; Moore and Chang, 1995). Studies from Sweden indicate an upsurge in cases of classic Kaposi's sarcoma in the 1970s, before the AIDS epidemic. The frequency of Kaposi's sarcoma in HIV-seronegative homosexual men is higher than expected, supporting the hypothesis that the etiologic agent can be sexually transmitted and is distinct from HIV. Sophisticated molecular studies identified the newly described Kaposi's sarcoma–associated herpesvirus in lesions from patients with Kaposi's sarcoma and in some AIDS-related B-cell lymphomas (Cesarman et al, 1995; Moore and Chang, 1995).

The typical cutaneous lesion appears as a subcutaneous, painless, nonpruritic nodule. Lesions are often pigmented and red to blue. Exophytic masses can occur, and they may present with bleeding or pain. Lymphedema is common, as would be expected from any lymphatic lesion (Volberding, 1990). Involvement of the lower extremities is common and may be associated with marked scrotal and penile edema.

Diagnosis is usually made by biopsy. However, once the patient has biopsy confirmation, additional lesions can be recognized based on their characteristic clinical appearance. Although three variants have been reported (spindle cell, anaplastic, and mixed), the mixed cellular variant is by far the most common type in AIDS patients (Volberding, 1990). Kaposi's sarcoma is characterized histologically by proliferation of abnormal vascular structures. Three diagnostic features include (1) vascular structures with slits lined by large malignant-appearing endothelial cells, (2) surrounding spindle cells, and (3) extravasated erythrocytes. Most authorities believe that the origin of the tumor is endothelial.

The natural history of AIDS-associated Kaposi's sarcoma is highly variable. Occasional patients have had spontaneous remissions or long intervals without progression. Others experience rapid deterioration (Volberding, 1990). Patients with constitutional symptoms such as fevers, night sweats, and weight loss do poorly. In the usual setting of HIV infection, Kaposi's sarcoma appears to progress rapidly, often with visceral involvement. Patients who have had previous opportunistic infections, anemia, low CD4 cell counts, or gastrointestinal or pulmonary disease appear to do especially poorly (Volberding, 1990). In contrast, patients with few small lesions and no evidence of opportunistic infection or constitutional symptoms do relatively well.

The optimal therapy is currently unclear for several reasons. First, the natural history of this tumor is highly variable. Second, no therapeutic agent has been proved to reduce the underlying immune deficit. Third, conventional cytotoxic therapy may cause further impairment of cellular immunity. Surgery is usually used for biopsy to confirm the diagnosis or for palliation of lesions that bleed or are uncomfortable. Radiation therapy has proved useful for symptomatic local disease with an optimal dose of approximately 2500 rad (Volberding, 1990). Alternating single-agent chemotherapy, with agents such as vinblastine and vincristine, is recommended for selected patients with favorable prognostic indicators (Chaisson and Volberding, 1995).

NON-HODGKIN'S LYMPHOMA

Non-Hodgkin's lymphoma was first associated with HIV infection in 1982. The CDC definition for AIDS (Centers for Disease Control and Prevention, 1992a) now includes patients with high-grade B-cell non-Hodgkin's lymphoma in the setting of documented HIV infection. The AIDS-associated non-Hodgkin's lymphoma closely resembles that associated with other immune deficiency states.

INVASIVE CERVICAL CARCINOMA

Cervical disorders are exceedingly common in HIV-seropositive women (Chaisson and Volberding, 1995). The prevalence of cervical lesions increases as immunosuppression progresses. Human papillomavirus coinfection appears to play a major role in the development of cervical atypia and squamous dysplasia. Thus, frequent evaluation, including cervical cytologic examination, colposcopy, and other indicated studies, is recommended for women with HIV infection.

Renal Disease

Renal disease is considered a "late syndrome" in patients with AIDS. However, whether there is a specific "AIDS-associated nephropathy" is still debatable (Chaisson and Volberding, 1995). The problem is that many patients with AIDS are at high risk for renal disease because of concomitant factors that have all been associated with renal disorders, such as hepatitis B infection, treatment with toxic drugs, fluid and electrolyte abnormalities, opportunistic infections, and malignancies.

In 1984, Rao and others described 11 AIDS patients with renal disease (Rao et al, 1984). These patients had a disease characterized by proteinuria, elevated serum creatinine levels, and focal and segmental glomerulosclerosis on biopsy. Although this disorder closely resembles heroin-associated nephropathy, only half the patients had a history of drug use. In a review of 75 consecutive AIDS patients in Miami, 43% had proteinuria (Pardo et al, 1984), and among 36 autopsy patients, 17 had renal abnormalities, including 5 with focal glomerulosclerosis and 12 with mesangial proliferation. (Pardo et al, 1984). This "AIDS-associated nephropathy" appears most frequently in the eastern United States, where there are large numbers of patients who have AIDS associated with intravenous drug use. In contrast, there are large numbers of patients with AIDS in San Francisco, Seattle, and other cities who have had little renal involvement compared with those in New York and Miami.

Renal dysfunction associated with HIV disease is usually diagnosed incidentally in patients with opportunistic infections and CD4+ cell counts less that 200/mm^3 (Chaisson and Volberding, 1995). The clinical course of AIDS-associated nephropathy is variable. Patients with other causes of renal dysfunction, such as nephrotoxic drugs or acute tubular necrosis, may improve. Others experience rapidly progressive clinical deterioration. Activation of cellular immunity through chronic dialysis may accelerate HIV abnormalities.

HIV, Semen, and Cervical Secretions

Direct contact with semen is important for the sexual transmission of HIV (Curran et al, 1988; Peterman et al, 1988). HIV has been isolated by co-cultivation of seminal cells and donor lymphocytes (Ho et al, 1984; Zagury et al, 1984). We found that asymptomatic and minimally symptomatic seropositive men shed HIV in their semen (Krieger et al, 1991a). The clinical stage of infection, counts of CD4+ cells in peripheral blood, and zidovudine treatment had minimal impact on seminal shedding. These findings are controversial because other studies suggest that shedding of HIV in semen occurs most often among men with low CD4+ cell counts in their blood and that antiretroviral therapy reduces shedding (Anderson et al, 1992). In recent studies, HIV was cultured from 36 (17%) of 215 semen specimens from 56 seropositive men and cytomegalovirus was cultured from 30% of the specimens (Krieger et al, 1995). The CD8+ cell count in peripheral blood was the best predictor of HIV shedding in semen. Shedding of HIV was more closely associated with concomitant shedding of cytomegalovirus than with the CD4+ count, and antiretroviral therapy had minimal influence on shedding of HIV. Lack of a strong relationship between CD4+ cell counts and HIV shedding may be explained in part by recent observation of large differences in virus load in the systemic compartment among subjects with similar CD4+ counts (SA Fiscus, RW Coombs, and associates, unpublished data). Differences in CD8+ cell counts may help resolve the controversy over the significance of systemic immunologic function, chiefly assessed by CD4+ counts, as a predictor for shedding of HIV in semen.

Cytomegalovirus is a viral cofactor suggested as potentially important for the development of AIDS. Cytomegalovirus seropositivity is very common among populations at risk for HIV, and cytomegalovirus is a frequent opportunistic agent in AIDS (Skolnick et al, 1988; Collier et al, 1990; Detels et al, 1994). Both viruses are shed in semen, and both infections are transmitted sexually. A recent study found that HIV-seropositive men with persistently positive semen for cytomegalovirus were more likely to develop AIDS than men whose semen was intermittently positive or those whose semen was persistently negative (Detels et al, 1994). Viral interactions in the male genital tract may also be important determinants of HIV shedding in semen. These results are consistent with the concepts that HIV may invade the male genital tract early in the course of infection and that viral shedding in the semen may be independent of the clinical stage of HIV infection. In these respects, HIV infection of the male reproductive tract may be similar to HIV infection of the central nervous system, another immunologically privileged site. These observations support recommendations for safe sexual practices by all persons infected with HIV regardless of the stage of infection or concurrent antiviral chemotherapy (Krieger et al, 1995).

Contact with cervicovaginal secretions of infected women is also believed to be important for the sexual transmission of HIV-1. In one study of HIV-seropositive commercial sex workers (Kreiss et al, 1986) cervical HIV DNA was detected in 40 (44%) of 92 women. The presence of cervical HIV was associated with cervical inflammation, suggesting that control of conditions associated with cervical inflammation might reduce the sexual transmission of HIV.

Other Urologic Manifestations

Other urologic manifestations in patients with AIDS and HIV infections reflect involvement of related organ systems. For example, bladder dysfunction may occur in patients with HIV-associated neurologic disorders. Similarly, urinary tract infections and chronic bacterial prostatitis have been described in some patients with HIV infections. In one study, bacterial prostatitis was diagnosed in 17 of 209 men hospitalized for treatment of HIV infections (Leport et al, 1989). The most common presentation was fever and irritative lower tract symptoms associated with bacteriuria. Other workers identified urinary tract infections in 22% of patients with AIDS (Kaplan et al, 1987).

Abnormalities on urinalysis are relatively common, including hematuria, pyuria, bacteriuria, and proteinuria. One study suggested that hematuria occurs in 25% of persons infected with HIV (Cespedes et al, 1995). Although hematuria may be related to many causes (see Table 19–3), genitourinary tumors appear to be uncommon, particularly in young men. Thus, complete urologic evaluation can be safely omitted in young men with asymptomatic microscopic hematuria (Cespedes et al, 1995).

HIV as a Blood-Borne Virus: Protecting Yourself and Your Staff

On the basis of the data discussed above and the documented potential for transmission to health care workers in occupational settings, we have modified our current practice to conform with uniform body substance precautions as recommended by the CDC (Centers for Disease Control and Prevention, 1987c). All patients are considered potentially infected with HIV. Uniform policies are then instituted to minimize the opportunity for transmission in the health care setting. The key concept is to avoid direct contact with potentially infected body substances. In urology, this means avoiding contact with blood, urine (which often contains blood), and semen.

We have three major policies for infection control. First, there should be no direct contact with blood, semen, urine, mucous membranes, or nonintact skin. Second, extraordinary care should be used to prevent injuries by sharp instruments during invasive procedures and operations. Phrases such as "knife back" or "needle back" are good ways to alert members of the operating team. "Recapping" (replacing the plastic container covering a needle) needles is especially dangerous and should not be done under any circumstance. Recapping accounted for one third of percutaneous exposures to health care workers in one recent study. Further reduction in injury rates will also require the development of puncture-resistant gloves and/or the redesign of needles and other sharp instruments (Chamberland et al, 1995). Third, health care workers with exudative skin lesions or weeping dermatitis should not perform surgery or assist with surgery or other invasive procedures. Disturbing case reports document the importance of these recommendations (Centers for Disease Control and Prevention, 1987d). For example, one health care worker had blood on her hands for 20 minutes during resuscitation of an AIDS patient. Although this health care worker had no other risk factors, she developed antibodies to HIV 16 weeks after the incident. In another case a phlebotomist was splattered with blood when the stopper flew off a vacuum tube from an HIV-positive patient. This woman had acne; she was wearing eyeglasses and gloves and immediately washed off the blood. Although she had no other risk factors, she became seropositive 9 months after exposure. A third case occurred when a technologist got blood on her hands and forearms during manipulation of a machine used to separate blood components. The technologist had dermatitis but no open lesions and became seropositive 3 months after the accident. These cases emphasize the potential for HIV transmission during diagnostic and therapeutic procedures.

Testing for HIV Infection

The issue of HIV testing has gone well beyond the medical arena. It affects the ability of patients to get insurance as well as many psychological and political issues. I consider basic concepts and generally accepted indications for HIV testing and then consider the case for wider testing in the health care setting.

Basic Concepts

Basic concepts underlie any consideration of testing for HIV infection. First, patients should not be denied access to necessary health care because of their HIV infection status. Second, test results, like all sensitive medical records, must remain confidential. This is difficult to ensure because many persons are interested in the test results and in some situations just agreeing to an HIV antibody test may have profoundly negative implications. Third, any HIV testing must be accompanied by adequate counseling. This means counseling before the tests are obtained and explanations of the reasons, the potential benefits, and the disadvantages of the test. In many states, written consent is required before testing. Fourth, I strongly believe that all testing should be voluntary. This means that the test should be discussed with the person before testing and that testing may be refused.

Generally Accepted Indications

Generally accepted indications for antibody testing include evaluation of blood and organs for tissue donation. In addition, most experts agree that persons at risk for HIV infection should be tested routinely. Such persons include those with a sexually transmitted disease or a history of intravenous drug use and others who consider themselves at risk of HIV infection. Physicians should routinely elicit a sexual history in patients, including a history of sexual contact with homosexual men, multiple unsafe heterosexual contacts, and any history of needle sharing or the use of intravenous drugs. In addition, testing should be recommended for persons who received unscreened blood transfusions after 1977; those with a history of any sexually transmitted disease, including hepatitis B; and those with a history of disease that might be associated with HIV infection, such as lymphopenia, unexplained elevation of hepatic enzyme levels, or positive status for hepatitis B markers (Rhame and Maki, 1989). Testing should be strongly encouraged for persons who have had sexual contact with any person who has tested positive for HIV or any person who is at high risk for HIV infection (Rhame and Maki, 1989).

The CDC has also recommended that HIV testing be done for all persons with active tuberculosis. Because a large fraction of persons infected with HIV will eventually develop AIDS, those with positive tuberculin tests should receive isoniazid prophylaxis unless there are major contraindications. This therapy should be initiated expeditiously because active tuberculosis may be the first sign of HIV-related disease. The CDC recommends testing for patients to whom health care workers have been exposed through injuries such as needlesticks. Testing is also recommended for selected women of reproductive age, particularly those living in communities with a high prevalence of HIV infection, and for children born to HIV-infected mothers.

Wider Indications for HIV Testing

Although 1 to 1.5 million Americans are infected with HIV (Centers for Disease Control and Prevention, 1987b, 1990, 1994), most infected persons do not know their status despite the fact that almost all will reveal a history of high-risk behaviors. The conclusion is that current efforts to make persons infected with HIV infection aware of their status are failing (Rhame and Maki, 1989). These data have led to a debate on the merits of wider testing for HIV infections.

Arguments Favoring Wider Testing

Knowledge of a person's antibody status may be of benefit to a person with an asymptomatic HIV infection. First, persons with asymptomatic HIV infections may be tested for tuberculosis before loss of delayed hypersensitivity and receive prophylactic therapy if necessary (Branson, 1995). Immunization is also recommended against influenza virus, *Streptococcus pneumoniae, Haemophilus influenzae,* and hepatitis B virus. Second, knowledge of the infection status may also confer additional benefits on an infected person (Rhame and Maki, 1989; Branson, 1995). Many persons who are infected with the disease do not recognize hazardous signs and symptoms and thus fail to seek health care promptly. Many infected persons do not recognize that HIV infection is a treatable condition. Early institution of antiviral chemotherapy may delay the onset of symptomatic disease. Third, patients should be afforded the opportunity for counseling in risk-reduction behavior. Fourth, HIV testing may identify potential subjects for research studies. Finally, wider use of HIV testing offers the potential benefit of early prophylaxis for health care workers after exposure to HIV. Reports of animal models describe the beneficial effects of zidovudine after exposure to retroviruses such as Rauscher murine leukemia virus and feline leukemia virus. If prophylaxis after exposure is accepted, then it should be initiated as soon after exposure as possible. In essence, the case for wider use of HIV testing is that HIV infection should be treated as much as possible like other infectious diseases.

Arguments Against Wider Testing

Several arguments may be advanced against wider use of HIV testing in the health care setting (Rhame and Maki, 1989). First, it has been stated that an aggressive testing program will drive persons at highest risk away from the health care system. The counterargument is that raising this issue with all patients will decrease the stigma of testing (Rhame and Maki, 1989). Second, a false-positive test could cause considerable disruption in a person's life. Using current screening criteria, a false-positive will occur rarely. False-negative tests can also occur during earliest phases of infection, but this is also exceedingly uncommon. The overwhelming majority of patients will have accurate test results. Thus, HIV antibody testing may be the most accurate test described in this text.

The practical problem with wider serologic testing for HIV is the indeterminate Western blot test. For example, during screening of Minnesota blood donors between 1985 and 1988; approximately 1 in 1000 uninfected persons had repeatedly reactive immunoassays and indeterminate Western blot tests. Thus, wider use of screening will increase the number of persons with such indeterminate results. In some studies 20% of normal persons had indeterminate Western blot tests for HIV. The implication is that Western blot should only be done for persons with repeatedly reactive ELISAs for HIV, and not as a routine screening test. The personal anguish and damage to relationships caused by uncertain test results for HIV infection may be considerable. It may be difficult to obtain insurance or find employment. Thus, advocates of wider use of HIV testing must be prepared to accept the substantial responsibility for persons with indeterminate results. The current recommendation is that persons at low risk have repeat tests in 6 months. If the repeat results are negative or indeterminate, the interpretation is that the person does not have an HIV infection. For persons at high risk, repeat testing should be continued indefinitely. It is possible that improved technology for culturing HIV from blood and more sensitive assays, such as the polymerase chain reaction, may soon become generally available to provide accurate estimates of the probability of infection in patients with indeterminate Western blots.

The final argument is that wider testing will result in widespread discrimination. Most discrimination related to HIV is irrational, despite substantial public sentiment to the contrary. "Because discrimination will subvert the good that wider HIV testing will produce, we must vigorously fight it" (Rhame and Maki, 1989).

REFERENCES

Anderson DJ, O'Brien TR, et al: Effects of disease stage and zidovudine therapy on the detection of human immunodeficiency virus type 1 in semen. JAMA 1992; 267:2769–2774.

Barre-Sinoussi F, Chermann JC, et al: Isolation of a T-lymphotropic retrovirus from a patient at risk for acquired immune deficiency syndrome (AIDS). Science 1983; 220:868–870.

Branson BM: Early intervention for persons infected with human immunodeficiency virus. Clin Infect Dis 1995; 20(suppl 1):S3–S22.

Buzelin F, Karam G, Moreau A, et al: Testicular tumor and the acquired immunodeficiency syndrome. Eur Urol 1994; 26(1):71–76.

Cameron DW, Simonsen JN, D'Costa LJ, et al: Female to male transmission of human immunodeficiency virus type 1: Risk factors for seroconversion in men. Lancet 1989; 2:403–407.

Centers for Disease Control and Prevention: Update: Revised Public Health Service definition of persons who should refrain from donating blood and plasma—United States. MMWR 1985; 34:547–548.

Centers for Disease Control and Prevention: Human immunodeficiency virus infection in the United States: A review of current knowledge. MMWR 1987a; 36(S6):(1S–48S).

Centers for Disease Control and Prevention: Human immunodeficiency virus infection in the United States. MMWR 1987; 36(S):6S.

Centers for Disease Control and Prevention: Recommendations for prevention of HIV transmission in health-care settings. MMWR 1987; 36(2S):3S–18S.

Centers for Disease Control and Prevention: Update: Human immunodeficiency virus infections in health care workers exposed to blood of infected patients. MMWR 1987d; 36:285–289.

Centers for Disease Control and Prevention: HIV prevalence estimates and AIDS case projections for the United States: Report based upon a workshop. MMWR 1990; 39(RR-16):1–31.

Centers for Disease Control and Prevention: 1993 Revised classification system for HIV infection and expanded surveillance case definition for AIDS among adolescents and adults. MMWR 1992a; 41(RR-17):1–19.

Centers for Disease Control and Prevention: Update: Acquired immunodeficiency syndrome—United States. MMWR 1992b; 42:547–557.

Centers for Disease Control and Prevention: US HIV and AIDS cases reported through December 1994. HIV/AIDS Surv Rep 1994; 6:1–39.

Cesarman E, Chang Y, Moore PS, et al: Kaposi's sarcoma-associated herpesvirus-like DNA sequences in AIDS-related body-cavity-based lymphomas. N Engl J Med 1995; 332:1186–1191.

Cespedes RD, Peretsman SJ, et al: The significance of hematuria in patients infected with the human immunodeficiency virus. J Urol 1995; 154:1455–1456.

Chaisson RE, Volberding: Clinical manifestations of HIV infection. *In* Mandell GL, ed: Principles and Practice of Infectious Diseases, 4th ed. New York, Churchill Livingstone, 1995, pp 1217–1252.

Chamberland M, Conley L, et al: Surveillance update: Health care workers with AIDS. (Abstract WAO 2.) Presented at the Fifth International Conference on AIDS, Montreal, Canada, 1989.

Chamberland M, Ward J, et al: Epidemiology and prevention of AIDS and HIV infection. *In* Mandell GL, Principles and Practice of Infectious Diseases, 4th ed. New York, Churchill Livingstone, 1995, pp 1174–1203.

Collier AC, Handsfield HH, et al: Cytomegalovirus infection in women attending a sexually transmitted diseases clinic. J Infect Dis 1990; 162:46–51.

Coombs R, Collier A, et al: Virologic markers or central nervous system HIV infection in HIV seropositive homosexual men without neurological symptoms. Presented at the Fifth International Conference on AIDS, Montreal, Canada, 1989.

Corey L: Therapy of HIV infection. *In* Mandell GL, ed: Principles and Practice of Infectious Diseases, 4th ed. New York, Churchill Livingstone, 1995.

Curran JW, Jaffe HW, et al: Epidemiology of HIV infection and AIDS in the United States. Science 1988; 239:610.

Detels R, Leach CT, et al: Persistent cytomegalovirus infection of semen increases risk of AIDS. J Infect Dis 1994; 169:766–768.

Dolin R, Keefer MC: Vaccines for HIV-1 infection. *In* Mandell GL, ed: Principles and Practice of Infectious Diseases, 4th ed. New York, Churchill Livingstone, 1995, 1294–1305.

Hasse AT: Lentiviruses: An overview. *In* Mandell GL, ed: Principles and Practice of Infectious Diseases, 4th ed. New York, Churchill Livingstone, 1995, 1584–1590.

Hirsch MS: Clinical Manifestations of HIV Infection in Adults in Industrialized Countries. New York, McGraw-Hill, 1990.

Ho DD, Schooley R, et al: HTLV-III in the semen and blood of a healthy homosexual man. Science 1984; 226:451–453.

Holmberg SD, Curran JW: The Epidemiology of HIV Infection in Industrialized Countries. New York, McGraw-Hill, 1990.

Jessamine PG, Plummer FA, et al: Human immunodeficiency virus, genital ulcers and the male foreskin: Synergism in HIV-1 transmission. Scand J Infect Dis Suppl 1990; 69:181–186.

Kaplan MS, Wechsler M, et al: Urologic manifestations of AIDS. Urology 1987; 30:441–443.

Kreiss J, Willerford DM, et al: Association between cervical inflammation and cervical shedding of human immunodeficiency virus DNA. J Infect Dis 1994; 170:1597–1601.

Kreiss JK, Koech D, et al: AIDS virus infection in Nairobi prostitutes. Spread of the epidemic to East Africa. N Eng J Med 1986; 314:414–418.

Krieger JN, Coombs RW, et al: Recovery of human immunodeficiency virus type 1 from semen: Minimal impact of stage of infection and current antiviral chemotherapy. J Infect Dis 1991a; 163:386–389.

Krieger JN, Coombs RW, et al: Fertility parameters in men infected with human immunodeficiency virus. J Infect Dis 1991b; 164:464–469.

Krieger JN, Coombs RW, et al: Seminal shedding of human immunodeficiency virus type 1 and human cytomegalovirus: Evidence for different immunological controls. J Infect Dis 1995; 171:1018–1022.

Kwan DJ, Lowe FC: Genitourinary manifestations of the acquired immunodeficiency syndrome. Urology 1995; 45(1):13–27.

Leibovitch I, Goldwasser B: The spectrum of acquired immune deficiency syndrome–associated testicular disorders. Urology 1994; 44(6):818–824.

Leport C, Rousseau F, et al: Bacterial prostatitis in patients infected with the human immunodeficiency virus. J Urol 1989; 141:334–336.

Masur H: Management of opportunistic infections associated with HIV infection. *In* Mandell GL, ed: Principles and Practice of Infectious Diseases, 4th ed. New York, Churchill Livingstone, 1995, pp 1280–1293.

Miles BJ, Melser M, et al: The urological manifestations of the acquired immunodeficiency syndrome. J Urol 1989; 142:771–773.

Moore PS, Chang Y: Detection of herpesvirus-like DNA sequences in Kaposi's sarcoma in patients with and those without HIV infection. N Engl J Med 1995; 332:1181–1185.

Moss AR: Predicting progression to AIDS. Br Med J 1988; 297:1067–1068.

Moss AR, Bachetti P: Natural history of HIV infection. AIDS 1989; 3:55–61.

Pardo V, Aldana M, et al: Glomerular lesions in the acquired immunodeficiency syndrome. Ann Intern Med 1984; 101:429–434.

Peterman TA, Stoneburner RL, et al: Risk of human immunodeficiency virus transmission from heterosexual adults with transfusion-associated infections. JAMA 1988; 259:55–58.

Piot P, Merson MH: Global perspectives on HIV infection and AIDS. *In* Mandell GL, ed: Principles and Practice of Infectious Diseases, 4th ed. New York, Churchill Livingstone, 1995, pp 1164–1174.

Polk BF, Fox R, et al: Predictors of the acquired immunodeficiency syndrome developing in a cohort of seropositive homosexual men. N Engl J Med 1987; 316:61–66.

Pudney J, Anderson D: Orchitis and human immunodeficiency virus type 1 infected cells in reproductive tissues from men with the acquired immune deficiency syndrome. Am J Pathol 1991; 139(1):149–160.

Quinn TC: Unique Aspects of Human Immunodeficiency Virus and Related Viruses in Developing Countries. New York, McGraw-Hill Information Services Company, 1990.

Randazzo RF, Hulette CM, et al: Cytomegaloviral epididymitis in a patient with the acquired immune deficiency syndrome. J Urol 1986; 136:1095–1097.

Rao TKS, Filippone EJ, et al: Associated focal and segmental glomerulosclerosis in the acquired immunodeficiency syndrome. N Engl J Med 1984; 310:669–673.

Rhame FS, Maki DG: The case for wider use of testing for HIV infection. N Engl J Med 1989; 320(19):1248–1254.

Schleupner C: Detection of HIV-1 infection. *In* Mandell GL, ed: Principles and Practice of Infectious Diseases, 4th ed. New York, Churchill Livingstone, 1995, pp 1253–1267.

Selwyn PA, Hartel D, et al: A prospective study of the risk of tuberculosis among intravenous drug users with human immunodeficiency virus infection. N Engl J Med 1989; 320(9):545–550.

Shevchuk M, de Silza M, et al: The male genital tract in AIDS. (Abstract 738.) J Urol, 1989; 141:354A.

Skolnick P, Kosloff B, et al: Bidirectional interactions between human immunodeficiency virus type 1 and cytomegalovirus. J Infect Dis 1988; 157:508–513.

Stamm W, Handsfield H, et al: The association between genital ulcer disease and acquisition of HIV infection in homosexual men. JAMA 1988; 260:1429–1433.

Stanley SK, Fauci AS: Immunology of AIDS and HIV infection. *In* Mandell GL, ed: Principles and Practice of Infectious Diseases, 4th ed. New York, Churchill Livingstone, 1995, pp 1203–1217.

Swartz DA, Harrington P, Wilcox R, et al: Candidal epididymitis treated with ketoconazole. N Engl J Med 1988; 319:1485.

Timmerman JM, Northfelt DW, et al: Malignant germ cell tumors in men infected with the human immunodeficiency virus: Natural history and results of therapy. J Clin Oncol 1995; 13(6):1391–1397.

Trauzzi SJ, Kay CJ, et al: Management of prostatic abscess in patients with human immunodeficiency syndrome. Urology 1994; 43(5):629–633.

Volberding PA: AIDS-Related Malignancies. New York, McGraw-Hill, 1990.

Walker BD, Chakrabarti S, et al: HIV-specific cytotoxic T lymphocytes in seropositive individuals. Nature 1987; 328:345–348.

Watkins BA, Klotman ME, Gallo RC: Human immunodeficiency viruses. *In* Mandell GL, ed: Principles and Practice of Infectious Diseases, 4th ed. New York, Churchill Livingstone, 1995; 1590–1606.

Wilkinson M, Carroll PR: Testicular carcinoma in patients positive and at risk for human immunodeficiency virus. J Urol 1990; 144:1157–1159.

Wilson WT, Frenkel E, et al: Testicular tumors in men with human immunodeficiency virus. J Urol 1992; 147(4):1038–1040.

Zagury D, Bernard J, et al: HTLV-III in cells cultured from semen of two patients with AIDS. Science 1984; 226:449–451.

ADDENDUM TO CHAPTER 19

When prepared, this chapter represented an up-to-the minute summary of HIV infection relevant to the practicing urologist. During more recent months, however, there was a major shift in our ideas of HIV pathogenesis and therapy. Antiretroviral targets that were entirely theoretical have become clinical tools. Some of this information is in the published literature; many more papers have been presented only at meetings or in published abstracts. After discussion with the Editors, it was decided to include the following update summarizing this new information and its major clinical implications.

OVERVIEW. For the first time in many years, most AIDS researchers are uncharacteristically upbeat (Stephenson, 1996). This mood reflects new insights into the immunopathology of HIV, leading to a new sense of direction regarding treatment. Three fundamental ideas form the basis for this new optimism. First, we now appreciate that HIV infection is a dynamic process characterized by high levels of viral replication. If viral replication is not suppressed, development of drug resistance can occur rapidly. Second, many investigators now accept the concept that measuring levels of virus, termed the "viral load," in the blood is the best predictor of disease progression. Third, there is a major shift from monotherapy with drugs of limited potency to combination therapy that includes new drugs that are considerably more powerful than previously available agents.

PROTEASE INHIBITORS. In large part the optimistic mood among AIDS researchers and clinicians is fueled by encouraging studies of some of these new drugs. In short-term studies, the protease inhibitors are at least 10-fold more potent than previously available drugs in reducing the HIV viral load among infected persons.

The HIV protease protein is essential for the virion's life cycle. The protease acts at a late phase of viral replication during assembly of new viral particles. The protease cleaves the gag-pol polyprotein into its component parts (Corey, 1995). Inhibition of the protease results in loss of the gag protein (p24), accumulation of unprocessed full-length constructs, and the emergence of "defective" HIV particles. A number of protease inhibitors have been developed, including several agents that have been evaluated clinically. These agents offer several advantages, particularly the ability to inhibit HIV replication in cells that are chronically infected by a mechanism that is distinct from the mechanism of action of the HIV reverse transcriptase inhibitors. Synergism between the reverse transcriptase inhibitors and the protease inhibitors has been readily demonstrated in vitro. Because the protease inhibitors constitute a class of agents that is different from the reverse transcriptase inhibitors, the toxicity profiles of these two classes of agents are very different, facilitating development of combination chemotherapy.

Clinical experience suggests that the HIV protease inhibitors are effective agents that are well tolerated by patients (Collier et al, 1996; Kelleher et al, 1996; Stephenson, 1996). Because of the need for new HIV therapeutics, the first available agent, saquinavir, received FDA approval in record time. On its heels came other protease inhibitors, such as ritonavir and indinavir. By lowering viral loads and boosting $CD4^+$ T lymphocyte counts, protease inhibitors are the most active agents ever brought to the clinic. Moreover, because there is only a distant relationship between HIV protease and human enzymes, selective inhibitors of HIV protease are expected to have little toxicity. Much hope is riding on this new class of drugs, particularly in combination regimens with the reverse transcriptase inhibitors.

Saquinavir is the prototype drug. It is poorly water soluble, incompletely absorbed after oral administration, difficult to synthesize, and comparatively ineffective when given as monotherapy. Nevertheless, the FDA approved saquinavir in record time, but only in combination with reverse transcriptase inhibitors. The FDA based its decision on studies combining saquinavir with either zalcitabine (ddC) or zidovudine (AZT). Estimates are that in about half of all patients who take saquinavir for 1 year, resistant HIV variants develop. Evidence suggests that the newly synthesized virions resistant to saquinavir are resistant to other protease inhibitors. Therefore, switching from one protease inhibitor to another on the emergence of resistance may be fruitless.

Several reports are summarized to provide a survey of progress as well as to emphasize the relatively short-term follow-up in current clinical series. Collier and associates studied the safety and efficacy of saquinavir, the first available HIV-protease inhibitor, given with reverse transcriptase agents compared with the safety and efficacy of a combination of two nucleosides alone in a double-blind trial (Collier et al, 1996). Of the 302 patients, 96% completed the 24-week study. In all three treatment groups, $CD4^+$ cell counts rose at first and then fell gradually. The normalized area under the curve for the $CD4^+$ count (a measure of positive immunologic response) was greater with the three-drug combination than with either saquinavir and zidovudine ($P = .017$) or ddC and AZT ($P < .001$). There were significantly greater reductions in plasma HIV with the three-drug combination than with the other regimens when peripheral-blood mononuclear cells were cultured for HIV and HIV RNA was assessed. There were no major differences in toxic effects among the three treatments. This study showed that combinations including a protease inhibitor reduced HIV replication and increased $CD4^+$ cell counts more than did treatment with AZT and either saquinavir or ddC.

Treatment with ritonavir, another protease inhibitor, resulted in significant increases in $CD4^+$, $CD8^+$, and CD4CD45RO lymphocytes after 1 week of therapy (Kelleher et al, 1996). Increases occurred in proliferative responses to phytohemagglutinin that correlated with duration of virus load (the amount of HIV in the blood plasma, measured as copies of viral RNA per milliliter of blood) suppression. In short-term studies (often 6 to 12 months or less), ritonavir nearly halved the death rate and the appearance of AIDS-related complications in patients with advanced disease (CD4+ cell counts < 100/ml) (Stephenson, 1996). Of 543 patients receiving ritonavir, 13% died or developed a new AIDS-related condition, compared with 27% of 547 patients on placebo. The mortality rate was 8.4% in the placebo group, in comparison with 4.8% in the ritonavir group. Side effects were modest: mostly nausea, vomiting, weakness, and diarrhea.

Studies of indinavir, a third protease inhibitor, found that indinavir caused striking reductions in viral load, especially when combined with two reverse transcriptase inhibitors. In an ongoing, placebo-controlled trial, HIV-positive patients who had high levels of virus in their blood despite previous

AZT therapy were randomized to three treatment regimens: indinavir alone, a triple-drug combination of indinavir and standard doses of AZT and 3TC, or standard doses of AZT and 3TC without the protease inhibitor. After 4 months, viral load dropped sharply to below the detection level of the viral RNA assay in 90% of 26 patients taking the three-drug regimen, in comparison with 40% of patients taking indinavir alone and none of the patients taking the AZT-3TC combination. $CD4^+$ cell counts increased by about 30 to 40/ml in the AZT-3TC group and by around 100/ml in both groups receiving indinavir. Although the three-drug combination resulted in profound reduction in viral load, low levels of HIV persisted. The concern is that if the drugs are discontinued or if the virus mutates, viral levels rise again. Two patients in the indinavir groups developed kidney stones but were able to remain in the study. According to the manufacturer, kidney stones are the most serious adverse effect observed so far in patients taking indinavir, appearing in about 2% to 3%.

COMBINATION ANTIRETROVIRAL THERAPY. Clearly the era of monotherapy for HIV infection is over; most interest is now centered on selecting optimal antiretroviral drug combinations (Stephenson, 1996). Nevertheless, a number of experts caution that while we are making advances toward the goal of transforming AIDS into a chronic disease whose effects can be largely held in check by treatment, long-term studies with greater numbers of patients are needed. Such caution reflects earlier experience with AZT, the first effective antiretroviral drug. The initially high hopes for AZT were generated by short-term studies showing that AZT appeared to extend life in HIV-infected patients. However, AZT proved to have only limited ability to reduce viral load. HIV with its high replication rate rapidly becomes resistant to AZT. AIDS researchers had a rude awakening in 1993: A 3-year study found that asymptomatic persons who began taking the drug in the early stages of HIV infection lived no longer than those who began treatment after the onset of AIDS. Researchers wary of premature enthusiasm also point to evidence that HIV can become resistant to the new protease inhibitors. Some suggest that this problem may not be inevitable if these potent drugs, in combination with other agents, can suppress levels of virus, dramatically forestalling development of resistance.

VIRAL RESISTANCE? One major question is whether development of drug resistance will limit the protease inhibitors' usefulness. For example, studies show that not only is indinavir most effective when used at high doses to suppress HIV viral replication but also resistance is more likely to develop in patients taking lower doses. Because HIV can replicate extremely rapidly, exposing the virus to a drug without greatly suppressing replication provides ample opportunity for the virus to develop resistance. The hope is that combination therapy will lower the HIV viral load sufficiently to limit the virus's opportunity to accumulate the mutations necessary for development of high-level drug resistance. Thus, protease inhibitor therapy may be appropriate only for patients who will be rigorous about taking their medications on a strict schedule exactly as prescribed.

Optimists point to the effective use of drug combinations in fending off the development of resistance and successfully treating tuberculosis and some cancers. Researchers hope that such a similar strategy may lead to success in treating patients with HIV infection. Only long-term studies can determine whether the beneficial effects of the new protease inhibitors will last. Most studies have monitored patients for up to 6 months or less. Available data suggest that a shift in the goal of antiretroviral therapy may be in order. The goal should be to lower the virus load as much as possible, preferably to undetectable levels, to limit resistance for as long as possible in as many patients as possible.

COSTS AND QUESTIONS. The recommended daily dose of saquinavir, the only currently available protease inhibitor, is 1800 mg taken as three 200-mg capsules three times daily. The wholesale acquisition cost of 1 year's worth of saquinavir therapy is $5800. There is evidence, however, that the recommended dose is suboptimal, and some patients will take more. Although saquinavir is a breakthrough drug, attention is quickly turning to ritonavir and indinavir, which appear to be even more potent.

Although progress is encouraging, prudent observers emphasize the short-term nature of the trials supporting the effectiveness of protease inhibitors. There is no way of knowing how long beneficial effects will last. If HIV does not become resistant to protease inhibitors in combination with the reverse transcriptase inhibitors and if patients tolerate long term treatment, HIV infection may become a treatable chronic disease. The cost, however, will be very high. Estimates are that combination antiviral therapy will cost $12,000 to $18,000 a year. Drugs needed to treat opportunistic infections and related conditions substantially add to that.

Physicians will likely treat patients much earlier during the infection than is now the case if studies find that drug combinations have the hoped-for outcome. Initiation of treatment with multiple drugs will be likely especially for patients who have high viral loads. The potential costs of the new drugs and combination therapy are expected to be considerable. Clinicians and patients are also faced with additional expenses for tests to monitor viral load, which now appears to be a more accurate way to predict the course of HIV infection than are measurements of $CD4^+$ cell counts (Sharp, 1996; Stazewski et al, 1996). Experts suggest that such tests, which are used extensively in research but have not yet been approved for marketing, could be used to stage HIV infection, assess the efficacy of treatment, and indicate whether the virus has developed resistance to drugs. Thus there is concern that the costs of these new therapeutic approaches might make them too expensive for many persons with HIV infection.

POSTEXPOSURE PROPHYLAXIS. These new developments have led to improved recommendations for management of exposure to HIV in the health care setting. Our infection control committee now recommends that after high-risk exposures, exposed health care workers receive a three-drug regimen incorporating both reverse-transcriptase inhibitors (both AZT and 3TC) and a protease inhibitor (currently indinavir). Treatment is instituted as soon as possible, preferably within 1 hour of exposure. The goal of therapy is to limit the potential for infection, or, failing that, to ensure that the infected health care worker will have the lowest possible viral load.

REFERENCES

Collier AC, Coombs RW, Schoenfeld DA, et al: Treatment of human immunodeficiency virus infection with saquinavir, zidovudine, and zalcitabine. AIDS Clinical Trials Group. N Engl J Med 1996; 334:1011–1017.

Corey L: Therapy of HIV infection. *In* Mandell GL, Bennett JE, Dolin R, eds: Mandell, Douglas and Bennett's Principles and Practice of Infectious Diseases, 4th ed. New York: Churchill-Livingstone, 1995, pp 1267–1280.

Kelleher AD, Carr A, Zaunders J, Cooper DA: Alterations in the immune response of human immunodeficiency virus (HIV)-infected subjects treated with an HIV-specific protease inhibitor, ritonavir. J Infect Dis 1996; 173:321–329.

Sharp D. Vancouver conference marks viral-load era of AIDS. Lancet 1996; 348:183.

Staszewski S, Loveday C, Picazo JJ, et al: Safety and efficacy of lamivudine-zidovudine combination therapy in zidovudine-experienced patients: A randomized controlled comparison with zidovudine monotherapy. Lamivudine European HIV Working Group. JAMA 1996; 276:111–117.

Stephenson J: New anti-HIV drugs and treatment strategies buoy AIDS researchers. JAMA 1996; 275:579–580.

20
COLOR ATLAS OF GENITAL DERMATOLOGY

David J. Margolis, M.D.
Alan J. Wein, M.D.

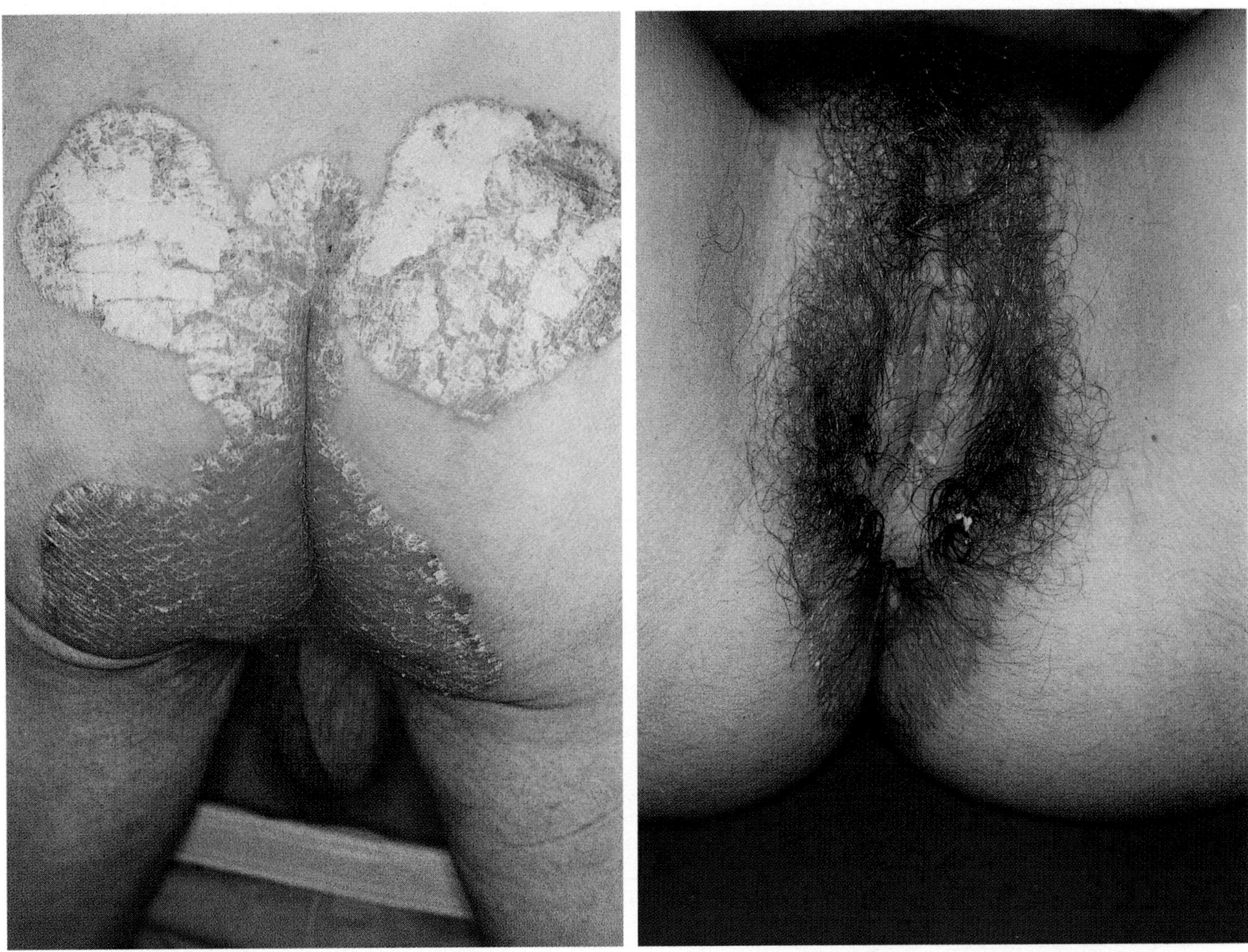

Figure 20–1. Psoriasis. Serpiginous erythematous plaque lesions with silvery scales. (From Callen JP, Greer DE, Hood AF, Paller AS: Color Atlas of Dermatology. Philadelphia, W.B. Saunders Company, 1993, p 320.)

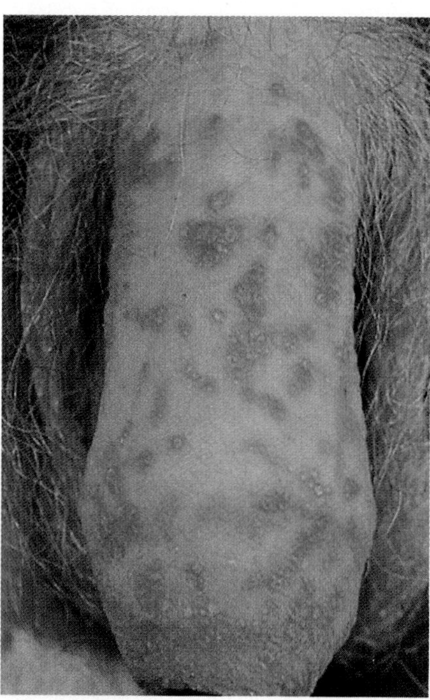

Figure 20–2. Lichen planus. Papules both individual and grouped on the shaft of the penis. The linearity of some of the lesions may be a response to local trauma. (From Korting GW: Practical Dermatology of the Genital Region. Philadelphia, W.B. Saunders Company, 1981, p 29.)

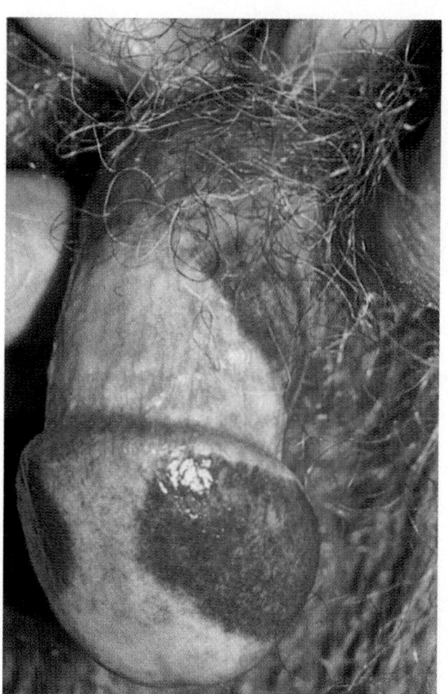

Figure 20–4. Plasma cell balanitis (Zoon's erythroplasia). Smooth tissue-paper–like erythematous lesion of the glans and shaft. (From Korting GW: Practical Dermatology of the Genital Region. Philadelphia, W.B. Saunders Company, 1981, p 159.)

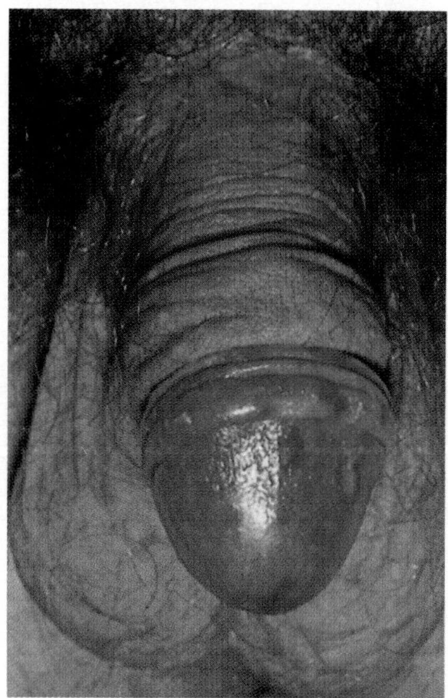

Figure 20–3. *Candida.* Superficially erosive erythematous lesion with fine scales on the glans of the penis. (From Korting GW: Practical Dermatology of the Genital Region. Philadelphia, W.B. Saunders Company, 1981, p 159.)

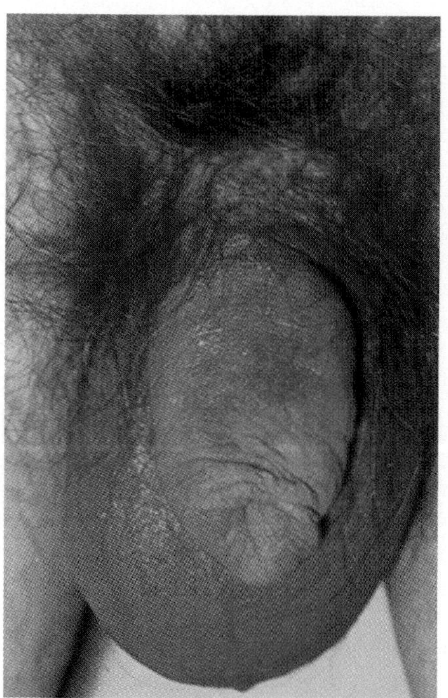

Figure 20–5. Cellulitis of the penis (Fournier's gangrene). Extensive edema and erythema associated with systemic complaints. (From Korting GW: Practical Dermatology of the Genital Region. Philadelphia, W.B. Saunders Company, 1981, p 37.)

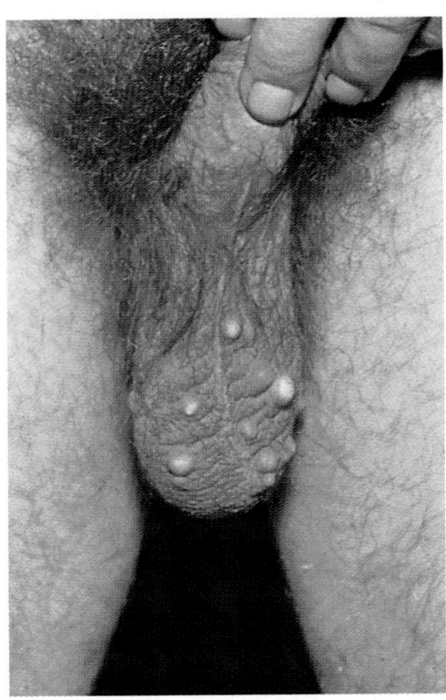

Figure 20–6. Sebaceous cyst. Large nodular or tumor-like structure. These cysts often have a central pore from which a keratin-containing compound can be expressed. (From Korting GW: Practical Dermatology of the Genital Region. Philadelphia, W.B. Saunders Company, 1981, p 115.)

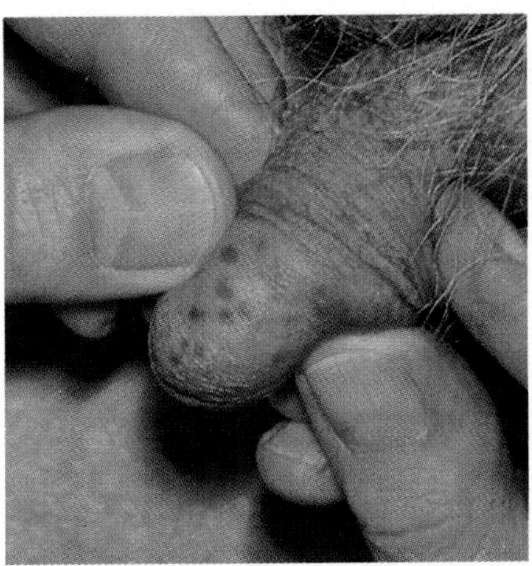

Figure 20–8. Lentigo. Small, evenly brown-pigmented macules of the glans. (From Korting GW: Practical Dermatology of the Genital Region. Philadelphia, W.B. Saunders Company, 1981, p 85.)

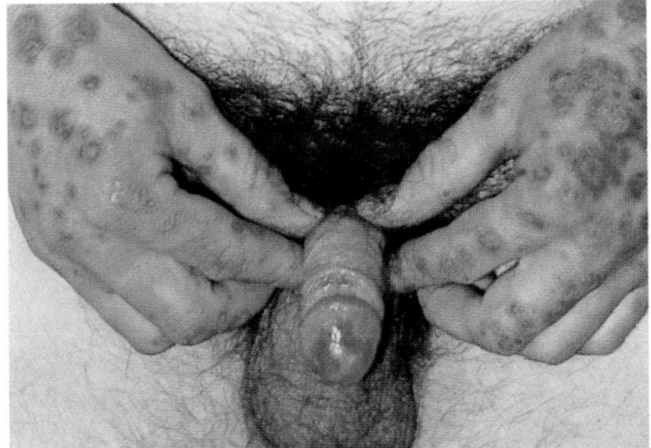

Figure 20–7. Erythema multiforme. Targetoid lesions of hands and penis. Lesions on friable tissue (e.g., glans, mucosal membranes) are prone to ulcerate. (From Korting GW: Practical Dermatology of the Genital Region. Philadelphia, W.B. Saunders Company, 1981, p 16.)

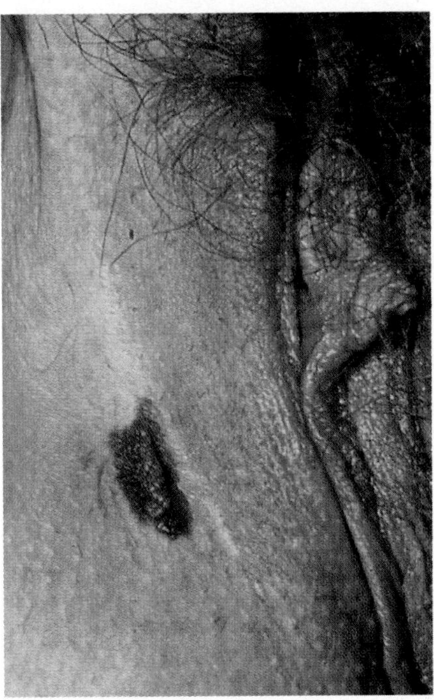

Figure 20–9. Compound nevus. Papular and macular brown lesion of the inguinal crease. (From Korting GW: Practical Dermatology of the Genital Region. Philadelphia, W.B. Saunders Company, 1981, p 121.)

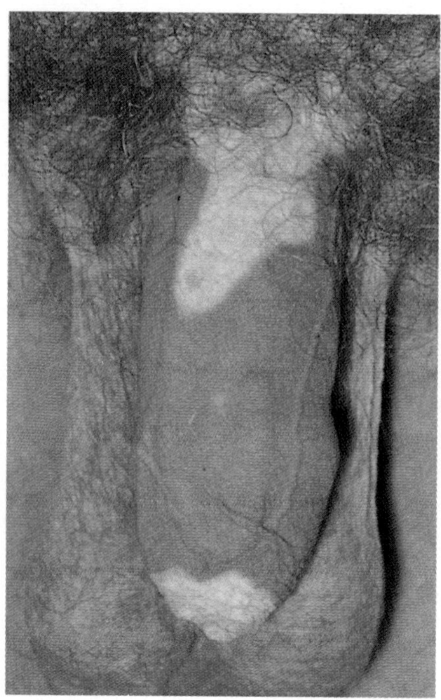

Figure 20–10. Vitiligo. Hypopigmented patches of vitiligo. The genital region is a common site of this disorder. (From Korting GW: Practical Dermatology of the Genital Region. Philadelphia, W.B. Saunders Company, 1981, p 88.)

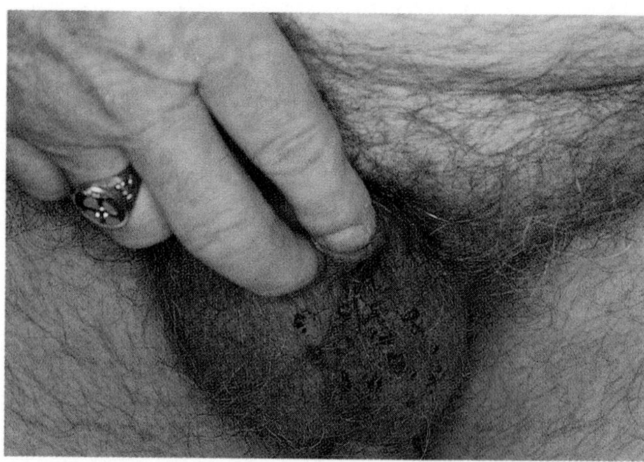

Figure 20–12. Angiokeratoma of Fordyce. Purplish vascular malformations of the scrotum. (From Callen JP, Greer DE, Hood AF, Paller AS: Color Atlas of Dermatology. Philadelphia, W.B. Saunders Company, 1993, p 328.)

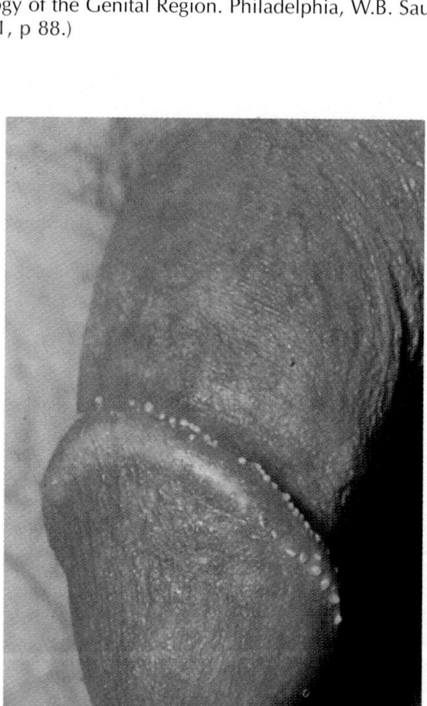

Figure 20–11. Pearly penile papules. Common papillomatous lesions, usually of the corona of the glans. They are often mistaken for verruca. (From Korting GW: Practical Dermatology of the Genital Region. Philadelphia, W.B. Saunders Company, 1981, p 5.)

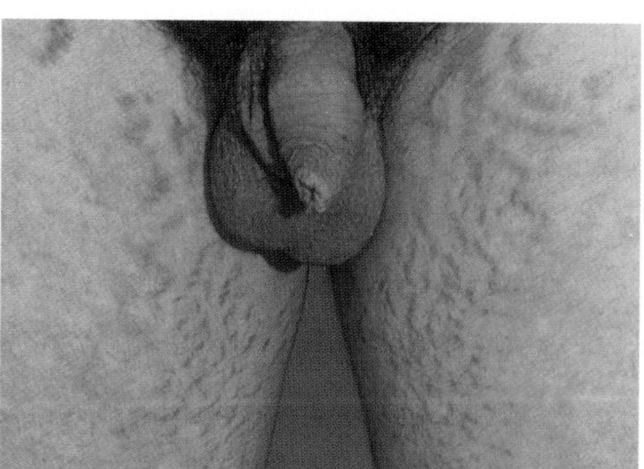

Figure 20–13. Striae. Atrophic lesion of the epidermis and dermis. The purple color of the lesion abates with time, but the atrophic nature of the lesion is permanent. These lesions can result from hormonal changes, from changes in body size, and from both topical and systemic use of glucocorticoid. (From Korting GW: Practical Dermatology of the Genital Region. Philadelphia, W.B. Saunders Company, 1981, p 70.)

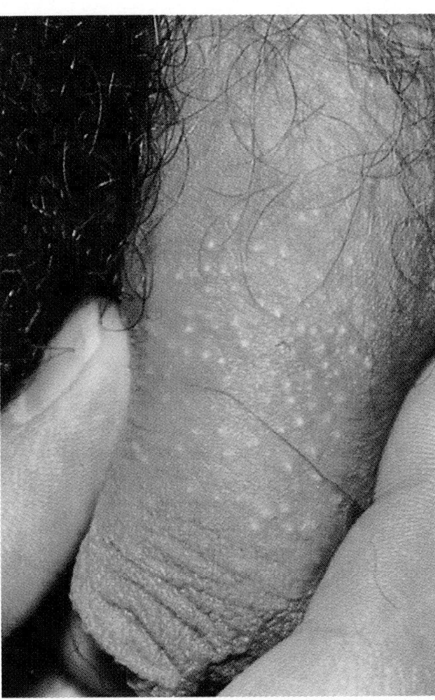

Figure 20–14. Ectopic sebaceous glans. Pin-sized papular lesions of the shaft of the penis, which are often mistaken for verruca. (From Callen JP, Greer DE, Hood AF, Paller AS: Color Atlas of Dermatology. Philadelphia, W.B. Saunders Company, 1993, p 3.)

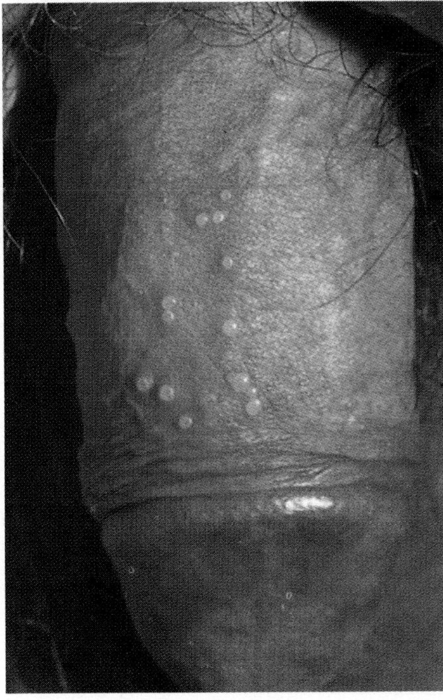

Figure 20–15. Herpes simplex virus. Umbilicated vesicle of the shaft, characteristic of early tissue infection. These lesions are often pustular and ulcerate during the course of the infection. (From Callen JP, Greer DE, Hood AF, Paller AS: Color Atlas of Dermatology. Philadelphia, W.B. Saunders Company, 1993, p 48.)

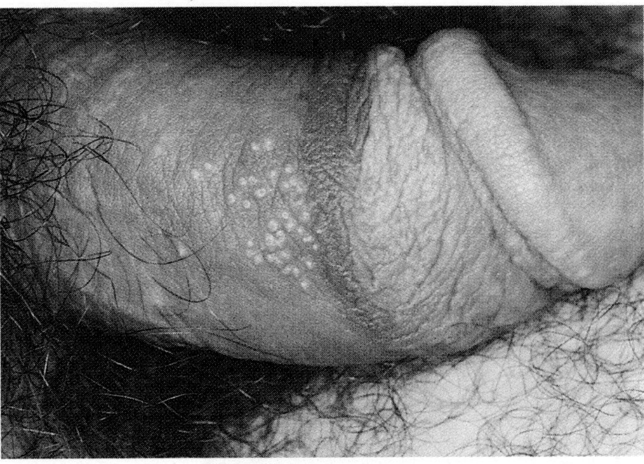

Figure 20–16. Molluscum contagiosum. Persistent umbilicated papules of the penile shaft. (From Callen JP, Greer DE, Hood AF, Paller AS: Color Atlas of Dermatology. Philadelphia, W.B. Saunders Company, 1993, p 328.)

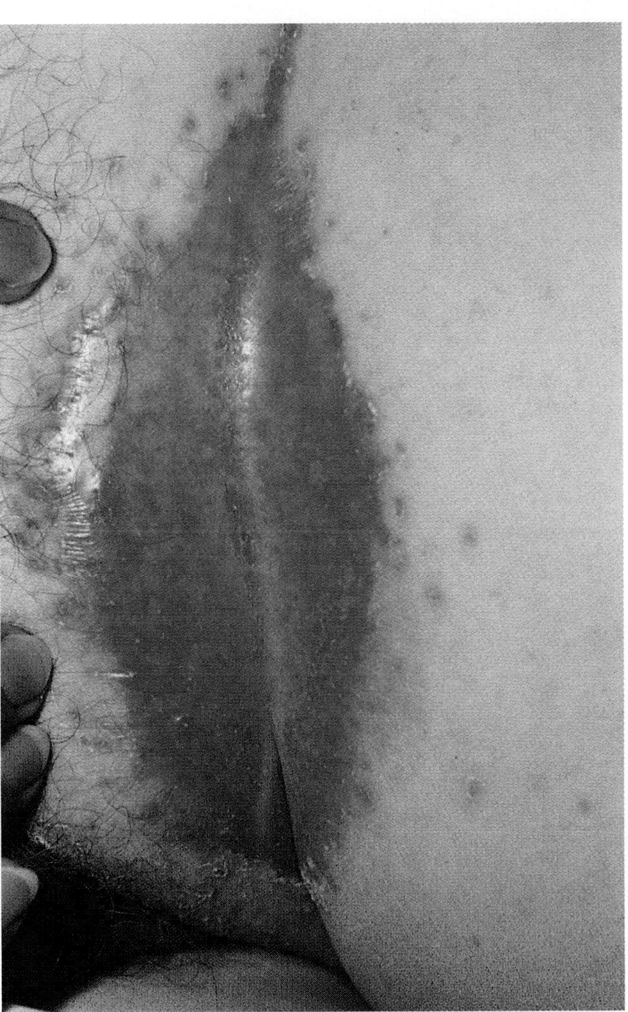

Figure 20–17. *Candida intertrigo.* Erythematous eruption with fine scales in an area of tissue maceration. Distinct individual satellite lesions are present. (From Callen JP, Greer DE, Hood AF, Paller AS: Color Atlas of Dermatology. Philadelphia, W.B. Saunders Company, 1993, p 318.)

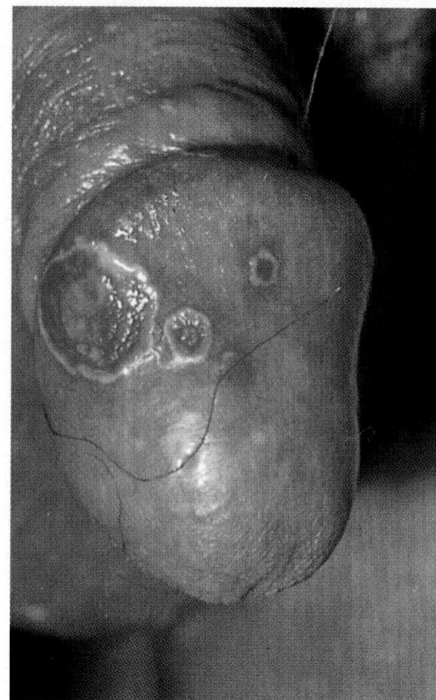

Figure 20–18. Circinate balanitis (Reiter's disease). Erosive circinate lesion of the glans penis. This condition may be difficult to differentiate from psoriasis. (From Callen JP, Greer DE, Hood AF, Paller AS: Color Atlas of Dermatology. Philadelphia, W.B. Saunders Company, 1993, p 160.)

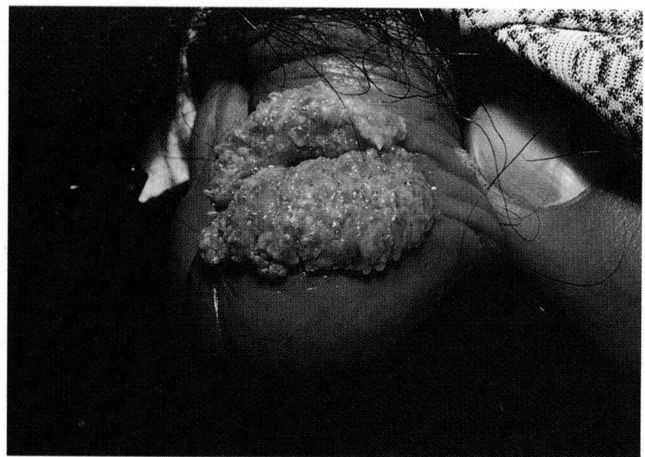

Figure 20–19. Verrucous carcinoma of the penis (Buschke-Löwenstein tumor). Exophytic warty lesion of squamous cell carcinoma, which has the histologic appearance of verruca vulgaris. (From Callen JP, Greer DE, Hood AF, Paller AS: Color Atlas of Dermatology. Philadelphia, W.B. Saunders Company, 1993, p 330.)

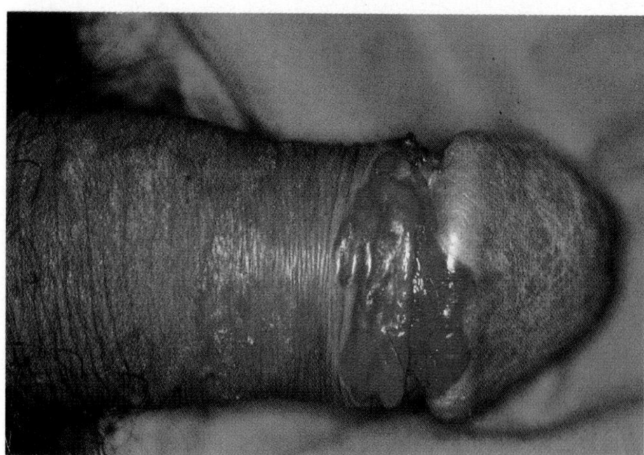

Figure 20–20. Erythroplasia of Queyrat. Squamous cell in situ on the glans penis. (From Callen JP, Greer DE, Hood AF, Paller AS: Color Atlas of Dermatology. Philadelphia, W.B. Saunders Company, 1993, p 330.)

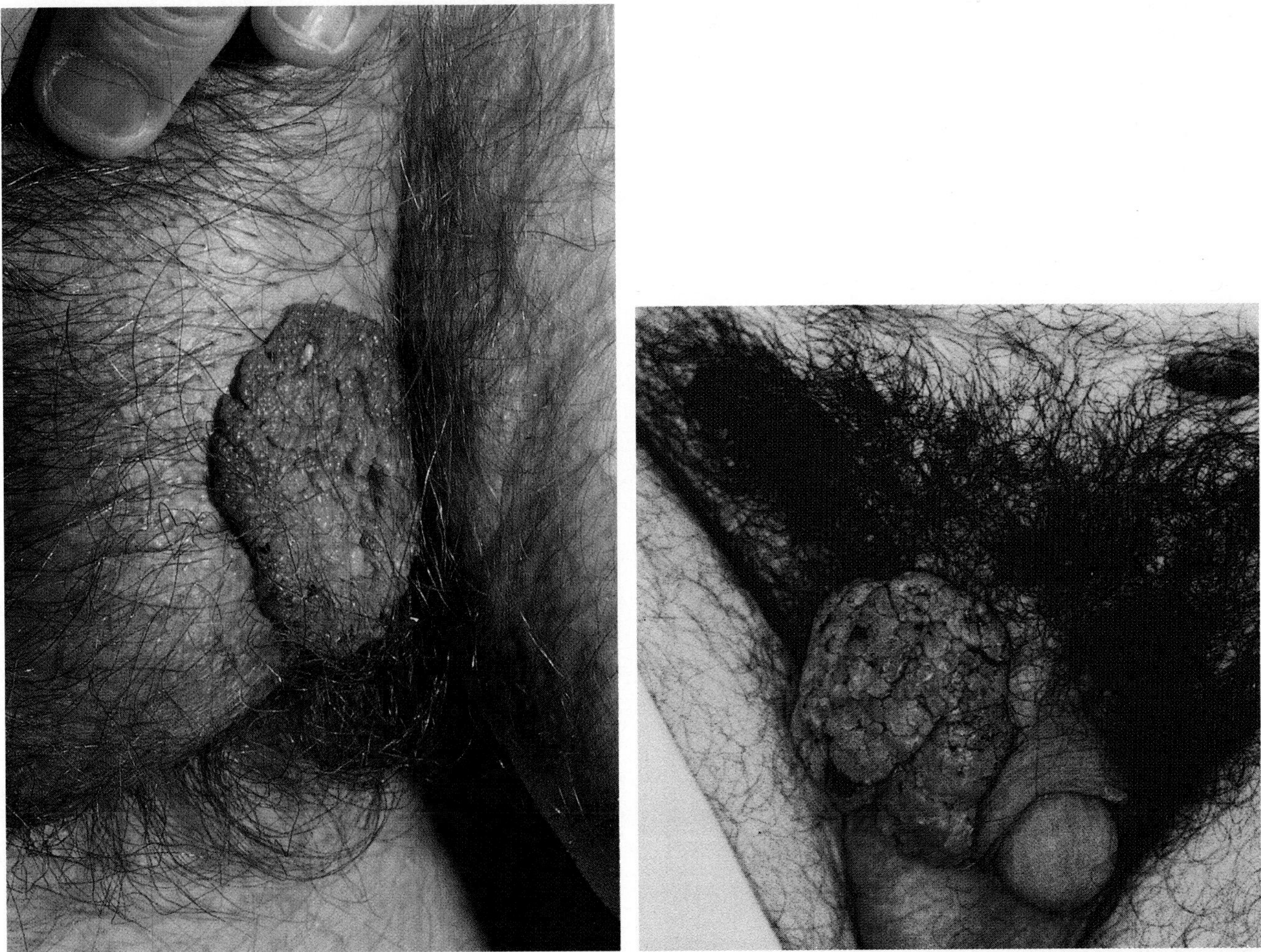

Figure 20–21. Condyloma acuminatum. Exophytic warty lesion of the genital region. (From Callen JP, Greer DE, Hood AF, Paller AS: Color Atlas of Dermatology. Philadelphia, W.B. Saunders Company, 1993, p 330.)

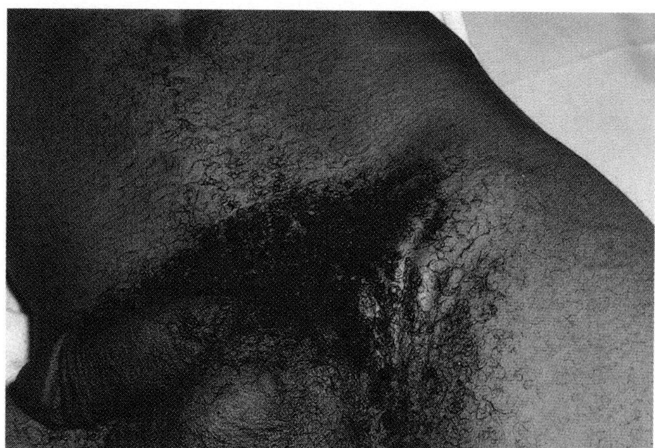

Figure 20–22. Lymphogranuloma venereum. Swollen bubo in the area of inguinal lymph nodes. (From Callen JP, Greer DE, Hood AF, Paller AS: Color Atlas of Dermatology. Philadelphia, W.B. Saunders Company, 1993, p 331.)

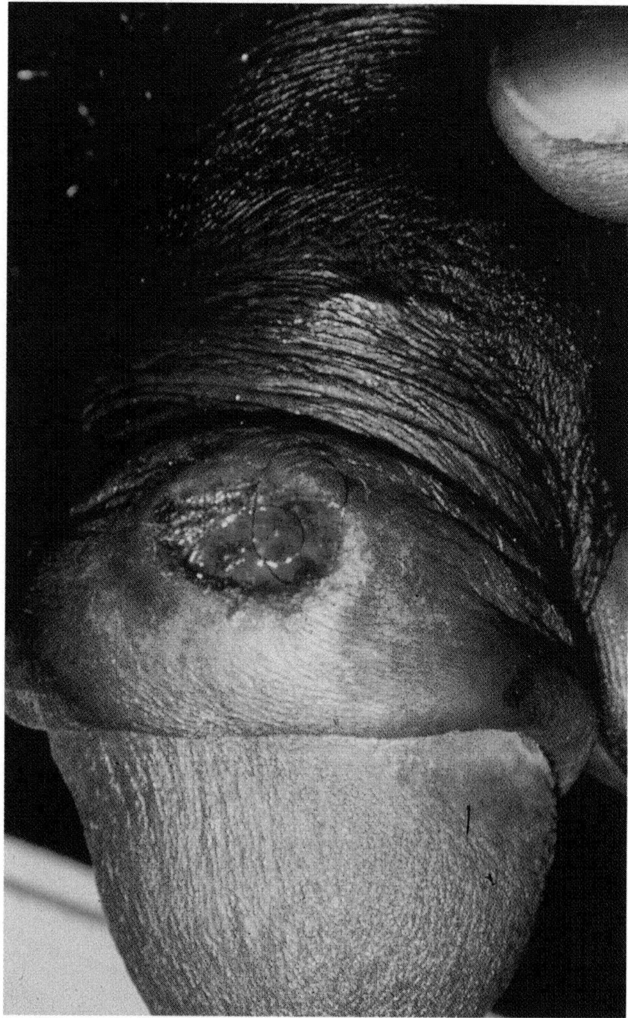

Figure 20–23. Chancre. Erosive volcano-like lesion with a hard border. (From Callen JP, Greer DE, Hood AF, Paller AS: Color Atlas of Dermatology. Philadelphia, W.B. Saunders Company, 1993, p 329.)

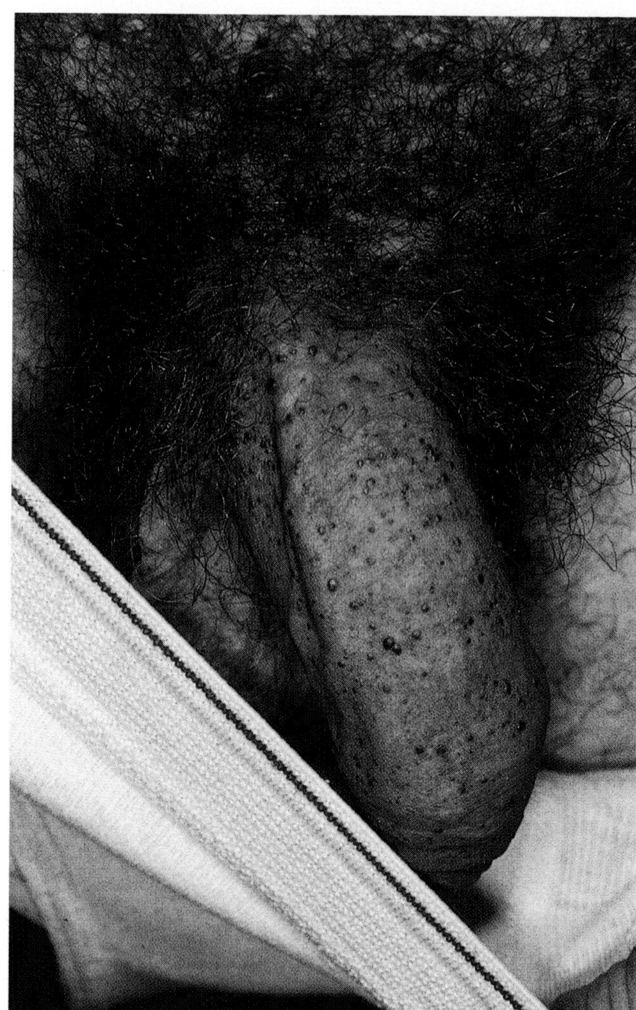

Figure 20–24. Fabry's disease (angiokeratoma corpus diffusum universale). Purplish vascular malformations of an uncommon glycogen storage disease. (From Callen JP, Greer DE, Hood AF, Paller AS: Color Atlas of Dermatology. Philadelphia, W.B. Saunders Company, 1993, p 327.)

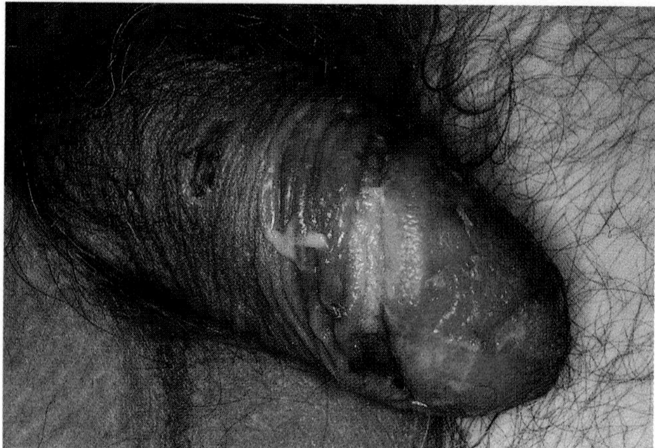

Figure 20–25. Fixed drug reaction. Deeply erythematous and sometimes erosive lesion related to a specific ingestant. (From Callen JP, Greer DE, Hood AF, Paller AS: Color Atlas of Dermatology. Philadelphia, W.B. Saunders Company, 1993, p 327.)

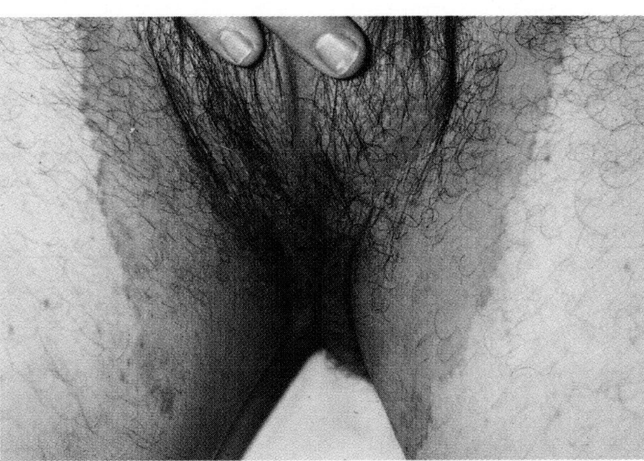

Figure 20–26. Tinea cruris. Typical lesions of dermatophyte infection, demonstrating chronic areas (hyperpigmented) and acute peripheral areas (linear area of erythematous papules). (From Callen JP, Greer DE, Hood AF, Paller AS: Color Atlas of Dermatology. Philadelphia, W.B. Saunders Company, 1993, p 318.)

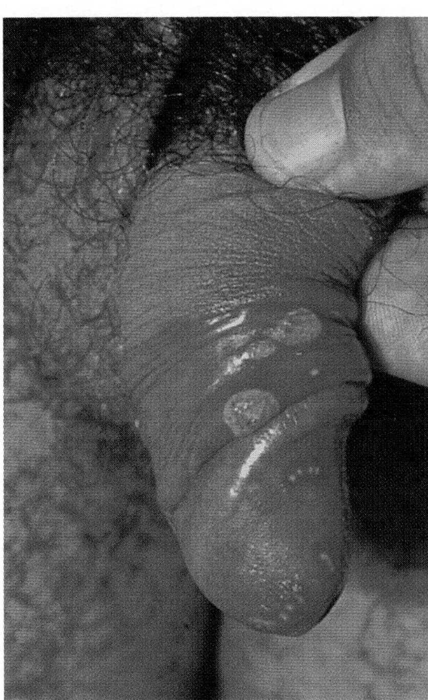

Figure 20–28. Chancroid. Soft, painful, erosive lesions. (From Callen JP, Greer DE, Hood AF, Paller AS: Color Atlas of Dermatology. Philadelphia, W.B. Saunders Company, 1993, p 177.)

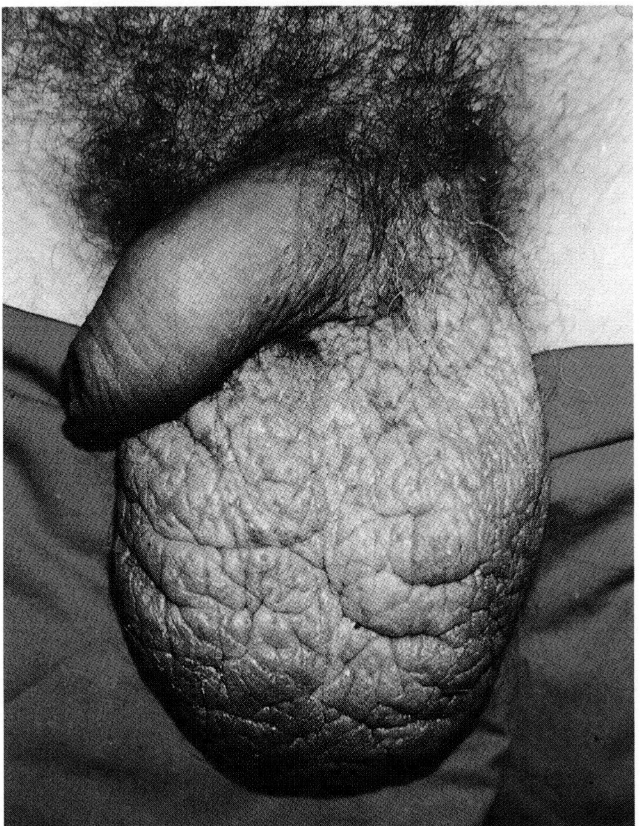

Figure 20–27. Lichen simplex chronicus. Thickened skin with accentuated skin folds and markings. (From Callen JP, Greer DE, Hood AF, Paller AS: Color Atlas of Dermatology. Philadelphia, W.B. Saunders Company, 1993, p 324.)

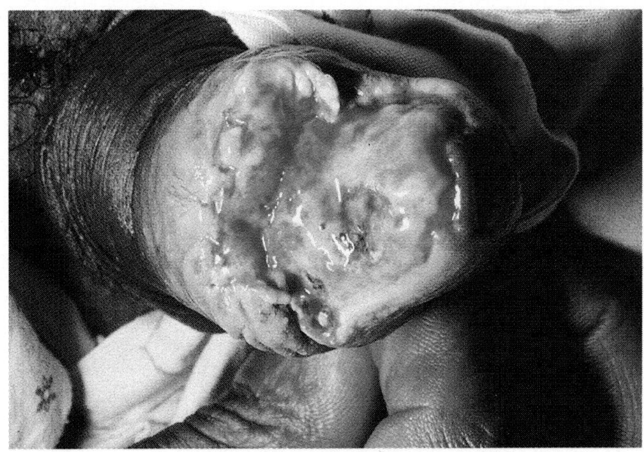

Figure 20–29. Granuloma inguinale. Irregularly shaped ulcer without inguinal adenopathy. (From Callen JP, Greer DE, Hood AF, Paller AS: Color Atlas of Dermatology. Philadelphia, W.B. Saunders Company, 1993, p 233.)

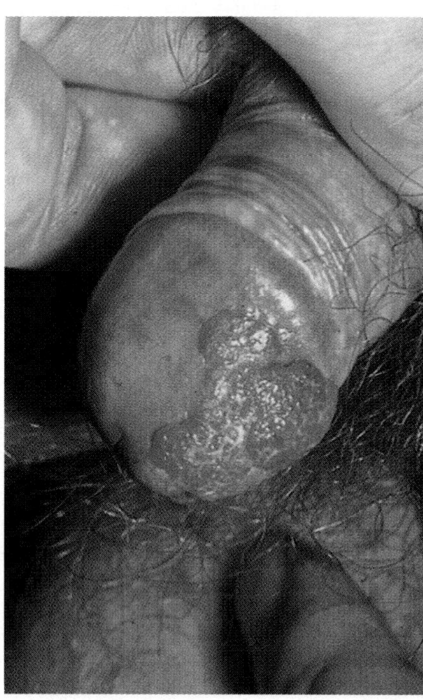

Figure 20–30. Squamous cell carcinoma. Exophytic erosive lesion, which may show signs of keratinization. (From Callen JP, Greer DE, Hood AF, Paller AS: Color Atlas of Dermatology. Philadelphia, W.B. Saunders Company, 1993, p 129.)

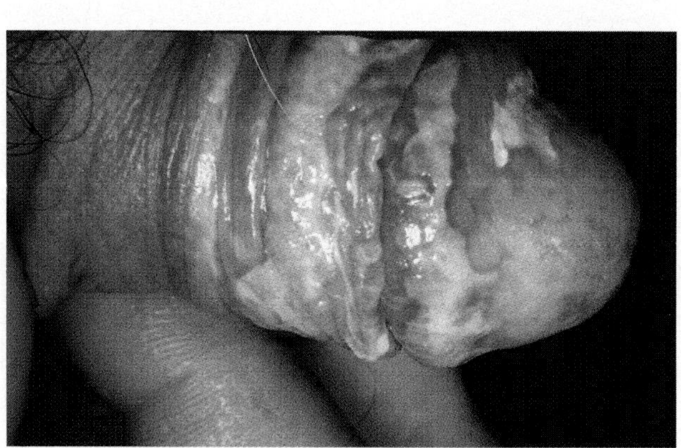

Figure 20–31. Lichen sclerosis et atrophicus (balanitis xerotica obliterans). Porcelain-like indurated lesions of the glans and shaft of the penis. (From Callen JP, Greer DE, Hood AF, Paller AS: Color Atlas of Dermatology. Philadelphia, W.B. Saunders Company, 1993, p 327.)

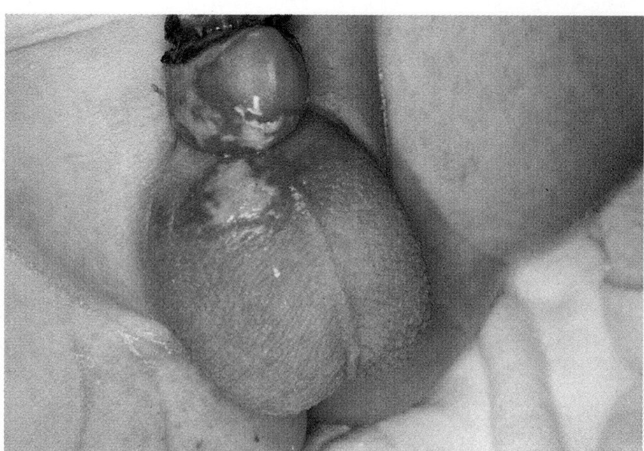

Figure 20–32. Penile pyoderma gangrenosum. Painful ulcers, often on an erythematous to violaceous base. (From Callen JP, Greer DE, Hood AF, Paller AS: Color Atlas of Dermatology. Philadelphia, W.B. Saunders Company, 1993, p 330.)

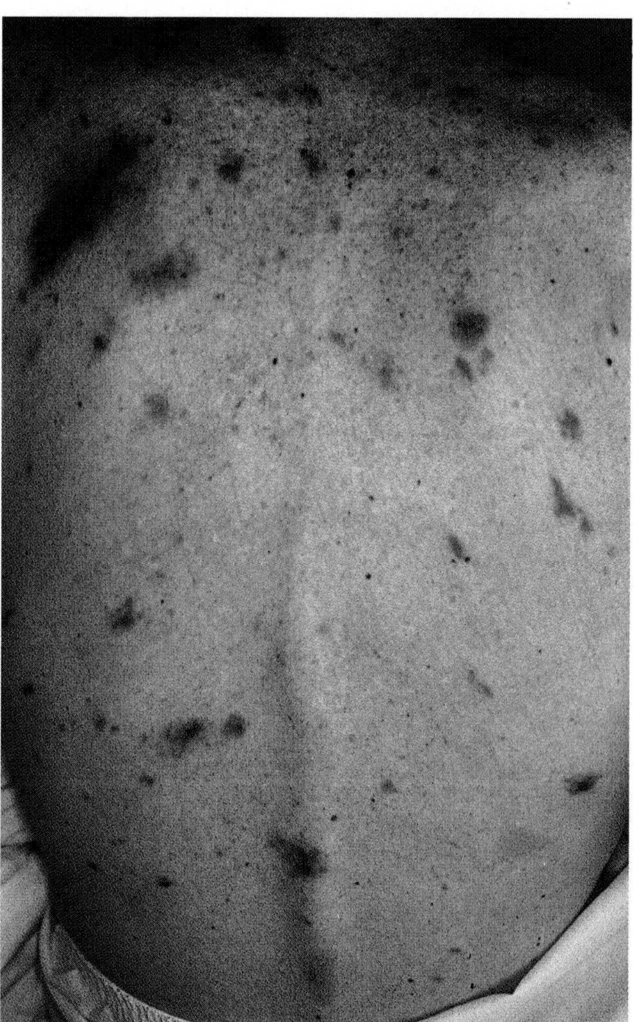

Figure 20–33. Kaposi's sarcoma. Macular lesions most frequently found on the lower extremities. (From Callen JP, Greer DE, Hood AF, Paller AS: Color Atlas of Dermatology. Philadelphia, W.B. Saunders Company, 1993, p 220.)

21 CUTANEOUS DISEASES OF THE MALE EXTERNAL GENITALIA

David J. Margolis, M.D.

Dermatology as a clinical discipline is involved with all aspects of the skin. For many dermatologic diseases, the diagnoses are made entirely by visual inspection and patient history. At times diagnosis is made by laboratory examination, by understanding the natural history of the disease, by repeated visual examination, and by repeated patient questioning. Very few cutaneous diseases occur only on the genital area. It is important to examine all cutaneous surfaces when diagnosing dermatologic illnesses. In general, diseases of the skin tend to present with similar symptoms and signs regardless of location.

Dermatologists try to use precise language to describe skin disease. The most common subjective symptom is pruritus (itching), although many patients also report pain and burning. The most common visual finding is erythema, a term used to describe redness. The quality and quantity of erythema are dependent on the disease process and the patient's background skin color. Skin lesions can also be brown, black, yellow, blue, and green. Common descriptive terms for skin lesions include *macule*, a flat lesion less than 0.5 cm; *patch*, a flat lesion more than 0.5 cm; *papule*, an elevated 0.5-cm lesion; *nodule*, a deeper-based papular lesion; *plaque*, a palpable lesion more than 0.5 cm; *vesicle*, a fluid-filled palpable lesion less than 0.5 cm; *pustule*, a pus-filled palpable lesion; *bulla* or *blister*, a fluid-filled lesion greater than 0.5 cm; *erosion*, a lesion representing only the loss of epidermis; *ulcer*, a lesion representing the loss of at least epidermis and superficial dermis; *hives*, or *urticaria*, circumscribed evanescent areas of cutaneous edema; *scale*, exfoliation of the superficial portions of the skin; and *crust*, scale with dried serum, pus, blood, or bacteria. Because of the mucosal nature of genital skin, papular and macular lesions may present as erosions.

Dermatologic diagnosis is often augmented by laboratory examinations. Skin biopsy is performed as an office-based procedure using punch biopsy blades. The histologic assessment of this specimen can be an invaluable diagnostic tool. Other techniques that could be useful for the diagnosis of genital lesions include the potassium hydroxide preparation, for cutaneous fungi such as *Candida* and dermatophyte; and the Tzanck preparation, for cutaneous viral infections such as molluscum contagiosum, varicella-zoster, and herpes simplex. For a more complete discussion of the language of dermatology and dermatologic techniques, the reader should obtain a general dermatology textbook.

Dermatologic therapy includes both systemic and topical compounds. The most frequently used systemic compounds are antibiotics, such as penicillins and tetracyclines; antifungals, such as ketoconazole and griseofulvin; antipruritics, such as hydroxyzine and diphenhydramine; and anti-inflammatory agents, such as glucocorticoid. The use of these agents should be guided by the perceived diagnosis and the clinical efficacy of the agent. Topical compounds are more frequently used by dermatologists than systemic agents but often seem to be difficult for nondermatologists to master. Topical agents are also available in the above-listed drug classes, and others can be destructive, such as liquid nitrogen and podophyllin. Topical agents are available in multiple vehicles such as creams, gels, lotions, ointments, and multiple strengths. Potency is influenced both by the vehicle—ointments are often the most potent—and by the steroid compound, but rarely by the percentage of the compound in the vehicle. The weakest efficacious therapeutic compound should always be used. Permanent cutaneous atrophy can occur with all topical steroids, especially in thin, often occluded, genital skin. Atrophy is less likely to occur with weaker steroid compounds than with the more potent products. It is good practice to become acquainted with a few corticosteroids of differing potency. High and maximally potent topical steroids are seldom required for the treatment of genital lesions, and a health care provider should use extreme caution when using a corticosteroid from this class. For potency rankings of corticosteroids the reader should refer to standard textbooks of dermatology and pharmaceuticals.

PAPULOSQUAMOUS DISORDERS

Papulosquamous disorders are scaling disorders on an erythematous base. The base can be a papule, macule, plaque, or patch (Table 21–1).

Psoriasis

Psoriasis (see Fig. 20–1) is a common illness that occurs worldwide and afflicts at least 1% of the population of the United States (Christophers and Sterry, 1993). It is hyperproliferation of the epidermis. It often begins by the third decade of life and is a chronic lifelong problem (Farber and Nall, 1974; Hensler and Christophers, 1985). The etiology of psoriasis is uncertain and most likely multifactorial. One third of affected individuals have a family history of this disease (Melski and Stern, 1981; Hensler and Christophers, 1985).

Lesions appear as red to pink plaques or patches covered with white to gray scale. However, scale may not be present in skin folds and on moist and mucosal surfaces. The diagnosis of genital psoriasis is greatly aided by the discovery of typical red scaling plaques elsewhere on the body. Lesions are most commonly noted on the elbows, knees, scalp, umbilicus, nails, and buttocks. Lesions may be pruritic and may occur as several morphologic varieties, including plaque-like, guttate, pustular, inverse, and nummular. The genital surfaces most commonly afflicted are hair-bearing structures and the perirectum. Psoriasis is also found on the glans

Table 21–1. DIFFERENTIAL DIAGNOSIS OF PAPULOSQUAMOUS LESIONS

Psoriasis
Seborrheic dermatitis
Dermatophyte infection
Erythrasma
Secondary syphilis
Pityriasis rosea
Discoid lupus
Mycosis fungoides
Lichen planus
Fixed drug reaction
Reiter's syndrome
Pityriasis versicolor
Bowen's disease
Extramammary Paget's disease

penis, where it is a common noninfectious dermatosis (Johnson, 1993). Genital involvement usually does not occur without nongenital disease.

Patients with genital psoriasis may note pruritus and tenderness in the location of a lesion. However, they often seek health care advice due to anxiety or concern about malignancy or sexually transmitted disease. For both clinical confirmation and patient comfort a diagnostic biopsy may be helpful (Weinrauch and Katz, 1986).

Psoriasis is a chronic lifelong disease with periods of exacerbation and remission. Improvement of genital lesions can occur with topical emollients but often requires low-potency topical steroids, which, on genital skin, should be used continuously for no more than 2 weeks. Prolonged use of topical steroids on thin and occluded (e.g., by skin folds) skin can result in cutaneous atrophy, the formation of striae, the proliferation of cutaneous fungi, and a skin dependency reaction. Other successful topical therapies include anthralin, calcipotriene, and tar. Patients with severe full-body disease may require systemic treatments, such as with methotrexate, etretinate, a psoralen, UVB, or cyclosporine (Greaves and Weinstein, 1995). These therapies are rarely required for local disease.

Lichen Planus

Lichen planus (see Fig. 20–2) is a pruritic inflammatory disease of the skin. It occurs on mucosal membranes and surfaces containing a mature stratum corneum. It occurs on the trunk, flexor aspects of limbs, oral mucosa, and the glans penis. The true frequency of this disease is not known, but it is relatively uncommon.

The characteristic lesion is a flat-topped violaceous polygonal papule. Patients commonly have multiple lesions that range from 2 to 5 mm in diameter and may coalesce to form larger or annular lesions. Linear configurations, as if in response to trauma, may also occur. Lesions on the glans penis may be ringlike but tend to be solitary and few. Lesions of lichen planus ulcerate, especially on macerated and mucosal surfaces.

The pathologic process is the result of T-cell interaction in the skin (Morhenn, 1986; Oliver and Winkelmann, 1993). Variants of lichen planus, often called lichenoid reactions, can occur in response to ingestants. The diagnosis of lichen planus on the skin is usually based on clinical observation unless lesions are ulcerated. These lesions often require histopathologic confirmation. The differential diagnosis of lichen planus includes secondary syphilis, Bowen's disease, psoriasis, Zoon's balanitis, and squamous cell carcinoma. These diagnostic possibilities must be excluded either on clinical grounds or with serologic or histologic evaluation.

Characteristically, lichen planus resolves spontaneously. Asymptomatic lesions do not require treatment. Patients require reassurance and emotional support regarding the benign and noninfectious nature of this ailment. Topical steroids may provide symptomatic relief. Systemic immunosuppressive agents, including corticosteroids, can successfully treat symptoms (Jemec and Baadsgaard, 1993; Oliver and Winkelmann, 1993) and may be necessary in severe oral lichen planus, but probably do not affect the course of the disease.

Lichen Nitidus

Lichen nitidus is an uncommon chronic inflammatory disease. It is characterized by very small flat-topped flesh-colored to pink or yellow-red papules. Lesions most commonly occur on the penis, lower abdomen, and arms. The lesions may appear follicular but are not. Lesions do occur in sites of local trauma. Rarely, as seen in lichen planus, lesions coalesce into larger lesions.

The cause of lichen nitidus is not known. Some authors believe that it may be a variant of lichen planus (Waisman, 1971; Aram, 1988). It has a distinctive histologic appearance. In the superficial dermis a dense infiltrate of lymphocytes, histiocytes, and melanophages forms a ball-like structure covered by thinned epidermis forming a clawlike covering.

These lesions usually spontaneously remit. Reassurance to the patient that he does not have a communicable disease such as a wart is very important. Otherwise, pharmacologic intervention is seldom required. Corticosteroids, psoralen-UVA, and etretinate have all been tried with varied results (Randle and Sander, 1986; Aram, 1988).

Reiter's Syndrome

Reiter's syndrome (see Fig. 20–15) is a systemic illness that involves several soft and hard tissues. The disease is much more common in men than in women (Tuncer et al, 1992). It is associated with a preceding urethritis—due to *Gonococcus* or *Chlamydia*—or enteritis—due to *Yersinia, Salmonella, Shigella, Campylobacter, Neisseria,* or *Ureaplasma* spp (Lahesmaa et al, 1991; Rahman et al, 1992). It is more common in individuals with human immunodeficiency virus (HIV) infection. This illness occurs as a triad of arthritis of a month's duration in association with urethritis, cervicitis or enteritis, and conjunctivitis. Iritis may also occur.

The cutaneous manifestations are similar to both plaquelike and pustular psoriasis. Individuals with Reiter's syndrome more commonly have HLA B27 than do individuals with psoriasis. Lesions commonly occur on the glans penis (circinate balanitis), are circinate, and are eroded. Similar lesions may occur on other mucosal membranes. Hyperkeratotic lesions of the hand and feet may occur (keratoderma blenorraghicum). Histologic examination of the cutaneous lesions cannot consistently differentiate the condition from psoriasis.

Fixed Drug Eruption

A fixed drug eruption (see Fig. 20–25) occurs in reaction to the parenteral administration of a medication. When an individual is rechallenged with this agent, then the lesion recurs in the same location. The medications most likely to cause this reaction are oral contraceptives, barbiturates, phenolphthalein, tetracycline, salicylates, and nonsteroidal anti-inflammatory agents (Thankappan and Zachariah, 1991).

Fixed drug eruptions of the genitalia are usually solitary, well-demarcated inflammatory plaques, which, like other genital lesions, may become erosive. Lesions are most frequently found on the shaft and glans of the penis and may be painful. Because of the location, and erosive and recurrent nature, the lesions are often misdiagnosed as herpetic. Postinflammatory hyperpigmentation is common in recurrent lesions. Lesions usually heal with topical care after the offending agent has been stopped.

Seborrheic Dermatitis

Seborrheic dermatitis is a very common dermatologic ailment. It is a cause of dandruff. It is usually found on the scalp, eyebrows, nasolabial folds, ears, and chest, but it can occur on the anus, penis, and pubic hair areas. This is a lifelong affliction with periods of exacerbation and remission (Webster, 1991). In immunocompromised hosts it can cover the entire skin surface.

Lesions are generally found on hair-bearing surfaces, have a red base, and often have a waxy yellow crust. Lesions may be pruritic and can be difficult to differentiate from psoriasis. Evaluation of extragenital skin sites is extremely helpful in making this distinction. A skin biopsy may be helpful to differentiate it from other papulosquamous illness. However, histopathologic examination is not pathognomonic. Although *Pityrosporon orbiculare* has been implicated as a causative organism for seborrheic dermatitis, the true cause of this disease is not known.

Treatment of seborrheic dermatitis includes frequent shampooing of involved hair-bearing areas. Shampoos should be used per the recommendations of the manufacturers. "Antidandruff" shampoos containing zinc, salicylic acid, selenium sulfide, tar, and ketoconazole can be used. The frequency of shampooing can be decreased once the affected site is no longer scaly. Topical antifungals and topical low-potency steroids may also be helpful. Caution should be exercised in the use of low-potency topical steroids. This is a lifelong disease, and prolonged use of topical steroids on genital skin can lead to local skin atrophy and skin dependence.

Lichen Sclerosis

Lichen sclerosis (see Fig. 20–31), also called lichen sclerosis et atrophicus, is a chronic dermatitis. It occurs commonly on genital skin and is believed to be more common in women than in men. The late stage of this disorder in men is called balanitis xerotica obliterans. The disease is usually limited to older men (Ledwig and Weigand, 1989). However, a histopathologic study of prepubertal boys requiring circumcision revealed that 4% to 14% of specimens had lichen sclerosis (Chalmers et al, 1984; Wright, 1994). The cause of this disorder is not well understood, although a recent study has implicated abnormal regulation of interleukin-1 (Clay et al, 1994). In patients with lichen sclerosis there is an unusually high prevalence of autoimmune diseases.

Lichen sclerosis can be asymptomatic but often causes severe itching and burning. Males may experience pain with urination or erection. The lesions are well-circumscribed porcelain white macules or plaques. Hyperkeratotic scale can occur. The epidermis is often atrophic, crinkles on examination, and is prone to shear injury resulting in ulceration. The lesions are most common on the moist skin of the foreskin, and in women the vulva and perianal area. As the disease becomes chronic, the dermis becomes sclerotic, resulting in an atrophic scar. As this process continues, destruction and contraction of the foreskin, clitoral prepuce, and vulva may occur. The disease can occur on other areas of the body. The most common nongenital sites of lichen sclerosis are the trunk, upper arms, chest, and abdomen. Squamous cell carcinoma has been reported in areas of lichen sclerosis.

The diagnosis of genital lichen sclerosis is often made by clinical findings. Histopathologic confirmation can be helpful. Histopathologic findings included basal cell layer vacuolation, epidermal atrophy, dermal edema, homogenization of collagen in the papillary dermis, focal perivascular infiltrate in the dermis, and plugging of the ostea of follicular and eccrine structures. The differential diagnosis includes vitiligo, postinflammatory hypopigmentation, and scar.

Most males are successfully treated by circumcision. In the past, medical treatment for this condition has been unsatisfactory. Topical treatments have included estrogen, progesterone, testosterone, antimicrobial and antifungal agents, and petrolatum. In controlled trials many of these agents have been shown to be no more effective than placebo (Sideri et al, 1994). High-potency topical steroids, which are usually not recommended for this area of the body, have been shown to be highly effective for this disorder in women (Dalziel and Wojnarowska, 1993). Topical steroids not only help alleviate symptoms but also stop and may reverse the disease process. The efficacy of these agents has not been thoroughly confirmed in men (Wright, 1994).

Miscellaneous Conditions

Lupus erythematosus and secondary syphilis can also present as papulosquamous lesions. Both these ailments should also be present on nongenital skin. Syphilis is discussed elsewhere. Lupus erythematosus is an autoimmune disease that can present with protean cutaneous manifestations with or without systemic involvement. Discoid lupus erythematosus, which presents without systemic findings, can present as red scaling macules. The resolution of these macules often results in atrophic and depigmented scars. Histologic examination with routine and immunofluorescent staining can be helpful in making the correct diagnosis. Treatment is dependent on the severity of the disorder but may involve intralesional or systemic glucocorticoids and antimalarials.

ECZEMATOUS OR ALLERGIC DERMATITIS

Eczematous or allergic dermatitis describes eruptions usually confined to the outer layer of skin. The skin appears red and weepy and often has crusts (Table 21–2). This section also includes other allergy-mediated processes.

Atopic Eczema

Eczema is a term used to describe a group of cutaneous illnesses that result in or are caused by damage to the

Table 21–2. DIFFERENTIAL DIAGNOSIS OF ECZEMATOUS DERMATITIS

Eczema
Allergic dermatitis
Seborrheic dermatitis
Intertrigo
Contact dermatitis
Irritant dermatitis
Balanoposthitis
Zoon's balanitis
Candidal-related illnesses
Impetigo
Herpes simplex
Herpes zoster
Drug reaction

epidermis. The damage to the epidermis results in the formation of red, scaling skin that weeps and forms yellow crusts. These ailments include atopic dermatitis, nummular eczema, neurodermatitis, and nonspecific dermatitis. A term commonly used in the gynecologic literature for this group of diseases is *squamous cell hyperplasia* or *hyperplastic dystrophy.* Unfortunately, many of these terms may represent diseases of different etiology, but because of similar clinical signs and symptoms, all these terms are often lumped together. None of these diseases are peculiar to the genital area.

Patients complain of itch. Usually the itch precedes the skin findings. The itch can be severe and is usually worse in the evening or when the patient is trying to relax, and scratching may occur without the patient's being aware of it. Patients may note an exacerbation of itch during periods of stress or in relationship to seasonal changes or allergens. Atopic dermatitis is very frequently associated with seasonal allergies, asthma, and a family history of these illnesses. Historically, patients have remissions and exacerbations.

Clinically, patients may present with a full spectrum of excoriation, localized edema, mild erythema, and scale. As the ailment becomes more chronic the skin markings become more pronounced, and the skin thickens (lichenifies) (see Fig. 20–27) and develops pigmentary changes. For the most part, the lesions do not have a precise border as seen in papulosquamous illnesses. The most common site of excoriation on the male genitalia is the scrotum. The rectum may be involved. Commonly patients concurrently have extragenital involvement.

The cause of eczema is not known. Atopic dermatitis has been thought to have an immunologic and genetic basis. In cases of severe disease a majority of patients have a personal or family history of allergic illnesses such as seasonal allergy and asthma (Hunter and Herd, 1994). In addition, these patients frequently have elevated circulating titers of immunoglobulin E (IgE) and defects of cell-mediated immunity (Cooper, 1994; Hunter and Herd, 1994). However, elevations in serum IgE levels are not specific to dermatologic patients with atopic dermatitis.

Successful treatments quench the patient's desire to scratch (Przybilla et al, 1994). Treatment is seldom successful if this desire is not stopped. A potential exacerbating factor such as an allergen or irritant must be eliminated from the patient's environment (Morren, 1994). Tight irritating clothing should be avoided. The affected skin should be gently treated. This is accomplished by infrequent bathing with tepid water, mild nonperfumed moisturizing soap, and minimal scrubbing or rubbing during the cleaning or drying process. A bland moisturizer should be used after gentle drying. Superficially infected areas may benefit from topical soaks. A topical bland moisturizer should be used after soaking, and soaking should be discontinued once the superficial infection has cleared. Topical steroids are often required to decrease the itch. If a topical steroid is used, it should be used for short periods of time under medical supervision. The weakest effective topical agent should be used, and superpotent topical steroids are almost never indicated. Prolonged use of a topical steroid on genital skin can cause pigmentary changes, atrophy of cutaneous structures, and a dependence-like syndrome.

Systemic agents may be needed. These agents include antihistamines and tricyclic antidepressants. Antidepressants are effective probably because of their antihistaminic properties, but chronic itching may also be a manifestation of depression (Van Moffaert, 1992). In addition, these oral agents may be effective because of their sedating properties. Systemic steroids are occasionally indicated for severe full-body disease.

Contact Dermatitis

Contact dermatitis is the skin's response to an externally applied agent. These reactions can be due to an irritant or an allergen. Clinically it can be difficult to differentiate between these two causes of contact dermatitis. Cutaneous reaction to irritation or allergy produces localized inflammation leading to scale and crust formation (Mozzannica, 1992). Severe reactions can cause blistering and tissue necrosis. Involved areas are often pruritic and may burn or sting.

Irritant dermatitis occurs almost immediately after exposure to the offending agent, which directly damages cutaneous tissues. Irritant dermatitis is a common industry-related problem where solvents, acid, and alkali are commonly used. Severe full-thickness wounds can occur. Irritants that commonly come in contact with the genital region include soaps and other cleansing products, spermicides and lubricants, perfumes, urogenital secretions, and feces. The intensity of the response may be modified by occlusion, rubbing, and scratching. The most important aspect of treatment is ensuring that the offending agent is removed from contact with the skin. Skin that is mildly to moderately irritated should be gently treated. The judicious use of low-potency topical steroids can be helpful. Severe reactions may require debridement and grafting.

Allergic dermatitis occurs because of an immune-mediated response to the topical application of a contactant. It is a type IV delayed hypersensitivity response. Therefore, the response may not occur until several days after exposure. Clinical findings vary with the intensity of the immune response, which is dependent on the cutaneous location of the application of the allergen, the allergen itself, the host's immune system, and the host's sensitization history. *Toxicodendron* dermatitis (poison ivy) is the archetype severe contact reaction. Nickel dermatitis is an example of a more modest and usually chronic contact allergic response. Common sensitizing agents applied to the genital skin include cleansing agents and disinfectants; lubricants and emollients;

spermicides and other topical ointments; perfumes and fragrances; latex and other types of rubber; clothing; dyes; and metals (nickel) (Le Sellin et al, 1991).

Removal of the offending agent is critical. However, identifying the offending agent can be difficult. Some clues may be present on other parts of the body (e.g., nickel dermatitis from a belt buckle, waistband snap, or watch band). Patch testing uninvolved skin to common antigens is often helpful. Topical corticosteroids and emollients can give symptomatic relief, but the health care provider should be certain that the topical agent chosen is not an allergen for the patient under treatment. Oral antihistamines may also give symptomatic relief. In case of severe allergic contact dermatitis, immunosuppressive agents such as oral corticosteroids may be required.

Table 21–3. DIFFERENTIAL DIAGNOSIS OF EROSIONS

Bullous pemphigoid
Pemphigus vulgaris
Pemphigus foliaceus
Zoon's balanitis
Behçet's syndrome
Contact dermatitis
Dermatitis herpetiformis
Porphyria cutanea tarda
Herpes zoster
Herpes simplex
Lymphangioma circumscriptum
Impetigo
Fixed drug eruption
Factitial
Innocent trauma
Benign familial pemphigus

Erythema Multiforme

Erythema multiforme (see Fig. 20–7) is a generalized skin disease (Raviglione et al, 1990; Roujeau, 1994; Roujeau and Stern, 1994). It is probably best thought of as a minor and major variant. The minor variant is represented by red 1- to 2-cm targetoid lesions. All cutaneous surfaces may be involved. The major variant, also called Stevens-Johnson syndrome, has targetoid lesions, blisters, and mucosal membrane involvement. Another disease often included in this classification is toxic epidermal necrolysis. This is manifested by the sloughing of the epidermis (mucosal and nonmucosal surfaces). Blisters are often present. All these reactions are most frequently caused by ingestants such as antibiotics and antiseizure medications (Roujeau, 1994; Roujeau and Stern, 1994). However, erythema multiforme, especially when recurrent, can be caused by infections (herpes simplex) and hormonal fluctuations.

For therapy to be successful the causative agent must be eliminated immediately. The denuded skin must be treated carefully and often requires the expertise of a burn unit. Systemic immunosuppression is controversial.

Other Drug Reactions

Drug-induced cutaneous reactions are very common. In most cases the mechanisms causing these reactions are unknown. Drug reactions can be a cause of almost any cutaneous reaction pattern on any part of the body. Except in unusual cases or fixed drug reactions, these reactions are not limited to the genital area. Readers interested in a comprehensive review of this subject should consult a textbook of dermatology.

VESICULOBULLOUS DISORDERS

Most vesiculobullous illnesses are uncommon. On genital skin the bullae are often evanescent, leaving behind erosions (Table 21–3).

Bullous Pemphigoid

Bullous pemphigoid is an immune-mediated blistering eruption. It is most common in the elderly population. For an unknown reason an IgG autoantibody is produced against a 230-kD protein in the lamina lucida. The antigen is called the bullous pemphigoid antigen and is important in anchoring the basal cell of the epidermis to the basement membrane. Typically, patients have large, tense blisters on several different cutaneous sites. Mucosal membranes may be involved. Diagnosis is facilitated by histologic examination, which should include both routine and immunofluorescent staining (Korman, 1993). Usually patients are treated with systemic immunosuppressive medication.

Pemphigus Vulgaris

Pemphigus vulgaris is an immune-mediated blistering eruption due to an IgG autoantibody directed against the cell surface of keratinocytes (Stanley, 1990). The disease may afflict all age groups but is most common after the fifth decade of life. Flaccid blisters occur on multiple body sites including mucosal membranes. Diagnosis is facilitated by histologic examinations, which should include both routine and immunofluorescent staining. Treatment with immunosuppressives is the mainstay of therapy.

Dermatitis Herpetiformis

Dermatitis herpetiformis is an immune-mediated blistering eruption due to IgA autoantibodies against the basement membrane. The lesion is an intensely painful burning pruritic papule or vesicle (Smith and Zone, 1993). Lesions are found most frequently on elbows, knees, buttocks, shoulders, and sacrum. A majority of patients suffer from an associated gluten-sensitive enteropathy. Histologic evaluation should include both routine and immunofluorescent staining. Most patients respond to dapsone. Strict adherence to a gluten-free diet can also be beneficial.

Hailey-Hailey Disease

Hailey-Hailey disease, or benign familial pemphigus, is an autosomal dominant vesicular eruption (Langenberg et al, 1992). It most commonly occurs in intertriginous areas.

The small vesicles, formed by the loss of keratinocyte cell adhesion, quickly denude because of frictional forces. These lesions become superinfected by bacteria and yeast. After superinfection the denuded areas crust. The cause of this disease is not known, but it is made worse by maceration, local friction, and bacterial superinfection. Histologic examination can be helpful to differentiate this disease from impetigo, pemphigus, intertrigo, and Darier's disease. Treatment options include local excision of involved tissues with grafting or secondary healing, topical antibiotics and drying agents, and systemic corticosteroids.

ULCERS

Ulcers are wounds that extend into the dermis. Cutaneous ulcers of the genital region are most commonly related to sexually transmitted diseases (Table 21–4).

Inflammatory Bowel Disease and Pyoderma Gangrenosum

Inflammatory bowel disease, or Crohn's disease, can involve the rectum and the genitalia. Most commonly this is noted as a fistula that extends directly from the bowel to the perirectal area. At presentation it is unusual for the afflicted individual not to be aware of a history of bowel disease. Treatment should be focused on good wound care and the bowel disease. However, Crohn's disease can also appear in a noncontiguous "metastatic" fashion in various body parts including the genitalia. These granulomatous lesions can be painful nodules, abscesses, and ulcers. It can be difficult to differentiated this disease process from pyoderma gangrenosum (see Fig. 20–32).

Pyoderma gangrenosum is a chronic, painful, ulcerating disease that is most frequently associated with Crohn's disease, ulcerative colitis, or collagen vascular disease. It can occur in the absence of an associated illness. Lesions tend to occur on the lower extremity but have been reported almost anywhere on the body (Bigler et al, 1995). Lesions frequently occur at the site of trauma. These wounds are very exudative and have a violaceous border. Lesions may begin as purple nodules or blisters. Treatment must include good wound care and frequently immunosuppression with either corticosteroids or cyclosporine.

Table 21–4. DIFFERENTIAL DIAGNOSIS OF ULCERS

Syphilis
Chancroid
Herpes simplex
Crohn's disease
Aphthous ulcer
Behçet's disease
Granuloma inguinale
Lymphogranuloma venereum
Factitial
Wegener's granulomatosis
Leukocytoclastic vasculitis

Factitia

Genitalia can be a site of nondecorative destructive self-induced lesions. These lesions are called factitial dermatitis or dermatitis artefacta. Most individuals who produce these lesions do so without full conscious awareness to satisfy a psychologic need (Koblenzer, 1987). These lesions usually take on the appearance of excoriations, papules, ulcers, or erosions. In the correct clinical setting, any lesion that is perfectly linear or represents a pattern that is not consistent with the anatomy of the skin or genitalia could be self-induced. All other diagnostic possibilities should be considered before finalizing this diagnosis. Treatment should explore the psychological reason for the creation of the lesion and include appropriate lesional skin care.

Innocent Trauma

Genitalia are commonly the site of innocent trauma. These lesions may be secondary to sexual practice (e.g., biting or subcutaneous insertion of foreign bodies), ornamentation (e.g., tattooing, piercing), or unusual cleansing techniques (e.g., cleaning with caustic agents). A thorough history is essential. Treatment is dependent on the lesion.

Behçet's Disease

Behçet's disease is a syndrome charaterized by oral and genital ulcers, uveitis, and non–mucous membrane skin lesions of unknown etiology. Individuals may suffer from aneurysms; arthritis; thrombophlebitis; and gastrointestinal, neurologic, and psychiatric problems. International criteria for this syndrome have been recently published (O'Neill et al, 1994). Oral ulceration is the primary criterion for this illness. Genital ulceration is one of four secondary criteria required for diagnosis. There appears to be geographic variation with respect to the severity of this illness, with persons in eastern Europe and Asia affected differently than those in North America and western Europe (O'Duffy, 1990, 1994).

Genital lesions occur in the majority of persons with this syndrome (Jorizzo et al, 1995). The lesions are painful and do not always occur concurrently with oral lesions or the other minor signs of this illness. These lesions can be described as either herpetiform, major (>1 cm), or minor (O'Duffy, 1994). Other causes of genital ulceration such as aphthous ulcers (Schreiner and Jorizzo, 1987), syphilis, herpes simplex, and chancroid must be thoroughly considered before confirming this diagnosis. The genital lesions are aphthous-like in that they tend to be superficial and circular to oval. They are also more likely to be more than 1 cm in diameter greater (major) than the oral lesions of this disease. The histopathologic appearance is often nonspecific, but inflammatory changes of leukocytoclastic or lymphocytic perivascular or perifollicular infiltrate or true vasculitis may be noted (Jorizzo et al, 1995).

The treatment of the genital lesions of Behçet's disease is both local and systemic. Local care includes moisture-retaining dressings, intralesional injection of corticosteroids, and topical anesthetics. Patients may also require systemic corticosteroids, azathioprine, cyclophosphamide, colchicine, cyclosporine, FK-506, hydroxychloroquine (plaquenil), or thalidomide (Gardner-Medwin et al, 1994; Sajjadi et al, 1994; O'Duffy, 1994).

Aphthous Ulcers

Aphthous ulcers are small, often painful, erosions most commonly found on the oral mucosa. Uncommonly, these lesions can be found on the penis and scrotum. The presence of lesions on the mouth and genitalia may be a forme fruste of Behçet's syndrome (Jorizzo et al, 1985). All other causes of genital ulcers should be considered before settling on this diagnosis.

MALIGNANCY

Squamous Cell Carcinoma in Situ

Squamous cell carinoma in situ (see Fig. 20–20) is also called Bowen's disease and erythroplasia of Queyrat. These lesions are sharply demarcated erythematous plaques. Lesions of keratinizing skin (Bowen's disease) often contain scale, whereas lesions of mucosal surfaces (erythroplasia of Queyrat) do not. The etiology of this disease is not fully understood but exposure to sunlight, exposure to arsenic and other carcinogens, and a history of papillomavirus have all been implicated (Richert et al, 1977; Ikenberg et al, 1983). As the name implies, the malignant clone of keratinocytes is fully localized in the epidermis. This lesion may be difficult to distinguish from benign papulosquamous lesions.

Clinically these lesions are often present for several months to years before they are brought to a physician's attention. The lesions may be pruritic and painful. Lesions are most often solitary and slowly enlarge to a size ranging from 1 to 10 cm.

Ultimately the diagnosis should be based on histologic examination of tissue. It may be necessary to perform several biopsies to confirm the diagnosis and demonstrate a lack of dermal invasion. Invasive lesions on mucosal surfaces are more prone to metastasis than lesions on other cutaneous surfaces.

Treatment for squamous cell carcinoma in situ involves tissue destruction. Destructive methods include cryotherapy, topical vesicants, laser destruction, and surgical excision (Gerber, 1994). Because of the risk of metastasis from invasive squamous carcinoma of mucosal surfaces, some authors feel that surgical excision with a 5-mm margin may be the best therapy (Bissada, 1992). This treatment is often curative and allows pathologic assessment of the entire lesion for an invasive component. Mohs' surgery has been successfully performed on this carcinoma.

Bowenoid Papulosis

Bowenoid papulosis of the genitalia occurs in sexually active men and women in the third and fourth decade of life (Patterson et al, 1986). Typically, lesions are multiple, erythematous papules less than 1 cm in diameter. Papules may coalesce to form plaques and may have a verrucous surface. There is a strong causal association between this disorder and human papillomavirus infection (Rosemberg et al, 1991; Schwartz and Janniger, 1995).

Bowenoid papulosis is histologically similar to carcinoma in situ. However, in this disease the atypical keratinocytes do not replace the entire epidermis but are randomly found throughout the epidermis. There is an increased risk of cervical neoplasia in female partners of men with Bowenoid papulosis, but in men the disease may regress without treatment (Eisen et al, 1983), and it has never been reported to progress to invasive squamous cell carcinoma. Because of the benign nature of the illness, treatment should be limited to careful follow-up and locally destructive methods such as electrodesiccation, cryotherapy, and vesicants (Gerber, 1994). Female partners of men with this disorder should be informed and followed in a fashion similar to that of other human papillomavirus disorders.

Kaposi's Sarcoma

Kaposi's sarcoma (see Fig. 20–33) is a rare neoplasm of endovascular cells. Twenty years ago it was primarily a sarcoma of the lower extremities of men of Mediterranean descent. However, infection with HIV-1 has increased the incidence of this malignancy 7000-fold (Miles, 1994). Recent studies have indicated an association between a herpesvirus and Kaposi's sarcoma (Moore and Chang, 1995). This association was noted in HIV- and non–HIV-infected individuals with Kaposi's sarcoma. The initial presentation of old world Kaposi's sarcoma is rarely on the genitalia of men, but 3% of men with acquired immunodeficiency syndrome and Kaposi's sarcoma may initially present with a genital lesion (Lowe et al, 1989).

The lesions of Kaposi's sarcoma are violaceous to light brown. These lesions can be macules, papules, or plaques, which can become confluent, covering large areas of skin. They may ulcerate. These lesions can cause venous and lymphatic obstruction resulting in significant local edema. Treatment of individual genital lesions may be necessary for anatomic (e.g., urethral obstruction) or cosmetic reasons. Modalities include intralesional injection of chemotherapeutic agents, radiation therapy, and local tissue destruction with laser, cryosurgery, or electrocoagulation. Systemic therapies are available (Gascon and Schwartz, 1994).

Pseudoepitheliomatous, Keratotic, and Micaceous Balanitis

Pseudoepitheliomatous, keratotic, and micaceous balanitis is a very uncommon lesion that occurs on the glans penis. Circumcised males typically present with a solitary slowly enlarging white thick hyperkeratotic plaque. A histologic examination is essential because this lesion must be differentiated from squamous cell carcinoma and verrucous carcinoma. Verrucous carcinoma has been reported concurrently, and some authors have speculated that this is a variant of verrucous carcinoma (Read and Abell, 1981; Bargman, 1985; Jenkins and Jakubovic, 1988). Histologically there is a hyperplastic epidermis with epithelial ridges that extend deeply into the dermis (Jenkins and Jakubovic, 1988). The lesion should be conservatively removed or destroyed and the patient followed closely (Read and Abell, 1981; Bargman, 1985).

Melanoma

Melanoma is an uncommon cutaneous malignancy that has been increasing in prevalence at a brisk rate (Armstrong and Kricker, 1994). Melanoma of the male genitalia is relatively uncommon (Olderbring and Mikulowski, 1987). Although melanoma has been described on the shaft of the penis and on the scrotum, it is most commonly found on the glans penis.

Genital melanoma usually presents as a macule or papule with an irregular border. The lesions may not be pigmented but usually contain shades of blue, red, black, and brown. Lesions may ulcerate. The diagnosis requires histopathologic confirmation. Prognosis is dependent on histopathologic and clinical criteria. Treatment is determined by the depth of the lesion and almost always includes at least a local excision of the full lesion.

Basal Cell Carcinoma

The most common cutaneous malignancy is basal cell carcinoma. The majority of these lesions occur on sun-exposed areas of persons with light complexions. Basal cell carcinoma of the male genitalia is distinctly uncommon. These lesions can occur on the penis (Kim et al, 1994) or the scrotum (Nahass et al, 1992). Lesions tend to be papular and pearly in color with telangiectasias. They frequently ulcerate. Lesions should be treated with local excision.

Verrucous Carcinoma

Verrucous carcinoma (see Fig. 20–19) or Buschke-Lowenstein tumor, is a variant of squamous cell carcinoma. It was originally thought to be a variant of condyloma acuminata. Verrucous carcinoma may account for as many as 24% of all tumors of the penis (Schwartz, 1995). The etiology of verrucous carcinoma is not known, but histologically it is often associated with warty changes. It has been associated with several serotypes of human papillomavirus including the "non"-oncogenic 6 and 11 (Schwarts, 1995) and is poorly associated with types 16 and 18 (Chan et al, 1994).

These tumors are most commonly located on the glans penis and appear as a fungating lesion. Verrucous carcinoma has also been described on the feet and mucosal membranes of the mouth and nose. In general, it is slow growing and mainly causes local damage. It is best treated with local excision or radiation therapy (Seixas et al, 1995).

Extramammary Paget's Disease

Extramammary Paget's disease is a rather uncommon tumor. Of the cases that have occurred outside the nipple the majority have been on the vulva or anus. The disease has been reported infrequently on the male genitalia (Perez et al, 1989; Weese et al, 1993). Between 10% and 30% of the cases of extramammary Paget's disease are associated with an underlying malignancy (Payne and Wells, 1994). Malignancies most often associated with extramammary Paget's disease of the male genitalia are of the urethra, bladder, rectum, or sweat glands.

Extramammary Paget's disease presents as a pruritic erythematous plaque. The plaques may become large and extend on more than one genital surface. The lesions can be excoriated and crusted. Extramammary Paget's disease must be differentiated from the benign papulosquamous diseases. Histopathologic confirmation of this lesion is essential. Biopsy of the lesion demonstrates vacuolated Paget cells, which must be differentiated from cells seen in lesions of squamous cell carcinoma and melanoma.

Treatment should include a complete evaluation for an underlying carcinoma. Any identified carcinoma should be treated. The site of extramammary Paget's disease should also be treated. Most frequently this involves definitive surgical removal of the plaque; however, radiation therapy and topical treatment with 5-fluorouracil have been used (Brierley and Stockdale, 1991; Reedy et al, 1991; Payne and Wells, 1994).

Cutaneous T-Cell Lymphoma

Cutaneous T-cell lymphoma is an uncommon lymphoproliferative malignancy of T-cell origin. Both Sézary syndrome and mycosis fungoides are included in this nosologic designation. The course of this disease is such that it begins as a nonspecific pruritus that clinically may mimic eczema, psoriasis, lichen simplex chronicus, or contact dermatitis. Patients may go on to develop fungating plaquelike lesions, erythroderma, ulcers, or erosions and hematologic involvement (Sézary syndrome). The course of this disease takes place over several years and may require long periods of observation and tissue biopsy before the correct diagnosis is made. It is associated with infection by an HIV (Ghosh et al, 1994). This disease may involve genital skin but has not been reported to exclusively involve this area.

INFECTIONS AND INFESTATIONS

Infections

Sexually transmitted disease such as herpes simplex, gonorrhea, granuloma inguinale, lymphogranuloma venereum, chancroid molluscum contagiosum, human papillomavirus, and syphilis are considered elsewhere.

Erythrasma

Erythrasma is a sharply bordered red to brown scaling eruption of the intertriginous areas. It is commonly noted in the crural area, between the scrotum and the thigh, and in the axilla. Groin lesions are frequently asymptomatic but may become pruritic and uncomfortable. Because of clinical findings it is frequently misdiagnosed as tinea cruris (Shidhuphak et al, 1985). A Wood's lamp can be helpful in distinguishing this disorder from tinea cruris. The causative bacterium is *Corynebacterium minutissimum*. This organism produces a porphyrin that produces a red fluorescence under Wood's light. The treatment of choice is oral erythromycin, although topical erythromycin and most antifungal creams may also be effective.

Trichomycosis

Trichomycosis is a bacterial infection of the hair in intertriginous areas (White and Smith, 1979). Infected patients usually suffer from hyperhidrosis. The causative organism is *Corynebacterium tenuis*. The organism causes discrete nodules on the hair. These nodules can vary in color from red to black to yellow. Treatment should center on alleviating the hyperhidrosis and using topical antibiotics such as clindamycin solution.

Balanoposthitis

Balanoposthitis is inflammation of the foreskin and glans penis. It occurs only in uncircumcised males. It is most frequently noted in individuals with poorly retractile foreskin, such as boys less then 5 years of age. Patients complain of redness, local edema, discharge, and pain or difficulty with urination.

The cause of balanoposthitis is often never ascertained; when the cause is discovered, it is somewhat dependent on the age of the afflicted individual. Boys tend to have bacterial infections (Kyriazi and Costenbader, 1991; Patrizi et al, 1994). The cause in men may be intertrigo, irritant dermatitis, maceration injury, or candidal or bacterial infection (Birley et al, 1993; Fornasa et al, 1994). To aid in identifying the cause of balanoposthitis, it can be helpful to question the patient about topical allergens or irritants and to obtain a potassium hydroxide preparation, Tzanck preparation, and fungal, bacterial, or viral culture. Biopsy is seldom required unless treatment is not successful. In these cases neoplastic diseases (Fernando and Wanas, 1991), psoriasis, Zoon's balanitis, and infectious processes, such as papillomavirus (Wikstrom et al, 1994), should be considered.

Treatment should be dictated by the cause. Treatment may include eliminating offending agents, good gentle skin care, topical antibiotics, topical antifungal agents, and for short periods of time the use of low-potency topical steroids. Retraction of the foreskin is helpful to allow the glans and prepuce to dry. Drying agents such as Castellani's paint can be helpful. Cases of recurrent balanoposthitis may require circumcision.

Hidradenitis Suppurativa

Hidradenitis suppurativa is a chronic suppurative disease of the apocrine gland–bearing areas of the body such as the groin, axilla, and buttocks. The disease can be associated with severe acne vulgaris and dissecting cellulitis of the scalp. It often begins after puberty or in young adulthood. Initial lesions are red nodules, papules, or cysts. Individual lesions can take on a "boil-like" appearance. Lesions can resolve without scarring, but scarring, fibrosis, keloid formation, and sinus tract formation are common. Mild cases may be difficult to differentiate from furunculosis. However, hidradenitis suppurativa tends to occur in patients with a history of acne vulgaris and tends to be more severe than furunculosis. In hidradenitis suppurativa, multiple lesions occur concurrently, tend to be recurrent and poorly responsive to antibiotics, and frequently develop sinus tract as a result of lesional rupture. Also hidradenitis suppurativa is usually confined to apocrine gland–bearing regions, and comedos form within the involved areas.

Hidradenitis suppurativa is not primarily an infectious disease. It occurs because of keratin plugging of follicles with associated inflammation of the apocrine gland (Attanoos et al, 1995). The plugged follicle swells and may become superinfected and/or rupture, causing a brisk inflammatory reaction in surrounding tissues. Irritation of the follicular pores by maceration and obesity often worsens the disease process. The disease is chronic but may wax and wane in severity. Even after the disease abates, secondary problems can persist because of sinus tract formation, lymphatic destruction, and lymphadenopathy.

Multiple treatment modalities exist. Treatment often begins with antibiotics such as tetracyclines and erythromycin. Oral and intralesional injections of glucocorticoid are helpful. Both these treatments work by decreasing inflammation. Isotretinoin can be helpful therapy, but long-term remissions are rare. For severe cases full excision of involved areas with either primary closure, secondary closure, or closure with grafting can result in long-term remissions (Banerjee, 1992; Lains et al, 1994). Success has also been reported with laser ablation (Lains et al, 1994) and radiation therapy to involved areas.

Folliculitis

Folliculitis denotes small red papules or pustules over a hair-bearing structure (Herman et al, 1991). It is commonly found in areas of the body with increased numbers of hair follicles such as the pubic area. Folliculitis can occur because of follicular irritation from external trauma or topically applied irritants, and from infection from staphylococcal species (Feingold, 1993), pseudomonal species, candidal species, and herpes simplex virus. External trauma can be from friction or pressure from clothing, shaving, and rubbing. These forces are exacerbated by local maceration from excessive sweating or perspiration. In general, lesions are discrete and not symptomatic. Treatment should include good skin care, removal of external irritants, and antimicrobial, antiviral, or antifungal therapy when indicated.

Furunculosis

A furuncle, or a boil, is a red, fluctuant, tender, often painful, perifollicular pustule or abscess. Lesions rapidly grow and may reach a size of up to 3 cm. There is often a central point from which pus can be expressed. Most frequently lesions occur because of localized cutaneous infection with *Staphylococcus aureus*. Incision and drainage can be helpful for larger lesions. All patients should receive either a topical or a systemic antistaphylococcal antibiotic, or both.

Erysipelas, Cellulitis, and Fournier's Gangrene

Erysipelas is a superficial infection of the skin generally not involving cutaneous layers deeper than the dermis. Cellulitis is a skin infection involving cutaneous layers as deep as the subcutaneous fat layer. A clinical finding that may aid in differentiating these two processes is that in erysipelas the skin at the border of the lesion is raised and sharply demarcated from normal skin. In cellulitis, the borders are indistinct and blurred. In addition, erysipelas is more common in newborns and the elderly. Clinically both these ailments present with edematous, red, warm skin and are uncommon in the genital region. Areas of skin breakdown can occur and either may represent the portal of entry of the causative bacteria or may be secondary to vesicle or blister formation from the infectious and inflammatory process.

Group A streptococcus is the most common causative organism for both disorders. *S. Aureus* may also cause cellulitis and rarely erysipelas. Patients often have fever and elevated white blood cell counts. Treatment should include good local skin care and systemic antibiotics that cover streptococcal and staphylococcal species.

Necrotizing fasciitis of the male genitalia, or Fournier's gangrene, is a life-threatening infection of deep cutaneous tissues and fascia. Although necrotizing fasciitis of other body sites is most commonly associated with toxin-producing group A streptococci, Fournier's gangrene most frequently is associated with mixed flora infections, which may include streptococcal species (Haury et al, 1975), but also other aerobic bacterial species, sometimes in combination with anaerobes (Melekos et al, 1983). This disorder is characterized by painful warm, red lesions that quickly become foul-smelling gangrenous necrotic lesions. Early on, the disease is similar to cellulitis; however, these patients tend to have blisters and to express more pain than is consistent with their physical examination. The infection can spread rapidly from the scrotum to the perineum and the abdominal wall. Patients are often severely ill. Early diagnosis is essential. Treatment should not be delayed and should include appropriate antibiotics and extensive debridement (Biswas et al, 1979).

Ecthyma Gangrenosum

Ecthyma gangrenosum is a necrotic cutaneous eruption related to pseudomonal sepsis (Kingston and Mackay, 1986). The lesion begins as tense grouped pseudomonas-containing vesicles on a violaceous base and rapidly progresses to a necrotic ulcer. It is most frequently located on the buttocks, inguinal crease, and lower extremities. It most frequently occurs in debilitated gravely ill persons and is associated with a high mortality rate. Immediate recognition of this lesion with institution of antipseudomonal antibiotics is essential. Debridement of the lesion may also be indicated.

Candidal Intertrigo

Infection of macerated skin folds is very common with *Candida* species (see Fig. 20–17). These yeast forms are commonly found in the lower gastrointestinal tract; therefore, they can easily spread to the rectum and intertriginous areas of the male genitalia. On examination the perirectal and intertriginous skin is found to be red. Fissures may be present in the reddened area. Small papules and pustules may be present in both the reddened areas and areas distal (satellite) to the initial lesion. All these lesions may be pruritic.

The diagnosis can be assisted by scraping infected skin and performing a KOH examination. After the KOH has had adequate time to digest keratin, the mycelia and spores of *Candida* should be apparent. Culture can be helpful but is seldom required for diagnosis. Candidal intertrigo should be differentiated from irritant intertrigo, seborrheic dermatitis, psoriasis, benign familial pemphigoid, and dermatophyte infection.

Removing the cause of the macerated skin is essential for successful treatment. This might include using talc or corn starch, using more-absorptive cotton-based clothing, and elevating skin to allow air drying. Appropriate topical antifungal therapy is also important. Occasionally oral agents are required.

Dermatophyte Infection

Tinea cruris is an infection of the crural areas of the genitalia with a dermatophyte (see Fig. 20–26). It is commonly called "jock itch." Dermatophytes are fungi that live primarily in the superficial layers of the epidermis. These same organisms are responsible for tinea corporis ("ringworm") and tinea unguium (nail disease). The most common dermatophytes that cause tinea cruris are *Trichophyton rubrum, Trichophyton mentagrophytes,* and *Epidermophyton floccosum* (Greer, 1994). Lesions are often reddish-brown with an elevated red border located in the crural area, the inner thigh, and the scrotum. The penis is seldom involved. Recurrent or chronic disease may result in postinflammatory hyperpigmentation.

Diagnosis can be confirmed with culture and by a KOH examination. The scraping should be on the active border of the lesion and reveals branching septate hyphae. Tinea cruris must be differentiated from erythrasma, psoriasis, and seborrheic dermatitis. The disease is often recurrent; care should be taken to treat only active disease and not postinflammatory hyperpigmentation. Treatment should focus on preventing skin maceration and the use of appropriate antifungal agents on the overt lesions and areas at risk (Chakrabarti et al, 1992). On rare occasions oral agents may be required for the treatment of dermatophyte infection of the groin.

Infestation

The two most common organisms causing infestation in humans are pediculosis pubis *(Phthirus pubis)*, which is covered elsewhere, and scabies *(Sarcoptes scabiei)*. Scabies is characterized by intensely pruritic, papular, and linear burrow-like lesions. It is most frequently found simultaneously on multiple areas of the body such as the fingerwebs; axillae; umbilicus; anus; flexure area of the arm, wrist, and leg; genitals; and areolae. The scalp and face are usually spared in the immunocompetent adult. The disease, even in the genital area, is so ubiquitous that it should always be considered in the differential diagnosis of pruritus not responsive to therapy (Hart, 1992). Pruritus is secondary to host sensitization to the mite and its feces and saliva.

A diagnosis is made by identifying the mite. This can be done by biopsy but is more easily made by scraping suspected lesions. The exfoliated skin can then be examined for the mite, its feces, and its eggs. Multiple effective treatments exist such as lindane, permethrin, precipitated sulfa, and crotamiton cream. Care must be taken to treat all the intimates of the patient to prevent reinfestation.

COMMON BENIGN DISORDERS SPECIFIC TO THE MALE GENITALIA

Pearly Penile Papules

Pearly penile papules (see Fig. 20–11) are a common disorder, found in as many as 30% of men (Rehbein, 1977). These lesions are most commonly seen in young adults, uncircumcised persons, and persons of African-American descent. The lesions are 1- to 2-mm flesh-colored to red papules that encircle the corona. They are not confluent but are often closely placed and may occur in more than one row.

Histologically the lesions are angiofibromas (Ackerman and Kronberg, 1973). Clinically, they can be confused with verruca, which should be easily differentiated on histopathologic review. Although it has been speculated that these lesions are of viral origin, human papillomavirus infection has not been demonstrated (Ferenczy et al, 1991). Lesions may abate with age (Rehbein, 1977) and generally treatment is not required. Lesions can be removed by locally destructive methods (Magid and Garden, 1989).

Angiokeratoma of Fordyce

Angiokeratomas of Fordyce (see Fig. 20–12) are commonly seen on the scrotum and glans and shaft of the penis of adult men. The lesions are small ectasias of dermal blood vessels. These lesions appear as red or purple 1- to 2-mm papules. Histopathologically these lesions are dilated venules and capillaries in the papillary dermis (Gioglio et al, 1992).

In general, these lesions are benign and are not a marker for systemic disease. Similar lesions can be seen in Fabry's disease (see Fig. 20–24), a rare glycogen storage disease and possibly in states of elevated venous pressures. Treatment of angiokeratomas is seldom required. An individual lesion may bleed (Taniguchi et al, 1994). Bleeding lesions can be controlled with electrodesiccation or topical coagulants.

Cysts

Cysts are benign invaginations of the normal components of skin. Cysts are found commonly on almost all cutaneous surfaces including the genitalia. They may increase in size because of accumulation of keratinous material or fluids produced by the cells that line the cyst. Cysts often become inflamed because of rupture of the cyst contents into surrounding tissue, local irritation of the cyst, or infection.

Medial raphe cyst is specific to the male genitalia. It is believed to be a developmental defect of embryonal tissue. These cysts are located near the glans penis and are lined by pseudostratified columnar epithelium (Asarch et al, 1979). If the cysts are bothersome, they should be surgically removed.

Epidermal cysts are the most common type of cyst found on the body. They are commonly found on the scrotum and more rarely on the shaft of the penis. Epidermal cysts are lined by well-developed stratified epithelium. These cysts may occur because of occluded hair follicles, local skin trauma, the inadvertent implantation of the epidermis in the dermis, and obstructed eccrine ducts. Epidermal cysts are firm and nodular, ranging in size from a few millimeters to centimeters. They are usually not tender and are flesh-colored. When epidermal cysts are inflamed they become red and malodorous. They often contain keratin, a cheesy material, which can be expressed from the cyst. Rupture of this material into the dermis surrounding a cyst is responsible for the brisk inflammatory response. Most cysts do not require treatment. Inflamed cysts may require incision and drainage. Cysts can be surgically removed for cosmetic reasons or because of recurrent episodes of rupture and inflammation. Definitive removal requires excising the entire cyst.

Penile Melanosis

Penile melanosis is a rare pigmented macule of the penis. The lesions have irregular borders, are large, and can vary from light brown and tan to black and blue. Clinically, they can be difficult to distinguish from melanoma. The lesions are most frequently found on the shaft and glans of the penis. They may occur in response to sunlight or the ingestion of photosenitizing agents.

Since it is critical that this lesion be differentiated from malignant melanoma, a histologic evaluation is often indicated. Full removal of this lesion may not be possible, so several biopsies from different lesional sites are often required. Histologic examination, with the exception of an increased number of melanocytes and an increase in basilar pigmentation, should not reveal any atypical melanocytic phenomena (Revuz and Clerici, 1989). Very few of these lesions have been followed, but the natural course of this lesion is felt to be benign (Konigsberg and Gray, 1976).

Sclerosing Lymphangitis

Sclerosing lymphangitis is a translucent cordlike lesion that occurs on the shaft or glans of the penis (Gharpuray and Tolat, 1991; Leventhal et al, 1993). It is seldom painful and usually flesh-colored but may appear slightly red. It is most commonly associated with vigorous sexual activity. Histologically thrombosed lymphatic vessels are noted. Thrombosis of these vessels is thought to be secondary to local trauma. Treatment is the avoidance of vigorous sexual activity. Sclerosing lymphangitis usually remits within several weeks.

Zoon's Balanitis

Zoon's, or plasma cell, balanitis (see Fig. 20–4) is seen only in uncircumcised men. It manifests as a lesion on the glans or prepuce. This patchlike lesion is usually solitary and red with distinct borders (Jolly et al, 1993). It may be erosive and can be as large as 2 cm. The lesion is usually asymptomatic, but chronic.

Zoon's balanitis must be differentiated from squamous cell carcinoma in situ and other forms of balanitis. Biopsy with routine histologic examination is very helpful (Souteyrand et al, 1981). Histologically there is a band of plasma cells in the dermis hugging the epidermis. Keratinocyte atypia should not be seen. Circumcision is the usual treatment, although it is not always successful.

Xerotica Obliterans

Balanitis xerotica obliterans is a clinical condition in which the foreskin becomes contracted and fixed over the glans penis. It is most commonly associated with lichen sclerosis but can be the end stage of other causes of balanoposthitis. Treatment is usually by circumcision.

COMMON BENIGN CUTANEOUS DISORDERS

Skin Tag

Skin tags, also called acrochordons, are very common flesh-colored pedunculated lesions. Lesions can be millimeters to several centimeters in size and can be pigmented. They most commonly occur in areas of skin folds. Histologically they represent a hyperplastic epidermis on a dermal stalk. Clinically they may become painful due to manipulation, local trauma, local pressure, or torsion. They may be viewed as cosmetically undesirable. Acrochordons require treatment only if painful or cosmetically undesirable. They can be surgically removed.

Seborrheic Keratosis

Seborrheic keratoses are "stuck-on" waxy or scaly, papular or nodular lesions most commonly found on the chest and back of persons after the fourth decade of life. The lesion may range from light brown to black and may be as large as several centimeters across. Patients may note that the lesions fall off and regrow. Differential diagnosis includes nevus, melanoma, and wart. Histologically there is hyperplasia of the epidermis. These lesions are usually painless but may become painful if they become inflamed. Seborrheic keratosis can be removed with topical application of liquid nitrogen or by mild surgical abrading of lesional skin.

Dermatofibroma

Dermatofibromas are firm nodules usually less than 2 cm in diameter most commonly found on the leg. The lesions are often yellow or red to flesh-colored. Lesions are benign and have a distinctive histologic pattern.

Neurofibroma

Neurofibromas are soft fleshy lesions that seldom are larger than a few centimeters. Lesions can be pedunculated and plexiform. Individuals with multiple lesions should be evaluated for neurofibromatosis.

Capillary Hemangioma

Capillary hemangiomas are tumor-like growths of blood vessels. They are often present at birth but may rapidly develop within the first few weeks of life. Lesions are often compressible, red, and smooth but may be verrucous and protuberant. The majority of capillary hemangiomas involute during childhood or early adolescence. This process is cosmetically more desirable than most surgical procedures. Capillary hemangiomas of the anogenital region can obstruct an orifice and bleed after local trauma, necessitating surgical intervention. In rare cases capillary hemangiomas can be the source of consumption coagulopathy, and they can be associated with other diseases.

Lymphangiectasia

Lymphangiectasia can occur because of congenital lymphedema or can be secondary to disease processes that cause chronic localized edema. In the genital region, secondary causes include sexually transmitted diseases. Clinically, lymphangiectasias appear as clear fluid-filled vesicles.

Lymphangioma Circumscriptum

Lymphangioma circumscriptum is an uncommon tumor of the lymph channels. It appears during childhood but may suddenly enlarge later in life. Histologically, tightly apposed to the epidermis is a dermis containing multiple dilated endothelium-lined lymph channels. Clinically, firm yellow compressible vesicles are noted. Surgical removal is complicated by a high rate of recurrence.

Acanthosis Nigricans

Acanthosis nigricans is a velvety, hyperpigmented, poorly demarcated, asymptomatic skin lesion most commonly found in skin fold areas. Patients are frequently bothered only by the "dirty appearance" of this skin lesion. At least five distinct clinical variants exist and have been associated with multiple factors (Matosuoka et al, 1993). These factors include heredity; endocrinopathies such as states of insulin resistance; obesity; medications such as niacin (Stals et al, 1994); and malignancy of the gastrointestinal tract, prostate, ovaries, and lungs (Matosuoka et al, 1993).

On clinical examination skin fold areas are covered with velvety mamillated brown plaques. Skin tags are frequently noted within these plaques. A work-up for associated factors is usually indicated. Patients should be reassured that their skin is not dirty and that the condition is not known to be contagious. There is no treatment for this condition.

Vitiligo

Vitiligo is a depigmentation of the skin in which sharply bordered patches of the skin become white. Patches can vary tremendously in size and shape. Before the onset of vitiligo, the affected skin should not have been involved in an inflammatory process, and in all other aspects, the affected skin appears normal. Perilesional skin appears normal. Vitiligo is a common condition that usually affects multiple body sites such as the face, chest, axilla, genital area, arms, and legs. Vitiligo of only the genital region occurs in less than 0.3% of the male population (Moss and Stevenson, 1981).

Vitiligo is believed to be of an autoimmune nature and is often associated with other autoimmune diseases such as diabetes mellitus and thyroid disease. Histologically the skin appears normal except for a lack of pigment-producing melanocytes. In the genital region it must be differentiated from post-inflammatory hypopigmentation and lichen sclerosis. Frequently, pigmentation recurs spontaneously. Treatment options include topical steroids, systemic steroids, topical UVB, skin grafting, bleaching, and cosmetic coverings. Supportive counseling may be necessary for extreme cases.

Post-inflammatory Pigment Changes

Both hyper- and hypopigmentation can occur as a sequela of an inflammatory dermatosis. These pigmentary alterations are more noticeable in persons with pigmented skin. The natural history of these lesions is that over several months the skin gradually returns to baseline color. The inflammatory dermatitis should first be treated to resolution; then the topical application of retinoids, corticosteroids, and hydroquinone may help to lighten areas of hyperpigmentation. Hypopigmented areas can be cosmetically covered.

Mole

Moles of the skin are more correctly termed *nevi.* A *nevus* is derived from a cluster of neuroectodermal cells. The cells are nondendritic melanocytes. Nevi are defined by the location of these cell clusters in the epidermis and dermis: junctional (cluster of cells between the epidermis and dermis); dermal (cluster of cells in the dermis); or compound (cluster of cells in both areas). Nevi can also be congenital and dysplastic (atypical).

Clinically, junctional nevi are usually flat, are tan to black, have a sharp border, and are less than 5 mm in diameter. Dermal nevi are usually papular and soft with sharp borders, tan to brown, and less than 5 mm in diameter. Clinically, compound nevi are similar to dermal nevi. Nevi should be differentiated from warts, seborrheic keratosis, freckles, Bowenoid papulosis, basal cell carcinoma, and melanoma. This differentiation often requires histologic examination, which should be encouraged for any lesion that is rapidly changing. Clinically recognizable stable lesions do not require biopsy or removal.

REFERENCES

Ackerman AB, Kronberg R: Pearly penile papules. Acral angiofibroma. Arch Dermatol 1973; 108:673–675.

Aram H: Association of lichen planus and lichen nitidus. Treatment with etretinate. Int J Dermatol 1988; 27:117.

Armstrong BK, Kricker A: Cutaneous melanoma. Cancer Surv 1994; 19–20, 219–240.

Asarch RG, Golitz LE, et al: Median raphe cysts of the penis. Arch Dermatol 1979; 115:1084–1086.

Attanoos RL, Appleton MAC, et al: The pathogenesis of hidradenitis suppurativa: A closer look at apocrine and apoeccrine glands. Br J Dermatol 1995; 133:254–258.

Banerjee AK: Surgical treatment of hidradenitis suppurativa. Br J Surg 1992; 79:863–866.

Bargman H: Pseudoepitheliomatous, keratotic, and micaceous balanitis. Cutis 1985; 35:77–79.

Bigler LR, Flint ID, et al: Painful ulcers of the scrotum. Pyoderma gangrenosum. Arch Dermatol 1995; 131:609–612.

Birley HD, Walker MM, et al: Clinical features and management of recurrent balanitis; association with atopy and genital washing. Genitourin Med 1993; 69:400–403.

Bissada NK: Conservative extirpative treatment of cancer of the penis. Urol Clin North Am 1992; 19:283.

Biswas M, Godec C, et al: Necrotizing infection of the scrotum. Urology 1979; 14:576–580.

Brierley JD, Stockdale AD: Radiotherapy: An effective treatment for extramammary Paget's disease. Clin Oncol 1991; 3:3–5.

Chakrabarti A, Sharma SC, et al: Isolation of dermatophytes from clinically normal sites in patients with tinea cruris. Mycopathologia 1992; 120:139–141.

Chalmers RJG, Burton PA, et al: Lichen sclerosus et atrophicus. Arch Dermatol 1984; 120:1025–1027.

Chan KW, Lam KY, et al: Prevalence of human papillomavirus types 16 and 18 in penile carcinoma: A study of 41 cases using PCR. J Clin Pathol 1994; 47:823–826.

Christophers E, Sterry W: Psoriasis. *In* Fitzpatrick TB, Eisen AZ, Wolff K, et al, eds: Dermatology in General Medicine. New York, McGraw-Hill, 1993, pp 489–514.

Clay FE, Cork MJ, et al: Interluekin 1 receptor antagonist gene polymorphism association with lichen sclerosus. Hum Genet 1994; 94:407–410.

Cooper KD: Atopic dermatitis: Recent trends in pathogenesis and therapy. J Invest Dermatol 1994; 102:128–137.

Dalziel KL, Wojnarowska F: Long-term control of vulval lichen sclerosus after treatment with a potent topical steroid cream. J Reprod Med 1993; 39:25.

Eisen RF, Bhawan J, et al: Spontaneous regression of bowenoid papulosis of the penis. Cutis 1983; 32:269.

Farber EM, Nall ML: The natural history of psoriasis in 5600 patients. Dermatologica 1974; 148:118.

Feingold DS: Staphylococcal and streptococcal pyodermas. Semin Dermatol 1993; 12:331–335.

Ferenczy A, Richart RM, et al: Pearly penile papules: Absence of human papillomavirus DNA by the polymerase chain reaction. Obstet Gynecol 1991; 78:118–122.

Fernando JJ, Wanas TM: Squamous carcinoma of the penis and previous recurrent balanitis: A case report. Genitourin Med 1991; 67:153–155.

Fornasa CV, Calabro A, et al: Mild balanoposthitis. Genitourin Med 1994; 70:345–346.

Gardner-Medwin JM, Smith NJ, et al: Clinical experience with thalidomide in the management of severe oral and genital ulceration in conditions such as Behçet's disease. Ann Rheum Dis 1994; 53:828–832.

Gascon P, Schwartz RA: Treatment of Kaposi's sarcoma. Dermatol Clin 1994; 12:451–456.

Gerber GS: Carcinoma in situ of the penis. J Urol 1994; 151:829–833.

Gharpuray MB, Tolat SN: Nonvenereal sclerosing lymphangitis of the penis. Cutis 1991; 47:421–422.

Ghosh SK, Abrams JT, et al: Human T-cell leukemia virus type I tax/rex DNA and RNA in cutaneous T-cell lymphoma. Blood 1994; 84:2263–2271.

Gioglio L, Porta C, et al: Scrotal angiokeratoma (Fordyce): Histopathological and ultrastructural findings. Histol Histopathol 1992; 7:47–55.

Greaves MW, Weinstein GD: Treatment of psoriasis. N Engl J Med 1995; 332:581–588.

Greer DL: An overview of common dermatophytes. J Am Acad Dermatol 1994; 31:S112–S116.

Hart G: Factors associated with pediculosis pubis and scabies. Genitourin Med 1992; 68:294–295.

Haury B, Rodeheaver G, et al: Streptococcal cellulitis of the scrotum and penis with secondary skin gangrene. Surg Gynecol Obstet 1975; 141:35–39.

Hensler T, Christophers E: Psoriasis of early and late onset: Characterization of two types of psoriasis vulgaris. J Am Acad Dermatol 1985; 13:450.

Herman LE, Harawi SJ, et al: Folliculitis, a clinicopathologic review. Pathol Annu 1991; 26:201–246.

Hunter JA, Herd RM: Recent advances in atopic dermatitis. Q J Med 1994; 87:323–327.

Ikenberg H, Gissmna L, et al: Human papillomavirus type-16 related DNA in genital Bowen's disease and in bowenoid papulosis. Int J Cancer 1983; 32:563.

Jemec GB, Baadsgaard O: Effect of cyclosporine on genital psoriasis and lichen planus. J Am Acad Dermatol 1993; 29:1048–1049.

Jenkins D, Jakubovic HR: Pseudoepitheliomatous, keratotic, micaceous balanitis. A clinical lesion with two histologic subsets: Hyperplastic dystrophy and verrucous carcinoma. J Am Acad Dermatol 1988; 18:419–422.

Johnson RA: Diseases and disorders of the anogenitalia of males. *In* Fitzpatrick TB, Eisen AZ, Wolff K, et al, eds: Dermatology in General Medicine. New York, McGraw-Hill, 1993, pp 1417–1462.

Jolly BB, Krishnamurty S, et al: Zoon's balanitis. Urol Int 1993; 50:182–184.

Jorizzo JL, Abernethy JL, et al: Mucocutaneous criteria for the diagnosis of Behçet's disease: An analysis of clinicopathologic data from multiple international centers. J Am Acad Dermatol 1995; 32:968–976.

Jorizzo JL, Taylor RS, et al: Complex aphthosis: A forme fruste of Behçet's syndrome? J Am Acad Dermatol 1985; 13:80.

Kim ED, Kroft S, et al: Basal cell carcinoma of the penis: Case report and review of the literature. J Urol 1994; 152:1557–1559.

Kingston ME, Mackay D: Skin clues in the diagnosis of life-threatening infections. Rev Infect Dis 1986; 8:1–11.

Koblenzer CS: Dermatitis artefacta. *In* Koblenzer CS, ed: Psychocutaneous Disease. Orlando, Fla, Grune & Stratton, 1987, pp 85–107.

Konigsberg HA, Gray GF: Benign and malignant melanoma of penis and male urethra. Urology 1976; 7:323–326.

Korman NJ: Bullous pemphigoid. Dermatol Clin 1993; 11:483–498.

Kyriazi NC, Costenbader CL: Group A beta-hemolytic streptococcal balanitis. Pediatrics 1991, 88:154–156.

Lahesmaa R, Skurnik M, et al: Molecular mimicry between HLA B27 and *Yersinia, Salmonella, Shigella,* and *Klebsiella* within the same region of HLA alpha 1-helix. Clin Exp Immunol 1991; 86:399–404.

Lains J, Marcusson JA, et al: Surgical treatment of chronic hidradenitis suppurativa: CO_2 laser stripping—secondary intention technique. Br J Dermatol 1994; 131:551–556.

Langenberg A, Berger TG, et al: Genital benign pemphigus presenting as condylomas. J Am Acad Dermatol 1992; 26:951–955.

Ledwig PA, Weigand DA: Late circumcision and lichen sclerosus et atrophicus of the penis. J Am Acad Dermatol 1989; 20:211–214.

Le Sellin J, Drouet M, et al: Allergy survey in genital contact dermatitis. Allerg Immunol 1991; 23:127–128.

Leventhal LC, Jaworsky C, et al: An asymptomatic penile lesion. Circular indurated lymphangitis of the penis with concurrent syphilis. Arch Dermatol 1993; 129:366–370.

Lowe FC, Lattimer DG, et al: Kaposi's sarcoma of the penis in patients with acquired immunodeficiency syndrome. J Urol 1989; 142:1475–1477.

Magid M, Garden JM: Pearly penile papules: Treatment with the carbon dioxide laser. J Dermatol Surg Oncol 1989; 15:552–554.

Matosuoka LY, Wortsman J, et al: Acanthosis nigricans. Clin Dermatol 1993; 11:21–25.

Melekos M, Asbach HW, et al: Idiopathic gangrene of the male external genitalia, with report of a case and review of the literature. Int Urol Nephrol 1983; 15:65–69.

Melski JW, Stern JS: The separation of susceptibility to psoriasis from age of onset. J Invest Dermatol 1981; 77:474.

Miles SA: Pathogenesis of HIV related Kaposi's sarcoma. Curr Opin Oncol 1994; 1:497–502.

Moore PS, Chang Y: Detection of herpesvirus-like DNA sequences in Kaposi's sarcoma in patients with and those without HIV infection. N Engl J Med, 1995; 332:1181–1185.

Morhenn VB: The etiology of lichen planus. J Dermatopathol 1986; 8:154.

Morren MA: Atopic dermatitis: Triggering factors. J Am Acad Dermatol 1994; 31:467–473.

Moss TR, Stevenson CJ: Incidence of male genital vitiligo. Report of a screening program. Br J Vener Dis 1981; 57:145–146.

Mozzanica N: Pathogenic aspects of allergic and irritant contact dermatitis. Clin Dermatol 1992; 10:115–121.

Nahass GT, Blauvelt A, et al: Basal cell carcinoma of the scrotum. J Am Acad Dermatol 1992; 26:574–578.

O'Duffy JD: Behçet's syndrome. N Engl J Med 1990; 322:326.

O'Duffy JD: Behçet's disease. Curr Opin Rheumatol 1994; 6:39–43.

Olderbring J, Mikulowski P: Malignant melanoma of the penis and male urethra. Cancer 1987; 59:581.

Oliver GF, Winkelmann RK: Treatment of lichen planus. Drugs 1993; 45:56–65.

O'Neill TW, Rigby N, et al: Validation of the International Study Group criteria for Behçet's disease. Br J Rheumatol 1994; 33:115–117.

Patrizi A, Costa AM, et al: Perianal streptococcal dermatitis associated with guttate psoriasis and/or balanoposthitis: A study of five cases. Pediatr Dermatol 1994; 11:168–171.

Patterson JW, Kao GF, et al: Bowenoid papulosis. A clinicopathologic study with ultrastructural observations. Cancer 1986; 57:823.

Payne WG, Wells KE: Extramammary Paget's disease of the scrotum. Ann Plast Surg 1994; 33:669–671.

Perez MA, LaRossa DD, et al: Paget's disease primarily involving the scrotum. Cancer 1989; 63:970.

Przybilla B, Eberlein-Konig B, et al: Practical management of atopic eczema. Lancet 1994; 343:1342–1346.

Rahman MU, Cheema MA, et al: Molecular evidence for the presence of chlamydia in the synovium of patients with Reiter's syndrome. Arthritis Rheum 1992; 35:521–529.

Randle HWI, Sander HM: Treatment of generalized lichen nitidus with PUVA. Int J Dermatol 1986; 25:330.

Raviglione MC, Pablos-Mendez A, et al: Clinical features and management of severe dermatological reactions to drugs. Drug Saf 1990; 5:39–64.

Read SI, Abell E: Pseudoepitheliomatous, keratotic, and micaceous balanitis. Cutis 1981; 117:435–437.

Reedy MB, Morales CA, et al: Paget's disease of the scrotum: A case report and review of current literature. Tex Med 1991; 87:77–79.

Rehbein HM: Pearly penile papules: Incidence. Cutis 1977; 19:54–57.

Revuz J, Clerici T: Penile melanosis. J Am Acad Dermatol 1989; 20:567–570.

Richert RR, Broadkin RH, et al: Bowen's disease. CA 1977; 27:160.

Rosemberg SK, Herman G, et al: Sexually transmitted papilloma viral infection in the male. VII: Is cancer of penis sexually transmitted? Urology 1991; 37:437–440.

Roujeau JC: The spectrum of Stevens-Johnson syndrome and toxic epidermal necrolysis: A clinical classification. J Invest Dermatol 1994; 102:28S–30S.

Roujeau JC, Stern RS: Severe adverse cutaneous reactions to drugs. N Engl J Med 1994; 331:1272–1285.

Sajjadi H, Scheilian M, et al: Low dose cyclosporin-A therapy in Behçet's disease. J Ocul Pharmacol 1994; 10:553–560.

Schreiner DT, Jorizzo JL: Behçet's disease and complex aphthosis. Dermatol Clin 1987; 5:769.

Schwartz RA: Verrucous carcinoma of the skin and mucosa. J Am Acad Dermatol 1995; 32:1–21.

Schwartz RA, Janniger CK: Bowenoid papulosis. J Am Acad Dermatol, 1995; 32:1–21.

Seixas AL, Ornellan AA, et al: Verrucous carcinoma of the penis: Retrospective analysis of 32 cases. J Urol 1995; 152:1476–1478.

Shidhuphak W, MacDonald E, et al: Erythrasma. Overlooked or misdiagnosed? Int J Dermatol 1985; 24:95–96.

Sideri M, Origoni M, et al: Topical testosterone in the treatment of vulvar lichen sclerosus. Int J Gynecol Obstet 1994; 46:53–56.

Smith EP, Zone JJ: Dermatitis herpetiformis and linear IgA bullous dermatosis. Dermatol Clin 1993; 11:511–526.

Souteyrand P, Wong E, et al: Zoon's balanitis. Br J Dermatol 1981; 105:195–199.

Stals H, Vercammen C, et al: Acanthosis nigricans caused by nicotinic acid: Case report and review of the literature. Dermatology 1994; 189:203–206.

Stanley JR: Pemphigus: Skin failure by autoantibodies. JAMA 1990; 264:1714–1717.

Taniguchi S, Inoue A, et al: Angiokeratoma of Fordyce: A cause of scrotal bleeding. Br J Urol 1994; 73:589–590.

Thankappan TP, Zachariah J: Drug-specific clinical pattern in fixed drug eruptions. Int J Dermat 1991; 30:867–870.

Tuncer T, Arman MI, et al: HLA B27 and clinical features of Reiter's syndrome. Clin Rheumatol 1992; 11:239–242.

Van Moffaert M: Psychodermatology: An overview. Psychodermatol Psychosomat 1992; 58:125–136.

Waisman M: Immunofluorescent studies in lichen nitidus. Arch Dermatol 1971; 107:200.

Webster G: Seborrheic dermatitis. Int J Dermatol 1991; 30:843–844.

Weese D, Murphy J, et al: Nd:YAG laser treatment of extramammary Paget's disease of the penis and scrotum. J Urol (Paris) 1993; 99:269–271.

Weinrauch L, Katz M: Psoriasis vulgaris of labium majus. Cutis 1986; 38:333.

White SW, Smith J: Trichomycosis pubis. Arch Dermatol 1979; 115:444–445.

Wikstrom A, von Krogh G, et al: Papillomavirus-associated balanoposthitis. Genitourin Med 1994; 70:175–181.

Wright JE: The treatment of childhood phimosis with topical steroid. Aust N Z J Surg 1994; 64:327–328.

22
Parasitic Diseases of the Genitourinary System*

Jerome Hazen Smith, M.S.(Anat.), M.Sc.Hyg., M.D.
Franz von Lichtenberg, M.D.

INTRODUCTION TO PARASITISM OF THE URINARY TRACT

Parasitic diseases are major health problems today, especially in developing countries, but the human urogenital tract is regularly affected by only a few species of parasites. Two are discussed in detail. *Schistosoma haematobium*, a digenetic blood fluke, causes severe urinary tract disease, and filarial roundworms of the genera *Wuchereria*, *Brugia*, and *Onchocerca* can give rise to funiculoepidydymitis, hydrocele, genital elephantiasis, "hanging groin" and chyluria. Genitourinary involvement due to other parasites (except sexually transmitted protozoa) is either subordinate to systemic manifestations or rare; only brief descriptions of these entities are given. Finally, proteinuria and renal failure may complicate endemic malaria, schistosomiasis, and other parasitic infections.

Millions of people harbor urogenital parasites; however, *symptomatic* infections are substantially less common. Therefore, parasitic *infection* must be clearly differentiated from parasitic *disease*, which constitutes a variable fraction of total prevalence, depending on intensity of infection and other complex pathogenic factors.

Whereas many infectious diseases are coming under better control, incidences of schistosomiasis and filariasis are increasing. Expansion of irrigation agriculture disseminates vector snails and concentrates human populations near new water impoundments and irrigated areas, enhancing transmission of schistosomiasis. Urban crowding in the tropics favors mosquito-host contact, which promotes transmission of filariasis.

At the same time, modern human mobility and jet travel bring "tropical diseases" into the offices of physicians far from endemic areas; these physicians have had increasingly briefer exposure to parasitic diseases in medical school and often lack familiarity with their management. The most important requirement for recognition of parasitic infections is still *awareness,* based on knowledge of common clinical presentations, pathogenesis, and geographic distribution of parasitic diseases (and parasitic life cycles). Therefore, evaluation must include *careful history taking,* including the question "Where have you been?" And there must be a competent *parasitology laboratory* with anatomic pathology

*Disseminated toxoplasmosis in renal transplant patients undergoing immunosuppressive therapy is discussed separately in Section III, Chapter 14, and trichomoniasis and sexually transmitted enteric protozoal diseases are discussed in Section IV, Chapter 18.

back-up, currently available in only a few health centers. If doctors do not consider parasitic diseases, they will bury more affected patients than they diagnose.

Management of systemic parasitic diseases may transcend the urogenital problem and must address the whole patient. Decisions on when and how to use parasiticidal drugs and/or surgical intervention require a thorough understanding of the patient's pathologic condition and current knowledge of the best available drugs for different parasites. Such information is often not found in standard textbooks, and consultation is advisable for physicians with limited experience. Such assistance can be obtained from key faculty of university- or government-sponsored health centers that maintain tropical disease training programs, including, in the continental United States, the Centers for Disease Control and Prevention in Atlanta,* which maintains both a laboratory consulting service and a drug repository for uncommon parasitic diseases, with liaisons to various state laboratories.

URINARY SCHISTOSOMIASIS

Definition and History

Schistosomiasis comprises a group of chronic diseases caused by schistosomes (blood flukes), a genus of digenetic parasitic trematodes. The paired adult male and female worms cohabitate the venous plexuses of the abdominal viscera. ***Schistosoma haematobium*** **worm pairs dwell principally in the perivesical venous plexus in humans** (other mammals are only sporadically infected) and cause urinary schistosomiasis (also known as bilharziasis and schistosomiasis haematobium). Schistosomiasis haematobium has scourged the great agricultural civilizations of the Middle East for millennia and is still a major cause of disease and death in these fertile areas. Egyptian physicians of the XIIth Dynasty (1900 B.C.) recognized the cardinal sign and symptom, hematuria and terminal dysuria, as a disease (Ruffer, 1910). Theodore Bilharz, a German pathologist working in Cairo in the late 1800s, first described worm pairs in mesenteric veins at autopsy and linked these to eggs found in human excreta. Clinical management and prognosis in urinary schistosomiasis differ, depending on *the stage* of the infection; therefore, understanding the disease's natural history is essential.

*Division of Parasitic Diseases, Center for Infectious Diseases, Centers for Disease Control and Prevention, Atlanta, Georgia 30333; telephone number (770) 488-7760.

Biology and Life Cycle

The **life cycle** of *S. haematobium*, like those of other digenetic trematodes, consists of a *sexual* reproductive phase, in which egg-laying, long-lived adult worms reside in the veins and venules of the definitive host, and *asexual* reproduction, represented by sporocyst development inside the specific intermediate host snail. The products both of sexual multiplication, the miracidia (which develop within eggs), and of asexual multiplication, the cercariae (which result from sporocysts), must migrate through fresh water to complete the cycle by penetrating the snail or the mammalian skin, respectively (Fig. 22–1). **Therefore, human infection is acquired by exposure to fresh (not salt) water that harbors the infected bulinid snails.**

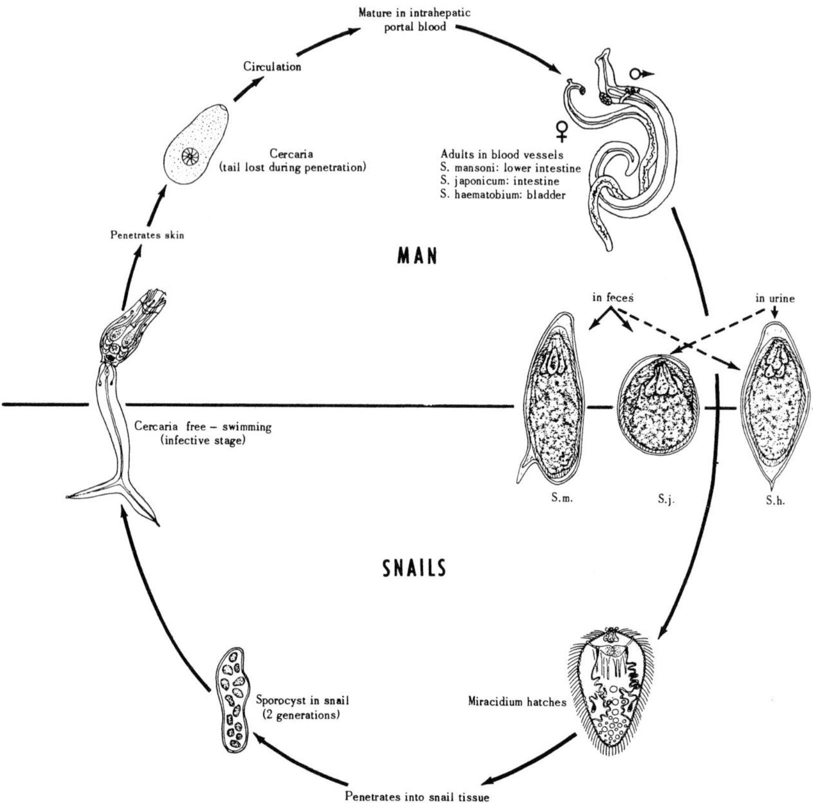

Figure 22–1. Life cycle of a schistosome. (From U.S. Department of Health and Human Services, Public Health Service Publications, U.S. Government Printing Office, Washington, DC, 1964.)

Oviposition (egg laying) by adult *S. haematobium* normally occurs in vesical and pelvic venules; these vessels are tributaries of the caval system but are connected to the portal venous system through hemorrhoidal collateral vessels. The worms measure about 1.5 cm in length, the male being lanceolate with a midline ventral fold (gynecophorous canal) that wraps around the slender, cylindrical female in permanent copula. Although worm pairs attach to endothelia by their acetabula and remain in intimate contact with the blood and endothelia of the vessels in which they nest, no clotting or inflammation occurs around them while they produce and deposit approximately 200 to 500 eggs per day. Worm pairs also lay eggs in the gut of experimental animals but lay more than twice the number of eggs per day in the urinary bladder than in the gut (Agnew et al, 1988). Thus during its estimated mean life span of 3.4 years (Wilkins et al, 1984) or 3 to 6 years (Butterworth et al, 1988), a single worm pair spawns 250,000 to 600,000 eggs; moreover, occasional worm pairs may persist as long as 30 years (de Gentile et al, 1988).

According to experimental data, 20% of the **eggs** erode into the lumina of the hollow viscera in which they are laid and are excreted in the urine or feces; the rest remain where deposited or are swept into the blood stream to microembolize the microvasculature of lungs, liver, and other sites (Cheever and Anderson, 1971). A portion of the eggs trapped in tissues (i.e., neither excreted nor microembolized) are destroyed by the host's granulomatous response. The remainder of the entrapped eggs become calcifically "mummified" and accumulate in the viscera at the rate of approximately 90 to 100 eggs per worm pair per day (Cheever et al, 1977).

S. haematobium eggs measure 80 × 150 μm, are ovoid, tan, thin-shelled, and terminally spined (Fig. 22–2), which differentiates them from laterally spined *Schistosoma mansoni* eggs. The only other schistosome that is pathogenic for humans and has terminally spined eggs, *Schistosoma intercalatum*, is rarely seen outside limited foci in the Republic of Zaire, Gabon, and Cameroon (Ratard and Greer, 1991); thus, terminally spined eggs in the urine, feces, or human tissue are diagnostic of *S. haematobium* infection.

Work in the early 1990s indicates that different species of the *S. haematobium* group (*S. intercalatum, S. mattheei,* and *S. bovis*) may hybridize in humans, experimental animals, and snails to produce parasites with different preferential sites of oviposition, cercarial shedding patterns, and fecundity (Kruger, 1990; Kruger and Evans, 1990; Mouahid et al, 1991; Ratard and Greer, 1991; De Clercq et al, 1994). Immunization with irradiated hybrid cercaria produces significant cross immunity throughout the *S. haematobium* group (Navarrete et al, 1994). Cross-mated *S. haematobium* and *S. mansoni* are viable with significant fecundity but differing patterns of distribution in experimental hosts (Khalil and Mansour, 1995).

Egg maturation begins in utero from a single oocyte, and it continues for several days after oviposition until the miracidium forms. Mature **miracidia** remain viable within eggs for less than 3 weeks (and probably infectious to snails for only 12 days); if not extruded into water within that period, they die, and the eggs degenerate. In active infection, all egg stages from immature through mature to degenerated and calcific are seen, whereas in cured or inactive infection, only degenerated (dark) or calcific eggs appear in the tissues or excreta.

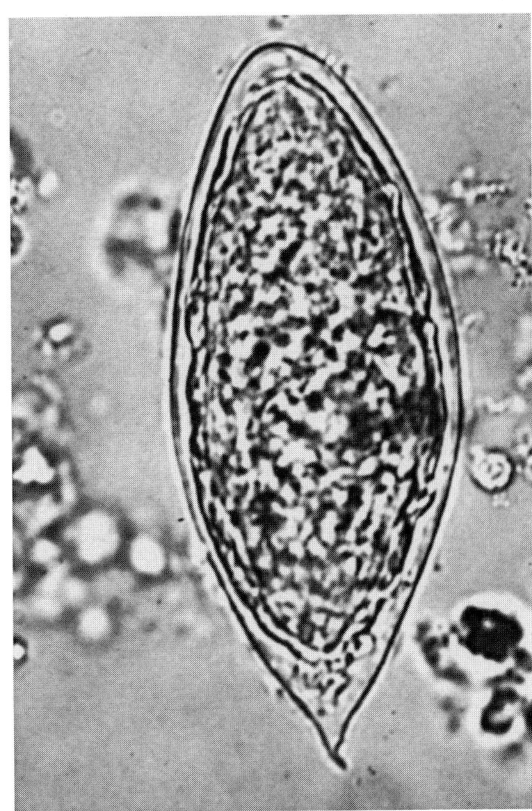

Figure 22–2. Egg of *Schistosoma haematobium,* as seen in urinary sediment. (Magnification, ×800.) (Courtesy of Dr. Steven Pan, Harvard School of Public Health.)

Upon deposition into fresh water, eggs osmotically swell, the shells break, and miracidia emerge as autonomous, short-lived, ciliated larvae that swim and seek hosts. Guided by phototropism and by snail trace minerals (Chernin, 1974), they find and enter snails of *Bulinus* species (e.g., *Bulinus truncatus* in Egypt, *B. globosus,* and *B. forskalii* in sub-Saharan Africa), migrate through their tissues, and transform into successive generations of **mother and daughter sporocysts**. Each miracidium develops into a mother sporocyst, which produces 20 to 40 daughter sporocysts, each of which in turn produces about 200 to 400 cercariae. The cercariae escape the daughter sporocyst, migrate to the snail's surface, and emerge into surrounding fresh water. This enormous, asexual multiplication from a single miracidium to 10^5 cercariae compensates for the attrition during aquatic parts of the life cycle.

Cercariae, shed by snails for several days or weeks, consist of a body (approximately 175 μm)—that is, an undifferentiated, but genotypically male or female miniature worm—and a forked muscular tail (approximately 220 μm), both covered by a protective glycocalyx. The tail propels the body through water by vibratory movements to find the human definitive host. Studies show that the mechanisms of cercarial host-finding differ between *S. haematobium* and *S. mansoni* (Haas, 1994). The cercariae penetrate *unbroken* skin; if they fail to penetrate skin within a few hours, they exhaust their glycogen, become lethargic, and die.

At penetration, the cercarial body becomes a **schistosomulum** by sloughing its glycocalyx and tail. The schistosomulum must undergo sudden radical adaptation to the new isotonic and isothermic environment; attendant mortality is up to two thirds of penetrating organisms. Surviving schistosomula, stimulated by the 37°C temperature and $NaHCO_3$ (Wiest et al, 1989), transform their trilaminate outer tegumental membrane into a multilaminate membrane characteristic of the adult worm (Hockley and McLaren, 1973). After a short rest in the dermis (Fig. 22–3), the schistosomulum begins its migratory, growth, pairing, and maturation processes, which in *S. haematobium* may require 80 to 110 days. Knowledge of migration routes is incomplete, but they are known to include interstitial spaces, blood, and lymph vessels; studies in experimental animals strongly indicate that lymphangioles of the skin provide the initial path for schistosomular migration (Bayssade-Dufour et al, 1994). Schistosomula congregate in the lung at 4 to 7 days and in the liver from the second week onward as growth of the worms accelerates. Finally, adults pair off and home in to sites where oviposition begins and, soon, ascends to the maximal egg-laying level, which is maintained until worm death.

Significant cellular and humoral **host responses** develop (Phillips and Colley, 1978; Warren, 1982; Butterworth, 1987; Butterworth et al, 1988) as schistosomula become adults; these responses partially abrogate (but do not eliminate) subsequent reinfection in experimental animals (Cheever et al, 1988a, 1988b) and human adults (but not children; Hagan et al, 1985b, 1987; Wilkins et al, 1987; Chandiwana et al, 1991; Woolhouse et al, 1991), via eosinophil-mediated killing (Hagan et al, 1985a, 1985b, 1991). These responses are ineffective against the adult worms, which, by themselves, do not produce significant disease in the host. Adult worms maintain an enduring balance with the host, even while schistosomula are decimated by host immunity to antigens cross-reacting with adult and egg antigens; this resistance to new infection is called *concomitant immunity* (Smithers and Terry, 1967).

In overview, the life cycle just described depends on so many fortuitous conjunctions that it should be easily broken, but it has proved remarkably hardy and has resisted many human attempts to interrupt it.

Distribution and Epidemiology

Cited prevalences of parasitic diseases have incredible magnitudes; 500 to 600 million people risk contracting schistosomiasis; 180 million for urinary schistosomiasis. Of the 200 million afflicted with schistosomiasis, 80 to 90 million are infected by *S. haematobium* (Peters and Gilles, 1977; Dittrich and Doehring, 1986; Koroltchouk et al, 1987; Mott, 1987). What proportion of infections are sufficiently heavy to cause clinical urinary schistosomiasis is uncertain, but some series indicate that 60% have schistosomal obstructive uropathy. Probably 60 million have significant hematuria, and 10 to 40 million have obstructive uropathy and other schistosomal sequelae and complications.

Transmission of *S. haematobium* occurs throughout the African continent, including the islands of Madagascar and Mauritius. In Southwest Asia, it is found in Southern Yemen, Yemen, Saudi Arabia, Lebanon, Syria, Turkey, Iraq, and Iran. All cases diagnosed outside these zones have been imported (Wright, 1973).

Within the vast endemic regions, prevalence and intensity

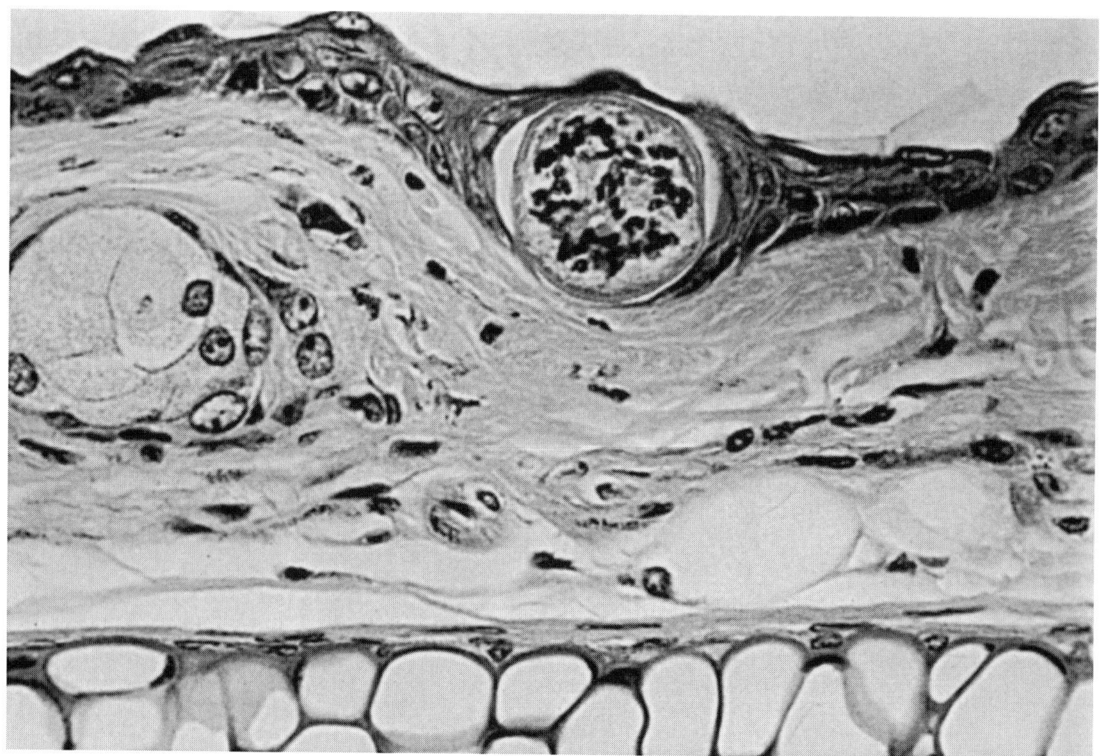

Figure 22–3. Schistosomulum traversing the epidermis of the mouse ear. (Magnification, ×800.)

of infection vary widely, as does the public health importance of the disease. Typically, these incidences are highest where irrigation agriculture is long established, such as in the Nile Valley and Delta. After 50 years of varied control efforts in the Nile Delta, prevalence of active *S. haematobium* has dropped from more than 50% to nearly 5% (Cline et al, 1989), but it is uncertain whether this results from public health efforts or alterations in snail habitat as a result of flood control by the Aswan Dam. The organism has apparently been eradicated in Israel and Cyprus. However, transmission is increasing in most endemic areas, especially around large water projects in Sudan and around the Aswan Dam and Lake Volta. Regional strains of *S. haematobium* may vary in "virulence" because of differences in vector snail species or other unknown parasite factors.

In endemic settings, first exposure usually occurs in preschool children (Perel et al, 1985) or during school age and is followed by repeated exposures. In communities in which swimming, bathing, or washing clothes is done in rivers or lakes that are the loci of exposure, infection may decline among adults; conversely, in fishermen, boatyard workers, and others with occupational water contact, exposure continues (Gilles et al, 1965). Sexual distribution, often biased toward men, depends partly on differences in water exposure.

Some acquired resistance has been demonstrated in humans after effective mass chemotherapy (Wilkins et al, 1984, 1987); resistance to repeat infection arises between 10 and 15 years of age and is stronger in women than in men, despite greater water exposure of women. This resistance may depend on host age (or perhaps duration of infection). Children produce nonprotective, "blocking" immunoglobulins M and G (IgM and IgG) antibodies to schistosomular surface antigens; these antibodies prevent the effect of concurrently emerging cellular and humoral protective immunity. Adults produce proportionately fewer "blocking" antibodies (Butterworth et al, 1988). CD4+ lymphocytes from infected and treated children (8 to 14 years of age) produced significantly higher amounts of interleukins-4 and -10 (IL-4 and IL-10) than comparably infected adults (>20 years of age); yet both groups produced comparable IFN (King et al, 1995); in addition, increasing IL-10 levels correlate with reciprocally decreased interferon (IFN) levels in humans infected with *S. haematobium* (Malhotra et al, 1995). In some heavily exposed groups, such as Sudanese canal-cleaners, remarkably little overt disease is found, and cohort studies of infected children show that infections stabilize while exposures continue (Bradley and McCullough, 1973; King et al, 1995). In fact, acquired immunity in humans is better documented for *S. haematobium* than for other schistosomes.

In both clinical and autopsy studies, the prevalence of infection and its intensity, as measured by egg excretion or tissue egg burden, are related (Smith et al, 1974b). Tissue egg burden, in turn, is related to the severity of the disease and to the frequency of complications. Autopsies in Nigeria (Edington et al, 1970; von Lichtenberg et al, 1971) and in Egypt (Smith et al, 1974a, 1975; Cheever et al, 1977, 1978) indicate that severe uropathy is uncommon when the frequency of infection in a population is below 30% but increases linearly after this threshold is exceeded. Moreover, community-based studies have shown that obstructive uropathy occurring during the active disease (see later discussion) is related to infection intensity (assessed by egg excretion) both in individual patients and in communities.

All of these caveats notwithstanding, careful epidemiologic studies have shown that schistosomiasis haematobium exhibits remarkable focality epidemiologically (Guyatt et al, 1994; Woolhouse et al, 1994), so that prevalence, incidence, and intensity of initial infection and reinfection after treatment not only are related to presence of snail habitat and level of infection (which varies seasonally and with compatibility of *S. haematobium* strain and snail species and strain) (Véra et al, 1990; Ratard et al, 1990; Adewunmi et al, 1991; Abdel-Wahab et al, 1993; Elias et al, 1994) but are also extraordinarily related to the kinds and extent of water contact (Akogun, 1990; Kloos et al, 1990; Chandiwana and Woolhouse, 1991; Sama and Ratard, 1994).

General Pathology and Pathogenesis

Disease development parallels parasite development within the host. Cercarial penetration and migration elicit immunologic reactions that cause swimmer's itch; this rarely brings patients to physicians. Similarly, adult worms per se produce no significant lesions.

Schistosomal disease results directly from schistosome *eggs* and from the *granulomatous* host response to them (von Lichtenberg et al, 1973; Kassis et al, 1978; Phillips and Colley, 1978; Garb et al, 1982; Warren, 1982; Cheever et al, 1985). The miracidia within eggs produce antigens that "leak" into surrounding interstitial spaces through pores in the egg shell (von Lichtenberg, 1964; Neill et al, 1988) (Fig. 22–4). The host responds to these antigens by forming granulomas ("pseudotubercles") around the egg—that is, an accumulation of macrophages, lymphocytes, and eosinophils (Fig. 22–5) that "sequester" that antigen locally (von Lichtenberg, 1962, 1964). The perioval granulomas of all schisto-

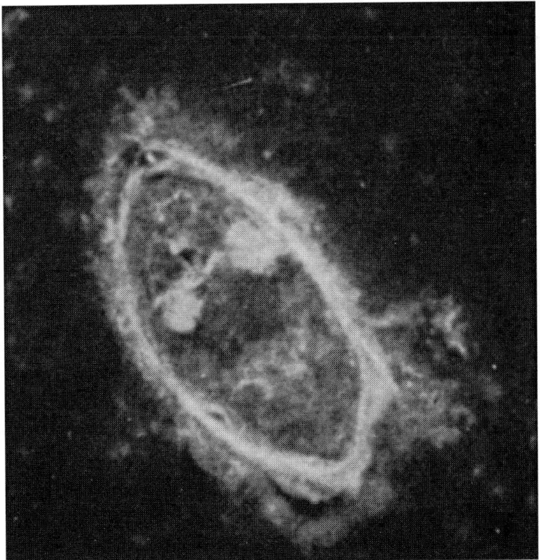

Figure 22–4. Egg of *Schistosoma mansoni* stained for soluble antigen by the direct immunofluorescence technique. Note positivity of apical glands and around eggshell in the granuloma center.

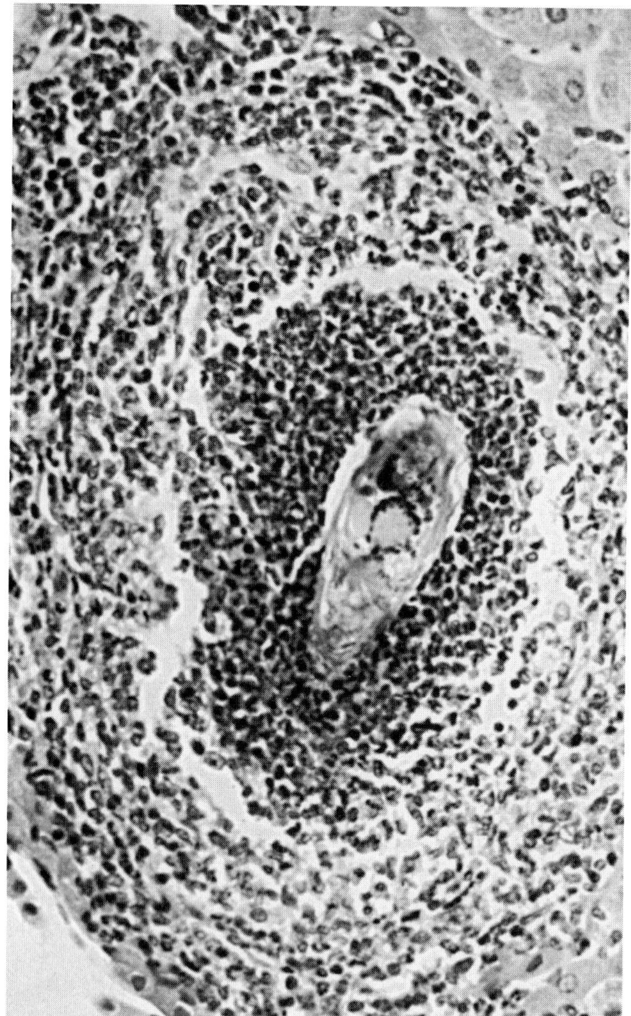

Figure 22–5. Early schistosome granuloma in the liver, showing mature miracidium and numerous granulocytes. (Magnification, ×420.)

somes are T-cell–dependent host responses (Kassis et al, 1978; Garb et al, 1982; Cheever et al, 1985) and are modulated by that system (Warren, 1973a; Hang et al, 1974); treatment eliminates such modulation in humans (Feldmeier et al, 1988). Humoral immunity manifests within the granuloma as antigen-antibody precipitates, the Hoeppli phenomenon (von Lichtenberg et al, 1966; Smith and von Lichtenberg, 1967), and there are circulating immune complexes (Manca et al, 1988), but the granuloma is a T-cell–mediated entity. Perioval granulomas enlarge and plateau at 8 days in the sensitized host, concomitant with egg maturation, and then slowly involute within 4 to 6 months (von Lichtenberg, 1962, 1973).

In patent human infections, all stages of granulomas are simultaneously present. In chronic schistosomiasis, after 5 to 6 weeks of oviposition, the granulomas formed around new eggs are smaller and less destructive; this is called *immune modulation* and results from increased antigen-specific suppressor T cells (OKT8) and decreased antigen-specific helper T cells (OKT4) (Khalil et al, 1987). It is now thought that in early *S. mansoni* infections of humans and experimental animals, granuloma formation may dominated by the TH^1 subset of T-lymphocytes, but the process soon becomes a TH^2 (CD3 + TcRγ/δ) subset–dominated granulomatous disease (Cai et al, 1995; Flores Villanueva et al, 1995; Rathore et al, 1995; Cayabyab and Harn, 1995); studies in human hepatosplenic schistosomiasis suggest that a greater number of subsets exist and that the system is even more complex (B. Doughty, personal communication). Patients with *urinary* schistosomiasis do, however, have high circulating levels of TNF and IL-2, indicative of high TH^1 activity (Raziuddin et al, 1992, 1993). In addition, in active *S. haematobium* infection, an inflammation, manifested by edema and increased eosinophils and plasma cells, diffuses between perioval granulomas.

S. haematobium adult worm pairs are widely distributed throughout the pelvic and mesenteric venous plexuses, but oviposition occurs chiefly in the pelvic lower urinary tract (Kamel et al, 1977; Cheever et al, 1977). The reason for such localization is unknown. *S. haematobium* concentrates oviposition in patches, probably because worm pairs have an affinity for each other's and/or previously deposited eggs (Edington et al, 1970; Smith et al, 1974a; Cheever et al, 1977). In experimental animals, the granulomagenicity of individual *S. haematobium* eggs lies between that of *S. mansoni* and *S. japonicum* (Erickson et al, 1971, 1974; von Lichtenberg et al, 1973; von Lichtenberg, 1973). *S. haematobium* eggs have terminal spines that differentiate them from other schistosomes (see Fig. 22–2), but egg distortion in histologic sections renders this feature useless. *S. haematobium* egg shells are not acid-fast, whereas *S. mansoni* and *S. japonicum* eggs are acid-fast; this feature differentiates the eggs in tissue sections from patients from areas where both *S. mansoni* and *S. haematobium* are coendemic (von Lichtenberg and Lindenberg, 1954; Rousset et al, 1962). *S. haematobium* deposits eggs in groups, rather than singly, and thus produces composite granulomas (Fig. 22–6) rather than unioval granulomas (see Fig. 22–5) (von Lichtenberg et al, 1971; Smith et al, 1974a; Smith and Christie, 1986). Studies of the *S. haematobium* egg granuloma in human ureters show that their ultrastructural features are similar to those of *S. mansoni* pseudotubercles in experimental animals (el-Shoura, 1993a, 1993b, 1994). Some *S. haematobium* eggs become calcific (Figs. 22–7 and 22–8), but artifactual decalcification may lead to underestimation of the proportion of eggs that are calcified (Cheever, 1986).

S. mansoni also lays eggs in the lower urinary tract, especially in heavy infections, but no lower urinary tract lesions have been ascribed solely to *S. mansoni* (Smith et al, 1974a; Cheever et al, 1978). The finding of *S. mansoni* eggs in the lower urinary tract should initiate an inquiry for possible hepatosplenic schistosomiasis. Experimental data suggest that heavy infections with *S. haematobium* may suppress T cell responses to *S. mansoni* (Feldmeier et al, 1981), but the severity of *S. mansoni* and *S. haematobium* infections was independent in humans (Smith et al, 1974a).

The spectrum of serious clinicopathologic syndromes ascribed to *S. haematobium* results from interaction of four factors: (1) intensity, (2) duration, (3) activity (in which the disease progresses from an active stage into an inactive, but still dangerous, stage) **and (4) focality** (egg deposition may randomly focus on a crucial anatomic site at any time during oviposition) of infection. These interacting factors determine the morbidity, mortality, and treatment of urinary schistosomiasis (Smith and Christie, 1986).

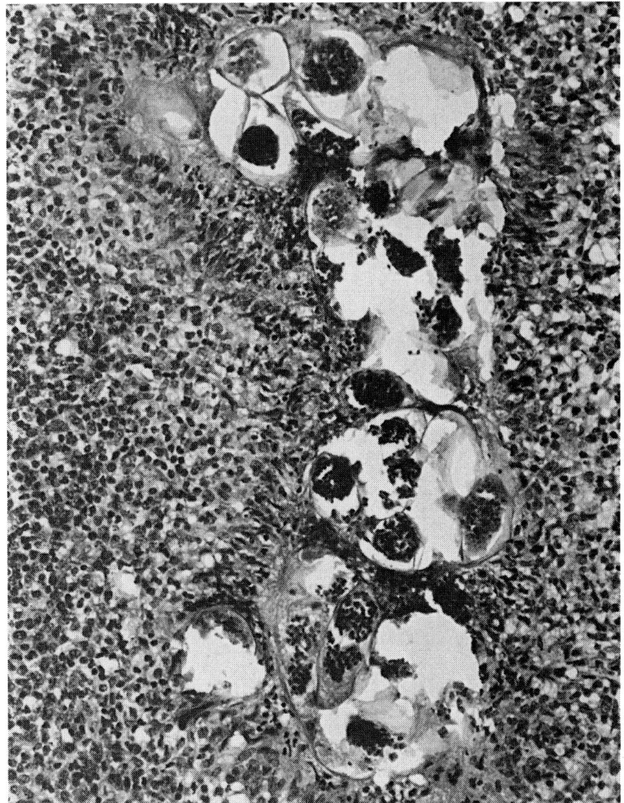

Figure 22–6. *Schistosoma haematobium* perioval granuloma. Numerous viable eggs are deposited in a small vein, which was destroyed by the subsequent host reaction, yielding a composite (multioval) granuloma composed of lymphocytes, macrophages, plasma cells, and eosinophils. (Hematoxylin-eosin stain; magnification, ×125.) (From Smith JH, Christie JD: Hum Pathol. 1986; 17:333.)

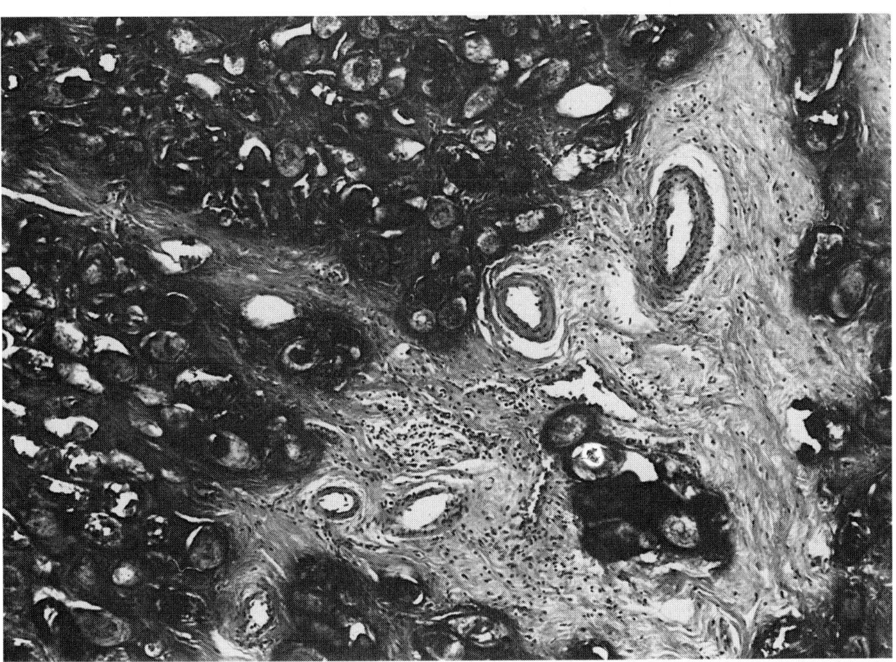

Figure 22–7. Microscopic section of sandy patch (i.e., chronic inactive urinary schistosomiasis) with numerous dead calcific eggs, scant cellular inflammatory infiltrate, and partially calcific fibrotic matrix. (Hematoxylin-eosin stain; magnification, ×125.) (Reproduced from Smith, J.H., and Christie, J.D.: Hum. Pathol., 17:333, 1986.)

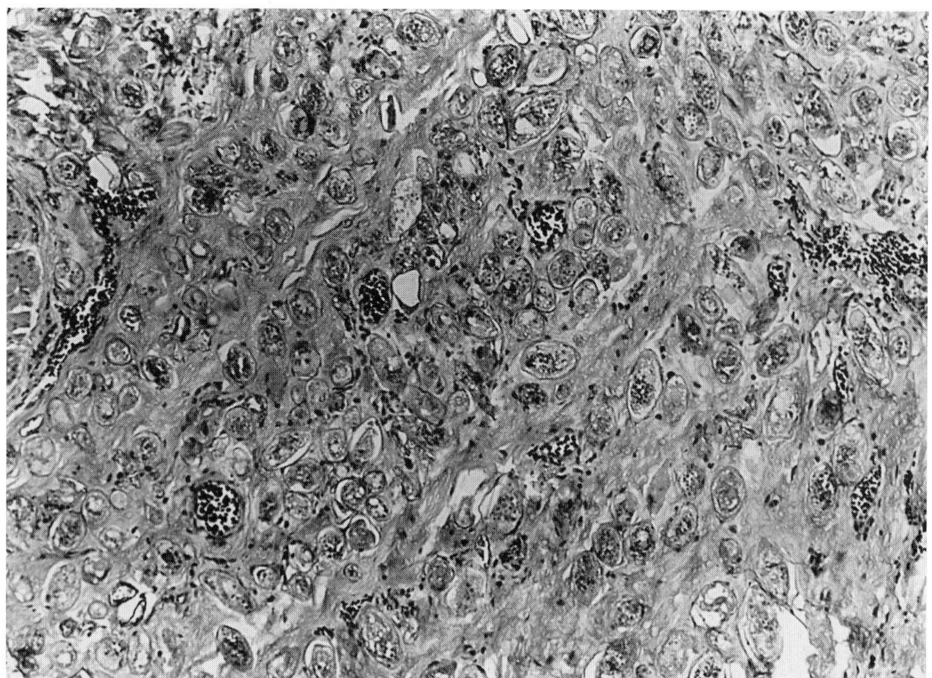

Figure 22–8. Sandy patch after decalcification, showing myriads of dead *Schistosoma haematobium* eggs in dense fibrotic matrix. Small, thin-walled vascular channels with erythrocytes lie within the fibrous tissue. The eggs contain partially degenerated embryos, which retain some morphologic integrity and intact nuclei. Compare the appearance of this decalcified section with that of the section shown in Figure 22–7, which is not decalcified. (Hematoxylin-eosin stain; magnification, ×125.) (From Smith JH, Christie JD: Hum Pathol 1986; 17:333.)

Progression (Activity) of the Disease

The form of *S. haematobium* lesions is highly variable (Makar, 1955; von Lichtenberg et al, 1971; Smith et al, 1974a; Cheever et al, 1978). In sites of *recent* oviposition, perioval granulomatous inflammation (see Fig. 22–6) results in large, bulky, hyperemic, and polypoid masses projecting into the lumen (Fig. 22–9). As oviposition at a site ceases, entrapped eggs are destroyed or calcified and inflammation wanes, being supplanted by fibrous tissue (see Figs. 22–7 and 22–8) to produce the sandy patches characteristic of chronic urinary schistosomiasis (Fig. 22–9). These patches have the appearance and consistency of fine golden-tan sand when incised (von Lichtenberg et al, 1971; Smith et al, 1974a; Smith and Christie, 1986).

In experimental studies of *S. haematobium* infection in chimpanzees, von Lichtenberg postulated that the spectrum of lesions formed a continuum from polypoid patch through fibrous patch to sandy patch and that this spectrum represented a progression; individual patches commencing at different times but evolving at similar rates would account for the heterogeneity of lesions encountered in the human disease (Sadun et al, 1970). Von Lichtenberg categorized the disease in four stages: early active, chronic active, late residual, and chronic inactive. This classification became a powerful tool in the understanding of the evolution of urinary schistosomiasis (Edington et al, 1970; von Lichtenberg et al, 1971; Smith et al, 1974a, 1975), and the progression was subsequently corroborated radiologically in humans (Young et al, 1974). The classification was simplified for clinical use into two stages: *active* and *inactive* (Lehman et al, 1973; Smith et al, 1975). A firm grasp of the biphasic nature of the disease is imperative in mastering the disease's morbidity, mortality, frequency of complications, epidemiology, treatment, and diagnosis (Table 22–1) (Smith and Christie, 1986).

Active urinary schistosomiasis (see Table 22–1) is characterized by viable adult worm pairs, sustained oviposition, and a vigorous granulomatous host response. On gross examination, the bladder shows sharply delimited, sessile (occasionally pedunculated) polypoid mucosal patches, covered by partly eroded hyperemic mucosa. Microscopic examination shows that the polypoid patch consists of scattered or massed composite granulomas separated by edematous granulation tissue diffusely infiltrated by eosinophils, lym-

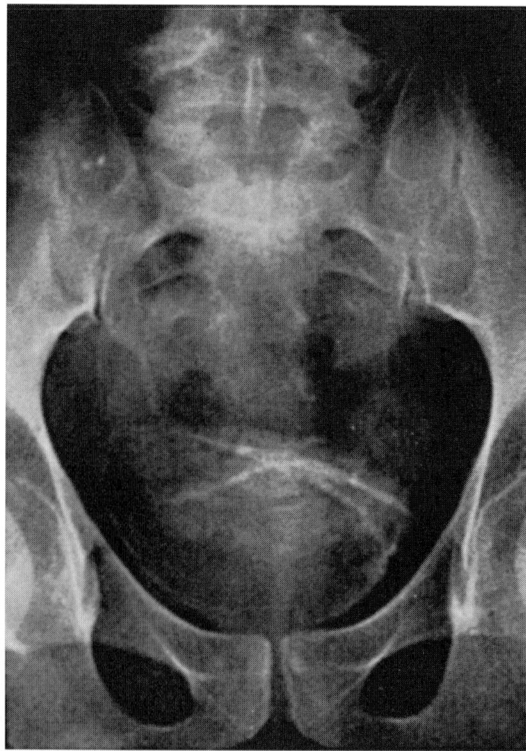

Figure 22–9. Plain x-ray film showing bladder calcification in a patient with *Schistosoma haematobium* infection.

Table 22–1. DIFFERENCES BETWEEN ACTIVE AND INACTIVE URINARY SCHISTOSOMIASIS

Feature	Active	Inactive
Adult worm pairs	+	−
Oviposition	+	−
Urinary egg excretion	+	−
Important in transmission	+	−
Granulomatous host response	+	−
Polypoid lesions	+ Possibly obstructive	Very rare
Sandy patches	+ in late active	+ Possibly obstructive
Schistosomal obstructive uropathy caused by:	Polypoid lesions	Sandy patches
Schistosomal ulceration	Uncommon	Common
Treatment	Chemotherapy	Surgical repair

phocytes, and plasma cells; adult worm pairs reside in small veins. Composite granulomas may be large and abscess-like, filled with eosinophils and viable eggs. In endemic areas, polypoid patches occur mainly in children through their early teens. Perioval granulomas and smaller lesions are scattered through interpolypoid mucosa. Polyps may obstruct ureters or rarely the bladder outlet. Ova are excreted in the urine in proportion to the *viable* egg (and worm) burden in lower urinary tract tissues but not in proportion to the *total* egg burden (Sadun et al, 1970; von Lichtenberg et al, 1971; Smith et al, 1974b; Cheever et al, 1975a, 1977; Kamel et al, 1977; Smith and Christie, 1986).

The active stage is diagnosed by examination of urine, and quantitation of urinary egg excretion estimates the intensity of current (but not past) infection and thus correlates, albeit imperfectly, with prognosis (Smith et al, 1974b; Cheever et al, 1975a). Although worms live only 3 to 4 years, the active stage of urinary schistosomiasis averages 12 to 13 years (Lehman et al, 1973; Smith et al, 1975), but activity wanes during later years. This infers that successive "crops" of worms infest the lower urinary tract during the course of endemic infection. Throughout the active stage, the calcific egg burden increases progressively, as worm burden decreases without change in worm fecundity (von Lichtenberg et al, 1971; Lehman et al, 1973; Cheever et al, 1977).

The active stage is epidemiologically important because of its role in transmission and is clinically important because it is during this stage that polypoid patches disappear within 35 days and obstructive sequelae can be dramatically ameliorated by chemotherapy alone (Lucas et al, 1966, 1969; Lehman et al, 1973; Doehring et al, 1985b, 1986a; Devidas et al, 1989). Effective chemotherapy iatrogenically converts active into inactive disease (Smith and Christie, 1986), unless the patient is reinfected (Pugh and Teesdale, 1984).

Inactive urinary schistosomiasis (see Table 22–1), which occurs after adult worms have died, is characterized by the absence of viable eggs in tissues or urine and the presence of "sandy patches": relatively flat, tan mucosal lesions of various depth, often less sharply defined than polypoid patches. Microscopic sandy patches consist of myriads of calcified eggs in a dense, irregular fibrous tissue matrix; scant or no inflammatory cells pervade these lesions. A variant of the sandy patch is the fibrous patch, in which more exuberant fibrous tissue widely separates the calcific eggs, resulting in a tough, keloid-like tissue. Sandy patches may be found late in the active stage and throughout the inactive stage. There is progressive increase in the proportion of inactive urinary schistosomiasis in the third and subsequent decades of life in endemic regions (Smith et al, 1975).

Urinary excretion of dead or calcific eggs during the inactive stage is rare and, when found, is not proportional to tissue egg burdens (Smith et al, 1974b; Cheever et al, 1975a; Patil et al, 1992). Calcific tissue egg burdens of more than 20,000 to 30,000 per gram are detectable radiologically (Cheever et al, 1975b). The clinicoradiologic term *calcified bladder* is a circumferential, thick, coalescent sandy patch that contains sufficient calcified eggs to appear as a shell-like radiopaque edge of the bladder on radiographs or as a cloudy veil on frontal projection. Calcific eggs contain copious antigen, which may stimulate a granulomatous response when the eggs are decalcified (Smith and von Lichtenberg, 1976). Clinically severe schistosomal disease may persist or become symptomatic for the first time during the inactive stage (Young et al, 1974; Smith et al, 1975, 1977a, 1977b; Cheever et al, 1975a, 1975b; Wallace, 1979; Al-Shukri and Alwan, 1983; Christie et al, 1986a, 1986b, 1986c; Patil et al, 1992).

Inactive urinary schistosomiasis plays no role in transmission, but in studies of morbidity and mortality, patients with inactive disease should not be categorized with uninfected controls (Smith and Christie, 1986). Diagnosis of inactive disease is made by demonstration of calcific *S. haematobium* eggs in biopsy specimens or radiographs (see section on diagnosis). Quantitative examination of urinary sediment at this stage is fruitless. Antischistosomal chemotherapy is also futile, and this stage can be treated only by appropriate surgical procedures. If sequelae (i.e., obstructive uropathy) persist after effective chemotherapy for active disease, the patient should be surgically treated for the iatrogenically induced inactive stage (Smith and Christie, 1986).

Intensity of Infection

Intensity of infection is assessed directly by quantitating the worm burden at autopsy (Kamel et al, 1977; Cheever et al, 1977) and indirectly by determining the tissue egg burden (Edington et al, 1970; Smith et al, 1974a; Cheever et al, 1977). Tissue egg burden is the mathematical product of the intensity of infection (number of worm pairs and hence the number of eggs deposited) and the duration of oviposition (Smith et al, 1975). **Analysis of tissue egg burdens has demonstrated that there is a direct relationship between the intensity of the infection and both the severity of disease and frequency of sequelae and complications** (Edington et al, 1970; Smith et al, 1974a; Cheever et al, 1978); this has been confirmed in clinical community-based studies (Abdel-Salam and Abdel-Fattah, 1977; Warren et al, 1979; Coopan et al, 1986). Tissue egg burdens also permit us to distinguish between lesions that occur incidentally in patients with urinary schistosomiasis and lesions that are *caused* by *S. haematobium* (Edington et al, 1970; Smith et al, 1974a). Moreover, analysis of correlation coefficients between tissue egg burden of the entire lower urinary tract and egg burdens of specific parts of the lower urinary tract or lower gut permits clinicians to distinguish schistosomal lesions, which are systematically related to intensifying infection, from ectopic oviposition, which does not regularly occur in all infected patients, as a function of overall intensity of infection (Smith and Christie, 1986).

Focalization of S. haematobium *Egg Deposition*

S. haematobium oviposition focuses in patches in chimpanzees and humans (Sadun et al, 1970; Cheever et al, 1978). In humans, the coefficients of variation of egg burden of different parts of the lower urinary tract decrease as the intensity and/or duration of the infection increases (Christie et al, 1986b); that is, in early infections, there are wide discrepancies between tissue egg burdens within the lower urinary tract, but these tend to decrease as duration and/or intensity of infection increases. In early active disease, oviposition may focus on and compromise a physiologically crucial site, such as the interstitial ureter. As the intensity and/or duration of infection increase, the probability of a "hit" at crucial sites increases (Christie et al, 1986b; Smith and Christie, 1986).

Patterns of Egg Accumulation over the Duration of the Disease

Because egg burden is the product of duration and rate of oviposition, the accumulation of eggs corresponds to the duration of oviposition, so that the number of eggs per gram of urinary tract serves as an independent variable approximating "time" to correlate with the accumulation of eggs in diverse parts of the urinary tract. This estimates rates of oviposition (slope) and the onset of oviposition (intercept) at each anatomic site. During active disease, rates of oviposition in all parts of the urinary tract are similar and higher than rates in other sites, such as the rectum, colon, and small intestine. Oviposition probably begins in the urinary bladder and then spreads centrifugally (Smith et al, 1975; Smith and Christie, 1986; Christie et al, 1986b, 1986c).

Within the lower urinary tract, three patterns of egg accumulation have been observed: apicocentric, basocentric, and combined. In the *apicocentric* pattern, oviposition begins and persists at the dome of the urinary bladder, spreading downward along the posterolateral walls, so that ureters and seminal vesicles are involved late or with heavy infections. In the *basocentric* pattern, oviposition begins in the basal regions (trigone and lower posterior wall of the urinary bladder and seminal vesicles), spreading centrifugally upward; seminal vesicles and interstitial ureters are involved early and with lower intensity infections. In the *combined* pattern, egg accumulation is randomly dispersed between apex and base; ureteral and bladder egg burdens become very high (Christie et al, 1986a, 1986b, 1986c). We presume that the differing patterns reflect obscure variations in perivesical venous plexus anatomy and/or adult worm behavior.

General Clinical Manifestations

Schistosomiasis haematobia progresses through five clinical stages: (1) "swimmer's itch" (schistosomal dermatitis), which relates to cercarial penetration; (2) acute schistosomiasis (also known as "Katayama fever"), which relates to the onset of oviposition; (3) early "active" urinary schistosomiasis, which relates to peak oviposition; (4) chronic active urinary schistosomiasis, which correlates with development of immunity to reinfection and/or attrition of worms; and (5) chronic inactive urinary schistosomiasis, in which infection no longer persists, but pathophysiologic aberrations slowly evolve into potentially lethal sequelae and complications.

SWIMMER'S ITCH. Swimmer's itch is a pruritic, macular (or, in rare instances, maculopapular) rash at the site of cercarial penetration. It occurs 3 to 18 hours after exposure to cercaria-infested fresh water and lasts a few hours to several days. Most endemic patients rarely give a history of swimmer's itch, but in one study, such a history predicted heavy infections as reliably as gross hematuria (Browning et al, 1984). Initially infected adults often suffer intensely pruritic rashes. This syndrome rarely leads to urologic consultation.

ACUTE SCHISTOSOMIASIS. Acute schistosomiasis is rarely found among endemic populations, but the first and presumably heavy exposure of a noninfected traveler may incur fever, lymphadenopathy, splenomegaly, eosinophilia, urticaria, and other manifestations of a serum sickness–like disease (Diaz Rivera et al, 1956; Warren, 1973a; Hiatt et al, 1979). Acute schistosomiasis generally occurs 3 to 9 weeks after infection, coinciding with the onset of egg laying and often preceding the occurrence of eggs in the urine, but it may be delayed for more than 4 months (Young et al, 1986). During initial migration and maturation, the host generates profound antibody responses to schistosomular antigens that cross-react with egg antigens. When oviposition begins, rapidly produced eggs "leak" antigens, which generates circulating antigen-antibody-complement complexes with preformed antibodies, mediating the Katayama fever. This syndrome may be fulminant in *S. japonicum* infection, probably as a result of *S. japonica*'s prodigious fecundity; it is rarely life-threatening in schistosomiasis haematobia.

Acute schistosomiasis often coincides with ectopic oviposition as worms meander toward the pelvic venous plexuses and become delayed or lost. Ectopic oviposition incites granulomas in such aberrant sites as thoracic, scrotal, or penile skin (Edington et al, 1975; El-Mofty and Nada, 1975; Obasi, 1986; Develoux et al, 1987), epididymis (Elem et al, 1989), or spinal cord and/or nerve roots, *before* eggs are discernible in urine or feces; such lesions can be diagnosed only as a result of a high index of suspicion and a congruous travel history; they are often espied only upon biopsy.

"ACTIVE" SCHISTOSOMIASIS. The infection enters the patent "active" stage, in which eggs are deposited in tissues, traverse the bladder or rectosigmoid mucosa, and are excreted in the urine (and less regularly in the feces). This prepatent period is usually 2 to 3 months but may last over 7 months (Young et al, 1986). The classic clinical presentation of "active" bilharziasis, *hematuria and terminal dysuria*, has been recognized for over 3000 years. In endemic foci, "active" disease usually arises in children or adolescents (Forsythe, 1969; Browning et al, 1984) by inconsequential hematuria and mild terminal dysuria. Dysuria may be minimal owing to light infection or patient stoicism; it is often prominent in patients from comfortably developed

Western countries. Dysuria may, in part, be due to coinfecting *Chlamydia trachomatis,* which has been reported in more than 40% of cases (Haberberger et al, 1993). Hematuria, pyuria, and proteinuria vary with the intensity of infection and may be used to measure infection intensity (see section on diagnosis). Hematuria may be sufficient to cause blood loss anemia (Wilkins et al, 1985b). Both serum alkaline and prostatic fraction of acid phosphatase may be elevated during active schistosomiasis in children (Kassim, 1988). Growth retardation, anemia, and impaired physical and academic performance have been documented; these rapidly reverse after successful treatment (Stephenson et al, 1985, 1989; Kvalsvig, 1986; Ndamba, 1986; Latham et al, 1990; Befidi-Mengue et al, 1992; Kimura et al, 1992; Prual et al, 1992; Ekanem et al, 1994). Yet in endemic regions, most patients sustain even complicated "active" urinary schistosomiasis without complaint and without seeking available medical attention. In highly endemic areas, nearly all youngsters eventually suffer dysuria and hematuria, and this becomes absorbed into a background of ills and hardships; indeed, hematuria in males may be seen as a sign of puberty.

After some years, active infection enters a more quiescent period (the **chronic active stage**), in which egg deposition and excretion continue at a lower magnitude and symptoms are less noticeable. Over 30% of light infections resolve spontaneously in some endemic areas (Rutasitara and Chimbe, 1985). However, although clinical disease is inapparent, silent obstructive uropathy develops throughout this phase, as sandy patches and fibrosis replace polypoid patches and the bladder and ureters undergo irreversible damage (vide infra). The slow, insidious evolution enables development of enormous hydroureters and hydronephroses with mild or no intervening symptoms, nonconcordant with the severity of damage. In heavily endemic areas, nonfunctioning kidneys are commonly found in apparently well patients who deny past renal colic. However, infected people from nonendemic regions usually have flank and loin pain commensurate with the obstructive uropathy. Among patients from endemic regions presenting for urologic intervention, 85% have recurrent renal colic, more than 80% have a history of recent and/or remote urinary schistosomiasis, 60% have dysuria, over 25% have had previous urologic surgery for schistosomal lesions, and gross hematuria and gross pyuria are present in 30% each; thus patients presenting to a urologist are usually symptomatic.

Chronic and/or recurrent urinary tract infections by *Salmonella* species, including *Salmonella typhi* and *S. paratyphi* (associated with intermittent bacteremic or septicemic episodes) are another infectious complication observed in patients with *active* urinary schistosomiasis. *Salmonella* bacilli rest in the apical invaginations of the schistosome tegument, where they are protected from immune injury and from administered antibiotics. They emerge from this sanctuary when conditions are favorable for their proliferation and consequently recolonize both the urine and blood (Farid et al, 1972; Young et al, 1973; Higashi et al, 1975; Bassily et al, 1976; Lambertucci et al, 1988). Patients with schistosomiasis and concomitant chronic salmonellosis appear seriously ill, suffer from profound weakness, and usually have intermittent fever, refractory anemia, and splenomegaly. Nephrotic syndrome, caused by immune-complex deposition in the renal glomerulus, may result from hypocomplementary mesangiocapillary, membranocapillary, or diffuse endocapillary proliferative glomerulonephritis (Farid et al, 1972; Higashi et al, 1975; Bassily et al, 1976; Lambertucci et al, 1988). These conditions often respond to antischistosomal drug treatment alone or in combination with antibiotics but not to antibiotic therapy alone.

CHRONIC INACTIVE SCHISTOSOMIASIS. As patients enter the *chronic inactive* phase, in which *viable* eggs are no longer detected in urine or tissues, most of the signs and symptoms are caused by sequelae and complications (see later discussion), rather than by the schistosomal infection itself. *Of patients with schistosomal obstructive uropathy (SOU), 40% to 60% present to urologists during the inactive stage of their disease* (Smith and Christie, 1986). During the inactive stage, SOU may worsen because contracting fibrous tissue tightens ureteral stenoses and increases ureteral atonicity with decreasing peristalsis. In one third to half of these patients, chronic or acute bacterial urinary tract infection (often including pyelonephritis) becomes superimposed upon their SOU.

Bacterial urinary tract infections associated with SOU are usually ascending infections predisposed by urinary stasis. They are usually caused by the same organisms, coliform bacteria, that cause ascending infections in patients without schistosomiasis. Lehman et al (1973) emphasized the marked vulnerability of schistosomiasis-damaged urinary tracts to iatrogenic infections, especially *Klebsiella* and *Pseudomonas* infections, related to cystoscopy or catheterization in patients in endemic regions. Clearly, such instrumentation in these patients must be hazarded only with stringent asepsis.

The clinical manifestations of urothelial malignancy in patients with urinary schistosomiasis are similar to those described in Section X, Chapter 77 (Urothelial Tumors of the Urinary Tract). Unique features of the bilharzial bladder cancer syndrome are noted in this chapter in the section Systematic Review of Primary Lesions, Sequelae, and Complications in Humans.

Diagnosis

Diagnostic objectives can be divided into four categories: diagnosing current or past infection with *S. haematobium* (and *S. mansoni*); determining the stage of infection (active or inactive); determining infection intensity; and evaluating the severity of sequelae and the presence of complications.

DIAGNOSIS OF INFECTION AND DETERMINATION OF ACTIVITY. The presence of terminally spined eggs in urinary sediment is diagnostic of active *S. haematobium* infection. In moderate to heavy infections, eggs are almost always present in a routine test of urinary sediment. In lighter infections, routine urinalysis does not always reveal eggs, and the measurement of sedimentation or filtration of larger volumes of urine, up to three consecutive 24-hour collections, is necessary. Because egg excretion follows a diurnal periodicity, with maximal egg excretion occurring between 10 A.M. and 2 P.M., a mid-day urine sample is most likely to contain eggs (Stimmel and Scott, 1956). Excretion of *viable* eggs of *S. haematobium* in the urine also indicates current activity of the infection, which necessitates schistosomacidal chemotherapy.

Eggs may be seen in rectal or bladder mucosal biopsy

specimens. If eggs are not found in several urine specimens, rectal biopsy should be attempted before bladder biopsy, because eggs are nearly as common in the rectum and the hazard of urinary tract infection is avoided. A squash preparation of the biopsy specimen between glass slides is preferable to histopathologic analysis, because its sensitivity is greater and it may permit a determination of egg viability. In many cases, urinary schistosomiasis is not suspected until histologic diagnosis is reported. The schistosome species may be confirmed by a Ziehl-Neelsen stain of the section (vide supra) or by quantitative examination of the sediment after digestion of a weighed aliquot of formalin-fixed (or fresh) tissue in a 4% potassium hydroxide solution (1 part tissue/10 parts solution) for 18 hours at 56°C. (Cheever, 1968). The latter procedure also quantitates the tissue egg burden.

Serologic and molecular biologic techniques have also been used in diagnosis of schistosomiasis. Many tests employed in the past (Kagan, 1974) have been replaced by the enzyme-linked immunosorbent assay (ELISA) techniques, but none provides more applicable information than the circumoval precipitation test, which uses *S. haematobium* eggs collected from patients' urine (Hillyer et al, 1981). However, preformed in vivo circumoval precipitates must be removed before their use (Koech et al, 1984). Eosinophiluria and serologic detection of urinary or serum eosinophilic proteins have been used to diagnose and estimate intensity of infection in endemic areas of *S. haematobium* infection (Eltoum et al, 1993; Reimert et al, 1993; Vennervald et al, 1994).

Development of schistosomal cDNA libraries may provide better antigens for serologic detection of "active" infection (Knight et al, 1986). Serologic tests performed with egg-derived antigens have shown high sensitivity-specificity for detecting *S. mansoni* infection (Janitschke et al, 1987), but most antigens produced do not differentiate between *S. haematobium* and *S. mansoni* (Idris and Ruppel, 1988, 1991). Serologic testing of urine confirms infection but, again, does not differentiate between schistosomes (Ripert et al, 1988). Specific *S. haematobium* egg antigens have been isolated and characterized (Hamburger et al, 1982; Hillyer and Pacheco, 1986; Sathe et al, 1991), but past serologic tests did not differentiate active and inactive disease. An *S. haematobium* species-specific serine protease inhibitor (Serpin) and its antibodies have been used for detection of active schistosomiasis haematobium, using both patient serum and patient urine, but is yet to be used in the field (Blanton et al, 1994; Li et al, 1995). Detection of antigenemia or antigenuria by using circulating anodic antigen (CAA) and/or circulating cathodic antigen (CCA) *diagnoses* active disease and *quantitates infection intensity* (Simpson and Smithers, 1985; Feldmeier et al, 1986; Maddison, 1987; de Jonge et al, 1990; van Lieshout et al, 1991; Barsoum et al, 1991; van Lieshout et al, 1992; Kremsner et al, 1994; van Lieshout et al, 1994); however, these reagents are not easily available commercially and they do not differentiate between *S. mansoni* and *S. haematobium*. **Immunologic testing is becoming the clinical diagnostic and epidemiologic tool of the day, but finding eggs remains the bedrock of diagnosis (Mott and Dixon, 1982), except in chronic inactive urinary schistosomiasis, in which egg excretion is uncommon and serologic, radiographic, and cystoscopic diagnoses are all superior (Patil et al, 1992).**

DETERMINATION OF INTENSITY OF INFECTION. The eggs of *S. haematobium* are easily counted by filtering urine through filter paper and staining the eggs with triketohydrindene hydrate (Ninhydrin) under controlled heat and humidity. The purple-stained eggs are then counted under low magnification, and the number of eggs per volume of urine or per 24 hours are calculated (Bell, 1963). Alternative methods, suitable for epidemiologic studies and clinical evaluation, are nucleopore filtration (Peters et al, 1976a, 1976b) or nylon mesh filtration (Mott, 1983), but neither filter is reusable (Klumpp and Southgate, 1986). Great care must be exercised in handling and transporting dried filters before examination (Rohde et al, 1985; Braun-Munzinger and Rohde, 1986). Substitution of Ninhydrin staining with in vivo trypan blue combines quantitation with viability testing (Feldmeier et al, 1979). The latter technique may be supplanted by using Nytrel filters with mercurochrome or iodine (Braun-Munzinger and Southgate, 1993a, 1993b, 1993c). Day-to-day egg excretion for individuals varies considerably, but it remains high in patients with heavy egg excretion and low in patients with light egg excretion (Warren et al, 1978) and may be used confidently to estimate intensity of infection in epidemiologic and individual patient care scenarios (Braun-Munzinger and Southgate, 1992). As noted before, *S. haematobium* egg excretion peaks between 10 A.M. and 2 P.M.; this circadian phenomenon reverses in night-shift workers without any variation induced by athletic activity or water loading (McMahon, 1976). Enumeration of eggs in a 24-hour urine sample is the least variable method for estimating *S. haematobium* infection intensity; however, these collections are often virtually impossible in endemic areas and in children, and so nucleopore or nylon mesh filtration of 10 ml of mid-day urine has become the standard technique for epidemiologic and clinical assessment. Findings of 1 to 100, 101 to 250 (or 350), and over 250 (or 350) eggs per 10 ml of mid-day urine correspond to light, moderate, and severe infections, respectively (Abdel-Salam and Ehsan, 1978). The number of eggs per 10 ml of urine has the best sensitivity and specificity of all estimates of intensity of current infection (Wilkins et al, 1979; Stephenson et al, 1984; Wilkins, 1986; Gigase et al, 1988).

Urinary protein excretion parallels egg excretion and peaks at noon; erythrocyte excretion is delayed about 6 hours, and white blood cell excretion is bimodal at noon and 6:00 P.M. (Doehring et al, 1985c). Screening infected young people in an endemic setting is easily done by dipstick method for detecting blood in the urine (Pugh et al, 1980). Whereas afternoon gross terminal hematuria (as an index of urinary schistosomiasis) has only 73% sensitivity but 97% specificity in endemic areas (Sarda et al, 1986), dipstick testing for hematuria has excellent sensitivity, approaching that for egg excretion (Wilkins et al, 1979; Stephenson et al, 1984; Sarda et al, 1985, 1986; Murare and Taylor, 1987; Coopan et al, 1987b; Gigase et al, 1988; Ngandu, 1988; Savioli et al, 1990; Taylor et al, 1990; Kiliku et al, 1991; Kaiser et al, 1992; Eltoum et al, 1992; Jemaneh et al, 1994; Robert et al, 1995). Dipstick testing for proteinuria has high sensitivity in some areas (Wilkins et al, 1979; Stephenson et al, 1984; Doehring et al, 1986b; Murare and Taylor, 1987; Savioli et al, 1990; Taylor et al, 1990; Kiliku et al, 1991;

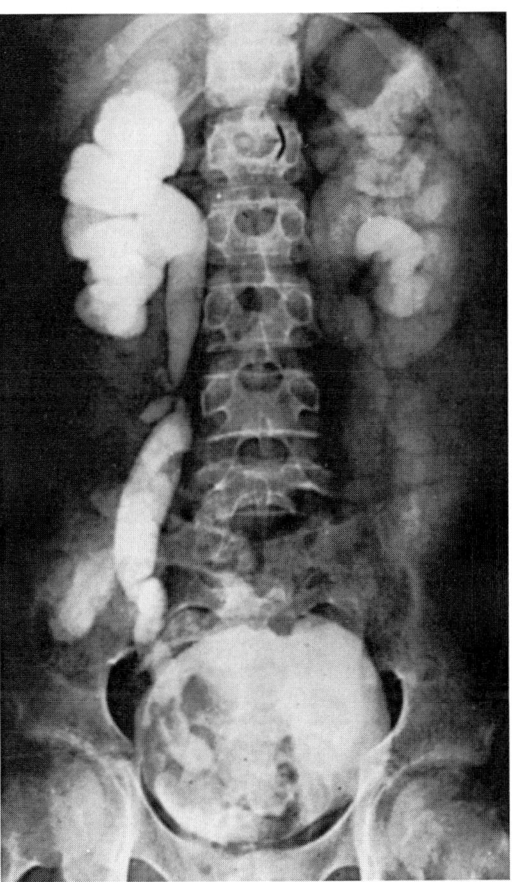

Figure 22–10. Intravenous urogram in a 15-year-old Egyptian boy with *Schistosoma haematobium* infection. Note the massive space-occupying lesion in the bladder and similar lesions in the right lower ureter.

Kaiser et al, 1992; Eltoum et al, 1992; Jemaneh et al, 1994; Robert et al, 1995), and noon urine samples with >1.0 g of protein usually have schistosomal obstructive uropathy (Doehring et al, 1985a) but lower proteinuria adds little more information than dipstick hematuria (Gigase et al, 1988). Proteinuria involves all classes of serum proteins as expected in bleeding into a lumen, as opposed to selective albuminuria seen in renogenic nephrotic syndromes, but rarely is enough to produce hypoalbuminemia and anasarca. Indeed, in endemic areas, all patients with more than 200 eggs per 10 ml of urine or a proteinuria count of more than 30 mg/dl should be treated promptly (Wilkins et al, 1979).

Urinary egg excretion measurement accurately estimates infection intensity during the early active and early chronic active stages but is imprecise in late chronic active and inactive cases (see section on pathology). Thus in older infections, patients with severe sequelae can excrete no eggs on multiple examinations when there are 10^6 eggs per gram of tissue (Smith et al, 1974b). Radiographic findings are better indices of severity than urinary egg counts in older age groups (Lehman et al, 1973).

DIAGNOSIS OF SEQUELAE AND COMPLICATIONS OF URINARY SCHISTOSOMIASIS. Radiography is *the* important diagnostic tool in evaluation of sequelae and complications. Urinary tract alterations resulting from schistosomiasis are not subtle and may be interpreted with ease by an alert physician. A plain x-ray film of the abdomen may reveal calcification within the urinary tract. The classic presentation of a calcified bladder, which looks like a fetal head in the pelvis, is pathognomonic of chronic urinary schistosomiasis (Fig. 22–10). The seminal vesicles, prostate, posterior urethra, distal ureters, and, in rare instances, the colon may also be calcified. The earliest radiographic changes appear to be striations in the ureters and renal pelvis (Hugosson, 1987), followed by linear calcifications in the ureters and bladder along with ureteral irregularities (Hugosson and Olsen, 1986).

Intravenous urography (von Lichtenberg and Swick, 1929), although not available in most endemic areas, should be included in the examination of individual office patients suspected of *S. haematobium* infection. Hydroureter, hydronephrosis, nonfunctioning kidney, ureteral stenosis, and bladder and ureteral filling defects such as polypoid lesions are readily observed in a standard urogram (Figs. 22–11, 22–12, and 22–13). In the presence of severe obstructive uropathy, delayed films are often needed to discern distended ureters and kidneys. If no visualization is attained, an infusion urogram can be done on a subsequent day. Postvoiding films may indicate bladder neck obstruction with retention. Fluoroscopy can differentiate tonic and atonic ureters (Husain et al, 1980; Abdel-Halim et al, 1985) and identify nonstenotic, immotile ureters (Umerah, 1981). The use of the cystourethrogram indicates the presence of vesicoureteric reflux, which occurs in 25% of infected ureters (Hanafy et al, 1975). Further details on the radiography of urinary schistosomiasis were given by Reeder and Palmer (1981).

Abdominal *ultrasonography* is a highly useful, cost-effective, and technically feasible method for detection of

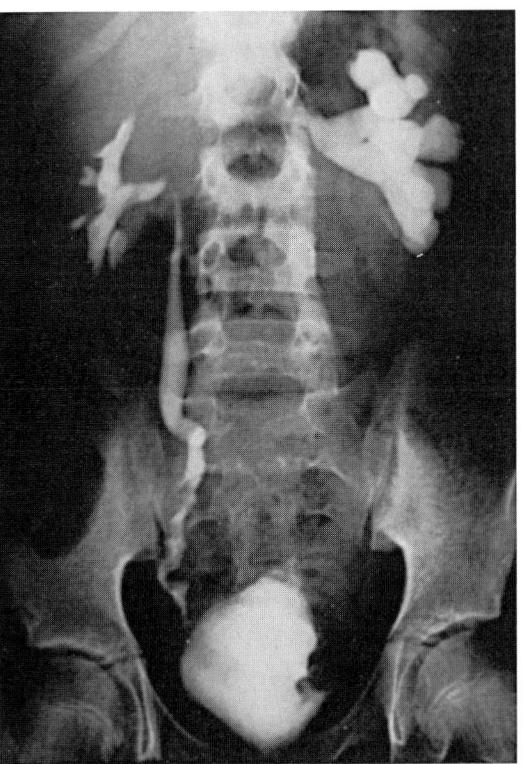

Figure 22–11. Intravenous urogram in another Egyptian boy, showing scalloping of the bladder and right lower ureter by schistosomal polypoid lesions.

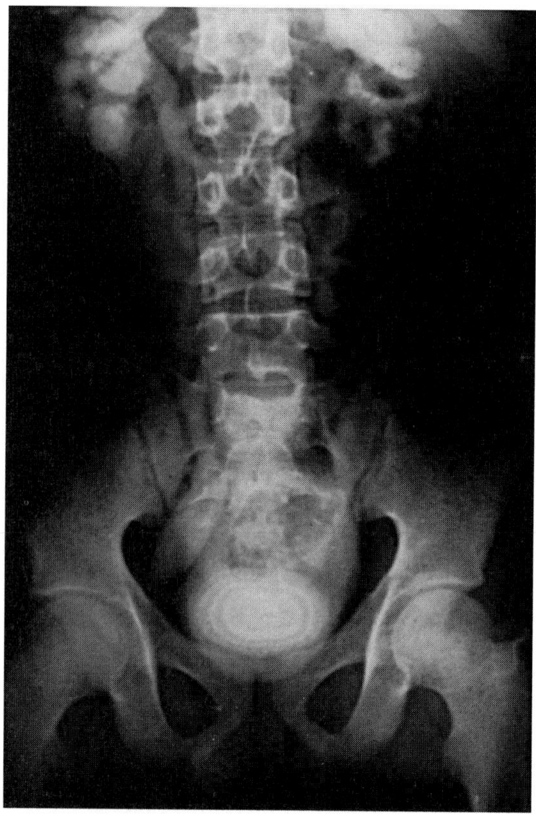

Figure 22–12. Intravenous pyelogram at $2\frac{1}{2}$ hours in a 23-year-old Egyptian farmer who was shedding numerous viable eggs of *Schistosoma haematobium* in the urine. Note hydronephrosis, poor excretory function, and unusually large, laminated bladder calculus. (Courtesy of Dr. Stuart Young, United States Naval Medical Research Unit No. 3, Cairo.)

focal thickening of the bladder wall and large polypoid lesions of the urinary tract (see Fig. 22–13), hydroureter, and hydronephrosis in endemic areas, and it detects heavily calcific sandy patches (Fig. 22–14) but does not show more lightly calcified sandy patches (Degremont et al, 1985; Doehring et al, 1985a; Burki et al, 1986; Dittrich and Doehring, 1986; Heurtier et al, 1986; Devidas et al, 1988; King et al, 1988a; Lamothe et al, 1988; Hatz et al, 1990a, 1990b, 1992; Laurent et al, 1990; Abdel-Wahab et al, 1992a, 1992b, 1993; Nafeh et al, 1992; Abdel-Wahab and Strickland, 1993; Strickland and Abdel-Wahab, 1993; Kardorff et al, 1994). Computed tomographic (CT) scans detect both obstructive uropathy and calcific lesions *in the urinary tract and the colon* (Aisen et al, 1983; Lautin et al, 1983; Jorulf and Linstedt, 1985; Schwarzbach and Genseke, 1987; al-Hindawi et al, 1990), and thus complement or substitute for intravenous pyelography.

In the past, cystoscopy was widely used in patients with urinary schistosomiasis (Makar, 1955). Many lesions are visually characteristic, and biopsy may be done simultaneously, but instrumentation of the urinary tract in schistosomiasis hazards serious and resistant urinary tract infections.

Renography by radioisotopic techniques has been used, particularly to evaluate treatment response, but this is an experimental rather than a diagnostic tool (Zahran, and Badr, 1980; Pawar and Abdel-Dayem, 1984; Geneseke et al, 1985; Bahar et al, 1988).

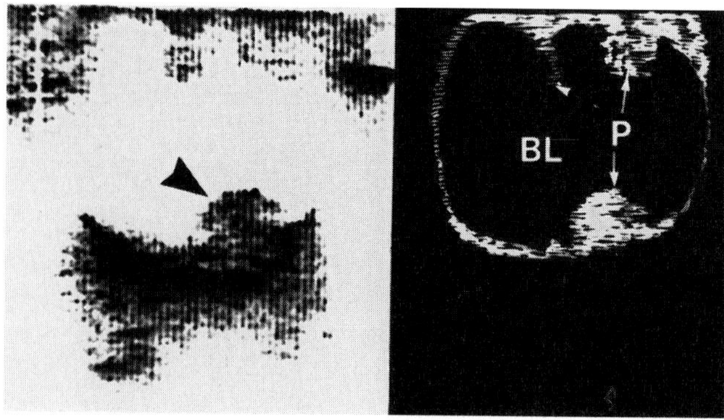

Figure 22–13. Ultrasonogram (*left*) of urinary bladder (BL) with schistosomal polyps (P and *arrows*) in a 13-year-old Egyptian schoolboy. (Courtesy of G. Thomas Strickland, M.D. From Strickland GT, Abdel-Wahab MF: Trans R Soc Trop Med Hyg 1993; 87:132.)

Pyelonephritis complicating urinary schistosomiasis is diagnosed with the same laboratory methods and criteria as in patients without urinary schistosomiasis. Microscopic pyuria is usually noted on urinalysis of patients with urinary schistosomiasis and does not necessarily imply concomitant bacterial urinary tract infection. Differential counts of urinary leukocytes show a preponderance of eosinophils and no peripheral blood neutrophilia in pure urinary schistosomiasis,

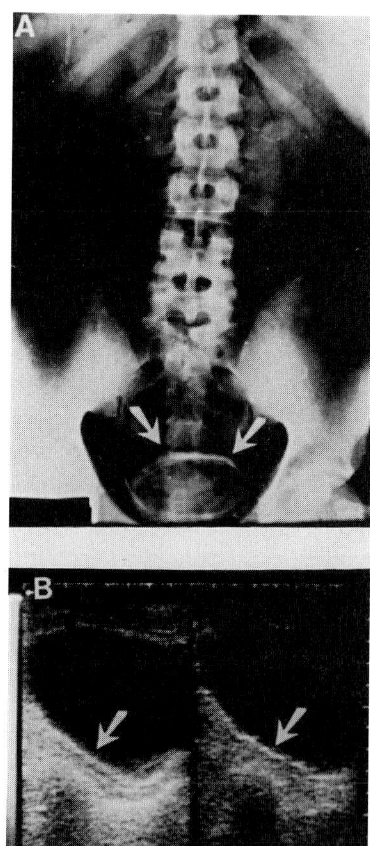

Figure 22–14. Bladder calcification in 30-year-old Egyptian farmer. *A,* Plain x-ray film of abdomen shows rim of calcification surrounding urinary bladder (*arrows*). *B,* Abdominal ultrasound shows bright line surrounding bladder with definite dark rim behind it (*arrows*). (Courtesy of G. Thomas Strickland, M.D. Abdel-Wahab MF, Ramzy I, Esmat G, et al: J Urol 1992; 148:346.)

whereas there is a preponderance of urinary neutrophils and peripheral blood neutrophilia with bacterial superinfection (Bhatt et al, 1984).

Treatment

Medical Management

Development of safe and effective antischistosomal drugs has simplified both the treatment and decision to treat schistosome infection. There is no valid reason to withhold medical treatment from persons with light or advanced infections, assuming that the indications and safeguards prescribed for the drugs are observed. Treatment should not be given without first defining the activity, sequelae, and complications present in the patient or without follow-up to assess response, to detect residual iatrogenic chronic inactive disease requiring surgical correction, and to teach patients to avoid re-exposure (Davis, 1982).

Of the schistosomes pathogenic for humans, *S. haematobium* is the most amenable to schistosomacidal chemotherapy. It responds well to metrifonate (Bilharcil), to hycanthone mesylate (Etrenol), to praziquantel (Biltricide), to niridazole (Ambilhar), and to oltipraz (Cook, 1982; Davis, 1982; Moczon and Swiderski, 1992). There is no need to use the toxic antimonial compounds. Treatment aims to reduce worm burden, even if not achieving total parasitologic cure. In endemic areas, there may be a rationale for leaving a few persisting worms, if concomitant immunity plays a role in resistance to reinfection. Schistosomacidal treatment should begin as early as possible, because lesion reversibility declines with progressive stages (von Lichtenberg, 1975). Both experimental and clinical data indicate that treatment during acute schistosomiasis (as in visitors to endemic areas) and in children during the early active stage prevents irreversible pathologic effects. Before sequelae of late infection are surgically treated, continued activity must be interdicted by schistosomacidal medication. More recent studies in endemic areas have explored the efficacy of certain "native" medicaments and their derivatives (Ndamba et al, 1994). Both the two principally used chemotherapeutic agents, metrifonate and praziquantel, are highly effective, and there seem to be little differences in efficacy in large-scale control programs (King et al, 1990).

METRIFONATE. This organophosphate compound is the drug of choice for *S. haematobium* infection in its endemic setting (Siongok et al, 1978; Feldmeier et al, 1982). When given by mouth, as 100-mg tablets, it slowly metabolizes to the anticholinesterase compound dichlorvos. Its presumed mode of action is to block the worm's cholinesterase, thereby paralyzing it. This action kills both *S. mansoni* and *S. haematobium* in the vesicle venous plexus, but neither organism is eliminated from the mesenteric plexus (Doehring et al, 1986c). At the same time, the patient's own plasma cholinesterase and erythrocyte cholinesterase levels are lowered, but they return to normal without clinical toxicity. Studies indicate that sensitivity of schistosome species is directly related to the acetylcholinesterase activity on its surfaces (Camacho et al, 1994). Only rarely have nausea, vomiting, and bronchospasm been reported as side effects. The recommended dose is 7.5 to 10 mg/kg body weight, given in three oral doses at intervals of 14 days (Webbe, 1987; Gilles, 1988). Similar results have been reported with 5 mg/kg body weight, given three times in 1 day (Aden-Abdi et al, 1987). Cure rates have generally been between 70% to 80%, and no major adverse reactions have been observed among the thousands of individuals treated (Feldmeier and Doehring, 1987). The only known contraindications concern pregnant patients and agricultural workers exposed to organophosphate insecticides (Webbe, 1987). Relapses are uncommon. There seems to be no obstacle to extending treatment to four or more doses, if advisable. Should overdose occur and cholinergic symptoms arise, atropine can be administered. Metrifonate has been used in large-scale antischistosomal chemotherapy in several control projects. It is safe and effective against *S. haematobium* infection but not against *S. mansoni* or *S. japonicum*. Its sole disadvantage is the need for multiple successive doses, which increases the risk of noncompliance (Aden-Abdi and Gustafsson, 1989) and limits applicability among people living nomadically or in poorly accessible places.

PRAZIQUANTEL. Praziquantel is the preferred drug in office practice. It interferes with the ion transport mechanism of the schistosome tegument, resulting in rapid fluxes of Ca^+ and Na^+ into the worms and sudden contraction of the parasite's musculature. Cure rates for *S. haematobium* infection are 83% to 100%; this is the drug of choice in combined *S. mansoni* and *S. haematobium* infections (Bassily et al, 1985; Mott et al, 1985). Animal toxicity studies have shown tolerance for well over 20 times the therapeutic level of the drug, and results of mutagenicity testing in various systems have been negative. Pharmacokinetics of the drug are similar in schistosome-infected and -noninfected people (Ofori-Adjei et al, 1988). In human trials, the drug has been nearly free of toxic side effects, and complaints have been limited to epigastric pain, abdominal discomfort, nausea, anorexia, diarrhea, dizziness, headache, and occasionally pruritus or urticariform eruptions and fever; these mild symptoms have lasted for less than 24 hours and may have been related to the death of worms. A *single* oral dose of 40 mg/kg is the recommended procedure for *S. haematobium* (McMahon and Kolstrup, 1979; Pugh and Teesdale, 1983, 1984; Webbe, 1987; Gilles, 1988); a dosage of 20 mg/kg is effective in reducing the intensity of *S. haematobium* infection (and 30 mg/kg for *S. mansoni*) but does not achieve cure (Taylor et al, 1988; King et al, 1989). The only contraindication known is pregnancy (Webbe, 1987). Higher or multiple doses may be required for *S. mansoni* or *S. japonicum*. Praziquantel is available in tablets of 600 mg for oral administration. Praziquantel and metrifonate have been licensed by the U.S. Food and Drug Administration. The Parasitic Disease Division (vide supra) can be consulted for use of these drugs.

It is clear that low-level infections are well tolerated by many persons and do not invariably produce symptomatic or silent obstructive uropathy. However, because a single space-occupying lesion in the ureter may obstruct urine flow and because of the hazard of serious ectopic lesions, evaluation of patients with continued active *S. haematobium* infection after treatment is advised. **Follow-up should be performed at 3-month intervals for at least 1 year to assess cure or reduction in egg excretion. Retreatment may be necessary.**

Surgical Management

The large number of different surgical procedures, employed in the treatment of various complications of urinary schistosomiasis, is enumerated in the section Systematic Review of the Primary Lesions, Sequelae, and Complications in Humans. In general, surgery is reserved for complications that have not responded to adequate medical treatment within a reasonable follow-up time (e.g., SOU) or for those mandating immediate intervention (e.g., hematocystis).

Although renal transplantation is not contraindicated in patients with urinary schistosomiasis (Weeden et al, 1982), its concomitant immunosuppression must be undertaken with reticence in patients returning to undersanitated regions, where there is great hazard of overwhelming infections (Smith and Christie, 1986). Patients with urinary schistosomiasis may serve as either transplant donors or recipients, provided that successful chemotherapy of active disease be achieved 2 months before receipt or donation; if not, the ureter may break down with new oviposition at the anastomotic site (Weeden et al, 1982; Hefty and McCorkell, 1986; Shokeir et al, 1992).

Prognosis

Considering the tens of millions of people affected with *S. haematobium*, many of whom have mild infections, the prognosis is generally good (Warren, 1973b). However, the morbidity and mortality of schistosomiasis are determined by the overall intensity and risk of reinfection. No mortality was observed where the prevalence of schistosomiasis and frequency and severity of SOU was low, as in Ibadan, Nigeria (Edington et al, 1970), but in Egypt, in which prevalence was 50% to 60%, mortality approached 10% (Smith et al, 1974a; Cheever et al, 1978). Among patients with severe disease or nonfunctioning kidneys, mortality may reach 50% in 2 to 5 years (Forsythe, 1969; Lehman et al, 1970; Smith et al, 1974a, 1975; Wilkins et al, 1985a).

Patients who die directly from SOU (bilateral end-stage hydronephrosis with fatal uremia) are young (in their 20s), have early-stage disease, heavy but not astronomic total egg burdens, and have high egg burdens in the gut, especially the appendix. Patients who die of complications of schistosomiasis, or in whom sequelae and complications contribute to but do not cause death, and those with severe schistosomal disease who die of unrelated causes are older (35 to 40 years of age) and have infections of longer duration with spectacular egg burdens, apically or diffusely distributed. This suggests that heavy, short infections with rapidly accumulating basally distributed egg burdens sustain early and severe morbidity and mortality due to SOU, whereas heavier but more slowly accumulated egg burdens, apically and diffusely distributed, produce severe disease that leaves the patient vulnerable to development of such complications as pyelonephritis and urothelial cancer (Smith et al, 1975; Christie et al, 1986a, 1986b, 1986c; Smith and Christie, 1986).

The prognosis for persons with demonstrable urinary tract lesions has improved with the newer and better antischistosomal drugs. In children, the active infection and polypoid lesions are readily treatable; these polyps and consequent obstructive uropathy usually completely resolve within 2 to 6 weeks after antischistosomal treatment.

Visitors to endemic foci (businessmen, tourists, etc.) have usually had single or few exposures and have relatively early stages of schistosomiasis that are responsive to therapy, even when egg excretion is high. A variant of this presentation is the incompletely treated early infection without follow-up that returns with recurrent symptoms.

For patients with later chronic stages in which obstructive uropathy is due to sandy patches and fibrosis, the prognosis is less clear. Some individuals tolerate advanced obstructive uropathy with little, if any, deterioration in renal function. Bacterial superinfection is a menacing prognostic event and should be treated as vigorously and as soon as possible. Older patients with bilateral obstructive uropathy, a contracted bladder, and bacterial superinfection have dismal prognoses, as do patients with bilharzial bladder cancer.

Prevention and Control

Individuals who avoid contact with water inhabited by snails infected with *S. haematobium* effectively prevent this infection. Travelers in endemic areas should be advised of the hazard of infected streams, rivers, ponds, and lakes and should avoid bathing in or otherwise using such water. If contaminated water is inadvertently contacted, brisk toweling of the skin, dry or with alcohol, after exposure may prevent cercarial penetration. Boiling of water kills cercariae. At present, no prophylactic drug is available.

Measures of control in endemic areas have utilized several approaches: destruction of the snail host, elimination of urine and fecal contamination of water, and reduction of contact with infected water. Obviously, in many endemic areas, such measures are expensive, unfeasible, or poorly tolerated by the local population. Therefore, mass therapy by drugs has been emphasized, and currently all major control campaigns include drug treatment as a major component, often age-directed and/or annual (King et al, 1990, 1991, 1992). Favorable short-term results have been reported, but their long-term effects may not be known for some time, and patient noncompliance (Aden-Abdi and Gustafsson, 1989) and reinfection (Etard et al, 1990) have proved significant compromising factors. Research has led to safe and effective vaccines in the laboratory through use of recombinant antigens, but use in humans has so far failed to reduce infection or disease (World Health Organization, 1974; Sher et al, 1989), yet the most current works are more promising (Bergguist, 1990; Harrison et al, 1990).

Systematic Review of the Primary Lesions, Sequelae, and Complications of *Schistosoma haematobium* Infection in Humans

Urethra, Prostate, Seminal Vesicles, and Bladder Outlet Obstruction

Prostatic oviposition is low and not associated with significant prostatitis or hypertrophy. No evidence of bladder outlet obstruction was associated with light or heavy *S.*

haematobium infections in autopsy studies (Smith et al, 1974a; Cheever et al, 1977, 1978). However, clinical studies consistently report cystoscopic (Fam, 1964), urodynamic (Sabha and Nilsson, 1988), and isotope clearance abnormalities (Zahran and Badr, 1980; Bahar et al, 1988) and high residual urine (up to 200 ml), which are evidence of functional bladder outlet obstruction in patients with severe inactive urinary schistosomiasis (Young et al, 1974; Abdel-Halim, 1984; Aslamazov, 1988); even though these patients had no benign prostatic hypertrophy, partial transurethral prostatic resection reversed the dilatation, trabeculation, and post-trigonal pouch formation. Bladder neck obstruction has also been successfully treated by urethral dilatation or excision of the trigonal plate.

S. haematobium oviposition in seminal vesicles has long been recognized (Grace and Aidaros, 1952; Makar, 1955). Egg burdens of seminal vesicles and the ejaculatory ducts are high and correlate well with infection intensity (Smith et al, 1974a; Smith and Christie, 1986). Oviposition in these structures commonly results in asymptomatic hematospermia (Corachan et al, 1994; Obel and Black, 1994) and ovispermia but rarely, if ever, causes male infertility (Cheever et al, 1977, 1978). Schistosome eggs, blood, or both may appear in the ejaculate before they appear in the urine, but eggs are rarely seen in prepubertal seminal vesicles. Egg accumulation in the seminal vesicles probably starts later than in the lower urinary tract, but, once started, it proceeds more rapidly, so that seminal vesicle egg burdens equal those of the lower ureters, at 20,000 to 30,000 eggs per gram of tissue (in both organs); above this level, the probability of ureteral obstruction increases markedly (Smith et al, 1975; Christie et al, 1986b, 1986c). Egg burdens in the seminal vesicles correlate well with their weight and volume, so seminal vesicle hypertrophy (which can be estimated by rectal examination) may be useful for screening adult males from endemic areas for SOU (Christie et al, 1986b, 1986c).

Other Male and Female Genital Organs

Surgically removed epididymis, ovaries, and fallopian tubes sometimes have high egg burdens (Gelfand et al, 1970, 1971; Edington et al, 1975; Wright et al, 1982), but their mean egg burdens in autopsy series are unimpressive (Smith et al, 1974a; Cheever et al, 1977, 1978; Smith and Christie, 1986); this indicates that these cases represent aberrant, ectopic, or atypically distributed oviposition rather than severe generalized schistosomiasis. Egg burdens of the uterus, vagina, and testes are even lower than those of epididymis, ovaries, and fallopian tubes (Cheever et al, 1977, 1978). Schistosomal involvement of the scrotal or penile skin has been noted previously. Schistosomal epididymitis commonly manifests as induration and enlargement with variable scrotal pain; surgery is often performed for suspicion of testicular tumor, and a bilharzioma is found (Elem et al, 1989).

Schistosomal cervicitis and vaginitis are often asymptomatic but may manifest similarly to other etiologies of cervicitis and vaginitis (Williams, 1967); routine Papanicolaou smear may reveal terminally spined eggs, biopsy may demonstrate non–acid-fast ova (Berry, 1966), or wet smear of cervical scrapings in 10% potassium hydroxide (KOH) may reveal *S. haematobium* eggs (Swart and van der Merwe, 1987). In heavy chronic schistosomal vaginitis (and, in rare instances, cervicitis) with sandy patches, the presenting complaint may be dyspareunia *of both partners*; however, it is rare, even in endemic regions, which is fortunate because no remedy is known. Schistosomal lesions of the vagina and cervix may predispose patients to acquisition of human immunodeficiency virus (HIV) infection and acquired immunodeficiency syndrome (AIDS), just as ulcerating sexually transmitted diseases (STDs) do (Feldmeier et al, 1994). Incomplete cervical stenosis resulting from fibrous and sandy patches may not become apparent until parturition, when cervical effacement without dilatation may necessitate cervicotomy or even cesarean section. More rarely, complete cervical stenosis results in retention of menses, necessitating cervicoplasty. At term in pregnancy, schistosome eggs have been found in the placenta and amniotic fluid (Sutherland et al, 1965), but there are no documented reports of fetal schistosomiasis. Maternal infection is associated with increased proportions of preterm deliveries and lower birth weights (Siegrist, and Siegrist-Obimpeh, 1992), and tubal schistosomiasis may be associated with increased incidence of tubal pregnancy (Okonofua et al, 1990; Ville et al, 1991). Ovarian egg deposition and granulomas have been associated with focal cortical stromal fibrosis, but when infertility is found in patients with schistosomiasis, other causes must first be ruled out (Williams, 1967).

Urinary Bladder

Schistosomal disease of the urinary bladder includes schistosomal polyposis (Fig. 22–15*A*), "contracted bladder" (Fig. 22–16), schistosomal ulceration (see Fig. 22–15*F*), urothelial hyperplasia (Figs. 22–17 and 22–18), metaplasia (Figs. 22–19, and 22–20; see also Fig. 22–15*D,F*), dysplasia, and the bilharzial bladder cancer syndrome (see Fig. 22–15*C*). The severity of schistosomal disease in the urinary bladder can be histologically graded (Table 22–2) (Edington et al, 1970), approximating tissue egg burden when tissue digestion is not available.

Schistosomal *polyposis* of the urinary bladder (see Fig. 22–15*A*) consists of multiple large, inflammatory polyps related to heavy localized egg burdens during the active stage of the disease (Smith et al, 1977d). Such polyps occasionally retain their polypoid nature into the inactive stage (Smith et al, 1974a, 1977d). They may obstruct urethral or ureteral orifices or bleed enough to produce large obstructive clots (hematocystis) and/or anemia. Polyps occurring near the bladder outlet may temporarily or completely obstruct bladder emptying, causing combinations of

Table 22–2. HISTOLOGIC GRADATION OF SCHISTOSOMAL URINARY BLADDER DISEASE

Grade	Criteria
1	Occasional eggs in lamina propria
2	Lamina propria filled with eggs, no involvement of detrusor muscle
3	Lamina propria filled with eggs, involvement of superficial third of detrusor muscle
4	Lamina propria filled with eggs, involvement of external two thirds of detrusor muscle

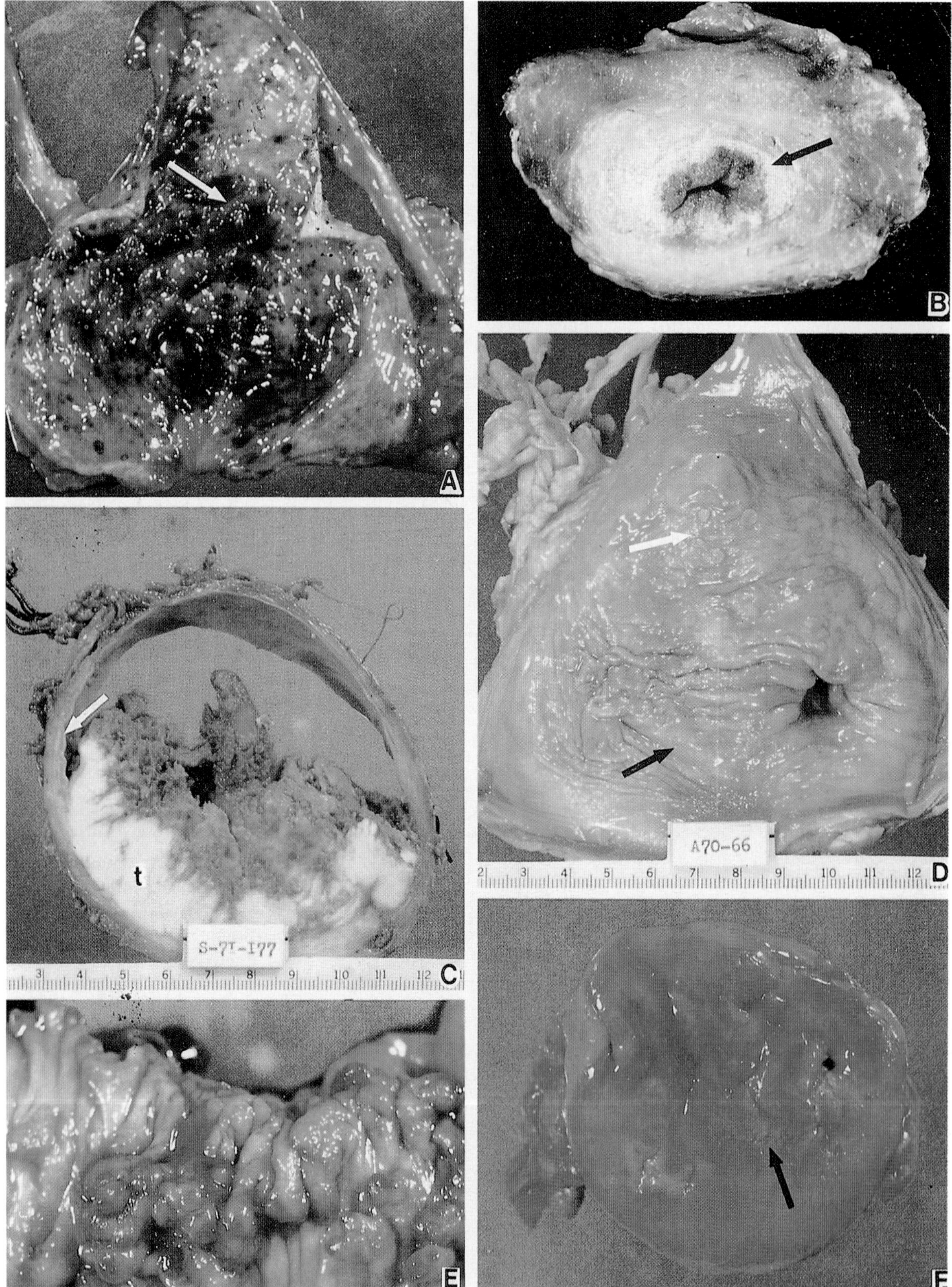

Figure 22–15 *See legend on opposite page*

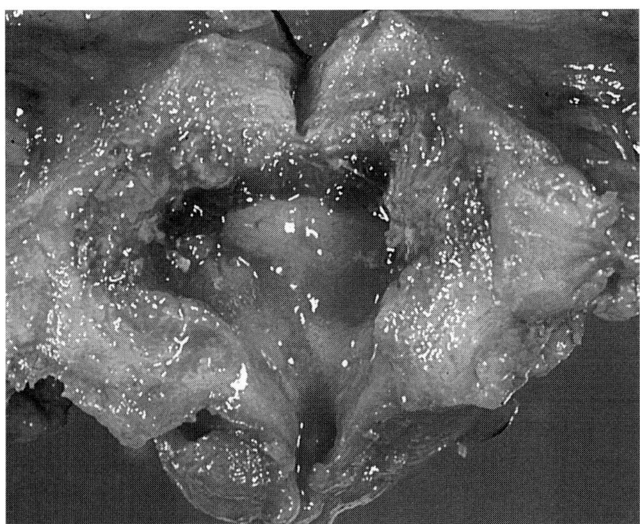

Figure 22–16. Urinary bladder opened with anterior Y-incision showing schistosomal contracted bladder. The prominent trigone is fibrotic. The detrusor muscle is thickened and fibrotic and contains sandy foci and active granulomas (i.e., chronic active disease). The vesical lumen is reduced to about 40 ml.

urinary retention and incontinence. Almost 60% of polypoid lesions of the urinary bladder in patients with schistosomiasis result from conditions other than schistosomiasis, such as polypoid cystitis (Smith et al, 1974a). Schistosomal polyposis of the lower urinary tract produces signs, symptoms, and laboratory findings of "active" urinary schistosomiasis and is treated chemotherapeutically, as noted previously. Obstructing polypoid lesions that are resistant to antischistosomal therapy may necessitate resection by either an open or a closed procedure.

The **schistosomal "contracted bladder"** syndrome occurs most frequently during the late chronic active stage, when egg burdens are highest. It manifests as constant, deep, hard, lower abdominal and pelvic pain; urgency; both diurnal and nocturnal frequency; and incontinence (Duvie, 1986). Oviposition is intense and involves the deepest levels of the detrusor muscle, but dense fibrous and sandy patches are also prominent. Whereas the trigone appears normal or minimally hyperemic and edematous, the detrusor muscle is indurated and thickened, as is the entire bladder wall, and the bladder lumen is reduced to as little as 50 ml of functional capacity (see Fig. 22–16). The chronically contracted bladder has been managed variously by vesical denervation, urinary shunting, cup-patch ileocystoplasty, and overdistention under anesthesia along with schistosomacidal chemotherapy.

Two types of schistosomal **bladder ulcers** occur (Smith et al, 1977a). Acute schistosomal ulceration may in rare instances present in the active stage, when a necrotic polyp sloughs into the urine. The more common chronic schistosomal ulceration (see Fig. 22–15*F*) is a sequela of heavy (greater than 250,000 eggs per gram of bladder tissue) infections, most commonly in the inactive (70%) or late chronic active (27.5%) stages. These lesions are associated with a constant "burning" micturition and deep, intense, and hard pelvic and suprapubic pain (often described as "burning" or "boring") radiating into the perineum or, if the trigone is involved, radiating into the glans penis. Patients often describe a perineal "heaviness" preceding the more intense lancinating pain. Over 90% of these patients have a history of previous urinary schistosomiasis, 20% have histories of previous sequelae and complications, and 10% have had previous surgical intervention for urinary schistosomiasis. Hematuria (gross hematuria in 35%) and pyuria (gross pyuria in 20%) are found in over half of patients.

Such ulcers begin at or near the posterior midsagittal line of the bladder, anywhere from the trigone to the anterior apex, but usually on the middle to upper posterior wall. They may extend vertically or horizontally or, in rare instances, both (the cruciate ulcer). Multiple midline lesions often coalesce. Beginning as superficial stellate (perpendicular crevasse-like) lesions of the mucosa, they later become deep, elongated ovoid ulcers. They are found mostly in young adult males (mean age, 29 years), which suggests that they result from rapidly accumulated egg burdens, but nothing else is known of their pathogenesis (Smith et al, 1977a).

Chronic deep bladder ulcers necessitate full-thickness excision (i.e., partial cystectomy); cauterization rarely produces either symptomatic relief or healing of the ulcer.

Urothelial hyperplasia (see Figs. 22–17 and 22–18) in humans is strongly associated with severe, but not mild, urinary schistosomiasis and is seen in all stages of the disease; however, it is even more strongly associated with bacterial urinary tract infection (Smith et al, 1974a). Urothelial metaplasia and dysplasia are strongly associated with severe *S. haematobium* infection, are more common in the inactive stages of the disease, and are more closely related to urinary schistosomiasis than to bacterial urinary tract infection (Smith et al, 1974a).

Figure 22–15. Macroscopic appearance of human urinary schistosomiasis. *A,* Urinary bladder opened with anterior Y-incision. The posterior and apical walls have many erythematous, granular, sessile, and pedunculated polyps (*arrow*), characteristic of the early active stage of urinary schistosomiasis. *B,* Coronal section through the apex of a formalin-fixed urinary bladder. The lamina propria has been expanded and is replaced by a yellow-tan, finely granular sandy patch (*arrow*), which is characteristic of chronic inactive foci. Small sandy patches are sprinkled through the fibrotic, atrophic detrusor muscle, and even in perivesical fat. The more superficial erythematous portion of the lamina propria contains some viable eggs with granulomatous response (chronic active stage of urinary schistosomiasis). *C,* Coronal section through the middle of a urinary bladder after formalin inflation and fixation. The lamina propria (*arrow*) has been replaced by a concentric sandy patch, most prominent at the margin of the exophytic, moderately differentiated squamous cell carcinoma. The bladder wall is attenuated except for the tumor. No evidence of recent oviposition was found in the lower urinary tract (chronic inactive stage of urinary schistosomiasis, usually found with the bilharzial bladder cancer syndrome). *D,* Urinary bladder opened with anterior Y-incision, showing several features of severe chronic inactive urinary schistosomiasis. The entire lamina propria has been replaced by a sandy patch. Foci of epidermidization are seen at or near the *white arrow.* The left ureteral orifice (right of field) is markedly dilated (the so-called golf-hole ureter of schistosomal uropathy). The right ureteral orifice (point of *black arrow*) is markedly stenotic. *E,* Rectosigmoid colon with polyposis. Numerous sessile and pedunculated polyps are seen. Many are erythematous, indicative of active oviposition with granuloma formation. Some have necrotic hemorrhagic tips. *F,* Mucosal surface of partial cystectomy specimen (4 × 5 cm ellipse) from a patient with the chronic inactive stage of the disease. There is a stellate chronic schistosomal ulcer. Despite the inactivity of the disease, these ulcers may bleed profusely. Pale mucoid flecks at the margin of the ulcer (*arrow*) are areas of adenoid (goblet cell) metaplasia.

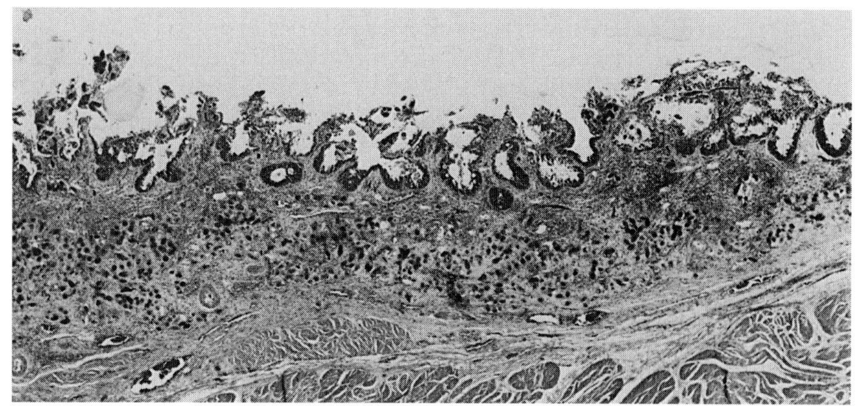

Figure 22–17. Urinary bladder lamina propria in grade 2, chronic active urinary schistosomiasis. There is moderate urothelial hyperplasia. The superficial lamina propria contains pale (viable) eggs and perioval granulomata (*arrows*), with a moderate and diffuse infiltrate of eosinophils, lymphocytes, and plasma cells. Deeper portions of the lamina propria contain dead calcific eggs in a fibrotic matrix. The superficial detrusor muscle is visible at the bottom of the field. (Hematoxylin-eosin stain; magnification, ×25.)

Urothelia in patients with **metaplasia** (see Figs. 22–15*D,F,* 22–19, and 22–20) exhibit either squamous or adenoid differentiation; the more common squamous metaplasia covers a spectrum from hyperplastic transitional epithelium to epidermization (Smith et al, 1974a). Another cause of urothelial squamous metaplasia, vitamin A deficiency, plays no role in metaplasia of schistosomal origin (Borel and Etard, 1988). **Dysplasia** often accompanies squamous metaplasia in a manner histologically comparable to the metaplasia/dysplasia/carcinoma-in-situ spectrum of the cervix uteri (Smith and Christie, 1986), and urothelial metaplasia and dysplasia commonly accompany schistosomal bladder cancer (Khafagy et al, 1972). However, dysplastic urothelium does not manifest low-molecular-weight cytokeratins (Tungekar et al, 1987), as does dysplastic uterine cervical metaplasia (Bobrow et al, 1986).

Urinary schistosomiasis has been linked to urothelial (bladder) cancer (see Fig. 22–15*C*) since the turn of the 20th century (Ferguson, 1911). **The bilharzial bladder cancer syndrome manifests with an early onset (40 to 50 years of age) and a high frequency of squamous cell carcinomas (60% to 90%) and adenocarcinomas (5% to 15%) and has been exhaustively documented from many regions endemic for *S. haematobium*** (El-Bolkainy et al, 1972, 1981; Cheever, 1978; Lucas, 1982; Al-Adnani and Salah, 1983; Elem and Purohit, 1983; Kitinya et al, 1986; Al-Shukri et al, 1987b; Thomas et al, 1990). However, unselected autopsy series from the same regions have shown similar frequencies of bladder cancer in patients with and without schistosomiasis (Edington et al, 1970; Smith et al, 1974a; Cheever et al, 1978) and have shown no relationship between bladder cancer and egg burdens in the lower urinary tract (Smith et al, 1974b; Lucas, 1982; Elem and Purohit, 1983).

Urothelial carcinogenesis is a multistep process (Hicks et al, 1982; Koroltchouk et al, 1987). Experimental work indicates that chronic bacterial infection, foreign bodies (including calcific *S. haematobium* eggs), and urinary concentration of experimentally given nitrosamines induce urothelial cancer (Hicks et al, 1980, 1982; Harzmann et al, 1983; Davis et al, 1984, 1985). Mucosal foreign bodies and calcific *S. haematobium* eggs focus the site of nitrosamine-induced experimental cancers (Hicks et al, 1980, 1982). Similarly, human bladder cancers originate in regions with the heaviest

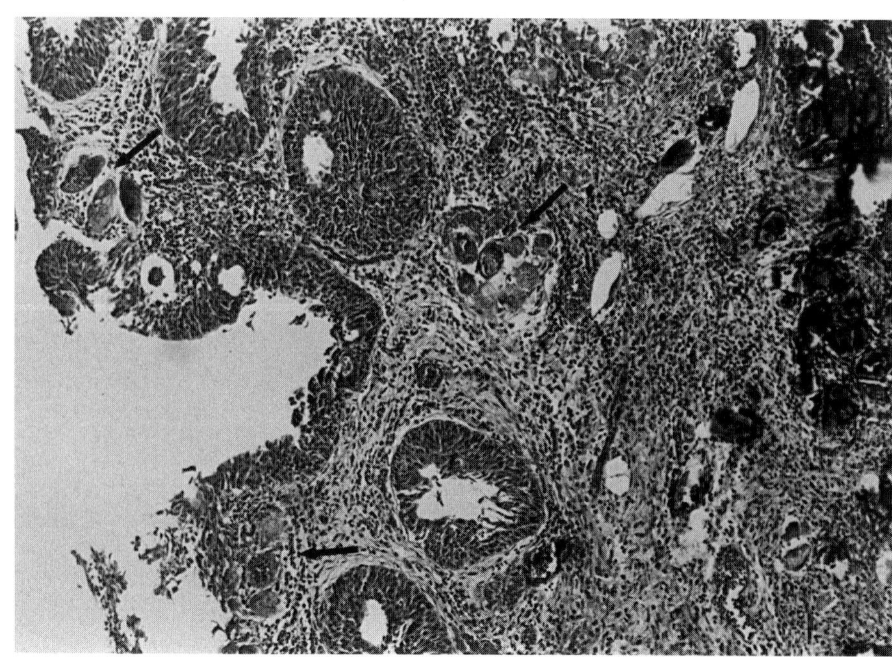

Figure 22–18. Higher magnification of the lamina propria of the bladder illustrated in Figure 22–17, showing urothelial hyperplasia (left of field), viable eggs (*arrows*), and sandy patch (upper right of field) with packed calcific eggs. (Hematoxylin-eosin stain; magnification, ×125.)

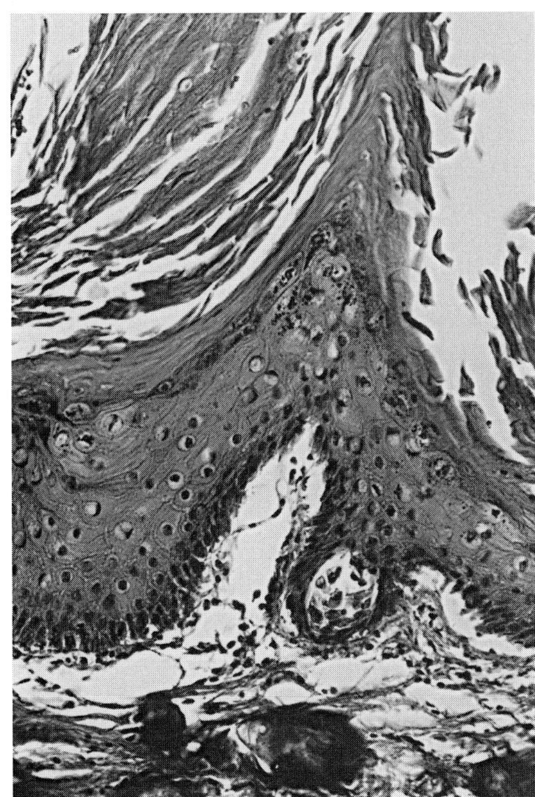

Figure 22–19. Area of epidermization seen in Figure 22–15*D*. All layers of skin (basal, spinous, granular, and corneal) are replicated in this example of the extreme end of the spectrum of squamous metaplasia. Skin appendages are absent. Calcific eggs are visible at the bottom of the field. (Hematoxylin-eosin stain; magnification, ×250.)

egg burdens, irrespective of the overall magnitude of the egg burden in the entire urinary tract (Christie et al, 1986a). Schistosomal obstructive uropathy predisposes to urinary tract infection (see later discussion) with bacteria that produce carcinogenic nitrosamines (El-Merzabani et al, 1979; Hicks et al, 1982; Abdel-Tawab et al, 1986). Nitrate, nitrite, and volatile N-nitroso compounds have been demonstrated in the urine of bilharzial bladder cancer patients (Tricker et al, 1991; Mostafa et al, 1994). Patients with both chronic urinary and hepatosplenic schistosomiasis also excrete high levels of carcinogenic tryptophan metabolites (Abul-Fadl and Khalafallah, 1961; Abdel-Tawab et al, 1986); in Egypt, many patients are coinfected. Urinary schistosomiasis stimulates production of beta-glucuronidase by the hyperplastic urothelium; this deconjugates inactive carcinogens, rendering them active (Fripp, 1988).

Moreover, bilharzial bladder cancer has been associated with certain T lymphocyte subsets and altered levels of various lymphokines in the urine (Raziuddin et al, 1991, 1992; Rosin et al, 1994a, 1994b), and some of these abnormalities appear to be associated with chromosomal instabilities in urothelial cells (Rosin and Anwar, 1992; Anwar and Rosin, 1993; Rosin et al, 1994a, 1994b). HLA-B16 and Cw2 antigens are related to bilharzial bladder cancer, but there is a negative correlation with HLA-A9 and its split Aw24 antigen (Wishahi et al, 1989).

Therefore, urinary schistosomiasis (1) is a co-carcinogen or promoter of urothelial cancer and sets the tumor location; (2) alters the histologic differentiation into squamous cell carcinoma by its direct metaplastic effect (Smith and Christie, 1986; Christie et al, 1986a); and (3) predisposes to bacterial infections that increase urinary carcinogens.

More than 40% of squamous cell carcinomas associated with urinary schistosomiasis are well-differentiated (grade 1) or perhaps verrucous carcinomas that are exophytic and carry a good prognosis. Most occur on the posterior (40% to 50%) and lateral walls (about 30%) of the bladder. Exophytic tumors constitute nearly 70% of bilharzial bladder cancers, whereas 25% are ulcerative endophytic tumors. More poorly differentiated bilharzial carcinomas, which carry a poorer prognosis, lose their ABO(H) blood group surface antigens (Halim et al, 1986) and produce low-molecular-weight cytokeratins (Fukushima et al, 1987; Tungekar et al, 1987, 1988b) and chorionic gonadotropin (Tungekar et al, 1988a). Urinary schistosomiasis increases the frequency of leiomyosarcomas of the bladder, which remain scarce; histological differentiation of leiomyosarcomas from the rare spindle cell type of squamous cell carcinomas has been simplified by immunoperoxidase techniques for keratin and myoglobin (Tungekar and Al-Adnani, 1986).

Bilharzial bladder cancer is usually diagnosed late in its course when necroturia, pain, or hemorrhage ensue or when

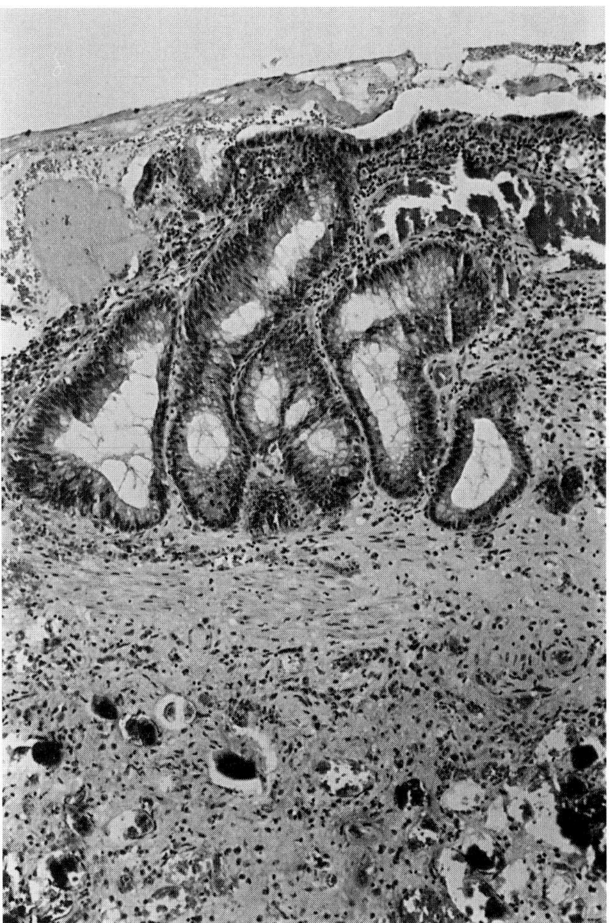

Figure 22–20. Area of adenoid (goblet cell) metaplasia shown in Figure 9–15*E*. Branching simple glands appear identical to colonic glands in chronic inflammatory states; goblet cells are numerous. Abortive formation of muscularis mucosa (*arrow*) is seen. (Hematoxylin-eosin stain; magnification, ×250.)

radiology or cystoscopy for other causes intervenes. Because the majority of these cancers are well-differentiated exophytic carcinomas that slough superficially necrotic tumor, necroturia is more common than in nonschistosomal bladder cancers. Focal lysis of concentric bladder calcification in pelvic radiographs (especially if the "hole" subsequently enlarges) is pathognomonic for bladder cancer in endemic regions. Cytologic criteria distinguishing cancers from schistosomiasis-induced atypia have been developed, so that patients may now be screened by urinary cytology (El-Bolkainy et al, 1982). Evaluation of urinary cytokeratins may provide another screening method, because they are shed into urine with cancer but not with schistosomiasis (Basta et al, 1988).

Treatment is frequently surgical and involves a radical anterior pelvic exenteration, if possible.

Urolithiasis

Ureteritis cystica calcinosa is associated with *S. haematobium* infection, especially heavy infections, and is not associated with pyelonephritis (Smith et al, 1974a; Cheever et al, 1978).

Urinary tract stone formation may complicate schistosomal stenoses in areas encompassed within the "stone belt," such as Egypt (Ghorab, 1962). In Egypt, ureterolithiasis, not nephrolithiasis, is more common in patients with *S. haematobium* infections than in controls (Smith et al, 1974a), and an association between pyelonephritis and urolithiasis was found (Smith et al, 1974a; Cheever et al, 1978). Studies in other *S. haematobium*–endemic areas have shown no correlation between urinary schistosomiasis and urolithiasis (Ibrahim, 1978; Cutajar, 1983; Elem, 1984). Therefore, the association in Egypt denotes an epidemiologic, rather than a pathogenetic, relationship (Smith and Christie, 1986).

Ureters and Schistosomal Obstructive Uropathy

The most common and dangerous sequelae of urinary schistosomiasis result from ureteral involvement (Makar, 1948, 1955; Edington et al, 1970; Lehman et al, 1973; Smith et al, 1974a; Cheever et al, 1978; Smith and Christie, 1986). Autopsy (Edington et al, 1970; Smith et al, 1974a; Cheever et al, 1977) and community-based (Forsythe, 1969; King et al, 1988a) studies have established that **hydroureter and hydronephrosis are related to the presence and intensity of *S. haematobium* infection**. SOU (Fig. 22–21; see also Figs. 22–10, 22–11, 22–12, and 22–15*D*) encompasses anatomic and/or functional stenoses, hydroureter, and hydronephrosis (Smith and Christie, 1986). SOU resembles other forms of obstructive uropathy (see Chapter 10, The Pathophysiology of Urinary Obstruction). Patients with *both* schistosomal hydroureter and hydronephrosis are more heavily infected than those with hydroureter alone (Smith et al, 1974a; Smith et al, 1977b). SOU is bilaterally asymmetric; patients with bilateral SOU have been found to have higher egg burdens than those with unilateral SOU (Smith et al, 1974a; Smith et al, 1977b).

Ureteral egg burdens correlate with egg burdens of the entire urinary tract and are highest at the distal end, adjacent to the bladder, progressively diminishing proximally, except

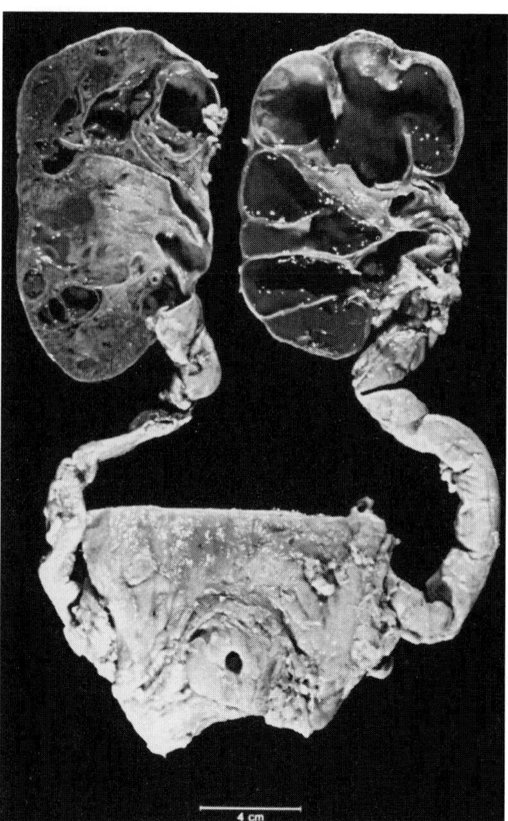

Figure 22–21. Schistosomal obstructive uropathy. The urinary bladder and ureters were fixed by inflation with formalin, and the bladder was sectioned coronally. The left hydroureter (right of the field) is dilated (external diameter, 2 cm) and thin-walled throughout its extravesicular course (interstitial ureteral stenosis is behind the bladder) and appears to be an atonic ureter; it is tortuous and kinked. The left kidney exhibits stage IV (end-stage) hydronephrosis with complete medullary and nearly complete cortical atrophy, and its pelvis is filled with sterile gelatinous rusty material; this is simple, uncomplicated hydronephrosis. The right ureter exhibits a moderately thick-walled hydroureter (probably tonic), with stage II to III hydronephrosis and complicating acute and chronic pyelonephritis. The patient died of septicemia secondary to the right renal pyelonephritis, and the urinary schistosomiasis is therefore classified as an underlying cause of death.

for uncommon focal involvement of the upper ureter in the "second or third lumbar" and "fifth lumbar" segmental lesions (Smith et al, 1974a; Smith et al, 1977b). Not surprisingly, schistosomal ureteral lesions are most common in interstitial and juxtavesical ureters (Fam, 1964; Smith et al, 1974a, 1977b; Cheever et al, 1978; Al-Shukri and Alwan, 1983; Al-Shukri et al, 1987a).

There are two components to SOU: (1) obstruction, which may be anatomic or functional, and (2) the result of obstruction upon the proximal ureter. Both components differ qualitatively and quantitatively in active and inactive stages. SOU in active disease has been studied principally in radiography and in community-wide analyses. SOU in more inactive stages has been analyzed mostly by urologists and pathologists in hospitalized patients.

In *active* schistosomiasis, ureteral oviposition and egg accumulation begins in the *lamina propria*, progressively encircles the ureter, and spreads outward into the muscle layers. Ureteral obstruction is most often caused by concentric or hemiconcentric polypoid lesions (which "girdle" the ureteral muscle) in the interstitial and adjacent extravesical ureter, although polypoid lesions in the urinary bladder may encroach upon the ureteral meatus and interstitial ureter. In addition, eggs perforate the ureteral urothelium, allowing backflow of acidic and saline-rich urine into ureteral interstitium, which results in ureteral muscular spasm (Ugaily-Thulesius et al, 1988). Ureteral hypotonia, absence or decrease in the frequency and amplitude of ureteral peristalsis, and delayed excretion are noted **even before radiologically demonstrable ureteral dilatation**, and delayed excretion occurs in over half of cases examined (Zahran and Badr, 1980; Umerah, 1981; Pawar and Abdel-Dayem, 1984; Abdel-Halim et al, 1985; Bahar et al, 1988). In active disease, the principal problem may be ureteral dysfunction rather than anatomic stenoses. In addition, vesicoureteral reflux is seen in 20% of patients (Hanafy et al, 1975; Umerah, 1981; Pawar and Abdel-Dayem, 1984). Nevertheless, modest colicky flank pain is often the only indication that early obstructive uropathy is developing (Lehman et al, 1973).

In **late chronic active** and **inactive** urinary schistosomiasis, anatomic obstruction is more prominent. Anatomic ureteral stenoses, with or without calculi, have been identified in up to 80% of obstructions (Makar, 1955; Fam, 1964; Lehman et al, 1973; Smith et al, 1974a, 1977b; Cheever et al, 1978; Al-Shukri and Alwan, 1983). In the remaining obstructions, the ureteral lumen is patent, often dilated, but the ureteral wall is rigid and fibrotic, and the adjacent proximal ureter is dilated and trabeculated, indicative of functional obstruction (Lehman et al, 1973; Smith et al, 1974a, 1977b; Cheever et al, 1978). These nonstenotic obstructions are caused by circumferential sandy patches, which concentrically obliterate all layers of ureteral muscle, producing an aperistaltic rigid dilated segment; peristalsis on either side of these segments is dyssynchronous, and urine flushes back and forth ineffectually (Smith et al, 1977b).

Obstruction may occur at the ureteral meatus ($<1\%$), interstitial ureter (10% to 30%), juxtavesical ureter (20% to 60%), lower third (pelvic) ureter (15% to 50%), or contiguous combinations of these areas (30% to 60%) (Makar, 1948, 1955; Gelfand, 1948; Fam, 1964; Smith et al, 1977b; Al-Shukri and Alwan, 1983). Sandy or fibrous patches around the ureteral orifices can produce incomplete or complete meatal stenosis or gaping incompetence, the so-called "golf-hole ureter." However, vesicoureteric reflux may be slightly less common (2% to 14%) than in the active stage.

The *results* of these obstructions are hydroureter and hydronephrosis. Anatomic configuration of ureteral muscle differs in the upper, middle, and lower thirds (Schneider, 1938), so that oviposition during *active* disease, encroaching upon superficial muscle, in the lower and upper thirds of the ureter compromises initially longitudinal and later circular muscle, lengthening, before dilating, those segments. Conversely, oviposition in the middle third initially weakens circular muscle, causing dilatation before elongation. Because oviposition decreases proximally and ureters are fixed at both ends and the pelvic brim, lengthening and dilatation first mold the hydroureter's "pelvic loop" and then the "abdominal loop" so typical of urinary schistosomiasis (Smith et al, 1977b).

Three types of hydroureter are associated with schistosomal obstruction: segmental (i.e., cylindrical or fusiform), tonic, and atonic (Smith et al, 1977b). **Segmental ureteral dilatations** constitute 25% of SOU; nearly 80% of these are in the lower ureter and are accompanied by concentric ureteral muscular obliteration by fibrosis and sandy patches; some are also accompanied by ureteral muscle hypertrophy proximal to an obstruction. Segmental lesions are rarely associated with important hydronephrosis; a rare ($<2\%$) variant involves the whole or most of the ureter (i.e., multisegmental) in concentric sandy patches, converting the entire ureter into a dilated, grittily indurated, rigid, and thick-walled tube that exhibits no peristalsis (Smith et al, 1977b). **Tonic hydroureter,** found in 25% to 30% of patients with SOU, is a dilated, tortuous, thick-walled, and trabeculated ureter with marked ureteral muscle hypertrophy and active, although retarded, peristaltic action. It involves the entire ureter proximal to an obstructive lesion, often a functional stenosis, and is often accompanied by significant hydronephrosis, which usually resolves after relief of obstruction (Smith et al, 1977b). **Atonic hydroureter,** seen in 35% of patients with SOU, is a markedly dilated, very tortuous, thin-walled ureter, without peristalsis and with atrophic fibrotic ureteral muscle. The entire ureter proximal to an obstruction is usually involved, often associated with advanced hydronephrosis; renal function recovery after obstruction removal is often not as good as with tonic hydroureters (Smith et al, 1977b).

Hydroureter usually precedes **hydronephrosis,** thus hydronephrosis represents the final stage in the succession of sequelae (Edington et al, 1970; Lehman et al, 1973; Smith et al, 1974a, 1977b; Cheever et al, 1978). Schistosomal hydronephrosis passes from progressive renal pelvic dilatation, then medullary atrophy to nearly total medullary effacement, before cortical atrophy ensues (Smith et al, 1974a, 1977b). This progression explains abrogation of tubular function (especially maximal urine concentration) before glomerular function compromise (Lehman et al, 1971, 1973). The 18-hour concentration test becomes abnormal early in schistosomal hydronephrosis, and this is the only routine renal function test that is impaired until obstructive uropathy becomes very severe. Elevation of urinary beta-2 microglobulin indicates cortical compromise (Coopan et al, 1987a).

Superimposed urinary tract infection similarly reduces urine concentration, and the effects of obstruction *and* infection on urinary concentration are additive (Lehman et al, 1971); these may even induce severe polyuria and a diabetes insipidus–like syndrome. The glomerular filtration rate and renal plasma flow are altered very late in the course of SOU (Wilkins et al, 1985a). Some patients with remarkably obstructed urinary tracts and severe bilateral hydronephrosis properly maintain creatinine clearance. This is a very precarious situation, and superimposed bacterial infection can initiate rapid deterioration of renal function, uremia, and death (Lehman et al, 1970). **Complete resolution of renal function occurs within 1 to 2 months of antischistosomal chemotherapy when obstruction is caused by active disease** (Lucas et al, 1966, 1969; Lehman et al, 1973). Similarly, renal function losses in severe hydronephrosis that result from "inactive" lesions may revert to normal after successful surgical intervention (Smith et al, 1977b), but the obstructive uropathy is not ameliorated by chemotherapy alone (King et al, 1988b).

Although severe SOU may be asymptomatic, most patients seeking urologic consultation have had recurrent renal colic or loin pain for varying periods, up to 40 years (Smith et al, 1977b; Wallace, 1979; Al-Shukri and Alwan, 1983; Fievet et al, 1987).

Residual ureteral stenosis after successful chemotherapy is usually amenable to surgical intervention; depending on the extent and location of the stricture, procedures involving excision or dilatation have been used. "Balloon dilatation" has reportedly proved effective with anatomic stenoses (Jacobsson et al, 1987); however, mechanical dilatation is frequently followed by repeat stenosis (Wishahi, 1987).

When the ureteral meatus, interstitial ureter, ureterovesical junction, or lower ureter is involved, a variety of plastic operations to reconstruct a functional valve are available. Most of these procedures are variants of the Leadbetter-Politano operation (Politano and Leadbetter, 1958; Leadbetter and Leadbetter, 1961). Although highly effective for some patients (Smith et al, 1977b; Al-Shukri and Alwan, 1983), other authors have noted restenoses (Wallace, 1979; Husain et al, 1980; Umerah, 1981), and some advocate full-length ureteric splints (Rady and Rady, 1987).

In long or multisegmental lesions, excision of the effected portion leaves inadequate residual ureter for reimplantation; Boari-Ockerbladt bladder flap, Boari-Kuss flap, ileal conduit, suprapubic intravesical ureterostomy, and ureteroileocystostomy with care to have an isoperistaltic direction of the ileal segment have been successfully employed in these cases (Wallace, 1979; Abdel-Halim, 1980, 1984; Al-Shukri and Alwan, 1983; Abu-Aisha et al, 1985). Isolated meatal stenosis may be amenable to simple meatoplasty (Al-Shukri and Alwan, 1983). When a ureter is hopelessly obstructed, nephrostomy is performed as a last resort, particularly in the presence of superimposed bacterial infection.

Complications of Schistosomal Obstructive Uropathy

Unselected autopsy studies indicate no association between urinary schistosomiasis per se and pyelonephritis (Edington et al, 1970; Smith et al, 1974a; Cheever et al, 1978) but document a marked increase in pyelonephritis in patients with severe SOU (Smith et al, 1974a; Cheever et al, 1978). Community-wide clinical studies have corroborated autopsy studies (Carter et al, 1970; Shokeir et al, 1972; Lehman et al, 1973; Laughlin et al, 1978; Warren et al, 1979; Hicks et al, 1982). SOU with pyelonephritis is even more common in the presence of histologic cystitis, bladder outlet obstruction, or bacterial cystitis (Smith et al, 1974a; Cheever et al, 1978).

Schistosomal infection in endemic populations is often additive to, and interrelated with, other pathologic urinary tract conditions, such as lower and upper urinary tract infections and obstruction due to prostatism or urinary stone formation. We conclude, therefore, that SOU, urolithiasis, bladder outlet obstruction, and bacterial cystitis all predispose to pyelonephritis and that patients with more risk factors for longer periods of time are at greater risk (Smith and Christie, 1986).

Xanthogranulomatous pyelonephritis, which represents a relatively anergic T cell response to various species of bacteria, can coexist with intact granulomas around *S. haematobium* eggs (Bazeed et al, 1989). No significant predilection for glomerulopathy, hypertensive nephropathy, or amyloidosis has been associated with *S. haematobium* infection in humans (Edington et al, 1970; Smith et al, 1974a; Sadigursky et al, 1976; Cheever et al, 1978), but there are occasional reports of nephrotic syndrome (with mesangioproliferative, membranoproliferative, or minimal change histopathology), which remits after successful treatment of the *S. haematobium* infection (Greenham and Cameron, 1980; Turner et al, 1987) or histologic changes without clinical disease (Beaufils et al, 1978). Glomerulonephritis has been induced in experimental *S. haematobium* infections (Sobh et al, 1991). The glomerulonephritis of *S. haematobium* and *Salmonella* coinfection were previously noted.

Gastrointestinal Tract

Schistosoma haematobium egg burdens progressively increase as the intestine is descended; the steepest increment occurs between the splenic flexure and the sigmoid colon (Smith et al, 1974a; Kamel et al, 1977; Cheever et al, 1977, 1978). Egg burdens of the sigmoid colon and rectum correlate well with overall infection intensity, so that these sites are "usual," rather than aberrant ectopic, loci of oviposition (Smith et al, 1975). Oviposition probably begins earlier but proceeds more slowly in the rectum and sigmoid colon than in the lower urinary tract (Smith et al, 1975); eggs may appear in the stool before the urine, but quantitative stool egg counts do not correlate with infection intensity.

Sandy patches in the rectum are associated with severe disease in the lower urinary tract (Lehman et al, 1973; Smith et al, 1974a), but sandy patches in the upper colon and ileum represent ectopic sites and are not prognostic of lower urinary tract compromise (Lehman et al, 1973; Smith et al, 1974a, 1975; Fataar et al, 1984a, 1984b, 1985).

In **schistosomal colonic polyposis** (see Fig. 22–15*E*), which occurs mostly in Egypt, sessile and/or pedunculated granulomatous masses cover inflamed mucosa. This condition yields abdominal pain, dysentery, finger clubbing and arthralgia (caused by new bone formation), anemia from blood loss, and protein-losing enteropathy (documented by [^{51}Cr] albumin excretion studies) with edema and anasarca (Lehman et al, 1968; El-Masry et al, 1986). Rectal polyposis occurs in *S. haematobium* infections without *S. mansoni* coinfection. Most rectal and sigmoid polyps contain eggs of both *S. mansoni* and *S. haematobium* (Lehman et al, 1973; Smith et al, 1977c; Cheever et al, 1978), but the colonic polyposis syndrome is provoked only by *S. mansoni* (Lehman et al, 1973; Smith et al, 1977c; Cheever et al, 1978). The frequency of colonic polyposis in Egypt, where coinfections with *S. haematobium* and *S. mansoni* afford possible cross-pairing, and its infrequency in Brazil, where only *S. mansoni* is found, suggests that *S. mansoni* males paired with *S. haematobium* female worms may produce the polyposis syndrome; such cross-pairing has been demonstrated in experimental animals (Khalil and Mansour, 1995).

Appendiceal egg burdens exceed those in adjacent gut in *S. haematobium*, but not *S. mansoni*, infections (Smith et al, 1974a, 1975); schistosomal appendicitis may become symptomatic during heavy infections (Edington et al, 1975; Duvie et al, 1987; Hodasi, 1988; Adebamowo et al, 1991), and mortality, directly from active schistosomiasis, is associated with (but not caused by) high appendiceal egg burdens

(Smith et al, 1975). Therefore, patients with schistosomal appendicitis should be carefully studied for SOU (Smith and Christie, 1986). Calcific appendices may appear on abdominal radiographs or computed axial tomographic (CAT) scans (Fataar and Satayanath, 1986).

Other Sites

Egg burdens of **hepatic** *S. haematobium* are often higher than those of *S. mansoni*, but Symmer's fibrosis and portal hypertension are not caused by *S. haematobium* infections (Edington et al, 1970; Smith et al, 1974a; Cheever et al, 1977; Kamel et al, 1978). Significant **pulmonary** *S. haematobium* egg burdens reflect overall infection intensity but develop late in the disease and do not induce pulmonary angiopathy or cor pulmonale (Edington et al, 1970; Smith et al, 1974a; Cheever et al, 1977, 1978).

Ectopic oviposition may occur during any stage of infection (including the prepatent period) and at any anatomic site (Gelfand, 1950; Alves, 1958). Schistosomal granulomas, sandy patches, and bilharziomas (see later discussion) are found in skin, pericardium, mediastinum (al-Fawaz et al, 1990; Ashour, 1990), mesenteries, gallbladder, thyroid, and adrenal glands, and may result from either aberrant oviposition or microembolization. These eggs rarely produce symptoms (Smith and Christie, 1986).

Bilharziomas are exuberant fibrogranulomatous masses induced by schistosome eggs deposited where they cannot escape into excreta. The large (occasionally up to 30 cm in diameter), resilient, lobulated tumors have pink-white cut surfaces flecked by tan to yellow milia. They often arise in the colorectal serosa, mesenteries, appendix, urinary bladder, female internal genitalia, and epididymis but can occur wherever ectopic oviposition is prolonged. When pedunculated, they may undergo torsion, simulating an acute abdominal or intrascrotal catastrophe.

Central nervous system involvement is rare but, when present, severe. It usually focuses on the lower spinal cord, producing space-occupying lesions, myelitis, or transverse myelitis (Wakefield et al, 1962; Marcial-Rojas Fiol, 1963; Bird, 1967; Ghaly and El-Banhawy, 1973; Scrimgeour and Gajdusek, 1985; Cosnett and Van Dellen, 1986). It may result from aberrant oviposition or microembolization via Batson's plexus (Smith and Christie, 1986). Ectopic oviposition may involve nerve roots, leptomeninges, or the spinal cord, evoking the diverse syndromes of radiculitis, simulated spinal cord tumor, or transverse myelitis. An important clinical feature is the sudden appearance, when infection is prepatent, mild, or latent (i.e., apparently inactive after a previously active clinical course); eggs may not be detectable in stool or urine. Diagnosis and treatment are extremely urgent, because motor deficits often progress rapidly to permanent paraplegia. A thorough clinical history, including records of exposure to schistosome-infected waters, is essential; significant spinal fluid eosinophilia occurs in more than half of patients. The spinal fluid contains circumoval precipitins (Yogore et al, 1975). **Negative results of urine or stool examinations do not rule out this diagnosis!**

Current recommendations for treatment are early laminectomy to relieve edema and cord compression and antischistosomal treatment with simultaneous corticosteroid suppression of inflammatory and immune responses, but outcome depends on the location and extent of fixed neural damage. Some patients respond to drug treatment alone; other patients sustain permanent deficits despite treatment. Schistosomal "mass lesions" in the brain may occur (Pollner et al, 1994) but are unusual in schistosomiasis haematobium, although they are often seen in schistosomiasis japonica.

In summary, *S. haematobium* produces highly variable lesions dependent on infection intensity, duration, activity, and focalization of oviposition. The disease evolves after infection ceases naturally or chemotherapeutically. Heavy infections regularly produce lower urinary tract lesions that yield significant morbidity and mortality. In addition, ectopic oviposition may unpredictably produce significant lesions in a few patients. Diagnosis of urinary schistosomiasis should include differentiation of species and determination of activity and severity. Treatment should include initial chemotherapy of active cases with follow-up in 2 to 3 months to ensure parasitologic cure and reassess the residual disease, principally schistosomal obstructive uropathy, and surgical remediation of such residual lesions. In addition, patients who have experienced severe urinary schistosomiasis should have long-term follow-up to ensure early intervention in developing urothelial cancer.

GENITAL FILARIASIS

Filarial diseases are classified as either lymphatic or nonlymphatic afflictions. ***Wuchereria bancrofti*** (which has periodic nocturnal, periodic diurnal, and, in the Pacific area, subperiodic variants) **accounts for 90% of cases of human *lymphatic* filariasis and is widespread throughout the tropics.** It is probably an exclusively human parasite without animal reservoirs. *Brugia malayi* and *B. timori* cause the remainder of human lymphatic filariasis, spontaneously (and in the laboratory) infect primates and domestic animals, and are confined to the Far East. **Nonlymphatic** filarial parasites (*Loa, Dipetalonema, Dirofilaria,* and *Mansonella* species) rarely cause urogenital manifestations, but *Onchocerca volvulus*, the agent of African river blindness, is known to cause massive inguinal lymphadenopathy, "hanging groin," and scrotal elephantiasis (see later discussion).

Lymphatic Filariasis

All lymphatic filaria are transmitted by mosquitoes, which inject larvae with salivary secretions when stinging the host; multiple injections over a prolonged period are necessary to produce disease. Clinical and pathologic manifestations differ in endemic and nonendemic human hosts, supposedly as a result of intrauterine exposure to filarial antigens in endemic populations (Ottesen, 1989). **In *patients from nonendemic areas,* acute hypersensitivity and/or febrile reactions associated with transitory lymphadenopathy, localized lymphangitis, genital edema, or hydrocele occur after long (2 to 3 years) prepatent periods.** Subsequent recrudescences result in funiculoepididymitis, orchitis, or lymphangitis. Such recurrences occur at irregular and lengthy intervals, related to excretion of exoantigens or death of adult worms residing in lymphangioles. Eventually damage accumulates, resulting in chyluria or permanent deformity (elephantiasis or hydrocele). Microfilaremia may occur during patent infections of patients from nonendemic areas, but microfilaremia is generally inversely proportional to pathologic sequelae; thus a variety of amicrofilaremic ("occult") filarial syndromes occur.

Most **patients from endemic areas** manifest microfilaremia but rarely develop pathologic sequelae, as described earlier. However, this scant proportion of endemic patients who develop pathologic sequelae accounts for the bulk of clinical disease (Ottesen, 1989).

Episodic or relentlessly progressive filariasis produces considerable patient anxiety and discomfort; it is frequently incapacitating, and only limited therapeutic recourses avail. It is comparable to leprosy in its socially stigmatizing aspect. However, minor and stationary filarial maladies, such as hydrocele, are usually ignored, and their public health importance is underestimated. Current prospects for control of filarial transmission remain dim in most endemic areas.

Biology and Life Cycle

The lymphatic filariae are elongated (100 × 0.3 mm for female *W. bancrofti*), viviparous nematodes. Their cycle proceeds from human to mosquito and back, through a sequence of larval molts. The most common urban vectors of *W. bancrofti* are the ubiquitous *Culex pipiens* complex, but filariae have adapted to a wide variety of *Culex*, *Anopheles*, *Aedes*, and *Mansonella* mosquitoes in different settings.

Female mosquitoes ingest microfilariae, first-stage larvae (Fig. 22–22), with their blood meals. These rapidly molt to become infective third-stage larvae and go to the mosquitoes' salivary glands. The infective larvae are injected into the dermis with the saliva during the next mosquito sting. While unable to traverse unbroken skin, the infective larvae can cross the normal conjunctiva or buccal mucosa (Ah et al, 1974b; Sullivan and Chernin, 1976); aquatic transmission from dead mosquitoes to humans may be a rare alternative pathway.

The prepatent period of human *Wuchereria* infections is unknown but is probably longer than that of *Brugia* (which ranges from 53 to 131 days in experimental animals), even though the larvae reach the host lung via the blood within minutes of inoculation. The last two larval molts occur in the lymphatics near the final nesting sites of the adult worms; these molts incite local inflammation and early, episodic clinical symptoms; similar bouts coincide with early mating.

Adult filaria prefer to live in the larger lymphatic vessels of human, more rarely in distended lymphatic capillaries or in the sinuses of lymph nodes. *W. bancrofti* adults have a predilection for periaortic, iliac, inguinal, and intrascrotal lymph vessels (and, uncommonly, subclavicular and axillary nodes, especially in the nonperiodic form), whereas *B. malayi* prefers inguinal and more distal lymphangioles (as well as axillary and epitrochlear groups), and *B. timori* commences in the inguinal nodes and subsequently involves progressively more distal lymphangioles (Partono, 1987). Occasionally, worms enter veins and embolize small pulmonary arteries, where their death evokes arteritis and pulmonary infarction similar to human infection with the dog heartworm *Dirofilaria immitis* (Beaver and Cran, 1974).

Most of the mature *Wuchereria* female is composed of the uterus, which contains all stages of embryos from eggs to mature microfilariae (Fig. 22–23). Microfilarial discharge into the blood is regulated by a feedback system that maintains a constant level of microfilaremia. There is, however, no constant relationship between worm number and level of microfilaremia. Indeed, microfilaremia is found in only 30% to 40% of all infections.

Transfer experiments have established that microfilariae live for several months. Thus, microfilarial periodicity is the

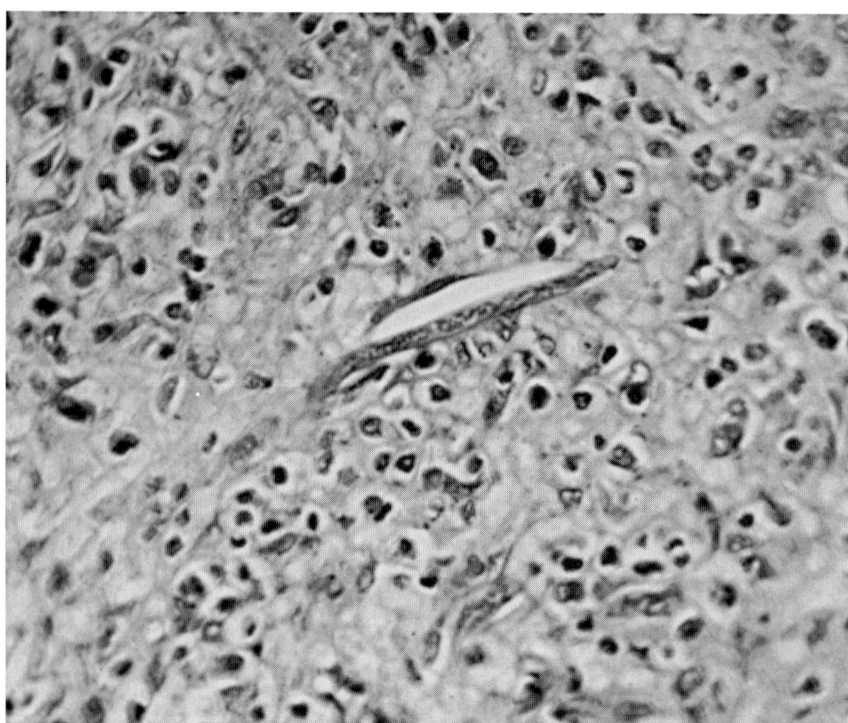

Figure 22–22. Microfilaria of *Wuchereria bancrofti* in splenic granuloma found at autopsy. Most of the surrounding cells are macrophages and eosinophils. (Magnification, ×380.)

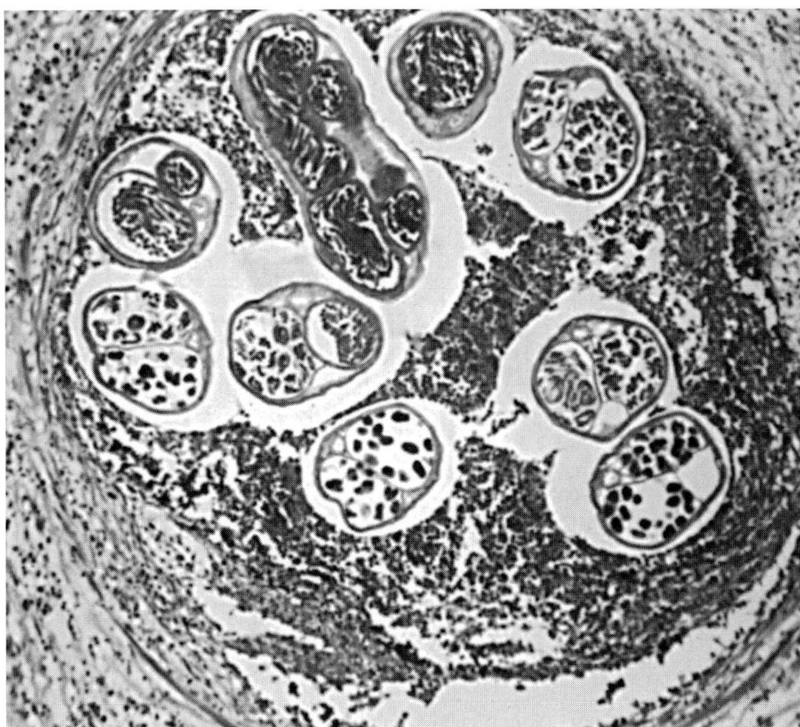

Figure 22–23. Intact, adult *Wuchereria bancrofti* female in acutely inflamed lymph vessel of epididymis. Note developmental stages of microfilariae in worm uterus. (Magnification, ×100.)

result, not of periodic release from adult females, but of release from parenchymal capillary beds (lung, spleen, etc.) into the peripheral circulation. A variety of drugs and anesthetics can quickly and temporarily alter this distribution. Research has not elucidated the regulatory mechanisms that produce the circadian rhythms of microfilaremia; however, the timing of peak microfilaremia in each endemic focus corresponds to the peak feeding period of local mosquito vectors.

Distribution and Epidemiology

Other than tropical parts of the continental United States and Australia, few tropical countries are free of *Wuchereria*. However, the prevalence of microfilaremia varies greatly, from sporadic in Puerto Rico to nearly 50% in parts of southern India. Neither percentage reflects the prevalence of infection, and the latter implies a near-holoendemic condition. In most endemic foci, both microfilaremia and filarial pathologic effects are more common among males, particularly urogenital lesions. Within each endemic country, bancroftian filariasis is concentrated in coastal plains and is less common and less severe in the highlands. Many of the small, flat archipelagos of the South Pacific are holoendemic, including the area east of the International Date Line, where subperiodic filariasis is common.

In contrast to *Wuchereria*, the distribution of *Brugia* is relatively focal and limited to rural populations of tropical Southeast Asia, extending from the western coast of India to New Guinea, the Philippines, and Japan. Both day- and night-stinging mosquitoes are involved in transmission, and a variety of circadian patterns of microfilaremia has been reported in different endemic foci (Sasa and Tanaka, 1972). Spontaneously infected jungle primates and other mammals are reservoir hosts.

Two patterns have been observed in the age distribution of microfilaremia: In some populations, there is a linear increase in prevalence into the fourth decade, and microfilaremia subsequently continues for as long as 14 years. In other foci, prevalence falls after patients' 20s or 30s; only sporadic microfilaremia persists in older age groups. The latter pattern prevails where transmission is moderate or low; the fall in microfilaremia often coincides with the onset of permanent pathologic alterations.

As already indicated, a large proportion of patients infected with filariae remain asymptomatic permanently, as shown by autopsy studies in which small numbers of live and dead worms are found in older patients with no history of clinical filariasis (Galindo et al, 1962). These minimal infections are urban and may well represent the most endemic infections, the symptomatic cases denoting the "tip of the iceberg." The most serious lesions are found in stable, agricultural, or fishing communities in which transmission continues for many years. Therefore, it is assumed that repetitive, prolonged exposure is necessary to induce elephantiasis or lymph scrotum.

Pathology and Pathogenesis

Epidemiologic findings and animal experiments clearly indicate that host reactions to microfilariae differ from those to adult worms. Experimentally, microfilaria-vaccinated hosts become amicrofilaremic, while adult worms develop normally and their uteri contain microfilariae (Wong et al, 1969). Longitudinal studies of experimental feline *Brugia* infections show that waning microfilaremia coincides with developing eosinophilia (Denham et al, 1972).

Although pathologic and clinical features differ between patients from endemic and nonendemic areas, significant humoral and cellular immune responses develop in both groups. Filaria-specific IgE titers rise, and IgE-eosinophil–mediated killing of microfilariae has been noted in vitro; parameters of T cell sensitization are also elevated. However, patients from endemic regions manifest IgG_4 blocking antibodies and antigen-specific suppressor T cells. The extent of immune down-regulation correlates with absence of pathologic sequelae and presence of microfilaremia. Moreover, individuals with hyperergic responses to filaria develop "occult" filarial syndromes, such as tropical eosinophilia or eosinophilic interstitial pneumonitis (Piessens, 1982; von Lichtenberg, 1987; Davis, 1989, and Ottesen, 1989). Despite advances in filarial immunopathology, such immune responses have not been proved to protect against repeated infection; both partial resistance to reinfection and partial enhancement have been demonstrated in different experimental systems (Ah et al, 1974a; Klei et al, 1974).

Human occult filariasis is characterized by circulating eosinophilia, eosinophilic infiltrates of affected lymph nodes or lung, and granulomas around damaged microfilariae. Microfilariae are often surrounded by stellate hyalin precipitates, Meyers-Kouvenaar (M-K) bodies, that resemble Splendore-Hoeppli phenomena and that contain antigen-antibody precipitates (Williams et al, 1969; Danaraj et al, 1966; Lie, 1962). Granulomas surrounding microfilariae occur in spleens of humans (see Fig. 22–22) and infected baboons (Orihel and Moore, 1975). Thus host reactivity to microfilariae ranges from delayed to reaginic hypersensitivity.

Adult worms elicit the significant urogenital lesions in lymphatic filariasis. The course of filariasis can be divided into the prepatent period, early established infection, and late infection. The manifestation further varies with the location of worms and interposition of complications.

The Prepatent Period

The prepatent period is known principally from experimental *Brugia* infections in cats, dogs, and birds, but a few tissue specimens from World War II soldiers in a comparable stage confirmed experimental studies (Wartman, 1947). Lesions are diffuse and poorly related to the number and size of developing worms; they probably represent responses to exoantigens, rather than somatic antigens. The lymph vessels harboring worms are dilated or varicose ("lymphangiectasis") but only mildly inflamed with a few eosinophils and lymphocytes. There is considerable edema, vasodilatation, and inflammatory infiltration of the tissues drained by the lymphatics, including hydrocele (von Lichtenberg, 1957). Lymph nodes are enlarged with lymphoreticular proliferation and eosinophilia, but the relationship of lymph nodal involvement and the edema is not clear. In *Brugia*-infected dogs, fragments of molted cuticle and egg shells were found in the infiltrate (Schacher and Sahyoun, 1967). In human biopsy specimens, adult worms are rarely found, but the character of areolar tissue and lymph nodal inflammation is distinctive. Most lesions of prepatent filariasis remit spontaneously or after treatment and appear to be reversible.

Early Established Infection

In contrast, lesions of established infection do not remit but either persist actively or yield significant scarring and lymphatic obstruction. Lesions may appear at worm nesting areas (funiculoepididymitis, orchitis, filarial lymphangitis, filarial abscess), in their lymphatic distribution (e.g., hydrocele, lymphadenitis, genital edema), or both. Dying or dead adult filariae are often detected in surgically excised tissue, which suggests that worm death provokes the filarial attack.

The lesions vary from nodular inflammation, simulating neoplasm, to suppuration, simulating acute bacterial disease (Fig. 22–24; see also Fig. 22–23). In both instances, the lymphatics within which the reaction centers become obliterated far beyond the site of the dying worms (von Lichtenberg, 1957).

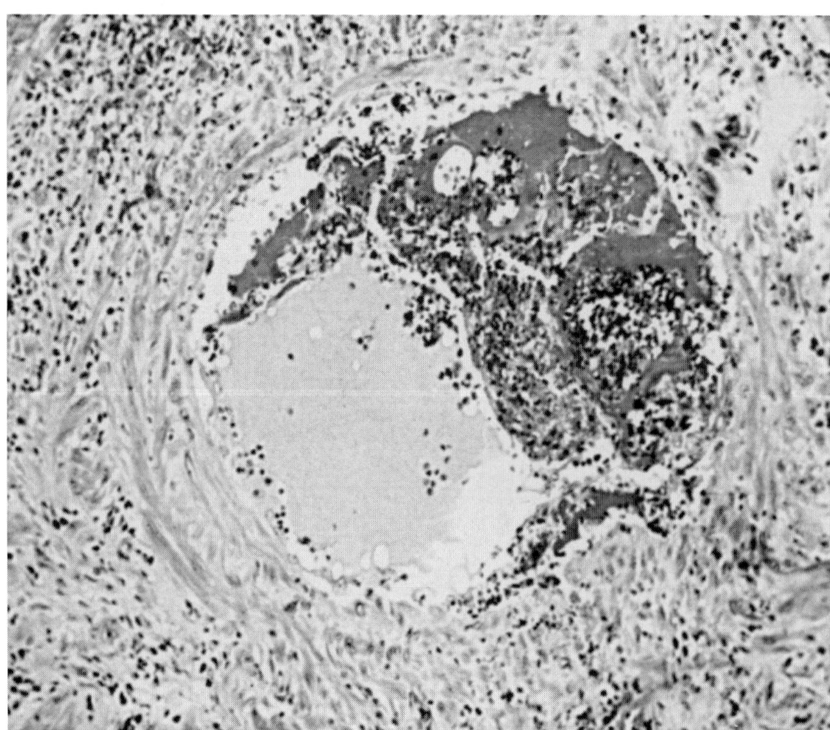

Figure 22–24. Inflamed lymph vessel of cord distant from site of adult filarial worm, showing diffuse inflammation and thrombosis with fibrin and red blood cells. (Magnification, ×100.)

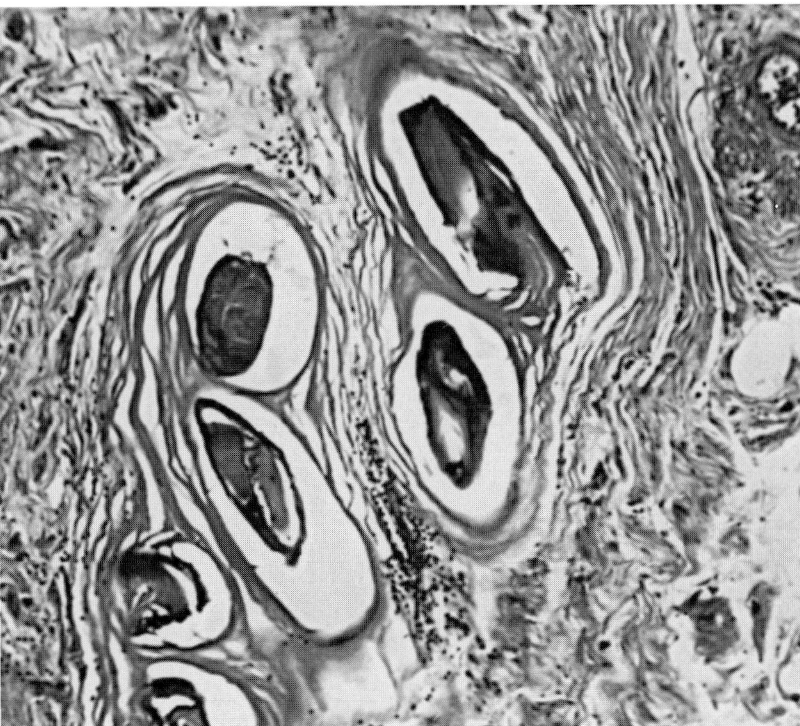

Figure 22–25. Coiled, calcified adult filaria with concentric fibrosis and minimal lymphoid infiltrate found in epididymis of a patient with hydrocele. (Magnification, ×200.)

Histologically, nodular lesions show massive granulomas around cuticular fragments or necrotic filaria. Similar but smaller granulomas can occur in the draining lymph nodes and, in the absence of filarial fragments, may be misdiagnosed as tuberculosis. The granulomatous response often affects one portion of a worm while adjacent worm segments appear intact or calcified or have a mild foreign body reaction (Fig. 22–25). Tissue eosinophilia is a useful diagnostic hint but may be absent. Surrounding and distant areolar tissues exhibit edema and primarily lymphoid infiltrates, often around blood vessels, or in lymphangiolar walls where infiltrates may protrude to form inflammatory polyps (polypoid lymphangitis). More violent reactions precipitate fibrin thrombi within lymphatics or microhemorrhages (see Figs. 22–23 and 22–24). Adjacent veins may also be inflamed and thrombosed (von Lichtenberg, 1957).

The most acute, exudative filarial lesions, especially subcutaneous, simulate fluctuant abscesses with rich, whitish purulent exudate (composed of variable mixtures of neutrophils and eosinophils) that surrounds a dying worm and is bacteriologically sterile (O'Connor and Hulse, 1935). The inflammatory process often ascends in a cordlike manner along a lymph vessel, with exudate found in remote branches and aggregates of granulocytes in regional lymph nodes. The worms have obviously lived innocuously before these inflammatory episodes, and the mechanism that initiates these "filarial attacks" is poorly understood.

Episodic filarial inflammation eventually abates, leaving obliterated lymphatics surrounded by poorly organized granulation and scar tissue. The nodules around dead worms shrink; with mild inflammation and calcific worms, scars may be only a few millimeters in size and difficult to detect except by tissue-clearing methods (Galindo et al, 1962). Conversely, after severe and continued smoldering inflammation, a palpable mass or indurated cord may develop. The consequences of lymphatic obstruction vary with the location of the obstruction (vide infra); their common feature is the accumulation of protein- and cholesterol-rich edema or hydrocele fluid associated with lymphoid infiltrates.

Late Infection

Neither the pathology nor the pathophysiology of filarial lymphatic obstruction is fully understood. Lymphangiographic studies reveal that initial obliteration of lymphatic vessels is bypassed by collateral formation; later, these collaterals become progressively obstructed, and, finally, deficient lymph drainage follows. Lymphatic obstruction is enhanced as adult filariae from successive reinfections settle in progressively more distal lymph vessels. Thus in primary feline *Brugia* infections, worms localize in the popliteal trunk; worms from subsequent infections lodge in more distal lymphatics, choking off collaterals (Ewert, 1971). Lymphangiograms in late filariasis show rich networks of intercommunicating lymph vessels extending through lymphedematous tissues into superficial dermal layers, but these drain poorly into the inguinofemoral and iliac trunks (Kanetkar et al, 1966; Cohen et al, 1961). It is yet uncertain whether normally present lymphaticovenous fistulae dilate in filariasis. Significant phlebosclerosis and phlebothrombosis probably contribute to developing lymphedema, especially in the spermatic cord, but their importance remains uncertain. Indeed, long-term treatment of filarial lymphedema and elephantiasis with the anticlotting agent coumarin has been reported to yield good results (Casley-Smith et al, 1993).

A relationship of lymphatic obstruction to filarial infection intensity has been proved in experimental *Brugia* infection (Ewert, 1971). Heavy infections of filariasis alone can produce lymphedema, but swelling and inflammation are exacerbated if the impaired extremity is exposed to virulent

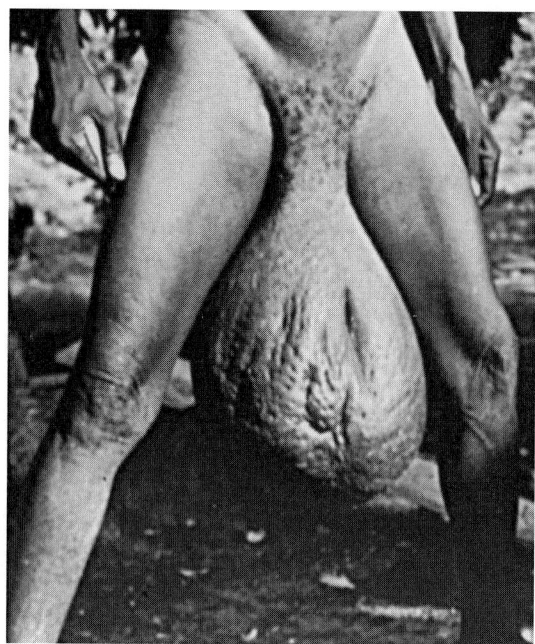

Figure 22–26. Huge hydrocele and scrotal elephantiasis. (Courtesy of Dr. B. H. Kean. From Zaiman H: A Pictorial Presentation of Parasites. Available from H. Zaiman, M.D., P.O. Box 543, Valley City, ND 58072.)

streptococcal superinfection (Bosworth and Ewert, 1975). Although bacteria play no role in chyluria and filarial hydrocele is rarely superinfected, elephantiasis and lymph scrotum are often superinfected. Thus bacterial superinfection is probably an important contributing factor, and after lymphedema has become established, it is unavoidable, especially in farmers or laborers. To further confirm the role of infection, it has been noted that classical elephantiasis can be prevented when patients with swollen limbs are instructed to use antiseptic soap and have access to antibiotics (Erik Ottesen, personal communication, 1995).

Preference of anatomic sites of bancroftian filaria has not been methodically studied in humans, especially in women, and the relationship of these predilections to pathologic consequences remain muddled. Serial autopsy studies of men show that the tail of the epididymis and the lower spermatic cord are the most constant locations of worms and often the only sites found to be affected in mild infections (Galindo et al, 1962). Correspondingly, funiculoepididymitis is the most common direct consequence of bancroftian filariasis, and hydrocele the most common indirect one. Thus far no filariae have been found in the cisterna chyli or thoracic duct.

Assuming that heavy infections saturate the preferred habitat and compel adult filariae to spread centrifugally to increasingly distant sites, saturation of inguinal lymphatic trunks (yielding scrotal edema) initiates encroachment into femoral lymphatics (causing elephantiasis of lower extremities and proximally to renal lymphangioles (producing lymph varices whose intrapelvic rupture causes chyluria). This hypothesis is bolstered by the greater frequency of these sequelae (except in epididymitis and hydrocele) in areas of high filarial transmission and in heavily infected individuals; however, direct proof is not available.

The outcome of permanent lymphatic obstruction is most simply portrayed by chyluria, in which protein- and lipid-rich lymph leaks into urine, rendering it cloudy or milky. In hydrocele, fluid is stored in the scrotal cavity, varying from clear, slightly viscid liquid (Fig. 22–26) to a milky or even cheesy material; prolonged retention of this fluid provokes chronic lymphoplasmocytic inflammation, rarely calcification, and fibrotic thickening of the tunica (Figs. 22–27 and 22–28). These secondary changes render the scrotal contents increasingly vulnerable to trauma with resultant minor bleeding and further calcium and cholesterol deposition (von Lichtenberg and Medina, 1957).

Likewise, the edema of filarial elephantiasis has high-protein and high-cholesterol content, which differentiates it from hydrostatic edema. Permanent lymphedema in the subcutaneous tissue and dermis is regularly accompanied by lymphoid cell infiltrates, often around dilated lymph vessels containing polypoid lymphangitis or thrombi. These ectatic vessels can be seen (with or without dye injection) when the dermis is thin, especially over the scrotum. Perivasculitis with thickening of blood vessels and, later, fibroblastic and epithelial proliferation ensue as the process continues. Plump fibroblasts deposit ground substance and gradually form thick, dense collagen. The epidermis may undergo pseudoepitheliomatous hyperplasia with hyperkeratosis and acquires

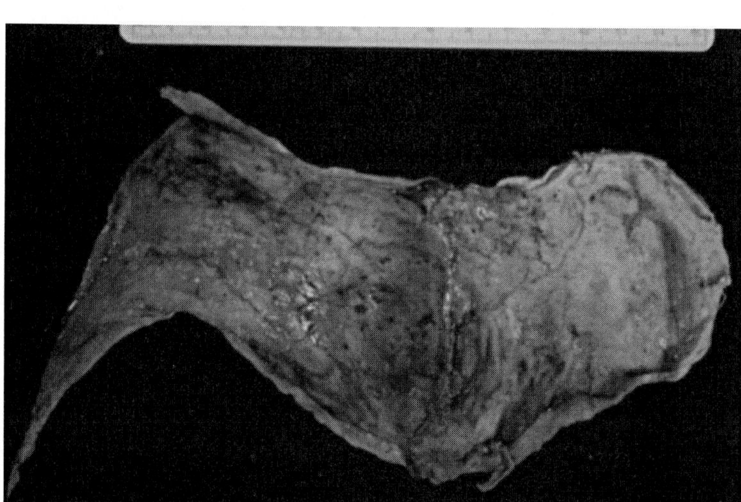

Figure 22–27. Excised hydrocele sac with marked fibrous thickening and focal calcification, plus recent focal hemorrhages.

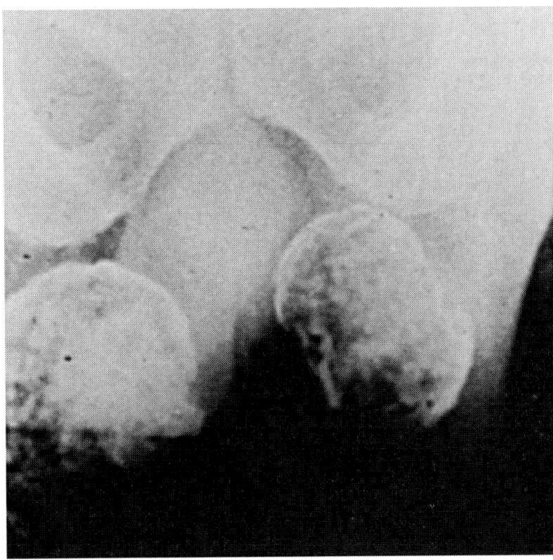

Figure 22–28. Bilateral intrascrotal calcifications in a filariasis patient. (Courtesy of Dr. B. H. Kean. Reproduced from Zaiman H: A Pictorial Presentation of Parasites. Available from H. Zaiman, M.D., P.O. Box 543, Valley City, ND 58072.)

the pachydermal appearance of elephantiasis (Fig. 22–29). Initially, the dermis is boggy but later becomes tough. Persistent unlimited connective tissue and epidermal growth produces grotesque penile, scrotal, or extremity enlargement. Bacterial or fungal superinfection leads to recurrent lymphangitis, erysipelas, chronic festering ulcer, or persisting fungal crusting, aggravating the ensconced vicious cycle.

Clinical Manifestations

Clinical lymphatic filariasis manifests as one of five forms, depending on the host's origin and immune responsiveness: (1) endemic normal, (2) asymptomatic microfilaremia, (3) filarial fevers (and symptomatic expatriates), (4) chronic pathology, and (5) tropical eosinophilia (von Lichtenberg, 1987; Ottesen, 1989). Superimposed upon these "archetypes" is the natural progression from prepatent through late infection.

Endemic Normal

Endemic normal patients have positive serologic or skin test reactivity to filarial antigens but no microfilaremia and no clinical evidence of filariasis. Their specific IgE antifilarial antibody levels are comparable with those of other "archetypal" groups but both significantly higher than that of asymptomatic microfilaremia and lower than that of tropical eosinophilia. Many such patients may be in the prepatent period.

Asymptomatic Microfilaremia

Asymptomatic microfilaremia patients have down-regulated effector immune responses. They develop both antigen-specific T-cell effector mechanisms and IgE antibodies, but these are made ineffective by filarial antigen-specific suppressor T cell subsets and blocking IgG_4 antibodies (Ottesen, 1989). Such individuals probably developed tolerance to filarial antigens in utero (Weil et al, 1983). In addition, generation of elevated levels of interleukin-12 (IL-12) has been noted in individuals with chronic microfilaremia (King et al, 1995).

Filarial Fevers and Chronic Pathology

Patients with filarial fevers and chronic pathology have prominent "effector-type" immune T cell and B cell responses but lack adequate down-regulating T cell responses and blocking antibodies. Patients with filarial fever sustain episodic fevers, lymphangitis/lymphadenitis, funiculoepididymitis, transient edema, and small acute hydroceles and are typically amicrofilaremic. Patients with chronic pathology have chronic hydroceles, fixed lymphedema, elephantiasis, chyluria, lymph scrotum, and so forth and are often amicrofilaremic. Thus the deficiency of down-regulation of filaria-specific "effector" responses lets those responses destroy filariae with consequent amicrofilaremia but, concomitantly, creates irreversible anatomic and pathophysiologic damage to the host. Expatriates, residing in endemic areas long enough to sustain repeated filarial infections, constitute one moiety of the "filarial fever" group; unlike patients with endemic "filarial fever" who inexorably progress to "chronic pathology," their disease abates, presumably because repatriation averts further infection. Thus lymphatic filarial *disease* affects only *filaria-infected* patients whose down-regulation of their "effector" immune responses are deficient.

Early established filariasis evolves from prepatent filariasis and progresses to the late chronic stage with a series of recurrently progressive lesions: hydrocele, funiculoepididymitis, orchitis, scrotal and penile elephantiasis, lymph scrotum, and chyluria. These partially revert upon treatment

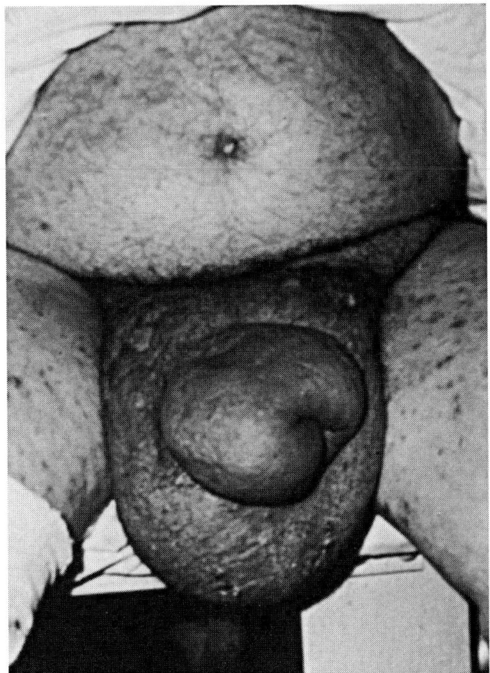

Figure 22–29. Elephantiasis of the penis and scrotum. (Courtesy of Dr. M. Wittner. Reproduced from Zaiman H: A Pictorial Presentation of Parasites. Available from H. Zaiman, M.D., P.O. Box 543, Valley City, ND 58072.)

or cessation of repeated exposure. Bancroftian filariasis initially centers in the epididymis and spreads centrifugally with continued duration and repeated infections. Brugian filariasis usually commences in lymphatics distal to the urogenital tract; thus urologic involvement is less common and occurs later in the progression of the disease.

FUNICULOEPIDIDYMITIS. Most symptomatic cases of filarial funiculoepididymitis appear before patients' fourth decade. The attack may be isolated with remission or may be repetitive and progressive. Although intrascrotal portions of the cord are favored, higher intra-abdominal portions can be involved. Local pain, often radiating to the testis or simulating ureteral colic, may be accompanied by systemic symptoms (fever, chills, and anorexia) and marked anxiety.

Palpably lumpy or cordlike swelling may mimic an intrascrotal tumor or torsion of the cord and may be accompanied by hydrocele or soft tissue edema. Granulocytemia with variable eosinophilia is common. Varicocele or thrombosis of the pampiniform plexus may complicate inflammation, augmenting pain and discomfort. Bacterial superinfection of acute filarial corditis, a rare but often lethal complication, brings exquisite pain, high fever, septic thrombophlebitis, and pyemia or endocarditis. A nonfilarial form of thrombophlebitis of the cord has also been reported from India (Castellani, 1931).

Prognosis of the funicular filarial attack is uncertain. Mild cases *may* involute spontaneously, but in an endemic setting, they more often augur future recurrences and/or the development of chronic lymphedema (Kazura et al, 1995). Because the disease frequently simulates clinical malignancy, many patients ultimately undergo operations, often with homolateral orchiectomy; the criteria for surgical intervention have not been formulated. Even in severe filarial funiculitis, the spermatic cord is usually intact and patent, unlike that in ascending bacterial infection; sterility due to filariasis is rare. We believe that a rational therapy of filarial funiculoepididymitis requires a thorough work-up differentiating malignant, filarial, and bacterial etiologies. Appropriate antibiotics should be prescribed for bacterial disease, and filariasis should be treated by surgical decompression or excision of filarial nodules, preserving the testis and cord. When funiculoepididymitis is recurrent, painful, and deforming or complicated by blood vessel involvement, more radical surgery is warranted. New approaches, such as funicular lymphangiography and lymph flow studies, are needed.

ORCHITIS. This complication is rare and has many features noted in the preceding section. It *may* simulate a rapidly developing testicular malignant tumor.

HYDROCELE. Differentiation of filarial from idiopathic hydrocele is difficult on either clinical or laboratory grounds; some features may permit an inferential judgment. Microfilariae or adult worms are rarely detected in the hydrocele fluid, but a milky or sediment-rich hydrocele fluid suggests a filarial origin. Hydrocele accompanied by nodules in the cord or epididymis and a history of travel to or residence in an endemic area augurs filariasis. Discovery of a thick, fibrous tunica, especially with cholesterol or calcium deposits, should prompt a diagnosis of filariasis; indeed, tunical calcification is so rare in idiopathic hydrocele that its presence strongly suggests infectious, especially filarial, etiology. Excision of the hydrocele sac—if possible, intact—is the treatment of choice; an alternative method is inversion with partial excision (Jachowski et al, 1962). Small hydroceles that do not enlarge can be ignored.

SCROTAL AND PENILE ELEPHANTIASIS AND LYMPH SCROTUM. Mild scrotal edema is not unusual during early infection or with established hydrocele. Penile edema is unusual, and the monstrous elephantine enlargements of the scrotum or penis depicted in textbooks occur largely in populations without access to medical care. Occasionally, such penile or scrotal lesions present to urologists for care (Sato et al, 1974). Elephantiasis of the limbs pose the difficult differential diagnosis between filarial and other etiologies (*elephantiasis nostras*), but genital elephantiasis is rarely due to other causes, such as malignancy, lymph node surgery, or radiation. The only treatment currently available is excision and plastic reconstruction by full-thickness skin grafting (Jantet et al, 1961); unless associated bacterial infection is present, surgical healing is usually decent, despite lymphorrhea during and after surgery. Because the physiologic derangement is not corrected by such procedures, recurrence is common (although systematic data on recurrence frequency are not available), and repeat operations are less successful and carry greater risk of local complications.

Lymph scrotum is profuse scrotal edema, with blistering and weeping of lymph spontaneously; this uncommon condition is practically pathognomonic of severe filarial infection. Because the moist intercrural area is easily superinfected by cutaneous or colonic bacteria or fungi, festering skin ulcers and/or systemic sepsis often ensue. Lymph scrotum is difficult to treat medically, but excision can be effective.

CHYLURIA. Chyluria occurs with or without microfilaremia, usually in young adults; it arises earlier in the natural history of filariasis than genital elephantiasis. Dying worms provoke lymphatic obstruction with proximal lymphangiolar dilatation. Rupture of a lymphatic varix into the urinary collecting system has been demonstrated by lymphangiography. One or more lymph fistulae occur most often near the renal calyces (Tani and Akisada, 1970). Chyluria may initially alarm patients but often is disregarded and may result in protein loss exceeding hepatic albumin synthesis, leading to hypoalbuminemia and anasarca; chyluria is usually intermittent, and protein loss is minor. It may spontaneously remit with bed rest and/or use of abdominal binders that increase intra-abdominal pressure enough to stop the leakage (Ahrens, 1970). Moreover, diagnostic retrograde lymphangiography curatively scleroses lymphatic fistulae in 48% of patients (Gandhi, 1976). Thus surgical correction is unnecessary in many cases; operative intervention is challenging because the varices are hard to identify and eliminate. Nephrectomy is rarely warranted.

Tropical Pulmonary Eosinophilia

Tropical pulmonary eosinophilia occurs in patients with a hyperreactive allergic response to microfilarial antigens and they are amicrofilaremic. This syndrome, variously named "occult" filariasis, eosinophilic lung, or Meyers-Kouvenaar syndrome, is characterized by marked, sustained peripheral eosinophilia only temporarily affected by corticosteroids but responsive to antifilarial drugs; absence of classic filarial lesions such as lymphedema or funiculoepididymitis; presence of lymphadenopathy that can be marked enough to simulate lymphoma; and striking pulmonary infiltrates, often associated with allergic manifestations, especially asthma (Danaraj et al, 1966; Lie, 1962). Patients develop very high levels of filaria-specific IgE and pulmonary reticulonodular densities on chest radiographs that reveal an eosinophilic interstitial pneumonitis on biopsy. Moreover, the basophils and mast cells of patients with tropical eosinophilia discharge histamine more vigorously when stimulated with microfilarial antigen than do cells of normal persons or of filaria-infected persons without the hypereosinophilic syndrome (Ottesen et al, 1979). The frequency of this syndrome varies markedly between endemic foci and is particularly predominant in southern India and in Singapore. Urologic manifestations are negligible.

Diagnosis

As in urinary schistosomiasis, distinction must be made between diagnosis of infection and diagnosis of disease.

Diagnosis of Infection

Findings of *Brugia* or *Wuchereria* microfilariae in peripheral blood, chylous urine, or hydrocele fluid are diagnostic. Species identification is based on the presence or absence of sheaths and on the number and position of nuclei in the caudal end (Taylor, 1960; Hunter et al, 1976). Samples must be taken when peak microfilaremia occurs (e.g., midnight, in the case of nocturnal periodic *W. bancrofti*). Peripheral blood is best examined by thick-drop technique with Giemsa stain. Concentration methods include filtration or centrifugation of hemolyzed blood. Direct observation by ultrasonography of adult filariae has been reported in lymph vessels of microfilaremic and otherwise asymptomatic patients, made possible by energetic movements of the worms ("filarial dance sign"), an important addition to the diagnostic armamentarium (Amaral et al, 1994). Furthermore, specific serodiagnostic tests for *W. bancrofti* infection are available at the Centers for Disease Control and Prevention, and an ELISA test evaluating IgG_4 antibody against recombinant filarial antigen has been field-tested with promising results (Dissanayake et al, 1994). Histologic finding of adult worms is a diagnostically definitive but insensitive technique, and lymphadenectomy may further compromise lymph drainage. Peripheral blood eosinophilia is not invariably present.

Recognition of Amicrofilaremic Filariasis

Amicrofilaremic disease occurs in four settings: (1) in early symptomatic cases, especially nonresidents exposed for the first time (military personnel, tourists); (2) in the late stages of filariasis, whether symptomatic or asymptomatic; (3) after treatment with a microfilaricide; and (4) as the distinctive syndrome, tropical pulmonary eosinophilia. Serologic test results are usually positive but do not differentiate among these four categories.

Diagnosis of Filarial Disease States

Careful history taking and physical examination are paramount in suggesting a filarial lymphedema, and yet all late filarial lesions have nonfilarial counterparts. Tuberculosis, schistosomiasis haematobium, and gonorrhea may produce funiculoepididymitis. Nonfilarial elephantiasis may result from malignancies, surgery, or x-irradiation, and there are idiopathic, infectious, and hereditary forms of lymphedema, some found in tropical areas without transmission of filaria. Idiopathic hydrocele with or without varicocele or hernia is common in tropical and nontropical areas, but hydrocele occurs at an earlier age and in greater frequency in areas of endemic filariasis (Jachowski et al, 1962).

Lymphangiography may distinguish filariasis from other causes of lymphatic obstruction, especially conditions with reduced numbers and competence of lymph vessels (Jantet et al, 1961). Also, plain x-ray films may reveal calcified worms, which are a diagnostic aid.

Treatment

Medical Management

Treatment of lymphatic filariasis has two objectives: (1) elimination of adult worms, which stops further progression of disease, and (2) abolition of microfilaremia, which interrupts vector-borne transmission. Most workers agree that persons with patent microfilaremia should be treated.

The *traditional* oral antimicrofilarial drug is diethylcarbamazine (DEC; Hetrazan, banocide), which promptly abolishes microfilaremia for at least several weeks. DEC *also* kills adult filariae, **but only at much higher dosages than are used for microfilariae,** and long-term low-dose treatment is reported to reduce the frequency of elephantiasis (Partono et al, 1981). In advanced filariasis, DEC has little effect on established pathology. Moreover, it causes allergic "Mazotti reactions" in patients treated for *Onchocerca volvulus* and similar, although milder, allergic side effects in patients with *Wuchereria* or *Brugia* species. Therefore, patients with high microfilarial counts should start with low doses of DEC (3 mg/kg body weight/day) and increase gradually to avoid severe symptoms. Otherwise, the recommended schedules are 6 mg/kg body weight/day for a total course of 72 mg/kg body weight for *W. bancrofti* and 4 mg/kg body weight/day for a total of 60 mg/kg body weight for *B. malayi*. Opinions vary regarding optimal scheduling and dosage. The schedule must be adjusted to the patient's reaction to the drug. Headache, fever, nausea, vomiting, and allergic manifestations occur, in addition to local pain and swelling over lymph nodes and along lymphatics. Generalized and allergic symptoms respond to antihistamines. The disadvantage of this regimen is that it requires *daily* treatment for nearly 2 weeks or more and repeated at 3- to 6-month intervals. This and its side effects often impair patient compliance.

Ivermectin in a single oral dose of 20 to 25 μg/kg body weight has proved to be an effective microfilaricide, comparable with DEC with fewer toxic and side reactions. Ivermectin will probably become the antimicrofilarial drug of choice, because of its convenience and low expense (Ottesen et al, 1990), but it must be repeated *at half-yearly intervals* to avert recurrent microfilaremia. **Ivermectin has *no* effect on adult filariae.**

In any case, most authorities now concur that an effective anti–adult filarial drug is the *desideratum* and, when available, will replace microfilaricides. Until that time, the reader is advised to turn to an experienced tropical medicine consultant or to the Parasitic Disease Section of the Center for Disease Control and Prevention, Atlanta, Georgia, which maintains a repository of antifilarial drugs and can furnish detailed information about their use. Hints for the nonsurgical therapy of chyluria are given elsewhere in this text.

Foot and skin care is very important in the management of lymphedema. To further confirm the role of infection, it has been noted that classical elephantiasis can be prevented when patients with swollen limbs are instructed to use antiseptic soap and have access to antibiotics (Ottesen, Erik; personal communication, 1995). Superimposed bacterial infections, particularly with streptococci, must be treated vigorously.

SURGICAL MANAGEMENT

Genital elephantiasis is often amenable to surgery. A variety of procedures have been devised to remove edematous and fibrous tissue and to reconstruct the scrotum or vulva. For local management, the reader is referred to the preceding sections dealing with specific complications.

Prognosis

ACUTE FILARIASIS IN THE RECENTLY INFECTED PATIENT

The experience in the World War II Pacific theater has shown that early filariasis can produce considerable physical and psychologic discomfort. The migratory nature of the tissue swellings, the marked itchiness, genital area localization, and uncertain prognosis frequently undermined the patient's self-confidence, particularly if he or she was familiar with the chronic deformities seen in endemic populations. However, long-term follow-up has revealed that incidentally infected patients rarely develop hydrocele or elephantiasis.

LATE CHRONIC STAGES

The prognosis of elephantiasis in patients receiving medical treatment is not known, although it is unusual for marked progression to continue. In some treated patients, elephantiasis continues to progress, whereas in other patients, a slow improvement has been noted.

Prevention and Control

DEC has been used as a prophylactic drug, given in a small monthly dose. Trials with prophylactic ivermectin have similar salutary effects. Major control methods include the use of residual insecticides, the use of domestic mosquito netting, and the reduction of mosquito-breeding sites.

Onchocerciasis

Onchocerca volvulus is the agent of African river blindness and of severe, debilitating, chronic dermatitis. Onchocerciasis is common throughout tropical Africa, and endemic foci also exist in Central and South America, with some regional variation in the clinical pattern. This filaria differs sharply from *Brugia* and *Wuchereria* in that (1) it is transmitted by black flies of the *Simulium* species, (2) adult worms inhabit subcutaneous tissue and cause palpable fibrous nodules in which they are encapsulated, and (3) microfilariae diffusely pervade the dermis (and the eye) but are not in the peripheral blood. Diagnosis and estimation of infection intensity are made by microscopic examination of skin snips immersed in normal saline for 20 to 30 minutes under a coverslip on a slide or (after air drying) with Giemsa stain.

In the late stages when blindness and atrophic dermatitis are the principal infirmities, onchocercal infection may produce "hanging groin" or scrotal elephantiasis. A few hanging groins have been successfully excised with good primary wound closure. Excised surgical specimens show atrophy and fibrosis in the inguinal lymph nodes with subcutaneous edema and fibrosis superimposed on the usual onchocercal dermatitis (Connor et al, 1970). The pathogenesis of "hanging groin" is uncertain, but the condition occurs in areas where *Wuchereria* or *Brugia* infection are not found (Connor et al, 1970). Onchocerciasis is occasionally accompanied by giant inguinal lymphadenopathy, which may be an antecedent to "hanging groin." Most patients with onchocercal "hanging groin" are from rural Africa, where prevention of infection is now a high priority in order to ensure continued and improved agriculture.

Therapy has been difficult in the past. Suramin is a toxic but effective adult filaricide without much action against microfilariae. Microfilaricide therapy with DEC is complicated by severe allergic immune responses to microfilariae dying in the skin and other sites (the Mazotti reaction). This, combined with the prolonged course of daily doses, has minimized patient compliance. A single oral dose of ivermectin (125 μg/kg body weight) has proved to be a successful onchocercal microfilaricide with few side reactions, which are easily controlled with antihistaminics (Aziz, 1982; Greene et al, 1985). Periodic ivermectin distribution has been successfully used for curbing *Onchocerca volvulus* transmission in a multinational campaign against African river blindness under the auspices of the World Health Organization, once again demonstrating that prevention is preferable to cure.

OTHER PARASITIC DISEASES OF THE GENITOURINARY TRACT

Grouped in this section are descriptions of parasitic infections that are rare or in which urogenital manifestations are overshadowed by processes in other organs. These include the other human schistosomes, principally *S. mansoni* and *S. japonica*; the intestinal helminth *Enterobius*; the larval tapeworm of hydatid disease; and *Entamoeba histolytica* with all of its protean manifestations. The remainder of parasites in this group can be considered medical curiosities. Urogenital trichomoniasis and sexually transmitted enteric protozoan diseases are discussed in Section IV, Chapters 18 and 19.

Schistosomiasis mansoni and japonica

Although *S. mansoni* eggs are regularly deposited in the bladder and pelvic organs, their numbers are rarely substantial; in Egypt, the *S. mansoni* egg load was <1% of the *S.*

haematobium egg burden. *S. mansoni* and *S. japonica* can produce chronic cervicitis, asymptomatic intrascrotal lumps, or, in rare instances, subcutaneous granulomas of the penile or perineal skin. Eggs deposited in the kidney and urogenital passages may be shed in the urine or ejaculate in small numbers. Such findings should direct attention to more substantial schistosomal lesions of the intestinal tract, liver, pulmonary vasculature, and central nervous system.

Pelvic Enterobiasis

The common intestinal pinworm *Enterobius vermicularis*, which is ubiquitous worldwide, occasionally migrates from its nocturnal swarming site, the anus, into the vagina upward, reaching the peritoneal cavity via the uterus and fallopian tubes. In that unnatural habitat, worm movement and egg laying may continue producing inflammation of the pelvic peritoneum with pain, fever, simulated acute appendicitis, or other lesions. Dead worms and eggs incite granulomas and adhesions; these granulomas grossly resemble miliary tubercles and may cause confusion until the eggs are identified (Symmers, 1950). Eggs of pinworms differ from those of schistosomes but occasionally show Hoeppli phenomena. It is unusual to find *Ascaris* eggs in the same pelvic location without severe peritonitis or perforation (Waller and Othersen, 1971). Thus the correct parasitologic diagnosis is important. Treatment of pelvic enterobiasis is simply effected with pyrvinium pamoate or other systemic antihelminthics.

Hydatid Disease

No part of the human anatomy is invulnerable to hydatid cysts, but renal hydatids occur in only about 2% of cases (Borrell and Barnes, 1933; Musacchio and Mitchell, 1966). The hydatid is the larval form of *Echinococcus granulosus*, whose definitive host is the dog and whose principal intermediate host is the sheep. The major endemic loci of hydatidosis are sheep-herding areas, such as Australia, Argentina, Greece, Spain, and the Middle East. Although many of these areas have made progress in preventing transmission, cysts may emerge in previously infected patients during their

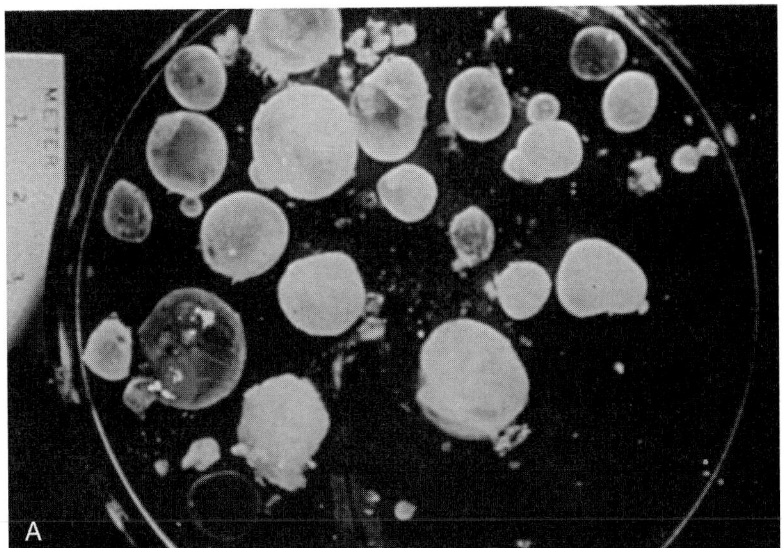

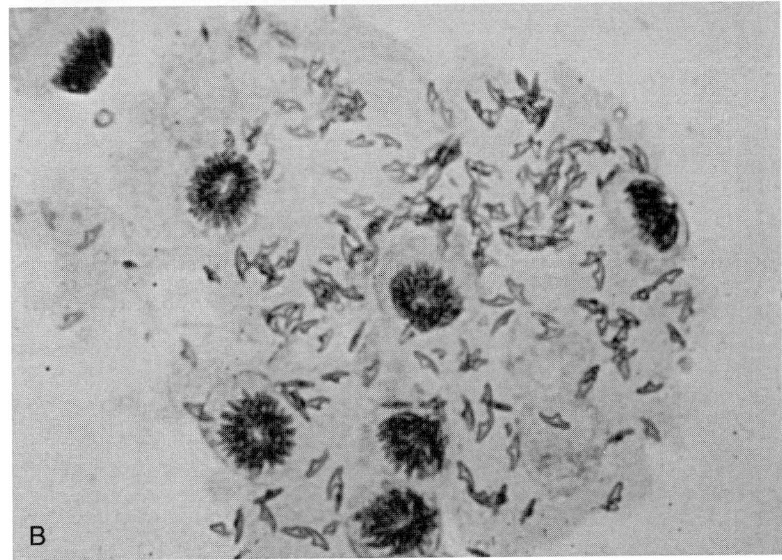

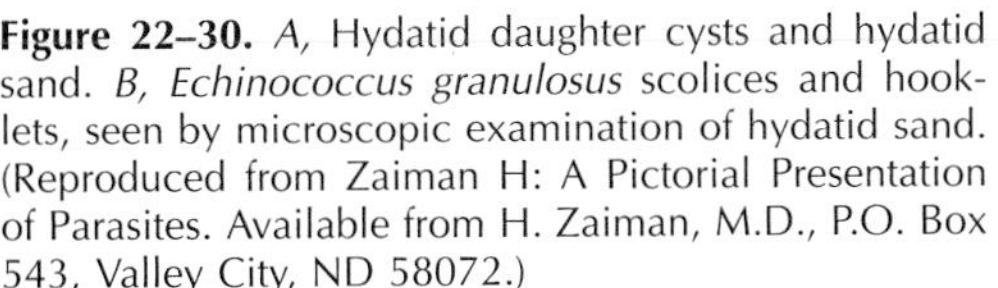

Figure 22–30. *A,* Hydatid daughter cysts and hydatid sand. *B, Echinococcus granulosus* scolices and hooklets, seen by microscopic examination of hydatid sand. (Reproduced from Zaiman H: A Pictorial Presentation of Parasites. Available from H. Zaiman, M.D., P.O. Box 543, Valley City, ND 58072.)

remaining lifetimes. In addition, feral life cycles lead to sporadic human cases in sites without sheep. Echinococcal cysts of other species are found in Alaska, Siberia, and parts of Europe *(E. multilocularis)* (Rausch, 1967) and in Central America *(E. vogeli)* (D'Alessandro et al, 1979). In each instance, humans acquire the cysts by accidentally eating eggs excreted in the feces of dogs or alternative feral hosts.

In the kidney or other urogenital sites, hydatid cysts evolve by the slow, asymptomatic, concentric growth over years and may invoke pressure symptoms or flank pain, depending on location and size. While viable and growing, the cyst wall is a thick, laminated polysaccharide parasite membrane on which the parasite's germinal epithelium is anchored (Fig. 22–30). The cyst is enveloped by a host fibrous shell with scant inflammatory reaction. Epithelial sprouts evaginate into the cyst, generating scolices and daughter cysts that may beget their own daughter cysts; each scolex constitutes a small, inverted tapeworm head recognizable by its crown of hooklets (see Fig. 22–30). Water-clear cyst fluid with a high protein and antigen content bathes germinal structures. Cysts can reach 20 cm in diameter but usually rupture earlier (Fig. 22–31).

The most common urologic presentation is of chronic dull flank or lower back discomfort from cystic pressure, rarely with microscopic hematuria. The cysts, being focal, seldom affect renal function. Diagnosis can be made by radiographs or CAT scans, which show a thick-walled, fluid-filled spherical cyst, often with a calcific cyst wall. When the radiographic appearance is not diagnostic, the Casoni skin test with hydatid fluid antigen or complement fixation and hemagglutination inhibition serologic testing (available through state laboratories or the Centers for Disease Control and Prevention) have proved useful. In most cases, diagnosis, *once suspected,* presents little difficulty. Treatment, if warranted, is by surgical excision; excision is elective, unless the cyst becomes superinfected by bacteria and constitutes a nidus of chronic urinary infection that is difficult to eradicate. Allergic manifestations of leaking or ruptured hydatid cysts may necessitate corticosteroids.

Rupture of cysts may be precipitous, attended by systemic anaphylaxis and spillage of cystic products into the peritoneum or the blood stream. New metastatic cysts may thus arise. Rupture into the renal pelvis occasions acute flank pain, followed by voiding of scolices or daughter cysts, with or without hematuria and/or obstruction of urinary passages (Borrell and Barnes, 1933; Musacchio and Mitchell, 1966). This unusual complication is diagnosed from the presence of scolices or single hooklets in the urinary sediment. The refringent 5-μm hooklets must be searched for carefully. Slow leakage results in the involution of the cyst, which fills with debris, cholesterol, daughter cysts, and "hydatid sand" composed of dead and/or viable scolices and hooklets and eventually calcifies.

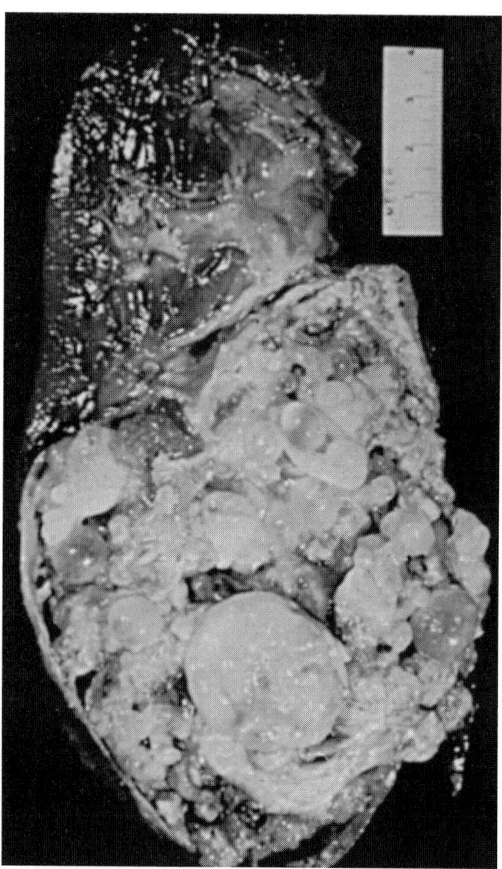

Figure 22–31. Echinococcosis of the human kidney.

Amoebiasis

In invasive infections by *Entamoeba histolytica,* the kidney is the fifth most common site of abscess localization (Brandt and Perez Tamayo, 1970). The abscess is invariably accompanied by other invasive lesions, particularly liver abscesses. The right kidney is more frequently involved. The pathologic lesion is like that in the liver. Hematuria may be a prominent manifestation, especially if the abscess induces renal vein thrombosis. The prognosis is often lethal, and medical therapy (metronidazole, emetine, or chloroquine) must be promptly instituted. **Surgery, if necessary, should be delayed until drug therapy has taken hold; otherwise, disastrous spread of amebic infection is likely (Grigsby, 1969).**

Amebic ulceration of the perineum (e.g., anal skin, scrotum, and penis) occurs in continuity with rectal ulcers or by fecal contamination of abraded skin. These lesions, although rare, are extremely destructive and can permanently deform the area (Engman and Meleney, 1931). Clinical awareness is important, because the lesions resemble bacterial or fusospirillary ulcers, but their undermined margins, necrotic and discolored surface, and indolence should lead to microscopic identification of amebae on trichrome or iron hematoxylin–stained smears of freshly collected necrotic exudate. These procedures are preferable to biopsy diagnosis. Such lesions are most likely in children in endemic areas where hygiene is poor and water scarce; most have or have had dysentery. Amebiasis of the urethra and bladder is usually part of devastating invasive amebiasis with other systemic lesions that bring the patient to a physician. Good reviews on the pathology (Brandt and Perez Tamayo, 1970), surgery (Grigsby, 1969), and medical management of amoebiasis (Powell, 1969; Barrett-Connor, 1972) are available.

Stray Parasites of the Urogenital Organs

Many nematode species that have migratory larvae or that can produce ectopic lesions have been detected in urine or urogenital organs; these include *Strongyloides stercoralis* in *Strongyloides* hyperinfection (Whitehill and Miller, 1944), *Toxocara canis* (visceral larva migrans) (Dent et al, 1965), and *Armillifer armillatus* (a primitive pentastomid acquired from reptiles, seen chiefly in Africa and Southeast Asia) (Cannon, 1942; Lindner, 1965; Hopps, 1971). Rare organisms that have at one time or another been reported in human urine are flies and insect larvae (Sanjurjo, 1970), and even fish: *Vandelia cirrhosa*, or Candiru, a small Amazonian catfish (Lins, 1945).

EFFECT OF PARASITIC INFECTIONS ON THE KIDNEY

Improving clinical laboratories in tropical countries have discovered greater frequencies of proteinuria and nephrosis-nephritis than are reported from temperate, industrialized countries. Children and young adults are particularly affected. Populations with a propensity for renal disease usually have diverse endemic infectious and parasitic diseases, including malaria, schistosomiasis, salmonellosis, leprosy, filariasis, hepatitis, and streptococcal infection. Thus it is difficult in individual cases or populations to ascribe the disease to a single agent. Even so, physicians must recognize nephropathy as an important health hazard in the tropics and must appropriately screen individuals belonging to high-risk groups, even if they are symptom free.

Some of the etiologic factors of tropical nephropathies are well defined. Malarial antigen and specific antibody globulin have been demonstrated in glomerular basement membranes of nephrotic children infected with *Plasmodium malariae* and in macaque and *Aotus* monkeys with primate malarias (Ward and Conran, 1969; Voller et al, 1973). Although not unique to quartan malaria, this nephropathy is more often associated with *P. malariae*, possibly because of its frequently long subclinical course. Glomerular damage in malarial nephrosis involves both the classic and alternate complement pathways. The chronic and progressive course of malarial nephrosis is relatively unresponsive to corticosteroid therapy. Affected patients have hyperglobulinemia and show distinctive serum protein clearance patterns (Soothill and Hendrickse, 1967). Eradication of quartan malaria in an endemic focus substantially decreases the number of cases of childhood nephrosis (Gilles and Hendrickse, 1963).

A relationship among proteinuria, nephropathy, and schistosomiasis mansoni has also been confirmed. Urinary protein excretion was significantly higher in schistosome-infected than in noninfected individuals in a malaria-free zone of Brazil, even though severe manifestations of schistosomiasis were uncommon (Lehman et al, 1975). Mesangial glomerular proliferation with focal membranous change is significantly increased in patients with *S. mansoni* infections with hepatosplenic disease: that is, severe infection with hepatic pipe stem fibrosis (Andrade et al, 1971; Andrade and Rocha, 1979). These changes (Fig. 22–32) have also been reproduced in chimpanzees (Cavallo et al, 1974) and in other experimental animals (Hillyer and Lewert, 1974). Renal failure ensues in relatively few patients. The pathogenesis of this entity remains uncertain, but circulating antigen of schistosome gut origin (von Lichtenberg et al, 1974) is detectable in experimental and human *S. mansoni* infection. Immunoglobulins and complement fractions (de Brito et al, 1971) and schistosome antigens (Moriearty and Brito, 1977; de Water et al, 1988) are deposited in the mesangium and in glomerular loops of human and experimental animals.

Similar findings appear with lepromatous leprosy, in which specific immune complexes have been found in the

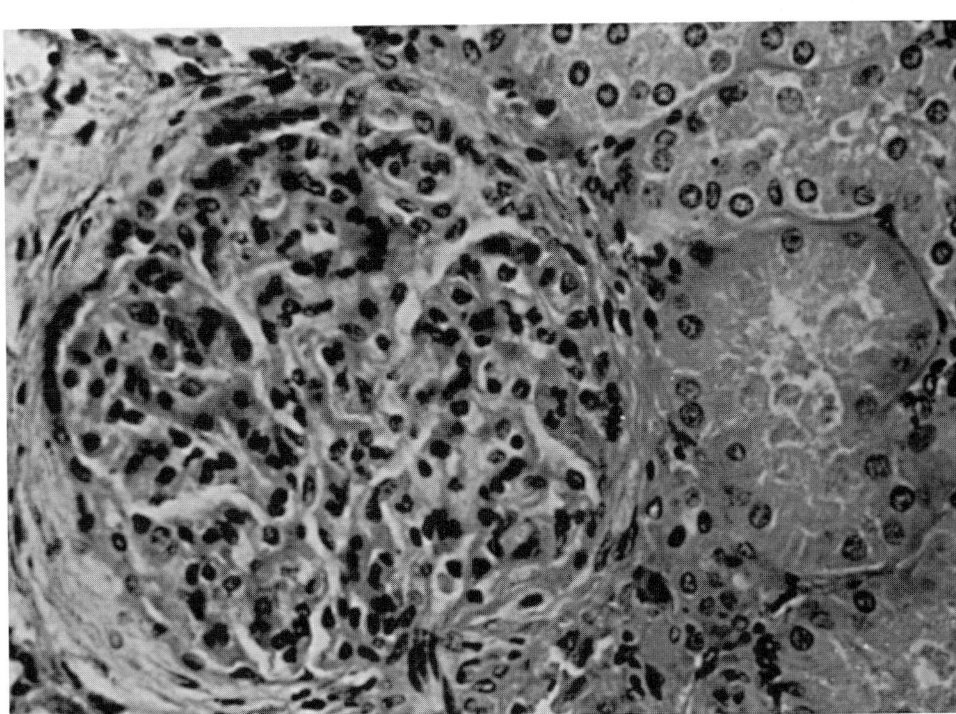

Figure 22–32. Glomerulus of experimental primate with schistosomal nephropathy. Note mesangial and capsular proliferation and neutrophils in glomerular loops. (Magnification, ×420.)

glomeruli (Moran et al, 1972); the antigen is reputedly the same protein-linked polysaccharide found in arterioles of erythema nodosum leprosum. Nephropathy with renal antigen-antibody complexes and electron micrographic abnormalities have been shown in *Dirofilaria*-infected dogs and in *Brugia*-infected hamsters (Klei et al, 1974) but have not yet been documented in chronic human filariasis. Nephritic kidney changes have been reported in cattle infected with *Trypanosoma congolense*, and marked proliferative nephritis was seen in macaques experimentally infected with *T. rhodesiense*; this renal lesion also involves both the classic and alternate complement pathway (Nagle et al, 1974). Disseminated intravascular coagulation rather than nephritis causes renal failure in human acute Rhodesian trypanosomiasis, but chronic Gambian sleeping sickness has not yet been studied nephrologically. Renal amyloidosis is a well-known complication of human and experimental leprosy and filariasis. Salmonella bacilli "hide" in the tegument of schistosomes (Young et al, 1973), emerging recurrently to produce septicemia and/or a hypocomplementary nephrotic syndrome (diffuse endocapillary proliferative glomerulonephritis), the so-called schistosomiasis-salmonellosis syndrome (Higashi et al, 1975), previously discussed with urinary schistosomiasis.

Thus in tropical countries, endemic parasitic infections are added to other causes of nephropathy that exist in temperate zones; a variety of nephropathies are often lumped under the label "tropical mesangiocapillary (membranoproliferative) glomerulonephritis." This subject has expanded greatly; the reader is referred to an excellent treatise (Sinniah et al, 1988).

REFERENCES

Urinary Schistosomiasis

Abdel-Halim RE: Ileal loop replacement and restoration of kidney function in extensive bilharziasis of the ureter. Br J Urol 1980; 52:280.

Abdel-Halim RE: Bilharzial uropathies and a scheme for primary medical care. Br J Urol 1984; 56:13.

Abdel-Halim RE, Al-Mashad S, Al-Dabbagh A: Fluoroscopic assessment of bilharzial ureteropathy. Clin Radiol 1985; 36:89.

Abdel-Salam E, Abdel-Fattah M: Prevalence and morbidity of *Schistosoma haematobium* in Egyptian children. A controlled study. Am J Trop Med Hyg 1977; 26:463.

Abdel-Salam E, Ehsan A: Cystoscopic picture of *Schistosoma haematobium* in Egyptian children correlated with intensity of infection and morbidity. Am J Trop Med Hyg 1978; 27:774.

Abdel-Tawab GA, Aboul-Azm T, Ebied SA, et al: The correlation between certain tryptophane metabolites and the N-nitrosamine content in the urine of bilharzial bladder cancer patients. J Urol 1986; 135:826.

Abdel-Wahab MF, Esmat G, Ramzy I, et al: *Schistosoma haematobium* infection in Egyptian school children: demonstration of both hepatic and urinary tract morbidity by ultrasonography. Trans R Soc Trop Med Hyg 1992a; 86:406.

Abdel-Wahab MF, Ramzy I, Esmat G, et al: Ultrasound for detecting *Schistosoma haematobium* urinary tract complications: comparison with radiographic procedures. J Urol 1992b; 148:346.

Abdel-Wahab MF, Strickland GT: Abdominal ultrasonography for assessing morbidity from schistosomiasis 2. Hospital studies. Trans R Soc Trop Med Hyg 1993; 87:135.

Abdel-Wahab MF, Yosery A, Narooz S, et al: Is *Schistosoma mansoni* replacing *Schistosoma haematobium* in the Fayoum? Am J Trop Med Hyg 1993; 49:697.

Abu-Aisha H, Reddy JJ, Hussain S, Balbeesi A: Long-term ureterostomy with suprapubic intravesical drainage used to bypass severe schistosomal obstructive uropathy-preliminary report. Urol Res 1985; 13:263.

Abul-Fadl MAM, Khalafallah AS: Studies of the urinary excretion of certain tryptophane metabolites in bilharziasis and its possible relation to bladder cancer in Egypt. Br J Cancer 1961; 15:479.

Adebamowo CA, Akang EE, Ladipo JK, Ajao OG: Schistosomiasis of the appendix. Br J Surg 1991; 78:1219.

Aden-Abdi Y, Gustafsson LL: Poor patient compliance reduces the efficacy of metrifonate treatment of *Schistosoma haematobium* in Somalia. Eur J Clin Pharmacol 1989; 36:161.

Aden-Abdi Y, Gustafsson LL, Elmi SA: A simplified dosage schedule of metrifonate in the treatment of *Schistosoma haematobium* infection in Somalia. Eur J Clin Pharmacol 1987; 32:437.

Adewunmi CO, Furu P, Christensen NO, Olorunmola F: Endemicity, seasonality and focality of transmission of human schistosomiasis in 3 communities in southwestern Nigeria. Trop Med Parasitol 1991; 42:332.

Agnew AM, Lucas SB, Doenhoff MJ: The host-parasite relationship of *Schistosoma haematobium* in CBA mice. Parasitology 1988; 97:403.

Aisen AM, Gross BH, Glazer GM: Computerized tomography of ureterovesical schistosomiasis. J Comput Assist Tomogr 1983; 7:161.

Akogun OB: Water demand and schistosomiasis among the Gumau people of Bauchi State, Nigeria. Trans R Soc Trop Med Hyg 1990; 84:548.

Al-Adnani MS, Salah KM: Schistosomiasis and bladder cancer in southern Iraq. J Trop Med Hyg 1983; 86:93.

al-Fawaz IM, al-Rasheed SA, al-Majed SA, Ashour M: Schistosomiasis associated with a mediastinal mass: Case report and review of the literature. Ann Trop Paediatr 1990; 10:293.

al-Hindawi M, Whitehorse GH, Al-Ansari AG, et al: Calcification of the large bowel in schistosomiasis demonstrated by computed tomography. Br J Radiol 1990; 63:357.

Al-Shukri S, Alwan MH: Bilharzial strictures of the lower third of the ureter: A critical review of 560 strictures. Br J Urol 1983; 55:477.

Al-Shukri S, Alwan MH, Nayef M: Ureteral strictures caused by bilharziasis. Z Urol Nephrol 1987a; 80:615.

Al-Shukri S, Alwan MH, Nayef M, Rahman AA: Bilharziasis in malignant tumors of the urinary bladder. Br J Urol 1987b; 59:59.

Alves W: The distribution of *Schistosoma* eggs in human tissues. Bull WHO 1958; 18:1092.

Anwar WA, Rosin MP: Reduction in chromosomal damage in schistosomiasis patients after treatment with praziquantel. Mutat Res 1993; 298:179.

Ashour M: Schistosomiasis associated with a mediastinal mass: Case report and review of the literature. Ann Trop Paediatr 1990; 10:293–297.

Aslamazov EG: Schistosomiasis of the bladder neck and proximal segment of the urethra. Urol Nefrol (Mosk) 1988; 1:34.

Bahar RH, Sabha M, Kouris K, et al: Chronic urinary schistosomiasis: patterns of abnormalities in radionuclide Tc-99 m DTPA diuretic renogram. APMIS 1988; (suppl 3):54–58.

Barsoum IS, Kamal KA, Bassily S, et al: Diagnosis of human schistosomiasis by detection of circulating cathodic antigen with a monoclonal antibody. J Infect Dis 1991; 164:1010.

Bassily S, Farid Z, Barsoum RS, et al: Renal biopsy in *Schistosoma-Salmonella* associated nephrotic syndrome. J Trop Med Hyg 1976; 79:256.

Bassily S, Farid Z, Dunn M, et al: Praziquantel for treatment of schistosomiasis in patients with advanced hepatosplenomegaly. Ann Trop Med Parasitol 1985; 79:629.

Basta MT, Attallah AM, Seddek MN, et al: Cytokeratin shedding in the urine: A biologic marker for bladder cancer? Br J Urol 1988; 61:116.

Bayssade-Dufour C, Vuong PN, Farhati K, et al: Speed of skin penetration and initial migration route of infective larvae of *Schistosoma haematobium* in *Meriones unguiculatus*. C R Acad Sci III, 1994; 317:529.

Bazeed MA, Nabeeh A, Atwan N: Xanthogranulomatous pyelonephritis in bilharzial patients: A report of 25 cases. J Urol 1989; 141:261.

Beaufils H, LeBon P, Auriol M, Danis M: Glomerular lesions in patients with *Schistosoma haematobium* infection. Trop Geo Med 1978; 30:183.

Befidi-Mengue RN, Ratard RC, D'Alessandro A, et al: The impact of *Schistosoma haematobium* infection and of praziquantel treatment on the growth of primary school children in Bertoua, Cameroon. J Trop Med Hyg 1992; 95:404.

Bell DR: A new method for counting *Schistosoma mansoni* eggs in faeces: With special reference to therapeutic trials. Bull WHO 1963; 29:525.

Bergguist, R: Prospects of vaccination against schistosomiasis. Scand J Infect Dis Suppl 1990; 76:60.

Berry A: A cytopathological and histopathological study of bilharziosis of the female genital tract. J Pathol Bacteriol 1966; 91:325.

Bhatt KM, Bhatt SM, Kanja C, Kyobe J: Urinary leukocytes in bladder schistosomiasis. E Afr Med J 1984; 61:449.

Bird AV: Spinal cord complications of bilharziasis. S Afr Med J 1967; 39:158.

Blanton RE, Licate LS, Aman RA: Characterization of a native and recombinant *Schistosoma haematobium* serine protease inhibitor gene product. Mol Biochem Parasitol 1994; 63:1.

Bobrow LG, Makin CA, Law S, Bodmer WF: Expression of low molecular weight cytokeratin proteins in cervical neoplasia. J Pathol 1986; 148:135.

Borel E, Etard JF: Vitamin A deficiency in a rural population of Mauritania and absence of a correlation with urinary schistosomiasis. Acta Trop 1988; 45:379.

Bradley DJ, McCullough FS: Egg output stability and the epidemiology of *Schistosoma haematobium*: II. An analysis of the epidemiology of endemic *S. haematobium*. Trans R Soc Trop Med Hyg 1973; 67:491.

Braun-Munzinger RA, Rohde R: False epidemiologic results from the bulk transport of dried filter papers in urinary schistosomiasis. Trop Med Parasitol 1986; 37:286.

Braun-Munzinger RA, Southgate BA: Repeatability and reproducibility of egg counts of *Schistosoma haematobium* in urine. Trop Med Parasitol 1992; 43:149.

Braun-Munzinger RA, Southgate BA: Egg viability in urinary schistosomiasis: I. New methods compared with available methods. J Trop Med Hyg 1993a; 96:22.

Braun-Munzinger RA, Southgate BA: Egg viability in urinary schistosomiasis: II. Simplifying modifications and standardization of new methods. J Trop Med Hyg 1993b; 96:71.

Braun-Munzinger RA, Southgate BA: Egg viability in urinary schistosomiasis: III. Repeatability and reproducibility of new methods. J Trop Med Hyg 1993c; 96:179.

Browning MD, Narooz SI, Strickland GT, et al: Clinical characteristics and response to therapy in Egyptian children infected with *Schistosoma haematobium*. J Infect Dis 1984; 149:998.

Burki A, Tanner M, Burnier E, et al: Comparison of ultrasonography, intravenous pyelography and cystoscopy in detection of urinary tract lesions due to *Schistosoma haematobium*. Acta Trop 1986; 43:139.

Butterworth AE: Immunity in human schistosomiasis. Acta Trop Suppl 1987; 12:31.

Butterworth AE, Fulford AJ, Dunne DW, et al: Longitudinal studies on human schistosomiasis. Philos Trans R Soc Lond (Biol) 1988; 321:495.

Cai Y, Langley JG, Smith DI, Boros DL: A cloned 38 kDa *Schistosoma mansoni* egg peptide induces TH1 type lymphocyte responses. Am J Trop Med Hyg 1995; 53:148.

Cayabyab M, Harn DA: Up-regulation of B7.2 expression on B cells correlates with the development of Th2 pathway in murine experimental schistosomiasis. Am J Trop Med Hyg 1995; 53:150.

Camacho M, Tarrab-Hazdai R, Espinoza B, et al: The amount of acetylcholinesterase on the parasite surface reflects the differential sensitivity of schistosome species to metrifonate. Parasitology 1994; 108:153–160.

Carter JP, Diab AS, Nasif S, et al: Bacteriologic and urinary findings in adolescent Egyptian males with and without urinary schistosomiasis. Am J Trop Med Hyg 1970; 73:211.

Chandiwana SK, Woolhouse ME: Heterogeneities in water contact patterns and the epidemiology of *Schistosoma haematobium*. Parasitology 1991; 103:363.

Chandiwana SK, Woolhouse ME, Bradley M: Factors affecting the intensity of reinfection with *Schistosoma haematobium* following treatment with praziquantel. Parasitology 1991; 102:73.

Cheever AW: Conditions affecting the accuracy of potassium hydroxide digestion techniques for counting *Schistosoma mansoni* eggs in tissues. Bull WHO 1968; 39:328.

Cheever AW: Schistosomiasis and neoplasia [Editorial]. J Natl Cancer Inst 1978; 61:13.

Cheever AW: Decalcification of schistosome eggs during staining of tissue sections: A potential source of diagnostic error. Am J Trop Med Hyg 1986; 35:959.

Cheever AW, Anderson LA: Rate of destruction of *Schistosoma mansoni* eggs in the tissues of mice. Am J Trop Med Hyg 1971; 20:62.

Cheever AW, Byram JE, Hieny S, et al: Schistosomiasis in B-cell depleted mice. Parasite Immunol 1985; 7:399.

Cheever AW, Duvall RH, Kuntz RE, et al: Resistance of capuchin monkeys to reinfection with *Schistosoma haematobium*. Trans Roy Soc Trop Med Hyg 1988a; 82:112.

Cheever AW, Kamel IA, Elwi AM, et al: *Schistosoma mansoni* and *Schistosoma haematobium* infections in Egypt: II. Quantitative parasitological findings at necropsy. Am J Trop Med Hyg 1977; 26:702.

Cheever AW, Kamel IA, Elwi AM, et al: *Schistosoma mansoni* and *Schistosoma haematobium* infections in Egypt: III. Extrahepatic pathology. Am J Trop Med Hyg 1978; 27:55.

Cheever AW, Kuntz RE, Moore JA, Huang TC: Pathology of *Schistosoma haematobium* infection in the capuchin monkey (*Cebus apella*). Trans Roy Soc Trop Med Hyg 1988b; 82:107.

Cheever AW, Torky AH, Shirbiney M: The relation of worm burden to passage of *Schistosoma haematobium* eggs in the urine of infected patients. Am J Trop Med Hyg 1975a; 24:284.

Cheever AW, Young SW, Shehata A: Calcification of *Schistosoma haematobium* eggs: Relation of radiologically demonstrable calcification to eggs in tissues and passage of eggs in urine. Trans R Soc Trop Med Hyg 1975b; 69:410.

Chernin E: Some host-finding attributes of *Schistosoma mansoni* miracidia. Am J Trop Med Hyg 1974; 23:320.

Christie JD, Crouse D, Kelada AS, et al: Patterns of *Schistosoma haematobium* egg distribution in the human lower urinary tract: III. Cancerous lower urinary tracts. Am J Trop Med Hyg 1986a; 35:759.

Christie JD, Crouse D, Pineda J, et al: Patterns of *Schistosoma haematobium* egg distribution in the human lower urinary tract: I. Non-cancerous lower urinary tracts. Am J Trop Med Hyg 1986b; 35:743.

Christie JD, Crouse D, Smith JH, et al: Patterns of *Schistosoma haematobium* egg distribution in the human lower urinary tract: II. Obstructive uropathy. Am J Trop Med Hyg 1986c; 35:752.

Cline BL, Richards FO, El Alamy MA, et al: 1983 Nile Delta schistosomiasis survey: 48 years after Scott. Am J Trop Med Hyg 1989; 47:56.

Cook JA: Treatment. *In* Nash TE (Moderator): Schistosome infection in humans: Perspectives and recent findings. Ann Intern Med 1982; 97:740.

Coopan RM, Naidoo K, Jialal I: Renal function in urinary schistosomiasis in Natal Province of South Africa. Am J Trop Med Hyg 1987a; 37:556.

Coopan RM, Schutte CH, Dingle CE, et al: Urinalysis reagent strips in the screening of children for urinary schistosomiasis in the RSA. S Afr Med J 1987b; 72:459.

Coopan RM, Schutte CH, Mayet FG, et al: Morbidity from urinary schistosomiasis in relation to intensity of infection in Natal Province of South Africa. Am J Trop Med Hyg 1986; 35:765.

Corachan M, Valls ME, Gascon J, et al: Hematospermia: A new etiology of clinical interest. Am J Trop Med Hyg 1994; 50:580.

Cosnett JE, Van Dellen JR: Schistosomiasis (Bilharzia) of the spinal cord: Case reports and clinical profile. Q J Med 1986; 61:1131.

Cutajar CL: The role of schistosomiasis in urolithiasis. Br J Urol 1983; 55:349.

Davis A: Management of the patient with schistosomiasis. *In* Jordan P, Webbe G, eds: Schistosomiasis, Epidemiology, Treatment and Control. London, William Heinemann Medical Books, 1982, pp 184–226.

Davis CP, Cohen MS, Anderson MD, et al: Urothelial hyperplasia and neoplasia: II. Detection of nitrosamines and interferon in chronic urinary tract infections in rats. J Urol 1985; 134:1002.

Davis CP, Cohen MS, Gruber MB, et al: Urothelial hyperplasia and neoplasia: Response to chronic urinary tract infections in rats. J Urol 1984; 132:1025.

De Clercq D, Rollinson D, Diarra A, et al: Schistosomiasis in Dogon country, Mali: identification and prevalence of the species responsible for infection in the local community. Trans R Soc Trop Med Hyg 1994; 88:653.

de Gentile L, Fayad M, Denis P, Lecastre MJ: Erratic localization and uncommon longevity of *Schistosoma haematobium*. Apropos of a case. J Urol 1988; 94:163.

Degremont A, Burnier E, Mendt R, et al: Value of ultrasonography in investigating morbidity due to *Schistosoma haematobium* infection. Lancet 1985; 1:662.

de Jonge N, Schommer G, Feldmeier H, et al: Mixed *Schistosoma haematobium* and *S. mansoni* infection: Effect of different treatments on the serum level of circulating anodic antigen (CAA). Acta Trop 1990; 48:25.

Develoux M, Blanc L, Vetter JM, Cenac A: Cutaneous schistosomiasis of the chest. Ann Dermatol Venereol 1987; 114:695.

Devidas A, Lamothe F, Develoux M, et al: Morbidity due to bilharziasis caused by *S. haematobium*. Relationship between bladder lesions observed by ultrasonography and cystoscopic and anatomo-pathologic lesions. Acta Trop 1988; 45:277.

Devidas A, Lamothe F, Develoux M, et al: Ultrasonographic assessment of the regression of bladder and renal lesions due to *Schistosoma haematobium* after treatment with praziquantel. Ann Soc Belg Med Trop 1989; 69:57.

Diaz Rivera RS, Ramos Morales F, Koppisch E, et al: Acute Manson's schistosomiasis. Am J Med 1956; 21:918.

Dittrich M, Doehring E: Ultrasonographical aspects of urinary schistosomiasis: Assessment of morphological lesions in the upper and lower urinary tract. Pediatr Radiol 1986; 16:225.

Doehring E, Ehrich JH, Bremer HJ: Reversibility of urinary tract abnormalities due to *Schistosoma haematobium* infection. Kidney Int 1986a; 30:582.

Doehring E, Ehrich JH, Reider F: Daily urinary protein loss in *Schistosoma haematobium* infection. Am J Trop Med Hyg 1986b; 35:954.

Doehring E, Ehrich JH, Reider F, et al: Morbidity in urinary schistosomiasis: Relation between sonographical lesions and pathological urine findings. Trop Med Parasitol 1985a; 36:145.

Doehring E, Poggensee U, Feldmeier H: The effect of metrifonate in mixed *Schistosoma haematobium* and *Schistosoma mansoni* infections in humans. Am J Trop Med Hyg 1986c; 35:323.

Doehring E, Reider F, Schmidt-Ehry G, Ehrich JH: Reduction in pathologic findings in urine and bladder lesions in infection with *Schistosoma haematobium* after treatment with praziquantel. J Infect Dis 1985b; 152:807.

Doehring E, Vester U, Ehrich JHH, Feldmeier H: Circadian variation of ova excretion, proteinuria, hematuria and leukocyturia in urinary schistosomiasis. Kid Int 1985c; 27:667.

Duvie SOA: Cup-patch ileocystoplasty in treatment of bilharzial contracted bladder. J R Coll Surg Edinb 1986; 31:56.

Duvie SOA, Diffang C, Guirguis MN: The effects of *Schistosoma haematobium* infestation on the vermiform appendix: The Nigerian experience. J Trop Med Hyg 1987; 90:13.

Edington GM, Nwabuebo I, Junaid TA: The pathology of schistosomiasis in Ibadan, Nigeria, with special reference to the appendix, brain, pancreas and genital organs. Trans R Soc Trop Med Hyg 1975; 69:153.

Edington GM, von Lichtenberg F, Nwabuebo I, et al: Pathologic effects of schistosomiasis in Ibadan, Western State of Nigeria: I. Incidence and intensity of infection; distribution and severity of lesions. Am J Trop Med Hyg 1970; 19:982.

Ekanem EE, Asindi AA, Ejezie GC, Antai-Otong OE: Effect of *Schistosoma haematobium* infection on the physical growth and school performance of Nigerian children. Cent Afr J Med 1994; 40:38.

El-Bolkainy MN, Chu EW, Ghoneim MA, Ibrahim AS: Cytologic detection of bladder cancer in rural Egyptian population infected with schistosomiasis. Acta Cytol 1982; 26:303.

El-Bolkainy MN, Ghoneim MA, Mansour MA: Carcinoma of the bilharzial bladder in Egypt: Clinical and pathological features. Br J Urol 1972; 44:561.

El-Bolkainy MN, Mokhtar NM, Ghoneim MA, Hussein MH: The impact of schistosomiasis on the pathology of bladder cancer. Cancer 1981; 48:2643.

Elem B: Urinary calculus in Zambia: Its incidence and relationship to *Schistosoma haematobium* infection and vesicovaginal fistula. Br J Urol 1984; 56:44.

Elem B, Patil PS, Lambert TK: Giant fibrous pseudotumor of the testicular tunics in association with *Schistosoma haematobium* infection. J Urol 1989; 141:376.

Elem B, Purohit R: Carcinoma of the urinary bladder in Zambia. A quantitative estimation of *Schistosoma haematobium* infection. Br J Urol 1983; 55:275.

Elias E, Daffalla A, Lassen JM, Madsen H, Christiansen NO: *Schistosoma haematobium* infection patterns in the Rahad Irrigation Scheme. Acta Trop 1994; 58:115–125.

El-Masry NA, Farid Z, Bassily S, et al: Schistosomal colonic polyposis: Clinical, radiological and parasitological study. J Trop Med Hyg 1986; 89:13.

El-Merzabani MM, El-Aaser AA, Zakhary NI: A study of the aetiologic factors of bilharzial bladder cancer in Egypt—I-nitrosamine and their precursors in urine. Europ J Cancer 1979; 15:287.

El-Mofty AM, Nada M: Cutaneous schistosomiasis. Egypt J Bilharz 1975; 2:23.

el-Shoura SM: Human bilharzial ureters: II. Cellular dynamic against deposited eggs. Ann Parasitol Hum Comp 1993a; 68:121.

el-Shoura SM: Human bilharzial ureters: III. Fine structure of the egg granuloma. Appl Parasitol 1993b; 34:265.

el-Shoura SM: Human bilharzial ureters: IV. Ultrastructural interaction between multinucleate giant cells and the parasite eggs. Appl Parasitol 1994; 35:257.

Eltoum IA, Sulaiman S, Ismail BM, et al: Evaluation of hematuria as an indirect screening test for schistosomiasis haematobium: A population-based study in the White Nile province. Sudan Acta Trop 1992; 51:151.

Eltoum IA, Sulaiman SM, Ismail BM, et al: Demonstration of urinary eosinophils in *Schistosoma haematobium*: A comparative study among three different stains. Biotech Histochem 1993; 68:146.

Erickson DG, Jones CE, Tang DB: *Schistosomiasis mansoni, haematobium,* and *japonica* in hamsters: Liver granuloma measurements. Exp Parasitol 1974; 35:425.

Erickson DG, von Lichtenberg F, Sadun EH, et al: Comparison of *Schistosoma haematobium*, *Schistosoma mansoni* and *Schistosoma japonica* infections in the owl monkey, *Aotus trivirgatus*. J Parasitol 1971; 57:543.

Etard JF, Borel E, Segala C: *Schistosoma haematobium* infection in Mauritania: Two years of follow-up after a targeted chemotherapy—A life-table approach of the risk of reinfection. Parasitology 1990; 100:399.

Fam A: The problem of the bilharzial ureter. Br J Urol 1964; 36:211.

Farid Z, Higashi GI, Bassily S, et al: Chronic salmonellosis, urinary schistosomiasis and massive proteinuria. Am J Trop Med Hyg 1972; 21:578.

Fataar S, Bassiony H, Hamed MS, et al: Radiographic spectrum of rectocolonic calcification from schistosomiasis. Am J Roentgenol 1984a; 142:933.

Fataar S, Bassiony H, Satayanath S, et al: Computerized tomography of schistosomal calcification of the intestine. Am J Roentgenol 1985; 144:75.

Fataar S, Jakob GS, Bassiony H, et al: Rectocolonic calcification due to schistosomiasis. A clinicoradiologic study. Dis Colon Rect 1984b; 27:164.

Fataar S, Satayanath S: The radiographic evaluation of appendiceal calcification due to schistosomiasis. Am J Trop Med Hyg 1986; 35:1157.

Feldmeier H, Bienzle U, Dietrich M: Combination of a viability test and a quantification method for *Schistosoma haematobium* eggs. Tropenmed Parasitol 1979; 30:417.

Feldmeier H, Doehring E: Clinical experience with metrifonate. Review with emphasis on its use in endemic areas. Acta Trop 1987; 44:357.

Feldmeier H, Doehring E, Daffalla AA, et al: Efficacy of metrifonate in urinary schistosomiasis: Comparison of reduction of *Schistosoma haematobium* and *S. mansoni* eggs. Am J Trop Med Hyg 1982; 31:1188.

Feldmeier H, Gastl GA, Poggensee U, et al: Immune response in chronic schistosomiasis haematobium and mansoni. Reversibility of alterations after anti-parasitic treatment with praziquantel. Scand J Immunol 1988; 28:147.

Feldmeier H, Kern P, Niel G: Modulation of in vitro lymphocyte proliferation in patients with schistosomiasis haematobium, schistosomiasis mansoni and mixed infection. Tropenmed Parasitol 1981; 32:237.

Feldmeier H, Krantz I, Poggensee G: Female genital schistosomiasis as a risk-factor for the transmission of HIV. Int J STD AIDS 1994; 5:368.

Feldmeier H, Nogueira-Queiroz JA, Peixoto-Queiroz MA, et al: Detection and quantification of circulating antigen in schistosomiasis by monoclonal antibody: II. The quantification of circulating antigens in human schistosomiasis mansoni and haematobium: Relationship to intensity of infection and disease status. Clin Exp Immunol 1986; 65:232.

Ferguson AR: Associated bilharziasis and primary malignant disease of the urinary bladder with observations on a series of 40 cases. J Pathol Bacteriol 1911; 16:76.

Fievet JP, Barnaud P, Moncada K, et al: Long-term surveillance of bilharzian ureterohydronephrosis. A 22-year follow-up. J Urol (Paris) 1987; 93:235.

Flores Villanueva PO, Zheng XX, Strom TB, Stadecker MJ: The IL-10/Fc fusion protein inhibits egg granuloma formation in schistosomiasis. Am J Trop Med Hyg 1995; 53:149.

Forsythe DM: A longitudinal study of endemic urinary schistosomiasis in a small East African community. Bull WHO 1969; 40:771.

Fripp PJ: *Schistosoma haematobium* and urinary beta-glucuronidase. Trans R Soc Trop Med Hyg 1988; 82:351.

Fukushima S, Ito N, el-Bolkainy MN, et al: Immunohistochemical observations of keratins, involucrin, and epithelial membrane antigen in urinary bladder carcinomas from patients infected with *Schistosoma haematobium*. Virchows Arch [A] 1987; 411:103.

Garb KS, Stavitsky AB, Olds GR, et al: Immune regulation in murine schistosomiasis japonica: Inhibition of in vitro antigen- and mitogen-induced cellular responses by splenocyte culture supernatants and purified fractions from serum of chronically infected mice. J Immunol 1982; 129:2752.

Gelfand M: Bilharzial affection of the ureter; Study of 110 consecutive necropsies showing vesicle bilharziasis. BMJ 1948; 1:1228–1230.

Gelfand M: Schistosomiasis in South Central Africa, a Clinicopathological Study. Cape Town, Juta, 1950.

Gelfand M, Ross CMD, Blair DM, et al: Schistosomiasis of the male pelvic organs. Severity of infection as determined by digestion of tissue and histologic methods in 300 cadavers. Am J Trop Med Hyg 1970; 19:779.

Gelfand M, Ross MD, Blair DM, Weber MC: Distribution and extent of schistosomiasis in female pelvic organs, with special reference to the genital tract, as determined at autopsy. Am J Trop Med Hyg 1971; 20:846.

Geneseke R, Hofs R, Otto HJ, Meinhard F: X-ray and nuclear medical studies in children with urinary bilharziasis. Radiol Diagn (Berlin) 1985; 26:575.

Ghaly AF, El-Banhawy A: Schistosomiasis of the spinal cord. J Pathol 1973; 111:57.

Ghorab MMA: Ureteritis calcinosa—A complication of bilharzial ureteritis and its relation to primary ureteric stone formation. Br J Urol 1962; 34:33.

Gigase PL, Mangelschots E, Bockaert R, et al: Simple indicators of prevalence and intensity of urinary bilharziasis in Chad. Ann Soc Belg Med Trop 1988; 68:123.

Gilles HM: Schistosomiasis update. Int J Dermatol 1988; 27:400.

Gilles HM, Lucas A, Linder R, et al: *Schistosoma haematobium* infection in Nigeria: III. Infection in boatyard workers at Epe. Ann Trop Med Parasitol 1965; 59:451.

Grace HK, Aidaros SM: The pathogenesis of intrapelvic schistosomiasis with special reference to bilharziasis of the seminal vesicles. J R Egypt Med Assn 1952; 35:613.

Greenham R, Cameron AH: *Schistosoma haematobium* and the nephrotic syndrome. Trans R Soc Trop Med Hyg 1980; 74:609.

Guyatt HL, Smith T, Gryseels B, et al: Aggregation in schistosomiasis: Comparison of the relationships between prevalence and intensity in different endemic areas. Parasitology 1994; 109:45.

Haas W, Haberl B, Schmalfuss G, Khayyal MT: *Schistosoma haematobium* cercarial host-finding and host-recognition differs from that of *S. mansoni*. J Parasitol 1994; 80:345.

Haberberger RL Jr, Mokhtar S, Badawy H, Abu-Elyazeed R: *Chlamydia trachomatis* associated with chronic dysuria among patients with *Schistosoma haematobium*. Trans R Soc Trop Med Hyg 1993; 87:671.

Hagan P, Blumenthal UJ, Chaudri M, et al: Resistance to reinfection with *Schistosoma haematobium* in Gambian children: Analysis of their immune responses. Trans R Soc Trop Med Hyg 1987; 81:938.

Hagan P, Blumenthal UJ, Dunn D, et al: Human IgE, IgG4 and resistance to reinfection with *Schistosoma haematobium*. Nature 1991; 349:243.

Hagan P, Moore PJ, Adjukiewicz AB, et al: In-vitro antibody-dependent killing of schistosomula of *Schistosoma haematobium* by human eosinophils. Parasite Immunol 1985a; 7:617.

Hagan P, Wilkins A, Blumenthal UJ, et al: Eosinophilia and resistance to *Schistosoma haematobium* in man. Parasite Immunol 1985b; 7:625.

Halim A, Javadpour N, Kasraeian A, Young JD: Cell surface antigen in bilharzial bladder tumors. Br J Urol 1986; 58:523.

Hamburger J, Lustigman S, Siongok TK, et al: Analysis and preliminary purification of glycoproteins isolated from eggs in the urine of patients with *Schistosoma haematobium* infection. J Immunol 1982; 129:1711.

Hanafy HM, Youssef TK, Saad SM: Radiologic aspects of bilharzial (schistosomal) ureter. Urology 1975; 6:118.

Hang LM, Boros DL, Warren KS: Induction of Immunologic hyporesponsiveness to granulomatous hypersensitivity in *Schistosoma mansoni* infection. J Infect Dis 1974; 130:515.

Harrison RA, Bickle QD, Kiare S, et al: Immunization of baboons with attenuated schistosomula of *Schistosoma haematobium*: Levels of protection induced by immunization with larvae irradiated with 20 and 60 krad. Trans R Soc Trop Med Hyg 1990; 84:89.

Harzmann R, Schubert GE, Gericke D, et al: Morphology of the urinary bladder following long-term experimental irritation of the urothelium. Urol Int 1983; 38:166.

Hatz C, Jenkins JM, Meudt R, et al: A review of the literature on the use of ultrasonography in schistosomiasis with special reference to its use in field studies: 1. *Schistosoma haematobium*. Acta Trop 1992; 51:1.

Hatz C, Mayombana C, de Savigny D, et al: Ultrasound scanning for detecting morbidity due to *Schistosoma haematobium* and its resolution following treatment with different doses of praziquantel. Trans R Soc Trop Med Hyg 1990a; 84:84.

Hatz C, Savioli, L, Mayombana C, et al: Measurement of schistosomiasis-related morbidity at community level in areas of different endemicity. Bull WHO 1990b; 68:777.

Hefty TR, McCorkell SJ: Schistosomiasis and renal transplantation. J Urol 1986; 135:1163.

Heurtier Y, Lamothe F, Develoux M, et al: Urinary tract lesions due to *Schistosoma haematobium* infection assessed by ultrasonography in a community based study in Niger. Am J Trop Med Hyg 1986; 35:1163.

Hiatt RA, Sotomayor ZR, Sanchez G, et al: Factors in the pathogenesis of acute schistosomiasis mansoni. J Infect Dis 1979; 139:659.

Hicks RM, Ismail MM, Walters CL, et al: Association of bacteriuria and urinary nitrosamine formation with *Schistosoma haematobium* infection in the Qalyub area of Egypt. Trans R Soc Trop Med Hyg 1982; 76:519.

Hicks RM, James C, Webbe G: Effect of *Schistosoma haematobium* and N-butyl-N(4-hydroxybutyl) nitrosamine on the development of urothelial neoplasia in the baboon. Br J Cancer 1980; 42:730.

Higashi GI, Farid Z, Bassily S, Miner WF: Nephrotic syndrome in schistosomiasis mansoni complicated by chronic salmonellosis. Am J Trop Med Hyg 1975; 24:713.

Hillyer GV, Pacheco E: Isolation and characterization of *Schistosoma haematobium* egg antigens. Am J Trop Med Hyg 1986; 35:777.

Hillyer GV, Ramzy RMR, El-Alamy MA, Cline BL: The circumoval precipitin test for the serodiagnosis of human schistosomiasis mansoni and haematobium. Am J Trop Med Hyg 1981; 30:121.

Hockley DJ, McLaren DJ: *Schistosoma mansoni*: Changes in the outer membrane of the tegument during development from cercaria to adult worm. Int J Parasitol 1973; 3:13.

Hodasi WM: *Schistosoma* appendicitis. Trop Doct 1988; 18:105.

Hugosson CO: Striation of the renal pelvis and ureter in bilharziasis. Clin Radiol 1987; 38:407.

Hugosson CO, Olsen P: Early ureteric changes in *Schistosoma haematobium* infection. Clin Radiol 1986; 37:501.

Husain I, Al Ali IH, Kinare AS: Evaluating bilharzial ureteropathy for surgery. Br J Urol 1980; 52:446.

Ibrahim A: The relationship between urinary bilharziasis and urolithiasis in the Sudan. Br J Urol 1978; 50:294.

Idris MA, Ruppel A: Diagnostic Mr31/32,000 *Schistosoma mansoni* proteins (Sm31/32): Reaction with sera from Sudanese patients infected with *S. mansoni* or *S. haematobium*. J Helminthol 1988; 62:95.

Idris MA, Ruppel A: Diagnostic Mr 31/32000 proteins of *Schistosoma mansoni* (Sm31/32) and *S. haematobium* (Sh31/32): Stability and reaction conditions for prospective field tests. J Helminthol 1991; 65:89.

Jacobsson B, Lindstedt E, Narasimham DL, et al: Balloon dilatation of bilharzial ureteral strictures. Br J Urol 1987; 60:28.

Janitschke K, Reinhold A, Bode L: Nitrocellulose dot-ELISA for serodiagnosis of schistosomiasis. Trans R Soc Trop Med Hyg 1987; 81:956.

Jemaneh L, Tedla S, Birrie H: The use of reagent strips for detection of urinary schistosomiasis infection in the middle Awash Valley, Ethiopia. East Afr Med J 1994; 71:679.

Jorulf H, Linstedt E: Urogenital schistosomiasis: CT evaluation. Radiology 1985; 157:745.

Kagan IG: Current status of serologic testing for parasitic disease. Hosp Pract 1974; 9:157.

Kaiser C, Bergel F, Doehring-Schwerdtfeger E, et al: Urine test strips: Reliability of semi-quantitative findings under tropical conditions. Pediatr Nephrol 1992; 6:145.

Kamel IA, Cheever AW, Elwi AM, et al: *Schistosoma mansoni* and *Schistosoma haematobium* infections in Egypt: I. Evaluation of techniques for recovery of worms and eggs at necropsy. Am J Trop Med Hyg 1977; 26:696.

Kamel IA, Elwi AM, Cheever AW, et al: *Schistosoma mansoni* and *Schistosoma haematobium* infections in Egypt: IV. Hepatic lesions. Am J Trop Med Hyg 1978; 27:931.

Kardorff R, Traoré M, Doehring-Schwerdtfeger E, et al: Ultrasonography of ureteric abnormalities induced by *Schistosoma haematobium* infection before and after praziquantel treatment. Br J Urol 1994; 74:703.

Kassim OO: Serum lysozyme and phosphatases in children with *Schistosoma haematobium* infections. J Trop Pediatr 1988; 34:248.

Kassis AI, Warren KS, Mahmoud AAF: The *Schistosoma haematobium* egg granuloma. Cell Immunol 1978; 38:310.

Khafagy MM, El-Bolkainy MN, Mansour MA: Carcinoma of the bilharzial bladder. A study of associated mucosal lesions in 86 cases. Cancer 1972; 30:150.

Khalil HM, Makled MK, El-Missiry AG, et al: Markers and subpopulations of T-lymphocytes in schistosomiasis. J Egypt Soc Parasit 1987; 17:325.

Khalil SB, Mansour NS: Worm development in hamsters infected with unisex and cross-mated *Schistosoma mansoni* and *Schistosoma haematobium*. J Parasitol 1995; 81:8.

Kiliku FM, Kimura E, Muhoho N, et al: The usefulness of urinalysis reagent strips in selecting *Schistosoma haematobium* egg positives before and after treatment with praziquantel. J Trop Med Hyg 1991; 94:401.

Kimura E, Moji K, Uga S, et al: Effects of *Schistosoma haematobium* infection on mental test scores of Kenyan school children. Trop Med Parasitol 1992; 43:155.

King CH, Keating CE, Muraka JF, et al: Urinary tract morbidity in schistosomiasis haematobium: Associations with age and intensity of infection in an endemic area of Coast Province, Kenya. Am J Trop Med Hyg 1988a; 39:361.

King CH, Lombardi G, Lombardi C, et al: Chemotherapy-based control of schistosomiasis haematobium: I. Metrifonate versus praziquantel in control of intensity and prevalence of infection. Am J Trop Med Hyg 1988b; 39:295.

King CH, Lombardi G, Lombardi C, et al: Chemotherapy-based control of schistosomiasis haematobium: II. Metrifonate vs. praziquantel in control of infection-associated morbidity. Am J Trop Med Hyg 1990; 42:587.

King CH, Muchiri EM, Ouma JH: Age-targeted chemotherapy for control of urinary schistosomiasis in endemic populations. Mem Inst Oswaldo Cruz 1992; 87:203.

King CH, Muchiri E, Ouma JH, Koech D: Chemotherapy-based control of schistosomiasis haematobium: IV. Impact of repeated annual chemotherapy on prevalence and intensity of *Schistosoma haematobium* infection in an endemic area of Kenya. Am J Trop Med Hyg 1991; 45:498.

King CH, Wiper DW III, De Stigter KV, et al: Dose-finding study for praziquantel therapy of *Schistosoma* haematobium in Coast Province, Kenya. Am J Trop Med Hyg 1989; 40:507.

King CL, Malhotra I, Koech D, et al: Immunity in human urinary schistosomiasis: Association of cellular responses with age and intensity of infection. Am J Trop Med Hyg 1995; 53:118.

Kitinya JN, Lauren PA, Eshelman LJ, et al: The incidence of squamous and transitional cell carcinomas of the urinary bladder in Northern Tanzania in areas of high and low levels of endemic *Schistosoma haematobium* infection. Trans R Soc Trop Med Hyg 1986; 80:1009.

Kloos H, Higashi G, Schinski VD, et al: Water contact and *Schistosoma haematobium* infection: A case study from an upper Egyptian village. Int J Epidemiol 1990; 19:749.

Klumpp RK, Southgate BA: Nytrel filters not reusable. Trans R Soc Trop Med Hyg 1986; 80:494.

Knight M, Simpson AJ, Bickle Q, et al: Adult schistosome cDNA libraries as a source of antigens for the study of experimental and human schistosomiasis. Mol Biochem Parasitol 1986; 18:235.

Koech DK, Hirata M, Shimada M, Wambayi E: Precipitates found around *Schistosoma haematobium* eggs from human urine prior to circumoval precipitin test. Ann Trop Med Parasitol 1984; 78:627.

Koroltchouk V, Stanley K, Stjernsward J, Mott K: Bladder cancer: Approaches to prevention and control. Bull WHO 1987; 65:513.

Kremsner PG, Enyong P, Krijger FW, et al: Circulating anodic and cathodic antigen in serum and urine from *Schistosoma haematobium*–infected Cameroonian children receiving praziquantel: A longitudinal study. Clin Infect Dis 1994; 18:408.

Kruger FJ: Frequency and possible consequences of hybridization between *Schistosoma haematobium* and *S. mattheei* in the Eastern Transvaal Lowveld. J Helminthol 1990; 64:333.

Kruger FJ, Evans AC: Do all human urinary infections with *Schistosoma mattheei* represent hybridization between *S. haematobium* and *S. mattheei*? J Helminthol 1990; 64:330.

Kvalsvig JD: The effects of schistosomiasis haematobium on the activity of school children. J Trop Med Hyg 1986; 89:85.

Lambertucci JR, Godoy P, Neves J, et al: Glomerulonephritis in *Salmonella–Schistosoma mansoni* association. Am J Trop Med Hyg 1988; 38:97.

Lamothe F, Develoux M, Devidas A, Sellin B: Echography in urinary bilharziosis. Apropos of 304 studies in Niger. Ann Radiol (Paris) 1988; 31:297.

Latham MC, Stephenson LS, Kurz KM, Kinoti SN: Metrifonate or praziquantel treatment improves physical fitness and appetite of Kenyan school boys with *Schistosoma haematobium* and hookworm infections. Am J Trop Med Hyg 1990; 43:170.

Laughlin LW, Farid Z, Mansour N, et al: Bacteriuria in urinary schistosomiasis in Egypt. A prevalence survey. Am J Trop Med Hyg 1978; 27:916.

Laurent C, Lamothe F, Develoux M, et al: Ultrasonographic assessment of urinary tract lesions due to *Schistosoma haematobium* in Niger after four consecutive years of treatment with praziquantel. Trop Med Parasitol 1990; 41:139.

Lautin EM, Becker RD, Fromowitz FB, Bezahler GH: Computed tomography of the lower urinary tract in schistosomiasis. J Comput Assist Tomogr 1983; 7:164.

Leadbetter GW Jr, Leadbetter WF: Ureteral re-implantation and bladder neck reconstruction. JAMA 1961; 175:349.

Lehman JS Jr, Farid Z, Bassily S: Mortality in urinary schistosomiasis. Lancet 1970; 2:822.

Lehman JS Jr, Farid Z, Bassily S, Kent DC: Hydronephrosis, bacteriuria, and maximal urine concentration in urinary schistosomiasis. Ann Intern Med 1971; 75:49.

Lehman JS Jr, Farid Z, Bassily S, et al: Intestinal protein loss in schistosomal polyposis of the colon. Gastroenterology 1968; 59:433.

Lehman JS Jr, Farid Z, Smith JH, et al: Urinary schistosomiasis in Egypt: Clinical, radiological, bacteriological and parasitological correlations. Trans R Soc Trop Med Hyg 1973; 67:384.

Li Z, King CL, Ogundipe JO, et al: Preferential recognition by human IgE and IgG4 of a species-specific *Schistosoma haematobium* serine protease inhibitor. J Infect Dis 1995; 171:416.

Lucas AO, Adeniyi-Jones CC, Cockshot WP, Gilles HM: Radiological changes after medical treatment of vesical schistosomiasis. Lancet 1966; 1:631.

Lucas AO, Akpom CA, Cockshot WP, Bohrer SP: Reversibility of schistosomiasis in children after specific treatment. Ann N Y Acad Sci 1969; 160:629.

Lucas S: Squamous cell carcinoma of the bladder and schistosomiasis. East Afr Med J 1982; 59:345.

Maddison SE: The present status of serodiagnosis and seroepidemiology of schistosomiasis. Diagn Microbiol Infect Dis 1987; 7:93.

Makar N: The bilharzial ureter. Some observation on the surgical pathology and surgical treatment. Br J Surg 1948; 36:148.

Makar N: Urologic Aspects of Bilharziasis in Egypt. Cairo, Societe Orientale de Publicite Press, 1955.

Malhotra IJ, Medhat A, Nafeh M, et al: Interleukin-10 regulates in vivo T-cell reactivity in human urinary schistosomiasis. Am J Trop Med Hyg 1995; 53:118.

Manca F, Cauda R, Laghi V, et al: Detection of parasite related antigens associated with conglutinin binding immune complexes in patients with *Schistosoma haematobium*. Trans R Soc Trop Med Hyg 1988; 82:254.

Marcial-Rojas Fiol RE: Neurologic complications of schistosomiasis: Review of the literature and report of two cases of transverse myelitis due to *S. mansoni*. Ann Intern Med 1963; 59:215.

McMahon JE: Circadian rhythm in *Schistosoma haematobium* egg excretion. Int J Parasit 1976; 6:373.

McMahon JE, Kolstrup N: Praziquantel: A new schistosomacide against *Schistosoma haematobium*. BMJ 1979; 2:1396.

Moczon T, Swiderski Z: *Schistosoma haematobium:* Histochemistry of glycogen phosphorylase a and glycogen branching enzyme in niridazole-treated females. Int J Parasitol 1992; 22:55.

Mostafa MH, Helmi S, Badawi AF, et al: Nitrate, nitrite and volatile N-nitroso compounds in the urine of *Schistosoma haematobium* and *Schistosoma mansoni* infected patients. Carcinogenesis 1994; 15:619.

Mouahid A, Moné H, Chaib A, Théron A: Cercarial shedding patterns of *Schistosoma bovis* and *S. haematobium* from single and mixed infections of Bulinus truncatus. J Helminthol 1991; 65:8.

Mott KE: A reusable polyamide filter for the diagnosis of *Schistosoma haematobium* infection by urine filtration. Bull Soc Path Exotic 1983; 76:101.

Mott KE: Epidemiological considerations for development of a schistosome vaccine. Acta Trop Suppl 1987; 12:13.

Mott KE, Dixon H: Collaborative study of antigens for immunodiagnosis of schistosomiasis. Bull WHO 1982; 60:729.

Mott KE, Dixon H, Osei-Tutu E, et al: Effect of praziquantel on hematuria and proteinuria in urinary schistosomiasis. Am J Trop Med Hyg 1985; 34:1119.

Murare HM, Taylor P: Hematuria and proteinuria during *Schistosoma haematobium* infection: Relationship to intensity of infection and the value of chemical reagent strips for pre- and post-treatment diagnosis. Trans R Soc Trop Med Hyg 1987; 81:426.

Nafeh MA, Medhat A, Swifae Y, et al: Ultrasonographic changes of the liver in *Schistosoma haematobium* infection. Am J Trop Med Hyg 1992; 47:225.

Navarrete S, Rollinson D, Agnew AM: Cross-protection between species of the *Schistosoma haematobium* group induced by vaccination with irradiated parasites. Parasit Immunol 1994; 16:19.

Ndamba J: Schistosomiasis: Its effects on the physical performance of school children in Zimbabwe. Cent Afr J Med 1986; 32:289.

Ndamba J, Nyazema N, Makaza N, et al: Traditional herbal remedies used for the treatment of urinary schistosomiasis in Zimbabwe. J Ethnopharmacol 1994; 42:125.

Neill PJG, Smith JH, Doughty B, Kemp WM: Ultrastructure of the *Schistosoma mansoni* egg. Am J Trop Med Hyg 1988; 39:52.

Ngandu NH: The use of Bayes' theorem and other indices of agreement in evaluating the use of reagent strips in screening rural schoolchildren for *Schistosoma haematobium* in Zambia. Int J Epidemiol 1988; 17:202.

Obasi OE: Cutaneous schistosomiasis in Nigeria. An update. Br J Dermatol 1986; 114:597.

Obel N, Black FT: Microscopic examination of sperm as the diagnostic clue in a case of *Schistosoma haematobium* infection. Scand J Infect Dis 1994; 26:117.

Ofori-Adjei D, Adjepon-Yamoah KK, Lindstrom B: Oral praziquantel kinetics in normal and *Schistosoma haematobium*-infected subjects. Ther Drug Monit 1988; 10:45.

Okonofua FE, Ojo OS, Odunsi OA, Odesanmi WO: Ectopic pregnancy associated with tubal schistosomiasis in a Nigerian woman. Int J Gynaecol Obstet 1990; 32:281.

Patil KP, Ibrahim AI, Shetty SD, et al: Specific investigations in chronic urinary bilharziasis. Urology 1992; 40:117.

Pawar HN, Abdel-Dayem HM: Diuretic renography and urodynamic pressure studies in evaluating dilated bilharzial ureters. A preliminary report. Clin Nucl Med 1984; 9:402.

Perel Y, Sellin B, Perel C, et al: Use of urine collectors for infants from 0 to 4 years of age in a mass survey of urinary schistosomiasis in Niger. Med Trop (Mars) 1985; 45:429.

Peters PA, Mahmoud AAF, Warren KS, et al: Field studies of a rapid accurate means of quantifying *Schistosoma haematobium* eggs in urine samples. Bull WHO 1976a; 54:159.

Peters PA, Warren KS, Mahmoud AAF: Rapid, accurate quantification of schistosome eggs via nucleopore filters. J Parasitol 1976b; 62:154.

Peters W, Gilles HM: A Color Atlas of Tropical Medicine and Parasitology. London, Wolfe Medical Publishers, 1977.

Phillips SM, Colley DG: Immunologic aspects of host responses to schistosomiasis: Resistance, immunopathology and eosinophil involvement. Prog Allergy 1978; 24:49.

Politano V, Leadbetter NF: An operative technique for correction of vesicoureteral reflux. J Urol 1958; 79:932.

Pollner JH, Schwartz A, Kobrine A, Parenti DM: Cerebral schistosomiasis caused by *Schistosoma haematobium*: Case report. Clin Infect Dis 1994; 18:354.

Prual A, Daouda H, Develoux M, et al: Consequences of *Schistosoma haematobium* infection on the iron status of school children in Niger. Am J Trop Med Hyg 1992; 47:291.

Pugh RNH, Bell DR, Gilles HM: Malumfasi endemic diseases research project XV. The potential medical importance of bilharzia in northern Nigeria: A suggested rapid, cheap and effective solution for control of *Schistosoma haematobium* infection. Ann Trop Med Parasitol 1980; 74:597.

Pugh RNH, Teesdale CH: Single-dose oral treatment in urinary schistosomiasis: A double-blind trial. BMJ 1983; 286:429.

Pugh RNH, Teesdale CH: Long term efficacy of single dose oral treatment in schistosomiasis haematobium. Trans R Soc Trop Med Hyg 1984; 78:55.

Rady MY, Rady AM: Full-length ureteric splintage in the management of bilharzial ureteric strictures. Br J Urol 1987; 59:297.

Ratard RC, Greer GJ: A new focus of *Schistosoma haematobium/S. intercalatum* hybrid in Cameroon. Am J Trop Med Hyg 1991; 45:332.

Ratard RC, Kouemeni LE, Bessala MM, et al: Human schistosomiasis in Cameroon: I. Distribution of schistosomiasis. Am J Trop Med Hyg 1990; 42:561.

Rathore A, Ricklan DE, Flores Villanueva PO, Stadecker MJ: In situ analysis of Th cell–regulatory B7 molecule expression in *Schistosoma mansoni* egg granulomas. Am J Trop Med Hyg 1995; 53:150.

Raziuddin S, Masihuzzaman M, Shetty S, Ibrahim A: Tumor necrosis factor alpha production in schistosomiasis with carcinoma of urinary bladder. J Clin Immunol 1993; 13:23.

Raziuddin S, Shetty S, Ibrahim A: T-cell abnormality and defective interleukin-2 production in patients with carcinoma of the urinary bladder with schistosomiasis. J Clin Immunol 1991; 11:103.

Raziuddin S, Shetty S, Ibrahim A: Phenotype, activation and lymphokine secretion by gamma/delta T lymphocytes from schistosomiasis and carcinoma of the urinary bladder. Eur J Immunol 1992; 22:309.

Reeder MM, Palmer PES: Schistosomiasis. *In* The Radiology of Tropical Diseases with Epidemiological, Pathological and Clinical Correlations. Baltimore, Williams & Wilkins, 1981, pp 83–156.

Reimert CM, Ouma JH, Mwanje MT, et al: Indirect assessment of eosinophiluria in urinary schistosomiasis using eosinophil cationic protein (ECP) and eosinophil protein X (EPX). Acta Trop 1993; 54:1.

Ripert C, Combe A, Daulouede S, et al: Detection with a monoclonal antibody of an antigen, characteristic of the genus, *Schistosoma*, excreted in the urine. Trop Med Parasitol 1988; 39:131.

Robert CF, Mauris A, Bouvier P, Rougemont A: Proteinuria screening using sulfosalicylic acid: Advantages of the method for the monitoring of prenatal consultations in West Africa. Soz Praventivmed 1995; 40:44.

Rohde R, Braun-Munzinger RA, Rasoloarison C: Potential false positive egg-counts through the reuse of polyamide filters in the diagnosis of urinary schistosomiasis. Trop Med Parasitol 1985; 36:143.

Rosin MP, Anwar W: Chromosomal damage in urothelial cells from Egyptians with chronic *Schistosoma haematobium* infections. Int J Cancer 1992; 50:539.

Rosin MP, Anwar WA, Ward AJ: Inflammation, chromosomal instability, and cancer: The schistosomiasis model. Cancer Res 1994a; 54:1929S.

Rosin MP, Saad el Din Zaki S, Ward AJ, Anwar WA: Involvement of inflammatory reactions and elevated cell proliferation in development of bladder cancer in schistosomiasis patients. Mutat Res 1994b; 305:283.

Rousset JJ, Houin R, Buttner A: Acido-alcoholo resistance de divers oeufs de schistosomas. Ann Parasit Hum Comp 1962; 37:866.

Ruffer MA: Note on the presence of *Bilharzia haematobium* in Egyptian mummies of the Twentieth Dynasty (1250–1000 B.C.). BMJ 1910; 1:16.

Rutasitara WK, Chimbe A: Spontaneous cure in schistosomiasis. East Afr Med J 1985; 62:408.

Sabha M, Nilsson T: Urodynamic evaluation of calcified bilharzial bladders. APMIS 1988; (suppl 3):50–53.

Sadigursky M, Kamel IA, Elwi AM, et al: Absence of schistosomal glomerulopathy in *Schistosoma haematobium* infection in man. Trans R Soc Trop Med Hyg 1976; 70:322.

Sadun EH, von Lichtenberg F, Cheever AW, et al: Experimental infection with *Schistosoma haematobium* in chimpanzees. Parasitologic, clinical, serologic, and pathological observations. Am J Trop Med Hyg 1970; 19:427.

Sama MT, Ratard RC: Water contact and schistosomiasis infection in Kumba, south-western Cameroon. Ann Trop Med Parasitol 1994; 88:629.

Sarda RK, Minjas JN, Mahikwano LF: Evaluation of indirect screening techniques for the detection of *Schistosoma haematobium* infection in an urban area, Dar es Salaam, Tanzania. Acta Trop 1985; 42:241.

Sarda RK, Minjas JN, Mahikwano LF: Further observations on the use of gross hematuria as an indirect screening technique for the detection of *Schistosoma haematobium* infection in school children in Dar es Salaam, Tanzania. J Trop Med Hyg 1986; 89:309.

Sathe BD, Pandit CH, Chanderkar NG, et al: Sero-diagnosis of schistosomiasis by ELISA test in an endemic area of Gimvi village, India. J Trop Med Hyg 1991; 94:76.

Savioli L, Hatz C, Dixon H, et al: Control of morbidity due to *Schistosoma haematobium* on Pemba Island: Egg excretion and hematuria as indicators of infection. Am J Trop Med Hyg 1990; 43:289.

Schneider W: Die Muskulatur der oberen harnableitenden Wege. Z Anat Entwicklungsgesch 1938; 109:187.

Schwarzbach C, Genseke R: Computerized tomography image of chronic urogenital bilharziasis in childhood and adolescence. Zeit Urol Nephrol 1987; 80:635.

Scrimgeour EM, Gadjusek DC: Involvement of the central nervous system in *Schistosoma mansoni* and *S. haematobium* infection. A review. Brain 1985; 108:1023.

Sher A, James SL, Correa-Oliveira R, et al: Schistosome vaccines: Current progress and future prospects. Parasitology 1989; 98(Suppl):S61.

Shokeir AA, Bakr MA, el-Daisty TA, et al: Urological complications following live donor kidney transplantation: Effect of urinary schistosomiasis. Br J Urol 1992; 70:247.

Shokeir AA, Ibrahim AM, Hamid MY, et al: Urinary bilharziasis in upper Egypt: II. A bacteriologic study. East Afr Med J 1972; 49:312.

Siegrist D and Siegrist-Obimpeh P: *Schistosoma haematobium* infection in pregnancy. Acta Trop 1992; 50:317.

Simpson AJ, Smithers SR: Schistosomes: Surface, egg and circulating antigens. Curr Top Microbiol Immunol 1985; 120:205.

Siongok TK, Ouma JH, Houser HB, Warren KS: Quantification of infection with *Schistosoma haematobium* in relation to epidemiology and selective population chemotherapy: II. Mass treatment with a single oral dose of metrifonate. J Infect Dis 1978; 138:856.

Smith JH, Christie JD: The pathobiology of *Schistosoma haematobium* infection in humans. Human Pathology 1986; 17:333.

Smith JH, Elwi A, Kamel IA, von Lichtenberg F: A quantitative post mortem analysis of urinary schistosomiasis in Egypt: I. Pathology and pathogenesis. Am J Trop Med Hyg 1974a; 23:1054.

Smith JH, Elwi A, Kamel IA, von Lichtenberg F: A quantitative post mortem analysis of urinary schistosomiasis in Egypt: II. Evolution and epidemiology. Am J Trop Med Hyg 1975; 24:806.

Smith JH, Kelada AS, Khalil A: Schistosomal ulceration of the urinary bladder. Am J Trop Med Hyg 1977a; 26:89.

Smith JH, Kelada AS, Khalil A, Torky AH: Surgical pathology of schistosomal obstructive uropathy: A clinicopathologic study. Am J Trop Med Hyg 1977b; 26:96.

Smith JH, Said MN, Kelada AS: Studies on schistosomal rectal and colonic polyposis. Am J Trop Med Hyg 1977c; 26:80.

Smith JH, Torky H, Kelada AS, Farid Z: Schistosomal polyposis of the urinary bladder. Am J Trop Med Hyg 1977d; 26:85.

Smith JH, Torky H, Mansour N, Cheever AW: Studies on egg excretion and tissue egg burden in urinary schistosomiasis. Am J Trop Med Hyg 1974b; 23:163.

Smith JH, von Lichtenberg F: The Hoeppli phenomenon in schistosomiasis: II. Histochemistry. Am J Pathol 1967; 50:993.

Smith JH, von Lichtenberg F: Tissue degradation of calcific *Schistosoma haematobium* eggs. Am J Trop Med Hyg 1976; 25:595.

Smithers SR, Terry RJ: Resistance to experimental infection with *Schistosoma mansoni* in rhesus monkeys induced by transfer of adult worms. Trans R Soc Trop Med Hyg 1967; 61:517.

Sobh MA, Moustafa FE, Ramzy RM, et al: *Schistosoma haematobium*–induced glomerular disease: An experimental study in the golden hamster. Nephron 1991; 57:216.

Stephenson LS, Latham MC, Kinoti SN, Odowri ML: Sensitivity and specificity of reagent strips in screening of Kenyan children for *Schistosoma haematobium* infection. Am J Trop Med Hyg 1984; 33:862.

Stephenson LS, Latham MC, Kurz KM, et al: Relationships of *Schistosoma haematobium*, hookworm and malarial infections and metrifonate treatment to growth of Kenyan school children. Am J Trop Med Hyg 1985; 34:1109.

Stephenson LS, Latham MC, Kurz KM, Kinoti SN: Single dose metrifonate or praziquantel treatment in Kenyan children: II. Effects on growth in relation to *Schistosoma haematobium* and hookworm egg counts. Am J Trop Med Hyg 1989; 41:445.

Stimmel CM, Scott JA: The regularity of egg output of *Schistosoma haematobium*. Tex Rpt Biol Med 1956; 14:440.

Strickland GT, Abdel-Wahab MF: Abdominal ultrasonography for assessing morbidity from schistosomiasis: 1. Community studies. Trans R Soc Trop Med Hyg 1993; 87:132.

Sutherland JC, Berry A, Hynd M, Proctor NSF: Placental bilharziasis. Report of a case. S Afr J Obstet Gynaecol 1965; 3:76.

Swart PJ, van der Merwe JV: Wet-smear diagnosis of genital schistosomiasis. S Afr Med J 1987; 72:631.

Taylor P, Chandiwana SK, Matanhire D: Evaluation of the reagent strip test for hematuria in the control of *Schistosoma haematobium* infection in school children. Acta Trop 1990; 47:91.

Taylor P, Murare HM, Manomano K: Efficacy of low dose of praziquantel for *Schistosoma mansoni* and *S. haematobium*. J Trop Med Hyg 1988; 91:13.

Thomas JE, Bassett MT, Sigola LB, Taylor P: Relationship between bladder cancer incidence, *Schistosoma haematobium* infection, and geographical region in Zimbabwe. Trans R Soc Trop Med Hyg 1990; 84:551.

Tricker AR, Mostafa MH, Spiegelhalder B, Preussmann R: Urinary nitrate, nitrite and N-nitroso compounds in bladder cancer patients with schistosomiasis (bilharzia). IARC Sci Publ 1991; (105):178–181.

Tungekar MF, Abdul-Sattar S, Al-Adnani MS: Expression of chorionic gonadotropin by schistosomiasis-associated squamous carcinomas of the bladder. Eur Urol 1988a; 14:30.

Tungekar MF, Al-Adnani MS: Sarcomas of the bladder and prostate: The role of immunohistochemistry and ultrastructure in diagnosis. Eur Urol 1986; 12:180.

Tungekar MF, Gatter KC, Al-Adnani MS: Schistosomiasis-associated squamous lesions of the bladder. Expression of low molecular weight cytokeratin proteins. Br J Urol 1987; 60:423.

Tungekar MF, Gatter KC, Al-Adnani MS: Immunohistochemistry of cytokeratin proteins in squamous and transitional cell lesions of the urinary tract. J Clin Path 1988b; 41:1288.

Turner I, Ibels LS, Alexander JH, Harrison A, Moir D: Minimal change glomerulonephritis associated with *Schistosoma haematobium* infection—Resolution with praziquantel treatment. Aust N Z J Med 1987; 17:596.

Ugaily-Thulesius L, Thulesius O, Sabha M: The effect of urothelial damage on ureteric motility. An ultrastructural and functional study. Br J Urol 1988; 62:19.

Umerah BC: Bilharzial hydronephrosis: A clinicoradiologic study. J Urol 1981; 126:164.

van Lieshout L, de Jonge N, Bassily S, Mansour MM, Deelder AM: Assessment of cure in schistosomiasis patients after chemotherapy with praziquantel by quantitation of circulating anodic antigen (CAA) in urine. Am J Trop Med Hyg 1991; 44:323.

van Lieshout L, De Jonge N, el-Masry NA, et al: Improved diagnostic performance of the circulating antigen assay in human schistosomiasis by parallel testing for circulation anodic and cathodic antigens in serum and urine. Am J Trop Med Hyg 1992; 47:463.

van Lieshout L, De Jonge N, el-Masry N, et al: Monitoring the efficacy of different doses of praziquantel by quantification of circulation antigens in serum and urine of schistosomiasis patients. Parasitology 1994; 108:519.

Vennervald BJ, Reimert CM, Ouma JH, et al: Morbidity markers for *Schistosoma haematobium* infection. Trop Geogr Med 1994; 46:239.

Véra C, Jourdane J, Sellin B, Combes C: Genetic variability in the compatibility between *Schistosoma haematobium* and its potential vectors in Niger. Epidemiological implications. Trop Med Parasitol 1990; 41:143.

Ville Y, Leruez M, Picaud A, et al: Tubal schistosomiasis as a cause of ectopic pregnancy in endemic areas? A report of three cases. Eur J Obstet Gynecol Reprod Biol 1991; 42:77.

von Lichtenberg F: Host response to eggs of *Schistosoma mansoni*: I. Granuloma formation in the unsensitized laboratory mouse. Am J Pathol 1962; 41:711.

von Lichtenberg F: Studies on granuloma formation: III. Antigen sequestration and destruction in the schistosome pseudotubercle. Am J Pathol 1964; 45:75.

von Lichtenberg F: Comparative histopathology of schistosome granulomas in the hamster. Am J Pathol 1973; 72:149.

von Lichtenberg F: Schistosomiasis as a world-wide problem: Pathology. J Toxicol Environ Health 1975; 1:175.

von Lichtenberg F, Edington GM, Nwabuebo I, et al: Pathologic effects of schistosomiasis in Ibadan, Western State of Nigeria: II. Pathogenesis of lesions of the bladder and ureters. Am J Trop Med Hyg 1971; 20:244.

von Lichtenberg F, Erickson DG, Sadun EH: Comparative histopathology of schistosome granulomas in the hamster. Am J Pathol 1973; 72:149.

von Lichtenberg F, Lindenberg M: An acid-fast substance in ova of *Schistosoma mansoni*. Am J Trop Med Hyg 1954; 3:1066.

von Lichtenberg F, Smith JH, Cheever AW: The Hoeppli phenomenon in schistosomiasis: I. Comparative pathology and immunopathology. Am J Trop Med Hyg 1966; 15:886.

von Lichtenberg A, Swick M: Klinische Prufung des Uroselectans. Klin Wochenschr 1929; 8:2089.

Wakefield GS, Carroll JD, Speed DE: Schistosomiasis of the spinal cord. Brain 1962; 85:535.

Wallace DM: Urinary schistosomiasis in Saudi Arabia. Ann R Coll Surg Eng 1979; 61:265.

Warren KS: The pathology of schistosome infections. Helminthol Abstr 1973a; 42:592.

Warren KS: Regulation of the prevalence and intensity of schistosomiasis in man. Immunology or ecology? J Infect Dis 1973b; 127:595.

Warren KS: Schistosomiasis: Host-pathogen biology. Rev Infect Dis 1982; 4:771.

Warren KS, Mahmoud AAF, Muraka JF, et al: *Schistosomiasis haematobium* in Coast Province, Kenya. Relationship between egg output and morbidity. Am J Trop Med Hyg 1979; 28:864.

Warren KS, Siongok TK, Houser HB, et al: Quantification of infection with *Schistosoma haematobium* in relation to epidemiology and selective population chemotherapy: I. Minimal number of daily egg counts in urine necessary to establish intensity of infection. J Infect Dis 1978; 138:849.

Webbe G: Treatment of schistosomiasis. Eur J Clin Pharm 1987; 32:433.

Weeden D, Hopewell JP, Moorhead JF, et al: Schistosomiasis in renal transplantation. Br J Urol 1982; 54:478.

Wiest PM, Kossman RJ, Tartakoff AM: Determinants of surface membrane maturation during the cercarial-schistosomule transformation of *Schistosoma mansoni*. Am J Trop Med Hyg 1989; 47:70.

Wilkins HA: Are measurements of intensity of infection or morbidity necessary to evaluate schistosomiasis control within PHC? Trop Med Parasitol 1986; 37:223.

Wilkins HA, Amnasi JH, Crawley JCW, Veall N: Isotope renography and urinary schistosomiasis: A study in a Gambian community. Trans R Soc Trop Med Hyg 1985a; 79:306.

Wilkins HA, Blumenthal UJ, Hagan RJ, et al: Resistance to reinfection after treatment of urinary schistosomiasis. Trans R Soc Trop Med Hyg 1987; 81:29.

Wilkins HA, Goll PH, Marshall TFC, Moore PJ: The significance of proteinuria and hematuria in *Schistosoma haematobium* infections. Trans R Soc Trop Med Hyg 1979; 73:74.

Wilkins HA, Goll PH, Marshall TFC, Moore PJ: Dynamics of *Schistosoma haematobium* infections in a Gambian community: III. Acquisition and loss of infection. Trans R Soc Trop Med Hyg 1984; 78:227.

Wilkins HA, Goll PH, Moore PJ: *Schistosoma haematobium* infections and hemoglobin concentrations in a Gambian community. Ann Trop Med Parasitol 1985b; 79:159.

Williams AO: Pathology of schistosomiasis of the uterine cervix due to *S. haematobium*. Am J Obstet Gynecol 1967; 98:784.

Wishahi M: The role of dilatation in bilharzial ureters. Br J Urol 1987; 59:405.

Wishahi M, el-Baz HG, Shaker ZA: Association of HLA-A, B, C and DR antigens and clinical manifestations of *Schistosoma haematobium* in the bladder. Eur Urol 1989; 16:138.

Woolhouse ME, Ndamba J, Bradley DJ: The interpretation of intensity and aggregation data for infections of *Schistosoma haematobium*. Trans R Soc Trop Med Hyg 1994; 88:520.

Woolhouse ME, Taylor P, Matanhire D, Chandiwana SK: Acquired immunity and epidemiology of *Schistosoma haematobium*. Nature 1991; 351:757.

World Health Organization: Immunology of Schistosomiasis. Memorandum of a meeting of investigators held in Nairobi, December 11–17, 1974.

Wright ED, Chiphangwe J, Hutt MSR: Schistosomiasis of the female genital tract. A histopathologic study of 176 cases from Malawi. Trans R Soc Trop Med Hyg 1982; 76:822.

Wright WH: Geographical distribution of schistosomes and their intermediate hosts. *In* Ansari N, ed: Epidemiology and Control of Schistosomiasis (Bilharziasis). Basel, S. Karger, 1973, pp 32–49.

Yogore MG Jr, Lewert RM, Reyes VA: Cerebral Schistosomiasis japonica in the Philippines: Immunoprecipitins in the Cerebrospinal Fluid. Paper presented at the Fiftieth Annual Meeting of the American Society of Tropical Medicine and Hygiene, New Orleans, Nov. 11, 1975.

Young D, Beland JE, Kloos H, et al: Schistosomiasis in an American medical investigator. J Clin Gastroenterol 1986; 8:589.

Young SW, Higashi GI, Kamel R: Interaction of Salmonellae and Schistosomiasis in host-parasite relations. Trans R Soc Trop Med Hyg 1973; 67:797.

Young SW, Khalid KH, Farid Z, Mahmoud AH: Urinary tract lesions of *Schistosoma haematobium* with detailed radiographic consideration of the ureter. Radiology 1974; 111:81.

Zahran MM, Badr MM: Study of bilharzial uropathy by means of hippuran I^{131} extended renography. Am J Trop Hyg 1980; 29:576.

Genital Filariasis

Ah HS, McCall JW, Thompson PE: Vaccination against experimental *Brugia pahangi* infection in dogs. Proc Third Int Cong Parasitol Munich, Germany 1974a; 3:1236–1237.

Ah HS, Klei TR, McCall JW, Thompson PE: *Brugia pahangi* infections in Mongolian jirds and dogs following the ocular inoculation of infective larvae. J Parasitol 1974b; 60:643.

Ahrens EH Jr: Clinical research on patients with chyluria. Jpn J Trop Med 1970; 11:53.

Amaral F, Dreyer G, Figuereido-Silva J, et al: Live adult worms detected by ultrasonography in human bancroftian filariasis. Am J Trop Med Hyg 1994; 50:753–757.

Aziz MA: Efficacy and tolerance of ivermectin in human onchocerciasis. Lancet 1982; 2:171.

Beaver PC, Cran IR: *Wuchereria*-like filaria in an artery, associated with pulmonary infarction. Am J Trop Med Hyg 1974; 23:869.

Bosworth W, Ewert A: The effect of streptococcus on the persistence of *Brugia malayi* and the production of elephantiasis in cats. Int J Parasitol 1975; 5:583.

Casley-Smith JR, Wang CT, Casley-Smith JR, Zi Hai C: Treatment of filarial lymphedema and elephantiasis with 5,6-benzo-alpha-pyrone (Coumarin). BMJ 1993; 307:1037.

Castellani A: Endemic funiculitis, brief general account. J Trop Med 1931; 34:373.

Cohen LB, Nelson G, Wood AM, et al: Lymphangiography in filarial lymphedema and elephantiasis. Am J Trop Med Hyg 1961; 10:843.

Connor DH, Morrison NE, Kerdel-Vegas F, et al: Onchocerciasis: Onchocerciasis dermatitis, lymphadenitis and elephantiasis in the Ubangi territory. Hum Pathol 1970; 1:553.

Danaraj TJ, Pacheco W, Shanmugaratnam K, Beaver PC: The etiology and pathology of eosinophilic lung (tropical eosinophilia). Am J Trop Med Hyg 1966; 19:181.

Davis BR: Filariasis. Dermatol Clin 1989; 7:313.

Denham DA, Ponnudurai T, Nelson GS, et al: Studies with *Brugia pahangi*: I. Parasitological observations on primary infections of cats (*Felis catus*). Int J Parasitol 1972; 2:239.

Dissanayake S, Zseng H, Dreyer G, et al: Evaluation of recombinant parasite antigen for the diagnosis of lymphatic filariasis. Am J Trop Med Hyg 1994; 50:727–734.

Ewert A: Distribution of developing and mature *Brugia malayi* in cats at various times after a single inoculation. J Parasitol 1971; 74:1039.

Galindo L, von Lichtenberg F, Baldizon C: Bancroftian filariasis in Puerto Rico: Infection pattern and tissue lesions. Am J Trop Med Hyg 1962; 11:739.

Gandhi GM: Role of lymphangiography in management of filarial chyluria. Lymphology 1976; 9:11.

Greene BM, Taylor HR, Cupp EW, et al: Comparison of ivermectin and diethylcarbamazine in treatment of onchocerciasis. N Engl J Med 1985; 313:133.

Hunter GW, Swartzwelder JC, Clyde DF: Morphology of the Filarioidea. *In* Hunter GW, Swartzwelder JD, Clyde DF, eds: Tropical Medicine, 5th ed. Philadelphia, WB Saunders Company, 1976, pp 492–494.

Jachowski LA, Gonzalez-Flores B, von Lichtenberg F: Filarial etiology of tropical hydroceles in Puerto Rico. Am J Trop Med Hyg 1962; 11:220.

Jantet GH, Taylor GW, Kinmonth JB: Operations for primary lymphedema of the lower limbs: Results after 1–9 years. J Cardiovasc Surg (Torino) 1961; 2:27.

Kanetkar AV, Deshmukh SM, Pradham RS, et al: Lymphangiographic patterns in filarial oedema of lower limbs. Clin Radiol 1966; 17:258.

Kazura J, Bockarie M, Alexander N, et al: Risk factors for acute morbidity in bancroftian filariasis. Am J Trop Med Hyg 1995; 53:100.

King CL, Hakimi J, Shata MT, Medhat A: IL-12 regulation of parasite antigen-driven IgE production in human helminth infections. J Immunol 1995; 155:454–461.

Klei TR, McCall JW, Malone JB, Thompson PE: Superinfections of *Brugia pahangi* in the Mongolian jird. Proc Third Int Cong Parasitol Munich, Germany, 1974; 2:617.

Lie KJ: Occult filariasis: Its relationship with tropical pulmonary eosinophilia. Am J Trop Med Hyg 1962; 11:646.

O'Connor FW, Hulse CR: Studies in filariasis: I. In Puerto Rico. Puerto Rico J Public Health Trop Med 1935; 11:167.

Orihel TC, Moore PJ: *Loa loa*: Experimental infection in two species of African primates. Am J Trop Med Hyg 1975; 24:606.

Ottesen EA: Filariasis now. Am J Trop Med Hyg 1989; 41(suppl):8.

Ottesen EA, Neva FA, Paranjare RS, et al: Specific allergic sensitization to filarial antigens in tropical eosinophilia syndrome. Lancet 1979; 1:1158.

Ottesen EA, Vijayasekaran V, Kumaraswami V, et al: A controlled trial of ivermectin and diethylcarbamazine in lymphatic filariasis. N Engl J Med 1990; 322:1113.

Partono F: The spectrum of disease in lymphatic filariasis. *In* Filariasis: Ciba Foundation Symposium, vol 127. New York, John Wiley & Sons, 1987; p 265.

Partono F, Purnomo, Oemijati S, Soewarta A: The long-term effects of repeated diethylcarbamazine administration with special reference to microfilaremia and elephantiasis. Acta Trop 1981; 38:217.

Piessens WF: Immunology of lymphatic filariasis and onchocerciasis. *In* Cohen S, Warren KS, eds: Immunology of Parasitic Disease, 2nd ed. Oxford, Blackwell Scientific Publications, 1982, pp 622–653.

Sasa M, Tanaka H: A new method for statistical analysis of the microfilarial periodicity survey data [Abstract 35]. *In* Japan-U.S. Cooperative Medical Science Program: Joint Conference on Parasitic Diseases, Hiroshima, July 18–20, 1972, pp 104–106.

Sato H, Otsuji Y, Maeda T, et al: A case of huge penile and scrotal elephantiasis [Abstract F 12]. *In* Japan-U.S. Cooperative Medical Science Program: Joint Conference on Parasitic Diseases, Unzen, Nagasaki, Japan, August 17–19, 1974.

Schacher JF, Sahyoun PF: A chronological study of the histopathology of filarial disease in cats and dogs caused by *Brugia pahangi*. Trans R Soc Trop Med Hyg 1967; 61:234.

Sullivan JJ, Chernin E: Oral transmission of *Brugia pahangi* and *Dipetalonema viteae* to adult and neonatal jirds. Int J Parasitol 1976; 6:75.

Tani S, Akisada M: Lymphographical findings of the lymphaticopelvic fistulization in filarial chyluria. Jpn J Trop Med 1970; 11:55.

Taylor AER: Studies on the microfilaria of *Loa loa*, *Wuchereria bancrofti*, *Brugia malayi*, *Dirofilaria immitis*, *Dirofilaria repens* and *Dirofilaria aethiops*. J Helminthol 1960; 34:13.

von Lichtenberg F: The early phase of bancroftian filariasis in the male. Pathologic study. J Mt Sinai Hosp 1957; 24:983.

von Lichtenberg F: Inflammatory responses to filarial connective tissue parasites. Parasitol 1987; 94:S101.

von Lichtenberg F, Medina R: Bancroftian filariasis in the etiology of funiculoepididymitis, periorchitis and hydrocele in Puerto Rico (statistical study of surgical and autopsy material over a 13-year period). Am J Trop Med Hyg 1957; 6:739.

Wartman WB: Filariasis in American Armed Forces in World War II. Medicine 1947; 26:333.

Weil GJ, Hussain R, Kumaraswami V, et al: Prenatal allergic sensitization to helminth antigens in offspring of parasite-infected mothers. J Clin Invest 1983; 71:1124.

Williams AO, von Lichtenberg F, Smith JH, Martinson FD: Ultrastructure of phycomycosis and associated Splendore-Hoeppli phenomenon. Arch Pathol 1969; 87:459.

Wong MM, Fredericks HJ, Ramachandran CP: Studies on immunization against *Brugia malayi* infection in the rhesus monkey. Bull WHO 1969; 40:493.

Other Parasitic Diseases of the Genitourinary Tract

Barrett-Connor L: Chemoprophylaxis of amoebiasis and trypanosomiasis. Ann Intern Med 1972; 77:797.

Borrell JH, Barnes JM: Renal manifestations of hydatid diseases. N Y State J Med 1933; 33:1390.

Brandt H, Perez Tamayo R: Pathology of human amoebiasis. Hum Pathol 1970; 1:351.

Cannon DA: Linguatulid infestation of man. Ann Trop Med Parasitol 1942; 36:160.

D'Alessandro RL: *Echinococcus vogeli* in man with a review of polycystic disease in Columbia and neighboring countries. Am J Trop Med Hyg 1979; 28:303.

Dent JH, Nichols RL, Beaver PC, et al: Visceral larva migrans; with a case report. Am J Pathol 1965; 32:777.

Engman MF, Meleney HE: Amoebiasis cutis. Arch Dermatol Syph 1931; 24:1.

Grigsby WP: Surgical treatment of amoebiasis. Surg Gynecol Obstet 1969; 128:609.

Hopps HC: Pentastomiasis. *In* Marcial-Rojas R, ed: Pathology of Protozoal and Helminthic Diseases. Baltimore, Williams & Wilkins, 1971, pp 970–989.

Lindner RR: Retrospective x-ray survey for *Porocephalus*. J Trop Med Hyg 1965; 68:155.

Lins EE: The solution of incrustations in the urinary bladder by a new method. J Urol 1945; 53:702.

Musacchio F, Mitchell N: Primary renal echinococcosis: A case report. Am J Trop Med Hyg 1966; 15:168.

Powell SJ: Drug therapy of amoebiasis. Bull WHO 1969; 40:953.

Rausch RL: On the occurrence and distribution of *Echinococcus* sp. (Cestoda, Taeniidae) and characteristics of their development in the intermediate host. Am J Parasitol 1967; 42:19.

Sanjurjo LA: Strongylosis. *In* Campbell MF, Harrison JH, eds: Campbell's Urology, 3rd ed. Philadelphia, WB Saunders Company, 1970, pp. 508–509.

Symmers W St C: Pathology of enterobiasis. AMA Arch Pathol 1950; 50:475.

Waller CE, Othersen HB Jr: Ascariasis: Surgical complications in children. Am J Surg 1971; 120:50.

Whitehill R, Miller HM: Infestations of the genitourinary tract by *Strongyloides stercoralis*. A case report. Bull Johns Hopkins Hosp 1944; 75:169.

Effect of Parasitic Infections on the Kidney

Andrade ZS, Andrade SG, Sadigursky M: Renal changes in patients with hepatosplenic schistosomiasis. Am J Trop Med Hyg 1971; 20:77.

Andrade ZS, Rocha H: Schistosomal glomerulopathy. Kidney Int 1979; 16:23.

Cavallo T, Galvanek EG, Ward PA, von Lichtenberg F: The nephropathy of experimental hepatosplenic schistosomiasis. Am J Pathol 1974; 76:433.

de Brito T, Gunji J, Camargo ME, et al: Glomerular lesions in experimental infection of *Schistosoma mansoni* in *Cebus apella* monkeys. Bull WHO, 1971; 45:419.

de Water R, Van Marck EAE, Fransen JAM, Deelder AM: *Schistosoma mansoni*: Ultrastructural localization of circulating anodic antigen and circulating cathodic antigen in mouse kidney glomerulus. Am J Trop Med Hyg 1988; 38:118.

Gilles HM, Hendrickse RG: Nephrosis in Nigerian children: Role of *Plasmodium malariae*; effect of antimalarial treatment. BMJ 1963; 2:27.

Higashi GI, Farid Z, Bassily S, Miner WF: Nephrotic syndrome in schistosomiasis mansoni complicated by chronic salmonellosis. Am J Trop Med Hyg 1975; 24:713.

Hillyer GV, Lewert RM: Studies on renal pathology in hamsters infected with *Schistosoma mansoni* and *Schistosoma japonica*. Am J Trop Med Hyg 1974; 23:404.

Klei TR, Crowell WA, Thompson PE: Ultrastructural glomerular changes associated with filariasis. Am J Trop Med Hyg 1974; 23:608.

Lehman JS, Mott KE, de Souza CAM, et al: The association of schistosomiasis mansoni and proteinuria in an endemic area. A preliminary report. Am J Trop Med Hyg 1975; 24:616.

Moran CJ, Ryder G, Turk JL, Waters MFR: Evidence for circulating immune complexes in lepromatous leprosy. Lancet 1972; 2:572.

Moriearty PL, Brito E: Elution of renal antischistosome antibodies in human schistosomiasis mansoni. Am J Trop Med Hyg 1977; 26:717.

Nagle RB, Ward PA, Lindsley HB, et al: Experimental infections with African trypanosomes: VI. Glomerulonephritis involving the alternate pathway of complement activation. Am J Trop Med Hyg 1974; 23:15.

Sinniah R, Churg J, Sobin L: Renal Disease: Classification and Atlas of Infectious and Tropical Diseases. Chicago, American Society of Clinical Pathologists Press, 1988, pp 1–264.

Soothill JF, Hendrickse RG: Some immunological studies of the nephrotic syndrome of Nigerian children. Lancet 1967; 2:629.

Voller A, Davies DR, Hutt MSR: Quartan malarial infections in *Aotus trivirgatus*, with special reference to renal pathology. Br J Exp Pathol 1973; 54:457.

von Lichtenberg F, Bawden MP, Shealey SH: Origin of circulating antigen from the schistosome gut. An immunofluorescent study. Am J Trop Med Hyg 1974; 23:1088.

Ward PA, Conran PB: Immunopathology of renal complications in simian malaria and human quartan malaria. Milit Med 1969; 134:1228.

Young SW, Higashi GI, Kamel R: Interaction of Salmonellae and schistosomiasis in host-parasite relations. Trans R Soc Trop Med Hyg 1973; 67:797.

23
FUNGAL INFECTIONS OF THE URINARY TRACT

Gilbert J. Wise, M.D.

THE OPPORTUNISTIC FUNGI

Candidal Infection

Historical Perspectives

The terms thrush, moniliasis, and yeast infection have been used interchangeably to describe a clinical entity caused by species of the fungus *Candida*, particularly *C. albicans*. Thrush (or white patches) has been known since the days of Hippocrates (Rippon, 1988, p 536). In 1890, Schmorl reported renal involvement in a patient with disseminated candidiasis. Rafin recognized candidal cystitis in 1910 but did not report his observation until 1927. Primary renal mycosis, presumably candidal, was reported by Lundquist in 1931 (Odds, 1988). In 1948, Moulder described cystoscopic findings of "thrush of the urinary bladder" in a 26-year-old male. By 1963, an additional 12 cases of candidal infection of the kidney had been reported (Hurley and Winner, 1963). Since then there have been increasing reports of clinical infections relating to *Candida* species, in part as a result of the increasing use of broad-spectrum antibiotics (Fisher et al, 1982).

Epidemiology and Predisposing Factors

During the decade 1980 to 1990, 344,610 infections were reported to the National Nosocomial Infections Surveillance System (Edwards, 1991). Fungi comprised 27,200 (7.9%), of which *Candida* accounted for 22,000 infections (6.2%).

In a study of 135 patients with candidemia, *C. albicans* was the most common species (51%), followed by *C. tropicalis* (25%), *C. parapsilosis* (12%), *Torulopsis glabrata* (9%), and other species (3%) (Komshian et al, 1989). An increase in incidence of fungemia caused by *Candida* and *Torulopsis* species has been observed in patients with neoplasia (Komshian et al, 1989). Candidal sepsis attack rates in this group rose from 4.6% in 1983 to 6.2% in 1986. The urinary tract was the portal of entry in 9 of 135 patients (7%). In a study of hospital-acquired fungemia, Klein and Watanakunakorn (1979) noted that positive urine culture for *Candida* species was observed for 18 of 31 patients (58%) before development of positive blood cultures, whereas urine cultures became positive in 20 of 25 patients (80%) after fungemia. Contributing factors in patients in whom fungemia developed included intravenous catheters (100%), antibiotic therapy (100%), and Foley catheter drainage (97%). Other predisposing conditions were surgery (69%) and genitourinary surgery (5%).

In an extensive review of urinary tract infections resulting from *C. albicans*, Fisher and associates (1982) cited diabetes mellitus, antibiotic administration, steroid therapy, urine flow turbulence, congenital anomalies, neurogenic bladder, indwelling catheters, and ileal conduits as factors that enhance the patient's vulnerability to these infections.

Hamory and Wenzel (1978) evaluated 98 hospital patients with significant candiduria (>10,000 to 15,000 colonies per milliliter). Patients in whom candiduria developed had longer urethral catheter drainage (12 versus 6 days) and had received antibiotic therapy for a longer time (16 versus 7 days) than noncandiduria patients. Primary diagnoses in this group included neoplasia, trauma, major surgery, cardiovascular disease, and renal stones.

Persistent candiduria in the critically ill surgical patient may portend disseminated infection with a mortality of 50% (Nassoura et al, 1993). Fungi, primarily *Candida,* account for 5% of infections in renal transplant patients (Paya, 1993).

Symptomatology

Candidal urinary tract infections can cause a variety of clinical symptoms and signs. The patient may be asymptomatic or may manifest signs of bladder irritability, namely, frequency, dysuria, and stranguria (with passage of fungal material). Pyuria, hematuria, or pneumaturia can occur. **Flank pain and symptoms of renal colic may be caused by the passage of fungal balls that obstruct the collecting system. Candidal infection may present as a classic pyelonephritis with flank pain, renal tenderness, and fever.** Fungal accretions may develop in the collecting system without overt clinical findings (Beilke and Kirmani, 1988; Sales and Mundy, 1973). Oliguria and anuria have been known to occur (Harbach et al, 1970). Other foci of infection may be present in the pharynx, esophagus, wound, intravenous catheter site, or genitalia. Recurrent fever in the patient who has been treated for bacterial infection may be caused by a secondary candidal infection.

Superficial Infection

Infection may develop around ileostomies and cutaneous pyelostomies (Schonebeck, 1986). Postoperative wound infections can occur with erythema and pustules in the incision site (Fig. 23–1) (Wise, 1989). Diagnosis can be established by identification of the fungus in exudate by smear or culture. If it is an isolated finding, this infection can be treated with topic antifungal agents such as nystatin, clotrimazole, or miconazole.

Vaginitis

C. albicans causes vulvovaginitis. Other *Candida* species that cause this clinical entity include *C. tropicalis, C. stellatoides,* and *C. parapsilosis* (Krieger, 1983). Antibacterial antibiotic therapy, oral contraceptives, pregnancy, and diabetes mellitus are predisposing factors. The patient may have a yellowish-white vaginal discharge and gray-white pseudomembranous exudate in the vagina and vulva. Pruritic symptoms are proportional to the number of organisms found in the vaginal discharge (Odds et al, 1988). Diagnosis can be established by microscopic detection of *Candida* species in vaginal exudate or by culture. The detection of candidal antigen in vaginal washings by latex agglutination test may be helpful in equivocal cases (Hopwood et al, 1985).

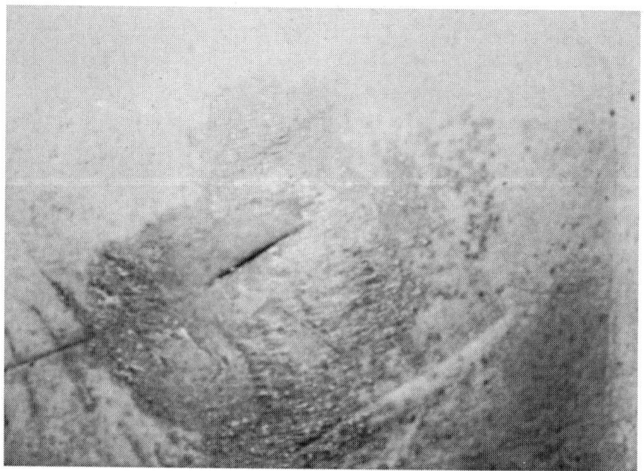

Figure 23–1. Incisional infection caused by *Candida albicans.* (From Wise GJ: AUA Update Series 1989; 8:195.)

Nystatin (100,000 units intravaginally for 14 days) has been the classic therapy. The numerous imidazole derivatives available today, which include butoconazole, clotrimazole, miconazole, terconazole, and tioconazole, provide a wide spectrum of topical agents that are efficacious for the treatment of vaginal candidiasis (The Medical Letter, 1994). Use of these agents in either cream, tablet, or suppository for 3 to 7 days has proved to be satisfactory treatment in most patients. **Oral fluconazole (single 150-mg dose) is as effective as intravaginal clotrimazole in the treatment of vulvovaginal candidiasis (Andersen et al, 1989).** Chronic infections have been more difficult to eradicate. Long-term therapy with ketoconazole (400 mg daily for 2 weeks followed by 100 mg daily for 6 months) has reduced the incidence of recurrent infection from 71.4% to 4.8%. However, recurrence developed with cessation of therapy (Sobel, 1986). Boric acid powder (600 mg in gelatin capsules) inserted vaginally each day for 2 weeks has been advocated as cost-effective therapy (Krieger, 1983).

Infection of the Genitalia

In a study of 135 unselected men, *C. albicans* was the most frequent isolate of "yeast" found in the coronal sulcus and meatus. Its incidence was similar in both circumcised (14%) and uncircumcised (17%) men; however, clinical manifestations of infection were greater in uncircumcised men (Davidson, 1977).

Candidal infection in a diabetic patient with an indwelling urethral catheter resulted in emphysematous cellulitis that involved the genital region. Despite systemic antifungal therapy, the patient died (Humayun and Maliwan, 1982).

Epididymitis has been an unusual manifestation of candidal infection. Two cases have been reported; one patient had the acquired immunodeficiency syndrome (AIDS) and was successfully treated with ketoconazole (200 mg/day for 6 weeks) (Swartz et al, 1988). The other patient was a diabetic who required an orchiectomy and subsequently received postoperative bladder irrigations of amphotericin B (Docimo et al, 1993). In both patients the urine cultures were positive for *C. albicans.*

A fungal abscess caused by *C. albicans* developed in a patient with a penile prosthesis. Removal of the prosthesis and treatment with intravenous amphotericin B were necessary to eradicate infection (Peppas et al, 1988).

Infection of the Bladder and Prostate

Candidal cystitis may occur in patients who require long-term urinary catheter drainage. Cystoscopy reveals gray-white patches on the bladder wall that are mixed with areas of mucosal edema and erythema (Hopfer, 1985; Rippon, 1988, p 554). A gray-white "snow effect" may obscure visualization. Microscopic examination of the exudate demonstrates inflammatory cells, among which yeast forms and

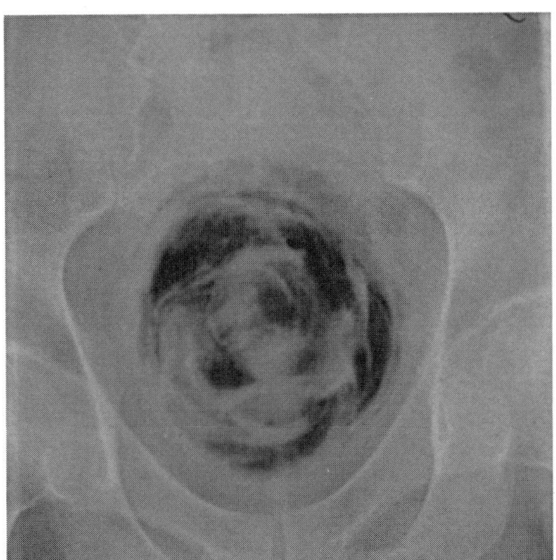

Figure 23–2. Radiographic appearance of large fungal bezoar in bladder of 48-year-old diabetic man.

pseudohyphae can be seen (Zincke et al, 1973). Accretions of the candidal pseudohyphae may develop with formation of fungus balls that may require surgical removal (Figs. 23–2 and 23–3) (Chisholm and Hutch, 1961; Harold et al, 1977). *C. albicans* caused a "perivesical" infection in a patient who underwent surgical correction of sigmoid diverticulitis. The infection was resolved with surgical drainage and intravenous fluconazole (100 mg twice daily for 10 days) (Sheynkin and Wise, 1995). Emphysematous cystitis caused by *C. albicans* has been reported in a 69-year-old insulin-dependent diabetic. Treatment consisted of bladder mucosal debridement followed by flucytosine (5-FC), 50 mg/kg every 6 hours, and ketoconazole, 200 mg/day; however, the patient expired from overwhelming infection (Singh and Lytle, 1983).

Prostatic emphysematosa secondary to *C. albicans* infection has been reported in diabetic patients. One patient with emphysematous prostatitis and cystitis was successfully treated by transurethral drainage of the prostate, suprapubic cystotomy, and 1 month of intravenous amphotericin B followed by ketoconazole (200 mg/day) (Bartkowski and Lanesky, 1988). A prostatic abscess caused by *C. tropicalis* was cured by transurethral drainage, suprapubic bladder drainage, intravenous amphotericin B (4 days) and oral fluconazole (200 mg/day for 6 weeks) (Yu and Provet, 1992) (Fig. 23–4). Surgical drainage and 6 weeks of intravenous amphotericin B (total dose 980 mg) resolved a prostatic abscess caused by *C. albicans* (Lentino et al, 1984).

Infection of the Ureter, Collecting System, and Kidney

An indwelling urinary catheter, diabetes mellitus, immune suppression, or obstructive uropathy enhances a patient's vulnerability to upper tract infection by a nonhematogenous route (Blum, 1966; Shelp et al, 1966). **In a retrospective study of 50 patients with genitourinary fungal infections, 25 patients (50%) had "complex" infections, as defined by upper tract involvement or a positive culture requiring intravenous antifungal therapy, or both; the other 25 (50%) had "simple" infections that were confined to the bladder and resolved with bladder irrigation with amphotericin B or catheter removal. The patients with complex infections had a higher incidence of obstructive uropathy (88% versus 20%). Fourteen (56%) required surgical intervention. Upper tract imaging was cited as essential in patients with complex genitourinary fungal infections (Wainstain et al, 1995).**

Fungal accretions known as fungal balls are known to cause ureteral obstruction (Keane at al, 1993) or renal pelvic obstruction (Stein et al, 1993). More than 50 cases of obstructive uropathy caused by fungal balls have been reported (Scerpella and Alhalel, 1994). *C. albicans* and *C. tropicalis* have been the most prevalent fungi. A *C. tropicalis* bladder infection has been reported to cause ureteral obstruction in a diabetic patient. Nephrostomies, oral ketoconazole (400 mg/day for 10 days), intravenous amphotericin B (30 mg/day for 6 weeks) and bladder irrigations with amphotericin B (45 mg/L at 100 ml/hour) eradicated the infection.

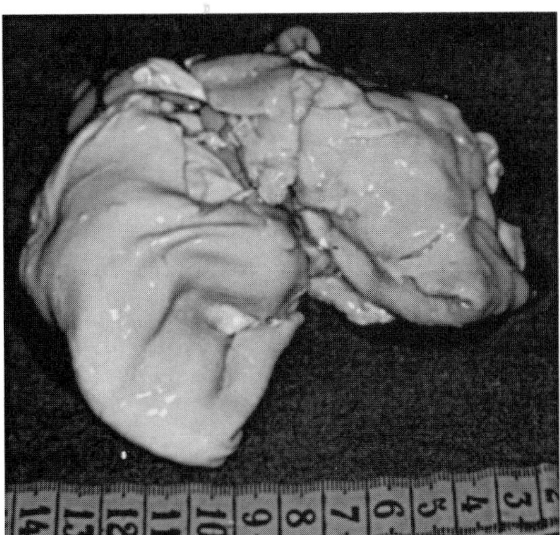

Figure 23–3. Large fungal bladder bezoar obtained by suprapubic removal.

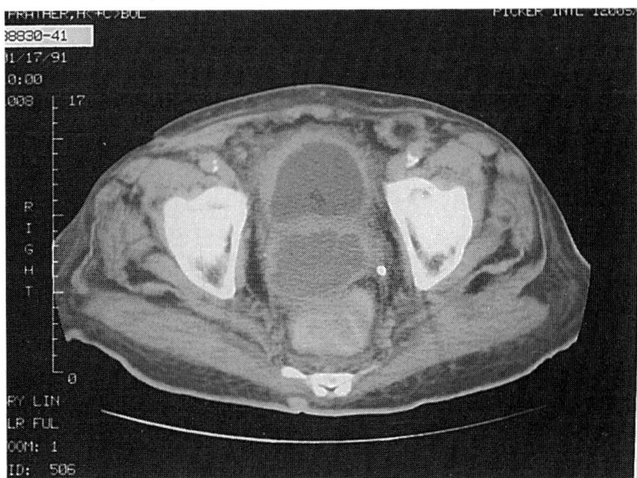

Figure 23–4. Computed tomographic scan demonstrating prostatic abscess cavity caused by *Candida*. (From Yu S, Provet J: J Urol 1992; 148:1536–1538.)

Criteria for success were documented by negative culture, biopsy, and resolution of obstruction (Gerridzen and Wesley-James, 1988).

Anuria caused by fungal accretion has been reported in a patient with a solitary kidney and an obstructed ureter caused by fungal accretion (Kocak et al, 1991). In rare cases, the obstruction may be bilateral (Harbach et al, 1970). Diagnosis is established by the identification of fungi in the urine, obstructive uropathy as documented by ultrasound or intravenous pyelogram, and often soft tissue densities within the renal pelvis, which represent fungal material (Stein et al, 1993). Treatment requires the use of nephrostomies, intravenous amphotericin B (total dose >850 mg), and direct irrigation of renal pelvis with amphotericin B (50 mg/L sterile water 40 ml/hour) (Bell et al, 1993; Scerpella and Alhalel, 1994). *C. albicans* infection of the ureter caused inflammation and stricture resulting in bilateral hydronephrosis (Lye et al, 1991).

Candidal pyocalix developed in a 58-year-old nondiabetic who required a long-term nephrostomy after percutaneous extraction of a renal stone. Amphotericin B irrigations through the nephrostomy tube (50 mg/24 hours), oral ketoconazole, and subsequent removal of the nephrostomy tube resolved the infection (Sonda and Amendola, 1985).

Candidal infection can cause pyelonephritis. Predisposing events have included candidal cystitis, ileal conduits (Schonebeck, 1986) and chronic neurogenic bladder disease (Sandin et al, 1991). Histologic findings in the renal pelvis may be similar to those in the bladder, namely, edema, erythema, and pseudoexudate (Hopfer, 1985). Candidal organisms have been found in association with renal pelvic lithiasis (Bhattacharya et al, 1982; Sales and Mundy, 1973).

Renal infection associated with obstructive uropathy causing fungemia was reported in three patients (Beilke and Kirmani, 1988). Treatment included renal irrigations (3.8 mg/hour) and intravenous administration of amphotericin B (850 to 1000 mg total dose) in conjunction with ureteral stent or nephrostomy. One patient received a 2-week course of 5-FC. Two of the three patients survived.

C. albicans and *C. tropicalis* have caused emphysematous pyelonephritis in diabetic patients who did not manifest urinary obstruction (Johnson et al, 1986; Seidenfeld et al, 1982). Nephrectomy was required in both patients.

Perinephric abscess secondary to *Candida* has been reported in 9 patients, most of whom were diabetics. Predisposing factors included surgery (including renal transplantation) and prolonged antibiotic therapy. Fever and flank pain were the most common clinical findings. Diagnosis was determined by ultrasonography and computed tomography (CT) scan. Positive urine cultures for *Candida* were noted in only 4 patients, whereas abscess aspirate or drainage yielded pure cultures in 9 patients. Treatment used surgical drainage in 5 patients and nephrectomy in 4 patients. Four patients received amphotericin B (590 to 1030 mg). There were no deaths that could be attributed to the perinephric abscess (High and Quagliarello, 1992). One report cites the development of a perinephric abscess in the transplanted kidney of a diabetic patient. Despite aggressive therapy with local bladder and systemic administration of amphotericin B, the infection progressed with rupture of the renal artery anastomosis, which necessitated graft removal (Pluemecke et al, 1992).

Systemic Candidal Infection

The kidney is second to the lung as a target organ for candidal infection in patients with fungemia (Luno and Tortoledo, 1985). **Genitourinary candidal infection may be the result or cause of systemic infection. Hematogenous renal infection can be unilateral in manifestation.** Experimental and clinical studies indicate that hematogenous candidal infection can cause pyelonephritis, abscess formation, papillary necrosis, and obstruction (Lehner, 1964; Hurley and Winner, 1963). Microscopic study demonstrates yeast forms or pseudohyphae in the glomeruli, interstitium, and tubules (Fig. 23–5). The proliferation of tubular pseudohyphae causes intrarenal obstructive uropathy. In later stages of hematogenous infection, larger fungal accretions develop that can cause obstruction of the renal collecting system (Hurley and Winner, 1963; Louria et al, 1962; Luno and Tortoledo, 1985).

Candidemia may occur synchronously or metachronously with staphylococcal or enterococcal infections (Meunier-Carpentier et al, 1981), or with bacteremia involving *Klebsiella, Serratia, Bacteroides, Enterobacter,* or *Proteus* species or *Escherichia coli* (Dyess et al, 1985). In a study of 83 patients with fungemia, Dyess and associates noted that 24 of 139 blood cultures (17%) were positive for bacteria before fungemia occurred, whereas 28 patients (20%) had synchronous bacterial and fungal positive blood cultures. The portal of entry of the fungus could be identified in only 38 of 83 patients (46%) in this study. The putative site of entry was the central venous line in 17 patients (45%), the urinary tract in 9 (24%), and the abdominal cavity or wound in 6 (16%).

The presence of candidemia in the surgical patient represents a significant risk. A retrospective study of 46 surgical patients with fungemia revealed that 26 (57%) died (Eubanks et al, 1993). Risk factors included renal failure, hepatic dysfunction, postoperative shock, and adult respiratory distress syndrome. Fifteen (32%) of the patients with fungemia had positive cultures from urine or catheter. Bacterial sepsis preceded or developed concomitantly in 15 (58%) of the 26 patients who died. The authors concluded that fungemia represents a failure of host resistance and that all critically

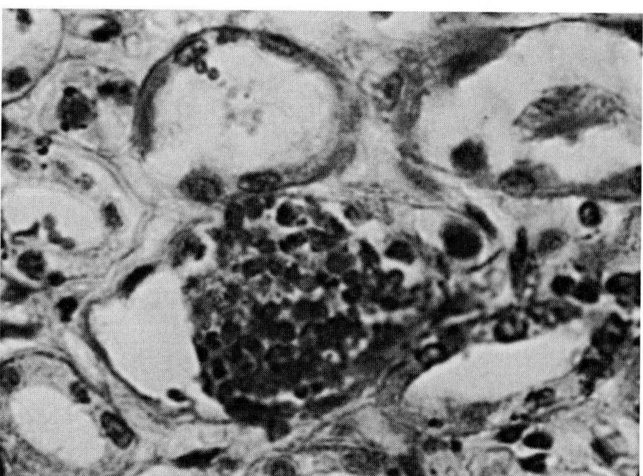

Figure 23–5. Candidal infection in renal peritubular vessel. Original magnification, × 900. (From Wise GJ: AUA Update Series 1989; 8[25]:195.)

ill surgical patients should receive oral antifungal prophylaxis (the drug and dosage were not specified).

Diagnosis of disseminated infection can be determined by culture of *Candida* species from other sites, such as wound, oropharynx, or gastrointestinal tract. Funduscopic study may demonstrate retinal exudate caused by candidal endophthalmitis (Kozinn et al, 1978).

Candidal Infection in Pediatric Patients

Indwelling intravascular catheters, treatment with antibacterial broad-spectrum antibiotics, prematurity, and low birth weight have been associated with the development of renal candidal infection in infants (Robinson et al, 1987). *C. albicans* has been the most prevalent organism, but *C. lusitaniae* has been reported as a cause of fungemia and urinary tract infection (Yinnon et al, 1992). Species differentiation is important because *C. lusitaniae* is known to have strains resistant to amphotericin B. Fungal infections occur in seriously ill infants, who may develop oliguria and anuria secondary to obstruction caused by fungal accretions (Bartone et al, 1988; Eckstein and Kass, 1982; Noe and Tonkin, 1982). Delay in diagnosis has resulted in a 50% mortality rate (Bartone et al, 1988; Noe and Tonkin, 1982). Examination of urine sediment may reveal *Candida* fungal elements. **Renal sonography is critical to the diagnosis; it often demonstrates hydronephrosis and fungal accretions within the collecting system. Percutaneous nephrostomy and the use of regional or systemic amphotericin B, or both, have increased survival dramatically.**

Candidal infections have developed in association with artificial sphincters in children. In two such cases, the infection was successfully treated with systemic amphotericin B. In only one patient was the artificial sphincter removed (Walterspiel et al, 1986).

Diagnostic Studies

Urine

Microscopic examination of the urine can reveal candidal fungi with budding forms or pseudohyphae (Fig. 23–6). Pyuria and hematuria may be present but are not specific findings. Urinary casts containing fungal material may be demonstrated by use of Papanicolau's stain; this observation is diagnostic of renal infection (Gregory et al, 1984). The use of fluorescence-labeled antibody for fungal antigens in urine has not proved efficacious to differentiate renal infection from bladder infection (Hall, 1980). *Candida* organisms can be cultured from the urine with a variety of laboratory media, including cystine-lactose-electrolyte-deficient medium, blood agar, and Sabouraud's agar with dextrose. Species differentiation is dependent on germ tube growth and carbohydrate fermentation (Hopfer, 1985).

Urinary candidal colony counts have been helpful in differentiating colonization from infection. Kozinn and associates (1978) reported that urine specimens obtained by clean catch or single catheterization from patients with histologically proven renal candidiasis had colony counts higher than 10,000 to 15,000/ml, whereas urine obtained from patients without renal infection had colony counts of 3500 ± 2500/ml. In the presence of indwelling urinary catheters, patients with renal candidiasis had colony counts of 64,000 ± 32,000/ml; in patients without renal candidiasis, colony counts were 72,000 ± 28,000/ml. These differences were not statistically different. Hence, **in the presence of indwelling urinary catheters, colony counts cannot be used to differentiate colonization from local or invasive infection.**

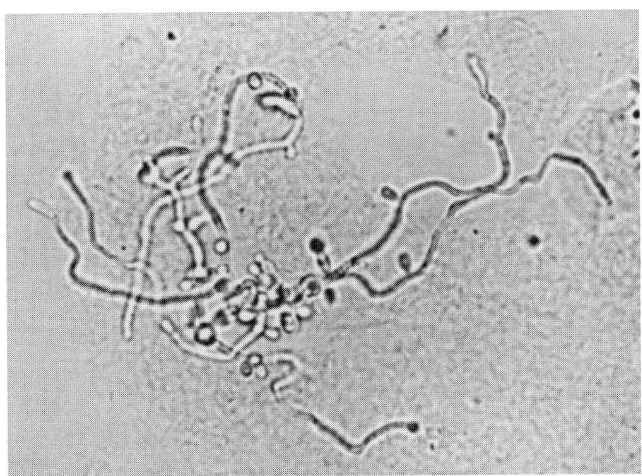

Figure 23–6. *Candida* organisms in urine demonstrating budding phase with pseudomycelia. Reduced from magnification of 100×. (From Wise GJ: J Urol 1972; 107:1043–1046. Copyright by Williams & Wilkins.)

Other laboratory and diagnostic methods, including blood, serologic, and imaging studies, should be used to differentiate local from systemic infection.

Blood and Serologic Studies

The presence of anemia in patients with candiduria is nondiagnostic for infection, because many of these patients have underlying disease that contributes to abnormality of the hemogram. In patients with histologically proven renal candidiasis, fungemia could be detected in fewer than one half (Kozinn et al, 1978); hence, blood cultures in themselves are not consistent markers of invasive infection. Although one positive blood culture is suggestive of disseminated infection, it may be transient, and a change of intravenous lines or discontinuation of hyperalimentation may prevent further episodes of fungemia (Klein and Watanakunakorn, 1979). The author has noted similar findings after removal of indwelling urethral catheters. However, persistence of positive *Candida* blood cultures, particularly in older patients or in association with positive bacterial blood cultures, has a poor prognosis (Dyess et al, 1985).

Whole cell agglutination, agar cell diffusion, latex agglutination, counterimmune electrophoresis, and radioimmune assay have been used to assess patient antibody response to candidal antigen. For a variety of reasons, including variability of antigen and inconsistency of patient response, these serologic tests have not been consistent or reliable markers for candidal infection (de Repentigny and Reiss, 1984; de Repentigny, 1992).

Suits and associates (1989) have used antibody-coated latex particles (CAND-TEC, Ramco Laboratory, Houston, Texas) as an adjunct in the evaluation of 98 patients, with or without catheters, who had persistent candiduria. A titer of 1:8 provided a sensitivity of 63% and a specificity of 84% in diagnosing multifocal infection in patients with candiduria. In another study, Ness and associates (1989) used the CAND-TEC in evaluation of 11 patients with invasive candidiasis as documented by multiple positive culture sites or tissue diagnosis. With a titer of 1:4 as positive, they found a sensitivity of 54.5% and a specificity of 29%; however, they noted that an elevated antigen titer correlated with a high creatinine level.

Other studies indicate that circulating *Candida* enolase by immunoassay can detect parenchymal candidal infection (Walsh et al, 1991). However, these assays are investigational in nature and are not available for clinical use.

Polymerase chain reaction (PCR) is a molecular biologic tool that rapidly and accurately identifies *Candida* (Buchman et al, 1990; Kan, 1993). In investigative studies, the use of PCR technique provided a 100% sensitivity and specificity for the detection of candiduria (Muncan and Wise, 1996). **There are no standardized laboratory studies that indicate whether candiduria involves an upper tract or invasive infection (Fisher et al, 1995). Diagnosis of upper tract or invasive infection is dependent on assessment of the total patient. The presence of fever, renal tenderness or pain, leukocytosis, funguria, and abnormal imaging studies (which indicate obstructive uropathy or compromised renal function) are indicative of upper tract infection.**

Radiographic and Imaging Studies

Candida species can form accretions, known as fungal balls or bezoars, that cause obstruction of the urinary collecting system, pelvis, ureter, or bladder. Cystography, intravenous pyelography, and retrograde pyelography often delineate filling defects (Beilke and Kirmani, 1988; Bhattacharya et al, 1982; Blum, 1966; Chisholm and Hutch, 1961; Shelp et al, 1966). Sonography also may demonstrate fungal material within the collecting system, particularly in pediatric patients (Aragona et al, 1985; Dembner and Pfister, 1977). Percutaneous nephrostomy has been used in the demonstration of filling defects in the collecting system (Fig. 23–7). Nephrostomy also provides access for collection of material for microscopic study or culture, drainage, and access for percutaneous removal of a fungal bezoar (Abramowitz et al, 1986; Bartone et al, 1988; Doemeny et al, 1988). In CT studies of the renal collecting system, the fungal accretion images as a mass lesion with less attenuation than a calculus (Doemeny et al, 1988).

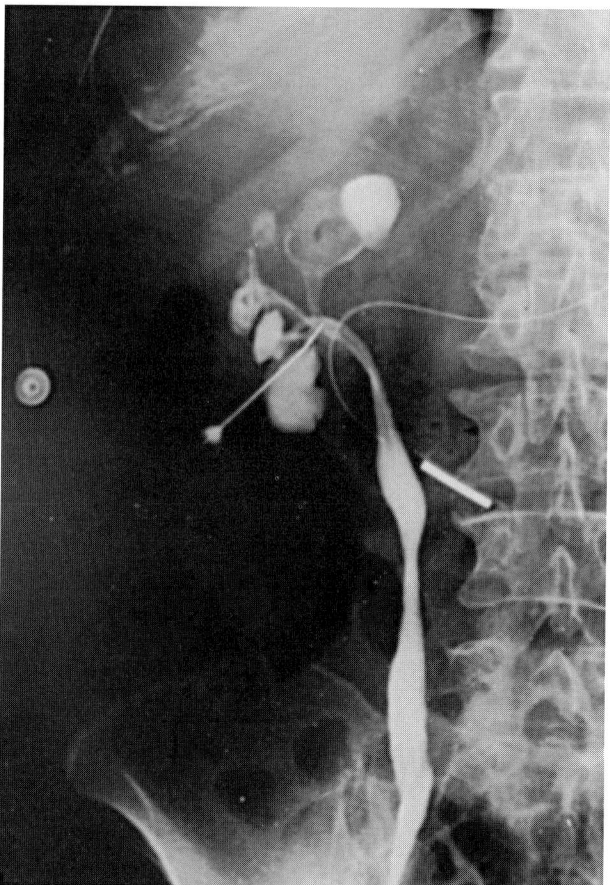

Figure 23–7. Antegrade nephrostogram demonstrating filling defect caused by fungal accretion. (From Wise GJ: AUA Update Series, 1989; 8[25]:197.)

Treatment Concepts

Candida species in the urine may be an isolated finding that may requires no treatment. **However, the persistence of candiduria requires evaluation and treatment.** The guidelines as described here and delineated in Figure 23–8 (Wise, 1990) should be followed.

Observation

The laboratory report of a single positive urine culture, irrespective of the count, should be reassessed. If *repeat* urine cultures are positive (>10,000 per uncatheterized or single-catheterized specimen), treatment is advisable. Treatment modalities are dependent on whether the infection is in the bladder, in the upper tracts, or disseminated. Before implementation of treatment the following steps should be taken.

Host Factors

Removal of an indwelling urinary catheter or intravenous line and improvement of nutritional status may ameliorate the potential for persistent candidal colonization or infection. Discontinuation of broad-spectrum antibiotics may be efficacious in reducing localized colonization (Urinary Tract Candidosis, 1988).

Irrigation with Antifungal Agents

Persistence of candiduria in the debilitated patient is not uncommon in clinical practice. If candiduria does not resolve after removal of the indwelling catheter (if present) or cessation of broad-spectrum antibiotic therapy, then irrigation of the bladder with amphotericin B is efficacious. The dosage and length of treatment can vary (Wong-Beringer et al, 1992; Sanford, 1993). Most studies have used a dose of 50 mg amphotericin B in 1000 ml of water or 5% dextrose in water administered at 42 ml/hour (1 L/day) (Jacobs et al, 1994).

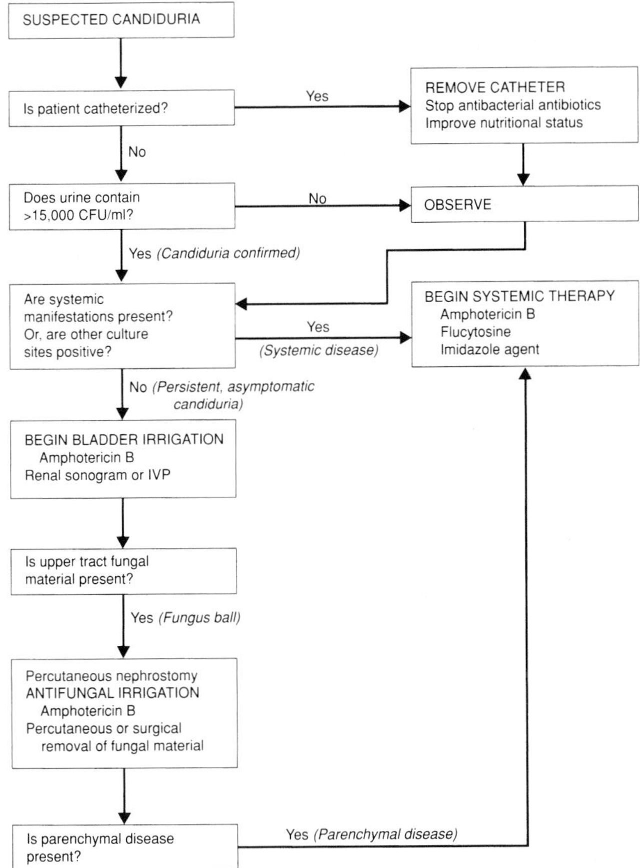

Figure 23–8. Guidelines for treatment of genitourinary candidal infection. CFU, colony-forming units; IVP, intraveneous pyelogram. (From Wise GJ: Amphotericin B in urologic practice. J Urol 1990; 144:215. Copyright by Williams & Wilkins.)

Bladder irrigations have resolved funguria in 80% to 92% of patients (Jacobs et al, 1994; Wise et al, 1982). Amphotericin B (100 mg/500 ml) given daily as a bladder irrigant has been efficacious in outpatient therapy (Cuetara et al, 1972). Miconazole (50 mg/liter of saline/day) in limited trials has been proved 80% effective when used as an antifungal bladder irrigant (Wise et al, 1987). Anecdotal observations have cited alkali (bicarbonate) as an antifungal bladder irrigant (Schonebeck, 1986), but no clinical studies have documented its effectiveness. Nystatin is similar in structure and pharmacologic effect to amphotericin B. Although nystatin is successful in isolated cases, poor colloidal dispersion properties have limited its use as a bladder irrigant (Wise, 1990).

Local or regional treatment (i.e., irrigation of the renal collecting system or bladder with an antifungal agent such as amphotericin B) should be used after correction of obstructive uropathy provided there is no invasive parenchymal or systemic infection, as demonstrated by absence of fever, toxicity, or elevated white count.

Localized renal pelvic and collecting system candidal infections have been treated successfully with amphotericin B irrigants with dose schedules similar to those used in bladder irrigations (Wise et al, 1982). Low-dose amphotericin B (10 to 24 mg/day for up to 15 days) has been advocated as a renal irrigation fluid in infants with localized upper tract candidiasis (Bartone et al, 1988.) Persistence of localized bladder or renal infection requires systemic therapy.

Systemic Treatment for Local Infection

The triazole fluconazole achieves high urine levels and it is effective in the treatment of urinary candidal infections (Urinary Tract Candidosis, 1988). Oral fluconazole (100 mg twice daily for 10 days) eradicated candiduria in 19 of 20 critically ill patients (Nassoura et al, 1993). **Fluconazole (100 mg orally twice daily for 10 days) was effective as amphotericin B irrigations (91.4% versus 94.2%; P = .322) in the treatment of bladder candidal infection (Muncan and Wise, 1995a).**

Intravenous liposomal amphotericin B in a dose range of 321 to 821 mg over 7 to 17 days has been successful in controlling candiduria in 4 patients (Ralph et al, 1991).

Clinical and laboratory evidence of multifocal or disseminated infection mandates systemic therapy.

Systemic Therapy for Invasive or Disseminated Infection

Clinical, laboratory, and radiographic evidence of disseminated infection indicates the need for systemic therapy. Three drug groups are now available for the treatment of systemic fungal infection: (1) amphotericin B, (2) 5-FC, and (3) the imidazoles and triazoles. Amphotericin B remains the gold standard for treatment of the patient with invasive or disseminated infection. A total dose of 6 mg/kg of body weight has been advocated as adequate in the critically ill surgical patient (Solomkin et al, 1982). Modified doses of amphotericin B have been used in patients with candidal urinary tract infections who were not acutely ill and did not manifest multisystem involvement (Medoff, 1987).

5-FC (150 mg/kg) can be used for localized candidal urinary tract infection. Because 5-FC can be administered by mouth, it is suitable for the treatment of ambulatory patients; however, candidal species may develop rapid drug resistance. Adverse effects include bone marrow depression. When used in conjunction with amphotericin B, 5-FC has a synergistic effect, and lower doses of amphotericin B may be used. Combined therapy with amphotericin B and 5-FC has been used in the treatment of cryptococcal infections (Graybill, 1988), but clinical studies of combined amphotericin B and 5-FC therapy in genitourinary infection are lacking.

The imidazoles, notably miconazole and ketoconazole, have proved effective in the treatment of systemic *Histoplasma capsulatum* and *Blastomyces dermatitidis* infections. However, the imidazoles are poorly excreted by the kidney and therefore have low urinary concentrations. The success rate in the treatment of urinary infection caused by *Candida* species and *Torulopsis* ranges from 40% to 50% (Graybill, 1988; Wise et al, 1985).

The triazoles (fluconazole and itraconazole) are chemically related to the imidazoles. Comparison between intravenous amphotericin B (0.5 to 0.6 mg/kg body weight per day) and fluconazole (400 mg/day) in the treatment of candidemia in non-neutropenic patients indicates comparable success (79% versus 70%; P = .22) (Rex et al, 1994). Isolated case reports have noted the successful use of fluconazole alone in the treatment of renal candidosis (Dave et al, 1989).

Pharmacologic guidelines are reviewed at the end of the chapter.

Percutaneous, Endoscopic, and Surgical Treatment

Most species of *Candida* develop pseudohyphae, which can produce fungal balls or accretions, resulting in obstruction of the collecting system, ureter, or bladder (Aragona et al, 1985; Beilke and Kirmani, 1988; Chisholm and Hutch, 1961; Eckstein and Kass, 1982; Shelp et al, 1966). Percutaneous nephrostomy has been used successfully in the management of patients with obstructive uropathy secondary to fungal material; the nephrostomy not only relieves the obstruction but also provides access for antifungal irrigation (Bartone et al, 1988). Furthermore, nephrostomy provides access for percutaneous identification and removal of fungal material from the renal pelvis (Abramowitz et al, 1986). Before the era of endourology, open surgical procedures with pyelotomy were necessary for identification and removal of fungal accretions from the renal collecting system (Bhattacharya et al, 1982; Leiter et al, 1982).

Torulopsis glabrata Infection

Introduction

***T. glabrata* is similar to *Candida* species in morphology, growth characteristics, clinical manifestations, and response to antifungal therapy.** There is controversy whether *Torulopsis* should be classified as *Candida glabrata*. However, *T. glabrata* does not develop pseudohyphae and differs slightly in morphology and metabolism. For these reasons, a separate taxonomic classification has been advocated (McGinnis et al, 1984).

Epidemiology and Predisposing Factors

Torulopsis fungi can exist as saprophytes in the oral cavity, alimentary canal, and respiratory tree. Whereas asymptomatic urinary colonization may exist (Frye et al, 1988), *Torulopsis* has caused fungemia and death in debilitated patients (Komshian et al, 1989). Diabetes mellitus, antibiotic therapy, surgery, and obstructive uropathy have been associated with *T. glabrata* infections of the kidneys and bladder (Frye et al, 1988; Kauffman and Tan, 1974).

Diagnosis

Diagnosis can be established by culture of the fungus from the urine, blood, or purulent material. Microscopic examination of the urine may reveal budding yeast forms without mycelia. Urinary colony counts may range from 1000 to more than 100,000/ml. There are no specific serologic studies that are indicative of invasive infection. Radiographic studies may demonstrate pre-existing disease, such as chronic (bacterial) pyelonephritis, calculi, obstructive uropathy, or perinephric collection.

Genitourinary Manifestations and Treatment

In upper tract disease, the patient may develop flank pain, fever, and leukocytosis (Frye et al, 1988). Obstructive uropathy must be corrected to control infection (Wise, 1984b; Bell et al, 1993). Systemic therapy is advocated, because renal infection has a high mortality rate (Kauffman and Tan, 1974). Renal microabscesses have been associated with *Torulopsis* septicemia (Minkowitz et al, 1963).

Torulopsis has been associated with perirenal abscesses (Khauli et al, 1983; Thompson and Brock, 1983; High and Quagliarello, 1992); perinephric abscesses have been treated successfully by surgical drainage with or without systemic amphotericin B (dose range of 590 to 2000 mg) (Khauli et al, 1983; Thompson and Brock, 1983). Successful treatment has been achieved by percutaneous aspiration and fluconazole (400-mg loading dose, followed by 100 mg/day for 8 weeks in one patient or 200 mg/for 7 days in another patient) (High and Quagliarello, 1992; Krcmery et al, 1994).

A pelvic abscess and fungemia caused by *T. glabrata* developed in a 43-year-old woman after a hysterectomy and right salpingo-oophorectomy for in situ cervical carcinoma. The patient responded to percutaneous drainage of the abscess and intravenous amphotericin B (total dose of 825 mg) (Wiesenfeld et al, 1994). Perivesical infection and abscess formation caused by *T. glabrata* have been reported. Surgical drainage or percutaneous drainage in combination with intravenous fluconazole (200 mg/day for 10 days) resolved the infections (Sheynkin and Wise, 1995).

T. glabrata cystitis can cause voiding symptoms (i.e., pyuria and hematuria) (Frye et al, 1988). The use of amphotericin B bladder irrigations (15 to 30 mg/day) and oral 5-FC (100 mg/day) has proved efficacious (Rohner and Tuliszewski, 1980; Siminovitch and Herman, 1984; Takeuchi and Tomoyoshi, 1983). Recalcitrant infections require systemic amphotericin B (total dose 600 to 2000 mg). Limited success has been achieved with ketoconazole in the treatment of *T. glabrata* urinary tract infections (Graybill et al, 1983).

Epididymo-orchitis has been reported in an elderly diabetic who had blood and urine cultures positive for *T. glabrata*. The patient's infection responded to surgical drainage of the scrotal abscess and systemic amphotericin B (dose not cited). Gram, periodic acid-Schiff, and Grocott stains confirmed the presence of *T. glabrata* in purulent fluid (Sheaff et al, 1995).

Aspergillosis

Introduction

Human infection caused by species of *Aspergillus* was described in the nineteenth century. By the mid-20th century, aspergilli were recognized as causing a variety of pulmonary illnesses, including asthma, allergic alveolitis, and cavitary aspergillomas. Primary extrapulmonary foci of aspergillar infection have caused cutaneous, naso-orbital, and genitourinary disease (Cross, 1987; Flechner and McAninch, 1981; Rippon, 1988, p 618).

Epidemiology and Predisposing Factors

More than 900 species of *Aspergillus* exist; fewer than 20 have been identified as etiologic fungi in human disease. The more common infecting fungi, in decreasing frequency, are *A. fumigatus*, *A. flavus,* and *A. niger.* Aspergilli are ubiquitous in the environment and can be found throughout the world in soil, decomposing vegetation, paint, chemical agents, medication bottles, refrigerators, and bird excreta.

Outbreaks of disease have been attributed to contaminated air conditioning systems, surgical theaters, dialysis fluid, and construction dust. Contamination of hospital environs has resulted in aspergillar endocarditis, meningitis, and osteomyelitis.

Disseminated *Aspergillus* is second to *Candida* and *Torulopsis* species as an opportunistic fungus that afflicts those patients debilitated by malignancy, diabetes mellitus, and immunosuppression. Renal transplant recipients who receive steroid therapy are at increased risk for invasive aspergillar infection (Gallis et al, 1975; Gustafson et al, 1983). Aspergillosis has been observed in a patient with AIDS (Asnis et al, 1988) and intravenous drug abuse (Halpern et al, 1992). Fatal aspergillosis has been reported in a bone marrow recipient who smoked marijuana (Hamadeh et al, 1988). Primary cutaneous infection caused by aspergilli has occurred at Hickman intravenous catheter sites (Allo et al, 1987).

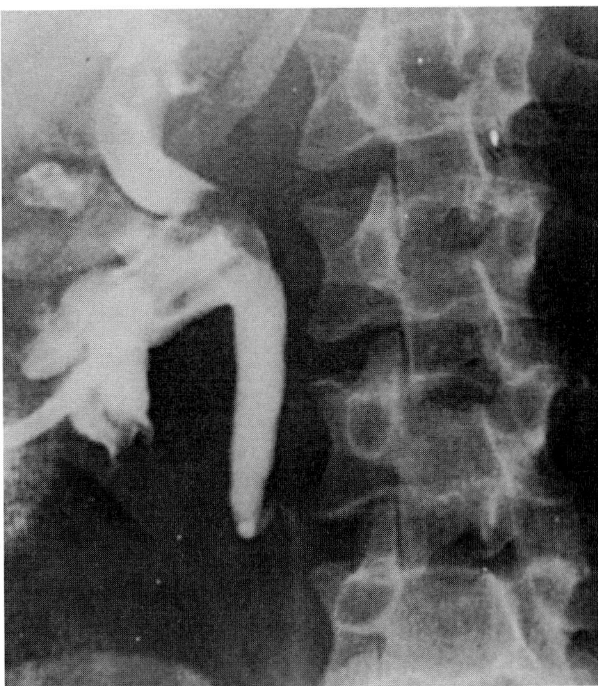

Figure 23–9. Nephrostogram demonstrating aspergillar bezoar. (From Irby PB, Stoller ML, McAninch JW: Fungal bezoars of the upper urinary tract. J Urol 1990; 143:447. Copyright by Williams & Wilkins.)

Renal Infection

Young and associates (1970) analyzed postmortem studies of 98 patients with aspergillosis. In most patients, the primary underlying diagnosis was leukemia or lymphoma. Aspergilli infected the pulmonary tract in 92 patients (94%), the gastrointestinal tract in 21 (23%), the brain in 19 (21%), the liver in 12 (13%), and the kidney in 12 (13%). The testes and adrenals were involved in one patient each. The infected kidneys demonstrated multiple small focal abscesses, vascular occlusion by fungi, and multiple renal infarcts. One kidney demonstrated papillary necrosis secondary to vascular occlusion. A retrospective analysis of these patients indicated that none had clinical manifestations of the renal disease. Hematuria and pyuria were noted but could not be correlated with renal aspergillar infection. In this series, six intravenous pyelographic studies demonstrated no abnormalities.

In clinical settings, patients with renal aspergillosis may present with flank pain, renal tenderness, and fever. Radiographic studies demonstrate filling defects within the collecting system that are unilateral or bilateral (Fig. 23–9). Primary renal aspergillar infection with obstructive uropathy has been reported in patients with diabetes mellitus or intravenous drug abuse (Flechner and McAninch, 1981; Godec et al, 1989; Melchior et al, 1972; Warshawsky et al, 1975). A renal pelvic aspergillar mycetoma has occurred in an otherwise healthy patient with a ureteropelvic junction obstruction (Eisenberg et al, 1977). **Renal aspergilloma or pseudotumor has been reported in patients with AIDS (Halpern et al, 1992; Piketty et al, 1993). The CT scan demonstrated a renal mass, and fungal elements were identified in the renal aspirate.** Intravenous amphotericin B and oral itraconazole were ineffective as initial management, so a nephrectomy was necessary.

Prostatic Infection

Prostatic aspergillar infection has been reported in four patients who presented with signs and symptoms of bladder outflow obstruction (Abbas et al, 1995). Predisposing medical conditions included prolonged use of antibiotics, diabetes mellitus, metastatic colon carcinoma, chronic steroid use, and indwelling bladder catheter. Diagnosis was established by identification of fungus in the prostatic tissue. Three of the four patients did well with surgical treatment alone (transurethral resection or open prostatectomy); the fourth patient received amphotericin B for 3 months.

Diagnosis

Aspergillar infection can be established by identification of the fungus in the urine or tissue removed from the infected organ. Methenamine silver or periodic acid-Schiff stain can demonstrate the fungus in tissue. *Aspergillus* species differ from *Mucor* species, which have broader, nonseptated branching hyphae. Tissue or excreted material can be cultured in Sabouraud's medium or brain-heart–enriched infusion broths (Cross, 1987).

In systemic aspergillar infection, blood cultures are often negative. Culture or biopsy of other lesions, such as skin, may document infection. Immune diffusion or radioimmunoassay serologic studies may be helpful in determining diagnosis (de Repentigny and Reiss, 1984; Rippon, 1988, p 642). The use of PCR amplification provides a more sensitive method to detect *Aspergillus* in blood and urine (Reddy et al, 1993).

Treatment

Combination therapy with 5-FC (8 g/day for 2 months) and amphotericin B (total dose >1.3 g) has been efficacious in treatment of recalcitrant pulmonary infections (Codish et al, 1979). The imidazoles have had an antagonistic effect when used with amphotericin B, whereas rifampin used in combination with amphotericin B has been efficacious in the treatment of aspergillar infections (Rippon, 1988, p 637). The newer triazole, itraconazole, may be an effective agent (Graybill, 1988).

In a review of 11 patients with aspergillomas involving 15 renal units, 8 patients were treated with systemic amphotericin B (dose range, 110 to 2500 mg), 6 of whom had insertion of ureteral stents, open pyelotomy, or nephrostomy in conjunction with amphotericin B irrigations. Three patients required nephrectomy (Bibler and Gianis, 1987).

Irby and associates (1990) treated three patients with bilateral renal aspergillar bezoars (Figs. 23–10 and 23–11). Urologic intervention was implemented in all patients with the use of retrograde catheters, ureteroscopic lavage, percutaneous nephrostomy, or open pyelotomy in conjunction with amphotericin B irrigations. Systemic amphotericin B was used in all patients. 5-FC was given to one patient, and rifampin was given to two patients. In one patient, itraconazole was used effectively. Two patients required nephrectomy for resolution of recalcitrant infection. Figure 23–12 presents an algorithm that delineates a treatment plan for renal aspergillar infection.

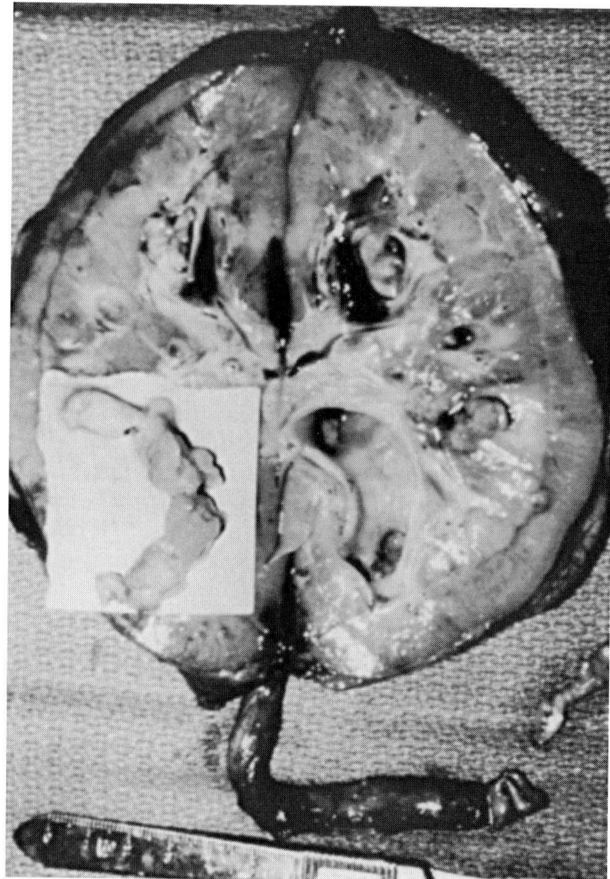

Figure 23–10. Gross specimen of kidney with aspergillar bezoar in collecting system. Renal parenchyma is spared. (From Irby PB, Stoller ML, McAninch JW: Fungal bezoars of the upper urinary tract. J Urol 1990; 143:447. Copyright by Williams & Wilkins.)

Cryptococcosis

Introduction

Cryptococcal genitourinary infection has been caused by one specific fungus, *Cryptococcus neoformans*. Cryptococcal infection has also been referred to as torulosis (Rippon, 1988, p 582). This nomenclature may be confused with that of a different fungus, *T. glabrata* (see previous section).

Epidemiology and Predisposing Factors

C. neoformans thrives in any environment inhabited by birds (particularly pigeons). Heavy fungal growth can be found in old attics, buildings, and barn lofts. After inhalation, the fungus may cause a pulmonary infection; this infection may be asymptomatic or it may develop into a virulent respiratory infection that mimics severe bacterial pneumonia, tuberculosis, malignancy, or other fungal infections. Often the pulmonary infection is self-limiting with residual pulmonary calcification and granulomas. **As in other fungal infections, compromise of the patient's immune system increases vulnerability for disseminated infection. Patients with AIDS are at increased risk to develop disseminated cryptococcal infection** (Kovacs et al, 1985; Scully et al, 1987; Chuck and Sande, 1989). The central nervous system (CNS) is the primary target of hematogenous spread with resultant meningitis, meningoencephalitis, or cryptococcoma.

Diagnosis

Cryptococcus can be identified in urine, cerebrospinal fluid (CSF), or other infected fluid following culture in Sabouraud's glucose agar medium. Direct examination of infected fluid with India ink stain may reveal budding yeast with capsule (Rippon, 1988, p 601). *C. neoformans* may be identified in tissue by periodic acid-Schiff or methenamine silver stain. Serum or CSF can be tested for capsular antigen

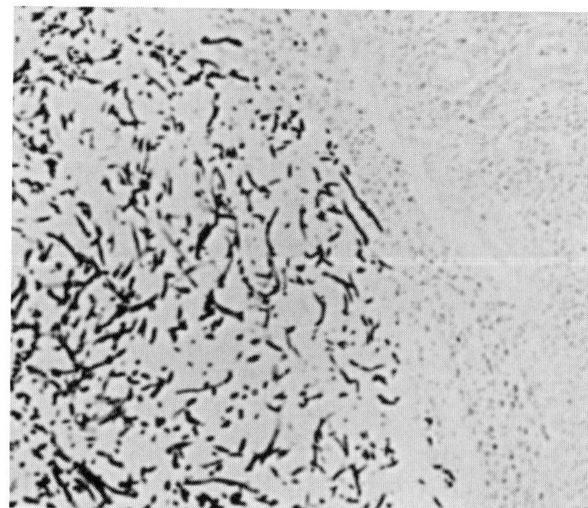

Figure 23–11. Photomicrograph of aspergillar mycelium limited to collecting system. Spared renal parenchyma is indicated. Hematoxylin and eosin with silver stain. (From Irby PB, Stoller ML, McAninch JW: Fungal bezoars of the upper urinary tract. J Urol 1990; 143:447. Copyright by Williams & Wilkins.)

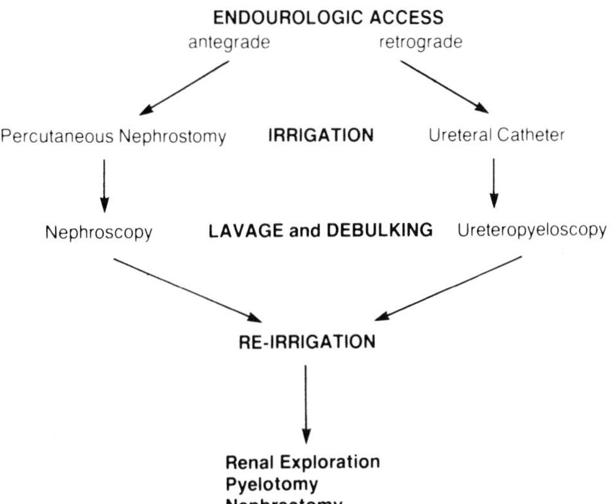

Figure 23–12. Algorithm for surgical management of upper tract fungal bezoars. (From Irby PB, Stoller ML, McAninch JW: Fungal bezoars of the upper urinary tract. J Urol 1990; 143:447. Copyright by Williams & Wilkins.)

by commercially available kits that utilize latex-coated capsule antibody (Rippon, 1988, p 600). **Cryptococcal antigen has also been found in urine of patients with AIDS (Chapin-Robertson et al, 1993).**

Adrenal Infection

Adrenal insufficiency secondary to cryptococcal infection was reported in a 72-year-old bird fancier (Shah et al, 1986). Adrenal biopsy revealed extensive caseating necrosis; the patient developed CNS infection and died despite antifungal therapy.

Renal Infection

In a pre-1980 postmortem study of 39 patients with disseminated cryptococcal infection, 20 (51%) had renal involvement, and 6 of the 23 male patients (26%) had prostatic infection (Salyer and Salyer, 1973). Renal findings revealed focal abscesses confined for the most part to the cortex; cryptococci also could be identified within the glomerulus. Urine cultures were obtained in 15 patients; only 6 (40%) yielded fungus.

Cryptococcal pyelonephritis has been reported in 4 patients, 3 of whom received long-term salicylate or steroid therapy; the fourth patient had lymphoma (Randall et al, 1968). All patients had hematuria, pyuria, and proteinuria before manifestation of CNS infection. Cryptococci were identified in the kidneys of all patients by either renal biopsy or postmortem study. The one surviving patient received amphotericin B (>1 g) administered over a 38-day period.

Cryptococcal pyelonephritis developed in a renal transplant patient. Despite intensive therapy with amphotericin B (0.51 g) and 5-FC (112.5 g), the patient died. Postmortem studies demonstrated cryptococci in the kidney (Hellman et al, 1981).

Prostate Infection

Cryptococcal prostatic lesions vary from small, chronic inflammatory changes to large granulomas with caseation (Salyer and Salyer, 1973). Before the era of AIDS, the clinical diagnosis of prostatic cryptococcal infection was rare. In a review of 12 cases of prostatic cryptococcosis, urinary symptoms were not noted in 8 patients but 4 presented with urinary retention. Five patients were treated with amphotericin B (total dose 1120 to 3400 mg), and 1 patient received 5-FC (total dose 116 g). There were 3 survivors (50%) among these 5 patients, whereas none of 6 untreated patients survived (Brock and Grieco, 1972). In 4 patients, the diagnosis was made by postmortem exam.

Other isolated case reports of prostatic cryptococcosis have been reported. One patient with cirrhosis underwent a transurethral resection of the prostate for correction of obstructive uropathy presumably caused by benign prostatic hypertrophy. Granulomatous changes with cryptococcus were noted on histologic study. The patient did well without antifungal therapy (Braman, 1981).

Prostatic cryptococcal infection has been observed in patients with immunosuppression resulting from causes other than AIDS, such as diabetes mellitus (Huyn and Reyes, 1982), lymphoma (King et al, 1990), and alcohol abuse (Hinchey and Someren, 1981). The first case of AIDS-related prostatic cryptococcal infection was noted in a 36-year-old homosexual man who presented with fever, headaches, abdominal discomfort, and voiding difficulties. The diagnosis of cryptococcal meningitis was made by examination of the CSF. Prostatic biopsy indicated cryptococci. A 6-week course of amphotericin B followed by 5-FC resolved the meningitis and prostatic infection (Lief and Sarfarazi, 1986).

In patients with AIDS, the prostate has become a reservoir for cryptococcus after treatment for cryptococcal meningitis (Larsen et al, 1989). Among 41 AIDS patients with cryptococcal meningitis who had been treated with systemic amphotericin B and 5-FC for 6 weeks, 9 patients developed positive urine cultures, of whom 4 had positive prostatic secretions for cryptococcus. The additional use of amphotericin B was not successful in eradicating infection. Fluconazole was successful in eradicating infection in 4 of 6 patients. In another study of 14 patients with prostatic cryptococcal infection, 7 responded after a median of 4 weeks (range, 1 to 27 weeks) of treatment with fluconazole. The other 7 patients continued to shed cryptococcuria (2 patients developed recurrent meningitis). The authors recommended that fluconazole be given at dose level of 200 to 600 mg/day (Bozzette et al, 1991). One report notes "resurgence" of *C. neoformans* on the urine despite 400 mg/day of fluconazole (Bailly et al, 1991). An abscess caused by *C. neoformans* has been reported in a 28-year-old AIDS patient. Diagnosis was established by CT scan and subsequent transperineal aspiration. Treatment with fluconazole (400 mg/day) and amphotericin B (40 mg/day) was unsuccessful. Transurethral drainage was refused, and the patient subsequently died from disseminated infection (Mamo et al, 1992).

Prostatic cryptococcosis can mimic adenocarcinoma. A 55-year-old patient with AIDS presented with prostatic nodules suggestive of prostate carcinoma. Ultrasound study de-

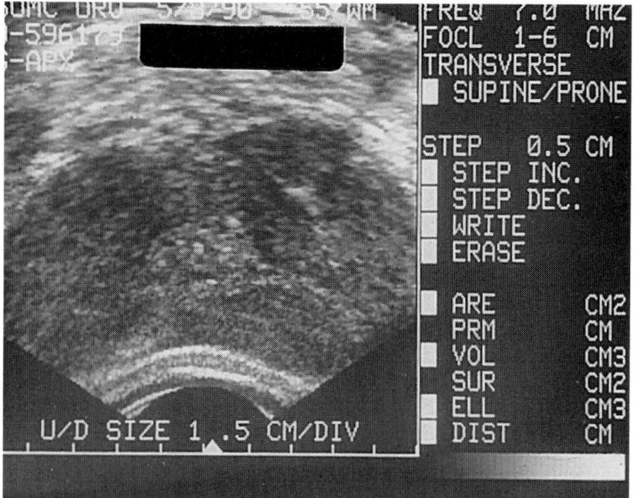

Figure 23–13. Transrectal ultrasonogram demonstrating findings in prostate with cryptococcosis. (From Adams JR, Mata JA, Culkin DJ, et al: Urology 1992; 39:289–291.)

picted hypoechoic peripheral zone lesions of the prostate (Fig. 23–13). Biopsy confirmed the presence of *Cryptococcus* (Fig. 23–14) (Adams et al, 1992).

Cryptococcal infection of the prostate requires systemic therapy. Fluconazole is the drug of choice, but dosage and length of treatment remain to be defined.

Genital Infection

Unusual manifestations of genital cryptococcal infection have been reported. An elderly patient on steroid therapy for chronic polychondritis developed an isolated epididymo-orchitis which was diagnosed by fine needle aspiration. Treatment consisted of epididymo-orchiectomy and systemic antifungal therapy (amphotericin B, ketoconazole, and 5-FC) (James and Lomax-Smith, 1991). **Penile cryptococcal infection has been observed in both non-AIDS (Perfect and Seaworth, 1985) and AIDS patients (Vapnek and McAninch, 1990). The lesions have varied from a glans ulcer to a large exophytic lesion that mimics a tumor or molluscum contagiosum (Concus et al, 1988).** Excisional biopsy and systemic therapy with amphotericin B (1 g) and 5-FC (100 mg/kg body weight for 6 weeks) have been successful in controlling infection.

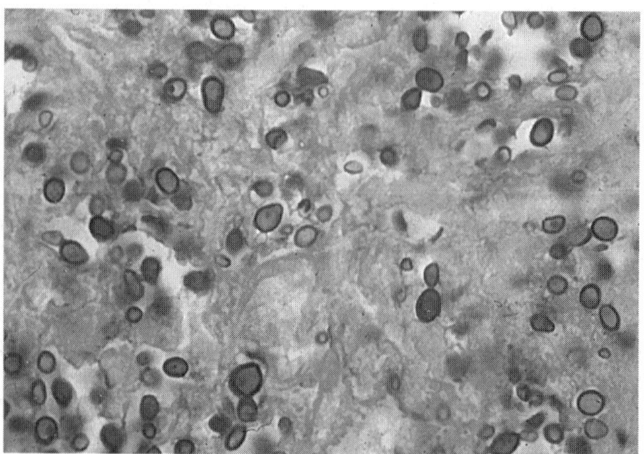

Figure 23–14. Photomicrograph depicting cryptococci in the prostate. Original magnification, × 900. (From Adams JR, Mata JA, Culkin DJ, et al: Urology 1992; 39:289–291.)

PRIMARY FUNGAL INFECTIONS

Blastomycosis

Epidemiology and Predisposing Factors

Described in 1894 by Gilchrist, blastomycosis has been known as Chicago disease because the first cluster of cases was identified in that region. The fungus *Blastomyces dermatitidis* is endemic in the Ohio, Missouri, and Mississippi river basins; it has been found also in the Great Lakes region and Canada and therefore has been known as North American blastomycosis. Cases have been reported in Africa, the Middle East, and Asia (Rippon, 1988, p 474). Four distinct fungal serotypes exist; the North American fungus primarily causes pulmonary infection, and the African isolates cause skin and bone lesions (Blastomycosis, 1989). South American blastomycosis is caused by a different fungus, *Paracoccidioides brasiliensis.*

The natural habitat and ecology of *B. dermatitidis* is not been well defined, but the fungus has a predilection for moist soil with high organic content (Rippon, 1988, p 476). One outbreak of blastomycosis occurred in a school where the children had visited a beaver pond (Klein et al, 1986).

Following inhalation of the fungal conidia (germ spores), a pulmonary infection may develop that is often subclinical and self-limiting. The infection often remains dormant but may disseminate by hematogenous or lymphatic routes to extrapulmonary sites such as the skin, bones, or genitourinary system. Isolated cutaneous lesions have occurred after laboratory accidents or bites by infected animals, particularly canines (Dismukes, 1986).

Blastomycosis has become more prevalent in immunocompromised patients. In a study of 185 patients with blastomycosis, 28 were found to have predisposing conditions that included long-term (>2 months) corticosteroid use, hematologic malignancy, solid tumor requiring cytotoxic or radiation therapy, solid organ or bone marrow transplantation, human immunodeficiency virus (HIV)–positive status, end-stage renal or hepatic disease, and pregnancy (Pappas et al, 1993).

Genitourinary Manifestations

Genitourinary involvement occurs in 15% to 30% of patients with systemic disease (Eickenberg et al, 1975; Inoshita et al, 1983; Malin et al, 1969). In one study of 51 patients with systemic blastomycosis, 11 patients (22%) had genitourinary involvement. The right or left epididymis was infected in 10 (91%) of these patients; the prostate was infected in 8 (73%); and the kidney, testis, and prepuce each had 1 lesion (9%) (Eickenberg et al, 1975).

Adrenal infection with clinical manifestations of Addison's disease has been described in patients who had exacerbation of systemic blastomycosis (Abernathy and Melby, 1962).

Conjugal transmission has been documented, in which the male developed *Blastomyces* infection of the prostate and epididymis and the female consort developed *Blastomyces* infection of the endometrium and fallopian tubes (Craig et al, 1970).

Patients with genitourinary blastomycosis may develop epididymal induration or prostatic symptoms (i.e., urinary frequency, hesitancy, nocturia, or even urinary retention). The patient may have an enlarged or fluctuant prostate. Systemic blastomycosis occurring with prostatic abscess has been reported (Bergner et al, 1981).

Diagnosis

Diagnosis is suggested by changes on chest x-ray studies and the development of a positive *Blastomyces* skin test. Serologic studies using complement fixation, immune diffusion, or enzyme-linked immunosorbent assay are useful laboratory adjuncts (Rippon, 1988, p 497).

Fungal stains may identify the *Blastomyces* "broad-neck" yeast forms in infected tissue (Fig. 23–15). Inflammatory and granulomatous reaction has been noted in prostate tissue removed for relief of obstructive uropathy (Inoshita et al, 1983).

Treatment

Genitourinary blastomycosis is a manifestation of disseminated disease that has required systemic amphotericin B in doses ranging from 1 to 3 g (Eickenberg et al, 1975; Inoshita et al, 1983). Prostatitis secondary to blastomycosis has been cured with 2 g systemic amphotericin B (Bissada et al, 1977). Chronic therapy with ketoconazole, an imidazole, has been advocated for patients with mild to moderate nonmeningeal forms of blastomycosis (Dismukes, 1986). Ketoconazole (400 mg/day) has been effective in isolated cases of cutaneous and prostatic blastomycosis (Inoshita et al, 1983). A patient with epididymal, pulmonary, and cutaneous infection secondary to blastomycosis was successfully treated with inguinal orchiectomy and long-term ketoconazole (200 mg/day for 1 year) (Short et al, 1983). The triazole, itraconazole (200 mg/day), has been effective in patients with pulmonary infection who have not responded to ketoconazole; fluconazole has not demonstrated clinical efficacy (Bradsher, 1992). None of the triazoles have been used in the treatment of genitourinary blastomycosis.

Coccidioidomycosis

Epidemiology and Predisposing Factors

Coccidioides immitis is a dimorphic fungus indigenous to the semiarid regions of the western United States, Mexico, and Central and South America. The fungus thrives in soil conditions that are inhibitory to competing organisms, namely, high temperature and increased salinity (Rippon, 1988, p 437).

Outbreaks of coccidioidomycosis have occurred in such groups as construction workers, farmers, and archaeologists exposed to dust containing the arthroconidia (germ cells) of the fungus. Urban outbreaks have been attributed to dust storms (Drutz, 1979). An increase in incidence has been ascribed to changes in climate such as prolonged drought followed by heavy rain (Jinadu et al, 1994).

After inhalation of the arthroconidia, an asymptomatic and transient pulmonary infection may develop. A more virulent infection occurs in some cases, with radiographic changes indicative of pulmonary infiltration or cavitation. The patient may manifest high fever, cough, night sweats, or pleuritic pain. An "allergic" reaction to the infection may develop in which the patient manifests erythema nodosum, also known as "valley bumps" or "valley fever." Fewer than 1% of patients develop extrapulmonary multiorgan dissemination. **Patients with increased skin pigmentation, pregnant women, and individuals who are younger than 5 years or older than 50 years of age have a higher risk of disseminated infection (Kuntze, 1988). Risk factors include steroid use, chemotherapy, malignancy, seropositivity for HIV (Einstein and Johnson, 1993), and AIDS (Abrams et al, 1984).**

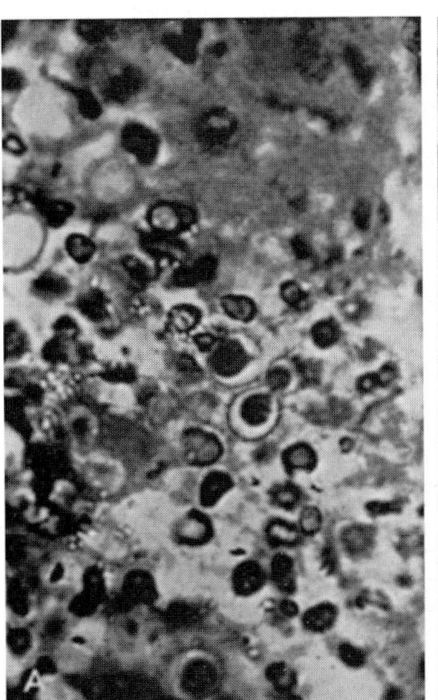

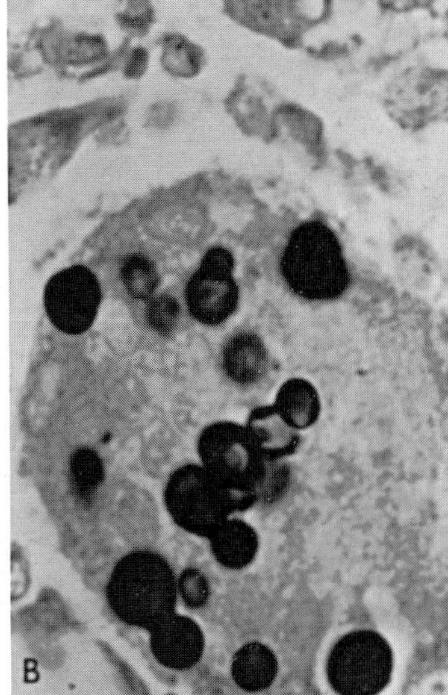

Figure 23–15. Blastomycosis. *A,* Budding yeast cell. The cytoplasm has shrunk from the side of the colorless wall but can be seen to be multinucleate. Hematoxylin and eosin stain; original magnification, × 440. *B,* Numerous yeast cells, some of which are budding, in a giant cell. Note the broad-based buds. Gomori methenamine silver stain; original magnification, × 440. (From Rippon JW: Medical Mycology, 3rd ed. Philadelphia, W. B. Saunders, 1988, p 492.)

Renal transplantation patients receiving immunosuppressive therapy have had dormant foci of infection develop into disseminated disease (Schroter et al, 1977). Previously, a positive coccidioidin skin test was a contraindication to renal transplantation (Conner et al, 1975; Galgiani, 1993); however, patients with a history of exposure may undergo successful transplantation with prophylactic antifungal therapy (Hall et al, 1993).

Genitourinary Manifestations

Postmortem studies in patients with disseminated coccidioidomycosis indicate involvement of the kidney in 35% to 60% of cases, the adrenal in 16% to 32% and the prostate in 6% (Kuntze et al, 1988).

The antemortem diagnosis of renal coccidioidal infection is difficult to establish. Radiographic findings may be similar to those of tuberculosis, with "moth-eaten calyces," infundibular stenosis, and renal calcification (Conner et al, 1975). Regression of lesions has been noted after systemic antifungal therapy (Kuntze et al, 1988). Coccidioiduria has been observed in 12 patients with chronic coccidioidomycosis; only 4 patients had proven genitourinary pathology that included granulomas and the characteristic coccidioidal spherules in kidney, epididymis, and prostate (Petersen et al, 1976).

Coccidioidal cystitis is a rare clinical entity. Two cases were reviewed; 1 patient had a concomitant vesicocolic fistula. Both patients had irritative voiding symptoms, pyuria, and associated hydronephrosis secondary to ureteral stricture (Fig. 23–16) (Kuntze et al, 1988). Treatment with systemic amphotericin B (2000 mg) and ketoconazole (200 mg/day for 1 year) was effective in one patient, and ketoconazole achieved resolution of infection in the other patient (Kuntze et al, 1988).

Prostatic infection is one of the more common manifestations of genitourinary coccidioidal infection. The patient may present with symptoms indicative of bladder outflow obstruction. Physical findings may reveal a boggy prostate or even induration suggestive of neoplasia (Price et al, 1982). Although expressed prostatic secretions or urine may yield positive cultures for *C. immitis*, diagnosis is usually established by identification of fungal spherules in tissue. Dissemination of infection has been reported in a patient undergoing transurethral resection of the prostate for "benign" disease (Wipf et al, 1983). Prostatic infection is usually a manifestation of multifocal or systemic disease; hence, systemic therapy with IV amphotericin B or the imidazoles, or both, is advocated (Sung et al, 1979).

A less frequent but clinically more apparent presentation of genitourinary coccidioidomycosis is scrotal infection. The patient may present with scrotal swelling, draining sinus, or indurated epididymis. Bilateral involvement may occur synchronously or metachronously. Often, there is concomitant prostatic disease (Chen, 1983). Urethrocutaneous fistula has been reported in a patient with epididymal and prostatic coccidioidal infection (Gottesman, 1974). The disease stabilized with debridement, orchiectomy, and short-term amphotericin B therapy.

Coccidioidal endometritis and salpingitis was reported in a patient who required chemotherapy for Hodgkin's disease. After total hysterectomy and bilateral salpingo-oophorectomy, the patient received systemic amphotericin B with a favorable outcome (Bylund et al, 1986).

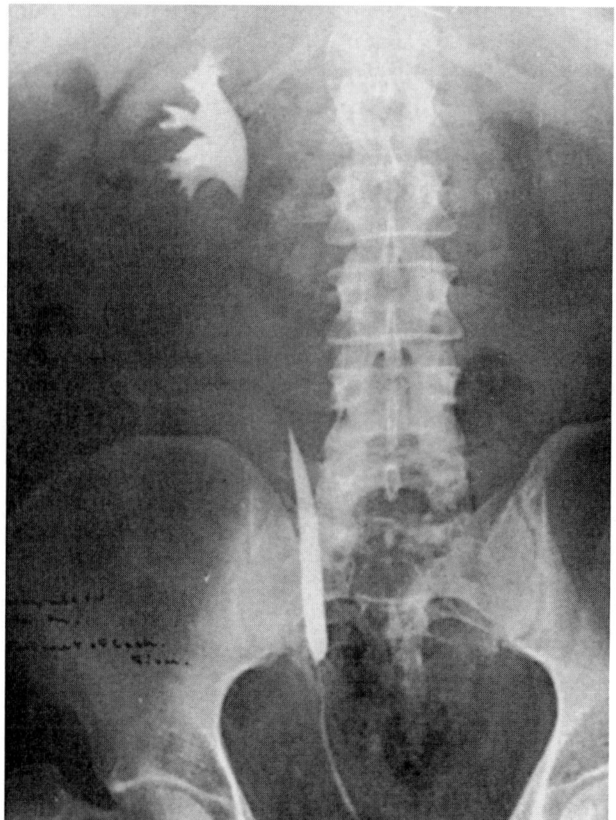

Figure 23–16. Retrograde pyelogram demonstrates ureteral stricture secondary to coccidioidal infection. (From Kuntze JR, Herman MK, Evans SG: Genitourinary coccidioidomycosis. J Urol 1988; 140:370. Copyright by Williams & Wilkins.)

Diagnosis

Knowledge of the patient's travel to endemic areas or environmental exposure should alert the urologist to potential infection. Skin tests and serologic studies (complement fixation [CF], immune diffusion [ID], and latex particle agglutination [LPA]) may provide laboratory evidence (Rippon, 1988, p 464; Einstein and Johnson, 1993).

Draining sinuses can be cultured for fungus on Sabouraud's medium. Tissue obtained by biopsy or at surgery can be stained with periodic acid-Schiff or methenamine silver to facilitate identification of the coccidioidal spherule (Fig. 23–17).

Treatment

Because genitourinary coccidioidal infection may be a manifestation of multiorgan disease, systemic therapy is advocated. Intravenous amphotericin B (total dose, 500 to 2500 mg) is the treatment of choice. Supplemental ketoconazole (200 mg/day) can be given for 1 year (Rippon, 1988, p 452). Isolated lesions, such as epididymal infections, may be treated by surgical excision alone. Preliminary data suggest that fluconazole (>400 mg/day) may be

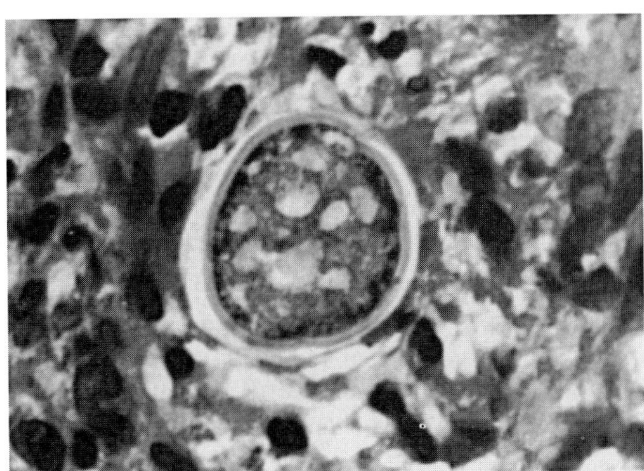

Figure 23–17. Photomicrograph demonstrates a mature coccidioidomycosis spherule with endospores. Hematoxylin and eosin stain; original magnification, × 500. (From Kuntze JR, Herman MK, Evans SG: Genitourinary coccidioidomycosis. J Urol 1988; 140:370. Copyright by Williams & Wilkins.)

efficacious for CNS infection. To date there are no studies citing the use of fluconazole in genitourinary infection.

Histoplasmosis

Epidemiology and Predisposing Factors

In 1905, S.T. Darling, a pathologist working in Panama, described pulmonary findings similar to those of tuberculosis. Subsequent studies by others indicated that this disease was caused by a fungus named *Histoplasma capsulatum* (Rippon, 1988, p 381).

Although the initial cases were identified in the tropics, the fungus has been found throughout the middle western and southern portions of the United States. *H. capsulatum* grows readily in soil of high nitrogen content that has been enriched by bird guano. **Outbreaks of the disease have occurred in individuals who work in chicken coops, infested caves, sills, and other bird areas. Major occurrences have been reported in association with construction sites and tree removal** (Drutz, 1979). In the United States, it has been estimated that 30 to 40 million people have been exposed to the fungus (Rippon, 1988, p 383; Rubin et al, 1959).

Inhalation of the fungal conidia may result in asymptomatic, self-limiting pulmonary infection. Diagnosis is made by chest x-ray changes (i.e., small pulmonary granulomas and calcification) and positive histoplasmin skin tests. Symptomatic infection develops in a small number of exposed individuals (< 5%) and is manifested by cough, fever, and hemoptysis. Radiographic studies may reveal pulmonary cavitation and mediastinal lymphadenopathy. Unless treated, the more virulent pulmonary infection becomes chronic, with increased chances of morbidity and mortality. **Disseminated and virulent disease has been known to occur in children and immunosuppressed individuals. Disseminated histoplasmosis has become an opportunistic infection in patients with AIDS** (Bonner et al, 1984; Wheat et al, 1992).

Genitourinary Manifestations

The liver, spleen, and lymph nodes are major sites of extrapulmonary histoplasmosis. However, the genitourinary tract is often involved in disseminated infection. **In a postmortem study of 17 patients with generalized histoplasmosis, the adrenal was infected in 14 patients (82%), the kidney in 3 (18%), and the prostate in 1 (6%)** (Rubin et al, 1959).

Addison's disease has been reported to occur with histoplasmosis. The diagnosis of adrenal involvement can be made by CT scan; the adrenals demonstrate change in size, calcification, low attenuation nodules, or areas of necrosis (Wilson et al, 1984).

Disseminated histoplasmosis has been reported in a female recipient of an infected kidney (Wong and Allen, 1992).

Obstructive uropathy was caused by disseminated histoplasmosis that caused sloughed papilla in a renal transplant recipient (Superdock et al, 1994). Percutaneous nephrostomy, long-term amphotericin B and itraconazole did not control the infection.

Superficial penile ulcers may develop in patients with disseminated infection. In one report, a patient with non–insulin-dependent diabetes mellitus had disseminated infection that caused hepato-splenomegaly and penile ulcer (Fig. 23–18). The putative exposure to the fungus was a train ride through the middle-western United States (Preminger et al, 1993). Despite treatment with intravenous amphotericin B, the patient died.

Isolated cutaneous *Histoplasma* lesions have been reported after direct inoculation by fungus; these lesions often heal spontaneously unless the patient is immunosuppressed (Cott et al, 1979).

Conjugal transmission has occurred. A woman developed an isolated labial lesion after sexual relations with her husband, who had disseminated disease and penile ulcers (Sills et al, 1973).

Epididymal histoplasmosis has been noted in two patients, one of whom developed paratracheal lymphadenopathy (Kauffman et al, 1981). In one patient, the epididymis was

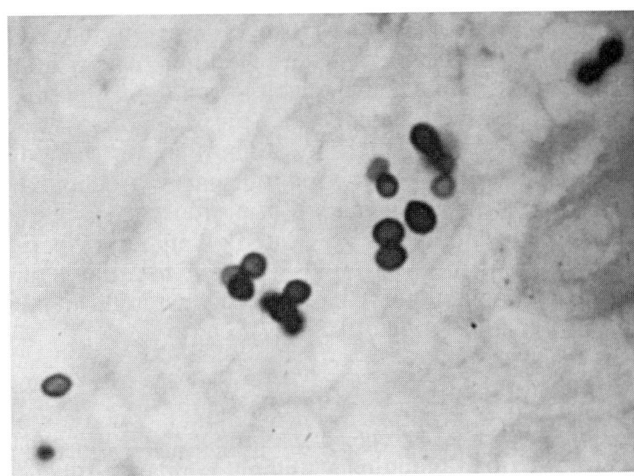

Figure 23–18. Photomicrograph of penile ulcer that demonstrates yeast-like forms of *Histoplasma capsulatum*. Methenamine silver stain, reduced from magnification of 500×. (From Wise GJ: AUA Update Series 1984; 3:4.)

filled with thick, purulent fluid; in the other patient, the epididymis was replaced by a granulomatous mass. The diagnosis was established by identification of the fungus in tissue. In both patients, surgical excision and drainage was the only treatment.

The *Histoplasma* fungus was identified in prostatic tissue removed by transurethral resection from a 65-year-old man with obstructive uropathy and pulmonary infiltrates. The patient received intravenous amphotericin B, but he died 6 months later; the precise cause of death was not ascertained (Orr et al, 1972). A prostatic abscess caused by *H. capsulatum* developed in a 39-year-old man with AIDS. Transurethral drainage and oral ketoconazole (600 mg/day) eradicated local infection (Marans et al, 1991).

Diagnosis

Changes on chest x-ray studies and conversion to positive histoplasmin skin tests often can determine exposure to *Histoplasma* fungus. However, immunosuppressed patients may have negative skin tests (Bonner et al, 1984). Culture of sputum, gastric washings, or abscess may yield the putative fungus. *H. capsulatum* may be identified in tissue specimens by methenamine silver or Giemsa's stain (Kauffman et al, 1981; Rippon, 1988, p 411).

In disseminated infection, peripheral blood smears may demonstrate intraleukocytic budding yeast (Henochowicz et al, 1985). Serologic studies (CF, ID, and LPA) have been helpful in establishing diagnosis and monitoring the course of disease (Rippon, 1988, p 410). However, antibody response may be muted in the immunosuppressed patient. The detection of *H. capsulatum* antigen in blood and urine by radioimmunoassay has been shown to be useful in diagnosis (Wheat et al, 1986).

Treatment

Disseminated histoplasmosis requires treatment with systemic amphotericin B. Relapse has been observed in patients who received less than 2 g of this therapy (Bradsher et al, 1982). The imidazoles, intravenous miconazole and oral ketoconazole, are not recommended as primary therapy in disseminated disease, but they may have a role in chronic therapy (Dismukes et al, 1983; Hawkins et al, 1981). **Maintenance therapy with amphotericin B or an oral agent such as itraconazole may be necessary to prevent relapse** (Wheat et al, 1992; Drew, 1993). Assessment of serum and urine *Histoplasma* polysaccharide antigen has been a useful marker for monitoring of treatment response in patients with AIDS and disseminated histoplasmosis (Wheat et al, 1992).

RARE AND UNUSUAL FUNGAL INFECTIONS

In the immunocompromised patient, fungal contaminants may become pathogens. These include species of *Fusarium, Trichosporon, Curvularia,* and *Alternaria* (Vartivarian et al, 1993; Morrison et al, 1993). Discussed here are unusual fungi that have caused infection in the genitourinary system.

Curvularia

A recurrent urinary tract infection was reported in a 5-year-old female without known predisposing or anatomic cause. Black specks in her urine were shown to be *Curvularia;* the infection resolved after hydration alone (Robson and Craver, 1994).

Fusarium

A diffuse erythematous skin rash developed in a 46-year-old male who required a bone marrow transplant for aplastic anemia. Biopsy of the skin reveal a fungus initially thought to be *Candida.* Despite treatment with amphotericin B (total dose 299 mg) and ketoconazole (500 mg), the patient died. Postmortem study revealed disseminated *Fusarium solani* involving the lungs, kidneys, spleen, lymph nodes, and testes. Extensive necrosis of the involved organs was caused by the predilection of the fungus for vascular structures (El-Ani, 1990).

Geotrichosis

Geotrichum candidum can be found in the sputum, feces, urine, and vaginal secretions of normal individuals. This fungus causes vaginitis that is often confused with candidal infection. Topical antifungal agents, such as nystatin, are effective treatment. (Rippon, 1988, p 715). Pulmonary infections may simulate tuberculosis or aspergillosis. Disseminated infection and multiorgan involvement with renal abscess and retroperitoneal lymph node infection have been reported in an immunocompromised patient (Kassamali et al, 1987).

G. candidum urinary tract infection was reported in a patient with renal stones and parathyroid adenoma. Amphotericin B (900 mg) stabilized but did not cure the infection (Drach et al, 1968).

Hansenula fabianii

Prostatic infection caused by *Hansenula fabianii* developed in a 57-year-old schizophrenic patient with chronic lymphocytic leukemia. Urethral instrumentation by the patient was the putative source of entry. The infection did not respond to ketoconazole but required a total dose of 2 g of intravenous amphotericin B (Dooley et al, 1990).

Paecilomyces

Paecilomyces can be found throughout the world in decaying vegetation. It is often associated with spoilage of canned and bottled fruits and vegetables. It is a common contaminant in the microbiology laboratory.

Paecilomyces fungi are characterized by broad-branching septate hyphae with characteristic spore-forming cells called phialides that can be identified in purulent material by Gram's stain. Endophthalmitis, endocarditis, and cellulitis have been usual foci of infection. A central venous catheter was the source of fungemia (*P. lilacinus*) in an 18-month-old, immunocompromised child with obstructive uropathy caused by a rhabdomyosarcoma of the prostate and bladder. The fungemia resolved after removal of the venous port and administration of intravenous amphotericin B (total dose

10 mg/kg) (Tan et al, 1992). One case of *Paecilomyces* pyelonephritis complicating nephrolithiasis has been reported; resolution of infection occurred with correction of obstructive uropathy alone (Sherwood and Dansky, 1983). Peritonitis caused by *P. variotti* was reported in four patients on continuous ambulatory peritoneal dialysis. Effective treatment required the removal of the Tenckhoff catheter and antifungal therapy, which included peritoneal irrigation (amphotericin B, 5 mg/L for 5 days); intravenous amphotericin B (1480 mg total dose); or ketoconazole (0.2 to 1.2 g/day for 10 days) (Marzec et al, 1993).

Treatment response by *Paecilomyces* has varied. Some species have been reported to be susceptible to amphotericin B, 5-FC, miconazole, ketoconazole, and itraconazole, but other variants been found resistant to amphotericin B, 5-FC, and fluconazole (Rippon, 1988, p 735; Marzec et al, 1993).

Paracoccidioidomycosis

P. brasiliensis causes a chronic granulomatous disease known as South American blastomycosis that can mimic tuberculosis or histoplasmosis. Indigenous to South America, it is a rare and unusual infection in the northern hemisphere. Clinical infection most often causes pulmonary or mucocutaneous disease. Disseminated infection may involve the lymphatic system, intestinal tract, liver, and spleen, although adrenal and testicular infection has been noted (Rippon, 1988, p 515). Ureteric involvement has been observed (Schonebeck, 1986). Diagnosis can be established by identification of the fungus in tissue or granulomatous material. Skin test and serologic studies utilizing CF or ID techniques are helpful in establishing diagnosis. Reactivation of pulmonary paracoccidioidomycosis has been reported in a male who required immune suppression for renal transplantation. The infection was controlled by amphotericin B (2 g given over 3 months), followed by ketoconazole (200 mg/day for 14 months) (Sugar et al, 1984).

Phycomycosis (Mucormycosis, Zygomycosis)

The taxonomic class Zygomycetes contains the family Mucoraceae with the genera *Rhizopus, Rhizomucor, Mucor,* and *Absidia*. Each genus includes species that can cause disease in humans (Rippon, 1988, p 681).

These fungi are worldwide in distribution and can readily be found in soil and in wild and domestic animals. Disease in humans may cause rhinocerebral infection that involves the sinus, pharynx, meninges, and brain. A fulminant clinical course has been reported in patients with diabetic acidosis. Pulmonary infection has been associated with hematologic malignancies, whereas gastrointestinal infection has been noted in malnourished children (Scully et al, 1988). Cutaneous infection and inguinal abscesses have been noted in renal transplantation patients.

Immune suppression may predispose the patient to disseminated zygomycosis that may involve the abdominopelvic organs. Renal involvement with and without associated disseminated disease has been reported (Dansky et al, 1978; Langston et al, 1973; Low et al, 1974; Prout and Goddard, 1960; Sane and Deshmukh, 1988; Santos et al, 1994). Renal zygomycosis (mucormycosis) may cause acute illness with signs of sepsis (i.e., fever, chills, tachycardia, and decreased urinary output) often associated with fungal-induced obstructive uropathy and renal infection (Figs. 23–19 and 23–20). Extensive renal involvement has developed in patients with AIDS (Vesa, 1992). Mucormycosis developed in the graft of a renal transplantation patient (Mitwalli et al, 1994). **Patients who require hemodialysis and receive deferoxamine are at increased risk for the development of disseminated mucormycosis (Boelaert, 1994; Boelaert et al, 1989).** Mucormycotic inguinal abscesses (*Rhizopus rhizopodoformis*) in a renal transplant were successfully treated with drainage and systemic amphotericin B and ketoconazole (Rippon, 1988, p 694). An isolated case of cutaneous infection of the vulva was reported in a diabetic patient who responded to surgical debridement alone (Scott et al, 1985).

Renal mucormycosis has required nephrectomy and systemic amphotericin B (total dose >1 g). Experience with the imidazoles in the treatment of this infection is limited. Lipid formulations of amphotericin B have had limited success in the treatment of rhinocerbral mucormycosis (Boelaert, 1994).

Penicillium

More than 900 species of *Penicillium* exist; most are nonpathogenic for humans, although some species have been

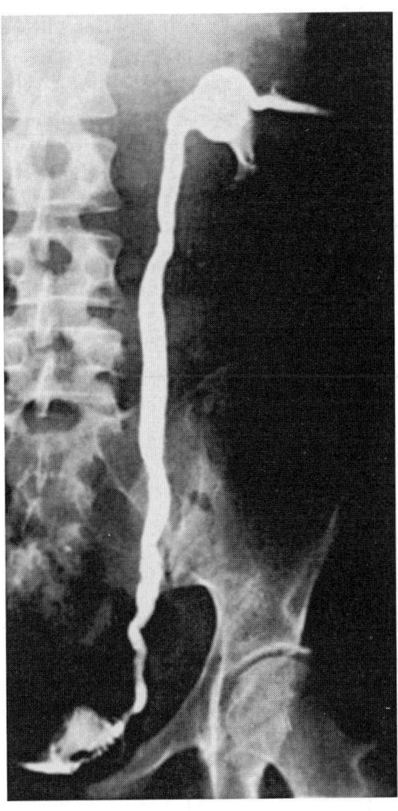

Figure 23–19. Contrast material injection of the percutaneous nephrostomy catheter, showing nonopaque filling defects in the renal pelvis and lower ureter caused by mucormycosis. (From Scully RE, Mark EJ, McNeely WF, McNeely BU: Case records of the Massachusetts General Hospital: Weekly clinicopathological exercise. N Engl J Med 1988; 319:631. Reprinted by permission of The New England Journal of Medicine.)

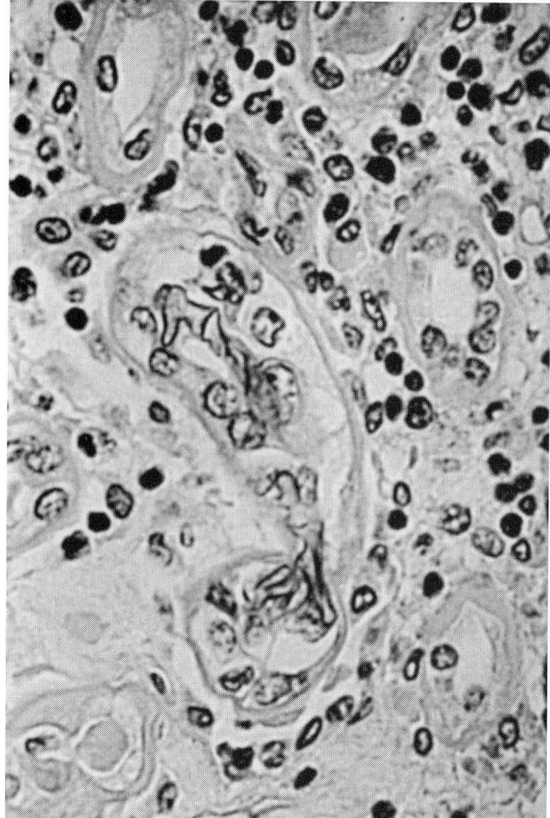

Figure 23–20. Renal medullary tubule containing fungal hyphae (mucormycosis), reduced from magnification of × 360. (From Scully RE, Mark EJ, McNeely WF, McNeely BU: Case records of the Massachusetts General Hospital: Weekly clinicopathological exercise. N Engl J Med 1988; 319:638. Reprinted by permission of The New England Journal of Medicine.)

known to cause external ear infection or bronchopulmonary penicilliosis. A bladder infection attributed to *P. glaucum* was reported in 1911 (Rippon, 1988, p 729). Another case of renal bladder urinary infection associated with *P. citrinum* occurred in a 56-year-old male with renal trauma. The patient received no treatment but would pass "balls of pink material in the voided urine." Urine material demonstrated mycelia, which grew readily on Sabouraud's medium. The patient subsequently died with the fungus present in the urinary tract, although it is uncertain whether this infection contributed to his death (Gilliam and Vest, 1951). Due to the rarity of *Penicillium* infection, there are insufficient data on treatment.

Pseudoallescheria boydii

Pseudoallescheria boydii is a ubiquitous soil fungus that has demonstrated pathogenicity for immunosuppressed patients. A renal fungoma (fungal ball) developed in a patient with chronic myelogenous leukemia (Schwartz, 1989).

Rhinosporidiosis

Rhinosporidium seeberi is indigenous to certain areas of India and Sri Lanka. The fungus can cause a chronic granulomatous inflammation that usually affects the anterior nares. Urethral infection may occur in males, usually 20 to 40 years old, with the development of a meatal pedunculated friable lesion that can mimic penile malignancy (Ravi et al, 1992). Female infection is less common. Diagnosis can be made by identification of fungus in resection tissue. Satisfactory treatment can be achieved by excision of the lesion (Sasidharan et al, 1987).

Sporotrichosis

Sporothrix schenckii can be found in soil or decaying vegetation. The fungus gains entry by means of skin trauma, such as thorn pricks or bites of animals or insects. Infection usually induces a chronic lymphocutaneous lesion. Dissemination may occur as a result of debilitation secondary to neoplasia, metabolic dysfunction, or steroid therapy. AIDS also has been cited as predisposing factor for disseminated infection (Bibler et al, 1986). Dissemination may involve bones, joints, sinuses, or meninges. Pulmonary changes may occur that mimic tuberculosis (Rippon, 1988, p 333).

Epididymal infection secondary to *S. schenckii* has occurred in association with systemic infection (Selman and Hampel, 1982). The fungus was identified in purulent fluid obtained from the scrotum. A renal transplant patient who had recurrent calculi and chronic ureteritis developed urinary sporotrichosis, which was diagnosed by histologic examination. No treatment was cited (Agarwal et al, 1994).

Diagnosis can be established by identification of fungus (cigar-shaped budding yeast forms) in tissue specimens (Bibler et al, 1986). The use of more sophisticated fluorescent antibody staining techniques can be helpful, as can serologic studies (Rippon, 1988, p 345).

Therapy with potassium iodide has been successful in treating cutaneous infection. In disseminated disease, intravenous amphotericin B or oral 5-FC may be used. Chronic therapy with fluconazole (200 to 400 mg/day for 3 to 6 months) has been successful in the treatment of lesions of the extremities (Castro et al, 1993); whereas itraconazole has been efficacious in the treatment of lymphocutaneous infection (Sharkey-Mathis et al, 1993). There are insufficient data to document the use of these drugs in genitourinary infection.

Tinea and *Trichosporon*

Infections by species of *Tinea (T. cruris, T. purpureum, T. rubrum)* are common causes of inguinal, scrotal, and crural infections that are manifested by itching, erythema, and scaling. Penile involvement is less frequent. Examination of skin scraping with potassium hydroxide and Sabouraud's culture establishes diagnosis (Kumar et al, 1981). A tinea infection of the umbilical region resulted in an urachal abscess in a healthy 27-year-old male. The cutaneous infection was successfully treated with topical ketoconazole preparation, but the abscess required surgical drainage (Thompson et al, 1994).

Fungi of the genus *Trichosporon (T. beigelii, T. capitatum)*, previously considered to cause innocuous superficial infections, have shown the capacity for invasive infection. *T. beigelii* has been identified in the urinary drainage systems of patients in an intensive care unit. Careful cleansing and change of drainage system resolved this outbreak (Stone and

Manasse, 1989). Disseminated infection, including a renal abscess, caused by *T. beigelii* was demonstrated by postmortem study in a 15-year-old bone marrow transplant recipient (Haupt et al, 1983).

ACTINOMYCETES

The actinomycetes have been considered as transitional forms between bacteria and fungi; however, their metabolic and morphologic characteristics classify them as higher forms of Monera (bacteria) (Rippon, 1988, p 15). Actinomyces are anaerobic, gram-positive, filamentous bacteria that often exist as saprophytes in the gastrointestinal tract or vagina. Pathogenicity may occur after trauma or dental procedures and usually develops as cervicofacial abscess. Microcolonies of these infections develop yellow pigmentations known as sulfur colonies (Scully et al, 1993).

Urogenital manifestations have included retroperitoneal abscess (Levine and Doyle, 1988), renal infections (Crosse et al, 1976; Patel et al, 1983), and renal-colic fistula (Yu et al, 1978). Pelvic infection associated with long-term use of intrauterine devices caused ureteric obstruction (Brown and Bancewicz, 1982). Actinomycotic vesicouterine fistula developed in an elderly woman with a vaginal pessary (Buckley et al, 1991). Primary bladder infection (Makar et al, 1992) and urachal infections (Ellis et al, 1979; Gotoh et al, 1988) have been reported. Intratesticular abscess has occurred in a patient with disseminated actinomycosis (Jani et al, 1990). Scrotal infection developed in a patient with actinomycotic perianal infection (Sarosdy et al, 1979). Actinomycosis has caused infection in a penile pilonidal sinus (Rashid et al, 1992). Prostatic infection occurred in a young male who had previous abdominal surgery (de Souza et al, 1985). Urethral infection has been associated with hypospadias repair (Weingärtner et al, 1992).

The identification of so-called sulfur granules in the infected tissue is characteristic of actinomycosis. A Gram's stain depicts gram-positive, rod-like, branching, filamentous structures (de Souza et al, 1985). **Treatment requires removal or debridement of infected tissue and the use of antibiotics. Intravenous penicillin (20 million units daily for 2 weeks) or oral ampicillin (1500 mg/day for 4 months) has been used for treatment of bladder infection (Makar et al, 1992).** Other effective antibiotics include tetracycline (Ellis et al, 1979), erythromycin (de Souza et al, 1985), and ciprofloxacin (Macfarlane et al, 1993).

ANTIFUNGAL THERAPEUTIC AGENTS

Amphotericin B

PHARMACOLOGY

Amphotericin B is a polyene antifungal agent with seven conjugated double bonds, an internal ester, a free carboxyl group, and a glycosidic side chain with primary amino groups (Walsh, 1987). It exerts fungicidal and fungistatic activity by binding to the ergosterol component of the fungal cell membrane, which results in disruption of internal cellular components, causing electrolytic flux (Medoff and Kobayashi, 1980). **For systemic effect, amphotericin B must be administered by intravenous injection.** The drug has a high protein-binding capacity and a prolonged half-life (15 days). Only 3% of the drug is excreted unchanged in the urine (Como and Dismukes, 1994). Placental tissue may serve as a reservoir for amphotericin B (Dean et al, 1994). **Local infections of the renal collecting system or bladder may be treated by irrigation with amphotericin B.**

ADVERSE EFFECTS

Intravenous use may induce systemic reactions, such as rigors, chills, and fever. Gigliotti and colleagues (1987) reported that pretreatment with ibuprofen (10 mg/kg) decreased the incidence of chills (from 87% to 49% of patients). Use of intravenous meperidine or dantrolene to control amphotericin B rigors has been reported (da Camara and Lane, 1987). Amphotericin B dosage must be decreased or its administration temporarily stopped in order to control these adverse effects. Intravenous corticosteroids (20 mg) given concomitantly with amphotericin B may control the rigors and chills.

Other adverse reactions ascribed to intravenous amphotericin B include generalized pain, headache, convulsions, localized phlebitis, anemia, and thrombocytopenia (Craven, 1982). Administration of heparin, use of large needles, and rotation of intravenous catheter sites are recommended to minimize the risk of phlebitis. Hearing loss also has been noted in isolated cases (Stamm et al, 1987).

Amphotericin B–related nephrotoxicity is characterized by hematuria, pyuria, cylindruria, proteinuria, and electrolyte imbalance (Branch, 1988). Amphotericin B may exacerbate the nephrotoxic effects of other agents, such as *cis*-platin (Walsh, 1987). This effect is more prevalent in elderly patients who have pre-existing renal disease. Electrolyte disturbances include potassium and magnesium depletion. Glomerular filtration rate decreases within 2 weeks of beginning therapy and usually stabilizes at 20% to 60% of baseline values with continued therapy (Branch, 1988; Medoff and Kobayashi, 1980). If renal function continues to deteriorate (on the basis of serum creatinine), therapy should be interrupted until renal function improves.

Clinical studies suggest that sodium supplementation with intravenous saline or ticarcillin disodium (which may be used to treat concomitant bacterial infections) and hydration reduce the risk of nephrotoxicity (Branch, 1988). **Hypertensive patients who are on salt-restricted diets or diuretics are at increased risk for renal toxicity.** The potassium wasting that accompanies use of amphotericin B can be corrected by potassium supplementation (usually by intravenous administration). The potassium-sparing diuretic amiloride may reduce potassium loss (Smith et al, 1988). Cardiac arrhythmias have been attributed to amphotericin B–induced potassium and magnesium depletion.

Amphotericin B in lipid complexes bind to the sites of the fungal cell membrane, with less potential for adverse effects (Wiebe and Degregorio, 1988). Liposomal amphotericin B was effective in the treatment of 4 patients with impaired renal function who had urinary tract infections caused by *C. albicans.* At dose levels of 50 mg/day, urine cultures became negative within 4 days. None of the patients had adverse effect usually ascribed to standard amphotericin B therapy (Ralph et al, 1991).

FUNGAL RESISTANCE TO AMPHOTERICIN B

Fungal resistance to amphotericin B is unusual. Fungal resistance has been noted in *P. boydii.* One potential genitourinary pathogen that has shown an increased tolerance to amphotericin B is *C. parapsilosis* (Seidenfeld et al, 1983).

Flucytosine

PHARMACOLOGY

5-FC is a fluorinated pyrimidine with a molecular weight of 129.1. The antifungal effect of 5-FC is caused by its conversion to 5-fluorouracil (5-FU) by cytosine deaminase, which is present in some fungal species but absent or present in low concentrations in mammalian cells. 5-FU is then converted to 5-fluorodoxyuridine monophosphate, which adversely affects fungal protein and DNA synthesis. It is readily absorbed by the gastrointestinal tract and widely distributed in a volume approximating the total body water. There is little binding to plasma proteins (Sande and Mandell, 1985). Serum half-life ranges from 3 to 5 hours, and there is good penetration into the CSF and other body fluids. Serum concentrations may reach as high as 70 to 80 μg/ml within 1 to 2 hours after a dose of 37.5 mg/kg. This far exceeds the minimal inhibitory concentration (MIC) of sensitive fungi. **The drug is excreted unchanged by filtration and may reach concentrations in urine of 200 to 500 μg/ml.**

Because the primary method of excretion is through the kidney, the dosage must be modified in the presence of renal disease. When first introduced, 5-FC was administered at doses of 50 mg/kg. A dose of 100 to 150 mg/kg is now advised (Harder and Hermans, 1975; Wise et al, 1980). 5-FC can be given every 6 hours; however, in the presence of renal insufficiency, the dosage should be modified in proportion to the degree of renal compromise and should be followed by assessment of serum levels of 5-FC. Because the drug can be cleared by dialysis, renal failure should not compromise its use when clinically indicated (Schonebeck, 1986).

ADVERSE EFFECTS OF FLUCYTOSINE

Nausea, vomiting, diarrhea, and enterocolitis can occur infrequently. Abnormalities in liver function have been noted in 5% of patients (Sande and Mandell, 1985). **Bone marrow depression may occur, with the development of anemia, leukopenia, and thrombocytopenia.** These toxic manifestations resolve if the drug is stopped, but one case of aplastic anemia has been associated with 5-FC (Meyer and Axelrod, 1974). The drug is interdicted during pregnancy, although it has been given to a pregnant woman during the second trimester without adverse effect in the fetus (Schonebeck and Segerbrand, 1973). **Successful management of urinary candidal infection has been reported to vary from 50% to 90%** (Harder and Hermans, 1975).

DRUG RESISTANCE TO FLUCYTOSINE

Primary resistance to 5-FC may occur in 10% of infections caused by *C. albicans*, but the rate may be as high as 30% with other *Candida* species. Secondary resistance was noted to occur in 6.2% of patients within 7 to 10 days of treatment. Fungal resistance to 5-FC has been attributed to lack of either cytosine deaminase or uridine monophosphate pyrophosphorylase, which controls the metabolism of 5-FU. Certain fungi may be deficient in permease, which enables 5-FC to cross the fungal membrane and interfere with intracellular metabolism (Medoff and Kobayashi, 1980).

Imidazoles and Triazoles

The imidazoles include clotrimazole, a topical agent; miconazole, an intravenous and intravesical agent; and ketoconazole, an oral agent. Econazole, another imidazole, is available in the United States as a topical antifungal agent. The primary mechanism of action of the imidazoles is inhibition of cytochrome P450, which regulates fungal ergosterol metabolism, a necessary function for cell membrane integrity.

The triazoles (itraconazole and fluconazole) are similar in chemical structure to the imidazoles, but they have a greater affinity for fungal cytochrome P450 enzymes than the imidazoles (Como and Dismukes, 1994).

DRUG INTERACTIONS

A number of drugs interact with the azoles. These include isoniazid, rifampin, cyclosporine, tolbutamide, and warfarin (see Table 23–4).

MICONAZOLE

Miconazole (Monistat) is available in 20-ml ampules at a drug concentration of 10 mg/ml (200 mg/ampule). This drug can be used intravenously by dissolving it in a 200-ml diluent of either normal saline or 5 per cent dextrose and water. For therapeutic effect, dosage may vary from 200 to 1200 mg given every 8 hours. The drug has been reported to be effective against a variety of fungi that can infect the genitourinary system, such as *Candida, Aspergillus,* and *Histoplasma* species. Toxic reactions, including anaphylaxis, cardiac arrhythmias, fever, chills, nausea, and anemia, have been noted. **Because miconazole is poorly excreted into the urine, it has a no role (when given intravenously) in the management of urinary fungal infections.** Miconazole can be used as a genitourinary irrigant (50 mg diluted in 1 liter of saline, administered by bladder catheter over 24 hours) in patients with candidal colonization or noninvasive infection (Wise et al, 1987).

KETOCONAZOLE

After oral administration, ketoconazole is absorbed from the gastrointestinal tract and reaches peak plasma concentration within 1 to 4 hours. **Absorption is limited if the patient has chlorhydria or uses the antacid cimetidine or ranitidine.** The drug is available in either 200-mg or 400-mg tablets. A 400-mg dose can achieve serum levels of 1.8 to 7.8 μg/ml, which exceeds the in vitro MIC of many *Candida (Torulopsis), Coccidioides, Cryptococcus, Aspergillus, Histoplasma,* and *Blastomyces* species. **Because of its poor renal excretion, ketoconazole has low urinary levels that may be insufficient to inhibit many fungal species; thus, it has a limited role in the treatment of fungi that**

may infect the urinary collecting system and bladder (Wise et al, 1985).

Ketoconazole's adverse effects may include headaches and skin rashes, but its most significant impact is on liver metabolism, with elevation of serum triglycerides and abnormal levels of liver enzymes. Ketoconazole interacts with mammalian steroid metabolism, which affects androgen metabolism (see Table 23–3).

In most patients with invasive fungal infection, an initial dose of 400 mg/day, with a gradual increase to 800 mg/day in divided doses, is recommended. Therapy may be required for many months (12 months or longer in disseminated coccidioidomycosis). In the pediatric age group, ketoconazole (7 to 10 mg/kg daily in divided doses) has been used with good results. Hepatotoxicity appears to be more prevalent in younger children. Because transplantation patients are prone to secondary fungal infections, imidazoles should be given cautiously in patients requiring cyclosporine. There is a drug interaction between cyclosporine and the imidazoles, and ketoconazole increases serum levels of cyclosporine (Trenk et al, 1987).

ITRACONAZOLE

Itraconazole is effective in the treatment of infections caused by *Aspergilla, Blastomyces, Coccidioides, Histoplasma,* and *Sporotrichosis* (Graybill, 1988; The Medical Letter, 1993). Absorption is enhanced when the drug is taken with food. The drug is lipophilic and achieves tissue levels two to three times higher than in serum; itraconazole has fewer adverse effects than ketoconazole. Recommended loading dose is 200 mg, three times daily for three days, followed by a dosage of 200 to 400 mg/day. The length of therapy is dependent on extent of infection (Como and Dismukes, 1994; The Medical Letter, 1993).

FLUCONAZOLE

Fluconazole can be administered by mouth or intravenously. Oral administration is not affected by the presence of food or gastric activity. This drug is water soluble and rapidly achieves high levels (10 μg/ml within 2 to 4 hours) in plasma, CSF, and urine (concentration may exceed 100 μg/ml). Fluconazole is efficacious in the treatment of urinary tract infections caused by *Candida, Torulopsis,* and *Cryptococcus.* **It is equally effective as bladder irrigation with amphotericin B in the treatment of bladder candidal infection** (Muncan and Wise, 1995a).

Isolated case reports have cited success in the use of fluconazole for treatment of renal infection (Dave et al, 1989).

Fluconazole may affect **the liver or steroidogenesis but to a lesser degree than the imidazoles.** Congenital anomalies were noted in an infant born to a woman who received

Table 23–1. GUIDELINES FOR PHARMACOTHERAPY OF MAJOR GENITOURINARY FUNGAL INFECTIONS

Disease	Site	Drug	Dosage*	Duration*
Aspergillosis	Kidney and collecting system	Amphotericin B	1.5 mg/kg/day IV ± 50 μg/ml, 40 ml/hour irrigation	6–18 weeks
		Itraconazole	200 mg p.o. bid	1 year?
	Prostate	Amphotericin B	1.5 mg/kg/day IV ± 50 μg/ml, 40 ml/hour irrigation	Unknown
		Itraconazole	200 mg p.o. bid	Unknown
Blastomycosis	Prostate	Ketoconazole	400 mg/day p.o.	>1 month
		Amphotericin B	1–3 g total dose IV	3 months
	Epididymis	Ketoconazole	400 mg p.o. daily	1 year
	Balanitis	Nystatin, clotrimazole	Topical cream or ointment	Not specified
		Fluconazole	150 mg/day p.o.	1 day
Candidiasis and *Torulopsis* infection	Vaginitis	Nystatin	100,000 units intravaginally	14 days
	Bladder	Fluconazole	150 mg p.o.	7 days
		Miconazole	200 mg intravaginally	3 days
		Amphotericin B	50 μg/ml, 40 ml/hour irrigation	4–14 days
		Miconazole	50 μg/ml, 40 ml/hour irrigation	5 days
		Fluconazole	400 mg loading, then 200 mg/day p.o.	14 days
	Kidney	Amphotericin B	1 g total dose IV ± 50 μg/ml, 40 ml/hour irrigation	Not specified
		Liposomal Amphotericin B?	320–820 (?) mg	7–17 days
	Prostate	Fluconazole	200 b.i.d.	6 weeks
Coccidioidomycosis	Kidney	Amphotericin B	>2 g IV	Not specified
	Prostate	Amphotericin B	2.5 g total dose IV	4 months
	Bladder	Amphotericin B + Ketoconazole	2 g total cose IV + 200 mg/day p.o.	1 year
Cryptococcosis	Prostate	Amphotericin B	1–3.4 g total dose IV	Not specified
		Flucytosine	100–150/mg/kg/day (normal renal function)	4–6 weeks
		Fluconazole	200 mg/day	2–6 months
Histoplasmosis	Renal	Amphotericin B	>2 g IV	Unknown
	Prostate	Ketoconazole	600 mg/day	Unknown
		Itraconazole?	200 mg/day	Unknown
Mucormycosis	Renal	Amphotericin B	>1 g IV	1 month

Adapted from Wise GJ, Silver DA: J Urol 1993; 149:1377–1378.

*Entries represent known dosage guidelines *only*. Specific therapy must be tailored to each patient; drug selection, dosage, and duration of treatment are determined by sensitivity testing, metabolic considerations, and clinical and laboratory evidence of improvement.

Table 23–2. AVAILABLE SYSTEMIC ANTIFUNGAL AGENTS AND THEIR COSTS

Agent	Proprietary Name and Maker	Form	Strength	Cost per Unit ($)*
Amphotericin B	Fungizone, Squibb	Powder for injection	50 mg	32.50–38.61†
Flucytosine	Ancobon, Hoffmann–La Roche	Capsule	230 mg	1.03
			500 mg	1.93
Miconazole	Monistat IV, Janssen	Solution for injection	200 mg ampule	40.08
Ketoconazole	Nizoral, Janssen	Tablets	200 mg	2.46
Fluconazole	Diflucan, Roerig	Solution for injection	200 mg in 100 ml normal saline	81.25
			400 mg in 100 ml normal saline	118.75
		Tablets	50 mg	4.38
			100 mg	6.88
Itraconazole	Sporanox, Janssen	Capsules	100 mg	4.92

Adapted from Como JA, Dismukes WE: N Engl J Med 1994; 330:263–272. Copyright 1994, Massachusetts Medical Society.
*The amounts represent the average cost to wholesalers as of December 1993. The actual cost to patients may vary considerably.
†More than one product is available.

fluconazole for systemic coccidioidomycosis (Lee et al, 1992).

Fungal drug resistance to fluconazole has been observed in patients with HIV who have required long-term treatment for esophageal candidiasis (Como and Dismukes, 1994). Fungal resistance has been reported in both immunocompetent patients and immunocompromised patients not previously treated with fluconazole (Goff et al, 1995; Iwen et al, 1995).

Guidelines for antifungal therapy are described in Table 23–1. Available systemic antifungal and costs are cited in Table 23–2. Common or serious adverse effects are noted in Table 23–3. Drug interactions involving oral azole drugs are listed in Table 23–4.

Table 23–3. COMMON OR SERIOUS ADVERSE EFFECTS OF SYSTEMIC ANTIFUNGAL DRUGS

Organ or System	Drug					
	Amphotericin B	*Flucytosine*	*Miconazole*	*Ketoconazole*	*Fluconazole*	*Itraconazole*
Gastrointestinal tract	Nausea, vomiting, anorexia	Nausea and vomiting (5% of patients), diarrhea, abdominal pain	Nausea and vomiting (<15% of patients)	Nausea and vomiting (<10% of patients), abdominal pain, anorexia	Nausea and vomiting (<5% of patients)	Nausea and vomiting (<10% of patients)
Skin	—	Rash	—	Pruritus, rash	Rash, possibly exfoliative (Stevens–Johnson syndrome)	Pruritus, rash
Liver	—	Asymptomatic rise of plasma ATA (7% of patients), hepatitis (rare)	—	Asymptomatic rise of plasma ATA (2%–10% of patients), hepatitis	Asymptomatic rise of plasma ATA (<1%–7% of patients), hepatitis	Asymptomatic rise of plasma ATA (<1%–5% of patients), hepatitis (rare)
Bone marrow	Anemia	Anemia (less common), leukopenia, thrombocytopenia	Anemia, leukopenia, thrombocytosis or thrombocytopenia	—	—	—
Kidney	Azotemia (80% of patients), renal, tubular acidosis, hypokalemia, hypomagnesemia	—	—	—	—	—
Endocrine system	—	—	Hyperlipidemia, hyponatremia	Adrenal insufficiency (rare), decreased libido, impotence, gynecomastia, menstrual irregularities	—	Hypokalemia, hypertension, edema, impotence
Other	Thrombophlebitis, headache, fever and chills	Confusion, headache	Phlebitis, fever, psychosis	Headache, fever and chills	Headache, seizure	Headache, dizziness

Adapted from Como JA, Dismukes WE: N Engl J Med 1994; 330:263–272. Copyright 1994, Massachusetts Medical Society.
ATA, aminotransferase.

Table 23–4. DRUG INTERACTIONS INVOLVING ORAL AZOLE ANTIFUNGAL DRUGS

Effect and Drug Involved	Azole Involved: *Clinically Important*	Azole Involved: *Potentially Important*
Decreased Plasma Concentration of Azole		
Decreased absorption of azole		
Antacids	Ketoconazole, itraconazole	
H_2-receptor–antagonist drugs	Ketoconazole, itraconazole	
Sucralfate		Ketoconazole
Increased metabolism of azole		
Isoniazid	Ketoconazole	
Phenytoin	Ketoconazole, itraconazole	
Rifampin	Ketoconazole, itraconazole	Fluconazole
Increased Plasma Concentration of Coadministered Drug		
Cyclosporin	Ketoconazole	Fluconazole, itraconazole
Digoxin		Itraconazole
Phenytoin	Ketoconazole, fluconazole	Itraconazole
Sulfonylurea drugs, especially tolbutamide		Ketoconazole, itraconazole, fluconazole
Terfenadine	Ketoconazole, itraconazole	
Astemizole	Ketoconazole, itraconazole	
Warfarin		Ketoconazole, itraconazole, fluconazole

Adapted from Como JA, Dismukes WE: N Engl J Med 1994; 330:263–272. Copyright 1994, Massachusetts Medical Society.

Other Treatment Modalities

Alkalinization

The ideal pH for growth of *Candida* fungi ranges from 5.1 to 6.4, which parallels that of urinary pH. Alkalinization of the urine has been cited as a method of resolving candiduria (Schonebeck, 1986). **These observations appear to be anecdotal, and no clinical studies have documented these findings.**

Allylamine

Derivatives of naftifine, such as allylamine, have demonstrated in vitro and in vivo antifungal activity. Their mechanism of action involves fungal inhibition of ergosterol biosynthesis. These drugs are still investigational (Rippon, 1986).

Transfer Factor

Transfer factor, derived from lymphocyte lysates, has been helpful in the treatment of generalized coccidioidomycosis, histoplasmosis, and chronic mucocutaneous candidosis (Schulkind and Ayoub, 1980). However, this treatment remains investigational.

Granulocyte-Macrophage Colony-Stimulating Factor

Granulocyte-macrophage colony-stimulating factor GM-CSF was used in conjunction with amphotericin B in the treatment of cancer patients with invasive fungal infections (*Aspergilla* pulmonary infection—2 patients; *Candida* pneumonia and disseminated infection—5 patients; disseminated sporotrichosis—1 patient). Six of eight patients had a cure or partial response. A capillary-leak syndrome developed in three patients, two of whom recovered (Bodey et al, 1993). There are no data on the use of GM-CSF in the treatment of genitourinary fungal infections.

REFERENCES

Abbas F, Kamal MK, Talati J: Prostatic aspergillosis. J Urol 1995; 153:748–750.

Abernathy RS, Melby JC: Addison's disease in North American blastomycosis. N Engl J Med 1962; 266:552–554.

Abramowitz J, Fowler JE Jr, Talluri K, et al: Percutaneous identification and removal of fungus ball from renal pelvis. J Urol 1986; 135:1232–1233.

Abrams DI, Robia M, Blumenfeld W, et al: Disseminated coccidioidomycosis in AIDS. N Engl J Med 1984; 310:986–987.

Adams JR, Mata JA, Culkin DJ, et al: Acquired immunodeficiency syndrome manifesting as prostate nodule secondary to cryptococcal infection. Urology 1992; 39:289–291.

Agarwal SK, Tiwari SC, Dash SC, et al: Urinary sporotrichosis in a renal allograft recipient. Nephron 1994; 66:485.

Allo MD, Miller J, Townsend T, Tan C: Primary cutaneous aspergillosis associated with Hickman intravenous catheters. N Engl J Med 1987; 317:1105–1108.

Andersen GM, Barrat J, Bergan T, et al: A comparison of single-dose oral fluconazole with 3-day intravaginal clotrimazole in the treatment of vaginal candidiasis. Br J Obstet Gynaecol 1989; 96:226–232.

Aragona F, Glazel GP, Pavanello L, et al: Upper urinary tract obstruction in children caused by Candida fungus balls. Eur Urol 1985; 11:188–191.

Asnis DS, Chitkara RK, Jacobson M, Goldstein JA: Invasive aspergillosis: An unusual manifestation of AIDS. N Y State J Med 1988; 88:653–655.

Bailly MP, Boibieux A, Biron F, et al: Persistence of *Cryptococcus neoformans* in the prostate: Failure of fluconazole despite high doses. J Infect Dis 1991; 164:435–436.

Bartkowski DP, Lanesky JR: Emphysematous prostatitis and cystitis secondary to *Candida albicans*. J Urol 1988; 139:1063–1065.

Bartone FF, Hurwitz RS, Rojas EL, et al: The role of percutaneous nephrostomy in the management of obstructing candidiasis of the urinary tract in infants. J Urol 1988; 140:338–341.

Beilke MA, Kirmani N: *Candida* pyelonephritis complicated by fungemia in obstructive uropathy. Br J Urol 1988; 62:7–10.

Bell DA, Rose SC, Starr NK, et al: Percutaneous nephrostomy for nonoperative management of fungal urinary tract infections. J Vasc Interv Radiol 1993; 4:311–315.

Bergner DM, Kraus SM, Duck GB, Lewis R: Systemic blastomycosis presenting with acute prostatic abscess. J Urol 1981; 126:132–133.

Bhattacharya S, Bryk D, Wise GJ: Renal pelvic filling defect in a diabetic woman. J Urol 1982; 127:751–753.

Bibler MR, Gianis JT: Acute ureteral colic from obstructing renal aspergilloma. Rev Infect Dis 1987; 9:790–794.

Bibler MR, Luber HJ, Glueck HI, Estes SA: Disseminated sporotrichosis in a patient with HIV infection after treatment for acquired factor VIII inhibitor. JAMA 1986; 256: 3125–3126.

Bissada NK, Finkbeiner AE, Redman JF: Prostatic mycosis: Nonsurgical diagnosis and management. Urology 1977; 9:327–328.

Blastomycosis—One disease or two? Lancet 1989; 1:25.

Blum JA: Acute monilial pyohydronephrosis: Report of a case successfully treated with amphotericin B continuous renal pelvis irrigation. J Urol 1966; 96:614–618.

Bodey GP, Anaissie E, Gutterman J, Vadhan-Raj S: Role of granulocyte-macrophage colony stimulating factor as adjuvant therapy for fungal infections in patients with cancer. Clin Infect Dis 1993; 17:705–707.

Boelaert JR: Mucormycosis (zygomycosis): Is there news for the clinician? J Infect Dis 1994; 28(Suppl 1):1–6.

Boelaert JR, Fenves AZ, Coburn JW: Mucormycosis among patients on dialysis. N Engl J Med 1989; 321:190–191.

Bonner JR, Alexander WJ, Dismukes WE, et al: Disseminated histoplasmosis in patients with acquired immunodeficiency syndrome. Arch Intern Med 1984; 144:2178–2181.

Bozzette SA, Larsen RA, Chiu J, et al: Fluconazole treatment of persistent cryptococcal neoformans prostatic infection in AIDS. Ann Intern Med 1991; 115:285–286.

Bradsher RW: Blastomycosis. Clin Infect Dis 1992; 14(Suppl 1):S82–S90.

Bradsher RW, Alford RH, Hawkins SS, Spickard WA: Conditions associated with relapse of amphotericin B treated disseminated histoplasmosis. Johns Hopkins Med J 1982; 150:127–131.

Braman RT: Cryptococcosis (torulosis) of the prostate. Urology 1981; 17:284–285.

Branch RA: Prevention of amphotericin B induced renal impairment. Arch Intern Med 1988; 148:2389–2394.

Brock DJ, Grieco MH: Cryptococcal prostatitis in a patient with sarcoidosis: Response to 5-fluorocytosine. J Urol 1972; 107:1017–1021.

Brown R, Bancewicz J: Ureteric obstruction due to pelvic actinomycosis. Br J Surg 1982; 69:156.

Buchman TG, Rossier M, Merz WG, Charache P: Detection of surgical pathogens by an in vitro DNA amplification: Part 1. Rapid identification of *Candida albicans* by in vitro amplification of a fungus-specific gene. Surgery 1990; 108:338–346.

Buckley P, McInerney PD, Stephenson TP: Actinomycotic vesico-uterine fistula from a wishbone pessary contraceptive device. Br J Urol 1991; 68:206–207.

Bylund DJ, Nanfro JJ, Marsh WL Jr: Coccidioidomycosis of the female genital tract. Arch Pathol Lab Med 1986; 110:232–235.

Castro LGM, Belda W Jr, Cuce LC, et al: Successful treatment of sporotrichosis with oral fluconazole: A report of three cases. Br J Dermatol 1993; 128:352–356.

Chapin-Robertson K, Bechtel C, Waycott S, et al: Cryptococcal antigen detection from the urine of AIDS patients. Diagn Microbiol Infect Dis 1993 17:197–201.

Chen KTK: Coccidioidomycosis of the epididymis. J Urol 1983; 130:978–979.

Chisholm ER, Hutch JA: Fungus ball (*Candida albicans*) formation in the bladder. J Urol 1961; 86:559–562.

Chuck SL, Sande MA: Infections with *Cryptococcus neoformans* in the acquired immunodeficiency syndrome. N Engl J Med 1989; 321:794–799.

Codish SD, Tobias JS, Hannigan M: Combined amphotericin B flucytosine therapy in *Aspergillus* pneumonia. JAMA 1979; 241:2418–2419.

Como JA, Dismukes WE: Oral azole drugs as systemic antifungal therapy. N Engl J Med 1994; 330:263–272.

Concus AP, Helfand RF, Imber MJ, et al: Cutaneous cryptococcosis mimicking molluscum contagiosum in a patient with AIDS. J Infect Dis 1988; 158:897–898.

Conner WT, Drach GW, Bucher WC Jr: Genitourinary aspects of disseminated coccidioidomycosis. J Urol 1975; 113:82–88.

Cott GR, Smith TW, Hinthorn DR, Liu C: Primary cutaneous histoplasmosis in immunosuppressed patients. JAMA 1979; 242:456–457.

Craig MW, Davey WN, Green RA: Conjugal blastomycosis. Am Rev Respir Dis 1970; 102:86–90.

Craven PG: Amphotericin B: An update. Drug Therapy 1982; 12:67–69.

Cross AS: Nosocomial aspergillosis: An increasing problem. J Nosocom Infect 1987; 4:6–9.

Crosse JEW, Soderdahl DW, Schamber DT: Renal actinomycosis. Urology 1976; 7:309–311.

Cuetara MM, Mallo N, Dalet F: Amphotericin B lavage in the treatment of candidal cystitis. Br J Urol 1972; 44:475–480.

da Camara CC, Lane TW: Dantrolene for amphotericin B induced rigors. (Letter.) Arch Intern Med 1987; 147:2220.

Dansky AS, Lynne CM, Politano VA: Disseminated mucormycosis with renal involvement. J Urol 1978; 119:275–277.

Dave J, Hickey MM, Wilkin EGL: Fluconazole in renal candidosis. (Letter.) Lancet 1989; 1:163–164.

Davidson F: Yeasts and circumcision in the male. Br J Vener Dis 1977; 53:121–122.

Dean JL, Wolf JE, Ranzini AC, Laughlin MA: Use of amphotericin B during pregnancy: Case report and review. Clin Infect Dis 1994; 18:364–368.

Dembner AG, Pfister RC: Fungal infection of the urinary tract: Demonstration by antegrade pyelography and drainage by percutaneous nephrostomy. Am J Roentgenol 1977; 129:415–418.

de Repentigny L: Serodiagnosis of candidiasis, aspergillosis, and cryptococcosis. Clin Infect Dis 1992; Suppl 1:S11–S22.

de Repentigny L, Reiss E: Current trends in immunodiagnosis of candidiasis and aspergillosis. Rev Infect Dis 1984; 6:301–312.

de Souza E, Katz DA, Dworzack DL, Longo G: Actinomycosis of the prostate. J Urol 1985; 133:290–291.

Dismukes WE: Blastomycosis: Leave it to Beaver. N Engl J Med 1986; 314:575–577.

Dismukes WE, Stamm AM, Graybill JR, et al: Treatment of systemic mycosis with ketoconazole: Emphasis on toxicity and clinical response in 52 patients. Ann Intern Med 1983; 98:13–20.

Docimo SG, Rukstalis DB, Rukstalis MB, et al: Candida epididymitis: Newly recognized opportunistic epididymal infection. Urology 1993; 41:280–282.

Doemeny JM, Banner MP, Shapiro MJ, et al: Percutaneous extraction of renal fungus ball. Am J Radiol 1988; 150:1331–1332.

Dooley DP, Beckius ML, McAllister CK, Jeffrey BS: Prostatitis caused by *Hansenula fabianii*. J Infect Dis 1990; 161:1040–1041.

Drach GW, Carlton CE, Chenault OW, Dykhuizen RF: Fungal superinfection: Geotrichosis of the urinary tract in association with parathyroid adenoma. J Urol 1968; 100:82–84.

Drew RH: Pharmacotherapy of disseminated histoplasmosis in patients with AIDS. Ann Pharmacother 1993; 27:1510–1518.

Drutz DJ: Urban coccidioidomycosis and histoplasmosis: Sacramento and Indianapolis. N Engl J Med 1979; 301:381–382.

Dyess DL, Garrison RN, Fry DE: Candidal sepsis. Implications of polymicrobial blood borne infection. Arch Surg 1985; 120:345–348.

Eckstein CW, Kass EJ: Anuria in a newborn secondary to bilateral ureteropelvic fungus balls. J Urol 1982; 127:109–110.

Edwards JE: Invasive *Candida* infections. Evolution of a fungal pathogen. N Engl J Med 1991; 324:1060–1062.

Eickenberg HU, Amin M, Lich R Jr: Blastomycosis of the genitourinary tract. J Urol 1975; 113:650–652.

Einstein HE, Johnson RH: Coccidioidomycosis: New aspects of epidemiology and therapy. Clin Infect Dis 1993; 16:349–356.

Eisenberg, RL, Hedgcock MW, Shanser JD: Aspergillus mycetoma of the renal pelvis associated with ureteropelvic junction obstruction. J Urol 1977; 118:466–467.

El-Ani AS: Disseminated infection caused by *Fusarium solani* in a patient with aplastic anemia. N Y State J Med 1990; 90:609–610.

Ellis LR, Kenny GM, Nellans RE: Urogenital aspects of actinomycosis. J Urol 1979; 122:132–133.

Eubanks PJ, de Virgilio C, Klein S, Bongard F: *Candida* sepsis in surgical patients. Am J Surg 1993; 166:617–619.

Fisher JF, Chev WH, Shadomy S, et al: Urinary tract infections due to *Candida albicans*. Rev Infect Dis 1982; 4:1107–1118.

Fisher JF, Newman CL, Sobel JD: Yeast in the urine: Solutions for a budding problem. Clin Infect Dis 1995; 20:183–189.

Flechner SM, McAninch JW: Aspergillosis of the urinary tract: Ascending route of infection and evolving patterns of disease. J Urol 1981; 125:598–601.

Frye KR, Donovan JM, Drach GW: *Torulopsis glabrata* urinary infections: A review. J Urol 1988; 139:1245–1249.

Galgiani JN: Markers of coccidioidomycosis before cardiac or renal transplantation and risk of recurrent infection. Transplantation 1993; 55:1422–1442.

Gallis HA, Berman RA, Cate TR, et al: Fungal infection following renal transplantation. Arch Intern Med 1975; 135:1163–1172.

Gerridzen RG, Wesley-James T: Acute ureteral obstruction from candidal cystitis requiring bilateral percutaneous nephrostomies. Urology 1988; 32:444–446.

Gigliotti F, Shenep JL, Lott L, Thornton D: Induction of prostaglandin synthesis as the mechanism responsible for the chills and fever produced by infusing amphotericin. Br J Infect Dis 1987; 156:784–789.

Gilliam JS, Vest SA: *Penicillium* infection of the urinary tract. J Urol 1951; 65:484–489.

Godec CJ, Mielnick A, Hilfer J: Primary renal aspergillosis. Urology 1989; 34:152–154.

Goff DA, Koletar SL, Buesching WJ, et al: Isolation of fluconazole-resistant *Candida albicans* from human immunodeficiency virus-negative patients never treated with azoles. Clin Infect Dis 1995; 20:77–83.

Gotoh S, Kura N, Nagahama K, et al: Actinomycosis of urachal remnants. J Urol 1988; 140:1534–1535.

Gottesman JE: Coccidioidomycosis of prostate and epididymis with urethrocutaneous fistula. Urology 1974; 4:311–314.

Graybill JR: Systemic fungal infections. Diagnosis and treatment. Infect Dis Clin North Am 1988; 2:805–825.

Graybill JR, Galgiani JN, Jorgensen JH, Strandberg DA: Ketoconazole therapy for fungal urinary tract infections. J Urol 1983; 129:68–70.

Gregory MC, Schumann GB, Schumann JL, Argyle JC: The clinical significance of candidal casts. Am J Kidney Dis 1984; 4:179–184.

Gustafson TL, Schaffner W, Lavely GB, et al: Invasive aspergillosis in renal transplant recipients: Correlation with corticosteroid therapy. J Infect Dis 1983; 148:230–238.

Hall KA, Copeland JG, Zukoski CF, et al: Markers of coccidioidomycosis before cardiac or renal transplantation and risk of recurrent infection. Transplantation 1993; 55:1422–1442.

Hall WJ: Study of antibody coated fungi in patients with funguria and suspected disseminated fungal infections in fungal pyelonephritis. J R Soc Med 1980; 73:567–569.

Halpern M, Szabo S, Hochberg E, et al: Renal aspergilloma: An unusual cause of infection in a patient with the acquired immunodeficiency syndrome. Am J Med 1992; 92:437–440.

Hamadeh R, Ardehali A, Locksley RM, York MK: Fatal aspergillosis associated with smoking contaminated marijuana in a marrow transplant patient. Chest 1988; 94:432–433.

Hamory BH, Wenzel RP: Hospital associated candiduria: Predisposing factors and review of the literature. J Urol 1978; 120:444–448.

Harbach LB, Burkholder GV, Goodwin WE: Renal candidiasis. A case of anuria. Br J Urol 1970; 42:258–264.

Harder EJ, Hermans PE: Treatment of fungal infections with flucytosine. Arch Intern Med 1975; 135:231–237.

Harold DL, Koff SA, Kass EJ: Candida albicans "fungus ball" in bladder. Urology 1977; 9:662–663.

Haupt HM, Merz WG, Beschorner WE, et al: Colonization and infection with *Trichosporon* species in the immunosuppressed host. J Infect Dis 1983; 147: 199–203.

Hawkins SS, Gregory DW, Alford RH: Progressive disseminated histoplasmosis: Favorable response to ketoconazole. Ann Intern Med 1981; 95:446–449.

Hellman RN, Hinrichs J, Sicard G, et al: Cryptococcal pyelonephritis and disseminated cryptococcosis in a renal transplant patient. Arch Intern Med 1981; 141:128–130.

Henochowicz S, Sanovic E, Pistole M, et al: Histoplasmosis diagnosed on peripheral blood smear from a patient with AIDS. JAMA 1985; 253:3148.

High KP, Quagliarello VJ: Yeast perinephric abscess: Report of a case and review. Clin Infect Dis 1992; 15:128–133.

Hinchey WW, Someren A: Cryptococcal prostatitis. Am J Clin Pathol 1981; 75:257–260.

Hopfer RL: Mycology of *Candida* infections. *In* Bodey GP, Fainstein V, eds: Candidiasis. New York, Raven Press, 1985, pp 1–12.

Hopwood V, Evans E, Carney J: Rapid diagnosis of vaginal candidosis by latex particle agglutination. J Clin Pathol 1985; 38:455–458.

Hughes CE, Harris C, Peterson LR, Gerding DN: Enhancement of the in-vitro activity of amphotericin B against *Aspergillus* spp. by tetracycline analogs. Antimicrob Agents Chemother 1984; 26:837–840.

Humayun H, Maliwan N: Emphysematous genital infection caused by *Candida albicans*. J Urol 1982; 128:1049–1050.

Hurley R, Winner HL: Experimental renal moniliasis in the mouse. J Pathol Bacteriol 1963; 86:75–82.

Huyn MT, Reyes CV: Prostatic cryptococcosis. Urology 1982; 20:622–623.

Inoshita T, Youngberg GA, Boelen LJ, Langston J: Blastomycosis presenting with prostatic involvement: Report of 2 cases and review of the literature. J Urol 1983; 130:160–162.

Irby PB, Stoller ML, McAninch JW: Fungal bezoars of the upper urinary tract. J Urol 1990; 143:447–451.

Itraconazole. The Medical Letter, January 22, 1993; 35:7–9.

Iwen PC, Kelly DM, Reed EC, Hinrichs SH: Invasive infection due to *Candida krusei* in immunocompromised patients not treated with fluconazole. Clin Infect Dis 1995; 20:342–347.

Jacobs LG, Skidmore EA, Cardoso LA, Ziv F: Bladder irrigation with amphotericin B for treatment of fungal urinary tract infections. Clin Infect Dis 1994; 18:313–318.

James CL, Lomax-Smith JD: Cryptococcal epididymoorchitis complicating steroid therapy for relapsing polychondritis. Pathology 1991; 23:256–258.

Jani AN, Casibang V, Mufarrij WA: Disseminated actinomycosis presenting as a testicular mass: A case report. J Urol 1990; 143:1012–1014.

Jinadu BA, Welch G, Talbot R, et al: Update: Coccidioidomycosis—California, 1991–1993. MMWR Morb Mortal Wkly Rep 1994; 43:421–423.

Johnson JR, Ireton RC, Lipsky BA: Emphysematous pyelonephritis caused by *Candida albicans*. J Urol 1986; 135:80–82.

Kan VL: Polymerase chain reaction for the diagnosis of candidemia. J Infect Dis 1993; 168:779–783.

Kassamali H, Anaissie E, Ro J, et al: Disseminated *Geotrichum candidum* infection. J Clin Microbiol 1987; 25:1782–1783.

Kauffman CA, Slama TG, Wheat LJ: *Histoplasma capsulatum* epididymitis. J Urol 1981; 125:434–435.

Kauffman CA, Tan JS: *Torulopsis glabrata* renal infection. Am J Med 1974; 57:217–224.

Keane PF, McKenna M, Johnston SR: Fungal bezoar causing ureteric obstruction. Br J Urol 1993; 72:247–248.

Khauli RB, Kalash S, Young JD Jr: *Torulopsis glabrata* perinephric abscess. J Urol 1983; 130:968–970.

King C, Finley R, Chapman SW: Prostatic cryptococcal infection. Ann Intern Med 1990; 113:720.

Klein BS, Vergeront JM, Weeks RJ, et al: Isolation of *Blastomyces dermatitidis* in soil associated with a large outbreak of blastomycosis in Wisconsin. N Engl J Med 1986; 314:529–534.

Klein JJ, Watanakunakorn C: Hospital acquired fungemia: Its natural course and clinical significance. Am J Med 1979; 67:51–58.

Kocak T, Tunc M, Karaman MI, et al: *Candida albicans* infection in solitary kidney presenting as anuria. Br J Urol 1991; 68:550.

Komshian SV, Uwaydah AK, Sobel JD, Crane LR: Fungemia caused by candidal species and *Torulopsis glabrata* in the hospitalized patient: Frequency, characteristics and evaluation of factors influencing outcome. Rev Infect Dis 1989; 11:379–390.

Kovacs JA, Kovacs AA, Polis M, et al: Cryptococcosis in the acquired immunodeficiency syndrome. Ann Intern Med 1985; 103:533–538.

Kozinn PJ, Taschdjian CL, Goldberg PK, et al: Advances in the diagnosis of renal candidiasis. J Urol 1978; 119:184–187.

Krcmery V, Trupl J, Kridl J, Danisovicova A: Renal abscess and fungemia due to *Torulopsis glabrata*: Successful treatment with drainage and fluconazole. Clin Infect Dis 1994; 18:116.

Krieger JN: Vaginitis. Current concepts of etiology, diagnosis and treatment. AUA Update Series 1983; 2(35, Part I):2–7.

Kumar B, Talwar P, Kaur S: Penile tinea. Mycopathologia 1981; 75:169–172.

Kuntze JR, Herman MH, Evans SG: Genitourinary coccidioidomycosis. J Urol 1988; 140:370–374.

Langston C, Roberts DA, Porter GA, Bennett WM: Renal phycomycosis. J Urol 1973; 109:941–944.

Larsen RA, Bozzette S, McCutchan A, et al: Persistent *Cryptococcus neoformans* infection of the prostate after successful treatment of meningitis. Ann Intern Med 1989; 111:125–128.

Lee BE, Feinberg M, Abraham JJ, Murthy ARK: Congenital malformations in an infant born to a woman treated with fluconazole. Pediatr Infect Dis J 1992; 12:1062–1064.

Lehner T: Systemic candidiasis and renal involvement. Lancet 1964; 1:1414–1416.

Leiter E, Whitehead ED, Desai SB: Fungus balls in renal pelvis. N Y State J Med 1982; 82:64–66.

Lentino JR, Zielinski A, Stachowski M, et al: Prostatic abscess due to *Candida albicans*. J Infect Dis 1984; 149:282.

Levine LA, Doyle CJ: Retroperitoneal actinomycosis: A case report and review of the literature. J Urol 1988; 140:367–369.

Lief M, Sarfarazi F: Prostatic cryptococcosis in acquired immune deficiency syndrome. Urology 1986; 28:318–319.

Louria DB, Stiff DP, Bennet B: Disseminated moniliasis in the adult. Medicine (Baltimore) 1962; 41:307–337.

Low AI, Tulloch AGS, England EJ: Phycomycosis of the kidney associated with transient immune defect and treated with clotrimazole. J Urol 1974; 111:732–734.

Luno MA, Tortoledo ME: Histologic identification and pathological patterns of disease due to *Candida*. *In* Bodey GP, Fainstein V, eds: Candidiasis. New York, Raven Press, 1985, p 13.

Lye WC, Lee EJC, Tung KH, Sinniah R: Bilateral ureteric strictures secondary to candidiasis. Br J Urol 1991; 67:551–552.

Macfarlane DJ, Tucker JG, Kemp RJ: Treatment of recalcitrant actinomycosis with ciprofloxacin. J Infect 1993; 27:177–180.

Makar AP, Michielsen JP, Boeckx GJ, Van Marck EA: Primary actinomycosis of the urinary bladder. Br J Urol 1992; 70:205–206.

Malin JM Jr, Anderson EE, Weber CH: North American blastomycosis of the urogenital tract. J Urol 1969; 102:754–757.

Mamo GJ, Rivero MA, Jacobs SC: Cryptococcal prostatic abscess associated with the acquired immunodeficiency syndrome. J Urol 1992; 148:889–890.

Marans HY, Mandell W, Kislak JW, et al: Prostatic abscess due to *Histoplasma capsulatum* in the acquired immunodeficiency syndrome. J Urol 1991; 145:1275–1276.

Marzec A, Heron LG, Pritchard RC, et al: *Paecilomyces variotti* in peritoneal dialysate. J Clin Microb 1993; 31:2392–2395.

McGinnis MR, Ajello L, Beneke ES, et al: Taxonomic and nomenclature evaluation of the genera *Candida* and *Torulopsis*. J Clin Microbiol 1984; 20:813–814.

Medoff G: Controversial areas in antifungal chemotherapy short course and antibiotic therapy with amphotericin B. Rev Infect Dis 1987; 9:403–407.

Medoff G, Kobayashi GS: Strategies in the treatment of systemic fungal infections. N Engl J Med 1980; 302:145–155.

Melchior J, Mebust WK, Valk WL: Ureteral colic from a fungus ball: Unusual presentation of systemic aspergillosis. J Urol 1972; 108:698–699.

Meunier-Carpentier F, Kiehn TE, Armstrong D: Fungemia in the immunocompromised host. Changing patterns, antigenemia, high mortality. Am J Med 1981; 71:363–370.

Meyer R, Axelrod JL: Fatal aplastic anemia resulting from flucytosine. JAMA 1974; 228:1573.

Minkowitz S, Koffler D, Zak FG: *Torulopsis glabrata* septicemia. Am J Med 1963; 34:252–255.

Mitwalli A, Malik GH, Al-Wakeel J, et al: Mucormycosis of the graft in a renal transplant patient. Nephrol Dial Transplant 1994; 9:718–720.

Morrison VA, Haake RJ, Weisdorf DJ: The spectrum of non-*Candida* fungal infections following bone marrow transplantation. Medicine (Baltimore) 1993; 72:78–89.

Moulder MK: Thrush of the urinary bladder: Case report. J Urol 1948; 59:420–426.

Mucormycosis. (Editorial.) Lancet 1986; 2:1362–1363.

Muncan P, Wise GJ: Comparison of fluconazole and bladder irrigations with ampB in patients with candiduria. (Abstract 773.) J Urol 1995; 153:422A.

Muncan P, Wise GJ: Early detection of candiduria in high risk patients by polymerase chain reaction. (Abstract 774.) J Urol 1996; 156:154–156.

Nassoura Z, Ivatury RR, Simon RJ, et al: Candiduria as an early marker of disseminated infection in critically ill surgical patients: The role of fluconazole therapy. J Trauma 1993; 35:290–294.

Ness MJ, Vaughan WP, Woods GL: *Candida* antigen latex test for detection of invasive candidiasis in immunocompromised patients. J Infect Dis 1989; 159:495–502.

Noe HN, Tonkin ILD: Renal candidiasis in the neonate. J Urol 1982; 127:517–519.

Odds FC: Candidiasis of the urinary tract. *In* FC Odds, ed: *Candida* and Candidosis. London, Bailliere Tindall, 1988.

Odds FC, Webster CE, Mayuranathan P, Simmons PD: *Candida* concentrations in the vagina and their association with signs and symptoms of vaginal candidosis. J Med Vet Mycol 1988; 26:277–283.

Oral fluconazole for vaginal candidiasis. The Medical Letter, September 16, 1994; 36:81

Orr WA, Mulholland SG, Walzak MP Jr: Genitourinary tract involvement with systemic mycosis. J Urol 1972; 107:1047–1050.

Pappas PG, Threlkeld MG, Besole GD, et al: Blastomycosis in immunocompromised patients. Medicine (Baltimore) 1993; 72:311–325.

Patel BJ, Moskowitz H, Hashmat A: Unilateral renal actinomycosis. Urology 1983; 21:172–174.

Paya CV: Fungal infections in solid-organ transplantation. Clin Infect Dis 1993; 16:677–688.

Peppas DS, Moul J, McLeod DG: *Candida albicans* corpora abscess following penile prosthesis placement. J Urol 1988; 140: 1541–1542.

Perfect JR, Seaworth BA: Penile cryptococcosis with review of mycotic infections of penis. Urology 1985; 25: 528–531.

Petersen EA, Friedman BA, Crowder ED, Rifkind D: Coccidioidouria: Clinical significance. Ann Intern Med 1976; 85:34–38.

Piketty C, George F, Weiss L, et al: Renal aspergilloma in AIDS. Am J Med 1993; 94:557–558.

Pluemecke G, Williams J, Elliott D, Paul LC: Renal transplant artery rupture secondary to *Candida* infection. Nephron 1992; 61:98–101.

Preminger B, Gerard PS, Lutwick L, et al: Histoplasmosis of the penis. J Urol 1993; 149:848–850.

Price MJ, Lewis EL, Carmalt JE: Coccidioidomycosis of prostate gland. Urology 1982; 19:653–655.

Prout GR Jr, Goddard AR: Renal mucormycosis. Survival after nephrectomy and amphotericin B therapy. N Engl J Med 1960; 263:1246–1248.

Ralph ED, Barber KR, Grant CWM: Liposomal amphotericin B: An effective nontoxic preparation for the treatment of urinary tract infections caused by *Candida albicans*. Am J Nephrol 1991; 11:118–122.

Randall RE Jr, Stacy WK, Toone EC, et al: Cryptococcal pyelonephritis. N Engl J Med 1968; 279:60–65.

Rashid A-MH, Williams RM, Parry D, Malone PR: Actinomycosis associated with pilonidal sinus of the penis. J Urol 1992; 148:405–406.

Ravi R, Mallikarjuna VS, Chaturvedi HK: Rhinosporidiosis mimicking penile malignancy. Urol Int 1992; 49:224–226.

Reddy LV, Kumar A, Kurup VP: Specific amplification of *Aspergilla fumigatus* DNA by polymerase chain reaction. Mol Cell Probes 1993; 7:121–126.

Rex JH, Bennet JE, Sugar AM, et al: A randomized trial comparing fluconazole with amphotericin B for the treatment of candidemia in patients without neutropenia. N Engl J Med 1994; 331:1325–1330.

Rippon JW: A new era in antimycotic agents. Arch Dermatol 1986; 122:399–402.

Rippon JW: Medical Mycology: The Pathogenic Fungi and the Pathogenic Actinomycetes, 3rd ed. Philadelphia, WB Saunders, 1988.

Robinson PJ, Pocock RD, Frank JD: The management of obstructive renal candidiasis in the neonate. Br J Urol 1987; 59:380–382.

Robson AM, Craver RD: Curvularia urinary tract infection. A case report. Pediatr Nephrol 1994; 8:83–84.

Rohner TJ Jr, Tuliszewski RM: Fungal cystitis: Awareness, diagnosis and treatment. J Urol 1980; 124:142–144.

Rubin H, Furcolow ML, Yates JL, Brasher CA: The course and prognosis of histoplasmosis. Am J Med 1959; 27:278–288.

Sales JL, Mundy HB: Renal candidiasis: Diagnosis and management. Can J Surg 1973; 16:139–143.

Salyer WR, Salyer DC: Involvement of the kidney and prostate in cryptococcosis. J Urol 1973; 109:695–698.

Sande MA, Mandell GL: Antimicrobial agents: Antifungal and antiviral agents. *In* Gilman AG, Goodman LS, Rall TW, Murad F, eds: The Pharmacologic Basis of Therapeutics, 7th ed. New York, Macmillan, 1985, pp 1219–1239.

Sandin KJ, Light JK, Holzman M, Donovan WH: *Candida* pyelonephritis complicating traumatic C5 quadriplegia: Diagnosis and management. Arch Phys Med Rehabil 1991; 72:243–246.

Sane SY, Deshmukh SS: Total renal infarct and perirenal abscess caused by phycomycosis. J Postgrad Med 1988; 34:44B–47B.

Sanford JP: The enigma of candiduria: Evolution of bladder irrigation with amphotericin B for management—From anecdote to dogma and a lesson from Machiavelli. Clin Infect Dis 1993; 16:145–147.

Santos J, Espigado P, Romero C, et al: Isolated renal mucormycosis in two AIDS patients. Eur J Clin Microbiol Infect Dis 1994; 13:430–432.

Sarosdy MF, Brock WA, Parsons CL: Scrotal actinomycosis. J Urol 1979; 121:256–257.

Sasidharan K, Subramonian P, Moni VN, et al: Urethral rhinosporidiosis: Analysis of 27 cases. Br J Urol 1987; 59:66–69.

Scerpella EG, Alhalel R: An unusual cause of acute renal failure: Bilateral ureteral obstruction due to *Candida tropicalis* fungus balls. Clin Infect Dis 1994; 18:440–442.

Schonebeck J: Fungal infections of the urinary tract. *In* Walsh PC, Gittes RP, Perlmutter AD, Stamey TA, eds: Campbell's Urology, 5th ed. Philadelphia, W. B. Saunders, 1986, pp 1025–1036.

Schonebeck J, Segerbrand E: *Candida albicans* septicaemia during first half of pregnancy successfully treated with 5-fluorocytosine. Br Med J 1973; 4:337–338.

Schroter GPJ, Bakshandeh K, Husberg BS, Weil R III: Coccidioidomycosis and renal transplantation. Transplantation 1977; 23:485–489.

Schulkind ML, Ayoub EM: Transfer factor and its clinical application. Adv Pediatr 1980; 27:89–115.

Schwartz DA: Organ-specific variation in the morphology of the fungomas (fungus balls) of *Pseudallescheria boydii*: Development within necrotic host tissue. Arch Pathol Lab Med 1989; 113:476–480.

Scott RA, Gallis HA, Livengood CH: Phycomycosis of the vulva. Am J Obstet Gynecol 1985; 153:675–676.

Scully RE, Mark EJ, McNeely WF, McNeely BU: Case records of the Massachusetts General Hospital. Weekly clinicopathological exercise. N Engl J Med 1987; 317:946–953.

Scully RE, Mark EJ, McNeely WF, McNeely BU: Case records of the Massachusetts General Hospital. Weekly clinicopathological exercise. N Engl J Med 1988; 319:629–640.

Scully RE, Mark EJ, McNeely WF, McNeely BU: Case records of the Massachusetts General Hospital. Weekly clinicopathological exercise. N Engl J Med 1993; 329:264–269.

Seidenfeld SM, Cooper BH, Smith JW, et al: Amphotericin B tolerance: A characteristic of *Candida parapsilosis* not shared by other *Candida* species. J Infect Dis 1983; 147:116–119.

Seidenfeld SM, LeMaistre CF, Setiawan H, Munford RS: Emphysematous pyelonephritis caused by *Candida tropicalis*. J Infect Dis 1982; 146:569.

Selman SH, Hampel N: Systemic sporotrichosis: Diagnosis through biopsy of epididymal mass. Urology 1982; 20:620–621.

Shah B, Taylor HC, Pillay I, et al: Adrenal insufficiency due to cryptococcosis. JAMA 1986; 256:3247–3249.

Sharkey-Mathis PK, Kauffman CA, Graybill JR: Treatment of sporotrichosis with itraconazole. Am J Med 1993; 95:279–285.

Sheaff M, Ahsan A, Badenoch D, Baithun S: A rare cause of epididymo-orchitis. Br J Urol 1995; 75:250–251.

Shelp WD, Wen SF, Weinstein AB: Ureteropelvic obstruction caused by *Candida* pyelitis in homotransplanted kidney. Arch Intern Med 1966; 117:401–404.

Sherwood JA, Dansky AS: *Paecilomyces* pyelonephritis complicating nephrolithiasis and review of *Paecilomyces* infections. J Urol 1983; 130:526–528.

Sheynkin YR, Wise GJ: Fungal infections of the perivesical space. J Urol 1995; 153:722–724.

Short KL, Harty JI, Amin M, Short LF: The use of ketoconazole to treat systemic blastomycosis presenting as acute epididymitis. J Urol 1983; 129:382–384.

Sills M, Schwartz A, Weg JG: Conjugal histoplasmosis: A consequence of progressive dissemination in the index case after steroid therapy. Ann Intern Med 1973; 79:221–224.

Siminovitch JMP, Herman GP: *Torulopsis glabrata* fungal cystitis. Urology 1984; 24:343–344.

Singh CR, Lytle WF Jr: Cystitis emphysematosa caused by *Candida albicans*. J Urol 1983; 130:1171–1173.

Smith SR, Galloway MJ, Reilly JT, Davies TJ: Amiloride prevents amphotericin B related hypokalemia in neutropenic patients. J Clin Pathol 1988; 41:494–497.

Sobel JD: Recurrent vulvovaginal candidiasis. A prospective study of the efficacy of maintenance ketoconazole therapy. N Engl J Med 1986; 315:1455–1458.

Solomkin JS, Flohr A, Simmons RL: *Candida* infections in surgical patients. Dose requirements and toxicity of amphotericin B. Ann Surg 1982; 195:177–185.

Sonda LP, Amendola MA: *Candida* pyocalix: Unusual complication of prolonged nephrostomy drainage. J Urol 1985; 134:722–724.

Stamm AM, Diasio RB, Dismukes WE, et al: Toxicity of amphotericin B plus flucytosine in 104 patients with cryptococcal meningitis. Am J Med 1987; 83:236–242.

Stein M, Laor E, Tolia BM, Reid RE: Unusual case of renal *Candida* fungus balls. Urology 1993; 41:49–51.

Stone J, Manasse R: Pseudoepidemic of urinary tract infections due to *Trichosporon beigelii*. Infect Control Hosp Epidemiol 1989; 10:312–315.

Sugar AM, Restrepo A, Stevens DA: Paracoccidioidomycosis in the immunosuppressed host: Report of a case and review of the literature. Am Rev Respir Dis 1984; 129:340–342.

Suits T, Wise GJ, Walters B: Candidal antigenemia. A prognostic determinant. J Urol 1989; 141:1381–1384.

Sung JP, Sun SSY, Crutchlow PF: Coccidioidomycosis of the prostate gland and its therapy. J Urol 1979; 121:127–128.

Superdock KR, Dummer JS, Koch MO, et al: Disseminated histoplasmosis presenting as urinary tract obstruction in a renal transplant unit. Am J Kidney Dis 1994; 23:600–604.

Swartz DA, Harrington P, Wilcox R: Candidal epididymitis treated with ketoconazole. N Engl J Med 1988; 319:1485.

Takeuchi H, Tomoyoshi T: *Torulopsis* infection extensively involving the urinary tract. Urology 1983; 22:173–175.

Tan TQ, Ogden AK, Tillman J, et al: *Paecilomyces lilacinus* catheter-related fungemia in an immunocompromised pediatric patient. J Clin Microb 1992; 30:2479–2483.

Thompson NP, Stoker DL, Springall RG: Urachal abscess as a complication of tinea corporis. Br J Urol 1994; 73:319.

Thompson WC, Brock JW: *Torulopsis glabrata* perinephric abscess: A case report. J Urol 1983; 130:529–530.

Trenk D, Brett W, Jähnchen E, Birnbaum D: Time course of cyclosporin/itraconazole interaction. (Letter.) Lancet 1987; 2:1335–1336.

Urinary tract candidosis. Lancet 1988; 2:1000.

Vapnek JM, McAninch JW: AIDS and the urologist. Infect Urol 1990; 3:101–107.

Vartivarian SE, Anaissie EJ, Bodey GP: Emerging fungal pathogens in immunocompromised patients: Classification, diagnosis, and management. Clin Infect Dis 1993; 17(Suppl 2):S487–S491.

Vesa J, Bielsa O, Arango O, et al: Massive renal infarction due to mucormycosis in an AIDS patient. Infection 1992; 20:234–236.

Wainstein MA, Graham RC Jr, Resnick MI: Predisposing factors of systemic fungal infections of the genitourinary tract. J Urol 1995; 154:160–163.

Walsh TJ: Recent advances in the treatment of systemic fungal infections. Methods Find Exp Clin Pharmacol 1987; 9:769–778.

Walsh TJ, Hathorn JW, Sobel JD, et al: Detection of circulating *Candida* enolase by immunoassay in patients with cancer and invasive candidiasis. N Engl J Med 1991; 324:1026–1031.

Walterspiel JN, Kaplan SL, Fishman I, Scott FB: Fungal infections associated with artificial urethral sphincters in children. J Urol 1986; 135:1245–1246.

Warshawsky AB, Keiller D, Gittes RF: Bilateral renal aspergillosis. J Urol 1975; 113:8–11.

Weingärtner K, Elsebach K, Bittinger A, et al: Paraurethral actinomycosis. Urol Int 1992; 49:179–180.

Wheat LJ, Connolly-Stringfield BS, Blair R, et al: Effect of successful treatment with amphotericin B on *Histoplasma capsulatum* variety capsulatum polysaccharide antigen levels in patients with AIDS and histoplasmosis. Am J Med 1992; 92:153–160.

Wheat LJ, Kohler RB, Tewari RP: Diagnosis of disseminated histoplasmosis by detection of *Histoplasma capsulatum* antigen in serum and urine specimens. N Engl J Med 1986; 314:83–88.

Whittaker RH: New concepts of kingdoms of organisms. Science 1969; 163:150–160.

Wiebe VJ, Degregorio MW: Liposome-encapsulated amphotericin B: A promising new treatment for disseminated fungal infections. Rev Infect Dis 1988; 10:1097–1101.

Wiesenfeld HC, Berg SR, Sweet RL: *Torulopsis glabrata* pelvic infection and fungemia. Obstet Gynecol 1994; 83:887–889.

Wilson DA, Muchmore KG, Tisdal RG, et al: Histoplasmosis of the adrenal glands studied by CT. Radiology 1984; 150:779–783.

Wipf MD, Scriven RR, Stewart SC: Coccidioidomycosis of the prostate: First case report of dissemination of disease after transurethral resection of prostate. (Abstract 666.) Presented at the American Urological Association Annual Meeting, Las Vegas, April 1983.

Wise GJ: Fungi in the genitourinary system. AUA Update Series 1984a; 3:1–7.

Wise GJ: Ureteral stent in management of fungal pyonephrosis due to *Torulopsis glabrata*. Urology 1984b; 24:128–129.

Wise GJ: Genitourinary candidal infection. AUA Update Series 1989; 8:194–200.

Wise GJ: Amphotericin B in urological practice. J Urol 1990; 144:215–223.

Wise GJ, Goldberg PE, Kozinn PJ: Do the imidazoles have a role in the management of genitourinary fungal infections? J Urol 1985; 133:61–64.

Wise GJ, Goldman WM, Goldberg PE, Rothenberg R: Miconazole: A cost-effective antifungal genitourinary irrigant. J Urol 1987; 138:1413–1415.

Wise GJ, Kozinn PJ, Goldberg PE: Flucytosine in the management of genitourinary candidiasis. Five years of experience. J Urol 1980; 124:70–72.

Wise GJ, Kozinn PJ, Goldberg PE: Amphotericin B as a urologic irrigant in the management of non-invasive candiduria. J Urol 1982; 128:82–84.

Wise GJ, Silver DA: Fungal infections of the genitourinary system. J Urol 1993; 149:1377–1388.

Wong SY, Allen DM: Transmission of disseminated histoplasmosis via cadaveric renal transplantation: Case report. Clin Infect Dis 1992; 14:232–234.

Wong-Beringer A, Jacobs RA, Guglielmo BJ: Treatment of funguria. JAMA 1992; 267:2780–2785.

Yinnon AM, Woodin KA, Powell KR: *Candida lusitaniae* infection in the newborn: Case report and review of the literature. Pediatr Infect Dis J 1992; 11:878–880.

Young RC, Bennett JE, Vogel CL, et al: Aspergillosis. The spectrum of disease in 98 patients. Medicine 1970; 49:147–173.

Yu HHY, Yim CM, Leong CH: Primary actinomycosis of kidney presenting with reno-colic fistula. Br J Urol 1978; 50:40.

Yu S, Provet J: Prostatic abscess due to *Candida tropicalis* in a nonacquired immunodeficiency syndrome patient. J Urol 1992; 148:1536–1538.

Zincke H, Furlow WL, Farrow GM: *Candida albicans* cystitis: Report of a case with special emphasis on diagnosis and treatment. J Urol 1973; 109:612–614.

24
GENITOURINARY TUBERCULOSIS

James G. Gow, M.D., Ch.M., F.R.C.S.

Since the mid-1970s, there has been a profound, if gradual, change in the manner in which genitourinary tuberculosis is managed. This change mirrors the approach taken by many disciplines in medicine. The ideology of optimism has given way to the ideology of concern, as the feeling that the future will always be better than the past has not been realized; yet is it not very rare for any future that is to span 20 years to be predictable? When it is considered that tuberculosis precedes recorded history, the results obtained in the modern treatment of all manifestations of the disease have been one of the outstanding achievements of this generation. Nevertheless, the concern is justified, because it is an undeniable fact that tuberculosis is increasing and that a reassessment of the current management is urgently required.

HISTORY

The disease known as consumption has been observed in humans for as long as 7000 years (Myers, 1952). The remains of ancient skeletons show the characteristic changes of tuberculosis, indicating that the disease affected humans about 4000 B.C., and it is known that it was a common disease in Egypt about 1000 B.C. (Morse et al, 1964). In 375 B.C., Hippocrates described phthisis, a lingering disease that becomes worse in winter, results in emaciation, and causes diarrhea in its terminal phase (Jenkins and Wolinsky, 1965). Galen, in A.D. 180, had considerable interest in consumption, and his methods of treatment were followed for the next 1500 years. In 1696, Wiseman wrote that "scrofula or the Kings-Evil was a difficult problem that confronted physicians and surgeons daily."

During the 1700s in Europe, tuberculosis infections reached epidemic proportions, and almost one fourth of the deaths in England at that time were caused by consumption (Colby, 1954; Flick, 1925). The infectious nature of the disease was established by Villemin, who showed in experiments carried out between 1865 and 1868 that tuberculosis could be transferred from humans or cattle to rabbits. In 1879, Cohnheim presented his elimination theory. According to his hypothesis, tubercle bacilli in the blood were eliminated in the urine, so that they lodged in a focus somewhere in the urinary tract. In March 1882, Koch announced that he had discovered the cause of tuberculosis; 3 weeks later, he published his first article, describing the pathogenesis of the disease and outlining Koch's postulates, which since have become the basis for studies of all infectious diseases. He had observed the organism in cases of the disease, he had grown the organism outside the body, and he had reproduced the disease in a susceptible host.

In 1885, Nocard isolated the avian form of the tubercle bacillus; in 1889, Smith described the bovine variety. The acid-fast nature of the bacillus was discovered by Ehrlich in 1882. Thirty years after Cohnheim's hypothesis, Ekehorn (1908) proposed his direct hematogenous theory, which suggested that the bacilli were transported like emboli to the renal capillaries, where they lodged and formed a tuberculous focus. According to his theory, the remainder of the kidney and the rest of the urinary tract were secondarily infected through the urine. This theory was accepted and formed the basis of the belief that tuberculosis could be treated by nephrectomy.

The pathogenesis of renal tuberculosis remained obscure until Medlar (1926) published his classic studies on 30 patients who had died from pulmonary tuberculosis, none of whom had any clinical evidence of genitourinary disease. He reviewed 100,000 serial sections from the kidneys of these patients. Microscopic lesions were found in these kidneys, almost all in the cortex and almost all bilateral. It was Medlar and associates (1949) who suggested that these pathologic changes should be termed *metastatic* rather than "secondary," because it was clear that the kidneys had become infected through the blood stream.

The next milestone was reached in 1935, when Coulaud succeeded in inducing primary tuberculous lesions in the renal cortex of rabbits; 2 years later, Wildbolz (1937), using the term *genitourinary tuberculosis*, emphasized that renal and epididymal tuberculosis did not constitute separate diseases but were local manifestations of the same blood-borne infection.

The greatest historical event was the discovery of the antituberculosis drugs, starting with streptomycin in 1943, followed by para-aminosalicylic acid in 1946, isoniazid in 1952, and rifampicin in 1966. These have been followed by the introduction of short-term courses of chemotherapy for all manifestations of the disease.

INCIDENCE

The incidence of new cases of tuberculosis is a good index of the progress of the disease. Although it does not reflect all the human suffering or the number of cases that require treatment, it reveals the trend of the problem and gives some idea of the effect of control measures. To be of value, any statistics must include a high proportion of all new cases, which can be detected only in countries with an efficient antituberculosis organization. Therefore, there will always be differences between reports from developed and developing countries. In the latter, the incidence is many times higher, a trend that has quickened since the advent of chemotherapy. Moreover, in developed countries, all forms of tuberculosis have tended to infect the older age groups, whereas in many developing countries the disease has continued to affect adolescents and young adults.

The World Health Organization has estimated that throughout the world there are 10 million new cases of all forms of tuberculosis each year, mostly in developing countries, where it continues to be a major problem. It is estimated that from 8 to 10 million people develop overt tuberculosis annually and 3 million die (Koch, 1991). In developed countries, the annual decline is about 12%, whereas in developing countries the decline has hardly been noticed (World Health Organization, 1981). Table 24–1

Table 24–1. INCIDENCE OF TUBERCULOSIS

Year	Total Number of Newly Notified, Previously Untreated Patients	Number With Genitourinary Disease
1983	3002	134
1988	2163	84
1993	2458	64

shows the reduction in the notification of all cases of pulmonary tuberculosis and genitourinary tuberculosis from 1983 to 1993 in Great Britain. Although the incidence of pulmonary tuberculosis has declined in the United Kingdom during the last two decades, that of nonpulmonary tuberculosis, apart from genitourinary tuberculosis, has remained static. Worldwide, the genitourinary form of the disease accounts for only 14% of the nonpulmonary manifestations, and only 20% of cases occur in the white population (Lane, 1982).

The consistently steady decline of the genitourinary manifestation of tuberculosis is almost certainly a result of effective chemotherapeutic treatment of the primary pulmonary focus. Nevertheless, new cases are always being seen, and urologists must be aware of the possible diagnosis. Compared with the incidence of 13 per 100,000 population in the United States and the United Kingdom, in some developing countries the incidence can be as high as 400 per 100,000 inhabitants (Lowell, 1976), a daunting prospect when it is realized that one patient with sputum-positive tuberculosis can affect as many as 30 other people, some of whom will undoubtedly develop the renal manifestation. The disease will continue to be a serious problem while so many cases remain undiagnosed and untreated. It is also significant for the urologist that, whereas in developed countries only 8% to 10% of patients with pulmonary tuberculosis develop renal tuberculosis, as many as 15% to 20% of patients in the underdeveloped countries are found with *Mycobacterium tuberculosis* in the urine (Freedman, 1979).

Although much more is known today about the incidence and treatment of tuberculosis, the ultimate goal of complete eradication remains in the distant future or until the identification of infected cases becomes more effective. Even in developed countries, it is estimated that it will take more than 30 years for the disease to be completely eradicated because of a small number of indigenous cases in remote areas and a few more that develop in the immigrant population. Figure 24–1 shows the expected deaths from tuberculosis by region.

EPIDEMIOLOGY

There is now general agreement that the annual tuberculosis infection rate is the best single indicator for evaluating the problem of tuberculosis and its trend in developed and developing countries and that it is an index expressing the importance of tuberculosis within the community (Styblo, 1980, 1989).

In developed countries, there is reliable evidence that (1) the incidence of tuberculosis has been falling since the turn of the century; (2) under present conditions, irrespective of any treatment, it is diminishing at the rate of 5% per annum; and (3) this decrease in infection rate is exponential (Sutherland, 1976). This means that under present conditions of human resistance and environment, the tubercule bacillus eventually will be eradicated (provided that the present balance against it is maintained), although eradication may take many decades.

The situation changes if the impact of modern chemotherapy is added to the natural regression rate. Although it is difficult to estimate the impact of chemotherapy on the overall tuberculosis situation, a conservative estimate is that case finding and treatment have accelerated the decrease in the incidence by about 7.8% annually. This percentage, when added to the yearly 5% natural decrease, results in a total fall in the risk of infection by more than 12% per annum, which will ultimately lead to a complete eradication. However, this goal may take longer than anticipated, because of the increase in resistant strains of organisms and the impact of the human immunodeficiency virus (HIV).

In developing countries, the situation is very different. In Lesotho and Uganda (World Health Organization, 1969) and

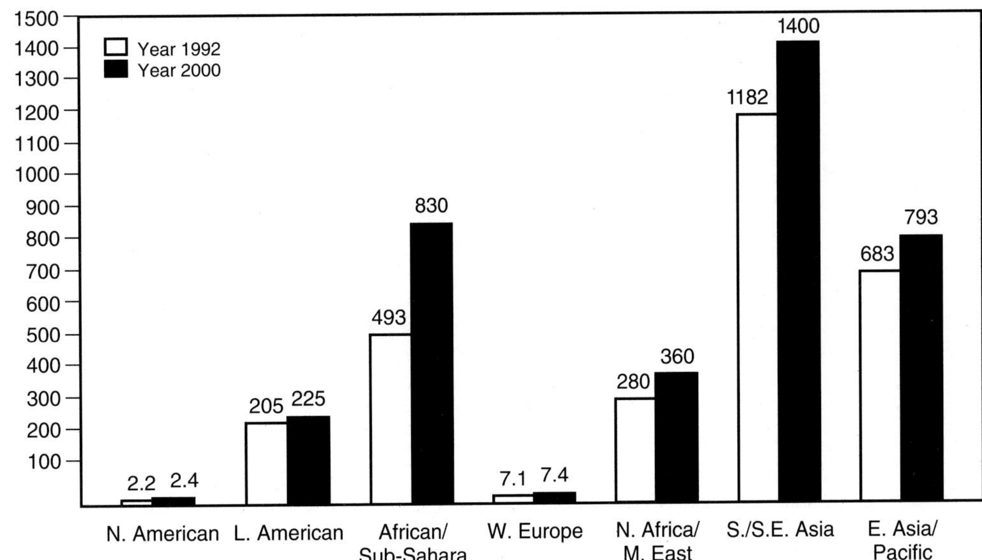

Figure 24–1. Deaths from tuberculosis per thousand: by region.

in Algeria and Tunis (Sutherland et al, 1971), there was little downward trend during a period of 10 years. The risk of infection remained at about 2.6%; this figure reflected a gradually increasing number of future cases. The disease, therefore, remains a major problem, because there is no tendency for self-elimination. It is estimated, accepting an annual risk of infection of 3%, that 26% of the population in these countries is infected by the age of 10 years and 45% by the age of 20 years. Between 2 and 3 million people die of tuberculosis in these countries each year.

It is a salutatory exercise to estimate the results if, in such countries, the annual infection rate could be decreased by 5%. If that were to happen, there would be a reduction of the risk of infection from 3% in 1980 to 0.7% in 2010 and an increase in the proportion of unaffected population from 55% to 68% (Styblo, 1980). An annual decrease of 14% would halve the incidence of tuberculosis in 5 years.

The two basic methods for planning efficient tuberculosis control are (1) bacille Calmette-Guérin (BCG) inoculation and (2) case finding and treatment. In developed countries, mass BCG vaccination is no longer important and has largely been discontinued, because economic considerations and complications are considered to outweigh any possible benefits, especially inasmuch as case finding and treatment have reached such a high degree of efficiency. The few cases that occur can be treated by the highly effective short-course regimens available. Furthermore, the vaccine does not protect the older population from the disease, and this is the main source of infection in the community.

In developing countries, BCG immunization may play a major part in the control of the disease if it can be effectively organized; for it to be efficient, the vaccination must be given soon after birth.

Case finding remains the major weakness of any antituberculosis program, and it is calculated that only one third of smear-positive cases are diagnosed (Farga, 1972). Also, any improvement will be difficult in the foreseeable future for reasons of population dispersal, poor transport, inadequate medical facilities, insufficient laboratories, poor socioeconomic conditions, chronic malnutrition, and the attitudes toward disease that vary from country to country. It is vital for the eventual control of the disease that this problem be tackled energetically, because, as noted previously, a single smear-positive patient can infect up to 30 additional persons. In the developing world, the necessary services are still totally inadequate, and economic facilities are just as much a problem as medical resources.

With modern short-course chemotherapy, treatment results are bound to be successful, provided the organisms are sensitive to the common antituberculosis drugs, and an improvement in the identification of smear-positive cases from 30% to 50% will make a considerable impact on the overall worldwide tuberculosis problem. With the use of effective drugs currently available, the rate at which patients can be rendered almost noninfectious is dramatic, because the organisms in the sputum of most patients with pulmonary disease are reduced to about one thousandth in 2 to 3 weeks. In patients with renal tuberculosis, it is almost impossible to isolate *M. tuberculosis* from the urine after 2 weeks of chemotherapy, so that at the end of this time they can be considered noninfectious. "Find, isolate, treat, and educate" should be the slogan that motivates all workers who are tackling the problem of tuberculosis in the developing countries, but the problems are formidable.

IMMUNOLOGY

The Immune Response

The development of any infectious disease depends on the reaction between the invasive properties of the pathogen and the immune response of the host. The immunologic response associated with an invading pathogen consists of recognition, responses, and reaction (Grange, 1980). The immune system consists of two main classes of lymphocytes, the T cells and the B cells. The T cells do not produce antibodies but synthesize lymphokines, which make macrophages more aggressive to the invading parasite. The B cells, however, develop into plasma cells, which rapidly produce antibodies. The two classes of cells are complementary, and both are essential for the rapid elimination of bacteria. However, these two factors vary in importance in response to different bacteria; in the case of *M. tuberculosis*, it is the cell-mediated response that is most important. The human immune response to infection by the tubercle bacillus is very effective; only about 5% of infected persons develop clinical, primary disease, and a further 5% develop postprimary disease later in life.

Bacille Calmette-Guérin

At a time when effective antibiotic therapy for tuberculosis is taken for granted, it is salutary to remember that the discovery of prophylactic measures against many infections (a more logical approach) antedated the discovery of powerful drugs by about 200 years. Early attempts to induce immunity against tuberculosis with tuberculin and various vaccines failed. It was not until Calmette and Guérin (1925) discovered the method of attenuating the virulence of *M. tuberculosis* by repeated subculture, eventually obtaining a permanently avirulent strain they called BCG, that any success was achieved. This vaccine, which has been given since its development in 1925, has a low but definite complication rate.

The degree of protection is variable, from 80% among urban schoolchildren in the United Kingdom and North American Indians to nil among schoolchildren in Georgia (United States) and in the southern Indian general population (Ten Dam et al, 1976). The reason for this variation is unknown.

It has been suggested that BCG acts not by preventing infection but by limiting the multiplication and spread of *M. tuberculosis*. Stanford and associates (1981) proposed that two different acquired mechanisms of cell-mediated response to mycobacteria exist, one of which confers good host protection and one of which does not. Early contact with environmental mycobacteria primes the host to respond in one of these two ways, the choice being determined by the species of *Mycobacterium* to which the host is first exposed. Once the host is primed, the pattern of response is established for life, and subsequent BCG vaccination merely boosts the established response. If the initial mycobacteria are those that prime the host with the less effective of the two mechanisms, the BCG confers little or no benefit. This hypothesis helps to explain the geographic variations of the efficacy of BCG. It is therefore essential that BCG preparations that activate macrophage-activating T lymphocytes be used.

Despite the variation of the response, the procedure is relatively safe and inexpensive. It is recommended that every effort be made to pursue the school vaccination program so that all tuberculin-negative children at the age of 11 or 12 years in developed countries can be inoculated with the appropriate BCG. In developing countries, the vaccine should be given as soon as possible after birth; otherwise, many children will die before the age of 13 years (Ten Dam and Hitze, 1980). If the subsequent level of tuberculin positivity is low, many workers recommend revaccination a few years later. However, there is a worldwide variation, and each region should carry out studies to identify the optimal time for vaccination.

The use of BCG remains controversial. In the first place, protection lasts for only 15 years. Second, a proportion of subjects in any age group will have been previously infected, and BCG cannot affect these individuals. Third, there is a chance of complications, including lymphadenitis, lupus vulgaris, and "BCG-itis." Fourth, the vaccine cannot influence the incidence of infection. It may not be able to protect against tuberculosis in older individuals, the main source of infection in the community (Fine, 1989). Fifth, it cannot be given in large quantities, because it can provoke severe allergic reaction. Because of these inconsistencies, some developed countries have already stopped mass BCG vaccination and have taken the view that the complications outweigh any possible benefits. However, this view is considered unwise, because epidemics of tuberculosis do occur and are not merely diseases of immigrants, chronic bronchitics, and alcoholics. The most recent epidemic was reported by Hill and Stevenson (1983), who published the details of an epidemic of 41 new tuberculous patients, only 7 of whom had been vaccinated with BCG.

Can BCG be improved? There is no absolute difference between avirulent environmental mycobacteria and virulent tubercle bacilli, and the protective antigens of mycobacteria are to be found among those common to all mycobacteria (Stanford and Grange, 1974). Therefore, it is illogical to develop vaccines for tubercle bacilli that are live, and the ideal vaccine could be a suspension of dead bacilli of a harmless environmental species. Such a species is *Mycobacteria vaccae*, which may prove a worthy successor to be given with, or instead of, BCG (Stanford and Grange, 1993).

Human Immunodeficiency Virus Infection and Tuberculosis

In many parts of the world, the epidemic of HIV infection has been blamed for the recent increase in tuberculosis, because these increases have occurred among groups in which the acquired immunodeficiency syndrome (AIDS) is common (Rieder et al, 1989).

Studies in New York showed that among patients with both tuberculosis and AIDS, almost two thirds had developed tuberculosis within 6 months of their diagnosis of AIDS. HIV infection is a cofactor with one of the highest risk ratios for the development of tuberculosis in people already infected with *M. tuberculosis* (Centers for Disease Control, 1987). Bloch and Snider (1990) reported that 2.6% of patients with AIDS in their survey had extrapulmonary tuberculosis.

It is recommended that all people infected with HIV should be tuberculin tested so that those who react to tuberculin can be offered treatment. It is also recommended that all people who contract tuberculosis should be offered HIV testing.

There is evidence that despite small differences, the underlying immunopathology of mycobacterial disease and other diseases, including HIV, is very similar (Grange et al, 1994). Immunotherapy for tuberculosis may also protect the individual from HIV. Preliminary observations of patients with HIV-related tuberculosis who received immunotherapy with *M. vaccae* are encouraging and suggest that such treatment benefits both diseases and may have global applications for future treatment (Grange and Stanford, 1994).

MYCOBACTERIA

In morphology, mycobacteria vary considerably from short cells to long filaments, which under certain conditions can show branching. The mycobacterium is 2.4 μm long and 0.2 to 0.5 μm wide. The mycobacterial cell has a thick wall that is separated from the cell membrane by a translucent zone. The organism has no true capsule or flagellum and is nonmotile and pathogenic. The cell wall itself is a complex structure composed of four layers. The innermost layer consists of murein (peptidoglycan), as in other bacteria, whereas the outer three layers are composed of ropelike complexes of peptides, polysaccharides, and lipids set in a homogenous matrix. The lipids account for 40% to 50% of the weight of the bacterium.

Tuberculous Mycobacteria

M. tuberculosis is the most virulent and infective of all mycobacteria, although the precise nature of this high virulence remains unknown (Barksdale and Kim, 1977). The cytoplasm of the mycobacterium does not differ essentially from that of other bacteria. *M. tuberculosis* is strictly aerobic and can multiply in air alveoli, whereas *Mycobacterium bovis* is partially anaerobic, a property that is used to help differentiate between the two. For example, *M. tuberculosis* will grow on the surface of an egg-enriched medium, whereas *M. bovis* is usually seen a few millimeters below the surface. It grows only within a restricted range of temperature, the optimum being 35°C, and on culture the first colonies are seen after 3 to 4 weeks. *M. bovis* is a much more important organism in underdeveloped countries because there is no pasteurization of milk.

Mycobacteria differ from other organisms in that they show different responses to antibiotic treatment. There are certain factors that may explain some of the difference. In the first place, mycobacteria are extremely slow growing. *Escherichia coli* and other common pathogens double in number every 20 minutes, whereas *M. tuberculosis* divides only once every 20 to 24 hours. Most antibiotics work only when the metabolic machinery is functioning, which means that the organisms are susceptible only when they are dividing; as long as they are not dividing, the metabolism does not become blocked by the antibiotic, and the mycobacteria survive in its presence.

The second factor that distinguishes the tuberculous infection from, for example, an *E. coli* infection is that there is effective cooperation between the antibiotic and the phagocytes in the latter case. Such organisms as *E. coli*, whose division may have been slowed or stopped, can be phagocytized. Once it is inside the cell, oxidative and lysosomal enzymes usually kill the phagocytized organism. This is not so in the case of *M. tuberculosis*, because that organism is resistant to the various intracellular killing mechanisms, certainly early in the infection before cellular immunity is fully developed. Therefore, *M. tuberculosis*, once it has been phagocytized, can survive and even travel around in the phagocytic cell. It is interesting that despite the lack of any significant humoral antibody response, phagocytes manage to ingest *M. tuberculosis*, possibly owing to the affinity between the waxy coat and the cell membrane lipids.

It is probably true that the concentration of most antibiotics is substantially lower inside phagocytes, and the intracellular pH may not favor some antibacterial drugs, because most are effective only at a particular pH. It is this population of *M. tuberculosis* that is susceptible to pyrazinamide, which enters phagocytes and is most active at a pH of 5.5 (see later section).

Another factor peculiar to *Mycobacteria* is that a proportion of the organisms (termed *persistors*) are able to become dormant and remain in tissues for a long time, even a lifetime, without dividing, and these are not susceptible to any antibiotic action. The nature of the mycobacteria that persist during apparently adequate chemotherapy or in the interval between infection and reactivation of disease remains a mystery, but they are important, because reactivation of the disease can occur many years after the original infection (Grange, 1991).

Finally, there is the well-known fact that *M. tuberculosis* is much more prone than most bacteria to developing resistance, especially if antibiotics are given singly.

Nontuberculous Mycobacteria

During the early 1950s, after it had become routine practice to culture *M. tuberculosis*, it was realized that other mycobacteria were important pathogens for humans, and a new concept about mycobacterial infection was reached. These organisms became known as nontuberculous mycobacteria (Wolinsky, 1979).

Mycobacteria are classified into two groups: human pathogens and human nonpathogens (Table 24–2). The organisms produce lesions similar to those of *M. tuberculosis*, but usually of lower virulence.

Nontuberculous mycobacteria rarely cause pathogenic changes in the genitourinary system. Only five cases of renal disease have been reported since 1956, two caused by *Mycobacterium kansasii* (Woods et al, 1956) and three by *Mycobacterium avium-intracellulare* (Pergament et al, 1974). Three cases of epididymitis have been recorded, all resulting from *Mycobacterium xenopi* (Hepper et al, 1971). One case of granulomatous prostatitis, caused by a combination of *M. kansasii* and *Mycobacterium fortuitum*, also has been reported (Lee et al, 1977).

Table 24–2. CLASSIFICATION OF MYCOBACTERIA

Human Pathogens	Human Nonpathogens
Mammalian tubercle bacilli (tuberculous complex)	Slow-growing
M. tuberculosis	*M. gordonae*
M. bovis (including BCG strain)	*M. gastri*
M. africanum	*M. terrae* complex
M. leprae	*M. flavescens*
Slow-growing potential pathogens	Rapid-growing
M. avium-intracellulare	*M. smegmatis*
M. scrofulaceum	*M. vaccae*
M. kansasii	*M. parafortuitum* complex
M. ulcerans	
M. marinum	
M. xenopi	
M. szulgai	
M. simiae	
Rapid-growing potential pathogen	
M. fortuitum complex	

BCG, bacille Calmette-Gúerin.

The principles of treatment, entailing intensive multidrug regimens, are the same as those for *M. tuberculosis* disease. However, because nontuberculous mycobacteria are often resistant to one or more of the first-line drugs, it is important to obtain an early, complete spectrum of drug sensitivities. Even so, treatment poses problems. There are many documented cases in which nontuberculous mycobacteria have been found in urine, none of which have caused any disease. Nevertheless, if sensitive organisms are found, it is prudent to give a 3- or 4-month intensive course of antituberculosis chemotherapy.

It is in these cases that combined treatment with *M. vaccae* and chemotherapy might be beneficial in the future.

PATHOGENESIS

To assess the progress of any tuberculous infection, it is important to differentiate between patients who have had no prior exposure to *M. tuberculosis* and those who have previously been infected. The former manifestation is called a primary focus or primary disease, and in this type of infection the mycobacterium lodges within the macrophage. At this stage, the macrophages have no capacity for controlling the disease. The organisms therefore multiply, but only at a slow rate because of their inherent capacity; hence, the condition resulting from the infection may require several weeks to become manifest. After the *M. tuberculosis* organisms have multiplied sufficiently, an inflammatory reaction occurs. In spite of this reaction, there is still little resistance to the multiplication of the bacteria, and rapid spread occurs, first by way of the lymphatics and then through the blood stream. Within about 4 weeks, however, the rate of multiplication decreases and the dissemination ceases. At this stage, two immunologic manifestations occur: (1) the individual shows evidence of delayed hypersensitivity, and (2) the macrophages acquire the ability to inhibit the multiplication of virulent *M. tuberculosis* (acquired cellular immunity).

PRIMARY AND SECONDARY TUBERCULOSIS

The difference between primary and secondary tuberculosis depends on the multiplication and spread of the infection (i.e., before the development of delayed hypersensitivity). Although the term *reactivation* is used for chronic tuberculosis, in some cases it is likely that dormant bacilli, through changed circumstances, begin to multiply and produce recurrence of the disease. Among these changed circumstances are debilitating disease, trauma, corticosteroid administration, immunosuppressive therapy, diabetes, and anemia. Genitourinary tuberculosis is caused by metastatic spread of organisms through the blood stream. Therefore, it produces the appearance of secondary tuberculosis, which can occur either by reactivation of old infection or by reinfection from an active case.

The initial lesion is characterized by destruction resulting from the inflammatory reaction that is caused by retained hypersensitivity. The disease is very slow to progress; if it does, it extends as necrosis of adjacent tissue develops, which, again, is caused by hypersensitive inflammation. Necrosis is the outstanding feature of renal tuberculosis, and the destruction it causes makes control of the disease more difficult. However, because the antituberculosis drugs enter renal cavities, there is no delay in the response to treatment.

PATHOLOGY

Tuberculosis of the Kidney

Renal tuberculosis is a secondary manifestation and is caused by a blood-borne metastatic organism; there is already a hypersensitive reaction produced by the previous primary infection in the lungs. The previous infection may have occurred many years before, after the inhalation of droplets of exhaled infected bronchial secretions. Most of these metastatic lesions heal, because the bacteremia is not intense. After a person has been infected, however, live *M. tuberculosis* organisms can be harbored anywhere in the body and can become reactivated if the appropriate circumstances occur.

If the organisms reach the kidney, they settle in the blood vessels, usually those close to the glomeruli, and cause microscopic foci that have the classic features of secondary tuberculosis. Polymorphonuclear leucocytes disappear early from the lesion. Macrophages appear, and a low-grade inflammatory reaction continues. Next, granulomas form. These consist of a central Langhans' giant cell surrounded by lymphocytes and fibroblasts. Because some immunity will have developed, the microscopic appearances are those of a more chronic lesion. Lymphocyte infiltration increases; macrophages appear in large numbers, many being transformed to epithelioid cells and others mediating the destruction of the phagocytized bacilli. The further course of the infection depends on the infecting dose, the virulence of the organism, and the resistance of the host. If the bacterial multiplication is checked, tubercles are replaced by fibrous tissue, but if they continue to multiply, they form further tubercles that coalesce and produce a central area of caseous necrosis. The factor that determines virulence in strains of *M. tuberculosis* is not known.

The healing process starts with the formation of reticula around the lesions, which eventually mature into fibrous tissue. Later, calcium salts are deposited, producing the classic calcified lesion, which is clearly visible on urography. In the kidney, these lesions eventually slough into parts of the collecting system and produce tuberculous bacilluria. They may go on increasing in size until they reach a papilla, which is invaded and destroyed. With further progress, a calyx is ulcerated, causing the typical ulcerocavernous lesion. The cavities usually are not large, and it is rare to see extensive cavitative destruction of renal tissue.

If the defense mechanisms of the body are powerful enough to control the infection, fibrous tissue reaction occurs. This causes strictures in the calyceal stem or at the pelviureteral junction. As a result, chronic abscesses form in the parenchymatous tissue and are always larger than urographic appearances suggest. Once a calyceal stem becomes stenosed, it is extremely rare for communication to be restored. Very occasionally, one moiety of a duplex kidney is involved. In every case in the author's experience, the disease has remained confined to the moiety originally infected; if surgery is required, it is never necessary to remove the whole kidney.

Renal Calcification

Calcification is becoming a growing hazard in renal tuberculosis. The incidence of calcification is slowly increasing, and its presence is assuming more importance in the management of renal tuberculosis (Antonio and Gow, 1975).

Between the early 1950s and 1964, 24% of patients had calcification somewhere in the renal tract (Gow, 1965), whereas in a survey taken between 1975 and 1988, 60% of patients showed some form of renal calcification. Marszalak and Dhai (1982), however, reported calcification in only 20% of 95 patients seen in their series between 1977 and 1980. The cause remains obscure, and there is no evidence to support different pathogeneses for tuberculous calcification and for discrete renal calculi. Occasionally, precipitating factors that are known to be associated with calculous disease, such as prolonged recumbency, high calcium intake, recurrent urinary tract infection, obstructive uropathy, and hypercalciuria, are found, but there is no common denominator. Twenty-eight percent of all large areas of calcification that were excised in one study had viable *M. tuberculosis* in the calcified matrix (Wong and Lan, 1980).

In the management of this complication, the aim should be to retain as much functioning renal tissue as possible. Small lesions can be kept under review on an annual basis and can continue to be managed conservatively, provided that there is no increase in size. This review should continue for 10 years or longer, because a sudden increase in size may occur that requires surgical intervention. However, most small calcified lesions remain unchanged for more than 20 years.

Larger areas of calcification (Fig. 24–2) should be excised,

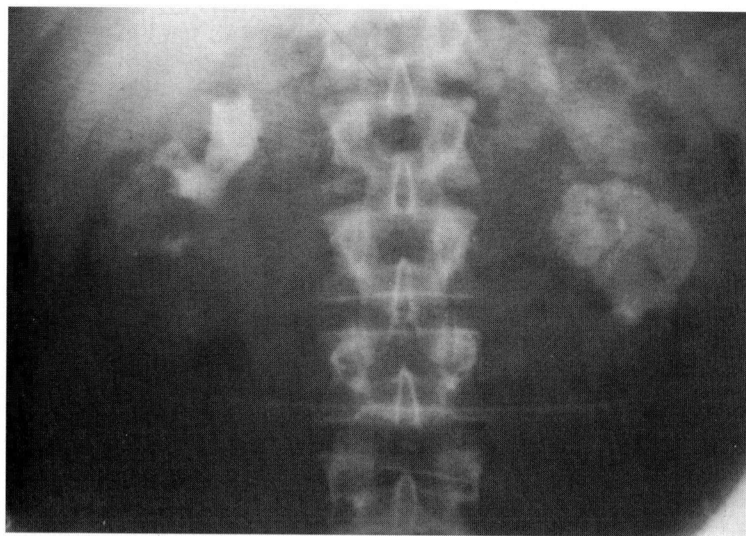

Figure 24–2. Moderate calcification in a tuberculous kidney.

and nonfunctioning kidneys with extensive calcification (Fig. 24–3) should be removed. Calcification or calculi occurring after completion of chemotherapeutic treatment should be managed in the same way as any other uncomplicated calcification in the renal tract.

Hypertension and Renal Tuberculosis

Many renal diseases have been associated with hypertension since Goldblatt and co-workers (1934) showed that obstruction of the renal artery of one kidney produced this disease. All of these associated renal diseases have one common factor, the reduction in the blood supply to part or the whole of the kidney. Because this is also a universal pathologic change in renal tuberculosis, it may be thought that the two conditions would be associated much more commonly than they are. Nesbit and Ratliff (1940) reported the first case of hypertension associated with renal tuberculosis that was cured by nephrectomy. An account of a study by Smith followed this in 1956. Since then, there have been many studies of different groups of patients with genitourinary tuberculosis. Braasch and co-workers (1940) reported a twofold increased incidence of hypertension in patients with severe renal tuberculosis, when compared with the incidence in all patients. These figures were confirmed by Flechner and Gow (1980). Hsiung and co-workers (1965) reported that of 30 patients treated by nephrectomy, 25 were greatly improved, but the long-term follow-up studies were inadequate. Schwartz and Lattimer (1967), however, reported that only 1 of 20 hypertensive patients showed any improvement in blood pressure.

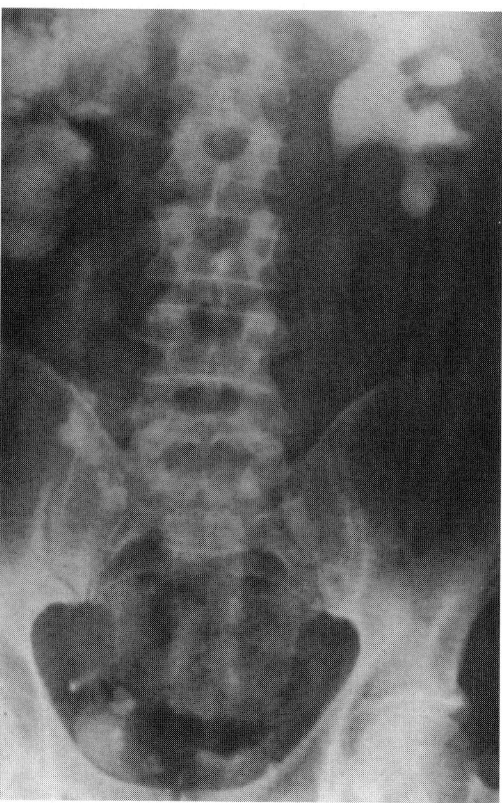

Figure 24–3. Extensive calcification. Note the quiescent disease in the right kidney and the calcification in the seminal vesicles.

In the series quoted by Flechner and Gow (1980), 64.7% of patients with unilateral nonfunctioning or poorly functioning kidneys had a fall in blood pressure after nephrectomy. These figures are consistent with those of Marks and Poutasse (1973) and Hsiung and associates (1965), so it is apparent that two thirds of patients with extensive unilateral tuberculous nephropathy achieve a substantial fall in blood pressure after nephrectomy. The results in this special group are far better than the rate of 25% that is generally accepted as the standard for hypertensive patients with other unilateral nephropathies. To what degree the extent of the disease is responsible can be predicted by the selective measurement of renal vein renin in unilateral tuberculous kidneys. This may be an important investigation before proceeding to nephrectomy in the doubtful case, because many patients with genitourinary tuberculosis have hypertension that is unrelated to the tuberculous disease. These patients should have medical treatment for the hypertension, combined with antituberculosis chemotherapy.

A review of recent cases of genitourinary tuberculosis in the author's series has shown that hypertension is now rarely seen except in patients in whom there is extensive destruction of renal tissue. There is no change in the suggested management of this complication.

Tuberculosis of the Ureter

Tuberculous ureteritis is always an extension of the disease from the kidney. Its effects are variable. The site most commonly affected is the ureterovesical junction. This is invariably secondary to extensive disease of the kidney and, if not recognized early, can rapidly cause complete destruction. The disease is seen only rarely in the middle third of the ureter. Very occasionally, the whole of the ureter is involved. In such patients, the kidney shows extensive disease, is often nonfunctioning, and is calcified (Fig. 24–4*A*). Nephroureterectomy is the only possible treatment.

Tuberculosis of the Bladder

Bladder lesions are without exception secondary to renal tuberculosis. The earliest forms of infection start around one or another ureteric orifice, which becomes red, inflamed, and edematous (see Fig. 24–4*B*). As the area of mild inflammation progresses, bullous granulations appear and may completely obscure the ureteric orifice (see Fig. 24–4*C*); if a retrograde pyelogram is required, endoscopic resection of these granulations is required for identification of the ureteric orifice.

Tuberculous ulcers may be present, but they are rare and are a late finding. They are irregular in outline and superficial, with a central, inflamed area usually surrounded by raised granulations. Initially, they are in close proximity to the ureteric orifices, but as the disease progresses they can appear in any part of the bladder (see Fig. 24–4*D*). Patchy cystitis with granulations on the fundus or the base is a late development. If the disease continues to progress, the inflammation spreads deep into the muscle, which is eventually replaced by fibrous tissue. This fibrosis starts around the ureteric orifice, which contracts and can either produce a stricture or become withdrawn, rigid, and dilated, assuming the classic golf-hole appearance (see Fig. 24–4*E, F*). These ureters are usually rigid in the lower third and always give rise to ureteric reflux. With modern chemotherapy, this is now a rare occurrence. Healed mucosal lesions have a stellate appearance that is caused by bands of fibrous tissue meeting at a central point, usually the site of the initial area of severe infection (see Fig. 24–4*G*).

Occasionally, the whole of the bladder is covered by angry, inflamed, velvety granulations with ulceration. If the disease reaches this stage, it is unlikely that, even with modern chemotherapy, there will be sufficient recovery of the bladder to ensure an adequate capacity with reasonable function (see Fig. 24–4*H*).

Tubercles are very infrequent, but if seen they are close to the ureteric orifices. Isolated tubercles that are visible away from the normal ureteric orifices must be assumed not to be caused by *M. tuberculosis* and are likely to be malignant; biopsy is essential in these patients.

In very extensive disease involving the ureter, bladder, and seminal vesicles, fistulas into the rectum are a rare complication (Patoir et al, 1969). Disease of this severity is now found only in developing countries where patients are neglected.

Tuberculosis of the Testis

Tuberculosis of the testis is almost always secondary to infection of the epididymis, which in most cases is bloodborne because of the extensive blood supply of the epididymis, particularly the globus minor (Macmillan, 1954). Tuberculous orchitis with no epididymal involvement is a very rare presentation. It is impossible to differentiate such a swelling from a tumor, and early exploration is therefore required if rapid response to antituberculosis chemotherapy does not occur.

Eleven percent of patients have a renal lesion at autopsy, which confirms the evidence of a direct hematogenous infection of these organs (Riehle and Jayavaman, 1982).

If the orchitis is secondary to a tuberculous epididymitis, the testicular lesion rapidly responds to chemotherapy after the epididymis has been removed, provided the destruction of testicular tissue is not extensive.

Tuberculosis of the Epididymis

Although for many years the route of infection of the epididymis was a source of controversy, it is now accepted that all the tuberculous foci in the epididymis are caused by metastatic spread of organisms through the blood stream. The disease usually starts in the globus minor, because it has a greater blood supply than other parts of the epididymis (Macmillan, 1954). Retrovasal migration of organisms may occur in acute epididymitis after prostatectomy, but abnormalities in the posterior urethra and extensive destructive lesions in tuberculous prostatitis are rarely seen. Furthermore, in a series of prostatic biopsies carried out by the author in 20 patients with proven tuberculous epididymitis, the author found only 1 patient with evidence of tuberculous infection. Although this evidence is not conclusive, because it is acknowledged that only small pieces of prostate were examined, it suggests that if the disease had been substantial enough to produce a tuberculous epididymitis, more than 1 of 20 patients would have been diseased.

Tuberculous epididymitis also may be associated with renal disease, but this is by no means universal. The renal focus is often microscopic, with the intravenous urogram appearing normal, and therefore only a small number of tubercle bacilli are excreted. Because of this, the chances of any organisms migrating up the vas deferens are remote. If this were a common route of infection, tuberculous epididymitis would be a frequent concomitant to severe tuberculous cystitis, in which *M. tuberculosis* organisms are constantly present in the urine, but in fact it is a rare occurrence.

Finally, tuberculous epididymitis may be the first and only presenting symptom of genitourinary tuberculosis, in cases in which an intravenous urogram shows a normal ureter and upper urinary tract and *M. tuberculosis* cannot be isolated from the urine. The diagnosis is made by culture of *M. tuberculosis* from a discharging sinus or after epididymectomy.

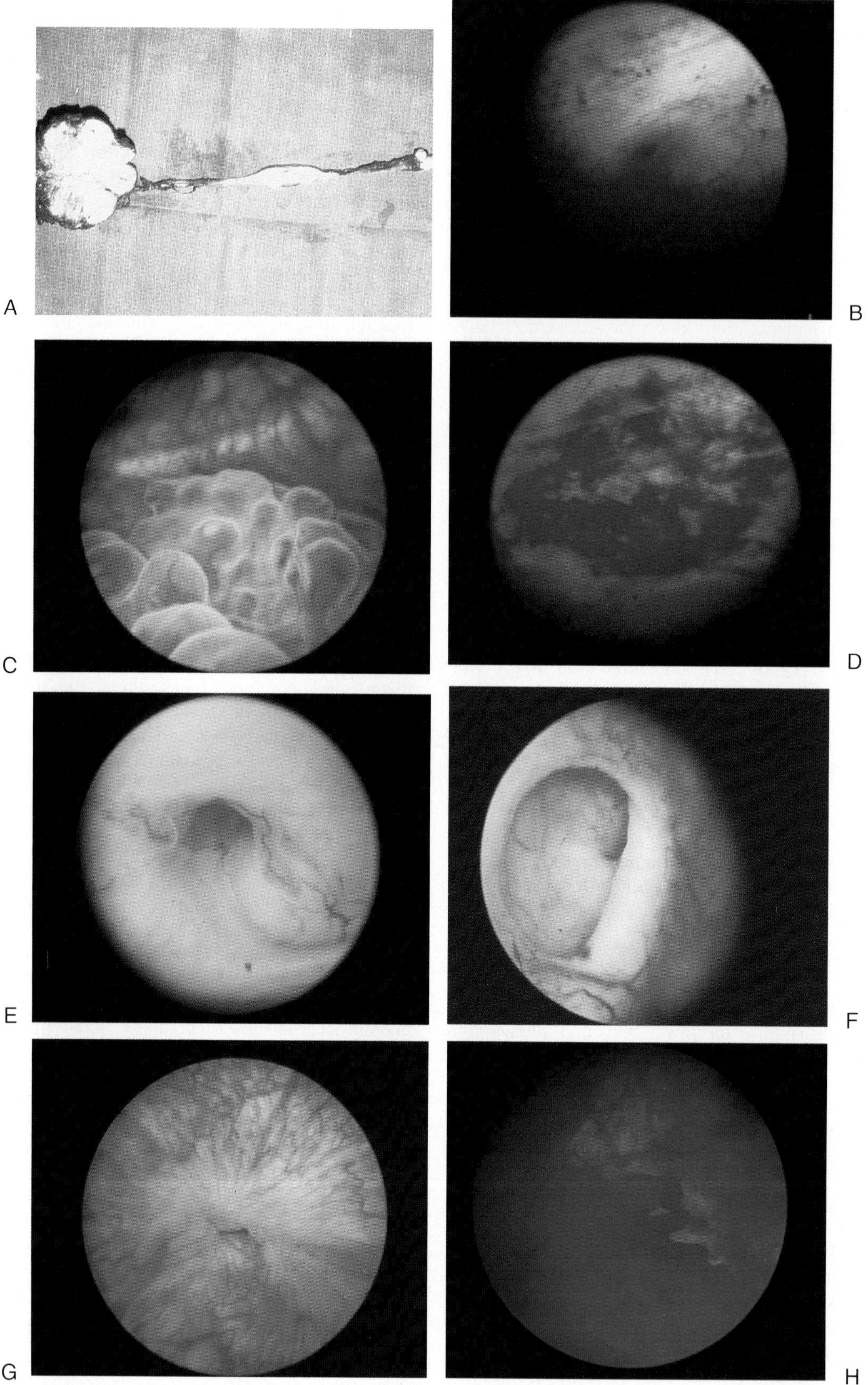

Figure 24–4. *A,* Extensive tuberculosis of the kidney and ureter with calcification and stricture formation. *B,* Acutely inflamed ureteric orifice. *C,* Tuberculous bullous granulations. *D,* Acute tuberculous ulcer. *E,* Tuberculous golf-hole ureter. *F,* Tuberculous golf-hole ureter, severely withdrawn. *G,* Healed tuberculous lesion. *H,* Acute tuberculous cystitis with ulceration.

As with other forms of tuberculosis, epididymitis is decreasing in incidence in the developed world but is still endemic in many other regions. The disease usually develops in young, sexually active males, and in 70% of patients there is a previous history of tuberculosis.

The usual presentation is a painful, inflamed scrotal swelling. The globus minor alone is affected in 40% of cases. In extensive disease, there may be generalized epididymal induration with beading of the palpable vas and even involvement of the testis, but this is now rare. In an earlier series (Ross et al, 1961) lesions were bilateral in 34% of cases, but today this presentation is unusual.

External injury causing severe tissue damage may reactivate a dormant or persisting organism in a previously unidentified tuberculous focus so that it produces a focus of active disease (Kretschmer, 1928). The presentation of tuberculous epididymitis and a history of trauma with a previous history of tuberculosis may have medicolegal importance. The author has seen two cases of tuberculous epididymitis occurring after scrotal trauma, one 32 years and the other 35 years after tuberculosis of the spine had been treated in infancy.

The management of tuberculous epididymitis may pose problems if *M. tuberculosis* bacteria cannot be isolated from the urine. In the acute phase, the inflammatory reaction involves the testis, so it is difficult to differentiate the lesion from acute epididymo-orchitis.

Occasionally, a discharging sinus may be found posteriorly. If there is no sinus and the *M. tuberculosis* organisms are absent from the urine, the disease should be observed during treatment with an appropriate antibiotic, such as co-trimoxazole. If no improvement occurs after 2 to 3 weeks, antituberculosis chemotherapy must be started. After an additional 3 weeks, if the lesion becomes nodular, firm, and painless, exploration of the testis is mandatory without delay; two patients presenting with seminoma in conjunction with tuberculosis have been reported (Gow, 1957, 1963).

Tuberculosis of the tunica vaginalis with no disease in the epididymis or testis rarely may present with the finding of multiple nodules on palpation (Kato, 1970).

Tuberculosis of the Prostate

Tuberculosis of the prostate is rare, and in many cases it is diagnosed by the pathologist or is found incidentally after a transurethral resection. Very rarely, in acute fulminating cases, the disease spreads rapidly, and cavitation may lead to a perineal sinus (Sporer and Auerback, 1978).

The route of infection is through the hematogenous spread of organisms, as in infection of the kidney. There is no evidence that infection is caused by continuous contact with urine from a kidney with active disease. Advanced lesions that destroy tissue can cause a reduction in the volume of semen, a sign that may help in diagnosis (Lattimer and Wechsler, 1978). On palpation, the gland is nodular, hardly ever tender, and rarely enlarged. Soft areas are extremely uncommon. After the diagnosis is confirmed, the patient should receive a full course of chemotherapy.

Genital Tuberculosis

The transmission of genital tuberculosis from male to female is very rare; Lattimer and co-workers (1954) could find only eight reports in the literature. This is surprising, because many men with genital tuberculosis have *M. tuberculosis* in the semen. More recently (Sutherland et al, 1982), a study was made of the husbands of 229 women with proven tuberculosis of the genital tract. Sixteen husbands had a past history of various types of tuberculosis. Urologic examination was performed on 128 husbands, and active genitourinary tuberculosis was found in 3.9%. As in these cases, the diagnosis of disease in the male may be made only after the lesion has appeared in the female partner. The lesions respond rapidly to chemotherapy.

Although this form of the disease is unlikely to be seen in the developed world, it does appear in developing countries. A painful, swollen inguinal gland in a woman, if it is proven to be tuberculous, should alert the clinician to a possible diagnosis of genital tuberculosis in the male partner.

Tuberculosis of the Penis

Tuberculosis of the penis is a very rare manifestation of the disease. By 1971, only 139 cases had been reported in the literature (Lal et al, 1971). Many years ago, it was not uncommonly seen as a complication of ritual circumcision, when it was the usual practice for the operators, many of whom had open pulmonary tuberculosis, to suck the circumcised penis (Lewis, 1946). Today, tuberculosis of the penis always occurs in adults and is primary or secondary, depending on the presence or absence of pulmonary tuberculosis.

Primary tuberculosis of the penis occurs after coital contact with organisms already present in the female genital tract or by contamination from infected clothing (Agarwalla et al, 1980; Narayana et al, 1976). In a rare instance, the penile lesion may be caused by reinoculation from the male partner through an infected ejaculate. Secondary penile tuberculosis occurs as a secondary manifestation of active pulmonary tuberculosis.

In most cases, the lesion appears as a superficial ulcer of the glans. Clinically, it is indistinguishable from malignant disease, although it can also progress to cause a tubercular cavernositis with involvement of the urethra (Veukataramaiah et al, 1982). Rarely, the lesion occurs as a solid nodule (Baskin and Mee, 1989) or as a cavernositis with ulceration (Ramesh and Vasanthi, 1989). The diagnosis is confirmed by biopsy. All lesions rapidly respond to antituberculosis chemotherapy.

Tuberculosis of the Urethra

Tuberculosis of the urethra is very rare. Symes and Blandy (1973) quoted only 16 cases from the literature. It is caused by spread from another focus in the genital tract. Its rarity is difficult to understand in view of the almost constant exposure of the urethra to infected urine. The presentation can be either acute or chronic. In the acute phase, there is a urethral discharge with involvement of the epididymis, prostate, and other parts of the renal tract. This diagnosis is not difficult, because organisms are always isolated. The initial treatment is intensive chemotherapy.

In the chronic condition, diagnosis is difficult, because the disease occurs as a urethral obstruction. The disease may be quiescent, but invariably there is a history of tuberculosis, even though it may have occurred many years previously. The management of this type of stricture is the same as for any other urethral stricture, and a course of antituberculosis treatment should be given as soon as the diagnosis is confirmed. The diagnosis may be apparent only after surgical treatment of the stricture has reactivated a dormant focus. Internal urethrotomy now has a definite place in the initial management of chronic tuberculous urethral strictures.

CLINICAL FEATURES

Tuberculosis in Developed Countries

The patient usually presents with vague urinary tract symptoms, and a careful history is important. This may not be easy, because the patient's memory about details is often confused and the length of illness uncertain. Furthermore, urologists are at a disadvantage because they rarely see more than a few cases a year and the diagnosis does not come readily to mind. Once the disease is suspected, a family history is important, not only for close members of the family but also for any other probable contacts. A history of previous tuberculosis in the patient also may be significant. After the diagnosis is made, all members of the family, as well as frequent visitors and contacts, should be examined. Urologists should always consider the diagnosis in a patient presenting with vague, long-standing urinary symptoms for which there is no obvious cause. When told of the diagnosis, most patients immediately realize that they have not been well for some time. A recurrent *E. coli* infection should also alert the urologist to the possibility of tuberculosis.

The incidence of tuberculosis is much higher among immigrants than in the native population. In Great Britain, the notification rate for nonpulmonary tuberculosis has been 70 to 80 times higher among immigrants from India than in the native white population (Innes, 1981). This probably results from a more virulent strain of *M. tuberculosis* and lower host resistance. It has been shown that the longer an immigrant lives in Great Britain before developing the disease, the more apt the disease is to be like the pattern seen in the native population (Davies, 1980). Tuberculosis in immigrants is much more a disease of the young, and only 4% of cases are genitourinary (Davies, 1980).

Tuberculosis in Developing Countries

Tuberculosis in developing countries is a much more acute disease than in developed regions, and it affects mostly children and young adults. Because of poor socioeconomic conditions and lack of control, the disease is prevalent and the risk of infection is serious. The genitourinary manifestation is becoming more widespread; in one survey in India, 20% of patients with pulmonary disease also had genitourinary lesions, many of which required surgical treatment.

Symptoms and Signs

The symptoms and signs of genitourinary tuberculosis vary in both intensity and duration. Age and sex incidence have remained unchanged over many years, with males predominating over females in a ratio of 2:1. Most patients are in the age group of 20 to 40 years, but recently, as with the pulmonary form of the disease, there has been a notable increase among patients aged 45 to 55 years and among those older than 70 years of age.

The patient usually complains of increasing painless frequency of micturition, at first only at night but later during the day as well, which has not responded to the usual antibiotic treatment. Urgency is uncommon unless there is extensive bladder involvement. The urine is normally sterile, and in a high proportion of patients it contains more than 20 pus cells per high-power field. However, in the author's series (Gow, 1976), 20% of patients did not have any abnormal pus cells in the urine. A superimposed infection is found in 20% of cases, 90% of which are caused by *E. coli*. Commonly, the symptoms are intermittent and have been present for some time before the patient seeks medical advice. However, the patient is invariably vague as to the precise time the symptoms actually started.

Overt hematuria, which is almost without exception total and intermittent, is present in only 10% of patients, but microscopic hematuria is present in up to 50% of patients. Renal and suprapubic pain is a rare presenting symptom and usually means extensive involvement of the kidney and bladder. Suprapubic pain is always accompanied by severe frequency of micturition. Ureteric colic is uncommon and occurs only if a small flake of calcification or a clot passes down the ureter.

Hemospermia was noted in only five cases in the author's series, and it is a rare presenting symptom (Gow, 1976). However, Yu and co-workers (1977) reported an 11% incidence in 65 tuberculosis patients reviewed during a period of 10 years. All of these patients had other clinical evidence of genitourinary tuberculosis. Tuberculosis should always be considered in patients who are seen with repeated attacks of hemospermia as the only presenting symptom, even if there is no other evidence of genitourinary tuberculosis.

Recurrent cystitis is also a warning sign. An *E. coli* infection that responds to antibiotics but recurs repeatedly should alert the urologist, because tuberculosis must be excluded in these cases. If the disease is not confirmed and the symptoms persist or recur, investigation should be conducted repeatedly, because *M. tuberculosis* is notoriously difficult to isolate from the urine when only small lesions are present.

In a few patients, the only presenting symptom is a painful testicular swelling. Because it is often difficult to differentiate between tuberculosis and nonspecific epididymo-orchitis in the absence of any radiologic changes and a cutaneous sinus, early-morning specimens of urine should be examined.

Rarely, the diagnosis is an incidental finding that is made after transurethral resection of the prostate when the pathologist reports foci of tuberculosis. There may or may not be evidence of disease elsewhere in the urinary tract, but all of these patients require the full course of antituberculosis chemotherapy.

The classic triad of lassitude, loss of weight, and anorexia is never seen in the early stages of the disease.

Finally, the fact that the presenting symptoms may be minimal in no way reflects the true nature of the disease, which can be advanced and of long standing even with very few symptoms. In many cases, the diagnosis is delayed because this pattern of presentation is not appreciated.

Tuberculosis in Children

Genitourinary tuberculosis has always been one of the most uncommon manifestations of the disease in children. There are two possible reasons. First, the incidence of renal complications is small in relation to the number of children with primary infection. Second, the symptoms of renal tuberculosis do not appear for 3 to 10 or more years after the primary infection (Ustvedt, 1947). It is therefore unlikely that the disease will be seen in a child younger than 10 years of age.

The clinical presentation varies. Some children have other forms of tuberculous lesions, others present with frequency of micturition and occasional hematuria, and another group presents with painful swelling of the epididymis. In children, pyuria is an almost constant finding, and red blood cells are frequently found, but the culture for nonspecific organisms is invariably sterile.

The treatment is the same course of chemotherapy that is given to adults, with a reduced dose according to the age of the child.

INVESTIGATIONS

Tuberculin Test

The tuberculin test is accomplished by intradermal injection of a protein-purified derivative of tuberculin. An inflammatory reaction develops at the site and reaches a maximum between 48 and 72 hours after injection. This reaction consists of a central indurated zone surrounded by an area of inflammation; it is assessed by measuring the diameter of the indurated area. The response is cell mediated through the T-lymphocyte mediator. The problem is to interpret the results accurately, because any expression of sensitivity is an individual peculiarity that depends on the person's ability to respond to the local concentration of the injection at that particular time. Such a response also may be modified by malignancy, nutritional deficiencies (e.g., iron, vitamin C), steroids, irradiation, and liver diseases. However, an indurated area larger than 10 mm in diameter is considered a positive reaction. Positive tests must be interpreted with caution, because nonspecific reactions do occur, probably because of the presence of mycobacteria other than *M. tuberculosis* or because of a previous injection with BCG.

A positive reaction is considered an indication that the person has been infected, provided that he or she has not been vaccinated with BCG, but it cannot be regarded as an indication of active tuberculous disease or that the symptoms are caused by tuberculosis. *M. tuberculosis* infection is far more common than tuberculous disease. Nevertheless, areas of 5 mm or less suggest little or no mycobacterial activity, and indicate a high degree of acquired immunity as a result of environmental mycobacteria, whereas reactions greater than 15 mm in diameter indicate a high degree of hypersensitivity, which probably reflects active disease (Youmans et al, 1975).

A positive test is of more help if it is known that a previous test was negative; in that case, the infection may be recent, and it is likely to produce a lesion that requires treatment.

Urine Examination

The urine is examined for red blood cells and pus cells, and the pH and concentration are noted. The urine is also cultured for nonspecific organisms that are tested for antibiotic sensitivities. Secondary bacterial infection is not common with tuberculosis and is found in only about 20% of cases. The usual organism is *E. coli*.

At least three, but preferably five, consecutive early-morning specimens of urine should be cultured, each onto two slopes: (1) a plain Löwenstein-Jensen culture medium to isolate *M. tuberculosis*, BCG, and the occasional nontuberculous mycobacteria; and (2) a pyruvic egg medium containing penicillin to identify *M. bovis*, which is partially anaerobic and grows below the surface of the culture medium. It is particularly important to collect all specimens into sterile containers, because unsterilized containers may be contaminated with environmental bacteria. *M. xenopi* is a common culprit because it is thermophilic and survives in hospital hot water systems.

Improvements in technique have allowed laboratories to dispense with routine guinea pig inoculations; in a series of 200 urinary specimens, 14 out of 41 specimens of urine were positive on culture although the animal inoculations were negative, whereas only 1 specimen was positive on animal inoculation with a negative culture result. The important technical advances appear to be the use of sulfuric acid to control contamination and the variety of media used (Marks, 1972). Pallen (1987) clearly demonstrated that animal inoculations offered no advantage over in vitro culture. There is now very little place for animal inoculation in isolating the mycobacterium.

Each specimen of urine should be inoculated as soon as possible after collection, because the longer the urine remains in contact with organisms, the less likely it is that the mycobacterium will grow. (Bjornesjo, 1956). Infections can be missed if specimens are collected and then pooled for culture studies 2 or 3 days later.

Sensitivity tests are always conducted if the cultures are positive, in order that the most effective course of chemotherapy can be started. The tests are performed on streptomycin, isoniazid, pyrazinamide, ethambutol, and rifampicin. It is unusual to find an organism that is resistant to these antibiotics, although initial resistance to one or more drugs is occasionally found. Most secondary infections are controlled by a combination of streptomycin and rifampicin; therefore, no other specific treatment need be started unless the organisms are still present 2 weeks after commencement of the antituberculosis course.

More modern diagnostic methods are now available and should be used whenever possible (Salfinger and Pfyffer, 1994). These include the luciferase technique and the fluorescence technique, in which specimens are stained with auramine or phodamine and examined by fluorescence micros-

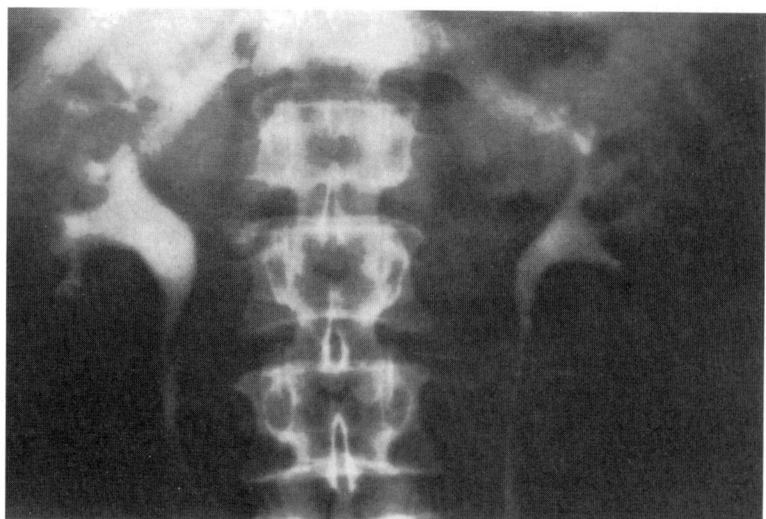

Figure 24–5. Distortion of the right upper pole calyx, with the typical stellate appearance.

copy. The latter method is said to increase the chance of detecting low numbers of organisms. The radiometric culture method is based on the release of radioactive carbon dioxide, which is detected by a special instrument. Growth of mycobacteria may be detected within 2 to 3 days. It can also be used for testing of drug susceptibility. However, it is very expensive, which reduces its use in routine diagnostic services.

The p-nitro-a-acetylamino-β hydroxyproprіophenole (NAP) test is used to differentiate *M. tuberculosis* from nontuberculous mycobacteria. The difference can be distinguished between the second and fifth days after the culture is started. Culture confirmation tests using DNA probes are now widely available for different mycobacteria and allow species specification within a few hours. Finally, high-performance liquid chromatography (HPLC) reveals qualitative and quantitative differences in the spectrum of mycolic acids present in the cell wall. This is a reliable criterion for identifying mycobacterial species, and HPLC offers rapid and easy identification.

Blood Analysis

A full blood count, erythrocyte sedimentation rate (ESR), and urea and electrolyte values are obtained in every case. In addition, if calcification is present, a complete biochemical assessment of calcium metabolism is performed. If the ESR is elevated, it should be measured at monthly intervals, because it gives some indication of response to treatment.

RADIOGRAPHY

Plain Radiographs

Straight x-ray films of the urinary tract are important because they may show calcification in the renal areas and in the lower genitourinary tract. Tuberculous ureteric calcification is very uncommon unless there is extensive renal calcification, but it must be distinguished from that seen in bilharziasis (schistosomiasis). In the former, all calcification is intraluminal and appears as a cast of the ureter, which is thickened and not dilated (Hartman et al, 1977). In schistosomiasis, the calcification is mural and the ureter is generally dilated and tortuous. Calcification rarely occurs in the bladder wall and seminal vesicles. A calcified psoas abscess can simulate renal calcification, and an intravenous urogram should be performed if there is any doubt of the diagnosis. Plain radiographs of the chest and spine are also performed to exclude any evidence of old or active pulmonary or spinal disease.

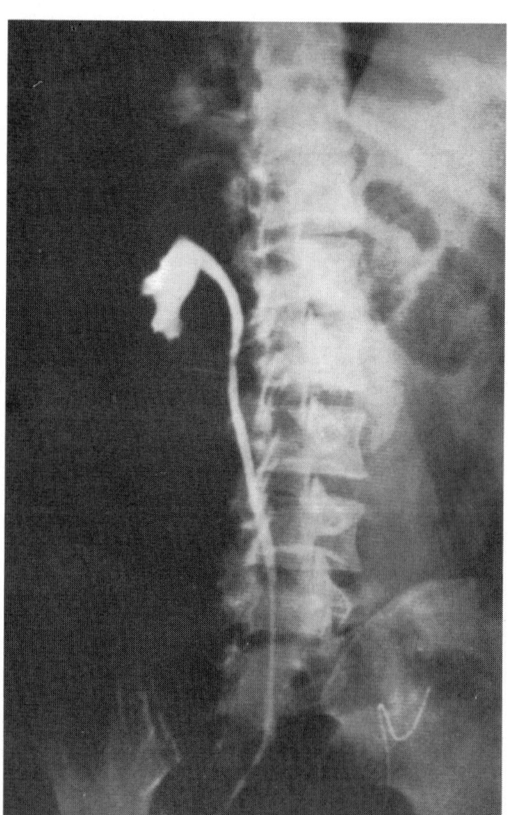

Figure 24–6. Occluded calyx.

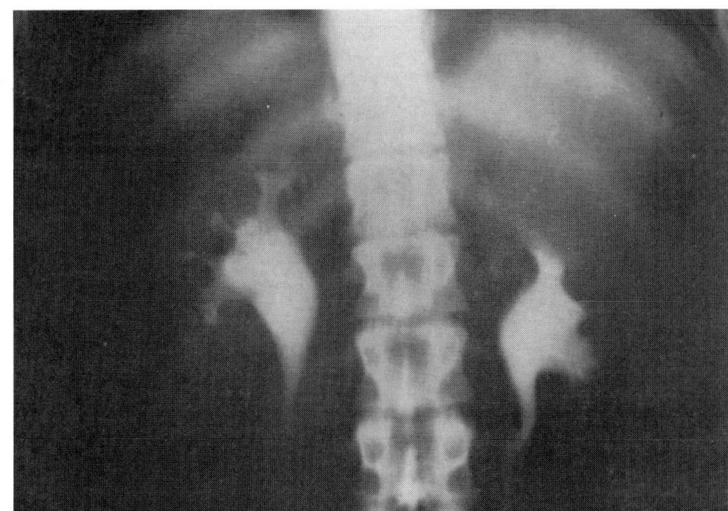

Figure 24–7. Multiple calyceal deformities.

Intravenous Urography

The introduction of the high-dose intravenous urogram has been a major advance in the investigation of renal tract pathology and is now standard practice. It has made retrograde pyelography a largely unnecessary, or a very infrequent, investigation in genitourinary tuberculosis. Tomography may be combined with an intravenous urogram if more precise information is required. In addition, image-intensified endoscopy allows a dynamic study of the diseased ureter, particularly at the pelviureteral junction. This functional information relating to ureteric peristalsis is an established part of the investigation of ureteric pathology, because it gives an indication of the extent of the disease, the peristaltic activity, the amount of fibrosis that is present, and the length of a stricture, particularly at the ureterovesical junction.

The renal lesion may appear as a distortion of a calyx (Fig. 24–5), as a calyx that is fibrosed and completely occluded (lost calyx) (Fig. 24–6; Sherwood, 1980), as multiple small calyceal deformities (Fig. 24–7), or as severe calyceal and parenchymal destruction (Fig. 24–8).

Calcification may be present. It is always associated with a calyceal lesion and can be minimal or extensive. Occasionally, one (Fig. 24–9) or, very rarely, both (Fig. 24–10)

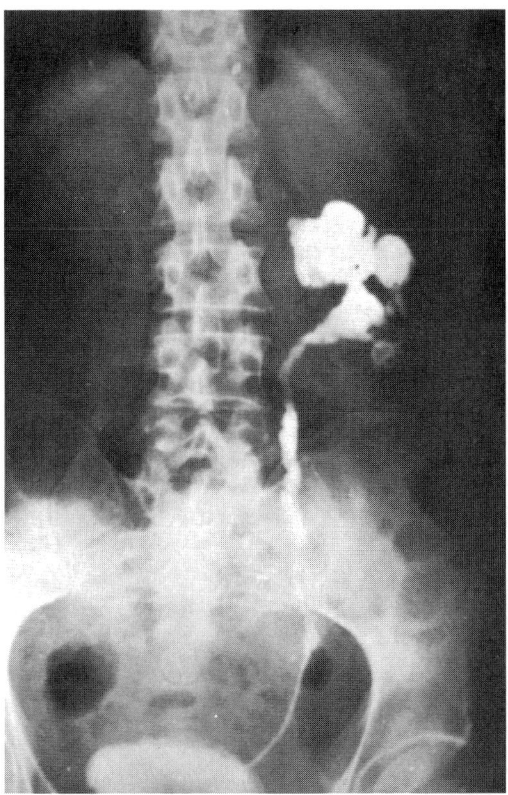

Figure 24–8. Severe calyceal and parenchymal destruction.

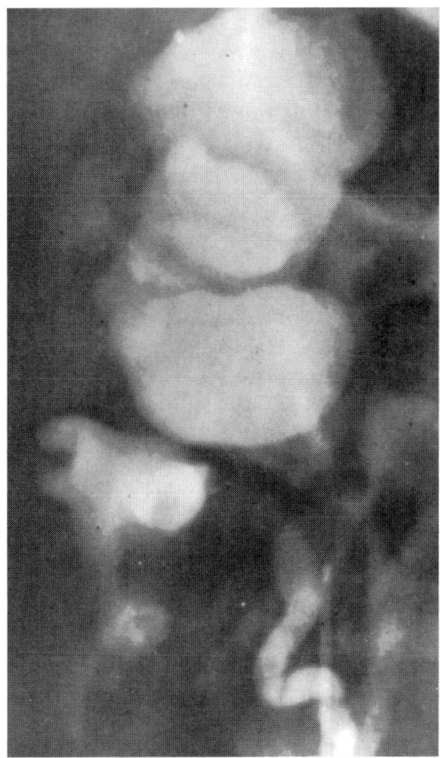

Figure 24–9. Involvement of one moiety of duplex kidney.

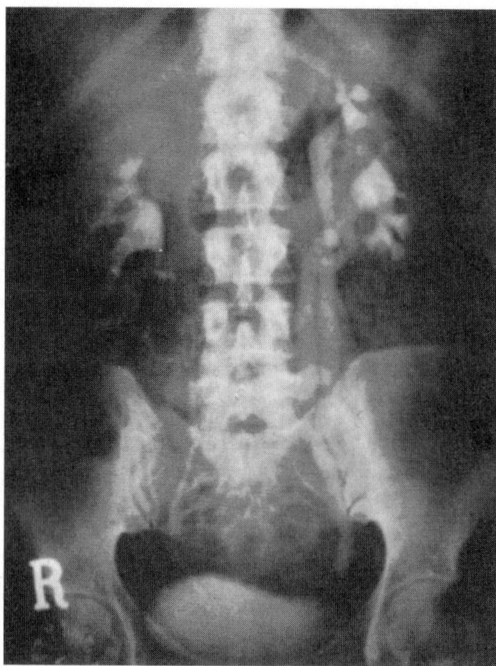

Figure 24–10. Involvement of both moieties of duplex kidney. Note also the stricture at the lower end of the ureter.

moieties of a duplex kidney are involved. Any renal calcification that is not discrete should alert the physician to the possibility of an underlying tuberculous infection.

A nonfunctioning or extensively diseased kidney indicates irreversible tuberculous disease. Tuberculous ureteritis is manifested by dilatation above a ureterovesical stricture or, if the disease is more advanced, by a rigid fibrotic ureter with multiple strictures.

The cystographic phase of the intravenous urogram can give valuable information about the condition of the bladder, which may be small and contracted (thimble bladder; Fig. 24–11) or irregular, with filling defects and bladder asymmetry.

Retrograde Pyelography

As noted previously, retrograde pyelography is now rarely necessary, but there are two indications for its use. The first is a stricture at the lower end of the ureter, where it is necessary to try to delineate (1) the length of the stricture and (2) the amount of obstruction and dilatation above the stricture. The examination is performed under direct vision using an image intensifier. The contrast agent should be introduced through a bulb-tipped catheter, Braasch or Chevassu, with the tip inserted into the ureteric orifice. As in intravenous urography, it is important to combine a dynamic study with the examination, so that ureteric function can be assessed.

The second indication for retrograde pyelography is ureteric catheterization, which may be required to obtain urine samples for culture from each kidney if it is not certain from which side the organisms are coming. In such cases, a 7-Fr catheter is passed into the renal pelvis. To increase the output of urine, furosemide (40 mg) is given one-half hour before the cystoscopy or, alternatively, mannitol (20 g) is infused intravenously during the examination.

Percutaneous Antegrade Pyelography

Percutaneous antegrade pyelography is becoming more important as an alternative to retrograde ureterography in the case of a large kidney. It is particularly useful in visualizing a nonfunctioning kidney or in determining the condition of all excretory pathways above an obstruction. It can be used to aspirate the contents of the renal pelvis so that they can be sent for diagnostic examination. This technique also can be used to aspirate the contents of tuberculous cavities in order to estimate the quantity of drugs that has penetrated the walls. Sometimes chemotherapeutic agents can be inoculated into the cavity by this method.

Arteriography

Arteriography is an invasive radiologic investigation that is of limited value and should never be considered as a method of routine evaluation in a patient with genitourinary tuberculosis. Occasionally, it may be used to assess the amount of renal parenchymal damage or to delineate arterial circulation if partial nephrectomy is being planned. Also, it can mark the precise area of destruction of a kidney, which is often more extensive than would be suggested by intravenous urography. Arteriography has one important application, when there is a possibility of coincidental renal tumor with tuberculosis. (I have seen seven such cases.)

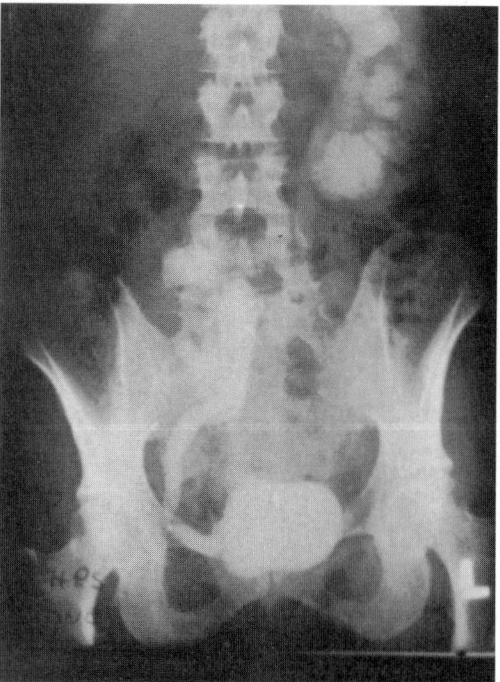

Figure 24–11. Contracted irregular bladder, with diseased left and right kidneys, the right being ectopic. Note stricture at the lower end of the right ureter.

Radioisotope Investigation

Renal scanning affords information on functional renal tissue and parenchymal abnormalities. It gives details regarding the extent of the disease. However, renal tuberculosis is well seen on intravenous urography, and it is doubtful whether radioisotope investigation can add anything to this investigation. Yet, it may be useful in assessing the response to treatment and the eventual optimal renal function.

Magnetic Resonance Imaging

This investigation has very little application in the management of genitourinary tuberculosis.

Cystoscopy

Endoscopy is not important in the diagnosis of genitourinary tuberculosis. It has some place, however, in assessing the extent of the disease or the response to chemotherapy. Occasionally, the appearance of the bladder suggests extensive tuberculosis, but no *M. tuberculosis* can be cultured from the urine and the upper urinary tract appears normal. In this situation, the most likely diagnosis is an acute interstitial cystitis. The procedure must always be performed under general anesthesia with a muscle relaxant to reduce the risk of hemorrhage. The phase of bladder filling should be performed under direct vision.

Ureteroscopy

Now that ureteroscopy has become a standard urologic procedure, it may be used to study the effect of the disease on the ureter and pelvis of the kidney, especially if the ureteric orifice has a golf-hole appearance and allows early passage of the instrument. Indications for the technique are rare, but it adds another dimension in the management of the disease.

Bladder Biopsy

Bladder biopsy is contraindicated in the presence of acute tuberculous cystitis and even if there are areas of inflammation, either in the bladder or close to the ureteric orifice, that are suggestive of tuberculosis. I have never seen a case in which a biopsy specimen was positive for tuberculosis and the urine was sterile. Biopsy is acceptable only in patients with tubercles or with ulcers some distance from a normal ureteric orifice, because a diagnosis of carcinoma must be excluded if such lesions are seen.

Ultrasonography

Ultrasound scan is of limited value in the initial investigations of genitourinary tuberculosis. It can be used to monitor kidney lesions found by an intravenous urogram during the period of chemotherapy. This noninvasive technique can show whether a cavity is increasing or decreasing in size, thus precluding repeated radiographic examinations. It also can be used to monitor the volume of a contracted bladder during treatment, which is of value to assess the need for bladder augmentation. Small, portable, battery-operated machines are now available that can be used to identify renal lesions in patients who live in areas where radiography is not available.

Computed Tomography

Computed tomography (CT) is of limited value in the early investigation of genitourinary tuberculosis because intravenous urography gives such accurate pictures. CT may help in the case of a difficult intrarenal lesion or if there is a possibility of a coexisting renal carcinoma. The subtleties of any ureteric change are better seen with a combination of a ureterogram and an image intensifier. CT scanning may be useful to delineate diseased seminal vesicles that were not originally thought to be infected (Premkumar and Newhouse, 1988).

MANAGEMENT

Setting

The management of genitourinary tuberculosis is presented in Figure 24–12. In developed countries, it is no longer necessary to treat patients in the hospital, except in special circumstances in which the disease is extensive, the symptoms are severe, and the home environment is inadequate for the care of the patient. In developing countries, however, it is usually essential to admit patients, at least for the first month, to ensure that the drugs are taken consistently. Then patients are seen weekly on an outpatient basis, liver function assessments are carried out, and the urine is inspected to note the color (it is brown if the patient has been taking the rifampicin regularly). If surgery is required, it is scheduled as a planned procedure, and the patient is admitted 6 weeks after the start of the intensive course of treatment.

The urologist should supervise the chemotherapy and not abdicate this responsibility by allowing drug regimens to be dictated by colleagues in other medical disciplines. Certainly, any problems should be discussed, especially if there are resistant strains of organisms, but the urologist should always be responsible for the overall management of the patient. Otherwise, severe, irreversible damage to the renal tract may occur, and kidneys may even be destroyed.

The aims of management are (1) to treat the active disease, (2) to make the patient noninfectious as soon as possible, (3) to preserve the maximal amount of renal tissue, and (4) to provide every member of the community with the best available treatment.

In developing countries, living conditions are poor, tuberculous infection is rife, malnutrition is common, and other diseases, such as malaria, gastroenteritis, and worm infestation, are endemic, so that resistance to an infection from *M. tuberculosis* is low. Although pulmonary tuberculosis is the

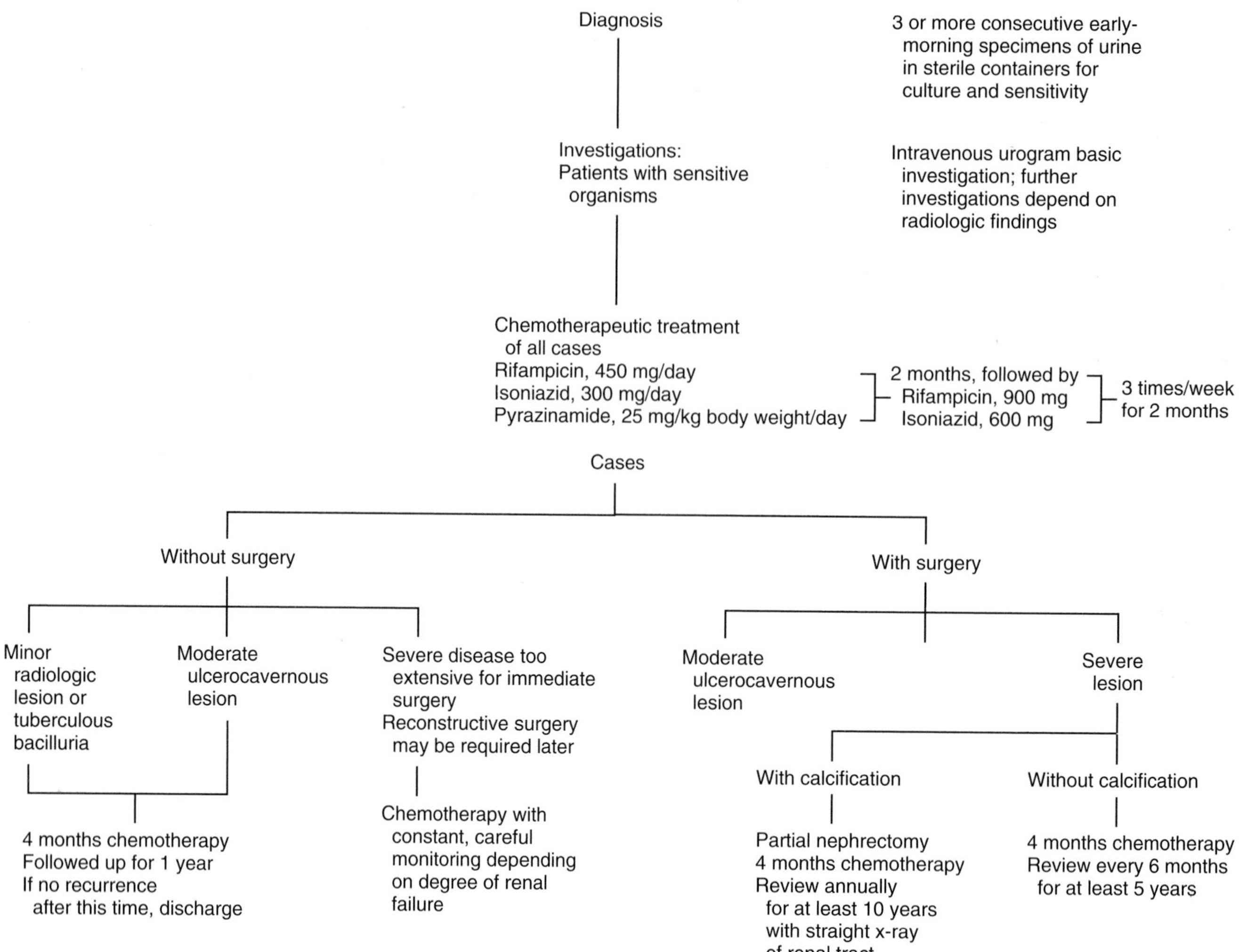

Figure 24–12. Management of genitourinary tuberculosis.

most common type, genitourinary tuberculosis is being seen more frequently in an acute form, and the physician always should be aware of this diagnosis. Management of the disease depends on the resources and facilities of the region, but hospital admission for surgical treatment is necessary for a high proportion of patients with genitourinary tuberculosis. In these countries, genitourinary tuberculosis is almost always seen in patients with the pulmonary form of the disease, very rarely as an isolated infection. The problems in these countries remain formidable. Radiographs and culture examinations are expensive, case finding is much more difficult, and infectious persons who are not diagnosed continue to spread the disease. Transportation is primitive, and the chemotherapeutic treatment, because of cost, is often less effective. Because of these factors, achievement of a noticeable improvement in the tuberculosis situation in many developing countries is hugely problematic.

Antituberculosis Drugs

Antituberculosis drugs are divided into three groups: primary agents, secondary agents, and minor agents (Table 24–3).

Primary Agents

Isoniazid

Isoniazid (isonicotinic acid hydrazide) was discovered in 1952. It is highly active against *M. tuberculosis* and inhibits most strains in a concentration of 0.05 to 0.2 μg/ml. The precise action is unknown. It has been postulated that it interferes with the biosynthesis of nucleic acids (Wimpenny,

Table 24–3. CLASSIFICATION OF ANTITUBERCULOSIS DRUGS

Classification	Agent	Activity
Primary agents	Rifampicin Isoniazid Pyrazinamide Streptomycin	Bacteriocidal
Secondary agents	Ethambutol Ethionamide Cycloserine	Bacteriostatic
Minor agents	Kanamycin Thioacetazone	Bacteriostatic

1967). It also inhibits the synthesis of mycolic acids in *M. tuberculosis* by affecting the enzyme mycolase synthetase, which is unique to mycobacteria. The inhibiting concentration against this enzyme is low and is comparable to the minimum inhibitory concentration (MIC) of the drugs against *M. tuberculosis* (Kucers and Bennett, 1979).

Some unchanged isoniazid is excreted by the kidneys, but most of it is excreted in the inactive form, acetylisoniazid. Seventy percent of all administered isoniazid is excreted by the kidneys (Mitchell et al, 1976). It is widely distributed in the body, and body tissue levels similar to serum levels are obtained. The drug readily penetrates caseous material and enters macrophages (Bennett et al, 1977). There is no cross-resistance with rifampicin.

Rifampicin

Rifampicin is one of a group of antibiotics that is isolated from *Streptomyces mediterranei.* It is highly active against *M. tuberculosis*; its MIC is 0.20 μg/ml. Rifampicin acts to inhibit bacterial RNA synthesis by interfering with DNA-directed RNA polymerase of sensitive bacteria (Hartmann et al, 1967). Rifampicin is lipid soluble and therefore enters macrophages. It is excreted in the urine; with a 600-mg oral dose, peak concentrations of 100 μg/ml are reached in the urine after 8 hours, and a lethal concentration for mycobacteria is detectable for 36 hours (Kunin et al, 1969).

Streptomycin

Streptomycin was isolated from *Streptomyces griseus* in 1944. It belongs to a group of antibiotics known as the aminoglycosides. The usual MIC for *M. tuberculosis* is 8 μg/ml. Like other aminoglycosides, it interferes with bacterial protein synthesis by its ability to bind to a particular protein or proteins of the 30 S unit of bacterial ribosomes so that faulty proteins are produced (Luzzatto et al, 1968). It penetrates the walls of tuberculous abscesses in lethal concentrations even in caseous material (Fellander et al, 1952). Streptomycin also rapidly diffuses into body tissues and is excreted by glomerular filtration. High concentrations are obtained in the urine (200 to 400 μg/ml after a 1-g intramuscular injection), and for a period of 24 hours after injection, the MIC of 8 μg/ml is retained.

Pyrazinamide

Pyrazinamide, a derivative of nicotinamide, was synthesized in 1952 and was shown to possess some activity against *M. tuberculosis*, especially in an acid medium. Its usual MIC is 20 μg/ml, but this is found only if the drug is tested in an acid medium with a pH of 5.5. The precise mechanism of action of pyrazinamide is unknown. Its metabolite, pyrozinoic acid, may be involved in the activity of pyrazinamide, and its activity is enhanced in an environment with a pH of less than 5.5. Pyrazinamide is excreted in the urine; urine concentration reaches a peak in 2 hours and then falls exponentially for 48 hours. Its half-life is 9 hours (Elland, 1969), but the lethal concentration is retained in the urine after a single dose of 1 g for a period of up to 36 hours (Stollmeyer et al, 1968).

Secondary and Minor Agents

Ethambutol was discovered in 1961 and was found to have a high degree of antituberculosis activity. MICs are between 1 and 2 μg/ml and rarely are higher than 5 μg/ml. Ethambutol is active against *M. tuberculosis* strains resistant to isoniazid and other commonly used antituberculosis drugs. It is well absorbed after oral administration, with a normal dose of 25 mg/kg of body weight. The peak serum level of about 5 μg/ml is reached in approximately 4 hours. About 80% is excreted in the urine as active unchanged drug, and this excretion occurs within 24 hours of administration. High concentrations of the active drug are obtained in the urine. Ethambutol appears to enter the cells of *M. tuberculosis* organisms. Its precise mechanism is not known, but it probably inhibits mycobacterial synthesis. It exerts its maximal inhibitory effect against mycobacteria at a neutral pH.

The other secondary agents and the minor agents kanamycin and thioacetazone are now very rarely used except in underdeveloped countries.

CHEMOTHERAPY

For many years, short courses of chemotherapy have constituted the normal method of treatment, because the irrefutable evidence obtained from treating many thousands of cases showed that to treat patients for longer than 9 months was wasteful in time, money, and resources. Although the clinical trials were carried out on patients with pulmonary tuberculosis, the results are equally applicable to the treatment of the genitourinary manifestation.

To appreciate the reason for adopting short-course treatment, it is necessary to understand the mechanisms of drug action and to study the thousands of patients who have been treated by various combinations since the mid-1970s.

Mechanisms of Drug Action

The mechanisms of short-course chemotherapy have been revealed by the experimental work on mice at the Pasteur Institute, the work of Professor Mitchison at his medical research unit, and a large number of cooperative clinical trials in many countries. Each of these trials was designed to compare the effectiveness of short-course regimens and, in addition, to assess the contribution of individual drugs (Fox, 1980).

Grosset (1978) summarized the experiments on mice as follows:

1. Pyrazinamide and rifampicin are very potent sterilizing drugs in experimentally infected mice.
2. The most important sterilizing combinations are isoniazid plus pyrazinamide and isoniazid plus rifampicin.
3. The addition of streptomycin or ethambutol makes little or no contribution to the sterilizing capacity of the two foregoing combinations.

On the basis of his experimental and clinical work, Mitchison (1980) suggested that there are four bacterial populations (Fig. 24–13). The first is a population of rapidly dividing bacilli, which are killed by all the bacteriocidal drugs. The second group consists of the intermittent metabolizers,

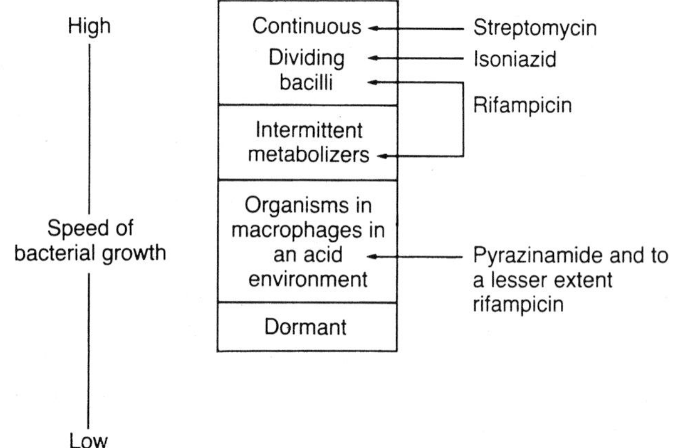

Figure 24–13. Bacterial populations within tuberculous lesions in humans. (Modified from Mitchison DA: Treatment of tuberculosis. J R Coll Phys 1980;14:91.)

which metabolize for periods of little more than a few hours. These are killed by rifampicin because of the speed with which its bacteriocidal action starts; they are not affected by other drugs, especially isoniazid, because there is a 1-day lag period before they begin to exert their bacteriocidal effect (Dickinson and Mitchison, 1981). The bacteria in the third group are those in the acid environment of macrophages. They are destroyed by pyrazinamide, whose activity is greatly enhanced in an acid medium. The last group consists of completely dormant organisms, or persistors, which are not affected by any of the antituberculosis drugs.

As a result of this hypothesis, various drug combinations have been studied, and it has been shown that combinations with isoniazid have the highest bacterial activity (Jindani et al, 1980). Isoniazid is therefore the key bacteriocidal drug, with rifampicin and pyrazinamide having definitive roles in sterilizing special populations.

The re-emergence of pyrazinamide as a vital drug is particularly gratifying. In the 1950s, it was relegated to the second line because of its toxicity, which was caused by the administration of unnecessarily high doses. It is a drug that has little value in preventing drug resistance, but it is an essential part of initial sterilizing regimens.

Streptomycin is occasionally added to make a quadruple combination, especially for the initial 2 months of intensive therapy. It is no longer necessary in drug-sensitive cases, however, because it has been shown to provide no additional benefit (Singapore Tuberculosis Service and British Medical Research Council, 1988).

Choice of Drug Regimens for Drug-Sensitive Infections

The British Thoracic Association (1980) showed unequivocally that for regimens not containing pyrazinamide there was a definite superiority of a 9-month duration over a 6-month duration. There is now abundant evidence, however, that many 6-month regimens are effective. The common factor in these regimens is the initial use of rifampicin, isoniazid, and pyrazinamide. In a combination of trials conducted in East Africa and Singapore and in a second study by the British Thoracic Association, a total of 422 patients were treated for 6 months, and only 4 patients (1%) relapsed bacteriologically (Fox, 1981). All of these patients received daily streptomycin, isoniazid, rifampicin, and pyrazinamide for the first 2 months, followed either by isoniazid, rifampicin, and pyrazinamide or by isoniazid and rifampicin for an additional 4 months. In addition, a trial in Hong Kong (Hong Kong Chest Service and British Medical Research Council, 1981) showed that the combination of streptomycin, isoniazid, rifampicin, and pyrazinamide, given three times a week for 6 months, was equally effective, because there was only 1% bacteriologic relapse.

Effectiveness of Regimens Shorter Than Six Months

There is growing evidence that regimens shorter than 6 months may also be effective. Mehrotra and associates (1981) showed that only 1% of patients treated with streptomycin, isoniazid, rifampicin, and pyrazinamide daily for 3 months, followed by rifampicin and isoniazid daily for 6 weeks, relapsed bacteriologically. This study may have wide implications for developing countries.

Regimens for Smear-Negative but Culture-Positive Disease

Most patients with genitourinary manifestations have negative smears but positive culture results. Two studies in Hong Kong (Chen, 1981; Girling, 1981) are significant. Both 2- and 3-month courses were inadequate; it was also doubtful whether 4 months would be sufficient, although patients given streptomycin, isoniazid, rifampicin, and pyrazinamide three times a week for 4 months did not show any relapses up to 8 months after cessation of treatment. A longer period of review is necessary before a definite opinion can be given. Treatment with the same four drugs given three times a week for 6 months did not produce any bacteriologic relapses.

A further study (Hong Kong Chest Service et al, 1989) confirmed this earlier work. It showed that, after treatment with isoniazid, rifampicin, and pyrazinamide for 2 months, followed by isoniazid and rifampicin for 2 months, the results were equally as effective as those of 6-month regimens. The 4-month regimen has now become standard for smear-negative patients treated in the Hong Kong Chest Service. Further confirmation of the success of this regimen and the importance of pyrazinamide is found in the publications of Howell and associates (1989) and Singapore Tuberculous Service and British Medical Research Council (1988).

For the treatment of pulmonary tuberculosis, evidence from these studies indicates that rifampicin, isoniazid, and pyrazinamide are the drugs of choice for the initial intensive treatment period, followed by rifampicin and isoniazid either continuously three times a week or twice a week, with the whole course to last 6 months. There is no place for ethambutol or other bacteriostatic drugs in the initial treatment of sensitive organisms. They should be considered only if drug resistance is suspected. Drug resistance to one drug is rare and to more than one very rare. If it occurs, special drug combinations are required.

In developing countries, this ideal may have to be relaxed and a lower success rate accepted. Supervision and compliance are more difficult, cost is a major factor, social and cultural traditions play important parts, and more patients fail to return for treatment. Despite the cost, rifampicin should be included in all regimens, because the length of the course can then be kept to a minimum; even if patients do fail to keep appointments, there is a greater chance of successful treatment and a consequent reduction of the rate of infection with rifampin. Nevertheless, infrequency of compliance and the irregular taking of drugs is a formula that can lead only to treatment failure and the emergence of resistant strains of *M. tuberculosis*.

Effects of Investigations on Genitourinary Disease

Certain aspects of genitourinary tuberculosis make it likely to respond equally well, if not better, to short-course chemotherapy. First, fewer organisms are involved in the renal form of the disease than in the pulmonary form, and these are discharged into the urine intermittently. Second, there are high concentrations of isoniazid, rifampicin, pyrazinamide, and streptomycin in the urine. Third, isoniazid and rifampicin pass freely into renal cavities in high concentration. Finally, all of these drugs reach adequate concentrations in the kidney, ureters, bladder, and prostate. The two recommended alternative regimens for genitourinary tuberculosis are shown in Figure 24–14.

All of the drugs should be administered in one dose; if they are given in divided doses, subtherapeutic levels may occur. My technique is to suggest that the drugs be taken together at night just before bedtime, with or without a milk drink, because this has been found to be the best way of achieving maximum patient tolerance (Israili et al, 1987).

2 months	2 months
Pyrazinamide 25 mg/kg body wt/day maximum dose 2 g daily	
Isoniazid 300 mg daily	600 mg 3 times a week
Rifampicin 450 mg daily	900 mg 3 times a week

2 months	2 months
Streptomycin 1 g daily	
Isoniazid 300 mg daily	
Rifampicin 450 mg daily	Isoniazid 600 mg 3 times a week
Pyrazinamide 25 mg/kg body wt/day maximum dose 2 g daily	Rifampicin 900 mg 3 times a week

Figure 24–14. Alternative regimens for treatment of genitourinary tuberculosis.

As has been stated, streptomycin adds nothing to the other three drugs in the initial phase; it is suggested, however, that it be given in cases of extensive disease with severe bladder symptoms because it has such a high concentration in the urine. The continuation phase is given three times a week for 2 months. The course should end after 4 months; more than 90% of patients are cured by that time. The author has had only one relapse among more than 200 patients treated with short-course regimens. It is far better to treat the very rare relapse when it occurs than to needlessly treat all patients, because recurrent organisms almost invariably remain sensitive to the four first-line drugs.

There are only two exceptions to this regimen of treatment. The first exception is the patient with a previous history of any form of tuberculosis who is undergoing renal transplantation. This patient should receive rifampicin (900 mg) and isoniazid (600 mg) three times a week for 1 year or longer, because with the administration of immunosuppressive drugs there is always the danger of reactivation of dormant bacilli.

The second exception is the patient who is receiving hemodialysis for end-stage renal tuberculosis. In this patient, rifampicin and isoniazid can be given in the normal dose, because they are largely metabolized in the liver and the part that remains unchanged is removed by the dialysate on the days of dialysis. The drugs should be given immediately after the dialysis is finished. Streptomycin is removed by dialysis, but because of its ototoxicity, it is recommended that daily blood concentration be estimated to ensure that the peak serum levels do not rise above 20 μg/ml. There are very few published data on patients undergoing dialysis who are also receiving pyrazinamide therapy. However, because this drug is largely metabolized in the liver, it should not be withdrawn from routine chemotherapy regimens, provided the liver function tests are carefully monitored.

Use of Steroids

Another approach to shortening the duration of chemotherapy was suggested by Tripathy (1978). He attempted to reduce the host resistance by means of steroids, so that the bacilli would become more vulnerable to the action of the antituberculosis drugs. After a 6-week course of prednisolone, however, there was no evidence that the steroids influenced the sterilizing activity of regimens that included isoniazid, rifampicin, and pyrazinamide.

Steroids may be useful in cases of acute tuberculous cystitis. Prednisolone, at least 20 mg three times per day given with the four antituberculous drugs for 4 weeks, helps to alleviate severe bladder symptoms and allows an earlier appraisal of subsequent management. This high dose of prednisolone is required because rifampicin reduces the effectiveness and bioavailability of prednisolone. McAllister and co-workers (1983) showed that when rifampicin is given with prednisolone, the amount of prednisolone available to the tissues is reduced by 66%.

Prospects for the Future

It is a true yet unpalatable fact that the present treatment of tuberculosis worldwide is inadequate. The number of new cases is rising, and resistant strains of organisms are increasing. One third of all cases treated in the New York City Survey in 1991 were resistant to one or more drugs (Frieden et al, 1993). To rely entirely on chemotherapy is to shut our eyes to this important evidence. A new approach is required, and further study of all forms of therapy is mandatory. There is an urgent need for ultra-short courses of chemotherapy, effective treatment for drug-resistant cases, and methods to prevent reactivation of tuberculosis in HIV-positive people.

Noncompliance is the greatest bar to the effective treatment of tuberculosis worldwide, but most patients do take their drugs for the first 2 months. After that time, more than 60% default, especially in the developing world, where tuberculosis is rife (Stanford and Grange, 1993). To achieve a reduction of treatment to 2 months would be a major advance. Only an immunotherapeutic approach is likely to achieve this aim, because all the common antituberculosis drugs act by disrupting one of the metabolic processes of the bacillus and have been proved to have suboptimal activity.

The present immunotherapy agent is an attenuated strain of mammalia *M. tuberculosis*, but this has many drawbacks, and recently an avirulent mycobacterium has been found to be effective (Stanford et al, 1990). A heat-killed suspension of *M. vaccae* has been found to possess all the required properties for immunotherapy (Grange and Stanford, 1994). Studies are being carried out in many parts of the world using short courses of chemotherapy together with one or more injections of *M. vaccae*, and the results are encouraging. Should this combined approach prove ultimately to be satisfactory, genitourinary tuberculosis could be treated by isoniazid, rifampicin, and pyrazinamide 3 times a week for 2 months, combined with one or more injections of *M. vaccae*. This would be a great advance, especially for the developing countries.

Chemoprophylaxis for Tuberculosis

Chemoprophylaxis is relevant only if clinical, nonproven pulmonary and genitourinary forms of tuberculosis are present at the same time. Isoniazid given alone for 12 months resulted in a 75% reduction in the incidence of culture-positive tuberculosis. Isoniazid, rifampicin, and pyrazinamide given together for 2 months, however, resulted in an 82% reduction in bacteriologically proven tuberculosis. Because compliance by patients is likely to be better for drugs that are taken for 8 weeks rather than 52, the three-drug regime is worthy of careful study (Snider et al, 1986). It may also be of value in people seropositive for HIV who are also tuberculin positive.

Follow-Up Management

Patients should be seen 3, 6, and 12 months after the course of chemotherapy has finished. At each review, three consecutive early-morning specimens of urine are examined and an intravenous urogram is performed. If radiographic results remain unchanged and the urine is consistently sterile, the patient is discharged with instructions to report back if there is any recurrence of previous urinary symptoms.

TOXICITY

Antituberculosis drugs do not often cause serious toxicity problems, but if they do, it is usually during the first few weeks of treatment. In a recent review (Hong Kong Chest Service et al, 1989), only 4% of patients had one or more drugs terminated because of toxicity. Mild toxicity occurs, but this rarely requires stopping the drugs, although the dose or frequency may have to be reduced. As soon as toxic reactions occur, they must be rapidly and efficiently managed; otherwise, there is the risk that the patient's treatment may be jeopardized and recovery prolonged.

The two main reactions are hypersensitivity to the antituberculosis drugs and jaundice.

Hypersensitivity

Although all of the antituberculosis drugs can produce hypersensitivity reactions, streptomycin, rifampicin, and thioacetazone are the most commonly involved. Only the first two are significant.

The clinical manifestation is a macular rash, which is irritable and accompanied by pyrexia. More general reactions may occur, including periorbital swellings, conjunctivitis, aching limbs, generalized lymphadenopathy, and, very rarely, Stevens-Johnson syndrome (British Medical Research Council, 1973).

Because the treatment regimens invariably use at least three drugs, it is important to determine as soon as possible which drug or drugs are causing the toxic reaction. A recently introduced test evaluates the drug-stimulating lymphocytic transformation rate (Umeki, 1989). The rate is measured by determining the uptake of tritiated thymidine by the patient's lymphocytes, which are cultured for 3 days in the presence and absence of each individual drug. When the degree of tritiated thymidine incorporation found in culture to which each drug has been added reaches more than 150% higher than the controls, desensitization should be started. Because this figure may be high, I believe that it is prudent to start desensitization at a lower figure, 100% to 125% higher than normal. This test reduces the application of challenge tests and enables all sensitive patients to benefit from an early desensitizing program.

Minor reactions can be treated by antihistamines and do not necessitate alteration in the course of treatment. If a reaction is severe, all drugs should be stopped until the symptoms have subsided. After the patient has recovered, management consists of (1) identification of the drug responsible for the reaction and (2) resumption of adequate chemotherapy as soon as possible. If a challenge test is required, the doses are outlined in Table 24–4 (Girling, 1982). Desensitization can be carried out rapidly by using a dose equal to or less than the first challenging dose, if necessary under steroid cover, but it should always be performed under the shield of antituberculosis drugs to which the patient is not hypersensitive.

Hepatotoxicity

Transient increases in liver enzyme concentrations occur during the early weeks of treatment with any antituberculosis

Table 24–4. CHALLENGE DOSES FOR DETECTING HYPERSENSITIVITY TO ANTITUBERCULOSIS DRUGS

Drug	Challenging Dose	
	Day 1	*Day 2*
Isoniazid	50 mg	300 mg
Rifampicin	75 mg	300 mg
Pyrazinamide	250 mg	1000 mg
Ethionamide	125 mg	375 mg
Cycloserine	125 mg	250 mg
Ethambutol	100 mg	500 mg
Streptomycin	125 mg	500 mg

Adapted from Girling, DJ: Drugs 1982; 23:56.

drug, and they are not significant because they soon return to normal (Baron and Bell, 1974). They must be distinguished from clinical hepatitis, however, which occurs in fewer than 1% of patients.

Because they are metabolized in the liver, combinations of the antituberculosis drugs pyrazinamide, rifampicin, and isoniazid were at first considered potentially toxic and more likely to produce jaundice than those combinations that included streptomycin and ethambutol, which are metabolized by the kidneys. Furthermore, pyrazinamide had gained a reputation for being hepatotoxic because it was given in very high doses when first used, and it is known that hepatitis is dose-related (McLeod et al, 1959). When pyrazinamide is used in combinations in dosages of less than 35 mg/kg of body weight daily, no unacceptable hepatotoxicity has been experienced. This statement is based on evidence from the treatment of thousands of patients in many countries (Fox, 1978).

If jaundice and associated symptoms occur, all drugs should be stopped. If the jaundice is caused by the drugs, recovery is usually rapid. After the patient has completely recovered, treatment with the same regimen usually can be resumed. However, liver function should be carefully monitored until the course is finished, and it may be wise to recommence treatment initially three times a week for 3 or 4 weeks.

Other Reactions

Other reactions to the drugs may occur infrequently. Isoniazid may cause urticarial rash and neurologic disturbances, which can be controlled by pyridoxine (20 mg daily); it is a wise precaution to give this drug if the daily dose of isoniazid exceeds 900 mg.

Rifampicin can give rise to gastrointestinal disturbances, to thrombocytopenic purpuras and the "flu syndrome," and, very rarely, to acute renal failure. Pyrazinamide can cause nausea, anorexia, and arthralgia. Streptomycin is ototoxic, but this is reversible if the drug is withdrawn immediately after the appearance of symptoms.

Ethambutol can cause retrobulbar neuritis and should be stopped if ocular changes occur. This reaction is always dose-related, so this drug must be carefully regulated. All symptoms disappear if the drug is immediately discontinued.

Rifampicin and the Contraceptive Pill

Rifampicin can result in the failure of oral contraceptive steroid therapy owing to changes in the kinetics of the estrogen component; these changes cause a rapid breakdown so that estrogen levels fall below the concentration required for contraception. Rifampicin also may cause disturbing menstrual disorders. Reimer and associates (1974) reported five pregnancies among 88 women receiving oral contraceptives who were being treated for tuberculosis with rifampicin. Of this group, 68 women had some menstrual changes. Efforts have been made to overcome this reaction by increasing the dose of estrogens, but the results have been too unpredictable because of individual variations in patient response. Some responses showed a fivefold shorter half-life of estrogen, whereas others had only a 1.5- to twofold reduction. It is suggested that female patients in the childbearing years adopt some other form of contraception while being treated with rifampicin, especially because the treatment is relatively short term and the metabolism of estrogens returns to normal within 3 to 4 weeks after the drug has been stopped.

Antituberculosis Drugs During Pregnancy

The diagnosis of tuberculosis of any form in a young woman is always a cause for anxiety, especially when pregnancy and the possible adverse effects of drugs are considered. Young women should be advised against pregnancy, if possible, until the treatment is completed. If the patient is already pregnant when the diagnosis is made, the risks to the patient versus those to the fetus must be assessed. Unless there is severe renal failure, in which case pregnancy should be terminated, the pregnancy is allowed to continue, because most reported fetal anomalies associated with these drugs have been caused by much higher doses than are used in humans. Rifampicin, in the series of Snider and co-workers (1980), produced an increased incidence of limb defects, but this result has not been confirmed. Moreover, there is very little evidence of any increased risk of toxemia or neonatal mortality in women with a history of renal tuberculosis, provided that renal function and blood pressure are normal. Because it is difficult to assess the toxicity of one drug when the treatment is a combination of three or more agents, it is advisable to give rifampicin three times a week rather than every day during the first 3 months of pregnancy and to add pyridoxine (20 mg daily) to the regimen as long as isoniazid is being taken. Streptomycin should never be given, because it is circulated in the placental blood and is ototoxic to the unborn child.

Antituberculosis Drugs in the Nursing Mother

Rifampicin is present in the nursing mother's milk but is not known to do any harm. Because there are also significant amounts of isoniazid in milk, with a consequent theoretical risk of neurotoxicity, both mother and baby should be given pyridoxine. Very little ethambutol is found in milk, so the risks of ocular toxicity are negligible.

Antituberculosis Drugs in Renal Failure

Streptomycin is excreted almost totally unchanged in the urine. In oliguric patients, its half-life is increased from the normal 2 to 3 hours to between 60 and 70 hours. Isoniazid is metabolized mostly in the liver; less than 25% is excreted unchanged in the urine. In oliguria, its half-life is hardly altered, remaining between 2 and 5 hours. Pyrazinamide has a half-life of 6 hours and is largely metabolized in the liver. Only 4% is excreted unchanged in the urine, and only in very severe renal failure does the dose need to be reduced (Stollmeyer et al, 1968). Ethambutol, like streptomycin, is excreted in the urine, 80% being unchanged. Because of its dose-related toxicity, it should be avoided in all cases of renal failure. In oliguria, its half-life is increased from between 2 and 4 hours to more than 15 hours.

The creatinine clearance (milliliters per minute) is the most accurate way to judge the best dose regimen in the presence of renal failure (Bennett et al, 1977). Table 24–5 shows the recommended doses in the presence of various degrees of renal insufficiency (Blythe, 1979). Streptomycin and ethambutol should never be used in the presence of tuberculous renal failure.

Topical Drugs

Topical agents have only a minor role in the management of genitourinary tuberculosis at the present time. In severe cystitis, a combination of 5% rifampicin and 1% isoniazid made up in normal saline can be used for slow irrigation of the bladder. Lidocaine should be added (10 ml of 1% lidocaine to each 100 ml of solution) because it helps to relieve severe bladder symptoms. If bladder fibrosis has already started, however, lidocaine can have no lasting effect. The same solution can be used to irrigate the pelvis of a kidney after repair of an obstruction at the pelviureteral junction and can be instilled into a closed renal abscess after the contents have been aspirated. A cream of the same combined concentration can be used as a dressing for discharging tuberculous sinuses, especially from the epididymis.

SURGERY

Surgical treatment has undergone many changes in the last 30 years. During recent years, there has been a steady increase in surgical procedures, which coincides with the introduction of short-course chemotherapeutic treatment. Surgery continues to play an important role in the modern philosophy of the management of genitourinary tuberculosis, and more than 80% of patients now require some operative procedure.

Excision of Diseased Tissue

Nephrectomy

The indications for nephrectomy are (1) a nonfunctioning kidney with or without calcification; (2) extensive disease involving the whole kidney, together with hypertension and pelviureteric obstruction; and (3) coexisting renal carcinoma. The last is a rare occurrence; however, if it is suspected, arteriograms should be carried out.

The management of nonfunctioning or severely diseased tuberculous kidneys is indisputable, and nephrectomy is mandatory. Kerr and co-workers (1969, 1970) recommended the removal of diseased organs. Wong and Lan (1980) reported that 89.3% of all nonfunctioning kidneys had been destroyed and required nephrectomy; in only 3 out of 28 cases was reconstruction possible.

It still can be argued that modern effective chemotherapy kills all organisms, apart from persistors; however, no such proof exists, and, in any case, it is never possible to salvage nonfunctioning kidneys. With short-course chemotherapy, it is advisable to remove a large focus and allow the drugs to destroy the residual mycobacteria, but it is also a sound surgical practice to excise a nonfunctioning and potentially dangerous organ. Short-course chemotherapy has altered the philosophy of surgical management of extensive disease of the genitourinary tract, but it is important that these lesions be explored, either to try to restore function or, more likely, to remove irreparable disease.

Flechner and Gow (1980) reviewed 300 cases of genitourinary tuberculosis. There were 73 patients with nonfunctioning or poorly functioning kidneys. In three of the four patients who did not have a nephrectomy, complications, flank sinuses, abscesses, and hypertension developed. Osterhage and co-workers (1980) investigated the activity of *M. tuberculosis* after efficient chemotherapy on the basis of histologic preparations of nephrectomy tissues. Despite sterile urine, 50% of their patients showed active tuberculosis. No cultures of the diseased tissues were taken, so an opinion based on histologic evidence may be suspect. Nevertheless, this is further evidence to support nephrectomy in extensive renal disease in patients undergoing short-course regimens.

Table 24–5. RECOMMENDED DOSES IN THE PRESENCE OF VARIOUS DEGREES OF RENAL INSUFFICIENCY

		Frequency of Administration in Relation to Creatine Clearance (ml/min)			
Drug	**Dose**	*>100 ml/min*	*80–50 ml/min*	*50–10 ml/min*	*<10 ml/min*
Streptomycin	1 g	1 × 24 hr	1 × 48 hr	1 × 72 hr	1 × 96 hr
Isoniazid	300 mg	1 × 24 hr	1 × 24 hr	1 × 36–48 hr	1 × 60–72 hr
Rifampicin	450 mg	1 × 24 hr	1 × 24 hr	1 × 24 hr	1 × 48 hr
Pyrazinamide	25 mg/kg body weight	1 × 24 hr	1 × 24 hr	1 × 24 hr	1 × 48 hr
Ethambutol	25 mg/kg body weight	1 × 24 hr	1 × 24 hr	1 × 48 hr	1 × 72 hr

Ureterectomy

Nephroureterectomy is rarely indicated. It is only required to remove as much as possible of the ureter with the kidney and transfix and ligate the lower end. I have had to reoperate on only one occasion out of more than 400 nephrectomies for removal of the ureter; this case involved a patient in whom a stone had formed. It is a rare complication and not an indication for ureterectomy.

Partial Nephrectomy

Partial nephrectomy is becoming less and less common and is now rarely carried out, because with modern chemotherapy the response of a local lesion in the kidney is rapid and effective. There are only two indications: (1) the localized polar lesion containing calcification that has failed to respond after 6 weeks of intensive chemotherapy, and (2) an area of calcification that is slowly increasing in size and is threatening to gradually destroy the whole kidney. Partial nephrectomy can never be justified in the absence of calcification.

Only a few points in the technique need emphasis. If possible, the artery to the area that is to be resected should be ligated. The capsule should be stripped from the renal cortex so that it can be used for strengthening the suture line in the final closure of the effect. All the vessels in the renal cortex and medulla are carefully and conscientiously ligated independently after being localized by frequent release of the clamp that is controlling the appropriate vessel. The calyces are closed by a continuous catgut or polyglycolic acid (Dexon) suture. The perirenal fat is carefully dissected off the kidney and retained so that it can be stitched over the suture line. The wound should be drained for a few days.

Cavernotomy

Cavernotomy has no place in the modern management of genitourinary tuberculosis because, with modern radiographic techniques, the contents of an abscess can be aspirated under the control of the image intensifier. This is a satisfactory method of treatment and largely obviates surgery. It also allows the instillation of antituberculosis drugs into the cavity and the aspiration of its contents, which can be cultured for viable organisms and from which the quantity of antituberculosis drugs can be estimated. If there is extensive calcification in the wall, a careful radiologic control must be exercised; otherwise, there may be a low but insidious extension that ultimately destroys the kidney. Once this process starts, a partial nephrectomy should be carried out.

Epididymectomy

The incidence of tuberculous epididymitis is declining, but exploration of the scrotum with a view to epididymectomy is still required. The main indication is a caseating abscess that is not responding to chemotherapy. Another indication is a firm swelling that has remained unchanged or has slowly increased in size despite the use of antibiotics and antituberculosis chemotherapy. The author has seen two unsuspected cases of seminoma of the epididymis presenting as tuberculous epididymitis; both patients died within a year (Gow, 1963).

Involvement of the testis is uncommon, and orchidectomy is required in only 5% of cases. Ligation of the contralateral vas is never needed; the author has seen a number of patients who have fathered children after unilateral epididymectomy for tuberculosis. The only serious complication is testicular atrophy, which occurs in 6% of patients. It is always confined to severe cases in which, because of the inflammation surrounding the cord, there is extreme difficulty in dissecting the globus major from the vascular pedicle. Epididymectomy should be performed through a scrotal incision. The globus minor is dissected first, followed by the body of the epididymis, and finally the globus major. The vas is then isolated and brought out in the groin through a separate stab incision to prevent the formation of a subcutaneous abscess.

Reconstructive Surgery

Ureteric Strictures

STRICTURE OF THE URETER. The most common site for tuberculous stricture is the ureterovesical junction; stricture may also occur at the pelviureteric junction and, rarely, in the middle third of the ureter. Very occasionally, it may involve the entire ureter and cause complete stenosis, fibrosis, and even calcification. If the whole ureter is involved, there is invariably extensive disease in the kidney; reconstructive surgery in this type of stricture is impossible.

PELVIURETERIC STRICTURES. Strictures at the level of the pelviureter are very uncommon; the author has seen only eight such cases. The probable explanation is that by the time the patient presents for treatment, the combination of an acute tuberculous infection with an obstruction at the pelviureteral junction has destroyed the greater part of the kidney.

The urologist confronted with genitourinary tuberculosis accompanied by kidney disease in which the kidney is functioning but in which there is pelviureteric obstruction should be prepared to relieve the obstruction at the earliest possible moment. A satisfactory method is to pass a double-J stent from the bladder after dilating the ureter. This stent can remain undisturbed, providing drainage is satisfactory, for up to 2 months or even longer. Sometimes insuperable difficulties are encountered that do not allow this technique. A percutaneous nephrostomy is then indicated, and the pelvis is irrigated with antituberculosis drugs. Progress of the stricture should be monitored by either a weekly ultrasound scan or one 25-minute film intravenous urogram. If the monitoring reveals significant deterioration, immediate surgery is performed. Surgery also may be required after the stent is removed, if an intravenous urogram shows that the pelviureteric obstruction has not improved.

Both the Anderson-Hynes technique and Culp technique give satisfactory results. The anastomosis is made over a silicone rubber (Silastic) stent, which is left in situ for 3 weeks. Pyelostomy is an essential part of the technique in cases in which a previous nephrostomy has not been performed; it not only allows free drainage but also permits instillation of antituberculosis drugs. The pyelostomy tube is clamped off the day after the Silastic stent is removed and is withdrawn after urine is shown to be draining satisfactorily. With this technique and modern chemotherapy, the chances of a secondary nephrectomy are small. A pyelostomy can be performed even in the presence of inflammation. If the inflammation is severe at the time of surgery, however, it is advisable to leave the stent in place for 5 to 6 weeks and to carry out instillation with antituberculosis drugs for a similar period. Very rarely, an intrapelvic stricture involving all the major calyces is present (Fig. 24–15). A reconstruction should be attempted by dissection of the sinus with the Gil-Vernet technique (1965) and restoration of the pelvis by bivalving the ureter and forming an anastomosis with the upper and lower dilated calyces.

STRICTURES OF THE MIDDLE THIRD OF THE URETER. Strictures at this level are very rare. Should they occur, the best method of treatment is by the Davis intubation ureterostomy technique (Davis et al, 1948; Smart, 1961) or by passage of a double-J stent from the bladder, if technically possible. Resolution is contingent on the integrity of some part of the urothelium; if this condition is met, the ureter regenerates around an indwelling tube over a stent or linear incision. The Silastic stent should be left in place for at least 6 weeks and can be brought out either through the skin or through the urethra. A double-J stent is a piece of equipment recommended for this operation. Recurrent stricture, however, is always likely to be a complication; all patients should be followed carefully, and an intravenous urogram should be performed at 3-month intervals for at least 12 months to guard against this serious complication.

STRICTURES OF THE LOWER END OF THE URETER. Strictures of the lower end of the ureter occur in approximately 9% of patients. These can be managed medically or by surgery.

Medical Management

If obstruction at the lower end of the ureter is present at the start of chemotherapy, careful observation is required.

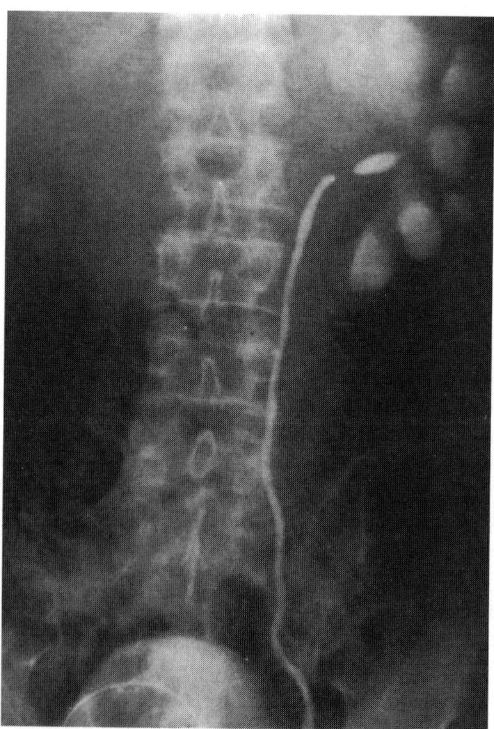

Figure 24–15. Multiple intrapelvic strictures with calyceal dilatation.

It is not necessary, however, to prescribe corticosteroids immediately. A number of these strictures result from edema, and they respond to chemotherapy. A recommended regimen is starting the patient on normal chemotherapy; performing an intravenous urogram, with one radiographic view at 25 minutes; taking a 17- by 14-inch picture at weekly intervals; and noting progress. If there is deterioration or no improvement after 3 weeks, corticosteroids (20 mg three times daily) should be given in addition to the other chemotherapy drugs. This is a large dose of steroids, but, as previously pointed out, rifampicin doubles the excretion of cortisone, and a much larger dose is needed to achieve the desired effect. The same management is continued with the weekly intravenous urogram; if there is deterioration or no improvement after a 6-week period, surgical reimplantation is carried out if an initial attempt at dilation has failed.

Ureteric Dilation

Endoscopic dilation has been referred to by many authors, but few large series of patients have been reviewed. Murphy and co-workers (1982) reported the results of the management of 97 strictures seen in 92 patients over a period of 25 years. Dilation was successful in 51 ureters (64%) and failed to relieve the strictures in 29. Dilation failed in 17 ureters because of technical difficulties. The dilation is performed under general anesthesia by passing either an 8-Fr Braasch catheter or two 5-Fr ureteric catheters up the affected side, or by a balloon catheter. The dilation is repeated every 2 weeks initially, later every 1 to 2 months, until the upper renal tract is stabilized; in Murphy's series, the mean number of dilations per patient was four. In view of the high failure rates and the number of general anesthesias required, this technique is not advocated except in special cases.

Surgical Management

Most ureteric strictures are less than 5 cm in length (Fig. 24–16) and commence in the intermural part of the bladder. The area of fibrosis is localized and, unless a large part of the ureter is involved, it is confined to the intermural part or an area just proximal to it. Above the fibrotic area there is often a dilated segment. Unless the stricture has been present for a considerable period, the muscle improves after the obstruction has been relieved and normal peristalsis recommences. These ureters should be reimplanted into the bladder. A reflux-preventing technique should be employed whenever possible, and for success to be guaranteed a submucous tunnel of at least 5 cm is necessary.

An accurate assessment of the length of the stricture and the function of the ureter is obtained by retrograde ureterography with the use of a bulb catheter, and the peristaltic function of the ureter is observed on an image intensifier. Cystoscopy is essential to study the bladder so that an area free from infection and fibrosis can be chosen for the reimplantation whenever it is necessary. The tuberculous infection is almost always localized to the area around the infected ureteric orifice, and there is no difficulty in reanastomosing the ureter into an area of bladder.

If the stricture is longer than 5 cm, a direct reimplantation cannot be achieved. In these cases, either a psoas hitch (Turner-Warwick, 1965) or a Boari flap procedure (Gow,

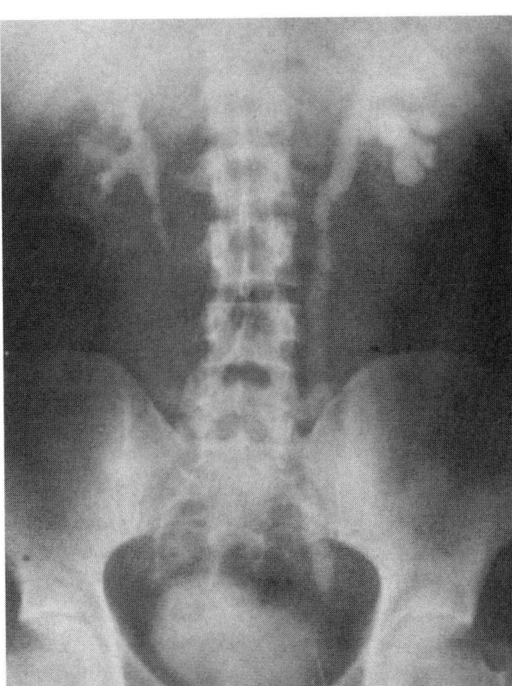

Figure 24–16. Stricture at the lower end of the ureter.

1968) may be necessary. Both give satisfactory results, provided that a reflux-preventing technique is used in the same way as for direct reimplantation. With the use of the latter technique, strictures as long as 14 to 15 cm can be excised and the remaining ureter reimplanted. If Boari's procedure is selected, it is helpful to distend the bladder by running in 200 to 500 ml of saline. In this way, the bladder flap can be accurately delineated and planned. A larger area of the bladder than would seem necessary is required, because there is always considerable contraction of the flap after the bladder is decompressed. The bladder and bladder flap are closed in two layers, and indwelling catheter drainage is maintained for 8 to 10 days. Some urologists advocate use of a stent through the anastomosis to the renal pelvis and out through the urethra. This is not considered necessary, and the author has experienced few complications without this addition to the technique. However, it remains a personal decision.

Two-layer closure is important, the first layer being continuous interlocking suture. Before final closure, the bladder is again distended with fluid so that any leaks can be identified and closed. The bladder flap and ureter are then sutured to the psoas muscle to avoid any kinking at the level of the ureterovesical flap. The wound is closed with drainage down to the anastomosis, which is removed after 4 to 5 days.

Ureteroureterostomy

If an extensive stricture involves one or both ureters, ureteroureterostomy can be performed, and either the longer of the two ureters can be anastomosed into the bladder or a Boari flap can be fashioned using a reflux-preventing technique. If, however, the bladder is diseased, a cutaneous ureterostomy is a suitable procedure. With modern chemotherapy, the risks are negligible.

Augmentation Cystoplasty

The urinary bladder, besides being a contractile organ for expelling urine, is also a reservoir. In determining the appropriate treatment, both of these aspects must be considered. The main symptoms that warrant consideration of an augmentation cystoplasty are an intolerable frequency of micturition, both day and night, together with pain, urgency, and hematuria. An intravenous urogram reveals a small, contracted, hypertonic bladder that normally empties completely. The appearance on cystoscopy is a diffuse velvet inflammation with a capacity of less than 100 ml. A superimposed secondary infection is invariably present in the initial stages. The word *augmentation* must be emphasized. The procedure is not a cystectomy, which should be reserved for carcinoma, interstitial cystitis, or total chemical or physical destruction of the bladder, but a method of increasing the bladder capacity while retaining as much of the bladder as possible. This is important if voiding is to be satisfactory; the average mural pressure of the cecum or colon is only 16 cm of water, which is insufficient force to empty the bladder. Hence, if very little bladder remains, voiding will depend entirely on abdominal pressure (Dounis and Gow, 1979; Gleason et al, 1972).

Many patients show deterioration of renal function caused by either reflux or obstruction. I agree with Kuss and coworkers (1970) that renal failure is no contraindication to surgery and that patients with a creatinine clearance of more than 15 ml/minute should be accepted for augmentation cystoplasty. There are many examples of patients with poor renal function who show marked improvement after this procedure, and the author knows of no case in which the renal function has deteriorated after surgery. Enuresis, incontinence, and psychiatric disturbances are contraindications to this procedure. If surgery is necessary in these cases, a urinary diversion is the only treatment.

The ileum was the first part of the bowel to be used, but the loop method that was employed frequently resulted in loop stagnation and a narrowing of the anastomosis. Even the patch ileocystoplasty advocated by Tasker (1953) failed to overcome all of the problems. The colon was the next part of the gastrointestinal tract to be tried, and even though there is significant ureteric reflux, this procedure still continues to give satisfactory results (Duff et al, 1970). Its advantages are a longer colonic mesentery, safer ureteral surgery, and complete extraperitoneal vesicocolic anastomosis, but it is essential to investigate the colon by a barium enema before surgery to exclude the presence of diverticular disease.

In 1965, Gil-Vernet advocated use of the cecum together with the terminal ileum. The technique using the cecum has certain advantages. Mucus discharge, infection, and residual urine are diminished, and if the urine has to be diverted, reimplantation into the ileum is a safe and reliable procedure, provided that an antireflux procedure, as suggested by Leadbetter (1951), is adopted. Because the ileocecal valve is competent in 80% of patients, the intussusception technique advocated by Hendren (1980) is not recommended. Splitting of the cecum also has disadvantages, because it then becomes a patch that reduces the voiding power of the cecal implant. Both colocystoplasty and cecocystoplasty are satisfactory methods, and the choice of the segment of bowel has not influenced the long-term results (Smith et al, 1977). The main advantage of the cecum is in reimplantation of the ureters, because the ileum can be used and reflux can more easily be prevented. In addition, there is no fashioning of the bowel, it is easily rotated, it is isoperistaltic, and there is very little absorption of solutes (Dounis et al, 1980).

All patients should have at least 4 weeks of extensive chemotherapy before surgery. Measurements of urethral flow rate are also an essential part of the preoperative preparation. A reduced flow rate in the female patient is treated by bladder neck dilatation, with incisions at the 3 o'clock and 9 o'clock positions, using the Otis urethrotome. In the male, either a transurethral resection or a bladder neck incision is performed. Either procedure should be performed 3 weeks before the augmentation. There is a fine line between retention and incontinence, and precise accuracy is difficult to achieve. Therefore, the resection must be carefully performed, and it may have to be repeated. It is better to repeat the procedure once, or even twice, rather than to have an incontinent patient. The Y-V-plasty suggested by Chan and associates (1980) is not recommended because it increases the risk of incontinence.

Certain aspects of the technique are worth emphasizing. A good bowel preparation is important. A combination of oral neomycin (1 g three times daily) and metronidazole (200 mg three times daily) for 48 hours before surgery, with a retention enema of 500 ml of povidone-iodine (5%) after a colonic washout, has given excellent results.

If a ureteroileal anastomosis is indicated, it should be performed before the vesicocolic anastomosis; otherwise, the technical difficulties may be insuperable. As little of the bladder as possible should be resected. Inflammation of the bladder is no contraindication to surgery, but a two-layer closure and the routine use of the omentum wrapped around the anastomosis reduce the complications. Gentamicin (160 mg intravenously) is given just before the bowel is resected.

Lower urinary tract infection is occasionally seen as a postoperative complication. It is often symptomless and difficult to eradicate, so that low-dose antibiotics taken continuously for 6 months or longer may be required.

Occasionally, patients present with a long-standing urinary diversion and wonder whether the normal anatomy can be restored. It may be possible, but a careful study of the defunctioned bladder is necessary to ensure that the disease is quiescent, that there is no bladder outlet obstruction, and that there is adequate detrusor activity. For this purpose, a full urodynamic profile is necessary.

The gastrocystoplasty, as advocated by Leong (1978), is a technique that requires further evaluation and a prolonged follow-up before it can be considered as an alternative to the proven methods. It has not proved to be any better than colocystoplasty or caecocystoplasty.

Urinary Diversion in Tuberculosis

Although in previous years urinary diversion was an accepted method of treatment in a few isolated cases, it is now rarely necessary. There are only three indications for permanent urinary diversion: (1) a history of psychiatric disturbance or obvious subnormal intelligence, (2) enuresis, and (3) intolerable diurnal symptoms with incontinence that has not responded to chemotherapy or bladder dilatation. Ileal or colonic conduits are both satisfactory methods.

Ureterosigmoid anastomosis is not recommended, because incontinence often occurs. The patient's control of fluid in the rectum should be determined before this procedure is carried out. Two hundred fifty milliliters of normal saline solution is run into the rectum, and the patient is asked to retain the fluid while ambulant for as long as possible. Unless there is complete control for more than 2 hours, ureterosigmoid anastomosis is contraindicated.

REFERENCES

Agarwalla B, Mohanty GP, Sahu LK, Rath RC: Tuberculosis of the penis: Report of two cases. J Urol 1980; 124:927.

Antonio D, Gow JG: Renal calcification in genitourinary tuberculosis: A clinical study. Int Urol Nephrol 1975; 7:289.

Barksdale L, Kim KS: Mycobacterium. Bacteriol Rev 1977; 41:217.

Baron ON, Bell JL: Serum enzyme changes in patients receiving antituberculous therapy with rifampicin or p-aminosalicylic acid plus isoniazid and streptomycin. Tubercle 1974; 55:115.

Baskin LS, Mee S: Tuberculosis of the penis presenting as a subcutaneous nodule. J Urol 1989; 141:1430.

Bennett WM, Singer I, Golper T, et al: Guidelines for drug therapy in renal failure. Ann Intern Med 1977; 86:754.

Bjornesjo KB: Tuberculostatic factor in normal human urine. Am Rev Tuberc Pulm Dis 1956; 73:967.

Block AB, Snider DE: Current impact of AIDs on tuberculosis in the United States. Am Rev Respir Dis 1990; (Suppl 2):A260.

Blythe WB: The management of intercurrent medical and surgical problems in the patient with chronic renal failure. *In* Earley LE, Gottschalk CW, eds: Strauss and Welt's Diseases of the Kidney, 3rd ed. Boston, Little, Brown and Company, 1979, p 523.

Braasch WF, Walters W, Hammer HJ: Hypertension and the surgical kidney. JAMA 1940; 115:1837.

British Medical Research Council: Co-operative controlled trial of standard regimen of streptomycin, P.A.S. and isoniazid and three alternative regimens of chemotherapy in Britain. Tubercle 1973; 54:99.

British Thoracic Association: Short course therapy in pulmonary tuberculosis. Lancet 1980; 1:1182.

Calmette A, Guérin C: Essai de premunition par le B.C.G. contra l'infection tuberculeuse de l'homme et des animaux. Presse Med 1925; 33:825.

Centers for Disease Control: Tuberculosis and AIDs: Connecticut. MMWR Morb Mortal Wkly Rep 1987; 36:133–135.

Chan SL, Ankerman GJ, Wright JE, et al: Caecocystoplasty in the surgical management of the small contracted bladder. J Urol 1980; 124:338.

Chen W: Hong Kong Chest Services, British Medical Research Council controlled trial of four three-times weekly regimens and a daily regimen all given for six months for pulmonary tuberculosis. 12th International Congress of Chemotherapy, Florence, 1981.

Cohnheim J: Die Tuberkulose von Standpunkte der Infectionskchre, Leipzig, 1879.

Colby GH: Tuberculous infections and inflammations of the urinary tract. *In* Campbell M, ed: Textbook of Urology, Vol I. Philadelphia, W. B. Saunders Company, 1954, p 525.

Coulaud MD: Etude experimentale de la tuberculose renale du lapin. J Urol (Paris) 1935; 39:572.

Davies PDO: Tuberculosis epidemiology and treatment. Hosp Update, p 777, August 1980.

Davis DM, Strong GH, Drake WM: Intubated ureterostomy: Experimental work and clinical results. J Urol 1948; 59:851.

Dickinson JM, Mitchison DA: Experimental models to explain the high sterilising activity of rifampicin in the chemotherapy of tuberculosis. Am Rev Respir Dis 1981; 123:367.

Dounis A, Gow JG: Bladder augmentation: A long term review. Br J Urol 1979; 51:264.

Duff FA, O'Grady JF, Kelly DJ: Colocystoplasty. Br J Urol 1970; 42:704.

Ekehorn G: Die Ausbreitumgswerse der Nieren tuberkulose in der tuberkulosen Niere. Folia Urol 1908; 2:412.

Elland GA: Absorption metabolism and excretion of pyrazinamide in man. Tubercle 1969; 50:144.

Farga V: The avenues of the Union. (Editorial.) Bull Int Union Tuberc 1972; 47:49.

Fellander M, Hiertoun T, Wallmark G: Studies on the concentration of streptomycin in the treatment of bone and joint tuberculosis. Acta Tuberc Scand 1952; 27:176.

Fine PEM: The B.C.G. story: Lessons from the past and implications for the future. Rev Infect Dis 1989; 11(Suppl 2):353.

Flechner SM, Gow JG: Role of nephrectomy in the treatment of non-functioning or very poorly functioning unilateral tuberculous kidney. J Urol 1980; 123:822.

Flick LF: Development of Our Knowledge of Tuberculosis. Lancaster, Pennsylvania, Wickersham Printing Company, 1925.

Fox W: The current status of short course chemotherapy. Bull Int Union Tuberc 1978; 53:268.

Fox W: Short course chemotherapy for tuberculosis. *In* Flenley DC, ed: Recent Advances in Respiratory Medicine, 2nd ed. Edinburgh, Churchill Livingstone, 1980, p 183.

Fox W: Whither short course chemotherapy. Br J Dis Chest, 1981; 75:331.

Freedman LR: *In* Earley LE, Gottschalk CW, eds: Strauss and Welt's Diseases of the Kidney, 3rd ed. Boston, Little, Brown and Company, 1979, p 859.

Frieden TR, Sterling T, Pablo-Mendez A, et al: The emergence of drug-resistant tuberculosis in New York City. N Engl J Med 1993; 328:521–526.

Gil-Vernet JM Jr: The ileocolic segment in urological surgery. J Urol 1965; 94:418.

Girling DJ: Hong Kong Chest Service/Tuberculosis Research Centre, Madras/British Medical Research Council Study of three-month and two-month regimens for smear-negative pulmonary tuberculosis. 12th International Congress of Chemotherapy. Florence, World Health Organization, 1981.

Girling DJ: Adverse effects of anti-tuberculous drugs. Drugs 1982; 23:56.

Gleason MD, Gittes RF, Bottaccini MR, Byrne JC: Energy balance of voiding after caecal cystoplasty. J Urol 1972; 108:259.

Goldblatt H, Lynch J, Hanzal RF, Summerville WW: Studies on experimental hypertension. J Exp Med 1934; 59:347.

Gow JG: Carcinoma of the epididymis. Urologia 1957; 24:594.

Gow JG: Seminoma of the epididymis. Urologia 1963; 30:589.

Gow JG: Renal calcification in genito-urinary tuberculosis. Br J Surg 1965; 52:283.

Gow JG: The results of the reimplantation of the ureter by the Boari technique. Proc R Soc Med 1968; 61:128.

Gow JG: Genito-urinary tuberculosis. *In* Blandy JP, ed: Urology. Oxford, Blackwell Scientific Publications, 1976.

Grange JM: Mycobacterial Disease, 1st ed. London, Edward Arnold, 1980, p 32.

Grange JM: The Mystery of the Mycobacterial Persistor. Tuber Lung Dis 1991; 73:249–251.

Grange JM, Stanford MD: Dogma and innovation in the global control of tuberculosis: Discussion paper. J R Soc Med 1994; 87:272–275.

Grange JM, Stanford JL, Rook JAW, et al. Tuberculosis and HIV: Light After Darkness. Thorax 1994; 49:537–539.

Grosset J: The sterilising value of rifampicin and pyrazinamide in experimental short-course chemotherapy. Tubercle 1978; 59:287.

Hartman GW, Segura JW, Hatter RR: *In* Witten DM, Myers GH, Utz DC, eds: Emmett's Clinical Urography, 4th ed. Philadelphia, W. B. Saunders Company, 1977, pp 898–921.

Hartmann G, Honikel KO, Knusel F, Nuesch J: The specific inhibition of the D.N.A.-directed R.N.A. synthesis b rifampicin. Biochem Biophys Acta 1967; 145:843.

Hendren WH: Re-operative ureteral reimplantation: Management of the difficult case. J Pediatr Surg 1980; 15:770.

Hepper NCG, Karlson AG, Learly FJ, Soule EH: Genito-urinary infection due to *Mycobacterium kansasii*. Mayo Clin Proc 1971; 46:387.

Hill JD, Stevenson DK: Tuberculosis in unvaccinated children, adolescents and young adults: A city epidemic. Br Med J 1983; 286:1471.

Hong Kong Chest Service, British Medical Research Council: Controlled trial of four thrice-weekly regimens and a daily regimen all given for six months for pulmonary tuberculosis. Lancet 1981; 1:171.

Hong Kong Chest Service, Tuberculosis Research Centre, Madras, and British Medical Research Council: A controlled trial of 3-month, 4-month and 6-month regimens of chemotherapy for sputum-smear-negative pulmonary tuberculosis. Am Rev Respir Dis 1989; 139:871–876.

Howell F, O'Laoide B, Kelly P, et al: Short course chemotherapy for pulmonary tuberculosis. Ir Med J 1989; 821:11–13.

Hsiung JC, Miao TC, Che'n CC: An investigation into hypertension due to renal tuberculosis. Chin Med J (Engl) 1965; 84:327.

Innes JA: Non-respiratory tuberculosis. J R Coll Physicians Lond 1981; 15:227.

Israili ZH, Rogers CM, El-Atlar H: Pharmacokinetics of anti-tuberculous drugs in patients. J Clin Pharmacol 1987; 27:78–83.

Jenkins DE, Wolinsky E: *In* Baum GR, ed: Textbook of Pulmonary Diseases. Boston, Little, Brown and Company, 1965, p 257.

Jindani A, Aber VR, Edwards EA, Mitchison DA: The early bacteriocidal activity of drugs in patients with pulmonary tuberculosis. Am Rev Respir Dis 1980; 121:939.

Kato T: A case of tuberculosis of the tunica vaginalis propria testis associated with hydrocele. Acta Urol Jpn 1970; 16:597.

Kerr WK, Gale GL, Peterson KSS: Reconstructive surgery for genito-urinary tuberculosis. J Urol 1969; 101:254.

Kerr WK, Gale GL, Struthers NW, et al: Prognosis in reconstructive surgery for urinary tuberculosis. Br J Urol 1970; 42:672.

Koch A, 1991. The global tuberculosis situation and the new control strategy of the World Health Organization. Tubercle 1991; 72:1–6.

Koch R: Die atilogie der Tuberkulose. Berl Klin Wochenschr 1882; 15:221.

Kretschmer HL: Tuberculosis of the epididymis. Surg Gynecol Obstet 1928; 47:652.

Kucers A, Bennett NMcK: The Rise of Antibiotics. London, William Heinemann Medical Books, 1979, p 805.

Kunin GM, Brandt D, Wood H: Bacteriologic structures of rifampicin, a new semi-synthetic antibiotic. J Infect Dis 1969; 119:132.

Kuss R, Bilker M, Camey M, et al: Indications and early and late results of intestinocystoplasty: A review of 185 cases. J Urol 1970; 103:53.

Lal MM, Sekhon GS, Dhall JC: Tuberculosis of the penis. J Indian Med Assoc 1971; 56:316.

Lane DJ: Extrapulmonary tuberculosis. Med Int 1982; 1:983.

Lattimer JK, Colmore HP, Sanger IS, et al: Transmission of genital tuberculosis from husband to wife via the semen. Annu Rev Tuberc 1954; 69:618–624.

Lattimer JK, Wechsler M: Genito-urinary tuberculosis. *In* Harrison JH, Gittes RF, Perlmutter AD, et al, eds: Campbell's Urology, 4th ed, Vol I. Philadelphia, W. B. Saunders Company, 1978.

Leadbetter WF: Consideration of problems incident to performance of uretero-enterostomy: Report of a technique. J Urol 1951; 65:818.

Lee LW, Burgler LW, Price EB, Cassidy E: Granulomatous prostatitis: Association isolation of *Mycobacerium fortuitum*, JAMA 1977; 237:2408.

Leong CH: Use of the stomach for bladder replacement and urinary diversion. Ann R Coll Surg Engl 1978; 60:283.

Lewis EL: Tuberculosis of the penis: A report of 5 new cases and a complete review of the literature. J Urol 1946; 56:737.

Lowell AN: Tuberculosis in the World. Publication No. CDC76-8317. Washington DC, US Department of Health, Education and Welfare, Public Health Service, Centers for Disease Control, 1976.

Luzzatto L, Apirian D, Schlessinger D: Mechanism of action of streptomycin, in *E. coli*: Interruption of the ribosome cycle at the initiation of protein synthesis. Proc Natl Acad Sci USA 1968; 60:873.

Macmillan EW: Blood supply of the epididymis in man. Br J Urol 1954; 26:60.

Marks J: Ending the routine guinea pig test. Tubercle 1972; 53:31.

Marks LS, Pontasse EF: Hypertension from renal tuberculosis: Operative cure predicted by renal vein renin. J Urol 1973; 109:149.

Marszalak WW, Dhia A: Genito-urinary tuberculosis. S Afr Med J 1982; 62:158.

McAllister WAC, Thompson PJ, Al-Habet SM, et al: Rifampicin reduces effectiveness and bioavailability of prednisolone. Br Med J 1983; 286:923.

McLeod MN, Hay D, Steward SM: The use of pyrazinamide plus isoniazid in the treatment of pulmonary tuberculosis. Tubercle 1959; 40:14.

Medlar EM: Cases of renal infection in pulmonary tuberculosis: Evidence of healed tuberculous lesions. Am J Pathol 1926; 2:401.

Medlar EM, Spain DM, Holliday RW: Post-mortem compared with clinical diagnosis of genito-urinary tuberculosis in adult males. J Urol 1949; 61:1078.

Mehrotra ML, Gautam KD, Chaube CK: Shortest possible acceptable effective ambulatory chemotherapy in pulmonary tuberculosis: Preliminary report. Am Rev Respir Dis 1981; 124:239.

Mitchell JR, Zimmerman HJ, Ishak KG, et al: Isoniazid, clinical spectrum, pathology and probable pathogenesis. Ann Intern Med 1976; 84:181.

Mitchison DA: Treatment of tuberculosis. J R Coll Phys Lond 1980; 14:91.

Morse D, Brothwell DR, Ucko PJ: Tuberculosis in ancient Egypt. Am Rev Respir Dis 1964; 90:524.

Murphy DM, Fallon B, Lane V, O'Flynn JD: Tuberculous stricture of ureter. Urology 1982; 20:382.

Myers JA: Chemotherapy in tuberculosis. (Editorial.) Dis Chest 1952; 22:598.

Narayana AS, Kelly DG, Duff FA: Tuberculosis of the penis. Br J Urol 1976; 48:274.

Nesbit RM, Ratliff RK: Hypertension associated with unilateral nephropathy. J Urol 1940; 43:427.

Osterhage HR, Fischer V, Hanbensak K: Positive histological tuberculous findings, despite stable sterility of the urine on culture. Eur Urol 1980; 6:116.

Pallen M: The inoculation of tissue specimens into guinea pigs in suspected cases of mycobacterial infection: Does it aid diagnosis and treatment. Tubercle 1987; 68:51–58.

Patoir G, Spy E, Cordier R: Trois cas de fistules vesico ou urethro-rectales tuberculeuses. J Urol Nephrol 1969; 75:210.

Pergament M, Gonzales R, Fraley EE: Atypical mycobacteriosis of the urinary tract: A case report of extensive disease caused by the Battey bacillus. JAMA 1974; 229:816.

Premkumar A, Newhouse J: Seminal vesicle tuberculosis: CT appearance. J Comput Assist Tomogr 1988; 12:676–677.

Ramesh V, Vasanthi R: Tuberculous cavernositis of the penis. Genitourin Med 1989; 65:58.

Rieder HL, Cauthen GM, Kelly GD, et al: Tuberculosis in the United States. JAMA 1989; 262:385–389.

Riehle RA, Jayavaman K: Tuberculosis of the testis. Urology 1982; 20:43.

Reimer D, Nocke-Finck L, Breuer H: Rifampicin and "pill" do not go well together. JAMA 1974; 227:608.

Ross JC, Gow JG, St Hill CA: Tuberculous epididymitis. Br J Urol 1961; 48:663.

Salfinger M, Pfyffer GE. The new diagnostic mycobacteriology laboratory. Eur J Clin Microbiol Infect Dis 1994; 13:961–979.

Schwartz DT, Lattimer JK: Incidence of arterial hypertension in 540 patients with renal tuberculosis. J Urol 1967; 98:651.

Sherwood T: Uroradiology. Oxford, Blackwell Scientific Publications, 1980.

Singapore Tuberculosis Service and British Medical Research Council: Five year follow-up of a clinical trial of 3 and 6 month regimes of chemotherapy, given intermittently in the continuation phase in the treatment of pulmonary tuberculosis. Am Rev Respir Dis 1988; 137:1147–1150.

Smart RW: An evaluation of intubation ureterotomy, with a description of surgical technique. J Urol 1961; 85:512.

Smith HW: Unilateral nephrectomy in hypertensive disease. J Urol 1956; 76:685.

Smith RB, Van Cangh P, Skinner DG, et al: Augmentation enterocystoplasty: A critical review. J Urol 1977; 118:35.

Smith T: A comparative study of bovine tubercle bacilli and of tubercle bacilli from sputum. J Exper Med 1898; 3:451.

Snider DR Jr, Caras GJ, Koplan JP: Preventive therapy with isoniazid: Cost-effectiveness of different methods of therapy. JAMA 1986; 255:1579–1583.

Snider DE Jr, Layde PM, Johnson MW, Lyle HA: Treatment of tuberculosis during pregnancy. Am Rev Respir Dis 1980; 122:65.

Sporer A, Auerback MD: Tuberculosis of the prostate. Urology 1978; 11:362.

Stanford JL, Bahr GM, Rook GAW, et al: Immunotherapy with *Mycobacterium vaccae* as an adjunct to chemotherapy in the treatment of pulmonary tuberculosis. Tubercle 1990; 71:87–93.

Stanford JL, Grange JM: The meaning and structure of species as applied to mycobacteria. Tubercle 1974; 55:143–152.

Stanford JL, Grange JM: New concepts for the control of tuberculosis in the twenty-first century. J R Coll Phys London 1993; 27:218–223.

Stanford J, Shield M, Rook G: How environmental mycobacteria may predetermine the protective efficacy of B.C.G. Tubercle 1981; 62:55.

Stollmeyer KD, Bean RE, Kubica GP: The absorption and excretion of pyrazinamide. Am Rev Respir Dis 1968; 98:70.

Styblo K: Recent advances in epidemiological research in tuberculosis. Adv Tuberc Res 1980; 20:1.

Styblo K: Overview and epidemiologic assessment of the current global tuberculosis situation with an emphasis on control in developing countries. Rev Infect Dis 1989; 2:(Suppl 2):S339–346.

Sutherland AM, Glen ES, MacFarlane JR: Transmission of genitourinary tuberculosis. Health Bull 1982; 40:2.

Sutherland I: Recent studies in the epidemiology of tuberculosis based on the risk of being infected by the tubercle bacillus. Adv Tuberc Res 1976; 19:1.

Sutherland I, Styblo K, Sampalik M, Bleiker MA: Annual risk of tuberculous infection in 4 countries, derived from the results of tuberculosis surveys in 1948–1952. Bull Int Union Tuberc Lung Dis 1971; 47:123.

Symes JM, Blandy JP: Tuberculosis of the male urethra. Br J Urol 1973; 45:432.

Tasker JH: Ileocystoplasty: A new technique. Experimental study with the report of a case. Br J Urol 1953; 25:349.

Ten Dam H, Hitze K: Does B.C.G. vaccination protect the newborn and your infants? Bull World Health Organ 1980; 58:37.

Ten Dam H, Tounan K, Hitze K, Guld J: Present knowledge of immunisation against tuberculosis. Bull World Health Organ 1976; 54:255.

Tripathy RC: Tuberculosis Chemotherapy Centre. Madras study of short course chemotherapy in pulmonary tuberculosis. Proceedings of the XXIVth World Conference of the International Union Against Tuberculosis, Brussels, September 5–9, 1978.

Turner-Warwick RT: The Psoas Hitch Procedure. (Film). London, Institute of Urology, 1965.

Umeki S: Adverse effects of antituberculous drugs and the significance of the measurement of the drug stimulating lymphocytic transformation rate. Jpn J Med Sci Biol 1989; 28:335–340.

Ustvedt HJ: The relation between renal tuberculosis and primary infection. Tubercle 1947; 28:22.

Veukataramaiah NR, Van Raalte JA, Dutla SN: Tuberculous ulcer of the penis. Postgrad Med J 1982; 50:59.

Villemin JA: *In* Tuberculosis in History. London: Baillière Tindall, 1949, p 139.

Wildbolz H: Ueber urogenical tuberkulose. Schweiz Med Wochenschr 1937; 67:1125.

Wimpenny JWT: Effect of isoniazid on biosynthesis on *Mycobacterium tuberculosis* var. *bovis* B.C.G. J Gen Microbiol 1967; 47:379.

Wiseman R: A Treatise of the Kings-Evil: Eight Chirurgical Treatises, 3rd ed. London, Tooke and Meredith, 1696.

Wolinsky E: Non-tuberculous mycobacteria and associated diseases. Am Rev Respir Dis 1979; 119:107.

Wong SH, Lan WY: The surgical management of non-functioning tuberculous kidneys. J Urol 1980; 124:187.

Woods LE, Butler VB, Pollak A: Human infection with the yellow acid fast bacillus: A report of fifteen additional cases. Am Rev Tuberc 1956; 73:917.

World Health Organization: The WHO-Assisted Tuberculosis Control Programme in Lesotho: Epidemiological Findings and an Evaluation of Two Different Case Finding Programmes. Nairobi, World Health Organization, 1969.

World Health Organization: Magnitude of the tuberculosis problem of the world. Wkly Epidemiol Rec 1981; 50:393.

Youmans GP, Paterson PY, Sommers HM: The Biological and Clinical Basis of Infectious Diseases. Philadelphia, W. B. Saunders Company, 1975, p 347.

Yu HHY, Wong KK, Lim TK, Leong CH: Clinical study of hemospermia. Urology 1977; 10:562.

V
URINE TRANSPORT AND VOIDING FUNCTION AND DYSFUNCTION

25
PHYSIOLOGY AND PHARMACOLOGY OF THE RENAL PELVIS AND URETER

Robert M. Weiss, M.D.

The function of the ureter is to transport urine from the kidney to the bladder. Under normal conditions, ureteral peristalsis originates with electrical activity at pacemaker sites located in the proximal portion of the urinary collecting system (Bozler, 1942; Constantinou, 1974; Gosling and Dixon, 1974; Shiratori and Kinoshita, 1961a; Tsuchida and Yamaguchi, 1977; Weiss et al, 1967). The electrical activity is then propagated distally and gives rise to the mechanical event of peristalsis, ureteral contraction, which propels the bolus of urine distally. Efficient propulsion of the urinary bolus is dependent on the ureter's ability to completely coapt its walls (Woodburne and Lapides, 1972). Urine passes into the bladder by means of the ureterovesical junction (UVJ), which under normal conditions permits urine to pass from the ureter into the bladder but not from the bladder into the ureter.

CELLULAR ANATOMY

The primary functional anatomic unit of the ureter is the ureteral smooth muscle cell. The cell is extremely small, approximately 250 to 400 μ in length and 5 to 7 μ in diameter. The *nucleus*, which is separated from the remainder of the cell by a nuclear membrane, is ellipsoid in shape and contains a dark-staining body, the *nucleolus*, and the genetic material of the cell. Surrounding the nucleus is the *cytoplasm* or *sarcoplasm*, which contains the structures involved in cell function. Frequently in close relation to the nucleus, *mitochondria* in the cytoplasm perform many of the nutritive functions of the cell.

Dispersed in the sarcoplasm are the contractile proteins *actin* and *myosin*. Depending on the local calcium (Ca^{2+}) concentration, they interact to produce contraction or relaxation. Any process that leads to an increase in the Ca^{2+} concentration in the region of the contractile proteins results in *contraction*; conversely, any process that decreases the Ca^{2+} concentration in the region of the contractile proteins results in *relaxation*. The actin is dispersed throughout the sarcoplasm in hexagonal clumps and is interspersed with the less numerous clumps of the more deeply staining myosin. Dark bands along the cell surface are referred to as attachment plaques. Along with dense bodies dispersed in the cytoplasm, they serve as attachment devices for the actin.

Around the periphery of the cell are numerous cavitary structures, some of which open to the outside of the cell, referred to as *caveolae* or pinocytic vesicles. Their exact function is not known, although they may serve a role in the nutritive functions of the cell or in the transport of ions across the cell membrane. A double-layer cell membrane surrounds the cell. The *inner plasma membrane* surrounds the entire cell, but the *outer basement membrane* is absent at areas of close cell-to-cell contact, referred to as *intermediate junctions*.

A

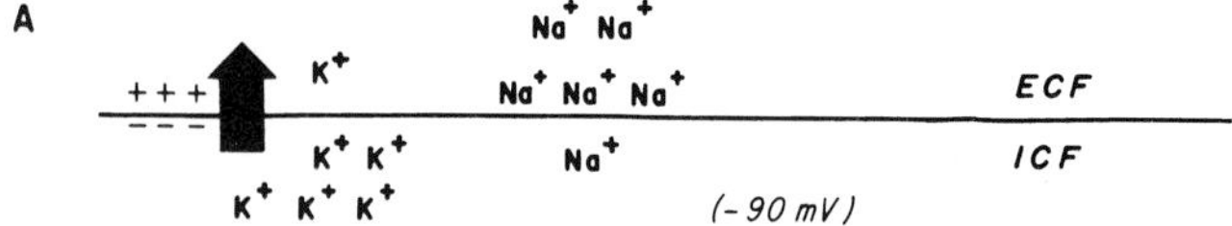

B

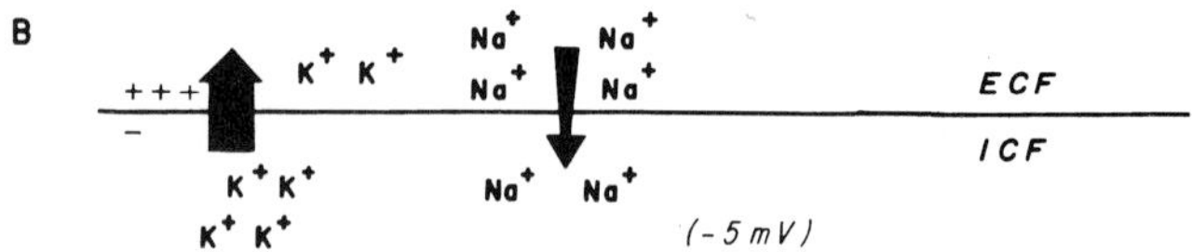

C

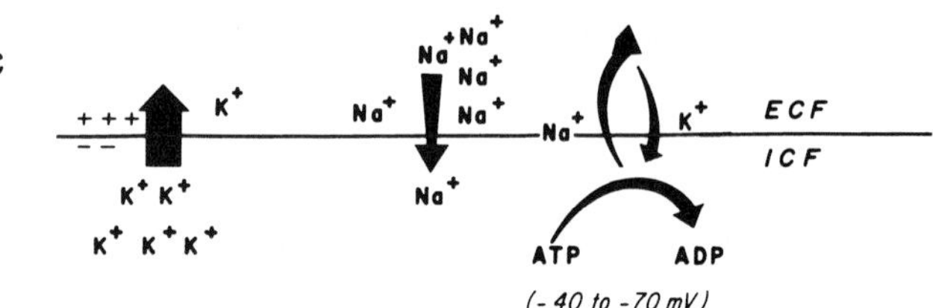

Figure 25–1. Ionic basis for resting membrane potential (RMP) in smooth muscle. In resting state, the concentration of potassium is greater on the inside than on the outside of the cell ($[K^+]_i > [K^+]_o$), whereas the opposite is true for sodium ($[Na^+]_o > [Na^+]_i$). *A,* Electrochemical changes that would occur if the membrane were permeable solely to K^+. K^+ would diffuse from the inside of the cell, where it is more concentrated, to the outside of the cell, where it is less concentrated. The outward movement of the positively charged K^+ ions would make the inside of the cell membrane negative with respect to the outside of the cell membrane. *B,* Electrochemical changes that would occur if the resting membrane were also permeable to Na^+. An inward movement of Na^+ along its concentration gradient would make the inside of the cell membrane less negative with respect to the outside of the cell membrane than is depicted in *A. C,* Pump mechanism for extruding Na^+ from within the cell against a concentration and electrochemical gradient. Inward movement of K^+ is coupled with an outward movement of Na^+. This mechanism helps to maintain a steady state of ion distribution across the cell membrane and a stable RMP. ECF, extracellular fluid; ICF, intracellular fluid. (From Weiss RM: Urology 1978; 12:114, with permission.)

ELECTRICAL ACTIVITY

The electrical properties of all excitable tissues depend on the distribution of ions on both the inside and the outside of the cell membrane and on the relative permeability of the cell membrane to these ions (Hodgkin, 1958). The ionic basis for electrical activity in ureteral smooth muscle has not been fully described; however, many of its properties resemble those in other excitable tissues.

Resting Potential

When a ureteral muscle cell is in a nonexcited or resting state, the electrical potential difference across the cell membrane, the transmembrane potential, is referred to as the *resting membrane potential (RMP)*. The RMP is determined primarily by the distribution of *potassium ions* (K^+) across the cell membrane and by the permeability of the membrane to potassium (Bennett and Burnstock, 1966; Hendrickx et al, 1975; Washizu, 1966). In the resting state, the potassium concentration on the inside of the cell is greater than that on the outside of the cell, $[K^+]_i > [K^+]_o$, and the membrane is preferentially permeable to potassium. Because of the tendency for the positively charged K^+ ions to diffuse from the inside of the cell, where they are more concentrated, to the outside of the cell, where they are less concentrated, an electrical gradient is created, with the inside of the cell membrane being more negative than the outside (Fig. 25–1*A*). The electrical gradient that is formed tends to oppose the further movement of K^+ ions outward across the cell membrane along its concentration gradient, and an equilibrium is reached. There is a greater concentration of K^+ on the inside of the membrane than on the outside, and the inside of the cell membrane is negative with respect to the outside of the cell membrane.

If the membrane in the resting state were permeable exclusively to K^+, the measured RMP of the ureteral smooth muscle cell would approximate -90 mV, the potassium equilibrium potential, as predicted by the *Nernst equation*:

$$E_k = -RT/nF\ (ln\ [K^+]_i/[K^+]_o)$$

where E_k is the potential difference attributable to the concentration difference of K^+ across the cell membrane; R is the molar gas constant; T is the absolute temperature; n is the number of moles; F is the Faraday constant; *ln* is the natural logarithm; and $[K^+]_i$ and $[K^+]_o$ are the potassium concentrations inside and outside of the cell, respectively (Nernst, 1908). However, in the ureter and in other smooth muscles, the *RMP* is considerably less than the potassium equilibrium potential, with values of *−33 to −70 mV*, the inside of the cell being negative with respect to the outside (Kobayashi, 1969; Kuriyama et al 1967; Washizu, 1966).

Studies from single isolated ureteral cells show spontaneous transient hyperpolarizations with the RMP transiently becoming more negative (Imaizumi et al, 1989). This phenomenon appears to be caused by spontaneous release of Ca^{2+} from the sarcoplasmic reticulum (SR) and activation of Ca^{2+}-dependent K^+ channels. Although the low resting potential of ureteral cells may be explained in part by a relatively small resting K^+ conductance (Imaizumi et al, 1989), it also may result from the contribution of other ions.

One such ion that could account for the relatively low RMP of the ureter and other smooth muscles is sodium (Na^+) (Kuriyama, 1963). In the resting state, the sodium concentration on the outside of the cell membrane is greater than that on the inside, $[Na^+]_o > [Na^+]_i$. If the resting membrane were somewhat permeable to Na^+, both the concentration and the electrical gradient would support an inward movement of sodium across the cell membrane, with a resultant decrease in the electronegativity of the inner surface of the cell membrane (see Fig. 25–1*B*).

If such an inward movement of Na^+ were to go unchecked, the RMP would decrease to a level lower than that actually observed, and the concentration gradient for Na^+ might become reversed. In order to maintain a steady-state ion distribution across the cell membrane with $[K^+]_o < [K^+]_i$ and $[Na^+]_o > [Na^+]_i$ and to prevent the transmembrane potential from becoming lower than the measured ureteral RMP, an active mechanism capable of extruding sodium from within the cell against a concentration and electrochemical gradient is required (see Fig. 25–1*C*). Such an outward Na^+ pump that is coupled with an inward movement of K^+ derives its energy requirements from the dephosphorylation of adenosine triphosphate (ATP) (Casteels, 1970). The presence of a Na^+ pump with characteristics of Na-K-ATPase has been demonstrated in numerous smooth muscles (Widdicombe, 1981). Na^+–Ca^{2+} exchange may also play a role in Na^+ extrusion, especially when the Na^+ pump is inhibited (Aickin, 1987; Aickin et al, 1987).

The dynamic processes illustrated in Figure 25–1 enable the ureter in its resting state to maintain a relatively low RMP. In addition to the mechanisms described, the distribution of chloride (Cl^-) ions across the cell membrane and the relative permeability of the membrane to Cl^- may be factors in the maintenance of the RMP in the ureter and other smooth muscles (Kuriyama, 1963; Washizu, 1966).

Action Potential

The transmembrane potential of an inactive or resting ureteral cell remains stable until it is excited by an external stimulus—electrical, mechanical (stretch), or chemical—or by conduction of electrical activity (*action potential*) from an already excited adjacent cell. When a ureteral cell is stimulated, *depolarization* occurs, with the inside of the cell membrane becoming less negative than it was before stimulation. If a sufficient area of the cell membrane is depolarized rapidly enough to reach a critical level of transmembrane potential, referred to as the *threshold potential*, a regenerative depolarization, or action potential, is initiated.

The changes that occur are diagrammatically depicted in Figure 25–2. If the stimulus is very weak, as shown by arrow *a*, the transmembrane potential may remain unchanged. A

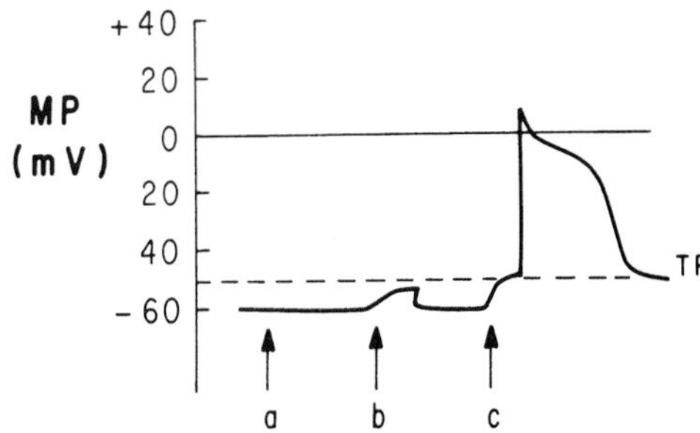

Figure 25–2. Response of ureteral transmembrane potential to stimuli. At arrow *a,* weak stimulus is applied that does not alter the resting membrane potential (RMP). At arrow *b,* subthreshold stimulus is applied, which decreases transmembrane potential but not to the level of the threshold potential (TP; *dashed line*). At arrow *c,* suprathreshold stimulus is applied, which decreases the transmembrane potential to TP and an action potential is initiated. (From Weiss RM: Urology 1978; 12:114, with permission.)

slightly stronger but yet subthreshold stimulus may result in an abortive displacement of the transmembrane potential but not to such a degree that an action potential is generated (arrow *b*). If the stimulus is strong enough to decrease the transmembrane potential to the threshold potential, the cell becomes excited and develops an action potential (arrow *c*). The action potential, which is the primary event in the conduction of the peristaltic impulse, has the capability to act as the stimulus for excitation of adjacent quiescent cells and, through a complicated chain of events, gives rise to the ureteral contraction.

When the ureteral cell is excited, its membrane loses its preferential permeability to K^+ and becomes more permeable *to* Ca^{2+} *ions,* which move inward across the cell membrane and give rise to the upstroke of the action potential (Imaizumi et al, 1989; Kobayashi, 1965, 1969; Lang, 1989, 1990; Vereecken et al, 1975a). As the positively charged Ca^{2+} ions move inward across the cell membrane, the inside of the membrane becomes less negative with respect to the outside and may even become positive at the peak of the action potential, a state referred to as *overshoot.* There is some evidence that Na^+ *ions* also may play a role in the upstroke of the ureteral action potential (Kobayashi, 1965; Kobayashi and Irisawa, 1964; Muraki et al, 1991; Vereecken et al, 1975b). The rate of rise of the upstroke of the ureteral action potential is relatively slow, 1.2 ± .06 V/second in the cat (Kobayashi, 1969). This compares with a 610 V/second rate of rise in cells of Purkinje's fibers in the dog heart (Draper and Weidmann, 1951) and a 740 V/second rate of rise in guinea pig skeletal muscle (Ferroni and Blanchi, 1965). The slow rate of rise in the upstroke of the ureteral action potential accounts for the slow conduction velocity in the ureter.

After reaching the peak of its action potential, the ureteral cell membrane maintains its potential for a period of time (*plateau of the action potential*) before the transmembrane potential returns to its resting level (*repolarization*) (Kuriyama et al, 1967). The plateau phase of the guinea pig action potential is superimposed, with multiple oscillations, a phenomenon not observed in the rat, rabbit, or cat (Fig. 25–3) (Bozler, 1938a). The plateau phase appears to depend on the persistence of an inward Ca^{2+} current and on Na^+ influx through a voltage-dependent Na^+ channel (Imaizumi

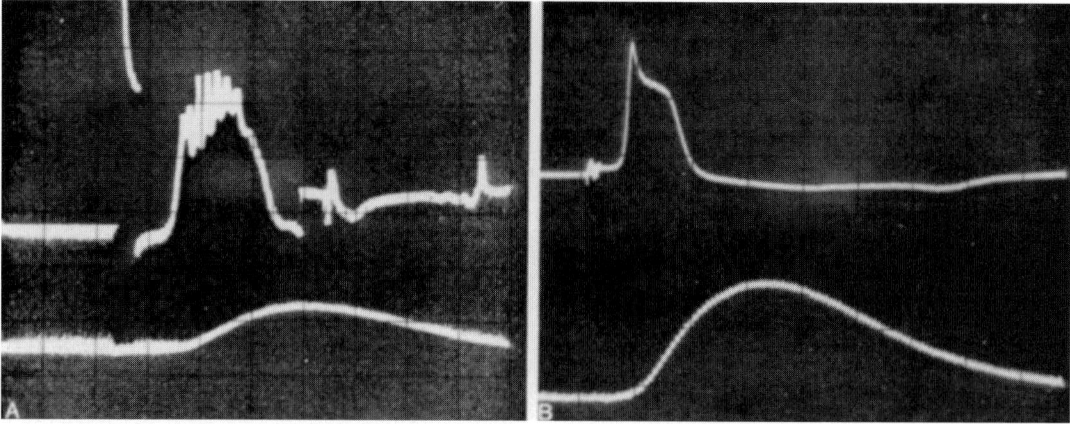

Figure 25–3. Intracellular recordings of ureteral action potentials *(upper tracings)* and isometric recordings of contractions *(lower tracings)* in response to electrical stimuli. Action potentials precede contractions. *A,* Guinea pig ureter; oscillations on plateau of action potential. *B,* Cat ureter; no oscillations on plateau of action potential. (From Weiss RM: Urology 1978; 12:114, with permission.)

et al, 1989; Kuriyama and Tomita, 1970; Shuba, 1978). The oscillations on the plateau of the guinea pig action potential appear to depend on the repetitive activation of an inward Ca^{2+} current (Kuriyama and Tomita, 1970) and of a Ca^{2+}-dependent K^+ current (Imaizumi et al, 1989). The activation of the Ca^{2+}-dependent K^+ current is mainly caused by Ca^{2+} release from the endoplasmic reticulum, which is triggered by the influx of extracellular Ca^{2+} through voltage-dependent Ca^{2+} channels. The increase in intracellular Ca^{2+} concentration during the upstroke and plateau of the action potential finally may activate the outward Ca^{2+}-dependent K^+ current to such a degree that repolarization occurs with return of the transmembrane potential to its resting level (Imaizumi et al, 1989). The *duration* of the *action potential* in the cat ranges from 259 to 405 milliseconds (Kobayashi and Irisawa, 1964).

In summary, the RMP of the ureteral cell is approximately −33 to −70 mV and is determined primarily by the distribution of K^+ ions across the cell membrane and the relatively selective permeability of the resting cell membrane to K^+. When excited by a suprathreshold stimulus, the membrane becomes less permeable to K^+ and more permeable to Ca^{2+}, which moves inward across the cell membrane and provides the ionic mechanism for the development of the upstroke of the action potential. After reaching the peak of its action potential, the membrane maintains a depolarized state (plateau of the action potential) for a period of time before the membrane potential of the activated cell returns to its resting level (repolarization). The plateau appears to be related to a persisting inward Ca^{2+} current and to an influx of Na^+. Repolarization of the membrane probably is related to a renewed increase in permeability to K^+.

Pacemaker Potentials and Pacemaker Activity

Electrical activity arises in a cell either spontaneously or in response to an external stimulus. If the activity arises spontaneously, the cell is referred to as a *pacemaker cell.* Pacemaker fibers differ from nonpacemaker fibers in that their transmembrane resting potential does not remain constant but rather undergoes a slow spontaneous depolarization (Fig. 25–4). If the spontaneously changing membrane potential reaches the threshold potential, the upstroke of an action potential occurs. Changes in the frequency of action potential development may result from a change in the level of the threshold potential, a change in the rate of slow spontaneous depolarization of the resting potential, or a change in the level of the resting potential.

Dixon and Gosling (Dixon and Gosling, 1973; Gosling, 1970; Gosling and Dixon, 1971, 1974) have provided morphologic evidence of specialized pacemaker tissue in the proximal portion of the urinary collecting system and described species differences. In species with a multicalyceal system, such as the pig and human, the "pacemaker cells" are located near the pelvicalyceal border (Dixon and Gosling, 1973). Bozler (1942), using small extracellular surface

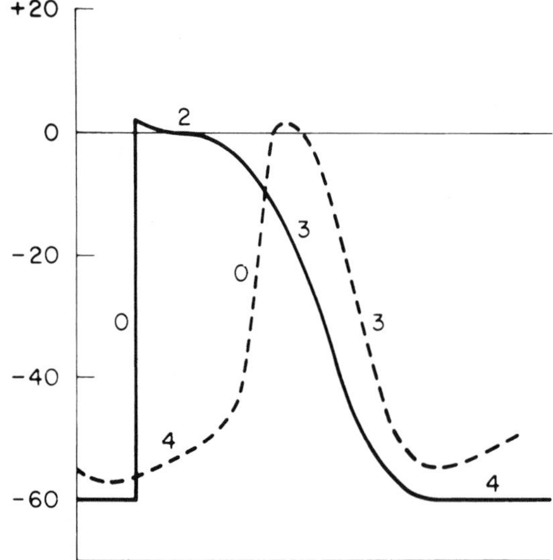

Figure 25–4. Schematic representation of pacemaker *(dashed line)* and nonpacemaker *(solid line)* action potentials: (0) upstroke or depolarization phase; (2) plateau phase; (3) repolarization phase; and (4) resting potential of nonpacemaker cell and spontaneous depolarization phase of pacemaker cell. Spontaneous decrease in transmembrane potential of pacemaker cell accounts for its spontaneous activity. (From Weiss RM: Urology 1978; 12:114, with permission.)

electrodes, demonstrated the characteristic slow spontaneous depolarization of pacemaker-type fibers in the proximal portion of the isolated ureter of a unicalyceal upper collecting system. In a multicalyceal kidney, Morita and associates (1981), using extracellular electrodes, recorded low-voltage potentials that appeared to be pacemaker potentials from the border of the minor calyces and the major calyx. They noted that the contraction rhythm varied in each calyx, a finding that is in accord with multiple pacemakers being present in the multicalyceal pig kidney (Constantinou et al, 1977).

Although the primary pacemaker for ureteral peristalsis is located in the proximal portion of the collecting system, other areas of the ureter may act as *latent pacemakers*. Under normal conditions, the latent pacemaker regions are dominated by activity arising at the primary pacemaker sites. If the latent pacemaker site is freed of its domination by the primary pacemaker, it, in turn, may act as a pacemaker. To demonstrate latent pacemaker sites, Shiratori and Kinoshita (1961b) transected the in vivo dog ureter at various levels. Before transection, peristaltic activity arose proximally from the primary pacemaker. After the ureter was transected at the ureteropelvic junction (UPJ), antiperistaltic waves of lower frequency than the previous normoperistaltic waves originated from the UVJ. Division of the ureter at the UVJ did not affect the normoperistaltic waves. After division of the midureter, the normoperistaltic waves in the upper segment remained unchanged, and the lower segment demonstrated antiperistaltic waves, which originated at the UVJ at a frequency less than that of the normoperistaltic waves in the upper segment. Thus it was demonstrated that cells at the UVJ of the dog may act as pacemaker cells if freed of control from the primary, proximally located pacemaker. Latent pacemaker activity also has been demonstrated at the UVJ of the rat (Tindall, 1972), and it is possible that other regions of the ureter also may show latent pacemaker activity.

Propagation of Electrical Activity

Excitable cells possess resistive and capacitative membrane properties similar to those of a cable or core conductor. The transverse resistance of the membrane is higher than the longitudinal resistance of the extracellular or intracellular fluid; this allows current resulting from a stimulus to propagate along the length of the fibers. The spread of current is referred to as electrotonic spread (Hoffman and Cranefield, 1960). The space constant (λ) determines the degree to which the electrotonic potential dissipates with increasing distance from an applied voltage. In a cable, this relation is expressed by the equation,

$$P = P_0 e^{-x/\lambda}$$

where χ is the distance from the applied voltage; P is the displacement of the membrane potential at χ; P_0 is the displacement of the membrane potential at the site of the applied voltage; *e* is the base of the natural logarithm; and λ is the space constant. The electrotonic potential decreases by 1/e in one space constant. The space constant of the guinea pig ureter, measured by extracellular stimulation, is 2.5 to 3.0 mm (Kuriyama et al, 1967).

The time constant τ_m is expressed by the formula,

$$\tau_m = RC$$

where R is the membrane resistance and C is the membrane capacity. A small displacement of potential is decreased by 1/e of its value in one time constant. The time constant of the guinea pig ureter, measured by extracellular stimulation, is 200 to 300 milliseconds (Kuriyama et al, 1967).

The ureter acts as a functional syncytium (Bozler, 1938b). Engelmann (1869, 1870) showed that stimulation of the ureter produces a contraction wave that propagates proximally and distally from the site of stimulation. Under normal conditions, electrical activity arises proximally and is conducted distally from one muscle cell to another across the areas of close cellular apposition referred to as *intermediate junctions* (Libertino and Weiss, 1972; Notley, 1970; Uehara and Burnstock, 1970). The similarity of these close cellular contacts to nexuses, which have been shown to be low-resistance pathways for cell-to-cell conduction in other smooth muscles (Barr et al, 1968), suggests that a similar mechanism for conduction may be present in the ureter. *Conduction velocity* in the ureter is *2 to 6 cm/second* (Ichikawa and Ikeda, 1960; Kobayashi, 1964; Kuriyama et al, 1967); it has been shown to vary with temperature and with the time interval between stimuli (van Mastrigt et al, 1986) and also with the pressure within the ureter (Tsuchiya and Takei, 1990). Conduction in the ureter is similar to that in cardiac tissue, even to the extent that the Wenckebach phenomenon (a partial conduction block) has been demonstrated in the ureter as it has in specialized cardiac fibers (Weiss et al, 1968).

CONTRACTILE ACTIVITY

The contractile event is dependent on the concentration of free sarcoplasmic Ca^{2+} in the region of the contractile proteins, actin and myosin. Any process that results in an increase in Ca^{2+} in the region of the contractile proteins favors the development of a contraction; any process that results in a decrease in Ca^{2+} in the region of the contractile proteins favors relaxation (Fig. 25–5).

Contractile Proteins

In skeletal muscle, Ca^{2+} appears to act as a derepressor. It is thought that in the relaxed state a regulator system, consisting of the proteins troponin and tropomyosin, prevents the interaction of actin and myosin (Fig. 25–6*A*). In the relaxed state, the troponin that is attached to the tropomyosin is inactive, and the tropomyosin prevents the interaction between actin and myosin. With activation, there is an increase in the sarcoplasmic Ca^{2+} concentration. The Ca^{2+} binds to the troponin, producing a conformational change that results in the displacement of tropomyosin, which in turn allows interaction of actin and myosin and the development of a contraction (see Fig. 25–6*B*).

In smooth muscle, on the other hand, Ca^{2+} appears to function as an activator. The most widely accepted theory suggests that phosphorylation of myosin is involved in the

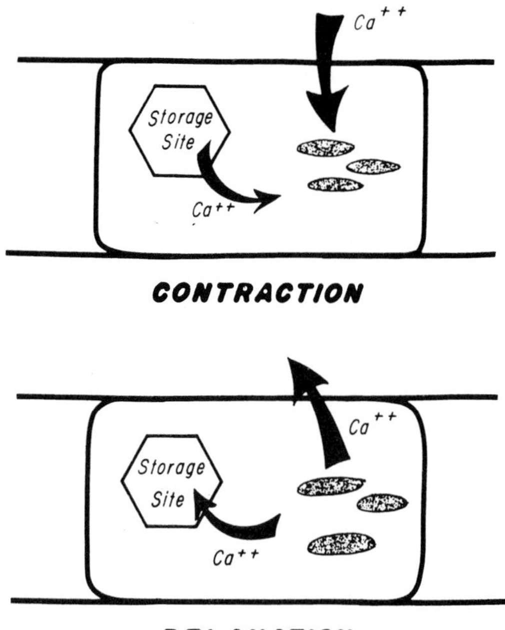

Figure 25–5. Schematic representation of calcium movements during contraction and relaxation. (From Weiss RM: Urology 1978; 12:114, with permission.)

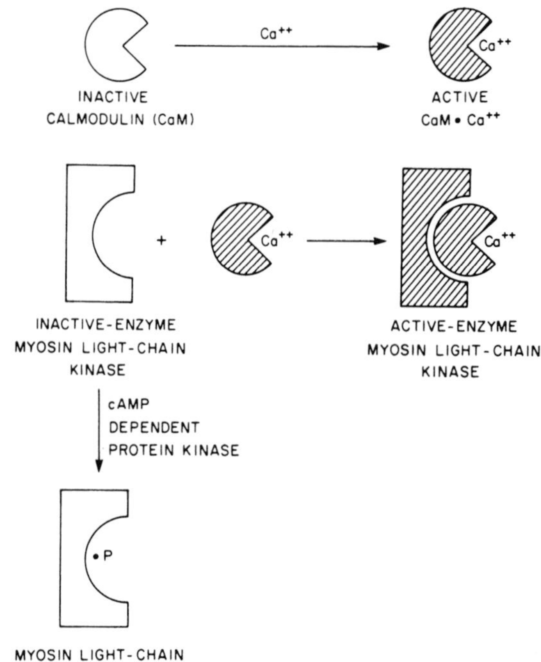

Figure 25–7. Schematic representation of contractile process in smooth muscle. Calmodulin is activated by Ca^{2+}. The activated calcium-calmodulin complex activates the enzyme myosin light-chain kinase, which phosphorylates the light chain of myosin. Phosphorylation of myosin light-chain kinase decreases the rate of activation of the enzyme by the calcium-calmodulin complex.

contractile process and that a troponin-like system does not constitute the primary regulatory mechanism, as it does in skeletal muscle. With excitation, there is a transient increase in the sarcoplasmic Ca^{2+} concentration from its steady-state concentration of 10^{-8} to 10^{-7} mol/L to a concentration of 10^{-6} mol/L or higher. At this higher concentration, Ca^{2+} forms an active complex with the *calcium-binding protein, calmodulin* (Cho et al, 1988; Watterson et al, 1976; Weiss et al, 1981). Calmodulin without Ca^{2+} is inactive (Fig. 25–7). The calcium-calmodulin complex activates a calmodulin-dependent enzyme, *myosin light-chain kinase* (see Fig. 25–7). The activated myosin light-chain kinase, in turn, catalyzes the phosphorylation of the 20,000-dalton light chain of myosin (Fig. 25–8). Phosphorylation of the *myosin light chain* allows activation by actin of myosin magnesium (Mg^{2+})–ATPase activity, leading to hydrolysis of ATP and the development of smooth muscle tension or shortening (Fig. 25–9). Actin cannot activate the ATPase activity of the dephosphorylated myosin light chain.

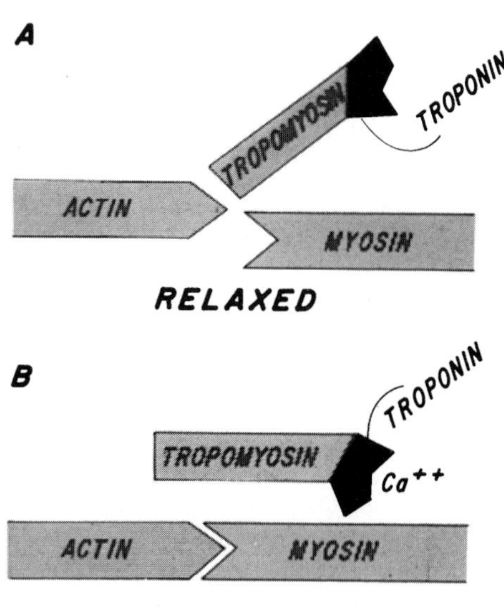

Figure 25–6. Schematic representation of contractile process in skeletal muscle. *A*, Relaxed state. *B*, Contracted state. (From Weiss RM: Urology 1978; 12:114, with permission.)

When the Ca^{2+} concentration in the region of the contractile proteins is low, the myosin light-chain kinase is not active, because calmodulin requires Ca^{2+} to activate the enzyme. This prevents activation of the contractile apparatus, because the myosin light chain cannot be phosphorylated, a process that must precede tension development. Furthermore, a phosphatase dephosphorylates the myosin light chain, thereby preventing actin activation of myosin ATPase activity, and relaxation results (Kamm and Stull, 1985).

Evidence indicates that phosphorylation of the enzyme myosin light-chain kinase by a cyclic adenosine monophosphate (cAMP)–dependent protein kinase decreases myosin light-chain kinase activity by decreasing the affinity of this enzyme for calmodulin (Adelstein et al, 1981).

Although most recent evidence supports the myosin phosphorylation theory of smooth muscle contractility, a minority opinion holds that regulation of contraction is linked primarily to actin and that phosphorylation is not the primary mechanism. Leiotonin, a protein similar to troponin, and calmodulin are thought to be involved in the contractile process.

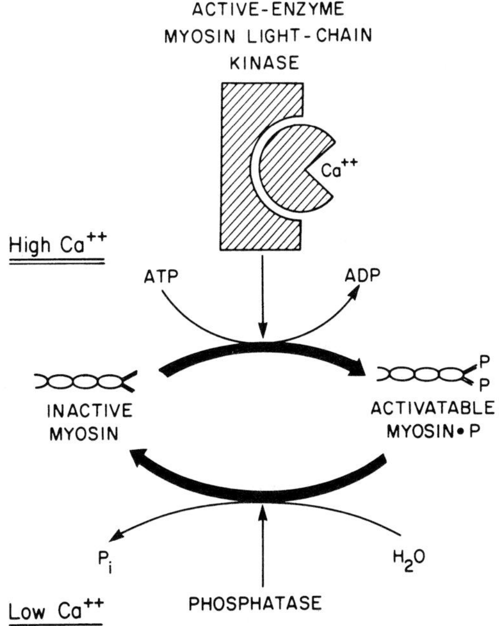

Figure 25–8. Schematic representation of the contractile process in smooth muscle. The activated enzyme, myosin light-chain kinase, catalyzes the phosphorylation of myosin. Myosin must be phosphorylated in order for actin to activate myosin ATPase.

Calcium and Excitation-Contraction Coupling

The mechanical event of ureteral peristalsis follows an electrical event to which it is related. The Ca^{2+} involved in the ureteral contraction is derived from two main sources. Because smooth muscle cells have a very small diameter, the inward movement of extracellular Ca^{2+} into the cell during the upstroke of the action potential provides a significant source of sarcoplasmic Ca^{2+} (see Fig. 25–5). L-type voltage-dependent Ca^{2+} channels play a role in this process (Brading et al, 1983; Maggi et al, 1994a; Yoshida et al, 1992). In response to an excitatory impulse, release of calcium from more tightly bound storage sites (i.e., the endoplasmic reticulum) also increases the Ca^{2+} concentration in the sarcoplasm.

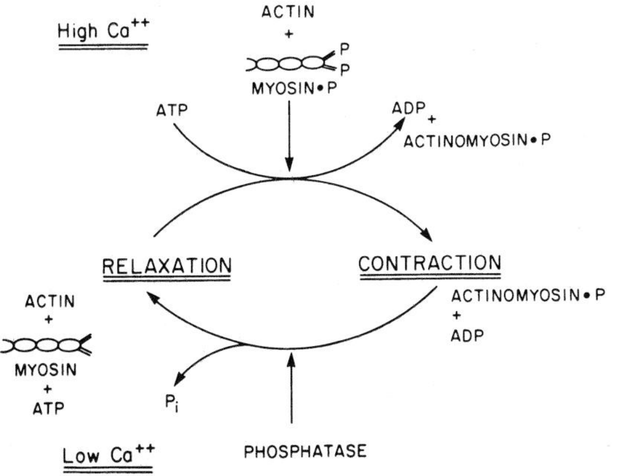

Figure 25–9. Schematic representation of the contractile process in smooth muscle. Actin activates ATPase activity of phosphorylated myosin. This allows interaction of actin and myosin with the development of a contraction.

Support for utilization of a dual source of Ca^{2+} in the ureter has been provided by Vereecken and co-workers (1975a), who noted that it took approximately 45 minutes for spontaneous contractions of isolated guinea pig ureters to cease after the tissue was placed in a Ca^{2+}-free medium. They interpreted this to indicate that some of the Ca^{2+} involved in the contractile process is derived from tightly bound intracellular stores. They also noted that recovery of the contractile response to electrical stimuli was almost immediate after the tissue was returned to a physiologic solution containing a normal concentration of Ca^{2+}. This suggests that free extracellular Ca^{2+} entering the cell during excitation also provides a source of Ca^{2+} for the contractile machinery. A similar conclusion was reached by Hong and associates (1985). Relaxation results from a decrease in the concentration of free sarcoplasmic Ca^{2+} in the region of the contractile proteins. The decrease in sarcoplasmic Ca^{2+} can result from uptake of Ca^{2+} into intracellular storage sites or from extrusion of Ca^{2+} from the cell.

Second Messengers

The functional response to a number of hormones, neurotransmitters, and other agents is mediated by second messengers. The agonist, or first messenger, interacts with a specific membrane-bound receptor (Alquist, 1948; Furchgott, 1964); the agonist-receptor complex then activates or inactivates an enzyme that leads to alteration of an amount of a second messenger within the cell. These *second messengers* include *cyclic AMP*, guanosine 3′,5′-monophosphate (*cyclic GMP* or cGMP), *Ca^{2+}, inositol 1,4,5-trisphosphate (IP_3)*, and *diacylglycerol (DG)*. They mediate the functional response to the agonist through a process that frequently involves protein phosphorylation.

Although relaxation of smooth muscle may occur independently of changes in cyclic nucleotides (Vesin and Harbon, 1974), cAMP is believed to mediate the relaxing effects of beta-adrenergic agonists in a variety of smooth muscles (Andersson, 1972; Kroeger and Marshall, 1974; Triner et al, 1971). According to this concept, a beta-adrenergic agonist, such as isoproterenol, serves as the first messenger and combines with a receptor on the outer surface of the cell membrane (Fig. 25–10). Isoproterenol itself does not enter the cell, but the beta-adrenergic agonist–receptor complex activates the enzyme *adenylyl cyclase* located on the inner surface of the cell membrane in close morphologic relation to the receptor. In the presence of Mg^{2+} and a guanine nucleotide, guanosine triphosphate (GTP), adenylyl cyclase catalyzes the conversion within the cell of ATP to cAMP:

$$\text{ATP} = \xrightarrow[\text{Mg}^{2+},\ \text{GTP}]{\text{adenylyl cyclase}} \text{cAMP}$$

A *guanine nucleotide–regulatory protein (G protein)* acts as a functional communicator between the agonist-receptor complex and the catalytic or active unit of the enzyme adenylyl cyclase. cAMP acts as a second, or internal, messenger of the response elicited by the beta-adrenergic ago-

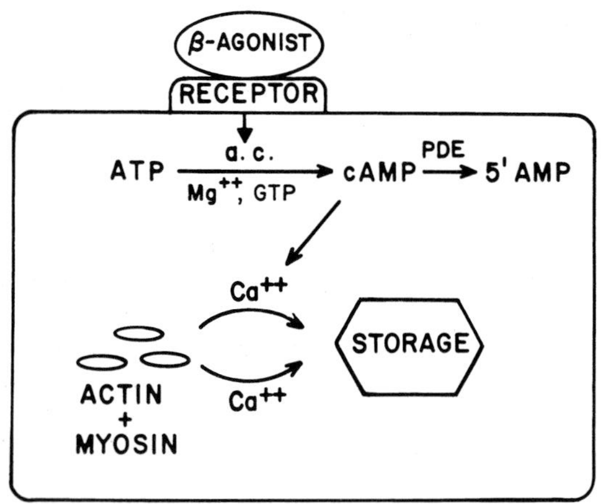

Figure 25–10. Schematic representation of the role of cyclic adenosine monophosphate (cAMP) in beta-adrenergic agonist-induced relaxation of smooth muscle. Agonist combines with receptor on the outer side of the cell membrane. The receptor-agonist complex, in turn, activates the enzyme adenylyl cyclase (a.c.) on the inner surface of the cell membrane, which, in the presence of magnesium (Mg^{2+}) and guanosine triphosphate (GTP), results in the conversion of adenosine triphosphate (ATP) to cAMP. cAMP is postulated to cause an increased uptake of Ca^{2+} into intracellular storage sites, with a resultant decrease in Ca^{2+} in the region of the contractile proteins, resulting in relaxation. cAMP also may have other actions (not shown) that inhibit the contractile process. The enzyme phosphodiesterase (PDE) degrades cAMP to 5′-AMP. (From Weiss RM: *In* Bergman H, ed: The Ureter. New York, Springer-Verlag, 1981, p 137, with permission.)

nist. It has been suggested that the increase in cAMP through activation of an enzyme (i.e., a protein kinase) and phosphorylation of proteins leads to the uptake of Ca^{2+} into intracellular storage sites (i.e., the endoplasmic reticulum), with the resultant decrease of free sarcoplasmic Ca^{2+} in the region of the contractile proteins (Andersson and Nilsson, 1972). The decrease in sarcoplasmic Ca^{2+} in the region of the contractile proteins leads to relaxation of the smooth muscle.

Levels of cAMP may be increased within the cell in two ways. One is by increasing synthesis, which involves activation of the enzyme adenylyl cyclase; the other is by decreasing degradation. The degradation of cAMP to 5′-AMP involves activation of an enzyme, a *phosphodiesterase*. Agents that either increase adenylyl cyclase activity (e.g., the beta-adrenergic agonist isoproterenol) or decrease phosphodiesterase activity (e.g., phosphodiesterase inhibitors such as theophylline and papaverine) may increase intracellular levels of cAMP and cause smooth muscle relaxation.

Weiss and associates (1977) have demonstrated both adenylyl cyclase and phosphodiesterase activities in the ureter. They have shown that isoproterenol stimulates adenylyl cyclase activity and theophylline inhibits phosphodiesterase activity. These two agents that relax ureteral smooth muscle would be expected to increase cAMP levels—isoproterenol by increasing synthesis and theophylline by decreasing degradation. These data suggest that isoproterenol and theophylline could exert their ureter-relaxing effects, at least in part, through the cyclase-phosphodiesterase system. Further support of a role for cAMP in smooth muscle relaxation can be derived from the finding that dibutyryl cAMP, which more readily diffuses into the intact cell and is less likely to be broken down by phosphodiesterase than is cAMP, has been shown to relax a variety of smooth muscles, including the ureter (Takago et al, 1971; Wheeler et al, 1990).

In addition to receptors and G proteins that are involved in stimulation of adenylyl cyclase and the formation of cAMP, as in the actions of beta-adrenergic agonists, other receptors and G proteins inhibit adenylyl cyclase activity (Londos et al, 1981). Some actions of alpha$_2$-adrenergic and muscarinic cholinergic agonists involve stimulation of these inhibitory G proteins, with subsequent inhibition of adenylyl cyclase activity.

Another cyclic nucleotide, cGMP, also can cause smooth muscle relaxation. cGMP is synthesized from GTP by the enzyme *guanylyl cyclase* and is degraded to 5′-GMP by a phosphodiesterase. Phosphodiesterase activity that can degrade both cAMP and cGMP has been demonstrated in the canine ureter, and various inhibitors can preferentially inhibit the breakdown of one or the other cyclic nucleotide (Weiss et al, 1981). Insulin has been shown to activate cAMP phosphodiesterase activity in the ureter (Weiss and Wheeler, 1988), and 8-bromo-cGMP has been shown to cause relaxation of a number of smooth muscles (Schultz et al, 1979), including the ureter (Cho et al, 1984).

Recently, *nitric oxide (NO)* has been shown to stimulate guanylyl cyclase activity and to cause smooth muscle relaxation (Dokita et al, 1991, 1994). *Nitric oxide synthase (NOS)* converts *L-arginine* to NO and L-citrulline in a reaction that requires nicotinamide-adenine-dinucleotide phosphate (NADPH). A *constitutive isoform of NOS (nNOS),* which is Ca^{2+} dependent, is present in neuronal tissues, and an *inducible isoform of NOS (iNOS),* which is NADPH dependent but Ca^{2+} independent, has been identified in ureteral smooth muscle (Smith et al, 1993). It is thought that with neuronal excitation there is an increase in calcium concentration within nerves, which leads to the synthesis of NO from L-arginine. NO released from the nerve activates the enzyme guanylyl cyclase in the smooth muscle cell, with the resultant conversion of GTP to cGMP and subsequent smooth muscle relaxation (Fig. 25–11).

It also is possible that a yet to be determined neurotransmitter is released from the neuron and stimulates NO production in the smooth muscle cell, which in turn leads to formation of cGMP and smooth muscle relaxation. NOS-containing nerves have been demonstrated in the human ureter (Stief et al, 1993), and NOS has been demonstrated in the pig UVJ (Phillips et al, 1995). NOS has been shown to colocalize with vasoactive polypeptide (VIP) and neuropeptide Y (NPY) in nerves supplying the lower human ureter (Smet et al, 1994). NOS does not appear to be present in adrenergic neurons. Furthermore, NO has been shown to be involved in nonadrenergic, noncholinergic induced relaxation of the pig UVJ (Hernández et al, 1995) and to inhibit ureteral contractility (Chiu et al, 1994).

Some actions of alpha$_1$-adrenergic and muscarinic cholinergic agonists and a number of other hormones, neurotransmitters, and biologic substances are associated with an increase in intracellular Ca^{2+} and are related to changes in inositol lipid metabolism. These agonists combine with a receptor on the cell membrane, and the agonist-receptor complex, in turn, activates an enzyme, *phospholipase C,* that leads to the hydrolysis of polyphosphatidylinositol 4,5-bisphosphate *(PIP_2)* with the formation of two second messengers, *IP_3 and DG* (Berridge, 1984) (Fig. 25–12). The

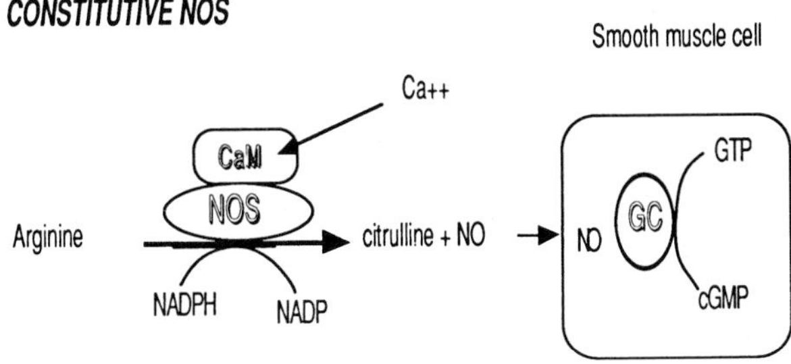

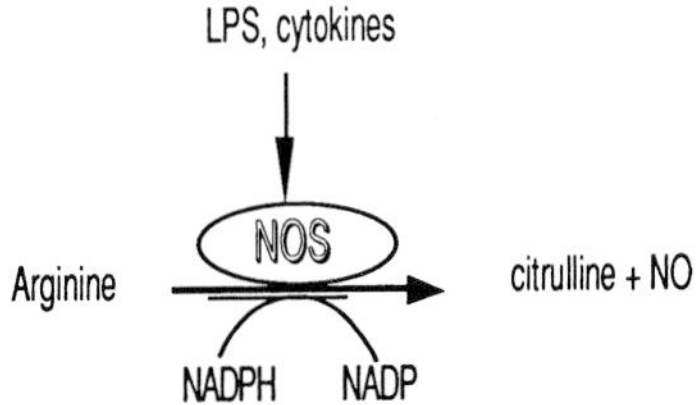

Figure 25–11. Schematic representation of the actions of inducible and constitutive nitric oxide synthase (NOS). CaM, calmodulin; GC, guanylyl cyclase; cGMP, cyclic guanosine monophosphate; GTP, guanosine triphosphate; LPS, lipopolysaccharide; NADP, oxidized form of nicotinamide-adenine-dinucleotide phosphate (NADPH).

activation of phospholipase C involves a G protein. IP_3 mobilizes Ca^{2+} from intracellular stores (i.e., endoplasmic reticulum) with initiation of a cascade of events through the calmodulin branch of the calcium messenger system. In smooth muscles, IP_3 is thought to be involved in brief contractile responses or in the initial phase of sustained responses (Park and Rasmussen, 1985).

The other second messenger, DG, binds to an enzyme, *protein kinase C (PKC),* causes its translocation to the cell membrane, and, by reducing the concentration of Ca^{2+} required for PKC activation, results in an increase in this enzyme's activity. The actions of PKC and therefore DG involve the phosphorylation of proteins (Nishizuka, 1984). The PKC branch of the calcium messenger system is thought to be responsible for the sustained phase of the contractile response in smooth muscle (Park and Rasmussen, 1985) and is responsive to hormone-induced changes in intracellular calcium. DG also activates the enzyme, phospholipase A, which serves as a source of arachidonic acid, the substrate for prostaglandin synthesis (Mahadevappa and Holub, 1983). Arachidonic acid, in turn, may stimulate guanylyl cyclase activity with the subsequent formation of cGMP (Berridge, 1984), and this would explain the Ca^{2+}-dependent increase in cGMP levels associated with muscarinic cholinergic and $alpha_1$-adrenergic agonist–induced contractions in smooth muscle. The observed increases in cGMP levels follow, rather than precede, the onset of contractions induced by these agonists.

In summary, a group of second messengers are involved in the transduction of the signal that is initiated when an agonist combines with a specific receptor on the cell membrane of the smooth muscle. This process of *signal transduction* ultimately results in the functional response to the agonist.

MECHANICAL PROPERTIES

Mechanical characteristics of muscle are commonly assessed by defining *force-length and force-velocity relations.* Isometric force-length measurements depend on the number of linkages between the contractile proteins, actin and myosin, that are brought into action during contraction. Force-velocity relations depend on the rate of formation and breakdown of linkages between the contractile proteins. Interventions may affect force-velocity relations, with or without affecting force-length relations (Sonnenblick, 1962). In addition to these methods of assessing mechanical properties of the ureter, the bidimensional nature of the ureter has lent itself to studies of pressure-length-diameter relations.

Force-Length Relations

Force-length relations express the association between the force developed by muscle when it is stimulated under isometric conditions and the resting length of the muscle at the time of stimulation. With stretching of the ureter (muscle lengthening), the resting force (i.e., the tension present when the muscle is not excited) increases at a progressive rate (Weiss et al, 1972). Force developed during isometric contraction also increases with elongation until a length is reached at which maximum contractile force is achieved. With further lengthening, developed force decreases (Thulesius et al, 1989; Weiss et al, 1972). The ureter at this length is overstretched, or beyond the peak of its force-length

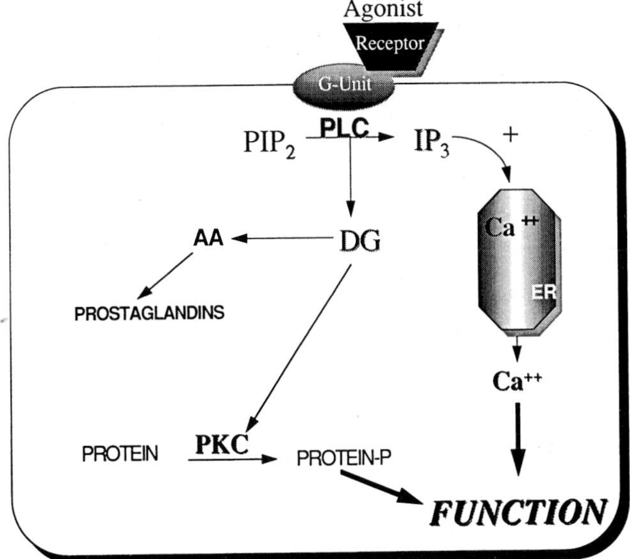

Figure 25–12. Schematic representation of the role of inositol lipid metabolism in smooth muscle function. The agonist combines with the receptor on the outer side of the cell membrane. The receptor-agonist complex in turn activates the enzyme phospholipase C (PLC), which leads to the hydrolysis of polyphosphatidylinositol 4,5-bisphosphate (PIP_2), with the formation of two second messengers, inositol 1,4,5-trisphosphate (IP_3) and diacylglycerol (DG). The activation of PLC involves a G protein. IP_3 mobilizes Ca^{2+} from intracellular stores (i.e., endoplasmic reticulum), and this leads to a functional response. DG binds to an enzyme, protein kinase C (PKC), which results in phosphorylation of proteins and a subsequent functional response. ER, endoplasmic reticulum; AA, arachidonic acid.

curve. Ureteral resting tension is high at the length at which maximum contractile force is developed.

Because the ureter is a *viscoelastic* structure (Weiss et al, 1972), the resting or contractile force developed at any given length depends on the direction in which change in length is occurring and the rate of change in length (Vereecken et al, 1973; Weiss et al, 1972). This is referred to as *hysteresis*; for the ureter, at any given length, resting force is less and contractile force is greater if the ureter is being allowed to shorten than if it is being stretched (Fig. 25–13).

When the ureter is stretched, resting force increases. If a new, longer length is kept constant after a stretch, changes occur that result in a decrease in resting force, or *stress relaxation* (Fig. 25–14) (Weiss et al, 1972). Within certain limits, when the ureter is stretched to a length beyond the peak of the force-length curve (i.e., to a length at which contractile force declines in the face of increasing muscle length), the degree of stress relaxation may be such that within a period of time the developed force no longer declines, even though the increased length is kept constant (Weiss et al, 1972). Stress relaxation can therefore be considered a compensatory mechanism of a viscoelastic structure in response to stretch.

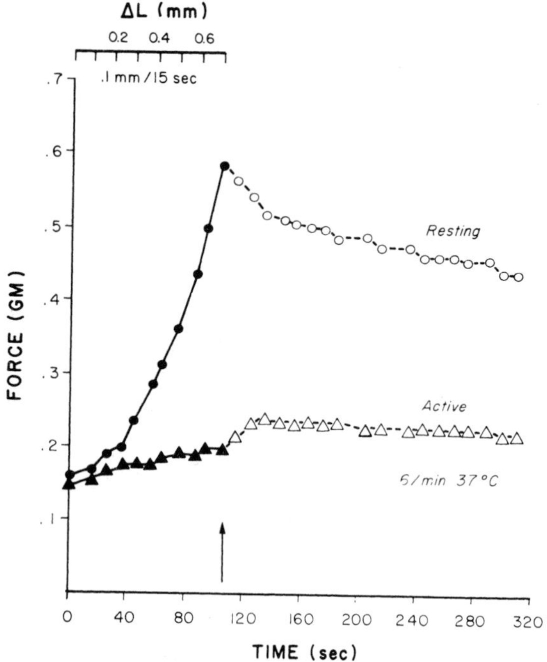

Figure 25–14. Stress relaxation. Resting and contractile (active) force of cat ureter (in grams) is shown on the ordinate, time from onset of stretching on the lower abscissa, and change in length (Δ L) on the left upper abscissa. Muscle is stretched by a given amount and then held at a fixed length. Filled data points and solid lines show data obtained during muscle lengthening; open data points and dashed lines show data obtained after stretching has ceased *(arrow)* and muscle is maintained at a constant length. Resting force decreases when muscle is held at a constant length following a stretch (stress relaxation). Contractile (active) force increases during this period of time. (From Weiss RM, Bassett AL, Hoffman BF: Am J Physiol 1972; 222:388, with permission.)

Force-Velocity Relations

Force-velocity curves depict the relation between the load and the velocity of shortening. A typical force-velocity curve, as predicted by Hill's equation for muscle shortening, has a hyperbolic configuration (Fig. 25–15) (Hill, 1938). From the force-velocity curve, the maximal velocity of shortening (V_{max}) can be extrapolated; this represents velocity of shortening at zero load (i.e., at isotonic conditions). V_{max} is determined by the level at which the force-velocity curve crosses the ordinate. V_{max} values in the ureter are in the range of 0.5 to 0.7 lengths/second (Biancani et al, 1984), which is in accord with observations in other smooth muscles (Aberg and Axelsson, 1965). The force-velocity curve intersects the abscissa at zero shortening—that is, at isometric conditions where the load is great. Shortening depends on the total load lifted, so that the ureter shortens to a lesser extent with heavier loads. At conditions near those of zero load, that is, conditions of free shortening (isotonic conditions), the in vitro guinea pig ureter shortens by 25% to 30% of its initial length (Biancani et al, 1984).

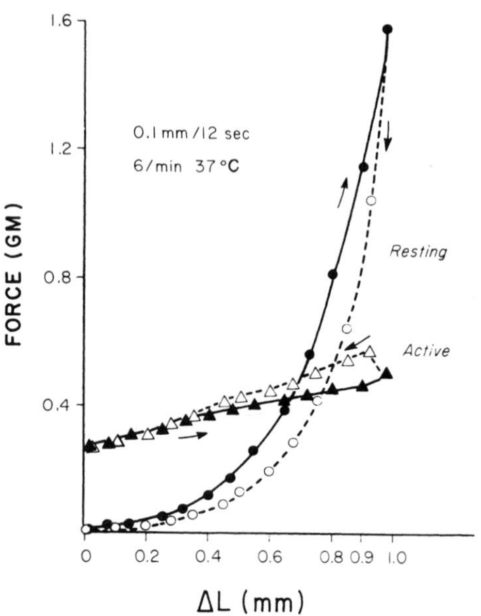

Figure 25–13. Hysteresis. Resting and contractile (active) force of cat ureter during muscle lengthening and shortening. Force (in grams) is shown on the ordinate, change in length (Δ L) on the abscissa. Closed data points and solid lines show data obtained during muscle lengthening. Open data points and dashed lines show data obtained during muscle shortening. Circles show resting force, and triangles show active or contractile force. Length and the direction of length change influence resting and contractile force. (From Weiss RM, Bassett AL, Hoffman BF: Am J Physiol 1972; 222:388, with permission.)

Pressure-Length-Diameter Relations

Because ureteral muscle fibers are arranged in a longitudinal, circumferential, and spiral configuration (Tanagho, 1971), longitudinal and diametral deformation of the ureter are inter-related. Simultaneous studies of length and diameter changes in response to an intraluminal pressure load are another means of assessing the mechanical properties of a tubular structure. After application of an intraluminal pressure, the ureter increases in both length and diameter, a process known as *creep* (Biancani et al, 1973). Deformation in response to a given intraluminal pressure load is greater

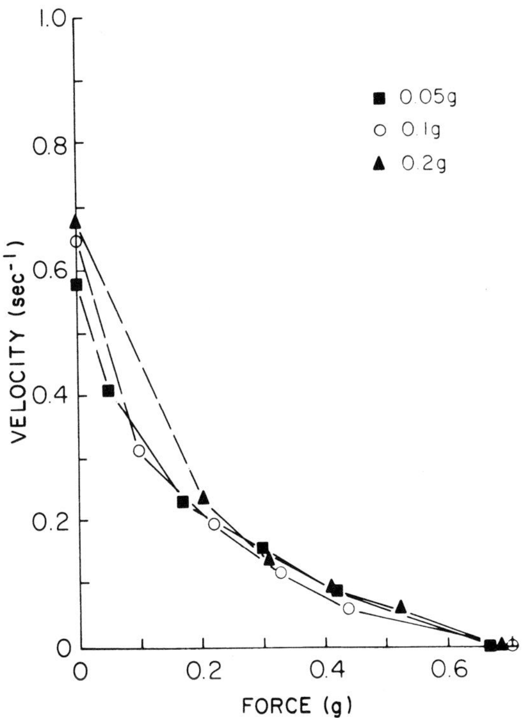

Figure 25–15. Force-velocity relation of guinea pig ureter. Specimens stretched by three different preloads (0.05, 0.1, and 0.2 g). The velocity of shortening on the ordinate is plotted as a function of the total load lifted on the abscissa. The maximal velocity of shortening (V_{max}) is obtained by extrapolation of the experimental curves to intersect the ordinate. Isometric force is given by data points at which velocity equals zero. (From Biancani P, Onyski JH, Zabinski MP, Weiss RM: J Urol 1984; 131:988. Copyright by Williams & Wilkins, 1984.)

in vitro than in vivo; this difference is partially negated if the in vivo preparation is pretreated with reserpine to suppress adrenergic influences (Fig. 25–16). Such data provide support for a role of the adrenergic nervous system in the control of ureteral function.

ROLE OF NERVOUS SYSTEM IN URETERAL FUNCTION

Some smooth muscles have a specific innervation of each muscle fiber, whereas other, syncytial-type smooth muscles lack discrete neuromuscular junctions and depend on a diffuse release of transmitter from a bundle of nerves with subsequent spread of excitation from one muscle cell to another (Burnstock, 1970). The ureter is a syncytial type of smooth muscle without discrete neuromuscular junctions (Burnstock, 1970).

As peristalsis may persist after transplantation (O'Conor and Dawson-Edwards, 1959) or denervation (Wharton, 1932), as spontaneous activity may occur in isolated in vitro ureteral segments (Finberg and Peart, 1970; Macht, 1916a; Malin et al, 1970), and as normal antegrade peristalsis continues after reversal of a segment of ureter in situ (Melick et al, 1961), it is apparent that ureteral peristalsis can occur without innervation. However, analysis of the data in the literature clearly indicates that the nervous system plays at least a modulating role in ureteral peristalsis. Morita and associates (1987) have provided evidence that the autonomic nervous system may influence urine transport through the ureter by affecting both peristaltic frequency and bolus volume. Catecholamine fluorescence and acetylcholine release studies indicate that the human ureter is supplied by both sympathetic (noradrenaline-containing) and parasympathetic (acetylcholine [ACh]–containing) neurons (DelTacca, 1978; Durante-Escalante, et al, 1969; Elbadawi and Schenk, 1969).

Parasympathetic Nervous System

Although the role of the parasympathetic nervous system in the control of ureteral peristalsis has not been well defined, muscarinic cholinergic receptors have been demonstrated in the ureter (Latifpour et al, 1989, 1990; Hernández et al, 1993), and acetylcholinesterase (AChE)–positive nerve fibers have been demonstrated in the equine ureter (Prieto et al, 1994). Furthermore, ACh has been shown to be released from isolated guinea pig, rabbit, and human ureters in response to electrical field stimulation (DelTacca, 1978) and this release is inhibited by the neural poison tetrodotoxin. These data suggest but do not prove that the parasympathetic nervous system has at least a modulatory role in the control of ureteral activity.

The prototypic cholinergic agonist is ACh, which serves as the neurotransmitter at (1) neuromuscular junctions of somatic motor nerves (nicotinic sites); (2) preganglionic parasympathetic and sympathetic neuroeffector junctions (nicotinic sites); and (3) postganglionic parasympathetic neuroeffector sites (muscarinic sites). ACh is synthesized from acetyl coenzyme A and choline in a reaction that is catalyzed by the enzyme choline acetyltransferase.

The ACh is stored in vesicles within the synaptic terminal; its release is dependent on the influx of Ca^{2+} into the

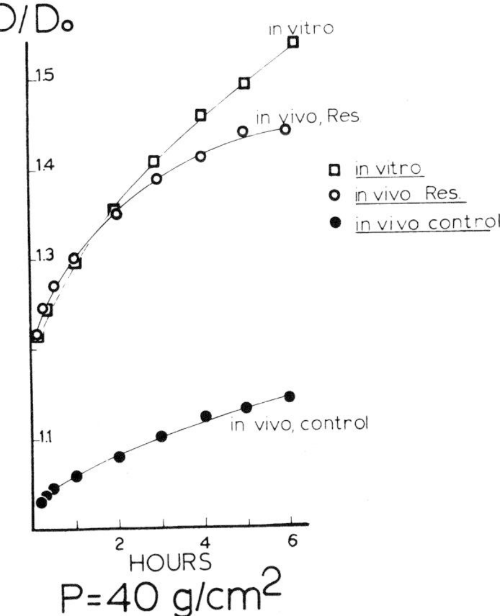

Figure 25–16. Pressure-diameter relations. An intraluminal pressure load of 40 g/cm² is applied to rabbit ureters, and change in diameter (D/D_0) is measured as a function of time. Squares show data obtained from in vitro ureters. Closed circles show data obtained in vivo. Open circles show data obtained in vivo from animals previously treated with reserpine. Open squares show data obtained in vitro. D_0, initial diameter; D, diameter during deformation.

terminal, which presumably causes vesicle fusion with the presynaptic terminal membrane, thereby expelling ACh into the synaptic cleft. ACh subsequently is hydrolyzed by AChE. The muscarinic effects of cholinergic agonists can be blocked by atropine. The effects of nicotinic agonists can be blocked by nondepolarizing ganglionic blocking agents or by high concentrations of the nicotinic agonist itself, which may cause ganglionic blockade by desensitization of receptor sites after an initial period of ganglionic stimulation.

Cholinergic Agonists

Cholinergic agonists, including ACh, methacholine (Mecholyl), carbamylcholine (carbachol), and bethanechol (Urecholine), in general have been observed to have an excitatory effect on ureteral function, that is, to increase the frequency and force of contractions (Barastegui, 1977; Boatman et al, 1967; Deane, 1967; Hernández et al, 1993; Hukuhara et al, 1964; Kaplan et al, 1968; Labay et al, 1968; Longrigg, 1974; Morita et al, 1986, 1987; Prieto et al, 1994; Rose and Gillenwater, 1974; Theobald, 1986; Vereecken, 1973). ACh also has been shown to increase the duration of the guinea pig and rat ureteral action potential (Ichikawa and Ikeda, 1960; Prosser et al, 1955) and the number of oscillations on the plateau of the guinea pig ureteral action potential (Ichikawa and Ikeda, 1960). The excitatory effects of cholinergic agonists may be related to an indirect release of catecholamines—as supported by the findings that the excitatory effects of Urecholine can be blocked by the alpha-adrenergic blocking agent phentolamine (Rose and Gillenwater, 1974) and that the increased frequency of canine ureteral peristalsis induced by ACh can be blocked by adrenalectomy (Labay et al, 1968)—or to a direct effect of the drug on muscarinic receptors (Hernández et al, 1993; Vereecken, 1973).

Nicotinic agonists, such as nicotine, tetramethylammonium, and dimethylphenylpiperazinium (DMPP), cause an initial stimulation of nicotinic receptors followed by desensitization of the receptor sites; the receptors then become unresponsive to nicotinic agonists and also to endogenous ACh, with resultant transmission blockade. Nicotine has been shown to have excitatory (Boyarsky et al, 1968), biphasic (Barastegui, 1977; Labay and Boyarsky, 1967; Macht, 1916a; Satani, 1919), and inhibitory (Prosser et al, 1955; Vereecken, 1973) actions on the ureter that may be dose-dependent.

Anticholinesterases

Anticholinesterases prevent hydrolysis of ACh by cholinesterases and thereby increase the duration and intensity of ACh action at both muscarinic and nicotinic receptor sites. With prolonged administration in high doses, they can result in desensitization blockade at nicotinic sites. The effects of anticholinesterases such as physostigmine and neostigmine parallel the excitatory effects of ACh and other parasympathomimetics on the ureter (Macht, 1916b; Prosser et al, 1955; Satani, 1919; Slaughter et al, 1945; Vereecken, 1973).

Parasympathetic Blocking Agents

Atropine is a competitive antagonist of the muscarinic effects of ACh. The inhibitory effects of atropine may be preceded by a transitory stimulatory effect on muscarinic receptors. Although atropine has been shown to inhibit the excitatory effects of parasympathomimetic agents (Barastegui, 1977; Boatman et al, 1967; Deane, 1967; Gould et al, 1955; Kaplan et al, 1968; Longrigg, 1974; Macht, 1916b; Vereecken, 1973) and of physostigmine (Macht, 1916b) on a variety of ureteral and calyceal preparations, the majority of studies have shown that atropine itself has little direct effect on ureteral activity in a number of species (Boatman et al, 1967; Butcher et al, 1957; Gibbs, 1929; Gould et al, 1955; Mazzella and Schroeder, 1960; Reid et al, 1976; Roth, 1917; Vereecken, 1973; Washizu, 1967), including humans (Kiil, 1957; Weinberg, 1962). Even when atropine has been observed to inhibit ureteral activity, its effects are frequently minimal and inconsistent (Hukuhara et al, 1964; Ross et al, 1967; Slaughter et al, 1945), providing little rationale for its use in the treatment of ureteral colic.

Reports of the direct effects on ureteral activity of two other parasympathetic blocking agents, methantheline (Banthine) and propantheline (Pro-Banthine), also have been inconsistent (Draper and Zorgniotti, 1954; Hanley, 1953; Kiil, 1957; Reid et al, 1976; Sierp and Draper, 1964; Weinberg, 1962).

Sympathetic Nervous System

The sympathetic nervous system appears to modulate ureteral activity, as evidenced by the demonstration of adrenergic receptors in the ureter (Latifpour et al, 1989, 1990), by the identification of catecholaminergic neurons in the ureter with the use of labeled tyrosine hydroxylase as a marker (Edyvane et al, 1994), and by the demonstration that catecholamines are released from the ureter (Weiss et al, 1978) and renal calyx (Longrigg, 1975) in response to electrical field stimulation.

The ureter contains excitatory alpha-adrenergic and inhibitory beta-adrenergic receptors (McLeod et al, 1973; Rose and Gillenwater, 1974; Tindall, 1972; Weiss et al, 1978), which have been demonstrated with receptor-binding techniques (Latifpour et al, 1989, 1990). Norepinephrine, primarily an alpha-adrenergic agonist (although it also can stimulate beta-adrenergic receptors), increases the force of electrically-induced ureteral contractions (Fig. 25–17) (Weiss et al, 1978). When administered in the presence of phentolamine (Regitine), an alpha-adrenergic blocking agent, norepinephrine decreases the force of ureteral contractions (see Fig. 25–17) (Weiss et al, 1978). A similar reversal of action occurs in the in vivo ureter (Kaplan et al, 1968; McLeod et al, 1973) and can be explained by norepinephrine's primary action on inhibitory beta-adrenergic receptors if the excitatory alpha-adrenergic receptors are blocked. Propranolol (Inderal), a beta-adrenergic antagonist, potentiates the increase in contractile force induced by norepinephrine (see Fig. 25–17) (Weiss et al, 1978). This can be explained by norepinephrine's acting more exclusively on excitatory alpha-adrenergic receptors if the inhibitory beta-adrenergic receptors are blocked. Furthermore, isoproterenol, a beta-adrenergic agonist, depresses contractility (Weiss et al, 1978). These data provide evidence for excitatory alpha-adrenergic and inhibitory beta-adrenergic receptors in the ureter; they are in accord with the findings of Deane (1967)

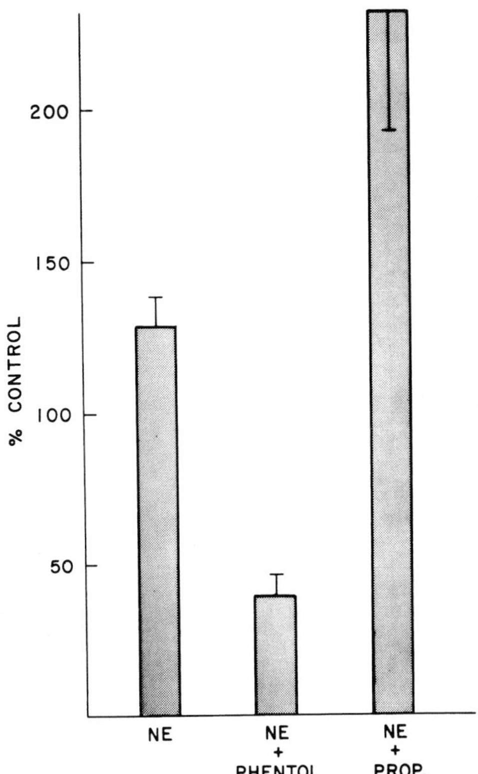

Figure 25–17. Effect of norepinephrine (NE) on electrically induced contractions of canine ureteral smooth muscle. One hundred per cent represents magnitude of control contractions. NE potentiation of contractility is inhibited by the alpha-adrenergic antagonist phentolamine (Phentol.) and increased by the beta-adrenergic antagonist propranolol (Prop.). (From Weiss RM: *In* Bergman H, ed: The Ureter. New York, Springer-Verlag, 1981, p 137, with permission.)

and Malin and co-workers (1968) on spontaneously-contracting, in vitro ureteral segments and with the observations of McLeod and associates (1973) and Rose and Gillenwater (1974) on in vivo ureters.

Further support for the presence of *excitatory alpha-adrenergic and inhibitory beta-adrenergic receptors in the ureter* includes the demonstration of adenylyl cyclase activity in the ureter (Weiss et al, 1977; Wheeler et al, 1986) and the finding that the ureters of rabbits depleted of catecholamines by the administration of reserpine undergo greater degrees of deformation when a given intraluminal pressure is applied than would result from application of the same pressure load to the ureters of normal animals (see Fig. 25–16) (Weiss et al, 1974). Last, electrical stimulation with high-intensity, high-frequency, short-duration stimuli has been shown to release neurotransmitter, presumably from intrinsic neural tissue within the wall of the ureter (Weiss et al, 1978) and renal calyx (Longrigg, 1975).

Adrenergic Agonists

Norepinephrine, the chemical mediator responsible for adrenergic transmission, is synthesized in the neuron from tyrosine. After its release from the nerve terminal, some of the norepinephrine combines with receptors in the effector organ, leading to a physiologic response. The greatest percentage of the norepinephrine is actively taken up (re-uptake or neuronal uptake) into the neuron. Neuronal re-uptake regulates the duration that norepinephrine is in contact with the innervated tissue and therefore the magnitude and duration of the catecholamine-induced response. Agents such as cocaine and imipramine (Tofranil), which inhibit neuronal uptake, potentiate the physiologic response to norepinephrine. The enzymes monoamine oxidase and catechol-*o*-methyltransferase provide degradative pathways for norepinephrine.

According to the general consensus, agents that activate alpha-adrenergic receptors, such as norepinephrine and phenylephrine, tend to stimulate ureteral activity (Boatman et al, 1967; Casteels et al, 1971; Deane, 1967; Gruber, 1928; Hannappel and Golenhofen, 1974; Hernández et al, 1992; Hukuhara et al, 1964; Kaplan et al, 1968; Macht, 1916a; Malin et al, 1968; McLeod et al, 1973; Reid et al, 1976; Rivera et al, 1992; Rose and Gillenwater, 1974; Tindall, 1972; Vereecken, 1973), and agents that activate beta-adrenergic receptors, such as isoproterenol and orciprenaline, tend to inhibit ureteral activity (Ancill et al, 1972; Deane, 1967; Finberg and Peart, 1970; Hannappel and Golenhofen, 1974; Hernández et al, 1992; Kiil and Kjekshus, 1967; Malin et al, 1968; McLeod et al, 1973; Reid et al, 1976; Rivera et al, 1992; Rose and Gillenwater, 1974; Tindall, 1972; Vereecken, 1973; Weiss et al, 1978). Tyramine, whose adrenergic-agonist effects result primarily from the release of norepinephrine from adrenergic terminals, also has a stimulatory effect on the upper urinary tract (Boyarsky and Labay, 1969; Finberg and Peart, 1970; Longrigg, 1974). The reported stimulatory effects of cocaine on ureteral activity (Boyarsky and Labay, 1969) may be explained by blockage of norepinephrine re-uptake into adrenergic nerve endings, with a resultant increase in the magnitude and duration of the effect of norepinephrine.

Adrenergic Antagonists

The alpha-adrenergic antagonists phentolamine (Regitine) and phenoxybenzamine (Dibenzyline) have been shown to inhibit the stimulatory effects of norepinephrine and other alpha-adrenergic agonists in a variety of preparations (Boatman et al, 1967; Casteels et al, 1971; Deane, 1967; Finberg and Peart, 1970; Gosling and Waas, 1971; Hannappel and Golenhofen, 1974; Hernández et al, 1992; Kaplan et al, 1968; Longrigg, 1974; McLeod et al, 1973; Rose and Gillenwater, 1974; Tindall, 1972; Vereecken, 1973; Weiss et al, 1978). The beta-adrenergic antagonist propranolol (Inderal) has been shown to block or attenuate the inhibitory effects of beta-adrenergic agonists, such as isoproterenol, in a variety of preparations (Casteels et al, 1971; Longrigg, 1974; McLeod et al, 1973; Reid et al, 1976; Rose and Gillenwater, 1974; Tindall, 1972; Vereecken, 1973; Weiss et al, 1978).

Peptidergic Agents in the Control of Ureteral Function

Tachykinins and *calcitonin gene-related peptide (CGRP)* are neurotransmitters released from peripheral endings of sensory nerves (Maggi, 1995). Tachykinins stimulate contractile activity, and CGRP inhibits contractile activity. Capsaicin-sensitive sensory nerves are located in the ureter (Dray et al, 1989; Maggi and Meli, 1988; Maggi et al, 1986) and contain the tachykinins known as *substance P, neurokinin A,* and *neuropeptide K* (Hua et al, 1985; Sann et al, 1992), as well as CGRP (Gibbins et al, 1985; Sann et al, 1992; Tamaki et al, 1992). *Capsaicin* in low doses inhibits ureteral activity, presumably by the release of CGRP, but in high doses it increases ureteral activity, presumably by release of the tachykinins neurokinin A, neuropeptide K, and substance P (Hua and Lundberg, 1986). The excitatory effects of the tachykinins are more prominent in the renal pelvis than in the ureter, and the inhibitory effects of CGRP are more prominent in the ureter than in the renal pelvis (Maggi et al, 1992b). The inhibitory actions on the ureter of the neurotransmitter CGRP, a 37-amino-acid-residue neuropeptide, appear to involve multiple mechanisms (Maggi and Giuliani, 1991; Maggi et al, 1994b). By opening ATP-sensitive K^+ channels, CGRP causes membrane hyperpolarization with a resultant blocking of voltage-sensitive Ca^{2+} channels that are involved in generation of the ureteral action potential and ureteral contraction (Maggi et al, 1994c; Meini et al, 1995; Santicioli and Maggi, 1994). CGRP-induced ureteral relaxation also may result from stimulation of adenylyl cyclase activity with a resultant increase in cAMP (Santicioli et al, 1995). The action of CGRP on the ureter may be regulated by an endopeptidase that can degrade the CGRP released from the sensory nerves (Maggi and Giuliani, 1994).

Histochemical studies show that the tachykinins and CGRP colocalize in the same nerves in the ureter (Hua et al, 1987). Peptidergic neurons containing *NPY and VIP* also are present in the ureter (Allen et al, 1990; Edyvane et al, 1992). Edyvane and associates (1994) have provided evidence of at least four, and possibly six, different immunohistochemical populations of nerve fibers in the human ureter. The predominant types include noradrenergic nerves containing NPY, neurons containing NPY and VIP, neurons containing substance P and CGRP, and neurons containing CGRP. Rare coexistences also were observed between CGRP and VIP, CGRP and NPY, and CGRP and tyrosine hydroxylase, a marker of noradrenergic neurons. These investigators demonstrated regional differences in the innervation of the ureter, with a more extensive innervation being noted in the lower than in the upper ureter.

Furthermore, two classes of mechanosensitive afferent fibers have been identified in the guinea pig ureter through the use of electrophysiologic techniques (Cervero and Sann, 1989). It would appear that one group of fibers responds to normal ureteral peristalsis, and the other is likely to be involved in the signaling of noxious events such as kidney stones and increased intraluminal pressures.

URINE TRANSPORT

Physiology of the Ureteropelvic Junction

At normal urine flows, the frequency of calyceal and renal pelvic contractions is greater than that in the upper ureter, and there is a relative block of electrical activity at the UPJ (Morita et al, 1981). At these flows, the renal pelvis fills; as renal pelvic pressure rises, urine is extruded into the upper ureter, which is initially in a collapsed state (Griffiths and Notschaele, 1983). Ureteral contractile pressures that move the bolus of urine are higher than renal pelvic pressures, and a closed UPJ may be protective of the kidney in dissipating backpressure from the ureter. As flow rate increases, the block at the UPJ ceases and a 1:1 correspondence between pacemaker and ureteral contractions develops (Constantinou and Hrynczuk, 1976; Constantinou and Yamaguchi, 1981).

With UPJ obstruction, there may be areas of narrowing or valve-like processes (Maizels and Stephens, 1980). In other instances, there is no gross narrowing at the UPJ, and abnormal propagation of the peristaltic impulse is a causative factor in the obstruction. In these instances, there appears to be a functional obstruction at the UPJ, inasmuch as a large-caliber catheter can be passed readily through the UPJ even though urine transport is inadequate. Murnaghan (1958) related the functional abnormality to an alteration in the configuration of the muscle bundles at the UPJ, and Foote and associates (1970) observed a decrease in musculature at the UPJ. Hanna (1978), in an electron microscopic study of severe UPJ obstructions, noted abnormalities in the musculature of the renal pelvis and disruption of intercellular relationships at the UPJ itself. Gosling and Dixon (1978) also observed histologic abnormalities in the dilated renal pelvis but were unable to confirm the alterations in the intercellular relationships at the UPJ. A vessel or adhesive band crossing the UPJ may potentiate the degree of dilatation in any of the forms of UPJ obstruction.

The differences in the reported findings suggest a spectrum of histopathology in the group of cases referred to as UPJ obstructions. It appears possible that, at least in some instances, disruption of cell-to-cell propagation of peristaltic activity results in impairment of urine transport across the UPJ.

One must consider input and output when predicting whether dilatation will occur; the effects of diuresis and obstruction appear to be complementary and additive with respect to the development of renal pelvic and calyceal dilatation. Some UPJs can handle urine flow regardless of the magnitude of diuresis, others cause ureteral dilatation at even the lowest flows, and still others can handle low flows but cause massive ureteral dilatation at high flows (Fig. 25–18).

Propulsion of Urinary Bolus

The theoretical aspects of the mechanics of urine transport within the ureter have been described in detail by Griffiths and Notschaele (1983); these are depicted in Figure 25–19. At normal flow rates, as the renal pelvis fills, a rise in renal pelvic pressure occurs, and urine is extruded into the upper ureter, which is initially in a collapsed state. The contraction wave originates in the most proximal portion of the ureter and moves the urine in front of it in a distal direction. The urine that had previously entered the ureter is formed into a bolus. In order to propel the bolus of urine efficiently, the contraction wave must completely coapt the ureteral walls (Griffiths and Notschaele, 1983; Woodburne and Lapides, 1972); the pressure generated by this contraction wave provides the primary component of what is recorded by intraluminal pressure measurements. The bolus that is pushed in front of the contraction wave lies almost entirely in a

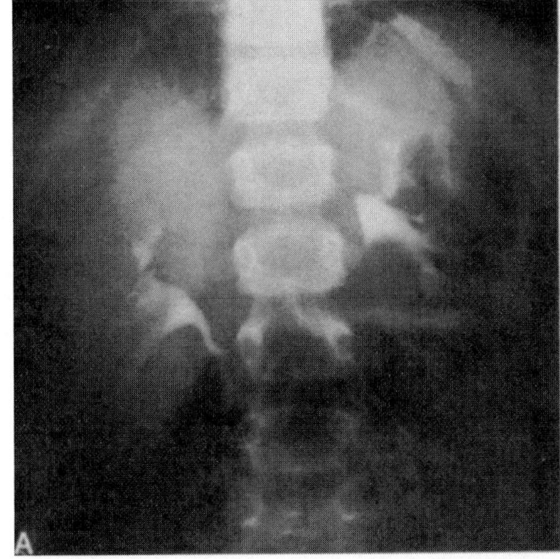

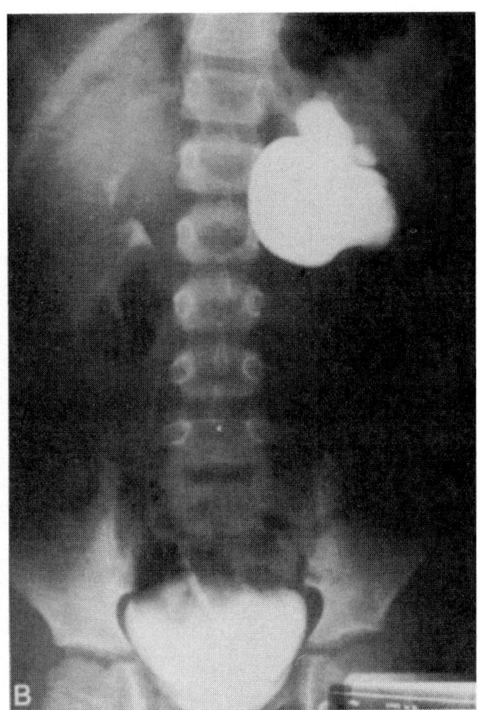

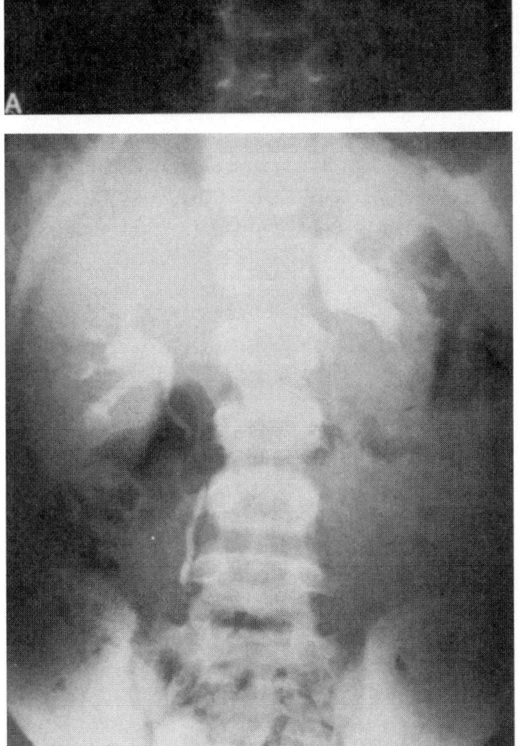

Figure 25–18. *A,* Intravenous pyelogram (IVP) shows essentially normal upper urinary tracts. *B,* Film from same child taken immediately after cardiac angiogram, which produces a massive diuresis. *C,* IVP 6 weeks after angiogram. (From Weiss RM: J Urol 1979; 121:401. Copyright by Williams & Wilkins, 1979.)

passive, noncontracting part of the ureter (Fung, 1971; Weinberg, 1974). Baseline or resting ureteral pressure is approximately 0 to 5 cm H_2O, and superimposed ureteral contractions ranging from 20 to 80 cm H_2O occur two to six times per minute (Kiil, 1957; Ross et al, 1972). The urine traverses the UVJ to enter the bladder; if it is functioning properly, the UVJ assures one-way transport of urine. The bolus is forced into the bladder by the advancing contraction wave, which then dissipates at the UVJ.

As with any tubular structure, the ureter can transport a set maximum amount of fluid per unit time. Under normal flows, in which bolus formation occurs, the amount of urine transported per unit time is significantly less than the maximum transport capacity of the ureter. At extremely high flows, such as those employed in standard perfusion studies (Whitaker, 1973), the ureteral walls do not coapt, and a continuous column of fluid is transported rather than a series of boluses.

If transport becomes inadequate, stasis of urine occurs, with resultant ureteral dilatation. *Inadequate transport can result either from too much fluid entering the ureter per unit time or from too little fluid exiting the ureter per unit time.* Both input and output must be considered in predicting whether ureteral dilatation will occur. For example, a minor degree of obstruction to outflow causes more dilatation at high-flow rates than at low-flow rates. Even a normal, nonobstructed ureter can impede urine transport if the rate of flow is great enough.

Changes in ureteral dimensions that occur in pathologic states may in themselves result in inefficient urine transport,

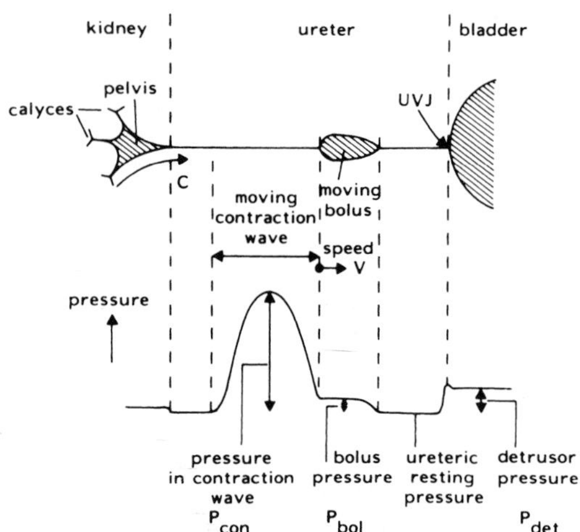

Figure 25–19. Schematic representation of a single bolus in the ureter moving away from the renal pelvis and toward the bladder. Arrow C indicates direction of bolus transport. Corresponding distribution of pressure within the urinary tract is shown in the lower tracing. (From Griffiths DJ, Notschaele C: Neurourol Urodynam 1983; 2:155, with permission.)

even if the contractile force of the individual fibers is unchanged. The *Laplace equation* expresses the relations between the variables that affect intraluminal pressure:

$$\text{Pressure} = (\text{Tension} \times \text{Wall Thickness}) \div \text{Radius}$$

An increase in ureteral diameter in itself can decrease intraluminal pressure and result in inefficient urine transport. Such dimensional changes may, at least theoretically, be deleterious (Griffiths, 1983).

Effect of Diuresis on Ureteral Function

With increasing urine flow rates, the initial response of the ureter is to increase peristaltic frequency. After the maximum frequency is achieved, further increases in urine transport occur by means of increases in bolus volume (Briggs et al, 1972; Constantinou et al, 1974; Morales et al, 1952). At relatively low flow rates, small increases in flow result in large increases in peristaltic frequency. At higher flow rates, relatively large increases in flow result in only small increases in peristaltic frequency. As flow rate continues to increase, several of the boluses coalesce, and finally the ureter becomes filled with a column of fluid and dilates. At these high flow rates, urine transport is through an open tube.

Effects of Bladder Filling and Neurogenic Vesical Dysfunction on Ureteral Function

Ureteral dilatation can result either from an increase in fluid input or from a decrease in fluid output from the ureter. Because there is no evidence that the UVJ relaxes (Weiss and Biancani, 1983), the relation between ureteral intraluminal pressure and intravesical pressure is important in determining the efficacy of urine passage across the UVJ into the bladder. In the normal ureter under normal physiologic rates of flow, ureteral contractile pressure exceeds intravesical pressure, resulting in passage of urine into the bladder. In the dilated, poorly contracting ureter or in the normal ureter at extreme flow rates, the ureter does not coapt its walls to form boluses, and the baseline pressure in the column of urine within the ureter must exceed intravesical pressure in order for urine to pass into the bladder.

The pressure within the bladder during the storage phase is of paramount importance in determining the efficacy of urine transport across the UVJ. This is the pressure that the ureter needs to work against for the longest period of time. During filling of the normal bladder, sympathetic impulses and the viscoelastic properties of the bladder wall inhibit the magnitude of the intravesical pressure rise (i.e., the tonus limb). With filling, the normal bladder maintains a relatively low intravesical pressure (McGuire, 1983), which facilitates transport of urine across the UVJ and prevents ureteral dilatation. In the noncompliant, fibrotic bladder and in some forms of neurogenic vesical dysfunction, the bladder is autonomous, and relatively small increases in bladder volume result in large increases in intravesical pressure with resultant impairment of ureteral emptying. The ureter initially responds to its decreased ability to empty by increasing its peristaltic frequency (Fredericks et al, 1972; Rosen et al, 1971; Zimskind et al, 1969). Ultimately, stasis occurs with the development of ureteral dilatation. The ureter has been shown to decompensate when intravesical pressure approaches 40 cm H_2O (McGuire et al, 1981).

Physiology of the Ureterovesical Junction

Griffiths (1983) has analyzed the factors involved in urine transport across the UVJ. Under normal conditions and at normal flow rates, the contraction wave, which occludes the ureteral lumen, propagates distally with the urine bolus in front of it. When the bolus reaches the UVJ, the pressure within the bolus must exceed intravesical pressure in order for the bolus of urine to pass across the UVJ into the bladder. Under these conditions, in which the contraction wave is able to coapt the ureteral wall and move the urinary bolus distally, the pressure generated by the contraction wave exceeds the pressure within the urinary bolus. As the bolus is ejected into the bladder, the distal ureter retracts within its sheaths; this telescoping of the ureter aids in decreasing UVJ resistance to flow and facilitates urine passage into the bladder (Blok et al, 1985). The UVJ does not relax (Weiss and Biancani, 1983).

Impediment of efficient bolus transfer across the UVJ into the bladder can occur if there is an obstruction at the UVJ, if intravesical pressure is excessive, or if flow rates are so high as to exceed the transport capacity of the normal UVJ. Under such conditions, in which the bolus of urine cannot pass freely into the bladder, the pressure within the bolus increases and may exceed the pressure in the contraction wave. This results in an inability of the contraction wave to completely occlude the ureter; there is retrograde flow of urine from the bolus, and only a fraction of the urinary bolus passes across the UVJ into the bladder. Griffiths (1983) has presented theoretical evidence to show that an exactly similar situation of impaired bolus transport across the UVJ would be expected if the ureter were wide or weakly contracting, even if the UVJ itself were completely normal. The wider and more weakly contracting the ureter, the lower the UVJ resistance must be in order not to interfere with bolus transport. The resistance to flow at the UVJ has been variously attributed to forces in the trigone (Tanagho et al, 1968) and to detrusor pressure (Coolsaet et al, 1982).

The theoretical considerations outlined by Griffiths (1983) have direct clinical implications. If the UVJ is obstructed (i.e., has an abnormally high resistance to flow) or if detrusor pressure is excessive, large boluses occurring at high-flow conditions are not completely discharged into the bladder, because the contraction wave pushing the bolus is forced open and intraureteric reflux occurs. Such obstruction at the UVJ can be detected by perfusion studies, as popularized by Whitaker (1973, 1979) (i.e., the Whitaker test). On the other hand, Griffiths' (1983) theory suggests that a similar breakdown of bolus discharge into the bladder can occur in the wide or weakly contracting ureter at high flow rates even if the UVJ is normal, and that such a condition would go undetected by a Whitaker test.

There is evidence that gravity may assist urine transport and that the erect position may aid urine transport across the UVJ, especially in individuals with dilated upper tracts (Schick and Tanagho, 1973). From a practical standpoint, George and associates (1984) suggested that bed rest may be deleterious to renal function in individuals with urinary retention and wide upper urinary tracts.

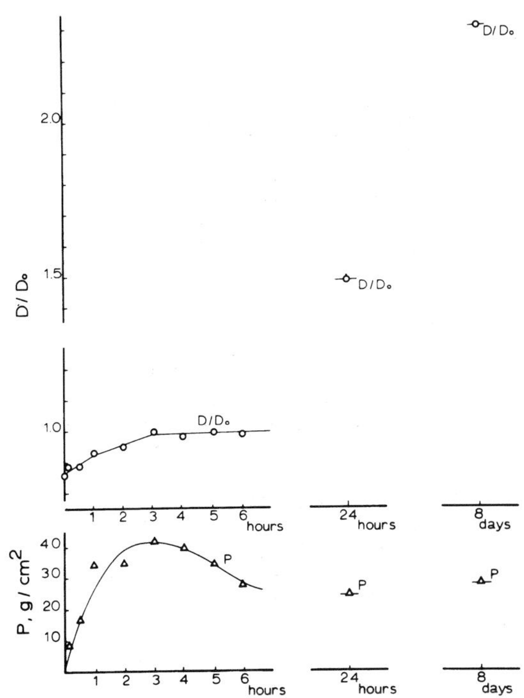

Figure 25–20. Changes in intraluminal pressure (P) and diameter subsequent to obstruction of rabbit ureter. Time from onset of obstruction is on the abscissa. Change in diameter (D/D_0) is on the upper ordinate, and P is on the lower ordinate. During the initial 3 hours of obstruction, P increased to a maximum and was associated with increase in diameter. Between 3 and 6 hours after onset of obstruction, P declined, although diametral deformation persisted. After 6 hours, P remained essentially unchanged, but diameter continued to increase. Each data point represents mean positive or negative standard error of mean. D_0, initial diameter; D, diameter during deformation. (Adapted from Biancani P, Zabinski MP, Weiss RM: Am J Physiol 1976; 231:393.)

PATHOLOGIC PROCESSES AFFECTING URETERAL FUNCTION

Effect of Obstruction on Ureteral Function

The effect of obstruction on ureteral function is dependent on the degree and duration of the obstruction, the rate of urine flow, and the presence or absence of infection. After the onset of obstruction, a backup of urine occurs within the urinary collecting system, along with an associated increase in baseline (resting) ureteral intraluminal pressure and an increase in ureteral dimensions, both length and diameter (Fig. 25–20) (Biancani et al, 1976; Rose and Gillenwater, 1973). The increase in ureteral intraluminal pressure is dependent on the continued production by the kidney of urine that cannot pass beyond the site of obstruction; the increase in ureteral dimensions results from the increased intraluminal pressure and the increased volume of urine retained within the ureter. A transient increase in the amplitude and frequency of the peristaltic contraction waves accompanies these initial dimensional and ureteral baseline pressure changes (Rose and Gillenwater, 1978). With time, as the ureter fills with urine, the peristaltic contraction waves become smaller and are unable to coapt the ureteral wall. Urine transport then becomes dependent on hydrostatic forces generated by the kidney (Rose and Gillenwater, 1973). Superimposed infection may result in a complete absence of contractions in the obstructed ureter and contributes to impairment of urine transport (Rose and Gillenwater, 1973).

Within a few hours after onset of obstruction, intraluminal baseline ureteral pressure reaches a peak and then declines to a level only slightly higher than the normal baseline pressure. During this time, dimensional changes remain stable (Biancani et al, 1976). The decrease in ureteral pressure can be attributed to changes in intrarenal hemodynamics, such as a reduction in renal blood flow (Vaughan et al, 1971), with resultant decreases in glomerular filtration rate and intratubular hydrostatic pressure (Gottschalk and Mylle, 1956). Fluid reabsorption into the venous and lymphatic systems and a decrease in wall tension also may play a role in the reduction in baseline ureteral pressure (Rose and Gillenwater, 1978). The persistence of dimensional changes in the face of a decrease in intraluminal pressure is dependent on the hysteretic properties of the viscoelastic ureteral structure (Fig. 25–21) (Biancani et al, 1973, 1976; Vereecken et al, 1973; Weiss et al, 1972).

As the obstruction persists, there is a gradual increase in ureteral length and diameter to considerable dimensions. This occurs even though ureteral pressure remains at a relatively low and constant level. This process, observed in viscoelastic structures, is referred to as creep (Biancani et al, 1973). A continued, albeit small, urine production is required for the continuing increase in intraureteral volume. Such changes account for the relatively low intrapelvic pressures clinically observed in the massively dilated, chronically obstructed upper urinary tract (Backlund et al, 1965; Djurhuus and Stage, 1976; Struthers, 1969; Vela-Navarrete, 1971) and in experimentally produced obstruction (Koff and Thrall, 1981a; Schweitzer, 1973; Vaughan et al, 1970). One

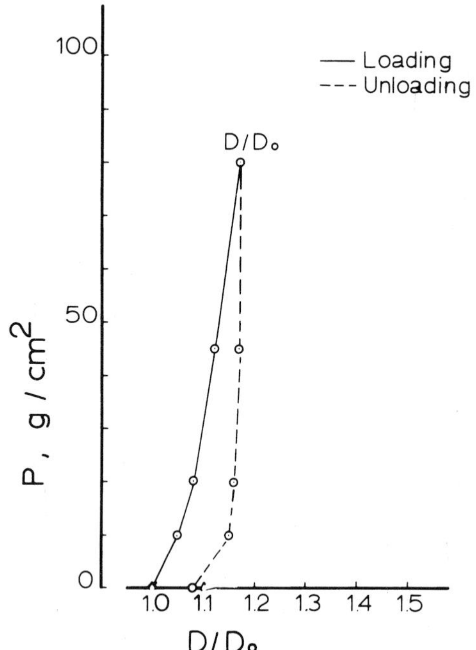

Figure 25–21. Demonstration of hysteretic properties of ureter showing that dimensional changes are dependent on intraluminal pressure and on the direction of change of that pressure. At comparable pressures, deformations are greater during ureteral emptying than during ureteral filling. Solid line shows data obtained during loading; dashed line, data obtained during unloading. D_0, initial diameter; D, diameter during deformation; P, intraluminal pressure in g/cm^2. (Adapted from Biancani P, Zabinski MP, and Weiss RM: Am J Physiol 1976; 231:393.)

could postulate that with prolonged complete obstruction, total cessation of urine output ultimately occurs. Subsequent decrease in ureteral dimensions would depend on whether urine is reabsorbed and on the mechanical properties of the ureter at that time.

In order to determine the effect of obstruction on the contractile properties of the ureter, a rabbit model in which the ureter was totally obstructed for 2 weeks was employed (Biancani et al, 1982; Hausman et al, 1979). After 2 weeks of obstruction, cross-sectional muscle area increased by 250%, ureteral length by 24%, and ureteral outer diameter by 100%. In addition to undergoing muscle hypertrophy, in vitro segments from obstructed ureters developed greater contractile forces, in both longitudinal and circumferential directions, than segments from control ureters (Fig. 25–22). Determinations of *stress (force per unit area of muscle)* provide a means of judging whether observed increases in developed force result from an increase in contractility or from an increase in muscle mass alone. The increases in force were associated with an increase in maximum active circumferential stress but no change in maximum active longitudinal stress (Fig. 25–23); because of this, the sum of the stresses (total stress) or overall contractility increased after 2 weeks of obstruction. In order to account for these differences in longitudinal and circumferential stresses subsequent to obstruction, rotation of muscle bundles must occur; otherwise, longitudinal and circumferential stresses would have increased equally. The rotation could result from the greater increase in diameter than in length that occurred after obstruction, from remodeling of the muscle fibers, or from both.

Therefore, after 2 weeks of obstruction, the dilated ureter is not mechanically decompensated but rather undergoes changes that result in an increase in contractility. Despite both the muscle hypertrophy and the increase in contractility, it is clinically and experimentally evident that the obstructed, dilated ureter is less able than the normal ureter to generate the contractile pressures required for urine transport (Rose and Gillenwater, 1973). The decrease in the ability to generate an intraluminal pressure despite an increase in contractility results from the increase in ureteral diameter that occurs after obstruction and can be explained by the Laplace relation (see previous section on propulsion of urinary bolus). Although contractility (stress) increases after 2 weeks of obstruction, the decrease in the ratio of ureteral wall thickness to radius resulting from the marked increase in intraluminal diameter and thinning of the muscle layer accounts for the decrease in pressure. A longer duration of obstruction or the presence of infection may alter these relations.

Estimates of intraluminal pressures as a function of diameter (pressure-diameter curves) can be calculated from in vitro circumferential force-length data (Fig. 25–24) (Biancani et al, 1982; Weiss and Biancani, 1982) and provide insight as to how obstruction interferes with urine transport. The validity of such calculations is supported by their correspondence to actual in vivo measurements (Biancani et al, 1976; Rose and Gillenwater, 1973). The obstructed ureter at in vivo dimensions has a higher resting (baseline) pressure and a lower contractile (active) pressure than does a control ureter. In the control ureter, the total (active plus passive or resting) pressure developed at all diameters exceeds the passive pressure shown by the horizontal dotted line, and therefore the generated active or contractile pressures are able to fully coapt the ureteral lumen and propel the urine bolus. In the obstructed ureter at diameters less than 3.3 mm, the passive pressure, as shown by the horizontal dotted line, exceeds the total pressure. The contraction ring therefore is incapable of contracting at smaller diameters, and the pressure in the whole ureter remains approximately uniform and equal to the passive pressure. The principal effect of the contraction wave in the obstructed, dilated ureter is to reduce slightly the ureteral volume and thereby raise slightly the overall resting pressure. Although the obstructed ureter is able to develop greater circumferential contractile forces than the control ureter, the expected intraluminal pressure generated by the obstructed ureter is little different from baseline pressure, and the contraction wave occurring during propagation of peristalsis is incapable of coapting the ureteral lumen and propelling the urine bolus in an effective manner.

The calculated active pressure in the obstructed ureter estimates the pressure that would develop if the whole ureter contracted simultaneously and uniformly throughout its whole length, rather than the pressure measured in a peristaltic contraction wave, which involves contraction of only a small segment of ureter at a given time. The fact that the calculated pressures in the obstructed ureter are, if anything, a slight overestimate of expected pressures only further supports the conclusion that the obstructed ureter is incapable of coapting its lumen and efficiently propelling the urine bolus. If, however, the urine were removed from the lumen of the ureter (for instance, by relief of obstruction), the ureter obstructed for 2 weeks would be able to immediately coapt its lumen and produce pressures comparable to those

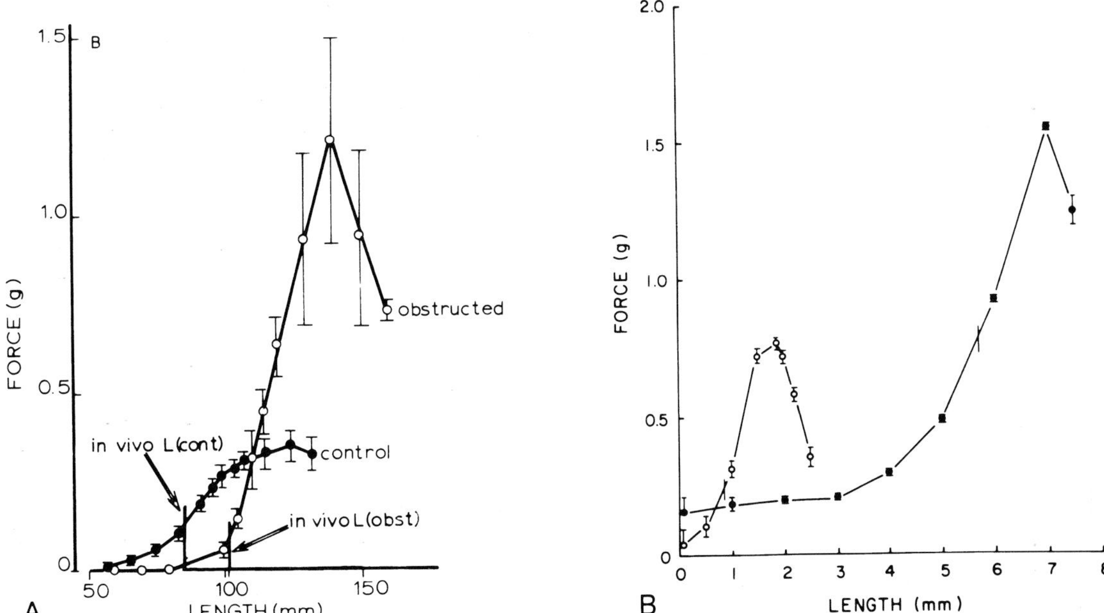

Figure 25–22. *A,* Active (contractile) longitudinal force-length relations of control *(closed circles)* and obstructed *(open circles)* rabbit ureters. Each data point represents mean plus or minus standard error of the mean. (From Hausman M, Biancani P, Weiss RM: Invest Urol 1979; 17:223. Copyright Williams & Wilkins, 1979.) *B,* Active (contractile) circumferential force-length relations of obstructed *(closed circles)* and control *(open circles)* ureteral rings. Vertical bars correspond to in vivo lengths of control and obstructed segments. (From Biancani P, Hausman M, Weiss RM: Am J Physiol 1982; 243:F204, with permission.)

of control ureters. This can be appreciated from Figure 25–24, in which the total pressure in the obstructed ureter at near-zero diameters is comparable to the total pressure in the control ureter at a similar diameter. Two weeks of obstruction therefore results in an increase in ureteral contractility but a decrease in contractile intraluminal pressures. This decrease in the ability to generate an active intraluminal pressure and to coapt the ureteral lumen impairs urine transport in the obstructed ureter.

Obstruction also has been shown to alter the hierarchic organization of the multiple coupled pacemakers that normally coordinate peristaltic activity (Constantinou and Djurhuus, 1981; Djurhuus and Constantinou, 1982). Such disruption causes discoordination of pelvic contractility, with

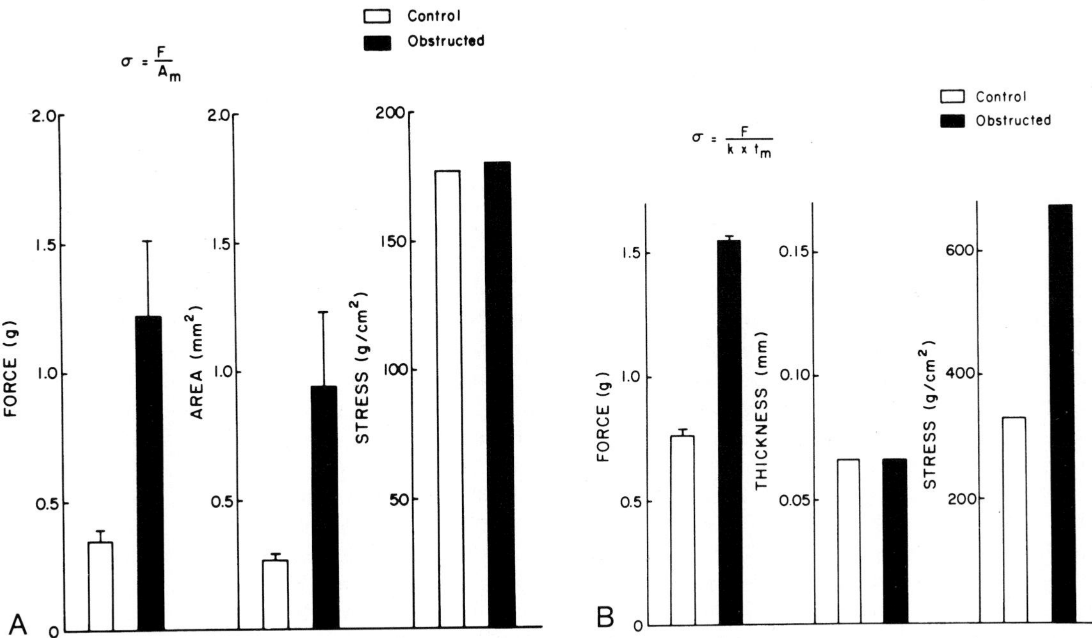

Figure 25–23. *A,* Longitudinal force, cross-sectional muscle area, and longitudinal stress at length of maximal active force development. *B,* Circumferential force, average muscle thickness, and circumferential stress at length of maximal active force development. σ, stress; F, force; A_m, cross-sectional muscle area; t_m, average thickness of muscle layer; K, a constant. (From Weiss RM, Biancani P: Urology 1982; 20:482, with permission.)

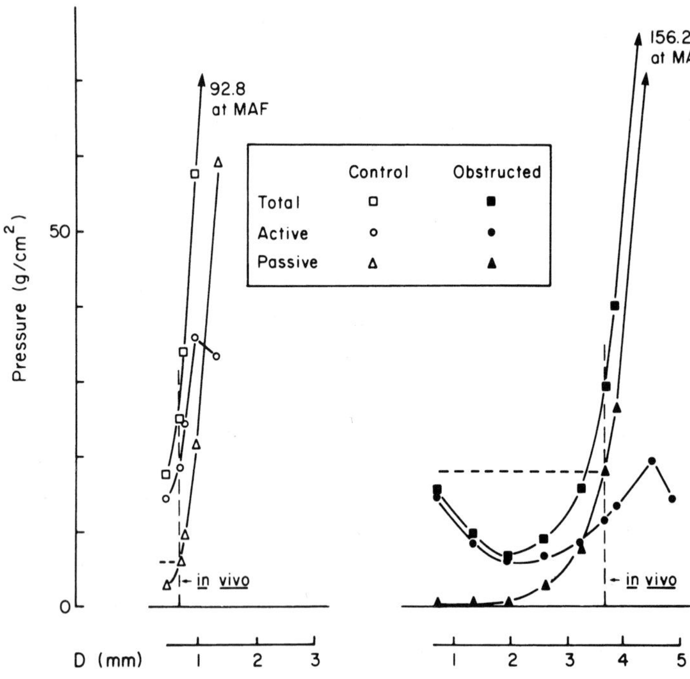

Figure 25–24. Relation between pressure and diameter in control and obstructed ureters. Calculated total, active, and passive pressures are shown as a function of intraluminal diameter (D). In vivo passive pressures are indicated by horizontal dashed lines and in vivo dimensions by vertical dashed lines. (Adapted from Biancani P, Hausman M, Weiss RM: Am J Physiol 1982; 243:F204.)

resultant incomplete emptying of the renal pelvis, which contributes to upper urinary tract dilatation.

Physiologic Methodologies for Assessing Clinical Obstruction

A variety of radiographic methodologies based on physiologic principles are employed in the evaluation and differentiation of upper urinary tract dilatation and obstruction. Description of these examinations, which include diuretic urograms, diuretic radionuclide renograms, and pulsed Doppler sonographic assessment of renal vascular resistance, is beyond the scope of this chapter (see Chapter 10). The best methods now available for differentiating obstructive from nonobstructive dilatation depend on assessment of the efficacy of urine transport. If transport becomes inadequate, urine stagnates and dilatation occurs. Dilatation is dependent on the *compliance* of the system and can result either from too much fluid entering the system per unit time or from too little fluid exiting the system per unit time. The properly functioning upper urinary tract should transport urine over the entire range of physiologically possible flow rates without undergoing marked deformational changes or increases in intraluminal pressure of a magnitude that would be deleterious to the function of the ureter, renal pelvis, or kidney.

Measurement of basal or resting intraluminal pressures does not help in differentiating obstructive from nonobstructive dilatation, because the pressures may be low even when obstruction is present (Backlund et al, 1965; Struthers, 1969; Vela-Navarrete, 1971). The values obtained vary with the state of hydration, the degree of renal function, the severity and duration of obstruction, and the compliance of the system. *Perfusion studies* are widely used in an attempt to differentiate dilated systems that are obstructed from those that are not obstructed (Backlund and Reuterskiöld, 1969a, 1969b; Reuterskiöld, 1969, 1970; Whitaker, 1973, 1978). The technique involves cannulating the dilated upper urinary tract and perfusing the system at a rate of 10 ml/minute. Pressures are measured after achievement of a steady-state condition, which occurs when an equilibrium is reached between the flows into and out of the system. Fluoroscopic monitoring aids in the interpretation of the data (Coolsaet et al, 1980; Whitfield et al, 1976). The basic hypothesis in perfusion studies is that if the dilated upper urinary tract can transport 10 ml/minute (a fluid load greater than it would ever be expected to handle during usual physiologic states) without an inordinate increase in pressure, any degree of obstruction that is present is not clinically significant. Whitaker and associates have concluded from a large clinical experience that under these flow conditions, a pressure of less than 15 cm H_2O correlates with a nonobstructive state, whereas pressures greater than 22 cm H_2O invariably correlate with clinically significant obstruction (Whitaker, 1978; Witherow and Whitaker, 1981). With this definition, minor degrees of obstruction could go undetected; however, the presumption is that if at high flows the hydrostatic pressure in the system is not at a level that would produce renal deterioration, then lower and more physiologic flows can be tolerated. The high flows are used to stress the system and thereby to detect the slightest propensity to obstruction. The interpretation of data obtained by perfusion studies is schematically shown in Figure 25–25.

In order to obtain relevant information, strict adherence to detail is required in the performance of perfusion studies. Care must be taken to ensure that an equilibrium state has been reached before making pressure measurements. Extrinsic factors that affect resistance to flow, such as needle size, length and compliance of extrinsic tubing, viscosity of perfusion fluid, temperature, and flow rate, must be considered when quantitative data are obtained (Toguri and Fournier, 1982). Furthermore, the bladder should be continuously drained to eliminate the bladder's effect on urine transport.

When performed and interpreted properly, perfusion studies may provide clinically relevant information in selected cases. The basic problem in the interpretation of data with this and other diagnostic methods is the definition of clinically relevant obstruction—that is, how much resistance to flow or increase in pressure is required to produce renal functional or anatomic deterioration as a function of time, taking into account the compliance of the system (Koff and Thrall, 1981b). Also, it is theoretically possible that the wide or weakly contracting ureter at high flow rates may interfere with bolus transport even if the UVJ is normal (Griffiths, 1983). Such an obstructive process would not be detected by perfusion studies (see previous discussion).

These theoretical considerations provide a rationale for ureteral tapering (Hendren, 1970), a procedure that has been shown to improve radiographic appearances, although the question remains as to whether it aids in preserving renal function when anatomic or functional obstruction does not exist. The Laplace relation provides a possible explanation for anticipated improvement in function resulting from tapering. With ureteral tapering, muscle thickness and the ability of the ureteral fibers to contract (stress) are unchanged. The decrease in radius resulting from tapering itself, according to the Laplace relation, could account for higher intraluminal pressures, which could improve urine transport. Therefore, the tapered ureter may coapt its walls more readily and

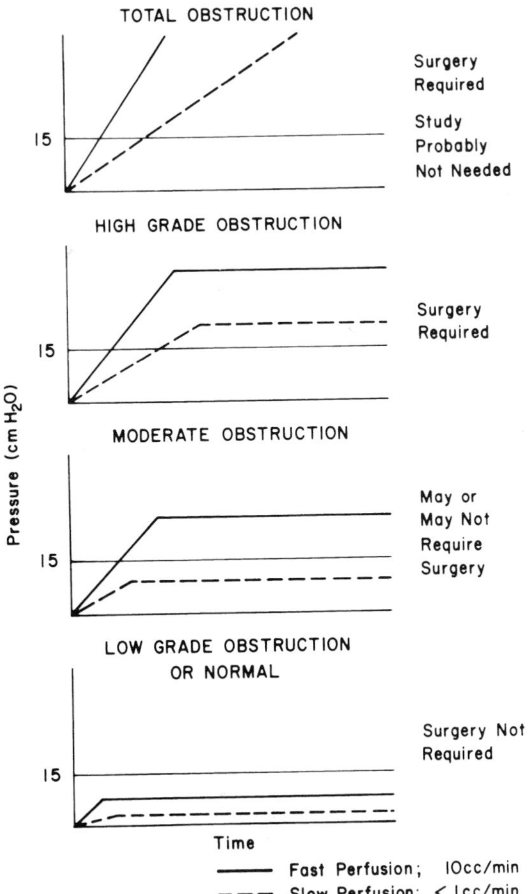

Figure 25–25. Schematic representation of data that can be obtained with perfusion studies. The fast perfusion rate, 10 ml/minute, would be used in the standard Whitaker test. The slow perfusion rate, less than 1 ml/minute, would be closer to more physiologic rates of flow. (From Weiss RM: J Urol 1979; 121:401. Copyright by Williams & Wilkins, 1979.)

generate higher intraluminal pressures even though the material itself has not changed (Weiss and Biancani, 1982). Although the possibility of deleterious effects of the wide, nonobstructed ureter remains controversial, such effects should be considered when interpreting data obtained with the present modalities for diagnosing obstruction and when determining management.

Relation Between Vesicoureteral Reflux and Ureteral Function

Factors that have been implicated in the development of vesicoureteral reflux include (1) anatomic and functional abnormalities at the UVJ, (2) inordinately high intravesical pressures, and (3) impaired ureteral function. The normal intravesical ureter is approximately 1.5 cm in length and takes an oblique course through the bladder wall. It is composed of an intramural segment surrounded by detrusor muscle and a submucosal segment that lies directly under the bladder urothelium (Tanagho et al, 1968). The relation between length and diameter of this intravesical segment of ureter appears to be a factor in the prevention of vesicoureteral reflux (Paquin, 1959). Reflux may occur if the intravesical tunnel is destroyed. Trigonal function also may be a factor in the prevention of vesicoureteral reflux. Tanagho and associates (1965) created vesicoureteral reflux in the cat by disruption of the trigone or by sympathectomy and, conversely, increased the pressure within the intravesical ureter by electrical stimulation of the trigone or by administration of intravenous epinephrine. The development of vesicoureteral reflux in individuals with bladder outlet obstruction and neurogenic vesical dysfunction provides evidence that increased intravesical pressures also may be a factor in certain instances of reflux.

Although an abnormality of the UVJ is the primary etiologic factor in most cases of reflux, decreased ureteral peristaltic activity can be a contributory factor. This may explain why a normal ureter may not reflux even if it is reimplanted into a bladder without a submucosal tunnel (Debruyne et al, 1978) or why a defunctionalized, refluxing ureter may cease to reflux after a proximal diversion is taken down (Teele et al, 1976; Weiss, 1979). The observation that vesicoureteral reflux may temporarily cease after ureteral electrical stimulation (Melick et al, 1966) further supports this possibility.

Even the mildest forms of vesicoureteral reflux are associated with a decreased frequency of ureteral peristalsis (Kirkland et al, 1971; Weiss and Biancani, 1983). Although this may offer further evidence that decreased peristaltic activity is a possible etiologic factor in the development of reflux, an alternative interpretation is that the decreased peristaltic activity reflects changes in ureteral or renal function resulting from the reflux. Finally, the success rate of antireflux procedures is lower with poorly functioning, dilated ureters, and although this may be related to technical factors, decreased peristaltic activity may be another reason for failure in many instances.

Studies in normal and mildly refluxing systems have shown that there is a high-pressure zone in the distal ureter, with a resultant pressure gradient across the UVJ (Weiss and Biancani, 1983). Although the cause of the UVJ gradient is not known, the weight of the fluid within the bladder compressing the intravesical ureter may be a factor. Another causative factor may be bladder or trigonal tension involving myogenic or neurohumoral mechanisms. With bladder filling, there is an increase in the amplitude of the high-pressure zone that is greater in nonrefluxing than in refluxing systems. With bladder filling, the resultant UVJ–bladder pressure gradient increases in nonrefluxing systems, whereas it decreases and may disappear in refluxing systems (Fig. 25–26) (Weiss and Biancani, 1983). This decrease in pressure gradient may correspond to the time when reflux occurs and may be related to lateralization of the ureteral orifice and shortening of the intravesical tunnel.

Effect of Infection on Ureteral Function

Infection within the upper urinary tract may impair urine transport. Pyelonephritis in the monkey has been associated with decreased peristaltic activity (Roberts, 1975). Furthermore, Rose and Gillenwater (1973) have shown that infection can potentiate the deleterious effects of obstruction on ureteral function. In 1913, Primbs showed that *Escherichia coli* and staphylococcal toxins inhibited contractions of in vitro guinea pig ureteral segments (Primbs, 1913). A number of studies have confirmed that bacterial and *E. coli* endotoxins can inhibit ureteral activity (Grana et al, 1965; King and Cox, 1972; Teague and Boyarsky, 1968), although these findings have not been universal (Struthers, 1976). Thulesius and Araj (1987) also failed to suppress ureteral activity with *E. coli* endotoxin but noted that growth supernatants from *E. coli, Pseudomonas aeruginosa*, and *Klebsiella pneumoniae* inhibited ureteral contractility. These investigators suggested that the inhibition of peristaltic activity was caused by an exotoxin.

In humans, irregular peristaltic contractions with an often decreased amplitude have been recorded with infection, and absence of activity has been noted in the more severe cases (Ross et al, 1972). Furthermore, ureteral dilatation has been reported to result from retroperitoneal inflammatory processes secondary to appendicitis, regional enteritis, ulcerative colitis, or peritonitis (Makker et al, 1972). Infection also may reduce the compliance of the intravesical ureter and permit reflux to occur in situations in which the UVJ is intrinsically of marginal competence (Cook and King, 1979).

Effect of Calculi on Ureteral Function

Factors that affect the spontaneous passage of calculi are (1) the size and shape of the stone (Ueno et al, 1977), (2) intrinsic areas of narrowing within the ureter, (3) ureteral peristalsis, (4) hydrostatic pressure of the column of urine proximal to the calculus (Sivula and Lehtonen, 1967), and (5) edema, inflammation, and spasm of the ureter at the site at which the stone is lodged (Holmlund and Hassler, 1965; Scheele, 1965).

In an attempt to understand the physiologic processes that contribute to or hinder the passage of stones through the ureter, Crowley and associates (1990) created acute ureteral obstruction with an intraluminal balloon catheter and measured intraluminal ureteral pressures and peristaltic activity above and below the acutely obstructed site. Peristaltic rate and baseline, peak, and delta (peak minus baseline) pressures increased proximal to the site of obstruction. In contrast, peristaltic rate remained unchanged distal to the obstruction, despite decreases in baseline, peak, and delta pressures. It was suggested that failure of transmission of effective peristalsis across the site of obstruction may hinder stone passage; however, this remains to be proved.

Two factors that appear to be most useful in facilitating stone passage are an increase in hydrostatic pressure proximal to a calculus and relaxation of the ureter in the region of the stone. In support of the theory that hydrostatic pressure facilitates stone passage, artificial concretions with holes were shown to move more slowly in the rabbit and dog ureter than those without holes (Sivula and Lehtonen, 1967). Furthermore, ureteral ligation proximal to a concretion, which decreases hydrostatic pressure by decreasing urine output and which decreases peristaltic activity proximal to a stone, hampers stone passage (Sivula and Lehtonen, 1967).

With respect to the potential facilitative effect of ureteral relaxation on stone passage, the spasmolytic agents phentolamine, an alpha-adrenergic antagonist, and orciprenaline, a beta-adrenergic agonist, have been shown to dilate the ureteral lumen at the level of an artificial concretion and thereby

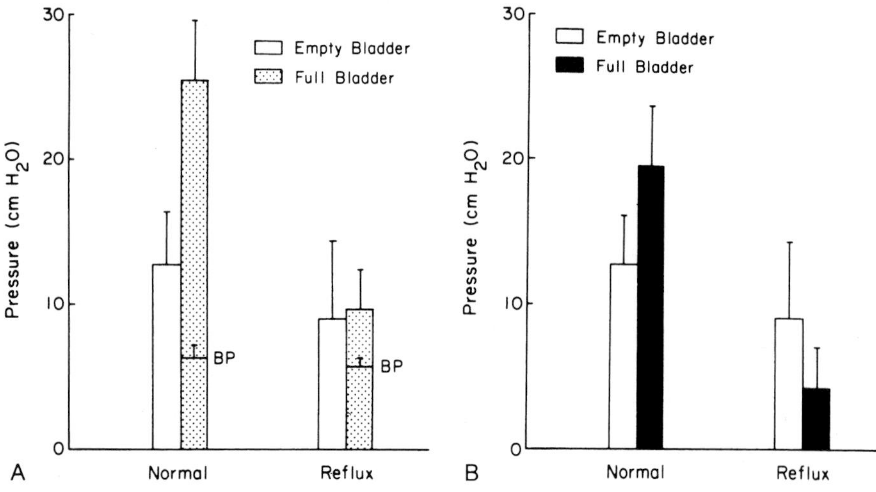

Figure 25–26. *A,* Ureterovesical junction pressures. Bladder pressure is approximately zero with the bladder empty and is labeled as BP with the bladder full. *B,* Pressure gradient across ureterovesical junction, obtained by subtracting bladder pressure from ureterovesical junction pressure. (From Weiss RM, Biancani P: J Urol 1983; 129:858. Copyright by Williams & Wilkins, 1983.)

to permit increased fluid flow beyond the concretion (Peters and Eckstein, 1975). Whether this spasmolytic effect would aid in stone passage has not been determined. In a human study, renal colic was relieved by meperidine in 83% of patients, by phentolamine in 63%, and by propranolol, a beta-adrenergic antagonist that presumably would interfere with the beta-adrenergic inhibitory actions of catecholamines, in 0% (Kubacz and Catchpole, 1972). Although these data suggest that drugs with spasmolytic effects on the ureter may relieve renal colic, whereas those with spasmogenic actions do not, no attempt was made to assess the efficacy of these agents in promoting stone passage.

Although the aforementioned pharmacologic data can be interpreted to imply that ureteral relaxation in the region of a concretion would aid in stone passage, a controlled study is not available. Such a study with an agent known to have strong relaxant effects on the ureter, such as theophylline (Green et al, 1987; Weiss et al, 1977), would be of value, but interpretation of the data may be difficult because of the marked variability of spontaneous stone passage in the clinical setting.

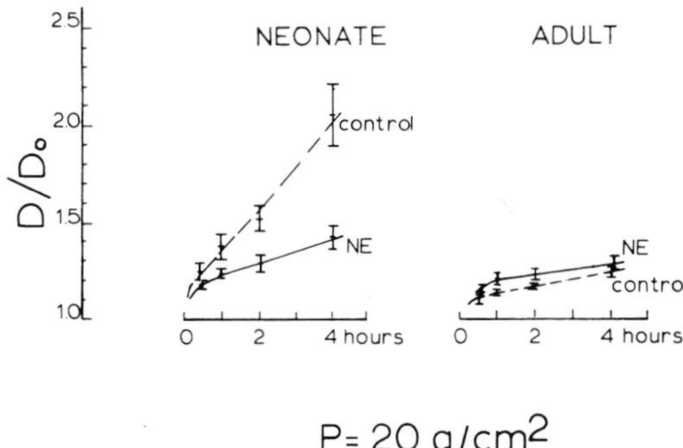

Figure 25–27. Changes in diameter of neonatal and adult rabbit ureteral segments as a function of time after application of a constant intraluminal pressure of 20 g/cm^2. Diametral deformation (D/D_0) of control neonatal ureters was significantly greater than that of control adult ureters. Norepinephrine (10^{-5} mol/L) decreased diametral deformation of neonatal ureters but had no significant effect on deformation of adult ureteral segments. D_0, initial diameter; D, diameter during deformation; P, intraluminal pressure. (From Akimoto M, Biancani P, Weiss RM: Invest Urol 1977; 14:297, with permission.)

EFFECT OF AGE ON URETERAL FUNCTION

Clinically, the response of the ureter to pathologic conditions seems to vary with age. More marked degrees of ureteral dilatation are observed in the neonate and young child than in the adult. Experimental data corroborating this clinical impression can be derived from observed age-dependent differences in the response of in vitro ureteral segments to an intraluminal pressure load. The neonatal rabbit ureter undergoes a greater degree of deformation in response to an applied intraluminal pressure than does the adult rabbit ureter (Akimoto et al, 1977). Furthermore, norepinephrine decreases diametral deformation of the neonatal rabbit ureter in response to an applied intraluminal pressure but has little effect on deformation of the adult rabbit ureter (Fig. 25–27). The in vitro neonatal rabbit ureter therefore appears to be more compliant and more sensitive to norepinephrine than does the adult rabbit ureter.

Age also affects the response of the ureter to beta-adrenergic agonists, with a decrease in the relaxant response to the beta-adrenergic agonist isoproterenol with aging (Wheeler et al, 1990). The relaxant response to beta-adrenergic agonists is related, in part, to levels of cAMP; it has been shown that with aging there is a decrease in the enzymatic activities involved in the synthesis of cAMP (Wheeler et al, 1986) but no change in the enzymatic activities involved in its degradation (Cho et al, 1988). These data suggest that the decrease in the ability of isoproterenol to relax the ureter with aging results from a decrease in the ability of isoproterenol to activate adenylyl cyclase, the enzyme involved in cAMP synthesis.

A progressive increase in ureteral cross-sectional muscle area is observed in the guinea pig between 3 weeks and 3 years of age. This is in accord with the findings of Cussen (1967), who noted in a human autopsy study in subjects ranging in age from 12 weeks of gestation to 12 years of age that there is a progressive increase in the ureteral population of smooth muscle cells and a small increase in the overall size of the individual smooth muscle cells. In addition, an irregular increase in the number of elastic fibers was observed with increasing age.

The contractility of the ureter also is affected by age. Maximal active force of isolated guinea pig ureteral segments increases between 3 weeks and 3 years of age (Fig. 25–28) (Hong et al, 1980). The increase in force developed between 3 weeks and 3 months of age seems to be attributable to an increase in contractility, because there is an associated increase in active stress (force per unit area of muscle). The increase in force that occurs between 3 months and 3 years of age can be explained by an increase in mass alone, because there is no change in active stress between these two age groups (see Fig. 25–28).

Although changes in the force-length relations of guinea pig ureter occur with age, the force-velocity relations do not change with age (Biancani et al, 1984). Therefore, although ureteral contractility increases during early development, as shown by an increase in force per unit area of muscle (stress), no significant change is apparent in the rate of the driving reactions that control the contractile process—that is, no change in shortening, velocity, work, or power.

EFFECT OF PREGNANCY ON URETERAL FUNCTION

Hydroureteronephrosis of pregnancy begins in the second trimester of gestation and subsides within the first month after parturition. It is more severe on the right side, and the ureteral dilatation does not occur below the pelvic brim. Roberts (1976) has presented a strong case in favor of obstruction as the etiologic factor in the development of hydroureteronephrosis of pregnancy, whereas other investigators have suggested a hormonal mechanism (van Wagenen and Jenkins, 1939).

Roberts (1976) emphasized the following: (1) elevated baseline ureteral pressures consistent with obstructive changes have been recorded above the pelvic brim in pregnant women, and these pressures decrease when positional

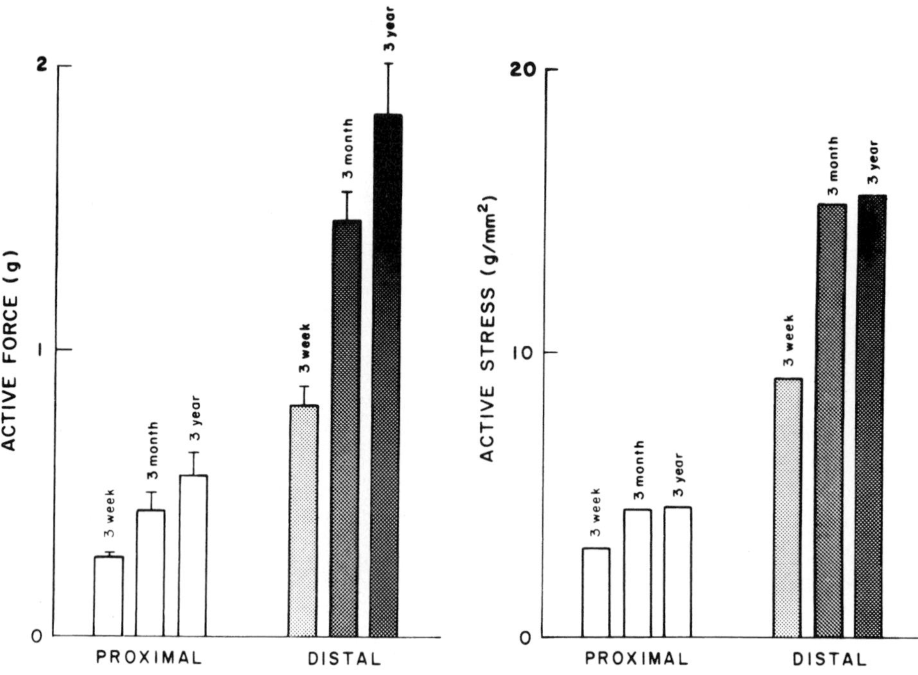

Figure 25–28. Maximal active (contractile) force and maximal active stress of proximal and distal guinea pig ureteral segments as a function of age.

changes permit the uterus to fall away from the ureters (Sala and Rubi, 1967); (2) normal ureteral contractile pressures recorded during pregnancy suggest that hormonally induced ureteral atony is not the prime factor in ureteral dilatation of pregnancy; (3) women whose ureters do not cross the pelvic brim (i.e., those with pelvic kidneys or ileal conduits) do not develop hydronephrosis of pregnancy; (4) hydronephrosis of pregnancy usually does not occur in quadrupeds, whose uterus hangs away from the ureters (Traut and Kuder, 1938); and (5) elevated ureteral pressures in the pregnant monkey return to normal if the uterus is elevated from the ureters at laparotomy or if the fetus and placenta are removed from the uterus.

Observed hormonal effects on ureteral function have been used to implicate a hormonal mechanism in the ureteral dilatation of pregnancy, although difficulties in interpretation arise from inconsistencies in the data. Several studies have shown an inhibitory effect of progesterone on ureteral function (Hundley et al, 1942; Kumar, 1962; Lubin et al, 1941). Progesterone has been noted to increase the degree of ureteral dilatation during pregnancy and to retard the rate of disappearance of hydroureter in postpartum women (Lubin et al, 1941). Other studies, however, have failed to demonstrate an effect of progesterone on ureteral activity in animals (McNellis and Sherline, 1967; Payne and Hodes, 1939) or in humans (Lapides, 1948; Schneider et al, 1953), and still others have failed to induce changes in ureteral activity in women through administration of estrogens, progesterone, or a mixture of these drugs (Clayton and Roberts, 1973; Marchant, 1972). Although some workers have noted that estrogens increase ureteral activity (Hundley et al, 1942), most have failed to observe an effect of estrogens in various animal models (Abramson et al, 1953; Payne and Hodes, 1939) or in humans (Kumar, 1962; Lubin et al, 1941; Schneider et al, 1953). Therefore, obstruction appears to be the primary factor in the development of hydronephrosis of pregnancy, although some evidence suggests that a combination of hormonal and obstructive factors is involved (Fainstat, 1963).

EFFECT OF DRUGS ON THE URETER

To assess the effects of drugs on the ureter, it is necessary to understand the anatomic, physiologic, and biochemical properties of the ureter, in addition to understanding the principles of drug action. For a drug to elicit a given response, it is necessary to achieve and maintain an appropriate concentration of that drug at its site of action. Factors that can influence achievement of an effective concentration of drug at a site of action are (1) the route of administration and cellular distribution of the drug; (2) the dosage of the drug administered; (3) the biotransformation, including metabolism and excretion, of the drug; (4) the binding of the drug to plasma and tissue proteins; and (5) the effects of age and disease on the absorption, distribution, metabolism, and elimination of the drug.

The literature contains considerable confusing and conflicting information concerning the effects of drugs on the ureter. To some extent, the discrepancies in the available data result from poorly controlled experimental procedures or attempts to compare dissimilar functional responses of the ureter to a given drug. To simplify the present section, no attempt is made to analyze the validity of each pharmacologic study or to rationalize discrepancies in the literature; rather, an overview is presented with an attempt to provide a consensus that, at times, may be prejudiced by personal bias. Furthermore, discussions of drugs related to the nervous system, pregnancy, and a variety of pathologic states have been included in earlier sections of this chapter. A more complete review of drug effects on the ureter is available (Weiss, 1982).

Histamine and Its Antagonists

Histamine has a dual action on smooth muscle; it may (1) release catecholamines from sympathetic nerve endings and (2) act directly on receptors within the smooth muscle. Excitatory effects of histamine on ureteral function have been demonstrated (Benedito et al, 1991; Boatman et al, 1967; Borgstedt et al, 1962; Boyarsky and Labay, 1967; Butcher et al, 1957; Sharkey et al, 1965; Struthers, 1973; Vereecken, 1973), a finding that may be species-dependent (Thackston et al, 1955; Tindall, 1972). Histamine's excitatory effect on the UVJ appears to be mediated by H_1 receptors, because it is partially inhibited by the *H_1-receptor antagonist, mepyramine,* but not by the *H_2-receptor antagonist, cimetidine* (Benedito et al, 1991). Furthermore, this excitatory effect of histamine on the sheep UVJ is partially blocked by scopolamine, suggesting an indirect stimulatory action of histamine on intramural parasympathetic nerves. The antihistamines diphenhydramine (Benadryl) and tripelennamine (Pyribenzamine) have been shown to inhibit the effects of histamine on the ureter (Boatman et al, 1967; Borgstedt et al, 1962; Butcher et al, 1957; Sharkey et al, 1965).

Narcotic Analgesics

Morphine has been reported to increase ureteral tone or the frequency and amplitude of ureteral contractions, or both, in a variety of preparations (Gruber, 1928; Hukuhara et al, 1964; Macht, 1916c; Slaughter et al, 1945; Vereecken, 1973). Several early studies using the hydrophorograph, which was more sensitive to changes in urine flow than to changes in actual ureteral peristalsis, suggested that morphine increases ureteral activity in humans (Carroll and Zingale, 1938; Ockerblad et al, 1935). However, more recent studies have failed to confirm these findings (Chen et al, 1957; Kiil, 1957; Weinberg and Maletta, 1961).

The contradictory findings concerning the effect of morphine on ureteral function are further compounded by the fact that other workers have failed to observe such an effect in various experimental preparations (Chen et al, 1957; Gould et al, 1955; Ross et al, 1967; Weinberg, 1962). Meperidine (Demerol) appears to have a similar excitatory effect on the activity of the intact dog ureter (Kaplan et al, 1968; Sharkey et al, 1968). However, Kiil (1957) failed to observe an effect of Demerol on ureteral peristalsis in humans. If only the effects on ureteral activity are considered, there is no basis to preferentially favor morphine or meperidine in the treatment of renal colic. Both agents may have ureteral spasmogenic effects that theoretically would detract from their value in the management of ureteral colic. They certainly do not have potentially valuable spasmolytic actions. Their efficacy in treating colic is dependent on their central nervous system actions, which decrease the perception of pain.

Prostaglandins

Prostaglandins are derived from fatty acids and have a variety of biologic actions in various systems of the body. Their effects vary with species, type of prostaglandin, endocrine status of tissue, experimental conditions, and origin of the smooth muscle. The primary prostaglandins, PGE_1, PGE_2, and $PGF_{2\alpha}$, are synthesized from the fatty acid *arachidonic acid* by enzymatic reactions that can be inhibited by *indomethacin* and aspirin.

Indomethacin has been employed in the management of ureteral colic (Flannigan et al, 1983; Holmlund and Sjöden, 1978; Jönsson et al, 1987). The beneficial effects probably result from indomethacin's inhibition of the prostaglandin-mediated vasodilatation that occurs subsequent to obstruction (Allen et al, 1978; Sjöden et al, 1982). The vasodilatation theoretically would result in an increase in glomerular capillary pressure and subsequent increase in pelviureteral pressure. Indomethacin, by reducing pelviureteral pressure and thus pelviureteral wall tension, may eliminate some of the pain of renal colic that is caused by distention of the upper urinary tract. A potential problem with the use of indomethacin for the treatment of renal colic is that prostaglandin-mediated vasodilatation aids in preserving renal function; therefore, indomethacin may provide pain relief, but it is potentially deleterious to renal function (W.S. McDougal, personal communication, 1992).

PGE_1 inhibits ureteral activity in the dog (Abrams and Feneley, 1976; Boyarsky et al, 1966; Wooster, 1971) and the guinea pig (Vermue and Den Hertog, 1987). PGE_1 inhibition of ureteral activity in the guinea pig is associated with an increase in cAMP levels (Vermue and Den Hertog, 1987). In the ureter, PGE_1 activates adenylyl cyclase, and this may account for the increase in cAMP (Wheeler et al, 1986). Johns and Wooster (1975) suggested that the inhibitory effects of PGE_1 on ureteral activity were dependent on the sequestration of Ca^{2+} at the inner surface of the cell membrane, with a resultant increase in outward conductance of K^+ and hyperpolarization of the membrane. Although some reports have indicated that PGE_2 relaxes the ureter (Vermue and Den Hertog, 1987), other reports describe an excitatory action of PGE_2 on the ureters of sheep (Thulesius and Angelo-Khattar, 1985) and humans (Angelo-Khattar et al, 1985; Cole et al, 1988) and on renal pelvic smooth muscle (Lundstam et al, 1985). In contrast to the inhibitory effects of PGE_1, *$PGF_{2\alpha}$* increases the frequency of ureteral peristalsis in the dog (Boyarsky and Labay, 1969). Indomethacin has been shown to inhibit the activity of sheep (Thulesius and Angelo-Khattar, 1985) and human (Angelo-Khattar et al, 1985; Cole et al, 1988) ureters and of renal pelvic smooth muscle (Lundstam et al, 1985).

Cardiac Glycosides

Ouabain, a cardiac glycoside, has an effect on ureteral activity that appears to be species-dependent. In the isolated cat ureter, ouabain produces a marked increase in contractility, which usually is followed by a late decrease in excitability (Weiss et al, 1970). In the guinea pig ureter, ouabain inhibits activity without a preliminary potentiation of contractility (Hendrickx et al, 1975; Washizu, 1968). The inhibitory effects of ouabain are accompanied by a shortening of the action potential duration, a decrease of the number of oscillations on the plateau of the guinea pig action potential, and a decrease in resting membrane potential.

Calcium Antagonists

Because Ca^{2+} is necessary for the development of the action potential and contraction of the ureter, agents that block the movement of Ca^{2+} into the cell would be expected to depress ureteral function. Voltage-dependent Ca^{2+} channel antagonist binding sites (receptors) have been demonstrated in the ureter, the density of which decreases with age (Yoshida et al, 1992). These dihydropyridine-sensitive, L-type, voltage-dependent Ca^{2+} calcium channels appear to provide the main inward current for generation of the ureteral action potential and the phasic contractile response (Aickin et al, 1984; Brading et al, 1983; Imaizumi et al, 1989; Lang, 1989; Shuba, 1977). The *dihydropyridine Ca^{2+} channel agonist, Bay K 8644,* has an excitatory effect on ureteral activity (Maggi et al, 1994a). The *Ca^{2+} channel blockers, verapamil, D-600* (a methoxy-derivative of verapamil), *diltiazem*, and *nifedipine,* have been shown to inhibit ureteral activity (Golenhofen and Lammel, 1972; Hertle and Nawrath, 1984; Hong et al, 1985; Maggi et al, 1994a; Sakanashi et al, 1985, 1986; Vereecken et al, 1975a). These inhibitory effects are accompanied by decreases in action potential duration, number of oscillations on the plateau of the guinea pig action potential, excitability, and rate of rise and amplitude of the action potential. High concentrations of verapamil and D-600 cause a complete cessation of electrical and mechanical activity.

Potassium Channel Openers

Potassium channel openers such as *cromakalin* and *BRL 38227* hyperpolarize smooth muscle membranes and inhibit renal pelvic and ureteral activity (Kotani et al, 1993; Maggi et al, 1994c). The inhibitory effects of cromakalin are prevented by glibenclamide, providing evidence that glibenclamide-sensitive K^+ channels are important in the generation of ureteral electrical activity (Maggi et al, 1994c). Activation of these K^+ channels may reduce the probability of the opening of voltage-sensitive Ca^{2+} channels that are important in the generation of the ureteral action potential and the contractile response (Cook and Quast, 1990).

Endothelins

Endothelins are potent vasoconstrictor peptides that exist in three isoforms, ET-1, ET-2, and ET-3. Endothelin binding sites (receptors) have been identified in the ureter (Eguchi et al, 1991; Latifpour et al, 1995), where they are primarily of the ET (A) subtype (Latifpour et al, 1995). Endothelins have been shown to initiate contractions in isolated guinea pig and porcine ureters (Eguchi et al, 1991; Maggi et al, 1992a).

Antibiotics

Ampicillin causes relaxation of the ureter and antagonizes the stimulatory effects of barium chloride, histamine, serotonin, and carbachol on the ureter, suggesting that its action is directly on the smooth muscle (Benzi et al, 1970b). Chloramphenicol, the isoxazolyl penicillins, and gentamicin also have spasmolytic effects on the ureter (Benzi et al, 1970a, 1971, 1973). The tetracyclines, on the other hand, potentiate the contractile effects of barium chloride on the ureter (Benzi et al, 1973).

This section has provided an assessment of the effects of the major classes of drugs on ureteral function. Many of the studies referred to were performed on animal models, and the extrapolation of the data to the intact human ureter is often difficult. In the clinical situation, the relatively sparse blood supply to the ureter limits the distribution of drugs to the ureter. In addition, many drugs with potential usefulness in the management of ureteral pathology have potential untoward side effects when used in concentrations required to affect the ureter.

ACKNOWLEDGMENT

The original work was supported in part by Public Health Service Grants DK-38311 and DK-47548 from the National Institutes of Health.

REFERENCES

Aberg AKG, Axelsson J: Some mechanical aspects of an intestinal smooth muscle. Acta Physiol Scand 1965; 64:15.

Abrams PH, Feneley RCL: The actions of prostaglandins on the smooth muscle of the human urinary tract *in vitro*. Br J Urol 1976; 47:909.

Abramson D, Caton WL Jr, Roly CC: The effect of relaxin on the excretion of Diodrast in the castrate hysterectomized rabbit. Am J Obstet Gynecol 1953; 65:644.

Adelstein RS, Pato MD, Conti MA: The role of phosphorylation in regulating contractile proteins. Adv Cyclic Nucleotide Res 1981; 14:361.

Aickin CC: Investigation of factors affecting the intracellular sodium activity in the smooth muscle of guinea-pig ureter. J Physiol (Lond) 1987; 385:483.

Aickin CC, Brading AF, Burdyga TV: Evidence for sodium-calcium exchange in the guinea-pig ureter. J Physiol (Lond) 1984; 347:411.

Aickin CC, Brading AF, Walmsley D: An investigation of sodium-calcium exchange in the smooth muscle of guinea-pig ureter. J Physiol (Lond) 1987; 391:325.

Akimoto M, Biancani P, Weiss RM: Comparative pressure-length-diameter relationships of neonatal and adult rabbit ureters. Invest Urol 1977; 14:297.

Allen JM, Rodrigo J, Kerlie DJ, et al: Neuropeptide Y (NPY)–containing nerves in mammalian ureter. Urology 1990; 35:81.

Allen JT, Vaughan ED Jr, Gillenwater JY: The effect of indomethacin on renal blood flow and ureteral pressure in unilateral ureteral obstruction in awake dogs. Invest Urol 1978; 15:324.

Alquist RP: Study of adrenotropic receptors. Am J Physiol 1948; 153:586.

Ancill RJ, Jackson DM, Redfern PH: The pharmacology of the rat ureter *in vivo.* Br J Pharmacol 1972; 44:628.

Andersson RGG: Cyclic AMP and calcium ions in mechanical and metabolic responses of smooth muscle: Influence of some hormones and drugs. Acta Physiol Scand (Suppl) 1972; 382:1.

Andersson R, Nilsson K: Cyclic AMP and calcium in relaxation in intestinal smooth muscle. Nature New Biol 1972; 238:119.

Angelo-Khattar M, Thulesius O, Nilsson T, et al: Motility of the human ureter, with special reference to the effect of indomethacin. Scand J Urol Nephrol 1985; 19:261.

Backlund L, Grotte G, Reuterskiöld A: Functional stenosis as a cause of pelvi-ureteric obstruction and hydronephrosis. Arch Dis Child 1965; 40:203.

Backlund L, Reuterskiöld AG: Activity in the dilated dog ureter. Scand J Urol Nephrol 1969a; 3:99.

Backlund L, Reuterskiöld AG: The abnormal ureter in children. Scand J Urol Nephrol 1969b; 3:219.

Barastegui CA: Motility of the rat ureter *in vitro:* Responses to cholinergic drugs. Rev Esp Fisiol 1977; 33:1.

Barr L, Berger W, Dewey MM: Electrical transmission at the nexus between smooth muscle cells. J Gen Physiol 1968; 51:347.

Benedito S, Prieto D, Rivera L, et al: Mechanisms implicated in the histamine response of the sheep ureterovesical junction. J Urol 1991; 146:184.

Bennett MR, Burnstock G: Application of the sucrose-gap method to determine the ionic basis of the membrane potential of smooth muscle. J Physiol (Lond) 1966; 183:637.

Benzi G, Arrigoni E, Sanguinetti L: Antibiotics and ureter. III: Chloramphenicol. Arch Int Pharmacodyn Ther 1970a; 185:329.

Benzi G, Arrigoni E, Sanguinetti L: Antibiotics and ureter. V: Gentamicin. Arch Int Pharmacodyn Ther 1971; 189:303.

Benzi G, Arrigoni E, Sanguinetti L: Effect of antibiotics on the ureter motor activity. Jpn J Pharmacol 1973; 23:599.

Benzi G, Bermudez E, Arrigoni E, Berte F: Antibiotics and the ureter. I: Ampicillin. Arch Int Pharmacodyn Ther 1970b; 183:159.

Berridge MJ: Inositol triphosphate and diacylglycerol as second messengers. Biochem J 1984; 220:345.

Biancani P, Hausman M, Weiss RM: Effect of obstruction on ureteral circumferential force-length relations. Am J Physiol 1982; 243:F204.

Biancani P, Onyski JH, Zabinski MP, Weiss RM: Force-velocity relationships of the guinea pig ureter. J Urol 1984; 131:988.

Biancani P, Zabinski MP, Weiss RM: Bidimensional deformation of acutely obstructed in vitro rabbit ureter. Am J Physiol 1973; 225:671.

Biancani P, Zabinski MP, Weiss RM: Time course of ureteral changes with acute and chronic obstruction. Am J Physiol 1976; 231:393.

Blok C, van Venrooij GEPM, Coolsaet BLRA: Dynamics of the ureterovesical junction: A qualitative analysis of the ureterovesical pressure profile in the pig. J Urol 1985; 134:818.

Boatman DL, Lewin ML, Culp DA, Flocks RH: Pharmacologic evaluation of ureteral smooth muscle: A technique of monitoring ureteral peristalsis. Invest Urol 1967; 4:509.

Borgstedt HH, Benjamin JA, Emmel VM: The role of histamine in ureteral function. J Pharmacol Exp Ther 1962; 136:386.

Boyarsky S, Labay P: Histamine analog effect on the ureter. Invest Urol 1967; 4:351.

Boyarsky S, Labay P: Ureteral motility. Annu Rev Med 1969; 20:383.

Boyarsky S, Labay P, Gerber C: Prostaglandin inhibition of ureteral peristalsis. Invest Urol 1966; 4:9.

Boyarsky S, Labay P, Pfautz CJ: The effect of nicotine upon ureteral peristalsis. South Med J 1968; 61:573.

Bozler E: The action potentials of visceral smooth muscle. Am J Physiol 1938a; 124:502.

Bozler E: Electric stimulation and conduction of excitation in smooth muscle. Am J Physiol 1938b; 122:614.

Bozler E: The activity of the pacemaker previous to the discharge of a muscular impulse. Am J Physiol 1942; 136:543.

Brading AF, Burdyga THV, Scripnyuk ZD: The effects of papaverine on the electrical and mechanical activity of the guinea pig ureter. J Physiol (Lond) 1983; 334:79.

Briggs ME, Constantinou CE, Govan DE: Dynamics of the upper urinary tract: The relationship of urine flow rate and rate of ureteral peristalsis. Invest Urol 1972; 10:56.

Burnstock G: Structure of smooth muscle and its innervation. *In* Bhlbring E, Brading AF, Jones AW, Tomita T, eds: Smooth Muscle. Baltimore, Williams & Wilkins, 1970, pp 1–69.

Butcher HR Jr, Sleator W Jr, Schmandt WL: A study of the peristaltic conduction mechanism in the canine ureter. J Urol 1957; 78:221.

Carroll G, Zingale FG: A clinical and experimental study of the effect of pancreatic tissue extracts on the ureter. South Med J 1938; 31:233.

Casteels R: The relation between the membrane potential and the ion distribution in smooth muscle cells. *In* Bhlbring E, Brading AF, Jones AW, Tomita T, eds: Smooth Muscle. Baltimore, Williams & Wilkins, 1970, pp 70–79.

Casteels R, Hendrickx H, Vereecken R: Effects of catecholamines on the electrical and mechanical activity of the guinea pig ureter. Br J Pharmacol 1971; 43:429P.

Cervero F, Sann H: Mechanically evoked responses of afferent fibres innervating the guinea-pig's ureter: An in vitro study. J Physiol (Lond) 1989; 412:245.

Chen PS, Emmel VM, Benjamin JA, Distefano V: Studies on the isolated dog ureter: The pharmacological action of histamine, levarterenol and antihistaminics. Arch Int Pharmacodyn Ther 1957; 110:131.

Chiu AW, Babayan RK, Krane RJ, Saenz de Tejada I: Effects of nitric oxide on ureteral contraction. J Urol 1994; 151:335A.

Cho YH, Biancani P, Weiss RM: Adenylyl and guanylyl nucleotide induced relaxation of ureteral smooth muscle. Fed Proc 1984; 43:353.

Cho YH, Wheeler MA, Weiss RM: Ontogeny of phosphodiesterase and of calmodulin levels in guinea pig ureter. J Urol 1988; 139:1095.

Clayton JD, Roberts JA: Radionuclide postpartum evaluation of the urinary tract during anovular therapy. Surg Gynecol Obstet 1973; 137:215.

Cole RS, Fry CH, Shuttleworth KED: The action of the prostaglandins on isolated human ureteric smooth muscle. Br J Urol 1988; 61:19.

Constantinou CE: Renal pelvic pacemaker control of ureteral peristaltic rate. Am J Physiol 1974; 226:1413.

Constantinou CE, Djurhuus JC: Pyeloureteral dynamics in the intact and chronically obstructed multicalyceal kidney. Am J Physiol 1981; 241:R398.

Constantinou CE, Grenato JJ Jr, Govan DE: Dynamics of the upper urinary tract: Accommodation in the rate and stroke volume of ureteral peristalsis as a response to transient alteration in urine flow rate. Urol Int 1974; 29:249.

Constantinou CE, Hrynczuk JR: Urodynamics of the upper urinary tract. Invest Urol 1976; 14:233.

Constantinou CE, Silvert MA, Gosling J: Pacemaker system in the control of ureteral peristaltic rate in the multicalyceal kidney of the pig. Invest Urol 1977; 14:440.

Constantinou CE, Yamaguchi O: Multiple-coupled pacemaker system in renal pelvis of the unicalyceal kidney. Am J Physiol 1981; 241:R412.

Cook NS, Quast U: Potassium channel pharmacology. *In* Cook NS, ed: Potassium Channels. Chichester, England, Ellis Horwood Series in Pharmaceutical Technology, 1990; pp 181–258.

Cook WA, King LR: Vesicoureteral reflux. *In* Harrison JH, Gittes RF, Perlmutter AD, et al, eds: Campbell's Urology, 4th ed. Philadelphia, W.B. Saunders, 1979, pp 1596–1634.

Coolsaet BLRA, Griffiths DJ, Van Mastrigt R, Duyl W AV: Urodynamic investigation of the wide ureter. J Urol 1980; 124:666.

Coolsaet BLRA, van Venrooij GEPM, Blok C: Detrusor pressure versus wall stress in relation to ureterovesical resistance. Neurourol Urodynam 1982; 1:105.

Crowley AR, Byrne JC, Vaughan ED Jr, Marion DN: The effect of acute obstruction on ureteral function. J Urol 1990; 143:596.

Cussen LJ: The structure of the normal human ureter in infancy and childhood: A quantitative study of the muscular and elastic tissue. Invest Urol 1967; 5:179.

Deane RF: Functional studies of the ureter: Its behavior in the domestic pig *(Sus scrofa domestica)* as recorded by the technique of Trendelenburg. Br J Urol 1967; 39:31.

Debruyne FMJ, Wijdeveld PGAB, Koene RAP, et al: Uretero-neo-cystomy in renal transplantation: Is an antireflux mechanism mandatory? Br J Urol 1978; 50:378.

DelTacca M: Acetylcholine content of and release from isolated pelviureteral tract. Naunyn Schmiedebergs Arch Pharmacol 1978; 302:293.

Dixon JS, Gosling JA: The fine structure of pacemaker cells in the pig renal calices. Anat Rec 1973; 175:139.

Djurhuus JC, Constantinou CE: Chronic ureteric obstruction and its impact on the coordinating mechanisms of peristalsis (pyeloureteric pacemaker system). Urol Res 1982; 10:267.

Djurhuus JC, Stage P: Percutaneous intrapelvic pressure registration in hydronephrosis during diuresis. Acta Chir Scand 1976; 473:43.

Dokita S, Morgan WR, Wheeler MA, et al: N^G-nitro-L-arginine inhibits non-adrenergic, non-cholinergic relaxation in rabbit urethral smooth muscle. Life Sci 1991; 48:2429.

Dokita S, Smith SD, Nishimoto T, et al: Involvement of nitric oxide and cyclic GMP in rabbit urethral relaxation. Eur J Pharmacol 1994; 269:269.

Draper JW, Zorgniotti AW: The effect of Banthine and similar agents on the urinary tract. N Y State J Med 1954; 54:77.

Draper MH, Weidmann S: Cardiac resting and action potentials recorded with an intracellular electrode. J Physiol (Lond) 1951; 115:74.

Dray A, Hankins MW, Yeats JC: Desensitization and capsaicin-induced release of substance P–like immunoreactivity from guinea-pig ureter *in vitro.* Neuroscience 1989; 31:479.

Durante-Escalante O, Labay P, Boyarsky S: The neurohistochemistry of mammalian ureter: A new combination of histochemical procedures to demonstrate adrenergic, cholinergic and chromaffin structures in ureter. J Urol 1969; 101:803.

Edyvane KA, Smet PJ, Trussell DC, et al: Patterns of neuronal colocalisation of tyrosine hydroxylase, neuropeptide Y, vasoactive intestinal polypeptide, calcitonin gene-related peptide and substance P in human ureter. J Auton Nerv Syst 1994; 48:241.

Edyvane KA, Trussell DC, Jonavicius J, et al: Presence and regional variation in peptide-containing nerves in the human ureter. J Auton Nerv Syst 1992; 39:127.

Eguchi S, Kozuka M, Hirose S, et al: Unique contractile action of endothelins on porcine isolated ureter and characterization of the endothelin-binding sites. Biomed Res 1991; 12:35.

Elbadawi A, Schenk AE: Innervation of the abdominopelvic ureter in the cat. Am J Anat 1969; 126:103.

Engelmann TW: Zur Physiologie des Ureters. Pfluegers Arch Gesamte Physiol Menschen Tiere 1869; 2:243.

Engelmann TW: Uber die electrische Erregung des Ureter, mit Bemerkungen uber die electrische Erregung im Allgemeinen. Pfluegers Arch Gesamte Physiol Menschen Tiere 1870; 3:247.

Fainstat T: Ureteral dilatation in pregnancy: A review. Obstet Gynecol Surg 1963; 18:845.

Ferroni A, Blanchi D: Maximum rate of depolarization of single muscle fiber in normal and low sodium solutions. J Gen Physiol 1965; 49:17.

Finberg JPM, Peart WS: Function of smooth muscle of the rat renal pelvis: Response of the isolated pelvis muscle to angiotensin and some other substances. Br J Pharmacol 1970; 39:373.

Flannigan GM, Clifford RPC, Carver RA, et al: Indomethacin: An alternative to pethidine in ureteric colic. Br J Urol 1983; 55:6.

Foote JW, Blennerhassett JB, Wigglesworth FW, MacKinnon KJ: Observations on the ureteropelvic junction. J Urol 1970; 104:252.

Fredericks CM, Anderson GF, Pierce JM: Electrical and mechanical responses of intact canine ureter to elevated intravesical pressure. Invest Urol 1972; 9:496.

Fung YC: Peristaltic pumping: A bioengineering model. *In* Boyarsky S, Gottschalk CW, Tanagho EA, Zimskind PD, eds: Urodynamics. New York, Academic Press, 1971, pp 177–198.

Furchgott RF: Receptor mechanisms. Annu Rev Pharmacol Toxicol 1964; 4:21.

George NJR, O'Reilly PH Jr, Barnard RJ, Blacklock NJ: Practical management of patients with dilated upper tracts and chronic retention of urine. Br J Urol 1984; 56:9.

Gibbins IL, Furness JB, Costa M, et al: Co-localization of calcitonin gene-related peptide-like immunoreactivity with substance P in cutaneous vascular and visceral sensory neurons of guinea-pig. Neurosci Lett 1985; 57:125.

Gibbs OS: The function of the fowl's ureter. Am J Physiol 1929; 87:594.

Golenhofen K, Lammel E: Selective suppression of some components of spontaneous activity in various types of smooth muscle by iproveratril (verapamil). Pfluegers Arch 1972; 331:233.

Gosling JA: Atypical muscle cells in the wall of the renal calix and pelvis with a note on their possible significance. Experientia 1970; 26:769.

Gosling JA, Dixon JS: Morphologic evidence that the renal calyx and pelvis control ureteric activity in the rabbit. Am J Anat 1971; 130:393.

Gosling JA, Dixon JS: Species variation in the location of upper urinary tract pacemaker cells. Invest Urol 1974; 11:418.

Gosling JA, Dixon JS: Functional obstruction of the ureter and renal pelvis: A histological and electron microscopic study. Br J Urol 1978; 50:145.

Gosling JA, Waas ANC: The behavior of the isolated rabbit renal calix and pelvis compared with that of the ureter. Eur J Pharmacol 1971; 16:100.

Gottschalk CW, Mylle M: Micropuncture study of pressures in proximal tubules and peritubular capillaries of the rat kidney and their relation to ureteral and renal venous pressures. Am J Physiol 1956; 185:430.

Gould DW, Hsieh ACL, Tinckler LF: Behavior of isolated water-buffalo ureter. J Physiol (Lond) 1955; 129:425.

Grana L, Kidd J, Idriss F, Swenson O: Effects of chronic urinary tract infection on ureteral peristalsis. J Urol 1965; 94:652.

Green DF, Glickman MG, Weiss RM: Preliminary results with aminophylline as smooth muscle relaxant in percutaneous renal surgery. J Endourol 1987; 1:243.

Griffiths DJ: The mechanics of urine transport in the upper urinary tract: II. The discharge of the bolus into the bladder and dynamics at high rates of flow. Neurourol Urodynam 1983; 2:167.

Griffiths DJ, Notschaele C: The mechanics of urine transport in the upper urinary tract: I. The dynamics of the isolated bolus. Neurourol Urodynam 1983; 2:155.

Gruber CM: The effect of morphine and papaverine upon the peristaltic and antiperistaltic contractions of the ureter. J Pharmacol Exp Ther 1928; 33:191.

Hanley HG: The electro-ureterogram. Br J Urol 1953; 25:358.

Hanna MK: Some observations on congenital ureteropelvic junction obstruction. Urology 1978; 12:151.

Hannappel J, Golenhofen K: The effect of catecholamines on ureteral peristalsis in different species (dog, guinea pig and rat). Pfluegers Arch 1974; 55:350.

Hausman M, Biancani P, Weiss RM: Obstruction induced changes in longitudinal force-length relations of rabbit ureter. Invest Urol 1979; 17:223.

Hendren WH: A new approach to infants with severe obstructive uropathy: Early complete reconstruction. J Pediatr Surg 1970; 5:184.

Hendrickx H, Vereecken RL, Casteels R: The influence of potassium on the electrical and mechanical activity of the guinea pig ureter. Urol Res 1975; 3:155.

Hernández M, Prieto D, Orensanz LM, et al: Nitric oxide is involved in the non-adrenergic, non-cholinergic inhibitory neurotransmission of the pig intravesical ureter. Neurosci Lett 1995; 186:33.

Hernández M, Prieto D, Simonsen U, et al: Noradrenaline modulates smooth muscle activity of the isolated intravesical ureter of the pig through different types of adrenoceptors. Br J Pharmacol 1992; 107:924.

Hernández M, Simonsen U, Prieto D, et al: Different muscarinic receptor subtypes mediating the phasic activity and basal tone of pig isolated intravesical ureter. Br J Pharmacol 1993; 110:1413.

Hertle L, Nawrath H: Calcium channel blockade in smooth muscle of the upper urinary tract: I. Effects on depolarization-induced activation. J Urol 1984; 132:1265.

Hill AV: The heat of shortening and the dynamic constants of 1 muscle. Proc R Soc Lond B Biol Sci 1938; 126:136.

Hodgkin AL: Ionic movements and electrical activity in giant nerve fibres. Proc R Soc Lond B Biol Sci 1958; 148:1.

Hoffman BF, Cranefield PF: Electrophysiology of the Heart. New York, McGraw-Hill, 1960.

Holmlund D, Hassler O: A method of studying the ureteral reaction to artificial concrements. Acta Chir Scand 1965; 130:335.

Holmlund D, Sjöden JG: Treatment of ureteral colic with intravenous indomethacin. J Urol 1978; 120:676.

Hong KW, Biancani P, Weiss RM: Effect of age on contractility of guinea pig ureter. Invest Urol 1980; 17:459.

Hong KW, Biancani P, Weiss RM: "On" and "off" responses of guinea pig ureter. Am J Physiol 1985; 248:C165.

Hua X-Y, Lundberg JM: Dual capsaicin effects on ureteric motility: Low dose inhibition mediated by calcitonin gene-related peptide and high dose stimulation by tachykinins? Acta Physiol Scand 1986; 128:453.

Hua X-Y, Theodorsson-Norheim E, Brodin E, et al: Multiple tachykinins (neurokinin A, neuropeptide K and substance P) in capsaicin-sensitive sensory neurons in the guinea pig. Regul Pept 1985; 13:1.

Hua X-Y, Theodorsson-Norheim E, Lundberg JM, et al: Co-localization of tachykinins and calcitonin gene-related peptide in capsaicin-sensitive afferents in relation to motility effects on human ureter in vitro. Neuroscience 1987; 23:693.

Hukuhara T, Nanba R, Fukuda H: The effects of the stimulation of extraureteral nerves on the ureteral motility of the dog. Jpn J Physiol 1964; 14:197.

Hundley JM Jr, Diehl WK, Diggs ES: Hormonal influences upon the ureter. Am J Obstet Gynecol 1942; 44:858.

Ichikawa S, Ikeda O: Recovery curve and conduction of action potentials in the ureter of the guinea pig. Jpn J Physiol 1960; 10:1.

Imaizumi Y, Muraki K, Watanabe M: Ionic currents in single smooth muscle cells from the ureter of the guinea pig. J Physiol (Lond) 1989; 411:131.

Johns A, Wooster MJ: The inhibitory effects of prostaglandin E_1 on guinea pig ureter. Can J Physiol Pharmacol 1975; 53:239.

Jönsson PE, Olsson AM, Petersson BA, Johansson K: Intravenous indomethacin and oxycone-papaverine in the treatment of acute renal colic: A double-blind study. Br J Urol 1987; 59:396.

Kamm KE, Stull JT: The function of myosin and myosin light chain kinase phosphorylation in smooth muscle. Annu Rev Pharmacol Toxicol 1985; 25:593.

Kaplan N, Elkin M, Sharkey J: Ureteral peristalsis and the autonomic nervous system. Invest Urol 1968; 5:468.

Kiil F: The Function of the Ureter and Renal Pelvis. Philadelphia, W.B. Saunders, 1957.

Kiil F, Kjekshus J: The physiology of the ureter and renal pelvis. *In* Proceedings of the Third International Congress on Nephrology, Washington, DC, 1966. 1967; 2:321.

King WW, Cox CE: Bacterial inhibition of ureteral smooth muscle contractility: I. The effect of common urinary pathogens and endotoxin in an in vitro system. J Urol 1972; 108:700.

Kirkland IS, Ross JA, Edmond P, Long WJ: Ureteral function in vesicoureteral reflux. Br J Urol 1971; 43:289.

Kobayashi M: Conduction velocity in various regions of the ureter. Tohoku J Exp Med 1964; 83:220.

Kobayashi M: Effects of Na and Ca on the generation and conduction of excitation in the ureter. Am J Physiol 1965; 208:715.

Kobayashi M: Effect of calcium on electrical activity in smooth muscle cells of cat ureter. Am J Physiol 1969; 216:1279.

Kobayashi M, Irisawa H: Effect of sodium deficiency on the action potential of the smooth muscle of ureter. Am J Physiol 1964; 206:205.

Koff SA, Thrall JH: Diagnosis of obstruction in experimental hydroureteronephrosis. Urology 1981a; 17:570.

Koff SA, Thrall JH: The diagnosis of obstruction in experimental hydroureteronephrosis: Mechanism for progressive urinary tract dilation. Invest Urol 1981b; 19:85.

Kontani H, Ginkawa M, Sakai T: A simple method for measurement of ureteric peristaltic function in vivo and the effects of drugs acting on ion channels applied from the ureter lumen in anesthetized rats. Jp J Pharmacol 1993; 62:331.

Kroeger EA, Marshall JM: Beta-adrenergic effects on rat myometrium: Role of cyclic AMP. Am J Physiol 1974; 226:1298.

Kubacz GJ, Catchpole BN: The role of adrenergic blockade in the treatment of ureteral colic. J Urol 1972; 107:949.

Kumar D: In vitro inhibitory effect of progesterone on extrauterine smooth muscle. Am J Obstet Gynecol 1962; 84:1300.

Kuriyama H: The influence of potassium, sodium, chloride on the membrane potential of the smooth muscle of taenia coli. J Physiol (Lond) 1963; 166:15.

Kuriyama H, Osa T, Toida N: Membrane properties of the smooth muscle of guinea-pig ureter. J Physiol (Lond) 1967; 191:225.

Kuriyama H, Tomita T: The action potential in the smooth muscle of the guinea pig taenia coli and ureter studied by the double sucrose-gap method. J Gen Physiol 1970; 55:147.

Labay P, Boyarsky S: The effect of topical nicotine on ureteral peristalsis. JAMA 1967; 200:209.

Labay PC, Boyarsky S, Herlong JH: Relation of adrenal to ureteral function. Fed Proc 1968; 27:444.

Lang RJ: Identification of the major membrane currents in freshly dispersed single smooth muscle cells of guinea-pig ureter. J Physiol (Lond) 1989; 412:375.

Lang RJ: The whole cell Ca^{2+} channel current in single smooth muscle cells of the guinea-pig ureter. J Physiol (Lond) 1990; 423:453.

Lapides J: The physiology of the intact human ureter. J Urol 1948; 59:501.

Latifpour J, Fukumoto Y, Weiss RM: Regional differences in the density and subtype specificity of endothelin receptors in rabbit urinary tract. Naunyn Schmiedebergs Arch Pharmacol 1995; 352:459.

Latifpour J, Kondo S, O'Hollaren B, et al: Autonomic receptors in urinary tract: Sex and age differences. J Pharmacol Exp Ther 1990; 253:661.

Latifpour J, Morita T, O'Hollaren B, et al: Characterization of autonomic receptors in neonatal urinary tract smooth muscle. Dev Pharm Ther 1989; 13:1.

Libertino JA, Weiss RM: Ultrastructure of human ureter. J Urol 1972; 108:71.

Londos C, Cooper DMF, Rodbell M: Receptor-mediated stimulation and inhibition of adenylate cyclases: The fat cell as a model system. Adv Cyclic Nucleotide Res 1981; 14:163.

Longrigg N: Autonomic innervation of the renal calyx. Br J Urol 1974; 46:357.

Longrigg N: Minor calyces as primary pacemaker sites for ureteral activity in man. Lancet 1975; 1:253.

Lubin S, Drexler LS, Bilotta WA: Post-partum pyeloureteral changes following hormone administration. Surg Gynecol Obstet 1941; 73:391.

Lundstam S, Jönsson O, Kihl B, Pettersson S: Prostaglandin synthetase inhibition of renal pelvic smooth muscle in the rabbit. Br J Urol 1985; 57:390.

Macht DI: On the pharmacology of the ureter: I. Action of epinephrine, ergotoxine and of nicotin. J Pharmacol Exp Ther 1916a; 8:155.

Macht DI: On the pharmacology of the ureter: II. Actions of drugs affecting the sacral autonomics. J Pharmacol Exp Ther 1916b; 8:261.

Macht DI: On the pharmacology of the ureter: III. Action of the opium alkaloids. J Pharmacol Exp Ther 1916c; 9:197.

Maggi CA: Tachykinins and calcitonin gene-related peptide (CGRP) as co-transmitters released from peripheral endings of sensory nerves. Prog Neurobiol 1995; 45:1.

Maggi CA, Giuliani S: The neurotransmitter role of CGRP in the rat and guinea-pig ureter: Effect of a CGRP antagonist and species related differences in the action of omega conotoxin on CGRP release from primary afferents. Neuroscience 1991; 43:261.

Maggi CA, Giuliani S: A thiorphan-sensitive mechanism regulates the action of both exogenous and endogenous calcitonin gene-related peptide (CGRP) in the guinea-pig ureter. Regul Pept 1994; 51:263.

Maggi CA, Giuliani S, Santicioli P: Effect of Bay K 8644 and ryanodine on the refractory period, action potential and mechanical response of the guinea-pig ureter to electrical stimulation. Naunyn Schmiedebergs Arch Pharmacol 1994a; 349:510.

Maggi CA, Giuliani S, Santicioli P: Multiple mechanisms in the smooth muscle relaxant action of calcitonin gene-related peptide (CGRP) in the guinea-pig ureter. Naunyn Schmiedeberg Arch Pharmacol 1994b; 350:537.

Maggi CA, Giuliani S, Santicioli P: Effect of cromakalim and glibenclamide on spontaneous and evoked motility of the guinea-pig isolated renal pelvis and ureter. Br J Pharmacol 1994c; 111:687.

Maggi CA, Meli A: The sensory-efferent function of capsaicin-sensitive sensory neurons. Gen Pharmacol 1988; 19:1.

Maggi CA, Santicioli P, delBianco E, Giuliani S: Local motor responses to bradykinin and bacterial chemotactic peptide formyl-methionyl-levcyl-phenylalanine (FMLP) in the guinea-pig isolated renal pelvis and ureter. J Urol 1992a; 148:1944.

Maggi CA, Santicioli P, Guiliani S, et al: The motor effect of the capsaicin-sensitive inhibitory innervation of the rat ureter. Eur J Pharmacol 1986; 126:333.

Maggi CA, Theodorsson E, Santicioli P, Giuliani S: Tachykinins and calcitonin gene-related peptides as co-transmitters in local motor responses produced by sensory activation in the guinea pig isolated renal pelvis. Neuroscience 1992b; 46:549.

Mahadevappa VG, Holub BJ: Degradation of different molecular species of phosphatidylinositol in thrombin-stimulated human platelets. J Biol Chem 1983; 258:5337.

Maizels M, Stephens FD: Valves of the ureter as a cause of primary obstruction of the ureter: Anatomic, embryologic, clinical aspects. J Urol 1980; 123:742.

Makker SP, Tucker AS, Izant RJ Jr, Heymann W: Nonobstructive hydronephrosis and hydroureter associated with peritonitis. N Engl J Med 1972; 287:535.

Malin JM Jr, Boyarsky S, Labay P, Gerber C: In vitro isometric studies of ureteral smooth muscle. J Urol 1968; 99:396.

Malin JM Jr, Deane RF, Boyarsky S: Characterization of adrenergic receptors in human ureter. Br J Urol 1970; 42:171.

Marchant DJ: Effects of pregnancy and progestational agents on the urinary tract. Am J Obstet Gynecol 1972; 112:487.

Mazzella H, Schroeder G: Ureteral contractility in the dog and the influence of drugs. Arch Int Pharmacodyn Ther 1960; 128:291.

McGuire EJ: Physiology of the lower urinary tract. Am J Kidney Dis 1983; 2:402.

McGuire EJ, Woodside JR, Borden TA, Weiss RM: Prognostic value of urodynamic testing in myelodysplastic patients. J Urol 1981; 126:205.

McLeod DG, Reynolds DG, Swan KG: Adrenergic mechanisms in the canine ureter. Am J Physiol 1973; 224:1054.

McNellis D, Sherline DM: The rabbit ureter in pregnancy and after norethynodrel-mestranol administration: A radiographic and histologic study. Obstet Gynecol 1967; 30:336.

Meini S, Santicioli P, Maggi CA: Propagation of impulses in the guinea-pig ureter and its blockade by calcitonin gene-related peptide (CGRP). Naunyn Schmiedebergs Arch Pharmacol 1995; 351:79.

Melick WF, Brodeur AE, Herbig F, Naryka JJ: Use of a ureteral pacemaker in the treatment of ureteral reflux. J Urol 1966; 95:184.

Melick WF, Naryka JJ, Schmidt JH: Experimental studies of ureteral peristaltic patterns in the pig: II. Myogenic activity of the pig ureter. J Urol 1961; 86:46.

Morales PA, Crowder CH, Fishman AP, Maxwell MH: The response of the ureter and pelvis to changing urine flows. J Urol 1952; 67:484.

Morita T, Ishizuka G, Tsuchida S: Initiation and propagation of stimulus from the renal pelvic pacemaker in pig kidney. Invest Urol 1981; 19:157.

Morita T, Wada I, Saeki H, et al: Ureteral urine transport: Changes in bolus volume, peristaltic frequency, intraluminal pressure and volume of flow resulting from autonomic drugs. J Urol 1987; 137:132.

Morita T, Wheeler MA, Weiss RM: Effects of noradrenaline, isoproterenol, acetylcholine on ureteral resistance. J Urol 1986; 135:1296.

Muraki K, Imaizumi Y, Watanabe M: Sodium currents in smooth muscle cells freshly isolated from stomach fundus of the rat and ureter of the guinea pig. J Physiol (Lond) 1991; 442:351.

Murnaghan GF: The dynamics of the renal pelvis and ureter with reference to congenital hydronephrosis. Br J Urol 1958; 30:321.

Nernst W: Zur theorie des elektrischen reizes. Arch Ges Physiol 1908; 122:275.

Nishizuka Y: The role of protein kinase C in cell surface signal transduction and tumor production. Nature 1984; 308:693.

Notley RG: The musculature of the human ureter. Br J Urol 1970; 42:724.

Ockerblad NF, Carlson HE, Simon JF: The effect of morphine upon the human ureter. J Urol 1935; 33:356.

O'Conor VJ Jr, Dawson-Edwards P: Role of the ureter in renal transplantation: I. Studies of denervated ureter with particular reference to ureteroureteral anastomosis. J Urol 1959; 82:566.

Paquin AJ Jr: Ureterovesical anastomosis: The description and evaluation of a technique. J Urol 1959; 82:573.

Park S, Rasmussen H: Activation of tracheal smooth muscle contraction: Synergism between Ca^{2+} and activators of protein kinase C. Proc Natl Acad Sci USA 1985; 82:8835.

Payne FL, Hodes PJ: The effect of the female hormones and of pregnancy upon the ureters of lower animals as demonstrated by intravenous urography. Am J Obstet Gynecol 1939; 37:1024.

Peters HJ, Eckstein W: Possible pharmacological means of treating renal colic. Urol Res 1975; 3:55.

Phillips JL, Wheeler MA, Weiss RM: Differential nitric oxide synthase (NOS) activity in developing fetal pig ureterovesical junction. FASEB J 1995; 9:A679.

Prieto D, Simonsen U, Martín J, et al: Histochemical and functional evidence for a cholinergic innervation of the equine ureter. J Auton Nerv Syst 1994; 47:159.

Primbs K: Untersuchungen uber die Einwirkung von Bakterientoxinen auf der uberlebenden Meerschweinchenureter. Z Urol Chir 1913; 1:600.

Prosser CL, Smith CE, Melton CE: Conduction of action potentials in the ureter of the rat. Am J Physiol 1955; 181:651.

Reid RE, Herman R, Teng C: Attempts at altering ureteral activity in the unanesthetized, conditioned dog with commonly employed drugs. Invest Urol 1976; 12:74.

Reuterskiöld AG: Ureteric pressure variations at different flow rates and varying bladder pressures in normal dogs. Acta Soc Med Upsal 1969; 74:94.

Reuterskiöld AG: The abnormal ureter in children: II. Perfusion studies on the refluxing ureter. Scand J Urol Nephrol 1970; 4:99.

Rivera L, Hernández M, Benedito S, et al: Mediation of contraction and relaxation by alpha- and beta-adrenoceptors in the ureterovesical junction of the sheep. Res Vet Sci 1992; 52:57.

Roberts JA: Experimental pyelonephritis in the monkey: III. Pathophysiology of ureteral malfunction induced by bacteria. Invest Urol 1975; 13:117.

Roberts JA: Hydronephrosis of pregnancy. Urology 1976; 8:1.

Rose JG, Gillenwater JY: Pathophysiology of ureteral obstruction. Am J Physiol 1973; 225:830.

Rose JG, Gillenwater JY: The effect of adrenergic and cholinergic agents and their blockers upon ureteral activity. Invest Urol 1974; 11:439.

Rose JG, Gillenwater JY: Effects of obstruction upon ureteral function. Urology 1978; 12:139.

Rosen DE, Constantinou CE, Sands JP, Govan DE: Dynamics of the upper urinary tract: Effects of changes in bladder pressure on ureteral peristalsis. J Urol 1971; 106:209.

Ross JA, Edmond P, Griffiths JM: The action of drugs on the intact human ureter. Br J Urol 1967; 39:26.

Ross JA, Edmond P, Kirkland IS: Behavior of the Human Ureter in Health and Disease. Edinburgh, Churchill Livingstone, 1972.

Roth GB.: On the movement of the excised ureter of the dog. Am J Physiol 1917; 44:275.

Sakanashi M, Kato T, Miyamoto Y, et al: Comparison of the effects of nifedipine on ureter and coronary artery isolated from the dog. Drug Res 1985; 35:584.

Sakanashi M, Kato T, Miyamoto Y, et al: Comparative effects of diltiazem and glycerol trinitrate on isolated ureter and coronary artery of the dog. Pharmacology 1986; 32:11.

Sala NL, Rubi RA: Ureteral function in pregnant women: II. Ureteral contractility during normal pregnancy. Am J Obstet Gynecol 1967; 99:228.

Sann H, Rössler W, Hammer K, Pierau Fr-K: Substance P and calcitonin gene-related peptide in the ureter of chicken and guinea-pig: Distribution, binding sites and possible functions. Neuroscience 1992; 49:699.

Santicioli P, Maggi CA: Inhibitory transmitter action of CGRP in guinea-pig ureter via activation of glibenclamide-sensitive K^+ channels. Br J Pharmacol 1994; 113:588.

Santicioli P, Morbidelli L, Parenti A, et al: Calcitonin gene-related peptide selectively increases cAMP levels in the guinea-pig ureter. Eur J Pharmacol 1995; 289:17.

Satani Y: Experimental studies of the ureter. Am J Physiol 1919; 49:474.

Scheele K: Die Spasmen bei Uretersteine. Z Urol 1965; 58:455.

Schick E, Tanagho EA: The effect of gravity on ureteral peristalsis. J Urol 1973; 109:187.

Schneider DH, Eichner E, Gordon MB: An attempt at production of hydronephrosis of pregnancy, artificially induced. Am J Obstet Gynecol 1953; 65:660.

Schultz K, Bohme E, Volker AWK, Schultz G: Relaxation of hormonally stimulated smooth muscular tissues by the 8-bromo derivative of cyclic GMP. Naunyn Schmiedebergs Arch Pharmacol 1979; 306:1.

Schweitzer FAW: Intrapelvic pressure and renal function studies in experimental chronic partial ureteric obstruction. Br J Urol 1973; 45:2.

Sharkey J, Boyarsky S, Catacutan-Labay P, Martinez J: The *in vivo* effects of histamine and Benadryl on the peristalsis of the canine ureter and plasma potassium levels. Invest Urol 1965; 2:417.

Sharkey J, Kaplan N, Newman HR, Elkin M: The role of potassium in ureteral physiology and pharmacology. Invest Urol 1968; 6:119.

Shiratori T, Kinoshita H: Electromyographic studies on urinary tract: II. Electromyography study on the genesis of peristaltic movement of the dog's ureters. Tohoku J Exp Med 1961a; 73:103.

Shiratori T, Kinoshita H: Electromyographic studies on urinary tract: III. Influence of pinching and cutting the ureters of dogs on their EMGs. Tohoku J Exp Med 1961b; 73:159.

Shuba MF: The effect of sodium-free and potassium-free solutions, ionic current inhibitors and ouabain on electrophysiological properties of smooth muscle of guinea-pig ureter. J Physiol (Lond) 1977; 264:837.

Shuba MF: The ionic nature of the excitation of the smooth muscle cells. *In* Kostyuk PG, ed: Recent Problems of the General Physiology of the Excitable Tissues. Kiev, Naukova Dumka, 1978, pp 39–46.

Sierp M, Draper JW: Peristalsis in the urinary tract: Experimental observations of the effect of various drugs on the musculature of the ureter. Ann N Y Acad Sci 1964; 118:7.

Sivula A, Lehtonen T: Spontaneous passage of artificial concretions applied in the rabbit ureter. Scand J Urol Nephrol 1967; 1:259.

Sjöden JG, Wahlberg J, Persson AEG: The effect of indomethacin on glomerular capillary pressure and pelvic pressure during ureteral obstruction. J Urol 1982; 127:1017.

Slaughter D, Johnson TV, Tobalowsky N, VanDuzen R: The effect of spasmolytic drugs on the isolated ureter. Tex Rep Biol Med 1945; 3:37.

Smet PJ, Edyvane KA, Jonavicius J, Marshall VR: Colocalization of nitric oxide synthase with vasoactive intestinal peptide, neuropeptide Y, tyrosine hydroxylase in nerves supplying the human ureter. J Urol 1994; 152:1292.

Smith SD, Wheeler MA, Nishimoto T, Weiss RM: The differential expression of nitric oxide synthase in guinea-pig urinary tract. J Urol 1993; 149:248A.

Sonnenblick EH: Force-velocity relations in mammalian heart muscle. Am J Physiol 1962; 202:931.

Stief CG, Taher A, Meyer M, et al: A possible role of nitric oxide (NO) in the relaxation of renal pelvis and ureter. J Urol 1993; 149:492A.

Struthers NW: The role of manometry in the investigation of pelviureteral function. Br J Urol 1969; 41:129.

Struthers NW: An experimental model for evaluating drug effects on the ureter. Br J Urol 1973; 45:23.

Struthers NW: The effect of *E. coli* and *E. coli* endotoxin on peristalsis in the canine ureter. Urol Res 1976; 4:107.

Takago K, Takayanagi I, Tomiyama A: Actions of dibutyryl cyclic adenosine monophosphate, papaverine, isoprenaline on intestinal smooth muscle. Jpn J Pharmacol 1971; 21:477.

Tamaki M, Iwanaga T, Sato S, Fujita T: Calcitonin gene-related peptide (CGRP)–immunoreactive nerve plexuses in the renal pelvis and ureter of rats. Cell Tissue Res 1992; 267:29.

Tanagho EA: Ureteral embryology, developmental anatomy and myology. *In* Boyarsky S, Gottschalk TW, Tanagho EA, Zimskind P, eds: Urodynamics. New York, Academic Press, 1971, pp 3–27.

Tanagho EA, Hutch JA, Meyers FH, Rambo ON Jr: Primary vesicoureteral reflux: Experimental studies of its etiology. J Urol 1965; 93:165.

Tanagho EA, Meyers FH, Smith DE: The trigone: Anatomical and physiological considerations: 1. In relation to the ureterovesical junction. J Urol 1968; 100:623.

Teague N, Boyarsky S: The effect of coliform bacilli upon ureteral peristalsis. Invest Urol 1968; 5:423.

Teele RL, Lebowitz RL, Colodny AH: Reflux into the unused ureter. J Urol 1976; 115:310.

Thackston LP, Price NC, Richardson AG: Use of antispasmodics in treatment of spastic ureteritis. J Urol 1955; 73:487.

Theobald RJ Jr: Changes in ureteral peristaltic activity induced by various stimuli. Neurourol Urodynam 1986; 5:493.

Thulesius O, Angelo-Khattar M: The effect of indomethacin on the motility of isolated sheep ureters. Acta Pharmacol Toxicol 1985; 56:298.

Thulesius O, Angelo-Khattar M, Sabha M: The effect of ureteral distension on peristalsis: Studies on human and sheep ureters. Urol Res 1989; 17:385.

Thulesius O, Araj G: The effect of uropathogenic bacteria on ureteral motility. Urol Res 1987; 15:273.

Tindall AR: Preliminary observations on the mechanical and electrical activity of the rat ureter. J Physiol (Lond) 1972; 223:633.

Toguri AG, Fournier G: Factors influencing the pressure-flow perfusion system. J Urol 1982; 127:1021.

Traut HF, Kuder A: Inflammation of the upper urinary tract complicating the reproductive period of woman: Collective review. Int Abstr Surg 1938; 67:568.

Triner L, Nahas GG, Vulliemoz Y, et al: Cyclic AMP and smooth muscle function. Ann N Y Acad Sci 1971; 185:458.

Tsuchida S, Yamaguchi O: A constant electrical activity of the renal pelvis correlated to ureteral peristalsis. Tohoku J Exp Med 1977; 121:133.

Tsuchiya T, Takei N: Pressure responses and conduction of peristaltic wave in guinea-pig ureter. Jpn J Physiol 1990; 40:139.

Uehara Y, Burnstock G: Demonstration of "gap junctions" between smooth muscle cells. J Cell Biol 1970; 44:215.

Ueno A, Kawamura T, Ogawa A, Takayasu H: Relation of spontaneous passage of ureteral calculi to size. Urology 1977; 10:544.

van Mastrigt R, van de Wetering J, Glerum JJ: Influence of temperature and stimulus interval variations on the propagation of contractions in the pig ureter. Urol Int 1986; 41:266.

van Wagenen G, Jenkins RH: An experimental examination of factors causing ureteral dilatation of pregnancy. J Urol 1939; 42:1010.

Vaughan ED Jr, Shenasky JH II, Gillenwater JY: Mechanism of acute hemodynamic response to ureteral occlusion. Invest Urol 1971; 9:109.

Vaughan ED Jr, Sorenson EJ, Gillenwater JY: The renal hemodynamic response to chronic unilateral ureteral occlusion. Invest Urol 1970; 8:78.

Vela-Navarrete R: Percutaneous intrapelvic pressure determinations in the study of hydronephrosis. Invest Urol 1971; 8:526.

Vereecken RL: Dynamical Aspects of Urine Transport in the Ureter. Acco, Louvain, 1973.

Vereecken RL, Derluyn J, Verduyn H: The viscoelastic behavior of the ureter during elongation. Urol Res 1973; 1:15.

Vereecken RL, Hendrickx H, Casteels R: The influence of calcium on the electrical and mechanical activity of the guinea pig ureter. Urol Res 1975a; 3:149.

Vereecken RL, Hendrickx H, Casteels R: The influence of sodium on the electrical and mechanical activity of the guinea pig ureter. Urol Res 1975b; 3:159.

Vermue NA, Den Hertog A: The action of prostaglandins on ureter smooth muscle of guinea pig. Eur J Pharmacol 1987; 142:163.

Vesin MF, Harbon S: The effects of epinephrine, prostaglandins, and their antagonists on adenosine cyclic 3′,5′-monophosphate concentrations and motility of the rat uterus. Mol Pharmacol 1974; 10:457.

Washizu Y: Grouped discharges in ureter muscle. Comp Biochem Physiol 1966; 19:713.

Washizu Y: Membrane potential and tension in guinea-pig ureter. J Pharmacol Exp Ther 1967; 158:445.

Washizu Y: Ouabain on excitation contraction in guinea pig ureter. Fed Proc 1968; 27:662.

Watterson DM, Harrelson WG Jr, Keller PM, et al: Structural similarities between the Ca^{2+}-dependent regulatory proteins of 3′,5′-cyclic nucleotide phosphodiesterase and actomyosin ATPase. J Biol Chem 1976; 251:4501.

Weinberg SR: Application of physiologic principles to surgery of the ureter. Am J Surg 1962; 103:549.

Weinberg SR: Ureteral function: I. Simultaneous monitoring of ureteral peristalsis. Invest Urol 1974; 12:103.

Weinberg SR, Maletta JJ: Measurement of peristalsis of the ureter and its relation to drugs. JAMA 1961; 175:109.

Weiss RM: Ureteral function. Urology 1978; 12:114.

Weiss RM: Clinical implications of ureteral physiology. J Urol 1979; 121:401.

Weiss RM: Effect of drugs on the ureter. *In* Bergman H, ed: The Ureter. New York, Springer-Verlag, 1981, pp 137–162.

Weiss RM: Pharmacology of the ureter. *In* Finkbeiner AE, Barbour GL, Bissada NK, eds: Pharmacology of the Urinary Tract and Male Reproductive System. New York, Appleton-Century-Crofts, 1982, pp 137–173.

Weiss RM, Bassett AL, Hoffman BF: Effect of ouabain on contractility of the isolated ureter. Invest Urol 1970; 8:161.

Weiss RM, Bassett AL, Hoffman BF: Dynamic length-tension curves of cat ureter. Am J Physiol 1972; 222:388.

Weiss RM, Bassett AL, Hoffman BF: Adrenergic innervation of the ureter. Invest Urol 1978; 16:123.

Weiss RM, Biancani P: A rationale for ureteral tapering. Urology 1982; 20:482.

Weiss RM, Biancani P: Characteristics of normal and refluxing ureterovesical junctions. J Urol 1983; 129:858.

Weiss RM, Biancani P, Zabinski MP: Adrenergic control of ureteral tonus. Invest Urol 1974; 12:30.

Weiss RM, Hardman JG, Wells JN: Resistance of a separated form of canine ureteral phosphodiesterase activity to inhibition by xanthines and papaverine. Biochem Pharmacol 1981; 30:2371.

Weiss RM, Vulliemoz Y, Verosky M, et al: Adenylate cyclase and phosphodiesterase activity in rabbit ureter. Invest Urol 1977; 15:15.

Weiss RM, Wagner ML, Hoffman BF: Localization of pacemaker for peristalsis in the intact canine ureter. Invest Urol 1967; 5:42.

Weiss RM, Wagner ML, Hoffman BF: Wenckebach periods of the ureter: A further note on the ubiquity of the Wenckebach phenomenon. Invest Urol 1968; 5:463.

Weiss RM, Wheeler MA: Insulin activation of cyclic AMP phosphodiesterase in intact ureteral segments. J Pharmacol Exp Ther 1988; 247:630.

Wharton LR: The innervation of the ureter, with respect to denervation. J Urol 1932; 28:639.

Wheeler MA, Cho YH, Hong KW, Weiss RM: Age-dependent alterations in beta-adrenergic receptor function in guinea-pig ureter. *In* Sperelakis N, Wood J, eds: Frontiers in Smooth Muscle Research, Vol 327. Progress in Clinical and Biological Research. New York, Alan R. Liss, 1990, pp 711–715.

Wheeler MA, Housman A, Cho YH, Weiss RM: Age dependence of adenylate cyclase activity in guinea pig ureter homogenate. J Pharmacol Exp Ther 1986; 239:99.

Whitaker RH: Methods of assessing obstruction in dilated ureters. Br J Urol 1973; 45:15.

Whitaker RH: Clinical assessment of pelvic and ureteral function. Urology 1978; 12:146.

Whitaker RH: The Whitaker test. Urol Clin North Am 1979; 6:529.

Whitfield HN, Harrison NW, Sherwood T, Williams DI: Upper urinary tract obstruction: Pressure flow studies in children. Br J Urol 1976; 48:427.

Widdicombe JH: The ionic properties of the sodium pump in smooth muscle. *In* Bhlbring E, Brading AF, Jones AW, Tomita T, eds: Smooth Muscle: An Assessment of Current Knowledge. London, Edward Arnold, 1981, pp 93–104.

Witherow RO, Whitaker RH: The predicative accuracy of antegrade pressure flow studies in equivocal upper tract obstruction. Br J Urol 1981; 53:496.

Woodburne RT, Lapides J: The ureteral lumen during peristalsis. Am J Anat 1972; 133:255.

Wooster MJ: Effects of prostaglandin E_1 on the dog ureter in vitro. J Physiol (Lond) 1971; 213:51P.

Yoshida M, Latifpour J, Weiss RM: Age-related changes in calcium antagonist receptors in rabbit ureter. Dev Pharmacol Ther 1992; 18:100.

Zimskind PD, Davis DM, Decaestecker JE: Effects of bladder filling on ureteral dynamics. J Urol 1969; 102:693.

26
PHYSIOLOGY AND PHARMACOLOGY OF THE BLADDER AND URETHRA

William D. Steers, M.D.

The bladder serves as a reservoir for the storage and periodic release of urine. The bladder is unique with regard to its myogenic properties as well as the complexity of its extrinsic neural regulation. Urine release is dependent on voluntary neural mechanisms that involve the brain and spinal cord (see reviews by Kuru, 1965; de Groat, 1975; de Groat and Steers, 1990). Although neural input plays a role in maintaining continence, urine storage relies also on the viscoelastic and myogenic properties of the bladder and urethra. Because of this complex myogenic and neurogenic regulation, the bladder and its outlet are exquisitely sensitive to metabolic disorders, neurologic disease, trauma, and drugs.

Bladder dysfunction is responsible for tremendous morbidity in the United States. It is estimated that 12 to 15 million individuals are incontinent of urine. One-half million individuals with spinal cord injury; 150,000 with Parkinson's disease (Aranda and Cramer, 1993); 200,000 following a cerebrovascular accident (Zhan, 1981); and 100,000 with multiple sclerosis manifested by some voiding abnormality. Progress on treating bladder dysfunction depends on understanding the myogenic and neural mechanisms regulating lower urinary tract function.

This chapter focuses on the physiologic, pharmacologic, and biomechanical mechanisms regulating urine storage and release. This review integrates continuing advances in smooth muscle physiology and pharmacology with basic and clinical studies of the bladder. Since the last review, our knowledge of sensory nerve and urethral function has greatly increased. The challenge is to exploit these basic concepts and apply them clinically.

BLADDER EPITHELIUM AND TRANSPORT PROPERTIES

In contrast to amphibians, the mammalian bladder functions as a reservoir for hypertonic urine. The mammalian bladder must be relatively impermeable to water. Although structural features of the urothelium support the concept of an impermeable membrane, physiologic experiments suggest otherwise. Ultrastructural studies have shown that the lumen of the bladder is lined by a transitional epithelium composed of at least three cell layers (Staehelin et al, 1972; Minsky and Chlapowski, 1978; Jacob et al, 1978). The innermost layer of the urothelium is formed by basal cells attached to a basement membrane. An intermediate layer consists of larger cells containing lysosomes and numerous cytoplasmic vesicles. The most superficial apical layer is composed of large hexagonal cells containing microfilaments and covered with a glycocalyx. An impermeable urothelium has been inferred from the presence of tight junctions between adjacent apical cells.

Transitional epithelium is thought to be impermeable based on the failure to demonstrate a net flux of ions or volume markers (Englund, 1956; Strohmeyer and Sack, 1966; Hicks, 1976). Other studies conclude that the bladder is permeable to ions. Kaupp (1856) showed that the volume and composition of urine changed when left in the bladder for 12 hours compared with hourly voiding. Similarly, Wickham (1964) demonstrated that the rabbit bladder transports small amounts of sodium but not calcium from urine to blood. In addition, instillation of amino acids into the bladder produces an increasing concentration gradient from the mucosal to serosal surfaces (Henderson and Weber, 1964). Sodium and amino acid gradients prove that mechanisms exist for transport of substances across the urothelium.

In vitro data demonstrate that the mammalian bladder possesses active ion transport systems. However, apical epithelial cells in the bladder are impermeable to water they actively transport sodium by means of different channels (Lewis, 1977; Eaton et al, 1984; Lewis and Hanrahan, 1985; Donaldson et al, 1989). Some sodium channels are aldosterone-sensitive, whereas other channels on epithelial cells do not respond to this mineralocorticoid. A third, less characterized, transport process relies on relatively unstable sodium/potassium channels. These channels are also found on cells lining renal collecting tubules, suggesting a functional similarity between the bladder and the distal nephron of the kidney (Lewis, 1986).

Sodium transport in the bladder can be altered by a variety of mechanical or chemical manipulations. For example, distention or urothelial disruption increases active sodium transport by apical cells. In addition, sodium channels can be altered by proteolytic enzymes in urine such as urokinase and kallikrein (Lewis, 1986). These enzymes decrease active sodium transport in apical cells, which may explain discrepancies between some in vivo and in vitro data (Lewis, 1986).

Sulfated polysaccharides covering apical cells, especially glycosaminoglycans, act as an epithelial barrier to small molecules. Disruption of this polysaccharide layer increases permeability to urea and has been linked to inflammatory or hypersensitivity disorders of the bladder, such as interstitial cystitis (Parsons et al, 1990). In models for interstitial cystitis, increased permeability to drugs has been shown (Gao et al, 1994). It is also possible that other substances such as prostaglandins have a cytoprotective role and affect urothelial permeability. Human bladder mucosa synthesizes a variety of prostaglandins that may influence bladder contractility and permeability (see Prostaglandins, Endothelins, and Hormones section) (Jeremey et al, 1987).

A consensus has not been reached concerning the physiologic role of active ion transport mechanisms in the bladder. One function may be in epithelial cell volume regulation during changes accompanying distention (Lewis, 1986; Donaldson et al, 1989). Because ion transport can occur in several directions, another role for this process may be to actively maintain urine hypertonicity. The extensive vascularity of the subepithelial region of the bladder has been used as evidence for this latter hypothesis. Subepithelial vasculature provides an increased blood flow to the mucosa compared with that to the detrusor muscle (Nemeth et al, 1977). Because an excess blood flow is not required for increased metabolism by epithelial cells, a subepithelial vascular network could function as a countercurrent exchanger to maintain a hypertonic urine (Hohlbrugger, 1987). In addition, the microvasculature of the bladder can change with disease. Following obstruction of the rat bladder lumenal diameters of intramural vessels increase and these vessels become more sensitive the alpha-adrenergic agonists (Boels et al, 1994).

Epithelial permeability could provide a mechanism for exposing smooth muscle to intravesical contents, thereby altering bladder contractility. Investigators have demon-

strated that intravesical instillations of antineoplastic drugs, anticholinergic agents (Obrink and Brunne, 1978; Brendler et al, 1989) and calcium channel antagonists (Mattiasson et al, 1989) influence detrusor muscle function and access systemic circulation. A better understanding of urothelial permeability may explain disorders such as interstitial cystitis and the means by which substances excreted in the urine or administered intravesically influence bladder sensation and contractility.

ANATOMY OF THE BLADDER AND URETHRA

The morphologic characteristics of the bladder and urethra provide a useful framework for understanding urine storage and release. However, attempts to explain function based solely on gross or microscopic anatomy have been unsuccessful. This section discusses the possible implications of anatomy on bladder function, but as will become clear in subsequent sections, a complete understanding of the lower urinary tract requires an integration of biochemical, pharmacologic, and neurobiologic principles.

The bladder has been divided into two components: a body lying above the ureteral orifices, and a base consisting of the posterior trigone, deep detrusor, and the anterior bladder wall (Elbadawi and Schenk, 1966). Grossly, the trigone represents the more superficial portion of the posterior bladder base and encompasses the ureteral orifices and internal urethral meatus.

Bladder Histology

Histologic examination of the bladder body reveals that myofibrils lack hierarchical organization. Myofibrils are arranged into fascicles of varying widths depending on the degree of bladder distention (Donker et al, 1982). This architecture differs from the discrete circular and longitudinal smooth muscle layers in the ureter or gastrointestinal tract.

The bladder outlet is composed of the bladder base, urethra, and external urethral sphincter (Fig. 26–1). The bladder base has a laminar architecture with a superficial longitudinal layer lying beneath the trigone. A muscle layer deep to the superficial layer is continuous with the detrusor (Tanagho, 1982; Dixon and Gosling, 1987; Zederic et al, 1996). The smaller muscle bundles of the deep muscle layer in the bladder base exhibit a predominantly circular orientation. However, the bladder base does not possess an anatomic sphincter. Some believe its morphology provides a functional basis for its role as sphincter.

Proximal Urethral Sphincter

The urethra begins at the internal meatus of the bladder and extends to the external meatus. In the male, four segments are readily identified. The preprostatic portion measures up to 1 cm in length and runs from the bladder neck to the prostate. The prostatic urethra travels throughout the length of the gland, terminating at its apex. The membranous urethra extends from the prostatic apex through the pelvic floor musculature until it becomes the bulbous urethra at the base of the penis. Finally, the penile urethra traverses the length of the penis. In women, the urethra extends throughout the distal third of the anterior vaginal wall from the bladder neck to the meatus. The urethra is composed of tissues that aid continence. A vascular subepithelial tissue in women maintains a urethral seal effect.

It is debatable whether the detrusor or trigonal muscles project into the proximal urethra (see Fig. 26–1). Embryo-

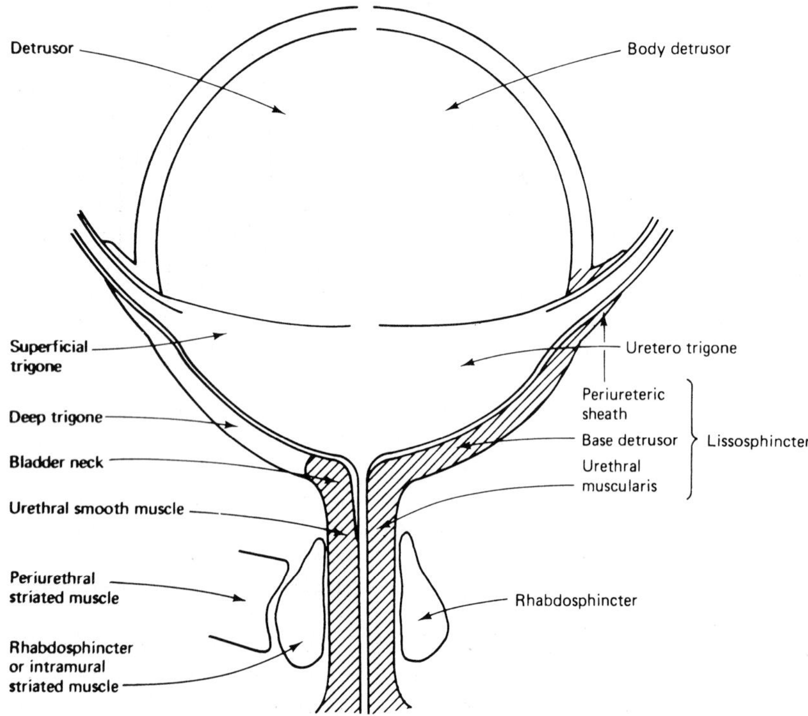

Figure 26–1. Anatomy of the bladder and its outlet as defined by Gosling and Dixon versus Elbadawi and co-workers. (From Torrens M, Morrison JFB: The Physiology of the Urinary Bladder, Berlin, Springer-Verlag, 1987, p 1.)

logic data support the concept of a separate origin for muscles of the bladder and urethra (Dixon and Gosling, 1987; Zederic et al, 1996). Histologically, studies show that the longitudinal muscle of the bladder base extends distally into the urethra to form an inner longitudinal layer (Hutch and Rambo, 1967; Tanagho, 1982). Examination of adult and fetal specimens shows that striated and smooth muscles coalesce in the urethra and interdigitate with the fibrous prostatic capsule (Oerlich, 1980).

On the other hand, Gosling and co-workers describe a complete ring of smooth muscle at the bladder neck in the male (Gosling et al, 1983). No such collar of muscle is identified in the female. The absence of this structure in women, and the maintenance of continence in men and some women with destruction or opening of the bladder neck argues that this region is not the principal site for urinary continence (Chapple et al, 1989).

The bladder neck serves an important function in reproduction. In men, the bladder neck allows anterograde ejaculation. This is accomplished through a rich noradrenergic innervation by sympathetic nerves. However, in women a sparse adrenergic innervation is identified in this region.

Intrinsic Distal Urethral Sphincter and External Striated Sphincter (Rhabdosphincter)

A thin smooth muscle layer extends along the entire urethra in the female and throughout the prostate and its capsule in the male (Dixon and Gosling, 1987; Tanagho, 1982). On the anterior surface of the male urethra, an outer layer of circularly oriented striated muscle forms a horseshoe configuration in the adult near the prostatic apex. This striated muscle develops as a complete ring in the fetus and neonate and forms the external urethral sphincter or rhabdosphincter. The periurethral striated muscles of the pelvic floor lie external to the rhabdosphincter (see Fig. 26–1). Despite the horseshoe configuration, stereographic recording of urethral pressure at the external sphincter during bladder filling increases uniformly along the entire circumference like an iris (Morita and Tsuchida, 1989). Norepinephrine or hypogastric nerve stimulation augments this pressure, suggesting a role for adrenergic receptors and sympathetic nerves in the function of the external urethral sphincter. Electromyographic (EMG) study by Kakizaki and co-workers (1991) of external sphincter shows that hypogastric nerve stimulation activates muscle cells.

The arrangement of muscle forming the distal sphincter of the female differs from that in the male. The female has an attenuated striated sphincter mechanism as well as additional muscular structures termed the *compressor urethrae* and *urethrovaginal sphincter* (De Lancey, 1989). The posterior wall remains rigid if there is adequate pelvic support from muscle and connective tissues. As in the male, the striated components are deficient posteriorly. This relative deficiency of periurethral striated musculature contributes to the difficulty in obtaining reliable external sphincter electromyography results during urodynamic studies in women. This attenuation of distal sphincteric muscles may contribute to urinary incontinence in females following resection of the bladder neck.

Investigators have correlated structure of the bladder outlet with its role in urine storage (Elbadawi and Schenk, 1966, Donker et al, 1982; Oerlich, 1980, 1983; Tanagho et al, 1989). Continence in males following resection of the bladder neck and radical prostatectomy is attributed to the activity of circular urethral smooth muscle fibers just beyond the prostatic apex and along the length of the membranous urethra. This region has been termed the *distal intrinsic urethral sphincter.* In females, continence is maintained through an active mechanism along the entire length of the urethra, although the midportion is the most important segment.

In women, urinary continence is maintained during elevations in intra-abdominal pressure by three processes. First, there is passive transmission of abdominal pressure to the proximal urethra. A guarding reflex involving an active contraction of striated muscle of the external urethral sphincter can transiently help continence (Enhorning, 1961; Tanagho, 1982). However, mere transmission of abdominal pressure to proximal urethra does not account for the entire increase in urethral pressure when actually measured during urodynamic monitoring (Constantinou and Govan, 1982; Petros and Ulmsten, 1993, 1995). Urethral pressure rises before cough transmission (Fig. 26–2). These findings implicate an active urethral continence (neural) in women (Constantinou and Govan, 1982). De Lancey proposes that abdominal pressure transmitted through the proximal urethra presses the anterior against the posterior wall. The posterior wall remains rigid if there is adequate pelvic support from muscle and connective tissues. More distally, based on morphologic data, De Lancey (1989) has postulated that the urethral attachments to the pubis (pubourethral) and vaginal connections to pelvic muscles and fascia actively change the position of the bladder neck and proximal urethra with voiding. This arrangement compresses the urethra against the pubis during bladder filling and straining. These attachments contain both fascia and smooth muscle (Oerlich, 1983; De Lancey, 1988, 1989). Thus, urinary continence results from the combination of passive anatomy and active muscle tone.

A greater role for striated muscles of the pelvis floor is postulated in women compared with men. The function of the external urethral sphincter has been explained by examining the properties of its striated muscle components. Striated muscles are characterized as slow type or twitch type (Table 26–1). Twitch type myofibrils can be further classified as slow and fast, based on functional and metabolic characteristics (Padykula and Gauthier, 1967). Slow-twitch fibers are relatively fatigue-resistant owing to high oxidative enzyme activity. In contrast, fast-twitch fibers may be fatigable or fatigue-resistant depending on the amount of oxidative enzyme activity (see Table 26–1).

The relative contributions of fast- and slow-twitch fibers to the external urethral sphincter is variable in the dog (Bazeed et al, 1982) and cat (Elbadawi and Atta, 1985). Gosling and co-workers (1981) present histochemical evidence in humans that striated muscle within the distal urethra is composed primarily of slow-twitch myofibrils in contrast to the periurethral striated muscles of the pelvic floor, which contain fast and slow fibers.

The predominance of slow-twitch fibers in the human external urethral sphincter is consistent with its role in maintaining tone. The external urethral sphincter provides greater

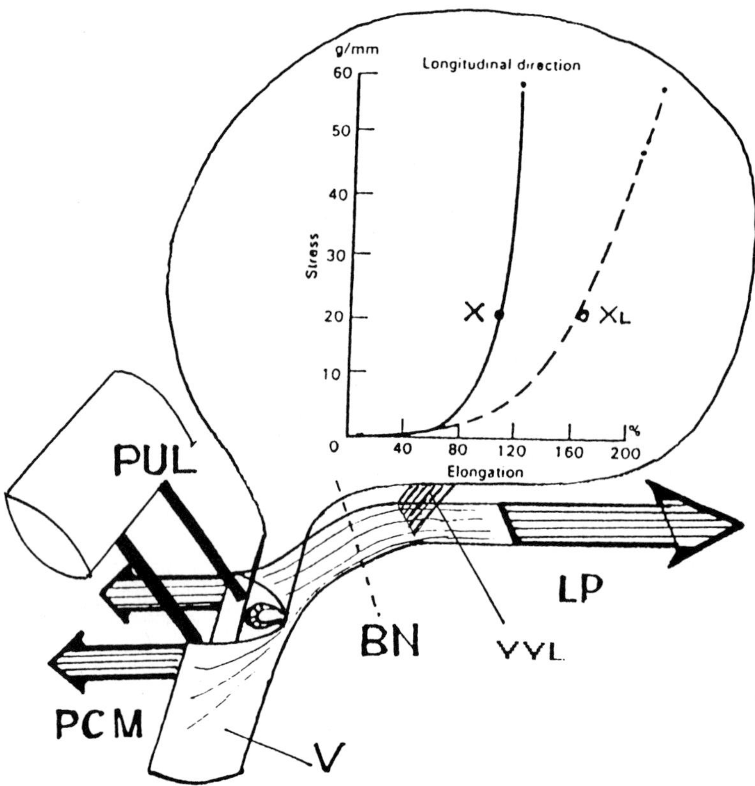

Figure 26–2. Influence of vaginal laxity of muscle force transmission and urinary continence. *(Inset)* Stress extension curve of vagina; X, normal elasticity; XL, vaginal laxity; PUL, pubourethral ligament; BN, bladder neck; LP, levator plate; V, vaginal hammock; PCM, pubococcygeous muscle; VVL, vaginal attachment to bladder base. Authors propose that an increase in urethral pressure prior to cough transmission proves that an active continence mechanism is involved in preventing stress urinary incontinence. (Reprinted by permission from Petros PE, Ulmsten U: An integral theory and its method for the diagnosis and management of female urinary incontinence. Scand J Urol Nephrol 1993; 27[Suppl 153]:1–93. Copyright 1993 Scandinavian University Press, Stockholm, Sweden.)

than 50% of the static urethral resistance (Tanagho et al, 1989). Moreover, the striated periurethral muscles of the pelvic floor are adapted for the rapid recruitment of motor units required during increases in abdominal pressure. Some authors have attempted to explain the success of some therapies for urinary incontinence, such as pelvic floor exercises or electrostimulation, on the basis of changes in the oxidative characteristics of striated muscle (Bazeed et al, 1982). Practically speaking, one cannot voluntarily contract the pelvic muscle several times a minute, 24 hours a day, which is the rate needed to alter muscle metabolism and structure. With striated sphincter dyssynergia, significant hypertrophy of this muscle is possible. Consistent with the notion that exercises do not increase external urethral sphincter function are reports that behavioral therapy and pelvic floor exercises are more effective in urge than stress urinary incontinence (Stein et al, 1995).

In addition to striated muscle, the external sphincter contains smooth muscle, which receives noradrenergic innervation. Investigators have shown that stimulation of the hypogastric nerve elicits myogenic potentials in the external urethral sphincter (Kakizaki et al, 1991). Whether this activity is the result of smooth or striated muscle is unclear. Because these potentials persist after alpha-adrenergic blockade, investigators postulate that it arises from striated muscle.

PROPERTIES OF SMOOTH AND STRIATED MUSCLE

Understanding voiding and continence requires knowledge of the contractile properties of detrusor and urethral smooth muscle. Many properties of bladder and urethral smooth muscle differ from those of striated muscle. Other variables, including differences between non-genitourinary smooth muscles, age, species, and hormonal environment, must also be considered when examining the physiology of smooth muscle.

The contractile properties of bladder smooth muscle cells

Table 26–1. CHARACTERISTICS OF MUSCLE CELLS

	Striated Muscle	Smooth Muscle
Ultrastructure	Sarcomere pattern No intermediate filaments	No sarcomere pattern Intermediate filaments Dense bodies
Contractile activity	Disinhibition of tropomyosin Sliding filaments Rapid contraction	Active myosin phosphorylation ? Sliding filaments Formation of "latch state"
Calcium regulation	Rapid Ca^{2+} influx via T-tubule	Voltage- and receptor-operated Ca^{2+} channels Release from internal stores

Table 26–2. CORRELATION OF BLADDER PRESSURE AND AFFERENT THRESHOLDS

	Intravesical Pressure ($cm\ H_2O$)
Cystometrogram parameters	
Filling	< 10
Capacity	< 10
Micturition	< 15
Afferent thresholds	
Pelvic nerve	6–27
Hypogastric nerve	6–41

are well suited for either urine storage or release. Filling the bladder at a slow physiologic rate maintains an intraluminal pressure of less than 10 cm of water (Klevmark, 1974) (Table 26–2). Acute denervation of the bladder does not appreciably alter this low filling pressure (Langley and Whiteside, 1951). This concept has been used to support the hypothesis that the intrinsic myogenic or viscoelastic properties of cellular and extracellular components are major contributors to low-pressure bladder filling and compliance (see Biomechanics section). Conversely, neural input is required for the rapid and sustained smooth muscle contraction accompanying voiding.

Gap Junctions

Gap junctions are a class of cellular connections that occur in smooth muscle. Gap junctions influence contractility and transfer of nutrients between muscle cells and allow electrical coupling between cells. It is postulated that gap junctions reduce intercellular resistance and allow muscle cells to function as a syncytium by promoting conduction of electrical signals and nutrients throughout the bladder.

Gap junctions are not found in bladder smooth muscle of humans but are present in other species (Dixon and Gosling, 1987). The absence of gap junctions implies a lack of electronic coupling, with a greater resistance to electrical current flow between muscle cells. It is possible that an extensive innervation with a 1:1 ratio between nerve endings and muscle fibers can compensate for this lack of coupling. Although histologic analysis of fiber distributions supports such a multi-unitary innervation of bladder muscle (Elbadawi and Schenk, 1966), ultrastructural examination fails to show that smooth muscle cells are innervated on a 1:1 basis (Elbadawi, 1982). In a detailed study by Gabella (1995), multiple neuromuscular junctions per bladder smooth muscle cell were noted in the rat. Although specialized neuromuscular junctions such as in striated muscle do not exist, some characteristics suggest adaptive contact between smooth muscle and nerve terminals with bladder characterized by bare axons, reductions in the gap between nerve and muscle, and accumulation of axonal vesicles at varicosities closest to the smooth muscle cell. This loose pattern of innervation is postulated to be adaptive for an organ in which intramural nerves cope with substantial structural deformation.

Contractile Proteins

A cyclic interaction between protein filaments is responsible for smooth muscle contraction. These contractile proteins are myosin, actin, and tropomyosin. The urinary bladder contains predominately α-actin and two isoforms of myosin—SM-1 and SM-2 (Chacko and Longhurst, 1994). Myosin is the major enzymatic constituent of thick filaments. It can be dissociated into two high molecular weight heavy chains and two lower molecular weight light chains. Thin filaments contain actin, tropomyosin, and an inhibitory protein known as caldesmon.

It is generally accepted that phosphorylation of the 20 KDa light chain of myosin by a Ca^{2+}/calmodulin-dependant myosin light chain kinase allows interaction between thick and thin filaments with subsequent force generation (Kamm and Stull, 1985, 1989; Steers, 1994). Certain aspects of smooth muscle contraction may also rely on phosphorylation of myosin heavy chains or intermediate filaments. It is hypothesized that a Ca^{2+}-calmodulin complex binds to a myosin light chain kinase (MLCK), which phosphorylates the light chain of myosin (Fig. 26–3). Phosphorylated myosin allows actin to activate a myosin Mg^{2+}-adenosinetriphosphatase (ATPase), which provides the energy for crossbridging between thick and thin filaments with subsequent smooth muscle contraction.

Although myosin phosphorylation represents the major mechanism for contraction, it does not completely account for force generation, thereby implicating other contractile mechanisms. Alternatively, thin filament actin regulation may rely on Ca^{2+} regulation involving caldesmon. Because caldesmon inhibits actomyosin-Mg-ATPase, it is also possible that reversal of caldesmon inhibition by a Ca^{2+} calmodulin messenger complex regulates smooth muscle contractility.

Smooth muscle relaxation occurs by dephosphorylation of the light chain of myosin. The shorter time course for myosin dephosphorylation relative to relaxation has been attributed to a dephosphorylated myosin crossbridge, known as a "latch state," which maintains force by another Ca^{2+}-dependent regulatory process. This secondary process is characterized by a greater sensitivity to Ca^{2+} than to MLCK. Phosphorylation of cytoskeleton proteins in intermediate filaments is also an important regulatory mechanism for a sustained contraction. Failure of these mechanisms or

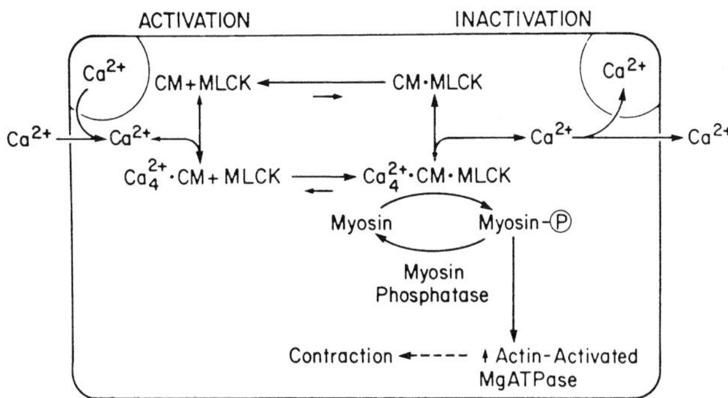

Figure 26–3. Chemomechanical transduction in smooth muscle. Calcium (Ca^{2+}) upon entering the myofibril *(left)*, or following its release from intracellular stores, activates the calmodulin (CM) + myosin light chain kinase (MLCK) complex. The activated Ca^{2+} CM + MLCK complex phosphorylates myosin, resulting in smooth muscle contraction. Biochemical analysis of bladder smooth muscle indicates that a similar scheme is operational in the detrusor. (From Kamm KE, Stull JT: Ann Rev Pharmacol Toxicol, 1985; 25:597.)

changes in the amount of contractile proteins may form the basis for poor detrusor contractility resulting in residual urine. If the contractile apparatus is dysfunctional, it is unlikely that drugs acting at membrane-bound receptors or electrostimulation could empty the bladder.

Calcium (Ca^{2+}) Mechanisms

Drugs or disorders that affect Ca^{2+} fluxes in smooth muscle influence detrusor function. Intracellular Ca^{2+} binds to a protein carrier calmodulin, which initiates the cascade of events necessary to phosphorylate myosin. The influx of Ca^{2+} required for activation of the contractile apparatus is regulated by two separate mechanisms—voltage-sensitive channels and receptor-operated channels. Three voltage-sensitive channels have been proposed: (1) channels susceptible to classic antagonists referred to as L-channels; (2) small transient current or T-channels; and (3) channels found on neurons termed N-channels (Miller, 1987). Recognition of multiple Ca^{2+} channels was based on the inability of such classic Ca^{2+} channel antagonists as nifedipine and verapamil to block Ca^{2+} entry into a cell and from single channel measurements using patch clamp techniques.

A second class of Ca^{2+} channels are receptor-operated. Receptor-operated or gated Ca^{2+} channels can raise the intracellular Ca^{2+}, depolarize the cell membrane, or elicit intracellular changes in second messengers in response to neurotransmitters and drugs. Binding of substrates to receptor-operated Ca^{2+} channels produces a detrusor or urethral contraction by the influx of extracellular Ca^{2+}.

In addition to influx of extracellular Ca^{2+}, Ca^{2+} is released from intracellular stores such as mitochondria and sarcoplasmic reticulum (Mostwin, 1985; Andersson et al, 1989). The release of Ca^{2+} from intracellular sites involves membrane-derived inositol phosphates. For example, muscarinic stimulation of the bladder hydrolyzes the phospholipid phosphatidylinositol biphosphate (PIP_2), leading to intracellular Ca^{2+} release. Activation of all three mechanisms—(1) voltage-operated Ca^{2+} channels, (2) receptor-operated Ca^{2+} channels, and (3) Ca^{2+} release from intracellular stores—has been associated with contraction of human bladder muscle (Fovaeus et al, 1987; Maggi et al, 1989b).

Munro and Wendt (1994) showed that Ca^{2+} released from sarcoplasmic reticulum in the bladder smooth muscle cell increases intracellular Ca^{2+}. However, most of the Ca^{2+} required for detrusor contraction results from influx of extracellular Ca^{2+} through voltage-gated channels. Relaxation of detrusor smooth muscle is accomplished by reducing intracellular Ca^{2+}. Ca^{2+} is either extruded out of the cell or sequestered by intracellular stores. Intracellular Ca^{2+} levels also regulate potassium (K^+) channels (see Potassium Mechanism section).

The spontaneous and agonist-mediated action potentials generated by bladder smooth muscle cells rely on an inward Ca^{2+} current. This produces an upward stroke in an action potential. Repolarization and the downward portion of the action potential corresponds to an outward K^+ current (Montgomery and Fry, 1992). This reliance of smooth muscle electrical activity on Ca^{2+}, as opposed to Na^+ as in nerves, allows selective use of toxins to distinguish myogenic from neurogenic contractions during pharmacologic experiments.

The concentration of intracellular Ca^{2+} does not directly correlate with force generation. For example, exposure of smooth muscle to K^+ causes a larger influx of extracellular Ca^{2+} than does exposure to muscarinic or alpha-adrenergic agonists. However, these latter stimuli generate a greater force than K^+ (Morgan et al, 1989). Wein and co-workers (1989) have used Ca^{2+}-sensitive fluorescent dyes to quantitate changes in intracellular Ca^{2+} concentration in bladder smooth muscle during contraction in vitro. These investigators found that the muscarinic agonist, bethanechol, produces a bladder contraction that is associated with a rise in intracellular Ca^{2+}. However, tension is maintained after intracellular Ca^{2+} levels return to baseline. Wein and co-workers (1989) and Munro and Wendt (1994) have both found that the final concentration of free intracellular Ca^{2+} does correlate with the magnitude of the contraction. The manner in which Ca^{2+} is measured, or regional intracellular concentration fluxes (waves), may explain the lack of correlation of muscle force development with Ca^{2+} levels.

The response of bladder smooth muscle to drugs that act on Ca^{2+} channels makes these agents candidates for treating bladder dysfunction (Mattiasson et al, 1989). Receptor-operated Ca^{2+} channels are subject to up-and-down regulation (Godfraind and Govoni, 1989). Molecular biologic and clinical studies suggest that certain Ca^{2+} antagonists exert greater activity in pathophysiologic than in physiologic conditions. Furthermore, trophic factors released by target tissues can alter the number or binding properties of selective antagonists to Ca^{2+} channels (Godfraind and Govoni, 1989). Therefore, the action of Ca^{2+} antagonists on the hypertrophied or denervated detrusor may not be predicted based on studies of normal smooth muscle (Saito et al, 1989). Unfortunately, Ca^{2+} channel blockers have not been clinically useful to treat bladder hyperactivity (Mattiason et al, 1989). However, neurogenic bladders rather than those demonstrating idiopathic instability respond to Ca^{2+} blockers.

Potassium (K^+) Mechanisms

A variety of K^+ channels are expressed by smooth muscle. ATP-sensitive (K_{ATP}) and Ca^{2+}-sensitive ($K_{Ca^{2+}}$) channels are found in smooth muscle. In the bladder, ATP-sensitive K^+ channels close with a rise in intracellular ATP. Opening K^+ channels causes efflux of K^+, hyperpolarization, and smooth muscle relaxation. The K^+ channel openers cromakalim, pinacidil, and nicorandil relax bladder muscle via this mechanism (Foster et al, 1989; Fujii et al, 1990). Other types of K^+ channels such as those influenced by Ca^{2+} levels are not expressed by human bladder muscle (Zhou et al, 1995). Unfortunately, K^+ channel openers have not been useful clinically to relax noncompliant bladders or abolish detrusor instability (Fovaeus et al, 1989).

In summary, the generation of electrical activity and contraction of smooth muscle in the bladder relies on Ca^{2+}. Nerves cause contraction of the bladder through chemomechanical transduction regulated through numerous intracellular processes. The increased level of free intracellular Ca^{2+} required for contraction can be regulated by voltage- or receptor-operated channels or

by the release of Ca^{2+} from intracellular organelles. K^+ efflux through K^+_{ATP} channels relaxes bladder smooth muscle. However, both Ca^{2+} channel blockers and K^+ channel openners have yet to provide a clinically important role in the treatment of bladder dysfunction. Understanding the relationship between intracellular Ca^{2+} and contractile activity is complex because of potential interaction with a variety of second messenger systems and methods used to measure intracellular events. It is hoped that these mechanisms will provide new opportunities for managing detrusor hypercontractility or hypocontractility using drugs that affect levels of intracellular Ca^{2+} or second messengers such as cyclic adenosine monophosphate (cAMP) (Morita et al, 1986) or inositol phosphates (e.g., diacylglycerate, PIP_2).

Energetics

Smooth muscle maintains tone with relatively little expenditure of energy. Studies have shown that a linear relationship exists between force and metabolism in bladder smooth muscle (Wendt and Gibbs, 1987). Furthermore, the rate of energy expenditure to develop a bladder contraction is only a half that associated with maintenance of an active contraction.

In addition to regulating channel function, adenosine triphosphate (ATP) generated from aerobic glycolysis and glucose metabolism provides the energy required for a bladder contraction (Levin et al, 1987; Wendt and Gibbs, 1987). Under certain conditions, fatty acid metabolism may also serve as an energy source for bladder contraction (Hypolite et al, 1989). This may correspond to clinical regional conditions in which nutrient supply to the bladder is impaired, such as after bilateral iliac artery bypass surgery or prolonged urinary retention.

Electromechanical Coupling and Stretch-Activated Channels

The maintenance of low pressure during filling has been attributed to the passive mechanical properties of the bladder resulting from elastic and plastic elements (Griffiths, 1988). With rapid filling, intravesical pressure rises abruptly then rapidly falls. **Phasic smooth muscles such as the detrusor develop an active myogenic response to unopposed stretch.** This contractile response occurs even in a denervated bladder because of the spontaneous electrical activity previously discussed. Muscle tone corresponds to the frequency of action potential generation (Brading, 1987). Wellner and Isenberg (1994) in a series of experiments using isolated, patch-clamped bladder smooth muscle cells have demonstrated the existence of stretch-activated nonselective cation channels (SAC). These channels regulate Ca^{2+} influx through L-type Ca^{2+} channels.

If isolated cells are rounded up, stretch fails to induce action potentials, suggesting that membrane conformation is important. Thus, the scaffolding provided by passive elements such as collagen and actin indirectly affects active myogenic properties. An active component also exists to bladder compliance or distensibility that helps maintain low ($<$40cm H_2O) filling pressures. The relaxation following stretch-induced action potentials and contractile activity can be the result of several mechanisms. β-adrenergic relaxation could participate in bladder relaxation during filling. However, β-blockers do not exert an influence in the filling portion of a cystometrogram. β-adrenergic relaxation would occur through an increase in intracellular cAMP. Other factors released by the bladder with stretch could also increase cAMP. Likely candidates include prostaglandins and parathyroid hormone-related peptide (PTHrp). In vivo (Yamamoto et al, 1992) and in vitro (Persson and Steers, 1994) stretch of bladder smooth muscle increases levels of PTHrp. PTHrp in turn relaxes bladder and urethral smooth muscles (Yamamoto et al, 1992; Persson and Steers, 1994). Stretch could also directly increase cAMP and elicit relaxation.

The electrophysiologic properties of the detrusor differ from those of urethral smooth muscle. Callahan and Creed (1981, 1985) have found that the frequencies of action potential generation evoked by stretching guinea pig smooth muscle are less regular in the urethra than in the bladder. In contrast, Nakayama and Brading (1993) found that the bladder dome exhibits spontaneous electrical activity but generates little tone. The urethra maintains tone in the absence of electrical activity. It is tempting to speculate that these electrophysiologic characteristics correspond to differences in function. The synchronous electrical behavior of the detrusor may facilitate complete bladder emptying, whereas asynchronous or absent urethral electrical activity promotes continence. Bladder emptying may be enhanced because the resting potential of bladder smooth muscle resides near threshold. Therefore, the distended bladder sits poised to contract upon the arrival of an appropriate neural signal.

These electrophysiologic characteristics of bladder smooth muscle suggest that the nervous system must exert strict control to prevent inadvertent contraction. The phasic nature and excitability of the stretched detrusor through stretch-activated channels (SACs) provide the bladder with an enhanced susceptibility to neural and hormonal control. Conditions, drugs, and circulating factors that alter the membrane threshold can predispose the bladder to hyper- or hypoactivity. The propensity for spontaneous activity most likely contributes in part to common finding of detrusor instability or hyperreflexia.

Passive Components: Connective Tissue

Collagen and elastin are the major connective tissue components in the urinary bladder. With aging, obstruction, or denervation, changes occur in the structure and isoform expression as well as collagen content. Changes in the expression of these proteins play an important role in the inability of the bladder to fill at low pressure, empty completely, and maintain continence with injury or disease (Ewalt et al, 1992; Shapiro et al, 1991).

Collagen exists throughout the adult bladder as either a loose network of bundles in the mucosa or sheets that cover muscle fascicles (Murakumo et al, 1995). Trabeculation of the bladder on cystoscopy represents increased collagen formation. Elastin is sparse throughout the bladder muscle layer, but forms dense networks around vessels and muscle fascicles.

Fibroblasts in the bladder secrete collagen (types I, III, and IV) (Coplen et al, 1994). With decreased bladder compliance there is an increase in extracellular matrix (Shapiro et al, 1991). Ewalt and co-workers (1992) have shown that **in patients with poor compliance, smooth muscle bundles are infiltrated with type III collagen and surrounded by increased amounts of types I and III as well as elastin. These changes in amount as well as distribution have been linked to alterations in bladder and renal function.**

BIOMECHANICS

Filling Mechanics

The viscoelastic behavior of the bladder and urethra depends on both neuromuscular and mechanical properties. Mechanical properties vary with the magnitude of stretch (distention), even in tissue deprived of ATP (e.g., postmortem). Mechanical properties are extremely sensitive to tissue structure and composition. As mentioned, in the bladder and urethra, collagen and elastin content have a profound influence on the viscoelastic properties when these tissues are subjected to stress (force per area). The human bladder is composed of roughly 50% collagen and 2% elastin. With injury, obstruction and denervation collagen content increases. When contractible protein content exceeds collagen, greater distensibility is achieved (compliance). Conversely, when collagen levels increase, compliance falls. Bladder compliance (C) is defined as the change in volume relative to the corresponding change in intravesical pressure:

$$\Delta V/\Delta p = C$$

A loss or decrease in compliance resulting from an alteration in bladder composition, or efferent neural input, can alter afferent firing and thereby the threshold for micturition. A loss of compliance alters wall tension. With increasing bladder volume, wall stress or tension *(T)* increases, as defined by Laplace's equation (Fig. 26–4). Laplace's equation states that

$$T = P_{ves}R/2d$$

In this equation, T is tension, P_{ves} is intravesical pressure, R is bladder radius, and d is wall thickness. During bladder filling, P_{ves} is relatively constant. With a fully distended bladder d is ignored relative to the other parameters unless a hypertrophied wall exists. **Thus, $T = P_{ves}R/2$ approximates tension in the full normal bladder.**

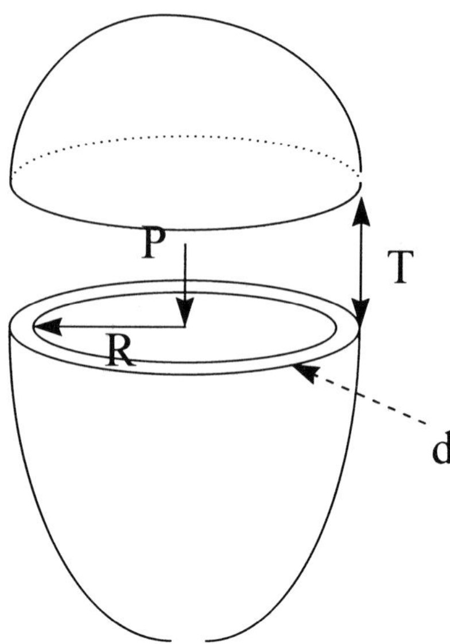

Figure 26–4. Laplace's equation describing wall tension (T) as a function of bladder radius (R), intravesical pressure (P), and wall thickness (D).

Voiding Mechanics

Intravesical pressure reflects the combined factors of abdominal (P_{abd}) and detrusor (P_{det}) pressures. Therefore,

$$P_{ves} = P_{det} + P_{abd}$$

Micturition relies on a neurally-mediated detrusor contraction causing P_{det} to rise without a significant change in P_{abd}.

To assess the strength of a detrusor contraction, P_{det} alone is an insufficient measure. A muscle can use energy to either generate force or shorten its length. Because the bladder is a hollow viscus, the force developed contributes to P_{det}, whereas the velocity of shortening relates to urine flow (Q). There is a trade-off between generating P_{det} and urine flow. This has been nicely reviewed by Griffiths (1988). If urethral resistance is high, as with obstruction, P_{det} can achieve substantial levels acutely (i.e., >60–90 cm H_2O). If urethral resistance is low, as in some women with sphincter insufficiency, P_{det} may be almost undetectable. In each instance the detrusor smooth muscle contractility may be identical despite vastly different values for P_{det}. The trade-off between P_{det} and *Q* resembles a curve for constant mechanical power (W) in which

$$W = P_{det} \times Q$$

Computer-based models have been developed to estimate the strength or contractility of the bladder. These relationships are important in assessing whether obstruction exists in the face of reduced contractility.

It would be very useful to assign a value for urethral resistance in a given patient. This resistance would be an objective measure of the degree of obstruction. Although various models with corresponding formulas have been proposed, none is agreed upon. One problem is that the urethra is a nonideal distensible tube. Some models based on energy balances have been used. Because energy cannot be created or destroyed, P_{det} must equal the energy dissipated (as heat) through kinetic energy (E) of urine flow. If $E = \delta V^2/2$, where δ is the density and V the velocity of urine during voiding, the equation can be manipulated to produce a resistance (R) factor that depends on flow rate (Q). If $V = Q/A$,

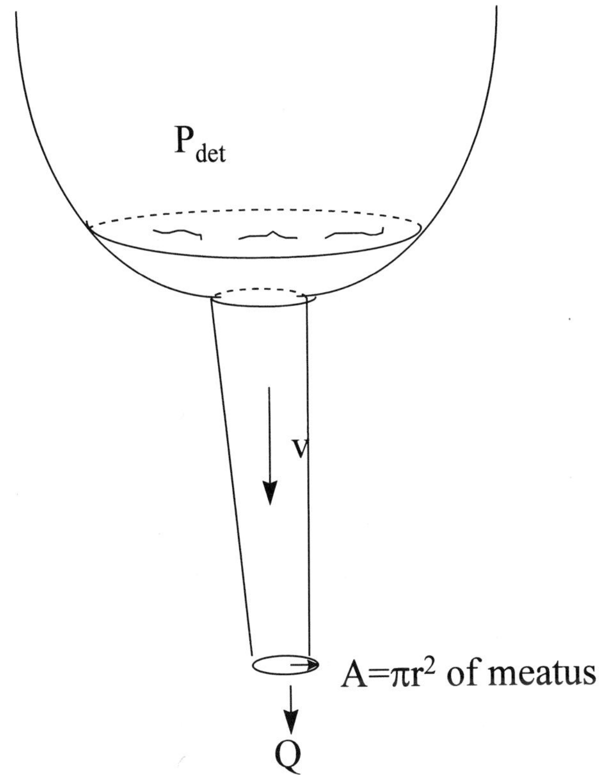

Figure 26–5. During voiding, urine flows through urethra at a varying velocity (V). The region of the outlet most influential in the flow rate (Q) is the urethral meatus in the absence of proximal obstruction. The area of the meatus (A), flow rate, and detrusor pressure (P_{det}) are used to approximate urethral resistance ($R = P_{det}/Q^2$). This estimate, however, fails to take into account nonideal conditions such as distensible urethral and nonlaminae flow.

where A corresponds to the area of the flow-controlling zone (i.e., the urethral meatus), manipulation gives the equation

$$R = P_{det}/Q^2$$

This is illustrated in Figure 26–5. **Thus, resistance varies with the inverse square of flow rate.** A distensible urethra is subjected to a flow-controlling region that governs impedance. Such a flow-controlling region exists in the distal urethra in women and men. During voiding, urethral closure pressure must be overcome by P_{det}. This is accomplished by the nervous system eliciting a coordinated detrusor contraction and urethral relaxation.

PERIPHERAL NEUROANATOMY

Coordinated and complete urine release depends on an intact innervation. Autonomic innervation to the urinary bladder accomplishes these tasks through parasympathetic and sympathetic pathways. In addition to autonomics, somatic nerves innervate the striated muscles of the bladder outlet (Elbadawi and Schenk, 1974). Coordinated voiding results from viscerosomatic integration between these autonomic and somatic pathways.

Parasympathetic Pathways to the Bladder

Parasympathetic input to the human bladder arises in the intermediolateral cell column of the second, third, and fourth sacral spinal cord segments (Fig. 26–6). The perikarya of preganglionic neurons and their dendrites are organized in a viscerotopic manner in the sacral spinal cord. This viscerotopic arrangement explains selective sparing of certain pelvic visceral functions following discrete lesions of the sacral spinal cord. Axon collaterals from a single preganglionic neuron branch out and synapse on up to 50 neurons throughout various regions of the sacral spinal cord (Morgan et al, 1991). Local neural networks coordinate pelvic visceral and somatic function during voiding, defecation, penile erection, ejaculation and lower limb movement. The sacral preganglionic axons projecting to the bladder are conveyed by the pelvic nerve (see Fig. 26–6). The pelvic nerve also contains postganglionic sympathetic fibers coursing from the chain ganglia. Synaptic connections between axons and ganglion

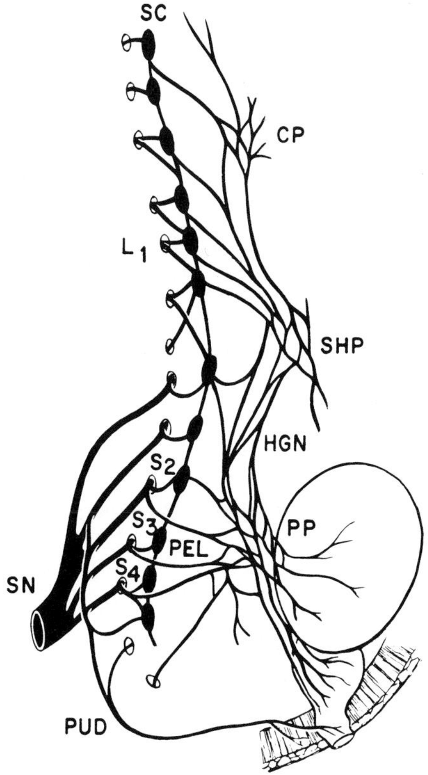

Figure 26–6. Diagram of innervation to the lower urinary tract. Thoracolumbar sympathetic outflow arises from T10–L2 spinal cord segments and travels by either lumbar splanchnic nerves or prevertebral ganglia (celiac, plexus, CP, superior hypogastric plexus, SHP). The hypogastric nerves (HGN) exit the hypogastric plexus to innervate ganglion cells in the pelvis. Alternatively, sympathetic outflow travels down the sympathetic chain (SC) and via the pelvic nerve to supply primarily the pelvic vasculature. Parasympathetic input to the bladder and urethra arises in the sacral (S2–S4) spinal cord and is conveyed by the pelvic nerve (PEL), which supplies ganglion cells in the pelvic plexus (PP) and bladder wall. Somatic neural input to the striated muscles of the urethra and pelvic floor originates in Onuf's nucleus from S2–S4 spinal cord segments. Somatic fibers are conveyed by the pudendal nerve (PUD). SN, sciatic nerve.

cells innervating the bladder occur in the pelvic plexus and on the surface of the bladder.

The pelvic plexus is a curvilinear network of nerves lying in the pelvic fascia on either side of the lower genitourinary tract and rectum. It can be injured following pelvic surgery to cause transient or permanent voiding dysfunction. This plexus serves as a relay center where preganglionic axons synapse on postganglionic neurons that innervate the bladder and urethra. The pelvic plexus is organized in some species in a viscerotopic manner, with neurons supplying the bladder often located in that portion of the plexus closest to the urinary tract (Keast et al, 1989a). In the human, a separate vesical plexus cannot be identified (Higgins and Gosling, 1989). Pelvic bladder neurons have been recently characterized using patch clamp techniques. These experiments reveal that bladder postganglionics are of high threshold and possess tetrodotoxin-sensitive Na^{2+} channels (Yoshimura and de Groat, 1992). Afferent axons from the bladder to the spinal cord may also synapse on pelvic ganglia.

Sympathetic Pathways to the Bladder

Sympathetic preganglionics arise from cells in the intermediolateral cell column and nucleus intercalus of the tenth thoracic to second lumbar spinal cord segments. At more rostral levels, preganglionic fibers exit the chain ganglia and pass along the lumbar splanchnic nerves toward the superior hypogastric plexus (see Fig. 26–6). The hypogastric plexus in turn lies on the great vessels at the level of the third lumbar to first sacral vertebrae and gives rise to the left and right hypogastric nerves. The hypogastric nerves contain postganglionic fibers from prevertebral ganglion neurons. Preganglionic axons in the hypogastric nerve pass through the prevertebral ganglia and synapse within the pelvic plexus or bladder wall.

Sympathetic fibers that enter the pelvic plexus may interact with sacral parasympathetic pathways or with postganglionic neurons from the sympathetic chain. Thus, the pelvic plexus serves as an integration and relay center for autonomic input to the bladder and other pelvic viscera.

Parasympathetic Pathways to the Urethra

Parasympathetic nerves exiting the sacral spinal cord are conveyed by the pelvic nerve and supply the urethra and prostate in males, and the urethra in females. Urethral nerves contain afferents responsible for reflexes that influence bladder filling and emptying, as outlined by Barrington (1931). Urethral nerves exit the pelvic ganglion and some branch off from the cavernous nerves. Thus, **the designation of "cavernous nerve" is a misnomer because branches of this nerve also supply the urethra. As a corollary, injury to the more proximal portion of these nerves may affect urethral function and contribute to sphincteric insufficiency and urinary incontinence after pelvic surgeries such as radical prostatectomy.**

Sympathetic Pathways to the Urethra

The sympathetic nerves supplying the urethra arise in the same regions of the spinal cord as those to the bladder. Noradrenergic input to the bladder is sparse. In contrast, noradrenergic postganglionic fibers are abundant around the vasculature and smooth muscle of the urethra. The hypogastric nerve provides the primary sympathetic input to the urethra (Creed, 1979; McGuire and Herlihy, 1979). In addition, noradrenergic fibers from the hypogastric nerve supply the external urethral sphincter (Kakizaki et al, 1991; Williams and Brading, 1992).

Somatic Pathways

Striated muscle forming the external urethral sphincter is innervated by the pudendal nerve. Motor axons in the pudendal nerve arise from the second, third, and fourth segments of the sacral spinal cord. These somatic motoneurons are located anterior to bladder preganglionics in a region termed *Onuf's nucleus.* Similar to sacral autonomic preganglionic neurons, cells within Onuf's nucleus are topographically organized depending on whether they supply the external urethral sphincter, striated muscles of the pelvic floor, or the anal sphincter (McKenna and Nadelhaft, 1985; Roppolo et al, 1985; Beattie et al, 1990). Cells within Onuf's nucleus are unique in that their properties and size more closely resemble autonomic neurons rather than other somatic motoneurons within the spinal cord (see Storage Reflexes section).

PHARMACOLOGY OF THE BLADDER AND PERIPHERAL AUTONOMIC GANGLIA

Communication between nerves and other nerves or tissues relies on a mixture of substances. Differential release of neurotransmitters or modulators depends on factors such as the frequency or pattern of stimulation. Transmission between different neural pathways, termed *crosstalk,* provides nerves with flexibility and safety (Burnstock, 1986a). For example, peripheral sympathetic and parasympathetic terminals as well as afferents and efferents communicate with one another. Such crosstalk provides a mechanism for peripheral coordination of neural function. For example, during voiding, nerves responsible for maintaining tone of the outlet are actively prevented from firing. Conversely, during filling, a reciprocal set of nerves keeps transmission in parasympathetics quiescent. Local substances and growth factors also affect the function, maintenance, and growth of nerves to the lower urinary tract.

When a neurotransmitter binds to a receptor on the bladder, a process of signal transduction generates second messengers, changes membrane conductances, and alters ionic channels in smooth muscle and nerve. These events are linked with synaptic transmission, neuronal excitability (Zucker and Lando, 1986), and smooth muscle contractility (Hoffmann, 1985). Primary regulators of signal transduction are membrane bound enzymes, which include guanylate cyclase, adenylate cyclase, phospholipase C, and phospholipase A_2. These effector enzymes regulate a variety of second messengers including Ca^{2+}-calmodulin, cGMP, cAMP, inositol phosphates, diacylglycerate, and arachidonic acid derivatives. Intracellular enzymes subsequently activate these second messengers and form phosphoprotein substrates known as kinases. Kinases phosphorylate a variety of substrates responsible for the relaxation and contraction of smooth muscle (Hoffmann, 1985) or the synthesis and release of transmitters (Zucker and Lando, 1986). The following sections discuss the mechanisms and functional implications of drugs, hormones, and autocrine and growth factors on neurotransmission in the peripheral nerves supplying the urinary tract.

Acetylcholine

Classically, preganglionic neurons release acetylcholine, which activates nicotinic (N) receptors on peripheral ganglion cells (see Fig. 26–6). Nicotinic ganglionic blockers abolish bladder contractions produced by electrical stimulation of the pelvic nerve (Learmonth, 1931) or sacral roots (Learmonth, 1931; Brindley, 1986; Brindley et al, 1986). Thus, excitatory input to the bladder is mediated by cholinergic neurons exiting the sacral spinal cord. These preganglionic fibers synapse on ganglion cells in the pelvic plexus or bladder wall. Blockade of autonomic transmission with nicotinic receptor antagonists is nonspecific and thus is not used clinically to abolish bladder activity.

Parasympathetic ganglion cells, which send axons to the bladder, also contain acetylcholine. Histochemical identification of postganglionic cholinergic nerves is accomplished by localization of enzymes involved in acetylcholine synthesis (choline acetyltransferase) or degradation (acetylcholinesterase). Acetylcholinesterase-positive fibers are found between human bladder smooth muscle fascicles and beneath the urothelium (Ek et al, 1977; Gosling et al, 1977; Kluck, 1980). On electron microscopy, cholinergic terminals are characterized by small, clear synaptic vesicles. In the bladder wall, nerve terminals and ganglionic cells containing these small, clear, presumably cholinergic vesicles have been identified (Gosling et al, 1977). Cholinergic nerves appear in the bladder before birth. In patients with idiopathic hypotonic bladders, acetylcholinesterase staining is reduced, which has been interpreted as a reduction of cholinergic innervation (Kinn et al, 1987). Acetylcholinesterase-staining fibers are also decreased following denervation or hypertrophy of the bladder (Ekstrom et al, 1986; Nilvebrant et al, 1989).

Electrical stimulation of nerves innervating the bladder or local administration of cholinergic agonists produces a bladder contraction and a rise in intravesical pressure. These effects are mediated by muscarinic (M) receptors because they are abolished by the muscarinic antagonist atropine (Fig. 26–7). In normal humans, intravenous atropine causes complete paralysis of the bladder (Collumbine et al, 1955), confirming the crucial role of cholinergic transmission in voiding. Drugs such as physostigmine that inhibit acetylcholine degradation by acetylcholinesterase enhance bladder contractions evoked by nerve stimulation or by cholinergic agonists (Benson et al, 1976b; Sibley, 1984). These effects are abolished by muscarinic antagonists (Nergardh and Boreus, 1972; Benson et al, 1976b; Sibley, 1984; Sjögren et al, 1982; Mostwin, 1986; Zappia et al, 1986).

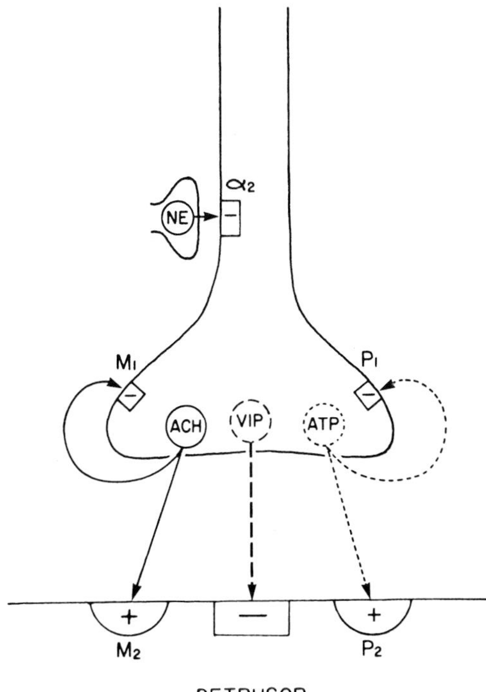

Figure 26–7. Diagram of possible transmitters in a cholinergic terminal innervating the bladder or urethra. Acetylcholine release activates M_2 receptors to elicit a contraction (+) or feedback that inhibits (−) further ACH release via M_1 receptors. Vasoactive intestinal polypeptide (VIP) is found in some cholinergic terminals. Release of adenosine triphosphate (ATP) from cholinergic terminals has been postulated to cause smooth muscle contraction via P receptors. Prejunctional activation of P_1 receptors may inhibit release of ATP. Norepinephrine (NE) release from adrenergic terminals in synaptic contact with a cholinergic varicosity can inhibit firing of cholinergic axon via alpha$_2$-adrenergic receptors. Not shown is possible prejunctional inhibition of ACH release by NPY. This "crosstalk" between different varicosities may ensure synchronous firing of a single neural pathway.

The desire to inhibit detrusor contractions in patients with unstable bladders and urge incontinence has led to a search for muscarinic agonists that are relatively selective for the bladder. Radioligand-binding studies confirm that the bladder body and base contain several subtypes of muscarinic receptors (Levin et al, 1982; Nilvebrant et al, 1985; Lepor et al, 1989; Wang et al., 1995). Muscarinic receptors are expressed by fetal bladders (Keating et al, 1990). Muscarinic receptors have been categorized into M_1, M_2, and M_3 subtypes based on their affinity for cholinergic ligands. In addition, molecular biological techniques have identified 5 molecular forms (m1–m5) of the muscarinic receptor (Bonner, 1989). In general, the m1, m2 and m3 molecularly-identified types of muscarinic receptors correspond to their ligand counterparts (M_1, M_2, and M_3), whereas the m4 and m5 receptors share different pharmacologic profiles. Within the central nervous system, cholinergic transmission is mediated by M_1 and M_2 receptors.

A close examination of muscarinic receptor mechanisms helps explain why once a detrusor contraction is initiated, it is nearly impossible to abort or inhibit it. **The human bladder is endowed with M_2 and M_3 receptors (Zappia et al, 1986; Wang et al, 1995)** (Figs. 26–7 and 26–8; Table

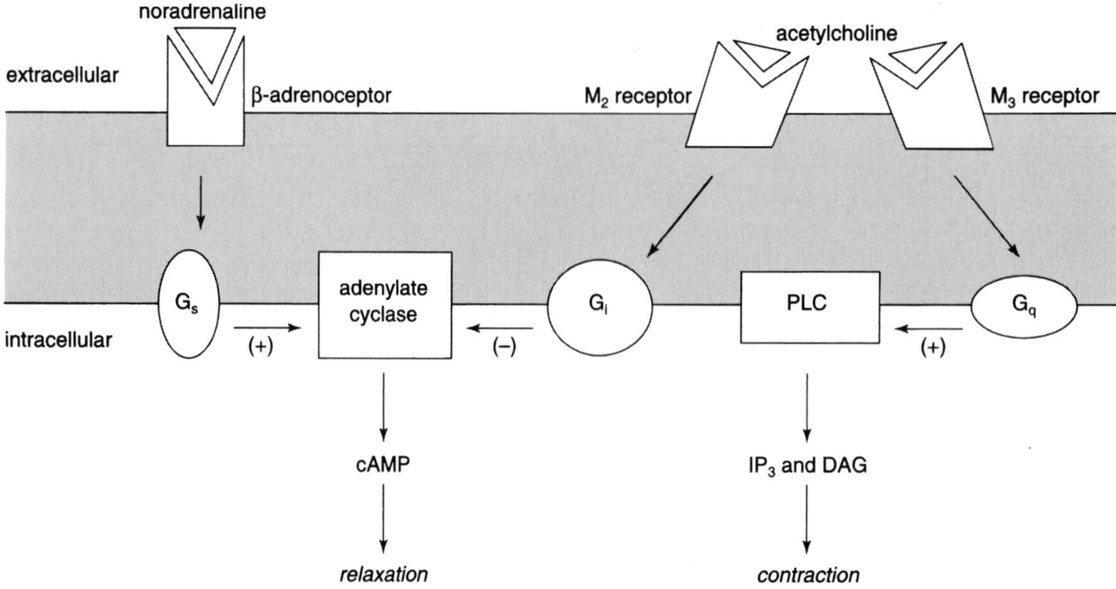

Figure 26–8. The balance between the relaxant and contractile state of smooth muscle depends on the prevailing parasympathetic and sympathetic drive. In this model, both muscarinic M_2 and M_3 receptors modulate the contractile state of the tissue. M_3 receptors mediate contraction, by coupling to the G protein G_q, mobilizing inositol (1,4,5)-trisphosphate (IP_3) and diacyglycerol (DAG) from phospholipase C (PLC) and, consequently, elevating intracellular Ca^{2+} levels. Stimulation of beta adrenoceptors causes relaxation by enhancement of adenylate cyclase activity, whereas activation of M_2 receptors, by coupling to G_i, inhibits this augmentation. (From Eglen RM, Reddy H, Watson N, Challiss RA: Trends Pharmacol Sci 1994; 15:114–119.)

26–3). Functional (Poli et al, 1992) and in vivo studies (Kondo and Morita, 1993) suggest that the M_3 subtype predominates in the human bladder. However, immunoprecipitation assays indicate that the M_2 type predominates (Wang et al, 1995). Regardless, it appears that contraction is mediated by the M_3 type in the human bladder (Wang et al, 1995). The action of M receptors is ultimately dependent on activation of G-proteins and intracellular calcium (see Fig. 26–8). In contrast, M_2 receptors are linked to voltage-gated calcium channels. Thus blocking one type may not completely abolish calcium mechanisms for contraction. The blockade of both muscarinic receptors M_2 and M_3 and calcium channels with the drug terodiline can abolish bladder contractions but results in cardiac toxicity. Despite the potential multiplicity of ligand or molecularly-defined muscarinic receptors, cholinergic agents that are relatively selective for bladder smooth muscle have not been readily identified (Nilvebrant et al, 1985; Zappia et al, 1986; Batra et al, 1987). More recently, investigators have reported on a novel muscarinic antagonist, tolterodine, which has less effect on salivary glands than on the bladder, thus reducing the side effect of dry mouth (Gillberg et al, 1994; Ekstrom et al, 1995). This selectivity, however, is not due to changes in binding properties.

Aside from different types of receptors, the binding properties of muscarinic receptors in the bladder are altered following smooth muscle hypertrophy or nerve injury (Lepor et al, 1989). Changes in muscarinic receptors can be rapid. For example, the binding affinity of muscarinic receptors increases within a few hours after bladder outlet destruction (Levin et al, 1988).

Pharmacologic activation of muscarinic receptors should theoretically be useful to enhance voiding. Yet, cholinergic agonists such as bethanechol cause simultaneous contraction of the bladder, bladder neck, and urethra, preventing coordinated and complete bladder emptying (Table 26–4) (Sogbein et al, 1984). In addition, cholinergic agonists would not be effective if residual urine or urinary retention were the result of defects in intracellular chemomechanical mechanisms.

Another reason bethanechol fails to help empty the bladder is that pelvic ganglion cells and their axons express both cholinergic and adrenergic receptors. Acting by a feedback mechanism, acetylcholine released by cholinergic axons in the bladder inhibits the further release of acetylcholine through M_2 or M_4 receptors (D'Agostino et al, 1986; Somogyi and de Groat, 1992; Alberts, 1995) (Figs. 26–9, 26–10). Activation of muscarinic receptors on adrenergic terminals in the bladder base and urethra inhibits norepinephrine release (Mattiasson et al, 1987; Somogyi et al, 1990) (Fig. 26–11; see Fig. 26–10). Lastly, bethanechol is poorly absorbed from the intestine, and subcutaneous and high oral doses are needed to achieve a pharmacologic effect. Although cholinergic agonists raise baseline bladder pressure and can increase maximal detrusor pressure, they do not completely evacuate the bladder. Furthermore, in neurogenic bladders cholinergic agonists decrease compliance and promote upper tract deterioration. Lastly, certain drugs such as furosemide can directly augment cholinergic responses (Okpukpara and Akah, 1990).

In contrast to cholinergic agonists, anticholinergics are widely used to treat voiding problems. The anticholinergics propantheline and oxybutynin are the most common agents used to treat detrusor hyperactivity. Unfortunately, these drugs do not always eliminate detrusor hyperreflexia (Jensen, 1981). The systemic side effects of these agents contribute to poor patient compliance. The possible reasons for the inability of antimuscarinics to prevent an unstable bladder condition are listed in Table 26–5.

Table 26–3. LOCALIZATION AND PHARMACOLOGIC EFFECTS OF PUTATIVE NEUROTRANSMITTERS/ MODULATORS IN THE HUMAN BLADDER AND URETHRA

Substance	Receptor	Location	In Vitro Effect
Postganglionic Efferent (Motor nerves)		D = detrusor B = base, bladder neck U = urethra	+ = contract, enhance − = relax, inhibit 0 = no effect
Acetylcholine	$M_2 > M_3$	D,B,U	+ D,B,U
Norepinephrine	$\alpha_{1A} > \alpha_{1D} > \alpha_2$	B,U	+ B,U
	$\beta_2 > \beta_1$	D,U	− D,U
ATP	P_{2X}	D,B,U	+ D
NPY	Y_2	B,U	− acetylcholine release
Efferent/Afferent			
VIP	cAMP	D,B,U	− D,U
Nitric Oxide (NO)	cGMP	D,B,U	0
Afferent (Sensory nerves)			
Substance P (SP)	$NK_2 > NK_1$	D,B,U	+ D,B,U
Neurokinin A (NKA)	NK_2	?	+ D,U
Neurokinin B (NKB)	NK_2	?	+ D,U
CGRP		B,U	0
Enkephalin (ENK)	$\mu > \delta$	D	− D
Bombesin		D	+ D
Galanin		D	− D
Neuromodulators/ Autocoids			
Bradykinin		D	+ D
Endothelinin-1,-2	ET-1, ET-3	D,U	+ D (ET-1, ET-3), + U (ET-1)
Angiotensin II	AT_1	D	+ D
$PGF_{2\alpha}$, PGE_1, PGE_2		D,B,U	+ D ($PGF_{2\alpha}$, $PGE_{1,2}$) + U ($PGF_{2\alpha}$)
Histamine	H_1	D	+ D
Serotonin	$5\text{-}HT_3$, $5\text{-}HT_1$, $5\text{-}HT_2$	D,U	− D ($5\text{-}HT_1$), + D, − U ($5\text{-}HT_2$)
Dopamine	D_1 or α_1	D,U	+ D,U

In some species, bladder contractions evoked by neural stimulation are not completely abolished by the muscarinic antagonist atropine (Zederic et al, 1996). This atropine resistance has been used to explain the failure of cholinergic antagonists such as propantheline and oxybutynin to control bladder hyperactivity. Previous experiments that demonstrated atropine resistance in specimens from human bladder have been discredited because atropine-insensitive contractions were probably evoked by direct smooth muscle stimulation rather than by the release of neurotransmitter (Sibley, 1984). Other data suggest that in humans atropine resistance may be limited to denervated or hypertrophied bladders or may be seen only with certain frequencies of stimulation of smooth muscle (Sjögren et al, 1982; Sibley, 1984). Thus, in conditions causing involuntary bladder contractions, noncholinergic excitatory mechanisms may play a role.

Table 26–4. REASONS WHY CHOLINERGIC AGONISTS (BETHANECHOL) DO NOT EMPTY THE BLADDER

1. Activation of muscarinic receptors in bladder neck and urethra (no coordination)
2. Defect in contractile proteins or signal transduction pathway
3. Inhibition of acetylcholine release from parasympathetic postganglionics via presynaptic mechanism
4. Ineffective pharmacologic dose
5. Participation of noncholinergic excitatory transmission in initiating bladder contraction. Cholinergic transmission maintains contraction.

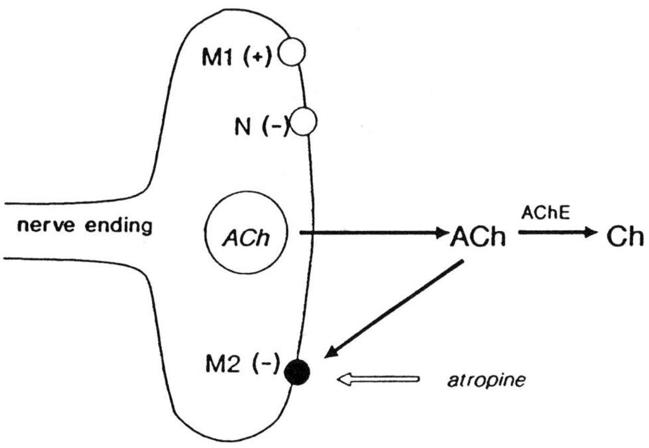

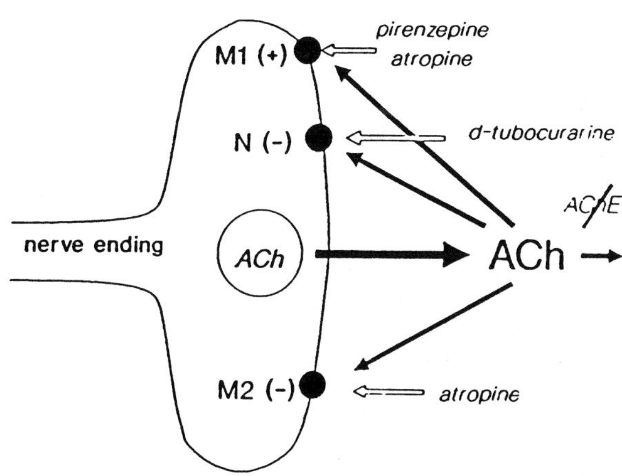

Figure 26–9. Cholinergic receptors and cholinergic post-ganglionic nerves in the rat bladder are modulated by endogenous ACh in normal and physostigmine-treated preparations. M_2-receptors are activated by ACh and untreated preparations. M_1, M_2, and nicotinic receptors are turned on after administration of physostigmine. (+), facilitory; (−), inhibitory; (●), activated; (o), inactive receptors; N, nicotinic; M, muscarinic receptors. (From Somogyi GT, de Groat WC: J Auton Nerv Sys 1992; 37:89–98.)

Norepinephrine

Learmonth (1931) showed that stimulation to the hypogastric nerve in humans contracted the bladder neck and trigone. On the other hand, Brindley (1986) noted that hypogastric nerve stimulation fails to contract or relax the bladder or urethra in humans. Some authors believe that hypogastric pathways facilitate urine storage by relaxing the detrusor and contracting the bladder outlet (Krane and Olsson, 1973;

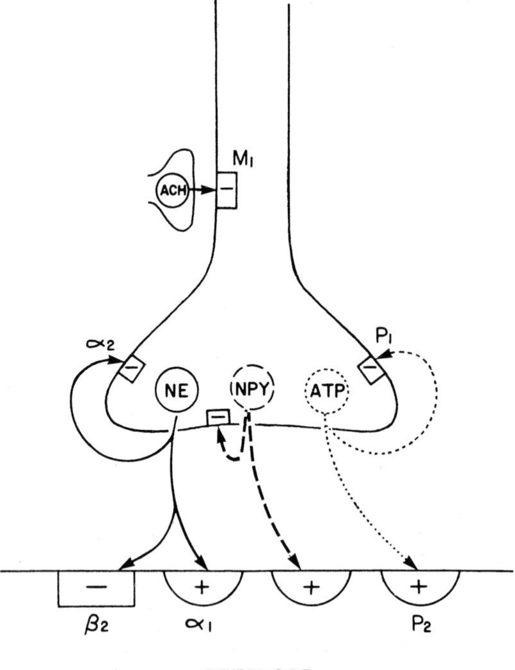

Figure 26–10. Diagram of possible transmitters in an adrenergic terminal supplying the bladder or urethra. Norepinephrine (NE) release can activate alpha$_1$-adrenergic receptors and produce contraction (+) or beta receptors and cause relaxation (−) of the detrusor. Feedback inhibition of NE release via alpha$_2$-receptors can also occur. Neuropeptide Y (NPY) can produce smooth muscle contraction (+), can inhibit acetylcholine release (not shown), or feedback can inhibit NE release. Adenosine triphosphate (ATP) can activate P$_2$ receptors in the detrusor, which elicit contraction (+) or inhibit (−) further ATP release via P$_1$ prejunctional receptors. Acetylcholine (ACH) release from terminals in synaptic contact with an adrenergic varicosity can inhibit firing of adrenergic axons by activation of M$_1$ receptors.

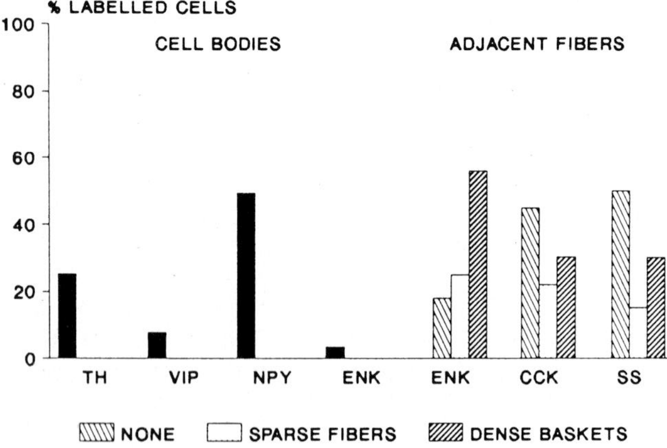

Figure 26–11. Percentages of retrogradely labeled bladder neurons in the pelvic ganglion of the rat, which are immunoreactive (IR) for vasoactive intestinal polypeptide (VIP), neuropeptide Y (NPY), enkephalin (ENK), cholecystokinin (CCK), and somatostatin (SS). Tyrosine hydroxylase (TH) immunoreactivity is used as a marker for noradrenergic neurons. The proportion of bladder neurons immunoreactive for various peptides and types of peptides varies among species. Note that the majority of neurons stain for NPY, which is probably in both cholinergic and adrenergic neurons. Dense ENK baskets surround most bladder neurons. Neuropeptides such as substance P or calcitonin gene–related peptide are found only in sensory neurons. (Modified from Keast JR, de Groat WC: J Comp Neurol 1989; 288:396.)

Table 26–5. LACK OF EFFICACY OF ANTIMUSCARINICS FOR UNSTABLE BLADDER CONTRACTIONS AND URGE INCONTINENCE

1. Noncholinergic excitatory transmission (e.g., ATP) in abnormal bladder
2. Involvement of afferents with release of noncholinergic transmitters affecting smooth muscle
3. Antimuscarinics increase acetylcholine and norepinephrine release through presynaptic mechanisms
4. Direct activation of intracellular signaling by pathologic process (e.g., increase in phospholipase C and calcium)
5. Altered membrane potential of the smooth muscle cell
6. Lack of pharmacologic levels in bladder tissue

McGuire, 1984) (see Fig. 26–18, later); others (Nordling, 1983) remain skeptical. Despite controversy regarding the precise role of sympathetic input to the bladder, peripheral noradrenergic mechanisms can potentially influence bladder function. Noradrenergics are likely to be involved in urinary continence during periods of stress or at volumes exceeding the normal micturition threshold.

Cholinergic neurons that originate in the thoracolumbar spinal cord provide excitatory input to norepinephrine-containing (adrenergic) ganglion cells within the hypogastric and pelvic plexuses, sympathetic chain ganglia, and the bladder wall (see Fig. 26–6). In some species, nonadrenergic pelvic ganglion cells receiving sympathetic preganglionics have been reported (Keast, 1995). Nevertheless, most postganglionics forming the sympathetic pathways account for noradrenergic varicosities within the bladder and urethra (Elbadawi et al, 1966; Ek et al, 1977; Sundin et al, 1977; Gosling and Dixon, 1983; Dixon and Gosling, 1987; Benson et al, 1979). Noradrenergic varicosities appear in the bladder shortly after birth (Levin et al, 1981). Noradrenergic fibers have also been observed in the striated muscle of the rhabdosphincter (Elbadawi and Schenk, 1974; Elbadawi and Atta, 1985). Compared with other species, noradrenergic innervation in the human bladder and urethra, especially in females, is sparse and is limited to the bladder base and proximal urethra (Ek et al, 1977; Sundin et al, 1977; Benson et al, 1979; Kluck, 1980). Sundin and co-workers (1977) rarely observed catecholamine-fluorescent varicosities in the human detrusor. Using electron microscopy, Gosling and Dixon (1983) observed nerve terminals characteristic of norepinephrine-containing vesicles containing small dense core inclusions lying in close proximity to intramural ganglia of the bladder. Noradrenergic terminals were also seen in the trigone. Although noradrenergic innervation is sparse, norepinephrine can be measured in superfusates from human bladder and urethra after electrical stimulation (Andersson, 1986).

Although data regarding the role of hypogastric pathways on lower urinary tract function are inconclusive, pharmacologic studies indicate that the bladder and urethra respond to adrenergic drugs (Nordling, 1983). Adrenergic receptors have been classified according to their responses to norepinephrine or structurally-related compounds. Postjunctional alpha receptor activation produces smooth muscle contraction, whereas stimulation of beta receptors causes relaxation (see Fig. 26–10, Table 26–3). The pre- and postjunctional effects of alpha agonists and antagonists led to a further subdividing of alpha receptors into alpha-1 and alpha-2 subtypes. Prejunctional alpha-2 receptors present on adrenergic (see Fig. 26–10) and cholinergic nerve terminals (see Figs. 26–7, 26–8) inhibit transmitter release, whereas postjunctional alpha-1 receptors mediate smooth muscle contraction. The alpha-1 receptors have been further subdivided, first based on agonists, then on cloning of the receptors, into α_{1A}, α_{1B}, and α_{1D} categories (Table 26–6) (Michel et al, 1995). Although $alpha_1$ blockers used clinically do not discriminate between these subtypes, nongenitourinary tissues may express predominately one type, offering a reduction in side effects for new alpha blockers used for urinary tract problems.

Electrical stimulation of muscle strips from human bladder body in vitro elicits contractile activity (Benson et al, 1976b; Sibley, 1984; Mattiasson et al, 1987). Failure of adrenergic antagonists to block electrically-evoked contractions indicates the lack of alpha-adrenergic receptor stimulation by release of endogenous norepinephrine. Alpha- and beta-adrenergic binding sites are found in human bladder (Nergardh and Boreus, 1972; Larson, 1979; Wein and Levin, 1979). These receptors are first expressed by the bladder in utero (Lee et al, 1993). In humans, beta-adrenergic agonists barely enhance bladder capacity during filling (Norlen et al, 1978). However, beta-adrenergic receptor agonists reduce the amplitude of uninhibited bladder contractions (Norlen et al, 1978; Jensen, 1981). Conversely, the beta receptor antagonists, such as propranolol, raise bladder pressure in patients with spinal cord injury (Kaplan and Nanninga, 1980). These studies support the notion that pharmacologic activation of beta-adrenergic receptors in abnormal bladders occasionally relaxes the smooth muscle of the body. This relaxation occurs through the intracellular action of cAMP (see Fig. 26–8).

Adenosine Triphosphate (ATP)

Preganglionic and postganglionic neurons contain purines that influence bladder function (Burnstock, 1986b). Neurons containing purine nucleotides and nucleosides, such as adenosine triphosphate (ATP) and adenosine (Senba et al, 1987) are found in the bladder and may influence contractility.

The pharmacologic actions of purines are mediated by purinergic receptors classified as P_1, P_2, preferentially recognizing adenosine and ATP, respectively (Table 26–7). P_2 receptors are further subclassifed into P_{2x}, P_{2y}, P_{2D}, P_{2u}, P_{2t}, and P_{2z} receptors based on agonist properties. In vitro experiments show that exogenous and endogenously released purinergic substances inhibit excitatory cholinergic transmission in the vesical ganglia (Akasu et al, 1984; Theobald and de Groat, 1989) (see Fig. 26–10, Table 26–3). This inhibition of synaptic transmission can be blocked by the P_1 antagonists theophylline and caffeine. Purinergic effects in the pelvic plexus differ from those at the neuroeffector junction where endogenous release of ATP or exogenous administration of purine analogues produces depolarization of bladder smooth muscle (Mostwin, 1986) and contraction (Burnstock, 1986b; Levin et al, 1986) via P_{2x} receptors (see Fig. 26–10, Table 26–7). Both pre- and postjunctional P_2 receptors occur in the human bladder (Palea et al, 1995).

Electrical stimulation of the pelvic nerve in animals produces a biphasic bladder contraction. Pharmacologic experiments indicate that the initial contraction is mediated by purines, whereas the second component is cholinergic. Levin and co-workers (1986) speculate that purinergic stimulation may initiate a bladder contraction while sustained bladder emptying by a cholinergic mechanism. Brading and Williams (1990) present evidence that in some species nerve-evoked bladder contraction is mediated by activation of P_2 purinoceptors, whereas acetylcholine merely modifies the excitability of smooth muscle. In the mouse and rat, P_{2y} receptors cause relaxation of the bladder in vitro through a G-protein mechanism. This relaxation can be increased by removal of the urothelium, suggesting a local excitatory mediator is released by the bladder lining. In vivo, ATP agonists raises bladder pressure and increase voided volumes in rats and cats (Theobald, 1995; Igawa et al, 1993a). These studies predict that exogenous purines would increase detrusor contractility. Hashimoto and Kokubun (1995) show that in rat bladder, 15% of the electrically-evoked contractions are due to activation of muscarinic receptors, whereas 50% from activation of 50% P_{2x} receptors, and 34% from P_{2z} receptor activity. Theobald (1995) compared purinergic and cholinergic components of the micturition contractions in cats in vivo and found that purinergic agonists cause a greater rise in bladder pressure than cholinergic agonists. Similarly, Chancellor and colleagues (1992) found that ATP generates greater force of bladder smooth muscle contraction than a cholinergic agonist. In neonates, the purinergic components of bladder contraction is even greater than in adults (Sneddon and McLees, 1992). However, others have shown that emptying is less complete with purinergic than cholinergic agonists (Igawa et al, 1993a). One explanation for mixed results is that these agents have opposing effects on the bladder outlet. In humans, the importance of purinergic contractions may be limited to disease. Investigators suggest that purinergic excitatory transmission may even play a role

Table 26–6. ALPHA ADRENOCEPTOR SUBTYPES IN URINARY TRACT BASED ON MOLECULAR CLONING

Receptor	α_{1A}	α_{1B}	α_{1D}
Structure	466 amino acids	515 amino acids	560 amino acids
Location in human	Chromosome 8	Chromosome 5	Chromosome 20
Agonist selectivity	(±) niguldipine 5–methyl-urapidil	None	Noradrenaline, methoxamine WB 4101
Sensitivity to chlorethylclonidine	±	+ + +	+ +

Table 26–7. PURINERGIC RECEPTOR SUBTYPES IN BLADDERS OF DIFFERENT SPECIES

Species	Type
Guinea pig	P2X
Mouse	P1, P2x, P2y
Rat	P1, P2x, P2y
Human	P2x

in detrusor instability and interstitial cystitis (Sjögren et al, 1982; Palea et al, 1993; Hoyle et al, 1989). It appears that histamine potentiates purinergic contractions (Patra and Westfall, 1994).

The concept that nonadrenergic, noncholinergic transmission contracts the bladder or relaxes the urethra has led to a search for other endogenous substances that influence voiding and continence function. Because neuropeptides function as transmitters in other viscera, their identification within the urinary tract has led investigators to examine their role in the neural control of the bladder (see Table 26–3, Fig. 26–7).

Vasoactive Intestinal Polypeptide (VIP)

VIP is often found in cholinergic neurons (see Fig. 26–7). VIP inhibits contractions of isolated smooth muscle from human bladders (Klarskov et al, 1984; Sjögren et al, 1985). VIP colocalizes with acetylcholinesterase-positive pelvic ganglion cells in the rat (Dail et al, 1986) and human (Van Poppel et al, 1988). In the cat, approximately 15% of bladder neurons are immunoreactive for VIP (Kawatani et al, 1986). In one detailed morphologic study, retrograde labeling of neurons in the rat pelvic ganglion was combined with immunohistochemical staining to determine the types of putative transmitters in ganglion cells innervating the bladder (Keast and de Groat, 1989) (see Fig. 26–11). Few bladder neurons showed VIP (8%) or ENK-immunoreactivity (3%) in contrast to the number of cells stained for neuropeptide Y (NPY) (49%).

VIP, CCK, and SP enhance cholinergic transmission in pelvic ganglia (Kawatani et al, 1986, 1989; Keast et al, 1989b). The slow onset and long duration of peptidergic responses is consistent with diffusion of neuropeptides between synapses rather than by direct presynaptic contact with preganglionic terminals. Enhancement of ganglionic transmission could facilitate sustained bladder emptying while inhibition may be used to turn off micturition, conserve transmitters, or prevent subthreshold excitatory transmitter release from ganglion. As for direct effects on smooth muscle, VIP fails to prevent cholinergic-induced bladder contractions. Nor does VIP given systemically alter the cystometrogram in humans (Klarskov et al, 1987). However, VIP is reduced in bladder of patients with detrusor instability and lower motoneuron disorders (Crowe et al, 1991; Milner et al, 1987) leading to speculation that a reduction in VIP elicits involuntary bladder interaction (Gu et al, 1983; de Groat and Kawatani, 1984). It is likely that this substance modulates neural function or acts centrally rather than directly affects smooth muscle (Blank et al, 1984).

Neuropeptide Y (NPY)

NPY exists in most noradrenergic neurons (Fig. 26–12; see Fig. 26–10) (Keast, 1995). NPY commonly colocalizes with tyrosine hydroxylase, a marker for adrenergic nerves, in bladder neurons (Keast and de Groat, 1989) and human lumbar ganglia (Jarvi and Pelto-Huikko, 1990). Some sympathetics contain NPY without norepinephrine, based on results of immunocytochemistry testing (Keast, 1995). Supporting the notion that NPY is found in noradrenergic pathways to the lower urinary tract, Mattiasson and associates (1985) showed that chemical sympathectomy, induced by 6-hydroxydopamine, eliminates NPY-immunoreactive fibers in the bladders of animals.

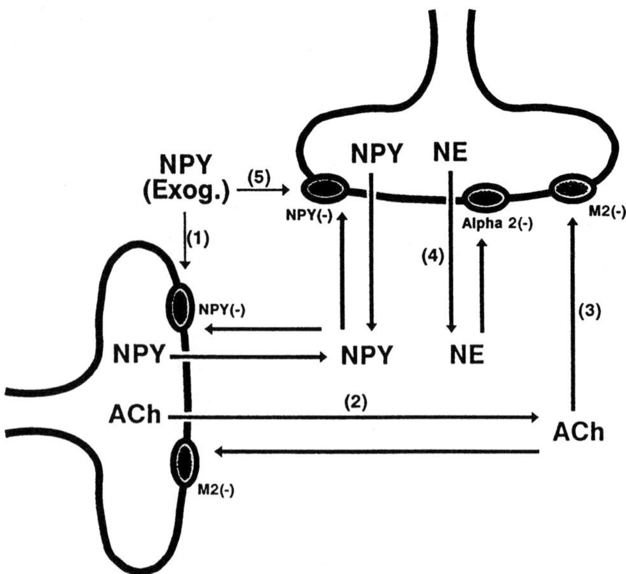

Figure 26–12. An example of crosstalk; implications for urine storage and release. Interactions between neuropeptide Y (NPY), norepinephrine (NE), and acetylcholine (ACh) in terminals in the bladder. NPY can directly inhibit release of ACh and NE from cholinergic and noradrenergic terminals by acting at prejunctional NPY (possibly Y-2) receptors. When exogenous NPY is greater than 0.1 μM, NPY binds to cholinergic terminals (step 1) to inhibit ACh release (step 2). This decreases inhibition in nearby terminals by ACh (step 3). Zoubek and co-workers (1993) proposed that this onset of micturition parasympathetic input could trigger release of NPY from cholinergic nerves. NPY could then lead to relaxing the outlet by prejunction inhibition of norepinephrine release from noradrenergic nerves. During bladder filling, sympathetic activity could release NPY from noradrenergic terminals and inhibit cholinergic pathways to the bladder, preventing involuntary detrusor contractions. (Tran LV, Somogyi GT, de Groat WC: Am J Physiol 1994; 266:R1411–R1417.)

Immunohistochemical staining of the human bladder reveals that NPY is the most prevalent of the neuropeptides including VIP, calcitonin gene-related peptide, substance P, and somatostatin (Crowe et al, 1991). NPY is found throughout the bladder, especially around blood vessels. In patients with lower motoneuron disorders of the bladder, NPY remains constant (Milner et al, 1987).

The role of a NPY on bladder function is complex. Pharmacologic studies reveal that NPY mediates (1) direct bladder smooth muscle contraction; (2) modulation of postjunctional effects of norepinephrine; (3) prejunctional inhibition of norepinephrine and purine release; (4) inhibition of acetylcholine release with subsequent decreased cholinergic contraction of the bladder after electrical stimulation (see Fig. 26–12) **(Zoubek et al, 1993); and (5) blockade of atropine-resistant bladder contractions (Lundberg et al, 1984)** (see Fig. 26–12).

Tachykinins

Substance P (SP) and the related tachykinins neurokinin A and neurokinin B are found in the urinary bladder. **Immu-**

nohistochemical staining of retrogradely labeled bladder neurons indicates that tachykinins are expressed in afferents (Maggi, 1995; Keast and de Groat, 1992). SP-containing axon terminals are found primarily in the lamina propria beneath bladder epithelium and surrounding vessels (Wakabayashi et al, 1993). Following presumed decentralization of the human bladder, SP immunoreactivity decreases (Crowe et al, 1991). This observation is in agreement with SP occurring in sensory nerves.

Tachykinins increase detrusor contractility, cause vasodilatation, and enhance mucosal permeability (Maggi et al, 1989a, 1989c). NK agonists cause plasma extravasation via a histamine-mediated mechanism in the bladder (Abelli et al, 1989b).

The physiologic effects of SP and related compounds are mediated by NK_1, NK_2, and NK_3 receptors (see Table 26–3) (Maggi et al, 1988a, 1988b). **The human bladder, based on results of radioligand binding studies, contains primary NK_2 receptors (Zeng, 1995).** The NK_2 receptor mediates bladder contraction. Agonist studies show a rank order potency of NKA > NKB > SP in the bladder (Dion et al, 1988; Maggi, 1995). SP released from afferents in the lamina propria of the bladder influences initiation of a micturition reflex (Maggi, 1995). In newborn animals, SP containing nerves can be destroyed by capsaicin treatment (Holzer-Petsche and Lembeck, 1984). This abolishes micturition, and muscle strips from these bladders demonstrate enhanced cholinergic contractions (Ziganshin et al, 1995). However, blockade of a NK_1 or NK_2 receptor in the adult does not abolish voiding in animals. Thus, SP or neurokinins are not thought to be the principal afferent transmitters responsible for voiding (Lecci et al, 1993).

SP and related tachykinins released from afferent terminals in the bladder can cause detrusor contractions. Following inflammation of the bladder, receptors for SP increase in the bladder and may augment vasomotor and contractile responses (Kushner et al, 1995). Potentially, these substances could modulate the micturition reflex, transmit pain sensation to the spinal cord, and thereby play a role in facilitating removal of irritative substances from the bladder (see Afferent Mechanisms section).

Calcitonin Gene–Related Peptide (CGRP)

Similar to SP and tachykinins, CGRP is found exclusively in bladder afferents. CGRP relaxes detrusor smooth muscle in the bladder neck and increases blood flow contractility in some species (Watts and Cohen, 1991; Maggi, 1995; Andersson et al, 1989). CGRP binding sites are expressed by human bladder mucosa (Edyvane and Marshall, 1990). In patients with lower motoneuron disorders, CGRP immunoreactivity in the detrusor is decreased (Crowe et al, 1986).

Although CGRP relaxes the guinea pig and dog bladder, it has no effect on detrusor contractions in humans (see Table 26–3) (Maggi, 1995). Like other peptides, the physiologic role for CGRP remains to be determined.

Opiates

Enkephalin-staining nerves represent both afferents and efferents in the bladder (de Groat and Kawatani, 1989). Enkephalinergic fibers are rarely found in the human bladder and probably arise from afferent or preganglionic nerves supplying intramural bladder ganglia (Kawatani et al, 1989).

Leucine enkephalin (L-ENK) inhibits cholinergic transmission by a heterosynaptic mechanism in the pelvic plexus, which is an effect blocked by the opiate antagonist naloxone (Simmonds et al, 1983; de Groat et al, 1986a). Both met- and leu-enkephalin reduce electrically-evoked contractions of human bladder muscle (see Table 26–3) (Klarskov, 1987). This effect is probably due to presynaptic inhibition of acetylcholine release. The opiate antagonist naloxone enhances electrically-induced contractions of bladder smooth muscle in vitro (Berggren et al, 1992). It has been suggested that endogenous opiates exert peripheral inhibitory effect in the bladder. However, the central effect of opiates is probably more significant (see Central Neuropharmacology section).

Vasopressin, Somatostatin, Bombesin, Angiotensin, and Neuromedin-U

Other less common neuropeptides are found in the lower urinary tract. The human bladder contains arginine vasopressin (AVP) (Holmquist et al, 1991). However, this substance exerts little effect on bladder smooth muscle contractility. This lack of effect is not surprising because specific AVP binding sites have not been found in the human bladder.

Somatostatin, bombesin, and neuromedin-U, galanin, and angiotensin II occur in the human bladder (Table 26–8) (Erspamer et al, 1981; Bauer et al, 1986; Domin et al, 1986; Saito et al, 1993; Maggi et al, 1987b; Crowe et al, 1986, 1991). Following presumed decentralization of the bladder, somatostatin immunoreactivity is unchanged (Crowe et al, 1991). This finding suggests that somatostatin exists in peripheral ganglia near the bladder. Bombesin, galanin, and angiotensin all contract human bladder smooth muscle. The effects of angiotensin II appear to be mediated by AT_1 receptors (Tanabe et al, 1993). In addition, galanin can inhibit electrically-evoked bladder contractions.

Nitric Oxide

The bladder contains few nitric oxide synthase-positive (NOS) or reduced nicotinamide-adenine dinucleotide phosphate (NADPH) diaphorase-staining nerves (Andersson and

Table 26–8. NEUROPEPTIDES IDENTIFIED IN THE HUMAN BLADDER

Peptide	Probable Origin
Calcitonin gene–related peptide	Sensory
Enkephalin	Preganglionic sensory
Galanin	
Neuropeptide Y	Pelvic ganglia
Neuromedin U	?
Somatostatin	Preganglionic/pelvic ganglia
Substance P	Sensory
Peptide histidine isoleucine	?
Vasoactive intestinal polypeptide	Sensory/pelvic ganglia

Persson, 1994; Vizzard et al, 1994). Nitric oxide nerves are predominately afferent. NO has little effect on bladder smooth contractility in the adult (Ehren et al, 1994). However, studies in fetal sheep reveal that stimulation of NO production with L-arginine increased bladder capacity (Mevorach et al, 1994). Conversely, inhibitors of NO synthesis increased low-amplitude bladder contractions in fetal bladders. NO has also been implicated in regulation of bladder activity after inflammation (see Afferent Mechanisms section).

GABA

Gamma-amino butyric acid (GABA) may influence synaptic transmission in the pelvic plexus and excitability of detrusor smooth muscle (Maggi et al, 1985a; 1985b; Araki, 1994). Although the effects of GABAminergic drugs are often attributed to a central action, GABA-synthesizing enzymes are found in small intensely fluorescent (SIF) cells in pelvic ganglia (Karhula et al, 1988). Because SIF cells may send axons to postganglionic neurons, it is possible that these cells modulate efferent activity to pelvic viscera. Indeed, GABA inhibits excitatory neural transmission in pelvic ganglia (Simmonds et al, 1983; Maggi et al, 1985c). Thus, GABAminergic drugs or endogenous release of GABA from SIF cells may regulate bladder function.

As for direct effects on the bladder, in vitro data reveal that GABA agonists reduce cholinergic contractions (Maggi et al, 1985b; Ferguson and Marchant, 1995). This effect has been attributed to an activation of K^+ channels through GABA receptor.

Serotonin

Serotonin (5-HT) may participate in the peripheral neural control of the bladder and urethra, although its central effects are probably more substantial. Immunocytochemical techniques demonstrate SIF cells in pelvic ganglia, which are immunoreactive for 5-HT. 5-HT immunoreactive fibers also surround ganglion cells (Nishimura et al, 1989).

Uncertainty regarding the effects of 5-HT on bladder function arises from the multiplicity of 5-HT receptors. As has happened with most receptors, 5-HT binding sites were first characterized using nonspecific then relatively specific ligands, leading to four subfamilies, namely, 5-HT_1, 5-HT_2, 5-HT_3, and 5-HT_4. Among the 5-HT_1 subfamily 5-HT_{1A}, 5-HT_{1B}, 5-HT_{1C}, and 5-HT_{1E} receptors were found. Molecular biologic methods then allowed identification of additional receptors whose functional significance is uncertain. These receptors include 5-HT_{1E}, 5-HT_{1F}, 5-HT_{5A}, 5-HT_{5B}, 5-HT_6, and 5-HT_7. The lack of selective 5-HT antagonists has hampered functional characterization of these receptors (Cohen, 1990). It is known, however, that 5-HT or its agonists primarily inhibit, and occasionally facilitate, cholinergic ganglionic transmission in pelvic ganglia (Saum and de Groat, 1973; Akasu et al, 1987; Nishimura et al, 1988). Furthermore, 5-HT facilitates neurally-evoked bladder contractions by increasing the release of acetylcholine from nerve terminals in the bladder wall. 5-HT has also been shown to contract the bladder body (Erspamer et al, 1981; Klarskov and Horby-Petersen, 1986) and relax the bladder neck (Hills et al, 1984). The excitatory effects on bladder smooth muscle are blocked by 5-HT_2 antagonists (Matsumura et al, 1968; Saum and de Groat, 1973; Holt et al, 1986; Watts and Cohen, 1991). In the human bladder, 5-HT potentiates electrical contractions at low concentration, possibly through 5-HT_3 receptor (see Table 26–3) (Corsi et al, 1991; Waikar et al, 1994). At high concentrations, 5-HT inhibits electrical contraction. This latter inhibitory action has been attributed to a 5-HT_1 receptor.

Prostaglandins, Endothelins, and Hormones

Prostaglandins are manufactured throughout the lower urinary tract and have been implicated in bladder contractility, inflammatory responses, and neurotransmission. Biopsies of human bladder mucosa contain prostaglandins PGI_2, PGE_2, $PGE_{2\alpha}$, and TXA. In decreasing order of potency, $PGF_{2\alpha}$, PGE, and PGE_2 contract the human detrusor (see Table 26–3) (Andersson, 1993). The slow onset of action for these substances suggests a modulatory role for prostaglandins. Some prostaglandins may effect neural release of transmitters, whereas others inhibit acetylcholinesterase activity. These actions provide mechanisms whereby prostaglandins could potentially augment the amplitude of cholinergic-induced detrusor contractions (Borda et al, 1982).

Attempts to use prostaglandins to facilitate voiding have had mixed results. Intravesical PGE_2 has been shown to enhance bladder emptying in women with urinary retention and patients with neurogenic voiding dysfunction (Bultitude et al, 1976; Desmond et al, 1980; Vadyanaathan et al, 1981; Tammela et al, 1987). Others have failed to find PGE_2 useful to facilitate complete evacuation of the bladder (Delaere et al, 1981; Wagner et al, 1985). Intravesical PGE_2 does produce urgency and involuntary bladder contractions (Schussler, 1990). Consistent with this finding, inhibition of prostaglandin synthesis with indomethacin reduces detrusor instability (Cardozo and Stanton, 1980). Finally, intravesical prostaglandins as well as estrogens have been used to treat hemorrhagic cystitis.

Like prostaglandins, endothelins are produced by many tissues, particularly the mucosa and vascular endothelium. In humans, endothelin immunoreactivity is localized in the bladder beneath transitional epithelium (Saenz de Tejada et al, 1992). Endothelin-1 and endothelin-3 contract isolated strips of bladder muscle (Maggi et al, 1990). Possibly like prostaglandins, endothelins may be released locally in response to bladder distention or inflammation and alter detrusor contractility.

Some locally released substances cause detrusor relaxation. Parathyroid hormone-related peptide (PTHrp) is manufactured by bladder smooth muscle. Stretch in vivo (Yamamoto et al, 1992) and in vitro (Persson and Steers, 1994) increases PTHrp. This peptide relaxes bladder smooth muscle in vitro. Slow or gradual distention could release local relaxants, thereby maintaining low filling pressures.

Differences in responses of human and animal bladders to the effect of drugs suggest that sex steroids play a role in detrusor contractility. It is not unusual for women to note changes in voiding, bladder pain, or continence at different times of their menstrual cycle. Sex steroids do not directly affect bladder contractility, but they modulate receptors and influence growth of bladder tissues. Estrogen receptors are expressed by the trigone in women (Iosif et al, 1981). Levin and associates (1980) noted that bladder body muscle from young female rabbits treated with estrogens possesses increased responsiveness to alpha-adrenergic, cholinergic, and purinergic agonists. An increase in alpha-adrenergic receptor density was also reported, which could explain the increased response to alpha agonists. Others have seen a decreased density of adrenergic and muscarinic receptors in the bladder following estrogen administration (Batra and Andersson, 1989; Shapiro, 1986). In contrast to the study by Levin, Elliot and associates (1992) showed that bladder smooth muscle from estrogen-treated rats exhibits decreased responses to cholinergic and electrically-induced contractions. Ekstrom and associates (1993) report that estrogen administration to ovariectomized rabbits unveil contractile responses with alpha-adrenergic agonists, whereas contracted and normal rabbit bladders demonstrated no response to these agents. In addition, progesterone increases electrical and cholinergic contractions. Exogenous estrogens and progesterones also induce NO synthase activity in bladders of female guinea pigs (Ehren et al, 1995). This latter effect is postulated to contribute to relief of detrusor instability with hormonal treatment. The proposed benefit of oral or intravaginal estrogens either alone or in combination with other drugs for the treatment of urinary incontinence in women suggests that sex steroids play a role in neural or myogenic responses of the lower urinary tract (Kurz et al, 1993).

PHARMACOLOGY OF THE URETHRA

Acetylcholine

In 1931 Barrington hypothesized that stimulation of pelvic nerve, in addition to evoking a bladder contraction, produces urethral relaxation. Indeed, urodynamic studies document a reduction in urethral pressure just before a bladder contraction (Scott et al, 1964; van Waalwijk et al, 1991). In support of the contention that this urethral relaxation is mediated by parasympathetic nerves, sacral root stimulation reduces urethral pressure (Torrens, 1978; McGuire and Herlihy, 1978). A clinical condition even exists in which this urethral relaxation can be urodynamically documented to cause stress urinary incontinence. *Urethral instability* was a term coined by McGuire (1978) to denote an involuntary drop in urethral pressure in the absence of a detrusor contraction. This occurs in rare patients in whom afferents from the bladder are intact and either motor nerves or smooth muscle contractility are impaired. Straining raises intravesical pressure, which triggers an afferent volley to the spinal cord with subsequent efferent discharge to the urethra. Because a detrusor contraction cannot occur, urethral relaxation occurs following a transient use in urethral pressure. Because postganglionic neurons mediating parasympathetic events are traditionally cholinergic, investigators initially postulated that acetylcholine may be responsible for reflex urethral relaxation. This is not the case.

Cholinergic innervation to the urethra has been supported by histochemical identification of acetylcholinesterase-staining fibers and ultrastructural data showing varicosities containing small clear vesicles in the human urethra (Ek et al, 1977; Gosling et al, 1977). Exogenous cholinergic agonists do not relax, but rather contract urethral smooth muscle in vivo (Ek et al, 1978; Yalla et al, 1977; Nergardh and Boreus, 1972) and in vitro (Ek et al, 1978). Therefore, parasympathetic pathways mediating urethral relaxation must rely on a noncholinergic transmitter. The current candidate for transmitter in the parasympathetic evoked urethral relaxation is NO (see Nitric Oxide section).

Norepinephrine

Substantial pharmacologic and physiologic evidence indicates that urethral tone and intraurethral pressure is influenced by alpha-adrenergic receptors. Radioligand binding reveals that alpha-1 and alpha-2 adrenoceptors are present in rabbit urethra (Yamaguchi et al, 1993). In female animals, the majority of alpha adrenoceptors are of the alpha-2 subtype (Andersson, 1993), whereas alpha-1 receptors predominate in the male.

Isolated human urethral smooth muscle contracts in response to alpha-adrenergic agonists (Nordling, 1983; Mattiasson et al, 1984; Awad et al, 1976; Yalla et al, 1977). This contraction is blocked by alpha$_1$-adrenergic antagonists. In vivo alpha-adrenergic antagonists lower intraurethral pressure. It has been shown that the alpha receptor in the urethras of rabbits, dogs, cats, and humans is of the 1C subtype (old 1A) (Testa et al, 1993; Chess-Williams et al, 1994). Likewise, hypogastric nerve stimulation and alpha$_1$-adrenergic agonists produce a rise in intraurethral pressure, which is blocked by alpha$_1$-adrenergic antagonists (Awad and Downie, 1976; Yalla et al, 1977). These findings provide the rationale for using alpha agonists to promote urine storage for decreased urethral resistance. Conversely, alpha antagonists facilitate urine release in conditions of functionally increased urethral resistance, such as benign prostatic hyperplasia.

Alpha$_2$-adrenergic antagonists increase the release of norepinephrine from urethral tissues through a presynaptic mechanism, but this does not affect the contractility of urethral smooth muscle in vitro (Mattiasson et al, 1984; Willette et al, 1990). The human urethra lacks postjunctional alpha$_2$-adrenergic receptors, although in vitro prejunctional activation of these receptors produces a feedback inhibition of norepinephrine release. Nordling in 1979 found that the alpha$_2$ agonist clonidine lowers intraurethral pressure in humans. This is likely to be the result of a central action whereby sympathetic tone is reduced.

Adrenergic drugs may exert a peripheral effect on lower urinary function through actions at pelvic ganglia or spinal cord. Pharmacologic and electrophysiologic data suggest that adrenergic nerves influence excitatory cholinergic transmission in pelvic ganglia (de Groat and Booth, 1980). de Groat and Booth (1980) have shown in the cat that hypogastric nerves inhibit excitatory cholinergic transmission in vesical ganglia by activation of alpha$_2$-adrenergic receptors (see Table 26–3, Fig. 26–10). Conversely, beta-adrenergic agonists facilitate transmission in vesical ganglia. Sympathetic modulation of synaptic transmission by adrenergic mechanisms has not been observed in all species (Mallory et al, 1989).

Beta-adrenergic blockers have been advocated for urinary incontinence due to inappropriate reflex urethral relaxation, because propranolol prevents the reduction in urethral pressure following sacral root stimulation (McGuire, 1978; McGuire and Herlihy, 1978). Unfortunately, beta-adrenergic antagonists are not particularly useful in treating bladder or urethral disorders (Castleden and Morgan, 1980; Naglo et al, 1981).

VIP

The human urethra contains VIP-immunoreactive fibers (Gu et al, 1984). Although VIP relaxes some smooth muscles, relaxation of urethra is an inconsistent finding (Sjögren et al, 1985). In vivo administration of VIP has no effect on urethral resistance (Klarskov et al, 1987). Although VIP is present in the urethra, it does not directly alter smooth muscle contractility.

NPY

NPY is found in the human urethra and external urethral sphincter. In patients with areflexic bladders, levels of NPY, as well as VIP, are increased in the striated sphincter compared with those with detrusor sphincter dyssynergia (Milner et al, 1987). The significance of this finding is unclear but probably reflects compensatory mechanisms.

Similar to bladder, NPY inhibits electrically-evoked contractions of the urethra (see Fig. 26–12). NPY also decreases norepinephine release from urethral tissue at low frequencies of electrical stimulation, but at high frequencies, norepinephrine release in increased (Zoubek et al, 1993). These observations are best explained by blockade of acetylcholine release by NPY, which would normally decrease norepinephrine release by a presynaptic mechanism. If NPY serves any significant role in the bladder outlet, it is to modulate norepinephrine and acetylcholine release, thereby modulating the urethral closure mechanisms.

Tachykinins

The urethra contains SP-immunoreactive varicosities. Similar to the bladder, tachykinins contract isolated urethral smooth muscle ($NK_A > NK_B >$ SP) (Maggi et al, 1988b). The rank order potency for these substances suggests that the contractile response of the human urethra is mediated by NK_2 receptors. Although SP and related peptides are probably involved in afferent transmission from the urethra, especially in response to irritative stimuli, release of these substances for afferent terminals could influence contractility and vascular permeability.

Nitric Oxide

NO has been closely linked to neurally mediated relaxation of the urethra. The urethras of many nonhuman species contain NADPH diaphorase-positive fibers or specifically stain for NO synthase (NOS).

Inhibition of NOS prevents neural-evoked relaxation of the urethra in vitro (Persson et al, 1993; Andersson and Persson, 1994). In vivo, inhibition of NOS prevents electrically-evoked relaxation of the urethra and external sphincter (Bennett et al, 1993; Parlani et al, 1993). If these findings are confirmed in humans, NOS inhibitors may be useful in conditions such as stress incontinence, whereas NOS activators or NO donors may relieve obstruction due to prostatism.

Prostaglandins and Hormones

Strips of human urethral smooth muscle contract in response to $PGF_{2\alpha}$ (Andersson et al, 1978). If this tissue is precontracted with norepinephrine, PGE and PGE_2 relax the strips. Consistent with this in vitro data, maximal urethral pressure falls following intraurethral PGE_2 (Andersson et al, 1978).

Hormones can affect adrenergic receptors in the urethra. For example, estrogens increase adrenergic receptors in the urethra (Callahan and Creed, 1985). Estrogens increase the response of urethral tissues to alpha-adrenergic agonists in vitro. Some clinicians have combined these agents in vivo to elevate urethral pressure in patients with stress incontinence (Wilson et al, 1987). It is not surprising that estrogens facilitate continence and enhance effects of alpha-adrenergic agonists. However, the clinical efficacy of the combined use of estrogen with alpha agonists has been questioned (Walter et al, 1978). The effect of estrogens on urinary continence in females probably reflects the multiple actions of this hormone on adrenergic receptors, vasculature, and urethral morphology.

Serotonin (5-HT)

Serotonin has been found in neuroendocrine cells along the urethra and in the prostate (Hanyu et al, 1987). In animals, 5-HT_2 and possibly 5-HT_3 agonists contract the urethra. If inflammatory conditions promote release of serotonin from paraurethral cells, irritative symptoms such as the urethral syndrome may arise owing to serotonergic mechanisms.

The 5-HT_2 antagonist ketanserin has been shown to reduce urethral pressure in humans (Horby-Petersen et al, 1985). However, the reduction in urethral pressure following ketanserin administration can also be the result of blockade of alpha-adrenergic receptors.

PHARMACOLOGY OF THE BRAIN AND SPINAL CORD

Pharmacologic experiments in animals, and occasional humans, provide insight into the potential roles of central neurotransmitters involved in the regulation of lower urinary tract function. Changes in rhythmic bladder activity or cystometrograms (CMG) have been used to gauge the effect of drugs in sites implicated in bladder function, including the locus coeruleus, pontine tegmentum, periaqueductal gray matter, and sacral spinal cord. Recent advances in our knowledge of that central mechanism responsible for micturition and effects of drugs have relied on intrathecal administration of agents to awake animals followed by CMGs. More sophisticated experiments rely on spinal cord slices or intact bladder-brain-cord in vitro preparations from neonatal animals. These experiments combined with immunohistochemical staining of the pontine micturition center (PMC) (Loewy et al, 1979; Sutin and Jacobowitz, 1988) or the sacral autonomic nucleus (Gibson et al, 1981; de Laverolle and LaMotte, 1982; Sasek et al, 1984; Kawatani et al, 1986) indicate that various transmitters influence voiding and urine storage. Although clinicians have exploited the action of peripherally acting drugs for voiding dysfunction, centrally acting drugs may also play an important therapeutic role. Unfortunately, specificity remains a problem.

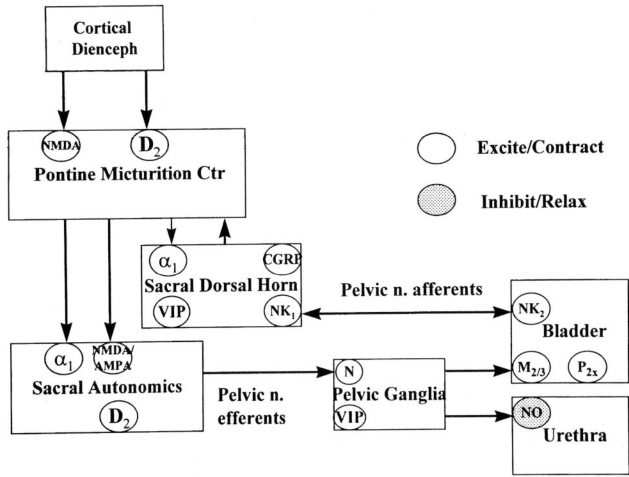

Figure 26–13. Neuropharmacology of voiding. Activation of central and peripheral receptors can induce bladder contractions. Release of substance P and neurokinins from pelvic nerve afferent fibers activate NK-1 receptors in the dorsal horn following pain or distention of the bladder. Release of these substances from afferent terminals in the bladder can cause a detrusor contraction through activation of NK-2 receptors. Stimulation of alpha-1, VIP, or CGRP receptors in the sacral dorsal horn facilitates micturition. The pontine micturition center (PMC) triggers voiding following administration of glutamate, which acts on NMDA receptors. Activation of dopamine (D_2) and muscarinic (M) receptors in the PMC also causes bladder contractions. Descending input from the brain stem can activate either alpha-1 or glutamate (NMDA + AMPA) receptors in the sacral spinal cord to facilitate micturition or initiate bladder contractions. Dopamine (D_2) can also elicit bladder contractions when given intrathecally or in spinal cord slice preparations. Acetylcholine released from preganglionics in the pelvic nerve activates nicotinic receptors (N) in the pelvic ganglia. Ganglionic transmission can also be augmented by the actions of VIP. Acetylcholine release from post-ganglionic nerves to the bladder activates M_2 or M_3 receptors, causing bladder contraction. In pathologic conditions, ATP release may elicit noncholinergic contractions by acting at P_{2x} receptors in the detrusor. Release of nitric oxide from pelvic nerve post-ganglionics relaxes the urethra during voiding.

Glutamate

Glutamate is a common neurotransmitter in the brain and spinal cord. Glutamate not only plays an essential role in normal neurotransmission, but is a key participant in neural plasticity associated with conditions such as ischemia, spinal cord injury, and chronic pain.

Glutamate receptors are categorized as N-methyl-D-aspartate (NMDA) or non-NMDA based on agonist properties. Non-NMDA receptors are subclassified into AMPA (D,L-α-amino-3-hydroxy-5-methyl-4-isoxazote) propionic acid and kianate receptors. **Glutamate is released from (1) visceral afferents in the dorsal horn of the spinal cord; (2) spinal interneurons; (3) descending projections from the pontine micturition center; and (4) neurons within the pons. Glutamate appears to facilitate bladder function at all of these sites under certain conditions** (Figs. 26–13, 26–14). The noncompetitive NMDA antagonist, MK801, blocks detrusor contractions elicited by electrical stimulation of the pontine micturition center (Yoshiyama et al, 1994). A similar effect is seen with GYKI-52460, an AMPA antagonist in urethane-anesthetized rats (Matsumoto et al, 1995a, 1995b). However, MK801 fails to inhibit detrusor contractions in spinalized animals. This data has led investigators to postulate that descending input from the brain responsible for voiding relies on binding of glutamate to both NMDA and AMPA receptors. Data from Araki and de Groat (1995) shows spinal cord slices from L6 of the neonatal rat; NMDA and AMPA receptors mediate excitatory inputs from interneurons to sacral preganglionic neurons rather than directly by descending axons.

In awake animals, MK801 enhances bladder contractions. MK801 also enhances bladder contractions in the neonate induced by perineal stimulation and unmasks distention-evoked contractions. Normally, distention of the bladder fails to trigger micturition in neonates of many species. To explain these findings, Matsumoto and co-workers (1995a, 1995b) suggest that glutamate neurons provide excitatory input to GABA neurons which in turn inhibit preganglionics to the bladder.

These findings raise several important caveats in reaching conclusions about centrally acting drugs and mechanisms. First, anesthesia activates or inhibits certain neural pathways responsible for micturition. Second, a receptor-specific drug acts at multiple sites, which may have opposing effects on visceral function. Last, transmitter mechanisms evolve during ontogeny and are profoundly altered following injury, disease, and aging.

Serotonin

Lumbosacral sympathetic and parasympathetic autonomic nuclei receive serotonergic (5-HT) projections from the raphe nuclei in the caudal brain stem (Loewy and Neil, 1981; Bowker et al, 1983). Electrical stimulation of 5-HT neurons in the raphe nuclei inhibits rhythmic bladder activity (McMahon and Spillane, 1982) (Fig. 26–15; see Fig. 26–14). Furthermore, systemic administration of the 5-HT precursor, 5-hydroxytryptophan, inhibits the parasympathetic micturition reflex, but facilitates a vesicosympathetic storage reflex. These findings are consistent with results of experiments by Ryall and de Groat (1972), which showed that microiontophoretic administration of 5-HT inhibits sacral preganglionic firing (see Fig. 26–15). On the other hand, application of 5-HT to thoracolumbar preganglionic neurons facilitates neural

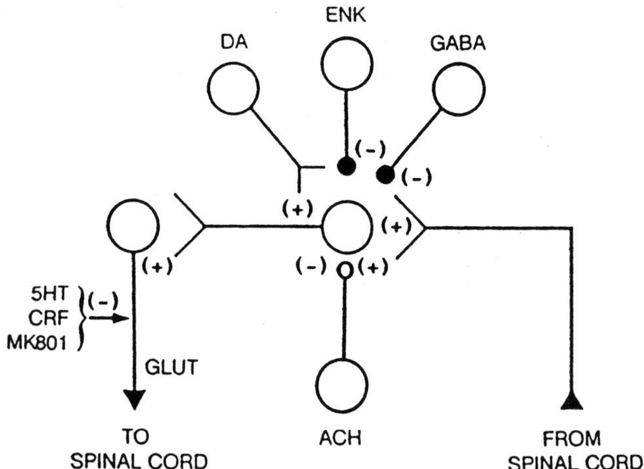

Figure 26–14. Influence of nerve transmitters in pontine on micturition based on studies in rats. Ascending input from the spinal cord reaches the periaqueductal gray matter, in the pons, providing excitatory input. This input is inhibited by GABA and enkephalins (ENK) neurons. Dopamine (DA) and acetylcholine (ACh) provide excitatory input to this region. Acetylcholine has inhibitory inputs as well. Serotonin (5-HT) corticotropin releasing factor (CRF) and MK-801 and NMDA antagonist inhibit descending input to the cord. Inhibition may occur at the descending limb or at interneurons in the sacral spinal cord. Exogenous opiates inhibit micturition through enkephalin receptors. Dopamine agonists given to Parkinson's patients facilitate micturition. Agents that block uptake of serotonin, such as imipramine, inhibit micturition in the sacral spinal cord by influencing descending inputs. (From de Groat WC: Urol Clin North Am 1993; 20[3]:383–401.)

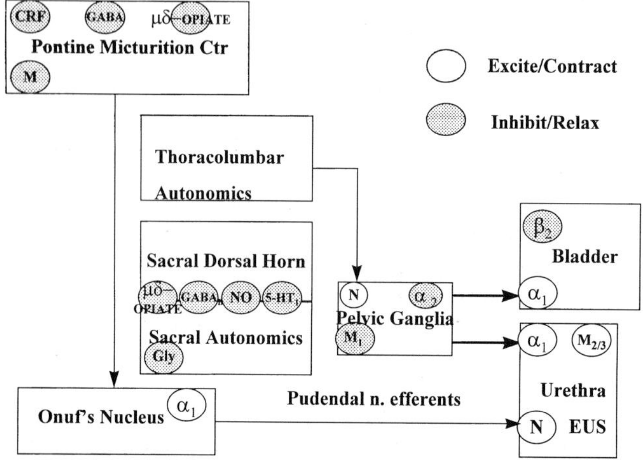

Figure 26–15. Neuropharmacology of continence. Activation of certain receptors in the central and peripheral nervous system inhibits reflex micturition and bladder contractility or increases urethral tone. In the pons, corticotropin releasing factor (CRF), norepinephrine, GABA, opiates, as well as acetylcholine inhibit micturition. Blockade of sacral alpha-1 receptors decreases neural input in the hypogastric and pudendal nerves to the external sphincter and urethra. Administration of M, opiate, GABA, nitric oxide (NO), and serotonin (5-HT) receptor agonists in the dorsal and ventral horns of the sacral spinal cord inhibits detrusor contraction. Norepinephrine, acting through alpha-1 receptors in the bladder and urethra, prevents urine loss, whereas its action at beta-2 receptors in the dome promote urine storage. Muscarinic (M_2) receptors in the longitudinal muscle of the urethra cause contraction and increase urethral resistance.

activity. Reserpine treatment, which depletes central 5-HT, as well as norepinephrine, causes bladder hyperreflexia (Maggi and Meli, 1983). Administration of mixed 5-$HT_{1C/2}$ agonists inhibits rhythmic bladder activity (Steers et al, 1992a). This effect has been attributed to a central action because inhibition of the micturition reflex was seen with blockade of efferent firing in the pelvic nerve and no change in ganglionic transmission.

Clinically, it is of interest that 5-HT-containing raphe neurons in the brain stem are quiescent during rapid eye movement (REM) sleep in humans, corresponding to periods of increased autonomic activity (Broughton, 1968). This time frame corresponds to the window for potential enuretic episodes. **The efficacy of tricyclics in the treatment of nocturnal enuresis may be explained in part by the blockade of 5-HT uptake, allowing increased levels of this transmitter to inhibit detrusor activity. Interestingly, childhood enuretics are more prone to urge incontinence during later adulthood (Foldspang and Mommsen, 1994). Depression has been associated with low levels of 5-HT or activity of 5-HT pathways. Therefore, it is not surprising that urge incontinence occurs more frequently in depressed individuals (Hafner et al, 1977; Walters et al, 1990). These observations provide circumstantial evidence that central serotonergic mechanisms play a crucial role in maintaining continence. Alteration in 5-HT may promote enuresis or urge incontinence. Drugs based on 5-HT may therefore be useful in these disorders.**

Despite investigations that propose a major role for serotonergic transmission on bladder function (Ryall and de Groat, 1972; de Groat et al, 1979; Morrison and Spillane, 1986; McMahon and Spillane, 1982), others have failed to demonstrate that intrathecal administration of 5-HT or the 5-HT_2 agonist methysergide alters the cystometrogram of unanesthetized rats (Durant et al, 1988b). In contrast, Espey and co-workers (1992) found that intrathecal methysergide decreased volume to micturition in awake cats, suggesting an inhibitory role for 5-HT in the sacral spinal cord. Hence, the role of endogenous 5-HT in the spinal cord on bladder function is complex, facilitating urine storage at some sites in the CNS and inhibiting or having no effect on micturition at others. Differences in species or in the distribution of 5-HT receptor subtypes may partially explain these findings.

Dopamine

Systemic administration of the dopamine precursor L-dopa following blockade of its peripheral metabolism produces bladder hyperactivity (Sillen et al, 1981; Ishizuka et al, 1994). Administration of L-dopa or the dopamine agonist apomorphine to Parkinson's patients reduces residual urines and increases urine flow rates (Benson et al, 1976a; Christmas et al, 1989). These data indicate that dopaminergic mechanisms can facilitate voiding.

Pharmacologic experiments in rats and cats implicate a central origin for dopaminergic facilitation of voiding. Sillen and co-workers (1982) propose that the site for dopaminergic facilitation resides within the pontine-mesencephalic (PMC) region of the brain (see Figs. 26–14, 26–15). However, Dray and Metsch (1983) have shown that injections of dopamine or apomorphine into the basal ganglia in the rat stimulate or inhibit bladder activity, depending upon the precise site of application. Furthermore, Roppolo and colleagues (1987) found that application of dopamine or apomorphine within the PMC of the cat increased the frequency of spontaneous bladder contractions and decreased bladder capacity (see Figs. 26–13, 26–14). In this latter study, the pharmacologic effects were prevented by haloperidol, a dopamine antagonist, indicating selective activation of dopamine receptors. Systemic apomorphine reduces the threshold for micturition (Kontani et al, 1990) in anesthetized rats. Ishizuka and colleagues show that L-dopa or apomorphine induces bladder hyperreflexia in awake rats (Ishizuka et al, 1994, 1995).

Dopaminergic transmission within the sacral spinal cord also influences lower urinary tract function (see Fig. 26–15). Dopaminergic neurons project to the spinal cord, yet their site of termination is unknown (Loewy et al, 1979). Durant and Yaksh (1988) have shown that intrathecal apomorphine, but not dopamine, induces micturition. Therefore, centrally acting dopamine agonists could provide a pharmacologic tool for emptying the bladder (Aranda and Cramer, 1993).

Norepinephrine

Brain stem neurons that contain norepinephrine project to interneurons in the dorsal horn and intermediolateral cell columns in the thoracolumbar and sacral spinal cord (Loewy et al, 1979). Thus, central noradrenergic mechanisms in the spinal cord may affect function of the bladder and sphincter by influencing afferent input or preganglionic neurons. Following hypogastric nerve transection in cats, intrathecal alpha$_1$-adrenergic antagonists, but not alpha$_2$ antagonists or beta-adrenergic agonists, prevent bladder contraction evoked by electrostimulation of the locus coeruleus (see Figs. 26–13, 26–14) (Yoshimura et al, 1988, 1990). Furthermore, catecholamine depletion followed by intrathecal administration of the alpha$_1$-adrenergic agonist phenylephedrine enhances voiding, whereas the alpha$_1$ blocker prazosin inhibits distention-induced bladder contractions (Yoshimura et al, 1988, 1990). Ishizuka and colleagues (1996) have shown that an intrathecal alpha antagonist, indoramin, prevents detrusor hyperreflexia induced by dopamine agonists. Danuser and Thor (1995) demonstrated that alpha-adrenergic antagonists can act centrally to inhibit both hypogastric and pudendal nerve outflow and thereby facilitate urine evacuation. Following spinal cord injury the alpha blocker terazosin increases compliance and improves continence (Swierzewski et al, 1994). Intrathecal clonidine, an alpha$_2$-adrenergic agonist, increases bladder capacity in humans and animals (Herman et al, 1988a; Espey et al, 1992). Other investigators (Durant et al, 1988a) find that activation of spinal alpha adrenoceptors with intrathecal norepinephrine inhibits rather than facilitates bladder activity. Furthermore, intrathecal alpha$_1$- and alpha$_2$-adrenergic blockers inhibit the external sphincter, but not micturition, in unanesthetized freely moving cats (Espey et al, 1992; Downie et al, 1991). These inconsistencies regarding the possible effects of spinal alpha adrenoceptors may be explained on the basis of species, different dosages, type of receptor, type of anesthesia or the preparations used (i.e., decerebrate versus intact). In the experiments by Durant and co-workers, hypogastric pathways were intact, permitting peripheral adrenergic inhibition of bladder function via sympathetic pathways. **Taken together, these observations suggest that alpha blockers can act centrally to either facilitate voiding or reduce bladder hyperactivity.**

In summary, the activities of the bladder and external sphincter are influenced by descending noradrenergic input from the locus coeruleus. Norepinephrine released from these pathways activates alpha$_1$- and alpha$_2$-adrenergic receptors in the sacral spinal cord, which inhibit the external sphincter and micturition, respectively. This is accomplished by the action of descending input on interneurons.

GABA/Glycine

GABA is an inhibitory amino acid transmitter at numerous sites within the central and peripheral nervous systems at other GABA-A or GABA-B receptors. Baclofen is a lipid-soluble form of GABA that penetrates the blood-brain barrier and activates GABA-B receptors. These two receptor types are distinguished by the selectivity of the GABA-A for the antagonist bicuculline. In general, GABA-B receptor agonists modulate presynaptic transmission, whereas GABA-A receptor agonists act postsynaptically in the spinal cord (Wu and Dun, 1992).

GABAminergic neurons have been identified in the sacral spinal cord and locus coeruleus (Iijima and Oktomo, 1988). Administration of the GABA-A agonist muscimol within the PMC of the cat (Roppolo et al, 1986) or intracerebroventricularly in the rat (Sillen et al, 1981) inhibits bladder activity (see Figs. 26–14, 26–15). These inhibitory effects can be abolished by bicuculline, indicating selective activation of the GABA-A receptor. Intracerebroventricular administration of baclofen inhibits L-dopa-induced bladder hyperactivity (Sillen et al, 1981, 1982).

Intrathecal administration of baclofen inhibits bladder activity and lowers urethral pressures in the dog (Magora et al, 1989), rat (Maggi et al, 1987a) and human (Nanninga et al, 1989; Steers et al, 1992b) (Fig. 26–16; see Figs. 26–14, 26–15). Not surprisingly, high doses of baclofen cause impotence and constipation. At the level of the spinal cord, GABA agonists also inhibit afferent nociceptive input from the bladder in rats (Abelli et al, 1989a; Araki and de Groat, 1995). Using a sixth lumbar to first sacral spinal cord slice, preparation from the neonatal rat identified interneurons that provide inhibitory input to sacral preganglionics. The inhibition was mediated primarily by GABA-A and glycine. It was concluded that either two separate interneurons provide inhibitory input to preganglionic neurons or one interneuron contains two transmitters in different terminals. Other investigators have shown that GABA-B receptors can also inhibit sacral preganglionic neurons (Todd and Sullivan, 1990). Not unexpectedly, systemic GABA-A antagonists enhance micturition reflexes (Kontani et al, 1987). These studies suggest that GABAminergic neurons at sites along the neuraxis could provide a mechanism for turning the positive feedback loop of urine storage into an "on-off" switch.

GABAminergic interneurons facilitate urine storage by inhibition of afferents and interneurons in the sacral spinal cord or supraspinal pathways. GABA-B receptors probably act presynaptically to inhibit afferent input to the

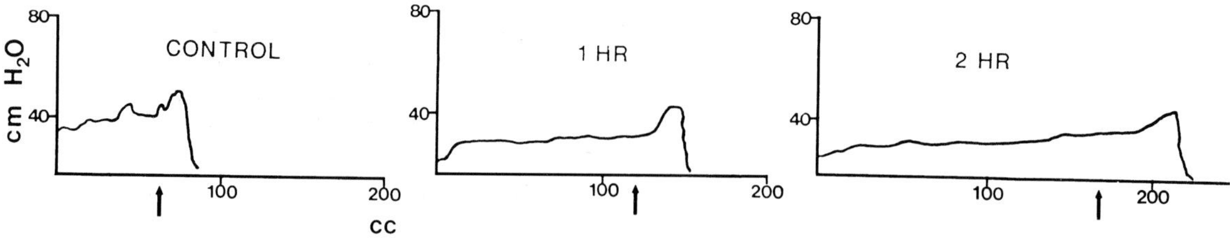

Figure 26–16. Effect of intrathecal baclofen bolus (50 mcg) on the cystometrogram in a patient with detrusor hyperreflexia resulting from partial spinal cord injury. Note the delay in first sensation and increased micturition threshold. Four months later, continuous intrathecal baclofen (400 mcg/day) produced a bladder capacity of 400 cc with low filling pressure. Data suggest that intrathecal drug administration may be a powerful pharmacologic tool for manipulating genitourinary function.

sacral spinal cord. GABA-B receptors probably mediate inhibition of sacral preganglionics.

Like GABA, glycine administration within the brain inhibits L-dopa-induced bladder hyperactivity (Sillen et al, 1981). In addition, glycine depresses firing of sacral preganglionic neurons (see Fig. 26–15) (de Groat, 1970). Effects on neural activity and bladder function can be blocked by the glycine receptor antagonist strychnine. These findings raise the possibility that some glycine-containing neurons inhibit micturition and promote urine storage.

Acetylcholine

Similar to glycinergic and GABAminergic neurons, cholinergic cells within the basal ganglia and brain stem inhibit bladder activity. The cholinomimetic carbachol applied within the basal ganglia of the rat (Dray and Metsch, 1983) or the PMC of the cat (Roppolo et al, 1987) produces atropine-sensitive inhibition of rhythmic bladder contractions (see Figs. 26–14, 26–15). However, Sillen and co-workers (1982) obtained a hyperactive bladder response with another muscarinic agonist, oxotremorine, following blockade of peripheral muscarinic receptors. Similarly, O'Donnell (1990) showed that bethanechol given to the brain enhances bladder activity in dogs.

Intrathecal carbachol has no effect on the CMG of the rat, although intrathecal atropine slightly reduces detrusor pressure (Durant et al, 1988b). Furthermore, iontophoretic application of acetylcholine has no effect on the firing of sacral preganglionic neurons (Ryall and de Groat, 1972). These data suggest that urine storage may be either facilitated or inhibited by different cholinergic neurons acting at supraspinal sites. Oral anticholinergics such as propantheline and oxybutynin probably do not achieve significant levels in the brain.

Opiates

Pharmacologic and immunocytochemical studies have provided an extensive body of information regarding the role of central enkephalinergic inhibitory mechanisms on lower urinary tract function. Enkephalinergic terminals are found in the PMC, dorsal horn of the spinal cord, surrounding sacral preganglionic neurons, and within Onuf's nucleus (de Groat et al, 1983; Booth et al, 1983; de Groat et al, 1986b). Intracerebroventricular or intrathecal administration of enkephalins or related opiates (dynorphin, endorphins, metorphamide, peptide E, or proenkephalin-A fragments) in intact animals depress bladder and external urethral sphincter function (see Figs. 26–14, 26–15) (Aoki et al, 1982; Lumb and Morrisson, 1987; Hisamitsu and de Groat, 1984; Dray and Metsch, 1984a, 1984b; Willmette et al, 1988; and reviews by Booth et al, 1985; de Groat et al, 1986a; Maggi and Meli, 1986). Likewise, intrathecal application of the opiate agonist morphine increases bladder capacity and causes urinary retention in humans (Aoki et al, 1982). In spinal cord–injured patients, intrathecal opiates depress bladder function but increase EMG activity recorded from the external urethral sphincter and increase maximal urethral pressures (Herman et al, 1988a, 1988b). The rapid development of tolerance with continuous intrathecal morphine prevents this therapy from being used to diminish detrusor hyperreflexia.

Opiate receptors have been categorized into at least three types: μ, δ, and κ (Mansour et al, 1988). Regional differences exist with respect to receptor subtype and effect on bladder function. In the cat brainstem, μ and δ opiate receptors regulate micturition threshold volume, whereas in the spinal cord, δ opiate receptor activation inhibits bladder function (Hisamitsu and de Groat, 1984) (Fig. 26–17). Sphincter reflexes are not affected by μ or δ opiate agonists, but are depressed by κ agonists. Knowledge of the effects of opiate receptor activation on bladder function may be clinically useful in avoiding drugs that produce urinary retention. For example, the analgesic morphine causes urinary retention in humans, whereas pentazocine, a κ agonist, does not have this side effect.

The role of endogenous enkephalins on bladder function has been examined using agents that antagonize or enhance the effect of these peptides (Roppolo et al, 1986; Thor et al, 1983; Booth et al, 1983, 1985). For example, thiorphan prevents the metabolism of enkephalins. When thiorphan is administered to animals, bladder activity is reduced. Furthermore, naloxone, an opiate antagonist, given centrally, increases spontaneous bladder contraction and decreases the micturition threshold volume. From the animal studies, it was suggested that endogenous opiates in the pons control the setting of a switch for bladder capacity and frequency of

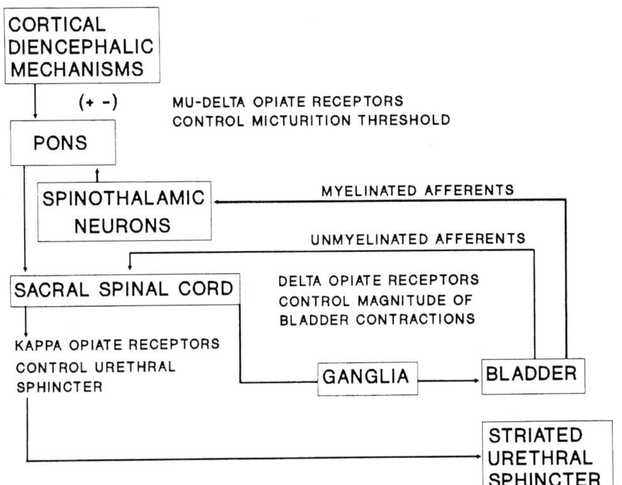

Figure 26–17. Diagram illustrating micturition reflex pathways and the possible role of enkephalinergic mechanisms based on studies in the cat. A supraspinal micturition reflex pathway that passes through the pons initiates voiding in response to activation of A-delta myelinated bladder afferents. Mu- and delta-opiate receptors in the pons may control micturition threshold and bladder capacity. In chronic spinal cats, a spinal micturition reflex is triggered by activation of unmyelinated C-fibers. Delta opiate receptors in the sacral cord control magnitude of bladder contractions. On the other hand, kappa-receptor activation depresses pudendal motoneuron firing and inhibits striated urethral sphincter. Kappa receptors in pelvic ganglia inhibit cholinergic transmission. (Modified from de Groat WC, Kawatani M: Neurourol Urodynam 1984; 4:291.)

isovolumetric contractions. In the sacral spinal cord, opiates control duration and amplitude of bladder contraction. The same observations have been made in neonates (Thor et al, 1990). In normal humans, naloxone increases intravesical pressure (Murray and Feneley, 1982). However, in patients with spinal cord lesions, naloxone exacerbates detrusor hyperreflexia (Vadyanaathan et al, 1981). Unfortunately, naloxone does not clinically facilitate bladder emptying.

Investigators postulate that endogenous enkephalinergic mechanisms in the brain and spinal cord promote continence by altering the threshold volume for voiding or by directly inhibiting micturition. Opiates also interact with tachykinins in the spinal cord and are involved with processing pain input from the lower urinary tract (Urban et al, 1994). The heterogeneity of opiate receptors offers the possibility of developing drugs with selective action on different parts of the voiding cycle. The different pharmacologic responses to opiates or opiate antagonists in intact versus spinalized subjects suggests a reorganization of enkephalinergic pathways following spinal cord injury (Thor et al, 1983). **Data regarding opiate mechanisms provide an attractive explanation for postoperative urinary retention. The combined effects of endogenous opiates and those given for analgesia act in the brain and spinal cord as well as peripheral ganglia to inhibit micturition.**

Neuropeptides

Because VIP, SP, CCK, corticotropin-releasing hormone (CRH), and somatostatin-containing neurons or fibers are found within the PMC and sacral spinal cord, there has been considerable interest in whether the central actions of these substances affect lower urinary tract function (Sokanaka et al, 1983; Sutin and Jacobowitz, 1988). Intracerebroventricular administration of SP does not antagonize excitatory effects of L-dopa or the inhibition of bladder activity by baclofen. On the other hand, intrathecal VIP and SP excites and inhibits micturition (Mallory and de Groat, 1987; Tiseo and Yaksh, 1989). Igawa and co-workers (1993b) found that intra-arterial and intrathecal VIP decreased micturition volume and bladder capacity as well as facilitated spontaneous bladder contraction. Thus, both peripheral and central actions of VIP are excitatory with regard to micturition. CRH neurons in the PMC of the rat appear to inhibit micturition, since intrathecal CRH antagonists block pontine-evoked bladder contractions (Pavcovich and Valentino, 1995).

The central regulation of urine storage and release relies on a balance of excitatory and inhibitory inputs with feedback mechanisms at different sites using many transmitter mechanisms in the neuraxis. It remains for the clinician to use this knowledge to develop improved drug therapies for lower urinary tract dysfunction. Recent biomedical advances, such as the development of pumps for intrathecal drug administration, provide methods for targeting pharmacologic therapy to central sites regulating bladder function.

VOIDING REFLEXES

The central mechanisms influencing urinary tract function are organized as a simple "on-off" switching circuit with a reciprocal relationship between the bladder and its outlet (see reviews by Kuru, 1965; de Groat, 1975; Morrison, 1987a, 1987b; de Groat and Steers, 1990). Depending on whether urine storage or release is desired, the integration of neuronal networks involved in lower urinary tract function requires both excitation and inhibition by the transmitters just discussed. Because urination is evoked by bladder filling, one could envision that significant inhibitory mechanisms are required to turn a positive feedback loop to a simple on-off switch.

Voiding results when mechanoreceptors in the bladder respond to a threshold tension (Iggo, 1955). Burst firing in afferents from bladder is followed by efferent firing conveyed by the pelvic nerve (de Groat and Ryall, 1969; Mallory et al., 1989). During voiding, hypogastric and pudendal neurons are inhibited (Garry, 1959; de Groat, 1975; Okada et al, 1975) (Fig. 26–18). Blockade of pudendal efferents does not abolish volitional voiding (Lapides et al, 1953). This integration of central neuronal pathways allows the bladder to empty completely at a low voiding pressure.

Previous investigators (Denny-Brown and Robertson, 1933; Lapides, 1953) argued that voiding resulted from a sacral spinal reflex because urination eventually resumes in patients with complete suprasacral spinal cord transection. **However it is now clear that a spinobulbospinal micturition reflex pathway that passes through the pons is responsible for urination in intact individuals (de Groat and Steers, 1990)** (Fig. 26–19). **Voiding following spinal cord transection results from a reorganization of sacral micturition reflex pathways (Thor et al, 1986; de Groat and Steers, 1990)** (Fig. 26–20).

Lesioning studies have shown that destruction of the neu-

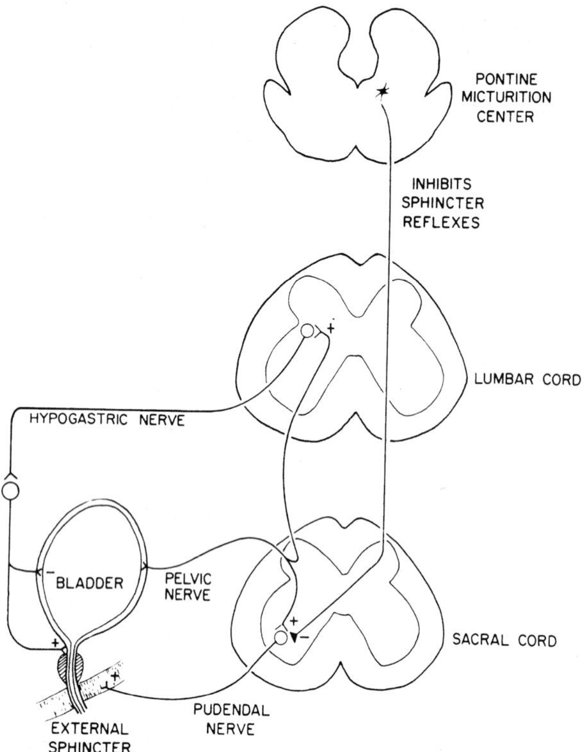

Figure 26–18. Representation of sphincter reflexes. Distention of bladder during filling produces low-level afferent firing, which triggers (1) hypogastric outflow to the bladder, and (2) pudendal outflow to the external urethral sphincter. Hypogastric pathways may promote urine storage by mediating relaxation (−) of bladder body via beta-adrenergic receptors and contraction (+) of the bladder base and urethra via alpha adrenoceptors. Hypogastric input may also inhibit ganglionic transmission in some species. During voiding, inhibition of hypogastric and pudendal pathways promotes complete bladder emptying. (Modified from de Groat WC, Booth AM: *In* Dyck PK, et al, eds: Peripheral Neuropathy, 2nd ed, Philadelphia, W. B. Saunders Company, 1984, p 289.)

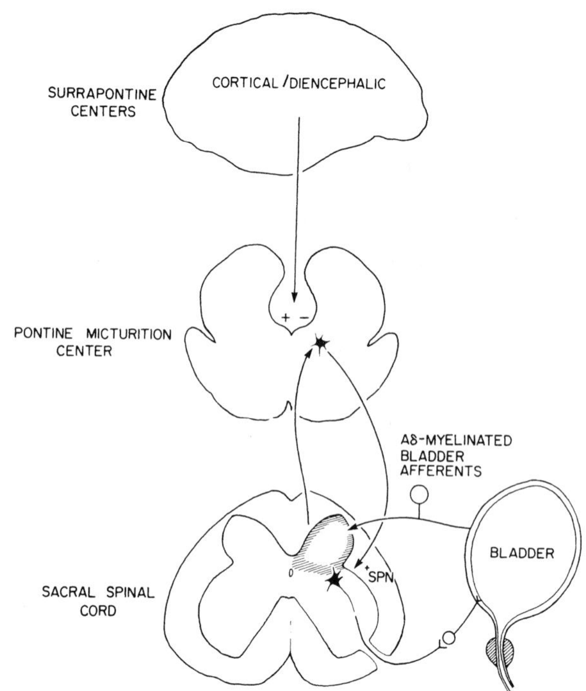

Figure 26–19. Schematic of supraspinal micturition reflex pathway. Bladder distention activates unmyelinated A-delta fiber afferents. Ascending input is relayed to a region of the pons termed the pontine micturition center (PMC). Depending on cortical input, excitatory descending input activates neurons in the sacral parasympathetic nucleus, which cause bladder contraction. Evidence for a spinobulbospinal pathway exists in the cat (de Groat and Ryall, 1969) and rat (Mallory et al, 1989).

raxis above the pons fails to eliminate involuntary micturition (Tang, 1955; Tang and Ruch, 1956; Kuru, 1965; Bradley and Conway, 1966) (Fig. 26–21). However, voluntary voiding in humans is abolished if connections between the frontal lobe, hypothalamus, or the paralobule and the brain stem are destroyed (Nathan, 1976). Positron emission tomography (PET) scanning of the brain in humans during voiding confirms that these regions are involved in micturition (Blok et al, 1995). Transection of the superior cerebellar peduncle or the neuraxis below the pons initially abolishes voiding in the rat (Mallory et al, 1989), cat (Tang and Ruch, 1956), and dog (Okada et al, 1975). Likewise, bilateral lesions in the rostral pons in the region of the locus coeruleus in cats (Griffiths et al, 1990) or in the dorsolateral tegmental nucleus in rats (Satoh et al, 1978) eliminates bladder contractions, whereas stimulation at these sites triggers micturition. In humans, pontine strokes have been associated with detrusor areflexia (Bors and Comarr, 1971; Zhan, 1981). These imaging and lesioning studies strengthen the concept that voiding depends on a spinobulbospinal reflex relayed through a region of the rostral brain stem referred to as the *pontine micturition center* (PMC) or Barrington's nucleus.

Electrophysiologic experiments are consistent with the notion of a spinobulbospinal micturition reflex. Stimulation

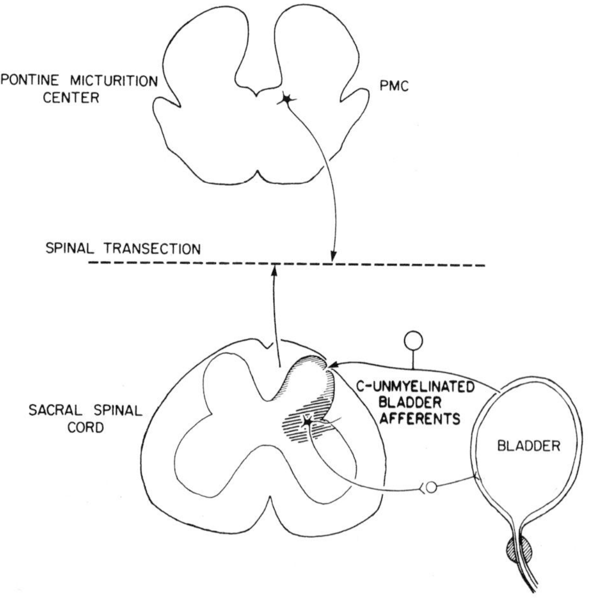

Figure 26–20. Schematic of spinal micturition reflex pathway in chronic spinal animals. Bladder distention activates unmyelinated C-fiber afferents in the cat (de Groat et al, 1981), which excite sacral preganglionic neurons (SPN) and trigger a bladder contraction. Reorganization of sacral spinal pathways leads to development of a spinal micturition reflex.

A

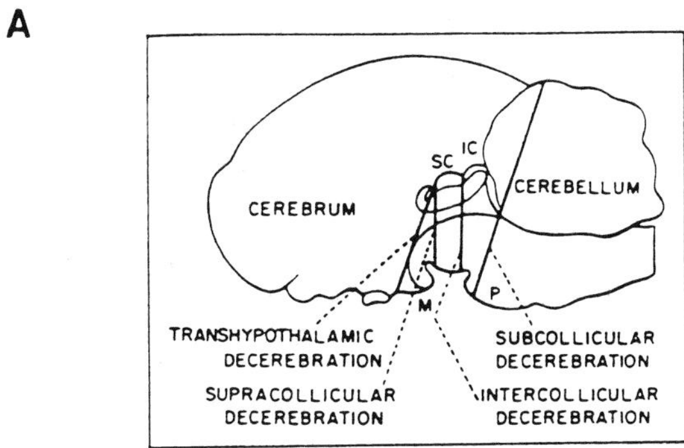

B

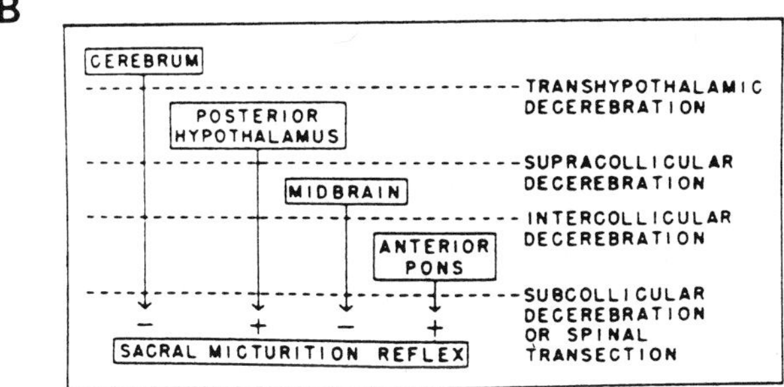

Figure 26–21. Results of progressive decerebration lesioning experiments on cystometrograms (CMG) (micturition threshold) in cats. *A*, level of lesion. *B*, effect on CMG. Subcollicular decerebration or spinal transection transiently eliminates bladder activity consistent with Barrington's earlier work (1931) suggesting a micturition center in the dorsal half of the anterior pons. Note that except for the posterior hypothalamus, other suprapontine centers tend to inhibit detrusor function. IC, infracollicular; SC, supracollicular; M, medulla; P, pons. (From Tang PC: J Neurophysiol 1955; 18:584.)

of myelinated (A-delta) bladder afferents in cats (de Groat et al, 1979) and rats (Mallory et al, 1989) elicits long latency reflex firing in sacral preganglionic neurons (see Fig. 26–19). The latencies for this central reflex (100 to 150 milliseconds) are similar in both species. Afferent stimulation also evokes negative field potentials in the pons with latencies of 40 to 60 milliseconds (de Groat, 1975; Noto et al, 1989). The sum of latencies for ascending (spinobulbar) and descending (bulbospinal) discharges approximates the latency for the entire central reflex in the cat and rat (de Groat, 1975; Mallory et al, 1989).

Anterolateral cordotomies performed in patients with chronic pain reveal that ascending routes responsible for transmitting bladder sensation and that trigger voiding travel in the lateral spinothalamic tract (Fig. 26–22) (Pool, 1954; Nathan and Smith, 1958; Nathan, 1976). Sectioning these pathways abolishes bladder sensation as well as voiding (Blok and Holstege, 1994).

Unit recordings in the locus coeruleus of the cat and rat (de Groat, 1975; Elam et al, 1986) or dorsolateral tegmentum of the rat have identified neurons that are activated by changes in intravesical pressure. Similarly, electrical and pharmacologic stimulation of the dorsolateral pons in the rat, dog, and cat produces burst activity in the pelvic nerve associated with a bladder contraction (de Groat, 1975; McMahon and Spillane, 1982; Holstege et al, 1986; Noto et al, 1989). These observations have helped localize the area of the pons containing a micturition center.

Stimulation and lesioning studies in the pontine tegmentum of the cat indicate that bladder contraction and sphincter relaxation may be regulated by separate brain stem regions (Holstege et al, 1986; Kruse et al, 1988; Griffiths et al, 1990) (Fig. 26–23). Electrical stimulation of a discrete dorsomedial (M) region in the pons elicits relaxation of anal and urethral striated sphincters. Furthermore, bilateral lesioning of this M region in cats produces urinary retention. However, the M region does not receive direct inputs from the sacral spinal cord. Rather, ascending sacral inputs, corresponding to pathways from the bladder, terminate in the ventrolateral periaqueductal gray area and from there project to the micturition center. Interestingly, the periadqueductal gray area plays an important role in pain processing. The M region (or PMC) receives input from various regions of the brain. The angulate gyrus, medial preoptic region of the hypothalamus bed nucleus of stria terminalis and amygdala all send projections to the M region (Blok and Holstege, 1994). These pathways form the anatomic and functional substrates for emotional or homeostatic influences on micturition.

Elimination of ascending or afferent input from the bladder has been used to influence the properties of the descending limit from the pons to sacral spinal cord (Kruse et al, 1991). From these experiments it was found that the pons can initiate bladder contractions and coordinate sphincter activity. The afferent feedback via the sacral dorsal roots was necessary to maintain large-amplitude micturition contractility of sufficient deviation to empty the bladder. These observations combined with pharmacologic data strongly suggest that the pons contains circuitry for switching between urine storage and release.

Stimulation of a more lateral (L) region produces both contraction and relaxation of the external urethral sphincter in cats and rats (Griffiths et al, 1990; Kruse et al, 1988). In addition, bilateral destruction of this L region induces bladder hyperactivity and urinary incontinence, whereas lesions

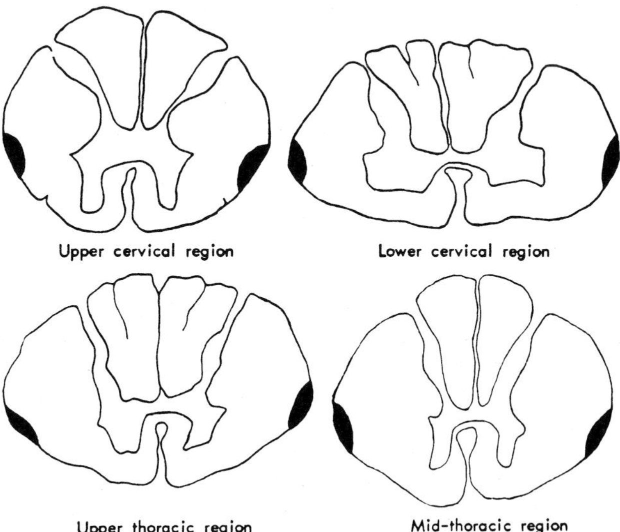

Figure 26–22. Regions of human spinal cord containing ascending tracts involved in micturition, as suggested from anterolateral cordotomies performed for chronic pain. Bilateral lesions of spinothalamic tracts produce loss of bladder sensation and micturition. (From Nathan PW, Smith MC: J Neurol Neurosurg Psychiatr, 1951; 14:278.)

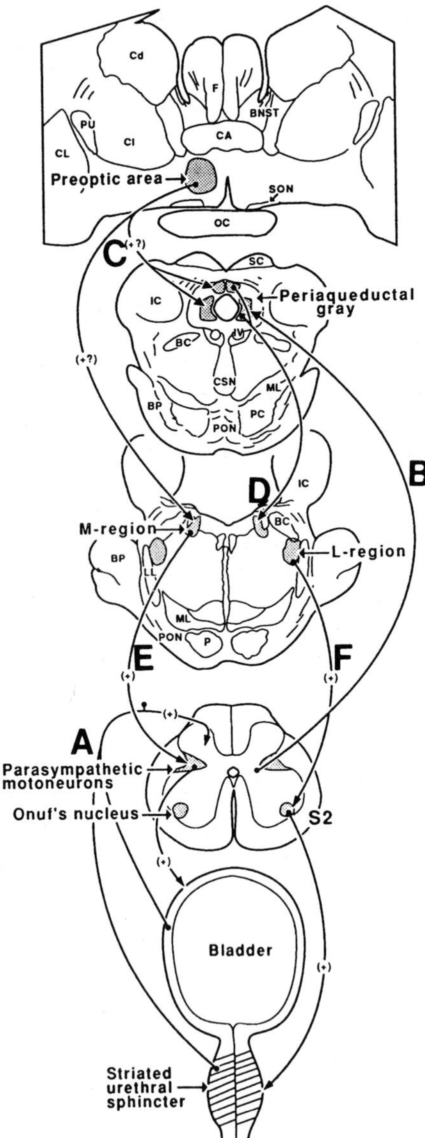

Figure 26–23. Representation of spinal and supraspinal structures involved in micturition based on retrograde tracing and electrophysiologic experiments. (A) Afferent input from the bladder and urethra travel in the pelvic nerve and synapses in the dorsal horn and commissure of the S2 spinal cord. (B) Ascending input to the periaqueductal gray matter of the pons. Periaqueductal gray matter functions as a sensory receiving area providing input (D) into the micturition center of the pons. Periaqueductal gray micturition center also receives descending input (C) from preoptic area of hypothalamus to the periqueductal M regions; impulses provide emotional and general autonomic modulation of voiding. (E) Descending input from the micturition region of the pons provides excitatory descending input from the micturition center of the pons to parasympathetic motoneurons in the sacral spinal cord. (F) Descending input from the L-region of the pons to the Onuf's nucleus in S2. (From Blok BFM, Holstege G: Direct projections from the periaqueductal gray to the pontine micturation center (M-region). Neurosci Lett 1994; 166:93–96.)

adjacent to the M and L areas fail to alter lower urinary tract function. However, a lack of coordination between the external urethral sphincter and the bladder during voiding (detrusor sphincter dyssynergia) (Fig. 26–24) is not seen with destruction of the M or L regions. These data confirm that a PMC facilitates bladder activity, whereas a more laterally located region in the pons is concerned with regulation of the pelvic floor muscles, which include those involved in urinary continence and voiding.

Descending projections from the PMC to the sacral spinal cord have been examined using retrograde axonal tracing and electrophysiologic techniques (Hida and Shimizu, 1982; Nadelhaft and Deveny, 1987). In the cat, these descending pathways terminate in regions containing bladder afferent terminals and dendritic projections from sacral preganglionic neurons (Nadelhaft et al, 1980; Morgan et al, 1981). In the rat, the PMC also sends descending projections in the ventral columns to the bulbocavernosus nucleus (corresponding to Onuf's nucleus). The previously described L region of the pons is situated adjacent to neurons that project to sphincter motor neurons in Onuf's nucleus in the sacral spinal cord (Holstege et al, 1986) (see Fig. 26–23).

Retrograde viral tracing methods have been used to label cells that synapse on sacral preganglionic neurons. Neurons in the paraventricular nucleus of the hypothalamus, the dorsolateral tegmental nucleus, locus coeruleus, and A_5 cell group of the pons have been identified after injection of an attenuated pseudorabies virus into pelvic ganglia of rats after

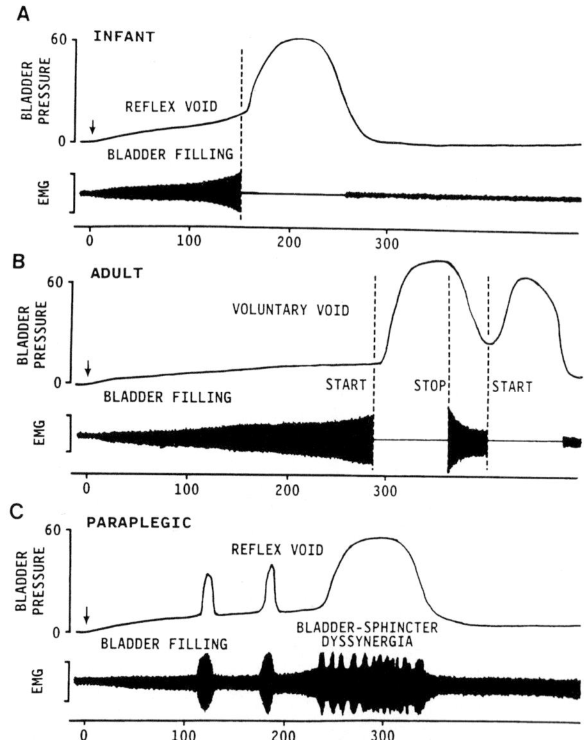

Figure 26–24. Examples of combined cystometrics (CMG) and external urethral sphincter (EUS) electromyograms (EMG) in infants, adults, and paraplegics. *A*, Voiding in infants is involuntary with reflex bladder contraction associated with decreased firing of EUS, EMG. *B*, In the adult, voluntary micturition is also associated with decreased EUS, EMG. *A* and *B* demonstrate a reciprocal relationship between micturition and striated sphincter pathways. *C*, Paraplegic patients demonstrate involuntary voiding with lack of coordination of EUS. Note bladder contractions at low volume (125,190 cc), with increase in EUS, EMG, which is referred to as bladder detrusor sphincter dyssynergia. Some paraplegics are also unable to sustain a detrusor contraction. (From de Groat WC, Steers WD: In Loewy AD, Spyer KM, eds: Central Regulation of Autonomic Functions, 1st ed. Oxford, Oxford University Press, 1990, p 314.)

bilateral hypogastric neural transection (Marson, 1995) (Fig. 26–25). These results indicate that input from various supraspinal sites directly regulates pelvic autonomic function.

Suprapontine areas of the brain involved in bladder function have been selectively examined in the cat, dog, and rat using lesioning and electrical or chemical stimulation techniques. These studies indicate that cortical, extrapyramidal, cerebellar, and brain stem sites can inhibit or facilitate voiding (Bradley and Scott, 1978; Morrison, 1987a, 1987b; Nishizawa et al, 1987).

Axonal tracing studies have also demonstrated direct hypothalamic projections passing through the median forebrain bundle to the PMC (Holstege, 1987), sacral autonomic centers (Saper et al, 1976; Swanson and Sawchenko, 1983) and Onuf's nucleus (Holstege, 1987) (see Figs. 26–23, 26–25). Electrical stimulation of the anterior and lateral hypothalamus induces bladder contractions and voiding, whereas stimulation of the posterior and medial hypothalamic regions inhibits bladder activity (Enoch et al, 1967a, 1967b; Morrison, 1987b). Viral tracing studies confirm that nuclei send projections to pontine regions, which regulate bladder and pelvic visceral function. These findings are consistent with the notion of hypothalamic regulation of autonomic function. Thus, it is not surprising that emotions or psychological stressors can have a profound influence on voiding. For example, psychogenic retention or anxiety are associated with nonrelaxation of the bladder neck or areflexia.

The spinobulbospinal micturition reflex is modulated by excitatory and inhibitory influences from regions of the brain rostral to the pons. The role of the basal ganglia, parietal frontal cortex, and cerebellum on micturition has been confirmed by urodynamic studies following selective lesioning (Tang and Ruch, 1956), cerebrovascular accident (Zhan, 1981; Tschida et al, 1983), epilepsy, intracranial aneurysms, and tumors (Barnett and Hyland, 1952). Although excitatory and inhibitory effects have been described for many sites within the brain, the net effect of lesions rostral to the pons is often hyperactivity of the bladder. This framework offers an explanation of why the unstable detrusor and urge incontinence are common clinical findings.

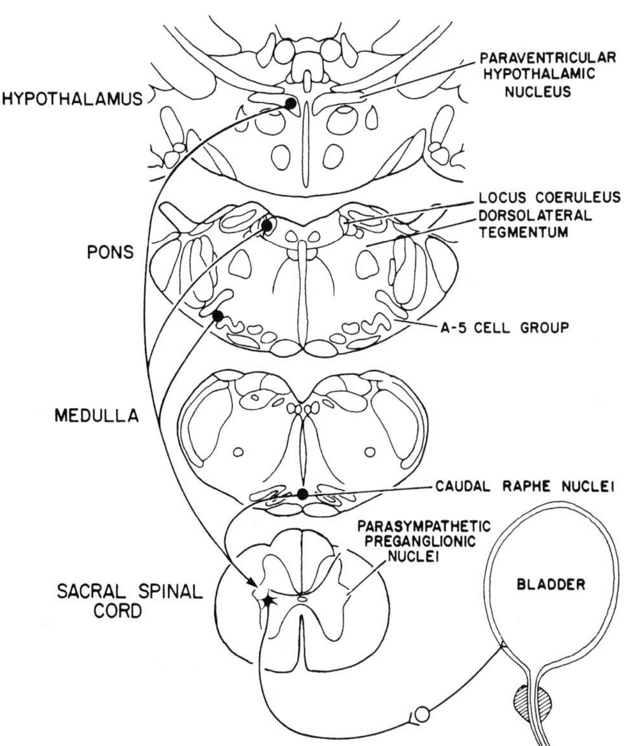

Figure 26–25. Summary diagram illustrating the regions of the brain that directly project to sacral preganglionic neurons. These centers were identified by peripheral injection of pseudorabies virus into pelvic ganglion of the rat which labels second-order neurons. Labeled regions are remarkably similar to those projecting to the thoracolumbar preganglionic neurons. (From Strack AM, Sawyer WB, Platt KB, Lowey AD: Brain Res 1989; 491:274.)

In summary, micturition results from a tension-activated reflex mediated by myelinated axons to the sacral spinal cord. Second-order neurons relay afferent input to periaqueductal gray areas in the pons, which transmits this signal to micturition (M) or storage (L) centers. These centers coordinate the bladder and its outlet. Descending axons synapse on interneurons that project to the sacral preganglionics responsible for bladder contraction and urethral relaxation as well as those mediating inhibition of pudendal motoneurons, which innervate the striated external urethral sphincter (rhabdosphincter).

STORAGE REFLEXES

Continence is maintained by active and passive mechanisms in the proximal (see the section on proximal and distal urethral sphincter regions (see Proximal Urethral Sphincter section and Intrinsic Distal Urethral Sphincter and External Striated Sphincter [Rhabdosphincter] section). During periods of stress or elevated abdominal pressure with a full bladder, the external urethral sphincter augments the urethral closure mechanism. Before the onset of voiding, urethral pressure falls. This relaxation of the urethra is conveyed by efferent fibers in the pelvic nerve. To store urine, this urethral reflex must be inhibited. The nervous system possesses substantial inhibitory mechanisms to prevent inadvertent triggering of a micturition reflex as well. This blockade of excitatory input to the bladder is especially important because the stretched detrusor smooth muscle sits poised near its threshold for firing. Two schemes can be envisioned to facilitate continence and store urine at low pressure. One scheme could rely on excitation of sphincter pathways innervating the bladder outlet, especially during increases in intra-abdominal pressure. Other mechanisms could prevent voiding by inhibition of the spinobulbospinal micturition reflex to the bladder and urethra. It appears both are operational.

Investigators have ascribed a storage role to hypogastric and pudendal nerves (see Fig. 26–18). Yet, acute transection or chemical blockade of sympathetic and pudendal nerves in humans does not produce poor bladder compliance or urinary incontinence (Bors and Comarr, 1971). Likewise, patients with dopamine β-hydroxylase deficiency who lack noradrenergic nerves are continent and have no voiding complaints (Gary and Robertson, 1994). In many species, these nerves influence bladder capacity and outlet resistance. For example, hypogastric input to the lower urinary tract is tonically active during bladder filling in the cat (Edvardsen, 1968; de Groat and Lalley, 1972). Hypogastric firing is initiated in part by a lumbosacral intersegmental spinal reflex. This storage reflex is triggered by pelvic nerve afferent fibers entering the sacral cord and ascending to thoracolumbar sympathetic preganglionic fibers (de Groat and Lalley, 1972) (see Fig. 26–18). The activity of sympathetic nerves represents a negative feedback mechanism whereby elevations in intravesical pressure trigger inhibitory input to the bladder and allow greater urine accommodation. During voiding, this hypogastric firing is switched off (Edvardsen, 1968; de Groat and Lalley, 1972). This reciprocal inhibition is influenced by a supraspinal site because it is prevented by thoracic spinal cord transection (de Groat and Lalley, 1972).

In addition to excitatory input to the bladder responsible for voiding, parasympathetic pathways paradoxically provide tonic inhibitory input. After acute transection of the pelvic nerve or sacral ventral roots, low-amplitude detrusor contractions develop. The significance of this parasympathetic inhibition is unclear, but may provide an additional mechanism for maintaining low-pressure filling of the bladder.

Reflex pathways to the external urethral sphincter (EUS) facilitate urine storage by (1) closure of the midurethra and (2) feedback inhibition of preganglionic input to the bladder and urethra (see Fig. 26–18). Urodynamic and EMG data indicate that a rise in maximal urethral pressure corresponds to increased EMG activity of the striated muscles of the pelvic floor. Pudendal motoneuron firing occurs when the bladder is filled to near capacity or following a sudden increase in intravesical pressure. This phenomenon has been termed the *guarding* or *continence* reflex and represents a somatic mechanism for increasing urethral resistance (Diokno et al, 1974; Blaivas et al, 1977). Voluntary overactivity of this reflex can result in obstruction of the lower urinary tract. Differentiating voluntary contraction of this sphincter from detrusor sphincter dyssynergia can be difficult. Rudy and Woodside (1991) found that close examination of the onset of sphincter activity relative to the rise in intravesical pressure can help distinguish a guarding reflex from true detrusor striated sphincter dyssynergia.

Conversely, during voiding, pudendal motoneurons in Onuf's nuclei are inactivated, thereby inhibiting the external urethral sphincter. Both direct hyperpolarization (inhibition) of pudendal motoneurons by descending inputs (L-region) (see Fig. 26–23), and presynaptic neuron mechanisms relying on afferent input from perineum or interneurons contribute to switching off the external sphincter (Fedirchuk et al, 1994).

The mechanisms responsible for this switching of reflexes from storage to voiding rely on axodendritic contacts between parasympathetic, sympathetic, and somatic pathways in the spinal cord. Pudendal motoneurons lie in a circumscribed region within the S_2 through S_4 sacral spinal cord, which, in humans, is termed *Onuf's nucleus*. In animal studies, some dendrites project dorsolaterally to the sacral preganglionic neurons in lateral lamina V (see Fig. 26–28) (McKenna and Nadelhaft, 1985; Roppolo et al, 1985; Thor et al, 1989; Beattie et al, 1990). Other dendrites project dorsomedially to the dorsal gray commissure or laterally into the ventrolateral funiculus. Dendrites receive descending input from the lateral pons and hypothalamus (Holstege et al, 1986; Griffiths et al, 1990) (see Fig. 26–23). In addition, longitudinal spinal cord sections reveal dense rostrocaudal projections distributed within Onuf's nucleus. Sensory projections from the urinary bladder terminate in the region of dorsal dendritic projects from Onuf's motoneurons. The location of these dendritic processes in the sacral spinal cord is consistent with the inhibition of the external sphincter that occurs with a rise in intravesical pressure.

Central inhibition of the spinobulbospinal micturition reflex is carried out at multiple levels of the neuraxis. Parasympathetic outflow to the bladder and urethra is prevented by various sacral inputs including recurrent inhibition from preganglionic axon collaterals, visceral afferent fibers from various pelvic organs, and somatic afferent fibers (de Groat et al, 1979). Pudendal afferent fibers from the perineum transiently block detrusor activity and provide the basis for treating incontinence with cutaneous electrical stimulators (de Groat, 1971; Sato and Schmidt, 1987). Likewise, visceral afferent input from rectal distention or probing the uterine cervix inhibits bladder activity (Sato and Schmidt, 1987). Spinal mechanisms for inhibition of bladder activity may be mediated by interneurons, which send axons to sacral preganglionic neurons. These mechanisms are useful in preventing micturition during sexual intercourse or defecation.

It is clear from the preceding discussion that the central nervous system possesses diverse switching mechanisms for regulating voiding and continence. During voiding, excitatory transmission to bladder and inhibitory input to the urethra occurs through parasympathetic pathways. Simultaneously, hypogastric and pudendal pathways are switched off.

AFFERENT MECHANISMS

Many if not all symptoms of bladder dysfunction are mediated by sensory pathways. Yet, until recently little attention has been paid to the afferents supplying the lower urinary tract. **Bladder afferent fibers convey mechanoreceptive input essential for voiding. These visceral afferent fibers also transmit sensations of bladder fullness, urgency, and pain. Visceral afferent fibers are capable of local transmitter release, which influences (1) cellular components of the immune system; (2) vascular permeability; (3) smooth muscle contractility; and (4) neurotransmission** (Fig. 26–26) **(Maggi and Meli, 1986; de Groat, 1987). These diverse pharmacologic and physiologic properties of afferent fibers may contribute to urologic disorders previously attributed to psychiatric illness or inflammatory disease such as urethral syndrome and interstitial cystitis.**

Afferent fibers projecting to the bladder travel in sympathetic and parasympathetic pathways. They are involved in triggering reflex phenomena such as urination and autonomic dysreflexia (see Voiding Reflexes). Sectioning sacral but not thoracolumbar dorsal roots results in urinary retention with loss of bladder sensation except for the vague feeling of pain with overdistention (Learmonth, 1931; Bors and Comarr, 1971). Thus, pain and the mechanoreceptive input tension that triggers micturition travels in the pelvic nerve. Many unmyelinated C-fiber afferent fibers are "silent" and fail to fire with a wide range of stimuli (Habler et al, 1990, 1993; Janig and Koltzenburg, 1990, 1992). Following inflammatory stimuli, these C-fibers become active (Habler et al, 1990, 1993; Janig and Koltzenburg, 1992; Yoshimura

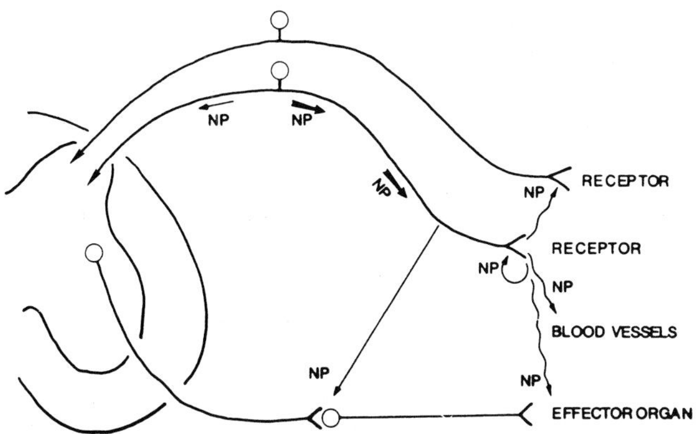

Figure 26–26. Diagram of possible peripheral roles for afferents termed the "afferent-efferent" hypothesis. Neuropeptides (NP) synthesized in dorsal root ganglion cells are transported centrally and peripherally. Electrical, mechanical, or chemical release of NP such as substance P or calcitonin gene–related peptide (CGRP) can exert a wide range of effects including alterations in vascular permeability, transmitter release, smooth muscle contractility, ganglionic transmission, and function of cellular components of the immune system. (From de Groat WC: Experientia 1987; 37:80.)

and de Groat, 1992). Likewise. sympathetic fibers in the hypogastric nerve transmit pain sensation to the central nervous system from the lower urinary tract.

Iggo (1955) found that bladder afferent fibers respond to tension rather than volume. Multiunit recording on bladder nerves confirms that bladder afferent nerves are quiescent during increases in volume but fire when a certain tension threshold is reached (McMahon, 1986). The intravesical pressure thresholds for A-delta afferent fibers range from 5 to 15 mm Hg, which correspond to pressures at which humans sense filling on a cystometrogram (Abrams et al, 1983) (see Table 26–2). Afferent fibers in the pelvic nerve respond to bladder distention in a graded fashion (Janig and Morrison, 1986). Janig and Morrison (1986), using single-fiber recording techniques, have shown that afferent firing occurs at pressures (tension) that induce micturition, whereas presumably painful (nociceptive) pressures produce greater rates of firing. Some authors propose that frequency-encoding is capable of differentiating between such mechanoreceptive and nociceptive input. Alternatively, some afferent fibers to the bladder may be unimodal and achieve specificity by varying the frequency of firing or encoding by the type of chemical transmitter. It is possible that specialized receptors in the bladder respond to different stimuli. However, in most species investigators have observed only free nerve endings running beneath urothelium or between smooth muscle fascicles (Fletcher and Bradley, 1968; Uemura et al, 1968; Gabella, 1995). Pacinian corpuscles are rarely seen. Fletcher and Bradley (1968) confirmed that free nerve endings in the bladder wall represent parasympathetic afferent terminals because they were eliminated with sectioning of the sacral dorsal roots.

Anatomic studies by Hulsebosch and Coggeshall (1982) have shown that sacral afferent fibers projecting to the sacral spinal cord are either lightly myelinated (A-delta) or unmyelinated (C-fiber). Conduction velocities of axons that originate in the dorsal root ganglia (DRG) are consistent with this morphologic heterogeneity (de Groat, 1975; de Groat et al, 1981; Mallory et al, 1989). Electrophysiologic studies have identified both fast-conducting (up to 30 meters per second) and slow-conducting (0.3 meters per second) fibers corresponding to lightly myelinated A-delta and unmyelinated C-fibers, respectively. Most DRG cells that supply the bladder are small, possess high thresholds to fire, and express tetrodotoxin-resistant Na^{2+} channels (de Groat et al, 1990b; Yoshimura and de Groat, 1992).

Characteristic patterns for bladder afferent fibers have been seen within lamina I, V, VII, and X in the sacral spinal cord (Fig. 26–27) (Morgan et al, 1981; Jansco and Maggi, 1987; Steers et al, 1991a). The distribution of these visceral afferent fibers in the pelvic nerve differs from that for somatic afferent fibers in the pudendal nerve (Fig. 26–28). Wheat germ agglutinin horseradish peroxidase (WGA-HRP) labeling of afferent fibers from the bladder shows that their projections form a thin shell around the dorsal horn (Morgan et al, 1981; Jansco and Maggi, 1987; Steers et al, 1991a). Furthermore, the terminal fields of these afferent fibers are found in regions containing neurons projecting to supraspinal centers and in the vicinity of dendritic projections from sacral parasympathetic neurons. This contrasts with afferent projections to the spinal cord that are located more centrally in the dorsal horn (see Fig. 26–27) (Roppolo et al, 1985; McKenna and Nadelhaft, 1985; Thor et al, 1989). Differences in terminations for pelvic and pudendal afferent fibers corresponds to separate ascending pathways and interneurons for visceral versus somatic inputs to the sacral spinal cord. Until recently, one limitation of dyes and lectins used to identify projections into the spinal cord has been the inability to cross synapses. Using retrograde viral tracers, such as pseudorabies and herpesviruses, has allowed identification of second- and third-order neurons within the central nervous

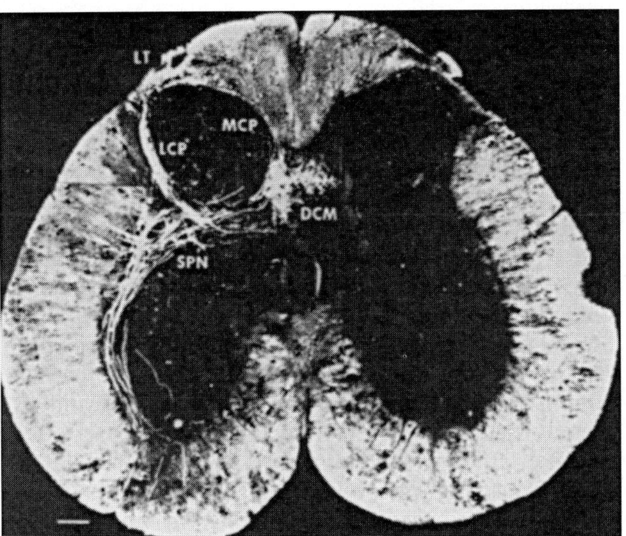

Figure 26–27. Combined labeling of afferents and preganglionic neurons in S2 spinal cord of the cat following application of horseradish peroxidase (HRP) to the pelvic nerve. Afferents enter Lissauer's tract (LT) and extend laterally into the lateral collateral pathway (LCP), which reaches areas of dendritic projections from preganglionic neurons in the sacral parasympathetic nucleus (SPN). Note the close proximity of afferent and efferent limbs for neurons forming the spinal micturition reflex pathway. Afferent collaterals extend medially in the medial collateral pathway (MCP) and dorsal gray commissure (DCM). Bar represents 200 microns. (From Morgan C, Nadelhaft I, de Groat WC: J Comp Neurol 1981; 201:417.)

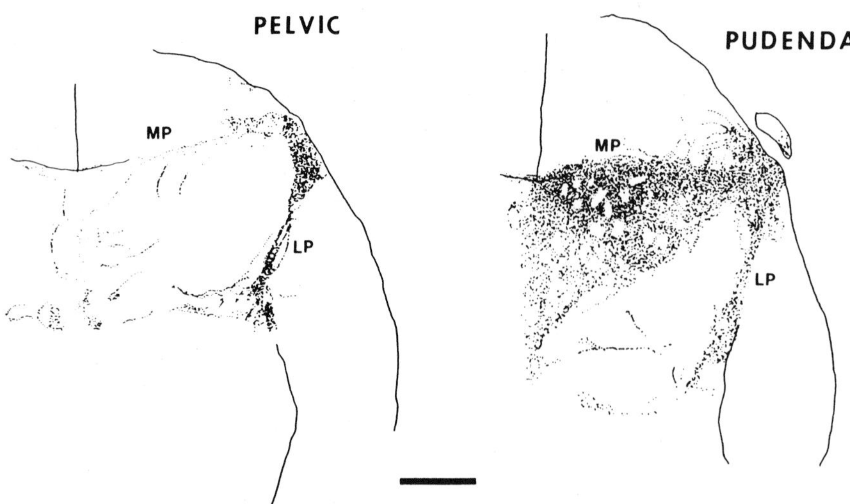

Figure 26–28. Comparison of central projections for visceral afferents in pelvic nerve with somatic afferents in pudendal nerve in S1 spinal cord of the rhesus monkey. Retrograde axonal transport of horseradish peroxidase (HRP) was used to label projections. HRP reaction product is found along the edge of dorsal horn in the medial collateral pathway (MP) and lateral collateral pathway (LP). Application of HRP to pudendal nerve results in diffuse central labeling in the dorsal horn. Labeling for bladder afferents in cat and rat resembles patterns seen following application of HRP to pelvic nerve. Bar corresponds to 400 microns. (From Roppolo JR, Nadelhaft I, de Groat WC: J Comp Neurol 1985; 234:486.)

system. Several groups have injected either the bladder or pelvic ganglia and found these retrograde viral tracers in areas such as the pontine micturition center known as Barrington's nucleus in the rat (see Fig. 26–25) (Marson, 1995).

SP, CGRP, VIP, L-ENK, NO synthase, and other peptides occur either singly or in various combinations within sacral dorsal root ganglia projecting to the bladder (see Table 26–8) **(de Groat, 1987; Gibson et al, 1986; Su et al, 1986; Keast and de Groat, 1992). Areas of the sacral spinal cord that receive nociceptive input contain SP as well as structurally-related peptides referred to as tachykinins and express tachykinin receptors (de Laverolle and LaMotte, 1982; Seybold, 1985). These areas also correspond to the sites of bladder afferent labeling using WGA-HRP.**

Subjecting an animal to painful stimuli (Yaksh et al, 1980) evokes the release of (SP) and other tachykinins from afferent terminals in the bladder and spinal cord (McMahon, 1986; Abelli et al, 1989a). Furthermore, central projections of SP and CGRP afferent fibers make axodendritic and axosomatic synapses on sacral preganglionic neurons (Peng et al, 1988). As previously mentioned, in the peripheral nervous system SP and tachykinins are expressed exclusively within afferent fibers. The neurotoxin capsaicin causes the release of SP, related tachykinins, and other neuropeptides such as CGRP from unmyelinated or lightly myelinated capsaicin-sensitive afferent nerves in the bladder (see reviews by Maggi and Meli, 1988; Holzer-Petsche, 1988). Exposing the bladder to topical or intravesical capsaicin produces smooth muscle contraction, which can be blocked by SP-antagonists or the neurotoxin tetrodotoxin (Maggi et al, 1984, 1986, 1988b; Ishizuka et al, 1995). SP is released from nerve terminals and mediates its effects through receptors (Maggi, 1995). Systemic capsaicin and related compounds such as resiniferatoxin produces a partial or complete degeneration of capsaicin-sensitive afferent nerves depending upon the dose, species, and age of the experimental animal (Maggi and Meli, 1988; Holzer-Petsche, 1988). Capsaicin and resiniferatoxin act at receptors located on afferent fibers. These vanilloid receptors may be altered in disease states. Systemic capsaicin treatment causes the near-complete loss of SP and CGRP-immunoreactivity in neonatal and adult rat and guinea pig bladders. The loss of SP fibers in neonatal rats is associated with urinary retention (Holzer-Petsche and Lembeck, 1984). Intrathecal capsaicin eliminates SP in the spinal cord and micturition (Durant et al, 1988b). Capsaicin treatment in adult rats elevates the volume threshold, but does not abolish voiding (Chen et al, 1993). This latter data suggests that capsaicin-sensitive afferent nerves may be essential for micturition early in development and may assume a modulatory role in the adult. A concentration-dependent reduction in first sensation and bladder capacity occurs in humans following acute administration of intravesical capsaicin. In patients with hypersensitive bladders or detrusor instability, intravesical capsaicin temporarily attenuates or eliminates symptoms (Fowler et al, 1992, 1994).

These findings suggest that SP and other tachykinins may play a role in mediating pain transmission from the bladder. Afferent nerves containing NO may also play a role in transmitting painful stimuli to the spinal cord (Dun et al, 1993). Although NOS inhibitors have no effect on normal micturition, following inflammation of the bladder these drugs reduce bladder activity (Rice, 1995).

To explore acute pain mechanisms in the bladder, a variety of stimuli have been used. Instillation of the irritants turpentine (McMahon and Abel, 1987), mustard oil (McMahon and Abel, 1987; Koltzenburg and McMahon, 1986), formalin (Birder et al, 1990; Dupont et al, 1994) and xylene (Abelli et al, 1989a) produces, behavioral responses indicative of pain. Dupont and colleagues have also used endotoxin and suture material to create chronic inflammatory states in the bladder. Others have tried autoimmunization to substances such as ovalbumin (Kim et al, 1991; Saban et al, 1994).

Chronic bladder pain can be the result of activation of afferent nerves that under normal conditions do not respond to physiologic stimuli. These postulated "silent afferents" are activated by repetitive, irritative stimuli (Bahns et al, 1986; Janig and Koltzenburg, 1992; Habler et al, 1990, 1993). Recent electrophysiologic studies on isolated sacral dorsal root ganglion cells have documented a population of very high threshold afferent neurons that possess tetrodotoxin-resistant sodium channels (Yoshimura and de Groat,

1992). These high-threshold neurons may correspond to the hypothesized "silent afferent." Following inflammatory stimuli in the bladder, the spontaneous activity of bladder afferent nerves increases while their mechanical thresholds decrease (Habler et al, 1993).

Long-term changes in C-fiber afferent nerves leading to chronic bladder pain may involve structural or biochemical alterations of sensory neurons. Proto-oncogene products such as c-fos coordinate signal transduction and act as a third messenger, linking short-term cellular messages to long-term responses that influence gene expression (Menetrey et al, 1989). This type of signal transduction may occur with acute or chronic nociceptive stimuli because an increase in c-fos expression in the spinal cord has been observed following painful stimuli (Cruz et al, 1994). Birder and co-workers (1990, 1991) have examined the expression of c-fos in the spinal cord in response to either overdistention or instillation of chemical irritants into the bladders of cats and rats. The c-fos immunoreactivity was observed in regions of the dorsal horn of the sacral spinal cord corresponding to areas receiving bladder afferent nerve input. Furthermore, irritant instillation rather than overdistention was a more potent stimulus for c-fos expression. On the other hand, minimal c-fos staining was seen in the upper lumbar cord, which receives sympathetic afferent nerve input from the bladder. This latter data is consistent with Learmonth's (1931) work regarding the selectivity and specificity of pain transmission from the bladder in humans. Based on lesioning data in humans, **Learmonth (1931) suggested that sacral afferent fibers process information regarding mucosal irritation, whereas thoracolumbar sensory nerves originating as high as T6 transmitted messages pertaining to overdistention.**

One result of the proto-oncogene changes could be long-term alterations in receptor expression, neurotransmitter production, or mechanisms regulating transmitter release. Indeed, tissue damage and/or inflammation up-regulates tachykinin receptors (NK_2) located on the peripheral projections of sensory nerves as well as NK_1 receptors in the sacral spinal cord (Helke et al, 1990; Lecci et al, 1994; Kushner et al, 1995; Sokolov et al, 1995). This up-regulation of tachykinin receptors may produce an increased susceptibility to SP released from afferent nerves in response to pain and sensed as urinary urgency.

Another possibility is that inflammation leads to an increase in the duration or excitability of afferent fibers and subsequent cellular changes that alter receptor expression. This scenario involves glutamate (NMDA, AMPA, and kianate receptors) and opiate receptor mechanisms (Urban et al, 1994). For example, Rice and McMahon (1994) have demonstrated that the NMDA receptor antagonist (AP-5) prevents hyperreflexia associated with chemical cystitis but has little effect on normal bladder function. Kakizaki and co-workers (1996) extended this observation to show that AMPA as well as NMDA receptors are involved in nociceptive processing.

What transduces acute inflammatory or painful stimuli into long-term structural or functional changes? Acutely, the signal can be the intensity or duration of neural firing. Another possibility is that cytokines and growth factors lead to afferent plasticity. Nerve growth factor (NGF) is a trophic signaling protein that maintains the structure and function of sensory and adrenergic neurons. Acute administration of NGF lowers the threshold for afferent firing (Lewin et al, 1993). Following chemical or mechanical inflammation of the rat bladder, both NGF messenger RNA and protein levels rise in the bladder (Oddiah et al, 1995; Wakabayashi et al, 1995; Dupont et al, 1994). NGF causes enlargement of bladder afferent nerves in the lumbar (L1/L2) and sacral (L6/S1) DRGs. Enlargement of these DRGs in other conditions such as spinal cord transection is associated with increased excitability and changes in channel properties of afferent nerves (Yoshimura et al, 1995). McMahon and colleagues (1994) have recently shown that 80% of retrogradely labeled bladder neurons in the rat DRG possesses tyrosine kinase (trk) receptors that bind NGF and mediate its actions (trkA). Therefore, if inflammatory stimuli or injury up-regulate NGF receptors on bladder afferent nerves or increases NGF, a lowering or increased sensitivity of bladder afferents may occur over the long term. The profuse sensory innervation of the lower urinary tract with its potential exposure to changes in urine pH, ionic strengths, dietary substances, and infectious agents may explain the common development of irritative disorders such as cystitis, prostatitis, and urethritis.

Researchers have also postulated that afferent nerves participate in peripheral motor, secretory and neuroimmune processes (de Groat, 1987) (see Fig. 26–26). Electrical or chemical stimulation of bladder afferent nerves releases neuropeptides, which alter epithelial permeability (Koltzenburg and McMahon, 1986; Abelli et al, 1989b), smooth muscle contractility (Maggi et al, 1984, 1986, 1988b; Kalbfleisch and Daniel, 1987), and neurotransmitter release from adjacent nerves (Maggi and Meli, 1986; de Groat, 1987). Neuropeptides found within afferent nerves such as SP, ENK, and VIP also alter the function or growth of lymphocytes, macrophages, fibroblasts, and smooth muscle cells in culture (Nilsson et al, 1985; Mitsuhashi and Payan, 1987; Lotz et al, 1988). The notion that peripheral afferent nerves merely convey sensory information is simplistic. These nerves also mediate peripheral motor, secretory, or neuroimmune functions, and participate in inflammatory processes in the bladder. In some individuals, afferent nerves are undoubtedly involved in chronic pain.

PATHOPHYSIOLOGY

Based upon the preceding physiologic and pharmacologic discussions regarding bladder and urethral function, it is becoming possible to explain the consequences of injury or disease on micturition at the cellular level. More importantly, future therapies will rely on specific cellular or molecular targets. However, the responses of the smooth muscle or the nervous system to various stimuli are still unpredictable due in part to their capacity for reorganization and remodeling by neural plasticity, trophic factors or neurohumoral interactions. Contrary to previous beliefs, the morphology, function, and transmitter expression of adult neurons are not static. A dependent relationship exists between a nerve and its target (e.g., smooth muscle) and surrounding tissues. These complex relationships explain some of the unpredictable results of therapy or responses to disease. This section describes some conditions in which reorganization of bladder pathways produces voiding dysfunction.

Supraspinal Lesions

Given the wide array of inputs to the pontine micturition center and descending projections to the sacral parasympathetic nucleus, it is not surprising that many disorders of the brain elicit disturbances in bladder function resulting in either urinary retention or incontinence. Critical to the understanding of the pathophysiology of these conditions is the recognition that the coordination of the bladder contraction and external urethral sphincter relaxation occurs in the pons through interactions in the M and L regions (see Voiding Reflexes). **If the pathology is limited to suprapontine sites, coordination of the bladder and sphincter should be preserved (Blaivas, 1982, 1988).**

Acute lesions in the brain such as a cerebrovascular accident or removal of a tumor are often associated with urinary retention (Zhan et al, 1981; Tschida et al, 1983; Barnett and Hyland, 1952). This may be due to interruption of cortical pathways from the paracentral lobule that facilitate voiding. Alternatively, lack of micturition can result from increased inhibitory transmission, possibly mediated by either GABA or opiate receptors in the pons or sacral spinal cord.

Cerebellar ataxia, hydrocephalus, brain tumors, and recovery from strokes are often associated with facilitation of micturition expressed as detrusor hyperreflexia and urge incontinence (Leach et al, 1982; Ahlberg et al, 1988; Blaivas, 1988). If endogenous opiates in the pons regulate the setpoint for bladder contractions it is tempting to speculate that changes in opiate mechanisms may contribute to low-volume induced bladder contractions. Alternatively, increased glutamate transmission mediated by both NMDA and AMPA receptors in the brain and spinal cord could facilitate micturition. The dynamic responses of the neurons or receptors to injury or disease, which is termed *neural plasticity*, plays a role in these conditions.

A perplexing condition is Parkinson's disease. As observed with many suprapontine disorders, detrusor hyperreflexia is common. However, pathology within the basal ganglia cause disturbances in motor function. The onset of motor events is often delayed. In patients with Parkinson's disease, involuntary contractions are of short duration, onset of a voluntary micturition contraction is delayed, and relaxation of the external urethral sphincter is slowed. These events are manifested as urgency, urge incontinence, hesitancy, and slow urinary stream, which is difficult to distinguish from prostatism.

Spinal Cord Transection

After suprasacral spinal cord transection in humans and animals, micturition is abolished, but it subsequently returns weeks to months later (see Figs. 26–22, 26–24). When bladder emptying returns, it often occurs at a low volume and is incomplete. Incomplete emptying is the result of lack of coordination of the bladder with the external urethral sphincter, which is termed *detrusor sphincter dyssynergia*, and/or a poorly sustained detrusor contraction (see Fig. 26–24). Lesions above spinal level T6 can also produce loss of coordination between the detusor and bladder neck. Voiding in chronic spinal cats and rats is mediated by a sacral reflex. This spinal reflex occurs with a short central delay, suggesting that few synapses occur within the spinal micturition pathway. In chronic spinal cats the afferent limb for the spinal micturition reflex consists of unmyelinated C-fibers, whereas in intact animals it is composed of myelinated A-delta fibers (de Groat et al, 1981). In contrast, the latencies for supraspinal and spinal micturition reflexes in the rat correspond to A-delta afferent fibers (Mallory et al, 1989). In humans, capsaicin, which is known to affect C-fiber afferent nerves, can abolish voiding in spinal cord–injured patients (Fowler et al, 1994). **This observation suggests that C-fiber afferent nerves trigger a spinal reflex after removal of supraspinal inputs. These data reinforce the concept that reorganization of micturition reflex pathways occurs following spinal cord injury (de Groat et al, 1990a).**

The stimulus for the development or unmasking of a spinal reflex is unclear. Kruse and colleagues (1994) showed that development of a spinal reflex after spinal cord injury is not dependent on afferent input from the bladder. Rats with urinary diversion still develop a spinal reflex and detrusor-sphincter dyssynergia. Thus, techniques such as "bladder training" by clamping a catheter and allowing the bladder to periodically distend in hope of promoting return of voiding are unfounded.

In many species urination by neonates is not dependent upon a spinobulbospinal reflex (Thor et al, 1986). Rather, voiding relies on an exteroceptive somatobladder reflex triggered by cutaneous stimulation of the perineum. This behavioral response occurs when the mother licks the perineum of her newborn to initiate voiding. Separation of the mother from her newborn produces urinary retention. This excitatory somatovisceral reflex in newborns is preserved following spinal cord transection in neonates, indicating its spinal organization. **Similarly in humans voiding can be initiated in infants by suprapubic or perineal stimulation. The re-emergence of an excitatory somatobladder reflex is exploited by paraplegics to facilitate bladder emptying ("trigger voiding") and supports the notion of reorganization of sacral spinal centers following spinal cord injury.** This is not to say that a supraspinal reflex is not present in newborns. Kruse and de Groat (1990) have shown that a pontine reflex is present in newborns, but not fully operational. Maturation of afferent or central pathways may be necessary to cause voiding to be regulated by the supraspinal reflex. This process takes 1 to 3 weeks to occur in animals. During this period, increases in SP and CGRP are seen in the bladder, which suggests maturation of bladder afferents (Iuchi et al, 1994).

During postnatal development the excitatory somato-bladder response diminishes and is replaced by an inhibitory reflex whereby stimulation of the sacral dermatomes prevents or delays a detrusor contraction (Sato and Schmidt, 1987; Sato et al, 1992). **The adult pattern of somatovisceral (skin to bladder) inhibition explains the clinical efficacy of techniques for urge incontinence such as acupuncture, electrostimulation, and pelvic floor exercises.**

Peripheral Injury

Transection of the pelvic nerve or injury to the pelvic plexus can occur during surgery. In addition, selective sacral root transection has been performed to interrupt reflex pathways and inhibit bladder activity. These neural injuries may elicit compensatory changes in the remaining pathways supplying the bladder.

Decentralization of the bladder triggers a variety of neuroanatomic, pharmacologic, and electrophysiologic changes. The degree to which these alterations arise explains why cystometrograms in some patients with injury to nerves supplying the bladder show flaccid hypotonic bladders, whereas other individuals with similar injuries develop poorly compliant, hypertonic bladders.

Ultrastructural studies suggest that sprouting of adrenergic terminals in the bladder and pelvic plexus occurs following decentralization (Elbadawi and Atta, 1989; Hanno et al, 1988). Sundin and co-workers (1977) also document increased fluorescent adrenergic fibers in the bladder following decentralization. Ekstrom and Elmer (1977) showed a fall and then a rise in acetyl co-transferase acting in the hemidenervated bladder. Furthermore, cholinergic terminals in the bladder are preserved following decentralization only if hypogastric pathways are preserved (Elbadawi et al, 1989).

Adrenergic innervation and sensitivity of the urethra to adrenergic drug changes following parasympathetic decentralization or obstruction (Koyanagi, 1979; Rohner et al, 1978). Alpha-adrenergic antagonists increase urethral flow rates and reduce residual urine volumes in patients with neurogenic bladders or obstruction (Krane and Olsson, 1973; Scott and Morrow, 1978; Caine, 1986).

Electrophysiologic data show that electrical stimulation of the hypogastric nerve in intact cats elicits a transient increase or no change in intravesical pressure. Following parasympathetic decentralization, hypogastric stimulation evokes atropine-sensitive bladder contractions (de Groat and Kawatani, 1989).

These data suggest that sympathetic pathways to the bladder are reorganized and become excitatory after removal of sacral preganglionic input (Fig. 26–29). One explanation is that preganglionic fibers in the hypogastric nerve provide innervation to cholinergic postganglionic neurons that lost preganglionic input from the pelvic nerve. **Furthermore, up-regulation of adrenergic mechanisms through excitatory hypogastric input could explain the failure of sacral rhizotomies performed for detrusor hyperreflexia to maintain a flaccid bladder. With regard to therapy, whereas anticholinergic drugs increase bladder compliance in the partially decentralized bladder, alpha-adrenergic blockers are sometimes of additional benefit in treating neurogenic dysfunction (Andersson, 1986).**

The stimulus for the reorganization of adrenergic mechanism may rely on production of growth factors. Following either unilateral decentralization or denervation of the bladder, the ipsilateral bladder undergoes hypertrophy (Ekstrom et al, 1986; Nilvebrant et al, 1989; Tuttle et al, 1994). The level of NGF, which promotes maintenance and growth of sensory and adrenergic nerves, increases in the bladder (Tuttle et al, 1994). NGF may be responsible for attempts at bladder re-innervation.

With injury, changes are not limited to the peripheral nerves or bladder. Following removal of the pelvic ganglia, changes in the sacral spinal cord also develop. NOS immunoreactivity increases in DRG cells labeled from the bladder (Vizzard et al, 1993, 1995). GAP-43, a marker for neuronal growth, increases in the dorsal horn and sacral parasympathetic nucleus (Tang et al, 1994). It has been postulated that regions of the CNS that express GAP-43 into adulthood are more likely to undergo neural plasticity. Sacral-dorsal horns and anatomic centers express low levels of GAP-43 in the adult.

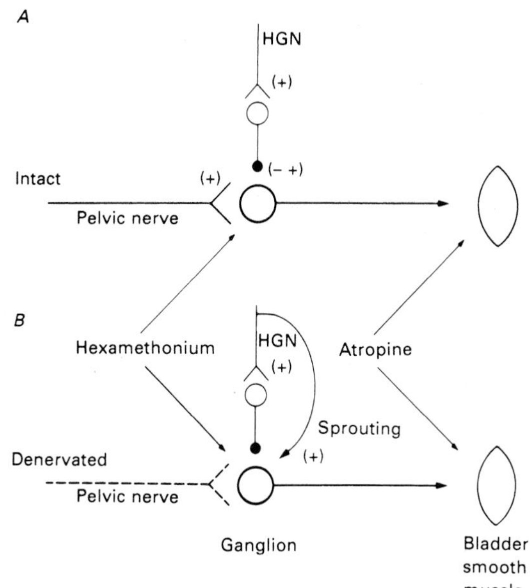

Figure 26–29. Schematic representation of possible reorganization of parasympathetic pathways following decentralization of the bladder. *A*, Stimulation of the hypogastric nerve (HGN) normally modulates parasympathetic transmission but has a minimal direct effect on the detrusor. *B*, Following pelvic nerve transection in the cat with intact HGN pathways, increased adrenergic fibers and maintenance of some cholinergic fibers in detrusor are observed (Elbadawi et al, 1989). HGN stimulation after pelvic nerve transection now evokes an atropine-sensitive bladder contraction. Postulated sprouting of HGN preganglionic fibers could explain anatomic, electrophysiologic, and pharmacologic results. (From de Groat WC, Kawatani M: J Physiol [Lond] 1989; 409:431.)

Obstruction

Bladder outlet obstruction often produces detrusor hypertrophy and bladder hyperactivity (Gosling and Dixon, 1983). Obstruction-induced detrusor instability with irritative voiding symptoms has been attributed to a denervation supersensitivity because increased contractile responses of the bladder smooth muscle to cholinergic agonists and electrical stimulation have been observed (Speakman et al, 1987). Molecular biologic techniques have also shown that alterations in detrusor contractility may result from changes in contractile proteins (Cher et al, 1990; Uvelius et al, 1989). Following obstruction, a wide variety of structural, pharmacologic, and physiologic changes occur in the lower urinary tract (Levin et al, 1990). These changes include alterations in neural function—especially those of bladder afferent nerves, as noted by changes in afferent neuropeptides are spinal responses to the NK antagonists (Ishizuka et al, 1994). Although the apparent density of nerve fibers in the bladder drops after urethral obstruction, perikarya for afferent and efferent nerves enlarge, suggesting that changes are occurring in these nerves (Steers and de Groat, 1988; Steers et al, 1991a). Alterations occur in neural networks in the central nervous system following obstruction of the lower urinary tract. A protein associated with axonal growth, GAP-43, increases in the sacral spinal cord in the same distribution as bladder afferent nerves (Steers et al, 1991a, 1996). This region is also more vigorously labeled using retrograde tracers following obstruction. Surprisingly, these changes mirror those that develop in spinalized animals. Thus, it is intriguing that electrophysiologic data indicate an enhancement of the spinal micturition reflex pathway (Steers and de Groat, 1988). Both patients with obstruction and those who are paraplegics develop poorly sustained involuntary bladder contractions. The mechanism for this neural plasticity in obstruction depends on signaling between the bladder and its innervation because these changes fail to develop if obstruction is preceded by denervation.

As previously mentioned, NGF rises in the bladder with denervation and inflammation. Thus, it is of interest that increases in NGF and possibly other neurotrophic factors in obstructed bladders are temporally related to a doubling of voiding frequency (Steers et al, 1989). Endogenous NGF antibody production prevents the obstruction-induced neuroanatomic and physicologic changes and the increase in voiding frequency (Steers et al, 1991b, 1996). These experiments demonstrate that NGF mediates neural changes and bladder hyperactivity. Thus, future therapies for bladder dysfunction could include manipulation of various growth factors (Buttyan et al, 1992) or their receptors that play a role in neural plasticity associated with bladder dysfunction.

SUMMARY

The bladder and its outlet have a dual function—urine storage and release. These events can be best understood by examining the myogenic and neurogenic mechanisms regulating the lower urinary tract. Bladder smooth contractility depends on access of contractile proteins to Ca^{2+}. Neurotransmitters and circulatory factors acting on membrane-bound receptors regulate smooth muscle contractility.

Voiding requires participation of both autonomic and somatic pathways. Switching between voiding and urine storage and the prevention of overactivity of the system requires integration and coordination of excitatory and inhibitory mechanisms and numerous feedback loops. These networks are operative over several levels of the neuraxis and are capable of significant plasticity following neuronal injury, aging, and disease. An understanding of the physiologic events mediating micturition and continence provides a rational basis for the management of lower urinary tract dysfunction.

REFERENCES

Abelli L, Conte B, Somma V, Maggi CA, Giuliani S, Meli A: A method for studying pain arising from the urinary bladder in conscious, freely moving rats. J Urol 1989a; 141:148.

Abelli L, Somma V, Maggi CA, et al: Effects of tachykinins and selective tackykinin receptor agonists on vascular permeability in the rat lower urinary tract: Evidence for the involvement of NK-1 receptors. J Auton Pharmacol 1989b; 9:253–263.

Abrams P, Fineley R, Torrens MJ: Urodynamics. Berlin, Springer-Verlag, 1983, p 229.

Ahlberg J, Norlen L, Blomstrand C, Wikkelso C: Outcome of shunt operation on urinary incontinence in normal pressure hydrocephalus predicted by lumbar puncture. J Neurol Neurosurg Psych 1988; 51:105–108.

Akasu T, Hasuo H, Tokimasa T: Activation of 5-HT_3 receptor subtypes causes rapid excitation of rabbit parasympathetic neurons. Br J Pharmacol 1987; 91:453.

Akasu T, Shinnick-Gallagher P, Gallagher JP: Adenosine mediates a slow hyperpolarizing synaptic potential in autonomic neurones. Nature 1984; 311:62.

Alberts P: Classification of the presynaptic muscarinic receptor subtype that regulates 3H-acetylcholine secretion in the guinia pig urinary bladder in vitro. J Pharmacol Exper Ther 1995; 274:458–468.

Andersson KE: Clinical relevance of some findings in neuroanatomy and neurophysiology of the lower urinary tract. Clin Sci 1986; 70(Suppl 14):215–325.

Andersson KE: Pharmacology of lower urinary tract smooth muscle and penile erectile tissues. Pharmacol Rev 1993; 45:253–307.

Andersson KE, Fovaeus M, Hedlund H, Sundler R: Muscarinic receptor stimulation of phosphoinositide hydrolysis in human urinary bladder. J Urol 1989; 141:324A.

Andersson KE, Persson K: Nitric oxide synthase and nitric oxide-mediated effects in lower urinary tract smooth muscles. World J Urol 1994; 12:274–280.

Andersson KE, Persson CGA, Alm P, Kullander S, Ulmsten U: Effects of acetylcholine, noradrenaline, and prostaglandins on the isolated, perfused human fetal urethra. Acta Physiol Scand 1978; 104:394–401.

Aoki M, Watanabe H, Naminki A, et al: Mechanism of urinary retention following intrathecal administration of morphine. Matsui 1982; 31:939.

Araki I: Inhibitory postsynaptic currents and the effects of GABA on visually identified sacral parasympathetic preganglionic neurons in neonatal rats. J Neurophysiol 1994; 72:2903–2910.

Araki I, de Groat WC: Patch clamp analysis of synaptic inputs to sacral parasympathetic preganglionic neurons. J Urol 1995; 153:459A.

Aranda B, Cramer P: Effects of apomorphine and L-dopa on the parkinsonian bladder. Neurourol Urodynam 1993; 12:203–209.

Awad SA, Downie JW: The effect of adrenergic drugs and hypogastric nerve stimulation on the canine urethra. Invest Urol 1976; 13:298.

Awad SA, Downie JW, Lywood DW: Sympathetic activity in the proximal urethra in patients with urinary obstruction. J Urol 1976; 115:545.

Bahns E, Ernsberger U, Janig W, Nelke A: Functional characteristics of lumbar visceral afferent fibers from the urinary bladder and urethra in the cat. Pflugers Arch 1986; 407:510.

Barnett HI, Hyland HH: Tumors involving the brain stem. Q J Med 1952; 21:265.

Barrington FJF: The component reflexes of micturition in the cat. Parts I and II. Brain 1931; 54:177.

Batra S, Andersson KE: Oestrogen-induced changes in muscarinic receptor density and contractile responses in the female rabbit urinary bladder. Acta Physiol Scand 1989; 137:135–141.

Batra S, Bjorklund A, Hedlund H, Andersson KE: Identification and characterization of muscarinic cholinergic receptors in the human urinary bladder and parotid gland. J Auton Nerv Sys 1987; 20:129.

Bauer FE, Christofides ND, Hacker GW, et al: Distribution of galanin immunoreactivity in the genitourinary tract of man and rat. Peptides 1986; 7:5.

Bazeed MA, Thuroff JM, Schmidt RA, Tanagho EA: Histochemical study of urethral striated muscle in the dog. J Urol 1982; 128:406.

Beattie MS, Li Q, Leedy MG, Bresnahan JC: Motoneurons innervating the external anal and urethral sphincters of the female cat have different patterns of dendritic arborization. Neurosci Lett 1990; 111:69.

Bennett BC, Vizzard MA, Booth AM, de Groat WC: Role of nitric oxide in reflex urethral sphincter relaxation during micturition. Soc Neurosci Abstr 1993; 19:511

Benson GS, McConnell JA, Wood JG: Adrenergic innervation of the human bladder body. J Urol 1979; 122:189.

Benson GS, Raezer DM, Anderson JR, et al: Effect of levodopa on urinary bladder. Urology 1976a; 17:24.

Benson GS, Wein AJ, Raezer DM, Corriere JN: Adrenergic and cholinergic stimulation and blockade of the human bladder base. J Urol 1976b; 116:174.

Berggren A, Rubenson A, Sillen U: Involvement of opioid mechanisms in peripheral motor control of detrusor muscle. Pharmacol Toxicol 1992; 71:179–184.

Birder LA, Roppolo JR, Iadarola MJ, de Groat WC: Spinal cord distribution of C-fos protein in visceral versus somatic models of chemical inflammation. Abstr Soc Neurosci 1990; 15:468.

Birder LA, Roppolo JR, Iadarola MJ, de Groat WC: Electrical stimulation of visceral afferent pathways in the pelvic nerve increases c-fos in the rat lumbosacral spinal cord. Neurosci Lett 1991; 129:193–196.

Blaivas JG: The neurophysiology of micturition: a clinical study of 550 patients. J Urol 1982; 127:958–966.

Blaivas JG: Neurologic dysfunctions. *In* Yalla S, McGuire E, Elbadawi A, Blaivas J, eds: Neurourology and Urodynamics: Principles and Practice. New York, Macmillan, 1988, pp 343–357.

Blaivas JG, Labib KL, Bauer SB, Retik AB: A new approach to electromyography of the external urethral sphincter. J Urol 1977; 117:773.

Blank MA, Anand P, Lumb BM, et al: Release of vasoactive intestinal polypeptide-like immunoreactivity from cat urinary bladder and sacral spinal cord during pelvic nerve stimulation. Dig Dis Sci 1984; 29:115.

Blok BFM, Holstege G: Direct projections from the periaqueductal gray to the pontine micturition center (M-region). An anterograde and retrograde tracing study in the cat. Neurosci Lett 1994; 166:93–96.

Blok BF, Willemsen AT, Holstege G: Mapping micturition control areas in the central nervous system with positron emission tomography (PET). Soc Neurosci Abstr 1995; 21:1872.

Boels PJ, Arner A, Malmqvist U, Uvelius B: Structure and mechanics of growing arterial microvessels from hypertrophied urinary bladder in rat. Pflugers Arch Eur J Physiol 1994; 426:506–515.

Bonner T: New subtypes of muscarinic acetylcholine receptors. Trends in Pharmacol 1989; 4(Suppl):11–14.

Booth AM, Hisamitsu T, Kawatani M, de Groat WC: Regulation of urinary bladder capacity by endogenous opioid peptides. J Urol 1985; 133:339.

Booth JR, Booth AM, de Groat WC: The effects of naloxone on the neural control of the urinary bladder of the cat. Brain Res 1983; 264:355.

Borda E, Conteras-Ortiz R, Gutinski R, Gimeno MF: In vitro effect of acetylcholine and bethanecol in the contractions of the human detrusor muscle. Influence of prostaglandins. Arch Inv Pharmacodyn Ther 1982; 259:31–39.

Bors E, Comarr AE: Neurological Urology. Baltimore, University Park Press, 1971.

Bowker RM, Westlund KN, Sullivan MC, et al: Descending serotonergic, peptidergic, and cholinergic pathways from raphe nuclei: A multiple transmitter complex. Brain Res 1983; 288:33.

Brading A: Physiology of bladder smooth muscle. *In* Torrens M, Morrison JFB, eds: The Physiology of the Lower Urinary Tract. Berlin, Springer-Verlag, 1987, pp 161–191.

Brading AF, Williams JH: Contractile responses of smooth muscle strips from rat and guinea pig urinary bladder to transmural stimulation: Effects of atropine and methylene ATP. Br J Pharmacol 1990; 99:493.

Bradley WE, Conway CJ: Bladder representation in the pontine-mesencephalic reticular formation. Exp Neurol 1966; 16:237.

Bradley WE, Scott FB: Physiology of the Urinary Bladder: *In* Harrison JH, Gittes RF, Pearlmutter AD, et al, eds: Campbell's Urology, 4th ed. Philadelphia, W.B. Saunders Company, 1978, pp 87–124.

Brendler CB, Radebaugh LC, Mohler JL: Topical oxybutinin chloride for relaxation of dysfunctional bladders. J Urol 1989; 141:1350.

Brindley GS: Sacral root and hypogastric plexus stimulators and what these implants tell us about autonomic actions on the bladder and urethra. Clin Sci 1986; 70:415.

Brindley GS, Polkey CE, Rushton DN, Cardozo L: Sacral anterior root stimulators for bladder control in paraplegia. The first 50 cases. J Neurol Neurosurg Psychiat 1986; 49:1104.

Broughton RJ: Sleep disorders: Disorders of arousal? Science 1968; 159:1070.

Bultitude MJ, Hills NH, Shuttleworth KE: Clinical and experimental studies on the action of prostaglandins and their synthesis inhibitors on detrusor muscle in vitro and in vivo. Br J Urol 1976; 48:631–637.

Burnstock G: The changing face of autonomic neurotransmission. Acta Physiol Scand 1986a; 126:67.

Burnstock G: Purines as cotransmitters in adrenergic and cholinergic neurones. *In* Hokfelt K, Fuxe K, Pernow B, eds: Progress in Brain Research. Amsterdam, Elsevier, 1986b, pp 193–203.

Buttyan R, Jacobs BZ, Blaivas J, Levin RM: Early molecular response to rabbit bladder outlet obstruction. Neurourol Urodynam 1992; 11:225–229.

Caine M: The present role of alpha adrenergic blockers in the treatment of prostatic hyperplasia. J Urol 1986; 136:1.

Callahan SM, Creed KE: Electrical and mechanical activity of isolated lower urinary tract of the guinea-pig. Br J Pharmacol 1981; 74:353.

Callahan SM, Creed KE: The effects of estrogens on spontaneous activity and responses to phenylephedrine of the mammalian urethra. J Physiol (Lond) 1985; 358:35.

Cardozo LD, Stanton SL: A comparison between bromocriptine and indomethacin in the treatment of detrusor instability. J Urol 1980; 123:399–401.

Castleden CM, Morgan B: The effect of beta-adrenoceptor agonists on urinary incontinence in the elderly. Br J Clin Pharmacol 1980; 10:619.

Chacko S, Longhurst P: Regulation of actomyosin and contraction in smooth muscle. World J Urol 1994; 12:292–297.

Chancellor MB, Kaplan SA, Blaivas JG: The cholinergic and purinergic components of detrusor contractility in a whole rabbit bladder model. J Urol 1992; 148:906–909.

Chapple CR, Helm CW, Blease S, et al: Asymptomatic bladder neck incompetence in nulliparous females. Br J Urol 1989; 64:357–361.

Chen C, Ma C, de Groat WC: Effects of capsaicin on micturition and associated reflexes in rats. Am J Physiol 1993; 265:R132–R138.

Cher ML, Kamm KE, McConnell JD: Stress generation and myosin phosphorylation in the obstructed bladder. J Urol 1990; 143:355A.

Chess-Williams R, Aston N, Couldwell C: Alpha-1A subtype mediates contraction of the rat urethra. J Auton Pharmacol 1994; 14:375–381.

Christmas TJ, Chapple CR, Kempster PA, et al: The role of subcutaneous apomorphine in the treatment of Parkinsonian voiding dysfunction. J Urol 1989; 141:327A.

Cohen ML: Canine, but not rat bladder contracts to serotonin via activation of 5-HT_2 receptors. J Urol 1990; 143:1032.

Collumbine H, McKee W, Creasey NH: The effects of atropine sulfate upon healthy male subjects. Q J Exp Physiol 1955; 30:309–319.

Constantinou CE, Govan DE: Spatial distribution and timing of transmitted and reflexly generated urethral pressures in healthy women. J Urol 1982; 127:964–977.

Coplen DE, Macarak EJ, Levin RM: Developmental changes in normal fetal whole bladder physiology. J Urol 1994; 151:1391–1395.

Corsi M, Pietra C, Toson G, et al: Pharmacological analysis of 5-hydroxytryptamine (5-HT) on electrically-induced contractions in the mouse urinary bladder. Br J Pharmacol 1991; 104:719–725.

Creed K: The role of hypogastric nerve in bladder and urethral activity of the dog. Br J Pharmacol 1979; 65:367.

Crowe R, Light K, Chilton CP, Burnstock G: Vasoactive intestinal polypeptide-somatostatin-and substance P-immunoreactive nerves in the smooth and striated muscle of the intrinsic external urethral sphincter of patients with spinal cord injury. J Urol 1986; 136:487.

Crowe R, Moss HE, Chapple CR, et al: Patients with lower motor spinal cord lesion: A decrease of vasoactive intestinal polypeptide, calcitonin gene-related peptide and substance P, but not neuropeptide Y and somatostatin-immunoreactive nerves in the detrusor muscle of the bladder. (Abstract.) J Urol 1991; 145:600–604.

Cruz F, Avelino A, Lima D, Coimbra A: Activation of c-fos proto-oncogene in the spinal cord following noxious stimulation of the urinary bladder. Somatosens Motor Res 1994; 11:319–325.

D'Agostino G, Kilbinger H, Chiari MC, Grana E: Presynaptic inhibitory muscarinic receptors modulating [^{3}H] acetylcholine release in the rat urinary bladder. J Pharm Exper Ther 1986; 239:522.

Dail WG, Minorsky N, Moll MA, Manzanares K: The hypogastric nerve pathway to penile erectile tissue and histochemical evidence supporting a vasodilatory role. J Auton Nerv Sys 1986; 15:341.

Danuser H, Thor KB: Inhibition of central sympathetic and somatic outflow to the lower urinary tract of the cat by the alpha-1 adrenergic receptor antagonist prazosin. J Urol 1995; 153:1308–1312.

de Groat WC: The effects of glycine, GABA and strychnine on sacral parasympathetic preganglionic neurons. Brain Res 1970; 18:542.

de Groat WC: Excitation and inhibition of sacral parasympathetic neurons by visceral and cutaneous stimuli in the cat. Brain Res 1971; 33:499.

de Groat WC: Nervous control of the urinary bladder in the cat. Brain Res 1975; 87:201.

de Groat WC: Neuropeptides in pelvic afferent pathways. Experientia 1987; 43:801.

de Groat WC, Booth AM: Inhibition and facilitation in parasympathetic ganglia of the urinary bladder. Fed Proc 1980; 39:2990.

de Groat WC, Booth AM, Krier J, et al: Neural control of the urinary bladder and large intestine. *In* Brooks C, Koizumi K, Sato A, eds: Integrative Function of the Autonomic Nervous System. Amsterdam, Elsevier/North Holland Biomed Press, 1979, 50–66.

de Groat WC, Kawatani M: Neural control of the urinary bladder: Possible relationship between peptidergic inhibitory mechanisms and detrusor instability. Neurourol Urodynam 1984; 4:285.

de Groat WC, Kawatani M: Reorganization of sympathetic preganglionic connections in cat bladder ganglia following parasympathetic denervation. J Physiol (Lond) 1989; 409:431.

de Groat WC, Kawatani M, Booth AM: Enkephalinergic modulation of cholinergic transmission in parasympathetic ganglia of the cat urinary bladder. *In* Hanin I, ed: Dynamics of Cholinergic Function. New York, Plenum, 1986a, pp 1007–1017.

de Groat WC, Kawatani M, Hisamitsu T, et al: The role of neuropeptides in the sacral autonomic reflex pathways of the cat. J Auton Nerv Sys 1983; 7:339.

de Groat WC, Kawatani M, Hisamitsu T, et al: Neural control of micturition: The role of neuropeptides. J Auton Nerv Sys (Suppl) 1986b; 369.

de Groat WC, Kawatani M, Hisamitsu T, et al: Mechanisms underlying the recovery of urinary bladder function following spinal cord injury. J Auton Nerv Sys 1990a; 30:S71–S78.

de Groat WC, Lalley PM: Reflex firing in lumbar sympathetic outflow to activation of vesical afferent fibers. J Physiol (Lond) 1972; 226:289.

de Groat WC, Nadelhaft I, Milne RJ, et al: Organization of the sacral parasympathetic reflex pathways to the urinary bladder and large intestine. J Auton Nerv Sys 1981; 3:135.

de Groat WC, Ryall RW: Reflexes to sacral parasympathetic concerned with micturition in the cat. J Physiol 1969; 200:87.

de Groat WC, Steers WD: Autonomic regulation of the urinary bladder and sexual organs. *In* Loewy AD, Spyer KM, eds: Central Regulation of the Autonomic Functions, 1st ed. Oxford, Oxford University Press, 1990, p 313.

de Groat WC, Wright FF, White G: A patch-clamp analysis of tetrodotoxin-sensitive and -resistant Na^{2+} currents in neurons isolated from sensory and parasympathetic ganglia of the adult rat. Abstr Soc Neurosci 1990b; 15:440.

Delaere KP, Thomas CM, Moonen WA, Debruyne FM: The value of intravesicle prostaglandin E_2 and $F_{2\alpha}$ in women with abnormalities of bladder emptying. Br J Urol 1981; 53:306–309.

De Lancey JOL: Structural aspects of urethrovesical function in the female. Neurourol Urodynam 1988; 7:509.

De Lancey JOL: Pubovesical ligaments: A separate structure from the urethral supports ("pubo-urethral ligaments"). Neurourol Urodynam 1989; 8:53.

de Laverolle NC, LaMotte CC: The human spinal cord: Substance P and met-Enkephalin immunoreactivity. J Neurosci 1982; 2:1369.

Denny-Brown D, Robertson EG: On the physiology of micturition. Brain 1933; 56:149.

Desmond AD, Bultitude MI, Hills NH, Shuttleworth KE: Clinical experience with intravesical prostaglandin E2. A prospective study in 36 patients. Br J Urol 1980; 52:357–366.

Diokno AC, Koff SA, Bender LF: Periurethral striated muscle activity in neurogenic bladder dysfunction. J Urol 1974; 112:743.

Dion S, Corcos J, Carmel M, et al: Substance P and neurokinins as stimulants of the human isolated urinary bladder. Neuropeptides 1988; 11:83–87.

Dixon J, Gosling J: Structure and innervation of human bladder. *In* Torrens M, Morrison JFB, eds: The Physiology of the Lower Urinary Tract. Berlin, Springer-Verlag, 1987, pp 3–22.

Domin J, Ghatei MA, Chohan P, Bloom SR: Characterization of neuromedin u-like immunoreactivity in rat, porcine, guinea-pig, and human tissue extracts using a specific radioimmunoassay. Biochem Biophys Res Commun 1986; 140:1127.

Donaldson PJ, Chen LK, Lewis SA: Effects of serosal axion composition on the permeability properties of rabbit urinary bladder. Am J Physiol 1989; 256:F1125.

Donker PJ, Droes JP, Van Alder BM: Anatomy of the musculature and innovation of the bladder and urethra. *In* Chisholm GO, Williams DI, eds: Scientific Foundations of Urology. Chicago, Year Book, 1982, pp 404–441.

Downie JW, Espey MJ, Gajewski JB: Alpha 2-adrenoceptors not imidazole receptors mediate depression of a sacral spinal reflex in the cat. Eur J Pharmacol 1991; 195:301–304.

Dray A, Metsch R: The basal ganglia and the control of urinary bladder motility in the rat. Soc Neurosci Abstr 1983; 9:952.

Dray A, Metsch R: Opioid receptor subtype invoked in the central inhibition of bladder motility. Eur J Pharmacol 1984a; 104:47.

Dray A, Metsch R: Inhibition of urinary bladder contractions by a special action of morphine and other opioids. J Pharmacol Exper Ther 1984b; 231:254.

Dun NJ, Dun SL, Wu SY, et al: Nitric oxide synthase immunoreactivity in the rat, mouse, cat and squirrel monkey spinal cord. Neuroscience 1993; 54:845–857.

Dupont M, Steers WD, McCarty R, Tuttle JB: Neural plasticity and alterations in nerve growth factor and norepinephrine in response to bladder inflammation. J Urol 1994; 151:284.

Durant PA, Lucas PC, Yaksh TL: Micturition in unanesthetized rats: Spinal versus peripheral pharmacology of the adrenergic system. J Pharm Exper Ther 1988a; 245:426.

Durant PAC, Yaksh TL: Drug effects on urinary bladder tone during spinal morphine-induced inhibition of the micturition reflex in unanesthetized rats. Anesthesiology 1988; 68:325.

Durant PA, Yaksh TL, Wicks WC: Micturition in unanesthetized rats: Effects of intrathecal capsaicin, 6-hydroxydopamine and 5, 6-dihydroxytryptamine on bladder function in unanesthetized rats. Brain Res 1988b; 451:301–308.

Eaton GC, Hamilton KL, Johnson KE: Intracellular acidosis blocks the basolateral Na-K pump in rabbit urinary bladder. Am J Physiol 1984; 247:F946.

Edvardsen P: Nervous control of the urinary bladder in cats, I. The collecting phase. Acta Physiol Scand 1968; 72:157.

Edyvane KA, Marshall VR: Neuropeptides in the human urinary tract. Neurourol Urodyn 1990; 9:346–347.

Ehren I, Hammarstrom M, Adolfsson J, Wiklund NP: Induction of calcium-dependent nitric oxide synthase by sex hormones in the guinea pig urinary bladder. Acta Physiol Scand 1995; 153:393–394.

Ehren I, Iverson H, Jansson O, et al: Localization of nitric oxide synthase activity in the human lower urinary tract and its correlation with neuroeffector responses. Urology 1994; 44:683–687.

Ek A, Alan P, Hendersson KE, Persson CG: Adrenergic and cholinergic nerves of the human urethra and urinary bladder. A histochemical study. Acta Physiol Scand 1977; 99:345.

Ek A, Andersson KE, Ulmsten U: The effects of norepinephrine and bethanecol on the human urethral closure pressure profile. Scand J Urol Nephrol 1978; 12:97–104.

Ekstrom B, Stahl M, Mattiasson A, et al: Effects of tolterodine on bladder function in healthy volunteers. J Urol 1995; 153:394(Abstract).

Ekstrom J, Elmer M: Choline acetyltransferase activity in the denervated urinary bladder of the rat. Acta Physiol Scand 1977; 101:58–62.

Ekstrom J, Iosif CS, Malmberg L: Effects of long-term treatment with estrogen and progesterone on in vivo muscle responses of the female rabbit urinary bladder and urethra to autonomic drugs and nerve stimulation. J Urol 1993; 150:1284–1288.

Ekstrom J, Malmberg L, Oberg S: Unilateral denervation of the rat urinary bladder and reinnervation: A predominance for ipsilateral changes. Acta Physiol Scand 1986; 127:223–231.

Elam K, Thoren P, Svensson TH: Locus coeruleus neurons and sympathetic nerves: Activation by visceral afferents. Brain Res 1986; 375:117.

Elbadawi A: Neuromorphologic basis of vesicourethral function. Histochemistry, ultrastructure, and function of intrinsic nerves of the bladder and urethra. Neurourol Urodynam 1982; 1:3.

Elbadawi A, Atta MA: Ultrastructural analysis of vesicourethral innervation: IV. Evidence for somatomotor plus autonomic innervation of the male feline rhabdosphincter. Neurourol Urodynam 1985; 4:23.

Elbadawi A, Atta MA: Intrinsic neuromuscular defects in the neurogenic bladder: X. Value and limitations of neurohistochemistry. Neurourol Urodyn 1989; 8:263–276.

Elbadawi A, Schenk EA: Dual innervation of the mammalian urinary bladder; a histochemical study of the distributions of cholinergic and adrenergic nerves. Am J Anat 1966; 119:405.

Elbadawi A, Schenk EA: A new theory of the innervation of the bladder musculature: IV. Innervation of the vesicourethral junction and external urethral sphincter. J Urol 1974; 111:613.

Elliot RA, Castleden CM, Miodrag A: The effect of in vivo oestrogen pretreatment on the contractile response of rat isolated detrusor muscle. Br J Pharmacol 1992; 107:766–770.

Englund SE: Observations on the migration of somal labelled substances between the urinary bladder and the blood in rabbit. Review of the literature. Acta Radiol 1956; 135(Suppl):1.

Enhorning G: Simultaneous recording of the intravesical and intraurethral pressures. Acta Chir Scand 1961; 276(Suppl):1.

Enoch DM, Kerr FWL: Hypothalamic vasopressor and vesicopressor pathways. *In* Functional Studies. Arch Neurol (Chicago) 1967a; 16:290.

Enoch DM, Kerr FWL: Hypothalamic vasopressor and vesicopressor pathways. II. Anatomical study of their course and connections. Arch Neurol (Chicago) 1967b; 16:307.

Erspamer V, Ronzoni G, Erspamer F: Effects of active peptides on the isolated muscle of the human urinary bladder. Invest Urol 1981; 18:302.

Espey MJ, Downie JW, Fine A: Effect of 5-HT receptor and adrenoceptor antagonists on micturition in conscious cats. Eur J Pharmacol 1992; 221:167–170.

Ewalt DH, Howard P, Blyth B: Is lamina propria matrix responsible for normal bladder compliance? J Urol 1992; 148:544–550.

Fedirchuk B, Downie J, Shefchyk SJ: Reduction of perineal evoked excitatory postsynaptic potentials in cat lumbar and sacral motoneurons during micturition. J Neurosci 1994; 14:6153–6159.

Ferguson DR, Marchant JS: Inhibitory actions of GABA on rabbit urinary bladder muscle strips: Mediation by potassium channels. Br J Pharmacol 1995; 115:81–83.

Fletcher TF, Bradley WD: Afferent nerve endings in the urinary bladder of the cat. Am J Anat 1968; 128:147.

Foldspang A, Mommsen S: Adult female urinary incontinence and childhood bedwetting. J Urol 1994; 152:85–88.

Foster CD, Fuju K, Kingdon J, Brading AF: The effect of cromakalim on the smooth muscle of the guinea pig urinary bladder. Br J Pharmacol 1989; 97:281.

Fovaeus M, Andersson K-E, Batra S, et al: Effects of calcium, calcium channel blockers and Bay K 8644 on contractions induced by muscarinic receptor stimulation of isolated bladder muscle from rabbit and man. J Urol 1987; 137:798.

Fovaeus M, Andersson KE, Hedlund H: The action of pinacidil in the isolated human bladder. J Urol 1989; 141:637.

Fowler C, Beck RO, Gerrard S, et al: Intravesical capsaicin for treatment of detrusor hyperreflexia. J Neurol Neurosurg Psych 1994; 57:169–173.

Fowler CJ, Jewkes D, McDonald WI: Intravesical capsaicin for neurogenic bladder dysfunction. Lancet 1992; 339:1239–1240.

Fujii K, Foster CD, Brading AF, Parekh AB: Potassium channel blockers and the effects of cromakalin on the smooth muscle of the guinea-pig bladder. Br J Pharmacol 1990; 99:779.

Gabella G: The structural relations between nerve fibers and muscle cells in the urinary bladder of the rat. J Neurocytol 1995; 24:159–187.

Gao X, Buffington CAT, Au J: Effect of interstitial cystitis on drug absorption from the urinary bladder. J Pharmacol Exper Ther 1994; 271:818–823.

Garry RC, Roberts TDM, Todd JK: Reflexes involving the external urethral sphincter in the cat. J Physiol (Lond) 1959; 149:653.

Gary T, Robertson D: Lessons learned from dopamine β-hydroxylase deficiency in humans. News Physiol Sci 1994; 9:35–39.

Gibson SJ, Polak JM, Arand P, et al: A VIP/PHI containing pathway links urinary bladder and sacral spinal cord. Peptides 1986; 7(Suppl):1205.

Gibson SJ, Polak JM, Bloom SR, Wall PD: The distribution of nine peptides in rat spinal cord with special emphasis on the substantia gelatenosa and on the area around the central canal (lamina x). J Comp Neurol 1981; 201:65.

Gillberg PG, Moderi AR, Sparf B: Tolterodine—A new agent with tissue effect selectivity for urinary bladder. (Abstract.) Neurourol Urodynam 1994; 13:435.

Godfraind T, Govoni S: Increasing complexity revealed in regulation of Ca^{2+} antagonist receptor. Trends Pharmacol Sci 1989; 10:120.

Gosling JA, Dixon JS: Detrusor morphology in relation to bladder outflow obstruction and instability. *In* Hinman F, ed: Benign Prostatic Hypertrophy. Berlin, Springer-Verlag, 1983, pp 666–671.

Gosling JA, Dixon JS, Critchley OD, Thompson SA: A comparative study of the human external sphincter and periurethral levator ani muscles. Br J Urol 1981; 53:35–41.

Gosling JA, Dixon JS, Humpherson JR: Functional Anatomy of the Urinary Tract. Edinburgh, Churchill Livingstone, 1983, p 1.

Gosling JA, Dixon JS, Lendon RG: The autonomic innervation of the human male and female bladder neck and proximal urethra. J Urol 1977; 118:302.

Griffiths D, Holstege G, Dalm E, de Wall H: Control and coordination of bladder and urethral function in the brainstem of the cat. Neurourol Urodynam 1990; 9:63.

Griffiths DF: Mechanics of micturition. *In* Yalla SV, McGuire EJ, Elbadawi A, Blaivas JG, eds: Neurourology and Urodynamics: Principles and Practice. New York, Macmillan, 1988, pp 96–105.

Gu J, Blank MA, Huang WM, et al: Peptide containing nerves in human urinary bladder. Urology 1984; 24:353.

Gu J, Restorick JM, Blank MA, et al: Vasoactive intestinal polypeptide in normal and unstable bladder. Br J Urol 1983; 55: 649.

Habler HJ, Janig W, Koltzenburg M: Activation of unmyelinated afferent fibers by mechanical stimuli and inflammation of the urinary bladder in the cat. J Physiol (Lond) 1990; 425:545

Habler HJ, Janig W, Koltzenburg M: Receptive properties of myelinated primary afferents innervating the inflammed urinary bladder of the cat. J Neurophysiol 1993; 69:395–405.

Hafner RJ, Stanton SL, Guy J: Psychiatric study of women with urgency and urgency incontinence. Br J Urol 1977; 49:211–214.

Hanno AG, Atta MA, Elbadawi A: Intrinsic neuromuscular defects in the neurogenic bladder: IX. Effects of combined parasympathetic decentralization and hypogastric neurectomy on neuromuscular ultrastructure of the feline bladder base. Neurourol Urodyn 1988; 7:93.

Hanrahan JW, Alles WP, Lewis SA: Single anion-selective channels in basolateral membrane of a mammalian tight epithelium. Proc Natl Acad Sci USA 1985; 82:7791.

Hanyu S, Iwanaga T, Kano K, Fujita I: Distribution of serotonin-immunoreactive paraneurons in the lower urinary tract of dogs. Am J Anat 1987; 180:349.

Hashimoto M, Kokubun S: Contribution of P2-purinoceptors to neurogenic contraction of rat urinary bladder smooth muscle. Br J Pharmacol 1995; 115:636–640.

Helke CJ, Krause JE, Mantyh PW, et al: Diversity in mammalian tachykinin peptidergic neurons: Multiple peptides, receptors, and regulatory mechanisms. Fed Am Soc Exper Biol 1990; 4:1606–1615.

Henderson CB, Weber WA: Amino acid transport across rat bladder. Can J Physiol Pharmacol 1964; 24:275.

Herman RM, Coombs DW, Saunders R, Weinberg MC: Intrathecal clonidine induces inhibition of micturition reflexes and spasticity in spinal cord patients made tolerant to spinal morphine. Abstr Neurosci Soc 1988a; 14:537.

Herman RM, Wainberg MC, del Guidice P, Wellscher MD. The effect of low dose intrathecal morphine on impaired micturition reflexes in human subjects with spinal cord lesions. Anesthesiology 1988b; 69:313.

Hicks RM: The mammalian urinary bladder: An accommodating organ. Biol Rev 1976; 50:215.

Hida T, Shimizu N: The interrelation between the laterodorsal tegmental area and lumbosacral segments of rats as studied by HRP method. Arch Histol Jpn 1982; 45:495.

Higgins JR, Gosling JA: Studies on the structure and intrinsic innervation of the normal human prostate. Prostate 1989; 2:5–16.

Hills J, Meldrum L, Klarskov P: A novel non-adrenergic, non-cholinergic nerve mediated relaxation of the pig bladder neck: An examination of possible neuro-transmitter candidates. Eur J Pharmacol 1984; 99:287.

Hisamitsu T, de Groat WC: Inhibitory effect of opioid peptides and morphine applied intrathecally and intracerebro-ventricularly on the micturition reflex in the cat. Brain Res 1984; 298:51.

Hoffmann F: The molecular basis of second messenger systems for regulation of smooth muscle contractility state of the art lecture. J Hypertension 1985; 3(Suppl 3):S3–S8.

Hohlbrugger G: Changes in hypo- and hypertonic sodium chloride induced by the rat urinary bladder at various filling stages. Eur Urol 1987; 13:83.

Holmquist F, Lundin S, Larsson B, et al: Studies on binding sites, contents, and effects of AVP in isolated bladde and urethra from rabbits and humans. Am J Physiol 1991; 261:R865–R874.

Holstege G: Some anatomical observations on the projections from the hypothalamus to brainstem and spinal cord: An HRP and autoradiographic tracing study in the cat. J Comp Neurol 1987; 260:98.

Holstege G, Griffiths D, de Wall H, Dalm E: Anatomical and physiological observations on supraspinal control of bladder and urethral sphincter muscles in the cat. J Comp Neurol 1986; 250:449.

Holt SE, Cooper M, Wyllie JH: On the nature of the receptor mediating the action of 5-hydroxytryptamine in potentiating responses of the mouse urinary bladder strip to electrical stimulation. Naunyn-Schmiedebergs Arch Pharmacol 1986; 334:333.

Holzer-Petsche U: Local effector functions of capsaicin-sensitive sensory nerve endings: involvement of tachykinins, calcitonin gene-related peptide and other neuropeptides. Neuroscience 1988; 18:739.

Holzer-Petsche U, Lembeck F: Systemic capsaicin treatment impairs the micturition in the rat. Br J Pharmacol 1984; 83:935–941.

Horby-Petersen J, Schmidt PF, Meyhoff HH, et al: The effects of a new serotonin receptor antagonist (Ketanserin) on lower urinary tract function in patients with prostatism. J Urol 1985; 133:1095.

Hoyle CV, Chapple C, Burnstock G: Isolated human bladder: Evidence for an adenine dinucleotide acting on P_{2x}-purinoceptors and for purinergic transmission. Eur J Pharmacol 1989; 174:115–118.

Hulsebosch CE, Coggeshall RE: An analysis of the axon populations in the nerves to the pelvic viscera in the rat. J Comp Neurol 1982; 211:1.

Hutch JA, Rambo OA: A new theory of the anatomy of the internal urinary sphincter and the physiology of micturition: III. Anatomy of the urethra. J Urol 1967; 97:696.

Hypolite JA, Haugaard N, Wein AJ, et al: Comparison of palmitic acid and glucose metabolism in the rabbit urinary bladder. Neurourol Urodynam 1989; 8:599.

Igawa Y, Mattiasson A, Andersson KE: Functional importance of cholinergic and purinergic neurotransmission for micturition contraction in the normal unanesthetized rat. Br J Pharmacol 1993a; 109:473–479.

Igawa Y, Persson K, Andersson KE, et al: Facilitory effect of vasoactive intestinal polypeptide on spinal and peripheral micturition reflex pathways in conscious rats with and without detrusor instability. J Urol 1993b; 149:884–889.

Iggo A: Tension receptors in the stomach and the urinary bladder. J Physiol (Lond) 1955; 128:593.

Iijima K, Oktomo K: Immunocytochemical study using a GABA antiserum for the demonstration of inhibitory neurons in the rat locus coeruleus. Am J Anat 1988; 181:43.

Iosif CS, Batra S, Ek A, Astedt B: Estrogen receptors in the human female lower urinary tract. Am J Obstet Gynecol 1981; 141:817–820.

Ishizuka O, Igawa Y, Lecci A, et al: Role of intrathecal tachykinins for micturition in unanesthetized rats with and without outlet obstruction. Br J Pharmacol 1994; 113:111–117.

Ishizuka O, Mattiasson A, Andersson KE: Neurokinin receptor antagonists on L-dopa induced bladder hyperactivity in normal conscious rats. J Urol 1995; 154:1548–1551.

Ishizuka O, Mattiasson A, Steers WD, Andersson KE: Stimulation of bladder activity by volume, L-dopa and capsaicin in normal conscious rats—effect of spinal alpha1 adrenoceptor blockade. Submitted 1996.

Iuchi H, Satoh Y, Ono K: Postnatal development of neuropeptide Y and calcitonin gene related peptide immunoreactive nerves in the rat urinary bladder. Anat Embryol 1994; 189:361–373.

Jacob J, Ludgate CM, Forder J, Tulloch WS: Recent observations of the ultrastructure of human urothelium I. Normal bladder of older subjects. Cell Tiss Res 1978; 193:543.

Janig W, Koltzenburg M: On the function of spinal primary afferents supplying colon and urinary bladder. J Auton Nerv Sys 1990; 30:S89–S96.

Janig W, Koltzenburg M: Pain arising from the urogenital tract. *In* Maggi CA, ed: The Autonomic Nervous System: Nervous Control of the Urogenital System. London, Harwook Academic Publishers, 1992, p 525.

Janig W, Morrison JFB: Functional properties of spinal visceral afferents supplying abdominal and pelvic organs, with special emphasis on visceral nociception. *In* Cervero F, Morrison JFB, eds: Visceral Sensation. Amsterdam, Elsevier, 1986, pp 87–114.

Jansco G, Maggi CA: Distribution of capsaicin-sensitive urinary bladder afferents in the rat spinal cord. Brain Res 1987; 418:371.

Jarvi R, Pelto-Huikko M: Localization of neuropeptide Y in human sympathetic ganglia: Correlation with met-enkephalin, tyrosine hydroxylase and acetylcholinesterase. Histochem J 1990; 22:87.

Jensen D: Pharmacological studies of uninhibited neurogenic bladder. Acta Neurol Scand 1981; 64:175.

Jeremey JY, Tsang V, Mikhaifidis H, et al: Eicosanoid synthesis by human urinary bladder mucosa: Pathological implications. Br J Urol 1987; 59:36.

Kakizaki H, Koyanagi T, Kato M: Sympathetic innervation of the male feline urethra rhabdosphincter. Neurosci Lett 1991; 129:165–167.

Kakizaki H, Yoshiyama M, de Groat WC: Role of NMDA and AMPA glutaminergic transmission in spinal c-fos expression after urinary tract irritation. Am J Physiol 1996; 270:R990–R996.

Kalbfleisch RE, Daniel EE: The role of substance P in the human urinary bladder. Arch Int Pharmacodyn 1987; 285:238.

Kamm KE, Stull JT: The function of myosin and myosin light chain kinase phosphorylation in smooth muscle. Annu Rev Pharmacol Toxicol 1985; 25:593.

Kamm KE, Stull JT: Regulation of smooth muscle contractile elements by second messengers. Annu Rev Physiol 1989; 51:299.

Kaplan PE, Nanninga JB: Augmentation of bladder contractility after beta-adrenergic blockade in spinal cord injured patients. Acta Neurol Scand 1980; 61:125.

Karhula T, Happola O, Joh T, Wu J-Y: Localization of L-glutamate decarboxylase immunoreactivity in the major pelvic ganglion and in the coeliac-superior mesenteric ganglion complex of the rat. Histochemistry 1988; 90:255.

Kaupp W: Uber die Aufsaugung van Hornbestandthilen in del Blase. Arch Physiol Heilk 1856; 15:125.

Kawatani M, Rutigliano M, de Groat WC: Selective facilitatory effects of vasoactive intestinal polypeptide on muscarinic mechanisms in sympathetic and parasympathetic ganglia of the cat. *In* Hanin I, ed: Dynamics of Cholinergic Function. New York, Plenum, 1986, pp 1057–1065.

Kawatani M, Shioda A, Nakai Y, et al: Ultrastructural analysis of enkephalinergic terminals in parasympathetic ganglia innervating the urinary bladder of the cat. J Comp Neurol 1989; 188:81–91.

Keast JR: Visualization and immunohistochemical characterization of sympathetic and parasympathetic neurons in the male rat major pelvic ganglion. Neuroscience 1995; 66:655–662.

Keast JF, Booth AM, de Groat WC: Distribution of neurons in the major pelvic ganglion of the rat which supply bladder, colon or penis. Cell Tiss Res 1989a; 156.

Keast JF, de Groat WC: Immunocytochemical characterization of pelvic neurons which project to the bladder, colon or penis in rats. J Comp Neurol 1989; 288:387.

Keast JR, de Groat WC: Segmental distribution and peptide content of primary afferent neurons innervating the urogenital organs and colon of male rats. J Comp Neurol 1992; 319:615–623.

Keast JR, Kawatani M, de Groat WC: Cholecystokinin has excitatory effects on transmission in vesical ganglia and on bladder contractility in cats. Soc Neurosci Abstr 1989b; 15:630.

Keating MA, Duckett J, Snyder HW, et al: The ontogeny of bladder function in the rabbit. J Urol 1990; 144:766–769.

Kim YS, Longhurst PA, Wein AJ, Levin RM: Effects of sensitization on female guinea pig urinary bladder function: In vivo and in vitro studies. J Urol 1991; 146:454–457.

Kinn A-C, Alm P, Lundgren G, Negardh A: Changes in cholinergic innervation and neuropharmacological properties in idiopathic hypotonic urinary bladders. Scan J Urol Nephrol 1987; 21:17.

Klarskov P: Enkephalin inhibits presynaptically the contractility of urinary tract smooth muscle. Br J Urol 1987; 59:31.

Klarskov P, Gerstenberg T, Hald T: Vasoactive intestinal polypeptide influence on lower urinary tract smooth muscle from human and pig. J Urol 1984; 131:1000.

Klarskov P, Holm-Bentzen M, Norgaard T, et al: Vasoactive intestinal polypeptide concentration in human bladder neck smooth muscle and its influence on urodynamic parameters. Br J Urol 1987; 60:113.

Klarskov P, Horby-Petersen J: Influence of serotonin on lower urinary tract smooth muscle in vitro. Br J Urol 1986; 58:507.

Klevmark B: Motility of the urinary bladder in cats during filling at physiologic rates: I. Intravesical pressure patterns studied by a new method of cystometry. Acta Physiol Scand 1974; 90:565.

Kluck P: The autonomic innervation of the human urinary bladder, bladder neck and urethra, a histochemical study. Anat Rec 1980; 198:439.

Koltzenburg M, McMahon SB: Plasma extravasation in the rat urinary bladder following mechanical, electrical and chemical stimuli: Evidence for a new population of chemosensitive primary sensory afferents. Neurosci Lett 1986; 72:352.

Kondo S, Morita T: A study of muscarinic cholinergic receptor subtypes in human detrusor muscle using radioligand binding techniques. Jpn J Urol 1993; 84:1255–1261.

Kontani H, Inoue T, Saki T: Effects of apomorphine on urinary bladder motility in anesthetized rats. Jpn J Pharmacol 1990; 52:59–67.

Kontani H, Kawabata Y, Koshiura R: In vivo effects of GABA on the urinary bladder contraction accompanying micturition. Jpn J Pharmacol 1987; 45:45–53.

Koyanagi T: Further observation on the denervation supersensitivity of the urethra in patients with chronic neurogenic bladders. J Urol 1979; 122:348.

Krane RJ, Olsson CA: Phenoxybenzamine in neurogenic bladder dysfunction: I. A theory of micturition. J Urol 1973; 110:650.

Kruse MN, Bennett B, de Groat WC: Effect of urinary diversion on the recovery of micturition reflexes after spinal cord injury in the rat. J Urol 1994; 151:1088–1091.

Kruse MN, de Groat WC: Micturition reflexes in decerebrate and spinalized neonatal rats. Am J Physiol 1990; 258:R1508–R1511.

Kruse MN, Mallory BS, Noto H, et al: Properties of the descending limb of the spinobulbospinal micturition reflex pathway in the cat. Brain Res 1991; 556:6–12.

Kruse M, Noto H, Roppolo J, de Groat WC: Pontine control of micturition in the rat. Abstr Soc Neurosci 1988; 14:537.

Kuru M: Nervous control of micturition. Physiol Rev 1965; 45:425.

Kurz C, Nagele F, Sevelda P, Enzelsberger H: Intravesical administration of estriol in sensory urge incontinence—a prospective study. Geburtshilfe Frauenheilkunde 1993; 53:535–538.

Kushner L, Chiu PY, Chen Y, et al: Effect of intravesical instillation of xylene on substance P and substance P receptor transcripts in rat urinary bladder. (Abstract.) Soc Neurosci Abstr 1995; 21:507.

Langley LL, Whiteside JA: Mechanism of accommodation and tone of urinary bladder. J Neurophysiol 1951; 14:147.

Lapides J: Observations on normal and abnormal bladder physiology. J Urol 1953; 70:74.

Larson JJ: Alpha and beta adrenoceptors in the detrusor muscle and bladder base of the pig and beta adrenoceptors in the detrusor muscle of man. Br J Pharmacol 1979; 65:215.

Leach G, Farsaii A, Kark P, Raz S: Urodynamic manifestations of cerebellar ataxia. J Urol 1982; 128:348–350.

Learmonth JR: A contribution to the neurophysiology of the urinary bladder in man. Brain 1931; 54:147

Lecci A, Giuliani S, Patacchini R, Maggi CA: Evidence against a peripheral role of tachykinins in the initiation of micturition reflex in rats. J Pharmacol Exper Ther 1993; 264:1327–1332.

Lecci A, Guiliani S, Santicioli P, Maggi CA: Involvement of spinal tachykinin NK1 and NK2 receptors in detrusor hyperreflexia during chemical cystitis in anesthetized rats. Eur J Pharmacol 1994; 259:129–135.

Lee JG, Macarak E, Coplen D, et al: Distribution and function of the adrenergic and cholinergic receptors in the fetal calf bladder during mid-gestational age. Neurourol Urodynam 1993; 12:599–607.

Lepor H, Gup D, Shapiro E, Baumann M: Muscarinic cholinergic receptors in normal and neurogenic human bladder. J Urol 1989; 142:869.

Levin RM, Chun AL, Kitada S, et al: Effect of contractile activity on muscarinic receptor density and the response to muscarinic agonists. J Pharmacol Exper Ther 1988; 247:624.

Levin RM, Haugaard N, Ruggieri MR, Wein AJ: Biochemical characterization of the rabbit urinary bladder. J Urol 1987; 137:782.

Levin R, Longhurst P, Monson F, et al: Effect of bladder outlet obstruction on the morphology, physiology, and pharmacology of the bladder. Prostate Suppl 1990; 3:9–26.

Levin RM, Malkowicz B, Jacobowitz D, Wein AJ: The ontogeny of the autonomic innervation and contractile response of the rabbit urinary bladder. J Pharmacol Exper Ther 1981; 219:250–257.

Levin RM, Ruggieri MR, Wein AJ: Functional effects of the purinergic innervation of the rabbit urinary bladder. J Pharmacol Exper Ther 1986; 236:452.

Levin RM, Shofer FS, Wein AJ: Estrogen-induced alterations in the autonomic responses of the rabbit urinary bladder. J Pharmacol Exper Ther 1980; 215:614–617.

Levin RM, Staskin DR, Wein AJ: The muscarinic cholinergic binding kinetics of the human urinary bladder. Neurourol Urodynam 1982; 1:221.

Lewin GR, Ritter AM, Mendell LM: Nerve growth factor induced hyperalgesia in the neonatal and adult rat. J Neurosci 1993; 13:2136–2148.

Lewis SA: A reinvestigation of the function of the mammalian urinary bladder. Am J Physiol 1977; 232:F187.

Lewis SA: The mammalian urinary bladder: It's more than accommodating. News Physiol Sci 1986; 1:61.

Lewis SA, Hanrahan JW: Apical and basolateral membrane ionic channels in rabbit urinary bladder epithelium. Plfugers Arch 1985; 405(Suppl):583.

Loewy AD, Neil JJ: The role of descending monoaminergic systems in the central control of blood pressure. Fed Proc 1981; 40:2778–2785.

Loewy AD, Saper CB, Baker RP: Descending projections from the pontine micturition center. Brain Res 1979; 172:533.

Lotz M, Vaughan JH, Carson DA: Effect of neuropeptides on production of inflammatory cytokines by human monocytes. Science 1988; 241:1218.

Lumb BM, Morrison JFB: An excitatory influence of dorsolateral pontine structure on urinary bladder motility in the rat. Brain Res 1987; 435:363.

Lundberg JM, Hua XY, Franco-Cereceda A: Effects of neuropeptide Y (NPY) on mechanical activity and neurotransmission in the heart, Vas deferens, and urinary bladder of the guinea pig. Acta Physiol Scand 1984; 121:325.

Maggi CA: Tachykinins and calcitonin gene related peptide (CGRP) as co-transmitters released from peripheral endings of sensory nerves. Prog Neurobiol 1995; 45:1–98.

Maggi CA, Barbanti G, Santicioli P, et al: Cystometric evidence that capsaicin-sensitive nerves modulate the afferent branch of micturition reflex in humans. J Urol 1989a; 142:150.

Maggi CA, Giuliani S, Pattachini R, et al: Multiple sources of calcium for contraction of the human urinary bladder muscle. Br J Pharmacol 1989b; 98:1021.

Maggi CA, Meli A: Reserpine-induced detrusor hyperreflexia: an in vivo model for studying smooth muscle relaxants at urinary bladder level. J Pharmacol Meth 1983; 10:79–81.

Maggi CA, Meli A: The role of neuropeptides in the regulation of the micturition reflex. J Auton Pharmacol 1986; 6:133.

Maggi CA, Meli A: The sensory-efferent function of capsaicin-sensitive sensory neurons. Gen Pharmacol 1988; 19:1.

Maggi CA, Parlani M, Astolfi M, et al: Neurokinin receptors in the rat lower urinary tract. J Pharmacol Exper Ther 1988a; 246:308–315.

Maggi CA, Patacchini R, Giuliani S, et al: Motor response of the isolated small intestine and urinary bladder to procine neuromedin-u. Br J Pharmacol 1990; 99:186.

Maggi CA, Patacchini R, Santicioli P, et al: Further studies on the motor response of the human isolated urinary bladder to tachykinins, capsaicin and electrical field stimulation. Gen Pharmacol 1989c; 20:663–669.

Maggi CA, Santicioli P, Borsini F, et al: The role of capsaicin-sensitive innervation of the rat urinary bladder in the activation of micturition reflex. Naunyn-Schmied Arch Pharmacol 1986; 332:276.

Maggi CA, Santicioli P, Giuliani S, et al: The effects of baclofen on spinal or supraspinal micturition reflexes in rats. Naunyn Schmied Arch Pharmacol 1987; 336:297.

Maggi CA, Santicioli P, Meli A: GABA-A and GABA-B receptors in detrusor strips from guinea pig bladder dome. J Auton Pharmacol 1985a; 5:55–64.

Maggi CA, Santicioli P, Meli A: GABA inhibits excitatory neurotransmission in rat pelvic ganglia. J Pharm Pharmacol 1985b; 37:349.

Maggi CA, Santicioli P, Meli A: The effects of topical capsaicin on rat urinary bladder motility in vivo. Eur J Pharmacol 1984; 103:41.

Maggi CA, Santicioli P, Patacchini R, et al: A potent modulator of excitatory neurotransmission in the human urinary bladder. Eur J Pharmacol 1987b; 143:135–137.

Maggi CA, Santicioli P, Patacchini R, et al: Contractile response of the human isolated urinary bladder to neurokinins: involvement of NK-2 receptors. Eur J Pharmacol 1988b; 145:335–340.

Magora F, Skazar N, Drenger B: Urodynamic studies after intrathecal administration of baclofen and morphine in dogs. J Urol 1989; 141:143.

Mallory B, de Groat WC: Effect of intrathecal substance P on micturition contractions in urethane anesthetized rats. Abstr Soc Neurosci 1987; 13:270.

Mallory B, Steers WD, de Groat WC: Electrophysiological study of micturition reflexes in the rat. Am J Physiol 1989; 257:R410.

Mansour A, Khalchaturian H, Lewis ME, et al: Anatomy of CNS opioid receptors. Trends Neurosci 1988; 11:308.

Marson L: Brain and spinal neurons identified in the female rat after injection of pseudorabies virus into the bladder body, base and external urethral sphincter. Soc Neurosci Abstr 1995; 21:1872.

Matsumoto G, Hisamitsu T, de Groat WC: Role of glutamate and nMDA receptors in the descending limb of the spinobulbospinal micturition reflex pathway of the rat. Neurosci Lett 1995a; 183:58–61.

Matsumoto G, Hisamitsu T, de Groat WC: Non-NMDA glutaminergic excitatory transmission in the descending limb of the spinobulbospinal micturition reflex pathway of the rat. Brain Res 1995b; 693:246–250.

Matsumura S, Taira N, Hashimoto M: The pharmacological behavior of the urinary bladder and its vasculature in the dog. Tohuku J Exp Med 1968; 96:247–258.

Mattiasson A, Andersson K-E, Elbadawi A, et al: Interaction between adrenergic and cholinergic nerve terminals in the urinary bladder of rabbit, cat and man. J Urol 1987; 137:1017.

Mattiasson A, Andersson K-E, Sjögren C: Adrenoceptors and cholinoceptors controlling noradrenaline release from adrenergic nerves in the urethra of rabbit and man. J Urol 1984; 131:1190.

Mattiasson A, Ekblad E, Sundler F, Uvelius B: Origin and distribution of neuropeptide Y, vasoactive intestinal polypeptide and substance P-containing fibers in urinary bladder of the rat. Cell Tiss Res 1985; 239:141.

Mattiasson A, Ekstrom B, Andersson KE: Effects of intravesical instillation of verapamil in patients with detrusor hyperactivity. J Urol 1989; 141:174–177.

McGuire EJ: Reflex urethral instability. Br J Urol 1978; 50:200.

McGuire EJ: Mechanisms of urethral continence and their clinical application. World J Urol 1984; 2:272.

McGuire EJ, Herlihy EL: Bladder and urethral responses to isolated sacral motor root stimulation. Invest Urol 1978; 16:219.

McGuire EJ, Herlihy EL: Bladder and urethral responses to sympathetic stimulation. Invest Urol 1979; 17:9.

McKenna KD, Nadelhaft I: The organization of the pudendal nerve in the male and female cat. J Comp Neurol 1985; 248:532.

McMahon SB: Sensory-motor integration in urinary bladder function. *In*

Cervero F, Morrison JFB, eds: Progress in Brain Research, vol 67. Amsterdam, Elsevier, 1986, pp 245–283.

McMahon SB, Abel C: A model for the study of visceral pain states: Chronic inflammation of the chronic decerebrate rat urinary bladder by irritant chemicals. Pain 1987; 28:109.

McMahon SB, Armanimi MP, Ling LH, Phillips HS: Expression and coexpression of trk receptors in subpopulations of adult primary sensory neurons projecting to identified peripheral targets. Neuron 1994; 12:1161–1171.

McMahon SB, Spillane K: Brainstem influences on the parasympathetic supply to the urinary bladder. Brain Res 1982; 234:237–249.

Menetrey D, Gannon A, Levine JD, Basbaum AI: Expression of c-fos protein in interneurons and projection neurons of the rat spinal cord in response to noxious somatic, articular and visceral stimulation. J Comp Neurol 1989; 285:177.

Mevorach RA, Bogaert GA, Kogan BA: Role of nitric oxide in fetal lower urinary tract function. J Urol 1994; 152:510–514.

Michel MC, Kenny B, Schwinn DA: Classification of alpha-1 adrenoceptor subtypes. Naunyn-Schmied Arch Pharmacol 1995; 352:1–10.

Miller RJ: Multiple calcium channels and neuronal function. Science 1987; 235:46.

Milner P, Crowe R, Burnstock G, Light JK: Neuropeptide Y and vasoactive intestinal polypeptide containing nerves in the intrinsic external urethral sphincter in the areflexic bladder compared to detrusor-sphincter dyssynergia in patients with spinal cord injury. J Urol 1987; 138:888.

Minsky BD, Chlapowski FJ: Morphometric analysis of the translocation of lumenal membrane between cytoplasm and cell surface of transitional epithelial cells during the expansion-contraction cycles of the mammalian urinary bladder. J Cell Biol 1978; 77:685.

Mitsuhashi M, Payan DG: The neurogenic effects of vasoactive neuropeptide on cultured smooth muscle cell lines. Life Sci 1987; 40:853.

Montgomery BSI, Fry CH: The action potential and net membrane currents in isolated human detrusor smooth muscle cells. J Urol 1992; 147:176–184.

Morgan CW, de Groat WC, Felkins LA, Zhang SJ: Axon collaterals indicate broad intraspinal role for sacral preganglionic neurons. Proc Natl Acad Sci USA 1991; 88:6888–6892.

Morgan C, Nadelhaft I, de Groat WC: The distribution of visceral primary afferents from the pelvic nerve within Lissauer's tract and the spinal gray matter and its relationship to sacral parasympathetic nucleus. J Comp Neurol 1981; 201:415.

Morgan KG, Papageorgion P, Jiang MJ: Pathophysiologic role of calcium in the development of vascular smooth muscle tone. Am J Cardiol 1989; 64:35F.

Morita T, Tsuchida S: Stereographic urethral pressure profile. Urol Int 1989; 39:199–204.

Morita T, Wheeler MA, Weiss RM: Relaxant effect of forskolin in rabbit detrusor smooth muscle: Role of cyclic AMP. J Urol 1986; 135:1293.

Morrison JFB: Reflex control of the lower urinary tract. *In* Torrens M, Morrison JFB, eds: The Physiology of the Urinary Bladder. Berlin, Springer-Verlag, 1987a, 194–235.

Morrison JFB: Bladder control: Role of higher levels of the central nervous system. *In* Torrens M, Morrison JFB, eds: The Physiology of the Lower Urinary Tract. Berlin, Springer-Verlag, 1987b, 238–274.

Morrison JFB, Spillane K: Neuropharmacological studies on descending inhibitory controls over micturition reflex. J Auton Nerv Sys 1986; (Suppl) 393–396.

Mostwin JL: Receptor operated calcium stores in smooth muscle of the guinea pig bladder. J Urol 1985; 133:900.

Mostwin JL: The action potential of guinea pig bladder smooth muscle. J Urol 1986; 135:1299.

Munro DD, Wendt IR: Effects of cyclopiazonic acid on calcium and contraction in rat bladder smooth muscle. Cell Calcium 1994; 15:369–380.

Murakumo M, Ushiki T, Abe K, et al: Three dimensional arrangement of collagen and elastin fibers in the human urinary bladder: A scanning electron microscopic study. J Urol 1995; 154:251–256.

Murray KH, Feneley RC: Endorphins—A role in lower urinary tract function? The effect of opioid blockade on the detrusor and urethral sphincter mechanisms. Br J Urol 1982; 54:638–640.

Nadelhaft I, Devenyi C: Pontine micturition center in rat revealed by retrograde transport of rhodamine-labelled beads injected into the sacral intermediolateral column. Abstr Neurosci Soc 1987; 13:734.

Nadelhaft I, Morgan C, de Groat WC: Localization of the sacral autonomic nucleus in the spinal cord of the cat by the horseradish peroxidase technique. J Comp Neurol 1980; 193:265.

Naglo AS, Negardh A, Boreus LO: Influence of atropine and isoprenaline on detrusor hyperactivity in children with neurogenic bladder. Scand J Urol Nephrol 1981; 15:97.

Nakayama S, Brading AF: Evidence for multiple open states of the Ca^{2+} channels in smooth muscle cells isolated from the guinea-pig detrusor. J Physiol 1993; 471:87–105.

Nanninga JB, Frost F, Penn R: Effect of intrathecal baclofen on bladder and sphincter function. J Urol 1989; 142:101.

Nathan PW: The central nervous connections of the bladder. *In* Williams DI, Chisholm GD, eds: Scientific Foundations of Urology. London, Heineman, 1976, pp 51–58.

Nathan PW, Smith MC: The centrifugal pathway for micturition within the spinal cord. J Neurol Neurosurg Psychiatr 1958; 21:177.

Nemeth CJ, Khan RM, Kirchner P, Adams P: Changes in canine bladder perfusion with distension. Invest Urol 1977; 15:149.

Nergardh A, Boreus LO: Autonomic receptor function in the lower urinary tract of man and cat. Scand J Urol Nephrol 1972; 6:32.

Nilsson J, van Euler AM, Dalsgaard C-J: Stimulation of connective tissue cell growth by substance P and substance K. Nature 1985; 315:61.

Nilvebrant L, Andersson K-E, Mattiasson A: Characterization of the muscarinic cholinoreceptors in the human detrusor. J Urol 1985; 134:418–423.

Nilvebrant L, Ekstrom J, Malinberg L: Muscarinic receptor density in the rat urinary bladder after unilateral denervation. Pharmacol Toxicol 1989; 64:150–151.

Nishimura T, Tokimasa T, Akasu T: 5-Hydroxytryptamine inhibits cholinergic transmission through 5-HT_{1A} receptor subtypes in rabbit vesical parasympathetic ganglia. Brain Res 1988; 442:399.

Nishimura T, Yoshida M, Nagatsu I, Akasu T: Frequency dependent inhibition of nicotinic transmission by serotonin in vesical pelvic ganglia of the rabbit. Neurosci Lett 1989; 103:179.

Nishizawa O, Sugaya K, Noto H, et al: Pontine urine storage center in the dog. Tohoku J Exp Med 1987; 153:77.

Nordling J: Effects of clonidine on urethral pressure. Invest Urol 1979; 16:289–291.

Nordling J: Influence of the sympathetic nervous system on lower urinary tract in man. Neurourol Urodynam 1983; 2:3.

Norlen L, Sundin T, Waagstein F: Beta adrenoceptor stimulation of the human urinary bladder in vivo. Acta Pharmacol Toxicol 1978; 43:26.

Noto H, Roppolo JR, Steers WD, de Groat WC: Excitatory and inhibitory influences on bladder activity elicited by electrical stimulation in the pontine micturition center in the rat. Brain Res 1989; 492:99.

Obrink A, Brunne G: Treatment of urgency by intravesical instillation of emepronium bromide in the urinary bladder. Scand J Urol Nephrol 1978; 12:215.

Oddiah D, McMahon SB, Rattray M: Inflammation produces up-regulation of neurotrophin messenger RNA levels in the bladder. Soc Neurosci Abstr 1995; 21:1534.

O'Donnell PD: Central actions of bethanecol on the bladder in dogs. J Urol 1990; 143:634.

Oerlich TM: The urethral sphincter muscle in the male. Am J Anat 1980; 158:229.

Oerlich TM: The striated urogenital sphincter muscle in the female. Anat Rec 1983; 205:223.

Okada H, Yamane M, Orchi K: The reciprocal activity between the pelvic nerves and external urethal sphincter muscles during micturition reflex in the dog. J Auton Nerv Sys 1975; 12:178.

Okpukpara JN, Akah PA: Furosemide potentiates acetylcholine and carbachol in contracting the rat urinary bladder. J Pharm Pharmacol 1990; 42:597–598.

Padykula HA, Gauthier GF: Morphological and cytochemical characteristics of fiber types in mammalian skeletal muscle. *In* Explanatory Concepts in Neuromuscular Dystrophy and Related Disorders. Amsterdam, Excerpta Medica International Congress Series 1967, No 147, pp 117–131.

Palea S, Arbitani W, Ostardo E, et al: Evidence for purinergic neurotransmission in human urinary bladder affected by interstitial cystitis. J Urol 1993; 150:2007–2012.

Palea S, Pietra C, Trist DG, et al: Evidence for the presence of both pre- and postjunctional P2-purinoceptor subtypes in human isolated urinary bladder. Br J Pharmacol 1995; 114:35–40.

Parlani M, Conte B, Manzini S: Nonadrenergic, noncholinergic inhibitory control of the rat external urethra sphincter: Involvement of nitric oxide. J Pharmacol Exp Ther 1993; 265:713–719.

Parsons CL, Boychuk D, Jones S, et al: Bladder surface glycosaminoglycans: An epithelial permeability barrier. J Urol 1990; 143:139.

Patra PB, Westfall DP: Potentiation of purinergic neurotransmission in guinea pig urinary bladder by histamine. J Urol 1994; 151:787–790.

Pavcovich LA, Valentino RJ: Regulation of micturition by corticotropin-releasing hormone (CRH) from Barrington's nucleus. Neurosci Lett 1995; 196:185–188.

Peng Y, Kohno J, Shinoda K, Shiotani Y: Interaction between sacral parasympathetic preganglionic neurons and substance P or calcitonin gene-related peptide terminals of the rat: An immunoelectron microscopic double staining analysis. J Electron Microsc 1988; 37:278.

Persson K, Alm P, Johansson K, et al: Nitric oxide synthase in pig lower urinary tract: Immunohistochemistry, NADPH diaphorase histochemistry and functional effects. Br J Pharmacol 1993; 110:521–530.

Persson K, Steers WD: Stretch increases secretion of PTHrp by cultured bladder smooth muscle cells. Neurourol Urodynam 1994; 13:406

Petros PE, Ulmsten U: An integral theory and its method for the diagnosis and management of female urinary incontinence. Scand J Urol Nephrol 1993; 27(Suppl 153):1–93.

Petros PE, Ulmsten U: Urethral pressure increase on effort originates from within the urethra and continence from musculovaginal closure. Neurourol Urodynam 1995; 14:337–350.

Poli E, Monica B, Zappia L, et al: Antimuscarinic activity of telenzepine on isolated human urinary bladder: A role for M1-muscarinic receptors. Gen Pharmacol 1992; 23:659–664.

Pool JL: The visceral brain of man. J Neurosurg 1954; 11:45.

Rice ASC: Topical spinal administration of a nitric oxide synthase inhibitor prevents the hyper-reflexia associated with a rat model of persistent visceral pain. Neurosci Lett 1995; 187:111–114.

Rice ASC, McMahon SB: Pre-emptive intrathecal administration of an NMDA receptor antagonist (AP-5) prevents hyper-reflexia in a model of persistent visceral pain. Pain 1994; 57:335–340.

Rohner T, Hannigan J, Sanford E: Altered in vitro adrenergic responses of dog detrusor muscle after chronic bladder outlet obstruction. Urology 1978; 11:357.

Roppolo JR, Mallory BS, Ragoowansi A, de Groat WC: Modulation of bladder function in the cat by application of pharmacological agents to the pontine micturition center. Soc Neurosci Abstr 1986; 12:645.

Roppolo JR, Nadelhaft I, de Groat WC: The organization of pudendal motoneurons and primary afferent projections in the spinal cord of the rhesus monkey revealed by horseradish peroxidase. J Comp Neurol 1985; 234:475.

Roppolo JR, Noto H, Mallory B, de Groat WC: Dopaminergic and cholinergic modulation of bladder reflexes at the level of the pontine micturition center in the cat. Soc Neurosci Abstr 1987; 13:733.

Rudy D, Woodside J: Non-neurogenic neurogenic bladder: The relationship between intravesical pressure and the external sphincter electromyogram. Neurourol Urodynam 1991; 10:169–176.

Ryall RW, de Groat WC: The microiontophoretic administration of noradrenaline, 5-hydroxytryptamine, acetylcholine and glycine on parasympathetic preganglionic neurones. Brain Res 1972; 37:345.

Saban R, Undem BJ, Keith I, et al: Differential release of prostaglandins and leukotrienes by sensitized guinea pig urinary bladder layers upon antigen challenge. J Urol 1994; 152:544–549.

Saenz de Tejada I, Mueller JD, de las Morenas A, et al: Endothelin in the urinary bladder. Synthesis of endothelin-1 by epithelia, smooth muscle and fibroblasts, suggests autocrine and paracrine cellular functions. J Urol 1992; 148:1290–1298.

Saito M, Gotoh M, Kato K, Kondo A: Denervation supersensitivity of the rabbit urinary bladder to calcium ion. J Urol 1989; 142:418.

Saito M, Kondo A, Kato T, Miyake K: Response of the human urinary bladder to angiotensins: A comparison between neurogenic and control bladders. J Urol 1993; 149:408–411.

Saper CB, Loewy AD, Swanson LW, Cowan WM: Direct hypothalamo-autonomic connections. Brain Res 1976; 117:305.

Sasek CA, Seybold VS, Elde RP: The immunohistochemical localization of nine peptides in the sacral parasympathetic nucleus and dorsal gray commissure in the rat spinal cord. Neuroscience 1984; 12:855.

Sato A, Sato Y, Suzuki A: Mechanism of the reflex inhibition of micturition contractions of the urinary bladder elicited by acupuncture-like stimulation in anesthetized rats. Neurosci Res 1992; 15:189–198.

Sato A, Schmidt RF: The modulation of visceral function by somatic afferent activity. Jpn J Physiol 1987; 37:1.

Satoh K, Tokyama M, Sakomoto T, et al: Descending projection of the nucleus tegmentalis laterodorsalis to the spinal cord: Studied by the HRP method following 6-hydroxy-DOPA administration. Neurosci Lett 1978; 8:9.

Saum WR, de Groat WC: The actions of 5-hydroxytryptamine on the urinary bladder and in vesical autonomic ganglia in the cat. J Pharmacol Exp Ther 1973; 185:70.

Schussler B: Comparison of mode of action of prostaglandin E_2 and sulprostone, a PGE_2 derivative on the lower urinary tract in healthy women. Urol Res 1990; 18:349–352.

Scott FB, Quesada EM, Cardus D: Studies on the dynamics of micturition: Observations in healthy men. J Urol 1964; 92:455–463.

Scott M, Morrow J: Phenoxybenzamine on neurogenic bladder dysfunction after spinal cord injury: I. Voiding dysfunction. J Urol 1978; 119:480.

Senba E, Daddona PF, Nagy JI: A subpopulation of preganglionic parasympathetic neurons in the rat containing adenosine deaminase. Neuroscience 1987; 20:487.

Seybold VS: Neurotransmitter receptor sites in the spinal cord. *In* Yaksh TL, ed: Spinal Afferent Processing. New York, Plenum Press, 1985, pp 117–139.

Shapiro E: Effect of estrogens on the weight and muscarinic cholinergic receptor density of the rabbit bladder and urethra. J Urol 1986; 135:1084–1087.

Shapiro E, Becich MJ, Perlman E, Lepor H: Bladder wall abnormalities in myelodysplastic bladders: A computer assisted morphometric analysis. J Urol 1991; 145:1024–1029.

Sibley GNA: A comparison of spontaneous and nerve-mediated activity in bladder muscle from man, pig and rabbit. J Physiol (Lond) 1984; 354:431.

Sillen U, Rubenson A, Hjalmas K: On the localization and mediation of central monoaminergic hyperactive bladder response induced by L-dopa in the rat. Acta Physiol Scand 1981; 112:137.

Sillen U, Rubenson A, Hjalmas K: Central cholinergic mechanisms in L-dopa induced hyperactive urinary bladder of the rat. Urol Res 1982; 10:239.

Simmonds WF, Booth AM, Thor KB, et al: Parasympathetic ganglia: Naloxone antagonizes inhibition by leucine-enkephaline and GABA. Brain Res 1983; 271:365.

Sjögren C, Andersson K-E, Husted S, et al: Atropine resistance of transmurally stimulated isolated human bladder muscle. J Urol 1982; 128:1368.

Sjögren C, Andersson KE, Mattiasson A: Effects of vasoactive intestinal polypeptide on isolated urethral and urinary bladder smooth muscle from rabbit and man. J Urol 1985; 133:136–140.

Sneddon P, McLees A: Purinergic and cholinergic contractions in adult and neonatal rabbit bladder. Eur J Pharmacol 1992; 214:7–12.

Sogbein SK, Downie JW, Awad SA: Urethral response during bladder contraction induced by subcutaneous bethanechol chloride: Elicitation of sympathetic reflex urethral constriction. J Urol 1984; 131:791.

Sokanaka M, Shiosaka S, Takatsuki K, Tohyana M: Evidence for the existence of a substance P containing pathway from the nucleus laterodorsalis tegmenti to the medial frontal cortex of the rat. Brain Res 1983; 259:123.

Sokolov A, Buffington RW, Burry RW, Wolfe SA: Neurogenic inflammation causes up-regulation of binding sites for 3H-substance P in cat urinary bladder. (Abstract.) Soc Neurosci Abstr 1995; 21:95.

Somogyi GT, de Groat WC: Modulation of the release of [3H] norepinephrine from the base and body of the rat urinary bladder by endogenous adrenergic and cholinergic mechanisms. J Pharmacol Exper Ther 1990; 255(1):204–210.

Somogyi GT, de Groat WC: Evidence for inhibitory nicotinic and facilitatory muscarinic receptors in cholinergic nerve terminals of the rat urinary bladder. J Auton Nerv Sys 1992; 37:89–98.

Speakman MJ, Brading AF, Gilpin CJ, Dixon SA: Bladder outflow obstruction—a cause of denervation supersensitivity. J Urol 1987; 138:1461.

Staehelin LA, Chlapowski FJ, Bonneville MA: Luminal plasma membrane of the urinary bladder. I. Three dimensional reconstruction from freeze-etch images. J Cell Biol 1972; 53:73.

Steers WD: Smooth muscle physiology. AUA Update 1994; 8:238–244.

Steers WD, Albo M, van Asselt E: Effects of serotonergic agonists on micturition and sexual function in the rat. Drug Devel Res 1992a; 27:361–375.

Steers WD, Ciambotti J, Etzel B, et al: Alterations in afferent pathways from the urinary bladder in response to partial urethral obstruction. J Comp Neurol 1991a; 310:401–410.

Steers WD, Creedon D, Tuttle JB: Immunity to NGF prevents afferent plasticity following hypertrophy of the urinary bladder. J Urol 1996; 155:379–385.

Steers WD, de Groat WC: Effect of bladder outlet obstruction on micturition reflex pathways in the rat. J Urol 1988; 140:864.

Steers WD, Kolbeck S, Creedon D, Tuttle JB: Nerve growth factor in the urinary bladder of the adult regulates neuronal form and function. J Clin Invest 1991b; 88:1709–1715.

Steers WD, Meythaler JM, Herrell D, et al: The effects of acute bolus and continuous intrathecal baclofen on genitourinary dysfunction in patients with disorders of the spinal cord. J Urol 1992b; 148:1849–1855.

Steers WD, Tuttle JB, Creedon DJ: Neurotrophic influence of the bladder following outlet obstruction: Implications for the unstable detrusor. Neurourol Urodynam 1989; 8:395.

Stein M, Discippio W, David M, Taub H: Biofeedback for the treatment of stress and urge incontinence. J Urol 1995; 153:641–643.

Strohmeger P, Sack H: Resorption redioactiv Markierter substanzen aus hornlose and isoliertec Duenndarmschlinge. Urol Int 1966; 21:538.

Su HC, Wharton J, Polak JM, et al: Calcitonin gene-related peptide immunoreactivity in afferent neurons supplying the urinary tract: Combined retrograde tracing and immunohistochemistry. Neuroscience 1986; 18:727.

Sundin T, Dahlstrom A, Norlen L, Svedmyr N: The sympathetic innervation and adrenoreceptor function of the human lower urinary tract in the normal state and after parasympathetic denervation. Invest Urol 1977; 14:322.

Sutin EL, Jacobowitz DM: Immunocytochemical localization of peptides and other neurochemicals in the rat laterodorsal tegmental nucleus and adjacent area. J Comp Neurol 1988; 270:243.

Swanson LW, Sawchenko PE: Hypothalamic integration: Organization of the paraventricular and supraoptic nuclei. Ann Rev Neurosci 1983; 6:269.

Swierzewski S, III, Gormley EA, Belville W, et al:The effect of terazosin on bladder function in the spinal cord injured patient. J Urol 1994; 151:951–954.

Tammela T, Kontturi M, Kaar K, Lukkarinen O: Intravesical prostaglandin E_2 for promoting bladder emptying after surgery for female stress incontinence. Br J Urol 1987; 60:43–46.

Tanabe N, Veno A, Tsujimoto G: Angiotensin II: Receptors in the rat urinary bladder smooth muscle: Type I subtype receptors mediate contractile responses. J Urol 1993; 150:1056–1059.

Tanagho EA: The ureterovesical junction: Anatomy and physiology. *In* Chishold GD, Williams DI, eds: Scientific Foundations of Urology. Chicago, YearBook Medical Publishers, 1982, pp 295–404.

Tanagho EA, Schmidt RA, Orvis BR: Neural stimulation for control of voiding dysfunction: Preliminary report in 22 patients with serious neuropathic voiding disorders. J Urol 1989; 142:340.

Tang LH, Erdman S, de Groat WC, Vizzard M: Increased expression of nitric oxide synthase and growth associated protein (GAP-43) in visceral neurons after nerve injury. Soc Neurosci Abstr 1994; 20:1498.

Tang PC: Levels of the brainstem and diencephalin controlling micturition reflex. J Neurophysiol 1955; 18:583.

Tang PC, Ruch TC: Localization of brainstem and diencephalic area controlling the micturition reflex. J Comp Neurol 1956; 206z; 213.

Testa R, Guarneri L, Ibba M, et al: Characterization of the alpha-1 adrenoceptor subtypes in the prostate and prostatic urethra of rat, rabbit, dog and man. Eur J Pharmacol 1993; 249:307–315.

Theobald RJ: Purinergic and cholinergic components of bladder contractility and flow. Life Sci 1995; 56:445–454.

Theobald RJ, de Groat WC: The effects of purine nucleotides on transmission in vesical parasympathetic ganglia of the cat. J Auton Pharmacol 1989; 9:167.

Thor KB, Blais DP, Kawatani M, et al: Postnatal development of opioid regulation of micturition in the kitten. Dev Brain Res 1990; 57:255–261.

Thor K, Morgan C, Nadelhaft I, et al: Organization of afferent and efferent pathways in the pudendal nerve of the cat. J Comp Neurol 1989; 288:263.

Thor K, Kawatani M, de Groat WC: Plasticity in reflex pathways to the lower urinary tract of the cat during postnatal development and following spinal cord injury. *In* Goldberger AG, Murray GM, eds: Development and Plasticity of the Mammalian Spinal Cord. Padova, Liviana Press, 1986, pp 65–80.

Thor KB, Roppolo JR, de Groat WC: Naloxone induced micturition in unanesthetized cats. J Urol 1983; 129:202.

Tiseo PJ, Yaksh TL: Response of normal and areflexic bladder to spinally administered primary afferent neurotransmitters in intact and chronic spinal rats. Abstr Soc Neurosci 1989; 15:216.

Todd AJ, Sullivan AC: Light microscopic study of the coexistency of GABA-like and glycine-like immunoreactivities in the spinal cord of the rat. J Comp Neurol 1990; 296:496–505.

Torrens MJ: Urethral sphincteric responses to stimulation of the sacral nerves in the human female. Urol Int 1978; 33:22.

Tschida S, Noto H, Yamaguchi O, Itoh M: Urodynamic studies on hemiplegic patients after cerebrovascular accident. Urology 1983; 21:315.

Tuttle JB, Steers WD, Albo M, Nataluk E: Neural input regulates tissue NGF and growth of the adult rat urinary bladder. J Auton Nerv Sys 1994; 49:147–158.

Uemura E, Fletcher TF, Dirks VA, Bradley WE: Distribution of sacral afferent axons in cat urinary bladder. Am J Anat 1968; 136:309.

Urban L, Thompson SW, Dray A: Modulation of spinal excitability: co-operation between neurokinin and excitatory amino acid neurotransmitters. Trends Neurosci 1994; 17:432–438.

Uvelius B, Arner A, Malmquist U: Contractile and cytoskeletal proteins in detrusor muscle from obstructed rat and human bladder. Neurourol Urodynam 1989; 8:396.

Vadyanaathan S, Rao MS, Chary KS, et al: Enhancement of detrusor reflex activity by naloxone in patients with chronic neurogenic bladder dysfunction. J Urol 1981; 126:500–502.

Van Poppel H, Stessons R, Baert L, et al: Vasoactive intestinal polypeptide innervation of human urinary bladder in normal and pathological conditions. Urol Int 1988; 43:205–210.

van Waalwijk Van Doorn ESC, Remmers A, Janknegt RA: Extramural ambulatory urodynamic monitoring during natural filling and normal daily activities: Evaluation of 100 patients. J Urol 1991; 146:124–131.

Vizzard M, Erdman S, de Groat W: The effect of rhizotomy on NADPH diaphorase staining in the lumbar spinal cord of the rat. Brain Res 1993; 607:349–353.

Vizzard MA, Erdman S, de Groat WC: Increased expression of neuronal nitric oxide synthase (NOS) in visceral neurons after nerve injury. J Neurosci 1995; 15:4033–4045.

Vizzard MA, Erdman S, Forstermann U, de Groat WC: Differential expression of nitric oxide synthase in neural pathways to the urogenital organs (urethra, penis, urinary bladder) of the rat. Brain Res 1994; 646:279–291.

Wagner G, Husslein P, Enzelsberger H: Is prostaglandin E_2 really of therapeutic value for postoperative urinary retention: results of a prospective randomized study. Am J Obstet Gynecol 1985; 151:375–379.

Waikar MV, Ford APDW, Clarke DE: Evidence for an inhibitory 5-HT4 receptor in urinary bladder of Rhesus and Cynomolgus monkeys. Br J Pharmacol 1994; 111:213–2128.

Wakabayashi Y, Buchan A, Kwok YN: Denervation and inflammation induced increase of low-affinity NGF receptor immunoreactivity in the rat urinary bladder. Soc Neurosci Abstr 1995; 21:1873.

Wakabayashi Y, Tomoyoshi T, Fujimiya M, et al: Substance P-containing axon terminals in the mucosa of the human urinary bladder: Pre-embedding immunohistochemistry using cryostat sections for electron microscopy. Histochem 1993; 100:401–407.

Walter S, Wolf H, Barlebo H, et al. Urinary incontinence in post-menopausal women treated with oestrogens: A double blind clinical trial. Urol Int 1978; 33:135.

Walters MD, Taylor S, Schoenfeld LS: Psychosexual study of women with detrusor instability. Obstet Gynecol 1990; 75:22–26.

Wang P, Luthin GR, Ruggieri MR: Muscarinic acetylcholine receptor subtypes mediating urinary bladder contractility and coupling to GTP binding proteins. J Pharmacol Exper Ther 1995; 273:959–966.

Watts SW, Cohen ML: Effect of bombesin, bradykinin, substance P and CGRP in prostate, bladder body and neck. Peptides 1991; 12:1057–1062.

Wein AJ, Hypolite JA, Ruggieri MR, Levin RM: Correlation of bladder contraction with calcium fluorescence using FURA-2. J Urol 1989; 141:325A.

Wein AJ, Levin RM: Comparison of adrenergic receptor density in the urinary bladder of man, dog and rabbit. Surg Forum 1979; 30:576.

Wellner MC, Isenberg G: Stretch effects on whole-cell currents of guinea-pig urinary bladder myocytes. J Physiol (Lond) 1994; 480:439–448.

Wendt IR, Gibbs CL: Energy expenditure of longitudinal smooth muscle of rabbit urinary bladder. Am J Physiol 1987; 252:C88–C96.

Wickham JEA: Active transport of sodium ion by mammalian bladder epithelium. Invest Urol 1964; 2:145.

Willette RN, Morrison A, Sapru HN, Reis DJ: Stimulation of opiate receptors in the dorsal pontine tegmentum inhibits reflex contraction of the urinary bladder. J Pharmacol Exper Ther 1988; 244:403.

Willette RN, Sauermelch CF, Hieble JP: Role of alpha-1 and alpha-2 adrenoceptors in the sympathetic control of the proximal urethra. J Pharmacol Exper Ther 1990; 252:706.

Williams JH, Brading A: Urethral sphincters: Normal function and changes in disease. *In* Daniel EE, Tomira T, Tschuida S, Wantanabe M, eds: Sphincters. Boca Raton, FL, CRC Press, 1992, pp 316–338.

Wilson PD, Faragher B, Butler B: Treatment with piperazine oestrone sulphate for genuine stress incontinence in post-menopausal women. Br J Obstet Gynecol 1987; 84:568.

Wu SY, Dun NJ: Presynaptic GABA-B receptor activation attenuates synaptic transmission to rat sympathetic neurons in vitro. Brain Res 1992; 572:94–102.

Yaksh TL, Jessell TM, Ganise R, et al: Intrathecal morphine inhibits substance P release from mammalian spinal cord in vivo. Nature 1980; 286:155.

Yalla SV, Rossier AB, Fam BA, et al: Functional contribution of autonomic innervation to urethral striated sphincter: Studies with parasympathomimetic, parasympatholytic, and alpha adrenergic blocking agents in spinal cord injury and control male subjects. J Urol 1977; 117:494.

Yamaguchi T, Kitada S, Osada Y: Role of adrenoceptors in the proximal urethral function of female and male rabbits using an in vitro model of isovolumetric pressure generation. Neurourol Urodynam 1993; 12:49–57.

Yamamoto M, Harm S, Grasser WA, Thiede MA: Parathyroid hormone-related protein in the rat urinary bladder: A smooth muscle relaxant produced locally in response to mechanical stretch. Proc Natl Acad Sci USA 1992; 89:5326–5330.

Yoshimura N, de Groat WC: Patch clamp analysis of afferent and efferent neurons that innervate the urinary bladder of the rat. (Abstract.) Soc Neurosci Abstr 1992; 18(59.7):127.

Yoshimura N, Sasa M, Ohno Y, et al: Contraction of the urinary bladder by central norepinephrine originating in the locus coeruleus. J Urol 1988; 139:423.

Yoshimura N, Sasa M, Yoshida O, Takaori S: Mediation of micturition reflex by central norepinephrine from the locus coeruleus in the cat. J Urol 1990; 143:840.

Yoshimura N, Yoshida O, de Groat WC: Regional differences in plasticity of membrane properties of rat urinary bladder afferent neurons following spinal cord injury. J Urol 1995; 153:262a.

Yoshiyama M, Roppolo JR, de Groat WC: Interactions between glutaminergic and monoaminergic systems controlling the micturition reflex in the urethane-anesthetized rat. Brain Res 1994; 639:300–308.

Zappia L, Cartella A, Potenzoni D, Bertaccini G: Action of pirenzepine on the human urinary bladder in vitro. J Urol 1986; 136:739.

Zederic SA, Levin RM, Wein AJ: Voiding function: Relevant anatomy, physiology, pharmacology, and molecular aspects. *In* Gillenwater JY, Grayhack J, Howards SS, Duckett J, eds: Adult and Pediatric Urology. St. Louis, C.V. Mosby, 1996, pp 1159–1219.

Zeng XP, Moore KH, Burcher E: Characterization of tachykinin NK_2 receptors in the human urinary bladder. J Urol 1995; 153:1680–1692.

Zhan A: Predictive correlation of urodynamic dysfunction and brain injury after cerebrovascular accident. J Urol 1981; 126:86.

Zhou Q, Satake N, Shibata S: The inhibitory mechanisms of nicorandel in isolated rat urinary bladder and femoral artery. Eur J Pharmacol 1995; 273:153–159.

Ziganshin AU, Ralevic V, Burnstock G: Contractility of the urinary bladder and vas deferens after sensory denervation by capsaicin treatment of newborn rats. Br J Pharmacol 1995; 114:166–170.

Zoubek J, Somogyi GT, de Groat WC: A comparison of inhibitory effects of neuropeptide Y on rat bladder, urethra, and vas deferens. Am J Physiol 1993; 265:R537–R543.

Zucker RS, Lando L: Mechanism of transmitter release: Voltage hypothesis and calcium hypothesis. Science 1986; 231:574–578.

27
PATHOPHYSIOLOGY AND CATEGORIZATION OF VOIDING DYSFUNCTION

Alan J. Wein, M.D.

The lower urinary tract functions as a group of interrelated structures whose joint function in the adult is to bring about efficient and low-pressure bladder filling, low-pressure urine storage with perfect continence, and periodic voluntary urine expulsion, again at low pressure. This chapter begins with a functional, physiologic, and pharmacologic overview of normal and abnormal lower urinary tract function. A simple way of looking at the pathophysiology of all types of voiding dysfunction is then presented, followed by a discussion of various systems of classification and categorization. Consistent with the author's philosophy and prior attempts to make the understanding, evaluation, and management of voiding dysfunction interesting and logical (Wein and Barrett, 1988), a functional and practical approach is favored.

NORMAL LOWER URINARY TRACT FUNCTION

Two-Phase Concept of Function

Whatever disagreements exist regarding the anatomic, morphologic, physiologic, pharmacologic, and mechanical details involved in both the storage and the expulsion of urine by the lower urinary tract, this author has always taken the rather simple-minded view that the "experts" would agree on certain points (Wein and Barrett, 1988). The first is that **the micturition cycle involves two relatively discrete processes:** (1) bladder filling and urine storage, and (2) bladder emptying. The second is that, whatever the details involved, **one can succinctly summarize these processes from a conceptual point of view as follows.**

Bladder filling and urine storage require

1. Accommodation of increasing volumes of urine at a low intravesical pressure and with appropriate sensation
2. A bladder outlet that is closed at rest and remains so during increases in intra-abdominal pressure.
3. The absence of involuntary bladder contractions

Bladder emptying requires

1. A coordinated contraction of the bladder smooth musculature of adequate magnitude
2. A concomitant lowering of resistance at the level of the smooth and striated sphincter.
3. The absence of anatomic (as opposed to functional) obstruction.

The **smooth sphincter** refers to the smooth musculature of the bladder neck and proximal urethra. This is a physiologic but not an anatomic sphincter, and one that is not under voluntary control. The **striated sphincter** refers to the striated musculature that is a part of the outer wall of the urethra in both the male and the female (intrinsic or intramural) and the bulky skeletal muscle group that surrounds the urethra at the level of the membranous portion in the male and the middle segment in the female (extrinsic or extramural). The extramural portion, the classically described "external urethral sphincter" is under voluntary control (see Chapter 26 and Zderic et al, 1995, for a detailed discussion).

Any type of voiding dysfunction must result from an abnormality of one or more of the factors listed above. This two-phase concept of micturition, with the three components of each related to either the bladder or the outlet, provides a logical framework for a functional categorization of all types of voiding dysfunction and disorders as related primarily to filling-storage or to emptying (see Tables 27–6 and 27–7). There are indeed some types of voiding dysfunction that represent combinations of filling-storage and emptying abnormalities. Within this scheme, however, these become readily understandable, and their detection and treatment can be logically described. Various aspects of physiology and pathophysiology are always related more to one phase of micturition than to another. All aspects of urodynamic and video-urodynamic evaluation can be conceptualized as to exactly what they evaluate in terms of either bladder or outlet activity during filling-storage or emptying (see Table 27–7). One can easily classify all known treatments for voiding dysfunction under the broad categories of whether they facilitate filling-storage or emptying and whether they do so by an action primarily on the bladder or on one or more of the components of the bladder outlet (see Tables 29–1 and 29–2). Finally, the individual disorders produced by various neuromuscular dysfunctions can be thought of in terms of whether they produce primarily storage or emptying abnormalities or a combination of these.

MECHANISMS UNDERLYING THE TWO PHASES OF FUNCTION

This section briefly summarizes pertinent points regarding the physiology of the various mechanisms underlying normal bladder filling-storage and emptying, abnormalities of which constitute the pathophysiologic mechanisms seen in the various types of dysfunction of the lower urinary tract. The information is consistent with that detailed by deGroat and colleagues (1993), Mundy and Thomas (1994), Zderic and associates (1995), and Chapter 26; additional references are provided only where particularly applicable.

Bladder Response During Filling

The normal adult bladder response to filling at a physiologic rate is an almost imperceptible change in intravesical pressure. **During at least the initial stages of bladder filling, after unfolding of the bladder wall from its collapsed state, this very high compliance (Δvolume/Δpressure) is due primarily to elastic and viscoelastic properties.** Elasticity allows the constituents of the bladder wall to stretch to a certain degree without any increase in tension. Viscoelasticity allows stretch to induce a rise in tension followed by a decay **(stress relaxation)** when the filling (stretch stimulus) slows or stops. There may also be an active component to the storage properties of the bladder. The mucosa and lamina propria are normally the most compliant layers of the bladder. Coplen and colleagues (1994) have hypothesized that the smooth muscle layer may have a chronic effect on compliance in the midportion of the cystometric filling curve through a complex interaction between muscle and extracellular matrix. This layer may acutely affect compliance in response to neurologic input as well (see below).

In the usual clinical setting, filling cystometry seems to show a slight increase in intravesical pressure, but Klevmark (1974, 1977) elegantly showed that this pressure rise is a function of the fact that filling is carried out at a greater than physiologic rate and that at physiologic filling rates there is essentially no rise in bladder pressure until bladder capacity is reached. Clinically, bladder compliance may be altered by (1) any process that alters the viscoelasticity or elasticity of the wall components, (2) filling the bladder at a rate exceeding the rate of stress relaxation, (3) filling the bladder beyond its limits of distensibility, and, perhaps, neurologic factors that modify the response of the smooth muscle component during filling. Significant alteration is seen most commonly in patients in whom the components of the bladder wall have been replaced or augmented by fibrosis, as in pancystitis secondary to long-term catheter drainage. Such a decrease in compliance is generally unresponsive to pharmacologic manipulation, hydraulic distention, or nerve section and most often requires augmentation cystoplasty for the bladder to achieve satisfactory reservoir function. One can also see the same effect clinically in association with some cases of neurologic decentralization and/or obstruction, and experimentally in response to obstruction or ischemia.

Does the nervous system affect the normal bladder response to filling? At a certain level of distention, spinal sympathetic reflexes facilitatory to bladder filling-storage are clearly evoked in animals, a concept developed over the years by deGroat and associates (1993), who have also cited indirect evidence to support such a role in humans. This inhibitory effect is thought to be mediated primarily by sympathetic modulation of cholinergic ganglionic transmission. Through such a reflex mechanism, two other possibilities exist for promoting filling-storage. The first involves stimulation of the predominantly alpha-adrenergic receptors in the area of the smooth sphincter, the net result of which would be to cause an increase in resistance in that area. The second consists of a neurally mediated stimulation of the predominantly beta-adrenergic receptors (inhibitory) in the bladder body smooth musculature. McGuire (1983) has also cited evidence for direct inhibition of detrusor motor neurons in the sacral spinal cord during bladder filling that is due to increased afferent pudendal nerve activity generated by receptors in the striated sphincter. Good evidence also seems to exist to support a strong tonic inhibitory effect of endogenous opioids on bladder activity at the level of the spinal cord, the parasympathetic ganglia, and perhaps the brain stem as well (deGroat and Kawatani, 1989). Such activity likely contributes to the lack of bladder contractile response during filling and may affect contractility during emptying as well. Bladder filling and wall distention may also release autocrine-like factors that themselves influence contractility (e.g., nitric oxide, prostaglandins, peptides).

Outlet Response During Filling

There is a gradual increase in urethral pressure during bladder filling, contributed to by at least the striated sphincteric element and perhaps by the smooth sphincteric element as well. The rise in urethral pressure seen during the filling phase of micturition can certainly be correlated with an increase in efferent pudendal nerve impulse frequency in cats and in humans (deGroat and Booth, 1984; deGroat, 1993) and at least in cats with an increase in efferent hypogastric nerve impulse frequency.

Although it seems logical and certainly compatible with neuropharmacologic, neurophysiologic, and neuromorphologic data to assume that the muscular component of the smooth sphincter also contributes to the change in urethral response during bladder filling, it is extremely difficult to prove this either experimentally or clinically. The direct and circumstantial evidence in favor of such a hypothesis has been summarized by Wein and Barrett (1988) and Elbadawi (1988). The passive properties of the urethral wall certainly deserve mention, as these undoubtedly play a large role in the maintenance of continence (Zinner et al, 1983). Urethral wall tension develops within the outer layers of the urethra; however, it is a product not only of the active characteristics of smooth and striated muscle but also of the passive characteristics of the elastic collagenous tissue that makes up the urethral wall. In addition, this tension must be exerted on a soft or plastic inner layer capable of being compressed to a closed configuration—the "filler material" representing the submucosal portion of the urethra. The softer and more plastic this area is, the less pressure required by the tension-producing area to produce continence.

Finally, whatever the compressive forces, the lumen of the urethra must be capable of being obliterated by a watertight seal. This "mucosal seal" mechanism explains why it requires less pressure to close an open end of a very thin walled rubber tube when the inner layer is coated with a fine layer of grease than when it is not, the latter case being much like scarred or atrophic urethral mucosa.

Voiding with a Normal Bladder Contraction

Although many factors are involved in the initiation of micturition, in adults it is intravesical pressure producing the sensation of distention that is primarily responsible for the initiation of voluntarily induced emptying of the lower urinary tract. Although the origin of the parasympathetic neural outflow to the bladder, the pelvic nerve, is in the sacral spinal cord, **the actual organizational center for the micturition reflex in an intact neural axis is in the brain stem,** and the complete neural circuit for normal micturition includes the ascending and descending spinal cord pathways to and from this area and the facilitory and inhibitory influences from other parts of the brain.

The final step in voluntarily induced micturition involves inhibition of the somatic neural efferent activity to the striated sphincter and an inhibition of all aspects of any spinal sympathetic reflex evoked during filling. Efferent parasympathetic pelvic nerve activity is ultimately what is responsible for a highly coordinated contraction of the bulk of the bladder smooth musculature. A decrease in outlet resistance occurs, with adaptive shaping or funneling of the relaxed bladder outlet. Besides the inhibition of any continence-promoting reflexes that have occurred during bladder filling, the change in outlet resistance may also involve an active relaxation of the smooth sphincter area through a noncholinergic nonadrenergic mechanism mediated by nitric oxide. The adaptive changes that occur in the outlet are also due at least in part to the anatomic interrelationships of the smooth muscle of the bladder base and proximal urethra. Other reflexes that are elicited by bladder contraction and by the passage of urine through the urethra may reinforce and facilitate complete bladder emptying. Superimposed on these autonomic and somatic reflexes are complex modifying supraspinal inputs from other central neuronal networks. These facilitatory and inhibitory impulses, which originate from several areas of the nervous system, allow the full conscious control of micturition.

Urinary Continence During Abdominal Pressure Increases

During voluntarily initiated micturition, the bladder pressure becomes higher than the outlet pressure and certain adaptive changes occur in the shape of the bladder outlet with consequent passage of urine into and through the proximal urethra. One could reasonably ask why such changes do not occur with increases in pressure that are similar in magnitude but that are produced by changes in only intra-abdominal pressure, such as straining or coughing. A coordinated bladder contraction does not occur in response to such stimuli, clearly emphasizing the fact that increases in total intravesical pressure are by no means equivalent to emptying ability. For urine to flow into the proximal urethra, not only must there be an increase in intravesical pressure, but the increase must also be a product of a coordinated bladder contraction, occurring through a neurally mediated reflex mechanism and associated with characteristic conformational and tension changes in the bladder neck and proximal urethral area.

A major factor in the prevention of urinary leakage during increases in intra-abdominal pressure is the fact that there is at least equal pressure transmission to this smooth sphincter area during such activity. This phenomenon was first described by Enhorning (1961) and has been confirmed in virtually every urodynamic laboratory since that time. For years most of us have written that during a cough, equal pressure transmission to the normal female urethra occurred because the urethra lay within the abdomen, above what we pictured as a horizontal plane of fascia and muscle separating the abdomen from the pelvis. When the urethra descended below this plane, the explanation continued, normal pressure transmission to it was lost and "genuine stress incontinence" occurred. DeLancey (1994) has been evolving an alternate hypothesis for years **(the "hammock hypothesis").** He clearly underscores the fact that **there is no unbroken layer of urogenital diaphragm through which the female urethra passes, nor is there a definite relationship between the position of the urethra and the occurrence of stress incontinence in the female.** His theory is that the effect of abdominal pressure increases on the normal urethra and pelvic floor depends primarily on the stability of the suburethral supportive layer (the connection of the endopelvic fascia and anterior vaginal wall to the arcus tendineus fasciae pelvis and striated levator ani muscles). If the supportive layer is firm, compression of the urethra by intra-abdominal pressure increases is rapid and effective. If the supportive layer is lax and/or movable, compression is not as effective.

A lack of suburethral support is not the entire explanation to stress incontinence. **Intrinsic competence of the bladder neck and proximal urethra at rest is necessary.** The increase in urethral closure pressure that is seen with increments in intra-abdominal pressure actually exceeds the extrinsic pressure increase, indicating that active muscular function, in addition to simple transmission of pressure, is also involved. Tanagho (1978) was the first to provide direct evidence that this additional increment in urethral closure pressure during straining involves a reflex increase in sphincter activity, a now commonly accepted urodynamic fact.

ABNORMALITIES OF FILLING/STORAGE AND EMPTYING: OVERVIEW

The pathophysiology of failure of the lower urinary tract to fill with or store urine adequately may be secondary to reasons related to the bladder, the outlet, or both. **Hyperactivity of the bladder during filling can be expressed as phasic involuntary contractions, as low compliance, or as a combination.** Involuntary contractions are most commonly seen in association with neurologic disease or after neurologic injury; however, they may also be associated with aging; inflammation or irritation of the bladder wall; or bladder outlet obstruction, or they may be idiopathic. Decreased compliance during filling may be secondary to neurologic injury or disease, usually at a sacral or infrasacral level, but may also result from any process that destroys the viscoelastic or elastic properties of the bladder wall.

Storage failure may also occur in the absence of hyperactivity, secondary to hypersensitivity or pain during filling. Irritation and inflammation can be responsible, as well as neurologic, psychological, or idiopathic causes. The classic clinical example is interstitial cystitis (see Chapter 17).

Decreased outlet resistance may result from any process that damages the innervation or the structural elements of the smooth or striated sphincter. This may occur with neurologic disease or injury, surgical or other mechanical trauma, or aging. Assuming the bladder neck and proximal urethra are competent at rest, lack of a stable suburethral supportive layer (see above) seems a plausible explanation of the primary factor responsible for genuine stress urinary incontinence in the female. Such failure can occur because of laxity or hypermobility, each resulting in a failure of the normal transmission of intra-abdominal pressure increases to the bladder outlet. The primary etiologic factors may be any of the causes of pelvic floor relaxation or weakness.

The treatment of filling-storage abnormalities is directed toward inhibiting bladder contractility; decreasing sensory input; mechanically increasing bladder capacity; or increasing outlet resistance, either continuously or just during increases in intra-abdominal pressure.

Absolute or relative failure to empty results from decreased bladder contractility (a decrease in magnitude or duration), increased outlet resistance, or both. Absolute or relative failure of bladder contractility may result from temporary or permanent alteration in one of the neuromuscular mechanisms necessary for initiating and maintaining a normal detrusor contraction. Inhibition of the voiding reflex in a neurologically normal individual may also occur—by a reflex mechanism secondary to painful stimuli, especially from the pelvic and perineal areas—or such an inhibition may be psychogenic. Non-neurogenic causes also include impairment of bladder smooth muscle function, which may result from overdistention, severe infection, or fibrosis.

Pathologically increased outlet resistance is generally seen in the male and is most often secondary to anatomic obstruction, but it may be secondary to a failure of coordination (relaxation) of the striated or smooth sphincter during bladder contraction. Striated sphincter dyssynergia is a common cause of functional (as opposed to fixed anatomic) obstruction in patients with neurologic disease or injury.

The treatment of emptying failure generally consists of attempts to increase intravesical pressure or facilitate the micturition reflex, to decrease outlet resistance, or both. If all else fails or the attempt is impractical, intermittent catheterization is an effective way of circumventing emptying failure.

CATEGORIZATION

Based on the data obtained from the neurourologic evaluation, a given voiding dysfunction can be categorized in an ever-increasing number of descriptive systems. The purpose of any classification system should be to facilitate understanding and management, and to avoid confusion among those who are concerned with the problem for which the system was designed. A good classification should serve as intellectual shorthand and should convey, in a few key words or phrases, the essence of a clinical situation. An ideal system for all types of voiding dysfunction would include or imply a number of factors. The first of these is the conclusions reached from urodynamic testing. Expected clinical symptoms should be able to be inferred. The approximate site and type of a neurologic lesion, or lack of one, would ideally also be implied. If the various categories accurately portray pathophysiology, treatment options should then be obvious, and a treatment "menu" should be evident. Most systems of classification for voiding dysfunction were formulated primarily to describe dysfunction secondary to neurologic disease or injury. The ideal system should be applicable to all types of voiding dysfunction. Most of the major systems or types of systems in use are reviewed, along with their advantages, disadvantages, and applicability. For a more detailed reference list, the reader may consult Wein and Barrett (1988).

Bors-Comarr Classification

Bors and Comarr (1971) made a remarkable contribution by logically deducing a classification system from clinical observation of their patients with traumatic spinal cord injury

(Table 27–1). **This system applies only to patients with neurologic dysfunction** and considers three factors: (1) the anatomic localization of the lesion, (2) the neurologic completeness or incompleteness of the lesion, and (3) a designation indicating whether lower urinary tract function is **balanced** or **unbalanced.** The latter terms are based solely on the percentage of residual urine relative to bladder capacity. **Unbalanced** signifies the presence of greater than 20% residual urine in a patient with an upper motor neuron (UMN) lesion or 10% in a patient with a lower motor neuron (LMN) lesion. This relative residual urine volume was ideally meant to imply coordination (synergy) or dyssynergia between the smooth and striated sphincters of the outlet and the bladder, during bladder contraction or during attempted micturition by abdominal straining or Credé. The determination of the completeness of the lesion is made on the basis of a thorough neurologic examination. The system erroneously assumes that the sacral spinal cord is the primary reflex center for micturition. **LMN** implies collectively the preganglionic and postganglionic parasympathetic autonomic fibers that innervate the bladder and outlet and originate as preganglionic fibers in the sacral spinal cord. The term is used in an analogy to efferent somatic nerve fibers, such as those of the pudendal nerve, which originate in the same sacral cord segment but terminate directly on pelvic floor striated musculature without the interposition of ganglia. **UMN** is used in a similar analogy to the somatic nervous system to describe those descending autonomic pathways above the sacral spinal cord (the origin of the motor efferent supply to the bladder).

In this system, **UMN bladder** refers to the pattern of micturition that results from an injury to the suprasacral spinal cord after the period of spinal shock has passed, assuming that the sacral spinal cord and the sacral nerve roots are intact and that the pelvic and pudendal nerve reflexes are intact. **LMN bladder** refers to the pattern resulting if the sacral spinal cord or sacral roots are damaged and the reflex pattern through the autonomic and somatic nerves that emanate from these segments is absent. This system implies that if skeletal muscle spasticity exists below the level of the lesion, the lesion is above the sacral spinal cord and is by definition a UMN lesion. This type of lesion is characterized by detrusor hyperreflexia during filling. If flaccidity of the skeletal musculature below the level of a lesion exists, an LMN lesion is assumed to exist, implying detrusor areflexia. Exceptions occur and are classified in a "mixed lesion" group characterized either by detrusor hyperreflexia with a flaccid paralysis below the level of the lesion or by detrusor areflexia with spasticity or normal skeletal muscle tone neurologically below the lesion level.

The use of this system is illustrated as follows. A UMN lesion, complete, unbalanced, implies a neurologically complete lesion above the level of the sacral spinal cord that results in skeletal muscle spasticity below the level of the injury. Detrusor hyperreflexia exists during filling, but a residual urine volume of greater than 20% of the bladder capacity is left after bladder contraction, implying obstruction in the area of the bladder outlet during the hyperreflexic detrusor contraction. This obstruction is generally due to striated sphincter dyssynergia, typically occurring in patients who are paraplegic and quadriplegic with lesions between the cervical and the sacral spinal cord. Smooth sphincter dyssynergia may be seen as well in patients with lesions above the level of T6, usually in association with autonomic hyperreflexia (see Chapter 29). An LMN lesion, complete, unbalanced, implies a neurologically complete lesion at the level of the sacral spinal cord or of the sacral roots, resulting in skeletal muscle flaccidity below that level. Detrusor areflexia results, and whatever measures the patient may use to increase intravesical pressure during attempted voiding are not sufficient to decrease residual urine to less than 10% of bladder capacity.

This classification system applies best to spinal cord injury patients with complete neurologic lesions after spinal shock has passed. It is difficult to apply to patients with multicentric neurologic disease and cannot be used at all for patients with non-neurologic disease. The system fails to reconcile the clinical and urodynamic variability exhibited by patients who, by neurologic examination alone, seem to have similar lesions. The period of spinal shock that immediately follows severe cord injury is generally associated with bladder areflexia, whatever the status of the sacral somatic reflexes. Temporary or permanent changes in bladder or outlet activity during filling-storage or emptying may occur secondary to a number of factors such as chronic overdistention, infection, and reinnervation or reorganization of neural pathways after injury or disease; such changes make it impossible to always accurately predict lower urinary tract activity solely on the basis of the level of the neurologic lesion. Finally, although the terms "balanced" and "unbalanced" are helpful, in that they describe the presence or absence of a certain relative percentage of residual urine, they do not necessarily imply the true functional significance of a lesion, which depends on the potential for damage to the lower or upper urinary tracts, and also on the social and vocational disability that results.

Table 27–1. BORS-COMARR CLASSIFICATION

Sensory Neuron Lesion
Incomplete, balanced
Complete, unbalanced
Motor Neuron Lesion
Balanced
Unbalanced
Sensory–Motor Neuron Lesion
Upper Motor Neuron Lesion
Complete, balanced
Complete, unbalanced
Incomplete, balanced
Incomplete, unbalanced
Lower Motor Neuron Lesion
Complete, balanced
Complete, unbalanced
Incomplete, balanced
Incomplete, unbalanced
Mixed Lesion
Upper somatomotor neuron, lower visceromotor neuron
Lower somatomotor neuron, upper visceromotor neuron
Normal somatomotor neuron, lower visceromotor neuron

Hald-Bradley Classification

Hald and Bradley (1982) described what they termed a simple neurotopographic classification (Table 27–2). A

Table 27–2. HALD-BRADLEY CLASSIFICATION

Suprasacral lesion
Suprasacral spinal lesion
Infrasacral lesion
Peripheral autonomic neuropathy
Muscular lesion

supraspinal lesion is characterized by synergy between detrusor contraction and the smooth and striated sphincters, but a defective inhibition of the voiding reflex exists. In patients with a supraspinal lesion in this classification, detrusor hyperreflexia generally occurs and sensation is usually preserved. However, depending on the site of the lesion, detrusor areflexia and defective sensation may be seen. A **suprasacral spinal lesion** is roughly equivalent to what is described as a UMN lesion in the Bors-Comarr classification. An **infrasacral lesion** is roughly equivalent to an LMN lesion. **Peripheral autonomic neuropathy** is most frequently encountered in the diabetic patient and is characterized by deficient bladder sensation, gradually increasing residual urine, and ultimate decompensation, with a loss of detrusor contractility. A **muscular lesion** can involve the detrusor itself, the smooth sphincter, or any portion, or all, of the striated sphincter. The resultant dysfunction is dependent on which structure is affected. Detrusor dysfunction is the most common and generally results from decompensation, following long-standing bladder outlet obstruction.

Bradley Classification

Bradley's "loop system" of classification is a primarily neurologic system based on a conceptualization of central nervous system control of the lower urinary tract that identifies four neurologic "loops" (Hald and Bradley, 1982). Dysfunctions are classified according to the loop affected.

Loop 1 consists of neuronal connections between the cerebral cortex and the pontine-mesencephalic micturition center; this coordinates voluntary control of the detrusor reflex. Loop 1 lesions are seen in conditions such as brain tumor; cerebrovascular accident or disease; and cerebral atrophy with dementia. The final result is characteristically detrusor hyperreflexia.

Loop 2 includes the intraspinal pathway of detrusor muscle afferents to the brain stem micturition center and the motor impulses from this center to the sacral spinal cord. Loop 2 is thought to coordinate and provide for a detrusor reflex of adequate temporal duration to allow complete voiding. Partial interruption by spinal cord injury results in a detrusor reflex of low threshold and in poor emptying with residual urine. Spinal cord transection of loop 2 acutely produces detrusor areflexia and urinary retention—spinal shock. After this has passed, detrusor hyperreflexia results.

Loop 3 consists of the peripheral detrusor afferent axons and their pathway in the spinal cord; these terminate by synapsing on pudendal motor neurons that ultimately innervate periurethral striated muscle. Loop 3 was thought to provide a neurologic substrate for coordinated reciprocal action of the bladder and striated sphincter. Loop 3 dysfunction could be responsible for detrusor–striated sphincter dyssynergia or involuntary sphincter relaxation.

Loop 4 consists of two components. Loop 4A is the suprasacral afferent and efferent innervation of the pudendal motor neurons to the periurethral striated musculature. Loop 4B consists of afferent fibers from the periurethral striated musculature that synapse on pudendal motor neurons in Onuf's nucleus—the segmental innervation of the periurethral striated muscle. In contrast to the stimulation of detrusor afferent fibers, which produces inhibitory postsynaptic potentials in pudendal motor neurons through loop 3, pudendal nerve afferents produce excitatory postsynaptic potentials in those motor neurons through loop 4B. These provide contraction of the periurethral striated muscle during bladder filling and urine storage. The related sensory impulses arise from muscle spindles and tendon organs in the pelvic floor musculature. Loop 4 provides volitional control of the striated sphincter. Abnormalities of the suprasacral portion result in abnormal responses of the pudendal motor neurons to bladder filling and emptying, manifested as detrusor–striated sphincter dyssynergia, and/or loss of the ability to voluntarily contract the striated sphincter.

The Bradley system is sophisticated and reflects the ingenuity and neurophysiologic expertise of its originator. For the neurologist, this method may be an excellent way to conceptualize the neurophysiology involved, assuming that there is in fact agreement on the existence and significance of all four loops. Most urologists find this system difficult to use for many types of neurogenic voiding dysfunction and not at all applicable to non-neurogenic voiding dysfunction. Urodynamically, it may be extremely difficult to test the intactness of each loop system, and multicentric and partial lesions are difficult to describe.

Lapides Classification

Lapides (1970) contributed significantly to the classification and care of the patient with neuropathic voiding dysfunction by popularizing a modification (Table 27–3) of a system originally proposed by McLellan in 1939. This remains one of the most familiar systems to urologists and nonurologists because it describes in recognizable shorthand the clinical and cystometric conditions of many types of neurogenic voiding dysfunction.

A **sensory neurogenic bladder** results from disease that selectively interrupts the sensory fibers between the bladder and spinal cord or the afferent tracts to the brain. Diabetes mellitus, tabes dorsalis, and pernicious anemia are most commonly responsible. The first clinical changes are described as those of impaired sensation of bladder distention. Unless voiding is initiated on a timed basis, varying degrees of bladder overdistention can result with resultant hypotonic-

Table 27–3. LAPIDES CLASSIFICATION

Sensory neurogenic bladder
Motor paralytic bladder
Uninhibited neurogenic bladder
Reflex neurogenic bladder
Autonomous neurogenic bladder

ity. With bladder decompensation, significant amounts of residual urine are found and, at this time, the cystometric curve generally demonstrates a large-capacity bladder with a flat high compliance low-pressure filling curve.

A **motor paralytic bladder** results from disease processes that destroy the parasympathetic motor innervation of the bladder. Extensive pelvic surgery or trauma may produce this. Herpes zoster has been listed as a cause as well, but recent evidence suggests that the voiding dysfunction seen with herpes is more related to a problem with afferent input (see Chapter 29). The early symptoms may vary from painful urinary retention to only a relative inability to initiate and maintain normal micturition. Early cystometric filling is normal but without a voluntary bladder contraction at capacity. Chronic overdistention and decompensation may occur in a large-capacity bladder with a flat, low-pressure filling curve; a large residual urine may result.

The **uninhibited neurogenic bladder** was described originally as resulting from injury or disease to the "corticoregulatory tract." The sacral spinal cord was presumed to be the micturition reflex center, and this corticoregulatory tract was believed to normally exert an inhibitory influence on the sacral micturition reflex center. A destructive lesion in this tract would then result in overfacilitation of the micturition reflex. Cerebrovascular accident, brain or spinal cord tumor, Parkinson's disease, and demyelinating disease are the most common causes in this category. The voiding dysfunction is most often characterized symptomatically by frequency, urgency, and urge incontinence; and urodynamically by normal sensation with an involuntary bladder contraction at low filling volumes. Residual urine is characteristically low unless anatomic outlet obstruction or true smooth or striated sphincter dyssynergia occurs. The patient generally can initiate a bladder contraction voluntarily but is often unable to do so during cystometry because sufficient urine storage cannot occur before detrusor hyperreflexia is stimulated.

Reflex neurogenic bladder describes the post–spinal shock condition that exists after complete interruption of the sensory and motor pathways between the sacral spinal cord and the brain stem. Most commonly, this occurs in traumatic spinal cord injury and transverse myelitis, but it may occur with extensive demyelinating disease or any process that produces significant spinal cord destruction as well. Typically, there is no bladder sensation and there is an inability to initiate voluntary micturition. Incontinence without sensation generally results because of low-volume involuntary bladder contraction. Striated sphincter dyssynergia is the rule. This type of lesion is essentially equivalent to a complete UMN lesion in the Bors-Comarr system.

An **autonomous neurogenic bladder** results from complete motor and sensory separation of the bladder from the sacral spinal cord. This may be caused by any disease that destroys the sacral cord or causes extensive damage to the sacral roots or pelvic nerves. There is inability to voluntarily initiate micturition, no bladder reflex activity, and no specific bladder sensation. This type of bladder is equivalent to a complete LMN lesion in the Bors-Comarr system and is also the type of dysfunction seen in patients with spinal shock. The characteristic cystometric pattern is initially similar to the late stages of the motor or sensory paralytic bladder, with a marked shift to the right of the cystometric filling curve and a large bladder capacity at low intravesical pressure. However, decreased compliance may develop, secondary either to chronic inflammatory change or to the effects of denervation/decentralization with secondary neuromorphologic and neuropharmacologic reorganizational changes. Emptying capacity may vary widely, depending on the ability of the patient to increase intravesical pressure and on the resistance offered during this increase by the smooth and striated sphincters.

These classic categories in their usual settings are usually easily understood and remembered, and this is why this system provides an excellent framework for teaching some fundamentals of neurogenic voiding dysfunction to students and nonurologists. Unfortunately, many patients' conditions do not exactly fit into one or another category. Gradations of sensory, motor, and mixed lesions occur, and the patterns produced after different types of peripheral denervation/decentralization may vary widely from those that are classically described. The system is applicable only to neuropathic dysfunction.

Urodynamic Classification

As urodynamic techniques have become more accepted and sophisticated, systems of classification have evolved based solely on objective urodynamic data (Table 27–4). Among the first to popularize this concept were Krane and Siroky (1984). When exact urodynamic classification is possible, this system provides a truly exact description of the voiding dysfunction that occurs. If a normal or hyperreflexic detrusor exists with coordinated smooth and striated sphincter function and without anatomic obstruction, normal bladder emptying should occur.

Detrusor hyperreflexia is most commonly associated with neurologic lesions above the sacral spinal cord. Striated sphincter dyssynergia is most commonly seen after complete suprasacral spinal cord injury, following the period of spinal shock. Smooth sphincter dyssynergia is seen most classically in autonomic hyperreflexia (see Chapter 29), when it is characteristically associated with detrusor hyperreflexia and striated sphincter dyssynergia.

Detrusor areflexia may be secondary to bladder muscle decompensation or to various other conditions that produce inhibition at the level of the brain stem micturition center, the sacral spinal cord, bladder ganglia, or bladder smooth muscle. Patients with a voiding dysfunction secondary to

Table 27–4. URODYNAMIC CLASSIFICATION

Detrusor Hyperreflexia (or Normoreflexia)
Coordinated sphincters
Striated sphincter dyssynergia
Smooth sphincter dyssynergia
Nonrelaxing smooth sphincter
Detrusor Areflexia
Coordinated sphincters
Nonrelaxing striated sphincter
Denervated striated sphincter
Nonrelaxing smooth sphincter

From Krane RJ, Siroky MB: Classification of voiding dysfunction: Value of classification systems. *In* Barrett DM, Wein AJ, eds: Controversies in Neuro-Urology. New York, Churchill Livingstone, 1984, pp 223–238.

detrusor areflexia generally attempt bladder emptying by abdominal straining, and their continence status and the efficiency of their emptying efforts are determined by the status of their smooth and striated sphincter mechanisms.

This classification system is easiest to use when detrusor hyperreflexia or normoreflexia exists. Thus, a typical T10 level paraplegic exhibits detrusor hyperreflexia, smooth sphincter synergia, and striated sphincter dyssynergia. When a voluntary or hyperreflexic contraction cannot be elicited, the system is more difficult to use, because it is not appropriate to speak of true sphincter dyssynergia in the absence of an opposing bladder contraction. There are obviously many variations and extensions of such a system. Such systems work well when total urodynamic agreement exists among classifiers. Unfortunately, there are many voiding dysfunctions that do not fit neatly into a urodynamic classification system that is agreed on by all "experts." As sophisticated urodynamic technology and understanding improve, this type of classification system may supplant some others in general use.

International Continence Society Classification

The classification system proposed by the International Continence Society (ICS) (Table 27–5) is in many ways an extension of a urodynamic classification system. The storage and voiding phases of micturition are described separately, and, within each, various designations are applied to describe bladder and urethral function (Abrams et al, 1990).

Normal bladder function during filling-storage implies no significant rises in detrusor pressure (stability). **Overactive detrusor function** indicates the presence of involuntary contractions. If this is due to neurologic disease, the term **detrusor hyperreflexia** is used; if not, the phenomenon is known as **detrusor instability. Bladder sensation** can be categorized only in qualitative terms as indicated. **Bladder capacity and compliance** (Δ volume/Δ pressure) are cystometric measurements. **Normal urethral function during filling-storage** indicates a positive urethral closure pressure (urethral pressure minus bladder pressure) even with increases in intra-abdominal pressure. **Incompetent urethral function during filling-storage** implies urine leakage in the absence of a detrusor contraction. This may be secondary to genuine stress incontinence, intrinsic sphincter dysfunction, or an involuntary fall in urethral pressure in the absence of a detrusor contraction (see Chapter 30).

Table 27–5. INTERNATIONAL CONTINENCE SOCIETY CLASSIFICATION

Storage Phase	Voiding Phase
Bladder Function	***Bladder Function***
Detrusor Activity	*Detrusor Activity*
Normal or stable	Normal
Overactive	Underactive
Unstable	Acontractile
Hyperreflexic	***Urethral Function***
Bladder Sensation	Normal
Normal	Obstructive
Increased or hypersensitive	Overactive
Reduced or hyposensitive	Mechanical
Absent	
Bladder Capacity	
Normal	
High	
Low	
Compliance	
Normal	
High	
Low	
Urethral Function	
Normal	
Incompetent	

Adapted from Abrams P, Blaivas JG, Stanton SL, Andersen JT: Int Urogynecol J 1990; 1:45.

During the voiding-emptying phase of micturition, normal detrusor activity implies voiding by a voluntarily initiated sustained contraction that can also be suppressed voluntarily. An **underactive detrusor** defines a contraction of inadequate magnitude or/and duration to empty the bladder within a normal time span. An **acontractile detrusor** is one that cannot be demonstrated to contract during urodynamic testing. **Areflexia** is defined as acontractility due to an abnormality of neural control, implying the complete absence of centrally coordinated contraction. **Normal urethral function during voiding** indicates opening before micturition to allow bladder emptying. An **obstructed urethra** is one that contracts against a detrusor contraction or fails to open (nonrelaxation) with attempted micturition. Contraction may be due to smooth or striated sphincter dyssynergia. **Striated sphincter dyssynergia** is a term that should be applied only when neurologic disease is present. A similar syndrome but without neurologic disease is called **dysfunctional voiding. Mechanical obstruction** is generally anatomic and caused by benign prostatic hyperplasia; urethral or bladder neck stricture; scarring or compression; or, rarely, kinking of a portion of the urethra during straining.

Voiding dysfunction in a classic T10 level paraplegic after spinal shock has passed would be classified as follows:

Storage phase—overactive hyperreflexic detrusor, absent sensation, low capacity, normal compliance, normal urethral closure function

Voiding phase—overactive obstructive urethral function, and possibly normal detrusor activity (actually, hyperreflexic)

The voiding dysfunction of a stroke patient with urgency incontinence would most likely be classified during storage as overactive hyperreflexic detrusor, normal sensation, low capacity, normal compliance, normal urethral closure function. During voiding the dysfunction would be classified as normal detrusor activity and normal urethral function, assuming that no anatomic obstruction existed.

The Functional System

Classification of voiding dysfunction can also be formulated on a simple functional basis (Tables 27–6 and 27–7), describing the dysfunction in terms of whether the deficit produced is primarily one of the filling-storage or the emptying phase of micturition (see Table 27–6) (Wein, 1981; Wein and Barrett, 1988). The genesis of such a system was

Table 27–6. FUNCTIONAL CLASSIFICATION

Failure to Store
- Because of bladder
- Because of outlet

Failure to Empty
- Because of bladder
- Because of outlet

proposed initially by Quesada and colleagues (1968). This type of system is an excellent alternative when a particular dysfunction does not readily lend itself to a generally agreed upon classification elsewhere. This simple-minded scheme assumes only that, whatever their differences, all "experts" would agree upon the two-phase concept of micturition (filling-storage and emptying) and upon the simple overall mechanisms underlying the normality of each phase (see above).

Storage failure results either because of bladder or outlet abnormalities or a combination. The bladder abnormalities very simply include involuntary bladder contractions, low compliance, and hypersensitivity. The outlet abnormalities can include only an intermittent or a continuous decrease in outlet resistance.

Emptying failure, likewise, can occur because of bladder or outlet abnormalities or a combination. The bladder side includes inadequate or unsustained bladder contractility, and the outlet side includes anatomic obstruction and sphincter(s) dyssynergia.

Failure in either category generally is not absolute but more often is relative. Such a functional system can easily be "expanded" and made more complicated to include etiologic or specific urodynamic connotations (see Table 27–7). However, the simplified system is perfectly workable and avoids argument in those complex situations in which the exact cause or urodynamic mechanism for a voiding dysfunction cannot be agreed on.

Proper use of this system for a given voiding dysfunction obviously requires a reasonably accurate notion of what the urodynamic data show. However, an exact diagnosis is **not** required for treatment. It should be recognized that some patients do not have only a discrete storage or emptying failure, and **the existence of combination deficits must be recognized to properly use this system** of classification. For instance, the classic T10 paraplegic after spinal shock generally exhibits a relative failure to store because of detrusor hyperreflexia and a relative failure to empty because of striated sphincter dyssynergia. With such a combination deficit, to use this classification system as a guide to treatment, one must assume that one of the deficits is primary and that significant improvement will result from its treatment alone, or that the voiding dysfunction can be converted primarily to a disorder of either storage or emptying by means of nonsurgical or surgical therapy. The resultant deficit can then be treated or circumvented. Using the same example, the combined deficit in a T10 paraplegic can be converted primarily to a storage failure by procedures directed at the dyssynergic striated sphincter; the resultant incontinence (secondary to detrusor hyperreflexia) can be circumvented (in a male) with an external collecting device. Alternatively, the deficit can be converted primarily to an emptying failure by pharmacologic or surgical measures designed to abolish or reduce the detrusor hyperreflexia, and the resultant emptying failure can then be circumvented with clean intermittent catheterization. Other examples of combination deficits include impaired bladder contractility with sphincter dysfunction, bladder outlet obstruction with detrusor hyperactivity, bladder outlet obstruction with sphincter malfunction, and detrusor hyperactivity with impaired contractility.

The major problem with the functional system is that not every voiding dysfunction can be reduced or converted primarily to a failure of storage or emptying. Additionally, although the functional classification of therapy that is a correlate of this scheme is entirely logical and complete, there is a danger of accepting an easy therapeutic solution and of thereby overlooking an etiology of a voiding dysfunction that is reversible at the primary level of causation. Nonneurogenic voiding dysfunctions, however, can be classified within this system, including those involving only the sensory aspect of micturition.

An additional advantage to the functional system is that the underlying concepts can be used repeatedly to simplify

Table 27–7. EXPANDED FUNCTIONAL CLASSIFICATION

Failure to Store
- ***Because of Bladder***
  - *Detrusor Hyperactivity*
    - Involuntary contractions
      - Neurologic disease, injury, or degeneration
      - Bladder outlet obstruction
      - Inflammation
      - Idiopathic
    - Decreased compliance
      - Neurologic disease
      - Fibrosis
      - Idiopathic
  - *Detrusor Hypersensitivity*
    - Inflammatory
    - Infectious
    - Neurologic
    - Psychologic
    - Idiopathic
- ***Because of Outlet***
  - Stress incontinence (hypermobility related)
  - Nonfunctional bladder neck–proximal urethra (intrinsic sphincter dysfunction)

Failure to Empty
- ***Because of Bladder***
  - Neurologic
  - Myogenic
  - Psychogenic
  - Idiopathic
- ***Because of Outlet***
  - *Anatomic*
    - Prostatic obstruction
    - Bladder neck contracture
    - Urethral stricture
    - Urethral compression
  - *Functional*
    - Smooth sphincter dyssynergia
    - Striated sphincter dyssynergia

Table 27–8. URODYNAMICS SIMPLIFIED*

	Bladder	Outlet
Filling-storage phase	P_{ves} P_{det} (FCMG)† DLPP	VLPP FLUORO UPP
Emptying phase	P_{ves} P_{det} (VCMG)‡	MUPP FLUORO EMG
	FLOW	
	RU	

*This functional conceptualization of urodynamics categorizes each study as to whether it examines bladder or outlet activity during the filling-storage or during the emptying phase of micturition. In this scheme uroflow and residual urine integrate the activity of the bladder and the outlet during the emptying phase.

†P_{ves} and P_{det} during a FCMG.

‡P_{ves} and P_{det} during a VCMG.

P_{ves}, Bladder pressure; P_{det}, detrusor pressure; FCMG, filling cystometrogram; DLPP, detrusor leak point pressure; UPP, urethral pressure profilometry; VLPP, Valsalva leak point pressure; VCMG, voiding cystometrogram; MUPP, micturitional urethral pressure profilometry; FLUORO, fluoroscopy of outlet during detrusor contraction; EMG, electromyography of periurethral striated musculature; FLOW, flowmetry; RU, residual urine.

many areas in neurourology. One logical extension makes urodynamics become more readily understandable (Table 27–8), whereas a different type of adaptation functions especially well as a "menu" for the categorization of all the types of treatment for voiding dysfunction (see Tables 29–1 and 29–2).

It is obvious that no type of system for classifying voiding dysfunction is perfect. Each offers something to every clinician, however, the amount being dependent on his or her level and type of training, interests, experience, and prejudices regarding the accuracy and interpretation of urodynamic data. The ideal approach to a given patient with voiding dysfunction remains a thorough neurourologic evaluation and an attempt at categorization in each system described. If the clinician can classify a given patient's voiding dysfunction in each system or can understand why this cannot be done, there is enough of a working knowledge to proceed with treatment. However, if the clinician is familiar with only one or two of these systems, a given patient does not fit these, and the reason is uncertain, the patient should certainly be studied further and the voiding dysfunction better characterized, at least before irreversible therapy is undertaken.

REFERENCES

Abrams P, Blaivas JG, Stanton SL, Andersen JT: The standardization of terminology of lower urinary tract function recommended by the International Continence Society. Int Urogynecol J 1990; 1:45.

Bors E, Comarr AE: Neurological Urology. Baltimore, University Park Press, 1971.

Coplen D, Macarek E, Levin RM: Developmental changes in normal fetal bovine whole bladder physiology. J Urol 1994; 151:1391.

DeGroat WC: Anatomy and physiology of the lower urinary tract. Urol Clin North Am 1993; 20(3):383.

DeGroat WC, Booth AM: Autonomic systems to the urinary bladder and sexual organs. *In* Dyck PJ, Thomas PK, Lambert EH, et al, eds: Peripheral Neuropathy. Philadelphia, W. B. Saunders Company, 1984, pp 285–299.

DeGroat WC, Booth AM, Yoshimura N: Neurophysiology of micturition and its modifications in animal models of human disease. *In* Maggi CA, ed: The Autonomic Nervous System, Vol 3. London, Harwood Academic Publishers, 1993, pp 227–290.

DeGroat WC, Kawatani M: Enkephalinergic inhibition in parasympathetic ganglia of the urinary bladder of the cat. J Physiol 1989; 413:13.

DeLancey JOL: Structural support of the urethra as it relates to stress urinary incontinence: The hammock hypothesis. Am J Obstet Gynecol 1994; 170:1713.

Elbadawi A: Neuromuscular mechanisms of micturition. *In* Yalla SV, McGuire EJ, Elbadawi A, Blaivas JG, eds: Neurourological Urodynamics: Principles and Practice. New York, Macmillan Publishing Company, 1988, pp 3–35.

Enhorning G: Simultaneous recording of intravesical and intraurethral pressure. Acta Chir Scand 1961; 276(suppl):1.

Hald T, Bradley WE: The Urinary Bladder: Neurology and Dynamics. Baltimore, Williams & Wilkins Company, 1982.

Klevmark B: Motility of the urinary bladder in cats during filling at physiological rates. I: Intravesical pressure patterns studied by new methods of cystometry. Acta Physiol Scand 1974; 90:565.

Klevmark B: Motility of the urinary bladder in cats during filling at physiologic rates. II: Effects of extrinsic bladder denervation on intramural tension and on intravesical pressure patterns. Acta Physiol Scand 1977; 101:176.

Krane RJ, Siroky MB: Classification of voiding dysfunction: Value of classification systems. *In* Barrett DM, Wein AJ, eds: Controversies in Neuro-Urology. New York, Churchill Livingstone, 1984, pp 223–238.

Lapides J: Neuromuscular, vesical and ureteral dysfunction. *In* Campbell MF, Harrison JH, eds: Urology. Philadelphia, W. B. Saunders Company, 1970, pp 1343–1379.

McGuire EJ: Physiology of the lower urinary tract. Am J Kidney Dis 1983; 2:402.

McLellan FC: The Neurogenic Bladder. Springfield, Ill, Charles C Thomas Company, 1939, pp 57–70, 116–185.

Mundy AR, Thomas PJ: Clinical physiology of the bladder, urethra and pelvic floor. *In* Mundy AR, Stephenson TP, Wein AJ, eds: Urodynamics: Principles, Practice, Application, 2nd ed. London, Churchill Livingstone, 1994, pp 15–28.

Quesada EM, Scott FB, Cardus D: Functional classification of neurogenic bladder dysfunction. Arch Phys Med Rehabil 1968; 49:692.

Steers WD, Barrett DM, Wein AJ: Voiding dysfunction: Diagnosis, classification, and management. *In* Gillenwater JY, Grayhack JT, Howards SS, Duckett JW Jr, eds: Adult and Pediatric Urology. Chicago, Year Book Medical Publishers, 1996, pp 1220–1326.

Tanagho EA: The anatomy and physiology of micturition. Clin Obstet Gynecol 1978, 5:3.

Wein AJ: Classification of neurogenic voiding dysfunction. J Urol 1981; 125:605.

Wein AJ, Barrett DM: Voiding Function and Dysfunction: A Logical and Practical Approach. Chicago, Year Book Medical Publishers, 1988.

Zderic SA, Levin RM, Wein AJ: Voiding function: Relevant anatomy, physiology, pharmacology and molecular aspects. *In* Gillenwater JY, Grayhack JT, Howards SS, Duckett JW Jr, eds: Adult and Pediatric Urology. Chicago, Year Book Medical Publishers, 1995, in press.

Zinner NR, Sterling AM, Ritter R: Structure and forces of continence. *In* Raz S ed: Female Urology. Philadelphia, W. B. Saunders Company, 1983, pp 33–41.

28
THE NEUROUROLOGIC EVALUATION

George D. Webster, M.B., Ch.B.
Karl J. Kreder, M.D.

The modalities available for the neurourologic evaluation of the patient with voiding dysfunction include the following:

- History
- Physical Examination
- Neurologic Examination
- Urinalysis
- Renal Function Studies
- Radiographic Evaluation
- Endoscopy
- Urodynamic Evaluation

In patients with uncomplicated urinary tract dysfunction, the neurourologic evaluation may be relatively simple, and many cases are managed after a history, physical examination, and basic laboratory evaluation alone. However, in more complex cases the full complement of tests available in the neurourologic armamentarium may be necessary. The general urologic examination is presented in Chapter 4; this chapter addresses the list of studies as it pertains to the patient with vesicourethral dysfunction, with particular emphasis on the urodynamic evaluation.

PATIENT HISTORY

Events Before the Commencement of Symptoms

Symptoms that date to childhood suggest a congenital origin. Past medical history should include careful questioning regarding any neurologic conditions such as spinal cord injury, low back pain, or previous spinal surgery. Neurologic conditions such as Parkinson's disease, cerebrovascular accident (CVA), multiple sclerosis, or degenerative conditions of the central nervous system are important, because these conditions commonly affect lower urinary tract function. Patients should be questioned about use of medicines, particularly those with anticholinergic, antidepressant, psychotropic, or alpha-blockade effect. Prior surgical history should include documentation of prior anti-incontinence surgery, prostatic surgery in males, or pelvic surgery. A family history should question for such disorders as epilepsy, Huntington's disease, and degenerative conditions of the central nervous system.

A 3-day voiding diary is one of the most helpful tools

in the assessment of voiding dysfunction. From such a record, the frequency, timing, and functional bladder capacity may be determined (Kassis and Schick, 1993; Diokno et al, 1987; McCormack et al, 1992).

Current Symptoms

Storage and Voiding Symptoms

Lower urinary tract symptoms (LUTS) have been divided into voiding (or obstructive) and irritative (or storage) categories. Voiding or obstructive symptoms are represented by hesitancy, straining to void, poor flow, terminal dribbling, and, ultimately, retention. Such symptoms may be caused not only by structural impediments to flow or functional bladder outlet obstruction (BOO) but also by poor detrusor contractility. The relative importance of individual symptoms is questionable, although hesitancy and weak stream have been nonspecifically correlated with urodynamic evidence of outlet obstruction (Bruskewitz et al, 1982; Christensen and Bruskewitz, 1990). The leading cause of BOO is benign prostatic hypertrophy (BPH). Although BPH is prevalent, it does not always lead to BOO, and similarly, even though BOO exists, the patient may not be troubled by LUTS. **In men with LUTS typical of those arising with prostate obstruction, objective evaluation confirms BOO in only 60% to 70%** (Abrams, 1995; Andersen, 1982). In the unobstructed group, the causes for the symptoms include poor detrusor contractility, bladder hyperactivity, and bladder hypersensitivity states.

Irritative or storage symptoms comprise urinary frequency, nocturia, urgency, and urge incontinence. These symptoms may represent the presence of detrusor hyperactivity, in which event they are termed instability symptoms. Patients who void more than eight times in a 24-hour period are generally considered to have excessive urinary frequency (Glenning, 1985). Frequency may have a number of causes: it may be secondary to excessive fluid intake, detrusor hyperactivity, small bladder capacity, or inadequate bladder emptying, or it may be psychogenic in nature. It may also result from pain or bladder hypersensitivity, as is seen frequently in inflammatory conditions and in patients with interstitial cystitis. Nocturia is the interruption of sleep by the urge to void. It has the same causes as diurnal frequency but may also occur in patients who mobilize fluid at night with resulting physiologic nocturnal diuresis. Urgency is the extreme desire to void, which if not heeded may result in incontinence, and it is typically associated with detrusor hyperactivity. Urgency that is secondary to pain is more typically associated with inflammatory conditions of the bladder, such as interstitial cystitis.

The symptom of the sensation of bladder pressure is difficult to quantify. It is the feeling that the urge to void will occur soon and is most commonly a result of bladder hypersensitivity states and of incomplete bladder emptying. Enuresis may be either nocturnal (urinary incontinence occurring only at night), or diurnal (occurring both day and night). Children with isolated nocturnal enuresis are unlikely to have significant voiding dysfunction. Patients with daytime incontinence or persistent nocturnal enuresis into adulthood are more likely to have some form of underlying voiding dysfunction.

Urinary incontinence is one of the most common and troublesome symptoms affecting both men and women. It may be categorized as occurring through the urethra or through an extraurethral channel such as a vesicovaginal fistula. Urethral urinary incontinence is further subdivided into that which occurs with an associated urge to void and that which occurs because of an increase in intra-abdominal pressure (stress incontinence). Urgency incontinence is caused by an involuntary bladder contraction and may have many causes, including neurologic disease, BOO, and senile and congenital causes. When an involuntary bladder contraction occurs, the bladder neck opens automatically and continence must be maintained by the volitional contraction of the distal sphincter mechanism (Fig. 28–1). If for any reason external sphincter contraction is delayed or deficient, incontinence occurs. Stress urinary incontinence occurs during increases in intra-abdominal pressure such as coughing, lifting, or sneezing. In women, it is most commonly associated with vesical neck hypermobility; however, some degree of intrinsic sphincter deficiency must coexist. In some patients, intrinsic sphincter deficiency alone is the cause, an entity previously called type III stress urinary incontinence. This entity may result from congenital causes such as myelomeningocele or epispadias, or it may be acquired after injury to the sacral spinal cord, urethral trauma, pelvic irradiation, or prior incontinence surgery; in men, it may develop after prostatectomy.

Overflow incontinence is the involuntary loss of urine associated with overdistention of the bladder. Overflow incontinence has a variety of clinical presentations, including that of stress incontinence or continuous dribbling-type incontinence. Overflow incontinence is secondary to poor bladder emptying caused by either impaired detrusor contractility or outflow obstruction. In men and women, impaired detrusor contractility may be secondary to medications, radical pelvic or spinal surgery, spinal cord injury, medical conditions such as diabetes, or myogenic injury from overdistention or from aging. In men, overflow incontinence secondary to BOO is commonly seen in cases of BPH, bladder neck obstruction, prostatic carcinoma, or urethral stricture. In women, BOO, though uncommon, can occur after anti-incontinence procedures, particularly sling cystourethropexy, or as the result of an anatomic derangement such as the presence of a large cystocele. In elderly persons, incontinence may have other causes, which can be remembered by the acronym DIAPPERS (delirium, infection, atrophic

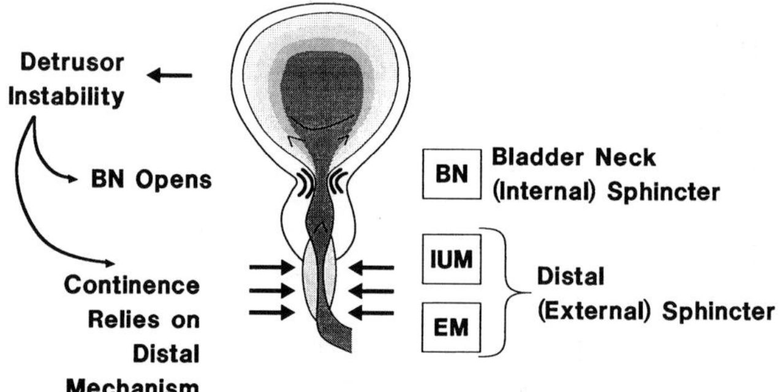

Figure 28–1. Schematic representation of the sphincter mechanism and the effect of an involuntary detrusor contraction. BN, bladder neck; IUM, intrinsic urethral mechanism; EM, extrinsic mechanism.

urethritis, pharmaceuticals, psychologic factors, endocrine disorders, restricted mobility, and stool impaction) (Resnick, 1990).

Scoring systems have been developed to quantify LUTS so as to assess the influence the symptoms have on the quality of life and the degree of bother they cause. Several scoring systems have been used in clinical research on BPH in the past, but their reliability and validity were never studied (Boyarsky et al, 1977; Madsen and Iversen, 1983). More recently, the American Urologic Association (AUA), collaborating with a team of experts in outcomes research, has developed a symptom score system known as the International Prostate Symptom Score (IPSS), and this has been validated formally using both clinimetric and psychometric principles (O'Leary, 1995; Barry et al, 1992). With the self-administered IPSS system, seven symptoms are scored from 0 to 5 (see Chapter 47). Symptoms are classified as mild (total score 0 to 7), moderate (total score 8 to 19), or severe (total score 20 to 35). To supplement the IPSS, two measures of disease-specific health status have also been developed. The Symptom Problem Index reflects how troublesome patients find their urinary symptoms, and the BPH Impact Index measures how much their urinary problems affect various domains of health (see Chapter 47). **Obviously, the symptoms being scored, although commonly seen in men with BPH, are not specific to BPH. Although the system tests the degree to which symptoms are present and bothersome, they do not reveal that the patient is obstructed or will benefit from prostatectomy.** Chancellor and colleagues (1994b) compared urodynamic findings and AUA symptom scores in 57 consecutive men and found no difference between obstructed symptomatic cases and unobstructed symptomatic cases (those with detrusor dysfunction). Despite these deficiencies, the BPH Impact Index has important uses. It helps determine the need for further evaluation, helps monitor surgical overuse, and effectively grades treatment outcome. This scoring system has been validated only for use in men with BPH and cannot be used in women.

Other symptoms that have relevance in the evaluation of the urologic patient include hematuria and urologic pain, including dysuria.

Sexual and Bowel Dysfunction

Sensory alterations in the genital or perianal area, fecal incontinence or constipation, difficulty in attaining and maintaining an erection, and disorders of ejaculation or orgasm may all be suggestive of impairment in the innervation of pelvic organs and the lower urinary tract.

PHYSICAL EXAMINATION

General Neurologic Examination

Evaluation of the patient with voiding dysfunction should include a general neurologic as well as a urologic physical examination. The neurologic portion of the examination can be divided into an assessment of general neurologic function (including mental status), examination of motor function, examination of sensory function, and assessment of reflexes.

Mental Status Examination

The mental status examination includes observation of the patient's general appearance. For instance, is the patient appropriately dressed, are the responses to questions appropriate, and are movements and actions appropriate for the situation? Orientation, memory, intellectual performance, insight, mood, speech, and thought content are all specific areas in the mental status examination that may need to be assessed.

Motor Examination

The motor examination primarily evaluates motor strength. In a patient complaining of weakness, the goals are threefold: (1) determine whether the weakness is focal or generalized; (2) establish whether the muscle weakness is organic or functional; and (3) isolate the cause of the paresis or plegia to either an abnormality of a lower or an upper motor neuron or one intrinsic to the muscle itself.

Sensory Examination

Patterns of sensory loss are important because they often follow the segmental distribution of one or more spinal nerve roots and therefore may help to localize the level of neurologic deficit (Fig. 28–2). It is helpful to remember that the anterior portions of the labia and scrotum are supplied by roots from the thoracolumbar spinal cord, whereas the posterior portions of the scrotum, the perianal area, and the posterior portions of the labia are supplied by sacral roots.

Assessment of Reflexes

The deep tendon reflexes are altered in most diseases of muscle and in those diseases that involve the peripheral nerves. Commonly tested muscle reflexes include the biceps (C5–6) and triceps (C7) in the upper extremity, and the quadriceps reflex (L3–4) and Achilles tendon reflex (L5–S2) in the lower extremity. Neurologic reflexes are those that are not present in neurologically normal patients, the best known of which is the Babinski reflex, elicited by stroking the plantar surface of the foot toward the great toe (Walton, 1989).

Cutaneous reflexes are motor responses to cutaneous stimuli. Perhaps the most useful cutaneous reflex in urology is the bulbocavernosus reflex, elicited by placing an examining finger in the patient's rectum and then either squeezing the glans penis, squeezing the clitoris, or pulling on an indwelling Foley catheter. **A normal bulbocavernosus reflex is** contraction of the anal sphincter and bulbocavernosus muscles in response to any of these maneuvers. This reflex is **primarily a test of the integrity of spinal cord segments S2 through S4 and is present in most normal individuals**; absence of this reflex may be an indication of a peripheral or segmental neurologic lesion (Bors and Blinn, 1959; Lapides and Bobbitt, 1956). Other cutaneous reflexes tested include the cremasteric (L1–2), abdominal (T6–L2), and anal (S2–5) reflexes.

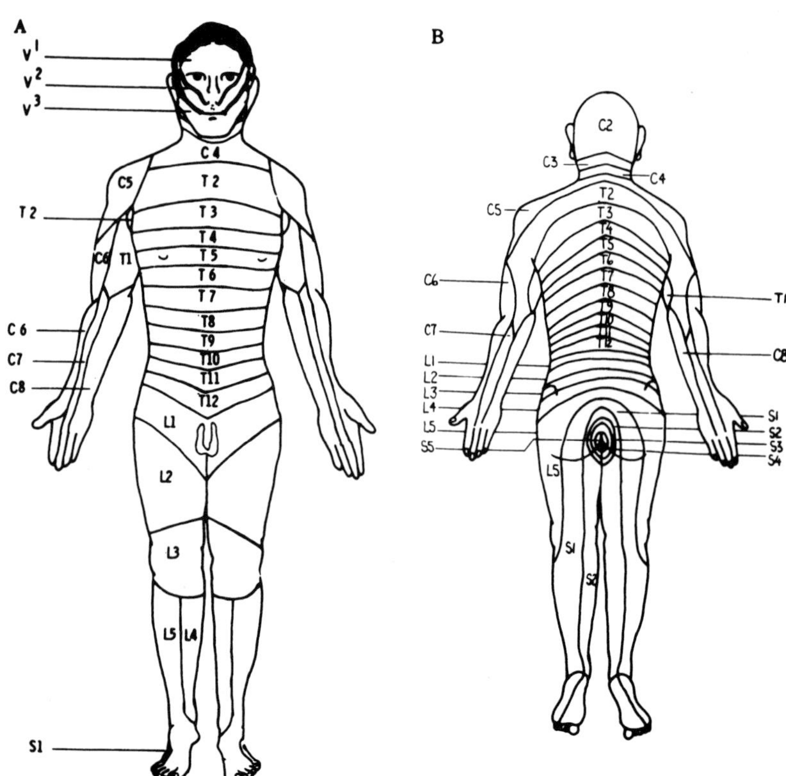

Figure 28–2. Sensory dermatome map used to help localize the level of neurologic deficit.

Urologic Examination

Examination of the Abdomen, Genitalia, and Vagina

The bladder cannot be palpated unless it is distended, and it is not evident on percussion unless it has a volume of more than 150 ml. A palpable bladder that is evident soon after the patient has voided is therefore suggestive of chronic urinary retention. In women, the pelvic examination assesses the general perineal skin condition and genital atrophy and documents vaginal hypermobility and prolapse, including cystocele, rectocele, enterocele, and uterine or vaginal cuff descent. The degree of vaginal wall hypermobility is assessed by having the patient strain or cough while retracting the opposing vaginal wall. Ideally, this examination should be repeated in the standing position to better identify the magnitude of uterine and vaginal prolapse.

Rectal Examination

In females, the rectal examination is performed to check for the presence of a rectal mass or fecal impaction and also to assess sphincter tone, sensation, and the bulbocavernosus reflex. The combined digital rectal and vaginal examination identifies the presence of enterocele. In males, the digital examination of the prostate is also performed to estimate size and detect abnormalities suggestive of malignancy.

URINE EXAMINATION

Urinalysis

Urine examination is indicated in all patients with symptoms or signs of urologic disease, and it takes on particular importance in the patient with lower urinary tract dysfunction in whom infection (symptomatic or asymptomatic) is common. The specimen is examined for color, appearance, and specific gravity, and reagent strips are used to assess pH, protein, glucose, hemoglobin, bacteria, and leukocytes. The nitrite test for bacteria is positive if there are bacteria in the urine that are capable of reducing nitrate to nitrite. A positive nitrite test suggests the presence of more than 100,000 organisms/ml. This test is positive only if coagulase-splitting bacteria are present; used alone, it is only 40% to 60% accurate (Kunin and de Groot, 1977). The leukocyte esterase test is a widely used chemical test that depends on the presence of esterase in granulocytic leukocytes. This test is an indication of pyuria and is positive even if the leukocytes have undergone degeneration. The test identifies those patients who have between 10 and 12 leukocytes per high-powered field in a centrifuged specimen (Bolann et al, 1989). This test does not necessarily detect bacteria in the urine but is only an indicator of pyuria. **For this reason, the leukocyte esterase test and the nitrite test are often combined to detect both bacteria and the presence of inflammation in the urine.** Particularly in patients with neurogenic bladder and in those with urinary stasis, cloudy urine is common, and although it may be a sign of infection, it is also frequently caused by the presence of amorphous phosphate (Williams and Kreder, 1995). Proteinuria may be a sign of renal impairment and may justify a 24-hour urine collection.

Microscopic Examination

The urine sediment is examined unstained for the presence of bacteria and leukocytes, which may suggest urinary tract infection; however, positive urine cultures are not obtained in more than 60% of patients who have pyuria. Urine cultures are performed to confirm the presence of an infection and to identify the offending organism. Microscopy may reveal red blood cells, leukocytes, and leukocyte, hyaline, or granular casts. The presence of even a few red blood cells in the urine is abnormal and warrants further evaluation; in patients with neurogenic bladder who are neurologically impaired, microhematuria may be the only sign of associated serious pathology. Microhematuria may result from catheter trauma in patients performing self-catheterization, and good judgment is crucial in knowing when and when not to investigate.

RENAL FUNCTION EVALUATION

Lower urinary tract dysfunction is a common cause of renal deterioration, and a range of studies is available to monitor the patient.

Urine Specific Gravity

Urine specific gravity is the simplest of all tests of renal function. The kidneys retain the ability to dilute urine until renal damage is quite severe, and even in a uremic patient it is still possible for the urine specific gravity to be in the range of 1.002 to 1.004. Concentrating ability, however, is severely impaired if the patient is unable to concentrate urine to a specific gravity greater than 1.010.

Serum Creatinine and Creatinine Clearance

Creatinine, a by-product of skeletal muscle metabolism, is produced each day in a relatively constant amount and therefore serum concentrations of creatinine are a direct reflection of renal function. Normal serum creatinine levels in adults are between 0.8 and 1.2 mg/dl, and in children, 0.4 to 0.8 mg/dl. Serum creatinine remains in the normal range until approximately one half of renal function has been lost. Serum creatinine level is relatively insensitive to dietary intake or hydration. It is routinely monitored in the evaluation and follow-up of patients with neurourologic disorders.

Because the production of creatinine is relatively stable and because creatinine is filtered by the glomerulus, its renal clearance is approximately equal to the glomerular filtration rate (GFR). It is an accurate and reproducible measure of renal function that can easily be performed on a 24-hour urine specimen and calculated by the following formula: Clearance = UV/P, where U is the concentration of creatinine in the urine (in mg/dl), P is the creatinine concentration in plasma (in mg/dl), and V is milliliters of urine excreted per minute for 24 hours. The resulting clearance is expressed in milliliters per minute, with a normal range being between 90 and 110. This test can be refined further by standardizing the ratio of muscle mass to body surface area using the following formula:

$$\frac{UV}{P} \times \frac{1.73\ \text{m}^2}{\text{estimated surface area}} = \text{corrected clearance.}$$

A corrected clearance of between 70 and 140 ml/minute is in the normal range.

Radionuclide Imaging

Any substance that is filtered by the glomerulus and not reabsorbed or excreted by the tubular cells is an ideal agent to quantify GFR. These studies are discussed later in this chapter.

RADIOLOGIC EVALUATION

Upper Urinary Tract

Several studies are commonly used to evaluate the status of the kidneys and ureters: renal sonography, excretory urography, and radioisotope studies.

Renal Ultrasonography

Renal ultrasound has become the primary upper urinary tract imaging technique in patients with neurourologic disorders. It accurately measures renal size and identifies parenchymal scarring, renal masses, and the features of obstruction. It should be performed in the hydrated patient with an empty bladder. Duplex or Doppler ultrasonography can be used to examine the renal veins or inferior vena cava for the presence of flow (Resnick and Rifkin, 1991).

Excretory Urography

For many years, excretory urography was the most widely performed diagnostic test in urology, but recently it has been supplanted by a variety of other radiographic studies in the initial evaluation and follow-up of patients with bladder dysfunction. It continues to be a valuable study of the structure of the upper urinary tract but has lost its historic screening role in such conditions as BPH (Abrams et al, 1976; Andersen et al, 1977).

Radioisotope Studies

Radioisotope studies are frequently used for the initial evaluation and follow-up of patients with vesicourethral dysfunction, particularly those with neurogenic origins. For this purpose, they have been suggested as the appropriate studies in the child with spinal dysraphism and the adult with spinal cord injury (Lloyd, 1989). Technetium-labeled diethylenetriaminepentaacetic acid (^{99m}Tc-DTPA) is used to identify renal function and test for obstruction. Technetium-labeled dimercaptosuccinic acid (^{99m}Tc-DMSA) is the preferred agent for imaging the renal parenchyma. Technetium-labeled mercaptoacetylglycineglycine-glycine (^{99m}Tc-MAG3) is excreted in one transit through the kidney and is used to measure renal blood flow and function (Russell and Duborsky, 1991; Eshima and Taylor, 1992). A variety of other agents enjoy popular use in some centers, and newer compounds continue to be developed.

Radiologic Follow-up in Neurogenic Dysfunction

Patients with lower urinary tract dysfunction may be at risk for deterioration of the upper urinary tracts. **McGuire and associates (1981) recognized that patients with a detrusor leak point pressure (LPP) of more than 40 cm H_2O were at increased risk for development of upper tract deterioration** (see later discussion)**. Bauer et al (1984) reported that detrusor sphincter dyssynergy was the most important factor in predicting the development of subsequent hydronephrosis. Galloway and colleagues (1991) devised a hostility score,** which included bladder compliance, detrusor contractility, reflux, detrusor LPP, and sphincter behavior, that correlates very well with subsequent upper tract deterioration. **It is logical to identify those patients at higher risk for upper tract damage and monitor them more closely with appropriate studies (ultrasound, urography, or renal scans), in order to institute timely intervention.** It is the authors' practice to obtain a baseline renal ultrasound study on all patients with a neurogenic bladder. In high-risk patients, follow-up ultrasound examination is carried out at 6 months, and if the upper tracts are stable, subsequent ultrasound studies are obtained at yearly intervals. Other radiologic studies are performed as indicated, and routine follow-up using such modalities is recommended by some (Lloyd, 1989).

Lower Urinary Tract

Cystography

Cystography is an important test of the lower urinary tract in patients with neurogenic dysfunction; it provides information regarding the anatomy of the bladder and urethra, reflux, presence of diverticula, and presence of stones, as well as a reasonable assessment of residual urine. Cystography is performed with the use of a radiographic contrast agent and may be performed at the time of urodynamic study (video-urodynamics) or as a separate test.

Radionuclide cystography is the most sensitive imaging method for detection of ureterovesical ureteroreflux. This technique requires less radiation exposure than conventional cystography. ^{99m}Tc-sulfurcolide or pertechnetate is instilled into the bladder through a catheter, and imaging is performed during bladder filling and voiding.

ENDOSCOPIC EXAMINATION

Endoscopic evaluation of the lower urinary tract is most helpful to detect anatomic or structural abnormalities (e.g., stricture) and urethral or vesical diverticula, stones, and so on. It is also indicated in the evaluation of hematuria. It cannot be used to diagnose functional (sphincteric) or prostatic obstruction and should not be used in place of urodynamics in this role. It is not indicated in the routine screening evaluation of patients with neurogenic bladder dysfunction nor in patients with BPH, in whom it has the same indications as in the general urologic population. Little or no correlation has been demonstrated between prostate size or length as assessed endoscopically, or between the presence of BOO and the endoscopic findings of trabeculation (Roehrborn et al, 1993).

FUNCTIONAL AND URODYNAMIC EVALUATION

Urodynamics has several clinical roles in the neurourologic evaluation. These include the characterization of detrusor function, evaluation of the bladder outlet, evaluation of voiding function, and diagnosis and characterization of neuropathy.

The Urodynamic Armamentarium

The urodynamic armamentarium includes uroflowmetry, cystometry, urethral pressure studies, pressure flow micturition studies, sphincter electromyography, video-urodynamic evaluation, and pharmacologic testing. The range of urodynamic testing is extensive, and although some patients may benefit from sophisticated testing, more limited techniques suffice in many cases. The challenge for the clinician is to determine which of these studies are necessary in order to characterize and treat an individual patient's voiding dysfunction. Although patients are usually evaluated in a laboratory setting, ambulatory testing is gaining in popularity (Robertson et al, 1994).

Patient Selection

Most patients with lower urinary tract dysfunction benefit from some form of urodynamic evaluation, but urodynamic studies are particularly helpful in certain groups. These include incontinent patients, patients with BOO, patients with voiding dysfunction secondary to neurogenic bladder, and some children who have complex voiding and incontinence problems.

Urinary incontinence in women with classic stress symptoms by history, who have no associated bladder instability symptoms nor voiding dysfunction and in whom an anatomic cause (urethrovesical or anterior vaginal wall hypermobility) can be identified, may require little or no further urodynamic evaluation before definitive therapy is undertaken. However, women with recurrent incontinence, urinary incontinence and associated voiding dysfunction, or marked bladder instability symptoms and associated neurologic disease, and those in whom an anatomic cause cannot be identified will certainly benefit from further urodynamic study. Incontinent males with non-neurogenic incontinence usually experience incontinence as a result of either radical or transurethral prostatectomy. Urodynamic studies are helpful in this group of patients to exclude significant bladder pathology (low compliance or detrusor hyperactivity) as a contributing cause of incontinence and to identify sphincteric weakness. Voiding problems related to BOO may be caused by structural outlet obstruction (BPH) or by poor detrusor contractility or inadequate sphincter relaxation. Patient history, physical examination, endoscopic findings, and radiologic studies cannot necessarily identify which is the cause of symptoms (Kreder and Webster, 1991).

Patients in whom urodynamic study is recommended include those who have symptoms of obstruction but also marked bladder instability symptoms, those with obstructive symptoms but no identifiable endoscopic cause, obstructed patients who also have neurologic disease, young men (<50 years) with obstructive symptoms, and those women who have obstructive voiding symptoms as their major complaint. In patients undergoing urodynamic study for suspected BOO, a pressure-flow study is performed; video-urodynamic study adds an anatomic dimension to the pressure-flow study, allowing identification of the site of obstruction.

All patients who have neurogenic bladder dysfunction should undergo urodynamic study in order to characterize the nature of the detrusor and sphincter problem and to determine prognosis and management. The study should be performed at the time of initial presentation and should be repeated periodically. The schedule of repetition is determined by the presence or absence of hostile features (e.g., low bladder compliance, detrusor sphincter dyssynergia, reflux), the attainment of clinical goals (e.g., continence, efficient emptying), the progress of the upper tracts and renal function, and the incidence of symptomatic urinary tract infections. In patients with spinal cord injury, the study performed soon after presentation often reveals detrusor areflexia, and it must be repeated after reflex activity has returned.

Children with isolated enuresis rarely have abnormalities that are identified by routine laboratory-based urodynamic investigations. Children with daytime urgency, urge incontinence, recurrent infections, reflux, or upper tract changes may be screened by noninvasive uroflow and electromyographic (EMG) studies and may require formal urodynamic evaluation. Invasive urodynamic studies are particularly difficult to perform in children, and interpretation is complicated by artifact and by the child's inability to cooperate. The child most frequently referred for study has persistent diurnal enuresis, and the most common finding is involuntary detrusor activity. The identification of sphincter hyperactivity in this group is marred by the irritative effects of catheterization. Urodynamic study is mandatory in the child with spinal dysraphism and ideally is performed during the hospitalization at birth to identify the degree of hostility on which urologic management depends (Perez and Webster, 1992; Perez et al, 1992; Galloway et al, 1991).

Patient Preparation and Precautions

Before a urodynamic study, the procedure should be explained to the patient, an adequate history obtained, physical examination completed, and a 3-day voiding diary completed. Information from the voiding diary is invaluable in determining the patient's customary functional capacity, daily urine output, and approximate filling volume, values that are necessary for cystometry. Although rarely injurious, urodynamic studies are invasive, and patients may be asked to sign a consent form.

Studies should be deferred in the presence of urinary tract infection and ideally should not be performed after recent instrumentation (cystoscopy). Many pharmacologic agents can significantly affect detrusor or sphincteric function, and either patients should stop these medications or their impact on the urodynamic study should be taken into account.

Parenteral antibiotic prophylaxis is necessary in patients with prosthetic heart valves, mitral valve prolapse, artificial joints, and so on (Dajani et al, 1990). Routine oral prophylactic antibacterial drugs are not necessarily given before urodynamic studies; however, those patients requiring multiple instrumentation or who are at high risk for urinary tract infection are usually treated for 24 to 48 hours after completion of the study. **Autonomic dysreflexia can be a life-threatening condition and should be considered in patients with high neurologic lesions (above T6) (Trop and Bennett, 1991). If the patient begins to experience autonomic dysreflexia as manifested by symptoms and hypertension during the course of a urodynamic study, the bladder should immediately be emptied and the patient may be treated with an antihypertensive (sublingual nifedipine or intravenous hydralazine) if the condition does not rapidly resolve.** In patients with a known diagnosis of autonomic dysreflexia, pretreatment is undertaken with administration of sublingual nifedipine (Thyberg et al, 1994) or an alpha-blocking agent (Chancellor et al, 1994a; Krum et al, 1992), or both.

Evaluation of the Detrusor (Storage Phase)

Cystometry

Cystometry is the measurement of intravesical bladder pressure during the course of bladder filling. Cystometry was first performed the 19th century, but its clinical value was not recognized until recently, with the development of the clinical science of urodynamics (Mosso and Pellicani, 1882; Perez and Webster, 1992). Cystometry is the cornerstone of the urodynamic evaluation.

Study Variables

There are a number of variables in the manner in which cystometry is performed, and these should be specified (Abrams et al, 1988; International Continence Society, 1977a, 1977b, 1980, 1981). All systems should be zeroed to atmospheric pressure, and for external transducers the reference point is the superior edge of the symphysis pubis. The patient must be awake, unsedated, and not taking any medications that could affect the functioning of the lower urinary tract. Bladder access may be accomplished by transurethral catheterization or, rarely, by the placement of a percutaneous suprapubic cystotomy tube. The filling medium may be either gas (carbon dioxide) or liquid (water, saline, or radiographic contrast material). The advantage of liquid cystometry is that the bladder is filled with a physiologic medium. Liquid also facilitates detection of urinary incontinence and allows cystometry to be followed by a voiding study. If contrast solution is used, a video-urodynamic study may be obtained. When fluid cystometry is performed, the temperature of the liquid infused should be at or near body temperature.

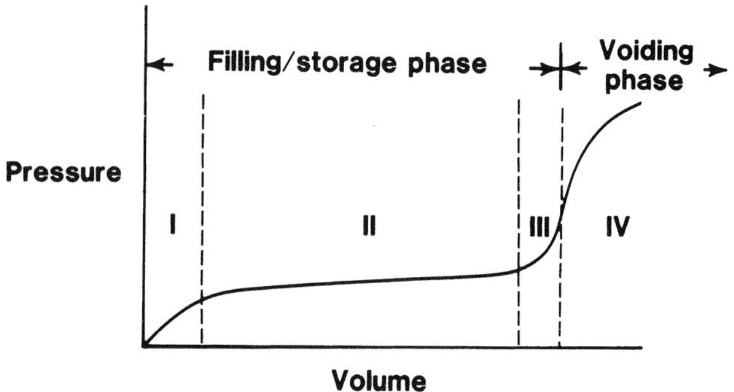

Figure 28–3. Schematically the normal cystometrogram has four phases: (I) an initial pressure rise to achieve resting bladder pressure; (II) the toner slim, which reflects the viscoelastic properties of the bladder wall; (III) bladder wall structures' achieving maximal elongation and a pressure rise caused by additional filling (this phase should not be encountered during cystometry); and (IV) the voiding phase, representing bladder contractility. (From Steers WD, Barrett DM, Wein AJ: Voiding dysfunction: Diagnosis, classification and management. *In* Gillenwater JY, Grayhack JT, Howards SS, Duckett JW, eds: Adult and Pediatric Urology, 3rd ed. St. Louis, Mosby–Year Book, 1996, Fig. 26B–1.)

Gas cystometry has its proponents, who suggest that it shortens the time necessary to perform the test because rapid fill rates are possible and that there are fewer problems of hygiene if incontinence occurs during this portion of the study (Bradley et al, 1968; Gleason and Reilly, 1979; Godec and Cass, 1979). However, the disadvantage of gas cystometry is that it is an unphysiologic medium and the rapid fill rates achieved may artifactually change the normal bladder response. A voiding study is not possible, and because gas is compressible, subtle changes in intravesical pressure may not be evident. Carbon dioxide, when dissolved, forms carbonic acid, which can irritate the bladder.

Cystometry may be performed with the patient supine, seated, or standing, in a laboratory or an ambulatory setting. In order for the results to be diagnostic, the symptoms being evaluated must be duplicated during the study. If cystometry is performed in the supine position alone, bladder instability may not be identified. Ideally, filling should be performed with the patient standing. Several provocative maneuvers are performed to try to "unmask" abnormalities of detrusor function (involuntary contractions) in patients in whom abnormalities are suspected but not present at slow or medium fill rates. These provocative maneuvers include fast-fill cystometry, posture change by erect filling, coughing, heel jouncing, jumping, running water, and hand washing (Papa Petros and Elmsten, 1993).

Bladder filling during cystometry may be achieved either by diuresis or by filling through a catheter; with the latter procedure, the filling rate should be specified. **Up to 10 ml/min filling is considered physiologic and is termed slow fill cystometry. Fill rates between 10 and 100 ml/min are considered medium fill cystometry, and rates greater than 100 ml/min are considered rapid filling cystometry. The fill rate selected is to some degree determined by the population being studied.** Children and those with known bladder hyperactivity require slow fill rates. A number of catheter arrangements are available for cystometry. A single-lumen catheter may be used to both fill and measure simultaneous pressure from a side port. Double- or triple-lumen single catheters are available to fill the bladder, monitor bladder pressure, and record pressure in the urethra simultaneously. Optimally, a two-catheter technique is used in which the filling catheter and the small (No. 4 Fr) pressure monitoring catheter are passed into the bladder side by side. This technique facilitates the performance of a pressure flow study after cystometry has been completed. The filling catheter is removed, leaving in place the small-caliber pressure-measuring catheter, around which voiding can occur without significant obstruction. Microtransducer-tipped catheters are also available.

NOMENCLATURE

During the course of cystometry, information is sought regarding the bladder's capacity and compliance, sensation, and the occurrence of involuntary contractions.

The term *capacity* must be qualified, because there are really three bladder capacities that can be measured. **The functional bladder capacity is best determined from a urinary diary and is the largest volume voided during the period recorded. It is important because it indicates the anticipated volume to which the bladder may be filled during cystometry.** The maximum cystometric capacity is the volume at which a patient with normal bladder sensation feels that micturition can no longer be delayed; it is usually slightly greater than the functional capacity. In patients with impaired bladder sensation, the maximum cystometric capacity cannot be determined, and it is simply the point at which the examiner terminates the study. The maximum anesthetic capacity is the volume of the bladder after filling under general, spinal, or epidural anesthesia. This capacity is rarely measured except in the evaluation of patients with suspected structurally reduced bladder capacity, such as occurs in some patients with interstitial cystitis. A reduced anesthetic capacity may be an indication for bladder augmentation surgery.

***Bladder compliance* is defined as the change in bladder pressure for a given change in volume. Compliance is calculated by dividing the volume change (V) by the detrusor pressure (P_{det}) during that change in bladder volume (compliance = V/P_{det}) and is expressed as ml/cm of H_2O.** Normal bladder compliance is high and is usually better approximated by ambulatory urodynamic assessment using physiologic bladder fill rates than by the fast fill rates

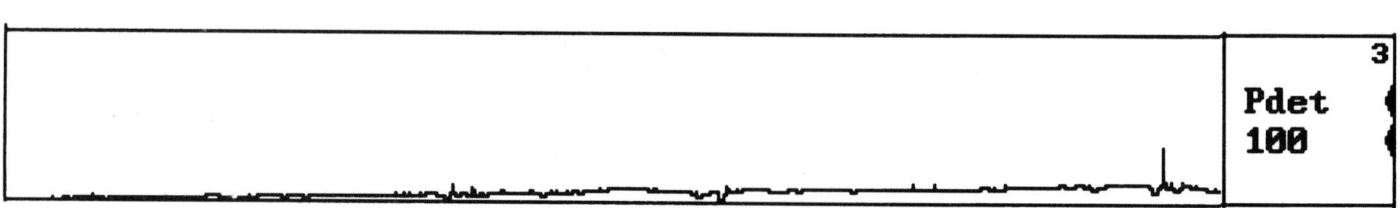

Figure 28–4. A cystometrogram showing a stable detrusor. P_{det}, detrusor pressure.

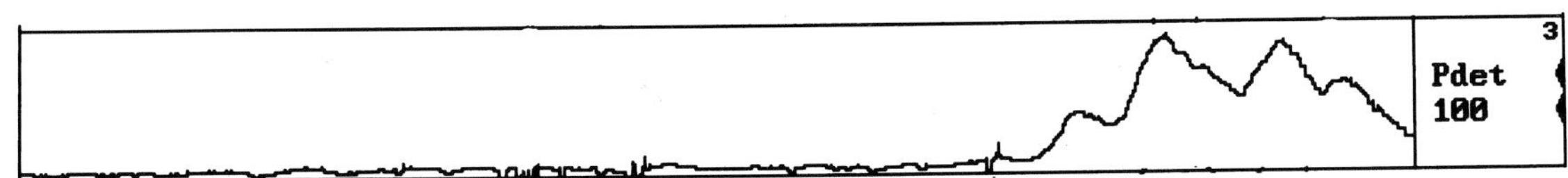

Figure 28–5. Cystometrogram of an unstable bladder, showing involuntary detrusor contraction despite the patient's attempt to delay micturition. P_{det}, detrusor pressure.

used in the laboratory setting. **In the laboratory, the normal pressure rise is less than 6 to 10 cm H_2O.** Webb and associates (1989) suggested that the decreased compliance recorded in patients undergoing medium fill cystometry is artifact (Webb et al, 1989). Bladder compliance in a group of patients with neurogenic bladder averaged 4.9 ± 2.7 ml/cm H_2O when measured cystometrically but 92 ± 12 ml/cm H_2O with ambulatory monitoring.

During filling cystometry, *bladder sensation* is evaluated by questioning the patient about the feeling of fullness of the bladder. Commonly, the patient is asked to indicate the first desire to void, normal desire to void (defined as the sensation that leads the patient to void at the next convenient time, but voiding can be delayed if necessary), strong desire to void, urgency, and pain. Pain during bladder filling is considered to be abnormal and is often associated with some form of cystitis.

Detrusor stability reflects the integrity of central nervous system control over bladder function. **An *unstable bladder* is one that can be demonstrated to contract either spontaneously or with provocative maneuvers during filling cystometry while the patient is attempting to inhibit micturition. *Detrusor hyperreflexia* implies a bladder that contracts involuntarily because of neurologic disease**. Detrusor instability is an unstable bladder contraction that occurs during cystometry in a patient without an identifiable neurologic lesion.

The Concept of Bladder Hyperactivity

The hyperactive bladder is one that demonstrates instability, hyperreflexia, or low compliance. The normal bladder, although capable of voluntary contraction, should not contract involuntarily even if provoked by some of the maneuvers mentioned previously, and is therefore termed stable (Figs. 28–3 and 28–4). The unstable bladder (overactive detrusor) contracts either spontaneously or on provocation during cystometric filling despite the fact that the patient is attempting to delay micturition (Fig. 28–5). Because cystometry is always performed with the understanding that the patient will delay micturition if at all possible, any bladder contraction under these circumstances is termed an involuntary one, and the bladder is then termed unstable.

Bladder instability may be asymptomatic but typically causes presenting symptoms of frequency, nocturia, urgency, and urge incontinence. Patients with urgency and urge incontinence in whom unstable detrusor contractions can be demonstrated on a urodynamic study are said to have motor urge incontinence. Patients in whom the same symptoms are present but who have a stable bladder on urodynamic studies are said to have sensory urgency. **It is probable that sensory and motor urgency are conditions in the same spectrum and that patients with sensory urgency are able to inhibit unstable contractions during the course of a urodynamic study (Creighton et al, 1991). However, during activities of normal living, when the patient is not focused on the bladder to the same degree, these unstable contractions are unmasked and manifest with symptoms.** Women with sensory urgency in whom the feeling of urge to void is accompanied by a feeling of threatened incontinence should be differentiated from those with bladder hypersensitivity states in whom the urgency is because of discomfort.

Bladder compliance is a reflection of the bladder's ability to accommodate increasing filling volumes. **Low bladder compliance implies a poorly distensible bladder in which the pressure/volume curve is steep and the pressure rise is rapid for low volume increases** (Fig. 28–6). Low bladder compliance may be seen in a number of clinical scenarios:

- Patients who have had a Foley catheter in place for a prolonged period, resulting in a combination of muscular hypertonia and mucosal and mural changes
- Patients with a defunctionalized bladder after a urinary diversion
- Patients with neurogenic bladder dysfunction, particularly if the lesion is in or distal to the conus medullaris
- Patients with clinical conditions such as tuberculosis or schistosomiasis, in which excessive collagen is deposited in the bladder wall after radiation therapy

High detrusor compliance can also be attributed to a number of clinical situations:

- Patients with prolonged and gradually progressive delayed voiding
- Patients with conditions that affect the sensory pathways of the detrusor, the most common being diabetic neuropathy and pernicious anemia
- Patients with spinal cord trauma, after which a period of "bladder shock" is usually seen for 6 to 8 weeks

Detrusor Leak Point Pressure. The detrusor LPP may be determined during cystometry and is an important variable in the evaluation of the patient with low bladder compliance. McGuire et al (1981) have demonstrated a significant risk

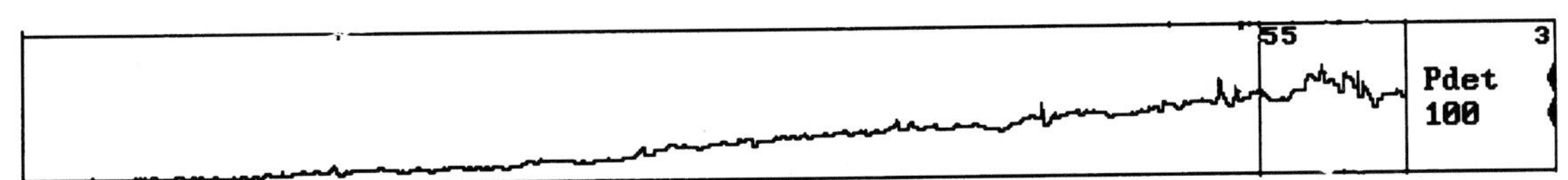

Figure 28–6. A cystometrogram depicting low bladder compliance. Pressure has risen to 55 cm H_2O during fill to 200 ml. P_{det}, detrusor pressure.

of upper tract deterioration if bladder storage occurs at sustained urodynamically measured detrusor pressures in excess of 40 cm H_2O, regardless of continence. The bladder outlet must not be occluded by the use of too large a catheter or by a Foley catheter balloon during the filling process, which is at approximately 25 ml/minute, depending on patient age. Indigo carmine or methylene blue can be added to the infusion medium to aid in identifying leakage. The detrusor LPP is the pressure at which urethral leak of urine is first identified (Fig. 28–7). It may be recorded from the P_{det} or the intravesical (P_{ves}) tracing, but in the latter case it is the increment in pressure from baseline. **In general, those patients with a detrusor LPP of more than 40 cm H_2O are at increased risk for upper tract deterioration, although any alteration in compliance, particularly in a child, must lead to more intensive follow-up** (McGuire et al, 1981; Ghoniem et al, 1990; Flood et al, 1994).

Factors That May Alter the Cystometrogram. A number of factors may alter the cystometrogram and lead to misinterpretation. These include an incompetent outlet, massive reflux, rapid fill, lack of patient cooperation, and substances irritative to the bladder. If a bladder outlet is incompetent, urine may leak around the filling catheter, and low bladder compliance may not be diagnosed because the bladder is never adequately filled. This problem most commonly occurs during cystometry in the spinal dysraphic child and in the elderly woman with profound intrinsic sphincter deficiency resulting from senile and other atrophic changes. In this scenario, the cystometrogram should be repeated using a Foley catheter for bladder filling and with the distended Foley balloon pulled down to occlude the bladder neck.

In patients with massive reflux, large volumes of the filling solution reflux into the dilated upper tracts, and a low capacity–low compliance detrusor may be missed because of the seemingly adequate capacity of the system. This problem is easier to identify during video-urodynamic study. If detrusor filling is too rapid, even a normal detrusor may appear to have low compliance; therefore, the identification of low compliance should be confirmed by repeated filling at a much slower fill rate. In addition, the terminal filling pressure should be considered to be that pressure recorded after filling has been stopped and the bladder has been allowed to accommodate.

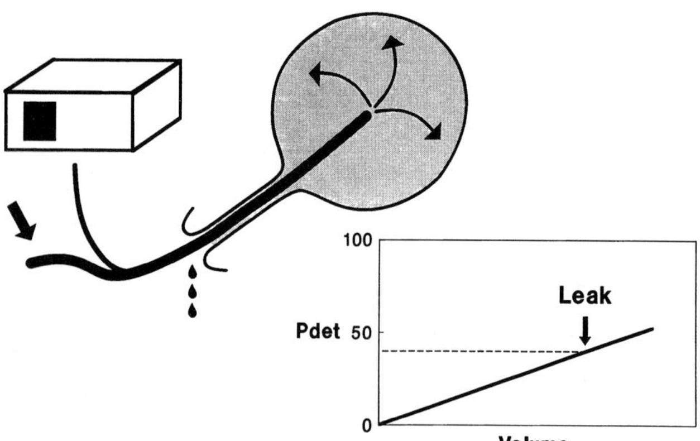

Figure 28–7. A schematic representation of the detrusor leak point pressure study. The urethral meatus is observed for urine leakage, and the pressure at which leakage occurs is the detrusor leak point pressure. P_{det}, detrusor pressure.

Implicit in the performance of successful cystometry is the patient's cooperation with and understanding of the goals of the study. This may be a particular problem with pediatric or mentally impaired patients, in whom "involuntary" contractions may not be what they seem! Urinary tract infection and indwelling catheters in bladder hypersensitivity states may result in the loss of bladder compliance, low cystometric capacity, and perhaps bladder instability that might not otherwise exist; therefore, every attempt should be made to clear infections before the performance of a urodynamic study. Those patients who are catheter-dependent ideally should be placed on clean intermittent catheterization for a period before the urodynamic study is undertaken.

Pharmacologic Tests

The bethanechol supersensitivity or bethanechol stimulation test was originally described by Lapides and colleagues (1962) and is performed in an attempt to identify a neurogenic origin in the patient with an acontractile bladder. It is based on the observation that after an organ is deprived of its nerve supply it develops hypersensitivity to the normal excitatory neurotransmitters for that organ. The cystometry is performed by infusion of liquid at a rate of 1 ml/second to a volume of 100 ml, at which time bladder pressure is measured. After two or three such infusions, an average value for end-fill pressure is obtained. After this, 2.5 mg bethanechol chloride is injected subcutaneously, and cystometry is repeatedly performed at a rate of 1 ml/second, filling to a volume of 100 ml, at 10, 20, and 30 minutes after the injection. A normal bladder shows an increase of less than 15 cm H_2O above the control value; the denervated bladder shows a response greater than 15 cm H_2O. A false-negative test may occur in patients who are obese and therefore receive too low a dose of bethanechol chloride. In order to decrease the number of false-negative responses, some have suggested increasing the dose of bethanechol chloride to 5 mg (Pavlakis et al, 1983). Other investigators believe that bethanechol should be administered on a weight basis (0.035 mg/kg) (Wein, 1992). False-positive results may occur in patients with detrusor hypertrophy, urinary tract infection, or azotemia. A positive bethanechol test suggests an interruption in the afferent or efferent peripheral or distal spinal innervation of the bladder.

The Ice Water Test

The ice water test has been reported to differentiate upper from lower motor neuron lesions. This test is performed by rapidly injecting the bladder with ice water; if the ice water is expelled from the bladder within 1 minute, the test is considered to be positive. The test is positive in approximately 97% of patients with complete suprasacral lesions and in 91% of those with incomplete suprasacral lesions; it is almost never positive in patients with lower motor neuron lesions. Approximately 75% of patients with multiple sclerosis, Parkinson's disease, or history of CVA have a positive ice water test. The test, as originally described by Bors and Blinn (1957), is performed after standard cystometry with the patient in the supine position. A total of 100 ml of sterile water at 0°C is rapidly instilled through the filling catheter while subtracted bladder pressure (P_{det}) is monitored. If the cystometric capacity was determined to be less than 200 ml, a volume corresponding to one half of the cystometric capacity is used. The cold fluid is left in the bladder for 1 minute. If a sustained bladder contraction is registered and fluid is expelled during this period, the test is considered positive. If no water escapes, despite sustained detrusor contraction of about the same magnitude as the micturition contraction, the test result is said to be falsely negative (Geirsson et al, 1993; 1994).

Evaluation of Voiding Function

Urodynamic evaluation of voiding function encompasses the use of uroflowmetry, pressure-flow studies, video-urodynamic study, and micturition urethral pressure studies. In addition, outlet function may be monitored electromyographically, and pressure-flow data may be analyzed mathematically.

Uroflowmetry

Uroflowmetry is the only noninvasive urodynamic test available. It is a reflection of the final result of the act of voiding and is therefore influenced by a number of variables. These include the effectiveness of the detrusor contraction, the completeness of sphincteric relaxation, and the patency of the urethra (absence of obstruction). Because of these variables, uroflowmetry cannot be used as a diagnostic study, but together with the measurement of residual urine, it provides an estimate of the effectiveness of the act of voiding and is a rapid and economic screening tool. **A low uroflow rate does not necessarily imply BOO; conversely, a normal or supernormal uroflow does not necessarily exclude it. Patients with abnormal uroflowmetry require more detailed evaluation to further elucidate the cause of their voiding problem.**

Equipment and Other Variables

The first uroflowmeters were described at the end of the 19th century and were based on the principle of air displacement, a system no longer used (Perez and Webster, 1992). Currently there are three widely used methods for flow rate measurement. The gravimetric method operates by measuring the weight of collected fluid or by measuring the hydrostatic pressure at the base of the collecting cylinder. The output signal is proportional to the weight of the fluid collected. The rotating disk method works by directing the voided urine onto a rotating disk. This fluid increases the inertia of the disk, and the power required to keep the disk rotating at a constant speed is measured and is proportional to the flow rate of the fluid. The electronic dipstick method uses a capacitance dipstick mounted on the collecting chamber, which changes its capacitance as the urine accumulates in the cylinder. The output signal is then proportional to the accumulated volume of urine.

The patient who presents for a uroflow study should be well hydrated with a reasonably full bladder. The most reliable and reproducible uroflow results are obtained when an adult voids between 200 to 400 ml. Abnormal uroflow rates with voided volumes of less than 150 ml are difficult to interpret unless uroflow nomograms or computer-based diagnostics are used. Uroflow studies should be performed in relative privacy, and the patient should be encouraged to void in as normal a fashion as possible, because many patients will try to "do their best" during the course of the study. The uroflowmetry tracing should be examined visually, because machine-read maximum urinary flow rates vary considerably owing to flow rate artifacts (Grino et al, 1993). The voided volume, the patient's position, the method of bladder filling (diuresis or catheter; transurethral or suprapubic), and the type of fluid should all be recorded.

Interpretation of Uroflowmetry Data

The International Continence Society has recommended the following definitions for evaluation of uroflowmetry (Abrams et al, 1988; Bates et al, 1979; International Continence Society, 1981). In patients with a continuous uroflow, the voided volume is the total volume expelled through the urethra. The maximum flow rate (Q_{max}) is the maximum measured rate of flow. The average flow rate is determined by dividing the voided volume by the flow time. This calculation is only meaningful if flow is continuous and without significant terminal dribbling. Flow time is the time over which measurable flow actually occurs, and time to maximum flow is the elapsed time from onset of flow to maximum flow. In patients with intermittent flow patterns, the same parameters are used to characterize continuous flow, except that in measuring flow time the interval between flow episodes is disregarded. These parameters are graphically illustrated in Figure 28–8*A* and *B*. The age, sex, voided volume, and circadian variability must also be taken into account (Drach et al, 1979, 1982; Jensen et al 1985; Drach and Steinbronn, 1986; Poulsen and Kirkeby, 1988; Golomb et al, 1992). Normal values for uroflowmetry are listed in Table 28–1 (Abrams and Torrens, 1979).

Peak flow rate varies with volume voided, and it is generally accepted that voided volumes of less than 150 ml generate inaccurate flow patterns and parameters (Siroky et al, 1979, 1980; Marshall et al, 1983; Drach et al, 1982). For this reason, several nomograms have been constructed to allow for the comparison of flow rates regardless of volume (Figs. 28–9 and 28–10) (Siroky et al, 1979; Abrams and Griffiths, 1979). Abrams (1995) commented that the sensitivity and specificity of flow rate nomograms are poor, especially for those constructed using data that do not have age-matched controls (e.g., the Siroky nomogram). Abrams suggested that currently employed uroflow data are insufficient to diagnose BOO, but that further work on the sensitivity and specificity of uroflow studies in relation to

Table 28–1. NORMAL VALUES FOR UROFLOWMETRY

Gender	Age (years)	Flow Rate (ml/second)
Males	<40	>22
	40–60	>18
	>60	>13
Females	<50	>25
	>50	>18

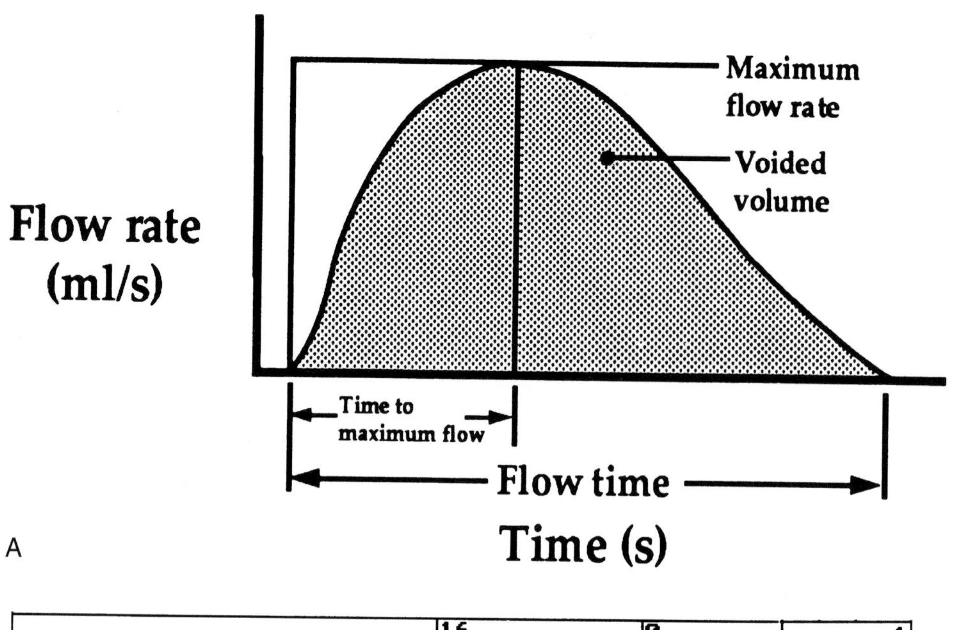

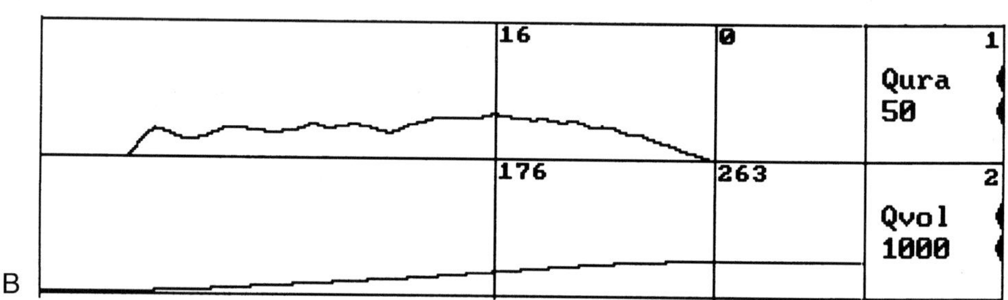

Figure 28–8. *A,* Schematic of a normal flow curve. Frequently measured variables are noted. *B,* A uroflow study in a 60-year-old man. Peak flow rate is 16 ml/second. Total volume voided is 263 ml.

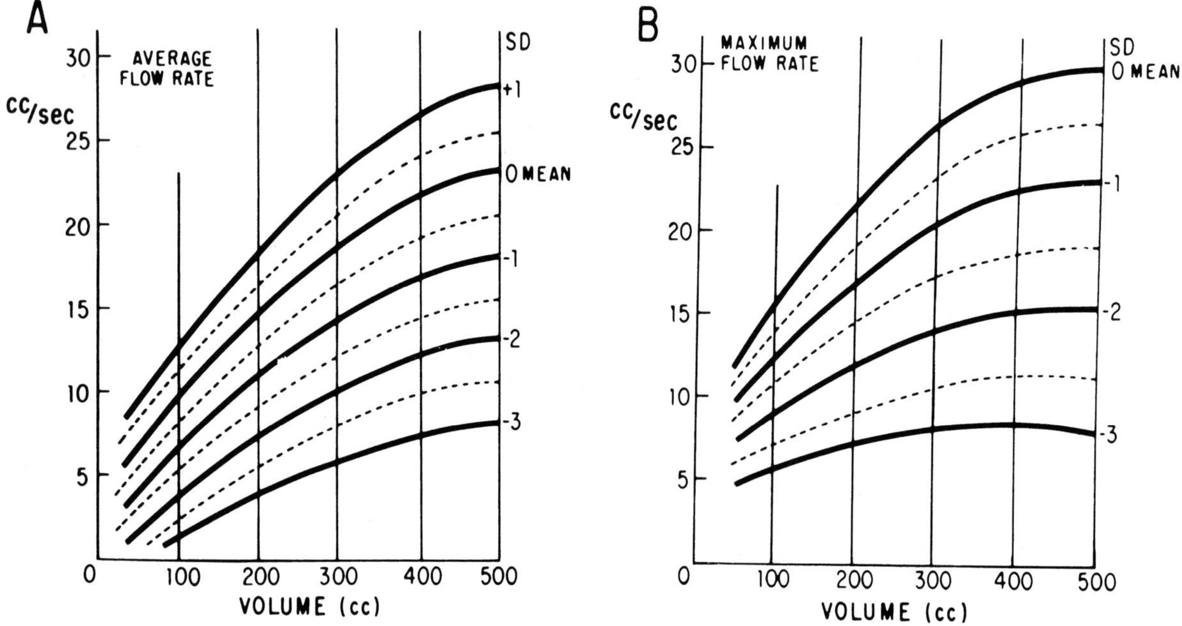

Figure 28–9. The Siroky nomogram facilitates comparison of flow rates regardless of volume voided. (From Siroky BM, Olsson CA, Krane RJ: J Urol 1979; 122:665.)

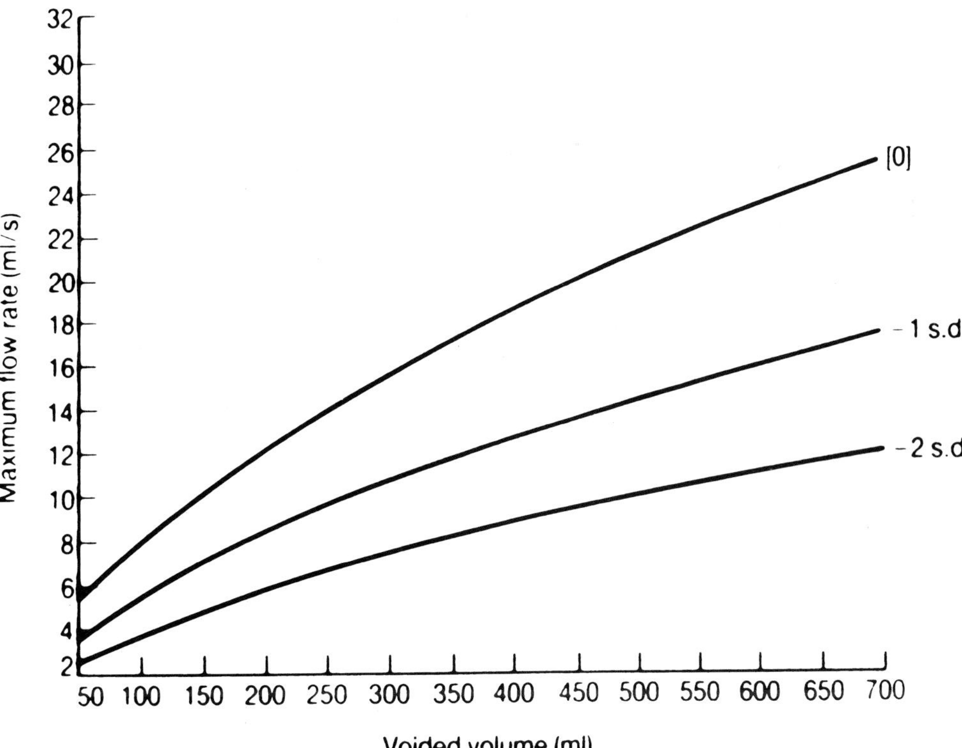

Figure 28–10. The Bristol nomogram popularly used for flow rate comparisons.

the maximum flow rate and shape of the curve may produce more reliable indicators of BOO.

Rollema (1983) has described the use of the computer-aided diagnostic uroflow classification (DUC) of free uroflow curves. The uroflow classification factor is derived by calculating the velocity of the contraction of the circumference in the bladder (DL/DT) from the flow rate (Q) and the instantaneous bladder volume (V). This calculation is made using the assumption of a spherical bladder and the absence of residual urine. The variable DL/DT 40 (value of DL/DT at 40 ml bladder contents) appears to discriminate between normal and impaired micturition and is included as part of the DUC software. DUC software may help to select patients for more sophisticated and invasive pressure-flow analysis in order to diagnose outflow obstruction. The software has a sensitivity rate of 91% in identifying patients who are ultimately found to be obstructed by pressure-flow analysis (Rollema, 1983; Rollema et al, 1994).

Several studies have addressed the ability of uroflowmetry or corrected uroflowmetry to predict the presence of outlet obstruction. Schäfer reported that only 75% of patients with obstruction according to the Siroky nomogram had outflow obstruction based on passive urethral resistance relation (PURR—computer assisted pressure flow relation), which is discussed in a later section (Schäfer, et al, 1988). Chancellor and co-workers, (1991), using the Abrams-Griffiths method, demonstrated that uroflowmetry could not differentiate between outflow obstruction and impaired detrusor contractility. Similarly, Neilsen and associates (1994), summarizing data collected by Jensen and Schou, demonstrated that uroflowmetry alone is insufficient to diagnose infravesical obstruction. Despite these misgivings, however, it continues to be an extensively used and noninvasive tool for the evaluation of patients with suspected outlet obstruction.

The maximum flow rate (Q_{max}) has been reported to predict surgical outcome in some patients undergoing prostatectomy for BPH. Jensen and associates (1984) reported that of 53 men undergoing prostatectomy based on clinical indications alone, those with a preoperative Q_{max} of less than 10 ml/second had a better overall subjective outcome on symptom score analysis. McLoughlin and co-workers (1990) reported on 108 men with prostatism who were studied urodynamically before and 1 year after surgery and concluded that a Q_{max} of less than 12 ml/second was a good indicator of obstruction, subjecting only 3% of patients to unnecessary transurethral prostatectomy. He went on to suggest that routine pressure-flow studies and cystometrograms were not indicated to identify men with BPH in need of prostatectomy, but to recommend screening of flow rate followed by further urodynamic testing in patients with a Q_{max} of more than 12 ml/second.

Pressure-Flow Micturition Studies

Because of the limitations of uroflowmetry in the evaluation of the patient with voiding problems, the simultaneous measurement of bladder pressure and flow rate throughout the micturition cycle is the next recourse in an attempt at accurate diagnosis. There are a number of variables that relate to such micturition studies. The indices measured may include intravesical pressure, rectal pressure, intraurethral pressure, sphincter electromyography, and urine flow rate (Fig. 28–11). Access to the bladder is most commonly by transurethral catheter, although suprapubic cystotomy is used by some. If the two-catheter system described for cystometry is used, then the filling catheter must be removed during voiding, and repeat voiding studies require catheter reinsertion. There are double- and triple-lumen cath-

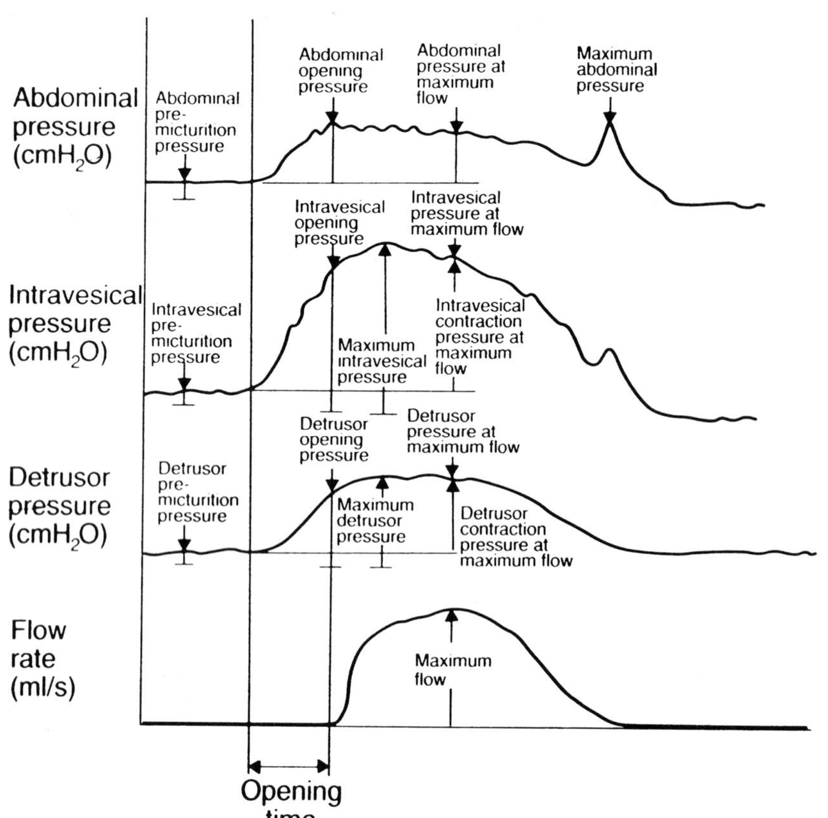

Figure 28–11. A schematic pressure flow study labeled with recommended terminology.

eter systems available to allow for filling and pressure monitoring, and these can be incorporated into one system of relatively small diameter. This is left in place during voiding, and if subsequent studies are necessary, no further instrumentation of the patient is required. If the catheter is larger than 8 Fr, however, it will to some degree obstruct the outlet and affect the pressure-flow recordings. The intra-abdominal pressure is most commonly measured by a balloon catheter in the rectum, although it may be placed in the vagina or in either an ileostomy or colostomy if the rectum has been surgically removed.

Many patients find it difficult to void in the setting of the urodynamic laboratory, where they may be required to void in an unfamiliar position, in the company of others, and encumbered and in discomfort because of the necessary catheters and electrodes. Every attempt should be made to replicate normal voiding conditions as closely as possible. Men should usually void in the standing position and women while seated on the commode. This ideal is not always possible, particularly in video-urodynamic studies, and interpretation of urodynamic results should take these factors into account. The reference point for zero pressure in preparing the extravesical transducer for recording is the level of the superior edge of the symphysis pubis.

International Continence Society Nomenclature

The International Continence Society has defined the following terms in the interpretation of pressure flow studies (see Fig. 28–11). The opening time is the time that elapses from the initial rise in detrusor pressure to the onset of flow. There is a time lag between these two events because urine must traverse the distance from the urethra to the flowmeter before recording can commence. Prolonged opening times may occur in cases of outlet obstruction. Premicturition pressure is the intravesical pressure just before the onset of the micturition contraction. Detrusor opening pressure is the detrusor pressure recorded at the onset of measured flow. It tends to be elevated in patients with intravesical obstruction, and pressures greater than 80 cm H_2O may indicate outflow obstruction. Detrusor pressure at maximum flow is the magnitude of the micturition contraction at a time when the flow rate is at its maximum. If this pressure is greater than 100 cm H_2O, it implies the presence of outlet obstruction even if the flow rate is normal (Gerstenberg et al, 1982). Maximum detrusor pressure is the maximum recorded regardless of flow. This pressure can exceed the pressure at maximum flow if the bladder is contracting isometrically against a closed sphincter. Detrusor contraction pressure at maximum flow is the difference between the pressure at maximum flow and the premicturition detrusor pressure. Isometric detrusor pressure is obtained by mechanical obstruction of the urethra or by active contraction of the distal sphincter mechanism during voiding. The micturition pressure rises as the detrusor continues to isometrically contract, and the magnitude of this isometric spike is a reflection of the reserve strength of the detrusor. Postmicturition contraction (after-contraction) is a reiteration of the detrusor contraction after flow has ceased, and its magnitude is typically greater than that of the micturition pressure at maximum flow. After-contractions are not well understood, but they seem to be more common in patients with unstable or hypersensitive bladders (Webster and Koefoot, 1983). Residual urine is the volume of urine

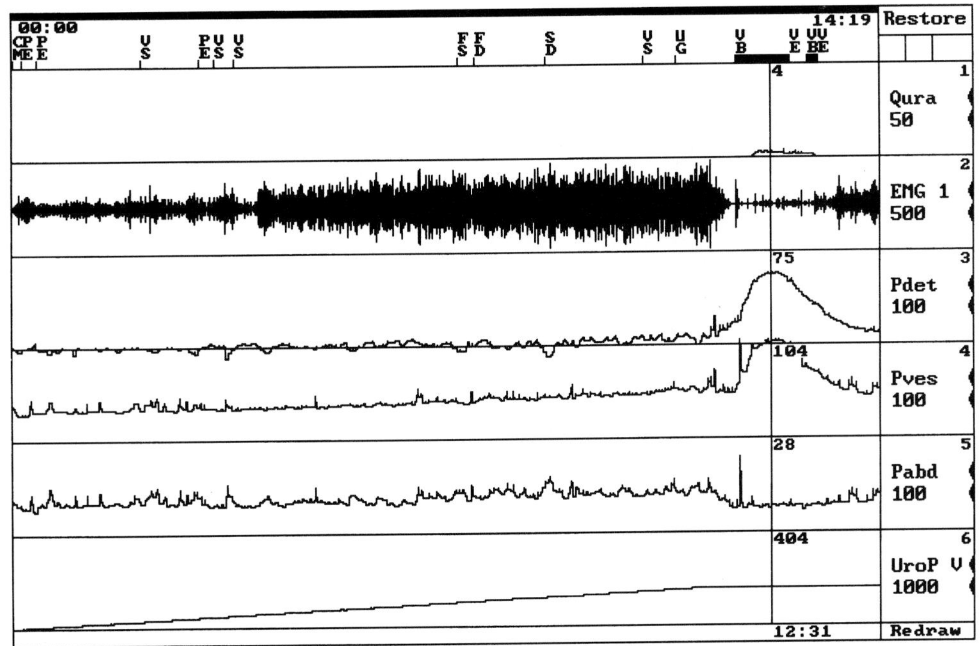

Figure 28–12. A typical micturition study showing an obstructed pressure flow portion. The initial filling cystometrogram reveals a normal stable bladder. During micturition a characteristic high-pressure (P_{det}, 75 cm H_2O), low-flow (Qura 4 ml/second) recording is obtained, indicating obstruction. Qura, urine flow rate; EMG, electromyogram; P_{det}, detrusor pressure; P_{ves}, vesicle pressure; P_{abd}, abdominal pressure; UroPV, filling volume.

remaining in the bladder immediately after micturition. Although the testing situation often leads to inefficient voiding and a falsely elevated residual urine, the absence of residual urine does not exclude intravesical obstruction or bladder dysfunction. A typical obstructed pressure-flow study is depicted in Figure 28–12.

The Concept of Detrusor Pressure

Bladder pressure recordings may be reported as P_{ves} or P_{det}. P_{ves} is the total pressure within the bladder and represents a summation of the pressure caused by bladder wall events and pressure from extravesical sources. **P_{det} more accurately measures bladder wall contractile events and is therefore the more critical pressure to monitor. P_{det} cannot be measured directly, but rather it is obtained by subtracting the abdominal pressure (P_{abd}) from the total bladder pressure (P_{ves}).** P_{abd} is recorded by a catheter in the rectum and is subtracted from the P_{ves} recorded by a small catheter left in the bladder during voiding (Fig. 28–13). This subtraction is performed electronically. Subtracted bladder pressure (P_{det}) measurements are particularly valuable in situations in which changes in P_{abd} would otherwise mask detrusor events (Webster and Older, 1980a). An example is the patient who voids primarily by Valsalva effort; in this patient, the pressure measured within the bladder is a sum of the bladder wall contraction and the contribution of abdominal straining. In order to determine how much of the contribution is from the detrusor itself, the component of abdominal straining or increased P_{abd} must be subtracted (Fig. 28–14). Another situation in which P_{abd} changes may mask detrusor events is during provocative cystometry. The provocative maneuvers used (e.g., coughing, position change, heel jouncing, jumping) may lead to increases in intra-abdominal pressure that would otherwise mask any detrusor response, and involuntary detrusor activity may be missed (Papa Petros and Elmsten, 1993).

P_{det} is the component of P_{ves} that is created by forces within the bladder wall alone. These forces are a combination of both active and passive forces. Active bladder wall forces include unstable or voluntary bladder contractions, and passive events are those that result from bladder elasticity. Changes in passive forces may be caused by loss of

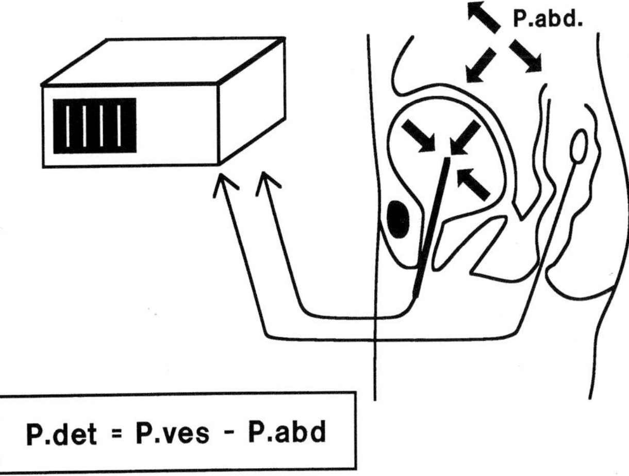

Figure 28–13. A schematic demonstrating the recording of detrusor pressure (P_{det}). The detrusor contribution to micturition is recorded by subtracting abdominal pressure (recorded as rectal pressure) from total intravesical pressure (P_{ves}).

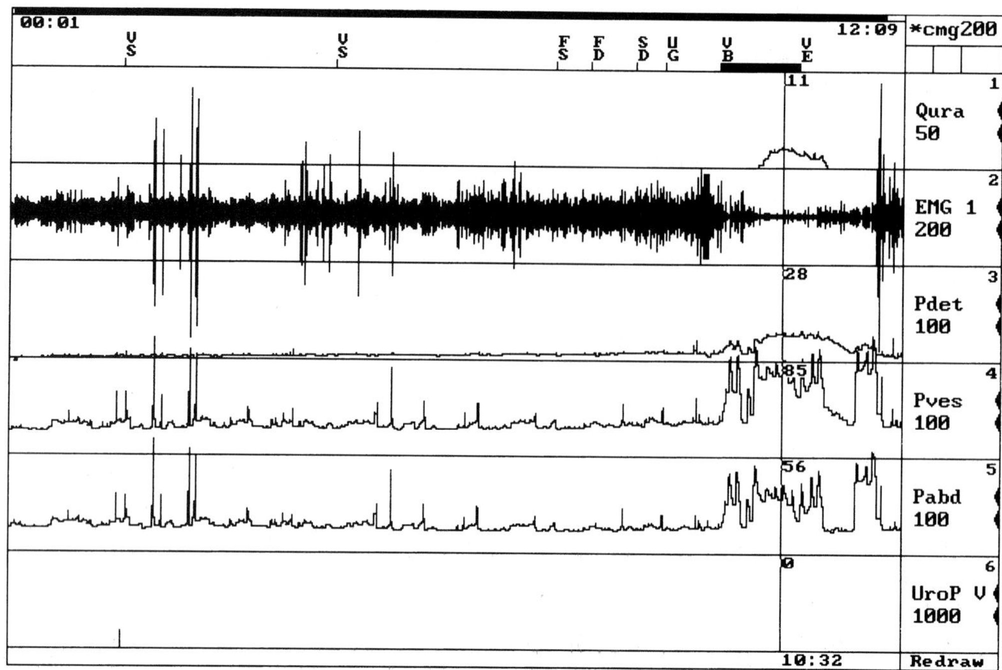

Figure 28–14. A multifunction urodynamic study showing the value of subtracted pressure measurement. During micturition abdominal straining masks the interpretation of the pressure recording. However, the subtracted detrusor pressure (P_{det}) trace demonstrates the detrusor contraction perfectly. Similarly, movement artifact during the filling cystometrogram mars interpretation of stability on the P_{ves} tracing.

bladder compliance as a result of bladder wall fibrosis; changes in active forces may result from muscular or neurogenic events. Differentiating between active and passive bladder forces may be difficult. Intravenous administration of anticholinergic medication may suppress bladder wall contractions but may not affect the loss of elasticity or other factors that cause low bladder compliance. Anesthesia also tends to suppress uninhibited contractions but not low bladder compliance.

Indications for Pressure-Flow Studies

Ideally pressure-flow studies should differentiate between patients with a low Q_{max} secondary to obstruction and those whose low Q_{max} is a result of poor detrusor contractility. They may also help identify those patients with high-pressure obstruction and normal flow rates. The obstruction may be structural and caused by BPH or functional and caused by proximal or distal sphincter dyssynergia. Similarly, poor detrusor contractility may be neurogenic, or it may be caused by decompensation, a myogenic event that can result from overdistention, aging, and collagenous replacement of detrusor muscle of other cause.

There is no consensus regarding a critical value for pressure and flow that is diagnostic for obstruction. Although there would be little argument that obstruction existed in a patient in whom P_{det} was 100 cm H_2O at Q_{max} of 10 ml/second, there would be less agreement regarding a patient with P_{det} of 50 cm H_2O and a flow rate of 10 ml/second. Recognizing this dilemma, Blaivas' posture is that obstruction is suggested by a pressure-flow study in which low flow occurs despite a detrusor contraction of adequate force, duration, and speed, regardless of the actual numerical values (Chancellor et al, 1991). Pressure-flow studies find their main use in the evaluation of men with prostatism; in those cases, the goal is to reduce the reported 30% to 40% misdiagnosis rate that exists if decisions are based on LUTS alone (Abrams and Feneley, 1978; Andersen, 1982). These studies should be performed only if the information obtained will affect major therapeutic decisions, or especially if surgical intervention is contemplated. **Strong indications for pressure-flow studies include prostatism in a patient with a history of neurologic disease such as CVA or Parkinson's disease, which are known to affect detrusor or sphincter function. They are indicated in patients with symptoms of prostatism who have normal flow rates (Q_{max} >12 to 15 ml/second) and in younger men with prostatism in whom an alternative functional diagnosis is more likely. We also believe they are strongly indicated in the man whose symptoms of prostatism are primarily those of bladder instability rather than flow disorder and in the man who has little endoscopic evidence of prostate occlusion.**

Voiding dysfunction is relatively common in women, but there is considerable confusion surrounding its cause and diagnosis. Urinary retention or a large postvoid residual volume in a woman is more commonly the result of poor detrusor contractility than BOO (Wheeler et al, 1990). In a large retrospective review of women with voiding complaints, obstruction was identified in only 2.7% to 8% of cases (Farrar, 1975; Massey and Abrams, 1988; Rees et al, 1976). Once again, however, pressure-flow study in the woman with suspected obstruction may be misleading. This is typified by those women with postcystourethropexy voiding dysfunction who undergo successful urethrolysis, in whom only 56% of those with a successful outcome had preoperative voiding pressures higher than 30 cm H_2O and uroflow rates less than 12 ml/second (Nitti and Raz, 1994).

Classic obstructive pressure-flow study results were obtained in only 33% of women before successful urethrolysis (Webster and Kreder, 1990).

URETHRAL RESISTANCE MODEL AND PRESSURE-FLOW PLOTS

In patients with very high micturition pressures and low simultaneous uroflowmetry, the diagnosis of outflow obstruction is relatively straightforward. The challenge is in those patients with equivocal results, in whom advanced urodynamic analysis of pressure-flow data finds its role.

Early attempts to quantify the degree of outflow obstruction based on urodynamic pressure-flow data modeled the urethra as a rigid tube. This was a false assumption, and therefore these early systems were inaccurate. All modern pressure-flow analysis methods are based on the Griffiths model of flow through collapsible or elastic tubes (Griffiths, 1971a, 1971b, 1973).

The basis of all techniques for pressure-flow analysis is the plotting of P_{det} against flow rate at each point in time throughout micturition; this is the pressure-flow loop, or the urethral resistance relation (URR) (Fig. 28–15). The important measurements from the pressure-flow loop include the opening pressure at the start of flow, the detrusor pressure at maximum flow ($P_{det}Q_{max}$), the closing pressure at the end of flow, and the minimum voiding detrusor pressure ($P_{det}Q_{min}$), which is usually at the end of voiding, when the voiding pressure is at its least and the outlet at its most relaxed. Relating $P_{det}Q_{max}$ to maximum flow rate (Q_{max}) gives the best diagnostic accuracy of BOO, and a variety of techniques have been used to manipulate this data.

Abrams-Griffiths Nomogram. By plotting the Q_{max} and $P_{det}Q_{max}$ measurements from the pressure-flow study on the Abrams-Griffiths nomogram (see Fig. 28–15), a diagnosis of obstruction, equivocal obstruction, or no obstruction can be made (Abrams, 1995). This simple use may be further refined for patients who fall into the equivocal group. In this event, if the minimum voiding pressure is higher than 40 cm H_2O, then obstruction is present. Or, alternatively, if a line is drawn joining the $P_{det}Q_{min}$ location and the $Q_{max}/P_{det}Q_{max}$ point and the slope is more than 2 cm H_2O/ml/second, then the patient is also obstructed. Abrams suggests that with these three techniques all patients can be categorized as obstructed or not. He further suggests that the degree of obstruction may be graded using the Abrams-Griffiths number (AG number) (Lim and Abrams, 1995). The AG number can be obtained by the formula AG number = $P_{det}Q_{max} - 2Q_{max}$, or by graphically projecting a line parallel to the upper line of the AG nomogram from the $P_{det}Q_{max}/Q_{max}$ point to the pressure axis. This AG number is evidently an estimate of $P_{det}Q_{min}$, and it provides a constant variable, allowing the examiner to grade the degree of obstruction before and after treatment (Lim and Abrams, 1995).

Schäfer Method. The linear passive urethral resistance relation (LPURR) is based on consideration of the urethra as a distensible tube with a flow controlling zone, which in the case of BPH is the proximal urethra (Schäfer, 1985). In this model, the urethra is seen as a passive or elastic tube that requires a certain amount of pressure to open; this is defined as the opening pressure (P_{muo}), which is the equivalent of the $P_{det}Q_{min}$ of the Abrams-Griffiths nomogram. The LPURR line is constructed in the same way as previously described on the prepared nomogram, linking the $P_{det}Q_{max}/Q_{max}$ point to the P_{muo} point (Schäfer, 1985, 1990, 1992) (Fig. 28–16). This method has gone through a number of modifications to get to this point. More recently, Schäfer (1993) has added a further continuous variable called the detrusor adjusted mean PURR factor (DAMPF). The DAMPF number is given by the intersection point of the LPURR line with the standard detrusor power curve, which is drawn onto a Schäfer nomogram.

Group-Specific Urethral Resistance Factor. The group-specific urethral resistance factor (URA) nomogram was constructed from results obtained from a large group of patients with and without BOO (Griffiths et al, 1989). Once

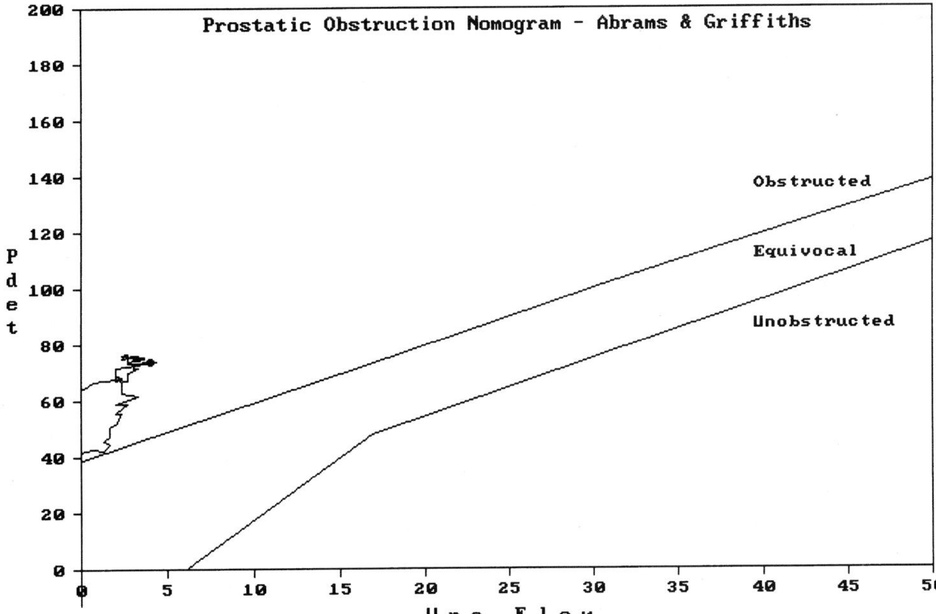

Figure 28–15. Detrusor pressure is plotted against flow rate throughout micturition on the Abrams-Griffiths nomogram. This plot is from the pressure flow study depicted in Figure 28–12 and confirms obstruction.

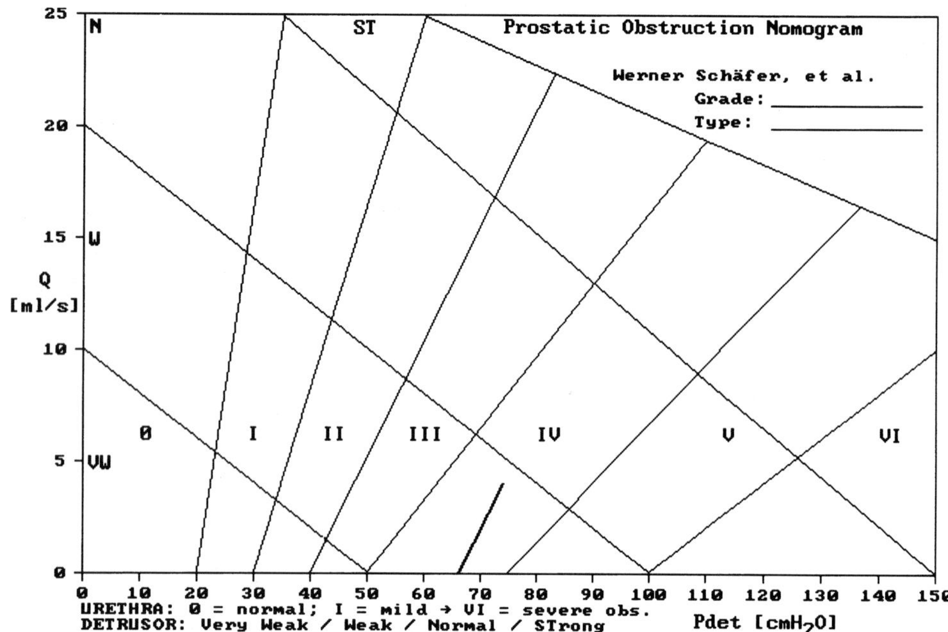

Figure 28–16. Information from the same pressure flow study (Figure 28–12) plotted on the Schäfer nomogram. The line connects P_{muo} (the pressure at commencement of flow) with the pressure at maximum flow. The "box" into which the line falls describes the magnitude of obstruction and the strength of the detrusor.

again, the patient is assigned a URA number according to the position of the $P_{det}Q_{max}/Q_{max}$ point on the URA nomogram. The URA number is similar to the AG number in that it reflects an estimate of $P_{det}Q_{min}$. Unlike the AG and LPURR lines, which are linear, the URA line is parabolic. This methodology has been further elaborated, refined, and reported by Rollema and van Mastrigt (Rollema et al, 1991; Rollema and van Mastrigt, 1992; van Mastrigt, 1984, 1987). It forms the basis of the CLIM computer program, which is an on-line measurement storage, analysis, and retrieval system for the processing of pressure-flow urodynamic data. The CLIM program stores in digital form the detrusor pressure and flow rate signals during voiding as well as the isometric detrusor pressure increase just before flow begins. The computer program determines the parameters.

Other computer-assisted data analysis techniques have been reported, including the three-parameter model developed by Spangberg and co-workers (1989) and the Chess classification recently proposed by Jonas and associates (1994). All of these techniques are based on the same pressure-flow loop, each has its proponents, and each continues to be modified. Protagonists of these methodologies propose that pressure-flow studies analyzed in this manner leave little doubt as to who is truly obstructed and who is not. The fact that these techniques are easy to use, simply by plotting the appropriate pressure-flow data on the nomogram, significantly improves the diagnostic efficacy of such studies. These nomograms have been developed for use in men with BOO caused by prostate enlargement and are not validated for use in women or in other situations.

Video-Urodynamics

The term video-urodynamics describes the technique in which the urodynamic parameters previously described in this chapter are displayed simultaneously with a fluoroscopic image of the lower urinary tract. Pioneering work in video-urodynamics began in the late 1950s (von Garrelts, 1956), and in recent years video-urodynamics has become the most sophisticated form of evaluation of patients with complex urinary tract dysfunction (Blaivas and Fisher, 1981; Webster and Older, 1980b).

Equipment and Technique

When video-urodynamics is performed, the cystometry and pressure-flow studies are conducted in the same manner as previously described. The only difference is that the study is conducted on a fluoroscopy table and the filling medium is a radiographic contrast. The amount of fluoroscopic screening is kept to a minimum to reduce radiation exposure; in practice, less than 20 seconds of total screening time is used. A tilting fluoroscopy table is ideal because it facilitates the placement of catheters and other manipulations with the patient in the supine position, initial filling cystometry may be performed with the patient supine, and the patient may then be tilted to the upright position for either repeat cystometry or the voiding study. The ideal table has commode seat attachments also to facilitate fluoroscopic screening of voiding in the seated position, which is ideal for women. Figure 28–17 is a block diagram depicting the basic video and urodynamic setup that allows both urodynamic and radiologic imaging data to be simultaneously projected onto a television monitor for real-time viewing and for videotape or digital storage for later review. With the recent introduction of digitalized imaging, advances are now largely software driven.

Clinical Applicability

The addition of simultaneous video enhances the urodynamic evaluation of all patients. However, because of the added hardware requirements, including space, lead-lined room, fluoroscopy table, and video monitoring equipment, the test tends to be available only in academic or medical centers and to be reserved for the investigation of more complex problems.

Complex Bladder Outlet Obstruction. Simultaneous fluoroscopic screening of the outlet during voiding and while pressure-flow data are being recorded helps to identify the site of the obstruction as being at either the bladder neck, the prostatic urethra, or the distal sphincter mechanism (Fig. 28–18). It is particularly useful in the identification of bladder neck dysfunction in young men with voiding problems and in identification of dyssynergia of the distal sphincter mechanism in neurogenic patients.

Evaluation of Incontinence. Fluoroscopic screening of the incontinent woman in the standing position helps identify the presence and degree of vesical neck hypermobility, the degree of proximal urethral weakness, and the degree and type of cystocele present. These factors all translate directly into treatment decisions. Video also improves the accuracy of Valsalva LPP measurement, which helps determine the degree of intrinsic sphincter deficiency (see later discussion).

Neurogenic Bladder Dysfunction. Although electronic urodynamics adequately evaluates detrusor function and identifies low bladder compliance and detrusor hyperreflexia, simultaneous video screening facilitates the diagnosis of proximal and distal sphincter dyssynergia and demonstrates the presence of reflux and bladder diverticula. It also aids in determination of the degree of hostility of the lower urinary tract.

Identification of Associated Pathology. In the patient with complex voiding dysfunction of whatever cause, the presence of reflux, bladder and urethral diverticula, fistula, stones, and so on are identified and characterized.

Micturitional Urethral Pressure Studies

At rest, the pressure within the urethra exceeds that within the bladder if the urethral pressure transducer is at the level of the sphincteric mechanism. At the onset of voiding, P_{det} rises (because of the micturition contraction) and intraurethral pressure falls. Voiding begins when the bladder pressure exceeds intraurethral pressure. **During voiding, bladder pressure and urethral pressure are the same (isobaric). If an obstruction exists in the urethra, the intraurethral pressure distal to the obstruction is less than that within the bladder or proximal to the obstruction** (Yalla et al, 1980). Theoretically, therefore, functional obstruction at the bladder neck or distal sphincter may be identified in this fashion. However, distortion artifact in micturitional urethral pressure profiles is considerable, and despite the use of radiopaque marks on the catheter and fluoroscopic screening to identify transducer position, the location of the urethral transducer is inexact.

Evaluation of the Bladder Outlet

Urethral Pressure Studies

Urethral pressure measurements were first described by Bonney in 1923 but were popularized by Brown and Wickham in 1969. The technique has since evolved, and currently the methods used to evaluate the outlet include the static

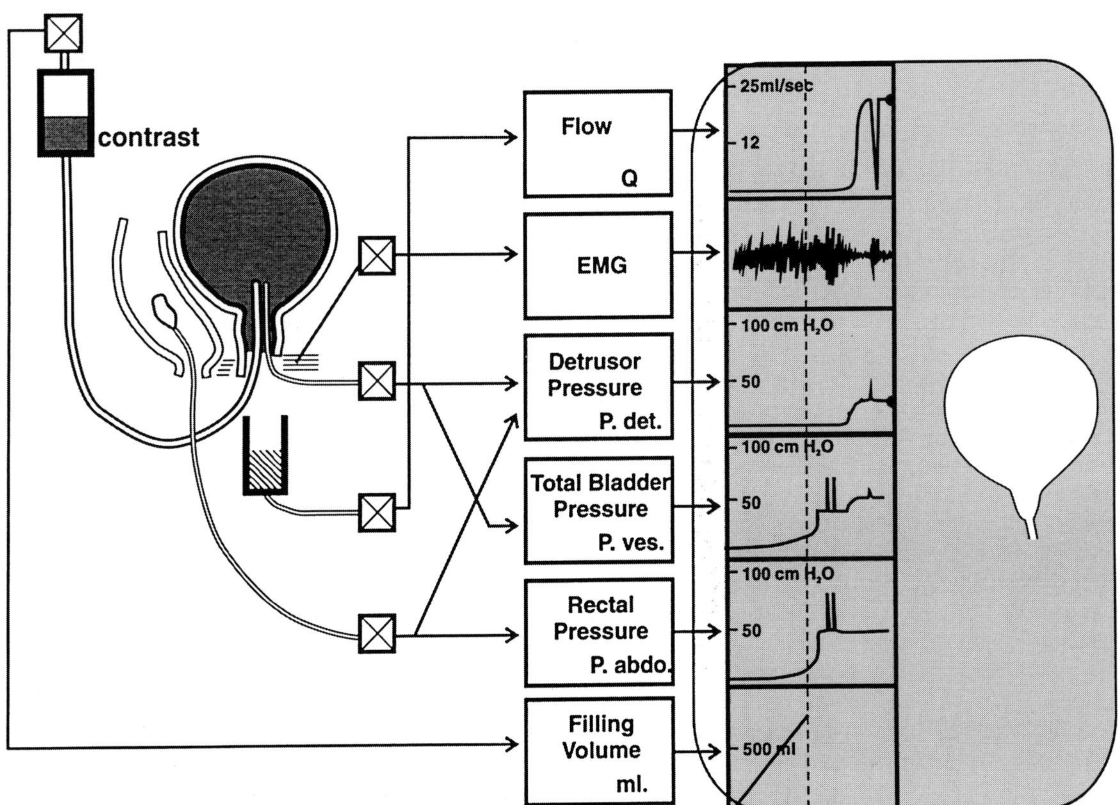

Figure 28–17. A block diagram depicting video-urodynamic evaluation. Electronic urodynamic data are projected onto the screen together with the simultaneously recorded cystogram.

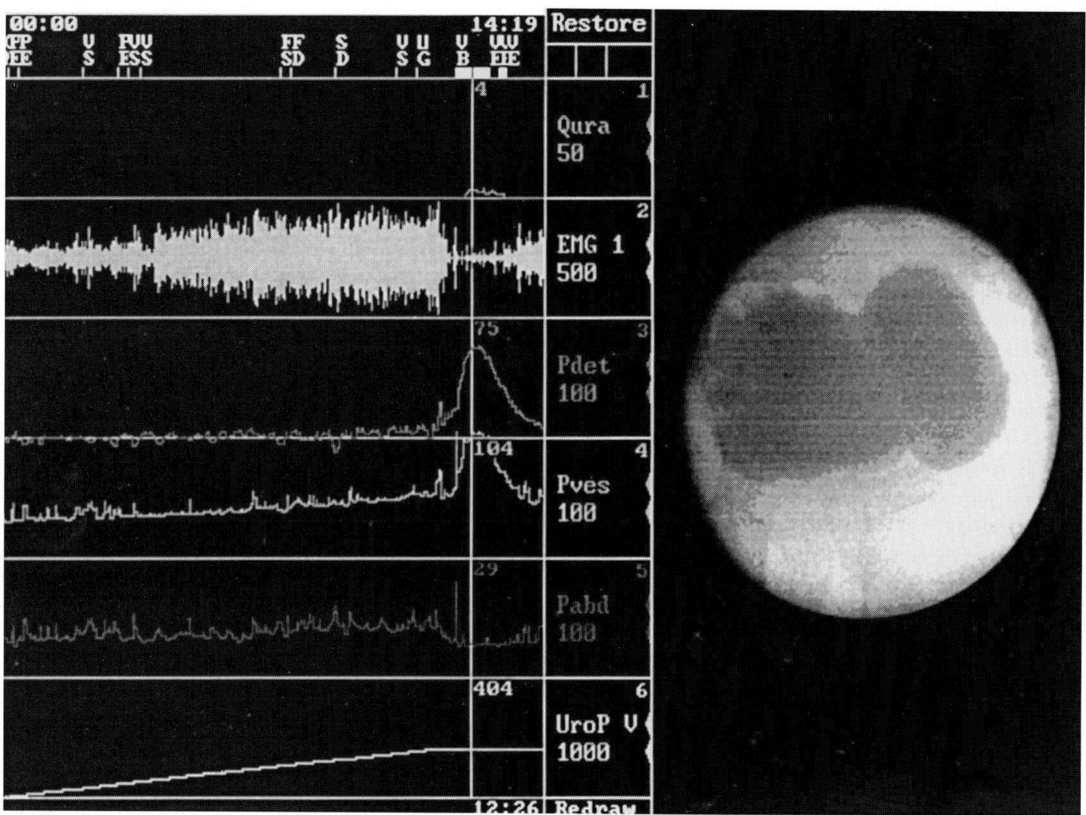

Figure 28–18. Video-urodynamic study of obstruction in a male patient. Pressure flow data show evidence of obstruction (high pressure, low flow) and the simultaneous video image (recorded at the vertical line) shows a poorly filled prostatic urethra and an obviously large diverticulum.

(resting) urethral pressure profile (UPP), the stress urethral pressure profile, and the Valsalva LPP.

URETHRAL PRESSURE PROFILOMETRY

The UPP is a recording of the intraluminal pressure along the length of the urethra. The study is performed during slow retraction of a catheter that has radially drilled side holes and is perfused with liquid. An automatic pulling device is used to advance the catheter at a rate of 0.5 mm/second. Bladder pressure should be measured simultaneously to exclude the effects of an associated detrusor contraction. Static URR has few proponents among current urologic urodynamicists. The study is used by some to help identify the presence of intrinsic sphincter deficiency in women with type III incontinence and in patients with neurogenic bladder dysfunction. In these groups, it may serve as an adjunct to confirm results obtained by Valsalva LPP study, cystography, or video-urodynamics. **The static UPP cannot diagnose stress urinary incontinence, and many women with low UPPs are continent and vice versa.** Likewise, it cannot be used to diagnose sphincter dyssynergia or BOO. Normal values for female urethral closure pressure decline with age; using the upper edge of the symphysis pubis as a zero reference, young women have maximum urethral closure pressures in excess of 65 cm H_2O, whereas in older (postmenopausal) women pressures are significantly lower.

The International Continence Society has defined the following parameters for referring to profiles measured in the storage phase (Abrams et al, 1988). Maximum urethral pressure is the maximum pressure of the measured profile. Maximum urethral closure pressure (MUCP) is the maximum difference between the urethral pressure and the intravesical pressure. Functional profile length is the length of the urethra along which the urethral pressure exceeds intravesical pressure (Fig. 28–19). Functional profile length on stress is the length over which the urethral pressure exceeds the intravesical pressure on stress. Pressure transmission ratio is the increment in urethral pressure on stress as a percentage of the simultaneously recorded increment in intravesical pressure. For stress profiles obtained during coughing, pressure transmission ratios can be obtained at any point along

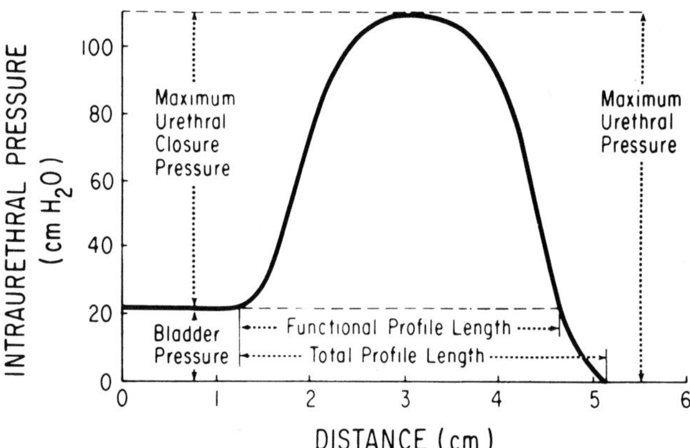

Figure 28–19. Schematic representation of urethral pressure profile with customarily measured variables.

the urethra. A pressure transmission ratio is calculated from the MUCP and is equal to urethral pressure rise at the point of the MUCP divided by the bladder pressure rise, times 100.

Stress Urethral Pressure Profiles

Stress UPPs monitor urethral pressure and bladder pressure simultaneously. They are performed as the profile catheter is withdrawn along the urethra during periods of intermittent stress (cough). Because the proximal portion of the female urethra is in an intra-abdominal position, "cough spikes" are transmitted to both the bladder and the portion of the urethra within the abdomen. If there is significant hypermobility of the urethrovesical junction and descent of the urethra carries it outside the intra-abdominal pressure zone, then pressure transmission does not occur (Enhorning, 1961; Bunne and Obrink, 1978). These studies are often recorded with subtraction of the intravesical pressure from the urethral pressure so that what is produced is the urethral closure pressure profile. Hence, it is a test of urethral position and has been used to imply that cystourethropexy will be successful in correcting the incontinence that is present. However, there are a number of problems with this study; it is technically difficult to perform, and movement artifact of the catheter during applied stress is commonplace.

Valsalva Leak Point Pressure

The abdominal or Valsalva LPP is that pressure required to cause leakage in the absence of a bladder contraction (McGuire et al, 1993; Wan et al, 1993). This study, recently popularized by McGuire, represents an alternative assessment of urethral function. The test is performed during cystometry (preferably with the patient standing) after the bladder has been filled to 150 to 200 ml. If the patient has significant detrusor instability during the performance of the cystometry, then the bladder is filled to half the cystometry capacity. The patient is then instructed to perform a slow Valsalva maneuver until urinary leakage occurs. If no urinary leakage is seen, the patient is asked to cough until incontinence occurs. The lowest pressure at which incontinence occurs is the abdominal LPP. In order to determine the abdominal or Valsalva LPP, the resting intravesical pressure is subtracted from the pressure at which leakage occurs (Fig. 28–20).

The Valsalva LPP, which appears reproducible, correlates well with the magnitude of incontinence, those patients with high-volume incontinence caused by intrinsic sphincter deficiency (type III incontinent women) having low LPPs. A number of factors may interfere with the study, including the presence of significant cystocele, detrusor instability, or involuntary contraction of the urethral sphincter during the test. The test has not yet been standardized with respect to catheter size, catheter location (bladder, vaginal, or rectal), and bladder volume, nor have normal values been established. In normal women, the Valsalva LPP should be infinity, because no incontinence should occur regardless of abdominal pressure. **A Valsalva LPP of less than 60 cm H_2O is evidence for the presence of significant intrinsic sphincter deficiency.** An LPP between 60 and 90 cm H_2O is equivocal but suggests some component of deficiency, and intrinsic sphincter deficiency is minimal with an LPP pressure higher than 90 cm H_2O (Heritz and Blaivas, 1995; Usui et al, 1995). McGuire has reported a study that compared the Valsalva LPP and maximum urethral pressure on UPP in incontinent patients and found them to be unrelated, further calling into question the value of UPP (McGuire et al, 1993).

Electrophysiologic Testing

Sphincter EMG studies the bioelectric potentials generated in the distal striated sphincter mechanism. Such studies are performed at two different levels of sophistication, each with distinct goals and requiring different instrumentation. The first, termed kinesiologic studies, are commonly performed in the urodynamic laboratory and simply **examine sphincter activity during bladder filling and voiding.** The second are **neurophysiologic tests,** which require considerable expertise and elaborate equipment and are designed to **examine the integrity of innervation of the muscle.**

Kinesiologic Studies

Kinesiologic studies may be performed with the use of a variety of electrodes and display methods. The signal may be recorded by surface electrodes (stick-on skin electrocardiographic electrodes) but preferably by hooked wire electrodes introduced into the periurethral muscle. The advantage of the latter is that their more proximate location to the muscle being recorded renders the information more interpretable. **Although in many patients the recordings obtained from the periurethral pelvic floor and the perianal sphincter are the same, dissimilar information may be obtained, particularly in patients with lower spinal cord injury and in those who have had pelvic surgery or have demyelinating disease** (Perkash, 1980). Hence, it is always preferable to record from the periurethral area. The signal is usually recorded onto a chart strip recorder, or the signal is amplified and recorded as sound on an audio monitor, or both. Chart strip recording of the signal shows characteristic changes in sphincter activity during bladder filling and voiding.

At the commencement of cystometry, before bladder filling begins, the patient is asked to demonstrate volitional

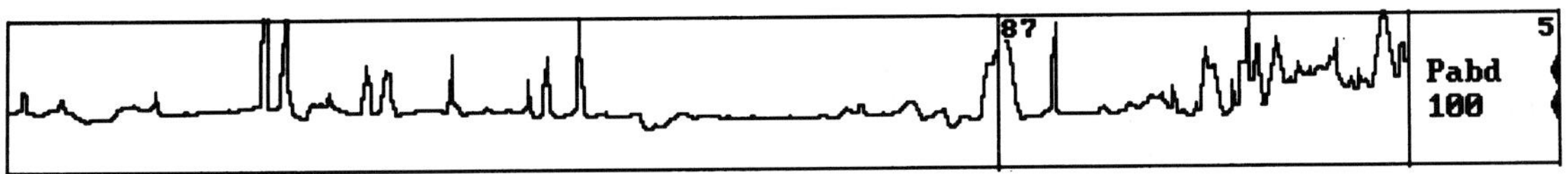

Figure 28–20. Valsalva leak point pressure (LPP) measurement may be recorded from the vesicle pressure (P_{ves}) or abdominal pressure (Pabd) tracing. In this recording, the patient was asked to perform a Valsalva maneuver, and the pressure at which leakage occurred from the urethra was recorded (87 cm H_2O). The Valsalva LPP is the increment of pressure over baseline pressure at which leakage occurs.

control of the sphincter by actively contracting and relaxing it. Ability to do this implies intact pyramidal tracts. Next, the bulbocavernosus reflex is tested by squeezing the glans penis or clitoris or pulling on the Foley catheter. A burst of EMG activity is a positive result and implies an intact sacral arc. Bladder filling is then commenced, and as it proceeds there is progressive **recruitment** of sphincter activity, demonstrated by increased amplitude and frequency of firing (see Fig. 28–12). During voiding, sphincter activity should cease, and failure to do so is termed detrusor-sphincter dyssynergia. **Detrusor-sphincter dyssynergia is diagnosed only in patients with neurologic disease and occurs commonly in patients with suprasacral spinal cord injury.** The inappropriate sphincter activity during voiding has a variety of patterns ranging from crescendo contraction to failure of relaxation (Fig. 28–21). Normal sphincter EMG activity has a recognizable audio quality, whereas in neurologic conditions abnormal EMG wave forms, which include complex polyphasic potentials, fibrillation potentials, and complex repetitive discharges, result in characteristic identifiable sounds. Many urodynamic investigators simultaneously monitor the chart strip and audio recordings for improved interpretability.

Deviations from the normal EMG pattern during a kinesiologic study do not necessarily imply the presence of neurologic disease and may occur simply as a result of technical recording difficulties. **Quite commonly, total electrical silence is not seen during the voiding study, but true detrusor sphincter dyssynergy should rarely be diagnosed in these circumstances. True detrusor striated sphincter dyssynergy is diagnosed only in patients who have neurologic disease.** Quite commonly, increased EMG activity during voiding is secondary to straining by the patient.

As stated previously, EMG activity should gradually increase during filling cystometry (recruitment) and then cease at the time of voiding. However, if the patient has an unstable bladder contraction during the course of filling cystometry, then the normal response of the external sphincter is to increase activity in an attempt to prevent incontinence. This should not be interpreted as detrusor sphincter dyssynergy.

Kinesiologic studies do not diagnose neuropathy but may characterize the effects of it. Their most important role is in the identification of abnormal sphincter activity in patients with neurogenic bladder dysfunction and in those with voiding dysfunction of behavioral origin. This is particularly important in patients with spinal cord injury or multiple sclerosis and in children with spinal dysraphism. These studies have little role to play in the routine urodynamic evaluation of incontinent or obstructed patients in whom neuropathy is not suggested by other clinical findings. In children

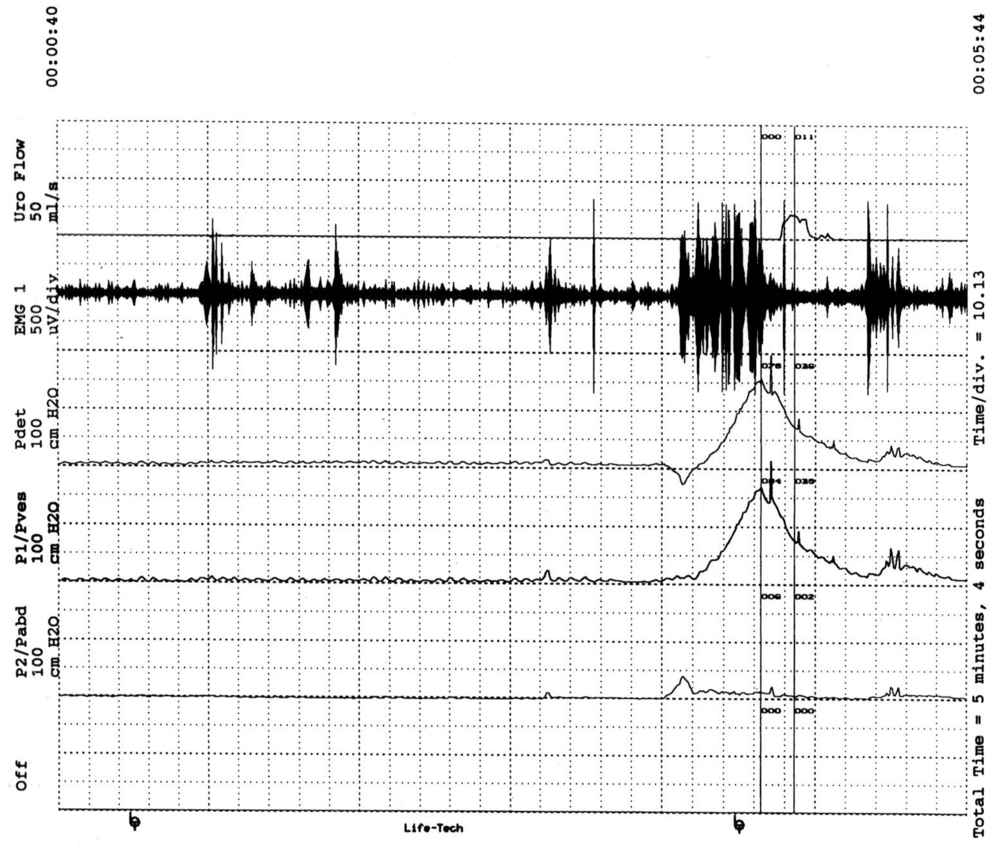

Figure 28–21. A filling cystometrogram in a man with complete suprasacral spinal cord injury. Detrusor hyperreflexia is demonstrated by the involuntary contraction, which is accompanied by a dyssynergic contraction of the external sphincter (see increased electromyographic activity). As the detrusor contraction is inhibited, the dyssynergic response in the sphincter decreases and flow occurs, but emptying is inefficient.

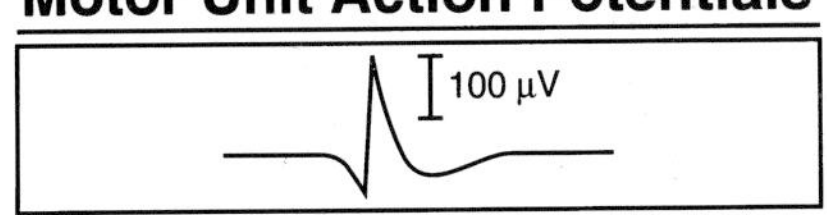

Normal Features

Characteristic configuration
Amplitude 50 - 300 µv
Duration 3 - 5 m.secs.
A Frequency 1 - 4 per sec.

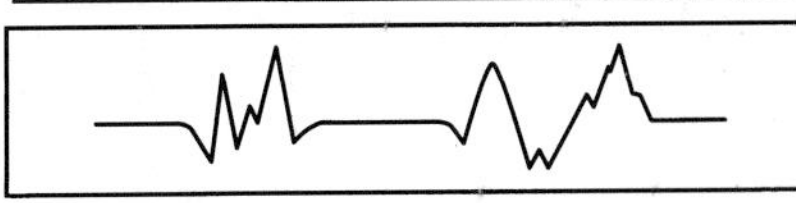

Abnormal Features

Increase in amplitude, duration, complexity of wave form.
Polyphasic potentials (>5 deflections)
Fibrillation potentials
Positive sharp waves
B Bizarre high frequency forms

Figure 28–22. *A,* Schematic of a normal motor unit action potential from the periurethral striated male sphincter. *B,* Schematic of an abnormal motor unit action potential, showing complex form.

with voiding dysfunction, EMG studies may reveal poor sphincter relaxation, termed sphincter or pelvic floor hyperactivity, which is probably of behavioral origin. Invasive EMG studies are not indicated in all children with voiding dysfunction (e.g., diurnal enuresis) and should be reserved for those with strong indications including upper tract changes. Poor pelvic floor or sphincter relaxation also occurs in neurologically normal women with voiding problems and is also probably behavioral; however, it may occur as a result of urethral irritative or pelvic pain causes.

Neurophysiologic Recordings

Neurophysiologic studies require more sophisticated instrumentation and investigator expertise and are **designed to actually diagnose and characterize the presence of neuropathy or myopathy.** Potentials generated during sphincter activity may be recorded with a specialized needle electrode inserted directly into the muscle to be tested, the individual wave forms being recorded on an oscilloscope. **Motor unit action potentials (MUAP) in health and disease differ, and, within certain limitations, the expert observer may use these studies to determine whether neuropathy is present.**

Normally, the MUAP recorded from the distal urethral sphincter muscle has a biphasic or triphasic wave form with an amplitude of 50 to 300 mV and a firing frequency of 10 to 100 discharges per second (Fig. 28–22*A*). Simplistically, when the motor neuron or nerve to a muscle is damaged, the muscle responds in a characteristic fashion. Those muscle fibers that have lost their nerve supply become reinnervated by adjacent healthy nerves, and the MUAP changes. The wave forms becomes larger in amplitude and increases in complexity and duration; these are termed polyphasic potentials (see Fig. 28–22*B*). These potentials are thought to represent the increased number of muscle fibers per motor unit which follows reinnervation. Normal muscle may have up to 15% of its activity in the form of such polyphasic potentials; however, when the amount of polyphasic activity is significantly greater than this, neuropathy is implied. Further refinement of study may imply whether the injury is ongoing or old.

Neurophysiologic studies are beyond the expertise of most urodynamic laboratories and are uncommonly indicated. Their role is in diagnosis of occult neuropathy or myopathy. **In the patient with overt neurologic findings who has bladder dysfunction, neurogenic bladder dysfunction can be deduced without further study. In such cases, kinesiologic study to identify the pattern of dysfunction is all that is indicated. MUAP studies find their role in the evaluation of the patient with bladder dysfunction of unknown cause in whom neuropathy is suspected.** They are also used in medicolegal situations in an attempt to correlate voiding symptoms and sexual dysfunction with prior injuries. It is important to recognize that these studies remain poorly standardized.

Nerve Conduction Studies

Nerve conduction studies are performed by the stimulation of a peripheral nerve and the monitoring of the time taken for a response to occur in its innervated muscle (Fig. 28–23). The time from stimulation to response is termed the "latency." **Nerve conduction studies are a test of the integrity of a reflex arc and can be relatively sensitive indicators of the presence of neurologic disease (Galloway et al, 1985). In urologic practice, these studies are most often performed as bulbocavernosus reflex latency determinations.** They require elaborate instrumentation and careful user interpretation. Abnormal responses occur in a variety of situations and are particularly diagnostic in patients with diabetes and peripheral neuropathies. In patients with conus

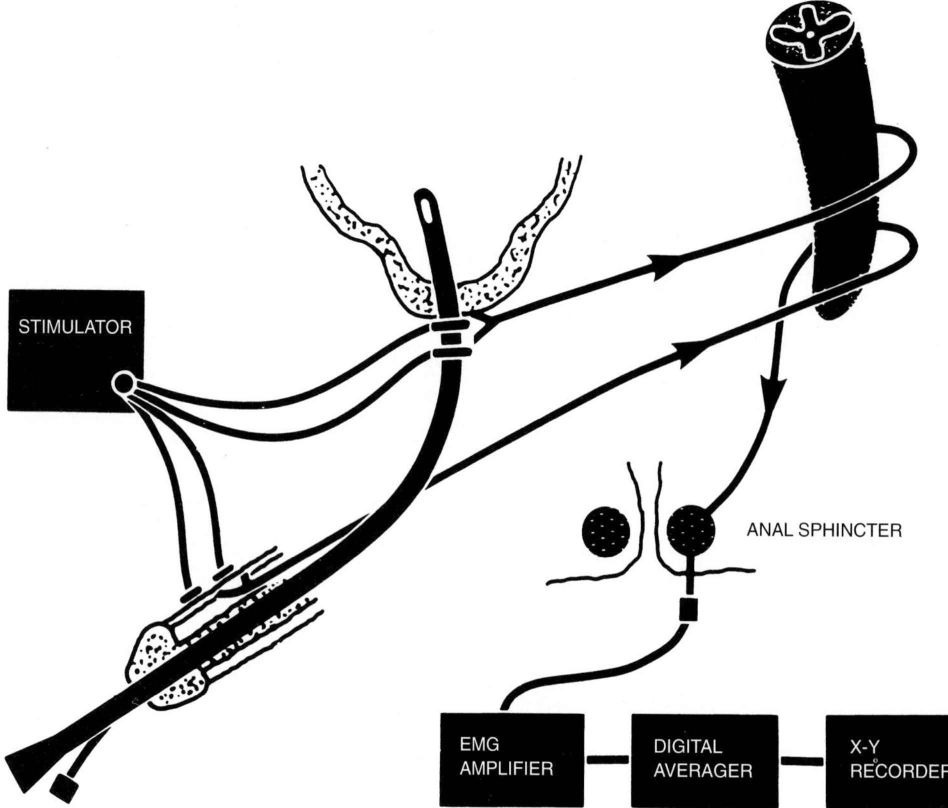

Figure 28–23. Schematic representation of nerve conduction studies performed to test the integrity of the sacral reflex arc.

medullaris or cauda equina lesions, normal, prolonged, or absent latencies may be found, and asymmetric responses are not uncommon. Patients with suprasacral lesions may have normal or low latencies (26 to 30 milliseconds) because of loss of inhibitory neural pathways from higher centers.

A variety of evoked response studies are used to test the integrity of peripheral, spinal, and central nervous pathways, and in urology these are performed as genitospinal and genitocortical evoked response recordings. They also require sophisticated instrumentation using averaging techniques, and their performance is confined to specialized centers.

REFERENCES

Abrams P: Objective evaluation of bladder outlet obstruction. Br J Urol 1995; 76:11–15.

Abrams P, Blaivas JG, Stanton SL, Andersen JT (International Continence Society Committee on Standardization of Terminology): The standardisation of terminology of lower urinary tract function. Scand J Urol Nephrol Suppl 1988; 114:5–19.

Abrams PH, Griffiths DJ: The assessment of prostatic obstruction from urodynamic measurements and from residual urine. Br J Urol 1979; 51:129–134.

Abrams PH, Torrens M: Urine flow studies. Urol Clin North Am 1979; 6:71–88.

Abrams PH, Feneley RCL: The significance of the symptoms associated with bladder outlet obstruction. Urol Int 1978; 33:171–174.

Abrams PH, Roylance J, Feneley RCL: Excretion urography in the investigation of prostatism. Br J Urol 1976; 48:681–684.

Andersen JT: Prostatism: Clinical, radiological and urodynamic aspects. Neurourol Urodyn 1982; 1:2–59.

Andersen JT, Jacobsen O, Strandgaard L: The diagnostic value of intravenous pyelography in infravesical obstruction in males. Scand J Urol Nephrol 1977; 11:225–230.

Bates P, Bradley WE, Glen E, et al: The standardization of terminology of lower urinary tract function. J Urol 1979; 121:551–554.

Barry MJ, Fowler FJ Jr, O'Leary MP, et al (AUA Measurement Committee): The American Urological Association symptom index for benign prostatic hyperplasia. J Urol 1992; 148:1549–1557.

Bauer SB, Hallett M, Khoshbin S, et al: Predictive value of urodynamic evaluation in newborns with myelodysplasia. JAMA 1984; 252:650–652.

Blaivas JG, Fisher DM: Combined radiographic and urodynamic monitoring: Advances in technique. J Urol 1981; 125:693–694.

Bolann BJ, Sandberg S, Digranes A: Implications of probability analysis for interpreting results of leukocyte esterase and nitrite test strips. Clin Chem 1989; 35:1663–1668.

Bonney V: On diurnal incontinence of urine in women. J Obstet Gynecol 1923; 30:358–365.

Bors EH, Blinn KA: Bulbocavernosus reflex. J Urol 1959; 82:128–130.

Bors EH, Blinn KA: Spinal reflux activity from the vesical mucosa in paraplegic patients. Arch Neruol Psychiatr 1957; 78:339–354.

Boyarsky S, Jones G, Paulson DF, et al: A new look at bladder neck obstruction by the Food and Drug Administration: Guidelines for investigation of benign prostatic hypertrophy. Trans Am Assoc Genitourin Surg 1977; 68:29–32.

Bradley W, Clarren S, Shapiro R, Wolfson J: Air cystometry. J Urol 1968; 100:451–458.

Brown M, Wickham JEA: The urethral pressure profile. Br J Urol 1969; 41:211–217.

Bruskewitz RC, Iversen P, Madsen PO: Value of postvoid residual urine determination in evaluation of prostatism. Urology 1982; 20:602.

Bunne G, Obrink A: Urethral closure pressure with stress: A comparison between stress incontinent and continent women. Urol Res 1978; 6:127–134.

Chancellor MB, Blaivis JG, Kaplan SA, Axelrod S: Bladder outlet obstruction versus impaired detrusor contractility: The role of uroflow. J Urol 1991; 145:810–812.

Chancellor MB, Erhard MJ, Hirsch IH, Stass WE Jr: Prospective evaluation of terazocin for the treatment of autonomic dysreflexia. J Urol 1994a; 151:111–113.

Chancellor MB, Rivas DA, Keeley FX, et al: Similarity of the American Urologic Association symptom index among men with benign prostate hyperplasia (BPH), urethral obstruction not due to BPH and detrusor hyperreflexia without outlet obstruction. Br J Urol 1994b; 74:200–203.

Christensen MM, Bruskewitz RC: Clinical manifestations of benign prostatic hyperplasia and indications for therapeutic intervention. Urol Clin N Am 1990; 17:509–516.

Creighton SM, Pearce JM, Robson I, et al: Sensory urgency: How full is your bladder. Br J Obstet Gynecol 1991; 98:1287–1289.

Dajani AS, Bisno AL, Chung KJ, et al: Prevention of bacterial endocarditis: Recommendations of the American Heart Association. JAMA 1990; 264:2919–2922.

Diokno AC, Wells TJ, Brink CA: Comparison of self-reported voided volume with cystometric bladder capacity. J Urol 1987; 137:698–700.

Drach GW, Layton TN, Binard WJ: Male peak urinary flow rate: Relationships to volume voided and age. J Urol 1979; 122:215–219.

Drach GW, Layton TN, Bottaccini MR: A method of adjustment of male peak urinary flow rate for varying age and volume voided. J Urol 1982; 128:960–962.

Drach GW, Steinbronn DV: Clinical evaluation of patients with prostatic obstruction: Correlation of flow rates with voided, residual or total bladder volume. J Urol 1986; 135:737–740.

Enhorning G: Simultaneous recording of infravesical and intraurethral pressure. Acta Chir Scand 1961; 276:1.

Eshima D, Taylor A Jr: Technetium-99 (^{99m}Tc) mercaptoacetyltriglicine: Update on the new ^{99m}Tc renal tubular function agent. Semin Nucl Med 1992; 22:61–73.

Farrar DJ, Whiteside CG, Osborne JL, et al: A urodynamic analysis of micturition symptoms in the female. Surg Gynecol Obstet 1975; 141:875.

Flood HD, Ritchey ML, Bloom DA, et al: Outcome of reflux in children with myelodysplasia managed by bladder pressure monitoring. J Urol 1994; 152:1574–1577.

Galloway NTM, Mekras JA, Helms M, Webster GD: An objective score to predict upper tract deterioration in myelodysplasia. J Urol 1991; 145:535–537.

Galloway NTM, Chisholm GD, McInnes A: Patterns and significance of the sacral evoked response (the urologist's knee jerk). Br J Urol 1985; 57:145–147.

Geirsson G, Fall M, Lindström S: The ice water test: A simple and valuable supplement to routine cystometry. Br J Urol 1993; 71:681–685.

Geirsson G, Lindström S, Fall M: Pressure, volume and infusion speed criteria for the ice water test. Br J Urol 1994; 73:498–503.

Gerstenberg TC, Andersen JT, Klarskov P, et al: High flow intravesical obstruction in men: Symptomatology, urodynamics and the results of surgery. J Urol 1982; 127:943–945.

Ghoneim GM, Roach MB, Lewis VH, Harmon EP: The value of leak pressure and bladder compliance in the urodynamic evaluation of meningomyelocele patients. J Urol 1990; 144:1440–1442.

Gleason D, Reilly B: Gas cystometry. Urol Clin North Am 1979; 6:85–88.

Glenning PP: Urinary voiding patterns of apparently normal women. Aust N Z J Obstet Gynecol 1985; 25:62–65.

Godec CJ, Cass AS: Rapid- and slow-fill gas cystometry. Urology 1979; 13:109–110.

Golomb J, Lindner A, Siegel Y, Korczak D: Variability and circadian changes in home uroflowmetry in patients with benign prostatic hyperplasia compared to normal controls. J Urol 1992; 147:1044–1047.

Griffiths DJ: Hydrodynamics of male micturition: I. Therapy of steady state flow through elastic walled tubes. Med Biol Eng 1971a; 7:201–215.

Griffiths DJ: Hydrodynamics of male micturition: II. Measurements of stream parameters and urethral elasticity. Med Biol Eng 1971b; 9:589–596.

Griffiths DJ: The mechanics of the urethra and of micturition. Br J Urol 1973; 45:497–507.

Griffiths D, van Mastrigt R, Bosch R: Quantification of urethral resistance and bladder function during voiding, with special reference to the effects of prostate size reduction on urethral obstruction due to benign prostatic hyperplasia. Neurourol Urodyn 1989; 8:17–27.

Grino PB, Bruskewtiz R, Blaivas JG, et al: Maximum urinary flow rate by uroflowmetry: Automatic or visual interpretation. J Urol 1993; 149:339–341.

Heritz DM, Blaivas JG: Reliability and specificity of the leak point pressure. J Urol 1995; 153:492A.

International Continence Society: First report on the standardization of terminology of lower urinary tract function. Scand J Urol Nephrol 1977a; 11:193–196.

International Continence Society: Second report on the standardization of terminology of lower urinary tract funtion. Br J Urol 1977b; 49:207–210.

International Continence Society: Third report on the standardization of terminology of lower urinary tract funtion. Br J Urol 1980; 52:348–350.

International Continence Society: Fourth report on the standardization of terminology of lower urinary tract function. Br J Urol 1981; 53:333–335.

Jensen KM-E, Bruskewitz RC, Iversen P, Madsen PO: Spontaneous uroflowmetry in prostatism. Urology 1984; 24:403–409.

Jensen KM-E, Jørgensen JB, Mogensen P: Reproducibility of uroflowmetry variables in elderly males. Urol Res 1985; 13:237–239.

Jonas U, Kramer G, Höfner K: The principles and clinical application of advanced urodynamic analysis for BPH. *In* Kurth KH, Newling DWW, eds: Benign Prostatic Hyperplasia. New York, Wiley-Liss, 1994; pp 141–156.

Kassis A, Schick E: Frequency-volume chart pattern in a healthy female population. Br J Urol 1993; 72:708–710.

Kreder KJ, Webster GD: Urodynamic assessment of bladder outlet obstruction. Probl Urol 1991; 5:386–396.

Krum H, Louis WJ, Brown DJ, Howes LG: A study of the alpha-1 adrenoceptor blocker prazocin in the prophylactic management of autonomic dysreflexia in high spinal cord injury patients. Clin Autonom Res 1992; 2:83–88.

Kunin CM, de Groot JE: Sensitivity of a nitrite indicator strip method in detecting bacturia in preschool girls. Pediatrics 1977; 60:244–245.

Lapides J, Bobbitt JM: Diagnostic value of bulbocavernosus reflex. JAMA 1956; 162:971–972.

Lapides J, Friend CR, Ajemian EP, Reus WF: A new test for neurogenic bladder. J Urol 1962; 88:245–247.

Lim CS, Abrams PH: The Abrams-Griffiths nomogram. World J Urol 1995; 13:34–39.

Lloyd LK: Monitoring the upper tracts in neurogenic bladder dysfunction. Probl Urol 1989;3:72.

Madsen PO, Iversen PA: A point system for selecting operative candidates. *In* Hinman F Jr, ed: Benign Prostatic Hypertrophy. New York, Springer-Verlag, 1983; pp 763–765.

Marshall VR, Ryall RL, Austin ML, Sinclair GR: The use of urinary flow rates obtained from voided volumes less than 150 mL in the assessment of voiding ability. Br J Urol 1983; 55:28–33.

Massey JA, Abrams PH: Obstructed voiding in the female. Br J Urol 1988; 61:36.

McCormack M, Infante-Rivard C, Schick E: Agreement between clinical methods of measurement of urinary frequency and functional bladder capacity. Br J Urol 1992; 69:17–21.

McGuire EJ, Fitzpatrick CC, Wan J, et al: Clinical assessment of urethral sphincter function. J Urol 1993; 150:1452–1454.

McGuire EJ, Woodside JR, Borden TA, Weiss RM: Prognostic value of urodynamic testing in myelodysplastic patients. J Urol 1981; 126:205–209.

McLoughlin J, Gill KP, Abel PD, Williams G: Symptoms versus flow rates versus urodynamics in the selection of patients for prostatectomy. Br J Urol 1990; 66:303–305.

Mosso O, Pellicani P: Sur les functions de la vessie. Arch Ital Biol 1882; 1:97–128.

O'Leary MP: Evaluating symptoms and functional status in benign prostate hyperplasia. Br J Urol 1995; 76:25–28.

Neilsen KK, Nording J, Hald T: Critical review of the diagnosis of prostatic obstruction. Neurourol Urodyn 1994; 13:201–217.

Nitti VW, Raz S: Obstruction following anti-incontinence procedures: Diagnosis and treatment with transvaginal urethrolysis. J Urol 1994; 152:93.

Papa Petros PE, Elmsten U: Tests for detrusor instability in women. Acta Obstet Gynecol Scand 1993; 72:661–667.

Pavlakis AJ, Siroky MB, Krane RJ: Neurogenic detrusor areflexia: Correlation of perineal electromyography and bethanechol chloride supresensitivity testing. J Urol 1983; 129:1182–1184.

Perez LM, Webster GD: The history of urodynamics. Neurourol Urodyn 1992; 11:1.

Perez LM, Khoury JM, Webster GD: The value of urodynamic studies in infants less than one year of age with spinal dysraphism. J Urol 1992; 148:584–587.

Perkash I: Urodynamic evaluation: Periurethral striated EMG vs. perianal striated EMG. Paraplegia 1980; 18:275–282.

Poulsen EU, Kirkeby HJ: Home-monitoring of uroflow in normal male adolescents: Relation between flow-curve, voided volume and time of day. Scand J Urol Nephrol Suppl 1988; 114:58–62.

Rees DLP, Whitefield HN, Islam AKMS, et al: Urodynamic findings in adult females with frequency and dysuria. Br J Urol 1976; 47:853.

Resnick MI, Rifkin MD: Ultrasonography of the Urinary Tract, 3rd ed. Baltimore, Williams & Wilkins, 1991.

Resnick NM: Initial evaluation of the incontinent patient. J Am Geriatr Soc 1990; 38:311–316.

Robertson AS, Griffiths CJ, Ramsden PD, Neal DB: Bladder function in healthy volunteers: Ambulatory monitoring and conventional urodynamic studies. Br J Urol 1994; 73:242–249.

Roehrborn CG, Kurth K, Leriche E, et al: Diagnostic recommendation for clinical practice. *In* Cockett ATK, Khoury S, Aso Y, et al, eds: The Second International Consultation on Benign Prostatic Hyperplasia: Proceedings. Jersey: Scientific Communication International, 1993, pp 291–293.

Rollema HJ: Uroflowmetry in males: Reference values and clinical applications of microprocessor controlled interpretation of urinary flow patterns. Proceedings of the Joint Meeting of the International Continence Society and Urodynamics Society, Aachen, West Germany, 1983.

Rollema HJ, Boender H, van der Beek C, et al: Value and validity of free uroflowmetry in prostatism: Comparison between nomograms. J Urol 1994; 151:324A.

Rollema HJ, van Mastrigt R: Improved indication and followup in transurethral resection of the prostate using the computer program CLIM: A prospective study. J Urol 1992; 148:111–116.

Rollema HJ, van Mastrigt R, Janknegt RA: Urodynamic assessment and quantification of prostatic obstruction before and after transurethral resection of the prostate: Standardization with the aid of the computer program. Urol Int 1991; 47:52–54.

Russell CD, Duborsky EV: Quantitation of renal function using MAG3. J Nucl Med 1991; 32:2061–2063.

Schäfer W: Urethral resistance? Urodynamic concepts of physiological and pathological outlet function during voiding. Neurourol Urodyn 1985; 4:161–201.

Schäfer W: Basic principles and clinical application of advanced analysis of bladder voiding function. Urol Clin North Am 1990; 17:553–566.

Schäfer W: Comparison of simple concepts of pressure/flow analysis: URA versus linear PURR and p/Q diagram. Neurourol Urodyn 1992; 11:397–398.

Schäfer W: A new concept for simple but specific grading of bladder outflow conditions independent from detrusor functions. J Urol 1993; 149:356A.

Schäfer W, Noppeney R, Rubben H, Lutzeyer W: The value of free flow rate and pressure/flow studies in the routine investigation of BPH patients. Neurourol Urodyn 1988; 7:219–221.

Siroky MB, Olsson CA, Krane RJ: The flow rate nomogram: I. Development. J Urol 1979; 122:665–668.

Siroky MB, Olsson CA, Krane RJ: The flow rate nomogram: II. Clinical correlations. J Urol 1980; 123:208–210.

Spangberg A, Terio H, Engberg A, Ask P: Qualification of urethral function based on Griffiths' model of flow through elastic tubes. Neurourol Urodyn 1989; 8:29–52.

Thyberg M, Ertzgaard P, Gylling M, Granerus G: Effect of nifedipine on cystometry-induced evaluation of blood pressure in patients with a reflex urinary bladder after high level spinal cord injury. Paraplegia 1994; 32:308–313.

Trop CS, Bennett CJ: Autonomic dysreflexia and its urologic implications: A review. J Urol 1991; 146:1461–1469.

Usui A, McGuire EJ, O'Connell HE, Aboseif S: Abdominal leak point pressures in stress incontinence. J Urol 1995; 153:493A.

van Mastrigt R: A computer program for on-line measurement, storage, analysis and retrieval of urodynamic data. Comput Prog Biomed 1984; 18:109–117.

van Mastrigt R: Urodynamic analysis using an on-line computer. Neurourol Urodyn 1987; 6:206–207.

von Garrelts B: Analysis of micturition: A new method of recording the voiding of the bladder. Acta Chir Scand 1956; 112:326–340.

Walton L: The motor system. *In* Essentials of Neurology, 6th ed. New York, Churchill Livingstone, 1989, pp 127–160.

Wan J, McGuire EJ, Bloom DA, Ritchey ML: Stress leak point pressure: A diagnostic tool for incontinent children. J Urol 1993; 150:700–702.

Webb RJ, Styles RA, Griffiths CJ, et al: Ambulatory monitoring of bladder pressures in patients with low compliance as a result of neurogenic bladder dysfunction. Br J Urol 1989; 64:150.

Webster GD, Older RA: Value of subtracted bladder pressure measurement in routine urodynamics. Urology 1980a; 16:656–660.

Webster GD, Older RA: Video urodynamics. Urology 1980b; 16:106–114.

Webster GD, Koefoot RB: The after contraction in urodynamic micturition studies. Neurourol Urodyn 1983; 2:213–218.

Webster GD, Kreder KJ: Voiding dysfunction following cystourethropexy: Its evaluation and management. J Urol 1990; 144:670.

Wein AJ: Neuromuscular dysfunction of the lower urinary tract. *In* Walsh PC, Retik AB, Stamey TA, Vaughn ED Jr, eds: Campbell's Urology, 6th ed. Philadelphia, W.B. Saunders Company, 1992, pp 573–642.

Wheeler JS Jr, Culkin DJ, Walter JS, et al: Female urinary retention. Urology 1990; 35:428.

Williams RD, Kreder KJ: Urologic laboratory examination. *In* Tanagho EA, McAninch JW, eds: Smith's General Urology. Norwalk, CT, 1995, pp 50–63.

Yalla SV, Sharma GVK, Barsaman EM: Micturitional static urethral pressure profile: A method of recording urethral pressure profile during voiding and the implications. J Urol 1980; 124:649–654.

29 NEUROMUSCULAR DYSFUNCTION OF THE LOWER URINARY TRACT AND ITS TREATMENT

Alan J. Wein, M.D.

This chapter begins by summarizing the available information on the types of voiding dysfunction that occur with specific neurologic and muscular diseases, injuries, or dysfunctions in the adult. It concludes with a detailed consideration of the various types of therapy available for these. Although most of the treatments are applicable to all types of voiding dysfunction, certain treatments and non-neuropathic dysfunctions are considered in much greater detail elsewhere in the text and are so indicated. Pediatric voiding dysfunction is specifically covered in Chapters 64 and 66.

GENERAL PATTERNS OF NEUROPATHIC VOIDING DYSFUNCTION

Discrete neurologic lesions generally affect the filling-storage and emptying phases of lower urinary tract function in a relatively consistent fashion, that fashion dependent on the area(s) affected, the physiologic function of the area(s), and whether the lesion is destructive or irritative. **Neurologic lesions above the brain stem that affect micturition generally result in involuntary bladder contractions with smooth and striated sphincter synergy.** Sensation and voluntary striated sphincter function are generally preserved. Areflexia may, however, occur, either initially or as a permanent dysfunction. **Patients with complete lesions of the spinal cord above spinal cord level S2, after they recover from spinal shock, generally exhibit involuntary bladder contractions without sensation, smooth sphincter synergy, but striated sphincter dyssynergia.** Patients with significant spinal cord trauma below that cord level generally do not manifest involuntary bladder contractions per se. Detrusor areflexia is the rule initially after spinal shock, and, depending on the type and extent of neurologic injury, various forms of decreased compliance during filling may occur. An open smooth sphincter area may result, but whether this is due to sympathetic or parasympathetic decentralization-defunctionalization (or both or neither) has never been settled (Wein and Barrett, 1988; Zderic et al, 1995). Various types of striated sphincter dysfunction may occur, but commonly the area retains a residual resting sphincter tone (not the same as dyssynergia) and is not under voluntary control. **The dysfunctions that occur with interruption of the peripheral reflex arc may be very similar to those of distal spinal cord injury.** Detrusor areflexia often develops, low compliance may result, the smooth sphincter area may be relatively incompetent, and the striated sphincter area may exhibit fixed residual tone not amenable to voluntary relaxation. True peripheral neuropathy can be motor or sensory with the usual expected sequelae, at least initially. Table 29–1 summarizes some features of many common types of voiding dysfunction due to neurologic disease or injury.

DISEASE AT OR ABOVE THE BRAIN STEM

Cerebrovascular Disease

Cerebrovascular disease is the third most common cause of death and one of the most common causes of disability in the United States and Europe. The prevalence of stroke in persons older than 65 years of age is cited as approximately 60 in 1000, and, in persons older than 75, 95 per 1000 (Khan et al, 1990). The annual incidence has been estimated at 6 to 12 per 1000 in individuals 65 to 74 years and at 40 per 1000 in those over 85 years. Of every 100 survivors, Arunabh and Badlani (1993) estimate only 10 are unimpaired, 40 have a mild residual, 40 are disabled, and 10 require institutionalization. Thrombosis, occlusion, and hemorrhage are the most common causes, leading to ischemia and infarction of variably sized areas in the brain, usually around the internal capsule. The effects on micturition depend on the location and size of the damage.

After the initial acute episode, urinary retention due to detrusor areflexia may occur. The neurophysiology of this "cerebral shock" is unclear. After a variable degree of recovery from the neurologic lesion, a fixed deficit may become apparent over a few weeks or months. The **most common long-term expression of lower urinary tract dysfunction after cerebrovascular accident (CVA) is detrusor hyperreflexia** (Wein and Barrett, 1988; Khan et al, 1990). Sensation is variable but generally intact, and thus the patient has urgency and frequency with hyperreflexia. The appropriate response is to try to inhibit the involuntary bladder contraction by forceful contraction of the striated sphincter. If this can be accomplished, only urgency and frequency result; if not, urgency with incontinence results. The exact acute and chronic incidence of any voiding dysfunction after CVA, and specifically of incontinence, is not readily apparent. Shortly after CVA, estimates of incontinence range from 44% to 83% (data cited by Arunabh and Badlani, 1993), with 70% to 80% of these regaining their continence over time. Incontinence is a poor prognostication of survival and of ultimate rehabilitation and functional independence. Detrusor areflexia may also exist.

Previous descriptions of the voiding dysfunction after CVA have all cited the preponderance of detrusor hyperreflexia with coordinated sphincter activity. It is difficult to reconcile this with the relatively high incontinence rate that occurs, even considering the fact that a percentage of these patients had an incontinence problem before the CVA. Tsuchida and co-workers (1983) and Khan and associates (1990) have made significant contributions in this area by correlating the urodynamic and computed tomographic (CT) pictures after CVA. There is general agreement on the fact that patients with lesions in only the basal ganglia or thalamus have normal sphincter function. This means that when an impending involuntary contraction or its onset is sensed, they can voluntarily contract the striated sphincter and abort or considerably lessen the effect of the abnormal micturition reflex. The majority of patients with involvement of the cerebral cortex and/or internal capsule are unable to forcefully contract the striated sphincter under these circumstances. Although the authors call this "uninhibited relaxation of the sphincter," it is really not, but certainly the term does imply that a profound abnormality exists in these patients in the cerebral-to-corticospinal circuitry that is necessary for voluntary control of the striated sphincter.

Detrusor hypocontractility or areflexia may persist after CVA. The exact incidence of areflexia as a cause of chronic voiding symptoms after CVA is uncertain. In our patient population it is very small, but some estimates place it as high as 20% (Arunabh and Badlani, 1993). **True detrusor–striated sphincter dyssynergia does not occur. Pseudodyssynergia may occur during urodynamic testing** (Wein and Barrett, 1982). This refers to an electromyographic (EMG) sphincter "flare" during filling cystometry secondary to attempted inhibition of an involuntary bladder contraction by contraction of the striated sphincter. Smooth sphincter function is generally unaffected by CVA. Poor flow rates and high residual urine volumes in a man with pre-CVA symptoms of prostatism generally indicate prostatic obstruction, but a urodynamic evaluation is advisable before committing

Table 29–1. MOST COMMON PATTERNS OF TYPICAL VOIDING DYSFUNCTIONS SEEN WITH VARIOUS TYPES OF NEUROLOGIC DISEASE OR INJURY

Disorder	Detrusor Activity	Compliance	Smooth Sphincter	Striated Sphincter	Other
Cerebrovascular accident	+	N	S	S ± VC	
Brain tumor	+	N	S	S	May have decreased sensation of lower urinary tract events.
Cerebral palsy	+	N	S	S D (25%) ± VC	
Parkinson's disease	+ I	N	S	S ± VC	
Shy-Drager syndrome	+ I	N D	O	S	Striated sphincter may exhibit denervation.
Multiple sclerosis	+ I − (5%–30%)	N	S	S D (30%–65%)	Dyssynergia figures refer to percentage of those with detrusor hyperreflexia.
Spinal cord injury					
Suprasacral	+	N	S	D	Smooth sphincter may be dyssynergic if lesion above T7.
Sacral	−	N D (may develop)	CNR O (may develop)	F	
Autonomic hyperreflexia	+	N	D	D	
Myelodysplasia	− +	N D (may develop)	O	F	Findings vary widely in different series. Striated sphincter commonly shows some evidence of denervation.
Tabes, pernicious anemia	I−	N I	S	S	Primary problem is loss of sensation. Detrusor may become decompensated secondary to overdistention.
Disc disease	−	N	CNR	S	Striated sphincter may show evidence of denervation and fixed tone.
Radical pelvic surgery	I−	D N	O	F	
Diabetes	I	N I	S	S	Sensory loss contributes, but there is a motor neuropathy as well.

Detrusor activity: I, impaired; +, involuntary contraction; −, areflexia. Compliance: N, normal; D, decreased; I, increased. Smooth sphincter: S, synergic; D, dyssynergic; O, open, incompetent at rest; CNR, competent, nonrelaxing. Striated sphincter: S, synergic; D, dyssynergic; ±VC, voluntary control may be impaired; F, fixed tone.

a patient to mechanical outlet reduction in order to exclude detrusor hyperactivity with impaired contractility (DHIC) as a cause of symptoms.

Other important modifying factors should be considered in the care of these patients. This is generally a problem of the elderly, some of whom have pre-existent lower urinary tract abnormalities. Previously the problems may have been manageable, but the additional difficulty may make the situation intolerable. As Andrews (1994) notes, other aspects of the brain damage can affect general rehabilitation and control of the lower urinary tract dysfunction. These may include cognitive impairment, dysphasia, inappropriate and aggressive behavior, impaired mobility, and low motivation. Finally, the entire voiding dysfunction may be adversely affected by treatment regimens that concentrate on detrusor hyperactivity alone (e.g., anticholinergic or antispasmodic therapy). Many such patients are depressed, and confusion and disorientation often results, which compounds the problem. Vigorous pharmacologic therapy of detrusor hyperreflexia may make these associated problems of mentation worse.

Dementia

Dementia is a poorly understood disease complex involving atrophy and the loss of gray and white matter of the brain, particularly of the frontal lobes. Problems with memory and the performance of tasks requiring intellectual mentation result. Associated conditions include widespread vascular disease, Alzheimer's disease, Pick's disease, Jakob-Creutzfeldt disease, syphilis, heat trauma, and encephalitis. When voiding dysfunction occurs, the result is generally incontinence. It is difficult to ascertain whether this is due to detrusor hyperreflexia with the type of disorder of voluntary striated sphincter control mentioned above or whether the incontinence reflects a situation in which the individual has simply lost the awareness of the desirability of voluntary urinary control. Even if they have voluntary sphincter control, such individuals may void when and where they please, because mentation fails to dictate why they should not. Such activity may be due to detrusor hyperreflexia or a normal, but inappropriately timed, micturition reflex. Treatment is obviously difficult without a desire for improvement. Additionally, anticholinergic therapy may be contraindicated in Alzheimer's disease if current theories about its cause are valid (cortical cholinergic loss).

Concussion

Generally, when voiding dysfunction occurs after a closed head injury, there is an initial period of detrusor areflexia followed by the appearance of hyperreflexic detrusor dysfunction (McGuire, 1984). This is an uncommon sequela of concussion, but when it occurs, similar considerations apply as to voiding dysfunction secondary to cerebrovascular disease.

Brain Tumor

Both primary and metastatic brain tumors have been reported to be associated with disturbances of bladder function. When dysfunction results, it is related to the localized area involved rather than to the tumor type. The areas most frequently involved with associated bladder dysfunction are the superior aspects of the frontal lobe (Blaivas, 1985). **When voiding dysfunction occurs, it generally consists of detrusor hyperreflexia and urinary incontinence.** These individuals may have a markedly diminished awareness of all lower urinary tract events and, if so, are totally unable even to attempt suppression of the micturition reflex. Smooth and striated sphincter activities are generally synergic. Pseudodyssynergia may occur during urodynamic testing.

Cerebellar Ataxia

The cerebellar ataxia group of diseases involves pathologic degeneration of the nervous system generally involving the cerebellum, but with a possible extension to the brain stem, spinal cord, and dorsal nerve roots (Leach et al, 1982). Poor coordination, depressed deep tendon reflexes, dysarthria, dysmetria, and choreiform movements result because of the cerebellar involvement. Voiding dysfunction is generally manifested by incontinence, generally associated with detrusor hyperreflexia and sphincter synergia. Retention or high residual urine volume may be seen as well. This is most commonly due to detrusor areflexia but may be associated with detrusor striated sphincter dyssynergia, presumably secondary to spinal cord involvement.

Normal Pressure Hydrocephalus

Normal pressure hydrocephalus is a disease of progressive dementia and ataxia occurring in patients with a normal spinal fluid pressure and distended cerebral ventricles but with no passage of air over the cerebral convexities by pneumoencephalography (Blaivas, 1985). When voiding dysfunction occurs, it is generally incontinence secondary to detrusor hyperreflexia with sphincter synergia.

Cerebral Palsy

Cerebral palsy (CP) is the rubric applied to a nonprogressive injury of the brain in the prenatal or perinatal period (some say up to 3 years) that produces neuromuscular disability and/or specific symptom complexes of cerebral dysfunction. The cause is generally infection or a period of hypoxia. Affected children exhibit delayed gross motor development, abnormal motor performance, altered muscle tone, abnormal posture, and exaggerated reflexes. Most children and adults with only CP have urinary control and what seems to be normal filling-storage and normal emptying. The incidence of voiding dysfunction is vague, since the few available series report mostly subcategorizations of those who present with symptoms. Andrews (1994) estimates that a third or more of children with CP are so affected. When an adult with CP presents with an acute or subacute change in voiding status, it is most likely unrelated to CP.

Reid and Borzyskowski (1993) described findings in 27 CP patients, aged 3 to 20 years, referred for voiding dysfunction. Incontinence (74%), frequency (56%), and urgency (37%) were the most common presenting symptoms, and detrusor hyperreflexia the most common urodynamic abnormality (87% of those undergoing urodynamics), with 25% of these exhibiting striated sphincter dyssynergia. Mayo (1992) reported on 33 CP patients referred for evaluation, of whom 10 were over the age of 20. Difficulty urinating was the predominant symptom in about half the patients, but half of these also had hyperreflexia and urgency when the bladder was full. The cause of the difficulty in voluntarily initiating micturition was thought to be a problem with relaxing the pelvic floor and not true striated sphincter dyssynergia. Incontinence was the major presenting symptom in the other half, associated in 14 of 16 with detrusor hyperreflexia but in all with normal voiding otherwise. Decreased sensation was reported in 17 of 23 patients under 20 years of age and in 4 of 10 over 20 years. The more serious manifestations, such as retention, were found only in the adults, causing the author to suggest that difficulty urinating may progress in adulthood. Although Reid and Borzyskowski (1993) note that incontinence can be significantly improved in most CP patients and that, in their experience, intellectual delay is not a barrier to successful management, one special problem that is encountered in some of these patients that makes their management very difficult is a severe degree of mental retardation, so that cooperation, evaluation, and treatment are virtually impossible. With such patients, sometimes the best that one can do is to check the upper tracts with renal ultrasonography and obtain an estimate of postvoid residual urine, either via catheterization or by ultrasonography, and proceed accordingly. **In those persons that exhibit signifi-**

cant dysfunction, the type of deficit that one would suspect from the urodynamic abnormalities most often seen seems to be localized anatomically above the brain stem and is commonly reflected by detrusor hyperreflexia and coordinated sphincters. However, spinal cord damage can occur also, and perhaps this accounts for those with CP who seem to have evidence of striated sphincter dyssynergia or evidence of a more distal type of neural axis lesion.

Parkinson's Disease

Parkinson's disease, a degenerative disorder, affects primarily the dopaminergic substantia nigra–corpus striatum pathway, resulting in a **relative dopamine deficiency and cholinergic predominance in the corpus striatum** and the loss of pigmented neurons in the substantia nigra with associated intracytoplasmic inclusions (Lewy bodies). Classic neurologic symptoms include bradykinesia, tremor, and skeletal rigidity. The prevalence in the United States is estimated at between 100 and 150 cases per 100,000 population, respectively, with the onset generally between the ages of 45 and 65 years, affecting men and women equally (Blaivas, 1985; Marsden, 1990; Sotolongo and Chancellor, 1993). **Voiding dysfunction occurs in 35% to 70% of patients.** Pre-existing detrusor or outlet abnormalities may exist, and the symptomatology may be affected by various types of treatment for the primary disease. When voiding dysfunction occurs, **symptoms generally (50% to 70%) consist of urgency, frequency, nocturia, and urge incontinence.** The remainder of patients have obstructive symptoms or a combination.

The most common urodynamic finding is detrusor hyperreflexia (Blaivas, 1985; Berger et al, 1990). **The smooth sphincter is synergic. There is some confusion regarding EMG interpretation.** Sporadic involuntary activity in the striated sphincter during involuntary bladder contraction may be detected in as many as 60% of patients; however, this does not cause obstruction and cannot be termed true dyssynergia, which generally does not occur (Berger et al, 1990; Sotolongo and Chancellor, 1993). Pseudodyssynergia may also occur, as well as a delay in striated sphincter relaxation at the onset of voluntary micturition, both of which can be urodynamically misinterpreted as true dyssynergia. Detection of poor voluntary striated sphincter control is important, as Staskin et al (1988) have shown it predisposes to an increased incidence of postprostatectomy incontinence. Impaired detrusor contractility may occur, in the form of either low amplitude or poorly sustained contractions, or a combination.

One significant problem in dealing with the male patient with Parkinson's disease is determining whether or not there is outlet obstruction secondary to prostatic enlargement and whether prostatectomy or other mechanical measures to decrease prostatic urethral resistance are indicated. It is important to note that the considerations under these circumstances are different than they are for a patient with voiding dysfunction after a CVA who also has outlet obstruction. Generally, detrusor contractility seems to be unimpaired in CVA patients with involuntary bladder hyperactivity, and, in the absence of dyssynergia (essentially nonexistent), poor flow rates and high residual urine volumes generally indicate prostatic obstruction. Outlet reduction in those patients with primarily obstructive symptoms is generally beneficial and is usually beneficial as well in those with irritative symptoms. In the latter group, improvement results because the functional bladder capacity increases, either as a result of a decrease in a residual urine volume or because the clinician feels more comfortable in treating these now-unobstructed patients with agents to decrease bladder contractility. **Male patients with Parkinson's disease and identical symptoms do not seem to fare as well as CVA patients after prostatectomy.** Poorly sustained bladder contractions, sometimes with slow sphincter relaxation, may occur consequent to the neurologic disease, and in such patients prostatectomy may result in no change or in a worsening of the voiding symptoms. Also, the type of sphincter control problem that predisposes to postprostatectomy incontinence in patients with Parkinson's disease (see above) is generally not seen in patients after stroke.

Christmas and co-workers (1988) demonstrated that the subcutaneous administration of a dopamine receptor agonist (apomorphine) can reliably and rapidly reverse parkinsonian "off" periods (periods of worsening symptoms mainly caused by the timing of previous medication doses and the unpredictable nature of motor fluctuations). By repeating videourodynamic studies during the motor improvement after apomorphine administration, bladder outlet obstruction secondary to benign prostatic hyperplasia (BPH) may be distinguished from voiding dysfunction secondary to the disease itself. The authors also point out that apomorphine might be useful in such patients who have severe off-phase voiding dysfunction with disabling nocturnal frequency and incontinence.

Shy-Drager Syndrome (Multiple System Atrophy)

The Shy-Drager syndrome is an uncommon neurologic disorder characterized clinically by orthostatic hypotension, anhydrosis, and differing degrees of cerebellar and parkinsonian dysfunction. In some prior discussions, it was listed as a form of atypical parkinsonism, with involvement not only of the extrapyramidal system (as is typical for parkinsonism) but also of the pyramidal and autonomic systems. Voiding and erectile dysfunction are common.

The neurologic lesions (cell loss and gliosis) have been identified in the cerebellum, substantia nigra, globus pallidus, caudate, putamen, inferior olives, intermediolateral columns of the spinal cord, and Onuf's nucleus (Kirby et al, 1986; Beck et al, 1994). Men and women are equally affected, with the onset in middle age. The disease is progressive and generally is associated with a poor prognosis.

The **initial urinary symptoms are urgency, frequency, and urge incontinence,** occurring up to 4 years before the diagnosis, as does erectile failure. **Detrusor hyperreflexia is frequently found, as one would expect from the central nervous system areas affected, but decreased compliance may occur, reflecting distal spinal involvement of the locations of the cell bodies of autonomic neurons innervating the lower urinary tract.** As the disease progresses, difficulty in initiating and maintaining voiding occurs, probably due to pontine and sacral cord lesions and generally is associated with a poor prognosis. Cystourethrography or videourodynamic studies generally reveal an **open bladder neck** (nonfunctional bladder neck and proximal urethra), and **many patients exhibit evidence of striated sphincter denervation** on motor unit electromyography. The **smooth and striated sphincter abnormalities predispose women to sphincteric incontinence and make prostatectomy hazardous in men.** Berger and co-workers (1990) have described a useful urodynamic differentiation of Shy-Drager syndrome from Parkinson's disease. Parkinsonian patients with voiding dysfunction generally have detrusor hyperreflexia and normal compliance. An open bladder neck is seen only in patients with Shy-Drager syndrome, excluding those patients with Parkinson's disease who have had a prostatectomy. EMG evidence of striated sphincter denervation is seen much more commonly in Shy-Drager syndrome.

The treatment of voiding dysfunction due to multiple system atrophy is difficult and seldom satisfactory. Treatment of detrusor hyperactivity during filling may worsen problems imitating voluntary micturition or worsen impaired contractility during emptying. Patients generally have sphincteric insufficiency, and rarely, therefore, is an outlet-reducing procedure indicated. Drug treatment of sphincteric incontinence may further worsen emptying problems. Generally, the goal in these patients is to facilitate storage, and clean intermittent catheterization (CIC) would often be desirable. Unfortunately, patients with advanced disease are often not candidates for CIC.

DISEASE PRIMARILY INVOLVING THE SPINAL CORD

Multiple Sclerosis

Multiple sclerosis (MS) is primarily a disease of young and middle-aged adults, with a predilection for women. Prevalence in the United States varies from 6 to 122 per 100,000 (Poser, 1994). The disease is due to focal neural demyelination, with relative axon sparing, which causes impairment of nerve conduction. The slowing of nerve conduction results in differing neurologic abnormalities that are subject to exacerbation and remission. Lesions (known as plaques) range from 1 mm to 4 cm and are scattered throughout the white matter of the nervous system (Chancellor and Blaivas, 1993). **The demyelinating process most commonly involves the posterior and lateral columns of the cervical spinal cord,** and it is thus not surprising that voiding dysfunction is so common. Autopsy studies have revealed almost constant evidence of demyelination in the cervical spinal cord, but involvement of the lumbar and sacral cord occurs in approximately 40% and 18%, respectively (Blaivas and Kaplan, 1988). Lesions also may occur in the cerebral cortex and midbrain, accounting for the intellectual deterioration and/or euphoria that may be seen as well (Kirby, 1994).

Of patients with MS, **50% to 90% complain of voiding symptoms at some time.** Lower urinary tract involvement may constitute the sole initial complaint or be part of the presenting symptom complex in up to 10% of patients, usually in the form of acute urinary retention of "unknown" cause or as an acute onset of urgency and frequency secondary to hyperreflexia. **Detrusor hyperreflexia is the most common urodynamic abnormality detected,** occurring in 50% to 99% of cases in reported series (Blaivas and Kaplan, 1988; Bemelmans et al, 1991; Chancellor and Blaivas, 1993; Sirls et al, 1994). **Of the patients with hyperreflexia, 30% to 65% have coexistent striated sphincter dyssynergia. Up to 60% of those with hyperreflexia may have impaired detrusor contractility** (Mayo and Chetner, 1992), a phenomenon that can considerably complicate treatment efforts. **Bladder areflexia may also occur**; reports of its frequency vary but generally average from 5% to 20%. Generally, the **smooth sphincter is synergic.** Chancellor and Blaivas (1993) reviewed urodynamic findings in multiple series of patients with MS and voiding dysfunction and summarize the incidence of three basic patterns: (1) detrusor hyperreflexia, striated sphincter synergia 26% to 50% (average 38%); detrusor hyperreflexia, striated sphincter dyssynergia 24% to 46% (average 29%); detrusor areflexia 19% to 40% (average 26%).

Because sensation is frequently intact in these patients, one must be careful to distinguish pseudodyssynergia from true striated sphincter dyssynergia. Blaivas and associates (1981) subcategorized striated sphincter dyssynergia and identified some varieties that are more worrisome than others. For instance, in a woman with MS, a brief period of striated sphincter dyssynergia during detrusor contraction (but one that does not result in excessive intravesical pressure during voiding, substantial residual urine volume, or secondary detrusor hypertrophy) may be relatively inconsequential, whereas those varieties that are more sustained—resulting in high bladder pressures of long duration—are most associated with urologic complications. Chancellor and Blaivas (1993) re-emphasize that the **most important parameters predisposing patients with MS to significant urologic complications** are (1) striated sphincter dyssynergia in men, (2) high detrusor filling pressure (>40 cm H_2O), and (3) an indwelling catheter.

Aggressive and anticipatory medical management can obviate most significant complications. Sirls and colleagues (1994) reported that only 7% (I calculate 10.4%) of their patients required surgical intervention because of failure of aggressive medical management and that none developed hydronephrosis on such therapy. The regimens used were (1) drugs to decrease detrusor hyperactivity plus CIC (57%), (2) such drugs alone (13%), (3) CIC alone (15%), and (4) behavioral therapy.

Miscellaneous Central Nervous System Diseases Causing Voiding Dysfunction Similar to That of Multiple Sclerosis

Lyme Disease

Associated neurologic symptoms fall broadly into three syndromes: (1) encephalopathy, (2) polyneuropathy, and (3) leukoencephalitis. Chancellor and colleagues (1993) described seven patients with lower urinary tract dysfunction. Five had detrusor hyperreflexia, none had dyssynergia, and two had detrusor areflexia. Follow-up 6 months to 2 years after treatment revealed residual urgency and frequency in three patients.

Hereditary Spastic Paraplegia

Hereditary spastic paraplegia is a genetically transmitted disorder, generally autosomal-dominant, less commonly autosomal-recessive, and rarely sex-linked. There is a pattern of central demyelination with axon loss and progressive lower extremity spasticity with or without muscle weakness. Bushman and associates (1993) reported three patients, two of whom had detrusor hyperreflexia (one with striated sphincter dyssynergia); one had significantly decreased compliance, and one was urodynamically normal except for a high maximal urethral pressure of uncertain significance.

Tropical Spastic Paraparesis

Tropical spastic paraparesis (TSP) is primarily a spinal cord disorder caused by a retrovirus (human T-cell lymphotropic virus type I [HTLV-I]) similar to the human immunodeficiency virus (HIV). Progressive lower-limb weakness and back pain are typically the primary complaints, but voiding dysfunction occurs in 60% or more of those affected. Eardley and associates (1991) describe two of six patients with detrusor areflexia and three of six with hyperreflexia, one of these with dyssynergia. Walton and Kaplan (1993) found four of their five patients had detrusor hyperreflexia and striated sphincter dyssynergia, whereas one had hyperreflexia and synergia. The type of voiding dysfunction depends on whether the damage is primarily to the descending spinal tracts to the sacral nuclei or to the sacral outflow.

Acquired Immunodeficiency Syndrome

A series of 11 acquired immunodeficiency syndrome (AIDS) patients with voiding dysfunction was reported by Khan and associates (1992). Urinary retention occurred in six. On urodynamic evaluation, three had detrusor hyperreflexia, four had areflexia, two had hypocontractile detrusors, and two had outlet obstruction secondary to BPH.

Spinal Cord Injury and Disease

Epidemiology, Morbidity, General Concepts

Spinal cord injury (SCI) may occur as a consequence of acts of violence; fracture or dislocation of the spinal column secondary to motor vehicle or diving accidents; vascular injuries; infection; disc prolapse; or sudden or severe hyperextension with other causes. Complete anatomic transection is rare, and the degree of neurologic deficit varies with the level and severity of the injury. **Spinal column (bone) segments are numbered by the vertebral level,** and these have a different relationship to the spinal cord segmental level at different locations. **The sacral spinal cord begins at about the spinal column level of T12–L1. The spinal cord terminates in the cauda equina at the spinal column level at approximately L2.** Multiple-level injuries may occur, and even with a single initial injury, cord damage may not be confined to a single cord segment and may extend cephalad, caudal, or both.

Stover and Fine (1987) reviewed the epidemiology and other general aspects of SCI. The annual rate is between 30 and 32 new spinal cord injuries per million persons at risk in the United States; the prevalence of SCI is approximately 906 per million. Motor vehicle injuries account for approximately half of all SCIs, followed by falls (approximately 21%), with acts of violence and sporting-related accidents each accounting for approximately 14% to 15%. The male-to-female ratio is 4:1. Neurologically incomplete quadriplegics constitute the largest group of SCI patients at the time of hospital admission (28%), followed by complete paraplegics (26%), complete quadriplegics (24%), and incomplete paraplegics (18%). Although earlier data (Hackler, 1977) indicated that renal disease was the major cause of death, at least in the paraplegic patient, a retrospective study of more than 5000 patients who sustained SCIs between 1973 and 1980 revealed that the leading causes of death were then pneumonia, accidents, and suicide (Stover and Fine, 1987). Septicemia, however, showed the highest ratio of actual-to-expected deaths for all age groups, followed by pulmonary emboli for patients younger than 55 years of age and by pneumonia for patients 55 years of age or older. Accidents, suicides, and cancer were the leading causes of death among paraplegics, whereas pneumonia was the leading cause of death among quadriplegics. These figures indicate, it is hoped, a distinct improvement in the urologic care of these patients.

Controlled and coordinated lower urinary tract function depends on an intact neural axis. Bladder contractility and the occurrence of reflex contractions depend on an intact sacral spinal cord and its afferent and efferent connections (see Chapter 26). **Generally, complete lesions above this area, but below the area of the sympathetic outflow, result in detrusor hyperreflexia, absent sensation below the level of the lesion, smooth sphincter synergia, and striated sphincter dyssynergia. Lesions above the spinal cord level of T7 or T8 (the spinal column level of T6) may result in smooth sphincter dyssynergia as well.** However, although the correlation between neurologic and urodynamic findings is good, it is not perfect, and a neurologic examination is no substitute for a urodynamic evaluation in these patients when one is determining risk factors and treatment (see below).

There is an impressive amount of literature that is continually building on the neurobiology of the spinal cord and its acute and chronic alteration after SCI. These topics are not specifically considered here, nor are the ramifications of this information relative to potential improvement of spinal cord function after injury. Sexual and reproductive dysfunction in the SCI patient is a topic that deserves much attention in the overall rehabilitation plan. Pertinent general concepts of sexual and reproductive function and their normalization in this special group of patients can be found in Chapters 38 to 40 and 41 to 43. Excellent specific reviews on sexual function can be found by Bennett and colleagues (1988), Stone and MacDermott (1989), and Smith and Bodner (1993); recommended reviews on fertility are by Linsenmeyer and Perkash (1991) and Seager and Halstead (1993).

Spinal Shock

After a significant SCI, a period of decreased excitability of spinal cord segments at and below the level of the lesion occurs, referred to as "spinal shock." There is absent somatic reflex activity and flaccid muscle paralysis below this level. Although classic teaching refers to generalized areflexia below the level of the lesion for days to months, Thomas and O'Flynn (1994) confirm that the most peripheral somatic reflexes of the sacral cord segments (the anal and bulbocavernosus reflexes) may never disappear, or, if they do, may return within minutes or hours of the injury.

Spinal shock includes a suppression of autonomic activity as well as somatic activity, and **the bladder is acontractile and areflexic. Radiologically, the bladder has a smooth contour with no evidence of trabeculation. The bladder neck is generally closed and competent** unless there has been prior surgery or in some cases of thoracolumbar and presumably sympathetic injury (Sullivan and Yalla, 1992). The smooth sphincter mechanism seems to be functional. **Some EMG activity may be recorded from the striated sphincter, and the maximal urethral closure pressure is lower than normal but still maintained at the level of the external sphincter zone; however, the normal guarding reflex is absent and there is no voluntary control** (Fam and Yalla, 1988).

Because sphincter tone exists, **urinary incontinence generally does not result** unless there is gross overdistention with overflow. In evolving lesions, every attempt should be made to preserve as low a bladder storage pressure as possible and to avoid any measures that might impair this. **Urinary retention is the rule,** and catheterization is necessary to circumvent this problem. Although virtually all would agree that intermittent catheterization (IC) is an excellent method of management during this period and advocate its use, Lloyd and colleagues (1986) report their own experience and cite that of others, both indicating no differences in outcome when a small-bore Foley catheter or suprapubic tube is used at this stage.

If the distal spinal cord is intact but is simply isolated from higher centers, there is generally a return of detrusor contractility. At first, such reflex activity is poorly sustained and produces only low pressure changes, but the strength and duration of such involuntary contractions increase, producing involuntary voiding, usually with incomplete bladder emptying. This return of reflex bladder activity is generally manifested by involuntary voiding between catheterizations and occurs along with the recovery of lower-extremity deep tendon reflexes. This period generally lasts 6 to 12 weeks in complete suprasacral spinal cord lesions but may last up to a year or two. It may last a shorter period of time in incomplete suprasacral lesions and only a few days in some patients.

Suprasacral Spinal Cord Injury

There is no agreement on the neurobiology of the development of reflex bladder contraction in response to bladder distention after suprasacral SCI. DeGroat and colleagues (1993) list four potential mechanisms for the synaptic reorganization in the cord that results in this reflex bladder activity: (1) elimination of bulbospinal inhibitory pathways (with emergency of vestigial reflex pathways); (2) strengthening of existing synapses or formation of new synaptic connections due to axonal collateral sprouting; (3) changes in synthesis, release, or action of neurotransmitters; and (4) alteration in afferent input from peripheral organs. **The characteristic pattern that results when a patient has a complete lesion above the sacral spinal cord is detrusor hyperreflexia, smooth sphincter synergia (with lesions below the sympathetic outflow), and striated sphincter dyssynergia** (Sullivan and Yalla, 1992; Thomas and O'Flynn, 1994). Neurologic examination shows spasticity of skeletal muscle distal to the lesion, hyperreflexic deep tendon reflexes, and abnormal plantar responses. There is impairment of superficial and deep sensation. Figures 29–1, 29–2, and 29–3 typify the cystourethrographic and urodynamic patterns.

The striated sphincter dyssynergia causes a functional obstruction with poor emptying and high detrusor pressure. Occasionally, incomplete bladder emptying may result from what seems to be a poorly sustained or absent detrusor contraction. This seems to occur more commonly in lesions close to the conus medullaris than with more cephalad lesions. This may result from a second occult lesion or may be due to locally functioning reflex arcs, which result in

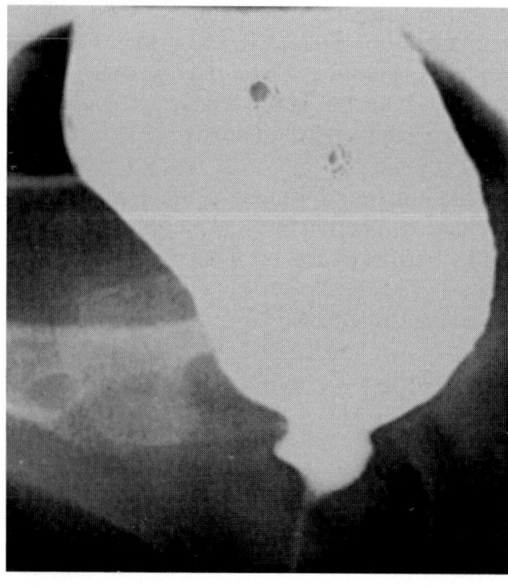

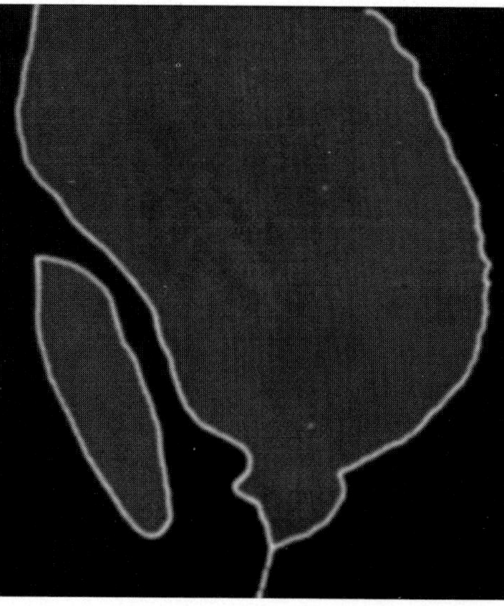

Figure 29–1. Cystourethrogram in a 19-year-old woman with detrusor–striated sphincter dyssynergia secondary to a complete spinal cord injury at vertebral level T11. Image taken during an involuntary bladder contraction with exaggerated bladder neck opening caused by the obstruction below. (From Nordling J, Olesen KP: Basic urographic and cystourethrographic patterns. *In* Pollack HM, ed.: Clinical Urography. Philadelphia, W. B. Saunders Company, 1990, p 1953.)

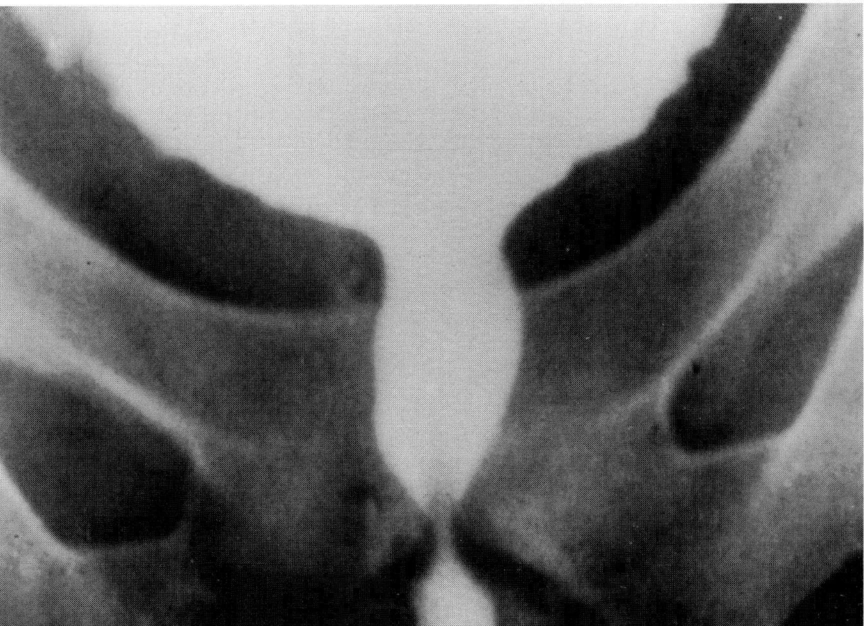

Figure 29–2. Typical cystourethrographic configuration of a synergic smooth sphincter and a dyssynergic striated sphincter in a man during a bladder contraction. (From Nanninga JB: Radiological appearances following surgery for neuromuscular diseases affecting the urinary tract. *In* Pollack HM, ed: Clinical Urography. Philadelphia, W. B. Saunders Company, 1990, p 2003.)

detrusor inhibition from strong striated pelvic floor muscle contraction, or to a loss of higher-center-mediated detrusor facilitation, which normally occurs after the initial increase in pressure during a bladder contraction (Thomas and O'Flynn, 1994). Once reflex voiding is established, it can be initiated or reinforced by the stimulation of certain dermatomes, as by tapping the suprapubic area (see the section on promotion or initiation of reflex contractions, under Treatment). The urodynamic consequences of the striated sphincter dyssynergia vary with severity (complete lesions generally worse than incomplete, continuous contraction during detrusor activity worse than intermittent) and anatomy (male worse than female).

Although treatment is considered fully in the final portion of this chapter, **from a functional standpoint the voiding dysfunction most commonly seen in suprasacral SCI represents both a filling-storage and an emptying failure.** Although the urodynamics are "safe" enough in some patients to allow only periodic stimulation of bladder reflex activity, many require some treatment. If bladder pressures are suitably low or if they can be made suitably low with nonsurgical or surgical management, the problem can be treated primarily as an emptying failure, and CIC can be continued, when practical, as a safe and effective way of satisfying many of the goals of treatment. Alternatively, external sphincterotomy can be used in men to lower the detrusor leak point to an acceptable level, thus treating the dysfunction primarily as one of emptying. The resultant storage failure can be obviated either by timed stimulation or with an external collecting device. In the dextrous SCI patient, the former approach using CIC is becoming predominant. Electric stimulation of the anterior sacral root with some form of deafferentiation is also a reality (see the section on electric stimulation to the nerve roots, under Treatment). As with all patients with neurologic impairment, a careful initial evaluation and periodic follow-up evaluation must be performed in order to identify and correct the following risk factors: bladder overdistention, high-pressure storage, high detrusor leak point pressure, vesicoureteral reflux, stone formation (lower and upper tracts), and complicating infection, especially in association with reflux.

Sacral Spinal Cord Injury

After recovery from spinal shock, there is generally a depression of deep tendon reflexes below the level of the lesion with differing degrees of flaccid paralysis. Sensation is generally absent below the lesion level. **Detrusor areflexia with high or normal compliance is the common initial result, but decreased compliance may develop,** a change seen in some neurologic lesions at or distal to the sacral spinal cord and most likely representing a complex response to neurologic decentralization (McGuire, 1984; Fam and Yalla, 1988). **There is surprisingly little consensus on the evolution of the appearance or function of the bladder neck or smooth sphincter area after sacral spinal cord damage. The classic outlet findings are described as a competent but nonrelaxing smooth sphincter and a striated sphincter that retains some fixed tone but is not under voluntary control.** Closure pressures are decreased in both areas (Sullivan and Yalla, 1992; Thomas and O'Flynn, 1994). However, the late appearance of the bladder neck may be "open" (Kaplan et al, 1991). **Attempted voiding by straining or the Credé maneuver results in "obstruction" at the bladder neck (if closed) or at the distal sphincter area by fixed sphincter tone** (Fam and Yalla, 1988; Thomas and O'Flynn, 1994). Figure 29–4 illustrates the typical cystourographic and urodynamic pictures of the late phases of such a complete lesion. Potential risk factors are those previously described, with particular emphasis on storage pressure, which can result in silent upper tract decompensation and deterioration in the absence of vesicoureteral reflux. The treatment of such a patient is generally directed toward producing or maintaining low-pressure storage while circumventing emptying failure with CIC when possible. Pharmacologic treatment and electric

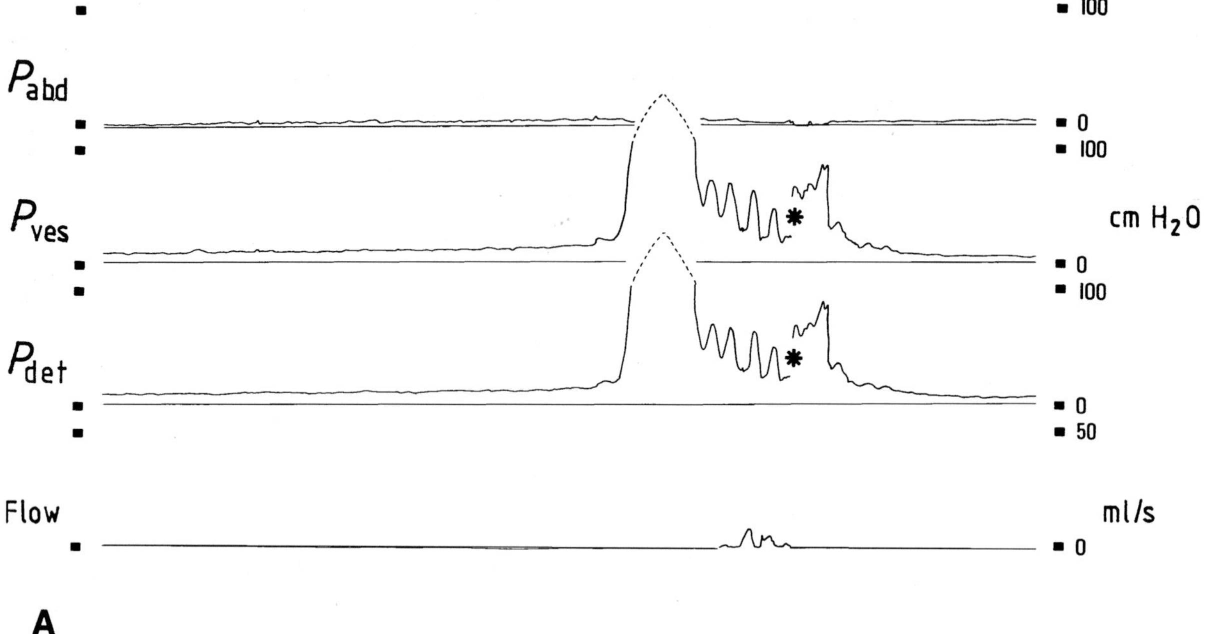

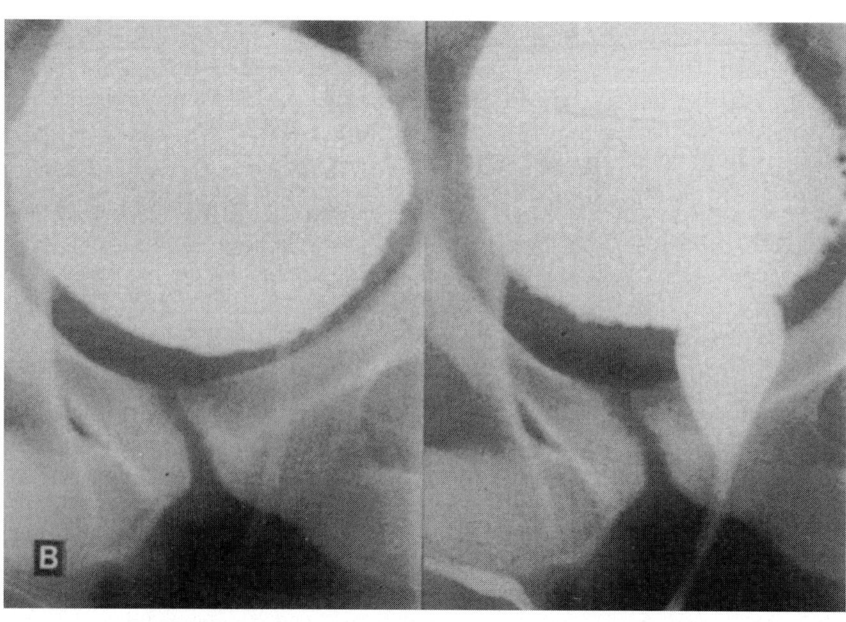

Figure 29–3. *B* shows video images at corresponding points of the urodynamic tracings in *A*. Detrusor hyperreflexia (P_{det} 150 cm H_2O) synergic bladder neck, dyssynergic striated sphincter. The asterisk represents a range change from a scale of 0 to 100 cm H_2O. (From Lawrence WT, Thomas DC: Urodynamic techniques in the neurologic patient. *In* O'Reilly PH, George NJR, Weiss RM, eds: Diagnostic Techniques in Urology. Philadelphia, W. B. Saunders Company, 1990, p 360.)

stimulation may be useful in promoting emptying in certain circumstances (see the section on therapy to facilitate bladder emptying, under Treatment).

Neurologic and Urodynamic Correlation

Although generally correct, the correlation between somatic neurologic findings and urodynamic findings in suprasacral and sacral SCI patients is not exact. A number of factors should be considered in this regard. First, whether a lesion is complete or incomplete is sometimes a matter of definition, and a complete lesion, somatically speaking, may not translate into a complete lesion autonomically, and vice versa. Multiple injuries may actually exist at different levels, even though what is seen somatically may reflect a single level of injury. Even considering these situations, however, all such discrepancies are not explained.

In a classic article, Blaivas (1982) correlated clinical and urodynamic data from 550 patients with voiding dysfunction. In 155 patients with complete and incomplete suprasacral neurologic lesions, physiologically normal voiding was seen in 41%. Detrusor–striated sphincter dyssynergia was demonstrated in 34%, and, surprisingly (and seemingly paradoxically), detrusor areflexia was noted in 25%. Other authors have noted detrusor areflexia with suprasacral SCI or disease, and the causes have been hypothesized as a coexistent distal spinal cord lesion or a disordered integration of afferent activity at the sacral root or cord level (Light et al, 1985; Beric and Light, 1992).

Detrusor–striated sphincter dyssynergia was found in 45% of 119 patients with suprasacral spinal cord lesions. None of 36 patients with supraspinal neurologic lesions had striated sphincter dyssynergia. **These data certainly support prior conclusions that coordinated voiding is regulated by neurologic centers above the spinal cord and that a diagnosis of striated sphincter dyssynergia implies a neurologic lesion that interrupts the neural axis between the pontine-mesencephalic reticular formation and the sacral spinal cord.** All 27 patients with neurologic lesions above the pons who were able to void did so synergistically—with relaxation of the striated sphincter preceding detrusor contraction. Twenty of these patients had detrusor hyperreflexia, but 12 of these 20 had voluntary control of the striated sphincter, **supporting a thesis of separate neural pathways governing voluntary control of the bladder and of the periurethral striated musculature.** Most of these patients with detrusor hyperreflexia secondary to lesions above the pons were able to voluntarily contract the striated sphincter, but without abolishing bladder contraction. This seems to indicate that the inhibition of bladder contraction by pudendal motor activity is not merely simple sacral reflex but, rather, a complex neurologic event. Twenty-two of these patients had evidence of either sacral or infrasacral neurologic impairment of bladder function with suprasacral control of striated sphincter function or vice versa; **this provides**

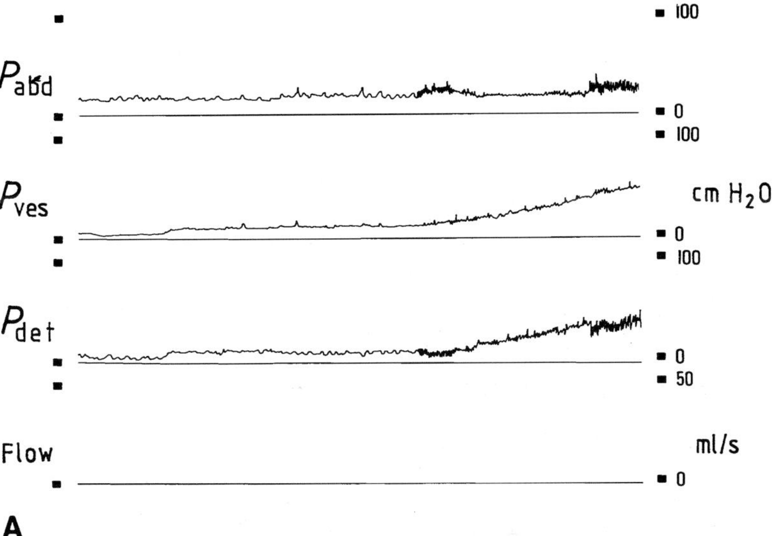

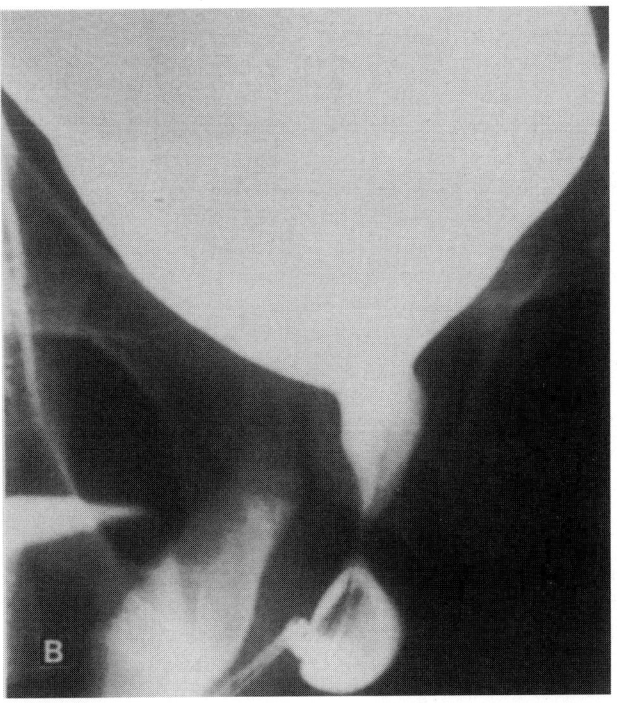

Figure 29–4. Simultaneous video and urodynamic study from a 28-year-old man whose bladder has been filled with 420 ml of contrast material. There is low compliance, the bladder neck is incompetent, and with straining the distal sphincter mechanism does not open—a pattern often seen in sacral spinal cord or efferent nerve root injury or disease. (From Lawrence WT, Thomas DG: Urodynamic techniques in the neurologic patient. *In* O'Reilly PH, George NJR, Weiss RM, eds: Diagnostic Techniques in Urology. Philadelphia, W. B. Saunders Company, 1990, p 362.)

a clinical correlate to the separate anatomic locations of the parasympathetic motor nucleus and the pudendal nucleus in the sacral spinal cord (see Chapter 26).

A subsequent study from the same center analyzed the results of urodynamic evaluation in 489 consecutive patients with either congenital or acquired SCI or disease and correlated these with the diagnosed neurologic deficit (Kaplan et al, 1991). Although there was a general correlation between the neurologic level of injury and expected vesicourethral function, it was neither absolute nor specific. Twenty of 117 cervical lesions exhibited detrusor areflexia; 42 of 156 lumbar lesions, detrusor–striated sphincter dyssynergia; and 26 of 84 sacral lesions, either detrusor hyperreflexia or detrusor–striated sphincter dyssynergia. The patients were further classified on the basis of the integrity of the sacral dermatomes (intact sacral reflexes or not). This helps to explain some, but not all, of the apparent discrepancies. Of the patients with suprasacral cord lesions who had detrusor areflexia, 84% also had abnormal sacral cord signs (absent bulbocavernosus reflex, lax anal sphincter tone, or sphincter EMG abnormalities indicative of lower motor neuron degeneration). All suprasacral cord lesion patients who had no evidence of sacral cord involvement had either detrusor hyperreflexia or detrusor–striated sphincter dyssynergia.

Patients were also classified according to the three most common neurologic causes of their lesion: trauma, myelomeningocele, and spinal stenosis. Of the 284 trauma patients, all with thoracic cord lesions had either detrusor hyperreflexia or detrusor–striated dyssynergia and negative sacral cord signs. In contrast, in patients with traumatic lesions affecting other parts of the spinal cord, there was a wide distribution of both urodynamic and sacral cord sign findings. For example, of patients with traumatic lumbar cord injury, 38% had detrusor areflexia and positive sacral cord signs, 25% had detrusor–striated sphincter dyssynergia and negative sacral cord signs, 25% had detrusor hyperreflexia and negative sacral cord signs, and 14% had either detrusor hyperreflexia or detrusor striated sphincter dyssynergia and negative sacral cord signs. Of 25 patients with lumbar myelomeningocele, 20 had either detrusor areflexia or detrusor–striated sphincter dyssynergia. All patients with lumbar myelomeningocele and detrusor areflexia had positive sacral cord signs. Of 48 patients with sacral myelomeningocele, 37 had detrusor areflexia and 35 had positive sacral cord signs. Of 54 patients with spinal stenosis, all those with cervical and thoracic cord lesions had either detrusor hyperreflexia or detrusor–striated sphincter dyssynergia and negative sacral cord signs. Patients with a lumbar cord stenosis had no consistent pattern of detrusor activity or sacral cord signs. An open bladder neck at rest was found in 21 patients. All had either lumbar or sacral spinal cord injury. Sixteen of these had sacral cord lesions and detrusor areflexia. Decreased bladder compliance was noted in 54 patients, 41 of whom had sacral cord injury and 43 of whom had detrusor areflexia.

These data make the point, as cogently as possible, that **management of the urinary tract in such patients must be based upon urodynamic principles and findings rather than inferences from the neurologic history and evaluation. Similarly, although the information regarding "classic" complete lesions is for the most part valid, one should not make neurologic conclusions solely on the basis of urodynamic findings.**

Autonomic Hyperreflexia

Autonomic hyperreflexia (autonomic dysreflexia) is a potentially fatal emergency unique to the SCI patient. An excellent source of information is the review by Trop and Bennett (1991). **Autonomic hyperreflexia represents an acute massive disordered autonomic (primarily sympathetic) response to specific stimuli in patients with SCI above the level of T6–T8 (the sympathetic outflow).** It is more common in cervical (60%) than in thoracic (20%) injuries. Onset after injury is variable—usually after spinal shock but maybe up to years after injury. Distal cord viability is a prerequisite.

Symptomatically, autonomic hyperreflexia is a syndrome of exaggerated sympathetic activity in response to stimuli below the level of the lesion. **The symptoms are pounding headache, hypertension, and flushing of the face and body above the level of the lesion with sweating. Bradycardia is a usual accompaniment, although tachycardia or arrhythmia may be present. Hypertension may be of varying severity,** from causing a mild headache before the occurrence of voiding to life-threatening cerebral hemorrhage or seizure.

The stimuli for this exaggerated response commonly arise from the bladder or rectum. Precipitation may be due to simple instrumentation, tube change, catheter obstruction, or clot retention and, in such cases, resolves quickly if the stimulus is withdrawn. Other causes or exacerbating factors may include fecal impaction, other gastrointestinal abnormality, long-bone fracture, and pressure sores. **Striated sphincter dyssynergia invariably occurs, and smooth sphincter dyssynergia is generally a part of the syndrome as well, at least in male patients. The pathophysiology is that of a nociceptive stimulation of afferent impulses that ascend through the cord and elicit reflex motor outflow, causing arteriolar, pilomotor, and pelvic visceral spasm, and sweating.** Normally, the reflexes would be inhibited by secondary output from the medulla, but because of the SCI, this does not occur below the lesion level. **Ideally, any endoscopic procedure in susceptible patients should be done with the patient under spinal anesthesia or carefully monitored general anesthesia.** Acutely, the hemodynamic effects of this syndrome may be managed with parenteral ganglionic or alpha-adrenergic blockade or with parenteral chlorpromazine. **Oral nifedipine has been shown to be capable of alleviating this syndrome when given sublingually during cystoscopy (10 to 20 mg) and of preventing it when given orally 30 minutes before cystoscopy (10 mg)** (Dykstra et al, 1987). This presumably prevents smooth muscle contraction through its calcium antagonist properties and thereby prevents the increase in peripheral vascular resistance normally seen with sympathetic stimulation. With a more noxious stimulation, that of electroejaculation, Steinberger and colleagues (1990) recommended oral prophylaxis with 20 mg of nifedipine, finding that this markedly lowered pressure rises during treatment. Chancellor and associates (1994) reported on the use of terazosin (a selective $alpha_1$-blocker) for long-term management (3-month study) and prophylaxis. A nightly dose of 5 mg reduced severity, while erectile function and blood pressure were unchanged. Prophylaxis, however, does not eliminate the need for careful monitoring during provocative procedures. There are patients with severe dysreflexia, intractable to urodynamic correction and oral prophylaxis. For these unfortunate patients, a number of ablative procedures have been utilized—sympathectomy, sacral neurectomy, rhizotomy, cordectomy, and dorsal root ganglionectomy (Trop and Bennett, 1991).

Vesicoureteral Reflux

Surprisingly little is written about vesicoureteral reflux in the SCI patient. The reported incidence varies between 17% and 25% of such patients (Thomas and Lucas, 1990) and is more common in suprasacral SCI. Contributing factors include elevated intravesical pressure during filling and emptying, and infection. Persistent reflux can lead to chronic renal damage and may be an important factor in the long-term survival of SCI patients. In the series of SCI patients reported by Hackler and colleagues (1965), persistent reflux was present in 60% of those dying of renal disease. In patients with only transient reflux over a 5- to 15-year period, the urogram was normal in 83%, or calyceal changes were only minimal.

The best initial treatment for reflux is to normalize lower urinary tract urodynamics as much as possible. If this fails, the question of whether to operate on such patients for correction of the reflux or to correct the reflux while performing another procedure (e.g., augmentation cystoplasty) is not an easy one, because correction of reflux in an often very thickened bladder may not be an easy task. Transureteroureterostomy for unilateral reflux is feasible, but even experienced urologists have had difficulties with ureteral calculi trapping, recurrent reflux, and obstruction at the vesicoureteral junction after such procedures in this difficult group of patients (Van Arsdalen and Hackler, 1983). Submucosal collagen injection may add a new dimension to the treatment of this difficult problem. One must also remember the potential artifact that significant reflux can introduce into urodynamic studies. Measured pressures at given inflow volumes may be less. The apparent significance of detrusor hyperactivity may thus be underestimated.

Spinal Cord Injury in Women

In SCI women, special difficulty is encountered because of the lack of an appropriate external collecting device. Suitable bladder reservoir function can usually be achieved either pharmacologically or surgically, and paraplegic women can generally master CIC. Although a few quadriplegic women can be trained to self-CIC, for the majority there is no practical alternative to indwelling catheterization (Lindan et al, 1987). McGuire and Savastano (1988) point out that indwelling catheter drainage on a long-term basis in women may not be, as is sometimes written, well tolerated, as significant incontinence around the catheter, and upper-tract changes, may develop. This area is discussed further in the section on continuous catheterization, under Treatment. For those SCI female patients who can assume CIC or who have around-the-clock medical or family care, creation of adequate bladder reservoir function is reasonable. For those not in this category, the alternatives are limited and difficult. Overall, however, female patients seem to suffer less morbidity and mortality from the urinary tract in SCI than do male patients of a similar age who have similar neurologic lesions. In particular, women seem to have less of a problem with outlet obstruction and with incontinence (Grainger et al, 1990).

Neurospinal Dysraphism

Neurospinal dysraphism is covered primarily in Chapter 65. However, certain considerations regarding the adult with these abnormalities should be mentioned.

McGuire and Denil (1991) point out that secondary to progress in the overall care of children with myelodysplasia, urologic dysfunction often becomes a problem of the adult with this disease. In their experience, **the typical myelodysplastic patient shows an areflexic bladder with an open bladder neck. The bladder generally fills until the resting residual fixed external sphincter pressure is reached, and then leakage occurs. Stress incontinence occurs also,** related to changes in intra-abdominal pressure. **A small percentage (10% to 15%) of patients demonstrate detrusor–striated sphincter dyssynergia,** but these patients show normal bladder neck function that, if detrusor reflex activity is controlled, is associated with continence. **They note that most myelodysplastic patients experience an improvement in continence after puberty,** but, at that age and after, they are less inclined than children to tolerate any degree of incontinence. In adult patients, the problems encountered in myelodysplastic children still exist but are often compounded by prior surgery, upper tract dysfunction, and one form of urinary diversion or another. In women, the problem generally is to increase urethral sphincter efficiency without causing a major enough increase in urethral closing pressure that will result in a change in bladder compliance. Periurethral injection therapy to achieve continence may replace the pubovaginal sling and artificial sphincter in this circumstance. They point out that continence in myelodysplastic men follows the same general rules as in women, and injectable materials may give good results in this group as well. When the urethra is very widely dilated and somewhat rigid, and neither procedure alone provides sufficient coaptation, it may be possible to combine a "prostatic sling" with periurethral collagen injection. Dry individuals, of course, are on intermittent self-catheterization.

It should be noted that "classic" may imply different urodynamic findings to different groups of clinicians, but nowhere is the failure of a neurologic examination to predict urodynamic behavior more obvious than in patients with myelomeningocele. For instance, Webster and colleagues (1986) have urodynamically classified a large number of myelomeningocele patients as follows: 62% had detrusor hyperreflexia, whereas 38% had detrusor areflexia, 30 of 34 of these having low compliance with high terminal filling pressure. Striated sphincter behavior was characterized as follows: true detrusor–striated sphincter dyssynergia in 15%, an apparently innervated but fixed nonrelaxing sphincter in 15%, and some evidence of striated sphincter denervation in 69%.

Voiding dysfunction secondary to sacral agenesis and dysgenesis may not present in childhood, and such patients may be referred for symptoms as mundane as incontinence or recurrent urinary infection. Jakobsen and co-workers (1985) reported seven such patients ranging in age from 10 to 51 years; delayed diagnosis of such voiding dysfunction was also reported by Yip and colleagues (1985). There is no characteristic abnormality, and the specific dysfunction is dependent on the level and extent of the neurologic injury.

The tethered cord syndrome occurs secondary to adhesions resulting from surgical management of distal spinal cord disorders or as a primary disorder. There is no typical dysfunction, and treatment must be based on contemporary urodynamic evaluation. Voiding dysfunction may not be present until the teenage years or later (Kaplan et al, 1988; Husmann, 1995).

Tabes Dorsalis, Pernicious Anemia

Although **syphilitic myelopathy** is disappearing as a major neurologic problem, involvement of the spinal cord dorsal columns and posterior sacral roots **can result in a loss of bladder sensation and large residual urine volumes and therefore be a cause of "sensory neurogenic bladder"** (see Chapter 27). Although this represents the "classic" tabetic bladder (Wheeler et al, 1986), Hattori and co-authors (1990) reported on some patients with only tabes as an obvious cause of their voiding dysfunction who had low compliance or detrusor hyperreflexia. **Another spinal cord cause of the classic "sensory bladder"** is the now-uncommon **pernicious anemia,** which produced this disorder by virtue of subacute combined degeneration of the dorsolateral columns of the spinal cord.

Poliomyelitis

When seen, voiding dysfunction in polio is that of a typical "motor neurogenic bladder," with urinary retention, detrusor areflexia, and intact sensation. The incidence of voiding dysfunction in patients with polio was reported as 4% to 42% (Bors and Comarr, 1971).

DISEASE DISTAL TO THE SPINAL CORD

Disc Disease and Spinal Stenosis

Disc Disease

Most disc protrusions compress the spinal roots in the L4–L5 or L5–S1 interspaces. Voiding dysfunction may occur as a result, and, when present, generally occurs with the usual clinical manifestations of low back pain radiating in a girdle-like fashion along the involved spinal root areas. Examination may reveal reflex and sensory loss consistent with nerve root compression.

One of the largest series of such patients is that reported by Sandre and associates (1987). After citing literature that recognizes **the incidence of voiding dysfunction in disc prolapse ranging from 1% to 18%,** they reviewed 82 patients with voiding dysfunction and disc prolapse. Their findings are similar to the descriptions seen in most global reviews (Appell, 1993) in that **the most consistent urodynamic finding was that of a normally compliant areflexic bladder associated with normal innervation or incomplete denervation of the perineal floor muscles.** The authors offer two possible hypotheses for the **lower incidence of decreased compliance in root damage secondary to disc prolapse as opposed to myelomeningocele.** The first possibility is that the lesion is primarily sensory; the second is that it simply represents a more incomplete lesion of the preganglionic parasympathetic fibers. Occasionally patients may show detrusor hyperreflexia, attributed to irritation of the nerve roots (O'Flynn et al, 1992).

Patients with voiding dysfunction generally present with difficulty voiding, straining, or urinary retention. It should be noted that **laminectomy may not improve bladder function,** and prelaminectomy urodynamic evaluation is therefore desirable, as it may be difficult postoperatively in these cases to separate causation of voiding dysfunction due to the disc sequelae from changes secondary to the surgery.

Spinal Stenosis

Spinal stenosis is a term applied to any narrowing of the spinal canal, nerve root canals, or intervertebral foramina. It may be congenital, developmental, or acquired. Compression of the nerve roots or cord by such a problem may lead to neuronal damage, ischemia, or edema. Spinal stenosis may occur without disc prolapse. Symptoms may range from those consequent to cervical spinal cord compression to a cauda equina syndrome, with corresponding urodynamic findings (Smith and Woodside, 1988). Back pain and lower extremity pain, cramping, and paresthesias related to exercise and relieved by rest are the classic symptoms of lumbar stenosis due to lumbar spondylosis and are believed to result from sacral nerve root ischemia. The urodynamic findings are dependent on the level and the amount of spinal cord or nerve root damage. Deen and colleagues (1994) reported subjective improvement in over 50% of such patients with bladder dysfunction who were treated by decompressive laminectomy. In cervical spondylitic spinal stenosis, detrusor hyperactivity or underactivity may occur, depending on whether the primary abnormality affecting the micturition neural axis is compression of the inhibitory reticulospinal tracts or myelopathy in the posterior funiculus, which carries proprioceptive sensation (Tammela et al, 1992). **Because there is no consistent pattern of dysfunction with any type of spinal stenosis, urodynamic studies again are the cornerstone of rational therapy.**

Radical Pelvic Surgery

Voiding dysfunction after pelvic plexus injury occurs most commonly after abdominoperineal resection and radical hysterectomy. **Lower urinary tract dysfunction after these procedures is reported in 10% to 60% of patients, and in 15% to 20% voiding dysfunction is permanent** (McGuire, 1984; Mundy, 1984). The injury may occur consequent to denervation or defunctionalization; tethering of the nerves or encasement in scar; direct bladder or urethral trauma; or bladder devascularization. Adjuvant treatment, such as chemotherapy or radiation, may play a role as well. The type of voiding dysfunction that occurs is dependent on the specific nerves involved, the degree of injury, and any pattern of reinnervation or altered innervation that results over time (see Chapter 26).

There is an abundant literature on the effects of parasympathetic decentralization on neuromorphology and neuropharmacology of the lower urinary tract in many animal models (see Wein and Barrett, 1988). Parasympathetic decentralization has been reported to lead to a marked increase in adrenergic innervation of the bladder in some experimental models, with the resultant conversion of the usual beta (relaxant) response of the bladder body in response to sympathetic stimulation to an alpha (contractile) effect (Sundin et al, 1977). Hanno and co-workers (1988) confirmed that, in the cat model, parasympathetic decentralization does result in adrenergic hyperinnervation of the detrusor, but that pelvic plexus neurectomy alone or parasympathetic decentralization plus hypogastric neurectomy yields no detectable increase in adrenergic innervation. In their experimental model, decentralization did result in synaptic reorganization in bladder wall ganglia with new cholinergic excitatory inputs from the hypogastric nerves. Koyanagi was the first to call attention to what he termed supersensitivity of the urethra to alpha-adrenergic stimulation in a similar group of patients with neurologic decentralization of the lower urinary tract, implying a similar change in adrenergic receptor function in the urethra after parasympathetic decentralization (Koyanagi et al, 1988). Nordling and co-authors (1981) described a similar change in women after radical hysterectomy and ascribed this change to damage to the sympathetic innervation of the lower urinary tract.

When permanent voiding dysfunction occurs after radical pelvic surgery, the pattern is generally one of a failure of voluntary bladder contraction, or impaired bladder contractility, with obstruction by what seems urodynamically to be residual fixed striated sphincter tone, which is not subject to voluntarily induced relaxation. Often, the smooth sphincter area is open and nonfunctional. Whether this is due to parasympathetic damage or terminal sympathetic damage or whether it results from the hydrodynamic effects of obstruction at the level of the striated sphincter is debated and unknown. **Decreased compliance is common in these patients, and this, with the "obstruction" caused by fixed residual striated sphincter tone, results in both storage and emptying failure.** These patients often experience leaking across the distal sphincter area and, in addition, are unable to empty the bladder, because although intravesical pressure may be increased, there is nothing that approximates a true bladder contraction. The patient often presents with urinary incontinence that is characteristically most manifest with increases in intra-abdominal pressure. This is usually most obvious in female patients, as the prostatic bulk in male patients often masks an equivalent deficit in urethral closure function. Alternatively, patients may present with variable degrees of urinary retention.

Urodynamic studies may show decreased compliance, poor proximal urethral closure function, loss of voluntary control of the striated sphincter, and a positive bethanechol supersensitivity test, that is, findings similar to those in Figure 29–4. **Upper-tract risk factors are related to intravesical pressure and the detrusor leak point pressure, and the therapeutic goal is always low-pressure storage with periodic emptying. The temptation to perform a prostatectomy should be avoided unless a clear demonstration of outlet obstruction at this level is possible.** Otherwise, prostatectomy simply decreases urethral sphincter function and thereby may result in the occurrence or worsening of sphincteric urinary incontinence. **Many of these dysfunctions are transient,** and the temptation to "do something" other than perform CIC early after surgery in these patients, especially in those with little or no preexistent history of voiding dysfunction, cannot be too strongly criticized. Our general practice in such patients is to discharge them on CIC and then have them return for a full urodynamic evaluation at a later date. Many of the changes after radical pelvic surgery are similar to those seen in sacral cord injury or disease. Sislow and Mayo (1990), in an excellent study on decreased bladder compliance after decentralization, noted a higher prevalence of this finding in patients who had undergone radical pelvic surgery than in those who had sustained conus–cauda equina injury.

Finally, it is certainly possible that at least some types of nonradical pelvic surgery, such as simple hysterectomy, are ultimately responsible for filling-storage or emptying abnormalities on the basis of neurologic damage (Parys et al, 1989). As the frequency of sophisticated preoperative and postoperative urodynamic evaluation in such patients increases, we can certainly expect to see more about this subject in the literature.

Herpes Zoster

Invasion of the sacral dorsal root ganglia and posterior nerve roots with herpes zoster virus **may produce urinary retention and detrusor areflexia days to weeks after the other primary viral manifestations** (Ryttov et al, 1985). Generally, painful cutaneous eruptions secondary to the virus are also present, but initially there may be just fever and malaise with perineal and thigh paresthesias and obstipation. Urinary incontinence secondary to detrusor hyperreflexia may also occur, but the pathophysiology is uncertain, unless related to nerve root irritation (Broseta et al, 1993). Cystoscopy may reveal vesicles in the bladder mucosa similar to those seen on the skin. Spontaneous resolution generally occurs in 1 to 2 months.

Diabetes Mellitus

Diabetes is the most common cause of peripheral neuropathy in Europe and North America. The clinical spectrum of associated voiding dysfunction has been well reviewed by Kaplan and Blaivas (1988), Kaplan and Te (1992), and Beck and colleagues (1994). Acute hyperglycemia decreases nerve function. Chronic hyperglycemia is associated with the loss of myelinated and unmyelinated fibers, wallerian degeneration, and blunted nerve fiber reproduction (Clark and Lee, 1995). The proposed mechanisms include (1) increased accumulation of polyols (sorbitol) from glucose through the aldose reductase pathway, ultimately resulting in decreased activity of Na-K-ATPase and (2) the formation of advanced glycosylation end products from glucose.

Neuropathy tends to develop in middle-aged and elderly patients with long-standing or poorly controlled diabetes. The exact incidence of voiding dysfunction is uncertain, as unselected patients generally do not complain of bladder symptoms. **If specifically questioned, anywhere from 5% to 50% report symptoms of voiding dysfunction.** In studies on selected diabetic patients, up to a third have urodynamically abnormal bladder function (Beck et al, 1994). Frimodt-Moller (1976) coined the term *diabetic cystopathy* to describe the involvement of the lower urinary tract by this disease. **The classic description of the neuropathy and its lower urinary tract effects is of a primarily sensory neuropathy,** which first causes the insidious onset of impaired bladder sensation. A gradual increase in the time interval between voiding results and may progress to the point at which the patient voids only once or twice a day without ever sensing any real urgency. If this continues, detrusor distention and decompensation ultimately occur. Detrusor contractility, therefore, is diminished on this basis. **Current evidence points to a sensory and motor neuropathy** as being involved in the pathogenesis, the motor aspect per se contributing to impaired detrusor contractility.

The typical urodynamic findings include impaired bladder sensation, increased cystometric capacity, decreased bladder contractility, impaired uroflow, and, later, increased residual urine. The main differential diagnosis is generally bladder outlet obstruction, as both conditions commonly produce a low flow rate. However, the flow pattern in diabetes is more commonly one of abdominal straining, and, of course, pressure-flow studies easily differentiate the two. Involuntary bladder contractions may also be seen. If due to diabetes and not to coincident abnormality (bladder outlet obstruction, detrusor instability), the cause must be neuropathic change outside the bladder. Smooth or striated sphincter dyssynergia generally are not seen in diabetic cystopathy but can easily be misdiagnosed on a poor or incomplete urodynamic study—abdominal straining alone will not open the bladder neck and produces pseudodyssynergia.

Early institution of timed voiding avoids the portion of the impaired detrusor contractility due to chronic distention and decompensation. Experimental studies are currently directed at inhibiting the proposed mechanisms by which hyperglycemia produces neuropathy (Clark and Lee, 1995). Pharmacologic or surgical treatment of late diabetic cystopathy is rarely successful (see treatment section), and CIC remains the best option.

Guillain-Barré Syndrome

Guillain-Barré syndrome is an inflammatory demyelinating disorder of the peripheral nervous system that may be life-threatening. It results from aberrant immune responses directed against peripheral nerve components (Hartung et al, 1995). Clinically it presents as an idiopathic polyradiculopathy, frequently after an infection or vaccination. Motor paralysis occurs first in the lower extremities and progresses cephalad. Autonomic neuropathy is a common complication. Cardiac arrhythmia, hyper- and hypotension, and bowel and sexual dysfunction may occur. Urinary retention occurred in 11% to 30% of those in the multiple series reviewed by Zochodne (1994). The urinary involvement is managed best by CIC while waiting and hoping for resolution.

OTHER RELATED CONDITIONS

Bladder Neck Dysfunction

Also called *smooth sphincter dyssynergia* and *proximal urethral obstruction,* bladder neck dysfunction is characterized by an incomplete opening of the bladder neck during voiding. Although cases were first described over a century ago, the condition was first fully characterized by Turner-Warwick and colleagues in 1973. **The dysfunction is found almost exclusively in young and middle-aged men, and characteristically they complain of long-standing obstructive and irritative symptoms** (Webster et al, 1980; Norlen and Blaivas, 1986; Wein and Barrett, 1988). These patients have often been seen by many urologists and have been diagnosed as having psychogenic voiding dysfunction because of a normal prostate on rectal examination, a negligible residual urine volume, and a normal endoscopic bladder appearance. The differential diagnosis concludes anatomic bladder neck contracture, benign prostatic hyperplasia (BPH), dysfunctional voiding (see below), prostatitis or prostatosis, neurogenic dysfunction, and low pressure and low flow (see below). **Objective evidence of outlet obstruction in these patients is easily obtainable by urodynamic study. Once obstruction is diagnosed, it can be localized at the level of the bladder neck** by videourodynamic study, cystourethrography during a bladder contraction, or micturitional urethral profilometry (see Chapter 28). **The diagnosis may also be made indirectly by the urodynamic findings of outlet obstruction in the typical clinical situation in the absence of urethral stricture, prostatic enlargement, or striated sphincter dyssynergia. Secondary detrusor instability is common;** Noble and colleagues (1994) cite the incidence as 50%.

The exact cause of this problem is unknown. Some have proposed that there is an abnormal arrangement of musculature in the bladder neck region so that coordinated detrusor contractions cause bladder neck narrowing instead of the normal funneling (Bates et al, 1975). The occurrence of this problem in young, anxious, and high-strung individuals and its partial relief by alpha-adrenergic blocking agents have prompted some to speculate that it may in some way be related to sympathetic hyperactivity. When prostatic enlargement develops in persons with this problem, a double obstruction results, and Turner-Warwick (1984) has applied the term *trapped prostate* to this entity. The lobes of the prostate cannot expand the bladder neck and therefore expand into the urethra. A patient so affected generally has a lifelong history of voiding dysfunction that has gone relatively unnoticed because he has always accepted this as normal, and exacerbation of these symptoms occurs during a relatively short and early period of prostatic enlargement. Although alpha-adrenergic blocking agents provide improvement in some patients with bladder neck dysfunction, definitive relief in the male patient is best achieved by bladder neck incision (see the section on treatment). In patients with this and a trapped prostate, marked relief is generally effected by a "small" prostatic resection or ablation that includes the bladder neck. Such patients often note afterward that they have "never" voided as well as after their treatment.

Similar bladder neck obstruction in female patients is quite rare. Diokno and co-workers (1984) clearly defined this entity in a small number of patients on the basis of video-urodynamic criteria. Even then, surgical treatment of this problem should be approached with caution, as sphincteric incontinence is a significant risk.

Low Pressure–Low Flow

Low-pressure–low-flow voiding occurs in younger men and is symptomatically characterized by frequency, hesitancy, and a poor stream. This entity is demonstrated on urodynamic assessment and with no endoscopic abnormalities. The patient generally notes marked hesitancy when attempting to initiate micturition in the presence of others, and some have therefore described this group as having an "anxious bladder." The estimate of the incidence of this problem in younger male patients referred for urodynamic assessment varies between 6% (Barnes et al, 1985) and 19% (George and Slade, 1979). My experience has been similar to those reports stating that **neither empirical pharmacologic treatment nor transurethral surgery has any consistent beneficial effect in this difficult group of patients.** Barnes and others (1985) suggested that these men are psychologically unusual, but in the direction of being obsessional rather than anxious. They suggest that these individuals have a lifelong tendency to overcontrol the process of micturition and are thus vulnerable to lower urinary tract symptoms under stress, and the authors recommend that a behavior modification program be considered.

Adult Enuresis

Monosynaptic nocturnal enuresis is a common disorder of childhood that occurs in approximately 20% of 4-year-olds, with an approximately 15% spontaneous cure rate annually (see Chapter 66). Epidemiologic studies in adults report a prevalence of 1% to 3% in 20-year-olds (Rittig et al, 1989). The pathophysiology is the same and seems to be associated with a lack of diurnal rhythmicity of plasma vasopressin, a phenomenon whose cause is not understood. This explains the beneficial effects of treatment with desmopressin in both children and adults with enuresis. This subject is more extensively considered in Chapter 41.

Non-Neurogenic–Neurogenic Bladder

The non-neurogenic–neurogenic bladder is likewise considered in Chapter 66 but is mentioned here because persons with a history of unexplained lower urinary tract dysfunction symptoms may not present to the urologist or be definitively diagnosed with this entity until adulthood. This syndrome, usually known as **dysfunctional voiding, or Hinman's syndrome, presents the unusual circumstance of what appears urodynamically to be involuntary obstruction at the striated sphincter level existing in the absence of demonstrable neurologic disease** (Hinman, 1986). It is very difficult to prove urodynamically that a person has this entity, and it should further be noted that the diagnoses in most of the patients reported have been made on the basis of only history, isolated flowmetry, isolated measurements of total intravesical pressure, and pelvic floor EMG activity (see Wein and Barrett, 1988). **Unequivocal demonstration** of this entity, in my opinion, **requires simultaneous pressure-flow-EMG evidence that bladder emptying occurs simultaneously with involuntary striated sphincter contraction in the absence of any element of abdominal straining,** either in an attempt to augment bladder contraction or as a response to discomfort during urination. Such reports do exist and confirm the existence of this syndrome. The cause is uncertain and may represent a persistent transitional phase in the development of micturitional control or persistence of a reaction phase to the stimulus of lower urinary tract discomfort during voiding, long after the initial program that caused this has disappeared (Jorgensen et al, 1982).

Retention in Women

Retention in women is an unusual entity whose potential causes are classically listed as neurologic, pharmacologic, anatomic, myopathic, and psychogenic. Noble and colleagues (1994) describe the evolution of a hypothesis regarding another organic cause—an isolated disorder of the striated sphincter, impairing its ability to relax. This sphincter dysfunction may result in detrusor areflexia or hyperactivity. Unfortunately, attempts to modify this primary sphincter abnormality and thereby break the retention cycle have not been successful. Treatment therefore reverts to the usual menu for emptying failure.

Postoperative Retention

Postoperative urinary retention is a well-recognized but poorly understood event. Its incidence is generally quoted overall as 4% to 25%. It occurs more frequently after lower urinary tract, perineal, gynecologic, and anorectal surgery. In the placebo arms of four trials of alpha-adrenergic blocker prophylaxis after these types of surgery, the incidence of postoperative retention ranged from 18.8% to 57% (Velanovich, 1992).

Contributing factors, which are not mutually exclusive, include

1. Traumatic instrumentation
2. Bladder overdistention
3. Diminished awareness of bladder sensation
4. Decreased bladder contractility
5. Increased outlet resistance
6. Decreased micturition reflex activity
7. Nociceptive inhibitory reflex
8. Pre-existent outlet pathology (BPH, for example)

Anesthesia and analgesia can contribute to factors 2, 3, 4, and 6. The idea of a nociceptive inhibitory reflex, initiated by pain or discomfort, is an attractive one, as a sympathetic efferent limb could directly affect factors 4, 5, and 6 (see Chapter 26).

Bladder decompression for 18 to 24 hours postoperatively decreased the incidence of retention in patients undergoing joint replacement surgery by 52% versus 27% (Michelson et al, 1988) and 65% versus 0% (Carpiniello et al, 1988), compared with intermittent catheterization. The incidence of urinary infection with continuous catheterization was no different in the study by Michelson and colleagues (15% versus 11%) and was less in the study by Carpiniello and associates (16% versus 43%), in which straight catheterization was carried out in the recovery room as well.

Alpha-adrenergic blockade seems effective prophylactically in decreasing the incidence of postoperative retention. Velanovich (1992) performed a meta-analysis on the use of phenoxybenzamine (POB) (only randomized placebo-controlled studies) and concluded that this agent reduced the occurrence by 29.1%. In a retrospective review of colorectal patients treated with and without POB, Goldman and colleagues (1988) found a 54.7% incidence of retention in patients not given POB versus a 19.2% incidence in those who were. The regimen for those not catheterized preoperatively was 10 mg orally the evening before and 1 hour before surgery, 2 hours after surgery, and 10 mg twice daily for 3 days. For those who were catheterized before the procedure, the regimen was 10 mg twice daily, initiated the day before catheter removal. The mechanism of action is uncertain. If an inhibitory nociceptive reflex is initiated, and this is similar to the sympathetic reflex elicited by bladder filling (see Chapter 26), the mechanism is multifactorial. Alternatively, the drug may act only on the outlet to decrease resistance (see treatment section), which may be pathologically increased by anxiety, pain, and other factors related to surgery. Whether other alpha blockers are as effective is uncertain. Cataldo and Senagore (1991) found that prazosin (Minipress; see the section on decreasing outlet resistance at the level of the smooth sphincter, under Treatment) in a dose of 1 mg on arrival to the surgical unit and every 12 hours thereafter for a total of four doses, was ineffective in patients undergoing anorectal surgery (40% retention versus 50% in a placebo group). Peterson and associates (1991), however, reported a positive effect with the same drug in a randomized but not placebo-controlled study in patients undergoing joint replacement surgery. The dose used was 2 mg before the procedure and every 12 hours throughout hospitalization. For those who also had an intraoperative catheter placed, the retention rates were 7% (drug) versus 75% (no drug). For those without intraoperative catheterization, the differences were less marked (36% versus 54%). Whether the differences in reported results between POB and prazosin are meaningful or not is uncertain. POB inhibits both alpha-1 and alpha-2 receptors (see Chapter 26), while prazosin is a relatively selective alpha-1 blocker. The doses of prazosin used do not seem as pharmacologic as those of POB. Any effect of the newer alpha-1 antagonists (terazosin, doxazosin) is as yet unknown.

Myasthenia Gravis

Any neuromuscular disease that affects the tone of the smooth or striated muscle of the distal sphincter mechanism can predispose a patient to a greater chance of urinary incontinence after even a well-performed transurethral or open prostatectomy. Myasthenia gravis is an autoimmune

Table 29–2. THERAPY TO FACILITATE BLADDER FILLING AND URINE STORAGE

Inhibiting Bladder Contractility, Decreasing Sensory Input, and/or Increasing Bladder Capacity	Increasing Outlet Resistance
Behavioral Therapy	***Physiotherapy and Biofeedback***
Timed bladder emptying	***Electric Stimulation***
Bladder training; biofeedback	***Pharmacologic Therapy***
Pharmacologic Therapy	Alpha-adrenergic agonists
Anticholinergic agents	Tricyclic antidepressants
Musculotropic relaxants	Beta-adrenergic antagonists, agonists
Calcium antagonists	Estrogens
Potassium channel openers	***Vesicourethral Suspension (Stress Urinary Incontinence)***
Prostaglandin inhibitors	***Nonsurgical Mechanical Compression***
Beta-adrenergic agonists	Periurethral polytef injection
Alpha-adrenergic antagonists	Periurethral collagen injection
Tricyclic antidepressants	Occlusive and supportive devices; urethral plugs
Dimethyl sulfoxide (DMSO)	***Surgical Mechanical Compression***
Polysynaptic inhibitors	Sling procedures
Therapy decreasing sensory input	Closure of the bladder outlet
Bladder Overdistention	Artificial urinary sphincter
Electric Stimulation (Reflex Inhibition)	***Bladder Outlet Reconstruction***
Acupuncture	**Circumventing the Problem**
Interruption of Innervation	Antidiuretic hormone–like agents
Central (subarachnoid block)	Diuretics
Sacral rhizotomy, selective sacral rhizotomy	Intermittent catheterization
Perivesical (peripheral bladder denervation)	Continuous catheterization
Augmentation Cystoplasty	Urinary diversion
	External collecting devices
	Absorbent products

Table 29–3. THERAPY TO FACILITATE BLADDER EMPTYING

Increasing Intravesical Pressure and/or Bladder Contractility
- ***External Compression, Valsalva Maneuver***
- ***Promotion or Initiation of Reflex Contractions***
  - Trigger zones or maneuvers
  - Bladder training, tidal drainage
- ***Pharmacologic Therapy***
  - Parasympathomimetic agents
  - Prostaglandins
  - Blockers of inhibition
    - Alpha-adrenergic antagonists
    - Opioid antagonists
- ***Reduction Cystoplasty***
- ***Electric Stimulation***
  - Directly to the bladder or spinal cord
  - To the nerve roots
  - Transurethral intravesical electrotherapy

Decreasing Outlet Resistance
- ***At a Site of Anatomic Obstruction***
  - *At the Level of the Prostate*
    - Pharmacologic
      - Decrease prostatic size
      - Decrease prostatic tone
    - Balloon dilatation
    - Intraurethral stent
  - *Urethral Stricture Repair or Dilatation*
- ***At the Level of the Smooth Sphincter***
  - Pharmacologic therapy
  - Transurethral resection or incision of the bladder neck
  - Y-V-plasty of the bladder neck
    - Alpha-adrenergic antagonists
    - Beta-adrenergic agonists
- ***At the Level of the Striated Sphincter***
  - *Biofeedback and Psychotherapy*
  - *Pharmacologic Therapy*
    - Skeletal muscle relaxants
      - Benzodiazepines
      - Baclofen
      - Dantrolene
  - *Surgical Sphincterotomy, Botulinum A Toxin*
  - *Urethral Overdilation*
  - *Urethral Stent*
  - *Pudendal Nerve Interruption*
- ***Alpha-Adrenergic Antagonists***

Circumventing the Problem
- Intermittent catheterization
- Continuous catheterization
- Urinary diversion

disease caused by autoantibodies to acetylcholine (ACh) nicotinic receptors. This leads to neuromuscular blockade and hence weakness in a variety of striated muscle groups. The incidence of incontinence after prostatectomy is indeed greatly increased in patients with this disease (Greene et al, 1974; Khan and Bhola, 1989).

TREATMENT OF NEUROMUSCULAR VOIDING DYSFUNCTION

This portion of the chapter considers the various therapies available for the treatment of voiding dysfunction. Only a discrete number of such therapies are available, and these are easily categorized on a functional "menu" basis according to whether they are used primarily to facilitate urine storage or emptying and according to whether their primary effect is on the bladder or on the outlet (Tables 29–2, 29–3). This basic outline is followed in this chapter.

Table 29–4. VOIDING DYSFUNCTION: GOALS OF MANAGEMENT

- Upper urinary tract preservation or improvement
- Absence or control of infection
- Adequate storage at low intravesical pressure
- Adequate emptying at low intravesical pressure
- Adequate control
- No catheter or stoma
- Social acceptability and adaptability
- Vocational acceptability and adaptability

The initial choice of a nonsurgical versus a surgical mode of management for a given problem is multifactorial. Although many urologists who lecture and write about the management of voiding dysfunction are associated primarily with one approach or another, all would doubtless agree on certain goals of management for voiding dysfunction (Table 29–4). As a corollary, absolute or relative indications for changing or augmenting a particular regimen exist, and, likewise, there is general agreement on these, although the relative importance of the indication for change might be disputed (Table 29–5). It should be remembered that the term *inadequate,* when applied to storage or emptying, implies not only completeness in terms of residual urine volume but also unacceptably high detrusor pressures.

In the planning of goals of therapy and reasons for change, the concept of a "hostility score," such as that of Galloway (1989), is attractive. This "hostility score" consists of five urodynamic characteristics—bladder compliance, hyperreflexia, dyssynergia, outlet resistance, and vesicoureteral reflux. Each is allocated a score of 0, 1, or 2. The best possible score is zero and implies normal compliance, no inappropriate detrusor activity, a synergic sphincter, a low leak pressure, and no reflux.

The results of treatment of voiding dysfunction are rarely perfect, and a very flexible approach must be adopted in choosing therapy. This approach must take into account the individual wishes of each patient and the family, and the practicality of each proposed solution for that particular patient (Table 29–6). Therapeutic decisions are thus made with the patient and with the family. In every case, within the limits of practicality, alternative methods of management, including reversibility and side effects that occur with some

Table 29–5. REASONS TO CHANGE OR AUGMENT A GIVEN REGIMEN

- Upper urinary tract deterioration
- Recurrent sepsis or fever of urinary tract origin
- Lower urinary tract deterioration
- Inadequate storage
- Inadequate emptying
- Inadequate control
- Unacceptable side effects
- Skin changes secondary to incontinence or collecting device

Table 29–6. PATIENT FACTORS TO CONSIDER IN CHOOSING THERAPY

Prognosis of underlying disease, especially if progressive or malignant
Limiting factors: inability to perform certain tasks (hand dexterity, ability to transfer)
Mental status
Motivation
Desire to remain catheter- or appliance-free
Desire to avoid surgery
Sexual activity status
Reliability
Educability
Psychosocial environment, interest, reliability, and cooperation of family
Economic resources
Age

regularity, the ultimate best and worst possible scenario, and frequency and extent of follow-up, should be discussed. **It has always been our subjective bias that the simplest, least destructive, and most reversible form of therapy that has a chance of satisfying the goals of treatment should be tried first.** A combination of therapeutic maneuvers, drugs, and surgery can sometimes be used to achieve a particular end, especially if these modalities act through different mechanisms and their side effects are not synergistic. There are circumstances and locales in which hospital resources and bed usage efficiency must also be considered, especially in this day and age when some health care systems and third-party payers have placed considerable financial restraints on health care.

THERAPY TO FACILITATE BLADDER FILLING AND/OR URINE STORAGE

(see Table 29–2)

Inhibiting Bladder Contractility, Decreasing Sensory Input, and/or Increasing Bladder Capacity

Behavioral Therapy

TIMED BLADDER EMPTYING

Although timed bladder emptying is not a sophisticated concept, like many used, it seems to work quite well in certain circumstances. The idea is to completely or partially empty the bladder on a frequent enough schedule so as to keep the intravesical pressure and volume below that at which storage failure results. This may involve only more frequent voiding with more limited fluid intake in a patient with detrusor hyperactivity, or it may involve CIC. Pharmacologic therapy to inhibit bladder contractility should always include timed bladder emptying.

BLADDER TRAINING; BIOFEEDBACK

Bladder training or retraining includes a regimen of detailed instruction about lower-tract function and control, coupled with a program to increase the interval between voidings. This may involve inhibition of phasic detrusor hyperactivity by pelvic floor muscle contraction, for which electromyographic and/or cystometric biofeedback may be useful. Mostly used for treatment of non-neurogenic frequency and urgency or urge incontinence, with or without detrusor instability, this is covered in more detail in Chapter 30.

Pharmacologic Therapy

ANTICHOLINERGIC AGENTS: GENERAL DISCUSSION

The major portion of the neurohumoral stimulus for physiologic bladder contraction is ACh-induced stimulation of postganglionic parasympathetic muscarinic cholinergic receptor sites on bladder smooth muscle (Chapter 26). **Atropine and atropine-like agents therefore depress normal bladder contractions and involuntary bladder contractions (IBC) of any cause** (Andersson 1988, 1993). In such patients **the volume to the first IBC is generally increased, the amplitude of the IBC decreased, and the capacity increased** (Jensen, 1981a). However, although the volume and pressure thresholds at which IBC is elicited may increase, **the "warning time"** (the time between the perception of an IBC about to occur and its occurrence) **and the ability to suppress are not increased. Thus, urgency and incontinence still occur unless such therapy is combined with a regimen of timed voiding or toileting.** Bladder compliance in normal persons and in those with detrusor hyperreflexia in whom the initial slope of the filling curve on cystometry is normal before the involuntary contraction, does not seem to be significantly altered. The effect of pure antimuscarinics in those patients who exhibit only decreased compliance has not been well studied. Outlet resistance, at least as reflected by urethral pressure measurements, does not seem to be clinically affected.

Although the antimuscarinic agents usually produce significant clinical improvement in patients with involuntary bladder contractions and associated symptoms, generally only partial inhibition results. In many animal models, atropine only partially antagonizes the response of the whole bladder to pelvic nerve stimulation and of bladder strips to field stimulation, although it does completely inhibit the response of bladder smooth muscle to exogenous cholinergic stimulation. Of the theories proposed to explain this phenomenon, which is called *atropine resistance,* the most attractive and most commonly cited is that a major portion of the neurotransmission involved in the final common pathway of bladder contraction is secondary to release of a transmitter other than ACh or norepinephrine (see Andersson, 1993; Chapter 26). Although the existence of atropine resistance in human bladder muscle is by no means agreed on, this concept is the most common hypothesis invoked to explain the clinical difficulty in establishing IBC with anticholinergic agents alone, and it is also invoked to support the rationale of treatment of such types of bladder activity with agents that have different mechanisms of action.

ANTICHOLINERGIC AGENTS: SPECIFIC DRUGS

Propantheline bromide (Pro-Banthīne, others) is the classically described oral agent for producing an antimuscarinic effect in the lower urinary tract. The usual adult oral dosage is 15 to 30 mg every 4 to 6 hours, although higher doses are often necessary. Propantheline is a quarternary ammonium compound, all of which are poorly absorbed after oral administration (Brown, 1990). **There seems to be little difference between the antimuscarinic effects of propantheline on bladder smooth muscle and those of other antimuscarinic agents** such as glycopyrrolate (Robinul), isopropamide (Darbid), anisotropine methylbromide (Valpin), methscopolamine (Pamine), homatropine, and others. Some of these agents, such as glycopyrrolate, have a more convenient dosage schedule (two to three times daily), but their clinical effects on the lower urinary tract seem to be indistinguishable. Although there are obviously many other considerations to account for the activity of a given dose of drug at its site of action, there is no oral drug available whose direct in vitro antimuscarinic binding potential approximates that of atropine better than the long-available and relatively inexpensive propantheline bromide (Levin et al, 1982; Peterson et al, 1990). There is a surprising lack of evaluable data on the effectiveness of propantheline for the treatment of bladder hyperactivity. As Andersson (1988) points out, there are reports of both great and poor efficacy of anticholinergic drugs for this indication. The Agency for Health Care Policy and Research (AHCPR) clinical practice guidelines (Urinary Incontinence Guideline Panel, 1992) lists five randomized controlled trials reviewed for propantheline, with 82% female patients. The percentage of cures (all figures refer to the percentage effect on the drug **minus** the percentage effect on placebo) are listed as 0% to 5%, reduction in urge incontinence as 0% to 53%, and the percentage of side effects and percentage of dropouts as 0% to 50% and 0% to 9% respectively.

Hyoscyamine (Cystospaz) **and hyoscyamine sulfate** (Levsin, Levsinex, Cystospaz-M) are reported to have about the same general anticholinergic actions and side effects as the other belladonna alkaloids. Hyoscyamine sulfate is available as a sublingual formulation (Levsin/SL)—a theoretical advantage—but controlled studies of its effects on bladder hyperactivity are lacking. **Glycopyrrolate** (Robinul) is a synthetic quarternary ammonium compound that is a potent inhibitor of both M_1 and M_2 receptors (see Chapter 26 for discussion of receptor subtypes), but with a preference for the M_2 subtype (Lau and Szilagyi, 1992). It is available as both an oral and a parenteral preparation; the latter is commonly used as an antisialagogue during anesthesia.

It would seem that an anticholinergic agent with a significant blocking action at ganglia as well as at the peripheral receptor level might be more effective in suppressing bladder contractility. Although **methantheline** (Banthīne) has a higher ratio of ganglionic blocking to antimuscarinic activity than does propantheline, the latter drug seems to be at least as potent in each respect, clinical dose for dose (Wein and Barrett, 1988). Methantheline does have similar effects on the lower urinary tract, and some clinicians still prefer it over other anticholinergic agents. Few real data are available regarding its efficacy.

A lack of selectivity is a major problem with all antimuscarinic compounds since they tend to affect parasympathetically innervated organs in the same order, with generally larger doses required to inhibit bladder activity than to affect salivary, bronchial, nasopharyngeal, and sweat secretions. The potential side effects of all antimuscarinic agents include inhibition of salivary secretion (dry mouth), blockade of the ciliary muscle of the lens to cholinergic stimulation (blurred vision for near objects), tachycardia, drowsiness, and inhibition of gut motility. Those agents that possess some ganglionic-blocking activity may also cause orthostatic hypotension and impotence at high doses (generally required for the nicotinic activity to manifest itself). Antimuscarinic agents are generally contraindicated in patients with narrow-angle glaucoma and should be used with caution in patients with significant bladder outlet obstruction, as complete urinary retention may be precipitated.

MUSCULOTROPIC RELAXANTS

Musculotropic relaxants fall under the general heading of direct-acting smooth muscle depressants, whose "antispasmodic" activity reportedly is directly on smooth muscle at a site that is metabolically distal to the cholinergic or other contractile receptor mechanism. Although **all the agents to be discussed do relax smooth muscle in vitro by papaverine-like (direct) activity, all have been found to possess variable anticholinergic and local anesthetic properties in addition. There is still a significant question as to how much of their clinical efficacy is due only to their atropine-like effect.** If in fact any of these agents do exert a clinically significant inhibitory effect that is independent of antimuscarinic action, there is a therapeutic rationale for combining their use with that of a relatively pure anticholinergic agent.

Oxybutynin chloride (Ditropan) is a moderately potent anticholinergic agent with a strong independent musculotropic relaxant activity and local anesthetic activity as well. Comparatively higher concentrations in vitro are necessary for the direct spasmolytic effects, which may be due to calcium channel blockade (Tonini et al, 1986). The recommended oral adult dose is 5 mg three or four times daily; the side effects are antimuscarinic and dose-related. Initial reports documented success in depressing detrusor hyperreflexia in patients with neurogenic bladder dysfunction; subsequent reports documented success in inhibiting other types of bladder hyperactivity as well (Andersson, 1988). A randomized double-blind placebo-controlled study comparing 5 mg of oxybutynin three times daily with placebo in 30 patients with detrusor instability was carried out by Moisey and colleagues (1980). Seventeen of 23 patients who completed the study with oxybutynin had symptomatic improvement, and 9 had evidence of urodynamic improvement—mainly an increase in maximal bladder capacity (MBC). Hehir and Fitzpatrick (1985) found that 16 of 24 patients with neuropathic voiding dysfunction secondary to myelomeningocele were cured or improved (17% dry, 50% improved) with oxybutynin treatment. The average bladder capacity increased from 197 to 299 ml (drug) versus 218 ml (placebo). Maximal bladder filling pressure decreased from 47 to 37 cm H_2O (drug) versus 45 cm H_2O (placebo). Thuroff and associates (1991) compared oxybutynin versus propantheline versus placebo in a group of patients with symptoms of instability and either detrusor instability or hyperreflexia. Oxybutynin (5 mg three times daily) performed best, but propantheline was used at a relatively low dose—15 mg three times daily. The rate of side effects was higher for oxybutynin at just about the level of the clinical and urodynamic improvement. The mean grade of improvement on a visual analogue scale was higher for oxybutynin (58.2%) versus propantheline (44.7%) and placebo (43.4%). The urodynamic volume at the first IBC was increased more with oxybutynin (51 versus 11.2 versus −9.7 ml), as was the change in maximal cystometric capacity (80.1 versus 48.9 versus 22.5 ml). Residual urine volume was also increased more (27.0 versus −2.2 versus −1.9 ml). The authors further subdivided their overall results into excellent (>75% improvement), good (50% to 74%), fair (25% to 49%), and poor (<25%). Their oxybutynin percentages were, respectively, 42%, 25%, 15%, and 18%. They compared their 67% rate of good to excellent results to seven other oxybutynin series in the literature and concluded that this compared favorably with the range of such results that they calculated from these studies (61% to 86%). The results of propantheline treatment were generally between those of oxybutynin and placebo but did not reach significant levels over placebo in any variable. Similar subdivision of propantheline results yielded percentages (see above) of 20%, 30%, 14%, and 36%. The authors compared their 50% ratio of good to excellent results in six other propantheline studies in the literature (30% to 57%) and concluded that their results were consistent with these. The AHCPR guideline (Urinary Incontinence Guideline Panel, 1992) lists six randomized controlled trials for oxybutynin; 90% of patients were female. The percentage of cures (all figures refer to the percentage effect on the drug *minus* the percentage effect on placebo) are listed as 28% and 44%; the percentage reduction in urge incontinence as 9% to 56%; and the percentage side effects and percentage dropouts as 2% to 66% and 3% to 45%, respectively.

Topical application of oxybutynin and other agents to normal or intestinal bladders has been suggested and implemented. This conceptually attractive form of alternative drug delivery, either by periodic intravesical instillation of liquid or timed-released pellets, awaits further clinical trials and the development of preparations specifically formulated for that purpose. Madersbacher and Jilg (1991) reviewed such usage with oxybutynin and presented data on 13 patients with complete suprasacral cord lesions on CIC. One 5-mg tablet was dissolved in 30 ml of distilled water and the solution instilled intravesically. Of the 10 patients who were incontinent, 9 remained dry for 6 hours. For the group the changes in bladder capacity and maximal detrusor pressure were statistically significant. Some of the more interesting data were in a figure that shows plasma oxybutynin levels in a group of patients in whom administration was intravesical or oral. The level following an oral dose rose to 7.3 ng/ml within 2 hours and then precipitously dropped to slightly less than 2 ng/ml at 4 hours. After intravesical administration, the level rose gradually to a peak of about 6.2 at 3.5 hours, but the level at 6 hours was still greater than 4 and at 9 hours was still between 3 and 4. Did the intravesically applied drug act locally or systemically? Weese and colleagues (1993) reported on using a similar dose of oxybutynin (5 mg in 30 ml of sterile water) to treat 42 patients with IBC who had either failed oral anticholinergic therapy (11) or had intolerable side effects (31). Twenty had hyperreflexia, 19 instability, and 3 bowel and/or bladder hyperactivity after augmentation. The drug was instilled two or three times daily for 10 minutes by catheterization. Twenty-one percent (9) dropped out because of inability to tolerate CIC or retain the solution properly, but there were no reported side effects. Fifty-five percent (18 of 33) of patients who were able to follow the protocol reported at least a moderate subjective improvement in incontinence and urgency. Nine patients became totally continent and experienced complete resolution of their symptoms; 18 improved patients experienced a decrease of 2.5 pads per day. There were no urodynamic data. Follow-up was 5 to 35 months (mean 18.4). The lack of side effects prompted some speculation about the mechanism. One possibility suggested was simply a more prolonged rate of absorption. Another more intriguing one was a decreased pass through the liver and therefore a decrease in metabolites, with the hypothesis that perhaps the metabolites and not the primary compound are responsible for the side effects.

With regard to the subject of hyperactivity in bowel-augmented or intestinal neobladders, Andersson and colleagues (1992) reviewed this phenomenon and its pharmacologic treatment. They note a few instances of positive results of agents given systemically. Locally applied agents were felt to offer more promise. A list of possibilities and their assessments was included. Pure anticholinergics have produced no good results either locally or systemically. Oxybutynin has shown poor results with systemic therapy and some good results with local therapy. Alpha agonists have shown no effect; beta agonists have shown no effects with local administration, and equivocal effects when administered subcutaneously, but the comment was made that such use will probably be limited by side effects. Other possibilities mentioned for future use included opioid agonists (diphenoxylate—a component of Lomotil—and loperamide), calcium antagonists, potassium channel openers, and NO donors.

Dicyclomine hydrochloride (Bentyl) is also reported to possess a direct relaxant effect on smooth muscle in addition to an antimuscarinic action. An oral dose of 20 mg three times daily in adults was reported to increase bladder capacity in patients with detrusor hyperreflexia (Fischer et al, 1978). Beck and associates (1976) compared the use of 10 mg of dicyclomine, 15 mg of propantheline, and placebo three times daily in patients with detrusor hyperactivity. The cure or improved rates, respectively, were 62%, 73%, and 20%. Awad and colleagues (1977) reported that 20 mg of dicyclomine three times daily caused resolution or significant improvement in 24 of 27 patients with IBC.

Flavoxate hydrochloride (Urispas) is a compound that has a direct inhibitory action on smooth muscle but very weak anticholinergic properties (see Andersson, 1988). Overall favorable clinical effects have been noted in some series of patients with frequency, urgency, and incontinence, and in patients with urodynamically documented detrusor hyperreflexia (Jonas et al, 1979). However, Briggs and colleagues (1980) reported essentially no effect on detrusor hyperreflexia in an elderly population. A similar conclusion was reached by Chapple and associates (1990) in a double-blind placebo-controlled cross-over study of the treatment of idiopathic detrusor instability with flavoxate. The recommended adult dosage is 100 to 200 mg three or four times daily. As with all agents in this group, a short clinical trial may be worthwhile. Reported side effects are few.

CALCIUM ANTAGONISTS

The role of calcium (Ca) as a messenger in linking extracellular stimuli to the intracellular environment is well established, including its involvement in excitation-contraction coupling in striated, cardiac, and smooth muscle (see Chapter 26; Andersson, 1993). The dependence of contractile activity on changes in cytosolic Ca levels varies from tissue to tissue, as do the characteristics of the Ca channels involved, but **interference with Ca inflow or intracellular release is a very potent potential mechanism for bladder smooth muscle relaxation.** Many experimental studies have confirmed the inhibitory effect of Ca antagonists on a variety of experimental models of spontaneous and induced bladder muscle strip and whole-bladder preparation activity, these results supporting the view that combined muscarinic receptor and Ca channel blockade might offer a more effective way of treating bladder hyperactivity than single-mechanism therapies presently available.

Terodiline is an agent with both Ca antagonist and anticholinergic properties. At low concentrations it has mainly an anticholinergic effect, whereas at higher concentrations a Ca-antagonistic effect becomes evident.

A number of clinical studies on the inhibitory action of terodiline on bladder hyperactivity have shown clinical effectiveness (see Abrams, 1990). Peters and the Multicentre Study Group (1984) reported the results of a multicenter study that ultimately included data from 89 patients (of an original 128) comparing terodiline and placebo in women with motor urge incontinence. The daily dose in this study was 12.5 mg in the morning and 25 mg at night. They concluded that terodiline was more effective than placebo but noted that this improvement was much more apparent on subjective assessment than on objective assessment of cystometric and micturition data. Sixty-three percent of patients preferred terodiline, regardless of treatment sequence. Although statistically significant objective results were recorded between terodiline and placebo, these were not very impressive. Tapp and associates (1989) reported on a double-blind placebo study, using a dose titration technique, that included 70 women with urodynamically proven detrusor instability and bladder capacities of less than 400 ml. Sixty-two percent of the 34 women in the terodiline group considered themselves improved, 38% unchanged. Of the 36 women in the placebo group, 42% considered themselves improved, 47% unchanged, and 11% worse, a statistically significant response in favor of the terodiline group with regard to the improvement percentage. Micturition variables of daytime frequency, daytime incontinence episodes, number of pads used, and average voided volumes were statistically changed in favor of terodiline, but the absolute changes were relatively small. Urodynamic data, although showing a trend in favor of terodiline in each parameter, showed no statistically significant differences in any category. Side effects were noted in a large number and with equal frequency in both groups after the dose titration phase. However, the incidence of anticholinergic side effects was higher in the drug group. The AHCPR guideline (Urinary Incontinence Guideline Panel, 1992) lists seven randomized controlled risks for terodiline; 94% of the patients were female. The percentage of cures (all figures refer to the percentage drug effect *minus* the percentage effect on placebo) is listed at 18% to 33%; the percentage reduction in urge incontinence as 14% to 83%; and the percentage of side effects and percentage of dropouts as 14% to 40% and 2% to 8%, respectively. Terodiline also exhibits an inhibitory effect on experimental hyperreflexia in the rabbit whole-bladder model, suggesting a possible role for local administration as well (Levin et al, 1993). More recent studies in women 18 to 80 years of age with urge incontinence showed a 70% decrease in the number of incontinent episodes per week compared with 9% for placebo (Norton et al, 1994) and, in women over 60 years of age with urge incontinence, a decrease of 64% in incontinence frequency versus 21% for placebo (Ouslander, 1993).

Terodiline is almost completely absorbed from the gastrointestinal tract and has a low serum clearance. The recommended dosage in adults is 25 mg twice daily, reduced to an initial dose of 12 mg twice daily in geriatric patients. The half-life is around 60 hours, and Abrams (1990) logically proposes, on this basis, a once-daily dose but emphasizes the necessity of dose titration for each patient. The common side effects seen with calcium antagonists (hypotension, facial flushing, headache, dizziness, abdominal discomfort, constipation, nausea, rash, weakness, and palpitations) have not been reported in the larger initial clinical studies with terodiline, side effects consisting primarily of those consequent to its anticholinergic action. However, **questions were raised about the occurrence of a rare arrhythmia (torsades de pointes) in patients taking terodiline simultaneously with antidepressants or antiarrhythmic drugs** (Connolly et al, 1991). Stewart and colleagues (1992) reported a prolongation of AT and QTc intervals and a reduction of heart rate in elderly patients taking 12.5 mg of terodiline twice daily. These were apparent after 1 week but not 1 day of therapy. They also reported four cases of polymorphic ventricular tachycardia in four patients (three over the age of 80 years) receiving the drug. They advised avoiding use of the drug in patients with cardiac disease requiring cardioactive drugs, hypokalemia, or in combination with other drugs that can prolong the QT interval such as tricyclic antidepressants or antipsychotics. After further other reports of apparent cardiac toxicity, the drug was voluntarily withdrawn by the manufacturer pending the results of further safety studies. The U.S. studies for Food and Drug Administration approval were likewise voluntarily halted by the manufacturer; there is currently activity directed toward their reinstitution. The problems were unfortunate, because the drug seemed quite effective and offered the additional advantages of a long half-life and the ability to titrate the dose for each patient, sometimes to a once-daily administration. Other Ca antagonist drugs have not been widely used to treat voiding dysfunction.

POTASSIUM CHANNEL OPENERS

Potassium (K) channel openers efficiently relax various types of smooth muscle by increasing K efflux, resulting in membrane hyperpolarization. Hyperpolarization reduces the opening probability of ion channels involved in membrane depolarization, and excitation is reduced (Andersson, 1992). There are some suggestions that bladder instability, at least that associated with infravesical obstruction and detrusor hypertrophy, might be secondary to supersensitivity to depolarizing stimuli. Theoretically, then, K channel openers might be an attractive alternative for the treatment of detrusor instability in such circumstances, without inhibiting the normal voluntary contraction necessary for bladder emptying (Malmgren et al, 1990). Pinacidil is such a compound that, in a concentration-dependent fashion, inhibits not only spontaneous myogenic contractions but also contractile responses induced by electric field stimulation and carbachol in isolated human detrusor (Fovaeus et al, 1989) and in normal and hypertrophied rat detrusor. Unfortunately, a preliminary study with this agent in a double-blind cross-over format showed no effect on symptom status in nine patients with detrusor instability and bladder outlet obstruction (Hedlund et al, 1990). Nurse and colleagues (1991) reported on the use of cromakalim, another potassium channel opener, in 17 patients with refractory detrusor instability or hyperreflexia or who had stopped other drug therapy because of intolerable side effects. Six out of 16 (35%) patients who completed the study showed a decrease in frequency and an increase in voided volume. Long-term observation was not possible since the drug was withdrawn because of reported adverse effects of high doses in animal toxicologic studies. Potassium channel openers are not at present very specific for bladder and are more potent in relaxing other tissues—hence their potential utility in the treatment of hypertension, asthma, and angina. If tissue-selective K-activator drugs can be developed, they may prove very useful for the treatment of detrusor instability. Side effects of pinacidil have been best studied and include headache, peripheral edema (25% to 50% and dose-related), weight gain, palpitations, dizziness, and rhinitis. Hypertrichosis and asymptomatic T-wave changes are also reported (30%). Fewer data are available on cromakalim, which can produce a dose-related headache, but rarely edema (Andersson, 1992).

Prostaglandin Inhibitors

Prostaglandins (PGs) are ubiquitous compounds that have been mentioned as having a potential role in excitatory neurotransmission to the bladder, in the development of bladder contractility or tension occurring during filling, in the emptying contractile response of bladder smooth muscle to neural stimulation, and even in the maintenance of urethral tone during the storage phase of micturition, as well as in the release of this tone during the emptying phase (see Andersson, 1993; Zderic et al, 1995; for discussion and references). There are multiple mechanisms whereby PG-synthesis inhibitors might decrease bladder contractility in response to various stimuli. However, objective evidence that this does occur clinically is scant.

Beta-Adrenergic Agonists

The presence of beta-adrenergic receptors in human bladder muscle has prompted attempts to increase bladder capacity with beta-adrenergic stimulation. Such stimulation can cause significant increases in the capacity of animal bladders, which contain a moderate density of beta-adrenergic receptors (see Zderic et al, 1995). In vitro studies show a strong dose-related relaxant effect of beta-2 agonists on the bladder body of rabbits, but little effect on the bladder base or proximal urethra. Terbutaline, in oral dosages of 5 mg three times daily, has been reported to have a "good clinical effect" in some patients with urgency and urgency incontinence, but no significant effect on the bladders of neurologically normal humans without voiding difficulty (Norlen et al, 1978). Although these results are compatible with those in other organ systems (beta-adrenergic stimulation causes no acute change in total lung capacity in normal humans while it does favorably affect patients with bronchial asthma), few adequate studies are available on the effects of beta-adrenergic stimulation in patients with detrusor hyperactivity. Lindholm and Lose (1986) used 5 mg of terbutaline three times daily in eight women with motor and seven with sensory urge incontinence. After 3 months of treatment, 14 patients claimed beneficial effects and 12 became subjectively continent. In 6 of 8 cases, the detrusor became stable on cystometry. Interestingly, the volume at which there was the first desire to void increased in the patients with originally unstable bladders from a mean of 200 to 302 ml, but the maximal cystometric capacity did not change. Nine patients had transient side effects, including palpitations, tachycardia, and/or hand tremor, and in three of these, side effects continued but were acceptable. In one patient the drug was discontinued because of severe adverse effects. Gruneberger (1984) reported that in a double-blind study, clenbuterol had a good therapeutic effect in 15 of 20 patients with motor urge incontinence. Unfavorable results of beta-agonist usage for bladder hyperactivity were published by Casteleden and Morgan (1980) and Naglo and associates (1981).

Alpha-Adrenergic Antagonists

Alpha-adrenergic blocking agents have also been used to treat both bladder and outlet abnormalities in patients with so-called autonomous bladders (Norlen, 1982). These include voiding dysfunctions resulting from myelodysplasia; sacral spinal cord or infrasacral neural injury; and radical pelvic surgery. Parasympathetic decentralization has been reported to lead to a marked increase in adrenergic innervation of the bladder, with a resultant conversion of the usual beta (relaxant) response of the bladder in response to sympathetic stimulation to an alpha (contractile) effect (see the section on changes after radical surgery) (Sundin et al, 1977). Although the alterations in innervation have been disputed, the alterations in receptor function have not. Koyanagi and colleagues (1988) showed urethral **supersensitivity to alpha-adrenergic stimulation in a group of patients with autonomous neurogenic bladders, implying that a change had occurred in adrenergic receptor function in the urethra** after parasympathetic decentralization. **Nordling and colleagues (1981a) described a similar phenomenon in women after radical hysterectomy** and ascribed this change to damage to the sympathetic innervation. **Decreased bladder compliance is often a clinical problem in such patients, and this, along with a fixed urethral sphincter tone, results in the paradoxical occurrence of both storage and emptying failure. Norlen (1982) has summarized the supporting evidence for the success of alpha-adrenolytic treatment in these patients.** Phenoxybenzamine (see the section on decreasing outlet resistance) is capable of increasing bladder compliance (increasing storage) and decreasing urethral resistance (facilitating emptying). Andersson and associates (1981) used prazosin (Minipress) in such patients and found that maximal urethral pressure during filling was decreased whereas "autonomous waves" were reduced. McGuire and Savastano (1985) reported that phenoxybenzamine decreased filling cystometric pressure in the decentralized primate bladder. More recently Amark and Nergardh (1991) reported that in children with myelodysplasia, alpha blockade decreased not only urethral tone but bladder tone and hyperactivity as well. Swierzewski and coworkers (1994) studied the use of a 5-mg daily dose of terazosin (Hytrin) in 12 SCI patients who were candidates for cystoplasty because of decreased bladder compliance. Detrusor compliance improved in all patients, and bladder pressure at capacity decreased by a mean of 36 cm H_2O. The maximal safe volume stored at a detrusor pressure of 40 cm H_2O increased by a mean of 157 ml.

Alpha-adrenergic blockade can decrease bladder contractility in patients with non-neurogenic voiding dysfunction as well. Jensen (1981a, 1981b, 1981c) reported an increase in "alpha-adrenergic effect" in bladders characterized as "uninhibited." Short- and long-term prazosin administration increased capacity and decreased the amplitude of contractions. Rohner and colleagues (1978) found that the normal beta response of canine bladder body smooth musculature was changed to an alpha response after bladder outlet obstruction. Perlberg and Caine (1982) studied bladder dome muscle from patients with obstructive prostatic hypertrophy and found an alpha-adrenergic response to noradrenalin stimulation (instead of the usual beta response) in 23% of 47 patients. They theorized that at least some of the symptomatic improvement in irritative symptoms in such patients treated with alpha-adrenergic antagonists is due to a direct effect on bladder muscle, rather than on outflow resistance, and hypothesized a potential relationship between the irritative symptoms of prostatism and this altered adrenergic response.

Tricyclic Antidepressants

Many clinicians have found tricyclic antidepressants, particularly imipramine hydrochloride (Tofranil, others), to be **especially useful agents for facilitating urine storage, both by decreasing bladder contractility and by increasing outlet resistance** (see Barrett and Wein, 1991). These agents have been the subject of a voluminous amount of highly sophisticated pharmacologic investigation to determine the mechanisms of action responsible for their varied effects (Baldessarini, 1990; Richelson, 1994). Most data have been accumulated as a result of trying to explain the antidepressant properties of these agents and thus primarily from central nervous system (CNS) tissue. The results, conclusions, and speculations inferred from the data are extremely interesting, but it should be emphasized that it is essentially unknown whether they apply to or have relevance for the lower urinary tract. **All these agents possess differing degrees of at least three major pharmacologic actions: (1) they have central and peripheral anticholinergic effects at some, but not all, sites; (2) in the presynaptic nerve ending they block the active transport system that is responsible for the reuptake of the released amine neurotransmitters norepinephrine and serotonin; and (3) they are sedatives,** an action that occurs presumably on a central basis but is perhaps related to antihistaminic properties (at H_1 receptors, though they also antagonize H_2 receptors to some extent). There is also evidence that they desensitize at least some alpha-2 adrenoceptors and some beta adrenoceptors. Paradoxically, they also have been shown to block some alpha and serotonin-1 receptors. **Imipramine has prominent systemic anticholinergic effects but has only a weak antimuscarinic effect on bladder smooth muscle** (Levin et al, 1983). **A strong direct inhibitory effect on bladder smooth muscle that is neither anticholinergic nor adrenergic does exist, however** (Olubadewo, 1980; Levin and Wein, 1984). This may be due to a local anesthetic-like action at the nerve terminals in the adjacent effector membrane, an effect that seems to occur also in cardiac muscle, or to an inhibition of the participation of Ca in the excitation-contraction coupling process (Malkowicz et al, 1987). Akah (1986) has provided supportive evidence in the rat bladder that desipramine, the active metabolite of imipramine, depresses the response to electric field stimulation by interfering with Ca movement (perhaps not only extracellular Ca movement but also internal translocation and binding). Direct evidence to suggest that the effect of imipramine on norepinephrine reuptake occurs on lower urinary tract tissue as well as brain tissue has been provided by Foreman and McNulty (1993) in the rabbit. An enhanced alpha-adrenergic effect in the smooth muscle of the bladder base and proximal urethra, where alpha receptors outnumber beta receptors, is generally considered to be the mechanism whereby imipramine increases outlet resistance. Attempting to correlate clinical effects with mechanisms of action, one might also postulate a beta-receptor-induced decrease in bladder body contractility if peripheral blockade of norepinephrine reuptake does occur there as well, due to the increased concentration of beta- over alpha-adrenergic receptors in that area.

Clinically, imipramine (Tofranil, others) seems to be effective in decreasing bladder contractility and in increasing outlet resistance (Cole and Fried, 1972; Mahony et al, 1973; Raezer et al, 1977; Tulloch and Creed, 1979; Castleden et al, 1981). Castleden and colleagues (1981) began therapy in elderly patients with detrusor instability with a single 25-mg nighttime dose of imipramine, which was increased every third day by 25 mg either until the patient was continent or had side effects, or until a dose of 150 mg was reached. Six of 10 patients became continent, and, in those who underwent repeated cystometry, bladder capacity increased by a mean of 105 ml and bladder pressure at capacity decreased by a mean of 18 cm H_2O. Maximal urethral pressure (MUP) increased by a mean of 30 cm H_2O. Although our subjective impression (Raezer et al, 1977) was that the bladder effects became evident only after days of treatment, some patients in the Castleden series became continent after only 3 to 5 days of therapy. Our usual adult dose for voiding dysfunction is 25 mg four times daily; less frequent administration is possible because of the drug's long half-life. Half that dose is given in elderly patients, in whom the drug half-life may be prolonged. In our experience, the effects of imipramine on the lower urinary tract are often additive to those of the atropine-like agents, and consequently a combination of imipramine and an antimuscarinic or an antispasmodic is sometimes especially useful for decreasing bladder contractility. If imipramine is used in conjunction with an atropine-like agent, it should be noted that the anticholinergic side effects of the drugs may be additive. It has been known for many years that imipramine is relatively effective in the treatment of childhood nocturnal enuresis. Doses for this range from 10 to 50 mg daily. Whether the mechanisms of action in the situation are the same as those for decreasing bladder contractility or increasing outlet resistance, or whether the antienuretic effect is more centrally mediated, is unknown. Korczyn and Kish (1979) have presented evidence that the antienuretic effect is neither on a peripheral anticholinergic basis nor on the same basis of whatever effects are responsible for the drug's antidepressant action. The antienuretic effect occurs soon after initial administration, whereas the antidepressant effects generally take 2 to 4 weeks to develop.

Doxepin (Sinequan) is another tricyclic antidepressant that was found to be more potent, using in vitro rabbit bladder strips, than other tricyclic compounds with respect to antimuscarinic and musculotropic relaxant activity (Levin and Wein, 1984). Lose and colleagues (1989) in a randomized double-blind cross-over study of female patients with involuntary bladder contractions and either frequency, urgency, or urge incontinence, found that this agent caused a significant decrease over control in nighttime frequency and nighttime incontinence episodes, and a near significant decrease in urine loss (pad-weighing test), and in the cystometric parameters of first sensation and MBC. The dosage of doxepin used was either a single 50-mg bedtime dose or this dose plus an additional 25 mg in the morning. The number of daytime incontinence episodes decreased in both doxepin and placebo groups, and the difference was not statistically significant. Doxepin treatment was preferred by 14 patients, whereas 2 preferred placebo; 3 patients had no preference. Of the 14 patients who stated a preference for doxepin, 12 claimed that they became continent during treatment and 2 claimed improvement; the 2 patients who preferred placebo claimed improvement. The AHCPR guidelines combine results for imipramine and doxepin, citing only three randomized controlled trials, with an unknown percentage of female patients. The percentage of cures (all figures refer to the percentage drug effect *minus* the percentage effect on placebo) are listed as 31%, the percentage reduction in urge incontinence as 20% to 77%, and the percentage of side effects as 0% to 70% (Urinary Incontinence Guideline Panel, 1992).

When used in the generally larger doses employed for antidepressant effects, the most frequent side effects of the tricyclic antidepressants are those attributable to their systemic anticholinergic activity (Baldessarini, 1990; Richelson, 1994). Allergic phenomena, including rash, hepatic dysfunction, obstructive jaundice, and agranulocytosis may also occur, but rarely. CNS side effects may include weakness; fatigue; a parkinsonian effect; a fine tremor noted most in the upper extremities; a manic or schizophrenic picture; and sedation, probably from an antihistaminic effect. Postural hypotension may also be seen, presumably on the basis of selective blockade (a paradoxical effect) of alpha-1-adrenergic receptors in some vascular smooth muscle. Tricyclic antidepressants can also cause excess sweating of obscure cause and a delay of orgasm, or orgasmic impotence, whose cause is likewise unclear. They can also produce arrhythmias and interact in deleterious ways with other drugs, so caution must be observed in their use in patients with cardiac disease (Baldessarini, 1990). Whether cardiotoxicity will prove to be a legitimate concern in patients receiving the smaller (than for treatment of depression) doses for lower urinary tract dysfunction remains to be seen but is a potential matter of concern. Consultation with a patient's internist or cardiologist is always helpful before instituting such therapy in questionable situations. The use of imipramine is contraindicated in patients receiving monoamine oxidase inhibitors, as severe CNS toxicity can be precipitated, including hyperpyrexia, seizures, and coma. Some potential side effects of the antidepressants may be especially significant for elderly patients, specifically weakness, fatigue, and postural hypotension. If imipramine or any of the tricyclic antidepressants is to be prescribed for the treatment of voiding dysfunction, the patient should be thoroughly informed of the fact that this is **not** the usual indication for this drug and that potential side effects exist. Reports of significant side effects (severe abdominal distress, nausea, vomiting, headache, lethargy, and irritability) after abrupt cessation of high doses of imipramine in children would suggest that the drug should be discontinued gradually, especially in patients receiving high doses.

Dimethyl Sulfoxide

Dimethyl sulfoxide (DMSO) is a relatively simple, naturally occurring organic compound that has been used as an industrial solvent for many years. It has multiple pharmacologic actions (membrane penetrant, anti-inflammatory, local analgesic, bacteriostatic, diuretic, cholinesterase inhibitor, collagen solvent, vasodilator) and has been used for the treatment of arthritis and other musculoskeletal disorders, generally in a 70% solution. The formulation for human intravesical use is a 50% solution. Sant (1987) has summarized the pharmacology and clinical usage of DMSO and has tabulated good to excellent results in 50% to 90% of a collected series of patients treated with intravesical instillation for interstitial cystitis. However, DMSO has not been shown to be useful in the treatment of detrusor hyperreflexia or instability or in any patients with urgency and/or frequency but without interstitial cystitis. The subject of interstitial cystitis and its treatment is considered in Chapter 17.

Polysynaptic Inhibitors

Baclofen (Lioresal) is discussed primarily along with agents that decrease outlet resistance secondary to striated sphincter dyssynergia. It has also been shown capable of depressing detrusor hyperreflexia secondary to a spinal cord lesion (Kiesswetter and Schober, 1975). Taylor and Bates (1979), in a double-blind cross-over study, reported it to be very effective also in decreasing daytime and nighttime urinary frequency and incontinence in patients with idiopathic instability. Cystometric changes were not recorded, however, and considerable improvement was also obtained in the placebo group. The intrathecal use of baclofen for treatment of detrusor hyperactivity is a potentially exciting area (see the section on decreasing outlet resistance), and further reports are awaited.

Increasing Bladder Capacity by Decreasing Sensory (Afferent) Input

Decreasing afferent input peripherally would be the ideal treatment for sensory urgency and for instability or hyperreflexia in a bladder with relatively normal elastic and/or viscoelastic properties in which the sensory afferents constituted the first limb in the abnormal micturition reflex. Maggi (1991, 1992, and references) has written extensively about the potential for treatment, specifically with reference to the properties of capsaicin, an irritant and algogenic compound obtained from hot red peppers that has highly selective effects on a subset of mammalian sensory neurons, including polymodal receptors and warm thermoreceptors (Dray, 1992). Systemic and topical capsaicin produces a reversible antinociceptive and anti-inflammatory action after an initially undesirable algesic effect. Local or topical application blocks C-fiber conduction and inactivates neuropeptide release from peripheral nerve endings, accounting for local antinociception and reduction of neurogenic inflammation. Systemic capsaicin produces antinociception by activating specific receptors on afferent nerve terminals in the spinal cord, and spinal neurotransmission is subsequently blocked by a prolonged inactivation of sensory neurotransmitter release. With local administration (intravesical) the potential advantage is a lack of systemic side effects. The actions are highly specific when applied locally—the compound affects primarily small-diameter nociceptive afferents, leaving the sensations of touch and pressure unchanged, although heat (not cold) perception may be reduced. Motor fibers are not affected (Craft and Porreca, 1992). The effects are reversible, although it is unknown whether initial levels of sensitivity are regained. Craft and Porreca (1992) list intravesical doses for the rat at 0.03 to 10.0 μmol/l for 15 to 30 minutes and, for the human, up to a 1- to 2-mmol/l dose.

Maggi (1992) reviewed the therapeutic potential of capsaicin-like molecules. Capsaicin-sensitive primary afferents (CSPA) innervate the human bladder, and intravesical instillation of capsaicin into human bladder produced a concentration-dependent decrease in the volume at first desire to void, decreased bladder capacity, and a warm burning sensation. Concentrations used were 0.01, 1.0, and 10 μmol/l, administered in ascending order at 10- to 15-minute intervals as constant infusions of 20 ml/min until micturition. Five capsaicin-treated patients with "hypersensitive disorders" reported either a complete disappearance (4) or marked attenuation (1) of their symptoms, beginning 2 to 3 days after administration and lasting 4 to 16 days. After that time symptoms gradually reappeared but were not worse. Fowler and colleagues (1994) reported on the use of capsaicin in 14 patients with detrusor hyperactivity, 12 with spinal cord disease. Low concentrations (0.1 to 10 μmol/l) had no effect on bladder capacity or hyperactivity. The dose suggested was 100 ml of either 1 mmol/l (0.3 g/l) or 2 mmol/l dissolved in 30% alcohol in saline introduced intravesically with a balloon catheter (to prevent urethral leakage) and left in place for 30 minutes. All patients with bladder sensation reported immediate suprapubic burning that lasted 5 to 10 minutes. All reported initial deterioration of their symptoms for a period of 1 to 14 days followed by clinical improvement or a return to their previous state. An improvement in some aspect of bladder behavior was seen in nine patients, great improvement (increase in bladder capacity from 127 to 404 ml with continence between CIC) in five. Systemic side effects did not occur. The longest follow-up was 20 months in a patient who was retreated at 3, 12, and 20 months. It is unclear from the report what the exact effects on compliance were, but the results certainly deserve the authors' designation of "promising" for the treatment of intractable hyperreflexia and incontinence and seem to confirm that capsaicin-sensitive afferents exist in the human bladder and become functionally significant in the detrusor hyperreflexia seen secondary to spinal disease.

Bladder Overdistention

Therapeutic overdistention involves prolonged stretching of the bladder wall using a hydrostatic pressure equal to systolic blood pressure. Smith (1981) originally summarized the experience at his center and detailed the technique used, a modification of the original cystodistention procedure described by Helmstein. **Improvement, when it occurs, is generally attributable to ischemic changes in the nerve endings or terminals in the bladder wall. Potential complications include bladder rupture (5% to 10%), hematuria, and retention.** Good to excellent results have been reported in the treatment of detrusor instability by Ramsden and colleagues (1976), but our impression is that this procedure is of little use in patients with storage failure secondary to neuropathic detrusor hyperactivity. Even in patients with detrusor instability, Jorgensen and co-workers (1985) reported a success rate of 1 out of 15 patients. In 27 patients with benign functional disease reported by Lloyd and colleagues (1992) (none with hyperreflexia), only 6 had a good response (zero of 6 with detrusor instability). This is also discussed in Chapter 17.

Electric Stimulation

Electric stimulation (ES) and neuromodulation are undergoing a revival and are discussed in three later sections, reflecting their use to facilitate storage by both inhibiting bladder contractility and increasing sphincter resistance, and to facilitate emptying by increasing detrusor contractility. **Applied through removable anal and vaginal devices and also peripherally through patch electrodes, ES has been used to facilitate storage by inhibiting bladder contractility** (see Wein and Barrett, 1988; Schmidt, 1989; Madersbacher, 1993; Fall and Madersbacher, 1994; for references). When effective, **this is primarily by an inhibitory pudendal–to–pelvic nerve reflex.** Cortical inhibition may also result, the mechanism of which is uncertain. In cats, this depression of bladder contractility also involves a pudendal-to-hypogastric reflex, with further inhibition mediated through a peripheral beta-adrenergic effect on the bladder smooth muscle. Such stimulation also increases sphincter resistance directly through pudendal nerve efferents to the striated sphincter, and, at least in cats, by a pudendal–to–hypogastric nerve reflex resulting in additional outlet closure through an alpha-adrenergic effect on the smooth musculature of the bladder neck and proximal urethra. **Neuromodulation** is a term that implies modification of the sensory and/or motor functions of the bladder through ES. For inhibition of bladder activity, stimulation is applied to the sacral roots resulting in excitation of pudendal afferents (and possibly efferents). The mode of action is still unclear, but modulation of reflex pathways to restore a "normal balance" is a general but deliberately vague summary statement gleaned from various authors.

There is much discordant opinion in the literature regarding the optimal parameters for ES for various indications, the sites of application, the criteria for patient selection, the necessity for chronic stimulation, the long-term cure or improvement rates, and the exact mechanism(s) involved. In no part of this section are parameters emphasized, and the interested reader is encouraged to consult the source document(s) for the details.

All concerned would probably agree that **successful use of ES to inhibit bladder contractility requires (1) a cooperative patient, (2) preservation of the morphology of the urinary tract, (3) preservation of the sacral spinal cord "reflex center," (4) a low degree of peripheral denervation of the pelvic floor musculature, and (5) the ability to voluntarily empty satisfactorily when the stimulus is turned off, or with CIC.** Ohlsson and associates (1989) reported on the results of anal and vaginal stimulation in 29 female patients with either idiopathic detrusor instability or an uninhibited overactive bladder, all of whom had failed to respond to conservative treatment. The stimulation was intermittent, with gradual increases in amplitude determined by patient adaptation. Treatment consisted of four segments of stimulation with intervals of 1 week between each application. All patients showed a significant increase in functional bladder capacity, and 11 of 29 reported a 30% decrease in the frequency of micturition. Two patients were unaffected by the usual stimulation used and responded well to stimulation delivered via a single needle bipolar electrode inserted directly into the pelvic nerve. Patients with neurologic disease of the central nervous system met with less successful results. Eriksen and colleagues (1989) reported on 48 women with idiopathic detrusor instability using an average of 7 treatments of 20 minutes each. Clinical and urodynamic cures were reported in approximately 50% of the population studied, with what was termed a significant improvement in another 33%. At a 1-year follow-up, a persisting positive therapeutic effect was found in 77% of the study group, and the urodynamic improvement seemed to continue. Using a stimulator that applied more or less continuous anal stimulation to women with various types of incontinence, this group reported initially optimistic results as well; using the same stimulator, Leach and Bavendam (1989) reported markedly contrasting negative results and recommended against its use. Petersen and colleagues (1994) reported no urodynamic efficacy of maximum functional ES of the anal sphincter in 13 patients with detrusor hyperreflexia, 12 with multiple sclerosis, and 2 with a history of myelitis. Subjectively, "good improvement" was reported in 2 patients and "improvement" in 8.

McGuire and associates (1983) reported on 16 patients with involuntary bladder contractions of differing cause who were treated with common perineal or posterior tibial patch electrode stimulation. Twelve patients initially were dry, 3 were improved, and 1 was "possibly improved." Vereecker and colleagues (1984) were unable to suppress hyperactivity by this method in patients with suprasacral spinal cord injury or disease.

Schmidt and Tanagho's technique (Schmidt, 1989) for neuromodulation to increase bladder capacity involves direct stimulation of the sacral roots. Percutaneous transcutaneous stimulation is used initially for a trial over 3 to 7 days. If successful, a permanent electrode and receiver implant is considered. Koldewijn and colleagues (1994) cite Schmidt as reporting in 1988 temporary trial stimulation in 1028 patients with an overall success rate (all indications) of 66%. In only 87 of these was a permanent stimulator implanted. In 1989 Schmidt reported a total permanent implant experience of 110 patients from 1981 to 1987. Of 29 with urgency incontinence, 79.3% were said to have experienced very significant symptom improvement. Corresponding numbers for 23 patients with postprostatectomy incontinence and pelvic dysfunction (dysfunctional voiding and/or pelvic pain) were 56.5% and 65.5%. Koldewijn and colleagues (1994) reported on the results of temporary neuromodulation in 57 patients with detrusor overactivity and/or urethral instability. A "perfect" result was achieved in 39%, moderate in 14%, slight in 18%, and none in 30%. Dijkema and associates (1993) report the results of an implanted prosthesis for neuromodulation for urge incontinence as a decrease in the number of incontinent episodes from 7.4 to 1.5 per day and an increase in the functional capacity from 135 to 227 ml. Potential problems related to permanent implantation include electrode migration or breakage, electric failure, pain, and loss or deterioration of the response with chronic stimulation. The exact incidences are difficult to ascertain.

Intravesical transurethral bladder stimulation has been pursued for initiating sensory awareness of bladder filling and stimulating detrusor contraction (see the discussion on ES to facilitate bladder contractility). This technique has also been found capable of increasing bladder capacity at low pressure, at least in pediatric patients with myelomeningocele (Kaplan et al, 1989). Decter and co-workers (1994) also reported a clinically significant improvement in end bladder filling pressure in 5 of 18 patients.

Acupuncture

Acupuncture therapy is mentioned for the sake of completeness and also because it represents a noninvasive modality with initially promising results. Philp and colleagues (1988) reported on patients who underwent acupuncture treatments weekly for 10 to 12 weeks. Of three patients with sensory urgency, none noted symptomatic improvement. Of 16 patients with idiopathic bladder instability, 3 had enuresis, 1 was cured, and 2 were unchanged. Of 13 patients with instability and diurnal symptoms, 10 showed significant symptomatic improvement, although cystometric bladder function changes were inconsistent. Geirsson and associates (1993) reported no success with this treatment (or transcutaneous stimulation of the posterior tibial nerve) in patients with interstitial cystitis. Some evidence exists suggesting that acupuncture may modify sensory afferent impulses at a spinal level, and there is other evidence suggesting that it raises the cerebrospinal fluid levels of endogenous opiates and that many of its effects can be reversed by the administration of narcotic antagonists. Although it may prove useful for bladder instability, it would be expected to have much less utility in the treatment of hyperreflexia.

Interruption of Innervation

CENTRAL (SUBARACHNOID BLOCK). Historically, this type of interruption was not used solely for urologic indications but, rather, to convert a state of severe somatic spasticity to flaccidity and to abolish autonomic hyperreflexia (see Wein and Barrett, 1988, for references). As a by-product, bladder hyperreflexia was converted acutely to areflexia. The flaccid bladder that resulted generally required additional therapy to empty, or required CIC. The obvious disadvantage of this type of procedure is a lack of selectivity, with unintended motor or sensory loss other than that related to the bladder. Impotence was very common in men, and in those patients with some residual motor or sensory function, these functions were often significantly altered or lost. Additionally, the conceptually simple result of an areflexic bladder, although it may be produced acutely, very often was not maintained on a long-term basis after decentralization. Decreased compliance often developed in such patients, resulting in significant storage problems.

PERIPHERAL (SACRAL RHIZOTOMY, SELECTIVE SACRAL RHIZOTOMY). In most cases, **bilateral anterior and posterior sacral rhizotomy or conusectomy converts a hyperreflexic bladder to an areflexic one.** This alone may be inappropriate therapy as it also adversely affects the rectum; anal and urethral sphincters; sexual function; and the lower extremities. **Selective nerve section was originally introduced as a treatment to increase bladder capacity by abolishing only the motor supply responsible for involuntary contractions** in an attempt to leave sphincter and sexual function intact. The initial use of this procedure followed the observation that the third anterior or ventral sacral root provided the dominant motor innervation of the human bladder. To enhance the clinical response and to minimize side effects, differential sacral rhizotomy should always be preceded by stimulation and blockade of the individual sacral roots with cystometric and sphincterometric control. Although technique refinements, such as percutaneous radio frequency–selective sacral rhizotomy and cryoneurolysis have occurred, there is still much argument about the place of these anterior rhizotomy procedures within a plan of treatment for detrusor hyperactivity. Torrens (1985) summarized successful results in collected groups of patients that ranged from 48% for idiopathic instability to 81% for patients classified as having a "paraplegic bladder." However, as he astutely pointed out, what is meant by a "success" varies from one series and one patient to another. When these procedures are used, they should certainly be preceded by urodynamic and urologic evaluation of the effects of selective nerve blocks before performance, especially in patients without fixed neurologic disease or injury. Even then, unintended effects on pelvic and lower extremity sensory or motor functions may occur, with disastrous medical and legal sequelae. Obtaining informed consent before such a procedure, in my opinion, should be the responsibility of an experienced neurosurgeon.

Both Tanagho and Schmidt (1988; Tanagho et al, 1989) **and Brindley** (1990) **have popularized the conception of deafferentation using dorsal or posterior rhizotomy to increase bladder capacity as part of their overall plan to simultaneously rehabilitate storage and emptying problems in patients with significant spinal cord injury or disease. These are patients in whom they have also used ES to alleviate emptying deficits** (see the appropriate subsection in the section on increasing intravesical pressure and/or bladder contractility). McGuire and Savastano (1984) also mentioned dorsal root ganglionectomy alone in such patients to increase bladder capacity.

Gasparini and colleagues (1992) report durability of the deafferentation response to selective dorsal sacral rhizotomy up to 64 months after section. The technique involves selecting nerve roots whose intraoperative stimulation provokes an adequate detrusor response. The dorsal and ventral components of these roots are then separated and the dorsal root(s) severed. An increase in bladder capacity from 148 to 377 ml was noted in 16 of 17 studied patients (24 in the original series) with an increase in the volume to the first contraction from 99 to 270 ml. A total of 14 patients were cured of incontinence, 2 improved, and 1 failed. Of 7 potent men, 2 experienced a decrease in erectile frequency but were still able to achieve penetration. Bowel and sphincter function were unaffected. Koldewijn and colleagues (1994) reported on the effects of intradural bilateral posterior root rhizotomies from S2 to S5 with implantation of an anterior root stimulator in a group of patients with suprasacral SCI. All showed persistent detrusor areflexia afterward, although 2 required subsequent secondary rhizotomy at the level of the conus. A majority showed decreased bladder compliance up to 5 days postoperatively, followed by a rapid increase thereafter. Brindley (1994a, 1994b) summarized the **advantages of bilateral posterior sacral rhizotomy in treating voiding dysfunction after SCI as (1) abolishing reflex incontinence, (2) improving low compliance, and (3) abolishing striated sphincter dyssynergia without altering resting tone.** Partial or selective procedures are considered only in such patients who retain some sensation or have excellent reflex erections.

PERIVESICAL (PERIPHERAL BLADDER DENERVATION). A number of procedures fall into the category of attempts to achieve a peripheral parasympathetic denervation. As is evident from neuroanatomic considerations, such attempts at best achieve primarily neurologic decentralization and partial peripheral denervation. It is interesting, however, to consider at this juncture the fact that many reported success rates for many of these procedures are high enough to make one wonder why the procedures are not used more frequently. Considering just the problem of bladder hyperactivity, there seems to be a number of reasons for this. First, many clinicians feel that more conservative methods (as opposed to surgery) are often successful in managing bladder hyperactivity with fewer side effects. In their hands, the success rates of peripheral bladder denervation are much lower in patients in whom vigorous but nonsurgical attempts at therapy have failed. Second, in many articles, there is little description of what "success" actually means. Finally, there is very little long-term follow-up for any of these procedures, and "postoperative assessment" usually means within a few months of the procedure.

Mundy (1985) has very nicely summarized surgical treatment of bladder hyperactivity up to that point in time. It is sometimes difficult in reading the literature to ascertain exactly what variety of phasic hyperactivity (hyperreflexia or instability) is being considered (or whether both are included in the treatment results). **Transvaginal partial denervation of the bladder** was originally described by Ingelman-Sundberg in 1959. This procedure has been used mostly for the treatment of refractory urge incontinence, and in the originator's hands, success rates of up to 80% have been achieved. Mundy (1985) cites these reports and reports of the successes of others in 50% to 65% of cases. Torrens (1985) cites the original work but simply states that "the technique has not found favor with other workers." **Cystolysis** is a term used to describe extensive perivesical dissection and mobilization with division of the superior vesical pedicle and the ascending branches of the inferior vesical pedicle. Although some initial reports were very promising for both relief of pain and hyperactivity (see Wein and Barrett, 1988, for references), it is interesting that there has been essentially nothing in the literature on this procedure since 1983, perhaps because the short-term optimism was replaced by nonpublished long-term pessimism.

Bladder transection involves a complete circumferential division of the full thickness of the bladder wall at a level just above the ureteric orifices, although Mundy (1985) felt that only the posterior part of the transection was of importance. Initial encouraging reports in the early 1970s were followed by longer-term reviews of larger series, all reporting success rates in excess of 50% for at least detrusor instability, using differing criteria. Mundy (1985) reviewed his large experience with transection in patients with detrusor instability and reported that of 104 patients with a follow-up of 1 to 5 years, 74% were cured, 14% were improved, and 12% were failures. Between 20 and 32 months, 10% of the group initially judged to have a satisfactory response suffered a relapse, giving a long-term subjective success rate of 65%. Only 35% of those who claimed to be symptomatically cured had reverted to stable detrusor behavior, however. Thus, Mundy wisely commented that a symptomatic cure does not necessarily mean a urodynamic one, and a symptomatic failure does not necessarily mean a urodynamic failure. Parsons and co-workers (1984) described endoscopic bladder transection in patients with phasic detrusor hyperactivity. Their early results were encouraging, but Lucas and Thomas (1987) reported essentially no change in 14 of 18 patients with intractable detrusor instability treated by this technique. Two achieved complete symptomatic relief, and two more were rendered continent but with the complaint of urgency and nocturia.

Transvesical infiltration of the pelvic plexuses with phenol aims to produce a chemical neurolysis whose results parallel those of the surgical approaches outlined above. Mundy (1985) and Torrens (1985) described the technique as being originated by Ewing and colleagues, who successfully treated 19 of 24 patients with MS. Blackford and associates (1984) reported a satisfactory response in 82% of women with refractory detrusor hyperreflexia and in 69% of women over the age of 55 with detrusor instability. For some reason, the response rate was much less satisfactory for detrusor instability in female patients younger than 55 years (14%). Cameron-Strange and Millard (1988) reported a 70% success rate in 11 patients with detrusor hyperreflexia secondary to MS. Although they achieved a 58% success rate in 29 patients with detrusor instability, Wall and Stanton (1989) report only a 29% significant response rate to therapy in a mixed group of 28 female patients with urge incontinence, only two of whom did not have instability, hyperreflexia, or low compliance. The potential risks include urinary retention and vaginal fistula. Chapple and associates (1991) reported success in only 2 of 18 patients with detrusor instability followed for 6 months and in 2 of 6 with hyperreflexia. Two fistulas resulted, one vesicouterovaginal and one vesicovaginal. They conclude, on reviewing their results and those of others, that subtrigonal phenol should be used in hyperreflexia only when no other treatment is possible.

To show how time tempers some views, in discussing the management of refractory urgency, Stephenson and Mundy stated in 1994, "The procedures popularized in the early 1980s intended to partially or totally denervate (or more correctly decentralize) the bladder have been abandoned. . . . Although some of these techniques had a high initial success rate in controlling incontinence and abolishing instability . . . the relapse rate within 18 months approached 100%. The advent of clam enterocystoplasty has revolutionized the treatment of the refractory group."

Augmentation Cystoplasty

The fact that augmentation cystoplasty has been accorded its own chapter (Chapter 107) emphasizes its importance in lower urinary tract reconstruction and in the treatment of refractory filling and/or storage problems of various causes. Suffice it to say here that **positive results have been obtained in 90% of patients with neurogenic lower urinary tract dysfunction and also in patients with contracted bladders secondary to other problems, such as tuberculous cystitis, for which the procedure was used initially.** Emptying failure afterward is a distinct possibility but can usually be predicted most of the time by careful preoperative urodynamic evaluation. The ability to perform CIC, or the means to have someone perform it, is essential. By the time this point in the treatment "menu" for filling and/or storage problems has been reached, urinary retention at low pressure is generally not an unreasonable result, and the main issue is therefore one of patient and family informed consent. Specific issues regarding augmentation cystoplasty are explicitly considered in Chapter 107 and include the type of procedure to be carried out (bowel versus autoaugmentation), the amount (if any) of bladder to be removed in different disease states, the effect of the loss of the bowel segment on the individual patient's physiology, and the question of whether to perform a simultaneous procedure on the bladder outlet, generally to increase its resistance.

Increasing Outlet Resistance

Physiotherapy and Biofeedback

Although pelvic floor exercises have not received the favorable attention which they deserve in the urologic literature as a successful modality of treatment in "anatomic" or "genuine" stress urinary incontinence, it has been increasingly obvious that the recent literature is remarkably consistent in describing at least a significant improvement rate in

50% to 65% of the patients so treated (Urinary Incontinence Guideline Panel, 1992). **For hypermobility-related stress incontinence in the female patient and for stress incontinence in the male patient, it is certainly worthwhile to try this as an initial or adjunctive form of treatment.** For patients with sphincteric incontinence secondary to a nonfunctional bladder neck and proximal urethra, it is conceptually doubtful whether significant improvement would occur in a majority of such patients; however, it is also certain that it can't hurt either, and such exercises may in fact allow the patient to be able to exert greater control over the detrusor reflex as well. Whether "bell and whistle" biofeedback adds to careful and periodic personal instruction and supervision has not yet been settled. Regardless, one must keep in mind that incontinence, assuming it is not related to lower-tract conditions that predispose to upper-tract damage, is the type of condition in which some (the author included) feel quite strongly that treatment should begin at the simplest level possible and that the patient, ultimately and ideally, should be the one to decide when improvement is satisfactory (not necessarily curative), and when "enough is enough." This subject is more completely discussed in Chapter 30.

Electric Stimulation

Intravaginal and anal ES have been used to treat storage failure by increasing outlet resistance as well as by decreasing bladder contractility (see the previous section on ES). The mechanism involves direct stimulation of the striated pelvic floor musculature through branches of the pudendal nerve, and additional urethral closure may be provided by a pudendal-to-hypogastric reflex that stimulates the smooth muscle of the bladder neck and proximal urethra through an alpha-adrenergic effect. Tanagho and Schmidt (1988) suggest that such chronic nerve stimulation results in a transformation of fast-twitch to slow-twitch striated muscle fibers, with an increase in sustained tension and fatigue resistance. In a review of available literature, we (Wein and Barrett, 1988) quoted **initial reported cure or improvement rates as high as 50% to 80%.** Eriksen and Eik-Nes (1989) reported the results of such treatment in 55 women with stress incontinence. Chronic ES was applied anally or vaginally for a median of 5 to 6 months. After therapy, 68% of patients achieved enough improvement so that a planned operation was canceled. At a 2-year follow-up, the success rate had been reduced to 56%. In 45 patients with high compliance who had used the device regularly for at least 3 months, the satisfaction rate at a 2-year follow-up was 72%. Bent and colleagues (1993) report on 14 patients with genuine stress incontinence treated with ES via intravaginal probe twice daily for 6 weeks. The subjective success rate, based on a questionnaire, was 71%. The pad test improved in 8 patients, incontinent episodes decreased in 6, and the number of pads per day decreased in 2. There were no statistically significant changes in urodynamic parameters, a finding not unique to this series. Schmidt and Tanagho's neuromodulation regimen (see the section on ES to inhibit bladder contractility) resulted in "very significant" symptom improvement in 23 men with postprostatectomy incontinence (Schmidt, 1989). ES regimens for sphincters are generally consciously or unconsciously combined with pelvic floor exercises and an increased awareness of lower urinary tract function. The contribution of each to improvement has been debated in view of the lack of urodynamic change. The use of ES to treat urinary incontinence is further discussed in Chapter 30.

Pharmacologic Agents

ALPHA-ADRENERGIC AGONISTS, GENERAL

The bladder neck and proximal urethra contain a preponderance of alpha-adrenergic receptor sites, which, when stimulated, produce smooth muscle contraction (see Chapter 26; Andersson, 1993). The static infusion urethral pressure profile is altered by such stimulation, which produces an increase in MUP and maximal urethral closure pressure (MUCP). Various orally administered pharmacologic agents that produce alpha-adrenergic stimulation are available. **Generally, outlet resistance is increased to a variable degree by such an action.** Potential side effects of all these agents include blood pressure elevation, anxiety, and insomnia due to stimulation of the CNS; headache; tremor; weakness; palpitations; cardiac arrhythmias; and respiratory difficulties. They all should be used with caution in patients with hypertension, cardiovascular disease, or hyperthyroidism.

EPHEDRINE, PSEUDOEPHEDRINE

Ephedrine is a noncatecholamine sympathomimetic agent that enhances the release of norepinephrine from sympathetic neurons and directly stimulates both alpha- and beta-adrenergic receptors. The oral adult dosage is 25 to 50 mg four times daily. Some tachyphylaxis develops to its peripheral actions, probably as a result of depletion or norepinephrine stores. **Pseudoephedrine,** a steroisomer of ephedrine, is used for similar indications with similar precautions. The adult dosage is 30 to 60 mg four times daily, and the 30-mg dose form is available in the United States without prescription. Diokno and Taub (1975) reported a "good to excellent" result in 27 of 38 patients with sphincteric incontinence treated with ephedrine sulfate. Beneficial effects were most often achieved in those with minimal to moderate wetting, and little benefit was achieved in patients with severe stress incontinence. A dose of 75 to 100 mg of norephedrine chloride has been shown to increase MUP and MUCP in women with urinary stress incontinence (Ek et al, 1978). At a 300-ml bladder volume, MUP rose from 82 to 110 cm H_2O, and MUCP rose from 63 to 93 cm H_2O. The functional profile length did not change significantly. Obrink and Bunne (1978), however, noted that 100 mg of norephedrine chloride twice daily did not improve severe stress incontinence sufficiently to offer it as an alternative to surgical treatment. They further noted in their group of 10 such patients that the MUCP was not influenced at rest or with stress at low or moderate bladder volumes. Lose and Lindholm (1984) treated 20 women with stress incontinence with norfenefrine, an alpha-agonist, given as a slow-release tablet. Nineteen patients reported reduced urinary leakage; 10 reported no further stress incontinence. MUCP increased in 16 patients during treatment, the mean rise being from 53 to 64 cm H_2O. It is interesting and perplexing that most patients reported an effect only after 14 days of treatment. The delay is difficult to explain on the basis of drug action, unless one postulates a change in the number of alpha receptors or in their sensitivity. It is obvious that there is a powerful placebo effect, for which the reasons are unknown, and, therefore, caution must be exercised in the evaluation of **all** modalities of therapy for sphincteric (and detrusor as well) incontinence.

Phenylpropanolamine

Phenylpropanolamine hydrochloride (PPA) shares the pharmacologic properties of ephedrine and is approximately equal in peripheral potency while causing less central stimulation. It is available in 25- and 50-mg tablets and in 75-mg timed release capsules and is a component of numerous proprietary mixtures, some marketed for the treatment of nasal and sinus congestion (usually in combination with an H_1-antihistamine drug) and some marketed as appetite suppressants. With doses of 50 mg three times daily, Awad and colleagues (1978) found that 11 of 13 female and 6 of 7 male patients with stress incontinence were significantly improved after 4 weeks of therapy. MUCP increased from a mean of 47 to 72 cm H_2O in patients with an empty bladder and from 43 to 58 cm H_2O in patients with a full bladder. With a capsule that contained 50 mg of PPA, 8 mg of chlorpheniramine (an antihistamine), and 2 mg of isopropamide (an antimuscarinic), Stewart and associates (1976) found that of 77 women with stress urinary incontinence, 18 were completely cured with one sustained-release capsule twice daily. Twenty-eight patients were "much better," 6 were "slightly better," and 25 were no better. In 11 men with postprostatectomy stress incontinence, the numbers in the corresponding categories were 1, 2, 1, and 7. The formulation of Ornade has now been changed, and each capsule of drug contains 75 mg of PPA and 12 mg of chlorpheniramine. Calliste and Linoskog (1987) reported on a group of 24 women with stress urinary incontinence treated with PPA or placebo (PL) with a cross-over after 2 weeks. Severity was graded 1 (slight) or 2 (moderate). Average MUCP overall increased significantly with PPA compared with PL (48 to 55 versus 48 to 49 cm H_2O). This was significant in grade 2 but not in grade 1 patients. The average number of leakage episodes per 48 hours was reduced significantly overall for PPA patients (from 5 to 1 versus 5 to 6). This was significant for grade 1 but not grade 2 patients. Subjectively 6 of 24 felt both PPA and PL were ineffective. Of 18 of 24 reporting a subjective preference, 14 preferred PPA and 4 PL. Improvements were rated subjectively as good, moderately good, and slight. Those obtained with PPA were significant compared with PL for the entire population and for both groups individually. The AHCPR guideline (Urinary Incontinence Guideline Panel, 1992) reports eight randomized controlled trials with PPA 50 mg twice daily for stress urinary incontinence in female patients. The percentage of cures (all figures refer to the percentage effect on drug *minus* the percentage effect on PL) are listed as 0% to 14%, the percentage reduction in incontinence as 19% to 60%, and the percentage of side effects and percentage of dropouts as 5% to 33% and 0% to 4.3%, respectively. There are potential complications of PPA. Baggioni and colleagues (1987) emphasized the possibility of blood pressure elevation, especially in patients with autonomic impairment. Liebson and associates (1987) found no cardiovascular or subjective adverse effects with doses of 25 mg three times daily or a 75-mg sustained-release preparation in a population of 150 healthy normal volunteers. Blackburn and colleagues (1989), in a larger series of healthy subjects and using multiple over-the-counter formulations, concluded that there was a statistically significant but clinically unimportant pressor effect in the first 6 hours after administration of PPA and this was greater with a sustained-release preparation. Caution should still be exercised in individuals known to be significantly hypertensive and in the elderly, whose pharmacokinetics may be altered.

Imipramine

The actions of imipramine have already been discussed in the section on inhibiting bladder contractility. **On a theoretical basis, an increase in urethral resistance might be expected if indeed an enhanced alpha-adrenergic effect was produced at this level because of an inhibition of norepinephrine reuptake.** Many clinicians have noted improvement in patients who were treated with imipramine primarily for reasons related to bladder hyperactivity but who had, in addition, some component of sphincteric incontinence. Gilja and associates (1984) reported a study of 30 women with stress incontinence treated with 75 mg of imipramine daily for 4 weeks. Twenty-one women subjectively reported continence. Mean MUCP for the group increased from 34.06 to 48.23 mm Hg.

Although some clinicians have reported spectacular cure and improvement rates with alpha-adrenergic agonists and agents that produce an alpha-adrenergic effect in the outlet of patients with sphincteric urinary incontinence, our own experience coincides with the experience of those who report that such treatment with such agents often produces satisfactory or some improvement in mild cases, but rarely total dryness in cases of severe or even moderate stress incontinence. A clinical trial, when possible, is certainly worthwhile, however, especially in conjunction with pelvic floor physiotherapy and/or biofeedback.

Beta-Adrenergic Antagonists and Agonists

Theoretically, beta-adrenergic blocking agents might be expected to "unmask" or potentiate an alpha-adrenergic effect, thereby increasing urethral resistance. Gleason and associates (1974) reported success in treating certain stress urinary incontinence patients with propranolol, using oral doses of 10 mg four times daily. The beneficial effect became manifest only after 4 to 10 weeks of treatment. Cardiac effects occur rather promptly after administration of this drug, but the hypotensive effects do not usually appear as rapidly, though it is difficult to explain such a long delay in the onset of the therapeutic effect on incontinence on this basis. Kaisary (1984) also reported success in treating stress incontinence with propranolol. Although such treatment has been suggested as alternative treatment to alpha agonists in patients with sphincteric incontinence and hypertension, few if any subsequent reports of such efficacy have appeared. Others have reported no significant changes in urethral profile pressures in normal women after beta-adrenergic blockage (Donker and Van der Sluis, 1976). Though 10 mg four times daily is a relatively small dose of propranolol, it should be recalled that the major potential side effects of the drug are related to its therapeutic beta-blocking effects. Heart failure may develop, as well as an increase in airway resistance, and asthma is a contraindication to its use. Abrupt discontinuation may precipitate an exacerbation of anginal attacks and rebound hypertension.

Beta-adrenergic stimulation is generally conceded to decrease urethral pressure (see Andersson, 1993 for references), but beta-2 agonists have been reported to **increase** the contractility of fast-contracting striated muscle fibers (extensor digitorum longus) from guinea pigs and suppress that of slow-contracting fibers (soleus) (Fellenius et al, 1980). Some beta agonists also stimulate skeletal muscle hypertrophy, fast-twitch fibers more than slow-twitch (Kim and Sainz, 1992). Clenbuterol, a selective beta-2 agonist, has been reported to potentiate, in a dose-dependent fashion, the field stimulation–induced contraction in isolated periurethral muscle preparation in the rabbit. The potentiation is greater than that produced by isoproterenol and is suppressed by propranolol (Kishimoto et al, 1991). These authors report an **increase** in urethral pressure with clinical use of clenbuterol and speculate on its promise for the treatment of sphincteric incontinence. Yamanishi and co-workers (1994) report an inotropic effect of clenbuterol and terbutaline on the fatigued striated urethral sphincter in female dogs, abolished by beta blockade. They also cite their own experience and that of others that suggest effectiveness of clenbuterol in the treatment of stress incontinence.

Estrogens

Although many studies in the literature lack objective evidence of a positive effect of estrogen therapy on stress incontinence in women, **such therapy certainly seems potentially capable of facilitating urinary storage in some postmenopausal patients by increasing the sum total of factors contributing to urethral outlet resistance.** The clinical experience of many support an augmentative or perhaps additive effect with alpha-adrenergic therapy in this regard. Whether this effect is related to changes in the autonomic innervation; changes in receptor content or metabolism of the smooth muscle; or changes in estrogen-binding sites or in the nonmuscular elements of the urethral wall or "muscosal seal" mechanism has not been settled. As this therapy is used exclusively in women with sphincteric incontinence, the reader is referred to Chapter 30 and to Wein (1995) for further detailed information.

Vesicourethral Suspension

Fixation of the vesicourethral junction in a physiologic position has been observed to correct genuine stress urinary incontinence in the female patient in 85% to 90% of those patients undergoing a first operation for this problem. The approach may be vaginal, retropubic, or laparoscopic. The procedure is rarely if ever used for other types of incontinence. The numerous variations of vesicourethral suspension are appropriately discussed in Chapters 32 and 33.

Nonsurgical Mechanical Compression

Periurethral Polytef or Collagen Injection

The injection of polytetrafluorethylene paste (polytef) periurethrally to increase urethral resistance was first reported by Berg (1973). This technique has been promoted and developed primarily by Politano and co-workers (see Wein and Barrett, 1988; Appell, 1990; for a summary of results). Highly purified bovine dermal collagen, lightly cross-linked with glutaraldehyde and dispersed in phosphate-buffered saline (Contigen) has likewise been injected into the submucosa of the bladder neck and proximal urethra with a similar rationale (see Appell, 1990; McGuire and Appell, 1994; for a summary of results). Autologous fat has been used as well (Santarosa and Blaivas, 1994). **The usual indications for periurethral bulking to increase outlet resistance are intrinsic sphincter deficiency and postprostatectomy incontinence.** A full chapter (Chapter 35) is devoted to this subject.

Occlusive and Supportive Devices; Urethral Plugs

Over the years, and especially more currently, there have appeared a number of nonsurgical urethral occlusive devices. Besides the time-honored penile clamp for postprostatectomy incontinence, these have been mostly for the treatment of female sphincter incontinence and have consisted of a variety of intravaginal devices to support or occlude the bladder neck and, more recently, to occlude the urethra. **Factors to be considered include not only "success" (in terms of a decrease in the number of incontinent episodes or the amount of fluid lost) but comfort, long-term safety (lack of pressure necrosis and infection), and ease of use.** Once again, it is useful to remember that patient satisfaction is the goal and not absolute dryness. At the time of this writing (1995) there are many devices in the trial stage, but none on the market that satisfy all the desirable criteria.

Surgical Mechanical Compression

Sling Procedures

The suburethral sling procedure was first reported by von Giordano in 1907 (see Wein and Barrett, 1988). Since that time a considerable number of procedures utilizing this principle have been described, employing autologous or alloplastic material. The **primary indication for sling surgery is intrinsic sphincter deficiency, but the procedure is quite effective in women with recurrent stress incontinence and pelvic floor weakness, especially after repeated unsuccessful surgeries.** Ed McGuire has written most extensively about this procedure and about the diagnosis and treatment of intrinsic sphincter dysfunction and deserves the credit for familiarizing the urologic public with these concepts. These are discussed fully by him in Chapter 34.

Closure of the Bladder Outlet

The primary indication for the drastic measure of closing the bladder outlet is intractable incontinence secondary to urethral necrosis due to long-term urethral

catheterization in the neurologically impaired woman. Trauma, infection, and fibrosis may also be responsible for irreparable urethral damage in both the male and the female patient. Our technique of combined abdominal and vaginal bladder neck closure was described by Levy and colleagues (1994), with success in 10 patients. Drainage was by a suprapubic tube. Eckford and associates (1994) reported an initial 54% continence rate using only a transvaginal closure (and suprapubic cystostomy) in women with MS; an additional 24% were rendered dry after a revision. Chancellor and co-workers (1994) used a pubovaginal sling to close the outlet in 14 women; greater tension than usual was applied. In 5 of these, an ileocystostomy and cutaneous urostomy (bladder chimney) were performed, in 2 a suprapubic tube was utilized, in 5 an augmentation cystoplasty was necessary, and in 2 only the sling was necessary.

Artificial Urinary Sphincter

Control of sphincteric urinary incontinence with implantable prosthetic devices has evolved rapidly over the past 20 years. Clearly the most significant contribution was the introduction by Scott and co-workers (1974) of a totally implantable artificial sphincter mechanism that could be used in adults and children of both sexes. The biomechanical evolution of this device and its current indications and usage are considered in Chapter 36. Silent upper-tract deterioration after genitourinary sphincter placement (or any procedure designed to increase outlet resistance) should be remembered as an increasingly recognized phenomenon for which post-treatment surveillance must be instituted. This may occur even if involuntary bladder contractions or decreased compliance was not present preoperatively.

Bladder Outlet Reconstruction

Reconstruction of the bladder outlet is one method of restoring sphincteric continence in patients with a fixed, open bladder outlet. This technique was introduced for the treatment of urinary incontinence by Hugh Hampton Young in 1907 and was subsequently modified by Dees, Leadbetter, and Tanagho. Procedures utilizing the Young-Dees principle involve construction of a neourethra from the posterior surface of the bladder wall and trigone. In the male patient, the prostatic urethra affords additional substance for closure and increase in outlet resistance. The Leadbetter modification involves proximal reimplantation of the ureters to allow more extensive tubularization of the trigone. Tanagho has described a procedure based on a similar concept but using the anterior bladder neck to create a functioning neourethral sphincter. Long-term success rates of between 60% and 70% have been reported (Tanagho, 1981; Leadbetter, 1985).

Circumventing the Problem

Antidiuretic Hormone–Like Agents

The synthetic antidiuretic hormone (ADH) peptide analogue 1-deamino-8-D-arginine-vasopressin (DDAVP) has been used for the symptomatic relief of refractory nocturnal enuresis in both children and adults (Norgaard et al, 1989; Rew and Rundle, 1989). The drug can conveniently be administered by intranasal spray at bedtime (dose 10 to 40 mg) and effectively suppresses urine production for 7 to 10 hours. Its clinical long-term safety has been established by continued use in patients with diabetes insipidus. Normal water-deprivation tests in the Rew and Rundle article would seem to indicate that long-term use does not cause depression of endogenous ADH secretion, at least in patients with nocturnal enuresis. Changes in diuresis during 2 months of treatment in an elderly group of six men and two women with increased nocturia and decreased ADH secretion were reported by Asplund and Oberg (1993). Nocturia decreased 20% (reported in milliliters) in men and 34% in females. However, the micturition number from 8 PM to 8 AM changed only from 4.3 to 4.5 in men and 3.5 to 2.8 in women, but the drug was not given until 8 PM. At present, this novel circumventive approach to the treatment of urinary frequency and incontinence has been largely restricted to those with nocturnal enuresis and diabetes insipidus. The fact that the drug seems to be much more effective than simple fluid restriction alone for the former condition is perhaps explained by relatively recent reports suggesting a decreased nocturnal secretion of ADH by such patients (Norgaard et al, 1989). Recently, suggestions have been made that DDAVP might be useful in patients with refractory nocturnal frequency and incontinence who do not fall into the category of primary nocturnal enuresis or decreased ADH secretion. Kinn and Larsson (1990) report that micturition frequency "decreased significantly" in 13 patients with MS and urge incontinence treated with oral tablets of desmopressin and that less leakage occurred. The actual approximate average change in the number of voidings during the 6 hours after drug intake was 3.2 to 2.5. Eckford and associates (1994) showed a numerically small but statistically significant decrease in nocturnal urinary frequency, nocturnal urine volume, and percentage of urine passed at night in a group of MS patients treated with DDAVP. After the study "the majority" continued to use the drug, but many for just "spot" usage—to avoid social inconvenience or during an exacerbation of their voiding symptoms.

Diuretics

Another circumventive pharmacologic approach is to give a rapidly acting loop diuretic 4 to 6 hours before bedtime. This, of course, assumes the nocturia is not due to obstructive uropathy. A randomized double-blind cross-over study on this approach using bumetanide in a group of 14 general practice patients was reported by Pedersen and Johansen (1988). Control nocturia episodes per week averaged 17.5; with placebo this decreased to 12 (!) and with drug to 8. Bumetanide was preferred to placebo by 11 of 14 patients. It would be interesting to see whether any drug companies pursue this avenue of treatment for the large number of patients with refractory nocturnal bladder storage problems, or for "spot" usage before some important event in patients with urgency and frequency with and without incontinence.

Intermittent Catheterization

Clean intermittent catheterization (CIC) has proved to be the most effective means of attaining a catheter-free

state in the majority of patients with acute spinal cord lesions. It is also an extremely effective method of treating the adult or child whose bladder fails to empty, especially when efforts to increase intravesical pressure and/or decrease outlet resistance have been unsuccessful. In those patients who have filling-storage failure due to bladder hyperactivity and/or sphincteric incontinence with adequate or inadequate emptying, CIC may also be used if the dysfunction can be converted solely or primarily to one of emptying by nonsurgical or surgical means (Wein and Barrett, 1988).

Intermittent catheterization has revolutionized the treatment of difficult cases of neuromuscular dysfunction of the lower urinary tract by providing a safe and effective method that preserves the independence of the patient to empty the lower urinary tract in cases in which continence has been produced by pharmacologically or surgically producing total or partial urinary retention. Without CIC, the success of augmentation cystoplasty or continent urinary diversion would never have been achieved, and all of us should feel a great debt to Jack Lapides for promoting and popularizing CIC (Lapides et al, 1972). Lapides deserves enormous credit for first applying the concept of self-CIC to large groups of patients with voiding dysfunction. He and his co-workers demonstrated the long-term efficacy and safety of such a program, and subsequently so have many others.

A cooperative, well-motivated patient or family is a requirement. The patient must have adequate hand control, or a family member must be willing to catheterize; in addition, adequate urethral exposure must be able to be obtained. An excellent consideration of factors involved in making a catheterization program work in the patient with functional limitation, as exists in many patients with neurogenic lower urinary tract dysfunction, is reported by Graham (1989). It is advantageous to have a special nurse who instructs the patients and families in the regimen; provides them with understandable written instructions to refresh their memory regarding technique, precautions, and danger signals; and provides continuing support for patients and families who call with questions or problems referable to their regimen. Teaching self-CIC requires an approach that communicates acceptance of the procedure by the instructor. Many patients are initially extremely reluctant to perform any procedure on themselves that involves the genitalia. Patients need a thorough explanation of the advantages of CIC along with assurances that it is simple and that it will not tie them to their houses or to an absolute time schedule. Additionally, proper selection of equipment for the patient's intelligence and financial level increases patient acceptance of and compliance with a self-CIC program. Patients who are reticent initially are continually amazed by the ease with which such a regimen is established. For adult male patients, a No. 14 or 16 Fr red rubber catheter is generally used. Patients with impaired fine motor skills may find stiffer plastic catheters easier to insert. A notable advantage of the red rubber catheters is their longevity. They can be reused indefinitely and boiled or microwaved for sterilization (Douglas et al, 1990). For female patients, disposable plastic catheters are recommended; they are inexpensive, very convenient, and can be obtained under many insurance plans. Red rubber catheters may also be used.

Complications to be watched for, and that we have seen, can include urethral false passages, bladder perforation, and silent deterioration of the upper urinary tracts. Bacteriuria is common, but symptomatic infection and antibiotic or antiseptic prophylaxis in this group of patients are not further considered here.

Continuous Catheterization

Indwelling urethral catheters are generally used for short-term bladder drainage, and such use of a small-bore catheter for a short time, when careful, does not, in our opinion and that of others, seem to adversely affect the ultimate outcome, at least insofar as this applies to initial bladder management in spinal cord injury (Lloyd et al, 1986).

Occasionally, more often in female patients, an indwelling catheter is a last-resort type of therapy for long-term bladder drainage. Virtually all such patients have bacteriuria after a certain period of time. A contracted fibrotic bladder may be the ultimate result. Bladder calculi may form on the catheter or on the retention balloon. Urethral complications are relatively uncommon in female patients, but bladder spasm may occur, producing urinary incontinence around the catheter. The temptation to use a larger-bore catheter with a larger-capacity balloon should be resisted, as the continuous use of such a drainage system combined with some pressure on the catheter may cause erosion of the bladder neck. A suprapubic catheter may be initially more comfortable and obviates urethral complications in the male patient, the main advantage of this type of continuous drainage over longer periods of time. **Use of a suprapubic catheter does not, however, obviate urethral leakage with detrusor contraction, nor does it provide better drainage in patients with sphincteric incontinence.** When blockage or dislodgment occurs, nursing personnel may be reluctant to change this type of catheter without physician assistance.

There is controversy, much of it recent, over whether long-term indwelling catheterization in the neurologically challenged population is associated with a poorer outcome with respect to either significant upper and lower urinary tract complications or quality of life. After CIC became a popular option, indwelling catheterization was discouraged for all but desperate situations, just on the basis of infection, and then on the basis of the occurrence of other urologic complications. The article by Jacobs and Kaufman (1978) was often cited to show that removal of an indwelling catheter in SCI men would prevent renal deterioration. What this article actually showed was that there were more renal and other urologic complications in patients with long-term (over 10 years) than in those with short-term (removed just after injury) use. Hackler (1982) reported accelerated renal deterioration in SCI patients managed with long-term suprapubic catheterization. McGuire and Savastano (1986) reported a poorer outcome in women with an indwelling urethral catheter than in those on CIC after 2 to 12 years. Of 13 in the former group, 54% had adverse changes on intravenous pyelography, as opposed to 0% in the latter group. Other urologic complications were also more frequent and severe in the former group.

Talbot and colleagues (1959) were among the first to suggest a relatively benign renal course for indwelling catheterization in the SCI patient. Dewire and associates (1992) reviewed the course of 32 quadriplegic patients managed with, and 25 without, an indwelling catheter. The groups were roughly comparable, and follow-up was for 10 years or more. The incidences of upper and lower urinary tract complications and renal deterioration were not significantly different. Chao and colleagues (1993) did a similar review on 32 SCI patients with an indwelling urethral (14) or suprapubic catheter (18) compared with 41 without. Follow-up was 20 years or more. Although the catheterized group had a higher prevalence of upper-tract scarring and caliectasis, no significant differences were found in other indices of renal function or in the prevalence of other urologic complications. Jackson and DeVivo (1992) reported on the results of indwelling catheterization in 108 women after SCI followed for 2 to 5 years (56), 6 to 9 years (31), and 10 or more years (21) after injury. Compared with their male population, the majority of whom were managed by condom drainage, there was no difference in upper- or lower-tract complications. Renal function was assessed by effective renal plasma flow, quantitated on a renal scan. Barnes and colleagues (1993) concluded that long-term suprapubic catheters were well tolerated by patients with neuropathic bladders. Based on the replies of 32 of 35 who expressed an opinion, 84% were satisfied. However, the follow-up was short (3 to 66 months, mean 23). In only 2 patients (of 12) assessable at over 2 years (exact length not specified) was there an increase in serum creatinine levels. Other problems, however, were apparent in the entire group. Recurrent catheter blockage occurred in 38%; recurrent symptomatic urinary infections in 23%; displaced catheters, requiring reinsertion in the operating room, in 15%; and urethral leakage (8 of 14 female patients with a suprapubic catheter alone, 6 of 16 male patients). Bladder neck closure to obviate the leakage has already been discussed.

Thus, the classic teaching that long-term continuous bladder catheterization in these patients should be avoided at all costs has been significantly challenged, at least for urethral catheterization. In the absence of a prospective randomized study or at least "cleaner" data, patient and family comfort, convenience, and quality of life must be strongly considered in this decision.

The development of carcinoma of the bladder in 6 of 59 patients with spinal cord injuries who had long-term indwelling catheters was reported by Kaufman and colleagues (1977). All were squamous cell lesions. Four of these patients had no obvious tumors visible at endoscopy, and the diagnosis was made by bladder biopsy. Five of these patients also had transitional cell elements in their tumor. Broecker and associates (1981) surveyed 81 consecutive SCI patients with an indwelling urinary catheter for more than 10 years. Although the investigators did not find frank carcinoma in any patients, they found squamous metaplasia of the bladder in 11 and leukoplakia in 1. Locke and co-authors (1985) noted 2 cases of squamous cell carcinoma of the bladder in 25 consecutive SCI patients catheterized for a minimum of 10 years. Bickel and colleagues (1991) reported 8 cases of bladder cancer in SCI men, although the denominator was uncertain. Four of these had been managed by indwelling catheterization for 7, 10, 14, and 19 years, respectively. All these had transitional cell carcinoma, whereas in the other 4, there were 2 cases of transitional and 2 of squamous cell carcinoma. In the series of Chao and associates (1993, see above), 6 patients developed bladder cancer, 3 of whom had indwelling catheters (3 of a total of 32). This issue is very worrisome, because such patients tend to "disappear" for long periods of time. **Periodic urinary cytologic examination and cystoscopy, perhaps with random biopsy, especially in patients with the new onset of gross hematuria, seem necessary in patients on long-term indwelling catheter drainage.**

Urinary Diversion

Although commonly employed in the past for the treatment of neurogenic voiding dysfunction, supravesical diversion is now rarely indicated in any patient with only voiding dysfunction. **Indications may include (1) progressive hydronephrosis and intractable upper-tract dilatation** (which may be due to obstruction at the ureterovesical junction caused by a trabeculated thick bladder or to vesicoureteral reflux that does not respond to conservative measures); **(2) recurrent episodes of urosepsis; and (3) intractable filling-storage or emptying failure when CIC is impossible.**

Continent diversion requires that the patient be able to perform CIC or that dependable assistance be available for this. The potential advantages of continent reservoir diversion are obvious, but they introduce the potential of upper-tract deterioration secondary to high-pressure storage, with or without vesicoureteral reflux. Continent diversion can be performed with anastomosis to a urethral stump, with at least the potential of less reliance on CIC. No further discussion of conduit or reservoir diversion is presented here, and the reader is referred to Chapters 100 to 103.

External Collecting Devices

Unfortunately, no optimal external collecting device has been approved for the female, primarily because of the difficulties of fixation and of leakproof collection. External collecting devices for the male (a condom or Texas catheter) are generally successful insofar as urine collection is concerned, but are unacceptable to many patients because of the visible equipment required and the leaks of often foul-smelling urine that can result. Since many patients with neurogenic lower urinary tract dysfunction have impairment of sensation, it is easy for these devices to cause severe pressure necrosis of the penis down to and including the urethra (Golji, 1981). A collecting device without a single discrete roller band or application ring offers at least a theoretical advantage for this reason. Maintaining an external urinary collecting device is a major problem in some SCI patients because of the inability to maintain a device during a vigorous voiding contraction, often associated with inadequate penile length, and because of recurrent lacerations of the penile skin, dictating temporary use of a Foley catheter. Van Arsdalen and co-authors (1981) described the use of a noninflatable penile prosthesis in this type of patient, with resultant ease of applying and maintaining such a device. This is particularly an advantage in those patients who are interested in a prosthesis for potency reasons as well. It should be noted, however, that the penile implant loss in these patients is much higher than in the general population (25% in this series). For similar problems due to a receding phallus, Binard and colleagues (1993) describe a "penoplasty."

Absorbent Products

A collection device of sorts, absorbent products represent a last resort for many patients. The ideal substance for absorptive padding is one that is highly permeable and absorbent. Immediately next to the patient is generally a layer of hydrophobic material, through which the urine passes into the absorbent pad, which is in turn surrounded by a waterproof material to keep clothing dry. Ideally, the hydrophobic material next to the skin keeps the patient relatively dry and reduces chafing as much as possible. An excellent review of the types of such devices available for males and females, as well as a review of external collecting devices and urethral compression devices and of skin care, can be found in the article by Jeter (1990) and the catalog available from her organization (Jeter, 1995).

THERAPY TO FACILITATE BLADDER EMPTYING (see Table 29–3)

Increasing Intravesical Pressure and/or Bladder Contractility

External Compression, Valsalva Maneuver

The Credé maneuver (manual) compression of the bladder) **is most effective in patients with decreased bladder tone who can generate an intravesical pressure greater than 50 cm H_2O with this maneuver and in whom outlet resistance is borderline or decreased** (Wein and Barrett, 1988). The technique of voiding by the openhanded Credé method involves placement of the thumb of each hand over the area of the anterior superior iliac spines and of the digits over the suprapubic area, with slight overlap at the fingertips. The slightly overlapped digits are then pressed into the abdomen and, when they have gotten behind the symphysis, pressed downward to compress the fundus of the bladder. Both hands are then pressed as deeply as possible into the real pelvic cavity. At times, the compression can be accomplished more efficiently by the use of the closed fist of one hand or by a rolled-up towel.

A similar increase in intravesical pressure may be achieved by abdominal straining (Valsalva maneuver). The proper technique involves sitting and letting the abdomen protrude forward on the thighs. During straining in this position, hugging of the knees and legs may be advantageous to prevent any bulging of the abdomen. To increase intravesical pressure in this manner requires voluntary control of the abdominal wall and diaphragmatic muscles. The Credé maneuver obviously requires adequate hand control. Straining at the time the Credé maneuver is applied is generally counterproductive because this increases intra-abdominal pressure and causes bulging of the abdominal wall, which then tends to lift the compressing hands off the fundus of the bladder. If the proper reflex arcs are intact, this also causes striated sphincter contraction. The Credé maneuver is obviously much easier in a patient with a lax, lean abdominal wall than in a person with a taut or obese one, and it is more readily performed in a child than in an adult.

Such "voiding" is unphysiologic and is resisted by the same forces that normally resist stress incontinence. Adaptive changes (funneling) of the bladder outlet generally do not occur with external compression maneuvers of any kind. As referred to previously, increases in outlet resistance may actually occur. If adequate emptying does not occur, other types of therapy to decrease outlet resistance may be considered; however, these may adversely affect urinary continence. **Vesicoureteral reflux is a relative contraindication** to external compression or Valsalva maneuver, especially in patients capable of generating a high intravesical pressure by doing so. The greatest likelihood of success with this mode of therapy (although some would say it should never be used) is in the patient with an areflexic and hypotonic or atonic bladder, and some outlet denervation (smooth or striated sphincter or both). Such a patient not uncommonly has stress incontinence as well. The continued use of external compression or Valsalva maneuver implies that the intravesical pressure between attempted voidings is consistently below that associated with upper-tract deterioration. This may be an erroneous assumption, and close follow-up and periodic evaluation are necessary to avoid this complication. The **most flagrant misuse of this form of management is in the patient with a decentralized or denervated bladder in whom decreased compliance during filling has already developed.** In such a patient, intravesical pressures that are greater than those necessary to cause upper-tract deterioration with minimal filling may develop silently, and external compression and Valsalva maneuver simply aggravate an already-dangerous situation.

Promotion or Initiation of Reflex Contractions

In most types of SCI or disease characterized by detrusor hyperreflexia, manual stimulation of certain areas within sacral and lumbar dermatomes may sometimes provoke a reflex bladder contraction (Wein and Barrett, 1988). Such "trigger voiding" is sometimes induced by pulling the skin or hair of the pubis, scrotum, or thigh; squeezing the clitoris; or digitally stimulating the rectum. According to the classic reference (Glahn, 1974), the most effective method of initiating a reflex contraction is rhythmic suprapubic manual pressure (seven or eight pushes every 3 seconds). Such activity is thought to produce a summation effect on the tension receptors in the bladder wall, resulting in an afferent neural discharge that activates the bladder reflex arc. Ideally, the contractions thus produced are sustained and of adequate magnitude. Patients potentially able to induce bladder contraction in such a way should be encouraged to find their own optimal "trigger points" and position for urination. To accomplish this, manual dexterity and either the ability to transfer to a commode or an external collecting device are required. If this type of patient has significant sphincter dyssynergia, such maneuvers may have to be combined with measures to decrease outlet resistance. This form of inducing bladder contraction is occasionally possible and desirable in patients with supraspinal disease and involuntary bladder contractions. If induced emptying can be carried out frequently enough so as to keep bladder volume and pressure below the threshold for activation of the micturition reflex and below the level dangerous for upper-tract deterioration, incontinence can be "controlled." This actually amounts to a form of timed voiding.

Some clinicians still feel that the establishment of a rhythmic pattern of bladder filling and emptying by maintaining a copious fluid intake and by periodically clamping and unclamping an indwelling catheter or by CIC can "condition" or "train" the micturition reflex. By focusing attention on the urinary tract and ensuring an adequate fluid intake, such regimens certainly are of benefit. It is also true that balanced lower urinary tract function can be achieved while a patient is on such a program (Opitz, 1984), but whether this is a cause-and-effect relationship is unknown and difficult to prove.

Pharmacologic Therapy

Parasympathomimetic Agents

Since a major portion of the final common pathway in physiologic bladder contraction is stimulation of parasympathetic postganglionic muscarinic cholinergic receptor sites, **agents that imitate the actions of acetylcholine (ACh) might be expected to be effective in treating patients who cannot empty because of inadequate bladder contractility.** ACh cannot be used for therapeutic purposes because of its action at central and ganglionic levels and because of its rapid hydrolysis by acetylcholinesterase and by butyrylcholinesterase (Taylor, 1990). Many ACh-like drugs exist, but **only bethanechol chloride (BC)** (Urecholine, Duvoid, others) **exhibits a relatively selective in vitro action on the urinary bladder and gut with little or no nicotinic action** (Taylor, 1990). BC is cholinesterase-resistant and causes an in vitro contraction of smooth muscle from all areas of the bladder (see Chapter 26; Zderic et al, 1995).

BC, or agents similar to it, has historically been recommended for the treatment of postoperative or postpartum urinary retention, but only if the patient is awake and alert and if there is no outlet obstruction. The recommended dose has been 5 to 10 mg subcutaneously. For over 45 years BC has been recommended for the treatment of the atonic or hypotonic bladder and has been reported to be effective in achieving "rehabilitation" of the chronically atonic or hypotonic detrusor (Sonda et al, 1979). BC has also been used to stimulate or facilitate the development of reflex bladder contractions in patients in spinal shock secondary to suprasacral spinal cord injury (Perkash, 1975).

Although BC has been reported to increase gastrointestinal motility and has been used in the treatment of gastroesophageal reflux, and although anecdotal success in specific patients with voiding dysfunction seems to occur, **there is little or no evidence to support its success in facilitating bladder emptying in series of patients in which the drug was the only variable** (Finkbeiner, 1985). In one set of trials, a pharmacologically active subcutaneous dose (5 mg) did not demonstrate significant changes in flow parameters or residual urine volume in (1) a group of women with a residual urine volume equal to or greater than 20% of bladder capacity but no evidence of neurologic disease or outlet obstruction; (2) a group of 27 "normal" women of approximately the same age; or (3) a group of patients with a positive BC supersensitivity test (Wein et al, 1980a, 1980b). This dose did increase cystometric filling pressure and also decreased bladder capacity threshold, findings previously described by others (Sonda et al, 1979). Short-term studies in which the drug was the only variable have generally failed to demonstrate significant efficacy in terms of flow and residual urine volume data (Barrett, 1981). Farrell and colleagues (1990) conducted a double-blind randomized trial that looked at the effects of two catheter management protocols and the effect of BC on postoperative retention after gynecologic incontinence surgery. They concluded that BC was not helpful at all in this setting. **Although BC is capable of eliciting an increase in bladder smooth muscle tension, as would be expected from in vitro studies, its ability to stimulate or facilitate a coordinated and sustained physiologic-like bladder contraction in patients with voiding dysfunction has been unimpressive** (Finkbeiner, 1985; Andersson, 1988).

It is difficult to find reproducible urodynamic data that support recommendations for the use of BC in any specific category of patients. Most, if not all, "long-term" reports in such patients are neither prospective nor double-blind and do not exclude the effects of other simultaneous regimens (such as treatment of urinary infection, bladder decompression, timed emptying, or other types of treatment affecting the bladder or outlet), an important observation to consider when reporting such drug studies. Whether repeated doses of BC or any cholinergic agonist can achieve a clinical effect that a single dose cannot is speculative, as are suggestions that BC has a different mode of action or effect on atonic or decompensated bladder muscle than on normal tissue. BC, administered subcutaneously, does cause an increased awareness of a distended bladder (Downie, 1984). This could facilitate more frequent emptying at lower volumes and thereby help to avoid overdistention.

As described in a recent article, O'Donnell and Hawkins (1993) administered 5 mg of BC subcutaneously to 10 neurologically intact male patients and made the following cystometric observations: Bladder volume at first desire to void (FDV) decreased (from 220 to 85 ml), MBC decreased (from 380 to 160 ml), FDV occurred at a higher pressure (5 versus 28 cm H_2O), and compliance was reduced. They concluded that BC affects the ability of the bladder to accommodate volume. Patients were comfortable at a resting bladder pressure of 20 cm H_2O (uncommon in their population), and the pressures at MBC were considerably higher than commonly seen under normal conditions. This suggested to them either that bladder pressure alone is not a significant factor in the perception of a sensation of FDV **or** that BC somehow alters the threshold at which the perception of desire to void occurs (since these patients showed a tolerance for increased intravesical pressure before FDV and at MBC). No agreement exists as to whether cholinergic stimulation produces an increase in urethral resistance (Wein et al, 1980a, 1980b). It would appear that pharmacologically active doses do in fact increase urethral closure pressure, at least in patients with detrusor hyperreflexia (Sporer et al, 1978). This would of course tend to inhibit bladder emptying. As to whether cholinergic agonists can be combined with agents to decrease outlet resistance to facilitate emptying and achieve an additive or synergistic effect, our own experience with such therapy, using even 200 mg of oral BC daily, has been extremely disappointing. Certainly, most clinicians would agree that a total divided daily dose of 50 to 100 mg rarely affects any urodynamic parameter at all.

The question of whether BC may be efficacious in a particular patient can be answered by a brief urodynamically controlled trial in which the institution of therapy is the only variable. In the laboratory, a functioning micturition reflex is an absolute requirement for the production of a sustained bladder contraction by a subcutaneous injection of the drug (Downie, 1984). Patients with incomplete lower motor neuron lesions constitute the most reasonable group for a trial of BC (Awad, 1985), although subcutaneous administration may be required. It is generally agreed that, at least in a "denervated" bladder, an oral dose of 200 mg is required to produce the same urodynamic effects as a subcutaneous dose of 5 mg (Diokno and Lapides, 1977).

The potential side effects of cholinomimetic drugs include flushing, nausea, vomiting, diarrhea, gastrointestinal cramps, bronchospasm, headache, salivation, sweating, and difficulty with visual accommodation (Taylor, 1990). Intramuscular and intravenous use can precipitate acute and severe side effects, resulting in acute circulatory failure and cardiac arrest, and is therefore prohibited. Contraindications to the use of this general category of drug include bronchial asthma, peptic ulcer, bowel obstruction, enteritis, recent gastrointestinal surgery, cardiac arrhythmia, hyperthyroidism, and any type of bladder outlet obstruction.

One potential avenue of increasing bladder contractility is cholinergic enhancement or augmentation. Such an action might be useful above or in combination with a parasympathomimetic agent. **Metoclopramide** (Reglan) is a dopamine antagonist with cholinergic properties. It has a central antiemetic effect in the chemoreceptor trigger zone and peripherally increases the tone of the lower esophageal sphincter, promoting gastric emptying. Its effects seem to be related to its ability to antagonize the inhibitory action of dopamine, to augment ACh release, and to sensitize the muscarinic receptors of gastrointestinal smooth muscle. Some data in the dog suggest that this agent can increase detrusor contractility (Mitchell and Venable, 1985), and there is one anecdotal case report of improvement of bladder function in a diabetic patient treated originally with this agent for gastroparesis (Nestler et al, 1983). **Cisapride** is a substituted synthetic benzamide that enhances the release of ACh in Auerbach's plexus (in the gastrointestinal tract). In 15 patients with complete SCI treated with 10 mg three times daily for 3 days, Carone and colleagues (1993) noted earlier and higher amplitude reflex contractions in those with hyperactive bladders; in those with hypoactive bladders there was a significant decrease in compliance. There was also increased activity of and decreased compliance of the anorectal ampulla with no alteration in striated sphincter activity. In another study in paraplegic patients, cisapride was found to decrease colonic transit time and maximal rectal capacity; an incidental decrease in residual urine was also noted (though only 51.5 to 27.7 ml) (Binnie et al, 1988).

PROSTAGLANDINS

The reported use of PGs to facilitate emptying is based upon **hypotheses that these substances contribute to the maintenance of bladder tone and bladder contractile activity** (see Chapter 26; Andersson, 1993; Zderic et al, 1995; for a complete discussion). **PGE_2 and PGF_{2a} cause an invitro and in vivo bladder contractile response. PGE_2 seems to cause a net decrease in urethral smooth muscle tone; PGF_{2a} causes an increase**. Bultitude and colleagues (1976) first reported that instillation of 0.5 mg PGE_2 into the bladders of female patients with differing degrees of urinary retention resulted in acute emptying and in improvement of longer-term emptying (several months) in two thirds of the patients studied (N = 22). Desmond and associates (1980) reported results with intravesical use of 1.5 mg of this agent (diluted with 20 ml of 0.2% neomycin solution) in patients whose bladders exhibited no contractile activity or in whom bladder contractility was relatively impaired. Twenty of 36 patients showed a strongly positive and 6 showed a weakly positive immediate response. Fourteen patients were reported to show prolonged beneficial effects; all but one of them had shown a strongly positive immediate response. Stratification of the data revealed that an intact sacral reflex arc was a prerequisite for any type of positive response. Tammela and co-workers (1987) reported that one intravesical administration of 10 mg of PGF_{2a} facilitated voiding in women who were in retention 3 days after surgery for stress urinary incontinence. The drug was administered in 50 ml of saline as a single dose and retained for 2 hours. It should be noted, however, that in these "successfully" treated patients, the average maximal flow rate was 10.6 ml/second with a mean residual urine volume of 107 ml and also that the authors state that "bladder emptying deteriorated in most patients on the day after treatment." Koonings and associates (1990) reported that daily intravesical PGF_{2a} and intravaginal PGE_2 reduced the number of days required for catheterization after stress incontinence surgery when compared with a control group receiving intravesical saline. Others, however, have reported negative results. Stanton and co-workers (1979) and Delaere and associates (1981) reported no success utilizing intravesical PGE_2 in doses similar to those reported above; Delaere and colleagues (1981) similarly reported no success using PGF_{2a} in a group of women with emptying difficulties of various causes. Wagner and associates (1985) used PGE_2 in doses of 0.75 to 2.25 mg and reported no effect on urinary retention in a group of patients after anterior colporrhaphy. There has been little recent activity in this area, a fact that generally means that clinicians have lost interest or that the initial optimistic results have not been confirmed. PGs have a relatively short half-life, and it is difficult to understand how any effects after a single application can last up to several months. If such does occur, it must be the result of a "triggering effect" on some as yet unknown physiologic or metabolic mechanism. Because of the number of conflicting positive and negative reports with various intravesical preparations, double-blind placebo-controlled studies would obviously be helpful to see whether there are circumstances in which PG usage can reproducibly facilitate emptying or treat postoperative retention. Potential side effects of prostaglandin usage include vomiting, diarrhea, pyrexia, hypertension, and hypotension (Rall, 1990).

BLOCKERS OF INHIBITION

DeGroat and co-workers (deGroat and Booth, 1984; deGroat, 1993; Chapter 26; Zderic et al, 1995) **have demon-**

strated a sympathetic reflex during bladder filling that, at least in the cat, promotes urine storage partly by exerting an alpha-adrenergic inhibitory effect on pelvic parasympathetic ganglionic transmission. Some have suggested that **alpha-adrenergic blockade, in addition to decreasing outlet resistance, may in fact facilitate transmission through these ganglia and thereby enhance bladder contractility.** On this basis, Raz and Smith (1976) first advocated a trial of an alpha-adrenergic blocking agent for the treatment of nonobstructive urinary retention. A complete discussion of postoperative retention, including the use of alpha blockers for its treatment, is presented earlier in this chapter.

Opioid Antagonists

Recent advances in neuropeptide physiology and pharmacology have provided new insights into lower urinary tract function and its potential pharmacologic alteration. **Endogenous opioids have been hypothesized to exert a tonic inhibitory effect on the micturiton reflex at various levels** (see Chapter 26; Zderic et al, 1995) **and agents such as narcotic antagonists therefore may offer possibilities for stimulating reflex bladder activity.** Thor and colleagues (1983) were able to stimulate a micturition contraction with naloxone, an opiate antagonist, in unanesthetized cats with chronic spinal cord injury. The effects, however, were transient, and tachyphylaxis developed. Vaidyanathan and associates (1981) reported that an intravenous injection of 0.4 mg of naloxone enhanced detrusor reflex activity in five of seven patients with neuropathic bladder dysfunction caused by incomplete suprasacral spinal cord lesions. The maximal effect occurred within 1 to 2 minutes after intravenous injection and was gone by 5 minutes. Murray and Feneley (1982) reported that the same dose of naloxone caused, in a group of patients with idiopathic detrusor instability, an increase in detrusor pressure at zero volume and at FDV; a decrease in the maximum cystometric capacity, and a worsening of the degree of instability. Galeano and co-workers (1986) reported that although naloxone increased bladder contractility in the cat with spinal cord injury, it also aggravated striated sphincter dyssynergia and spasticity—a potential problem in the treatment of emptying failure. Wheeler and associates (1987) noted no significant cystometric changes in a group of 15 spinal cord injury patients after intravenous naloxone, whereas 11 showed decreased perineal EMG activity. Although an intriguing area, the concept of reversing an inhibitory opioid influence to stimulate reflex bladder activity is of little practical use at present.

Reduction Cystoplasty

Myogenic decompensation of the bladder with persistently large amounts of residual urine may arise as a result of neurogenic problems or intravesical obstruction, may exist with megacystitis, or may have an unknown cause. **The anatomy and pathology of myogenic decompensation have suggested surgical treatment to some, as the chronic overstretching affects mainly the upper free part of the bladder, and as the nerve and vessel supply enter primarily from below, resection of the dome does not influence the function of the spared bladder base and lower bladder body** (Klarskov et al, 1988). When the detrusor is underactive rather than acontractile, partial cystectomy has been performed with successful results (Kinn, 1985; Klarskov et al, 1988). Because of limited success, Kinn recommends that such surgery be combined with radical incision of the bladder neck in male patients, rarely in female patients. Of Klarskov's 11 patients, three were termed subjectively cured. One went on to supravesical diversion, and five were on CIC either regularly or periodically. Hanna (1982) suggested a different concept in bladder remodeling that conceptually seemed to make more sense than just resection of the upper part of the detrusor. This procedure involved creating a laterally based mucosa-free detrusor pedicle flap and wrapping this flap around the body of the bladder, thus doubling the muscle bulk while reducing the bladder size. Bukowski and Perlmutter (1994) reported the results of a similar procedure in 11 boys with prune belly syndrome. Interpretation of the data was complicated, but they concluded that the operation "has helped to improve voiding and minimize infection during early childhood but it does not seem to decrease bladder capacity or improve voiding dynamics in the long term." Whether the risk/benefit ratio of these procedures, in view of their success rate, justifies their use over CIC is debatable.

Electric Stimulation

Directly to the Bladder or Spinal Cord

Clinical trials of direct ES of the bladder originated in 1940 but met with only partial success and intermittent enthusiasm since that time (see Wein and Barrett, 1988). **Direct ES was most effective in patients with hypotonic and areflexic bladders.** Initial success, defined as a low postvoid residual urine volume with sterile urine, was achieved in only 50% to 60% of patients, and **secondary failure often supervened, usually related to fibrosis, bladder erosion, electrode malfunction, or other equipment malfunction. The spread of current to other pelvic structures whose stimulus thresholds are lower than that of the bladder often resulted in abdominal, pelvic, and perineal pain; a desire to defecate or defecation; contraction of the pelvic and leg muscles; and erection and ejaculation in male patients. It was also noted that the increase in intravesical pressure was generally not coordinated with bladder neck opening or with pelvic floor relaxation and that other measures to accomplish these ends could be necessary.** Direct ES of the sacral spinal cord was also performed as an attempt to take advantage of the remaining motor pathways to initiate micturition. Although some short-term success was noted, many of the side effects seen with direct bladder stimulation occurred as well, since the stimulus, applied in this way, was also unphysiologic. Enthusiasm for both these approaches has waned considerably, and resurrection seems unlikely.

To the Nerve Roots

For the last 25 years Brindley (see Brindley, 1993, for history) and Tanagho and Schmidt (summarized in Tanagho and Schmidt, 1988, and Tanagho et al, 1989) have pursued neurostimulation for the treatment of voiding dysfunction.

The use of ES for storage disorders and for pelvic floor dysfunction has been covered, and this section concentrates exclusively on the use of anterior root ES to facilitate emptying. The Brindley device is the one most commonly used. **Prerequisites for such usage** are described by Madersbacher and Fischer (1993) as **(1) intact neural pathways between the sacral cord nuclei of the pelvic nerve and the bladder, and (2) a bladder that is capable of contracting. The chief application is in patients with inefficient or no reflex micturition after SCI. Simultaneous bladder and striated sphincter stimulation is obviated by sacral posterior rhizotomy, usually complete, which also (1) eliminates reflex incontinence and (2) improves low bladder compliance,** if present (Brindley, 1994a). The stimulation sequences and parameters themselves and their neurophysiologic consequences lead to less striated sphincter dyssynergia, even without posterior rhizotomy, than in reflex micturition in an SCI patient. Complete sacral deafferentiation is usually performed, however, the exception listed by Brindley being patients who have genital sensation or useful reflex erections. Electrodes are applied intradurally to sacral roots 2, 3, and 4, but the pairs can be activated independently. **The detrusor is usually innervated chiefly by S3 and to a smaller extent by S2 and/or S4. Rectal stimulation is via all three roots equally. Erectile stimulation is chiefly by S2 with a small contribution from S3 and none from S4.** Micturition, defecation, and erection programs are possible, with stimulus patterns set specifically for each patient (Brindley, 1994a).

Brindley (1994b) carefully reviewed the experience in the first 500 patients treated with his prosthesis with a total follow-up, at that time, of 2033.5 years. Of the total, 2 patients were lost to follow-up and 21 had died. Of the deaths, 2 were from septicemia (1 definitely unrelated to the implant and the specifics of the other unmentioned) and 1 was from related renal failure; the causes of 5 were unknown. Ninety-five operations were required for repair, 6 stimulators removed (4 infected), and 2 awaiting repair. In 45 patients the stimulator was believed to be intact but not used for various reasons. In all others, the stimulators were in use (411 for micturition and in most for defecation, and in 13 for defecation alone), and the users reported being "pleased." Upper-tract deterioration was reported in only 2 of 365 patients who were fully deafferentiated and in 10 of 135 who were incompletely or not deafferentiated. Two of these 10 had impaired renal function and one died of this.

Extradural stimulation has been used by Tanagho's group (Tanagho and Schmidt, 1988; Tanagho et al, 1989; Schmidt, 1989). They reported on the treatment of 19 patients with serious and refractory neuropathic voiding disorders. Extensive dorsal rhizotomy was performed, and a stimulator implanted on the ventral component of S3 or S4 with selective peripheral neurotomy (Tanagho et al, 1989). In 8 patients (42%) complete success was achieved with reservoir function, continence, and low-pressure–low-residual voiding with ES. Ten patients qualified as a partial success, regaining reservoir function and achieving continence.

These techniques are still in a phase of evolution but hold much promise for the future.

Intravesical Electrostimulation

Intravesical electrotherapy is an old technique that has been resurrected with some very interesting and promising results. Madersbacher (1993) describes his concept of the basis for this therapy as follows: **In patients with incomplete central or peripheral nerve lesions—and only these patients are suitable for this method—at least some nerve pathways between the bladder and cerebral centers are preserved but are too weak to be efficient under normal circumstances.** Intravesical electrostimulation (IVES) is based on the activation of specific mechanoreceptors in the bladder wall. With depolarization of these receptors, activation of the intramural motor system is said to occur, resulting in small local muscle contractions that further depolarize the receptor cells. As soon as this local motor reaction reaches a certain strength, vegetative afferentation begins, meaning that stimuli travel along afferent pathways to the corresponding cerebral structures with the occurrence of sensation. This in time reinforces efferent pathways, and their stimuli create centrally induced and more coordinated and stronger detrusor contractions. Ebner and colleagues (1992) **simply conceptualize the mechanism as involving an artificial activation of the normal micturition reflex and further suggest that repeated activation of this pathway may "upgrade" its performance during voluntary micturition.**

Children with congenital neurogenic bladder dysfunction, who have never experienced the urge to void, require a biofeedback system to realize the nature and meaning of this new sensation induced by IVES. This exteroceptive stimulation is also important for other groups of patients, as it signals detrusor contractions and whether and to what degree voluntary detrusor control is or has become possible and, by demonstrating progress, serves as positive feedback.

The technique involves direct intraluminal monopolar ES with a special catheter equipped with a stimulation electrode. Saline is used as the current-leading fluid medium in the bladder. Exteroceptive reinforcement is achieved by visual recording of detrusor contractions on a water manometer connected to the stimulation catheter. An intensive bladder-training program has to be combined with IVES and must be highly individualized. It must be remembered that only patients with an incomplete spinal cord lesion and with receptors still capable of reactivity and with a detrusor still capable of contractility will benefit from this technique. The achievement of conscious control requires, in addition, an intact cortex. Madersbacher (1993) has used this technique in patients with incomplete SCI and other incomplete central or peripheral lesions of bladder innervation; in pediatric patients with congenital neurogenic lower urinary tract dysfunction; and in patients, especially children, with non-neurogenic dysfunctional voiding. Only patients with preserved pain sensation in sacral dermatomes S2–S4 improved with this technique. The technique is time-consuming, as stimulation must be performed on a daily basis over weeks and months, with an individual treatment time of about 90 minutes. Kaplan and Richards (1988) reported on such therapy in myelodysplastic children, carrying out the treatment for 60 minutes (during a 90-minute catheterization), 3 to 5 days a week for 15 to 30 daily sessions. Of 62 patients evaluated, 42 completed at least one series of treatment. "Success" was defined differently for infants than for older children. For instance, this result implied a decrease in filling pressure, an increase in the quality of bladder contraction, and a decrease in residual urine. For older children, this type of result implied a heightened awareness of detrusor contractions before and during a contraction, maintenance of low-pressure filling, effectively emptying detrusor contractions with low residual, and either a conscious urinary control or timely enough sensory input to allow CIC for continence. Of children who initially had some detrusor contraction on initial evaluation, 80% achieved some or all of the success parameters. Of those with no initial detrusor activity, 33% achieved some success. Other reports have been less optimistic. Lyne and Bellinger (1993) reported the results of IVES treatment in 17 patients with neurologic dysfunction, 10 with myelomeningocele, and 2 with lipomeningocele. Ultimately all patients showed detrusor contraction during therapy (12 did so initially), but results related to increased bladder capacity and improved continence were disappointing. Five patients showed minor positive changes in continence. After the completion of therapy in 12 patients who had serial cystometry, 5 experienced an increase in capacity (14% to 158%) and 4 a decrease (7% to 37%). Decter and associates (1994) used IVES in 25 patients with neurogenic voiding dysfunction. After IVES the number of patients who manifested contraction on stimulation increased from 18 to 24, the number who sensed contraction during stimulation increased from 3 to 12. However, cystometry showed a greater than 20% increase in the age-adjusted bladder capacity in only 6 of 18 patients with serial studies and clinically significant improvements in end filling pressures in 5 of these. A telephone questionnaire revealed that 10 of 18 patients or parents perceived an improvement in bladder function, but the authors state, "The limited urodynamic benefits our patients achieved have not materially altered the daily voiding regimen and, because of these factors, we are not enrolling any new patients in our . . . program."

This technique is certainly controversial. Some question the theoretical basis and the definitions of **success** applied to patients treated. Further answers await study and usage by others.

Decreasing Outlet Resistance

At a Site of Anatomic Obstruction

The topics here properly include the treatment of prostatic obstruction and urethral stricture disease, and their discussion is appropriately found in Chapters 47 to 50 and 107.

At the Level of the Smooth Sphincter

Pharmacologic Therapy

Whether or not one believes that there is significant innervation of the bladder and proximal urethral smooth musculature by postganglionic fibers of the sympathetic nervous system, one must acknowledge the existence of alpha-adrenergic and beta-adrenergic receptor sites. The smooth muscle of the bladder base and proximal urethra contains predominantly alpha-adrenergic receptors, though beta receptors are present. The bladder body contains both varieties of adrenergic receptors, with the beta variety more common (see Chapter 26; Zderic et al, 1995)

Krane and Olsson (1973) were among the first to promote the concept of a physiologic internal sphincter partially controlled by tonic sympathetic stimulation of contractile alpha-adrenergic receptors in the smooth musculature of the bladder neck and proximal urethra. Further, they hypothesized that **some obstructions at this level during bladder contraction are a result of inadequate opening of the bladder neck and/or of an inadequate decrease in resistance in the area of the proximal urethra.** They also theorized and presented evidence that **alpha-adrenergic blockade could be useful in promoting bladder emptying in such a patient** with an adequate detrusor contraction but without anatomic obstruction or detrusor–striated sphincter dyssynergia. They and many others (see Wein and Barrett, 1988) have confirmed **the utility of alpha blockade in the treatment of what is now usually referred to as *smooth sphincter* or *bladder neck dyssynergia* or *dysfunction.*** Successful results, usually defined as an increase in flow rate, a decrease in residual urine, and an improvement in upper-tract appearance (where pathologic), could often be correlated with an objective decrease in urethral profile closure pressure.

One would expect success with such therapy to be most evident in patients without detrusor–striated sphincter dyssynergia, as reported by Hachen (1980). Mobley (1976), however, reported a startling 86% subjective success rate in 21 patients with a reflex neurogenic bladder, with a corresponding success rate of 66% in what was termed ***flaccid*** and 57% in what was termed ***autonomous*** neurogenic bladder dysfunction, success being defined as postvoid residual urine volume consistently less than 100 ml. Scott and Morrow (1978), on the other hand, noted excellent results with phenoxybenzamine (POB) therapy in 9 of 10 patients with a flaccid bladder and a flaccid external sphincter and in a single patient with upper motor neuron (UMN) bladder with intact sympathetic innervation, but in only 8 of 21 patients with hyperreflexia and autonomic dysreflexia, and in none of six patients with a UMN bladder and sympathetic denervation (lesion between T10 and L2).

Although most would agree that alpha-adrenergic blocking agents exert their favorable effects on voiding dysfunction by affecting the smooth muscle of the bladder neck and proximal urethra, **some information in the literature suggests that they may decrease striated sphincter tone as well,** and other information suggests that they may exert some of their effects on at least the symptoms of voiding dysfunction by decreasing bladder contractility (see previous discussion). Much of the confusion relative to whether or not alpha-adrenergic blocking agents have a direct (as opposed to indirect) inhibitory effect on the striated sphincter relates to the interpretation of clinical observations and experimental data referable to their effect on urethral pressure in the region of the urogenital diaphragm and on EMG activity in the periurethral striated muscle of this area. One cannot tell by pressure tracings alone whether decreased resistance in this area of the urethra is secondary to a decrease in smooth or striated muscle activity. Nanninga and colleagues (1977) found that the EMG activity of the external sphincter decreased after phentolamine administration in three paraplegic patients and attributed this effect to a direct inhibition of sympathetic action on the striated sphincter. Nordling and co-authors (1981b) demonstrated that clonidine and POB (both of which pass the blood-brain barrier) decreased urethral pressure and EMG activity from the area of the striated sphincter in five normal women, but that phentolamine (which does not pass the blood-brain barrier) also decreased urethral pressure in this area and yet had no effect on EMG activity. They concluded that (1) the effect of phentolamine was due to smooth muscle relaxation alone; (2) the effect of clonidine, and possibly POB, was elicited mostly through centrally induced changes in striated urethral sphincter tonus; and (3) these agents also had an effect on the smooth muscle component of urethral pressure. None of the three drugs, however, affected the reflex rise in either urethral pressure or EMG activity seen during bladder filling, and none decreased the urethral pressure or EMG activity response to voluntary contraction of the pelvic floor striated musculature. Gajewski and colleagues (1984) concluded that alpha blockers do not influence the pudendal nerve–dependent urethral response in the cat through a peripheral action, but that at least prazosin can significantly inhibit this response at a central level. Thind and associates (1992) reported on the effects of prazosin on static urethral sphincter function in 10 healthy female patients. They found a reduction—predominantly in the midurethral area—and hypothesized that the response was due to a decrease in both smooth and striated sphincter, the latter as a result of a reduced somatomotor output from the CNS. Clinically, Chancellor and associates (1994) found that terazosin, a selective $alpha_1$ antagonist, had little or no effect on striated sphincter function in SCI patients.

Alpha-adrenergic blocking agents have also been used to treat both bladder and outlet abnormalities in patients with so-called autonomous bladders—such as those with myelodysplasia; sacral spinal cord or infrasacral neural injury; and voiding dysfunction after radical pelvic surgery (Wein and Barrett, 1988). Decreased bladder compliance is a common clinical problem in such patients, and this, along with a fixed urethral sphincter tone, results in the paradoxical occurrence of both storage and emptying failure. The treatment of such patients with alpha blockers to decrease urethral resistance (and increase bladder compliance) has been discussed (see the section on alpha blockers to decrease bladder contractility [increase capacity]).

Phenoxybenzamine (Dibenzyline) was the alpha-adrenolytic agent originally used for the treatment of voiding dysfunction. POB and phentolamine have blocking properties at both alpha-1 and alpha-2 receptor sites. The initial adult dosage of this agent is 10 mg per day, and the usual daily dose for voiding dysfunction is 10 to 20 mg. Daily doses larger than 10 mg are generally divided and given every 8 to 12 hours. After discontinuation, the effects of administration may persist for days, since the drug irreversibly inactivates alpha receptors and the duration of the effect depends on the rate of receptor resynthesis (Hoffman and Lefkowitz, 1990). Potential side effects include orthostatic hypotension, reflex tachycardia, nasal congestion, diarrhea, miosis, sedation, nausea, and vomiting (secondary to local irritation). Those who still use POB for long-term therapy should be aware that it has mutagenic activity in the Ames test and that repeated administration to animals can cause peritoneal sarcomas and lung tumors (Hoffman and Lefkowitz, 1990). Further, the manufacturer has indicated a dose-related incidence of gastrointestinal tumors in rats (see Physicians' Desk Reference, 1995), the majority of which were in the nonglandular portion of the stomach. Although this agent has been in clinical use for some 30 years without clinically apparent oncologic associations, one must now consider the potential medicolegal ramifications of long-term therapy, especially in younger persons.

Prazosin hydrochloride (Minipress) is a potent selective $alpha_1$ antagonist (Hoffman and Lefkowitz, 1990), and its clinical use to lower outlet resistance has already been mentioned. The duration of action is 4 to 6 hours; therapy is generally begun in daily divided doses of 2 to 3 mg. The dose may be very gradually increased to a maximum of 20 mg daily, though seldom has anyone used more than 9 to 10 mg daily for voiding dysfunction. The potential side effects of prazosin are consequent to its $alpha_1$ blockade. Occasionally, there occurs a "**first-dose phenomenon,**" a symptom complex of faintness, dizziness, palpitation, and, infrequently, syncope, thought to be due to acute postural hypotension. Its incidence can be minimized by restricting the initial dose of the drug to 1 mg and administering this at bedtime. Other side effects associated with chronic prazosin therapy are generally mild and rarely necessitate withdrawal of the drug.

Terazosin (Hytrin) and **doxazosin** (Cardura) are two of the latest in the series of highly selective postsynaptic $alpha_1$ blockers. They are readily absorbed with high bioavailability and a long plasma half-life, enabling their activity to be maintained over 24 hours after a single oral dose (Taylor, 1989; Lepor, 1990). Their use has been recently promoted in the treatment of voiding dysfunction secondary to BPH, consequent to the $alpha_1$ receptor content of prostatic stroma and capsule. Their side effect profile is similar to that of prazosin. Daily doses range from 1 to 10 mg given generally at bedtime—a convenient advantage over a three-times-daily dosage schedule. Terazosin is said to have a similar affinity for $alpha_1$ receptors in genitourinary as in vascular tissue and a fourfold greater selectivity for $alpha_1$ receptors than doxazosin (Wilde et al, 1993a). **Alfluzosin** is a new agent that is reported to be a selective and competitive antagonist of $alpha_1$-mediated contraction of prostate capsule, bladder base, and proximal urethral smooth muscle. It is said to be more specific for such receptors in the genitourinary tract than in vasculature, raising the possibility that voiding may be facilitated by doses that have minimal vasodilation effects, minimizing postural hypotension (Wilde et al, 1993b). The drug requires three-times-daily dosing (7.5 to 10 mg total).

Thus, agents with alpha-adrenergic–blocking properties at various levels of neural organization have been utilized in patients with very varied types of voiding dysfunction–functional outlet obstruction, urinary retention, decreased compliance, and detrusor instability and/or hyperreflexia. Our own experience would suggest that a trial of such an agent is certainly worthwhile, as the effect or noneffect will become obvious in a matter of days and the pharmacologic side effects are of course reversible. However, our results with such therapy for non-BPH-related voiding dysfunction have been somewhat less spectacular than those of at least some other investigators.

Transurethral Resection or Incision of the Bladder Neck

Emmett performed the first transurethral bladder neck resection for neurogenic lower urinary tract dysfunction in

1937, and for years this procedure represented the first line of surgical treatment in such patients with poorly balanced bladder function (Wein and Barrett, 1988). The operation was originally performed primarily in two types of patients: (1) those with weak or absent detrusor contractions, and (2) those with anatomic or functional obstruction at the level of the bladder neck and/or proximal urethra, which prevented emptying either with abdominal straining or with a sustained detrusor contraction.

More refined urodynamic techniques have resulted in the realization that **dyssynergia at the level of the bladder neck or proximal urethra is uncommon, both in patients with neurologic disease and in those without. The prime indication for transurethral resection or incision of the bladder neck is the demonstration of true obstruction at the bladder neck or proximal urethra by combining urodynamic studies with either fluoroscopic demonstration of failure of opening of the smooth sphincter area or a micturitional profile showing that the pressure falls off sharply at some point between the bladder neck and the area of the striated sphincter.**

In the past, it was felt by some that another category for which this procedure was useful was that of a patient with sacral spinal cord lesion and an areflexic bladder who could achieve a measurable increase in intravesical pressure by straining or the Credé maneuver but who could not empty adequately with these methods (Wein et al, 1976). It is our feeling that such a procedure in this type of patient simply creates a form of graded stress incontinence, and that other alternatives for adequate emptying should be sought first.

Bladder neck or smooth sphincter dyssynergia has been previously discussed, and it is this entity, which **occurs almost exclusively in male patients, that is the most common indication for the current performance of transurethral incision or resection of the bladder neck.** The preferred technique at this time is incision of the bladder neck at the 5 o'clock and/or 7 o'clock position, a single full-thickness incision extending from the bladder base down to the level of the verumontanum. As Turner-Warwick (1984) originally described this technique, it involves deepening the incision until pinpoints of reflected light reveal minute interstitial fat globules between the latticework of the residual prostatic capsule fibers. Turner-Warwick reports the incidence of diminished ejaculate volume to be only 10% with this technique, and in less than 5% of these patients does he report absent ejaculate. Most people would place the incidence of retrograde or diminished ejaculation somewhere between the reported incidences of 15% and 50%. Other techniques of resection include a limited resection of dorsal tissue from the 3 o'clock to the 9 o'clock position, a resection further limited to the posterior lip, and a thorough circumferential resection of all tissue in male patients between the internal orifice and the verumontanum.

Y-V-Plasty of the Bladder Neck

It would seem reasonable to recommend Y-V-plasty only when a bladder neck resection or incision was desired and an open surgical procedure was simultaneously required to correct a concomitant disorder. This procedure, although certainly an established one, is in reality a revision of only the anterior bladder neck, as the posterior bladder neck is untouched. Since it is rarely carried out at this time, there is little information on whether it actually achieved, or was capable of achieving, the same urodynamic results as transurethral resection or incision.

At the Level of the Striated Sphincter

Biofeedback and Psychotherapy

The dysfunctional voider has been mentioned previously in the context of voiding dysfunction with the characteristics of striated sphincter dyssynergia, but in a neurologically normal individual. For this type of person, a urodynamic display of external sphincter EMG activity can facilitate clinical improvement in a strongly motivated patient capable of understanding the instructions of biofeedback training (Wein and Barrett, 1988).

Pharmacologic Therapy

There is no class of pharmacologic agents that will selectively relax the striated musculature of the pelvic floor. Three different types of drugs have been used to treat voiding dysfunction secondary to outlet obstruction at the level of the striated sphincter: the benzodiazepines, dantrolene, and baclofen. All are characterized under the general heading of antispasticity drugs (Cedarbaum and Schleifer, 1990). Baclofen and diazepam exert their actions predominantly within the CNS, whereas dantrolene acts directly on skeletal muscle. Unfortunately, there is no completely satisfactory form of therapy for the alleviation of skeletal muscle spasticity. Although these drugs are capable of providing variable relief in given circumstances, their efficacy is far from complete, and troublesome muscle weakness, adverse effects on gait, and a variety of other side effects minimize their overall usefulness as treatments of spasticity (Cedarbaum and Schleifer, 1990). **Glycine and gamma-aminobutyric acid (GABA) have been identified as the major inhibitory transmitters in the spinal cord** (Bloom, 1990). Evidence favors glycine as the mediator of intraspinal postsynaptic inhibition and the most likely inhibitory transmitter in the reticular formation. GABA appears to mediate presynaptic inhibition within the spinal cord and the inhibitory actions of local interneurons in the brain. The specific substrate for spinal cord inhibition consists of the synapses located in the terminals of the primary afferent fibers. GABA is the transmitter secreted by these synapses and activates specific receptors, resulting in a decrease in the amount of excitatory transmitter related by impulses from primary afferent fibers, consequently reducing the amplitude of the excitatory postsynaptic potentials. The inhibitory action of GABA in the brain is through an increase in chloride conductance with hyperpolarization of the membrane.

BENZODIAZEPINES. The benzodiazepines **potentiate the action of GABA at both presynaptic and postsynaptic sites in the brain and spinal cord** (Davidoff, 1985; Lader, 1987). When GABA recognition sites are activated, increased chloride conductance across the neuronal membrane is responsible for the inhibitory effects. The benzodiazepines increase the affinity of the GABA receptor sites on CNS membranes, and the increased binding increases the frequency with which the chloride channels open in response to a given amount of GABA. Presynaptic inhibition is augmented, and it is thought that this reduces the release of excitatory transmitters from afferent fibers and thereby reduces the gain of the stretch reflex and flexor reflex in patients with spasticity. This is a postulated mechanism of action of the muscle relaxant properties of at least diazepam (Davidoff, 1985).

Benzodiazepines are extensively used for the treatment of anxiety and related disorders (Shader and Greenblatt, 1992), although pharmacologically they can also be classified as centrally acting muscle relaxants. The generalized anxiety disorder that is responsive to pharmacotherapy with these agents is characterized by unrealistic and/or excessive anxiety and worry about life circumstances. Specific symptoms can be related to motor tension, autonomic hyperactivity (frequent urination can be a manifestation of this, as well as nausea, vomiting, diarrhea, and abdominal distress), and excessive vigilance. Other common usages have included treatment of insomnia, stress-related disorders, muscle spasm, and epilepsy, and preoperative sedation (Lader, 1987). Side effects include nonspecific CNS depression—manifested as sedation, lethargy, drowsiness, a feeling of slowing of thought processes, ataxia, and decreased ability to acquire or store information (Shader and Greenblatt, 1993). Some feel that any muscle relaxation effect in clinically used doses is due to the CNS depressant effects and cite a lack of clinical studies showing any advantages of these agents over placebo or aspirin in this regard (Baldessarini, 1990). Effective total daily doses of diazepam (Valium, others), the most widely used agent of this group, range from 4 to 40 mg. Other benzodiazepine anxiolytic agents include chlordiazepoxide, (Librium, others), clorazepate (Tranxene), prazepam (Centrax), halazepam (Paxipam), clonazepam (Klonopin), lorazepam (Ativan, others), oxazepam (Serax), and alprazolam (Xanax).

Few references are available that provide evaluable data on the use of any of the benzodiazepines in the treatment of functional obstruction at the level of the striated sphincter. Favorable and unfavorable opinions, however, are commonly expressed, at least in regard to diazepam. We have not found the recommended oral doses of diazepam to be effective in controlling the classic type of detrusor–striated sphincter dyssynergia secondary to neurologic disease. **If the cause of incomplete emptying in a neurologically normal patient is obscure and the patient has urodynamically what appears to be inadequate relaxation of the pelvic floor striated musculature (dysfunctional voiding, occult neuropathic bladder, the Hinman syndrome, e.g.), a trial of such an agent may be worthwhile.** The rationale for use is either that of relaxation of the pelvic floor striated musculature during bladder contraction, or of such relaxation's removing an inhibitory stimulus to reflex bladder activity. Improvement under such circumstances may simply be due, however, to the antianxiety effect of the drug, or to the intensive explanation, encouragement, and modified biofeedback therapy that usually accompanies such treatment in these patients.

BACLOFEN. Baclofen (Lioresal) depresses monosynaptic and polysynaptic excitation of motor neurons and interneurons in the spinal cord and was originally thought to function as a GABA agonist (Davidoff, 1985; Cedarbaum and Schleifer, 1990). However, its electrophysiologic and pharmacologic profile is quite different from that of GABA. Although its effects superficially resemble those of GABA, some specific GABA inhibitors (e.g., bicuculline) do not antagonize the actions of baclofen. Baclofen does not cause depolarization of primary afferent nerve terminals, and there is no evidence that baclofen increases chloride conduction, the most prominent action of GABA. Since both GABA and baclofen can produce some effects that are insensitive to blockade by classic GABA antagonists, two classes of GABA receptors have been proposed, a (the classic receptor) and b receptors. **Baclofen does not bind strongly or specifically to classic $GABA_a$ receptors but does to b-type receptors in brain and spinal membranes.** Currently, **it is felt that activation of the GABA receptor by baclofen causes a decrease in the release of excitatory transmitter(s) onto motor neurons by increasing the threshold for excitation of primary afferent terminals in the spinal cord.** This may occur by increasing potassium conductance or/and by inhibiting calcium influx. **Baclofen's primary site of action is the spinal cord,** but it is also reported to have activity at more rostral sites in the CNS. Milanov (1991) states that, like a GABA b agonist, it suppresses excitatory neurotransmitter(s) release, but it also has direct GABAergic activity. Its effect on the reduction of spasticity is caused primarily by normalizing interneuron activity and decreasing motor neuron activity (perhaps secondary to normalizing interneuron activity) (Milanov, 1991).

Baclofen has been found useful in the treatment of skeletal spasticity due to a variety of causes (especially MS and traumatic spinal cord lesions) (Cedarbaum and Schleifer, 1990). Determination of the optimal dose in individual patients requires careful titration. Treatment is started at an initial dose of 5 mg twice daily, and the dose is increased every 3 days up to a maximal daily dose of 20 mg four times daily. With reference to voiding dysfunction, Hachen and Krucker (1977) found a daily oral dose of 75 mg ineffective in patients with striated sphincter dyssynergia due to traumatic paraplegia, whereas they found a daily intravenous dose of 20 mg highly effective. Florante and colleagues (1980) reported that 73% of their patients with voiding dysfunction secondary to acute and chronic spinal cord injury showed lower striated sphincter responses and decreased residual urine volumes after baclofen treatment, but only with an average daily oral dose of 120 mg. Potential side effects of baclofen include drowsiness, insomnia, rash, pruritus, dizziness, and weakness. It may impair ability to walk or stand and is not recommended for the management of spasticity due to cerebral lesions or disease. Sudden withdrawal has been shown to provoke hallucinations, anxiety, and tachycardia; hallucinations during treatment, which have been responsive to reductions in dosage, have also been reported (Roy and Wakefield, 1986).

Drug delivery often frustrates adequate pharmacologic treatment and baclofen is a good example of this. GABA's hydrophilic properties prevent its crossing the blood-brain barrier in sufficient amounts to make it therapeutically useful. For oral use the more lipophilic analogue, baclofen, was developed. However, its passage through the barrier is likewise limited, and it has proved to be a generally insufficient drug, when given orally, to treat severe somatic spasticity and micturition disorders secondary to neurogenic dysfunction (Kums and Delhaas, 1991). **Intrathecal infusion**

bypasses the blood-brain barrier. Cerebrospinal fluid levels 10 times higher than with oral administration are achieved with infusion amounts 100 times less than those taken orally (Penn et al, 1989). **Direct administration into the subarachnoid space by an implanted infusion pump has shown promising results for not only skeletal spasticity, but striated sphincter dyssynergia and bladder hyperactivity as well.** Nanninga and associates (1989) reported on such administration to seven patients with intractable spasticity. All patients experienced a general decrease in spasticity, and the amount of striated sphincter activity during bladder contraction decreased; six showed an increase in bladder capacity. Four previously incontinent patients were able to stay dry with CIC. The action on bladder hyperactivity is not unexpected, given its spinal cord mechanism of action, and this inhibition of bladder contractility when administered intrathecally may in fact prove to be its most important benefit. Using an external pump to initially test response, Laubser and colleagues (1991) studied nine spinal injury patients with refractory spasticity. Eight showed objective improvement in functional abilities; three of seven studied urodynamically showed an increase in bladder capacity. Kums and Delhaas (1991) reported on nine para- or quadriplegic (secondary to trauma or MS) with intractable muscle spasticity treated with intrathecal baclofen. After a successful test period through an external catheter, a drug delivery system was implanted and connected to a spinal catheter. Doses per 24 hours ranged from 74 to 840 μg. Patients were studied before and 4 to 6 weeks after the initiation of therapy. The mean residual urine volume fell from 224 to 110 ml ($P = .01$), mean urodynamic bladder capacity rose from 162 to 263 ml ($P < .005$), and pelvic floor spasm decreased at both baseline and at MBC ($P <$ .005 and .025, respectively). Three subjects became continent. Additionally, CIC was no longer complicated by adductor spasm. Bushman and colleagues (1993) reported an increase in bladder storage in three persons with hereditary spastic paraplegia tested with intrathecal baclofen. Tolerance to intrathecal baclofen with a requirement for increasing doses may prove to be a problem with long-term chronic use, and studies are under way to investigate this.

DANTROLENE. Dantrolene (Dantrium) exerts its effects by a **direct peripheral action on skeletal muscle** (Davidoff, 1985; Cedarbaum and Schleifer, 1990). **It is thought to inhibit the excitation-induced release of calcium ions from the sarcoplasmic reticulum of striated muscle fibers, thereby inhibiting excitation-contraction coupling and diminishing the mechanical force of contraction.** The blockade of calcium release is not complete, however, and contraction is not completely abolished. It reduces reflex more than voluntary contraction, probably because of a preferential action on fast-type, compared with slow-type, skeletal muscle fibers. It has been shown to have therapeutic benefits for chronic spasticity associated with CNS disorders. The drug has been reported to improve voiding function in some patients with classic detrusor–striated sphincter dyssynergia and was initially reported to be very successful in doing so (Murdock et al, 1976). Therapy in adults is recommended to begin at a dose of 25 mg daily, and this is gradually increased by increments of 25 mg every 4 to 7 days to maximal oral dose of 400 mg given in four divided doses. Hackler and colleagues (1980) achieved improvement in voiding function in approximately half their patients treated with dantrolene but found that such improvement required oral doses of 600 mg daily. Although no inhibitory effect on bladder smooth muscle seems to occur (Harris and Benson, 1980), the generalized weakness that dantrolene can induce is often significant enough to compromise its therapeutic effects. Other potential side effects include euphoria, dizziness, diarrhea, and hepatotoxicity. Fatal hepatitis has been reported in approximately 0.1% to 0.2% of patients treated with the drug for 60 days or longer, and symptomatic hepatitis may occur in 0.5% of patients on treatment for more than 60 days, whereas chemical abnormalities of liver function are noted in up to 1%. The risk of hepatic injury is twofold greater in female patients (Ward et al, 1986). One agreed-upon use of dantrolene is to acutely manage malignant hyperthermia, a rare hereditary syndrome characterized by vigorous contraction of skeletal muscle precipitated by excess release of calcium from the sarcoplasmic reticulum, generally in response to neuromuscular blocking agents or inhalational anesthetics. Virtually all hospital pharmacies stock parenteral dantrolene for this purpose.

BOTULINUM TOXIN. Botulinum toxin (an inhibitor of ACh release at the neuromuscular junction of striated muscle) **has been injected directly into the striated sphincter for the treatment of dyssynergia** (Dykstra and Sidi, 1990). Injections carried out weekly for 3 weeks achieved a duration of effect averaging 2 months. The number of patients tested was small, and more information is needed regarding parameters of success and side effects. Fowler and colleagues (1992) injected six women with difficult voiding and/or retention secondary to abnormal myotonus-like EMG activity in the striated urethral sphincter. Although no patient improved voiding (attributed to the type of repetitive discharge activity), three patients developed transient stress incontinence, indicating that the sphincter muscle had indeed been weakened.

Surgical Sphincterotomy

Therapeutic destruction of the external urethral sphincter was first performed in 1936, but the first large clinical series was not reported until 1958 by J. C. Ross and colleagues (Wein and Barrett, 1988). **The primary indication for this procedure was and still is detrusor–striated sphincter dyssynergia in a male patient when other types of management have been unsuccessful or are not possible.** A substantial improvement in bladder emptying occurs in 70% to 90% of cases (Wein et al, 1976). Upper-tract deterioration is rare after successful sphincterotomy; vesicoureteral reflux, if present preoperatively, often disappears because of decreased bladder pressures and a reduced incidence of infection in a catheter-free patient with a low residual urine volume. An external collecting device is generally worn postoperatively, although total dripping incontinence or severe stress incontinence should be unusual unless the proximal sphincter mechanism (the bladder neck and proximal urethra) has been compromised—by prior surgical therapy, the neurologic lesion itself, or as a secondary effect of the striated sphincter dyssynergia (presumably a hydraulic effect on the bladder neck itself).

The 12 o'clock sphincterotomy, originally proposed by Madersbacher and Scott (1975), **remains the procedure of**

choice for a number of reasons, which have been confirmed and commented upon by others. The anatomy of the striated sphincter is such that its main bulk is anteromedial. The blood supply is primarily lateral, and thus there is less chance of significant hemorrhage with a 12 o'clock incision. There is some disagreement about the rate of postoperative erectile dysfunction in those individuals who preoperatively have erections. Estimates of dysfunction when the 3 o'clock and 9 o'clock techniques are used vary from 5% to 30%, but whatever the true figure is, it is clear that most would agree that this complication is far less common (approximately 5%) with incision in the anteromedial position. Other complications may include significant hemorrhage (5% to 20%) and urinary extravasation. Sphincterotomy can be performed by use of a knife electrode or by resection with a loop electrode. Laser ablation may also be used. The incision must extend from the level of the verumontanum at least to the bulbomembranous junction. Gradual deepening of the incision allows good visual control and minimizes the chance of significant hemorrhage and extravasation. When early failure occurs, it is generally attributable to an inadequate surgical procedure (either not deep enough or not extensive enough), inadequate detrusor function, or unrecognized bladder neck obstruction.

Recent reports have questioned the long-term efficacy of sphincterotomy. Santiago (1993) reported late failure requiring reoperation in 10 of 25 SCI patients. Vapnek and colleagues (1994) reported that of 13 cervical and 3 thoracic SCI patients undergoing sphincterotomy 3 months to 8 years previously, only 8 of 16 were still on condom catheter drainage, and these had a significantly shorter follow-up (16 months average) than those who converted to an indwelling suprapubic catheter (39 months). Late failure may occur because of fibrosis somewhere along the extent of the sphincterotomy, a change in detrusor function, the development of prostatic obstruction, or a change in neurologic status such that smooth sphincter dyssynergia develops (Lockhart and Pow-Sang, 1989). It should be remembered that outcome parameters after sphincterotomy to judge success or failure should include detrusor leak point pressure, renal function, urosepsis, upper-tract appearance, vesicoureteral reflux, autonomic hyperreflexia, need for catheterization, and sexual function. Residual urine volume per se does not always indicate the success or failure of the procedure.

Urethral Overdilation

Urethral overdilation to No. 40 to 50 Fr in females patients can achieve the same objective as external sphincterotomy in male patients (Wein and Barrett, 1988) but is rarely performed because of the lack of a suitable external collecting device. In young boys, when sphincterotomy is contemplated, a similar stretching of the posterior urethra can be accomplished through a perineal urethrostomy, obviating or postponing the need for normal sphincterotomy. Wang and associates (1989) reported the results of urethral dilation with urethral sounds or balloon procedures to No. 22 to 28 Fr in 11 myelodysplastic children with high intravesical pressures refractory to other traditional forms of management. After dilation, the intravesical pressures decreased and upper-tract function and bladder compliance improved. There was no discernible effect on continence function. These observations indicate that compliance in these patients can be improved by a decrease in outlet resistance, and producing a decrease in outlet resistance in this fashion did not result in any deterioration in urinary control over what was present preoperatively.

Balloon dilation of the external urethral sphincter was reported by Werbrouck and colleagues (1990). Using balloon dilation to No. 90 Fr at 3 atm, Chancellor and associates (1994) compared balloon dilation (20 patients), sphincterotomy (15), and stent placement (26) (see below) in the treatment of striated sphincter dyssynergia. A significant decrease in detrusor leak point pressure and residual urine occurred in all three groups. Bladder capacity remained constant and, renal function stabilized or improved; autonomic hyperreflexia likewise improved. Balloon dilation and stent placement were associated with a significantly shorter surgery and hospitalization and less of a decrease in hemoglobin levels. In the dilation group, three developed recurrent obstruction (at 3, 8, and 12 months), one had bleeding requiring transfusion, and one developed a 1-cm bulbar stricture. In the sphincterotomy group there were two cases of bleeding requiring transfusion, two cases of stricture with obstruction, and one case of erectile dysfunction. In the stent group, three had migration requiring adjustment (one replaced, two with a second overlapping stent), and two developed bladder neck obstruction requiring transurethral incision.

Urethral Stent Prosthesis

Shah and co-workers (1990) suggested the use of a permanent urethral stent to bypass the sphincter area, drawing on the British experience with urethral stricture disease. Chancellor and Rivas (1995) report the multicenter North American data with the use of the Urolume stent in 153 patients at 15 centers. A significant decrease in detrusor leak pressure and residual urine volume occurred. Eighteen percent of patients required more than one procedure to adequately cover the sphincter with the prosthesis. Three months afterward, hyperplasia within the lumen was seen in 42 patients (33.3%). Of these, the ingrowth was labeled minor in 36, moderate in 5, and marked in 1. Ten devices were removed (7 for migration) and 7 were replaced. Thirteen patients developed bladder neck obstruction requiring treatment (4 with alpha blockers, 7 with incision, 2 with CIC). When removal was required (in 4) this was not a problem up to 12 months. Rivas and colleagues (1994) concluded that in comparison with sphincterotomy, a stent prosthesis is as effective, easier, less morbid, and less expensive. Long-term follow-up is necessary. The device is under consideration for approval by the Food and Drug Administration.

Pudendal Nerve Interruption

Relief of obstruction at the level of the striated sphincter can also be achieved by pudendal neurectomy, first described in 1899 by Rocket (Wein and Barrett, 1988). **This method is seldom used today because of the potential for undesirable effects consequent to even a unilateral nerve section.** Bilateral nerve section results in an extremely high rate of male impotence and may result in fecal and severe stress urinary incontinence. In the rare instance of usage, therapeutic assessment of the results of a block should certainly precede the formal procedure, which should be performed only unilaterally.

Circumventing the Problem

Intermittent catheterization, continuous catheterization, and conduit- and reservoir-type supravesical urinary diversion have already been discussed as methods of circumventing filling and storage failure. A similar discussion of each is applicable for emptying failure.

Acknowledgment

The author expresses his utmost appreciation to Rosemarie Larmer for her forbearance and expertise in typing and editing this chapter.

REFERENCES

Abrams P: Terodiline in clinical practice. Urology 1990; 36(suppl):60.

Akah PA: Tricyclic antidepressant inhibition of the electrical evoked responses of the rat urinary bladder strip—effect of variation in extracellular Ca concentration. Arch Int Pharmacodyn 1986; 284:231.

Amark P, Nergardh A: Influence of adrenergic agonists and antagonists on urethral pressure, bladder pressure and detrusor hyperactivity in children with myelodysplasia. Acta Pediatr Scand 1991; 80:824.

Andersson KE: Current concepts in the treatment of disorders of micturition. Drugs 1988; 35:477.

Andersson KE: Clinical pharmacology of potassium channel openers. Pharmacol Toxicol 1992; 70:244.

Andersson KE: Pharmacology of lower urinary tract smooth muscles and penile erectile tissues. Pharmacol Rev 1993; 45:253.

Andersson K, Ek A, Hedlund H, et al: Effects of prazosin on isolated human urethra and in patients with lower neuron lesions. Invest Urol 1981; 19:39.

Andersson KE, Hedlund H, Mansson W: Pharmacologic treatment of bladder hyperactivity after augmentation and substitution enterocystoplasty. Scand J Urol Nephrol 1992; 142(Suppl):42–46.

Andrews I: Bladder disorders in brain damage. *In* Rushton DN, ed: Handbook of Neuro-Urology. New York, Marcel Dekker, 1994, pp 253–279.

Appell RA: Injectables for urethral incompetence. World J Urol 1990; 8:208.

Appell RA: Voiding dysfunction and lumbar disc disorders. Prob Urol 1993; 7(1):35–40.

Arunabh MB, Badlani G: Urologic problems in cerebrovascular accidents. Probl Urol 1993; 7(1):41–53.

Asplund R, Oberg H: Desmopressin in elderly subjects with increased nocturnal diuresis: A two month treatment study. Scand J Urol Nephrol 1993; 27:77.

Awad SA: Clinical use of bethanechol. J Urol 1985; 134:523.

Awad SA, Bryniak S, Downie JW, Bruce AW: The treatment of the uninhibited bladder with dicyclomine. J Urol 1977; 117:161.

Awad S, Downie J, Kiruluta H: Alpha adrenergic agents in urinary disorders of the proximal urethra. I: Stress incontinence. Br J Urol 1978; 50:332.

Baggioni I, Onrot J, Stewart CK, Robertson D: The potent pressor effect of phenylpropanolamine in patients with autonomic impairment. JAMA 1987; 258:236.

Baldessarini RJ: Drugs and the treatment of psychiatric disorders. *In* Gilman AG, Rall TW, Nies AS, Taylor P, eds. Goodman and Gilman's The Pharmacological Basis of Therapeutics, 8th ed. New York, Pergamon Press, 1990, pp 383–435.

Barnes DG, Shaw PJR, Timoney AG, Tsokos N: Management of the neuropathic bladder by suprapubic catheterization. Br J Urol 1993; 72:169.

Barnes JC, Harrison G, Murray K: Low pressure/low flow voiding in younger men: Psychological aspects. Br J Urol 1985; 57:414.

Barrett DM: The effects of oral bethanechol chloride on voiding in female patients with excessive residual urine: A randomized double-blind study. J Urol 1981; 126:640.

Barrett D, Wein AJ: Voiding dysfunction: Diagnosis, classification and management. *In* Gillenwater JY, Grayhack JT, Howards SS, Duckett JW, eds: Adult and Pediatric Urology, 2nd ed. St Louis, Mosby–Year Book Medical Publishers, 1991, pp 1001–1099.

Bates CP, Arnold EP, Griffiths DJ: The nature of the abnormality in bladder neck obstruction. Br J Urol 1975; 47:651.

Beck RP, Amausch T, King C: Results in testing 210 patients with detrusor overactivity incontinence of urine. Am J Obstet Gynecol 1976; 125: 593.

Beck R, Fowler CJ, Mathias CJ: Genitourinary dysfunction in disorders of the autonomic nervous system. *In* Rushton DN, ed: Handbook of Neuro-Urology. New York, Marcel Dekker, 1994, pp 281–301.

Bemelmans B, Hommes O, VanKerrebroeck P, et al: Evidence for early lower urinary tract dysfunction in clinically silent multiple sclerosis. J Urol 1991; 145:1219.

Bennett CJ, Seager SW, Vasker EA, McGuire EJ: Sexual dysfunction and electroejaculation in men with spinal cord injury: A review. J Urol 1988; 139:453.

Bent AE, Sand PK, Ostergard DR, Brubaker CT: Transvaginal electrical stimulation in the treatment of genuine stress incontinence and detrusor instability. Int Urogynecol J 1993; 4:9.

Berg S: Polytef augmentation urethroplasty. Arch Surg 1973; 107:379.

Berger Y, Salinas J, Blaivas J: Urodynamic differentiation of Parkinson disease and the Shy-Drager syndrome. Neurourol Urodynam 1990; 9: 117.

Beric A, Light JK: Function of the conus medullaris and cauda equina in the early period following spinal cord injury and the relationship to recovery of detrusor function. J Urol 1992; 148:1845.

Beyer et al (p. 11)

Bickel A, Culkin DJ, Wheeler JS Jr: Bladder cancer in spinal cord injury patients. J Urol 1991; 146:1240.

Binard JE, Persky L, DeLeary G, et al: Penoplasty for receding phallus: A new surgical technique to prevent dislodging of external collecting device. J Am Paraplegia Soc 1993; 16:204.

Binnie N, Creasey G, Edmond P, Smith A: The action of cisapride on the chronic constipation of paraplegia. Paraplegia 1988; 26:151.

Blackburn GL, Morgan JP, Lavin PT, et al: Determinants of the pressor effect of phenylpropanolamine in healthy subjects. JAMA 1989; 261:3267.

Blackford HN, Murray K, Stephenson TP, Mundy AR: Results of transvesical infiltration of the pelvic plexuses with phenol in 116 patients. Br J Urol 1984; 56:647.

Blaivas JG: The neurophysiology of micturition: A clinical study of 550 patients. J Urol 1982; 127:958.

Blaivas JG: Non-traumatic neurogenic voiding dysfunction in the adult. AUA Update Series 1985; 4:1–15.

Blaivas JG, Kaplan SA: Urologic dysfunction in patients with multiple sclerosis. Semin Urol 1988; 8:159.

Blaivas JG, Sinha HP, Zayed AA, Labib KB: Detrusor sphincter dyssynergia. J Urol 1981; 125:541.

Bloom FE: Neurohumoral transmission and the central nervous system. *In* Gilman AG, Rall TW, Nies AS, Taylor P, eds: Goodman and Gilman's The Pharmacological Basis of Therapeutics, 8th ed. New York, Pergamon Press, 1990, pp 244–268.

Bors E, Comarr, AE: Neurological Urology. Baltimore, University Park Press, 1971.

Briggs RS, Casteleden CM, Asher MJ: The effect of flavoxate on uninhibited detrusor contractions and urinary incontinence in the elderly. J Urol 1980; 123:656.

Brindley GS: Control of the bladder and urethral sphincters by surgically implanted electrical stimulation. *In* Chisholm GD, Fair WB, eds: Scientific Foundations of Urology. Chicago, Year Book Medical Publishers, 1990, pp 336–339.

Brindley GS: History of the sacral anterior root stimulator, 1969–1982. Neurourol Urodyn 1993; 12:481.

Brindley GS: Electrical stimulation in vesico-urethral dysfunction: General principles; practical devices. *In* Mundy AR, Stephenson TP, Wein AJ, eds: Urodynamics: Principles, Practice, Application. London, Churchill Livingstone, 1994a, pp 481–488, 489–493.

Brindley GS: The first 500 patients with sacral anterior root implants: General description. Paraplegia 1994b; 32:795.

Broecker BH, Klein FA, Hackler RH: Cancer of the bladder in spinal cord injury patients. J Urol 1981; 125:196.

Broseta E, Osca JM, Moosa J, et al: Urological manifestations of herpes zoster. Eur Urol 1993; 24:244.

Brown JH: Atropine, scopolamine and related antimuscarinic drugs. *In* Gilman AG, Rall TW, Nies AS, Taylor P, eds: Goodman and Gilman's The Pharmacological Basis of Therapeutics, 8th ed. New York, Pergamon Press, 1990, pp 150–165.

Bukowski TP, Perlmutter AD: Reduction cystoplasty in the prune belly syndrome: A long term follow up. J Urol 1994; 152:2113.

Bultitude M, Hills N, Shuttleworth K: Clinical and experimental studies on the action of prostaglandins and their synthesis inhibitors on detrusor muscle in vitro and in vivo. Br J Urol 1976; 48:631.

Bushman W, Steers W, Meythaler J: Voiding dysfunction in patients with spastic paraplegia: Urodynamic evaluation and response to continuous intrathecal baclofen. Neurol Urodyn 1993; 12:163.

Calliste L, Lindskog M: Phenylpropanolamine in treatment of female stress urinary incontinence. Urology 1987; 30:398.

Cameron-Strange A, Millard RJ: Management of refractory detrusor instability with transvesical phenol injection. Br J Urol 1988; 62:323.

Carone R, Vercella D, Bertapelli P: Effects of cisapride on anorectal and vesicourethral function in spinal cord injured patients. Paraplegia 1993; 31:125.

Carpiniello VL, Cendron M, Altman HG, et al: Treatment of urinary complications after total joint replacement in elderly females. Urology 1988; 32:186.

Casteleden CM, George CF, Renwick AG, Asher MJ: Imipramine—a possible alternative to current therapy for urinary incontinence in the elderly. J Urol 1981; 125:218.

Castelden CM, Morgan B: The effect of beta adrenoceptor agonists on urinary incontinence in the elderly. Br J Clin Pharmacol 1980; 10:619.

Cataldo PA, Senagore AJ: Does alpha sympathetic blockade prevent urinary retention following anorectal surgery? Dis Colon Rectum 1991; 34: 1113.

Cedarbaum JM, Schleifer LS: Drugs for Parkinson's disease, spasticity, and acute muscle spasms. *In* Gilman AG, Rall TW, Nies AS, Taylor P, eds: Goodman and Gilman's The Pharmacological Basis of Therapeutics, 8th ed. New York, Pergamon Press, 1990, pp 463–484.

Chancellor MB, Blaivas, JG: Multiple sclerosis. Prob Urol 1993; 7(1):15–33.

Chancellor MB, Erhard JM, Hirsch IH, Stass WE Jr: Prospective evaluation of terazosin for the treatment of autonomic dysreflexia. J Urol 1994; 151:111.

Chancellor MB, Erhard MJ, Kilholma P, et al: Functional urethral closure with pubovaginal sling for destroyed female urethra after long term catheterization. Urology 1994; 43:499.

Chancellor MB, Erhard MJ, Rivas DA: Clinical effect of alpha-1 antagonism by terazosin on external and internal urinary sphincter function. J Am Parapl Soc 1994; 16:207.

Chancellor MB, McGinnis DE, Sherot PJ, et al: Urinary dysfunction in lyme disease. J Urol 1993; 149:26.

Chancellor MB, Rivas DA: Current management of detrusor-sphincter dyssynergia. Urol 1995; (8):291–324.

Chao R, Clowers D, Mayo ME: Fate of upper tracts in patients with indwelling catheter after spinal cord injury. Urology 1993; 42:259.

Chapple CR, Parkhouse H, Gardener C, Mulroy EJG: Double blind, placebo controlled, crossover study of flavoxate in the treatment of idiopathic detrusor instability. Br J Urol 1990; 66:491.

Chapple CR, Hampson SJ, Turner-Warwick RT, Worth PHL: Subtrigonal phenol ingestion. How safe and effective is it? Br J Urol 1991; 68:483.

Christmas TJ, Chapple CR, Lees AJ, et al: Role of subcutaneous apomorphine in Parkinsonism voiding dysfunction. Lancet 1988; 2:1451.

Clark CMJ, Lee DA: Prevention and treatment of the complications of diabetes mellitus. N Engl J Med 1995; 332:1210.

Cole A, Fried F: Favorable experiences with imipramine in the treatment of neurogenic bladder. J Urol 1972; 107:44.

Connolly MJ, Astridge PS, White EG, et al: Torsade de pointes ventricular tachycardia and terodilene. Lancet 1991; 338:344.

Craft RM, Porreca F: Treatment parameters of desensitization to capsaicin. Life Sci 1992; 51:1767.

Davidoff RA: Antispasticity drugs: Mechanisms of action. Ann Neurol 1985; 17:107.

Decter RM, Snyder P, Laudermilch C: Transurethral electrical bladder stimulation: A follow up report. J Urol 1994; 152:812.

Deen HG, Zimmerman RS, Swanson SK, Larson TR: Assessment of bladder function after lumbar decompressive laminectomy for spinal stenosis: A prospective study. J Neurosurg 1994; 80:971.

DeGroat WC: Anatomy and physiology of the lower urinary tract. Urol Clin North Am 1993; 20:383–401.

DeGroat WC, Booth AM: Autonomic systems to the urinary bladder and sexual organs. *In* Dyck PJ, Thomas PK, Lambert EH, et al, eds: Peripheral Neuropathy. Philadelphia, WB Saunders Company, 1984, pp 285–299.

DeGroat WC, Booth AM, Yoshimura N: Neurophysiology of micturition and its modification in animal models of human disease. *In* Maggi CA, ed: The Autonomic Nervous System, vol 3. London, Harwood Academic Publishers, 1993, pp 227–290.

Delaere KPJ, Thomas CMG, Moonen WA, Debruyne FMJ: The value of intravesical prostaglandin F_{2alpha} and E_2 in women with abnormalities of bladder emptying. Br J Urol 1981; 53:306.

Desmond A, Bultitude M, Hills N, Shuttleworth KED: Clinical experience with intravesical prostaglandin E_2: A prospective study of 36 patients. Br J Urol 1980; 53:357.

Dewire DM, Owns RS, Anderson GA, et al: A comparison of the urological complications associated with long term management of quadriplegics with and without chronic indwelling urinary catheters. J Urol 1992; 147:1069.

Dijkema HE, Wein EH, Mijs PT, Janknegt RA: Neuromodulation of sacral nerves for incontinence and voiding dysfunction. Eur Urol 1993; 24: 72.

Diokno AC, Hollander JB, Bennett CJ: Bladder neck obstruction in females: A real entity. J Urol 1984; 132:294.

Diokno AC, Lapides J: Action of oral and parenteral bethanechol on decompensated bladder. Urology 1977; 10:23.

Diokno A, Taub M: Ephedrine in treatment of urinary incontinence. Urology 1975; 5:624.

Donker P, Van der Sluis C: Action of beta adrenergic blocking agents on the urethral pressure profile. Urol Int 1976; 31:6.

Douglas C, Burke B, Kessler OL, et al: Microwave: Practical cost effective method for sterilizing urinary catheters in the home. Urology 1990; 35:219.

Downie J: Bethanechol chloride in urology—A discussion of issues. Neurourol Urodyn 1984; 3:211.

Dray A: Mechanism of action of capsaicin like molecules on sensory neurons. Life Sci 1992; 51:1759.

Dykstra DD, Sidi AA: Treatment of detrusor–striated sphincter dyssynergia with botulinum A toxin. Arch Phys Med Rehabil 1990; 71:24.

Dykstra D, Sidi AA, Anderson LL: The effect of nifedipine on cystoscopy induced autonomic hyperreflexia in patients with high spinal cord injuries. J Urol 1987; 138:1155.

Eardley I, Fowler CJ, Nagendron K, et al: The neurourology of tropical spastic paraparesis. Br J Urol 1991; 68:598.

Ebner A, Jiang C, Lindstrom S: Intravesical electrical stimulation—An experimental analysis of its mechanism of action. J Urol 1992; 148: 920.

Eckford SB, Kohler-Ockmore J, Feneley RCL: Long term follow up of transvaginal urethral closure and suprapubic cystotomy for urinary incontinence in women with multiple sclerosis. Br J Urol 1994a; 74:319.

Eckford SD, Swami KS, Jackson SR, Abrams PH: Desmopressin in the treatment of nocturia and enuresis in patients with multiple sclerosis. Br J Urol 1994b; 74:733.

Ek A, Andersson KE, Gullberg B, Ulmster K: The effects of long term treatment with norephedrine on stress incontinence and urethral pressure profile. Scand J Urol Nephrol 1978; 12:105.

Eriksen BC, Bergmann S, Eik-Nes SH: Maximal electrical stimulation of the pelvic floor in female idiopathic detrusor instability and urge incontinence. Neurourol Urodynam 1989; 8:219.

Fall M, Madersbacher H: Peripheral electrical stimulation. *In* Mundy AR, Stephenson TP, Wein AJ, eds: Urodynamics: Principles, Practice, Application. London, Churchill Livingtone, 1994, pp 495–520.

Fam B, Yalla SV: Vesicourethral dysfunction in spinal cord injury and its management. Semin Neurol 1988; 8:150.

Farrell SA, Webster RD, Higgins LM, Steeves RA: Duration of postoperative catheterization: A randomized double-blind trial comparing two catheter management protocols and the effect of bethanechol chloride. Int Urogynecol J 1990; 1:132.

Fellenius E, Hedberg R, Holmberg E, et al: Functional and metabolic effects of terbutaline and propranolol in fast and slow contracting skeletal muscle in vitro. Acta Physiol Scand 1980; 109:89.

Finkbeiner AE: Is bethanechol chloride clinically effective in promoting bladder emptying? A literature review. J Urol 1985; 134:443.

Fischer C, Diokno A, Lapides J: The anticholinergic effects of dicyclomine hydrochloride in uninhibited neurogenic bladder dysfunction. J Urol 1978; 120:328.

Florante J, Leyson J, Martin B, Sporer A: Baclofen in the treatment of detrusor sphincter dyssynergy in spinal cord injury patients. J Urol 1980; 124:82.

Foreman MM, McNulty AM: Alterations in K(+) evoked release of 3-H-norepinephrine and contractile responses in urethral and bladder tissues induced by norepinephrine reuptake inhibition. Life Sc 1993; 53:193.

Fovaeus M, Andersson KE, Hedlund H: The action of pinacidil in the isolated human bladder. J Urol 1989; 142:637.

Fowler CJ, Beck RO, Gerrard S, et al: Intravesical capsaicin for treatment of detrusor hyperreflexia. J Neurol Neurosurg Psychiatry 1994; 57:169.

Fowler CJ, Betts C, Christmas T, et al: Botulinum toxin in the treatment of chronic urinary retention in women. Br J Urol 1992; 70:387.

Frimodt-Moller C: Diabetes cystopathy: I. A clinical study on the frequency of bladder dysfunction in diabetics. Dan Med Bull 1976; 23:267.

Gajewski J, Downie J, Awad S: Experimental evidence for a central nervous system site of action in the effect of alpha adrenergic blockers on the external urethral sphincter. J Urol 1984; 133:403.

Galeano C, Jubelin B, Biron L, Guenette L: Effect of naloxone on detrusor-sphincter dyssynergia in chronic spinal cat. Neurol Urodyn 1986; 5:203.

Galloway NTM: Classification and diagnosis of neurogenic bladder dysfunction. Probl Urol 1989; 3:1.

Gasparini ME, Schmidt RA, Tanagho EA: Selective sacral rhizotomy in the management of the reflex neuropathic bladder: A report on 17 patients with long term follow up. J Urol 1992; 148:1207.

Geirsson G, Want YH, Lindstrom S, Fall M: Traditional acupuncture and electrical stimulation of the posterior tibial nerve. Scand J Urol Nephrol 1993; 27:67.

George NJR, Slade N: Hesitancy and poor stream in younger men without outflow tract obstruction—the anxious bladder. Br J Urol 1979; 51:506.

Gilja I, Radej M, Kovacic M, Parazajades J: Conservative treatment of female stresses incontinence with imipramine. J Urol 1984; 132:909.

Glahn BE: Neurogenic bladder in spinal cord injury: Management of patients. Urol Clin North Am 1974; 1:163.

Gleason D, Reilly R, Bottaccini M, Pierce MJ: The urethral continence zone and its relation to stress incontinence. J Urol 1974; 112:81.

Goldman G, Kahn PJ, Kashton H, et al: Prevention and treatment of urinary retention and infection after surgical treatment of the colon and rectum with alpha adrenergic blockers. Surg Gynecol Obstet 1988; 166:447.

Golji H: Complications of external condom drainage. Paraplegia 1981; 19:189.

Graham C: Making a catheterization program work in patients with functional limitations. Probl Urol 1989; 3:54.

Grainger R, O'Flynn JD, Fitzpatrick JM: Urological follow up of 124 women following spinal cord injury. World J Urol 1990; 7:212.

Greene LF, Ghosh MK, Howard FM: Transurethral prostatic resection in patients with myasthenia gravis. J Urol 1974; 112:226.

Gruneberger A: Treatment of motor urge incontinence with clenbuterol and flavoxate hydrochloride. Br J Obstet Gynecol 1984; 91:275.

Hachen H: Clinical and urodynamic assessment of alpha adrenolytic therapy in patients with neurogenic bladder function. Paraplegia 1980; 18:229.

Hachen H, Krucker V: Clinical and laboratory assessment of the efficacy of baclofen on urethral sphincter spasticity in patients with traumatic paraplegia. Eur Urol 1977; 3:237.

Hackler R: A 25 year prospective mortality in the spinal cord injury patient: Comparison with the long term living paraplegia. J Urol 1977; 117: 486.

Hackler RH: Long term suprapubic cystotomy in spinal cord injury patients. Br J Urol 1982; 54:120.

Hackler R, Broecker B, Klein F, Brady S: A clinical experience with dantrolene sodium for external urinary sphincter hypertonicity in spinal cord injured patients. J Urol 1980; 124:78.

Hackler RH, Dillon JJ, Bunk RC: Changing concepts on the preservation of renal function in the paraplegic. J Urol 1965; 94; 107.

Hanna MK: New concept in bladder remodeling. Urology 1982; 19:6.

Hanno AEG, Atta MA, Elbadawi A: Intrinsic neuromuscular defects in the neurogenic bladder. IX: Effects of combined parasympathetic decentralization and hypogastric neurectomy on neuromuscular ultrastructure of the feline bladder base. Neurourol Urodynam 1988; 7:93.

Harris JD, Benson GS: Effect of dantrolene on canine bladder contractility. Urology 1980; 16:229.

Hartung HP, Pollard JD, Harvey GK, Toykaku C: Immunopathogenesis and treatment of the Guillain-Barré syndrome—Parts 1 and 2. Muscle Nerve 1995; 18:137, 154.

Hattori T, Yasuda K, Kitak K, Hirayama K: Disorders of micturition on tabes dorsalis. Br J Urol 1990; 65:497.

Hedlund H, Mattiasson A, Andersson KE: Lack of effect of pinacidil on detrusor instability in men with bladder outlet obstruction. J Urol 1990; 143:369A.

Hehir M. Fitzpatrick JM: Oxybutynin and the prevention of urinary incontinence in spina bifida. Eur Urol 1985; 11:254.

Hinman F Jr: Non-neurogenic neurogenic bladder (the Hinman syndrome)—15 years later. J Urol 1986; 136:769.

Hoffman BB, Lefkowitz RJ: Adrenergic receptor antagonists. *In* Gilman AG, Rall TW, Nies AS, Taylor P, eds: Goodman and Gilman's The Pharmacological Basis of Therapeutics, 8th ed. New York, Pergamon Press, 1990, pp 221–243.

Husmann DA: Occult spinal dysraphism (the tethered cord) and the urologist. AUA Update Series 1995; 14:78–83.

Ingleman-Sundberg A: Partial denervation of the bladder. A new method for the treatment of urge incontinence and similar conditions in women. Acta Gynecol Scand 1959; 38:487–502.

Jacobs SC, Kaufman JM: Complications of permanent bladder catheter drainage in spinal cord injury patients. J Urol 1978; 119:740.

Jackson AB, DeVivo M: Urological long term follow up in women with spinal cord injuries. Arch Phys Med Rehabil 1992; 73:1029.

Jakobsen H, Holm BM, Hald T: Neurogenic bladder dysfunction in sacral agenesis and dysgenesis. Neurourul Urodynam 1985; 4:99.

Jensen D Jr: Pharmacological studies of the uninhibited neurogenic bladder. Acta Neurol Scand 1981a; 64:175.

Jensen D Jr: Altered adrenergic innervation in the uninhibited neurogenic bladder. Scand J Urol Nephrol 1981b; 60:61.

Jensen D Jr: Uninhibited neurogenic bladder treated with prazosin. Scand J Urol Nephrol 1981c; 15:229.

Jeter KF: Managing intractable urinary incontinence with absorbent products, devices, and procedures. Probl Urol 1990; 4:124.

Jeter KF, ed: Resource Guide of Incontinence Products and Service. Union, SC, Help for Incontinent People (HIP) (PO Box 544), 1995.

Jonas U, Petri E, Kissal J: The effect of flavoxate on hyperactive detrusor muscle. Eur Urol 1979; 5:106.

Jorgensen L, Mortensen SO, Colstrup H, Andersen JT: Bladder distention in the management of detrusor instability. Scand J Urol Nephrol 1985; 19:101.

Jorgensen TM, Djurhuus JC, Schroder HD: Idiopathic detrusor sphincter dyssynergia in neurologically normal patients with voiding abnormalities. Eur Urol 1982; 8:107.

Kaisary AU: Beta adrenoceptor blockade in the treatment of female stress urinary incontinence. J Urol (Paris) 1984; 90:351.

Kaplan SA, Blaivas JG: Diabetic cystopathy. J Diabetes Complications 1988; 2:133.

Kaplan SA, Chancellor MB, Blaivas JG: Bladder and sphincter behavior in patients with spinal cord lesions. J Urol 1991; 146:113.

Kaplan SA, Te A: Bladder dysfunction in diabetes. Probl Urol 1992; 6(4):659–668.

Kaplan WE, McLone DG, Richards I: The urological manifestations of the tethered spinal cord. J Urol 1988; 140:1285.

Kaplan WE, Richards I: Intravesical bladder stimulation in myelodysplasia. J Urol 1988; 140:1282.

Kaplan WE, Richards TW, Richards I: Intravesical transurethral bladder stimulation to increase bladder capacity. J Urol 1989; 142:600.

Kaufman JM, Fam B, Jacobs SC, et al: Bladder cancer and squamous metaplasia in spinal cord injury patients. J Urol 1977; 118:967.

Khan Z, Bhola A: Urinary incontinence after transurethral resection of prostate in myasthenia gravis patients. Urology 1989; 34:168.

Khan Z, Singh V, Yang WL: Neurogenic bladder in acquired immune deficiency syndrome. Urology 1992; 40:289.

Khan Z, Starer P, Yang WC, Bhola A: Analysis of voiding disorders in patients with cerebrovascular accidents. Urology 1990; 32:256.

Kiesswetter H, Schober W: Lioresal in the treatment of neurogenic bladder dysfunction. Urol Int 1975; 30:63.

Kim YS, Sainz RD: Beta-adrenergic agonists and hypertrophy of skeletal muscles. Life Sci 1992; 50:397.

Kinn, AC: The lazy bladder—Appraisal of surgical reduction. Scand J Urol Nephrol 1985; 19:93.

Kinn AC, Larsson PO: Desmopressin: A new principle for symptomatic treatment of urgency and incontinence in patients with multiple sclerosis. Scand J Urol Nephrol 1990; 24:109.

Kirby R: Non-traumatic neurogenic bladder dysfunction. *In* Mundy AR, Stephenson TP, Wein AJ, eds: Urodynamics: Principles, Practice, Application. London, Churchill Livingstone, 1994, pp 365–373.

Kirby R, Fowler R, Gosling J, Bannister R: Urethrovesical dysfunction in progressive autonomic failure with multiple system atrophy. J Neurol Neurosurg Psychiatry 1986; 49:554.

Kishimoto T, Morita T, Okamiya Y: Effect of clenbuterol on contractile response in periurethral striated muscle of rabbits. Tohoku J Exp Med 1991; 165:243.

Klarskov P, Holm-Bentzen M, Larsen S, et al: Partial cystectomy for the myogenous decompensated bladder with excessive residual urine. Scand J Urol Nephrol 1988; 22:251.

Koldewijn E, Van Kerrebroeck PEV, Rosier PF, et al: Bladder compliance after posterior sacral root rhizotomies and anterior sacral root stimulation. J Urol 1994; 151:955.

Koldewijn EK, Rosier PF, Meuleman JH, et al: Predictors of success with neuromodulation in lower urinary tract dysfunction: Results of trial stimulation in 100 patients. J Urol 1994; 152:2071.

Koonings P, Bergman A, Ballard CA: Prostaglandins for enhancing detrusor function after surgery for stress incontinence in women. J Reprod Med 1990; 35:1.

Korczyn AD, Kish I: The mechanism of imipramine in enuresis nocturna. Clin Exp Pharmacol Physiol 1979; 6:31.

Koyanagi T, Morita H, Taniguchi K, et al: Neurogenic urethra: Clinical relevance of isolated neuropathic dysfunction of the urethra and the denervation supersensitivity of the urethra revisited. Eur Urol 1988; 15:77.

Krane R, Olsson C: Phenoxybenzamine in neurogenic bladder dysfunction: I. A theory of micturition. J Urol 1973; 110:650.

Kums JJM, Delhaas EM: Intrathecal baclofen infusion in patients with spasticity and neurogenic bladder disease. World J Urol 1991; 9:99.

Lader M: Clinical pharmacology of benzodiazepines. Ann Rev Med 1987; 38:19.

Lapides J, Diokno A, Silber S, Lowe B: Clean intermittent self-catheterization in the treatment of urinary tract disease. J Urol 1972; 107:458.

Lau W, Szilagyi M: A pharmacological profile of glycopyrrolate: Interactions at the muscarinic acetylcholine receptor. Gen Pharmacol 1992; 23:1165.

Laubser PG, Narayan RK, Sadin KJ: Continuous infusion of intrathecal baclofen: Long term effects on spasticity in spinal cord injury. Paraplegia 1991; 29:48.

Leach, GE, Bavendam TG: Prospective evaluation of the Inconton transrectal stimulator in women with urinary incontinence. Neurourol Urodynam 1989; 8:231.

Leach GE, Farsaii A, Kark P, Raz S: Urodynamic manifestations of cerebellar ataxia. J Urol 1982; 128:348.

Leadbetter GW Jr: Surgical reconstruction for complete urinary incontinence: A 10 to 22 year follow up. J Urol 1985; 133:205.

Lepor H: Role of long acting selective alpha-1 blockers in the treatment of benign prostatic hyperplasia. Urol Clin North Am 1990; 17:651.

Levin RM, Scheiner S, Zhao Y, Wein AJ: The effect of terodiline on hyperreflexia (in vitro) and the in vitro response of isolated strips of rabbit bladder to field stimulation, bethanechol and KCl. Pharmacology 1993; 46:346.

Levin RM, Staskin D, Wein AJ: The muscarinic cholinergic binding kinetics of the human urinary bladder. Neurourol Urodyn 1982; 1:221.

Levin RM, Staskin DR, Wein AJ: Analysis of the anticholinergic and musculotropic effects of desmethylimipramine on the rabbit urinary bladder. Urol Res 1983; 11:259.

Levin RM, Wein AJ: Comparative effects of five tricyclic compounds on the rabbit urinary bladder. Neurourol Urodyn 1984; 3:127.

Levy JB, Jacobs JA, Wein AJ: Combined abdominal and vaginal approach for bladder neck closure and permanent suprapubic tube: Urinary diversion in the neurologically impaired woman. J Urol 1994; 152:2081.

Liebson I, Bigelow G, Griffiths RR, Funderbuck M: Phenylpropanolamine: Effects on subjective and cardiovascular variables at recommended over-the-counter dose levels. J Clin Pharmacol 1987; 27:685.

Light JK, Faganel J, Beric A: Detrusor areflexia in supraspinal spinal cord injuries. J Urol 1985; 134:295.

Lindan R, Leffler EJ, Bodner D: Urological problems in the management of quadriplegic women. Paraplegia 1987; 25:381.

Lindholm P, Lose G: Terbutaline (Bricanyl) in the treatment of female urge incontinence. Urol Int 1986; 41:158.

Linsenmayer TA, Perkash I: Infertility in men with spinal cord injury. Arch Phys Med Rehabil 1991; 72:747.

Lloyd LK, Kuhlemeier LV, Fine PR, Stover SL: Initial bladder management in spinal cord injury: Does it make a difference? J Urol 1986; 135:523.

Lloyd SN, Lloyd SM, Rogers K, et al: Is there still a place for prolonged bladder distention? Br J Urol 1992; 70:382.

Locke JR, Hall DE, Walzer Y: Incidence of squamous cell carcinoma in patients with long term catheter drainage. J Urol 1985; 133:1034.

Lockhart JL, Pow-Sang JM: Indications and problems with external urethral sphincterotomy. Probl Urol 1989; 3:44.

Lose G, Jorgensen L, Thunedborg P: Doxepin in the treatment of female detrusor overactivity: A randomized double-blind crossover study. J Urol 1989; 142:1024.

Lose G, Lindholm D: Clinical and urodynamic effects of norfenefrine in women with stress incontinence. Urol Int 1984; 39:298.

Lucas MG, Thomas DG: Endoscopic bladder transection for detrusor instability. Br J Urol 1987; 59:526.

Lyne CJ, Bellinger MF: Early experience with transurethral electrical bladder stimulation. J Urol 1993; 150:697.

Madersbacher H: Neurostimulation for functional (neurogenic) detrusor and sphincter dysfunction. Eur Urol Update Series 1993; 21(13):98.

Madersbacher H, Fischer J: Sacral anterior root stimulation: Prerequisites and indications. Neurourol Urodyn 1993; 12:489.

Madersbacher H, Jilg G: Control of detrusor hyperreflexia by the intravesical instillation of oxybutynin hydrochloride. Paraplegia 1991; 29:84.

Madersbacher H, Scott FB: Twelve o'clock sphincterotomy. Urol Int 1975; 30:75.

Maggi CA: Capsaicin and primary afferent neurons: From basic science to human therapy? J Auton Nerv Syst 1991; 33:1.

Maggi CA: Therapeutic potential of capsaicin-like molecules. Life Sci 1992; 51:1777.

Mahony D, Laferte F, Mahoney J: Observations on sphincter augmenting effect of imipramine in children with urinary incontinence. Urology 1973; 2:317.

Malkowicz SB, Wein AJ, Ruggieri MR, Levin RM: Comparison of calcium antagonist properties of antispasmodic agents. J Urol 1987; 138:667.

Malmgren A, Andersson KE, Fovaeus M, Sjogren C: Effects of cromakalim and pinacidil on normal and hypertrophied rat detrusor in vitro. J Urol 1990; 143:828.

Marsden C: Parkinson's disease. Lancet 1990; 335:948.

Mayo ME: Lower urinary tract dysfunction in cerebral palsy. J Urol 1992; 147:419.

Mayo ME, Chetner MP: Lower urinary tract dysfunction in multiple sclerosis. Urology 1992; 39:67.

McGuire EJ: Clinical evaluation and treatment of neurogenic vesical dysfunction. *In* Libertino J, ed: International Perspectives in Urology, vol 11. Baltimore, Williams & Wilkins Company, 1984.

McGuire EJ, Appell RA: Transurethral collagen injection for urinary incontinence. Urology 1994; 43:413.

McGuire EJ, Denil J: Adult myelodysplasia. AUA Update Series 1991; 10(Lesson 38):298–303.

McGuire E, Savastano JA: Urodynamic findings and clinical status following vesical denervation procedures for control of continence. J Urol 1984; 132:87.

McGuire E, Savastano J: Effect of alpha adrenergic blockade and anticholinergic agents on the decentralized primate bladder. Neurourol Urodyn 1985; 4:139.

McGuire EJ, Savastano J: Comparative urological outcome in women with spinal cord injury. J Urol 1986; 135:730.

McGuire EJ, Shi-Chun Z, Horwinski ER: Treatment for motor and sensory detrusor instability by electrical stimulation. J Urol 1983; 129:78.

Michelson JD, Lotke PA, Steinberg ME: Urinary bladder management after total joint replacement surgery. N Engl J Med 1988; 319:321.

Milanov IG: Mechanisms of baclofen action on spasticity. Acta Neurol Scand 1991; 85:305.

Mitchell WC, Venable DD: Effects of metoclopromide on detrusor function. J Urol 1985; 134:791.

Mobley D: Phenoxybenzamine in the management of neurogenic vesical dysfunction. J Urol 1976; 116:737.

Moisey C, Stephenson T, Brendler C: The urodynamic and subjective results of treatment of detrusor instability with oxybutynin chloride. Br J Urol 1980; 52:472.

Mundy AR: Pelvic plexus injury. *In* Mundy AR, Stephenson TP, Wein AJ, eds: Urodynamics: Principles, Practice, Application. London, Churchill Livingstone, 1984, pp 273–277.

Mundy AR: The surgical treatment of detrusor instability. Neurourol Urodynam 1985; 4:357.

Murdock M, Sax D, Krane R: Use of dantrolene sodium in external sphincter spasm. Urology 1976; 8:133.

Murray KHA, Feneley RCL: Endorphins, a role in urinary tract function? The effect of opioid blockade on the detrusor and urethral sphincter mechanisms. Br J Urol 1982; 54:638.

Naglo AS, Nergardh A, Boreus LO: Influence of atropine and isoprenaline on detrusor hyperactivity in children with neurogenic bladder. Scand J Urol Nephrol 1981; 15:97.

Nanninga JB, Frost F, Penn R: Effect of intrathecal baclofen on bladder and sphincter function. J Urol 1989; 142:101.

Nanninga J, Kaplan P, Lal S: Effect of phentolamine on peripheral muscle EMG activity in paraplegia. Br J Urol 1977; 49:537.

Nestler JE, Stratton MA, Hakin CA: Effect of metoclopromide on diabetic neurogenic bladder. Clin Pharmacol 1983; 2:83.

Noble JG, Lemieux MC, Fowler CJ: Non-urological obstructed voiding and retention. *In* Rushton DN, ed. Handbook of Neuro-Urology. New York, Marcel Dekker, 1994, pp 209–231.

Nordling J, Meyhoff H, Hald T: Urethral denervation supersensitivity to noradrenaline after radical hysterectomy. Scand J Urol Nephrol 1981a; 15:21.

Nordling J, Meyhoff H, Hald T: Sympatholytic effect on striated urethral sphincter. A peripheral or central nervous system effect? Scand J Urol Nephrol 1981b; 15:173.

Norgaard JP, Rillig S, Djurhuus JC: Nocturnal enuresis: An approach to treatment based on pathogenesis. J Pediatr 1989; 114:705.

Norlen L: Influence of the sympathetic nervous system on the lower urinary tract and its clinical implications. Neurourol Urodynam 1982; 1:129.

Norlen LJ, Blaivas JG: Unsuspected proximal urethral obstruction in young and middle-aged men. J Urol 1986; 135:972.

Norlen L, Sundin T, Waagstein F: Beta-adrenoceptor stimulation of the human urinary bladder in vivo. Acta Pharmacol Toxicol 1978; 43:5.

Norton P, Karrom M, Wall LL, et al: Randomized double blind trial of terodiline in the treatment of urge incontinence in women. Obstet Gynecol 1994; 84:386.

Nurse D, Restorick J, Mundy A: The effect of cromkalim on the normal and hyperreflexic human detrusor muscle. Br J Urol 1991; 68:27.

Obrink A, Bunne G: The effect of alpha adrenergic stimulation in stress incontinence. Scand J Urol Nephrol 1978; 12:205.

O'Donnell P, Hawkins WH: Effects of subcutaneous bethanechol on bladder sensation during cystometry. Urology 1993; 41:452.

O'Flynn KJ, Murphy R, Thomas DG: Neurogenic bladder dysfunction in lumbar intervertebral disc prolapse. Br J Urol 1992; 69:38.

Ohlsson BL, Fall M, Frankenberg-Sommars D: Effects of external and direct pudendal nerve maximal electrical stimulation in the treatment of the uninhibited overactive bladder. Br J Urol 1989; 64:374.

Olubadewo J: The effect of imipramine on rat detrusor muscle contractility. Arch Int Pharmacodyn Ther 1980; 145:84.

Opitz JL: Treatment of voiding dysfunction in spinal cord injured patients. *In* Barrett DM, Wein AJ, eds: Controversies in Neuro-Urology. New York, Churchill Livingstone, 1984, pp 437–452.

Ouslander JG: Effects of terodilene on urinary incontinence among older non-institutionalized women. J Am Geriatric Soc 1993; 41:915.

Parsons KF, Macher DG, Woolfender ICA, et al: Endoscopic bladder transection. Br J Urol 1984; 56:625.

Parys B, Haylen B, Hutton J, Parsons K: The effects of simple hysterectomy on vesicourethral function. Br J Urol 1989; 64:594.

Pedersen PA, Johansen PB: Prophylactic treatment of adult nocturia with bumetanide. Br J Urol 1988; 62:145.

Penn RD, Savoy SM, Corcos D: Intrathecal baclofen for severe spinal spasticity. Engl J Med 1989; 320:1517.

Perkash I: Intermittent catheterization and bladder rehabilitation in spinal cord injury patients. J Urol 1975; 114:230.

Perlberg S, Caine M: Adrenergic response of bladder muscle in prostatic obstruction. Urology 1982; 10:524.

Peters D, Multicentre Study Group: Terodiline in the treatment of urinary frequency and motor urge incontinence, a controlled multicentre trial. Scand J Urol Nephrol 1984; 87(suppl):21.

Petersen MS, Collins DN, Selakovich WG, Finkbeiner AE: Postoperative urinary retention associated with total hip and knee arthroplasties. Clin Orthop Rel Research 1991; 269:102.

Petersen T, Just-Christensen JE, Kousgaard P, et al: Anal sphincter maximum functional stimulation in detrusor hyeprreflexia. J Urol 1994; 152:1460.

Peterson JS, Patton AJ, Noronha-Blob L: Mini-pig urinary bladder function: Comparisons of in vitro anticholinergic responses and in vivo cystometry with drugs indicated for urinary incontinence. J Auton Pharmacol 1990; 10:65.

Philp T, Shaw P, Worth P: Acupuncture in the treatment of bladder instability. Br J Urol 1988; 61:490.

Physician's Desk Reference. Oradell, NJ, Medical Economics Co., 1995.

Poser CM: The epidemiology of multiple sclerosis: A general overview. Ann Neurol 1994; 36 (S2):S180.

Raezer DM, Benson GS, Wein AJ, et al: The functional approach to the management of the pediatric neuropathic bladder: A clinical study. J Urol 1977; 117:649.

Rall TW: Oxytocin, prostaglandins, ergot alkaloids and other drugs; toxolytic agents. *In* Gilman AG, Rall TW, Nies AS, Taylor P, eds: Goodman and Gilman's The Pharmacological Basis of Therapeutics, 8th ed. New York, Pergamon Press, 1990, pp 933–953.

Ramsden PD, Smith JC, Dunn M, Ardan GM: Distention therapy for the unstable bladder: Later results including an assessment of repeat distention. Br J Urol 1976; 48:623.

Raz S, Smith RB: External sphincter spasticity syndrome in female patients. J Urol 1976; 115:443.

Reid CJD, Borzyskowski M: Lower urinary tract dysfunction in cerebral palsy. Arch Dis Child 1993; 68:739.

Rew DA, Rundle JSH: Assessment of the safety of regular DDAVP therapy on primary nocturnal enuresis. Br J Urol 1989; 63:352.

Richelson E: Pharmacology of antidepressants—Characteristics of the ideal drug. Mayo Clinic Proc 1994; 69:1069.

Rittig S, Knudsen UB, Jonter M, et al: Adult enuresis: The role of vasopressor and atrial natriuretic peptide. Scand J Urol Nephrol 1989; 125(suppl):79.

Rivas DA, Chancellor MB, Bagley D: Prospective comparison of external sphincter prosthesis and external sphincterotomy in men with spinal cord injury. J Endouro 1994; 8:89.

Rohner T, Hannigan J, Sanford E: Altered in vitro adrenergic responses of dog detrusor muscle after chronic bladder outlet obstruction. Urology 1978; 11:357.

Roy CW, Wakefield IR: Baclofen pseudopsychosis: Case report. Paraplegia 1986; 24:318.

Ryttov N, Aagaard J, Hertz J: Retention of urine in genital herpetic infection. Urol Int 1985; 40:22.

Sandre S, Fanciullacci F, Politi P, Zonallo A: Urinary disorders in intervertebral disc prolapse. Neurourol Urodynam 1987; 6:11.

Sant G: Intravesical 50% dimethylsulfoxide in the treatment of interstitial cystitis. Urology 1987; 4(Suppl):17.

Santarosa RP, Blaivas JG: Periurethral injection of autologous fat for the treatment of sphincteric incontinence. J Urol 1994; 151:607.

Santiago JA: Sphincterotomy failure. J Am Paraplegia Soc 1993; 16:164.

Schmidt R: Experience with neurostimulation in urology. Prob Urol 1989; 3(1):135:146.

Scott FB, Bradley W, Timm GW: Treatment of urinary incontinence by an implantable prosthetic urinary sphincter. J Urol 1974; 112:75.

Scott M, Morrow J: Phenoxybenzamine in neurogenic bladder dysfunction after spinal cord injury. I: Voiding dysfunction. J Urol 1978; 119:480.

Seager SW, Halstead LS: Fertility options and success after spinal cord injury. Urol Clin North Am 1993; 20:543–548.

Shader RI, Greenblatt DJ: Use of benzodiazepines in anxiety disorders. N Engl J Med 1993; 328:1398.

Shah PJR, Milroy EJ, Timoney AG, Elden A: Permanent external striated sphincter stents in spinal injured patients. Neurourol Urodynam 1990; 9:311.

Sislow JG, Mayo ME: Reduction of bladder wall compliance following decentralization. J Urol 1990; 144:945.

Sirls LT, Zimmern PE, Leach GE: Role of limited evaluation and aggressive medical management in multiple sclerosis: A review of 113 patients. J Urol 1994; 151:946.

Smith AY, Woodside JR: Urodynamic evaluation of patients with spinal stenosis. Urology 1988; 32:474.

Smith EM, Bodner DR: Sexual dysfunction after spinal cord injury. Urol Clin North Am 1993; 20:535–542.

Smith JC: The place of prolonged bladder distention in the treatment of bladder instability and other disorders. Br J Urol 1981; 53:283.

Sonda L, Gershon C, Diokno A: Further observations on the cystometric and uroflowmetric effects of bethanechol chloride on the human bladder. J Urol 1979; 122:775.

Sotolongo JR, Chancellor M: Parkinson's disease. Probl Urol 1993; 7(1):54–67.

Sporer A, Leyson J, Martin B: Effects of bethanechol chloride on the external urethral sphincter in spinal cord injury patients. J Urol 1978; 120:62.

Stanton SL, Cardozo LD, Ken-Wilson R: Treatment of delayed onset of spontaneous voiding after surgery for incontinence. Urology 1979; 13:494.

Staskin DS, Varde Y, Siroky MB: Postprostatectomy continence in the parkinsonian patient: The significance of poor voluntary sphincter control. J Urol 1988; 140:117.

Steinberger RE, Ohl DA, Bennett CJ, et al: Nifedipine pretreatment for autonomic dysreflexia during electroejaculation. Urology 1990; 36:228.

Stephenson TP, Mundy AR: The urge syndrome. *In* Stephenson TP, Mundy AR, Wein AJ, eds. Urodynamics, Principles, Practice, Application. London, Churchill Livingstone, 1994, pp 263–275.

Stewart B, Borowsky L, Montague D: Stress incontinence: Conservative therapy with sympathomimetic drugs. J Urol 1976; 115:558.

Stewart DA, Taylor J, Ghosh S, et al: Terodiline causes polymorphic ventricular tachycardia due to reduced heart rate and prolongation of QT interval. Eur J Clin Pharmacol 1992; 42:577.

Stone AR, MacDermott JP: Sexual dysfunction: The neurologically impaired patient. Probl Urol 1989; 3:147.

Stover SL, Fine PR: Epidemiology and economics of spinal cord injury. Paraplegia 1987; 25:225.

Sullivan M, Yalla SV: Spinal cord injury and other forms of myeloneuropathies. Probl Urol 1992; 6(4):643–658.

Sundin T, Dahlstrom A, Norlen L, Svednyr N: The sympathetic innervation and adrenoreceptor function of the human lower urinary tract in the normal state and after parasympathetic denervation. Invest Urol 1977; 14:322.

Swierzewski S, Gormley EA, Belville WD, et al: The effect of terazosin on bladder function in the spinal cord injured patient. J Urol 1994; 151:951.

Talbot HS, Mahony EM, Jaffee SR: The effects of prolonged urethral catheterization. 1: Persistence of normal renal structure and function. J Urol 1959; 81:138.

Tammela T, Heiskari M, Lukkarinen O: Voiding dysfunction and urodynamic findings in patients with cervical spondylotic spinal stenosis compared with the severity of the disease. Br J Urol 1992; 70:144.

Tammela T, Kontturi M, Kaar K, Lukkarinen O: Intravesical prostaglandin F_2 for promoting bladder emptying after surgery for female stress incontinence. Br J Urol 1987; 60:43.

Tanagho EA: Bladder neck reconstruction for total urinary incontinence: Ten years of experience. J Urol 1981; 1215:321.

Tanagho EA, Schmidt RA: Electrical stimulation in the clinical management of the neurogenic bladder. J Urol 1988; 140:1331.

Tanagho EA, Schmidt RA, Orvis BR: Neural stimulation for control of voiding disorders: A preliminary report in 22 patients with serious neuropathic voiding disorders. J Urol 1989; 142:340.

Tapp A, Fall M, Norgaard J, et al: Terodiline: A dose titrated, multicenter study of the treatment of idiopathic detrusor instability in women. J Urol 1989; 142:1027.

Taylor MC, Bates CP: A double-blind crossover trial of baclofen: A new treatment for the unstable bladder syndrome. Br J Urol 1979; 51:505.

Taylor P: Cholinergic agonists. *In* Gilman AG, Rall TW, Nies AS, Taylor P, eds: Goodman and Gilman's The Pharmacological Basis of Therapeutics, 8th ed. New York, Pergamon Press, 1990, pp 122–130.

Taylor SH: Clinical pharmacotherapeutics of doxazosin. Am J Med 87(suppl 2A):25, 1989.

Thind P, Lose G, Colatrue H, Andersson KE: The effect of alpha adrenoceptor stimulation and blockade on the static urethral sphincter function in healthy females. Scand J Urol Nephrol 1992; 26:219.

Thomas DG, Lucas MG: The urinary tract following spinal cord injury. *In* Chisolm GD, Fair WR, eds: Scientific Foundations of Urology. Chicago, Year Book Medical Publishers, 1990, pp 286–299.

Thomas DG, O'Flynn KJ: Spinal cord injury. *In* Mundy AR, Stephenson TP, Wein AJ, eds: Urodynamics: Principles, Practice, Application. London, Churchill Livingstone, 1994, pp 345–358.

Thor KB, Roppolo JR, deGroat WC: Naloxone induced micturition in unanesthetized paraplegic cats. J Urol 1983; 129:202.

Thuroff J, Burke B, Ebner A, et al: Randomized double-blind multicentre trial on treatment of frequency, urgency and incontinence related to detrusor hyperactivity: Oxybutynin vs propantheline vs placebo. J Urol 1991; 145:813.

Tonini M, Rizzi CA, Perrucca E, et al: Depressant action of oxybutynin on the contractility of intestinal and urinary tract smooth muscle. J Pharm Pharmacol 1986; 39:103.

Torrens MJ: The role of denervation in the treatment of detrusor instability. Neurol Urodynam 1985; 4:353.

Trop CS, Bennett CJ: Autonomic dysreflexia and the urological implications: A review. J Urol 1991; 146:1461.

Tsuchida S, Noto H, Yamaguchi O, Itoh M: Urodynamic studies in hemiplegic patients after cerebrovascular accidents. Urology 1983; 21:315.

Tulloch AGS, Creed KE: A comparison between propantheline and imipramine on bladder and salivary gland function. Br J Urol 1979; 51:359.

Turner-Warwick R: Bladder outflow obstruction in the male. *In* Mundy AR, Stephenson TP, Wein AJ, eds: Urodynamics: Principles, Practice, Application. London, Churchill Livingstone, 1984, pp 183–204.

Turner-Warwick RT, Whiteside CG, Worth PHL, et al: A urodynamic view of the clinical problems associated with bladder neck dysfunction and its treatment by endoscopic incision and trans-trigonal posterior prostatectomy. Br J Urol 1973; 44:45.

Urinary Incontinence Guideline Panel: Urinary Incontinence in Adults: Clinical Practice Guideline. AHCPR Publication No 92-0038. Rockville, Md, Agency for Health Care Policy and Research, Public Health Service, US Department of Health and Human Services, March 1992.

Vaidyanathan S, Rao M, Chary KSN: Enhancement of detrusor reflex activity by naloxone in patients with chronic neurogenic bladder dysfunction. J Urol 1981; 126:500.

Van Arsdalen KN, Hackler RH: Transureterostomy in spinal cord injury patients for persistent vesicoureteral reflux: 6 to 14 year follow up. J Urol 1983; 129:1117.

Van Arsdalen KN, Klein FA, Hackler RH, Brady SM: Penile implants in spinal cord injury patients for maintaining external appliances. J Urol 1981; 126:331.

Vapnek JM, Couillard DR, Stone AR: Is sphincterotomy the best management of the spinal cord injured bladder? J Urol 1994; 151:961.

Velanovich V: Pharmacologic prevention and treatment of postoperative urinary retention. Infect Urol 1992; 3(May/June):87.

Vereecker RL, Das RJ, Grisar P: Electrical sphincter stimulation in the treatment of detrusor hyperreflexia of paraplegia. Neurourol Urodyn, 1984; 3:145.

Wagner G, Husstein P, Enzelsberger H: Is prostaglandin E_2 really of therapeutic value for postoperative urinary retention? Results of a prospectively randomized double-blind study. Am J Obstet Gynecol 1985; 151:375.

Wall LL, Stanton SL: Transvesical phenol injection of pelvic nerve plexuses in females with refractory urge incontinence. Br J Urol 1989; 63:645.

Walton GW, Kaplan SA: Urinary dysfunction in tropical spastic paraparesis: Preliminary urodynamic survey. J Urol 1993; 150:930.

Wang SC, McGuire EJ, Bloom DA: Urethral dilation in the management of urologic complications of myelodysplasia. J Urol 1989; 142:1504.

Ward A, Chaffman MO, Sorkin EM: Dantrolene. A review of its pharmacodynamic and pharmacokinetic properties and therapeutic use in malignant hyperthermia, the neuroleptic syndrome and an update of its use in muscle spasticity. Drugs 1986; 32:130.

Webster GD, El-Mahrovky A, Stone AR, Zakrzewski C: The urological evaluation and management of patients with myelodysplasia. Br J Urol 1986; 58:261.

Webster GD, Lockhart JL, Older RA: The evaluation of bladder neck dysfunction. J Urol 1980; 123:196.

Weese DL, Roskamp DA, Leach GE, Zimmern PE: Intravesical oxybutynin chloride: Experience with 42 patients. Urology 1993; 41:527.

Wein AJ: Pharmacologic management of voiding dysfunction. *In* Raz S, ed: Female Urology. Philadelphia, W. B. Saunders Company, 1996, pp 283–318.

Wein AJ, Barrett DM: Etiologic possibilities for increased pelvic floor electromyography activity during bladder filling. J Urol 1982; 127:949.

Wein AJ, Barrett DM: Voiding Function and Dysfunction—A Logical and Practical Approach. Chicago, Year Book Medical Publishers, 1988.

Wein A, Malloy T, Shofer F, et al: The effects of bethanechol chloride on urodynamic parameters in normal women and in women with significant residual urine volumes. J Urol 1980a; 124:397.

Wein AJ, Raezer DM, Benson GS: Management of neurogenic bladder dysfunction in the adult. Urology 1976; 8:432.

Wein A, Raezer D, Malloy T: Failure of the bethanechol supersensitivity test to predict improved voiding after subcutaneous bethanechol administration. J Urol 1980b; 123:202.

Werbrouck P, Baert L, Binard JE, et al: Balloon dilation of the external urethral sphincter: A clinical study. J Am Paraplegia Soc 1990; 13:13.

Wheeler JS, Culken DJ, Ottara RJ, Canning JR: Bladder dysfunction and neurosyphilis. J Urol 1986; 136:903.

Wheeler JS Jr, Robinson CJ, Culkin DJ, Nemchausky BA: Naloxone efficacy in bladder rehabilitation of spinal cord injury patients. J Urol 1987; 137:1201.

Wilde M, Fitton A, McTavish D: Afluzosoin—A review of its pharmacodynamic and pharmacokinetic properties and its therapeutic potential in BPH. Drugs 1993b; 45:410.

Wilde M, Fitton A, Sorkin E: Terazosin—A review of its pharmacodynamic and pharmacokinetic properties and therapeutic potential in BPH. Drugs Aging 1993a; 3:258.

Yamaniski T, Yasuda K, Togo M, et al: Effects of beta-2 stimulants on contractility and fatigue of canine urethral sphincter. J Urol 1994; 151:1066.

Yip C, Leach GE, Rosenfeld DS, et al: Delayed diagnosis of voiding dysfunction: Occult spinal dysraphism. J Urol 1985; 134:694.

Zderic SA, Levin RM, Wein AJ: Voiding function: Relevant anatomy, physiology, pharmacology and molecular aspects. *In* Gillenwater JY, Grayhack J, Howards SS, Duckett JW, eds: Adult and Pediatric Urology, 3rd ed. Chicago, Mosby-Year Book Medical Publishers, 1996, pp 1159–1220.

Zochodne DW: Autonomic involvement in Guillain-Barré syndrome: A review. Muscle Nerve 1994; 17:1145.

30

URINARY INCONTINENCE: PATHOPHYSIOLOGY, EVALUATION, TREATMENT OVERVIEW, AND NONSURGICAL MANAGEMENT

Jerry G. Blaivas, M.D.
Lauri J. Romanzi, M.D.
Dianne M. Heritz, M.D.

The lower urinary tract has but two functions: the storage and timely expulsion of urine. The bladder fills with urine from the kidneys, and when the urge to void is felt, micturition normally can be postponed until a socially convenient time. During micturition, the sphincter relaxes and the bladder contracts and empties. When the lower urinary tract fails to maintain its storage function, urinary incontinence ensues. **The bladder neck and the proximal urethra function as a sphincter, but an anatomic sphincter cannot be seen with the naked eye, nor is it apparent under the careful scrutiny of the microscope or in the gross anatomy laboratory.** There is no valve, as there is in the heart. Rather, **the sphincteric action results from an integrated interaction between smooth and striated muscle, other soft tissue components such as collagen and elastin, and a mucosal seal.** The bladder neck and the proximal urethra retain sphincteric function throughout life unless damaged by disease or surgery or by the slow pull of gravity on its musculofascial supports.

OVERVIEW OF PHYSIOLOGY AND PATHOPHYSIOLOGY OF MICTURITION

Normal voiding is accomplished by activation of the micturition reflex (Fig. 30–1). The **first recorded event is sud-**

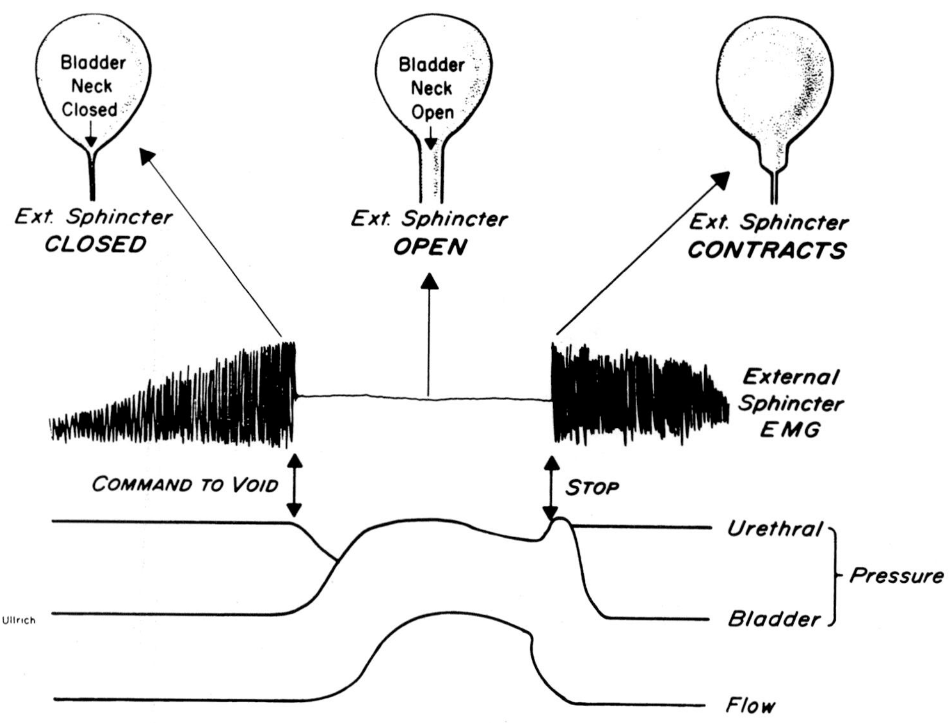

Figure 30–1. Physiology of micturition. See text for details. EMG, electromyogram. (From Blaivas JG: Pathophysiology of lower urinary tract dysfunction. Clin Obstet Gynecol 1985, 12:297.)

den and complete relaxation of the striated sphincteric muscles, characterized by complete electrical silence of the sphincter electromyogram (EMG) (Tanagho and Miller, 1970; Blaivas, 1982). **This is followed almost immediately by a rise in detrusor pressure and a concomitant fall in urethral pressure as the bladder and proximal urethra become isobaric** (Yalla et al, 1980; Blaivas, 1988b). **The vesical neck and urethra open, and voiding ensues. Voluntary interruption of the stream is accomplished by a sudden contraction of the striated periurethral musculature, which, through a reflex mechanism, shuts off the detrusor contraction, aborting micturition.**

The micturition reflex is normally under voluntary control and is organized in the rostral brain stem (the pontine micturition center). It requires integration and modulation by the parasympathetic and somatic components of the sacral spinal cord (the sacral micturition center) and the thoracolumbar sympathetic components (Bradley and Conway, 1966; Blaivas, 1982; Morrison, 1987b; deGroat and Steers, 1990).

Neurologic lesions above the pons usually leave the micturition reflex intact. Many affected patients have no voiding dysfunction at all. When micturition is affected, there is generally a loss of voluntary control of the micturition reflex (Blaivas, 1982). In these patients, micturition is physiologically normal—there is a coordinated relaxation of the sphincter during detrusor contraction—but the patient has simply lost the ability to either prevent or initiate voiding (Blaivas, 1982; Tsuchida et al, 1983; Reding et al, 1987; Khan et al, 1990). There is great variability in the degree of the patient's awareness of, control of, and concern about micturition (Andrew and Nathan, 1964; Andrew et al, 1966; Blaivas, 1982; Morrison, 1987b). Some patients have either no awareness or no concern and simply void involuntarily. Some patients can sense the impending onset of an involuntary detrusor contraction and are able to voluntarily contract the sphincter and abort the detrusor contraction before it starts (Fig. 30–2). Such patients usually complain of urgency but not urge incontinence. Others are aware of the involuntary detrusor contraction and can contract the striated sphincter, but this does not abort the detrusor contraction, and incontinence ensues (Fig. 30–3). In addition to urinary urgency, these patients also complain of urge incontinence. Still others can contract the sphincter during an involuntary detrusor contraction and abort the stream but not the detrusor contraction. As soon as they relax the sphincter, incontinence occurs. Some patients with supraspinal neurologic lesions develop detrusor areflexia or an acontractile detrusor, but the neurophysiologic pathways responsible for this have not been well described.

Interruption of the neural pathways connecting the pontine micturition center to the sacral micturition center usually results in detrusor external sphincter dyssynergia or other manifestations of poor coordination of the micturition reflex, such as weak, poorly sustained detrusor contractions (McGuire and Brady, 1979; Blaivas et al, 1981; Blaivas, 1982; Rudy et al, 1988). **Detrusor–external sphincter dyssynergia (DESD) is characterized by involuntary contractions of the striated musculature of the urethral sphincter during an involuntary detrusor contraction** (Fig. 30–4). **It is seen exclusively in patients with neurologic lesions between the brain stem (pontine micturition center) and the sacral spinal cord (sacral micturition center).** These lesions include traumatic spinal cord injury, multiple sclerosis, myelodysplasia, and other forms of transverse myelitis.

Sacral neurologic lesions have a variable effect on micturition, depending on the extent to which the neurologic injury affects the parasympathetic, sympathetic, and somatic systems (Gerstenberg et al, 1980; Blaivas and Barbalias, 1983; Yalla and Andriole, 1984; Wheeler et al, 1986; McGuire et al, 1988). **In complete parasympathetic le-**

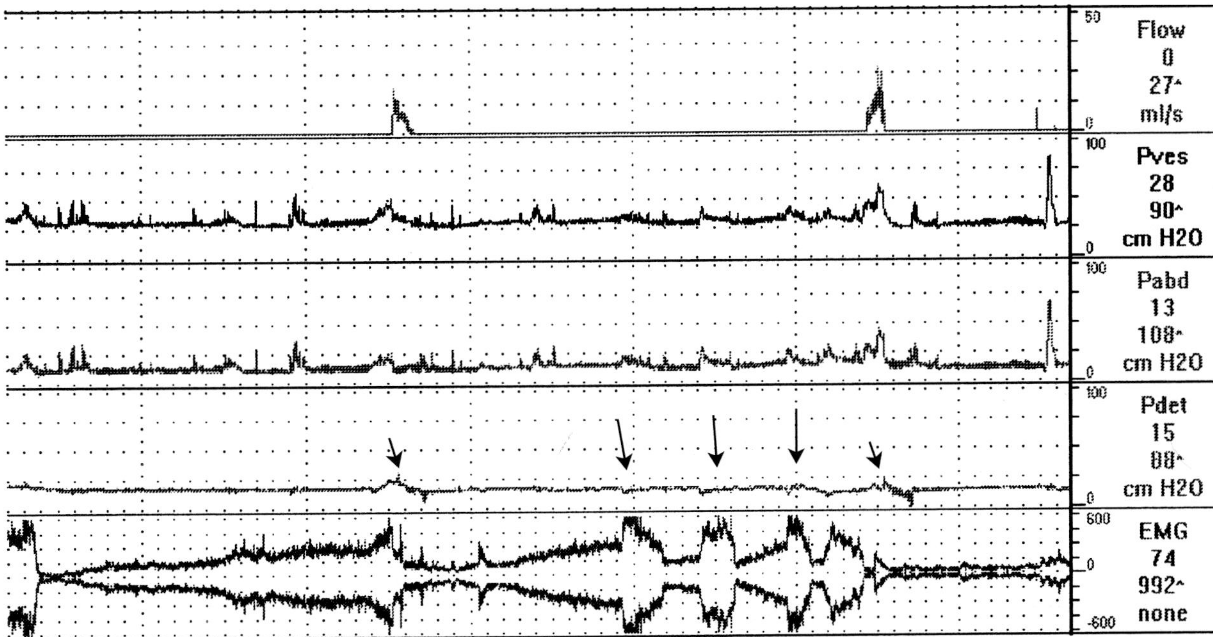

Figure 30–2. Involuntary detrusor contractions with voluntary control of the micturition reflex. Urodynamic tracing demonstrates multiple low pressure involuntary detrusor contractions (marked by the *small arrows*), which the patient perceived as an urge to void with only a few seconds' warning. She was aware of each contraction and was able to voluntarily contract her sphincter. When she was instructed to void, she relaxed the sphincter and voided normally. When instructed to try to prevent incontinence, she contracted the sphincter and aborted the detrusor contractions (*large arrows*).

sions, the bladder is areflexic and the patient is in urinary retention. In many cases, there is also the gradual onset of low compliance, which is characterized by a steep rise in detrusor pressure during bladder filling. **When, in addition to a parasympathetic lesion, there is also a sympathetic lesion, the proximal urethra loses its sphincteric function** (Fig. 30–5). Clinically, this results in incomplete bladder emptying (caused by the acontractile detrusor) and sphincteric incontinence (caused by the nonfunctioning proximal urethra) (Gerstenberg et al, 1980; Blaivas and Barbalias, 1983; Yalla and Andriole, 1984).

Somatic neurologic lesions affect pudendal afferent and efferent nerves (Blaivas et al, 1982). In addition to loss of perineal and perianal sensation, these lesions abolish the bulbocavernosus reflex and impair the ability to voluntarily contract the urethral and anal sphincters. Sacral neurologic

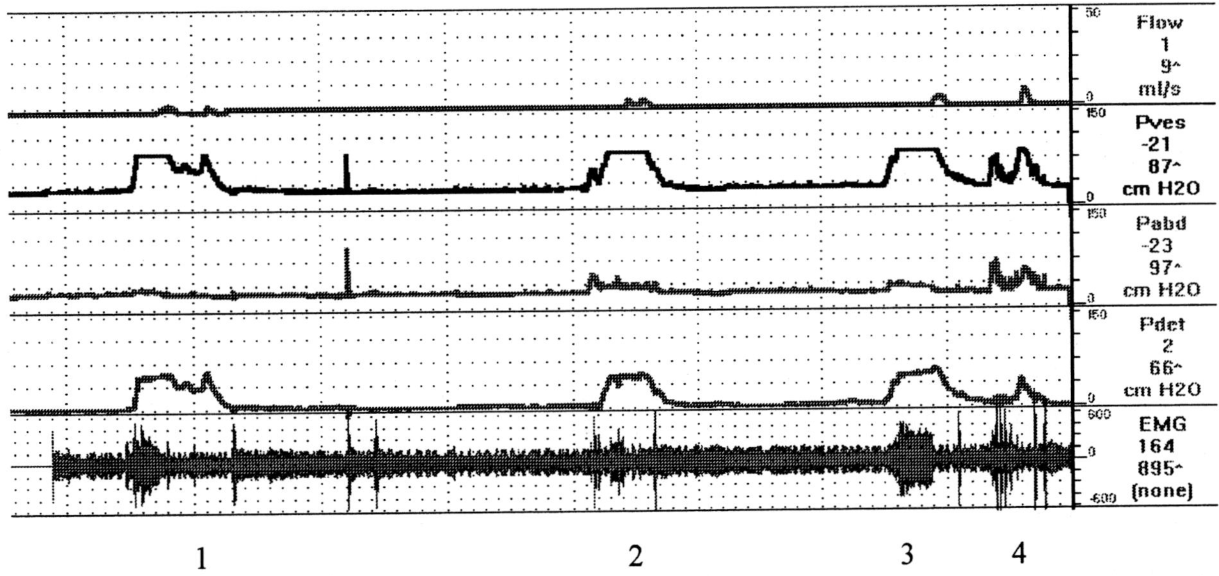

Figure 30–3. Detrusor hyperreflexia resulting from a supraspinal neurologic lesion in a 39-year-old man with multiple sclerosis. Urodynamic tracing demonstrates three hyperreflexic detrusor contractions (1, 2, and 3). He perceived each contraction as an urge to void and contracted his sphincter in an attempt to abort the stream. He could delay the onset of flow for over 20 seconds, but when the sphincter fatigued, he voided involuntarily. At the end of the study, he voided voluntarily (4).

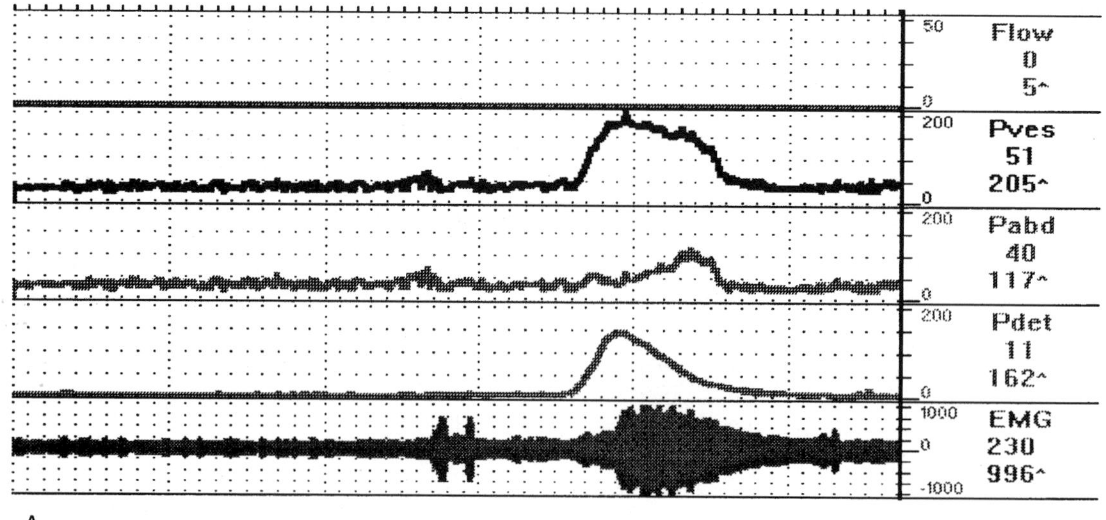

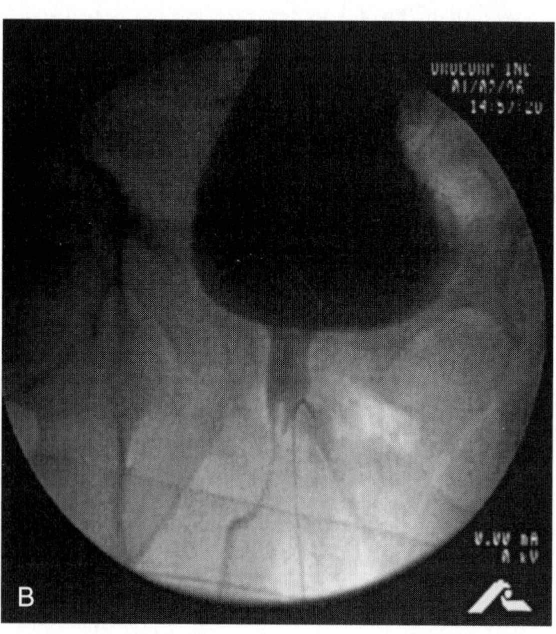

Figure 30–4. Detrusor–external sphincter dyssynergia (type 3) in a 53-year-old man with an arteriovenous malformation of the thoracic spine. *A*, Urodynamic tracing. There is a crescendo-decrescendo increase in sphincter EMG activity during an involuntary detrusor contraction over 150 cm H_2O. *B*, Voiding cytourethrogram exposed at point 1 shows complete obstruction at the membranous urethra by the contracting sphincter.

lesions are caused by herniated discs, diabetic neuropathy, multiple sclerosis, and spinal cord tumors. They are also commonly encountered after extensive pelvic surgery such as abdominoperineal resection of the rectum and radical hysterectomy (Gerstenberg et al, 1980; Blaivas and Barbalias, 1983; Chang and Fan, 1983; Yalla and Andriole, 1984; McGuire et al, 1988).

DEFINITION AND CLASSIFICATION OF INCONTINENCE

Simply stated, urinary incontinence is the involuntary loss of urine. In women, it is common and rarely caused by serious medical conditions; in men, it is uncommon and almost always the consequence of a serious underlying condition, prior surgery, or injury. From a clinical perspective, **incontinence denotes a symptom, a sign, and a condition** (Abrams et al, 1988). The **symptom** indicates the patient's (or caregiver's) statement of involuntary urine loss; the **sign** is the objective demonstration of urine loss; and the **condition** is the underlying pathophysiologic process as demonstrated by clinical or urodynamic techniques.

Incontinence may be urethral or extraurethral. Extraurethral incontinence is caused by urinary fistula or ectopic ureter. These conditions are discussed in detail elsewhere in this volume and are not recounted here.

Two generic conditions cause urethral incontinence: bladder abnormalities and sphincter abnormalities (Wein, 1981; Blaivas, 1985c; Wein and Barrett, 1988) (Table 30–1). Cognitive abnormalities, such as Alzheimer's disease, and physical immobility, such as in Parkinson's disease, although not directly causing incontinence, are important comorbid conditions that greatly exacerbate the clinical problem. Other contributing factors include urinary tract infection, atrophic vulvovaginitis, fecal impaction, and fluid

Table 30–1. CONDITIONS CAUSING URETHRAL INCONTINENCE

Bladder Abnormalities	Sphincter Abnormalities
Detrusor overactivity Detrusor instability Detrusor hyperreflexia Low bladder compliance Urinary fistula	Urethral hypermobility Intrinsic sphincter deficiency

overload resulting from such conditions as heart failure, venous insufficiency, diabetes insipidus, and inappropriate antidiuretic hormone (ADH) syndrome. Although other comorbid factors such as autonomically active medications, endocrinopathies, and psychologic factors have also been implicated, in our experience these are very rare (Resnick et al, 1989; O'Donnell, 1991).

Bladder abnormalities causing urinary incontinence include detrusor overactivity and low bladder compliance (Abrams et al, 1988). **Detrusor overactivity** is a generic term for **involuntary detrusor contractions. Detrusor hyperreflexia** denotes involuntary detrusor contractions that result from a neurologic condition. **Detrusor instability** denotes involuntary detrusor contractions that do not result from a neurologic disorder. When it is uncertain whether the condition is of neurologic origin, the term **detrusor overactivity** should be used. **Low bladder compliance** describes an abnormal volume/pressure relationship wherein there is a high incremental rise in detrusor pressure during bladder filling.

Sphincter abnormalities are different in men and women. **In men, sphincter abnormalities are most commonly caused by anatomic disruption after prostate surgery** (Fig. 30–6) or occasionally by trauma or neurologic abnormalities. In women, sphincter abnormalities may be classified in two ways: from a functional or an anatomic viewpoint. These are complementary ways of assessing sphincteric incontinence in women and are not mutually exclusive. **From a functional viewpoint, there are two generic types of sphincteric incontinence: urethral hypermobility** (Fig. 30–7) **and intrinsic sphincter deficiency** (Fig. 30–8) (Jeffcoate and Roberts, 1952; Hodgkinson, 1953, 1965; Green, 1962; McGuire and Herlihy, 1977; Blaivas, 1988b; Wein and Barrett, 1988; Yang et al, 1991, 1993; McGuire et al, 1993a; Sanders et al, 1994; Mostwin et al, 1995). **In urethral hypermobility, the basic abnormality is a weakness of pelvic floor support.** Because of this weakness, there is rotational descent of the vesical neck and proximal urethra during increases in abdominal pressure. If the urethra opens concomitantly, stress urinary incontinence ensues. Urethral hypermobility is often present in women who are not incontinent (Versi et al, 1986). Thus the mere presence of urethral hypermobility is not sufficient to make a diagnosis of a sphincter abnormality unless incontinence is also demonstrated.

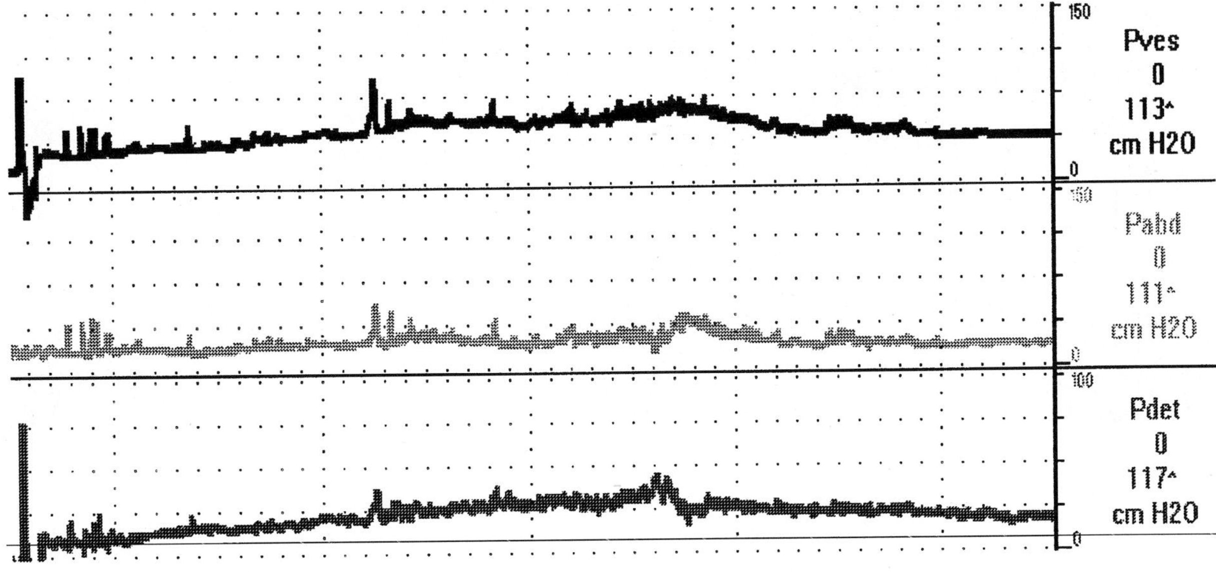

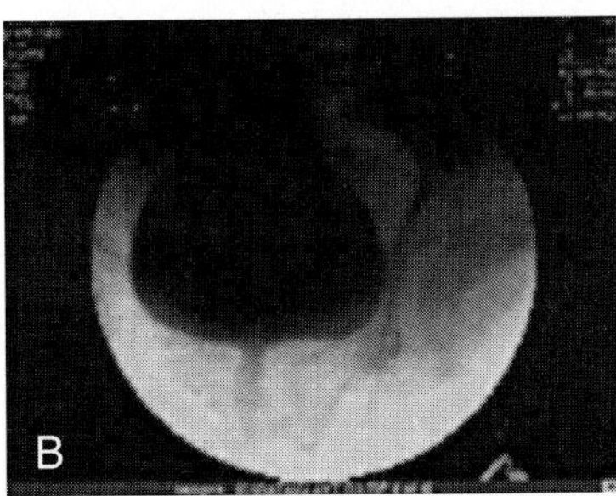

Figure 30–5. Parasympathetic, sympathetic, and somatic decentralization resulting in low bladder compliance, detrusor areflexia, and intrinsic sphincter deficiency in a 58-year-old man with traumatic (thoracolumbar) paraplegia, with resultant low bladder compliance and intrinsic sphincter deficiency. *A,* Urodynamic tracing. Detrusor pressure at point 1 is 42 cm H_2O at a bladder volume of 530 ml. *B,* Voiding cystourethrogram exposed at the same point shows an open vesical neck.

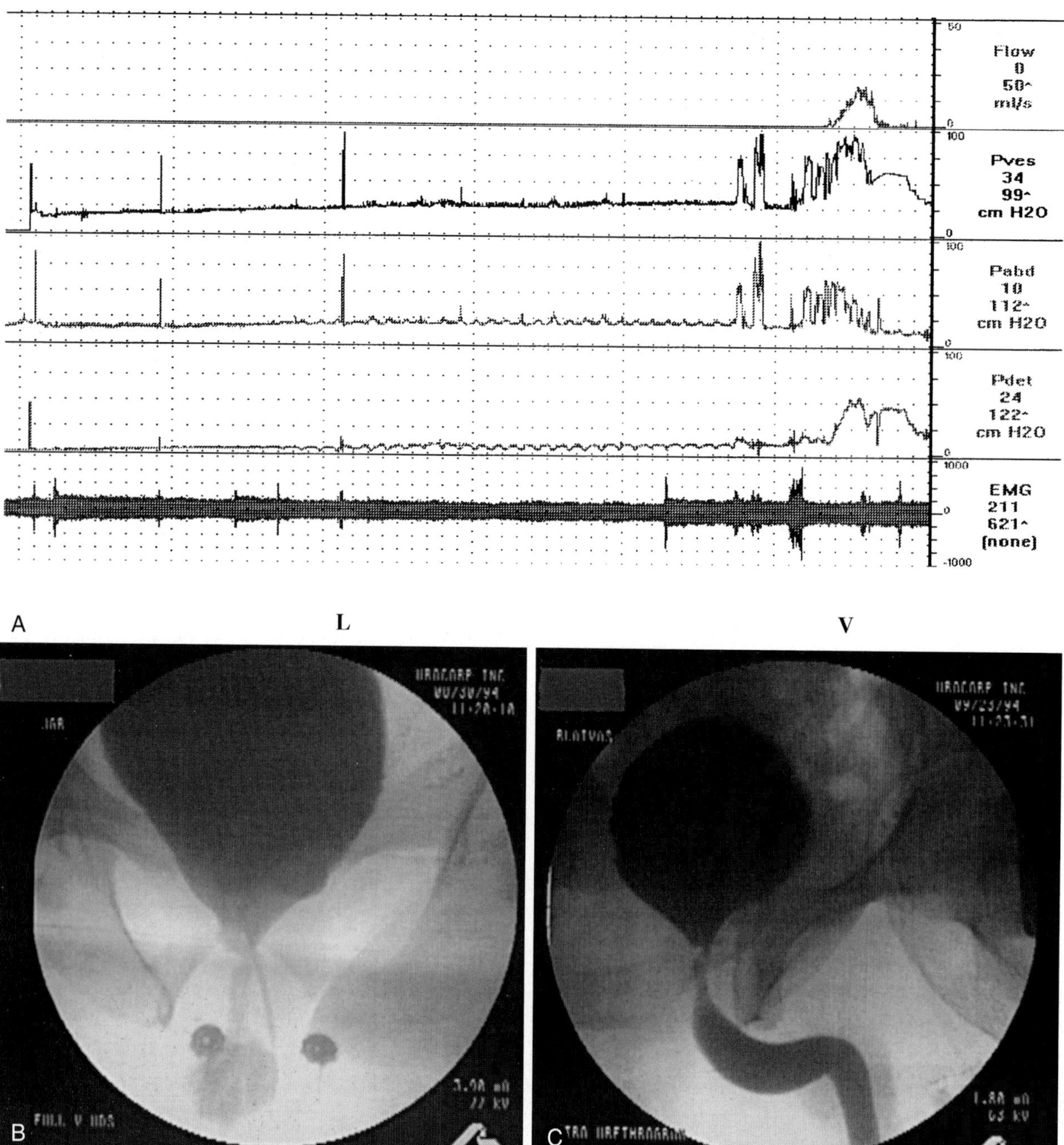

Figure 30–6. Postprostatectomy sphincteric incontinence in a 59-year-old man 18 months after radical prostatectomy. *A,* Urodynamic tracing demonstrates an abdominal leak point pressure of 40 cm H_2O (point L). The patient voided with a voluntary detrusor contraction at point V. *B,* Radiograph exposed at point L reveals sphincteric incontinence. *C,* Radiograph exposed at point V during voluntary micturition.

Intrinsic sphincteric deficiency (ISD) denotes an intrinsic malfunction of the urethral sphincter itself. In its most overt form (type III stress incontinence), it is characterized by an open vesical neck at rest and a low Valsalva leak point pressure (Blaivas and Olsson, 1988; McGuire et al, 1993a). The concept of ISD is a relatively new one, and the clinical definition has not yet met the test of time. **We believe that sphincteric incontinence that is unaccompanied by urethral descent or rotation is a manifestation of ISD, even if the vesical neck is radiologically closed at rest and if the leak point pressure is not low.** In addition, all patients with sphincteric incontinence might be considered to have some degree of ISD, because the normal urethra is intended to remain closed no matter what the degree of stress or rotational descent. **Overt ISD is usually the result of previous surgery for incontinence or a neurologic lesion involving the thoracolumbar outflow,** but it may be seen in elderly women for no apparent reason (Aho et al, 1969; McGuire et al, 1976, 1980, 1988; Fowler et al, 1978; Al-Mefty et al, 1979; Barbalias and Blaivas, 1983; Blaivas, 1983; Kirby, 1986; Salinas et al, 1986; Blaivas and Olsson, 1988). A complete list of the causes of ISD is presented in Table 30–2. **Urethral hypermobility and ISD may (and often do) coexist in the same patient.**

An anatomic classification of stress incontinence, which is complementary to the one cited earlier is presented as follows (Blaivas and Olsson, 1988):

TYPE 0. The patient complains of a typical history of stress incontinence, but no urinary leakage is demonstrated during the clinical and urodynamic investigation. At videourodynamic study, the vesical neck and proximal urethra are closed at rest and situated at or above the lower end of the symphysis pubis. During stress, the vesical neck and proximal urethra descend and open, assuming an anatomic configuration similar to that seen in types I and II stress urinary incontinence (SUI), to be described. Failure to demonstrate incontinence is probably caused by momentary voluntary contraction of the external urethral sphincter during the examination.

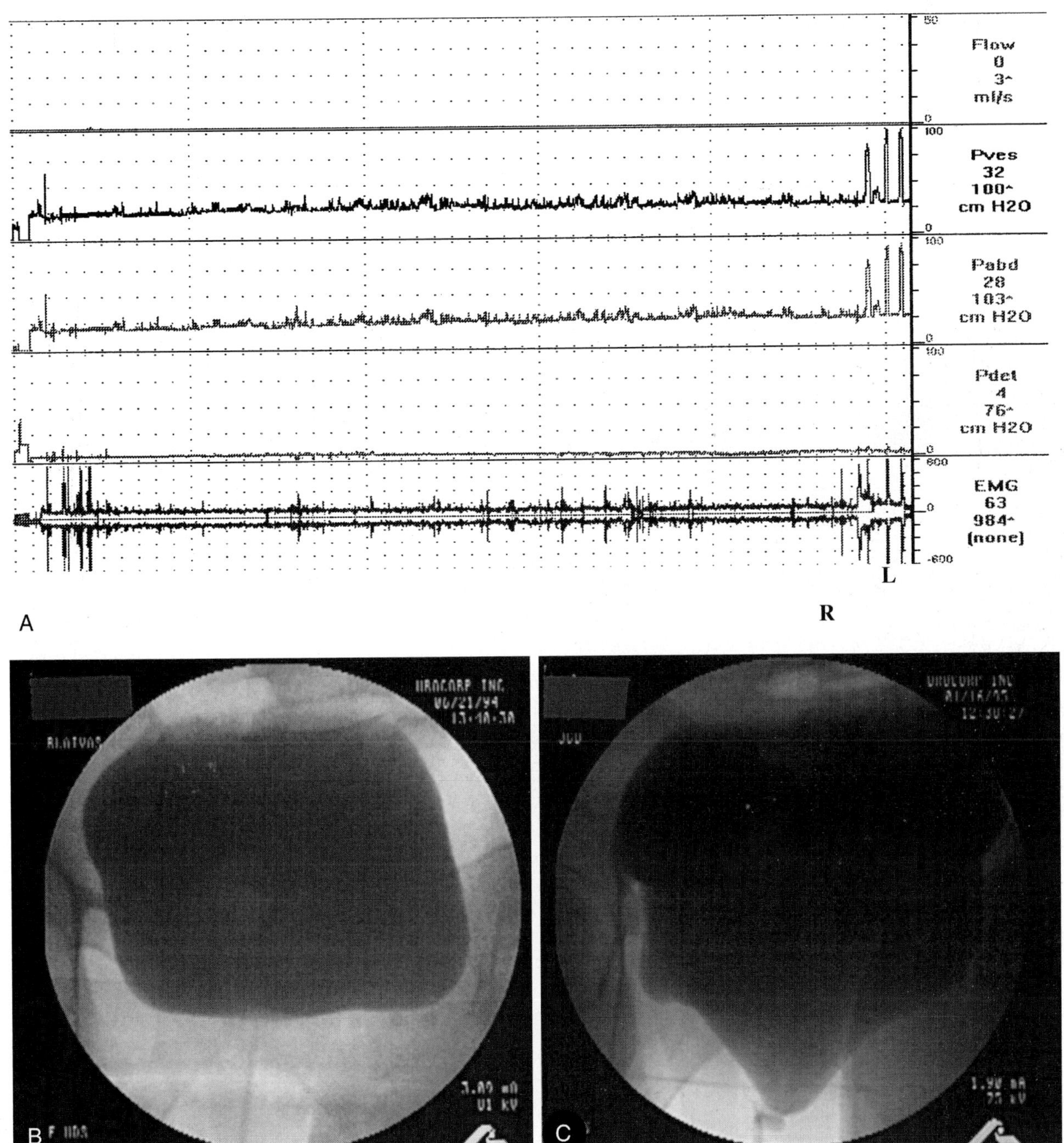

Figure 30–7. Sphincteric incontinence resulting from urethral hypermobility (type 2 stress incontinence) in a 51-year-old woman with a chief complaint of urinary stress incontinence. *A,* Urodynamic tracing demonstrates a stable bladder. Leak point pressure (point L) is 100 cm H_2O. *B,* Radiograph obtained at point R shows a closed bladder neck situated at the midpoint of the pubis. *C,* Radiograph obtained at point L demonstrates urinary incontinence resulting from urethral hypermobility.

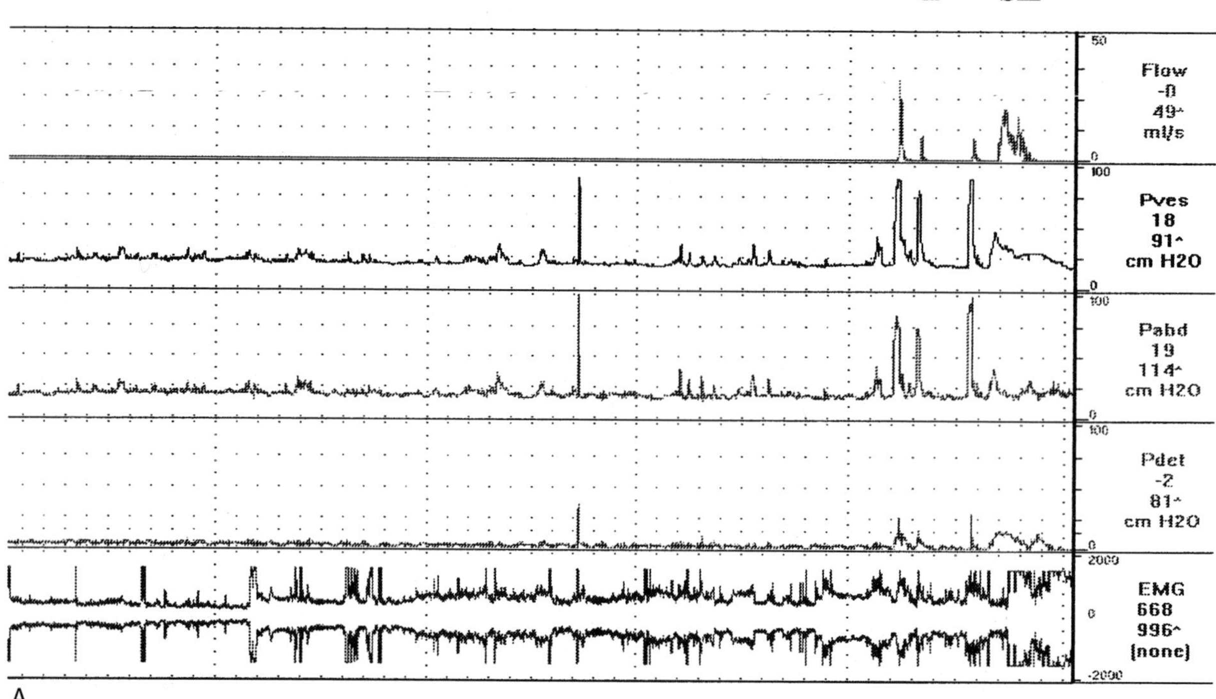

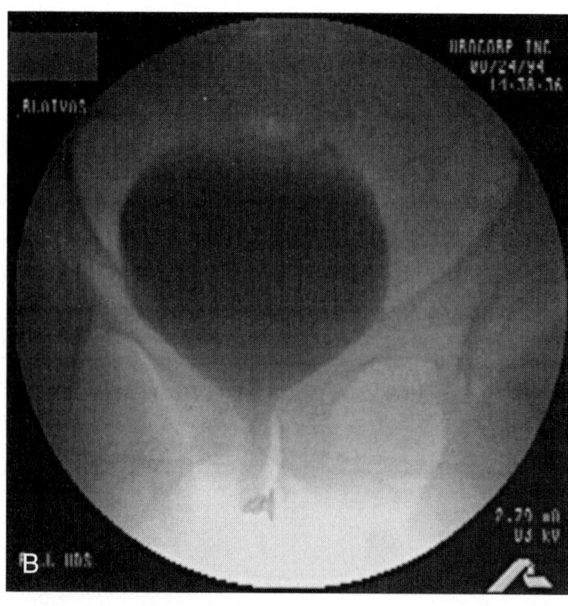

Figure 30–8. Sphincteric incontinence resulting from intrinsic sphincter deficiency (type III stress incontinence) and stress hyperreflexia in a 70-year-old woman. *A,* Urodynamic tracing shows a leak point pressure of 45 cm H_2O (point L) and several stress-induced involuntary detrusor contractions (stress hyperreflexia) at a bladder volume of 150 ml (point SH). *B,* Radiograph exposed at point L demonstrates urinary leakage at a leak point pressure of 40 cm H_2O. There is opening of the vesical neck without rotational descent.

Table 30–2. CAUSES OF INTRINSIC SPHINCTER DEFICIENCY

Previous Pelvic Surgery	*Neurologic Conditions*
Anti-incontinence surgery	Myelodysplasia
Urethral diverticulectomy	Anterior spinal artery syndrome
Radical hysterectomy	Lumbosacral neurologic conditions
Abdominoperineal resection of the rectum	Shy-Drager syndrome
Urethrotomy	*Aging Versus Hypoestrogenic States*
Resection or incision of the vesical neck	

TYPE I. The vesical neck is closed at rest and situated above the inferior margin of the symphysis (Fig. 30–9). During stress, the vesical neck and proximal urethra open and descend less than 2 cm, and urinary incontinence is apparent during periods of increased abdominal pressure. There is a small or no cystocele.

TYPE IIA. The vesical neck is closed at rest and situated above the inferior margin of the symphysis pubis (see Fig. 30–7). During stress, the vesical neck and proximal urethra open, and there is rotational descent characteristic of a cystourethrocele. Urinary incontinence is apparent during periods of increased intra-abdominal pressure.

TYPE IIB. The vesical neck is closed at rest and situated at or below the inferior margin of the symphysis pubis. During stress, there may or may not be further descent, but the proximal urethra opens and incontinence ensues.

TYPE III. The vesical neck and proximal urethra are open at rest in the absence of a detrusor contraction (see Fig. 30–8). The proximal urethra no longer functions as a sphincter. There is obvious urinary leakage, which may be

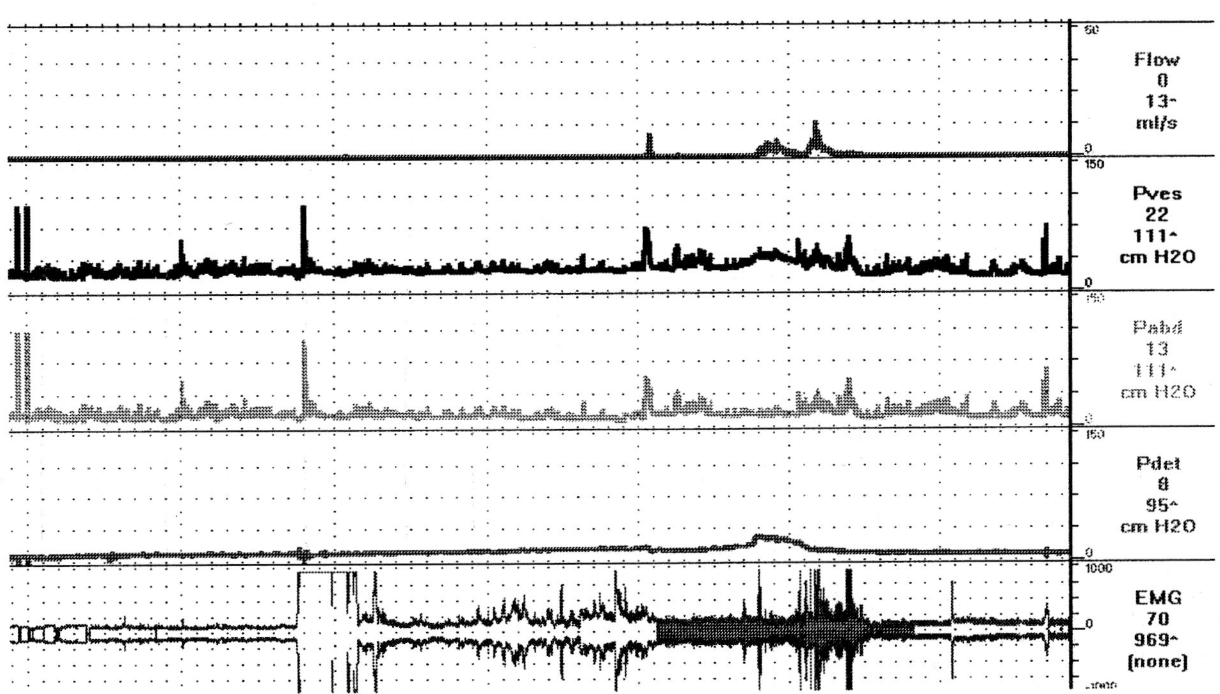

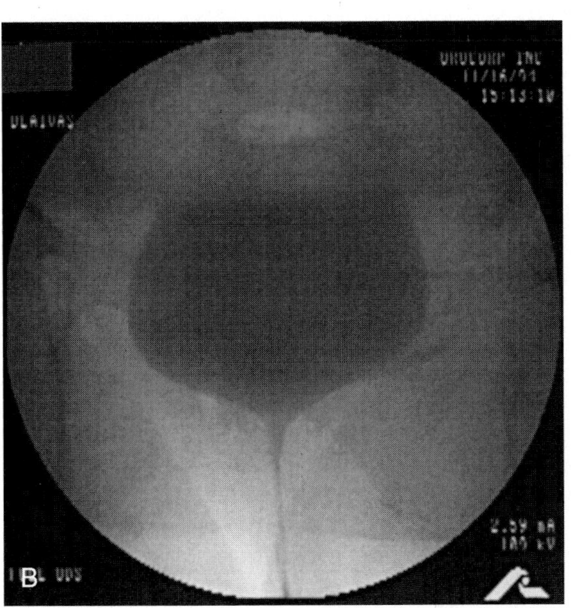

Figure 30–9. Type I stress incontinence in a 56-year-old woman. *A,* Urodynamic tracing. Valsalva leak point pressure = 70 cm H_2O at point L. *B,* Radiograph exposed at point L demonstrates stress incontinence with minimal urethral descent.

gravitational in nature or associated with minimal increases in intravesical pressure.

PHYSIOLOGY AND PATHOPHYSIOLOGY

The unique properties of the bladder and sphincter that are responsible for continence are listed in Table 30–3. **During bladder filling, detrusor pressure remains nearly constant because of a special property of the bladder known as *accommodation*** (Klevmark, 1974). Accommodation accounts for the nearly flat cystometric curve that is seen during normal bladder filling. In experimental animals (cats, dogs, rabbits, rats, and mice), accommodation is unaffected by acute neurologic impairments achieved by sacral and suprasacral spinal cord transection, sacral nerve root section, decerebration, ganglionic blockade, or administration of cholinergic agonists or antagonists (Tang and Ruch, 1955; Ruch and Tang, 1967; Klevmark, 1974, 1977). When accommodation is impaired, low bladder compliance results. *Compliance* refers to the change in bladder volume for a change in detrusor pressure. From a clinical perspective, it may be thought of as a measure of "stiffness" of the bladder wall and is calculated by dividing the change in bladder volume by the change in detrusor pressure that occurred during that change in volume ($\Delta V/\Delta P$ = bladder compliance). Bladder compliance is expressed in milliliters per centimeters of H_2O (Abrams et al, 1988). Low compliance is manifested as a steep rise in detrusor pressure during bladder filling (see Fig. 30–5).

Low bladder compliance may be caused by changes in the elastic and viscoelastic properties of the bladder, changes in detrusor muscle tone, or combinations of the two (McGuire et al, 1981; Ghoneim et al, 1989; Steinkohl and Leach, 1989; Zoubek et al, 1989; McGuire, 1994). **Elastic and viscoelastic abnormalities are due primarily to changes in extracellular matrix (ECM).** ECM is composed of four generic types of macromolecules: (1) collagens, (2) elastins, (3) proteoglycans, and (4) glycoproteins. The first two components, collagen and elastin, account for the structural support of the tissue; the proteoglycans and glycoproteins fill interstices. There is evidence that ECM has an important regulatory and facilitative role in cell behavior, affecting such domains as cell shape, movement, adhesion, migration, invasion, organization, differentiation, and aging (Labat-Robert et al, 1990; Schnaper and Kleinman, 1993). **Collagen is the most abundant of the structural proteins in the ECM of the bladder wall** (Bradley et al, 1965; Swaiman and Bradley, 1967; Kondo and Susset, 1974; Susset et al, 1978), **and an increased collagen content is thought to be the basic abnormality in decreased bladder wall compliance.** The clinical causes of low bladder compliance are listed in Table 30–4. However, low bladder compliance, by itself, does not usually result in urinary incontinence unless there are concomitant sphincteric abnormalities.

Normally, the bladder and sphincter are under voluntary control (Denny-Brown and Robertson, 1933; Lapides et al, 1955, 1957; Blaivas et al, 1981). The details of neural regulation of the lower urinary tract are discussed in Chapter 26; only the relevant clinical correlates are presented here. **Detrusor overactivity (involuntary detrusor contractions) may be of neurologic origin (detrusor hyperreflexia)** (Andrew and Nathan, 1964; Andrew et al, 1966; Dam et al, 1976; Hebjorn et al, 1976; Yalla et al, 1976, 1977; Blaivas et al, 1979a; Beck et al, 1981; Blaivas et al, 1981, 1982; Goldstein et al, 1982; Leach et al, 1982; Siroky and Krane, 1982; Awad and McGinnis, 1983; Pavlakis et al, 1983; Tsuchida et al, 1983; Awad et al, 1984; Andersen, 1985; Blaivas, 1985b; Madersbacher, 1986; Salinas et al, 1986; Berger et al, 1987; Morrison, 1987; Reding et al, 1987; Rudy et al, 1988; Bemelmans et al, 1991; Eardley et al, 1991; Kaplan et al, 1991; Mayo and Chetner, 1992; Mayo, 1992; Chancellor and Blaivas, 1993; Reid and Borzyskowski, 1993; Sotolongo and Chancellor, 1993; Beck et al, 1994; German et al, 1995), **idiopathic** (Hebjorn et al, 1976; Blaivas et al, 1981; Blaivas, 1985a; Abrams et al, 1988; Massey and Abrams, 1988; Wein and Barrett, 1988), **or caused by a variety of other clinical conditions (detrusor instability), such as urethral obstruction** (Fig. 30–10),

Table 30–4. CAUSES OF LOW BLADDER COMPLIANCE

Neurogenic	Increased Collagen
Myelodysplasia	Tuberculous cystitis
Shy-Drager syndrome	Radiation-induced cystitis
Thoracolumbar spinal cord injury	Interstitial cystitis
Radical hysterectomy	Chronic indwelling catheter
Abdominoperineal resection of the rectum	Prostatic obstruction

Table 30–3. PROPERTIES OF THE BLADDER AND SPHINCTER THAT PROMOTE CONTINENCE

Bladder	Sphincter
Accommodation	Coaptation
Compliance	Mucosal seal
Capacity	Inner wall softness
Neural control	Compression
	Extracellular matrix
	Collagen
	Elastin
	Urethral smooth muscle
	Urethral striated muscle
	Anatomic support
	Transmission of Pabd pressure
	Neural control

Table 30–5. CAUSES OF DETRUSOR OVERACTIVITY

Detrusor Hyperreflexia	Detrusor Instability
Supraspinal Neurologic Lesions	Idiopathic urethral obstruction
Stroke	Benign prostatic hyperplasia
Parkinson's disease	Bladder stones
Hydrocephalus	Bladder tumor
Brain tumor	Bladder infection
Multiple sclerosis	Sphincteric incontinence
Suprasacral Spinal Lesions	
Spinal cord injury	
Multiple sclerosis	
Spina bifida	
Transverse myelitis	

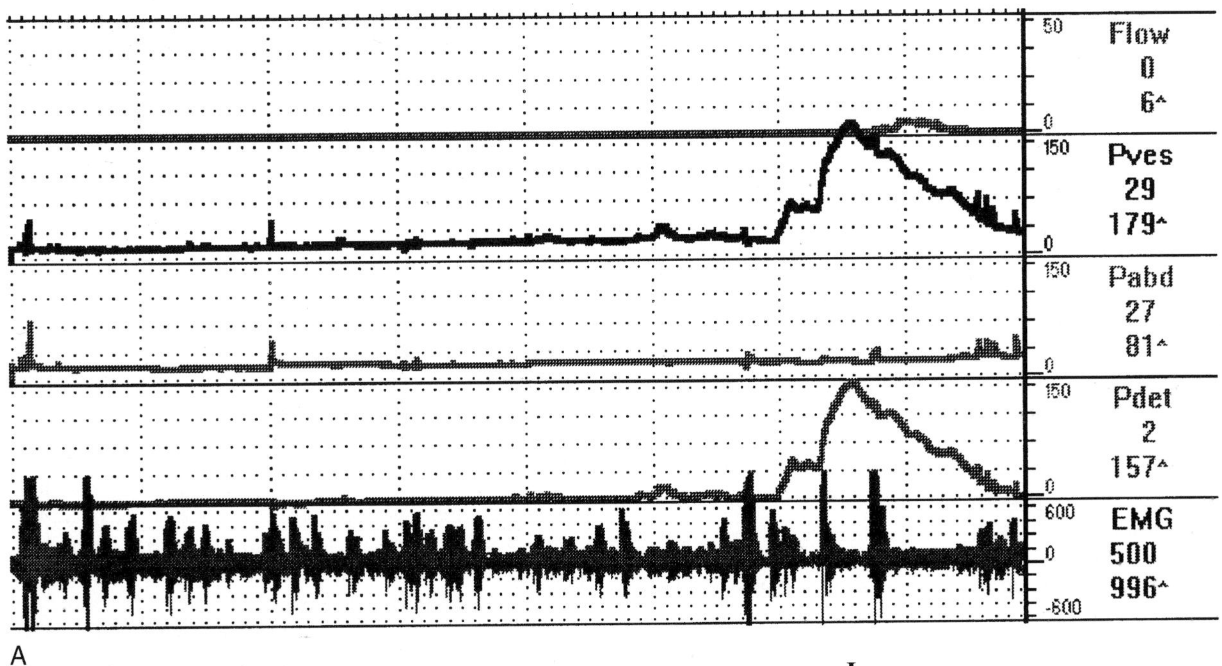

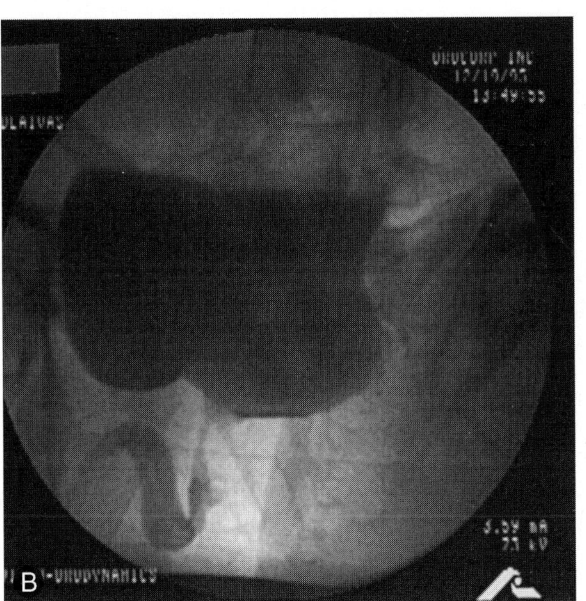

Figure 30–10. Detrusor instability associated with prostatic urethral obstruction. *A,* Urodynamic tracing demonstrates an involuntary detrusor contraction to over 150 cm H_2O and a uroflow of 4 ml/s. *B,* Radiograph exposed at point I demonstrates a narrowed prostatic urethra and a bladder diverticulum.

listed in Table 30–5 (Turner-Warwick et al, 1973; Hebjorn et al, 1976; Blaivas et al, 1981; Andersen, 1982; Awad and McGinnis, 1983; Blaivas, 1985a; Coolsaet and Block, 1986; Blaivas, 1988a; Blaivas and Olsson, 1988; Resnick et al, 1989; Fantl et al, 1990; Brading and Turner, 1994). Elbadawi and colleagues (1993; Elbadawi, 1995) demonstrated ultrastructural changes in patients with detrusor overactivity (dysfunction ultrastructural pattern) that are thought to result in a diminished electrical resistance between detrusor muscle cells and hence a hyperexcitable state that results in involuntary detrusor contractions.

From a clinical standpoint, **the bladder neck/proximal urethra normally functions as a sphincter in both sexes, but anatomically there is no identifiable sphincter as such. Rather, a unique admixture of smooth and striated muscle** (Wesson, 1920; Uhlenhuth, 1953; Hutch, 1965, 1966, 1967, 1972; Woodburne, 1968; Tanagho et al, 1969; Donker et al, 1976; Gosling and Dixon, 1979, 1987; Oelrich, 1983; Turner-Warwick, 1983; Gosling, 1985; Myers, 1991), **intracellular matrix, and mucosal factors** (Zinner et al, 1980) **account for the functional counterparts of a sphincter.** The principles underlying the functional components of the sphincter are (1) watertight apposition of the urethral lumen, (2) compression of the wall around the lumen, (3) structural support to keep the proximal urethra from moving during increases in pressure, (4) a means of compensating for abdominal pressure changes (pressure transmission), and (5) neural control.

The mechanism by which the urethra maintains a watertight seal has not been well defined. Zinner and associates

(1980), in a series of experiments performed on mechanical models of a urethra, concluded that there are at least three urethral wall factors that promote continence: (1) wall tension or external compression, (2) inner wall softness, and (3) a filler material beneath the mucosa that helps to deform the mucosal folds into apposition. The actual shape of the lumen of the sphincteric part of the urethra during bladder filling is difficult to define because there is no obvious way of looking at it. Histologic cross sections of the urethra show that the urethra is not simply a closed tube; rather, there are numerous mucosal folds, between which are potential spaces for urine leakage. Zinner and associates (1980) proposed that a mucous lining, analogous to stopcock grease, provides the stickiness that enables coaptation of these mucosal folds. The softer the lining is, the better apposition can be achieved. In women, estrogen and a cushion effect of the submucosal vasculature have been suggested as ancillary factors (Raz et al, 1972; Tulloch, 1974).

External compression of the urethral lumen is achieved by (1) smooth and striated muscle tone, (2) phasic contractions of the smooth and striated musculature, (3) elastic and viscoelastic properties of the ECM, (4) mechanical factors related to pressure transmission of abdominal pressure, and (5) structural (anatomic) support of the posterior urethral wall; this support serves as a backboard against which the urethra is compressed during increases in abdominal pressure. The commonly held view is that loss of structural support results in varying degrees of descent of the vesical neck and urethra and that the resultant urethral hypermobility is the proximate cause of stress incontinence (Hodgkinson, 1953, 1965; Green, 1962, 1968; McGuire et al, 1976; Hodgkinson et al, 1978; Blaivas, 1988b; Walters and Jackson, 1990). On the basis of such anatomic considerations, a classification of stress incontinence according to the degree and type of urethral descent was described by Green (1962). Minimal descent was termed type 1 stress incontinence, and rotational descent was termed type 2 (Green, 1962; McGuire et al, 1976; Blaivas, 1988b). Other investigators suggested that the physiologic mechanism underlying stress incontinence is unequal transmission of abdominal pressure to the bladder and urethra; when vesical pressure exceeds urethral pressure, incontinence ensues (Graver and Tanagho, 1974; McGuire and Herlihy, 1977; Constantinou and Govan, 1982; Westby et al, 1982; Constantinou, 1985; Bump et al, 1988a; Rosensweig et al, 1991).

More recent investigations have challenged this concept. **In a series of elegant magnetic resonance imaging studies of the pelvic floor, stress incontinence was found to occur when there was unequal movement of the anterior and posterior walls of the vesical neck and proximal urethra during stress; the urethral lumen is literally pulled open as the posterior wall moves away from the anterior wall** (Yang et al, 1991, 1993; Sanders et al, 1994; Mostwin et al, 1995) (Fig. 30–11). Furthermore, ultrasound imaging of the vesical neck and proximal urethra, in both normal and stress-incontinent patients, demonstrated that opening (funneling) of the vesical neck was the common denominator underlying stress incontinence, not urethral hypermobility (Sanders et al, 1994; Mostwin et al, 1995). According to Mostwin and colleagues (1995):

> ***It is the* relative, *not the* absolute, *position of the urethra with respect to the pubis that may contribute to urethral opening in stress incontinence. The length and strength of the subpubic fascial complex may vary in patients. In those with shorter, stronger anterior fascial support, only a small loss of suburethral support may be sufficient to permit distraction (of the anterior and posterior urethral walls) during rotational descent.***

These findings have important clinical implications that support our contention that **the primary goal of surgery for sphincteric incontinence in the female is twofold: to prevent urethral descent and to provide a backboard against which the vesical neck and proximal urethra can be compressed during increases in abdominal pressure** (Blaivas, 1988b).

A detailed discussion of the anatomy of the anterior vaginal wall and its musculofascial support is beyond the scope of this chapter. Conceptually, however, it is clear that **the vesical neck and urethra are supported by a "hammock" of tissue that more or less suspends these structures from the pubis and pelvic sidewalls and prevents their descent during increases in abdominal pressure** (Mengert, 1936; Ricci et al, 1947; Zacharin, 1963, 1985; Milley and Nichols, 1971; Lawson, 1974; Donker et al, 1976; Wilson et al, 1983; Delancey, 1986, 1988a, 1988b, 1989; Nichols and Randall, 1989; Wijma et al, 1991; Yang et al, 1991, 1993; Fu et al, 1995; Mostwin et al, 1995; Weber and Walters, 1995). The attachment of the distal urethra to the pubis (the pubourethral ligament) is a dense, white, fibrous structure that is mostly very strong, but the part that recedes beneath the pubis and into the pelvis fans out and is much weaker (Zacharin, 1985; Mostwin et al, 1995). **The posterior support of the proximal urethra is a musculofascial structure of varying strength. When it becomes weakened, it allows the rotational descent that defines urethral hypermobility and contributes to the genesis of sphincteric incontinence.**

Conceptually, the entire pelvic support structure can be considered a sheet or hammock of musculofascial tissue, attached to the bony pelvis, through which there are openings for the urethra, vagina, and rectum. From a clinical perspective, there are no consistent landmarks that define the structures whose names abound in the anatomic and surgical literature. We find the anatomic concepts from which these names are derived appealing; however, when these structures are viewed through the vagina, at the time of surgery, we have never seen a pubocervical ligament, a urethropelvic ligament, a vesicopelvic ligament, or any of the other named structures—with two notable exceptions. The pubourethral ligament that attaches the distal portion of the urethra to the pubis has always been visible (and palpable) as a strong, white, fibrous band, and the arcus tendineus has been observed in many, but certainly not all, patients through a retropubic incision lateral to the vesical neck and urethra.

A summary of the clinical causes of abnormalities of urethral compression and support is presented in Table 30–6.

SYMPTOMS, SIGNS, AND CONDITIONS OF INCONTINENCE

(Table 30–7)

1. **Urge incontinence:** The symptom urge incontinence is the patient's complaint of involuntary loss of urine associ-

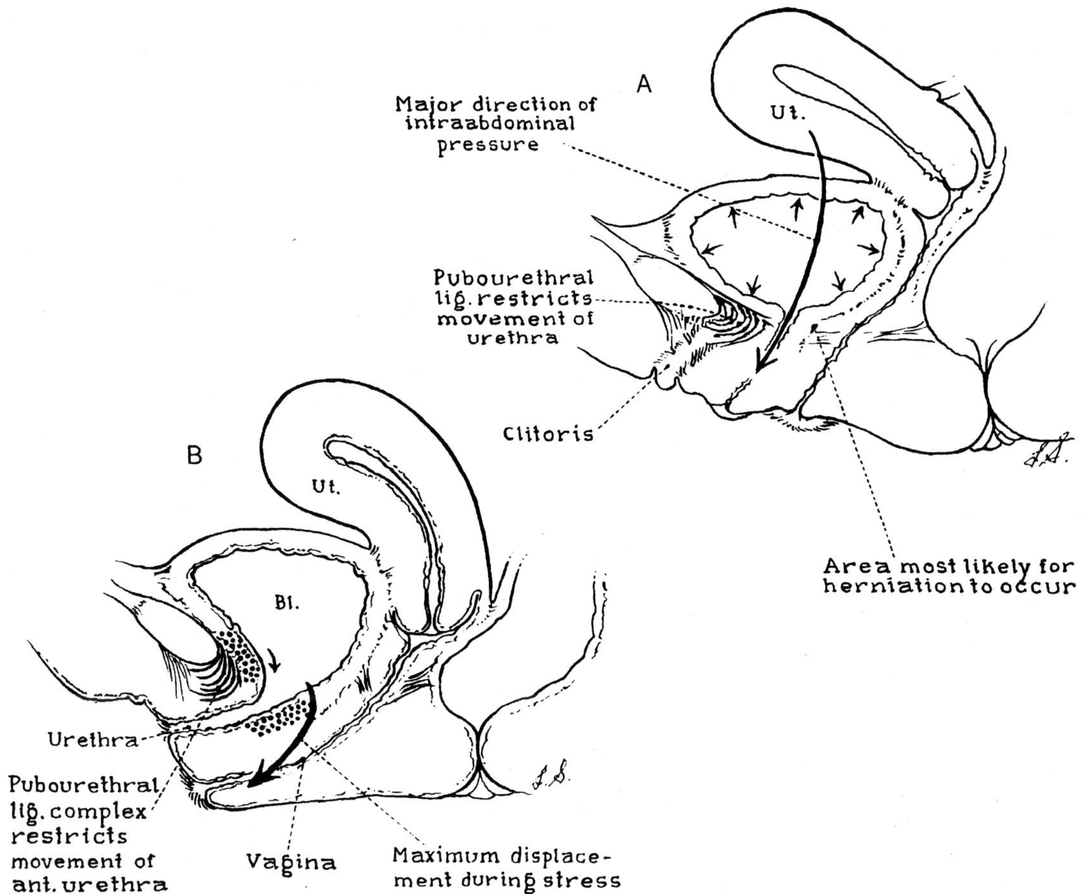

Figure 30–11. Proposed mechanism of sphincteric incontinence resulting from urethral hypermobility. *A,* Normally, the vesical neck and proximal urethra are held in place by the pubourethral ligaments and their proximal extensions. *B,* In patients with urethral hypermobility, during increases in abdominal pressure, posterior support is more deficient than anterior support. The posterior urethral wall moves more than the anterior urethral wall. Hence the net result is that the urethra is pulled open and incontinence ensues. (From Mostwin JL, Yang A, Sanders R, Genadry R: Urol Clin North Am 1995; 22[3]:539–549.)

ated with a sudden, strong desire to void (urgency). The sign urge incontinence is the observation of involuntary urinary loss from the urethra synchronous with an uncontrollable urge to void. The condition is due to detrusor overactivity.

2. **Stress incontinence:** The symptom is the patient's complaint of involuntary loss of urine during coughing, sneezing, or physical exertion such as sport activities, sudden changes of position, and so forth. The sign is the observation of loss of urine from the urethra synchronous with coughing, sneezing, or physical exertion. The condition is caused by sphincter abnormalities or detrusor overactivity provoked by such physical activity. The latter condition is called *stress hyperreflexia*.

Table 30–6. CLINICAL CAUSES OF LOSS OF URETHRAL COMPRESSION AND SUPPORT

Loss of Urethral Compression	Loss of Urethral Support
Neurologic	Levator (hammock) weakness
Anterior spinal artery syndrome	Childbirth
Radical hysterectomy	Trauma
Myelodysplasia	Surgery
Abdominoperineal resection of the rectum	Hypoestrogenic states
Structural scarring from urethral surgery	Aging

3. **Unconscious incontinence:** The symptom is the involuntary loss of urine that is unaccompanied by either urge or stress. The sign is the observation of loss of urine without the patient's awareness of urge or stress. The condition may be caused by detrusor overactivity, sphincter abnormalities, overflow, or extraurethral incontinence.

4. **Continuous leakage:** The symptom is the patient's complaint of a continuous involuntary loss of urine. The sign is the observation of a continuous urinary loss. The condition may be caused by sphincter abnormalities or extraurethral incontinence

5. **Nocturnal enuresis:** The symptom is the patient's complaint of urinary loss that occurs only during sleep. There is no corresponding sign. The condition may be caused by a sphincter abnormality, detrusor overactivity, or extraurethral incontinence.

6. **Postvoid dribble:** The symptom is the patient's complaint of a dribbling loss of urine that occurs after voiding. The sign is the observation of a dribbling loss of urine that occurs after voiding. The condition underlying postvoid dribble has not been adequately defined but is thought to be retained urine in the urethra distal to the sphincter in men

Table 30–7. SYMPTOMS, SIGNS, AND CONDITIONS CAUSING URINARY INCONTINENCE

Symptom	Condition	Medical/Surgical Causes
Urge incontinence	Detrusor overactivity	Idiopathic Neurogenic Urinary tract infection Bladder cancer Outlet obstruction
Stress incontinence	Sphincter hypermobility Intrinsic sphincter deficiency	Pelvic floor relaxation Prior urethral, bladder, or pelvic surgery Neurogenic
Unaware incontinence	Detrusor overactivity Sphincter abnormality Extraurethral incontinence	Idiopathic Neurogenic Prior urethral, bladder, or pelvic surgery Vesico-, uretero-, or urethrovaginal fistula Ectopic ureter
Continuous leakage	Sphincter abnormality Impaired detrusor contractility Extraurethral incontinence	Neurogenic Prior urethral, bladder, or pelvic surgery Ectopic ureter Urinary or vaginal fistula
Nocturnal enuresis	Sphincter abnormality Detrusor overactivity	Idiopathic Neurogenic Outlet obstruction
Postvoid dribble	Postsphincteric collection of urine	Idiopathic Urethral diverticulum
Extraurethral incontinence	Vesico-, uretero-, or urethrovaginal fistula Ectopic ureter	Trauma: surgical, obstetric, other Congenital

and retained urine in the vagina or in a urethral diverticulum in women.

7. **Overflow incontinence:** Overflow incontinence is a commonly used descriptive term. It is not a symptom, but the sign is the observation of incontinence accompanied by urinary retention. The condition may be caused by detrusor instability or sphincteric malfunction accompanied by either impaired detrusor contractility or bladder outlet obstruction.

DIAGNOSTIC EVALUATION

Diagnostic evaluation of urinary incontinence commences with a thorough history taking, physical examination, and routine laboratory studies, including urinalysis, urine culture, and renal function tests. Positive urine culture results should prompt treatment with culture-specific antibiotics, but patients with persistent bacteriuria or recurrent infections may require invasive testing while taking antibiotics. Hematuria should be evaluated by urinary cytologic studies, intravenous pyelography, and cystourethroscopy.

The sine qua non for a precise diagnosis is that the urinary incontinence is actually witnessed by the examiner. It makes little difference whether the urinary loss is demonstrated during physical examination, at cystoscopy, at cystometry, or by radiography, because the observations and measurements of an astute clinician are usually sufficient for establishing the correct diagnosis.

Urologic History

The history begins with a detailed account of the precise nature of the patient's symptoms. Each symptom should be characterized and quantified as accurately as possible (Romanzi et al, 1995). **When more than one symptom is present, the patient's assessment of the relative severity of each should be noted.** The patient should be asked how often he or she urinates during the day and night and how long he or she can comfortably wait between urinations. It should be determined why voiding occurs as often as it does. Is it because of a severe urge, or is it merely out of convenience or an attempt to prevent incontinence? The severity of incontinence should be graded. Does the patient lose a few drops or saturate the outer clothing? Are protective pads worn? Do they become saturated? How often are they changed? Is the patient aware of the act of incontinence, or does he or she just find himself or herself wet? Is there a sense of urgency first? If so, how long can micturition be postponed? Does urge incontinence occur? Does stress incontinence occur during coughing, during sneezing, while the patient rises from a sitting to standing position, or only during heavy physical exercise? If the incontinence is associated with stress, is urine lost only for an instant during the stress, or is there uncontrollable voiding? Is the incontinence positional? Does it ever occur in the lying or sitting positions? Is there difficulty initiating the stream, necessitating pushing or straining to start? Is the stream weak or interrupted? Is there postvoid dribbling? Has the patient ever been in urinary retention?

In order to document the nature and severity of urinary incontinence, a micturition diary (Fig. 30–12) **and a pad test are most useful.** Conceptually, a pad test provides a semiobjective measurement of urine loss over a given period of time. A number of pad tests have been described (Abrams et al, 1988; Hahn and Fall, 1991), but none has met with widespread approval, mainly because of poor test-retest validation (Christensen et al, 1986; Lose et al, 1986). The simplest pad test can be done by having the patient change his or her pads every 6 hours for one representative 24-hour period while he or she is taking phenazopyridine (Pyridium; 200 mg tid). The amount of staining on the pads is a rough estimate of the severity of the incontinence. Alternatively, the pads can be weighed and the total weight, minus the weight of an unused pad, recorded in the patient's record as an estimate of the volume of urine loss (1 g equals approximately 1 ml of urine). **We believe the pad test is very useful and recommend that, once it is completed, the patient simply be asked to state whether it was representative of his or her expected degree of incontinence** or

Voiding Diary

Name: ______________________________ Date: ________________

Time of Urge to Void	Strength of Pain or Urge	Time of Actual Void	Voided Volume	Incontinence (S, U, or W) (see below)	Amount of Leakage (Large = L, Medium = M, Small = S)
1.					
2.					
3.					
4.					
5.					
6.					
7.					
8.					
9.					
10.					
11.					
12.					
13.					
14.					
15.					
16.					
17.					

Urgency is the feeling that you have to urinate badly.

Incontinence is the loss of urine control before reaching the bathroom.
S = Stress Incontinence is wetting or leakage at times of coughing, sneezing, or with physical activity, etc.
U = Urge Incontinence is wetting or leakage because of urgency.
W = Unaware Incontinence is wetting without conscious awareness of when it happens.

Figure 30–12. Incontinence diary, to be completed over a 24-hour period. This is usually done with a concomitant 24-hour pad test.

was better or worse than usual. If the patient states that the urinary loss was unusually large or small, that information is recorded, and, if appropriate, the pad test is repeated.

The main purpose of these tests is to grossly quantify the relative severity of the incontinence so that it can be determined whether the symptoms are being accurately reproduced during subsequent examinations. Although there may be great variability in the actual data accumulated by these instruments, simply asking the patient whether the diary and pad test are representative of a "good" or "bad" day usually suffices for clinical purposes.

Past Medical History

The patient should be queried specifically about neurologic conditions that are known to affect bladder and sphincteric function, such as multiple sclerosis, spinal cord injury, diabetes, myelodysplasia, stroke, and Parkinson's disease. In this regard, it is important to ask about double vision, muscular weakness, paralysis or poor coordination, tremor, numbness, and tingling sensation. A history of prostate surgery, vaginal surgery, or previous surgical repair of incontinence should suggest the possibility of sphincteric injury (Mc-

Guire, 1980; Staskin et al, 1985; McGuire et al, 1987; Awad et al, 1988; Blaivas, 1988b; Blaivas and Jacobs, 1991; Morgan et al, 1995). Abdominoperineal resection of the rectum (Smith and Ballantyne, 1968; Gerstenberg et al, 1980; Mundy, 1982; Blaivas and Barbalias, 1983; Chang and Fan, 1983; Yalla and Andriole, 1984; McGuire et al, 1988) or radical hysterectomy (Smith and Ballantyne, 1968; Forney, 1980; Mundy, 1982; Woodside and McGuire, 1982) may be associated with neurologic injury to the bladder and sphincter. Radiation therapy may cause a reduced bladder capacity and/or low bladder compliance.

Medications are a rare cause of urinary incontinence. Sympatholytic agents such as clonidine, phenoxybenzamine, terazosin, and doxazosin may cause or worsen stress incontinence. Sympathomimetics and tricyclic antidepressants such as ephedrine, pseudoephedrine, or imipramine may increase bladder outlet obstruction and contribute to urinary retention and overflow incontinence.

Physical Examination

The physical examination should focus on detecting anatomic and neurologic abnormalities that contribute to urinary incontinence. The nature of the incontinence should be determined by examining the patient with a full bladder, as discussed in the later section on eyeball urodynamics.

The neurourologic examination begins by observing the patient's gait and demeanor as he or she first enters the office. A slight limp or lack of coordination, an abnormal speech pattern, facial asymmetry, or other abnormalities may be subtle signs of a neurologic condition.

The abdomen and flanks should be examined for masses, hernias, and a distended bladder. Rectal examination discloses the size and consistency of the prostate. The sacral dermatomes are evaluated by assessing anal sphincter tone and control, perianal sensation, and the bulbocavernosus reflex. With the physician's finger in the patient's rectum, the patient is asked to squeeze as if in the middle of urinating and trying to stop. A lax or weakened anal sphincter or the inability to voluntarily contract and relax are signs of neurologic damage, but some patients simply do not know or do not understand how to contract these muscles, whereas others may be too embarrassed to comply with the instructions. **The bulbocavernosus reflex is checked by suddenly squeezing the glans penis or clitoris and feeling (or seeing) the anal sphincter and perineal muscles contract. Alternatively, the reflex may be initiated by suddenly pulling the balloon of a Foley catheter against the vesical neck. The absence of this reflex in a man is almost always associated with a neurologic lesion, but the reflex is not detectable in up to 30% of otherwise normal women** (Blaivas, 1981).

In women a vaginal examination should be performed with the bladder both empty (to check the pelvic organs) and full (to check for incontinence and prolapse) (Romanzi et al, 1995). With the bladder comfortably full in the lithotomy position, the patient is asked to cough or strain in an attempt to reproduce the incontinence. **The degree of urethral hypermobility is assessed by the Q-tip test** (Crystle et al, 1971; Montz and Stanton, 1986; Bergman and Bhatia, 1987; Walters and Diaz, 1987). The Q-tip test was devised as a method to differentiate type I stress incontinence from type II stress incontinence at a time when bead chain cystourethrograms were routinely used for this purpose. It is performed by inserting a well-lubricated sterile cotton-tipped applicator gently through the urethra into the bladder. Once in the bladder, the applicator is withdrawn to the point of resistance, which is at the level of the vesical neck. The resting angle from the horizontal is recorded. The patient is then asked to strain, and the degree of rotation is assessed. Hypermobility is defined as a resting or straining angle of greater than 30 degrees from the horizontal and is equivalent to stress incontinence type II, provided that incontinence is demonstrated.

The anterior vaginal wall is examined first with the patient in the lithotomy position. The posterior blade from a split vaginal speculum is inserted and retracted posteriorly. If a metal speculum is used, it should be warmed with water. The patient is instructed to strain and cough, to assess for bladder, urethral, and cervical mobility and stress incontinence. Reduction of the cystocele (either manually or with a pessary) may be necessary to demonstrate stress incontinence.

After the anterior vaginal wall has been examined, the blade is rotated and the anterior vagina gently retracted. The posterior vaginal wall and vault are examined for the presence of a rectocele or an enterocele. As the speculum is slowly withdrawn, a transverse groove separating an enterocele from a rectocele below may be visible. A finger inserted into the rectum can "tent up" a rectocele but not an enterocele. The perineal body and vaginal rectal septum are examined by palpating the septum through the vagina and rectum. Pelvic floor strength is assessed by use of a clinical rating scale, outlined later in the section on assessment of patients for pelvic floor exercises (Hahn et al, 1993; McIntosh et al, 1993).

If incontinence is not demonstrated in the lithotomy position, and in patients with known or suspected prolapse, the examination is repeated in the standing position. The patient should be positioned standing in front of the examiner with one foot elevated on a short stool and again asked to cough and strain.

Patients who present for evaluation with a pessary in place should be examined both with and without the pessary in the vagina. With the pessary in place, she should be checked for stress incontinence with a full bladder; without the pessary, the degree of prolapse should be assessed. Not infrequently, patients with significant prolapse have seemingly good support even after many hours without pessary support, and maneuvers other than ambulation may be necessary to demonstrate the defect after pessary removal. Alternatively, the patient may leave the office without the pessary in place and return after the prolapse descends in the course of her daily activities. The vagina should be examined for any erosions or pudendal nerve injury from an ill-fitting pessary. Pudendal nerve injury is associated with paravaginal and perianal anesthesia, absence of the bulbocavernosus reflex, decreased anal sphincter tone, and worsening prolapse (Blaivas et al, 1979a; Bruskewitz, 1983; Snooks et al, 1984).

Urodynamic Evaluation

The purpose of urodynamic investigation is (1) to determine the precise etiology of the patient's incontinence

(McGuire et al, 1980), **(2) to evaluate detrusor function and determine the likelihood of voiding dysfunction after treatment of incontinence, (3) to determine the degree of pelvic floor prolapse (in female) and the need for correction of anatomic abnormalities, and (4) to identify urodynamic risk factors for the development of upper urinary tract deterioration.** Urodynamic risk factors include DESD, low bladder wall compliance, bladder outlet obstruction, and vesicoureteral reflux (McGuire et al, 1981; Blaivas and Barbalias, 1984; Ghoneim et al, 1989; Zoubek et al, 1989).

Urodynamic techniques range from simple "eyeball urodynamics" to sophisticated multichannel synchronous video/pressure/flow/EMG studies. **We believe that synchronous multichannel videourodynamics offer the most comprehensive, artifact-free means of arriving at a precise diagnosis,** and we perform them routinely when urodynamics are indicated. **When multichannel studies are not routinely performed, they should be considered under the following circumstances: (1) when results of simpler diagnostic tests have been inconclusive; (2) when empirical treatments have proved unsuccessful; (3) when the patient complains of incontinence but it cannot be demonstrated clinically; (4) in symptomatic patients who have previously undergone corrective surgery; (5) in patients who have previously undergone radical pelvic surgery,** such as abdominoperineal resection of the rectum or radical hysterectomy; **and (6) in patients with known or suspected neurologic disorders** that might interfere with bladder or sphincter function (myelodysplasia, spinal cord injury, multiple sclerosis, herniated disc, cerebrovascular accident, Parkinson's disease, and Shy-Drager syndrome).

Urodynamics is discussed in more detail in Chapter 28; only the relevant clinical features are presented here.

"EYEBALL URODYNAMICS"

"Eyeball urodynamics" is performed with the patient in the lithotomy position immediately after uroflow. A Foley catheter is inserted and postvoid residual urine measured. A regional neurologic examination is performed as outlined earlier. A 60-ml catheter-tipped syringe is connected to the Foley catheter and its barrel removed. Water or saline is then poured in through the open end of the syringe and allowed to drip into the bladder by gravity. As the water level in the syringe falls, its meniscus represents the vesical pressure, which can be estimated in centimeters of water above the symphysis pubis. When the water level in the syringe falls to the level of the catheter tip, it is refilled.

During bladder filling, the patient is told to neither void nor try to inhibit micturition but to simply report the sensations to the examiner. When the urge to void is perceived, the patient is asked whether that is the usual feeling experienced when he or she needs to urinate. Decreased sensations may be subtle signs of an underlying neuropathy (Wyndaele, 1993). Changes in vesical pressure are apparent as a slowing down in the rate of fall or a rise in the level of the fluid meniscus. A rise in pressure may be caused by a detrusor contraction, an increase in abdominal pressure, or low bladder wall compliance. As soon as a change in pressure is noted, the examiner should attempt to determine the cause. Visual inspection usually belies abdominal straining, but in doubtful cases, the abdomen should be palpated. In most instances, the cause of the rise in vesical pressure will be obvious, but when there is doubt, formal cystometry with rectal pressure monitoring is necessary.

Any sudden rise in pressure that is accompanied by an urge to void or by incontinence is indicative of an involuntary detrusor contraction. In some instances, the etiology of the patient's incontinence is easily discernible as the patient voids uncontrollably around the catheter during an involuntary detrusor contraction. If involuntary detrusor contractions do not occur, the bladder is filled until the patient feels comfortably full. The bladder is left full, and the catheter removed. The presence or absence of gravitational urinary loss is noted. The patient is asked to cough and bear down with gradually increasing force in order to determine the ease with which incontinence may be produced. In women, the introitus is observed for signs of cystourethrocele, rectocele, enterocele, and uterine prolapse.

Incontinence that occurs during stress is not always caused by sphincter abnormalities. In some patients, the stress initiates a reflex detrusor contraction. This condition has been termed **stress hyperreflexia**. Thus it is important to determine whether the leakage is accompanied by descent of the bladder base and urethra. **Furthermore, it should be noted whether the leakage stops as soon as the stress is over or whether the patient actually continues to void uncontrollably. In the former case, the condition is stress incontinence; in the latter, it is stress hyperreflexia. If the patient has leakage that is clearly accompanied by descent of the bladder base and proximal urethra (a cystourethrocele) and the leakage stops as soon as the cough or strain is over, the condition is type I or II stress incontinence. If the leakage occurs without descent, or with minimal provocation, the patient probably has intrinsic sphincteric deficiency (type III stress incontinence)** (Blaivas, 1988b).

If a female patient complains of urinary incontinence but it has not been demonstrated, the examination should be repeated with the patient in the standing position. It is best performed by having the patient stand with one foot on a small stool. The examiner sits beside her and performs the vaginal examination while the patient coughs and strains. If the examiner is still unable to demonstrate the incontinence, the patient is given a prescription for a urinary dye, such as Pyridium, and asked to wear incontinence pads and tampons, which she changes every 2 hours for a single representative day. She is instructed to bring the stained pads and tampons with her to the next office visit. The amount and location of the staining may help to determine the site and degree of urinary loss. It is axiomatic that **under ordinary circumstances, no patient should undergo invasive or irreversible treatment until the etiology of the incontinence has been clearly demonstrated.**

LABORATORY URODYNAMICS

Laboratory urodynamics relies on the same general principles as "eyeball urodynamics"; however, the measurements of pressure and flow are recorded electronically rather than visually. In addition, other physiologic parameters, such as sphincter EMG, are impossible to evaluate without electron-ics. Fluoroscopic evaluation of the lower urinary tract is another valuable diagnostic tool that is not possible without sophisticated equipment. The main advantage of laboratory urodynamics is the ability to record and display multiple parameters simultaneously. Not only does this provide a more precise understanding of physiology, but the individual findings serve as a check against one another to minimize the likelihood of misinterpretation.

Cystometry

From a technical standpoint, **cystometry is the graphic representation of vesical pressure as a function of bladder volume. It is used to assess detrusor activity, sensation, capacity, and compliance** (Blaivas et al, 1982; Abrams et al, 1988; Blaivas and Olsson, 1988). According to the International Continence Society, **detrusor activity may be either normal or overactive** (Abrams et al, 1988). **The overactive detrusor is characterized by involuntary detrusor contractions**, which may be spontaneous or provoked by rapid filling, changes in position, coughing, or other triggering maneuvers. When involuntary detrusor contractions are caused by neurologic disorders, the condition is called **detrusor hyperreflexia**. In the absence of a demonstrable neurologic etiology, the proper term to describe involuntary detrusor contractions is **detrusor instability**. Bladder sensation may be described as normal, absent, hypersensitive, or hyposensitive. Bladder compliance is defined as Δ volume/Δ pressure (ml/cm H_2O) on a cystometric curve (Abrams et al, 1988).

The bladder is filled at a rate that is determined by the patient's symptoms. In most instances, medium-fill cystometry is appropriate (filling rates between 10 and 100 ml/min), but slower rates may be advisable in patients with sensory urge syndromes (Abrams et al, 1988). The rest of the cystometric examination is performed as described in the section on "eyeball urodynamics." **The main disadvantage of "eyeball urodynamics" and one-channel cystometry is that it may be very difficult to detect the presence of small-magnitude detrusor contractions and to differentiate detrusor contractions from increases in usual pressure that result from abdominal straining.** Electronic cystometry overcomes this problem because vesical, abdominal, and detrusor pressure can be measured separately. This enables the detection of detrusor contractions that might otherwise be masked by the effects of abdominal pressure on the vesical pressure tracing.

Urinary Flow Rate

Urinary flow rate is a composite measure of the interaction between the pressure generated by the detrusor and the resistance offered by the urethra. Thus **a low uroflow may result from either bladder outlet obstruction or impaired detrusor contractility** (Chancellor et al, 1991). Moreover, **a normal uroflow may be seen in patients with urethral obstruction** if they generate detrusor pressure high enough to overcome the increased urethral resistance (Gerstenberg et al, 1982). **To distinguish between obstruction and impaired detrusor contractility, it is necessary to measure detrusor pressure and uroflow simultaneously, as discussed later** (Griffiths, 1980, 1988; Schäfer, 1985; Blaivas and Olsson, 1988; Schäfer et al, 1989). Thus a normal uroflow does not necessarily mean that the detrusor is normal, nor does it mean that the patient will be able to void normally after corrective surgery for incontinence.

Cystogram and Voiding Cystourethrogram

Radiologic visualization of the lower urinary tract during bladder filling and voiding is **useful for determining the site of bladder outlet obstruction, the integrity of the sphincter mechanism, and the presence of vesicoureteral reflux, bladder diverticula, and trabeculations of the bladder wall** (Shapiro and Raz, 1983; Blaivas, 1988b; Grischke et al, 1991). Fluoroscopic monitoring during filling, voiding, and provocative maneuvers such as straining or coughing is far preferable to static films. In general, when these studies cannot be performed at the same time as urodynamic evaluation, it is better to perform the urodynamic studies first so that the functional status of the bladder and urethra are known at the time of radiologic examination.

Leak Point Pressure

A leak point pressure is **conceptually useful for two types of patients: those with stress incontinence and those with low compliance.** In patients with low compliance, the **detrusor leak point pressure** is measured by filling the bladder and determining the vesical pressure at which there is leakage from the urethra (without increasing abdominal pressure). McGuire documented the deleterious effects that a high detrusor leak point pressure has on the upper urinary tracts; leak point pressures greater than 40 cm H_2O result in hydronephrosis or vesicoureteral reflux in 85% of myelodysplastic patients (McGuire et al, 1981).

In patients with stress incontinence, **the Valsalva leak point pressure** appears to be a good index of sphincteric function (McGuire et al, 1993a), but the test is relatively new and more studies are needed to establish normal values and optimal technique (Decter and Harpster, 1992). The technique is as follows: The bladder is filled either until the patient is comfortably full or to a preset volume. The patient is asked to perform a Valsalva maneuver gradually, increasing the intravesical pressure until urinary leakage is seen at the meatus or by radiography. Vesical and abdominal pressure are measured, and the Valsalva leak point pressure is defined as the lowest vesical pressure that causes leakage.

Conceptually, women with low leak point pressures have ISD. Patients who do not exhibit leakage with the Valsalva maneuver probably have a "good" intrinsic sphincter mechanism, but the effect of voluntary striated muscle control during the Valsalva maneuver has not been studied well enough to determine whether there are false-negative results.

Sphincter Electromyography

EMG is the measurement and display of electrical activity recruited from the striated muscles of the urethral or anal sphincter or from the perineal floor muscles. Sphincter EMG plays a dual role: In an indirect way, it provides kinesiologic information about the urethral sphincter and the pelvic floor muscles, and it also provides objective data about the integrity of the innervation to these muscles and the synchronization between detrusor and external sphincter. In order to objectively evaluate innervation, it should be performed by an experienced examiner using needle electrodes and oscilloscopic or audio control (Blaivas et al, 1977, 1979b; Nordling and Meyhoff, 1979; Blaivas and Fisher, 1981; Anderson, 1983; Blaivas, 1983; Snooks et al, 1984; Lose et al, 1985; Blaivas, 1988b; Smith et al, 1989; Fowler, 1991).

URETHRAL PRESSURE PROFILOMETRY

Despite an abundant literature on urethral profilometry, **it is our opinion that routine measurement of urethral pressures is neither necessary nor useful in the evaluation of incontinence** (Blaivas et al, 1982). A number of new techniques that measure pressure transmission ratios from bladder to urethra during increases in intra-abdominal pressure have been described, but their clinical applicability have yet to be proved (Versi, 1990; Rosenzweig et al, 1991; Sorensen et al, 1991; Versi et al, 1991; Richardson and Ramahi, 1993). The micturitional static urethral pressure profile as described by Yalla and associates (1980, 1981a, 1981b) is a useful means of pinpointing the site of urethral obstruction, but is not necessary for routine evaluation.

Synchronous Multichannel Urodynamic Studies

Synchronous measurement and display of urodynamic parameters with radiographic visualization of the lower urinary tract is the most precise diagnostic tool for evaluating disturbances of micturition (Bates and Corney, 1971; McGuire and Herlihy, 1977; Webster and Older, 1980; Blaivas and Fisher, 1981; Blaivas, 1988b; Brubaker and Sand, 1990). In these studies, radiographic contrast is used as the infusant for cystometry. Depending on the level of sophistication required, other urodynamic parameters such as abdominal pressure, urethral pressure, uroflow, and sphincter electromyographic characteristics may be recorded as well. There are important advantages to synchronous video/pressure flow studies over conventional single-channel urodynamics and over conventional cystography and voiding cystourethrography. By simultaneously measuring multiple urodynamic variables, the clinician gains a better insight into the underlying pathophysiologic process. Moreover, because all variables are visualized simultaneously, it is possible to better appreciate their interrelationships and identify artifacts with ease.

Table 30–8. TREATMENT GUIDELINES

Condition	Treatment
Detrusor Overactivity	
Detrusor instability and detrusor hyperreflexia	Treat underlying condition (urethral obstruction, infection, bladder stones, bladder cancer, spinal cord tumors, spinal disc disease, etc.) Anticholinergics and/or musculotropic relaxants and/or tricyclic antidepressants (+/− intermittent catheterization) Behavior modification Electrical stimulation Biofeedback Augmentation cystoplasty (+/− intermittent catheterization) Continent urinary diversion
Low bladder compliance	Anticholinergics and/or Musculotropic relaxants and/or Tricyclic antidepressants and/or (+/− intermittent catheterization) Augmentation cystoplasty (+/− intermittent catheterization) Continent urinary diversion
Sphincteric Incontinence	
Urethral hypermobility	Alpha-adrenergic sympathetic agonists Biofeedback Electrical stimulation Urethropexy Pubovaginal sling
Intrinsic sphincter deficiency	Alpha-adrenergic sympathetic agonists Biofeedback Electrical stimulation Periurethral injections • Collagen • Autologous fat • Polytetrafluoroethylene Pubovaginal sling

TREATMENT OVERVIEW

Treatment of incontinence should be predicated on a clear understanding of the underlying physiology (Table 30–8).

Involuntary Detrusor Contractions

The **ideal approach** to the treatment of urinary incontinence caused by involuntary detrusor contractions is to **eliminate the underlying etiology**. Although this is rarely possible when the cause is neurologic or idiopathic, **in the majority of patients with urethral obstruction, the symptoms of detrusor instability are ameliorated after the obstruction has been cured. Urethral obstruction is rare in women and usually caused by previous pelvic surgery. Urethrolysis, with or without resuspension of the vesical neck, is reportedly effective in about 60% of women who develop detrusor instability after operations for stress incontinence** (Lockhart et al, 1984; McGuire et al, 1989; Webster and Kreder, 1990a; Foster and McGuire, 1993; Nitti and Raz, 1994a). **In women with mixed stress and urge incontinence, if the stress incontinence is the primary problem, successful repair is associated with cure of the urge incontinence in 50% to 75% of patients** (McGuire et al, 1987; Awad et al, 1988; Blaivas and Jacobs, 1991). **In men, urethral obstruction is usually caused by benign prostatic hypertrophy, and symptomatic relief of detrusor instability is expected in more than two thirds of men who undergo transurethral prostatic resection (TURP)** (Abrams, 1977, 1985; Abrams et al, 1979; Cumming and Chisholm, 1992; Gormley et al, 1993).

When it is not possible to treat the underlying etiology, the basic treatment is to abolish the involuntary detrusor

contractions. This may be accomplished by medications (Holmes et al, 1989; Mostwin, 1990; Wein, 1995), **behavior modification, electrical stimulation, and biofeedback** (to be discussed). When these conservative techniques fail, denervation procedures have been recommended, but there is little documentation of efficacy, and many of the techniques are associated with considerable morbidity (Nordling et al, 1986; Ramsay et al, 1992; McGuire et al, 1993b). Some patients with detrusor instability also have incomplete bladder emptying. Although first described in the elderly as detrusor hyperactivity with impaired contractility (DHIC) by Resnick and Yalla (1987), in our experience this condition is quite common and spans all ages. It is usually more difficult to treat, and patients may require adjunctive intermittent catheterization.

In the great majority of patients with refractory detrusor instability, augmentation enterocystoplasty is effective, provided that the intestine is detubularized, but many require intermittent self-catheterization (Linder et al, 1983; Webster, 1987; Luangkhot et al, 1991; Robertson et al, 1991). There have been reports of successful outcomes after detrusor myectomy (Cartwright and Snow, 1989, 1995) and other forms of "autoaugmentation."

Anticholinergics and Musculotropic Relaxing Agents

Anticholinergics are competitive inhibitors of acetylcholine that block the muscarinic effects. Musculotropic relaxants possess direct relaxing effects on smooth muscle, and most possess anticholinergic properties as well. If fully effective, these drugs would result in abolition of the involuntary detrusor contractions; however, this rarely occurs. Partial efficacy results in increase in the volume to the first involuntary detrusor contraction, a decrease in its amplitude, and an increase in bladder capacity. In many patients, however, the time between the first significant urge and the onset of the involuntary detrusor contraction (the "warning time") is unchanged, and the ability to suppress it is unchanged. Thus, symptomatic detrusor overactivity may persist unless the anticholinergic/antispasmodic therapy is combined with behavior modification such as timed bladder emptying (Wein, 1995).

All the active drugs must be given in an adequate dosage to ensure a physiologic effect. In practice, the dosage may be increased every 3 to 5 days until the patient exhibits clinical improvement or until untoward side effects occur. Common side effects consist of dry mouth, blurred vision, and constipation. In some patients, the drug may be so effective that the patient is unable to void at all and must be managed with intermittent self-catheterization. The two most commonly used drugs are propantheline bromide (Pro-Banthine) and oxybutynin chloride (Ditropan). Propantheline is usually begun at 7.5 to 15 mg orally four times a day; dosages as high as 105 mg four times a day are sometimes needed because of the erratic absorption of the drug. Oxybutynin is usually begun at 2.5 to 5 mg three to four times a day, and it is rarely necessary to exceed 10 mg per dose (Wein, 1995). See Chapter 29 for a complete discussion.

Tricyclic Antidepressants

Imipramine (Tofranil) is the prototype tricyclic antidepressant. The exact mode of action has not been clearly demonstrated, but it exerts a direct relaxant effect on bladder smooth muscle and has sympathomimetic and central effects as well (Wein, 1995). Although many of the side effects are anticholinergic, it does not exert a major or even moderate anticholinergic effect on bladder smooth muscle. The usual starting dosage is 25 mg per day, given at bedtime. Unlike the anticholinergics, imipramine builds up a blood level over a period of several weeks. Its effect may not be apparent for at least that length of time. The dose is increased by 25 mg per week (up to a maximum of about 150 mg) until the patient is clinically well or has anticholinergic side effects. However, if it must be discontinued, it should be tapered over several weeks lest a severe rebound depression occur. See Chapter 29 for a complete discussion.

Rehabilitative Techniques: Behavior Modification, Pelvic Floor Exercises, Biofeedback, and Electrical Stimulation

All these techniques may be applicable for the treatment of detrusor instability and are discussed in detail later in this chapter.

Sphincter Abnormalities

In general, surgical treatment of sphincteric incontinence is far more successful than nonsurgical treatment.

Non-Surgical Treatment

Biofeedback, electrical stimulation, and behavior modification have all been reported to cause improvement in 30% to 75% of patients; "cure" is usually reported in about 10%, but long-term data confirming these claims are sorely lacking. Medical treatment has been largely confined to agents with an alpha-adrenergic agonist action (Wein, 1995) and to estrogens.

A complete discussion of the nonhormonal aspects of medical treatment of stress incontinence can be found in Chapter 29. Surgical treatment consists of periurethral injection, transvaginal operations, retropubic urethropexy, colposuspensions, "needle suspensions," and pubovaginal sling and are discussed in detail elsewhere in this volume.

Estrogens in the Treatment of Incontinence

Estrogens were used for the treatment of urinary incontinence as early as 1941 (Salmon et al, 1941), but debate regarding their efficacy, site of action, route of administration, and dosage persists to the present time. In both animals and humans, there is a high concentration of estrogen receptors in the urethra (Iosif et al, 1981; Batra and Iosif, 1983; Fantl et al, 1988). Estrogens appear to affect the urinary bladder by enhancing alpha-adrenergic receptor density and sensitivity (Caine and Raz, 1975; Hodgson et al, 1978; Levin et al, 1980, 1981; Larsson et al, 1984), by enhancing neuronal sensitivity and transmitter metabolism, and by exerting trophic effects on urethral mucosa, submucosa, and pelvic floor/periurethral collagen (Fantl et al, 1988; Bump et al, 1988b; Versi et al, 1988). Bump and Friedman reported that sex hormone replacement therapy with estrogen, but not testosterone, enhanced the urethral sphincter mechanism in the castrated female baboon by effects that were unrelated to skeletal muscle. They suggested that these effects might also result from changes in the urethral mucosa, submucosal vascular plexus, and connective tissue (Bump and Friedman, 1986). After menopause, urethral pressure parameters normally decrease somewhat (Rud, 1980), and although this is generally conceded to be related in some way to lower estrogen levels, whether the actual changes occur in smooth muscle, blood circulation, supporting tissues, or the mucosal seal mechanism is still largely a matter of speculation. Versi and colleagues (1988) described a positive correlation between skin collagen content, which does decline with declining estrogen status, and parameters of the urethral pressure profile; this correlation suggests that estrogen effect on the urethra may be predicted, at least in part, by changes in the collagen component.

A daily dose of 2.5 mg conjugated estrogens was demonstrated to improve stress incontinence and increase urethral pressures in 65% of postmenopausal women treated (Raz et al, 1973). Another regimen (2 g of daily intravaginal conjugated estrogen cream) led to 60% improvement or cure rates in a small series of postmenopausal women. Favorable response was correlated with increased urethral closure pressure and increased pressure transmission ratios (Bhatia et al, 1989). Karram and Bhatia (1989) administered estrogens, either oral or vaginal, to women with premature ovarian failure and no lower urinary tract complaints; they found no change in cystometric parameters other than a significant increase in the pressure transmission ratio to the proximal and midurethra of women using vaginal estrogens only. Other researchers have found favorable therapeutic effect on patients with urinary frequency, urgency, and urge incontinence (Walter et al, 1978; Hilton and Stanton, 1983; Samisoe et al, 1985).

In view of the favorable response noted in these clinical trials it is not unreasonable to try estrogen replacement therapy in peri- and postmenopausal patients with minimal to moderate stress incontinence, as well as those with urgency symptoms. When any woman is treated with estrogen, however, the need for concomitant progesterone therapy must be assessed. Unopposed oral or transdermal estrogen therapy in a woman who has not previously undergone hysterectomy is a well-established risk factor for endometrial cancer. In general, women with a history of breast cancer, particularly those whose tumors are estrogen receptor positive, are not candidates for hormonal manipulation. Whether low dose vaginal cream entails a similar risk remains undetermined.

The effect of progesterone on the lower urinary tract is poorly understood. In a bioassay of rabbit bladder specimens (Rosenzweig et al, 1995), estrogen receptors were found in highest density in urethral epithelium and urethral and bladder smooth muscle. Androgen receptors were found in high concentrations in urethral and bladder epithelium but not in the smooth muscle, and progesterone receptors were not demonstrated to any appreciable degree. However, the rabbits had not been primed with estrogen, which is known to be a necessary step in order to demonstrate progesterone receptors in other organs. Thus, although the focus of hormone therapy trials for incontinence have focused on estrogens, the interaction among estrogens, androgens, and the priming of progesterone receptors may shed light on the variable results found by various investigators.

Urethral Hypermobility (Stress Incontinence Types IIA and IIB)

The basic principles of surgical treatment are to prevent the abnormal descent of the urethra that occurs during increases in abdominal pressure and to provide a backboard against which the urethra is compressed during increases in abdominal pressure. This may be accomplished with any of the standard "urethropexy operations," such as the Marshall-Marchetti-Krantz or Burch, the "needle bladder neck suspension procedures" (modified Pereyra procedures) or creation of a pubovaginal sling (Aldridge, 1942; Burch, 1961, 1963, 1968; TeLinde, 1963; Lapides, 1970, 1974; Backer and Probst, 1971; Tanagho and Smith, 1971, 1972; Flocks and Boldus, 1973; Nichols and Milley, 1973; Stamey, 1973, 1980; Beck et al, 1974; Pelosi et al, 1976; Stanton et al, 1976, 1982; Tanagho, 1976; Green, 1977; Zacharin, 1977, 1983; Cobb and Ragde, 1978; Corr and Shapiro, 1978; McGuire and Lytton, 1978; Stanton and Cardozo, 1979; Raz, 1981, 1990; de-Kock and de-Klerk, 1982; Ingelman-Sundberg, 1982; Iosif, 1982, 1983; Parnell et al, 1982, 1984; Mattingly and Davis, 1984; Schaeffer and Stamey, 1984; Hadley et al, 1985; Pow-Sang et al, 1986; Schmidbauer et al, 1986; Gittes and Loughlin, 1987; McGuire et al, 1987; Brubaker and Sand, 1988; Langer et al, 1988, 1990; Mainprize and Drutz, 1988; Siegel and Raz, 1988; Van Geelen et al, 1988; Bergman et al, 1989; Blaivas and Chancellor, 1989; Hilton and Mayne, 1989; Karram and Bhatia, 1989; Korda et al, 1989; Little et al, 1989; Raz et al, 1989; Bent, 1990; Blaivas, 1990; Kelly et al, 1990; Knespl, 1990; Lockhart et al, 1990; Thunedborg et al, 1990; Webster and Kreder, 1990a; Winter, 1990; Blaivas and Jacobs, 1991; Kursh, 1991; Morgan et al, 1995; Stothers et al, 1995). **Although all these procedures have a comparable short-term success rate of about 75% to 95%, long-term data are sorely lacking. We believe that the retropubic procedures (Burch, Marshall-Marchetti-Krantz) and the fascial pubovaginal sling offer a clear superiority over the needle suspensions and vaginal procedures** (Iosif, 1983; Van Geelen et al, 1988; Bergman et al, 1989). The role of collagen, autologous fat, polytef, and other implantable substances is currently under investigation, but preliminary data suggest that the injectables have an unacceptably low success rate in patients with hypermobility (Santiago et al, 1989; Santarosa and Blaivas, 1991; Herschorn et al, 1992; Appell, 1994; Ganabathi and Leach, 1994; Kageyama et al, 1994; McGuire and Appell, 1994).

Intrinsic Sphincter Deficiency (Stress Incontinence Type III)

In type III SUI, the proximal urethra no longer functions adequately as a sphincter. Because the problem is not one of abnormal descent, the usual suspension operations for SUI are often unsuccessful. **A sphincter prosthesis is theoretically ideal and reportedly has excellent results when inserted by experienced surgeons but, in our judgment,**

has an unacceptably high complication rate in patients who have undergone multiple prior operations (Diokno et al, 1984, 1987; Scott, 1985; Goldwasser et al, 1987; Appell, 1988; Fishman et al, 1989; Aliabadi and Gonzalez, 1990; Parulkar and Barrett, 1990; Duncan et al, 1992; Wang and Hadley, 1992). **In these patients, a pubovaginal sling is the operation of choice** (Aldridge, 1942; Beck et al, 1974; Wheeless et al, 1977; Corr and Shapiro, 1978; McGuire and Lytton, 1978; McGuire et al, 1987; Woodside, 1987; Blaivas and Olsson, 1988; Blaivas and Chancellor, 1989; Blaivas, 1990; Blaivas and Jacobs, 1991; Morgan et al, 1995). **The periurethral injection of collagen, autologous fat, polytef, and other implantable substances shows great promise** and is currently under clinical investigation (Santiago et al, 1989; Santarosa and Blaivas, 1991; Herschorn et al, 1992; Appell, 1994; Ganabathi and Leach, 1994; Kageyama et al, 1994; McGuire and Appell, 1994).

Types 0 and I Stress Incontinence

In types 0 and I stress incontinence, the relative contributions of hypermobility and ISD may be difficult to assess. An estimation of the pressure necessary to induce incontinence, such as the abdominal or Valsalva leak point pressure, is the most useful diagnostic technique currently available to make this distinction. Treatment should be based on the underlying abnormality as described earlier.

Stress Incontinence Associated with Urethral Diverticulum

The preoperative evaluation of patients with urethral diverticulum should include a careful assessment for stress urinary incontinence. **When both are present, they should be repaired at the same time,** according to the principles outlined earlier. It should be recognized that during the vaginal dissection, the vesical neck supports may become weakened, and iatrogenic stress incontinence may ensue. To prevent this, the surgeon should consider making an intraoperative decision to correct the potential anatomic condition whenever necessary.

Stress Incontinence Associated with Vesicovaginal or Urethrovaginal Fistula

Whenever there is urinary incontinence associated with a vesicovaginal or urethrovaginal fistula, a careful evaluation should be undertaken to ensure that the patient does not have sphincteric incontinence in addition to the fistula. If sphincteric incontinence is documented, **it should be repaired at the same time as the fistula repair.**

Stress Incontinence Associated with Urinary Frequency, Urgency, and Urge Incontinence

Approximately 30% to 50% of women with stress incontinence also complain of urinary frequency, urgency, and/or urge incontinence (McGuire et al, 1976; Webster et al, 1984; Sand et al, 1987; Blaivas and Olsson, 1988; Couillard and Webster, 1995). In addition to the routine work-up, these patients should undergo careful evaluation, including urinary cytologic studies and cystourethroscopy, to rule out such conditions as carcinoma in situ of the bladder, bladder stones, and interstitial cystitis. **When the stress symptoms predominate and stress incontinence is objectively demonstrated, surgical repair usually (50% to 70%) alleviates all the symptoms** (Blaivas and Jacobs, 1988; McGuire et al, 1987, 1993a; Awad et al, 1988). **However, when the other symptoms predominate or when the degree of stress incontinence seems minimal in comparison to the severity of the urge symptoms, repair of the stress incontinence may not be helpful at all and may even intensify the patient's symptoms** (Meyhoff et al, 1981, 1983). Whenever there is doubt, it is most reasonable to proceed with noninvasive medical treatment of the frequency and urgency symptoms before consideration of surgical therapy of stress incontinence.

Postprostatectomy Incontinence

Urinary incontinence is an uncommon complication after routine prostatectomy, but it is encountered at least temporarily in the majority of men after radical prostatectomy and is a persistent problem in at least 5% to 10% (Rudy et al, 1984; Leach and Yun, 1992; Fowler et al, 1993, 1995). In most patients, the symptoms are transitory and subside within several week to several months. Optimal treatment is prevention, and prevention is best attained by careful attention to patient selection and to surgical technique. **Patients at higher risk for developing postprostatectomy incontinence for benign disease include those with preoperative incontinence, those with neurologic conditions, those who have undergone abdominoperineal resection of the rectum, and those who undergo surgery shortly after being treated for an acute infection of the lower urinary tract. The risk factors for those undergoing radical prostatectomy include all those just listed, but, in addition, there is a further risk for those with bulky disease, particularly at the apex, and those who have undergone prior radiation therapy or previous prostatic surgery.**

The diagnosis and treatment of postprostatectomy incontinence is, in our judgment, more difficult than a review of the literature might suggest. Conceptually, postprostatectomy incontinence can be caused by sphincter malfunction, detrusor abnormalities, or urinary retention with overflow. Detrusor abnormalities include involuntary detrusor contractions, impaired or absent detrusor contractility, and low bladder compliance. From a diagnostic standpoint, most patients who complain of constant, dribbling, gravitational, or stress-induced incontinence have sphincteric malfunction, and most who complain of urinary frequency, urgency, and urge incontinence have involuntary detrusor contractions. However, there may be considerable overlap between these two conditions, and both may coexist in the same patient. **In most series, sphincteric abnormalities are present in about 75% of patients, but coexistent detrusor abnormalities (detrusor instability and/or low compliance) are seen in about half of the patients with sphincter abnormalities. Detrusor abnormalities alone are seen in about 15%** (Rudy et al, 1984; Leach et al, 1987; Foote et al, 1991; Leach and Yun, 1992; Chao and Mayo, 1995; Goluboff et al, 1995). A complete list of the causes of postprostatectomy incontinence is presented in Table 30–9.

In most men, postprostatectomy sphincteric incontinence subsides spontaneously in the first few weeks to months after surgery. **For persistent incontinence, conservative therapies such as alpha-adrenergic agonists, biofeedback, electrical stimulation, and behavior modification should be tried, but for incontinence that persists longer than a year after surgery, surgical treatment is generally the only reasonable long-term solution** unless the patient prefers to manage the problem with absorbent pads, condom catheters, a penile clamp, or an indwelling catheter.

The most successful surgical treatment is the implantation of a sphincter prosthesis, which has a reported success rate of 80% to 90% (Scott et al, 1973; Furlow and Barrett, 1985; Leach et al, 1987; Fishman et al, 1989; Gundian et al, 1989; Mark and Light, 1989; Scott, 1989; Zimmern and Leach, 1989; Kreder and Webster, 1991; Light and Reynolds, 1992; Montague, 1992; Perez and Webster, 1992; Brito et al, 1993; Leo and Barrett, 1993; Ghoneim et al, 1994). The role of periurethral injections is still under investigation. Although short-term success has been reported in up to 85% of men, most of that success has been described in terms of a reduction in the number of pads worn (Appell, 1994; McGuire and Appell, 1994). In our experience, after radical prostatectomy, only about 10% of men have experienced a meaningful response that had lasted more than several months, even after repeated injections. After TURP, the results appear to be somewhat better.

PELVIC FLOOR EXERCISES, BIOFEEDBACK, ELECTRICAL STIMULATION, AND BEHAVIOR MODIFICATION

Pelvic floor exercises, biofeedback, electrical stimulation, and behavior modification are rehabilitative therapies that may be used singly or in combination. They have been described for the treatment of a variety of conditions, including urinary incontinence caused both by sphincteric abnormalities and by detrusor overactivity. Optimal patient care mandates that these therapies be tailored to the needs of the individual patient, but not all patients are good candidates for these interventions. Many patients are unwilling or unable to comply with established treatment regimens, preferring surgery or pharmacotherapy instead. However, **for motivated patients who are willing to pursue the rigors of long-term treatment, a reasonable degree of improvement can be expected. Although there is a paucity of data on long-term therapy, effective treatment probably requires a lifetime commitment.** As with the treatment of any other chronic condition that has an inevitable toll on lifestyle and self-perception, encouragement, close follow-up, and flexibility are as important to a successful treatment as any individual therapeutic method.

All these treatments are based on common physiologic principles designed to (1) inhibit the onset of involuntary detrusor contractions, (2) abort unstable detrusor contractions before they cause incontinence, (3) strengthen the sphincter mechanism, and (4) convert periurethral and levator ani striated muscle fibers from fast-twitch (type 2) to slow-twitch (type 1) fibers.

Involuntary detrusor contractions can be inhibited through at least 3 neural mechanisms:

1. Central neural pathways that mediate voluntary control of the bladder. The neural pathways subserving this function have not been well defined, but cortical-hypothalamic-pontine and medullopontine sites have been proposed (Gjone and Setekleiv, 1963; Kuru, 1965; Bradley et al, 1974; Fall et al, 1978c; Blaivas, 1982; Morrison, 1987b; deGroat et al, 1989; deGroat and Steers, 1990). **These are the mechanisms by which micturition is voluntarily delayed, without contraction of the striated sphincter, once the urge to void is felt** (Denny-Brown and Robertson, 1933; Langworthy et al, 1940; Lapides et al, 1955, 1957). It has been proposed that these pathways can be "retrained" through the use of behavior modification therapies (Frewen, 1978, 1979, 1980, 1982; Elder and Stephenson, 1980; Jarvis, 1980, 1981, 1982a, 1982b; Jarvis and Millar, 1983; Fantl et al, 1991).

2. Central neural pathways that mediate voluntary control of the striated sphincter. These are neuronal connections between the frontal cortex and the pudendal nucleus (Kuru, 1965; Bradley et al, 1974; Blaivas, 1982; Morrison, 1987b; deGroat et al, 1989; deGroat and Steers, 1990). **Contraction of the striated sphincter not only interrupts the urinary stream but also inhibits the onset of or shuts off the detrusor contraction once it starts** (Yalla et al, 1976, 1978; Fall et al, 1977b, 1977c; Blaivas, 1982; Lindstrom et al, 1983; Lindstrom and Sudsuang, 1989). **It does not appear to matter whether this is accomplished through volitional control or electrical stimulation; contraction of the sphincter causes a reflexive inhibition of the detrusor. This is another pathway that can be "retrained"** with behavioral modification or by electrical stimulation and pelvic floor exercises.

3. Reflex (cutaneous) stimulation of the perineum and anal dilatation. These cause inhibition of detrusor contraction (Fall et al, 1977b, 1977c; Yalla et al, 1978; Lindstrom et al, 1983; Morrison, 1987a; Lindstrom and Sudsuang, 1989). These reflexes are mediated via pelvic and pudendal nerve afferent nerves that activate inhibitory sympathetic nerves to the detrusor and central pathways that

Table 30–9. ETIOLOGY OF POSTPROSTATECTOMY INCONTINENCE

Sphincteric Incontinence
Postsurgical anatomic damage
Postsurgical neurologic damage
Neurologic disorders
Detrusor Instability
Urinary tract infection
Occult carcinoma of the bladder
Bladder stones
Retained sutures
Urethral obstruction
Anastomotic stricture
Vesical neck contracture
Detrusor Hyperreflexia
Low Bladder Compliance

inhibit preganglionic detrusor motor neurons (Lindstrom et al, 1983; Lindstrom and Sudsuang, 1989). **These are the pathways that are involved with direct electrical stimulation of the pelvic floor** (Figs. 30–13, 30–14).

Strengthening of the striated muscles of the sphincter is accomplished by repetitive aerobic and anaerobic exercise. The conversion of fast- to slow-twitch striated muscle fibers has been demonstrated by chronic stimulation of anterior sacral roots, and it has been suggested that prolonged, forceful contractions induced by voluntary effort can induce a similar transformation (Bazeed et al, 1982). Fast-twitch muscle fibers respond to exercise by becoming hypertrophic, and hypertrophied muscles generate more force. Theoretically, this is best accomplished by rapid, forceful, repetitive contractions. Slow-twitch fibers appear to respond better to sustained maximal voluntary contractions. Pelvic floor exercises, biofeedback, and electrical stimulation may be used to induce both types of muscle contractions, but it is not known whether any one of these techniques is more effective at accomplishing these goals than another. However, **from a clinical perspective, two of the most important determinants of success or failure are patient motivation and compliance. For this reason, regimens that incorporate scheduled exercise programs with routine monitoring by a therapist are more likely to achieve successful results.** All these rehabilitative techniques are essentially no different than other exercise programs: If not done regularly, they are ineffective. Moreover, no matter how effective the program, once it is discontinued, the beneficial effects are likely to be short-lived.

Pelvic Floor Exercises and Biofeedback

Pelvic floor exercises (PFEs) entail the voluntary contraction of the pelvic muscles. Biofeedback displays auditory and/or visual correlates of pelvic muscle contraction, which may be used both as an aid to teach proper muscle isolation and to record the strength and duration of muscle contractions in order to document a baseline and monitor the patient's progress and compliance. In this regard, biofeedback, by itself, is not therapy; it can only be used in conjunction with PFEs. Biofeedback may be accomplished by monitoring EMG activity from the pelvic floor and abdominal muscles or by monitoring vaginal and abdominal pressure.

PFEs are typically done by the patient on a daily or every-other-day basis with office evaluation at regular intervals. PFE regimens generally involve rapid and sustained contractions in order to strengthen both the fast and slow twitch fibers found in the levator musculature. **Instructing patients in the performance of PFEs is a hands-on effort, requiring individual instruction in order to ensure isolation of the proper muscle group.** In a demonstration of quick instruction during urodynamic testing, Bump and co-workers (1991) found that 25% of the women actually made a distinct

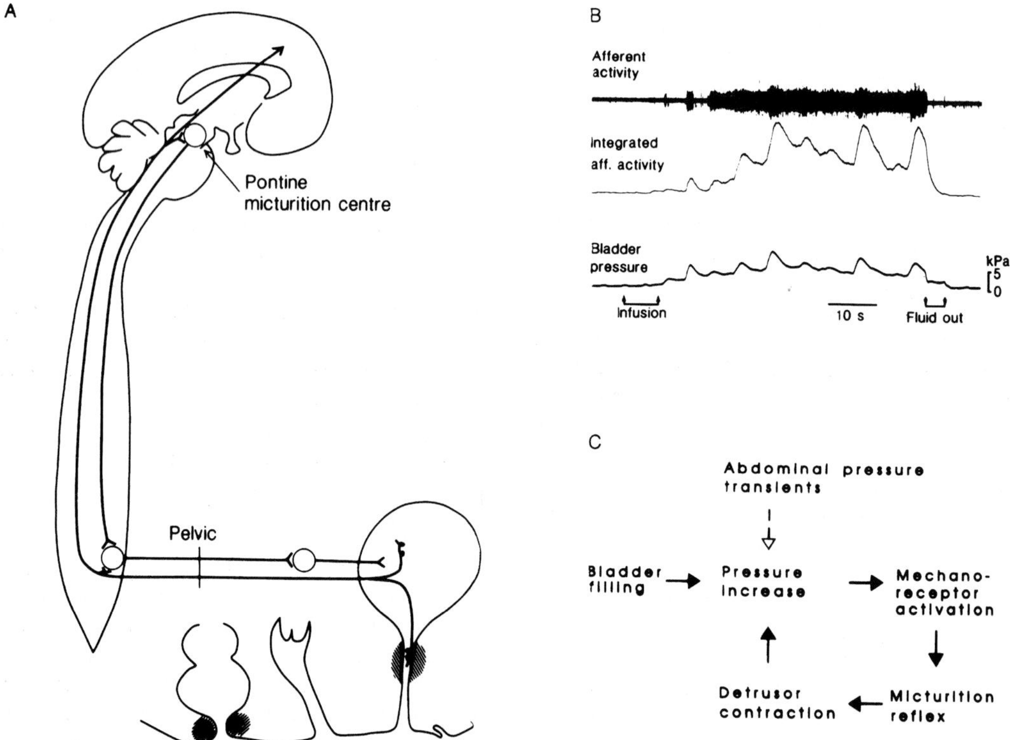

Figure 30–13. *A,* The micturition reflex involves afferent sympathetic input to the pontine micturition center from bladder wall stretch receptors, which in turn generate efferent motor output to the bladder via the pelvic (parasympathetic) nerves. *B,* Coordinate activity between afferent stretch receptor input and reflex detrusor contraction activity in the cat during bladder filling. The top tracing depicts the raw afferent activity (analogous to an EMG), and the middle tracing depicts integrated afferent activity from the mechanoreceptors in the bladder. The bottom tracing is of vesical pressure. *C,* Once the micturition reflex is initiated, the detrusor contraction enhances afferent input from stretch receptors, facilitating a self-perpetuated contraction and complete micturition. (From Fall M, Lindstrom S: Urol Clin North Am 1991; 18:394.)

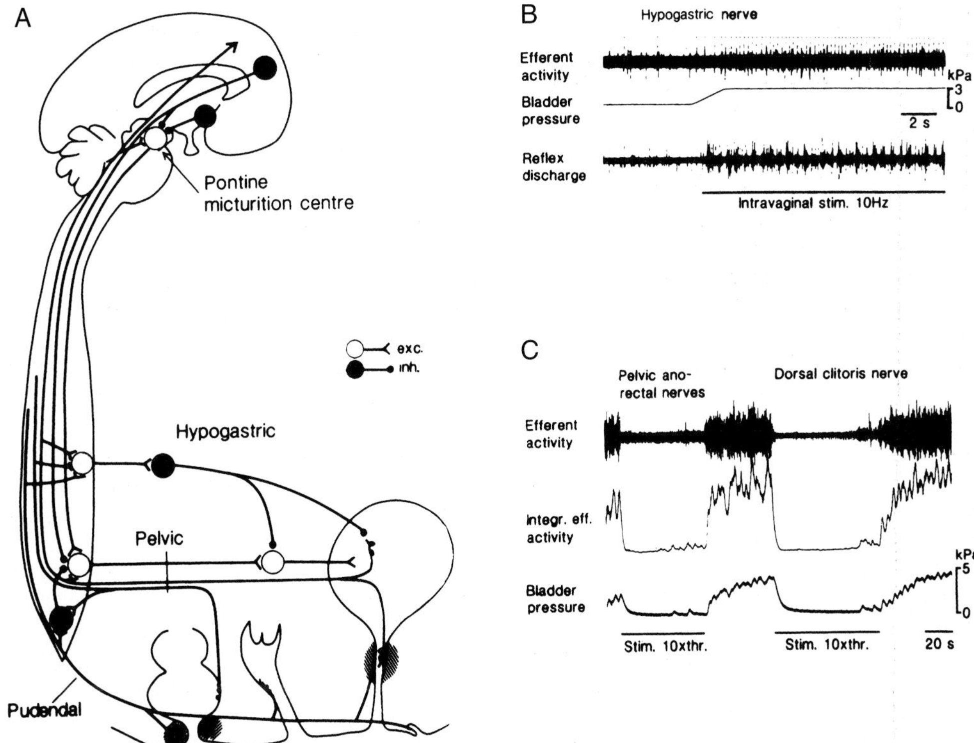

Figure 30–14. *A,* Bladder filling and continence are facilitated by reflex activation of the hypogastric (sympathetic) nerve plexes, which leads to intrinsic bladder sphincter contraction and concomitant detrusor relaxation. Detrusor inhibition is also activated by anal dilatation (pelvic nerve) and clitoral or penile stimulation (pudendal nerve). *B,* A demonstration of pudendal nerve stimulation in the cat. A 10-Hz current for intravaginal electrical stimulation (*bottom*) leads to increased hypogastric output (*top*). (From Fall M, Lindstrom S: Urol Clin North Am 1991; 18:395.)

Valsalva effort, which, if practiced regularly, may actually worsen pelvic floor tone and incontinence.

Patient Assessment

Before initiating rehabilitative therapies, **a detailed assessment of the pelvic floor muscles should be performed. The patient should be instructed in the anatomy and function of the pelvic floor;** in this regard, pelvic floor models or diagrams may prove useful. With two examining fingers in the vagina, the levator muscles are located at the 5- and 7-o'clock positions just superior to the hymeneal ring. The patient is instructed to contract these muscles. To assist in proper muscle group isolation, various verbal cues can be tried, such as "squeeze as if you were trying to stop your urine stream" or "as if you were trying to prevent flatus" or "pull the examining fingers up into the vagina." **A correctly performed pelvic floor contraction is demonstrated by cephalad retraction of the perineum and anus, posterior rotation of the clitoris, and anterior displacement of the examining fingers.** Many patients unfamiliar with this maneuver initially contract the abdominal wall and/or contract the buttocks or lower extremity adductors rather than the levator musculature (Bo et al, 1988; Bump et al, 1991; Boucier and Juras, 1995). Once the patient is able to contract the muscles properly, she is asked to contract as strongly as possible for as long as possible in order to assess baseline pelvic floor function. This maximal effort is then rated according to a pelvic muscle rating scale.

A variety of pelvic muscle rating scales have been published (Hahn et al, 1993; McIntosh et al, 1993). We use a modification of a scale, first published in 1986 by Worth and associates with a subsequent modification by Brink and coworkers (1994) (Fig. 30–15). This scale incorporates objective data (duration of the contraction) and semiobjective data (anterior vaginal wall displacement and palpable strength of contraction) obtained during digital pelvic evaluation.

Once awareness and function of the muscle groups have been established, the patient is instructed to perform a series of "quick flick," maximal, and sustained contractions as part of a daily exercise regimen. Patients are encouraged to return for regular follow-up in order to monitor their progress and compliance. **In addition to physical examination and muscle testing (either manually or with pressure and/or EMG monitoring), voiding diaries and pad tests are repeated at the follow-up visits.**

History

First described by Arnold Kegel in 1948, active rehabilitation of the levator musculature, or **"Kegel exercises," have utility as both primary and adjunctive therapy.** In his initial description, Kegel described the use of a perineometer that measured vaginal pressure and provided a method of biofeedback. His regimen involved pelvic floor contractions for 20-minute periods three times daily. After using this method in 64 women with stress incontinence, he stated that "there have been no failures when the condition was due primarily to relaxation or atrophy of the anterior vaginal muscles and the patient had at least partial control at times." In subsequent studies, **he claimed a cure rate of**

PELVIC MUSCLE RATING SCALE: (/9)

	1	2	3	4
Pressure:	none	weak	moderate	strong
Duration:	none	<1 sec	1-5 sec	>5 sec
Displacement:	none	slt.ant.	whole ant.	gripped

Figure 30–15. Pelvic muscle rating scale used to assess levator function. It incorporates objective and semi-objective parameters (pelvic floor contraction pressure and duration and anterior displacement of the vaginal axis) during routine bimanual pelvic examination.

over 80% in more than 600 women, but methods of follow-up were not described (Kegel, 1948, 1951).

Current Applications

Subsequent studies have claimed cure/improvement rates ranging from 50% to 80% with the use of PFEs. Satisfaction is high among patients motivated to undertake the therapy (Henalla et al, 1988, 1989; Bo et al, 1990; Mouritsen et al, 1991; Bo and Larsen, 1992; Elia and Bergman, 1993; Cammu and Van Nylen, 1995). There does not appear to be a correlation between a successful outcome and patient weight, age, or parity; severity of incontinence; or urodynamic diagnosis (Worth et al, 1986; Henalla et al, 1988; Mouritsen et al, 1991; Bo and Larsen, 1992a, 1992b; Elia and Bergman, 1993; McIntosh et al, 1993; Cammu and Van Nylen, 1995). Mouritsen and colleagues (1991) found that women with a positive estrogen status were five times more likely to be cured than those who were hypoestrogenic. Henalla and colleagues (1988) found that improvement was correlated with a shorter duration of incontinence symptoms, but Bo and Larsen (1992a, 1992b) found no such correlation.

Adjunctive Modification

Biofeedback is often used with PFEs in an effort to maximize treatment outcome. Originally, Kegel treated all PFE patients with a form of biofeedback, the perineometer. However, this device could not distinguish pelvic floor contractions from abdominal straining and, for this reason, is no longer widely used. Improved perineometers, with vaginal and rectal pressure balloons, vaginal and rectal probe EMG, and concentric needle EMG units, are used today.

The utility of concomitant biofeedback and PFEs has been demonstrated by a number of investigators. Bo and associates (1990) showed that stress-incontinent women undergoing PFEs for 6 months with intensive interval coaching by a physiotherapist had a subjective cure rate of 60%, in comparison with 17% of their uncoached counterparts. These results were corroborated by objective data from pad tests and urethral closure pressure. Burgio and co-workers (1986), in a series of 24 stress-incontinent women, had similar results. Completing biweekly training sessions, half of the patients used biofeedback from a rectal pressure transducer, and the other half were coached with digital palpation by a physiotherapist only. Biofeedback patients documented a 76% decrease in incontinent episodes on diary, whereas those without biofeedback showed a 51% decrease at the 6-month follow-up. Susset and associates (1990) demonstrated an increased clinical response in stress-incontinent women who used PFE and a portable air-filled vaginal probe home biofeedback device. Patients exercised with the probe in place for 20 minutes twice daily. After 6 weeks, there was an 80% subjective cure rate, 87% of pad test results were negative, and there was a 3- to 14-fold increase in intravaginal pressure generated on pelvic floor contraction. McIntosh and co-workers (1993) used PFEs with vaginal probe EMG biofeedback and documented improvement in 66% of stress-incontinent women, 33% of women with detrusor instability, and 50% of women with mixed incontinence. Fecal incontinence was reduced in 63% of those reporting this as a concomitant problem.

A less elaborate method of biofeedback is the use of weighted vaginal cones, which are inserted into the vagina and held in place by voluntary contraction of the pelvic muscles. These are commercially available as a set of five identical-looking cones of gradually increasing weight. The standard regimen involves using the heaviest cone that can be retained for 1 minute of ambulation. This cone is then held in the vagina for 15 minutes twice daily. The next heaviest cone is tested on a weekly basis, and changed when it can be retained for 1 minute of ambulation. The only way to retain the cone is by proper pelvic floor contraction; Valsalva maneuvers lead to expulsion. In a 1-month vaginal cone exercise regimen followed by 30 stress-incontinent women awaiting surgery, 70% were cured or experienced dramatic improvement and only 37% actually went on to have the planned surgical procedure (Peattie et al, 1988).

In one of the largest biofeedback series, 170 stress-incontinent women underwent a course of physiotherapist-supervised PFEs done four to six times daily for an average of 5 months. The initial post-treatment cure rate was 23%; 48% improved, and the remaining patients experienced no change (Hahn et al, 1993). On questionnaire follow-up 2 to 7 years after training, 25% had subsequently elected surgical therapy. Of the nonoperated patients, 11% were subjectively cured, 44% had improved, 31% had experienced no change, and 14% were worse off. Hahn and associates noted that the patients who elected surgery had more severe incontinence both subjectively and on pad testing before beginning the exercise program. In another 5-year follow-up study of 48 women who had undergone a similar biofeedback/exercise regimen, the initial cure/improvement rate was 54%. After 5 years, however, 13 patients (27%) had elected surgery because of incontinence and/or prolapse. In the remaining 35 women, a 58% cure/improvement rate was found (Cammu and Van Nylen, 1995).

The frequency of home exercises in these studies varied, ranging from one session every other day to six times daily. The most common regimen involved 20-minute sessions two to three times daily for 3 to 6 months. Post-therapy maintenance regimens and follow-up schedules have not been tested. We instruct patients that **there is no "end point" for exercise therapy. As with any other exercise program, one can expect a deterioration if exercises are abandoned. We advise a maintenance schedule of 20 minutes daily or, at minimum, every other day, with office follow-up every 3 months, at which time a subjective evaluation and a pelvic muscle rating scale evaluation are obtained.**

The vast majority of research with PFEs has been done with stress-incontinent women. Few studies have documented improvement in adults with detrusor instability (Mouritsen et al, 1991; Burns et al, 1993; Kjolseth et al, 1993; McIntosh et al, 1993; Schneider et al, 1994). There is also a dearth of evidence as to the utility of PFE in the preventive treatment of continent women. Despite Kegel's early enthusiasm for the prophylactic use of PFEs, little has been done to identify and treat continent women who may benefit. In a preliminary randomized study of 24 continent nulliparous women with no clinical evidence of pelvic floor disorder or defect, Thorp and colleagues (1994) found no difference in pelvic floor strength between exercisers and nonexercising controls. Exercisers received detailed instruction at the first visit and performed the exercises three times daily for 6 weeks. Controls were not instructed in PFEs and also returned in 6 weeks for evaluation. Both digital scale and anal or vaginal EMG recordings showed no significant change in either group. However, in view of the fact that evidence of stress incontinence has been documented to occur with surprising frequency even among healthy nulliparous women, including college athletes, we can expect further research directed to the utility of PFEs for women of all age groups and continence categories (Wolin, 1969; Nygaard et al, 1994).

Other Methods of Biofeedback

Cystometric biofeedback has been used as the biofeedback monitor to treat detrusor overactivity. In one of the earliest series, Wear and co-workers (1979) used cystometric biofeedback to treat a small group of eight men and women with pelvic pain, urinary incontinence, and/or retention. **The cystometric tracing was used to provide visible biofeedback (detrusor contraction), and the patients were coached during the sessions with a focus on developing voluntary control of the periurethral musculature.** Half of the patients noted significant reduction in symptoms. In a series of 27 women with detrusor instability, Cardozo and associates (1978) undertook a program of biofeedback bladder reeducation carried out during cystometrics. Participants underwent hour-long cystometric sessions at weekly intervals for 4 to 8 weeks in which an audible and visible biofeedback unit registered increases in bladder pressure. Eighty-two percent of patients reported subjective cure or improvement, and cystometrograms showed a 46% decrease in the provocation of involuntary detrusor contractions and a 52% reduction in demonstrable urge incontinence. Although a 5-year follow-up examination of these women did not document a high rate of persistent therapeutic effect among those initially cured or improved, the authors believed that it remained "worth trying in a highly motivated group of women with a mild to moderate detrusor instability and a good insight into their bladder problems" (Cardozo and Stanton, 1984). As with PFEs, a dissipation of therapeutic effect might be anticipated in the absence of a maintenance program, and further research in this area is needed. Cystometric biofeedback has also been utilized with and without adjunctive PFE in the treatment of childhood bladder dysfunction (Kjolseth et al, 1993, 1994).

Electrical Stimulation

Since Caldwell introduced the concept of electrical stimulation for the treatment of urinary incontinence in 1963, there have been many favorable reports as to its feasibility, but only since the 1980s has the intensity of activity in clinical and basic research increased. Although it offers a promising avenue of therapy, at present **there is no single "most effective method." Effective stimulation parameters have not been standardized, nor has the site of optimal electrode stimulation been determined.** It is not clear whether electrodes need to be implanted or whether surface ones will suffice. Various types of electrodes have been used, including anal or vaginal probe–mounted band electrodes, implanted cuff or wire electrodes, and cutaneous surface electrodes to provide retrograde stimulation of the pudendal nerve and pudendal/pelvic nerve reflex arc, as well as antegrade sacral anterior root stimulation.

Despite these shortcomings, a realistic interpretation of reported results suggests that **some degree of improvement can be expected in approximately 35% to 60% of patients so treated** (Caldwell, 1963; Godec et al, 1975, 1976; Sotiropolous et al, 1976; Fall et al, 1977a, 1977b, 1977c, 1986; Plevnik and Janez, 1979; McGuire et al, 1983; Fall, 1984; Plevnik et al, 1986; Eriksen and Mjolnerod, 1987; Bent et al, 1989; Henalla et al, 1989; Leach and Bavendam, 1989; Ohlsson, 1989; Green and Laycock, 1990; Olah et al, 1990; Lamhut et al, 1992; Zollner-Nielsen and Samuelsson, 1992; Caputo et al, 1993; Geirsson et al, 1993; Ishigooka et al, 1993; Fall and Lindstrom, 1994; Schiotz, 1994).

From a physiologic standpoint, **electrical stimulation can promote continence in one of two ways: by causing contraction of the sphincteric and/or pelvic floor muscles or by a reflex inhibition of the detrusor. The former is theoretically useful in controlling incontinence caused by sphincteric malfunction, the latter for detrusor instability or hyperreflexia.** Because **the threshold for afferent stimulation is generally lower than that for efferent stimulation,** selection of appropriate parameters can result in reflex contraction of the striated muscles of the urethral sphincter and/or the other pelvic floor muscles without direct muscle stimulation. In some patients, contraction of these muscles elicits a neural reflex that results in inhibition of detrusor contraction. Increasing the electrical current to above the threshold for efferent stimulation results in direct stimulation of the motor axon, which results in an immediate contraction of the appropriate muscle. In addition, a delayed reflex contraction appears with a latency of approximately 35 to 40 milliseconds. At the present time, clinical trials of vaginal, perineal, rectal, and posterior tibial nerve surface electrodes are ongoing. In addition, implantable devices for stimulating the sacral nerve roots are being evaluated. These may be positioned either percutaneously via the sacral foramen or by intradural or extradural surgical exposure of the appropriate nerve roots.

Fundamentals of Electricity

Ohm's law (current = voltage/resistance) describes the flow of electrons (current) as a function of the relationship between the force that makes charged particles move (voltage) and capacity of the substance to which current is being applied to store charge and resist opposition to the movement of charged particles (resistance). In the human body, resistance is situated in the tissue adjacent to the electrode, and voltage and current can be varied via the delivery system. To reduce the potential for thermal injury, voltage is fixed and current is adjustable in most commercially available stimulators. Current is delivered in a series of interrupted pulses, usually in a bidirectional (biphasic) wave form. The number of pulses per second is called the frequency, denoted by Hertz (Hz); one pulse per second = 1 Hz. Pelvic floor muscle contraction requires a high stimulation frequency in the range of 50 to 100 Hz, whereas the bladder inhibition reflex system responds best at 5 to 10 Hz (Erlandson et al, 1977a; Fall et al, 1977a, 1977b, 1977c).

Effective stimulation depends on a number of factors, including excitability of the nerve, stimulation threshold, conduction speed, and the proximity of the stimulating electrode to the nerve. The conduction speed of nerve fibers increases with fiber width and degree of myelination. Group A fibers are the largest and most thickly myelinated; they are involved in motor function and sensory (touch, pressure, temperature) perception. Group B fibers are minimally myelinated and of moderate diameter and are found in the autonomic system, serving visceral organs in a motor and sensory capacity. Group C fibers are small, unmyelinated, and transmit current at the slowest speed; they function primarily in somatic pain reflex responses.

History

Electrical stimulation for the treatment of incontinence was first described by Caldwell in 1963 in the "Preliminary Communications" section of the Lancet. Using implanted electrodes attached to a radiofrequency generator, two women, one with a 23-year history of fecal incontinence and the other with a 20-year history of urinary urge incontinence, were reportedly cured.

In 1977, Fall and colleagues (1977a, 1977b, 1977c) reported an elegant series of feline and human studies, elucidating the physiologic mechanisms of action and optimal stimulation parameters for therapeutic electrical stimulation. In parts I and II of the series, it was determined that intravaginal stimulation accomplished closure of the feline urethra and inhibition of detrusor activity and that these responses could be elicited independently of each other. In the remaining studies, carried out with female human volunteers, it was determined that urethral closure was maximal at frequencies of 20 to 50 Hz (part III) and bladder inhibition was effected best at 10 Hz (part IV). In part V, differences in response to conduction and general anesthesia were observed; these differences were such that a role for electrical stimulation in patients with lower motor neuron lesions was proposed. In the final segment (part VI) of this series, a prototype of a commercially available intravaginal stimulation device was successfully tested in women with stress, urge, and mixed incontinence. Stress incontinence necessitated 4 to 9 months of therapy to effect significant clinical improvement, whereas patients with urge incontinence noted significant improvement within 3 months of treatment.

Chronic Electrical Stimulation Therapy

Most long-term treatment protocols have used anal or vaginal probe–mounted electrodes. Patients underwent stimulation ranging from 6 to 24 hours daily, for 1 to 36 months (Godec et al, 1976; Sotiropolous et al, 1976; Fall et al, 1977b, 1986; Fall, 1984; Eriksen and Mjolnerod, 1987). Studies were carried out almost exclusively with participants who suffered stress, urge, and mixed incontinence; a few trials included patients with neurogenic bladder dysfunction (Godec et al, 1975, 1976; Sotiropolous et al, 1976; Ishigooka et al, 1993). Cure, improvement, and failure rates covered a wide range; subjects suffering detrusor instability demonstrated a greater likelihood to respond to therapy than did those with stress incontinence. Follow-up ranged from 1 month to several years, but there were few comparable data, nor are there long-term follow-up reports documenting the degree to which successful therapy is persistent.

Maximal Electrical Stimulation Therapy

In one of the earliest studies using maximal electrical stimulation (MES), Plevnik and Janez (1979) treated 98 men and women with stress, urge, and neurogenic incontinence, using anal or vaginal probe–mounted electrodes. The regimen involved one to three treatment sessions lasting only 15 to 20 minutes, and the results were encouraging; three patients with mixed incontinence remained cured 1 year after only one treatment session. The authors proposed that MES appeared to be more efficient and simpler to apply in many types of urinary incontinence than is chronic (long-term) stimulation. About 10 years later, Eriksen et al (1989) used weekly or biweekly MES sessions to treat 48 women with detrusor instability, noting an 85% cure/improved rate just after therapy and 77% at 1-year follow-up. As with long-term therapy, the majority of MES studies have been done with patients with stress, urge, or mixed incontinence, using anal and/or vaginal probe–mounted electrodes.

Regimens have ranged from 15- to 20-minute sessions carried out anywhere from twice daily to once weekly, with a total number of sessions ranging from 1 to 84. On review of the literature, no regimen appears optimal. For instance, Bent and associates (1989) treated a group of women with stress and urge incontinence for 15 minutes twice daily for 6 weeks. At 6-week follow-up, they reported comparable cure/improvement rates for patients with stress (9%/78%) and urge (8%/61%) incontinence. Ohlsson and co-workers (1989) treated patients with idiopathic detrusor instability or uninhibited overactive bladder in a series of four weekly 20-minute sessions and, at 10-month follow-up, found 40% of the idiopathic and 53% of the uninhibited patients to be cured. Caputo and associates (1993) treated patients with stress, urge, and mixed incontinence in a series of six weekly 15-minute sessions, reporting cure/improvement in 80% of stress-, 63% of urge-, and 67% of mixed-incontinence patients on follow-up ranging from 2 to 12 months. In addition, 58% of surgical candidates opted to forgo surgery after completing MES therapy. Schiotz (1994) treated stress-incontinent women for 20 minutes per day over a 1-month period, resulting in 12% cure, 33% improvement, and 65% failure rates, and one third of patients elected to forgo surgical treatment.

In a multicenter placebo-controlled trial of stress-incontinent women, Richardson and Ramahi (1993) noted a 73% cure/improved rate after 20 weeks of 15-minute sessions of intravaginal stimulation performed daily or every other day. **As with chronic electrical stimulation therapy, response rates for stress, urge, and mixed incontinence vary greatly with MES, and further study is necessary to evaluate optimization of therapeutic regimens for various categories of incontinence and bladder dysfunction** (Plevnik and Janez, 1979; Plevnik et al, 1986; Bent et al, 1989; Eriksen et al, 1989; Ohlsson et al, 1989; Lamhut et al, 1992; Zollner-Nielsen and Samuelsson, 1992; Caputo et al, 1993; Richardson and Ramahi, 1993; Schiotz, 1994).

MES has also been used to treat neurogenic bladder; response rates have ranged from 75% cured to a 20% increase in the number of incontinent episodes (Plevnik and Janez, 1979; Lamhut et al, 1992; Zollner-Nielsen and Samuelsson, 1992; Ishigooka et al, 1993). Sensory urgency (interstitial cystitis) has also been shown to respond; two studies showed cure rates of 38% and 53% (Eriksen et al, 1989; Zollner-Nielsen and Samuelsson, 1992). Childhood enuresis resulted in cure/improvement rates of 36%/43% after 1 month of daily MES sessions (Plevnik et al, 1986). Further research application in these areas is needed, inasmuch as all the initial results have been promising.

Interferential Therapy

Interferential electrical stimulation (IFT) is another method of delivering current to the pelvic floor in which either two or four external patch or suction cup electrodes are used. The electrodes are placed in such a way that stimulation results in two perpendicular high-frequency (2 to 4 kHz) currents that cross, or "interfere," at the level of the pelvic floor. Despite these high frequencies, perceptible stimulation occurs only in the area of interference, because of increased current impedance across the area of the pelvis. The currents are set at slightly different intensities, and this difference becomes the low-frequency therapeutic interferential current (e.g., a 10-Hz difference becomes a 10-Hz current for pelvic floor stimulation).

The advantage to interferential therapy is the lack of invasiveness; no devices are placed within the vagina or rectum, and no needles are implanted. This method is routinely used by many pelvic floor physiotherapists, almost exclusively outside the United States (Wilson et al, 1987; Henalla et al, 1989; Green and Laycock, 1990; Olah et al, 1990). The most common electrode placement involves two electrodes above the inguinal ligament and two applied to the inner thigh near the groin. Using an intravaginal pressure sensor, Green and Laycock (1990) demonstrated that this was the least effective method; the greatest pelvic floor contractions were demonstrated when two electrodes were placed just lateral and anterior to the anus. In a comparison of weighted vaginal cones with IFT, Olah and co-workers (1990) demonstrated no significant difference in subjective or objective improvement between the two experimental groups; however, the cup electrodes were placed in the standard, and possibly least effective, position (two inguinal, two adductor). In a comparison of PFE with and without adjunctive IFT, Wilson and colleagues (1987) showed significant increases in vaginal pressure in the PFE/IFT group with no improvement in the PFE-only group. However, in a comparison of PFE, IFT, and local Premarin cream, PFE alone resulted in the most improvement (65%), as opposed to IFT alone (32%) and local estrogen cream alone (12%) (Henalla et al, 1989). Thus, although its use is encouraging in view of patient comfort and compliance, there is no consensus as to the efficacy of IFT at this time.

Transcutaneous Electrical Nerve Stimulation

The acupuncture points for the bladder are located over the peroneal (L5) and posterior tibial (S1) nerves, and it was suggested that detrusor instability could be successfully treated with acupuncture (Pigne et al, 1985). This report generated interest in the possibility of enhancing the response with electrical stimulation, and transcutaneous electrical nerve stimulation (TENS) therapy of the posterior tibial nerve has been tried in patients with detrusor instability, neurogenic bladder, and/or interstitial cystitis with both encouraging and discouraging results (McGuire et al, 1983). TENS applied suprapubically has been demonstrated to treat both ulcerative and nonulcerative interstitial cystitis successfully (Fall and Lindstrom, 1994).

Behavioral Therapy

Also called bladder training, habit training, bladder drill, and bladder re-education, **behavioral modification is an effective form of treatment for the symptoms of urinary frequency, urgency, and urge incontinence. There are a number of different behavioral techniques, but all rely on the same general principles of "teaching" the patient to regain control of the bladder and sphincter** (Frewen, 1978, 1979, 1980, 1982; Elder and Stephenson, 1980; Jarvis, 1980, 1981, 1982a, 1982b; Jarvis and Millar, 1983; Fantl et al, 1991; Chaikin et al, 1993). Some of the principles are quite simple. For example, for any degree of urinary incontinence, fluid restriction decreases the urine output and therefore decreases the amount of urine available to cause incontinence. In most programs, the patient keeps a voiding diary and voids by the clock at predetermined intervals, depending on the results of the previous week's diary. The patient is also instructed in PFEs and told to contract the sphincter whenever it is necessary to delay micturition in order to comply with the predetermined voiding schedule. Success in therapy usually requires 8 to 12 weeks of treatment.

Detrusor Instability

In treating detrusor instability, it is most useful to base the particulars of biofeedback therapy on the results of the urodynamic evaluation. If detrusor instability was demonstrable during cystometry, much useful information can be gleaned. **About half of the patients perceive an urge before the onset of an unstable detrusor contraction and are able to contract the sphincter, abort the stream, and abort the detrusor contraction** (Blaivas, 1982). **For these patients, treatment is fairly straightforward. They are instructed to void at the end of the longest intervoiding interval that, according to the previous week's diary, would have prevented urgency or incontinence. Thereafter, the intervoiding interval is increased by 15 minutes per week,** provided that they were successful during the previous week. The goal of treatment is to attain a continent intervoiding interval of 3 to 4 hours.

Treatment is more difficult if the patient is unaware of the impending unstable detrusor contraction, if it cannot be aborted, or if he or she is unable to contract the sphincter voluntarily. In such a patient, biofeedback may be useful for teaching PFEs and control; in addition, short-term anticholinergic drug therapy may supplement the behavior modification program. Anticholinergics may be gradually withdrawn after bladder function is normalized (Frewen, 1979; Mahady and Begg, 1981; Holmes et al, 1983).

In one of the earliest series, Frewen (1979) treated 50 patients with detrusor instability with in-patient bladder training for 10 days, adjunctive short-term pharmacotherapy, and monthly outpatient follow-up. Results were encouraging, with an 82% short-term cure rate that was maintained (80%) at 1-year follow-up. In a comparison of bladder drill alone with standard drug therapy, Jarvis (1981) found a post-treatment continence rate of 84% of bladder drill patients, as opposed to 56% of the drug therapy group at 3-month follow-up.

To ascertain whether response to therapy varies with urodynamic diagnosis, Holmes and colleagues (1983) evaluated 56 patients with urge syndromes and categorized them in terms of detrusor instability, urge symptoms without cystometric detrusor instability, and urge syndrome caused by decreased bladder compliance. All participants undertook identical programs of bladder training. Anticholinergic therapy was used initially and withdrawn at 3 months. The initial overall cure/improvement rate was 85%. However, at 1- to 5-year follow-up, differences in therapeutic persistence became evident. The patients without demonstrable detrusor instability and normal compliance maintained a high level of relief, but among patients with urodynamically demonstrated detrusor instability and/or decreased bladder compliance, the relapse rate was 43%. Conversely, Mahady and Begg (1981) treated 48 patients, all with cystometric evidence of detrusor instability, with behavioral therapy, short-term pharmacotherapy, and adjunctive psychotherapy. At 4-year follow-up, a 90% subjective cure rate and a 77% rate of cystometric detrusor stability were found.

Interstitial Cystitis

The voiding symptoms of interstitial cystitis, or sensory urgency, have also been successfully treated with behavioral therapy (Jarvis, 1982a, 1982b; Chaikin et al, 1993). **Behavioral therapy in this group focuses on desensitization and a gradual and purposeful increase in the intervoiding interval until the patient senses bladder fullness and an urge to void only at normal volumes. The technique is similar to that of detrusor instability protocols, whereby the patient keeps a daily bladder diary and maintains a set intervoiding interval, which is increased at weekly intervals.** Adjunctive PFE has also been utilized to reduce sensations of urgency and, conversely, to aid in reduction of the confounding discoordinate voiding that so often accompanies this syndrome.

Using an inpatient bladder drill protocol only, Jarvis (1982a, 1982b) demonstrated a 60% cure rate at 6-month follow-up. In a 3-month outpatient treatment series of timed void diaries, fluid intake manipulation, and adjunctive PFE, Chaikin and co-workers (1993) demonstrated 88% success in a group of 42 women with refractory interstitial cystitis. This type of therapy is labor intensive for both patient and physician or therapist, requiring a high level of motivation and frequent follow-up in the outpatient setting.

Incontinence in the Frail Elderly

Various categories of behavioral therapy have found practical application in the reduction of incontinence among the frail elderly (Burgio et al, 1985; Hadley, 1986; Ouslander et al, 1988; Hu et al, 1989). **Incontinence in this age group is much more likely to be multifaceted in etiology, with impaired mental status, diminished physical mobility, fecal impaction, and neurologic conditions often compounding primary urologic dysfunctions** such as detrusor instability or sphincteric incontinence. In these patients, cognitive abnormalities and/or lack of motivation severely limit the efficacy of behavioral interventions, and it is often necessary to enlist the aid of caregivers or family members to assist in diary keeping and prompted voiding. Sometimes, very simple interventions such as raising the height of a chair to enable a person to rise and get to the bathroom easily will suffice (Finlay et al, 1983). In addition, many patients have nocturnal polyuria resulting from a variety of factors, including venous insufficiency, congestive heart failure, dependent edema, poorly timed diuretic use, inappropriate oral intake of fluids in the evening, and a reversal of the normal nocturnal antidiuretic hormone secretion. Most of these conditions can be reversed with fairly simple behavioral interventions based on logic.

Using adjunctive cystometric biofeedback, Burgio and associates (1985) demonstrated an 82% to 94% reduction in incontinent episodes among a group of elderly stress- and urge-incontinent outpatients. Utility among the institutional elderly has also been demonstrated (Ouslander et al, 1988; Hu et al, 1989).

REFERENCES

Abrams PH: Prostatism and prostatectomy: The value of urine flow rate measurement in the pre-operative assessment for operation. J Urol 1977; 117:70.

Abrams PH: Motor urge incontinence and bladder outlet obstruction. Neurourol Urodynam 1985; 4:317–328.

Abrams PH, Blaivas JG, Stanton SL, Andersen JT: Standardisation of lower urinary tract function. Neurourol Urodynam 1988; 7:403.

Abrams PH, Farrar DJ, Turner-Warwick RT, et al: The results of prostatectomy: A symptomatic and urodynamic analysis of 152 patients. J Urol 1979; 121:640–642.

Aho AJ, Auranen A, Personen K: Analysis of cauda equina symptoms in patients with lumbar disc prolapse. Acta Chir Scand 1969; 135:413.

Aldridge AH: Transplantation of fascia for relief of urinary stress incontinence. Am J Obstet Gynecol 1942; 44:398.

Aliabadi H, Gonzalez R: Success of the artificial urinary sphincter after failed surgery for incontinence. J Urol 1990; 143:987–990.

Al-Mefty O, Kandzari S, Fox JL: Neurogenic bladder and tethered cord syndrome. J Urol 1979; 122:112.

Andersen JT: Prostatism: Clinical, radiologic, and urodynamic aspects. Neurourol Urodynam 1982; 1:241–293.

Andersen JT: Disturbances of bladder and urethral function in Parkinson's disease. Int Urol Nephrol 1985; 17(1):35.

Anderson RS: Increased motor unit fibre density in the external anal sphincter in genuine stress incontinence: A single fibre EMG study. Neurourol Urodynam 1983; 2:45.

Andrew J, Nathan PW: Lesions of the anterior frontal lobes and disturbances of micturition and defecation. Brain 1964; 87:233.

Andrew J, Nathan PW, Spanos NC: Disturbances of micturition and defecation due to aneurysms of anterior communicating or anterior cerebral arteries. J Neurosurg 1966; 24:1.

Appell RA: Techniques and results in the implantation of the artificial urinary sphincter in women with type III stress incontinence by a vaginal approach. Neurourol Urodynam 1988; 7:613.

Appell RA: Collagen injection therapy for urinary incontinence. Urol Clin North Am 1994; 21:177–186.

Awad SA, Downie JW, Sogbein SK, et al: Relationship between neurologic and urologic status in patients with multiple sclerosis. J Urol 1984; 132:499.

Awad SA, Flood HD, Acker KL: The significance of prior anti-incontinence surgery in women who present with urinary incontinence. J Urol 1988; 140:514–517.

Awad SA, McGinnis RH: Factors that influence the incidence of detrusor instability in women. J Urol 1983; 130(1):114–115.

Backer MH Jr, Probst RE: The Pereyra procedure. A favorable report of 80 operations. Obstet Gynecol 1971; 38:225–231.

Barbalias GA, Blaivas JG: Neurologic implication of the pathologically open bladder neck. J Urol 1983; 129:780–782.

Bates CP, Corney LE: Synchronous cine/pressure/flow cytography: A method of routine urodynamic investigation. Br J Radiol 1971; 44:44.

Batra SC, Iosif CS: Female urethra: A target for estrogen action. J Urol 1983; 129:418.

Bazeed MA, Thuroff JW, Schmidt RA: Effect of chronic electrostimulation of the sacral roots on the striated urethral sphincter. J Urol 1982; 128:1357.

Beck P, Grove D, Arnusch D, Harvey J: Recurrent urinary stress incontinence treated by the fascia lata sling procedure. Am J Obstet Gynecol 1974; 120:613–621.

Beck PR, Warren KG, Whitman P: Urodynamic studies in female patients with multiple sclerosis. Am J Obstet Gynecol 1981; 139:273–276.

Bemelmans EI, Hommes O, VanKerrebroeck P, et al: Evidence for early lower urinary tract dysfunction in clinically silent multiple sclerosis. J Urol 1991; 145:1219.

Bent AE: Management of recurrent genuine stress incontinence. Clin Obstet Gynecol 1990; 33:358–366.

Bent AE, Sand PK, Ostergard DR: Transvaginal electrostimulation in the therapy of genuine stress incontinence and detrusor instability. Neurourol Urodynam 1989; 8:363.

Berger Y, Blaivas JG, DeLarocha ER, Salinas JM: Urodynamic findings in Parkinson's disease. J Urol 1987; 138:836.

Bergman A, Ballard CA, Koonings PP: Comparison of three different surgical procedures for genuine stress incontinence: Prospective randomized study. Am J Obstet Gynecol 1989; 160:1102.

Bergman A, Bhatia NN: Urodynamic appraisal of the Marshall-Marchetti test in women with stress urinary incontinence. Urology 1987; 29:458–462.

Bhatia NN, Bergman AM, Karram MM: Effects of estrogen on urethral function in women with urinary incontinence. Am J Obstet Gynecol 1989; 160:176.

Blaivas JG: The bulbocavernosus reflex in urology: A prospective study of 299 patients. J Urol 1981; 126:197.

Blaivas JG: The neurophysiology of micturition: A clinical study of 550 patients. J Urol 1982; 127:958.

Blaivas JG: Sphincter electromyography. Neurourol Urodynam 1983; 2:269–288.

Blaivas JG: Non-traumatic neurogenic voiding dysfunction in the adults: Part II. Multiple sclerosis and diabetes mellitus with bibliography. AUA Update Series 1985a; 4:Lesson 11.

Blaivas JG: Non-traumatic neurogenic voiding dysfunction in the adult: Part II. Physiology and approach to therapy. AUA Update Series 1985b; 4:Lesson 11.

Blaivas JG: Pathophysiology of lower urinary tract dysfunction. Urol Clin North Am 1985c; 12:215–225.

Blaivas JG: Pathophysiology and differential diagnosis of benign prostatic hyperthophy. Urology 1988a; 32(6):5–11.

Blaivas JG: Techniques of evaluation. *In* Yalla SV, McGuire EJ, Elbadawi A, Blaivas JG, eds: Neurourology and Urodynamics: Principles and Practice. New York, Macmillan, 1988b, chapter 10.

Blaivas JG: Pubovaginal sling procedure. *In* Whitehead ED, ed: Current Operative Urology. Philadelphia, J.B. Lippincott Company, 1990, pp 93–101.

Blaivas JG, Awad SA, Bissada N, et al: Urodynamic procedure: Recommendations of the Urodynamic Society 1. Procedures that should be available for routine urologic practice. Neurourol Urodynam 1982; 1:51.

Blaivas JG, Barbalias GA: Characteristics of neural injury after abdominal perineal resection of the rectum. J Urol 1983; 129:84.

Blaivas JG, Barbalias GA: Detrusor external sphincter dyssynergia in men with multiple sclerosis: An ominous urologic condition. J Urol 1984; 131:94.

Blaivas JG, Bhimani G, Labib KB: Vesicourethral dysfunction in multiple sclerosis. J Urol 1979a; 122:342–347.

Blaivas JG, Chancellor M: Complicated stress urinary incontinence. Semin Urol 1989; 7:103–116.

Blaivas JG, Fisher DM: Combined radiolographic and urodynamic monitoring: Advances in techniques. J Urol 1981; 125:693–694.

Blaivas JG, Jacobs BZ: Pubovaginal fascial sling for the treatment of complicated stress urinary incontinence. J Urol 1991; 145:1214.

Blaivas JG, Kaplan SA: Urologic dysfunction in patients with multiple sclerosis. Urology 1988; 8:159.

Blaivas JG, Labib KB, Bauer SB, Retik AB: A new approach to electromyography of the external urethral sphincter. J Urol 1977; 117:773–777.

Blaivas JG, Olsson CA: Stress incontinence: Classification and surgical approach. J Urol 1988; 139:737.

Blaivas JG, Scott M, Labib KB: Urodynamic evaluation as a test of sacral cord function. Urology 1979b; 9:692.

Blaivas JG, Sinha HP, Zayed AAH, Labib KB: Detrusor–external sphincter dyssynergia. J Urol 1981; 125:541.

Bo K, Hagen RH, Kvarstein B, et al: Pelvic floor muscle exercise for the treatment of female stress urinary incontinence: III. Effects of two different degrees of pelvic floor muscle exercises. Neurourol Urodynam 1990; 9:489–502.

Bo K, Larsen S: Pelvic floor muscle exercise for the treatment of female stress urinary incontinence: Classification and characterization of responders. Neurourol Urodynam 1992a; 11:497–507.

Bo K, Oesid S, Kvarstein B, et al: Knowledge about and ability to correct pelvic floor exercises in women with stress urinary incontinence. Neurourol Urodynam 1988; 7:26.

Boucier AP, Juras JC: Non-surgical therapy for stress incontinence. Urol Clin North Am 1995; 22:613.

Brading AF, Turner WH: The unstable bladder: Towards a common mechanism. Br J Urol 1994; 73:3–8.

Bradley WE, Chou S, Markland C, Swaiman K: Biochemical assay technique fibrosis. Invest Urol 1965; 3:59.

Bradley WE, Conway CJ: Bladder representation in the pontine-mesencephalic reticular formation. Exp Neurol 1966; 16:237.

Bradley WE, Timm GW, Scott FB: Innervation of the detrusor muscle and urethra. Urol Clin North Am 1974; 1:3.

Brink CA, Wells TJ, Sampselle CM, et al: A digital test for pelvic muscle strength in women with urinary incontinence. Nurs Res 1994; 43:352–356.

Brito G, Mulcahy JJ, Mitchell ME, Adams MC: Use of a double cuff AMS 800 urinary sphincter for severe stress urinary incontinence. J Urol 1993; 149:283–285.

Brubaker LT, Sand PK: Surgical treatment of stress urinary incontinence; a comparison of the Kelly plication, Marshall-Marchetti-Krantz, and Pereyra procedures. (Letter.) Obstet Gynecol 1988; 72:820–821.

Brubaker L, Sand PK: Cystometry, urethrocystometry and videocystourethrography. Clin Obstet Gynecol 1990; 33(2):315–324.

Bruskewitz R: Female incontinence: Signs and symptoms. *In* Shlomo R, ed: Female Urology. Philadelphia, W.B. Saunders Company, 1983, p 45.

Bump RC, Fantl JA, Hurt WG: Dynamic urethral pressure profilometry pressure transmission ratio determinations after continence surgery: Understanding the mechanisms of success, failure and complications. Obstet Gynecol 1988a; 72:870.

Bump RC, Friedman CI: Intraluminal urethral pressure measurements in the female baboon: Effects of hormonal manipulation. J Urol 1986; 136:508.

Bump RC, Friedman CI, Copeland WE Jr: Non-neuromuscular determinants of intraluminal urethral pressure in the female baboon: Relative importance of vascular factors. J Urol 1988b; 139:162.

Bump RC, Hurt WG, Fantl JA, et al: Assessment of Kegel pelvic muscle exercise performance after brief verbal instruction. Am J Obstet Gynecol 1991; 165:322–329.

Burch JC: Urethrovaginal fixation to Cooper's ligament for correction of stress urinary incontinence, cystocele and prolapse. Am J Obstet Gynecol 1961; 81:281–290.

Burch JC: Urethrovaginal fixation to Cooper's ligament in the treatment of cystocele and stress incontinence. Progr Gynecol 1963; 4:591–600.

Burch JC: Cooper's ligament urethrovesicle suspension for stress incontinence. Am J Obstet Gynecol 1968; 100:764.

Burgio KL, Robinson JC, Engel BT: The role of biofeedback in Kegel exercise training for stress urinary incontinence. Am J Obstet Gynecol 1986; 154:58–64.

Burgio KL, Whitehead WE, Engel BT: Urinary incontinence in the elderly; Bladder-sphincter biofeedback and toileting skills training. Ann Intern Med 1985; 104:507–515.

Burns PA, Pranikoff K, Nochajski TH, et al: A comparison of effectiveness of biofeedback and pelvic muscle exercise treatment of stress incontinence in older community-dwelling women. J Gerontol 1993; 48:M167–M174.

Caine M, Raz S: Some clinical implications of adrenergic receptors in the urinary tract. Arch Surg 1975; 110:247.

Caldwell KPS: The electrical control of sphincter incompetence. Lancet 1963; 2:174–175.

Cammu H, Van Nylen M: Pelvic floor muscle exercises: 5 years later. Urology 1995; 45:113–8.

Caputo TM, Benson JT, McClellan E: Intravaginal maximal electrical stimulation on the treatment of urinary incontinence. J Repro Med 1993; 38:667–671.

Cardozo LD, Abrams PH, Stanton SL, et al: Idiopathic bladder instability treated by biofeedback. Br J Urol 1978; 50:521–523.

Cardozo LD, Stanton SL: Biofeedback: A 5-year review. Br J Urol 1984; 56:220.

Cartwright PC, Snow BW: Bladder autoaugmentation: Early clinical experience. J Urol 1989; 142:505.

Cartwright PC, Snow BW: Bladder autoaugmentation. Adv Urol 1995; 8:273.

Chaikin DC, Blaivas JG, Blaivas ST: Behavioral therapy for the treatment of refractory interstitial cystitis. J Urol 1993; 149:1445–1448.

Chancellor MB, Blaivas JG: Multiple sclerosis. Probl Urol 1993; 7(1):15–33.

Chancellor MB, Blaivas JG, Kaplan SA, Axelrod S: Bladder outlet obstruction versus impaired detrusor contractility: Role of uroflow. J Urol 1991; 145:810.

Chang PL, Fan HA: Urodynamic studies before and after abdominoperineal resection of the rectum for carcinoma. J Urol 1983; 130:948.

Chao R, Mayo ME: Incontinence after radical prostatectomy: Detrusor or sphincter causes. J Urol 1995; 154:16–18.

Christensen SJ, Colstrup H, Hertz JB, et al: Inter- and intra-departmental variations of the perineal pad-weighing test. Neurourol Urodynam 1986; 5:23.

Cobb OE, Ragde H: Correction of female stress incontinence. J Urol 1978; 120:418.

Constantinou CE: Resting and stress urethral pressures as a clinical guide to the mechanism of continence in the female patient. Urol Clin North Am 1985; 12:247.

Constantinou CE, Govan DE: Spatial distrubution and timing of transmitted and reflexly generated urethral pressures in healthy women. J Urol 1982; 127:964.

Coolsaet BRLA, Blok C: Detrusor properties related to prostatism. Neururol Urodynam 1986; 5:435.

Corr CA, Shapiro SR: Use of fascia lata in urology. Urology 1978; 11:507–509.

Couillard DR, Webster GD: Detrusor instability. Urol Clin North Am 1995; 22:593–612.

Crystle C, Charme L, Copeland W: Q-Tip test in stress urinary incontinence. Obstet Gynecol 1971; 38:313.

Cumming JA, Chisholm GD: Changes in detrusor innervation with relief of outflow tract obstruction. Br J Urol 1992; 69:7–11.

Dam AM, Hebjorn S, Hal TL: Neurological disorders and detrusor hyperreflexia. Acta Neurol Scand 1976; 54:415–422.

Decter RM, Harpster L: Pitfalls in determination of leak point pressure. J Urol 1992; 148:588–591.

deGroat WC, Booth AM, Krier J, et al: Neural control of the urinary bladder and large intestine. *In* McBrooks C, Koizumi K, Sato A, eds: Integrative Functions of the Autonomic Nervous System. Amsterdam, Elsevier Biomedical, 1989, Chapter 4.

deGroat WC, Steers WD: Autonomic regulation of the urinary bladder and sex organs. *In* Loewy AD, Spyer, KM, eds: Central Regulation and Autonomic Functions. London, Oxford University Press, 1990, pp 310–333.

de-Kock ML, de-Klerk JN: The suprapubic approach in the surgical treatment of female stress incontinence. S Afr Med J 1982; 62:686–688.

Delancey JOL: Correlative study of paraurethral anatomy. Obstet Gynecol 1986; 68:91–97.

Delancey JOL: Structural aspects of the extrinsic continence mechanism. Obstet Gynecol 1988a; 72:296–301.

Delancey JOL: Structural aspects of urethrovesical function in the female. Neurourol Urodynam 1988b; 7:509–520.

Delancey JOL: Pubovesical ligament: A separate structure from urethral supports ("pubo-urethral ligaments"). Neurourol Urodynam 1989; 8:53–62.

Denny-Brown D, Robertson EG: On the physiology of micturition. Brain 1933; 56:149.

Diokno AC, Hollander HB, Alderson TP: Artificial urinary sphincter for recurrent female urinary incontinence: Indications and results. J Urol 1987; 138:778.

Diokno AC, Sonda LP, MacGregor RJ: Long-term followup of the artificial urinary sphincter. J Urol 1984; 131:1084–1086.

Donker PJ, Droes J, van Ulden BM: Anatomy of the musculature and innervation of the bladder and the urethra. *In* Williams DI, Chisolm GD, eds: Scientific Foundations of Urology. London, William Heinemann Medical Books, 1976, p 32.

Duncan HJ, Nurse DE, Mundy AR: Role of the artificial urinary sphincter in the treatment of stress incontinence in women. Br J Urol 1992; 69:141–143.

Eardley L, Fowler CJ, Nagendron K, et al: The neurourology of tropical spastic paraparesis. Br J Urol 1991; 68:598.

Elbadawi A: Pathology and pathophysiology of detrusor in incontinence. Urol Clin North Am 1995; 22:499–512.

Elbadawi A, Yalla SV, Resnick NM: Structural basis of geriatric voiding dysfunction: III. Detrusor overactivity. J Urol 1993; 150:1668.

Elder DD, Stephenson TP: An assessment of the Frewen regimen in the treatment of detrusor dysfunction in females. Br J Urol 1980; 52:467–471.

Elia G, Bergman A: Pelvic muscle exercises: When do they work? Obstet Gynecol 1993; 81:283–286.

Eriksen BC, Bergmann S, Eik-ness FH: Maximal electrostimulation of the pelvic floor in female idiopathic detrusor instability and urge incontinence. Neurol Urodyn 1989; 8:219–230.

Eriksen BC, Bergmann S, Mjolnerod OK: Effect of anal electrostimulation with the "Incontan" device in women with urinary incontinence. Br J Obstet Gynaecol 1987; 94:147–156.

Eriksen BC, Mjolnerod OK: Changes in urodynamic measurements after successful anal electrostimulation in female urinary incontinence. Br J Urol 1987; 59:45–49.

Erlandson BE, Fall M, Carlsson CA, et al: Mechanisms for closure of the human urethra during intravaginal electrical stimulation. Scand J Urol Nephrol 1977a; (suppl 44, pt V):49–53.

Erlandson BE, Magnus, F, Sundin T: Intravaginal electrical stimulation. Clinical experiments on urethral closure. Scand J Urol Nephrol 1977b; (suppl 44, pt III):31–39.

Fall M: Does electrostimulation cure urinary incontinence? J Urol 1984; 131:664–667.

Fall M, Ahlstrom K, Carlsson CA, et al: Contelle: Pelvic floor stimulator for female stress-urge incontinence—A multicenter study. Urology 1986; 27:282–287.

Fall M, Erlandson BE, Carlsson CA, et al: The effect of intravaginal electrical stimulation on the feline urethra and urinary bladder. Neuronal mechanisms. Scand J Urol Nephrol 1977a; (suppl 44, pt II):19–31.

Fall M, Erlandson BE, Nilson AE, et al: Long-term intravaginal electrical stimulation in urge and stress incontinence. Scand J Urol Nephrol 1977b; (suppl 44, pt VI):55–63.

Fall M, Erlandson BE, Sundin T, et al: Intravaginal eletrical stimulation. Clinical experiments on bladder inhibition. Scand J Urol Nephrol 1977c; (suppl 44, pt IV):41–47.

Fall M, Lindstrom S: Transcutaneous electrical nerve stimulation in classical and nonulcer interstitial cystitis. Urol Clin North Am 1994; 21:131–139.

Fantl JA, Wyman JF, Anderson RL, et al: Post-menopausal urinary incontinence: Comparison between non-estrogen supplemented and estrogen supplemented women. Obstet Gynecol 1988; 71:823.

Fantl JA, Wyman JF, McClish DK, Bump RC: Urinary incontinence in community dwelling women: Clinical, urodynamic, and severity characteristics. Am J Obstet Gynecol 1990; 162(4):946–951.

Fantl JA, Wyman JF, McClish DK, et al: Efficacy of bldder training in older women with urinary incontinence. JAMA 1991; 265:609–613.

Finlay OE, Bayles TB, Rosen C, Milling J: Effects of chair design, age and cognitive status on moblity. Age Aging 1983; 12:329–335.

Fishman IJ, Shabsigh R, Scott FB: Experience with the artificial urinary sphincter model AS800 in 148 patients. J Urol 1989; 141:307–310.

Flocks RH, Boldus R: The surgical treatment and prevention of urinary incontinence associated with disturbance of the internal urethral sphincteric mechanism. J Urol 1973; 109:279–285.

Foote J, Yun S, Leach GE: Post prostatectomy incontinence: Pathophysiology, evaluation and management. Urol Clin North Am 1991; 18:229–241.

Forney JP: The effect of radical hysterectomy on bladder physiology. Am J Obstet Gynecol 1980; 138:374.

Foster HE, McGuire EJ: Management of urethral obstruction with transvaginal urethrolysis. J Urol 1993; 150:1448–1451.

Fowler CJ: Pelvic foor neurophysiology. Methods Clin Neurophysiol 1991; 2:1–24.

Fowler FJ Jr, Barry MJ, Lu-Yao G, et al: Patient reported complications and follow up treatment after radical prostatectomy. The national Medicare experience: 1988–1990 (updated June 1993). Urology 1993; 42:622–629.

Fowler FJ Jr, Barry MJ, Lu-Yao G, et al: Effect of radical prostatectomy for prostate cancer on patient quality of life: Result from a Medicare survey. Urology 1995; 45:1007–1015.

Fowler JW, Bremner DN, Moffat LEF: The incidence and consequence of damage to the parasympathetic nerve supply to the bladder after abdomino-perineal resection of the rectum for carcinoma. Br J Urol 1978; 50:95.

Frewen WK: An objective assessment of the unstable bladder of psychosomatic origin. Br J Urol 1978; 52:367–368.

Frewen WK: Role of bladder training in the treatment of the unstable bladder in the female. Urol Clin North Am 1979; 6:273–277.

Frewen WK: The management of urgency and frequency of micturition. Br J Urol 1980; 52:367–368.

Frewen WK: A reassessment of bladder training in detrusor dysfunction in the female. Br J Urol 1982; 54:372.

Fu X, Siltberg H, Johnson P, Ulmsten U: Viscoelastic properties and muscular function of the human anterior vaginal wall. Int Urogynecol J 1995; 6:229–234.

Furlow WF, Barrett DM: Recurrent or persistent urinary incontinence in patients with the artificial urinary sphincter. Diagnostic considerations and management. J Urol 1985; 133:792–795.

Ganabathi K, Leach GE: Periurethral injection techniques. Atlas Urol Clin North Am 1994; 2:101–109.

Geirsson G, Wang YH, Lindstrom S, et al: Traditional acupuncture and electrical stimulation of the posterior tibial nerve. Scand J Urol Nephrol 1993; 27:67–70.

German K, Bedwani J, Davies J, et al: Physiological and morphometric studies into pathophysiology of detrusor hyperreflexia in neuropathic patients. J Urol 1995; 153:1678–1683.

Gerstenberg TC, Andersen JT, Klarskov P, et al: High flow infravesical obstruction. J Urol 1982; 127:943.

Gerstenberg TC, Nielsen ML, Clausen S, et al: Bladder function after abdominoperineal resection of the rectum for anorectal cancer: Urodynamic investigation before and after operation in a consecutive series. Ann Surg 1980; 191:81.

Ghoneim GM, Bloom DA, McGuire EJ, Stewart KL: Bladder compliance in meningomyelocele children. J Urol 1989; 141:1404.

Ghoneim GM, Lapeyrolerie J, Sood OP, Thomas R: Tulane experience with management of urinary incontinence after placement of an artificial urinary sphincter. World J Urol 1994; 12:333–336.

Gittes RF, Loughlin KR: No-incision pubovaginal suspension for stress incontinence. J Urol 1987; 138:568–570.

Gjone R, Setekleiv J: Excitatory and inhibitory bladder responses to stimulation in the cerebral cortex in the cat. Acta Physiol Scand 1963; 59:337.

Godec C, Cass AS, Ayala GF: Bladder inhibition with functional electrical stimulation. Urology 1975; 6:663–666.

Godec C, Cass AS, Ayala GF: Electrical stimulation for incontinence. Urology 1976; 7:388–397.

Goldstein I, Siroky MB, Sax DS, Krane RJ: Neuro-urologic abnormalities in multiple sclerosis. J Urol 1982; 128:541.

Goldwasser B, Furlow WL, Barrett DM: The model AS 800 artificial urinary sphincter: Mayo Clinic experience. J Urol 1987; 137:668–671.

Goluboff ET, Chang DT, Olsson CA, et al: Urodynamics and the etiology of post prostatectomy urinary incontinence: The initial Columbia experience. J Urol 1995; 153:1034–1037.

Gormley EA, Griffiths DJ, McCracken PN, et al: Effect of transurethral resection of the prostate on detrusor instability and urge incontinence in elderly males. Neurourol Urodynam 1993; 12:445.

Gosling JA: The structure and function of the female lower urinary tract and pelvic floor. Urol Clin North Am 1985; 12:207.

Gosling JA, Dixon JS: Light and electron microscopic observations on the human external urethral sphincter. J Anat 1979; 129:216.

Gosling JA, Dixon JS: Structure and innervation in the human. *In* Torrens M, Morrison JFB, eds: The Physiology of the Lower Urinary Tract. London, Springer-Verlag, 1987.

Graver P, Tanagho EA: Effect of abdominal pressure rise on the urethral pressure profile. Invest Urol 1974; 12:57.

Green RC, Laycock J: Objective methods for evaluation of interferential therapy in the treatment of incontinence. Trans Biomed Eng 1990; 37:615–623.

Green TH: Development of a plan for the diagnosis and treatment of urinary stress incontinence. Am J Obstet Gynecol 1962; 83:632.

Green TH Jr: The problem of urinary stress incontinence in the female: An appraisal of its current status. Obstet Gynecol Survey 1968; 23:603.

Green TH Jr: Selection of vaginal or suprapubic approach in operative treatment of urinary stress incontinence. Clin Obstet Gynecol 1977; 20:881–901.

Griffiths DJ: Urodynamics: The Mechanics of Hydrodynamics of the Lower Urinary Tract. Medical Physics Handbooks, vol 4. Bristol, England, Hilger, 1980.

Griffiths DJ: The mechanics of micturition. *In* Yalla SV, Elbadawi A, McGuire E, Blaivas JG, eds: The Principles and Practice of Neurourology and Urodynamics. New York, Macmillan, 1988, chapter 5.

Grischke EM, Anton H, Stolz W, et al: Urodynamic assessment and lateral urethrocystography. A comparison of two diagnostic procedures for female urinary incontinence. Acta Obstet Gynecol Scand 1991; 70:225–229.

Gundian JC, Barrett DM, Parulkar BG: Mayo Clinic experience with use of the AMS800 artificial urinary sphincter for urinary uncontinence following radical prostatectoomy. J Urol 1989; 142(6):1459–1461.

Hadley EC: Bladder training and related therapies for urinary incontinence in older people. JAMA 1986; 256:372–379.

Hadley HR, Zimmern PE, Staskin DR, Raz S: Transvaginal needle bladder neck suspension. Urol Clin North Am 1985; 12:291–303.

Hahn I, Fall M: Objective quantification of stress urinary incontinence: A short, reproducible, provocative pad-test. Neurourol Urodynam 1991; 10:475.

Hahn I, Milsom I, Fall M, et al: Long-term results of pelvic floor training in female stress urinary incontinence. Br J Urol 1993; 72:421–427.

Hebjorn S, Andersen JT, Walter S, Dam AM: Detrusor hyperreflexia; A survey on its etiology and treatment. Scand J Urol Nephrol 1976; 10:103–109.

Henalla SM, Hutchins CJ, Robinson P, et al: Non-operative methods in the treatment of female genuine stress incontinence of urine. J Obstet Gynecol 1989; 9:222–225.

Henalla SM, Kirwan P, Castleden CM, et al: The effect of pelvic floor exercises in the treatment of genuine urinary stress incontinence in women at two hospitals. Br J Obstet Gynaecol 1988; 95:602–606.

Herschorn S, Radomski SB, Steele DJ: Early experience with intraurethral collagen injections for urinary incontinence. J Urol 1992; 148:1797–1800.

Hilton P, Mayne CJ: The Stamey endoscopic bladder neck suspension: A clinical and urodynamic evaluation including an actuarial follow-up over four years. Neurourol Urodynam 1989; 8:336–337.

Hilton P, Stanton SL: The use of intravaginal estrogen cream in genuine stress incontinence. Br J Obstet Gynaecol 1983; 90:940.

Hodgkinson CP: Relationships of the female urethra and bladder in urinary stress incontinence. Am J Obstet Gynecol 1953; 65:560.

Hodgkinson CP: Stress urinary incontinence in the female. Surg Gynecol Obstet 1965; 120:595.

Hodgkinson CP, Doub H, Kelly W: Urethrocystograms: Metallic bead-chain urethrocystography in preoperative and postoperative evaluation of gynecologic urologic problems. Clin Obstet Gynecol 1978; 21:725.

Hodgson BT, Dumas S, Bolling DR, et al: Effect of estrogen on sensitivity of rabbit bladder and urethra to phenylephrine. Invest Urol 1978; 16:67.

Holmes DM, Montz FJ, Stanton SLL: Oxybutinin versus propantheline in the management of detrusor instability. A patient-regulated variable dose trial. Br J Obstet Gynaecol 1989; 96:607–612.

Holmes DM, Stone AR, Bary PR, et al: Bladder training—3 years on. Br J Urol 1983; 55:660–664.

Hu TW, Igou JF, Kaltreider DL, et al: A clinical trial of a behavioral therapy to reduce urinary incontinence in nursing homes. JAMA 1989; 261:2656–2662.

Hutch JA: A new theory of the anatomy of the internal urinary sphincter and the physiology of micturition. Invest Urol 1965; 3:36.

Hutch JA: A new theory of the anatomy of the internal urinary sphincter and the physiology of micturition II: The base plate. J Urol 1966; 96:182–188.

Hutch JA: A new theory of the anatomy of the internal urinary sphincter and the physiology of micturition IV: The urinary sphincter mechanism. J Urol 1967; 96:705–712.

Hutch JA: Anatomy and Physiology of the Bladder, Trigone and Urethra. London, Butterworths Appleton-Century-Crofts, 1972.

Ingelman-Sundberg A: Operative treatment of female urinary incontinence. Ann Chir Gynaecol 1982; 71:208–220.

Iosif CS: Retropubic colpourethrocystopexy. Urol Int 1982; 37:125–129.

Iosif CS: Results of various operations for urinary stress incontinence. Arch Gynecol 1983; 233:93–100.

Iosif CS, Batra S, Ek A, Astedt B: Estrogen receptors in the human female lower urinary tract. Am J Obstet Gynecol 1981; 141:817.

Ishigooka M, Hashimoto T, Izumiya K, et al: Electrical pelvic floor stimulation in the management of urinary incontinence due to neuropathic overactive bladder. Front Med Biol Eng 1993; 5:1–10.

Jarvis GJ: A controlled trial of bladder drill and drug therapy in the management of detrusor instability. Br J Urol 1981; 53:565–566.

Jarvis GJ: Bladder drill for the treatment of enuresis in adults. Br J Urol 1982a; 545:118–119.

Jarvis GJ: The management of urinary incontinence due to primary vesical sensory urgency by bladder drill. Br J Urol 1982b; 54:374–376.

Jarvis GJ: A controlled trial of bladder drill and drug therapy in the management of detrusor instability. Br J Urol 1983; 55:660–664.

Jarvis GJ, Millar DR: Controlled trial of bladder drill for detrusor instability. BMJ 1980; 281:1322–1322.

Jeffcoate TNA, Roberts H: Observations on stress incontinence of urine. Am J Obstet Gynecol 1952; 64:721.

Kageyama S, Kawabe K, Suzuki K, et al: Collagen implantation for post prostatectomy incontinence: Early experience with a transrectal ultrasonographically guided method. J Urol 1994; 152:1473–1475.

Kaplan SA, Chancellor MB, Blaivas JG: Bladder and sphincter behavior in patients with spinal cord injuries. J Urol 1991; 146:113.

Karram MM, Bhatia NN: Transvaginal needle bladder neck suspension procedures for stress urinary incontinence: A comprehensive review. Obstet Gynecol 1989; 73:906–914.

Kegel AH: Progressive resistance exercise in the functional restoration of the perineal muscles. Am J Obstet Gynecol 1948; 56:238–248.

Kegel AH: Physiologic therapy for urinary stress incontinence. JAMA 1951; 7:915–917.

Kelly MJ, Nielsen KK, Roskamp DA, et al: Long-term follow-up of the Raz bladder neck suspension for the correction of female stress urinary incontinence. Neurourol Urodynam 1990; 9:231–232.

Khan Z, Starer P, Yang WC, Bhola A: Analysis of voiding disorders in patients with cerebrovascular accidents. Urology 1990; 32:256.

Kirby RS: Autonomic failure and the role of the sympathetic nervous system in the control of lower urinary tract function. Clin Science 1986; 70(14):45S–50S.

Kirby RS, Fowler R, Gosling J, Bannister R: Urethrovesical dysfunction in progressive autonomic failure with multiple system atrophy. J Neurol Neurosurg Psychiatry 1986; 49:554.

Kjolseth DK, Knudsen KM, Madsen B, et al: Urodynamic biofeedback training for children with bladder-sphincter dyscoordination during voiding. Neurourol Urodynam 1993; 12:211–221.

Kjolseth DK, Madsen B, Knudsen KM, et al: Biofeedback treatment of children and adults with idiopathic detrusor instability. Scand J Urol Nephrol 1994; 28:243–247.

Klevmark BJ: Motility of the urinary bladder in cats during filling at physiologic rates: I. Intravesical pressure patterns studied by a new method of cystometry. Acta Physol Scand 1974; 90:565.

Klevmark BJ: Motility of the urinary bladder in cats during filling at physiological rates: II. Effects of extrinsic bladder denervation on intramural tension and on intravesical pressure patterns. Acta Physiol Scand 1977; 101:176.

Knespl J: The Cobb-Ragde method of a simplified correction of female stress incontinence. Cesk Gynekol 1990; 55:268–269.

Kondo A, Susset JG: Viscoelastic properties of bladder: II. Comparative studies in normal and pathologic dogs. Invest Urol 1974; 11(6):459–465.

Korda A, Peat B, Hunter P: Experience with Silastic slings for female urinary incontinence. Aust N Z J Obstet Gynaecol 1989; 29:150–154.

Kreder KJ, Webster GD: Evaluation and management of incontinence after implantation of the urinary sphincter. Urol Clin North Am 1991; 18:375–381.

Kursh ED: What factors influence the outcome of a no-incision endoscopic urethropexy? J Urol 1991; 145:223A.

Kuru M: Nervous control of micturition. Physiol Rev 1965; 45:425.

Labat-Robert J, Bihari-Varga M, Robert L: Extracellular matrix. (Review.) FEBS Lett 1990; 268(2):386–393.

Lamhut P, Jackson TW, Wall LL: The treatment of urinary incontinence with electrical stimulation in nursing home patients: A pilot study. JAGS 1992; 40:48–52.

Langer R, Golan A, Ron-El R, et al: Colposuspension for urinary stress incontinence in premenopausal and postmenopausal women. Surg Gynecol Obstet 1990; 171:13–16.

Langer R, Ron-El R, Bukovsky I, Caspi E: Colposuspension in patients with combined stress incontinence and detrusor instability. Eur Urol 1988; 14:437–439.

Langworthy OR, Kolb LC, Lewis LG: Physiology of Micturition. Baltimore, Williams & Wilkins, 1940.

Lapides J: Simplified operation for stress incontinence. Trans Am Assoc Genitourin Surg 1970; 62:12–16.

Lapides J: Operative technique for stress urinary incontinence. Urology 1974; 3:657–660.

Lapides J, Gray HO, Rawling JC: Function of striated muscles in control of urination. Surg Forum 1955; 6:611.

Lapides J, Sweet RB, Lewis LW: Role of striated muscle in urination. J Urol 1957; 77:247–250.

Larsson B, Andersson KE, Batra S, et al: Effects of estradiol on norepinephrine induced contraction, alpha adrenoreceptor number and norepinephrine content in the female rabbit urethra. J Pharmacol Exp Ther 1984; 22:557.

Lawson JON: Pelvic anatomy: Pelvic floor muscles. Ann R Coll Surg 1974; 54:244–252.

Leach GE, Bavendam TG: Prospective evaluation of the Incontan transrectal stimulator in women with urinary incontinence. Neurourol Urodynam 1989; 8:231–235.

Leach GE, Farsaii A, Kark P, Raz S: Urodynamic manifestations of cerebellar ataxia. J Urol 1982; 128:348.

Leach GE, Yip C, Donovan BJ: Post prostatectomy incontinence: The influence of bladder dysfunction. J Urol 1987; 138:574–578.

Leach GE, Yun SK: Post prostatectomy incontinence, parts I and II. Neurourol Urodynam 1992; 11:91–105.

Leo ME, Barrett DM: Success of the narrow-backed cuff design of the AMS 800 artificial urinary sphincter. Analysis of 144 patients. J Urol 1993; 150:1412–1414.

Levin RM, Jacobowitz D, Wein AJ: Autonomic innervation of rabbit urinary bladder following estrogen administration. Urology 1981; 17:449.

Levin RM, Shofer FS, Wein AJ: Estrogen-induced alterations in the autonomic responses of the rabbit urinary bladder. J Pharmacol Exp Ther 1980; 215:614.

Light JK, Reynolds JC: Impact of the new cuff design on reliability of the AS 800 artificial urinary sphincter. J Urol 1992; 147:609–611.

Linder A, Leach GE, Raz S: Augmentation cystoplasty in the treatment of neurogenic bladder dysfunction. J Urol 1983; 129:491.

Lindstrom S, Fall M, Carlsson CA, et al: The neurophysiologic basis of bladder inhibition in response to intravaginal electrical stimulaton. J Urol 1983; 129:405.

Lindstrom S, Sudsuang TG: Functionally specific bladder reflexes from pelvic and pudendal nerve branches. An experimental study in the cat. Neurourol Urodynam 1989; 8:392.

Little NA, Juma S, Raz S: Surgical treatment of stress urinary incontinence. Semin Urol 1989; 7:86–102.

Lockhart JL, Ellis GF, Helal M, Pow-Ang JM: Combined cytourethropexy for the treatment of type 3 and complicated female urinary incontinence. J Urol 1990; 143:722–725.

Lockhart JL, Vorstman B, Politano VA: Anti-incontinence surgery in females with detrusor instability. Neurourol Urodynam 1984; 3:201–207.

Lose G, Gammelgaard J, Jorgensen TJ: The one-hour pad-weighing test: Reproducibility and the correlation between the test result, start volume in the bladder and the diuresis. Neurourol Urodynam 1986; 5:17.

Lose G, Tanko, Colstrup H, Andersen JT: Urethral sphincter elelctromyography with vaginal surface electrodes: A comparison with sphincter electromyography recorded via periurethral, coaxial, anal sphincter needle and perineal surface electrodes. J Urol 1985; 133:815–818.

Luangkhot R, Peng B, Blaivas JG: Ileocystoplasty fo the management of refractory neurogenic bladder: Surgical technique and urodynamic findings. J Urol 1991; 146:1340.

Madersbacher H: Striated sphincter dyssynergia. Neurourol Urodynam 1986; 5:307.

Mahady UW, Begg BM: Long-term symptomatic and cystometric cure of the urge incontinence syndrome using a technique of bladder re-education. Br J Obstet Gynaecol 1981; 88:1038–1043.

Mainprize TC, Drutz HP: The Marshall-Marchetti-Krantz procedure: A critical review. Obstet Gynecol Surv 1988; 43:724–729.

Mark JL, Light JK: Management of urinary incontinence after prostatectomy with artificial urinary sphincter. J Urol 1989; 142:302–306.

Massey JA, Abrams PH: Obstructed voiding in the female. Br J Urol 1988; 61:36.

Mattingly RF, Davis LE: Primary treatment of anatomic stress urinary incontinence. Clin Obstet Gynecol 1984; 27:445–458.

Mayo M: Lower urinary tract dysfunction in cerebral palsy. J Urol 1992; 147:419.

Mayo ME, Chetner MP: Lower urinary tract dysfunction in multiple sclerosis. Urology 1992; 39:67.

McGuire EJ: Urodynamic findings in patients after failure of stress incontinence operations. *In* Zinner NR, Sterling AM, eds: Female Incontinence. New York, Alan R. Liss, 1980, pp 351–360.

McGuire EJ: Editorial: Bladder compliance. J Urol 1994; 151:965–966.

McGuire EJ, Appell RA: Transurethral collagen injection for urinary incontinence. Urology 1994; 43:413–415.

McGuire EJ, Bennett CJ, Konnak JA, et al: Experience with pubovaginal slings for urinary incontinence at University of Michigan. J Urol 1987; 138:525.

McGuire EJ, Brady S: Detrusor-sphincter dyssynergia. J Urol 1979; 121:774.

McGuire EJ, Fitzpatrick CC, Wan J, et al: Clinical assessment of urethral sphincter function. J Urol 1993a; 150:1452.

McGuire EJ, Herlihy E: The influence of urethral position on urinary continence. Invest Urol 1977; 15:205.

McGuire EJ, Letson W, Wang S: Transvaginal urethrolysis after obstructive urethral suspension procedures. J Urol 1989; 142:1038–1039.

McGuire EJ, Lytton B: The pubovaginal sling in stress urinary incontinence. J Urol 1978; 119:82.

McGuire EJ, Lytton B, Kohorn EI, Pepe V: Stress urinary incontinence. Obstet Gynecol 1976; 47:255.

McGuire EJ, Lytton B, Pepe V, Kohorn EI: The value of urodynamic testing in stress urinary incontinence. J Urol 1980; 124:256.

McGuire EJ, Ritchey ML, Wan JH: Surgical therapy of uncontrollable detrusor contractility. *In* Kursh ED, McGuire EJ, eds: Female Urology. Philadelphia, J.B. Lippincott Company, 1993b, p 119.

McGuire EJ, Shi-Chun Z, Horwinski R, et al: Treatment of motor and sensory detrusor instability by electrical stimulation. J Urol 1983; 129:78–79.

McGuire EJ, Woodside JR, Borden TA, et al: The prognostic significance of urodynamic testing in myelodysplastic patients. J Urol 1981; 125:205.

McGuire EJ, Yalla SV, Elbadawi A: Abnormalities of vesicourethral function following radical pelvic extirpative surgery. *In* Yalla SV, McGuire EJ, Elbadawi A, Blaivas JG, eds: The Principles and Practice of Neurourology and Urodynamics. New York, Macmillan, 1988, pp 331–337.

McIntosh LJ, Frahm JD, Mallett VT, et al: Pelvic floor rehabilitation in the treatment of incontinence. J Repro Med 1993; 38:662–666.

Mengert WF: Mechanics of uterine support and position. Am J Obstet Gynecol 1936; 31:775–782.

Meyhoff HH, Walter S, Gerstenberg T, et al: Incontinence surgery in females with motor urge incontinence. Prog Clin Biol Res 1981; 78;347–350.

Meyhoff HH, Walter S, Gerstenberg TC, et al: Incontinence surgery in female motor urge incontinence. Acta Obstet Gynecol Scand 1983; 62:365–368.

Milley PS, Nichols DH: The relationship between the pubourethral ligaments and the urogenital diaphragm in the human female. Anat Rec 1971; 170:281.

Montague DK: The artificial urinary sphincter (AS 800): Experience in 166 consecutive patients. J Urol 1992; 147:380–382.

Montz FJ, Stanton SL: Q-tip test in female urinary incontinence. Obstet Gynecol 1986; 67:259.

Morgan JE, Heritz DM, Stewart FE, et al: The polypropylene pubovaginal sling for the treatment of recurrent stress urinary incontinence. J Urol 1995; 154:1013–1015.

Morrison JFB: Reflex control of the lower urinary tract. *In* Torrens M, Morrison JFB, eds: The Physiology of the Lower Urinary Tract. London, Springer-Verlag, 1987a, pp 193–236.

Morrison JFB: Bladder control: Role of higher levels of the central nervous system. *In* Torrens M, Morrison JFB, eds: The Physiology of the Lower Urinary Tract. London, Springer-Verlag, 1987b, pp 237–274.

Mostwin JL: Effects of pharmaceuticals on bladder function. Curr Sci 1990; 580:584.

Mostwin JL, Yang A, Sanders R, Genadry R: Radiography, sonography, and magnetic resonance imaging for stress incontinence. Urol Clin North Am 1995; 22(3):539–549.

Mouritsen L, Frimodt-Moller C, Moller M: Long-term effect of pelvic floor exercises on female urinary incontinence. Br J Urol 1991; 68:32–37.

Mundy AR: An anatomic explanation for bladder dysfunction following rectal and uterine surgery. Br J Urol 1982; 54:504.

Myers RP: Male urethral sphincteric anatomy and radical prostatectomy. Urol Clin North Am 1991; 18:211–227.

Nichols DH, Milley PS: Identification of pubourethral ligaments and their role in transvaginal surgical correction of stress incontinence. Am J Obstet Gynecol 1973; 115:123–128.

Nichols DH, Randall CL: Anatomy of the living. *In* Vaginal Surgery, 3rd ed. Baltimore, Williams & Wilkins, 1989, pp 1–45.

Nitti VW, Raz S: Obstruction following antiincontinence procedures: Diagnosis and treatment with transvaginal urethelysis. J Urol 1994; 152:93–98.

Nordling J, Meyhoff HH: Disssociation of urethral and anal sphincter activity in neurogenic bladder dysfunction. J Urol 1979; 122:352–355.

Nordling J, Steven K, Meyhoff HH: Subtrigonal phenol injection: Lack of effect in the treatment of detrusor instability. Neurourol Urodynam 1986; 5:449.

Nygaard IE, Thompson FL, Svengalis SL, et al: Urinary incontinence in elite nulliparous athletes. Obstet Gynecol 1994; 84:183–187.

O'Donnell PD: The pathophysiology of incontinence in the elderly. Adv Urol 1991; 4:129.

Oelrich TM: The striated urogenital sphincter muscle in the female. Anat Rec 1983; 205:223–232.

Ohlsson BL, Fall M, Frankenberg-Sommar S: Effects of external and direct pudendal nerve maximal electrical stimulation in the treatment of the uninhibited overactive bladder. Br J Urol 1989; 64:374–380.

Olah KS, Bridges N, Denning J, et al: The conservative management of patients with symptoms of stress incontinence: A randomized, prospective study comparing weighted vaginal cones and interferential therapy. Am J Obstet Gynecol 1990; 162:87–92.

Ouslander JG, Blaustein J, Connor A, et al: Habit training and oxybutynin for incontinence in nursing home patients: A placebo controlled trial. JAGS 1988; 36:40–46.

Parulkar BG, Barrett DM: Application of the AS 800 artificial sphincter for intractable urinary incontinence in females. Surg Gynecol Obstet 1990; 171:131–138.

Parnell JP, Marshall VF, Vaughan ED: Primary management of urinary stress incontinence by the Marshall-Marchetti-Kranz vesicourethropexy. J Urol 1982; 127:679.

Parnell JP, Marshall VF, Vaughan ED: Management of recurrent urinary stress incontinence by the Marshall-Marchetti-Krantz vesicourethropexy. J Urol 1984; 132:912.

Pavlakis AJ, Siroky MB, Goldstein I, Krane RJ: Neurourologic findings in Parkinson's disease. J Urol 1983; 129:80–83.

Peattie AB, Plevnik S, Stanton SL: Vaginal cones: A conservative method of treating genuine stress incontinence. Br J Obstet Gynaecol 1988; 95:1049–1053.

Pelosi MA, Langer A, Sama JC, et al: Treatment of urinary stress incontinence. Use of dermal graft in the sling procedure. Obstet Gynecol 1976; 47:377–379.

Perez LM, Webster GD: Successful outcome of artificial urinary sphincters in men with postprostatectomy urinary incontinence despite adverse implantation features. J Urol 1992; 147:1166–1170.

Pigne A, De Goursac C, Barrat J: Acupuncture and unstable bladder. *In* Proceedings of the 15th Annual Meeting of the International Continence Society, London, 1985, pp 186–187.

Plevnik S, Janez J: Maximal electrical stimulation for urinary incontinence. Urology 1979; 14:638–646.

Plevnik S, Janez J, Vrtacnik P, et al: Short-term electrical stimulation: Home treatment for urinary incontinence. World J Urol 1986; 4:24–26.

Pow-Sang JM, Lockhart JL, Suarez A, et al: Female urinary incontinence: Preoperative selection, surgical complications and results. J Urol 1986; 136:831.

Ramsay IN, Clancy S, Hilton P: Subtrigonal phenol injections in the treatment of idiopathic detrusor instability in the female—A long term urodynamic follow-up. Br J Urol 1992; 69:363.

Raz S: Modified bladder neck suspension of the vesical neck for urinary incontinence. Urology 1981; 18:82.

Raz S: Vaginal surgery for stress incontinence. J Am Geriatr Soc 1990; 38:345–347.

Raz S, Caine M, Ziegler M: The vascular component in the production of urethral pressure. J Urol 1972; 108:93.

Raz S, Siegel AL, Sjort JL, et al: Vaginal wall sling. J Urol 1989; 141:43.

Raz S, Ziegler M, Caine M: The role of female hormones in stress incontinence. *In* Proceedings of the 16th Congress of the Societé Internationale d'Urologie, Paris, vol 1, 1973, p 397.

Reding MJ, Winter SW, Hochrein WA, et al: Urinary incontinence after unilateral hemispheric stroke: A neurologic-epidemiologic perspective. J Neuro Rehab 1987; 1:25.

Reid CJD, Borzyskowski M: Lower urinary tract dysfunction in cerebral palsy. Arch Dis Child 1993; 68:739.

Resnick NM, Yalla SV: Detrusor hyperactivity with impaired contractile function: An unrecognized but common cause of incontinence in elderly patients. JAMA 1987; 257:3076.

Resnick NM, Yalla SV, Laurino E: The pathophysiology of urinary incontinence among institutionalized elderly persons. N Engl J Med 1989; 320:1–7.

Ricci JV, Lisa JR, Thom CH, Kron WL: The relationship of the vagina to adjacent organs in reconstructive surgery: A histologic study. Am J Surg 1947; 74:387–410.

Richardson DA, Ramahi A: Reproducibility of pressure transmission ratios in stress incontinent women. Neurourol Urodynam 1993; 12:123–130.

Robertson AS, Davies JB, Webb RJ, Neal DE: Bladder augmentation and replacement: Urodynamic and clinical review of 25 patients. Br J Urol 1991; 68:590–597.

Rosenzweig BA, Bhatia NM, Nelson AL: Dynamic urethral pressure profile transmission ration: What do the numbers mean? Obstet Gynecol 1991; 77:586.

Rosenzweig BA, Bolina PS, Birch L, et al: Location and concentration of estrogen, progesterone, and androgen receptors in the bladder and urethra of the rabbit. Neurourol Urodynam 1995; 14:87–96.

Romanzi LR, Heritz DM, Blaivas JG: Preliminary assessment of the incontinent woman. Urol Clin North Am 1995; 22:513–520.

Ruch TC, Tang PC: The higher control of the bladder. *In* Boyarsky S, ed: The Neurogenic Bladder. Baltimore, Williams & Wilkins, 1967, chapter 13.

Rud T: Urethral pressure profile in continent women from childhood to old age. Acta Obstet Gynecol Scand 1980; 59:331.

Rudy DC, Awad SA, Downie JW: External sphincter dyssynergia: An abnormal continence reflex. J Urol 1988; 140:105–110.

Rudy DC, Woodside JR, Jeffrey R, et al: Urodynamic evaluation of incontinence in patients undergoing modified Campbell radical retropubic prostatectomy: A prospective study. J Urol 1984; 132:708–711.

Salinas JM, Berger Y, De la Rocha RE, Blaivas JG: Urological evaluation in the Shy-Drager syndrome. J Urol 1986; 135:741–743.

Salmon UJ, Walter RL, Geist SH: The use of estrogen in the treatment of dysuria and incontinence in post-menopausal women. Am J Obstet Gynecol 1941; 42:845.

Samisoe G, Jansson I, Mellstrom D, et al: Occurrence, nature and treatment of urinary incontinence in a 70-year-old female population. Maturitas 1985; 7:335.

Sand PK, Hill RC, Ostergard DO: Supine urethroscopic and standing cystometry as screening methods for the detection of detrusor instability. Obstet Gynecol 1987; 70:57.

Sanders RC, Genadry R, Yang A, et al: Imaging the female urethra. Ultrasound Q 1994; 12:167.

Santarosa RP, Blaivas JG: Periurethral injection of autologous fat for the treatment of sphincteric incontinence. J Urol 1994; 151:607–611.

Santiago Gonzales de Garibay AS, Castro Morrondo J, Castillo Jimeno JM, et al: Endoscopic injection of autologous adipose tissue in the treatment of female incontinence. Arch Esp Urol 1989; 42:143–147.

Schäfer W: Urethral resistance? Urodynamic concepts of physiological and pathological bladder outlet function during voiding. Neurourol Urodynam 1985; 4:161.

Schäfer W, Waterbar F, Langen PH, Deutz FJ: A simplified graphical procedure for detailed analysis of detrusor and outlet function during voiding. Neurourol Urodynam 1989; 8:405.

Schaeffer AJ, Stamey TA: Endoscopic suspension of vesical neck for urinary incontinence. Urology 1984; 23:484–494.

Schiotz HJ: One month maximal electrostimulation for genuine stress incontinence in women. Neurourol Urodynam 1994; 13:43–50.

Schmidbauer CP, Chiang H, Raz S: Surgical treatment for female geriatric incontinence. Clin Geriatr Med 1986; 2:59–76.

Schnaper HW, Kleinman HK: Regulation of cell function by extracellular matrix. (Review.) Pediat Nephrol 1993; 7(1):96–104.

Schneider MS, King LR, Surwit RS: Kegel exercises and childhood incontinence: A new role for an old treatment. J Pediat 1994; 124:91–92.

Scott FB: The use of the artificial sphincter in the treatment of urinary incontinence in the female patient. Urol Clin North Am 1985; 12:305.

Scott FB: The artificial urinary sphincter: Experience in adults. Urol Clin North Am 1989; 16:105–117.

Scott FB, Bradley WE, Timm GW: Treatment of urinary incontinence by implantable prosthetic sphincter. Urology 1973; 1:252–259.

Shapiro RA, Raz S: Clinical applications of the radiologic evaluation of female incontinence. *In* Raz S, ed: Female Urology. W.B. Saunders Company, 1983, pp 123–136.

Siegel AL, Raz S: Surgical treatment of anatomical stress incontinence. Neurourol Urodynam 1988; 7:569–583.

Siroky MB, Krane RJ: Neurological aspects of detrusor-sphincter dyssynergia, with reference to the guarding reflex. J Urol 1982; 127:953–957.

Smith ARB, Hosker GL, Warrell DW: The role of partial denervation of the pelvic floor in the aetiology of genitourinary prolapse and stress incontinence of urine: A neurophysiological study. Br J Obstet Gynaecol 1989; 96:24–28.

Smith PH, Ballantyne B: The neuroanatomic basis for denervation of the urinary bladder following major pelvic surgery. Br J Surg 1968; 55:929.

Snooks SJ, Barnes PRH, Swash M: Abnormalities of the innervation of the voluntary anal and urethral sphincters in incontinence: An electrophysiologic study. J Neurol Neurosurg Psychol 1984; 47:1269–1273.

Sorensen S, Waechter PB, Constantinou CE, et al: Urethral pressure and pressure variations in healthy fertile and postmenopausal women with unstable detrusor. Neurourol Urodynam 1991; 10(5):483–492.

Sotiropolous A, Yeaw S, Lattimer JK: Management of urinary incontinence with electronic stimulation: Observations and results. J Urol 1976; 116:747–750.

Sotolongo JR, Chancellor M: Parkinson's disease. Probl Urol 1993; 7(l):54–67.

Stamey TA: Endoscopic suspension of the vesical neck for urinary incontinence. Surg Gynecol Obstet 1973; 136:547–554.

Stamey TA: Clinical and roentgenographic evaluation of endoscopic suspension of the vesical neck for urinary incontinence in females: Report on 203 consecutive patients. Ann Surg 1980; 192:465.

Stanton SL, Cardozo LD: A comparison of vaginal and suprapubic surgery in the correction of incontinence due to urethral sphincter incompetence. Br J Urol 1979; 51:497–499.

Stanton SL, Hertogs K, Cox C, et al: Colposuspension operation for genuine stress incontinence, a five-year study. *In* Proceedings of the XII Annual Meeting of the International Continence Society, vol 12, 1982, pp 94–96.

Stanton SL, Williams LE, Ritchie D: The colposuspension operation for urinary incontinence. Br J Obstet Gynaecol 1976; 83:890–895.

Staskin DR, Zimmern PE, Hadley HR, Raz S: The pathophsyiology of stress incontinence. Urol Clin North Am 1985; 12:271.

Steinkohl WB, Leach GE: Urodynamic findings in interstitial cystitis. Urology 1989; 34:399–401.

Stothers L, Chopra A, Raz S: Vaginal reconstructive surgery for female incontinence and anterior vaginal-wall prolapse. Urol Clin North Am 1995; 22:641–655.

Susset JG, Galea G, Read L: Biofeedback therapy for female incontience due to low urethral resistance. J Urol 1990; 143:1205–1208.

Susset JG, Servot-Viguier D, Lamy F, et al: Collagen in 155 human bladders. Invest Urol 1978; 16(3):204–206.

Swaiman KF, Bradley WE: Quantification of collagen in the wall of the human urinary bladder. J Appl Phys 1967; 22:122.

Tanagho EA: Colpocystourethropexy: The way we do it. J Urol 1976; 116:751–753.

Tanagho EA, Meyers FH, Smith DR: Urethral resistance: Its components and implications—1. Smooth muscle components. Invest Urol 1969; 7:136.

Tanagho EA, Miller ER: Initiation of voiding. Br J Urol 1970; 42:175.

Tanagho EA, Smith DR: Clinical evaluation of a surgical technique for the

correction of complete urinary incontinence. Trans Am Assoc Genitourin Surg 1971; 63:103–112.
Tanagho EA, Smith DR: Clinical evaluation of a surgical technique for the correction of complete urinary incontinence. J Urol 1972; 107:402–411.
Tang PC, Ruch TC: Non-neurogenic basis of bladder tone. Am J Phys 1955; 181:249.
TeLinde RW: The urethral sling operation. Clin Obstet Gynecol 1963; 6:206–219.
Thorp JM, Stephenson H, Jones LH: Pelvic floor (Kegel) exercises—A pilot study in nulliparous women. Int Urogynecol J 1994; 5:86–89.
Thunedborg P, Fischer-Rasmussen W, Jensen SB: Stress urinary incontinence and posterior bladder suspension defects—Results of vaginal repair versus Burch colposuspension. Acta Obstet Gynecol Scand 1990; 69:55.
Tsuchida S, Noto H, Yamaguchi O, Itoh M: Urodynamic studies in hemiplegic patients after cerebrovascular accidents. Urology 1983; 21:315.
Tulloch AGS: The vascular contribution to intraurethral pressure. Br J Urol 1974; 46:659.
Turner-Warwick R: The sphincter mechanisms: Their relation to prostatic enlargement and its treatment. *In* Hinman F Jr, ed: Benign Prostatic Hypertrophy. New York, Springer-Verlag, 1983, p 809.
Turner-Warwick R, Whiteside CG, Arnold EP, et al: A urodynamic view of prostatic obstruction and prostatectomey. Br J Urol 1973; 45:631.
Uhlenhuth E: Problems in the Anatomy of the Pelvis. Philadelphia, J.B. Lippincott Company, 1953.
Van Geelen JM, Theeuwes AGM, Eskes TKAB, Martin CB Jr: The clinical and urodynamic effects of anterior vaginal repair and Burch colposuspension. Am J Obstet Gynecol 1988; 159:137–144.
Versi E: Discriminant analysis of urethral pressure profilometry data for the diagnosis of genuine stress incontinence. Br J Obstet Gynaecol 1990; 97:251–259.
Versi E, Cardozo LD, Brincat M, et al: Correlation of urethral physiology and skin collagen in postmenopausal women. Br J Obstet Gynaecol 1988; 95:147.
Versi E, Cardozo, LD, Cooper DJ: Urethral pressures: Analysis of transmission pressure ratios. Br J Urol 1991; 68:266–270.
Versi E, Cardozo LD, Studd JW, et al: Clinical assessment of urethral sphincter function. BMJ 1986; 292:166.
Walter S, Wolf H, Barleto H, et al: Urinary incontinence in post-menopausal women treated with estrogens. Urol Int 1978; 33:135.
Walters MD, Diaz K: Q-Tip test: A study of continent and incontinent women. Obstet Gynecol 1987; 70(2):208–211.
Walters MD, Jackson GM: Urethral mobility and its relationship to stress incontinence in women. J Repro Med 1990; 35(8):777–784.
Wang Y, Hadley HR: Experience with the artificial sphincter in the irradiated patients. J Urol 1992; 147:612–613.
Wear JB, Wear RB, Cleveland C: Biofeedback in urology using urodynamics: Preliminary observations. J Urol 1979; 121:464–468.
Webster GD: Achieving the goals of bladder reconstruction by enterocystoplasty. Probl Urol 1987; 1:337.
Webster GD, Kreder KJ: Voiding dysfunction following cystourethropexy: Its evaluation and management. J Urol 1990b; 144:670–673.
Webster GD, Older RA: Video urodynamics. Urology 1980; 16:106–114.
Webster GD, Sihelnik SA, Stone AR: Female urinary incontinence: The incidence, identification and characteristics of detrusor instability. Neurourol Urodynam 1984; 3:325.
Wein AJ: Classification of neurogenic voiding dysfunction. J Urol 1981; 125:605.
Wein AJ: Pharmacology of incontinence. Urol Clin North Am 1995; 22(3):557–578.
Wein AJ, Barrett DM: Voiding Function and Dysfunction: A Logical and Practical Approach. St. Louis, Year Book Medical Publishers, 1988.
Wesson MB: Anatomical, embryological and physiological studies of the trigone and neck of the bladder. J Urol 1920; 4:279–317.
Westby M, Asmussen M, Ulmsten U: Location of maximum intraurethral pressure related to urogenital diaphragm in the female subject as studied by simultaneous urethrocystometry and voiding urethrocystography. Am J Obstet Gynecol 1982; 144:408–412.
Wheeler JS Jr, Culkin DJ, O'Hara RJ, Canning JR: Bladder dysfunction and neurosyphilis. J Urol 1986; 136:903–905.
Wheeless CR Jr, Wharton LR, Dorsey JH, TeLinde RW: The Goebell-Stoeckel operation for universal cases of urinary incontinence. Am J Obstet Gynecol 1977; 128:546–549.
Wijma J, Tinga DJ, Visser GH: Perineal ultrasonography in women with stress incontinence and controls: The role of the pelvic floor muscles. Gynecol Obstet Invest 1991; 32:176.
Wilson PD, Al-Samarrai T, Deakin M, et al: An objective assesment of physiotherapy of female genuine stress incontinence. Br J Obstet Gynaecol 1987; 94:575–582.
Wilson PD, Dixon JS, Brown ADG, et al: Posterior pubo-urethral ligaments in normal and genuine stress incontinent women. J Urol 1983; 130:802–805.
Winter CC: Review of an 8-year experience with modifications of endoscopic suspension of the bladder neck for female stress urinary incontinence. (Letter; Comment.) J Urol 1990; 144:1481–1482.
Wolin KG: Stress incontinence in young, healthy, nulliparous female subjects. J Urol 1969; 101:545–549.
Woodburne RT: Anatomy of the bladder outlet. J Urol 1968; 100:474–487.
Woodside JR: Pubovaginal sling procedure for the management of urinary incontinence after urethral trauma in women. J Urol 1987; 138:527–528.
Woodside JR, McGuire EJ: Detrusor hypotonicity as a late complication of a Wertheim hysterectomy. J Urol 1982; 127:1143.
Worth AM, Dougherty MC, McKey PL: Development and testing of the circumvaginal muscles rating scale. Nurs Res 1986; 35:166.
Wyndaele JJ: Is impaired perception of bladder filling during cystometry a sign of neuropathy? Br J Urol 1993; 71:270–273.
Yalla SV, Andriole G: Vesicourethral dysfunction following pelvic visceral ablative surgery. J Urol 1984; 132:A503.
Yalla SV, Blunt KJ, Fam BA, et al: Detrusor-urethral sphincter dyssynergia. J Urol 1977; 118:1026.
Yalla SV, Blute R, Waters W, et al: Urodynamic evaluation of prostatic enlargements with micturitional vesicourethral static pressure profiles. J Urol 1981a; 125:685.
Yalla SV, DiBenedetto M, Blunt KJ, et al: Urethral striated sphincter response to electro-bulbocavernosus stimulation. J Urol 1978; 119:406.
Yalla SV, Rossier AB, Fam B: Dyssynergic vesicourethral responses during bladder rehabilitation in spinal cord injury patients: Effects of suprapubic percussion, Credé method and bethanechol chloride. J Urol 1976; 115:575.
Yalla SV, Sharma GVRK, Barsamian EM: Micturitional urethral pressure profile during voiding and the implications. J Urol 1980; 124:649.
Yalla SV, Walters WB, Snyder H, et al: Urodynamic localization of isolated bladder neck obstruction in men: Studies with micturitional vesicourethral static pressure profiles. J Urol 1981b; 125:677.
Yang A, Mostwin JL, Genadry R, et al: Patterns of prolapse demonstrated with dynamic fastscan—MRI reassessment of conventional concepts of pelvic floor weakness. Neurourol Urodynam 1993; 12:310.
Yang A, Mostwin JL, Rosenshein N, et al: Dynamic evaluation of pelvic floor descent using fastscan MRI and cinematic display. Radiology 1991; 179:25.
Zacharin RF: The suspensory mechanism of the female urethra. J Anat Lond 1963; 97:423–427.
Zacharin RF: Abdominoperineal urethral suspension: A ten-year experience in the management of recurrent stress incontinence of urine. Obstet Gynecol 1977; 50:1–8.
Zacharin RF: Abdominoperineal urethral suspension in the management of recurrent stress incontinence of urine—A 15 year experience. Obstet Gynecol 1983; 62:644–654.
Zacharin RF: Pelvic Floor Anatomy and the Surgery of Pulsion Enterocele. New York, Springer-Verlag, 1985.
Zimmern PE, Leach GE: Treatment of incontinence in men. Semin Urol 1989; 7:124–132.
Zinner NR, Sterling AM, Ritter RC: Role of inner urethral softness and urinary continence. Urology 1980; 16:115.
Zollner-Nielsen M, Samuelsson SM: Maximal electrical stimulation of patients with frequency, urgency and urge incontinence. Acta Obstet Gynecol Scand 1992; 71:629–630.
Zoubek J, McGuire EJ, Noll F, Delancey JOL: Late occurrence of urinary tract damage in patients successfully treated with radiation for cervical carcinoma. J Urol 1989; 141:1347.

31 GERIATRIC INCONTINENCE AND VOIDING DYSFUNCTION

Neil M. Resnick, M.D.
Subbarao V. Yalla, M.D.

Urinary incontinence is a major problem for elderly people. It afflicts 15% to 30% of older individuals living at home, one third of those in acute-care settings, and half of those in nursing homes (Resnick and Ouslander, 1990; Urinary Incontinence Guideline Panel, 1996). It predisposes to perineal rashes, pressure ulcers, urinary tract infections, urosepsis, falls, and fractures (Resnick and Ouslander, 1990; Urinary Incontinence Guideline Panel, 1996). It is associated with embarrassment, stigmatization, isolation, depression, and risk of institutionalization (Herzog et al, 1989; Wyman et al, 1990). And it cost more than $16 billion to manage in America in 1994 (Urinary Incontinence Guideline Panel, 1996), exceeding the amount devoted to dialysis and coronary artery bypass surgery combined.

Providers and older patients alike often neglect incontinence or dismiss it as a normal part of growing older (Branch et al, 1994), but it is abnormal at any age (Resnick, 1988; Herzog and Fultz, 1990; Urinary Incontinence Guideline Panel, 1996). Although its prevalence increases, at no age does incontinence affect the majority of individuals—even over the age of 85 years (Wetle et al, 1995; Resnick et al, unpublished). Moreover, the reason for its increased prevalence in the elderly population appears to be the diseases and functional impairments that become more likely with growing older rather than age itself (Resnick et al, 1988; Herzog and Fultz, 1990; Wetle et al, 1995; Resnick et al, unpublished). Regardless, incontinence is usually treatable and often curable at all ages—even in frail, elderly—(Ouslander and Schnelle, 1995; Resnick, 1988), but the approach must differ significantly from that used in younger patients.

THE IMPACT OF AGE ON INCONTINENCE

At any age, continence depends on not only the integrity of lower urinary tract function but also the presence of adequate mentation, mobility, motivation, and manual dexterity. Although incontinence in younger patients is rarely associated with deficits outside the urinary tract, such deficits are found commonly in older patients. It is crucial to detect them, both because they exacerbate and occasionally even cause incontinence in the elderly and because the design of an efficacious intervention requires that they be addressed.

In addition, the lower urinary tract changes with age, even in the absence of disease. Data from continent elderly people are sparse, and longitudinal data virtually nonexistent, but bladder contractility, capacity, and the ability to postpone voiding appear to decline in both sexes, whereas urethral length and maximal closure pressure probably decline with age in women (Diokno et al, 1988; Resnick, 1988; Resnick et al, 1995). The prostate enlarges in most men and appears to cause urodynamic obstruction in half (Resnick et al, 1995). In both sexes, the prevalence of involuntary detrusor contractions increases whereas the postvoiding residual (PVR) volume probably increases to no more than 50 to 100 ml (Diokno et al, 1988; Resnick, 1988; Resnick et al, 1995). In addition, elderly people often excrete most of their fluid intake at night, even in the absence of venous insufficiency, renal disease, heart failure, or prostatism (Kirkland et al, 1983). This fact, coupled with an age-associated increase in sleep disorders, leads to one to two episodes of nocturia in the majority of healthy elderly people (Brocklehurst et al, 1968; Diokno et al, 1986; Resnick, 1988). Finally, at the cellular level, detrusor smooth muscle develops a "dense band pattern" characterized by dense sarcolemmal bands with depleted caveolae (Elbadawi et al, 1993a, 1993b). This depletion may mediate the age-related decline in bladder contractility. In addition, an incomplete "dysjunction pattern" develops, characterized by scattered protrusion junctions, albeit not in chains; these changes likely underlie the high prevalence of involuntary detrusor contractions (see below) (Resnick et al, in press-a; Elbadawi et al, in press).

None of these age-related changes cause incontinence, but they do predispose to it. This predisposition, coupled with the increased likelihood that an older person will encounter an additional pathologic, physiologic, or pharmacologic insult, explains why elderly people are so likely to become incontinent. The implications are equally important. The onset or exacerbation of incontinence in an older person is likely to be due to precipitant(s) **outside** the lower urinary tract that are amenable to medical intervention. Furthermore, **treatment of the precipitant(s) alone may be sufficient to restore continence even if there is coexistent urinary tract dysfunction.** For instance, flare of hip arthritis in a woman with age-related detrusor overactivity may be sufficient to convert her urinary urgency into incontinence. Treatment of the arthritis—rather than the involuntary detrusor contractions—will not only restore continence but also lessen pain and improve mobility. These principles provide the rationale in the older patient for adding to the established lower urinary tract causes of incontinence a set of transient causes as well. Because of their frequency, ready reversibility, and association with morbidity beyond incontinence, the transient causes are discussed first.

TRANSIENT INCONTINENCE

Incontinence is transient in up to one third of community-dwelling elderly people and up to half of acutely hospitalized patients (Resnick, 1988; Herzog and Fultz, 1990). Although most of the transient causes lie outside the lower urinary tract, three points warrant emphasis. First, the risk of incontinence's developing from a transient cause is increased if, in addition to physiologic changes in the lower urinary tract, the older person also suffers from pathologic changes. Anticholinergic agents are more likely to cause overflow incontinence in people with a weak or obstructed bladder, whereas excess urine output is more likely to cause urge incontinence in people with detrusor overactivity and/or impaired mobility (Fantl et al, 1990; Diokno et al, 1991). Second, although termed *transient,* these causes of incontinence may persist if left untreated and cannot be dismissed merely because incontinence is longstanding. Third, similar to the situation for established causes (see below), identification of "the most common cause" is of little value. The likelihood of each cause depends on the individual, the clinical setting (community, acute hospital, nursing home), and the referral pattern. Moreover, geriatric incontinence is rarely due to just one of these causes. Trying to disentangle which of the multiple abnormalities as *the* cause is more useful for metaphysics than clinical practice.

The causes of transient incontinence can be recalled easily using the mnemonic *DIAPPERS* (misspelled with an extra *P*; Table 31–1). In the setting of **delirium** (an acute and fluctuating confusional state due to virtually any drug or acute illness), incontinence is merely an associated symptom that abates once the underlying cause of confusion is identified and treated. The patient needs medical rather than bladder management (Resnick, 1988).

Symptomatic urinary tract **infection** causes transient incontinence when dysuria and urgency are so prominent that the older person is unable to reach the toilet before voiding. Asymptomatic infection, which is much more common in elderly people, does not cause incontinence (Brocklehurst et al, 1968; Baldassare and Kaye, 1991; Ouslander el al, 1995; Resnick, 1988). Because illness can present atypically in older patients, however, incontinence is occasionally the only atypical symptom of a urinary tract infection. Thus, if otherwise asymptomatic bacteriuria is found on the initial evaluation, it should be treated and the result recorded in the patient's record to prevent future futile therapy.

Atrophic urethritis and/or **vaginitis** frequently causes lower urinary tract symptoms, including incontinence. As many as 80% of elderly women attending an incontinence clinic have atrophic vaginitis, characterized by vaginal mucosal atrophy, friability, erosions, and punctate hemorrhages (Robinson, 1984). Incontinence associated with this entity usually is associated with urgency and occasionally a sense of "scalding" dysuria, mimicking a urinary tract infection, but both symptoms may be unimpressive. In demented persons, atrophic vaginitis may present as agitation. Atrophic vaginitis also can exacerbate or even cause stress incontinence.

The importance of recognizing atrophic vaginitis is that it responds to low-dose estrogen (e.g., 0.3 to 0.6 mg of conjugated estrogen per day, orally or vaginally) (Urinary

Table 31–1. CAUSES OF TRANSIENT INCONTINENCE

Delirium (confusional state)
Infection—urinary (only symptomatic)
Atrophic urethritis and/or vaginitis
Pharmaceuticals
Psychological problem, especially severe depression (effect on incontinence rare)
Excess urine output (e.g., congestive heart failure, hyperglycemia)
Restricted mobility
Stool impaction

Adapted from Resnick NM: *Med Grand Rounds* 1984; 3:281–290.

Incontinence Guideline Panel, 1996). Moreover, as with transient incontinence from other causes, treatment has other benefits; in the case of atrophic urethritis, treatment ameliorates dyspareunia and reduces the frequency of recurrent cystitis (Resnick, 1988; Raz and Stamm, 1993). Symptoms remit in a few days to several weeks, but the intracellular response takes longer (Semmens et al, 1985). The duration of therapy has not been well established. One approach is to administer a low dose of estrogen daily for 1 to 2 months and then taper it. Many patients can be weaned to a dose given as infrequently as 2 to 4 times per month. After 6 months, estrogen can be discontinued entirely in some patients, but recrudescence is common. Because the dose is low and given briefly, its carcinogenic effect is likely slight, if any. However, if long-term treatment is required, progestin probably should be added if the patient has a uterus. Hormone treatment is contraindicated for women with a history of breast cancer. For those without such a history, mammography should be performed before initiating hormone therapy. There is a 20% to 40% increased risk of breast cancer among women using estrogen daily for more than 5 years, and progestin therapy does not reduce it (Colditz et al, 1995). Fortunately, such high-dose, frequent, and long-term therapy is rarely required for incontinence.

Pharmaceuticals are one of the most common causes of geriatric incontinence, precipitating leakage by a variety of mechanisms (Table 31–2). Experts often cite dosages and serum levels below which side effects are uncommon. Unfortunately, such rules are of limited use in the elderly patient because they are generally derived from studies of healthy younger people who have no other diseases and take no other medications. Of note, many of these agents also are used in the treatment of incontinence, underscoring the fact that most medications are "double-edged swords" for the elderly.

Long-acting sedative-hypnotics, whose half-life can exceed 100 hours, are associated with not only incontinence but also falling, hip fractures, driving accidents, depression, and confusion. Alcohol causes similar problems, but for a variety of reasons, physicians frequently fail to identify alcohol use by older people as a source of symptoms, including incontinence. Sequelae of alcohol abuse are often absent or attributed to other causes. In addition, because of age-related alterations in the pharmacokinetics and pharmacodynamics of alcohol disposal, as well as interactions with other commonly used drugs, as few as one or two drinks can pose a problem for older persons.

Because anticholinergic agents are prescribed so often for older people and are used even without prescription (e.g., older antihistamines used for allergies, coryza, and insomnia), they are important to ask about. They cause or contribute to incontinence in several ways. In addition to provoking overt urinary retention, these agents often induce subclinical retention. The resultant decrease in functional bladder capacity allows bladder capacity to be reached more quickly, exacerbating incontinence due to detrusor overactivity as well as that due to functional impairment. By increasing residual volume, anticholinergic agents also can aggravate leakage due to stress incontinence. Additionally, many of these drugs decrease mobility (e.g., antipsychotics that induce extrapyramidal stiffness) and precipitate confusion. Finally, several agents intensify the dry mouth that many elderly people already suffer owing to an age-related decrease in salivary gland function; the resultant increased fluid intake contributes to incontinence. Attempts should be made to discontinue anticholinergic agents, or to substitute ones with less anticholinergic effect (e.g., desipramine for amitriptyline, haloperidol for chlorpromazine). Bethanechol may be useful for nonobstructed patients whose urinary retention is associated with use of an anticholinergic that cannot be discontinued (Everett, 1975).

In men with asymptomatic prostatic obstruction, alpha-adrenergic agonists can provoke acute retention. Particularly problematic are nonprescribed decongestants. They often contain an (anticholinergic) antihistamine and are frequently taken with a nonprescribed hypnotic, all of which are also

Table 31–2. COMMONLY USED MEDICATIONS THAT MAY AFFECT CONTINENCE

Type of Medication	Examples	Potential Effects on Continence
Sedatives or hypnotics	Long-acting benzodiazepines (e.g., diazepam, flurazepam)	Sedation, delirium, immobility.
Alcohol		Polyuria, frequency, urgency, sedation, delirium, immobility.
Anticholinergics	Propantheline, oxybutynin, glycopyrrolate, dicyclomine, disopyramide, older antihistamines	Urinary retention, overflow incontinence, delirium, impaction.
Antipsychotics	Thioridazine, haloperidol	Anticholinergic actions, sedation, rigidity, immobility.
Antidepressants	Amitriptyline, desipramine	Anticholinergic actions, sedation.
Antiparkinsonians	Trihexyphenidyl, benztropine mesylate (not L-dopa or selegiline)	Anticholinergic actions, sedation.
Narcotic analgesics	Opiates	Urinary retention, fecal impaction, sedation, delirium.
α-Adrenergic antagonists	Prazosin, terazosin	Urethral relaxation may precipitate stress incontinence in women.
α-Adrenergic agonists	Nasal decongestants	Urinary retention in men.
Calcium channel blockers	All	Urinary retention; nocturnal diuresis due to fluid retention.*
Potent diuretics	Furosemide, bumetanide	Polyuria, frequency, urgency.
Angiotensin-converting enzyme (ACE) inhibitors	Captopril, enalapril, lisinopril	Drug-induced cough can precipitate stress incontinence in women and in some men with prior prostatectomy.
Vincristine		Urinary retention.

*Dihydropyridine class of calcium channel blockers.

Adapted from Resnick NM: Geriatric medicine. *In* Isselbacher KJ, Braunwald E, Wilson JD, et al, eds: Harrison's Principles of Internal Medicine. New York, McGraw-Hill, 1994, p. 34.

antihistamines. Because older individuals often fail to mention nonprescribed agents to a physician, urinary retention due to use of a decongestant, nose drops, and a hypnotic may result in premature or even unnecessary prostatectomy.

By blocking receptors at the bladder neck, alpha-adrenergic antagonists (many antihypertensives) may induce stress incontinence in older women (Mathew et al, 1988), in whom urethral length and closure pressure decline with age. Since hypertension affects half of older people, the use of these agents will increase, now that clinical trials have proved that treatment of both diastolic and isolated systolic hypertension reduces the risk of stroke and cardiovascular morbidity and mortality (Resnick, 1996). Before considering interventions for stress incontinence in such women, one should substitute an alternative agent and re-evaluate the incontinence.

Calcium channel blockers also can cause incontinence. As smooth muscle relaxants, they may increase residual volume and occasionally lead to overflow incontinence, particularly in obstructed men with coexisting detrusor weakness. The dihydropyridine class of these agents (e.g., nifedipine, nicardipine, isradipine, nimodipine) also can cause peripheral edema, which can exacerbate nocturia and nocturnal incontinence.

Angiotensin converting enzyme inhibitors (ACEIs) are prescribed increasingly for age-associated conditions such as myocardial infarction, congestive heart failure, and hypertension. Since the risk of developing an ACEI-induced cough increases with age, these agents may exacerbate what otherwise would be minimal stress incontinence in older women.

Psychological causes of incontinence have not been well studied in any age group but probably are less common in older than in younger people. Initial intervention is properly directed at the psychological disturbance, usually depression or lifelong neurosis. Once the psychological disturbance has been treated, persistent incontinence warrants further evaluation.

Excess urine output commonly contributes to or even causes geriatric incontinence. Causes include excessive fluid intake; diuretics (including theophylline-containing fluids, lithium, and alcohol); metabolic abnormalities (e.g., hyperglycemia and hypercalcemia); and disorders associated with fluid overload, including congestive heart failure, peripheral venous insufficiency, hypoalbuminemia (especially in malnourished debilitated elderly people), and drug-induced peripheral edema associated with nonsteroidal anti-inflammatory drugs (NSAIDs) and dihydropyridine calcium channel blockers. Excess output is a likely contributor when incontinence is associated with nocturia.

Restricted mobility commonly contributes to geriatric incontinence. It can result from numerous treatable conditions including arthritis, hip deformity, deconditioning, postural or postprandial hypotension, claudication, spinal stenosis, heart failure, poor eyesight, fear of falling, stroke, foot problems, drug-induced disequilibrium or confusion, or being restrained in a bed or chair (Resnick, 1996). A careful search often identifies these or other correctable causes. If not, a urinal or bedside commode may still improve or resolve the incontinence.

Finally, **stool impaction** is implicated as a cause of urinary incontinence in up to 10% of older patients seen in acute hospitals or referred to incontinence clinics (Resnick, 1988); the mechanism may involve stimulation of opioid receptors (Hellstrom and Sjoqvist, 1988). Patients present with urge or overflow incontinence and typically have associated fecal incontinence as well. Disimpaction restores continence.

These eight reversible causes of incontinence should be assiduously sought in every elderly patient. In one series of hospitalized elderly patients, when these causes were identified, continence was regained by most of those who became incontinent in the context of acute illness (Resnick, 1988). Regardless of their frequency, their identification is important in all settings because they are easily treatable and contribute to morbidity beyond incontinence.

ESTABLISHED INCONTINENCE

Lower Urinary Tract Causes

If incontinence persists after transient causes have been addressed, the lower urinary tract causes should be considered. These are similar to the causes in younger individuals, but there are several significant differences.

Detrusor overactivity (DO) is the most common type of lower urinary tract dysfunction in incontinent elderly people of either sex (Resnick, 1988; Resnick et al, 1989). DO is associated with increased spontaneous activity of detrusor smooth muscle and with specific changes at the cellular level. Termed the *dysjunction pattern,* these changes include widening of the intercellular space and replacement of normal (intermediate) muscle cell junctions by novel *protrusion* junctions and ultraclose abutments connecting cells together in chains. These junctions and abutments may mediate a change in cell coupling from a mechanical to an electric mechanism, which could facilitate propagation of heightened smooth muscle activity and provide the "final common pathway" by which such spontaneous cellular contractions result in involuntary contraction of the entire bladder (Elbadawi et al, 1993c, in press).

A distinction is generally made between DO that is associated with a central nervous system lesion (detrusor hyperreflexia) and that which is not (detrusor instability). In older patients the distinction is often unclear, because involuntary detrusor contractions may be due to normal aging, a past stroke (even if clinically inapparent), or urethral incompetence or obstruction—even in a patient with Alzheimer's disease. There is still no reliable way to determine the source of such contractions. This obviously complicates treatment decisions. It also suggests that DO coexisting with urethral obstruction or stress incontinence is less likely to resolve postoperatively than in younger individuals without other reasons for DO (Resnick, 1988; Gormley, 1993).

Traditionally, DO has been thought to be the primary urinary tract cause of incontinence in demented patients. Although this is true, it is also the most common cause in nondemented patients, and the three studies that have examined it failed to find an association between cognitive status and DO (Castleden et al, 1981; Resnick et al, 1989; Dennis et al, 1991). This lack of association likely reflects the fact that in elderly people there are multiple causes of DO unrelated to dementia, including cervical disk disease or spondylosis, Parkinson's disease, stroke, subclinical urethral obstruction or sphincter incompetence, and age itself. Moreover, demented patients also may be incontinent due to the transient causes discussed above. Thus, it is no longer tenable to ascribe incontinence in demented persons a priori to DO.

DO in elderly patients exists as two physiologic subsets—one in which contractile function is preserved and one in which it is impaired (Resnick and Yalla, 1987). The latter condition is called detrusor hyperactivity with impaired contractility (DHIC) and is the most common form of DO in the elderly (Resnick et al, 1989; Elbadawi et al, 1993c). Recent evidence suggests that DHIC may represent the coexistence of DO and bladder weakness rather than a separate entity (Elbadawi et al, 1993c). Nonetheless, DHIC has several implications. First, since the bladder is weak, urinary retention develops commonly in these patients, and DHIC must be added to outlet obstruction and detrusor underactivity as a cause of retention. Second, even in the absence of retention, DHIC mimics virtually every other lower urinary tract cause of incontinence. For instance, if the involuntary detrusor contraction is triggered by or occurs coincident with a stress maneuver, and the weak contraction (often only 2 to 6 cm H_2O) is not detected, DHIC will be misdiagnosed as stress incontinence or urethral instability (Resnick et al, in press-a). Alternatively, since DHIC may be associated with urinary urgency, frequency, weak flow rate, elevated residual urine, and bladder trabeculation, in men it may mimic urethral obstruction (Brandeis et al, 1990). Third, bladder weakness often frustrates anticholinergic therapy of DHIC since urinary retention is induced so easily. Thus, alternative therapeutic approaches are often required (see the section on therapy).

Stress incontinence is the second most common cause of incontinence in older women. As in younger women, it is usually due to pelvic muscle laxity. A less common cause is intrinsic sphincter deficiency (ISD) or type 3 stress incontinence (McGuire, 1981; Blaivas and Olsson, 1988). The prevalence of ISD may be lower than thought, however, because the diagnosis is often based solely on documenting a urethral closure pressure less than 20 cm H_2O. Since urethral pressure falls with age, this finding does not establish the presence of ISD. Moreover, since urethral pressure normally decreases with detrusor contraction, leakage coinciding with low urethral pressure can be seen in patients with DHIC in whom the low pressure contraction is missed.

When it occurs, ISD is usually due to operative trauma. But a milder form also occurs in older women, resulting only from urethral atrophy superimposed on the age-related decline in urethral pressure. Instead of leaking with any bladder volume, such women leak at higher amounts (e.g., >200 ml). Many become dry if bladder volume is kept below this level.

A rare cause of stress incontinence in older women is urethral instability, in which the sphincter paradoxically relaxes in the absence of apparent detrusor contraction (McGuire, 1978). However, most older women thought to have this condition actually have DHIC (Resnick et al, in press-a).

In men, stress incontinence is usually due to sphincter damage caused during prostatectomy. In both sexes, stress-associated leakage also can occur in association with urinary retention, but in this situation leakage it is not due to outlet incompetence.

Outlet obstruction is the second most common cause of incontinence in older men, although most obstructed men are not incontinent. With age, urethral elasticity decreases in most women and in a small proportion of them—in whom it may be compounded by fibrotic changes associated with atrophic vaginitis—moderate urethral stenosis may occur. Frank outlet obstruction is as rare in older women as in younger women. When present it is usually due to kinking associated with a large cystocele or to obstruction after bladder neck suspension. Rarely, bladder neck obstruction or a bladder calculus is the cause.

Detrusor underactivity is usually idiopathic. In the absence of obstruction or overt neuropathy, it is characterized at the cellular level by widespread degenerative changes of both muscle cells and axons, without accompanying regenerative changes (Elbadawi et al, 1993b). When it causes incontinence, detrusor underactivity is associated with overflow incontinence (<10% of geriatric incontinence) (Diokno et al, 1988; Resnick, 1988; Resnick et al, 1989). Owing to the age-related decline in sphincter strength, however, the PVR volume in women with overflow incontinence is often lower than in younger women. A mild degree of bladder weakness occurs quite commonly in older individuals. Although insufficient to cause incontinence, it can complicate treatment of other causes (see the section on therapy).

Causes Unrelated to the Lower Urinary Tract ("Functional" Incontinence)

"Functional" incontinence is often cited as a distinct type of geriatric incontinence and attributed to deficits of cognition and mobility. This concept is problematic for several reasons. First, *functional incontinence* implies that urinary tract function is normal, but studies of both institutionalized and ambulatory elderly people reveal that normal urinary tract function is the exception, even in continent subjects, and is rarely observed in incontinent patients (Ouslander et al, 1986; Resnick, 1988; Resnick et al, 1989; Resnick et al, in press-a). Second, incontinence is not inevitable with either dementia or immobility. We found that 17% of the most severely demented institutionalized residents (mean age, 89 years) were continent; more impressive, if they could merely transfer from a bed to a chair, nearly *half* were *continent* (Resnick et al, 1988). Third, since functionally impaired persons are the most likely to suffer from factors causing transient incontinence (Brocklehurst et al, 1966a, 1966b; Resnick et al, 1988; DuBeau et al, 1995; Skelly and Flint, 1995), a diagnosis of functional incontinence may result in failure to detect reversible causes of incontinence. Finally, functionally impaired persons may still have obstruction or stress incontinence and benefit from targeted therapy (Resnick, 1988; Resnick et al, 1989; Gormley et al, 1993; DuBeau and Resnick, 1995).

Nonetheless, the importance of functional impairment as a factor *contributing* to incontinence should not be underestimated, since incontinence is also affected by environmental demands, mentation, mobility, manual dexterity, medical factors, and motivation. Although lower urinary tract function is rarely normal in such persons, these factors are important to keep in mind because small improvements in each may markedly ameliorate both incontinence and functional status.

In fact, once one has excluded causes of transient incontinence and serious underlying lesions, addressing causes of functional impairment often obviates the need for further investigation.

DIAGNOSTIC APPROACH

Evaluation

The evaluation should identify transient and established causes of incontinence, assess the patient's environment and available support, and detect uncommon but serious conditions that may underly incontinence, including lesions of the brain and spinal cord, carcinoma of the bladder or prostate, hydronephrosis, bladder calculi, detrusor-sphincter dyssynergia, and decreased bladder compliance. Assessment must be tailored to the individual's clinical status and goals and be tempered by the realization that not all detected conditions can be cured; that simple interventions may be effective even in the absence of a diagnosis; and that for many elderly persons, diagnostic tests are themselves often interventions. Because the evaluation generally requires a comprehensive approach, it should be conducted over several visits to ease the burden and obviate further evaluation in those who respond to simple measures.

History

In addition to the assessment outlined in Chapter 4, evaluation of the older patient should search for transient causes of incontinence (including nonprescribed medications) and functional impairment. It should be augmented by medical records, as well as input from caregivers. Functional assessment focuses on both basic activities of daily living (ADLs: e.g., transferring from a bed, walking, bathing, toileting, eating, and grooming) and more advanced *instrumental* activities of daily living (IADLs: e.g., shopping, cooking, driving, managing finances, using the telephone). The assessment is accomplished by using a questionnaire, which can be completed by the patient or caregiver before the evaluation, and by objective evaluation of the patient from the beginning of the encounter, noting affect, mobility, ability to sit and rise from a chair, ability to provide a coherent history, and amount of time and assistance required to dress and undress.

Of course, as for younger persons, it also is important to characterize the voiding pattern and the type of incontinence. Although the clinical type of incontinence most often associated with DO is urge incontinence, *urge* is neither a sensitive nor a specific symptom; it is absent in 20% of older patients with DO, and the figure is higher in demented patients (Resnick, 1989). *Urge* is also reported commonly by patients with stress incontinence, outlet obstruction, and overflow incontinence.

A better term for the symptom associated with DO is *precipitancy,* which can be defined in two ways. For patients with no warning of imminent urination (*reflex* or *unconscious* incontinence), the abrupt gush of urine in the absence of a stress maneuver can be termed *precipitant leakage,* and it is almost invariably due to DO. For those who do sense a warning, it is of less value to focus on the leakage, since the presence and volume of leakage in this situation depend on bladder volume, amount of warning, toilet accessibility, the patient's mobility, and whether the individual can overcome the relative sphincter relaxation accompanying detrusor contraction (Dyro and Yalla, 1986). Instead, precipitancy should be defined as the **abrupt *sensation*** that urination is imminent, **whatever the interval or amount of leakage that follows**; defined in these two ways, precipitancy is both a sensitive and a specific symptom (Resnick, 1990).

As with the situation for urgency, other symptoms ascribed to DO also can be misleading in the older person unless explored carefully. Urinary frequency (>7 diurnal voids) is common (Brocklehurst et al, 1968; Diokno et al, 1986; Resnick, 1988) and may be due to voiding habit, preemptive urination to avoid leakage, overflow incontinence, sensory urgency, a stable but poorly compliant bladder, excessive urine production, depression, anxiety, or social reasons (Resnick, 1990). Conversely, incontinent persons may severely restrict their fluid intake so that even in the presence of DO they do not void frequently. Thus, the significance of urinary frequency—or its absence—can be determined only in the context of more information.

Nocturia also can be misleading unless it is first defined (e.g., two episodes may be normal for the person who sleeps 10 hours but not for one who sleeps 4) and then approached systematically (Table 31–3). The three general reasons for nocturia—excessive urine output, sleep-related difficulties, and urinary tract dysfunction—can be differentiated by careful questioning and a voiding diary that includes voided volumes (Table 31–4). One inspects the record of voided volumes to determine the functional bladder capacity (the largest single voided volume) and compares the capacity to the volume of each nighttime void. For instance, if the

Table 31–3. CAUSES OF NOCTURIA

Volume-Related
Age-related
Excess intake or alcohol
Diuretic, caffeine, theophylline
Endocrine or metabolic
Diabetes mellitus or insipidus
Hypercalcemia
Peripheral edema
Congestive heart failure
Low albumin states
Peripheral vascular disease
Drugs (e.g., lithium, NSAIDs, nifedipine)
Sleep-Related
Insomnia
Pain
Dyspnea
Depression
Drugs
Lower Urinary Tract–Related
Small bladder capacity
Detrusor hyperactivity
Prostate-related
Overflow incontinence
Decreased bladder compliance
Sensory urgency

NSAIDs, nonsteroidal anti-inflammatory drugs.
Adapted from Resnick NM: Gerontology 1990; 36(suppl 2):8–18.

Table 31–4. SAMPLE VOIDING RECORD

Date	Time	Volume Voided (ml)	Are You Wet or Dry?	Approximate Volume of Incontinence	Comments
4/5	3:50 pm	240	Wet	Slight	
	6:05 pm	210	Dry		
	8:15 pm	150	Dry		
	10:20 pm	150	Wet	15 ml	Running water
	10:30 pm	30	Dry		Bowel movement
4/6	3:15 am	270	Dry		
	6:05 am	300	Dry		
	7:40 am	200	Dry		
	9:50 am	?	Dry		
	11:20 am	200	Dry		
	12:50 pm	180	Dry		
	1:40 pm	240	Dry		
	3:35 pm	160	Wet	Slight	
	6:00 pm	170	Wet	Slight	Running water
	8:20 pm	215	Wet	Slight	
	10:25 pm	130	Dry		

Voiding diary of an incontinent 75-year-old man. Urodynamic evaluation excluded urethral obstruction and confirmed a diagnosis of detrusor hyperactivity with impaired contractility. However, note the 24-hour urine output of nearly 3 liters because of the belief that drinking 10 glasses of fluid per day was "good for my health." (Patient did not mention this until queried about the voiding record.) Given the typical voided volume of 150 to 250 ml and a measured postvoid residual volume of 150 ml, excess fluid intake was overwhelming his usual bladder capacity of 400 ml (150 + 250 ml). Although uninhibited bladder contractions were present, the easily reversible volume component of the problem—coupled with the risk of precipitating urinary retention with an anticholinergic agent—prompted treatment with volume restriction alone. After daily urinary output dropped to 1500 ml, frequency abated and incontinence resolved.

Adapted from DuBeau CE, Resnick NM: Urol Clin North Am 1991; 18:243–256.

functional bladder capacity is 400 ml and each of three nightly voids is approximately 400 ml, the nocturia is due to excessive production of urine at night. If the volume of most nightly voids is much smaller than bladder capacity, nocturia is due to either (1) a sleep-related problem (the patient voids since she is awake anyway) or (2) a problem with the lower urinary tract. Like excess urine output, sleep-related nocturia may also be due to treatable causes, including age-related sleep disorders, pain (e.g., bursitis, arthritis), dyspnea, depression, caffeine, or a short-acting hypnotic (e.g., triazolam). Bladder-related causes of nocturia are displayed in Table 31–3. Whatever the cause, the nocturnal component of incontinence is generally remediable.

The symptoms of "prostatism" also warrant comment. Owing to the high prevalence of medication use, altered fluid excretion, constipation, and DHIC, as well as the impairment of bladder contractility that accompanies aging, "prostatic" symptoms are less specific in older men than in younger men (DuBeau and Resnick, 1991).

Finally, patients or their caregivers should be asked which voiding symptom is most bothersome. For example, although a woman may have both stress and urge incontinence, the urge component may be her worst problem and should become the focus of evaluation and treatment. A man with "prostatism" may be most bothered by nocturia (DuBeau et al, 1995), which may be remedied without any consideration of his prostate (see Table 31–4). Failure to address symptom bother can lead to frustration for patient and provider alike.

Voiding Record

One of the most helpful components of the history is the voiding diary. Kept by the patient or caregiver for 48 to 72 hours, the diary records the time of each void and incontinent episode. No attempt is made to alter voiding pattern or fluid intake. Many formats have been proposed; a sample is shown in Table 31–4.

To record voided volumes at home, individuals use a measuring cup, coffee can, pickle jar, or other large-mouthed container. Information regarding the volume voided provides an index of functional bladder capacity and, together with the pattern of voiding and leakage, can suggest the cause of leakage. For example, incontinence occurring only between 8 AM and noon may be caused by a morning diuretic. Incontinence that occurs at night in a demented man with congestive heart failure, but not during a 4-hour nap in his wheelchair, is likely due to neither dementia nor prostatic obstruction but to postural diuresis associated with his heart failure. A woman with volume-dependent stress incontinence may leak only on the way to void after a full night's sleep, when her bladder contains more than 400 ml—more than it ever does during her continent waking hours. A patient may also void frequently because of polyuria.

The voiding record should also guide therapy. For instance, in a patient with DO or prostatic obstruction, excess nocturnal excretion may result in nocturnal incontinence, which is more severe and troublesome than daytime leakage; successful therapy must address the excess excretion. By contrast, another patient with the same urinary dysfunction and excretion—but with the ability to hold more urine when asleep—might be bothered more by daytime leakage. Shifting nocturnal excretion to the daytime will *exacerbate* his problem.

Targeted Physical Examination

Like the history, the physical examination is essential to detect transient causes, comorbid disease, and functional impairment. In addition to the standard neurourologic examination, one should check for signs of neurologic disease more common in the older person—such as delirium, dementia, stroke, Parkinson's disease, cord compression, and neuropathy (autonomic or peripheral)—as well as for atrophic vaginitis and general medical illnesses such as heart failure and peripheral edema. The rectal examination checks for fecal impaction, masses, sacral reflexes, symmetry of the gluteal creases, and prostate consistency and nodularity; as noted in Chapter 47, the palpated size of the prostate is unhelpful. Many neurologically unimpaired elderly patients are unable to volitionally contract the anal sphincter, but if they can it is evidence against a spinal cord lesion. The absence of the anal wink is not necessarily pathologic in the elderly patient, nor does its presence exclude an underactive detrusor (due to diabetic neuropathy, for example).

Stress Testing and Postvoid Residual Volume Measurement

Several caveats apply to performing the stress test and measuring the PVR in older patients. Stress testing is performed optimally when the bladder is full and the patient is relaxed (check the gluteal folds to corroborate) and in as close to the upright position as possible. The cough or strain should be vigorous and *single,* so one can determine whether leakage coincides with the increase in abdominal pressure or follows it. Stress-related leakage can be missed if any of these conditions is not met. Delayed leakage typical of stress-induced DO should be differentiated from leakage typical of stress incontinence, which is instantaneous and ceases as abdominal pressure declines. To be useful diagnostically, leakage must replicate the symptom for which help is sought, since many older women have incidental but not bothersome leakage of a few drops. The test should not be performed if the patient has an abrupt urge to void since this is usually due to an involuntary detrusor contraction that will lead to a falsely positive stress test. Falsely negative tests occur when the patient fails to cough vigorously or to relax the perineal muscles, the bladder is not full, or the test is performed in the upright position in a woman with a large cystocele (which kinks the urethra). If performed correctly the stress test is reasonably sensitive and quite specific (>90%) (Hilton and Stanton, 1981; Diokno, 1990; Kong et al, 1990).

After the stress test, the patient is asked to void into a receptacle and the PVR is measured. If the stress test was negative, the history suggests stress incontinence, *and* the combined volume of the void and PVR is less than 200 ml, the bladder should be filled with sterile fluid so that the stress test can be repeated at an adequate volume. There is no need to repeat a positive stress test or to repeat it in a woman whose history is negative for stress-related leakage; the sensitivity of the history for stress incontinence—unlike its specificity—exceeds 90% (Diokno et al, 1987; Jensen et al, 1994), making the likelihood of stress incontinence remote in this situation.

Optimally, the PVR is measured within 5 minutes of voiding. Measuring it after an intentional void is better than after an incontinent episode, since many patients are able to partially suppress the involuntary contraction during the episode and more than the true PVR remains. In cognitively impaired patients this may not be possible. Nonetheless, since the resulting artifact will lead to a falsely elevated PVR, a low value is still useful. The PVR will also be spuriously high if measurement is delayed (especially if the patient's fluid intake was high or included caffeine), the patient was inhibited during voiding, or there is discomfort due to urethral inflammation or infection. It will be spuriously low if the patient augmented voiding by straining (most important in women), if the catheter is withdrawn too quickly, and if the woman has a cystocele that allows urine to "puddle" beneath the catheter's reach. Of note, relying on the ease of catheterization to establish the presence of obstruction can be misleading, since difficult catheter passage may be caused by urethral tortuosity, a "false passage," or catheter-induced spasm of the distal sphincter, whereas catheter passage may be easy even in obstructed men (Klarskov et al, 1987).

Two other tests should be mentioned. The cotton swab test for pelvic floor laxity is of little value in determining the cause of a patient's leakage and has a high false-negative rate in elderly women (DuBeau and Resnick, 1991). The Bonney (or Marshall) test is also of limited usefulness in the elderly patient because vaginal stenosis is common and may lead to a false-positive result by precluding accurate finger placement. Furthermore, even if the test is performed correctly, a false-positive result may occur if the first episode of leakage was due to a cough-induced detrusor contraction, which, having emptied the bladder, does not recur during bladder base elevation.

Laboratory Investigation

As part of the laboratory investigation (Resnick, 1990; Resnick and Ouslander, 1990; DuBeau and Resnick, 1991; Urinary Incontinence Guideline Panel, 1996), one should check the blood urea nitrogen and creatinine levels, do a urinalysis and urine culture, and measure the PVR in all patients. Serum sodium, calcium, and glucose levels should be measured in patients with confusion. If the voiding record suggests polyuria, serum glucose and calcium levels (and albumin levels, to allow calculation of free calcium levels in sick or malnourished patients) should be determined. Sterile hematuria suggests partially or recently treated bacteriuria, malignancy, or calculus. But one must also bear in mind tuberculosis, since elderly people—particularly institutionalized residents—are an unappreciated reservoir of this infection (Stead, 1985). Finally, it is important to recognize when evaluating renal function that the age-related decline in glomerular filtration rate—30% by the 8th decade—is not associated with an increase in creatinine levels because of a concomitant decrease in muscle mass; thus, normal creatinine levels do not imply a normal glomerular filtration rate.

Empirical Diagnostic Categorization

After transient and serious causes have been addressed, the optimal diagnostic strategy for persistent incontinence is unknown (Resnick and Ouslander, 1990; Urinary Incontinence Guideline Panel, 1996). "Bedside" cystometry has been proposed, but its utility is limited because it misses low-pressure contractions of DHIC; its feasibility and accuracy are low in frail elderly patients (Ouslander et al, 1992); and detected DO may be either incidental and unrelated to leakage, or due to urethral obstruction or incompetence and warrant different therapy. The following approach (Resnick, 1995), although still unproved, is relatively noninvasive, accurate, cost-effective, and easily tolerated. A similar approach forms the basis for the U.S. Agency for Health Care Policy and Research Clinical Practice Guideline (Urinary Incontinence Guideline Panel, 1996), as well as the Minimum Data Set/Resident Assessment Instrument that we designed and validated for use in all American nursing homes (Resnick and Baumann, 1991; Resnick and Baumann, in press; Resnick et al, in press-b).

The first step is to identify patients with overflow incontinence (e.g., PVR ≥450 ml). Because obstruction and underactive detrusor cannot be differentiated clinically, further assessment is warranted for those in whom it would affect therapy, whereas catheterization should be used for the rest. For the remaining 90% to 95% of patients, the next step depends on their sex. Because obstruction is rare in women, the differential diagnosis is generally between stress incontinence and DO in the absence of previous bladder neck suspension or prolapsing cystocele. If the contemplated intervention is nonoperative, this distinction usually can be made on clinical grounds alone, informed by the caveats mentioned earlier.

Stress incontinence is uncommon in men and presents with a characteristic drip, similar to that of a leaky faucet, that is exacerbated by standing or straining. Thus, the usual problem in men is differentiating DO from obstruction. Uroflowmetry is helpful, but only if peak flow is normal (e.g., >12 ml/second for a voided volume of 200 ml); the age-related decrease in bladder contractility means that a normal unstrained flow rate—together with a PVR less than 100 ml—effectively excludes obstruction in an older man (DuBeau and Resnick, 1992). The next step is to search for hydronephrosis in men whose PVR exceeds 200 ml and to decompress those in whom it is found (DuBeau and Resnick, 1992). Further evaluation is also reasonable for men without hydronephrosis who are appropriate candidates and would be amenable to surgery if obstructed. For the rest, it seems sensible to treat those with urge incontinence for presumed DO, provided they are compliant and can be taught signs of incipient urinary retention; bladder relaxants should be avoided in those with significantly elevated PVR (e.g., ≥150 ml). A similar approach is advocated for cognitively impaired men who can be closely observed (e.g., institutionalized residents) (Resnick and Baumann, 1996, in press). Men without urge incontinence, those who fail empirical therapy, and those who are cognitively impaired and less supervised, should be evaluated further if findings would affect therapy.

Urodynamic Testing

Although its precise role in elderly people is unclear, multichannel urodynamic evaluation is probably warranted when diagnostic uncertainty may affect therapy and when empirical therapy has failed and other approaches would be tried. Because conditions that closely mimic obstruction and stress incontinence are so common in elderly people—including altered fluid excretion, medication use, detrusor hyperactivity, and DHIC (Brandeis et al, 1990)—urodynamic corroboration of the diagnosis is strongly recommended if surgery will be performed (Resnick and Baumann, 1991; Urinary Incontinence Guideline Panel, 1996; Resnick and Baumann, 1996, in press). Whatever its role, however, urodynamic evaluation of even frail elderly patients is reproducible, safe, and feasible (Resnick et al, 1987, 1989).

THERAPY

As with the diagnostic approach, treatment must be individualized because factors outside the lower urinary tract so often affect feasibility and efficacy. For instance, although both may have DO that can be managed successfully, a severely demented and bedfast woman must be treated differently from one who is ambulatory and cognitively intact. This section and Table 31–5 outline several treatments for each condition and provide guidance for their use. It is assumed that serious underlying conditions, transient causes of incontinence, and functional impairments have already been addressed. It cannot be overemphasized that successful treatment of established incontinence, especially in the elderly patient, is usually multifactorial and must address factors beyond the urinary tract.

Detrusor Overactivity

The initial approach to DO is to identify and treat its reversible causes. Unfortunately, many of its causes are not amenable to specific therapy or a cause may not be found, so treatment usually must be symptomatic. Simple measures, such as adjusting the timing or amount of fluid excretion (see Table 31–4) or providing a bedside commode or urinal are often successful. If not, the cornerstone of treatment is behavioral therapy. If the patient can cooperate, bladder training regimens extend the voiding interval (Burgio and Burgio, 1986; Hadley, 1986; Fantl et al, 1991). For instance, if the voiding record documents incontinence when the interval exceeds 3 hours, the patient is instructed to void every 2 hours and suppress urgency in between. Once dry, the patient can extend the interval by half an hour and repeat the process until a satisfactory result or continence is achieved. Patients need not follow this regimen at night since nighttime improvement parallels daytime success. Biofeedback may be added (Baigis-Smith et al, 1989; Burgio and Engel, 1990), but its marginal benefit is unclear.

For cognitively impaired patients, *prompting voiding* is used. Asked every 2 hours whether they need to void, patients are escorted to the toilet if the response is affirmative. Positive verbal reinforcement is employed, and negative comments are avoided. Prompted voiding reduces incontinence frequency in nursing homes by roughly 50%, and leakage can be virtually eliminated during daytime hours in one third of residents (Hu et al, 1989; Engel et al, 1990; Schnelle, 1990). The latter group can be identified within 3 days. When prompted *hourly* to void, they urinate into a toilet or commode more than two thirds of the time that they indicate the need to do so, or they become continent on more than 80% of checks. Response is maintained when the prompting interval is increased to 2 hours. Half of the remaining patients also improve with prompting, but they are still wet more than once during the daytime. For the quarter of patients who do not respond to prompting at baseline, little benefit is obtained by further prompting. Importantly, the response does not correlate with the degree of

Table 31–5. STEPWISE APPROACH TO TREATMENT*

Condition	Clinical Type of Incontinence†	Treatment
Detrusor overactivity with normal contractility (DO)	Urge	1. Bladder retraining or prompted voiding regimens. 2. ± bladder relaxant medication (anticholinergic, smooth muscle relaxant, calcium channel blocker), if needed and not contraindicated. 3. Indwelling catheterization alone often unhelpful because detrusor "spasms" often increase, leading to leakage around the catheter. 4. In selected cases, induce urinary retention pharmacologically and add intermittent or indwelling catheterization.‡
Detrusor hyperactivity with impaired contractility (DHIC)	Urge§	1. If bladder empties adequately with straining, behavioral methods (as above) ± bladder relaxant medication (low doses; especially feasible if sphincter incompetence coexists). 2. If residual urine >150 ml, augmented voiding techniques** or intermittent catheterization (± bladder relaxant medication). If neither feasible, undergarment or indwelling catheter.‡
Stress incontinence	Stress	1. Conservative methods (weight loss if obese; treatment of cough or atrophic vaginitis; physical maneuvers to prevent leakage [e.g., have patient tighten pelvic muscles, cross legs]; rarely, use of pessary or tampon). 2. If leakage threshold ≥150 ml identified, adjust fluid excretion and voiding intervals. 3. Pelvic muscle exercises ± biofeedback or weighted intravaginal "cones." 4. Imipramine (or doxepin) or alpha-adrenergic agonists—± estrogen—if not contraindicated. 5. Surgery (urethral suspension, or compression ["sling"], periurethral bulking injections, artificial sphincter).
Urethral obstruction	Urge or overflow¶	1. Conservative methods (including adjustment of fluid excretion, bladder retraining or prompted voiding) if hydronephrosis, elevated residual urine, recurrent symptomatic UTI, and gross hematuria have been excluded. 2. Bladder relaxants if DO coexists, PVR is small, and surgery is not desired or feasible. 3. Alpha-adrenergic antagonists, finasteride, antiandrogens, and/or LHRH analogues if not contraindicated and patient either prefers them or is not surgical candidate. 4. Surgery (incision, prostatectomy).
Underactive detrusor	Overflow	1. If duration unknown, decompress for several weeks and perform voiding trial. 2. If cannot void, PVR remains large, or retention is chronic, try augmented voiding techniques** ± alpha-adrenergic antagonist, but only if some voiding possible; bethanechol rarely useful unless bladder weakness due to anticholinergic agent that cannot be discontinued. 3. If fails, or voiding not possible, intermittent or indwelling catheterization.‡

*These treatments should be initiated only after adequate toilet access has been ensured, contributing conditions have been treated (e.g., atrophic vaginitis, heart failure), fluid management has been optimized, and necessary or exacerbating medications have been stopped. For additional details, recommendations, and drug doses, see text.

†*Urge:* Leakage in absence of stress maneuvers and urinary retention, usually preceded by *abrupt* onset of need to void.

Stress: Leakage that coincides *instantaneously* with stress maneuvers, in absence of urinary retention.

Overflow: Frequent leakage of small amounts associated with urinary retention.

‡UTI prophylaxis can be used for recurrent symptomatic UTIs, but only if catheter is not indwelling.

§But may also mimic stress or overflow incontinence.

¶Also can cause postvoid "dribbling" alone, which is treated conservatively (e.g., by sitting to void and allowing more time, "double voiding," and by gently "milking" the urethra after voiding).

**Augmented voiding techniques include Credé (application of suprapubic pressure) and Valsalva (straining) maneuvers, and "double" voiding. They should be performed only *after* voiding has begun.

UTI, urinary tract infection; PVR, postvoiding residual; LH, luteinizing hormone; RH, releasing hormone.

Adapted from Resnick NM: Voiding dysfunction and urinary incontinence. *In* Beck C, ed: Geriatric Review Syllabus. New York, American Geriatrics Society, 1991, pp 141–154.

dementia. In addition, these results were obtained without drugs, and urodynamic evaluations were not performed (Schnelle, 1990; Ouslander et al, 1995). Tailoring the regimen to the cause and pattern of incontinence should further improve outcome.

The voiding record also can be helpful if it reveals that nocturnal incontinence correlates with nocturnal diuresis. If due to systolic congestive heart failure, it should improve with diuretic therapy. If due to peripheral edema in the absence of heart failure and hypoalbuminemia (i.e., venous insufficiency), it should respond to pressure gradient stockings. If not associated with peripheral edema, it may respond to alteration of the pattern of fluid intake or the administration of a rapidly acting diuretic in the late afternoon or early evening (Pedersen and Johansen, 1988). For patients with DHIC whose voiding record and PVR suggest that involuntary detrusor contractions are provoked only at high bladder volumes, catheterization at bedtime removes the residual urine, thereby increasing functional bladder capacity and restoring both continence and sleep.

Drugs augment behavioral intervention but do not supplant it, since they generally do not abolish involuntary contractions. There are few data on efficacy or toxicity in the elderly population. Available studies show similar efficacy for most drugs—except flavoxate, which fares poorly in controlled trials (Urinary Incontinence Guideline Panel).

Thus, the choice of drug (Table 31–6) should be based on factors unrelated to bladder function. Propantheline is best avoided in demented patients and those taking other anticholinergics. A calcium channel blocker may be preferred for persons with associated hypertension, angina pectoris, or cardiac diastolic relaxation. Orthostatic hypotension often precludes the use of imipramine and nifedipine, but a tricyclic antidepressant may be optimal for a patient without orthostatic hypotension who also requires pharmacotherapy for depression. Medications with rapid onset of action, such as oxybutynin, can be employed prophylactically if incontinence occurs at predictable times. Combining low doses of two agents with complementary actions, such as oxybutynin and imipramine, occasionally maximizes benefits and minimizes side effects. Intravesical instillation of several of these agents is also effective, but useful only if self-catheterization is feasible. Vasopressin has little efficacy in the elderly patient (Dequecker, 1965; Asplund and Åberg, 1993). Because of the high prevalence of contraindications to its use (e.g., renal insufficiency, heart failure), the risk of inducing hyponatremia and fluid retention (Seiler et al, 1992), and its considerable expense, the use of 1-deamino-8-D-arginine-vasopressin in the elderly patient should await results of further studies.

Regardless of which bladder relaxant is used, urinary retention may develop. PVR and urine output should be monitored, especially in DHIC in which the detrusor is already weak. Subclinical urinary retention also may develop, reducing functional bladder capacity and attenuating or even reversing the drug's benefit. Thus, if incontinence worsens as the dose is increased, PVR should be remeasured. Another reason for drug failure is excess fluid ingestion engendered by anticholinergic-induced xerostomia. For patients whose incontinence defies other remedies (such as those with DHIC), inducing urinary retention and using intermittent catheterization may be viable if catheterization is feasible. Other remedies for urge incontinence, including electric stimulation (Chapters 29 and 30) and selective nerve blocks, are successful in selected situations but have not been studied adequately in elderly patients.

Adjunctive measures, such as pads and special undergarments, are invaluable if incontinence proves refractory. Many types are now available, allowing the recommendation to be tailored to the individual's problem (Brink and Wells, 1986; Snow, 1988; Brink, 1990). Most are included in an illustrated catalog (HIP, PO Box 544, Union, SC 29379). For bedridden individuals a launderable bed pad may be preferable; for those with a stroke, a diaper or pants that can be opened using the good hand may be preferred. For ambulatory patients with large gushes of incontinence, wood pulp–containing products are usually superior to ones containing polymer gel, since the gel generally cannot absorb the large amount and rapid flow, whereas the wood pulp product can easily be doubled up if necessary. Optimal products for men and women differ because of the location of the "target zone" of the urinary loss. Finally, the choice is influenced by the presence of fecal incontinence.

Condom catheters are helpful for men, but they are associated with skin breakdown, bacteriuria, and decreased motivation to become dry (Johnson, 1983; Jayachandran et al, 1985; Ouslander and Schnelle, 1995), and they are not feasible for the older man with a small or retracted penis. Recently, external collecting devices have been devised for institutionalized women (Johnson et al, 1990), but whether they will adhere adequately in more active women remains to be determined. Indwelling urethral catheters are not recom-

Table 31–6. BLADDER RELAXANT MEDICATIONS USED TO TREAT URGE INCONTINENCE*

Medication Class, Name, and Dosage	Comments
Smooth Muscle Relaxant	
Flavoxate 300–800 mg daily (100–200 mg po tid–qid)†	Has not proved effective in placebo-controlled trials.
Calcium Channel Blocker	
Diltiazem 90–270 mg daily (30–90 mg po qd–tid) Nifedipine 30–90 mg daily (10–30 mg po qd–tid)	No controlled trial data. Most useful for the patient with other indication for drug (e.g., hypertension, angina pectoris, or abnormalities of cardiac diastolic relaxation).
Anticholinergic	
Propantheline 15–150 mg daily (7/.5–30 mg po tid–5×/day)‡	Use with particular caution in demented patients and in patients taking other anticholinergic agents.
Combination Smooth Muscle Relaxant and Anticholinergic	
Oxybutynin 5–20 mg daily (2.5–5 mg po tid–qid)§ Dicyclomine 30–90 mg daily (10–30 mg po tid)	These medications, which have rapid onset of action, can be employed prophylactically if incontinence occurs at predicatable times. They can also be used continuously.
Antidepressants¶	
Doxepin 25–75 mg daily (10–25 mg po qd–tid) Imipramine 25–100 mg daily (10–25 mg po qd–qid)	May be particularly helpful in women with coexistent stress incontinence. Orthostatic hypotension often precludes their use, but a tricyclic antidepressant may be preferred for a depressed incontinent patient without orthostatic hypotension.

*All drugs should be started at the lowest dose and increased slowly until encountering maximal benefit or intolerable side effects. All are given in divided doses, except the antidepressants, which may be given as a single daily dose.

†Some uncontrolled reports suggest that doses up to 1200 mg per day may be effective with tolerable side effects; efficacy has not been supported by randomized controlled trials at any dose.

‡Higher doses are occasionally tolerated and effective; should be given in the *fasting* state.

§May also be applied intravesically in patients who can use intermittent catheterization.

¶May be given as single daily dose of 25–100 mg.

Adapted from Resnick NM: Lancet 1995; 346:94–99.

mended for DO because they usually exacerbate it. If they must be used (e.g., to allow healing of a pressure sore), a small catheter with a small balloon is preferable to avoid leakage around the catheter; such leakage almost invariably results from bladder contractions rather than a catheter that is too small. Increasing catheter and balloon size only aggravates the problem and may result in urethral erosion and sphincter incompetence. If spasms persist, drugs such as oxybutynin can be tried. More potent anticholinergic agents, such as belladonna suppositories, should be avoided in the elderly patient.

Stress Incontinence

Urethral hypermobility, the most common cause of stress incontinence in older women, may be improved by weight loss if the patient is obese, by postural maneuvers (Norton and Baker, 1994), by therapy of precipitating conditions such as atrophic vaginitis or cough (e.g., due to an angiotensin-converting enzyme inhibitor), and (rarely) by insertion of a pessary (Suarez et al, 1991; Zeitlin and Lebherz, 1992). If the voiding diary reveals that leakage is volume-dependent, it may be improved by adjusting fluid excretion and voiding intervals to keep bladder volume below this threshold. However, if the threshold is less than 150 to 200 ml, this strategy is generally not sufficient alone.

Pelvic muscle exercises can decrease incontinence substantially in motivated and cognitively intact older women trained to perform them 30 to 200 times daily (Wells, 1990; Wells et al, 1991; Urinary Incontinence Guideline Panel, 1996; Burns et al, 1993). Unfortunately, such exercises must be pursued indefinitely, efficacy is limited for severe incontinence, only 10% to 25% of women become fully continent, and many older women are unable or unmotivated to follow such regimens. Adding vaginal cones, biofeedback, or electric stimulation likely enhances efficacy, but their marginal benefit is unclear (Burgio and Engel, 1990; Urinary Incontinence Guideline Panel, 1996; Burns et al, 1993). Urethral plugs are still under development.

If not contraindicated by other conditions, treatment with an alpha-adrenergic agonist such as sustained-release phenylpropanolamine (PPA, 25 to 100 mg twice daily) may be added and is often beneficial for women, especially when administered with estrogen (Wells et al, 1991; Urinary Incontinence Guideline Panel, 1996). PPA and estrogen may work for women with sphincter deficiency as well. PPA is inexpensive, available without a prescription, and contained in many diet pills. Moreover, it is often tolerated in those with uncomplicated hypertension (Beck et al, 1992). However, the physician should prescribe the dose and guide the choice of preparation, since some capsules also contain agents such as chlorpheniramine in doses that can be troublesome for elderly patients. Imipramine, with beneficial effects on the bladder and the outlet, is a reasonable alternative for patients with evidence of both stress and urge incontinence. But it should be used only if symptoms as well as signs of postural hypotension have been excluded.

If these methods fail or are unacceptable, further evaluation of the urinary tract may be warranted. If urethral hypermobility is confirmed, surgical correction is successful in the majority of selected elderly patients (Resnick, 1988; Ericksen et al, 1990; Griffith-James and Abrams, 1990; Nitti et al, 1993). If intrinsic sphincter deficiency (ISD) is diagnosed instead, it can be corrected with a different procedure (pubovaginal sling) (Blaivas and Jacobs), but the morbidity is higher and precipitation of chronic retention is more likely than with correction of urethral hypermobility. The influence of coincident DO on the outcome in older women has been inadequately investigated for either type of stress incontinence. Other treatments for sphincter incompetence include periurethral bulking injections and insertion of an artificial sphincter, but reported experience with these approaches in persons over the age of 75 years is still limited, and so is long-term follow-up.

For men in whom these interventions fail, prostheses such as condom catheters or penile clamps may be useful, but most require substantial cognitive capacity and manual dexterity and are often poorly tolerated. Penile sheaths (e.g., McGuire prosthesis or adhesive underwear liners) are an alternative. As discussed above, pads and undergarments are used as adjunctive measures. However, in these cases, polymer gel pads are frequently successful because the gel can more readily absorb the smaller amount of leakage. Some products can be flushed down the toilet, a feature that is convenient for ambulatory persons.

Outlet Obstruction

For older men, conservative management of outlet obstruction often suffices. In the absence of urinary retention, modification of fluid excretion and voiding habits may be effective. If not, alpha-adrenergic antagonists are useful and generally well tolerated; they are actually beneficial for men with systolic (not diastolic) congestive heart failure. However, their use requires caution. With age, cardiac output depends less on cardioacceleration than on adequate ventricular filling. Unfortunately, the left ventricle also becomes stiffer, necessitating higher filling pressure. Thus, alpha blockers—which decrease preload as well as afterload—can result in symptomatic hypotension in older men, particularly those whose age-related ventricular hypertrophy is exacerbated by hypertension or aortic stenosis. Medical consultation should be sought before prescribing an alpha blocker to such individuals.

The 5α-reductase inhibitor finasteride is another alternative, but fewer men appear to benefit, the effect is more modest, and the benefit is more delayed (Gormley et al, 1992). Devices and surgical approaches, as well as the approach to obstruction in women, are discussed elsewhere. Of note, DO probably resolves less often after removal of obstruction in older patients than in younger ones. But incontinence may still improve, even in cognitively impaired persons (Eastwood and Smart, 1985; Gormley et al, 1993). In addition, less extensive resection or ablation often suffices for frail, elderly men, in whom recurrence of symptoms with adenoma regrowth years later is often not an issue. This fact, coupled with surgical techniques that now permit resection or ablation under local anesthesia, has made surgery increasingly feasible for this population.

Underactive Detrusor

Management of detrusor underactivity is directed at reducing the residual volume, eliminating hydronephrosis (if pres-

Table 31–7. REMOVING AN INDWELLING URETHRAL CATHETER

Correct reversible causes of urinary retention fecal impaction; pelvic and or perineal pain; and use of anticholinergic, alpha-adrenergic agonist, or calcium channel blocker medications. If an anticholinergic antidepressant or antipsychotic agent cannot be stopped, consider switching to one with less or no anticholinergic side effects, or consider adding bethanechol. Addition of an alpha-adrenoceptor antagonist may be helpful but is unproved in women.

Treat delirium, depression, atrophic vaginitis, or urinary tract infection, if present.

Record urinary output at intervals of 6–8 hours for 2 days to establish a pattern of baseline urine excretion.

Remove the catheter at a time that permits accurate recording of urine output and allows postvoiding recatheterization; clamping the catheter before removal is not necessary and can be dangerous.

Reinsert the catheter *only:*

- After the patient voids, to determine postvoiding residual (PVR) volume; or
- After the expected bladder *volume* (based on records of urine output—not the time since the catheter was removed—exceeds a preset limit (e.g., 600–800 ml); or
- If the patient is uncomfortable and unable to void despite ensured privacy and maneuvers performed to encourage voiding (e.g., running water, tapping suprapubic area, or stroking inner thigh).

If the patient voids and the PVR volume is

- Greater than 400 ml—reinsert the catheter and evaluate further, if appropriate.*
- 100–400 ml—watch for delayed retention and evaluate further, if appropriate.*
- Less than 100 ml—watch for delayed retention.

If the patient is unable to void, refer for evaluation, if appropriate.* If not, patient requires permanent catheterization.

*Further evaluation is appropriate when the patient and physician feel that if a surgically correctable condition were found (e.g., urethral obstruction), an operation would be preferable to chronic catheterization or the other options described in the text.

Modified from Resnick NM: Incontinence. *In* Beck C, ed: Geriatric Review Syllabus. New York, American Geriatrics Society, 1991, pp 141–154.

ent), and preventing urosepsis. The first step is to use indwelling or intermittent catheterization to decompress the bladder for up to a month (at least 7 to 14 days), while reversing potential contributors to impaired detrusor function (fecal impaction and medications). If an indwelling catheter has been inserted, it should then be removed (Table 31–7). If decompression does not fully restore bladder function, augmented voiding techniques (such as double voiding and implementation of the Credé [application of suprapubic pressure during voiding] or Valsalva maneuver) may help if the patient is able to initiate a detrusor contraction or if there is coexistent stress incontinence. Bethanechol (40 to 200 mg per day in divided doses) is occasionally useful in a patient whose bladder contracts poorly because of treatment with anticholinergic agents that cannot be discontinued (e.g., a tricyclic antidepressant). In other patients, bethanechol may decrease the PVR if sphincter function and local innervation are normal, but evidence for its efficacy is equivocal, and residual volume should be monitored to assess its effect (Downie, 1984; Finkbeiner, 1985).

On the other hand, if after decompression the detrusor is acontractile, these interventions are apt to be fruitless and the patient should be started on intermittent catheterization or an indwelling urethral catheter. For patients at home, intermittent self-catheterization is preferable and requires only clean, rather than sterile, catheter insertion. The patient can purchase two or three of these catheters inexpensively. One or two are used during the day and another is kept at home. The catheters are cleaned daily, allowed to air dry at night, and sterilized periodically, and may be reused repeatedly. Antibiotic or methenamine prophylaxis against urinary tract infection is probably warranted if the patient gets more than an occasional symptomatic infection or has an abnormal heart valve (Chawla et al, 1988; Warren, 1990). Intermittent catheterization in this setting is generally painless, safe, inexpensive, and effective and allows patients to carry on with their usual daily activities. For debilitated patients, however, intermittent catheterization is usually less feasible, although sometimes possible (Hunt and Whitaker, 1990). If intermittent catheterization is used in an institutional setting, sterile rather than clean technique should be employed until studies document the safety of the latter.

Unfortunately, despite the benefits and proven feasibility of intermittent catheterization (Bennett and Diokno, 1984; Bakke et al, 1992), most elderly people choose indwelling catheterization instead. As in younger people, complications of chronic indwelling catheterization include renal inflammation and chronic pyelonephritis (Warren et al, 1994),

Table 31–8. PRINCIPLES OF INDEWELLING CATHETER CARE

Maintain sterile, closed gravity drainage system:

- Secure the catheter to upper thigh or abdomen to avoid urethral irritation and contamination. Rotate the site of attachment every few days.
- Empty the bag every 8 hours.
- Do not routinely irrigate the catheter.
- Do not clamp or kink the drainage tubing, and keep the collection bag below bladder level at all times.
- Avoid frequent cleaning of the urethral meatus; washing with soap and water once daily is sufficient; periurethral application of antimicrobial creams is ineffective.

If "bypassing" occurs in the absence of obstruction, it is likely due to a bladder spasm, which can be minimized by using the smallest balloon that will keep the catheter in place and by treating with a bladder relaxant medication if necessary.

Infection prophylaxis, as well as treatment of asymptomatic bacteriuria, is fruitless and usually leads to the emergence of resistant organisms.

Surveillance cultures are unnecessary and potentially misleading since bacteriuria is universal, frequently changing, and often polymicrobial.

If symptomatic urinary tract infection (UTI) develops, change the catheter before obtaining a culture specimen, since cultures obtained through the old catheter may reflect organisms colonizing encrustations rather than the infecting organism. Pending culture results, antibiotic treatment should include coverage of common uropathogens, as well as uncommon ones such as *Providencia stuartii* and *Morganella morganii.*

If catheter obstruction occurs frequently, and urine cultures reveal *P. stuartii* or *Proteus mirabilis,* antibiotic treatment may reduce the frequency of obstruction but induces emergence of resistant organisms. In the absence of urea-splitting organisms, consider urine acidification if urine output is normal (at low output, acidification may increase blockage due to uric acid crystals). If frequent blockage persists, consider using a silicon catheter.

In the absence of obstruction and symptomatic UTI, there is no consensus on the best time to change the catheter. Some persons form material that frequently clogs the lumen; their catheter probably should be changed often enough to reduce such obstruction. Other individuals can use the same catheter for years, but it is customary to change it every 1–2 months. For patients who are difficult to catheterize, the catheter can be changed less frequently if it remains patent, and complication-free.

Adapted from Resnick NM: Voiding dysfunction and urinary incontinence. *In* Beck C, ed: Geriatric Review Syllabus. New York, American Geriatrics Society, 1991, pp 141–154.

bladder and urethral erosions, bladder stones, and cancer, as well as urosepsis (Warren, 1990). Principles of catheter care are summarized in Table 31–8.

When indicated, indwelling catheters can be extremely effective, but their use should be restricted. They are indicated in the acutely ill patient to monitor fluid balance, in the patient with a nonhealing pressure ulcer, for temporary bladder decompression in patients with acute urinary retention, and in the patient with overflow incontinence refractory to other measures. Even in long-term care facilities, they are probably indicated for only 1% to 2% of patients.

SUMMARY

Regardless of age, mobility, mentation, or institutionalization, incontinence is never normal. By attenuating physiologic reserve, aging increases the likelihood of becoming incontinent in the setting of additional physiologic, pharmacologic, or pathologic insults. Since many of these problems lie outside the urinary tract, so too must the diagnostic and therapeutic focus. However, such a strategy—coupled with a multifactorial, creative, persistent, and optimistic approach—increases the chances of a successful outcome and generally rewards patient and physician alike.

REFERENCES

Asplund R: Åberg H: Desmopressin in elderly subjects with increased nocturnal diuresis. A two-month treatment study. Scand J Urol Nephrol 1993; 27:77–82.

Baigis-Smith J, Jakovac Smith DA, Rose M, Newman DK: Managing urinary incontinence in community-residing elderly persons. Gerontologist 1989; 29:229–233.

Bakke A, Brun OH, Hoisæter PÅ: Clinical background of patients treated with clean intermittent catheterization in Norway. Scand J Urol Nephrol 1992; 26:211–217.

Baldassare JS, Kaye D: Special problems in urinary tract infection in the elderly. Med Clin North Am 1991; 75:375–390.

Beck RA, Mercado DL, Seguin SM, et al: Cardiovascular effects of pseudoephedrine in medically controlled hypertensive patients. Arch Intern Med 1992; 152:1242–1245.

Bennett CJ, Diokno AC: Clean intermittent self-catheterization in the elderly. Urol 1984; 24:43–45.

Blaivas JG, Jacobs BZ: Pubovaginal fascial sling for the treatment of complicated stress urinary incontinence. J Urol 1991; 145:1214–1218.

Blaivas JG, Olsson CA: Stress incontinence: Classification and surgical approach. J Urol 1988; 139:727–731.

Branch LG, Walker LA, Wetle TT, et al: Urinary incontinence knowledge among community-dwelling people 65 years of age and older. J Am Geriatr Soc 1994; 42:1257–1262.

Brandeis GB, Yalla SV, Resnick NM: Detrusor hyperactivity with impaired contractility (DHIC): The great mimic. J Urol 1990; 143:223A.

Brink CA: Absorbent pads, garments, and management strategies, J Am Geriatr Soc 1990; 38:368–373.

Brink CA, Wells TJ: Environmental support for incontinence: Toilets, toilet supplements, and external equipment. Clin Geriatr Med 1986; 2:829–840.

Brocklehurst JC, Dillane JB: Studies of the female bladder in old age. I: Cystometrograms in non-incontinent women. Gerontol Clin 1966a; 8:285–305.

Brocklehurst JC, Dillane JB: Studies of the female bladder in old age. II: Cystometrograms in 100 incontinent women. Gerontol Clin 1966b; 8:306–319.

Brocklehurst JC, Dillane JB, Griffiths L, Fry J: The prevalence and symptomatology of urinary infection in an aged population. Gerontol Clin 1968; 10:242–253.

Burgio KL, Burgio LD: Behavior therapies for urinary incontinence in the elderly. Clin Geriatr Med 1986; 2:809–827.

Burgio KL, Engel BT: Biofeedback-assisted behavioral training for elderly men and women. J Am Geriatr Soc 1990; 38:338–340.

Burns PA, Pranikoff K, Nochajski TH, et al: A comparison of effectiveness of biofeedback and pelvic muscle exercise treatment of stress incontinence in older community-dwelling women. J Gerontol 1993; 48:M167–M174.

Castleden CM, Duffin HM, Asher MJ: Clinical and urodynamic studies in 100 elderly incontinent patients. BMJ 1981; 282:1103–1105.

Chawla JC, Clayton CL, Stickler DJ: Antiseptics in the longterm urological management of patients by intermittent catheterization. Br J Urol 1988; 62:289–294.

Colditz GA, Hankinson SE, Hunter DJ, et al: The use of estrogens and progestins and the risk of breast cancer in postmenopausal women. N Engl J Med 1995; 332:1589–1593.

Dennis PJ, Rohner TJ, Hu TW, et al: Simple urodynamic evaluation of incontinent elderly female nursing home patients. A descriptive analysis. Urology 1991; 37:173–179.

Dequecker J: Drug treatment of urinary incontinence in the elderly. Gerontol Clin 1965; 7:311–317.

Diokno AC: Diagnostic categories of incontinence and the role of urodynamic testing. J Am Geriatr Soc 1990; 38:300–305.

Diokno AC, Brock BM, Brown M, Herzog AR: Prevalence of urinary incontinence and other urological symptoms in the non-institutionalized elderly. J Urol 1986; 136:1022–1025.

Diokno AC, Brown MB, Brock BM, et al: Clinical and cystometric characteristics of continent and incontinent noninstitutionalized elderly. J Urol 1988; 140:567–571.

Diokno AC, Brown MB, Herzog AR: Relationship between use of diuretics and continence status in the elderly. Urol 1991; 38:39–42.

Diokno AC, Wells TJ, Brink CA: Urinary incontinence in elderly women: Urodynamic evaluation. J Am Geriatr Soc 1987; 35:940–946.

Downie JW: Bethanechol chloride in urology—a discussion of issues. Neurourol Urodyn 1984; 3:211–222.

DuBeau CE, Resnick NM: Evaluation of the causes and severity of geriatric incontinence: A critical appraisal. Urol Clin North Am 1991; 18:243–256.

DuBeau CE, Resnick NM: Controversies in the diagnosis and management of benign prostatic hypertrophy. Adv Intern Med 1992; 37:55–83.

DuBeau CE, Resnick NM: Urinary incontinence and dementia: The perils of guilt by association. J Am Geriatr Soc 1995; 43:310–311.

DuBeau CE, Yalla SV, Resnick NM: Screening elderly men with voiding symptoms for outlet obstruction: Utility of urine flow rate. J Am Geriatr Soc 1993; 41:SA12.

DuBeau CE, Yalla SV, Resnick NM: Most bothersome symptom in men presenting prostatism: Implications for outcomes research. J Am Geriatr Soc 1995; 43:985–993.

Dyro FM, Yalla SV: Refractoriness of urethral striated sphincter during voiding: Studies with afferent pudendal reflex arc stimulation in male subjects. J Urol 1986; 135:732–736.

Eastwood HD, Smart CJ: Urinary incontinence in the disabled elderly male. Age Ageing 1985; 14:235–239.

Elbadawi A, Yalla SV, Hailemariam S, Resnick NM: Structural basis of geriatric voiding dysfunction. VI: Validation and update of diagnostic criteria in 71 detrusor biopsies. J Urol, in press.

Elbadawi A, Yalla SV, Resnick NM: Structural basis of geriatric voiding dysfunction. I: Methods of a correlative study, and overview of the findings. J Urol 1993a: 150:1650–1656.

Elbadawi A, Yalla SV, Resnick NM: Structural basis of geriatric voiding dysfunction. II: Aging detrusor: Normal vs. impaired contractility. J Urol 1993b; 150:1657–1667.

Elbadawi A, Yalla SV, Resnick NM: Structural basis of geriatric voiding dysfunction. III: Detrusor overactivity. J Urol 1993c; 150:1668–1680.

Engel BT, Burgio LD, McCormick KA: Behavioral treatment of incontinence in the long-term care setting. J Am Geriatr Soc 1990; 38:361–363.

Eriksen BC, Hagen B, Eik-Nes SH: Long-term effectiveness of the Burch colposuspension in female urinary stress incontinence. Acta Obstet Gynecol Scand 1990; 69:45–50.

Everett HC: The use of bethanechol chloride with tricyclic antidepressants. Am J Psychiat 1975; 132:1202–1204.

Fantl JA, Wyman JF, McClish DK: Efficacy of bladder training in older women with urinary incontinence. JAMA 1991; 265:609–613.

Fantl JA, Wyman JF, Wilson M, et al: Diuretics and urinary incontinence in community-dwelling women. Neurourol Urodyn 1990; 9:25–34.

Finkbeiner A: Is bethanechol chloride clinically effective in promoting bladder emptying? A literature review. J Urol 1985; 134:443–449.

Gormley EA, Griffiths DJ, McCracken PN, et al: Effect of transurethral resection of the prostate on detrusor instability and urge incontinence in elderly males. Neurourol Urodyn 1993; 12:445–453.

Gormley GJ, Stoner E, Bruskewitz RC, et al: The effect of finasteride in men with benign prostatic hyperplasia. N Engl J Med 1992; 327:1185–1191.

Griffith-Jones MD, Abrams PH: The Stamey endoscopic bladder neck suspension in the elderly. Br J Urol 1990; 65:170–172.

Hadley E: Bladder training and related therapies for urinary incontinence in older people. JAMA 1986; 256:372–379.

Hellstrom PM, Sjoqvist A: Involvement of opioid and nicotinic receptors in rectal and anal reflex inhibition of urinary bladder motility in cats. Acta Physiol Scand 1988; 133:559–562.

Herzog AR, Diokno AC, Fultz NH: Urinary incontinence: Medical and psychosocial aspects. Ann Rev Gerontol Geriatr 1989; 9:74–119.

Herzog AR, Fultz NH: Prevalence and incidence of urinary incontinence in community-dwelling populations. J Am Geriatr Soc 1990; 38:273–281.

Hilton P, Stanton SL: Algorithmic method for assessing urinary incontinence in elderly women. BMJ 1981; 282:940–942.

Hu T-W: Impact of urinary incontinence on health care costs. J Am Geriatr Soc 1990; 38:292–295.

Hu T-W, Igou JF, Kaltreider DL: A clinical trial of a behavioral therapy to reduce urinary incontinence in nursing homes. JAMA 1989; 261:2656–2662.

Hunt GM, Whitaker RH: A new device for self-catheterization in wheelchair-bound women. Br J Urol 1990; 66:162–163.

Jayachandran S, Moopan UMM, Kim H: Complications from external (condom) urinary drainage devices. Urology 1985; 25:31–34.

Jensen JK, Nielsen FR Jr, Ostergard DR: The role of patient history in the diagnosis of urinary incontinence. Obstet Gynecol 1994; 83:904–910.

Johnson DE, Muncie HL, O'Reilly JL, Warren JW: An external urine collection device for incontinent women. J Am Geriatr Soc 1990; 38:1016–1022.

Johnson ET: The condom catheter: Urinary tract infection and other complications. South Med J 1983; 76:579–582.

Kirkland JL, Lye M, Levy DW, Banerjee AK: Patterns of urine flow and electrolyte excretion in healthy elderly people. BMJ 1983; 287:1665–1667.

Klarskov P, Andersen JT, Asmussen CF, et al: Symptoms and signs predictive of the voiding pattern after acute urinary retention in men. Scand J Urol Nephrol 1987; 21:23–28.

Kong TK, Morris JA, Robinson JM, Brocklehurst JC: Predicting urodynamic dysfunction from clinical features in incontinent elderly women. Age Ageing 1990; 19:257–263.

Mathew TH, McEwen J, Rohan A: Urinary incontinence secondary to prazosin. Med J Aust 1988; 148:305–306.

McGuire EJ: Reflex urethral instability. Br J Urol 1978; 50:200–204.

McGuire EJ: Urinary Incontinence. New York: Grune & Stratton, 1981.

Nitti VW, Bregg KJ, Sussman EM, Raz S: The Raz bladder neck suspension in patients 65 years old and older. J Urol 1993; 149:802–807.

Norton PA, Baker JE: Postural changes can reduce leakage in women with stress urinary incontinence. Obstet Gynecol 1994; 84:770–774.

Ouslander JG, Colling J, the PURT study group: Use of simple urodynamic tests in nursing homes. Neurourol Urodyn 1992; 11:159–160.

Ouslander JG, Hepps K, Raz S, Su H-L: Genitourinary dysfunction in a geriatric outpatient population. J Am Geriatr Soc 1986; 34:507–514.

Ouslander JG, Schapira M, Schnelle JF, et al: Does eradicating bacteriuria affect the severity of chronic urinary incontinence in nursing home residents? Ann Intern Med 1995; 122:749–754.

Ouslander JG, Schnelle JF: Incontinence in the nursing home. Ann Intern Med 1995; 122:438–449.

Ouslander JG, Schnelle JF, Uman G, et al: Predictors of successful prompted voiding among incontinent nursing home residents. JAMA 1995; 273:1366–1370.

Pedersen PA, Johansen PB: Prophylactic treatment of adult nocturia with bumetanide. Br J Urol 1988; 62:145–147.

Raz R, Stamm WE: A controlled trial of intravaginal estriol in postmenopausal women with recurrent urinary tract infections. N Engl J Med 1993; 329:753–756.

Resnick NM: Voiding dysfunction in the elderly. *In* Yalla SV, McGuire EJ, Elbadawi A, Blaivas JG, eds: Neurourology and Urodynamics: Principles and Practice. New York, MacMillan Publishing Company, 1988, pp 303–330.

Resnick NM: Noninvasive diagnosis of the patient with complex incontinence. Gerontology 1990; 36(suppl. 2):8–18.

Resnick NM: Initial evaluation of the incontinent patient. J Am Geriatr Soc 1990; 38:311–316.

Resnick NM: Geriatric Medicine. *In* Isselbacher K, Braunwald E, Wilson JD, et al, eds: Harrison's Principles of Internal Medicine, 14th ed. McGraw-Hill, in press.

Resnick NM: Urinary incontinence. Lancet 1995; 346:94–99.

Resnick NM, Baumann M, Scott M, et al: Risk factors for incontinence in the nursing home: A multivariate study. Neurourol Urodyn 1988; 7:274–276.

Resnick NM, Baumann MM: Urinary incontinence and indwelling catheter. *In* Morris JN, Hawes C, eds: Minimum Data Set Training Manual and Resource Guide. Natick, Mass, Eliot Press, 1991, pp F24–F31.

Resnick NM, Baumann MM: Urinary Incontinence. *In* Morris JN, Lipsitz LA, eds: Quality Care for the Nursing Home Resident. St Louis: C. V. Mosby Company, in press.

Resnick NM, Brandeis GH, Baumann MM, et al: Misdiagnosis of urinary incontinence in nursing home women: Prevalence and a proposed solution. Neurourol Urodyn, in press-a.

Resnick NM, Brandeis GH, Baumann MM, Morris JN: A national assessment strategy for urinary incontinence in nursing home residents: Reliability and validity of the Minimum Data Set and Resident Assessment Protocol. Neurourol Urodyn, in press-b.

Resnick NM, Elbadawi A, Yalla SV: Age and the lower urinary tract: What is normal? Neurourol Urodyn 1995; 14:577–579.

Resnick NM, Ouslander JG, eds: National Institutes of Health Consensus Development Conference on Urinary Incontinence. J Am Geriatr Soc 1990; 38:263–386.

Resnick NM, Scherr PA, Wetle T, et al: Urinary incontinence and urgency among older persons in a geographically-defined community. Unpublished.

Resnick NM, Yalla SV: Detrusor hyperactivity with impaired contractile function. An unrecognized but common cause of incontinence in elderly patients. JAMA 1987; 257:3076–3081.

Resnick NM, Yalla SV, Laurino E: Feasibility, safety and reproducibility of urodynamics in the elderly. (Abstract.) J Urol 1987; 137:189A.

Resnick NM, Yalla SV, Laurino E: The pathophysiology and clinical correlates of established urinary incontinence in frail elderly. N Engl J Med 1989; 320:1–7.

Robinson JM: Evaluation of methods for assessment of bladder and urethral function. *In* Brocklehurst JC, ed: Urology in the Elderly. New York, Churchill Livingstone, 1984, pp 19–54.

Schnelle JF: Treatment of urinary incontinence in nursing home patients by prompted voiding. J Am Geriatr Soc 1990; 38:356–360.

Seiler WO, Stähelin HB, Hefti U: Desmopressin reduces night urine volume in geriatric patients: Implication for treatment of the nocturnal incontinence. Clin Investig 1992; 70:619.

Semmens JP, Tsai CC, Semmens EC, Loadholt CB: Effects of estrogen therapy on vaginal physiology during menopause. Obstet Gynecol 1985; 66:15–18.

Skelly J, Flint AJ: Urinary incontinence associated with dementia. J Am Geriatr Soc 1995; 43:286–294.

Snow TL: Equipment for prevention, treatment, and management of urinary incontinence. Top Geriatr Rehab 1988; 3:58–77.

Stead WW: Tuberculosis as an endemic and nosocomial infection among the elderly in nursing homes. N Engl J Med 1985; 312:1483–1487.

Suarez GM, Baum NH, Jacobs J: Use of standard contraceptive diaphragm in management of stress urinary incontinence. Urology 1991; 37:119–122.

Urinary Incontinence Guideline Panel: Urinary Incontinence in Adults: Clinical Practice Guideline, No. 2, 1996 Update. AHCPR Publication No. 96-0682. Rockville, Md, Agency for Health Care Policy and Research, Public Health Service, US Department of Health and Human Services, 1996.

Warren JW: Urine collection devices for use in adults with urinary incontinence. J Am Geriatr Soc 1990; 38:364–367.

Warren JW, Muncie HL, Hebel JR, Hall-Craggs M: Long-term urethral catheterization increases risk of chronic pyelonephritis and renal inflammation. J Am Geriatr Soc 1994; 42:1286–1290.

Wells TJ: Pelvic (floor) muscle exercises. J Am Geriatr Soc 1990; 38:333–337.

Wells TJ, Brink CA, Diokno AC, et al: Pelvic muscle exercise for stress urinary incontinence in elderly women. J Am Geriatr Soc 1991; 39:785–791.

Wetle TT, Scherr P, Branch LG, et al: Difficulty with holding urine among older persons in a geographically-defined community: Prevalence and correlates. J Am Geriatr Soc 1995; 43:349–355.

Wyman JF, Harkins SW, Fantl JA: Psychosocial impact of urinary incontinence in the community-dwelling population. J Am Geriatr Soc 1990; 38:282–288.

Zeitlin MP, Lebherz TB: Pessaries in the geriatric patient. J Am Geriatr Soc 1992; 40:635–639.

32 VAGINAL RECONSTRUCTIVE SURGERY FOR INCONTINENCE AND PROLAPSE

Shlomo Raz, M.D.
Lynn Stothers, M.D.
Ashok Chopra, M.D.

The objective of surgery to treat the clinical entities of stress urinary incontinence and prolapse is to restore coordinated support to all of the pelvic organs. To achieve this goal, a precise understanding of the anatomy of the female pelvis that results in functional unity of the pelvic floor is required. In the discussion that follows, surgical anatomy is described: the fascial and ligamentous structures that the urologist must identify, isolate, and make use of in reconstruction. Specific surgical techniques to treat the clinical manifestations that result from loss of coordinated pelvic support—namely, stress urinary incontinence and pelvic prolapse—are then reviewed. Finally, potential complications related to vaginal pelvic reconstructive surgery are discussed.

ANATOMY OF PELVIC SUPPORT

The maintenance of continence and the prevention of female pelvic prolapse rely on a precise anatomic relationship of all the pelvic organs. As such, the bony pelvis provides a framework from which the supporting elements in the pelvis are derived, and upon which all pelvic structures ultimately depend. Although many radiologic techniques and **anatomic diagrams depict pelvic anatomy in two dimensions, it is the three-dimensional relationships in space that allow each of the component parts to work individually and in concert, producing the integrated behaviors of pelvic support and continence.** Failure of one of the components of this delicate balance does not invariably produce stress incontinence or prolapse because of compensatory effects of the other components. This balance may explain the phenomenon whereby many patients with urethral and bladder prolapse can be totally asymptomatic and only a small percentage have stress urinary incontinence. Likewise, surgical procedures to repair stress urinary incontinence may result in pelvic prolapse. For example, Wiskind and colleagues found 26.7% of patients developed genital prolapse requiring corrective surgery following colposuspension (Wiskind et al, 1992). Therefore, the successful surgical treatment of pelvic disorders requires the clinician to consider all the pelvic organs and their interdependent anatomic relationships.

Pelvic Diaphragm, Levator Muscle, and Levator Fascia

The bony pelvis is the scaffolding from which the pelvic diaphragm and perineal musculature arise, providing a floor of support on which the pelvic organs rest. The pelvic diaphragm is divided into the levator ani and coccygeus muscles. **The levator ani with its component parts, the pubococcygeus, iliococcygeus, and ischiococcygeus muscles, can be viewed as the major inferior support of the urethra, vagina, and rectum.** The proximal half of the vagina lies horizontally over the levator plate (Fig. 32–1).

The levator ani muscle is depicted in anatomy texts as a broad thin sheet that takes rise from bony structures in the pelvis as well as tendinous condensations. Anteriorly the levator ani arises from the pubic bone lateral to the symphysis pubis. Posteriorly, it arises from the inner surface of the ischial spine. Between these points, the levator ani originates from the "arcuate line," which is a condensation of the obturator fascia (the tendinous arc). **When viewed from above, looking down into the retropubic space, the fascial thickening of the tendinous arc can be seen extending on either side of the pelvic floor from the posterior-inferior pubic ramus to the ischial spines** (Fig. 32–2). The tendinous arc is an important anatomic support in the pelvis because it forms the common insertion point for the obturator internus and levator ani musculature. Although anatomic drawings reveal that the levator muscle has a continuous insertion along the tendinous arc, three-dimensional magnetic resonance imaging (MRI) has shown that the insertion

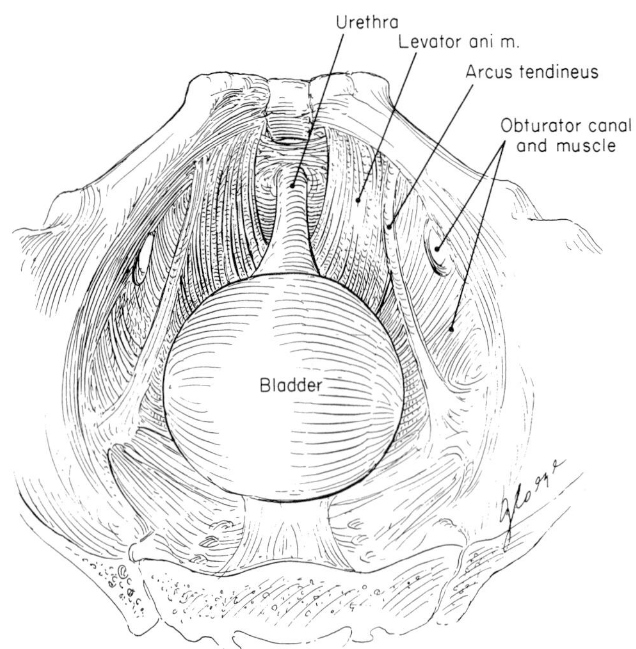

Figure 32–2. Abdominal view of the levator ani and the tendinous arc. Note the relationship of the bladder and urethra to the levator muscle. As viewed from inside the pelvis, the levator ani muscle has a hammock shape. Note that the levator has insertion points onto both the right and the left sides of the symphysis pubis anterior to the urethra. Clinical correlate: This area of the levator is incorporated into the most anterior sutures of the anterior vaginal wall sling.

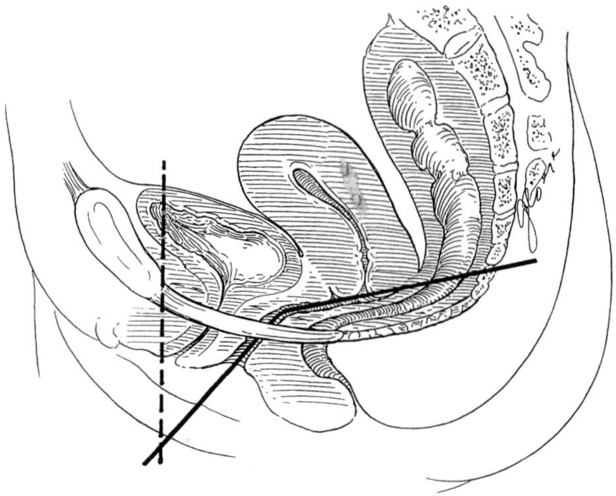

Figure 32–1. The anatomy of the female pelvic diaphragm is shown in sagittal view with the patient in the standing position. The pelvic floor is shown extending between the symphysis pubis to the sacrum. In its anterior portion, it is composed of the levator fascia, whereas in its posterior aspect, it is made up of the levator muscular plate. The proximal half of the vagina rests almost horizontally over the levator plate, forming a posterior angle of approximately 110 degrees with the distal half of the vagina. The distal half of the vaginal canal has an angle of inclination of approximately 45 degrees with the vertical axis (shown by the dotted line).

may be fenestrated (Stothers and Raz, 1995) (Fig. 32–3). The clinical implication of this finding is not yet known but is hypothesized to be a potential source of inherent weakness in the pelvic floor in some patients.

From the tendinous arc, fibers of the levator muscle extend posteriorly and inferiorly to unite with fibers from the opposite side, creating the shape of a hammock. In its anterior portion, the hammock of the levator muscle forms a U-shaped hiatus and is referred to as the **pubococcygeus muscle**. It is through this hiatus where the vagina, rectum, and urethra exit the pelvis. The pubococcygeus muscle sends a number of muscle fibers into this U-shaped hiatus. Around the urethra, they form its external sphincter. More inferiorly, the fibers fuse anterior to the rectum, forming part of the perineal support deep to the perineal body. The U-shaped pubococcygeus muscle has been referred to by some authors as the "pubovisceral" muscle (Lawson, 1974). This portion of the levator muscle can be appreciated during physical examination of the pelvis as a bulky muscular ridge on both the right and the left lateral sidewalls of the vagina superior to the hymen. With contraction, the pubovisceral muscle elevates the rectum, vagina, and urethra anteriorly and aids in compression of their associated lumens. The **iliococcygeus** portion of the levator muscle arises from the tendinous arc as a broad, thin sheet whose fibers unite in the median raphe posterior to the rectum. More posteriorly, the iliococcygeus borders with the sacrospinous ligament and the coccygeal muscle. Microscopically the levator muscle contains both type I and type II (fast-twitch) fibers compared with the fibers forming the external urethral sphincter, which contain only type I (slow-twitch) fibers. The anatomic loca-

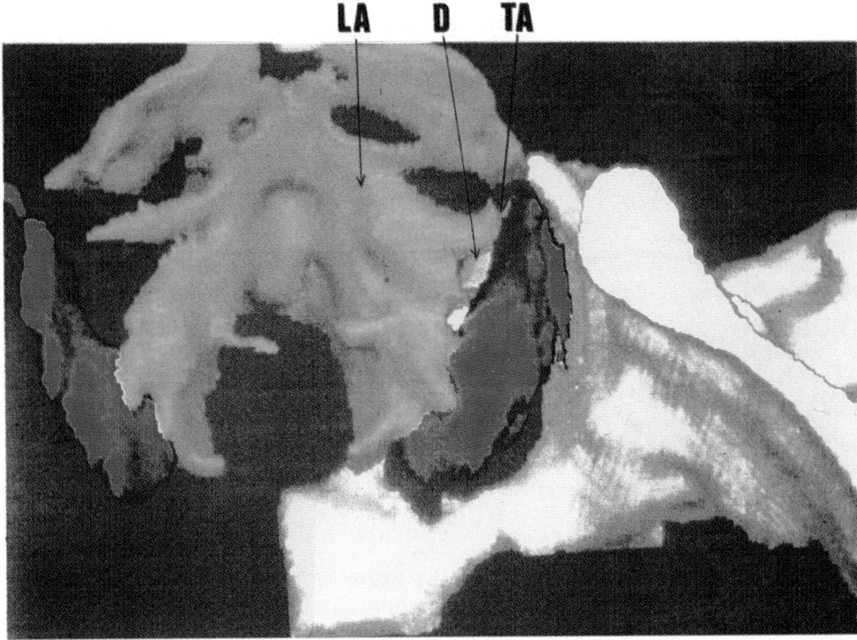

Figure 32–3. Three-dimensional magnetic resonance image of the levator ani muscle (LA) as viewed from inside the female pelvis. The symphysis pubis and the bony pelvis are shown in relationship to the levator ani and obturator internus muscles on the right. Note the fenestrated insertion of the levator ani along the tendinous arc (TA) resulting in defects (D).

tion of the levator along with its fast-twitch fibers suggests that functionally the levator may actively assist in urethral closure at times of increased abdominal pressure (Gosling et al, 1981).

Textbooks of anatomy and cadaver dissection agree that there is a strong broad lining of fascia inside the pelvis that covers the pelvic organs. This fascia is commonly referred to as the endopelvic fascia (Fig. 32–4). The authors describe the endopelvic fascia as only one component of the levator fascia. The name *endopelvic* implies that this fascia exists only on the inside of the pelvis. Enhanced MRI with the use of rectal and vaginal coils, however, demonstrates that the levator fascia has an important extrapelvic component (Stothers and Raz, 1995). The extrapelvic component is not seen from inside the abdomen and covers the vaginal side of the bladder and urethra. The vaginal side of the levator fascia and the abdominal side come together laterally in the pelvis, similar to two leaves, which fuse together attaching the urethra, bladder, and vagina to the tendinous arc. Therefore, **the levator fascia is a single structure, with two component parts, an intrapelvic (abdominal) leaf and an extrapelvic (vaginal) leaf, which come together laterally, fusing into a common insertion along the tendinous arc** (Fig. 32–5). The abdominal leaf is known as the endopelvic fascia. The vaginal leaf is known as the periurethral fascia at the level of the urethra and as the perivesical fascia at the level of the bladder base. **Contained within the two sides or leaves of the levator fascia are the pelvic organs to which it provides support: the urethra, bladder, vagina, and uterus**.

Specialized **regions of condensation occur in the levator fascia forming critical ligamentous supports to maintain the relationships between the urethra, bladder, vagina, and uterus within the bony pelvis.** The names given to the different areas of specialization are only a matter of location, and it should be emphasized that all are components or regions of the larger levator fascia. Surgically, however, they are described as separate structures to make use of them during surgical reconstruction of the female pelvis with stress incontinence and/or prolapse.

A frequent point of confusion revolves around the concept of the difference between the levator *musculature*

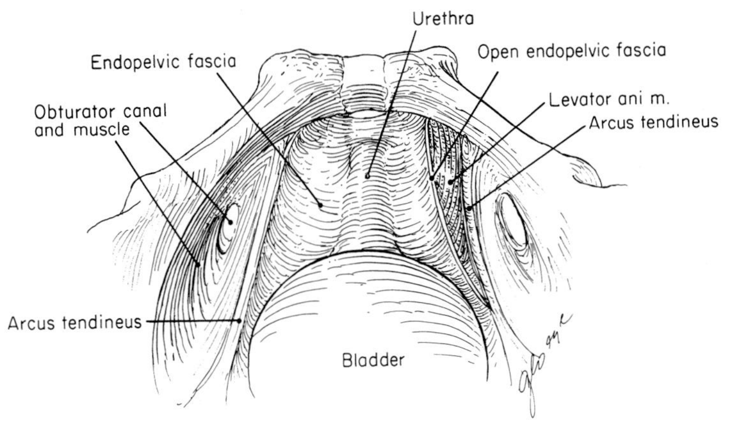

Figure 32–4. A view of the inside of the pelvis showing the pelvic viscera covered by the intrapelvic component of the levator fascia, referred to as the endopelvic fascia. The extrapelvic component of the levator fascia cannot be seen from inside the pelvis. The endopelvic fascia is opened on the right side, revealing the levator ani muscle.

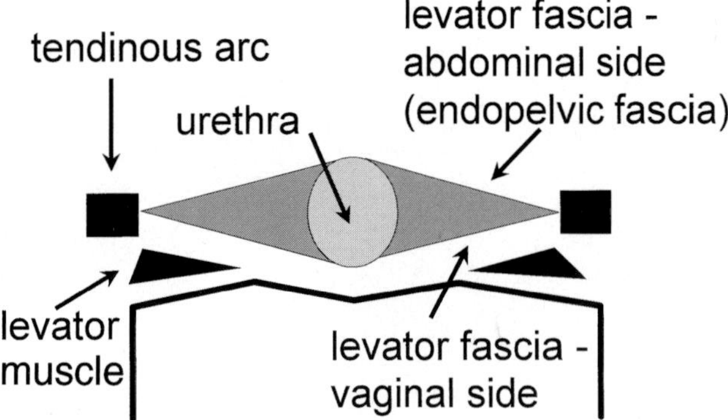

Figure 32–5. The levator fascia has two components: an abdominal side (the endopelvic fascia) and a vaginal side. The vaginal side of the levator fascia is referred to as the periurethral fascia at the level of the urethra and bladder neck. At the level of the bladder base, the vaginal side of the levator fascia is referred to as the perivesical fascia.

and the levator ***fascia.*** Figure 32–6 shows the levator muscle in a three-dimensional MRI reconstruction of a female patient with pelvic relaxation and stress incontinence. This view is taken during a relaxed state with the patient in lithotomy position. The wide separation of the levator musculature underneath the pubis can be noted. Anteriorly the levator joins in the midline, beneath the symphysis at the level of the midurethra, and has insertion points on the inferior ramus of the pubis. The levator also comes together in the perineum at the level of the central tendon. A large hiatus in the muscle exists between these two points. **In the hiatus between the extensions of the levator musculature is the levator fascia. The levator fascia has four specialized condensations that are used during surgical reconstruction of the female pelvis: the pubourethral ligaments, the urethropelvic ligaments, the vesicopelvic fascia, and the cardinal ligaments.** The levator fascia, and not the levator musculature itself, provides support to the bladder neck and urethra, maintaining their position during times of increased abdominal pressure.

Pubourethral Ligament

The pubourethral ligament is a specialized condensation of the levator fascia that anchors the urethra to the inferior ramus of the symphysis pubis. It is the female equivalent of the puboprostatic ligaments in the male. The ligament is dense and triangular-shaped, arising from a relatively narrow origin on the inferior ramus of the symphysis, fanning out to a broader attachment on the urethra itself. Microscopically the pubourethral ligament is composed of dense connective tissue with scattered smooth muscle bundles associated with cholinergic autonomic nerve endings (Wilson et al, 1983).

The point of attachment of the pubourethral ligament to the urethra results in a functional division of the urethra into three areas. The point at which the pubourethral ligament attaches to the urethra identifies this area as the **midurethra.** The region of the midurethra occupies approximately 40% of the total urethral length and is associated not only with the pubourethral ligament but also with the striated urethral sphincter muscle and the urethropelvic ligaments (DeLancey, 1986). The urethra proximal to this is referred to on urodynamic fluoroscopy as the area of the bladder neck and **proximal urethra**. The proximal urethra is visualized during retropubic surgery and occupies 20% of the total urethral length (DeLancey, 1986). The remaining 40% of the urethral length distal to the midurethra is seen during vaginal surgical approaches. The paraurethral structures adjacent to the **distal urethra** include the region of the urogenital diaphragm and the bulbocavernosus muscle (DeLancey, 1986). It is important to remember that when performing retropubic surgery, only the proximal third of the urethra is seen. Although the pubourethral ligament does not provide support to the bladder neck, it does stabilize and support the midurethral area. **Weakness of the pubourethral ligament permits posterior and inferior movement of the midurethra with increases in intra-abdominal pressure**. The pubourethral ligament is divided from a vaginal approach during some surgical techniques to correct urinary retention: allowing for urethrolysis in the retropubic space. The skeletal muscle fibers of the external urethral sphincter are found just distal to the pubourethral ligament.

Urethropelvic Ligaments

The urethropelvic ligaments are composed of the regions of the levator fascia that attach and support the urethra and bladder neck to the tendinous arc. The urethropelvic ligaments have two component leaves—an abdominal leaf of endopelvic fascia and a vaginal leaf of periurethral fascia—which envelop the urethra and support and attach it to the tendinous arcs on both sides of the pelvis. This anatomic arrangement anchors the urethra and bladder neck to the inner pelvis, providing elastic support at times of increased abdominal pressure. **Weakness of the urethropelvic ligament is present in patients with anatomic stress urinary incontinence**.

The urethropelvic ligament is an anatomic and a surgical structure; it can be dissected, isolated, detached, and exposed; it can be found to be weak or strong, detached or firmly attached to the tendinous arc. The urethropelvic ligaments can be exposed surgically from either an abdominal or a vaginal approach. Whether viewed from above in the pelvis or below from the perineum, the urethropelvic ligament is one anatomic structure that can be visualized surgically and seen on MRI (Fig. 32–7). The urethropelvic ligament can be partially detached from its insertion point onto the tendinous arc. This is done during vaginal approaches to isolate the urethropelvic ligament for the correction of stress urinary incontinence because of its **major role in the support of the bladder neck and proximal urethra.**

Vesicopelvic Fascia

The vesicopelvic fascia is the region of the levator fascia that attaches and supports the bladder base to the tendinous arc and the pelvic sidewall (Fig. 32–8). Similar to the urethropelvic ligaments, the vesicopelvic fascia has **two sides or leaves,** which envelop the bladder and provide lateral support within the pelvis to the bladder base. **The abdominal side (endopelvic fascia) and the vaginal side**

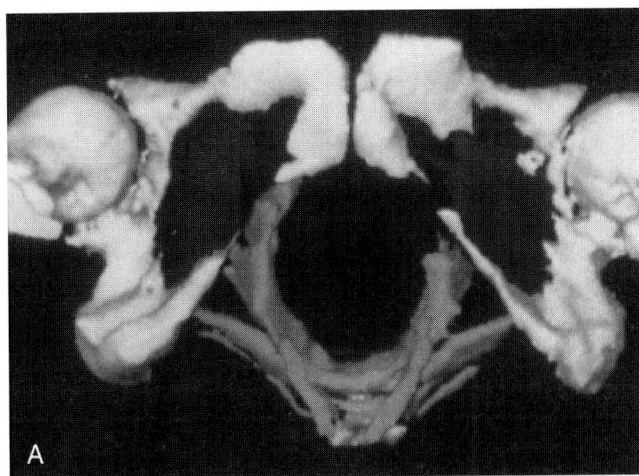

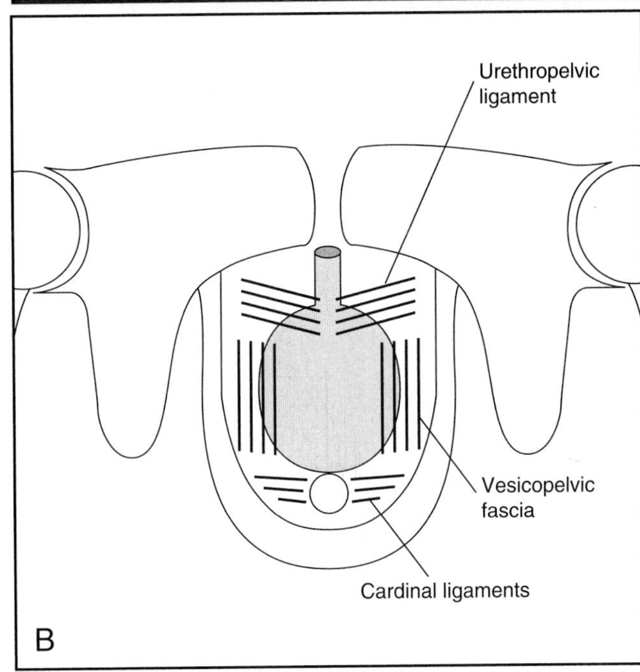

Figure 32–6. *A,* three-dimensional magnetic resonance scan in a patient with pelvic prolapse and stress urinary incontinence. The patient is in lithotomy position. The pelvic bones and femoral heads are seen laterally with the symphysis pubis anterior. The obturator musculature is shown filling the obturator foramen on both sides of the pelvis. The complex shape of the *levator ani musculature* is seen originating anteriorly and extends posteriorly, forming the shape of a hammock. There is a widened hiatus in the hammock of the levator muscle between which the regions of the levator fascia are found. *B,* Diagrammatic representation of *A* showing the regions of the levator fascia found within the hiatus of the levator muscle.

(perivesical fascia) come together to insert into the tendinous arc.

The term *pubocervical fascia* used in medical texts is equivalent to the terms *periurethral* and *perivesical fascia.* As such, the pubocervical fascia describes only the vaginal leaf of the levator fascia. The term *pubocervical fascia* can be confusing because it signifies different anatomic structures to different surgeons. As its name implies, the pubocervical fascia is so named because the vaginal leaf of the levator fascia extends between the pubis symphysis posteriorly to its insertion onto the cervix.

Vesicopelvic fascial defects result in cystocele formation. Comparing video-urodynamic studies with dynamic MRI in patients with significant cystocele, two defects in the vesicopelvic fascia can be found. These defects are known as **central and lateral defects**. The central portion of the vesicopelvic fascia, in the region of the midline overlying the bladder base, is lax in patients with a central vesicopelvic fascial defect (Richardson et al, 1981). In others, a purely lateral descent of the tendinous arc in the area of the vesicopelvic fascia is seen resulting in a sliding hernia of the bladder base and vesicopelvic fascia. When defects in the vesicopelvic fascia exist, whether central or lateral, hypermobility of the urethropelvic ligaments may also be seen. **The most common clinical observation is that of a combined lateral and central defect with lateral descent of the tendinous arc together with relaxation of the central region in the area of the bladder base.**

Cardinal Ligaments

The cardinal ligaments are the most posterior condensation of the levator fascia (Fig. 32–9). They are not totally separate structures; rather, they are continuous with the vesicopelvic fascia. MRI reveals that the cardinal ligaments come together in the midline in their area of reflection onto the lateral aspects of the cervix. The cardinal ligaments extend from the uterine isthmus to the lateral pelvic wall. They are thick and triangular and contain the uterine arteries.

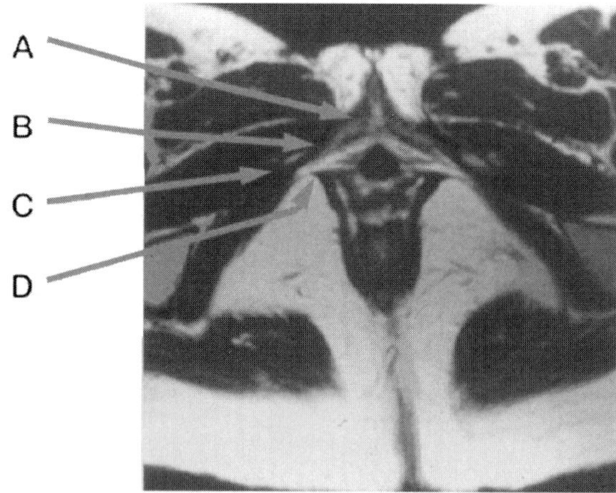

Figure 32–7. Transverse magnetic resonance scan of the female pelvis showing the urethropelvic ligament. The region of the midurethra is seen. The area just superior to the pubourethral ligament is seen (A). The two leaves of the urethropelvic ligament (vaginal side B and the abdominal side D) come together to insert into the tendinous arc labeled C.

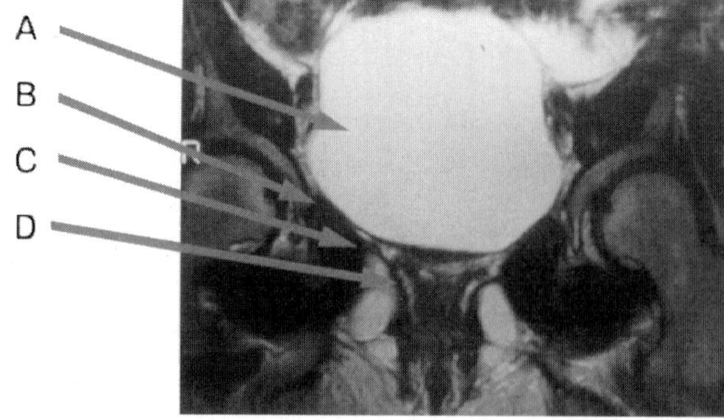

Figure 32–8. Magnetic resonance imaging of the female pelvis in the coronal plane reflecting the standing position. The bladder, *A,* is supported by the vesicopelvic fascia, *B,* which can be seen inserting into the tendinous arc, *C.* The periurethral fascia, *D,* is seen adjacent to the urethra. Note the closed bladder neck and the absence of contrast within the urethral lumen.

Posteriorly, they are fused with the sacrouterine ligaments. The anterior extensions of the cardinal ligaments fuse as previously described with the vesicopelvic fascia.

The cardinal ligaments and sacrouterine complex are not important for continence per se, but they do play a role in the support of the bladder base and vaginal apex and the pathophysiology of cystocele. **Surgically the cardinal ligaments form the base of the rectangle of levator fascia responsible for bladder support (urethropelvic ligaments, vesicopelvic fascia, and cardinal ligaments)** (Fig. 32–10). During vaginal hysterectomy, the cardinal ligaments can be demonstrated surgically when they are separated from their cervical attachment. **Weakness or separation of the cardinal and sacrouterine ligaments leads to the clinical correlate of cystocele,** and their reapproximation is necessary for adequate surgical correction of grade 4 cystocele. Weakness when the uterus is in place may result in **uterine hypermobility and uterine prolapse,** whereas separation after hysterectomy results in **enterocele** formation.

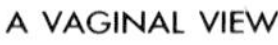

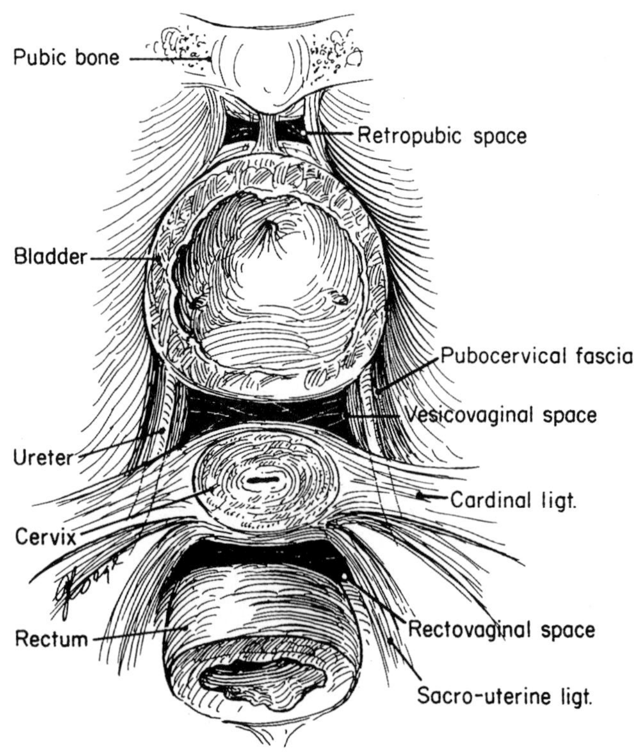

Figure 32–9. The cardinal and sacrouterine ligaments provide support to the cervix and indirectly to the bladder base. The retropubic, vesicovaginal, and rectovaginal spaces are seen at the level of the cervix. (From Raz S: Atlas of Transvaginal Surgery, Philadelphia, W. B. Saunders Company, 1992.)

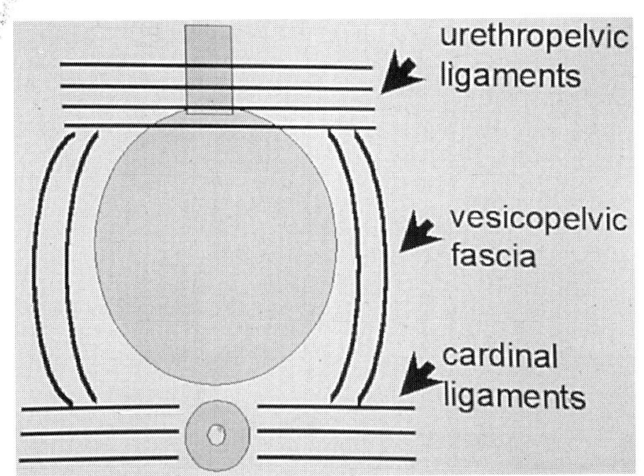

Figure 32–10. The urethropelvic ligaments, vesicopelvic fascia, and cardinal ligaments support the bladder and bladder neck, forming a rectangle of support in a patient without cystocele.

Posterior Vaginal Support

A complex fascial and muscular arrangement provides support to the vagina, rectum, perineum, and anal sphincter (Fig. 32–11). **Two levels of muscular support** can be identified: (1) the pelvic floor (**levator musculature**, particularly its pubococcygeus portion) and (2) the **urogenital diaphragm** (bulbocavernosus, superficial and deep transverse perineal muscles, external anal sphincter, and central perineal tendon).

In the normally supported patient in the erect position, the proximal two thirds of the vagina is 110 degrees from horizontal, compared with the distal third, which is 45 degrees compared with a vertical line (see Fig. 32–1). The transition from the proximal to distal half occurs at the point where the vagina crosses the pelvic floor, reflecting the degree of support of the levator musculature and the urogenital diaphragm. As such, the proximal half of the vagina is practically in a horizontal plane, resting over the levator plate. Vaginal support is derived from the cardinal ligaments and tendinous arc in the proximal and midthird, respectively. The distal third of the vagina is intimately related to the levator muscles and perineal body (DeLancey, 1992).

When **pelvic floor relaxation** occurs, the normal proximal and distal orientation of the vagina in the standing position are lost (Fig. 32–12). The **levator plate relaxes and becomes convex instead of horizontal, the levator hiatus enlarges, and the normal proximal vaginal orientation disappears. The distal half of the vagina is no longer 45 degrees from the vertical.** The vagina is now relaxed downward and posteriorly and is no longer in a high supported horizontal position. Herniation of the rectum may ensue.

In a patient with damage to the second level of muscular support (the perineal or urogenital diaphragm), the vaginal introitus is wider, and the distance between the urethra and posterior fourchette is greater. Different degrees of perineal tear may be seen: minimal, when only a small separation of the perineum occurs; to a severe degree, when the perineal structures have disappeared and the vaginal wall reaches the anterior rectal wall. Surgical reconstruction of the posterior vaginal wall should (1) correct rectocele formation by reinforcement of the attenuated prerectal and pararectal fasciae, (2) repair the defect of the levator muscles by narrowing the size of the levator hiatus, providing a horizontal support for the proximal half of the vagina, and (3) repair the urogenital diaphragm (perineal musculature), providing a normal introital size and improved vaginal support.

Vaginal Dome and Uterine Support

The most important supporting structures of the uterus are the **sacrouterine, broad, and cardinal ligaments** (previously described). The sacrouterine ligaments are posteriorly located and run from the cervix to either side of the sacrum. At the level of the cervix, they fuse with the posterior aspect of the cardinal ligaments. The broad ligaments

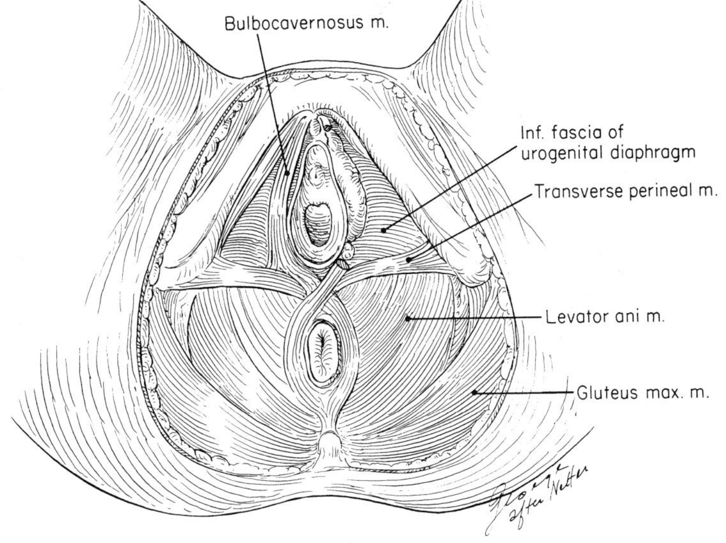

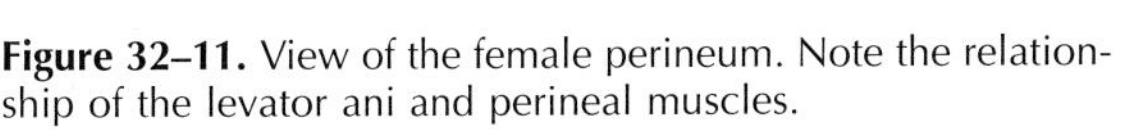
Figure 32–11. View of the female perineum. Note the relationship of the levator ani and perineal muscles.

are two superiorly located folds of peritoneum attaching the lateral walls of the uterus to the lateral pelvic wall. They contain the fallopian tubes, round ligaments, ovarian ligaments, and ovarian vessels.

DeLancey (1993) has identified **three biomechanical principles that contribute to support of the uterus and vagina in the normal female pelvis, preventing genital prolapse.** The first contributing factor is the support given to the uterus by the condensations of the levator fascia as previously described. A second support is provided by the levator ani musculature, which constricts the lumen of vagina, maintaining a closed lumen on which the pelvic organs rest. The compressed vaginal lumen is easily appreciated on MRI images of the pelvis in which the vagina has a characteristic H shape in cross section. Finally, a third form of support, referred to as a flap valve, results from the coordinated action of the first two factors. The supported and closed walls of the vaginal lumen compress against each other during times of increased abdominal pressure, thereby pinning the vagina in place against the pelvic floor.

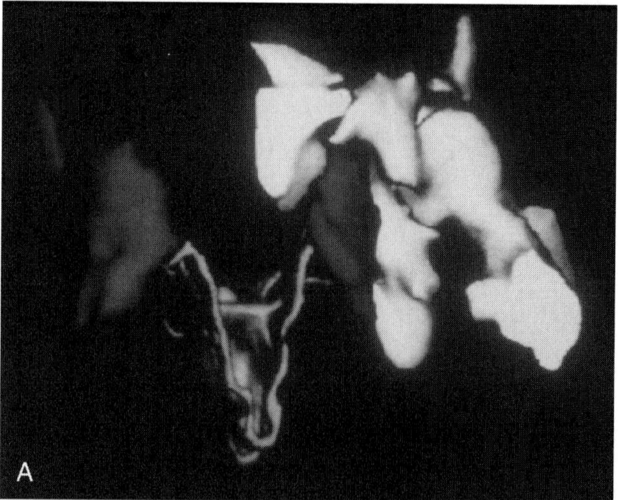

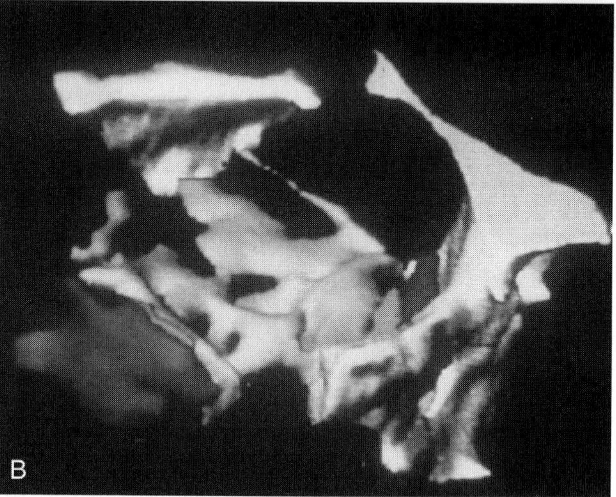

Figure 32–12. An anterior view of the pelvis in a patient with pelvic floor relaxation *(A)* compared with the normal, slightly concave pelvic floor seen in *(B)*.

VAGINAL SURGERY FOR STRESS INCONTINENCE

Preoperative Considerations

The presence of pelvic floor relaxation and symptoms of stress urinary incontinence alone is not enough to warrant surgical therapy. Urinary incontinence may limit daily activities (Stothers and Raz, 1996), cause social isolation (Fonda et al, 1995), or cause financial hardship (Ekelund et al, 1993) and negatively affect the psychologic well-being of the patient (Diokno, 1995). **Surgery for stress incontinence is indicated in motivated patients with significant loss of urine, creating a social or hygienic problem.** Once a decision for surgical management is made, three factors must be considered to plan a comprehensive pelvic reconstruction: **(1) type and severity of stress incontinence; (2) degree of associated cystocele; and (3) presence of other pelvic floor abnormalities, such as enterocele, uterine hypermobility, and rectocele** that must be corrected at the time of stress incontinence surgery. Despite technical differences in the various vaginal techniques, all share common surgical goals depending on the type of stress urinary incontinence. **With anatomic incontinence,** hypermobility of the midurethral segment and bladder neck exists, and **the goal of surgery is to reposition the bladder neck and urethra in a supported retropubic position. When intrinsic sphincter dysfunction is diagnosed, the goal of surgery is to provide increased urethral resistance by improving urethral coaptation and compression.** When interpreting the success rate of any particular operation for stress urinary incontinence, a successful outcome should be based on the ability of the treatment to have a positive impact on the patient's quality of life.

Measuring Outcomes Before and After Treatment of Stress Incontinence

Outcomes research is the branch of clinical epidemiology that measures the effectiveness of treatment interventions through a broad range of outcomes focusing on patient-centered and societal-centered concerns. This represents an expanded viewpoint of measuring the success of treatment and includes the patient's physical, social, and emotional functioning; patient satisfaction and expectations; quality of life; and cost-effectiveness and benefit resulting from a cure or improvement in urinary incontinence. Numerous tools to measure and scale outcomes such as quality of life and patient satisfaction have been developed and are reported in the literature. Before implementation, each questionnaire should undergo a sophisticated process to establish its reliability and validity. A discussion of this is beyond the scope of this chapter, but numerous excellent references are available (Woodward and Chambers, 1981; McDowell and Newell, 1987; Sackett et al, 1991).

An example of a scoring system that aims to quantify traditional outcomes of stress incontinence surgery in addition to quality of life is provided by the SEAPI incontinence classification system (Raz and Erickson, 1992). The system is analogous to the TNM system for tumor staging, and each aspect of the score is graded between 0 and 3. Zero indicates no symptom, problem, or abnormality, and 1, 2, and 3 indicate correspondingly increasing symptoms. When applicable, the practitioner can assign both a subjective and an objective score to a given patient. Five domains are covered by the SEAPI score and are represented in the score name: *S* for stress activity–related incontinence, *E* for emptying ability, *A* for anatomy, *P* for protection, and *I* for inhibition (Table 32–1). In addition to a pretreatment and post-treatment SEAPI score, the authors use the SEAPI quality of life score, which has been validated in patients with stress incontinence (Raz et al, 1996b; Stothers and Raz, 1996). The self-administered quality of life score covers numerous domains, including emotional well-being, interpersonal relationships, work, financial factors, physical health, recreation, and overall satisfaction with life, all as they relate to incontinence. Other modified validated quality of life scales that are specific to women with incontinence include the Urogenital Distress Inventory and the Incontinence Impact Questionnaire (Schumaker et al, 1994; Wyman et al, 1987).

Table 32–1. SEAPI STAGING SYSTEM

Subjective According to Patient Historical Factors	
S Stress-related leakage	0 = No urine loss
	1 = Loss with strenuous activity
	2 = Loss with moderate activity
	3 = Loss with minimal activity, or gravitational incontinence
E Emptying ability	0 = No obstructive symptoms
	1 = Minimal symptoms
	2 = Significant symptoms
	3 = Voiding only in dribbles or urinary retention
A Anatomy	0 = No descent during strain
	1 = Descent, not to introitus
	2 = Descent through introitus with strain
	3 = Through introitus without strain
P Protection	0 = Never used
	1 = Used only for certain occasions
	2 = Used daily for occasional accidents
	3 = Used continually for frequent accidents or constant leaking
I Inhibition	0 = No urgency incontinence
	1 = Rare urgency incontinence
	2 = Urgency incontinence once a week
	3 = Urgency incontinence at least once a day
Objective Based on Physical Examination Findings and Urodynamic Parameters	
S Stress-related leakage	Observe for leak during Valsalva and cough
	0 = No leak
	1 = Leak at >80 cm H_2O
	2 = Leak at 30–80 cm H_2O
	3 = Leak at <30 cm H_2O
E Emptying ability	Postvoid residual should be verified by repeat measurement
	0 = 0–60 ml
	1 = 61–100 ml
	2 = 101–200 ml
	3 = >200 ml or unable to void
A Anatomy	Position of bladder neck relative to symphysis during cough or Valsalva seen on lateral cystogram
	0 = Above symphysis with strain
	1 = <2 cm below symphysis with strain
	2 = >2 cm below symphysis with strain
	3 = >2 cm below symphysis at rest
P Protection	0 = Never used
	1 = Used only for certain occasions
	2 = Used daily for occasional accidents
	3 = Used continually for frequent accidents or constant leaking
I Inhibition	Involuntary rise in pressure during cystometry
	0 = No pressure rise
	1 = Rise late in filling (>500 ml)
	2 = Medium fill rise (150–500 ml)
	3 = Early rise (<150 ml)

From Raz S, Eriksen D: SEAPI Incontinence Classification System. Neurol Urodynam 1992; 11:187.

Table 32–2. DIAGNOSTIC MEASURES USED IN THE ASSESSMENT OF STRESS URINARY INCONTINENCE

International Continence Society Pad Test
Administration of phenazopyridine hydrochloride
Voiding diary
Valsalva leak point pressure
Marshall's test
Voiding cystourethrogram
Multichannel videourodynamics

Various other methods of measuring outcomes of stress incontinence therapies reported in the literature are shown in Table 32–2. Further guidelines and definitions of outcomes relating to incontinence are provided by the International Continence Society (International Continence Society Committee, 1992; Proceedings of the International Continence Society, 1994). The Pyridium pad test as described by the International Continence Society and quantitative weighing of pads to detect urinary leakage have been compared by Wall and colleagues (1990) and Victor (1990). Wall and colleagues studied 23 normal volunteers without stress urinary incontinence, comparing them with 18 women with urodynamically proven stress incontinence, using the pad test. The authors found that in the group with stress incontinence, all 18 had positive Pyridium pad tests and positive pad weight gains of greater than 1.0 g. However, 52% of healthy volunteers had a positive Pyridium pad test. The mean pad weight gain in the volunteer group was 0.1 g. Therefore, the Pyridium pad test had a high false-positive rate in continent volunteers and would be misleading as an outcome measure if pad weighing tests were not performed.

Surgical Techniques

The **contemporary techniques of needle bladder neck suspension** have arisen as modifications of the first description by Pereyra in 1959. They **vary in (1) their potential use of graft or suture material, (2) the location and number of sutures in the urethropelvic ligament, (3) their use of single-pronged or double-pronged needle carriers, and (4) the extent of periurethral dissection** (Fig. 32–13). The following techniques of needle bladder neck suspension are performed in isolation *only* when stress urinary incontinence occurs without significant cystocele, rectocele, or other forms of pelvic relaxation.

Historical Background

In 1959, Pereyra presented a simplified vaginal approach to suspend the urethropelvic ligament, obviating the need

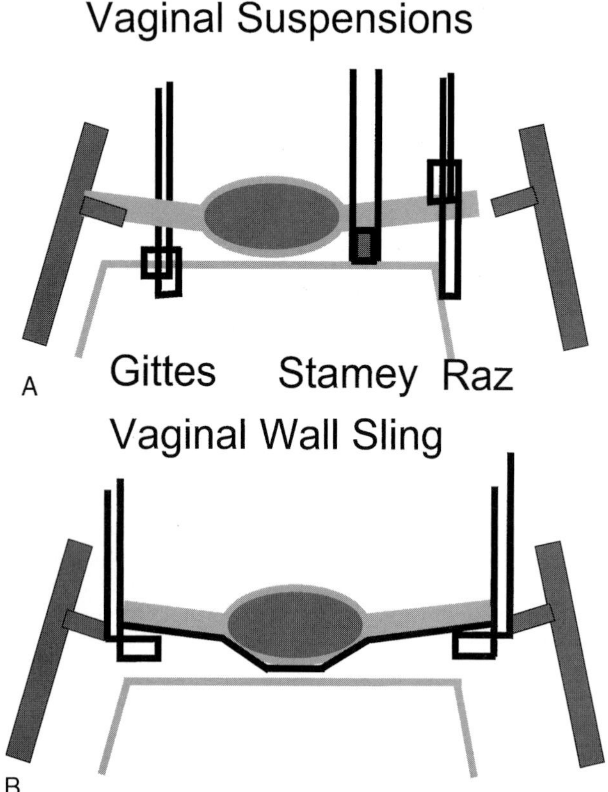

Figure 32–13. Diagrammatic comparison of vaginal procedures used for the correction of stress urinary incontinence and prolapse. *A,* Comparison of the various procedures noting the depth and distance of suture placement from both the urethra and the insertion of the levator fascia into the tendinous arc (shown as a square anchoring either end of the levator fascia). *B,* Diagrammatic representation of the anterior vaginal wall sling.

for an open abdominal procedure. The technique used a special angulated, partly hollow cannula, with a needle stylet. A T-shaped incision was made over the anterior vaginal wall, and periurethral dissection in the area of the bladder neck was undertaken without entering the retropubic space. Under fingertip control, the operator passed the Pereyra cannula through the abdominal wall and retropubic space, delivering the tip into the vaginal incision. Advancement of the needle stylet, which exited the cannula at a point of angulation, passed a second needle tip into the vagina. Both the cannula and the needle stylet were provided with an eye to carry both ends of a vaginally placed absorbable suture up through the abdominal wall when the instrument was withdrawn. Repeating the procedure on the contralateral side supported the urethropelvic ligament bilaterally. Following the clinical observation that recurrent stress incontinence could result from sutures pulling out of the urethropelvic ligament, Pereyra and Lebherz (1967), Stamey (1973), and Raz (1981) described modifications that improved clinical outcome. Following are the indications, techniques, and results of the surgical procedures themselves.

Stamey Needle Bladder Neck Suspension

The endoscopic needle suspension of Stamey was described in 1973. Stamey's description was important in that it was the first procedure described to use the cystoscope to place sutures precisely at the bladder neck. In contrast to the Raz and Gittes needle suspensions, the procedure incorporates a knitted Dacron graft to buttress either side of the urethra and aid in the prevention of suture pull-out. It is indicated for the correction of stress incontinence in the absence of significant cystocele.

Surgical Technique

Excellent descriptions of the surgical technique have been given by Stamey (1992). The patient is prepared in the lithotomy position and the bladder emptied with a Foley catheter. An incision is made in the anterior vaginal wall in the form of a T, and dissection is carried out over the glistening periurethral fascia. Continued lateral dissection is carried out until the operator can place a fingertip into the incision such that it rests against the bladder neck on either side of the catheter. This permits adequate exposure for the placement of the Dacron pledget. Two suprapubic stab wounds are made on each side of the lower abdomen, and the anterior rectus fascia is exposed. The single-pronged Stamey needle is then inserted into the medial edge of one of the suprapubic wounds and passed through the rectus fascia, adjacent to the periosteum, under fingertip control. The needle is advanced into the vaginal incision, passing alongside the bladder neck and through the periurethral fascia. The Foley catheter is removed, and cystoscopy is carried out with the needle in position to confirm correct placement. One end of a No. 2 nylon suture is threaded through the needle and then transferred suprapubically. The needle is passed a second time on the ipsilateral side to allow for placement of the Dacron arterial graft as described in Figure 32–14. A second suture and graft are placed in a similar fashion on the contralateral side. The vaginal wound should be irrigated with antibiotic solution, then closed, giving full attention to adequate burying of the grafts. A vaginal pack is placed following which the suspension sutures are tied, without tension, such that the knots rest against the rectus fascia.

Results

A synopsis of contemporary case series with 50 or greater patients is shown in Table 32–3. Eighty-two percent of 192 respondents were found to be improved after the Stamey needle suspension compared with their preoperative status when a mail-in questionnaire was used as an outcome measure (Walker and Texter, 1992). Patient satisfaction following the Stamey needle suspension has been measured by Walker and Texter (1992), who reported 65% of respondents would be willing to undergo the procedure again. In their study, prior Marshall-Marchetti-Krantz procedure, concomitant abdominal hysterectomy, respiratory disease, and obesity were found to lower the long-term cure rate.

Potential Complications

Complications particular to the Stamey needle suspension include long-term erosion of suture and bolster material into the urinary tract, which can occur up to 36 months after the procedure (Bihrle and Tarantino, 1990). Of patients undergo-

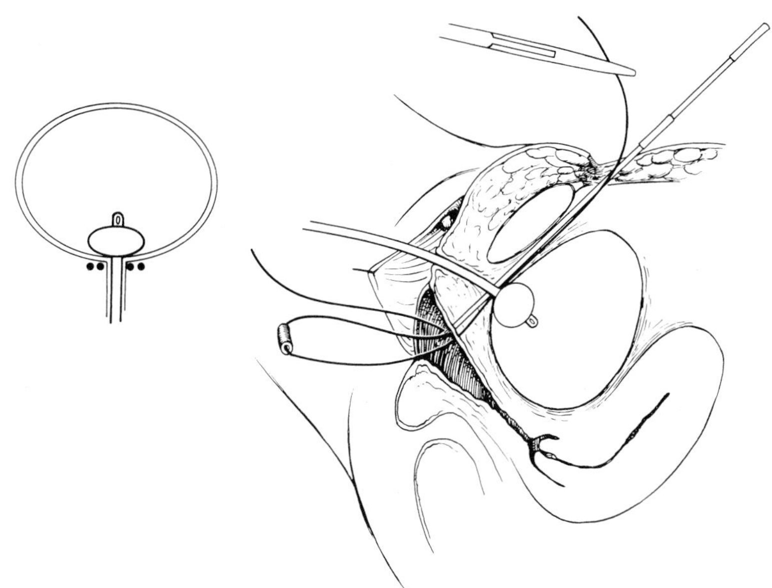

Figure 32–14. The Stamey needle is passed for a second time, 1 cm laterally on the ipsilateral side, and its position is confirmed once again cystoscopically. The vaginal end of the suture is placed through a 10 mm × 5 mm Dacron arterial graft and then through the eye of the needle. The Dacron graft is visually guided into the area of the urethrovesical junction while the needle is withdrawn for the second time. The procedure is repeated on the contralateral side, resulting in two Dacron grafts located on either side of the urethrovesical junction, which should be symmetric in location.

ing the procedure, 1% to 2% have been reported to require removal of one of the sutures for pain or infection. Long-term urinary retention may occur if sutures are tied too tight, and loosening of the nylon loop under local anesthesia has been reported to result in voiding without recurrence of stress incontinence (Araki et al, 1990).

Raz Bladder Neck Suspension

In 1981, Raz presented a modification of the Pereyra needle suspension that improved exposure and anchoring of sutures into the urethropelvic ligament. An inverted U-shaped incision in the anterior vaginal wall was developed to create increased exposure. The retropubic space was opened to (1) afford the opportunity for retropubic urethrolysis; (2) allow fingertip guidance of the needle, thereby avoiding perforation of the bladder or urethra; and (3) permit placement of a pair of permanent helical sutures into the urethropelvic ligament, incorporating both its vaginal and abdominal sides. Subsequent modifications led to the development of the anterior vaginal wall sling, which has replaced the Raz bladder neck suspension at the authors' institution. As originally described, the Raz bladder neck suspension is best suited to patients with anatomic incontinence due to urethral and bladder neck hypermobility (subjective SEAPI scores of S = 1 or 2) with minimal (grade I) or no cystocele.

Technique

A detailed description of the technique has been given by Raz (1992) and is summarized in Figure 32–15. The two polypropylene (Prolene) sutures that form the Raz bladder neck suspension are incorporated into the Raz anterior vaginal wall sling, which is detailed in a subsequent section.

Results

A retrospective review of 206 patients undergoing the Raz bladder neck suspension at the University of California, Los Angeles (UCLA), were reported in 1992 with a mean follow-up of 15 months (Raz et al, 1992). Ninety percent of patients were believed to demonstrate a successful outcome (S0–1; E0; A0; P0–1). Of importance was the observation that preoperative subjective severity of stress incontinence (S

Table 32–3. CONTEMPORARY SERIES REPORTING ON THE STAMEY NEEDLE SUSPENSION FOR STRESS URINARY INCONTINENCE

Author	Study Design	No. of Patients	Follow-up	Cured According to Author's Definition	Comments
Stamey, 1980	Case series	203	All >6 months	91%	
Hermieu et al, 1994	Uncontrolled observational study	55	21 months mean	76%	16% of patients had combined SUI and urge incontinence
Valle Gerhold et al, 1993	Uncontrolled observational study	51	35 months mean	60%	
Hilton and Mayne, 1991	Uncontrolled observational study	100	27 months	53% 76%	Aged <65 years Aged >65 years Uses actuarial life-table analysis
Ralph and Tamussino, 1991	Uncontrolled observational study	70	16 months	70%	
Ashken, 1990	Uncontrolled observational study	100		80%	Pad test for outcome measure

SUI, stress urinary incontinence.

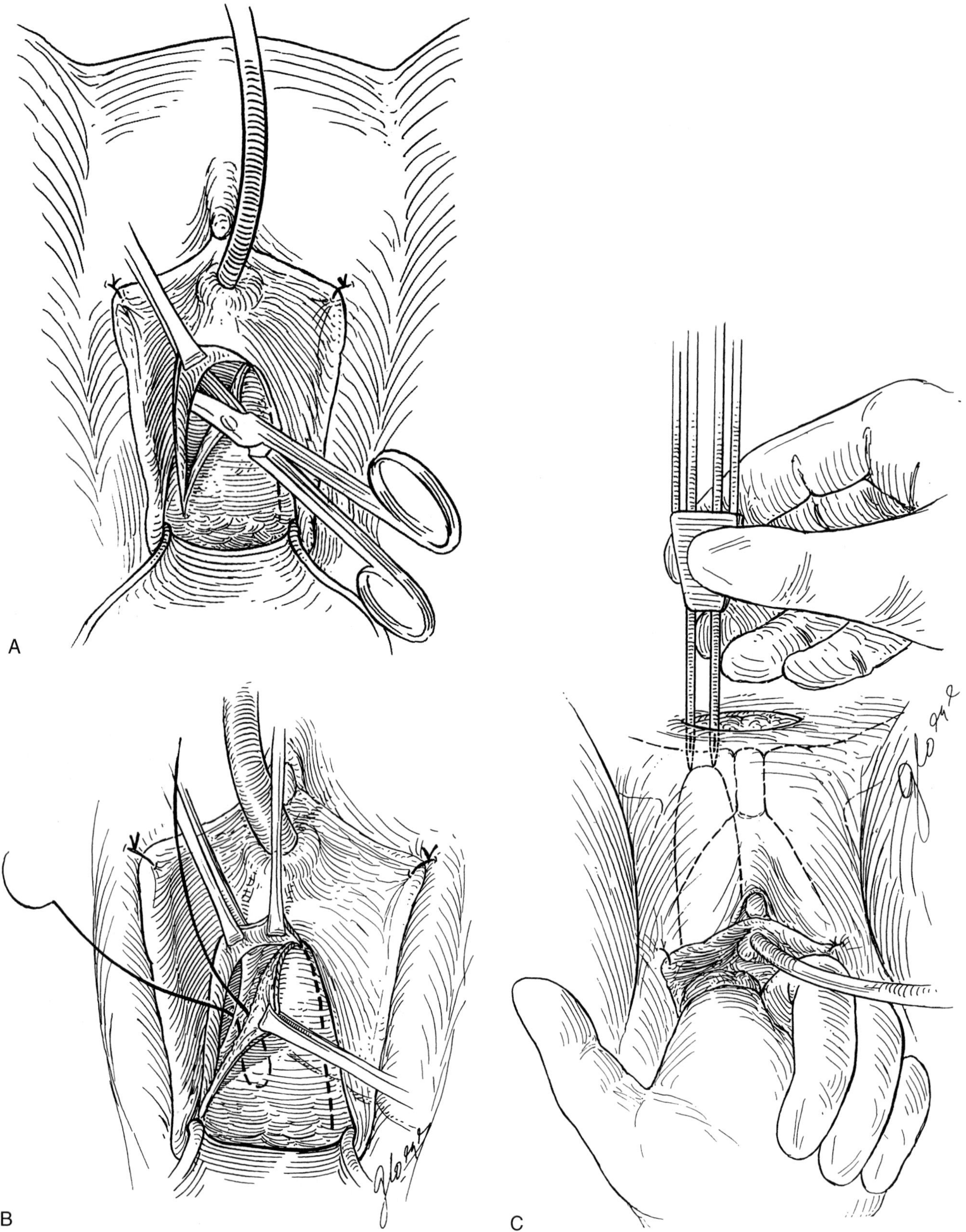

Figure 32–15. *A,* Raz bladder neck suspension. An inverted U-shaped incision is made in the anterior vaginal wall, with the base of the U at a point midway between the bladder neck and the external urethral meatus. The legs of the U extend just proximal to the bladder neck. The vaginal wall is dissected off the glistening surface of the periurethral fascia, and the retropubic space is entered by detaching the urethropelvic ligament off the tendinous arc. *B,* A No. 1 Prolene suture is placed to encompass the urethropelvic ligament and the vesicopelvic fascia, which underlies the vaginal wall. Note that these sutures should include the whole depth of the ligament to provide a secure anchor for the suture. A similar suture is placed on the contralateral side. *C,* A 1-cm midline incision is made transversely just above the pubic bone and carried down to the rectus fascia. The double-pronged needle is placed in the suprapubic wound, just cephalad to the pubic bone. With a finger in the retropubic space, the operator guides the needle out through the vaginal incision, and the suture is transferred by retraction of the needle. After both Prolene sutures are transferred, cystoscopy is carried out, and the vaginal incisions are closed. Following this, a vaginal pack is placed and the Prolene sutures are tied down without undue tension, and the wound is closed. (From Raz S: Female Genitourinary Dysfunction and Reconstruction. Philadelphia; W. B. Saunders Company, 1996.)

level, as measured by the SEAPI score) was predictive of recurrent stress incontinence. Stratifying the results for degree of incontinence preoperatively, patients reported cure of stress urinary incontinence in 95%, 93%, and 65% for mild (S1), moderate (S2), and severe (S3) degrees of incontinence preoperatively. Other contemporary retrospective case series report 65% to 95% of patients cured of stress incontinence (Naudin et al, 1992; Pastor et al, 1992; Nitti et al, 1993; Deliveliotis et al, 1994; Golomb et al, 1994).

An outcome analysis using mailed questionnaires found 77% of 106 patient respondents were satisfied with the outcome of the modified Pererya bladder neck suspension at 25 months mean follow-up (Korman et al, 1994). Forty-seven percent of questionnaire respondents reported cure (no urine leakage under any circumstance), and 64% were improved, compared with their preoperative status. Contrary to the reports of case series, this outcome study found more frequent postoperative failures in the elderly and in those with higher irritative symptom scores.

Potential Complications

Overall the Raz bladder neck suspension is well tolerated by patients, and more than 95% are discharged from hospital on the first postoperative day. Short-term complications are rare but may include vaginal spotting, urinary tract infection, or urinary irritative symptoms. Potential long-term complications include de novo urgency incontinence (7.5%), secondary prolapse such as enterocele (6%), prolonged retention (2.5%), and suprapubic pain (3%) (Raz et al, 1992).

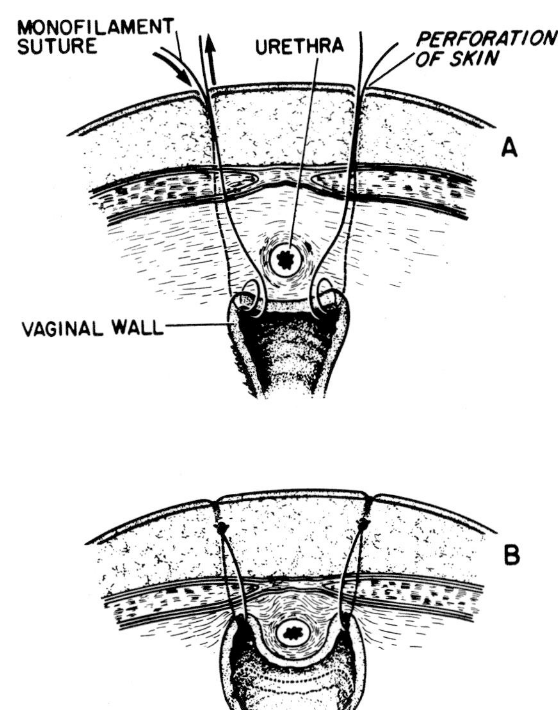

Figure 32–16. *A* and *B,* No incision (Gittes) transvaginal bladder neck suspension.

Gittes Needle Bladder Neck Suspension

In 1987, Gittes and Loughlin described their modification of the Pereyra needle suspension, simplifying the technique by obviating the need for vaginal incisions. To achieve support of the bladder neck, suspension sutures placed into the vaginal wall become incorporated over time, creating an "autologous pledget." Gittes and Loughlin (1987) have elegantly described the mechanism through which this occurs. Vaginal suspension sutures placed under slight traction cut through the vaginal wall and eventually become buried and encased in scar tissue. This scar extends from around the suture to the vaginal wall in the form of a band, thereby linking the suture material to the vaginal wall. Superiorly the suspension sutures are anchored over the rectus fascia. Together a two-link chain is created, connecting the vaginal wall to the rectus fascia and subsequently preventing hypermobility of the bladder neck at times of increased intra-abdominal pressure.

Surgical Technique

Gittes and Loughlin (1987) have carefully described the technique (Fig. 32–16), which begins with the patient in the dorsal lithotomy position and the bladder drained through a urethral Foley catheter. Two stab incisions are made on either side lateral to the midline at the upper border of the symphysis pubis. The Stamey needle is passed through the medial aspect of one of the suprapubic stab wounds such that the tip of the needle scrapes the posterior aspect of the pubic bone. The anterior vaginal wall at the level of the bladder neck is simultaneously elevated with the operator's second hand pressing upward just lateral to the Foley catheter balloon. The needle is directed from above, toward the intravaginal fingertip. Once the needle tip is palpable by the intravaginal fingertip, the needle is advanced through the vaginal wall and out through the introitus. Cystoscopic examination confirms that the needle has not perforated the bladder. Gentle rocking of the needle may allow the operator to observe an indentation in the bladder wall, which identifies the site of needle passage. Once correct positioning of the needle is confirmed, one end of a No. 2 Prolene suture is passed through the eye of the needle, and the needle is withdrawn to deliver one end to the suprapubic wound. A second pass of the needle on the ipsilateral side is performed 1 cm lateral to the initial pass under fingertip control. (This allows a 1-cm bridge of fascia to remain over which the ipsilateral suture is tied.) The site where the second pass perforates the vaginal tissues should be within 1 cm of the initial pass so as to avoid tenting up a large amount of vaginal tissues at the completion of the procedure. Cystoscopy is repeated to confirm that the needle has not penetrated the bladder. The free vaginal end of the Prolene suture is threaded temporarily through a Mayo needle, and two or three helical bites of vaginal tissue are taken at varying angles. The Mayo needle is unthreaded, and the suture end is threaded through the eye of the Stamey needle already placed. The Stamey needle is withdrawn, and the two ends of the suspension suture are held with a clamp for later tying. A second suture is placed in a similar fashion on the contralateral side. A suprapubic cystotomy is placed at the completion of the procedure. The sutures are tied without undue tension in their respective suprapubic wounds. Knot tension is equivalent to that for fascial stitches elsewhere. The skin wounds are covered with an adhesive bandage after umbilication of the skin is eliminated by pulling the puncture site up with small tooth forceps.

Results

Reported success rates for cure of stress urinary incontinence vary between 66% and 94% depending on the length of follow-up and the authors' definition of cure (Benson et al, 1990; Loughlin et al, 1990; Kursh et al, 1991; Kursh, 1992; Zerbib et al, 1992; Conquy et al, 1993). Gittes and Loughlin reported an 87% cure of stress urinary incontinence in their initial report in 1987. In 1990, Loughlin and co-workers reported a modification of the technique in which patients with and without the autologous pledget bites were compared. Cure rates of 86% and 75% were reported for those with and without the autologous pledget bites. In 1992, Kursh evaluated factors that influenced the long-term outcome of the no-incision urethropexy, finding that a statistically significant decrease in success rate was seen with worsening degrees of preoperative incontinence. Women with type 1 stress incontinence had excellent outcome (97% cure rate), whereas those with type 3 stress incontinence had only a 45% cure rate. Postmenopausal women had a statistically poorer outcome regardless of exogenous estrogen intake.

Nonrandomized retrospective group comparisons that compare the no-incision urethropexy with other needle suspensions have found similar continence in short-term follow-up (Kil et al, 1991; Conquy et al, 1993).

Potential Complications

An overall 9.8% complication rate has been reported by Loughlin and co-workers (1990). Specific complications may include prolonged urinary retention (7%), suprapubic pain or cellulitis, vaginitis, suture infection with abscess formation, and genitofemoral nerve entrapment (Summers and Meyers, 1989; Loughlin et al, 1990; Kursh, 1992).

Raz Vaginal Wall Sling

In 1992, Raz developed a new surgical technique for the treatment of stress urinary incontinence caused by intrinsic sphincter dysfunction or anatomic incontinence. Its development followed an increased understanding of female pelvic floor anatomy together with clinical observations related to failures of bladder neck suspension procedures.

McGuire (1981) observed that patients presenting with primary stress urinary incontinence had only a 6% incidence of poor urethral function. This percentage increased to 30% in those who had failed one bladder neck suspension and 75% following two or more failed bladder neck suspensions. Subsequently, high failure rates of bladder neck suspension procedures were reported in patients with severe forms of preoperative incontinence (Raz et al, 1992). It became clinically apparent that the diagnosis of anatomic incontinence preoperatively did not eliminate the possibility of potentially coexisting or subsequently unmasked intrinsic sphincter dysfunction. Although stress incontinence is separated into anatomic incontinence and intrinsic sphincter dysfunction types for the purpose of classification, features of both conditions may occur in any given patient, and separation between the two may be difficult (McGuire, 1994).

New anatomic principles also contributed to the development of the anterior vaginal wall sling, including (1) a need to correct a defect of midurethral support, (2) a better understanding of the levator musculature as it envelops the urethra just distal to the pubourethral ligaments, and (3) evidence to suggest that the bladder neck is not the most important mechanism of continence. Examples to support this last principle include the observations that up to 30% of postmenopausal women have an open bladder neck on a straining cystogram without any incontinence and that Y-V-plasty does not produce stress incontinence. Most bladder neck suspension procedures elevate the bladder neck, creating a valvular effect, but do not have an impact on the midurethral area. In the authors' opinion, in many if not most patients, the most important area of continence is the midurethra.

The surgical goals of the anterior vaginal wall sling are (1) to provide elastic support to the midurethra and bladder neck and (2) to create a strong hammock of vaginal wall and underlying tissues, which provides a backboard against which the urethra can be compressed and supported. The procedure is indicated for patients with stress urinary incontinence (SEAPI S1–3) due to anatomic incontinence or intrinsic sphincter dysfunction with minimal (grade 1) or no cystocele. When stress incontinence is found with more severe forms of cystocele, the degree of anterior vaginal wall prolapse dictates the procedure of choice (Fig. 32–17).

Surgical Technique

After induction of spinal or general anesthesia, the patient is placed in the dorsal lithotomy position with the use of candy cane stirrups having the feet protected by foam boots. The lower abdomen and perineum are prepared with an iodine-based solution and sterile draping is applied, being careful to exclude the anus from the operative field. A 30-degree weighted vaginal speculum and silk labial retraction sutures are used for exposure.

A suprapubic catheter is next inserted. The curved Lowsley retractor is inserted through the urethra and positioned against the anterior bladder and abdominal wall 3 cm superior to the symphysis pubis. The assistant palpates for the tip of the retractor and makes a stab incision just wide enough to allow passage of the instrument through the abdominal wall. The operator grasps the end of an unlubricated No. 16 Fr Foley catheter within the jaws of the Lowsley retractor, following which the instrument is withdrawn deliv-

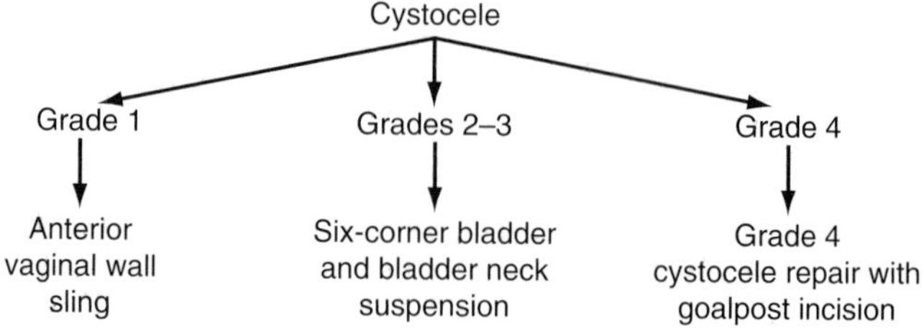

Figure 32–17. Suggested clinical pathway for surgical treatment of anterior vaginal wall prolapse.

ering the end of the catheter out through the urethra. A tonsil clamp is placed on the tip of the catheter to push it back into the bladder, and the assistant inflates the balloon. Irrigation confirms intravesical positioning of the catheter, and the suprapubic tube is left on slight traction to achieve hemostasis and prevent leakage during the procedure. The bladder is then drained through a second No. 16 Fr Foley catheter placed per urethra.

To aid in exposure of the anterior vaginal wall, an Allis clamp is placed in the midline just below the urethral meatus to provide upward retraction. Saline is used to infiltrate the anterior vaginal wall to develop tissue planes, which facilitates dissection. Using a forceps to retract the bladder medially, the operator makes two oblique incisions, which extend from the level of the midurethra to 3 cm beyond the level of the bladder neck. These are 1 cm medial to the folded margin of the anterior vaginal wall throughout their entire length. Making the incisions too lateral results in difficulty closing the incisions because of the natural folding of the anterior vaginal wall. Locating the incisions too medial results in difficult dissection and a greater potential for entering the bladder. An Allis clamp is added at the periurethral end of each incision, and upward retraction is provided by the assistant (Fig. 32–18*A*).

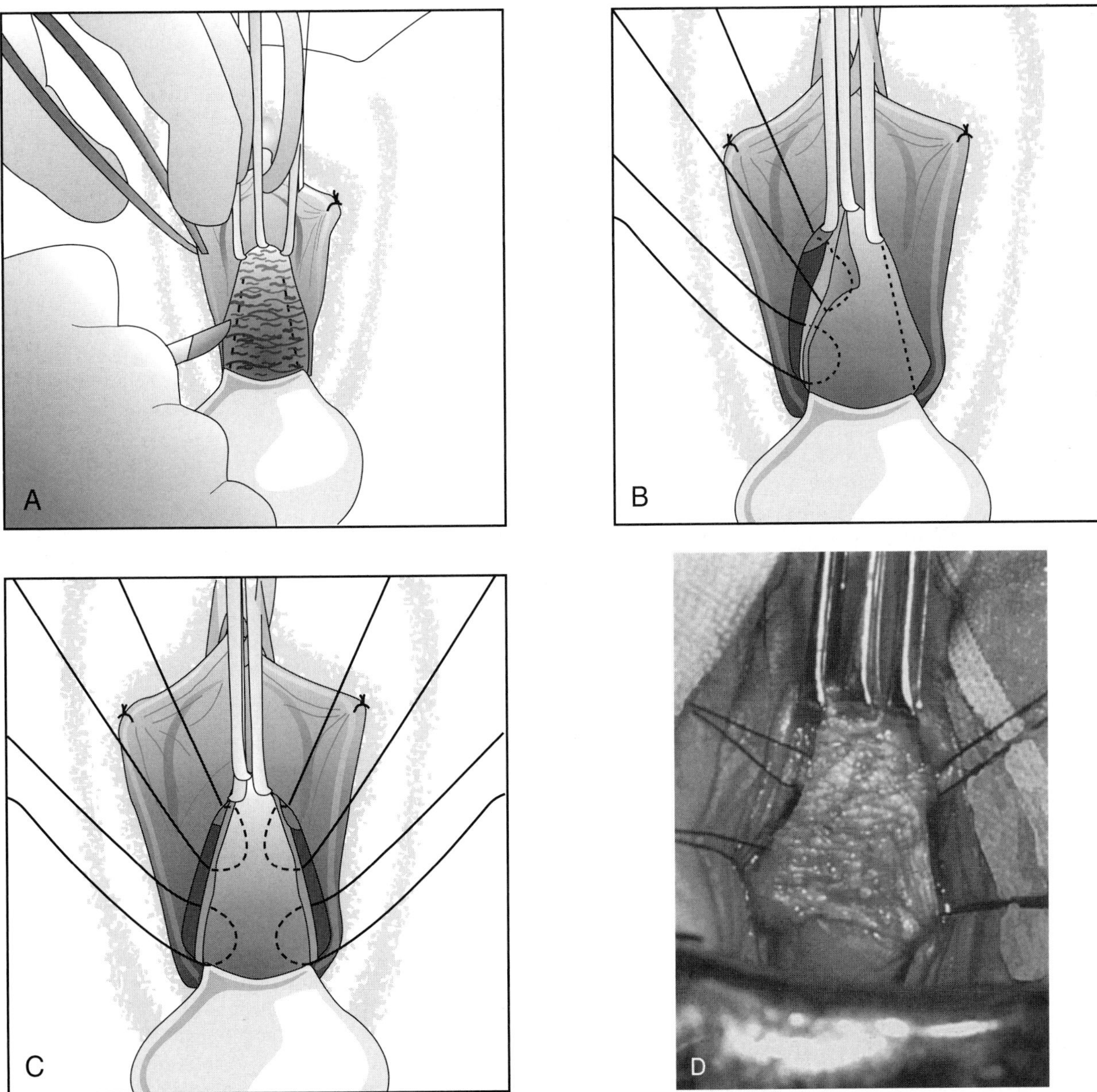

Figure 32–18. Raz vaginal wall sling. *A,* Two oblique incisions are made in the anterior vaginal wall, and upward retraction is provided by Allis clamps. *B,* Positioning of the proximal and distal Prolene sutures shown are on the patient's right. The proximal No. 1 Prolene suture is placed in a manner equivalent to that of the Raz bladder neck suspension. It incorporates helical bites of the vesicopelvic fascia underlying the vaginal wall and the urethropelvic ligament. The distal No. 1 Prolene suture incorporates the levator ani musculature as it inserts into the midurethral segment, the medial edge of the urethropelvic ligament, and the anterior vaginal wall without epithelium. *C,* Diagrammatic representation of the two pairs of No. 1 Prolene suture, which create a hammock of support once transferred to the retropubic space by the double-pronged needle carrier. *D,* Correct positioning of the four sutures in a patient before transfer with the double-pronged needle.

Sharp dissection is carried out laterally over the surface of the glistening periurethral fascia along the corridor between the levator ani muscle inferiorly and the vaginal side of the urethropelvic ligament superiorly. When this dissection is completed correctly, a finger inserted into the incision can palpate the levator muscle inferiorly and the urethropelvic ligament superiorly. Where these two structures come together, palpated by the tip of the finger, is the tendinous arc. At the level of the bladder neck, the retropubic space is entered with the use of the curved Mayo scissors. The closed blades enter the retropubic space and are then opened, exposing and detaching the urethropelvic ligament from the tendinous arc. Once the retropubic space has been opened, the operator's index finger is inserted, and all adhesions along the proximal urethra and bladder neck are bluntly released. Adequate urethrolysis should permit a finger entering the retropubic space from either incision to palpate the inner surface of the pubic bone and the pubourethral ligament.

First, the proximal pair of Prolene sutures is placed as in the Raz bladder neck suspension. To begin, several helical passes are made, keeping the needle parallel to the vaginal wall, to incorporate the vesicopelvic fascia underlying the vaginal wall. This adds to support and corrects mild (grade 1) cystocele. Then, several helical passes of the same suture are placed into the urethropelvic ligament at the level of the bladder neck. To achieve this, the long Russian forceps are extended into the retropubic space and opened, and gentle medial retraction is applied to expose the edge of the urethropelvic ligament. A second Prolene suture is placed in a similar manner on the contralateral side.

Before the distal pair of Prolene sutures is placed, the surgeon begins with long Russian forceps opened widely in the retropubic space. Gentle downward traction is applied, keeping the open forceps parallel to the floor, creating an open triangular window in the retropubic space. At the apex of the triangle is the levator musculature and the posterior pubourethral ligament. Medial is the edge of the urethropelvic ligament and laterally the vaginal wall. The floor of the triangle is parallel to the cardinal ligaments. With the assistant providing upward traction on the Allis clamps, the surgeon incorporates several passes of the levator muscle and the ipsilateral edge of the urethropelvic ligament. To obtain an adequate amount of levator tissue, the needle must be placed deep into the retropubic space. The levator should be visualized on the arc of the needle. The forceps is repositioned to put downward traction on the anterior vaginal wall in the area of the midurethra and to incorporate several helical bites of the underlying periurethral fascia. As in placing sutures into the vesicopelvic fascia, it is important to keep the needle parallel with the vaginal wall to prevent suture material from entering the urethra. The arc of the needle should not cross the midline but should include a generous amount of tissue (Fig. 32–18*B*).

After the four Prolene sutures are in place, one can visualize a rectangle of support for the bladder neck and midurethra (Fig. 32–18*C* and *D*). A small suprapubic stab wound is made transversely just above the superior margin of the pubic bone and carried down to the level of the underlying rectus fascia. The double-pronged ligature carrier is placed in the suprapubic wound, just cephalad to the symphysis pubis. With the surgeon's index finger in the retropubic space and under direct digital control, the needle is passed through the vaginal incision. Correct needle placement is critical to avoid postoperative pain and injury to the bladder. The needle should pass in the midline, close to the pubic bone through an immobile portion of the rectus fascia. The Prolene sutures are individually transferred suprapubically by way of the ligature carrier.

Cystoscopy is performed after injection of indigo carmine intravenously by the anesthetist. Inspection with 30- and 70-degree lenses is done to ensure that no bladder perforation occurred, that the suprapubic catheter is in position, and that ureteric efflux of indigo carmine is present bilaterally. With the suspension sutures pulled upward, the vaginal examination should now reveal the anterior vaginal wall to be lifted into a supported retropubic position.

The vaginal wall is closed with a running, locking, 2-0 polyglycolic acid suture. A vaginal pack, impregnated with antibiotic cream, is inserted into the vagina. The suspending sutures are tied independently with multiple knots snug onto the underlying rectus fascia without tension, and then one end is tied to its neighbor for extra security. After tying the Prolene sutures, a cystoscope sheath in the urethra should demonstrate elastic support and should not feel fixed in position. The skin edges overlying the Prolene sutures are loosened with a forceps to prevent dimpling of the skin, which can cause suprapubic discomfort. The suprapubic wound is closed with a subcuticular 4-0 absorbable suture, and Steri-Strips are applied. The suprapubic tube is taped on gentle traction over a folded gauze, and both the suprapubic tube and the urethral catheter are left to straight drainage (Stothers et al, 1996).

Postoperative Care

This procedure is currently performed on an outpatient basis. Within 6 to 20 hours postoperatively, the patient is prepared for discharge. The vaginal pack and urethral catheter are removed, and the suprapubic tube is plugged. The patient should maintain the suprapubic catheter taped on slight traction over a folded gauze to prevent leakage around the tube. The patient is asked to try to void per urethra and to check her own postvoid residual urines. Oral antibiotics, stool softeners, and oral analgesics are given to the patient to use after discharge. Antibiotics are continued while the suprapubic tube is in place. The suprapubic catheter is removed in the office once the postvoid residuals are consistently less than 50 ml.

Results

Early clinical outcome of 160 women who underwent the sling with a median follow-up of 17 months has been reported (Raz et al, 1996; Stothers et al, 1995). Clinically, 95 had intrinsic sphincter dysfunction and 65 anatomic incontinence classified preoperatively. A total of 152 patients were considered cured of stress urinary incontinence at last follow-up and had clinical SEAPI scores of S0–1, E0, A0, P0–1. Eight patients were considered failures and had recurrent incontinence, which was unrelated to instability and required further therapy. Regression models and time to failure analysis revealed the results in anatomic incontinence and intrinsic sphincter dysfunction groups to be similar.

Quality of life scores were significantly improved in both anatomic incontinence and intrinsic sphincter dysfunction (Stothers et al, 1995; Raz et al, 1996; Stothers and Raz, 1996).

Potential Complications

De novo urgency incontinence (7.5%), secondary prolapse such as enterocele (6%), prolonged retention (2.5%), and suprapubic pain (3%) have been reported (Raz et al, 1996; Stothers et al, 1996).

VAGINAL SURGERY FOR PROLAPSE

Multiple factors influence the development and progression of pelvic prolapse (Table 32–4). Differences in pelvic architecture, inherent quality of the pelvic musculature, and character of tissue response to injury are significant. Neurogenic or congenital factors play a role as demonstrated by the incidence of prolapse in nulliparous multiple sclerosis and spina bifida patients (Youngblood, 1993). Trauma from childbirth may contribute to prolapse through increases in progesterone and cortisol during pregnancy, which soften pelvic supports. In addition, the weight of a full-term pregnancy may lead to symptoms initially limited to the term of pregnancy itself (Copeland, 1993).

The interrelatedness of the various forms of pelvic prolapse need to be emphasized. **Although correction of anterior, posterior, uterine, and vault defects is described separately, the surgeon should not consider these procedures in isolation; rather, they should be performed together in patients to establish functional unity of the pelvic organs** (Nichols and Genadry, 1993; Timmons and Addison, 1993; Raz, 1996). This discussion is limited to surgical therapies for pelvic prolapse; however, nonoperative therapy is often indicated in patients who have minimal symptoms or who pose a surgical risk. This therapy may involve changes in activities, treatment of constipation (and other circumstances that increase intra-abdominal pressure), Kegel exercises, pessaries, and hormonal replacement.

Table 32–4. ETIOLOGIC FACTORS CONTRIBUTING TO UROGENITAL PELVIC PROLAPSE

- Congenital
  - Spina bifida
- Acquired
  - Pregnancy
  - Trauma
    - Childbirth
    - Episiotomy
    - Postsurgical
      - Radical pelvic urologic/gynecologic surgery
      - Hemorrhoidectomy
      - Rectal fistula repair
  - Menopause
  - Chronic increases in intra-abdominal pressure
    - Cough/chronic respiratory disease
    - Constipation
    - Bladder outlet obstruction
    - Heavy lifting
  - Ascites
  - Neurogenic
    - Multiple sclerosis
  - Pelvic mass
  - Obesity
  - Smoking
  - Strenuous physical activity

Table 32–5. CLINICAL GRADING OF COMPONENTS OF PELVIC PROLAPSE

Type of Prolapse	Grade	Clinical Finding
Cystocele	1	Descent of bladder base toward introitus with straining
	2	Descent of bladder base to the level of the introitus with straining
	3	Descent of bladder base outside the introitus with straining
	4	Bladder base outside introitus at rest
Uterine prolapse	1	Descent of cervix toward introitus with straining
	2	Descent of cervix to the level of the introitus with straining
	3	Cervix outside introitus with straining
	4	Cervix outside introitus at rest
Perineal separation/ lacerations	1	Separation of the fourchette and perineal skin
	2	Separation of muscles and fascia of perineal body
	3	Separation of perineal body and anal sphincter
	4	Separation of anal sphincter and exposure of rectal lumen
Rectocele	Low	Separation of the levator ani and bulbocavernosus from the perineal body
	Mid	Bulging of rectum into the vagina above the levator hiatus Separation of pararectal and prerectal fascia
	High	Bulging of rectum into the upper vaginal vault Frequently associated with an enterocele

Anterior Vaginal Wall Prolapse

Definition and Classification

A cystocele is present when the bladder base descends below the inferior ramus of the symphysis pubis either at rest or with straining. Although cystoceles are classically graded according to degree of anterior wall descent (Table 32–5), they may be further defined by the location of the primary anatomic defect. **An isolated central cystocele is found when the vesicopelvic fascia spanning the levator hiatus becomes attenuated without compromise of lateral support** (Fig. 32–19). Central cystoceles account for 5% to 15% of all cystoceles. **Lateral cystoceles occur when weakness or disruption of lateral attachments of the vesicopelvic or cardinal ligaments to pelvic sidewall is found.** These cystoceles account for 70% to 80% of all anterior vaginal wall prolapse (Macer, 1978). Combinations of lateral and central defects also occur and are especially common in

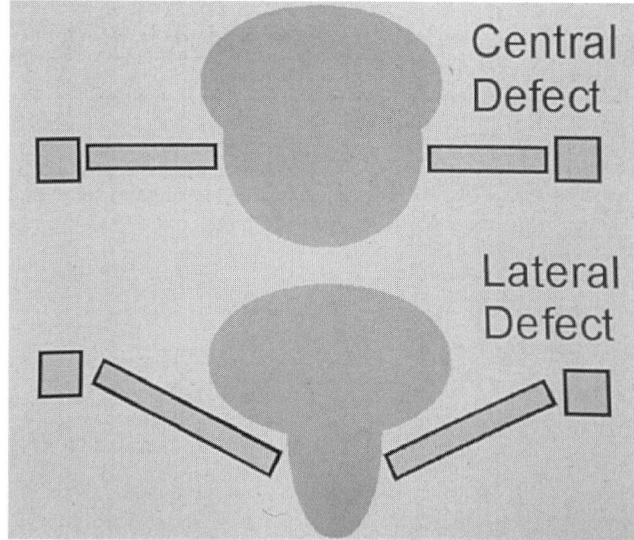

Figure 32–19. The defects found in cystocele formation are depicted diagrammatically. A central defect is shown in the top of the diagram, where the area of fascial weakness is located in the midline region of the vesicopelvic fascia. A lateral defect is shown below where the area of weakness is located at the lateral attachments of the vesicopelvic fascia to the tendinous arc of the obturator.

patients with higher grades of prolapse. Several authors also discuss the transverse defect secondary to disruption of the fascial attachments to the pericervical fascia (Nichols and Randall, 1991). It is important to remember that a cystocele reflects one specific aspect of pelvic prolapse. For example, up to 60% of patients with grade 3 cystoceles are found to have other forms of concomitant pelvic prolapse (e.g., rectocele, enterocele, uterine prolapse, vaginal vault prolapse); 95% of patients with grade 4 cystocele have concomitant forms of pelvic prolapse (Raz, unpublished data).

Symptoms

Grade 1 and 2 cystoceles are frequently asymptomatic, becoming problematic only in association with urethral hypermobility and stress incontinence. Larger cystoceles, however, are frequently symptomatic, with common complaints including dyspareunia and vaginal bulging. Raz and colleagues reported on 29 patients with grade 4 cystocele, finding that the chief complaint of the patient was, in decreasing frequency, **a painful vaginal mass, a painless vaginal mass, recurrent urinary tract infections, back pain, renal failure, staghorn calculi, and an inability to walk** (Raz et al, 1995). **Retention of urine may occur because of kinking at the bladder neck**; this scenario is often found when the urethra has been fixed in place by previous surgery. To minimize the obstructive effect, many patients manually reduce their cystocele to facilitate emptying. **Silent hydronephrosis** secondary to ureteral obstruction may occur. Patients with grade 4 cystocele frequently delay seeking treatment for prolapse. Stothers and associates found the mean time taken for patients to seek treatment once they had become aware of the presence of grade 4 cystocele was 5.6 years (Stothers et al, 1996).

Diagnosis and Evaluation

Physical examination of the patient is best performed with a full bladder. Evaluation in the **standing position** reveals a mass descending toward the introitus. In the supine position, the patient must be examined both at rest and with straining to determine the severity of anterior vaginal wall defect (Shull, 1993). **In addition to determining the grade of cystocele, the anatomic defects contributing to the cystocele (i.e., lateral and/or central) should be documented** (see Fig. 32–19). If the source of the prolapse is uncertain, examination with a half-speculum, a vaginal defect analyzer, or a wooden tongue blade is often helpful (Richardson, 1976). With the half-speculum supporting the central bladder base, loss of the lateral vaginal supports (the H configuration) may be found, suggesting a lateral defect. Likewise, if support of the lateral vaginal wall alone results in reduction of the cystocele, a lateral defect is said to be present (Baden and Walker, 1992). A central defect may be revealed when the surgeon demonstrates central prolapse despite mechanical support of the lateral attachments. Of note, a lateral defect is much more likely to be accompanied by urethral descent, vaginal eversion, and uterine hypermobility (Raz et al, 1992). Although central and lateral defects may occur in isolation, they frequently coexist, as in the case of grade 4 cystocele. **After determining the defects in anatomic support, it is important to examine the patient after reduction of the cystocele. This maneuver often reveals otherwise hidden stress incontinence and urethral and bladder neck hypermobility, particularly when grade 4 cystocele is present.** Gardy and colleagues have stated that symptoms of stress incontinence do not reliably indicate the presence or absence of urethral dysfunction in patients with cystoceles (Gardy et al, 1991). **To avoid the complication of postoperative stress incontinence, consideration should always be given to bladder neck support when cystocele repair is undertaken in the presence of malposition or hypermobility of the urethra or bladder neck.**

If video-urodynamics are not available, a voiding cystourethrogram done in the standing position with both resting and straining films is useful to help grade the severity of cystocele defect, demonstrate hypermobility of the urethra, demonstrate stress incontinence, and document postvoid residual urine (Raz et al, 1992; Raz, 1996). **With a full bladder, cystography in the standing position often upgrades the severity of cystocele compared with the supine physical examination.** Radiologically, with an isolated central cystocele, the urethra maintains a normal relationship with the pubic symphysis and the posterior wall of the bladder. With lateral defects, this relationship between urethra and pubis is lost, and a greater portion of the bladder prolapses (Raz et al, 1992). Grading of cystocele severity is shown in Table 32–5.

Renal ultrasound should be included in the presence of grade 4 cystocele to rule out silent hydronephrosis. A urine culture often reveals bacteriuria. Urodynamics may aid the surgeon preoperatively because bladder dysfunction may vary from the simple presence of stress incontinence with low grades of cystocele to bladder outlet obstruction and urgency incontinence with more severe defects. Gardy and colleagues described 33 patients with large cystoceles (Gardy et al, 1991). In her review, 32 out of 33 patients had symptoms or urodynamic evidence of stress incontinence, 18 patients had significant residual urines, and 24 patients had urgency incontinence.

Operative Strategy

Three primary types of cystocele repair are described in the literature: the transabdominal suspension procedures, the Kelly plication/anterior colporrhaphy and its modifications, and the transvaginal suspension procedures.

Until the work of Richardson in 1976, it was believed by most surgeons that midline defects were the cause of most cystoceles. As such, anterior repair and its modifications remained the standard for repair. In 1976, Richardson published his landmark paper in which he described the various types and locations of fascial defects involved in the pathogenesis of cystoceles. In his experience, **70% to 80% of all cystoceles resulted from damage to the lateral support**. With this finding in mind, Richardson described his results with a technique of transabdominal suspension aimed specifically at repairing the lateral defect (Richardson et al, 1981). Other authors have followed his lead and used various techniques of transabdominal and transvaginal suspension techniques for cystocele repair secondary to weakness of lateral support. Despite the predominance of lateral defects associated with cystoceles, however, central defect repairs (i.e., Kelly plication/anterior colporrhaphy) remain the most common procedures performed for cystocele repair. A brief discussion of the techniques of transabdominal cystocele repair and anterior colporrhaphy/Kelly plication follows.

Transabdominal approaches allow fixation of the vaginal wall to the lateral pelvic sidewall. As such, they are used for patients with lateral defects. Patients with central defects should be repaired transvaginally because the plication or reapproximation of the vesicopelvic fascia and cardinal ligaments required to repair a central defect cannot be achieved transabdominally. **The two primary procedures for transabdominal cystocele repair are the Burch colposuspension and the paravaginal repair described by Richardson and colleagues** (1981). These two techniques differ primarily in the location of the suspension. In the Burch suspension, the vaginal wall and fascia are apposed to Cooper's ligaments; in the paravaginal repair, the vaginal wall and fascia are approximated to the obturator fascia.

The Kelly-type plication with anterior colporrhaphy (anterior repair) involves midline plication of the vesicopelvic fascia and is, as such, ideally suited for repair of central defects. Kelly initially described his procedure in 1912 as a procedure for the treatment of incontinence (not cystocele). In his description, the vaginal wall was incised in the midline with lateral dissection of the vaginal wall for 2 to 2.5 cm at the level of the bladder neck. The "lateral tissues" were reapproximated with silk or linen with bites of 1.5 cm of tissue. Of historical interest, in Kelly's follow-up, 80% of his 20 patients had improved continence. His paper did not comment on anatomic resolution of bladder prolapse.

The **anterior colporrhaphy** in a similar fashion involves exposure of the vesicopelvic fascia with reapproximation and plication in the midline with absorbable sutures. In distinction, the dissection and repair are not limited to the area of the bladder neck but rather involve the entire anterior vaginal wall to the level of the cardinal ligaments. **Anterior colporrhaphy is ideally suited to repair isolated central defects. Of note, because of the high incidence of postoperative incontinence after anterior colporrhaphy (up to 40%) many surgeons have modified their techniques to include a urethral suspension procedure** (Beck et al, 1991). **The anterior colporrhaphy does not treat lateral defects commonly found with cystoceles.**

Transvaginal approaches allow for correction of all grades of cystocele. The goals of surgery are determined by the presence of anatomic defects in the anterior vaginal wall: **Central defects are repaired by plication or reapproximation of the vesicopelvic fascia and the cardinal ligaments. Lateral defects are repaired by suspension of the vesicopelvic ligament and urethropelvic and cardinal/sacrouterine ligament complex toward the anterior abdominal wall. For combined defects (classically grade 4 cystocele), both central and lateral defect repairs through a transvaginal technique are used**.

The authors' current techniques of repair represent an evolution in understanding of cystocele development and reflect concerns with (1) predominance of lateral defects in patients with cystocele (70%–80%), (2) a desire to correct coexistent stress incontinence (Raz et al, 1989), and (3) limiting the onset of de novo postoperative stress incontinence (up to 40%). Because of the focus on the role of the midurethral complex and interest in treating potentially hidden intrinsic sphincteric deficiency, **the authors routinely incorporate the vaginal wall sling in cystocele repairs.**

The following two sections discuss techniques of repair for patients with one of two types of defects: (1) moderate (grade 2–3) cystocele with a predominantly lateral defect treated by the six-corner suspension and (2) grade 4 cystocele (central and lateral defects). A symptomatic grade 1 cystocele with stress urinary incontinence should be treated by a surgical technique directed at correction of the stress urinary incontinence. The reader is referred to sources in the references for in-depth description of isolated central defect repair (anterior colporrhaphy).

Transvaginal Surgical Procedures to Correct Cystocele

Six-Corner Suspension for Stress Incontinence and Moderate Cystocele

TECHNIQUE. The patient is placed in the lithotomy position, and the vagina is prepared and draped as in the anterior vaginal wall sling. Two oblique incisions are made from the level of the vaginal cuff (paracervical area if the uterus is present) to the level of the midurethra. The vesicopelvic fascia is exposed by lateral dissection with the Metzenbaum scissors. At the level of the midurethra, the retropubic space is entered by advancing the closed, curved Mayo scissors pointing toward the ipsilateral shoulder of the patient. The scissors are opened, exposing the urethropelvic ligament and the retropubic space. This results in a similar exposure to the vaginal wall sling with the exception that the lateral attachments of the vesicopelvic fascia over the bladder base are displayed to the level of the cardinal ligaments.

Three sutures of No. 1 Prolene are placed on each side

(Fig. 32–20). Each suture incorporates multiple passes through the tissues. The proximal suture is placed at the level of the vaginal vault to incorporate the vesicopelvic fascia and the cardinal ligaments. This suture should be of such strength that the patient can be rocked on the table with tension on the suture. The middle and distal sutures are applied as for the vaginal wall sling. Next a small suprapubic puncture is made, and the double-pronged ligature carrier is passed under direct fingertip control through the retropubic space, exiting in the vaginal incision. The Prolene sutures are transferred individually to the suprapubic incision, following which indigo carmine is administered and cystoscopy carried out. As with the vaginal wall sling, cystoscopy confirms the patency of the ureters by visualization of blue efflux from each orifice and ensures correct positioning of the suprapubic tube and an absence of Prolene suture within the bladder. Finally, anterior tension is placed on the sutures to ensure that adequate anatomic reduction is achieved. The vaginal incisions are closed with a 2-0 polyglycolic acid (Vicryl) running interlocking suture, and a vaginal pack is inserted. The Prolene suspension sutures are next tied sequentially to themselves and their ipsilateral mates. **It is important to tie the Prolene sutures without tension to avoid postoperative urinary retention.** The suprapubic site is irrigated with povidone-iodine (Betadine) solution, and the wound is closed with 4-0 Vicryl.

POSTOPERATIVE CARE. Both urethral and suprapubic catheters are left to gravity until the next postoperative morning, when the Foley catheter and vaginal pack are removed, and the suprapubic catheter is clamped. The patient is allowed to void immediately postoperatively, and postvoid residual urines are measured. When the residual is consistently less than 50 ml, the suprapubic tube is removed.

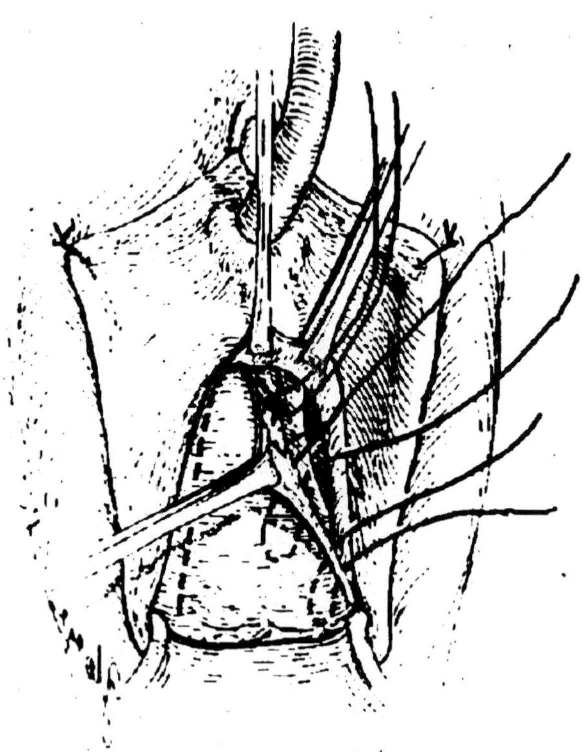

Figure 32–20. The six-corner suspension demonstrating the position of the line of incision (patient's right) and the sutures before transfer (shown on the patient's left side). Note that the most inferior pair of sutures is placed at the level of the vaginal cuff (if there was a prior hysterectomy) or cervix. The two anterior Prolene sutures are placed in the same manner as the vaginal wall sling.

Repair of Grade 4 Cystocele with Combined Central and Lateral Defects, with the Goalpost Incision

Grade 4 cystocele implies prolapse of the bladder outside the introitus at rest. **Generally, this defect involves three specific problems: urethral hypermobility, a lateral defect, and a central defect.** These three defects are repaired in one operation.

TECHNIQUE. Repair of a grade 4 cystocele is begun with placement of a suprapubic tube and a urethral Foley catheter with the patient in lithotomy position. The anterior vaginal wall is infiltrated with saline, and a "goalpost" incision is made with the arms distal and the incision extending proximally to the level of the vaginal cuff or paracervical area. This incision creates an island of vaginal wall tissue, which is used to create a hammock of support for the urethra (Fig. 32–21*A*). The dissection is begun in the midline, removing the vaginal wall to expose the underlying vesicopelvic fascia (Fig. 32–21*B*). Care must be taken not to perforate the bladder during this part of the dissection. The entire bladder base is exposed, and dissection is continued laterally until the attachments of the vesicopelvic fascia into the tendinous arc are encountered. **Before entering the retropubic space, the operator should identify the following landmarks, which indicate the margins of the dissection: (1) the junction of the periurethral fascia with the tendinous arcs distally, (2) the junction of the bladder with the midline peritoneal folds (if prior hysterectomy) or cervix proximally, and (3) the attachment of the vesicopelvic fascia to the tendinous arc laterally** (see Fig. 32–21*B*). During this dissection, careful attention should be paid to the possibility of a coexistent enterocele, and, if indicated, enterocele repair should proceed at this stage. The retropubic space is entered, exposing the urethropelvic ligament in a manner similar to that of the vaginal wall sling. The midurethral and lateral defects can now be repaired with Prolene sutures while the central defect is closed with absorbable mattress sutures. First, a proximal set of helical No. 1 Prolene sutures is used to incorporate the freed lateral edge of the urethropelvic ligament, the vesicopelvic fascia, and the cardinal/sacrouterine ligaments. A second set of No. 1 Prolene sutures is placed to include the freed lateral edge of the urethropelvic ligament, the levator complex at its inserts into the midurethra, and the "island" of vaginal wall excluding the epithelium (Fig. 32–21*C*). **De novo stress incontinence may occur postoperatively if the urethra is left with poor support** (Raz et al, 1991). A suprapubic puncture is made, and the four Prolene sutures are passed to the rectus fascia with the double-pronged ligature carrier. The Prolene sutures are not tied at this time. These maneuvers constitute the repair of the lateral defect and the modified vaginal sling. They provide support for the lateral defect, the bladder neck, and the urethra.

Attention is then turned to the central defect. The central defect is reduced with a small folded Dexon mesh and held in place by the Haney retractor until the mattress sutures are

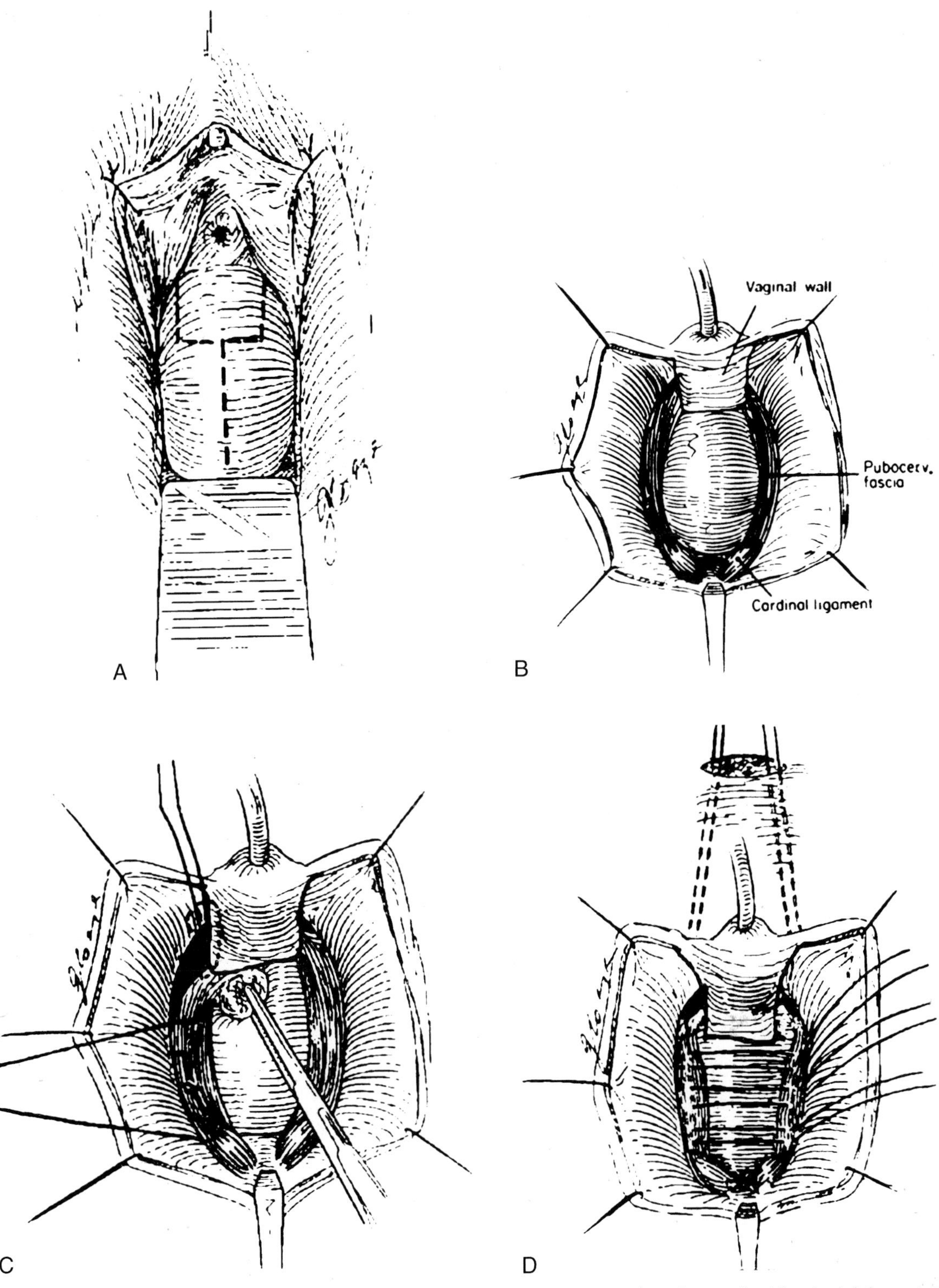

Figure 32–21. The technique for repair of grade 4 cystocele using a goalpost incision to repair lateral, central, midurethral defects. *A,* The incision for a grade 4 cystocele is shown. The goalpost incision facilitates central dissection over the cystocele (the midline "post" portion of the incision), while the arms of the goalpost provide exposure to the urethropelvic ligament and create an "island" of tissue for the sling. *B,* The anatomic boundaries following completed dissection. *C,* Placement of No. 1 Prolene sutures for the repair of the lateral defect and modified vaginal wall sling (before transfer). *D,* Repair of the central defect with horizontal mattress sutures (mesh not depicted).

placed. A single 2-0 polyglycolic acid suture is placed distally to reapproximate the cardinal ligaments. These two maneuvers not only reduce the central defect but also expose the infolded edges of the vesicopelvic fascia into which the mattress sutures are placed. Multiple mattress sutures of 2-0 Vicryl are used to reapproximate the infolded edges of the vesicopelvic fascia and tied down, thereby burying the folded Dexon mesh (Fig. 32–21*D*). The central defect is now corrected.

Indigo carmine is administered, and cystoscopy is carried out as in the vaginal wall sling. The excess vaginal wall is excised, and the edges of the vaginal wall are closed with a running interlocking 2-0 Vicryl suture. A vaginal pack is placed. Lastly the Prolene suspension sutures are tied down without tension against the rectus fascia, and the suprapubic wound is closed with 4-0 subcuticular Vicryl suture.

POSTOPERATIVE CARE. Postoperative care is similar to that for the six-corner suspension.

COMPLICATIONS. Many complications of cystocele repair can be avoided at the time of surgery by careful anatomic dissection and intraoperative cystoscopy. The most frequent complications include de novo urgency incontinence (14%), de novo stress incontinence (2%), and recurrent cystocele. Urinary retention, ureteral obstruction, inadvertent cystotomy, and significant bleeding rarely occur (Raz et al, 1991; Stothers et al, 1995).

Posterior Vaginal Wall Prolapse: Rectocele and Perineal Repair

Definition and Pathophysiology

A rectocele, or herniation of the rectum into the vagina, is the result of a defect in the supporting fascia of the rectum. The layers of this fascial support include the prerectal fascia, the pararectal fascia, and the rectovaginal septum. Perineal body defects represent an abnormality of the structure of the perineal body generally encountered following vaginal delivery or episiotomy (see Table 32–5).

Symptoms

Symptoms of isolated defects in the posterior wall are related to problems with bowel function and intercourse. Perineal body defects are generally asymptomatic; signs, when present, may include incontinence of liquid stool, flatus, or interference with intercourse. Symptoms associated with a rectocele include a sensation of fullness in the vagina, a mass bulging through the entroitus, and dyspareunia. **Constipation** can be a significant problem; occasionally, patients manually reduce their rectocele to improve bowel emptying.

Diagnosis

The diagnosis of a posterior wall defect is made on physical examination. Inspection reveals **perineal body defects**, which are associated with a widened or gaping introitus and a decreased distance between the anus and the posterior aspect of the vagina. A rectocele is manifest as a **bulge extending from the posterior wall of the vagina**. This may be well seen with a Sims speculum or half-speculum placed anteriorly, supporting the anterior vaginal wall and bladder while the patient strains. **Digital examination** with one finger in the vagina and one finger in the rectum **reveals attenuation of the dividing fascia**. With both rectocele and perineal body defects, loss of the normal right-angle configuration of the lower and upper vagina is seen. When the patient is examined in the lithotomy or supine position, the vagina assumes a straight orientation rather than the normal posterior orientation directed toward the sacrum. Advancements in the techniques of defecography and dynamic rectal radiologic examinations have aided in the understanding of the pathophysiology of rectoceles and are used by some authors in the diagnosis and classification of posterior vault defects (Mellgren et al, 1994; Wiersma et al, 1994; Sentovich et al, 1995).

Surgical Treatment

Adequate repair of a rectocele incorporates three goals: (1) plication of the prerectal and pararectal fascia, (2) reconstruction of the levator hiatus, and (3) repair of the perineal body. These maneuvers together reconstruct the rectovaginal septum and restore the levator plate. The goal of reconstruction of the perineal body is to reanchor the muscles of the lower vagina and perineum and thus to restore support to the lower vagina and introitus.

The patient undergoes a lower bowel preparation with oral laxatives and enemas and is administered preoperative intravenous antibiotics. The patient is placed in the dorsal lithotomy position, and the rectum is packed with a Betadine-soaked gauze and isolated from the operative field with double draping. A Foley catheter is placed and the bladder retracted upward with a Deaver retractor. **Use of an anterior retractor helps prevent excessive vaginal wall tissue excision, which could result in vaginal stenosis.** A ring retractor is applied to the perineum with hooks aiding in lateral exposure of the vaginal vault (Raz, 1992).

To expose the perineal body for repair, two Allis clamps are applied to the posterior margin of the introitus at the 5-o'clock and 7-o'clock positions. With the use of a V-shaped incision, a triangular flap of the mucocutaneous junction is excised (Fig. 32–22*A*). Next, two Allis clamps are used to grasp the rectocele, and the posterior vaginal wall is infiltrated with saline solution. An inverted V incision is made just through the epithelium at the level of the rectocele. Sharp dissection with Metzenbaum scissors is used to develop the plane between the herniated rectal wall and the vaginal wall, exposing the attenuated prerectal fascia. This dissection hugs the vaginal wall to avoid injury to the rectum. The dissection extends laterally to expose the pararectal fascia and is carried to the level of the apex of the vagina. The isolated triangle of vaginal wall is then excised (Fig. 32–22*B*).

At this point, attention is turned toward reconstruction. The rectum is retracted downward with a Deaver retractor, which reduces the rectocele and facilitates reapproximation of the pararectal and prerectal fascia. A running interlocking 2-0 Vicryl suture begins at the apex of the vaginal incision and is carried down to the level of the levator hiatus. This suture incorporates the edges of the vaginal wall and a generous bite of the right and left pararectal fascia as well

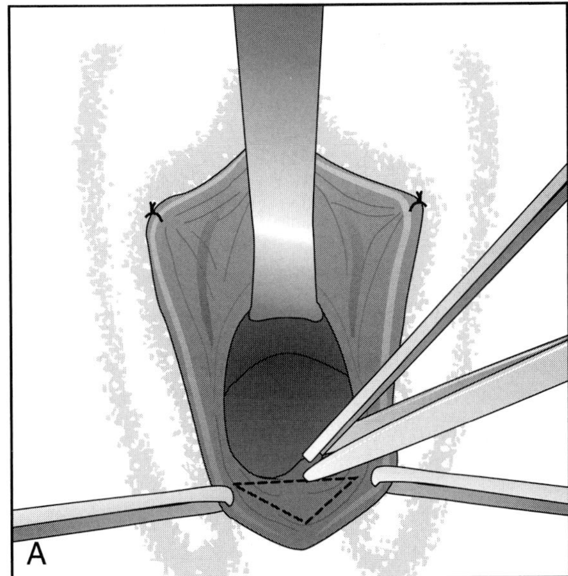

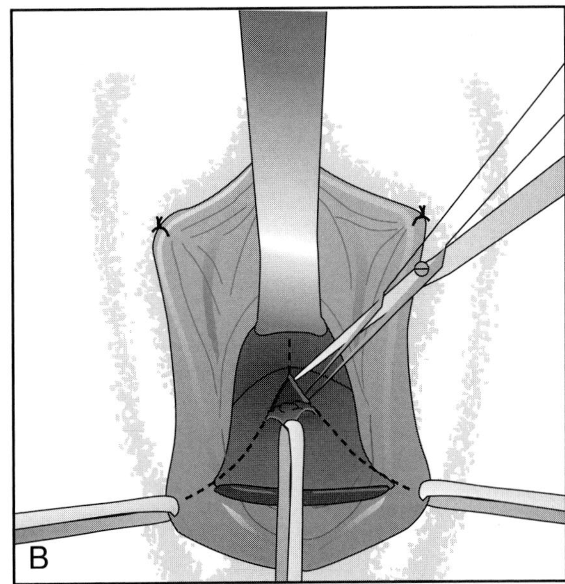

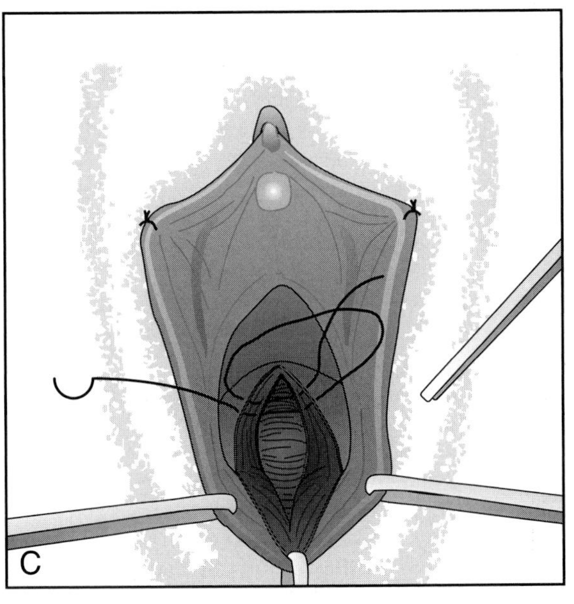

Figure 32–22. Rectocele and perineal body repair. *A,* Excision of mucocutaneous junction. Note that the two Allis clamps are placed so that when they are brought together in the midline, the introitus readily admists two fingers. *B,* Following the inverted V–shaped incision made over the rectocele, lateral dissection is carried out to expose the pararectal fascia. Slight traction is applied by the Allis clamps to facilitate the lateral dissection. In the case in which the rectocele continues toward the apex of the vagina, the incision should be extended toward the apex of the vagina in the midline. Following dissection, excision of the island of posterior vaginal wall tissue is completed. *C,* Repair of posterior wall of vagina with a small bite of vaginal wall and large bite of pararectal and prerectal fascia. The rectal wall is initially retracted downward by a posteriorly placed Deaver retractor (not shown), which facilitates exposure of the pararectal fascia and protects the rectal wall.

as the prerectal fascia (Fig. 32–22*C*). The levators are included in the distal one third of the closure, which is carried down to the transverse perineal incision.

Finally, the perineal body is reconstructed. One or two horizontal mattress sutures of 2-0 Vicryl are used to approximate the bulbocavernosus muscles, the transverse perineal muscles, and the levator complex. **Restoration of the normal axis of the vagina should be noted at the completion of the procedure, and the posterior floor should have a smooth contour.** The perineal skin is closed with a running 4-0 Vicryl suture, and a vaginal pack is placed for 12 to 24 hours.

Enterocele and Prolapse of the Vaginal Vault

Definition and Classification

An enterocele is defined as a herniation of the peritoneum and its contents at the level of the vaginal apex. Although this form of prolapse may occur in isolation, 75% of cases are associated with some degree of vault prolapse.

Enteroceles are classically divided into four types (Nichols, 1992). **Congenital enteroceles** result from failure of fusion of the layers of peritoneum at the level of the rectovaginal septum. In this situation, there is no cystocele or rectocele. **Traction enteroceles** occur when prolapse of the vaginal vault or uterus pulls the peritoneum caudally. **Pulsion enteroceles** exist when chronic pressure is exerted on the vault of the vagina (Zacharin, 1980). This pressure creates a hernia sac and often pushes the vaginal vault in a caudad fashion. As such, pulsion enteroceles represent a sliding-type hernia with the vaginal vault and anterior vaginal wall sliding on the anterior surface of the rectum (Sanz, 1988). This type of enterocele is unusual in patients with a uterus, and therefore prolapse of the uterus is rarely associated. **Iatrogenic enteroceles** follow a surgically induced change in vaginal axis, leaving the cul-de-sac unprotected. This type of enterocele is classically seen after colposuspension; indeed, **the incidence of enterocele after the Burch**

procedure may be as high as 26.7% (Stanton and Cardozo, 1979; Wiskind et al, 1992). To avoid secondary prolapse, the cul-de-sac should be closed at the time of the Burch colposuspension.

The authors use an alternative classification of enteroceles based on anatomic findings at the time of physical examination because these findings eventually determine the course of treatment. The majority of enteroceles occur in the post-hysterectomy patient, and thus the authors divide patients into categories based on the presence or absence of vault prolapse. **Simple enteroceles** exist when there is no vault prolapse and the cuff is well supported. No cystocele or rectocele is found. **Complex enteroceles** are associated with vault or uterine prolapse. The cuff is poorly supported, and prolapse may include either the anterior wall of the vagina (cystocele) or the posterior wall (rectocele) (Lee, 1993; Raz et al, 1993).

Symptoms

Enteroceles are minimally symptomatic until descent reaches the grade 2 hymenal level (Baden and Walker, 1992). At this point, the patient may begin to complain of a sensation of **fullness in the perineal area. Dyspareunia, vaginal discomfort, and low back discomfort accentuated in the standing position** are common. Rarely, complications of **bowel obstruction** may be found. If rectocele and cystocele are coexisting problems, constipation and urinary complaints may also be present.

Diagnosis and Evaluation

Diagnosis of an enterocele is made based on physical examination. Observation of the introitus may reveal a bulging mass. Bimanual examination may reveal a herniating sac at the apex of the vagina. During the rectovaginal examination, straining often reveals an impulse of the enterocele sac against the fingertip. This mass classically is found posterior to the cervix (in cases of hysterectomy, this sac is found at the apex of the vagina). Bimanual examination also often reveals thickness of the high rectal-vaginal septum. Difficulty may be encountered in differentiating an enterocele from a high rectocele; indeed, these conditions are often found together. When attempting to establish this differential diagnosis, it is helpful to appreciate that the posterior vaginal wall is approximately 8 to 9 cm in length from its apex to the level of the hymen. With some degree of accuracy, the wall can be divided into segments of 3 cm each. The proximal 3 cm is the cul-de-sac floor, the middle 3 cm is the rectum, and the distal 3 cm is the perineal body (Baden and Walker, 1992). Classically, if both an enterocele and a high rectocele are present, a small furrow is seen dividing the two. A half-speculum should be placed on the posterior vaginal wall and slowly withdrawn as the patient is asked to bear down. This maneuver usually reveals the site of the hernia.

Radiographic examination with a kidney, ureter, and bladder film may reveal bowel gas in the prolapsing mass. A stress **voiding cystourethrogram rules out the bladder as a source of the mass**.

Surgical Therapy

Five principles are involved in enterocele repair: (1) Identify the probable cause of the enterocele, (2) mobilize and excise the entire sac with ligation as cephalad as possible to preserve vaginal depth, (3) approximate and secure the cardinal and sacrouterine ligaments in the midline, (4) support the vaginal cuff (through sacrospinous fixation or vault suspension), and **(5) correct concurrent prolapse** (rectocele, cystocele, perineal separation).

The authors prefer the vaginal approach because it allows broader treatment of the many manifestations of vaginal prolapse (e.g., repair of cystocele, rectocele, bladder neck suspension). **If a vaginal approach is chosen, the surgical procedure of choice depends on the presence or absence of associated vault prolapse** (Fig. 32–23). The abdominal approach is appropriate if coexistent pathology mandates an intrapelvic view of the anatomy.

VAGINAL REPAIR OF A SIMPLE ENTEROCELE

The patient is prepared and draped as for rectocele repair, and enterocele repair proceeds as depicted in Figure 32–24. The enterocele is grasped with two Allis clamps, and normal saline is injected to facilitate dissection. A vertical incision is performed in the vaginal wall over the bulging hernia (Fig. 32–24*A*). (When there is significant descent of the uterus, or the cervix alone is present, the enterocele repair is performed in conjunction with hysterectomy.) After the vaginal wall is incised and dissected laterally, the peritoneal hernia sac is defined and separated from the vaginal wall, bladder, and rectum through sharp dissection. The sac is opened, and its contents are reduced to facilitate definition of the peritoneum and the neck of the hernia sac (Fig. 32–24*B*). A small, moist laparotomy pad is temporarily inserted into the peritoneal cavity to protect the bowel during obliteration of the enterocele.

To close the apex of the vault, two modified McCall sutures (Wall, 1994) and two purse-string sutures are placed (Fig. 32–24*C*, *D*). After all sutures have been carefully placed, the purse-string sutures are tied in a proximal-to-distal direction, thus obliterating the space of Douglas. The remainder of the peritoneal sac is suture-ligated at its base and excised. The excess vaginal wall is excised and then closed with a running 2-0 Vicryl suture, incorporating the area of underlying repair to eliminate any dead space. It is important that the preplaced sutures that included the sacrouterine complex, the prerectal fascia, and rectal wall (the modified **McCall sutures), be tied last** because these elevate the cuff away from the operator, making subsequent closure of the vaginal wall difficult. A vaginal packing is placed for 24 hours.

VAGINAL REPAIR OF COMPLEX ENTEROCELES

ENTEROCELE AND MODERATE CYSTOCELE WITH MAINLY LATERAL DEFECT. The first steps of the operation are similar to those for simple enterocele repair. After completion of the enterocele repair, the vaginal wall is not closed. The anchoring sutures of the sacrouterine and cardinal complex are left tagged on a clamp after being tied. At this point, the procedure becomes identical to that

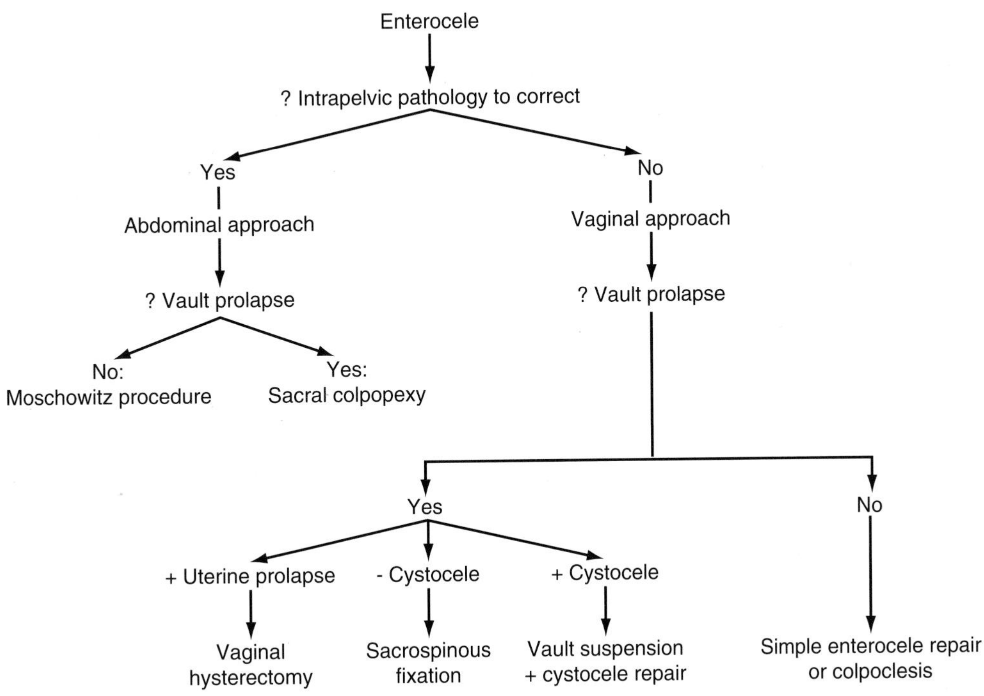

Figure 32–23. Suggested clinical pathway to evaluate and select operative therapy for enterocele.

for repair of cystocele with lateral defect, and the reader is referred to that section for illustrations of the repair.

ENTEROCELE WITH GRADE 4 CYSTOCELE. If the cystocele is severe (grade 4), the surgeon begins with a goalpost incision in the anterior vaginal wall. The bladder base is exposed, and the retropubic space is opened as described for grade 4 cystocele repair. The enterocele sac is now dissected from the posterior aspect of the bladder, the sac opened, and the intra-abdominal contents reduced. Two purse-string and two McCall sutures are applied to the vault as in a simple enterocele repair. The purse-string sutures are tied in a sequential fashion, thus closing the cul-de-sac. The sacrouterine and cardinal ligament sutures are tagged with a clamp. The excess peritoneal sac is excised, and grade 4 cystocele repair is completed as previously described.

Sacrospinalis Fixation of Vault Prolapse

In cases of massive vaginal vault prolapse, when there is limited cardinal and uterosacral ligament strength, the transvaginal sacrospinalis vaginal suspension is a suitable procedure for restoration of a functional vagina. **The authors restrict the use of this procedure for patients with vault prolapse without concomitant cystocele** (no surgery required to the anterior vaginal wall). Because of the potential for bowel injury, patients who undergo this repair must have proper bowel preparation and perioperative intravenous antibiotics.

SURGICAL TECHNIQUE. The patient is placed in a dorsal lithotomy position. The lower abdomen and vagina are prepared and draped in a sterile fashion. The rectum is packed with Betadine-impregnated lubricated gauze and then isolated from the operative field. The bladder is drained with a suprapubic cystostomy or a urethral catheter. A ring retractor is positioned, and the hooks are applied to the vaginal introitus.

A longitudinal incision is made over the enterocele sac extending to the posterior vaginal wall. The enterocele sac is exposed and dissected free from the vaginal, bladder, and rectal walls. In the posterior vaginal wall, dissection is carried out laterally over the prerectal fascia. Either the right or left rectal pillar is penetrated to expose the pararectal space and the coccygeus muscle, which overlies the sacrospinous ligament (Fig. 32–25). Deep retractors such as the Breisky-Navratil are required to retract the rectum medially and displace the bladder and peritoneum anteriorly. Loose areolar tissue is pushed to one side, and the pelvic surface of the coccygeus muscle is identified running posterolaterally from the ischial spine toward the sacrum. Buried within this muscle is the sacrospinalis ligament. **It is unnecessary, difficult, and potentially dangerous to dissect the coccygeus muscle from the sacrospinous ligament.**

The **sacrospinalis ligaments** run between the ischial spine and the lateral side of the sacrum in close proximity to a number of vital vessels and nerves. **The pudendal nerve and vessels are located just under the ischial spine, and any suture applied to the sacrospinous ligament should be placed 1 to 2 cm medial to the ischial spine to avoid injury to these structures. Sutures applied higher than the level of the ischial spine run the risk of injury to the sciatic nerve as it courses beneath the piriformis muscle.**

With the use of a long needle holder, Deschamps ligature carrier, or a Mayo hook, two threads of No. 1 Vicryl are passed through the substance of the coccygeus muscle and the sacrospinal ligament at the predetermined point, 1 cm apart. Gentle traction on the free ends of the suture tests the strength of the anchor and essentially allows rocking of the patient over the operating table. It is necessary only to fix

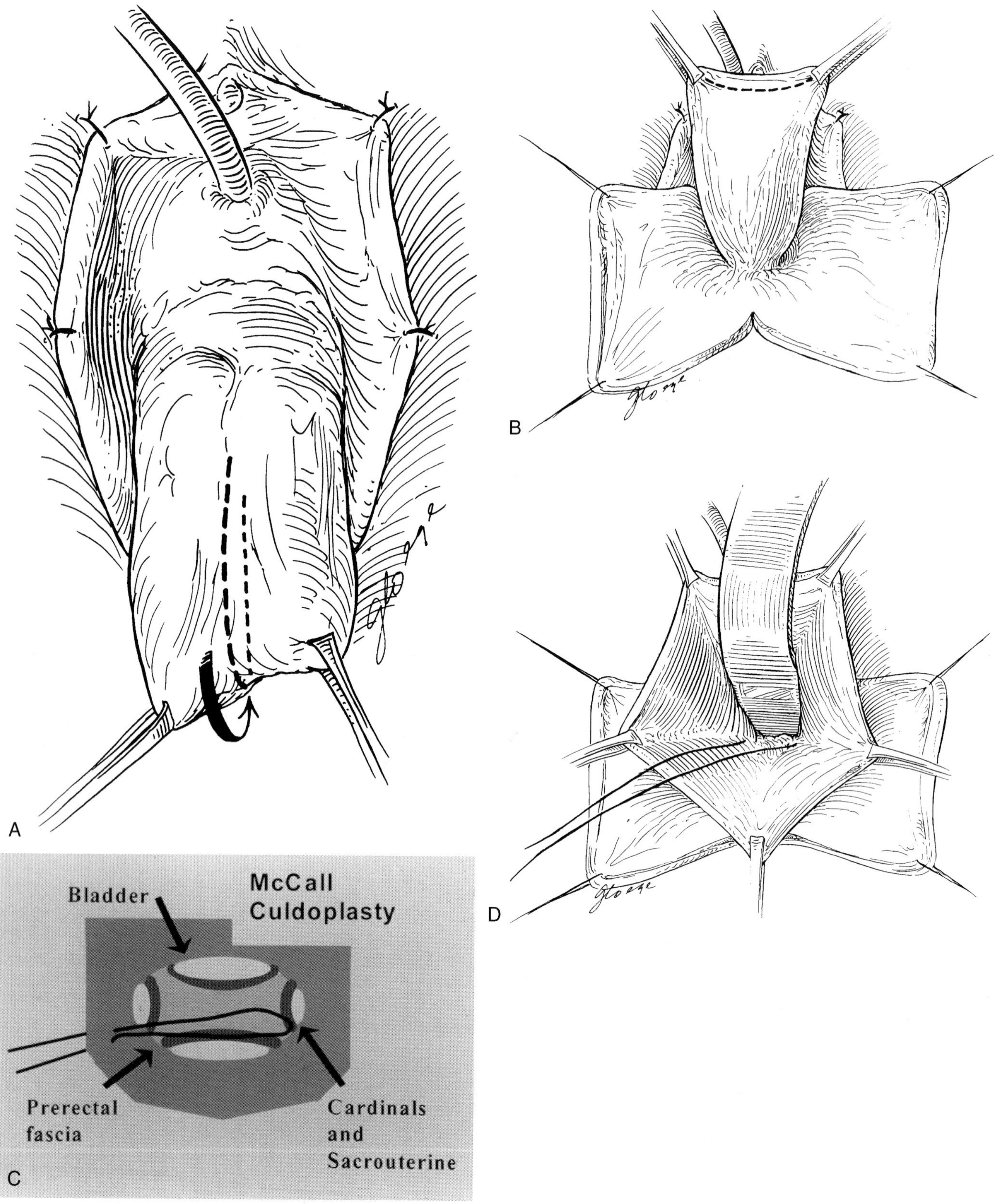

Figure 32–24. Surgical correction of a simple enterocele. *A,* Depiction of vertical incision and retraction of the enterocele with Allis clamps. *B,* After the vaginal wall is incised and dissected laterally, the peritoneal hernia sac is defined and separated from the vaginal wall, bladder, and rectum, using blunt and sharp dissection. The dotted line indicates the site where the sac is opened, following which any adhesions of the bowel are dissected free. *C,* A small lap pad is placed into the peritoneal cavity and a hand-held Deaver retractor used to protect the small bowel during the placement of the McCall sutures. Diagrammatic depiction of the McCall suture, which incorporates both sacrouterine/cardinal complexes and the prerectal fascia. The sutures are initially transferred from the vaginal lumen, through the vaginal wall into the peritoneal sac through the sacrouterine ligaments and back outside to the vaginal lumen. The sutures are secured with a clamp to be tied later. They are intended to provide depth and support to the vaginal cuff, relying on the strength of the sacrouterine ligaments. *D,* Two purse-string sutures of No. 1 Vicryl are placed proximal to the McCall sutures to close the peritoneal sac. They incorporate the prerectal fascia posteriorly, the sacrouterine and cardinal complex laterally, and the bladder base anteriorly. It is important to maintain protection of the bladder base and trigone during placement of the sutures, which close the pouch of Douglas.

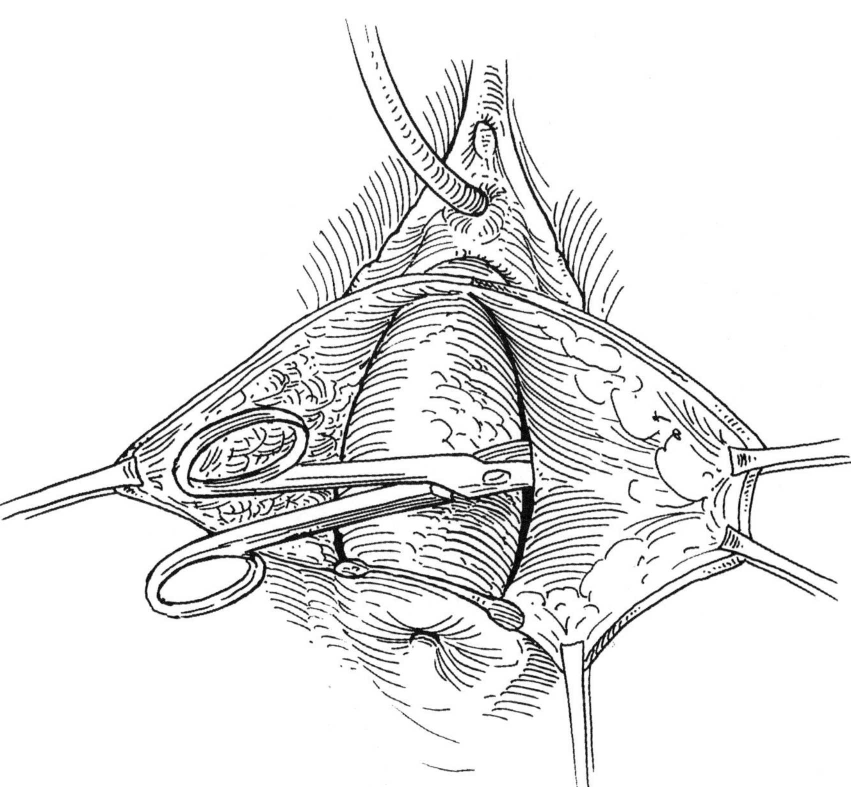

Figure 32–25. Sacrospinous fixation to correct vault prolapse with a vaginal approach. A longitudinal incision is made in the posterior vaginal wall, exposing the prerectal fascia. Either the right or the left rectal pillar, which separates the rectovaginal space from the pararectal space, is penetrated by blunt or sharp dissection as shown. The pararectal space is beneath the peritoneum and above the levator floor. The opening in the rectal pillar is widened, exposing the superior surface of the pelvic diaphragm, including the coccygeus muscle, which contains the sacrospinal ligament.

the vault to either the right or the left sacrospinous ligament. The two free ends of the sutures are left on a clamp for use at the end of the operation.

Attention is now turned to the enterocele sac, which is opened. Two purse-string sutures are applied as in a simple enterocele repair and left untied. Rather than excise the redundant vaginal wall, it is left in situ, and the ends of the two sutures in the sacrospinous ligament are individually passed through the full thickness of the vaginal wall at the dome with the use of a free needle with the threads emerging on the ipsilateral epithelial side. The two sutures are placed in healthy vaginal tissue that is not traversed by an incision or suture line with a distance of 1 to 2 cm between the two. The sacrospinous ligament sutures are temporarily left untied and secured with a clamp. The purse-string sutures are now tied down to close the vault. **The previously placed sutures in the sacrospinous ligament are tied, with the vaginal vault being directed under finger guidance to the uppermost position, where a square knot of the suspension sutures affixes it to the sacrospinous ligament on one side.** Patients are cared for postoperatively as for enterocele repair, and vaginal intercourse is restricted for 12 weeks (Chopra et al, 1996).

COMPLICATIONS. Significant bleeding can be encountered if the levator is damaged or if the pudendal vessels are penetrated. A branch of the internal iliac venous system can be injured as well. **Pudendal nerve injury** may occur if the sutures are placed too laterally; the **sciatic nerve** may be injured if sutures are placed too cephalad (in the area of the piriformis). Another potential complication is **rectal injury** during the dissection or retraction of the pararectal space (this surgery should be performed under a complete lower bowel preparation and parenteral antibiotics). Successful primary repair of a small rectal enterotomy has been reported (Sauer and Klutke, 1995). **Ureteric injury** may occur because of the severe distortion of pelvic anatomy associated with significant prolapse. Postoperatively, some patients may complain of low back pain radiating to the back of the thigh following the procedure. This is a self-limiting phenomenon that should respond to analgesics and time. **Vaginal narrowing** (7%) and **pelvic cellulitis** (2%) may occur (Backer, 1992).

OUTCOME. Recurrent prolapse of the vaginal dome may occur because of tissue laxity or poor anchoring of the vaginal dome into the sacrospinous ligament itself. Rates of recurrent vault prolapse are reported between 0 and 20% (Backer, 1992; Carey and Slack, 1994; Holley et al, 1995; Sauer and Klutke, 1995). Dyspareunia is rare (Carey and Slack, 1994). In long-term follow-up (median 42 months), Holley and co-workers found enterocele formation in 6% and rectoceles in 17% of patients treated with sacrospinalis fixation (Holley et al, 1995). Although recurrent sacrospinalis fixation has been reported in cases of recurrent vault prolapse, an abdominal approach should be considered.

Abdominal Repairs of Enterocele and Vault Prolapse

MOSCHCOWITZ'S PROCEDURE. The Moschcowitz procedure was initially designed to treat rectal prolapse by securing the rectum to the relatively fixed vagina (Moschcowitz, 1912). The identical logic has been used to fix the vagina in place by securing it to the rectum. Unfortunately the rectum is frequently not well secured in place. The goal of the Moschcowitz procedure is to **close the cul-de-sac through placement of a series of purse-string sutures with the use of abdominal exposure**.

The patient is placed in the frog-leg or abdominoperineal position, and laparotomy is performed. If the uterus is present, it is grasped and pulled forward to expose the pouch of Douglas. If the uterus is absent, the posterior wall of the vagina is grasped with Allis clamps and held anteriorly under traction. Starting at the base of the sac, purse-string sutures of No. 2-0 Vicryl are placed to close the cul-de-sac of Douglas, incorporating any remnants of the uterosacral ligaments, serosa of the vagina, lateral peritoneum, and superficial serosal surface of the rectum. The sutures are then successively tied without excessive tension. Special care is taken to avoid ureteral injury. Modifications of this technique include two concentric series of purse-strings that close the cul-de-sac on either side of the rectum rather than in the midline (Thompson, 1992) and laparoscopic approaches.

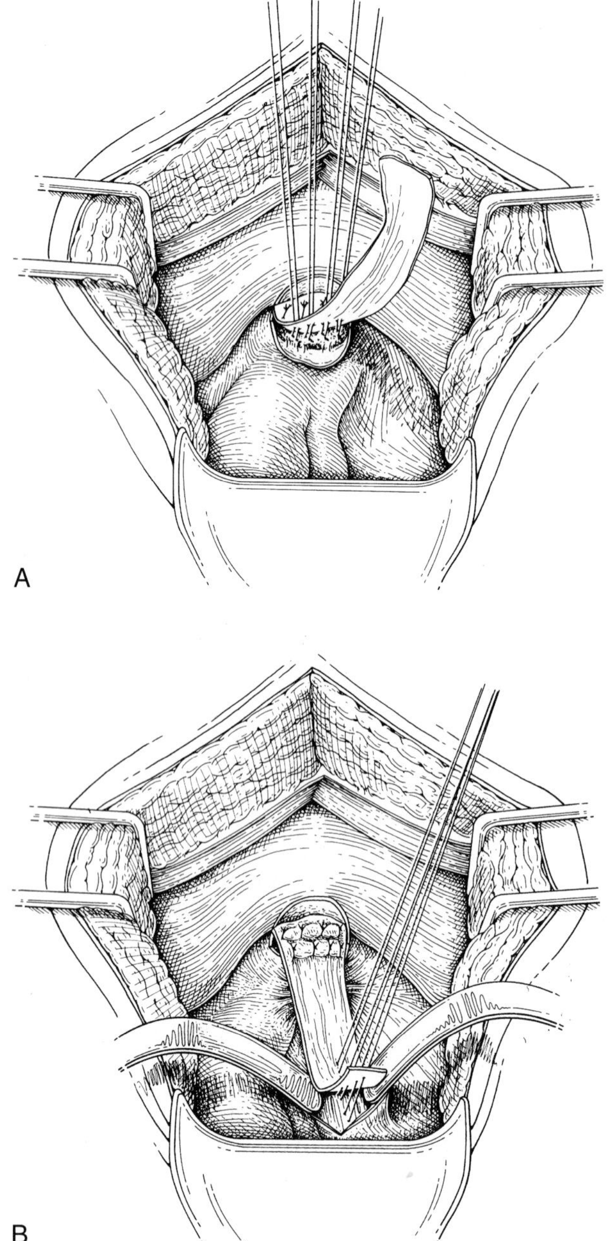

Figure 32–26. Abdominal approach to the correction of vault prolapse as described by Nichols. *A*, Following closure of the cul-de-sac, using the Moschcowitz technique, the fascial graft is attached to the vaginal apex with interrupted 2-0 Vicryl suture. The graft, now attached to the vaginal apex, is measured and trimmed such that sutures placed into the anterior sacral fascia result in the graft being taut. *B*, The posterior parietal peritoneum over the sacrum is incised longitudinally below the level of S3. The periosteum is exposed, taking care to avoid injury to the presacral blood vessels. Several permanent interrupted sutures are placed 1 cm apart overlying the S3 and S4 vertebrae. These are secured to the graft, resulting in support of the vaginal apex. Care should be taken not to constrict the sigmoid colon. (From Thompson JD, Rock JA, eds: Te Linde's Operative Gynecology, 7th ed. Philadelphia, J. B. Lippincott, 1992, pp 882–883.)

SACROCOLPOPEXY. Transabdominal vault suspension techniques include sacrocolpopexy, in which **the vault or uterus is fixed or directed to the sacrum at the S3–S4 level**. This technique may be performed with the use of a graft of rectus fascia or synthetic material if there is inadequate length to appose the vaginal vault directly to the sacral promontory. **If concurrent repair of cystocele or rectocele is planned, these should be performed first transvaginally because repair of these lesions after colpopexy is technically difficult**. Finally, it is vital that the surgeon accurately assess the presence or absence of perineal or rectal abnormalities because failure to repair these may compromise the long-term results of the repair.

One technique of repair is described by Nichols (1992) and depicted in Figure 32–26. The bladder is drained with a Foley catheter, following which laparotomy is performed with the patient in the dorsal lithotomy position. A rectus fascial graft measuring 2 × 10 cm is harvested for later use. The peritoneal cavity is entered, a self-retaining retractor placed, and the bowel packed out of the field. The vaginal apex is grasped with two Allis clamps and gentle superior traction placed. The peritoneum overlying the vaginal apex is incised, and the bladder and rectum are sharply dissected away, exposing at least a 3 × 4 cm area of vaginal wall. With one hand in the vagina to aid exposure, four figure-of-eight Tevdek sutures are placed in the full thickness of the vaginal wall from one lateral fornix to the other. These sutures are left untied until both free ends of each suture are placed through one end of the fascial graft (Fig. 32–26*A*). Tying the sutures then secures one end of the graft. A second row of 2-0 Vicryl sutures is placed through the graft into the posterior vaginal wall for further security. Closure of the cul-de-sac is next performed with the use of the Moschcowitz technique. **This technique may be modified as a hemi-Moschcowitz on either side of the colon to avoid constriction of the sigmoid colon.** The parietal peritoneum over the sacrum is next opened longitudinally in the midline from the promontory to a point caudal to S3. The sacral fascia is exposed taking care to avoid the presacral vessels. The free end of the graft is secured to the presacral fascia without tension (Fig. 32–26*B*). Finally, **after closure of the anterior peritoneum, attention is turned toward suprapubic colpopexy** (Burch, 1961), **which minimizes the potential for postoperative stress incontinence.**

Uterine Prolapse

Hysterectomy is the second most common operation performed on women in the United States following cesarean section. In 1988, the National Center for Health Statistics reported that 578,000 hysterectomies were performed in the United States, of which 23% were performed through a vaginal approach (Copeland, 1993). Most urologic surgeons have some familiarity with techniques of abdominal hysterectomy, specifically as involved in anterior exenterative surgery. Uterine prolapse, however, is particularly suited to transvaginal hysterectomy. This section specifically addresses this indication for vaginal hysterectomy and does not take into account confounding factors such as bleeding or dysplasia or nonoperative forms of therapy.

Definition and Classification

Uterine prolapse is said to be present when there is uterine descent at rest or with straining. It is classified by grade in a fashion similar to that for cystocele (see Table 32–5). Increasing degrees of severity occur as structural supports in the pelvis fail. Initially, weakness of the uterosacral ligaments allows anterior movement of the cervix, and the position of the uterus over the levator plate is compromised. The axis of the uterus changes with the corpus swinging backward on a relatively fixed transverse axis. When this occurs, the intra-abdominal pressure falls on the anterior surface of the uterus, thus further exacerbating the retroversion and leading to the development of prolapse. Stress on the cardinal ligaments encourages prolapse by loss of the support over the levator plate.

Symptoms

Patients with grades 1 to 2 uterine prolapse may be **asymptomatic**. When symptomatic, **back pain**, classically aggravated by standing and decreasing in the recumbent position, may develop. With more severe grades of uterine prolapse, the patient often presents with a history of a **mass per vagina, pelvic pain, dyspareunia, urinary retention**, or associated **incontinence**.

Diagnosis

The diagnosis is established on physical examination by observing uterine descent at rest or with straining. Cervical erosions may be present when the cervix is exposed beyond the introitus. **The term *fourth-degree prolapse* or *procidentia* is used when the uterus extends outside the introitus. Progressive hydronephrosis has been reported in association with procidentia in 2% to 92% of cases** (Thompson, 1992). This renal dysfunction is **insidious in its onset**, and patients may present with **recurrent pyelonephritis, upper tract calculi, or signs of renal failure**.

Imaging modalities such as ultrasound may be required to fully evaluate upper tract function, particularly when procidentia is found. Pelvic ultrasound may also be used when uterine fibroids are present to assess their size and location.

Vaginal Hysterectomy

Indications

Many patients with prolapse will be seen by the physician for urinary complaints of incontinence, instability, or retention. Most will have a variety of anatomic defects, including cystocele, urethrocele, rectocele, and enterocele. These patients require a comprehensive plan of reconstruction. **Isolated repair of a cystocele or suspension of the bladder neck may aggravate pre-existing uterine prolapse**.

Whether or not hysterectomy is performed in the presence of a prolapsed uterus depends on the patient's symptoms, degree of prolapse, and desire to maintain fertility. Mildly symptomatic patients may require no therapy at all. Patients with severe prolapse, moderate prolapse and associated enterocele, or moderate prolapse and large cystocele and those with significant discomfort compose the ideal population for hysterectomy.

Contraindications

Specific contraindications to transvaginal hysterectomy include size disproportions (i.e., enlarged uterus, stenotic vagina), obliteration of the cul-de-sac, adnexal tumors, pelvic inflammatory disease, and malignancy of the uterus or ovaries (extrafascial vaginal hysterectomy may be done in selected patients with low-grade tumors of the uterus) (Nichols, 1989; Copeland, 1993). A history of endometriosis of unknown extent may be considered an absolute contraindication. To these contraindications, one must add the patient who has a strong desire to maintain fertility.

Surgical Technique

Pelvic examination under anesthesia should immediately precede hysterectomy to confirm earlier impressions regarding size of the uterus, mobility, position of the posterior cul-de-sac, and length and strength of the cardinal/uterosacral ligaments (Nichols, 1989). The clinician, at this time, appreciates the marked increase in relaxation of the ligamentous support during anesthesia. Minimal traction often reveals descent that is not clinically apparent in the awake patient. Attentive bimanual examination often reveals other pathology germane to the planned operation (i.e., enterocele, rectocele, cystocele, urethral hypermobility, perineal body laxity). The bony structure of the pelvis should be assessed to obtain some estimation of the degree of technical difficulty of transvaginal delivery of the uterus.

The patient is prepared and draped in the dorsal lithotomy position, and a tenaculum is used to grasp the cervix. If bladder neck suspension or cystocele repair is planned, a suprapubic tube is inserted at this point. A urethral catheter is inserted following which normal saline is injected around the cervix to help create cleavage planes.

A circumferential incision is made 1 cm proximal to the cervix and anterior dissection begun. It is important to note that sharp dissection of the bladder from the cervix is safer than blunt stripping. This dissection may be aided by anterior traction on the bladder and dissection with the scissors pointing toward the uterus. As the vesicoperitoneal fold is approached, the peritoneum becomes apparent. On occasion, the operator enters the wrong plane in attempting to stay as far away from the bladder as possible. This error is particularly likely if the initial incision has been made too close to the cervical os. In these instances, the surgeon may inadvertently mistake the peritoneum for the undersurface of the bladder. In a similar fashion, the posterior peritoneal fold is exposed as described in Figure 32–27*A*. The posterior peritoneum is opened sharply and the cul-de-sac explored through a small peritoneotomy for unsuspected adhesions, carcinoma, or other pathology. At times, the operator may have difficulty identifying the posterior cul-de-sac. In these instances, it is often advisable to begin the hysterectomy in an extraperitoneal fashion, initially severing the uterosacral and caudal portions of the cardinal ligaments close to the cervix. This maneuver allows the uterus to descend, providing better visualization. Once the posterior peritoneum is opened, the cardinal ligament and uterine artery are taken in suture ligatures on either side (Fig. 32–27*B*). Note that the uterine vessels should be ligated separately. The ends of the suture ligatures are left long and anchored to the grooves in the retractor ring. **Any traction on the cardinal ligaments implies traction on the uterine vessels. This maneuver brings the ureters closer to the operator's field.**

At this point, the uterus should be markedly mobile because the round ligaments provide little resistance to movement. **If free descent of the uterus does not occur, the surgeon should consider confounding factors, such as ventral fixation, endometriosis, adhesions, carcinoma, size disproportion, and fibrosis.**

The surgeon should next evert the uterus and open the

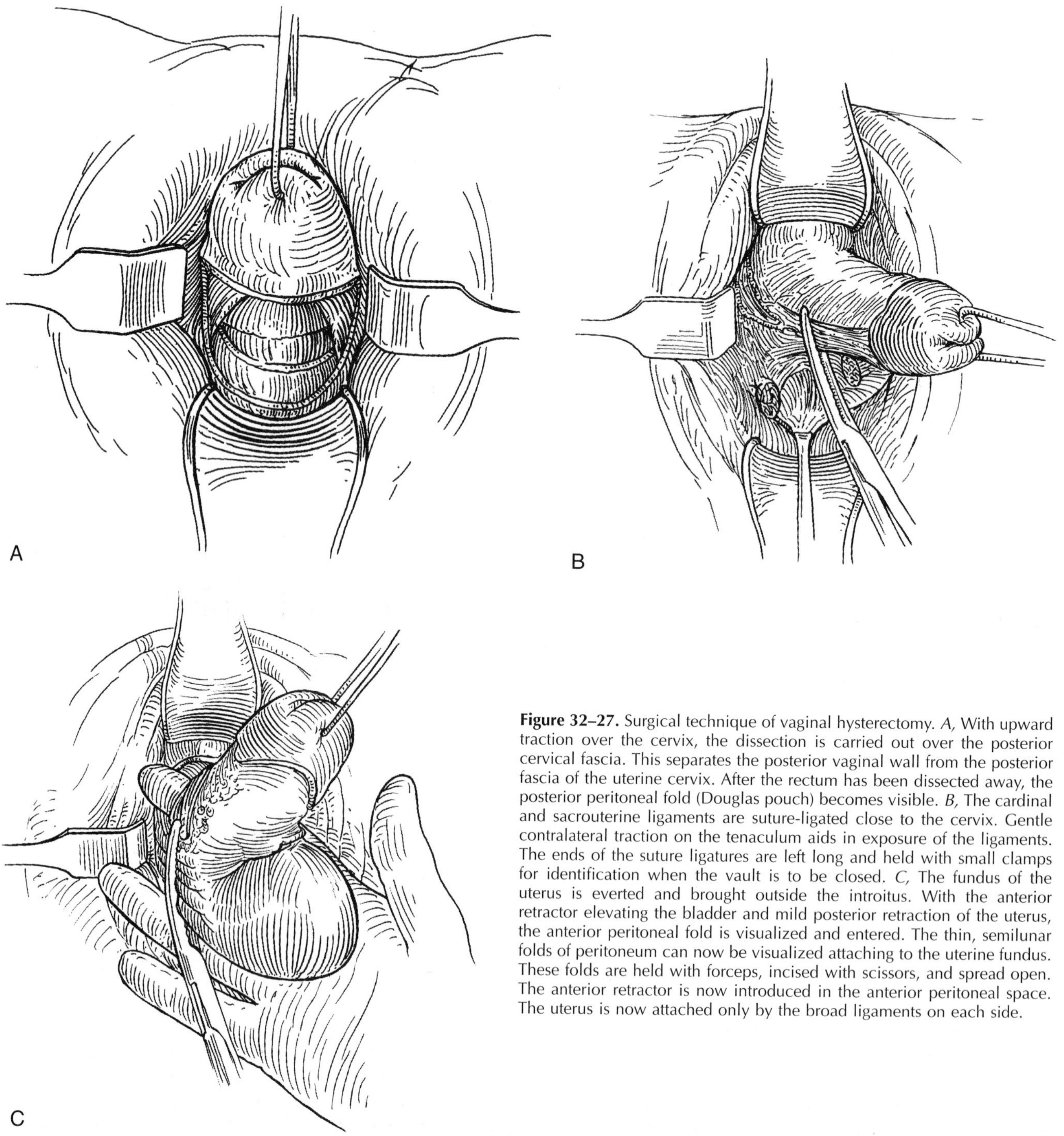

Figure 32–27. Surgical technique of vaginal hysterectomy. *A,* With upward traction over the cervix, the dissection is carried out over the posterior cervical fascia. This separates the posterior vaginal wall from the posterior fascia of the uterine cervix. After the rectum has been dissected away, the posterior peritoneal fold (Douglas pouch) becomes visible. *B,* The cardinal and sacrouterine ligaments are suture-ligated close to the cervix. Gentle contralateral traction on the tenaculum aids in exposure of the ligaments. The ends of the suture ligatures are left long and held with small clamps for identification when the vault is to be closed. *C,* The fundus of the uterus is everted and brought outside the introitus. With the anterior retractor elevating the bladder and mild posterior retraction of the uterus, the anterior peritoneal fold is visualized and entered. The thin, semilunar folds of peritoneum can now be visualized attaching to the uterine fundus. These folds are held with forceps, incised with scissors, and spread open. The anterior retractor is now introduced in the anterior peritoneal space. The uterus is now attached only by the broad ligaments on each side.

anterior peritoneum as shown in Figure 32–27*C*. This portion of the procedure entails the risk of inadvertent entry into the bladder. As such, it is advantageous to insert a finger over the fundus of the uterus to tent the anterior peritoneum. In this fashion, an incision can be made over the operator's finger, allowing safe entry.

Further parametrial ligation is undertaken to the level of the peritoneal folds (see Fig. 32–27*C*). The broad ligaments and their contents are suture-ligated, and the uterus is removed. Three pedicles are identified on each side: the broad ligaments, the cardinal ligaments, and the uterine arteries. Closure of the cul-de-sac is now completed by placing two purse-string sutures and two McCall culdoplasty sutures as previously described for simple enterocele repair. The tags on the broad ligaments and uterine arteries are tied in the midline, following which the purse-string sutures are gently tied. If simultaneous vaginal surgery is planned, it is now performed. The vaginal mucosa is closed with a running 2-0 Vicryl suture, following which the McCall sutures are tied last.

COMPLICATIONS

The Centers for Disease Control report that the overall complication rate associated with vaginal hysterectomy is 24.5% compared with 42.5% in patients undergoing abdominal hysterectomy (Dicker et al, 1982). The most commonly encountered complications include febrile illness (15.3%), bleeding requiring transfusion (8.3%), and unintended major surgical procedures (5.1%) (Dicker et al, 1982). **So long as the uterus is freely movable, the technical difficulty of the hysterectomy increases with increasing degree of prolapse owing to lack of consistent anatomy.**

Bladder and ureteral injury are less common during vaginal hysterectomy compared with abdominal hysterectomy (Hofmeister and Woifgram, 1962; Thompson, 1992a). Ureteral fistula (0.09%–0.5%), cystotomy (0.5%), and bladder fistulas (0.05%–0.6%) rarely occur. **The importance of anterior retraction of the bladder cannot be overemphasized; this maneuver protects the bladder, trigone, and ureters.**

POTENTIAL COMPLICATIONS OF VAGINAL SURGERY

The potential complications of transvaginal surgery are classified as intraoperative, postoperative, early, or late (Table 32–6). **The vast majority of complications are preventable, particularly when the operator is aware of the hazards and risk factors in any given patient based on his or her preoperative history, physical examination, and preoperative diagnostic tests.** Should a complication arise, early recognition and appropriate intervention can minimize any sequelae.

Table 32–6. CLASSIFICATION OF THE POTENTIAL COMPLICATIONS RELATED TO TRANSVAGINAL SURGERY

Intraoperative

- Hemorrhage
- Misplacement of suture or graft material
- Urethral injury
- Ureteral injuries
  - Ligation
  - Incision
  - Crush or clamp
  - Cautery/burn
- Bladder injuries
  - Incision/perforation
  - Suture related
  - Cautery/burn
- Small bowel injuries
  - Incision/perforation
  - Suture related
  - Cautery/burn
- Rectal injury
  - Incision/perforation
  - Suture related
  - Cautery/burn
- Neurologic injury
  - Motor
    - Pudendal nerve
    - Obturator nerve
    - Sciatic nerve
    - Peroneal nerve palsy
    - Femoral neuropraxia
    - Pudendal nerve
  - Sensory
    - Ilioinguinal
    - Genitofemoral
  - Lower limb compartment syndromes
  - Bladder denervation

Postoperative

- Early
  - Vaginal bleeding/discharge
  - Urinary tract infection (upper/lower)
  - Pain
    - Suprapubic
    - Vaginal
    - Rectal
  - Bladder dysfunction
    - Urinary retention
    - Recurrent stress urinary incontinence
    - De novo urgency incontinence
  - Infection of suture/graft material
  - Pelvic infection/abscess formation
  - Bladder/ureteral fistula formation
  - Embolism/thromboembolism/pulmonary embolism
- Late
  - Vaginal shortening
  - Vaginal stenosis
  - Dyspareunia
  - Osteitis pubis
  - Recurrent stress urinary incontinence
    - Enterocele
    - Cystocele
    - Rectocele
    - Uterine prolapse
    - Vault prolapse
  - Erosion of suture/graft material into vagina/urinary tract

Preoperative Considerations and Patient Preparation

A careful preoperative history should include the **known preoperative risk factors associated with the complications of vaginal surgery, including a past medical history of prior pelvic surgery, pelvic abscess, pelvic inflammatory disease, radiation, endometriosis, or pelvic malignancy, which increase the likelihood of pelvic scarring**

and adhesions. A knowledge of previous surgical procedures and their associated complications allows the surgeon to anticipate and avoid a recurrence of such problems.

In addition to a detailed pelvic and abdominal examination, a careful inspection of the neurologic status and respiratory and cadiovascular systems is completed. Patients with valvular abnormalities should receive prophylaxis against endocarditis according to the recommendations of the American Heart Association. **Patients with urogenital atrophy because of estrogen deficiency may be given hormone replacement therapy preoperatively.** Estrogens without progestin may be given to women without a uterus. When the patient has not had a hysterectomy, estrogens and progestins are advocated (Copeland, 1993). **Range of motion of the lower limbs is noted, and any physical abnormality that would prevent proper lithotomy positioning is noted because this contraindicates vaginal surgery**.

Both gynecologic and urologic indications for prophylactic antibiotics should be considered by the surgeon. **Gram-positive and -negative aerobes and anaerobes are indigenous to the vagina, and their relative contributions to the overall flora may change with the patient's age, sexual activity, and time of menstruation.** Bacteroides, streptococcus, and the coliforms are frequent pathologic organisms. Prophylactic antibiotics should always be given when vaginal hysterectomy is planned, because randomized, placebo-controlled trials have shown a decrease in febrile infection from 25% to 5% in patients receiving antibiotics (Hirsch, 1985).

Once the patient enters the operating room, **correct lithotomy positioning is critical to surgical exposure and prevention of complications**. After the feet are well padded and suspended in stirrups, the pelvis is pulled forward until the buttocks project slightly over the edge of the operating table. This ensures free mobility of the weighted vaginal speculum and produces a lumbar kyphosis, which makes the pelvic organs more accessible to the surgeon. Correct positioning of the hips can prevent femoral nerve palsy, which can occur when the hips are severely flexed and abducted.

It is prudent for the operator to remain alert to alterations in anatomy that may occur when instruments are applied to aid in exposure. For example, traction applied to the cervix with a tenaculum may distort the adjacent relationships of the bladder, ureters, and rectum. **During vaginal surgery, a symmetric approach should be maintained during dissection, frequently alternating from one side to another to avoid anatomic distortion.** Asymmetry may result in poor exposure, which can increase blood loss and result in loss of anatomic landmarks.

Specific Complications

Bleeding

Significant pelvic hematomas occur in less than 2% of patients; intraoperative bleeding requiring transfusion is exceedingly rare. A frequent cause of intraoperative bleeding is dissection in the wrong fascial plane, such as perforation of the urethropelvic ligament rather than dissection over its glistening surface during exposure. Bleeding may also occur when the retropubic space is entered if the point of entry is made too close to the urethra with subsequent injury to the periurethral vessels. Precise suture placement or the temporary placement of a pack into the retropubic space facilitates exposure and provides hemostasis. **Temporary packing is always preferable to the excessive use of electrocautery on the delicate tissues of the urethra, bladder, and ureter, which are easily injured by thermal burns.** Before closing any vaginal incisions, hemostasis should be achieved; excessive bleeding within the retropubic space should never be relied on to stop with simple closure of the vaginal wall. If packing does not control bleeding, transvaginal tamponade may be achieved by inflating a Foley balloon with 50 to 60 ml of water positioned over gauze packing in the vagina until hemostasis is achieved (Katske and Raz, 1987).

Postoperative spotting may occur for several weeks following vaginal surgery and is usually self-limited. If small amounts of vaginal bleeding persist, temporary placement of a vaginal pack generally is all that is required. **Significant postoperative hemorrhage within the retropubic space or peritoneal cavity is exceedingly rare and is heralded by hypotension, tachycardia, and a falling hematocrit in the absence of significant vaginal bleeding.** If this occurs, prompt resuscitation with fluids or transfusion (or both) is undertaken, and computed tomography scanning may help to locate the hematoma. If such bleeding persists, angiography with embolization or transabdominal exploration through a midline laparotomy incision may be required. The source of the bleeding should be isolated and suture-ligated. When the source is obscure, bilateral ligation of the internal iliac arteries may achieve hemostasis.

Neurologic Injury

Motor nerve injury ranges from minor (neurapraxia), requiring several weeks to recover, to the more serious forms of axonotmesis, which may take months to recover. **The most common motor nerve injury following vaginal surgery occurs to the common peroneal nerve, which can be compressed against the fibula head by improperly placed leg stirrups. Femoral, saphenous, and sciatic nerve injury may all result from improper positioning of the patient with hyperflexion of the hips** (Angermeir and Jordon, 1994). Femoral nerve injury results when the femoral nerve is compressed against the inguinal ligament, and saphenous nerve injury is created by stretching of the nerve against the medial aspect of the knee. **The obturator nerve may become compressed as it exits the obturator foramen, or it can be injured directly through lateral dissection within the retropubic space**. The sciatic nerve may be stretched or compressed as it exits the sciatic notch, or it may be entrapped in sutures placed near the internal iliac artery. **Pudendal nerve injury may follow sacrospinalis vault fixation**.

The most common sensory nerve injuries occur to the ilioinguinal and genitofemoral nerves, resulting in suprapubic and ipsilateral medial inner thigh pain. This complication has been reported to occur in 1% to 10% of patients following needle suspension procedures (Diaz et al, 1984; Stothers and Raz, 1996) and is prevented by transfer of sutures directly in the midline, passing the needle close to the pubis through the fixed region of the rectus fascia.

Bladder Injury

Bladder injury may result from misplaced or deep operative incisions over the anterior vaginal wall, misplaced sutures, perforation during suture transfer with the use of the double-pronged needle carrier, excessive electrocautery, or extreme medial displacement of the scissors when entering the retropubic space. Risk factors for bladder injury include a prior history of vaginal or pelvic surgery, radiation exposure, the period during grade 4 cystocele repair or reoperation for stress urinary incontinence, and existence of atrophic tissues secondary to hormonal deprivation. **Preventive measures include precise sharp dissection over the vesicopelvic fascia, transferring of sutures with the double-pronged needle carrier under fingertip control, and an adherence to important anatomic landmarks.** Cystotomy may be signified by gross hematuria through the urethral catheter or may be uncovered by the use of intraoperative indigo carmine and cystoscopy. If this occurs, any suture material that has perforated the bladder should be immediately removed, and the integrity of the ureters should be documented with retrograde pyelograms, if necessary. Any opening in the bladder should be immediately repaired in two layers while adhering to the principles of vesicovaginal fistula repair. The integrity of the bladder closure should be demonstrated after 10 days of drainage with a cystogram before catheter removal. The outcome of ten cystotomies during vaginal surgery with immediate closure and completion of the procedure disclosed no postoperative sequelae as reported by Hadley and Myers (1989).

Delayed recognition of suture material in the bladder may present as persistent urinary tract infection, bladder stone formation, or irritative voiding symptoms. If found, the suture material may be removed from the bladder with endoscopic scissors (Raz, 1992). An unrecognized bladder injury resulting in a vesicovaginal fistula may be repaired through a vaginal approach (Raz, 1992, Stothers and Raz, 1996).

Ureteral Injury

Injury to the ureter during vaginal surgery is reported to occur in between 0.1% and 1.5% of all cases (Mann et al, 1988; Raz, 1992). The incidence of ureteral injury during vaginal approaches to correct stress urinary incontinence alone is less than 0.1%. Only 20% to 30% present intraoperatively, whereas the remainder are recognized postoperatively. **Known preoperative risk factors for ureteral injury during vaginal surgery include a history of endometriosis, prior pelvic or vaginal surgery, and presence of pelvic prolapse (enterocele, large cystocele, or uterine procidentia).** Intraoperative recognition and repair of ureteral injury significantly decrease the incidence of postoperative renal loss compared with delayed recognition and repair (Thompson, 1992).

Intraoperatively the ureter may be injured through various mechanisms, including electrocautery, ligation, incision, crush, or clamping. During dissection, the position of the bladder neck and trigone should be verified by palpation of the balloon on the urethral Foley catheter. Intraoperative incisional injuries should be closed over an indwelling stent with the use of 4-0 or 5-0 interrupted absorbable sutures in a tension-free manner; a retropubic drain left should be in situ as with bladder injury. It is important to exit the drain through the lower abdomen and not the vagina, which minimizes the risk of secondary ureterovaginal fistula formation. Complete ligation, crush, or clamping injuries are best repaired with a ureteroureterostomy or ureteral reimplantation, which is most easily performed transabdominally. Incomplete clamp or suture injuries occur when the clamp or suture is removed within 30 minutes and the integrity of the ureter shown through retrograde pyelography. In these cases, a double-J stent may be inserted and should remain in place for a minimum of 10 days. Partial crush injuries, during which the tissue has remained avascular for greater than 30 minutes, are best repaired by excision of the avascular area and reimplantation and reconstruction as described for complete crush injuries.

The majority of ureteral insults present postoperatively with any combination of flank pain, costovertebral angle tenderness, fever, paralytic ileus, abdominal pain, vaginal drainage of urine, anuria, or an increased serum creatinine. The **diagnosis requires a high index of suspicion** and should be confirmed by intravenous urography. If the injury is incomplete with only partial transection, the urogram may be normal. If a high clinical index of suspicion remains in the face of a normal urogram, retrograde pyeloureterography may confirm the diagnosis. If a guide wire can be passed, a double-J stent may be placed as the first therapeutic maneuver. If complete ureteral obstruction is diagnosed, a temporary percutaneous nephrostomy tube is placed. Spontaneous resolution of ureteral obstruction may occur, but failure to resolve requires endoscopic balloon dilation, endoscopic ureteral incision, or open reconstructive repair.

Infection

Infection of sutures and other permanent graft materials results from vaginal contamination and should occur in less than 1% of patients if careful technique is used. Pain and swelling in the suprapubic area should alert the surgeon to a potential infection at the site of suspension sutures, which may require wound drainage or suture removal should antibiotic therapy be unsuccessful.

Lower urinary tract infections are common in the first month following any vaginal surgery and generally respond to a short course of oral antibiotics. A persistent lower urinary tract infection may be the presenting complaint when erosion of suture and bolster material occurs into the urinary tract, causing symptoms as delayed as 2 to 36 months following the procedure (Bihrle and Tarantino, 1990).

Postoperative Pain

Postoperative suprapubic pain may be related to suspension sutures and generally subsides with several weeks of decreased physical activity. **Persistent suprapubic pain** is reported in 0.01% to 16% of patients and **is often idiopathic in nature but may also be caused by cellulitis, subcutaneous abscess formation, osteitis pubis (in operations in which sutures are anchored to the bone), ilioinguinal nerve entrapment, muscle entrapment, vigorous overtying of sutures, or placement of sutures through a mobile portion of the rectus fascia** (Kelly et al, 1991; Raz, 1992). If conservative measures fail, removal of permanent sutures through the suprapubic wound may result in relief but risks subsequent return of stress urinary incontinence.

Vaginal Stenosis or Shortening

Vaginal stenosis or shortening may result from excessive plication of the vaginal epithelium during closure or secondary scarring following hematoma formation in the anterior vaginal wall. A history of new onset of dyspareunia, pelvic pain, or vaginal pain and the finding of foreshortening on physical examination confirm the diagnosis. Mild shortening or stenosis may be treated with longitudinal relaxing incisions in the lateral vaginal wall with transverse closure. Severe shortening or stenosis may require reconstruction with the use of free skin grafts or a pedicle flap from the adjacent labia.

Bladder Dysfunction

Temporary voiding dysfunction is common after pelvic reconstructive surgery, and changes in voiding patterns, including obstructive voiding symptoms and mild bladder irritability, should be explained to the patient preoperatively. The majority of patients with voiding dysfunction have resolution of symptoms within a short period of time; however, persistent voiding dysfunction should prompt reinvestigation.

Although transient urinary retention may occur in up to 41% of patients after bladder neck suspension procedures, the incidence of prolonged retention following vaginal approaches has been reported to be less than 5% (Raz, 1992). Temporary urinary retention in the immediate postoperative period resolves in the majority of patients with the use of a suprapubic or clean intermittent self-catheterization. Retention persisting longer than 6 months postoperatively is rare (McGuire et al, 1989; Foster and McGuire, 1993). Urethral obstruction may result from extraluminal (scarring or a retroperitoneal hematoma), intramural (misplaced sutures or graft material), or intraluminal (sutures crossing the urethra) causes and may present in one of three ways: complete retention, obstructive voiding symptoms, or irritative symptoms such as de novo detrusor instability. Continued intermittent catheterization, cutting or removing permanent suture material, transvaginal urethrolysis, or urethrolysis and placement of an infrapubic Martius flap are treatment options and are individualized in each patient (Raz, 1992; Foster and McGuire, 1993; Stothers et al, 1995).

De novo stress urinary incontinence may result as a complication of cystocele repair or repair of vault prolapse when concomitant bladder neck suspension is not performed (Harris and Bent, 1990). **Persistent or recurrent stress incontinence** following bladder neck suspension or sling procedures requires complete urodynamic evaluation and usually reoperation. The most common cause of persistent stress incontinence is recurrent or persistent malposition and hypermobility of the bladder neck and urethra. In this case, reoperation with proper suture placement should correct the problem. When the cause is intrinsic sphincteric dysfunction, corrective measures include sling procedures, injection of urethral bulking agents, or artificial urinary sphincters.

Secondary Prolapse

Secondary enterocele or genital prolapse is reported in 6% to 25% of patients postoperatively and is generally treated by reoperation if the patient is symptomatic. Conservative treatment includes the use of a pessary. Despite adequate initial repair, this complication may occur in the setting of poor-quality tissues, after multiple prior procedures, or after pelvic infection or hematoma formation.

Careful patient selection with attention to preoperative planning and surgical detail prevents most of the potential complications of vaginal surgery and allows the patient to enjoy the benefits of such an approach: short hospital stay, early postoperative recovery, a low incidence of complications, and simultaneous repair of multiple pelvic problems. A global approach to pelvic floor defects results not only in stabilization of the pelvic floor but also in a functional unity of the pelvic organs, maximizing the function of each within the confines of the pelvis.

REFERENCES

Anatomy of Pelvic Support

DeLancey JOL: Correlative study of paraurethral anatomy. Obstet Gynecol 1986; 68:91–97.

DeLancey JOL: Anatomic aspects of vaginal eversion after hysterectomy. Am J Obstet Gynecol 1992; 166:1717–1728.

DeLancey JOL: Anatomy and biomechanics of genital prolapse. Clin Obstet Gynecol 1993; 36:897–909.

Gosling JA, Dixon JS, Critchley HOD, Thompson S: A comparative study of the human external sphincter and periurethral levator ani muscles. Br J Urol 1981; 53:35–41.

Lawson JO: Pelvic anatomy: I. Pelvic floor muscles. Ann R Coll Surg Engl 1974; 54:244.

Richardson AC, Edmonds PB, Williams NL: Treatment of stress urinary incontinence due to paravaginal fascial defect. Obstet Gynecol 1981; 57:357–362.

Stothers L, Raz S: The anatomy of female continence. Published abstracts of the Western Section American Urologic Association, 1995, p 118.

Wilson PD, Dixon JS, Brown DG, Gosling JA: Posterior pubo-urethral ligaments in normal and genuine stress incontinence women. J Urol 1983; 130:802–805.

Wiskind AK, Creighton SM, Stanton SL: The incidence of genital prolapse after the Burch colposuspension. Am J Obstet Gynecol 1992; 167:399–405.

Vaginal Surgery for Stress Incontinence

Araki T, Takamoto H, Hara T, et al: The loop-loosening procedure for urination difficulties after Stamey suspension of the vesical neck. J Urol 1990; 144(2 Pt I):319–322, discussion 322–323.

Ashken NM: Follow-up results with the Stamey operation for stress incontinence of urine. Br J Urol 1990; 65:168–169.

Benson JT, Agosta A, McClellan E: Evaluation of a minimal-incision pubovaginal suspension as an adjunct to other pelvic-floor surgery. Obstet Gynecol 1990; 75:844–847.

Bihrle W 3d, Tarantino AF: Complications of retropubic bladder neck suspension. Urology 1990; 35:213–214.

Conquy S, Zerbib M, Younes E, et al: Retrospective comparative study of three surgical procedures in the treatment of urinary stress incontinence in women: Apropos of 119 patients treated from 1985 to 1990. J Urol 1993; 99:169.

Deliveliotis C, et al: Treatment of stress urinary incontinence by the Raz vaginal colpopexy. Prog Urol 1994; 4:974–976.

Diokno AC: Epidemiology and psychosocial aspects of incontinence. Urol Clin North Am 1995; 22:481–485.

Ekelund P, Grimby A, Milsom I: Urinary incontinence: Social and financial costs high. BMJ 1993; 306:1344.

Fonda D, Woodward M, D'Astoli M, Chin WF: Sustained improvement of subjective quality of life in older community-dwelling people after treatment of urinary incontinence. Age Ageing 1995; 24:283–286.

Gittes RF, Loughlin KR: No incision pubovaginal suspension for stress incontinence. J Urol 1987; 138:568.

Golomb J, Goldwasser B, Mashiach S: Raz bladder neck suspension in women younger than sixty-five years compared with elderly women: Three years' experience. Urology 1994; 43:40–43.

Griffith-Jones NW, Abrams PH: The Stamey endoscopic bladder neck suspension in the elderly. Br J Urol 1990; 65:170–172.

Hermieu JF, Van Glabeke E, Patard JJ, et al: Endoscopic retropubic colpopexy for stress urinary incontinence in women (Stamey's operation): 55 cases. Prog Urol 1994; 4:63–69.

Hilton P, Mayne CJ: The Stamey endoscopic bladder neck suspension: A clinical and urodynamic investigation, including actuarial follow-up over four years. Br J Obstet Gynaecol 1991; 91:1141–1149.

International Continence Society Committee on Standardisation of Technology: Seventh report on the standardisation of terminology of lower urinary tract function: Lower urinary tract rehabilitation techniques. Scand J Urol Nephrol 1992; 26:99–106.

Kil PJ, Hoekstra JW, van der Meijden AP, et al: Transvaginal ultrasonography and urodynamic evaluation after suspension operations: Comparison among the Gittes, Stamey and Burch suspensions. J Urol 1991; 146:132–136.

Korman IU, Sirls LT, Kirkemo AK: Success rate of modified Pereyra bladder neck suspension determined by outcomes analysis. J Urol 1994; 152:1453–1457.

Kursh ED: Factors influencing the outcome of a no-incision endoscopic urethropexy. Surg Gynecol Obstet 1992; 175:254.

Kursh ED, Angell AH, Resnick MI: Evolution of endoscopic urethropexy: Seven-year experience with various techniques. Urology 1991; 37:428.

Loughlin KR, Whitmore WF 3d, Gittes RF, Richie JP: Review of an 8-year experience with modifications of endoscopic suspension of the bladder neck for female stress urinary incontinence. J Urol 1990; 143:44–45.

McDowell I, Newell C: Measuring Health. Oxford, Oxford University Press, 1987.

McGuire EJ: Urodynamic findings in patients after failure of stress incontinence operations. *In* Zinner N, Sterling A, eds: Female Incontinence: Proceedings of the first joint meeting of the International Continence Society and the Urodynamics Society. New York, AR Liss, 1981, pp 351–360.

McGuire EJ: Urethral dysfunction. *In* Kursh ED, McGuire EJ, eds: Female Urology. Philadelphia, JB Lippincott, 1994, pp 163–174.

Naudin M, Hauzeur C, Schulman CS: Raz' method of bladder suspension and treatment of cystocele in urinary stress incontinence. Acta Urol Belg 1992; 60:67–75.

Nitti VW, Bregg KJ, Sussman EM, Raz S: The Raz bladder neck suspension in patients 65 years old and older. J Urol 1993; 149:802–807.

Pastor Sempere F, Cisnal Monsalve JN, Chicote Perez F, et al: Treatment of stress urinary incontinence in women, by the Raz technique—results. Arch Espan Urol 1992; 45:59–61.

Pereyra AJ: A simplified surgical procedure for the correction of stress incontinence in women. West J Surg Obstet Gynecol 1959; 67:223.

Pereyra AJ, Lebherz TB: Combined urethrovesical suspension and vaginal urethroplasty for correction of urinary stress incontinence. Obstet Gynecol 1967; 30:537.

Proceedings of the International Continence Society 24th annual meeting, Prague, 1994 (Abstracts). Neurourol Urodynam 1994; 13:345–500.

Ralph G, Tamussino K: Endoscopic bladder neck suspension—Clinical, urodynamic and radiologic results. Geburtsh Frauenheilk 1991; 51(10):830–833.

Raz S: Modified bladder neck suspension for female stress incontinence. Urology 1981; 17:82–85.

Raz S: Female Urology, 2nd ed. Philadelphia, W. B. Saunders Company, 1996.

Raz S, Erickson DR: SEAPI QMM Incontinence Classification System. Neurourol Urodynam 1992; 1:187–199.

Raz S, Stothers L, Young G, et al: Vaginal wall sling for anatomic incontinence and intrinsic sphincter damage—efficacy and outcome analysis. J Urol 1996; 156(1):166–170.

Raz S, Sussman EM, Erickson DB, et al: The Raz bladder neck suspension: Results in 206 patients. J Urol 1992; 148:845–850.

Sackett DL, Haynes RD, Guyatt HG, Tugwell P: Clinical Epidemiology: A Basic Science for Clinical Medicine, 2nd ed. Boston, Little, Brown, 1991.

Schumaker SA, Wyman JF, Uebersax JS, et al: Health related quality of life measures for women with urinary incontinence: The Incontinence Impact Questionnaire and the Urogenital Distress Inventory. Quality of Life Research 1994; 3:291–306.

Stamey TA: Endoscopic suspension of the vesical neck for urinary incontinence. Surg Gynecol Obstet 1973; 136:547.

Stamey TA: Endoscopic suspension of the vesical neck for urinary incontinence in females: Report of 203 consecutive patients. Ann Surg 1980; 192:465.

Stamey TA: Urinary incontinence in the female. *In* Walsh PC et al, eds: Campbell's Urology, 6th ed. Philadelphia, W. B. Saunders Company, 1992.

Stamey TA, Schaeffer AJ, Condy M: Clinical and roentgenographic evaluation of endoscopic suspension of the vesical neck for urinary incontinence. Surg Gynecol Obstet 1975; 140:355–361.

Stothers L, Chopra A, Raz S: Vaginal wall sling for anatomic incontinence and intrinsic sphincter damage—efficacy and outcome analysis. J Urol 1995; 153:525a.

Stothers L, Raz S, Chopra A: Anterior vaginal wall sling. *In* Raz S, ed: Female Urology, 2nd ed. Philadelphia, W. B. Saunders, 1996, pp 395–398.

Stothers L, Raz S: The reliability, validity and gender differences in a quality of life score for urinary incontinence. Abstracts of the American Urologic Association Meeting, Orlando, 1996.

Summers JL, Myers G: Complications of Gittes procedure. Presented at the North Central Section Meeting of the American Urologic Association, Chicago, 1989.

Valle Gerhold J, Murillo Perez C, Timon Garcia A, et al: Experience with endoscopic urethrocervicopexy: Long-term results. Acta Urol Espan 1993; 17:595–597.

Victor A: Pad weighing test—a simple method to quantitate urinary incontinence. Ann Med 1990; 22:443–447.

Walker GT, Texter JH Jr: Success and patient satisfaction following the Stamey procedure for stress urinary incontinence. J Urol 1992; 147:1521–1523.

Wall LL, Wang K, Robson I, Stanton SL: The Pyridium pad test for diagnosing urinary incontinence: A comparative study of asymptomatic and incontinent women. J Reprod Med 1990; 35:682–684.

Woodward C, Chambers L: Guide to Questionnaire Construction. Canadian Public Health Association, 1981.

Wyman JF, Harkins SW, Choi SC, et al: Psychosocial impact of urinary incontinence in women. Obstet Gynecol 1987; 70(3, Pt 1):378–381.

Zerbib M, Younes E, Conquy S, et al. Treatment of urinary stress incontinence in women by percutaneous cervico-cystoplexy. J Urol (Paris) 1992; 98(2):93–97.

Zimmern PE, Leach G: Bladder neck suspension using the modified Pereyra-Raz procedure in the treatment of stress urinary incontinence in women. J Urol 1991; 97:309-319.

Vaginal Surgery for Prolapse: Anterior Vaginal Wall Prolapse

Baden WE, Walker J: Surgical Repair of Vaginal Defects. Philadelphia, J. B. Lippincott, 1992.

Beck RP, McCormick S, Nordstrom L, et al: A 25 year experience with 519 anterior colporrhaphy procedures. Obstet Gynecol 1991; 78:1011–1018.

Copeland LJ: Textbook of Gynecology. Philadelphia, W. B. Saunders Company, 1993.

Gardy M, Kozminski M, DeLancey J, et al: Stress incontinence and cystoceles. J Urol 1991; 145:1211-1213.

Kelly HA: Urinary incontinence in women without manifest injury to the bladder. Surg Gynecol Obstet 1912; 18:444.

Macer G: Transabdominal repair of cystocele, a 20 year experience, compared with the traditional vaginal approach. Am J Obstet Gynecol 1978; 45:116–120.

Nichols DH, Genadry RR: Pelvic relaxation of the posterior compartment. Curr Opin Obstet Gynecol 1993; 5:458.

Nichols DH, Randall CL: Surgery for pelvic floor disorders. Surg Clin North Am 1991; 71:927–946.

Raz S: Female Genitourinary Dysfunction and Reconstruction. Philadelphia, W. B. Saunders Company, 1996.

Raz S, Chopra A, Stothers L: Outcome of surgical treatment for grade four cystocele. Published abstracts of the Western Section of the American Urologic Association, 1995, p 124.

Raz S, Erickson D, Sussman E: Operative repair of rectocele, enterocele and cystocele. Adv Urol 1992; 5:121–144.

Raz S, Golomb J, Klutke C: Four corner bladder and urethral suspension for moderate cystocele. J Urol 1989; 142:712–715.

Raz S, Little NA, Juma S, Sussman EM: Repair of severe anterior vaginal wall prolapse (grade IV cystourethrocele). J Urol 1991; 146:988–992.

Richardson AC: A new look at pelvic relaxation. Am J Obstet Gynecol 1976; 126(5):568–573.

Richardson AC, Edmonds PB, Williams NL: Treatment of stress urinary incontinence due to paravaginal fascial defect. Obstet Gynecol 1981; 57:357.

Shull B: Clinical evaluation of women with pelvic support defects. Clin Obstet Gynecol 1993; 36:939.

Stothers L, Chopra A, Raz S: Vaginal reconstructive surgery for female incontinence and anterior vaginal-wall prolapse. Urol Clin North Am 1995; 22:641–655.

Stothers L, Chopra A, Raz S: Outcome of surgical treatment for grade four cystocele. Abstracts of the Canadian Urologic Association, Victoria, British Columbia, Canada, 1996.

Thompson JD: Urinary stress incontinence. *In* Thompson JD, Rock JA, eds: Te Linde's Operative Gynecology, 7th ed. Philadelphia, J. B. Lippincott, 1992.

Timmons MC, Addison WA: Pelvic relaxation involving the middle compartment. Curr Opin Obstet Gynecol 1993; 5:452–457.

Youngblood JP: Paravaginal repair for cystourethrocele. Clin Obstet Gynecol 1993; 36:960–966.

Vault Prolapse and Enterocele/Rectocele and Perineal Body Repair

Backer MH Jr: Success with sacrospinous suspension of the prolapsed vaginal vault. Surg Gynecol Obstet 1992; 175:419–420.

Baden WE, Walker J: Surgical Repair of Vaginal Defects. Philadelphia, J. B. Lippincott, 1992.

Burch JC: Urethrovaginal fixation to Cooper's ligament for correction of stress incontinence, cystocele and prolapse. Am J Obstet Gynecol 1961; 81:281.

Carey MP, Slack MC: Transvaginal sacrospinous colpopexy for vault and marked uterovaginal prolapse. Br J Obstet Gynaecol 1994; 101:536–540.

Chopra A, Raz S, Stothers L: Enterocele and vault prolapse. *In* Raz S ed: Female Urology, 2nd ed. Philadelphia, W. B. Saunders, 1996, 465–473.

Feldman GB, Bimbaum SJ: Sacral colpopexy for vaginal vault prolapse. Obstet Gynecol 1979; 53:399.

Hofineister FJ: Prolapsed vagina. Obstet Gynecol 1973; 42.

Holley RL, Varner RE, Gleason BP, et al: Recurrent pelvic support defects after sacrospinous ligament fixation for vaginal vault prolapse. J Am Coll Surg 1995; 180:444–448.

I-Iiller RI: Repair of enterocele with preservation of the vagina. Am J Obstet Gynecol 1952; 64:301.

Jeffcoate TNA: Posterior colporrhaphy. Am J Obstet Gynecol 1959; 77:490.

Leach GE, Zimmern P, Staskin D, et al: Surgery for pelvic prolapse. Semin Urol 1986; 4:43–50.

Lee RA: Vaginal hysterectomy with repair of enterocele, cystocele, and rectocele. Clin Obstet Gynecol 1993; 36:967–975.

McCall NI: Posterior culdoplasty. Obstet Gynecol 1957; 10:95.

Mellgren A, Bremmer S, Johansson C, et al: Decography: Results of investigations in 2816 patients. Dis Colon Rectum 1994; 37:1133–1141.

Moschcowitz AV: The cure of prolapse of the rectum. Surg Gynecol Obstet 1912; 15:721.

Nichols DH: Types of enterocele and principles underlying choice of operation for repair. Obstet Gynecol 1972; 40(2):257–273.

Nichols DH: Enterocele and massive eversion of the vagina. *In* Thompson JD, Rock JA, eds: Te Linde's Operative Gynecology, 7th ed. Philadelphia, J. B. Lippincott, 1992.

Raz S: Atlas of Transvaginal Surgery. Philadelphia, W. B. Saunders Company, 1992.

Raz S, Nitti VW, Bregg KJ: Transvaginal repair of enterocele. J Urol 1993; 149:724–730.

Richardson AC: The rectovaginal septum revisited: Its relationship to rectocele and its importance in rectocele repair. Clin Obstet Gynecol 1993; 36:976–983.

Sanz L: Gynecological Surgery. New York, Medical Economics Books, 1988.

Sauer HA, Klutke CG: Transvaginal sacrospinous ligament fixation for treatment of vaginal prolapse. J Urol 1995; 154:1008–1012.

Sentovich SM, Rivela LJ, Christensen MA, Blatchford GJ: Simultaneous dynamic proctography and peritoneography for pelvic floor disorders. Dis Colon Rectum 1995; 38:912–915.

Stanton SL, Cardozo LD: Results of colposuspension operation for incontinence and prolapse. Br J Obstet Gynaecol 1979; 86:693.

Thompson JD: Relaxed vaginal outlet, rectocele, fecal incontinence, and rectovaginal fistula. *In* Thompson JD, Rock JA, eds: Te Linde's Operative Gynecology, 7th ed. Philadelphia, J. B. Lippincott, 1992.

Wiersma TG, Mulder CJ, Reeders JW, et al: Dynamic rectal examination (defecography). Baillieres Clin Gastoenterol 1994; 8:729.

Wiskind AK, Creighton SM, Stanton SL: The incidence of genital prolapse after the Burch colposuspension. Am J Obstet Gynecol 1992; 167:399–404.

Zacharin RF: Pulsion enterocele: Review of functional anatomy of the pelvic floor. Obstet Gynecol 1980; 55:135.

Vaginal Hysterectomy

Copeland LJ: Textbook of Gynecology. Philadelphia, W. B. Saunders Company, 1993.

Dicker RC, Greenspan JR, Strauss LT, et al: Complications of abdominal and vaginal hysterectomy among women of reproductive age in the United States. Am J Obstet Gynecol 1982; 144:841.

Hofmeister FJ, Woifgram RL: Methods of demonstrating measurement relationships between vaginal hysterectomy ligatures and the ureters. Am J Obstet Gynecol 1962; 83:938–948.

Nichols D: Vaginal Surgery, 3rd ed. Baltimore, Williams & Wilkins, 1989.

Randall CL, Nichols DH: Surgical treatment of vaginal inversion. Obstet Gynecol 1971; 38:327.

Thompson JD: Hysterectomy. *In* Thompson JD, Rock JA, eds: Te Linde's Operative Gynecology, 7th ed. Philadelphia, J. B. Lippincott, 1992a.

Thompson JD: Malposition of the uterus. *In* Thompson JD, Rock JA, eds: Te Linde's Operative Gynecology, 7th ed. Philadelphia, J. B. Lippincott, 1992b.

Wall LL: A technique for modified McCall culdoplasty at the time of abdominal hysterectomy. J Am Coll Surg 1994; 178:507–509.

Potential Complications of Vaginal Surgery

Angermeir KW, Jordon GH: Complications of the exaggerated lithotomy position: A review of 177 cases. J Urol 1994; 151:866.

Araki T, Takamoto H, Hara T, et al: The loop-loosening procedure for urination difficulties after Stamey suspension of the vesical neck. J Urol 1990; 144(2 Pt I):319–322, discussion 322–323.

Bihrle W 3d, Tarantino AF: Complications of retropubic bladder neck suspension. Urology 1990; 35:213–214.

Copeland LJ: Textbook of Gynecology. Philadelphia, W. B. Saunders Company, 1993.

Diaz DL, Fox BM, Walzak MP, et al: Endoscopic vesicourethropexy. Urology 1984; 24:321.

Foster HE, McGuire EJ: Management of urethral obstruction with transvaginal urethrolysis. J Urol 1993; 150:1448–1451.

Hadley PR, Myers RC: Complications of vaginal surgery. Proceedings of the Western Section of the American Urological Association, 1989, p 32.

Harris TA, Bent AE: Genital prolapse with and without urinary incontinence. J Reprod Med 1990; 35:792–798.

Hirsch HA: Prophylactic antibiotics in obstetrics and gynecology. Am J Med 1985; 78:170.

Katske FA, Raz S: Use of Foley catheter to obtain transvaginal tamponade. Urology 1987; 18 May.

Kelly MJ, Zimmern PE, Leach GE: Complications of bladder neck suspension procedures. Urol Clin North Am 1991; 18:339.

Larsen EH, Gasser TC, Madsen PO: Antimicrobial prophylaxis in urologic surgery. Urol Clin North Am 1986; 13:591.

Madsen PO, Larsen EH, Dorflinger T: The role of antibacterial prophylaxis in urologic surgery. Urology 1985; 26:38.

Mann WJ, Arato M, Patsner B, Stone ML: Ureteral injuries in an obstetrics and gynecology training program: Etiology and management. Obstet Gynecol 1988; 72:82–85.

McGuire EJ, Letson W, Wang S: Transvaginal urethrolysis after obstructive urethral suspension procedures. J Urol 1989; 142:1037–1039.

Raz S: Complications of vaginal surgery. *In* Raz S, ed: Atlas of Transvaginal Surgery. Philadelphia, W. B. Saunders Company, 1992.

Stothers L, Broseta E, Chopra A, Raz S: The Martius flap techniques in the surgical management of iatrogenic urinary obstruction following anti-incontinence procedures. Published abstracts of the Western Section American Urologic Association, 1995, p 126.

Stothers L, Raz S: Vaginal repair of vesicovaginal fistula. *In* Raz S, ed: Female Urology, 2nd ed. Philadelphia, W. B. Saunders Company, 1996.

Thompson JD: Operative injuries to the ureter: Prevention, recognition and management. *In* Thompson JD, Rock JA, eds: Te Linde's Operative Gynecology, 7th ed. Philadelphia, J. B. Lippincott, 1992, pp 749–783.

33
RETROPUBIC SUSPENSION SURGERY FOR FEMALE SPHINCTERIC INCONTINENCE

George D. Webster, M.B., Ch.B.
Joseph M. Khoury, M.D.

INDICATIONS FOR ABDOMINAL REPAIR OF STRESS URINARY INCONTINENCE

The treatment of urinary incontinence in women must be tailored to the individual patient. Once evaluation has identified the contributing etiologies, the patient should be exposed to the various conservative managements before being considered for surgery. Conservative options include fluid management; pharmacologic therapy including re-estrogenization; and pelvic floor rehabilitation, including pelvic floor exercises, biofeedback, and perhaps electrical stimulation. In patients whose condition is refractory to such treatments, surgical options may be considered, at which point a wide array of choices exists. The initial choice is between procedures designed to correct anatomic relaxation and urethral hypermobility and those designed for the correction of intrinsic sphincter deficiency, which may coexist with hypermobility. This chapter does not address patients with significant intrinsic sphincter deficiency, for whom a sling procedure is customarily performed vaginally.

Urethral hypermobility may be surgically corrected via vaginal or abdominal approach, and selection of technique is largely based on the surgeon's preference and prior experience. In a review of results of various procedures reported by Spencer and O'Connor, there was certainly no significant difference in the outcome between the 35 series of cases that were roughly equally divided between Marshall-Marchetti-Krantz (MMK), Burch and Pereyra (and its modifications), and Stamey procedures (Spencer and O'Connor, 1987). The mean cure rate for the population as a whole was approximately 90%. Indeed, however, such reports demand critical review, because the patient populations included and the modifications to surgical techniques employed render such comparison questionable. However, recognizing these data and the fact that abdominal and retropubic procedures require longer hospitalization and are less cost-effective, it may be suggested that specific indications be fulfilled for their performance (Green et al, 1986; Stanton, 1990; Forneret and Leach, 1985).

Certain unequivocal indications have been established for an abdominal approach, the most obvious being that patient who requires a concomitant abdominal surgical procedure that cannot be performed vaginally. This may include a hysterectomy, enterocele repair, or vaginal cuff suspension by sacral colpopexy when these, by their nature, are deemed inappropriate for vaginal performance. In some cases, vaginal access is precluded because of associated hip disease or reduced vaginal capacity or abnormality, and these may too indicate an abdominal approach. It has been suggested that an abdominal approach is particularly well suited for women who have had previous failed vaginal procedures to correct their incontinence, and in whom fixation of tissues owing to fibrosis make repeated vaginal surgery more difficult, especially for mobilization of the vesicourethral junction (Appell, 1993). This is not a universally accepted philosophy; techniques do exist that allow for the safe lysis of retropubic adhesions by a vaginal approach in conjunction with the needle suspension procedure (Ramon et al, 1991). In patients who have had prior failed surgical procedures for anatomic incontinence, one must suspect a significant element of intrinsic sphincter deficiency, even if recurrent urethral hypermobility is also evident. Results of a leak-point pressure study and a videourodynamic study help confirm the degree to which intrinsic sphincter deficiencies (ISD) coexist, but results may well indicate a need for a sling, periurethral bulking agent, or artificial urinary sphincter rather than an abdominal cystourethropexy. It is also suggested that the abdominal approach be considered in patients with medical problems associated with frequently increased intra-abdominal pressure (e.g., obstructive pulmonary disorders) or those who participate in strenuous occupations or athletic activity, the implication being that the abdominal repair gives greater security (Appell, 1993). The disadvantage of an abdominal procedure is that it does not give the opportunity to correct associated vaginal prolapse or pathology, which frequently coexists in patients with vesical neck hypermobility. Although lateral defect cystocele and enterocele lend themselves also to abdominal repair, central defect cystocele, rectocele, and introital deficiency do not. Abdominal repair is complicated by obesity and may make the complication of deep venous thrombosis more common.

Two of the important factors to be considered when deciding upon choice of surgical approach are the reported results and complications of each procedure, as judged from the scientific literature (Jarvis, 1994). Unfortunately, comparison of series is made difficult by lack of standardization in reporting and the fact that truly randomized clinical trials do not exist. Jarvis suggests that the following list of factors be considered in comparing different series:

- Do all the patients have genuine stress incontinence and no other urologic pathology?
- Is the procedure primary or repeat surgery?
- Does selection bias exist?
- Is the operative technique standard?
- Is follow-up subjective or objective?
- How long is the minimum follow-up?
- Is the outcome measure defined?

Not unimportant are the surgeon's philosophy and prejudices, which are generally dictated by prior success and failure. For the surgeon who has minimal experience in training with vaginal repairs, the transvaginal approach to incontinence surgery may yield disappointing results and increased risk of complications. On the other hand, retropubic cystourethropexy, such as those described herein, are reliable procedures that have stood the test of time, offering satisfying outcomes when properly performed, and, most important, being familiar to most urologists.

RETROPUBIC SURGICAL PROCEDURES FOR GENUINE STRESS URINARY INCONTINENCE IN WOMEN

Various abdominal procedures have been reported in the past, most of these being variations on a theme. The three most common variants are considered: The MMK procedure, Burch colposuspension, and paravaginal fascial repair, also termed *vagino-obturator shelf repair.*

Marshall-Marchetti-Krantz Cystourethropexy

In 1949, Marshall and co-workers described their retropubic vesicourethral suspension in 50 patients, 38 of whom had symptoms of stress urinary incontinence, and in these 25 had failed prior gynecologic operations for urinary incontinence. Of historic note is that their first patient was a 54-year-old man who had undergone abdominoperineal resection of the rectum, resulting in urinary retention and necessitating transurethral resection of the prostate, which culminated in total urinary incontinence. They described a simple suprapubic procedure by which the vesical outlet was suspended to the pubis, resulting in urinary continence for close to 4 years (Marshall et al, 1949). Their procedure has undergone a number of modifications; however, the principle remains the same, which is essentially to elevate the proximal urethra and bladder neck by anchoring it to the cartilaginous portion of the symphysis pubis.

The MMK cystourethropexy is best performed with the patient in the supine position with the legs abducted in a modified dorsal lithotomy position using stirrups, which allow access to the vagina during the procedure (Fig. 33–1*A–D*). A urethral Foley catheter is inserted, and the abdomen is entered through a Pfannenstiel or lower abdominal midline incision. The rectus muscles are separated in the midline, and the anterior peritoneal reflection is swept off the bladder to give access to the retropubic space. The space is carefully dissected, teasing away retropubic fat and identifying retropubic veins, which are cauterized and severed. The bladder neck, anterior vaginal wall, and urethra are identified and dissected in this manner. The bladder neck is generally easy to identify, but confirmation is obtained by gentle traction on the Foley catheter to observe where the Foley balloon makes contact. In patients who have had previous vaginal or retropubic operations, the dissection may be tedious, but it is important to take down all old retropubic adhesions, particularly in the face of a prior failed repair. If difficulty is encountered, the bladder may be partially filled or opened to identify its limits, and an assistant's examining finger in the vagina may help to identify the vaginal wall. As originally described, No. 1 chromic catgut sutures were used to suspend the paraurethral anterior vaginal wall to the back of the symphysis pubis. Marshall described three pairs of sutures being placed on each side of the urethra, the most proximal pair being at the level of the bladder neck. Each suture takes a double bite through the paraurethral fascia and anterior vaginal wall (excluding mucosa) close to, but not through, the urethra, and each suture is passed into

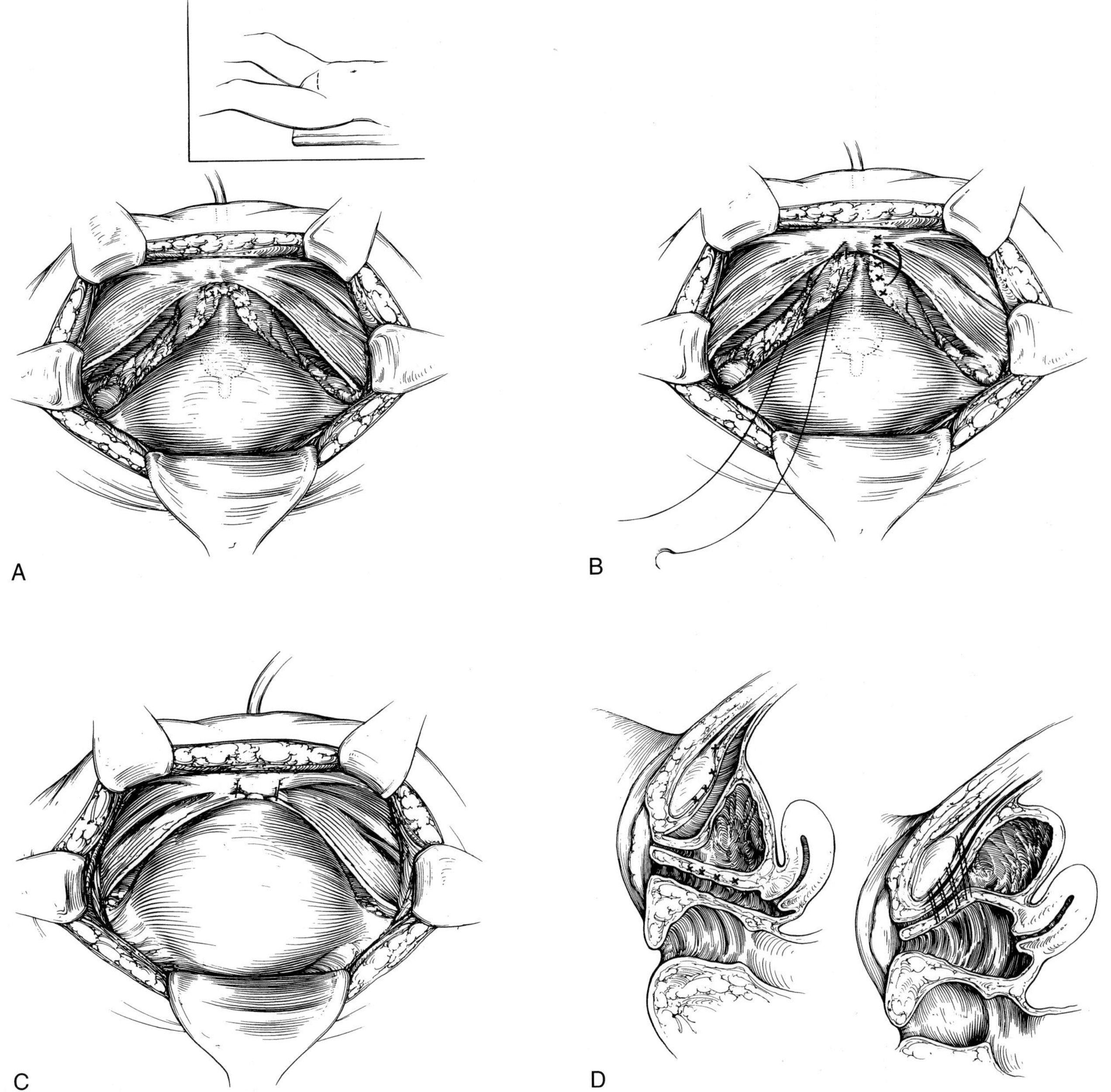

Figure 33–1. *A (inset),* Position and incision used for abdominal cystourethropexy. Pelvic dissection demonstrates pelvic sidewalls with Cooper's ligament and tendinous arc (*white line,* accentuated for clarity in illustration). *B,* Suture placement for Marshall-Marchetti-Krantz (MMK) procedure. *C,* Vaginal wall approximated to retrosymphysis. *D,* Sagittal representation following MMK urethropexy.

an appropriate portion of the cartilaginous portion of the symphysis. All six sutures are inserted, and while an assistant elevates the anterior vaginal wall, each suture is individually tied, starting with the more distal pair. The proximal, or bladder neck suture frequently needs to be passed through the insertion of the rectus abdominis muscle. In some cases, the synchondrosis of the pubis is poorly developed, in which case the sutures are passed through the periosteum. This is often difficult to achieve; if this problem is encountered, it may be more appropriate to select another procedure such as a Burch or paravaginal repair, which ensures more secure fixation. Numerous modifications of the original procedure have been reported, as described by Marshall, using different types of suture material and more or fewer sutures to achieve the goals of the vesicourethral suspension.

A suction drain may be placed in the retropubic space, and the abdominal wall is closed in the routine fashion. The Foley catheter is removed on the third to fifth postoperative day, and the suction drain is removed generally on the second or third day, when minimal output is noted.

The most frequent postoperative problem encountered is that of delayed return of voiding. A postvoid residual urine check is routinely made following removal of the catheter; if the volume is significant (more than 100 ml), a postvoid self-intermittent catheterization program is instituted until normal voiding ensues. In most situations, this is achieved within 7 days of surgery, and the patient has usually been discharged by this time. Provided that the surgeon is careful to exclude patients who had pre-existing voiding difficulties, it is unusual for postoperative urinary retention to be prolonged. With good patient selection and good operative technique most authors report an 80% to 96% long-term success rate with the MMK procedure (Marshall et al, 1949; Grout and O'Conor, 1972; McDuffie et al, 1981; Parnell et al, 1982; Colombo et al, 1994). Jarvis, performing a metanalysis of 15 series including 2460 patients, reported an 88.2% subjective cure rate. Objective cure rates in a smaller series were similar (Jarvis, 1994).

Burch Colposuspension

In 1961, Burch reported on his experience with the Cooper's ligament repair (Burch, 1961). He was dissatisfied with the fixation of the vaginal wall to the symphysis pubis as described by Marshall, and in his first seven patients, he attached the paravaginal fascia to the "white line" of the pelvis, the arcus tendineus, to which the obturator internus muscle and fascia and pubovesical muscle attach to the pelvic side wall. Still hampered by insecure fixation, Burch changed his point of suspension to the iliopectineal ligaments, which are thick bands of fibrous tissue running along the superior surfaces of the superior rami of the pubic bones.

The Burch retropubic colposuspension, which has undergone few modifications since its original description, is appropriate only if the patient has adequate vaginal mobility and capacity to allow the lateral vaginal fornices to be elevated toward and approximated to Cooper's ligament on either side. The supine, low, modified dorsal lithotomy position is again optimal, and the procedure is similar to the MMK operation, except for the extent of dissection and the location of suture placement. It is important to identify the lateral limits of the bladder as it reflects off the vaginal wall, because it is only in this manner that one can avoid inadvertent suturing of the bladder itself. Dissection over the bladder neck and urethra is avoided. Using careful technique, and sometimes by incision of the endopelvic fascia, the lateral bladder wall may be "rolled off" the vaginal wall, venous bleeding from the large vaginal veins being controlled by suture ligature. To aid in the identification of the lateral margin of the bladder, it is helpful to displace the balloon of the Foley catheter into the lateral recess, where it can be easily palpated through the bladder wall. This degree of extensive dissection is not always necessary, but in reoperated cases, it does ensure correct suture placement for ideal suspension.

Cooper's (iliopectineal) ligaments are identified beneath the lateral margins of the incision, and their examination confirms that they will give very good support for the suspension suture. Adipose tissue on the lateral pelvic wall is teased away, because it does not promote adhesion of the elevated vagina, which is necessary for the prolonged success of the operation. Because of the risks of sutures traversing the bladder wall and inadvertent ligation of a ureter, some surgeons advise routine opening of the bladder by midline cystotomy and even placement of ureteral catheters. Others recommend the use of methylene blue instilled through the Foley catheter before initiating the operation, so that if a bladder injury does occur intraoperatively it may be readily recognized. Sutures are of No. 1 polyglycolic acid, and their placement is facilitated by the elevation of the dissected anterolateral vaginal wall into the field by either the surgeon's left vaginal-examining fingers or by the assistant (Fig. 33–2*A* and *B*). The bladder is retracted to the opposite side, using a narrow-blade Deaver retractor. Two to four sutures are placed on each side, each suture taking a good bite of fascia and vaginal wall, taking care not to pass through the vaginal mucosa. The most distal suture is at the level of the bladder neck and is placed approximately 2 cm lateral to it (some place the distal sutures at the midurethral level). Subsequent sutures are placed proximal to the level of the bladder neck, at about 1-cm intervals. These sutures pick up a portion of Cooper's ligament, although the most distal suture at times cannot be brought through Cooper's ligament, and therefore instead picks up pubic periosteum and the fibrous insertion of the rectus muscle.

The highly vascular vaginal wall may bleed profusely during suture placement, and often large vaginal veins need to be undersewn, but most bleeding ceases once the sutures are tied and the vagina is suspended. To facilitate tying the sutures, the assistant elevates the appropriate portion of the vaginal wall as each suture is tied, commencing with the more distal pair. It is important to note that no attempt is made to tie these sutures tightly. In most cases the anterolateral vaginal wall does not approximate Cooper's ligament, and free suture material is seen between the vagina and ligaments. The object of the operation is to approximate this vaginal wall to the lateral pelvic wall, where it will heal and promote adhesion formation. Once the sutures have been tied, a broad support for the urethra and the bladder neck is seen to have been created; however, the urethra, although suspended, is not compressed behind the symphysis pubis, and one can usually insert an examining finger between it and the synchondrosis of the pubis.

A suction drain may be left in the retropubic space, to be removed on the second or third postoperative day when there is minimal drainage. The urethral Foley catheter remains until the third to fifth postoperative day, and the same program as is used with the MMK operation of checking for residual urine and clean intermittent catheterization is instituted if necessary, until residual urine is usually less than 100 ml.

An advantage of the Burch procedure is that it simultaneously corrects lateral defect cystourethrocele. It corrects urinary incontinence by the repositioning of the vesicourethral region within the abdomen, but does not compress the urethra. Stanton and Cardozo reported an 84.2% cure rate using the colposuspension operation for patients who had undergone previous incontinence surgery, and an overall cure rate of 86% at 2 years (Stanton and Cardoza, 1979). Likewise, others have documented similar success rates, ranging from 63% to 89% with longer follow-up time ranging between 3 and 7 years (Stanton, 1990; Van Geelen et al, 1988; Galloway et al, 1987; Gillon and Stanton, 1984; Benson, 1988; Hebertsson and Iosif, 1993; Kjølhede and Ryden, 1994). A metanalysis by Jarvis reported a subjective cure rate of 90.7% in 1320 patients and an 83.9% objective cure rate in 1773 patients (Jarvis, 1994). The range was from 59% to 100% and the series with the longest follow-up period showed a subjective continence rate of 62.5% at 5 years.

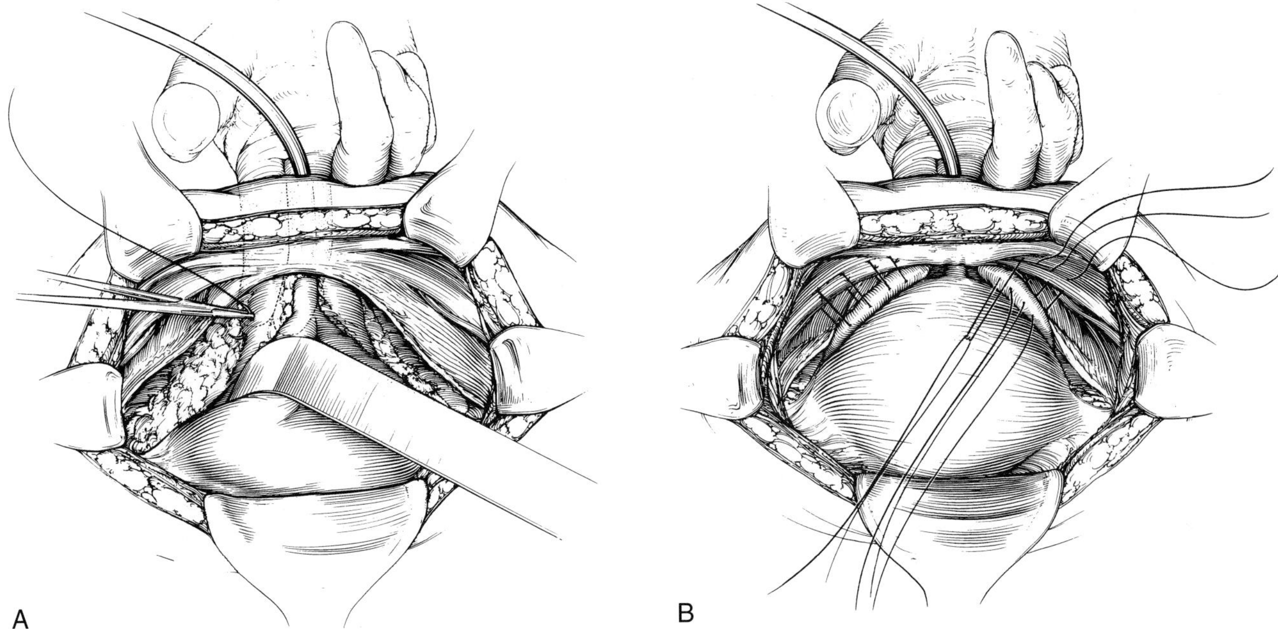

Figure 33–2. *A,* Suture placement for Burch colposuspension. Digital elevation of the vaginal wall and medial retraction of the bladder facilitate placement of the vaginal suture. *B,* Suture ligation is facilitated by vaginal elevations. Note that the vaginal wall does not approximate Cooper's ligament.

When the results were assessed for primary or previous surgery, a 94% continence is recorded when it was a primary procedure and 84% when it was secondary.

Paravaginal Fascial Repair

The paravaginal fascial repair and its variants have enjoyed a resurgence of interest recently, although they are less widely performed than the MMK or Burch procedure. Its origins date to the early writings of a gynecologist, George R. White, as early as 1909, who described the importance of the "white line" (arcus tendineus) as an integral structure supporting the proximal urethra and bladder base to the pelvic wall, and the development of paravaginal fascial tears predisposing to cystocele formation. Although White performed the paravaginal repair using a vaginal approach, he envisioned that performing the procedure abdominally would be easier to correct the fascial defect (White, 1909, 1912). In 1976, Richardson and coworkers described their retropubic approach, which was soon followed by other modifications (Richardson et al, 1976; Turner-Warwick, 1986).

Like the MMK and Burch colposuspension, the patient is positioned using low lithotomy, as previously described. If there are prevesical and retropubic adhesions from a prior cystourethropexy, they are sharply incised and the dissection is facilitated by placing two fingers of the surgeon's left hand in the vagina. The bladder and urethra are not mobilized from the vaginal attachments. The vaginal wall in the region of the bladder neck is identified and three interrupted No. 1 polyglycolic acid sutures are placed at approximately 1-cm intervals through the paravaginal fascia and vaginal wall (excluding vaginal mucosa) beginning at the urethrovesical junction, and continuing for approximately 3 cm proximal to it. These sutures are then passed through the adjacent obturator fascia and underlying muscle at the site of the arcus tendineus fascia (Fig. 33–3). Richardson describes a more extensive reattachment of the lateral vaginal sulcus with its overlying fascia to the arcus tendineus fasciae pelvis from the back of the lower edge of the symphysis pubis to the ischial spine, using six to eight sutures placed at 1-cm intervals.

This fixation leaves the urethral axis in an anatomic position, easily allowing three fingerbreadths between the retro-

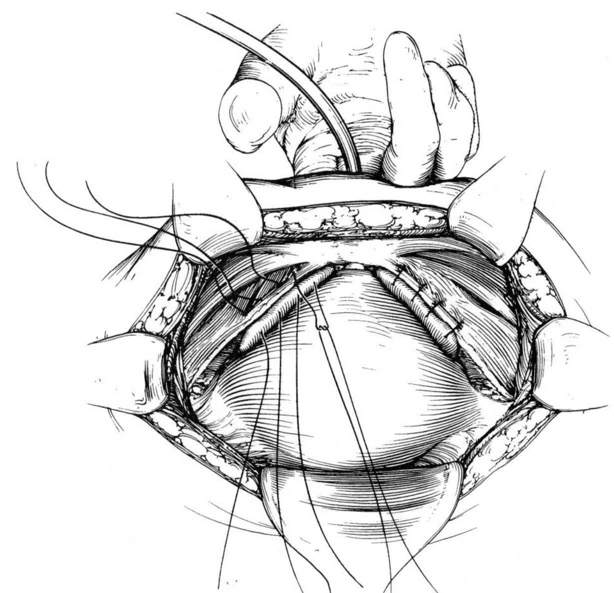

Figure 33–3. Suture placement for the paravaginal fascial repair approximates the vaginal wall to the tendinous arc on the sidewall of the pelvis. The number of sutures placed on each side varies.

symphysis and the proximal urethra, and therefore avoiding overcorrection but providing secure fixation and preventing rotational descent. Postoperative urine drainage is by either a percutaneous suprapubic cystocatheter or by a Foley catheter, as in the MMK or Burch procedure. Suction drains are used, depending on the extent of the surgical dissection, and are usually removed on postoperative days 2 or 3, when drainage is minimal. On day 3, a voiding trial may commence, and a similar program as used with the MMK and Burch operation of checking for residual urine is employed and clean intermittent catheterization is instituted if necessary. Outcome reports are not as plentiful as for the MMK and Burch procedures but the long-term success rate with the paravaginal fascial repair and its variant, the vagino-obturator shelf repair, appears to be between 90% and 95% (Richardson et al, 1981; Shull and Baden, 1989). Its more extensive dissection and fixation predicts a higher risk of ureteral injury and the risk of obturator nerve injury is ever-present.

Laparoscopic Retropubic Cystourethropexy

Reviewing the evolution of surgical procedures to correct genuine stress urinary incontinence, there is a definite effort to achieve the goals of cystourethropexy using minimally invasive techniques. Transvaginal needle suspensions, originally described by Pereyra (1959) and modified by others (Stamey, 1980; Raz, 1981; Gittes and Laughlin, 1987) are an attempt to reduce the morbidity associated with an open abdominal procedure. Van Caillie and Schuessler first described the laparoscopic approach for the correction of stress urinary incontinence using a modified MMK technique (Van Caillie and Schuessler, 1991). Likewise, Liu reported on 58 patients who underwent a laparoscopic Burch procedure for the treatment of genuine stress urinary incontinence (Liu, 1993). His overall success rate, with follow-up ranging from 6 to 22 months, was approximately 95% with a complication rate of 8.5%. According to Liu, the advantages of the laparoscopic retropubic colposuspension over the more traditional abdominal approach included easy access to the space of Retzius, better visibility of the operative field, minimal intraoperative blood loss, and minimal postoperative requirement for analgesia as well as shortened hospital stay and recovery period. Polascik and co-workers compare the operative technique of laparoscopic colposuspension with a traditional open Burch cystourethropexy to treat women with genuine stress urinary incontinence (Polascik et al, 1995). Those women who underwent laparoscopic Burch repair required less postoperative analgesia and had a shorter hospital stay and a more expedient return to normal activity when compared with those who underwent open Burch colposuspension. No statistical difference exists in the continence rate between the two groups, although the patients undergoing laparoscopic repair were followed for a shorter time than those patients who had open repair (20.8 months and 35.6 months, respectively). In summary, laparoscopic surgical approaches to treat genuine stress urinary incontinence seem to offer minimal morbidity and shorter hospital stays with comparable short-term success rates when compared with the open surgical technique.

COMPLICATIONS OF RETROPUBIC REPAIRS

As with any major abdominal or pelvic surgical procedure, early postoperative complications that may occur include pulmonary atelectasis and infection, wound infection or dehiscence, abscess formation, bladder fistula or leaks, and ureteral obstruction or fistula. Because pelvic surgery may predispose patients to deep venous thrombosis and pulmonary embolus, those patients at increased risk should be considered for intermittent pneumatic compression stockings, minidose heparin, and early ambulation. The reported incidence of these problems is relatively low. In a review of the literature by Mainprize and Drutz, the most common postoperative complications in 2712 MMK procedures were wound problems and urinary infections, resulting in 5.5% and 3.9% of all complications, respectively (Mainprize and Drutz, 1988). Osteitis pubis was a complication in 2.5%, and direct surgical injury to the urinary tract occurred in 1.6%. Ureteral obstruction has been reported rarely after Burch colposuspension, and usually it results from ureteral kinking after elevation of the vagina and bladder base, although direct suture ligation of the ureter can occur. In more difficult cases in which prior pelvic surgery has resulted in fibrosis, a cystotomy may allow the surgeon to dissect the proximal urethra and bladder base from the retrosymphysis and vaginal wall under direct vision and reduce the chance of injury to these organs.

Other complications more specific to retropubic surgery for genuine stress urinary incontinence include postoperative voiding difficulty, detrusor instability, and other vaginal vault abnormalities.

Postoperative Voiding Difficulty

Postoperative voiding difficulty after any type of cystourethropexy is not uncommon and may arise because of pre-existing detrusor dysfunction, or perhaps because of denervation because of extensive perivesical dissection. In most cases, however, it is the result of overcorrection of the urethral axis owing to sutures being inappropriately placed or excessively tightened. Sutures may also transfix the urethra or distort it. Preoperatively, at-risk patients may be identified by their history of prior voiding dysfunction or episodes of urinary retention. Certainly, these patients or those with documented inefficient bladder emptying by postvoid residual urine check should undergo a urodynamic micturition study in an attempt to elaborate the problem. Preoperative urodynamic features that may herald post-cystourethropexy voiding problems include bladders of large capacity, high compliance, and poor sensation. Women with such bladders generally fail to generate a good micturition contraction; they void with poor flow and empty inefficiently, often using Valsalva effort. These women should be counseled carefully preoperatively about the potential for postoperative voiding difficulty and the possible need for self-intermittent catheterization. Their incontinence should be of sufficient magnitude that its correction offsets the risk of need for self-catheterization. Following surgery, if return of normal voiding is significantly delayed, a urodynamic study again is indicated to determine whether outlet obstruction or detrusor dysfunction is the cause. Women with post-cystourethropexy voiding problems who have obstruction often do not exhibit the classic urodynamic features of outlet obstruction. However, the history of postoperative voiding symptoms and associated new-onset bladder irritative symptoms, and the finding of a retropubically angulated and fixed urethra generally indicate that obstruction does exist. In such cases, revision of the cystourethropexy, releasing the urethra into a more anatomic position, resolves voiding symptoms in up to 90% of cases (Nitti and Raz, 1994; Webster and Kreder, 1990).

The metanalysis of MMK procedures by Jarvis (1994) reported an incidence of 3.6% for postoperative voiding problems. This incidence can certainly be higher if the surgery is inexpertly performed, which is particularly prone to occur when the vesicourethral angle is overcorrected in the presence of mild to moderate cystocele. In such cases the cystocele tends to "drape" over the fixed bladder neck resulting in a distortional obstruction. Following Burch colposuspension, the incidence of voiding disorders is reported as 3% by Eriksen and co-workers (1990), but higher numbers are reported by others including Mundy (1983) with 12%, Galloway and co-workers (1987) with 16%, and Hilton and Stanton (1983) with 32%. Little chance of overcorrection of the urethral axis is found following paravaginal fascial repair, because the procedure aims only to restore normal anatomy, and so it most likely has the lowest obstruction rate, although there is insufficient data to support this.

Bladder Instability

Bladder instability commonly accompanies anatomic stress urinary incontinence, and its incidence preoperatively has been reported to be as high as 30% in patients undergoing either their first correction or repeated operations (McGuire, 1981). Prevailing philosophy suggests that preoperative bladder instability does not contraindicate cystourethropexy, provided that anatomic stress incontinence has been demonstrated. In the majority of cases, the instability symptoms resolve following surgical repair and do not have a significant impact on the outcome of these operations (McGuire, 1988; Awad et al, 1988). In such cases it is customary to first try a course of anticholinergic therapy, because in a few cases, resolution of the urge component may leave the patient continent and not requiring cystourethropexy. For those in whom postoperative bladder instability symptoms persist, management should include anticholinergic therapy and behavioral modification. Only in rare cases is surgical management such as augmentation cystoplasty indicated.

As noted earlier, bladder instability symptoms arising de novo following cystourethropexy may be related to obstruction. This premise is supported by the frequent coexistence of these symptoms with impaired voiding following suspension procedures and by the fact that urethrolysis freeing the urethra from an obstructed position usually resolves both symptoms (Webster and Kreder, 1990; Raz, 1981). Bladder instability has been recorded in 3.4%, 14%, 17%, and 18% of patients undergoing Burch colposuspension (Stanton and Cardoza, 1979; Lose et al, 1987; Steel et al, 1985; Cardoza et al, 1979). The incidence following the MMK procedure was as low as 0.9% in the metanalysis of 15 series of MMKs reported by Mainprize and Drutz (1988). However, Parnell and co-workers reported that 28.5% of patients developed postoperative "irritative symptoms" (Parnell et al, 1982).

Vaginal Prolapse

Vaginal prolapse other than cystocele has been reported following retropubic cystourethropexy. The reported incidence of enterocele after the Burch procedure varies between 3% and 17% and is most likely caused by an alteration in vaginal depth and axis, aggravating posterior vaginal wall weakness (Burch, 1961; Langer et al, 1988). Wiskind and co-workers noted that 27% of patients who had undergone a Burch colposuspension developed prolapse requiring surgery for rectocele (22%), enterocele (11%), uterine prolapse (13%), and cystocele (2%) (Wiskind et al, 1992). Prophylactic obliteration of the cul-de-sac of Douglas is sometimes considered when performing retropubic cystourethropexy to avoid enterocele formation. Prophylactic simultaneous hysterectomy does not enhance the outcome of cystourethropexy and should be performed only when uterine pathology exists, and this may include uterine disease or marked uterine descensus (Langer et al, 1988; Kiilholma et al, 1993).

REFERENCES

Appell RA: Retropubic procedures for female stress incontinence. *In* Webster GD, Kirby R, King L, Goldwasser B, eds: Reconstructive Urology. Oxford, Blackwell Scientific Publishers, 1993, pp 887–894.

Awad SA, Flood HD, Acker KL: The significance of prior anti-incontinence surgery in women who present with urinary incontinence. J Urol 1988;140:514.

Benson R: Retropubic vesicourethropexy—success or failure? Am J Obstet Gynecol 1988; 35:665–669.

Burch JC: Urethrovaginal fixation to Cooper's ligament for correction of stress incontinence, cystocele, and prolapse. Am J Obstet Gynecol 1961; 81:281–290.

Cardoza LD, Stanton SL, Williams JE: Detrusor instability following surgery for genuine stress incontinence. Br J Urol 1979; 51:204–207.

Colombo M, Scalambrino S, Maggioni A, Milani R: Burch colposuspension vs. modified Marshall-Marchetti-Krantz urethropexy for primary genuine stress urinary incontinence: A prospective, randomized clinical trial. Am J Obstet Gynecol 1994; 171:1573–1579.

Eriksen BC, Hagen B, Eik-Nes SH, et al: Long term effectiveness of the Burch colposuspension in female urinary stress incontinence. Acta Obstet Gynaecol Scand 1990; 69:45–50.

Forneret E, Leach GE: Cost-effective treatment of female stress urinary incontinence: Modified Pereyra bladder neck suspension. Urology 1985; 25:365.

Galloway NTM, Davies N, Stephenson TP: The complications of colposuspension. Br J Urol 1987; 60:122–124.

Gillon G, Stanton SL: Long-term follow-up of surgery for urinary incontinence in elderly women. Br J Urol 1984; 56:478–481.

Gittes RF, Laughlin KR: No-incision pubovaginal suspension for stress incontinence. J Urol 1987; 138:568.

Green DF, McGuire EJ, Lytton B: A comparison of endoscopic suspension of the vesical neck vs. anterior urethropexy for the treatment of stress urinary incontinence. J Urol 1986; 136:1205.

Grout D, O'Conor VJ: Long-term results of suprapubic vesicourethropexy. J Urol 1972; 107:610–612.

Hebertsson G, Iosif CS: Surgical results and urodynamic studies 10 years after retropubic colpourethrocystopexy. Acta Obstet Gynecol Scand 1993; 72:298–301.

Hilton P, Stanton SL: A clinical and urodynamic assessment of the Burch colposuspension for genuine stress incontinence. Br J Obstet Gynecol 1983; 90:934–939.

Jarvis GJ: Stress incontinence. *In* Mundy AR, Stephenson TP, Wein AJ, eds: Urodynamics: Principles, Practice and Application, 2nd ed. New York, Churchill Livingstone, 1994, pp 299–326.

Kiilholma P, Makinen J, Chancellor MB, et al: Modified Burch colposuspension for stress urinary incontinence in females. Surg Gynecol Obstet 1993; 176:111–115.

Kjølhede P, Ryden G: Prognostic factors and long-term results of the Burch colposuspension. Acta Obstet Gynecol Scand 1994; 73:642–647.

Langer R, Ron-El R, Neuman M, et al: The value of simultaneous hysterectomy during Burch colposuspension for stress urinary incontinence. Obstet Gynecol 1988; 72:866–869.

Liu CY: Laparoscopic retropubic colposuspension (Burch procedure)—a review of 58 cases. J Reprod Med 1993; 38(7):526–530.

Lose G, Jorgennsen L, Mortensen SO, et al: Voiding difficulties after colposuspension. Obstet Gynecol 1987; 69:33–38.

McDuffie RW, Litin RB, Blundun KE: Urethrovesical suspension (Marshall-Marchetti-Krantz). Am J Surg 1981; 141:297–298.

McGuire EJ: Urodynamic findings in patients after failure of stress incontinence operations. Prog Clin Biol Res 1981; 78:351.

McGuire EJ: Bladder instability in stress urinary incontinence. Neurourol Urodynam 1988; 7:563.

Mainprize TC, Drutz HP: The Marshall-Marchetti-Krantz procedure: A critical review. Obstet Gynecol Surv 1988; 43:724.

Marshall FV, Marchetti AA, Krantz KE: The correction of stress incontinence by simple vesicourethral suspension. Surg Gynecol Obstet 1949; 88:509–518.

Mundy AR: A trial comparing the Stamey bladder neck suspension with a colposuspension for the treatment of stress incontinence. Br J Urol 1983; 55:687–690.

Nitti VW, Raz S: Obstruction following anti-incontinence procedures: Diagnosis and treatment with transvaginal urethrolysis. J Urol 1994; 152:93.

Parnell JP, Marshall VF, Vaughn ED: Primary management of urinary stress incontinence by the Marshall-Marchetti-Krantz vesicourethropexy. J Urol 1982; 127:679–682.

Pereyra AJ: A simplified surgical procedure for the correction of stress incontinence in women. West J Surg Obstet Gynecol 1959; 67:223–226.

Polascik TJ, Moore RG, Rosenberg MT, Kavoussi LR: Comparison of laparoscopic and open retropubic urethropexy for treatment of stress urinary incontinence. Urology 1995; 45:647–652.

Ramon J, Mekras JA, Webster GD: Transvaginal needle suspension procedures for recurrent stress incontinence. Urology 1991; 38:519–522.

Raz S: Modified bladder neck suspension for female stress incontinence. Urology 1981; 17:82.

Richardson AC, Edmonds PB, Williams NL: Treatment of stress urinary incontinence due to paravaginal fascial defect. Obstet Gynecol 1981; 57:357–363.

Richardson AC, Lyon J, Williams NL: A new look at pelvic relaxation. Am J Obstet Gynecol 1976; 126:568.

Shull BL, Baden WF: A six year experience with paravaginal defect repair for stress urinary incontinence. Am J Obstet Gynecol 1989; 160:1432–40.

Spencer JR, O'Connor VJ: Comparison of procedures for stress urinary incontinence. AUA Update 1987; 6:1–7.

Stamey TA: Endoscopic suspension of the vesical neck for urinary incontinence in females. Ann Surg 1980; 192:465.

Stanton SL: Suprapubic approaches for stress incontinence in women. J Am Geriatr Soc 1990; 38:348–351.

Stanton SL, Cardoza LD: Results of the colposuspension operation for incontinence and prolapse. Br J Obstet Gynecol 1979; 86:693–697.

Steel SA, Cox C, Stanton SL: Long term follow-up of detrusor instability following the colposuspension operation. Br J Urol 1985; 58:138.

Turner-Warwick R: The Turner-Warwick vagino-obturator shelf urethral-repositioning procedure. *In* Debruyne FMJ, Van Kerrenbroech PEUAM, eds: Practical Aspects of Urinary Incontinence. Dordrecht, Martinus Nijhoff, 1986, pp 100–104.

Van Caillie TG, Schuessler W: Laparoscopic bladder neck suspension. J Laparo Endosc Surg 1991; 1:169–173.

Van Geelen JM, Theeuwes AGM, Eskes TKAB, Martin CB: The clinical and urodynamic effects of anterior vaginal repair and Burch colposuspension. Am J Obstet Gynecol 1988; 159:137–144.

Webster JD, Kreder KJ: Voiding dysfunction following cystourethropexy: Its evaluation and management. J Urol 1990; 144:670–673.

White GR: Cystocele, a radical cure by suturing lateral sulci of vagina to white line of pelvic fascia. JAMA 1909; 53:1707–1711.

White GR: An anatomic operation for the cure of cystocele. Am J Obstet Dis Women Child 1912; 65:286.

Wiskind AK, Creighton SM, Stanton SL: The incidence of genital prolapse after the Burch colposuspension. Am J Obstet Gynecol 1992;167:399–405.

34
PUBOVAGINAL SLINGS

Edward J. McGuire, M.D.
Helen E. O'Connell, M.D.

Pubovaginal slings are increasingly recognized as a robust form of treatment for stress urinary incontinence (SUI) especially when it is due to intrinsic sphincter deficiency. Several series of women treated with pubovaginal rectus fascial slings present evidence of prolonged follow-up and durable efficacy (Jeffcoate, 1956; McGuire et al, 1987; Blaivas and Jacobs, 1991; Swierzewski et al, 1994). Slings formed from other materials are durable (Beck et al, 1988; Morgan et al, 1985), although synthetic materials are associated with significant morbidity. Since the early descriptions of pubovaginal slings, the indications for their use and methods of patient selection have been refined, as have the choice and length of material used and the operative technique.

HISTORY OF PUBOVAGINAL SLINGS

Von Giordano is credited with the first sling (Blaivas, 1994), which involved wrapping a gracilis graft around the urethra. Goebel used pyramidalis slings in children (Deming, 1926), and Frangenheim (1914) used rectus abdominus muscle and fascia. Te Linde (1934) quoted Stoeckel, one of the German originators of slings, as noting that the material used was unimportant to the outcome, which depended on a high urethral position and attachment of the sling to abdominal muscles. In Britain, Aldridge (1942) used fascial slings in conjunction with vaginal plastic operations, and Millin and Read (1948) used long fascial strips and achieved good results in patients with urethral hypermobility.

Development of Specific Indications for Slings

Until the 1970s, the standard operation for SUI was an anterior colporrhaphy. Several early reports suggested that this was an inadequate treatment for at least some forms of SUI. Aldridge (Millin and Read, 1948) and Jeffcoate (1956) suggested that slings should be used when "something more than an anterior colporrhaphy" was needed. Incontinence due to neurogenic causes, or associated with a marked degree of genital prolapse, was regarded as a contraindication to sling procedures (Millin and Read, 1948).

FAILURE OF PRIOR OPERATIONS AND TYPE III STRESS URINARY INCONTINENCE (INTRINSIC SPHINCTER DEFICIENCY). During the 1970s a number of investigators independently recognized that SUI could occur without urethral hypermobility, even after an operation resulted in a "well-supported" urethra. Robertson (1974) described the "stovepipe" urethra as one with poor closure characteristics. Green (1962) and Hodgkinson (1970) independently described the radiologic appearance of a well-supported urethra that nevertheless leaked with increased abdominal pressure. Both treated patients who failed standard suspension procedures with slings.

McGuire (1981) compared the urodynamic and radiographic findings in 414 women with SUI who had never had surgery with 234 women who developed recurrent or persistent SUI after surgery (Table 34–1). Most women with primary SUI had normal intrinsic sphincter function and mild to gross urethral hypermobility (types I and II SUI). Type III SUI, or a poorly closed proximal urethra, was quite

Table 34–1. TYPES OF STRESS URINARY INCONTINENCE IN 648 WOMEN

Previous Surgery Status	Number	Type I (%)	Type II (%)	Type III (%)
Never had an operation	414	131 (31)	230 (55)	53 (13)
Failed anterior colporrhaphy	143	8 (5)	100 (70)	35 (25)
Failed retropubic suspension	15	0	10 (67)	5 (33)
Failed multiple operations	76	3 (4)	16 (21)	57 (75)
Total failed	234	11 (5)	126 (54)	97 (41)
Overall total	648	142 (22)	356 (56)	150 (23)

unusual in this group (13%). By contrast, in the 234 women in whom an operation had failed, type III was much more common. After a single failed procedure, urethral hypermobility was still the most common finding, but 25% had type III SUI, usually without any urethral mobility. In those women whose operation had failed more than once, 75% demonstrated type III SUI. This suggests that type III SUI is associated with operative failure. Patients with type III SUI identified by videourodynamic testing who were treated with a pubovaginal sling had an SUI cure rate of 91% (McGuire and Lytton, 1978) at a mean of 2.3 years. These findings suggest that preoperative identification of type III SUI is valuable to select the appropriate operative procedure.

CURRENT METHODS TO IDENTIFY TYPE III SUI. The lowest abdominal pressure required to induce leakage is the *abdominal leak point pressure* (ALPP), or *stress* or *Valsalva* leak point pressure (Wan et al, 1993). Intrinsic sphincter deficiency (ISD) can be identified by testing the ALPP (McGuire et al, 1993), since that measurement correlates with the videourodynamic diagnosis. The majority of patients (76%) with type III SUI have an ALPP of 0 to 60 cm H_2O, although a further 25% of patients with type III SUI have ALPPs between 60 and 90 cm H_2O.

INDICATIONS FOR PUBOVAGINAL SLING SURGERY

Conditions Best Treated by a Sling

INTRINSIC SPHINCTER DEFICIENCY AND URETHRAL HYPERMOBILITY—SLINGS VERSUS COLLAGEN. A pubovaginal sling is the treatment of choice when both urethral hypermobility and ISD are present. Collagen and other injectables that are used to treat ISD have uncertain long-term efficacy and are probably not effective for urethral hypermobility (O'Connell et al, 1995).

Because of the difference in the magnitude of the procedures, it is difficult to compare success rates for the slings and collagen. At a mean of 3 years follow-up, a sling has a success rate of approximately 90% for curing SUI (Jeffcoate, 1956; Hohenfellner and Petri, 1980; McGuire et al, 1987; Blaivas and Jacobs, 1991; Swierzewski et al, 1994) compared with collagen cure rates closer to 65% at a shorter interval (O'Connell et al, 1995).

INTRINSIC SPHINCTER DEFICIENCY AND CYSTOCELE. The combined problem of a cystocele and SUI is not uncommon, but surprisingly little has been written about it. In a series of 65 women with various forms of genital prolapse (McGuire et al, 1991), 53 had urodynamic evidence of SUI, often without SUI symptoms. When a cystocele or other form of genital prolapse is the presenting complaint, urethral function should be evaluated urodynamically with the cystocele reduced (Ghoniem et al, 1994) because significant urethral dysfunction may be present in the absence of SUI symptoms. This is more likely to occur with grade III cystoceles (Ghoniem et al, 1994). The pubovaginal sling in this setting is useful for urethral dysfunction and to simultaneously provide support for the cystocele repair.

INTRINSIC SPHINCTER DEFICIENCY ASSOCIATED WITH A URETHRAL DIVERTICULUM. Before excision of a urethral diverticulum, urethral function should be evaluated because of a high incidence of concomitant urethral dysfunction. Swierzewski and McGuire (1993) identified ISD in five of 14 cases of diverticulum, and urethral hypermobility in a further two patients. All seven patients underwent combined diverticulum excision and pubovaginal sling. At follow-up over a mean of 17 months, no patient had developed recurrent SUI. These findings differ from those reported in other recent series, in which 22% developed SUI after urethral diverticulectomy despite a concomitant needle suspension (Bass and Leach, 1991). This difference may be related to the presence of ISD as a preexisting condition, or perhaps the ISD was induced by the diverticulectomy.

FAILED PRIOR NEEDLE OR RETROPUBIC SUSPENSION. When slings have been used to treat women with unclassified recurrent SUI, success rates have been as high as 98% (Beck et al, 1988). There are few data on the comparative efficacy of standard suspensions in such patient populations.

INTRINSIC SPHINCTER DEFICIENCY IN NEUROGENIC CONDITIONS SUCH AS MYELODYSPLASIA. Slings are an effective treatment of neurogenic ISD (McGuire et al, 1986, 1987; Gormley et al, 1994). Apart from the frequent need in neurogenic conditions to perform intermittent catheterization, the principles governing the choice of treatment are the same as for non-neurogenic patients. When there is another indication for surgery, for example, poor compliance in addition to ISD, it adds little to an augmentation cystoplasty to perform a concomitant sling (Gormley et al, 1994).

Indications Favoring Sling Use

VIGOROUS ATHLETES, OBESE PATIENTS, PATIENTS WITH CHRONIC OBSTRUCTIVE PULMONARY DISEASE. Slings are very durable, with few reported cases of late sling failure. For that reason, patients who exert considerable abdominal pressure such as vigorous athletes, obese patients, and those with chronic obstructive pulmonary disease are suitable candidates for a sling.

SLINGS IN RECONSTRUCTION—URETHRAL LOSS. Total urethral dysfunction or tissue loss can occur in a number of circumstances including prolonged Foley catheterization (Chancellor et al, 1994), urethrovaginal fistula repair (Blaivas and Jacobs, 1991), urethral diverticulum excision, urethral injury from a pelvic fracture (Woodside, 1987; Gormley et al, 1994), and repeated SUI operations, or, more rarely, from complicated vaginal delivery. In these situations, the sling can be used to reinforce a urethral repair and other reconstructive efforts including Martius grafts, or vaginal flap reconstruction or gracilis flap (Blaivas, 1991; Blaivas and Jacobs, 1991). Blaivas (1991) reported an 85% continence rate for a series of 46 such patients treated with slings and other reconstructive techniques, although six patients required more than one procedure to achieve continence.

SLING MATERIALS

Autologous Materials

RECTUS FASCIA—SLING STRENGTH, LENGTH, VASCULARIZATION. Rectus fascia is a durable and robust material, although the evidence of its strength is historical and not experimental. There are few data on the ideal dimensions for slings although when very short slings (1 × 3 cm) were used in children, proximal urethral compression at rest was less reliably created (Gormley et al, 1994). The use of sling sutures as an extension of the sling has enabled sling length to be reduced somewhat without any apparent reduction in efficacy (Gormley, 1994; O'Connell et al, 1996). Blaivas (1994) noted that even after a number of retropubic operations, it was always possible to obtain a satisfactory strip of rectus fascia. Although synthetic materials have been used in an effort to shorten procedure time, there is little evidence that that is the case. Experiments with nonpedicled fascial slings indicate that at 3 months the sling is embedded in surrounding tissue that provides a vascular supply to the sling (Lampel et al, 1993).

FASCIA LATA. Fascia lata is efficacious (Beck et al, 1988), with a cure rate as high as 98% reported for a series of women with unspecified types of "recurrent" SUI. Morbidity with fascia lata slings is low, although pulmonary embolus and deep venous thrombosis have been reported (Beck et al, 1988), as have complications related to the thigh incision (Peters and Thornton, 1980). In a direct comparison with polytetrafluoroethylene slings, no statistically significant difference in cure rate or morbidity was observed (Ogundipe et al, 1992). Fascia lata has not been directly compared with rectus fascia.

VAGINAL WALL. At a mean follow-up of 23.9 months, a 94.4% SUI cure rate was reported (Juma et al, 1992). Full-thickness vaginal wall has been found to be strong, able to withstand a greater load than partial-thickness wall, but not as strong as Gore-Tex (Winters et al, 1995). In a recent nonrandomized series of 33 women comparing pubovaginal fascial slings with modified vaginal wall slings, no significant difference in outcome was revealed (Golomb et al, 1995).

OTHER AUTOLOGOUS MATERIALS. A variety of other human tissues have been used to wrap or sling the urethra. These include pyramidalis muscle, round ligament, gracilis, levator ani, adductors and biceps, and external oblique fascia.

Synthetic Materials: Mersilene and Polypropylene

Although Mersilene (Dacron) slings have been associated with cure rates as high as 92% (Williams and Te Linde, 1961), significant morbidity, including suprapubic abscesses, sling erosion into the bladder (Melnick and Lee, 1976), and delayed transection of the urethra (Melnick and Lee, 1976) have been reported. Polypropylene slings have been associated with complications (Morgan et al, 1985), including 16 cases of a "totally sloughed urethra" resulting in total incontinence. Considering the excellent outcome when native substances are used and the severity of complications associated with synthetic materials, there seems no compelling reason to use the latter materials.

Nonsynthetic Materials

Lyophilized dura mater and *porcine dermis* are nonsynthetic "biocompatible" materials that have been used to avoid the complications associated with synthetic slings (Faber et al, 1978; Iosif, 1987). These materials are expensive, appear to offer no advantage over fascia, and may be absorbed with time (Lampel et al, 1993).

PREOPERATIVE DETAIL: INFORMED CONSENT ISSUES, OUTCOME, INCLUDING COMPLICATIONS

STRESS URINARY CONTINENCE CURE. Although a long-term cure rate of approximately 90% can be expected for all forms of SUI, if incontinence occurs postoperatively, a fluoroscopic urodynamic study should be used to identify the cause, that is, a urethral or bladder problem. If SUI is present with no urethral mobility, collagen may cure residual SUI. If urethral mobility is present, another sling may be required. A history of something "giving way" is often present in the latter circumstance.

DETRUSOR-RELATED LEAKAGE. Detrusor overactivity present preoperatively disappeared postoperatively in approximately two thirds of patients treated with slings (McGuire and Lytton, 1978). Persistent or de novo detrusor instability may be a problem after a sling, as after any operation for SUI.

RETENTION AND VOIDING DYSFUNCTION. An issue to emphasize in informed consent is that return of normal voiding may be delayed, and, until that occurs, intermittent catheterization may be required. The routine practice of intermittent catheterization allows patients to be discharged on day 1 to 4 (mean day 3). Average times to voiding vary from 16 (Iosif, 1987) to 28 days (Swierzewski et al, 1994). Factors that may impair the return of voiding function include high sling tension, poor detrusor function, additional surgery such as a rectocele or cystocele repair, and temporary overdistention from too long an interval between intermittent catheterizations.

Long-standing inability to void is an unusual problem. In a most recent series (O'Connell et al, 1996) only three patients required permanent catheterization, and in two this was an expected outcome. Nevertheless, the adoption of unusual voiding postures and a slow stream commonly occur for periods after sling surgery even if bladder emptying is complete. A common problem before the return of normal voiding is poor emptying with a large residual volume and concomitant urge incontinence. Anticholinergic medication can be used without a fear that this will delay the return of normal voiding function.

When poor voiding is associated with evidence of outlet obstruction, for example, urge incontinence, palpable urethral hypersuspension, urodynamic evidence with a high voiding pressure, poor flow rate, or poor proximal urethral opening, urethrolysis may be necessary (Foster and McGuire, 1993).

NEED FOR THROMBOEMBOLIC PROPHYLAXIS. In none of the recent series reporting pubovaginal slings using rectus fascia has a thromboembolic complication been reported, as distinct from the experience with fascia lata (Beck et al, 1988), the older rectus fascial sling series (Sloan and Barwin, 1973), and, rarely, synthetic slings (Morgan et al, 1985). Patients now mobilize early, and the operation is of short duration (30 to 45 minutes). Thus, only in patients with identifiable risk factors are prophylactic measures used.

PREOPERATIVE ANTIMICROBIALS. A single dose of broad-spectrum intravenous antibiotic is administered so as to achieve a satisfactory blood level at the time of surgery. At the time of catheter removal and during the first few days of intermittent catheterization, patients take oral antibiotics.

OPERATIVE PROCEDURE

ANESTHESIA. Most patients have sling surgery performed under general anesthesia, though regional anesthesia can be used according to the preference of the patient and anesthesiologist.

POSITION. The patient is placed in the modified lithotomy position with the feet placed squarely in the boots of the Allen stirrups (Edgewater Medical Systems, Cleveland, Ohio) in a way that ensures there is no pressure on the calf. A foam support is placed between the lateral aspect of the calf and the stirrup. The hips are gently flexed to allow simultaneous vaginal and abdominal approaches. A weighted vaginal speculum is placed as well as a No. 18 Fr Foley catheter, which is clamped.

ABDOMINAL APPROACH. The pubovaginal sling has two components—vaginal and retropubic, which can be performed simultaneously or sequentially. In adults an 8- to 9-cm Pfannenstiel incision (Fig. 34–1) is made 4 cm above the top edge of the pubic symphysis or along a pre-existing Pfannenstiel scar. The rectus fascia is incised and the leaves of fascia are mobilized up and down to permit easy incision closure. A 9 × 1.5 to 2 cm sling is harvested from the lower leaf of the rectus fascia (the upper leaf can also be used) (see Fig. 34–1). A wider strip of fascia may be used in reconstructive cases so as to broadly reinforce a deficient urethral wall. The sling is oversewn at each end with heavy absorbable suture (e.g., polydioxanone sulfate, polyglactin). The sutures are placed perpendicular to the direction of the fascial fibers; two or three bites of the sling are taken, and the sutures are kept long.

Entry to the retropubic space is gained via blunt dissection

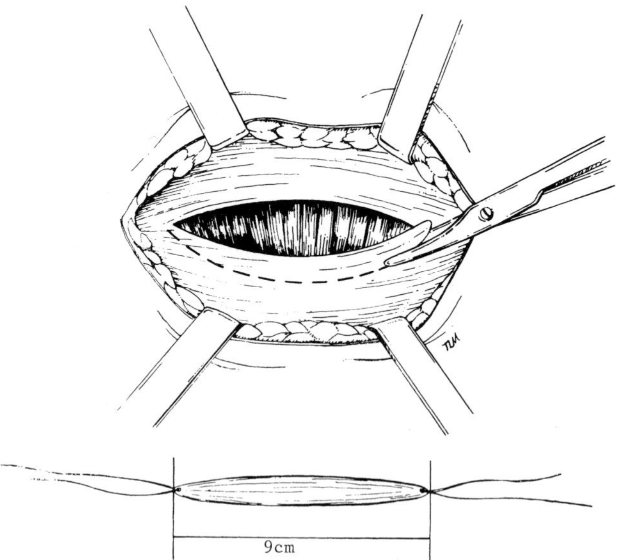

Figure 34–1. A 9 × 1.5 to 2 cm sling is harvested from a lower leaf of rectus fascia and sutured at each end.

after opening the transversalis fascia lateral to the recti as they insert on the symphysis. The recti are retracted medially close to their insertion on the pubis exposing a triangular defect that leads to the retropubic space.

VAGINAL APPROACH. A midline or inverted U incision is made overlying 2 to 3 cm of the proximal urethra. The vaginal mucosa is lifted off the underlying periurethral fascia. Entry to the retropubic space from below is started with sharp dissection, with the scissors parallel to the perineum, and developed further with blunt dissection (Fig. 34–2). In this way using a bimanual technique, a finger placed in the vaginal incision can touch a finger passing down from the abdominal incision. A long curved clamp is passed from the abdominal incision through the retropubic space guided by a finger below, the tip of the clamp passing

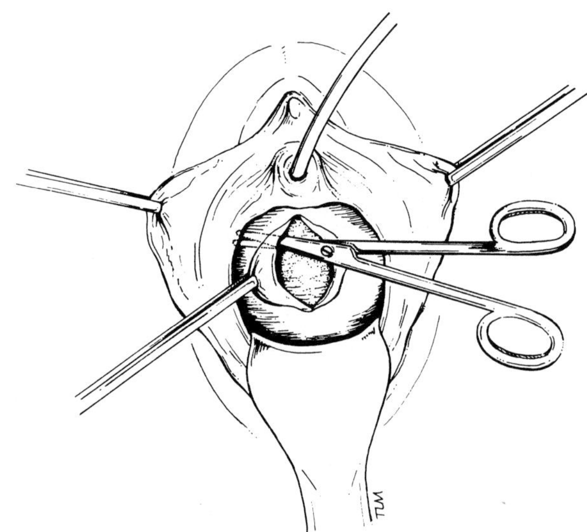

Figure 34–2. Entry to the retropubic space lateral to periurethral fascia is gained from vaginal incision. Note that the scissor tips are passed into the retropubic space with the scissors nearly parallel to the perineum.

into the vaginal incision (Fig. 34–3). The clamp then grasps the sling sutures and the sling is brought up on each side into the abdominal incision.

BLADDER INJURY. If the bladder is palpably adherent high on the posterior surface on the pubic symphysis, a Stamey needle may be used to convey the sling sutures. The Stamey needle is guided carefully along the periosteum of the pubis staying as high as possible under the pubis. If there is a high index of suspicion of bladder injury or if hematuria occurs, cystoscopy is performed with a 70-degree lens with the clamp or Stamey needle in situ. An injury typically occurs in the area described by the 11 through 2 o'clock positions, near the dome of the bladder. If an instrument is seen, it is removed and replaced in a slightly different position following the same principles.

ADJUSTMENT OF SLING POSITION. The sling is pulled up on each side, and after ensuring that it is lying symmetrically and is flat, the middle of the sling is secured to the underlying periurethral fascia with a 3-0 polyglactin suture. The sling sutures are then brought through separate stab wounds in the inferior leaf of the rectus fascia to be tied to each other after the fascia is closed.

WOUND CLOSURE. The rectus fascia is closed with a heavy polyglactin continuous suture from either end with a figure-of-eight suture in the middle. The vaginal wound is closed with a 2-0 chromic catgut continuous suture.

ADJUSTMENT OF SLING TENSION. Sling tension is adjusted according to the condition being treated. For the treatment of pure urethral hypermobility, tension is required to stop motion only. If ISD is present, the sling needs to effect urethral closure. If the ISD is very severe, the sling needs to be reasonably tight to achieve closure. Placement of a finger under the knot while the sutures are tied prevents excessive tension. Urethral motion can be evaluated during the sling operation, by pulling on the catheter while the sling sutures are held taut. A vaginal pack is used for 12 to 24 hours.

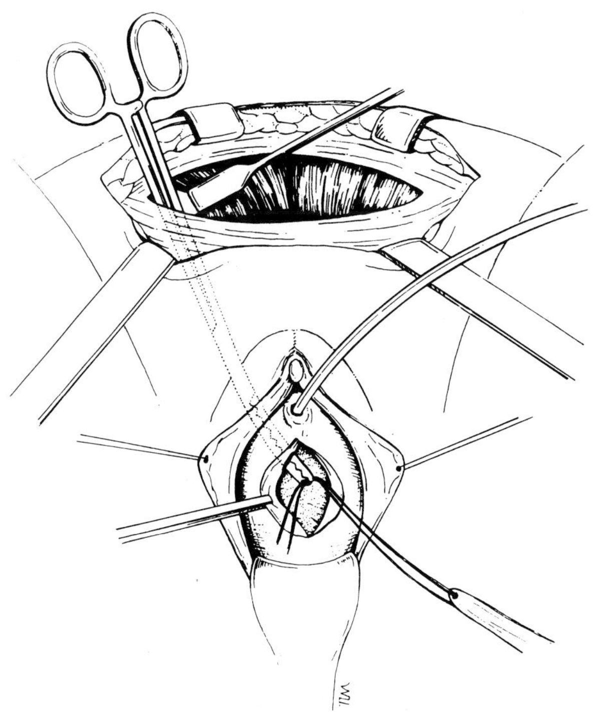

Figure 34–3. A long curved clamp is passed from the abdominal wound (through the triangular defect lateral to the rectus abdominis muscle) into the vaginal incision where it grasps the sling sutures.

OPERATING TIME AND BLOOD LOSS. When abdominal and vaginal components are performed synchronously, the operation takes 30 to 40 minutes. The blood loss is minimal, typically about 50 to 100 ml.

POSTOPERATIVE TREATMENT

EARLY POSTOPERATIVE CARE. On the first postoperative day, the vaginal pack is removed. A few doses of an intravenous opiate are usually, though not universally, required postoperatively. Patients are encouraged to ambulate as early as possible. In the first 4 postoperative weeks, patients are asked not to lift any heavy weights, especially lifting in association with stooping, for example, opening the garage door, but they may walk as tolerated. After this patients return to normal activity. At about 3 weeks, when the vaginal suture line has healed, intercourse can be recommenced as tolerated.

LATE POSTOPERATIVE CARE. One appointment at around 3 to 4 weeks postoperatively may be all that is required in addition to some inquiries (by telephone) about intermittent catheterization, urgency and urge incontinence, hematuria, unilateral wound pain, and vaginal discharge during that time—problems that are almost always short-term and self-limiting. The unilateral pain that commonly occurs temporarily is due to the sling and is relieved by relaxing the recti, for example, lying down and bending the knees.

PREGNANCY AND DELIVERY. There is little information in the literature about this topic, but in our experience normal vaginal delivery or cesarean section are feasible without damage to the sling.

REFERENCES

Aldridge AH: Transplantation of fascia for relief of urinary stress incontinence. Am J Obstet Gynecol 1942; 44:398.

Bass JS, Leach GE: Surgical treatment of concomitant urethral diverticulum and SUI. Urol Clin North Am 1991; 18:365.

Beck RP, McCormick S, Nordstrom L: The fascia lata sling procedure for treating recurrent genuine stress incontinence of urine. Obstet Gynecol 1988; 72:699.

Blaivas JG: Treatment of female incontinence secondary to urethral damage or loss. Urol Clin North Am 1991; 18:355.

Blaivas JG: Pubovaginal slings. *In* Kursh ED, McGuire EJ, eds: Female Urology. Philadelphia, J. B. Lippincott Company, 1994, p 235.

Blaivas JG, Jacobs BZ: Pubovaginal fascial sling for the treatment of complicated stress urinary incontinence. J Urol 1991; 145:1214–1218.

Chancellor MB, Erhard MJ, Kiilholma PJ, et al: Functional urethral closure with pubovaginal sling for destroyed female urethra after long-term urethral catheterization. Urol 1994; 43:499.

Deming CL: Transplantation of the gracilis muscle for incontinence of urine. JAMA 1926; 86:822–825.

Faber P, Beck L, Heidenreich J: Treatment of urinary stress incontinence in women with the lyodura sling. Urol Int 1978; 33:117–119.

Foster HE, McGuire EJ: Management of urethral obstruction with transvaginal urethrolysis. J Urol 1993; 150:1448.

Frangenheim P: Zur operativen Behandlung der Inkontinenz der Männlichen Harnrohre. Verh Dtsch Ges Chir 1914; 43:149.

Ghoniem GM, Walters F, Lewis V: The value of the vaginal pack test in large cystoceles. J Urol 1994; 152:931–934.

Golomb J, Goldwasser B, Mashiach S: Comparison of suspended pubovaginal sling and modified vaginal wall sling for sphincteric incompetence. (Abstract 1184.) J Urol 1995; 153.

Gormley EA, Bloom DA, McGuire EJ, Ritchey ML: Pubovaginal slings for the management of urinary incontinence in female adolescents. J Urol 1994; 152:822.

Green TH: Development of a plan for the diagnosis and treatment of urinary stress incontinence. Am J Obstet Gynecol 1962; 83:632.

Hodgkinson CP: Stress urinary incontinence—1970. Am J Obstet Gynecol 1970; 108:1141–1168.

Hohenfellner R, Petri E: Sling procedures. *In* Stanton SL, Tanagho EA, eds: Surgery of Female Incontinence. Berlin, Springer-Verlag, 1980, pp 67–71.

Iosif CS. Porcine corium sling in the treatment of urinary stress incontinence. Arch Gynecol Obstet 1987; 240:131–136.

Jeffcoate TNA: The results for the Aldridge sling operation for stress urinary incontinence. J Obstet Gynaecol 1956; 63:36–39.

Juma S, Little NA, Raz S: Vaginal wall sling: Four years later. Urology 1992; 39:424–428.

Lampel A, Fokaefs E, Hohenfellner M, et al: Experimental comparison of pedicled versus non-pedicled fascial slings. (Abstract.) J Urol 1993; vol 149.

McGuire EJ: Urodynamic findings in patients after failure of stress urinary incontinence operations. Prog Clin Biol Res 1981; 78:351–360.

McGuire EJ, Bennett CJ, Konnak JA, et al: Experience with pubovaginal slings for urinary incontinence at the University of Michigan. J Urol 1987; 138:525–526.

McGuire EJ, Fitzpatrick CC, Wan J, et al: Clinical assessment of urethral sphincter function. J Urol 1993; 150:1452.

McGuire EJ, Gardy M, Elkins T, De Lancey JOL: Treatment of incontinence with pelvic prolapse. Urol Clin North Am 1991; 18:349.

McGuire EJ, Lytton B: Pubovaginal sling procedure for stress incontinence. J Urol 1978; 119:82.

McGuire EJ, Wang C, Usitalo H, Savastano J: Modified pubovaginal sling in girls with myelodysplasia. J Urol 1986; 135:94.

Melnick I, Lee RE: Delayed transection of the urethra by Mersilene tape. Urology 1976; 8:580.

Millin T, Read CD: Stress urinary incontinence of urine in the female. Postgrad Med J 1948; 24:51–56.

Morgan JE, Farrow GA, Stewart FE: The Marlex sling operation for the treatment of recurrent stress urinary incontinence: A 16 year review. Am J Obstet Gynecol 1985; 151:224–226.

O'Connell HE, McGuire EJ, Aboseif SR, Gudziak MR: Pubovaginal slings in 1994. (Abstract.) J Urol 1996; 155:10–13

O'Connell HE, McGuire EJ, Aboseif SR, Usui A: Transurethral collagen therapy in women. J Urol 1995; 154:1463–1465.

Ogundipe A, Rosenzweig BA, Blumenfeld D, Bhatia NN: Modified suburethral sling procedures for treatment of recurrent or severe stress urinary incontinence. Surg Gynecol Obstet 1992; 175:173–176.

Peters AW, Thornton NW: Selection of primary operative procedure for stress urinary incontinence. Am J Obstet Gynecol 1980; 137:53–55.

Robertson JR: Ambulatory gynecologic urology clinic. Obstet Gynecol 1974; 17:261.

Sloan WR, Barwin BN: Stress incontinence of urine: A retrospective study of the complications and late results of simple suprapubic suburethral fascial slings. J Urol 1973; 110:533.

Swierzewski SJ, Castilla JA, Faerber G, McGuire EJ: The pubovaginal sling for tertiary type III stress urinary incontinence, long term results and outcomes. (Abstract 768.) J Urol 1994; 151:419A.

Swierzewski SJ, McGuire EJ: Pubovaginal sling for treatment of female SUI complicated by urethral diverticulum. J Urol 1993; 149:1012–1014.

Te Linde RW: The modified Goebell-Stoeckel operation for urinary incontinence. South Med J 1934; 27:193–197.

Wan J, McGuire EJ, Bloom DA, Ritchey ML: Stress leak point pressure: A diagnostic tool for incontinent children. J Urol 1993; 150:700–702.

Williams TJ, Te Linde RW: The sling operation for urinary incontinence using Mersilene ribbon. Obstet Gynecol 1961; 19:241–245.

Winters JC, Rackley RR, Kambie H, Appell RA: The biomechanical properties of the vaginal wall. (Abstract 1191.) J Urol 1995; vol 153.

Woodside JR: Pubovaginal sling procedure for the management of urinary incontinence after urethral trauma in women. J Urol 1987; 138:527.

35 PERIURETHRAL INJECTION THERAPY

Rodney A. Appell, M.D.

Surgical procedures designed to restore the urethra to its proper resting position and to keep it there during excursions in abdominal pressure (P_{abd}) do not resolve incontinence related to intrinsic sphincter dysfunction (ISD). To obviate that problem, surgeons have performed slings or have implanted artificial sphincters to compress the urethra, but increasing urethral resistance to P_{abd} may result in a parallel increase in detrusor pressure (P_{det}) with untoward effects on bladder compliance leading to upper tract damage. **One does not wish to increase resistance to P_{det} just to obviate stress incontinence produced by increases in P_{abd}. Injectable materials** can be used successfully in patients with ISD because they dramatically **improve the ability of the urethra to resist increases in P_{abd}** without changing voiding pressure or the P_{det} at the time of leakage.

PATIENT SELECTION

Injectables are not a panacea for all types of incontinence. Strict criteria exist for their consideration as a treatment modality. They are most suitable for patients with ISD and normal detrusor muscle function.

The activity precipitating the urinary leakage is important. **Patients who leak in the supine position, have bed wetting, or leak with a sensation of urinary urgency do not have genuine stress urinary incontinence** and need to be investigated for ISD. Urodynamic studies are performed to evaluate possible bladder causes of incontinence and to evaluate urethral function, which is easily ascertained by measuring **abdominal leak point pressure (ALPP) (i.e., the P_{abd} required to drive urine through the continence mechanism).** This corresponds to urethral opening pressure. Low ALPP (<65 cm H_2O) resulting in urinary leakage implies ISD. ALPP appears to be related to the grading or severity of incontinence reported by the patient and is less variable and easier to perform than urethral pressure profilometry. **Videourodynamics reveals an open bladder outlet at rest in the absence of a detrusor contraction, which is the true definition of ISD.** The ideal patient for the use of injectables is one with poor urethral function (ISD), normal bladder capacity and compliance, and good anatomic support. **Contraindications to injectables** include active urinary tract infection, untreated detrusor hyperreflexia, or known hyperactivity to the proposed injectable agent.

Adult Males

Leakage demonstrable with coughing, straining, or exercise is sufficient to judge that ISD is present in men. Urodynamic investigation is performed to rule out detrusor causes of incontinence. Bladder neck contracture must be recognized and addressed before injectable therapy, and previous radiation therapy may limit the ability to do suburothelial bulking without rupture of the urothelium, thus reducing the ability to coapt the walls of the urethra. To be effective, injectable material must be injected in the urethra superior to the external sphincter. The depth of injection is also critical, because the injectable material must deform the urethra mucosa so that it closes the urethral lumen.

Adult Females

Injectables are most suitable for patients with pure ISD. Therefore, the physical examination is essential to ascertain if associated prolapse and urethral hypermobility are present. A pelvic examination that shows no urethral mobility with straining or coughing in conjunction with a positive "*stress test,*" wherein leakage is seen to occur when the patient strains in the upright position with 200 ml in the bladder, constitutes presumptive evidence of ISD. The **cotton-swab test** is useful, with an **angle of greater than 30 degrees signifying urethral hypermobility** (Chrystle et al, 1971; Appell and Ostergard, 1992). Radiographically, the presence of an open bladder neck and proximal urethra in the absence of a detrusor contraction implies the presence of ISD. Urodynamic investigation is performed to rule out possible detrusor causes of incontinence, as well as to obtain ALPP. This measurement of the abdominal pressure required to induce leakage is a confirmatory step. Patients best suited for suspension operations and, therefore, unsuited for injection therapy are those with urethral hypermobility and high ALPP. **Patients with combined ISD and hypermobility are better served with** alternative surgical therapy such as the **artificial urinary sphincter or a sling procedure.**

Pediatric Males and Females

In these patients, although the etiology of the ISD may be different (e.g., myelodysplasia instead of postsurgical effects), the criteria of adequate bladder capacity, lack of detrusor dysfunction, and lack of anatomic abnormality (hypermobility) in the presence of ISD indicate the best candidates.

INJECTABLE MATERIALS

Historical Chronology

The technique of periurethral and intraurethral injection of material to increase outflow resistance in patients with urinary incontinence is not new. The first report (Murless, 1938) involved 20 patients and described the injection of a sclerosing solution (sodium morrhuate or cod liver oil) into the anterior vaginal wall. An inflammatory response developed with secondary scarring and resultant compression of the incompetent urethra. Cure or improvement was reported in 17 patients; however, the complications included pulmonary infarction and cardiorespiratory arrest. Quackels (1955) reported two patients successfully treated with periurethral paraffin injection without complications. Sachse (1963) treated 31 patients with another sclerosing agent, Dondren, and 12 of 24 men with postprostatectomy incontinence and 4 of 7 women were reported as cured. Again, however, pulmonary complications constituted the major drawback.

Polytetrafluoroethylene (PTFE)

The first report of the use of PTFE paste in a glycerol base (polytef; Urethrin) by Berg (1973) described three women with surgically induced ISD who experienced resolution of symptoms, although two of the three required a repeat injection. The only complication was asymptomatic bacteruria in one patient. The use of PTFE injection for incontinence was promulgated in the United States by Politano and associates at the University of Miami for many years (Politano et al, 1974; Lewis et al, 1984; Kaufman et al, 1984; Vorstman et al, 1985). However, this procedure did not attain universal acceptance despite reports from various other centers demonstrating its efficacy (Heer, 1977; Lampante et al, 1979; Lim et al, 1983; Schulman et al, 1983; Deane et al, 1985; Appell, 1990a). These and other studies were extensively reviewed for efficacy and safety by the **Department of Technology Assessment of the American Medical Association (Cole, 1993), which concluded that PTFE injection is a reasonably effective treatment for incontinence** and technically easy to perform. But because of migration of particles (Malizia et al, 1984) and granuloma formation (Mittleman and Marraccini, 1983), **the safety of the product remains uncertain.** Despite these findings, there have been no reports of untoward sequelae in humans. In addition, this product has had so many reports (listed earlier) of such great success in so many different types of incontinence problems that they have been treated with incredulity by many physicians. A current investigation into the efficacy and safety of PTFE injections for incontinence due only to ISD has begun under monitoring by the United States Food and Drug Administration, and it is hoped that this will clarify many of these concerns with respect to efficacy and safety.

Glutaraldehyde Cross-Linked Bovine Collagen (GAX-Collagen)

Bovine dermal collagen has long been recognized as a **biocompatible biomaterial** primarily in the form of resorbable sutures and hemostatic agents. **Cross-linking with glutaraldehyde results in** a fibrillar collagen with **resistance to collagenase digestion** and significantly enhances persistence with stabilization preventing syneresis. For this reason, overcorrection is not necessary or desirable with GAX-collagen implants. The volume does not undergo rapid shrinkage soon after injection because of the formation of this compact fibrous structure, which promotes incorporation into surrounding host connective tissue with additional production and deposition of new host collagen within the implant (DeLustro et al, 1991). This material **does not cause granuloma formation,** and migration of particles to distant body sites does not appear in autopsied individuals (DeLustro et al, 1991). GAX-collagen is a highly purified 35%

suspension of bovine collagen in a phosphate buffer containing at least 95% type I collagen and 1% to 5% type III collagen prepared by selective hydrolysis of the nonhelicoidal amino terminal and carboxy terminal segments (telopeptides) of the collagen molecules, which has the effect of decreasing the antigenicity (DeLustro et al, 1990) and increasing the duration of the implant within the human body by increasing its resistance to collagenase (McPherson et al, 1986). GAX-collagen is biocompatible and biodegradable and elicits only a minimal inflammatory reaction without foreign body reaction (Canning et al, 1988). **GAX-collagen begins to degrade in 12 weeks and is completely degraded in 19 months,** yet the transformation of the injected material into living connective tissue (Remacle and Marbaix, 1988) explains its ability to maintain its effectiveness in nearly 80% of those who have attained continence (Appell, 1994a). Despite United States Food and Drug Administration approval for the treatment of ISD in males and females in the later part of 1993, **GAX-collagen** does have the potential for eliciting an allergic reaction and, although it is **more compatible than PTFE in biologic systems,** it is considerably more expensive and requires more treatment sessions to attain continence; thus the search continues for a better injectable.

Autologous Injectables

Concerns over the negative aspects of PTFE and GAX-collagen discussed earlier have led to attempts to use autologous materials such as blood and fat.

Autologous blood appears to have no lasting quality. In one small study of 14 women (Appell, 1994b), 30 ml of blood from an antecubital vein in a heparinized syringe was used. Within two treatment sessions each patient was rendered continent; however, the duration of continence lasted only between 10 and 17 days, with the resultant recommendation that in questionable cases, the inexpensive injection of autologous blood under local anesthesia in an office setting can answer the question whether other injectables are worth the expense and effort for that individual patient.

Autologous fat provides the advantages of ready availability and biocompatibility and is easily obtainable via liposuction. First reported by Gonzalez de Garibay and co-workers (1989) in 10 women, a follow-up report at 1 year after a single injection in 15 women and 5 men noted "good" results in 33% of the women and in none of the postprostatectomy men (Gonzalez de Garibay et al, 1991), an **efficacy that does not compare favorably with PFTE or GAX-collagen.** The reason for this appears to be the result of the ultimate fate of the injected fat: Only a very small proportion remains viable, because neovascularity is never adequately achieved at the center of the graft to maintain its long-term viability. Some fat integrates as a graft, but only 10% to 20% survives overall, with 60% lost in only 3 weeks after injection (Bartynski et al, 1990) because of destruction of the normal adipocyte architecture (Nguyen et al, 1990). For this reason the potential advantages of autologous fat over other injectables must be tempered against the uncertain outcome.

Silicone Polymers

Macroplastique or Bioplastique denotes textured polydimethyl-siloxane macroparticles (>100 microns) suspended within a bioexcretable carrier hydrogel of polyvinylpyrrolidone (povidone [PVP]), wherein the solid particle content is 33% of the total volume. Henly and co-workers (1995) compared migratory and histologic tendencies of solid silicone macrospheres to smaller silicone particles in dogs. Nuclear imaging revealed that small particles were disseminated throughout the lung, kidney, brain, and lymph nodes 4 months after injection, whereas only one episode of large particle migration to the lung occurred without associated inflammation. More recently, a number of presentations of early favorable results have been reported (Buckley et al, 1992; Patterson et al, 1993; Iacovou et al, 1993; Buckley et al, 1993a) with fewer injection treatments than PTFE, GAX-collagen, or autologous fat. However, the concerns over migration of particles and the adverse publicity over silicone gel implants will likely limit the use of this material in the United States.

INTRAURETHRAL INJECTION TECHNIQUES

The techniques used to inject the varying materials are not difficult, even when the substance requires some special instrumentation, such as liposuction before autologous fat injection (Ganabathi and Leach, 1994). However, it is essential to perform precise placement of the material to ensure an optimal result. The **injections** (Appell, 1994a) can be **performed suburothelially** through a needle placed directly through a cystourethroscope (transurethral injection) or periurethrally with a spinal needle or specialty injector inserted percutaneously and positioned in the suburothelial space while observing the manipulation endoscopically per urethra or via ultrasound probe per vagina in females (Appell, 1996) or per rectum in males (Kageyama et al, 1994). Thus, **regardless of the technique used, the implant is placed within the wall of the urethra (intraurethral),** optimally in the lamina propria. The cause of the incontinence, the tissue at the injection site, and the plane of delivery of the injectable substance affect the treatment results. **Nearly every patient can be injected under local anesthesia,** which has the added advantage of allowing the patient to stand and perform a few provocative maneuvers immediately after the injection in an attempt to cause urinary leakage, which can then be addressed before the patient is released from treatment.

The methods of injection should not pose great difficulty to the urologist comfortable with transurethral surgery. Precise localization of the site of deposition of the material is essential to ensure an optimal response. Men are injected through the transurethral approach, and females are injected by either approach. This author performs more periurethral injections in females, because this approach decreases bleeding complications, which hamper visualization and extrusion of the injected material.

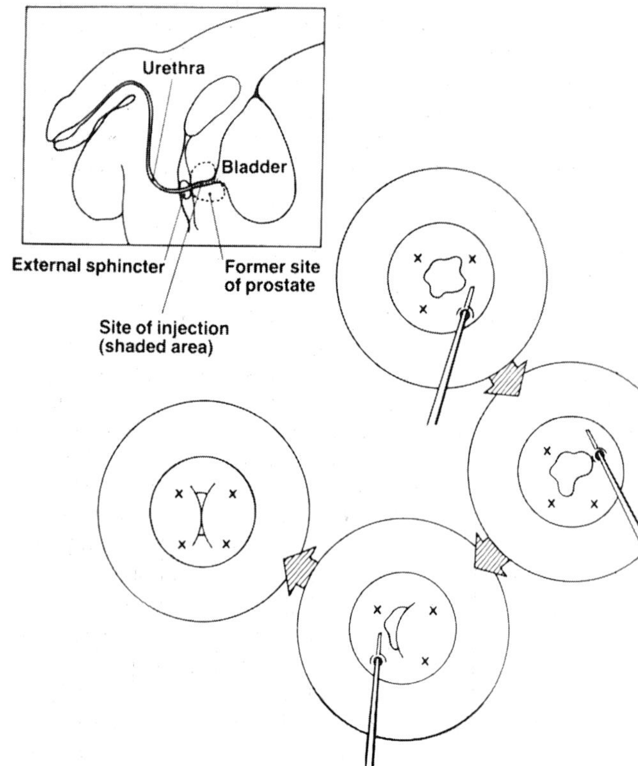

Figure 35–1. Schematic representation of transurethral circumferential injection in a postprostatectomy male. (From McGuire EJ, Appell RA: Contemp Urol 1991; 3[11]:19.)

Males

Male patients are positioned in a semilithotomy position, and the surgical field is prepared in the usual sterile fashion. If local anesthesia is employed, which the author prefers, it is used in the form of 2% lidocaine jelly intraurethrally 10 minutes before instrumentation. Anesthesia may be augmented by a perineal prostatic block with 5 to 10 ml of 1% plain lidocaine, but the author has frequently found this unnecessary. In some patients, preoperative sedation may also benefit. A 21-Fr cystoscopic sheath is employed using a 0-degree or 30-degree lens. When using GAX-collagen, it is provided in a 3.0 ml Luer-Lok syringe containing 2.5 ml of injectable material. The syringe attaches to a 5-Fr injection catheter containing a 1.5-cm 20-gauge needle at the tip. Most men are injected transurethrally under cystoscopic vision.

The **postprostatectomy** urethra is frequently scarred and less pliant; thus, **several needle positions are frequently needed** in order **to deposit sufficient material** to produce urethral coaptation. The **needle must be positioned proximal to the external sphincter,** because injection into the sphincter has been associated with sphincter spasm and failure (Appell, 1994a). The author prefers to complete the injection in four quadrants after localization of the appropriate level in the proximal urethra. The needle is advanced under the urethral mucosa with the **beveled portion of the needle facing the urethral lumen to allow for layering of the material.** The injectable material is then delivered, creating a bleb under the urethral mucosa, which protrudes into the urethral lumen. This is performed in a circumferential manner in four quadrants, creating a bleb in each quadrant (Fig. 35–1). After completion, the urethral mucosa is completely coapted and creates the appearance of an obstructed urethra. **Extrusion of the injectable agent into the urethral lumen as the needle is withdrawn may occur;** however, loss of injected material is minimal and inconsequential with most substances, with the exception of PTFE, in which case the loss may be significant. Apparently there is no loss whatsoever with silicone macrospheres. The **loss of additional material is diminished by preventing advancement of the cystoscope proximal to the injection sites.** If material extravasation occurs in all quadrants during injection, the procedure should be terminated and rescheduled after 4 weeks.

Due to the difficulty of localizing the injection in men via cystoscopy, a newer method of injecting GAX-collagen is being employed, using a **suprapubic approach.** This approach has been described employing a flexible cystoscope (Klutke, 1995) placed through a suprapubic cystotomy or using a small ureteroscope with a 5-Fr working channel (Pintauro, 1995). These methods have the advantage of direct visualization of the bladder neck and the injection of material into more supple, less scarred material. The author employs this technique using a 14-Fr pediatric endoscope, used formerly for PTFE injections, or a pediatric cystoscope (Winters and Appell, 1996). The patient is positioned in the modified lithotomy position and flexible cystoscopy is carried out, simultaneously filling the bladder. Following this, a percutaneous suprapubic punch is carried out, placing a guide wire within the bladder. A sheath may be used, but commonly the cystoscope can be advanced over the guide wire into the bladder. A small red rubber catheter or the flexible cystoscope can be used to assist in localization of the bladder neck. This approach offers an excellent view of the bladder neck and proximal urethra (Fig. 35–2). In the author's experience, fewer injection sites are needed because the non-scarred bladder neck tissue readily remodels as the material is injected. Therefore, it is not uncommon to be able to

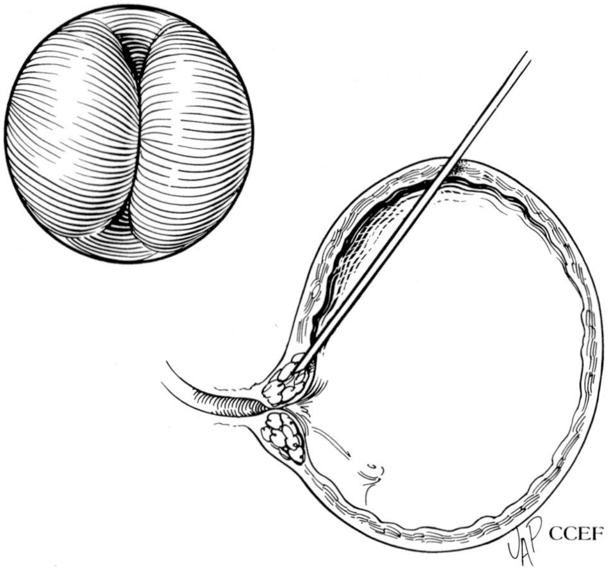

Figure 35–2. Antegrade injection in the male.

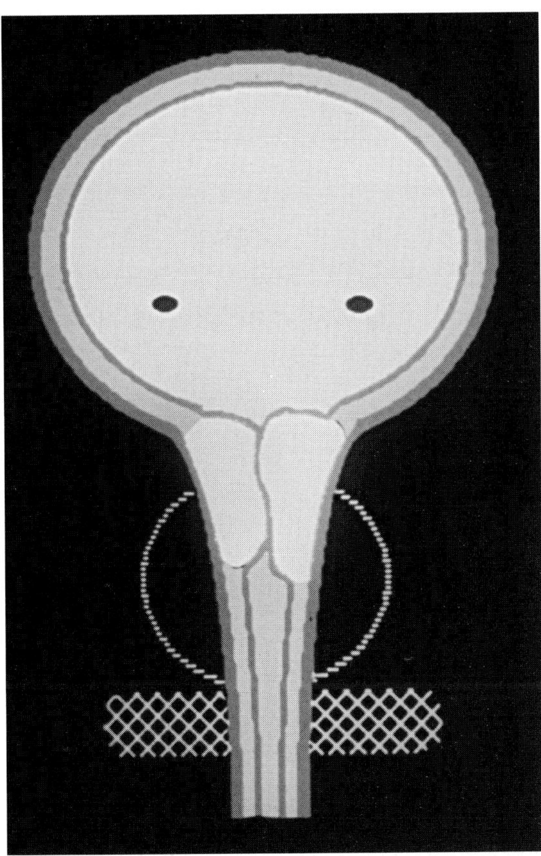

Figure 35–3. Schematic representation of cushion of injectable material just below the bladder neck. (From Appell RA: Adv Urol 1992; 5:145.)

complete an injection using two or three injection sites. The needle is placed just under the urethral mucosa at the level of the bladder neck and advanced proximally. The bladder neck closes off completely as the material is injected (Fig. 35–3). Injection stops after the bladder neck closes off, the two sides meeting in apposition near the midline. It is optional to place a small suprapubic tube to avoid the possible necessity of urethral catheterization.

To be effective, injectable material must be injected in the urethra superior to the external sphincter. Most certainly the injectable material must not be placed in the bulbous urethra where the cuff of the artificial sphincter is placed, because **injectables work at the level of the continence zone at the neck of the bladder** (i.e., the intra-abdominal urethral segment). In the treatment of postprostatic resection incontinence, the injection is in the proximal membranous urethra and laterally beside the verumontanum to give the impression of replacing "apical" tissue, and the urethra should visually appear obstructed at the conclusion of the injection. Injections in patients after radical prostatectomy are more difficult, especially in irradiated tissue or those with more scarification, and considerable practice is needed to reach correct tissue depth with the needle.

Females

Females may be injected by a transurethral technique (O'Connell and McGuire, 1995) via a needle inserted percutaneously through the wall of the urethra while observing needle placement directly by cystoscopy (Appell, 1990b), or transvaginally with the needle placed through the biopsy port of an ultrasound probe (Appell, 1996). Maneuvers to help in localization of the needle tip are useful, such as preinjecting during the periurethral technique with methylene blue to enable the surgeon to place the implant more accurately (Neal et al, 1995). In either case, the patients are placed in the lithotomy position and prepped in the usual sterile fashion. Topical 2% lidocaine jelly is used in the urethra and 20% benzocaine in the vestibule. The periurethral tissues are infiltrated with 2 to 4 ml 1% plain lidocaine injected at the 3-o'clock and 9-o'clock positions. Use of a female sound to straighten the urethra may be helpful in "removing" the curve upward of the urethra at the level of the bladder neck and to guide placement of the periurethral injection of lidocaine. It is **most important to emphasize that the material injected should be positioned at the bladder neck and proximal urethra** (see Fig. 35–3). Placement too distally ultimately is doomed to failure.

In the transurethral approach, a 0-degree lens is used. The endoscope is placed at the midurethra, and the needle is advanced in the 4-o'clock position. The point of submucosal insertion is immediately beyond the midurethra and advanced proximally to the level of the bladder neck. The material is then injected, and the urethral mucosa can be seen to gradually protrude to the midline. It is **important to inject slowly to allow the tissue to adequately accommodate the material.** When the mucosal bleb reaches the midline, the needle is withdrawn while continuing to slowly inject. The needle is then repositioned in the 8-o'clock position and the injection is performed until the urethral mucosal blebs again approximate into the midline, **creating the appearance of an obstructed prostatic urethra in the male.**

In the periurethral approach (which the author prefers to minimize intraurethral bleeding and extravasation of the injectable substance), the goal of creating urethral mucosal coaptation is the same. After infiltration of the periurethral tissues, the appropriately gauged needle (with GAX-collagen this is accomplished with a 20- or 22-gauge standard spinal needle) with the obturator in place is inserted into the periurethral tissue at the 4-o'clock position. **The needle should be positioned within the lamina propria;** in this plane the needle **advances with minimal resistance.** During advancement of the needle, urethroscopy is performed to monitor placement of the needle at the level of the bladder neck. It is quite easy to hold the endoscope with one hand while advancing the needle with the other hand. Gentle rocking of the needle assists in confirming the proper location and depth of the needle tip. Once this is confirmed, the material is injected, creating a mucosal bleb just as in the transurethral technique. Once the mucosal bleb meets the midline, the needle is repositioned in the 8-o'clock position and the injection carried out on the contralateral side (Fig. 35–4*A–C*). If extravasation occurs, the needle is repositioned in a more anterior location and the injection repeated. Once the appearance of obstruction is created by urethral coaptation, the procedure is terminated (Winters and Appell, 1995).

To avoid instrumenting the urethra and run the risk of compressing the freshly placed implant by the endoscope, transvaginal ultrasound-guided injections have been demon-

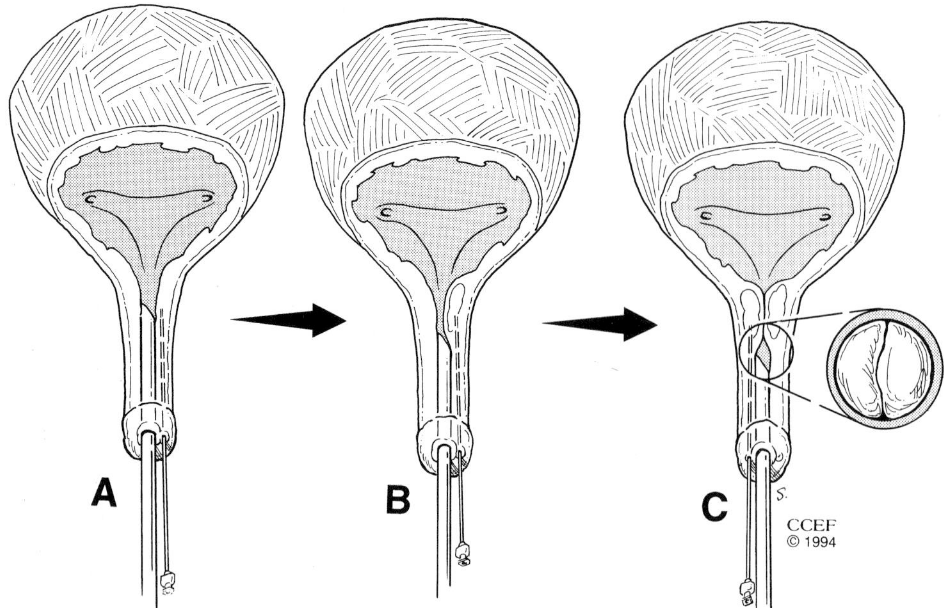

Figure 35–4. *A,* Appearance of the urethra before treatment. *B,* Periurethral needle positioned in the proximal urethra below the bladder neck. Note submucosal location within the lamina propria. *C,* Urethra after injection. (From Winters JC, Appell RA: Urol Clin N Am 1995; 22:673.)

strated to work equally as well (Appell, 1996). Using a multiplanar probe with a biopsy port (the standard transrectal ultrasound probe for prostate examination and biopsy) passed vaginally, the open bladder neck can be identified (Fig. 35–5*A*), the needle (same one used for transurethral injection) placed accurately through the biopsy port, and the injection followed through closure of the bladder neck (see Fig. 35–5*B*) by longitudinal (sagittal) scanning.

Regardless of the technique of injection chosen, the goal is closure of the bladder outlet such that there is mucosal apposition, as evidenced endoscopically (Fig. 35–6*A* and *B*).

Pediatrics

The techniques are identical to those used in adults. Williams needles as small as 3.7 Fr are available for the less viscous injectable implants (e.g. GAX-collagen).

POSTOPERATIVE CARE

Perioperative antibiotic coverage for 2 to 3 days is recommended even when the preprocedure urinalysis is normal. Most patients are able to void fairly easily or by Valsalva technique following the procedure. However, **if urinary retention occurs, clean intermittent catheterization should be utilized** with a 10-Fr to 14-Fr catheter. **Indwelling catheters should be avoided** in patients undergoing implantation because this promotes molding of the intraurethral material around the catheter. Although rarely necessary, if long-term catheterization is needed, the author recommends suprapubic cystotomy until voiding has again been initiated. Scheduled repeated injection treatment sessions for those requiring more implant should be scheduled based upon the desired period of time for the substance used. For example, GAX-collagen can be reinjected within 1 week (however, the

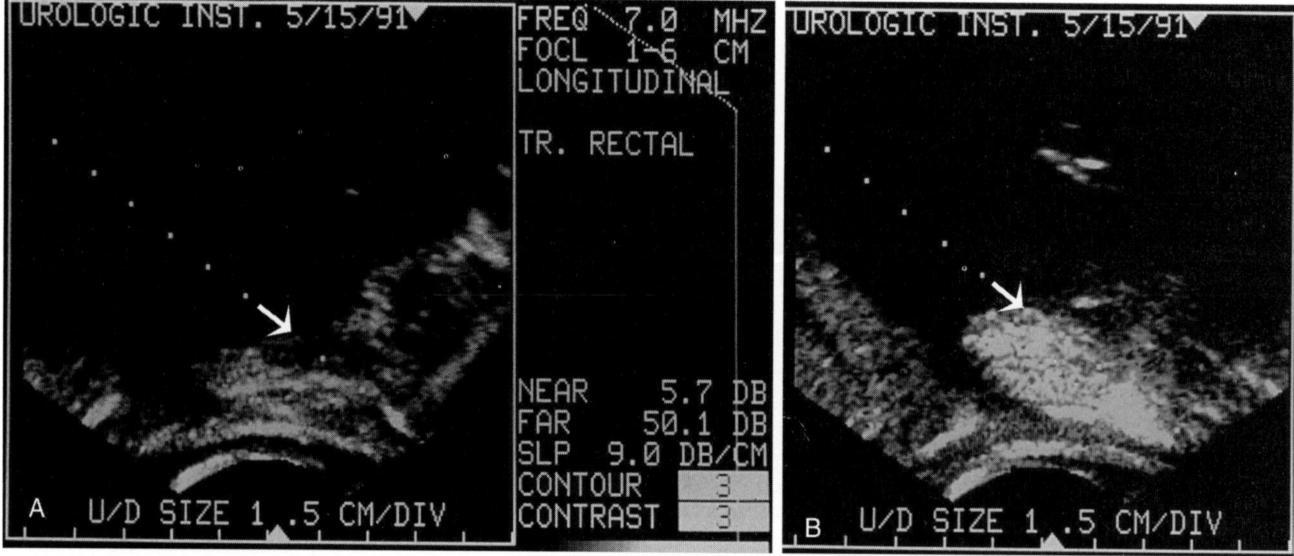

Figure 35–5. *A,* Transvaginal ultrasound identification of bladder neck *(white arrow). B,* Ultrasonogram of bladder neck after injection (glutaraldehyde cross-linked bovine [GAX]-collagen used in this patient; note hyperechoic appearance of injected GAX-collagen).

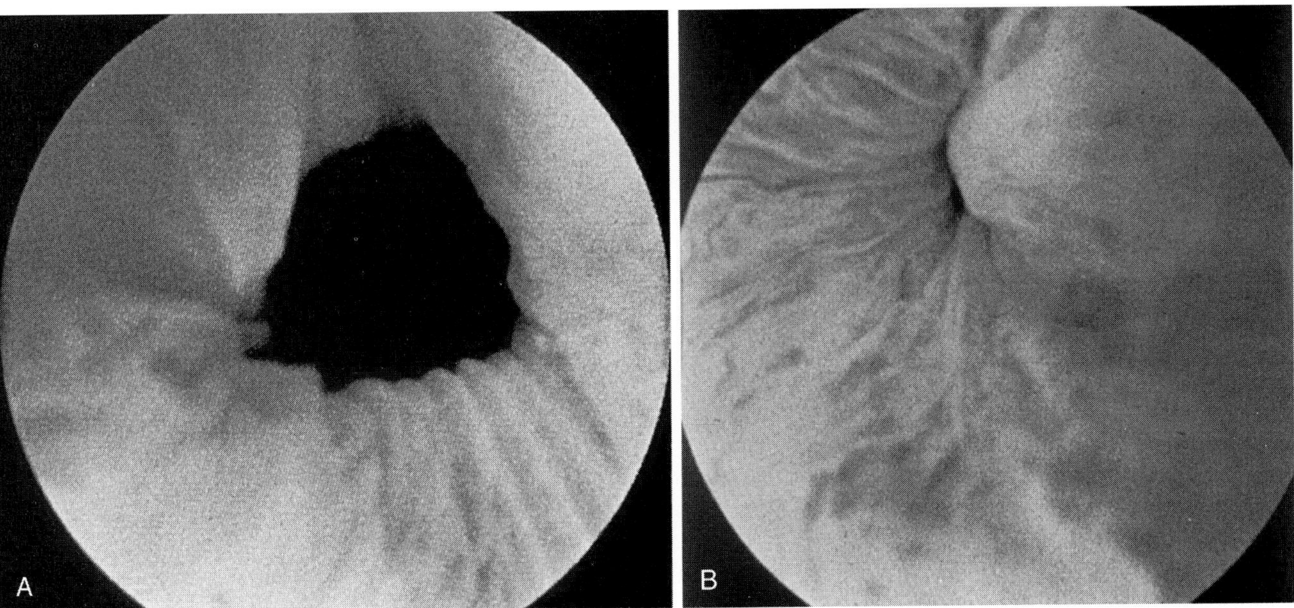

Figure 35–6. *A,* Endoscopic appearance of bladder neck from mid-urethra in ISD female. *B,* Same view following injection. (From Winters JC, Appell RA: Periurethral injection of collagen in the treatment of intrinsic sphincteric deficiency in the female patient. Urol Clin N Am 1995; 22:673.)

author prefers to wait 4 weeks), whereas with PTFE a wait of at least 4 months is recommended because of syneresis possibly resulting in improved coaptation and continence with time.

EFFICACY OF INJECTABLE TREATMENT

As a preface to this section it must be stated that **there are no controlled, long-term follow-up reports available on any substance in male, female, or pediatric patients.** In fact, it is difficult to glean information in any of these groups as to etiology of the incontinence. For example, many groups report their results of the use of injectables in stress incontinence without differentiating between patients with hypermobility, those with ISD, and those with both. Among males, those with incontinence following prostatic resection are not distinguished from those who have had a radical prostatectomy, let alone by which approach (retropubic or perineal). Very little information has emerged in the way of objective reporting; rather, reports are mostly subjective patient statements of cure, improvement, or failure. In addition, mixed techniques of injection and instrumentation are often intertwined. Sadly, the author is among the investigators who have failed to report the data as cleanly as "true" science requires. All of this means that **results are really a combination of anecdotal reporting mixed with conjecture,** speculation, and the hope that the truth is involved. In evaluating the results of intraurethral injections these procedures are compared with slings and the artificial sphincter. Having stated this, it appears that injectables are very helpful for some incontinent patients. Recently, primarily because of the fact that it was used in the North American GAX-Collagen Study, a subjective grading of incontinence (Table 35–1) is used in evaluating treatment success and failure. Improvement is noted when there appears to be a decrease in the grade of incontinence, as stated by the patient. Cure includes those patients with "social continence," a term coined by F. Brantley Scott and co-workers (1973), meaning that any perceived wetting by the patient is controlled with the use of tissues or a small minipad. Patients rendered dry or socially continent are considered successful in evaluation of these results. If one also includes as cured those dry individuals who must empty their bladders with self-catheterization, results may appear astounding for slings, the artificial sphincter, and injectables. With these criteria, **sling surgery is successful in 81% to 98% (Blaivas, 1991); sphincter surgery is successful in over 90% regardless of whether the abdominal (Light and Scott, 1985), transvaginal (Appell, 1988), or bulbous urethral (Scott, 1989) approach is utilized; PTFE injections are successful in 70% to 95% (Appell, 1990a); GAX-collagen is successful in 64% to 95% (Appell, 1990b); fat is successful in 70% to 90% (Ganabathi and Leach, 1994); and silicone macrospheres are successful in 70% to 82% (Buckley et al, 1992, 1993a).** Because all of these procedures appear to have comparable success rates, the question arises as to the reasons for lack of universal acceptance of injectables. **Two major disadvantages** to the use of injectables are recognized (Appell, 1992): (1) the **inability to determine the quantity of material needed** for an individual patient; and (2) the **safety of nonautologous products** for injection with respect to migration, foreign body reaction, and immunologic effects.

Table 35–1. INCONTINENCE GRADING SYSTEM

Grade 0	Continent
Grade I	Patient loses urine with sudden increase in P_{abd} but not supine
Grade II	Patient loses urine with physical stress (walking, changing from a reclining to a standing position, sitting up in bed)
Grade III	Patient with total incontinence; urine loss unrelated to physical activity and/or position

Males

Thus far there has been a single report (Patterson et al, 1993) of the use of silicone macrospheres for postprostatic resection incontinence where 43% were rendered continent, 19% improved, and 38% were unchanged. Autologous fat injection has demonstrated very poor results in postprostatectomy incontinence so that it cannot be recommended (Santarosa and Blaivas, 1994).

PTFE has been shown to achieve improvement or dryness in 88% of males for treatment of incontinence following transurethral resection of the prostate for benign disease and in 67% of males incontinent after radical prostatectomy (Politano, 1992). In this large series of 720 men, there were no major complications noted. Three diabetics did develop a perineal abscess requiring incision and drainage.

The first clinical trial of GAX-collagen involved 16 men with postprostatectomy incontinence (Shortliffe et al, 1989). Nine were reported as cured or improved with an average injected volume of 28.4 ml per patient, which is of import considering the significant expense of this injectable agent. A recent cost analysis report (Stothers et al, 1995) concluded that GAX-collagen is a less cost-effective means of treatment of postprostatectomy incontinence than the artificial sphincter. **Results** of the North American GAX-Collagen Study Group (McGuire and Appell, 1994) **of 134 postprostatectomy patients and 17 men rendered incontinent when treated with radiation for their malignancy showed that only 22 men (16.5%) regained continence following GAX-collagen injections,** although 78.7% were dry or significantly improved at 1 year of follow-up. Of 60 of these men followed for 2 years, 47% were improved and 25% cured (Appell et al, 1994a). Once improved, the probability of remaining so for 1 year was 71% and for two years, 60%. Those attaining continence required an average of 33 ml and 2.7 injection sessions. It is important to note that **of the 134 postprostatectomy incontinent males in the study, 17 were incontinent following prostatic resection and 15 of 17 were dry at 1 year, demonstrating rather poor results (only 7 dry) in postradical prostatectomy incontinence** (C.R. Bard, Inc., personal communication). It must be remembered that in this trial all patients with ISD were included, even those with other problems contributing to their incontinence, including detrusor causes.

Females

In women, the results of PTFE paste for incontinence have been relatively good, at least in the short term (Cole, 1993). The most recent report (Buckley et al, 1993b) of women followed for 21 to 72 months (mean 49 months) is less encouraging, with a success rate of only 38% and the occurrence of late local side effects such as fibrosis in the urethra and bladder granuloma balls in 15%, indicating a need for a more inert substance.

Recent reports with autologous fat have shown less than impressive results (Cervigni and Panei, 1993; Santarosa and Blaivas, 1994). Santarosa and Blaivas (1994) reported on 12 women with ISD of whom 83% were improved subjectively, but this improvement appeared to drop precipitously at 1 year. In addition, the role of injectables in urethral hypermobility is not reliable or efficacious (Blaivas, et al, 1994). Therefore, although autologous fat injections seem to work reasonably well for ISD, the long-term follow-up requires further assessment, because it appears that autologous fat undergoes a rapid rate of reabsorption owing to its high water content.

The first report of silicone particles used for incontinence in women appeared in 1992 and was encouraging with a short-term cure rate of 82% in 84 patients (Buckley et al, 1992). When the follow-up ran to 14 months the cure rate was 70% (Buckley et al, 1993a). Obviously, more and longer trials are necessary to determine the true efficacy using this injectable agent.

The most widely used injectable at present is GAX-collagen. The summary of the North American multicenter clinical investigation was presented in 1994 (Appell et al, 1994b). A group of 127 women with ISD were followed for 1 year and 88 were followed for 2 years. Of the patients followed for 2 years, 46% were dry and another 34% "socially continent," meaning significantly improved with management for urinary leakage by a single minipad or tissues. This was accomplished with a rise in ALPP of 40 cm H_2O. Continent women received a mean volume of 18.4 ml of GAX-collagen implanted over a mean of 2.1 ($\pm$ 1.5) treatment sessions. Once attaining continence, 77% remain dry and do not require repeated injection. It had previously been reported that 55% of women could regain continence after a single treatment session (Appell, 1990c). These multicenter results have been supported by other worldwide independent studies (Herschorn et al, 1992; Striker and Haylen, 1993; Swami et al, 1994; Goldenberg and Warkentin, 1994; Richardson et al, 1995) and compare favorably with results obtained using slings and the artificial sphincter for ISD (Appell, 1992). Although the success and efficacy of collagen implantation for females with ISD has been reproduced in these series, debate exists about the efficacy of GAX-collagen in patients with type II hypermobility of the vesicourethral junction, genuine anatomic stress urinary incontinence. Eckford and Abrams (1991) treated 25 females with stress urinary incontinence and reported 80% cured or improved 36 months after injection with GAX-collagen, again with markedly improved ALPP. However, 90% of the women had prior surgery, and it is difficult to determine from the paper whether these patients had type II stress urinary incontinence or ISD. In addition, 72% required retreatment, and it is difficult to accept the 36-month follow-up from the first injection and an 80% cure rate. Herschorn and co-workers (1992) reported equal success rates among patients with type II stress incontinence and patients with ISD; however, the number of injections and the amount of material injected were higher in patients with anatomic urinary incontinence. It has also been documented that elderly female patients with anatomic incontinence do well with the injections of GAX-collagen (Faerber, 1995). This contrasts with the 17 patients from the North American multicenter trial with hypermobility, wherein the early 82.3% success was short-lived, because all 17 patients required bladder neck suspension surgery within 2 years of the initial "dryness" (Press and Badlani, 1995).

Pediatrics

Reports of the use of injectables in children are sparse. Vorstman and co-workers (1985) reported on 11 children (nine girls and two boys) injected with PTFE. Of the four girls with myelodysplasia or sacral agenesis, 50% were rendered dry and required intermittent catheterization to empty. The other five girls and the two boys had ISD due to previous surgery and the success rate was 85.7%. Appell (1992) reported on 14 children treated with GAX-collagen. Seventy-five percent of six boys and all of the eight girls were rendered continent; however, the volume of material needed was significant (31.8 ml for the boys and 14.5 ml for the girls. ALPP rose 56.5 cm H_2O in the boys and 23.6 cm H_2O in the girls. Wan and co-workers (1992) treated eight children with GAX-collagen with an 88% cure rate at 14 months. More recently, the Cleveland Clinic experience (Ross et al, 1995) in treating seven children with GAX-collagen for ISD was presented, in which four of seven are reported to be dry but the other three had no benefit from multiple injections, and **it appears that the children who do benefit have large bladder capacities and moderate (as opposed to severe) ISD.**

COMPLICATIONS

Perioperative complications associated with periurethral injections are uncommon. The rate of *urinary retention* in patients undergoing PTFE injections is approximately 20% to 25% (Politano, 1982). These patients may require a transient period of catheterization. In the multicenter United States clinical trial of GAX-collagen injections, transient urinary retention developed in approximately 15% of patients (Bard PMAA Submission, 1990). In these patients, indwelling catheters are avoided because they promote molding of the GAX-collagen around the catheter, resulting in a failure. Therefore, if intermittent catheterization is not feasible, suprapubic trochar cystotomy should be performed.

Irritative voiding symptoms develop in 20% of patients following injection of PTFE, but they resolve after several days (Schulman et al, 1983), and urinary tract infection is stated at 2% (Lim et al, 1983). With GAX-collagen, only 1% of patients experienced irritative voiding symptoms, whereas 5% had a urinary tract infection (Bard PMAA Submission, 1990). Patients following PTFE have been noted to develop fever with negative blood and urine culture results at a rate of about 25%. This also resolves after a few days and probably indicates a mild allergic response, especially in the 5% who also report perineal discomfort that spontaneously resolves (Politano, 1978, 1982).

During injection, perforation and extravasation of the injected material can occur if the mucosa is disrupted. This may also result in minor urethral bleeding. Although the transurethral technique is mandatory in the male, the complications of bleeding and extrusion of the injectable material are eliminated by injecting via the periurethral approach in the female. With GAX-collagen, extravasation is generally not a problem because the material is easily flushed away in the urinary stream. However, during injection of PTFE, any extrusion of material can be problematic because it may be difficult to remove from the lumen.

Regardless of the material, the act of repeated injection into the urethra may result in some other minor complications, which are all rapid to resolve. Expansion of the data from the multicenter GAX-collagen study really covers all conceivable problems from injectables (Table 35–2).

SAFETY

When PTFE is injected, the acute reaction following injection is a histiocytic and giant cell response with an ingrowth of fibroblasts among the small PTFE particles. Although this creates a compression of the tissue at the injection site (Stone and Arnold, 1967), subsequently, foreign body giant cells and granuloma formation are seen at the site of injection with encapsulation of the material. After injection of PTFE, the particles are noted to be found within lymphatics and blood vessels. Particles have also been found 1 year after injection in the pelvic lymph nodes, lungs, brain, kidneys, and spleen of animal models (Malizia et al, 1984;

Table 35–2. ADVERSE EVENTS REPORTED DURING A MULTICENTER STUDY OF 382 PATIENTS TREATED WITH GAX-COLLAGEN

	Treatment-Related		Non–Treatment-Related	
Adverse Event	***Events n (%)***	***Patients n (%)***	***Events n (%)***	***Patients n (%)***
Urinary retention	36 (15)	31 (8)	2 (1)	1 (<1)
Urinary tract infection	14 (6)	14 (4)	92 (38)	63 (16)
Hematuria	8 (3)	8 (2)	0	0
Injection site injury	5 (2)	5 (1)	0	0
Urinary outlet obstruction	2 (1)	2 (<1)	5 (2)	4 (1)
Accidental injury, urinary	3 (1)	3 (1)	0	0
Pain at injection site	3 (1)	3 (1)	0	0
Balanitis	1 (<1)	1 (<1)	4 (2)	3 (1)
Urinary urgency	1 (<1)	1 (<1)	1 (<1)	1 (<1)
Urethritis	1 (<1)	1 (<1)	0	0
Epididymitis	1 (<1)	1 (<1)	0	0
Bladder spasm	1 (<1)	1 (<1)	0	0
Abscess injection site	1 (<1)	1 (<1)	0	0
Vaginitis	1 (<1)	1 (<1)	0	0
Application site reaction	0	0	1 (<1)	1 (<1)
Vesicovaginal fistula	0	0	1 (<1)	1 (<1)

From CR Bard Company, Product Monograph, Submission of USFDA for IDE G850010, 1990.

Vandenbossche et al, 1994). In humans, reports of PTFE particle migration to the lungs have been documented in two patients, the first report by Mittleman and Marraccini (1983) describing a PTFE granuloma in the lung of a patient 2 years after injection, and another case has been reported with an apparent clinically significant febrile response (Claes et al, 1989). A PTFE granuloma has also been reported to mimic a cold thyroid nodule several months after injection (Sanfilippo et al, 1980). No adverse clinical events were attributable to these findings by Mittelman and Marraccini (1983) or Sanfilippo and co-workers (1980). However, the first clinically significant case of migration of PTFE following injection therapy involved the report by Claes and co-workers (1989). Their patient had received injections of PTFE for urinary incontinence 3 years before presenting with unexplained fevers associated with new lung lesions. A bronchial lavage and lung biopsy revealed PTFE granulomas with surrounding inflammation.

The major concern associated with the use of PTFE particles is that following particle migration there is foreign body granuloma formation, and this has the potential to be carcinogenic, because sarcoma formation has been induced in rats and mice following implantation of material similar to PTFE (Oppenheimer et al, 1958) and chondrosarcoma of the larynx 6 years after PTFE injections for the treatment of vocal cord paralysis has been reported (Hakky et al, 1989). **It is important to note that no case of carcinogenesis has been identified** following widespread use of this material for over 30 years in laryngeal and urethral augmentation procedures. A complete review (Dewan, 1992) concluded that PTFE does not have any carcinogenic potential. Only three cases of malignancy adjacent to PTFE implants have been reported, and no cause-and-effect relationship has been demonstrated (Lewy, 1976; Montgomery 1979; Hakky et al, 1989). However, the fear of this potential problem has caused many to reserve the use of PTFE for older patients, and recently, PTFE for injection has been removed from the marketplace by the United States Food and Drug Administration, although they have allowed a long-term study to begin comparing PTFE and GAX-collagen for efficacy and safety.

GAX-collagen, as stated, **is both biocompatible and biodegradable. The low concentration of glutaraldehyde minimizes the immunoreactivity and cytotoxicity** of the implant and, therefore, this substance elicits no foreign body reaction as it becomes incorporated into the host tissue (Ford et al, 1984). A minimal inflammatory response has been associated with the injection of GAX-collagen, but **no granuloma formation is present** (DeLustro et al, 1986). GAX-collagen begins to degrade in 12 weeks; however, neovascularization and deposition of fibroblasts with host collagen formation occurs within the implant (Stegman et al, 1987). The GAX-collagen completely degrades within 10 to 19 months (Canning et al, 1988) and there are no reports of particle migration of the collagen material as it is transformed into living connective tissue (Remacle and Marbaix, 1988). Because of the minimal inflammatory response and no evidence of migration, GAX-collagen is the most widely used bulk-enhancing agent for the treatment of incontinence in adults and children.

Safety of GAX-collagen is further enhanced by the use of a **dermal skin test** with the more immunogenic non–cross-linked bovine collagen. Although those with a positive skin test results can conceivably not suffer from injection with the less immunogenic GAX-collagen, this is not advised. Positive skin tests in the multicenter study amounted to less than 1% of males and less than 4% of females (Appell et al, 1994a, 1994b). This is important because there have been legal claims by patients who had collagen injections for soft tissue augmentation (facial plastic surgery techniques) of signs and symptoms of collagen vascular disorders such as dermatomyositis. Despite these claims, **there has been no evidence to link injections of bovine collagen with any disorder (Appell, 1992).** The patient population has, thus far, actually had a lower incidence of such disorders than would be expected in the general population (DeLustro et al, 1991), and no plaintiffs have been able to garner support during litigation.

THE PRESENT AND FUTURE ROLES OF INJECTABLES FOR INCONTINENCE

In the properly selected patient, periurethral injections offer excellent treatment results for patients with ISD. Patients with no anatomic hypermobility and ISD in the presence of a stable bladder of adequate capacity appear to be the most satisfactory candidates for periurethral injections. GAX-collagen is the most widely used injectable, because it has been shown to be both biocompatible and biodegradable. No reports of particle migration have emerged with this material, and repeat injections can be performed safely under local anesthesia. Autologous fat is an alternative in periurethral injectable, particularly in patients who have had positive skin test results to the collagen material.

The treatment response in females with these procedures is similar to that for surgical procedures to correct ISD, and the complications are minimal. Although long-term reports of results (>5 years) for all of these procedures are scarce in the literature, injected patients have been followed for only short periods of time, and the data available do not take into consideration **reinjection rates, which run as high as 22% with collagen at 2 years after attaining dryness** (Winters and Appell, 1995). This factor affects the cost of this therapy. In males, the success rate of intraurethral injections does not approach that of the artificial urinary sphincter to date. On the other hand, there are minimal perioperative complications associated with the use of injectables

In selected elderly and less mobile female patients with anatomic incontinence, recent data suggest that collagen may be useful. The use of periurethral injections in the treatment of ISD certainly has a role in the treatment in the properly selected patient. Periurethral injections allow treatment of incontinence in patients who are poor surgical candidates and may be denied other forms of therapy.

Injectables must be considered to be in the developmental stages, and their roles in the management of incontinence still need to be defined more precisely, as must development of new, nonmigrating, safe, and technically simple-to-use injectables. **The optimal substance has to be inert and nondegradable. It must encapsulate and remain where injected, and neither lose bulk nor gain it** (syneresis). **It**

must not be too viscous so that it can be injected with standard cystoscopic equipment used for other purposes under local anesthesia in an outpatient setting to help keep the procedure safe and cost effective. In addition, more accurate techniques for determining the quantity of material to inject in an individual must be developed to achieve the optimal result in a single treatment session. This "wish list" for injectable therapy is not beyond our ability to develop.

REFERENCES

Appell RA: Collagen injections. *In* Raz S, ed: Female Urology, 3rd ed. Philadelphia, W.B. Saunders Company, 1996; pp 399–405.

Appell RA: Collagen injection therapy for urinary incontinence. Urol Clin North Am 1994a; 21:177–182.

Appell RA: The periurethral injection of autologous blood. Presented at the American Urogynecologic Society Annual Meeting, Toronto, 1994b.

Appell RA, McGuire EJ, DeRidder PA, et al: Summary of effectiveness and safety in the prospective, open, multicenter investigation of contigen implant for incontinence due to intrinsic sphincteric deficiency in males. J Urol 1994a; 151(Part 2):271A.

Appell RA, McGuire EJ, DeRidder PA, et al: Summary of effectiveness and safety in the prospective, open, multicenter investigation of contigen implant for incontinence due to intrinsic sphincteric deficiency in females. J Urol 1994b; 151(Part 2):418A.

Appell RA: Use of collagen injections for treatment of incontinence and reflux. Adv Urol 1992; 5:145–165.

Appell RA: Commentary: Periurethral polytetrafluoroethylene (polytef™) injection. *In* Whitehead ED, ed: Current Operative Urology 1990. Philadelphia, J.B. Lippincott Company, 1990a, pp 63–66.

Appell RA: Injectables for urethral incompetence. World J Urol 1990b; 8:208-211.

Appell RA: New developments: Injectables for urethral incompetence in women. Int Urogynecol J 1990c; 1:117–119.

Appell RA: Technique and results in the implantation of the artificial urinary sphincter in women with type III stress urinary incontinence by a vaginal approach. Neurourol Urodyn 1988; 7:613–619.

Appell RA, Ostergard D: Practical urodynamics. Illustrated Medicine, Female Urology Series 1992; 2:4–9.

Bard CR Inc: PMAA submission to United States Food and Drug Administration for IDE #G850010, 1990.

Bartynski J, Marion MS, Wang TD: Histopathologic evaluation of adipose autografts in a rabbit ear model. Otolaryngol 1990; 102:314.

Berg S: Polytef augmentation urethroplasty: Correction of surgically incurable urinary incontinence by injection technique. Arch Surg 1973; 107:379–381.

Blaivas JG: Treatment of female incontinence secondary to urethral damage or loss. Urol Clin North Am 1991; 18:355–363.

Blaivas JG, Herwitz D, Santarosa RP, et al: Periurethral fat injection for sphincteric incontinence in women. J Urol 1994; 151(Part 2):419A.

Buckley JF, Lingham K, Lloyd SN, et al: Injectable silicone macroparticles for female urinary incontinence. J Urol 1993a; 149(Part 2):402A.

Buckley JF, Lingham K, Meddings RN, Scott R: Injectable teflon paste for female stress incontinence: Long-term followup and results. J Urol 1993b; 149(Part 2):418A.

Buckley JF, Scott R, Meddings R, et al: Injectable silicone microparticles: A new treatment for female stress incontinence. J Urol 1992; 147(Part 2):280A.

Canning DA, Peters CA, Gearhart JR, Jeffs RD: Local tissue reaction to glutaraldehyde cross-linked bovine collagen in the rabbit bladder. J Urol 1988; 139:258–259.

Cervigni M, Panei M: Periurethral autologous fat injection for type III stress urinary incontinence. J Urol 1993; 149(Part 2):403A.

Chrystle CD, Charme LS, Copeland WE: Q-Tip test in stress urinary incontinence. Obstet Gynecol 1971; 39:313–315.

Claes H, Stroobants D, van Meerbeek J, et al: Pulmonary migration following periurethral polytetrafluoroethylene injection for urinary incontinence. J Urol 1989; 142:821–822.

Cole HM (ed): Diagnostic and therapeutic technology assessment (DATTA). JAMA 1993; 269:2975–2980.

Deane AM, English P, Hehir M, et al: Teflon injection in stress incontinence. Br J Urol 1985; 57:78–80.

DeLustro F, Condell RA, Nguyen MA, McPherson JM: A comparative study of the biologic and immunologic response to medical devices derived from dermal collagen. J Biomed Mater Res 1986; 20:109–120.

DeLustro F, Dasch J, Keefe J, Ellingsworth L: Immune response to allogeneic and xenogeneic implants of collagen and collagen derivatives. Clin Orthop 1990; 260:263–279.

DeLustro F, Keefe J, Fong AT, Jolivette DM: The biochemistry, biology, and immunology of injectable collagens: Contigen™ Bard® collagen implant in treatment of urinary incontinence. Pediatr Surg Int 1991; 6:245–251.

Dewan PA: Is injected polytetrafluoroethylene (polytef) carcinogenic? Br J Urol 1992; 69:29–33.

Eckford SD, Abrams P: Para-urethral collagen implantation for female stress incontinence. Br J Urol 1991; 68:586–589.

Faerber GJ: Endoscopic collagen injection therapy for elderly women with type I stress urinary incontinence. J Urol 1995; 153(Part 2):527A.

Ford CN, Martin CW, Warren TF: Injectable collagen in laryngeal rehabilitation. Laryngoscope 1984; 95:513–518.

Ganabathi K, Leach GE: Periurethral injection techniques. Atlas Urol Clin North Am 1994; 2:101–109.

Goldenberg SL, Warkentin MJ: Periurethral injection for patients with stress urinary incontinence. J Urol 1994; 151(Part 2):479A.

Gonzalez de Gariby AS, Castillo-Jimeno JM, Villanueva-Perez PI: Treatment of urinary stress incontinence using paraurethral injection of autologous fat. Arch Esp Urol 1991; 44:595–600.

Gonzalez de Gariby AS, Castro-Morrondo JM, Castro-Jimeno JM: Endoscopic injection of autologous adipose tissue in the treatment of female incontinence. Arch Esp Urol 1989; 42:143–146.

Hakky M, Kolbusz R, Reyes CV: Chondrosarcoma of the larynx. Ent J 1989; 68:60–62.

Heer H: Die behandlung der harnin-kontinenz mit der Teflon-paste. Urol Int 1977; 32:295–302.

Henly DR, Barrett DM, Weiland TL, et al: Particulate silicone for use in periurethral injections: Local tissue effects and search for migration. J Urol 1995; 153:2039–2043.

Herschorn S, Radomski SB, Steele DJ: Early experience with intraurethral collagen injection for urinary incontinence. J Urol 1992; 148:1797–1800.

Iacovou J, Lemberger J, James M, Kockelbergh R: Periurethral silicone microimplants for the treatment of simple stress incontinence: A one year follow-up. J Urol 1993; 149(Part 2):402A.

Kageyama S, Kawabe K, Susuki K, et al: Collagen implantation for post-prostatectomy incontinence: Early experience with a transrectal ultrasonographically guided method. J Urol 1994; 152:1473–1475.

Kaufman M, Lockhart JL, Silverstein MJ, Politano VA: Transurethral polytetrafluoroethylene injection for post-prostatectomy urinary incontinence. J Urol 1984; 132:463–464.

Klutke K: Personal communication, 1995.

Lampante L, Kaesler FP, Sparwasser H: Endourethrale submukose tefloninjektion zur erzielung von harninkontinenz. Aktuelle Urologie 1979; 10:265–272.

Lewis RI, Lockhart JL, Politano VA: Periurethral polytetrafluoroethylene injection in incontinent female subjects with neurogenic bladder disease. J Urol 1984; 131:459–462.

Lewy RB: Experience with vocal cord injection. Ann Otol Rhinol Laryngol 1976; 85:440–450.

Light JK, Scott FB: Management of urinary incontinence in women with the artificial urinary sphincter. J Urol 1985; 134:476–478.

Lim KB, Ball AJ, Feneley RCL: Periurethral teflon injection: A simple treatment for urinary incontinence. Br J Urol 1983; 55:208–210.

McGuire EJ, Appell RA: Transurethral collagen injection for urinary incontinence. Urology 1994; 43:413–415.

McPherson JM, Sawamura S, Armstrong R: An examination of the biologic response to injectable glutaraldehyde cross-linked collagen implants. J Biomed Mater Res 1986; 20:93–97.

Malizia AA Jr, Reiman JM, Myers RP, et al: Migration and granulomatous reaction after periurethral injection of polytef (Teflon). JAMA 1984; 251:3277–3281.

Mittleman RE, Marraccini JV: Pulmonary teflon granulomas following periurethral teflon injection for urinary incontinence. Arch Pathol Lab Med 1983; 107:611–612.

Montgomery WW: Laryngeal paralysis—Teflon injection. Ann Otol 1979; 88:647–657.

Murless BC: The injection treatment of stress incontinence. J Obstet Gynaecol Br Em 1938; 45:67–73.

Neal ED Jr, Lahaye ME, Lowe DC: Improved needle placement technique in periurethral collagen injection. Urology 1995; 45:865–866.

Nguyen A, Krystyna AP, Bouvier JN: Comparative study of survival of autologous adipose tissue taken and transplanted by different techniques. Plast Reconstr Surg 1990; 85:378.

O'Connell HE, McGuire EJ: Transurethral collagen therapy in women. J Urol, 1995; 154:1463–1465.

Oppenheimer BS, Oppenheimer ET, Stout AP, et al: The latent period in carcinogenesis by plastics in rats and its relation to the presarcomatous stage. Cancer 1958; 11:204–213.

Patterson PJ, Buckley JF, Smith M, Kirk D: Injectable silicone macroparticles for post-prostatectomy incontinence. J Urol 1993; 149(Part 2):235A.

Pintauro, W: Personal communication, 1995.

Politano VA: Transurethral polytef injection for post-prostatectomy urinary incontinence. Br J Urol 1992; 69:26–28.

Politano VA: Periurethral polytetrafluoroethylene injection for urinary incontinence. J Urol 1982; 127:439–442.

Politano VA: Periurethral teflon injection for urinary incontinence. Urol Clin North Am 1978; 5:415–422.

Politano VA, Small MP, Harper JM, Lynne CM: Periurethral teflon injection for urinary incontinence. J Urol 1974; 111:180–183.

Press SM, Badlani GH: Injection therapy for urinary incontinence. AUA Update Series 1995; 14:14–20.

Quackels R: Deux incontinence apris adenonectomie queries par injection de paraffine dans de perinee. Acta Urol Belg 1955; 23:259–262.

Remacle M, Marbaix E: Collagen implants in the human larynx. Arch Otorhinolaryngol 1988; 245:203–209.

Richardson TD, Kennelly MJ, Faerber GJ: Endoscopic injection of glutaraldehyde cross-linked collagen for the treatment of intrinsic sphincteric deficiency in women. Urology 1995; 46:378–381.

Ross JR, Kay R, Appell R: Preliminary results of periurethral collagen injection for the treatment of urinary incontinence in children. Presented at the 69th Annual Meeting of the North Central Section, AUA, Minneapolis, 1995.

Sachse H: Treatment of urinary incontinence with sclerosing solutions, indications, results, complications. Urol Int 1963; 15:225–244.

Sanfilippo F, Shelburne J, Ingram P: Analysis of a polytef granuloma mimicking a cold thyroid nodule 17 months after laryngeal injection. Ultrastruc Pathol 1980; 1:471–475.

Santarosa RP, Blaivas JG: Periurethral injection of autologous fat for the treatment of sphincteric incontinence. J Urol 1994; 151:607-611.

Schulman CC, Simon J, Wespes E, Germeau F. Endoscopic injection of teflon for female urinary incontinence. Eur Urol 1983; 9:246–247.

Scott FB: The artificial urinary sphincter experience in adults. Urol Clin North Am 1989; 16:105–117.

Scott FB, Bradley WE, Timm GW: Treatment of urinary incontinence by an implantable prosthetic sphincter. Urology 1973; 1:252–259.

Shortliffe LM, Freiha FS, Kessler R, et al: Treatment of urinary incontinence by the periurethral implantation of glutaraldehyde cross-linked collagen. J Urol 1989; 141:538–541.

Stegman S, Chu S, Bensch K, Armstrong R: A light and electron microscopic evaluation of Zyderm and Zyplast implants in aging human facial skin: A pilot study. Arch Dermatol 1987; 123:1644–1649.

Stone JW, Arnold GE: Human larynx injected with Teflon paste: Histologic study of innervation and tissue reaction. Arch Otolaryngol 1967; 86:550–562.

Stothers L, Chopra A, Ras S: A cost-effectiveness and utility analysis of the artificial urinary sphincter and collagen injection in the treatment of post-prostatectomy incontinence. J Urol 1995; 153(Part 2):278A.

Striker P, Haylen B: Injectable collagen for type 3 female stress incontinence: The first 50 Australian patients. Med J Aust 1993; 158:89–91.

Swami SK, Eckford SD, Abrams P: Collagen injections for female stress incontinence: Conclusions of a multistage analysis and results. J Urol 1994; 151(Part 2):479A.

Vandenbossche M, Delhobe O, Dumortier P, et al: Endoscopic treatment of reflux: Experimental study and review of Teflon and collagen. Eur Urol 1994; 23:386.

Vorstman B, Lockhart JL, Kaufman MR, Politano VA: Polytetrafluoroethylene injections for urinary incontinence in children. J Urol 1985; 133:248–250.

Wan J, McGuire EJ, Bloom DA, Ritchey ML: The treatment of urinary incontinence in children using glutaraldehyde cross-linked collagen. J Urol 1992; 147:127–130.

Winters JC, Appell RA: Collagen injection therapy in the treatment of urinary incontinence. Techn Urol 1996; 2:59–64.

Winters JC, Appell RA: Periurethral injection of collagen in the treatment of intrinsic sphincteric deficiency in the female patient. Urol Clin North Am 1995; 22:673–678.

36 IMPLANTATION OF THE ARTIFICIAL GENITOURINARY SPHINCTER IN MEN AND WOMEN

David M. Barrett, M.D.
Mark R. Licht, M.D.

Urinary incontinence is a major health and social problem. It is estimated that millions of men and women in this country have difficulty with urinary control. **Loss of urine can result from a large variety of medical ailments involving primary illness of a number of different organ systems. A subset of patients with urinary incontinence leak urine because of an incompetent or absent sphincter mechanism.** Urine loss in these patients is often quite severe and debilitating. Treatment for these patients can take the form of external collection devices, medical or surgical therapy to improve or restore sphincteric function, or urinary diversion. **The artificial genitourinary sphincter (AGUS) is an implantable prosthetic device that can restore urinary control in patients with sphincteric incontinence.**

HISTORY OF THE DEVICE

Prosthetic devices for the treatment of severe urinary incontinence have been in existence since the 1960s. The earliest implantable devices achieved continence by passive bulbous urethral compression; however, pressure control was a major problem. Insufficient pressure led to persistent incontinence, whereas excessive pressure contributed to frequent urethral erosion (Giesy et al, 1981).

Although there were anecdotal attempts to develop an active compression device, the first reliable artificial sphincter (AS-721)* was implanted by Scott in 1972 (Scott et al, 1974). The device was made of Dacron-reinforced silicone elastomer and stainless steel. It consisted of an inflatable cuff, two pumps connecting the cuff with a fluid reservoir filled with either isotonic saline or contrast material, and directional valves to fill and empty the cuff. The valves were engineered to maintain the pressure within the system at 70 to 80 cm H_2O and the reservoir was implanted within the abdomen to help maintain low pressure during stress. **This device had the advantage of delivering consistent physiologic tissue compression pressures and was designed to open, allowing for normal voiding or the passage of a catheter. The cuff could be implanted around the bulbous urethra or the bladder neck and, therefore, the device could be used in both males and females. The large number of components, however, made implantation of the device complex and increased the risk of technical or mechanical failures.**

Further developmental improvements in the artificial sphincter were made over the next decade. Components were consolidated and a pressure-regulating balloon replaced the valve system for controlling the amount of pressure applied to the tissues. Different pressure balloons were manufactured to deliver a range of preset pressures (51–60, 61–70, 71–80, and 81–90 cm H_2O) that could be selected, based on the clinical situation and site of cuff placement. The silicone components of the device were dip-coated to reduce the incidence of leaks, and the cuff was changed to dip-coated all-silicone rubber from the earlier Dacron-reinforced design to improve efficiency. The model AS-791/792, introduced in 1979, incorporated all of the above design improvements. It consisted of a pressure-regulating balloon/reservoir, a cuff, and a deflation pump. When pressurized, the cuff provided continuous closing pressure to the underlying urethra or bladder neck. Compression of the pump opened the cuff by transferring all of the cuff fluid through a unidirectional valve into the balloon reservoir (Fig. 36–1). The control assembly contained a delayed refill resistor that slowly repressurized the cuff under balloon pressure over 3 to 5 minutes to allow time for voiding. Model AS-791/792 did not have a deactivation mechanism; thus, once implanted, constant pressure was delivered to the inflatable cuff except during the short period when the cuff was emptied to allow for voiding. **Constant cuff pressure during healing after implantation led to a relatively high rate of early cuff erosion. This led to the concept of primary deactivation (Barrett and Furlow, 1981) wherein the three components of the device are implanted at one operation but not connected. Two to three months later the device is "activated" by inserting the control assembly and pressurizing the cuff.** Data analysis revealed a dramatic drop in cuff erosion following the introduction of the delayed activation concept (Motley and Barrett, 1990).

*American Medical Systems, Minnetonka, MN.

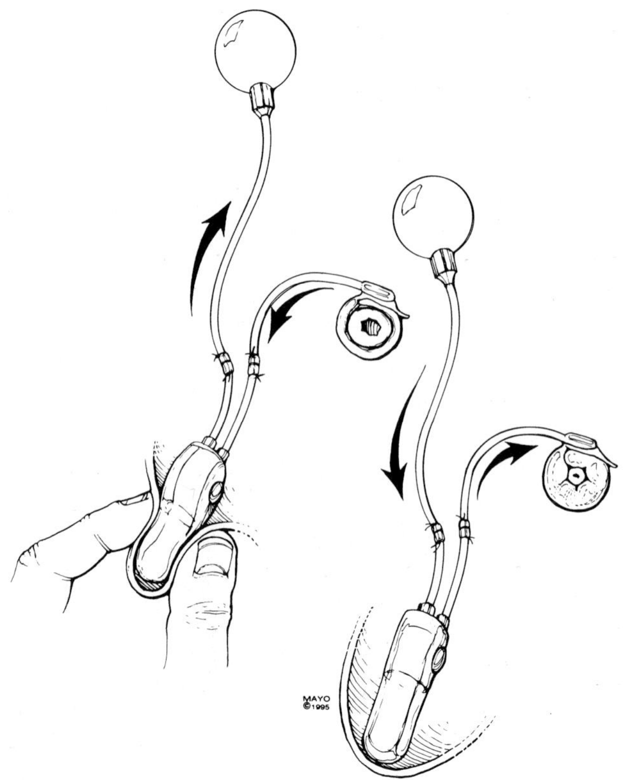

Figure 36–1. Functioning of the AS 800 artificial sphincter. Pressure on the pump transfers fluid out of the cuff to the pressure balloon. The cuff then refills passively. (Copyright by the Mayo Clinic, 1995.)

CURRENT MODEL

The AS-800, introduced in 1982, is the current model of the AGUS. Although similar to the AS-791, it incorporated several new design elements. The control assembly and refill resistor were joined with the deflation pump as one single component. A deactivation button was also installed in the control pump to facilitate externally controlled nonsurgical delayed activation and complete control by physician and patient over periods of cuff compression (Furlow and Barrett, 1985). The cuff was further improved by surface-treating it to decrease the incidence of cuff leaks. **In 1987 the narrow-backed cuff design was introduced to improve the transmission of cuff pressure to the underlying tissues and to decrease the incidence of tissue pressure atrophy and cuff erosion.** Several reports have confirmed the improved mechanical reliability of the model AS-800 with this new cuff design (Light and Reynolds, 1992; Leo and Barrett, 1993). The most recent modification is color-coded kink-resistant tubing to further improve ease of implantation and device reliability.

PATIENT SELECTION

Sphincteric Incompetence

Not all patients with urinary incontinence are candidates for an AGUS. Incontinence can result from detrusor dysfunction, sphincteric dysfunction, neurologic diseases, structural changes in the bladder or outlet due to trauma, surgery, or radiation, or any combination of these abnormalities. **The AGUS was specifically designed for use in patients with either sphincteric absence or incompetence.**

Postsurgical Incontinence

Urinary incontinence is a major complication of radical perineal or retropubic prostatectomy and occurs after transurethral prostatectomy as well. These patients are all good candidates for AGUS implantation. The bulbous urethra is the most common site for cuff placement, and the results are consistently good. **A minimum of 6 months should be allowed between the time of radical prostatectomy and AGUS placement because postprostatectomy incontinence can dramatically improve during this period. In addition, unless contraindicated, patients should have had a trial of anti-cholinergic and/or alpha-sympathomimetic medication along with pelvic floor exercises.** Patients rendered incontinent after urethral reconstructive surgery are also candidates for an AGUS. Bladder neck cuff placement is often necessary in these patients.

Congenital Disorders

A number of congenital disorders result in loss of urinary sphincter function. The most common of these is myelomeningocele. Sacral agenesis and extrophy-epispadias are less common congenital causes of sphincteric incontinence. After upper urinary tract and urodynamic evaluation, these patients may also benefit from AGUS implantation. **Many of these patients are also unable to empty their bladders completely, and thus additional measures are often required after AGUS implantation to ensure regular complete voiding. The bladder neck is often the optimal site for cuff placement because chronic intermittent self-catheterization is often required postoperatively.** In children, the bladder neck is the only site for cuff placement.

Post-Traumatic Effects; Neurogenic Bladder

Patients with sphincteric incontinence due to neurologic disease or injury, including spinal cord injury and pelvic fracture, are candidates for an AGUS, assuming that associated detrusor compliance and contractility abnormalities can be satisfactorily managed.

Contraindications

Few definite contraindications to AGUS implantation are identified. **Patients with low-volume detrusor hyperreflexia or instability are poor candidates for AGUS implantation because bladder contractions override sphincteric resistance, resulting in incontinence, and increased voiding pressures can risk upper tract damage.** Similarly at risk are patients with decreased compliance and a small functional bladder capacity. Through a combination of pharmacologic management, neurologic blockade, or additional surgical procedures such as augmentation cystoplasty, many of these patients may become suitable candidates for an AGUS.

Patients with sphincteric incompetence and decreased detrusor contractility with high residual urine volumes were formerly excluded from AGUS implantation. Because intermittent, clean self-catheterization has been shown not to lead to an increase in complications in patients with an AGUS in place (Barrett and Furlow, 1984), these patients have since been considered as candidates for AGUS implantation.

Other contraindications to AGUS implantation include active stone disease or recurrent bladder tumors that would require frequent instrumentation and increase the risk of cuff erosion. **Unstable recurrent urethral stricture disease or a urethral diverticulum at the level of the potential cuff site is also a contraindication to AGUS implantation.** Active urinary, genital, or perineal infection must be cleared before AGUS implantation, as should other systemic infectious sources. **Skin excoriations or severe dermatitis as a result of chronic urine contact are best managed with an indwelling Foley catheter for several days to weeks in advance of implantation to reduce the bacterial count on the skin and promote healing.** For an optimal result, the patient must also have adequate manual dexterity, must be motivated and cooperative, and must have enough intelligence to understand the workings of the device. Patients who lack any of these basic physical or cognitive skills are poor candidates for implantation of this mechanical prosthetic device.

Females with hypermobility-related stress urinary incontinence are generally not candidates for an AGUS and should instead be first considered for a bladder neck suspension procedure. **Intrinsic sphincter deficiency (ISD) in females due to birth trauma, aging, or prior vaginal or pelvic surgery or radiation is also best managed primarily with vaginal reconstructive procedures to increase outlet resistance and not AGUS implantation. Females with ISD due to neurogenic deficits who respond poorly to conventional surgery may be best suited for AGUS implantation.** In females, the bladder neck is the only site of cuff placement. All female patients should be instructed in clean intermittent catheterization before sphincter implantation. This is important if the patient develops postoperative retention or requires pharmacotherapy and catheterization to optimize continence.

PATIENT EVALUATION

All patients who are being considered as candidates for AGUS implantation should undergo urodynamic and endoscopic evaluation designed to quantitate voiding function and identify anatomic abnormalities that could jeopardize the long-term efficacy of the sphincter. **Even patients with**

an outwardly obvious cause for incontinence should be thoroughly evaluated to exclude coincident abnormalities that may preclude success with an implanted sphincter.

Bladder, Upper Tract Disorders

These are best evaluated with excretory urography and voiding cystourethrography. Upper tract stone disease must be completely treated before sphincter implantation. Vesicourethral reflux that was not clinically significant in a patient with total incontinence may lead to upper tract deterioration after placement of an AGUS increases resting and voiding intravesical pressure. **Reflux of grade 2 or higher should be corrected either before or at the time of AGUS implantation.**

Urodynamics

Filling cystometry is the preferred study; however, patients with more complex voiding problems may require further evaluation with pressure-flow studies or videourodynamics. Involuntary detrusor contractions can overcome sphincter cuff pressure and lead to incontinence after AGUS implantation. Similarly, poor detrusor compliance can cause persistent incontinence, and can also lead to adverse upper tract changes. Either medical therapy or surgical therapy must result in a stable, low-pressure bladder before AGUS implantation. Urodynamic identification of patients with atonic large-capacity bladders may influence the decision as to cuff site, because these patients will likely have to perform self-catheterization after surgery. If urodynamically significant detrusor–external sphincter dyssynergia is present, a decision must be made to either perform sphincterotomy before sphincter placement or to institute intermittent self-catheterization postoperatively.

Cystourethroscopy

Cystourethroscopy is recommended to identify urethral and bladder defects such as false passages, strictures, diverticulum, contracture, and foreign body. All such abnormalities should be appropriately managed and considered stable before implantation. **Bladder neck contractures after radical prostatectomy that have been incised should remain open for at least 3 months before implantation and should easily accept passage of at least a 14-Fr catheter.** Retrograde urethrography may also be indicated in patients with a history of recurrent urethral strictures, pelvic trauma, and/or urethral reconstruction. Distal or mid-bulbous urethral stricture disease or reconstruction may prevent implantation of the cuff at this level, and an alternative site should be chosen. **Visual inspection of the urethral mucosa can also give some indication of the health and vascularity of the tissues, which is particularly important in patients with a history of previous pelvic radiation therapy or trauma.**

PREOPERATIVE MANAGEMENT

The patient's expectations and motivations should be assessed. Occasionally, patients have unrealistic expectations about the AGUS. Patients must be informed of the mechanical nature of the device and the possibility of occasional postoperative stress incontinence. **They must accept the fact that additional surgery may be necessary at some time to make adjustments or repairs for mechanical malfunction and that in the event of periprosthetic infection, the components of the device will have to be removed.**

Female patients of childbearing age must be forewarned that although an implanted AGUS is not a contraindication to pregnancy, an elective cesarean section may be indicated to minimize the risk of damage to the bladder neck and its surrounding cuff. In addition, deactivation of the AGUS is recommended during the last trimester of pregnancy to reduce pressure on the cuff and decrease the subsequent risk of erosion (Barrett and Parulkar, 1989).

Antibiotics and Skin Preparation

Infection is a potentially devastating complication of prosthetic surgery. Strict measures are taken to minimize the risk of bacterial seeding of the device at the time of implantation. **All patients must have a documented negative urine culture result before surgery.** Patients are advised to take an antiseptic shower the night before surgery. Male patients having bladder neck cuff placement are instructed to perform a limited lower bowel preparation the night before surgery, and all female patients perform a standard vaginal douche preparation on the morning of surgery. Patients are admitted to the hospital on the morning of surgery.

Staphylococcus epidermidis is responsible for 35% to 80% of all genitourinary prosthetic infections (Carson, 1989; Blum, 1989). Other gram-positive skin organisms as well as gram-negative urinary tract pathogens also commonly cause prosthetic infection. **Therefore, parenteral broad-spectrum antibiotics consisting of an aminoglycoside such as gentamicin and the glycopeptide vancomycin are first administered on-call to the operating room.** Hair removal from the lower abdomen, genitals, and perineum is done just before surgery, and a full 10-minute iodophor skin scrub is performed. Members of the surgical team wear sterile hoods, and personnel traffic in and out of the operating room is kept to a minimum to decrease the risk of contamination. Antibiotic irrigation solution is used liberally throughout the procedure.

Patient Positioning

Male patients undergoing placement of a bladder neck cuff are positioned supine on the operating room table with their legs slightly abducted. A rectal tube is placed to facilitate identification of the rectum. Patients in whom a bulbous urethral cuff will be implanted are placed in the dorsal lithotomy position to expose the perineum. A 12-Fr Foley catheter is inserted in all male patients. Female patients are positioned in a dorsal lithotomy position and an iodoform-impregnated gauze is used to pack the vagina in patients undergoing an abdominal approach to aid in the identification of the plane between the vagina and the bladder neck. A 16-Fr Foley catheter is placed in the bladder per urethrum.

OPERATIVE TECHNIQUE

Male Bulbous Urethral Cuff

In the male patient, the bulbous urethra is the most common site of cuff implantation. Basic principles outlined here pertain to all subsequently described operative approaches. The device needs to be carefully protected from contamination and injury during implantation. Therefore, it should be handled only as often as absolutely necessary and should not be placed in prolonged contact with surgical sponges, which may shed fibers. The device should be kept clear of blood and tissue that might otherwise enter the tubing and cause later malfunction. Only silicone rubber–shod clamps should be used on the tubing to prevent damage that could result in a leak. Clamps placed on the tubing should be closed only to the first click to avoid crush injury. Care should also be taken when using suture needles around tubing or device components, because an unrecognized inadvertent needle stick injury can result in a slow leak. **Although saline can be used to fill the AGUS, the authors strongly recommend using iso-osmotic contrast material. Radiographic confirmation of device function and component location is much easier when contrast medium fills the system.**

Cuff Placement

A vertical midline incision is made in the perineum over the bulbous urethra. The deeper layers of the perineum are carefully divided with sharp and blunt dissection until the bulbocavernosus muscle is reached. A Young retractor is used to gain exposure superiorly and a Gelpi retractor provides lateral exposure. Care is taken to avoid the vascular fatty planes of the perineum. If possible, dissection should take place in the plane around the bulbocavernosus muscle and not directly on the bulb of the urethra to reduce the risk of cuff erosion. The urethra is circumferentially dissected off the tunica albuginea of the corporal bodies for a length of 2 cm to accommodate the width of the cuff (Fig. 36–2*A*). **Care is taken not to injure the urethra where it is attached to the septum of the corporal bodies at the 12 o'clock position. This is the most difficult point in the dissection and the site where most urethral injuries occur.** If the urethra is injured, it may be possible to close the defect primarily with 4–0 or 5–0 absorbable suture, and the cuff may then be placed at a different site during the same operation. If a large injury is sustained and the repair is questionable, a catheter should be left in place and the procedure abandoned. **If a urethral injury is suspected, it can be further evaluated by removing the catheter and injecting antibiotic solution down the urethra using a bulb syringe. Any fluid leakage confirms a urethral injury.**

The authors no longer measure the circumference of the urethra for cuff size selection. Although a 4.0-cm cuff size has recently been introduced, the authors routinely implant a 4.5-cm narrow-backed cuff around the bulbous urethra. The empty cuff is passed tab-first behind the urethra, the tubing is passed through the cuff opening, and the cuff is snapped into place by gentle opposing traction applied to the tab and tubing (see Fig. 36–2*B*). The tubing attached to the cuff should be directed toward the side where the pump and reservoir balloon will be inserted, and a shod clamp is placed near the end of the tubing (see Fig. 36–2*C*).

Reservoir Placement

A small transverse incision is then made in the lower abdomen over the rectus muscle on the side where the pump and reservoir will be located. In general, this should be on the side of hand dominance. Once the anterior rectus fascia is exposed, it is vertically incised for approximately 2 cm and a pocket is bluntly created beneath the belly of the rectus muscle, extraperitoneally, to allow placement of the balloon reservoir. The reservoir tubing is brought out through a separate stab incision in the anterior rectus fascia. The reservoir is then filled with 22 cc of iso-osmotic contrast medium and a shod clamp is placed near the end of the tubing to prevent fluid loss. **A 61- to 70-cm H_2O pressure**

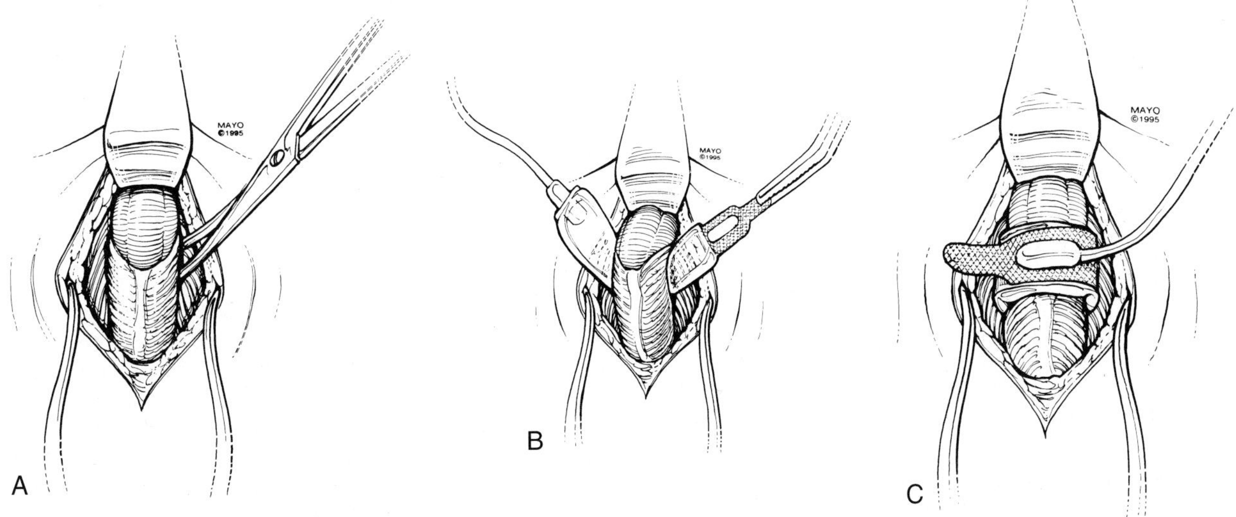

Figure 36–2. *A,* Dissection around the bulbous urethra. *B,* Passing the cuff behind the dissected urethra. *C,* Completion of cuff placement. (*A, B,* and *C,* copyright by the Mayo Clinic, 1995.)

balloon reservoir is used in most patients. In high-risk patients with evidence of tissue ischemia due to prior surgery or radiation, the 51- to 60-cm H_2O pressure reservoir is used to minimize tissue pressure ischemia. After assuring that the inflated balloon is well-accommodated within the rectus pocket, the fascial defect is closed with a running absorbable suture.

Pump Placement

A long clamp is passed down over the pubis to the perineal incision in the plane superior to the rectus fascia but inferior to Scarpa's fascia. The cuff tubing is grasped and guided up into the abdominal wound. A lateral subcutaneous hemiscrotal pouch is then created in the soft tissue plane superior to Scarpa's fascia using sequential Hegar dilators up to No. 15. The pouch is extended down to the most dependent portion of the scrotum. The pump is then placed in the pouch with the activation/deactivation button facing laterally and easily palpable against the skin. Once the pump is in position, a Babcock clamp is placed around it and the scrotal skin to prevent proximal migration during tubing connection.

All of the appropriate tubing connections are then made. Color-coded tubing has simplified this step. The cuff tubing is connected to the pump tubing with a right-angle connector to prevent kinking. The balloon tubing and the pump tubing are connected with a straight connector. Connectors are either tied in place with 2–0 Prolene suture or are assembled with the quick-connect set. Tubing length should be controlled to avoid a large amount of redundancy. All clamps are then taken off the tubing and the cuff is allowed to pressurize. The authors do not pressurize the cuff as a separate step after it is placed around the urethra. **Once the device has been tested and allowed to adequately cycle, it is deactivated with the cuff left in the open position.** The incisions are then closed in layers with absorbable suture and sterile mild-pressure dressings are applied.

Male Bladder Neck Cuff

Cuff Placement

A lower abdominal midline incision is made and carried down through the rectus and the transversalis fascia. The retropubic space is then bluntly developed. The peritoneal cavity need not be entered. A plane is then bluntly created around the bladder neck cephalad to the endopelvic fascia and caudad to the ureteral entrance to the bladder at the trigone (Fig. 36–3*A*). With the Foley catheter in place, the demarcation between the bladder neck and the proximal urethra can be palpated. **With a combination of sharp and blunt dissection, a plane is then established posterior to the bladder neck and anterior to the rectum.** Palpation of the rectal tube may facilitate identification of this plane. This portion of the dissection should be performed carefully and methodically to avoid injury to the rectum, bladder, or urethra. **The width of the plane should be 2 cm to allow unrestricted placement of the cuff.** A tape is then passed around the bladder neck and the bladder is filled with a mixture of methylene blue and antibiotic solution to identify small tears that have occurred during dissection. These can be closed in two layers with 3–0 or 4–0 absorbable suture. **However, if a rectal injury is sustained, this should be closed primarily and the procedure abandoned until a later date.** The bladder neck is then measured circumferentially with the measuring strap (Fig. 36–3*B*). If a 12-Fr Foley catheter is used it does not need to be removed before measurement. A size 8- to 14-cm cuff is usually required for adult males. The cuff is then passed around the bladder neck and snapped into place. The cuff tubing is passed through the belly of one rectus muscle as well as the anterior abdominal wall fascia on the side of the patient where the pump will be placed. The tubing should pierce the fascia and enter the subcutaneous tissue approximately 4 to 5 cm above the pubic symphysis. A shod clamp is placed at the end of the tubing and closed to one click.

Reservoir Placement

The pressure balloon reservoir is placed in the prevesical space. Its tubing is brought out through the rectus muscle near the cuff tubing and is clamped. **A 61- to 70-cm H_2O pressure reservoir is routinely used in most patients; however, if a larger size cuff is needed, the 71- to 80-cm H_2O pressure balloon may be used.** The anterior abdominal wall fascia is then closed in the midline with absorbable suture. The balloon is then filled with 22 ml of iso-osmotic contrast medium.

Pump Placement

Hegar dilators are used to create a lateral hemiscrotal pocket for the pump in a similar fashion to the description above for the bulbous urethral cuff. The pump is placed in a dependent portion of the scrotum with the deactivation/activation button laterally positioned for easy access through the skin. Tubing connections are then made between the AGUS components using straight connectors that are either tied in place with 2–0 Prolene suture, or are joined using the quick-connect set. The device is tested and cycled, and then deactivated with the cuff in the open position (Fig. 36–3*C*). The incision is closed in layers with absorbable suture.

Female Bladder Neck Cuff

Although the bladder neck is the only site of cuff placement in women, the operation can be performed via two different surgical approaches. The transabdominal approach was described first and is similar to implantation of a bladder neck cuff in male patients (Scott, 1985). The transvaginal approach was developed subsequently (Abbassian, 1988; Appell, 1988; Hadley, 1991). **The transabdominal approach allows for easier anterior dissection of the bladder neck, whereas the transvaginal approach enables the surgeon to perform the urethrovaginal dissection under direct vision.** The choice of surgical approach is optional and is usually determined by the surgeon's degree of familiarity with the anatomy and techniques of transvaginal surgery.

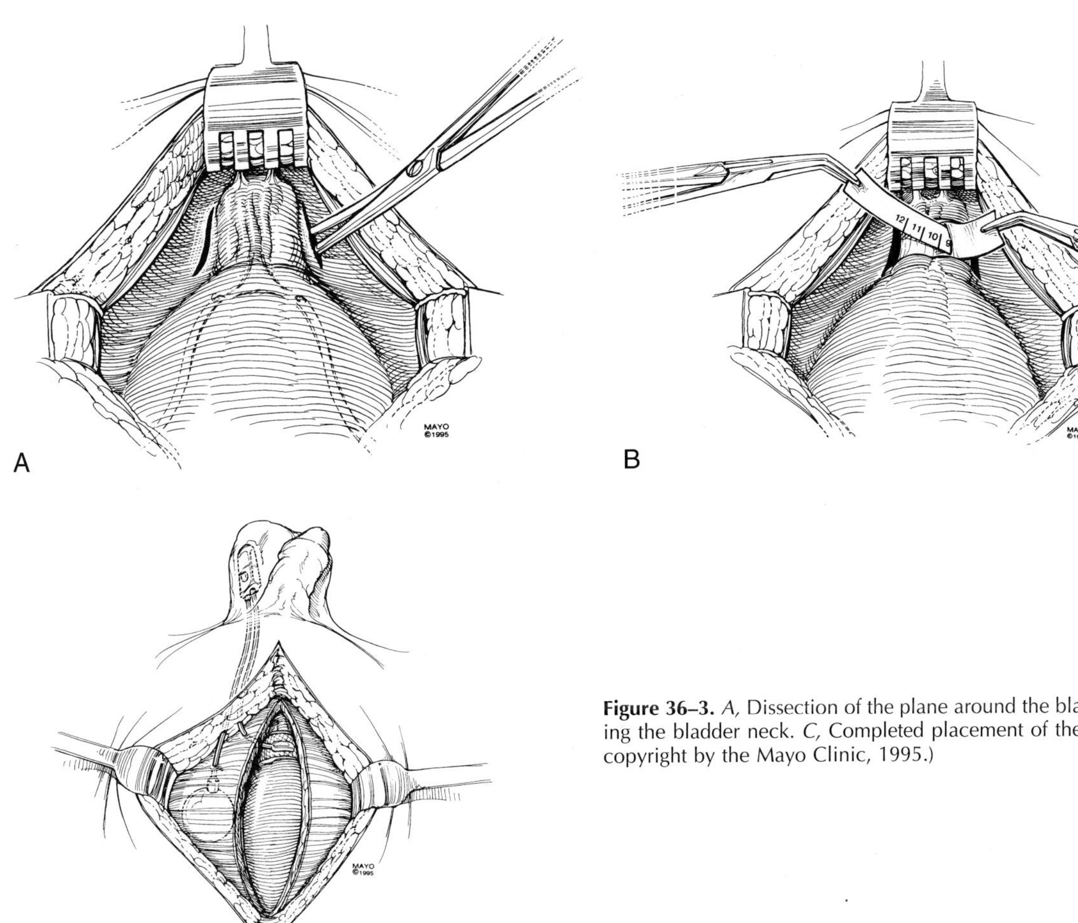

Figure 36–3. *A,* Dissection of the plane around the bladder neck. *B,* Measuring the bladder neck. *C,* Completed placement of the device. (*A, B,* and *C,* copyright by the Mayo Clinic, 1995.)

Abdominal Approach

A Pfannenstiel or lower midline incision is made and carried down into the retropubic space to expose the bladder neck. The peritoneal cavity is not opened. The vesicovaginal plane is then established at a point superior to the endopelvic fascia and caudad to the entrance of the ureters into the trigone (Fig. 36–4*A*). Palpation of the Foley catheter and the vaginal pack aids in identifying this plane between the urethra and vagina. **Patients who have had previous retropubic or bladder neck surgery may have significant scarring in this area and the plane may be difficult to establish. In these cases, it may be necessary to open the bladder to facilitate dissection.** The cystotomy must be made in the anterior midline, away from the bladder neck, to avoid the risk of future cuff erosion through the closure suture line. Palpation of the anterior vaginal wall with a finger in the vagina may also help to better define the plane. Circumferential dissection of the bladder neck should be approximately 2 cm in width to allow unrestricted placement of the cuff. **Once this step is completed, the bladder is filled with methylene blue antibiotic solution to identify bladder tears. These can be closed water-tight with a two-layer closure using absorbable suture. Vaginal wall injuries can also be closed primarily with absorbable suture.** The bladder neck is then measured with the calibrated measuring strap after the Foley catheter has been removed (see Fig. 36–3*B*). **In most women this measures between 6 and 8 cm.** Sizing is critically important because too small a cuff can lead to prolonged retention, whereas an oversized cuff does not adequately compress and close the bladder neck. A measurement of greater than 10 cm is uncommon and may represent dissection in a wide, soft tissue plane around the bladder neck. The properly sized cuff is passed beneath the bladder neck and snapped in place (see Fig. 36–3*C*). The cuff tubing is then passed through the rectus muscle and anterior rectus fascia near the internal inguinal ring on the side of the abdomen corresponding to the side of subsequent pump placement. The balloon is placed in the prevesical space and its tubing is also routed up through the rectus muscle next to the cuff tubing. A 61- to 70-cm H_2O balloon is routinely used and is filled with 22 ml of iso-osmotic contrast material. **Using a Hegar dilator, a pocket is developed in the subcutaneous tissue of the labia majora for the pump. The pump is placed in a dependent portion of the labia where it can be easily operated.** Tubing connections are made between the components of the device with either tie-on or quick-connect connectors. A Jackson-Pratt drain may be left in the retropubic space if necessary. The device is then cycled and the cuff is left open in the deactivated position and the incision is closed in layers with absorbable suture (Fig. 36–4*B*).

Transvaginal Approach

The labia minora are sutured to the skin laterally and a posterior weighted speculum is placed in the vagina for

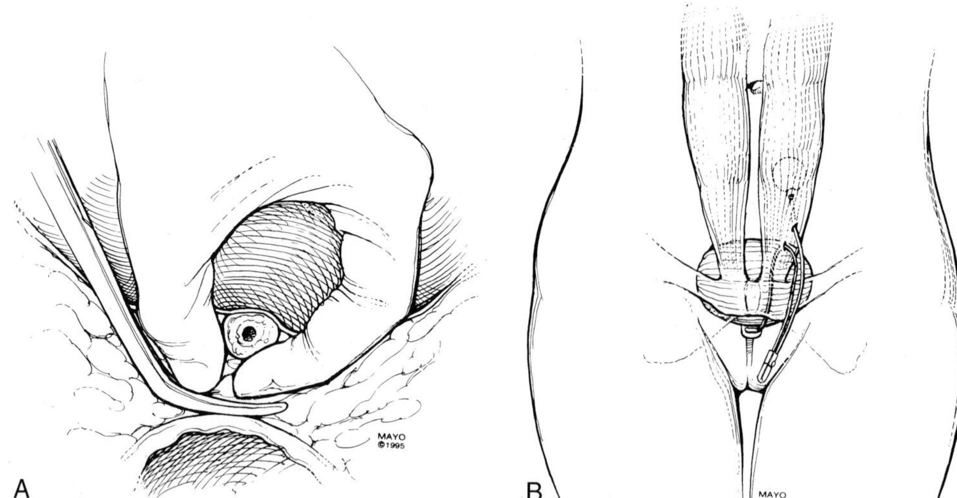

Figure 36–4. *A,* Dissection of the vesicovaginal plane. *B,* Location of components after AGUS implantation. (*A* and *B,* copyright by the Mayo Clinic, 1995.)

exposure. **An inverted U-shaped incision is made in the anterior vaginal wall. The apex of the incision is midway between the bladder neck and the urethral meatus** (Fig. 36–5*A*). The vaginal wall is dissected off the urethra back to the level of the bladder neck (Fig. 36–5*B*). The retropubic space is entered on either side of the bladder neck at the underside of the pubic bone. The endopelvic fascia is swept laterally off the pubic bone. This dissection should be done sharply if scar is encountered from prior bladder neck suspension procedures. After the retropubic space is entered and the endopelvic fascia is reflected, the bladder neck and proximal urethra are bluntly mobilized off the underside of the pubis. This portion of the dissection is not done under direct vision, and care must be taken not to inadvertently enter the bladder neck or the urethra anteriorly. Injury to the dorsal vein complex at this location can result in significant bleeding, which may be difficult to control. Prior retropubic suspension procedures or bladder neck surgery can cause dense scarring of the anterior urethra, making the dissection quite difficult. In these cases, one author describes making a second crescent-shaped incision above the external urethral meatus and then sharply dissecting a midline plane between the urethra and the underside of the pubic bone (Hadley, 1991). Once the bladder neck and urethra have been completely mobilized, the Foley catheter is removed and the measuring strap is placed around the bladder neck. The appropriate-size cuff is then snapped into place (Fig. 36–5*C*). Cystoscopy can then be performed to confirm appropriate cuff site at the bladder neck distal to the ureteral orifices. A transverse suprapubic incision is made and is carried down to the rectus fascia. This is opened in the midline, and a 61- to 70-cm H_2O balloon reservoir is placed in the prevesical space. **Under fingertip guidance, the cuff tubing is passed up into the abdominal incision using a needle in a fashion similar to the needle passage during a bladder neck suspension procedure.** A subcutaneous pocket is created in the dependent portion of the labia majora for the pump. After the balloon is filled with 22 ml of iso-osmotic contrast material, all components of the device are connected using one of the standard tubing connection methods. The device

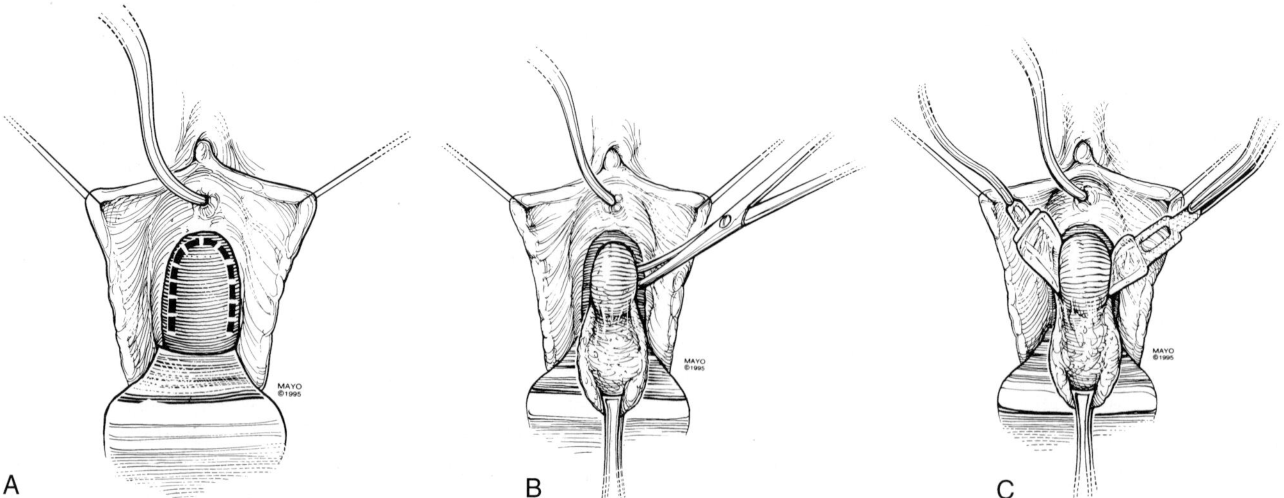

Figure 36–5. *A,* Site of incision on anterior vaginal wall. *B,* Dissection of the vaginal wall of the bladder neck. *C,* Cuff placement. (*A, B,* and *C,* copyright by the Mayo Clinic, 1995.)

is cycled and the cuff is left in the open, deactivated position. The abdominal and vaginal incisions are closed in layers using absorbable suture. An antibiotic-soaked vaginal pack is placed and the Foley catheter is reinserted into the bladder.

Bladder Neck Cuff Placement in Children

The bladder neck is the only site of cuff implantation in both male and female children. Most of these children have myelodysplasias and most likely require clean intermittent self-catheterization postoperatively. The child must be able to demonstrate the manual dexterity and emotional maturity to perform intermittent catheterization before implantation. **The usual minimal age for sphincter implantation is 6 years for boys and 8 to 9 years for girls.**

AGUS implantation in children follows the same preoperative preparation and intraoperative technique as in adults with a bladder neck cuff. A lower abdominal midline incision is made after the child has been placed in a supine, slightly bent-knee position. Dissection is carried out in an extraperitoneal plane. **The urethral and vaginal tissues are more fragile in prepubertal females and require meticulous dissection. A special cutter clamp may be necessary to develop the plane between the bladder neck anteriorly and the vaginal wall or rectum posteriorly. Occasionally, the bladder must be opened to facilitate the dissection. In children, the usual cuff size is 6 to 8 cm. A low-pressure, 61- to 70-cm H_2O pressure balloon is used because higher pressures in children may lead to significant tissue atrophy and cuff erosion.** The reservoir is placed in the prevesical space and the pump is positioned in either the scrotum or within the labia majora. A small Jackson Pratt bulb suction drain may be placed in the retropubic space.

The only usual revision needed with growth is lengthening of the pump tubing into the scrotum or labia. The placement of an AGUS with subsequent alteration of voiding mechanics need not be associated with change in renal function or growth. Scott and co-workers (1987) demonstrated adequate renal growth in their series of pediatric AGUS patients. Careful long-term follow-up with voiding cystourethrogram and urodynamics studies, with the possible need for lifetime intermittent catheterization, is required to avoid upper tract dysfunction and damage (Light and Scott, 1984; Scott et al, 1986).

AGUS Placement Along with Intestinal Segments for Bladder Reconstruction and Replacement

In patients with neurogenic bladders, detrusor hyperreflexia and/or decreased compliance often accompany sphincteric incompetence. Enterocystoplasty (Chapter 102) alone can increase bladder capacity and decrease intravesical pressure; however, acceptable continence is not always achieved. **Combining augmentation cystoplasty with AGUS placement can result in urinary continence with decreased risk of upper tract deterioration in patients with neurogenic bladders. The usual surgical approach is to complete the augmentation first, and then implant the AGUS.** In general, the authors bivalve the bladder in a clamshell configuration for augmentation. Care must be taken when anastamosing the bowel segment to the bladder to allow space in the area of the bladder neck for the cuff to be placed without impinging on any of the suture lines. The cuff is placed around the bladder neck using the standard technique described earlier. A suprapubic catheter is left in place for 14 to 21 days after surgery. A 14- to 16-Fr Foley catheter is also left in place, but this should be removed after 48 hours to prevent pressure on the recently dissected bladder neck.

Continent urinary diversion has become an acceptable form of bladder replacement after cystectomy. In several reports, the AGUS cuff has been placed directly around bowel segments of intestinal neobladders and urinary undiversions (Burbige, et al, 1987; Light, 1989). The combination of a low-pressure, highly compliant urinary reservoir and a 5.5- to 6-cm cuff placed directly around the bowel through a mesenteric window and the use of a low-pressure balloon (51–60 or 61–70 cm H_2O) has led to an improved success rate and minimized erosion (Light, 1989). Mitrofanoff and co-workers (1992) described use of an AGUS cuff as a continence mechanism in a failed appendicovesicostomy, providing a continent cutaneous diversion. The authors substituted a subcutaneous injection chamber for the pump mechanism to be able to increase the fluid volume in the system as necessary to maintain sufficient cuff pressure as tissue atrophy occurs.

Placement Along with a Penile Prosthesis

The treatment of prostate cancer has resulted in a large group of patients with simultaneous post-treatment impotence and urinary incontinence. Prosthetics can play a role in the management of both of these conditions. **A penile prosthesis and an AGUS can be implanted either simultaneously or in a two-stage approach with operations a few months apart. In the two-stage approach, either the penile prosthesis or the AGUS can be implanted first.**

Advantages of simultaneous implantation include risk of only one interval of anesthesia, decreased overall discomfort, and shorter total hospital stay. In addition, in a second stage procedure the surgeon has to be careful not to injure the tubing or components of the initial implant. Simultaneous procedures, however, can be more technically demanding. **With simultaneous implantation, in the event of infection of even one of the components of either prosthesis, it is difficult to avoid spread to other components.** In fact, early reports of simultaneous prosthetic implantation showed high rates of fistula and abscess formation (Graham et al, 1982). The corporeal and periurethral dissection and mobilization required during combined implantation were felt by some to be excessive and to significantly increase the risk of ischemia with subsequent erosion and infection.

For simultaneous procedures, the authors recommend implanting the sphincter first. The components should be connected and the cuff deactivated before introducing the penile prosthesis. If a multicomponent penile prosthesis is chosen, the procedures can be accomplished through a low transverse suprapubic incision. If a bulbous urethral cuff is implanted, a midline perineal incision is also made. The reservoirs are individually placed in pockets under each rectus muscle. The pumps are placed in separate subcutanous tunnels in the dependent portion of each hemiscrotum. The authors suggest placement of a small-caliber suction drain in the subcutaneous tissue to help prevent hematoma formation. Semirigid rod and unicomponent inflatable penile prostheses are inserted through a dorsal subcoronal penile incision.

In a two-stage approach, a preliminary radiograph helps to define the location of previously implanted prosthetic components. To further decrease the risk of component or tubing injury, a new incision away from the previous line of dissection should be made. Electrocautery on cutting current is used for dissection because it will not damage silicone components.

A review of combined implantation of an AGUS and a penile prosthesis revealed a satisfactory continence rate of 95% with a functional penile implant rate of 98% (Parulkar and Barrett, 1989). Only 2 of 52 patients in the study who received the AS 800 sphincter along with a prosthesis experienced cuff erosion.

Replacement After Partial or Total Explantation

Revision or explantation of components of the AGUS is sometimes clinically necessary. Replacement of individual components is most often accomplished with minor corrective surgery. Replacement of the device after removal for infection or cuff erosion can often be quite challenging. In the case of a bulbous urethral cuff, a new cuff can be inserted around a more distal segment of the urethra. **For the bladder neck in both males and females, the same site may be used, but because of technical difficulty, placement of another cuff cannot be guaranteed.** If no infection is present at explantation, the authors have used either a silicone strap or a tailored piece of omentum to wrap the plane around the bladder neck to facilitate later redissection. During replacement of the AGUS after infection, the pump and reservoir should be relocated to different sides of the scrotum/labia and abdomen, respectively.

When a cuff is changed for resizing or a balloon reservoir is changed to increase or decrease the pressure within the system, tubing from the new component must be connected to the existing tubing using tie-on connectors. If placement of a tandem urethral cuff is clinically indicated, this can be accomplished by adding the new tubing into the circuit with a stainless steel Y-connector.

POSTOPERATIVE CARE

Hospital Care

Hospital stay for patients with a bulbous urethral cuff is 2 days; with bladder neck placement, it is 2 to 3 days longer. **Swelling and edema can occur at the pump site in the scrotum or labia. To help reduce postoperative edema, ice packs are applied to the pump site for the first 24 to 48 hours.** Traction on the Foley catheter should be avoided, particularly in patients with a bladder neck cuff, because traction can put undue pressure against the cuff. **In most cases, the catheter is removed on the morning after implantation. Some patients report immediate improvement in urinary control, which is the result of increased urethral resistance from edema at the cuff site. This is usually transient, and patients are incontinent again in a few days. Most patients are able to urinate without difficulty. If a patient is unable to void, intermittent catheterization with a small-caliber catheter is necessary until spontaneous voiding occurs.** Prolonged catheterization through a recently implanted cuff significantly increases the risk of urethral cuff erosion.

If a Jackson-Pratt drain was placed during surgery, it should be removed as soon as possible. Preoperative broad-spectrum intravenous antibiotics are continued throughout the patient's hospital stay. Ambulation is not limited, and patients start on a regular diet shortly after surgery. **While in the hospital, patients are instructed on how to gently pull the pump down in the scrotum or labia once a day to avoid upward migration of the pump as capsule formation occurs.**

Discharge Instructions

Patients are continued on oral antibiotics consisting of a cephalosporin for 2 weeks after surgery. They may shower daily and can take a bath 5 days after surgery. They are restricted from driving and heavy lifting for 2 to 6 weeks, depending on the surgical approach. Patients are advised to abstain from sexual activity until the device is activated. Patients with a bulbous urethral cuff are cautioned to avoid undue compression of the perineum from sitting for long periods of time. **Permanent restrictions include riding a bicycle or exercise bike with a standard saddle seat, and horseback riding.**

Incontinence is expected to persist during the deactivation period, and some form of protection should be worn until the device is activated. **The authors have discouraged the use of penile clamps and have advised patients to use diapers or a condom catheter.**

Patients are made aware of the signs and symptoms of infection and are instructed to contact their surgeon immediately if these are experienced. Patients should wear a Medic-Alert bracelet that notes their AGUS, so that if a medical emergency necessitates placement of a urethral catheter, the treating physician will know to deactivate the cuff.

Activation and Use

In the authors' experience, patients are ready for activation in 6 to 8 weeks, regardless of cuff site. Scrotal or labial tenderness has generally subsided by that time and the abdominal and perineal incisions are well healed. Activation of the device is performed in the office by applying firm pressure to the pump to compress it. The deactivation pin will "pop" into the activated position, allowing fluid to circulate through the pump. Activation

can be monitored by deflate and inflate radiographs, which confirm filling of the cuff after activation.

Patient instruction on device function usually begins before implantation. After activation, however, patients are given a direct demonstration of the means by which to cycle the device. Patients must demonstrate the independent ability to compress the pump to open the cuff and void. Patients are told that after the cuff is deflated, recompression takes 3 to 5 minutes. Although bladder emptying may occur in less time, full continence returns only after the cuff is fully inflated. Patients with reduced flow rates may require a second pumping of the cuff to adequately empty their bladder.

Many patients are dry at night and do not require cuff compression for continence. These patients are instructed in the method used to deactivate the device at night. Deactivation reduces the risk of ischemia to the underlying urethra or bladder neck and helps delay tissue atrophy. Patients who cannot fully empty their bladder and require intermittent self-catheterization are instructed to deflate the sphincter cuff before inserting the catheter into the bladder.

POSTOPERATIVE COMPLICATIONS

Hematoma

Hematoma is the most common minor complication of AGUS implantation. These subcutaneous collections most often occur in the labia or scrotum along the path of blunt dilation, and if large enough, can displace the pump into an unfavorable location for external manipulation. **Most small hematomas resolve spontaneously, whereas an occasional large hematoma needs to be drained to prevent discomfort and enhance healing.**

Retention

Urinary retention after AGUS implantation usually occurs in the immediate postoperative period as a result of edema. **The sphincter mechanism, though, should first be checked to confirm that the cuff is deactivated in the open position.** Most patients, regardless of cuff location, begin to void after one or two catheterizations with a 10- or 12-Fr catheter.

Urinary retention after cuff activation may be the result of recurrent proximal obstruction from stricture disease or bladder neck contracture. This should be evaluated with retrograde urethrography and cystourethroscopy studies. Treatment can be performed endoscopically with the cuff deactivated. If the need arises for elective prolonged bladder drainage, a suprapubic tube should be inserted under fluoroscopic guidance to safely void the sphincter components.

Urinary retention in patients with neurogenic voiding dysfunction may represent a change in bladder function, and urodynamic evaluation is necessary before instituting treatment. Cuff erosion infrequently presents as urinary retention.

Infection

Periprosthetic infection can present early after AGUS implantation, or months or years later. The overall infection rate for primary AGUS implants is approximately 1% to 3% (Carson, 1989). With reoperation, the infection rate significantly increases. **Early infections are most often due to bacterial contamination at the time of implantation with either skin or airborne organisms. Late infections are usually due to indolent colonization with less virulent organisms, or gram-negative organisms of urinary tract origin. All patients who have undergone prosthetic implantation should take antibiotic prophylaxis before dental or surgical procedures to avoid hematogenous bacterial seeding of the device.**

Infection can present subtle signs and symptoms such as pain, mild swelling and induration, or erythema of the pump or cuff site. Patients with purulent infections, however, can present with fever, abscess formation with drainage from incision sites, pump erosion through the scrotal skin, or cuff erosion. **Treatment of periprosthetic infection most often requires removal of the entire sphincter device. Although drainage of the infected pyogenic process around a sphincter component can be attempted with drains and instilled antibiotic solutions, most devices still must be removed for ultimate resolution of the infection.** Reimplantation can be attempted 3 to 6 months later with an increased risk of infection and cuff erosion. Mild inflammatory skin changes can be safely treated with oral antibiotics and often do not progress to frank purulent infection.

Mechanical Malfunction

Design modifications incorporated into the AS 800 AGUS have significantly decreased the incidence of mechanical malfunction. Improvements have specifically addressed earlier deficiencies regarding tubing kinks, system leaks, and control pump malfunction. However, there are no solid long-term data available to help predict device longevity. This is due in part to the many different successive models of the device that have been implanted over the last 20 years. **Although the exact longevity of the current AS 800 device cannot be predicted, it appears that the 5-year reliability rate is greater than 90%.**

Cuff Erosion

The ability of the cuff to provide satisfactory occlusion pressure is the key to achieving continence with an AGUS. It is a delicate balance, however, between adequate pressure and excessive pressure, which can lead to tissue ischemia with subsequent cuff erosion. **Properly selected balloon pressure and cuff size, careful dissection around the urethra, and deactivation during healing have decreased the incidence of cuff erosion. The introduction of the narrow-backed cuff has also contributed to the current low rate of cuff erosion. Cuff erosion can also occur as a result of periprosthetic infection.**

Cuff erosion can occur at any time, but is most common 3 to 4 months after implantation. **Cuff erosion in the imme-**

diate postoperative period before activation is due to an unrecognized iatrogenic urethral injury. Symptoms of cuff erosion include pain and swelling in the perineum or scrotum, pain referred to the tip of the penis, recurrent incontinence, urinary tract infection, and bloody urethral discharge. Cystourethroscopy confirms the clinical suspicion. Confirmation of erosion mandates cuff removal. If no infection is present, a stainless steel plug can be used to cap the tubing to the cuff. After 3 months and a negative preoperative evaluation, a new cuff can be placed. Gross infection requires explantation of the entire device. A silicone catheter should be left in place for 3 to 6 weeks to allow the urethra to completely heal. An 18-Fr catheter is used for bladder neck erosions, whereas a 12- to 14-Fr catheter is appropriate for bulbous urethral erosions. Strictures are surprisingly rare after cuff erosion (Motley and Barrett, 1990).

Recurrent or Persistent Incontinence

Persistent incontinence after device activation, or recurrent incontinence after successful AGUS implantation, requires a systematic diagnostic approach to define the problem (Fig. 36–6). **The three most common etiologies are mechanical failure, tissue atrophy, and cuff erosion or periprosthetic infection.**

Inadvertent cuff deactivation is common and is easily treated by cycling the device. Mechanical failure due to fluid loss can be evaluated first with an inflate/deflate abdominal radiograph. Determining the site of the leak, however, requires surgical exploration. **In the authors' experience, the most common site for leakage is the lower surface of the cuff.** This is exposed first via a perineal incision. If the cuff is not the source of the problem, then the other components are examined in a systematic fashion. The tubing connectors are the next most common site of leakage, followed by the balloon reservoir. The pump is the least frequent site of a leak. Once the site has been discovered, the appropriate components can be individually replaced. If fluid loss is confirmed preoperatively and no distinct site is found during surgical exploration, the authors recommend replacing the entire device.

Tissue pressure atrophy is the natural result of cuff compression over time. Although the narrow-backed cuff design has compensated for this problem to some degree, tissue atrophy is still a significant cause of recurrent incontinence. A history of progressive decrease in device function as well as an increased number of pumps needed to empty the cuff are clues to the presence of atrophy. Urodynamic evaluation with leak point pressure measurement, as well as cystoscopy revealing poor cuff occlusion, confirms the diagnosis. Treatment involves surgical modification of the device. Compensation for atrophy can be achieved by one of three methods. Balloon reservoir pressure can be increased to the next higher category. This should be performed first in patients with a bladder neck cuff, because the reservoir is easier to reach than the cuff. Reduction in cuff size is another option, and the cuff should be reduced in size initially by 0.5 cm. With a bulbous urethral cuff, placement of a tandem cuff at a site distal to the primary cuff can correct the incontinence.

Urodynamic evaluation may also reveal involuntary detrusor contractions, which can be managed with pharmacologic therapy, or poor bladder compliance, which may require surgery to correct. Cuff erosion can be detected cystoscopically and should be managed as described in the previous section. Clinical signs of infection associated

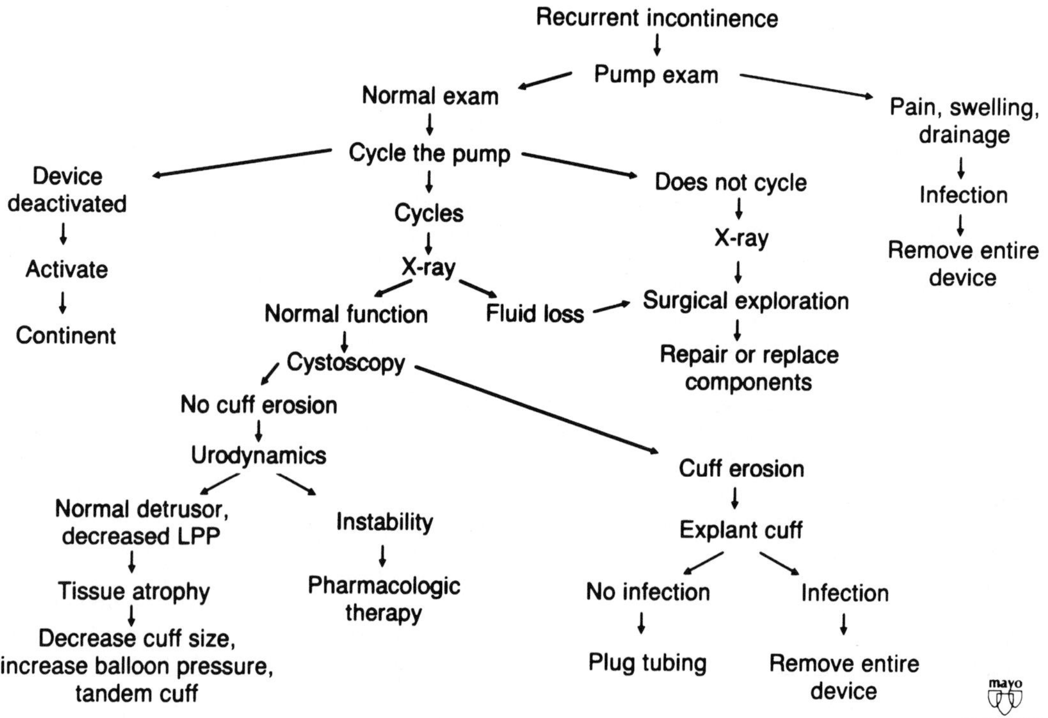

Figure 36–6. The evaluation of incontinence after AGUS implantation. (Copyright by the Mayo Clinic, 1995.)

with recurrent incontinence require institution of intravenous antibiotics and often result in device explantation. **Female patients who present with continuous incontinence after AGUS implantation should be further evaluated to rule out a vesicovaginal fistula, which may have resulted from an unrecognized intraoperative injury.**

RESULTS

Overall Experience

A number of reports have presented data on the success of the AS 800 AGUS in treating sphincteric incontinence. Goldwasser and co-workers (1987) reported on 109 AGUS patients. Satisfactory continence was achieved in 83% with 21% of patients requiring reoperation. The study by Fishman and co-workers (1989) reported 90% satisfactory continence in 148 patients.

Two large series have appeared in the literature since the introduction of the narrow-backed cuff design in 1987. Light and Reynolds (1992) reported on 126 patients of whom 95% had obtained satisfactory continence. No patient experienced a cuff erosion, whereas 19% of patients experienced tissue atrophy that required reoperation. Researchers at Mayo Clinic (Leo and Barrett, 1993) reviewed results in 144 patients. The satisfactory continence rate for the series was 92%. The rate of cuff erosion was 2%, and no patient required reoperation for incontinence due to inadequate cuff compression as a result of tissue atrophy.

Postprostatectomy Incontinence

The most common indication for AGUS implantation is incontinence following prostate surgery. Gundian and co-workers (1993) reported on 64 patients who received an AGUS after either transurethral resection of the prostate or open prostatectomy. Among all patients, 90% felt that their incontinence had improved, and 87% were either very satisfied or moderately satisfied with the device. Revision for inadequate cuff compression resulting from tissue atrophy accounted for 43% of the 21 surgical revisions. Device malfunction accounted for five revisions, or 24%. Four cuff erosions occurred in three patients, and no patient experienced periprosthetic infection. These data were accumulated before the introduction of the narrow-backed cuff design.

In another study, Gundian and co-workers (1989) reviewed the Mayo Clinic results with AGUS implantation in 117 patients with incontinence after radical retropubic prostatectomy. Of these patients, 83% were dry (two pads or less), whereas 6% were improved but required three pads. Among all patients, 90% believed that the AGUS had markedly improved their level of continence. In this series, which also was conducted before introduction of the new cuff design, tissue atrophy and cuff erosion were significant complications. The infection rate was 2.5% in this series.

Implantation in Females

Bladder neck cuff placement of the AGUS has been successfully used to treat both congenital and acquired sphincteric incontinence in females. Parulkar and Barrett (1990) reported on AGUS implantation in 24 women. At a mean follow-up of 40 months, 83.3% had improvement in continence. A review of the Baylor experience (Fishman, 1994) in 239 patients followed for up to 9 years found that 86% were socially continent. Only 12 patients required surgery to revise the device, and 7% had explantation due to infection.

Two series report the results of AGUS implantation via a transvaginal approach. Appell (1988) reported on 34 patients, 19 of whom had 3 years of follow-up. All of these patients are completely dry. Three patients required surgical revision, two for tissue atrophy and one for connector leak. No patient has experienced cuff erosion or infection. Hadley (1991) reported a 93% continence rate in 14 patients. These patients were dry and required no more than one pad per day. There have been no infections, cuff erosions, or patients complaining of urgency incontinence in this series.

Implantation in Children

Decter and co-workers (1988) reported on 16 patients with exstrophy and epispadias, 13 of whom had undergone a prior failed bladder neck reconstruction procedure. The continence rate was 90% in the 10 patients who still had an active device. A study on AGUS implantation in 46 children with congenital urinary incontinence (Gonzalez et al, 1989) revealed an 85% satisfactory continence rate in the 40 patients with functioning sphincters at a mean follow-up of 25 months. Bosco and co-workers (1991) reviewed the long-term results of AGUS implantation in 36 children. Among this group, 27 of the 36 sphincters were still in place at 5 years' follow-up. They found that 84% and 62% of patients were completely continent at 2 and 5 years, respectively. **They found no difference in success rates between boys and girls, although girls who had a prior bladder neck operation had a higher rate of cuff erosion.**

In another study, Barrett and co-workers (1993) reported on 61 AGUS implantations in 59 children and young adults, 46 of whom had incontinence resulting from myelodysplasia. At a mean follow-up of 43 months, 80% had good rate of return to continence, whereas continence was considered to be fair in another 14%. Augmentation cystoplasty was necessary in 20 patients to overcome problems of increased detrusor contractility, decreased compliance, or both.

Two series specifically looked at combination AGUS implantation and augmentation cystoplasty in children. Strawbridge and co-workers (1989) reported on 18 children. All 18 were continent and 15 required intermittent self-catheterization to empty their bladder. All six patients in whom the AGUS was implanted prior to the augmentation procedure developed decreased bladder compliance with incontinence over time, and upper tract deterioration occurred in two patients. More recently, Light and co-workers (1995) found a 50% infection rate in children who underwent simultaneous augmentation cystoplasty and AGUS placement, compared with a 9.5% incidence when the procedures were staged. The authors recommend placing the AGUS first and then performing the augmentation at a later date.

FUTURE CONSIDERATIONS

The AS 800 is a safe, reliable mechanical device with proven efficacy for the treatment of sphincteric incontinence in men, women, and children. Constant design modification and manufacturing improvement have made the current sphincter the state-of-the-art prosthetic implant for the management of incontinence. Future improvements should focus on more even distribution of pressure to the bladder neck or urethra to further decrease the incidence of tissue atrophy. We can expect to see an expanding role for the AGUS in conjunction with continent urinary diversion and as primary therapy for post-prostatectomy incontinence.

REFERENCES

Abbassian A: A new operation for insertion of the artificial urinary sphincter. J Urol 1988; 140:512–513.

Appell RA: Techniques and results in the implantation of the artificial urinary sphincter in women with Type III stress urinary incontinence by a vaginal approach. Neurourol Urodyn 1988; 7:613–619.

Barrett DM, Furlow WL: Incontinence, intermittent self-catheterization and the artificial genitourinary sphincter. J Urol 1984; 132:268–269.

Barrett DM, Furlow WL: Implantation of a new semi-automatic artificial genitourinary sphincter: Experience with patients utilizing a new concept of primary and secondary activation. Prog Clin Biol Res 1981; 78:375–386.

Barrett DM, Parulkar BG: The artificial sphincter (AS-800) experience in children and young adults. Urol Clin North Am 1989; 16:119–132.

Barrett DM, Parulkar BG, Kramer SA: Experience with AS 800 artificial sphincter in pediatric and young adult patients. Urology 1993; 42:431–435.

Blum MD: Infections of genitourinary prostheses. Infect Dis Clin North Am 1989; 3:259–274.

Bosco PJ, Bauer SB, Colodny AH, et al: The long-term results of artificial sphincters in children. J Urol 1991; 146:396–399.

Carson CC III: Infections in genitourinary prostheses. Urol Clin North Am 1989; 16:139–147.

Decter RM, Roth DR, Fishman IJ, et al: Use of the AS 800 device in extrophy and epispadias. J Urol 1988; 140:1202–1203.

Fishman IJ: Female incontinence and the artificial urinary sphincter. *In* Seidmon EJ, Hanno PM, eds: Current Urologic Therapy 3. Philadelphia, W.B. Saunders Company, 1994, pp 312–315.

Fishman IJ, Shabsigh R, Scott FB: Experience with the artificial urinary sphincter model AS 800 in 148 patients. J Urol 1989; 141:307–310.

Furlow WL, Barrett DM: The artificial urinary sphincter: Experience with the AS 800 pump-control assembly for single-stage primary deactivation and activation—a preliminary report. Mayo Clin Proc 1985; 60:255–258.

Giesy JD, Barry JM, Fuchs EF, Griffith LD: Initial experience with the Rosen incontinence device. J Urol 1981; 125:794–795.

Goldwasser B, Furlow WL, Barrett DM: The model AS 800 artificial urinary sphincter: Mayo Clinic experience. J Urol 1987; 137:668–671.

Gonzalez R, Koleilat N, Austin C, Sidi AA: The artificial sphincter AS 800 in congenital urinary incontinence. J Urol 1989; 142:512–515.

Graham SD Jr, Carson CC III, Anderson EE: Long-term results with the Kaufman prosthesis. J Urol 1982; 128:328–330.

Gundian JC, Barrett DM, Parulkar BG: Mayo Clinic experience with the AS 800 artificial urinary sphincter for urinary incontinence after transurethral resection of prostate or open prostatectomy. Urology 1993; 41:318–321.

Gundian JC, Barrett DM, Parulkar BG: Mayo Clinic experience with use of the AMS 800 artificial urinary sphincter for urinary incontinence following radical prostatectomy. J Urol 1989; 142:1459–1461.

Hadley RH: The artificial sphincter in the female. Prob Urol 1991; 5:123–133.

Leo ME, Barrett DM: Success of the narrow-backed cuff design of the AMS 800 artificial urinary sphincter: Analysis of 144 patients. J Urol 1993; 150:1412–1414.

Light JK, Lapin S, Vohra S: Combined use of bowel and the artificial urinary sphincter in reconstruction of the lower urinary tract: Infectious complications. J Urol 1995; 153:331–333.

Light JK, Reynolds JC: Impact of the new cuff design on reliability of the AS 800 artificial urinary sphincter. J Urol 1992; 147:609–611.

Light JK, Scott FB: The artificial sphincter in children. Br J Urol 1984; 56:54–57.

Mitrofanoff P, Bonnet O, Annoot MP, et al: Continent urinary diversion using an artificial urinary sphincter. Br J Urol 1992; 70:26–29.

Motley RC, Barrett DM: Artificial urinary sphincter cuff erosion; experience with reimplantation in 38 patients. Urology 1990; 35:215–218.

Parulkar BG, Barrett DM: Application of the AS 800 artificial sphincter for intractable urinary incontinence in females. Surg Gynecol Obstet 1990; 171:131–138.

Parulkar BG, Barrett DM: Combined implantation of artificial sphincter and penile prosthesis. J Urol 1989; 142:732–735.

Scott FB, Bradley WE, Timm GW: Treatment of urinary incontinence by an implantable prosthetic urinary sphincter. J Urol 1974; 112:75–80.

Scott FB, Fishman IJ, Shabsigh R: The impact of the artificial urinary sphincter in the neurogenic bladder on the upper urinary tracts. J Urol 1986; 136:636–642.

Scott FB, Fishman IJ, Shotland Y: Experience with simultaneous implantation of inflatable penile prosthesis and artificial urinary sphincter in 72 patients. J Urol 1987; 137:374a.

Strawbridge LR, Kramer SA, Castillo OA, Barrett DM: Augmentation cystoplasty and the artificial genitourinary sphincter. J Urol 1989; 142:297–301.

37 SURGERY FOR VESICOVAGINAL AND URETHROVAGINAL FISTULA AND URETHRAL DIVERTICULUM

Gary E. Leach, M.D.
Brett A. Trockman, M.D.

VESICOVAGINAL FISTULA

Background

Urinary fistula to the vagina has been described since the beginning of the written record (Zacharin, 1988). **In developed nations, these fistulas are usually unfortunate complications of gynecologic or other pelvic surgery;** they often result in extreme distress for both the patient and physician. Historically, birth trauma accounted for most vesicovaginal fistulas, and it remains the major cause of urinary fistulas in many underdeveloped nations with limited medical resources (Zacharin, 1988). Fortunately, modern obstetric care has made complicated labor a relatively rare cause of vesicovaginal fistulas in this country.

The history of the surgical treatment of obstetric fistulas is fascinating and instructive. Before the efforts of surgeons such as James Marion Simms practicing in the mid to late 1800s, urinary fistulas were generally considered to be irreparable, with the affected individual doomed to a life of incontinence (Falk and Tancer 1954, Zacharin 1988). Through their innovations in surgical technique and probably most importantly their **routine use of postoperative catheter drainage of the bladder,** they were the first to demonstrate that surgical treatment of urinary fistulas offered a reasonable chance for cure. Even today, surgeons working at dedicated fistula hospitals in Third World countries treat thousands of women with obstetric fistulas and continue to make substantial contributions to our understanding and management of this devastating condition (Zacharin, 1988; Arrowsmith, 1994; Elkins, 1994).

Etiology

In industrialized nations, **gynecologic surgery is the most common cause of vesicovaginal fistulas with either abdominal or vaginal hysterectomy associated with about 75% of genitourinary fistulas** (Lee et al, 1988; Symmonds, 1984; Tancer, 1992). Vesicovaginal fistulas after hysterectomy have been suggested to result from tissue necrosis and erosion as a consequence of inadvertent suture placement between the vaginal cuff and the posterior aspect of the bladder (Zimmern et al, 1994). Unrecognized surgical trauma to the bladder during hysterectomy may also result in urine extravasation and urinoma formation. The urinoma then dependently drains through the vaginal cuff, creating the fistula (Kursh et al, 1988). A review of 43 patients with vesicovaginal or urethrovaginal fistulas by Goodwin and Scardino in 1980 identified gynecologic surgery as the cause of the fistula in 32 of the patients. In 1992, Tancer reported on 151 genital fistulas of the lower urinary tract. A total of 137 (91%) were postsurgical, with 125 occurring after gynecologic surgery. Total hysterectomy was the most common antecedent procedure, accounting for 110 (73%) of the fistulas, with 99 of the hysterectomies performed transabdominally. Factors that may increase the risk of vesicovaginal fistula after hysterectomy include prior uterine surgery (including cesarean section), endometriosis, and prior pelvic radiation therapy.

Other causes of vesicovaginal fistula include urologic or gastrointestinal pelvic surgery, birth trauma, malignancy, radiation, and, rarely, infection, including urinary tuberculosis (Ba-Thike et al, 1992). Symmonds estimated that only 5% of over 800 vesicovaginal fistulas treated at the Mayo Clinic over 30 years were of obstetric origin (Symmonds, 1984). Erosion of foreign bodies, including pessaries, has also resulted in vesicovaginal fistula formation (Goldstein et al, 1990).

Clinical Features

Most patients with vesicovaginal fistula present with continuous discharge of urine from the vagina after gynecologic or other pelvic surgery. The genitourinary fistula may become clinically apparent in the immediate postoperative period but **more commonly becomes evident several days to weeks after the offending surgery.** The possibility of urinary extravasation and impending vesicovaginal fistula should also be considered in patients with a complicated course after hysterectomy, including the development of prolonged paralytic ileus, excessive postoperative pain, or hematuria (Kursh et al, 1988). In some patients with large vesicovaginal fistulas, nearly all urine is lost through the fistula, producing total incontinence; in others, the vaginal urine loss may be minimal and accompanied by an otherwise normal voiding pattern. Vesicovaginal fistula should be suspected also in patients with a history of pelvic malignancy and/or pelvic irradiation who spontaneously develop increased vaginal discharge. Vesicovaginal fistulas have been noted as long as 20 years after pelvic irradiation (Grahm, 1965; Raz et al, 1992).

Evaluation

The differential diagnosis of vaginal urine loss includes incontinence resulting from urethral or bladder dysfunction, ureteral ectopia, ureterovaginal fistula, and urinary fistula to the uterus. After pelvic surgery, excessive vaginal drainage of watery fluid that is not urine may be confused with a true urinary fistula. Postoperative vaginal drainage of peritoneal fluid or, more rarely, from an abnormal fallopian tube communication with the vaginal cuff may simulate a urinary fistula (Leach et al, 1987). Vaginal infection or a draining pelvic abscess may also generate excessive vaginal discharge that must be distinguished from a urinary fistula.

Once a vesicovaginal fistula is suspected, a thorough vaginal examination should be performed. **After hysterectomy, the fistula is usually located at the vaginal cuff.** When the fistula is not clearly identified at routine vaginal examination, several maneuvers can be used to help confirm the presence of a urinary fistula and identify its location. At times, an oral Pyridium test may be used to confirm that the vaginal drainage is indeed urine. A tampon is placed into the vagina, and the patient is given oral Pyridium. The tampon is examined several hours later, with orange staining of the tampon confirming the presence of a genitourinary fistula. A positive result on an oral Pyridium test only confirms the presence of a fistula but does not localize its site. When the fistula site is difficult to identify, vaginal examination while simultaneously distending the bladder with stained fluid or during cystoscopy may help localize the fistula. When the vaginal examination reveals continuous drainage of unstained urine, a supravesical urinary fistula should be suspected. An algorithm for the evaluation of a suspected genitourinary fistula is provided in Figure 37–1.

Cystoscopy may help identify the vesicovaginal fistula and characterize its size and location, especially in relation to the trigone. The presence of multiple fistulas must also be noted during cystoscopy. **A biopsy of the fistula site should be performed in a patient with a history of pelvic malignancy, because the therapeutic approach may be altered by the finding of recurrent malignancy.**

Cystography or voiding cystourethrography may be useful to identify or confirm the presence of a vesicovaginal fistula and assess for other abnormalities including anterior vaginal wall prolapse (Fig. 37–2). Rarely, vaginography may be needed to confirm the diagnosis of vesicovaginal fistula. The vaginogram is performed by injecting contrast material into the vagina through a Foley catheter with a large balloon, occluding the vaginal introitus (Zimmern et al, 1994). Intravenous pyelography is usually performed to assess the status of the upper tracts, because **ureterovaginal fistulas have been associated with vesicovaginal fistulas in up to 10% of cases** (Symmonds, 1984). Radiograghic evidence of partial or complete ureteral obstruction may indicate the presence of a ureterovaginal fistula. However, ureteral dilatation is not always associated with ureterovaginal fistulas. Thus, intravenous pyelography may not be adequate to identify or localize the fistula. **Retrograde pyelography is the most likely study to accurately localize the site of a ureterovaginal fistula and should be performed whenever one is suggested clinically or when the intravenous pyelogram inadequately demonstrates ureteral anatomy.**

Treatment

Conservative Management

Most vesicovaginal fistulas come to the attention of the urologist several days or weeks after the causative gynecologic or pelvic surgery. Once the diagnosis has been confirmed, a trial of conservative therapy should be implemented, including continuous uninterrupted catheter drainage of the bladder and appropriate treatment of any infection. Bladder spasms should be controlled with oral anticholinergics. Although the success rate of a short course

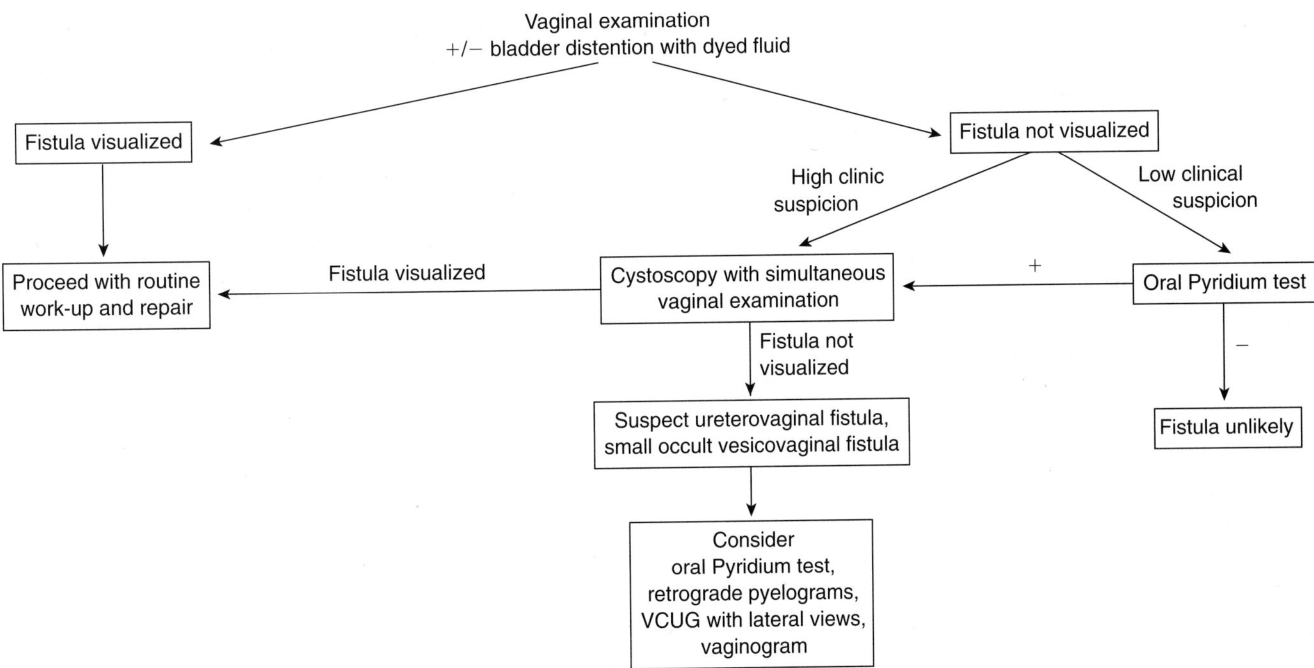

Figure 37–1. Suggested algorithm for evaluation of suspected vesicovaginal fistula.

of conservative management has not been well documented, a small portion of patients, probably those with the smallest fistulas, may be cured with catheter drainage alone. Tancer (1992) noted spontaneous closure in 3 of 151 patients with vesicovaginal fistulas treated with catheter drainage alone. Often, the patient has already undergone a prolonged unsuccessful trial of catheter drainage before referral to the urologist. In these cases, further conservative management with catheter drainage alone is unlikely to result in spontaneous closure of the fistula.

Transvaginal or transvesical electrocoagulation of the epithelial lining of the fistula tract has been advocated as a minimally invasive therapy for very small vesicovaginal fistulas (O'Connor, 1980; Stovsky et al, 1994). Stovsky and colleagues reported cure in 11 of 17 (73%) of women with vesicovaginal fistulas that were 1 to 3 mm in size treated with electrocoagulation of the fistula tract and a minimum of 2 weeks of Foley catheter drainage. Care must taken when using this technique to avoid increasing the size of the fistula tract. For this reason, the authors recommended using a pediatric bugbee electrode and minimal coagulation current. This technique should be attempted only on small, mature, and well-epithelialized fistula tracts.

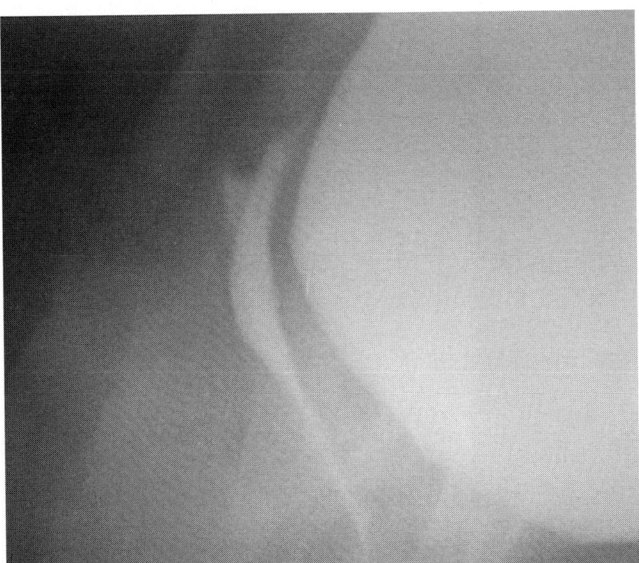

Figure 37–2. Lateral cystogram demonstrating a vesicovaginal fistula with contrast material entering the vagina via the fistula tract. (From Zimmern PE, Ganabathi K, Leach GE: Atlas Urol Clin North Am 1994; 2:87–99.)

Surgical Therapy

General Principles

The first attempt at closure of a vesicovaginal fistula has the best chance of success. Consequently, no compromises should be made when planning the initial repair. Multiple factors must be considered when planning a vesicovaginal fistula repair, including the etiology and duration of the fistula, the quality of the tissues available for repair, and probably most importantly the experience and training of the surgeon. Basic surgical principles should be closely followed. All suture lines should be tension-free, uninfected, and dry. **When the repair is tenuous, interposition of a well-vascularized graft is recommended** (Wein et al, 1980a; Raz et al, 1992; Zimmern et al, 1994). Careful consideration of all of these factors maximizes the chance for a successful surgical repair.

Historically, a 3- to 6-month waiting period between the development of a postoperative vesicovaginal fistula and an attempt at surgical closure has been recommended to allow for inflammation to subside (O'Connor and Sokol, 1951;

O'Connor, 1980; Wein et al, 1980a). More recently, a much more timely approach to surgical repair has been advocated without an enforced "waiting period." **Several authors have reported excellent results with almost immediate repair of postsurgical vesicovaginal fistulas** (Persky et al, 1979; Zimmern et al, 1986; Wang and Hadley, 1990; Raz et al, 1992; Blaivas et al, 1995). Early surgical repair has obvious psychologic and psychosocial advantages for the unfortunate woman with a urinary fistula, who is often a relatively young, active individual in otherwise good health. However, **clinical judgment must be used when determining the timing of repair in complicated cases, including those associated with radiation, infection, or extensive tissue loss.**

Preoperative Preparation

Preoperatively, estrogen replacement therapy may be helpful to improve the vascularity and general quality of the vaginal tissues before repair (Barnes et al, 1977; Jonas and Petri, 1984; Raz et al, 1992). Antiseptic vaginal douches are advised the morning of surgery, and prophylactic broad-spectrum antibiotics should be administered preoperatively. Informed consent including careful explanation of the expected postoperative course and possible complications should also be obtained and documented.

Surgical Approaches

Abdominal, vaginal, and combined abdominal/vaginal approaches have been described for the repair of vesicovaginal fistulas. **The approach selected is dependent on many factors, but is probably best determined by the experience and training of the surgeon.** For surgeons comfortable with vaginal surgery, the vaginal approach is generally more expedient and results in less morbidity; it usually provides for a more rapid recovery. The abdominal approach may be more familiar to the surgeon who infrequently treats this disorder and has the advantage of allowing for simultaneous ureteral reimplantation or bladder augmentation if needed. The abdominal approach is also recommended when the fistula site cannot be adequately visualized and exposed vaginally. Regardless of the approach selected, vascularized interposition grafts may be required in selected cases to reinforce the repair.

Vaginal Approach

The vaginal approach is the authors' preferred approach for vesicovaginal fistula repair. **The technique involves creation of an anterior vaginal wall flap, tension-free multilayer closure of the fistula without excision of the tract, and appropriate use of vascularized interposition grafts.** The patient is placed in the exaggerated lithotomy position. A 24-Fr suprapubic catheter is placed using the Lowsley tractor (Zeidman et al, 1988). A Foley catheter is also placed per urethra. In cases where the fistula lies in close proximity to the ureteral orifices, cystoscopy and ureteral stent placement are recommended. Exposure and visualization may be enhanced by use of a ring retractor and a headlight. In patients with a small vaginal vault, a posterolateral relaxing incision directed toward the ischial tuberosity may further improve exposure (Fig. 37–3).

The fistula tract is catheterized from the vaginal side with a small Foley or Fogarty catheter. A ring retractor with elastic stays and traction on the catheter optimize exposure of the fistula tract (Fig. 37–4*A*). A U-shaped incision is made after infiltrating the vaginal wall with saline. The apex of the U is adjacent to the fistula tract with the base of the flap usually oriented anteriorly for treatment of the most common fistulas located at the vaginal cuff. Posteriorly based flaps may also be used, depending on the location of the fistula. The vaginal wall flap is mobilized by dissection on the relatively avascular shiny white inner surface of the vaginal wall. **The fistula tract is circumscribed but not excised, leaving the scarred margins to provide secure anchoring tissue for the closure.** In the authors' experience, excision of the tract increases the size of the fistula and may decrease the strength of the closure. The vaginal wall is mobilized away from the edges of the fistula, and a small portion of vaginal wall opposite the flap is excised to allow for subsequent advancement of the vaginal wall flap beyond the fistula repair site (see Fig. 37–4*B*). The margins of the fistula tract may be trimmed slightly before performing the first layer of closure (see Fig. 37–4*C*). The fistula tract is closed transversely with 3-0 polyglycolic acid (PGA) suture, taking full thickness of the vaginal wall and partial thickness of the underlying bladder wall (see Fig. 37–4*D*). A second layer of closure is accomplished with a vertically oriented inverting 3-0 PGA suture carefully placed in the perivesical fascia (see Fig. 37–4*E*). The integrity of the first two layers of closure may be checked by instilling dyed fluid into the bladder. The third layer of closure is completed by advancing the vaginal wall flap over the repair site and securing it in

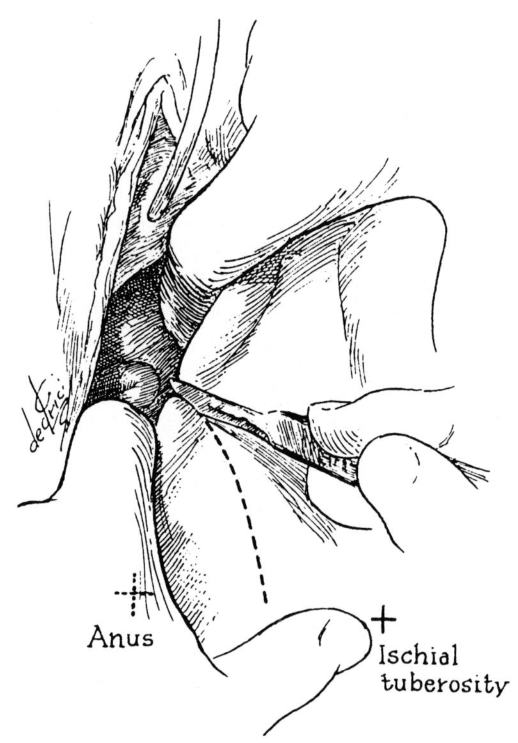

Figure 37–3. Posterior lateral relaxing incision to improve exposure of upper vagina. (From Zimmern PE, Ganabathi K, Leach GE: Atlas Urol Clin North Am 1994; 2:87–99.)

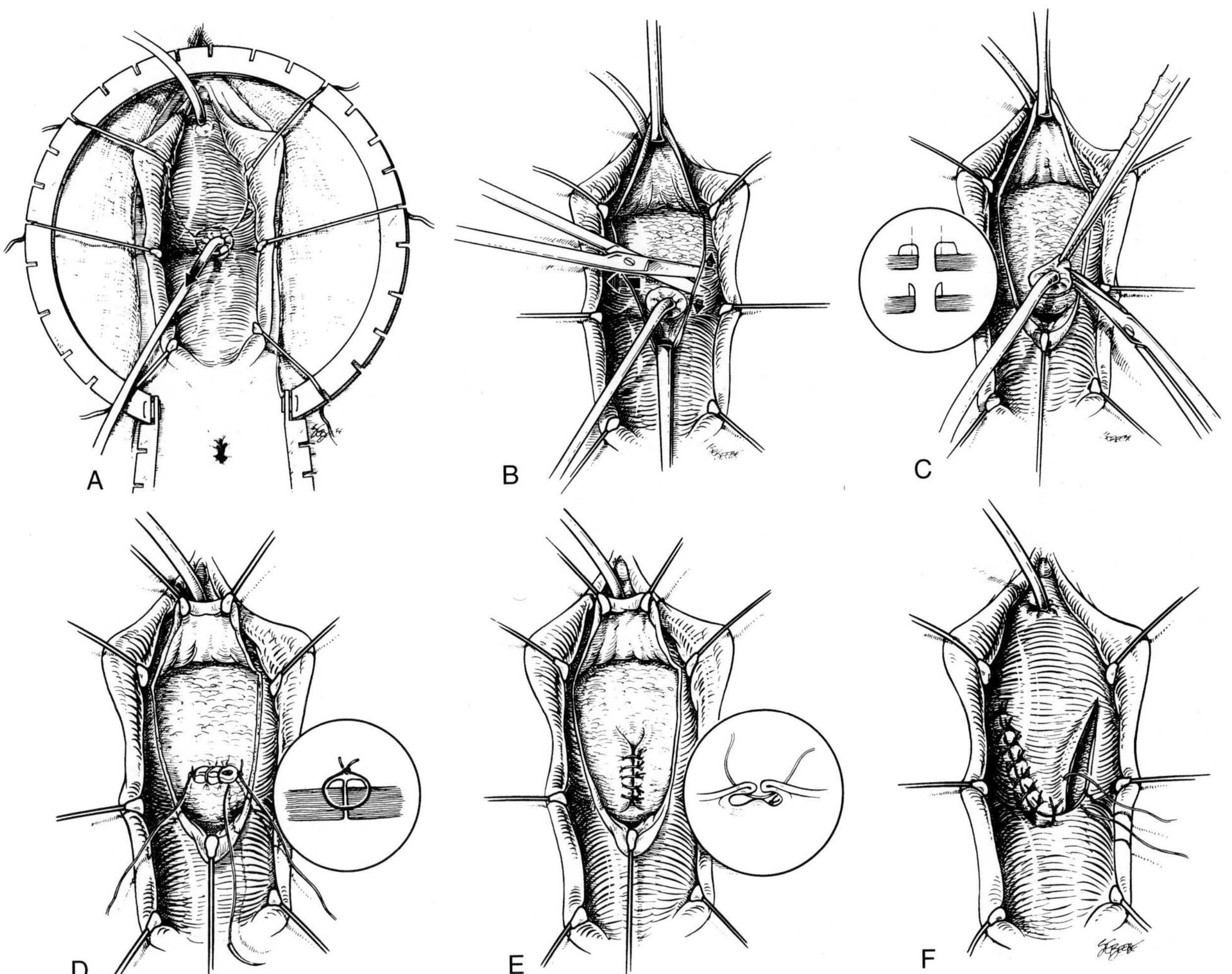

Figure 37–4. *A,* Ring retractor and traction on the catheter placed through the fistula tract enhance exposure. *B,* After the vaginal wall flap is mobilized, the lateral vaginal wall adjacent to the fistula is mobilized away from the fistula tract. *C,* The margins of the fistula tract are carefully trimmed before closure. *D,* The fistula is closed with running 3-0 absorbable suture. *E,* The perivesical fascia is closed vertically over the fistula tract, using absorbable suture. *F,* The final layer of closure is completed by advancing the vaginal wall flap over the repair site and securing it in place with absorbable sutures. (From Zimmern PE, Ganabathi K, Leach GE: Atlas Urol Clin North Am 1994; 2:87–99.)

place with an absorbable suture (see Fig. 37–4*F*). An antibiotic-soaked vaginal pack is inserted and both the urethral and suprapubic catheters are placed to drainage.

If there is any concern about the quality of vaginal tissues or integrity of the closure or in cases associated with prior radiation therapy or previous failed repairs, a Martius labial fat pad graft can be used to reinforce the fistula closure before advancing the vaginal wall flap and completing the repair (Martius, 1928; Raz et al, 1992; Zimmern et al, 1994; Blaivas et al, 1995). A Martius graft is obtained by making a vertical incision over the labia majora, exposing the deep labial fat pad. **The fat pad is mobilized starting anteriorly, preserving the pudendal vascular supply, which enters posteriorly** (Fig. 37–5*A*). After completely mobilizing the fat pad on its posterior vascular pedicle, a tunnel is made medially from the labia to the vagina. The Martius graft is then carefully passed through the tunnel without tension and secured over the fistula repair site with absorbable sutures (see Fig. 37–5*B*). The vaginal wall flap is advanced and sutured in place, as previously described. The labial incision is closed over a small Penrose drain with two layers of absorbable sutures.

In some cases of very proximal vesicovaginal fistulas, the repair site may be beyond the reach of a Martius labial fat pad graft. In those instances, alternative interposition grafts may be used, such as peritoneal or gracilis muscle flaps. A peritoneal flap is obtained by extending the vaginal flap dissection to the level of the peritoneal reflection. The peritoneum is freed from the posterior aspect of the bladder and advanced to cover the first two layers of closure (Raz et al, 1993). The use of a gracilis muscle flap is described under the section on treatment of complicated vesicovaginal fistulas.

The technique of partial colpoclesis described by Latzko offers another alternative for repair of the proximal vaginal vault fistula (Latzko, 1942). The vaginal epithelium around the fistula site is excised, and the colpoclesis is accomplished with several layers of absorbable sutures approximating the anterior to the posterior vaginal wall, obliterating the upper vagina. The technique does not involve excision of the fistula tract or suture placement through the bladder wall; therefore, ureteral reimplantation should almost never be required (Tancer, 1992). Although vaginal vault depth is compromised somewhat by partial colpoclesis, the technique does

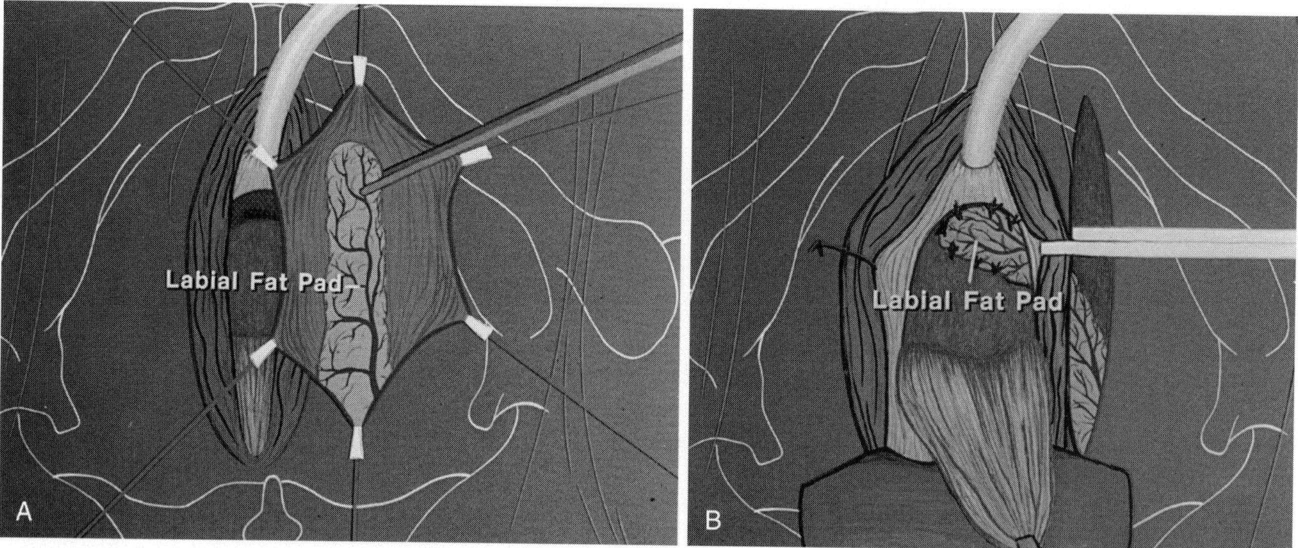

Figure 37–5. *A,* The Martius labial fat pad graft is mobilized, preserving the blood supply entering posteriorly. *B,* The Martius labial fat pad graft is passed through the labial tunnel and secured over the fistula repair site with absorbable suture. (From Zimmern PE, Ganabathi K, Leach GE: Atlas Urol Clin North Am 1994; 2:87–99.)

not appear to significantly impair sexual function (Raz et al, 1992).

The vast majority of vesicovaginal fistulas can be successfully repaired in one operation using the vaginal approach (Goodwin and Scardino, 1980; Wang and Hadley, 1990; Raz et al, 1992; Tancer, 1992). Raz and co-workers reported successful closure of 64 of 69 cases of vesicovaginal fistula (60% of which had failed one to three prior repairs) using a similar vaginal technique (Raz et al, 1992).

Abdominal Approach

The abdominal approach may be used to treat all types of vesicovaginal fistulas and is the preferred approach when concomitant ureteral reimplantation or bladder augmentation is required. O'Connor and Sokol (1951) reported the earliest large experience with abdominal transvesical repair of vesicovaginal fistulas. The technique involves bisection of the bladder to the level of the fistula. Ureteral catheters may be placed to help identify the ureteral orifices and protect them from injury during the repair. The bladder is widely mobilized from the vagina to allow closure in separate layers. The fistula is then completely excised, and further mobilization of the posterior wall of the bladder is performed if necessary (Fig. 37–6). The vagina and bladder are then closed in separate layers with absorbable sutures. A suprapubic catheter is placed before completing the bladder closure. This technique can be performed extraperitoneally; however, in difficult cases, midline transperitoneal exposure is recommended to allow for reinforcement of the repair with an omental pedicle graft. Wein and co-workers (1980b) recommended basing the omental graft on the right gastroepiploic artery, which is usually larger than the left. The omental pedicle must be long enough to reach the pelvis without tension. To obtain adequate length, mobilization of the omentum from the transverse colon and ligation and division of the short gastric branches may be required. Absorbable sutures should be used for ligation of vessels on the omental side to avoid potential complications resulting from contact of urine with permanent suture material. Once the omental pedicle is adequately mobilized, it is secured in position between the vaginal and bladder suture lines. When bladder augmentation is required, the large or small bowel augmenting segment is anastomosed to the bivalved bladder, including the site of repair. The closure is then routinely reinforced with an omental pedicle graft. Abdominal trans-

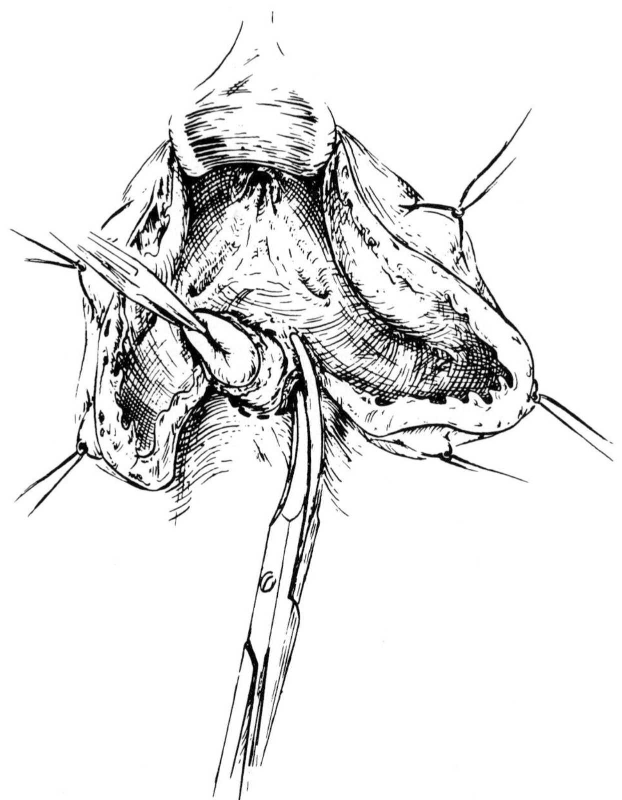

Figure 37–6. The bladder is bisected to the level of the fistula and the fistula tract is sharply excised. (From O'Connor VJ Jr: J Urol 1980; 123:367–369.)

vesical repair of vesicovaginal fistulas has been reported in modern series to result in cure rates of at least 85% (Landes, 1979; O'Connor, 1980; Wein, 1980a; Udeh, 1985; Gil-Vernet et al, 1989; Blaivas et al, 1995).

COMPLICATED VESICOVAGINAL FISTULAS

Complicated vesicovaginal fistulas include giant vesicovaginal fistulas larger than 5 cm in diameter that are usually of obstetric origin, multiply recurrent vesicovaginal fistulas, and fistulas associated with radiation therapy. Giant vesicovaginal fistulas are frequently associated with destruction of the trigone, bladder neck, and urethra. Numerous techniques have been described to repair and reconstruct these challenging anatomic defects, including the use of Martius labial fat pad grafts, anterior or posterior bladder flaps, rectus or gracilis muscle flaps, and myocutaneous flaps (Leadbetter, 1964; Patil et al, 1980; Tanago, 1981; Menchaca et al, 1990; Blaivas, 1991; Raz et al, 1992; Candiani et al, 1993; Tancer, 1993). The length, vascularity, and proximity of the gracilis muscle make it a useful adjunct in genitourinary reconstruction.

The gracilis muscle is mobilized after making a skin incision over the course of the muscle from the medial condyle of the femur to a point approximately 2 cm below the inferior border of the pubic symphysis. Distally, the tendinous portion of the muscle is identified and divided and held with stay sutures. Dissection continues proximally, carefully avoiding injury to the blood and vascular supplies, and entering laterally about 8 to 10 cm from the origin of the muscle. Once the muscle is adequately mobilized, a tunnel is made to the vagina under the skin and superficial fascia of the upper thigh and the labium. The tunnel is widened enough to accommodate the muscle, avoiding excessive constriction of the blood supply. The muscle is then passed through the tunnel and secured over the fistula repair site with absorbable sutures. The vaginal epithelium is closed over the muscle flap, again avoiding excessive tension. In some cases, vaginal closure over the muscle may not be possible and the muscle may be safely left exposed and allowed to epithelialize (Patil et al, 1980). The thigh wound is closed with absorbable sutures over a Penrose drain.

Pelvic radiation therapy is complicated by vesicovaginal fistula formation in a small percentage of patients and may increase the chance of vesicovaginal fistula after any subsequent surgery (Grahm, 1965; Strockbine et al, 1970; Raz et al, 1992). **Radiation-induced tissue damage and vascular changes decrease the chance of spontaneous closure and postoperative healing** (Öbrink and Bunne, 1978; Raz et al, 1992). Sound clinical judgment must be used to determine when the local tissues are in optimal condition for surgical closure. **Before proceeding with repair, the fistula site should be biopsied to rule out recurrent malignancy. The bladder capacity should also be assessed preoperatively to determine the need for concomitant bladder augmentation.**

When bladder capacity is adequate, a vaginal approach may be used. This approach avoids the complications associated with surgery in a previously irradiated abdomen. The technique is essentially the same as in nonirradiated vesicovaginal fistulas, with adherence to proper surgical principles and technique being of critical importance. Martius labial fat pad grafts have been used successfully to reinforce the repair; however, use of a gracilis muscle flap obtained from outside the field of radiation may be advisable in selected cases (Öbrink and Bunne, 1978). Externalized ureteral stents may also be used selectively to maximize urinary drainage during the early healing period.

Postoperative Care

Postoperative care is similar for both vaginal and abdominal vesicovaginal fistula repair. Adequate uninterrupted bladder drainage is probably the most critical aspect of postoperative management. To prevent bladder spasms that may compromise the repair, belladonna and opium suppositories are usually administered for the first 24 hours postoperatively, followed by oral anticholinergic agents until the catheters are removed. Oral antibiotics are also usually administered while catheters are in place. Patients usually do not experience excessive pain postoperatively and are encouraged to begin ambulation on the first postoperative day. **Uninterrupted catheter drainage is continued until a voiding cystourethrogram is performed at 10 to 14 postoperative days to confirm closure of the fistula.** Oral anticholinergics should be stopped 24 hours before performing the voiding cystourethrogram. Once the integrity of the closure is confirmed and the patient demonstrates the ability to void with minimal postvoid residual volumes, the suprapubic catheter is removed. Oral estrogen replacement is provided to postmenopausal women to promote vaginal healing. To prevent trauma to the repair during the healing process, the patient is advised to avoid the use of tampons and refrain from sexual activity for at least 2 months postoperatively.

Complications

Complications after vesicovaginal fistula repair include those common to abdominal or vaginal surgery. Complications specific to vesicovaginal fistula repair include recurrent fistula formation, ureteral injury, and vaginal stenosis with associated dyspareunia. New or recurrent fistulas identified in the immediate postoperative period should be managed conservatively with adequate bladder drainage and observation. If the fistula persists, secondary fistula repair may be undertaken after allowing for resolution of postoperative inflammation. A vaginal approach may be repeated successfully in the majority of cases (Raz et al, 1992). Significant ureteral obstruction is a rare complication of vesicovaginal fistula repair. When significant ureteral obstruction does occur, it should be managed using standard endoscopic, percutaneous, or open techniques. Rarely, in severely symptomatic cases of vaginal stenosis, vaginal relaxing incisions or split-thickness skin grafting may be required to increase the capacity of the vaginal vault.

URETHROVAGINAL FISTULA AND COMPLETE URETHRAL RECONSTRUCTION

Anatomic defects of the female urethra span a spectrum from the small urethrovaginal fistula causing vaginal voiding to loss of the entire urethra and bladder neck, causing total incontinence. **These anatomic defects of the female urethra are usually rare complications of prior gynecologic or urologic surgery, with anterior colporrhaphy and urethral diverticulectomy the most common antecedent procedures** (Patil et al, 1980; Blaivas, 1989). Modern obstetric care has made birth trauma a rare cause of urethral defects in developed nations; however, as with vesicovaginal fistulas, **complications of obstructed labor remain the major cause of urethral injury in underdeveloped nations** (Elkins, 1994; Arrowsmith, 1994).

The repair of urethrovaginal fistulas is usually accomplished transvaginally by techniques similar to those for the transvaginal repair of vesicovaginal fistulas (Webster et al, 1984; Leach, 1991). The surgical repair of complete urethral loss is a more complex surgical challenge. A multitude of techniques for urethral reconstruction have been described (Leadbetter, 1964; Flocks and Boldus, 1973; Hendren, 1980; Patil et al, 1980; Tanago, 1981; Blaivas, 1989). Most of these techniques employ some form of bladder or vaginal flap. Both bladder and vaginal flap urethral reconstructions have a high rate of postoperative incontinence unless a simultaneous anti-incontinence procedure is performed (Blaivas, 1989). **Accurate preoperative assessment of the extent of urethral loss, as well as identification of concomitant urethral hypermobility or intrinsic sphincter deficiency, are critical to planning a successful urethral reconstruction.**

Preoperative Evaluation

In patients who are not totally incontinent, a complete voiding history helps identify components of stress or urge incontinence. A history of multiple previous vaginal or pelvic surgeries increases the chance of severe scarring and intrinsic sphincter deficiency. A thorough physical examination is needed to assess the extent of urethral loss, the location and size of any urethrovaginal fistula, the degree of urethral support during straining, and the quality of the surrounding vaginal tissue. The presence of atrophic vaginitis should be noted and treated with estrogen before reconstruction.

Careful urethroscopy with a 20-Fr female cystoscope usually confirms the diagnosis of a urethrovaginal fistula. When confirmation is difficult, simultaneous vaginal exposure with a speculum may aid in visual identification of the fistula (Leach, 1991). Cystoscopy is essential to assess involvement of the bladder neck or trigone. **When the trigone is involved, upper tract screening with a renal ultrasound examination or intravenous pyelogram is recommended.** A voiding cystourethrogram performed under fluoroscopic control with the patient in the standing position and with adequate voiding views may be useful to identify the urethral defect, exclude vesicovaginal fistula, and demonstrate urethral hypermobility and/or leakage of contrast material across the bladder neck with stress. Urodynamic studies may be used selectively to assess bladder function or document intrinsic sphincter deficiency.

In general, symptomatic small- to moderate-size urethrovaginal fistulas can be managed with urethrovaginal fistula repair, assuming that a tension-free closure can be obtained. Very distal urethrovaginal fistulas may be managed with an extended meatotomy (Lamensdorf et al, 1977). Complete urethral reconstruction is required for patients with very large urethrovaginal fistulas or extensive urethral loss. **The results of the preoperative evaluation will determine the need for a simultaneous anti-incontinence procedure.** Preoperative preparation is similar to that for transvaginal vesicovaginal fistula repair.

Operative Technique

Urethrovaginal Fistula Repair

The patient is placed in lithotomy position. A 14-Fr urethral catheter and a 24-Fr suprapubic catheter are inserted using a Lowsley tractor. After infiltrating the anterior vaginal wall with plain saline, an inverted-U incision is made with the apex just proximal to the urethrovaginal fistula (Fig. 37–7*A*). An anterior vaginal wall flap is raised, with the wide base of the flap at the bladder neck. **The dissection should be performed in the relatively avascular plane below the vaginal epithelium on the shiny white interior surface of the vaginal wall.** When the dissection proceeds too deeply, excessive bleeding or bladder perforation may occur. At this point, if treatment of symptomatic urethral hypermobility or intrinsic sphincter deficiency is needed, the vaginal dissection may be carried laterally and the endopelvic fascia perforated laterally in preparation for a bladder neck suspension or pubovaginal sling. Full descriptions of bladder neck suspension and pubovaginal sling procedures are found in Chapters 32–34.

The fistula is circumscribed but not excised and the scarred margins are used to provide a secure closure of the fistula tract (see Fig. 37–7*B*). Similar to their experience with the repair of vesicovaginal fistulas, the authors believe that excision of the tract only increases the size of the fistula and may decrease the strength of the closure. The margins of the fistula are freed from surrounding scar tissue to allow tension-free closure. Just distal to the fistula, a portion of the vaginal epithelium is removed to allow adequate vaginal wall flap advancement and avoid overlapping suture lines during closure. The fistula is closed with a running locked 4-0 absorbable suture (see Fig. 37–7*C*). A second layer of closure is accomplished with interrupted Lembert-type sutures of 3-0 absorbable material in the periurethral fascia. These two layers should result in a watertight closure without tension.

When there is concern about the quality of vaginal tissues or integrity of the closure, a Martius labial fat pad graft can be used to reinforce the fistula closure (Webster et al, 1984; Leach, 1991).

The anterior vaginal flap is the final layer of closure. The vaginal wall flap can be advanced over the Martius graft, avoiding overlapping suture lines (see Fig. 37–7*D*). The vaginal closure is completed with a running locked absorbable suture. A small Penrose drain is placed deep in the labial wound, and the labial incision is closed in layers. Both the urethral and suprapubic catheters are placed to drainage and an antibiotic-soaked vaginal pack is inserted.

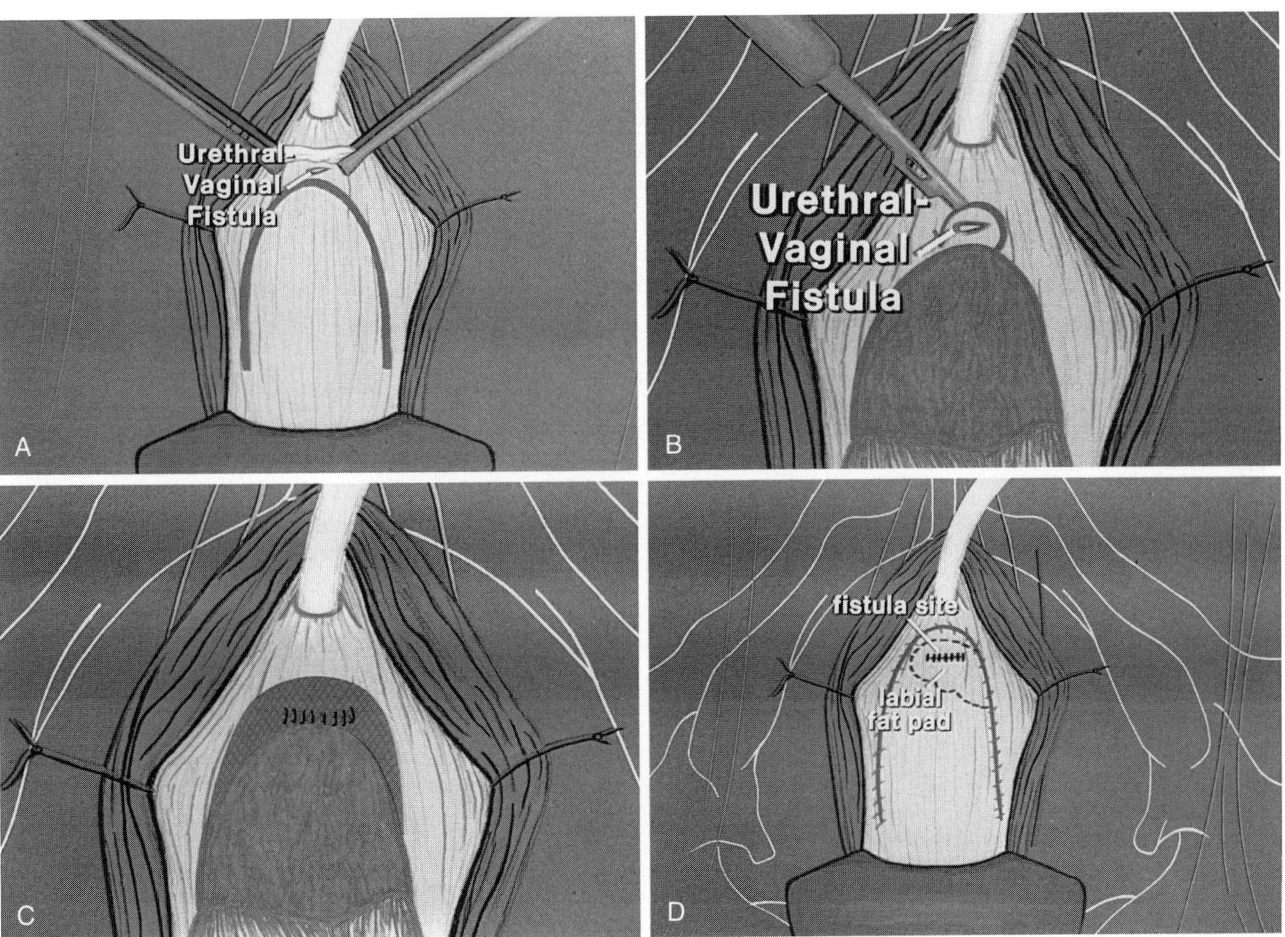

Figure 37–7. *A,* An inverted-U anterior vaginal wall incision is made with the apex just proximal to the urethrovaginal fistula. *B,* The urethrovaginal fistula is circumscribed but not excised. *C,* Fistula tract is closed with running 3-0 absorbable suture. *D,* The vaginal flap is advanced over the fistula repair site to complete the closure. (From Leach GE: Urol Clin North Am 1991; 18:409–413.)

Urethral Reconstruction

Large defects in the female urethra present a challenging urologic problem. Many transabdominal, transvaginal, and abdominovaginal approaches have been described for urethral reconstruction. The abdominal approaches generally incorporate either a posterior bladder flap as described by Young (1922) and later modified by Dees (1949) and Leadbetter (1964), or an anterior bladder flap as described by Tanagho (1981). The abdominal approach allows for omental interposition to reinforce the repair and is especially indicated when ureteral reimplantation is required. The utility of the vaginal approach for urethral reconstruction has been well-described (Goodwin and Scardino, 1980; Patil et al, 1980; Webster et al, 1984; Zimmern et al, 1985; Blaivas, 1989, 1991; Leach, 1991; Elkins et al, 1992). This approach may be used to successfully repair all types of urethral and bladder neck defects with the obvious advantage of avoiding a transabdominal procedure. Although transvaginal construction of an anterior bladder tube has been described (Elkins et al, 1992), most investigators have used vaginal flaps to transvaginally reconstruct the urethra, usually in conjunction with a Martius labial fat pad interposition graft (Goodwin and Scardino, 1980; Webster et al, 1984; Blaivas, 1989, 1991; Zimmern et al, 1985). The authors use a technique similar to that described by Blaivas in 1989.

Vaginal Flap Urethral Reconstruction

The patient is placed in the lithotomy position. A 20- to 24-Fr suprapubic Foley catheter is placed using the modified Lowsley tractor. A 14-Fr urethral Foley catheter is placed and the balloon overinflated enough to prevent passage through the bladder neck. In most cases, an inverted-U vaginal incision is used with its apex just proximal to the meatus of the damaged urethra and its base at the bladder neck (Blaivas, 1989).

The neourethra is then created by making two parallel incisions starting on each side of the meatus extending distally (Fig. 37–8*A*). Flaps are then mobilized laterally to medially, allowing tubularization of the mobilized flaps around the 14-Fr catheter. The flaps are approximated in the midline with 4-0 absorbable suture forming the neourethra (see Fig. 37–8*B*). The suture line is then reinforced with a Martius graft, as described in the repair of urethrovaginal fistulas (see Fig. 37–8*C*). The vagina and labia are closed with absorbable sutures (see Fig. 37–8*D*). If a pubovaginal sling has been used, it should be secured with minimal tension to the abdominal fascia or pubic tubercle before closing the vagina. The suprapubic and urethral catheters are placed to drainage, and an antibiotic-soaked vaginal pack is inserted.

As in all reconstructive surgery, anatomic considerations

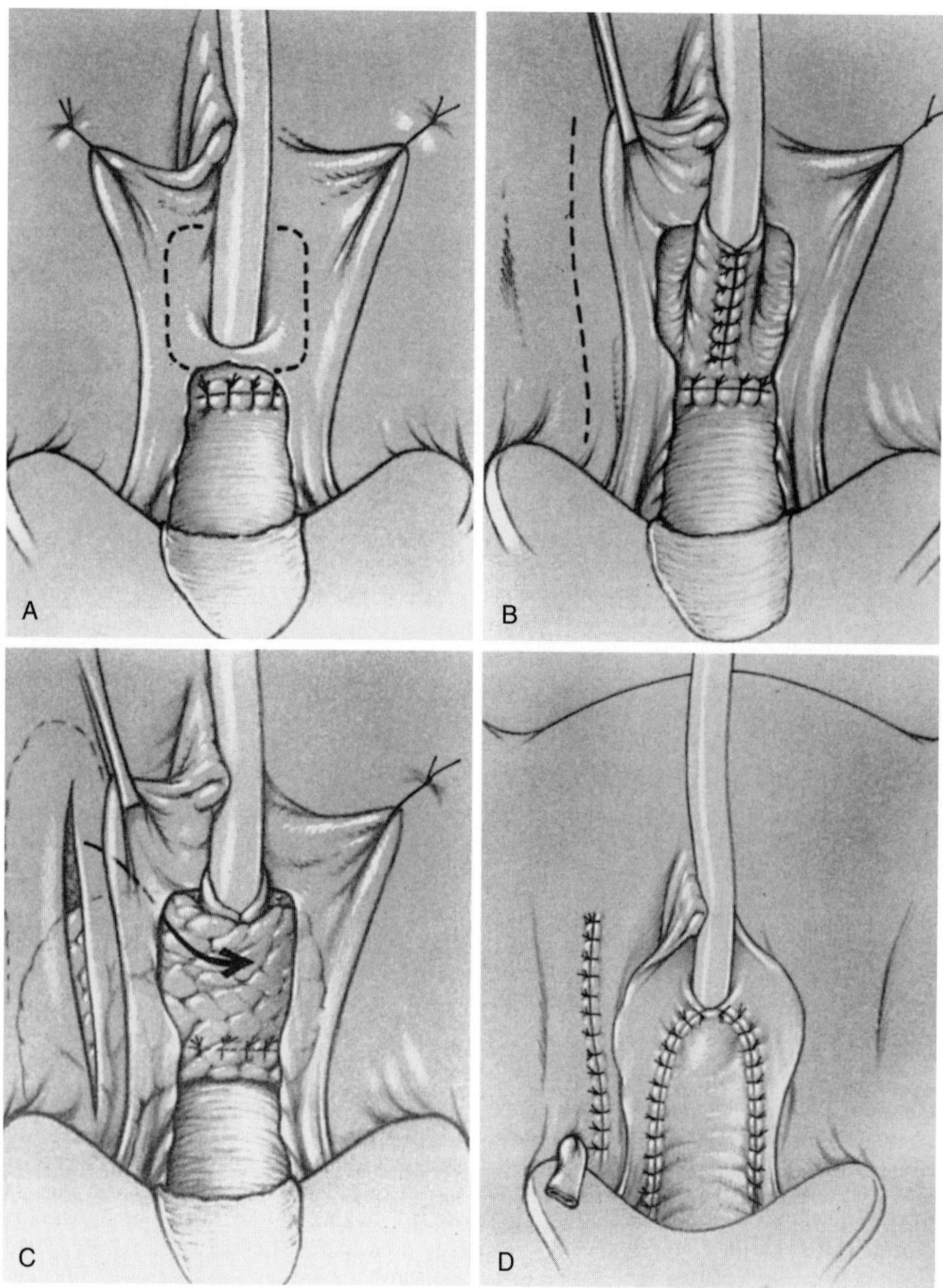

Figure 37–8. *A,* After closure of a bladder neck fistula in this patient (horizontal suture line), the neourethra is created by making lateral vaginal incisions around the catheter. *B,* The vaginal flaps are mobilized lateral to medial and tubularized over the 14-Fr catheter forming the neourethra. *C,* A Martius labial fat pad graft is secured over the neourethra. *D,* The vagina and labia are closed to complete the urethral reconstruction. (From Blaivas JG: J Urol 1989; 141:542–545.)

may make modifications of the usual technique necessary. A modified vaginal flap urethral reconstruction using a meatal-based vaginal flap rotated distally has also been successful (Fig. 37–9) (Blaivas, 1991). At times, inadequate vaginal wall tissue may prevent reapproximation of the vaginal wall over the reinforced neourethra. In these cases, epithelial ingrowth should eventually close the defect without undue risk to the repair (Blaivas, 1991). Alternative means of suture line reinforcement include labial-cutaneous, gracilis, and perineal artery–based flaps (Hendren, 1980; Patil et al, 1980; Mitchell et al, 1982; Nolan et al, 1991). In selected cases with severe tissue loss, the neourethra may be constructed from the cutaneous portion of a gracilis or perineal artery–based myocutaneous flap.

In some severely debilitated patients with extensive tissue loss, the most practical alternative may be transvaginal closure of the bladder neck with creation of a continent catheterizable stoma to the bladder or placement of a suprapubic tube (Zimmern et al, 1985).

Postoperative Management

Postoperative care is similar to that for vesicovaginal fistula repair, including appropriate use of preoperative antibiotics and anticholinergics to prevent bladder spasms. **Uninterrupted catheter drainage is maintained for 7 to 10 days, after which the urethral catheter is removed and a voiding cystourethrogram is performed via the suprapubic catheter.** Anticholinergics should be discontinued 24

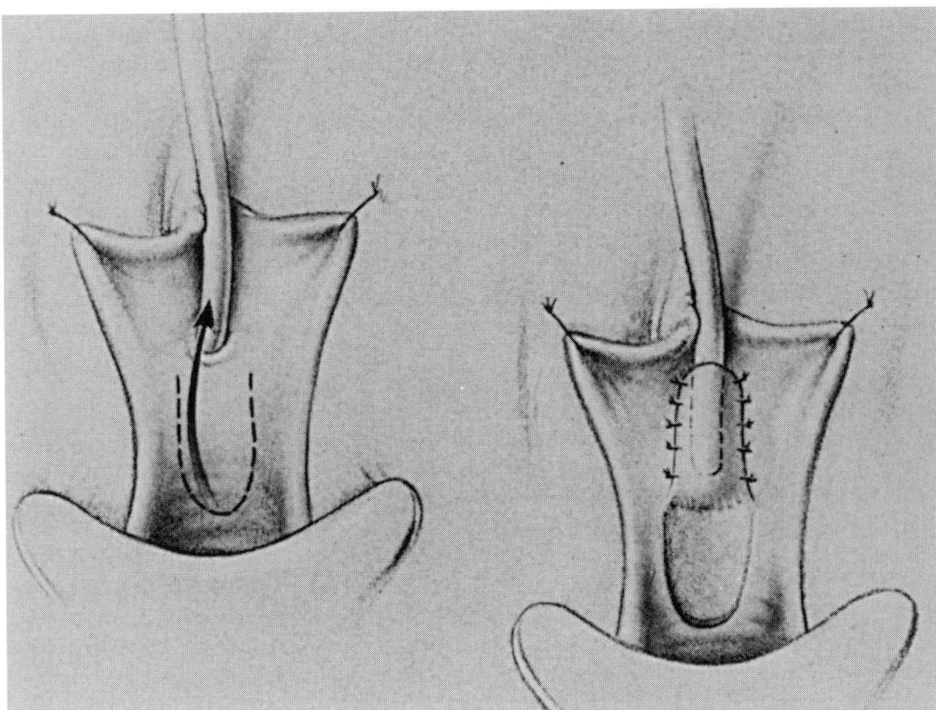

Figure 37–9. Meatal-based vaginal flap urethral reconstruction. (From Blaivas JG: Urol Clin North Am 1991; 18:355–363.)

hours before performing the voiding cystourethrogram. **When extravasation is noted, the urethral catheter is not replaced, and the suprapubic tube is placed to drainage.** The study is then repeated in 1 to 2 weeks.

Complications

Urinary retention or elevated postvoid residuals are a more common problem after urethral reconstruction, especially if a simultaneous anti-incontinence procedure was performed. When the patient is unable to void or elevated postvoid residuals are noted on the postoperative voiding cystourethrogram, the suprapubic catheter is not removed but is intermittently opened to drain the residual urine. Intermittent catheterization through the reconstructed urethra should be avoided in the early postoperative period. Within a few weeks, most patients are able to void adequately, and the suprapubic catheter is removed. When long-term intermittent catheterization is required, as often occurs after simultaneous pubovaginal sling placement, it should not be initiated until healing of the reconstructed urethra is complete.

Urinary incontinence after urethral reconstruction may be a consequence of stress incontinence, detrusor instability, or urethral fistula formation. As previously mentioned, careful preoperative evaluation helps select patients requiring a simultaneous anti-incontinence procedure, minimizing the risk of postoperative stress incontinence. However, if stress incontinence occurs, it should be evaluated and treated in the standard fashion. Periurethral injections may be useful for treatment of selected cases of postoperative stress incontinence (Lockhart et al, 1988; Ganabathi and Leach, 1994). Persistent urge incontinence may be related to outlet obstruction and should be fully evaluated. Blaivas (1989) reported restoration of continence in 9 of 10 patients undergoing vaginal flap urethral reconstruction. Six patients underwent one procedure, two patients required a subsequent pubovaginal sling for intrinsic sphincteric deficiency, and one patient required a subsequent vesicovaginal fistula closure.

A new or recurrent urethrovaginal fistula identified in the immediate postoperative period is managed conservatively with suprapubic drainage and observation. If the fistula persists, fistula repair may be undertaken after allowing at least 2 to 3 months for resolution of postoperative inflammation.

Urethral Diverticulum

The diagnosis of female urethral diverticulum has become much more common over the last several decades, mainly because of heightened clinical awareness and suspicion. Hey reported the first case of female urethral diverticulum in 1805. The entity continued to be only rarely reported until 1956, when Davis and Cian diagnosed 50 female cases using positive-pressure urethrography. Despite the increased awareness of urethral diverticulum in recent years, **this disorder continues to be routinely overlooked during the evaluation of women with lower urinary tract symptoms** (Roehrborn, 1988; Boyd, 1993; Ganabathi et al, 1994a). A high index of clinical suspicion coupled with appropriate clinical, radiologic, and endoscopic evaluation facilitate prompt diagnosis and appropriate treatment of female urethral diverticulum.

Incidence

The reported incidence of female urethral diverticulum varies from 1.4% to 5% (Anderson, 1967; Aldridge et al, 1978; Robertson, 1978). Because many urethral diverticula are asymptomatic, the true incidence is not known and may be higher. Aldridge and co-workers found urethral diverticula in 1.4% of women with stress urinary incontinence.

Female urethral diverticula are most commonly diagnosed in the third through sixth decades, with a mean age at diagnosis of about 45 years (Ganabathi et al, 1994a). The diagnosis has also been made rarely in neonates and young females (Lee, 1984). The incidence in black women has been suggested to be two to six times the incidence in the white population (Davis and Robinson, 1970), although Ganabathi and co-workers (1994a) found no racial predilection in 63 women they treated for urethral diverticulum.

Etiology

Several theories have been proposed to explain the etiology and pathogenesis of female urethral diverticulum. A few reports have suggested that most urethral diverticula are congenital in origin, although **most authors suggest the majority of urethral diverticula are acquired.**

Although few urethral diverticula have been found in children, some evidence does support the argument for a congenital origin in some cases, especially those occurring in the pediatric population. Congenital urethral diverticula have been postulated to arise from (1) a remnant of Gartner's duct; (2) faulty union of primordial folds; (3) "cell rests"; (4) vaginal wall cysts of müllerian origin; (5) congenital dilatation of periurethral cysts; or (6) in association with blind-ending ureters (Ratner et al, 1949; Nel, 1955; Ginsberg and Genadry, 1984; Orikasa et al, 1990; Ganabathi et al, 1994b). Silk and Lebowitz (1969) suggested that an anterior urethral diverticulum they treated represented an aborted attempt at urethral duplication. Mesonephric adenocarcinoma has been reported in two urethral diverticula, suggesting an origin from remnants of Gartner's ducts (Lee and Keller, 1977). The presence of paneth cell metaplasia in a number of diverticula also supports a congenital etiology in some cases (Niemic et al, 1989).

Although some urethral diverticula are likely to be congenital in origin, the majority are probably acquired. Several theories have been advanced to explain the development of acquired urethral diverticula. Historically, urethral trauma from childbirth was thought to be responsible for most urethral diverticula (McNally, 1935). However, more recent studies have shown that 15% to 20% of women with urethral diverticula are nulliparous, making this theory unlikely (Lee, 1984). Urethral trauma from instrumentation and obstruction from distal urethral or meatal strictures have also been postulated to be etiologic factors in the formation of urethral diverticulum, but these theories are now generally rejected.

The most widely accepted theory of urethral diverticulum formation implicates infection of the periurethral glands. Once infected, the periurethral glands become obstructed, dilate, and rupture into the urethral lumen, creating the diverticulum. This explanation was first proposed by Routh in 1890 and was supported by Huffman's detailed description of the female paraurethral ducts in 1948. The periurethral glands are tubuloalveolar structures usually located posterolaterally along the distal two thirds of the urethra, with the majority draining into the distal one third of the urethra (Huffman, 1948). Urethral diverticula are formed when the periurethral glands become infected and obstructed, forming cystic structures that rupture into the urethral lumen. The most commonly cultured organisms are *Escherichia coli*, gonococci, and *Chlamydia*, although various organisms have been cultured from the diverticulum or catheterized urine specimen (Peters and Vaughan, 1976; Rózsahegyi et al, 1981; Ganabathi et al, 1994b).

Pathologically, the diverticulum is a "false diverticulum" consisting of mostly fibrous tissue. In many cases an epithelial lining may not be present, probably as the result of chronic inflammation. This chronic inflammation within the diverticulum may also result in marked fibrosis and adherence of the diverticular wall to surrounding structures and spontaneous drainage into the vagina. **The periurethral glands are located within the periurethral fascia.** Therefore, all urethral diverticula are contained within this fascia as well. This is an important point, because **the periurethral fascia can usually be preserved during the dissection of the diverticulum and used to reinforce the repair.**

Associated Complications

Female urethral diverticula may be complicated by infection, stones, bladder outlet obstruction, and malignancy. Infection may be acute or chronic and may result in abscess. About one third of patients present with recurrent urinary tract infections (Ganabathi et al, 1994a). **An infected diverticulum may be the source of recurrent urinary tract infections but otherwise may be relatively asymptomatic.** In other cases, the infected diverticulum may be acutely inflamed and painful and associated with systemic symptoms of bacterial infection requiring transvaginal aspiration.

Stone formation within urethral diverticula is reported to occur in 1% to 10% of cases (Leach and Bavendam, 1987; Aragona et al, 1989; Hansen et al, 1989). Urinary stasis and chronic infection are responsible for calculi formation. Malignancy is a rare complication of urethral diverticulum, but should be suspected in the presence of recurrent hematuria, induration on palpation, noncalcified filling defects within the diverticulum on voiding cystourethrography, or a visible lesion seen at the diverticular communication site on urethroscopy. Fewer than 70 cases of urethral diverticular carcinoma have been reported in the English literature (Thomas and Maguire, 1991; Catalona and Jones, 1992; Clayton et al, 1992; Ganabathi et al, 1994b). **Adenocarcinoma is by far the most common histologic type,** followed by transitional cell carcinoma, which together account for 80% of the reported malignancies. Although squamous cell carcinoma is the most common histologic type of female urethral malignancy, it is less commonly found in female urethral diverticula (Wishard et al, 1963; Clayton et al, 1992; Ganabathi et al, 1994b). Endometriosis has also been reported in female urethral diverticula (Palagiri, 1978). Thirteen cases of nephrogenic adenoma arising in urethral diverticula have also been reported, and great care must taken to differentiate this benign lesion from adenocarcinoma. Wide local excision is recommended for localized diverticular carcinoma, although more radical surgical therapy may be required in some patients with more extensive disease. Radiation therapy may be used alone for poor surgical candidates or in combination with surgical therapy in selected cases (Patanaphan et al, 1983).

Urinary incontinence is frequently associated with a urethral diverticulum. Incontinence may be a sequel to urine loss from the diverticulum itself with stress maneuvers (paradoxical incontinence), genuine stress urinary incontinence, or urge incontinence. Ganabathi and co-workers (1994a) reported stress urinary incontinence as an initial symptom in 62% of women with urethral diverticula. A voiding cystourethrogram or videourodynamics study demonstrating loss of contrast material across the bladder neck with straining strongly suggests the presence of concomitant genuine stress urinary incontinence that may require simultaneous repair.

Presentation

The presenting symptoms of a urethral diverticulum have classically been described as the three Ds (**d**ysuria, postvoid **d**ribbling, and **d**yspareunia). However, the symptoms of urethral diverticulum are quite variable, with many completely asymptomatic diverticula found incidentally. **Urinary frequency, urgency, and dysuria are the most common symptoms, occurring in about 50% of patients.** Recurrent urinary tract infections occur in 40% of patients. About 25% of patients report postvoid dribbling, and about 10% report dyspareunia. Other less frequent symptoms include hematuria and anterior vaginal wall pain and swelling (Bass and Leach, 1991; Ganabathi et al, 1994a).

The symptoms of a urethral diverticulum may easily be confused with those of various other disorders associated with irritative voiding symptoms, including interstitial cystitis, detrusor instability, or carcinoma in situ. **Urethral diverticulum should be considered in a patient with persistent lower urinary tract symptoms unresponsive to therapy.** Once the diagnosis is suspected, an appropriate evaluation should be performed.

A careful physical examination frequently reveals the diverticulum. Telinde made the diagnosis on physical examination alone in 63% of cases (Davis and Te Linde, 1958). Pelvic examination should include careful palpation of the urethra. An anterior vaginal wall mass may be identified. Compression of the mass, which is often tender, may express urine or purulent or bloody material from the urethral meatus. In some cases, the diverticulum may be recognized only as an area of point tenderness along the urethra. Distinct firmness or induration of the mass may indicate the presence of a stone or neoplasm.

Not all anterior vaginal wall masses represent diverticula. Therefore, the full differential diagnosis of anterior vaginal wall or periurethral masses should be considered, including Skene's gland abscess, ectopic ureterocele, Gartner's duct cyst, müllerian remnant cyst, vaginal wall inclusion cyst, and urethral or vaginal neoplasm (Dmochowski et al, 1994). The pelvic examination should also include careful assessment of urethral hypermobility and other significant prolapse into the vagina that may require simultaneous repair at the time of diverticulectomy.

To aid in the accurate preoperative assessment and evaluation of urethral diverticula, Leach and co-workers (1993) proposed a standardized classification system. This classification system accounts for various important pretreatment factors and allows for more meaningful comparison of results between different series. Each letter of the L/N/S/C3 classification system represents a different characteristic of urethral diverticula.

L = **L**ocation
N = **N**umber
S = **S**ize
C3 = **C**onfiguration, **C**ommunication, and **C**ontinence

Table 37–1 provides the preoperative L/N/S/C3 classification for 63 cases of urethral diverticula treated at the authors' institution.

Endoscopic, Radiographic, and Urodynamic Evaluation

When evaluating female urethral pathology, including diverticula, cystourethroscopy is preferably performed using a short beaked female urethroscope and 0-degree lens. A urethrotome sheath may also be used if a female urethroscope is not available (Redman, 1990). Urethroscopy should be carefully performed in an attempt to locate the diverticular communication site and assess for associated neoplasm. Simultaneous digital compression of the anterior vaginal wall during urethroscopy may cause purulent material to be expressed into the urethral lumen, allowing identification of the communication site. The degree of urethral hypermobility may also be assessed endoscopically.

Various other imaging techniques have been used to evaluate urethral diverticula. **A properly performed voiding cystourethrogram is the most helpful imaging study when evaluating urethral diverticulum** (Fig. 37–10*A*). At the authors' institution, they have found that voiding cystourethrography has accurately identified the diverticulum in 95% of cases. The study should be performed under fluoroscopic control with the patient standing. **The presence of filling defects within the diverticulum may suggest the possibility of stones, tumor, or inflammatory mass** (see Fig. 37–10*B*). **An air-fluid level may be seen and usually indicates that the diverticulum is much larger than the portion visualized with contrast medium.** The voiding cystourethrogram may also provide additional information

Table 37–1. PREOPERATIVE CLASSIFICATION OF FEMALE URETHRAL DIVERTICULUM (L/N/S/C3) IN 63 WOMEN

Location (No.)	No.	Configuration (No.)	Communication (No.)	Continence (No.)
Proximal beneath bladder neck (9)	Single	Multiloculated (22)	Proximal urethra (16)	Completely continent (26)
Proximal urethra (7)	Multiple	Single (41)	Midurethra (35)	Stress incontinence only (30)
Midurethra (36)		Saddle-shaped (14)	Distal urethra (12)	Urge incontinence only (3)
Distal urethra (11)				Stress and urge incontinence (4)

From Ganabathi K, Leach GE, Zimmern PE, Dmochowski RR: J Urol 1994; 152:1445–1452.

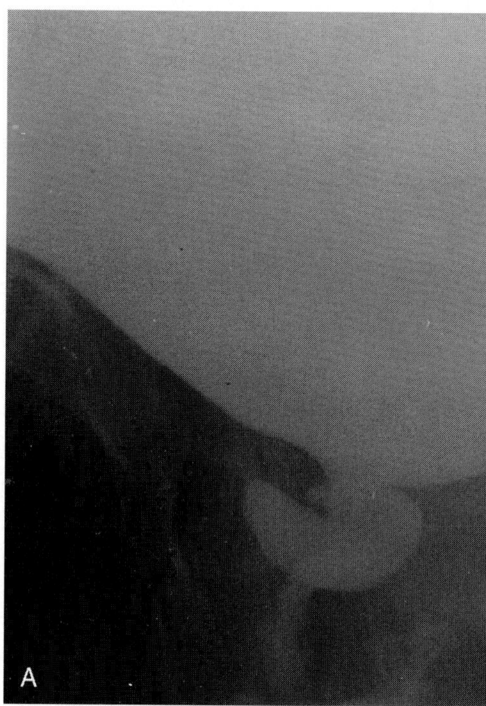

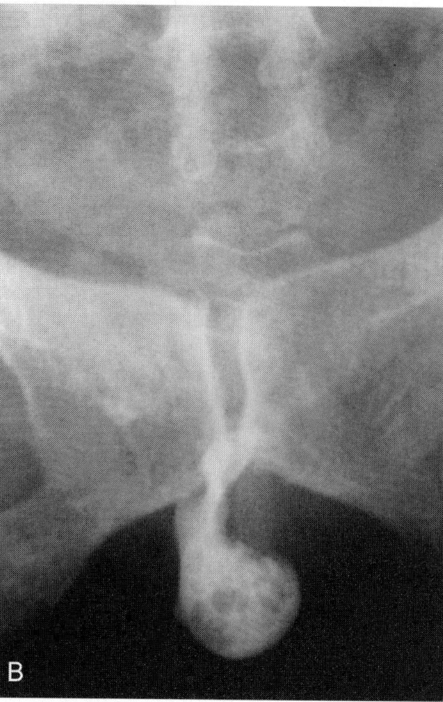

Figure 37–10. *A,* Voiding cystourethrogram demonstrating saddle-shaped urethral diverticulum at the midurethra. *B,* Stones within a urethral diverticulum represented as multiple filling defects within the diverticulum on the post-void view of a voiding cystourethrogram. (From Leach GE, Bavendam TG: Urology 1987; 30:407–415.)

regarding the degree of urethral hypermobility and competency of the bladder neck.

Retrograde positive-pressure urethrography using a double-balloon catheter has a reported accuracy of 90% and may be useful in selected cases where a suspected diverticulum cannot be demonstrated on a high-quality voiding cystourethrogram (Davis and Cian, 1956; Anderson, 1967). However, retrograde positive-pressure urethrography is technically difficult to perform and is usually painful, often requiring the use of general or regional anesthesia. Fortunately, this study is rarely required, because high-quality voiding cystourethrography usually demonstrates the diverticulum (Ganabathi et al, 1994a).

Intravenous pyelography may show the diverticulum on the postvoid film and is helpful in delineating the upper tracts and excluding an ectopic ureterocele. **To avoid misdiagnosis and inadvertent excision of an ectopic ureterocele, intravenous pyelography is recommended before diverticulectomy** (Blacklock et al, 1982). Ultrasonography (suprapubic, perineal, and vaginal) has also been used to investigate urethral diverticulum (Thomas and Maguire, 1991; Clayton et al, 1992; Ganabathi et al, 1994a). Transvaginal ultrasonography has successfully identified a diverticulum not demonstrated on voiding cystourethrography and may supplant retrograde positive-pressure urethrography in this situation (Ganabathi et al, 1994a).

Urodynamic studies should be considered in patients with symptoms of stress urinary incontinence or bladder dysfunction. Genuine stress urinary incontinence was urodynamically documented in 72% of women presenting with symptoms of stress incontinence (Ganabathi et al, 1994a). **In these cases, a simultaneous anti-incontinence procedure is recommended at the time of urethral diverticulectomy.** Patients with detrusor instability may require prolonged anticholinergic therapy to control irritative symptoms.

Surgical Therapy

Multiple open surgical and endoscopic approaches have been described for the treatment of urethral diverticula. Lapides (1979) described transurethral saucerization of urethral diverticulum by incising the floor of the urethra over the diverticulum using a knife electrode. Spencer and Streem (1987) used a similar endoscopic technique using a pediatric resectoscope and Collin's knife to treat an anterior diverticulum. In general, endoscopic incision should be reserved for distal diverticula, because more proximal incision of the urethral wall may compromise continence. Spence and Duckett (1970) described a marsupialization procedure for the treatment of urethral diverticula. The technique essentially creates a generous meatotomy, which may result in vaginal voiding. The reported incidence of incontinence after this procedure is low (Roehrborn, 1988). However, as with endoscopic saucerization, **overzealous incision or treatment of mid- or proximal diverticula with this technique may compromise continence.**

Numerous techniques for transvaginal excision have also been described. Lee (1984) reinforced the urethral closure with the periurethral fascia in a vest-over-pants fashion. Downs (1987) excised and closed the urethral communication, then marsupialized the proximal portion of the diverticulum into the vagina to avoid an extensive subtrigonal dissection. Edwards and Beebe (1955) and Parks (1965) incised the distal urethral floor during removal of the diverticulum and then reconstructed the urethra in layers.

Historically, several methods have been described to define or expose the diverticulum before its dissection. Hunner (1938) and Young (1938) passed sounds through the mouth of the diverticulum. Moore (1952) inserted a Foley catheter into the diverticulum, whereas Wear (1976) transurethrally passed a Fogarty embolectomy catheter into the diverticulum before dissection. Hyams and Hyams (1939) opened the diverticulum transvaginally and packed it with gauze before excision. Both blood products and a silicone mixture have been transvaginally injected into the diverticulum and allowed to form a coagulum or cast to aid in dissection of the sac (Hirschorn, 1964; O'Connor and Kropp, 1969). Ellik (1957) reported transvaginal incision of the diverticulum and packing the sac with Oxycel, allowing the subsequent reaction and fibrosis to obliterate the diverticulum; however, this technique did not always effectively treat loculated diverticula. Most contemporary authors suggest that these sometimes cumbersome maneuvers to define the diverticulum are unnecessary (Leach et al, 1987; Raz et al, 1992; Ganabathi et al, 1994a).

The authors prefer a transvaginal approach to excision of the diverticulum, using a vaginal flap (Moore, 1952; Benjamin et al, 1974; Leach et al, 1986; Raz et al, 1992; Leach and Ganabathi, 1994). This technique allows **complete excision of the diverticulum and a secure three-layer closure without overlapping suture lines.** When required, a simultaneous procedure to improve urethral support may also be performed using this technique, with minimal complications as a result.

Preoperative Care

Preoperative preparation is similar to that for other vaginal surgery. Preoperative patient counseling should include discussion of possible complications of urethral diverticulectomy including infection, bleeding, recurrent diverticulum, urethrovaginal fistula, and urinary incontinence. Because many diverticula are infected, a short course of oral antibiotics immediately before surgery may be advisable. Patients are usually admitted on the day of the surgery and receive prophylactic parenteral antibiotics before the procedure

The patient is placed in the lithotomy position and the Lowsley tractor is used to place a large suprapubic catheter. A ring retractor and posterior weighted vaginal retractor aid in exposure. After infiltrating the anterior vaginal wall with saline, a U-shaped incision is made with the apex just distal to the diverticulum (Fig. 37–11*A*). When genuine stress urinary incontinence is to be treated concomitantly, lateral dissection on the white shiny inner surface of the anterior vaginal wall is performed at the level of the bladder neck toward the pubic bone. With the bladder empty, the endopelvic fascia is then sharply or bluntly perforated laterally, and the retropubic space is developed with blunt dissection. The bladder neck suspension sutures are placed, using 1-0 Prolene sutures and taking large helical bites of the anterior vaginal wall, which exclude epithelium at the level of the bladder neck and avoid the diverticulum (Fig. 37–12). **In some cases of very large proximal diverticula, it may not be possible to place the bladder neck suspension sutures without entering the diverticulum. In this situation, bladder neck suspension should not be attempted at the time of diverticulectomy and should be performed as a secondary procedure if needed.** A small suprapubic incision is made and the suspension sutures passed anteriorly under fingertip control with a modified Pereyra ligature carrier. Cystoscopy should then be performed to exclude bladder or ureteral injury or the presence of suture material within the bladder. When bone fixation is used to suprapubically anchor the suspension sutures (Leach, 1988), the sutures should be passed through the pubic tubercles before proceeding with the diverticulectomy to minimize the risk of osteitis pubis. Swierzewski and McGuire (1993) have also described simultaneous pubovaginal sling at the time of diverticulectomy. The sling was placed after excision of the diverticulum and closure of the urethral defect. However, simultaneous use of a fascial sling may increase the risk of erosion of the sling into the delicate urethral closure.

The next step in performing the diverticulectomy is mobilization of the anterior vaginal wall flap. The flap is mobilized proximally by dissecting directly on the white shiny inner surface of the vaginal wall (see Fig. 37–11*B*). **Careful dissection in the proper plane prevents premature violation of the periurethral fascia or diverticulum itself.** The anterior vaginal wall flap is then reflected proximally, exposing the diverticulum. The periurethral fascia is then incised transversely (see Fig. 37–11*C*). **Sharp dissection allows proximal and distal flaps of periurethral fascia to be developed and reflected off of the underlying diverticulum** (see Fig. 37–11*D*). Again, care must be taken to maintain the proper plane because premature entry into the diverticulum makes subsequent dissection more difficult. The diverticulum is dissected circumferentially down to its urethral communication (see Fig. 37–11*E*). When the communication site is difficult to identify, urethroscopy may be performed and a small pediatric curved sound passed under vision per urethra through the diverticular communication. Palpation of the sound in the diverticulum then helps direct further dissection. **The diverticulum including its communication site with the urethra is completely excised** (see Fig. 37–11*F*). In cases of very large diverticula, complete dissection of the sac may result in extensive dissection under the trigone, risking injury to the bladder base or ureters. In these situations, it may be advisable to leave the most proximal portion of the sac in place. The inner surface may then be electrocauterized to destroy any epithelial elements. Care should also be taken to **avoid excessive excision of urethral wall, thus risking excessive tension on the urethral closure.** The Foley catheter is visible through the often sizable urethral defect. If necessary, additional weak attenuated urethral wall may be excised to healthy tissue. The urethral defect is then closed vertically without tension using a running 4-0 PGA suture incorporating both mucosal and muscular layers of the urethral wall (see Fig. 37–11*G*). After ensuring hemostasis, the periurethral fascia is reapproximated transversely with a 3-0 PGA suture constituting the second layer of closure (see Fig. 37–11*H*). Sutures should be appropriately placed to avoid dead space under the periurethral fascia. **When the first two layers of closure are tenuous, a Martius fat pad graft may be used to reinforce the closure in selected cases.** The third and final layer of closure is the vaginal wall, which is closed with a running 2-0 absorbable suture (see Fig. 37–11*I*). When placed, the bladder neck suspension sutures are tied with minimal tension and the suprapubic incision closed with absorbable sutures. An antibiotic-soaked vaginal pack is placed and both the suprapubic and urethral catheters are placed to sterile drainage.

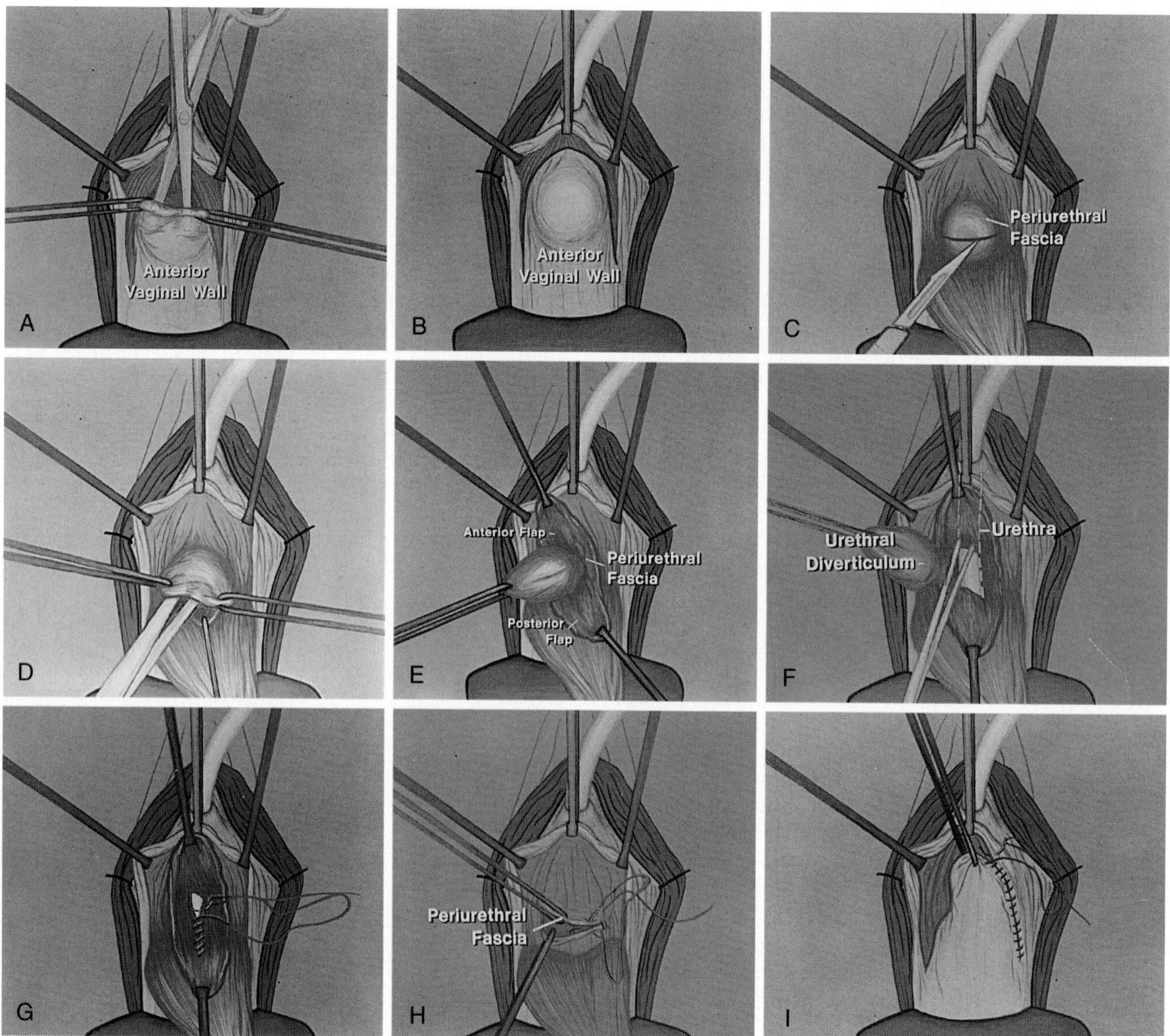

Figure 37–11. *A,* Inverted-U vaginal wall incision with the apex extending distal to the diverticulum. *B,* Anterior vaginal wall flap mobilized proximally. *C,* Periurethral fascia incised transversely. *D,* Periurethral fascia sharply mobilized off underlying diverticulum. *E,* Diverticulum is dissected to its communication with the urethra. *F,* The diverticulum, including its communication site, is excised, exposing the urethral catheter. *G,* The urethral defect is closed with 4-0 absorbable suture. *H,* The periurethral fascia is reapproximated with 3-0 absorbable suture. *I,* The vaginal wall is closed with absorbable sutures. (From Leach GE, Ganabathi K: Atlas Urol Clin North Am 1994; 2:73–85.)

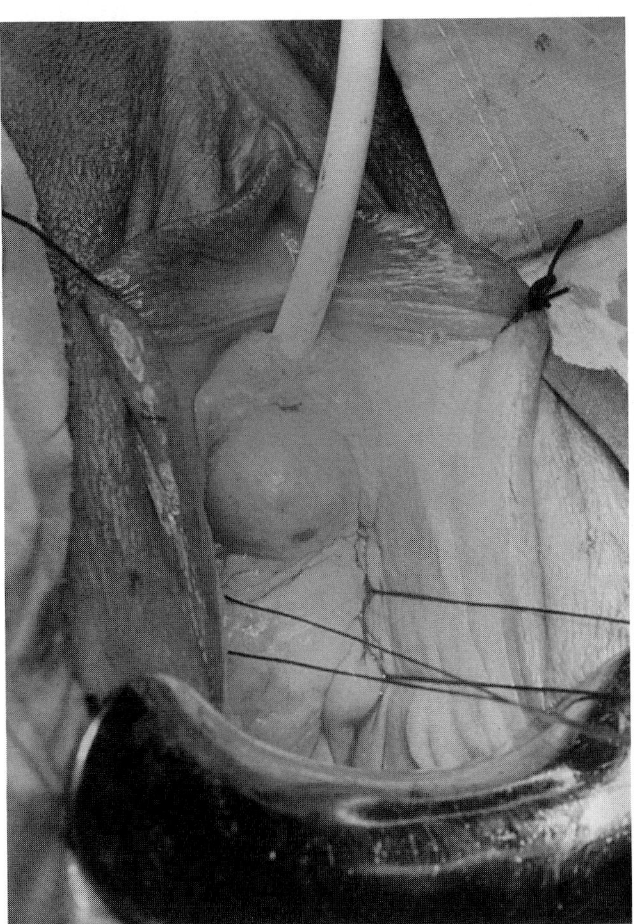

Figure 37–12. Placement of bladder neck suspension sutures prior to urethral diverticulectomy in a patient with a combined problem of stress urinary incontinence and urethral diverticulum. (From Leach GE, Ganabathi K: Atlas Urol Clin North Am 1994; 2:73–85.)

Postoperative Care

Parenteral antibiotics are continued for 24 hours postoperatively, followed by oral antibiotics until catheters are removed. Belladonna and opium suppositories, followed by oral anticholinergics, are used to prevent bladder spasms. The vaginal pack is removed on the first postoperative day. A voiding cystourethrogram is performed 7 and 10 days postoperatively after a vaginal examination has demonstrated a well-vascularized vaginal flap and intact suture lines. Anticholinergics should be discontinued 24 hours before the voiding study. The contrast study is performed by removing the urethral catheter and filling the bladder via the suprapubic catheter. The urethra is carefully observed fluoroscopically during voiding. **When extravasation is observed, the patient is asked to stop voiding, the suprapubic catheter is placed to drainage, and the study is repeated in 1 week.** The urethral catheter is not replaced. In the authors' experience, extravasation is noted on the first study in about 50% of patients. When no extravasation is seen and the patient empties well without excessive postvoid residual, the suprapubic tube is removed. When the postvoid residual is more than 100 ml, the suprapubic catheter is left in place and intermittently unclamped to drain the residual urine. Once adequate emptying has been documented, the suprapubic tube is removed.

Results and Complications

The authors have reported the results of the described vaginal flap technique of urethral diverticulectomy in 56 women (Ganabathi et al, 1994a). Twenty-seven patients underwent combined urethral diverticulectomy and bladder neck suspension. At a mean follow-up interval of 70 months, 86% of patients were relieved of their presenting complaint. Two small distal recurrent diverticula occurred and were successfully treated by endoscopic saucerization. No urethral strictures were encountered. Twenty-two percent of women who underwent combined diverticulectomy and bladder neck suspension and 10% of women who underwent diverticulectomy alone had minimal urinary incontinence (fewer than 2 pads/day) at a mean follow-up period of nearly 7 years. No infectious complications developed in the 27 patients undergoing the combined procedure. The complications of 703 women undergoing urethral diverticulectomy reported in the literature since 1956 are shown in Table 37–2.

Table 37–2. COMPLICATIONS OF DIVERTICULECTOMY FROM PUBLISHED SERIES SINCE 1956 IN 872 WOMEN

Reference	No. Women	Follow-up (mos.)	No. Urethrovaginal Fistula (%)	No. Recurrent Diverticulum (%)	No. Stress Incontinence (%)	No. Urethral Stricture (%)	No. Recurrent Urinary Tract Infections (%)
Wharton and Telinde	58	Not available	4 (7)		1 (1.7)	3 (5.2)	5 (8.6)
Davis and Telinde	84	Not available		10 (11.9)			11 (13.1)
MacKinnon et al	130	Not available	7 (5.4)	2 (1.5)	Several		13 (10)
Boatwright and Moore	48	Not available	4 (8.3)		2 (4.2)	1 (2.1)	
Hoffman and Adams	60	Not available	1 (1.7)		4 (6.7)	1 (1.7)	
Ward	24	Not available	2 (8.3)	7 (29.2)	3 (12.5)		
Davis and Robinson	98	Not available	4 (4.1)	1 (1)			
Pathak and House	42	Not available					3 (7.1)
Benjamin et al	30	Not available	1 (3.3)	1 (3.3)	1 (3.3)		
Peters and Vaughan	32	24	3 (6.3)	8 (25)			10 (31.3)
Ginsburg and Genadry	52	12–240	1 (1.9)	13 (25)		1 (1.9)	
Rózsahegyi et al	50	Not available	1 (2)			1 (2)	
Lee RA	108	24–204	1 (0.9)	10 (9.3)	16 (15)	2 (1.9)	
Ganabathi et al	56	6–136	1 (1.8)	2 (3.6)	9 (16.1)	0 (0)	0 (0)

From Ganabathi K, Leach GE, Zimmern PE, Dmochowski RR: J Urol 1994; 152:1445–1452.

REFERENCES

Aldridge CW, Beaton JH, Nanzig RP: A review of office urethroscopy and cystometry. Am J Obstet Gynecol 1978; 131:432–435.

Anderson MJF: The incidence of diverticula in the female. J Urol 1967; 98:96–98.

Aragona F, Mangano M, Artibani W, et al: Stone formation in female urethral diverticulum: Review of the literature. Int Urol Nephrol 1989; 21:621–625.

Arrowsmith SD: Genitourinary reconstruction in obstetric fistulas. J Urol 1994; 152:403–406.

Barnes R, Hadley H, Johnston O: Transvaginal repair of vesicovaginal fistulas. Urology 1977; 10:258.

Bass JS, Leach GE: Surgical treatment of concomitant urethral diverticulum and stress urinary incontinence. Urol Clin North Am 1991; 18:365–373.

Ba-Thike K, Than-Aye, Nan-Oo: Tuberculous vesicovaginal fistula. Int J Gynecol Obstet 1992; 37:127–130.

Benjamin J, Elliot L, Cooper J, et al: Urethral diverticulum in adult female: Clinical aspects, operative procedure, and pathology. Urology 1974; 3:1–7.

Blaivas JG: Vaginal flap urethral reconstruction: An alternative to the bladder flap neourethra. J Urol 1989; 141:542–545.

Blaivas JG: Treatment of female incontinence secondary to urethral damage or loss. Urol Clin North Am 1991; 18:355–363.

Blaivas JG, Heritz DM, Romanzi LJ: Early versus late repair of vesicovaginal fistulas: Vaginal and abdominal approaches. J Urol 1995; 153:1110–1113.

Blacklock ARE, Shaw RE, Geddes JR: Late presentation of ectopic ureter. Br J Urol 1982; 54:106–110.

Boatwright DC, Moore V: Suburethral diverticula in the female. J Urol 1963; 89:581.

Boyd SD, Raz S: Ectopic ureter presenting in midline urethral diverticulum. Urology 1993; 41(6):571–574.

Candiani P, Austoni E, Campiglio GL, et al: Repair of a recurrent urethrovaginal fistula with an island bulbocavernous musculocutaneous flap. Plast Reconstr Surg 1993; 92:1393–1396.

Catalona S, Jones I: Transitional cell carcinoma in a urethral diverticulum. Aust N Z Obstet Gynaecol 1992; 32:85–86.

Clayton M, Siami P, Guinan P: Urethral diverticular carcinoma. Cancer 1992; 70:665–670.

Davis BL, Robinson DG: Diverticula of the female urethra: Assay of 120 cases. J Urol 1970; 104:850.

Davis HJ, Cian LG: Positive pressure urethrography: A new diagnostic method. J Urol 1956; 75:753–757.

Davis HJ, Te Linde RW: Urethral diverticula: An assay of 121 cases. J Urol 1958; 80:34–39.

Dees JE: Congenital epispadias with incontinence. J Urol 1949; 62:513.

Dmochowski RR, Ganabathi K, Zimmern PE, Leach GE: Benign female periurethral masses. J Urol 1994: 152:1943–1951.

Downs RA: Urethral diverticula in females: Alternative surgical treatment. Urology 1987; 29:201–203.

Edwards EA, Beebe RA: Diverticula of the female urethra. Obstet Gynecol 1955; 5:729.

Elkins TE: Surgery for the obstetric vesicovaginal fistula: A review of 100 operations in 82 patients. Am J Obstet Gynecol 1994; 170:1108–1120.

Elkins TE, Ghosh TS, Tagoe GA, Stocker R: Transvaginal mobilization and utilization of the anterior bladder wall to repair vesicovaginal fistulas involving the urethra. Obstet Gynecol 1992; 79:455–460.

Ellik M: Diverticulum of the female urethra: A new method of ablation. J Urol 1957; 77:234.

Falk HC, Tancer ML: Vesicovaginal fistula: An historical survey. Obstet Gynecol 1954; 3:337–341.

Flocks RH, Boldus R: The surgical treatment and prevention of urinary incontinence associated with disturbance of the internal urethral sphincter mechanism. J Urol 1973; 109:279–285.

Ganabathi K, Leach GE: Periurethral injection techniques. Atlas Urol Clin North Am 1994; 2:101–109.

Ganabathi K, Leach GE, Zimmern PE, Dmochowski RR: Experience with the management of urethral diverticulum in 63 women. J Urol 1994a; 152:1445–1452.

Ganabathi K, Sirls L, Zimmern PE, Leach GE: Operative management of female urethral diverticulum. *In* McGuire E, ed: Advances in Urology. Chicago, C.V. Mosby Company, 1994b, pp 199–228.

Gil-Vernet JM, Gil-Vernet A, Campos JA: A new surgical approach for treatment of complex vesicovaginal fistula. J Urol 1989; 141:513–516.

Ginsberg DS, Genadry R: Suburethral diverticulum in the female. Obstet Gynecol Surv 1984; 39:1–7.

Goldstein I, Wise GJ, Tancer ML: A vesicovaginal fistula and intravesical foreign body: A rare case of the neglected pessary. Am J Obstet Gynecol 1990; 163:589–591.

Goodwin WE, Scardino PT: Vesicovaginal and ureterovaginal fistulas: A summary of 25 years of experience. J Urol 1980; 123:370–374.

Grahm JB: Vaginal fistulas following radiotherapy. Surg Gynecol Obstet 1965; 120:1019–1030.

Hansen BJ, Horby J, Brynitz S, et al: Calculi in female urethral diverticulum. Int Urol Nephrol 1989; 21:617–620.

Hendren WH: Construction of female urethra from vaginal wall and a perineal flap. J Urol 1980; 123:657–664.

Hey W: Practical Observations in Surgery. Philadelphia, J. Humphries, 1805.

Hirschorn RC: A new surgical technique for urethral diverticula in women. J Urol 1964; 92:206–209.

Hoffman MJ, Adams WE: Recognition and repair of urethral diverticula: A report of 60 cases. Am J Obstet Gynecol 1965; 92:106.

Huffman AB: The detailed anatomy of the paraurethral ducts in the adult human female. Am J Obstet Gynecol 1948; 55:86.

Hunner GL: Calculus formation in a urethral diverticulum in women. Urol Cut Rev 1938; 42:336.

Hyams JA, Hyams MN: New operative procedures for treatment of diverticulum of female urethra. Urol Cut Rev 1939; 43:573.

Jonas U, Petri E: Genitourinary fistulae. *In* Stanton SL, ed: Clinical Gynecologic Urology. St. Louis, C.V. Mosby Company, 1984, pp 238–255.

Kursh ED, Morse RM, Resnik MI, Persky L: Prevention and development of a vesicovaginal fistula. Surg Gynecol Obstet 1988; 166:409–412.

Lamensdorf H, Compere DE, Begley GF: Simple surgical correction of urethrovaginal fistula. Urology 1977; 10:152–153.

Landes RR: Simple transvesical repair of vesicovaginal fistula. J Urol 1979; 122:604–606.

Lapides J: Transurethral treatment of urethral diverticula in women. J Urol 1979; 121:736–738.

Latzko W: Postoperative vesicovaginal fistulas: Genesis and therapy. Am J Surg 1942; 58:211–228.

Leach GE: Bone fixation technique for transvaginal needle suspension. Urology 1988; 31:388–390.

Leach GE: Urethrovaginal fistula repair with Martius labial fat pad graft. Urol Clin North Am 1991; 18:409–413.

Leach GE, Bavendam TG: Female urethral diverticula. Urology 1987; 30:407–415.

Leach GE, Ganabathi K: Urethral diverticulectomy. Atlas Urol Clin North Am 1994; 2:73–85.

Leach GE, Schmidbauer CP, Hadley HR, et al: Surgical treatment of female urethral diverticulum. Semin Urol 1986; 4:33–42.

Leach GE, Sirls LT, Ganabathi K, et al: L N S C3; a proposed classification system for female urethral diverticula. Neurourol Urodyn 1993; 12:523–531.

Leach GE, Yip CM, Donovan BJ, Raz S: Tubovaginal leakage: An unusual cause of incontinence. J Urol 1987; 137:287–288.

Leadbetter GW Jr: Surgical correction of total urinary incontinence. J Urol 1964; 91:261.

Lee AL, Symmonds RE, Williams TJ: Current status of genitourinary fistula. Obstet Gynecol 1988; 72:313–319.

Lee RA: Diverticulum of the urethra: Clinical presentation, diagnosis, and management. Clin Obstet Gynecol 1984; 27:490.

Lee TG, Keller F: Urethral diverticulum: Diagnosis by ultrasound. AJR Am J Roentgenol 1977; 128:690–691.

Lockhart JL, Walker RD, Vorstman B, Politano VA: Periurethral polytetrafluoroethylene injection following urethral reconstruction in female patients with urinary incontinence. J Urol 1988; 140:51–52.

MacKinnon M, Pratt JH, Pool TL: Diverticulum of the female urethra. Surg Clin North Am 1959; 39:953.

Martius H: Die operative Wiedeherstellung der volkommen fehlenden Harnrohre und des Schiessmuskels derselben. Zentralbl Gynak 1928; 52:480.

McNally A: Diverticula of the female urethra. Am J Surg 1935; 28:177.

Menchaca A, Akhyat M, Gleicher N, et al: Rectus abdominis muscle flap in a combined abdominovaginal repair of difficult vesicovaginal fistulae: A report of three cases. J Reprod Med 1990; 35:565–568.

Mitchell ME, Hensle TW, Crooks KK: Urethral reconstruction in the young female using a perineal pedicle flap. J Ped Surg 1982; 17:687–694.

Moore TD: Diverticulum of the female urethra. An improved technique of surgical excision. J Urol 1952; 68:611–616.

Nel J: Diverticulum of female urethra. J Obstet Gynaecol Br Commonw 1955; 62:90.

Niemic TR, Mercer LJ, Stephens JK, et al: Unusual urethral diverticulum lined with colonic epithelium with paneth cell metaplasia. Am J Obstet Gynecol 1989; 160:186–188.

Nolan JF, Stillwell TJ, Barttelbort SW, Sands JP: Gracilis interposition in fistulas following radiotherapy for cervical cancer: A retrospective study. J Urol 1991; 146:843–844.

Öbrink A, Bunne G: Gracilis interposition in fistulas following radiotherapy for cervical cancer. Urol Int 1978; 33:370–376.

O'Connor VJ Jr: Review of experience with vesicovaginal fistula repair. J Urol 1980; 123:367–369.

O'Connor VJ Jr, Kropp KA: Surgery of the female urethra. *In* Glennn JF, Boyce WH, eds: Urologic Surgery. New York, Harper and Row, 1969.

O'Connor V, Sokol J: Vesicovaginal fistula from the standpoint of the urologist. J Urol 1951; 66:367–369.

Orikasa S, Metoki R, Ishikawa H, et al: Congenital urethral and vesical diverticula allied to blind ending ureters. Urology 1990; 35:137–141.

Palagiri A: Urethral diverticulum with endometriosis. Urology 1978; 11:271.

Patanaphan V, Prempree T, Sewchand W, et al: Adenocarcinoma arising in female urethral diverticulum. Urology 1983; 22:259–264.

Parks J: Section of the urethral wall for correction of urethrovaginal fistula and urethral diverticula. Am J Obstet Gynecol 1965; 93:683.

Pathak UN, House MJ: Diverticulum of the female urethra. Obstet Gynecol 1970; 36:789.

Patil U, Waterhouse K, Laungauni G: Management of 18 difficult vesicovaginal and urethrovaginal fistulas with modified Ingelman-Sundberg and Martius operations. J Urol 1980; 123:653–656.

Perlmutter S, Huang AB, Hon M, Subuddhi MK: Sonographic demonstration of calculi within a urethral diverticulum. Urology 1993; 42:735–737.

Persky L, Herman G, Guerrier K: Nondelay in vesicovaginal fistula repair. Urology 1979; 13:273–275.

Peters WH, Vaughan ED Jr: Urethral diverticulum in the female. Obstet Gynecol 1976; 47:549.

Ratner M, Ritz I, Siminovitch M: Diverticulum of the female urethra with multiple calculi. Can Med Assoc J 1949; 60:510.

Raz S, Bregg K, Nitti VW, Sussman E: Transvaginal repair of vesicovaginal fistula using a peritoneal flap. J Urol 1993; 150:56–59.

Raz S, Little NA, Juma S: Female urology. *In* Walsh PC, Retik AB, Stamey TA, eds: Campbell's Urology, 6th ed. Philadelphia, W.B. Saunders Company, 1992, pp 2782–2828.

Redman J: Female urologic techniques. Urol Clin North Am 1990; 17:5–8.

Robertson JR: Genitourinary Problems in Women. Springfield, IL, Charles C Thomas, 1978.

Roehrborn CG: Longterm follow up study of the marsupialization technique for urethral diverticula in women. Surg Gynecol Obstet 1988; 167:191–196.

Routh A: Urethral diverticulum. Br Med J 1890; 1:361.

Rózsahegyi J, Magasi P, Szule E: Diverticulum of the female urethra: A report of 50 cases. Acta Chir Hung 1981; 25:33–38.

Silk MR, Lebowitz JM: Anterior urethral diverticulum. J Urol 1969; 101:66.

Spence HM, Duckett JW: Diverticulum of the female urethra: Clinical aspects and presentation of a simple operative technique for cure. J Urol 1970; 104:432–437.

Spencer WF, Streem SB: Diverticula of the female urethra roof managed endoscopically. J Urol 1987; 138:147–148.

Stovsky MD, Ignatoff JM, Blum MD, et al: Use of electrocoagulation in the treatment of vesicovaginal fistulas. J Urol; 152:1443–1444.

Strockbine MF, Hancock JE, Fletcher GH: Complications in 831 patients with squamous cell carcinoma of the intact uterine cervix treated with 3,000 rads or more whole pelvis radiation. AJR 1970; 108:239–304.

Swierzewski SJ III, McGuire EJ: Pubovaginal sling for treatment of female stress urinary incontinence complicated by urethral diverticulum. J Urol 1993; 149:1012–1014.

Symmonds RE: Incontinence: Vesical and urethral fistulas. Obstet Gynecol 1984; 27:499–514.

Tanagho EA: Bladder neck reconstruction for total urinary incontinence: 10 years of experience. J Urol 1981; 125:321–326.

Tancer ML: Observations on prevention and management of vesicovaginal fistula after total hysterectomy. Surg Gynecol Obstet 1992; 175:501–506.

Tancer ML: A report of thirty-four instances of urethrovaginal and bladder neck fistulas. Surg Gynecol Obstet 1993; 177:77–80.

Thomas RB, Maguire B: Adenocarcinoma in a female urethral diverticulum. Aust N Z J Obstet Gynaecol 1991; 869–871.

Torres S, Quattlebaum R: Carcinoma in urethral diverticulum. South Med J 1972; 65:1374–1376.

Udeh FN: Simple management of difficult vesicovaginal fistulas by anterior transvesical approach. J Urol 1985; 133:591–593.

Wang Yu, Hadley R: Nondelayed transvaginal repair of high-lying vesicovaginal fistula. J Urol 1990; 144:34–36.

Ward JN: Technique to visualize the urethra in female patients. Surg Gynecol Obstet 1989; 168:278.

Wear JB: Urethral diverticulectomy in females. Urol Times 1976; 4:2–3.

Webster GD, Sihelnik SA, Stone AR: Urethrovaginal fistula: A review of the surgical management. J Urol 1984; 132:460–462.

Wein AJ, Malloy TR, Carpiniello VL, et al: Repair of vesicovaginal fistula by a suprapubic transvesical approach. Surg Gynecol Obstet 1980a; 150:57–60.

Wein AJ, Malloy TR, Greenberg SH, et al: Omental transposition as an aid in genitourinary reconstructive procedures. J Urol 1980b; 20:473–477.

Wharton LR Jr, Telinde RW: Urethral diverticulum. Obstet Gynecol 1956; 7:503.

Wishard WN, Nourse NH, Mertz JHO: Carcinoma in diverticulum of the female urethra. J Urol 1963; 89:431.

Young HH: Treatment of urethral diverticulum. South Med J 1938; 31:1043–1047.

Young HH: An operation for the cure of incontinence associated with epispadias. J Urol 1922; 7:1.

Zacharin RE: Obstetric Fistula. New York, Springer-Verlag, 1988.

Zeidman EJ, Chiang H, Alarcon A, Raz S: Suprapubic cystotomy using Lowsley retractor. Urology 1988; 23:54–55.

Zimmern PE, Ganabathi K, Leach GE: Vesicovaginal fistula repair. Atlas Urol Clin North Am 1994; 2:87–99.

Zimmern PE, Hadley HR, Leach GE, et al: Transvaginal closure of the bladder neck and placement of a suprapubic catheter for destroyed urethra after longterm indwelling catheter. J Urol 1985; 134:554.

Zimmern PE, Schmidbauer CP, Leach GE, et al: Vesicovaginal and urethrovaginal fistulae. Semin Urol 1986; 4:24–29.

INDEX

Note: Page numbers in *italics* refer to illustrations; page numbers followed by t refer to tables.